2009
E D I T I O N
D E L M A R

NURSE'S
DRUG
HANDBOOK

THE INFORMATION STANDARD
FOR PRESCRIPTION DRUGS AND
NURSING CONSIDERATIONS

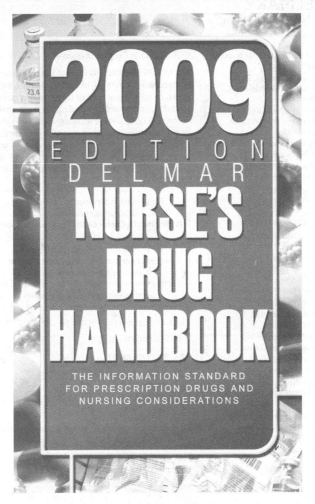

2009 EDITION

DELMAR

NURSE'S DRUG HANDBOOK

THE INFORMATION STANDARD
FOR PRESCRIPTION DRUGS AND
NURSING CONSIDERATIONS

George R. Spratto, PhD
Dean Emeritus and Professor
School of Pharmacy
West Virginia University
Morgantown, West Virginia

Adrienne L. Woods, MSN, ARNP, NP-C
Nurse Practitioner
Primary Care at the
Department of Veterans Affairs Medical
and Regional Office Center
Wilmington, Delaware

DELMAR
CENGAGE Learning

2009 Edition Delmar Nurse's Drug Handbook™

George R. Spratto, PhD
Adrienne L. Woods, MSN, ARNP, NP-C

Vice President, Career and Professional Editorial:
Dave Garza

Director of Learning Solutions:
Matthew Kane

Senior Acquisitions Editor:
Maureen Rosener

Managing Editor:
Marah Bellegarde

Senior Product Manager:
Debra Myette-Flis

Editorial Assistant:
Meaghan O'Brien

Vice President, Career and
Professional Marketing:
Jennifer McAvey

Senior Marketing Manager:
Michele McTighe

Production Director:
Carolyn S. Miller

Senior Content Project
Manager: Stacey Lamodi

Senior Art Director:
Jack Pendleton

Senior Product Manager,
Digital Solutions Group:
Mary Colleen Liburdi

Technology Project Manager:
Erin Zeggert

Web/Systems Developer:
Vince Nicotina

Library of Congress Control Number: 2008902076

ISBN-13: 978-1-4283-6106-5

ISBN-10: 1-4283-6106-5

Delmar Cengage Learning
5 Maxwell Drive
Clifton Park, NY 12065-2919
USA

Cengage Learning products are represented in Canada by Nelson Education, Ltd.

For your lifelong learning solutions, visit
delmar.cengage.com

Visit our corporate website at **www.cengage.com**

Notice to the Reader
Publisher does not warrant or guarantee any of the products described herein or perform any independent analysis in connection with any of the product information contained herein. Publisher does not assume, and expressly disclaims, any obligation to obtain and include information other than that provided to it by the manufacturer. The reader is expressly warned to consider and adopt all safety precautions that might be indicated by the activities described herein and to avoid all potential hazards. By following the instructions contained herein, the reader willingly assumes all risks in connection with such instructions. The publisher makes no representations or warranties of any kind, including but not limited to, the warranties of fitness for particular purpose or merchantability, nor are any such representations implied with respect to the material set forth herein, and the publisher takes no responsibility with respect to such material. The publisher shall not be liable for any special, consequential, or exemplary damages resulting, in whole or part, from the readers' use of, or reliance upon, this material.

Printed in the United States of America
1 2 3 4 5 XX 10 09 08

Table of Contents

Notice to the Reader

The monographs in this edition of the *Delmar Nurse's Drug Handbook*™ are the work of two distinguished authors: George R. Spratto, PhD, Dean Emeritus and Professor of Pharmacology of the School of Pharmacy at West Virginia University, Morgantown, West Virginia, and Adrienne L. Woods, MSN, ARNP, NP-C, Nurse Practitioner, Primary Care at the Department of Veterans Affairs Medical and Regional Office Center, Wilmington, Delaware.

The publisher and the authors do not warrant or guarantee any of the products described herein or perform any independent analysis in connection with any of the product information contained herein. The publisher and the authors do not assume and expressly disclaim any obligation to obtain and include information other than that provided by the manufacturer.

The reader is expressly warned to consider and adopt all safety precautions that might be indicated by the activities described herein and to avoid all potential hazards. By following the instructions contained herein, the reader willingly assumes all risks in connection with such instructions.

The publisher and the authors make no representations or warranties of any kind, including but not limited to the warranties of fitness for a particular purpose or merchantability nor are any such representations implied with respect to the material set forth herein, and the publisher and the authors take no responsibility with respect to such material. The publisher and the authors shall not be liable for any special, consequential, or exemplary damages resulting, in whole or in part, from the reader's use of, or reliance upon, this material.

The authors and publisher have made a conscientious effort to ensure that the drug information and recommended dosages in this book and companion web site are accurate and in accord with accepted standards at the time of publication. However, pharmacology and therapeutics are rapidly changing sciences, so readers are advised, before administering any drug, to check the package insert provided by the manufacturer for the recommended dose, for any contraindications for administration, and for any added warnings and precautions. This recommendation is especially important for new, infrequently used, or highly toxic drugs.

Preface

The *Delmar Nurse's Drug Handbook*™ is a trusted resource used by nursing students, practicing nurses, and other health care professionals. Each annual edition provides updates affecting thousands of bits of information and introduces monographs of drugs recently approved by the FDA and marketed by the drug manufacturers. Drug information changes rapidly, including the development of new drugs, new uses for established drugs, revised and new administration routes (dosage forms), newly identified side effects and drug interactions, and changes in dosing and use recommendations based on feedback from health care professionals, researchers, and consumers. Nurses and other health care professionals depend on this handbook to provide the latest information on drug therapy, guidelines for monitoring efficacy of the therapy, and recommendations for teaching the client and family about important aspects of the drug therapy.

ORGANIZATION OF CONTENT

The **2009 Nurse's Drug Handbook CD-ROM** is a dynamic reference tool providing you with monographs for over 180 of the most commonly prescribed medications wherever and whenever you need them. See also the "Quick Reference to Technology Tools."

Chapter 1 contains individual drug monographs in alphabetical order by generic name. Newly marketed drugs are also included in Chapter 1. The purpose and meaning of each of the components of a monograph are described under "Using the Drug Monographs." See also the "Quick Reference Guide to a Drug Monograph."

Chapter 2 includes general information on important therapeutic or chemical classes of drugs. The classes are listed alphabetically. Consult the Table of Contents for a listing of the therapeutic/chemical classes included in Chapter 2. Each class begins with a list of drugs for which a monograph appears in Chapter 1 as well as the Nurse's Drug Handbook Online Database (www.delmarnursesdrughandbook.com/2009). The information provided in the class applies to all drugs listed for the class. For complete knowledge of a specific drug, consult the class information in Chapter 2 as well as the appropriate monograph in Chapter 1.

The **Color Photo Quick Reference Guide** is a color insert that provides rapid identification of 74 most-commonly prescribed drugs. Products shown in the guide are identified by a camera icon 📷 in the drug name area of the related monograph in Chapter 1. Actual-sized tablets and capsules, with their strengths listed, are organized alphabetically by generic name. Each product is also labeled with its trade name and the name of the manufacturer.

The **Appendices** provide additional information to assist in administering drugs and monitoring drug therapy. A complete listing of the appendices is provided in the Table of Contents. Appendices are revised annually, as appropriate, to reflect the latest available information.

The FDA has added a boxed warning to prescribing information for numerous drugs whose side effects can be life-threatening and in some cases have resulted in death. In this handbook, these "Black Box Warnings" are indicated by a black box icon ■ following the drug name and by the black box icon and highlighted content in the "Special Concerns" portion of the monograph.

Two indexes are found in the back of the handbook. The **IV Index** lists IV drugs by generic name and trade name. The **General Index** is extensively cross-referenced: each generic drug name entry includes the major trade name(s) entry in pa-

rentheses and each trade name entry is followed by the generic drug name in pa-
rentheses. This is helpful when you or the client can only remember one name of
the drug prescribed (especially by another provider). Each page of the general index
contains a key identifying boldface as the generic drug name, italics as the therapeutic drug class, regular type as the trade name, and capitals as the name of combination drugs.

USING THE DRUG MONOGRAPHS

The following components are described in the order in which they appear in
the monographs. All components may not appear in each monograph but are represented where appropriate and when information is available. Refer also to the
"Quick Reference Guide to a Drug Monograph," with explanatory notes for the purpose and use of each component.

Drug Name: The generic drug name is the first item in the name block (in color at
the beginning of each monograph). One or more icons may follow the drug name:

■   Black box to indicate that the FDA has issued a boxed warning about po-
      tentially dangerous or life-threatening side effects

℮   Ear to indicate that sound-alike drug names may be linked to medication
      errors

📷   Camera to indicate that the oral form of a drug is shown in the Visual
      Identification Guide

IV   IV to indicate that the drug can also be given by IV

Phonetic Pronunciation: Pronunciation guide for generic name to assist in master-
ing often complex names.

Classification: Defines the type of drug or the class under which the drug is listed.
A classification or descriptor is provided for each drug name in Chapter 1. If the
drug class is new and/or only a few drugs are available in the class at the time of
printing the handbook, the classification will not appear in Chapter 2. It will be added at a later date as more drugs in the class reach the market.

Pregnancy Category: Lists the FDA pregnancy category (A, B, C, D, or X) assigned
to the drug (pregnancy categories are defined in Appendix 4).

Trade Name: Trade names are identified as OTC (over-the-counter, no prescription
required) or Rx (prescription). If numerous forms of the drug are available, the trade
names are preceded by identifying the dosage form. Trade names available only in
Canada are identified by a maple leaf icon leaf ♣.

Controlled Substance: If the drug is controlled by the U.S. Federal Controlled Substances Act, the schedule in which the drug is placed (C-I, C-II, C-III, C-IV, C-V) follows the trade name listing. See Appendix 3 for a listing of controlled substances in
both the United States and Canada.

Combination Drug: This heading at the top of the name block indicates that the
drug is a combination of two or more drugs in the same product. Additional combination drugs are listed in Appendix 8, Commonly Used Combination Drugs.

The following components may appear in the body of a drug monograph.

Cross Reference: "See also..." directs the reader to the classification entry in Chapter 2 that matches the classification of the drug being reviewed or to another drug
in Chapter 1. General information about the drugs in the class is provided in Chapter 2.

General Statement: This appears in a few drug monographs but is more common
in the class entries in Chapter 2. Information about the drug class and/or anything
specific or unusual about a group of drugs is presented. Information may also be
presented about the disease(s) or condition(s) for which the drugs are indicated.

Uses: Approved therapeutic uses for the drug are listed. Some investigational uses
are also listed for selected drugs.

Content: For combination drugs, provides the generic name and amount of each
drug in the combination product.

Action/Pharmacokinetics: The action portion describes the proposed mechanism(s) by which a drug achieves its therapeutic effect. Not all mechanisms of action are known, and some are self-evident, as when a hormone is administered as a replacement. The pharmacokinetics portion lists critical information, if known, about the rate of drug absorption (including, when known, the percent bioavailable), distribution, time for peak plasma levels or peak effect, minimum effective serum or plasma level, biological half-life, duration of action, metabolism, and excretion route(s). Metabolism and excretion routes may be important for clients with systemic liver disease, kidney disease, or both.

Many drugs bind to plasma proteins. If a client is prescribed two or more drugs that bind to plasma proteins, there is the potential for altered effects (either increased or decreased) because of competition for binding sites. It may be necessary to change the dose of one or more of the drugs to improve the therapeutic action. The percent of the drug bound to plasma proteins is included when known.

The half-life (the time required for half the drug to be excreted or removed from the blood, serum, or plasma—t½) is important in determining how often a drug is to be administered and how long the client is to be assessed for side effects. Therapeutic levels indicate the desired concentration, in serum or plasma, for the drug to exert its beneficial effect and are helpful in predicting the onset of side effects or the lack of effect. Drug therapy is often monitored in this manner (e.g., antibiotics, theophylline, phenytoin, amiodarone).

Contraindications: Disease states or conditions in which the drug should not be used are noted. The safe use of many of the newer pharmacologic agents during pregnancy, lactation, or childhood has not been established. As a general rule, the use of drugs during pregnancy is contraindicated unless the benefits of drug therapy are determined to far outweigh the potential risks.

Special Concerns: Numerous drugs have life-threatening or dangerous side effects that may lead to organ/system damage and possibly death. The FDA provides boxed warnings with the prescribing information for these drugs to alert health care professionals to the potential for serious side effects. A black box icon ■ and highlighted content in this section of the monograph draw attention to the warning information. This section also covers considerations for use with pediatric, geriatric, pregnant, or lactating clients. Situations and disease states when the drug should be used with caution are also listed.

Side Effects: Undesired or bothersome effects the client may experience while taking a particular agent are described. The most common side effects (shown in color) are listed first for quick reference, followed by a complete list of side effects organized by the body organ or system affected. Nearly all potential side effects are listed. In any given clinical situation; however, a client may experience no side effects, one or two side effects, or several side effects. If potentially life-threatening, the side effect is displayed in *bold italic* type.

OD **Overdose Management**: When appropriate, this section provides a list of the symptoms observed following an overdose (Symptoms) as well as treatment approaches and/or antidotes for the overdose (Treatment).

Drug Interactions: Alphabetical listing of drugs and herbals that may interact with the drug under discussion. The study of drug interactions is an important area of pharmacology that changes constantly. Because of the significant increase in the use of herbal products, interactions of medications with herbals are included in this section if known or suspected. These interactions are designated by the icon H . The listing of drug/drug and drug/herbal interactions is far from complete; therefore, listings in this handbook are to be considered only as general cautionary guidelines.

Drug interactions may result from a number of different mechanisms: (1) additive or inhibitory effects; (2) increased or decreased metabolism of the drug; (3) increased or decreased rate of elimination; (4) decreased absorption from the GI tract;

and (5) competition for or displacement from receptor sites or plasma protein binding sites. Drug interactions may manifest themselves in a variety of ways; however, an attempt has been made throughout the handbook to describe these interactions whenever possible as an increase (↑) or a decrease (↓) in the effect of the drug, and a reason for the change. It is important to realize that any side effects that accompany the administration of a particular agent may be increased as a result of a drug or herbal interaction.

Laboratory Test Considerations: The manner in which a drug may affect laboratory test values is presented. Some of the effects are caused by the therapeutic or toxic effects of the drugs; others result from interference with the testing method itself. The laboratory considerations are described as increased (↑) or false positive (+) values and as decreased (↓) or false negative (-) values. Also included, when available, are drug-induced changes in blood or urine levels of endogenous substances (e.g., glucose, electrolytes, and so on).

How Supplied: The various dosage forms available for the drug and amounts of the drug in each of the dosage forms are presented. Such information is important as one dosage form may be more appropriate for a client than another. This information also allows the user to ensure the appropriate dosage form and strength is being administered.

Dosage: The dosage form and route of administration (in color) is followed by the disease state or condition (in italics and color) for which the dosage is recommended. This is followed by the adult and pediatric doses, when available. The listed dosage is to be considered as a general guideline; the exact amount of the drug to be given is determined by the provider. However, one should question orders when dosages differ markedly from the accepted norm.

Nursing Considerations: The guidelines provided in this section are designed to help the practitioner in applying the nursing process to pharmacotherapeutics to ensure safe practice. When applicable this section begins with an ear icon ⓒ denoting that either generic and/or trade name(s) of the drug being discussed sound similar to one or more other drugs. Caution must be exercised to ensure that the correct drug is being used as many drug names do sound similar. In each monograph the following sections are provided when applicable.

- *Administration/Storage*: Guidelines for preparing medications for administration, administering the medication, things to be aware of during administration and storage and disposal of the medication. Guidelines for administration by IV are indicated by an icon ▐IV▌.
- *Assessment*: Guidelines for monitoring/assessing the client before, during, and after prescribed drug therapy.
- *Interventions*: Additional guidelines for specific nursing actions related to the drug being administered.
- *Client/Family Teaching*: Guidelines to promote education, active participation, understanding, and adherence to drug therapy by the client and/or care givers. Precautions about the drug therapy are also noted for communication to the client/care giver.
- *Outcomes/Evaluate*: Desired outcomes of the drug therapy and client response. These will help determine the effectiveness and positive therapeutic outcome of the prescribed drug therapy.

Notes on Assessment and Interventions. The following tasks are critical in assessing the client for drug therapy and for planning the interventions needed to undertake the therapy:

- Gather physical data and client history
- Assess specific physiologic functions likely to be affected by the drug therapy
- Determine specific laboratory tests needed to monitor the course of the drug therapy

- Identify sensitivities/interactions and conditions that may preclude a particular drug therapy
- Document specific indications for therapy and describe symptom characteristics related to this condition
- Know the physiologic, pharmacologic, and psychologic effects of the drug and how these may affect the client and impact the nursing process
- Know side effects that can arise as a result of drug therapy and be prepared with appropriate nursing interventions
- Monitor the client for side effects and document/report them to the provider. Severe side effects generally require dosage modification or discontinuation of the drug.
- Ensure client safety when receiving drug therapy

When taking the nursing history, place emphasis on the client's ability to read and to follow directions. Language barriers must be identified and appropriate written translations should be provided to promote adherence to the drug therapy. In addition, client lifestyle, culture, income, availability of health insurance, and access to transportation are important factors that may affect adherence with therapy and follow-up care. Appendix 13 discusses cultural aspects of medication therapy.

The assessment should include the potential for the client being/becoming pregnant, and if a mother is breastfeeding her infant.

The age and orientation level of the client, whether learned from personal observation or from discussion with close friends or family members, can be critical in determining potential relationships between drug therapy and/or drug interactions.

Including these factors in the nursing assessment will assist all members of the health care team to determine the type of pharmacotherapy, drug delivery system, and monitoring and follow-up plan best suited to a particular client to promote the highest level of adherence.

Notes on Client/Family Teaching: Specific understandable information for the client is provided for each drug. Client/family teaching assists the client/family to recognize side effects and avoid potentially dangerous situations, and alleviates anxiety associated with starting and maintaining drug therapy.

Details on administration are included to enhance client understanding and adherence. Side effects that require medical intervention are included, as are recommendations for minimizing the side effects for certain medications (e.g., take medication with food to decrease GI upset, or take at bedtime to minimize daytime sedative effects).

The proper education of clients is one of the most challenging aspects of nursing. The instructions must be tailored to the needs, awareness, and sophistication of each client. For example, clients who take medication to lower blood pressure should assume responsibility for taking their own blood pressure or having it taken and recorded.

Clients should carry identification listing the drugs currently prescribed. They should know what they are taking and why, and develop a mechanism to remind themselves to take their medication as prescribed. Clients should always carry this drug list with them whenever they go for a checkup or seek medical care, and it should be updated by providers at each visit. The drug list may also be shared with the pharmacist if there is a question concerning drugs prescribed, if the client is considering taking an over-the-counter medication, or if the client has to change pharmacies.

The records, especially blood pressure readings, should be shared with the health care provider to ensure accurate evaluation of the response to the prescribed drug therapy. This may also alert the provider to any drug/food/herbal consumption by the client that they did not prescribe, were not aware of, or that may interfere with (i.e., potentiate or antagonize) the current pharmacologic regimen. The provider may also encourage the client to call with any questions or concerns about the drug therapy to discourage stopping therapy or self-medicating.

Remember: The components described previously are covered for all drugs or drug classes. When drugs are presented as a group (as in Chapter 2), the information for each component is given only once for the group. Check each component for information relevant to all drugs covered in the class. Note that many of the drug monographs in Chapter 1 are cross-referenced to the general information in Chapter 2 or to another drug appearing in Chapter 1. Critical information or information relevant to a specific drug is provided in the individual drug monograph in Chapter 1 under appropriate headings, such as Additional Contraindications or Additional Side Effects. These are **in addition to** and **not instead of** the entry in Chapter 2, which is referenced and must be consulted.

NURSE'S DRUG HANDBOOK ONLINE DATABASE

Please join us on the web at www.delmarnursesdrughandbook.com/2009 for full monographs of less commonly used drugs, links to pharmaceutical companies and related sites, drug headlines, drug administration guidelines, and bonus drug monographs which include information on additional drugs in use as well as drugs that have been removed from the market. The website is updated with new and removed drugs periodically. For more information and updates, visit the Food and Drug Administration website at www.fda.gov.

Enjoy the benefits of the Delmar Nurse's Drug Handbook Online Database absolutely free! With your purchase of the *Delmar Nurse's Drug Handbook*, you are entitled to a searchable database of drugs by a number of categories 24 hours a day and 7 days a week. This edition of the database has been redesigned to make it easier to search. You will enjoy the same great drug information in a more user-friendly environment. You can even bookmark your most frequently referenced drugs. For convenient portability of drug information found on the Database website, just choose the drugs you wish to download to your Personal Digital Assistant (PDA) and hook it up to your computer. Accessible anytime and anywhere, the combination of the *Delmar Nurse's Drug Handbook* and Delmar Nurse's Drug Handbook Online Database is the greatest value for drug information available today!

To access the Delmar Nurse's Drug Handbook Online Database, go to the website printed on the inside front cover of this book and follow the instructions provided on the website.

Acknowledgments

We would like to extend our thanks and appreciation to the Delmar Cengage Learning team who works so diligently to ensure that the manuscript process flows smoothly and to keep us on the appropriate time schedule. Team members include Matthew Kane, Director of Learning Solutions; Maureen Rosener, Senior Acquisitions Editor; Deb Myette-Flis, Senior Product Manager; Stacey Lamodi, Senior Content Project Manager; Jack Pendleton, Senior Art Director; Mary Colleen Liburdi, Senior Product Manager, Digital Solutions Group; Erin Zeggert, Technology Project Manager; and Vince Nicotina, Web/Systems Developer.

George Spratto extends a special thanks to Dr. Matthew Blommel of the West Virginia Center for Drug and Health Information, West Virginia University, who assisted in researching information on new and existing drugs. Greatest appreciation and love go to his wife, Lynne, as well as son Chris and his family—daughter-in-law Mary Alice and grandchildren Patrick Santopietro and Victoria Santopietro and son Gregg and his family—daughter-in-law Kim and grandchildren Alexandra and Dominic, all of whom make the work of this project worthwhile by their unfailing support and encouragement.

Adrienne Woods would like to extend her appreciation to her colleagues and friends at the VA and VANA. To her husband, Howard, who always finds time and energy to keep it all together. She thanks him for all his patience, caring, love, and understanding. To her children, Katy and Nate, she extends thanks for enduring hectic schedules, dirty/lost uniforms, and a few missed soccer tournaments/games/college games and matches. Finally, thanks to Fudge, her German short hair pointer, and Oreo, their kitty, for their patience and undying affection.

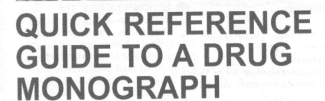

QUICK REFERENCE GUIDE TO A DRUG MONOGRAPH

1 GENERIC NAME OF DRUG: One or more icons may be found here: black box (side effects warning), camera (photo), ear (sound-alike drug), IV (drug can be given IV).

Nadolol

(NAY-doh-lohl) ←

CLASSIFICATION(S): ←
Beta-adrenergic blocking agent
PREGNANCY CATEGORY: C ←

Rx: Corgard
🍁**Rx:** Apo-Nadol, Novo-Nadolol, ratio-Nadolol

SEE ALSO *BETA-ADRENERGIC BLOCKING AGENTS.*
USES
(1) Hypertension, either alone or with other drugs (e.g., thiazide diuretic). (2) Long-term management of angina pectoris. *Investigational:* Prophylaxis of migraine, ventricular arrhythmias, aggres-si...

---

2 PHONETIC PRONUNCIATION of the generic name.

3 CLASSIFICATION: Defines the type of drug or the class under which the drug is listed.

4 PREGNANCY CATEGORY: Assigned by the FDA. Defined in Appendix 4.

5 TRADE NAMES: names by which a drug is marketed. If numerous forms of the drug are available, the trade names are identified by form. **Rx** denotes prescription drugs. **OTC** denotes over-the-counter, nonprescription drugs **CANADIAN** trade names are indicated by a maple leaf.

7 APPROVED THERAPEUTIC USES: Some investigational uses are also listed for selected drugs.

6 CONTROLLED SUBSTANCES: If the drug is controlled by the U. S. Federal Controlled Substances Act, the schedule in which the drug is placed follows the trade name listing. Controlled substance schedules are placed after Rx drugs. (ex: **C-II**) (See Appendix 3.)
CROSS REFERENCE (for selected drugs): "See also ..." directs the reader to the classification entry in Chapter 2 or to other parts of Chapter 1 that give a complete profile of the drug.

ACTION/KINETICS
Action
Manifests both beta$_1$- and beta$_2$-adrenergic blocking activity.
Pharmacokinetics
Peak serum concentration: 3–4 hr. t½: 20–24 hr (permits once-daily dosage).

9 MAXIMUM PLASMA LEVELS: Achieved at therapeutic doses.

Time to peak plasma levels: 2.5–4 hr. Peak effect: 9–12 hr. t½ of active metabolite: 22.5–30 hr. Excreted mainly (80%) in the urine. **Plasma protein binding:** More than 99%.
CONTRAINDICATIONS
Lactation.
SPECIAL CONCERNS

SPECIAL CONCERNS
■ Nortriptyline may increase the risk of suicidal thinking and behavior in children and adolescents with major depressive disorder and other psychiatric disorders.■
SIDE EFFECTS
Most Common
Nausea, decreased libido, impotence, insomnia, malaise, anxiety, nervousness.
See *Beta-Adrenergic Blocking Agents* for

LABORATORY TEST CONSIDERATIONS
↓ Urinary 5-HIAA.
OD OVERDOSE MANAGEMENT
Symptoms: Drowsiness, slurred speech. Possible obtundation, seizures, dystonic reaction of the head and neck. CV symptoms arrhythmias. *Treatment:* Es-

tion may worsen hypo...
DRUG INTERACTIONS
Antihypertensive agents / ↑ Antihypertensive effect
*Carb... / ↑ ... clear-

8 ACTION/KINETICS: The **Mechanism of Action** is stated when known. **Pharmacokinetics:** Critical information about the rate of drug absorption, distribution, time for peak plasma levels or peak effect, minimum effective serum or plasma level, duration of action, metabolism, and excretion route(s). Metabolism and excretion routes may be important for clients with systemic liver disease, kidney disease, or both.

10 BIOLOGICAL HALF-LIFE: The time required for half the drug to be excreted or removed from the blood, serum, or plasma.

11 PLASMA PROTEIN BINDING: The extent to which a drug is bound to plasma protein, when applicable.

12 CONTRAINDICATIONS: Lists disease states or conditions in which the drug should not be used.

13 SPECIAL CONCERNS: When appropriate, the FDA Black Box Warning is included. Considerations for use with caution in pediatric, geriatric, pregnant, or lactating clients, and in unique situations or disease states.

14 SIDE EFFECTS: The most common side effects are listed first for quick reference, followed by the complete list of side effects organized by body organ or system affected. If potentially life-threatening, the side effect is ***bold-italic.***

15 LABORATORY TEST CONSIDERATIONS: The manner in which the drug may affect laboratory test values is presented as increased values (↑) or false positive values (+) decreased values (↓) or false negative values (-). Also included, when available, are drug-induced changes in blood or urine levels of endogenous substances.

16 OVERDOSE MANAGEMENT: Symptoms observed following an overdose or toxic reaction and treatment approaches and/or antidotes for the overdose.

DRUG INTERACTIONS: Alphabetical listing of drugs and herbals that may interact with the drug. ↑ increase, ↓ decrease, → leading to.

tabolism

H *St. John's wort* / Possible ↓ olanza-pine plasma levels R/T ↑ metabolism.

HOW SUPPLIED

Capsules: 10 mg, 25 mg, 50 mg, 75 mg; *Oral Solution:* 10 mg base/5 mL.

HOW SUPPLIED

Nasal Spray: 2 mg/mL (200 mcg/inh).

DOSAGE

- **NASAL SPRAY**

  Endometriosis.

200 mcg into one nostril in the morning and 200 mcg into the other nostril at night (400 mcg twice a day may be required for some women).

NURSING CONSIDERATIONS

❧ Do not confuse Noroxin with Floxin or Neurontin (an anticonvulsant).

ADMINISTRATION/STORAGE

IV 1. Premedicate with antiemetics, including 5-HT₃ blockers with or without dexamethasone. Prehydration is not required.

2. Increase the infusion time from 2

24 GUIDELINES FOR ADMINISTRATION BY IV

ASSESSMENT

1. Document indications for therapy and characteristics of S&S. List other agents trialed and outcome. List drugs prescribed to ensure none interact unfavorably.

termine pregnant.

CLIENT/FAMILY TEACHING

1. Take 1 hr before or 2 hr after meals, with a glass of water; food decreases drug absorption. Antacids should not be taken with or for 2 hr after dosing. Take at evenly spaced intervals, generally response.

OUTCOMES/EVALUATE

- Negative culture reports
- Symptomatic improvement

18 HERBALS: Known or suspected drug interactions with herbal products.

19 HOW SUPPLIED: Dosage forms and amounts of the drug in each of the dosage forms. One dosage form may be more appropriate for a client than another. This information also allows the user to ensure the appropriate dosage form and strength is being administered.

20 DOSAGE: The dosage form (in color) and/or route of administration is followed by the disease state or condition (in italics and color) for which the dosage is recommended.

21 NURSING CONSIDERATIONS: Guidelines to help the practitioner in applying the nursing process to pharmacotherapeutics to ensure safe practice and patient safety.

22 SOUND ALIKE WARNINGS

23 ADMINISTRATION/STORAGE: Guidelines for preparing medications for administration, administering the medication, and proper storage and disposal of the medication.

25 ASSESSMENT: Guidelines for monitoring/assessing client before, during, and after prescribed drug therapy.

26 CLIENT/FAMILY TEACHING: Guidelines to promote education, active participation, understanding, and adherence to drug therapy by the client and/or family members. Precautions about drug therapy are also noted for communication to the client/family.

27 OUTCOMES/EVALUATE: Desired outcomes of the drug therapy and client response.

INTERVENTIONS (FOR SELECTED DRUGS): Guidelines for specific nursing actions related to the drug being administered.

CD-ROM

Delmar's 2009 Nurse's Drug Handbook CD-ROM is a dynam reference tool providing you with drug information wherever and whenever you need it!

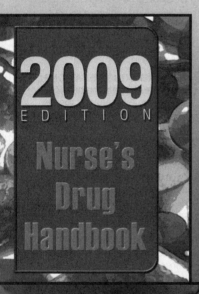

Key Features

- Easy download to your desktop to keep 195 of th Most Commonly Prescribe Drugs at your fingertips.
- Flexible search capabilities allow you to search by generic or trade name or entire drug information.
- Easy to read drug informatic has all of the great feature of the Nurse's Drug Handbook and allows for printing.

Version 1.0
ISBN 10: 1-
ISBN 13: 97
Technical Su
1-800-648-74
Monday-Frida
8:30 am to 5:3
E-mail: delmar.

Search

Acetaminophen

Pick One: ◉ Search
           ○ Search

DELMAR
NURSE'S
DRUG
HANDBOOK
COMPANION C

Online Database

With Delmar's 2009 Nurse's Drug Handbook Online Database, you can access the latest drug information for over 1,000 drug monographs in a new, more user friendly web environment. The database allows you to search by drug classification as well as generic and trade names, create custom folders of drug information, and even download selected information to a personal digital assistant (PDA) for remote use.

Key Features

- Flexible search capabilities allow you to search by name only or the entire drug information.
- Narrow your online search to account for over-the-counter, IV, or prescription medications.
- View your results by generic or trade name.
- Select and download drug monographs to your personal digital assistant (PDA) for customizable and convenient portability of essential information

PDA Downloads

Select and download drug monographs to your personal digit[al] assistant (PDA) for customizable and convenient portability o[f] essential information.

Key Features

- Entire database of drugs available for easy download to you[r] PDA device.
- Drug information available in Windows® Pocket PC or Palm® operating systems.
- Download as many drugs and as many times as you like.

chapter 1

A–Z Listing of Drugs

A

Abacavir sulfate ■
(uh-**BACK**-ah-veer)

CLASSIFICATION(S):
Antiviral, nucleoside reverse transcriptase inhibitor
PREGNANCY CATEGORY: C
Rx: Ziagen.

SEE ALSO *ANTIVIRAL DRUGS*.

USES
Treat HIV-1 infection in combination with other antiretroviral drugs (e.g., lamivudine and zidovudine). Do not add as a single agent when antiretroviral regimens are changed due to loss of virologic response.

ACTION/KINETICS

Action
Synthetic nucleoside analog. Converted intracellularly to the active carbovir triphosphate which inhibits the activity of HIV-1 reverse transcriptase by competing with the natural substrate deoxyguanosine-5'-triphosphate and by incorporation into viral DNA. Prevents the formation of the 5' to 3'-phosphodiester linkage essential for DNA chain elongation; thus, viral DNA growth is terminated. Cross resistance in vitro has been seen to lamivudine, didanosine, and zalcitabine.

Pharmacokinetics
Rapidly and extensively absorbed after PO use. Bioavailability of the tablet is about 80%. Not significantly metabolized by cytochrome P450 enzymes but it is metabolized by alcohol dehydrogenase in the liver and excreted in both the urine and feces. **Plasma protein binding:** About 50% bound to plasma proteins.

CONTRAINDICATIONS
Lactation. The safety, efficacy, and pharmacokinetic properties have not been determined in clients with severe hepatic impairment; do not use abacavir in clients with a Child-Pugh score from 10–15. Reintroduction to clients with a prior history of a hypersensitivity reaction to abacavir.

SPECIAL CONCERNS
■ (1) Hypersensitivity reactions. Serious and sometimes fatal hypersensitivity reactions are possible (See Side Effects). Hypersensitivity is a multi-organ clinical syndrome usually associated with 2 or more of the following groups:
• Constitutional, including achiness, fatigue, or generalized malaise
• Fever
• GI, including abdominal pain
• N&V
• Rash
• Respiratory, including cough, dyspnea, or pharyngitis
Discontinue as soon as hypersensitivity reaction is suspected. Permanently discontinue if hypersensitivity cannot be ruled out, even when other diagnoses are possible. Following a hypersensitivity reaction, never restart abacavir or any abacavir-containing product because more severe symptoms can occur within hours and may include life-threatening hypotension and death. Reintroduction of abacavir or any other abacavir-containing product, even in clients who have no identified history or unrecognized symptoms of hypersensitivity to abacavir therapy, can result in serious or fatal hypersensitivity reactions. Such reactions can occur

within hours. (2) Lactic acidosis and severe hepatomegaly. Lactic acidosis and severe hepatomegaly with steatosis (may be fatal) may occur following use of nucleoside analogs alone or in combination (including abacavir and other antiretroviral drugs). Efficacy for long-term suppression of HIV RNA or disease progression have not been determined. Not a cure for HIV infection; clients may continue to show illnesses associated with HIV infection, including opportunistic infections. Not shown to reduce the risk of transmission of HIV to others through sexual contact or blood. May show cross resistance with other nucleoside reverse transcriptase inhibitors. A poor response may be observed when abacavir is combined with lamivudine and tenofovir; this combination is not recommended.■ There is the potential for cross-resistance between abacavir and other nucleoside reverse transcriptase inhibitors. Safety and efficacy have not been determined in children 3 months to 13 years of age.

SIDE EFFECTS

Most Common

N&V, malaise/fatigue, dreams/sleep disorders, headache, migraine, abdominal pain/gastritis, diarrhea, fever/chills.

Hypersensitivity: Fever, skin rash, fatigue, N&V, diarrhea, abdominal pain, malaise, lethargy, myalgia, arthralgia, edema, SOB, pharyngitis, dyspnea, cough, paresthesia, lymphadenopathy, conjunctivitis, mouth ulcerations, erythema multiforme, maculopapular/urticarial rash, *life-threatening hypotension, liver failure, renal failure, death; fatal hypersensitivity reactions.* **GI:** N&V, diarrhea, loss of appetite, pancreatitis. **Body as a whole:** Redistribution/accumulation of body fat, including central obesity, dorsocervical fat enlargement (buffalo hump), peripheral/facial wasting, breast enlargement, and 'cushinoid appearance.' Malaise, fatigue, fever, chills, skin rashes. **Miscellaneous:** *Severe hepatomegaly with steatosis (may be fatal),* lactic acidosis, pancreatitis, insomnia, other sleep disorders, headache. *Stevens-Johnson syndrome and toxic epidermal necrolysis, especially in combination with drugs known to cause these effects.*

LABORATORY TEST CONSIDERATIONS

↑ LFTs, ALT, AST, CPK, GGT, creatinine, glucose. Hypertriglyceridemia, hyperamylasemia. Leukopenia, anemia, neutropenia, thrombocytopenia.

DRUG INTERACTIONS

Ethanol / ↓ Excretion of abacavir → ↑ exposure

Methadone / ↑ Methadone clearance; may need to ↑ dose in some clients

HOW SUPPLIED

Oral Solution: 20 mg/mL; *Tablets:* 300 mg.

DOSAGE

- **ORAL SOLUTION; TABLETS**
  Treat HIV-1 infection.

Adults: 300 mg twice a day with other antiretroviral drugs. **Pediatric, 3 months to 16 years:** 8 mg/kg twice a day, not to exceed 300 mg twice a day, in combination with other antiretroviral drugs. Use the following doses in hepatic impairment: **Child-Pugh score 7–9:** 200 mg twice a day. To enable dose reduction, use abacavir oral solution, 10 mL twice a day. Do not use in those with a Child-Pugh score of 10–15.

NURSING CONSIDERATIONS

ADMINISTRATION/STORAGE

1. Give with/without food.
2. Do not restart after hypersensitivity reaction. More severe symptoms will occur within hours; may include life-threatening hypotension or death.
3. Store at 20–25°C (68–77°F). Do not freeze, may be refrigerated.

ASSESSMENT

1. List reasons for therapy, other agents trialed.
2. Get electrolytes, renal, and LFTs; assess for liver enlargement, steatosis, lactic acidosis, opportunistic infections.
3. Assess for hypersensitivity reactions, even if alternative diagnosis possible. Once experienced, never resume therapy with abacavir.
4. If d/c and no hypersensitivity reactions, may reintroduce cautiously if medical care readily accessible.
5. Report hypersensitivity reactions to the Abacavir Hypersensitivity Registry

---

Bold Italic = life threatening side effect   ■ = black box warning   ♣ = Available in Canada

at 1-800-270-0425 Monday thru Friday 8 am to 8 pm.

6. Several products contain abacavir. Before starting abacavir, review medical history for prior exposure to any abacavir-containing product to avoid reintroduction in a client with a history of hypersensitivity to abacavir.

CLIENT/FAMILY TEACHING

1. Take with or without food and with other antiretroviral agents.

2. Review guide accompanying product; report any S&S of allergic reactions (fever, severe fatigue, skin rash, N&V, diarrhea or abdominal pain) and stop drug.

3. Does not prevent or cure disease; works to lower viral count.

4. If allergic reaction experienced, never restart—may be fatal.

5. Practice safe sex, drug does not prevent disease transmission.

6. Use reliable birth control; do not breastfeed.

7. Keep all F/U visits, labs and exams.

OUTCOMES/EVALUATE

Suppression of HIV RNA; increase in CD4 counts

Abatacept [IV]

(ah-**BAY**-tah-sept)

CLASSIFICATION(S):
Immunomodulator
PREGNANCY CATEGORY: C
Rx: Orencia.

USES

Reduce signs and symptoms, slow progression of structural damage, and improve physical function in adults with moderate to severe rheumatoid arthritis who have had an inadequate response to one or more disease-modifying antirheumatic drugs (such as methotrexate or tumor necrosis factor antagonists). Used alone or with other disease-modifying antirheumatic drugs.

ACTION/KINETICS

Action

Inhibits T-lymphocyte activation; activated T-lymphocytes are implicated in the pathogenesis of rheumatoid arthritis. Decreases serum levels of soluble interleukin-2 receptor, interleukin-6, rheumatoid factor, C-reactive protein, metalloproteinase-3, and tumor necrosis factor-alpha (relationship of these biological markers to rheumatoid arthritis is not known).

Pharmacokinetics

$t\frac{1}{2}$, **terminal:** 8–25 days in rheumatoid arthritis clients. Is a trend toward higher clearance with increasing body weight.

CONTRAINDICATIONS

Hypersensitivity to abatacept or any of its components. Use with TNF antagonists or anakinra. Use of live vaccines concurrently with abatacept or within 3 months of its discontinuation. Lactation.

SPECIAL CONCERNS

Concomitant use of abatacept and tissue necrosis factor (TNF) antagonists result in more infections (including serious infections) compared with use of TNF antagonists alone. Use with caution in the elderly. Use with caution in clients with a history of recurrent infections, underlying conditions that may predispose these clients to infections, or chronic, latent, or localized infections. Clients with COPD treated with abatacept developed side effects more frequently as well as exacerbation of their COPD; use with caution in such clients. A higher rate of infections may occur in abatacept-treated clients. Safety and efficacy have not been established in children.

SIDE EFFECTS

Most Common

Headache, URTI, nasopharyngitis, nausea.

Infections: URTI, bronchitis, herpes zoster, pneumonia, localized infection, sinusitis, influenza, rhinitis, herpes simplex, cellulitis, diverticulitis, acute pyelonephritis. **GI:** Dyspepsia. **CNS:** Dizziness, headache. **CV:** Hypertension. **Respiratory:** Cough, nasopharyngitis. **Malignancies:** Lung cancer, lymphoma, myelodysplastic syndrome, melanoma; cancer of the skin, breast, bile duct, bladder, cervix, endometrium, ovary, prostate, kidney, thyroid, and uterus.

Acute infusion reaction: Dizziness, headache, hypertension, hypotension, dyspnea, nausea, flushing, urticaria, cough, hypersensitivity, pruritus, rash, wheezing. **Miscellaneous:** Back pain, pain in extremity, rash, UTI, hypersensitivity reactions, worsening of COPD in COPD clients.

DRUG INTERACTIONS

Anakinra / Concomitant use is not recommended

Tissue necrosis factor antagonists / ↑ Risk of serious infections and no significant additional efficacy over use of TNF antagonists alone; do not use together

HOW SUPPLIED

Powder for Injection, Lyophilized: 250 mg.

DOSAGE

• **IV INFUSION**

Moderate to severe rheumatoid arthritis.

Adults, less than 60 kg: 500 mg. **Adults, 60–100 kg:** 750 mg. **Adults, over 100 kg:** 1 gram. Given as a 30 min IV infusion.

NURSING CONSIDERATIONS

ASSESSMENT

1. List reasons for therapy, other disease modifying antirheumatic drugs (DMARDs) failed, extent of disease, ROM, level of mobility.
2. Identify all drugs prescribed/OTC to ensure none interact.
3. Monitor CBC, renal, LFTs. Assess for any evidence of infection (skin, urine, lungs).
4. Perform TB test; CXR to ensure no lung disease. Avoid in those with COPD.

CLIENT/FAMILY TEACHING

1. Used to help slow joint destruction in rheumatoid arthritis when other agents have failed.
2. Avoid crowds, sick people and vaccinations-live (up to 3 mo after stopping drug) while on therapy.
3. Report lack of response, headaches, runny nose or dizziness; Use caution.
4. Avoid activities that require mental alertness until drug effects realized.
5. Given by IV infusion over 30 min at varying times. Ensure able to complete scheduled therapy.

6. Report fever, chills, non-healing wound, burning with urination, night sweats, Wt loss, wheezing, cough, skin rash, itching, flushing or shingles.
7. Practice reliable contraception; stop drug if pregnancy suspected.
8. Some receiving this drug have developed cancer, at this time, relationship is unknown.

OUTCOMES/EVALUATE

• ↓ Progression of joint damage
• Improved physical function.

Abciximab   IV
(ab-**SIX**-ih-mab)

CLASSIFICATION(S):
Antiplatelet drug
PREGNANCY CATEGORY: C
Rx: ReoPro.

USES

Adjunct to percutaneous coronary intervention (PCI) to prevent cardiac ischemic complications in clients undergoing PCI and in those with unstable angina not responding to conventional therapy when PCI is planned within 24 hr. Used with aspirin and heparin. *Investigational:* Early treatment of acute MI.

ACTION/KINETICS

Action

Binds to a glycoprotein receptor on human platelets, thus inhibiting platelet aggregation by preventing the binding of fibrinogen, von Willebrand factor, and other adhesive molecules to receptor sites on activated platelets.

Pharmacokinetics

t^1_2, **after IV bolus/infusion:** 10 min initially and a second phase half-life of about 30 min. **Recovery of platelet function:** About 48 hr, although the drug remains in the circulation bound to platelets for up to 15 days. Following IV infusion, free drug levels in the plasma decrease rapidly for about 6 hr and then decline at a slower rate.

CONTRAINDICATIONS

Due to a potential for drug-induced bleeding, abciximab is contraindicated as follows: History of CVA (within 2

---

years) or CVA with a significant residual neurologic deficit; active internal bleeding; within 6 weeks of GI or GU bleeding of clinical significance; bleeding diathesis; within 7 days of administration of oral anticoagulants unless the PT is less than 1.2 times control; thrombocytopenia (less than 100,000 cells/μL); within 6 weeks of major surgery or trauma; intracranial neoplasm; arteriovenous malformation or aneurysm; severe uncontrolled hypertension; presumed or documented history of vasculitis; use of IV dextran before PCI or intent to use it during PCI; hypersensitivity to murine proteins.

SPECIAL CONCERNS

Assess benefits versus the risk of increased bleeding in clients who weigh less than 75 kg, are 65 years of age or older, have a history of GI disease, and are receiving thrombolytics and heparin. Conditions also associated with an increased risk of bleeding in the angioplasty setting and which may be additive to that of abciximab: PCI within 12 hr of onset of symptoms for acute MI, PCI lasting more than 70 min, and failed PCI. Use with caution during lactation and when abciximab is used with other drugs that affect hemostasis, including thrombolytics, oral anticoagulants, NSAIDs, dipyridamole, and ticlopidine. Safety and efficacy have not been determined in children.

SIDE EFFECTS

Most Common
Back/chest pain, bleeding, hypotension, N&V, headache, bradycardia, puncture site pain, abdominal pain.
Bleeding tendencies: *Major bleeds, including intracranial hemorrhage.* Minor bleeding, including spontaneous gross hematuria/hematemesis. Loss of hemoglobin. **CV:** Hypotension, bradycardia, atrial fibrillation/flutter, vascular disorder, pulmonary edema, incomplete or ***complete AV block***, VT, weak pulse, palpitations, nodal arrhythmia, limb embolism, thrombophlebitis, intermittent claudication, pericardial effusion, pseudoaneurysm, AV fistula, ventricular arrhythmia. **GI:** N&V, abdominal pain, diarrhea, dry mouth, dyspepsia, enlarged abdomen, ileus, gastroesophageal reflux. **Hematologic:** Thrombocytopenia, anemia/hemolytic anemia, leukocytosis, petechiae. **CNS:** Hypesthesia, confusion, abnormal thinking, agitation, anxiety, dizziness, ***coma, brain ischemia***, insomnia. **Respiratory:** Pleural effusion, pleurisy, pneumonia, rales, bronchitis, bronchospasm, ***PE***, rhonchi. **Musculoskeletal:** Myopathy, cellulitis, myalgia, muscle contraction/pain. **GU:** UTI, urinary retention, abnormal renal function, dysuria, frequent micturition, cystalgia, incontinence, prostatitis. **Dermatologic:** Pruritus, pallor, increased sweating, bullous eruption. **Ophthalmic:** Diplopia, abnormal vision. **Miscellaneous:** Pain, peripheral edema, development of human antichimeric antibody, dysphonia, abscess, asthenia, incisional pain, wound abscess, cellulitis, peripheral coldness, injection site pain, diabetes mellitus, hypertonia, inflammation, immunogenicity, hypersensitivity reactions including ***anaphylaxis***.

LABORATORY TEST CONSIDERATIONS

Hyperkalemia.

DRUG INTERACTIONS

Anticoagulants / ↑ Risk of bleeding
[H] *Bromelain* / Possible ↑ bleeding risk
Dipyridamole / ↑ Risk of bleeding
[H] *Evening primrose oil* / Possible ↑ antiplatelet effect
[H] *Feverfew* / Possible ↑ antiplatelet effect
[H] *Garlic* / Possible ↑ antiplatelet effect
[H] *Ginger* / Possible ↑ antiplatelet effect
[H] *Ginkgo biloba* / Possible ↑ antiplatelet effect
[H] *Ginseng* / Possible ↑ antiplatelet effect
[H] *Grapeseed extract* / Possible ↑ antiplatelet effect
NSAIDs / ↑ Risk of bleeding
Ticlopidine / ↑ Risk of bleeding

HOW SUPPLIED

Injection: 2 mg/mL.

DOSAGE

• **IV BOLUS FOLLOWED BY IV INFUSION**

Prevention of cardiac ischemic complications with concomitant use of heparin and aspirin.

IV bolus: 0.25 mg/kg 10–60 min before the start of the intervention, followed by **continuous IV infusion:** 0.125 mcg/kg/min (to a maximum of 10 mcg/min) for 12 hr. Those with unstable angina not responding to usual therapy and who require PCI within 24 hr may be given abciximab, 0.25 mg/kg IV bolus, followed by an 18–24 hr IV infusion of 10 mcg/min, ending 1 hr after the PCI.

NURSING CONSIDERATIONS

ADMINISTRATION/STORAGE

[IV] 1. Stop infusion after 12 hr; avoids prolonged platelet receptor blockade effects.

2. Inspect visually for particulate matter prior to administration; do not use if visibly opaque particles noted. Use aseptic procedures.

3. Arterial access site care is important to prevent bleeding. Only the anterior wall of the femoral artery should be punctured. Avoid femoral vein sheath placement unless needed. While the vascular sheath is in place, maintain clients on complete bed rest with the head of the bed 30° or less and the affected limb restrained in a straight position. If needed medicate clients for back/groin pain as needed.

4. Following sheath removal, apply pressure to the femoral artery for at least 30 min using either manual compression or a mechanical device for hemostasis. Apply a pressure dressing following hemostasis. Maintain the client on bed rest for 6–8 hr after sheath removal or discontinuation of the drug, or 4 hr following discontinuation of heparin, whichever is later. Remove the pressure dressing prior to ambulation.

5. The following conditions may be associated with an increased risk of bleeding and may be additive with the effect of abciximab in the angioplasty setting: PCI within 12 hr of onset of symptoms for acute MI, prolonged PCI (lasting more than 70 min), and failed PCI.

6. Stop continuous infusion with failed PCIs; no evidence effective in such situations.

7. Stop abciximab and heparin immediately if serious bleeding occurs not controlled by compression.

8. If symptoms of an allergic reaction or anaphylaxis occur, stop infusion immediately; institute treatment. Have epinephrine, dopamine, theophylline, antihistamines, and corticosteroids for immediate use.

9. For the bolus injection withdraw the appropriate amount of drug into a syringe. Filter through a sterile, nonpyrogenic, low-protein-binding 0.2- or 5-μm filter into syringe; give bolus 10–60 min before procedure.

10. For continuous infusion withdraw the appropriate amount of drug into a syringe. Inject into a container of sterile 0.9% NSS or D5W. Filter either upon admixture using a sterile, nonpyrogenic, low–protein-binding 0.2- or 5-μm filter or upon administration using an in-line, sterile, nonpyrogenic low–protein-binding 0.2- or 0.22-μm filter. Discard any unused drug at the end of the infusion.

11. Give through separate IV line with no other medications added to solution. No incompatibilities have been noted with glass bottles or PVC bags or IV sets.

12. Use the following guidelines to minimize the risk of bleeding:
- When abciximab is started 18–24 hr before PCI, maintain the APTT between 60 and 85 seconds during the abciximab and heparin infusion period.
- During PCI, maintain the ACT between 200 and 300 seconds.
- If anticoagulation is continued in these clients following PCI, maintain the APTT between 55 and 75 seconds.
- Check the APTT or ACT prior to arterial sheath removal. Do not remove the sheath unless APTT is 50 seconds or less or ACT is 175 seconds or less.

13. Store vials at 2–8°C (36–46°F); do not freeze or shake vials.

ASSESSMENT

1. Obtain a thorough nursing history; note indications/goals of therapy.
2. Note any history of CVA, bleeding disorders, recent episodes of bleeding, trauma, or surgery.
3. List other agents prescribed/OTC and when last consumed to prevent any bleeding potential.
4. Monitor PT, INR, PTT, CBC, VS, and EKG. Check platelet count 2–4 hr after initial bolus and again in 24 hr.

INTERVENTIONS

1. If undergoing PCI will receive a bolus of abciximab (0.25 mg/kg) 10–60 min before procedure followed by a continuous IV infusion (10 mcg/min) for 12 hr.
2. Insert separate IV lines with saline locks for blood draws.
3. Observe during infusion; anaphylaxis may occur at any time.
4. Administer 325 mg aspirin orally 2 hr before procedure and prepare heparin bolus and infusion for administration.
5. Observe for any bleeding sites: catheter sites, needle punctures, GI, GU, and retroperitoneal sites. Remove tape/dressings gently.
6. If serious bleeding develops (not controlled with pressure), stop infusions of abciximab and heparin.
7. Complete bedrest while vascular access sheath in place. Restrain limb straight and raise HOB no more than 30 degrees. Stop heparin infusion at least 4 hr before sheath removal. Palpate/monitor distal pulses of involved extremity.
8. Apply pressure for 30 min over femoral artery once sheath is removed. When hemostasis evident, apply pressure dressing with sandbag and check frequently for bleeding. Monitor hematoma for enlargement. Enforce bedrest 6–8 hr after infusion completed and sheath removed.

CLIENT/FAMILY TEACHING

1. Review indications, what to expect, clinical management, and anticipated results.
2. Review risks with therapy, e.g., bleeding from intracranial hemorrhage, which may be lethal, or bloody urine/vomit; may require blood/platelet transfusions.
3. Report fever, chills, rash, or other adverse effects. It may take longer to stop bleeding and pressure will be applied to bleeding sites to help stop the flow.
4. Drug may cause formation of human antichimeric antibody, which may cause hypersensitivity reactions, low platelets, or diminished response on re-administration.

OUTCOMES/EVALUATE

Prevention of abrupt coronary vessel closure with associated ischemic complications

Acamprosate calcium
(a-**CAMP**-pro-sayt)

CLASSIFICATION(S):

Antialcoholic drug
PREGNANCY CATEGORY: C
Rx: Campral.

USES

Maintenance of abstinence from alcohol in those with alcohol dependence who are abstinent at beginning of treatment. Use of acamprosate should be part of a comprehensive management program that includes psychosocial support.

ACTION/KINETICS

Action

The mechanism is not fully understood. Acamprosate may interact with glutamate and GABA neurotransmitter systems centrally and may restore the normal balance between neural excitation and inhibition which is altered during chronic alcohol exposure. Not known to cause alcohol aversion and does not cause a disulfiram-like reaction if alcohol is ingested.

Pharmacokinetics

About 11% is bioavailable after PO ingestion. Steady-state plasma levels reached in about 5 days. **Steady-state peak plasma levels after usual daily doses:** 350 ng/mL 3–8 hr after dosing. Administration with food decreases bioavailability but is not clinically significant; no dosage adjustment is required. The drug is not metabolized; the major route of excretion is through the urine. **t½, terminal:** 20–33 hr. **Plasma protein binding:** Negligible.

CONTRAINDICATIONS

Use in severe renal impairment (C$_{CR}$ 30 mL/min or less). Previous hypersensitivity to acamprosate.

SPECIAL CONCERNS

Efficacy of acamprosate has not been shown in those who have not undergone detoxification and not achieved abstinence from alcohol prior to beginning acamprosate treatment. Efficacy in promoting abstinence from alcohol in polysubstance abusers has not been assessed adequately. Use of the drug does not eliminate or diminish alcohol withdrawal symptoms. Although rare, there is an increased risk of suicidal ideation, suicidal attempts, and completed suicides. Use with caution during lactation. Safety and efficacy have not been established in children.

SIDE EFFECTS

Most Common

Diarrhea, N&V, flatulence, pruritus, insomnia, dizziness.

Side effects listed are those with a frequency of 0.1% or more. **CNS:** Insomnia, depression, anxiety/nervousness, dizziness, paresthesia, abnormal thinking, amnesia, headache, decreased libido, somnolence, tremor, abnormal dreams, agitation, apathy, confusion, convulsion, hallucinations, hostility, hyperesthesia, increased libido, migraine, neuralgia, neurosis, *suicidal ideation, suicidal attempt,* vertigo, withdrawal syndrome. **GI:** Diarrhea, anorexia, dry mouth, N&V, flatulence, abdominal pain, constipation, dyspepsia, increased appetite, dysphagia, eructation, esophagitis, gastritis, gastroenteritis, *GI hemorrhage, pancreatitis, rectal hemorrhage,* hematemesis, hepatitis, liver cirrhosis. **CV:** Hypertension, palpitation, syncope, vasodilation, angina pectoris, *hemorrhage, MI,* hypotension, phlebitis, postural hypotension, tachycardia, varicose vein. **Hematologic:** Anemia, ecchymosis, eosinophilia, lymphocytosis, thrombocytopenia. **Respiratory:** Bronchitis, increased cough, dyspnea, pharyngitis, rhinitis, asthma, epistaxis, pneumonia. **Musculoskeletal:** Arthralgia, myalgia, leg cramps. **Dermatologic:** Pruritus, sweating, rash, alopecia, dry skin, eczema, exfoliative dermatitis, maculopapular rash, urticaria, vesiculobullous rash. **GU:** Impotence, abnormal sexual function, metrorrhagia, urinary frequency/incontinence, UTI, vaginitis. **Body as a whole:** Asthenia, accidental injury, pain, peripheral edema, weight gain, avitaminosis, diabetes mellitus, gout, thirst, weight loss, chills, flu syndrome, infection, abscess, allergic reaction, fever, malaise. **Ophthalmic:** Abnormal vision, amblyopia. **Otic:** Deafness, tinnitus. **Miscellaneous:** Taste perversion, back pain, chest pain, hernia, intentional injury, intentional overdose, neck pain.

LABORATORY TEST CONSIDERATIONS

Abnormal LFTs. ↑ AST, ALT, alkaline phosphatase, creatinine, lactic dehydrogenase. Bilirubinemia, hyperglycemia, hyperuricemia.

HOW SUPPLIED

Tablets, Delayed-Release: 333 mg.

DOSAGE

• **TABLETS, DELAYED-RELEASE**

Maintenance of abstinence from alcohol.

Two 333 mg tablets (total of 666 mg) 3 times per day. With moderate renal impairment (C$_{CR}$ of 30–50 mL/min), begin with one 333 mg tablet 3 times per day.

NURSING CONSIDERATIONS

ADMINISTRATION/STORAGE

1. Begin acamprosate treatment as soon as possible after alcohol withdrawal, when client achieved abstinence, and maintain treatment if client relapses.

2. Use care in dose selection in elderly due to possible decreased renal function.

ASSESSMENT

1. Note history of alcohol use, desire to stop and if alcohol free or detoxified prior to starting therapy.

2. Monitor VS, I&O, renal and LFTs; reduce dose with renal dysfunction.

3. Identify support system and willingness to attend counselling/support programs to ensure positive outcome.

Bold Italic = life threatening side effect   ■ = black box warning   ✦ = Available in Canada

CLIENT/FAMILY TEACHING
1. Take 3 times per day with/without food. Continue even with relapse and report to provider.
2. Avoid friends/locations that encourage drinking behaviors.
3. Use caution/avoid activities that require mental alertness until drug effects realized; may experience impairment of motor skills, judgment and thinking.
4. Report adverse side effects or lack of response. Report all depression and suicide thoughts immediately.
5. Practice reliable birth control; report if pregnant or breastfeeding.
6. Keep regularly scheduled meetings and counselling/support sessions to ensure abstinence.

OUTCOMES/EVALUATE
Maintenance of alcohol abstinence

Acarbose
(ah-**KAR**-bohs)

CLASSIFICATION(S):
Antidiabetic, oral; alpha-glucosidase inhibitor
PREGNANCY CATEGORY: B
Rx: Precose.
✤**Rx:** Prandase.

SEE ALSO *ANTIDIABETIC AGENTS: HYPOGLYCEMIC AGENTS.*

USES
(1) Alone as an adjunct to diet to treat type 2 diabetes mellitus in those whose hyperglycemia is not managed by diet alone. (2) With a sulfonylurea, insulin, or metformin when diet plus either acarbose or a sulfonylurea do not control diabetes.

ACTION/KINETICS
Action
Causes a competitive, reversible inhibition of pancreatic alpha-amylase and membrane-bound intestinal alpha-glucosidase hydrolase enzymes. This causes delayed glucose absorption resulting in a smaller increase in blood glucose following meals. Glycosylated hemoglobin levels are decreased in those with NIDDM. Additive effect with sulfonylureas due to different mechanism of action (the drug does not enhance insulin secretion).

Pharmacokinetics
Approximately 65% of an oral dose of acarbose remains in the GI tract, which is the site of action. **Peak plasma levels of active drug:** About 1 hr. Metabolized in the GI tract by both intestinal bacteria and intestinal enzymes. Acarbose and metabolites that are absorbed are excreted in the urine.

CONTRAINDICATIONS
Diabetic ketoacidosis, cirrhosis, IBD, colonic ulceration, partial intestinal obstruction or predisposition to intestinal obstruction, chronic intestinal diseases associated with marked disorders of digestion or absorption, conditions that may deteriorate as a result of increased gas formation in the intestine. In significant renal dysfunction (serum creatinine >2 mg/dL). Severe, persistent bradycardia. Lactation.

SPECIAL CONCERNS
Safety and efficacy have not been determined in children. Acarbose, alone, does not cause hypoglycemia; however, sulfonylureas and insulin can lower blood glucose sufficiently to cause symptoms or even life-threatening hypoglycemia. Loss of BG control may occur during stress, such as fever, trauma, infection, and surgery.

SIDE EFFECTS
Most Common
Flatulence, diarrhea, abdominal pain.
GI: Flatulence, diarrhea, abdominal pain. GI side effects may be severe and may be confused with paralytic ileus. **Miscellaneous:** Skin rash and edema (rare).

LABORATORY TEST CONSIDERATIONS
↑ Serum transaminases (especially long-term use with doses up to 300 mg 3 times/day). Small ↓ in hematocrit. ↓ Serum calcium. Low plasma vitamin B_6 levels.

OD OVERDOSE MANAGEMENT
Symptoms: Flatulence, diarrhea, abdominal discomfort. *Treatment:* Reduce dose; symptoms will subside.

A

DRUG INTERACTIONS

Charcoal / ↓ Acarbose effect; do not use together

Digestive enzymes / ↓ Acarbose effect; do not use together

Digoxin / ↓ Serum digoxin levels

Insulin / ↑ Hypoglycemia; possible severe hypoglycemia

Sulfonylureas / ↑ Hypoglycemia; possible severe hypoglycemia

HOW SUPPLIED

Tablets: 25 mg, 50 mg, 100 mg.

DOSAGE

• TABLETS

Type 2 diabetes mellitus.

Individualized, depending on effectiveness and tolerance, but not to exceed 100 mg 3 times per day. **Adults, initial:** 25 mg 3 times per day with the first bite of each main meal. Some may benefit from more gradual dose titration by starting with 15 mg once a day and then increasing to 25 mg twice a day. **Maintenance:** Increase dose to 50 mg 3 times per day. Some may benefit from 100 mg 3 times per day. The dosage can be adjusted at 4- to 8-week intervals. **Recommended maximum daily dose:** 50 mg 3 times per day for clients weighing less than 60 kg and 100 mg 3 times per day for those weighing more than 60 kg.

NURSING CONSIDERATIONS

ADMINISTRATION/STORAGE

1. Start with low dose; reduces GI side effects and helps determine minimum effective dose.

2. If dose missed, take usual dose at start of next main meal.

ASSESSMENT

1. List reasons for therapy, age at symptom onset, other agents trialed and outcome.

2. Note any cirrhosis, chronic intestinal diseases, or disorders of digestion/absorption. Avoid if serum creatinine >2 mg/dL.

3. Obtain baseline Ht, Wt, CBC, HbA1c, BS, electrolytes, U/A, renal and LFTs; assess for B_6 deficiency. Monitor HbA1c and LFTs q 3 months.

4. Initiate/titrate acarbose based on BS results. Ideally, measure 1-hr postprandial plasma glucose level to determine effective dose.

5. May enhance glycemic control with a sulfonylurea, but may also be used alone.

CLIENT/FAMILY TEACHING

1. Take three times daily with first bite of each meal. May be used with insulin or other oral agents. If dose missed and meal completed then skip dose and take at next meal.

2. Delays digestion of ingested carbohydrates (glucose); used in addition to diet.

3. Caloric restrictions and weight loss, especially in obese, must be continued to control BS and prevent complications of diabetes; continue regular daily exercise. Complete diabetes education classes to enhance success.

4. Most common side effects are of GI origin (abdominal discomfort, diarrhea, gas); should subside in frequency and intensity with continued use.

5. Monitor glucose (finger sticks) and record to assess response and provider review.

6. Loss of glucose control may result when exposed to stress, such as fever, trauma, infection, or surgery. In this event, temporary insulin therapy may be needed.

7. Do not use candy bars to counteract hypoglycemia; use Lifesavers™, glucose tablets/gel or lactose.

OUTCOMES/EVALUATE

Control of BS with NIDDM; A1c <7

Acetaminophen (APAP, Paracetamol)

(ah-**SEAT**-ah-**MIN**-oh-fen)

CLASSIFICATION(S):

Non-narcotic analgesic

PREGNANCY CATEGORY: B

OTC: Caplets/Caplets Extended-Release: Aspirin Free Anacin Maximum Strength, Aspirin Free Pain Relief, Genapap Extra Strength, Genebs Extra Strength Caplets, Pa-

---

Bold Italic = life threatening side effect   ■ = black box warning   ♣ = Available in Canada

nadol, Panadol Junior Strength, Tapanol Extra Strength, Tylenol 8 Hour, Tylenol Extended Relief. **Capsules:** Dapacin. **Drops:** Aspirin Free Anacin Maximum Strength, Children's Dynafed Jr., Children's Mapap, Dolono, Extra Strength Dynafed E.X., Infantaire, Infants' Pain Reliever, Liquiprin Drops for Children. **Elixir:** Aceta, Apra, Dolono, Genapap Children's, Mapap Children's, Oraphen-PD, Ridenol, Silapap Children's, Tylenol Children's. **Gelcaps/Geltabs:** Aspirin Free Anacin Maximum Strength, Tapanol Extra Strength, Tylenol 8 Hour, Tylenol Extra Strength. **Oral Liquid/Syrup:** Chloraseptic Sore Throat, Comtrex Maximum Strength Sore Throat, Halenol Children's, Panadol Children's, Silapap Children's, Tempra 2 Syrup, Tylenol Extra Strength, Tylenol Sore Throat Daytime, Tylenol Sore Throat Maximum Strength. **Oral Solution:** Acetaminophen Drops, Apacet, Genapap Infants' Drops, Mapap Infant Drops, Panadol Infants' Drops, Silapap Infants, Tempra 1, Tylenol Infants' Drops, Uni-Ace. **Capsules, Sprinkle:** Feverall Children's, Feverall Junior Strength. **Suppositories:** Acephen, Children's Feverall, Feverall Suppositories, Infant's Feverall, Junior Strength Feverall, Neopap. **Tablets, Chewable/Dispersible:** Apacet, Children's Genapap, Children's Pain Reliever Suspension, Children's Panadol, Children's Tylenol Soft Chews, Tempra 3, Tylenol Caplets, Tylenol Children's, Tylenol Children's Meltaways, Tylenol Extra Strength GoTabs. **Tablets:** Aceta, Aspirin Free Pain Relief, Genapap, Genapap Extra Strength, Genebs, Genebs Extra Strength, Mapap Extra Strength, Mapap Regular Strength, Maranox, Panadol, Redutemp, Tempra, Tylenol Extra Strength, Tylenol Extra Strength for Arthritis Pain, Tylenol Junior Strength, Tylenol Regular Strength, UN-Aspirin Extra Strength. **Tablets, Extended-Release:** Tylenol Arthritis. **Tablets, Oral Disintegrating:** Tylenol Meltaways Jr. ♣**OTC: Caplets:** Atasol, Atasol Forte. **Oral Liquid/Syrup:** Atasol, Childrens Acetaminophen Elixir Drops, Pediatrix, Tempra, Tempra

Children's Syrup. **Oral Solution:** Atasol, Children's Acetaminophen Oral Solution, PMS-Acetaminophen, Pediatrix. **Oral Suspension:** Tylenol Children's Suspension, Tylenol Infants' Suspension. **Suppositories:** Abenol 120, 325, 650 mg. **Tablets, Chewable:** Children's Chewable Acetaminophen, Tempra, Tylenol Junior Strength Chewable Tablets Fruit. **Tablets:** A.F. Anacin, A.F. Anacin Extra Strength, Apo-Acetaminophen, Atasol, Atasol Forte, Extra Strength Acetaminophen, Regular Strength Acetaminophen, Tylenol Tablets 325 mg, 500 mg.

Acetaminophen, buffered

OTC: Bromo Seltzer Effervescent Granules.

USES

(1) Control of pain due to headache, earache, dysmenorrhea, arthralgia, myalgia, musculoskeletal pain, arthritis, immunizations, teething, tonsillectomy. (2) To reduce fever in bacterial or viral infections. (3) As a substitute for aspirin in upper GI disease, aspirin allergy, bleeding disorders, clients on anticoagulant therapy, and gouty arthritis. *Investigational:* In children receiving DPT vaccination to decrease incidence of fever and pain at injection site. Addition of acetaminophen to strong opioids and/or coanalgesics in cancer clients may ease pain and improve well-being without major side effects.

ACTION/KINETICS

Action

Decreases fever by (1) a hypothalamic effect leading to sweating and vasodilation and (2) inhibits the effect of pyrogens on the hypothalamic heat-regulating centers. May cause analgesia by inhibiting CNS prostaglandin synthesis; however, due to minimal effects on peripheral prostaglandin synthesis, acetaminophen has no anti-inflammatory or uricosuric effects. Does not cause any anticoagulant effect or ulceration of the GI tract. Antipyretic and analgesic effects are comparable to those of aspirin.

= see color insert   H = Herbal   IV = Intravenous   = sound alike drug

Pharmacokinetics

Peak plasma levels: 30–120 min. **t½:** 45 min–3 hr. **Therapeutic serum levels** (analgesia): 5–20 mcg/mL. Metabolized in the urine as glucuronide and sulfate conjugates. However, an intermediate hydroxylated metabolite is hepatotoxic following large doses of acetaminophen. The extended-relief product uses a bilayer system that allows the outer layer to release acetaminophen rapidly while the inner layer is designed to release the remainder of the dose more slowly. This allows prolonged relief of symptoms. The buffered product is a mixture of acetaminophen, sodium bicarbonate, and citric acid that effervesces when placed in water. It also has a high sodium content (0.76 grams per ¾ capful). **Plasma protein binding:** Approximately 25%.

CONTRAINDICATIONS

Renal insufficiency, anemia. Clients with cardiac or pulmonary disease are more susceptible to acetaminophen toxicity.

SPECIAL CONCERNS

Toxicity, including serious liver damage (hepatocyte necrosis) and apoptosis, may occur with doses not far beyond labeled dosing, especially when using high doses and when taking more than one product containing acetaminophen and with moderate amounts of alcohol. Use with caution in pregnancy. Consult a physician before use if more than three alcoholic drinks per day are consumed.

SIDE EFFECTS

Most Common

Few when taken in usual therapeutic doses. GI upset in some.

Chronic and even acute toxicity can develop after long symptom-free usage. **Hematologic:** Methemoglobinemia, ***hemolytic anemia***, neutropenia, thrombocytopenia, pancytopenia, leukopenia. **Allergic:** Urticarial and erythematous skin reactions, skin eruptions, fever. **Miscellaneous:** CNS stimulation, hypoglycemic coma, jaundice, drowsiness, glossitis. Possible liver damage in those who consume three or more alcoholic drinks daily.

OD OVERDOSE MANAGEMENT

Symptoms: May be no early specific symptoms. Within first 24 hr: N&V, diaphoresis, anorexia, drowsiness, confusion, liver tenderness, cardiac arrhythmias, low BP, jaundice, acute hepatic and renal failure. Within 24–48 hr, increased AST, ALT, bilibrubin, PT levels. After 72–96 hr, peak hepatotoxicity with death possible due to liver necrosis. *Treatment:* Initially, induction of emesis, gastric lavage, activated charcoal. Oral *N*-acetylcysteine is said to reduce or prevent hepatic damage by inactivating acetaminophen metabolites, which cause liver toxicity.

DRUG INTERACTIONS

Alcohol, ethyl / Chronic use → ↑ toxicity of larger therapeutic doses of acetaminophen

Barbiturates / ↑ Potential of hepatotoxicity R/T ↑ liver breakdown of acetaminophen

Carbamazepine / ↑ Potential of hepatotoxicity R/T ↑ liver breakdown of acetaminophen

Charcoal, activated / ↓ Absorption of acetaminophen when given as soon as possible after overdose

Diuretics, loop / ↓ Effect R/T ↓ renal prostaglandin excretion and ↓ plasma renin activity

Hydantoins (including Phenytoin) / ↑ Potential of hepatotoxicity R/T ↑ liver breakdown of acetaminophen

Isoniazid / ↑ Potential of hepatotoxicity R/T ↑ liver breakdown of acetaminophen

Lamotrigine / ↓ Serum lamotrigine levels → ↓ effect

H *Milk thistle* / Helps prevent acetaminophen liver damage

NSAIDs / ↑ Risk of hypertension in women

Oral contraceptives / ↑ Liver breakdown of acetaminophen → ↓ t½

Propranolol / ↑ Effect R/T ↓ liver breakdown

Rifampin / ↑ Hepatotoxicity potential R/T ↑ liver breakdown of acetaminophen

Smoking / Possible ↓ serum acetaminophen levels R/T ↑ hepatic metabolism

---

Bold Italic = life threatening side effect   ■ = black box warning   ✦ = Available in Canada

Sulfinpyrazone / ↑ Hepatotoxicity potential R/T ↑ liver breakdown of acetaminophen

Zidovudine / ↓ Zidovudine effect R/T ↑ nonhepatic or renal clearance

HOW SUPPLIED

Acetaminophen *Caplets/Caplets Extended-Release:* 160 mg, 500 mg, 650 mg; *Capsules:* 325 mg, 500 mg; *Capsules, Sprinkle:* 80 mg, 160 mg; *Drops:* 80 mg/0.8 mL; *Elixir:* 80 mg/2.5 mL, 80 mg/5 mL, 120 mg/5 mL, 160 mg/5 mL; *Gelcaps:* 500 mg; *Geltabs:* 650 mg; *Liquid:* 160 mg/5 mL, 166.6 mg/5 mL, 500 mg/15 mL; *Solution:* 80 mg/1.66 mL, 100 mg/mL; *Suppositories:* 80 mg, 120 mg, 125 mg, 300 mg, 325 mg, 650 mg; *Tablets:* 325 mg, 500 mg, 650 mg; *Tablets, Chewable:* 80 mg, 160 mg, 500 mg; *Tablets, Dispersible:* 80 mg; *Tablets, Extra Strength:* 650 mg.; *Tablets, Oral Disintegrating:* 160 mg.

Acetaminophen, buffered *Granules, Effervescent:*

DOSAGE

• **CAPLETS; CAPSULES; CAPSULES, SPRINKLE; ELIXIR; GELCAPS; ORAL LIQUID/SYRUP; ORAL SOLUTION; SYRUP; TABLETS; TABLETS, CHEWABLE; TABLETS, DISPERSIBLE**

Analgesic, antipyretic.

Adults: 325–650 mg q 4 hr; doses up to a maximum of 1 gram q 6 hr may be used. **Pediatric:** Doses given 4–5 times per day. **Up to 3 months:** 40 mg/dose; **4–11 months:** 80 mg/dose; **1–2 years:** 120 mg/dose; **2–3 years:** 160 mg/dose; **4–5 years:** 240 mg/dose; **6–8 years:** 320 mg/dose; **9–10 years:** 400 mg/dose; **11 years:** 480 mg/dose. **12–14 years:** 640 mg/dose. **Over 14 years:** 650 mg/dose. *Alternative pediatric dose:* 10–15 mg/kg q 4 hr.

• **CAPLETS, EXTENDED-RELIEF**

Analgesic, antipyretic.

Adults: 2 caplets (1,300 mg) q 8 hr, up to 6 per day.

• **CAPLETS, EXTENDED-RELIEF; GELTABS**

Adults, 18 years and older: 1,300 mg (2 caplets or 2 geltabs) q 8 hr, up to 6 caplets or geltabs/day.

• **SUPPOSITORIES**

Analgesic, antipyretic.

Adults: 650 mg q 4 hr, not to exceed 4 grams/day for up to 10 days. Clients on long-term therapy should not exceed 2.6 grams/day. **Pediatric, 3–11 months:** 80 mg q 6 hr. **1–3 years:** 80 mg q 4 hr; **3–6 years:** 120–125 mg q 4–6 hr, with no more than 720 mg in 24 hr. **6–12 years:** 325 mg q 4–6 hr with no more than 2.6 grams in 24 hr. Given as needed while symptoms persist.

• **TABLETS, EXTENDED-RELEASE**

Adults and children over 12 years: 1,300 mg (2 tablets) q 8 hr, up to 6 tablets/day.

• **GRANULES, EFFERVESCENT**

Analgesic, antipyretic.

Adult, usual: 1 or 2 three-quarter capfuls are placed into an empty glass; add half a glass of cool water. May be taken while fizzing or after settling. Can be repeated q 4 hr as required or directed by provider.

• **TABLETS, ORAL DISINTEGRATING**

Analgesic, antipyretic.

Children, 6–8 years of age: 320 mg (2 tablets) q 4 hr, up to 10 per day; **9–10 years of age:** 400 mg (2½ tablets) q 4 hr, up to 12½ tablets per day; **11 years of age:** 480 mg (3 tablets) q 4 hr, up to 15 tablets per day; **12 years of age:** 640 mg (4 tablets) q 4 hr, up to 20 tablets per day.

NURSING CONSIDERATIONS

ADMINISTRATION/STORAGE

1. Do not exceed 4 grams/24 hr in adults and 75 mg/kg/day in children.
2. Do not take for >5 days for pain in children, 10 days for pain in adults, or more than 3 days for fever in adults or children without consulting provider.
3. Store suppositories below 27°C (80°F).
4. Take ER product with water; do not crush, chew, or dissolve before swallowing.
5. Bubble gum flavored OTC pediatric products (liquid and chewable tablets) are available to treat fever and/or pain.

ASSESSMENT

1. Note reasons for therapy, prescribed dosage, and expected outcomes.
2. With long-term therapy, monitor CBC, renal, LFTs.

📷 = see color insert   H = Herbal   IV = Intravenous   ℝ = sound alike drug

A

3. Document presence of pain/fever. Rate pain, noting type, onset, location, duration, and intensity.

4. Check urine for occult blood and albumin; assess for nephritis.

CLIENT/FAMILY TEACHING

1. Do not combine products containing acetaminophen, many of which are OTC. Read labels on all OTC products consumed.

2. Review with parents the difference between concentrated dropper dose formulation and teaspoon dose formulation.

3. Take as directed with food or milk to decrease GI upset.

4. S&S of acute toxicity that require immediate reporting include N&V or abdominal pain. Bluish coloration of skin/nailbeds or complaints of SOB, weakness, headache, or dizziness are S&S of methemoglobinemia caused by lack of oxygen and require immediate attention.

5. Report paleness, weakness, and heart beat skips; S&S of hemolytic anemia.

6. SOB, fast, weak pulse; cold extremities; unexplained bleeding, bruising, sore throat, fatigue, feeling clammy or sweaty; or low temperatures may also be symptoms of chronic poisoning; report.

7. Abdominal pain, yellow discoloration of skin and eyes, dark urine, itching, or clay-colored stools may indicate liver toxicity.

8. Phenacetin, the major active metabolite, may cause urine to become dark brown or wine-colored.

9. Headache and minor pain relievers containing combinations of salicylates, acetaminophen, and caffeine may be no more beneficial than aspirin alone.

10. Report any unexplained pain or fever that persists for longer than 3–5 days.

11. Avoid alcohol- may cause toxicity. Not for regular use with any form of liver disease.

OUTCOMES/EVALUATE

- ↓ Fever
- Relief of pain

—**COMBINATION DRUG**—

Acetaminophen and Codeine phosphate

(ah-**SEAT**-ah-**MIN**-oh-fen, **KOH**-deen)

CLASSIFICATION(S):
Non-narcotic/narcotic analgesic combination
PREGNANCY CATEGORY: C
Rx: Tylenol with Codeine, Vopac, **C-III**

SEE ALSO *ACETAMINOPHEN* AND *CODEINE PHOSPHATE.*

USES
Relief of mild to moderately severe pain.

CONTENT
Each Tylenol with Codeine No. 3 Tablet contains: Acetaminophen (non-narcotic analgesic), 300 mg and Codeine phosphate (narcotic analgesic), 30 mg. Each Tylenol with Codeine No. 4 Tablet contains Acetaminophen, 300 mg, and Codeine phosphate, 60 mg. Each 5 mL of Tylenol with Codeine Elixir (oral solution) contains: Acetaminophen, 120 mg and Codeine phosphate, 12 mg. Each Vopac Capsule contains Acetaminophen, 650 mg and Codeine phosphate, 30 mg.

ACTION/KINETICS

Action
Acetaminophen may cause analgesia by inhibiting CNS prostaglandin synthesis. The mechanism of morphine is believed to involve decreased permeability of the cell membrane to sodium, which results in diminished transmission of pain impulses and therefore analgesia.

Pharmacokinetics
Both are well absorbed after PO. Acetaminophen, plasma **t½:** 1–4 hr; codeine plasma **t½:** 2.5–3 hr. Acetaminophen is metabolized mainly in the liver and excreted in the urine. Codeine is metabolized in the liver and excreted in the urine.

CONTRAINDICATIONS
Renal insufficiency, anemia. Those with cardiac or pulmonary disease are more susceptible to acetaminophen toxicity. During labor when delivery of a premature infant is expected. Hypersensitivity to any component of the product.

SPECIAL CONCERNS
Tablets contain sodium metabisulfite that may cause allergic-type reactions including anaphylaxis and life-threatening or less severe asthmatic episodes in susceptible individuals. Use with caution in the elderly, debilitated, in those with severe hepatic or renal impairment, hypothyroidism, Addison's disease, and prostatic hypertrophy or urethral stricture. Acetaminophen toxicity, including serious liver damage and apoptosis, may occur with doses not far beyond labeled dosing. Consult a provider before use if more than three alcoholic drinks per day are consumed. Clinically significant amounts of codeine may appear in breast milk in individuals abusing codeine. Safety and efficacy of the tablets have not been determined in children. Safety and efficacy of the elixir (oral solution) has not been determined in children 3 years of age and younger.

SIDE EFFECTS
Most Common
Lightheadedness, dizziness, sedation, shortness of breath, N&V, respiratory depression (high doses of codeine).
See *Acetaminophen* and *Narcotic Analgesics* for a complete list of possible side effects. Codeine can produce drug dependence of the morphine type and thus has the potential to be abused. Psychological and physical dependence, as well as tolerance, can result upon repeated use.

OD OVERDOSE MANAGEMENT
SEE ALSO *ACETAMINOPHEN* AND *NARCOTIC ANALGESICS*.

DRUG INTERACTIONS
See also *Acetaminophen* and *Narcotic Analgesics*.
Anticholinergics / Possible paralytic ileus
CNS Depressants (other narcotic analgesics, antipsychotics, antianxiety drugs, alcohol) / Additive CNS depression

HOW SUPPLIED
See Content.

DOSAGE
- **ELIXIR (ORAL SOLUTION)**
  Mild to moderately severe pain.
Adults: 15 mL (360 mg acetaminophen and 36 mg codeine phosphate) q 4 hr. **Children, 7–12 years of age:** 10 mL (240 mg acetaminophen and 24 mg codeine phosphate) 3–4 times per day. **Children, 3–6 years of age:** 5 mL (120 mg acetaminophen and 12 mg codeine phosphate) 3–4 times per day.
- **TABLETS**
  Mild to moderately severe pain.
Adults, acetaminophen: 200–1,000 mg is the single dose range; maximum daily dose: 4,000 mg. **Adults, codeine:** 15–60 mg is the single dose range; maximum daily dose: 360 mg. Doses may be repeated q 4 hr.
- **TABLETS (VOPAC)**
  Mild to moderately severe pain.
Adults: $\frac{1}{2}$–2 tablets q 4 hr, up to 6 tablets per day.

NURSING CONSIDERATIONS
ADMINISTRATION/STORAGE
1. Adult doses of codeine higher than 60 mg do not give commensurate relief of pain but do prolong analgesia and are associated with a significant increase in the incidence of side effects.
2. Store tablets from 15–30°C (59–86°F). Dispense in a tight, light-resistant container.

ASSESSMENT
1. List reasons for therapy, onset, duration, characteristics of symptoms; rate pain level, list other drugs trialed/outcome.
2. Assess CBC, renal and LFTs; for hypothyroidism, CAD, BPH, asthma, seizures- may preclude therapy or require lower dosage.
3. With cough, determine co-morbidities, fever, change in sputum color/amount, leukocytosis, need for CXR/ATX.

CLIENT/FAMILY TEACHING
1. Take as directed with full glass of water. May take with food/ milk if GI upset.

---

2. Do not drive/perform activities that require mental alertness until drug effects realized; may cause dizziness, drowsiness.
3. For constipation, increase fluid and fiber intake to offset.
4. Store away from bedside; out of reach of children. Do not exceed prescribed dose.
5. Do not stop suddenly with prolonged use, may experience withdrawal.
6. Keep all F/U appointments. Report adverse side effects or lack of desired effects.

OUTCOMES/EVALUATE
Control of pain/cough

Acetazolamide   IV ©
(ah-set-ah-**ZOE**-la-myd)

CLASSIFICATION(S):
Anticonvulsant, carbonic anhydrase inhibitor
PREGNANCY CATEGORY: C
🍁**Rx:** Apo-Acetazolamide.

Acetazolamide sodium

SEE ALSO *ANTICONVULSANTS* AND *DIURETICS*.

USES
(1) Adjunct in the treatment of edema due to CHF or drug-induced edema. (2) Absence (petit mal), especially in children) and unlocalized seizures. (3) Open-angle, secondary, or acute-angle closure glaucoma when delay of surgery is desired to lower IOP. (4) Prophylaxis or treatment of acute mountain sickness in climbers attempting a rapid ascent or in those susceptible to mountain sickness even with gradual ascent.

ACTION/KINETICS
Action
Sulfonamide derivative possessing carbonic anhydrase inhibitor activity. Anticonvulsant effects may be due to (1)

inhibition of carbonic anhydrase in the CNS, which increases carbon dioxide tension resulting in a decrease in neuronal conduction, and (2) systemic acidosis. As a diuretic, the drug inhibits carbonic anhydrase in the kidney, which decreases formation of bicarbonate and hydrogen ions from carbon dioxide, thus reducing the availability of these ions for active transport. Use as a diuretic is limited because the drug promotes metabolic acidosis, which inhibits diuretic activity. This may be partially circumvented by giving acetazolamide on alternate days. Also reduces intraocular pressure.

Pharmacokinetics
Absorbed from the GI tract and widely distributed throughout the body, including the CNS. **Tablets: Onset,** 60–90 min; **peak:** 1–4 hr; **duration:** 8–12 hr. **Sustained-release capsules: Onset,** 2 hr; **peak:** 3–6 hr; **duration:** 18–24 hr. **Injection (IV): Onset,** 2 min; **peak:** 15 min; **duration:** 4–5 hr. Eliminated mainly unchanged through the kidneys.

CONTRAINDICATIONS
Low serum sodium and potassium levels. Renal and hepatic dysfunction. Hyperchloremic acidosis, adrenal insufficiency, suprarenal gland failure, hypersensitivity to thiazide diuretics, cirrhosis. Chronic use in noncongestive angle-closure glaucoma.

SPECIAL CONCERNS
Use with caution in the presence of mild acidosis, advanced pulmonary disease, and during lactation. Increasing the dose does not increase effectiveness but may increase the risk of drowsiness or paresthesia. Safety and efficacy have not been established in children.

SIDE EFFECTS
Most Common
Anorexia, dizziness, lightheadedness, blurred vision, pruritus, GI upset, headache, weakness.
GI: Anorexia, GI upset, N&V, melena, constipation, alteration in taste, diarrhea. **GU:** Hematuria, glycosuria, urinary frequency, renal colic/calculi, crystalluria, polyuria, phosphaturia, decreased/absent libido, impotence. **CNS:** *Seizures,* weakness, malaise, lighthead-

---

Bold Italic = life threatening side effect   ■ = black box warning   🍁 = Available in Canada edness, fatigue, nervousness, drowsiness, depression, dizziness, disorientation, confusion, ataxia, tremor, headache, tinnitus, flaccid paralysis, lassitude, paresthesia of the extremities. **Hematologic: Bone marrow depression,** thrombocytopenic purpura, thrombocytopenia, **hemolytic anemia,** leukopenia, pancytopenia, agranulocytosis. **Dermatologic:** Pruritus, urticaria, skin rashes, erythema multiforme, **Stevens-Johnson syndrome, toxic epidermal necrolysis,** photosensitivity. **Miscellaneous:** Weight loss, weakness, fever, acidosis, electrolyte imbalance, transient myopia, blurred vision, hepatic insufficiency. NOTE: Side effects similar to those produced by sulfonamides may also occur.

OD OVERDOSE MANAGEMENT
Symptoms: Drowsiness, anorexia, N&V, dizziness, ataxia, tremor, paresthesias, tinnitus. *Treatment:* Emesis or gastric lavage. Hyperchloremic acidosis may respond to bicarbonate. Administration of potassium may also be necessary. Observe carefully and give supportive treatment.

DRUG INTERACTIONS
SEE ALSO DIURETICS
Amphetamine / ↑ Amphetamine effect by ↑ renal tubular reabsorption
Cyclosporine / ↑ Cyclosporine levels → possible nephrotoxicity and neurotoxicity
Diflunisal / Significant ↓ in IOP with ↑ side effects
Ephedrine / ↑ Ephedrine effect R/T ↑ renal tubular reabsorption
Lithium carbonate / ↓ Lithium effect R/T ↑ renal excretion
Methotrexate / ↓ Methotrexate effect R/T ↑ renal excretion
Primidone / ↓ Primidone effect R/T ↓ GI absorption
Pseudoephedrine / ↑ Pseudoephedrine effect by ↑ renal tubular reabsorption
Quinidine / ↑ Quinidine effect by ↑ renal tubular reabsorption
Salicylates / Accumulation and toxicity of acetazolamide (including CNS depression and metabolic acidosis). Also, acidosis due to ↑ CNS penetration of salicylates

HOW SUPPLIED
Acetazolamide: *Capsules, Extended-Release:* 500 mg; *Tablets:* 125 mg, 250 mg.
Acetazolamide sodium: *Powder for Injection:* 500 mg.

DOSAGE
• **CAPSULES, EXTENDED-RELEASE; IV; TABLETS**
Epilepsy.
Adults/children: 8–30 mg/kg/day in divided doses. Optimum daily dosage: 375–1,000 mg (doses higher than 1,000 mg do not increase therapeutic effect).
Adjunct to other anticonvulsants.
Initial: 250 mg/day; dose can be increased up to 1,000 mg/day in divided doses if necessary.
Glaucoma, simple open-angle.
Adults: 250–1,000 mg/day in divided doses. Doses greater than 1 gram/day do not increase the effect.
Glaucoma, secondary or acute congestive (closed-angle).
Adults, short-term therapy: 250 mg q 4 hr or 250 mg twice a day. **Adults, acute therapy:** 500 mg followed by 125–250 mg q 4 hr using tablets. For extended-release capsules, give 500 mg twice a day in the morning and evening. IV therapy may be used for rapid decrease in intraocular pressure. **Pediatric:** 5–10 mg/kg/dose IM or IV q 6 hr or 10–15 mg/kg/day in divided doses q 6–8 hr using tablets.
Acute mountain sickness.
Adults: 500 mg 1–2 times per day of tablets or extended-release capsules. During rapid ascent, 1 gram/day is recommended.
Diuresis in CHF.
Adults, initial: 250–375 mg (5 mg/kg) once daily in the morning. If the client stops losing edema fluid after an initial response, do not increase doses; rather, skip medication for a day to allow the kidney to recover. The best diuretic effect occurs when the drug is given on alternate days or for 2 days alternating with a day of rest.
Drug-induced edema.
Adults: 250–375 mg once daily for 1 or 2 days. Most effective if given every other day or for 2 days followed by a

A

day of rest. **Children:** 5 mg/kg/dose PO or IV once daily in the morning.

NURSING CONSIDERATIONS

Do not confuse acetazolamide with acetohexamide (oral antidiabetic).

ADMINISTRATION/STORAGE

1. Changeover from other anticonvulsant therapy should be gradual.
2. Acetazolamide tablets may be crushed and suspended in a cherry, chocolate, raspberry, or other sweet syrup. Do not use vehicles containing glycerin or alcohol.
3. Tolerance after prolonged use may necessitate dosage increase.
4. Do not administer the extended-release dosage form as an anticonvulsant; used only for glaucoma and acute mountain sickness.
5. With mountain sickness prophylaxis, initiate dosage 1–2 days before ascent and continue for at least 2 days while at high altitudes.
6. Due to possible differences in bioavailability, do not interchange brands.
IV 7. IV administration is preferred; IM administration is painful due to alkalinity of solution.
8. For direct IV use, administer over at least 1 min. For intermittent IV use, further dilute in dextrose or saline solution and infuse over 4–8 hr. Reconstitute each 500-mg vial with at least 5 mL of sterile water for injection.
9. Refrigerate reconstituted solution at 28° C (36–46° F). Use within 12 hr; contains no preservative.

ASSESSMENT

1. Note reasons for therapy, onset/characteristics of symptoms.
2. Review I&O, CBC, electrolytes, uric acid, and glucose. Assess for liver/renal dysfunction.
3. List drugs prescribed to ensure no interactions.
4. With glaucoma, note baseline ophthalmic exam and intraocular pressures; assess for visual effects.
5. Perform CV/pulmonary assessment with CHF history. Obtain VS and weight.

CLIENT/FAMILY TEACHING

1. Taking drug with food may decrease GI upset/irritation.
2. Assess drug effects before undertaking tasks that require mental alertness.
3. Increases voiding frequency; take early to avoid interrupting sleep.
4. Use only as directed. If prescribed every other day, record to ensure adherence.
5. Increase fluids (2–3 L/day) to prevent urine crystals/stone formation.
6. May increase blood glucose levels. Monitor FS and report increases; diabetes agent may need adjustment. Avoid high-sodium foods.
7. Report if nausea, dizziness, rapid weight gain, muscle weakness, cramps, or any changes in the color/consistency of stools occur.
8. Report for F/U visits and labs; may need potassium replacement.

OUTCOMES/EVALUATE

- ↓ Seizure activity
- ↓ Intraocular pressure
- ↓ CHF-associated edema
- Prevention of mountain sickness

Acetylcysteine   IV
(ah-see-till-**SIS**-tay-een)

CLASSIFICATION(S):
Mucolytic

PREGNANCY CATEGORY: B

Rx: Acetadote, Mucomyst.

✦Rx: Parvolex.

USES

(1) Adjunct in the treatment of chronic emphysema, emphysema with bronchitis, chronic asthmatic bronchitis, tuberculosis, bronchiectasis, primary amyloidosis of lung, acute bronchopulmonary disease (bronchitis, pneumonia, tracheobronchitis). Oral solution only. (2) Routine care of clients with tracheostomy, pulmonary complications after thoracic or CV surgery, use during anesthesia, atelectasis due to mucus obstruction, and in posttraumatic chest conditions. (3) Pulmonary complications of cystic fibrosis. (4) Diagnostic bronchial studies. (5) Antidote in acetaminophen poisoning to reduce or prevent hepatotoxicity. Give within the first 10 hr after

exposure. *Investigational:* As an ophthalmic solution for dry eye. As an enema to treat bowel obstruction due to meconium ileus or equivalent. Alzheimer's disease to increase reasoning skills.

ACTION/KINETICS

Action

Reduces the viscosity of purulent and nonpurulent pulmonary secretions and facilitates their removal by splitting disulfide bonds. Action increases with increasing pH (peak: pH 7–9). Also reduces liver injury due to acetaminophen overdose by maintaining or restoring glutathione levels or by acting as an alternate substrate for the reactive metabolite of acetaminophen.

Pharmacokinetics

Onset, inhalation: Within 1 min; **by direct instillation:** immediate. **Time to peak effect:** 5–10 min.

CONTRAINDICATIONS

Sensitivity to drug.

SPECIAL CONCERNS

Use with caution during lactation, in the elderly, and in clients with asthma.

SIDE EFFECTS

Most Common

Bronchial/tracheal irritation, N&V, rash, stomatitis.

Respiratory: Increased incidence of bronchospasm in clients with asthma. Increased amount of liquefied bronchial secretions, which must be removed by suction if cough is inadequate. Bronchial and tracheal irritation, tightness in chest, bronchoconstriction. **GI:** N&V, stomatitis. **Miscellaneous:** Rashes, fever, drowsiness, rhinorrhea.

DRUG INTERACTIONS

Acetylcysteine is incompatible with antibiotics and should be administered separately.

HOW SUPPLIED

Injection: 20%; *Oral Solution:* (as sodium) 10%, 20%.

DOSAGE

• **10% OR 20% ORAL SOLUTION: NEBULIZATION, DIRECT APPLICATION, OR DIRECT INTRATRACHEAL INSTILLATION**

Nebulization into face mask, tracheostomy, mouth piece.

1–10 mL of 20% solution or 2–10 mL of 10% solution 3–4 times per day.

Closed tent or croupette.

Up to 300 mL of 10% or 20% solution/treatment.

Direct instillation into tracheostomy.

1–2 mL of 10% or 20% solution q 1–4 hr.

Percutaneous intratracheal catheter.

1–2 mL of 20% solution or 2–4 mL of 10% solution q 1–4 hr by syringe attached to catheter.

Instillation to particular portion of bronchopulmonary tree using small plastic catheter into the trachea.

2–5 mL of 20% solution instilled into the trachea by means of a syringe connected to a catheter.

Diagnostic procedures.

2–3 doses of 1–2 mL of 20% or 2–4 mL of 10% solution by nebulization or intratracheal instillation before the procedure.

Acetaminophen overdose.

PO, loading dose: 140 mg/kg; **maintenance dose:** 70 mg/kg 4 hr after the loading dose and q 4 hr thereafter for a total of 17 doses.

• **IV**

Acetaminophen overdosage.

Loading dose: 150 mg/kg in 200 mL of D5W given over 15 minutes; **maintenance dose 1:** 50 mg/kg in 500 mL of D5W given over 4 hr; **maintenance dose 2:** 100 mg/kg in 1,000 mL of D5W given over 16 hr. To avoid fluid overload, reduce the volume of D5W in clients weighing less than 50 kg and in those with a restriction on fluid intake.

NURSING CONSIDERATIONS

ADMINISTRATION/STORAGE

1. Use nonreactive plastic, glass, or stainless steel for administration.

2. For PO use to treat acetaminophen overdosage: Dilute 10% or 20% solution with diet cola or other diet soft drinks to final concentration of 5%. If given via gastric tube or Miller-Abbott tube, water may be used as the diluent. Freshly prepare solutions and use within 1 hr. Remaining undiluted solutions may be stored in the refrigerator for up to 96 hr.

A

3. For use as a mucolytic, the 10% solution may be used undiluted. Use either water for injection or saline to dilute the 20% solution.

4. May administer via face mask, face tent, oxygen tent, head tent, or by positive-pressure apparatus.

5. Administer with compressed air for nebulization. Hand nebulizers are contraindicated.

6. After prolonged nebulization, dilute the last fourth of the medication with sterile water to prevent drug concentration.

7. Solution may develop a light purple color; does not affect action.

8. Closed bottles of oral solution remain stable for 2 years when stored at 20°C (68°F). Store open bottles at 2–8°C (36–46°F) and use within 96 hr. Once opened, record time/date to prevent use beyond 96 hr. Store unopened vials of oral solution from 15–30°C (59–86°F).

9. Incompatible with antibiotics; administer separately.

10. Have suction available for removal of increased secretions.

IV 11. IV acetylcysteine is incompatible with rubber and metals, especially iron, copper, and nickel.

12. Stability and safety of acetylcysteine not determined when mixed with other drugs.

13. Store unopened vials of IV solution from 20–25°C (68–77°F). Reconstituted solution stable for 24 hr at controlled room temperature. Single-dose vials are preservative-free; discard any unused portion.

ASSESSMENT

1. Note pulmonary findings; determine when spasms occur.

2. List conditions likely to cause congestion and wheezing.

3. Identify previous approaches (successful and unsuccessful) used to treat symptoms.

4. Determine smoking status. If currently taking antibiotics, do not administer together.

5. With acetaminophen overdosage, document time of ingestion. Administer drug within 8–10 hr following overdose to protect from hepatoxicity and death.

Monitor LFTs and acetaminophen levels. May administer IV especially if vomiting.

INTERVENTIONS

1. With bronchospasm, have bronchodilator, (i.e., isoproterenol for HFN) readily available.

2. Position to facilitate removal of secretions. If unable to cough up secretions, provide suction.

3. Monitor VS, electrolytes, and I&O.

4. Wash face following nebulization treatments; may cause face to become sticky.

CLIENT/FAMILY TEACHING

1. Use as directed; do not exceed prescribed dosage.

2. Report changes in sputum color, consistency, characteristics or new onset fever.

3. Nauseous odor when treatment begins will become less noticeable as therapy continues.

4. Avoid any triggers that may stimulate bronchospasm (i.e., cigarette smoke, dust, chemicals, cold air).

5. Attend smoking cessation classes and support groups to help stop smoking.

6. Report lack of desired response, adverse side effects, or worsening of symptoms.

OUTCOMES/EVALUATE

• Improved airway exchange with ↓ viscosity; mobilization and expectoration of secretions

• ↓ Acetaminophen levels and associated liver toxicity

Acyclovir (Acycloguanosine) **IV** ©

(ay-**SYE**-kloh-veer, ay-**SYE**-kloh-**GWON**-oh-seen)

CLASSIFICATION(S):
Antiviral
PREGNANCY CATEGORY: B
Rx: Zovirax.

✦Rx: Apo-Acyclovir, Gen-Acyclovir, Nu-Acyclovir.

SEE ALSO *ANTIVIRAL DRUGS.*

USES
PO. (1) Initial and recurrent genital herpes in immunocompromised and nonimmunocompromised clients. (2) Prophylaxis of frequently recurring genital herpes infections in nonimmunocompromised clients. (3) Treatment of chickenpox in children ranging from 2 to 18 years of age. (4) Acute treatment of herpes zoster (shingles). **Parenteral.** (1) Mucosal and cutaneous herpes simplex virus types 1 and 2 infections in immunocompromised clients. (2) Shingles in immunocompromised clients. (3) Herpes simplex encephalitis. (4) Neonatal herpes simplex infections. **Topical.** (1) To decrease healing time and duration of viral shedding in initial herpes genitalis. (2) Limited non-life-threatening mucocutaneous HSV infections in immunocompromised clients. No beneficial effect in recurrent herpes genitalis or in herpes labialis in nonimmunocompromised clients. (3) Recurrent herpes labialis in adults and children 12 years and older. *Investigational:* Cytomegalovirus and HSV infection following bone marrow or renal transplantation; herpes simplex ocular infections; herpes simplex proctitis; herpes simplex labialis; herpes simplex whitlow; herpes zoster encephalitis; disseminated primary eczema herpeticum; herpes simplex–associated erythema multiforme; infectious mononucleosis; and varicella pneumonia.

ACTION/KINETICS
Action
Converted by HSV-infected cells to acyclovir triphosphate, which interferes with HSV DNA polymerase, thereby inhibiting DNA replication.

Pharmacokinetics
Systemic absorption is slow from the GI tract (although therapeutic levels are reached) and following topical administration. Food does not affect absorption. **Peak levels after PO:** 1.5–2 hr. Widely distributed in tissues and body fluids. The half-life and total body clearance depend on renal function. $t^{1/2}$, **PO, C_{CR} >80 mL/min/1.73 m^2:** 2.5 hr. Metabolites and unchanged drug (up to 85%) are excreted through the kidneys. Reduce dosage in clients with impaired renal function.

CONTRAINDICATIONS
Hypersensitivity to formulation. Use of the cream or ointment in the eyes, nose, or mouth. Use to prevent recurrent HSV infections.

SPECIAL CONCERNS
Use with caution during lactation or with concomitant intrathecal methotrexate or interferon. Geriatric clients have higher plasma levels than young adults and thus a higher incidence of side effects (especially N&V, dizziness, and CNS effects); dosage may need to be reduced in geriatric clients with renal impairment. Safety and efficacy of PO form not established in children less than 2 years of age. Safety and efficacy of the cream or ointment not established in children 12 years and younger. Prolonged or repeated doses in immunocompromised clients may result in emergence of resistant viruses. Use of oral acyclovir does not eliminate latent HSV and is not a cure.

SIDE EFFECTS
Most Common
IV: N&V, inflammation/phlebitis at injection site, itching, rash, hives, increased BUN or creatinine.
PO: N&V, headache, diarrhea, malaise.
Topical: Mild pain with transient burning/stinging, pruritus.

• **After PO or Parenteral use**
GI: Diarrhea, GI distress, N&V, sore throat, taste of drug, constipation, abdominal pain, flatulence. **CNS:** Aggressive behavior, agitation, ataxia, coma, confusion, delirium, dizziness, encephalopathy, hallucinations, paresthesia, psychosis, *seizure,* somnolence, tremors, headache. **Hematologic:** Leukocytoclastic vasculitis, leukopenia, lymphadenopathy. **Hepatic:** Elevated LFTs, hepatitis, hyperbilirubinemia, jaundice. **Renal:** *Fatal renal failure, fatal thrombotic thrombocytopenic purpura or hemolytic uremic syndrome in immunocompromised clients,* in-

A

creased BUN or creatinine, hematuria. **Dermatologic:** Alopecia, erythema multiforme, photosensitive rash, pruritus, rash, ***Stevens-Johnson syndrome, toxic epidermal necrolysis,*** urticaria. **Hematologic:** Anemia. **Musculoskeletal:** Myalgia. **Ophthalmologic:** Visual abnormalities. **Miscellaneous:** Anaphylaxis, ***angioedema,*** fever, pain, peripheral edema.

• **Additional symptoms after parenteral use.**

At injection site: Inflammation/phlebitis at site, itching, rash, hives. **CV:** Hypotension. **CNS:** Anorexia. Encephalopathic changes, including lethargy, obtundation, tremors, agitation, confusion, hallucination, ***seizures, coma,*** jitters, headache. **Hematologic:** Hematuria, neutropenia, thrombocytopenia, thrombocytosis, leukocytosis, neutrophilia, ***DIC,*** hemolysis. **Dermatologic:** Tissue necrosis following infusion into extravascular tissues. **Miscellaneous:** Elevated transaminases.

• **Additional symptoms after PO use**

CNS: Decreased consciousness, malaise. **Hematologic:** Thrombocytopenia.

• **Cream**

Dry lips/skin, desquamation, cracked lips, pruritus, skin flakiness, stinging/burning on skin. Also, ***angioedema, anaphylaxis,*** contact dermatitis, eczema, inflammation at application site.

OD **OVERDOSE MANAGEMENT**

Symptoms: Precipitation in renal tubules may occur when the solubility (2.5 mg/mL) in the intratubular fluid is exceeded. **After parenteral use:** Overdose has resulted with bolus injections, inappropriately high doses, and in those whose fluid and electrolyte balance was not properly monitored. Increased BUN and serum creatinine, followed by ***renal failure.*** **After PO use:** Agitation, ***coma, seizures,*** lethargy. *Treatment:* Hemodialysis (a 6-hr hemodialysis results in a 60% decrease in plasma acyclovir levels); peritoneal dialysis is less effective.

DRUG INTERACTIONS

Hydantoins / ↓ Hydantoin plasma levels

Mycophenolate mofetil / ↑ Acyclovir

AUC, peak concentration, and time to reach maximum concentration; ↓ acyclovir t½ and renal clearance

Probenecid / ↑ Bioavailability and half-life of acyclovir → ↑ effect

Theophyllines / ↑ Theophylline plasma levels; monitor plasma levels and side effects

Valproic acid / ↓ Valproic acid plasma levels

Zidovudine / Severe lethargy and drowsiness

HOW SUPPLIED

Capsules: 200 mg; *Cream:* 5%; *Injection:* 50 mg/mL; *Powder for Injection:* 500 mg/vial; *Powder for Injection, Lyophilized:* 500 mg/vial: 200 mg/5 mL; *Tablets:* 400 mg, 800 mg.

DOSAGE

• **CAPSULES; SUSPENSION; TABLETS**

Initial, genital herpes.

200 mg q 4 hr 5 times per day for 10 days.

Chronic suppressive therapy for recurrent genital herpes.

400 mg twice a day, 200 mg 3 times per day, or 200 mg 5 times per day for up to 12 months.

Intermittent therapy for genital herpes.

200 mg q 4 hr 5 times per day for 5 days. Start therapy at the first symptom/sign of recurrence.

Herpes zoster, acute treatment.

800 mg q 4 hr 5 times per day for 7–10 days.

Chickenpox.

Adults and children over 40 kg: 800 mg 4 times per day for 5 days. **Children, 2 years and older, 40 kg or less:** 20 mg/kg (of the suspension) 4 times per day for 5 days. A single dose should not exceed 800 mg. Begin therapy at the earliest sign/symptom.

• **IV INFUSION**

Mucosal and cutaneous herpes simplex in immunocompromised clients.

Adults: 5 mg/kg infused at a constant rate over 1 hr, q 8 hr (15 mg/kg/day) for 7 days. **Children less than 12 years of age:** 10 mg/kg infused at a constant rate over 1 hr q 8 hr for 7 days.

Varicella-zoster infections (shingles) in immunocompromised clients.

Bold Italic = life threatening side effect   ■ = black box warning   ✤ = Available in Canada

Adults: 10 mg/kg infused at a constant rate over 1 hr q 8 hr for 7 days. **Children less than 12 years of age:** 20 mg/kg infused at a constant rate over at least 1 hr q 8 hr for 7 days.

Herpes simplex encephalitis.

Adults: 10 mg/kg infused at a constant rate over at least 1 hr q 8 hr for 10 days. **Children less than 12 years of age and greater than 3 months of age:** 20 mg/kg infused at a constant rate over at least 1 hr q 8 hr for 10 days.

Neonatal HSV infections.

Children, birth–3 months: 10 mg/kg infused at a constant rate over 1 hr q 8 hr for 10 days. Doses as high as 15 mg/kg or 20 mg/kg infused at a constant rate over 1 hr q 8 hr have also been used.

• **CREAM, 5%**

Recurrent herpes labialis.

Adults and children 12 years and older: Apply 5 times per day for 4 days.

NURSING CONSIDERATIONS

℞ Do not confuse Zovirax with Zyvox (an antibiotic).

ADMINISTRATION/STORAGE

1. Do not exceed recommended dosage, frequency, or length of treatment. Adjust dosage based on estimated C_{CR}.

2. Store ointment in dry place at room temperature.

3. Adjust both PO and parenteral dose and/or dosing interval in acute or chronic renal impairment.

4. May use suspension to treat varicella zoster infections.

IV 5. Prepare IV solution by dissolving contents of the 500- or 1,000-mg vial in 10 or 20 mL sterile water for injection, respectively (final concentration of 50 mg/mL). Infusion concentrations of 7 mg/mL or lower are recommended; thus, the calculated dose must be added to an appropriate IV solution at the correct volume. Reconstituted solution should be used within 12 hr. Avoid bacteriostatic water containing benzyl alcohol or parabens; causes precipitate.

6. Administer infusion over 1 hr to prevent renal tubular damage; do not administer by rapid or bolus IV, IM, or SC injections.

7. Accompany IV infusion by hydration (3 L/day) to prevent precipitation in renal tubules (crystalluria).

8. If refrigerated, reconstituted solution may show a precipitate which dissolves at room temperature.

ASSESSMENT

1. List reasons for therapy; assess skin lesions noting location, size, distribution and number.

2. Monitor CBC, electrolytes, renal and LFTs closely, especially with IV therapy and if immunocompromised.

3. With chickenpox or herpes zoster, institute appropriate precautions for all susceptible individuals (i.e., pregnant women, immunocompromised clients, and those who have not had chickenpox [may check titer if unknown]).

CLIENT/FAMILY TEACHING

1. Drug is not a cure; use only to help manage symptoms. Virus may remain latent for lifetime or may emerge periodically to cause S&S. Drug will not prevent disease transmission to others or prevent reinfection. Most effective when started at first S&S of outbreak.

2. Wash area with soap and water 3–4 times per day and dry well. Adequately cover all lesions with topical acyclovir as ordered; do not exceed dosage, frequency of application or treatment time. Wear loose-fitting clothing and cotton underwear.

3. Report any burning, stinging, itching, and rash when applying.

4. Complete all exams/tests to rule out presence of other STDs. Return if lesions recur.

5. Apply ointment with a finger cot or rubber glove to prevent transmission of infection to other body sites.

6. Use condoms for sexual intercourse to prevent reinfections while undergoing treatment. Abstain during acute outbreaks (lesions present) and use condoms at all other times.

7. Total dose and dosage schedule differ depending on whether the infection is initial or chronic and whether intermittent therapy regimen is being used. Follow prescribed dosage guidelines, dosage combinations (i.e., with zidovudine) and duration of treatment.

📷 = see color insert   **H** = Herbal   **IV** = Intravenous   ℞ = sound alike drug

A

8. Consume 2–3 L/day of fluids, especially during parenteral therapy; prevents renal toxicity/crystalluria.

9. Females need annual Pap test; increased risk of cervical cancer may be associated with genital herpes.

10. Do not exceed dosage or share medications. With shingles, take tablets as directed, cover any open draining lesions to prevent disease transmission, avoid contact with children that have not had chicken pox, and pregnant women as fetuses may be vulnerable to the disease.

OUTCOMES/EVALUATE

• Less severe and less frequent herpes outbreaks
• Crusting and healing of herpetic lesions
• ↓ Pain with shingles outbreak

Adalimumab ■
(**ay**-dah-**LIM**-you-mab)

CLASSIFICATION(S):
Immunomodulator
PREGNANCY CATEGORY: B
Rx: Humira.

USES
(1) Reduce signs and symptoms of rheumatoid arthritis, including major clinical response, inhibiting the progression of structural damage, and improving physical function in adults with moderate to severe rheumatoid arthritis. May be used alone or in combination with methotrexate or other disease-modifying antirheumatic drugs. (2) Reduce signs and symptoms of active arthritis, including the progression of structural damage, and improving physical function in those with psoriatic arthritis May be used alone or with disease-modifying antirheumatic drugs. (3) Reduce signs and symptoms of active ankylosing spondylitis. (4) Reduce signs and symptoms and inducing and maintaining clinical remission in adults with moderate to severe active Crohn's disease who have had an inadequate response to conventional therapy. Also,

for those who have lost response to or are intolerant to infliximab. *Investigational:* Plaque psoriasis.

ACTION/KINETICS

Action

Tissue necrosis factor (TNF) is a naturally occurring cytokine involved in normal inflammatory and immune responses. TNF plays an important role in the pathologic inflammation and joint destruction in rheumatoid arthritis. Adalimumab binds specifically to tumor necrosis factor (TNF)-alpha and blocks its interaction with p55 and p75 cell surface TNF receptors. This results in a rapid decrease in levels of the acute phase reactants of inflammation and erythrocyte sedimentation rate and serum cytokines.

Pharmacokinetics

Maximum serum levels: 131 hr following a single SC injection of 40 mg. Absolute bioavailability is 64%. **Mean steady-state trough levels:** About 5 mcg/mL. **t½, terminal:** 2 weeks. Clearance is lower in clients 40 to 75 years of age and older. Methotrexate reduces adalimumab apparent clearance.

CONTRAINDICATIONS

Hypersensitivity to adalimumab or components of the product. Administration of live vaccines. Use in active infections, including chronic or localized infections. Lactation.

SPECIAL CONCERNS

■ Tuberculosis (frequently disseminated or extrapulmonary at clinical presentation), invasive fungal infections, and other opportunistic infections have been seen in clients receiving adalimumab. Some of these infections have been fatal. Antituberculosis treatment of clients with latent tuberculosis reduces the risk of reactivation in those receiving adalimumab. However, active tuberculosis has developed in clients receiving adalimumab whose screening for latent tuberculosis was negative. Evaluate clients for tuberculosis risk factors and test for latent tuberculosis infection prior to initiating adalimumab and during treatment. Monitor clients receiving adalimumab for signs and symptoms of active tuberculosis, in-

---

Bold Italic = life threatening side effect   ■ = black box warning   ♣ = Available in Canada

cluding those who tested negative for latent tuberculosis infection.■ Use with caution in the elderly, in those with pre-existing or recent-onset CNS demyelinating disorders, in those with active infections or a history of recurrent infection, in underlying conditions that may predispose to infections, or in those who have resided in regions where tuberculosis and histoplasmosis are endemic. Simultaneous use with other TNF-blocking drugs is discouraged. Safety and efficacy have not been determined in children. The frequency of serious infection and malignancy is higher for those 65 years of age and older; use with caution in this population.

SIDE EFFECTS

Most Common

Injection site reactions (erythema and/or itching, hemorrhage, pain, swelling), headache, sinusitis, URTI, rash.

Body as a whole: Serious infections (including opportunistic infections) and *sepsis*, especially in those also receiving immunosuppressants. Fever, lymphomas, adenoma, tuberculosis (miliary, lymphatic, peritoneal, pulmonary), lupus-like syndrome (due to development of autoantibodies), septic arthritis, prosthetic and postsurgical infections. Cancers, including breast, skin, urogenital, colon-rectum, uterine-cervical, prostate, melanoma, gallbladder-bile ducts. Reactivation of hepatitis B virus. **Allergic:** Rash, *anaphylaxis*, fixed and/or nonspecific drug reaction, urticaria, angioneurotic edema. **Injection site:** Erythema, itching, hemorrhage, pain, swelling, clinical flare reaction, rash. **GI:** N&V, abdominal pain, cholecystitis, cholelithiasis, esophagitis, gastroenteritis, GI disorder, *GI hemorrhage, hepatic necrosis.* **Respiratory:** Pneumonia, URTI, bronchitis, sinusitis, flu syndrome, asthma, bronchospasm, dyspnea, lung disorder, decreased lung function, pleural effusion, interstitial lung disease (including pulmonary fibrosis). **CNS:** Confusion, headache, multiple sclerosis, paresthesia, *subdural hematoma*, tremor. **CV:** Hypertension, arrhythmia, atrial fibrillation, CV disorder, chest pain, CHF, worsening of CHF, coronary artery disorder, *MI, cardiac arrest,* hypertensive encephalopathy, palpitation, pericardial effusion, pericarditis, syncope, tachycardia, vascular disorder, leg thrombosis, cutaneous vasculitis. **Hematologic:** Agranulocytosis including *aplastic anemia*, granulocytopenia, leukopenia, lymphoma-like reaction, pancytopenia, polycythemia, thrombocytopenia. **GU:** UTI, hematuria, pyelonephritis, cystitis, kidney calculus, menstrual disorder, ketosis. **Dermatologic:** Erysipelas, cellulitis, herpes zoster, cutaneous vasculitis. **Musculoskeletal:** Arthritis, bone disorder, bone fracture (not spontaneous), bone necrosis, joint disorder, muscle cramps, myasthenia, pyogenic arthritis, synovitis, tendon disorder. **Miscellaneous:** Accidental injury, back pain, dehydration, abnormal healing, peripheral edema, pain in extremities, pelvic pain, thorax pain, parathyroid disorder, cataract, paraproteinemia.

LABORATORY TEST CONSIDERATIONS

↑ Alkaline phosphatase. Hypercholesterolemia, hyperlipidemia, hematuria.

OD OVERDOSE MANAGEMENT

Treatment: In case of overdose, monitor for signs and symptoms of side effects. Begin appropriate symptomatic treatment immediately.

DRUG INTERACTIONS

Anakinra / Coadministration with anakinra → increased risk of serious infections, neutropenia, pancytopenia (including aplastic anemia) and hypersensitivity reactions (including anaphylaxis)

Immunosuppressants / Possible development of malignancies and/or infections

Methotrexate / ↓ Adalimumab clearance after single and multiple dosing; dosage adjustment may be needed

HOW SUPPLIED

Injection: 40 mg/0.8 mL.

DOSAGE

• **SC**

Rheumatoid arthritis, psoriatic arthritis, ankylosing spondylitis.

40 mg every other week SC. Clients not taking methotrexate may benefit more by increasing the dosing frequency to

40 mg every week. Methotrexate, glucocorticoids, salicylates, NSAIDs, analgesics, or other disease-modifying antirheumatic drugs may be continued during adalimumab therapy.

Crohn's disease.

Adults, initial: 160 mg at week 0 (can be given as 4 injections in 1 day or as 2 injections per day for 2 consecutive days), and 80 mg at week 2, followed by a maintenance dose of 40 mg every other week beginning at week 4. Aminosalicylates, corticosteroids and/or immunomodulatory drugs (e.g., 6-mercaptopurine, azathioprine) maybe continued during adalimumab therapy. Use of adalimumab for Crohn's disease has not been studied beyond 1 year.

NURSING CONSIDERATIONS

ADMINISTRATION/STORAGE

1. During treatment, methotrexate, glucocorticoids, salicylates, NSAIDs, analgesics, and other antirheumatic drugs may be continued.
2. Syringe needle cover is made of latex; if sensitive to latex do not handle the product.
3. Discard unused portions remaining in the vial/syringe; no preservative in product.
4. Refrigerate at 2–8°C (36–46°F). Do not freeze.
5. Protect vial/prefilled syringe from exposure to light. Store in original carton until administered.

ASSESSMENT

1. Note reasons for therapy, joints affected, presenting symptoms, other agents trialed/failed.
2. Assess carefully for evidence of chronic/local infections. Look for latent tuberculosis infection with a tuberculin skin test. Begin treatment of latent TB prior to adalimumab therapy. Discontinue if a serious infection develops.
3. Use cautiously in elderly and those with pre-existing or recent-onset CNS demyelinating disorders, recurrent infections or those who have resided in regions endemic with TB or histoplasmosis.
4. Observe client perform first injection after instruction.

CLIENT/FAMILY TEACHING

1. Used to preserve joint structure and stability. Methotrexate, glucocorticoids, salicylates, NSAIDs, analgesics, and other prescribed antirheumatic drugs may be continued during treatment.
2. May self-administer drug after proper training in injection technique. Review procedures for storage (refrigerate in original container), reconstitution, inspection, withdraw, administration, site rotation, and disposal of syringes. Instruct clients using the prefilled syringes or pen to inject the full amount in the syringe (0.8 mL) which provides the full 40 mg dose.
3. Always rotate sites for self-injection which include the thigh, abdomen, or upper arm. Give new injections at least one inch from the old site and never into areas where the skin is tender, bruised, red, or hard.
4. May experience rash, pain, or swelling at injection site. A cool moist compress should relieve. If no relief or S&S worsen, report.
5. Any evidence of dizziness, infection, numbness or tingling, weakness of legs or vision problems as well as facial swelling, chest pain, increased cough, fever, SOB, rash, or joint pains require medical evaluation.
6. Avoid immunizations with live vaccines.
7. Review risks of therapy related to lymphoma, serious infections, and lupus–like symptoms.
8. If sensitive to latex do not handle the needle cover of the syringe.

OUTCOMES/EVALUATE

↓ Joint pain/swelling; delayed structural damage with RA

Adefovir dipivoxil ■
(ah-**DEH**-foh-veer)

CLASSIFICATION(S):
Antiviral
PREGNANCY CATEGORY: C
Rx: Hepsera.

SEE ALSO *ANTIVIRAL DRUGS.*

USES

Chronic hepatitis B in adults with evidence of active viral replication and evidence of persistent increases of ALT or AST.

ACTION/KINETICS

Action

A prodrug that is phosphorylated to the active metabolite, adefovir diphosphate, by cellular kinases. Adefovir diphosphate inhibits HBV DNA polymerase by competing with the natural substrate deoxyadenosine triphosphate. This causes DNA chain termination after being incorporated into viral DNA.

Pharmacokinetics

59% absorbed PO. **Peak plasma level:** 18.4 ng/mL after 0.6–4 hr (median = 1.75 hr). May be taken without regard for food. $t^{1}/_{2}$, **terminal:** About 7.5 hr. Modify dose in those with renal impairment. Excreted in the urine.

CONTRAINDICATIONS

Hypersensitivity to any of the product components. Lactation.

SPECIAL CONCERNS

■ (1) Severe acute exacerbations of hepatitis have been reported in those who have discontinued anti-hepatitis B therapy, including use of adefovir dipivoxil. Closely monitor hepatic function in such clients. If appropriate, resumption of anti-hepatitis B therapy may be warranted. (2) In those at risk of or having underlying renal dysfunction, chronic use of adefovir dipivoxil may cause nephrotoxicity. Closely monitor these clients for renal function and adjust dose as needed. (3) HIV resistance may emerge in chronic hepatitis B clients with unrecognized or untreated HIV infection treated with anti-hepatitis B therapies, including adefovir dipivoxil, that may have activity against HIV. (4) Lactic acidosis and severe hepatomegaly with steatosis, including death, have been reported with the use of nucleoside analogs alone or in combination with other antiretrovirals.■ Use with caution in elderly clients due to a greater frequency of decreased renal or cardiac function as a result of concomitant disease or other drug therapy. Safety and efficacy have not been determined in children.

SIDE EFFECTS

Most Common

Asthenia, headache, abdominal pain, nausea, flatulence, diarrhea, dyspepsia.

Hepatic: Severe acute exacerbation of hepatitis in clients who have discontinued anti-hepatitis B therapy. *Severe hepatomegaly with steatosis, hepatic failure,* abnormal liver function. **GI:** N&V, flatulence, diarrhea, dyspepsia, abdominal pain. **GU:** Nephrotoxicity, renal failure, renal insufficiency. **Respiratory:** Increased cough, pharyngitis, sinusitis. **Dermatologic:** Pruritus, rash. **Miscellaneous:** Lactic acidosis, asthenia, headache, fever. **Side effects in pre- and post-liver transplantation clients. GI:** Abdominal pain, diarrhea, flatulence, N&V. **GU:** Renal failure, ↑ creatinine, renal insufficiency. **Dermatologic:** Pruritus, rash. **Respiratory:** Increased cough, pharyngitis, sinusitis. **Hepatic:** Abnormal liver function, hepatic failure, ↑ AST and ALT. **Miscellaneous:** Asthenia, fever, headache.

LABORATORY TEST CONSIDERATIONS

↑ ALT, AST, creatine kinase, amylase, serum creatinine. Glycosuria, hematuria.

OD OVERDOSE MANAGEMENT

Symptoms: GI side effects. *Treatment:* Monitor for evidence of toxicity. Provide standard supportive treatment as needed. Hemodialysis will remove a portion of the dose.

DRUG INTERACTIONS

Drugs that reduce renal function or compete for active tubular secretion / ↑ Serum levels of adefovir or coadministered drugs

Ibuprofen / ↑ C_{max}, AVG, and urinary recovery of adefovir

HOW SUPPLIED

Tablets: 10 mg.

DOSAGE

- **TABLETS**

  Chronic hepatitis B.

Adults: 10 mg once daily without regard to food. Adjust dose as follows in clients with impaired renal function: C_{CR} **20–49 mL/min:** 10 mg q 48 hr; C_{CR} **10–19 mL/min:** 10 mg q 72 hr; **hemo-**

dialysis clients: 10 mg q 7 days following dialysis.

NURSING CONSIDERATIONS

ADMINISTRATION/STORAGE

Store in original container from 15–30°C (59–86°F).

ASSESSMENT

1. Note onset, characteristics of S&S and contacts. Assess HIV risks/test results.
2. List drugs prescribed/consumed to ensure none interact.
3. Obtain baseline viral load, renal and LFTs, BS, CK, amylase, and U/A; monitor for liver/renal failure; reduce dose with renal dysfunction.
4. To monitor fetal outcomes of pregnant women exposed to Hepsera, register patients with the pregnancy registry by calling 1-800-258-4263.

CLIENT/FAMILY TEACHING

1. Take as directed once daily.
2. Review enclosed patient literature before starting therapy and with each refill. Do not stop suddenly: severe acute exacerbation of hepatitis may occur.
3. Report as scheduled for F/U labs and evaluation.
4. May experience weakness, headaches, and GI upset; report any unusual/adverse S&S.
5. Does not cure disease but controls it; must continue to practice safe behaviors.

OUTCOMES/EVALUATE

↓ Viral replication in hepatitis B; improved LFTs

Adenosine   **IV**

(ah-**DEN**-oh-seen)

CLASSIFICATION(S):

Antiarrhythmic
PREGNANCY CATEGORY: C
Rx: Adenocard, Adenoscan.

SEE ALSO *ANTIARRHYTHMIC DRUGS*.

USES

Conversion to sinus rhythm of PSVT, including that associated with accessory bypass tracts (Wolff-Parkinson-White syndrome). If clinically advisable, try appropriate vagal maneuvers (e.g., Valsalva maneuver) prior to use. *Investigational:* With thallium-201 tomography in noninvasive assessment of clients with suspected CAD who cannot exercise adequately prior to being stress-tested. Adenosine is not effective in converting rhythms other than PSVT.

ACTION/KINETICS

Action

Found naturally in all cells of the body. It slows conduction time through the AV node, interrupts the reentry pathways through the AV node, and restores normal sinus rhythm in paroxysmal supraventricular tachycardia (PSVT). May cause a transient slowing of ventricular response immediately after use. Increases HR and PR interval.

Pharmacokinetics

Onset, after IV: 34 sec. **t½:** Less than 10 sec (taken up by erythrocytes and vascular endothelial cells). **Duration:** 1–2 min. Exogenous adenosine becomes part of the body pool and is metabolized mainly to inosine and AMP.

CONTRAINDICATIONS

Second- or third-degree AV block or sick sinus syndrome (SSS) (except in clients with a functioning artificial pacemaker), atrial flutter, atrial fibrillation, ventricular tachycardia. History of MI or cerebral hemorrhage.

SPECIAL CONCERNS

At time of conversion to normal sinus rhythm, new rhythms (PVC, PACs, sinus bradycardia, skipped beats, varying degrees of AV block, sinus tachycardia) lasting a few seconds may occur. Use with caution in the elderly as severe bradycardia and AV block may occur and in clients with asthma due to possibility of bronchoconstriction. Safety and efficacy as a diagnostic agent have not been determined in clients less than 18 years of age.

SIDE EFFECTS

Most Common

Facial flushing, shortness of breath/dyspnea, chest pressure, headache, lightheadedness.

Bold Italic = life threatening side effect   ■ = black box warning   ✦ = Available in Canada

CV: Short lasting first-, second-, or *third-degree heart block; cardiac arrest,* sustained ventricular tachycardia, sinus bradycardia, ST-segment depression, sinus exit block, sinus pause, arrhythmias, T-wave changes, hypertension. Prolonged asystole, nonfatal MI, transient increase in BP, *ventricular fibrillation.* Facial flushing, chest pain, sweating, palpitations, hypotension (may be significant). **CNS:** Lightheadedness, dizziness, numbness, headache, blurred vision, apprehension, paresthesia, drowsiness, emotional instability, tremors, nervousness. **GI:** Nausea, metallic taste, tightness in throat. **Respiratory:** SOB or dyspnea, urge to breathe deeply, chest pressure or discomfort, cough, hyperventilation, nasal congestion. **GU:** Urinary urgency, vaginal pressure. **Miscellaneous:** Pressure in head, burning sensation, neck and back pain, weakness, blurred vision, dry mouth, ear discomfort, pressure in groin, scotomas, tongue discomfort, discomfort (tingling, heaviness) in upper extremities, discomfort in throat, neck, or jaw.

DRUG INTERACTIONS

H *Aloe; Buckthorn bark/berry; Cascara sagrada bark; Rhubarb root; Senna pod and leaf* / Possible ↑ adenosine effect

Caffeine / Competitively antagonizes adenosine effect

Carbamazepine / ↑ AV block

Digoxin / Possibility of ventricular fibrillation (rare)

Dipyridamole / Potentiates adenosine effect

Smoking (nicotine) / ↑ CV effects of adenosine; lower doses may be needed

Theophylline / Competitively antagonizes adenosine effect

Verapamil / Possibility of ventricular fibrillation (rare)

HOW SUPPLIED

Injection: 3 mg/mL.

DOSAGE————————

- **IV BOLUS (ONLY), RAPID**
   Antiarrhythmic.

Adults, initial: 6 mg over 1–2 sec. If the first dose does not reverse the PSVT within 1–2 min, 12 mg should be given as a rapid IV bolus. The 12-mg dose may be repeated a second time, if necessary. Doses greater than 12 mg are not recommended. **Children, less than 50 kg, initial:** 0.05–0.1 mg/kg as a rapid IV bolus given either centrally or peripherally; follow by a saline flush. If conversion of PSVT does not occur within 1–2 min, additional bolus injections can be given at increasing doses of 0.05–0.1 mg/kg. Continue this until sinus rhythm is established or a maximum single dose of 0.3 mg/kg is given. Doses greater than 12 mg are not recommended. **Children, 50 kg or over:** Give the adult dose.

NURSING CONSIDERATIONS

ADMINISTRATION/STORAGE

IV 1. Can be stored at room temperature; crystallization may result if refrigerated. If crystals form, dissolve by warming to room temperature. Solution must be clear when administered.

2. Discard any unused portion; contains no preservatives.

3. Administer directly into a vein over 1–2 sec. If given into IV line, introduce in most proximal line and follow with rapid saline flush.

ASSESSMENT

1. Note reasons for therapy, onset of symptoms, ECG confirmation of arrhythmia.

2. Monitor rhythm strips closely for evidence of varying degrees of AV block and increased arrhythmias during conversion to sinus rhythm; usually only transient due to short half-life of adenosine.

3. Monitor BP and pulse. Report complaints of numbness, tingling in the arms, blurred vision, or apprehensiveness; may be indication to discontinue therapy.

4. Document chest pressure, SOB, heaviness of the arms, palpitations, or dyspnea. Note any history of MI/CVA; drug contraindicated; may cause bronchoconstriction with asthma.

5. In stasis dermatitis assess extremities and note findings.

CLIENT/FAMILY TEACHING

1. Drug helps restore heart to a normal, slower rhythm when given IV.

A

2. Avoid caffeine; report if prescribed theophylline, digoxin, or dipyridamole.
3. Facial flushing is common temporary side effect of therapy. Report chest pain, numbness/tingling, increased SOB or other adverse side effects.

OUTCOMES/EVALUATE
- Conversion of PSVT to NSR
- Symptomatic relief with stasis dermatitis

Albuterol (Salbutamol) ©

(al-**BYOU**-ter-ohl)

CLASSIFICATION(S):
Sympathomimetic
PREGNANCY CATEGORY: C
Rx: AccuNeb, ProAir HFA, Proventil, Proventil HFA, Ventolin, Ventolin HFA, VoSpire ER.
✦Rx: Airomir, Gen-Salbutamol Respirator Solution, Gen-Salbutamol Sterinebs P.F., Novo-Salmol Tablets, Nu-Salbutamol Solution, PMS-Salbutamol, Rhoxal-salbutamol, ratio-Salbutamol HFA.

SEE ALSO SYMPATHOMIMETIC DRUGS.

USES
Inhalation: (1) Prophylaxis and relief of bronchospasm in reversible obstructive airway disease. (2) Acute attacks of bronchospasm (inhalation solution). (3) Prophylaxis of exercise-induced bronchospasm.
 Syrup: Relief of bronchospasm in adults and children 2 years and older with reversible obstructive airway disease.
 Tablets and Extended-Release Tablets: Relief of bronchospasm in adults and children 6 years and older with reversible obstructive airway disease.
 Investigational: Nebulized albuterol as an adjunct to treat serious acute hyperkalemia in renal failure.

ACTION/KINETICS
Action
Stimulates beta-2 receptors of the bronchi, leading to bronchodilation. Causes less tachycardia and is longer-acting than isoproterenol. Has minimal beta-1 activity. Available as an inhaler that contains no chlorofluorocarbons (Proventil HFA).

Pharmacokinetics
Onset, PO: 15–30 min; **inhalation,** within 5 min. **Peak effect, PO:** 2–3 hr; **inhalation,** 60–90 min (after 2 inhalations). **Duration, PO:** 4–8 hr (up to 12 hr for extended-release); **inhalation,** 3–6 hr. Metabolites and unchanged drug excreted in urine and feces.

CONTRAINDICATIONS
Aerosol for prevention of exercise-induced bronchospasm and tablets are not recommended for children less than 12 years of age. Use during lactation.

SPECIAL CONCERNS
Syrup and solution for inhalation are indicated for children 2 years and older; tablets (including extended-release) are for use in children 6 years of age and over; aerosol for use in children 4 years of age and over (12 years and over for Proventil). AccuNeb has not been studied for treating acute bronchospasms. May delay preterm labor. Large IV doses may aggravate preexisting diabetes mellitus and ketoacidosis.

ADDITIONAL SIDE EFFECTS
Most Common
Headache, N&V, palpitations/tachycardia, tremor, bronchospasm.
GI: Diarrhea, dry mouth, appetite loss or stimulation, epigastric pain. **CNS:** Hyperkinesia, excitement, nervousness, tension, tremor, dizziness, vertigo, weakness, drowsiness, restlessness, headache, insomnia, malaise, emotional lability, fatigue, lightheadedness, nightmares, disturbed sleep, aggressive behavior, irritability. **Respiratory:** Cough, wheezing, dyspnea, bronchospasm, dry throat, pharyngitis, throat irritation, bronchitis, epistaxis, hoarseness (especially in children), nasal congestion, increase in sputum. **CV:** Palpitations, tachycardia, BP changes, hypertension, tight chest, chest pain/discomfort, angina. **Hypersensitivity** (may be immediate): Urticaria, *angioedema,* rash, *bron-*

Bold Italic = life threatening side effect   ■ = black box warning   ✦ = Available in Canada

chospasm. **Miscellaneous:** Flushing, sweating, bad or unusual taste, change in smell, muscle cramps/spasm, pallor, teeth discoloration, conjunctivitis, dilated pupils, difficult urination, voice changes, *oropharyngeal edema*.

OD OVERDOSE MANAGEMENT
SEE ALSO SYMPATHOMIMETIC DRUGS
Symptoms: Seizures, anginal pain, hypertension, hypokalemia, tachycardia (rate may increase to 200 beats/min).

DRUG INTERACTIONS
H *Fir needle oil; Pine needle oil* / ↑ Risk of bronchospasm

HOW SUPPLIED
Inhalation Aerosol: 90 mcg/inh; *Inhalation Solution:* 0.021% (0.63 mg/3 mL), 0.042% (1.25 mg/3 mL), 0.083% (2.5 mg/3 mL), 0.5% (1.25 mg/3 mL); *Syrup:* 2 mg/5 mL; *Tablets:* 2 mg, 4 mg; *Tablets, Extended-Release:* 4 mg, 8 mg.

DOSAGE————————————
• **INHALATION AEROSOL**
Bronchodilation.
Adults and children over 4 years of age (12 and over for Proventil): 180 mcg (2 inhalations) q 4–6 hr. In some clients 1 inhalation (90 mcg) q 4 hr may be sufficient. **Maintenance (Proventil only):** 180 mcg (2 inhalations) 4 times per day.
Prophylaxis of exercise-induced bronchospasm.
Adults and children over 4 years of age (12 and over for Proventil): 180 mcg (2 inhalations) 15 min before exercise.
• **INHALATION SOLUTION**
Bronchodilation.
Adults and children over 12 years of age: 2.5 mg 3–4 times per day by nebulization (dilute 0.5 mL of the 0.5% solution with 2.5 mL sterile NSS and deliver over 5–15 min). **Children, 2–12 years of age (15 kg or over), initial:** 2.5 mg (1 UD vial) 3–4 times per day by nebulization. **Children weighing less than 15 kg who require less than the 2.5 mg dose (i.e., less than a full UD vial):** Use the 0.5% inhalation solution. Give over about 5–15 min.
• **ACCUNEB**

Relief and prophylaxis of bronchospasms.
Initial, children 2–12 years: 1.25 mg or 0.63 mg given 3–4 times per day, as needed, by nebulization. Do not give more frequently. Administer over about 5–15 min.
• **SYRUP**
Bronchodilation.
Adults and children over 14 years of age, usual initial: 2–4 mg (5–10 mL) 3–4 times per day, up to a maximum of 8 mg 4 times per day. In geriatric clients and those sensitive to β–adrenergic stimulation, restrict initial dose to 2 mg (5 mL) 3 or 4 times per day; adjunct individually thereafter. **Children, over 6–12 years, initial:** 2 mg (5 mL) 3–4 times per day; **then,** increase as necessary to a maximum of 24 mg/day in divided doses. **Children, 2–6 years, initial:** 0.1 mg/kg 3 times per day, not to exceed 2 mg (5 mL) 3 times per day; **then,** increase as necessary up to 0.2 mg/kg 3 times per day, not to exceed 4 mg (10 mL) 3 times per day.
• **TABLETS**
Bronchodilation.
Adults and children over 12 years of age, initial: 2 or 4 mg 3–4 times per day; **then,** increase dose as needed up to a maximum of 8 mg 4 times per day, as tolerated. In geriatric clients or those sensitive to beta agonists, start with 2 mg 3–4 times per day; increase dose gradually, if needed, to a maximum of 8 mg 3–4 times per day, not to exceed 32 mg/day in adults and children over 12 years of age. **Children, 6–12 years of age, usual, initial:** 2 mg 3–4 times per day; **then,** if necessary, increase the dose in a stepwise fashion to a maximum of 24 mg/day in divided doses.
• **VOSPIRE ER TABLETS**
Bronchodilation.
Adults and children over 12 years of age: 8 mg q 12 hr; in some clients (e.g., low adult body weight), 4 mg q 12 hr may be sufficient initially and then increased to 8 mg q 12 hr, depending on the response. The dose can be increased stepwise and cautiously (under provider supervision) to a maximum of 32 mg/day in divided doses q 12 hr.

Children, 6–12 years of age: 4 mg q 12 hr. The dose can be increased step-wise and cautiously (under provider supervision) to a maximum of 24 mg/day in divided doses q 12 hr.

NURSING CONSIDERATIONS

℞ Do not confuse albuterol with atenolol (a beta-blocker); Ventolin with Benylin (expectorant); or Volmax with Flomax (an alpha-adrenergic blocker).

ADMINISTRATION/STORAGE

1. The aerosol and inhalation powder are indicated for children 4 years and older (12 years and older for Proventil); the solution for inhalation is indicated for children 2 years and older.
2. Clients maintained on the tablets or syrup may be switched to the extended-release tablets. For example, the administration of one 4 mg extended-release tablet q 12 hr is comparable to one 2 mg tablet q 6 hr.
3. When given by nebulization, use either a face mask or mouthpiece. Use compressed air or oxygen with a gas flow of 6–10 L/min; a single treatment lasts from 5 to 15 min.
4. When given by IPPB, the inspiratory pressure should be from 10 to 20 cm water, with the duration of treatment ranging from 5 to 20 min depending on the client and instrument control.
5. The MDI may also be administered on a mechanical ventilator through an adapter.
6. Take extended-release tablets whole with the aid of liquids; do not chew or crush. The outer coating of Volmax Extended-Release Tablets is not absorbed and is excreted in the feces; empty outer coating may be seen in the stool.
7. Contents of the MDI container are under pressure. Do not store near heat or open flames and do not puncture the container.
8. Proventil HFA and Ventolin HFA contain hydrofluoroalkane as the propellant rather than chlorofluorocarbons.
9. AccuNeb, either 0.63 mg/3 mL or 1.25 mg/3 mL is intended for relief of bronchospasm in children 2–12 years of age with asthma. AccuNeb has not been studied in the setting of acute attacks of bronchospasms.
10. Store Volmax tablets refrigerated at 2–8°C (36–46°F).
11. Store canisters from 15–30°C (59–86°F). Failure to use within this temperature range may result in improper dosing. For optimum results, bring the canister to room temperature before use. Shake well before using.

ASSESSMENT

1. Obtain history; assess EKG and CNS status.
2. Document PFTs, CXR, lung sounds. Note anxiety; may contribute to air hunger.
3. Assess symptom characteristics, onset, duration, frequency, and any precipitating factors.
4. Determine if able to self-administer medication. Assess environmental/home issues.
5. Monitor pulmonary status (i.e., breath sounds, VS, peak flow, or ABGs).
6. Observe for allergic responses.

CLIENT/FAMILY TEACHING

1. Take as directed; do not exceed prescribed dose.
2. Maintain calm, reassuring approach. Do not leave client/child unattended if acutely short of breath; should improve 30–60 min after therapy.
3. Practice how to inhale through nose and exhale with pursed lips or diaphragmatic breathing; prolongs expiration and keeps the airways open longer, thus reducing the work of breathing.
4. Review how to use: Do not put lips around inhaler; go two fingerbreadths away before attempting to activate and inhale. May use a spacer to facilitate inhalation. Attend instruction on correct method for administration.
5. A spacer used with the MDI may enhance drug dispersion. Always thoroughly rinse mouth and equipment with water following each use to prevent oral fungal infections.
6. When using inhalers, do not use other albuterol inhalation medication unless specifically prescribed. If a steroid (Vanceril) inhaler is also prescribed, use this 20–30 min after albuterol to permit better lung penetration.

---

7. Establish dosing regimens that fit lifestyle, i.e., 1–2 puffs q 6 hr or 4 puffs 4 times per day; usual dosing is q 4–6 hr with an as-needed order, or before exercise. Check peak flows, call if requiring more puffs more frequently than prescribed or if drug dose used previously does not provide relief. Report lack of response, chest pain, dizziness, weakness, heart palpitations, significant drop in peak flow readings, changes in sputum color/amount.

8. Use caution, may cause dizziness/drowsiness.

9. To check inhaler content, place in glass of water: full inhalers sink, empty inhalers float and half-full inhalers are partially submerged. Check to ensure you do not run out of medication.

OUTCOMES/EVALUATE
Improved breathing patterns/airway exchange

Aldesleukin ▪️**IV** (Interleukin-2: IL-2)
(al-des-**LOO**-kin)

CLASSIFICATION(S):
Antineoplastic, miscellaneous
PREGNANCY CATEGORY: C
Rx: Proleukin.

SEE ALSO *ANTINEOPLASTIC AGENTS.*

USES
(1) Metastatic renal cell carcinoma in adults 18 years of age and older. (2) Metastatic melanoma in adults. *Investigational:* In combination with highly active antiretroviral therapy to treat HIV clients. In combination for treatment of cutaneous T cell lymphoma.

ACTION/KINETICS
Action
Aldesleukin possesses the biologic activity of human native IL-2, even though it is not identical. The drug produces several immunologic effects including (1) activation of cellular immunity with profound lymphocytosis, (2) eosinophilia and thrombocytopenia, (3) production of cytokines (including tissue necrosis factor, IL-2, gamma interferon), and (4) inhibition of tumor growth. The exact antitumor effect is not known.

Pharmacokinetics
High plasma levels reached after a short IV infusion; rapidly distributed to the extravascular, extracellular space. Rapidly cleared from the circulation by both glomerular filtration and peritubular extraction; metabolized in the kidneys with little or no active form excreted through the urine. **t½, distribution:** 13 min; **t½, elimination:** 85 min.

CONTRAINDICATIONS
Hypersensitivity to IL-2 or any components of the product. Abnormal thallium stress test or pulmonary function tests. Organ allografts. Use in either men or women not practicing effective contraception. Lactation.

Retreatment is contraindicated in those who have experienced the following during a previous course of therapy: Sustained ventricular tachycardia; uncontrolled or unresponsive cardiac rhythm disturbances; recurrent chest pain with ECG changes that are consistent with angina or MI; intubation required for more than 72 hr; pericardial tamponade; renal dysfunction requiring dialysis for more than 72 hr; coma or toxic psychosis lasting more than 48 hr; seizures that are repetitive or difficult to control; ischemia or perforation of the bowel; and GI bleeding requiring surgery.

SPECIAL CONCERNS
■ (1) Use has been associated with capillary leak syndrome (CLS). CLS results in hypotension and reduced organ perfusion that may result in death (See Side Effects). Restrict therapy to clients with normal cardiac and pulmonary function as defined by thallium stress testing and formal pulmonary function testing. Use extreme caution in those with normal thallium stress tests and pulmonary function tests who have a history of prior cardiac or pulmonary disease. (2) Withhold use in those who develop moderate to severe lethargy or somnolence; continued use may result in coma. (3) CLS may be associated with cardiac arrhythmias (supraventricular

---

and ventricular), angina, MI, respiratory insufficiency requiring intubation, GI bleeding or infarction, renal insufficiency, edema, and mental status changes. (4) Aldesleukin treatment is associated with impaired neutrophil function (reduced chemotaxis) and with an increased risk of disseminated infection, including sepsis and bacterial endocarditis. Adequately treat preexisting bacteria prior to initiation of therapy.■ Symptoms may worsen in unrecognized or untreated CNS metastases. Use of medications known to be nephrotoxic or hepatotoxic may further increase toxicity to the kidney and liver caused by aldesleukin. May increase the risk of allograft rejection in transplant clients. Safety and efficacy have not been established in children less than 18 years of age.

SIDE EFFECTS

Most Common

Fever, chills, rigors, GI side effects, hypotension, sinus tachycardia, mental status changes, pruritus/erythema, N&V, diarrhea, pulmonary congestion/dyspnea, oliguria/anuria, anemia/thrombocytopenia.

Side effects are frequent, often serious, and sometimes fatal. The frequency and severity of side effects are usually dose-related and schedule-dependent. Incidence of side effects is greater in PS 1 clients than in PS 0 clients. The side effects listed have an incidence of 1% or greater. **Capillary leak syndrome (CLS):** Results from extravasation of plasma proteins and fluid into the extracellular space with loss of vascular tone. This results in a drop in mean arterial BP within 2–12 hr after the start of treatment and reduced organ perfusion that may be severe and result in death. CLS causes hypotension, hypoperfusion, and extravasation that leads to edema and effusion. *CLS may be associated with supraventricular and ventricular arrhythmias MI,* angina, respiratory insufficiency requiring intubation, GI bleeding or infarction, renal insufficiency, and changes in mental status. **CV:** Hypotension (sometimes requiring vasopressor therapy), sinus tachycardia, *arrhythmias (atrial, junctional, supraventricular, ventricular),* bradycardia, PVCs, PACs, myocardial ischemia, *MI, cardiac arrest, CHF,* myocarditis, endocarditis, gangrene, *stroke, pericardial effusion, thrombosis.* **Respiratory:** Pulmonary congestion/edema, dyspnea, *respiratory failure,* tachypnea, pleural effusion, wheezing, apnea, pneumothorax, hemoptysis. **GI:** N&V, diarrhea, stomatitis, anorexia, *GI bleeding* (sometimes requiring surgery), dyspepsia, constipation, *intestinal perforation,* intestinal ileus, pancreatitis. **CNS:** Changes in mental status (may be an early indication of bacteremia or early bacterial sepsis), dizziness, sensory dysfunction, disorders of special senses (speech, taste, vision), syncope, motor dysfunction, *coma, seizure.* **GU:** Oliguria or anuria, proteinuria, hematuria, dysuria, impaired renal function requiring dialysis, urinary retention/frequency. **Hepatic:** Jaundice, ascites, hepatomegaly. **Hematologic:** Anemia, thrombocytopenia, leukopenia, coagulation disorders, leukocytosis, eosinophilia. **Dermatologic:** Pruritus, erythema, rash, dry skin, exfoliative dermatitis, purpura, petechiae, urticaria, alopecia. **Musculoskeletal:** Arthralgia, myalgia, arthritis, muscle spasm. **Electrolyte and other disturbances:** Hypomagnesemia, acidosis, hypocalcemia/-kalemia, hypophosphatemia, hyperuricemia, hypoalbuminemia/-proteinemia, hyponatremia, hyperkalemia, alkalosis, hypo-/hyperglycemia, hypocholesterolemia, hypercalcemia, hypernatremia/-phosphatemia. **Miscellaneous:** Fever, chills, pain (abdominal, chest, back), fatigue, malaise, weakness, edema, infection (including the injection site, urinary tract, catheter tip, phlebitis, sepsis), weight gain/loss, headache, conjunctivitis, reactions at the injection site, allergic reactions, hypothyroidism.

LABORATORY TEST CONSIDERATIONS

↑ BUN, bilirubin, serum creatinine, transaminase, alkaline phosphatase. See also *Electrolyte and other disturbances* under Side Effects.

OD OVERDOSE MANAGEMENT
Symptoms: See *Side Effects.* Exceeding the recommended dose may cause a more rapid onset of toxicity. *Treatment:* Side effects will usually reverse if the drug is stopped, especially because the serum half-life is short. Continuing toxicity is treated symptomatically. Life-threatening side effects have been treated by the IV administration of dexamethasone (which may result in loss of the therapeutic effectiveness of aldesleukin).

DRUG INTERACTIONS
Aminoglycosides / ↑ Risk of kidney toxicity
Antihypertensives / Potentiate hypotension due to aldesleukin
Asparaginase / ↑ Risk of hepatic toxicity
Cardiotoxic agents / ↑ Risk of cardiac toxicity
Corticosteroids / Concomitant use may ↓ antitumor effectiveness of aldesleukin (although corticosteroids ↓ aldesleukin side effects)
Cytotoxic chemotherapy / ↑ Risk of myelotoxicity
Doxorubicin / ↑ Risk of cardiac toxicity
Hepatotoxic drugs / ↑ Risk of liver toxicity
Indinavir / ↑ Indinavir plasma levels R/T ↓ liver breakdown
Indomethacin / ↑ Risk of kidney toxicity
Methotrexate / ↑ Risk of hepatic toxicity
Myelotoxic agents / ↑ Risk of myelotoxicity
Nephrotoxic agents / ↑ Risk of kidney toxicity
Psychotropic drugs (e.g., analgesics, antiemetics, narcotics, sedatives, tranquilizers) / Possible alteration of CNS function

HOW SUPPLIED
Powder for Injection: 22 million international units/vial (18 million international units/mL when reconstituted).

DOSAGE
- **IV INFUSION, INTERMITTENT**
  Metastatic renal cell carcinoma in adults and metastatic melanoma.
Each course of treatment consists of two 5-day treatment cycles separated by a rest period. **Adults:** 600,000 international units/kg (0.037 mg/kg) given q 8 hr by a 15-min IV infusion for a maximum of 14 doses. Following 9 days of rest, repeat schedule for another 14 doses, for a maximum of 28 doses per course as tolerated. *NOTE:* Due to toxicity, clients may not be able to receive all 28 doses (median number of doses given is 20 during the first course of therapy for renal cell carcinoma and 18 during the first course of therapy for metastatic melanoma).
  Retreatment for metastatic renal cell carcinoma and metastatic melanoma.
Evaluate for a response about 4 weeks after completion of a course of therapy and again just prior to the start of the next treatment course. Give additional courses only if there is evidence of some tumor shrinkage following the last course and retreatment is not contraindicated (see preceding *Contraindications*). Separate each treatment course by at least 7 weeks from the date of hospital discharge.

NURSING CONSIDERATIONS
ADMINISTRATION/STORAGE
IV 1. Undertake dose modification for toxicity by withholding/interrupting dose rather than reducing dose to be given.
2. *Permanently discontinue* therapy for the following toxicities:
- CV: Sustained VT, uncontrolled/unresponsive cardiac rhythm disturbances, recurrent chest pain with ECG changes indicating angina or MI, pericardial tamponade
- Pulmonary: Intubation >72 hr
- Renal: Dialysis >72 hr
- CNS: Coma or toxic psychosis >48 hr; repetitive/difficult to control seizures
- GI: Bowel ischemia/perforation, GI bleeding requiring surgery
3. Consult product information for withheld and subsequent doses of aldesleukin, as well as guidelines for discontinuing therapy.
4. Reconstitute vials aseptically with 1.2 mL sterile water; each mL will contain 18 million international units (1.1 mg) of aldesleukin. Solutions should be clear and colorless to slightly yellow.

---

5. The vial is for single use only; discard any unused portion. Not for use with transplants; risk of allograft rejection.
6. During reconstitution, direct sterile water at the side of the vial. Swirl contents gently to avoid foaming. *Do not shake vial.*
7. Reconstituted drug may be diluted in 50 mL of D5W and infused over 15 min.
8. Use plastic bags for more consistent drug delivery. Do *not* use in-line filters.
9. Due to increased aggregation, do not reconstitute using bacteriostatic water or 0.9% NaCl injection.
10. Dilution with albumin can alter pharmacology of aldesleukin. Do not mix with other drugs.
11. After reconstitution, drug stable for 48 hr if stored at room temperature or 2–8°C (36–46°F). Administer within 48 hr of reconstitution; bring solution to room temperature before infusing. Do not freeze.
12. Undiluted drug stable for 5 days if refrigerated in 1-mL B-D syringes.
13. Drug compatible with glass, PVC (preferred), or polypropylene syringes.

ASSESSMENT

1. Note any liver/renal dysfunction; cardiac, pulmonary, or CNS impairment.
2. Determine the following baseline parameters prior to therapy and daily during drug use: CBC, blood chemistries, renal and LFTs, and CXRs. Obtain baseline PFTs with ABGs.
3. Screen with a thallium stress test to document normal ejection fraction and unimpaired wall motion. If minor abnormalities in wall motion noted, a stress echocardiogram may help to exclude significant CAD.
4. Assess for any S&S of infection. Obtain cultures to R/O any potential sources. Preexisting bacterial infections must be treated prior to initiation of therapy, as intensive treatment may cause impaired neutrophil function and an increased risk of disseminated infection leading to sepsis and bacterial endocarditis.
5. All those with in-dwelling central lines should receive antibiotic prophylaxis against *Saccharomyces aureus*.

INTERVENTIONS

1. Initiate in a closely monitored environment where VS and I&O are assessed often.
2. Assess cardiac function daily by clinical examination and assessment of VS. Those with chest pain, murmurs, gallops, irregular rhythm, or palpitations should be further assessed with an ECG and CPKs. If ischemia or CHF evident, get a repeat thallium or cardiolyte stress test.
3. Perform daily CV evaluations to identify early S&S of drug toxicity. Monitor for symptoms of CLS characterized by hypotension and hypoperfusion, altered mental status, and decreased urine output. Mental status changes are usually transient but should be evaluated carefully. Alterations in urinary output may signal renal toxicity. Monitor for dehydration, liver or renal failure. Stop infusion and transport to ICU for intubation and dialysis if progressive toxicity evident.

CLIENT/FAMILY TEACHING

1. Report any persistent chest/abdominal pain/discomfort, unusual bruising or bleeding, fatigue, confusion, or ↑ SOB.
2. Review list of drug side effects and note those (SOB, palpitations, blood in sputum, confusion, chest pain, or impaired vision) requiring immediate intervention.
3. Practice reliable contraception.
4. Avoid any OTC drugs unless specifically ordered.

OUTCOMES/EVALUATE

Disease regression with evidence of ↓ tumor size and spread

Alefacept
(a-**LE**-fa-sept)

CLASSIFICATION(S):
Immunosuppressant
PREGNANCY CATEGORY: B
Rx: Amevive.

USES

Adults with moderate to severe chronic plaque psoriasis who are candidates for systemic therapy or phototherapy.

ACTION/KINETICS
Action
Alefacept interferes with lymphocyte activation by specifically binding to the lymphocyte antigen, CD2, and inhibiting LFA-3/CD2 interaction. Activation of T lymphocytes involving the interaction between LFA-3 on antigen-presenting cells and CD2 on T lymphocytes plays a role in the pathophysiology of chronic plaque psoriasis. Alefacept also reduces subsets of CD2+ T lymphocytes, probably by bridging between CD2 on target lymphocytes and immunoglobulin Fc receptors on cytotoxic cells, such as natural killer cells. The drug reduces circulating total CD4+ and CD8+ T lymphocyte counts. CD2 also is expressed at low levels on the surface of natural killer cells and certain bone marrow B lymphocytes. Thus, the potential exists for alefacept to affect the activation and numbers of cells other than T lymphocytes.

Pharmacokinetics
Following IM use, 63% was bioavailable. **t½, elimination:** 270 hr.

CONTRAINDICATIONS
Lactation. Use in children. Use in clients infected with HIV (alefacept may accelerate disease progression or increase complications of HIV). Initiation of therapy in clients with a CD4+ T lymphocyte count below normal. Known hypersensitivity to alefacept or any of its components.

SPECIAL CONCERNS
Alefacept induces dose-dependent reductions in circulating CD4+ and CD8+ T lymphocyte counts. It may also increase the risk of malignancies, increase the risk of serious infections, and cause serious hypersensitivity reactions. Use with caution in the elderly. Do not administer to clients receiving phototherapy due to the possibility of excessive immunosuppression.

SIDE EFFECTS
Most Common
Chills, pharyngitis, dizziness, increased cough, nausea, pruritus, myalgia, injection site pain/inflammation, accidental injury.

The most serious side effects are lymphopenia, malignancies, serious infections requiring hospitalization, and hypersensitivity reactions. **CV:** CV events, including coronary artery disorder and **MI. GI:** Hepatic injury, including asymptomatic transaminase elevations, fatty infiltration of the liver, hepatitis, *decompenstion of cirrhosis with liver failure, and acute liver failure*. **Body as a whole:** Pruritus, myalgia, chills, accidental injury, CD4+ lymphocyte levels below 250 cells/mcL, hypersensitivity reactions, treatment-emergent malignancies (e.g., basal or squamous cell cancer of the skin, lymphoma, Hodgkin's disease). **Infections:** Necrotizing cellulitis, peritonsillar abscess, postoperative and burn wound infection, toxic shock, pneumonia, appendicitis, preseptal cellulitis, cholecystitis, gastroenteritis, herpes simplex infection. **Injection site reactions:** Pain, inflammation, bleeding, edema, nonspecific reaction, mass, skin hypersensitivity. **Miscellaneous:** Pharyngitis, dizziness, increased cough, nausea, headache, injection site pain/inflammation.

OD OVERDOSE MANAGEMENT
Symptoms: Chills, headache, arthralgia, sinusitis. *Treatment:* Closely monitor for effects on total lymphocyte count and CD4+ lymphocyte count.

DRUG INTERACTIONS
Use of alefacept with other immunosuppressants may result in excessive immunosuppression; do not use together

HOW SUPPLIED
Powder for Injection, Lyophilized: 15 mg.

DOSAGE
- **IM**
  Plaque psoriasis.
Adults: 15 mg once weekly IM for a total of 12 weeks. An additional 12-week course may be started provided that the CD4+ T lymphocyte counts are within the normal range and a minimum of a 12-week interval has passed since the previous course of treatment.

A

NURSING CONSIDERATIONS

ADMINISTRATION/STORAGE

1. Withhold if CD4⁺ T lymphocyte counts <250 cells/mcL. Discontinue if they remain below 250 cells/mcL for 1 month.

2. For IM use reconstitute the 15 mg lyophilized powder with 0.6 mL of the supplied diluent (sterile water for injection). Keep needle pointed at the sidewall of vial and slowly inject diluent into the alefacept vial. Some foaming will occur (this is normal). To avoid excess foaming, do not shake or vigorously agitate. Swirl contents gently during dissolution. Dissolution usually takes less than 2 minutes. Use aseptic techniques. Do not reconstitute for IM with any other diluent; reconstituted solution for IM use contains 15 mg/0.5 mL.

3. Do not add other medications to alefacept solutions.

4. Do not filter reconstituted solution during preparation/administration.

5. Reconstituted solution should be clear and colorless to slightly yellow. Do not use if it is discolored or cloudy or if undissolved material remains.

6. Use the reconstituted solution immediately or within 4 hr if stored at 2–8°C (36–46°F). Discard if not used within 4 hr of reconstitution.

7. For IM use, remove the needle used for reconstitution and attach the other supplied needle. Withdraw 0.5 mL of the alefacept solution into the syringe; note that some foam or bubbles may remain in the vial.

8. Inject the full 0.5 mL of solution. Rotate sites so a different site is used for each injection. Give new injections at least 1 inch from an old site and never into areas where the skin is tender, bruised, red, or hard.

9. Refrigerate the lyophilized powder from 2–8° C (36–46° F). Protect from light. Keep in the drug/diluent pack until time of use.

ASSESSMENT

1. Note reasons for therapy, other agents trialed, outcome; describe/document presentation/photographs.

2. Monitor CBC, CD4⁺ T lymphocyte counts, renal and LFTs.

3. Assess carefully for any evidence of infection or malignancy.

CLIENT/FAMILY TEACHING

1. Used to treat individuals with severe chronic plaque psoriasis that are candidates for systemic therapy or phototherapy.

2. Therapy administered once a week for 12 weeks. If CD4⁺ T lymphocyte counts are normal, another 12-week course may be administered after a 12-week rest/break.

3. Report adverse side effects and evidence of infection immediately.

4. Keep all F/U visits for labs and for evaluation of response to medication.

5. Practice reliable contraception; report if pregnancy suspected. Biogen maintains a registry for studying drug effects during pregnancy; enroll at 1-866-263-8483 Mon-Fri 8:30 am to 8 pm.

OUTCOMES/EVALUATE

Control of chronic plaque psoriasis; clearing of lesions

Alemtuzumab
(**ah**-lem-**TOOZ**-uh-mab)

CLASSIFICATION(S):
Monoclonal antibody
PREGNANCY CATEGORY: C
Rx: Campath.

USES

Treatment of B-cell chronic lymphocytic leukemia in clients previously treated with alkylating agents and who have failed fludarabine therapy.

ACTION/KINETICS

Action

Recombinant DNA-derived humanized monoclonal antibody. Binds to CD52, a nonmodulating antigen, that is present on the surface of nearly all B and T lymphocytes, a majority of monocytes, macrophages, NK cells, and a subpopulation of granulocytes. Probably acts by lysis of leukemic cells following cell surface binding.

Pharmacokinetics

t½, mean: 11 hr after the first 30 mg dose and 6 days after the last 30 mg dose.

CONTRAINDICATIONS

Active systemic infections, underlying immunodeficiency (e.g., seropositive for HIV), or known Type I hypersensitivity or anaphylactic reaction to alemtuzumab or any of its components. Immunization of clients who have recently received the drug. Lactation.

SPECIAL CONCERNS

■ Administer under the supervision of a health care provider experienced in the use of antineoplastic therapy. (1) Serious and possible fatal pancytopenia/marrow hypoplasia, autoimmune idiopathic thrombocytopenia, and autoimmune hemolytic anemia may occur (See Side Effects). Do not give single doses >30 mg or cumulative doses >90 mg/week because these doses are associated with a higher incidence of pancytopenia. (2) Serious, and in some cases fatal, infusion reactions possible. Carefully monitor clients during infusions and discontinue if indicated. Gradual escalation to the recommended maintenance dose is required at the initiation of therapy and after interruption of therapy for at least 7 days. (3) Serious, sometimes fatal, bacterial, viral, fungal, and protozoan infections have been reported. Use prophylactic approach (See Administration/Storage) to decrease (but not eliminate) *Pneumocystis carinii* pneumonia and herpes virus infections.■ Due to immunosuppression by the drug, do not immunize with live viral vaccines clients who have recently received alemtuzumab. Safety and efficacy have not been determined in children.

SIDE EFFECTS

Most Common

Neutropenia, rigors, fever, anemia, thrombocytopenia, nausea, rash.

Infusion-related: Hypotension, rigors, drug-related fever, N&V, SOB, bronchospasm, chills, rash, fatigue, urticaria, dyspnea, pruritus, headache, diarrhea, syncope, pulmonary infiltrates, *acute respiratory distress syndrome, respiratory arrest*, cardiac arrhythmias, *MI, and cardiac arrest*. **GI:** N&V, diarrhea, stomatitis, ulcerative stomatitis, mucositis, abdominal pain, dyspepsia, constipation. **CNS:** Headache, dysesthesias, dizziness, insomnia, depression, tremor, somnolence. **CV:** Hypotension, tachycardia, SVT, hypertension. **Hematologic:** *Myelosuppression*, profound lymphopenia, bone marrow aplasia, hypoplasia, *severe/fatal autoimmune anemia*, thrombocytopenia, neutropenia, purpura, pancytopenia, purpura. **Respiratory:** Dyspnea, cough, bronchitis, pneumonitis, pneumonia, pharyngitis, bronchospasm, rhinitis, epistaxis. **Musculoskeletal:** Skeletal pain, myalgias, back/chest pain. **Dermatologic:** Rash (including maculopapular, erythematous), urticaria, pruritus, increased sweating. **Miscellaneous:** Opportunistic bacterial, viral, fungal, and protozoan infections (may be fatal), rigors, fever, fatigue, anorexia, *sepsis*, asthenia, edema, peripheral edema, herpes simplex, malaise, moniliasis, temperature change sensation.

LABORATORY TEST CONSIDERATIONS

Interference with diagnostic serum tests that use antibodies.

HOW SUPPLIED

Solution for Injection: 30 mg/mL.

DOSAGE

- **IV ONLY**

  B-cell chronic lymphocytic leukemia.

Initial: 3 mg/day given as a 2-hr infusion. When the 3 mg dose is tolerated (Grade 2 or less infusion-related toxicities), escalate the dose to 10 mg and continue as tolerated. When the 10 mg dose is tolerated, initiate maintenance dose of 30 mg/dose given 3 times per week on alternate days for 12 weeks or less. Escalation to 30 mg can usually be done in 3–7 days. Single doses greater than 30 mg or weekly doses greater than 90 mg are associated with an increased incidence of pancytopenia.

NURSING CONSIDERATIONS

ADMINISTRATION/STORAGE

IV 1. Do not give as IV push/bolus.
2. Withdraw correct amount of drug from ampule into syringe. To prepare

---

A

the 3 mg dose, withdraw 0.1 mL into a 1 mL syringe calibrated in increments of 0.1 mL. To prepare the 10 mg dose, withdraw 0.33 mL into a 1 mL syringe calibrated in increments of 0.1 mL. To prepare the 30 mg dose, withdraw 1 mL in either a 1 or 3 mL syringe calibrated in 0.1 mL increments. Inject into 100 mL sterile 0.9% NaCl or D5W. Gently invert bag to mix the solution. Discard syringe. Use within 8 hr afer dilution.

3. Do not use if particulate matter is present or solution discolored. Do not shake prior to use.

4. Do not add any drugs or simultaneously infuse any other drug through the same IV line.

5. Alemtuzumab contains no preservative; use within 8 hr of dilution. Store solutions at room temperature or refrigerate. Protect from light. Prior to dilution, store ampule at 2–8°C (36–46°F). Do not freeze. Discard if ampule has been frozen. Protect from direct sunlight.

6. To minimize infusion-related effects, premedicate prior to first dose, at dose escalations, and as needed. Premedication consists of diphenhydramine, 50 mg, and acetaminophen, 650 mg, each given 30 min prior to alemtuzumab. If severe infusion-related symptoms occur, give hydrocortisone, 200 mg.

7. To minimize risk of serious opportunistic infections, anti-infectives may be given. One regimen is trimethoprim/sulfamethoxazole DS twice a day 3 times per week and famciclovir (or equivalent) 250 mg twice a day upon starting therapy. Continue prophylaxis for 2 months after completion of therapy or until CD4+ count is 200 or more cells/microliter (whichever occurs later).

8. Discontinue during serious infection, serious hematologic toxicity, or other serious toxicity, until problem resolved. Permanently discontinue if autoimmune anemia or thrombocytopenia occurs. If severe neutropenia or thrombocytopenia occurs, use the following dose modification and reinitiation therapy protocol:

• For first occurrence of ANC <250/ mcL and/or platelet count 25,000/ mcL or less, withhold therapy. When ANC is 500/mcL or more and platelet count is 50,000/mcL or more, resume therapy at the same dose. If delay between dosing is 7 days or more, start therapy at 3 mg and escalate to 10 mg and then 30 mg as tolerated.

• For second occurrence of ANC <250/ mcL and/or platelet count 25,000/ mcL or less, withhold therapy. When ANC is 500/mcL or more and platelet count is 50,000/mcL or more, resume therapy at 10 mg. If dosing delay is 7 days or more, initiate therapy at 3 mg and escalate to 10 mg only.

• For a third incidence of ANC <250/ mcL and/or platelet count 25,000/ mcL or less, stop therapy permanently.

• If there is a ↓ ANC and/or platelet count of 50% or less of baseline value in those who started therapy with a baseline ANC of 500/mcL or less and/or a baseline platelet count of 25,000/mcL or less, withhold therapy. When ANC and platelet counts return to baseline value(s), resume therapy. If the dosing delay is 7 days or more, start therapy at 3 mg and escalate to 10 mg and then to 30 mg as tolerated.

ASSESSMENT

1. Note reasons for therapy, disease characteristics, physical condition; list fludarabine failure/other alkylating agents used.

2. Premedicate with diphenhydramine 50 mg and acetaminophen 650 mg 30 min before infusion, at dose escalations, and as indicated. Hydrocortisone 200 mg may help decrease infusion-related events.

3. Administer over 2 hr. Monitor CBCs and platelets closely. Follow guidelines under administration for resuming therapy if ANC depressed or CD4 count <200 cells/mcL.

4. Assess for evidence of infections; monitor VS and assess skin, urine, and lungs frequently. Follow infection prophylaxis under administration. Drug is extremely toxic; requires close observation.

Bold Italic = life threatening side effect   ■ = black box warning   ✦ = Available in Canada

CLIENT/FAMILY TEACHING
1. Used to treat CLL in those who have failed to respond to fludarabine and other alkylating agents.
2. Once maintenance dose of 30 mg has been reached, drug is given 3 times/week (over 2 hrs) on alternating days for up to 12 weeks. If the ANC or platelets drop, the dose may be modified.
3. Avoid live viral vaccines during therapy R/T drug-induced immunosuppression.
4. Report any adverse side effects immediately; drug is highly toxic.
5. Women of child-bearing age and men of reproductive potential should practice reliable contraception during treatment and for a minimum of 6 months after therapy. Consider egg/sperm harvesting prior to therapy.

OUTCOMES/EVALUATE
Control of malignant cell proliferation in B-cell CLL

Alendronate sodium
(ay-**LEN**-droh-nayt)

CLASSIFICATION(S):
Bone growth regulator, bisphosphonate
PREGNANCY CATEGORY: C
Rx: Fosamax.

USES
Daily dosing: (1) Prevent osteoporosis in women who are at risk of developing osteoporosis and to maintain bone mass and reduce the risk of future fracture. (2) Treat osteoporosis in postmenopausal women to increase bone mass and reduce the incidence of fractures, including those of the hip and spine. (3) Increase bone density in men with osteoporosis. (4) Glucocorticoid-induced osteoporosis in men and women receiving daily dosage equivalent to 7.5 mg or greater of prednisone and who have low bone mineral density. Used with adequate amounts of calcium and Vitamin D. (5) Paget's disease of bone in those with alkaline phosphatase at least two times the upper limit of normal or for those who are symptomatic or at risk for future complications from the disease. **Weekly dosing:** Treatment or prevention of postmenopausal osteoporosis in women or osteoporosis in men.

ACTION/KINETICS
Action
Binds to bone hydroxyapatite and inhibits osteoclast activity, thereby preventing bone resorption. Appears to reduce fracture risk and reverse the progression of osteoporosis. Does not inhibit bone mineralization.
Pharmacokinetics
Well absorbed orally and initially distributed to soft tissues, but then quickly redistributed to bone. Not metabolized; excreted through the urine. **$t\frac{1}{2}$, terminal:** Believed to be more than 10 years, due to slow release from the skeleton.

CONTRAINDICATIONS
In hypocalcemia. Severe renal insufficiency (C_{CR} less than 35 mL/min). Use of hormone replacement therapy with alendronate for osteoporosis in postmenopausal women. Use of the PO solution in clients at increased risk of aspiration. Lactation.

SPECIAL CONCERNS
Use with caution in those with upper GI problems, such as dysphagia, symptomatic esophageal diseases, gastritis, duodenitis, or ulcers. Safety and effectiveness have not been determined in children. Some elderly clients may be more sensitive to the drug effects. Rarely, visual and auditory hallucinations when client switched from daily to weekly use of alendronate.

SIDE EFFECTS
Most Common
Abdominal pain, dyspepsia, nausea, constipation, diarrhea.

GI: Flatulence, acid regurgitation, esophageal ulcer, dysphagia, abdominal pain/distention, gastritis, constipation, diarrhea, dyspepsia, N&V. **Miscellaneous:** Musculoskeletal/back pain, pain, headache, taste perversion, rash and erythema (rare), glaucoma, accidental injury, edema, flu–like symptoms, osteonecrosis of the jaw.

LABORATORY TEST CONSIDERATIONS
↓ Serum calcium and phosphate.

OD OVERDOSE MANAGEMENT

Symptoms: Hypocalcemia, hypophosphatemia, upset stomach, heartburn, esophagitis, gastritis, ulcer. *Treatment:* Consider giving milk or antacids to bind the drug.

DRUG INTERACTIONS
Antacids / ↓ Absorption of alendronate
Aspirin / ↑ Risk of GI side effects
Calcium supplements / ↓ Absorption of alendronate
Naproxen / ↑ Risk of drug-induced gastric ulcers
Ranitidine / ↑ Bioavailability of alendronate (significance not known)

HOW SUPPLIED
Oral Solution: 70 mg as base (0.93 mg/mL); *Tablets:* 5 mg, 10 mg, 35 mg, 40 mg, 70 mg.

DOSAGE

• **ORAL SOLUTION; TABLETS**

Prevention of osteoporosis in postmenopausal women.
One 35 mg tablet once weekly or one 5 mg tablet once daily.

Treatment of osteoporosis in postmenopausal women.
One 70 mg tablet once weekly, one 10 mg tablet once daily, or 1 bottle of 70 mg oral solution once weekly.

Osteoporosis in men.
One 70 mg tablet once weekly, one 10 mg tablet once daily, or 1 bottle of 70 mg oral solution once weekly.

Glucocorticoid-induced osteoporosis.
One 5 mg tablet once daily for men and women. For postmenopausal women not receiving estrogen, the recommended dose is one 10 mg tablet daily. Also give clients adequate amounts of calcium and vitamin D.

Paget disease of the bone.
40 mg once daily for 6 months for both men and women.

NURSING CONSIDERATIONS

ADMINISTRATION/STORAGE

1. To facilitate stomach delivery and reduce esophagus irritation, do not lie down for at least 30 min following administration.
2. Due to possible interference with absorption, at least 30 min should elapse before taking antacids or calcium supplements.
3. Retreatment for Paget's disease may be considered following a 6-month posttreatment evaluation in clients who have relapsed, based on increases in serum alkaline phosphatase. Retreatment may also be appropriate for those who failed to normalize serum alkaline phosphatase.
4. If dietary intake is insufficient, give supplemental calcium and vitamin D when used for glucocorticoid-induced osteoporosis or Paget's disease. A product called Fosamax Plus D containing alendronate sodium 70 mg and vitamin D_3, 2,800 international units, is available to treat osteoporosis in postmenopausal women and to increase bone mass in men with osteoporosis.
5. No dosage adjustment needed for the elderly.
6. Store tablets and oral solution in a tight container from 15–30° C (59–86° F). Do not freeze oral solution.

ASSESSMENT
1. Note reasons for therapy: osteoporosis prevention/treatment in postmenopausal women, steroid-induced osteoporosis, or Paget's disease. Note symptoms, onset, and physical changes.
2. Obtain baseline calcium, phosphate, electrolytes, liver and renal function studies; correct any calcium or vitamin D deficiencies, monitor periodically.
3. Note any history of GI problems (i.e., gastritis, dysphagia, duodenitis, or ulcers).
4. Document bone mineral density (BMD) studies and/or skeletal x-rays.
5. Assess for fractures; manage to prevent further injury and loss of function.
6. With Paget's disease, monitor baseline S&S and alkaline phosphatase.

CLIENT/FAMILY TEACHING
1. Osteoporosis usually occurs after age 40 and is a systemic skeletal disease characterized by low bone mass due to a higher amount of bone resorbed than

---

formed; may be induced by chronic steroid therapy at any age.

2. Take as prescribed. Benefit seen only when each tablet is taken with 6–8 oz of plain water first thing in the morning at least 30 min before the first food, beverage, or medication of the day. Remain upright. Waiting >30 min will improve absorption. Taking with juice or coffee will markedly reduce absorption. Once weekly therapy may enhance compliance.

3. Do not chew or crush tablets; take whole. Do not lie down after taking drug; wait at least 30 min. Do not take aspirin or aspirin-containing products unless approved by provider.

4. If dietary intake is inadequate, take calcium with vitamin D supplements. Regular daily weight bearing exercise encouraged for all.

5. Do not drink alcoholic beverages or smoke while taking this drug.

6. If used for steroid-induced osteoporosis or Paget's disease, take calcium (500 mg) and vitamin D daily, especially if dietary intake or sun exposure is inadequate.

OUTCOMES/EVALUATE
- Prevention of osteoporosis and bone resorption (↓ bone turnover)
- Increased bone mass
- Inhibition of kyphosis and pain R/T bone fracture or deformity
- ↓ Pain; ↓ Serum alkaline phosphatase levels with Paget's disease

Alfentanil hydrochloride

(al-**FEN**-tah-nil)

CLASSIFICATION(S):
Narcotic analgesic
PREGNANCY CATEGORY: C
Rx: Alfenta, **C-II**

SEE ALSO NARCOTIC ANALGESICS.

USES
(1) **Continuous infusion:** As an analgesic with nitrous oxide/oxygen to maintain general anesthesia. (2) **Incremen-**tal doses: Adjunct with barbiturate/nitrous oxide/oxygen to maintain general anesthesia. (3) **Anesthetic induction:** As primary agent when ET intubation and mechanical ventilation are necessary. (4) Analgesic component for monitored anesthesia care.

ACTION/KINETICS
Pharmacokinetics
Onset: Immediate. **t½:** 1–2 hr (after IV use).

CONTRAINDICATIONS
Use during labor and in children less than 12 years of age.

SPECIAL CONCERNS
Use with caution during lactation.

SIDE EFFECTS
Most Common
N&V, hyper-/hypotension, arrhythmias, tachycardia, chest wall rigidity.
See *Narcotic Analgesics.* Bradycardia, postoperative confusion, blurred vision, hypercapnia, shivering, and **asystole**. Neonates with respiratory distress syndrome have manifested hypotension with doses of 20 mcg/kg.

ADDITIONAL DRUG INTERACTIONS
Fluconazole / ↑ Alfentanil plasma levels due to ↓ liver breakdown
⬛ *Indian snakeroot* / Potentiation of alfentanil effects
⬛ *Kava kava* / Potentiation of alfentanil effects

HOW SUPPLIED
Injection: 0.5 mg/mL.

DOSAGE
Individualize dosage and titrate to desired effect according to body weight, physical status, underlying disease states, use of other drugs, and type and duration of surgical procedure and anesthesia.

- **IV**
  Continuous infusion to attenuate response to laryngoscopy and intubation (assisted or controlled ventilation).

Initial for induction: 50–75 mcg/kg; **maintenance, with nitrous oxide/oxygen:** 0.5–3 mcg/kg/min (average infusion rate: 1–1.5 mcg/kg/min). Following the induction dose, reduce the infusion rate requirement by 30–50% for the first hour of maintenance. The total

A

dose depends on the duration of the procedure.

Induction of anesthesia (assisted or controlled ventilation).

Initial for induction: 130–245 mcg/kg; give slowly over 3 min; **maintenance:** 0.5–1.5 mcg/kg/min. If a general anesthetic is used for maintenance, the concentration of inhalation agents should be reduced by 30–50% for the first hour

Incremental injection to attenuate response to laryngoscopy and intubation (assisted or controlled ventilation).

Initial for induction: 20–50 mcg/kg; **maintenance:** 5–15 mcg/kg q 5–20 min, up to a total dose of 75 mcg/kg.

Anesthetic adjunct, incremental injection, spontaneously breathing or assisted ventilation.

Initial for induction: 8–20 mcg/kg; **maintenance:** 3–5 mcg/kg q 5–20 min (or 0.5–1 mcg/kg/min, up to a total dose of 8–40 mcg/kg).

Monitored anesthesia care, for sedated and responsive spontaneously breathing clients.

Initial for induction: 3–8 mcg/kg; **maintenance:** 3–5 mcg/kg every 5–20 min (or 0.25–1 mcg/kg/min, up to a total dose of 3–40 mcg/kg). Infusions may be continued until the end of the procedure.

NOTE: If there is a lightening of general anesthesia or the client manifests signs of surgical stress, the rate of administration of alfentanil may be increased to 4 mcg/kg/min or a bolus dose of 7 mcg/kg may be used. If the situation is not controlled following three bolus doses over 5 min, an inhalation anesthetic, a barbiturate, or a vasodilator should be used. If signs of lightening anesthesia are noted within the last 15 min of surgery, a bolus dose of 7 mcg/kg should be given rather than increasing the infusion rate. A potent inhalation anesthetic may be used as an alternative.

NURSING CONSIDERATIONS

© Do not confuse fentanyl with either Anafranil (an antidepressant) or sufentanil (opioid analgesic).

ADMINISTRATION/STORAGE

IV 1.   Individualize drug dosage for each client and for each use:
- Reduce dosage for elderly or debilitated clients.
- For those who are more than 20% above ideal body weight, base dosage on lean body weight.
- Individualize selection of preanesthetic medication.

2. Neuromuscular-blocking drugs should be compatible with client condition.

3. Use a tuberculin-type syringe to assure accuracy when giving small volumes of drug.

4. The injectable form may be reconstituted with either NSS, D5W/NSS, RL solution, or D5W. Direct IV administration over 1½–3 min. For continuous IV administration dilute 20 mL of alfentanil in 230 mL diluent to provide a solution of 40 mcg/mL.

5. Discontinue infusion 10–15 min prior to the end of surgery.

6. Protect from light. Store at room temperature from 15–25° C (59–77° F).

ASSESSMENT

1. Note any history of drug hypersensitivity reactions. Those with chronic opioid use may become tolerant to alfentanil.

2. Obtain baseline weight and VS.

3. Report any muscular rigidity before giving next dose.

4. Assess respiratory and CV status continuously during therapy; note oxygen saturations.

CLIENT/FAMILY TEACHING

1. May experience dizziness, drowsiness, and orthostatic hypotension.

2. Avoid alcohol or any CNS depressants for at least 24 hr following drug administration.

OUTCOMES/EVALUATE

- Induction/maintenance of anesthesia
- Facilitation of intubation and mechanical ventilation

Bold Italic = life threatening side effect   ■ = black box warning   ✦ = Available in Canada

Alfuzosin hydrochloride ©

(al-fue-**ZO**-sin)

CLASSIFICATION(S):
Treat benign prostatic hypertrophy (alpha-1 receptor antagonist)
PREGNANCY CATEGORY: B
Rx: Uroxatral.

USES
Signs and symptoms of benign prostatic hyperplasia.

ACTION/KINETICS

Action
Selective antagonist of postsynaptic alpha-1 adrenergic receptors located in various areas of the prostate. Blockade of these receptors causes relaxation of smooth muscle in the bladder neck and prostate, resulting in an improvement in urine flow and a reduction in symptoms of BPH.

Pharmacokinetics
About 49% is bioavailable after PO dosing. **Maximum levels:** 8 hr after multiple dosing. Absorption is 50% lower under fasting conditions; thus, take immediately following a meal. Extensively metabolized by the liver principally by CYP3A4, with only 11% excreted unchanged in the urine. Metabolites and unchanged drug are excreted in the feces (69%) and urine (24%). $t\frac{1}{2}$, **elimination:** 10 hr. **Plasma protein binding:** 82–90%.

CONTRAINDICATIONS
Hypersensitivity to alfuzosin or any component of the product. Use with moderate to severe hepatic impairment. Concomitant use with itraconazole, ketoconazole, ritonavir, other alpha-adrenergic blockers, or another potent inhibitor of CYP3A4. Treatment of hypertension. Use in children or in women.

SPECIAL CONCERNS
Postural hypotension, with or without symptoms, may develop within a few hours of taking alfuzosin. Thus, use with caution in clients with symptomatic hypotension or who have had a hypotensive response to other drugs. Use with caution in severe renal insufficiency.

SIDE EFFECTS

Most Common
Dizziness, headache, fatigue, URTI.
CV: Hypotension (with or without dizziness), syncope, tachycardia. **GI:** Abdominal pain, dyspepsia, constipation, nausea. **Respiratory:** URTI, bronchitis, sinusitis, pharyngitis. **Body as a whole:** Headache, fatigue, dizziness, pain. **Miscellaneous:** Impotence, rash, chest pain, priapism.

OD OVERDOSE MANAGEMENT
Symptoms: Hypotension. *Treatment:* Restoration of BP and normalization of HR by keeping client supine. If this is inadequate, consider IV fluids. If needed, vasopressors can be given. Monitor renal function; support as needed. Dialysis may not be effective.

DRUG INTERACTIONS
Atenolol / ↑ Risk of significant ↓ in mean BP and mean HR
Diltiazem / ↑ Risk of hypotension
Cimetidine / ↑ Alfuzosin C_{max} and AUC
Itraconazole / ↑ Alfuzosin plasma levels R/T inhibition of CYP3A4 metabolizing enzyme
Ketoconazole / ↑ Alfuzosin plasma levels R/T inhibition of CYP3A4 metabolizing enzyme
Ritonavir / ↑ Alfuzosin plasma levels R/T inhibition of CYP3A4 metabolizing enzyme

HOW SUPPLIED
Tablets, Extended-Release: 10 mg.

DOSAGE
• **TABLETS, EXTENDED-RELEASE**
Benign prostatic hyperplasia.
10 mg daily immediately after the same meal each day.

NURSING CONSIDERATIONS
© Do not confuse Uroxatral with either Oxytrol (an anticholinergic) or Roxanol (an opoid analgesic).

ADMINISTRATION/STORAGE
1. Do not chew/crush tablets.
2. Store between 15–30°C (59–86°F). Protect from light and moisture.

A

ASSESSMENT

1. Note reasons for therapy, characteristics of S&S. List other drugs used for BPH and outcome.
2. Note drugs currently prescribed to ensure none interact.
3. Monitor BP. Document DRE and PSA to R/O prostatic pathology.

CLIENT/FAMILY TEACHING

1. Take as directed after the same meal each day.
2. Do not chew, break, or crush extended release tablets.
3. Avoid tasks that require mental alertness until drug effects realized; may experience dizziness, drowsiness and headaches.
4. May experience drop in BP with sudden change in position; change positions slowly and use caution.
5. Report lack of response, chest pain, or adverse side effects. Keep all F/U visits to evaluate drug response.

OUTCOMES/EVALUATE

Improved stream; ↓ nocturia

Aliskiren   ■
(a-lis-**KYE**-ren)

CLASSIFICATION(S):

Direct renin inhibitorC (first trimester); D (second and third trimester),
Rx: Tekturna.

USES

Treatment of hypertension alone or with other antihypertensive drugs.

ACTION/KINETICS

Action

Renin cleaves angiotensinogen to form angiotensin I (inactive); angiotensin I is converted to the active angiotensin II by angiotensin converting enzyme (ACE) and non-ACE pathways. Angiotensin II is a powerful vasoconstrictor. It also promotes aldosterone secretion and sodium reabsorption. Together these effects increase BP. Aliskiren is a direct renin inhibitor, decreasing plasma renin activity and inhibiting the conversion of angiotensinogen to angiotensin I.

Pharmacokinetics

Poorly absorbed; bioavailability is about 2.5%. t ½, **accumulation:** 24 hr. **Peak plasma levels:** 1-3 hr. High fat meals significantly decrease absorption from the GI tract. Metabolized by CYP3A4. About 25% excreted in the urine unchanged.

CONTRAINDICATIONS

Lactation.

SPECIAL CONCERNS

■ Use in pregnancy. When used in pregnancy during the second and third trimester, drugs that act on the renin-angiotensin system can cause injury and even death to the developing fetus. When pregnancy is detected, discontinue aliskiren as soon as possible.■ Use with caution in impaired renal function. Safety and efficacy have not been determined in children.

SIDE EFFECTS

Most Common

Diarrhea, abdominal pain, dyspepsia, gastroesophageal reflux, rash.

GI: Diarrhea, abdominal pain, dyspepsia, gastroesophageal reflux. **CNS:** Dizziness, headache. **CV:** Hypotension. **Respiratory:** Increased cough, nasopharyngitis, URTI. **Musculoskeletal:** Back pain. **Body as whole:** *Angioedema* of the face, extremities, lips, tongue, glottis, and/or larynx; rash, gout, fatigue. **Miscellaneous:** Renal stones.

LABORATORY TEST CONSIDERATIONS

↑ Creatine kinase, serum K, BUN, creatinine, serum uric acid. Small ↓ H&H.

OD OVERDOSE MANAGEMENT
Symptoms: Hypotension (most likely). *Treatment:* Initiate supportive treatment.

DRUG INTERACTIONS

Atorvastatin / ↑ Aliskiren C_{max} and AUC about 50% after multiple dosing
Furosemide / ↓ Furosemide AUC and C_{max} 30% and 50% respectively
Irbesartan / ↓ Aliskiren C_{max} up to 50% after multiple dosing
Ketoconazole / Significant ↑ plasma aliskiren levels after 200 mg ketoconazole twice daily

---

Bold Italic = life threatening side effect   ■ = black box warning   ♣ = Available in Canada

HOW SUPPLIED
Tablets: 150 mg, 300 mg.

DOSAGE————————————
- **TABLETS**
  Hypertension.

Initial: 150 mg once daily. The daily dose may be increased to 300 mg in those whose BP is not adequately controlled. Doses above 300 mg are not more effective but do increase the incidence of diarrhea.

NURSING CONSIDERATIONS

ADMINISTRATION/STORAGE
1. May be given with other antihypertensives, most commonly diuretics and an angiotensin receptor blocker (e.g., valsartan).
2. The antihypertensive effect is usually reached within 2 weeks.
3. If angioedema occurs, promptly discontinue aliskiren and provide appropriate therapy and monitoring until complete and sustained resolution of the symptoms has occurred.
4. Store from 15-30°C (59-86°F). Protect from moisture.

ASSESSMENT
1. Note reasons for therapy, presenting symptoms, other agents trialed, outcome.
2. Record ECG, VS, and weight. Determine if pregnant.
3. Monitor CBC, electrolytes, renal and LFTs. Reduce dose or avoid use with impaired renal function.

CLIENT/FAMILY TEACHING
1. For BP lowering, take at the same time each day. Use caution, may cause low BP effects and dizziness.
2. Maintain healthy diet; limit intake of caffeine; avoid alcohol, salt substitutes, or high Na and high K foods.
3. Stop drug and report if pregnancy suspected; may cause fetal harm.
4. Immediately report/seek help if swelling of the eyes, face, extremities, lips, or tongue, difficulty in breathing/swallowing noted.
5. Any persistent dry cough, flu-like symptoms, rash, fatigue, SOB, diarrhea, or unusual side effects should be reported immediately. Keep record of home BP readings for provider review.

OUTCOMES/EVALUATE
↓ BP; hypertension control

Allopurinol   Ⓘⓥ Ⓒ
(al-oh-**PYOUR**-ih-nohl)

CLASSIFICATION(S):
Antigout drug
PREGNANCY CATEGORY: C
Rx: Aloprim for Injection, Zyloprim.
✿Rx: Apo-Allopurinol.

USES
IV: Management of clients with leukemia, lymphoma, and solid tumor malignancies in whom cancer chemotherapy causes elevations of serum and urinary uric acid levels and who cannot tolerate PO therapy.

PO: (1) Primary or secondary gout (acute attacks, tophi, joint destruction, nephropathy, uric acid lithiasis). (2) Clients with leukemia, lymphoma, or other malignancies in whom drug therapy causes elevations of serum and urinary uric acid. Recurrent calcium oxalate calculi where daily uric acid excretion exceeds 800 mg/day in males and 750 mg/day in females.

Investigational: Mixed with methylcellulose as a mouthwash to prevent stomatitis following fluorouracil administration. Reduce granulocyte suppressant effect of fluorouracil. Prevent ischemic reperfusion tissue damage. Reduce the incidence of perioperative mortality and postoperative arrhythmias in coronary artery bypass surgery. Reduce rates of *Helicobacter pylori*-induced duodenal ulcers and treatment of hematemesis from NSAID-induced erosive esophagitis. Alleviate pain due to acute pancreatitis. Treatment of American cutaneous leishmaniasis and against *Trypanosoma cruzi*. Treat Chagas' disease. As an alternative in epileptic seizures refractory to standard therapy.

ACTION/KINETICS

Action
Allopurinol and its major metabolite, oxipurinol, are potent inhibitors of xan-

A

thine oxidase, an enzyme involved in the synthesis of uric acid. Results in decreased uric acid levels. Also allopurinol increases reutilization of xanthine and hypoxanthine for synthesis of nucleotide and nucleic acid by acting on the enzyme hypoxanthine-guanine phosphoribosyltransferase. The resultant increases in nucleotides cause a negative feedback to inhibit synthesis of purines and a decrease in uric acid levels.

Pharmacokinetics
Peak plasma levels, after PO: 1.5 hr for allopurinol and 4.5 hr for oxipurinol. **Onset, after PO:** 2–3 days. **$t^{1/2}$, after PO** (allopurinol); 1–3 hr; **$t^{1/2}$** (oxipurinol): 12–30 hr. **Peak serum levels after PO, allopurinol:** 2–3 mcg/mL; **oxipurinol:** 5–6.5 mcg/mL (up to 50 mcg/mL in clients with impaired renal function). **Maximum therapeutic effect, after PO:** 1–3 weeks. Well absorbed from GI tract, metabolized in liver, excreted in urine and feces (20%).

CONTRAINDICATIONS
Hypersensitivity to drug. Clients with idiopathic hemochromatosis or relatives of clients suffering from this condition. Children except as an adjunct in treatment of neoplastic disease. Severe skin reactions on previous exposure. To treat asymptomatic hyperuricemia.

SPECIAL CONCERNS
Use with caution during lactation and in clients with liver or renal disease. In children use has been limited to rare inborn errors of purine metabolism or hyperuricemia as a result of malignancy or cancer therapy.

SIDE EFFECTS
Most Common
Rash, N&V, renal failure/insufficiency.
Dermatologic: Pruritic maculopapular skin rash (may be accompanied by fever and malaise). Vesicular bullous dermatitis, eczematoid dermatitis, pruritus, urticaria, onycholysis, purpura, lichen planus, **Stevens-Johnson syndrome, toxic epidermal necrolysis**. Skin rash has been accompanied by hypertension and cataract development. **Allergic:** Fever, chills, leukopenia, eosinophilia, arthralgia, skin rash, pruritus, N&V, nephritis. **GI:** N&V, diarrhea, GI bleed-

ing, splenomegaly, intestinal obstruction, flatulence, constipation, proctitis, gastritis, dyspepsia, abdominal pain (intermittent). **CNS:** Agitation, cerebral infarction, coma, dystonia, change in mental status, myoclonus, paralysis, seizures, **status epilepticus**, tremor, twitching. **Hematologic:** Leukopenia, eosinophilia, thrombocytopenia, anemia, bone marrow suppression, leukocytosis, **DIC**, marrow aplasia, neutropenia, pancytopenia. **Hepatic:** Hepatomegaly, cholestatic jaundice, **hepatic necrosis, liver failure**, hyperbilirubinemia, jaundice, granulomatous hepatitis. **Neurologic:** Headache, peripheral neuropathy, paresthesia, somnolence, neuritis. **CV:** Bradycardia, **cardiorespiratory arrest**, CV disorder, decreased venous pressure, abnormal ECG, flushing, **heart failure, hemorrhage, stroke,** hyper/hypotension, **septic shock, ventricular fibrillation**, thrombophlebitis, necrotizing angiitis, hypersensitivity vasculitis. **GU:** Renal failure/insufficiency, hematuria, abnormal kidney function, oliguria, UTI. **Respiratory:** Apnea, mucositis, pharyngitis, **ARDS, respiratory failure**, respiratory insufficiency, increased respiratory rate, **pulmonary embolus**. **Metabolic:** Abnormal electrolytes, glycosuria, hyper/hypocalcemia, hyperglycemia, hyper/hypokalemia, hyper/hyponatremia, hyperphosphatemia, hyperuricemia, hypomagnesemia, lactic/metabolic acidosis, water intoxication. **Miscellaneous:** Ecchymosis, headache, blast crisis, edema, cellulitis, chills, diaphoresis, enlarged abdomen, hypervolemia, hypotonia, infection, pain, tumor lysis syndrome, arthralgia, epistaxis, taste loss, acute attacks of gout, fever, myopathy, renal failure, uremia, alopecia.

LABORATORY TEST CONSIDERATIONS
↑ ALT, AST, alkaline phosphatase, serum cholesterol. ↓ Serum glucose.

DRUG INTERACTIONS
ACE inhibitors / ↑ Risk of hypersensitivity reactions
Al salts / ↓ Allopurinol effect
Ampicillin / ↑ Risk of drug-induced skin rashes
Anticoagulants, oral / ↑ Anticoagulant

Bold Italic = life threatening side effect   ■ = black box warning   ✦ = Available in Canada

effect R/T ↓ liver breakdown
Azathioprine / ↑ Azathioprine effect R/T ↓ liver breakdown
Chlorpropamide / ↑ t½ of chlorpropamide → hypoglycemia
Cyclophosphamide / ↑ Risk of bleeding or infection due to ↑ drug myelosuppressive effects
Cyclosporine / ↑ Cyclosporine levels
Iron preparations / Allopurinol ↑ hepatic iron concentrations
Mercaptopurine / ↑ Mercaptopurine effects and toxicity R/T ↓ liver breakdown
Theophylline / Allopurinol ↑ plasma drug levels → possible toxicity
Thiazide diuretics / ↑ Risk of hypersensitivity reactions to allopurinol
Uricosuric agents / ↓ Effect of oxipurinol R/T ↑ rate of excretion

HOW SUPPLIED

Injection: 500 mg/30 mL; *Tablets:* 100 mg, 300 mg.

DOSAGE

- **IV INFUSION**
  Lower serum uric acid in leukemia, lymphoma, or solid malignancies.
  Adults: 200–400 mg/m²/day, to a maximum of 600 mg/day. **Children, initial:** 200 mg/m²/day.

- **TABLETS**
  Gout/hyperuricemia.
  Adults: 200–300 mg/day for mild gout and 400–600 mg/day for moderately severe tophaceous gout, not to exceed 800 mg/day. Minimum effective dose: 100–200 mg/day.
  Prevention of uric acid nephropathy during vigorous treatment of neoplasms.
  Adults: 600–800 mg/day for 2–3 days (with high fluid intake).
  Prophylaxis of flare-up of acute gouty attacks.
  Initial: 100 mg/day; increase by 100 mg at weekly intervals to achieve serum uric acid level of 6 mg/100 mL or less.
  Hyperuricemia associated with malignancy.
  Pediatric, 6–10 years of age: 300 mg/day either as a single dose or 100 mg 3 times per day; **under 6 years of age:** 150 mg/day in three divided doses.

Recurrent calcium oxalate calculi.
200–300 mg/day in one or more doses (dose may be adjusted according to urinary levels of uric acid).
To ameliorate granulocyte suppressant effect of fluorouracil.
600 mg/day.
Reduce perioperative mortality and postoperative arrhythmias in coronary artery bypass surgery.
300 mg 12 hr and 1 hr before surgery.
Reduce relapse rates of H. pylori-induced duodenal ulcers; treat hematemesis from NSAID-induced erosive gastritis.
50 mg 4 times per day.
Alleviate pain due to acute pancreatitis.
50 mg 4 times per day.
Treat American cutaneous leishmaniasis and T. cruzi.
20 mg/kg for 15 days.
Treat Chagas' disease.
600–900 mg/day for 60 days.
Alternative to treat epileptic seizures refractory to standard therapy.
300 mg/day, except use 150 mg/day in those less than 20 kg.

- **MOUTHWASH**
  Prevent fluorouracil-induced stomatitis.
  20 mg in 3% methylcellulose (1 mg/mL compounded in the pharmacy).

NURSING CONSIDERATIONS

🕮 Do not confuse allopurinol with apresoline (an antihypertensive) or Zyloprim with ZORprin (aspirin).

ADMINISTRATION/STORAGE

1. Keep urine slightly alkaline to prevent uric acid stone formation.
2. Transfer from colchicine, uricosuric agents, and/or anti-inflammatory agents to allopurinol should be made gradually by decreasing the dosage of one and increasing the dosage of allopurinol until a normal serum uric acid level is achieved.
3. Reduce PO dose as follows in impaired renal function: creatinine clearance (C_{CR}) <10 mL/min: 100 mg 3 times per week; C_{CR} 10 mL/min: 100 mg every other day; C_{CR} 20 mL/min: 100 mg/day;

C_{CR} 40 mL/min: 150 mg/day; C_{CR} 60 mL/min: 200 mg/day.

4. Do not reuse in those who develop a severe reaction.

IV 5. For either adults or children, give daily dose as a single infusion or in equally divided infusions at 6-, 8-, or 12-hr intervals at concentration not to exceed 6 mg/mL.

6. Whenever possible, administer 24–48 hr before start of chemotherapy known to cause tumor cell lysis (including corticosteroids).

7. Do not mix allopurinol with or administer through the same IV port with agents which are incompatible (see package insert).

8. Dissolve contents of each 30 mL vial with 25 mL of sterile water for injection. Then, dilute to the desired concentration with 0.9% NaCl or D5W injection (do not use sodium bicarbonate-containing solutions); administer over 30–60 min.

9. Store reconstituted solution at 20–25°C (68–77°F); begin administration within 10 hr after reconstitution.

10. Do not refrigerate either the reconstituted and/or diluted product.

ASSESSMENT

1. Take complete drug history; identify any drugs that may interact unfavorably.

2. Note reasons for therapy, type, onset of S&S, any previous allopurinol use. List location, severity, and frequency of gout attacks; joint size, swelling, color, deformity, pain.

3. If female and of childbearing age, or if nursing, avoid allopurinol.

4. Assess for idiopathic hemochromatosis; precludes therapy.

5. Take colchicine with allopurinol for acute flare, especially during first 6 weeks of therapy.

6. Monitor CBC, uric acid, liver and renal function studies. Reduce dose with renal dysfunction; x-ray joint.

CLIENT/FAMILY TEACHING

1. Take with food or immediately after meals to lessen gastric irritation. Consume at least 10–12 8-oz glasses of fluid/day to prevent stone formation.

2. When used IV, ensure sufficient fluid intake to yield a daily urinary output of at least 2 L in adults; maintain neutral, or preferably, a slightly alkaline urine (pH >7)

3. Monitor weight with N&V or other signs of gastric irritation; report persistent weight loss.

4. Skin rashes may start after months of therapy; stop therapy if drug-related.

5. Do not take iron salts; high iron concentrations may occur in liver.

6. Avoid excessive intake of vitamin C; may cause kidney stones.

7. Avoid caffeine and alcoholic beverages; decreases allopurinol effect.

8. Keep food diary to identify any triggers; may avoid foods high in purine which include sardines, roe, salmon, scallops, anchovies, organ meats.

9. Minimize exposure to UV light due to increased risk of cataracts; report vision changes. May experience drowsiness.

10. Keep F/U visits to evaluate serum and urinary uric acid levels.

OUTCOMES/EVALUATE

- ↓ Uric acid levels (6 mg/dL)
- ↓ Joint pain and inflammation
- ↓ Frequency of gout attacks
- Inhibition of stomatitis following fluorouracil therapy

Almotriptan maleate©
(**AL**-moh-**trip**-tin)

CLASSIFICATION(S):
Antimigraine drug (serotonin 5-HT$_1$ receptor agonist)
PREGNANCY CATEGORY: C
Rx: Axert.

USES
Acute treatment of migraine, with and without aura, in adults. Use only where there is a clear diagnosis of migraine.

ACTION/KINETICS
Action
As an agonist, binds to 5-HT$_{1D}$, 5-HT$_{1B}$, and 5-HT$_{1F}$ receptors on the extracerebral, intracranial blood vessels that become dilated during a migraine head-

ache, as well as on nerve terminals in the trigeminal system. Activation of these receptors causes cranial vessel vasoconstriction, inhibition of neuropeptide release, and reduced transmission in trigeminal nerve pathways.

Pharmacokinetics

Well absorbed after PO use; **onset:** 30 min; **peak plasma levels:** 1–3 hr. **t½, mean:** 3–4 hr. Metabolized in the liver; metabolites and unchanged drug (40%) are excreted mainly in the urine. **Plasma protein binding:** Approximately 35%.

CONTRAINDICATIONS

Use to prevent migraine or in management of hemiplegic or basilar migraine. Use in those with ischemic heart disease (angina pectoris, history of MI, documented silent ischemia) or who have symptoms or findings consistent with ischemic heart disease, coronary artery vasospasm (including Prinzmetal's variant angina), or other significant underlying CV disease. Use when unrecognized coronary artery disease is predicted by presence of risk factors such as hypertension, hypercholesterolemia, smoking, diabetes, strong family history of CAD, females with surgical or physiologic menopause, or males over 40 years of age unless a CV evaluation shows individual is reasonably free of CAD or ischemic myocardial disease. Use in uncontrolled hypertension, within 24 hr of treatment with another 5-HT₁ agonist or an ergotamine-containing or ergot-type medication (e.g., dihydroergotamine, methysergide). Use in children less than 18 years of age.

SPECIAL CONCERNS

Use with caution during lactation and in diseases that may alter the absorption, metabolism, or excretion of the drug, such as impaired hepatic or renal function. Safety and efficacy have not been determined in children less than 18 years of age or for cluster headaches (present in an older, predominantly male population). Safety has not been established for treating more than 4 headaches in a 30-day period.

SIDE EFFECTS

Most Common

Drowsiness, dry mouth, headache, nausea, paresthesia, dizziness.

CV: *Acute MI, disturbances of cardiac rhythm, death, cerebral hemorrhage, subarachnoid hemorrhage, stroke, hypertensive crisis, ventricular fibrillation,* peripheral vascular ischemia, transient myocardial ischemia, ventricular tachycardia, coronary artery vasospasm, vasodilation, palpitations, colonic ischemia (with abdominal pain and bloody diarrhea). **CNS:** Somnolence, drowsiness, dizziness, headache, tremor, vertigo, anxiety, hypesthesia, restlessness, CNS stimulation, insomnia, shakiness. **GI:** N&V, dry mouth, abdominal cramps or pain, diarrhea, dyspepsia. **Body as a whole:** Paresthesia, asthenia, chills, back pain, chest pain, neck pain, fatigue, rigid neck. **Musculoskeletal:** Myalgia, muscular weakness. **Respiratory:** Pharyngitis, rhinitis, dyspnea, laryngismus, sinusitis, bronchitis, epistaxis. **Dermatologic:** Diaphoresis, dermatitis, erythema, pruritus, rash. **Ophthalmic:** Conjunctivitis, eye irritation. **Miscellaneous:** Ear pain, hyperacusis, taste alteration, dysmenorrhea. Sensations of tightness, pain, and heaviness in the precordium, throat, neck, and jaw.

LABORATORY TEST CONSIDERATIONS

↑ Serum creatine phosphokinase. Hyperglycemia.

DRUG INTERACTIONS

Clarithromycin / Possible ↑ almotriptan levels R/T inhibition of CYP3A4

Dihydroergotamine / Possible additive vasospastic effects; do not use within 24 hr of each other

Erythromycin / Possible ↑ almotriptan levels

Itraconazole / Possible ↑ almotriptan AUC and plasma levels R/T inhibition of CYP3A4

Ketoconazole / Possible ↑ almotriptan levels R/T inhibition of CYP3A4

MAO inhibitors / ↓ Almotriptan clearance

Methysergide / Possible additive vasospastic effects; do not use within 24 hr of each other

Nefazodone / Possible ↑ almotriptan

A

levels R/T inhibition of CYP3A4
Nelfinavir / Possible ↑ almotriptan levels R/T inhibition of CYP3A4
Ritonavir / Possible ↑ almotriptan levels R/T inhibition of CYP3A4
Selective serotonin reuptake inhibitors / Rarely, weakness, hyperreflexia, and incoordination
Troleandomycin / Possible ↑ almotriptan levels R/T inhibition of CYP3A4
Verapamil / ↑ plasma levels of almotriptan

HOW SUPPLIED
Tablets: 6.25 mg, 12.5 mg.

DOSAGE

• **TABLETS**

Migraine headache.
Adults: Single dose of either 6.25 or 12.5 mg (more effective). Choice of dose is on an individual basis. If the headache returns, dose may be repeated after 2 hr, but give no more than 2 doses in a 24-hr period. In either hepatic or renal impairment, do not exceed a daily dose of 12.5 mg over a 24-hr period; use an initial dose of 6.25 mg.

NURSING CONSIDERATIONS

Ⓒ Do not confuse Axert with Antivert (antiemetic/antimotion sickness).

ADMINISTRATION/STORAGE
1. If first dose does not produce response, reconsider diagnosis of migraine before giving a second dose.
2. Safety of treating an average of more than 4 headaches in a 30-day period has not been studied.
3. For those with hepatic or renal impairment, do not exceed a maximum daily dose of 12.5 mg and a starting dose of 6.25 mg.

ASSESSMENT
1. Review symptom characteristics; ensure not hemiplegic or basilar migraine type of headaches. Have neurologist evaluate if unclear.
2. Note drugs currently prescribed to ensure none interact. List those taken within the past 24 h and ensure no other serotonin agonist or ergotamine derivatives prescribed
3. Assess for CAD, uncontrolled HTN, and cardiac risk factors. Obtain EKG, re-

nal and LFTs; check for renal dysfunction.

CLIENT/FAMILY TEACHING
1. Take only as directed for migraine headaches; do not share medications with another person regardless of symptoms; do not use for other types of headaches.
2. Drug acts to shrink swollen blood vessels surrounding the brain that cause migraine headaches. Keep a headache diary and identify factors/foods/events that surround migraine headaches.
3. If headache returns, may repeat dose in 2 hr unless otherwise instructed due to renal dysfunction. Do not exceed 2 tablets in 24 hr.
4. Use caution if driving or performing activities that require mental alertness; may cause dizziness or drowsiness.
5. Store away from heat, light, and moisture; store in a safe place.
6. Avoid known triggers, i.e., chocolate, cheese, citrus fruit, caffeine, alcohol, missing sleep or meals, etc.
7. Report unusual side effects, chest pain/heaviness, new onset jaw, throat or neck pain, intolerance, or lack of response.
8. Keep all F/U appointments to evaluate response to therapy.

OUTCOMES/EVALUATE
Resolution of migraine headaches

Alprazolam   Ⓒ
(al-**PRAYZ**-oh-lam)

CLASSIFICATION(S):
Antianxiety drug, benzodiazepine
PREGNANCY CATEGORY: D
Rx: Alprazolam Extended-Release, Alprazolam Intensol, Niravam, Xanax, Xanax XR, **C-IV**
✤Rx: Apo-Alpraz, Apo-Alpraz TS, Gen-Alprazolam, Novo-Alprazolam, Nu-Alpraz, Xanax TS, ratio-Alprazolam.

SEE ALSO *TRANQUILIZERS/ ANTIMANIC DRUGS/HYPNOTICS.*

USES
Immediate-Release Tablets, Orally Disintegrating Tablets and Intensol:

(1) Anxiety. (2) Anxiety associated with depression with or without agoraphobia. **Immediate- and Extended-Release Tablets, Orally Disintegrating Tablets:** Panic disorder with or without agoraphobia. *Investigational:* Agoraphobia with social phobia, depression, PMS.

ACTION/KINETICS
Action
Reduces anxiety by increasing or facilitating the inhibitory neurotransmitter activity of GABA. The skeletal muscle relaxant effect may be due to enhancement of GABA-mediated presynaptic inhibition at the spinal level as well as in the brain stem reticular formation.

Pharmacokinetics
Onset: Intermediate. **Peak plasma levels:** PO, 8–37 ng/mL after 1–2 hr. **t½:** 12–15 hr. Sublingual absorption is as rapid as PO use; completeness of absorption is comparable. Metabolized to alpha-hydroxyalprazolam, an active metabolite. **t½:** 12–15 hr. Excreted in urine. **Plasma protein binding:** 80%.

CONTRAINDICATIONS
Use with itraconazole or ketoconazole. Acute narrow-angle glaucoma.

SIDE EFFECTS
Most Common
Drowsiness, ataxia, confusion.
See *Tranquilizers, Antimanic Drugs,* and *Hypnotics* for a complete list of possible side effects.

ADDITIONAL DRUG INTERACTIONS
Azole antifungal drugs, clarithromycin, erythromycin, protease inhibitors, or SSRIs decrease the metabolism of alprazolam. Decrease the dose of alprazolam by 50 to 75%.

H Possible lethargy and disorientation when combined with kava kava.

HOW SUPPLIED
Oral Solution (Intensol): 1 mg/mL; *Tablets, Extended-Release:* 0.5 mg, 1 mg, 2 mg, 3 mg; *Tablets, Immediate-Release:* 0.25 mg, 0.5 mg, 1 mg, 2 mg; *Tablets, Oral Disintegrating:* 0.25 mg, 0.5 mg, 1 mg, 2 mg.

DOSAGE
• **ORAL SOLUTION; TABLETS, IMMEDIATE-RELEASE; TABLETS, ORAL DISINTEGRATING**
  Anxiety disorders.

Adults, initial: 0.25–0.5 mg 3 times per day; **then,** titrate to needs of client at intervals of 3–4 days in increments of no more than 1 mg/day, with total daily dosage not to exceed 4 mg. **In elderly or debilitated, initial:** 0.25 mg 2–3 times per day; **then,** adjust dosage to needs of client.

• **TABLETS, EXTENDED-RELEASE; TABLETS, IMMEDIATE-RELEASE; TABLETS, ORAL DISINTEGRATING**
  Panic disorders (use Niravam, Xanax, Xanax XR).

Immediate-Release Tablets, Oral Disintegrating Tablets: Adults, initial: 0.5 mg 3 times per day; increase dose as needed, every 3–4 days in increments of no more than 1 mg/day up to a maximum of 10 mg/day (mean dose: 5–6 mg/day). **Extended-Release Tablets: Adults, initial:** 0.5 mg–1 mg once daily. **Total daily dose:** 3–6 mg/day.
  Agoraphobia with social phobia.
Adults: 2–8 mg/day.
  PMS.
0.25 mg 3 times per day.

NURSING CONSIDERATIONS
@ Do not confuse alprazolam with lorazepam (anti-anxiety drug) or Xanax with Zantac (H-2 receptor blocker).

ADMINISTRATION/STORAGE
1. Do not decrease daily dose more than 0.5 mg over 3 days if therapy terminated or dose decreased.
2. Reduce dosage in elderly and debilitated clients. Starting dose of immediate-release and intensol is 0.25 mg given 2 or 3 times per day. Increase dose gradually if needed. For extended-release tablets, begin with 0.5 mg once a day; gradually increase if needed and tolerated.
3. To switch therapy from immediate-release to extended-release tablets, start with a once-daily dose of the extended-release product equal to the total daily dose of the immediate-release tablets.
4. Avoid abrupt discontinuation due to the possibility of withdrawal. When discontinuing therapy or decreasing the daily dose, reduce dosage gradually. It is recommended the daily dose be de-

A

creased by no more than 0.5 mg q 3 days; some clients may require an even slower dosage reduction. If significant withdrawal symptoms develop, reinstitute the previous dosing schedule and try a less rapid discontinuation schedule.

5. Store from 15–30°C (59–86°F) protected from moisture.

ASSESSMENT

1. Note reasons for therapy, other agents trialed and outcome.

2. With anxiety, evaluate/compare before and after therapy initiated.

3. Monitor CBC, liver and renal function during prolonged therapy.

CLIENT/FAMILY TEACHING

1. Do not chew, crush, or break the extended-release tablet.

2. Mix Intensol oral solution with liquids or semi-solid foods such as water, juices, soda, or soda-like beverages, applesauce, and puddings. Use the calibrated dropper provided. Draw up the required amount, squeeze the dropper contents into the liquid or semi-solid food, and stir gently for a few seconds.

3. Just before giving orally-disintegrating tablets, remove the tablet from the bottle with dry hands. Immediately place the tablet on top of the tongue where it will disintegrate and be swallowed with saliva. Giving with a liquid is not necessary. If only one-half of a scored tablet is used, discard the unused portion of the tablet immediately as it may not remain stable. Discard any cotton included in the bottle and reseal the bottle tightly to prevent introduction of moisture that may cause tablet disintegration.

4. May take tablets with milk or food to decrease GI upset.

5. Include extra fluids and bulk in the diet to minimize constipation.

6. Avoid activities that require mental alertness; may cause drowsiness.

7. Rise slowly to prevent lightheadedness or fainting.

8. Seek appropriate psychological therapy as prolonged use may cause dependence. Taper dose with prolonged use.

9. Use support devices as needed, especially at night; elderly tend to become confused. Store drug away from bedside to prevent overdose.

10. Avoid smoking, alcohol consumption, or any other CNS depressants without provider approval.

OUTCOMES/EVALUATE

• Positive behaviors with phobias
• ↓ Anxiety/restlessness; control of panic disorder
• Improvement in PMS symptoms

Alteplase, recombinant   **IV**

(**AL**-teh-playz)

CLASSIFICATION(S):
Thrombolytic, tissue plasminogen activator
PREGNANCY CATEGORY: C
Rx: Activase, Cathflo Activase.
✤Rx: Activase rt-PA.

USES

Activase. (1) Improvement of ventricular function following AMI, including reducing the incidence of CHF and decreasing mortality. (2) Acute ischemic stroke, after intracranial hemorrhage has been excluded by CT scan or other diagnostic imaging. (3) Acute pulmonary embolism (confirm diagnosis by pulmonary angiography or noninvasive procedures as lung scanning).

Cathflo Activase. Restoration of function to central venous access devices that have become occluded by a blood clot or thrombus.

Investigational: Unstable angina pectoris.

ACTION/KINETICS

Action

Alteplase, a tissue plasminogen activator, binds to fibrin in a thrombus, causing a conversion of plasminogen to plasmin. This conversion results in local fibrinolysis and a decrease in circulating fibrinogen.

Pharmacokinetics

Within 10 min following termination of an infusion, 80% of the alteplase has been cleared from the plasma by the liver. The enzyme activity of alteplase is 580,000 international units/mg. **t½, initial:** 4 min; **final:** 35 min (elimination phase).

CONTRAINDICATIONS

When used for AMI or pulmonary embolism: Active internal bleeding, history of CVA, within 2 months of intracranial or intraspinal surgery or trauma, intracranial neoplasm, AV malformation or aneurysm, bleeding diathesis, severe uncontrolled hypertension.

When used for acute ischemic stroke: Symptoms of intracranial hemorrhage on pretreatment evaluation, suspected subarachnoid hemorrhage, recent intracranial surgery or serious head trauma, recent previous stroke, history of intracranial hemorrhage, uncontrolled hypertension (above 185 mm Hg systolic or above 110 Hg diastolic) at time of treatment, active internal bleeding, seizure at onset of stroke, intracranial neoplasm, AV malformation or aneurysm, bleeding diathesis.

SPECIAL CONCERNS

Use with caution in the presence of recent GI or GU bleeding (within 10 days), subacute bacterial endocarditis, acute pericarditis, significant liver dysfunction, concomitant use of oral anticoagulants, diabetic hemorrhagic retinopathy, septic thrombophlebitis or occluded arteriovenous cannula (at infected site), lactation, mitral stenosis with atrial fibrillation. Since fibrin will be lysed during therapy, careful attention should be given to potential bleeding sites such as sites of catheter insertion and needle puncture sites. Use with caution within 10 days of major surgery (e.g., obstetrics, coronary artery bypass) and in clients over 75 years of age. Safety and efficacy have not been established in children. *NOTE:* Doses greater than 150 mg have been associated with an increase in intracranial bleeding.

Use Cathflo Activase with caution in presence of suspected infection in a catheter.

SIDE EFFECTS

Most Common

GU bleeding, ecchymosis, strokes, N&V, fever, hypotension.

Bleeding tendencies: *Internal bleeding* (including the GI and GU tracts and intracranial or retroperitoneal site). Superficial bleeding (e.g., gums, sites of recent surgery, venous cutdowns, arterial punctures). Ecchymosis, epistaxis. **CV:** Bradycardia, hypotension, cardiogenic shock, arrhythmias, *heart failure, cardiac arrest/tamponade, myocardial rupture*, recurrent ischemia, reinfarction, mitral regurgitation, pericardial effusion, pericarditis, venous thrombosis and embolism, electromechanical dissociation, cholesterol embolism. **Allergic:** Rash, *laryngeal edema, orolingual angioedema, anaphylaxis*. **GI:** N&V. **Miscellaneous:** Fever, urticaria, pulmonary edema, cerebral edema. **Due to accelerated infusion:** *Strokes, hemorrhagic stroke*, nonfatal stroke. Incidence increases with age.

OD OVERDOSE MANAGEMENT

Symptoms: Bleeding disorders. *Treatment:* Discontinue therapy immediately as well as any concomitant heparin therapy.

DRUG INTERACTIONS

Abciximab / ↑ Risk of bleeding
Aspirin / ↑ Risk of bleeding
Dipyridamole / ↑ Risk of bleeding
Heparin / ↑ Risk of bleeding, especially at arterial puncture sites
Nitroglycerin / ↓ Alteplase concentrations → ↓ thrombolytic effect
Vitamin K antagonists / ↑ Risk of bleeding

HOW SUPPLIED

Powder for Injection: 50 mg, 100 mg; *Single-patient vial (Cathflo Activase):* 2 mg.

DOSAGE

- **IV INFUSION ONLY**

  AMI, accelerated infusion.

Weight >67 kg: 100 mg as a 15-mg IV bolus, followed by 50 mg infused over the next 30 min and then 35 mg infused over the next 60 min. **Weight <67 kg:** 15 mg IV bolus, followed by 0.75 mg/kg infused over the next 30 min (not to exceed 50 mg) and then

0.50 mg/kg infused over the next 60 min (not to exceed 35 mg). The safety and efficacy of this regimen have only been evaluated using heparin and aspirin concomitantly.

AMI, 3-hr infusion.
100 mg total dose subdivided as follows: 60 mg (34.8 million international units) the first hour with 6–10 mg given in a bolus over the first 1–2 min and the remaining 50–54 mg given over the first hour; 20 mg (11.6 million international units) over the second hour and 20 mg (11.6 million international units) given over the third hour. **Clients less than 65 kg:** 1.25 mg/kg given over 3 hr, with 60% given the first hour with 6–10% given by direct IV injection within the first 1–2 min; 20% is given the second hour and 20% during the third hour. Doses of 150 mg have caused an increase in intracranial bleeding.

Pulmonary embolism.
100 mg over 2 hr; heparin therapy should be instituted near the end of or right after the alteplase infusion when the partial thromboplastin or thrombin time returns to twice that of normal or less.

Acute ischemic stroke.
0.9 mg/kg (maximum of 90 mg) infused over 60 min with 10% of the total dose given as an initial IV bolus over 1 min. Doses greater than 0.9 mg/kg may cause an increased incidence of intracranial hemorrhage. Use with aspirin and heparin during the first 24 hr after onset of symptoms has not been investigated.

Restoration of function to central venous access device.
2 mg in 2 mL of solution for clients weighing 30 kg or more; for those weighing between 10 and 30 kg, use a dose of 1 mg/mL solution equivalent to 110% of the volume of the catheter's internal lumen but not more than 2 mg. A second dose may be instilled if the catheter is not functioning 120 min after the first dose.

NURSING CONSIDERATIONS
ADMINISTRATION/STORAGE
IV 1. Initiate alteplase therapy as soon as possible after onset of symptoms of acute MI and within 3 hr after the onset of stroke symptoms.

2. For acute MI, nearly 90% of clients also receive heparin concomitantly with alteplase and either aspirin or dipyridamole during or after heparin therapy.

3. Reconstitute with only sterile water for injection without preservatives immediately prior to use. The reconstituted preparation contains 1 mg/mL and is a colorless to pale yellow transparent solution.

4. Using an 18-gauge needle, direct the stream of sterile water into the lyophilized cake. Leave product undisturbed for several minutes to allow dissipation of any large bubbles.

5. If necessary, the reconstituted solution may be further diluted immediately prior to use in an equal volume of 0.9% NaCl injection or D5W injection to yield a concentration of 0.5 mg/mL. Dilute by gentle swirling or slow inversion.

6. Either glass bottles or PVC bags may be used for administration.

7. Stable for up to 8 hr following reconstitution or dilution; stability will not be affected by light.

8. Do not use 50-mg vials if vacuum is not present (100-mg vials do not contain a vacuum). Reconstitute 50-mg vials with a large-bore needle (e.g., 18 gauge) directing stream of sterile water into lyophilized cake. For the 100-mg vial, use provided transfer device for reconstitution.

9. Use infusion device for administration. Do not add any other medications to the line. Anticipate 3 lines for access (1–alteplase; 1–heparin and other drugs such as lidocaine; 1–blood drawing and transfusions).

10. Store lyophilized alteplase at room temperatures not to exceed 30°C (86°F) or under refrigeration between 2–8°C (36–46°F).

11. Have emergency drugs (especially aminocaproic acid) and resuscitative equipment available.

ASSESSMENT
1. Note any history of hypertension, internal bleeding, PUD, or recent surgery.

---

2. Document onset/characteristics of chest pain and/or stroke symptoms; note deficits and monitor.

3. Assess/document overall physical condition; note CV and neurologic findings, weight, and ECG.

4. Obtain drug history. List those currently taking; note any anticoagulants/antiplatelets.

5. Obtain baseline hematologic parameters, type and cross, coagulation times, cardiac marker panel, renal, and LFTs.

INTERVENTIONS

1. Carefully review/follow instructions for drug reconstitution. Review contraindications before initiating therapy and document if accelerated or 3 hr infusion is prescribed.

2. Observe in a closely monitored environment; obtain VS, review and document monitor strips.

3. Anticipate and assess for reperfusion reactions such as:

- Reperfusion arrhythmias usually of short duration; may include accelerated idioventricular rhythm and sinus bradycardia.
- Reduction of chest pain
- Return of the elevated ST segment to near baseline levels
- Smaller Q waves

4. Check all access sites for any evidence of bleeding. During IV therapy, arterial sticks require 30 min of manual pressure followed by application of a pressure dressing. In event of any uncontrolled bleeding, terminate alteplase and heparin infusions and report.

5. Monitor neuro status; document status every 15–30 min during infusion.

6. During treatment of stroke, note CT or MRI results.

7. During treatment for pulmonary embolism, ensure that the PTT or PT is no more than twice that of normal before heparin therapy is added.

8. Keep on bed rest; observe for S&S of abnormal bleeding (hematuria, hematemesis, melena, CVA, cardiac tamponade, ↑ HR, ↓ BP).

9. Obtain appropriate postinfusion labs (cardiac marker, platelets, H&H, PTT, ECG) as directed.

CLIENT/FAMILY TEACHING

1. Review goals of therapy and inherent risks during acute coronary artery occlusion and/or stroke.

2. To be effective, therapy should be instituted within 3 hr of stroke and 4–6 hr of MI S&S.

3. Report any chest pain, SOB, N&V, heart palpitations or other adverse effects.

4. Encourage family members to learn CPR.

OUTCOMES/EVALUATE

- Lysis of thrombi with reperfusion of ischemic cardiac and/or cerebral tissue
- ↓ Infarct size with restoration of coronary perfusion and improved ventricular function (↑ CO, ↓ incidence of CHF, ↓ mortality)

Altretamine (Hexylmethyl-melamine)

(all-**TRET**-ah-meen)

CLASSIFICATION(S):
Antineoplastic, miscellaneous
PREGNANCY CATEGORY: D
Rx: Hexalen.

SEE ALSO *ANTINEOPLASTIC AGENTS.*

USES
Alone in the palliative treatment of persistent or recurrent ovarian cancer after first-line cisplatin- or alkylating agent-based combination therapy.

ACTION/KINETICS

Action
The mechanism of action is unknown, although metabolism of the drug is required for cytotoxicity.

Pharmacokinetics
Well absorbed following PO ingestion; undergoes rapid demethylation in the liver, yielding the principal metabolites–pentamethylmelamine and tetramethylmelamine. **Peak plasma levels:** 0.5–3 hr. **t½:** 4.7–10.2 hr. Metabolites are excreted mainly through the kidneys.

CONTRAINDICATIONS

Preexisting bone marrow depression or severe neurologic toxicity, although the drug has been used safely in clients with preexisting cisplatin neuropathies. Lactation.

SPECIAL CONCERNS

■ (1) Give only under the supervision of a physician experienced in the use of antineoplastic drugs. (2) Monitor peripheral blood counts at least monthly before beginning each course of therapy and as clinically indicated. (3) Due to the possibility of altretamine-induced neurotoxicity, perform neurologic exams regularly during use.■ Safety and effectiveness have not been determined in children. High daily doses may result in gradual onset of N&V.

SIDE EFFECTS

Most Common

N&V, peripheral sensory neuropathy, anemia.

GI: N&V. **Neurologic:** Peripheral sensory neuropathy, fatigue, anorexia, seizures. **CNS:** Mood disorders, disorders of consciousness, ataxia, dizziness, vertigo. **Hematologic:** Leukopenia, thrombocytopenia, anemia. **Miscellaneous:** *Hepatic toxicity*, skin rash, pruritus, alopecia.

LABORATORY TEST CONSIDERATIONS

↑ Serum creatinine, BUN, alkaline phosphatase.

DRUG INTERACTIONS

Cimetidine / ↑ Altretamine t½ and toxicity R/T inhibition of drug metabolism
MAO inhibitors / Severe orthostatic hypotension, especially in clients over the age of 60 years.

HOW SUPPLIED

Capsules: 50 mg.

DOSAGE

- **CAPSULES**
  Ovarian cancer.
  260 mg/m^2/day given either for 14 or 21 consecutive days in a 28-day cycle. The total daily dose is given as four divided doses PO after meals and at bedtime.

NURSING CONSIDERATIONS

ADMINISTRATION/STORAGE

Discontinue temporarily (for 14 or more days) and restart at 200 mg/m^2/day if any of the following occur:

- GI intolerance unresponsive to symptomatic treatment.
- WBCs <200/mm^3 or granulocyte count <1,000/mm^3.
- Platelet count <75,000/mm^3.
- Progressive neurotoxicity. Discontinue if neurologic symptoms fail to stabilize on a reduced dosage schedule.

ASSESSMENT

1. Identify disease onset, S&S; note all previous therapies.
2. Note neurologic findings; monitor regularly.
3. Assess CBC and LFTs.

INTERVENTIONS

1. Anticipate neurotoxicity as a side effect of drug therapy; assess neurologic status prior to starting therapy and before each subsequent course.
2. Give pyridoxine to reduce severity of neurotoxic effects.
3. Monitor peripheral blood counts monthly, prior to the initiation of each course of therapy and as clinically indicated.

CLIENT/FAMILY TEACHING

1. Take with food or milk or after meals to decrease nausea.
2. Report any adverse S&S, such as tingling, decreased sensation, dizziness, and N&V; may need to decrease or discontinue therapy.
3. Practice barrier contraception; may cause fetal damage.
4. Report unusual side effects and for monthly hematologic studies.

OUTCOMES/EVALUATE

Control of tumor growth and spread

Amantadine hydrochloride
(ah-**MAN**-tah-deen)

CLASSIFICATION(S):
Antiviral, antiparkinson drug
PREGNANCY CATEGORY: C
Rx: Symmetrel.

Bold Italic = life threatening side effect   ■ = black box warning   ✤ = Available in Canada

✣Rx: Endantadine, Gen-Amanta-dine.

SEE ALSO *ANTIVIRAL DRUGS.*

USES

(1) Prophylaxis of influenza A viral infections when early vaccination is not feasible or if vaccine is contraindicated or not available. (2) Treatment of uncomplicated respiratory tract infection caused by influenza A virus strains, especially if given early in the illness. (3) Symptomatic treatment of idiopathic parkinsonism and parkinsonism syndrome resulting from encephalitis, carbon monoxide intoxication, or cerebral arteriosclerosis. For parkinsonism, is usually used concomitantly with other agents, such as levodopa and anticholinergic agents. (4) Drug-induced extrapyramidal reactions.Amantadine is recommended for prophylaxis in the following situations:

- High risk clients vaccinated after flu outbreak has begun; may take up to 2 weeks for immunity.
- Unvaccinated caretakers of high-risk clients during peak flu activity.
- High-risk clients who are expected to have inadequate antibody response to flu vaccine (e.g., HIV).
- High-risk clients who should not be vaccinated or those who wish to avoid the flu.

ACTION/KINETICS

Action

As an antiviral, amantadine may prevent the release of infectious viral nucleic acid into the host cell by interfering with the function of the transmembrane domain of the viral M2 protein. It may also prevent virus assembly during virus replication. The drug reduces symptoms (70–90% effective) of viral infections if given within 24–48 hr after onset of illness. For parkinsonism, the mechanism is unknown but amantadine may (1) enhance cellular concentrations of dopamine by increasing the release or decreasing reuptake of dopamine into presynaptic neurons, (2) stimulate the dopamine receptor itself, or (3) drive the postsynaptic dopaminergic system to a more dopamine sensi-tive state. The drug decreases extrapyramidal symptoms, including akinesia, rigidity, tremors, excessive salivation, gait disturbances, and total functional disability.

Pharmacokinetics

Well absorbed from GI tract. **Peak blood levels:** 4 hr. **Onset:** 48 hr. **Peak serum concentration:** 0.2 mcg/mL after 1–4 hr. **t½:** Approximately 15 hr; elimination half-life increases two- to threefold when C_{CR} <40 mL/min/1.73 m^2. Renal clearance is reduced and plasma levels increased in otherwise healthy clients, aged 65 years and older. Ninety percent excreted unchanged in urine.

CONTRAINDICATIONS

Hypersensitivity to drug. Use in those with untreated angle closure glaucoma. Lactation.

SPECIAL CONCERNS

Use with caution in clients with liver and renal disease, history of epilepsy (possible increased seizure activity), CHF (possible worsening of CHF), peripheral edema, orthostatic hypotension, recurrent eczematoid dermatitis, psychosis or severe psychoneurosis, in clients taking CNS stimulant drugs, and in those exposed to rubella. Safe use in children less than 1 year has not been established. Abrupt withdrawal in Parkinson's clients may cause a parkinsonian crisis.

SIDE EFFECTS

Most Common

Nausea, dizziness, lightheadedness, insomnia.

GI: N&V, dry mouth, constipation, diarrhea, dysphagia. **CNS:** Dizziness, lightheadedness, insomnia, depression, anxiety, irritability, hallucinations, confusion, ataxia, headache, somnolence (may be sudden and uncontrolled), nervousness, dream abnormality, agitation, psychosis, euphoria, slurred speech, abnormal thinking, amnesia, suicidal attempt, *suicide,* suicidal ideation, **coma, convulsion**, stupor, delirium, hypo-/hyperkinesia, hypertension, delusions, aggressive behavior, paranoid reaction, manic reaction, gait abnormalities, paresthesia, EEG changes, tremor. **CV:** Or-

---

thostatic hypotension, CHF, hypertension, **cardiac arrest**, arrhythmias (including **malignant arrhythmias**), hypotension, tachycardia. **Dermatologic:** Pruritus, skin rash, diaphoresis, livedo reticularis, eczematoid dermatitis. **Hematologic:** Leukocytosis, leukopenia, neutropenia. **Respiratory:** *Acute respiratory failure*, pulmonary edema, tachypnea, dyspnea, dry nose. **Ophthalmic:** Mydriasis, punctuate subepithelial or other corneal opacity, corneal edema, decreased visual acuity, sensitivity to light, optic nerve palsy, oculogyric episodes. **Body as a whole:** Fatigue, weakness. **Miscellaneous:** Anorexia, urinary retention, decreased libido, keratitis, muscle contractions, **neuroleptic malignant syndrome.**

LABORATORY TEST CONSIDERATIONS
↑ CPK, BUN, serum creatinine, alkaline phosphatase, LDH, bilirubin, GGT, AST, ALT.

OD OVERDOSE MANAGEMENT
Symptoms: Arrhythmia, tachycardia, hypertension, pulmonary edema, respiratory distress, renal dysfunction. CNS effects include insomnia, anxiety, aggressive behavior, hypertonia, hyperkinesia, tremor, confusion, disorientation, depersonalization, fear, delirium, hallucinations, psychotic reactions, lethargy, somnolence, **coma, seizures,** hyperthermia.
Treatment:
- Gastric lavage or induction of emesis followed by supportive measures.
- Ensure that client is well hydrated; give IV fluids if necessary.
- To treat CNS toxicity: Slow IV physostigmine, 1–2 mg given q 1–2 hr in adults or 0.5 mg at 5–10-min intervals (maximum of 2 mg/hr) in children.
- Sedatives and anticonvulsants may be given if needed; antiarrhythmics and vasopressors may also be required. Force fluids and if necessary, give IV.
- Administration of urine acidifying drugs may increase the elimination of amantadine.

- Monitor BP, pulse, respiration, and temperature. Monitor blood electrolytes, urine pH, and urinary output.
- Exercise care if giving adrenergic drugs, such as isoproterenol, since the dopaminergic activity of amantadine may induce malignant arrhythmias.

DRUG INTERACTIONS
Acidic drugs / ↑ Elimination of amantadine
Anticholinergics / Additive anticholinergic effects (including hallucinations, confusion), especially with trihexyphenidyl and benztropine
H *Belladonna leaf/root* / ↑ Anticholinergic effect
CNS stimulants / May ↑ CNS and psychic effects of amantadine; use cautiously together
H *Henbane leaf* / ↑ Anticholinergic effects
Hydrochlorothiazide/triamterene combination / ↓ Urinary excretion of amantadine → ↑ amantadine plasma levels
Levodopa / Effects potentiated by amantadine
H *Pheasant's eye herb* / ↑ Amantadine effect
Quinidine/Quinine / ↓ Renal amantadine clearance
H *Scopolia root* / ↑ Amantadine effect
Thiazide diuretics / ↑ Plasma amantadine levels
Thioridazine / Worsening of tremors in the elderly with Parkinson's disease
Triamterene / ↑ Plasma amantadine levels
Trimethoprim/Sulfamethoxazole / ↓ Amantadine renal clearance → ↑ plasma levels

HOW SUPPLIED
Capsules: 100 mg; *Syrup:* 50 mg/5mL; *Tablets:* 100 mg.

DOSAGE————————
- **CAPSULES; SYRUP; TABLETS**
  Uncomplicated influenza A viral illness.

Adults, 13–64 years: 200 mg/day as a single or divided doses twice daily. A 100 mg daily dose has been used as prophylaxis in healthy adults who are not at high risk for flu-related complications but this dose is not as effective as the 200 mg daily dose for prophylaxis. **Adults, over 65 years:** 100 mg once daily. **Children, 1–9 years:** 4.4–8.8 mg/kg/day up to a maximum of 150 mg/day in one or two divided doses (use syrup); **9–12 years:** 100 mg twice daily. Decrease dose in renal impairment as follows: C_{CR} **30–50 mL/min:** 200 mg the first day and 100 mg/day thereafter; C_{CR} **15–29 mL/min:** 200 mg the first day and 100 mg on alternate days thereafter; C_{CR} **less than 15 mL/min or in hemodialysis clients:** 200 mg q 7 days.

Parkinsonism.

Use as sole agent, usual: 100 mg twice a day, up to 400 mg/day in divided doses, if necessary. **Use with other antiparkinson drugs:** 100 mg 1–2 times per day.

Drug-induced extrapyramidal symptoms.

100 mg twice daily. (Up to 300 mg/day may be required in some.) Reduce dose in impaired renal function.

NURSING CONSIDERATIONS

@ Do not confuse amantadine with memantine (Alzheimer's drug).

ADMINISTRATION/STORAGE

1. Protect capsules from moisture.
2. Dispense in a tight container with a child-resistant closure.
3. For influenza A prophylaxis, start before or immediately after exposure; continue for 10 or more days after exposure. If used with vaccine, give for 2–4 weeks after vaccine given.
4. When treating viral illness, start as soon as possible after symptoms begin and for 24–48 hr after symptoms disappear.
5. Reduce dose to 100 mg/day for persons with active seizure disorders R/T increased risk of seizure frequency with 200 mg daily dose.
6. Reduce dose in clients age 65 or older. Dose may need to be reduced in clients with CHF, peripheral edema, orthostatic hypotension, or impaired renal function.

ASSESSMENT

1. Obtain history; note evidence of seizures, CHF, and renal insufficiency.
2. With seizure disorder reduce dosage to prevent breakthrough seizures. With an increase in seizure activity, take precautions and reduce dosage to 100 mg/day to prevent loss of seizure control.
3. Monitor I&O; observe clients with renal impairment for crystalluria, oliguria, and increased BUN or creatinine levels; ensure adequate hydration.
4. With Parkinson's disease, following loss of drug effectiveness, benefits may be regained by increasing dosage or discontinuing the drug for several weeks and then reinstituting.

CLIENT/FAMILY TEACHING

1. To prevent insomnia give last dose several hours before bedtime.
2. Do not drive or work where alertness is important until drug effects realized; can affect vision, concentration, and coordination. Rise slowly from prone position; low BP may occur. Lie down if dizzy/weak to relieve symptoms.
3. Report diffuse patchy discoloration or skin mottling. Discoloration lessens when legs elevated; usually fades completely within weeks after stopping drug.
4. With flu protection report if S&S do not improve or worsen. Report any exposure to rubella; drug may increase disease susceptibility.
5. Susceptible individuals (elderly, immunocompromised) should avoid crowds during flu season, receive annual flu shot and the pneumonia vaccine.
6. Report any psychologic changes such as confusion, mental status changes, nervousness, or depression as well as any persistent, or new symptoms.
7. Avoid alcohol or any other unprescribed OTC products.
8. Clients with parkinsonism: do not stop drug abruptly; may take up to 2 weeks to notice any improvement.
9. With seizure disorders, report any early S&S of seizure activity; dosage may require adjustment.

OUTCOMES/EVALUATE
- ↓ Drug-induced extrapyramidal S&S
- Improved motor control; ↓ tremor
- Influenza A prophylaxis; ↓ spread of infection to high-risk individuals during outbreaks

Ambrisentan ■
(am-bree-**SEN**-tan)

CLASSIFICATION(S):
Endothelin receptor antagonist
PREGNANCY CATEGORY: X
Rx: Letairis.

USES
To improve exercise capacity and delay clinical worsening in those with pulmonary arterial hypertension with WHO class II or III symptoms.

ACTION/KINETICS

Action
In clients with pulmonary arterial hypertension, plasma endothelin-1 (ET-1) levels are increased as much as 10-fold and correlate with increased mean right atrial pressure and disease severity. Two receptor types, ET_A (cause vasoconstriction and cell proliferation) and ET_B (cause vasodilation and antiproliferation) mediate the effects of ET-1. Ambrisentan is a highly selective antagonist ET_A antagonist and presumably prevents the effects of endothelin-1 on this receptor subtype.

Pharmacokinetics
Rapidly absorbed. **Peak levels**: 2 hr. Elimination is mostly by nonrenal pathways. **t½, effective**: 9 hr. **Plasma protein binding**: 99%.

CONTRAINDICATIONS
Use in moderate to severe impaired hepatic function. Use in women who are or who may become pregnant. Use during breast feeding.

SPECIAL CONCERNS
■ (1) Potential liver injury. Ambrisentan can cause elevation of liver aminotransferases (ALT, AST) to at least 3 times the upper limit of normal (ULN). Ambrisentan treatment was associated with aminotransferase elevations of more than 3 times the ULN in 0.8% of clients in 12-week trials and 2.8% of clients in long-term, open-label trials of up to 1 year. One case of aminotransferase elevations of more than 3 times the ULN has been accompanied by bilirubin of more than 2 times the ULN. Because these changes are a marker for potentially serious liver injury, serum aminotransferase levels (and bilirubin if aminotransferase levels are elevated) must be measured prior to initial of treatment and then monthly. (2) In the postmarketing period with another endothelin receptor antagonist (bosentan), rare cases of unexplained hepatic cirrhosis were reported after prolonged (more than 12 months) therapy. In at least one case with bosentan, a late presentation (after more than 30 months of treatment) included pronounced elevations in aminotransferases and bilirubin levels accompanied by nonspecific symptoms, all of which resolved slowly over time after discontinuation of the suspect drug. This case reinforces the importance of strict adherence to the monthly monitoring schedule for the duration of treatment. (3) Elevations in aminotransferases require close attention. Generally avoid ambrisentan in clients with elevated aminotransferases (more than 3 times the ULN) at baseline because monitoring liver injury may be more difficult. If liver aminotransferase elevations are accompanied by clinical symptoms of liver injury (such as nausea, vomiting, fever, abdominal pain, jaundice, or unusual lethargy or fatigue) or increases in bilirubin of more than 2 times the ULN, stop treatment. There is no experience with the reintroduction of ambrisentan in these circumstances. (4) Contraindicated during pregnancy. Ambrisentan is very likely to produce serious birth defects if used by pregnant women, as this effect has been seen consistently when it is administered to animals. Pregnancy must therefore be excluded before the initiation of treatment with ambrisentan and prevented thereafter by the use of at least 2 reliable methods of contraception, unless the client has had a tubal steril-

---

ization or Copper T 380A IUD or levo-norgestrel 20 mcg/day (LNg 20) IUD inserted, in which case no other contraception is needed. Obtain monthly pregnancy tests. (5) Because of the risks of liver injury and birth defects, ambrisentan is available only through a special restricted distribution program called the Letairis Education and Access Program (LEAP), by calling 1-866-664-5327. Only prescribers and pharmacies registered with LEAP may prescribe and distribute ambrisentan. In addition, ambrisentan may be dispensed only to clients who are enrolled in and meet all conditions of LEAP.■ Use with caution in mild impaired hepatic function. Safety and efficacy have not been determined in children.

SIDE EFFECTS
Most Common
Peripheral edema, headache, palpitations, nasal congestion.

GI: Constipation, abdominal pain. **Hepatic:** Liver damage. **CNS:** Headache. **CV:** Palpitations. **Respiratory:** Nasal congestion, dyspnea, nasopharyngitis, sinusitis. **Body as a whole:** Peripheral edema (more common in the elderly), flushing.

LABORATORY TEST CONSIDERATIONS
↑ ALT, AST. ↓ H&H.

DRUG INTERACTIONS
Cyclosporine / Use with caution R/T cyclosporine being a strong CYP3A inhibitor; may cause ↑ ambrisentan exposure

Ketoconazole / Use with caution R/T ketoconazole being a strong CYP3A inhibitor; may cause ↑ ambrisentan exposure

Omeprazole / Use with caution R/T omeprazole being a strong CYP2C19 inhibitor; may cause ↑ ambrisentan exposure

HOW SUPPLIED
Tablets: 5 mg, 10 mg.

DOSAGE
- **TABLETS**
  Pulmonary arterial hypertension.
Adults, initial: 5 mg once daily with or without food. Consider increasing the dose to 10 mg once daily if 5 mg is tolerated.

NURSING CONSIDERATIONS
ADMINISTRATION/STORAGE
1. Use in women of childbearing potential **only** after a negative pregnancy test. Treat only those women who are using two reliable methods of contraception unless the client has had a tubal sterilization or a Coppre T 380A IUD or LNg 20 IUD inserted. Obtain pregnancy tests monthly in women of childbearing potential who are taking ambrisentan.
2. Carefully follow the guidelines for enrolling clients in the Letairis Education and Access Program (LEAP) @ 1-866-664-5327.
3. Store from 15-30°C (59-86°F).

ASSESSMENT
1. Note reasons for therapy, other agents trialed, when diagnosed, stage of pulmonary artery hypertension.
2. List drugs currently prescribed to ensure none interact adversely.
3. Ensure not pregnant; perform pregnancy test on all females of childbearing potential.
4. After initial labs, monitor LFTs and pregnancy tests monthly; H&H after 1 and 3 months and then periodically to assess for any deficiencies. CXR, ABGs, and PFTs as indicated.

CLIENT/FAMILY TEACHING
1. Review medication guide for safe drug administration. Do not split, chew, or crush ambrisentan tablets. Take exactly as directed. May increase dose as directed by provider if no adverse side effects.
2. Drug has two significant concerns: potential for serious liver damage and fetal damage. It is only administered through the Letairis Education and Access Program (LEAP). All adverse drug reactions should also be reported to LEAP by the provider.
3. Drug is not a cure but may improve clinical symptoms of disease. Report all side effects and any changes in breathing or exercise tolerance.
4. Practice reliable contraception; use at least 2 reliable methods of contraception unless had a tubal sterilization or copper T 380A IUD or LNg 20 IUD

inserted. Drug will cause major birth defects.

5. Continue all other therapies prescribed by pulmonologist. Keep all scheduled monthly lab and provider F/U as scheduled.

OUTCOMES/EVALUATE
• Improved exercise tolerance
• ↓ Pulmonary artery pressure

Amifostine IV
(am-ih-**FOS**-teen)

CLASSIFICATION(S):
Cytoprotective drug
PREGNANCY CATEGORY: C
Rx: Ethyol.

USES
(1) To decrease cumulative renal toxicity due to repeated use of cisplatin in clients with advanced ovarian cancer or in those with non-small-cell lung cancer. (2) Postoperative radiation-induced dry mouth in clients with head and neck cancer where the radiation port includes a significant part of the parotid glands. *Investigational:* Protect lung fibroblasts from damage by paclitaxel. Prevent or reduce cisplatin-induced neurotoxicity and cyclophosphamide-induced granulocytopenia. Prevent or reduce toxicity of radiation therapy to other areas.

ACTION/KINETICS
Action
Amifostine, an organic thiophosphate prodrug, is dephosphorylated by alkaline phosphatase in tissue to the active free thiol metabolite. The thiol metabolite reduces the toxic effects of cisplatin. The ability to protect normal tissues differentially is due to the higher capillary alkaline phosphatase activity, higher pH, and better vascularity of normal tissues compared with tumor tissue. This results in a more rapid generation of the active thiol metabolite as well as greater uptake into tissues. The higher levels of the thiol metabolite in normal tissues bind to, and thus detoxify, reactive metabolites of cisplatin; the thiol

metabolite can also scavenge free radicals that may be generated in tissues exposed to cisplatin.

Pharmacokinetics
Rapidly cleared from the plasma. **$t^{1/2}$, distribution:** less than 1 min; **$t^{1/2}$, elimination:** about 8 min. The thiol metabolite is further broken down to a disulfide metabolite that is less active.

CONTRAINDICATIONS
Hypersensitivity to aminothiol compounds or mannitol. Use in hypotensive or dehydrated clients, in those on antihypertensive therapy that cannot be terminated for 24 hr, and in clients receiving chemotherapy for malignancies that are potentially curable (e.g., certain malignancies of germ cell origin). Use in clients receiving definitive radiotherapy, except during a clinical trial. Lactation.

SPECIAL CONCERNS
Safety has not been determined in clients over 70 years of age or in those with preexisting CV or cerebrovascular conditions, such as ischemic heart disease, arrhythmias, CHF, or history of stroke or transient ischemic attacks. Use with caution in clients where N&V or hypotension may be more likely to have serious consequences. Safety and efficacy have not been determined in children.

SIDE EFFECTS
Most Common
N&V, skin rashes, feeling of warmth, chills, fever, dizziness.

CV: Transient decrease in BP, hypotension. **GI:** Severe N&V. **CNS:** Dizziness, somnolence; rarely, reversible loss of consciousness or seizures. **Hypersensitivity:** Mild skin rash, fever, chills, dyspnea, urticaria, rigors, erythema multiforme; rarely, *Stevens-Johnson syndrome, toxic epidermal necrolysis, anaphylaxis* (hypoxia, *laryngeal edema,* chest tightness, *cardiac arrest).* **Miscellaneous:** Flushing or feeling of warmth, chills or feeling of coldness, hiccoughs, fever, sneezing, hypocalcemia.

DRUG INTERACTIONS
Amifostine may cause hypotension in clients receiving antihypertensive drugs or other drugs that may potentiate hypotension.

Bold Italic = life threatening side effect   ■ = black box warning   ♣ = Available in Canada

HOW SUPPLIED

Powder for Injection, Lyophilized: 500 mg (anhydrous).

DOSAGE

- **IV INFUSION**

  Decrease cumulative renal toxicity with chemotherapy.

  Initial: 910 mg/m^2 given once daily as a 15-min IV infusion, starting within 30 min prior to cisplatin chemotherapy.

  Reduce dry mouth in postoperative radiation treatment for head and neck cancer.

  200 mg/m^2 given once daily as a 3 min IV infusion, starting 15 to 30 min before standard fraction radiation therapy.

  NOTE: Select dosage carefully in the elderly due to greater frequency of hepatic, renal, or cardiac function and of concomitant disease or other drug therapy.

NURSING CONSIDERATIONS

ADMINISTRATION/STORAGE

IV 1. The 15-min infusion is better tolerated than longer duration infusions.

2. Keep supine during administration; monitor BP every 5 min.

3. Stop infusion if systolic BP decreases significantly from recommended baseline values. If BP returns to normal within 5 min and the client has no symptoms, the infusion may be restarted so the full dose of amifostine can be given. If the full dose of amifostine cannot be given, the dose for subsequent cycles should be 740 mg/m^2.

4. To reconstitute add 9.5 mL of 0.9% NaCl injection (other solutions not recommended). Reconstituted solution contains 500 mg amifostine/10 mL and is stable for 5 hr at room temperature (25°C; 77°F) or up to 24 hr under refrigeration (2–8°C; 36–46°F).

ASSESSMENT

1. Note type of malignancy, onset, duration of symptoms, other agents trialed, anticipated dose and duration of cisplatin therapy.

2. List drugs currently prescribed; ensure none interact.

3. Obtain baseline VS, calcium, renal and LFTs; monitor throughout therapy. Those at risk of hypocalemia (e.g., ne-phrotic syndrome) or after multiple doses, give calcium supplements. Hydrate well and ensure not hypotensive. Monitor VS, I&O and keep supine during 15 min infusion checking BP every 5 min.

4. Review/follow manufacturer's guidelines for interrupting infusion due to decreased SBP and suggested dose for readmission.

5. Give an antiemetic, including dexamethasone (20 mg IV) and a serotonin 5HT$_3$ receptor antagonist, prior to and with amifostine.

CLIENT/FAMILY TEACHING

1. Given to protect kidneys during repeated cisplastin therapy.

2. Stop BP medications 24 hr prior to therapy; ensure well hydrated.

3. Chills, flushing, dizziness, somnolence, hiccups, and sneezing may occur.

4. Stay supine during infusion.

OUTCOMES/EVALUATE

↓ Renal toxicity with cisplatin chemotherapy

Amikacin sulfate ■ IV

(am-ih-**KAY**-sin)

CLASSIFICATION(S):

Antibiotic, aminoglycoside

PREGNANCY CATEGORY: D

Rx: Amikin.

SEE ALSO *ANTI-INFECTIVE DRUGS* AND *AMINOGLYCOSIDES.*

USES

(1) Short-term treatment of gram-negative bacterial infections including *Pseudomonas, Escherichia coli, Proteus, Providencia, Klebsiella, Enterobacter, Serratia,* and *Acinetobacter.* (2) For infections due to gentamicin or tobramycin resistant strains of *Providencia rettgeri, P. stuartii, Serratia marcescens,* and *Pseudomonas aeruginosa.* Infections include bacterial septicemia (including neonatal sepsis); serious infections of the respiratory tract, bones, joints, skin, soft tissue, and CNS (including meningitis); intra-abdominal infections (including peritonitis); burns; postoperative infections

---

(including postvascular surgery). Also, serious complicated and recurrent infections of the urinary tract. (3) May be used as initial therapy in certain situations in the treatment of known or suspected staphylococcal disease. *Investigational:* Intrathecal or intraventricular use. As part of multiple drug regimen for *Mycobacterium avium* complex (commonly seen in AIDS clients).

ACTION/KINETICS

Action

Its spectrum is somewhat broader than that of other aminoglycosides, including *Serratia* and *Acinetobacter* species, as well as certain staphylococci and streptococci. Effective against both penicillinase- and non-penicillinase-producing organisms.

Pharmacokinetics

Peak therapeutic serum levels: IM, 16–32 mcg/mL. **t½:** 2–3 hr. Toxic serum levels: >35 mcg/mL (peak measured after 1 hr) and >10 mcg/mL (trough measured before next dose).

CONTRAINDICATIONS

Concurrent use of nephrotoxic agents or diuretics.

SPECIAL CONCERNS

■ See *Aminoglycosides* in Chapter 2.■
Use with caution in premature infants and neonates. Neurotoxicity and nephrotoxicity may occur.

SIDE EFFECTS

Most Common

Arthralgia, oliguria, hearing loss/deafness, loss of balance, apnea, acute muscle paralysis.

See *Aminoglycosides* for a complete list of possible side effects.

HOW SUPPLIED

Injection: 250 mg/mL; *Pediatric Injection:* 50 mg/mL.

DOSAGE

• **IM (PREFERRED); IV**

Adults, children, and older infants: 15 mg/kg/day in two to three equally divided doses q 8–12 hr for 7–10 days; **maximum daily dose:** 15 mg/kg.

Uncomplicated UTIs.

250 mg twice a day; **newborns:** loading dose of 10 mg/kg followed by 7.5 mg/kg q 12 hr.

Use in neonates.

Initial: Loading dose of 10 mg/kg; **then,** 7.5 mg/kg q 12 hr. Lower doses may be safer during the first 2 weeks of life.

Intrathecal or intraventricular use.

8 mg/24 hr.

As part of multiple drug regimen for M. avium complex.

15 mg/kg/day IV in divided doses q 8–12 hr.

In clients with impaired renal function.

Normal loading dose of 7.5 mg/kg; **then** monitor administration by serum level of amikacin (35 mcg/mL maximum) or creatinine clearance rates. Duration of treatment: **Usual:** 7–10 days.

NURSING CONSIDERATIONS

ADMINISTRATION/STORAGE

IV 1. Add 500-mg vial to 200 mL of sterile diluent (NSS or D5W).

2. Administer over 30- to 60-min period for adults.

3. Administer to infants in prescribed fluid amount over 1–2 hr.

4. Store colorless liquid no longer than 2 years at room temperature.

5. Potency not affected if solution turns light yellow.

ASSESSMENT

1. Note reasons for therapy; C&S results. Assess weight, hydration status, U/A, renal and LFTs.

2. Obtain audiometric assessment with high doses or prolonged use.

3. Note vestibular dysfunction; monitor for 8th CN impairment R/T elevated peak drug levels.

CLIENT/FAMILY TEACHING

1. Report lack of response; adverse side effects. Consume fluids to ensure hydration.

2. Report alterations in hearing, vision, ambulation.

3. S&S of superinfection (black furry tongue, loose, foul smelling stools, vaginal itching) require evaluation.

OUTCOMES/EVALUATE

• Resolution of infection

• Therapeutic drug levels (peak 30–35 mcg/mL; trough <8 mcg/mL)

Amiodarone hydrochloride

■

(am-ee-**OH**-dah-rohn)

CLASSIFICATION(S):
Antiarrhythmic, class III
PREGNANCY CATEGORY: D
Rx: Cordarone, Pacerone.
✱**Rx:** Cordarone I.V., Gen-Amiodarone, Novo-Amiodarone, Rhoxal-amiodarone, ratio-Amiodarone.

SEE ALSO *ANTIARRHYTHMIC DRUGS.*

USES

PO and IV: Use should be reserved for life-threatening ventricular arrhythmias unresponsive to other therapy, such as recurrent ventricular fibrillation and recurrent, hemodynamically unstable ventricular tachycardia. During or after treatment with amiodarone injection, clients may be transferred to PO amiodarone therapy. Reserve IV use for acute treatment until the client's ventricular arrhythmias are stabilized (usually 48–96 hr); may be given IV for longer periods if needed. *Investigational:* Conversion of atrial fibrillation and maintenance of sinus rhythm, supraventricular tachycardia, IV for AV nodal reentry tachycardia.

ACTION/KINETICS

Action

Blocks sodium channels at rapid pacing frequencies, causing an increase in the duration of the myocardial cell action potential and refractory period, as well as alpha- and beta-adrenergic blockade. The drug decreases sinus rate, increases PR and QT intervals, results in development of U waves, and changes T-wave contour. After IV use, amiodarone relaxes vascular smooth muscle, reduces peripheral vascular resistance (afterload), and increases cardiac index slightly. No significant changes are seen in left ventricular ejection fraction after PO use.

Pharmacokinetics

Absorption is slow and variable but food increases the rate and extent of absorption. **Maximum plasma levels:** 3–7 hr after a single dose. **Onset:** Several days up to 1–3 weeks. Drug may accumulate in the liver, lung, spleen, and adipose tissue. **Therapeutic serum levels:** 0.5–2.5 mcg/mL. t½, biphasic, initial: 2.5–10 days; final t½: 26–107 days. Effects may persist for several weeks or months after therapy is terminated. **Therapeutic serum levels:** 0.5–2.5 mcg/mL; **toxic serum levels:** >2.5 mcg/mL. Neither amiodarone nor its major metabolite, desethylamiodarone, is dialyzable. Excreted primarily through the bile. **Plasma protein binding:** 96% is bound to plasma proteins.

CONTRAINDICATIONS

Marked sinus bradycardia due to severe sinus node dysfunction, second- or third-degree AV block unless a functioning pacemaker is available, cardiogenic shock, and when bradycardia has caused syncope except when used with a pacemaker. Known hypersensitivity to the drug or any of its components, including iodine. Lactation. Use in children is not recommended.

SPECIAL CONCERNS

■ (1) Amiodarone is intended for use only in clients with the indicated life-threatening arrhythmias because its use is accompanied by substantial toxicity. (2) Amiodarone has several potentially fatal toxicities, the most important of which is pulmonary toxicity (hypersensitivity pneumonitis or interstitial/alveolar pneumonitis) that has resulted in clinically manifest disease rates as high as 10% to 17% in some series of clients with ventricular arrhythmias given doses around 400 mg/day, and as abnormal diffusion capacity without symptoms in a much higher percentage of clients. Pulmonary toxicity has been fatal approximateley 10% of the time. (3) Liver injury is common with amiodarone, but is usually mild and evidenced only by abnormal liver enzymes. Overt liver disease can occur, however, and has been fatal in a few cases. Like other antiarrhythmics, amiodarone can exacerbate the arrhythmia, e.g., by making the arrhythmia less well tolerated or more difficult to reverse.

This has occurred in 2% to 5% of clients in various series, and significant heart block or sinus bradycardia has been seen in 2% to 5%. All of these events should be manageable in the proper clinical setting in most cases. Although the frequency of such proarrhythmic events does not appear greater with amiodarone than with many other agents used in this population, the effects are prolonged when they occur. (4) Even in clients at high risk of arrhythmic death, in whom the toxicity of amoidarone is an acceptable risk, amiodarone poses major management problems that could be life-threatening in a population at risk of sudden death, so that every effort should be made to utilize alternative agents first. (5) The difficulty of using amiodarone effectively and safely itself poses a significant risk to clients. Clients with the indicated arrhythmias must be hospitalized while the loading dose of amiodarone is given, and a response generally requires at least one week, usually two or more. Because absorption and elimination are variable, maintenance-dose selection is difficult, and it is not unusual to require dosage decrease or discontinuation of treatment. (6) The time at which a previously controlled life-threatening arrhythmnia will recur after discontinuation or dose adjustment is unpredictable, ranging from weeks to months. The client is obviously at great risk during this time and may need prolonged hospitalization. Attempts to substitute other antiarrhythmic agents when amiodarone must be stopped will be made difficult by the gradually, but unpredictably, changing amiodarone body burden. A similar problem exists when amiodarone is not effective; it still poses the risk of an interaction with whatever subsequent treatment is tried.■ Although not recommended for use in children, minimize the potential for the drug to leach out di-(2-ethylhexyl)phthalate (DEHP) from IV tubing during administration to children (DEHP may alter development of the male reproductive tract when given in high amounts). The drug may be more sensitive in geriatric clients, especially in thyroid dysfunction. Carefully monitor the IV product in geriatric clients and in those with severe left ventricular dysfunction. May cause fatal hepatocellular necrosis after administration of a much higher loading dose and at a rate much faster than the product's labeling. Use with caution with drugs that may cause hypokalemia and/or hypomagnesemia.

SIDE EFFECTS
Most Common
After PO use: CHF, cardiac arrhythmias, malaise, fatigue, tremor, involuntary movements, poor coordination, peripheral neuropathy, paresthesias, photosensitivity, N&V, constipation, anorexia, pulmonary inflammation.

After IV use: Hypotension, bradycardia, AV block, CHF, ventricular tachycardia, nausea, fever, injection site reactions. Adverse reactions, some potentially fatal, are common with doses greater than 400 mg/day. **Respiratory:** Pulmonary infiltrates or fibrosis, interstitial/alveolar pneumonitis, hypersensitivity pneumonitis, alveolitis, pulmonary inflammation or fibrosis, ***ARDS (after parenteral use)***, lung edema, cough and progressive dyspnea, ***bronchiolitis obliterans organizing pneumonia***, bronchospasm, hemoptysis, hypoxia, pleuritis, ***possibly fatal respiratory disorders***, wheezing. Oral use may cause a clinical syndrome of cough and progressive dyspnea accompanied by functional, radiographic, gallium scan, and pathologic data indicating pulmonary toxicity. **CV:** ***Worsening of arrhythmias, paroxysmal ventricular tachycardia***, proarrhythmias, symptomatic bradycardia, sinus arrest, SA node dysfunction, AV block, ***CHF***, edema, hypotension (especially with IV use), venous thrombosis, phlebitis, thrombophlebitis, ***cardiac conduction abnormalities, coagulation abnormalities, cardiac arrest (after IV use)***. IV use may result in atrial fibrillation, nodal arrhythmia, prolonged QT interval, sinus bradycardia, ***ventricular fibrillation, heart arrest***. **Hepatic:** Abnormal LFTs, overt liver disease, nonspecific hepatic disorders, cholestatic hepatitis, cirrhosis, hepatitis, steatohe-

---

patitis (with cumulative doses), **fatal hepatocellular necrosis, hepatic failure**. **CNS:** Malaise, tremor, lack of coordination, fatigue, ataxia, paresthesias, peripheral neuropathy, abnormal involuntary movements, sleep disturbances, dizziness, insomnia, headache, decreased libido, abnormal gait, hallucinations, confusion, disorientation, delirium, pseudotumor cerebri. **Hematologic: Hemolytic anemia, aplastic anemia**, thrombocytopenia, neutropenia, pancytopenia. **GI:** N&V, constipation, diarrhea, anorexia, abdominal pain, abnormal taste and smell, abnormal salivation, **pancreatitis**. **Hepatic:** Cholestatic jaundice, cirrhosis, hepatitis. **Musculoskeletal:** Myopathy, muscle weakness, rhabdomyolysis. **Ophthalmologic:** Ophthalmic abnormalities, including optic neuropathy and/or optic neuritis (may progress to permanent blindness). Papilledema, corneal degeneration, photosensitivity, eye discomfort, scotoma, lens opacities, macular degeneration. Corneal microdeposits (asymptomatic) in clients on therapy for 6 months or more, photophobia, dry eyes, visual disturbances, blurred vision, halos. **Dermatologic:** Photosensitivity, pruritus, solar dermatitis, blue discoloration of skin, rash, alopecia, spontaneous ecchymosis, erythema, erythema multiforme, exfoliative dermatitis, pigment changes, flushing, skin sloughing, **Stevens-Johnson syndrome, fatal toxic epidermal necrolysis**. **At injection site:** Cellulitis, edema, erythema, necrosis, pain, phlebitis, pigment changes, skin sloughing, thrombophlebitis, venous thrombosis. **Miscellaneous:** Hypothyroidism or hyperthyroidism, thyroid tumors, myopathy, vasculitis, fever, flushing, epididymitis, impotence, angioedema, cellulitis, syndrome of inappropriate ADH secretion, necrosis. IV use may cause abnormal kidney function, pain, **Stevens-Johnson syndrome**, respiratory syndrome, **fatal 'gasping syndrome' in neonates following IV use of benzyl alcohol-containing solutions, anaphylactic/anaphylactoid reactions,** and **shock**.

LABORATORY TEST CONSIDERATIONS
↑ AST, ALT, GGT. Alteration of thyroid function tests (↑ serum T_4, ↓ serum T_3), abnormal LFTs.

OD OVERDOSE MANAGEMENT
Symptoms: Bradycardia, hypotension, **disorders of cardiac rhythm, cardiogenic shock,** AV block, hepatoxicity. *Treatment:* Institute supportive treatment. Monitor cardiac rhythm and BP. Use a beta-adrenergic agonist or pacemaker to treat bradycardia; treat hypotension due to insufficient tissue perfusion with a vasopressor or positive inotropic agents. Cholestyramine may hasten the reversal of side effects by increasing elimination. Drug is not dialyzable.

DRUG INTERACTIONS
Anesthetics, volatile / ↑ Sensitivity to the myocardial depressant and conduction effects of halogenated inhalational anesthetics
Anticoagulants / ↑ PT → bleeding disorders
Atazanavir / ↑ Amiodarone levels → ↑ risk of amiodarone toxicity
Azithromycin / Potential for prolonged QTc interval and QT dispersion and dizziness
Azole antibiotics / ↑ Risk of QT-prolongation
Beta-adrenergic blocking agents / ↑ Bradycardia and hypotension
Calcium channel blockers / ↑ Risk of AV block with verapamil or diltiazem or hypotension with all calcium channel blockers
Cholestyramine / ↑ Elimination of amiodarone → ↓ serum levels and half-life
Cimetidine / ↑ Serum levels of amiodarone
Cyclosporine / ↑ Plasma drug levels → elevated creatinine levels (even with ↓ cyclosporine doses)
Dextromethorphan / Chronic use of PO amiodarone (>2 weeks) impairs dextromethorphan metabolism
Digoxin / ↑ Serum digoxin levels → toxicity; reduce digoxin dose by 50% or discontinue
Disopyramide / ↑ QT prolongation → possible arrhythmias; reduce disopy-

A

ramide dose

Fentanyl / Possibility of hypotension, bradycardia, ↓ CO

Flecainide / ↑ Plasma flecainide levels → toxicity; reduce flecainide dose

Fluoroquinolones / ↑ Risk of life-threatening cardiac arrhythmias, including torsades de pointes R/T prolongation of the QT-interval

Grapefruit juice / ↑ AUC by 50% and peak plasma amiodarone levels by 84% R/T inhibition of CYP3A4 metabolism of amiodarone; stop using grapefruit juice when starting amiodarone therapy

Hydantoins / ↑ Hydantoin levels → toxicity; also, ↓ amiodarone serum levels

Indinavir / ↑ Plasma levels of amiodarone due to ↓ breakdown by liver → ↑ risk of toxicity

Iohexol (contrast media) / ↑ QTc in clients taking amiodarone and undergoing cardiac catheterization

Itraconazole / ↑ Risk of life-threatening cardiac arrhythmias, including torsades de pointes

Lidocaine / Sinus bradycardia after PO amiodarone; seizures R/T ↑ lidocaine levels with concomitant IV amiodarone

Macrolide antibiotics (e.g., azithromycin) / ↑ Risk of life-threatening cardiac arrhythmias, including torsades de pointes

Methotrexate / Chronic use of PO amiodarone (>2 weeks) ↓ methotrexate metabolism → toxicity

Nelfinavir / ↑ Amiodarone levels → ↑ risk of amiodarone toxicity

Phenytoin / ↑ Serum phenytoin levels → toxicity; also, ↓ amiodarone levels

Procainamide / ↑ Serum procainamide levels → toxicity; reduce procainamide dose

Pyridoxine / ↑ Amiodarone-induced photosensitivity

Quinidine / ↑ Quinidine toxicity, including fatal cardiac arrhythmias; reduce quinidine dose

Rifampin / ↓ Serum levels of amiodarone and its active metabolite due to ↑ liver breakdown

Ritonavir / ↑ Levels of amiodarone → ↑ risk of amiodarone toxicity

Rosuvastatin / Possible ↑ serum transaminase levels

Simvastatin / Possible severe myopathy/rhabomyolysis with elevated creatine kinase

H   *St. John's Wort* / ↓ Amiodarone levels R/T ↑ metabolism by CYP3A4

Theophylline / ↑ Serum theophylline levels → toxicity (effects may not be seen for 1 week and may last for a prolonged period after amiodarone is discontinued)

Thioridazine / ↑ Risk of life-threatening cardiac arrhythmias, including torsades de pointes

Vardenafil / ↑ Risk of life-threatening cardiac arrhythmias, including torsades de pointes

Warfarin / ↑ PT; ↓ warfarin dose by 30-50%. Effect may persist for months after amiodarone discontinuation

Ziprasidone / ↑ Risk of life-threatening cardiac arrhythmias, including torsades de pointes

HOW SUPPLIED

Injection: 50 mg/mL; *Tablets:* 100 mg, 200 mg, 400 mg.

DOSAGE————————————

Due to the drug's side effects, unusual pharmacokinetic properties, and difficult dosing schedule, administer amiodarone in a hospital only by physicians trained in treating life-threatening arrhythmias. Loading doses are required to ensure a reasonable onset of action.

• **IV INFUSION**

  Life-threatening ventricular arrhythmias (e.g., ventricular fibrillation or hemodynamically unstable ventricular tachycardia).

Loading dose, first rapid: 150 mg over the first 10 minutes (15 mg/min). **Then, slow loading dose:** 360 mg over the next 6 hr (1 mg/min). **Maintenance dose:** 540 mg over the remaining 18 hr (0.5 mg/min). After the first 24 hr, continue maintenance infusion rate of 0.5 mg/min (720 mg/24 hr). This may be continued with monitoring for 2 to 3 weeks.

Once arrhythmias have been suppressed, the client may be switched to PO amiodarone. The following is intended only as a guideline for PO amiodarone dosage after IV infusion. **IV infu-**

sion less than 1 week: Initial daily dose of PO amiodarone, 800–1,600 mg. **IV infusion from 1 to 3 weeks:** Initial daily dose of PO amiodarone, 600–800 mg. **IV infusion longer than 3 weeks:** Initial daily dose of PO amiodarone, 400 mg.

- **TABLETS**

  Life-threatening ventricular arrhythmias (e.g., ventricular fibrillation or hemodynamically unstable ventricular tachycardia).

Loading dose: 800–1,600 mg/day for 1–3 weeks (or until initial response occurs); **then**, reduce dose to 600–800 mg/day for 1 month. **Maintenance dose:** 400 mg/day (as low as 200 mg/day or as high as 600 mg/day may be needed in some clients). Give in divided doses with meals for total daily doses of 1,000 mg or higher or when GI intolerance occurs.

NURSING CONSIDERATIONS

ADMINISTRATION/STORAGE

1. Correct K$^+$ or Mg$^+$ deficiencies before therapy since antiarrhythmics may be ineffective or arrhythmogenic with hypokalemia.
2. When initiating therapy, gradually discontinue other antiarrhythmic drugs.
3. To minimize side effects, determine lowest effective dose; if side effects occur; reduce dose.
4. If dosage adjustments required, monitor client for extended time frame R/T long and variable half-life of drug and the difficulty in predicting time needed to achieve new steady-state plasma drug level.
5. Administer daily PO doses of 1,000 mg or more in divided doses with meals.
6. If additional antiarrhythmic therapy required, initial dose of such drugs should be about one-half usual recommended dose.
7. Review labeling for PO formulation, esp. safety and efficacy, before switching route of administration from IV or PO.
IV 8. For first rapid loading dose, add 3 mL amiodarone IV (150 mg) to 100 mL D5W for concentration of 1.5

mg/mL; infuse at rate of 100 mL/10 min. For slower loading dose, add 18 mL amiodarone IV (900 mg) to 500 mL of D5W for concentration of 1.8 mg/mL.
9. IV concentrations of amiodarone greater than 3 mg/mL in D5W cause high incidence of peripheral vein phlebitis; concentrations of 2.5 mg/mL or less are not as irritating. For infusions greater than 1 hr, the IV concentration should not exceed 2 mg/mL unless central venous catheter used.
10. Because amiodarone adsorbs to PVC, IV infusions exceeding 2 hr must be given in glass or polyolefin bottles containing D5W.
11. Cordarone I.V. has been found to leach out plasticizers, such as DEHP, which can adversely affect male reproductive tract development in fetuses, infants, and toddlers. Cordarone I.V. is not indicated to treat arrhythmias in pediatric clients.
12. Amiodarone IV in D5W is incompatible with aminophylline, cefamandole nafate, cefazolin sodium, mezlocillin sodium, heparin sodium, and sodium bicarbonate.
13. Store the injection at room temperature protected from light.

ASSESSMENT

1. Note indications for therapy. Check if taking other antiarrhythmic drugs.
2. Assess quality of respirations and breath sounds; note cardiac status, EKG, and CV findings. Monitor for hepatic and pulmonary toxicity.
3. Note baseline VS and perfusion (skin temperature, color). Document ABGs; assess for circulatory impairment and hypotension.
4. Assess vision before therapy; monitor.
5. Monitor thyroid studies (drug inhibits conversion of T_4 to T_3). May require replacement therapy with prolonged use.
6. Obtain CBC, electrolytes (esp K$^+$ and Mg$^+$), CXR, renal and LFTs.
7. During administration, observe for increased PR and QRS intervals, increased arrhythmias, and HR <60 bpm. Obtain ECG, document rhythm strips; note EPS findings.

A

8. Reduce dosages of digoxin, warfarin, quinidine, procainamide, and phenytoin if administered with amiodarone.

CLIENT/FAMILY TEACHING

1. Drug is used to control heart beat irregularities, take as directed.
2. Report if crystals develop on skin, producing bluish color, so dosage can be adjusted.
3. Avoid direct exposure to sunlight. Wear protective clothing, sunglasses, and a sunscreen if exposed.
4. Report side effects, especially any abnormal swelling, bleeding, or bruising.
5. Painful breathing, wheezing, fever, coughing, or SOB are S&S of pulmonary problems; require prompt attention.
6. Report CNS symptoms such as tremor, lack of coordination, numbness, and dizziness.
7. Complaints of headaches, depression, or insomnia as well as any change in behavior such as decreased interest in personal appearance or apparent hallucinations may require a change in therapy.
8. Have periodic eye exams; small yellow-brown granular corneal deposits may develop during prolonged therapy. Visual changes require prompt eye evaluation.
9. Requires lab studies and close medical evaluation; drug is highly toxic and may stay in system for months after stopping.
10. Health care professionals who dispense Cordarone are required to provide medication guides to clients; these should not be used as substitutes for counseling regarding the risks and benefits of the drug.

OUTCOMES/EVALUATE

- Termination/control of arrhythmias
- Serum drug levels within therapeutic range (0.5–2.5 mcg/mL)

Amitriptyline hydrochloride ■ ©
(ah-me-**TRIP**-tih-leen)

CLASSIFICATION(S):
Antidepressant, tricyclic
PREGNANCY CATEGORY: C
🍁**Rx:** Apo-Amitriptyline.

SEE ALSO *ANTIDEPRESSANTS, TRICYCLIC.*

USES

(1) Relief of symptoms of depression, including depression accompanied by anxiety and insomnia. (2) Chronic pain due to cancer or other pain syndromes. (3) Prophylaxis of cluster and migraine headaches. *Investigational:* Pathologic laughing and crying secondary to forebrain disease, bulimia nervosa, antiulcer agent, enuresis. Adjunct analgesic for phantom limb pain, migraine, chronic tension headaches, diabetic neuropathy, tic douloureux, cancer pain, peripheral neuropathy with pain, postherpetic neuralgia, arthritic pain. Dermatologic disorders (chronic urticaria and angioedema, nocturnal pruritus in atopic eczema).

ACTION/KINETICS

Action

Amitriptyline is metabolized to an active metabolite, nortriptyline. Has significant anticholinergic and sedative effects with moderate orthostatic hypotension. Very high ability to block serotonin uptake and moderate activity with respect to norepinephrine uptake.

Pharmacokinetics

Effective plasma levels of amitriptyline and nortriptyline: Approximately 110–250 ng/mL. **Time to reach steady state:** 4–10 days. t½: 31–46 hr. Up to 1 month may be required for beneficial effects to be manifested.

CONTRAINDICATIONS

Use in children less than 12 years old

SPECIAL CONCERNS

■ Antidepressants increase the risk of suicidal thinking and behavior (suicidality) in short-term studies in children and adolescents with major depressive disorders and other psychiatric disorders. Anyone considering the use of amitriptyline or any other antidepressant in a child or adolescent must balance this risk with the clinical need. Clients who are started on therapy should be observed closely for clinical worsening, suicidality, or unusual changes in behavior. Families and caregivers should be advised of the need for close observation and communication with the prescriber. Amitriptyline is not approved for use in pediatric clients. Analysis of short-term (4–16 weeks) placebo-controlled trials in children and adolescents with major depressive disorder, obsessive-compulsive disorder, or other psychiatric disorders have revealed a greater risk of adverse reactions representing suicidal thinking or behavior during the first few months of treatment in those receiving antidepressants. The average risk of such reactions in such clients receiving antidepressants was 4%, twice the placebo risk of 2%. No suicides occurred in these trials.■

SIDE EFFECTS
Most Common
Sedation, dry mouth, blurred vision, constipation, mydriasis, urinary retention, disturbance of accommodation.
See *Antidepressants, Tricyclic* for a complete list of possible side effects.

ADDITIONAL DRUG INTERACTIONS
Guanethidine and similar drugs / Antihypertensive effect may be blocked
H *St. John's Wort* / ↓ Blood levels of amitriptyline and its metabolite
Smoking / ↓ Amitriptyline levels R/T ↑ hepatic metabolism; possible ↓ efficacy

HOW SUPPLIED
Tablets: 10 mg, 25 mg, 50 mg, 75 mg, 100 mg, 150 mg.

DOSAGE
• **TABLETS**
Antidepressant.
Adults (outpatients): 75 mg/day in divided doses; may be increased to 150 mg/day. *Alternate dosage:* **Initial,** 50–100 mg at bedtime; **then,** increase by 25–50 mg, if necessary, up to 150 mg/day. **Hospitalized clients: initial,**

100 mg/day; may be increased to 200–300 mg/day. **Maintenance: usual,** 40–100 mg/day (may be given as a single dose at bedtime). **Adolescent and geriatric:** 10 mg 3 times per day and 20 mg at bedtime up to a maximum of 100 mg/day.
Chronic pain.
50–100 mg/day.
Analgesic adjunct.
75–300 mg/day.
Dermatologic disorders.
10–50 mg/day.

NURSING CONSIDERATIONS
◎ Do not confuse amitriptyline with nortriptyline (also a tricyclic antidepressant).

ADMINISTRATION/STORAGE
1. Initiate dosage increases late in afternoon or bedtime.
2. Sedative effects may be manifested before antidepressant effects.
3. When satisfactory improvement is noted, reduce the dose to the lowest effective amount. Continue three or more months to lessen the possibility of relapse.

ASSESSMENT
1. Note indications, onset, characteristics/extent of S&S; list other agents trialed.
2. Monitor mental status, CBC, electrolytes, EKG, renal and LFTs.
3. Assess I&O, weights, VS, and bowel elimination patterns.

CLIENT/FAMILY TEACHING
1. Take with food; minimizes gastric upset.
2. Do not drive or operate hazardous machinery until drug effects realized; causes high degree of sedation.
3. May take entire dose at bedtime if sedation evident during waking hours.
4. Rise slowly from lying to sitting position to reduce low BP drug effects.
5. Wear sunscreen; avoid prolonged sun exposure.
6. Urine may appear blue-green in color; harmless. May experience dry mouth. Report urinary retention or constipation; increase fluids/bulk in diet to offset.

7. Beneficial antidepressant effects may not be noted for 30 days.

8. Elderly clients may be at increased risk for falls; start low doses, use precautions, and observe closely.

OUTCOMES/EVALUATE

- ↓ Symptoms of depression
- Control of incontinence
- Enhanced pain control with chronic pain management
- Relief of insomnia/itching

Amlodipine
(am-**LOH**-dih-peen)

CLASSIFICATION(S):
Calcium channel blocker
PREGNANCY CATEGORY: C
Rx: Amvaz, Norvasc.

SEE ALSO CALCIUM CHANNEL BLOCKING AGENTS.

USES
(1) Hypertension alone or in combination with other antihypertensives. (2) Chronic stable angina alone or in combination with other antianginal drugs. (3) Vasospastic (Prinzmetal's variant) angina alone or in combination with other antianginal drugs.

ACTION/KINETICS
Action
Inhibits influx of calcium through the cell membrane, resulting in a depression of automaticity and conduction velocity in cardiac muscle. Decreases SA and AV conduction and prolongs AV node effective and functional refractory periods. Slight decrease in HR. Possible slight decrease in myocardial contractility. CO is increased; moderate decrease in peripheral vascular resistance.

Pharmacokinetics
Peak plasma levels: 6–12 hr. **t½, elimination:** 30–50 hr. 90% metabolized in the liver to inactive metabolites; 10% excreted unchanged in the urine. **Plasma protein binding:** About 93%.

CONTRAINDICATIONS
Use with grapefruit juice.

SPECIAL CONCERNS
Use with caution in clients with CHF and in those with impaired hepatic function or reduced hepatic blood flow. Safety and efficacy have not been determined in children.

SIDE EFFECTS
Most Common
Edema, palpitations, dizziness/lightheadedness, headache, fatigue/lethargy, flushing.

CNS: Headache, fatigue, lethargy, somnolence, dizziness, lightheadedness, sleep disturbances, depression, amnesia, psychosis, hallucinations, paresthesia, asthenia, insomnia, abnormal dreams, malaise, anxiety, tremor, hand tremor, hypoesthesia, vertigo, depersonalization, migraine, apathy, agitation, amnesia. **GI:** Nausea, abdominal discomfort, cramps, dyspepsia, diarrhea, constipation, vomiting, dry mouth, thirst, flatulence, dysphagia, loose stools. **CV:** Peripheral edema, palpitations, hypotension, syncope, bradycardia, unspecified arrhythmias, tachycardia, ventricular extrasystoles, peripheral ischemia, *cardiac failure*, pulse irregularity, increased risk of MI. **Dermatologic:** Dermatitis, rash, pruritus, urticaria, photosensitivity, petechiae, ecchymosis, purpura, bruising, hematoma, cold/clammy skin, skin discoloration, dry skin. **Musculoskeletal:** Muscle cramps, pain, or inflammation; joint stiffness or pain, arthritis, twitching, ataxia, hypertonia. **GU:** Polyuria, dysuria, urinary frequency, nocturia, sexual difficulties. **Respiratory:** Nasal or chest congestion, sinusitis, rhinitis, SOB, dyspnea, wheezing, cough, chest pain. **Ophthalmic:** Diplopia, abnormal vision, conjunctivitis, eye pain, abnormal visual accommodation, xerophthalmia. **Miscellaneous:** Tinnitus, flushing, sweating, weight gain, epistaxis, anorexia, increased appetite, taste perversion, parosmia.

ADDITIONAL DRUG INTERACTIONS
Diltiazem ↑ Plasma levels of amlodipine → further ↓ BP
Grapefruit juice / ↑ Plasma amlodipine levels
Indinavir + Ritonavir / ↑ Amlodipine

AUC R/T inhibition of CYP3A4 metabolism of amlodipine

HOW SUPPLIED
Tablets: 2.5 mg, 5 mg, 10 mg.

DOSAGE

- **TABLETS**

  Hypertension.

  Adults, usual, individualized: 5 mg/day, up to a maximum of 10 mg/day. Titrate the dose over 7–14 days.

  Chronic stable or vasospastic angina.

  Adults: 5–10 mg, using the lower dose for elderly clients and those with hepatic insufficiency. Most clients require 10 mg.

NURSING CONSIDERATIONS

Do not confuse amlodipine with amiloride (a diuretic) or Norvasc with Navane (an antipsychotic).

ADMINISTRATION/STORAGE
1. Food does not affect bioavailability of amlodipine.
2. Elderly clients, small/fragile clients, or those with hepatic insufficiency may be started on 2.5 mg/day. May also use this dose when adding amlodipine to other antihypertensive therapy.
3. Can be given safely with ACEI, beta-blockers, nitrates (long-acting), nitroglycerin (sublingual), or thiazides.

ASSESSMENT
1. Note reasons for therapy, history of CAD or CHF, angina. Monitor carefully with angina as CCBs may cause increase in frequency/intensity of pain with severe CAD initially and with dose increase.
2. Review list of drugs prescribed to prevent interactions.
3. Monitor VS, ECG, CBC, renal and LFTs. Reduce dose in elderly and clients with liver dysfunction.

CLIENT/FAMILY TEACHING
1. Take as directed, once daily. May take with/without meals; food helps decrease stomach upset. Avoid grapefruit juice; increases drug concentrations.
2. Report S&S of chest pain, SOB, dizziness, swelling of extremities, irregular pulse, or altered vision immediately. Keep record of BP and pulse.

3. Use NTG SL for angina as directed; report lack of response.
4. Use caution, may experience light-headedness or dizziness.
5. Ask for generic; cost savings.

OUTCOMES/EVALUATE
- Desired BP control
- ↓ Frequency/intensity of angina

COMBINATION DRUG

Amlodipine besylate and Benazepril hydrochloride

(am-**LOH**-dih-peen, beh-**NAYZ**-eh-prill)

CLASSIFICATION(S):
Antihypertensive
PREGNANCY CATEGORY: D
Rx: Lotrel.

SEE ALSO *AMLODIPINE* AND *BENAZEPRIL HYDROCHLORIDE*.

USES
Hypertension (not indicated for initial therapy).

CONTENT
Amlodipine besylate (*calcium channel blocker*), 2.5 mg, 5 mg, or 10 mg with benazepril hydrochloride (*ACE inhibitor*), 10 mg, 20 mg, or 40 mg with the following available combinations: 2.5/10 mg, 5/10 mg, 5/20 mg, 5/40 mg, 10/20 mg, and 10/40 mg.

ACTION/KINETICS

Action
Benazepril (and its active metabolite benazeprilat) inhibit angiotensin-converting enzyme resulting in decreased plasma angiotensin II, which leads to decreased vasopressor activity and decreased aldosterone secretion. Amlodipine inhibits the transmembrane influx of calcium ions into vascular smooth muscle and cardiac muscle, resulting in a depression of automaticity and conduction velocity. There is a reduction of both supine and standing BP, with no compensatory tachycardia.

A

Pharmacokinetics

Absorption of either drug is not affected by food. **Peak plasma levels, amlodipine:** 6–12 hr; **benazepril and benazeprilat:** 0.5–2 hr and 1.5–4 hr, respectively. Amlodipine is metabolized in the liver and excreted through the urine. Benazepril and metabolites are excreted through the urine. $t\frac{1}{2}$, **elimination, amlodipine:** 2 days; **benazeprilat:** 10–11 hr.

CONTRAINDICATIONS

Hypersensitivity to benazepril, to any other ACE inhibitor, or to amlodipine. Lactation.

SPECIAL CONCERNS

■ When used in pregnancy during the second and third trimesters, ACE inhibitors can cause injury and even death to the developing fetus. When pregnancy is detected, discontinue the ACE inhibitor as soon as possible.■ Use amlodipine with caution in clients with severe aortic stenosis and in severe renal or hepatic disease. In clients with CHF, with or without associated renal insufficiency, benazepril may cause excessive hypotension. Safety and efficacy have not been determined in children.

SIDE EFFECTS

Most Common

Cough, hypotension, edema (dependent, *angioedema*, facial edema), headache, dizziness.

See *Amlodipine* and *Benazepril hydrochloride* for a complete list of possible side effects.

LABORATORY TEST CONSIDERATIONS

↑ Serum creatinine (especially in those with renal insufficiency, those pretreated with a diuretic, and those with renal artery stenosis). ↑ Serum bilirubin, uric acid.

DRUG INTERACTIONS

See *Amlodipine* and *Benazepril hydrochloride*.

HOW SUPPLIED

See Content.

DOSAGE

• **CAPSULES.**
  Hypertension.
One 2.5/10, 5/10, 5/20, 5/40, 10/20, or 10/40 capsule daily. For the small, elderly, frail, or hepatically impaired, initial amlodipine dose is 2.5 mg.

NURSING CONSIDERATIONS

ADMINISTRATION/STORAGE

1. To minimize dose-independent hazards, it is usually appropriate to begin Lotrel therapy only after a client has:
• failed to achieve the desired antihypertensive effect with one or the other monotherapy, or
• demonstrated inability to achieve adequate antihypertensive effect with amlodipine therapy without developing edema.
2. Store from 15–30°C (59–86°F).

ASSESSMENT

1. List reasons for therapy, other agents trialed, outcome.
2. Monitor VS, EKG, CBC, K+, renal and LFTs.
3. Note culture, risk factors, CAD, CHF, if renal artery stenosis; assess for pregnancy.

CLIENT/FAMILY TEACHING

1. Lotrel is a combination of two drugs in one capsule to better control BP.
2. Record BP, weight and report adverse effects.
3. If swelling of extremities/face, cough, SOB, dizziness, abdominal pain, dark urine, yellowing of skin, persistent sore throat occur- report.
4. Use reliable contraception; stop drug/report if pregnant.
5. Keep BP log for provider review.

OUTCOMES/EVALUATE

Control of BP

Amoxapine   ■
(ah-**MOX**-ah-peen)

CLASSIFICATION(S):
Antidepressant, tricyclic
PREGNANCY CATEGORY: C

SEE ALSO *ANTIDEPRESSANTS, TRICYCLIC*.

USES

(1) Endogenous and psychotic, as well as neurotic or reactive depressions. (2) Depression accompanied by anxiety or agitation.

ACTION/KINETICS

Action

In addition to its effect on monoamines, this drug also blocks dopamine receptors. Significant anticholinergic effects, moderate sedation, and slight orthostatic hypotensive effect.

Pharmacokinetics

Metabolized to the active metabolites 7-hydroxy- and 8-hydroxyamoxapine. **Peak blood levels:** 90 min. **Effective plasma levels:** 200–500 ng/mL. **Time to reach steady state:** 2–7 days. **t½:** 8 hr; t½ of major metabolite: 30 hr. Excreted in urine.

CONTRAINDICATIONS

High dose levels in clients with a history of convulsive seizures. During acute recovery period after MI. Use in children less than 16 years of age.

SPECIAL CONCERNS

■ Antidepressants increase the risk of suicidal thinking and behavior (suicidality) in short-term studies in children and adolescents with major depressive disorders and other psychiatric disorders. Anyone considering the use of amoxapine or any other antidepressant in a child or adolescent must balance this risk with the clinical need. Clients who are started on therapy should be observed closely for clinical worsening, suicidality, or unusual changes in behavior. Families and caregivers should be advised of the need for close observation and communication with the prescriber. Amoxapine is not approved for use in pediatric clients. Analysis of short-term (4–16 weeks) placebo-controlled trials in children and adolescents with major depressive disorder, obsessive-compulsive disorder, or other psychiatric disorders have revealed a greater risk of adverse reactions representing suicidal thinking or behavior during the first few months of treatment in those receiving antidepressants. The average risk of such reactions in such clients receiving antidepressants was 4%, twice the placebo risk of 2%. No suicides occurred in these trials.■ Safe use during lactation not established.

SIDE EFFECTS

Most Common

Headache, nausea, sweating, dry mouth, sleepiness, insomnia, diarrhea, constipation, blurred vision.

See *Antidepressants, Tricyclic* for a complete list of possible side effects. Also, Tardive dyskinesia. Overdosage may cause seizures (common), neuroleptic malignant syndrome, testicular swelling, impairment of sexual function, and breast enlargement in males and females. Also, renal failure may be seen 2–5 days after overdosage.

HOW SUPPLIED

Tablets: 25 mg, 50 mg, 100 mg, 150 mg.

DOSAGE

- **TABLETS**

  Antidepressant.

Adults, individualized, initial: 50 mg 2–3 times per day. Can be increased to 100 mg 2–3 times per day during first week. Due to sedation, do not use doses greater than 300 mg/day unless this dose has been ineffective for at least 14 days. **Maintenance:** 300 mg as a single dose at bedtime. **Hospitalized clients refractory to antidepressant therapy and who have no history of convulsive disorders:** Up to 150 mg 4 times per day. **Geriatric, initial:** 25 mg 2–3 times per day. If necessary and tolerated, increase to 50 mg 2–3 times per day after first week. **Maintenance:** Up to 300 mg/day at bedtime.

NURSING CONSIDERATIONS

ADMINISTRATION/STORAGE

Maintain therapy at the lowest dose that will maintain remission. If symptoms reappear, increase the dose to the earlier level until symptoms are controlled.

ASSESSMENT

1. Note reasons for therapy, onset/characteristics of symptoms, and other agents trialed.
2. Obtain baseline ECG, electrolytes, renal and LFTs; monitor. Reduce dose with organ impairment and with frail, elderly client.

CLIENT/FAMILY TEACHING

1. Take with food; minimizes gastric upset.

---

2. Take entire dose at bedtime if daytime sedation experienced.

3. Report early CNS S&S of tardive dyskinesia, i.e., slow repetitive movements or other adverse side effects; may require dose adjustment.

4. Report side effects R/T overdosage, especially seizures, that require immediate medical care. Increased depression or suicide ideations require immediate reporting; keep all F/U visits.

OUTCOMES/EVALUATE
- Improved coping mechanisms
- Control of depression; ↓ anxiety

Amoxicillin (Amoxycillin)
(ah-mox-ih-**SILL**-in)

CLASSIFICATION(S):
Antibiotic, penicillin
PREGNANCY CATEGORY: B
Rx: Amoxil, Amoxil Pediatric Drops, DisperMox, Polymox, Trimox.
♣Rx: Apo-Amoxi, Gen-Amoxicillin, Lin-Amox, Novamoxin, Nu-Amoxi.

SEE ALSO *ANTI-INFECTIVE DRUGS* AND *PENICILLINS*.

USES
1. Ear, nose, and throat infections due to *Streptococcus* species (α– and β–lactamase-negative only), *S. pneumoniae, Staphylococcus* species, or *Haemophilus influenzae*.
2. GU infections due to *Escherichia coli, Proteus mirabilis,* or *Enterococcus faecalis*.
3. Skin and skin structure infections due to *Streptococcus* species (α– and β–hemolytic strains only), *Staphylococcus* species, or *E. coli*.
4. Lower respiratory tract infections due to *Streptococcus* species (α– and β–hemolytic strains only), *S. pneumoniae, Staphylococcus* species, or *H. haemophilus*.
5. Acute uncomplicated (anogenital and urethral) gonococcal infections due to *Neisseria gonorrhoeae*.

6. In combination with omeprazole or lansoprazole and clarithromycin or metronidazole to treat duodenal ulcers by eradicating *Helicobacter pylori*.

ACTION/KINETICS
Action
Semisynthetic broad-spectrum penicillin closely related to ampicillin. Binds to penicillin-binding proteins (PBP-1 and PBP-3) in the cytoplasmic membranes of bacteria, thus inhibiting cell wall synthesis. Cell division and growth are inhibited. Destroyed by penicillinase, acid stable, and better absorbed than ampicillin.

Pharmacokinetics
From 50 to 80% of a PO dose is absorbed from the GI tract. **Peak serum levels, PO:** 4–11 mcg/mL after 1–2 hr. **t½:** 60 min. Mostly excreted unchanged in urine.

ADDITIONAL CONTRAINDICATIONS
Use of the 875 mg tablet in clients with a GFR less than 30 mL/min.

SPECIAL CONCERNS
Safe use during pregnancy has not been established. Effectiveness of oral contraceptives may be decreased.

SIDE EFFECTS
Most Common
Hypersensitivity, N&V, gastritis, stomatitis.

See *Penicillins* for a complete list of potential side effects.

HOW SUPPLIED
Capsules: 250 mg, 500 mg; **Powder for Oral Suspension:** 50 mg/mL, 125 mg/5 mL, 200 mg/5 mL, 250 mg/5 mL, 400 mg/5 mL; **Tablets:** 500 mg, 875 mg; **Tablets, Chewable:** 125 mg, 200 mg, 250 mg, 400 mg; **Tablets for Oral Suspension:** 200 mg, 400 mg, 600 mg.

DOSAGE
- **CAPSULES; ORAL SUSPENSION; TABLETS; TABLETS, CHEWABLE**
  Susceptible infections of ear, nose, throat, GU tract, skin and soft tissues. Mild to moderate infections.
Adults and children 40 kg and over: 500 mg q 8 hr or 500 mg q 12 hr. **Children three months and older and less than 40 kg:** 20 mg/kg/day in divided doses q 8 hr or 25 mg/kg/day in divided doses q 12 hr.

Bold Italic = life threatening side effect   ■ = black box warning   ♣ = Available in Canada

Severe infections.

Adults and children 40 kg and over: 875 mg q 12 hr or 500 mg q 8 hr. **Children three months and over and less than 40 kg:** 45 mg/kg/day in divided doses q 12 hr or 40 mg/kg/day in divided doses q 8 hr. For children, do not exceed the maximum adult dose.

Infections of the lower respiratory tract.

Adults and children 40 kg and over: 500 mg q 8 hr or 875 mg q 12 hr. **Children 3 months and older and under 40 kg:** 40 mg/kg/day in divided doses q 8 hr or 45 mg/kg/day in divided doses q 12 hr.

Prophylaxis of bacterial endocarditis: dental, oral, respiratory tract, or esophageal; moderate-risk clients undergoing GU/GI procedures.

Adults: 2 grams (50 mg/kg for children) PO 1 hr prior to procedure.

Eradicate H. pylori infections.

The following regimens using amoxicillin may be used: (1) A 14 day regimen including: Amoxicillin, 1,000 mg twice a day with meals; clarithromycin, 500 mg twice a day with meals; and either omeprazole, 20 mg twice a day with meals or lansoprazole, 30 mg twice a day with meals. A product, Prevpac, contains lansoprazole, clarithromycin, and amoxicillin. (2) A 14 day course of therapy consisting of amoxicillin, 1,000 mg twice a day with meals; metronidazole, 500 mg twice a day with meals; and omeprazole, 20 mg twice a day before meals. (3) A 14 day course of therapy consisting of amoxicillin, 1,000 mg twice a day with meals and at bedtime; clarithromycin, 500 mg twice a day; and ranitidine bismuth citrate, 400 mg twice a day with meals and at bedtime.

Gonococcal infections, uncomplicated urethral, endocervical, or rectal infections.

Adults: 3 grams as a single PO dose. **Children, over 2 years (prepubertal):** 50 mg/kg amoxicillin combined with 25 mg/kg probenecid as a single dose.

Early Lyme disease (localized or disseminated).

500 mg 3 times per day for 14–21 days.

Anthrax (postexposure prophylaxis following confirmed or suspected exposure to Bacillus anthracis).

Adults: 500 PO 3 times per day. **Children, less than 9 years of age:** 80 mg/kg/day PO divided into 2–3 doses. Continue prophylaxis until exposure has been excluded. If exposure is confirmed and vaccine is available, continue prophylaxis for 4 weeks and until 3 doses of vaccine have been given or for 30-60 days if vaccine is unavailable.

NURSING CONSIDERATIONS

ADMINISTRATION/STORAGE

1. Child's dose should not exceed maximum adult dose.
2. Clients with GFR of 10-30 mL/min should receive 250 or 500 mg q 12 hr, depending on severity of infection. Those with GFR <10 mL/min should receive 250 or 500 mg q 24 hr, depending on infection severity. Those on hemodialysis should receive 250 or 500 mg q 24 hr, depending on infection severity; should receive an additional dose both during and at end of dialysis.
3. Dry powder stable at room temperature for 18–30 months; reconstituted suspension stable 1 week at room temperature and 2 weeks at 2–8°C (36–46°F).

ASSESSMENT

1. List reasons for therapy; C&S results. Identify onset, symptoms, severity, location, other associated factors.
2. Assess for previous reactions to penicillins, cephalosporins or other antibiotics.
3. Obtain/monitor CBC, renal, and LFTs.

CLIENT/FAMILY TEACHING

1. Take entire prescription; don't stop if feeling 'better'; creates antibiotic resistance.
2. For school-age child space evenly over 24-hr period; give before school, upon arrival home, at bedtime.
3. Chewable tablets available for children; may be taken with food.
4. If using tablet for oral suspension (DisperMox), mix 1 tablet in about 10 mL of water. Drink entire mixture, rinse with small amount of water, and drink

---

🔲 = see color insert   **H** = Herbal   **IV** = Intravenous   ℂ = sound alike drug

A

contents to ensure entire dose is taken. Do not chew or swallow tablets.

5. Place pediatric drops directly on child's tongue to swallow. May add drops to formula, milk, fruit juice, water, ginger ale or cold drinks; must be taken immediately and consumed completely.

6. Report unusual symptoms, i.e., ↑ bruising/bleeding, sore throat, rash, diarrhea, worsening of symptoms, or lack of response.

OUTCOMES/EVALUATE

- Resolution of infection; symptomatic improvement
- Therapeutic peak serum drug levels (4–11 mcg/mL)

─── **COMBINATION DRUG** ───

Amoxicillin and Potassium clavulanate

(ah-mox-ih-**SILL**-in, poh-**TASS**-ee-um klav-you-**LAN**-ayt)

CLASSIFICATION(S):
Antibiotic, penicillin

PREGNANCY CATEGORY: B

Rx: Amoclan, Augmentin, Augmentin ES-600, Augmentin XR.

✚Rx: Apo-Amoxi-Clav, Clavulin, ratio-Amoxi Clav.

SEE ALSO *ANTI-INFECTIVE DRUGS* AND *PENICILLINS*.

USES

Augmentin. For beta-lactamase-producing strains of the following organisms: (1) Lower respiratory tract infections, otitis media, and sinusitis caused by *Haemophilus influenzae* and *Moraxella catarrhalis*. (2) Skin and skin structure infections caused by *Staphylococcus aureus, Escherichia coli,* and *Klebsiella*. (3) UTI caused by *E. coli, Klebsiella* species, and *Enterobacter*.

Augmentin ES-600. Recurrent or persistent acute otitis media in pediatric clients due to *Streptococcus pneumoniae* (penicillin MICs less than or equal

to 2 mcg/mL), *H. influenzae* (including β-lactamase-producing strains), or *M. catarrhalis* (including β-lactamase-producing strains) characterized by the following risk factors: Antibiotic exposure for acute otitis media within the preceding 3 months and **either** 2 years of age or younger or daycare attendance. Do not use Augmentin ES-600 to treat acute otitis media due to *S. pneumoniae* with penicillin MIC at least 4 mcg/mL.

Augmentin XR. Community-acquired pneumonia or acute bacterial sinusitis due to confirmed or suspected β–lactamase-producing pathogens, including *H. influenzae, M. catarrhalis, H. parainfluenzae, K. pneumoniae,* methicillin-susceptible *S. aureus,* or *S. pneumoniae* with reduced susceptibility to penicillin. Do not use to treat *S. pneumoniae* with penicillin MIC of 4 mcg/mL or more.

NOTE: Mixed infections caused by ampicillin-susceptible organisms and β–lactamase-producing organisms susceptible to amoxicillin/clavulanate should not require an additional antibiotic.

CONTENT

Powder for Oral Suspension: '125' Powder for Oral Suspension: 125 mg amoxicillin and 31.25 mg potassium clavulanate/5 mL. *'200' Powder for Oral Suspension:* 200 mg amoxicillin and 28.5 mg potassium clavulanate/5 mL. *'250' Powder for Oral Suspension:* 250 mg amoxicillin and 62.5 mg potassium clavulanate/5 mL. *'400' Powder for Oral Suspension:* 400 mg amoxicillin and 57 mg potassium clavulanate/5 mL; *Augmentin ES:* 600 mg amoxicillin (as trihydrate) and 42.9 mg clavulanic acid/5 mL.
Tablets: '250' Tablet: 250 mg amoxicillin and 125 mg potassium clavulanate. *'500' Tablet:* 500 mg amoxicillin and 125 mg potassium clavulanate. *'875' Tablet:* 875 mg amoxicillin and 125 mg potassium clavulanate.
Tablets, Chewable: '125' Chewable Tablet: 125 mg amoxicillin and 31.25 mg potassium clavulanate. *'200' Chewable Tablet:* 200 mg amoxicillin and 28.5 mg potassium clavulanate. *'250' Chewable Tablet:* 250 mg amoxicillin and 62.5 mg

---

Bold Italic = life threatening side effect   ▉ = black box warning   ✚ = Available in Canada potassium clavulanate. '400' Chewable Tablet: 400 mg amoxicillin and 57 mg potassium clavulanate.

Tablets, Extended-Release: 1,000 mg amoxicillin and 62.5 mg potassium clavulanate.

ACTION/KINETICS

Action

For details, see Amoxicillin. Potassium clavulanate inactivates lactamase enzymes, which are responsible for resistance to penicillins. Effective against microorganisms that have manifested resistance to amoxicillin.

Pharmacokinetics

For potassium clavulanate: **Peak serum levels:** 1–2 hr. **t½:** 1 hr.

CONTRAINDICATIONS

Use in those with a history of amoxicillin/clavulanate potassium-associated cholestatic jaundice or hepatic dysfunction. Use of Augmentin XR in severe renal impairment (C_{CR} less than 30 mL/min) and in hemodialysis clients.

SPECIAL CONCERNS

The effect of oral contraceptives may be decreased. Use with caution in hepatic dysfunction. Safety and efficacy of Augmentin XR has not been established in children less than 16 years of age.

SIDE EFFECTS

See Amoxicillin and Penicillins.

HOW SUPPLIED

See Content.

DOSAGE

AUGMENTIN

• ORAL SUSPENSION; TABLETS; TABLETS, CHEWABLE

Susceptible infections.

Adults, usual and children over 40 kg: One 500-mg tablet q 12 hr or one 250-mg tablet q 8 hr. Adults unable to take tablets can be given the 125-mg/5 mL or the 250-mg/5 mL suspension in place of the 500-mg tablet or the 200-mg/5 mL or 400-mg/5 mL suspension can be given in place of the 875-mg tablet. **Children less than 3 months old:** 30 mg/kg/day amoxicillin in divided doses q 12 hr. Use of the 125-mg/5 mL suspension is recommended. **Children over 3 months old:** 200 mg/5 mL or 400 mg/5 mL q 12 hr. Or, 125 mg/5 mL or 250 mg/5 mL q 8 hr.

Recurrent or persistent acute otitis media, sinusitis, lower respiratory tract infections, severe infections in children 3 months and older.

45 mg/kg/day of amoxicillin in divided doses q 12 hr or 40 mg/kg/day amoxicillin in divided doses q 8 hr. For less severe infections, use 25 mg/kg/day in divided doses q 12 hr or 20 mg/kg/day in divided doses q 8 hr.

Respiratory tract and severe infections.
Adults: One 875-mg tablet q 12 hr or one 500-mg tablet q 8 hr.

AUGMENTIN ES-600

• ORAL SUSPENSION

Recurrent or persistent acute otitis media in children.

Children, 3 months and older: 90 mg/kg/day amoxicillin in divided doses q 12 hr for 10 days. Experience is not available for pediatric clients weighing more than 40 kg or for adults.

AUGMENTIN XR

• TABLETS, EXTENDED-RELEASE

Acute bacterial sinusitis.

2 tablets (2 grams amoxicillin) q 12 hr for 10 days.

Community acquired pneumonia.

2 tablets (2 grams amoxicillin) q 12 hr for 7–10 days.

NURSING CONSIDERATIONS

ADMINISTRATION/STORAGE

1. Both '250' and '500' tablets contain 125 mg clavulanic acid; therefore, two '250' tablets are not the same as one '500' tablet. The 250-mg tablet and the 250-mg chewable tablet do not contain the same amount of potassium clavulanate and are thus not interchangeable. The 250-mg tablet should not be used until children are over 40 kg.

2. Two Augmentin 500 mg tablets are not equivalent to one Augmentin XR tablet because Augmentin XR contains 62.5 mg clavulanic acid while each Augmentin 500 mg tablet contains 125 mg clavulanic acid. The XR tablet provides an extended time course of plasma amoxicillin levels compared with the immediate-release tablets.

3. Pediatric formulations are available in fruit flavors for oral suspension and chewable tablets. These formulations

---

A

allow twice-daily dosing; more convenient than three-times daily dosing; and incidence of diarrhea is significantly reduced.

4. The 200- and 400-mg suspensions and chewable tablets contain aspartame; do not use with phenylketonuria.

ASSESSMENT

1. List reasons for therapy; C&S results. Identify onset, symptoms, severity, location, other associated factors.

2. Assess for previous reactions to penicillins, cephalosporins, or other antibiotics.

3. Obtain/monitor CBC, renal, and LFTs.

CLIENT/FAMILY TEACHING

1. Take as directed; complete entire prescription.

2. May take without regard for meals; absorption of potassium clavulanate enhanced if taken just before a meal. To lessen stomach upset, take with food.

3. Do not chew or crush; swallow tablets whole. Consume fluids to ensure adequate hydration.

4. Report side effects, i.e., rash, persistent diarrhea, lack of response, worsening of symptoms after 48–72 hr.

5. Refrigerate reconstituted suspension; discard after 10 days.

6. Return as scheduled for follow-up.

OUTCOMES/EVALUATE

Resolution of infection; symptomatic improvement

Amphetamine mixtures ■ ⬚

(am-**FET**-ah-meen)

CLASSIFICATION(S):
CNS stimulant
PREGNANCY CATEGORY: C
Rx: Adderall XR, Adderall, Amphetamine Salt Combo, **C-II**

SEE ALSO *AMPHETAMINES AND DERIVATIVES.*

USES

(1) Attention deficit/hyperactivity disorder (ADHD) in children over 3 years of age, along with other remedial approaches. Use with the following symptoms: Moderate to severe distractibility, short attention span, hyperactivity, emotional lability, and impulsivity. Learning disability and abnormal EEG may or may not be present; a diagnosis of CNS dysfunction may or may not be warranted. (2) Narcolepsy in adults and children over 6 years of age.

ACTION/KINETICS

Action

Thought to act on the cerebral cortex and reticular activating system by releasing norepinephrine from central adrenergic neurons. Adderall contains equal amounts of dextroamphetamine sulfate, dextroamphetamine saccharate, amphetamine sulfate, and amphetamine aspartate monohydrate in each dosage form.

Pharmacokinetics

Completely absorbed in 3 hr. **Peak effects:** 2–3 hr. **Duration:** 4–24 hr. **Therapeutic blood levels:** 5–10 mcg/dL. **t½, if urine pH is 5.6 or less:** 7– 8 hr; **t½, if urine pH is alkaline:** 18.6–33.6 hr. For every one unit increase in urinary pH, there is an average 7 hr increase in plasma t½. Metabolized in the liver and excreted in urine.

CONTRAINDICATIONS

Use in children less than 3 years of age for attention deficit disorders, in children less than 6 years of age for narcolepsy, or in children or adults with a structural cardiac abnormality due to the possibility of sudden death. Use as an appetite suppressant.

SPECIAL CONCERNS

■ Amphetamines have a high potential for abuse. Administration of amphetamines for prolonged periods of time may lead to drug dependence and must be avoided. Particular attention should be paid to the possibility of subjects obtaining amphetamines for nontherapeutic use or distribution to others, and the drugs should be prescribed or dispensed sparingly.■ Extended-release amphetamine has not been studied in children less than 6 years of age. *NOTE:* Adderall XR has been removed from the Canadian market due to concerns about sudden deaths, heart-relat-

---

Bold Italic = life threatening side effect   ■ = black box warning   ✦ = Available in Canada

ed deaths, and strokes in children and adults taking recommended doses.

SIDE EFFECTS
Most Common
Decreased appetite, upset stomach, insomnia, increased anxiety, irritability.
See *Amphetamine and Derivatives* for a complete list of possible side effects.

HOW SUPPLIED
Capsules, Extended Release: 5 mg, 10 mg, 15 mg, 20 mg, 25 mg, 30 mg; *Tablets:* 5 mg, 7.5 mg, 10 mg, 12.5 mg, 15 mg, 20 mg, 30 mg.

DOSAGE
- **CAPSULES, EXTENDED-RELEASE; TABLETS**
    Attention deficit/hyperactivity disorders in children.

3–5 years, initial: 2.5 mg/day; increase by 2.5 mg/day at weekly intervals until optimum dose is achieved (usual range 0.1–0.5 mg/kg/dose each morning). **6 years and older, initial:** 5 mg 1–2 times per day; increase in increments of 5 mg/day at weekly intervals until optimum dose is achieved (only rarely will doses exceed a total of 40 mg/day). For the extended release capsules, start with 10 mg once daily in the morning; increase in increments of 10 mg/day at weekly intervals, up to a maximum of 30 mg/day.

Attention-deficit/hyperactivity disorder in adults.
20 mg/day with or without food.

Narcolepsy.
Adults and children over 12 years, initial: 10 mg/day; increase in increments of 10 mg/day at weekly intervals until optimum dosage is achieved. **Children, 6–12 years, initial:** 5 mg/day; increase in increments of 5 mg/day until optimum dosage is achieved. For all ages, use immediate-release products. Give the first dose on awakening with additional 1–2 doses at intervals of 4–6 hr.

NURSING CONSIDERATIONS
ADMINISTRATION/STORAGE
1. Take extended-release capsules whole or sprinkle contents on applesauce. If applesauce used, take immediately (do not store). Do not chew applesauce sprinkled with amphetamine beads.
2. Take extended-release capsules upon awakening. Avoid afternoon doses R/T possibility of insomnia.
3. Those taking divided doses of immediate-release amphetamine may be switched to amphetamine extended-release at the same total daily dose taken once daily. Titrate at weekly intervals to effective and tolerable doses.
4. When possible, interrupt therapy occasionally to determine the need for continued therapy.

ASSESSMENT
1. Review CNS/neurologic status before starting therapy.
2. Document symptom type, onset, pretreatment findings, and/or educational testing results.
3. Determine if pregnant.
4. Monitor ht/weight, BP; assess CBC, chemistry profile, urinalysis, and ECG.

CLIENT/FAMILY TEACHING
1. For attention deficit disorders (ADD) or narcolepsy, give the first dose on awakening with additional one or two doses given at intervals of 4–6 hr. Give the last dose 6 hr before bedtime. Extended release product administered once daily upon awakening. The correct dose must be given at the right time; never give doses more than 2 hours late, unless told otherwise by the provider. Never double doses. It is safer for a child to skip a dose than inadvertantly be given two doses.
2. Take with water; do not take with milk, juice, or antacids.
3. Report changes in mood or affect, including S&S of impaired thinking. Also report headaches, extremity weakness or chest pain/SOB immediately.
4. Do not use caffeine/caffeine-containing products. Avoid OTC preparations containing caffeine or other stimulants.
5. Avoid using heavy machinery/driving until drug effects realized.
6. Keep weight records; report excessive loss. Store safely; has potential for abuse.
7. Drink 2.5 L/day; increase intake of high-fiber foods/fruits to decrease constipation.

A

8. Chew sugarless gum/candies and rinse mouth frequently with nonalcoholic mouth rinses for dry mouth.

9. Children receiving amphetamines may have growth retarded. Drug should periodically be discontinued (i.e. during the summer) by provider to allow growth to proceed normally and to evaluate the need for continued drug therapy.

10. Keep F/U visits to evaluate response and assess dose adequacy, and any adverse side effects.

OUTCOMES/EVALUATE

- Improved attention span/concentration/grades
- ↓ Episodes of narcolepsy
- Therapeutic serum levels 5–10 mcg/dL

Amphotericin B ■ⅣⒸ desoxycholate

(am-foe-**TER**-ih-sin)

CLASSIFICATION(S):
Antibiotic, antifungal
PREGNANCY CATEGORY: B
Rx: Amphocin, Fungizone Intravenous.

SEE ALSO *ANTI-INFECTIVE DRUGS.*

USES

Drug is toxic; used mainly for clients with progressive and potentially fatal fungal infections. **Parenteral:** (1) Systemic, potentially fatal life-threatening invasive fungal infections, including aspergillosis; cryptococcosis; North American blastomycosis; systemic candidiasis; coccidiodomycosis; histoplasmosis; sporotrichosis; zygomycosis including mucormycosis caused by *Mucor, Rhizopus,* and *Absidia* species. (2) Infections due to susceptible species of *Conidiobolus* and *Basidiobolus.* (3) Secondary therapy to treat American mucocutaneous leishmaniasis. *Investigational:* Prophylaxis of fungal infection in bone marrow transplantation; treatment of primary amoebic meningoencephalitis due to *Naegleria fowleri;* subconjunctival or intra-

vitreal injection in ocular aspergillosis; bladder irrigation for candidal cystitis; chemoprophylaxis for low dose IV, intranasal, or nebulized administration in immunocompromised clients at risk of aspergillosis; intrathecally in severe meningitis unresponsive to IV therapy; intra-articularly or IM for coccidioidal arthritis.

ACTION/KINETICS

Action

Binds to sterols in the cell membrane causing a change in membrane permeability leading to leakage of a variety of intracellular components. Fungistatic or fungicidal depending on the level of drug in body fluids and susceptibility of the fungus. Can also bind to cholesterol in the mammalian cell leading to cytotoxicity.

Pharmacokinetics

Peak plasma levels: 0.5–2 mcg/mL. **t½, initial:** 24 hr; **second phase:** 15 days. Slowly excreted by the kidneys. Kinetics differ in adults and children. **Plasma protein binding:** 90%.

CONTRAINDICATIONS

Hypersensitivity to drug unless the condition is life-threatening and amenable only to amphotericin B therapy. Use to treat noninvasive forms of fungal disease such as oral thrush, vaginal candidiasis, and esophageal candidiasis in clients with normal neutrophil counts. Lactation.

SPECIAL CONCERNS

■ Use primarily for progressive and potentially fatal fungal infections. Not used to treat noninvasive fungal disease, including oral thrush, vaginal candidiasis, and esophageal candidiasis in clients with normal neutrophil counts.■ The bone marrow depressant effects may result in increased incidence of microbial infection, delayed healing, and gingival bleeding. Although used in children, safety and efficacy have not been determined. Use with caution in clients receiving leukocyte transfusions.

SIDE EFFECTS

Most Common

Hypotension, headache, epigastric pain, normocytic anemia, muscle/joint pain, tachypnea.

Bold Italic = life threatening side effect   ■ = black box warning   ✤ = Available in Canada

GI: Anorexia, N&V, diarrhea, dyspepsia, cramping, epigastric pain, acute liver failure, hepatitis, melena, jaundice, hemorrhagic gastroenteritis. **CNS:** Headache, convulsions, tinnitus, vertigo (transient), peripheral neuropathy, encephalopathy, neurologic symptoms. **CV:** Hypotension, **cardiac arrest, cardiac failure, ventricular fibrillation**, arrhythmias, hypertension. **Dermatologic:** Rash, especially maculopapular, pruritus. **Hematologic:** Normochromic anemia, normocytic anemia (most common), **agranulocytosis**, coagulation defects, thrombocytopenia, leukopenia, eosinophilia, leukocytosis. **GU:** Decreased renal function, azotemia, hyposthenuria, renal tubular acidosis, nephrocalcinosis. **Respiratory:** Tachypnea, **shock**, pulmonary edema, hypersensitivity pneumonitis, dyspnea, bronchospasm, wheezing. **Ophthalmic:** Visual impairment, diplopia. **Miscellaneous:** Hearing loss, fever (with chills, shaking) occurring within 15 to 20 min after starting treatment, malaise, weight loss, pain at injection site (with or without phlebitis or thrombophlebitis), generalized pain (including muscle and joint pain), flushing, **anaphylaxis** and other allergic reactions.

LABORATORY TEST CONSIDERATIONS
↑ AST, ALT, GGT, LDH, alkaline phosphatase, serum creatinine, BUN, bilirubin. Hypomagnesemia, hyperkalemia, hypokalemia, hypercalcemia, acidosis, hypoglycemia, hyperglycemia, hypermyalesmia, hyperuricemia, hypophosphatemia. Abnormal serum electrolytes, liver function, renal function.

OD **OVERDOSE MANAGEMENT**
Symptoms: Cardiopulmonary arrest. *Treatment:* Discontinue therapy, monitor clinical status, and provide supportive therapy.

DRUG INTERACTIONS
Aminoglycosides / Additive nephrotoxicity and/or ototoxicity
Antineoplastic drugs / ↑ Risk for renal toxicity, bronchospasm, and hypotension
Azole antifungals / ↑ Risk of fungal resistance to amphotericin B
Corticosteroids, Corticotropin / ↑ Risk of hypokalemia → cardiac dysfunction
Cyclosporine / ↑ Risk of renal toxicity
Digitalis glycosides / ↑ Risk of hypokalemia → ↑ incidence of digitalis toxicity
Flucytosine / ↑ Risk of flucytosine toxicity due to ↑ cellular uptake or ↓ renal excretion
Nephrotoxic drugs / ↑ Risk of nephrotoxicity
Skeletal muscle relaxants, surgical (e.g., succinylcholine, d-tubocurarrine) / ↑ Muscle relaxation due to amphotericin B–induced hypokalemia
Tacrolimus / ↑ Serum creatinine levels
Thiazides / ↑ Electrolyte depletion, especially potassium
Zidovudine / ↑ Risk of myelotoxicity and nephrotoxicity

HOW SUPPLIED
Powder for Injection: 50 mg (as desoxycholate).

DOSAGE
• **IV**
Test dose by slow IV infusion.
1 mg in 20 mL of D5W injection should be infused over 20 to 30 min to determine tolerance.
Severe and rapidly progressing fungal infection.
Initial: 0.25–0.3 mg/kg over 2 to 6 hr. *NOTE:* In impaired cardiorenal function or if a severe reaction to the test dose, initiate therapy with smaller daily doses (e.g., 5–10 mg). Depending on client status, the dose may be increased gradually by 5–10 mg/day to a final daily dose of 0.5–0.7 mg/kg, not to exceed 1.5 mg/kg/day.
Aspergillosis.
1–1.5 mg/kg/day for a total dose of 3.6 grams.
Blastomyces, Histoplasmosis.
0.5–0.6 mg/kg/day for 4 to 12 weeks.
Candidiasis, Coccidioidomycosis.
0.5–1 mg/kg/day for 4 to 12 weeks.
Cryptococcus.
0.5–0.7 mg/kg/day for 4 to 12 weeks.
Mucormycosis.
1–1.5 mg/kg/day for 4 to 12 weeks.
Rhinocerebral phycomycosis.
0.25–0.3 mg/kg/day, up to 1–1.5 mg/kg/day, for a total dose of 3 to 4 grams.

A

Sporotrichosis.
0.5 mg/kg/day, up to 2.5 grams total dose.
Leishmaniasis.
0.5 mg/kg/day given on alternate days for 14 doses (not recommended as primary therapy).
Prophylaxis of fungal infections in bone marrow transplants.
0.1 mg/kg/day.
Paracoccidioidomycosis.
0.4–0.5 mg/kg/day by slow IV infusion for 4 to 12 weeks.

NURSING CONSIDERATIONS

€ Do not confuse amphotericin B desoxycholate with amphotericin B lipid-based.

ADMINISTRATION/STORAGE

IV 1. The following approaches may decrease severe side effects:
- Give aspirin, acetaminophen, antihistamines, and antiemetics before infusion and maintain sodium balance.
- Give on alternate days to decrease anorexia and phlebitis.
- Small doses of IV corticosteroids before infusion may decrease febrile reactions.
- Adding a small amount of heparin (500–2,000 units) to infusion, removing the needle after infusion, rotating the infusion sites, giving through a large central vein, and using a pediatric scalp-vein may decrease the incidence of thrombophlebitis.
- Meperidine, 25–50 mg IV, may decrease duration of shaking, chills, and fever that may occur.

2. *Preparation of amphotericin B desoxycholate:* To obtain initial concentration of 5 mg/mL, rapidly inject 10 mL sterile water (without a bacteriostatic agent) directly into lyophilized cake, using a sterile 20-gauge needle. Shake vial immediately until colloidal solution clear. To obtain infusion solution of 0.1 mg/mL, further dilute 1:50 with D5W with a pH of 4.2 or above.
3. Determine pH of each container of dextrose injection before use (pH usually >4.2). If pH <4.2, add 1 or 2 mL of buffer to dextrose injection before used to dilute concentrated amphotericin B

solution. Preferred buffer is dibasic sodium phosphate (anhydrous), 1.59 grams; monobasic sodium phosphate (anhydrous), 0.96 gram; and water for injection which is diluted to 100 mL. Sterilize buffer before adding to dextrose injection. Sterilize either by filtration through a bacterial retentive stone, mat, or membrane or by autoclaving for 30 min at 15 lb pressure and 121°C (249.8°F).
4. Strict aseptic technique must be used in preparation; contains no bacteriostatic agent.
5. **Do not** dilute or reconstitute with saline solution or mix with other drugs or electrolytes. If given through an existing IV line, flush with D5W prior to and after infusion.
6. Do not use initial concentrate if any precipitate is present.
7. Protect from light during administration. Loss of drug activity during administration is likely negligible if the solution is exposed for 8 hr or less.
8. Initiate therapy in the most distal veins. When administered peripherally, changing sites with each dose may decrease phlebitis.
9. *Storage/stability of amphotericin B desoxycholate:* Vials should be refrigerated and protected from light. After reconstitution concentrate may be stored in the dark at room temperature for 24 hr or under refrigeration for 1 week. Discard any unused solution. Use diluted solutions promptly after preparation. Protect from light during administration.

ASSESSMENT

1. Note any allergy to amphotericin B, adverse effects, hypersensitivity reactions.
2. Obtain cultures and/or histologic studies prior to systemic therapy.
3. Note mental status and age and reasons for therapy.
4. Describe characteristics of any severe systemic infections/lesions requiring therapy. Different organisms require different lengths of treatment, i.e. sporotrichosis may require 9 mo of IV therapy, whereas topical lesions may require only 2–4 weeks.

Bold Italic = life threatening side effect   ■ = black box warning   ♣ = Available in Canada

5. List drugs prescribed; ensure none interact unfavorably.

6. Monitor CBC, K+, Mg+, renal and LFTs, and cultures during therapy. Stop therapy; report any adverse effects. Monitor for bleeding.

INTERVENTIONS

1. Ensure correct drug form prepared for administration; IV form in D5W only.

2. Note results of 1-mg test dose (1 mg in 20 mL D5W over 20–30 min).

3. Premedicate with antipyretics, antihistamines, corticosteroids, and/or antiemetic drugs to reduce side effects. Rashes, fevers, and chills may occur.

4. Infuse slowly, monitor VS every 15–30 min during first dose; interrupt infusion for adverse effects.

5. Monitor I&O; report change in output; cloudy urine.

6. Weigh twice weekly; assess for malnutrition/dehydration.

7. Anticipate hypokalemia with digoxin therapy. Observe for toxicity, muscle weakness and monitor K^+, Mg^+, digoxin levels.

CLIENT/FAMILY TEACHING

1. GI effects reduced by antihistamine or antiemetic drug before therapy and taking drug before mealtime. Try small frequent meals if diarrhea occurs.

2. Report anorexia, N&V, headache, rashes, fever, chills or other adverse effects.

3. Consume 2.5 L/day of fluids to prevent toxic kidney effects. Report decrease in I&O, extreme weight loss.

4. Therapy usually requires long-term treatments (6–11 weeks) to ensure adequate response and to prevent relapse.

5. Report neurologic S&S such as ringing in ears, blurred vision, or dizziness.

6. Guidelines for therapy with creams and lotions:

- Does not stain skin when rubbed into skin.
- Any discoloration of fabric caused by cream or lotion may be removed by washing with soap and water.
- Discoloration of clothing caused by ointment may be removed with a standard cleaning fluid.

- Report any worsening of condition, lack of response, itching, burning, or rash.

- Do not apply a tight dressing; may promote yeast growth.

7. Keep all F/U appointment to evaluate response to therapy.

OUTCOMES/EVALUATE

- Resolution of fungal infection
- Reduction in number of skin lesions
- Symptomatic improvement

Amphotericin B ▪Ⅳ◎ Lipid-Based

CLASSIFICATION(S):
Antibiotic, antifungal

PREGNANCY CATEGORY: B
Rx: Abelcet, AmBisome, Amphotec.

SEE ALSO *ANTI-INFECTIVE DRUGS AND AMPHOTERICIN B DESOXYCHOLATE*

USES

Drug is toxic; use mainly for clients with progressive and potentially fatal fungal infections. Lipid products decrease the severe renal toxicity of amphotericin B and are indicated for use in clients with renal impairment when amphotericin B can not or should not be used. (1) **Abelcet:** Systemic invasive fungal infections in those refractory to conventional amphotericin B desoxycholate therapy or when renal impairment or toxicity precludes use of the desoxycholate product. (2) **AmBisome:** Treatment of infections due to *Aspergillus, Candida,* or *Cryptococcus;* empirical treatment in febrile, neutropenic clients with presumed fungal infection; cryptococcal meningitis in HIV-infected clients; visceral leishmaniasis. (3) **Amphotec:** Treatment of invasive aspergillosis.

ACTION/KINETICS

Action
See *Amphotericin B desoxycholate.*

Pharmacokinetics
Lipid-based products increase the circulation time and alter the biodistribution of amphotericin. Since lipid-based drugs stay in the circulation longer, they can localize and attain higher con-

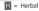

centrations in areas with increased capillary permeability (e.g., inflammation, infection, solid tumors). Importantly, the three amphotericin lipid-based products have different physical and chemical properties that affect their use, pharmacokinetic properties, and side effects. Each of the products has a long terminal t½ and varies depending on the product (about 6.3–6.8 hr for AmBisome, 27.5–28.3 hr for Amphotec, and about 173.4 hr for Abelcet).

CONTRAINDICATIONS
See *Amphotericin B desoxycholate*.

SPECIAL CONCERNS
■ Use primarily for progressive and potentially fatal fungal infections. Not used to treat noninvasive fungal disease, including oral thrush, vaginal candidiasis, and esophageal candidiasis in clients with normal neutrophil counts.■ Use with caution in impaired renal function.

SIDE EFFECTS
Most Common
Chills, fever, hypotension, tachycardia, N&V, dyspnea.

• **Common to all products**
CV: Hypotension, hypertension, *cardiac arrest,* chest pain, tachycardia. **GI:** N&V, diarrhea, abdominal pain, *GI hemorrhage.* **CNS:** Headache, anxiety, confusion, insomnia, leukoencephalopathy. **Respiratory:** *Respiratory failure,* dyspnea, respiratory disorder, hypoxia, increased cough, epistaxis, lung disorder, pleural effusion, rhinitis. **Hematologic:** Thrombocytopenia, anemia, leukopenia. **Dermatologic:** Rash, pruritus, sweating. **Infusion reactions:** Fever, shaking, chills, hypotension, anorexia, N&V, headache, tachypnea. **Miscellaneous:** Chills, fever, *multiple organ failure, sepsis, anaphylactic reaction,* infection, pain, kidney failure, asthenia, back pain, hematuria.

• **Reported for Abelcet**
CV: *Cardiac failure, MI, cardiomyopathy,* arrhythmias, including *ventricular fibrillation.* **GI:** Melena, dyspepsia, cramping, epigastric pain. **CNS:** Convulsions, peripheral neuropathy, transient vertigo, encephalopathy, *CVA,* extrapyramidal syndrome and other neurologic

symptoms. **Hematologic:** Coagulation defects, leukocytosis, eosinophilia. **GU:** Oliguria, decreased renal function, anuria, renal tubular acidosis, impotence, dysuria. **Respiratory:** Bronchospasm, wheezing, asthma, pulmonary edema, hemoptysis, *pulmonary embolus,* tachypnea, pleural effusion. **Hepatic:** Hepatitis, jaundice, *acute liver failure,* veno-occlusive liver disease, hepatomegaly, cholangitis, cholecystitis. **Dermatologic:** Maculopapular rash, exfoliative dermatitis, erythema multiforme. **Musculoskeletal:** Myasthenia, bone pain, muscle pain, joint pain. **Ophthalmic:** Visual impairment, diplopia. **Otic:** Deafness, tinnitus, hearing loss. **Miscellaneous:** Malaise, weight loss, reaction at injection site (including inflammation, anaphylactoid and other allergic reactions), *shock,* thrombophlebitis, anorexia, acidosis.

• **Reported for AmBisome**
CV: Arrhythmia, atrial fibrillation, bradycardia, cardiomegaly, *hemorrhage,* postural hypotension, valvular heart disease, vascular disorder, flushing, veno-occlusive disease. **GI:** Anorexia, constipation, dry mouth/nose, dyspepsia, dysphagia, eructation, fecal incontinence, *GI hemorrhage,* hemorrhoids, gum/oral hemorrhage, hematemesis, hepatocellular damage, hepatomegaly, mucositis, rectal disorder, stomatitis, ulcerative stomatitis. **CNS:** Agitation, *coma, convulsions,* cough, depression, dysesthesia, dizziness, hallucinations, nervousness, paresthesia, somnolence, abnormal thinking, tremor. **Hematologic:** Coagulation disorder, ecchymosis, fluid overload, petechia, agranulocytosis. **GU:** Abnormal renal function, acute renal failure, dysuria, toxic nephropathy, urinary incontinence, vaginal hemorrhage, hemorrhagic cystitis. **Respiratory:** Asthma, atelectasis, hemoptysis, hiccough, hyperventilation, flu-like symptoms, lung edema, pharyngitis, pneumonia, sinusitis, cyanosis, hypoventilation, pulmonary edema. **Dermatologic:** Alopecia, dry skin, herpes simplex, inflammation at injection site, purpura, skin discoloration, skin disorder/ulcer, urticaria, vesiculobullous

---

Bold Italic = life threatening side effect   ■ = black box warning   ✦ = Available in Canada

rash. **Musculoskeletal:** Arthralgia, bone pain, dystonia, myalgia, rigors. **Ophthalmic:** Conjunctivitis, dry eyes, eye hemorrhage. **Miscellaneous:** Enlarged abdomen, cellulitis, cell-mediated immunological reaction, face edema, graft-vs-host disease, malaise, neck pain, angioedema, erythema.

• Reported for Amphotec

CV: Postural hypotension, *hemorrhage*, *shock*, arrhythmia, atrial fibrillation, bradycardia, CHF, phlebitis, supraventricular tachycardia, syncope, vasodilation, veno-occlusive liver disease, ventricular extrasystoles. **GI:** Dry mouth, hematemesis, jaundice, stomatitis, anorexia, bloody diarrhea, constipation, dyspepsia, fecal incontinence, GI disorder, gingivitis, glossitis, *hepatic failure*, melena, mouth ulceration, oral moniliasis, rectal disorder. **CNS:** Dizziness, somnolence, abnormal thinking, tremor, agitation, depression, *convulsions*, hallucinations, hypertonia, nervousness, neuropathy, paresthesia, psychosis, speech disorder, stupor. **Hematologic:** Coagulation disorder, ecchymosis, hypochromic anemia, leukocytosis, petechia. **GU:** Dysuria, oliguria, urinary incontinence/retention, urinary tract disorder. **Dermatologic:** Maculopapular rash, acne, alopecia, petechial rash, skin discoloration/disorder, skin nodule/ulcer, urticaria, vesiculobullous rash. **Respiratory:** Apnea, asthma, hyperventilation, hemoptysis, lung edema, pharyngitis, sinusitis. **Musculoskeletal:** Arthralgia, myalgia. **Ophthalmic:** Eye hemorrhage, amblyopia. **Otic:** Deafness, ear disorder, tinnitus. **Miscellaneous:** Peripheral edema, weight gain or loss, acidosis, dehydration, enlarged abdomen, facial edema, mucous membrane disorder, accidental injury, allergic reaction, *death*, hypothermia, immune system disorder, injection site inflammation/pain/reaction, neck pain.

LABORATORY TEST CONSIDERATIONS
Those common to all products
↑ ALT, AST, creatine, BUN, alkaline phosphatase. Hyperbilirubinemia, hypokalemia, hypomagnesemia, hyperglycemia, hypernatremia, hypocalcemia,

hypervolemia. Abnormal liver function tests.

Those for Abelcet
Hyperkalemia, hypercalcemia, ↑ LDH, hyperamylasemia, hypoglycemia, hyperuricemia, hyperphosphatemia.

Those for AmBisome
↑ Amylase, LDH, NPN. ↑ or ↓ Prothrombin. Hyperchloremia, hyperkalemia, hypermagnesemia, hyperphosphatemia, hyponatremia, hypophosphatemia, hypoproteinemia.

Those for Amphotec
↑ LDH, gamma glutamyl transpeptidase, fibrinogen. ↓ Prothrombin, thromboplastin. Hypophosphatemia, hyponatremia, hyperkalemia, hyperlipemia, hypoglycemia, hypoproteinemia, albuminuria, glycosuria.

OD **OVERDOSE MANAGEMENT**
SEE ALSO *AMPHOTERICIN B DESOXYCHOLATE.*

DRUG INTERACTIONS
See *Amphotericin B desoxycholate.*

HOW SUPPLIED
Abelcet: *Suspension for Injection (as lipid complex):* 100 mg/20 mL.
AmBisome: *Powder for Injection (as liposomal):* 50 mg.
Amphotec: *Powder for Injection (as cholesteryl):* 50 mg, 100 mg.

DOSAGE ————————————
ABELCET
• **IV**
Systemic fungal infections.
5 mg/kg/day prepared as a 1 mg/mL infusion and given at a rate of 2.5 mg/kg/hr. For children and those with CV disease, dilute the drug to a final concentration of 2 mg/mL. If the infusion exceeds 2 hr, mix the contents by shaking the infusion bag. Do not use an in-line filter.
AMBISOME
• **IV**
Empirical fungal infections.
3 mg/kg/day using a controlled infusion device over about 2 hr. Can reduce infusion time to 60 min if well tolerated or increase if client is uncomfortable.
Infections due to Aspergillus, Candida, Cryptococcus.
3–5 mg/kg/day prepared as a 1–2 mg/mL infusion and given initially over

2 hr. Can reduce infusion time to 60 min if well tolerated or increase if client is uncomfortable. For infants and small children, infusion concentrations of 0.2–0.5 mg/mL may be better. A micron or more in-line filter may be used.

Cryptococcal meningitis in HIV.
6 mg/kg/day using a controlled infusion device over 2 hr. Can reduce infusion time to 60 min if well tolerated or increase if client is uncomfortable.

Leishmaniasis.
3 mg/kg/day on days 1 through 5, 14, and 21 to immunocompetent clients; repeat course may be given if parasite is not eradicated. Give 4 mg/kg/day on days 1 through 5, 10, 17, 24, 31, and 38 to immunosuppressed clients; if parasite is not eradicated, seek expert advice regarding further therapy.

AMPHOTEC
• **IV**
Systemic fungal infections.
3–4 mg/kg/day prepared as a 0.6 mg/mL (range: 0.16–0.83 mg/mL) infusion given at a rate of 1 mg/kg/hr. Give a test dose of 1.6–8.3 mg infused over 15–30 min. Do not filter or use an inline filter.

NURSING CONSIDERATIONS

℗ Do not confuse amphotericin B lipid-based with amphotericin B desoxycholate.

ADMINISTRATION/STORAGE

IV 1.   The following approaches may decrease severe side effects:
• Give aspirin, acetaminophen, antihistamines, and antiemetics before infusion and maintain sodium balance.
• Give on alternate days to decrease anorexia and phlebitis.
• Small doses of IV corticosteroids before infusion may decrease febrile reactions.
• Adding small amount of heparin (500–2,000 units) to infusion, removing the needle after infusion, rotating the infusion sites, giving through a large central vein, and using a pediatric scalp-vein may decrease incidence of thrombophlebitis.

• Meperidine, 25–50 mg IV, may decrease duration of shaking, chills, and fever that may occur.
2. *Preparation of amphotericin B lipid complex (Abelcet):* Shake vial gently until there is no yellow sediment at the bottom. Withdraw appropriate dose from the required number of vials into one or more sterile 20-mL syringes using an 18-gauge needle. Remove needle from each syringe filled with liposomal amphotericin B and replace with a 5-micron filter needle. Each filter needle is used for just one vial. Insert filter needle on the syringe into an IV bag containing D5W and empty syringe contents into the bag. The infusion concentration should be 1 mg/mL. For pediatric clients and those with CV disease, the drug may be diluted with D5W to a final infusion concentration of 2 mg/mL.
3. *Preparation of liposomal amphotericin B (AmBisome):* Add 12 mL of sterile water for injection to each vial to yield 4 mg/mL. Immediately shake vial vigorously for 30 sec to completely disperse drug until yellow, translucent suspension is formed. After calculating dose, withdraw appropriate amount of reconstituted suspension into a sterile syringe. Attach 5 micron filter provided and inject syringe contents through the filter needle into an appropriate volume of D5W for final concentration of 1 to 2 mg/mL.
4. *Preparation of amphotericin B cholesteryl (Amphotec):* Reconstitute only with sterile water for injection. Using sterile syringe and 20–gauge needle, rapidly add the following volumes to the vial to provide a liquid containing 5 mg/mL. Shake gently by hand, rotating vial until all solids have dissolved (fluid may be opalescent or clear). For 50 mg/vial add 10 mL sterile water; 100 mg/vial add 20 mL sterile water. For infusion, further dilute to final concentration of about 0.6 mg/mL (range 0.16–0.83 mg/mL).
5. Strict aseptic technique must be used in preparation; contains no bacteriostatic agent.
6. Do not dilute or reconstitute with saline solution or mix with other drugs

or electrolytes. If given through an existing IV line, flush with D5W before and after infusion.

7. Do not use initial concentrate if any precipitate is present.

8. Protect from light during administration. Loss of drug activity during administration is likely negligible if the solution is exposed for <8 hr.

9. Initiate therapy in the most distal veins. When administered peripherally, changing sites with each dose may decrease phlebitis.

10. *Storage/stability of amphotericin B lipid complex (Abelcet):* Prior to admixture store at 2–8°C (36–46°F). Protect from exposure to light; do not freeze. Keep in the carton until used. Admixture may be stored for up to 48 hr at 2–8°C (36–46°F) and an additional 6 hr at room temperature.

11. *Storage/stability of liposomal amphotericin B (AmBisome):* Store unopened vials at 2–8°C (36–46°F), without freezing. Keep product in the carton until used. Store reconstituted product concentrate at 2–8°C (36–46°F) for up to 24 hr. Do not freeze. Use within 6 hr of dilution with D5W. Discard any unused drug.

12. *Storage/stability of amphotericin B cholesteryl (Amphotec):* Store unopened vials at 15–30°C (59–86°F). After reconstitution, refrigerate at 2–8°C (36–46°F) and use within 24 hr; do not freeze. After further dilution with D5W, store in refrigerator at 2–8°C (36–46°F); use within 24 hr.

ASSESSMENT

1. Check for any allergy to amphotericin, adverse effects, hypersensitivity reactions.

2. Assess mental status; note age and reasons for therapy.

3. Describe characteristics of systemic infections requiring therapy. Different organisms require different lengths of treatment time.

4. List drugs prescribed; ensure none interact unfavorably.

5. Monitor CBC, renal and LFTs, cultures during therapy. Stop therapy/report any adverse effects. Monitor for bleeding, progressive liver and kidney dys-

function. The lipid form is generally used with kidney impairment.

INTERVENTIONS

1. Ensure correct form prepared for administration.

2. Premedicate with antipyretics, antihistamines, corticosteroids, and/or antiemetic drugs to reduce side effects. Rashes, fevers, and chills may occur.

3. Infuse slowly until response identified. May increase infusion time if well tolerated or decrease if not tolerated according to manufacturers' guidelines and orders.

4. Monitor VS every 15–30 min during first dose; interrupt infusion for adverse effects.

5. Monitor I&O; report change in output, cloudy urine. Weigh twice weekly; assess for malnutrition/ dehydration.

6. Assess for hypokalemia with digoxin therapy; and hyponatremia with this therapy. Observe for toxicity/muscle weakness and monitor K^+, Na, Mg^+, and digoxin levels.

7. Identify and protect those that are severely immunocompromised.

CLIENT/FAMILY TEACHING

1. Reduce GI effects with an antihistamine or antiemetic before drug therapy; administer before mealtime. Try small frequent meals if diarrhea occurs.

2. Report any anorexia, N&V, headache, rashes, fever, or chills.

3. Consume fluids as directed to prevent dehydration and further toxic kidney effects. Report any changes in I&O and extreme weight loss.

4. Therapy usually requires long-term treatments to ensure adequate response (eradication of organism) and prevent relapse.

5. Report neurologic symptoms such as ringing in ears, blurred vision, or dizziness.

6. Fever reaction may diminish with prolonged therapy, muscle pain/aches may be R/T low potassium.

7. Report any bleeding, bruising, or soft tissue swelling as well as vertigo or hearing loss. Keep all F/U lab and provider visits.

OUTCOMES/EVALUATE

• Resolution of fungal infection

- Eradication of parasites
- Symptomatic improvement

Ampicillin oral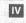
(am-pih-**SILL**-in)

CLASSIFICATION(S):
Antibiotic, penicillin
PREGNANCY CATEGORY: B
Rx: Principen.
♣Rx: Novo-Ampicillin.

Ampicillin sodium, parenteral

PREGNANCY CATEGORY: B
Rx: Ampicillin sodium.

SEE ALSO *ANTI-INFECTIVE DRUGS AND PENICILLINS.*

USES
(1) Respiratory tract infections due to non-penicillinase-producing *Haemophilus influenzae*, penicillinase (injection only) and non-penicillinase-producing staphylococci, and streptococci, including *Streptococcus pneumoniae*. (2) GI infections due to *Shigella, Salmonella typhosa* and other salmonella, *E. coli, P. mirabilis*, and enterococci. (3) GU infections due to *E. coli, P. mirabilis, Shigella, S. typhosa* and other salmonella, enterococci, and non-penicillinase-producing *Neisseria gonorrhoeae*. (4) Use of the injection only for bacterial meningitis due to *Neisseria meningitides, E. coli, Listeria monocytogenes* and Group B streptococci. Addition of an aminoglycoside may enhance effectiveness against gram negative bacteria. (5) Use of the injection only for septicemia and endocarditis due to *Streptococcus* species, penicillin G susceptible staphylococci, enterococci, *E. coli, P. mirabilis*, and *Salmonella*. Addition of an aminoglycoside may enhance effectiveness when treating streptococcal endocarditis.

ACTION/KINETICS

Action
Synthetic, broad-spectrum antibiotic suitable for gram-negative bacteria.

Acid resistant, destroyed by penicillinase.

Pharmacokinetics
Absorbed more slowly than other penicillins. From 30 to 60% of PO dose absorbed from GI tract. **Peak serum levels; PO:** 1.8–2.9 mcg/mL after 2 hr; **IM,** 4.5–7 mcg/mL. **t½:** 80 min–range 50–110 min. Partially inactivated in liver; 25–85% excreted unchanged in urine.

SIDE EFFECTS
Most Common
Hypersensitivity, N&V, gastritis, stomatitis.

See *Penicillins* for a complete list of potential side effects.

ADDITIONAL DRUG INTERACTIONS
Allopurinol / ↑ Skin rashes
Oral contraceptives / ↓ Effect of ampicillin

HOW SUPPLIED
Ampicillin oral: *Capsules (trihydrate):* 250 mg, 500 mg; *Powder for Oral Suspension (trihydrate):* 125 mg/5 mL, 250 mg/5 mL.

Ampicillin sodium, parenteral: *Powder for Injection:* 250 mg, 500 mg, 1 gram, 2 grams.

DOSAGE

• AMPICILLIN ORAL: CAPSULES, ORAL SUSPENSION; AMPICILLIN SODIUM: IM, IV

Respiratory tract and soft tissue infections.

PO, 20 kg or more: 250 mg q 6 hr; **less than 20 kg:** 50 mg/kg/day in equally divided doses q 6–8 hr. **IV, IM, 40 kg or more:** 250–500 mg q 6 hr; **less than 40 kg:** 25–50 mg/kg/day in equally divided doses q 6–8 hr.

Enterococcal endocarditis.

12 grams/day IV either continuously or in equally divided doses q 4 hr plus 1 mg/kg gentamicin, IM or IV, q 8 hr for 4–6 weeks.

Bacterial meningitis.

Adults and children: 150–200 mg/kg/day in divided doses q 3 to 4 hr. Initially give IV drip, followed by IM q 3 to 4 hr.

Bacterial endocarditis prophylaxis (dental, oral, or upper respiratory tract procedures).

Bold Italic = life threatening side effect   ■ = black box warning   ♣ = Available in Canada

Clients at moderate risk or those unable to take PO medications: **Adults, IM, IV:** 2 grams 30 min prior to procedure; **children:** 50 mg/kg, 30 min prior to procedure. Clients at high risk: **Adults, IM, IV:** 2 grams ampicillin plus gentamicin, 1.5 mg/kg, given 30 min before procedure followed in 6 hr by ampicillin, 1 gram IM or IV, or amoxicillin, 1 gram PO. **Children, IM, IV:** Ampicillin, 50 mg/kg, plus gentamicin, 1.5 mg/kg, 30 min prior to procedure followed in 6 hr by ampicillin, 25 mg/kg IM or IV, or amoxicillin, 25 mg/kg PO.

Septicemia.

Adults/children: 150–200 mg/kg/day, IV for first 3 days, then IM q 3–4 hr.

GI and GU infections, other than N. gonorrhoeae.

Adults/children, more than 20 kg: 500 mg PO q 6 hr. Use larger doses, if needed, for severe or chronic infections. **Children, less than 20 kg:** 100 mg/kg/day q 6 hr.

N. gonorrhoeae infections.

PO: Single dose of 3.5 grams given together with probenecid, 1 gram. **Parenteral, Adults/children over 40 kg:** 500 mg IV or IM q 6 hr. **Children, less than 40 kg:** 50 mg/kg/day IV or IM in equally divided doses q 6 to 8 hr.

Urethritis in males caused by N. gonorrhoeae.

Parenteral, males over 40 kg: Two 500 mg doses IV or IM at an interval of 8 to 12 hr. Repeat treatment if necessary. In complicated gonorrheal urethritis, prolonged and intensive therapy is recommended.

Prophylaxis for neonatal Group B streptococcal disease.

If culture is positive or risk factors are present, give 2 grams IV during labor; then, 1 gram IV q 4 hr until delivery. In preterm, premature rupture of membranes in Group B negative women, give 2 grams ampicillin IV q 6 hr plus erythromycin, 250 mg IV, q 8 hr for 48 hr; then, amoxicillin, 250 mg plus erythromycin base, 333 mg, q 8 hr PO for 5 days.

NURSING CONSIDERATIONS
ADMINISTRATION/STORAGE
1. Reconstituted PO solution stable for 7 days at room temperature, not exceeding 25°C (77°F); 14 days refrigerated.
2. For IM use, dilute only with sterile or bacteriostatic water for injection.
3. If the C_{CR} <10 mL/min, dosing interval should be increased to 12 hr.
IV 4. After reconstitution for IM or direct IV administration, solution **must be used within the hour.**
5. For IVPB, ampicillin may be reconstituted with NaCl injection.
6. Once reconstituted, give IV slowly over at least 10–15 min.
7. For IV, check compatibility and length of time drug retains potency in a particular solution. Use within one hr.

ASSESSMENT
1. List characteristics of S&S. Identify onset, severity, location, other associated factors.
2. Note history of sensitivity/reactions to this or related drugs.
3. Monitor CBC, cultures, renal and LFTs.
4. IM route may be painful; rotate/document sites.
5. Monitor urinary output and K^+ levels, especially in elderly.

CLIENT/FAMILY TEACHING
1. Take 1 hr before or 2 hr after meals; food may interfere with absorption.
2. Review method for administration/ storage. Consume fluids; ensure adequate hydration.
3. Take for prescribed number of days even if symptoms subside. Report adverse effects or if S&S do not improve or worsen during therapy.
4. Ampicillin chewable tablets should not be swallowed whole.
5. Do not save for future use or share with family members/friends who have similar symptoms.
6. May decrease effectiveness of oral contraceptives; use additional contraception during therapy.
7. Report any 'ampicillin rashes'; a dull, red, itchy, flat or raised rash occurs more often with this drug than with

other penicillins; usually benign. If late skin rash develops with symptoms of fever, fatigue, sore throat, generalized lymph node swelling, and enlarged spleen, a heterophil antibody test may be ordered to rule out mononucleosis.

OUTCOMES/EVALUATE
- Resolution of infection; symptomatic improvement
- Negative culture reports

—COMBINATION DRUG—

Ampicillin sodium/ Sulbactam sodium **IV**
(am-pih-**SILL**-in, sull-**BACK**-tam)

CLASSIFICATION(S):
Antibiotic, penicillin
PREGNANCY CATEGORY: B
Rx: Unasyn.

SEE ALSO *ANTI-INFECTIVE DRUGS* AND *PENICILLINS*.

USES
Infections caused by beta-lactamase-producing strains of the following: (1) Skin and skin structure infections caused by *Staphylococcus aureus*, *Escherichia coli*, *Klebsiella* species (including *K. pneumoniae*), *Proteus mirabilis*, *Bacteroides fragilis*, *Enterobacter* species, and *Acinetobacter calcoaceticus*. (2) Intra-abdominal infections caused by *E. coli*, *Klebsiella* species (including *K. pneumoniae*), and *Bacteroides* (including *B. fragilis*) and *Enterobacter*. (3) Gynecologic infections caused by *E. coli* and *Bacteroides* (including *B. fragilis*). NOTE: Mixed infections caused by ampicillin-susceptible organisms and beta-lactamase-producing organisms are susceptible to this product; thus, additional antibiotics do not have to be used.

CONTENT
Powder for Injection Solution: 1 gram ampicillin sodium/0.5 gram sulbactam sodium, 2 grams ampicillin sodium/1 gram sulbactam sodium, or 10 grams ampicillin sodium/5 grams sulbactam sodium.

ACTION/KINETICS
Action
For details, see *Ampicillin oral*. Sulbactam is present in this product because it irreversibly inhibits beta-lactamases, thus ensuring activity of ampicillin against beta-lactamase-producing microorganisms. Thus, sulbactam broadens the antibiotic spectrum of ampicillin to those bacteria normally resistant to it.

Pharmacokinetics
Peak serum levels, after IV infusion: 15 min. t$\frac{1}{2}$, **both drugs:** about 1 hr. From 75–85% of both drugs are excreted unchanged in the urine within 8 hr after administration.

SPECIAL CONCERNS
Safety and efficacy in children 1 year of age and older have not been established for intra-abdominal infections or for IM administration.

SIDE EFFECTS
Most Common
Hypersensitivity, N&V, gastritis, stomatitis.
See *Penicillins* for a complete list of potential side effects. **At site of injection:** Pain and thrombophlebitis. **GI:** Diarrhea, N&V, flatulence, abdominal distention, glossitis. **CNS:** Fatigue, malaise, headache. **GU:** Dysuria, urinary retention. **Miscellaneous:** Itching, chest pain, edema, facial swelling, erythema, chills, tightness in throat, epistaxis, substernal pain, mucosal bleeding, candidiasis.

LABORATORY TEST CONSIDERATIONS
↑ AST, ALT, alkaline phosphatase, LDH, creatinine, BUN; also, ↑ basophils, eosinophils, lymphocytes, monocytes, platelets. ↓ Serum albumin and total proteins, H&H, RBCs, WBCs, and platelets. Presence of RBCs and hyaline casts in urine.

OD **OVERDOSE MANAGEMENT**
Symptoms: Neurologic symptoms, including **convulsions.** *Treatment:* Both ampicillin and sulbactam may be removed by hemodialysis.

HOW SUPPLIED
See *Content*.

DOSAGE————————
- **IM; IV**

Bold Italic = life threatening side effect   ■ = black box warning   ✤ = Available in Canada

All infections.
Adults: 1 gram ampicillin/0.5 gram sulbactam to 2 grams ampicillin/1 gram sulbactam q 6 hr, not to exceed 4 grams sulbactam daily. Doses must be decreased in renal impairment. **Children, over 40 kg:** Use adult doses; total sulbactam dose should not exceed 4 grams/day. **Children, one year and older but less than 40 kg:** 300 mg/kg/day (200 mg ampicillin/100 mg sulbactam) in divided doses q 6 hr.

NURSING CONSIDERATIONS
ADMINISTRATION/STORAGE
1. For IM use: reconstitute with sterile water for injection or 0.5% or 2% lidocaine HCl injection.
2. Must use solutions for IM administration **within 1 hr** of preparation.
 3. After reconstitution, solutions should stand so that any foaming will dissipate; inspect vial to ensure dissolution.
4. For IV use, mix reconstituted drug with any of the following: D5W, D5W/45% NaCl, 10% invert sugar, RL injection, 0.9% NaCl, M/6 sodium lactate injection, or sterile water for injection.
5. Give by slow injection over 10–15 min or, if mixed with 50–100 mL of diluent, over 15–30 min.
6. If aminoglycosides are also prescribed, administer each separately (1 hr apart) because ampicillin will inactivate aminoglycosides.

ASSESSMENT
1. List type, onset, characteristics of S&S.
2. Note sensitivity/reactions to this drug or related drugs.
3. Monitor CBC, cultures, renal and LFTs. With impaired renal function, reduce dose.
4. During first 30 min of IV therapy, monitor closely for S&S of hypersensitivity reactions.
5. Ensure adequately hydrated. Assess for diarrhea and S&S of superinfection.

CLIENT/FAMILY TEACHING
1. Use additional form of birth control if using hormone pills.
2. IM injections extremely painful; expect some discomfort. Report if S&S

worsen, diarrhea, vaginal itching occurs or symptoms do not improve.
3. Report any adverse effects including skin rash; if accompanied by fatigue, sore throat and enlarged spleen and lymph nodes (a heterophil antibody test may be ordered to rule out mononucleosis).

OUTCOMES/EVALUATE
- Resolution of infection
- Symptomatic improvement

Amprenavir ■
(am-**PREH**-nah-vir)

CLASSIFICATION(S):
Antiviral, protease inhibitor
PREGNANCY CATEGORY: C
Rx: Agenerase.

USES
In combination with other antiretroviral drugs for the treatment of HIV-1 infections. Use the oral solution only when amprenavir capsules or other protease inhibitor formulations are not therapeutic options.

ACTION/KINETICS
Action
Inhibitor of HIV-1 protease. Binds to the active site of HIV-1 protease, thus preventing the processing of viral gag and gag-pol polyprotein precursors. Results in formation of immature noninfectious viral particles.

Pharmacokinetics
Rapidly absorbed after PO. High fat meals decrease absorption and should be avoided. **Peak levels:** 1–2 hr after a single dose. The PO solution is 14% less bioavailable than the capsules necessitating a difference in dosing (see Dosage). Metabolized in the liver by the CYP3A4 enzyme system. Excreted mainly in the urine with minimal amounts excreted in the feces. **t½:** 7.1–10.6 hr.

CONTRAINDICATIONS
Use with bepridil, dihydroergotamine, ergotamine, midazolam, rifampin, and triazolam. Lactation. Due to large amounts of propylene glycol ingestion and possible toxicity, do not use the

---

 = see color insert   = Herbal   = Intravenous   ℚ = sound alike drug

solution in infants, children less than 4 years of age, pregnancy, in liver or kidney failure, or in those treated with disulfiram or metronidazole. Concomitant use of amprenavir oral solution and ritonavir oral solution due to large amount of propylene glycol in amprenavir and alcohol in ritonavir oral solutions; they compete for the same metabolic pathways. Use of amprenavir oral solution in clients with hepatic failure. Use of flecainide or propafenone if amprenavir and ritonavir are given together.

SPECIAL CONCERNS

■ Due to large amounts of propylene glycol ingestion and possible toxicity, do not use the solution in infants, children less than 4 years of age, pregnancy, in liver or kidney failure, and in those treated with disulfiram or metronidazole. Use the oral solution only when amprenavir capsules or other protease inhibitors are not therapeutic options.■ Use with caution in those with moderate or severe impaired hepatic function and in the elderly. Safety and efficacy have not been determined in children less than 4 years of age. Use with caution in combination with sildenafil. Amprenavir is a sulfonamide; thus, there is potential for cross-sensitivity between drugs in the sulfonamide class. Possibility of resistance/cross-resistance among protease inhibitors.

SIDE EFFECTS

Most Common

Diarrhea/loose stools, N&V, oral/perioral/peripheral paresthesia, rash, depression/mood disorders.

GI: N&V, diarrhea or loose stools, abdominal pain/discomfort, taste disorders. **CNS:** Depression, mood disorders. **Dermatologic** Maculopapular rash, pruritus, oral/perioral paresthesia, peripheral paresthesia, *Stevens-Johnson syndrome*. **Metabolic:** New onset diabetes mellitus, exacerbation of preexisting diabetes mellitus, hyperglycemia, diabetic ketoacidosis. **Miscellaneous:** Spontaneous bleeding in clients with hemophilia A and B. Redistribution/accumulation of body fat, including central obesity, dorsocervical fat enlargement, peripheral wasting, breast enlargement, 'cushinoid' appearance, oral/perioral/peripheral paresthesia.

LABORATORY TEST CONSIDERATIONS

Hypercholesterolemia, hyperglycemia, hypertriglyceridemia. ↑ Total cholesterol and triglycerides when used with ritonavir.

DRUG INTERACTIONS

Abacavir / Possible ↑ amprenavir C_{max}, AUC, and C_{min}

Aldesleukin / Possible ↑ amprenavir levels

Amiodarone / Serious or life-threatening interactions; monitor levels

Antacids / ↓ Amprenavir absorption; take amprenavir at least 1 hr before or after antacids

Bepridil / Possible serious or life-threatening effects (including arrhythmias); do not use together

Calcium channel blockers / ↑ Levels of all calcium channel blockers when given with amprenavir

Carbamazepine / ↓ Amprenavir levels R/T ↑ liver metabolism; also, possible ↑ carbamazepine plasma levels

Cimetidine / ↑ Plasma amprenavir levels

Clarithromycin / Possible ↑ amprenavir's C_{max}, AUC, and C_{min} and ↓ plasma clarithromycin C_{max}

Cyclosporine / ↑ Cyclosporine levels; possible ↑ amprenavir levels

Delavirdine / ↑ Amprenavir AUC and peak plasma levels and ↓ delavirdine AUC and peak plasma levels; do not give together

Dexamethasone / ↓ Amprenavir levels

Didanosine (buffered product only) / ↓ Amprenavir levels; take at least 1 hr before or after buffered didanosine

Disulfiram / ↑ Risk of toxicity from propylene glycol if used with amprenavir oral solution; do not use together

Efavirenz / ↓ Amprenavir serum levels

Ergot alkaloids / Possible serious or life-threatening effects (e.g., peripheral vasospasm, ischemia of extremities); do not use together

Erythromycin / Possible ↑ plasma amprenavir levels and ↓ plasma erythromycin levels

Ethanol / Large amount of ethanol and propylene glycol may compete for

---

Bold Italic = life threatening side effect ■ = black box warning ✦ = Available in Canada

same metabolic pathway; do not use together

Fentanyl / ↑ Fentanyl plasma levels and half-life; monitor closely

Grapefruit juice / Possible slight ↓ in amprenavir peak plasma levels; probably not clinically important

HMG-CoA reductase inhibitors (atorvastatin, lovastatin, simvastatin) / ↑ Serum levels of HMG-CoA reductase inhibitors → ↑ activity or toxicity (e.g., myopathy, including rhabdomyolysis)

Indinavir / ↑ Plasma amprenavir levels and ↓ plasma indinavir levels

Itraconazole / Possible ↑ plasma levels of both drugs

Ketoconazole / Possible ↑ plasma levels of both drugs

Lidocaine (systemic) / Serious or life-threatening interactions; monitor levels

Loratidine / ↑ Plasma loratidine levels

Methadone / Possible ↓ levels of both drugs

Metronidazole / ↑ Risk of toxicity from propylene glycol if used with amprenavir oral solution; do not use together

Midazolam / Possible serious or life-threatening effects; do not use together

Nelfinavir / Possible ↓ amprenavir C_{max} and ↑ C_{min}; ↑ nelfinavir C_{max}, AUC, and C_{min}

Nevirapine / ↓ Amprenavir serum levels

Oral contraceptives / ↓ Effectiveness of oral contraceptives; use alternate contraceptive measures; also, ↓ amprenavir AUC and C_{min}

Phenobarbital / ↓ Amprenavir levels R/T ↑ liver metabolism

Phenytoin / ↓ Amprenavir levels R/T ↑ liver metabolism

Pimozide / ↑ Risk of serious and/or life-threatening reactions (e.g., cardiac arrhythmias)

Quinidine / Serious or life-threatening interactions; monitor levels

Rifabutin / ↓ Amprenavir AUC (15%) and ↑ rifabutin AUC (193%); decrease rifabutin dosage by at least one-half

Rifampin / ↓ Amprenavir C_{max} by 70% and AUC by 82% R/T ↑ liver metabolism

Ritonavir / ↑ Amprenavir AUC and C_{min} and ↓ ritonavir C_{max}, AUC, and C_{min}; reduce amprenavir capsule dose when given with ritonavir capsules

Saquinavir / Possible ↑ saquinavir C_{max} and ↓ its AUC and C_{min}; ↓ amprenavir C_{max}, AUC, and C_{min}

Sildenafil / ↑ Risk of sildenafil side effects, including hypotension, visual changes, and priapism R/T ↓ liver metabolism; ↓ sildenafil dosage

H *St. John's wort* / Possible ↑ amprenavir metabolism by CYP3A4 → ↓ amprenavir levels and clinical efficacy

Tacrolimus / Possible ↑ tacrolimus levels; ↑ amprenavir levels

Tadalafil / ↑ Risk of tadalafil side effects, including hypotension, visual changes, and priapism R/T ↓ liver metabolism; ↓ tadalafil dosage

Trazodone / ↑ Trazodone plasma levels; monitor closely and adjust dosage as needed

Triazolam / Possible serious or life-threatening effects; do not use together

Tricyclic antidepressants(amitriptyline, imipramine) / Serious or life-threatening interactions; monitor levels

Vardenafil / ↑ Risk of vardenafil side effects, including hypotension, visual changes, and priapism R/T ↓ liver metabolism; ↓ vardenafil dosage

Warfarin / Possible ↑ plasma warfarin levels; monitor INR if used together

Zidovudine / ↑ Amprenavir and zidovudine plasma levels

HOW SUPPLIED

Capsules: 50 mg; *Oral Solution:* 15 mg/mL.

DOSAGE————————

• **CAPSULES**

HIV-1 infection.

Adults and adolescents, aged 13–16 years old: 1,200 mg (eight 150 mg capsules) twice a day in combination with other antiretroviral drugs. **Children, 4–12 years old or aged 13–16 years old with weight less than 50 kg:** 20 mg/kg twice a day or 15 mg/kg 3 times per day, up to a maximum of 2,400 mg daily in combination with other antiretroviral drugs. Give capsules at a dose of 450 mg twice a day to clients with a Child-Pugh score from 7–9; give capsules at a dose of 300 mg twice a day to those with a Child-Pugh score from 10–15.

- **ORAL SOLUTION**
  HIV-1 infection.

Children, 4–12 years old or aged 13–16 years old with weight less than 50 kg: 22.5 mg/kg (1.5 mL/kg) twice a day or 17 mg/kg (1.1 mL/kg) 3 times per day, up to a maximum of 2,800 mg daily in combination with other antiretroviral drugs. **Children, 13–16 years old with weight 60 or more kg or 16 or more years old:** 1,400 mg twice daily. Adults with a Child-Pugh score from 5–8 should receive a reduced dosage of amprenavir oral solution of 513 mg (34 mL) twice daily, and adults with a Child-Pugh score from 9–12 should receive a dose of 342 mg (23 mL) of amprenavir oral solution twice a day. Switch clients from amprenavir oral solution to capsules as soon as they are able to take the capsule formulation.

NOTE: Capsules and oral solution are **not** interchangeable on a mg per mg basis.

NURSING CONSIDERATIONS
ADMINISTRATION/STORAGE
1. If amprenavir and ritonavir are used together, the dosage is: amprenavir, 1,200 mg, with ritonavir, 200 mg, once daily or amprenavir, 600 mg, with ritonavir, 100 mg twice daily.
2. Store at 25°C (77°F).

ASSESSMENT
1. List disease onset, previous agents used and all diseases under treatment.
2. Note evidence of sulfa allergy; potential for cross-sensitivity.
3. Identify all drugs prescribed/consumed to ensure none interact; do medication reconciliation at each visit.
4. Monitor CBC, chemistry panel, lipids, renal and LFTs; adjust dose with liver dysfunction.
5. Ensure not pregnant.

CLIENT/FAMILY TEACHING
1. Take at least 1 hr before or after antacids or didanosine. May be taken with or without food; avoid high fat meals.
2. Take every day as prescribed in combination with other antiretroviral drugs.

3. Do not exchange capsule dose for solution dose as solution is less bioavailable.
4. Do not take supplemental Vitamin E; the Vitamin E content of amprenavir capsules and oral solution exceeds the Reference Daily Intake (RDI) and may predispose one to easy bleeding/bruising.
5. If using hormonal contraceptives, use alternate contraceptive measures.
6. Drug does not cure or prevent disease, only controls symptoms. Always practice safe sex/barrier protection.
7. Do not alter dose or stop therapy without consulting provider. If dose is missed, take as soon as possible and return to the normal schedule. If dose skipped, do not double the next dose.
8. If also taking viagra, may be at an increased risk for low BP, visual changes, and sustained erection.
9. May cause a redistribution of body fat with enlargement centrally and at the back of the neck; may also cause or aggravate diabetes. Report severe nausea or diarrhea and any other unusual adverse effects. Keep F/U visits to monitor drug response and effects.

OUTCOMES/EVALUATE
Treatment of HIV infections; ↓ viral load; ↑ CD_4 counts

Anagrelide hydrochloride
(an-**AG**-greh-lyd)

CLASSIFICATION(S):
Antiplatelet drug
PREGNANCY CATEGORY: C
Rx: Agrylin.

USES
Reduce elevated platelet count and the risk of thrombosis in thrombocythemia, secondary to myeloproliferative disorders; also to reduce associated symptoms, including thrombo-hemorrhagic events.

Bold Italic = life threatening side effect   ■ = black box warning   ♣ = Available in Canada

ACTION/KINETICS

Action

May act to reduce platelets by decreasing megakaryocyte hypermaturation; possible disruption in the postmitotic phase of megakaryocyte development and a reduction in megakaryocyte size and ploidy. Does not cause significant changes in white cell counts or coagulation parameters. Inhibits platelet aggregation at higher doses than needed to reduce platelet count.

Pharmacokinetics

Peak plasma levels: 5 ng/mL at 1 hr. **t½:** 1.3 hr; **terminal t½:** About 3 days. Maximum drug levels and total drug exposure in clients 7–14 years old were about one-half the values in clients 16–86 years old. Food modestly (14%) reduces bioavailability but increased total exposure by 20%. Extensively metabolized in liver and excreted in urine and feces.

CONTRAINDICATIONS

Lactation. Severe hepatic impairment.

SPECIAL CONCERNS

Use with caution in known or suspected heart disease and in impaired renal function. AUC (serum) levels may increase 8-fold in those with moderate hepatic impairment; use lower doses in these clients. Use with caution in severe hepatic impairment (Child-Pugh score from 10 to 15). Safety and efficacy have not been determined in those less than 16 years of age.

SIDE EFFECTS

Most Common

Palpitations, headache, asthenia, dizziness, diarrhea, nausea, abdominal pain, dyspnea, flatulence, edema.

CV: CHF, palpitations, chest pain, tachycardia, arrhythmias, angina pectoris, postural hypotension, hypertension, CVD, vasodilation, migraine, syncope, *MI, cardiomyopathy, CHB, fibrillation, CVA, pericarditis, hemorrhage, heart failure, pericardial effusion, thrombosis*, cardiomegaly, AF. **GI:** Diarrhea, abdominal pain, pancreatitis, gastric/ duodenal ulcers, N&V, flatulence, anorexia, dyspepsia, constipation, GI distress, *GI hemorrhage*, gastritis, melena, aphthous stomatitis, eructation. **Respi-ratory:** Rhinitis, pharyngitis, cough, epistaxis, respiratory disease, sinusitis, pneumonia, bronchitis, asthma, pulmonary infiltrate, *pulmonary fibrosis, pulmonary hypertension, pleural effusion*, pulmonary infiltrates, dyspnea. **CNS:** Headache, *seizures*, dizziness, paresthesia, depression, somnolence, confusion, insomnia, nervousness, amnesia, migraine, asthenia. **Musculoskeletal:** Arthralgia, myalgia, leg cramps. **Dermatologic:** Pruritus, skin disease, alopecia, rash, urticaria. **Hematologic:** Anemia, thrombocytopenia, ecchymosis, lymphadenoma, lymphadenopathy. **GU:** Dysuria, hematuria. **Body as a whole:** Fever, flu symptoms, chills, photosensitivity, dehydration, malaise, asthenia, edema, peripheral edema, pain. **Ophthalmic:** Amblyopia, abnormal vision, visual field abnormality, diplopia. **Miscellaneous:** Back/chest pain, tinnitus.

LABORATORY TEST CONSIDERATIONS

↑ Liver enzymes.

OD OVERDOSE MANAGEMENT

Symptoms: Thrombocytopenia. *Treatment:* Close clinical monitoring. Decrease or stop dose until platelet count returns to the normal range.

DRUG INTERACTIONS

Amrinone / Exacerbation of effects

Aspirin / Less inhibition (slight) of platelet aggregation when given with single 1 mg doses of anagrelide compared with aspirin alone

Cilostazol / Exacerbation of effects

CYP1A2 inhibitors (e.g., theophylline) / Limited inhibition of CYP1A2 by anagrelide; potential for interaction with other products sharing the same clearance mechanism

H *Evening primrose oil* / Potential for ↑ antiplatelet effect

H *Feverfew* / Potential for ↑ antiplatelet effect

H *Garlic* / Potential for ↑ antiplatelet effect

H *Ginger* / Potential for ↑ antiplatelet effect

H *Ginkgo biloba* / Potential for ↑ antiplatelet effect

H *Ginseng* / Potential for ↑ antiplatelet effect

Grapeseed extract / Potential for ↑ antiplatelet effect
Milrinone / Exacerbation of effects

HOW SUPPLIED
Capsules: 0.5 mg, 1 mg.

DOSAGE

• **CAPSULES**
Thrombocythemia.
Adults, initial: 0.5 mg 4 times per day or 1 mg twice a day. Maintain for one week or more. **Children, initial:** 0.5 mg per day. **Then,** in both children and adults adjust to lowest effective dose to maintain platelet count less than 600,000/mcL and ideally to the normal range. Do not increase the dose by more than 0.5 mg/day in any 1 week. Maintenance dose is not expected to be different between adults and children. **Maximum dose:** 10 mg/day or 2.5 mg in single dose. Most respond at a dose of 1.5 to 3 mg/day. In those with moderate hepatic impairment (Child-Pugh score from 7 to 9), start with 0.5 mg/day and maintain for a minimum of 1 week with careful monitoring of CV effects. Do not exceed a dosage increment of more than 0.5 mg/day in any 1 week.

NURSING CONSIDERATIONS

ADMINISTRATION/STORAGE
1. Initiate under close medical supervision.
2. Platelet count usually responds within 7-14 days. The time to complete response (i.e., platelet count less than or equal to 600,000/mcL) ranged from 4–12 weeks.
3. Store from 15–30°C (59–86°F).

ASSESSMENT
1. List etiology, onset, duration of thrombocythemia.
2. Note any CAD, liver or renal dysfunction; document CV assessment, monitor closely.
3. Monitor VS, CBC, renal and LFTs; check platelets every 2 days during first week and then weekly thereafter until stabilized. Monitor for adverse CV effects if used with moderate hepatic impairment.
4. Determine if pregnant.

CLIENT/FAMILY TEACHING
1. Take as directed. Keep all F/U visits to monitor labs/assess response.
2. Used to lower platelet counts; increases usually occur within 4 days after therapy stopped.
3. Practice reliable contraception; may cause fetal harm.
4. Report palpitations, fever/chills, SOB, dizziness, chest/abdominal pain, or unusual bruising/bleeding.

OUTCOMES/EVALUATE
Reduction in platelet counts; ↓ risk of thrombosis

Anakinra
(**an**-ah-**KIN**-rah)

CLASSIFICATION(S):
Antiarthritic drug
PREGNANCY CATEGORY: B
Rx: Kineret.

USES
Decrease signs and symptoms and slow the progression of structural damage in moderate-to-severe active rheumatoid arthritis in clients 18 and older who have failed 1 or more disease modifying antirheumatic drugs (DMARD). Can be used alone or with DMARDs (except tissue necrosis factor blocking drugs).

ACTION/KINETICS

Action
Interleukin-1 (IL-1) production is induced by inflammation. IL-1 degrades cartilage due to its induction of the rapid loss of proteoglycans, as well as stimulation of bone resorption. Anakinra blocks the biologic activity of IL-1 by competitively inhibiting IL-1 binding to the interleukin-1 type I receptor found in many tissues and organs. Thus, symptoms of rheumatoid arthritis improve.

Pharmacokinetics
Is 95% bioavailable. **Maximum plasma levels:** 3–7 hr. **t½, terminal:** 4–6 hr. Plasma clearance decreased 70–75% in those with severe or end-stage renal disease.

CONTRAINDICATIONS

Known hypersensitivity to *E. coli-* derived proteins. Use of live vaccines concurrently with anakinra.

SPECIAL CONCERNS

Associated with an increased incidence of serious infections (especially when used with etanercept). Safety and efficacy have not been determined in immunosuppressed clients, in those with chronic infections, when used with blocking agents, or with use for juvenile rheumatoid arthritis. Vaccination may not be effective in those receiving anakinra. Use with caution during lactation, in treating geriatric clients, and in those with impaired renal function. Safety and efficacy for use in clients with juvenile rheumatoid arthritis have not been determined. Elderly clients may be more sensitive to the drug effects.

SIDE EFFECTS

Most Common

Injection site reaction, worsening of RA, URTI, headache, nausea, diarrhea, sinusitis, arthralgia, flu-like symptoms, abdominal pain.

Injection site reactions: Erythema, ecchymosis, inflammation, pain. **Body as a whole:** Increased incidence of serious infections (especially those with asthma), including cellulitis, pneumonia, bone and joint infections, bacterial pneumonia. Other infections, including URTI, sinusitis, flu-like symptoms. Also, malignancies, headache. Rarely, hypersensitivity reactions. **Hematologic:** Neutropenia. **GI:** Nausea, diarrhea, abdominal pain. **Musculoskeletal:** Worsening of RA, bone and joint infections, arthralgia.

LABORATORY TEST CONSIDERATIONS

↓ Total WBC, platelets, and absolute neutrophil blood counts. Small ↑ mean eosinophil differential percentage. Possible development of anti-anakinra antibodies after 12 months of use.

DRUG INTERACTIONS

Use with adalimumab may result in hypersensitivity reactions, hematololgic events, and serious infections.

HOW SUPPLIED

Injection, Single-Use: 100 mg/0.67 mL.

DOSAGE

• **SC**

Rheumatoid arthritis.

100 mg/day SC.

NURSING CONSIDERATIONS

ADMINISTRATION/STORAGE

1. Give at same time every day.
2. Before administration, visually inspect for particulate matter or discoloration; do not use if evident.
3. Give only one dose/day (i.e., entire contents of 1 prefilled glass syringe). Discard any unused portion; no preservative in product.
4. Store in refrigerator at 2–8°C (36–46°F); do not freeze or shake. Protect from light.

ASSESSMENT

1. Note reasons for therapy, extent, characteristics of disease, other agents trialed/failed; rate pain level.
2. List drugs taking; ensure none interact. Do not administer with TNF blocking agents or to those with juvenile RA.
3. Assess for any evidence of infection before and during therapy; stop drug and report if evident.
4. Monitor CBC, renal and LFTs; Assess joints, evaluate degree of function; note improvements/loss of mobility.

CLIENT/FAMILY TEACHING

1. Review drug insert/guidelines. Perform self injection after instruction. Inject anakinra daily, at same time each day, into the tissues as ordered.
2. Drug comes in single dose syringe and requires refrigeration. Check expiration date, protect from light, heat, and do **not** shake or freeze.
3. Store safely out of reach; dispose of needles and do not reuse needles.
4. Injection site reactions may occur; usually lasting 1–2 weeks. Rotate sites, report any pain, inflammation, bruising at sites.
5. Avoid immunizations with live vaccines.
6. Stop drug and report if any infection suspected. Drug highly toxic; has been associated with increased incidence of serious infections.
7. Anticipate frequent lab visits (q 1 mo x 3 months then q 3 months) for CBC

and to be evaluated regularly by rheumatologist.

OUTCOMES/EVALUATE
Control of RA progression; ↓ joint pain; ↓ bone erosion in those unresponsive to 1 or more DMARDs

Anastrozole
(an-**AS**-troh-zohl)

CLASSIFICATION(S):
Antineoplastic, hormone
PREGNANCY CATEGORY: D
Rx: Arimidex.

SEE ALSO *ANTINEOPLASTIC AGENTS.*

USES
(1) First-line treatment in postmenopausal women with advanced or locally advanced breast cancer whose disease is hormone receptor positive or hormone receptor unknown. (2) Advanced breast cancer in postmenopausal women with progression of the disease following tamoxifen therapy. (3) Adjuvant treatment of postmenopausal early breast cancer that is hormone receptor positive. *NOTE:* Clients with negative tumor estrogen receptors and those who do not respond to tamoxifen are rarely helped by anastrozole.

ACTION/KINETICS
Action
Growth of many breast cancers is due to stimulation of estrogen receptors by estrogens. In postmenopausal women the main source of circulating estrogen is conversion of androstenedione to estrone by aromatase in peripheral tissues with further conversion to estradiol. Anastrozole is a nonsteroidal aromatase inhibitor that significantly decreases serum estradiol levels. Has no effect on formation of adrenal corticosteroids or aldosterone.

Pharmacokinetics
Well absorbed from the GI tract; food does not affect the extent of absorption. $t\frac{1}{2}$, **terminal:** About 50 hr in postmenopausal women. Steady-state levels reached in about 7 days of once daily dosing. Metabolized by the liver and both unchanged drug (about 10%) and metabolites are excreted through the urine. **Plasma protein binding:** 40%.

SPECIAL CONCERNS
Causes changes in circulating levels of progesterone, androgen, and estrogens. Use with caution during lactation. Safety and efficacy have not been determined in children.

SIDE EFFECTS
Most Common
GI disturbances, hot flushes, vasodilation, nausea, asthenia, back pain, pain, peripheral edema, bone pain, increased cough, dyspnea, headache.
GI: N&V, diarrhea, constipation, abdominal pain, anorexia, dry mouth, increased appetite, GI disturbances, anorexia, GI disorder, dyspepsia. **CNS:** Headache, paresthesia, dizziness, depression, somnolence, confusion, insomnia, anxiety, nervousness, hypertonia, lethargy, mood disturbances. **CV:** Hypertension, vasodilation, ischemic CV disease, *venous thromboembolic events, DVT events, ischemic CV event, MI,* angina pectoris, hypertension, thrombophlebitis. **Musculoskeletal:** Asthenia, back/bone pain, myalgia, arthralgia, arthrosis, arthritis, osteoporosis, joint pain/stiffness, pathological fracture, fracture (hip, spine, wrist). **Respiratory:** Dyspnea, increased cough, pharyngitis, sinusitis, bronchitis, rhinitis. **Dermatologic:** Hot flushes, rash, sweating, hair thinning, pruritus, erythema multiforme, *Stevens-Johnson syndrome (rare).* **GU:** Vaginal hemorrhage, UTI, breast pain, vaginal dryness, vaginal bleeding during first few weeks after changing from hormone therapy, breast pain, vulvovaginitis, vaginal discharge, endometrial cancer. **Hematologic:** Anemia, leukopenia, leukorrhea. **Body as a whole:** Pain, edema, weight gain or loss, flu syndrome, fever, asthenia, malaise, accidental injury, infection. **Miscellaneous:** Peripheral edema, lymphedema, pelvic/chest/neck pain, infection, tumor flare, increased appetite, cataracts.

Bold Italic = life threatening side effect   ■ = black box warning   ✦ = Available in Canada

LABORATORY TEST CONSIDERATIONS
↑ GGT, AST, ALT, alkaline phosphatase, total and LDL cholesterol.

HOW SUPPLIED
Tablets: 1 mg.

DOSAGE
- **TABLETS**

  First-line treatment of advanced or locally advanced breast cancer. Advanced breast cancer following tamoxifen therapy. Adjuvant treatment of early breast cancer.

  1 mg daily.

NURSING CONSIDERATIONS

ADMINISTRATION/STORAGE
1. Glucocorticoid or mineralocorticoid therapy is not required.
2. For first-line therapy, continue treatment until tumor regression evident.
3. For adjuvant treatment of early breast cancer, treatment is long-term (up to 5 years).
4. Dosage adjustment not necessary with hepatic or renal dysfunction.

ASSESSMENT
1. Note disease progression, last tamoxifen therapy; rate pain level.
2. Obtain/monitor BP, CBC, renal and LFTs, and pregnancy test.

CLIENT/FAMILY TEACHING
1. Take as directed at same time daily; usually on empty stomach 1 hr before or 3 hr after meals. Consume fluids; ensure adequate hydration.
2. Use reliable birth control; may cause fetal harm and impair fertility.
3. Report unusual side effects, increased SOB/pain.
4. May experience vaginal bleeding esp. during first two weeks of change over from other hormonal therapy; report continued bleeding immediately. May experience rash, hot flashes, itching, and skin lesions.

OUTCOMES/EVALUATE
Control of malignant cell proliferation

Antihemophilic factor (AHF, Factor VIII) ⟨IV⟩ **A**
(an-tie-hee-moh-**FILL**-ick)

CLASSIFICATION(S):
Antihemophilic agent

PREGNANCY CATEGORY: C
Rx: Advate, Alphanate, Bioclate, Helixate FS, Hemofil M, Hyate: C (Porcine), Koate-DVI, Kogenate FS, Monarc-M, Monoclate-P, ReFacto, Recombinate.

USES
(1) Control of bleeding in clients suffering from hemophilia A (Factor VIII deficiency and acquired Factor VIII inhibitors). These products temporarily replace the missing clotting factor in order to correct or prevent bleeding episodes or to perform surgery. AHF is safe and effective for use in children of all ages, including neonates. *NOTE:* Not effective in controlling bleeding due to von Willebrand's disease. (2) Perioperative management of hemophilic clients. (2) ReFacto only: Short-term prophylaxis to decrease frequency of spontaneous bleeding episodes. (3) Hyate C only: Treatment and prevention of bleeding in congenital hemophilia A clients with antibodies to human Factor VIII. Also, for previously nonhemophilic clients with spontaneously acquired inhibitors to human Factor VIII.

ACTION/KINETICS

Action
Plasma protein (Factor VIII) accelerates the conversion of Factor X to activated Factor X which converts prothrombin to thrombin. Thrombin then converts fibrinogen to fibrin resulting in clot formation. *NOTE:* The potency and purity of preparations vary but each lot is standardized. Details on the package should be noted.

Pharmacokinetics
t½: 10–18 hr. One AHF unit is the activity found in 1 mL of normal pooled hu-

man plasma. *NOTE:* ReFacto is albumin free which reduces the risk of viral transmission.

CONTRAINDICATIONS

Use of monoclonal antibody-derived AHF in clients hypersensitive to bovine, hamster, or mouse protein or to murine or porcine factor.

SPECIAL CONCERNS

Since AHF is prepared from human plasma, there is a risk of transmitting hepatitis or AIDS. However, the products are carefully prepared and tested. Koate DVI has not been studied in children and limited studies have been conducted with Alphanate.

SIDE EFFECTS

Most Common

Chills, N&V, irritation at injection site, drowsiness, headache.

CNS: Headache, somnolence, drowsiness, lethargy, fatigue, dizziness, jittery feeling, asthenia. **CV:** Increased bleeding tendency, flushing, angina pectoris, tachycardia, chest discomfort, slight hypotension, acute hemolytic anemia, hyperfibrinogenemia. **GI:** N&V, constipation, stomach ache, diarrhea, anorexia, taste changes, gastroenteritis, abdominal pain. **Dermatologic:** Rash, flushing of face, acne, increased perspiration. **Musculoskeletal:** Myalgia, muscle weakness. **Respiratory:** Nose bleeds, rhinitis, dyspnea, coughing. **Hematologic:** Forearm bleeding following venipuncture, anemia, infected hematoma, forehead bruises, permanent venous access catheter complications. Acute thrombocytopenia (rare) with Hyate: C. **Ophthalmic:** Blurred vision, eye disorder, abnormal vision. **Allergic:** Nausea, fever, hives, chills, urticaria, wheezing, hypotension, chest tightness, stinging at infusion site, hypotension, *anaphylaxis*. **Miscellaneous:** Irritation at injection site, sore throat, cold feet; tingling in arm, ear, and face; fever, chills, urticaria, depersonalization, adenopathy, cold sensation, finger pain. Antibodies may form to the mouse protein found in AHF derived from monoclonal antibodies. Approximately 10% of clients develop inhibitors to Factor VIII, which leads to a significantly decreased re-

sponse. Antihemophilic factor contains traces of blood group A and B isohemagglutins. These may cause **intravascular hemolysis** in clients with types A, B, or AB blood. **Both hepatitis and AIDS may be transmitted from AHF prepared from human plasma**.

HOW SUPPLIED

Powder for Injection: Wide range of concentrations, depending on product.

DOSAGE

• **IV ONLY**

Individualized, depending on severity of bleeding, degree of deficiency, body weight, the presence of inhibitors of Factor VIII, and the level of Factor VIII desired. *NOTE:* AHF levels may rise 2% to 2.5% for every unit of AHF per kilogram administered. The following formula provides a guide for dosage calculation: Expected Factor VIII increase (in % of normal): AHF/international units administered × 2 divided by body weight (in kg). Dosages given are only guidelines. Also, AHF/IU required = body weight (kg) x desired Factor VIII increased (% normal) x 0.5.

Mild hemorrhage.

Minor episodes usually subside with a single infusion of 10 international units/kg if a level of 20% to 30% of normal is obtained. Dosage should not be repeated until further bleeding occurs.

Minor surgery, moderate hemorrhage.

AHF levels should be raised to 30–50% of normal. **Initial:** 15–25 international units/kg; **maintenance, if necessary:** 10–15 international units/kg q 8–12 hr.

Severe hemorrhage involving vital organs.

Increase AHF levels to 80–100% of normal. **Initial:** 40–50 international units/kg. **maintenance:** 20–25 international units/kg q 8–12 hr.

Major surgery.

Raise AHF levels to 80–100% of normal. Administer 1 hr before surgery; check Factor VIII level before surgery. Repeat injections may be given q 6–12 hr. AHF levels should be maintained at 30% of normal for a healing period of at least 10–14 days.

Dental extraction.

Factor VIII level should be increased to 60–80% immediately before the procedure. A single infusion plus PO antifibrinolytic therapy within 1 hr is sufficient in about 70% of cases.

NURSING CONSIDERATIONS
ADMINISTRATION/STORAGE

IV 1. Factor VIII concentrates may be given on a regular schedule to prevent bleeding.

2. AHF is labile inactivated within 10 min at 56°C and within 3 hr at 49°C. Store vials at 2–8°C (36–46°F). Check expiration date. **Do not freeze.**

3. Generally do not store products stabilized with sucrose (e.g., Helixate FS) at room temperature. Refrigerate at all times from 2–8°C (36–46°F). However, Kogenate FS may be stored at room temperature for up to 3 months, although it is still recommended that it be refrigerated. Do not return products stored at room temperature to refrigeration.

4. Warm concentrate and diluent to room temperature before reconstitution.

5. Place one needle in the concentrate to act as an airway and then aseptically with a syringe and needle add the diluent to the concentrate.

6. Gently agitate/roll vial containing diluent and concentrate to dissolve the drug. **Do not shake vigorously.**

7. Administer within 3 hr of reconstitution to avoid incubation if contamination occurs with mixing.

8. Do not refrigerate after reconstitution; active ingredient may precipitate out.

9. Keep reconstituted drug at room temperature during infusion; at lower temperature, precipitation of active ingredients may occur.

10. Administer IV using a plastic syringe (solutions stick to glass syringes). Administer at rate of 2 mL/min, although rates up to 10 mL/min can be used if necessary. If pulse rate increases significantly, reduce rate or discontinue administration.

11. There are a large number of products available. It is important to note the actual AHF units, which are indicated on the vial.

12. Give ReFacto 2 or more times a week for short-term prophylaxis to prevent or reduce the frequency of spontaneous musculoskeletal hemorrhage in those with hemophilia A. In children, shorter dosage intervals or higher doses may be necessary.

13. Store from 2–8°C (35–46°F) except for Hyate: C. Do not freeze.

ASSESSMENT

1. Note blood type. Clients with A, B, and AB are more prone to hemolytic reactions.

2. Identify recent trauma or injury; assess joints carefully.

3. List drugs prescribed; ensure none interact unfavorably.

4. Note baseline hematologic parameters and Factor VIII levels. May develop Factor VIII inhibitors which lead to decreased drug response. Monitor VS, H&H, coagulation studies and factor levels before and during therapy; obtain Coombs' test during therapy.

INTERVENTIONS

1. Document baseline VS; monitor q 5–15 min during infusion. If tachycardia and hypotension occur, slow IV and report.

2. Premedicate (usually diphenhydramine) to reduce allergic S&S.

3. Should only be administered in a center with specially trained personnel familiar with drug therapy and labs equipped to monitor factor levels.

4. Document I&O; assess urine for quantity, color, occult blood.

5. To control spontaneous bleeding, 5% of normal Factor VIII must be present. For moderate bleeding or prior to surgery, 30–50% must be present and for severe bleeding associated with trauma or major surgery, 80–100% of the normal Factor VIII level must be present.

6. Give the first dose 1 hr before surgery, and the second dose (1/2 of the first dose) 5–8 hr after surgery. Maintain Factor VIII levels at 30% of normal for 10–14 days postoperatively.

7. Slow infusion and report if headaches, flushing, numbness, back/joint

pain, visual disturbances, or chest constriction occur.

CLIENT/FAMILY TEACHING
1. Review method for storing/administering AHF at home.
2. If product prepared from human plasma identify rare but associated potential risks, such as hepatitis and HIV. Heat treated or monoclonal antibody preparations may decrease risk.
3. Avoid any drugs/OTC agents that may alter clotting (i.e., ASA, NSAIDS).
4. Increase knowledge level concerning disease process and hereditary transmission. Identify areas necessary to ensure compliance.
5. Reinforce safety measures related to sports, work, risk taking, and sexual activity. Report any unusual bleeding or adverse side effects immediately.
6. Identify local support groups that may assist to understand and cope with this disease.

OUTCOMES/EVALUATE
• Prevention and control of bleeding with hemophilia A
• Promotion of normal clotting mechanisms
• Coagulation times and Factor VIII levels within desired range

Apomorphine hydrochloride
(ey-poe-**MOR**-feen)

CLASSIFICATION(S):
Antiparkinson drug (dopamine receptor agonist)
PREGNANCY CATEGORY: C
Rx: Apokyn.

USES
Acute, intermittent treatment of acute hypomobility, 'off' episodes ('end-of-dose wearing off' and unpredictable 'on/off' episodes) associated with advanced Parkinson's disease. Used as an adjunct to other drugs.

ACTION/KINETICS
Action
Apomorphine is a dopamine receptor agonist. The precise mechanism to treat Parkinsonism is not known but may involve stimulation of postsynaptic dopamine D_2 receptors in the caudate-putamen in the brain. *NOTE:* If apomorphine is used with carbidopa/levodopa, the levodopa pharmacokinetics are not changed; however, motor response differences are significant. Also, the threshold levodopa concentration required to improve motor response was reduced significantly if used with apomorphine leading to an increased duration of action.

Pharmacokinetics
Rapidly absorbed; **time to peak levels after SC:** 10–60 min. **Mean t½, terminal:** About 40 min. Cytochrome P450 enzymes appear to play a minor role in the metabolism of apomorphine.

CONTRAINDICATIONS
Use in those with hypersensitivity to the drug or sodium metabisulfite. IV use. Use with $5HT_3$ antagonists (e.g., alosetron, dolasetron, granisetron, ondansetron, palonosetron) due to the possibility of severe hypotension and loss of consciousness. Lactation.

SPECIAL CONCERNS
Use with caution in those with hypokalemia, hypomagnesemia, bradycardia, concomitant use with other drugs that prolong the QTc interval, genetic predisposition to prolongation of the QT interval, known CV and cerebrovascular disease, or in those with mild to moderate hepatic or renal impairment. Safety and efficacy have not been determined in children. Serious side-effects (including those that may be life-threatening) are more common in geriatric clients.

SIDE EFFECTS
Most Common
N&V, postural hypotension, yawning, dyskinesias, somnolence, dizziness, edema, hallucinations, chest pain, increased sweating, flushing, pallor, rhinorrhea.
GI: N&V, constipation, diarrhea. **CV:** Chest pain/pressure, QT prolongation and potential for proarrhythmic effects, postural hypotension, CHF, angina, *MI, cardiac arrest and/or sudden death.* **CNS:** Somnolence, dizziness, insomnia, hallucinations, confusion, headache, de-

---

Bold Italic = life threatening side effect   ■ = black box warning   ♥ = Available in Canada pression, anxiety, falling asleep during activities of daily living. **Musculoskeletal:** Dyskinesia or exacerbation of existing dyskinesia, arthralgia, limb/back pain, spontaneous hypomobility. **GU:** Prolonged, painful erections; UTI. **Respiratory:** Rhinorrhea, pneumonia, dyspnea. **Body as a whole:** Edema, swelling of extremities, increased sweating, flushing, pallor, fatigue, weakness, dehydration, increased risk of falls. **Injection site reactions:** Bruising, granuloma, pruritus. **Miscellaneous:** Yawning, worsening of Parkinson's disease. Rarely, motivation for apomorphine abuse or a psychosexual reaction (including increased libido, priapism, atypical sexual behavior, heightened libido).

DRUG INTERACTIONS

5HT₃ Antagonists (e.g., alosetron, dolasetron, granisetron, ondansetron, palomosetron) / Profound hypotension and loss of consciousness; do not use apomorphine with any of these drugs
Antihypertensive drugs / ↑ Possibility of hypotension, MI, serious pneumonia, serious falls, bone/joint injuries
Butyrophenones / ↓ Effect of apomorphine R/T dopamine antagonist effect of butyrophenone
Metoclopramide / ↓ Effect of apomorphine R/T dopamine antagonist effect of metoclopramide
Phenothiazines / ↓ Effect of apomorphine R/T dopamine antagonist effect of phenothiazine
Thioxanthines / ↓ Effect of apomorphine R/T dopamine antagonist effect of thioxanthine
Vasodilators / ↑ Possibility of hypotension, MI, serious pneumonia, serious falls, bone/joint injuries

HOW SUPPLIED

Injection: 10 mg/mL.

DOSAGE

• **SC ONLY**
  Parkinson's disease.
Always express the dose of apomorphine in mL to avoid confusion. Doses greater than 0.6 mL (6 mg) are not recommended. Titrate the dose on the basis of effectiveness and tolerance starting at 0.2 mL (2 mg) and up to a maximum recommended dose of 0.6 mL (6 mg). Give

clients in an 'off' state a 0.2 mL (2 mg) test dose in a setting where BP can be closely monitored. Check both supine and standing BP predose and at 20, 40, and 60 min post dose. Those who develop clinically significant orthostatic hypotension to the test are not candidates for treatment with apomorphine. If the client tolerates the 0.2 mL (2 mg) dose and responds, the starting dose is 0.2 mL (2 mg) used on an as needed basis to treat existing 'off' episodes. If needed, the dose can be increased in 0.1 mL (1 mg) increments every few days on an outpatient basis.

For those who tolerate the test dose of 0.2 mL (2 mg) but achieve no response, give a dose of 0.4 mL (4 mg) at the next 'off' period, but no sooner than 2 hr after the initial test dose of 0.2 mL (2 mg). Check both supine and standing BP predose and at 20, 40, and 60 min post dose. If the client tolerates a test dose of 0.4 mL (4 mg) the starting dose should be 0.3 mL (3 mg) used on an as needed basis to treat existing 'off' episodes. If necessary, increase the dose in 0.1 mL (1 mg) increments every few days on an outpatient basis. If a client does not tolerate a test dose of 0.4 mL (4 mg), give a test dose of 0.3 mL (3 mg) during a separate 'off' period, no sooner than 2 hr after the test dose of 0.4 mg). Check both supine and standing BP predose and at 20, 40, and 60 min post dose. If the client tolerates the 0.3 mL (3 mg) dose, the starting dose should be 0.2 mL (2 mg) used on an as needed basis to treat existing 'off' episodes. If needed, and the 0.2 mL (2 mg) dose is tolerated, the dose can be increased to 0.3 mL (3 mg) after a few days. In such a client, the dose should ordinarily not be increased to 0.4 mL (4 mg) on an out-patient basis.

Most clients respond to 0.3 mL to 0.6 mL (3 to 6 mg). There is no evidence that doses greater than 0.6 mL (6 mg) give an increased effect and such doses are not recommended. The average frequency of dosing is 3 times per day. There is limited experience with single doses greater than 0.6 mL (6 mg), dosing more than 5 times per day, or with total daily doses greater than 2 mL (20 mg).

If a single dose of apomorphine is ineffective for a particular 'off' period, do not give a second dose for that 'off' episode. The safety and efficacy of a second dose for a single 'off' episode has not been systematically studied.

Clients who have an interruption in therapy of more than a week should be restarted on a 0.2 mL (2 mg) dose and gradually titrated to effect.

NURSING CONSIDERATIONS

ADMINISTRATION/STORAGE

1. *To avoid confusion, always express the dose in mL; do not give doses greater than 0.6 mL (6 mg).*
2. Clients and caregivers must be given detailed instructions in the preparation and administration of apomorphine. Pay particular attention to correct use of dosing pen.
3. Give apomorphine with an antiemetic (usually trimethobenzamide, 300 mg 3 times/day PO). Start trimethobenzamide 3 days before the initial dose of apomorphine; continue at least during the first two months of therapy. DO NOT use $5HT_3$ antagonist antiemetics (e.g., dolasetron, granisetron, ondansetron, palonosetron).
4. For clients with mild to moderate renal impairment, reduce testing dose and subsequently the starting dose to 0.1 mL (1 mg).
5. Use caution in clients with mild to moderate hepatic impairment due to the increased C_{max} and AUC in these people.
6. Store from 15–30°C (59–86°F).

ASSESSMENT

1. Identify frequency of hypomotility episodes.
2. List all drugs prescribed/consumed; ensure none interact unfavorably. Drug contains sodium metabisulfite; assess for sensitivity. Any $5HT_3$ antagonist (ondansetron etc.) should not be used with this drug due to serious adverse effects.
3. Assess mental status and neurologic evaluations. Ensure test doses performed and documented by provider.
4. Monitor BP, EKG, renal and LFTs. Reduce dose with renal impairment; monitor labs.

CLIENT/FAMILY TEACHING

1. Used to treat loss of control of body movements during a hypomobility phase with advanced Parkinson's disease. Does not prevent these occurrences but helps to improve them once they occur.
2. Dose determined by provider by performing test dose during 'off' period.
3. Drug administered just under the skin by a needle. After careful instruction and return demonstration, you or your care provider may administer at home. Drug is dosed in milliliters; do not confuse with milligrams as you may overdose. All directions and dosages will be written out for you to follow.
4. Read/review patient information sheet that comes with each new refill—for any changes and new information. Call provider to clarify dosage and answer questions.
5. The prefilled glass cartridges used in the injector pen may be set to administer a certain dose. If the cartridge contains only a partial dose you can still set the device for the full dose but you will need to 're-arm' the device and dial in the correct amount of the remaining dose in order to administer the correct amount. Keep a record of how many doses you have delivered for each cartridge to prevent situation from recurring; share with provider.
6. Prep site and rotate injection sites (stomach, upper arms or upper legs) each time; report any adverse site reactions. Use ice before and after injection at site to reduce chances of swelling, redness, pain, itching, bruising or soreness.
7. Drug may cause dizziness, fainting, or drowsiness; avoid activities that require mental alertness; report if persistent.
8. Change positions slowly to prevent sudden drop in BP resulting in dizziness or fainting.
9. Do not change dose without provider approval. Do not use drug if cloudy, green or contains particles; should be

clear and colorless; if not return for a replacement.

10. Avoid consuming alcohol and any other CNS depressants.

11. May experience worsening of symptoms, hallucinations, depression, headaches, yawning, runny nose and swelling of hands, arms, legs, and feet; report if persistent/bothersome.

12. Report chest pain, SOB, fast heartbeats, severe N&V immediately.

13. Store drug in a safe place at room temperature away from children.

14. Keep all F/U visits and labs; bring log of drug dose/usage and concerns/side effects.

OUTCOMES/EVALUATE

Improvement in mobility and body control during hypomobility phase with advanced Parkinson's disease

Aprepitant
(ah-**PREH**-pih-tant)

CLASSIFICATION(S):
Antiemetic
PREGNANCY CATEGORY: B
Rx: Emend.

USES

(1) Antiemetic in combination with other antiemetics to prevent acute and delayed N&V associated with initial and repeat courses of highly emetogenic cancer chemotherapy, including high-dose cisplatin. (2) Antiemetic in combination with other antiemtic agents to prevent N&V associated with initial and repeat courses of moderately emetogenic cancer chemotherapy. (3) Prevention of postoperative N&V. Has not been studied for treatment of N&V.

ACTION/KINETICS

Action

A selective, high-affinity antagonist of human substance P/neurokinin 1 (NK_1) receptors in the brain. It augments the antiemetic action of ondansetron and dexamethasone and inhibits both the acute and delayed phases of cisplatin-induced emesis.

Pharmacokinetics

Absolute bioavailability is about 60–65%. **Peak plasma levels**: 4 hr. Undergoes extensive metabolism primarily by CYP3A4 with minor metabolism by CYP1A2 and CYP2C19. Excreted in both the urine and feces. **$t\frac{1}{2}$, terminal:** 9–13 hr. **Plasma protein binding:** More than 95%.

CONTRAINDICATIONS

Use with astemizole, cisapride, pimozide, or terfenadine (inhibition of CYP3A4 could cause elevated plasma levels of these drugs). Hypersensitivity to any component of the product. Chronic continuous use to prevent N&V. Lactation.

SPECIAL CONCERNS

Has not been studied for treatment of established N&V. Use with caution in clients receiving concomitant drugs that are primarily metabolized via CYP3A4 as aprepitant inhibits this enzyme system, resulting in elevated plasma levels of these drugs and possible toxicity. Use with caution in severe hepatic insufficiency. Safety and efficacy have not been determined in children.

SIDE EFFECTS

Most Common

When used with highly emetogenic chemotherapy: Asthenia/fatigue, anorexia, constipation, diarrhea, N&V, hiccups, dehydration, dizziness, headache.

When used with moderately emetogenic chemotherapy: Fatigue, headache, constipation, dyspepsia, nausea, stomatitis, neutropenia, alopecia.

CNS: Fatigue, dizziness, headache, insomnia, anxiety disorder, confusion, depression, peripheral neuropathy, rigors, sensory neuropathy, tremor. **GI:** N&V, anorexia, constipation, diarrhea, abdominal pain, heartburn, gastritis, epigastric discomfort, dyspepsia, stomatitis, acid reflux, deglutition disorder, taste disturbance, dry mouth, dysgeusia, dysphagia, eructation, flatulence, increased salivation, obstipation. **CV:** Hot flush, *DVT,* hypertension, hypotension, *MI,* palpitations, *pulmonary embolism*, tachycardia. **Dermatologic:** Flushing, alopecia, acne, diaphoresis, rash. **Respi-**

ratory: Hiccups, pharyngolaryngeal pain, cough, dyspnea, lower RTI, nasal secretion, pharyngitis, pneumonitis, respiratory insufficiency, URTI, vocal disturbance. **Hematologic:** Neutropenia, anemia, febrile neutropenia, thrombocytopenia. **GU:** Dysuria, pelvic pain, UTI, renal insufficiency. **Musculoskeletal:** Arthralgia, back pain, muscular weakness, musculoskeletal pain, myalgia. **Metabolic:** Decreased appetite, diabetes mellitus, edema, hypokalemia, weight loss. **Ophthalmic:** Conjunctivitis. **Otic:** Tinnitus. **Body as a whole:** Dehydration, asthenia, fever, mucous membrane disorder, malaise, *septic shock*. **Miscellaneous:** Candidiasis, herpes simplex, neoplasm (benign, malignancy, unspecified), *non-small cell lung carcinoma.*

LABORATORY TEST CONSIDERATIONS
↑ Alkaline phosphatase, AST, ALT, BUN, creatinine, leukocytes. ↓ Hemoglobin, WBCs. Erythrocyturia, hyperglycemia, hyponatremia, leukocyturia.

DRUG INTERACTIONS
Alprazolam / ↑ Alprazolam plasma levels R/T inhibition of CYP3A4
Carbamazepine / ↓ Aprepitant plasma levels R/T increased metabolism by CYP3A4
Clarithromycin / ↑ Aprepitant plasma levels R/T inhibition of CYP3A4; use with caution
Dexamethasone / ↑ Dexamethasone AUC, peak levels, and t½ R/T inhibition of CYP3A4; reduce dexamethasone dose by 50%
Diltiazem / ↑ Aprepitant plasma levels R/T inhibition of CYP3A4; use with caution
Docetaxel / ↑ Docetaxel plasma levels R/T inhibition of CYP3A4
Etoposide / ↑ Etoposide plasma levels R/T inhibition of CYP3A4
Ifosfamide / ↑ Ifosfamide plasma levels R/T inhibition of CYP3A4
Imatinib / ↑ Imatinib plasma levels R/T inhibition of CYP3A4
Irinotecan / ↑ Irinotecan plasma levels R/T inhibition of CYP3A4
Itraconazole / ↑ Aprepitant plasma levels R/T inhibition of CYP3A4; use together with caution

Ketoconazole / ↑ Aprepitant plasma levels R/T inhibition of CYP3A4; use together with caution
Methylprednisolone / ↑ Methylprednisolone AUC, peak levels, and t½ R/T inhibition of CYP3A4; reduce IV methylprednisolone dose by 25% and PO dose by 50%
Midazolam / ↑ Midazolam AUC, peak plasma levels, and t½ R/T inhibition of CYP3A4
Nefazodone / ↑ Aprepitant plasma levels R/T inhibition of CYP3A4; use together with caution
Nelfinavir / ↑ Aprepitant plasma levels R/T inhibition of CYP3A4; use together with caution
Oral contraceptives / ↓ Oral contraceptive effectiveness; use alternative or backup contraceptive methods during treatment and for 1 month after the last dose
Paclitaxel / ↑ Paclitaxel plasma levels R/T inhibition of CYP3A4
Paroxetine / ↓ AUC and C_{max} of both drugs
Phenytoin / ↓ Aprepitant plasma levels R/T increased metabolism by CYP3A4; also, ↓ phenytoin plasma levels R/T induction of CYP2C9
Pimozide / ↑ Pimozide plasma levels R/T inhibition of CYP3A4; do not use together
Rifampin / ↓ Aprepitant plasma levels R/T increased metabolism by CYP3A4
Ritonavir / ↑ Aprepitant plasma levels R/T inhibition of CYP3A4; use together with caution
Tolbutamide / ↓ Tolbutamide plasma levels R/T induction of CYP2C9
Triazolam / ↑ Triazolam plasma levels R/T inhibition of CYP3A4
Troleandomycin / ↑ Aprepitant plasma levels R/T inhibition of CYP3A4; use together with caution
Vinblastine / ↑ Vinblastine plasma levels R/T inhibition of CYP3A4
Vincristine / ↑ Vincristine plasma levels R/T inhibition of CYP3A4
Vinorelbine / ↑ Vinorelbine plasma levels R/T inhibition of CYP3A4
Warfarin / ↓ Warfarin plasma levels R/T induction of CYP2C9; closely monitor INR

HOW SUPPLIED
Capsules: 40 mg, 80 mg, 125 mg.

DOSAGE

• CAPSULES
Antiemetic, highly emetogenic cancer chemotherapy.

Day 1: Aprepitant, 125 mg, 1 hr prior to chemotherapy; dexamethasone, 12 mg PO 30 min prior to chemotherapy; and, ondansetron, 32 mg IV 30 min prior to chemotherapy. **Days 2 and 3:** Aprepitant, 80 mg and dexamethasone, 8 mg PO in the morning. **Day 4:** Only dexamethasone, 8 mg PO, in the moring.

Antiemetic, moderately emetogenic cancer chemotherapy.

Day 1: Aprepitant, 125 mg, 1 hr prior to chemotherapy; dexamethasone, 12 mg PO, 30 min prior to chemotherapy; and, ondansetron, 8 mg PO 30–60 min prior to chemotherapy followed by a second 8 mg capsule 8 hr after the first dose. **Days 2 and 3:** Only aprepitant, 80 mg, in the morning.

Prevention of postoperative N&V.

40 mg within 3 hr prior to induction of anesthesia.

NURSING CONSIDERATIONS

ADMINISTRATION/STORAGE
1. The PO dexamethasone doses should be reduced approximately 50% when coadministered with aprepitant. The IV methylprednisolone dose should be reduced approximately 25% and the PO methylprednisolone dose reduced by approximateley 50% when coadministered with aprepitant.
2. Store bottles and blisters from 20–25°C (68–77°F). Keep the desiccant in the original bottle.

ASSESSMENT
1. Identify type of malignancy and chemotherapy prescribed; note other agents trialed and outcome.
2. List drugs prescribed; ensure none interact.
3. Give with other antiemetics and corticosteroid. Not for use over 3 days per chemo cycle.
4. Assess mental status. Monitor CBC, renal and LFTs during therapy.

CLIENT/FAMILY TEACHING
1. Take as directed: first dose 1 hour before start of chemotherapy with other antiemetics and a corticosteroid. Will need to use an additional antiemetic drug for break through vomiting. This drug is part of a regimen that has been found to help alleviate N&V associated with prescribed chemotherapy. Will take a lower dose on days 2 and 3 following the chemotherapy with or without food.
2. Consume plenty of fluids to ensure adequate hydration.
3. Practice reliable nonhormonal contraception.
4. Report adverse effects or lack of response. Use caution when performing tasks that require mental alertness; may cause dizziness and drowsiness esp. in higher doses.
5. May require medication to relieve headaches and constipation; report if evident or persistent. Avoid all OTC preparations or herbals without provider approval.

OUTCOMES/EVALUATE
Prevention/control of chemotherapy induced N&V

Argatroban   **IV**
(are-**GAT**-roh-ban)

CLASSIFICATION(S):
Anticoagulant, thrombin inhibitor
PREGNANCY CATEGORY: B
Rx: Acova.

USES
(1) Prophylaxis or treatment of thrombosis in heparin-induced thrombocytopenia (HIT). (2) Anticoagulant in those with or at risk for heparin-induced thrombocytopenia undergoing percutaneous coronary intervention.

ACTION/KINETICS

Action
A synthetic, direct thrombin inhibitor derived from L-arginine. Reversibly binds to the thrombin active site and does not require antithrombin III for antithrombotic activity. Acts by inhibiting

thrombin-catalyzed or induced reactions, including fibrin formation; activation of coagulation factors V, VIII, and XIII; protein C; and platelet aggregation. Inhibits both free and clot-associated thrombin. The small molecule provides the needed anticoagulant effect without worsening hypercoagulable states. Has little or no effect on trypsin, Factor Xa, plasmin, and kallikrein. Does not interact with heparin-induced antibodies.

Pharmacokinetics

Distributes mainly in the extracellular fluid. Steady state reached, by IV infusion, in 1–3 hr and is continued until infusion is stopped. Metabolized in the liver by CYP3A4/5. $t^{1}/_{2}$, **terminal:** 39–51 min. Excreted in the feces, primarily through biliary excretion.

CONTRAINDICATIONS

Overt major bleeding, hypersensitivity to the product or any of its components. Concomitant use of heparin. Lactation.

SPECIAL CONCERNS

Use with caution in hepatic disease and in disease states and circumstances with an increased danger of hemorrhage, including severe hypertension, immediately following lumbar puncture, spinal anesthesia, major surgery (especially the brain, spinal cord, or eye), congenital or acquired bleeding disorders, and GI lesions (e.g., ulcerations). Hemorrhage can occur at any site in the body. Safety and efficacy have not been determined in children less than 18 years of age.

SIDE EFFECTS

Most Common

Chest pain, hypotension, N&V, headache, bleeding episodes.

Bleeding: Major hemorrhagic events, including GI, GU/hematuria, decreased H&H, multisystem hemorrhage and DIC, limb and below the knee amputation stump, *intracranial hemorrhage*, *retroperitoneal hemorrhage*. Minor hemorrhagic events, including GI, GU/hematuria, groin, hemoptysis, brachial. Intracranial bleeding in clients with acute MI started on argatroban and streptokinase. **Allergic:** Airway reactions (coughing, dyspnea), rash, bullous eruption, vasodilation. **GI:** Diarrhea, N&V, GERD, abdominal pain, *GI hemorrhage:* **CV:** Hypotension, aortic stenosis, *cardiac arrest, VT, MI, coronary thrombosis, myocardial ischemia, coronary occlusion, arterial thrombosis*, cerebrovascular/vascular disorder, bradycardia, angina pectoris, atrial fibrillation. **Respiratory:** Dyspnea, pneumonia, coughing, lung edema. **GU:** UTI, abnormal renal function. **Miscellaneous:** Fever, pain, infection, abdominal pain, back pain, chest pain, headache, *sepsis*.

LABORATORY TEST CONSIDERATIONS

Coadministration of argatroban and warfarin produces a combined effect on laboratory measurement of INR. However, concurrent therapy exerts no additional effect on vitamin K-dependent Factor Xa activity, compared with warfarin monotherapy.

OD OVERDOSE MANAGEMENT

Symptoms: Major/minor bleeding events. *Treatment:* Discontinue argatroban or decrease infusion dose. Anticoagulation parameters usually return to baseline within 2–4 hr after discontinuing the drug. Reversal may take longer in hepatic impairment. No specific antidote is available. Provide symptomatic and supportive therapy.

DRUG INTERACTIONS

Concomitant use with antiplatelet drugs, thrombolytics, and other anticoagulants ↑ risk of bleeding (prolongation of PT and INR).

HOW SUPPLIED

Injection: 100 mg/mL.

DOSAGE

• **IV INFUSION**

Heparin-induced thrombocytopenia (HIT) or heparin-induced thrombocytopenia and thrombosis syndrome (HITTS).

Adults, initial, without hepatic impairment: 2 mcg/kg/min as a continuous IV infusion. The infusion rate depends on body weight (see package insert). After the initial dose, adjust dose as clinically indicated, not to exceed 10 mcg/kg/min, until the steady state aPTT is 1.5–3 times initial baseline value, not to exceed 100 seconds.

Percutaneous coronary intervention in HIT/HITTS.

Adults, initial: Start a continuous infusion at 25 mcg/kg/min and a bolus of 350 mcg/kg given via a large bore IV line over 3–5 min. Check activated clotting time (ACT) 5–10 min after the bolus dose is completed. If the ACT is greater than 450 seconds, decrease the infusion rate to 15 mcg/kg/min and check the ACT 5–10 min later. Once an ACT between 300 and 450 sec has been reached, continue this infusion for the duration of the procedure. In the event of dissection, impending abrupt closure, thrombus formation during the procedure, or inability to achieve or maintain ACT over 300 sec, give additional bolus doses of 150 mcg/kg and increase the infusion dose to 40 mcg/kg/min. Check ACT after each additional bolus or change in infusion rate.

Impaired hepatic function (for all uses).

Adults, initial, moderate hepatic impairment: 0.5 mcg/kg/min, based on about a 4-fold decrease in argatroban clearance compared with normal hepatic function.

NURSING CONSIDERATIONS

ADMINISTRATION/STORAGE

 IV 1. Discontinue all parenteral anticoagulants before giving argatroban.

2. If argatroban is begun after cessation of heparin, allow sufficient time for effects of heparin on aPTT to decrease before starting argatroban therapy.

3. To prepare IV infusion: Dilute in 0.9% NaCl, D5W, or LR injection to a final concentration of 1 mg/mL. Dilute each 2.5 mL vial 100-fold by mixing with 250 mL of diluent.

4. Mix reconstituted solution by repeated inversion of the diluent bag for 1 min. After preparation, solution may be briefly hazy R/T formation of microprecipitates; dissolves rapidly upon mixing.

5. If prepared correctly, pH of IV solution is 3.2–7.5.

6. Use of argatroban and warfarin results in prolongation of INR beyond that caused by warfarin alone. Measure INR daily if argatroban and warfarin are given together. Generally, with doses of argatroban of 2 mcg/kg/min or less, argatroban can be discontinued when the INR is greater than 4 on combined therapy. After argatroban is discontinued, repeat INR measurement in 4–6 hr. If the repeat INR is below the desired range, resume argatroban infusion and repeat the procedure daily until the desired therapeutic range on warfarin alone is reached.

7. For doses of argatroban greater than 2 mcg/kg/min, the relationship of INR on warfarin alone to the INR of both drugs given together is less predictable. Thus, temporarily reduce dose of argatroban to 2 mcg/kg/min. Repeat INR on argatroban and warfarin 4–6 hr after reducing argatroban dose and follow process outlined above for giving argatroban at doses of 2 mcg/kg/min or less.

8. Argatroban is a clear, colorless to pale yellow, slightly viscous solution. Discard vial if the solution is cloudy or an insoluble precipitate is observed.

9. Prepared solutions stable at 15–30°C (59–85°F) for 24 hr at ambient indoor light. Prepared solutions are stable for 48 hr or less when stored at 2–8°C (36–46°F) in the dark. Do not expose prepared solutions to direct sunlight.

ASSESSMENT

1. Note reasons for therapy: thrombosis prophylaxis or treatment. List all drugs prescribed/consumed; ensure none interact.

2. Review history; note conditions that may preclude drug therapy. Note active bleeding sites/disorders.

3. Stop heparin therapy. Obtain and monitor weight, INR, PT/PTT, CBC, and LFTs. Lower dosage with liver dysfunction.

4. Observe closely for evidence of abnormal bleeding or adverse effects. Perform routine vascular checks.

CLIENT/FAMILY TEACHING

1. Review goals of therapy and potential bleeding risks.

2. Report unusual oozing or bleeding sites and wet bandages or bedding.

3. Use soft bristled tooth brush, electric razor and avoid IM shots and contact sports

4. Encourage family members to learn CPR.

OUTCOMES/EVALUATE

Inhibition/treatment of thrombus formation with HIT

Aripiprazole
(ah-rih-PIP-rah-zohl)

CLASSIFICATION(S):
Antipsychotic
PREGNANCY CATEGORY: C
Rx: Abilify, Abilify Discmelt.

USES
(1) Schizophrenia, including maintaining stability in clients who had been symptomatically stable on other antipsychotic drugs for periods of 3 months or longer and are no longer using them. (2) Acute manic and/or mixed episodes associated with bipolar disorder. (3) IM for agitation associated with schizophrenia or bipolar disorder (manic or mixed).

ACTION/KINETICS
Action
Mechanism not known with certainty but likely due to high affinity for dopamine D_2 partial agonist) and D_3 receptors as well as $5-HT_{1A}$ (partial agonist) and antagonist activity at $5-HT_{2A}$ receptors. Low incidence of sedation and orthostatic hypotension.

Pharmacokinetics
Well absorbed (87% bioavailable). **Peak plasma levels:** 3–5 hr. A high fat meal will delay the T_{max}. **$t\frac{1}{2}$, elimination:** 75 hr for extensive metabolizers and 146 hr for poor metabolizers. Metabolized by CYP2D6 and CYP3A4 enzymes in the liver. Excreted through both the feces (about 55%) and urine (about 25%). **Plasma protein binding:** >99% bound to plasma proteins.

CONTRAINDICATIONS
Lactation. Use in those with dementia-related psychosis. Use of alcohol.

SPECIAL CONCERNS
■ Elderly clients with dementia-related psychosis treated with atypical antipsychotic drugs are at an increased risk of death, compared with placebo. Analyses of placebo-controlled trials (modal duration, 10 weeks), in these individuals revealed a risk of death in the drug-treated clients of between 1.6 to 1.7 times that seen in placebo-treated clients. Over the course of a typical 10-week controlled trial, the rate of death in drug-treated clients was about 4.5% compared with a rate of about 2.6% in the placebo group. Although the causes of death were varied, most of the deaths appeared to be either cardiovascular (e.g., heart failure, sudden death) or infections (e.g., pneumonia) in nature. Aripiprazole is not approved for the treatment of clients with dementia-related psychosis.■ Long-term efficacy has not been established. Use with caution in history of MI, ischemic heart disease, heart failure, conduction abnormalities, cerebrovascular disease, or conditions that predispose to hypotension (e.g., dehydration, hypovolemia, antihypertensive drug treatment). There is an increased risk of hyperglycemia and diabetes. Use with caution in conditions that may contribute to an increase in body temperature and in those at risk for aspiration pneumonia. Safety and efficacy in psychosis associated with dementia, in psychosis associated with Alzheimer's disease, or in children and adolescents have not been evaluated.

SIDE EFFECTS
Most Common
Headache, agitation, insomnia, dyspepsia, constipation, N&V, drowsiness/sedation/somnolence.

Neuroleptic Malignant Syndrome: Hyperpyrexia, muscle rigidity, altered mental status, autonomic instability, rhabdomyolysis, acute renal failure. **CNS:** Tardive dyskinesia, seizures, somnolence, headache, anxiety, insomnia, lightheadedness, akathisia, dyskinesia, tremor, depression, nervousness, hostility, manic reaction, abnormal gait, confusion, cogwheel rigidity, dystonia, twitch, im-

---

potence, bradykinesia, decreased or increased libido, panic attack, impaired memory, stupor, amnesia, hyperactivity, depersonalization, hypokinesia, restless leg syndrome, dysphoria, neuropathy, increased reflexes, slowed thinking, hyperkinesia, hyperesthesia, hypotonia, oculogyric crisis, suicidal thought, *suicide*. **GI:** N&V, constipation, increased salivation, anorexia, gastroenteritis, dysphagia, flatulence, gastritis, tooth caries, gingivitis, hemorrhoids, gastroesophageal reflux, *GI hemorrhage*, periodontal abscess, tongue edema, fecal incontinence, colitis, rectal hemorrhage, stomatitis, mouth ulcer, cholecystitis, fecal impaction, oral moniliasis, cholelithiasis, eructation, intestinal obstruction, peptic ulcer. **CV:** Hypertension, tachycardia, hypotension, bradycardia, palpitation, *hemorrhage, MI, CVA, cardiac arrest, heart failure*, prolonged QT interval, atrial fibrillation, AV block, myocardial ischemia, phlebitis, DVT, angina pectoris, extrasystoles. **Hematologic:** Ecchymosis, anemia, hypochromic anemia, leukopenia, leukocytosis, lymphadenopathy, thrombocytopenia, iron deficiency anemia. **Musculoskeletal:** Muscle cramps, arthralgia, bone pain, myasthenia, arthritis, arthrosis, muscle weakness, spasm, bursitis. **Body as a whole:** Asthenia, fever, weight gain or loss, flu syndrome, peripheral edema, chills, bloating, diabetes mellitus, edema, dehydration, thirst. **Metabolic:** Hyperglycemia, sometimes associated with ketoacidosis, hyperosmolar coma, or *death*. **Respiratory:** Rhinitis, coughing, chest tightness, dyspnea, pneumonia, asthma, epistaxis, hiccup, laryngitis. **Dermatologic:** Dry skin, rash, pruritus, sweating, skin ulcer, acne, vesiculobullous rash, eczema, alopecia, psoriasis, seborrhea. **GU:** Urinary incontinence, cystitis, leukorrhea, urinary frequency/urgency/retention, hematuria, dysuria, amenorrhea, abnormal ejaculation, vaginal hemorrhage, vaginal moniliasis, kidney failure, uterine hemorrhage, menorrhagia, kidney calculus, nocturia, polyuria. **Ophthalmic:** Blurred vision, conjunctivitis, dry eye, eye pain, cataract, blepharitis. **Otic:** Ear pain, tinnitus,

otitis media. **Miscellaneous:** Accidental injury, chest/neck/jaw pain, jaw tightness, enlarged abdomen, neck rigidity, pelvic pain, hypothyroidism, altered taste.

LABORATORY TEST CONSIDERATIONS
↑ CPK, AST, ALT, BUN, alkaline phosphatase, creatinine, LDH. Hypercholesterolemia, hyper/hypoglycemia, hypokalemia, hyperlipemia, hyponatremia, bilirubinemia.

DRUG INTERACTIONS
Carbamazepine / ↑ Aripiprazole clearance → ↓ blood levels R/T induction of CYP3A4 enzymes; double the aripiprazole dose
Fluoxetine / ↓ Aripiprazole metabolism → ↑ blood levels R/T inhibition of CYP2D6 enzymes; reduce aripiprazole dose to one-half the usual dose to 20 or 30 mg
Ketoconazole / ↓ Aripiprazole metabolism → ↑ blood levels R/T inhibition of CYP3A4 enzymes; reduce aripiprazole to one-half the usual dose
Paroxetine / ↓ Aripiprazole metabolism → ↑ blood levels R/T inhibition of CYP2D6 enzymes; reduce aripiprazole to one-half the usual dose
Quinidine / ↓ Aripiprazole metabolism → ↑ blood levels R/T inhibition of CYP2D6 enzymes; reduce aripiprazole to one-half the usual dose

HOW SUPPLIED
Injection: 7.5 mg/mL; *Oral Solution:* 1 mg/mL; *Tablets:* 2 mg, 5 mg, 10 mg, 15 mg, 20 mg, 30 mg; *Tablets, Orally Disintegrating:* 10 mg, 15 mg.

DOSAGE————————
• **ORAL SOLUTION; TABLETS; TABLETS, ORALLY DISINTEGRATING**
Schizophrenia.
Initial and target dose: 10 or 15 mg/day given on a once-a-day schedule. **Effective dose range:** 10–30 mg/day. Do not make dosage increases before 2 weeks, the time required to reach steady state. **Maintenance:** Has been used for periods up to 6 months. Periodically assess to determine the need for maintenance treatment.
Bipolar disorder.
Initial: 30 mg once daily; may be reduced to 15 mg once daily based on

tolerability. No data to support use beyond 6 weeks.

- **INJECTION (IM ONLY)**
  Agitation associated with schizophrenia or bipolar mania.

Initial: 9.75 mg; **dose range:** 5.25–15 mg. If agitation persists following the initial dose, cumulative doses up to 30 mg/day may be given. The safety of total daily doses greater than 30 mg or injections given more frequently than q 2 hr has not been adequately evaluated. If ongoing therapy is indicated, PO aripiprazole in a dose range from 10–30 mg/day should replace the injection as soon as possible.

NURSING CONSIDERATIONS

❦ Do not confuse aripiprazole with lansoprazole (proton pump inhibitor).

ADMINISTRATION/STORAGE

1. If switching from other antipsychotics, minimize period of overlapping antipsychotic administration.
2. Oral solution can be given on a mg-per-mg basis in place of the 5, 10, 15, or 20 mg tablets strengths. Clients receiving 30 mg tablets should receive 25 mg of the solution.
3. To administer the injection, draw up the required volume of solution as follows: 0.7 mL for the 5.25 mg dose, 1.3 mL for the 9.75 mg dose, and 2 mL for the 15 mg dose. Inject slowly deep in the muscle mass.
4. Do not give the injection IV or SC.
5. Store the injection, tablets, and oral solution between 15–30°C (59–86°F).
6. Opened bottles of solution can be used for up to 6 months after opening if refrigerated.
7. Protect the injection from light by storing in the original container. Keep in carton until time of use.

ASSESSMENT

1. Identify behaviors/conditions requiring management, other agents trialed and outcome.
2. List drugs prescribed; ensure no interactions or dosage adjustments needed.
3. Assess mental status and evidence/history of CAD, hypo/hypertension. Use cautiously with CAD, seizure history, or

conditions that lower seizure threshold e.g., Alzheimer's dementia.

4. Monitor VS, ECG, I&O, cholesterol panel, BS, electrolytes, CPK, renal, LFTs and for evidence of diabetes.
5. Aripiprazole has been given for up to 26 weeks, although it can be used for longer-term efficacy; assess clients periodically to determine need for maintenance therapy.

- DSM III/IV-TR criteria for schizophrenia: delusions, conceptual disorganization, hallucinatory behavior, excitement, grandiosity, suspiciousness/persecution, and hostility.
- PANSS (Positive and Negative Syndrome Scale) should include 7+ symptoms of schizophrenia: blunted affect, emotional withdrawal, poor rapport, passive apathetic withdrawal, difficulty with abstract thinking, lack of spontaneity/flow of conversation, stereotypical thinking).

CLIENT/FAMILY TEACHING

1. Take with or without food once daily.
2. Do not split the orally disintegrating tablets.
3. With diabetes, each mL of Abilify oral solution contains 400 mg of sucrose and 200 mg of fructose.
4. Avoid activities that require mental alertness until drug effects realized; may impair judgment, thinking, or motor skills.
5. Change positions slowly; prevents sudden drop in BP.
6. Practice reliable contraception, report if pregnancy suspected.
7. Avoid alcohol, CNS depressants, OTC agents, strenuous exercise, exposure to extreme heat, overheating, or dehydration.
8. May cause esophageal dysmotility-may cause aspiration; use caution.
9. Do not add any medications or OTC agents without provider approval due to the potential for strong drug interactions.
10. Immediately report any S&S of NMS (neuroleptic malignant syndrome): increased temperature, muscle rigidity, irregular heart rate/BP, arrhythmias or severe diaphoresis.

Bold Italic = life threatening side effect   ■ = black box warning   ✤ = Available in Canada

11. Report any movements that become involuntary, slow, repetitive, rhythmical (tardive dyskinesia) in select or groups of muscles; may become irreversible.

12. Prescriptions will be for small amounts to prevent overdose and for the smallest dose and shortest duration of treatment needed. Psychiatric therapy and evaluation should be regular and ongoing.

OUTCOMES/EVALUATE
- Improvement in PANSS and DSM III/IV-TR schizophrenia criteria
- Evidence of improved behavioral and emotional presentation
- ↓ Delusions/suspiciousness and hostility

Armodafinil
(ar-moe-**DAF**-in-il)

CLASSIFICATION(S):
Analeptic
PREGNANCY CATEGORY: C
Rx: Nuvigil, **C-IV**

USES
(1) Improve wakefulness in clients with excessive sleepiness associated with narcolepsy. (2) Improve wakefulness in clients with excessive sleepiness associated with obstructive sleep apnea-hypopnea syndrome (OSA). Used in conjunction with continuous positive airway pressure. (3) Improve wakefulness in those with excessive sleepiness associated with shift-work sleep disorder (SWSD).

ACTION/KINETICS
Action
Precise mechanism is unknown. The drug has wake-promoting effects similar to amphetamine or methylphenidate, although the pharmacology is not identical to that of sympathomimetic amines. Modafinil, a similar drug, produces psychoactive and euphoric effects, as well as alterations in mood, perception, thinking, and feelings. *NOTE:* Armodafinil is the R isomer of racemic modafinil.

Pharmacokinetics
Readily absorbed after PO use. **Peak plasma levels:** About 2 hr in the fasted state. **Apparent steady state:** Reached within 7 days. Time to reach T_{max} may be delayed from 2-4 hr in the fed state. Metabolized by liver enzymes, including CYP3A4 and CYP3A5. **t½, terminal:** About 15 hr. 80% excreted in the urine. Clearance may be reduced in geriatric clients. **Plasma protein binding:** Approximately 60%, mainly to albumin.

CONTRAINDICATIONS
Hypersensitivity to armodafinil or modafinil or any component of the product. Use not recommended in those with a history of left ventricular hypertrophy or with mitral valve prolapse who have experienced mitral valve prolapse syndrome when previously receiving CNS stimulants.

SPECIAL CONCERNS
Use with caution in those with a history of psychosis, depression, mania; in those with a recent history of MI or unstable angina; and, during lactation. The abuse potential is likely to be similar to that of modafinil. Safety and efficacy have not been determined in children younger than 17 years.

SIDE EFFECTS
Most Common
Headache, nausea, dry mouth, insomnia, dizziness, anxiety, diarrhea.
GI: Nausea, diarrhea, dry mouth, dyspepsia, upper abdominal pain, constipation, loose stools, vomiting. **CNS:** Headache, dizziness, insomnia, anxiety, fatigue, depression, agitation, depressed mood, disturbance in attention, migraine, nervousness, parestheisa, tremor. Persistent sleepiness, mania, delusions, hallucinations, *suicidal ideations.* **CV:** Palpitations, increased HR, small increases in mean systolic and diastolic BP and pulse rate. **Dermatologic:** Rash, including *Stevens-Johnson syndrome;* contact dermatitis, hyperhidrosis. **Metabolic/Nutritional:** Anorexia, decreased appetite. **Body as a whole:** Fatigue, angioedema, *anaphylactoid reactions,* multiorgan hypersensitivity reactions. **Miscellaneous:**

Dyspnea, flu-like illness, pain, polyuria, pyrexia, seasonal allergy, thirst.

LABORATORY TEST CONSIDERATIONS
↑ GGT, alkaline phosphatase.

OD OVERDOSE MANAGEMENT
Symptoms: Similar to modafinil, including excitation, agitation, insomnia, slight or moderate increase in hemodynamic parameters. *Treatment:* No specific antidote exists. Provide supportive treatment, including CV monitoring. If there are no contraindications, consider gastric lavage.

DRUG INTERACTIONS
Alcohol / Avoid concomitant use
Carbamazepine / Possible ↓ armodafinil levels R/T ↑ metabolism by CYP3A4/5
Clomipramine / ↑ Clomipramine levels R/T inhibition of CYP2C19
Contraceptives, steroidal / Possible ↓ efficacy of steroidal contraceptives during and for 1 month after armodafinil co-administration; use of alternative methods of contraception recommended
Cyclosporine / ↓ Cyclosporine levels; monitor levels and adjust dose
Diazepam / ↑ Diazepam levels R/T ↓ metabolism by CYP2C19
Erythromycin / Possible ↑ armodafinil levels R/T ↓ metabolism by CYP3A4/5
Ethinyl estradiol / ↓ Systemic exposure to ethinyl estradiol; dose adjustment may be needed
Ketoconazole / Possible ↑ armodafinil levels R/T metabolism by CYP3A4/5
MAO inhibitors / Use caution when using together
Midazolam / ↓ Midazolam levels R/T ↑ metabolism by CYP3A4/5
Omeprazole / ↑ Omeprazole levels R/T inhibition of CYP2C19
Phenobarbital / Possible ↓ armodafinil levels R/T ↑ metabolism by CYP3A4/5
Phenytoin / ↑ Phenytoin levels R/T inhibition of CYP2C19; dose reduction may be needed
Propranolol / ↑ Propranolol levels R/T inhibition of CYP2C19; dose reduction may be needed
Rifampin / Possible ↓ armodafinil levels R/T ↑ metabolism by CYP3A4/5
Triazolam / ↓ Triazolam levels R/T ↑ metabolism by CYP3A4/5

Warfarin / Possible interaction; monitor PT and INR more frequently

HOW SUPPLIED
Tablets: 50 mg, 150 mg, 250 mg.

DOSAGE
- **TABLETS**
  Obstructive sleep apnea-hypopnea syndrome, narcolepsy.
150 or 250 mg as a single dose in the morning. There is no evidence that the 250 mg/day dose confers additional benefit over the 150 mg/day for those with obstructive sleep apnea-hypopnea syndrome.
  Shift-work sleep disorder.
150 mg/day given about 1 hr before the start of the client's work shift.

NURSING CONSIDERATIONS
ADMINISTRATION/STORAGE
1. The efficacy for more than 12 weeks has not been evaluated.
2. Periodically re-evaluate long-term usefulness in each client.
3. Reduce dose in those with severely impaired hepatic function.
4. Store from 20-25°C (68-77°F).

ASSESSMENT
1. Note onset, characteristics of sleepiness episodes. Identify how often it interferes with normal functioning/work, any associated problems/accidents.
2. List drugs prescribed to ensure none interact or require dosage adjustments.
3. Reduce dose with liver dysfunction and in the elderly.
4. Obtain ECG, monitor BP; do not use with LVH, MVP, recent MI, ischemic ECG changes, chest pain, or arrhythmias.
5. Assess for any evidence or history of mental health issues; may aggravate. Observe for S&S of abuse (e.g., drug-seeking behaviors, increased usage).
6. Discontinue at the first sign of rash.

CLIENT/FAMILY TEACHING
1. May take with or without food in the morning unless otherwise directed.
2. Drug is used to promote wakefulness. It can cause psychoactive and euphoric effects similar to those with other controlled substances as well as depression.
3. May alter judgement, thinking, motor skills and cause dizziness. Do not

---

engage in activities that require mental alertness until drug effects realized.

4. With narcolepsy and obstructive sleep apnea, take as a single dose in the a.m. With shift work sleep disorder, drug should be taken approximately 1 hour prior to the start of the work shift.

5. Use additional protection to avoid pregnancy.

6. Avoid alcohol; do not take any OTC agents unless approved.

7. Immediately report any blisters, hives, mouth sores, peeling skin, rash, trouble swallowing or breathing.

8. Stop drug and report any unusual rash, chest pain, adverse side effects; report lack or desired response. Keep all F/U appointments to evaluate response to therapy and side effects.

OUTCOMES/EVALUATE

- ↑ Daytime wakefulness with narcolepsy
- Improved wakefulness with SWSD and OSA

Asparaginase ■ IV ⓒ
(ah-**SPAIR**-ah-jin-ays)

CLASSIFICATION(S):
Antineoplastic, miscellaneous
PREGNANCY CATEGORY: C
Rx: Elspar.
✤**Rx:** Kidrolase.

SEE ALSO *ANTINEOPLASTIC AGENTS.*

USES
Acute lymphocytic leukemia (ALL) in children; mostly used in combination with other drugs in the induction of remissions of the disease. Not to be used as the sole induction agent unless combination therapy is deemed inappropriate. Not recommended for maintenance therapy.

ACTION/KINETICS

Action
Neoplastic cells are unable to synthesize sufficient asparagine, an amino acid, to meet their metabolic needs. The supply of asparagine is further decreased by the enzyme asparaginase, which breaks down asparagine to aspartic acid and ammonia. Asparaginase interferes with synthesis of DNA, RNA, and protein and is cell-cycle specific for the G_1 phase of cell division.

Pharmacokinetics
Time to peak plasma levels, after IM: 14–24 hr. $t\frac{1}{2}$, **after IV:** 8–30 hr; **after IM:** 39–49 hr. Accumulates in plasma and tissue, and a small amount (1%) appears in CSF. Excretion is unknown. More toxic in adults than in children.

CONTRAINDICATIONS
Previous anaphylactic reactions to asparaginase. Pancreatitis (acute hemorrhagic pancreatitis has been fatal in some instances when asparaginase has been given) or a history of pancreatitis. Lactation.

SPECIAL CONCERNS
■ It is recommended that asparaginase be administered to clients only in a hospital setting under the supervision of a physician who is qualified by training and experience to administer cancer chemotherapeutic agents, because of the possibility of severe reactions, including anaphylaxis and sudden death. The physician must be prepared to treat anaphylaxis at each administration of the drug. In the treatment of each client, the physician must weigh carefully the possibility of achieving therapeutic benefit versus the risk of toxicity.■ Use with caution in presence of liver dysfunction. Due to the possibility of an increased risk of hypersensitivity, institute retreatment with great care.

SIDE EFFECTS

Most Common
N&V (may be severe), anorexia, abdominal cramps, swelling at injection site, headache, malaise, drowsiness.

GI: N&V, anorexia, abdominal cramps, *pancreatitis (sometimes fulminant)*, *acute hemorrhagic pancreatitis*. **CNS:** Depression, somnolence, drowsiness, coma, confusion, fatigue, malaise, agitation, mild to severe hallucinations, headache, irritability, Parkinson–like syndrome with tremor and a progressive increase in muscle tone (rare). **Hematologic:** Marked leukopenia, bone marrow depression (rare). Depression of

---

clotting factors (factors V, VII, VIII, IX); rarely, **intracranial hemorrhage and fatal bleeding**. **Hypersensitivity:** Skin rashes, urticaria, arthralgia, respiratory distress, **acute anaphylaxis, death**. **Renal:** Azotemia, proteinuria (rare), acute renal shutdown, **fatal renal insufficiency**. **Hepatic:** Hepatotoxicity, fatty changes in the liver. **Miscellaneous:** Hyperglycemia with glucosuria and polyuria. Marked hypoalbuminemia associated with peripheral edema, malabsorption syndrome, **fatal hyperthermia**, chills, fever, mild weight loss, uric acid nephropathy.

LABORATORY TEST CONSIDERATIONS
↑ Blood ammonia, BUN, glucose, serum uric acid, AST, ALT, alkaline phosphatase, bilirubin (direct and indirect). ↓ Serum albumin, cholesterol (total and esters), plasma fibrinogen, circulating lymphoblasts. ↑ or ↓ Total lipids. Interference with interpretation of thyroid function tests.

DRUG INTERACTIONS
Methotrexate / Asparaginase ↓ effect of methotrexate; do not use methotrexate with or following asparaginase
Prednisone / Even though used with asparaginase, may cause ↑ toxicity
Vincristine / Even though used with asparaginase, may cause ↑ toxicity; ↑ hyperglycemic effect

HOW SUPPLIED
Powder for Injection, Lyophilized: 10,000 international units.

DOSAGE
• **IM; IV**
When used as the sole agent for induction.
Adults and children: 200 international units/kg/day IV for 28 days.
Regimen I for ALL in children.
Prednisone: 40 mg/m²/day PO in three divided doses for 15 days, followed by tapering of dosage as follows: 20 mg/m²/day for 2 days, 10 mg/m²/day for 2 days, 5 mg/m²/day for 2 days, 2.5 mg/m²/day for 2 days, and then discontinue. Vincristine sulfate: 2 mg/m² IV once weekly on days 1, 8, and 15. The maximum single dose should not exceed 2 mg. Asparaginase: 1,000 international units/kg/day IV for 10 successive days beginning on day 22.
Regimen II for ALL in children.
Prednisone: 40 mg/m²/day PO in three divided doses for 28 days with the total daily dose to the nearest 2.5 mg; then, discontinue gradually over 14 days. Vincristine sulfate: 1.5 mg/m² IV weekly for four doses on days 1, 8, 15, and 22. The maximum single dose should not exceed 2 mg. Asparaginase: 6,000 international units/m² IM on days 4, 7, 10, 13, 16, 19, 22, 25, and 28. When remission is obtained with either regimen, appropriate maintenance therapy should be instituted. Do not use asparaginase for maintenance therapy.

NURSING CONSIDERATIONS
℘ Do not confuse asparaginase with pegaspargase (antineoplastic drug).

ADMINISTRATION/STORAGE
1. Give intradermal skin test (0.1 mL of a 20-international units/mL solution) at least 1 hr before initial administration of drug and when 1 week or more has elapsed between treatments. Observe for at least 1 hr for wheal/erythema that indicates a positive reaction. A negative skin test reaction does not preclude possibility of an allergic reaction.
2. A desensitization procedure, with increasing amounts of asparaginase may be carried out in those hypersensitive to the drug (1 international unit, then double dose q 10 min until total dose for day or reaction occurs).
3. Due to the unpredictability of side effects, initiate treatment only in hospitalized clients.
4. To prevent uric acid nephropathy, give allopurinol, increase fluid intake, and alkalinize the urine.
5. Do not use asparaginase as sole induction agent unless combined regimen is not possible due to toxicity or because client is refractory.
6. For IM use, reconstitute by adding 2 mL NaCl injection to the 10,000-unit vial. Use within 8 hr and only if clear. Give no more than 2 mL at a single injection site.
7. Handle the drug with care; is a contact irritant.

8. Have emergency equipment readily available during each administration; a severe hypersensitivity reaction is more likely to occur with this drug.

9. Store both the lyophilized product and reconstituted solution at 2–8°C (36–46°F). Discard reconstituted solution after 8 hr (sooner if cloudy).

IV 10. Follow administration guidelines carefully.

11. For IV use: reconstitute the 10,000-unit vial with either 5 mL sterile water or NaCl injection. Give solution by direct IV administration within 8 hr following reconstitution. For infusion, dilute solutions with NaCl injection or D5W. Infuse through the side arm of an already running infusion of sodium chloride injection or D5W over at least 30 min and within 8 hr of reconstitution only if solution is clear.

ASSESSMENT

1. Note reasons for therapy, leukemia history, baseline labs and VS. May cause mild lymphocyte suppression. Nadir: 7–10 days; recovery 14 days.

2. Determine intradermal skin test performed initially and after a 2 week or more interval between doses. (Repeated doses increase hypersensitivity reactions).

3. Increase fluids and add allopurinol to reduce uric acid levels from tumor necrosis.

4. Monitor neurologic status, LFTs, CBC, uric acid, glucose, amylase, and lipase levels; check for S&S of pancreatitis/allergic reactions.

5. Assess cardiopulmonary function; document ECG and CXR q 2 weeks.

INTERVENTIONS

1. Expect to administer antiemetic prior to drug therapy.

2. Give vincristine and prednisone before asparaginase to reduce the toxic effects.

3. Asparaginase administration 9–10 days before or within 24 hr after methotrexate (MTX) may reduce the GI and hematologic effects of MTX.

4. Weigh weekly, monitor I&O; assess for any evidence of renal failure. Alkalinization of the urine and allopurinol therapy may help prevent urate stone formation.

5. Observe for peripheral edema R/T hypoalbuminemia triggered by asparaginase.

6. Monitor for hyperglycemia, glycosuria, and polyuria, all of which may be precipitated by asparaginase. Have IV fluids and regular insulin available; stop therapy.

CLIENT/FAMILY TEACHING

1. Report stomach pain and N&V: S&S of pancreatitis.

2. Report any sudden increase in SOB, coughing, feet swelling, frequent urination, increased thirst, or fever.

3. Consume 2–3 L/day of fluids to prevent dehydration.

4. May cause drowsiness, even several weeks after administration; do not drive a car or operate hazardous machinery.

5. Report shakiness or unusual body movements; a Parkinson-like condition may be precipitated by drug.

6. Avoid immunizations and contact with child who has recently taken poliovirus vaccine. Avoid crowds, especially during flu season. Consider pneumococcal vaccine and annual flu shot.

7. Practice reliable contraception; drug is teratogenic.

8. Do not take any aspirin-containing compounds, NSAIDs, or alcohol; may cause GI bleeding.

OUTCOMES/EVALUATE

• Improved hematologic parameters
• Inhibition of malignant cell proliferation

Aspirin ■
(Acetylsalicylic acid, ASA)

(ah-**SEE**-till-sal-ih-**SILL**-ick **AH**-sid)

CLASSIFICATION(S):
Nonsteroidal anti-inflammatory drug, analgesic, antipyretic
PREGNANCY CATEGORY: C
OTC: Gum Tablets: Aspergum.

Caplets/Tablets: Arthritis Foundation Pain Reliever, Empirin, Genprin, Genuine Bayer Aspirin Caplets and Tablets, Maximum Bayer Aspirin Caplets and Tablets, Norwich Extra Strength, Norwich Regular Strength. **Tablets, Chewable:** Bayer Children's Aspirin, St. Joseph Adult Chewable Aspirin. **Tablets, Enteric-Coated:** Ecotrin Adult Low Strength, Ecotrin Caplets and Tablets, Ecotrin Maximum Strength Caplets and Tablets, Extra Strength Bayer Enteric 500 Aspirin, Halfprin 81, Heartline, Regular Strength Bayer Enteric Coated Caplets, ½ Halfprin. **Tablets, Extended-Release:** Bayer Low Adult Strength, Extended Release Bayer 8-Hour Caplets.

Rx: Easprin, ZORprin.

♣OTC: Asaphen, Asaphen E.C., Entrophen, MSD Enteric Coated ASA, Novasen.

Aspirin, buffered
PREGNANCY CATEGORY: C

OTC: Caplets: Asprimox, Asprimox Extra Protection for Arthritis Pain, Extra Strength Bayer Plus Caplets. **Caplets/Tablets:** Arthritis Pain Formula, Asprimox Extra Protection for Arthritis Pain, Bayer Buffered Aspirin, Buffered Aspirin, Bufferin Extra Strength, Buffex, Cama Arthritis Pain Reliever, Tri-Buffered Bufferin Caplets and Tablets. **Tablets, Coated:** Adprin-B, Ascriptin, Ascriptin A/D, Ascriptin Extra Strength, Asprimox, Bufferin, Extra-Strength Adprin-B. **Tablets, Effervescent:** Alka-Seltzer Extra Strength with Aspirin, Alka-Seltzer with Aspirin, Alka-Seltzer with Aspirin (Flavored).

SEE ALSO *NONSTEROIDAL ANTI-INFLAMMATORY DRUGS*

USES
Analgesic: (1) Pain from integumentary structures, myalgias, neuralgias, arthralgias, headache, dysmenorrhea, and similar types of pain. (2) Gout. (3) May be effective in less severe postoperative and postpartum pain; pain secondary to trauma and cancer.

Antipyretic, Anti-Inflammatory: Arthritis, osteoarthritis, SLE, acute rheumatic fever, gout, and many other conditions. Mucocutaneous lymph node syndrome (Kawasaki disease).

Cardiovascular: Despite the increased risk of GI bleeding, low-dose aspirin should be used for the following CV events:
1. Reduce risk of death and nonfatal stroke in those who have had an ischemic stroke or TIA; also combined with dipyridamole for this purpose.
2. Reduce risk of vascular mortality with suspected acute MI.
3. Reduce the combined risk of recurrent MI and death after an MI or unstable angina.
4. Reduce risk of MI and sudden death in chronic stable angina.
5. Pre-existing need for aspirin following coronary artery bypass grafting, PTCA, or carotid endarterectomy.
6. Used with ticlopidine as adjunctive therapy to reduce development of subacute stent thrombosis.
7. *Investigational:* Reduce risk of heart problems in healthy adults with a small risk of heart attack and no history of CV disease. Includes men over 40 years of age, postmenopausal women, and younger people with risk factors including, smoking, diabetes, hypertension, and high cholesterol.

Chronic use to prevent cataract formation; low doses to prevent toxemia of pregnancy; in pregnant women with inadequate uteroplacental blood flow. Reduce colon cancer mortality (low doses). Low doses of aspirin and warfarin to reduce risk of a second heart attack. In addition to treatment for CV risk factors, may reduce risk of dying from heart attack or stroke significantly.

ACTION/KINETICS
Action
Exhibits antipyretic, anti-inflammatory, and analgesic effects. The antipyretic effect is due to an action on the hypothalamus, resulting in heat loss by vasodilation of peripheral blood vessels and promoting sweating. The anti-inflammatory effects are probably mediated through inhibition of cyclo-oxygenase,

---

Bold Italic = life threatening side effect   ■ = black box warning   ♣ = Available in Canada

which results in a decrease in prostaglandin (implicated in the inflammatory response) synthesis and other mediators of the pain response. The mechanism of action for the analgesic effects of aspirin is not known fully but is partly attributable to improvement of the inflammatory condition. Aspirin also produces inhibition of platelet aggregation by decreasing the synthesis of endoperoxides and thromboxanes—substances that mediate platelet aggregation. Large doses of aspirin (5 grams/day or more) increase uric acid secretion, while low doses (2 grams/day or less) decrease uric acid secretion. However, aspirin antagonizes drugs used to treat gout.

Pharmacokinetics

Rapidly absorbed after PO administration. Is hydrolyzed to the active salicylic acid. **Blood levels for arthritis and rheumatic disease:** Maintain 150–300 mcg/mL. **Blood levels for analgesic and antipyretic:** 25–50 mcg/mL. **Blood levels for acute rheumatic fever:** 150–300 mcg/mL. Tinnitus occurs at serum levels above 200 mcg/mL and serious toxicity above 400 mcg/mL. **t½:** Aspirin, 15–20 min; salicylic acid, 2–20 hr, depending on the dose. Salicylic acid and metabolites are excreted by the kidney. The bioavailability of enteric-coated salicylate products may be poor. The addition of antacids (buffered aspirin) may decrease GI irritation and increase the dissolution and absorption of such products. **Plasma protein binding:** As active salicylic acid, 70–90%.

CONTRAINDICATIONS

Hypersensitivity to salicylates. Clients with asthma, hay fever, or nasal polyps have a higher incidence of hypersensitivity reactions. Severe anemia, history of blood coagulation defects, in conjunction with anticoagulant therapy. Salicylates can cause congestive failure when taken in the large doses used for rheumatic diseases. Vitamin K deficiency; 1 week before and after surgery. In pregnancy, especially the last trimester as the drug may cause problems in the newborn child or complications during delivery. In children or teenagers with chicken-pox or flu due to possibility of development of Reye's syndrome.

Controlled-release aspirin is not recommended for use as an antipyretic or short-term analgesic because adequate blood levels may not be reached. Also, controlled-release products are not recommended for children less than 12 years of age and in children with fever accompanied by dehydration.

SPECIAL CONCERNS

■ Do not use in children or teenagers with chickenpox or flu symptoms due to the possibility of Reye's syndrome, a rare but serious illness.■ Use with caution during lactation and in the presence of gastric or peptic ulcers, in mild diabetes, erosive gastritis, bleeding tendencies, in cardiac disease, and in liver or kidney disease. Aspirin products now carry the following labeling: 'It is especially important not to use aspirin during the last three months of pregnancy unless specifically directed to do so by a doctor because it may cause problems in the newborn child or complications during delivery.' There is increased potential for stomach bleeding in clients 60 years of age and older, in clients who have had prior ulcers or bleeding, and in those who take an anticoagulant when taking more than one product containing an NSAID, when taken with moderate amounts of alcohol, or when taken for longer than directed.

SIDE EFFECTS

Most Common

Dyspepsia, nausea, epigastric discomfort. The toxic effects of the salicylates are dose-related.

GI: Dyspepsia, heartburn, anorexia, nausea, occult blood loss, epigastric discomfort, *massive GI bleeding, potentiation of peptic ulcer.* Possible stomach bleeding in those who ingest three or more alcoholic drinks/day. **Allergic:** *Bronchospasm, asthma-like symptoms, anaphylaxis,* skin rashes, angioedema, urticaria, rhinitis, nasal polyps. **Hematologic:** Prolongation of bleeding time, thrombocytopenia, leukopenia, purpura, shortened erythrocyte survival time, decreased plasma iron levels. **Mis-**

cellaneous: Thirst, fever, dimness of vision.

NOTE: Use of aspirin in children and teenagers with flu or chickenpox may result in the development of Reye's syndrome. Also, dehydrated, febrile children are more prone to salicylate intoxication.

OD OVERDOSE MANAGEMENT

Symptoms: **Symptoms of Mild Salicylate Toxicity (Salicylism):** At serum levels between 150 and 200 mcg/mL. **GI:** N&V, diarrhea, thirst. **CNS:** Tinnitus (most common), dizziness, difficulty in hearing, mental confusion, lassitude. **Miscellaneous:** Flushing, sweating, tachycardia. Symptoms of salicylism may be observed with doses used for inflammatory disease or rheumatic fever. **Symptoms of Severe Salicylate Poisoning:** At serum levels over 400 mcg/mL. **CNS:** Excitement, confusion, disorientation, irritability, hallucinations, lethargy, stupor, *coma, respiratory failure, seizures.* **Metabolic:** Respiratory alkalosis (initially), respiratory acidosis and metabolic acidosis, dehydration. **GI:** N&V. **Hematologic:** Platelet dysfunction, hypoprothrombinemia, increased capillary fragility. **Miscellaneous:** *Hyperthermia, hemorrhage, CV collapse, renal failure,* hyperventilation, pulmonary edema, tetany, hypoglycemia (late).

Treatment: Mild Toxicity:

1. If the client has had repeated administration of large doses of salicylates, document and report evidence of hyperventilation or complaints of auditory or visual disturbances (symptoms of salicylism).

2. Severe salicylate poisoning, whether due to overdose or accumulation, will have an exaggerated effect on the CNS and the metabolic system:

- Clients may develop a salicylate jag characterized by garrulous behavior. They may act as if they were inebriated.
- Convulsions and coma may follow.

3. When working with febrile children or the elderly who have been treated with aspirin, maintain adequate fluid intake. These clients are more susceptible to salicylate intoxication if they are dehydrated.

4. The following treatment approaches may be considered for treatment of *acute salicylate toxicity:*

- Initially induce vomiting or perform gastric lavage followed by activated charcoal (most effective if given within 2 hr of ingestion).
- Monitor salicylate levels and acid-base and fluid and electrolyte balance. If required, administer IV solutions of dextrose, saline, potassium, and sodium bicarbonate as well as vitamin K.
- Seizures may be treated with diazepam.
- Treat hyperthermia if present.
- Alkaline diuresis will enhance renal excretion. Hemodialysis is effective but should be reserved for severe poisonings.
- If necessary, administer oxygen and artificial ventilation

DRUG INTERACTIONS

ACE inhibitors / ↓ Effect of ACE inhibitors possibly due to prostaglandin inhibition; also, significantly higher mortality rate using doses of aspirin of at least 325 mg/day

Acetazolamide / ↑ CNS toxicity of salicylates; also, ↑ excretion of salicylic acid in alkaline urine

Alcohol, ethyl / ↑ Chance of GI bleeding caused by salicylates

Alteplase, recombinant / ↑ Risk of bleeding

Aminosalicylate / Possible ↑ effect of PAS due to ↓ excretion by kidney or ↓ plasma protein binding

Ammonium chloride / ↑ Effect of salicylates by ↑ renal tubular reabsorption

Antacids / ↓ Salicylate levels in plasma due to ↑ rate of renal excretion

Anticoagulants, oral / ↑ Effect of anticoagulant by ↓ plasma protein binding and plasma prothrombin

Antirheumatics / Both are ulcerogenic and may cause ↑ GI bleeding

Ascorbic acid / ↑ Effect of salicylates by ↑ renal tubular reabsorption

Beta-adrenergic blocking agents / Salicylates ↓ action of beta-blockers, possibly due to prostaglandin inhibition

---

Charcoal, activated / ↓ Absorption of salicylates from GI tract

Clopidogrel / ↑ Risk of life-threatening or major bleeding events in high-risk clients with recent ischemic stroke or transient ischemic attacks

Corticosteroids / Both are ulcerogenic; also, corticosteroids may ↓ blood salicylate levels by ↑ breakdown by liver and ↑ excretion

Dipyridamole / Additive anticoagulant effects

H *Feverfew* / Possible ↑ antiplatelet effect

Furosemide / ↑ Risk of salicylate toxicity due to ↓ renal excretion; also, salicylates may ↓ effect of furosemide in clients with impaired renal function or cirrhosis with ascites

H *Garlic* / Possible ↑ antiplatelet effect

H *Ginkgo biloba* / Possible ↑ effect on platelet aggregation → bleeding episodes

H *Ginseng* / Possible ↓ effect on platelet aggregation

Griseofulvin / ↓ Salicylate levels

Heparin / Inhibition of platelet adhesiveness by aspirin may result in bleeding tendencies

Hypoglycemics, oral / ↑ Hypoglycemia R/T ↓ plasma protein binding and ↓ excretion

Ibuprofen / Cardioprotective effects of low dose aspirin may be negated or ↓ with concomitant ibuprofen use

Indomethacin / Both are ulcerogenic → ↑ GI bleeding

Insulin / Salicylates ↑ Hypoglycemic effect of insulin

Methionine / ↑ Effect of salicylates by ↑ renal tubular reabsorption

Methotrexate / ↑ Methotrexate effect by ↓ plasma protein binding; also, salicylates block drugs' renal excretion

Nitroglycerin / Combination may result in unexpected hypotension

Nizatidine / ↑ Serum levels of salicylates

NSAIDs / Additive ulcerogenic effects; also, aspirin may ↓ serum levels of NSAIDs

Phenytoin / ↑ Phenytoin effect by ↓ plasma protein binding

Probenecid / Salicylates inhibit uricosuric activity of probenecid

Sodium bicarbonate / ↓ Effect of salicylates by ↑ rate of excretion

Spironolactone / Aspirin ↓ Diuretic drug effect

Sulfinpyrazone / Salicylates inhibit uricosuric drug activity

Sulfonamides / ↑ Sulfonamides effect R/T displacement from plasma proteins

Valproic acid / ↑ Valproic effect R/T ↓ plasma protein binding

HOW SUPPLIED

Acetylsalicylic Acid. *Gum:* 227.5 mg; *Suppositories:* 120 mg, 200 mg, 300 mg, 600 mg; *Tablets:* 325 mg, 500 mg; *Tablets, Chewable:* 81 mg; *Tablets, Delayed-Release:* 81 mg; *Tablets, Enteric-Coated:* 81 mg, 165 mg, 325 mg, 500 mg, 650 mg, 975 mg; *Tablets, Extended-Release:* 650 mg, 800 mg.

Acetylsalicylic Acid, Buffered. *Caplets:* 325 mg; *Tablets:* 325 mg, 500 mg; *Tablets, Coated:* 325 mg, 500 mg; *Tablets, Effervescent:* 325 mg, 500 mg.

DOSAGE

• **CAPLETS; GUM; SUPPOSITORIES; TABLETS; TABLETS, CHEWABLE; TABLETS, COATED; TABLETS, DELAYED-RELEASE; TABLETS, EFFERVESCENT; TABLETS, ENTERIC-COATED**

Analgesic, antipyretic.

Adults: 325–500 mg q 3 hr, 325–600 mg q 4 hr, or 650–1,000 mg q 6 hr. As an alternative, the adult chewable tablet (81 mg each) may be used in doses of 4–8 tablets q 4 hr as needed. **Pediatric:** 65 mg/kg/day (alternate dose: 1.5 grams/m^2/day) in divided doses q 4–6 hr, not to exceed 3.6 grams/day. Alternatively, the following dosage regimen can be used: **Pediatric, 2–3 years:** 162 mg q 4 hr as needed; **4–5 years:** 243 mg q 4 hr as needed; **6–8 years:** 320–325 mg q 4 hr as needed; **9–10 years:** 405 mg q 4 hr as needed; **11 years:** 486 mg q 4 hr as needed; **12–14 years:** 648 mg q 4 hr.

Arthritis, rheumatic diseases.

Adults: 3.2–6 grams/day in divided doses.

Juvenile rheumatoid arthritis.

60–110 mg/kg/day (alternate dose: 3 grams/m^2/day) in divided doses q 6–8

---

hr. When initiating therapy at 60 mg/kg/day, dose may be increased by 20 mg/kg/day after 5–7 days and by 10 mg/kg/day after another 5–7 days.

Acute rheumatic fever.

Adults, initial: 5–8 grams/day. **Pediatric, initial:** 100 mg/kg/day (3 grams/m²/day) for 2 weeks; **then,** decrease to 75 mg/kg/day for 4–6 weeks.

Reduce risk of death and nonfatal stroke following ischemic stroke or TIA.

50–325 mg/day.

Reduce risk of vascular mortality in suspected acute MI.

Initial: 160–162.5 mg, **then** daily for 30 days. Consider subsequent prophylactic therapy.

Reduce combined risk of recurrent MI and death in those with a previous MI or unstable angina or to reduce risk of MI and sudden death in those with chronic stable angina.

75–325 mg/day.

Pre-existing need for aspirin following coronary artery bypass grafting, PTCA, carotid endarterectomy.

Dosage varies by procedure.

Kawasaki disease.

Adults: 80–180 mg/kg/day during the febrile period. After the fever resolves, the dose may be adjusted to 10 mg/kg/day.

NOTE: Aspirin Regimen Bayer 81 mg with Calcium contains 250 mg calcium carbonate (10% of RDA) and 81 mg of acetylsalicylic acid for individuals who require aspirin to prevent recurrent heart attacks and strokes.

NURSING CONSIDERATIONS

ADMINISTRATION/STORAGE

1. Enteric-coated tablets or buffered tablets are better tolerated by some.
2. Take with full glass of water to prevent lodging in the esophagus.
3. Have epinephrine available to counteract hypersensitivity reactions should they occur. Asthma caused by hypersensitivity reaction to salicylates may be refractory to epinephrine, so antihistamines should also be available for parenteral and PO use.

ASSESSMENT

1. Take complete drug history; note any hypersensitivity. Individuals allergic to tartrazine should not take aspirin. If salicylates not tolerated well in the past may suddenly have an allergic or anaphylactoid reaction.
2. For pain, rate and determine the type, location, and pattern of pain, if unusual, or if recurring. Note effectiveness of aspirin if previously used for pain and dose used.
3. Identify any asthma, hay fever, ulcer disease or nasal polyps.
4. Note age; avoid drug if under the age of 12. Assess for chickenpox or the flu.
5. Test stool and urine for blood; monitor renal, LFTs and CBC routinely during high-dose and chronic therapy.
6. Determine if diagnostic tests scheduled. Drug causes irreversible platelet effects. Anticipate 4–7 days for body to replace these once drug is discontinued; hence no salicylates one week prior to procedure.
7. Note history of peptic ulcers or bleeding tendencies. Obtain bleeding parameters with prolonged use.
8. Review drugs currently prescribed/OTC for drug interactions.
9. The therapeutic serum level of salicylate is 150–300 mcg/mL for adult and juvenile rheumatoid arthritis and acute rheumatic fever. Reassure that higher dosage is needed for anti-inflammatory effects.

CLIENT/FAMILY TEACHING

1. Take as directed. To reduce gastric irritation or lodging in the esophagus, administer with meals, milk, a full glass of water, or crackers and remain upright for at least 20–30 min.
2. Do not take if product is off-color or has a strange odor. Note expiration date.
3. Report toxic effects: ringing in the ears, difficulty hearing, dizziness or fainting spells, unusual increase in sweating, severe abdominal pain, or mental confusion.
4. Potentiates effects of antidiabetic drugs. Monitor FS and report low sug-

---

ars. Avoid high alcohol ingestion; may cause GI bleeding.

5. When administering for antipyretic effect, follow temperature administration parameters:

- Obtain temperature 1 hr after administering to assess outcome.
- With marked diaphoresis, dry client, change linens, provide fluids, and prevent chilling.

6. Cardiac clients on large doses should report symptoms of CHF.

7. Tell dentist and other HCPs you are taking salicylates.

8. Before purchasing other OTC preparations, read labels for salicylate content and notify provider noting quantity used per day.

9. Salicylates should be administered to children only upon specific medical order R/T risk of Reye's syndrome.

10. If child refuses medication or vomits it, consider suppositories or acetaminophen.

11. Dehydrated children who have a fever are especially susceptible to aspirin intoxication from even small doses. Report gastric irritation/pain; may be S&S of hypersensitivity or toxicity.

12. Sodium bicarbonate may decrease the serum level of aspirin, reducing its effectiveness.

13. Report unusual bruising or bleeding. Large doses may increase PT and should be avoided. Aspirin and NSAIDs may interfere with blood-clotting mechanisms (antiplatelet effects) and are usually discontinued 1 week before surgery to prevent increased risk of bleeding.

14. Avoid indiscriminate use; store appropriately.

OUTCOMES/EVALUATE

- Relief of pain/discomfort; Improved joint mobility/function
- ↓ Fever; ↓ Vascular mortality
- ↓ Inflammation
- Prophylaxis of MI/TIA

Atazanavir sulfate   A

(ah-**tah**-zah-**NAH**-veer)

CLASSIFICATION(S):
Antiretroviral agent, protease inhibitor
PREGNANCY CATEGORY: B
Rx: Reyataz.

USES
In combination with other antiretroviral drugs for HIV-1 infections.

ACTION/KINETICS

Action
Atazanavir is an azapeptide HIV-1 protease inhibitor that selectively inhibits the virus-specific processing of viral Gag and Gag-Pol polyproteins in HIV-1 infected cells, thus preventing formation of mature virions.

Pharmacokinetics
Readily absorbed; T_{max}: 2.5 hr. Food enhances bioavailability and reduces pharmacokinetic variability. Steady state is reached between 4 and 8 days. Is extensively metabolized by CYP3A. Metabolites and unchanged drug are excreted in the feces (79%) and urine (13%). $t\frac{1}{2}$, **elimination:** 7 hr at steady-state after a 400 mg/day dose with a light meal. $t\frac{1}{2}$ increases in clients with impaired hepatic function. **Plasma protein binding:** 86%.

CONTRAINDICATIONS
Use in clients with severe hepatic insufficiency (Child-Pugh C). Use with drugs (e.g., ergot derivatives, midazolam, pimozide, triazolam) that are highly dependent on CYP3A for clearance and for which increased plasma levels are associated with serious and/or life-threatening events. Various degrees of cross-resistance among protease inhibitors seen. Lactation. Use in pediatric clients below 3 months of age due to the possibility of kernicterus.

SPECIAL CONCERNS
Concentration- and dose-dependent prolongation of the PR interval in ECGs has been observed. Use with caution in clients with moderate hepatic impairment and in the elderly. Cross-resis-

tance among protease inhibitors has been observed.

SIDE EFFECTS

Most Common

N&V, jaundice/scleral icterus, myalgia, rash, headache, abdominal pain, diarrhea.

Many side effects occur when atazanavir is combined with other antiviral drugs. **CNS:** Headache, depression, dizziness, insomnia, peripheral neurologic symptoms, abnormal dreams/gait, agitation, amnesia, anxiety, confusion, convulsions, decreased libido, emotional lability, hallucinations, hostility, hyperkinesia, hypesthesia, increased reflexes, nervousness, psychosis, sleep disorder, somnolence, suicide attempt, twitch. **GI:** N&V, jaundice, scleral icterus, abdominal pain, diarrhea, acholia, anorexia, aphthous stomatitis, colitis, constipation, dental pain, dyspepsia, enlarged abdomen, esophageal ulcer, esophagitis, flatulence, gastritis, gastroenteritis, GI disorder, hepatitis, hepatomegaly, hepatosplenomegaly, increased appetite, liver damage, liver fatty deposit, mouth ulcer, pancreatitis, peptic ulcer. **Metabolic:** New-onset diabetes mellitus, exacerbation of pre-existing diabetes mellitus, hyperglycemia, diabetic ketoacidosis, *lactic acidosis syndrome (when used with nucleoside analogs),* dehydration, dyslipidemia, gout, lipohypertrophy, obesity, weight decrease/gain. Redistribution/accumulation of body fat, including central obesity, dorsocervical fat enlargement (buffalo hump), peripheral/facial wasting, breast enlargement, cushingoid appearance. **CV:** Increased bleeding, including spontaneous skin hematomas and hemarthrosis in hemophilia type A and B; prolongation of PR interval. *Heart arrest,* heart block, hypertension, myocarditis, palpitation, syncope, vasodilation. **GU:** Abnormal urine, amenorrhea, crystalluria, decreased male fertility, gynecomastia, hematuria, impotence, kidney calculus/failure/pain, menstrual disorder, oliguria, pelvic pain, polyuria, proteinuria, urinary frequency, UTI. **Musculoskeletal:** Bone/extremity pain, muscle atrophy, myalgia, myasthenia, myopathy, arthralgia. **Respiratory:** Dyspnea, hiccough, hypoxia, increased cough. **Dermatologic:** Alopecia, cellulitis, dermatophytosis, dry skin, eczema, nail disorder, pruritus, seborrhea, urticaria, vesiculobullous rash, ecchymosis, purpura, sweating. **Otic:** Otitis, tinnitus. **Body as a whole:** Rash, fatigue, fever, lipodystrophy, pain, allergic reaction, angioedema, asthenia, burning sensation, edema, heat sensitivity, infection, malaise, pallor, peripheral edema. **Miscellaneous:** Photosensitivity, taste perversion, back/chest pain, dysplasia, substernal chest pain, immune reconstitution syndrome (inflammatory response to indolent or residual opportunistic infections.)

LABORATORY TEST CONSIDERATIONS

↑ ALT, AST, total bilirubin, amylase, lipase, creatine kinase, total cholesterol, triglycerides. ↓ Hemoglobin, neutrophils, platelets.

OD OVERDOSE MANAGEMENT

Symptoms: Jaundice, PR interval prolongation. *Treatment:* General supportive measures, including monitoring of VS and ECG. Emesis or gastric lavage. Activated charcoal. Dialysis is unlikely to be beneficial.

DRUG INTERACTIONS

Antacids and buffered drugs / ↓ Atazanavir plasma levels; give atazanavir 2 hr before or 1 hr after these medications

Atenolol / Possible prolongation of PR interval; use together with caution

Antiarrhythmics (e.g., amiodarone, systemic lidocaine, quinidine) / Possible serious/life-threatening side effects; monitor carefully if given together

Antidepressants, tricyclic / Possible ↑ tricyclic levels

Benzodiazepines / Potential for serious/life-threatening prolonged or increased sedation or respiratory depression; do not use together

Bepridil / Possible prolongaton of PR interval; do not use together

Buffered drugs / ↓ Atazanavir plasma levels

Calcium channel blockers (e.g., diltiazem, felodipine, nicardipine, nifedipene, verapamil) / Possible prolongation of PR interval; dose reduction may be needed

---

Bold Italic = life threatening side effect   ■ = black box warning   ✦ = Available in Canada

Clarithromycin / ↑ Clarithromycin levels → QTc prolongation; consider a 50% dose reduction; also, significant ↓ in the active 14-OH clarithromycin

Didanosine, buffered formulation only / ↓ Atazanavir levels; take atazanavir 2 hr before or 1 hr after buffered didanosine

Ergot derivatives / Potential for serious/life-threatening acute ergot toxicity; do not use together

Fluticasone (with or without ritonavir) / Significant ↑ plasma fluticasone levels→ significantly ↓ plasma cortisol levels

H₂ receptor antagonists / ↓ Atazanavir plasma levels → ↓ therapeutic effect and resistance; give atazanavir as far apart as possible from H₂-receptor antagonists

HMG-CoA reductase inhibitors (e.g., atorvastatin, lovastatin, simvastatin)/ ↑ HMG-CoA reductase inhibitor serum levels → ↑ toxicity, including rhabdomyolysis; do not use together

Immunosuppressants (e.g., cyclosporine, sirolimus, tacrolimus) / ↑ Plasma levels of the immunosuppressant; monitor carefully

Indinavir / Both associated with indirect hyperbilirubinemia; do not use together

Irinotecan / ↑ Irinotecan toxicity R/T ↓ metabolism; do not use together

Itraconazole / Use with caution with atazanavir/ritonavir due to possible ↑ in atazanavir AUC and C_max

Ketoconazole / Use with caution with atazanavir/ritonavir due to possible ↑ in atazanavir AUC and C_max

Nevirapine / ↓ Atazanavir exposure; do not use together

Oral contraceptives (ethinyl estradiol and norethindrone) / ↑ Levels of hormones; use with caution and use lowest effective dose of each oral contraceptive component

PDE5 inhibitors (e.g., sildenafil, tadalafil, vardenafil) / ↑ PDE5 inhibitor side effects, including hypotension, visual changes, and priapism; use with caution at reduced doses

Pimozide / ↑ Pimozide serum levels and toxicity such as cardiac arrhythmias; do not use together

Proton pump inhibitors / Significant ↓ in atazanavir levels and ↓ therapeutic effect

Rifabutin / ↑ Rifabutin levels; reduce dose up to 75%

Rifampin / ↓ Atazanavir plasma levels and AUC by 90%; do not use together

 St. John's wort / ↓ Atazanavir plasma levels → ↓ effect R/T possible ↑ metabolism by CYP3A4 enzymes; do not use together

Sildenafil / ↑ Sildenafil-associated side effects, including hypotension, visual changes, and priapism; use together with caution

Trazodone (with or without ritonavir) / Significant ↑ plasma trazodone levels→ significantly ↓ plasma cortisol levels

Tricyclic antidepressants (TCA) / ↑ TCA levels; monitor levels

Voriconazole / Do not use with atazanavir; data not available on use together

Warfarin / Possible serious and/or life-threatening bleeding; monitor INR

HOW SUPPLIED

Capsules: 100 mg, 150 mg, 200 mg, 300 mg (all as the base).

DOSAGE

- **CAPSULES**

  HIV-1 infections.

Antiretroviral-experienced clients: 300 mg plus 100 mg ritonavir both once daily with food. **Antiretroviral-naive clients:** 400 mg (2 x 200 mg capsules) once daily with food. Consider a dose reduction to 300 mg of atazanavir for those with moderate hepatic insufficiency (Child-Pugh score from 7–9).

NURSING CONSIDERATIONS

ADMINISTRATION/STORAGE

1. Do not coadminister atazanavir and efavirenz without ritonavir.

2. If given with didanosine buffered products, give with food 2 hr before or 1 hr after didanosine.

3. Atazanavir without ritonavir is not recommended for treatment-experienced clients with prior virologic failure.

4. Safety and efficacy of atazanavir with ritonavir in doses greater than 100 mg once daily have not been determined. Use of higher ritonavir doses is not rec-

ommended as they may alter the safety profile of atazanavir (e.g., cardiac effects, hyperbilirubinemia).

5. In treatment-naive clients who receive efavirenz and atazanavir, the recommended dose of atazanavir is 300 mg with ritonavir 100 mg, and efavirenz, 600 mg.

6. When given with tenofovir disoproxil fumarate, give atazanavir 300 mg, with ritonavir, 100 mg, and tenofovir, 300 mg (all as a single daily dose with food). Atazanavir should not be given with tenofovir without ritonavir.

ASSESSMENT

1. Note disease onset, characteristics of S&S, other agents trialed, outcome.

2. List drugs prescribed; ensure none interact.

3. Assess EKG for prolonged PR interval. Monitor HIV RNA and LFTs; reduce dose with dysfunction. Observe for any new onset diabetes.

CLIENT/FAMILY TEACHING

1. Take with food to improve drug function and with other antiretroviral therapy; always used in combination therapy. Take as directed, do not skip or double doses.

2. Do not take any unprescribed or OTC meds/herbals without provider consent. Avoid St. Johns Wort and Viagra—may cause adverse reactions.

3. Report dizziness/lightheadedness as EKG may be needed; may prolong PR interval.

4. Drug may cause changes in body fat distribution/accumulation.

5. Does not prevent disease transmission or STDs; use protection. Report yellowing of skin/eyes; may cause bilirubin elevations.

6. May cause photosensitivity reaction; wear protective clothes/sunscreen—avoid prolonged exposure.

OUTCOMES/EVALUATE

Management of HIV infection; ↓ HIV-RNA

Atenolol

(ah-**TEN**-oh-lohl)

CLASSIFICATION(S):

Beta-adrenergic blocking agent
PREGNANCY CATEGORY: C
Rx: Tenormin.
♣Rx: Apo-Atenol, Gen-Atenolol, Novo-Atenol, Nu-Atenol, PMS-Atenolol, Rhoxal-atenolol, ratio-Atenolol.

SEE ALSO BETA-ADRENERGIC BLOCKING AGENTS.

USES

(1) Hypertension (either alone or with other antihypertensives such as thiazide diuretics). (2) Long-term treatment of angina pectoris due to coronary atherosclerosis. (3) Acute MI. *Investigational:* Prophylaxis of migraine, alcohol withdrawal syndrome, situational anxiety, ventricular arrhythmias, prophylactically to reduce incidence of supraventricular arrhythmias in coronary artery bypass graft surgery.

ACTION/KINETICS

Action

Combines reversibly with beta-adrenergic receptors to block the response to sympathetic nerve impulses, circulating catecholamines, or adrenergic drugs. Predominantly beta-1 blocking activity. Has no membrane stabilizing activity or intrinsic sympathomimetic activity.

Pharmacokinetics

Low lipid solubility. **Peak blood levels:** 2–4 hr. **t½:** 6–9 hr. 50% eliminated unchanged in the feces. Geriatric clients have a higher plasma level than younger clients and a total clearance value of about 50% less.

SPECIAL CONCERNS

Dosage not established in children.

SIDE EFFECTS

Most Common

Dizziness, fatigue, nausea, bradycardia, hypotension, vertigo.

See *Beta-Adrenergic Blocking Agents* for a complete list of possible side effects.

HOW SUPPLIED

Injection: 0.5 mg/mL; *Tablets:* 25 mg, 50 mg, 100 mg.

A

DOSAGE
- **TABLETS**

Hypertension.

Initial: 50 mg/day, either alone or with diuretics; if response is inadequate, 100 mg/day. Doses higher than 100 mg/day will not produce further beneficial effects. Maximum effects usually seen within 1–2 weeks.

Angina.

Initial: 50 mg/day; if maximum response is not seen in 1 week, increase dose to 100 mg/day (some clients require 200 mg/day).

Alcohol withdrawal syndrome.

50–100 mg/day.

Prophylaxis of migraine.

50–100 mg/day.

Ventricular arrhythmias.

50–100 mg/day.

Prior to coronary artery bypass graft surgery.

50 mg/day started 72 hr prior to surgery. *NOTE:* Adjust dosage in cases of renal failure to 50 mg/day if C_{CR} is 15–35 mL/min/1.73 m^2 and to 50 mg every other day if C_{CR} is less than 15 mL/min/1.73 m^2.

- **IV**

Acute myocardial infarction.

Initial: 5 mg over 5 min followed by a second 5-mg dose 10 min later. Begin treatment as soon as possible after client arrives at the hospital. In clients who tolerate the full 10-mg dose, give a 50-mg tablet 10 min after the last IV dose followed by another 50-mg dose 12 hr later. **Then,** 100 mg/day or 50 mg twice a day for 6–9 days (or until discharge from the hospital).

NURSING CONSIDERATIONS

🕮 Do not confuse atenolol with albuterol (sympathomimetic) or with timolol (beta-blocker). Do not confuse Tenormin with Tenoretic (atenolol plus chlorthalidone).

ADMINISTRATION/STORAGE
1. With hemodialysis, give 25 or 50 mg in the hospital after each dialysis. Give under supervision; significant decreases in BP may occur.

IV 2. For IV use, may be diluted in NaCl injection, dextrose injection, or both.
3. If any question in using IV atenolol, eliminate IV administration and use tablets, 100 mg once daily or 50 mg twice a day for 7 or more days.

ASSESSMENT
1. Identify reasons for therapy, type, onset of symptoms.
2. Note history of diabetes, pulmonary disease, or cardiac failure.
3. List drugs prescribed; ensure none interact.
4. Assess VS, EKG, and lung sounds.

CLIENT/FAMILY TEACHING
1. Take at same time each day. May take with food if GI upset occurs.
2. May mask symptoms of low blood sugar in those with diabetes.
3. A beta blocker drug lowers BP and heart rate, controls angina, and may decrease mortality from recurrent MI. With angina, do not stop abruptly; may cause anginal attack.
4. Report adverse effects or changes in mood or affect, especially severe depression and/or fatigue.
5. May enhance sensitivity to cold, dress accordingly.
6. With initiation of therapy or change in dosage stress importance of F/U for evaluation of drug response. Keep log of HR and BP at different times during the day for provider review.
7. Practice reliable contraception.

OUTCOMES/EVALUATE
- ↓ BP; ↓ HR
- ↓ Frequency of anginal attacks
- Prevention of repeat infarction

—— **COMBINATION DRUG** ——

Atenolol and Chlorthalidone 🕮
(ay-**TEN**-oh-lol, klor-**THAL**-i-done)

CLASSIFICATION(S):
Antihypertensive
PREGNANCY CATEGORY: D
Rx: Tenoretic.

SEE ALSO *ATENOLOL AND BETA-ADRENERGIC BLOCKING AGENTS.*

USES
Treatment of hypertension (not for initial therapy).

CONTENT
Tenoretic 50: Atenolol (beta-adrenergic blocking agent), 50 mg and chlorthalidone (diuretic), 25 mg. *Tenoretic 100:* Atenolol, 100 mg and chlorthalidone, 25 mg.

ACTION/KINETICS
Action
Atenolol is a beta$_1$-selective beta-adrenergic receptor blocking agent without membrane stabilizing or intrinsic sympathomimetic activities. At higher doses, atenolol inhibits beta$_2$-adrenergic receptors, mainly located in the bronchial and vascular musculature. Chlorthalidone is a diuretic that acts at the cortical diluting segment of the ascending limb of Henle's loop of the nephron. Both sodium and chloride excretion are increased. The antihypertensive effects of these drugs is additive.

Pharmacokinetics
Bioavailability is not affected when these two drugs are given together. Absorption of atenolol is rapid and consistent, but incomplete. **Peak plasma levels, atenolol:** 2–4 hr. **Peak effect, atenolol:** 2–4 hr; **duration:** 24 hr. **t½, elimination, atenolol:** 6–7 hr. Atenolol is excreted mostly unchanged in the urine. **Onset, chlorthalidone:** Within 2 hr. **Plasma protein binding:** From 6–16% of atenolol is bound to plasma proteins.

CONTRAINDICATIONS
Sinus bradycardia, heart block greater than first degree, cardiogenic shock, overt cardiac failure, anuria, untreated pheochromocytoma, hypersensitivity to the product or to sulfonamide-derived drugs.

SPECIAL CONCERNS
Use with caution in CHF controlled by digitalis and/or diuretics, in diabetics, in impaired renal or hepatic function, in those with bronchospastic disease who do not respond to or cannot tolerate other antihypertensive treatment, and when using anesthetic agents that may depress the myocardium. Exacerbation of angina pectoris and, in some cases, MI may occur following abrupt cessation of therapy with certain beta-adrenergic blocking agents in clients with coronary artery disease. Use with caution during lactation and pregnancy. Safety and efficacy have not been determined in children.

SIDE EFFECTS
Most Common
Cold extremities, dizziness, tiredness, depression, dyspnea, orthostatic hypotension, N&V.

See *Atenolol* and *Beta-Adrenergic Blocking Agents* for a complete list of possible side effects for Atenolol. **Chlorthalidone. CV:** Orthostatic hypotension. **GI:** Anorexia, gastric irritation, vomiting, cramping, constipation, jaundice, pancreatitis. **CNS:** Vertigo, paresthesia, xanthopsia. **Hematologic:** Leukopenia, agranulocytosis, thrombocytopenia, *aplastic anemia.* **Hypersensitivity:** Purpura, photosensitivity, rash, urticaria, vasculitis, *toxic epidermal necrolysis.* **Metabolic:** Hyperglycemia, glycosuria, hyperuricemia. **Miscellaneous:** Muscle spasm, weakness, restlessness.

DRUG INTERACTIONS
Antihypertensive drugs / Hypotension and/or marked bradycardia leading to vertigo, syncope, or postural hypotension
Calcium channel blockers / Possible bradycardia and heart block and ↑ left ventricular end diastolic pressure
Clonidine / Exacerbation of rebound hypertension after withdrawal of clonidine
Indomethacin / ↓ Hypotensive effects of atenolol
Lithium / ↑ Risk of lithium toxicity R/T ↓ lithium clearance

HOW SUPPLIED
See Content.

DOSAGE
• **TABLETS**
Hypertension (not for initial therapy).
Initial: One Tenoretic 50 tablet once a day. If an optimal response is not reached, increase the dose to one Tenoretic 100 tablet given once a day. Adjust the dose in cases of severe renal

---

Bold Italic = life threatening side effect   ■ = black box warning   ✚ = Available in Canada

function as follows: C_{CR}, 15–35 mL/min/1.73m²: 50 mg daily of atenolol; C_{CR}, less than 15 mL/min/1.73m²: 50 mg atenolol every other day.

NURSING CONSIDERATIONS

🕯 Do not confuse Tenoretic with Tenormin (atenolol alone).

ADMINISTRATION/STORAGE
Store from 20–25° C (68–77° F). Dispense in well-closed, light-resistant containers.

ASSESSMENT
1. List reasons for therapy, disease onset, other therapies trialed, outcome.
2. Monitor EKG, electrolytes, renal and LFTs; adjust dose with dysfunction.
3. Identify drugs prescribed to ensure none interact.
4. Assess for asthma, diabetes, depression, sulfonamide sensitivity, myasthenia; conditions that may preclude therapy.

CLIENT/FAMILY TEACHING
1. Take in a.m. and swallow tablet whole with a full glass of water; do not crush or chew.
2. Drug contains a beta blocker and a diuretic in one pill to better control BP.
3. With diabetes, may alter blood sugar control; monitor carefully.
4. May cause dizziness, drowsiness; assess response before undertaking activities that require mental alertness.
5. Record BP and pulse for provider review.
6. Practice reliable contraception; may harm fetus.
7. Use protection if sun exposed and avoid prolonged outings.
8. Report SOB, palpitations, sexual dysfunction and other adverse effects.
9. Keep all F/U appointments; do not stop drug suddenly without provider approval.

OUTCOMES/EVALUATE
Control of BP

Atomoxetine HCl ■
(**AT**-oh-mox-eh-teen)

CLASSIFICATION(S):
Drug for attention-deficit/hyperactivity disorder
PREGNANCY CATEGORY: C
Rx: Strattera.

SEE ALSO SELECTIVE SEROTONIN REUPTAKE INHIBITORS

USES
Attention-deficit/hyperactivity disorder (ADHD) as categorized by DSM-IV-TR.

ACTION/KINETICS

Action
Mechanism not known but thought to be related to selective inhibition of presynaptic norepinephrine transport, thus increasing levels of norepinephrine in nerve synapses.

Pharmacokinetics
Rapidly absorbed after PO use with absolute bioavailability of 63% in extensive metabolizers and 94% in poor metabolizers. High fat meals decrease the rate of absorption; in children and adolescents, administration with food results in a 9% lower C_{max}. **Maximum plasma levels:** 1–2 hr. Metabolized by the cytochrome P450 2D6 (CYP2D6) pathway. Those with reduced activity of this pathway (about 7% of Caucasians and 3% of African Americans) have higher plasma levels. **t½:** About 5 hr. Greater than 80% excreted in the urine and 17% in the feces. **Plasma protein binding:** About 98%.

CONTRAINDICATIONS
Hypersensitivity to atomoxetine or other product constituents. Use with a monoamine oxidase inhibitor (MAOI) or within 2 weeks after discontinuing an MAOI. Use in narrow angle glaucoma due to ↑ risk of mydriasis.

SPECIAL CONCERNS
■ Atomoxetine increased the risk of suicidal ideation in short-term studies in children or adolescents with ADHD. Anyone considering the use of atomoxetine in a child or adolescent must balance this risk with the clinical need.

A

Closely monitor clients who are started on therapy for suicidality (suicidal thinking and behavior), clinical worsening, or unusual changes in behavior. Advise families and caregivers of the need for close observation and communication with the prescribing health care provider. Atomoxetine is approved for ADHD in children and adults. It is not approved for major depressive disorder. The average risk of suicidal ideation in children and adolescents receiving atomoxetine was 0.4% compared with none in placebo-treated clients. No suicides occurred in trials.■ Safety and efficacy have not been determined in children younger than 6 years of age. Efficacy has not been evaluated systematically beyond 9 weeks of use and safety beyond 1 year of treatment. Use with caution in hypertension, tachycardia, CV, or cerebrovascular disease or with pressor agents due to drug-induced increases in BP and HR. Use with caution in any condition that predisposes to hypotension and during lactation. Discontinue in clients who develop jaundice or lab evidence of liver injury.

SIDE EFFECTS

Most Common

Dyspepsia, N&V, fatigue, decreased appetite, dizziness, mood swings.
CNS: Aggression, hostility, irritability, somnolence, dizziness, paresthesia, sinus headache, abnormal dreams, sleep disorder, insomnia and/or middle insomnia, sedation, depression, tremor, headache, mood swings, crying, tearfulness, early morning awakening. **GI:** N&V, dyspepsia, decreased appetite, upper abdominal pain, diarrhea, dry mouth, flatulence, constipation, viral gastroenteritis, *severe liver injury*. **CV:** Postural hypotension, increased BP, sinus tachycardia, tachycardia, palpitations, hot flushes, peripheral vascular instability and/or Raynaud phenomenon (new onset or worsening of preexisting). **Hypersensitivity:** Angioneurotic edema, urticaria, rash. **Respiratory:** Cough, rhinorrhea, sore throat, sinusitis, nasal/sinus congestion, nasopharyngitis, URTI. **Dermatologic:** Dermatitis, flushing, pruritus, increased sweating,

peripheral coldness. **GU:** Urinary retention, ejaculatory failure and/or ejaculation disorder, impotence, urinary hesitation, difficulty in micturition, dysmenorrhea, delayed menses, irregular menstruation, abnormal orgasm, prostatitis, erectile disturbance. **Body as a whole:** Fatigue and/or lethargy, pyrexia, rigors, flu, decreased appetite, weight loss, anorexia, arthralgia, myalgia. **Miscellaneous:** Mydriasis, ear infection, chest/back pain, decreased libido, paresthesias.

OD OVERDOSE MANAGEMENT

Symptoms: Agitation, abnormal behavior, GI symptoms, hyperactivity, somnolence, mydriasis, tachycardia, dry mouth. *Treatment:* Establish an airway. Monitor cardiac and vital signs. Provide symptomatic and supportive care. Gastric emptying and repeated activated charcoal may prevent systemic absorption. Dialysis is not likely to be beneficial.

DRUG INTERACTIONS

Albuterol / Potentiation of CV effects of albuterol
Fluoxetine / ↑ Atomoxetine AUC and C_{max}; consider dosage reduction
MAOIs / Possible serious, and sometimes fatal, reactions, including hyperthermia, rigidity, myoclonus, autonomic instability, extreme agitation, delirium, and coma; do not use together
Midazolam / ↑ Midazolam AUC
Paroxetine / ↑ Atomoxetine AUC and C_{max}; consider dosage reduction
Pressor drugs / Possible effects on BP; give with caution
Quinidine / ↑ Atomoxetine AUC and C_{max}; consider dosage reduction

HOW SUPPLIED

Capsules: 10 mg, 18 mg, 25 mg, 40 mg, 60 mg, 80 mg, 100 mg.

DOSAGE

- **CAPSULES**

    ADHD.

Adults and children/adolescents over 70 kg, initial: Total daily dose of 40 mg. May increase after a minimum of 3 days to a target total daily dose of about 80 mg given either as a single dose in the a.m. or as evenly divided doses in the morning and late afternoon/early evening. After 2–4 weeks,

---

Bold Italic = life threatening side effect   ■ = black box warning   ✦ = Available in Canada

dose may be increased to a maximum of 100 mg in those who have not achieved an optimal response. **Children and adolescents up to 70 kg, initial:** Total daily dose of about 0.5 mg/kg. May be increased after a minimum of 3 days to a target total daily dose of about 1.2 mg/kg given either as a single dose in the a.m. or as evenly divided doses in the morning and late afternoon/early evening. No additional benefit is noted for doses higher than 1.2 mg/kg/day. Do not exceed a maximum daily dose of 1.4 mg/kg or 100 mg, whichever is less.

NURSING CONSIDERATIONS

ADMINISTRATION/STORAGE

1. Take with or without food.
2. Periodically evaluate the long-term usefulness for each client.
3. Atomoxetine may be discontinued without the dose being tapered.
4. For moderate hepatic insufficiency (Child-Pugh Class B), reduce initial and target doses to 50% of the normal dose. For severe hepatic insufficiency (Child-Pugh Class C), reduce initial and target doses to 25% of the normal dose.
5. For children and adolescents up to 70 kg who have been given fluoxetine, quinidine, or paroxetine, initiate dosage at 0.5 mg/kg/day and only increase to the usual target dose of 1.2 mg/kg/day if symptoms fail to improve after 4 weeks and initial dose is well tolerated. Those over 70 kg who have been given fluoxetine, quinidine, or paroxetine, initiate dosage at 40 mg/day and only increase to the usual target dose of 80 mg/day if symptoms fail to improve after 4 weeks and the initial dose is well tolerated.
6. Store at controlled room temperature between 15–30°C (59–86°F).

ASSESSMENT

1. Note age at diagnosis of ADHD, chronicity/severity and type of symptoms, social/academic, or occupational impairment. Ensure no psychosis, environmental triggers, or undiagnosed psychiatric disorders.
2. Complete history, physical exam, list DSM IV-TR characteristics. Perform LFTs if itchy skin, dark urine, jaundice, tenderness in the right-upper abdominal quadrant, or unexplained flu-like symptoms.
3. Monitor VS, HT, and WT; may impair growth and weight gain during long-term therapy; may need to interrupt therapy in children who are not growing or gaining weight satisfactorily.
4. List drugs prescribed to ensure none interact (e.g., Prozac, Paxil, quinidine).
5. May increase HR and BP; assess EKG and use cautiously with HTN, cardio/cerebrovascular diseases.
6. Adjust dosage with liver dysfunction. Drug metabolized by cytochrome P450 pathway (CYP2D6).

CLIENT/FAMILY TEACHING

1. Take with or without food. If dose missed, take as soon as possible but do not take more than the prescribed total daily dose in any 24-hr period.
2. Use caution driving or operating machinery until drug effects realized.
3. Do not take any other prescribed, OTC, herbal, or dietary supplements without provider approval. Albuterol therapy may increase BP and heart rate.
4. May experience emotional upset, abdominal pain, GI upset, dry mouth; should subside with continued therapy. Report weight loss/loss of appetite.
5. Swelling of lips, face, rash, and itching are S&S of allergic reaction and require immediate treatment.
6. May inhibit sexual functioning and cause urinary retention/hesitancy; report if bothersome.
7. Ensure psychosocial intervention, lab F/U, and regular monitoring of growth in children.

OUTCOMES/EVALUATE

- Ability to sit quietly and concentrate
- ↓ Hyperactivity/impulsive behaviors

A

Atorvastatin calcium

(ah-**TORE**-vah-**stah**-tin)

CLASSIFICATION(S):
Antihyperlipidemic, HMG-CoA reductase inhibitor
PREGNANCY CATEGORY: X
Rx: Lipitor.

SEE ALSO *ANTIHYPERLIPIDEMIC AGENTS— HMG-COA REDUCTASE INHIBITORS.*

USES
(1) Adjunct to diet to decrease elevated total and LDL cholesterol, apo-B, and triglyceride levels and to increase HDL cholesterol in primary hypercholesterolemia (including heterozygous familial and nonfamilial) and mixed dyslipidemia (including Frederickson type IIa and IIb). (2) Adjunct to other lipid-lowering treatments to reduce total and LDL cholesterol in homozygous familial hypercholesterolemia. (3) Primary dysbetalipoproteinemia (Frederickson type III) in those who do not respond adequately to diet. (4) Adjunct to diet to treat elevated serum triglyceride levels (Frederickson type IV). (5) Adjunct to diet to reduce total and LDL cholesterol and apo-B levels in boys and postmenarchal girls 10–17 years of age with heterozygous familial hypercholesterolemia; used after a trial of diet therapy if the following are present: (a) LDL cholesterol remains 190 mg/dL or higher or (b) LDL remains 160 mg/dL or higher AND there is a positive family history of premature CV disease or two or more other CVD risk factors are present. (6) Reduce the risk of nonfatal MI, fatal and nonfatal stroke, revascularization procedures, hospitalization for CHF, and angina in clients with clinically evident coronary heart disease. (7) Reduce the risk of MI and stroke and the risk for revascularization procedures and angina in adults without clinically evident coronary heart disease but with multiple risk factors for coronary heart disease, including age, smoking, hypertension, low HDL-C, or a family history of early coronary heart disease. (8) Reduce the risk of stroke and MI in type 2 diabetics who show no evidence of coronary heart disease but with other risk factors, including retinopathy, albuminuria, smoking, or hypertension.

ACTION/KINETICS
Action
Competitively inhibits HMG-CoA reductase; this enzyme catalyzes the early rate-limiting step in the synthesis of cholesterol. Thus, cholesterol synthesis is inhibited/decreased. Decreases cholesterol, triglycerides, VLDL, and LDL and increases HDL.

Pharmacokinetics
Absolute bioavailability is about 14%. Undergoes first-pass metabolism by CYP3A4 enzymes to active metabolites. **$t^{1/2}$:** 14 hr. Plasma levels are not affected by renal disease but they are markedly increased with chronic alcoholic liver disease. Metabolized in the liver to active metabolites. Decreases in LDL cholesterol range from 35–40% (10 mg/day) to 50–60% (80 mg/day). Less than 2% excreted in the urine. **Plasma protein binding:** More than 98%.

CONTRAINDICATIONS
Active liver disease or unexplained persistently high LFTs. Use with grapefruit juice. Pregnancy, lactation.

SPECIAL CONCERNS
Safety and efficacy have not been determined in children less than 18 years of age.

SIDE EFFECTS
Most Common
Headache, asthenia, abdominal pain/cramps, infection, diarrhea, sinusitis, pharyngitis, myalgia, arthralgia, back pain, rash/pruritus, flu syndrome.

See also *Antihyperlipidemic Agents— HMG-CoA Reductase Inhibitors for a complete list of possible side effects.* **GI:** Altered LFTs (usually within the first 3 months of therapy), abdominal pain/cramps, diarrhea, flatulence, dyspepsia. **CNS:** Headache, paresthesia, asthenia, insomnia. **Musculoskeletal:** Myalgia, leg pain, back pain, arthritis, arthralgia. **Respiratory:** Sinusitis, bronchitis, pharyngitis, rhinitis. **Miscellaneous:** Infec-

---

tion, rash, pruritus, allergy, influenza, flu syndrome, accidental trauma, peripheral edema, chest pain, alopecia, asthenia.

ADDITIONAL DRUG INTERACTIONS

Antacids / ↓ Atorvastatin levels

Clarithromycin / ↑ Atorvastatin plasma levels; possibility of severe myopathy or rhabdomyolysis

Colestipol / ↓ Atorvastatin levels

Digoxin / ↑ Digoxin levels after 80 mg atorvastatin R/T ↑ digoxin absorption

Diltiazem / ↑ Plasma atorvastatin levels → ↑ risk of myopathy

Erythromycin / ↑ Atorvastatin levels; possibility of severe myopathy or rhabdomyolysis

Nefazodone / ↑ Risk of myopathy

Oral contraceptives / ↑ Plasma levels of norethindrone and ethinyl estradiol

Protease inhibitors (e.g., nelfinavir, ritonavir) / ↑ Atorvastatin levels → ↑ risk of myopathy

Verapamil ↑ Risk of myopathy

LABORATORY TEST CONSIDERATIONS

↑ CPK (due to myalgia).

HOW SUPPLIED

Tablets: 10 mg, 20 mg, 40 mg, 80 mg.

DOSAGE

- **TABLETS**

  Hypercholesterolemia (heterozygous familial and non-familial) and mixed dyslipidemia (Fredrieksen types IIa and IIb).

  Initial: 10–20 mg once daily (40 mg/day for those who require more than a 45% reduction in LDL cholesterol); **then,** a dose range of 10–80 mg once daily may be used. Individualize therapy according to goal of therapy and response.

  Homozygous familial hypercholesterolemia.

  Initial: 10–80 mg/day. Used as an adjunct to other lipid-lowering treatments, such as LDL apheresis.

  Heterozygous familial hypercholesterolemia in children 10–17 years of age.

  Initial: 10 mg/day; **then,** individualize dosage to a maximum of 20 mg/day. Adjust dosage at 4–week or more intervals.

  Prophylaxis of CV disease.

  Adults: 10 mg/day.

NURSING CONSIDERATIONS

ADMINISTRATION/STORAGE

1. Give as single dose at any time of the day, with or without food.

2. Determine lipid levels within 2–4 weeks; adjust dosage accordingly.

3. For additive effect, may be used in combination with a bile acid binding resin. Do not use atorvastatin with fibrates.

4. Store tablets from 20–25°C (68–77°F).

ASSESSMENT

1. Note reasons for therapy, other comorbidities, onset, duration of disease, other agents/measures trialed.

2. Obtain baseline cholesterol profile and LFTs. Monitor LFTs at 6 and 12 weeks after starting therapy and with any dosage change, then semiannually thereafter. If ALT or AST exceed 3 times the normal level, reduce dose or withdraw drug. Assess need for liver biopsy if elevations remain after stopping drug therapy.

3. Review dietary habits, weight, and exercise patterns; identify life-style changes needed.

CLIENT/FAMILY TEACHING

1. Helps to lower blood cholesterol and fat levels, which have been proven to promote CAD.

2. Take at same time each day with or without food; avoid alcohol.

3. Continue dietary restrictions of saturated fat and cholesterol, regular exercise and weight loss in the overall goal of lowering cholesterol levels. See dietician for additional dietary recommendations.

4. Do not add other drugs or OTC agents without provider approval.

5. Report any unexplained muscle pain, weakness, or tenderness, especially if accompanied by fever or malaise.

6. Use UV protection (i.e., sunglasses, sunscreens, clothing/hat) to prevent photosensitivity. Avoid prolonged exposure to direct or artificial sunlight.

7. Practice reliable birth control; may cause fetal damage.

8. Report for lab studies to evaluate effectiveness and need for dosage adjustments.

OUTCOMES/EVALUATE
Reduction in total and LDL cholesterol levels

Atracurium besylate

(ah-trah-**KYOUR**-ee-um)

CLASSIFICATION(S):
Skeletal muscle relaxant, nondepolarizing
PREGNANCY CATEGORY: C
Rx: Tracrium Injection.

SEE ALSO *NEUROMUSCULAR BLOCKING AGENTS.*
USES
(1) Skeletal muscle relaxant during surgery. (2) Adjunct to general anesthesia. (3) Assist in ET intubation. *Investigational:* Treat seizures due to drugs or electrically induced.
ACTION/KINETICS
Action
Prevents acetylcholine effects by competing for the cholinergic receptor at the motor end plate. May also release histamine, leading to hypotension.
Pharmacokinetics
Onset: Within 2 min. **Peak effect:** 1–2 min. **Duration:** 20–40 min with balanced anesthesia. Recovery from blockade under balanced anesthesia begins about 20–35 min after injection; recovery is usually 95% complete within 60–70 min after injection. **t½:** 20 min. Recovery occurs more rapidly than recovery from *d*-tubocurarine, metocurine, and pancuronium. Metabolized in the plasma.
CONTRAINDICATIONS
In clients with myasthenia gravis, Eaton-Lambert syndrome, electrolyte disorders, bronchial asthma.
SPECIAL CONCERNS
■ Should be used only by those skilled in airway management and respiratory support. Have equipment and personnel immediately available for endotracheal intubation and support for ventilation. Have anticholinesterase reversal drugs immediately available.■ Use with caution during labor and delivery and when significant histamine release would be dangerous (e.g., CV disease, asthma). Safety and efficacy have not been determined during lactation. Children up to 1 month of age may be more sensitive to the effects of atracurium. No known effect on pain threshold or consciousness; use only with adequate anesthesia.
ADDITIONAL SIDE EFFECTS
Most Common
Skin flushing, itching, wheezing, bronchial secretions, hives, increased HR, increased mean arterial pressure.
CV: Flushing, tachycardia, increased mean arterial pressure. **Dermatologic:** Rash, urticaria, reaction at injection site. **Musculoskeletal:** Prolonged block, inadequate block. **Respiratory:** Dyspnea, laryngospasm. **Hypersensitivity:** Allergic reactions. Other side effects may be due to histamine release and include flushing, erythema, wheezing, urticaria, itching, bronchial secretions, BP and HR changes.
ADDITIONAL DRUG INTERACTIONS
Acetylcholinesterase inhibitors / Muscle relaxation is inhibited and neuromuscular block is reversed
Aminoglycosides / ↑ Muscle relaxation
Corticosteroids / Prolonged weakness
Enflurane / ↑ Muscle relaxation
Halothane / ↑ Muscle relaxation
Isoflurane / ↑ Muscle relaxation
Lithium / ↑ Muscle relaxation
Phenytoin / ↓ Effect of atracurium
Procainamide / ↑ Muscle relaxation
Quinidine / ↑ Muscle relaxation
Succinylcholine / ↑ Onset and depth of muscle relaxation
Theophylline / ↓ Effect of atracurium
Trimethaphan / ↑ Muscle relaxation
Verapamil / ↑ Muscle relaxation
OD **OVERDOSE MANAGEMENT**
Symptoms: Hypotension, enhanced pharmacologic effects. *Treatment:* CV support. Ensure airway and ventilation. An anticholinesterase reversing agent (e.g., neostigmine, edrophonium, pyridostigmine) with an anticholinergic

agent (e.g., atropine, glycopyrrolate) may be used.

HOW SUPPLIED

Injection: 10 mg/mL.

DOSAGE

- **IV BOLUS ONLY**

Intubation and maintenance of neuromuscular blockade.

Adults and children over 2 years, initial: 0.4–0.5 mg/kg as IV bolus. **maintenance:** 0.08–0.1 mg/kg. The first maintenance dose is usually required 20–45 min after the initial dose. Give maintenance doses every 15–25 min under balanced anesthesia, slightly longer under isoflurane or enflurane anesthesia.

Following use of succinylcholine for intubation under balanced anesthesia.

Initial: 0.3–0.4 mg/kg; if using potent inhalation anesthetics, further reductions may be required.

Use in neuromuscular disease, severe electrolyte disorders, or carcinomatosis.

Consider dosage reductions where potentiation of neuromuscular blockade or difficulty with reversal have been noted.

Use after steady-state enflurane or isoflurane anesthesia established.

0.25–0.35 mg/kg (about one third less than the usual initial dose).

Use in infants 1 month to 2 years of age under halothane anesthesia.

0.3–0.4 mg/kg. More frequent maintenance doses may be required.

- **IV INFUSION**

Balanced anesthesia.

IV infusion: 9–10 mcg/kg until the level of neuromuscular blockade is reestablished; **then,** rate of infusion is adjusted according to client needs (usually 5–9 mcg/kg/min although some clients may require as little as 2 mcg/kg/min and others as much as 15 mcg/kg/min).

For cardiopulmonary bypass surgery in which hypothermia is induced.

Reduce rate of infusion by 50%.

NURSING CONSIDERATIONS

ADMINISTRATION/STORAGE

1. Hypomotility IM administration may cause tissue irritation.

2. Use only by those skilled in airway management and respiratory support. Equipment and personnel must be available immediately for intubation and support of ventilation. Have anticholinesterase reversal agents immediately available.

3. Reduce initial dose to 0.25–0.35 mg/kg if used with steady-state enflurane or isoflurane (smaller reductions with halothane).

4. Reduce dosage with myasthenia gravis or other neuromuscular diseases, electrolyte disorders, or carcinomatosis.

5. Prepare infusion solutions by admixing atracurium with either D5W/0.9% NaCl, D5W, or 0.9% NaCl. Do *not* mix with alkaline solutions, including LR injection.

6. Maintenance doses by continuous infusion of a diluted solution can be given to clients age 2 to adulthood.

7. Solutions containing 0.2 or 0.5 mg/mL can be stored either under refrigeration or at room temperature for 24 hr without significant loss of potency.

8. To preserve potency, refrigerate the drug at 2–8°C (36–46°F).

ASSESSMENT

1. Note reasons for therapy, expected duration, other agents/therapies trialed.

2. Use peripheral nerve stimulator to assess neuromuscular response and recovery intraoperatively.

3. Obtain baseline ECG, VS, lab studies; monitor. May cause vagal stimulation resulting in bradycardia, hypotension, arrhythmias. IV atropine may be used for bradycardia.

4. Should only be used on short-term basis and in continuously monitored environment. Drug blocks effect of acetylcholine at myoneural junction; prevents neuromuscular transmission.

5. Reassure once drug wears off may resume talking/moving.

CLIENT/FAMILY TEACHING

1. During administration, client may be able to see and hear things in the immediate environment but will not be able to move or talk. Resolves once drug discontinued.

2. Monitor breathing machine and set alarms, protect eyes with patches or drops.

3. May be fully conscious, aware of surroundings and conversations. Drug does not affect pain threshold or anxiety; will receive analgesics/antianxiety agents regularly.

4. Once drug stopped all movement, breathing and talking will return.

OUTCOMES/EVALUATE
- Skeletal muscle paralysis
- Facilitation of ET intubation; tolerance of mechanical ventilation
- Control of electrically/pharmacologically induced seizures

Atropine sulfate IV
(**AH**-troh-peen)

CLASSIFICATION(S):
Cholinergic blocking drug
PREGNANCY CATEGORY: C
Rx: AtroPen, Atropair, Atropine Sulfate Ophthalmic, Atropine-1 Ophthalmic, Isopto Atropine Ophthalmic, Sal-Tropine.
✤Rx: Minims Atropine.

SEE ALSO *CHOLINERGIC BLOCKING AGENTS.*

USES
PO: (1) Adjunct in peptic ulcer treatment. (2) Relieve pylorospasm, small intestine hypertonicity, and colon hypermotility. (3) Relax biliary and ureteral colic spasm and bronchial spasms. (4) Decrease tone of the detrusor muscle of the urinary bladder in treating urinary tract disorders. (5) Preanesthetic to control salivation and bronchial secretions. (6) Control rhinorrhea of acute rhinitis or hay fever. (7) Has been used for parkinsonism but more effective drugs are available.

Parenteral: (1) Restore cardiac rate and arterial pressure during anesthesia when vagal stimulation, due to intraabdominal surgical traction, causes a sudden decrease in pulse rate and cardiac action. (2) Decrease degree of AV heart block when increased vagal tone is a major factor in the conduction defect (e.g., due to digitalis). (3) Overcome severe bradycardia and syncope due to hyperactive carotid sinus reflex. (4) Relax upper GI tract and colon during hypertonic radiography. (5) Antidote (with external cardiac massage) for CV collapse from toxicity due to cholinergic drugs, pilocarpine, physostigmine, or isofluorophate. (6) Treat anticholinesterase poisoning from organophosphates; antidote for mushroom poisoning due to muscarine. (7) Poisoning by susceptible organophosphorus nerve agents having cholinesterase activity; also, poisoning due to organophosphorus or carbamate insecticides. (8) Control the crying and laughing episodes in clients with brain lesions. (9) Treat closed head injuries that cause acetylcholine to be released or be present in CSF, which causes abnormal EEG patterns, stupor, and neurological symptoms. (10) Relieve hypertonicity of uterine muscle. (11) As a preanesthetic or in dentistry to decrease secretions.

Ophthalmologic: Cycloplegic refraction or pupillary dilation in acute inflammatory conditions of the iris and uveal tract. *Investigational:* Treatment and prophylaxis of posterior synechiae; pre- and postoperative mydriasis; treatment of malignant glaucoma.

ACTION/KINETICS
Action
Blocks acetylcholine effects on postganglionic cholinergic receptors in smooth muscle, cardiac muscle, exocrine glands, urinary bladder, and the AV and SA nodes in the heart. Ophthalmologically, blocks acetylcholine effects on the sphincter muscle of the iris and the accommodative muscle of the ciliary body. This results in dilation of the pupil (mydriasis) and paralysis of the muscles required to accommodate for close vision (cycloplegia).

Pharmacokinetics
Peak effect: *Mydriasis,* 30–40 min; *cycloplegia,* 1–3 hr. **Recovery:** Up to 12 days. **Duration, PO:** 4–6 hr. **t½:** 2.5 hr. Metabolized by the liver although 30–50% is excreted through the kidneys unchanged.

ADDITIONAL CONTRAINDICATIONS

Ophthalmic use: Infants less than 3 months of age, primary glaucoma or a tendency toward glaucoma, adhesions between the iris and the lens, geriatric clients and others where undiagnosed glaucoma or excessive pressure in the eye may be present, in children who have had a previous severe systemic reaction to atropine.

SPECIAL CONCERNS

Use with caution in infants, small children, geriatric clients, diabetes, hypo- or hyperthyroidism, narrow anterior chamber angle, individuals with Down syndrome.

SIDE EFFECTS

Most Common

Systemic use: Dry mouth, urinary hesitancy, headache, flushing, constipation, heartburn, N&V.

Ophthalmic use: Blurred vision, stinging, increased intraocular pressure.

See *Cholinergic Blocking Agents* for a complete list of possible side effects.

Ophthalmic: Blurred vision, stinging, increased intraocular pressure, contact dermatitis. Long-term use may cause irritation, photophobia, eczematoid dermatitis, conjunctivitis, hyperemia, or edema.

OD OVERDOSE MANAGEMENT

Treatment: Ocular Overdose: Eyes should be flushed with water or normal saline. A topical miotic may be necessary.

HOW SUPPLIED

Autoinjector: 0.25 mg, 0.5 mg/0.7 mL, 1 mg/0.7 mL, 2 mg/0.7 mL; *Injection:* 0.05 mg/mL, 0.1 mg/mL, 0.3 mg/mL, 0.4 mg/mL, 0.5 mg/mL, 0.8 mg/mL, 1 mg/mL; *Ophthalmic Ointment:* 1%; *Ophthalmic Solution:* 0.5%, 1%; *Tablets:* 0.4 mg.

DOSAGE

• **TABLETS**

Anticholinergic or antispasmodic.

Adults: 0.3–1.2 mg q 4–6 hr. **Pediatric, over 41 kg:** same as adult; **29.5–41 kg:** 0.4 mg q 4–6 hr; **18.2–29.5 kg:** 0.3 mg q 4–6 hr; **10.9–18.2 kg:** 0.2 mg q 4–6 hr; **7.3–10.9 kg:** 0.15 mg q 4–6 hr; **3.2–7.3 kg:** 0.1 mg q 4–6 hr.

Prophylaxis of respiratory tract secretions and excess salivation during anesthesia.

Adults: 2 mg.

Parkinsonism.

Adults: 0.1–0.25 mg 4 times per day.

• **IM; IV; SC**

Anticholinergic.

Adults, IM, IV, SC: 0.4–0.6 mg q 4–6 hr.

Pediatric, SC: 0.01 mg/kg, not to exceed 0.4 mg (or 0.3 mg/m²).

Treatment of toxicity from cholinesterase inhibitors.

Adults, IV, initial: 2–4 mg; **then,** 2 mg repeated q 5–10 min until muscarinic symptoms disappear and signs of atropine toxicity begin to appear. **Pediatric, IM, IV, initial:** 1 mg; **then,** 0.5–1 mg q 5–10 min until muscarinic symptoms disappear and signs of atropine toxicity appear.

Treatment of mushroom poisoning due to muscarine.

Adults, IM, IV: 1–2 mg q hr until respiratory effects decrease.

Treatment of organophosphate poisoning.

Adults, IM, IV, Initial: 1–2 mg; **then,** repeat in 20–30 min (as soon as cyanosis has disappeared). Dosage may be continued for up to 2 days until symptoms improve.

Arrhythmias.

Pediatric, IV: 0.01–0.03 mg/kg.

Prophylaxis of respiratory tract secretions, excessive salivation, succinylcholine- or surgical procedure-induced arrhythmias.

Pediatric, up to 3 kg, SC: 0.1 mg; **7–9 kg:** 0.2 mg; **12–16 kg:** 0.3 mg; **20–27 kg:** 0.4 mg; **32 kg:** 0.5 mg: **41 kg:** 0.6 mg.

• **ATROPEN**

Organophosphorous or carbamate poisoning.

Adults and children weighing more than 90 lbs (and generally over 10 years of age): 2 mg. **Children weighing 40–90 lbs (generally 4–10 years of age):** 1 mg. **Children weighing 15–40 lbs (generally 6 months-4 years of age):** 0.5 mg.

• **OPHTHALMIC SOLUTION**

Uveitis.

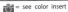 = see color insert   H = Herbal   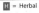 = Intravenous   ℗ = sound alike drug

A

Adults: 1–2 gtt instilled into the eye(s) up to 4 times/day. **Children:** 1–2 gtt of the 0.5% solution into the eye(s) up to 3 times per day.

Refraction.

Adults: 1–2 gtt of the 1% solution into the eye(s) 1 hr before refraction. **Children:** 1–2 gtt of the 0.5% solution into the eye(s) twice a day for 1–3 days before refraction.

• **OPHTHALMIC OINTMENT**
For mydriasis/cycloplegia.

Instill a small amount into the conjunctival sac up to 3 times per day.

NURSING CONSIDERATIONS

ADMINISTRATION/STORAGE

1. After instillation of ophthalmic ointment, compress lacrimal sac by digital pressure for 1–3 min to decrease systemic effects.

2. Have physostigmine available in the event of overdose.

3. Use the AtroPen Auto-injector as soon as symptoms of organophosphorus or carbamate poisoning appear. In moderate to severe poisoning, use of more than 1 AtroPen may be required until atropinization (e.g., flushing, mydriasis, tachycardia, dry mouth and nose) is achieved.

4. Do not use more than 3 AtroPen injections unless under supervision of trained medical provider.

5. In severe poisonings due to organophosphorus nerve agents or carbamate insecticides, it may be desirable to give an anticonvulsant (e.g., diazepam) concomitantly if seizures are suspected in an unconscious client (since classic tonic-clonic jerking may not be seen). Administration of a cholinesterase reactivator (e.g., pralidoxime chloride) may be helpful.

6. See package insert for AtroPen to determine number of AtroPen auto-injectors to use based on symptoms observed.

7. Administer AtroPen as follows:

• Snap grooved end of the plastic sleeve down and over the yellow safety cap. Remove AtroPen from plastic sleeve. Do not put fingers on the green tip.

• Firmly grasp AtroPen with the green tip pointed down.

• Pull off the yellow safety cap with the other hand.

• Aim and firmly jab the green tip straight down (a 90° angle) against the outer thigh. The AtroPen device will activate and deliver the drug. It is permissible to inject through clothing but be sure pockets at the injection site are empty. Very thin clients and small children should also be injected into the thigh but before giving the injection, bunch up the thigh to provide a thicker area for injection.

• Hold auto-injector firmly in place for at least 10 sec to allow injection to finish.

• Remove AtroPen and massage injection site for several seconds. If the needle is not visible, check to be sure the yellow safety cap has been removed; repeat the above steps but press harder.

8. Store AtroPen auto-injector from 15–30°C (59–86°F). Do not freeze and protect from light.

IV 9. May give by direct IV undiluted or may dilute in up to 10 mL sterile water and administer at 0.6–1 mg over 1 min.

10. Do not add to any existing IV solution. May give through 3-way stop cock, Y connection, or injection port.

11. Dose is dependent on condition being treated and age of recipient. See drug insert.

12. Store unopened at room temperature 15–30°C (59–86°F) in airtight, light resistant container.

ASSESSMENT

1. Note reasons for therapy, onset, characteristics of S&S. Review underlying presentation/history and update regularly.

2. Check for glaucoma before ophthalmic administration; may precipitate an acute crisis.

3. Obtain VS and ECG; monitor CV status during IV therapy.

A

CLIENT/FAMILY TEACHING

1. Review indications for drug use, frequency of use and route of administration.
2. When used in the eye, vision will be temporarily impaired. Close work, operating machinery, or driving a car should be avoided until drug effects have worn off.
3. Do not blink excessively; wait 5 min before instilling other drops. Stop eye drops and report if eye pain, conjunctivitis, rapid pulse/palpitations or dizziness occurs.
4. Drug impairs heat regulation; avoid strenuous activity in hot environments; wear sunglasses.
5. Males with enlarged prostate may experience urinary retention and hesitancy; void before use.
6. Increase fluids and add bulk to diet to ensure hydration and diminish constipating effects.
7. Drug inhibits salivation; use sugarless candies and gums to decrease dry mouth symptoms.
8. Use caution, may experience dizziness, confusion, or visual problems. Report all adverse side effects.

OUTCOMES/EVALUATE

- ↑ HR
- Desired pupillary dilatation
- ↓ GI activity; ↓ Salivation
- Reversal of muscarinic effects of anticholinesterase agents

---

Azacitidine

(ay-za-**SYE**-ti-deen)

CLASSIFICATION(S):

Antineoplastic (DNA demethylation agent)
PREGNANCY CATEGORY: D
Rx: Vidaza.

USES

Myelodysplastic syndrome with the following subtypes: (a) Refractory anemia or refractory anemia with ringed sideroblasts (if accompanied by neutropenia or thrombocytopenia or requiring transfusions), (b) refractory anemia with excess blasts, (c) refractory anemia with excess blasts in transformation, and (d) chronic myelomonocytic leukemia.

ACTION/KINETICS

Action

Antineoplastic effect due to demethylation or hypomethylation of DNA and by direct cytotoxicity on abnormal hematopoietic cells in the bone marrow. The cytotoxic effects cause death of rapidly dividing cells, including cancer cells that are no longer responsive to normal growth control mechanisms. Nonproliferating cells are relatively insensitive to azacitidine.

Pharmacokinetics

Rapidly absorbed after SC administration. **Peak plasma levels:** 30 min. Bioavailability is 89%. Metabolized by the liver. **t½, mean:** 41 min. Excreted in the urine; **elimination t½:** About 4 hr.

CONTRAINDICATIONS

Known hypersensitivity to azacitidine or mannitol. Those with advanced malignant hepatic tumors. Lactation.

SPECIAL CONCERNS

Safety and efficacy have not been determined in children.

SIDE EFFECTS

Most Common

N&V, anemia, thrombocytopenia, pyrexia, leukopenia, diarrhea, fatigue, injection site erythema, constipation, neutropenia, ecchymosis.

GI: N&V, diarrhea, constipation, anorexia, abdominal distension/tenderness/pain (including upper abdominal pain), gingival bleeding, oral mucosal petechiae, stomatitis, dyspepsia, hemorrhoids, loose stools, dysphagia, tongue ulceration, mouth hemorrhage, diverticulitis, *GI hemorrhage,* melena, perirectal abscess. **CNS:** Headache, dizziness, anxiety, decreased appetite, depression, confusion, insomnia, syncope, hypoesthesia, convulsions, *intracranial hemorrhage.* **CV:** *Cardiac murmur, tachycardia,* hypotension, atrial fibrillation, *cardiac failure, CHF, cardiorespiratory arrest, congestive cardiomyopathy,* orthostatic hypotension. **Respiratory:** Cough, dyspnea, pharyngitis, epistaxis, nasopharyngitis, exertional dyspnea, URTI, productive cough, crackles in

A

the lung, rhinorrhea, rales, pneumonia, wheezing, decreased breath sounds, pleural effusion, rhonchi, postnasal drip, sinusitis, atelectasis, exacerbated dyspnea, hemoptysis, lung infiltration, pneumonitis, respiratory distress. **Dermatologic:** Erythema, pallor, skin lesion, rash, pruritus, increased sweating, night sweats, urticaria, skin nodule, dry skin, pyoderma gangrenosum, pruritic rash, skin induration. **Hematologic:** Anemia, neutropenia, thrombocytopenia, leukopenia, febrile neutropenia, ecchymosis, petechiae, lymphadenopathy, hematoma, postprocedural hemorrhage, aggravated anemia, agranulocytosis, bone marrow depression, splenomegaly. **Injection site:** Erythema, pain, bruising, injection-site reaction, pruritus, swelling, granuloma, pigmentation changes. **Musculoskeletal:** Arthralgia, pain in limb, myalgia, muscle cramps, aggravated bone pain, muscle weakness, neck pain. **Metabolic:** Peripheral swelling/edema, decreased weight, pitting edema, hypokalemia. **Hepatic:** Cholecystectomy, cholecystitis, **hepatic coma.** **GU:** Dysuria, UTI, renal failure, renal tubular acidosis, hematuria, loin pain. **Infections:** Abscess limb, bacterial infection, blastomycosis, *Klebsiella* sepsis, streptococcal pharyngitis, injection-site infection, *Klebsiella* pneumonia, staphylococcal bacteremia/infection, sepsis, toxoplasmosis. **Body as a whole:** Pyrexia, fatigue, weakness, rigors, aggravated fatigue, lethargy, malaise. **Miscellaneous:** Back/chest/chest wall pain, pain, herpes simplex, cellulitis, transfusion reaction, postprocedural pain, ***anaphylactic shock,*** hypersensitivity, catheter-site hemorrhage, dehydration, general physical health deterioration, leukemia cutis, systemic inflammatory response syndrome.

LABORATORY TEST CONSIDERATIONS
↑ Serum creatinine, hypokalemia.

HOW SUPPLIED
Powder for Injection, Lyophilized: 100 mg.

DOSAGE
- **SC**
  Myelodysplastic syndrome.

Initial: 75 mg/m² daily for 7 days, every 4 weeks. The dose may be increased to 100 mg/m² if no beneficial effect is seen after 2 treatment cycles and if no toxicity other than N&V has occurred.

NURSING CONSIDERATIONS
ADMINISTRATION/STORAGE
1. Premedicate for N&V.
2. Treat for a minimum of 4 cycles; however, complete or partial response may require more than 4 treatment cycles. Treatment may continue as long as client continues to benefit.
3. If unexplained reductions in serum bicarbonate levels to <20 mEq/L occur, reduce dosage by 50% on next course.
4. If unexplained elevations of BUN or serum creatinine occur, delay next cycle until values return to normal or baseline and reduce dose by 50% on next treatment course.
5. Reconstitute aseptically with 4 mL sterile water for injection. Inject diluent slowly into vial. Invert vial 2 to 3 times and rotate gently until a uniform suspension occurs (will be cloudy). Reconstituted suspension will contain 25 mg/mL azacitidine.
6. Divide doses greater than 4 mL into 2 syringes. Inject into separate sites. Rotate sites for each injection (thigh, abdomen, or upper arm). Give new injections at least one inch from an old site and never into areas where the site is tender, bruised, red, or hard.
7. For delayed administration, reconstituted drug may be kept in the vial or drawn into a syringe.
8. To provide a homogeneous suspension, resuspend the contents by inverting the syringe 2 to 3 times and gently rolling the syringe between the palms for 30 sec immediately prior to administration.
9. Azacitidine is a cytotoxic drug; exercise caution when handling and preparing azacitidine. If reconstituted drug comes into contact with the skin, wash with soap and water immediately and thoroughly. If the drug comes into contact with mucous membranes, flush thoroughly with water.

Bold Italic = life threatening side effect   ■ = black box warning   ✦ = Available in Canada

10. Store unreconstituted vials from 15–30°C (59–86°F). The reconstituted product may be held at room temperature for up to 1 hr but must be administered within 1 hr after reconstitution.

11. Reconstituted drug may be refrigerated up to 8 hr. After removal from refrigerator, allow the suspension to equilibrate to room temperature for up to 30 min before administration.

12. Discard unused portions of each vial properly. Do not save any unused drug for later use.

ASSESSMENT

1. Note disease onset, subtype, other agents trialed and outcome.

2. Obtain baseline CBC, renal and LFTs; monitor prior to each cycle. Review drug literature for dosage adjustments (delay or reduction of dose), based on hematologic response calculated on Nadir counts of ANC, platelets, and bone marrow biopsy cellularity at time of nadir.

3. Do not use in those with hypersensitivity to azacitidine or mannitol or with advanced malignant hepatic tumors.

4. Monitor renal function closely, esp. in the elderly. Renal tubular acidosis (serum bicarbonate <20 mEq/L) in association with alkaline urine and hypokalemia (K^+ <3 mEq/L) may be fatal. Report any changes in renal function and hold drug; excreted primarily by the kidneys.

5. Review and follow administration guidelines carefully.

CLIENT/FAMILY TEACHING

1. Used to treat resistant types of leukemia; usually administered subcutaneously, once a day for 7 days and repeated every 4 weeks as long as benefit evident.

2. Drug therapy can be very toxic so blood tests must be performed before and after each treatment cycle and therapy adjusted or discontinued based on these lab results.

3. Males and females should both practice reliable contraception; drug may cause fetal harm.

4. Identify candidates for egg or sperm harvesting; drug may cause infertility.

5. Report changes in urine output/color, skin or stool color changes, fever, sore throat, severe muscle aches, abnormal bruising/bleeding or any other adverse effects. Keep regular visit/lab schedule.

OUTCOMES/EVALUATE

Improved hematologic parameters; inhibition of malignant cell proliferation

Azathioprine
(ay-zah-**THIGH**-oh-preen)

CLASSIFICATION(S):
Immunosuppressant

PREGNANCY CATEGORY: D

Rx: Azasan, Imuran.

✤**Rx:** Apo-Azathioprine, Gen-Azathioprine, ratio-Azathioprine.

USES

(1) As an adjunct to prevent rejection in renal homotransplantation. (2) In adult clients meeting criteria for classic or definite rheumatoid arthritis as defined by the American Rheumatism Association. Restrict use to clients with severe, active, and erosive disease that is not responsive to conventional therapy. *Investigational:* Chronic ulcerative colitis, generalized myasthenia gravis, to control the progression of Behçet's syndrome (especially eye disease), Crohn's disease (low doses).

ACTION/KINETICS

Action

Antimetabolite that is quickly split to form mercaptopurine. To be effective, must be given during the induction period of the antibody response. The precise mechanism in depressing the immune response is unknown, but it suppresses cell-mediated hypersensitivities and alters antibody production. Inhibits synthesis of DNA, RNA, and proteins and may interfere with meiosis and cellular metabolism. The mechanism for its effect on autoimmune diseases is not known. The anuric client manifests increased effectiveness and toxicity (up to twofold).

Pharmacokinetics
Readily absorbed from the GI tract. **Onset:** 6–8 weeks for rheumatoid arthritis. **t½:** 3 hr.

CONTRAINDICATIONS
Treatment of rheumatoid arthritis in pregnancy or in clients previously treated with alkylating agents. Pregnancy and lactation.

SPECIAL CONCERNS
■ Chronic immunosuppression with azathioprine increases the risk of neoplasia. Physicians using this drug should be familiar with this risk as well as with the mutagenic potential to both men and women and with possible hematologic toxicities.■ Hematologic toxicity is dose-related and may occur late in the course of therapy; may be more severe in renal transplant clients undergoing rejection. Although used in children, safety and efficacy have not been established.

SIDE EFFECTS
Most Common
GI toxicity (severe N&V, diarrhea), fever, rash, malaise, myalgias, leukopenia.
Hematologic: Leukopenia, thrombocytopenia, macrocytic anemia, ***severe bone marrow depression,*** selective erythrocyte aplasia. **GI:** N&V, diarrhea, abdominal pain, steatorrhea. **CNS:** Fever, malaise. **Miscellaneous:** *Increased risk of carcinoma,* severe infections (fungal, viral, bacterial, and protozoal), and *hepatotoxicity* are major side effects. Also, skin rashes, alopecia, myalgias, increase in liver enzymes, hypotension, negative nitrogen balance.

OD OVERDOSE MANAGEMENT
Symptoms: Large doses may result in ***bone marrow hypoplasia,*** bleeding, infection, and death. *Treatment:* Approximately 45% can be removed from the body following 8 hr of hemodialysis.

DRUG INTERACTIONS
ACE inhibitors / ↑ Risk of severe leukopenia
Allopurinol / ↑ Azathioprine effects R/T ↓ liver breakdown
Anticoagulants / ↓ Anticoagulant effect
Balsalazide / ↑ Rate of leukopenia in Crohn's disease clients R/T inhibition of thiopurine-metabolizing enzyme

Corticosteroids / Possible muscle wasting after prolonged therapy
Cyclosporine / ↑ Plasma cyclosporine levels
H *Echinacea* / Do not give with azathioprine
Mesalamine / ↑ Rate of leukopenia in Crohn's disease clients R/T inhibition of thiopurine-metabolizing enzyme
Methotrexate / ↑ Plasma levels of the active metabolite, 6-mercaptopurine
Sulfasalazine / ↑ Rate of leukopenia in Crohn's disease clients R/T inhibition of thiopurine-metabolizing enzyme
Tubocurarine / ↓ Tubocurarine (and other nondepolarizing neuromuscular blocking agents) effects

HOW SUPPLIED
Powder for Injection: 100 mg (as sodium); *Tablets:* 25 mg, 50 mg, 75 mg, 100 mg.

DOSAGE
• **IV; TABLETS**
Use in renal homotransplantation.
Adults and children, initial: 3–5 mg/kg (120 mg/m²), 1–3 days before or on the day of transplantation. **maintenance:** 1–3 mg/kg (45 mg/m²) daily.
Rheumatoid arthritis.
Adults and children, tablets, initial: 1 mg/kg (50–100 mg); **then,** increase dose by 0.5 mg/kg/day after 6–8 weeks and thereafter q 4 weeks, up to maximum of 2.5 mg/kg/day. **maintenance:** lowest effective dose. Dosage should be reduced in clients with renal dysfunction.
Myasthenia gravis.
2–3 mg/kg/day. However, side effects occur in more than 35% of clients.
To control progression of Behcet's syndrome.
2.5 mg/kg/day.
Crohn's disease.
75–100 mg/day.

NURSING CONSIDERATIONS
Ⓒ Do not confuse Imuran with Imdur (an antianginal drug).

ADMINISTRATION/STORAGE
1. For rheumatoid arthritis, a therapeutic response may not be observed for 6–8 weeks.

Bold Italic = life threatening side effect   ■ = black box warning   ✦ = Available in Canada

2. May be discontinued abruptly, but delayed effects are possible.

3. When used with allopurinol, reduce dose of azathioprine by 25–33% of the usual dose.

IV 4. Reconstitute drug (100 mg) with 10 mL of sterile water for injection and use within 24 hr. Further dilution with NSS or 0.9% NaCl is usually made; infusion time ranges from 5 min to 8 hr.

ASSESSMENT

1. Note reasons for therapy; include preassessment data. Check for drug interactions.

2. With RA assess joint for functional level: ROM, swelling, erythema, temperature, stiffness, and active synovitis.

3. With transplant procedures, protect from visitors or staff who may carry infectious organisms.

4. Monitor CBC, renal and LFTs. Observe for S&S bleeding abnormalities or hepatic dysfunction. Stop drug/report if jaundiced or abnormal LFTs.

5. Assess I&O and weigh daily. Report decreases in urine volume, C_{CR}, oliguria or symptoms of kidney transplant rejection.

CLIENT/FAMILY TEACHING

1. If GI upset occurs, give in divided doses or take with food.

2. Take only as directed and do not skip or stop drug without approval; increase fluid intake.

3. Practice reliable contraception during and for 4 months following therapy.

4. Report bruising, bleeding, S&S of infection, fever, rash, abdominal pain, yellow eyes or skin, itching, and/or clay-colored stools.

5. Must take this medication for life to prevent transplant rejection.

6. Avoid crowds or contact with anyone who has taken oral poliovirus vaccine recently or persons with active infections.

7. When used for RA, improvement in joint pain, swelling, and stiffness may take 6–12 weeks. Should be considered refractory if no beneficial effect is noted after 12 weeks.

OUTCOMES/EVALUATE

- Prevention of organ transplant rejection

- Suppression of cell-mediated immunity

- With RA ↓ joint pain and inflammation with improved mobility

Azithromycin **IV**

(ah-**zith**-roh-**MY**-sin)

CLASSIFICATION(S):

Antibiotic, macrolide

PREGNANCY CATEGORY: B

Rx: AzaSite Ophthalmic Solution, Zithromax, Zmax.

✸Rx: Z-Pak.

SEE ALSO *ANTI-INFECTIVE DRUGS.*

USES

Adults, Oral: (1) Acute bacterial exacerbations of COPD due to *Hemophilus influenzae, Moraxella catarrhalis,* or *Streptococcus pneumoniae.* (2) Those who can take PO therapy for mild community-acquired pneumonia (CAP) due to *C. pneumoniae, M. pneumoniae, S. pneumoniae,* or *H. influenzae.* (3) Genital ulcer disease in men due to *Haemophilus ducreyi.* (4) As an alternative to first-line therapy to treat streptococcal pharyngitis or tonsillitis due to *Streptococcus pyogenes.* (5) PO for uncomplicated skin and skin structure infections due to *S. aureus, Staphyloccus pyogenes,* or *Streptococcus agalactiae.* Abscesses usually require surgical drainage. (6) Urethritis and cervicitis due to *C. trachomatis* or *Neisseria gonorrhoeae.* (7) Alone or with rifabutin for prophylaxis of disseminated *Mycobacterium avium* complex disease in advanced HIV infection. (8) Treatment of disseminated MAC disease in combination with ethambutol in advanced HIV infection. (9) Acute bacterial sinusitis due to *H. influenzae, M. catarrhalis,* or *Streptococcus pneumoniae.*

Adults, IV: (1) Required initial IV therapy in CAP due to *S. pneumoniae, Chlamydia pneumoniae, Mycoplasma pneumoniae, S. pneumoniae, H. influenzae, M. catarrhalis, Legionella pneumophila,* and *Staphylococcus aureus.* (2) Initial IV therapy in PID due to *Chlamydia trachomatis, N. gonorrhoeae,* or *Myco-*

---

plasma hominis. If anaerobic organisms are suspected of contributing to the infection, an antimicrobial with anaerobic activity may be added to the regimen. *Investigational: Helicobacter pylori* infections, *Bartonella* infections, Lyme disease, toxoplasmosis, babesiosis, granulomavinguinale, cryptosporidiosis. *NOTE:* Zmax is approved only for the treatment of acute bacterial sinusitis and community-acquired pneumonia.

Children, Oral: (1) Acute otitis media due to *H. influenzae, M. catarrhalis,* or *S. pneumoniae* in children over 6 months of age. (2) Acute bacterial sinusitis in children 6 months and older due to *H. influenzae, M. catarrhalis,* or *S. pneumoniae.* (3) CAP due to *C. pneumoniae, H. influenzae, M. pneumoniae,* or *S. pneumoniae* in children over 6 months of age who can take PO therapy. (4) Pharyngitis/tonsillitis due to *S. pyogenes* in children over 2 years of age who cannot use first-line therapy. Penicillin IM is the usual drug of choice to treat *S. pyogenes* infections and for prophylaxis of rheumatic fever. Azithromycin is often effective to eradicate susceptible strains of *S. pyogenes* from the nasopharynx; perform susceptibility tests when clients are treated with azithromycin.

Ophthalmic: Bacterial conjunctivitis due to coryneform group G, *Haemophilus influenzae, Staphylococcus aureus, Streptococcus mitis* group, and *Streptococcus pneumoniae.*

Investigational: Uncomplicated gonococcal pharyngitis of the cervix, urethra, and rectum caused by *N. gonorrhoeae.* Gonococcal pharyngitis due to *N. gonorrhoeae.* Chlamydial infections due to *C. trachomatis. Helicobacter* infections, *Bartonella* infection, Lyme disease, toxoplasmosis, babesiosis, granuloma inguinale, cryptosporidiosis.

ACTION/KINETICS
Action
A macrolide antibiotic derived from erythromycin. Acts by binding to the P site of the 50S ribosomal subunit and may inhibit RNA-dependent protein synthesis by stimulating the dissociation of peptidyl t-RNA from ribosomes.

Pharmacokinetics
Rapidly absorbed and distributed widely throughout the body. Food increases the absorption of azithromycin. **Time to reach maximum concentration:** 2.2 hr. **t½, terminal:** 68 hr. A loading dose will achieve steady-state levels more quickly. Mainly excreted unchanged through the bile with a small amount being excreted through the kidneys. The ophthalmic solution is formulated in a system that enhances retention time of the drug on the surface of the eye allowing for administration of fewer drops for effective treatment.

CONTRAINDICATIONS
Hypersensitivity to azithromycin, any macrolide antibiotic, or erythromycin. In clients who are not eligible for outpatient PO therapy (e.g., known or suspected bacteremia, immunodeficiency, functional asplenia, nosocomially acquired infections, geriatric or debilitated clients). Use with pimozide. IV use in children less than 16 years of age.

SPECIAL CONCERNS
Use with caution in clients with impaired hepatic or renal function and during lactation. Possible cardiac arrhythmias and torsades de pointes development if azithromycin used in those at increased risk for prolonged cardiac repolarization. Safety and efficacy for acute otitis media have not been determined in children less than 6 months of age or for pharyngitis/tonsillitis in children less than 2 years of age.

SIDE EFFECTS
Most Common
Abdominal pain/discomfort, N&V, anorexia, diarrhea/loose stools, injection site reactions (local inflammation, pain), pruritus, rash, vaginitis.
GI: N&V, diarrhea, loose stools, abdominal pain, dyspepsia, anorexia, gastritis, flatulence, melena, mucositis, oral moniliasis, taste perversion, cholestatic jaundice, *pseudomembranous colitis.* In children, gastritis, constipation, and anorexia have also been noted. **CNS:** Dizziness, headache, somnolence, fatigue, vertigo. In children, hyperkinesia, agitation, nervousness, insomnia, fever, and malaise have also been noted. **CV:**

Bold Italic = life threatening side effect   ■ = black box warning   ✦ = Available in Canada

Chest pain, palpitations, QT-interval prolongation, **ventricular arrhythmias (including ventricular tachycardia and torsades de pointes in clients with prolonged QT intervals observed with other macrolides). GU:** Monilia, nephritis, vaginitis. **Allergic:** Angioedema, photosensitivity, rash, **anaphylaxis. Hematologic:** Leukopenia, neutropenia, decreased platelet count. **Miscellaneous:** Superinfection, pruritus, rash, bronchospasm, local IV site reactions (inflammation, pain). In children, pruritus, urticaria, conjunctivitis, and chest pain have been noted.

LABORATORY TEST CONSIDERATIONS

↑ Serum CPK, potassium, ALT, GGT, AST, serum alkaline phosphatase, bilirubin, BUN, creatinine, blood glucose, LDH, and phosphate.

DRUG INTERACTIONS

SEE ALSO DRUG INTERACTIONS FOR ERYTHROMYCINS

Al– and Mg–containing antacids / ↓ Peak serum levels of azithromycin but not the total amount absorbed

Amiodarone / Possible dizziness and prolonged QTc interval and QT dispersion

Atovaquone / Possible ↓ peak serum levels of azithromycin in pediatric HIV-infected clients

Cyclosporine / ↑ Serum cyclosporine levels R/T ↓ metabolism → ↑ risk of nephrotoxicity and neurotoxicity

HMG-CoA reductase inhibitors / ↑ Risk of severe myopathy/rhabdomyolysis

Phenytoin / ↑ Serum phenytoin levels R/T ↓ metabolism

Pimozide / Possibility of sudden death

HOW SUPPLIED

Ophthalmic Solution: 1%; Powder for Injection, Lyophilized: 500 mg; Powder for Oral Suspension: 100 mg/5 mL (when reconstituted), 167 mg/5 mL (extended-release microspheres), 200 mg/5 mL (when reconstituted), 1 gram/packet; Tablets: 250 mg, 500 mg, 600 mg.

DOSAGE

• **ORAL SUSPENSION; TABLETS**

Adults: Mild to moderate acute bacterial exacerbations of COPD, mild CAP, second-line therapy for pharyngitis/ tonsillitis; uncomplicated skin and skin structure infections.

Adults and children over 16 years of age: 500 mg as a single dose on day 1 followed by 250 mg once daily on days 2–5 for a total dose of 1.5 grams. For acute bacterial exacerbations of COPD, can also give 500 mg/day for three days. For CAP, a single 2 gram dose of Zmax may be given.

Acute bacterial sinusitis.

Adults: 500 mg once daily for 3 days or 2 grams as a single dose of Zmax.

Nongonococcal urethritis and cervicitis due to C. trachomatis or genital ulcer disease due to H. ducreyi.

1 gram given as a single dose.

Prevention of disseminated MAC infections.

1,200 mg once weekly; may be combined with rifabutin.

Treatment of disseminated MAC infections.

600 mg/day in combination with ethambutol, 15 mg/kg.

Gonococcal urethritis/cervicitis due to N. gonorrhoeae.

2 grams given as a single dose.

Uncomplicated gonococcal infections of the cervix, urethra, and rectum due to N. gonorrhoeae.

1 gram given as a single dose plus a single dose of 400 mg PO cefixime, 125 mg IM ceftriaxone, 500 mg PO ciprofloxacin, or 400 mg PO ofloxacin.

Uncomplicated gonococcal pharyngitis.

1 gram given as a single dose plus a single dose of 125 mg IM ceftriaxone, 500 mg ciprofloxacin, or 400 mg ofloxacin.

Chlamydial infections caused by C. trachomatis.

1 gram given as a single dose.

• **ORAL SUSPENSION**

Otitis media or CAP in children 6 months and older.

Children, 6 months and older weighing at least 5 kg, 5-day regimen: 10 mg/kg as a single dose (not to exceed 500 mg) on day 1, followed by 5 mg/kg (not to exceed 250 mg/day) on days 2 through 5. **Children, 6 months and older weighing at least 5 kg, 3-day**

regimen for otitis media: 10 mg/kg/day. **Children, 6 months and older weighing at least 5 kg, 1-day regimen for otitis media:** 30 mg/kg as a single dose.

Pharyngitis/tonsillitis in children.
Children: 12 mg/kg once daily for 5 days, not to exceed 500 mg/day.

Chlamydial infections in children caused by C. trachomatis.
Children 45 kg or more, and less than 8 years of age; or over 8 years of age: 1 gram given as a single dose.

Acute bacterial sinusitis, children 6 months and older.
Children, 6 months and older: 10 mg/kg once daily for 3 days.

• **ORAL SUSPENSION FOR EXTENDED RELEASE**

Acute bacterial sinusitis, CAP.
One dose of 2 grams taken at least 1 hr before or 2 hr after a meal.

• **IV**

CAP.
Adults: 500 mg IV as a single daily dose for at least 2 days followed by a single daily dose of 500 mg PO to complete a 7- to 10-day course of therapy.

PID.
Adults: 500 mg IV as a single daily dose for 1 or 2 days followed by a single daily dose of 250 mg PO to complete a 7-day course of therapy.

• **OPHTHALMIC SOLUTION**

Bacterial conjunctivitis.
Initial: 1 drop in the affected eye(s) 2 times per day, 8–12 hr apart for the first 2 days; **then,** 1 drop in the affected eye(s) once daily for the next 5 days.

NURSING CONSIDERATIONS

ADMINISTRATION/STORAGE

1. Tablets and oral suspension can be taken with or without food; however, there is increased tolerability when tablets are taken with food (can be taken with milk). Zmax should be taken at least 1 hr prior to or 2 hr after a meal.
2. To prepare the single 1 gram packet, thoroughly mix the entire contents of the packet with about 60 mL of water. Drink the entire contents immediately; add an additional 60 mL of water, mix, and drink to ensure complete con-

sumption of dosage. The packet is not for pediatric use.
3. To prepare the 2 gram dose bottle, reconstitute with 60 mL water. Shake well before dispensing. Consume the suspension within 12 hr.
IV 4. Infuse IV at a rate of 1 mg/mL over 3 hr or 2 mg/mL over 1 hr; do not give as a bolus or IM.
5. Prepare the initial solution by adding 4.8 mL sterile water for injection to the 500 mg vial; shake the vial until all of the drug is dissolved. It is recommended that a standard 5 mL (nonautomated) syringe be used to ensure the exact amount of 4.8 mL is delivered. Each mL of reconstituted solution contains 100 mg azithromycin. To obtain a concentration range of 1 to 2 mg/mL, transfer 5 mL of the 100-mg/mL solution into the appropriate amount of any of the following: 0.9% or 0.45% NaCl, D5W, RL solution, D5/0.45% NaCl with 20 mEq KCl, D5/RL solution, D5/0.3% NaCl, D5/0.45% NaCl, Normosol-M in D5%, or Normosol-R in D5%.
6. Reconstituted solution for injection is stable for 24 hr if stored below 30°C (86°F) or for 7 days refrigerated at 5°C (41°F).
7. Store unopened bottle of ophthalmic solution from 2–8°C (36–46°F). Once bottle is opened, store from 2–25°C (36–77°F) for up to 14 days; discard after 14 days.

ASSESSMENT

1. Note history of sensitivity to erythromycins and any previous therapy.
2. List indications for therapy, onset/characteristics of symptoms, other agents/remedies trialed.
3. Assess for prolonged QT interval; note EKG, and culture results.
4. List drugs prescribed; may cause an increase in concentrations of certain drugs (digoxin, carbamazepine, cyclosporine, dilantin).
5. Test sexually active for gonorrhea and syphilis at time of diagnosis. Ensure appropriate drug therapy instituted if necessary.
6. Obtain CBC, liver/renal function studies and cultures when warranted.

CLIENT/FAMILY TEACHING

1. Tablets may be taken with food or milk to improve tolerability. Food decreases absorption; take 1 hr before or 2–3 hr after a meal.

2. Finish all medication unless otherwise directed.

3. Avoid ingesting Al- or Mg-containing antacids simultaneously with azithromycin.

4. Notify provider if N&V or diarrhea is excessive or debilitating.

5. Avoid sun exposure and use protection when outside.

6. Report lack of response/unusual side effects. May cause drowsiness or dizziness; use caution.

7. With STDs, encourage sexual partner to seek medical evaluation and treatment to prevent re-infections. Use condoms during intercourse throughout therapy.

OUTCOMES/EVALUATE

Resolution of S&S of infection; Negative cultures

Bacitracin intramuscular ■ⓒ
(bass-ih-**TRAY**-sin)

CLASSIFICATION(S):
Antibiotic, miscellaneous
PREGNANCY CATEGORY: C
Rx: Baci-IM.

Bacitracin ointment
PREGNANCY CATEGORY: C
Rx: Baciguent.

Bacitracin ophthalmic ointment
PREGNANCY CATEGORY: C
Rx: AK-Tracin.

SEE ALSO *ANTI-INFECTIVE DRUGS*.

USES

Parenteral: Limited to the treatment of staphylococcal-induced pneumonia or empyema in infants.

Topical Ointment: Aid to prevent infection in minor cuts, scrapes, burns, and wounds.

Ophthalmic Ointment: Superficial ocular infections of the conjunctiva or cornea (e.g., conjunctivitis, keratitis, keratoconjunctivitis, corneal ulcers, blepharitis, blepharoconjunctivitis, acute meibomianitis, and dacryocystitis) involving species of *Staphylococcus, S. aureus, Streptococcus, S. pneumoniae, S. pyogenes, Corynebacterium, Neisseria, N. gonorrhoeae*, and beta-hemolytic streptococci. Do not use topical antibiotics in deep-seated ocular infections or in those that are likely to become systemic.

ACTION/KINETICS

Action

Interferes with synthesis of cell wall, preventing incorporation of amino acids and nucleotides. Is bactericidal, bacteriostatic, and active against protoplasts. Not absorbed from the GI tract. When given parenterally, drug is well distributed in pleural and ascitic fluids. High nephrotoxicity. Systemic use is restricted to infants (see *Uses*). Carefully evaluate renal function prior to, and daily, during use.

Pharmacokinetics

Peak plasma levels: IM, 0.2–2 mcg/mL after 2 hr. From 10–40% is excreted in the urine after IM administration.

CONTRAINDICATIONS

Hypersensitivity or toxic reaction to bacitracin. Pregnancy. Epithelial herpes simplex keratitis, vaccinia, varicella, mycobacterial eye infections, fungal dis-

B

eases of the eye. Concomitant use of nephrotoxic drugs.

SPECIAL CONCERNS

■ IM use may cause renal failure due to tubular and glomerular necrosis. Restrict use to infants with staphylococcal pneumonia and empyema due to susceptible organisms. Use only where laboratory facilities are adequate and constant supervision is possible. Carefully determine renal function prior to, and daily, during therapy. Do not exceed the recommended daily dose, and maintain fluid intake and urinary output at proper levels to avoid renal toxicity. If renal toxicity occurs, discontinue the drug. Avoid the concurrent use of other nephrotoxic drugs, especially streptomycin, kanamycin, polymyxin B, colistin, and neomycin.■ Ophthalmic ointments may retard corneal epithelial healing. Prolonged or repeated use may result in bacterial or fungal overgrowth of nonsusceptible organisms leading to a secondary infection. Use topical ointment with caution during pregnancy.

SIDE EFFECTS

Most Common

After IM use: N&V, skin rashes, pain at injection site.

After topical use: Skin rashes.

After ophthalmic use: Transient burning, stinging, itching, irritation.

• **IM**

N&V, skin rashes, pain at injection site, albuminuria, cylindruria, azotemia. *Nephrotoxicity due to tubular and glomerular necrosis, renal failure.*

• **Topical**

Allergic contact dermatitis, skin rashes, superinfection.

• **Ophthalmic**

Transient burning, stinging, itching, irritation, inflammation, angioneurotic edema, urticaria, vesicular and maculopapular dermatitis.

DRUG INTERACTIONS

Aminoglycosides / Additive nephrotoxicity and neuromuscular blocking activity

Anesthetics / ↑ Neuromuscular blockade → possible muscle paralysis

Neuromuscular blocking agents / Additive neuromuscular blockade → possible muscle paralysis

HOW SUPPLIED

Bacitracin intramuscular: *Powder for Injection:* 50,000 units/vial.

Bacitracin ointment : 500 units/gram.

Bacitracin ophthalmic ointment : 500 units/gram.

DOSAGE

• **IM ONLY**

Staphylococcal-induced pneumonia or empyema in infants.

Infants, 2.5 kg and below: 900 units/kg/day in 2–3 divided doses; **infants over 2.5 kg:** 1,000 units/kg/day in 2–3 divided doses.

• **TOPICAL OINTMENT**

Prophylaxis of topical infections.

Apply small amount equal to the surface area of a fingertip 1–3 times per day after cleaning affected area. Do not use for more than 1 week.

• **OPHTHALMIC OINTMENT**

Acute ophthalmic infections.

½ in. in lower conjunctival sac q 3–4 hr until improvement occurs. Reduce treatment before the drug is discontinued.

Mild to moderate ophthalmic infections.

½ in. 2–3 times per day.

NURSING CONSIDERATIONS

🕲 Do not confuse bacitracin with Bactroban (topical anti-infective).

ADMINISTRATION/STORAGE

1. When used IM, maintain adequate fluid intake; PO or parenterally.

2. Give IM in upper outer quadrant of buttocks; alternate sides, avoid multiple injections to same region R/T transient pain after injection.

3. For IM use: dissolve in NaCl injection containing 2% procaine HCl. Ensure bacitracin concentration is not <5,000 units/mL or >10,000 units/mL. Do not use diluents containing parabens. Reconstitution of 50,000 unit vial with 9.8 mL of diluent results in concentration of 5,000 units/mL.

4. Refrigerate unconstituted drug at 2–8°C (36–46°F). Solutions stable for 1 week if stored the same as the unreconstituted drug.

Bold Italic = life threatening side effect   ■ = black box warning   ♣ = Available in Canada

5. Do not mix with glycerin or other polyalcohols that cause drug to deteriorate.

6. When used topically: may cover affected area with sterile bandage.

ASSESSMENT

1. Note reasons for therapy, onset, characteristics of S&S, clinical presentation, culture results.

2. List experiences with this type of infection (esp. ocular), agents used, and outcome.

3. Recurrent ophthalmic infections should be cultured and carefully assessed by ophthalmologist.

INTERVENTIONS

1. Monitor renal function studies; maintain adequate I&O with parenteral therapy.

2. Test urine pH daily; pH should be kept at 6 or greater; decreases renal irritation. Have $NaHCO_3$ or other alkali available if pH <6.

3. Do not administer with topical or systemic nephrotoxic drug.

CLIENT/FAMILY TEACHING

1. Apply topically as directed. Cleanse area thoroughly before applying bacitracin as wet dressing or ointment.

2. Do not use topical ointment near eyes, nose, mouth, or mucous membranes.

3. With eye ointment place a ribbon inside eye lid and close eyes; lightly press the inner corner of the eye for 60 seconds. Avoid contact of tube with the eye and wash hands before and after application.

4. Report lack of response, rash, fever, stinging, itching, changes in vision, or unusual side effects. Keep all F/U appointments.

OUTCOMES/EVALUATE

- Resolution of S&S of infection
- Restoration of skin integrity

Baclofen   ■

(**BAK**-low-fen)

B

CLASSIFICATION(S):

Skeletal muscle relaxant, centrally-acting

PREGNANCY CATEGORY: C

Rx: Kemstro, Lioresal, Lioresal Intrathecal.

✦**Rx:** Apo-Baclofen, Gen-Baclofen, Lioresal Intrathecal, Lioresal Oral, Nu-Baclo, PMS-Baclofen, ratio-Baclofen.

SEE ALSO *SKELETAL MUSCLE RELAXANTS, CENTRALLY ACTING.*

USES

PO. Multiple sclerosis (flexor spasms, pain, clonus, and muscular rigidity) and diseases and injuries of the spinal cord associated with spasticity. Not effective for the treatment of cerebral palsy, stroke, parkinsonism, or rheumatic disorders. *Investigational:* Trigeminal neuralgia, tardive dyskinesia, intractable hiccoughs.

 Intrathecal. Severe spasticity of spinal cord of cerebral origin in clients unresponsive to PO baclofen therapy or who have intolerable CNS side effects.

 Investigational: Trigeminal neuralgia; intractable hiccoughs; reduce choreiform movements in Huntington's chorea; reduce rigidity in parkinsonism; reduce spasticity in cerebral lesions, cerebral palsy, or rheumatic disorders; reduce spasticity in CV stroke; acquired periodic alternating nystagmus; acquired pendular nystagmus; reduce number of gastroesophageal reflux episodes; Tourette syndrome in children; prophylaxis of migraine, neuropathic pain; reduce spasticity in children with cerebral palsy.

ACTION/KINETICS

Action

Related chemically to GABA, an inhibitory neurotransmitter. May act by combining with the $GABA_B$ receptor subtype. It increases threshold for excitation of primary afferent nerves and decreases the release of excitatory amino acids from presynaptic sites. May also

B

act at certain brain sites. Has CNS depressant effects.

Pharmacokinetics

After PO use, baclofen is rapidly and extensively absorbed. **Peak serum levels, PO:** 2–3 hr. **Therapeutic serum levels:** 80–400 ng/mL. **t½, PO:** 3–4 hr. **Onset after intrathecal bolus:** 30–60 min; **peak effect after intrathecal bolus:** 4 hr; **duration after intrathecal bolus:** 4–8 hr. **t½ after bolus lumbar injection of 50 or 100 mcg:** 1.5 hr over the first 4 hr. **Onset after intrathecal continuous infusion:** 6–8 hr; **peak effect after intrathecal continuous infusion:** 24–48 hr. 70–80% is eliminated unchanged by the kidney.

CONTRAINDICATIONS

Hypersensitivity. PO to treat rheumatic disorders, spasm resulting from Parkinson's disease, stroke, cerebral palsy. Intrathecal product for IV, IM, SC, or epidural use.

SPECIAL CONCERNS

■ Abrupt withdrawal after intrathecal use may result in high fever, altered mental status, exaggerated rebound spasticity, and muscle rigidity; rarely advances to rhabdomyolysis, multiple organ system failure, and death. Those at greatest risk include those with communication difficulties, history of baclofen withdrawal, or injuries at level of T-6 or above.■ Use during lactation only if potential benefit outweighs the potential risk. Safe use of the oral product for children under 12 years of age and of the intrathecal product for children under 4 years of age not established. Use with caution in impaired renal function, in those with autonomic dysreflexia and where spasticity is used to sustain an upright posture and balance in locomotion; in those with psychotic disorders, schizophrenia, or confusional states as worsening of these conditions has occurred following PO use. Geriatric clients may be at higher risk for developing CNS toxicity, including mental depression, confusion, hallucinations, and significant sedation. Due to serious, life-threatening side effects after intrathecal use, physicians must be trained

and educated in chronic intrathecal infusion therapy.

SIDE EFFECTS

Most Common After PO use: Drowsiness, hypotension, dizziness, headache, insomnia, fatigue, confusion, nausea, constipation, urinary frequency.

After intrathecal use: Hypotonia, somnolence, dizziness, convulsions, constipation, N&V, headache, paresthesia.

• **PO**

CNS: Drowsiness, dizziness, lightheadedness, weakness, lethargy, fatigue, confusion, headaches, insomnia, euphoria, excitement, depression, paresthesia, muscle pain, coordination disorder, tremor, rigidity, dystonia, ataxia, strabismus, dysarthria, slurred speech, *seizures* (rare). Hallucinations following abrupt withdrawal. **CV:** Hypotension, chest pain, syncope (rare), palpitations. **GI:** N&V, constipation, dry mouth, anorexia, taste disorder, abdominal pain, diarrhea. **GU:** Urinary frequency, enuresis, urinary retention, dysuria, impotence, inability to ejaculate, nocturia, hematuria (rare). **Dermatologic:** Rash, pruritus, excessive perspiration. **Respiratory:** Nasal congestion, dyspnea (rare). **Ophthalmic:** Nystagmus, miosis, mydriasis, diplopia, blurred vision. **Miscellaneous:** Ankle edema, weight gain, weakness.

• **Intrathecal**

Spasticity of spinal origin. **CNS:** Dizziness, somnolence, paresthesia, headache, *convulsion,* confusion, speech disorder, coma, ***death,*** insomnia, anxiety, depression, abnormal tremor, thinking, agitation, hallucinations. **GI:** N&V, constipation, dry mouth, diarrhea, anorexia, increased salivation. **GU:** Urinary retention, impotence, urinary incontinence, urinary frequency, impaired urination. **CV:** Hypotension, hypertension. **Miscellaneous:** Accidental injury, asthenia, amblyopia, pain, peripheral edema, dyspnea, hypoventilation, fever, urticaria, anorexia, diplopia, dysautonomia, hypertonia, back pain, pruritus, asthenia, chills, pneumonia.

LABORATORY TEST CONSIDERATIONS

↑ AST, alkaline phosphatase, blood glucose.

Bold Italic = life threatening side effect   ■ = black box warning   ✚ = Available in Canada

B

OD OVERDOSE MANAGEMENT

Symptoms: Symptoms after PO use include vomiting, drowsiness, muscular hypotonia, muscle twitching, accommodation disorders, respiratory depression, seizures, coma. Symptoms after intrathecal use include drowsiness, dizziness, lightheadedness, somnolence, respiratory depression, rostral progression of hypotonia, *seizures, loss of consciousness leading to coma (for up to 24 hr).*

Treatment: After PO use:
- Induce vomiting (only if the client is alert and conscious) followed by gastric lavage.
- If the client is not alert and conscious, undertake only gastric lavage making sure the airway is secured with a cuffed ET tube.
- Maintain an adequate airway.
- Atropine may be used to improve HR, BP, ventilation, and core body temperature.

Treatment: After intrathecal use:
- Remove residual solution from the pump as soon as possible.
- Intubate the client who has respiratory depression until the drug is eliminated.
- IV physostigmine (total dose of 1–2 mg given over 5–10 min) may be tried, with caution.
- Can withdraw 30–60 mL of CSF to decrease baclofen levels (provided that lumbar puncture is not contraindicated).

DRUG INTERACTIONS

CNS depressants / Additive CNS depression
MAO Inhibitors / ↑ CNS depression and hypotension
Tricyclic antidepressants / Muscle hypotonia

HOW SUPPLIED

Kit (Intrathecal): 0.05 mg/mL, 0.5 mg/mL, 2 mg/mL; *Tablets:* 10 mg, 20 mg; *Tablets, Oral Disintegrating:* 10 mg, 20 mg.

DOSAGE————————————————

- **TABLETS; TABLETS, ORAL DISINTEGRATING**

  Muscle relaxant, spasticity.

Adults, initial: 5 mg 3 times per day for 3 days; **then,** 10 mg 3 times per day for 3 days, 15 mg 3 times per day for 3 days, and 20 mg 3 times per day for 3 days. Additional increases in dose may be required but do not exceed 20 mg 4 times per day. **Children (treatment of spasticity), initial:** 10–15 mg/kg/day in 3 divided doses. Titrate to a maximum of 40 mg/day if less than 8 years of age and to a maximum of 80 mg/day if more than 8 years of age.

  Trigeminal neuralgia.

50–60 mg/day.

  Tardive dyskinesia.

40 mg/day used in combination with neuroleptics.

- **INTRATHECAL**

  Initial screening bolus for severe spasticity of spinal cord of cerebral origin.

50 mcg/mL given into the intrathecal space by barbotage over a period of not less than 1 min. The client is observed for 4–8 hr for a positive response consisting of a decrease in muscle tone, frequency, and/or severity of muscle spasms. If the response is not adequate, a second bolus dose of 75 mcg/1.5 mL, 24 hr after the first bolus dose, can be given with the client observed for 4–8 hr. If the response is still inadequate, a final bolus screening dose of 100 mcg/2 mL can be given 24 hr later.

  Postimplant dose titration for severe spasticity of spinal cord of cerebral origin.

To determine the initial daily dose of baclofen following the implant for intrathecal use, double the screening dose that gave a positive response and give over a 24-hr period. However, if the effectiveness of the bolus dose lasted for more than 12 hr, the daily dose should be the same as the screening dose but delivered over a period of 24 hr. After the first 24 hr, the dose can be increased slowly by 10–30% increments only once each 24 hr until the desired effect is reached.

  Maintenance therapy for severe spasticity of the spinal cord of cerebral origin.

The maintenance dose may need to be adjusted during the first few months of

B

intrathecal therapy. The daily dose may be increased by 10% to no more than 40% daily. If side effects occur, the daily dose may be decreased by 10–20%. Daily doses for long-term continuous infusion have ranged from 12 to 1,500 mcg (usual maintenance is 300–800 mcg/day). Use the lowest dose producing optimal control.

Reduce spasticity of cerebral palsy in children.

25, 50, or 100 mcg.

NURSING CONSIDERATIONS

ADMINISTRATION/STORAGE

1. If no beneficial effects noted, withdraw drug slowly.
2. Check manufacturer's manual for specific instructions/precautions for programming implantable intrathecal infusion pump and refilling reservoir.
3. Prior to intrathecal pump implantation, clients must show positive response to a bolus dose of baclofen in screening trial.
4. If no significant clinical response to increases in daily dose given intrathecally, check pump for proper function and catheter for patency.
5. During long-term intrathecal treatment, approximately 10% of clients become tolerant to increasing doses. If this occurs, a drug "holiday" consisting of a gradual decrease of intrathecal baclofen over a 2-week period can be considered. Alternate methods to treat spasticity must be undertaken. After a few days, sensitivity may return. To avoid possible side effects or overdose, discontinue alternative medication slowly.
6. Filling of the reservoir for intrathecal use must be performed by fully trained/qualified personnel. Refill intervals must be carefully calculated to avoid reservoir depletion.
7. Use extreme caution when filling an FDA-approved implantable pump equipped with an injection port (i.e., that allows direct access to the intrathecal catheter). Direct injection into the catheter through the access port may result in a life-threatening overdose of baclofen.

8. For screening purposes, intrathecal baclofen, either 10 mg/20 mL or 10 mg/5 mL, must be diluted with sterile preservative-free NaCl for injection, to a concentration of 50 mcg/mL for bolus administration. For maintenance, baclofen must be diluted with sterile preservative-free NaCl for injection USP for clients who require concentrations other than 500 mcg/mL (i.e., the 10 mg/20 mL product) or 2,000 mcg/mL (i.e., the 10 mg/5 mL product).

ASSESSMENT

1. List reasons and goals for therapy, other agents trialed, pre-treatment findings.
2. With epilepsy assess for clinical S&S of disease. Obtain EEG at regular intervals; assess for reduced seizure control.
3. Obtain initial renal and LFTs; assess for diabetes.
4. Must closely monitor clients in fully equipped/staffed facility during both the intrathecal screening phase and dose-titration period following intrathecal implant. Resuscitative equipment should be readily available.
5. Ensure free from S&S of infection. Systemic infection may alter response to screening trials, (during pump implantation) lead to surgical complications, and interfere with pump dosing rate.
6. Assess for level of useful spasticity (e.g., to aid in transfers or to maintain posture) as rigidity is important for gait in some clients.
7. In those who require hypertonicity to stand upright, to maintain balance when walking, or to increase functionality, baclofen may be contraindicated; interferes with this coping mechanism.

INTERVENTIONS

1. Report evidence of hypersensitivity reaction.
2. Monitor BP, blood sugar, weight, LFTs, urine output.
3. If no improvement within 6–8 weeks, drug should be withdrawn gradually.
4. For clients with an intrathecal pump:
- Calculate pump refill interval to prevent empty reservoir and return of severe spasticity.

Bold Italic = life threatening side effect   ■ = black box warning   ✦ = Available in Canada

- Access pump reservoir percutaneously. Refill/program by one specifically trained in this procedure.
- When filling pumps with injection ports permitting direct access to the catheter, use care as an injection directly into the catheter can cause lethal overdose. In this event, immediately remove any residual drug from the pump and follow guidelines for *Treatment* under *Overdose Management*.
- When dose requirements suddenly escalate, assess for catheter kinks or dislodgement.
- When programming for increased dosage, e.g., at bedtime, the flow rate should be programmed to change 2 hr before desired effect.

CLIENT/FAMILY TEACHING

1. Take orally with meals/snack to avoid gastric irritation. Report if GI S&S are severe/persistent.
2. To prevent constipation, increase fluids and roughage in diet.
3. Dizziness/drowsiness may occur; use caution. May take several weeks of therapy before improvement occurs.
4. Monitor/record weight/I&O; note frequency/amount of each voiding; report any swelling (edema).
5. May alter insulin requirements.
6. Report impotence; change of drug/dosage may be required. Do not stop abruptly; must be tapered off over 1–2 weeks.
7. Avoid OTC agents, antihistamines, cough remedies, CNS depressants, alcohol use.
8. With the intrathecal pump:
- Once screening trials completed, 'baclofen pump' will be surgically placed in the abdominal wall and attached to an implanted lumbar intrathecal catheter. Proper postop site care, S&S of infection that require immediate reporting will be reviewed.
- Maintain log identifying when spasms are greatest; facilitates proper pump programming to ensure optimal control of spasticity and discomfort.

- Identify symptoms requiring immediate medical intervention.
- Report as scheduled (usually monthly with maintenance) to ensure proper reservoir drug levels and prevent loss of effect or air entering the reservoir.
- Drowsiness, dizziness, and lower extremity weakness may occur; report if persistent/progressive; dose may require adjustment.
- Those refractory to increasing doses may require hospitalization for 'drug holiday;' consists of *gradual reduction* of intrathecal baclofen over a 2-week period and alternative therapy with other agents. Sensitivity to baclofen usually returns after several days and may be resumed intrathecally at the initial continuous dose.

9. Keep all F/U appointments to ensure no adverse events or loss of control.

OUTCOMES/EVALUATE

- Improved muscle tone and involuntary movements; ↓ muscle spasticity and pain
- ↓ Painful/disabling symptoms permitting ↑ functioning level

Balsalazide disodium
(bal-**SAL**-ah-zide)

CLASSIFICATION(S):
Ulcerative colitis drug
PREGNANCY CATEGORY: B
Rx: Colazal.

USES
Treatment of mild to moderately active ulcerative colitis, including children 5 years of age and older.

ACTION/KINETICS
Action
Delivered intact to the colon where it is cleaved by bacteria to release equimolar amounts of mesalamine, the active portion of the molecule. Exact mechanism unknown but the drug may act locally to diminish inflammation by blocking production of arachidonic acid metabolites in the colon.

Pharmacokinetics
Designed to be delivered to the colon as an intact prodrug. Absorption is low and variable. Metabolites and parent drug are mainly excreted in the feces. **Plasma protein binding:** 99%.

CONTRAINDICATIONS
Hypersensitivity to salicylates, components of balsalazide capsules, or balsalazide metabolites.

SPECIAL CONCERNS
There may be worsening of symptoms of ulcerative colitis in some clients. Use with caution in those with known renal dysfunction, history of renal disease, and during lactation. Those with pyloric stenosis may have prolonged gastric retention of balsalazide capsules. Safety and efficacy have not been determined in children less than 5 years of age.

SIDE EFFECTS
Most Common
Adults: Headache, abdominal pain, N&V, diarrhea, arthralgia, respiratory tract infection.
Children: Headache, upper abdominal pain, abdominal pain, vomiting, diarrhea, nasopharyngitis, pyrexia, ulcerative colitis.
GI: N&V, diarrhea, abdominal pain, rectal bleeding, flatulence, dyspepsia, frequent stools, dry mouth, constipation, cramps, bowel irregularity, aggravated ulcerative colitis, enlarged abdomen, diarrhea with blood, diverticulosis, epigastric pain, eructation, fecal incontinence, abnormal feces, gastroenteritis, giardiasis, glossitis, hemorrhoids, melena, benign neoplasm, pancreatitis, ulcerative stomatitis, tenesmus, tongue discoloration. **Hepatic:** Hepatic toxicity, jaundice, cholestatic jaundice, cirrhosis, hepatocellular damage, abnormal liver function, *liver necrosis, liver failure*. **CNS:** Headache, insomnia, dizziness, aphasia, dysphonia, abnormal gait, hypertonia, hypoesthesia, paresis, generalized spasm, tremor, anxiety, depression, nervousness, somnolence. **CV:** Bradycardia, DVT, hypertension, leg ulcer, palpitations, pericarditis. **Respiratory:** Respiratory infection, rhinitis, pharyngitis, coughing, sinusitis, bronchospasm, dyspnea, hemoptysis. **Dermatologic:** Alopecia, angioedema, dermatitis, dry skin, erythema nodosum, erythematous rash, pruritus, pruritus ani, psoriasis, skin ulceration. **Hematologic:** Anemia, eosinophilia, granulocytopenia, leukocytosis, leukopenia, lymphadenopathy, lymphoma-like disorder, lymphopenia, *hemorrhage,* thrombocytopenia. **GU:** Menstrual disorder, UTI, hematuria, interstitial nephritis, micturition frequency, polyuria, pyuria. **Musculoskeletal:** Myalgia, arthritis, back pain, pain, arthritis, arthropathy, leg stiffness. **Ophthalmic:** Conjunctivitis, iritis, abnormal vision. **Otic:** Earache/infection, tinnitus. **Body as a whole:** Fatigue, fever, myalgia, flu-like disorder, viral infection, asthenia, chills, edema, hot flushes, malaise. **Miscellaneous:** Epistaxis, abnormal hepatic function, abscess, infection, moniliasis, weight increase/decrease, parosmia, taste perversion, chest pain.

LABORATORY TEST CONSIDERATIONS
↑ Bilirubin, AST, ALT, amylase, GGT, creatine phosphokinase, LDH, alkaline phosphatase, plasma fibrinogen. ↓ Immunoglobulins. Hypocalcemia, hypokalemia, hypoproteinemia. Increased/decreased prothrombin.

DRUG INTERACTIONS
The use of PO antibiotics might interfere with the release of mesalamine in the colon.

HOW SUPPLIED
Capsules: 750 mg.

DOSAGE
- **CAPSULES**
  Ulcerative colitis.
Adults: Three 750 mg capsules 3 times per day (total daily dose of 6.75 grams) for 8 weeks. Some require treatment for 12 weeks or less. Safety and efficacy beyond 12 weeks have not been determined. **Children, 5–17 years of age:** Either three 750 mg capsules 3 times per day (total daily dose of 6.75 grams) for up to 8 weeks or 1 capsule (750 mg) three times daily (total daily dose of 2.25 grams) for up to 8 weeks. Use in children for more than 8 weeks has not been evaluated.

Bold Italic = life threatening side effect   ■ = black box warning   ✚ = Available in Canada

NURSING CONSIDERATIONS

ADMINISTRATION/STORAGE
Store from 15–30°C (59–86°F).

ASSESSMENT
1. Note character/frequency of stools. Assess abdomen for bowel sounds, distension, pain/tenderness.
2. List other agents trialed, outcome.
3. Monitor CBC, renal and LFTs; assess for liver dysfunction/toxicity. Note history of pyloric stenosis.

CLIENT/FAMILY TEACHING
1. Take as directed (3 capsules 3 times per day) to control bowel movements. Report if S&S do not improve after 6–8 weeks.
2. Alternatively, the drug may be given by carefully opening the capsule and sprinkling the contents on applesauce. The entire drug/applesauce mixture should be swallowed immediately; the contents may be chewed.
3. Practice reliable contraception; avoid drug if nursing.
4. May experience headaches, N&V, diarrhea, abdominal pain and fatigue; report if persistent.
5. Report prolonged abdominal pain, skin rash/hives, breathing problems, yellowing of eyes/skin; may cause liver toxicity. Have labs and colon studies as scheduled; F/U with provider.

OUTCOMES/EVALUATE
- Control of abnormal/frequent liquid stools with ulcerative colitis
- ↓ Diarrhea/abdominal pain with ulcerative colitis

Basiliximab ■ IV
(**bah**-zih-**LIX**-ih-mab)

CLASSIFICATION(S):
Immunosuppressant
PREGNANCY CATEGORY: B
Rx: Simulect.

USES
Prophylaxis of acute organ rejection in renal transplantation, including children. Used as part of an immunosuppressive regimen that includes cyclosporine and corticosteroids in adults and children.

ACTION/KINETICS
Action
An interleukin–2 (IL–2) receptor antagonist which is a monoclonal antibody produced by recombinant DNA technology. Acts as an immunosuppressant by binding to and blocking the IL–2 receptor α–chain which is selectively expressed on the surface of activated T–lymphocytes. This competitively inhibits IL–2–mediated activation of lymphocytes which is a critical pathway in the cellular immune response involved in allograft rejection.

Pharmacokinetics
To be effective, serum levels must exceed 0.2 mcg/mL. At the recommended dosing regimen, the mean duration of basiliximab saturation of IL–2Rα was 36 days. **t½, terminal, adults and adolescents:** 7.2 days; **t½, terminal, children:** 11.5 days.

CONTRAINDICATIONS
Lactation.

SPECIAL CONCERNS
■ Should be prescribed only by physicians experienced in immunosuppressive therapy and management of organ transplant clients. Have complete information available for follow-up. Manage clients in facilities equipped and staffed with adequate lab and supportive medical resources.■ Increased risk for developing opportunistic infections and lymphoproliferative disorders. Possible severe acute hypersensitivity reactions within 24 hr of use with both first and subsequent doses.

SIDE EFFECTS
Most Common (greater than 10%)
Headache, tremor, insomnia, acne, N&V, constipation, diarrhea, abdominal pain, dyspepsia, dyspnea, URTI, anemia, pain, peripheral edema, fever, viral infection, hypertension, UTI.

The incidence of side effects following basiliximab is no greater than placebo groups; however, 99% of clients in both groups reported side effects. Those with an incidence of 3% or greater are listed. **GI:** Constipation, N&V, diarrhea, abdominal pain, dyspepsia, moniliasis,

B

enlarged abdomen, flatulence, GI disorder, gastroenteritis, GI hemorrhage, gum hyperplasia, melena, esophagitis, ulcerative stomatitis. **CNS:** Headache, tremor, dizziness, insomnia, hypoesthesia, neuropathy, paresthesia, agitation, anxiety, depression. **CV:** Angina pectoris, cardiac failure, chest pain, abnormal heart sounds, aggravated hypertension, hypotension, arrhythmia, atrial fibrillation, tachycardia, vascular disorder. **GU:** Dysuria, UTI, impotence, genital edema, bladder disorder, hematuria, frequent micturition, oliguria, abnormal renal function, renal tubular necrosis, ureteral disorder, urinary retention. **Respiratory:** Dyspnea, URTI, coughing, rhinitis, pharyngitis, bronchitis, bronchospasm, abnormal chest sounds, pneumonia, pulmonary disorder, pulmonary edema, sinusitis. **Dermatologic:** Surgical wound complications, acne, cysts, herpes simplex, herpes zoster, hypertrichosis, pruritus, rash, skin disorder, skin ulceration. **Musculoskeletal:** Leg pain, back pain, arthralgia, arthropathy, bone fracture, cramps, hernia, myalgia. **Hematologic:** Hematoma, anemia, *hemorrhage,* purpura, thrombocytopenia, thrombosis, polycythemia. **Metabolic:** Acidosis, weight increase, dehydration, diabetes mellitus, fluid overload. **Ophthalmic:** Cataract, conjunctivitis, abnormal vision. **Miscellaneous:** Pain, peripheral edema, fever, viral infection, leg edema, asthenia, accidental trauma, chest pain, increased drug level, facial edema, fatigue, infection, malaise, generalized edema, rigors, *sepsis, hypersensitivity reactions (including anaphylaxis).*

LABORATORY TEST CONSIDERATIONS
↑ NPN, glucocorticoids. Albuminuria, hyper/hypokalemia, hyper/hypoglycemia, hyperuricemia, hypophosphatemia, hyper/hypocalcemia, hyperlipemia, hypercholesterolemia, hypoproteinemia, hypomagnesemia.

DRUG INTERACTIONS
H Do not give echinacea with basiliximab.

HOW SUPPLIED
Powder for Injection: 10 mg, 20 mg.

DOSAGE
• **IV BOLUS; IV INFUSION, CENTRAL OR PERIPHERAL ONLY**
Prevent kidney transplant rejection.
Adults: Two 20-mg doses; give the first 20 mg within 2 hr prior to transplant surgery and the second 20 mg dose 4 days after transplantation. **Children, <35 kg:** Two doses of 10 mg each. **Children, 35 kg and higher:** Two doses of 20 mg each. Space the doses as in adults. Withhold the second dose if complications occur (e.g., severe hypersensitivity).

NURSING CONSIDERATIONS
ADMINISTRATION/STORAGE
IV 1. To reconstitute: Add 5 mL of sterile water for injection to powder vial (20 mg/5 mL). Shake gently to dissolve.
2. After reconstitution, solution should be colorless and clear to opalescent. If particulate matter present or solution colored, do not use.
3. Reconstituted solution is isotonic. May be given as bolus injection or diluted to a volume of 50 mL with NSS or D5W and infused over 20–30 min.
4. Do not add/infuse other drugs simultaneously through same IV line.
5. Use reconstituted solution immediately. If not used immediately, store at 2–8°C (36–46°F) for 24 hr or at room temperature for 4 hr. Discard if not used within 24 hr.

ASSESSMENT
1. Used in conjunction with cyclosporine and corticosteroids.
2. Given as 2 doses: infuse the first dose 2 hr prior to transplant surgery, give the 2nd dose 4 days after transplantation.
3. Assess carefully for evidence of infection. Monitor labs/serum drug levels.
4. Have medications available for treatment of hypersensitivity reactions; Withhold second dose if hypersensitivity reactions occur.

CLIENT/FAMILY TEACHING
1. Report any fever, chills, fatigue, or sore throat; usually precedes more serious infection.
2. Taken with cyclosporine and steroids. May increase risk of opportunistic

---

Bold Italic = life threatening side effect   ■ = black box warning   ♣ = Available in Canada

infections and lymphoproliferative disorders. Keep all F/U appointments; report adverse side effects.

3. Avoid vaccinations for 2 weeks following last dose. Avoid crowds and persons with known infections.

4. Practice reliable contraception.

OUTCOMES/EVALUATE
- Prophylaxis of renal transplant rejection
- Serum drug levels of >0.2 mcg/mL

BCG, Intravesical ■

CLASSIFICATION(S):
Antineoplastic, miscellaneous
PREGNANCY CATEGORY: C
Rx: TICE BCG, TheraCys.

USES
(1) Treatment and prophylaxis of carcinoma in situ (CIS) of the urinary bladder. (2) Prophylaxis of primary or recurrent stage Ta and/or T1 papillary tumors after transurethral resection. (3) Intravesical use to treat CIS in the absence of an associated invasive cancer of the bladder in the following situations: (a) primary treatment of CIS with or without papillary tumors after transurethral resection; (b) secondary treatment of CIS in those failing to respond or relapsing after intravesical therapy with other agents; (c) primary or secondary treatment of CIS for those with medical contraindications to radical surgery.

ACTION/KINETICS
Action
BCG promotes a local acute inflammatory and subacute granulomatous reaction with macrophage and lymphocyte infiltration in the urothelium and lamina propria of the urinary bladder. Precise mechanism is unknown but the anti-tumor effect seems to be T-lymphocyte dependent.

CONTRAINDICATIONS
TheraCys, TICE BCG: Stage TaG1 papillary tumors unless there is a high risk of tumor recurrence. Positive Mantoux test, unless there is evidence of an active TB infection. Active tuberculosis.

Use as an immunizing agent to prevent TB. Use in presence of a urinary tract infection or fever. Lactation. **TheraCys:** Immunosuppressed clients with congenital or acquired immune deficiencies, whether due to concurrent disease (e.g., AIDS, leukemia, lymphoma), cancer therapy (e.g., cytotoxic drugs, radiation), or immunosuppressive therapy (e.g., corticosteroids) due to the possibility of a systemic BCG infection. **TICE BCG:** Papillary tumors of stages higher than T1; concurrent infections.

SPECIAL CONCERNS
■ BCG contains live, attenuated mycobacteria; there is the potential risk for transmission; thus, prepare, handle, and dispose of as a biohazardous material. BCG infections have been reported in health care workers, primarily from exposure resulting from accidental needle sticks or skin penetrations during preparation of BCG for administration. Nosocomial infections have been reported in immunosuppressed clients receiving parenteral drugs that were prepared in areas in which BCG was prepared. BCG is capable of dissemination when administered by the intravesical route, and serious infections, including fatal infections, have been reported in clients receiving intravesical BCG.■ BCG infection of aneurysms and prosthetic devices is possible, although risk is small. Safety and efficacy have not been established in children.

SIDE EFFECTS
Most Common
Dysuria, urinary urgency/frequency, nocturia, urinary incontinence, UTI, fever, flu-like symptoms, abdominal pain, local pain.

GU: Dysuria, cystitis, urinary urgency/frequency, hematuria, nocturia, urinary incontinence, UTI, foreign material in urine, renal toxicity, genital pain, contracted bladder, genital inflammation/abscess. **GI:** Diarrhea, N&V, anorexia, weight loss. **Hematologic:** Anemia, leukopenia, coagulopathy. **Musculoskeletal:** Arthralgia, myalgia, arthritis, rigors. **Respiratory:** Pulmonary infection. **Body as a whole:** Fever, flu-like symptoms, chills, malaise, fatigue, allergy,

B

systemic infection, hypersensitivity reactions. **Miscellaneous:** Abdominal pain, cramps/pain, liver involvement, cardiac involvement, headache, dizziness, skin rash.

DRUG INTERACTIONS

Antimicrobial therapy / Possible interference with effectiveness of TICE BCG
Bone marrow depressants / Possible impaired response to BCG
Immunosuppressants / Possible impaired response to BCG
Radiation / Possible impaired response to BCG

HOW SUPPLIED

Powder for Suspension, Lyophilized: 1– 8 x 10^8 CFU (TICE BCG), 10.5 +/- 8.7 x 10^8 CFU (TheraCys).

DOSAGE

- **INTRAVESICALLY**
  Carcinoma in situ of the urinary bladder.

Allow 7–14 days to elapse if bladder catheterization has been traumatic or after bladder biopsy or transurethral resection before giving BCG.

THERACYS

Instill 81 mg BCG (dry weight) into the bladder once a week for 6 weeks. Follow with maintenance therapy, consisting of 1 dose given at 3, 6, 12, 18, and 24 months after initial treatment.

TICE BCG

One vial (about 50 mg) suspended in 50 mL preservative-free saline and instilled into the bladder once a week for 6 weeks. Schedule may be repeated if tumor remission has not been achieved. For both products, retain in bladder for 2 hr and then void in a seated position to avoid splashing of urine.

NURSING CONSIDERATIONS

ADMINISTRATION/STORAGE

1. Product contains viable attenuated mycobacteria. Handle as biohazardous substance; use aseptic technique. If cannot be prepared in biocontainment hood, the person preparing product should wear gloves, mask, and gown to avoid inadvertent exposure to broken skin or inhalation of BCG organisms. Product should not be handled by individuals with an immunologic deficiency.

2. Reconstitute and dilute immediately before use. Any delay between reconstitution and administration must not exceed 2 hr.

3. For *TheraCys:* do not remove rubber stopper from the vial. Reconstitute contents of 1 vial with 3 mL of diluent provided. Shake gently until a fine, even suspension results. Further dilute in an additional 50 mL of sterile, preservative-free saline provided to a final volume of 53 mL.

4. For *TICE BCG:* draw 1 mL of sterile preservative-free 0.9% NaCl into small (e.g., 3 mL) syringe. Add to 1 vial of TICE BCG to resuspend. Gently swirl vial until a homogenous suspension obtained. Dispense cloudy BCG suspension into the top end of a catheter-tip syringe containing 49 mL of sterile, preservative-free 0.9% NaCl. Gently rotate syringe. Do not filter contents.

5. Instruct not to drink fluids for 4 hr before treatment. Empty bladder prior to instillation.

6. Instill suspension into the bladder slowly by gravity flow, via the catheter. Do not force the flow.

7. During first hour following instillation, have client lie for 15 min each in the prone and supine positions and on each side. Client can then be up but must retain the suspension for another hr (i.e., total of 2 hr).

8. Maintain adequate hydration.

9. After usage, place all equipment and materials used for product instillation into the bladder into plastic bags (usually red) labeled 'Infectious Waste' and dispose of properly as biohazardous waste.

10. Disinfect urine voided for 6 hr after instillation with equal volume of 5% sodium hypochlorite solution; (undiluted household bleach) allow to stand for 15 min before flushing.

ASSESSMENT

1. Note symptom onset, cysto/TUR, and staging results.

2. Avoid in immunocompromised individuals.

Bold Italic = life threatening side effect   ■ = black box warning   ✦ = Available in Canada

3. Handle and mix carefully away from other parenteral drugs; drug contamination may occur.

4. Dispose of all equipment used to administer product according to institutional guidelines for hazardous waste.

CLIENT/FAMILY TEACHING

1. Used to treat bladder cancer. Contains a viable mycobacteria and should be handled as a biohazard; can make others ill.

2. Do not drink fluids for 4 hr before treatment. Empty bladder prior to instillation. Retain for 2 hr in the bladder before expelling.

3. Sit on toilet seat and void to prevent splashing. Disinfect urine for up to 6 hr after instillation with equal volumes of bleach; wait 15 min before flushing to ensure deactivation of bacteria.

4. Report increase in symptoms associated with blood in the urine, rash, fever/chills, increased frequency/urgency, painful urination, or flu-like symptoms.

5. Any development of cough after BCG treatment requires immediate reporting; may signal a toxic systemic infection.

6. Report for F/U evaluations and cystogram to evaluate drug response.

OUTCOMES/EVALUATE

Control/resolution of bladder cancer

Beclomethasone dipropionate

(be-kloh-**METH**-ah-zohn)

CLASSIFICATION(S):

Glucocorticoid

PREGNANCY CATEGORY: C

Rx: Aerosol Inhaler: QVAR. **Spray:** Beconase AQ.

♣Rx: Inhalation Aerosol: QVAR. **Nasal Aerosol or Spray:** Apo-Beclomethasone, Gen-Beclo AQ, Nu-Beclomethasone, Rivanase AQ, ratio-Beclomethasone AQ. **Topical:** Propaderm.

SEE ALSO *CORTICOSTEROIDS.*

USES

Nasal Aerosol Spray: (1) Prevent recurrence of nasal polyps following surgical removal. (2) Relief of symptoms of seasonal or perennial allergic and nonallergic (vasomotor) rhinitis.

Respiratory inhalant (QVAR): (1) Maintenance treatment of asthma as a prophylaxis in clients 5 years and older. (2) For asthmatics who require systemic corticosteroids when adding an inhalation product may reduce or eliminate the need for systemic corticosteroids.

ACTION/KINETICS

Pharmacokinetics

$t\frac{1}{2}$, **after intranasal:** 0.5 hr. $t\frac{1}{2}$, **after inhalation:** 2.8 hr; 44% is bioavailable. Rapidly inactivated by the liver, resulting in few systemic effects. Excreted in the feces (about 60%) and urine (12%). **Plasma protein binding:** 87%.

CONTRAINDICATIONS

Status asthmaticus, acute episodes of asthma, hypersensitivity to drug or aerosol ingredients.

SPECIAL CONCERNS

Safe use during lactation and in children under 5 years of age not established.

SIDE EFFECTS

Most Common

Pharyngitis, rhinitis, nasal congestion, sinusitis, coughing, viral infection.

Respiratory: Pharyngitis, URTI, rhinitis, sinusitis, nasal congestion, coughing, dysphonia, bronchospasm, sneezing, chest congestion, bronchitis, respiratory disorder. Rarely, ulceration of the nasal mucosa and nasal septum perforation. **GU:** Dysmenorrhea. **Hypersensitivity:** Angioedema, urticaria. **Body as a whole:** Viral infection, flu-like syndrome, pain, fever, rigors. **Miscellaneous:** Taste alteration, earache, back pain, increased asthma symptoms, rectal hemorrhage, lacrimation, arthralgia, depression, skin discoloration, UTI, lymphadenopathy.

HOW SUPPLIED

Aerosol Inhaler: 40 mcg/inh, 80 mcg/inh; *Nasal Spray:* 0.042% (42 mcg/actuation).

DOSAGE

AEROSOL INHALER (QVAR)

Asthma, chronic.

B

Adults and adolescents: If previous therapy was bronchodilators alone, start with 40–80 mcg twice a day. The highest recommended dose is 320 mcg twice a day. If previous therapy was inhaled corticosteroids, start with 40–160 mcg twice a day. The highest recommended dose is 320 mcg twice a day. **Children, 5–11 years of age:** If previous therapy was bronchodilators alone or if previous therapy was inhaled corticosteroids, start with 40 mcg twice a day. The highest recommended dose is 80 mcg twice a day.

NASAL SPRAY (BECONASE AQ)

Allergic or nonallergic rhinitis, prophylaxis of nasal polyps.

Adults and children 12 years or older: 1 or 2 (42 to 84 mcg) nasal inhalations in each nostril twice a day (total dose: 168–336 mcg/day). **Children 6–11 years of age:** Start with 1 nasal inhalation in each nostril twice a day (168 mcg). Those not responding adequately or those with more severe symptoms may use 2 sprays in each nostril twice a day (336 mcg/day). **Maximum daily dose:** 2 sprays in each nostril twice a day (336 mcg/day). **Maintenance:** Once adequate control is achieved, decrease dose to 1 spray in each nostril twice a day.

NURSING CONSIDERATIONS

ADMINISTRATION/STORAGE

1. For nasal use, symptoms usually improve in a few days but relief may not be seen in some for up to 2 weeks. Do not continue therapy beyond 3 weeks if symptoms do not improve. For nasal polyps, treatment may be required for several weeks or more before a beneficial result assessed. Recurrence of nasal polyps can occur after stopping treatment.

2. Improvement usually observed within 1–4 weeks after beginning therapy. Consider tapering to lowest effective dose once desired effect is reached.

3. To prevent explosion of contents under pressure, do not store or use near heat or open flame, or throw into a fire or incinerator. Keep secure from children.

4. If canister is cold, therapeutic effect may be decreased. Shake well before using.

5. Once canister removed from moisture-protected package, use within 6 months.

6. If on systemic steroids, transfer to beclomethasone may be difficult because recovery from impaired adrenal function may be slow.

ASSESSMENT

1. Note any sensitivity to corticosteroids or fluorocarbon propellants.

2. Document allergy and congestion history, presenting symptoms, mucosa presentation, PFTs, ENT, and pulmonary findings.

CLIENT/FAMILY TEACHING

1. Use regularly as prescribed to ensure desired effect.

2. With nasal spray, activate new sprayer by pushing down on the pump 6 times. If pump has not been used for 7 days or more, must prime again. Insert tip into one nostril while pressing closed the other nostril. Slowly inhale while pushing down pump. Aim toward the outer eye and not the inside nose to decrease nasal irritation while inhaling. Shake and repeat steps in the other nostril. Wash cap and tip of activator in warm water and allow to air dry.

3. Review use, care, and storage of inhaler. Rinse out mouth and wash mouthpiece, spacer, sprayer; dry after each use.

4. A spacer may facilitate oral administration. Review video/instruction to ensure proper use.

5. To administer with an inhaler:
- Shake metal canister thoroughly immediately prior to use.
- Exhale as completely as possible.
- Place spacer/mouthpiece into the mouth and tighten lips around it.
- Inhale fully through the mouth while pressing the metal canister down with forefinger.
- Hold breath as long as possible.
- Remove spacer/mouthpiece.
- Exhale slowly.
- A minimum of 60 sec must elapse between inhalations.

Bold Italic = life threatening side effect   ■ = black box warning   ✦ = Available in Canada

6. Not to be used for acute asthma attacks but used regularly to prevent attacks.

7. Follow prescribed therapy; may take 1–4 weeks for any improvement to be realized.

8. To check inhaler content, place in a glass of water: full inhalers sink, empty inhalers float, and half-full inhalers are partially submerged.

9. Report signs of adrenal insufficiency (i.e., muscular pain, lassitude, and depression) even if respiratory function has improved. S&S such as hypotension and weight loss are indications that the dosage of systemic steroid should be boosted temporarily, and then withdrawn more gradually.

10. More than 1 mg in adults or more than 500 mcg in children may precipitate hypothalamic-pituitary axis depression, resulting in adrenal insufficiency. Do not overuse inhaler or exceed prescribed dosage.

11. Report any symptoms of localized oral infections. Gargling and rinsing after treatments, rinsing of the spacer and/or administration port may help prevent infections. May require antifungal meds and possibly discontinuation of drug if occur.

12. If also receiving bronchodilators by inhalation (i.e., Albuterol), use the bronchodilator first to open the airways and then use beclomethasone. Increases penetration of steroid.

13. For those receiving systemic steroid therapy, initiate beclomethasone therapy *very* slowly, withdrawing the systemic steroids as ordered. The benefit of inhaled steroids is a much lower dose, since it goes to target organ and does not require weaning. Once systemic steroid is withdrawn, keep supply of PO glucocorticoids and take immediately if subjected to unusual stress.

14. Carry ID with diagnosis, treatment, and possible need for systemic glucocorticoids, in the event of exposure to unusual stress. Keep regular F/U appointments to evaluate response.

15. Identify/practice relaxation techniques during stressful situations.

OUTCOMES/EVALUATE
- Control of asthma S&S (↓ wheezing, dyspnea)
- Relief of rhinitis
- Prophylaxis of nasal polyp recurrence

Benazepril ■ ⓒ
hydrochloride
(beh-**NAYZ**-eh-prill)

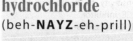

CLASSIFICATION(S):
Antihypertensive, ACE inhibitor
PREGNANCY CATEGORY: D
Rx: Lotensin.

SEE ALSO *ANGIOTENSIN-CONVERTING ENZYME INHIBITORS.*

USES
Hypertension, alone or in combination with other antihypertensives, especially thiazides. *Investigational:* Nondiabetic neuropathy. Heart failure, post MI, high coronary disease risk, diabetes, chronic kidney disease, and recurrent stroke prevention.

ACTION/KINETICS
Action
Benazepril (and its active metabolite benazeprilat) inhibit angiotensin-converting enzyme resulting in decreased plasma angiotensin II, which leads to decreased vasopressor activity and decreased aldosterone secretion (which contributes to sodium and fluid retention). Increased prostaglandin synthesis may also contribute to the antihypertensive action. Both supine and standing BPs are reduced with mild-to-moderate hypertension with an increased cardiac output and no compensatory tachycardia. Also an antihypertensive effect in clients with low-renin hypertension.

Pharmacokinetics
Food does not affect the extent of absorption. Almost completely converted to the active benazeprilat, which has greater ACE inhibitor activity. Is about 37% or more bioavailable. **Onset:** 1 hr. **Duration:** 24 hr. **Peak plasma levels, benazepril:** 30–60 min. **Peak plasma levels, benazeprilat:** 1–2 hr if fasting

---

and 2–4 hr if not fasting. **t½, benazeprilat:** 10–11 hr. **Peak reduction in BP:** 2–4 hr after dosing. **Peak effect with chronic therapy:** 1–2 weeks. About 20% benazeprilat excreted through the urine and 11–12% excreted in the bile. **Plasma protein binding:** About 96.7%.

CONTRAINDICATIONS
Hypersensitivity to benazepril or any other ACE inhibitor.

SPECIAL CONCERNS
■ When used in pregnancy during the second and third trimesters, ACE inhibitors can cause injury and even death to the developing fetus. When pregnancy is detected, discontinue the ACE inhibitor as soon as possible.■ Use with caution during lactation. Safety and effectiveness have not been determined in children.

SIDE EFFECTS
Most Common
Headache, dizziness, fatigue, somnolence/drowsiness, nausea, cough, postural dizziness.
CNS: Headache, dizziness, fatigue, anxiety, insomnia, drowsiness, nervousness. **GI:** N&V, constipation, abdominal pain, gastritis, melena, pancreatitis. **CV:** Symptomatic hypotension, postural hypotension/dizziness, syncope, angina pectoris, palpitations, peripheral edema, ECG changes. **Dermatologic:** Flushing, photosensitivity, pruritus, rash, diaphoresis. **GU:** Decreased libido, impotence, UTI. **Respiratory:** Cough, asthma, bronchitis, dyspnea, sinusitis, bronchospasm. **Neuromuscular:** Paresthesias, arthralgia, arthritis, asthenia, myalgia. **Hematologic:** Occasionally, eosinophilia, leukopenia, neutropenia, decreased hemoglobin. **Miscellaneous:** *Angioedema,* which may be associated with involvement of the tongue, glottis, or larynx, hypertonia, proteinuria, hyponatremia, infection.

LABORATORY TEST CONSIDERATIONS
↑ Serum creatinine, BUN, serum potassium. ↓ Hemoglobin. ECG changes.

DRUG INTERACTIONS
Diuretics / Excessive ↓ in BP
Lithium / ↑ Serum lithium levels with ↑ risk of lithium toxicity

Potassium-sparing diuretics, potassium supplements / ↑ Risk of hyperkalemia

HOW SUPPLIED
Tablets: 5 mg, 10 mg, 20 mg, 40 mg.

DOSAGE
• **TABLETS**
Hypertension in clients not receiving a diuretic.
Adults, initial: 10 mg once daily; **maintenance:** 20–40 mg/day given as a single dose or in two equally divided doses. Total daily doses greater than 80 mg have not been evaluated. **Children, 6 years and older, initial:** 0.2 mg/kg once daily as monotherapy. Doses above 0.6 mg/kg (in excess of 40 mg daily) have not been studied.
Hypertension in clients receiving a diuretic.
Initial: 5 mg/day. C_{CR} <30 mL/min/1.73 m^2. Start with 5 mg/day; **maintenance:** titrate dose upward until BP is controlled or to a maximum total daily dose of 40 mg.

NURSING CONSIDERATIONS
© Do not confuse Lotensin with lovastatin (antihyperlipidemic).
ADMINISTRATION/STORAGE
1. Base dosage adjustment on measuring peak (2–6 hr after dosing) and trough responses. Increase dose or give divided doses if once-daily dosing doesn't provide adequate trough response. Several weeks may be required to reach maximal effects.
2. If BP not controlled by benazepril alone, add a diuretic.
3. If receiving diuretic, discontinue the diuretic, if possible, 2–3 days before beginning benazepril therapy.
4. For children who cannot swallow tablets or for whom the calculated dosage does not correspond to the available tablet strength, a suspension can be made. To prepare 150 mL of a 2 mg/mL suspension: Add 75 mL Ora-Plus oral suspending vehicle to an amber polyethylene terephthalate bottle containing 15 benazepril 20 mg tablets; shake for at least 2 minutes. Allow suspension to stand for a minimum of 1 hr. After the standing time, shake suspension for a minimum of 1 additional min-

ute. Add 75 mL Ora-Sweet oral syrup to the bottle and shake suspension to disperse. Refrigerate from 2–8°C (36–46°F) for up to 30 days in the polyethylene bottle with a child-resistant screw-cap closure. Shake suspension before each use.

ASSESSMENT

1. Note previous experience with this class of drugs; list other agents trialed.
2. Review diet, weight loss, exercise, and life-style changes necessary to control BP.
3. Monitor CBC, electrolytes, renal (especially in geriatric clients) and LFTs. Check urine for protein.

CLIENT/FAMILY TEACHING

1. Take as directed. May take with or without food. Do not chew or crush; swallow tablets whole.
2. May be dizzy, faint, or lightheaded during first few days of therapy; use caution.
3. Avoid concomitant administration of potassium-sparing diuretics/supplements/salt substitutes; may lead to increased K⁺ levels.
4. Report headache, fatigue, dizziness, drowsiness, mouth sores, rash, sore throat, swelling of hands/feet, chest pain and cough.
5. Use birth control; report if pregnancy suspected.
6. Bring record of BP taken at different times during the day.
7. Avoid OTC products without provider approval.

OUTCOMES/EVALUATE

Desired BP control

Benzonatate

(ben-**ZOH**-nah-tayt)

CLASSIFICATION(S):

Antitussive, nonnarcotic
PREGNANCY CATEGORY: C
Rx: Tessalon Perles.

USES

Symptomatic relief of cough.

ACTION/KINETICS

Action

Anesthetizes stretch receptors in respiratory passages, lungs, and pleura reducing their activity and decreasing the cough reflex at its source. No inhibitory effect on the respiratory center in the doses recommended.

Pharmacokinetics

Onset: 15–20 min. **Duration:** 3–8 hr.

CONTRAINDICATIONS

Hypersensitivity to benzonatate or related drugs such as procaine and tetracaine.

SPECIAL CONCERNS

May cause severe hypersensitivity reactions (bronchospasm, laryngospasm, CV collapse) from sucking or chewing the capsule instead of swallowing it (may be related to local anesthesia). Use with caution during lactation. Safety and efficacy have not been determined in children less than 10 years of age.

SIDE EFFECTS

Most Common

GI upset, nausea, constipation, drowsiness, dizziness, nasal congestion, headache.

Hypersensitivity reactions: *Bronchospasm, laryngospasm, CV collapse.* **GI:** Nausea, GI upset, constipation, temporary local anesthesia of the oral mucosa resulting in *choking.* **CNS:** Sedation, headache, dizziness, mental confusion, visual hallucinations. **Dermatologic:** Pruritus, skin eruptions. **Miscellaneous:** Nasal congestion, sensation of burning in the eyes, 'chilly' sensation, numbness of the chest.

OD OVERDOSE MANAGEMENT

Symptoms: Oropharyngeal anesthesia if capsules are chewed or dissolved in the mouth. CNS stimulation, including restlessness, tremors, and clonic convulsions followed by profound CNS depression. *Treatment:* Evacuate gastric contents followed by copious amounts of activated charcoal slurry. Due to depressed cough and gag reflexes, efforts may be needed to protect against aspiration of gastric contents and orally administered substances. Treat convulsions with a short-acting IV barbiturate.

B

Do not use CNS stimulants. Support of respiration and CV-renal function.

HOW SUPPLIED
Capsules: 100 mg, 200 mg.

DOSAGE
• **CAPSULES (PERLES)**
Antitussive.
Adults and children over 10 years of age: 100–200 mg 3 times per day, up to a maximum of 600 mg/day.

NURSING CONSIDERATIONS

ADMINISTRATION/STORAGE
Store from 15–30° C (59–86° F).

ASSESSMENT
1. Identify cough onset, characteristics of S&S, including sputum production/color, fever, travel, exposure to sick individuals. List drugs trialed, outcome.
2. Note sensitivity to benzonatates: procaine or tetracaine.
3. Not for use during pregnancy.
4. Assess lung sounds, VS, characteristics of secretions/breathing patterns, oxygen saturation, and CXR.

CLIENT/FAMILY TEACHING
1. Take only as directed and with plenty of fluids. Swallow perles whole without chewing or crushing to avoid local anesthetic effect on oral mucosa and to prevent choking.
2. Avoid tasks that require alertness until drug effects realized.
3. Do not change positions suddenly-may have sudden drop in BP; take appropriate precautions if dizziness or drowsiness occur. Avoid alcohol and CNS depressants during therapy.
4. Report if symptoms intensify or do not improve after 5 days. Avoid all triggers/irritants such as dust, smoke, strong odors, and fumes. Keep all F/U appointments.

OUTCOMES/EVALUATE
Control of persistent cough.

Benztropine mesylate
(BENS-troh-peen)   **IV**

CLASSIFICATION(S):
Anti-Parkinsonian drug, cholinergic blocking drug
PREGNANCY CATEGORY: C
Rx: Cogentin.
✤**Rx:** Apo-Benztropine.

SEE ALSO *CHOLINERGIC BLOCKING AGENTS.*

USES
(1) Adjunct to treat parkinsonism (all types). (2) Reduce severity of extrapyramidal effects in phenothiazine or other antipsychotic drug therapy (not effective in tardive dyskinesia).

ACTION/KINETICS
Action
Synthetic anticholinergic possessing antihistamine and local anesthetic properties.

Pharmacokinetics
Onset, PO: 1–2 hr; **IM, IV:** Within a few minutes. Effects are cumulative; long-acting (24 hr). **Full effects:** 2–3 days. Low incidence of side effects.

CONTRAINDICATIONS
Use in children under 3 years of age.

SPECIAL CONCERNS
Geriatric and emaciated clients cannot tolerate large doses. Certain drug-induced extrapyramidal symptoms may not respond to benztropine.

SIDE EFFECTS
Most Common
Headache, blurred vision, constipation, mydriasis, dizziness, dry mouth, tachycardia, urinary retention, nausea.
See *Cholinergic Blocking Agents* for a complete list of possible side effects. Also, sudden, uncontrolled somnolence.

HOW SUPPLIED
Injection: 1 mg/mL; *Tablets:* 0.5 mg, 1 mg, 2 mg.

DOSAGE
• **TABLETS**
Parkinsonism.
Adults: 1–2 mg/day (range: 0.5–6.5 mg/day).

Bold Italic = life threatening side effect   ■ = black box warning   ✤ = Available in Canada

Idiopathic parkinsonism.
Adults, initial: 0.5–1 mg/day, increased gradually to 4–6 mg/day, if necessary.
Postencephalitic parkinsonism.
Adults: 2 mg/day in one or more doses.
Drug-induced extrapyramidal effects.
Adults: 1–4 mg 1–2 times per day.
• **IM; IV (RARELY)**
Acute dystonic reactions.
Adults, initial: 1–2 mg; **then,** 1–2 mg PO twice a day usually prevents recurrence. Clients can rarely tolerate full dosage.

NURSING CONSIDERATIONS
ADMINISTRATION/STORAGE
1. When used as replacement for or supplement to other antiparkinsonism drugs, substitute or add gradually.
2. For difficulty swallowing tablets, may crush tablets and mix with a small amount of food or liquid.
3. Some may benefit by taking entire dose at bedtime while others are best treated by taking divided doses, 2–4 times per day.
4. Initiate therapy with low dose (e.g., 0.5 mg) and increase in increments of 0.5 mg at 5–6-day intervals. Do not exceed 6 mg/day.
IV 5. May give IV undiluted at a rate of 1 mg over 1 min.

ASSESSMENT
1. List symptoms, onset, other agents trialed, outcome.
2. Note if phenothiazines or TCAs are being used; may cause paralytic ileus.
3. Elderly require lower dosage. Monitor mental status and assess for depression or mood changes.
4. Assess for tolerance, tardive dyskinesia with prolonged therapy, may require dosage/drug change.

INTERVENTIONS
1. Monitor I&O. Assess for urinary retention and bowel sounds; especially with limited mobility.
2. Inspect skin at regular intervals for evidence of skin changes.
3. Observe for extrapyramidal symptoms, i.e., drooling, muscle spasms, shuffling gait, muscle rigidity, and pill rolling.

4. If excitation or vomiting occurs, withdraw drug temporarily and resume at lower dose.

CLIENT/FAMILY TEACHING
1. Review goals of therapy (control of parkinsonian symptoms, i.e., improved gait and balance and less rigidity and involuntary movements; control of extrapyramidal symptoms, i.e., less drooling, muscle spasms, shuffling gait, or pill rolling).
2. With once-a-day dosing take at bedtime to minimize side effects; if taking more often take after meals.
3. Use caution when performing tasks that require mental alertness; drug has a sedative effect and may also cause drop in BP with sudden changes in position.
4. It usually takes 2–3 days for drug to exert desired effect. Take as ordered unless side effects occur; these usually subside with continued drug use.
5. Avoid strenuous activity and increased heat exposure. Plan rest periods during the day as ability to tolerate heat will be reduced and heatstroke may occur.
6. Report any difficulty in voiding or inadequate emptying of the bladder.
7. Avoid alcohol, OTC agents, and other CNS depressants.
8. Do not stop drug abruptly; requires gradual reduction in dose over one week to prevent withdrawal symptoms.

OUTCOMES/EVALUATE
• ↓ Involuntary movements and rigidity with improved gait and balance
• Control of extrapyramidal side effects of antipsychotic agents

Betamethasone
(bay-tah-**METH**-ah-zohn)

CLASSIFICATION(S):
Glucocorticoid
PREGNANCY CATEGORY: C
Rx: Celestone.

📷 = see color insert   **H** = Herbal   **IV** = Intravenous   ℂ = sound alike drug

Betamethasone dipropionate

Rx: Topical: Alphatrex, Augmented Betamethasone Dipropionate, Diprolene, Diprolene AF, Diprosone, Teladar.

♣Rx: Topical: Diprolene Glycol, Diprosone, Taro-Sone, ratio-Topilene, ratio-Topisone.

Betamethasone sodium phosphate and Betamethasone acetate

Rx: Celestone Soluspan.
♣Rx: Betaject.

Betamethasone valerate

Rx: Topical: Beta-Val, Ectosone Regular, Luxiq, Psorion Cream, Valisone, Valisone Reduced Strength.

♣Rx: Topical: Betaderm, Celestoderm-V, Celestoderm-V/2, Prevex B, ratio-Ectosone.

SEE ALSO CORTICOSTEROIDS.

ADDITIONAL USES

(1) Prevention of respiratory distress syndrome in premature infants. (2) Betamethasone dipropionate cream, lotion, and ointment can be used to treat atopic dermatitis in children younger than 12 years of age.

ACTION/KINETICS

Action

Causes low degree of sodium and water retention, as well as potassium depletion.

Pharmacokinetics

The injectable form contains both rapid-acting and repository forms of betamethasone (mixture of betamethasone sodium phosphate and betamethasone acetate). Long-acting. **t½:** over 300 min.

CONTRAINDICATIONS

Replacement therapy in any acute or chronic adrenal cortical insufficiency due to weak sodium-retaining effects.

SPECIAL CONCERNS

Safe use during pregnancy and lactation not established.

HOW SUPPLIED

Betamethasone: *Syrup:* 0.6 mg/5 mL.
Betamethasone dipropionate: *Cream:* 0.05%; *Gel:* 0.05%; *Lotion:* 0.05%; *Ointment:* 0.05%; *Spray:* 0.1%.
Betamethasone sodium phosphate and betamethasone acetate: *Injection:* 3 mg/mL each of sodium phosphate and of acetate.
Betamethasone valerate: *Cream:* 0.01%, 0.05%, 0.1%; *Foam:* 0.12%; *Lotion:* 0.1%; *Ointment:* 0.1%.

DOSAGE

BETAMETHASONE

• **SYRUP**

Initial: 0.6–7.2 mg/day; individualize dosage.

BETAMETHASONE SODIUM PHOSPHATE AND BETAMETHASONE ACETATE

• **IM**

Initial: 0.5–9 mg/day (dose ranges are ⅓–½ the PO dose given q 12 hr.) In life-threatening situations, dosages exceeding the usual dose may be acceptable; may be in multiple doses.

• **INTRA-ARTICULAR; INTRABURSAL; INTRALESIONAL**

Bursitis, peritendinitis, tenosynovitis.
1 mL intrabursally.
Rheumatoid arthritis and osteoarthritis.
0.25–2 mL intra-articularly, depending on size of the joint (1–2 mL for very large joints; 1 mL for large joints; 0.5–1 mL for medium joints; and, 0.25–0.5 mL for small joints).
Foot disorders, bursitis.
0.25–0.5 mL under heloma durum or heloma molle; 0.5 mL under calcaneal spur or over hallux rigidus or digiti quinti varus.
Tenosynovitis or periostitis of cuboid.
0.5 mL.
Acute gouty arthritis.
0.5–1 mL.

• **INTRADERMAL**

Dermatologic conditions.

0.2 mL/cm², not to exceed 1 mL/week.
BETAMETHASONE DIPROPIONATE, BETA-
METHASONE VALERATE
• CREAM; FOAM; GEL; LOTION; OINT-
MENT; TOPICAL SPRAY
Apply sparingly to affected areas and
rub in lightly.

NURSING CONSIDERATIONS

ADMINISTRATION/STORAGE
1. Avoid injection into deltoid; SC tissue atrophy may occur.
2. Intralesional use indicated for keloids; localized hypertrophic, infiltrated,
inflammatory lesions of lichen planus,
psoriatic plaques, granuloma annulare,
and lichen simplex chronicus; discoid
lupus erythematosus; necrobiosis lipoidica diabeticorum; alopecia areata.

ASSESSMENT
1. List reasons for therapy, type, onset,
location, characteristics of S&S and clinical presentation.
2. List agents trialed; outcome. With
joints, assess ROM, swelling, erythema
and pain level.
3. Monitor uric acid level with gout.

CLIENT/FAMILY TEACHING
1. Review appropriate method for administration. Wash hands before and after application.
2. Report S&S of infection, i.e., increased fever, any redness, odor, or purulent wound drainage. Avoid exposure
to those with contagious diseases.
3. Cover lesions to avoid sunburn.
4. Do not overuse joint after injection;
may further injure joint.
5. Record weight; report sudden
weight gain (>5 lbs/week), swelling of
limbs, blood in stools, severe abdominal
pain, bruising or lack of response.
6. Keep all F/U appointments to evaluate response to therapy.

OUTCOMES/EVALUATE
• ↓ Pain/inflammation; ↑ mobility
• Prevention of respiratory distress
syndrome in premature infants
• Improved skin integrity; healing of le-
sions

Betaxolol hydrochloride
(beh-**TAX**-oh-lohl)

CLASSIFICATION(S):
Beta-adrenergic blocking agent
PREGNANCY CATEGORY: C
Rx: Betoptic, Betoptic S, Kerlone.

SEE ALSO *BETA-ADRENERGIC
BLOCKING AGENTS.*

USES
PO: Hypertension, alone or with other
antihypertensive agents (especially
thiazide diuretics).
   Ophthalmic: (1) Ocular hypertension. (2) Chronic open-angle glaucoma,
alone or in combination with other antiglaucoma drugs.

ACTION/KINETICS
Action
Inhibits beta-1-adrenergic receptors
(beta-2 receptors inhibited at high
doses). Has some membrane stabilizing
activity but no intrinsic sympathomimetic activity. Low lipid solubility. Reduces the production of aqueous humor, thus reducing IOP. No effect on
pupil size or accommodation.
Pharmacokinetics
$t^{1/2}$: 14–22 hr. Metabolized in the liver
with most excreted through the urine;
about 15% is excreted unchanged.

SPECIAL CONCERNS
Use with caution during lactation. Safety and effectiveness have not been determined in children. Geriatric clients
are at greater risk of developing bradycardia.

SIDE EFFECTS
Most Common
After ophthalmic use: Brief discomfort,
tearing, headaches.
See *Beta-Adrenergic Blocking Agents* for
a complete list of side effects.

HOW SUPPLIED
Ophthalmic Solution: 0.5%; *Ophthalmic
Suspension:* 0.25%; *Tablets:* 10 mg, 20
mg.

DOSAGE
• **TABLETS**
  Hypertension.

Initial: 10 mg once daily either alone or with a diuretic. If desired effect is not reached, may increase dose to 20 mg; doses higher than 20 mg will not increase the therapeutic effect. In geriatric clients the initial dose should be 5 mg/day.

• **OPHTHALMIC SOLUTION; SUSPENSION**

Ocular hypertension; chronic open-angle glaucoma.

Adults, usual: 1–2 gtt twice a day. If used to replace another drug, continue the drug being used and add 1 gtt of betaxolol twice a day. Discontinue the previous drug the following day. If transferring from several antiglaucoma drugs being used together, adjust one drug at a time at intervals of not less than 1 week. The agents being used can be continued and add 1 gtt betaxolol twice a day. The next day another agent should be discontinued. The remaining antiglaucoma drug dosage can be decreased or discontinued depending on client response.

NURSING CONSIDERATIONS

ADMINISTRATION/STORAGE

1. Full antihypertensive effect usually observed within 7 to 14 days.
2. As PO dose increased, HR decreases.
3. Discontinue PO therapy gradually over 2-week period.
4. Shake ophthalmic suspension well before use.
5. Store ophthalmic products at room temperature; not to exceed 30°C (86°F).

ASSESSMENT

1. Note reasons for therapy, frequency/characteristics of symptoms, other agents trialed.
2. Monitor lung sounds, weight, EKG, VS. With glaucoma check eye exam and pressures.

CLIENT/FAMILY TEACHING

1. Review appropriate method/indications for therapy; take/use as directed. Do not stop suddenly.
2. May mask S&S of hypoglycemia, and cause increased cold sensitivity.
3. Avoid OTC agents without approval.
4. With HTN, monitor BP and record; report adverse effects.

5. With eye therapy, review instillation procedure. Wear sunglasses, avoid sun exposure; may cause photophobia.
6. Use caution, may cause dizziness or drowsiness. Change positions slowly; prevents sudden drop in BP.
7. Report SOB, wheezes, confusion, rash, unusual bruising/bleeding, slow pulse, cold hands/feet.

OUTCOMES/EVALUATE

• ↓ BP (PO)
• ↓ Intraocular pressure (ophthalmic)

Bevacizumab
(bev-ah-**CIZ**-yoo-mab)

CLASSIFICATION(S):
Antineoplastic, monoclonal antibody
PREGNANCY CATEGORY: C
Rx: Avastin.

USES

(1) With IV 5-fluorouracil-based chemotherapy for first-line treatment of metastatic carcinoma of the colon or rectum. (2) With IV 5-fluorouracil for second-line treatment of metastatic colorectal cancer. (3) WIth carboplatin and paclitaxel for initial systemic treatment of unresectable, locally advanced, recurrent, or metastatic nonsquamous, non–small cell lung cancer. *Investigational:* Metastatic renal cell carcinoma.

ACTION/KINETICS

Action

Bevacizumab is a recombinant, humanized, monoclonal IgG$_1$ antibody that binds to and inhibits the biologic activity of human vascular endothelial growth factor (VEGF). Binding of bevacizumab to VEGF prevents the interaction of VEGF to its receptor on the surface of endothelial cells. It is believed this results in reduction of microvascular growth and inhibition of metastatic disease progression.

Pharmacokinetics

t½: About 20 days. **Time to reach steady state:** 100 days.

B

CONTRAINDICATIONS

Use within 28 days following major surgery. Lactation.

SPECIAL CONCERNS

■ (1) Bevacizumab use can result in development of GI perforation and wound dehiscence, which can be fatal. GI perforation, sometimes associated with intra-abdominal abscess, occurred throughout treatment with bevacizumab (i.e., was not correlated to duration of exposure). The incidence of GI perforation in those receiving bolus-IFL (125 mg/m^2 irinotecan IV, 500 mg/m^2 5-fluorouracil, and 20 mg/m^2 leucovorin IV given once weekly for 4 weeks q 6 weeks) with bevacizumab was 2%. The typical presentation reported was abdominal pain associated with symptoms such as constipation and vomiting. Include GI perforation in the differential diagnosis of clients receiving bevacizumab presenting with abdominal pain. Permanently discontinue bevacizumab in those with GI perforation or wound dehiscence requiring medical intervention. The appropriate interval between termination of bevacizumab and subsequent elective surgery required to avoid the risks of impaired wound healing/wound dehiscence has not been determined. (2) Serious and, in some cases, fatal hemoptysis has occurred in clients with nonsmall cell lung cancer treated with chemotherapy and bevacizumab. In a small study, the incidence of serious or fatal hemoptysis was 31% in clients with squamous histology and 4% in clients with adenocarcinoma receiving bevacizumab as compared with no cases in clients treated with chemotherapy alone. Do not administer bevacizumab to clients with recent hemoptysis.■ Safety in clients with clinically significant CV disease has not been adequately evaluated. There is the potential for immunogenicity. Use with caution in clients with known hypersensitivity to bevacizumab or any component of the drug product. Severe side effects occur at a higher incidence in geriatric clients. There is an increased risk of serious arterial thromboembolic events, including CVA, cerebral infarction, MI, TIAs, angina, and fatal arterial thrombotic events in those receiving bevacizumab plus chemotherapy; risk factors include history of arterial thromboembolism before drug exposure and age 65 years and older. Safety and efficacy in children have not been evaluated. Side effects may be more severe in geriatric clients.

SIDE EFFECTS

Most Common

URTI, pain, asthenia, dyspnea, epistaxis, exfoliative dermatitis, headache, hypertension, N&V, abdominal pain, anorexia, constipation, diarrhea, stomatitis.

Most serious: *CHF, GI perforation/wound healing complications, serious and nonserious hemorrhagic events, arterial thromboembolic events, thromboembolism, hypertensive crises, nephrotic syndrome.* **Infusion reaction:** Hypertension, *hypertensive crisis* associated with neurologic signs and symptoms, wheezing, oxygen desaturation, *grade 3 hypersensitivity*, chest pain, headaches, rigors, diaphoresis. **GI:** Diarrhea, abdominal pain, anorexia, constipation, N&V, stomatitis, dyspepsia, flatulence, *GI hemorrhage*, dry mouth, colitis, anastomotic ulceration, *intestinal necrosis, mesenteric venous occlusion,* intestinal obstruction. **CV:** Hypertension, *DVT, intra-abdominal thrombosis, MI, CVA, fatal arterial thrombotic events, thromboembolism,* TIAs, CHF, angina, syncope, hypotension. **Hematologic:** Leukopenia, neutropenia, thrombocytopenia, pancytopenia. **CNS:** Dizziness, headache, confusion, abnormal gait. **Respiratory:** Dyspnea, epistaxis, URTI, voice alteration. **Dermatologic:** Alopecia, dry skin, exfoliative dermatitis, nail disorder, skin discoloration, skin ulcer. **GU:** Proteinuria, vaginal hemorrhage, urinary frequency/urgency, ureteral stricture. **Body as a whole:** Asthenia, pain, weight loss, myalgia. **Miscellaneous:** Syncope, taste disorder, excess lacrimation, minor gum bleeding, polyserositis, impaired fertility.

LABORATORY TEST CONSIDERATIONS

Proteinuria, hypokalemia, bilirubinemia, hyponatremia.

B

HOW SUPPLIED
Injection: 25 mg/mL, 100 mg/vial, 400 mg/vial.

DOSAGE
• **IV INFUSION**
Metastatic colon or rectal carcinoma.
5 mg/kg once every 14 days until disease progression is detected.

NURSING CONSIDERATIONS
ADMINISTRATION/STORAGE
IV 1. To prepare: Withdraw necessary amount of drug for a dose of 5 mg/kg; dilute in total volume of 100 mL 0.9% NaCl injection. Discard any unused portion; product contains no preservatives.
2. Do not give or mix bevacizumab infusions with dextrose solutions.
3. Give only as IV infusion; do **not** give as IV push or bolus.
4. If first infusion (given over 90 min) is well tolerated, the second infusion may be given over 60 min. If the 60-min infusion is well tolerated, all subsequent infusions may be given over 30 min.
5. Permanently discontinue bevacizumab in those who develop GI ulceration, wound dehiscence requiring medical intervention, serious bleeding, nephrotic syndrome, or hypertensive crisis.
6. Discontinue temporarily in those with evidence of moderate to severe proteinuria pending further evaluation and with severe hypertension not controlled with medical management.
7. Suspend bevacizumab at least several weeks before elective surgery. Do not resume bevacizumab until surgical incision is fully healed.
8. Refrigerate bevacizumab vials from 2–8°C (36–46°F). Diluted solutions for infusion may be stored at the same temperature as vials for up to 8 hr. Protect from light. Store in the original carton until time of use. Do not freeze or shake.

ASSESSMENT
1. Note reasons for therapy, disease onset, physical condition, extent of illness.
2. Drug impairs wound healing, may cause dehiscence and/or GI perforation and hemorrhage; monitor for abdominal pain, constipation, and vomiting.

Assess wound/surgical site; discontinue drug with any complications.
3. Monitor BP weekly to ensure no drug included HTN. Stop if hypertensive crisis occurs.
4. Assess for proteinuria; monitor urines for worsening. Temporarily stop therapy. Assess 24 hr urine with 2+ protein readings to prevent nephrotoxicity. Stop drug permanently with evidence of nephrotic syndrome.
5. Assess during infusion for evidence of reaction; interrupt infusion and treat symptoms.
6. Document cardiac status; assess for ventricular dysfunction. Drug may induce/worsen CHF; stop infusion, monitor carefully.
7. Monitor those over 65 years for increased incidence of adverse effects.
8. Wait at least 28 days after major surgery ensuring that the incision is fully healed, to initiate therapy. Drug half life is 20 days. If surgery planned in future, stop therapy for at least 1 month before.

CLIENT/FAMILY TEACHING
1. Used to treat cancer that spread in the colon or rectum or in combo for other cancers; extremely powerful-can cause many side effects.
2. With any surgery, drug will impair wound healing and may also cause GI bleeding.
3. Monitor/record BP readings and urine dip tests for protein.
4. Practice barrier contraception; drug will harm fetus.
5. Once therapy stopped, drug may stay in system for up to a month or more.
6. Report constipation, abdominal pains, calf pain, SOB, chest pain, opening of wound, bleeding or any unusual side effects immediately. Keep F/U visits to prevent adverse outcome and to monitor drug effects.

OUTCOMES/EVALUATE
Inhibition of malignant cell proliferation
Prevention of serious drug side effects

Bold Italic = life threatening side effect   ▅ = black box warning   ♣ = Available in Canada

Bicalutamide

(**buy**-kah-**LOO**-tah-myd)

CLASSIFICATION(S):
Antineoplastic, antiandrogen
PREGNANCY CATEGORY: X
Rx: Casodex.

SEE ALSO *ANTINEOPLASTIC AGENTS.*

USES
Treatment of advanced prostate cancer in combination with a leutinizing hormone-releasing hormone analog.

ACTION/KINETICS

Action
Nonsteroidal antiandrogen that competitively inhibits the action of androgens by binding to cytosolic androgen receptors in target tissues. The drug increases bone mineral density and reduces fat accumulation when used as monotherapy.

Pharmacokinetics
Well absorbed after PO; food does not affect the rate or amount absorbed. Metabolized in the liver, and both parent drug and metabolites are eliminated in the urine and feces. **t½:** 5.8 days. **Mean steady-state concentration in prostatic cancer:** 8.9 mcg/mL.

CONTRAINDICATIONS
Pregnancy. Use in women.

SPECIAL CONCERNS
Use with caution in clients with moderate to severe hepatic impairment and during lactation. Safety and efficacy have not been established in children.

SIDE EFFECTS

Most Common
Hot flashes, generalized pain, back pain, asthenia, pelvic pain, constipation, nausea, diarrhea, dyspnea, infection, peripheral edema, nocturia, hematuria, abdominal pain, anemia, dizziness.

GI: Constipation, N&V, diarrhea, anorexia, dyspepsia, rectal hemorrhage, dry mouth, melena, flatulence, dysphagia, GI disorder, periodontal abscess, GI carcinoma, hepatotoxicity. **CNS:** Dizziness, paresthesia, insomnia, anxiety, depression, decreased libido, hypertonia, confusion, neuropathy, somnolence, nervousness. **GU:** Gynecomastia, breast pain, nocturia, hematuria, UTI, impotence, urinary incontinence/frequency, impaired urination, dysuria, urinary retention/urgency, hydronephrosis, urinary tract disorder. **CV:** Hot flashes (most common), hypertension, angina pectoris, CHF, *MI, cardiac arrest,* coronary artery disorder, syncope. **Metabolic:** Peripheral edema, hyperglycemia, weight loss or gain, dehydration, gout, edema. **Musculoskeletal:** Myasthenia, arthritis, myalgia, bone pain, leg cramps, pathologic fracture. **Respiratory:** Dyspnea, increased cough, pharyngitis, bronchitis, pneumonia, rhinitis, lung disorder, asthma, epistaxis, sinusitis, interstitial pneumonitis, pulmonary fibrosis. **Dermatologic:** Rash, sweating, dry skin, pruritus, alopecia, herpes zoster, skin carcinoma, skin disorder. **Hematologic:** Anemia, hypochromic and iron deficiency anemia. **Body as a whole:** General pain, back pain, asthenia, pelvic/abdominal/chest pain, flu syndrome, edema, neoplasm, fever, neck pain, chills, *sepsis.* **Miscellaneous:** Infection, bone pain, headache, hernia, cyst, specified cataract, diabetes mellitus.

LABORATORY TEST CONSIDERATIONS
↑ Alkaline phosphatase, creatinine, AST, ALT, bilirubin, BUN, liver enzyme tests. ↓ Hemoglobin, white cell count.

DRUG INTERACTIONS
Bicalutamide may displace coumarin anticoagulants from their protein-binding sites, resulting in an increased anticoagulant effect.

HOW SUPPLIED
Tablets: 50 mg.

DOSAGE

• **TABLETS**

Prostatic carcinoma.

50 mg (1 tablet) once daily (morning or evening) in combination with an LHRH analog with or without food.

NURSING CONSIDERATIONS

ADMINISTRATION/STORAGE
1. Take at same time daily.
2. Start at same time as LHRH analog.

ASSESSMENT

1. Note reasons for therapy, onset/duration of symptoms, staging results, and other agents/therapies trialed.
2. Monitor renal, LFTs, CBC, PSA. (If transaminases increase 2x normal, stop drug.)
3. If on warfarin, monitor PT/INR; can displace from protein binding sites.

CLIENT/FAMILY TEACHING

1. Take at same time each day; used with LHRH analog (i.e., goserelin implant or leuprolide depot).
2. Side effects requiring immediate attention: hemorrhage, urinary retention, yellow skin, fracture, respiratory distress, persistent/severe diarrhea.
3. May experience hot flashes, breast enlargement and pain; drug-related hair loss should regrow following therapy.
4. Periodic PSA, CBC, liver and renal function required to assess response.

OUTCOMES/EVALUATE

• Symptomatic improvement
• Reduction of serum PSA and inhibition of tumor growth

Bimatoprost
(by-**MAH**-toh-prost)

CLASSIFICATION(S):
Antiglaucoma drug
PREGNANCY CATEGORY: C
Rx: Lumigan.

USES
Reduce elevated intraocular pressure in open angle glaucoma or ocular hypertension.

ACTION/KINETICS

Action
Selectively mimics the effects of the naturally occurring prostamides. Lowers IOP by increasing outflow of aqueous humor through the trabecular network and uveoscleral routes.

Pharmacokinetics
Onset: About 4 hr after first administration. **Maximum effect:** About 8–12 hr.

SPECIAL CONCERNS
Has not been evaluated to treat angle closure, inflammatory, or neovascular glaucoma. May cause increased pigmentation and growth of eyelashes. May increase the amount of brown pigment in the iris and darken the eyelid skin; changes may be permanent. Bacterial keratitis, due to contamination of the product, is possible. Use with caution in active intraocular inflammation, in aphakic or pseudophakic clients with a torn posterior lens capsule, in those with known risk factors for macular edema, and during lactation. Safety and efficacy have not been determined in children.

SIDE EFFECTS
Most Common
Conjunctival hyperemia, growth of eyelashes, ocular pruritus.
Ophthalmic: Conjunctival hyperemia, growth of eyelashes, ocular pruritus/burning/dryness, visual disturbances, foreign body sensation, eye pain/discharge, pigmentation of the periocular skin, blepharitis, cataract, superficial punctuate keratitis, eyelid erythema, ocular irritation, eyelash darkening, tearing, photophobia, allergic conjunctivitis, asthenopia, increases in iris pigmentation, conjunctival edema, iritis. **Systemic:** Infections, headache, abnormal LFTs, asthenia, hirsutism.

HOW SUPPLIED
Ophthalmic Solution: 0.03%.

DOSAGE
• **OPHTHALMIC SOLUTION**
  Elevated IOP.
1 gtt in the affected eye(s) once daily in the evening.

NURSING CONSIDERATIONS

ADMINISTRATION/STORAGE
Store in the original container at 15–25°C (59–77°F).

ASSESSMENT
1. Note reasons for therapy, other agents trialed, pressure readings; used with open angle glaucoma or ocular hypertension.
2. Assess eye for inflammation, exudate, pain, level of vision. Note iris color.

Bold Italic = life threatening side effect   ■ = black box warning   ✤ = Available in Canada

3. Monitor LFTs; drug may alter levels.

CLIENT/FAMILY TEACHING

1. Use once daily as directed, more frequent use may decrease eye pressure lowering effect.

2. Do not let tip of eyedropper come in contact with eye or surrounding tissue. If contact suspected rinse well, do not share eyedroppers.

3. May be used together with other topical eye drug products to lower IOP. If more than 1 eye drop used, administer at least 5 min apart.

4. Remove contact lenses prior to instillation; may be reinserted 15 min after drug administration. Bimatoprost contains benzalkonium chloride which may be absorbed by soft contact lenses.

5. May cause irreversible pigmentation changes to iris (brown color) and skin around the eye and lid. May cause increased eyelash growth; may be of concern if only one eye is being treated.

6. Report any unusual/intolerable side effects. Keep all F/U appointments to evaluate response to treatment. Do not drive or perform hazardous functions until vision clears.

OUTCOMES/EVALUATE

Reduction of IOP

Biperiden hydrochloride [IV]

(bye-**PER**-ih-den)

CLASSIFICATION(S):

Cholinergic blocking drug, antiparkinson drug

PREGNANCY CATEGORY: C

Rx: Akineton.

SEE ALSO *ANTIPARKINSON DRUGS* **AND** *CHOLINERGIC BLOCKING AGENTS.*

USES

(1) Parkinsonism, especially of the postencephalitic, arteriosclerotic, and idiopathic types. (2) Drug-induced (e.g., phenothiazines) extrapyramidal manifestations.

ACTION/KINETICS

Action

Synthetic anticholinergic. Tremor may increase as spasticity is relieved. Slight respiratory and CV effects.

Pharmacokinetics

Time to peak levels: 60–90 min. **Peak levels:** 4–5 mcg/L. **t½:** About 18–24 hr. Tolerance may develop.

ADDITIONAL CONTRAINDICATIONS

Children under 3 years of age.

SPECIAL CONCERNS

Use with caution in older children.

SIDE EFFECTS

Most Common

Agitation, blurred vision, constipation, dizziness, drowsiness, lightheadedness, dry mouth/nose/throat, nausea, nervousness, GI upset.

See *Cholinergic Blocking Agents* for a complete list of possible side effects. Also, muscle weakness, inability to move certain muscles.

HOW SUPPLIED

Injection: 5 mg/mL (as lactate); *Tablets:* 2 mg.

DOSAGE

- **TABLETS**

  Parkinsonism.

  Adults: 2 mg 3–4 times per day, to a maximum of 16 mg/day.

  Drug-induced extrapyramidal effects.

  Adults: 2 mg 1–3 times per day. Maximum daily dose: 16 mg.

- **IM; IV**

  Drug-induced extrapyramidal effects.

  2 mg. Repeat q 30 min until symptoms improve, but not more than 4 consecutive doses in 24 hr.

NURSING CONSIDERATIONS

ADMINISTRATION/STORAGE

[IV] 1. May give undiluted by direct IV at rate not exceeding 2 mg over at least 1 min.

2. Place in recumbent position during IV administration; may experience euphoria, postural hypotension, and/or loss of coordination.

3. Store in tightly closed, light resistant container at 15–30°C (59–86°F).

ASSESSMENT

1. Note reasons for therapy, characteristics of S&S, other agents trialed, out-

---

B

come. Note degree of involuntary movements, muscle spasms/rigidity and drooling.

2. Elderly clients should receive lower doses.

3. Assess for urinary retention, constipation.

4. List drugs taking to prevent unfavorable interactions.

CLIENT/FAMILY TEACHING

1. Review goals of therapy (control of parkinsonian symptoms, i.e., improved gait and balance and less rigidity and involuntary movements; control of extrapyramidal symptoms, i.e., less drooling, muscle spasms, shuffling gait, or pill rolling).

2. Take after meals to avoid gastric irritation. Do not stop abruptly.

3. Do not use antacids or antidiarrheal for 1–2 hr after taking drug.

4. Avoid activities that require mental alertness until drug effects realized. May cause dizziness, drowsiness, blurred vision. Change positions slowly to prevent sudden drop in BP.

5. Avoid overheating; drug reduces perspiration.

6. Record stools; increase intake of fluids, fruit juices, and fiber to avoid constipation; report urinary difficulty.

7. Report adverse effects/loss of response; dose may require adjustment.

8. Use sugarless gum/candies, rinse mouth often to control dry mouth effects.

OUTCOMES/EVALUATE

- ↓ Involuntary movements and rigidity with improved gait and balance
- Control of drug-induced (phenothiazine) extrapyramidal manifestations (i.e., ↓ muscle rigidity and drooling)

Bisoprolol fumarate ©

(BUY-soh-proh-lol)

CLASSIFICATION(S):
Beta-adrenergic blocking agent
PREGNANCY CATEGORY: C
Rx: Zebeta.
✦Rx: Monocor.

SEE ALSO *BETA-ADRENERGIC BLOCKING AGENTS.*

USES
Hypertension alone or in combination with other antihypertensive agents. *Investigational:* Angina pectoris, SVTs, PVCs.

ACTION/KINETICS

Action
Inhibits beta-1-adrenergic receptors and, at higher doses, beta-2 receptors. No intrinsic sympathomimetic activity and no membrane-stabilizing activity.

Pharmacokinetics
$t\frac{1}{2}$: 9–12 hr. Over 90% of PO dose is absorbed. Approximately 50% is excreted unchanged through the urine and the remainder as inactive metabolites; a small amount (less than 2%) is excreted through the feces.

SPECIAL CONCERNS
Use with caution during lactation. Safety and efficacy have not been determined in children. Due to selectivity for beta-1 receptors, it may be used with caution in clients with bronchospastic disease who do not respond to, or who cannot tolerate, other antihypertensive therapy.

SIDE EFFECTS

Most Common
Dizziness, fatigue, headache, diarrhea, rhinitis, URTI, cough, peripheral edema.
See *Beta-Adrenergic Blocking Agents* for a complete list of possible side effects.

HOW SUPPLIED
Tablets: 5 mg, 10 mg.

DOSAGE

- **TABLETS**
  Antihypertensive.
Dose must be individualized. **Adults, initial:** 5 mg once daily (in some, 2.5 mg/day may be appropriate). **Maintenance:** If the 5-mg dose is inadequate, the dose may be increased to 10 mg/day and then, if needed, to 20 mg once daily. In impaired renal (C_{CR} <40 mL/min) or hepatic function (hepatitis or cirrhosis), initially give 2.5 mg with caution in titrating the dose upward.

NURSING CONSIDERATIONS
© Do not confuse bisoprolol with bitolterol (a sympathomimetic drug). Also,

---

Bold Italic = life threatening side effect   ■ = black box warning   ✦ = Available in Canada

do not confuse Zebeta with DiaBeta (an oral hypoglycemic).

ADMINISTRATION/STORAGE
1. Food does not affect bioavailability; may give without regard to meals.
2. Bisoprolol is not dialyzable; dose adjustments not required if undergoing hemodialysis.
3. Dosage adjustment not necessary in the elderly.

ASSESSMENT
1. Note reasons for therapy, previous agents used, outcome.
2. Monitor CBC, glucose, electrolytes, renal and LFTs; reduce dose with dysfunction. Assess for lower extremity edema and JVD.
3. Once baseline parameters determined, monitor BP in both arms while lying, sitting, and standing.
4. Check EKG and CXR. Assess heart/lung sounds and note any arrhythmias.

CLIENT/FAMILY TEACHING
1. Take as directed at same time with/without food.
2. Use caution; may cause dizziness/drowsiness. Change positions slowly to avoid sudden drop in low BP.
3. Do not stop suddenly without provider knowledge. Avoid OTC drugs without approval.
4. With diabetes, monitor FS closely. Report weakness or fatigue; drug does not block dizziness and sweating as signs of hypoglycemia.
5. Report lack of response or adverse side effects. Keep log of BP and pulse for provider review.

OUTCOMES/EVALUATE
- ↓ BP; relief of angina
- Stable cardiac rhythm

—*COMBINATION DRUG*—

Bisoprolol fumarate and Hydrochlorothiazide
(**BUY**-soh-**proh**-lol, **hy**-droh-klor-oh-**THIGH**-ah-zyd)

B

CLASSIFICATION(S):
Antihypertensive
PREGNANCY CATEGORY: C
Rx: Ziac.

SEE ALSO *BISOPROLOL FUMARATE AND HYDROCHLOROTHIAZIDE.*

USES
First-line therapy for management of mild to moderate hypertension.

CONTENT
Ziac-2.5 mg/6.25 mg: Biosprolol fumarate *(beta-adrenergic blocking agent),* 2.5 mg and hydrochlorothiazide *(thiazide diuretic),* 6.25 mg. *Ziac-5 mg/6.25 mg:* Bisoprolol fumarate, 5 mg and hydrochlorothiazide, 6.25 mg. *Ziac-10 mg/6.25 mg:* Bisoprolol fumarate, 10 mg and hydrochlorothiazide, 6.25 mg.

ACTION/KINETICS
Action
Bisoprolol is a beta$_1$-selective adrenergic blocking drug with no significant membrane stabilizing or intrinsic sympathomimetic action. At higher doses, it also inhibits beta$_2$-adrenergic receptors located in bronchial and vascular musculature. Hydrochlorothiazide is a diuretic that increases excretion of sodium and chloride in approximately equal amounts. The antihypertensive effects are additive.

Pharmacokinetics
Both drugs are well absorbed; absorption is not affected whether the drug is taken with or without food. The bioavailability of bisoprolol is about 80% while the bioavailability of hydrochlorothiazide is 65–75%. **Peak plasma levels, bisoprolol:** 3 hr; **hydrochlorothiazide:** 2.5 hr. **t½, elimination, bisoprolol:** 7–15 hr; **hydrochlorothiazide:** 4–10 hr. About 50% of bisoprolol is ex-

---

creted unchanged in the urine. Hydrochlorothiazide is excreted mainly in the urine. **Plasma protein binding:** About 30% of bisoprolol and 40–68% of hydrochlorothiazide are bound to plasma proteins.

CONTRAINDICATIONS

Use in cardiogenic shock, overt cardiac failure, second or third degree heart block, marked sinus bradycardia, anuria, hypersensitivity to either drug or to other sulfonamide-derived drugs. Lactation.

SPECIAL CONCERNS

Continued depression of the myocardium with beta-blockers may precipitate heart failure. Use with caution in peripheral vascular disease, in clients with bronchospastic disease and who do not respond to or tolerate other antihypertensive treatment. Safety and efficacy have not been determined in children.

SIDE EFFECTS

Most Common

Cough, fatigue, dizziness, headache, myalgia, diarrhea.

See *Bisoprolol fumarate* and *Hydrochlorothiazide* for a complete list of possible side effects.

LABORATORY TEST CONSIDERATIONS

↑ Uric acid, serum triglycerides.

DRUG INTERACTIONS

See *Bisoprolol fumarate* and *Hydrochlorothiazide*.

HOW SUPPLIED

See Content.

DOSAGE

- **TABLETS**

  Hypertension.

Initial: One 2.5/6.25 mg tablet once daily; dose may be increased q 14 days to a maximum of two 10/6.25 mg tablets once daily.

NURSING CONSIDERATIONS

ADMINISTRATION/STORAGE

Store from 20–25° C (68–77° F). Dispense in tight containers.

ASSESSMENT

1. List reasons for therapy, disease onset, other agents trialed, outcome.
2. Assess for sulfonamide sensitivity; monitor EKG, electrolytes, Mg, renal and LFTs.

3. Determine any CAD, CHF, or lung disease.

CLIENT/FAMILY TEACHING

1. Ziac is a combination of two drugs (beta blocker and diuretic) in one pill to better control BP.
2. May cause dizziness, use caution operating machinery until drug effects realized.
3. With diabetes, monitor FS closely; may mask low glucose symptoms.
4. Record BP and pulse; report any difficulty breathing, low heart rate, swelling of extremities or adverse effects.
5. Keep all F/U appointments to evaluate response.

OUTCOMES/EVALUATE

Control of BP

Bitolterol mesylate ©
(bye-**TOHL**-ter-ohl)

CLASSIFICATION(S):

Bronchodilator

PREGNANCY CATEGORY: C

Rx: Tornalate.

SEE ALSO *SYMPATHOMIMETIC DRUGS.*

USES

Prophylaxis and treatment of bronchial asthma and reversible bronchospasms. May be used with theophylline or steroids.

ACTION/KINETICS

Action

Prodrug converted by esterases to the active colterol. Colterol combines with beta-2-adrenergic receptors, producing dilation of bronchioles. Minimal beta-1-adrenergic activity.

Pharmacokinetics

Onset following inhalation: 2–4 min. **Time to peak effect:** 30–60 min. **Duration:** 5–8 hr.

SPECIAL CONCERNS

Safety has not been established for use during lactation and in children less than 12 years of age. Use with caution in ischemic heart disease, hypertension, hyperthyroidism, diabetes mellitus, cardiac arrhythmias, seizure disorders, or in

---

Bold Italic = life threatening side effect   ■ = black box warning   ✦ = Available in Canada

those who respond unusually to beta-adrenergic agonists. There may be decreased effectiveness in steroid-dependent asthmatic clients. Hypersensitivity reactions may occur.

SIDE EFFECTS
Most Common
Nervousness/tension, headache, lightheadedness, tremor, palpitations, tachycardia, dizziness/vertigo, N&V, cough, dry throat/pharyngitis.

See *Sympathomimetic Drugs* for a complete list of possible side effects. Also, **CNS:** Hyperactivity, hyperkinesia, lightheadedness, tremor, dizziness, vertigo, nervousness, tension, headache, insomnia. **CV:** PVCs, palpitations, tachycardia, hypertension, chest tightness/pain/discomfort, angina. **Respiratory:** Dry throat, throat irritation, pharyngitis, cough, dyspnea, bronchospasm. **Miscellaneous:** N&V, flushing.

LABORATORY TEST CONSIDERATIONS
↑ AST. ↓ Platelets, WBCs. Proteinuria.

DRUG INTERACTIONS
Additive effects with other beta-adrenergic bronchodilators.

HOW SUPPLIED
Solution for Inhalation: 0.2%.

DOSAGE
- **SOLUTION FOR INHALATION**
  Bronchospasm.
Adults and children over 12 years of age: Continuous flow nebulization: **Usual:** 2.5 mg (1.25 mL); **decreased dose:** 1.5 mg (0.75 mL); **increased dose:** 3.5 mg (1.75 mL). Intermittent flow nebulization: **Usual:** 1 mg (0.5 mL); **decreased dose:** 0.5 mg (0.25 mL); **increased dose:** 1.5 mg (0.75 mL). Maximum daily dose: 8 mg with an intermittent flow nebulization system or 14 mg with a continuous flow nebulization system. *NOTE:* Usual frequency is 3 times per day; can increase to 4 times per day but interval between treatments should be 4 hr or more.

NURSING CONSIDERATIONS
Ⓒ Do not confuse bitolterol with bisoprolol (a beta-adrenergic blocking agent).

ADMINISTRATION/STORAGE
1. For adults and children over 12 years of age, administer solution for inhalation during a 10- to 15-minute period. Adjust the treatment period by varying the amount of diluent (normal saline solution) placed in the nebulizer with the drug. The total volume of medication plus diluent is usually 2 to 4 mL.
2. Up to 1 mL of solution for inhalation (0.2%, 2 mg) can be given with intermittent flow system to those severely obstructed.
3. Do not store drug above 49°C (120°F).

ASSESSMENT
1. Note reasons for therapy, age at onset, presenting symptoms, PFTs, peak flow, CXR, and pulmonary findings.
2. List other agents trialed and outcome.

CLIENT/FAMILY TEACHING
1. Review use, care, storage of equipment. Rinse mouth; wash mouthpiece, chamber, and tubing; dry after each use.
2. Do not exceed prescribed dosage; seek medical assistance if symptoms worsen. Check peak flows, report changes and if dose of drug used previously does not provide relief.
3. Use caution, may experience dizziness/drowsiness.
4. Report chest pain, breathing difficulty, fever, change in sputum color/amt, tremor, irregular heartbeat, lack of response. Keep regular F/U appointment.

OUTCOMES/EVALUATE
- Improved airway exchange with ↓ airway resistance
- Asthma/bronchospasm prophylaxis

Bivalirudin   IV
(**by**-val-ih-**ROO**-din)

CLASSIFICATION(S):
Anticoagulant, thrombin inhibitor
PREGNANCY CATEGORY: B
Rx: Angiomax.

SEE ALSO *ANTICOAGULANTS.*

USES

(1) As an anticoagulant with aspirin in clients with unstable angina undergoing percutaneous transluminal coronary angioplasty (PTCA). (2) As an anticoagulant in those undergoing percutaneous coronary intervention. (3) Use for clients with, or at risk of, heparin-induced thrombocytopenia or heparin-induced thrombocytopenia and thrombosis syndrome who are undergoing percutaneous coronary intervention. *NOTE:* Aspirin is intended to be used concomitantly for all indications.

ACTION/KINETICS

Action

Direct-acting thrombin inhibitor by binding to both the catalytic site and to the anion-binding exosite of circulating and clot-bound thrombin. Binding to thrombin is reversible. When bound to thrombin, all effects of thrombin are inhibited, including activation of platelets, cleavage of fibrinogen, and activation of the positive amplification reactions of thrombin. Advantages over heparin include activity against clot-bound thrombin, more predictable anticoagulation, and no inhibition by components of the platelet release reaction.

Pharmacokinetics

$t^{1/2}$, **after IV:** 25 min. $t^{1/2}$ is increased in clients with renal impairment. Metabolized in the liver with about 20% excreted unchanged in the urine.

CONTRAINDICATIONS

Use in active major bleeding, cerebral aneurysm, intracranial hemorrhage. IM use.

SPECIAL CONCERNS

Reduce dose in moderate to severe impaired renal function. Increased risk of hemorrhage with GI ulceration or hepatic disease. Hypertension may increase risk of cerebral hemorrhage. Use with caution following recent surgery or trauma and during lactation. Safety and efficacy not established when used with glycoprotein IIb/IIIa inhibitors, in clients with unstable angina who are not undergoing PTCA, in those with other acute coronary syndromes, or in children. Use with caution when bivalirudin is used as the antithrombin during brachytherapy procedures as there is an increased risk of thrombus formation. Elderly clients may experience more bleeding events than younger clients.

SIDE EFFECTS

Most Common

N&V, back pain, pain, hypotension, hypertension, headache, pelvic pain, injection-site pain, insomnia, anxiety, bradycardia, abdominal pain, dyspepsia, fever, urinary retention, nervousness.

Bleeding: Major side effect is bleeding with possibility (infrequent) of *major hemorrhage*, including *fatal bleeding*, *intracranial hemorrhage* and *retroperitoneal hemorrhage*. Most bleeding occurs at the site of arterial puncture; however, hemorrhage can occur at any site. **CV:** Hypo/hypertension, bradycardia, syncope, vascular anomaly, angina pectoris, *thrombus formation during PCI with and without intracoronary brachytherapy (may be fatal), ventricular fibrillation*. **GI:** N&V, dyspepsia, abdominal pain, dyspepsia. **CNS:** Headache, insomnia, anxiety, nervousness, cerebral ischemia, confusion, facial paralysis. **Dermatologic:** Hematoma, pain at injection site. **GU:** Urinary retention, kidney failure, oliguria. **Miscellaneous:** Back/pelvic/chest pain, injection site pain, fever, lung edema, infection, hypersensitivity/allergic reactions, *sepsis*.

LABORATORY TEST CONSIDERATIONS

Prolongation of aPTT, activated clotting time, thrombin time, and PT.

OD **OVERDOSE MANAGEMENT**

Symptoms: Possible bleeding episodes. *Treatment:* Discontinue the drug and monitor closely for signs of bleed. No known antidote. Bivalirudin is hemodialyzable.

DRUG INTERACTIONS

Coadministration of bivalirudin with heparin, warfarin, thrombolytics, or GPIIb/IIIa inhibitors was associated with an increased risk of major bleeding events.

HOW SUPPLIED

Powder for Injection, Lyophilized: 250 mg/vial.

DOSAGE

• **IV ONLY**

Bold Italic = life threatening side effect   ■ = black box warning   ♣ = Available in Canada

Percutaneous coronary intervention or percutaneous transluminal coronary angioplasty.

Adults: IV bolus dose of 0.75 mg/kg followed by an infusion of 1.75 mg/kg/hr for the duration of the PCI procedure. Five minutes after the bolus dose has been given, an activated clotting time should be performed and an additional bolus of 0.3 mg/kg should be given if needed. Continuation of the bivalirudin infusion following PCI for up to 4 hr postprocedure is optional. After 4 hr, an additional IV infusion may be initiated at a rate of 0.2 mg/kg/hr for up to 20 hr if needed. Use with aspirin (300–325 mg/day).

Clients with moderate renal impairment (C_{CR} of 30–59 mL/min) should receive 1.75 mg/kg/hr. If the C_{CR} is <30 mL/min, reduce the infusion rate to 1 mg/kg/hr. If the client is on hemodialysis, reduce the infusion to 0.25 mg/kg/hr. No reduction in the bolus dose is needed.

Heparin-induced thrombocytopenia or heparin-induced thrombocytopenia and thrombosis syndrome.

Adults: IV bolus of 0.75 mg/kg followed by a continuous infusion at a rate of 1.75 mg/kg/hr for the duration of the procedure.

NURSING CONSIDERATIONS

ADMINISTRATION/STORAGE

$\boxed{\text{IV}}$ 1. Initiate just prior to PTCA.

2. To reconstitute: add 5 mL sterile water to each 250 mg vial; gently swirl until material dissolved. Each reconstituted vial is further diluted in 50 mL of D5W or 0.9% NaCl for final concentration of 5 mg/mL.

3. Adjust dose according to client weight.

4. If the low-rate infusion (i.e., 0.2 mg/kg/hr) is needed, reconstitute the 250 mg vial with 5 mL of sterile water and further dilute in 500 mL of D5W or 0.9% NaCl for a final concentration of 0.5 mg/mL.

5. Do not mix with any other medications before administration.

6. The following drugs resulted in haze formation, microparticulate formation, or gross precipitation: Alteplase, amiodarone HCl, amphotericin B, chlorpromazine HCl, diazepam, prochlorperazine edisylate, reteplase, streptokinase, and vancomycin HCl. Do not give in the same IV line with bivalirudin.

7. Do not use if preparation contains particulate matter.

8. Do not freeze reconstituted or diluted drug.

9. Store reconstituted drug at 2–8°C (36–46°F) for up to 24 hr. Diluted drug (0.5–5 mg/mL) stable at room temperature for up to 24 hr.

ASSESSMENT

1. Note reasons for/method of therapy (bolus/infusion).

2. List history of cerebral aneurysm, intracranial hemorrhage, recent GI bleed or surgery. Monitor cardiac/neurologic status during therapy; report deficits.

3. Monitor VS, ECG, CBC, bleeding parameters, renal, LFTs; reduce dose with renal dysfunction. Assess carefully for any bleeding or hemorrhage at all access sites.

CLIENT/FAMILY TEACHING

1. Review procedure, and reasons for therapy during PTCA.

2. Report adverse effects or unusual bruising/bleeding. New onset SOB, chest pain, or edema warrant evaluation. Avoid aspirin or drugs used to treat swelling or pain (NSAIDs).

3. Incorporate lifestyle changes related to smoking cessation, alcohol reduction, diet and exercise into daily routine.

4. Avoid jostling or activities that may cause injury. Use electric razor, soft toothbrush, and nightlight to prevent injury.

5. Encourage family members to learn CPR.

OUTCOMES/EVALUATE

Anticoagulation during angioplasty

Bleomycin sulfate ■ IV (BLM)

(blee-oh-**MY**-sin)

B

CLASSIFICATION(S):
Antineoplastic, antibiotic
PREGNANCY CATEGORY: D
Rx: Blenoxane.

SEE ALSO *ANTINEOPLASTIC AGENTS.*

USES

Palliative treatment of cancers listed, either used alone or in combination. (1) Squamous cell carcinoma of the head and neck, including mouth, tongue, tonsil, nasopharynx, oropharynx, sinus, palate, lip, buccal mucosa, gingiva, epiglottis, skin, and larynx. Carcinoma of the skin, penis, cervix, and vulva. (2) Lymphomas, including Hodgkin's and non-Hodgkin's. (3) Testicular carcinoma, including embryonal cell, choriocarcinoma, and teratocarcinoma. (4) Sclerosing agent to prevent or treat malignant pleural effusions associated with cancer. *Investigational:* Mycosis fungoides, osteosarcoma, AIDS-related Kaposi sarcoma. Also, in children for palliative treatment of lymphomas, testicular carcinoma, germ cell tumors, and sclerosis of pleural effusions.

ACTION/KINETICS

Action

Mixture of cytotoxic glycopeptide antibiotics that likely inhibit DNA synthesis with less inhibition of RNA and protein synthesis. Most effective in the G_2 and M phases of cell division. Drug currently used is mostly a mixture of bleomycin A_2 and B_2. Relatively low bone marrow depressant activity; localizes in certain tissues. Is an important component of some combination regimens.

Pharmacokinetics

Peak plasma levels (after 4–5 days of therapy): 50 ng/mL. **$t^{1/2}$, distribution, after IV:** 10–20 min. **Peak blood levels, after IM:** 30–60 min with levels that are about one-third that of IV. **$t^{1/2}$, elimination, C_{CR} less than 35 mL/min:** About 2 hr; half-life increases exponentially as C_{CR} decreases below 35 mL/min. Two-thirds excreted in the urine as active bleomycin.

CONTRAINDICATIONS

Hypersensitivity or idiosyncratic reactions to bleomycin. Lactation. Renal or pulmonary diseases. Pregnancy.

SPECIAL CONCERNS

■ (1) Administer under the supervision of a qualified physician experienced in the use of cancer chemotherapeutic drugs. Appropriate management of therapy and complications is possible only when adequate diagnostic and treatment facilities are readily available. (2) Pulmonary fibrosis is the most severe toxic effect; most often seen as pneumonitis that may progress to fibrosis. Incidence is higher in geriatric clients and in those receiving >400 units total dose (but toxicity has occurred in young clients and in those treated with low doses). (3) Severe idiosyncratic reactions seen in about 1% of lymphoma clients; symptoms include hypotension, mental confusion, fever, chills, and wheezing.■ Safety and efficacy have not been determined in children. When used in combination with other antineoplastic drugs, pulmonary toxicity may occur at lower doses.

SIDE EFFECTS

Most Common

Pneumonitis, fever, chills, photosensitivity, N&V, weight loss, skin rash, darkening/thickening of skin, swollen fingers, changes in fingernails/toenails, colored bumps on fingertips/elbows/palms.

Pulmonary: Pneumonitis, *pulmonary fibrosis*, especially in older clients, acute chest pain syndrome, pain after intrapleural administration. **Hypersensitivity/Idiosyncratic reactions:** Hypotension, fever, chills, mental confusion, and wheezing in about 1% of lymphoma clients. **Integumentary and mucous membranes:** Erythema, rash, striae, vesiculation, hyperpigmentation, skin tenderness, hyperkeratosis, alopecia, pruritus, stomatitis, skin toxicity, darkening/thickening of skin, swollen fingers, changes in fingernails/toenails, colored bumps on fingertips/elbows/

Bold Italic = life threatening side effect   ■ = black box warning   ♣ = Available in Canada

palms, scleroderma-like skin changes. **GI:** N&V, anorexia, weight loss. **Body as a whole:** Chills, fever, vomiting, anorexia, weight loss that may persist long after termination of the drug, phlebitis, malaise, photosensitivity. **Miscellaneous:** Renal and hepatic toxicity, pain at tumor site.

NOTE: Use of bleomycin in combination with other antineoplastics may result in vascular toxicities, including cerebral arteritis, **CVA, MI,** thrombotic microangiopathy, Raynaud phenomenon.

DRUG INTERACTIONS

Digoxin / ↓ Digoxin levels
Filgrastim / ↑ Risk of pulmonary toxicity
Oxygen / ↑ Risk for pulmonary toxicity
Phenytoin / ↓ Phenytoin levels

HOW SUPPLIED

Powder for Injection: 15 units, 30 units.

DOSAGE

• **IM; IV; SC**

  Hodgkin's disease.

Initial: 0.25–0.5 units/kg (10–20 units/m²) IV, IM, or SC once or twice weekly. **Maintenance:** After a 50% response, give 1 unit/day or 5 units/week IM or IV. Due to pulmonary toxicity, give doses greater than 400 units with great caution.

  Squamous cell carcinoma, non-Hodgkin's lymphoma, testicular carcinoma.

0.25–0.5 units/kg (10–20 units/m²) IV, IM, or SC once or twice a week. Due to the possibility of anaphylaxis, give lymphoma clients 2 units or less for the first two doses; if no acute reaction occurs, follow the regular dosage schedule.

• **INTRAPLEURAL INJECTION**

  Malignant pleural effusion.

60 units given as a single bolus dose by a thoracostomy tube following drainage of excess pleural fluid and confirmation of complete lung expansion.

NURSING CONSIDERATIONS

ADMINISTRATION/STORAGE

1. For IM or SC use: Reconstitute drug with 1–5 mL (15-unit vial) or 2–10 mL (30-unit vial) 0.9% NaCl, sterile water, or bacteriostatic water for injection.
2. For intrapleural use: Dissolve 60 units in 50–100 mL of 0.9% NaCl and give through a thoracostomy tube following drainage of excess pleural fluid and confirmation of complete lung expansion. Drainage from chest tube should be as minimal as possible before instillation of bleomycin. Clamp thoracostomy tube after instillation. Move from supine to left and right lateral positions several times during the next 4 hr, followed by removal of the clamp to reestablish suction.
3. Do not reconstitute with D5W or other dextrose-containing dilutions; loss of potency.
4. Hodgkin's disease and testicular tumors should respond within 2 weeks; squamous cell cancers require at least 3 weeks.
5. Bleomycin is stable for 24 hr at room temperature (14 days if refrigerated) in NaCl.
6. For IV use: Reconstitute contents of 15- or 30-unit vial with 5 or 10 mL, respectively, of 0.9% NaCl. Administer IV slowly over 10 min. Do not reconstitute with D5W or other dextrose-containing solutions.

ASSESSMENT

1. Note reason for therapy, onset, symptom characteristics, method of administration.
2. Obtain baseline VS, CBC, LFTs, and PFTs. Assess/monitor for basilar crackles, cough, dyspnea, and tachypnea; dose-related symptoms of pulmonary toxicity.
3. Note and avoid adhesive on the skin; drug accumulates in keratin and may discolor epithelium.
4. If receiving digoxin, monitor levels.
5. Clients with lymphoma may initially receive two test doses of 2 units each to assess for idiosyncratic response.
6. May cause mild granulocyte suppression. Nadir: 10 days; recovery: 14 days.

CLIENT/FAMILY TEACHING

1. Report S&S of idiosyncratic reaction (hypoxia, fever, chills, confusion); *may occur with lymphoma.*
2. Fever 3–6 hr after treatment is common; may use acetaminophen. Avoid aspirin or ibuprofen type of analge-

sics—may cause bleeding. Use soft bristled tooth brush and electric razor.

3. Avoid vaccinations during therapy.

4. Practice safe contraception.

5. Report abnormal mouth/skin rashes or side effects; may lose hair.

6. Smoking may aggravate pulmonary symptoms. Report changes in breathing or increased coughing.

7. Keep all F/U appointments to evaluate response and for adverse effects.

OUTCOMES/EVALUATE
- ↓ Tumor size/spread
- Prevention/control of malignant pleural effusion

Bortezomib   IV
(bor-**TEZ**-oh-mib)

CLASSIFICATION(S):
Antineoplastic, proteasome inhibitor
PREGNANCY CATEGORY: D
Rx: Velcade.

SEE ALSO *ANTINEOPLASTIC AGENTS.*

USES
(1) Multiple myeloma in those who have received at least 1 prior therapy and have shown disease progression on the last therapy. (2) Mantle cell lymphoma in those who have received at least 1 prior therapy.

ACTION/KINETICS
Action
A reversible inhibitor of the chymotrypsin-like activity of the 26S proteasome (large protein that degrades ubiquitinated proteins) in mammalian cells. The ubiquitin-proteasome pathway plays an essential role in regulating the intracellular concentration of specific proteins, thus maintaining homeostasis within cells. Inhibition of the 26S proteasome affects multiple signaling cascades within the cell. This disruption of normal homeostasis can lead to cell death. Bortezomib causes a delay in tumor growth in multiple myeloma clients.

Pharmacokinetics
Primarily metabolized by cytochrome P450 enzymes 3A4, 2D6, 2C19, 2C9, and 1A2; the major metabolic pathway is deboronation. **t½, elimination:** 40–103 hr after the 1 mg/m^2 dose and 76–108 hr after the 1.3 mg/m^2 dose. **Plasma protein binding:** Average of 83% over the concentration range of 100 to 1,000 ng/mL.

CONTRAINDICATIONS
Hypersensitivity to the drug, boron, or mannitol. Lactation.

SPECIAL CONCERNS
Use with caution and closely monitor in impaired hepatic and renal function. Safety and efficacy have not been determined in children.

SIDE EFFECTS
Most Common
Asthenia, dizziness, lightheadedness, peripheral neuropathy, N&V, anorexia, diarrhea, constipation, malaise, weakness, blurred vision, cough, insomnia, psychiatric disorders, thrombocytopenia, dysesthesia, paresthesia, anemia, headache, injection site irritation.

GI: N&V, abdominal pain, diarrhea, decreased appetite, anorexia, constipation, abdominal pain, dyspepsia, dysgeusia, ascites, dysphagia, fecal impaction, ***hemorrhagic gastritis, GI hemorrhage,*** hematemesis, paralytic ileus, small/large intestine obstruction, paralytic intestinal obstruction, large intestine perforation, stomatitis, melena, acute pancreatitis. **Hepatic:** Hepatitis, ***acute liver failure.*** **Hematologic:** Thrombocytopenia, anemia, neutropenia. **CNS:** Asthenic conditions (including vertigo), peripheral neuropathy, headache, insomnia, dizziness, anxiety, ataxia, coma, dizziness, agitation, lightheadedness, confusion, psychotic disorders, ***suicidal ideation,*** dysarthria, dysautonomia, cranial palsy, ***grand mal seizures, hemorrhagic stroke,*** motor dysfunction, spinal cord compression, TIA. **CV:** Aggravated atrial fibrillation, hypotension, atrial flutter, cardiac amyloidosis, ***cardiac arrest, CHF, CVA, MI, pulmonary embolism, DIC,*** DVT, myocardial ischemia, pericardial effusion, peripheral embolism, pulmonary edema/

Bold Italic = life threatening side effect   ■ = black box warning   ♣ = Available in Canada

hypertension, ventricular tachycardia; subdural hematoma; acute development of or exacerbation of CHF and/or new onset of decreased left ventricular ejection fraction. **Hypersensitivity: Anaphylaxis,** hypersensitivity, immune complex mediated hypersensitivity. **Musculoskeletal:** Arthralgia, bone pain, back pain, muscle cramps, myalgia. **Respiratory:** Dyspnea, URTI, lower RTI, cough, pneumonia, nasopharyngitis, *acute respiratory distress syndrome,* atelectasis, worsening COPD, dyspnea, exertional dyspnea, epistaxis, hemoptysis, hypoxia, lung infiltration, pleural effusion, pneumonitis, respiratory distress, *respiratory failure,* acute diffuse infiltrative pulmonary disease (rare). **GU:** Renal calculus, bilateral hydronephrosis, bladder spasm, hematuria, urinary incontinence, urinary retention, acute and chronic renal failure, proliferative glomerular nephritis. **Dermatologic:** Pruritus, rash. **Body as a whole:** Fatigue, malaise, weakness, dehydration, edema, herpes zoster, paresthesia and dysesthesia, pyrexia, rigors, reactivation of herpes virus infection. **Miscellaneous:** Pain in limb, edema in lower limb, dysgeusia, blurred vision, portal vein thrombosis, tumor lysis syndrome, bacteremia, skeletal fracture, injection site irritation, tumor lysis syndrome. Rarely, reversible posterior leukoencephalopathy syndrome, including symptoms of seizures, hypertension, headache, lethargy, confusion, blindness, and other visual/neurological symptoms.

LABORATORY TEST CONSIDERATIONS
↑ Liver enzymes. Hyperbilirubinemia.

OD OVERDOSE MANAGEMENT
Symptoms: Acute onset of symptomatic hypotension and thrombocytopenia with possible fatal outcomes. *Treatment:* There is no specific antidote. Monitor vital signs and give appropriate supportive care.

DRUG INTERACTIONS
Antihypertensives / Possible potentiation of hypotension; adjust antihypertensive dose as needed
CYP3A4 inhibitors or inducers / Closely monitor for toxicity or reduced efficacy when bortezomib is coadministered with drugs that are inducers or inhibitors of cytochrome CYP3A4
CYP2A19 substrates / Inhibition of 2C19 isoenzyme activity → ↑ exposure to drugs that are substrates for this isoenzyme
Hypoglycemics, oral / Possible hypo- or hyperglycemia; monitor blood glucose levels closely

HOW SUPPLIED
Powder for Injection, Lyophilized: 3.5 mg.

DOSAGE
* **IV BOLUS**
    Multiple myeloma, Mantle cell lymphoma.

Adults: 1.3 mg/m^2/dose given as a 3- to 5-second IV bolus twice weekly for 2 weeks (i.e., days 1, 4, 8, and 11) followed by a 10-day rest period (days 12 to 21). Separate consecutive doses by at least 72 hr.

NURSING CONSIDERATIONS
ADMINISTRATION/STORAGE
IV 1. Give under the supervision of a provider experienced in the use of antineoplastic therapy.
2. Withhold at the onset of any grade 3 nonhematological or grade 4 hematological toxicity, excluding neuropathy. May restart therapy once toxic symptoms have resolved but at a 25% reduced dose (i.e., 1.3 mg/m^2/dose reduced to 1 mg/m^2/dose; 1 mg/m^2/dose reduced to 0.7 mg/m^2/dose).
3. The following are dose modifications for bortezomib-related neuropathic pain and/or peripheral sensory neuropathy:
* Grade 1 (paresthesias and/or loss of reflexes) without pain or loss of function: No action required.
* Grade 1 with pain or grade 2 (interference with function but not with activities of daily living): Reduce dose to 1 mg/m^2.
* Grade 2 with pain or grade 3 (interference with activities of daily living): Withhold therapy until toxicity resolves. When toxicity resolves, reinitiate with a reduced bortezomib dose of 0.7 mg/m^2 and change treatment schedule to once weekly.

B

- Grade 4 (permanent sensory loss that interferes with function): Discontinue bortezomib.

4. For treatment beyond eight cycles, doses may continue to be given on a three-week cycle or given once weekly on days 1, 8, 15, and 22, followed by no treatment on days 23–35.

5. Reconstitute each vial with 3.5 mL of NSS, NaCl injection.

6. Use caution during handling and preparation. Use gloves and other protective clothing to prevent skin contact.

7. Store unopened vials at controlled room temperature from 15–30°C (59–86°F) protected from light.

8. When reconstituted, drug may be stored from 15–30°C (59–86°F). Give within 8 hr of reconstitution. May store reconstituted drug in original/syringe prior to administration. Product may be stored up to 8 hr in a syringe; however, the total storage time for the reconstituted drug must not exceed 8 hr when exposed to normal indoor lighting.

ASSESSMENT

1. Note reasons for therapy, other two therapies and dates administered, and documented progression of multiple myeloma after those therapies.

2. Carefully assess nutritional status, hydration level to prevent adverse effects. Monitor renal, LFTs, CBC and VS: with HTN may require dosage adjustment for BP meds, increased fluid intake and steroids to manage hypotensive effects.

3. Before therapy, may need to administer drugs for diarrhea and nausea as therapy may cause N&V, diarrhea, and/or constipation.

4. Assess for history/presence of peripheral neuropathy; if new or worsening symptoms, stop drug and report as dose and schedule may need adjustment.

CLIENT/FAMILY TEACHING

1. Drug administered IV; used to prevent progression of cancerous cells.

2. Consume plenty of fluids to ensure adequate hydration.

3. Avoid activities that require mental alertness until drug effects realized;

may cause dizziness, faintness, lightheadedness, fatigue, and blurred vision.

4. Report any neuropathy: burning sensation, numbness, pins and needles sensation, loss of sensation, or discomfort in any extremity.

5. Practice reliable contraception during therapy.

6. Report new onset S&S /adverse effects. Keep F/U visits to evaluate drug response.

OUTCOMES/EVALUATE

Inhibition of malignant cell proliferation

Bosentan ■
(boh-**SEN**-tan)

CLASSIFICATION(S):
Vasodilator, endothelin receptor antagonist
PREGNANCY CATEGORY: X
Rx: Tracleer.

USES

To improve exercise ability and decrease the rate of worsening in pulmonary arterial hypertension in those with WHO Class III or IV symptoms. *Investigational:* Prevention of digital ulcers in systemic sclerosis. *NOTE:* Because of potential liver injury and to decrease the chance as much as possible for fetal exposure, bosentan may be prescribed only through the Tracleer Access Program.

ACTION/KINETICS

Action

Endothelin-1 (ET-1) is a neurohormone whose effects are mediated by binding to ET_A and ET_B receptors in the endothelium and smooth muscle. ET-1 levels are increased in plasma and lung tissue of clients with pulmonary arterial hypertension. Bosentan is a specific and competitive antagonist at endothelin receptor types ET_A and ET_B, thus improving pulmonary arterial hypertension.

Pharmacokinetics

Absolute bioavailability is about 50%. **Maximum plasma levels:** 3–5 hr. Metabolized in the liver by CYP3A4 and

CYP2C9 to three metabolites, one of which is active. Steady state reached in 3–5 days. Excreted in the bile. **t½, terminal:** About 5 hr. **Plasma protein binding:** More than 98%.

CONTRAINDICATIONS

Use in moderate or severe liver abnormalities or elevated aminotransferases >3 times ULN. Pregnancy, use with cyclosporine A or glyburide. Hypersensitivity to bosentan or any component of the medication. Lactation.

SPECIAL CONCERNS

■ (1) Potential liver injury: Bosentan causes at least a 3-fold (ULN) elevation of liver aminotransferases (ALT and AST) in about 11% of clients, accompanied by elevated bilirubin in a small number of cases. Because these changes are a marker for potential serious liver injury, serum aminotransferase levels must be measured prior to initiation of treatment and then monthly. To date, in a setting of close monitoring, elevations have been reversible, within a few days to 9 weeks, either spontaneously or after dose reduction or discontinuation, and without sequelae. (2) Elevations in aminotransferases require close attention. Avoid using bosentan in clients with elevated aminotransferases (greater than 3 times ULN) at baseline because monitoring liver injury may be more difficult. If liver aminotransferase elevations are accompanied by clinical symptoms of liver injury (e.g., abdominal pain, fever, jaundice, nausea, unusual lethargy or fatigue, vomiting) or increases in bilirubin greater than or equal to 2 times ULN, stop treatment. There is no experience with the reintroduction of bosentan in these circumstances. (3) Pregnancy: Bosentan is very likely to produce major birth defects if used by pregnant women; this effect has been seen consistently when it is administered to animals. Therefore, pregnancy must be excluded before the start of treatment with bosentan and prevented thereafter by the use of a reliable method of contraception. Do not use hormonal contraceptives, including oral, injectable, transdermal, and implantable contraceptives, as the sole means of contraception because these may not be effective in clients receiving bosentan. Therefore, effective contraception through additional forms of contraception must be practiced. Obtain monthly pregnancy tests. (4) Because of potential liver injury and in an effort to make the chance of fetal exposure to bosentan as small as possible, bosentan may be prescribed only through the bosentan access program by calling 1-866-228-3546. Adverse reactions also can be reported directly via this number.■ Use with caution in those with mildly impaired liver function. Safety and efficacy have not been determined in children.

SIDE EFFECTS

Most Common

Headache, nasopharyngitis, flushing, abnormal hepatic function, lower limb edema, hypotension, dyspepsia, edema. **CV:** Hypotension, palpitations, edema, lower limb edema, pulmonary hypertension. **GI:** Abnormal hepatic function, hepatotoxicity, dyspepsia. **CNS:** Headache, fatigue. **Dermatologic:** Flushing, pruritus, rash. **Respiratory:** Nasopharyngitis. **Metabolic:** Edema, lower limb edema. **Miscellaneous:** Anemia, hypersensitivity.

LABORATORY TEST CONSIDERATIONS

↑ Liver transferases (AST, ALT). Dose-related ↓ in H & H.

DRUG INTERACTIONS

Contraceptives, hormonal (oral, injectable, implantation, transdermal) / Possible contraceptive failure R/T ↑ liver metabolism of hormones by CYP3A4; clients should use additional methods of contraception

Cyclosporine A / ↑ Bosentan trough levels by about 30-fold and steady-state levels by 3–4 fold; ↓ Cyclosporine A levels by about 50%; **Do not give together**

Glyburide / ↓ Glyburide levels by about 40% and bosentan levels by about 30%. Also, ↑ risk of elevated liver aminotransferases. **Do not give together.**

Ketoconazole / ↑ Bosentan levels by about 2-fold

Sildenafil / ↓ Sildenafil levels and t½ R/T ↑ metabolism by CYP3A4

Simvastatin (and other statins) / ↓ Statin levels by about 50% R/T ↑ hepatic metabolism by CYP3A4; monitor statin levels and adjust statin dose accordingly

Warfarin / ↓ S-warfarin and R-warfarin levels 29% and 38% respectively

HOW SUPPLIED

Tablets: 62.5 mg, 125 mg.

DOSAGE

- **TABLETS**

    Pulmonary arterial hypertension.

Initial: 62.5 mg twice a day for 4 weeks. **Then,** increase to maintenance dose of 125 mg twice a day. In those with a body weight less than 40 kg and who are over 12 years of age, the recommended initial and maintenance doses are 62.5 mg twice a day.

NURSING CONSIDERATIONS

ADMINISTRATION/STORAGE

1. Use the following guidelines for dosage adjustment and monitoring in clients who develop aminotransferase abnormalities:

- If ALT/AST levels are >3 and 5 or less times ULN, confirm by another aminotransferase test. If confirmed, stop treatment and monitor aminotransferase levels at least every 2 weeks. If levels return to pretreatment values, continue or reintroduce the treatment as appropriate (see below).
- If ALT/AST levels are >5 and 8 or less times ULN, confirm by another aminotransferase test. If confirmed, stop treatment and monitor aminotransferase levels at least every 2 weeks. Once levels return to pretreatment values, consider reintroduction as described below.
- If ALT/AST levels are >8 times ULN, stop treatment and do not consider bosentan reintroduction.

2. If bosentan reintroduced, begin again with the starting dose. Check aminotransferase levels within 3 days and thereafter.

3. If aminotransferase levels are accompanied by N&V, fever, abdominal pain, jaundice, unusual lethargy, fatigue (i.e., symptoms of liver injury) or increases in bilirubin 2 or more times ULN, stop drug.

4. To avoid potential for clinical deterioration after abrupt discontinuation, reduce dose gradually (i.e., 62.5 twice a day for 3–7 days).

ASSESSMENT

1. Note reasons for therapy, other agents trialed, when diagnosed, stage of pulmonary artery hypertension.

2. List drugs currently prescribed to ensure none interact adversely; drug is highly protein bound.

3. Ensure not pregnant; perform pregnancy test on all females of childbearing potential.

4. After initial labs, monitor LFTs and pregnancy tests monthly; H&H after 1 and 3 mo and then q 3 mo to assess for any deficiencies. CXR, ABGs, and PFTs as indicated.

CLIENT/FAMILY TEACHING

1. Review bosentan medication guide for safe drug administration. Take twice a day as directed; increase dosage after 4 weeks upon provider recommendation.

2. Drug has two significant concerns: potential for serious liver damage and fetal damage. It is only administered through the Tracleer Access Program (TAP) at 1-866-228-3546 and follow directions. All adverse drug reactions should also be reported directly to this number by the provider.

3. Drug is not a cure but may improve clinical symptoms of disease. Report all side effects and any changes in breathing or exercise tolerance.

4. Practice reliable contraception; use an additional form of contraception with the hormonal form as drug will cause major birth defects.

5. Continue all other therapies prescribed by pulmonologist. Keep all scheduled monthly lab visits and provider as scheduled.

OUTCOMES/EVALUATE

- Improved exercise tolerance
- ↓ Pulmonary artery pressure

Bold Italic = life threatening side effect   ■ = black box warning   ✦ = Available in Canada

Botulinum Toxin, Type A ©

(**bot**-you-**LIE**-num **TOX**-in)

CLASSIFICATION(S):
Botulinum toxin
PREGNANCY CATEGORY: C
Rx: Botox, Botox Cosmetic.

USES

Botox only: (1) Cervical dystonia in adults to decrease the severity of abnormal head position and neck pain. (2) Severe primary emotional axillary hyperhidrosis inadequately managed with topical agents, including prescription antiperspirants. (3) Strabismus and blepharospasm associated with dystonia, including benign essential blepharospasm or VII nerve disorders in clients 12 years and older. **Botox Cosmetic only:** Temporary improvement in the appearance of moderate to severe glabellar (frown) lines between the eyebrows associated with corrugator or procerus muscle activity in those 65 years or younger. *Investigational:* Hemifacial spasms, spasmodic torticollis, oromandibular dystonia, spasmodic dysphonia, writer's cramp, and focal task-specific dystonia. Treatment of head and neck tremor unresponsive to other drug therapy. Is an orphan drug used to treat dynamic muscle contracture in pediatric cerebral palsy.

ACTION/KINETICS

Action

The product is a sterile, lyophilized form of purified botulinum toxin type A produced from *Clostridium botulinum* type A grown in a medium containing casein hydrolysate and yeast extract. The toxin blocks neuromuscular conduction by binding to receptor sites on motor nerve terminals, entering the nerve terminals, and inhibiting acetylcholine release. The mechanism to treat hyperhidrosis is due to inhibition of release of acetylcholine temporarily blocking the nerves in the underarm that stimulate sweating. When given IM, the toxin produces a partial chemical denervation of the muscle, resulting in a localized reduction in muscle activity.

CONTRAINDICATIONS

Infection at the proposed injection site(s). Use for glabellar lines in children.

SPECIAL CONCERNS

Use with caution in those with peripheral motor neuropathic diseases (e.g., amyotropic lateral sclerosis, motor neuropathy) or neuromuscular junctional disorders (e.g., myasthenia gravis, Lambert-Eaton syndrome). Since the product contains albumin, there is an extremely remote risk for transmission of viral diseases or Creutzfeldt-Jakob disease. Use with caution in the presence of inflammation at the injection site(s), when excessive weakness or atrophy is present in target tissue(s), or in clients taking drugs that interfere with neuromuscular transmission. Formation of neutralizing antibodies may reduce the effectiveness by inactivating the biological activity. Reduced blinking from injection of the orbicularis muscle can cause corneal exposure, persistent epithelial defect, and corneal ulceration, especially in those with VII nerve disorders. Use with caution during lactation. Safety and efficacy have not been determined in children less than 16 years of age.

SIDE EFFECTS

Most Common

When used for cervical dystonia: Dysphagia, URTI, neck pain, headache.
When used for primary axillary hyperhidrosis: Injection site pain and hemorrhage, nonaxillary sweating, infection, pharyngitis, flu syndrome, headache, fever, neck/back pain, pruritus, anxiety.
When used for glabellar lines: Headache, respiratory infection, flu syndrome, blepharoptosis, nausea.

- **Botox**
When used to treat blepharospasm, the most frequent side effects are ptosis, superficial punctuate keratitis, and eye dryness. When used to treat strabismus, side effects include ptosis and vertical deviation. Other side effects include: **GI:**

B

Nausea, oral dryness. **CNS:** Dizziness, speech disorder, drowsiness. **CV:** Rarely, arrhythmia, *MI*. **Respiratory:** Increased cough, flu syndrome, rhinitis, dyspnea. **Dermatologic:** Skin rash, including erythema multiforme, urticaria, and psoriaform eruption, pruritus, allergic reaction. **Ophthalmic:** Ptosis, diplopia. **Local:** Soreness at injection site, localized pain, tenderness, bruising, weakness of adjacent muscles. **Miscellaneous:** Back pain, hypertonia, hypersensitivity (including anaphylaxis).

• **Botox Cosmetic**
CNS: Headache, dizziness, paresthesia, anxiety, twitch, syncope. **GI:** Dyspepsia, tooth disorder, abdominal pain, diarrhea, loss of appetite, vomiting, abnormal liver function. **Respiratory:** Infection, bronchitis, sinusitis, pharyngitis, dyspnea, sinus infection, laryngitis, rhinitis. **Dermatologic:** Erythema, ecchymosis, skin tightness/irritation, erythema multiforme, urticaria, psoriaiform eruption. **Ophthalmologic:** Blurred vision, retinal vein occlusion, glaucoma, vertigo with nystagmus. **Otic:** Decreased hearing, ear noise and localized numbness. **Miscellaneous:** Pain in the face, erythema/pain/edema at injection site, muscle weakness, back pain, UTI, hypertension, accidental injury, flu-like syndrome, infection, allergic reaction, brachial plexopathy, focal facial paralysis, ***anaphylaxis,*** myasthenia gravis.

OD OVERDOSE MANAGEMENT
Symptoms: Signs and symptoms are not apparent immediately after injection. If accidental injection or oral ingestion occurs, monitor for several weeks for signs or symptoms of systemic weakness or muscle paralysis. *Treatment:* An antitoxin is available in the event of immediate knowledge of an overdose or misinjection. Contact Allergan Pharmaceuticals at 1-800-433-8871 from 8 a.m. to 4 p.m. Pacific Time or 714-246-5954 at other times for a recorded message.

DRUG INTERACTIONS
Effect of botulinum toxin may be potentiated by aminoglycosides or any other drug that interferes with neuromuscular transmission (e.g., curare-like drugs).

HOW SUPPLIED
Powder for Injection, Vacuum Dried: 100 units of *Clostridium botulinum* toxin type A neurotoxin complex.

DOSAGE
• **INJECTION**
Cervical dystonia (Botox only).
Clients with a known history of tolerating the toxin: The mean dose administered in the phase 3 study was 236 units (range: 198–300 units) and was divided among the affected muscles. Individualize both initial and subsequent doses based on the client's head and neck position, localization of pain, muscle hypertrophy, client response, and history of side effects. **Clients without prior use, initial:** Start with a lower dose and adjust based on individual response. Limiting the total dose injected into the sternocleidomastoid muscles to 100 units or less may decrease the occurrence of dysphagia.
Primary emotional axillary hyperhidrosis (Botox only).
Using a 30-gauge needle, 50 units of botulinum toxin type A (2 mL) is injected intradermally in 0.1–0.2 mL aliquots to each axilla evenly distributed in multiple sites (10–15) about 1–2 cm apart. Give repeated injections when the clinical effect of a previous injection diminishes.
Blepharospasm (Botox only).
Using a sterile 27- to 30-gauge needle, inject 1.25–2.5 units (0.05–0.1 mL at each site) of reconstituted solution. Injections are made into the medial and lateral pretarsal orbicularis oculi of the upper lid and into the lateral pretarsal orbicularis oculi of the lower lid. Avoid medial lower lid injections. Do not exceed a cumulative dose of more than 200 units in a 30-day period.
Strabismus (Botox only).
The volume should be between 0.05–0.15 mL per muscle.
• **IM ONLY**
Glabellar lines (Botox Cosmetic only).
Reconstitute with 0.9% sterile saline (nonpreserved); solution will be 4 units/0.1 mL. Total treatment dose: 20 units in 0.5 mL. Give IM only. Duration is about 3–4 months. Injection intervals

---

Bold Italic = life threatening side effect   ■ = black box warning   ♣ = Available in Canada

should be no more than every 3 months; use lowest effective dose.

NURSING CONSIDERATIONS

℞ Do not confuse Botulinum Toxin, Type A with Botulinum Toxin, Type B.

ADMINISTRATION/STORAGE

1. Safe and effective use depends on proper storage of the product, selection of the correct dose, and proper reconstitution and administration.

2. The following information relates to *Botox:*

- To reconstitute the vacuum-dried powder for injection, use 0.9% NaCl without a preservative. Draw up proper amount of diluent into appropriate size syringe; slowly inject the diluent into vial. Inject gently as bubbling or similar violent agitation denatures the toxin. Mix the toxin with saline by gently rotating the vial. Record date and time of reconstitution on the designated label space. Administer within 4 hr of reconstitution.

- Discard vial if vacuum does not pull the diluent into the vial.

- The usual injection volume is 0.1 mL. To obtain 10 unit/0.1 mL, add 1 mL of diluent, for 5 units/0.1 mL, add 2 mL diluent, for 2.5 units/0.1 mL, add 4 mL diluent, and for 1.25 units/0.1 mL, add 8 mL of diluent. The diluent should be 0.9% NaCl injection.

- Injection volume in excess of intended dose is expelled through the needle into an appropriate waste container to ensure patency of the needle and to confirm there is no syringe-needle leakage.

- For superficial muscles use a 25-, 27-, or 30-gauge needle. Use a longer 22-gauge needle for deeper musculature. Use a new, sterile needle and syringe to enter the vial on each occasion for dilution or removal of the toxin.

- Localization of the involved muscles with electromyographic guidance may be helpful.

- Improvement usually begins within the first 2 weeks after injection with maximum benefit noted at about 6 weeks postinjection. Most clients will return to pretreatment status by 3 months posttreatment.

- Do not exceed the recommended dose/frequency of administration since risks are not known. If accidental injection or PO ingestion occurs, monitor client for several days (on an outpatient basis) for S&S of systemic weakness or muscle paralysis.

- For the elderly, start at the low end of the dosing range.

- Clients with smaller neck mass and those who require bilateral injections into the sternocleidomastoid muscle are at greater risk to develop dysphagia. Limiting the dose may decrease the occurrence.

- Injections into the levator scapulae may increase the risk of URTIs and dysphagia.

- When used for blepharospasm, the initial effect is seen within 3 days and reaches a peak in 1–2 weeks. Each treatment lasts about 3 months after which injections can be repeated. Little beneficial effect is observed from injecting more than 5 units per site. To avoid ecchymosis, apply pressure at the injection site immediately after the injection.

3. The following information relates to *Botox Cosmetic:*

- Injection intervals are no more often than every three months using the lowest effective dose. Safety/efficacy of more frequent dosing has not been evaluated.

- To dilute, use a 21-gauge, 2.5 inch needle and an appropriate syringe (preferably tuberculin). Draw up a total of 2.5 mL of 0.9% sterile saline. Insert the needle at a 45°angle and slowly inject into the vial.

- Discard vial if a vacuum does not pull the diluent into the vial. Gently rotate the vial and record the date and time of reconstitution on the space on the label.

- Draw at least 0.5 mL of the reconstituted toxin into the sterile syringe; expel any air bubbles in the syringe barrel.

B

- Remove the needle used to reconstitute the product and attach a 30-gauge needle. Confirm patency of the needle.
- Store the vacuum-dried product at or below -5°C (23°F). Give within 4 hr after vial removed from the freezer and reconstituted. During the 4-hr period, store the reconstituted toxin at 2–8°C (36–46°F).
- The reconstituted toxin should be clear, colorless, and free of particulate matter.

ASSESSMENT

1. Note reasons for therapy, extent of neck rigidity/jerking, positional dysfunction, pain level, associated characteristics, other agents/therapies trialed.
2. Assess carefully for evidence/history of neuropathic, neurologic, or neuromuscular disorders.
3. For use/administration only by those individuals trained to administer.
4. Review associated risk factors to ensure client understanding. Drug contains albumin which may present the remote risk of disease transmission of Creutzfeldt-Jakob disease (CJD).

CLIENT/FAMILY TEACHING

1. Drug has many uses: may be used to relieve abnormal muscle spasms/contractures of the head and neck, or spasticity of extremities permitting more controlled movement, improved posture, and increased activity. Also, if other therapies fail, has been used to decrease excessive underarm sweating. There are forms to decrease frown lines and skin wrinkles.
2. Do not perform activities that require mental alertness until drug effects realized; may cause drowsiness. Resume activity slowly and carefully following administration.
3. The clostridium bacteria (A) that makes the toxin is not being injected directly; a sterilized by-product of the bacteria is utilized. May experience slight sting with injections.
4. Report any swallowing problems, SOB, respiratory disorders/infections, injection site abnormalities, facial drooping, weakness.

5. Effects usually last up to 3 mo; repeat injections may be required.
6. Practice reliable contraception.
7. For *Botox Cosmetic* the injection intervals are no more often than every three months using the lowest effective dose and administered by a qualified individual.
8. An antitoxin is available in the event of significant overdose or misinjection. Contact Allergan Pharmaceuticals at 1-800-433-8871 from 8 a.m. to 4 p.m. Pacific Time or the CDC at 1-800-311-3435 (1-404-639-2888 nights and weekends). The antitoxin would need to be administered within 20 hr of overdosage.

OUTCOMES/EVALUATE

- Relief of painful muscle spasms/contractures permitting improved posture, movement, and activity
- Smoothing of wrinkles/frown lines
- Relief of hyperhidrosis

Botulinum Toxin, Type B ©
(**bot**-you-**LIE**-num **TOX**-in)

CLASSIFICATION(S):
Botulinum toxin
PREGNANCY CATEGORY: C
Rx: Myobloc.

USES
Treatment of cervical dystonia to reduce the severity of abnormal head position and neck pain.

ACTION/KINETICS

Action
The product is a sterile liquid formulation of a purified neurotoxin derived from fermentation of *Clostridium botulinum* type B. It acts to produce flaccid paralysis by inhibiting acetylcholine release at the neuromuscular junction.

SPECIAL CONCERNS
Use with caution in those with peripheral motor neuropathic diseases (e.g., amyotropic lateral sclerosis, motor neuropathy) or neuromuscular junctional disorders (e.g., myasthenia gravis, Lam-

---

Bold Italic = life threatening side effect   ■ = black box warning   ♣ = Available in Canada

B

bert-Eaton syndrome). Since the product contains albumin, there is an extremely remote risk for transmission of viral diseases or Creutzfeldt-Jakob disease. The effect of giving different botulinum neurotoxin serotypes at the same time or within less than 4 months of each other is unknown; neuromuscular paralysis may be potentiated by coadministration or overlapping administration of different botulinum toxin serotypes. Use with caution during lactation. Safety and efficacy have not been determined in children.

SIDE EFFECTS
Most Common
Dry mouth, dysphagia, dyspepsia, pain at the injection site.
GI: N&V, GI disorder, glossitis, stomatitis, tooth disorder. **CNS:** Dizziness, neck pain related to cervical dystonia, headache, torticollis, pain related to cervical dystonia or torticollis, migraine, anxiety, tremor, hyperesthesia, somnolence, confusion. **Respiratory:** Increased cough, rhinitis, dyspnea, lung disorder, pneumonia. **Musculoskeletal:** Arthralgia, back pain, myasthenia, arthritis, joint disorder. **GU:** UTI, cystitis, vaginal moniliasis. **Dermatologic:** Pruritus, ecchymosis. **Ophthalmic:** Amblyopia, abnormal vision. **Otic:** Otitis media, tinnitus. **Body as a whole:** Infection, pain, flu syndrome, accidental injury, fever, chills, malaise, viral infection. **Miscellaneous:** Injection site pain, peripheral edema, hypercholesterolemia, taste perversion, allergic reaction, chest pain, hernia, abscess, cyst, neoplasm, vasodilation.

DRUG INTERACTIONS
Effect of botulinum toxin may be potentiated by aminoglycosides or any other drug that interferes with neuromuscular transmission (e.g., curare-like drugs).

HOW SUPPLIED
Solution for Injection: 5,000 units/mL.

DOSAGE
• **INJECTION**
  Cervical dystonia.
Clients with a history of tolerating botulinum toxin, initial: 2,500–5,000 units divided among the affected muscles. **Clients without a history of tolerating botulinum toxin:** Use a lower initial dose. Individualize subsequent dosing based on individual client response.

NURSING CONSIDERATIONS
@ Do not confuse Botulinum Toxin, Type B with Botulinum Toxin, Type A.

ADMINISTRATION/STORAGE
1. Duration of effect in those responding to the toxin is between 12 and 16 weeks at doses of 5,000 units or 10,000 units.
2. Administration of the toxin should only be by physicians familiar and experienced in assessing and managing clients with cervical dystonia.
3. Units of biological activity of botulinum toxin, type B cannot be compared or converted into units of any other botulinum toxin.
4. If a client ingests drug or is accidentally overdosed, monitor for up to several weeks for S&S of systemic weakness or paralysis.
5. Increased incidence of dysphagia with increased dose in the sternocleidomastoid muscle.
6. Incidence of dry mouth may increase when toxin used in the splenius capitis, trapezius, and sternocleidomastoid muscles.
7. Store under refrigeration at 2–8°C (36–46°F) for up to 21 months. Do not freeze or shake.
8. After dilution with normal saline, use within 4 hr; product does not contain a preservative.

ASSESSMENT
1. Note reasons for therapy, level of pain, extent of abnormal head/neck positioning, and other agents/therapies trialed.
2. Assess for any evidence/history of neuropathic, neurologic, or neuromuscular disorders.
3. For use/administration only by those individuals trained to administer.
4. Do not use within 4 mo of any other botulinum toxin serotype.
5. Review associated risk factors to ensure client understanding. Drug contains albumin which may present the

B

remote risk of disease transmission of CJD.

CLIENT/FAMILY TEACHING
1. Used to release abnormal muscle spasms/contractures permitting more controlled movements, mobility, and freedom.
2. The clostridium bacteria (B) that makes the toxin is not being injected directly; a sterilized by-product of the bacteria is utilized. May experience a slight sting with injections and dryness of mouth.
3. Do not perform activities that require mental alertness until drug effects realized, may experience dizziness, anxiety, confusion. Resume activity slowly and carefully following administration.
4. Report any swallowing problems, SOB, respiratory disorders/infections, injection site abnormalities, facial drooping, or weakness.
5. Effects usually last from 12–16 weeks; reinjection may be necessary to reattain desired results.
6. Practice reliable contraception.
7. An antitoxin is available in the event of significant overdose or misinjection. Contact Elan Pharmaceuticals at 1-888-638-7605, or the CDC at 1-800-311-3435 (1-404-639-2888 nights and weekends). The antitoxin would need to be administered within 20 hr of overdosage.

OUTCOMES/EVALUATE
Relief of painful neck spasms/contractures with cervical dystonia

Bretylium tosylate IV
(breh-**TILL**-ee-um **TOZ**-ill-ayt)

CLASSIFICATION(S):
Antiarrhythmic, class III
PREGNANCY CATEGORY: C
Rx: Bretylium tosylate in D5W.

USES
(1) Life-threatening ventricular arrhythmias that have failed to respond to first line antiarrhythmics (e.g., lidocaine). (2) Prophylaxis and treatment of ventricular fibrillation. For short-term use only. *Investigational:* Second-line drug (after lidocaine) for advanced cardiac life support during CPR.

ACTION/KINETICS
Action
Inhibits catecholamine release at nerve endings by decreasing excitability of the nerve terminal. Initially there is a release of norepinephrine, which may cause tachycardia and a rise in BP; this is followed by a blockade of release of catecholamines. Also increases the duration of the action potential and the effective refractory period, which may assist in reversing arrhythmias.

Pharmacokinetics
Peak plasma concentration and effect: 1 hr after IM. Antifibrillatory effect within a few minutes after IV use. Suppression of ventricular tachycardia and ventricular arrhythmias takes 20–120 min, whereas suppression of PVCs does not occur for 6–9 hr. **Therapeutic serum levels:** 0.5–1.5 mcg/mL. **$t^{1/2}$, terminal:** 6.9–8.1 hr. **Duration:** 6–8 hr. Up to 80% of drug is excreted unchanged in the urine after 24 hr. **Plasma protein binding:** 0–8%.

CONTRAINDICATIONS
Severe aortic stenosis, severe pulmonary hypertension.

SPECIAL CONCERNS
Safety and efficacy in children have not been established. Dosage adjustment required in impaired renal function.

SIDE EFFECTS
Most Common
Hypotension, postural hypotension, N&V (especially after rapid IV)
CV: Hypotension (including postural hypotension), transient hypertension, increased frequency of PVCs, bradycardia, precipitation of anginal attacks, initial increase in arrhythmias, sensation of substernal pressure. **GI:** N&V (especially after rapid IV administration), diarrhea, abdominal pain, hiccoughs. **CNS:** Vertigo, dizziness, lightheadedness, syncope, anxiety, paranoid psychosis, confusion, mood swings. **Miscellaneous:** Renal dysfunction, flushing, hyperthermia, SOB, nasal stuffiness, diaphoresis,

---

conjunctivitis, erythematous macular rash, lethargy, generalized tenderness.

OD OVERDOSE MANAGEMENT

Symptoms: Marked hypertension followed by hypotension. *Treatment:* Treat hypertension with nitroprusside or another short-acting IV antihypertensive. Treat hypotension with appropriate fluid therapy and pressor agents such as norepinephrine or dopamine.

DRUG INTERACTIONS

Catecholamines (dopamine, norepinephrine) / ↑ Catecholamine pressor effect; closely monitor BP

Digoxin / Bretylium may aggravate toxicity R/T initial release of norepinephrine

Procainamide, Quinidine / Concomitant use ↓ inotropic effect of bretylium and ↑ hypotension

HOW SUPPLIED

Injection: 50 mg/mL; *Injection in D5W:* 2 mg/mL, 4 mg/mL.

DOSAGE

- **IV INFUSION**

  Immediate, life-threatening ventricular arrhythmias.

Adults: 5 mg/kg by rapid IV injection of undiluted drug. If ventricular fibrillation persists, increase dose to 10 mg/kg and repeat as necessary.

  Acute ventricular fibrillation in children.

5 mg/kg/dose IV followed by 10 mg/kg at 15–30 min intervals up to a maximum total dose of 30 mg/kg. **Maintenance:** 5–10 mg/kg/dose q 6 hr.

  For continuous suppression of ventricular arrhythmias.

1–2 mg/minute of the diluted solution by continuous IV infusion. Alternatively, infuse 5–10 mg/kg of the diluted solution over more than 8 min q 6 hr.

  Other ventricular arrhythmias.

Adults: 5–10 mg/kg of diluted drug by IV infusion over more than 8 min. More rapid infusion may cause N&V. Give subsequent doses at 1 to 2 hr intervals if the arrhythmia persists. **Maintenance:** Give same dose q 6 hr or a constant infusion of 1 to 2 mg/min. **Children:** 5–10 mg/kg/dose q 6 hr.

- **IM**

  Other ventricular arrhythmias.

Adults: 5–10 mg/kg of undiluted solution followed, if necessary, by the same dose at 1–2-hr intervals; **then,** give same dosage q 6–8 hr.

NURSING CONSIDERATIONS

ADMINISTRATION/STORAGE

1. For IM, use drug undiluted.
2. Rotate injection sites; give no more than 5 mL of drug at any site to avoid atrophy, necrosis, fibrosis, vascular degeneration, or inflammation.
3. Keep supine; observe for postural hypotension.
4. Start oral antiarrhythmic as soon as possible.

IV 5. For IV infusion: Bretylium compatible with D5W, 0.9% NaCl, D5W/0.45% NaCl, D5W/0.9% NaCl, D5W/RL, 5% NaHCO$_3$, 20% mannitol, 1/6 molar sodium lactate, RL, CaCl$_2$ (54.5 mEq/L) in D5W, and KCl (40 mEq/L) in D5W.
6. For direct IV: Give undiluted over 15–30 sec, may repeat in 15–30 min if symptoms persist. May further dilute 500 mg in 50 mL and infuse over 10–30 min.

ASSESSMENT

1. Note reasons for therapy, pretreatment ECG, VS.
2. If taking digitalis, may aggravate digitalis toxicity.

INTERVENTIONS

1. Monitor VS and rhythm strips; dose titrated on response.
2. To reduce N&V, administer IV slowly over 10 min while supine. Once infusion complete keep supine until BP stabilized.
3. Supervise once ambulation permitted; may experience lightheadedness/vertigo.
4. Causes fall in supine BP within 1 hr of IV administration. If SBP <75 mm Hg, anticipate need for pressor agents.
5. If clients develop side effects, stay to reassure and reorient as needed.

CLIENT/FAMILY TEACHING

1. Used to convert abnormal heart rhythm to a normal rhythm.
2. Do not change positions suddenly; may experience sudden drop in BP causing dizziness.

B

3. Report any chest pain or SOB immediately.

OUTCOMES/EVALUATE
- Termination of life-threatening ventricular arrhythmia, stable cardiac rhythm
- Serum drug levels (0.5–1.5 mcg/mL)

Brinzolamide ophthalmic suspension
(brin-**ZOH**-lah-myd)

CLASSIFICATION(S):
Antiglaucoma drug
PREGNANCY CATEGORY: C
Rx: Azopt.

USES
(1) Treat elevated IOP in ocular hypertension or open-angle glaucoma in adults and children over 2 years of age. (2) Prevent postoperative increase in IOP in clients undergoing argon laser trabeculoplasty.

ACTION/KINETICS
Action
Inhibits carbonic hydrase in the ciliary processes of the eye, thus decreasing aqueous humor production and reducing intraocular pressure (IOP).

Pharmacokinetics
Is absorbed into the systemic circulation following ocular use. It can then distribute to RBCs. Eliminated unchanged mainly through the urine.

CONTRAINDICATIONS
Use in severe renal impairment (C_{CR} less than 30 mL/min). Concomitant use with oral carbonic anhydrase inhibitors. Lactation.

SPECIAL CONCERNS
Is a sulfonamide; thus, similar side effects can occur. Use with caution in hepatic impairment. Safety and efficacy have not been determined in children.

SIDE EFFECTS
Most Common
Blurred vision; bitter, sour, or unusual taste.

Ophthalmic: Blurred vision following dosing, blepharitis, dry eye, foreign body sensation, hyperemia, ocular discharge, ocular discomfort, ocular keratitis, ocular pain, ocular pruritus, rhinitis, conjunctivitis, diplopia, eye fatigue, keratoconjunctivitis, keratopathy, lid margin crusting or sticky sensation, tearing, hypertonia. **GI:** Bitter, sour, or unusual taste; nausea, diarrhea, dry mouth, dyspepsia. **CNS:** Headache, dizziness, somnolence (especially in children). **Miscellaneous:** Dermatitis, allergic reactions, alopecia, chest pain, dyspnea, kidney pain, pharyngitis, urticaria.

DRUG INTERACTIONS
Possible additive effects with oral carbonic anhydrase inhibitors.

HOW SUPPLIED
Ophthalmic Suspension: 1%.

DOSAGE
- **OPHTHALMIC SUSPENSION**
  Increased IOP.
1 gtt in the affected eye(s) three times per day.

NURSING CONSIDERATIONS
ADMINISTRATION/STORAGE
1. Shake well before use.
2. May be used with other topical ophthalmic products to lower IOP. If more than one topical drug is used, give drugs at least 10 min apart.
3. Store between 4–30°C (39–86°F).

ASSESSMENT
1. Note eye exam, IOP, other agents trialed/outcome; assess for sulfonamide sensitivity.
2. Obtain renal and LFTs; do not use with severe impairment.

CLIENT/FAMILY TEACHING
1. Shake well, wash hands, administer as directed. If other agents prescribed, wait at least 10 min before using next agent.
2. Do not permit tip of container to touch the eye or surrounding structures; contamination may occur.
3. Use care operating machinery/car; may temporarily blur vision after dosing.
4. If more than one topical ophthalmic drug being used, administer at least 10 min apart.

Bold Italic = life threatening side effect   ■ = black box warning   ✦ = Available in Canada

B

5. Report any S&S of infection, eye trauma, or surgery.

6. Benzalkonium chloride, the preservative in the product, may be absorbed by soft contact lenses. Remove lenses during administration; wait 15 min to reinsert.

OUTCOMES/EVALUATE
↓ IOP

Bromfenac ophthalmic solution
(**BROME**-fen-ak)

CLASSIFICATION(S):
Nonsteroidal anti-inflammatory drug, ophthalmic use
PREGNANCY CATEGORY: C
Rx: Xibrom.

USES
Treat postoperative inflammation and reduction of ocular pain in clients who have undergone cataract removal.

ACTION/KINETICS
Action
Ophthalmic NSAID that blocks prostaglandin synthesis by inhibiting cyclooxygenase 1 and 2. By inhibiting prostaglandin production, inflammation is reduced.

Pharmacokinetics
Achieves very low plasma concentrations.

CONTRAINDICATIONS
Known hypersensitivity to any ingredient in the formulation.

SPECIAL CONCERNS
Contains sodium sulfite that may cause severe allergic reactions, including anaphylaxis, in susceptible clients. May show cross-sensitivity to aspirin, phenylacetic acid derivatives, and other NSAIDs; use with caution in those who have demonstrated sensitivities to these drugs. May slow or delay healing. Use with caution in clients with complicated ocular surgery, corneal denervation, corneal epithelial defects, diabetes mellitus, ocular surface diseases, rheumatoid arthritis, or repeat ocular surgeries during a short period of time due to the possibility of increased corneal adverse effects that may be sight threatening. Use with caution during lactation. Safety and efficacy have not been demonstrated in children below the age of 18 years.

SIDE EFFECTS
Most Common
Burning/stinging upon instillation, ocular irritation.
Ophthalmic: Abnormal sensation in the eye, conjunctival hyperemia, ocular irritation, burning/stinging upon instillation, eye pain/pruritus/redness, iritis, corneal thinning/erosion/ perforation, epithelial breakdown, keratitis, increased bleeding of ocular tissue (including hyphemia) in conjunction with ocular surgery. **Miscellaneous:** Headache.

DRUG INTERACTIONS
Use with topical corticosteroids may ↑ potential for healing problems.

HOW SUPPLIED
Ophthalmic Solution: 0.09%.

DOSAGE
- **OPHTHALMIC SOLUTION**
  Postoperative inflammation after cataract removal.
  1 drop applied to the affected eye(s) two times daily beginning 24 hr after cataract surgery; continue through the first 2 postoperative weeks.

NURSING CONSIDERATIONS
ADMINISTRATION/STORAGE
1. Use more than 24 hr before surgery or beyond 14 days postsurgery may increase risk for occurrence and severity of corneal adverse events.
2. Store from 15–25°C (59–77°F).

ASSESSMENT
1. Note surgery date and status of eye health; list other agents prescribed to ensure none interact.
2. List allergy/sensitivity to NSAIDs, ASA or derivatives. Drug contains sodium sulfite. Assess site for post op bleeding or delayed healing of ocular tissue.
3. Document other medical conditions that may require cautious use of therapy (i.e. RA, DM, asthma, or recurrent ocular surgeries).

CLIENT/FAMILY TEACHING
1. Drug instilled into the operative eye twice a day for up to two weeks after surgery. Use care to wash hands before instilling and do not let dropper tip come in contact with mucosa. Do not use beyond stated time; may experience adverse corneal events.
2. With evidence of eye tissue breakdown immediately stop use of topical NSAIDs and report; must be closely monitored for corneal health.
3. May experience burning/stinging, mild pain, redness, itching and drainage.
4. Avoid use during pregnancy, use reliable measures to prevent pregnancy.
5. Keep all F/U appointments; report any unusual/persistent side effects or change in vision.

OUTCOMES/EVALUATE
↓ Postoperative inflammation after cataract removal

Budesonide
(byou-**DES**-oh-nyd)

CLASSIFICATION(S):
Glucocorticoid
PREGNANCY CATEGORY: B
Rx: **Capsules**: Entocort EC. **Inhalation**: Pulmicort Flexhaler, Pulmicort Respules, Pulmicort Turbuhaler. **Intranasal**: Rhinocort Aqua.
✤Rx: Entocort, Gen-Budesonide AQ, Pulmicort Nebuamp, Rhinocort Turbuhaler.

SEE ALSO *CORTICOSTEROIDS*.
USES
(1) **Entocort EC:** Treatment and maintenance (up to 3 months) of clinical remission of mild-to-moderate active Crohn's disease involving the ileum and/or ascending colon. (2) **Pulmicort Flexhaler:** Prophylaxis and maintenance treatment of asthma in clients 6 years and older, including those requiring PO corticosteroid therapy for asthma. (3) **Pulmicort Respules:** Prophylaxis of and maintenance treatment of asthma in children and infants 6 months to 8 years. (4) **Pulmicort Tur-**

buhaler: Maintenance treatment of asthma as prophylaxis in adults and children 6 years of age and older; also for those requiring oral corticosteroid therapy for asthma. (5) **Rhinocort Aqua:** Treat symptoms of seasonal or perennial allergic rhinitis in adults and children 6 years of age and older.

ACTION/KINETICS
Action
Exerts a direct local anti-inflammatory effect with minimal systemic effects when used intranasally.
Pharmacokinetics
Entocort EC capsules contain micronized budesonide which has been coated to prevent release in the stomach. Budesonide is released in the intestine resulting in decreased inflammation by a local action. When taken PO, not absorbed into the body. Exceeding the recommended dose may result in suppression of hypothalamic-pituitary-adrenal function. About 34% bioavailable (doubled by compromised liver function). **Onset, nasal spray:** 10 hr. t½: 2–3 hr. Rapidly metabolized by CYP3A liver enzymes. Excreted through both urine and feces. **Plasma protein binding:** 85–90% over a concentration range of 1–100 ng/mL.

CONTRAINDICATIONS
Hypersensitivity to the drug. Untreated localized nasal mucosa infections. Lactation. Use in children less than 6 years of age or for acute or life-threatening asthma attacks, including status asthmaticus.

SPECIAL CONCERNS
Use with caution in clients already on alternate-day corticosteroids (e.g., prednisone); in clients with active or quiescent tuberculosis infections of the respiratory tract, or in untreated fungal, bacterial infections or systemic viral infections; or ocular herpes simplex. Use with caution in clients with recent nasal septal ulcers, recurrent epistaxis, nasal surgery, or trauma. Avoid exposure to chickenpox or measles.

SIDE EFFECTS
Most Common
Inhalation Powder: Headache, URTI, flu-like symptoms, sinusitis, pharyngitis,

back pain/pain, bronchospasm, cough, epistaxis.

Inhalation Suspension: URTI, rhinitis, nasal congestion, otitis media/ear infection, epistaxis.

Oral: Headache, tremor, rash, acne, fainting.

Respiratory: Nasopharyngeal irritation, nasal irritation, pharyngitis, increased cough, hoarseness, nasal pain, burning, stinging, dryness, epistaxis, bloody mucus, rebound congestion, **bronchial asthma,** occasional sneezing attacks (especially in children), rhinorrhea, reduced sense of smell, throat discomfort, ulceration of the nasal mucosa, sore throat, dyspnea, localized infections of nose and pharynx with *Candida albicans,* wheezing (rare). **CNS:** Lightheadedness, headache, nervousness. **GI:** Nausea, loss of sense of taste, bad taste in mouth, dry mouth, dyspepsia. **Miscellaneous:** Watery eyes, *immediate and delayed hypersensitivity reactions,* moniliasis, facial edema, rash, pruritus, herpes simplex, alopecia, arthralgia, myalgia, contact dermatitis (rare).

OD OVERDOSE MANAGEMENT

Symptoms: Symptoms of hypercorticism, including menstrual irregularities, acneiform lesions, and cushingoid features (all are rarely seen, however). *Treatment:* Discontinue the drug slowly using procedures that are acceptable for discontinuing oral corticosteroids.

DRUG INTERACTIONS

Cimetidine / Slight ↓ in budesonide clearance and an ↑ in its oral bioavailability; also, ↓ metabolism of budesonide by CYP3A4 liver enzymes → ↑ systemic levels of budesonide

Clarithromycin / ↓ Metabolism of budesonide by CYP3A4 liver enzymes → ↑ systemic levels of budesonide

Erythromycin / ↓ Metabolism of budesonide by CYP3A4 liver enzymes → ↑ systemic levels of budesonide

Grapefruit juice / ↑ Systemic levels of budesonide 2-fold

Itraconazole / ↓ Metabolism of budesonide by CYP3A4 liver enzymes → ↑ systemic levels of budesonide

Ketoconazole / ↑ Systemic levels of budesonide more than sevenfold R/T ↓ metabolism by CYP3A4 liver enzymes

Ritonavir / ↓ Metabolism of budesonide by CYP3A4 liver enzymes → ↑ systemic levels of budesonide

HOW SUPPLIED

Capsules: 3 mg; *Inhalation Powder (Flexhaler):* 90 mcg/inh, 180 mcg/inh; *Inhalation Powder (Turboinhaler):* 200 mcg/inh; *Inhalation Suspension (Respules):* 0.25 mg/mL, 0.5 mg/mL; *Nasal Spray:* 32 mcg/spray.

DOSAGE

- **CAPSULES**

    Crohn's disease.

Adults: 9 mg once daily in the a.m. for up to 8 weeks. If the disease recurs, another 8-week course may be given. Once symptoms are controlled, give 6 mg once daily for maintenance of clinical remission for up to 3 months. If symptom control is still maintained at 3 months, attempt to taper to complete cessation.

- **PULMICORT RESPULES**

    Prophylaxis and maintenance treatment of asthma.

Children 12 months to 8 years old: If previous therapy was bronchodilators alone: 0.5 mg total daily dose given either once or twice daily in divided doses (maximum daily dose: 0.5 mg). If previous therapy was inhaled corticosteroids: 0.5 mg total daily dose given either once or twice daily in divided doses (maximum daily dose: 1 mg). If previous therapy was oral corticosteroids: 1 mg total daily dose given either as 0.5 mg twice a day or 1 mg daily (maximum daily dose: 1 mg).

- **PULMICORT TURBUHALER**

    Prevention or treatment of asthma.

Adults, initial, if previous therapy was bronchodilators alone: 200–400 mcg twice a day, not to exceed 400 mcg twice a day. **Adults, initial, if previous therapy was inhaled corticosteroids for well controlled mild to moderate asthma:** 200–400 mcg (1–2 inhalations) once daily either in the morning or evening. Do not exceed 800 mcg twice a day. **Adults, initial, if previous therapy was oral corticosteroids:**

400–800 mcg twice a day, not to exceed 800 mcg twice a day. **Children, over 6 years old, if previous therapy was bronchodilators alone:** 200 mcg twice a day, not to exceed 400 mcg twice a day. **Children, over 6 years old, if previous therapy was inhaled corticosteroids:** 200 mcg twice a day, not to exceed 400 mcg twice a day. **Children over 6 years old, if previous therapy was oral corticosteroids:** Do not give more than 400 mcg twice a day in children.

• AQUA NASAL SPRAY (RHINOCORT AQUA)

Seasonal and perennial allergic rhinitis.

Adults and children 6 years and older, initial: 1 spray/nostril (64 mcg/day) once daily. **Maximum:** 2 sprays/nostril (128 mcg/day) once daily for children 6–11 years and 4 sprays/nostril (256 mcg) once daily for adults and children 12 years and older. Maximum benefit seen in 2 weeks. After the maximum effect is obtained, reduce the maintenance dose to the smallest amount required to control symptoms.

NURSING CONSIDERATIONS

ADMINISTRATION/STORAGE

1. Clients with Crohn's disease involving ileum/ascending colon have been switched from PO prednisolone to budesonide with no S&S of adrenal insufficiency. Begin tapering of prednisolone with initiation of budesonide.

2. Turbuhaler contains no chlorofluorocarbon propellants; drug delivered by client's inhalation.

3. Turbuhaler does not require spacer; delivers about twice the amount of drug per inhalation to the airway as metered dose inhalers.

4. Pulmicort Respules may be used in children as young as 12 months. In symptomatic children not responding to nonsteroidal therapy, a starting dose of 0.25 mg using Respules may be tried.

5. Administer Pulmicort Respules using a jet nebulizer connected to an air compressor with an adequate air flow, equipped with a mouthpiece or suitable face mask. Ultrasonic nebulizers are not suitable. Do not administer with other nebulizable medications.

6. Once the desired clinical effect is achieved using Respules, consider tapering to the lowest effective dose.

7. For those not responding adequately when using the Respules, consider giving the total daily dose as a divided dose if a once-daily dosing schedule was followed.

8. Store Pulmicort Respules and Pulmicort Turbuhaler from 20–25° C (68–77° F). Store Respules upright, protected from light. When an envelope has been opened, the shelf life of the unused Respules is 2 weeks, when protected. After opening the aluminum foil envelope, return the unused Respules to the aluminum foil envelop to protect from light. Use opened Respules promptly; gently shake using a circular motion before use. Do not freeze.

9. Store Entocort EC capsules from 15–30°C (59–86°F) in a tightly closed container.

10. Store Rhinocort Aqua from 20–25°C (68–77°F) with valve up. Protect from light. Shake gently before use. Do not spray in the eyes. Do not freeze. Discard after 120 sprays following initial priming.

ASSESSMENT

1. With oral budesonide, monitor moderate to severe liver disease clients for increased S&S of hypercorticisim. Dose reduction may be required.

2. Note reasons for therapy, onset/characteristics of S&S, other agents trialed/outcome.

3. List drugs prescribed; ensure none interact unfavorably.

4. Assess VS, nasal integrity, PFTs and lung sounds.

CLIENT/FAMILY TEACHING

1. Review method/frequency for administration of prescribed agent. Review video/instruction for proper inhalation guidelines.

2. Rinse mouth (especially children) and equipment thoroughly after each use to prevent oral fungal infections.

3. Prior to using nasal form, clear nasal passages of secretions. If nasal passages

---

Bold Italic = life threatening side effect   ■ = black box warning   ✦ = Available in Canada

are blocked, use decongestant first unless <2 y.o.

4. Maximum benefit usually not seen for 3–7 days, although a decrease in symptoms can be seen within 24 hr. Report if no improvement within 3 weeks.

5. Shake canister well before administering. Store valve down and away from areas of high humidity. Once Al pouch opened, use/discard within 6 months. Prime unit before use with Pulmicort Turbuhaler. Store respules upright protected from light; gently shake before use, discard open envelopes after 2 weeks.

6. Prior to using nasal spray gently shake container and prime the pump by actuating 8 times. If not used for 2 consecutive days, reprime with 1 spray or until a fine mist appears. If not used for more than 14 days, rinse the applicator and reprime with 2 sprays or until a fine mist appears.

7. Avoid individuals with chickenpox or communicable diseases.

8. Symptoms of hoarseness may be evident; should subside upon completion of therapy.

9. Take capsules whole; do not chew, crush, or break. Take once daily in the a.m.; avoid grapefruit juice.

10. Drug is a steroid; chronic use in excessive amounts may lead to adverse systemic reactions. Keep all F/U appointments.

11. Identify triggers/avoid irritants to control symptoms.

12. Report chest pain, lower extremity swelling, severe headaches, respiratory infections, or increased bruising/bleeding.

OUTCOMES/EVALUATE
- Relief of nasal congestion/allergic manifestations
- Asthma prophylaxis
- Crohn's disease remission

Bumetanide ■ IV ©
(byou-**MET**-ah-nyd)

CLASSIFICATION(S):
Diuretic, loop
PREGNANCY CATEGORY: C
Rx: Bumex.
♣Rx: Burinex.

SEE ALSO *DIURETICS, LOOP.*

USES
(1) Edema associated with CHF, nephrotic syndrome, hepatic disease. (2) Adjunct to treat acute pulmonary edema. Especially useful in clients refractory to other diuretics. *Investigational:* Treatment of adult nocturia. Not effective in males with prostatic hypertrophy.

ACTION/KINETICS
Action
Inhibits reabsorption of both sodium and chloride in the proximal tubule and the ascending loop of Henle. Possible activity in the proximal tubule to promote phosphate excretion.

Pharmacokinetics
Onset, PO: 30–60 min. **Peak effect, PO:** 1–2 hr. **Duration, PO:** 4–6 hr (dose-dependent). **Onset, IV:** Several minutes. **Peak effect, IV:** 15–30 min. **Duration, IV:** 3.5–4 hr. **t½:** 1–1.5 hr. The t½ decreases from 6 hr at birth to 2.4 hr at one month of age. Metabolized in the liver although 45% excreted unchanged in the urine.

CONTRAINDICATIONS
Anuria. Hepatic coma or severe electrolyte depletion until condition improved/corrected. Hypersensitivity to drug. Lactation.

SPECIAL CONCERNS
■ Potent diuretic; excess amounts can cause profound diuresis with water and electrolyte depletion. Individualize dosage; monitor carefully.■ Safety and efficacy in children under 18 have not been established. Geriatric clients may be more sensitive to the hypotensive and electrolyte effects and are at greater risk for developing thromboembolic problems and circulatory collapse. SLE

B

may be activated or made worse. Clients allergic to sulfonamides may show cross sensitivity to bumetanide. Sudden changes in electrolyte balance may cause hepatic encephalopathy and coma in clients with hepatic cirrhosis and ascites.

SIDE EFFECTS

Most Common

Dizziness, hypotension, headache, nausea, muscle cramps, encephalopathy in those with preexisting liver disease.

Electrolyte and fluid changes: Excess water loss, **dehydration,** electrolyte depletion including hypokalemia, hypochloremia, hyponatremia, hypovolemia, thromboembolism, *circulatory collapse.* **Otic:** Tinnitus, reversible and irreversible hearing impairment, deafness, vertigo (with a sense of fullness in the ears). **CV:** *Reduction in blood volume may cause circulatory collapse and vascular thrombosis and embolism, especially in geriatric clients.* Hypotension, ECG changes, chest pain. **CNS:** Asterixis, encephalopathy in those with preexisting liver disease, vertigo, headache, dizziness. **GI:** Upset stomach, dry mouth, N&V, diarrhea, GI pain. **GU:** Premature ejaculation, difficulty maintaining erection, renal failure. **Musculoskeletal:** Arthritic pain, weakness, muscle cramps, fatigue. **Hematologic:** Agranulocytosis, thrombocytopenia. **Allergic:** Pruritus, urticaria, rashes. **Miscellaneous:** Sweating, hyperventilation, rash, nipple tenderness, photosensitivity, pain following parenteral use.

LABORATORY TEST CONSIDERATIONS

Alterations in LDH, AST, ALT, alkaline phosphatase, creatinine clearance, total serum bilirubin, serum proteins, cholesterol. Changes in hemoglobin, PT, hematocrit, WBCs, platelet and differential counts, phosphorus, carbon dioxide content, bicarbonate, and calcium. ↑ Urinary glucose and protein, serum creatinine. Also, hyperuricemia, hypochloremia, hypokalemia, azotemia, hyponatremia, hyperglycemia.

OD **OVERDOSE MANAGEMENT**

Symptoms: Profound loss of water, electrolyte depletion, dehydration, decreased blood volume, *circulatory collapse (possibility of vascular thrombosis and embolism).* Symptoms of electrolyte depletion include: Anorexia, cramps, weakness, dizziness, vomiting, and mental confusion. *Treatment:* Replace electrolyte and fluid losses and monitor urinary and serum electrolyte levels. Emesis or gastric lavage. Oxygen or artificial respiration may be necessary. General supportive measures

HOW SUPPLIED

Injection: 0.25 mg/mL; *Tablets:* 0.5 mg, 1 mg, 2 mg.

DOSAGE

- **TABLETS**

  Edema.

Adults: 0.5–2 mg once daily; if response is inadequate, a second or third dose may be given at 4–5-hr intervals up to a maximum of 10 mg/day.

- **IM; IV**

  Edema.

Adults: 0.5–1 mg; if response is inadequate, a second or third dose may be given at 2–3-hr intervals up to a maximum of 10 mg/day. Initiate PO dosing as soon as possible.

NURSING CONSIDERATIONS

@ Do not confuse Bumex with Buprenex (narcotic analgesic).

ADMINISTRATION/STORAGE

1. Recommended PO schedule is on alternate days or for 3–4 days with a 1- to 2-day rest period in between.

2. Bumetanide, at a 1:40 ratio of bumetanide: furosemide, may be ordered if allergic to furosemide.

3. Reserve IV or IM for those in whom PO use is not practical or absorption from the GI tract is impaired.

IV 4. In severe chronic renal insufficiency, a continuous infusion (12 mg over 12 hr) may be more effective and cause fewer side effects than intermittent bolus therapy.

5. Prepare solutions fresh for IM or IV; use within 24 hr.

6. Ampules may be reconstituted with D5W, NSS, or RL solution.

7. Administer IV solutions slowly over 1–2 min.

Bold Italic = life threatening side effect   ■ = black box warning   ♣ = Available in Canada

ASSESSMENT

1. List reasons for therapy; pretreatment findings.
2. Note sulfonamide allergy; may be cross sensitivity.
3. Monitor electrolytes, I&O, renal and LFTs; assess for ↓ K⁺.
4. Review history; note any hearing impairment, lupus, or thromboembolic events. Assess hearing; check for ototoxicity, especially if receiving other ototoxic drugs.
5. *NOTE:* 1 mg of bumetanide is equivalent to 40 mg of furosemide.
6. Monitor VS. Rapid diuresis may cause dehydration and circulatory collapse (especially in elderly). Hypotension may occur when administered with antihypertensives.

CLIENT/FAMILY TEACHING

1. Take early in day to prevent nighttime voidings. With alternate-day therapy, keep written record/calendar to ensure proper therapy and no overdosage.
2. Do not perform activities that require mental alertness until drug effects realized. Change positions slowly to prevent sudden drop in BP causing dizziness.
3. Review dietary requirements such as reduced sodium and high potassium; see dietitian PRN. May take with food to reduce GI upset.
4. Record weights; report any sudden weight gain (>3 lbs/day or 5 lbs/week), swelling in the hands or feet.
5. Report unusual side effects or hearing loss.
6. Keep all F/U appointment to evaluate labs and response to therapy.

OUTCOMES/EVALUATE

↓ Peripheral and sacral edema; enhanced diuresis

Buprenorphine hydrochloride
(byou-pren-**OR**-feen)

CLASSIFICATION(S):
Narcotic agonist/antagonist
PREGNANCY CATEGORY: C
Rx: Buprenex, Subutex, **C-III**

SEE ALSO *NARCOTIC ANALGESICS.*

USES

Injection: Moderate-to-severe pain.
Tablets: Treat opioid dependence.

ACTION/KINETICS

Action

Semisynthetic opiate possessing both narcotic agonist and antagonist activity. Partial agonist at the mu opioid receptor and an antagonist at the kappa opioid receptor. A 0.3 mg parenteral dose is equivalent to 10 mg morphine in respiratory depressant and analgesic effects.

Pharmacokinetics

IM, onset: 15 min; **Peak effect:** 1 hr; **Duration:** 6 hr. **t½:** 2–3 hr. May also be given IV with shorter onset and peak effect. Is about equipotent with naloxone as a narcotic antagonist.

CONTRAINDICATIONS

Lactation. Use of the tablets in children less than 16 years of age.

SPECIAL CONCERNS

Use of the injection in children less than 2 years of age has not been established. Safety and efficacy of the tablets have not been established in children below 16 years of age. Use with caution in clients with compromised respiratory function, in the elderly or debilitated, CNS depression or coma, toxic psychoses, acute alcoholism, delirium tremens, kyphoscoliosis, in head injuries, in impairment of liver or renal function, Addison's disease, prostatic hypertrophy, biliary tract dysfunction, urethral stricture, myxedema, and hypothyroidism. Administration to individuals physically dependent on narcotics may result in precipitation of a withdrawal syndrome. Use may obscure diagnosis or clinical course of those with acute abdominal conditions.

SIDE EFFECTS
Most Common
Following use of tablets: Headache, insomnia, N&V, abdominal pain, constipation, pain, infection, chills, rhinitis, sweating, asthenia, vasodilation, withdrawal syndrome.

Following use of injection: Hypotension, sedation, dizziness, vertigo, sweating, N&V, miosis, hypoventilation.

• **Injection**
CNS: Sedation, dizziness, vertigo, dreaming, psychosis, weakness, fatigue, nervousness, confusion, headache, euphoria, slurred speech, depression, paresthesia, malaise, depersonalization, tremors, hallucinations, coma, dysphoria, agitation, seizures. **GI:** N&V, constipation, dyspepsia, loss of appetite, flatulence, dry mouth, cytolytic hepatitis and hepatitis with jaundice in addicts, diarrhea. **Ophthalmic:** Miosis, blurred/double vision, conjunctivitis, visual abnormalities, amblyopia (rare). **CV:** Hypotension, bradycardia, hypertension, tachycardia, Wenckebach block. **Respiratory:** Decreased respiratory rate (especially after IV use), cyanosis, dyspnea, apnea (rare). **Dermatologic:** Sweating, rash, pruritus, flushing/warmth, injection site reaction, pallor, urticaria (rare). **Miscellaneous:** Urinary retention, chills, tinnitus, acute and chronic hypersensitivity.

• **Tablets**
CNS: Headache, insomnia. **GI:** N&V, abdominal pain, constipation, diarrhea. **Body as a whole:** Asthenia, chills, infection, pain, vasodilation, sweating. **Miscellaneous:** Back pain, withdrawal syndrome, rhinitis.

DRUG INTERACTIONS
Barbiturate anesthetics / ↑ Respiratory and CNS depression of buprenorphine
Benzodiazepines / Coma and death possible with concomitant IV use of both drugs by addicts
CNS depressants (alcohol, benzodiazepines, general anesthetics, narcotic analgesics, phenothiazines, sedative/hypnotics, tranquilizers) / Additive CNS depression

CYP3A4 inducers (carbamazepine, phenobarbital, phenytoin, rifampin) / Possible increased clearance of buprenorphine; monitor carefully
CYP3A4 inhibitors (azole antifungals, macrolide antibiotics, protease inhibitors) / Use caution; specific data not available

HOW SUPPLIED
Injection: Equivalent to 0.3 mg/mL buprenorphine; *Tablets, Sublingual:* 2 mg, 8 mg.

DOSAGE
• **IM; SLOW IV**
Analgesia.
Clients over 13 years of age: 0.3 mg (1 mL) given over 2 min q 6 hr; repeat once (up to 0.3 mg) if needed, 30–60 min after initial dose. **Children, 2–12 years of age:** 2–6 mcg/kg q 4–6 hr. Do not give single doses greater than 6 mcg/kg.

• **TABLETS, SUBLINGUAL**
Opioid dependence.
Adults: 12–16 mg given as a single daily dose.

NURSING CONSIDERATIONS
Do not confuse Buprenex with Bumex (diuretic).

ADMINISTRATION/STORAGE
1. Not all children may clear buprenorphine faster than adults. Thus, fixed interval or 'round the clock' dosing should not be undertaken until proper interdose interval has been established.
2. Some pediatric clients may not need to be remedicated with the injection for 6–8 hr.
3. When using injection, have naloxone to reverse drug-induced respiratory depression.
4. Avoid storing injection in excessive heat and light. Do not freeze.
5. Place sublingual tablets under the tongue until dissolved. For doses requiring more than 2 tablets, place all tablets under the tongue at once. If client cannot fit more than 2 tablets comfortably, place 2 tablets at a time under the tongue until dissolved. Swallowing tablets whole will reduce bioavailability.
6. Clients must undergo induction of therapy. Prior to induction, determine

---

type of opioid dependence, time since last opioid use, and degree/level of opioid dependence.

7. An adequate maintenance dose, titrated to clinical effect, should be achieved as rapidly as possible to prevent opioid withdrawal syndrome. In one induction regimen, clients received buprenorphine, 8 mg on day 1 and 16 mg on day 2. From day 3 onward, they received buprenorphine/naloxone tablets at the same buprenorphine dose as on day 2. Induction was achieved in 3 or 4 days.

8. In those taking heroin or other short-acting opioids, give buprenorphine during the initiation of induction at least 4 hr after the individual last used opioids (or when the first signs of withdrawal appear).

9. Preferred medication for maintenance treatment is buprenorphine/naloxone.

10. As part of the comprehensive treatment plan, the decision should be made to discontinue buprenorphine (or buprenorphine/naloxone) therapy after a period of maintenance or brief stabilization. Taper buprenorphine dose at the end of treatment.

IV 11. Do not mix with solutions containing diazepam or lorazepam.

12. May be mixed with solutions containing haloperidol, glycopyrrolate, scopolamine hydrobromide, hydroxyzine chloride, or droperidol.

13. May be mixed with isotonic saline, RL solution, and D5W/0.9% NaCl.

14. May be administered undiluted IV, over 3–5 min.

15. To prescribe Subutex, prescribers must enroll in a program via a special DEA number. Call 1-800-287-2728.

ASSESSMENT

1. Note reasons for therapy, characteristics of S&S, intensity/pain level. Monitor VS and level of consciousness.

2. Those with opioid dependence should undergo induction of therapy. Prior to induction, determine type of dependence, the time since last opioid use, and degree/level of opioid dependence. Observe for 2 hr and assess need for additional dosing.

3. Asses for any respiratory depression; drug contraindicated.

4. Report head injuries immediately.

5. If receiving narcotics, observe for withdrawal symptoms.

6. Assess for liver or renal dysfunction, diseases of the biliary tract, or BPH.

CLIENT/FAMILY TEACHING

1. May cause drowsiness, dizziness, low BP effects. Avoid activities that require mental alertness.

2. Cough and deep breathe every 2 hr to prevent lung collapse esp. when used for post-op pain.

3. Avoid alcohol. Report any CNS changes, adverse effects, or allergic S&S.

4. With opioid dependence, follow therapy guidelines. stay in recovery program to ensure freedom from dependence.

OUTCOMES/EVALUATE

Relief of pain; Treatment of opioid dependence

Bupropion hydrochloride ■ⓒ📷
(byou-**PROH**-pee-on)

CLASSIFICATION(S):
Antidepressant, miscellaneous; smoking deterrent (Zyban)
PREGNANCY CATEGORY: B
Rx: Budeprion SR, Budeprion XL, Wellbutrin, Wellbutrin SR, Wellbutrin XL, Zyban.

USES
(1) Treatment of major depressive episodes (immediate-release, extended-release, and sustained-release). (2) Major depressive episodes in those with a history of seasonal affective disorder (bupropion XL). (3) Aid to stop smoking (Zyban only); may be combined with a nicotine transdermal system. *Investigational:* Bupropion: Attention deficit hyperactivity disorder. Bupropion SR: Neuropathic pain, enhancement of weight loss.

B

ACTION/KINETICS

Action

Mechanism of action is not known; the drug does not inhibit MAO and it only weakly blocks neuronal uptake of epinephrine, serotonin, and dopamine. However, its action is believed to be mediated by noradrenergic and/or dopaminergic mechanisms. Exerts moderate anticholinergic and sedative effects, but only slight orthostatic hypotension.

Pharmacokinetics

Peak plasma levels, Wellbutrin SR and Zyban: 3 hr; **peak plasma levels, Wellbutrin XL:** 5 hr. **t½, terminal, immediate-release:** 8–24 hr. **Time to steady state:** Within 8 days. Significantly metabolized by a first-pass effect through the liver to both active and inactive metabolites. Can induce drug-metabolizing enzymes. During chronic use the plasma levels of two active metabolites may be higher than bupropion. Excreted through both the urine (87%) and the feces (10%). Zyban is a sustained-release formulation. **Plasma protein binding:** 84% at concentrations up to 200 mcg/mL.

CONTRAINDICATIONS

Hypersensitivity to bupropion or any ingredients. Seizure disorders; presence or history of bulimia or anorexia nervosa due to the higher incidence of seizures in such clients. Concomitant use of an MAO inhibitor. Use in clients undergoing abrupt discontinuation of alcohol and sedatives, including benzodiazepines. Use in clients who have shown an allergic response to bupropion or other components of the various products. Wellbutrin, Wellbutrin SR, Wellbutrin XL, and Zyban all contain bupropion; do not use together. Lactation.

SPECIAL CONCERNS

■ Antidepressants increased the risk of suicidal thinking and behavior (suicidality) in short-term studies in children and adolescents with major depressive disorder and other psychiatric disorders. Anyone considering the use of bupropion or other antidepressants in a child or adolescent must balance this risk with the clinical need. Closely observe clients who are started on therapy for clinical worsening, suicidality, or unusual changes in behavior. Advise families and caregivers of the need for close observation and communication with the prescriber. Bupropion is not approved for use in children.

Short-term (4–16 weeks), placebo-controlled trials of various antidepressant drugs in children and adolescents with major depressive disease, obsessive compulsive disorders, or other psychiatric disorders revealed a greater risk of adverse reactions representing suicidal thinking or behavior during the first few months of treatment in those receiving antidepressants. The average risk of such events in clients receiving antidepressants was 4%, twice the placebo risk of 2%. No suicides occurred in these trials.

Although Zyban is not indicated for the treatment of depression, it contains the same active ingredient as the antidepressant bupropion medications Wellbutrin, Wellbutrin SR, and Wellbutrin XL.■

Use with extreme caution in clients with cranial trauma, with drugs that lower the seizure threshold (e.g., alcohol use; addiction to opiates, cocaine, or stimulants; use of OTC stimulants and anorectics, antipsychotics, other antidepressants, theophylline, systemic steroids; diabetes treated with oral hypoglycemics or insulin); and, situations that might cause seizures (e.g., abrupt cessation of a benzodiazepine, CNS tumor, severe hepatic cirrhosis).

Adults and children with major depressive disease may show worsening of their depression and/or the emergence of suicidal ideation and behavior or unusual changes in behavior, whether or not they are taking antidepressants.

Use with extreme caution in severe hepatic cirrhosis (do not exceed 150 mg every other day). Use with caution and in lower doses in clients with liver or kidney disease and in those with a recent history of MI or unstable heart disease. Hypersensitivity reactions are possible characterized by pruritus, urticaria,

---

Bold Italic = life threatening side effect   ■ = black box warning   ✦ = Available in Canada

angioedema, dyspnea and, rarely, erythema multiform, Stevens-Johnson syndrome, and anaphylaxis.

Safety and efficacy have not been established in clients less than 18 years of age.

SIDE EFFECTS

Most Common

Agitation, anxiety, constipation, dizziness, headache/migraine, insomnia, tremor, sedation, excessive sweating, anorexia, dry mouth, N&V.

Listed are side effects for IR and SR forms with an incidence of 0.1% or greater.

• **Immediate-Release**

CNS: Agitation/restlessness, headache/migraine, dizziness, tremor, sedation, anxiety, insomnia, confusion, disturbed concentration, akinesia/bradykinesia, hostility, impaired sleep quality, sensory disturbance, anxiety, cutaneous temperature disturbance, *seizures*, akathisia, pseudoparkinsonism, delusions, euphoria, ataxia/incoordination, myoclonus, dyskinesia, dystonia, mania/hypomania, decreased/increased libido, hallucinations, decreased sexual function, depression, vertigo, dysarthria, impaired memory, depersonalization, psychosis, dysphoria, mood instability, paranoia, formal thought disorder, frigidity, vertigo. **GI:** Dry mouth, constipation, N&V, anorexia, diarrhea, increased/decreased appetite, dyspepsia, stomatitis, dysphagia, increased salivary flow, thirst disturbance, toothache, bruxism, gum irritation, oral edema, liver damage, jaundice. **CV:** Tachycardia, cardiac arrhythmias, hyper/hypotension, palpitations, syncope, edema, chest pain, ECG abnormalities. **Dermatologic:** Excessive sweating, rash, pruritus, nonspecific rashes, alopecia, dry skin. **GU:** Menstrual complaints, impotence, urinary frequency/retention, nocturia, gynecomastia, vaginal irritation, testicular swelling, UTI, painful erection, retarded ejaculation. **Musculoskeletal:** Arthritis, muscle spasms. **Respiratory:** Upper respiratory complaints, bronchitis, SOB, dyspnea. **Ophthalmic:** Blurred vision, mydriasis, visual disturbance. **Body as a whole:** Weight gain/loss, edema, fatigue, fever/chills, flu-like symptoms, nonspecific pain. **Miscellaneous:** Auditory disturbance, gustatory disturbance, changes in hormone levels.

• **Sustained-Release**

CNS: Headache/migraine, insomnia, dizziness, nervousness, tremor, anxiety, agitation, CNS stimulation, irritability, somnolence, paresthesia, decreased memory, abnormal coordination, decreased libido, depersonalization, dysphoria, emotional lability, hostility, hyperkinesia, hypertonia, hypesthesia, *seizures, suicidal ideation*. **GI:** Dry mouth, N&V, constipation, anorexia, diarrhea, abdominal pain, dysphagia, bruxism, gastric reflux, gingivitis, glossitis, dyspepsia, flatulence, increased salivation, mouth ulcers, stomatitis, thirst, abnormal liver function, jaundice. **CV:** Flushing, hot flashes, palpitations, postural hypotension, *stroke,* tachycardia, vasodilation. **Dermatologic:** Excessive sweating, rash, pruritus, urticaria, maculopapular rash, ecchymosis, acne, dry skin. **GU:** Urinary frequency/urgency, vaginal hemorrhage, UTI, impotence, polyuria, prostate disorder, inguinal hernia. **Musculoskeletal:** Myalgia, arthralgia, arthritis, twitch, leg cramps, musculoskeletal chest pain. **Respiratory:** Pharyngitis, increased cough, sinusitis. **Ophthalmic:** Amblyopia, abnormal accommodation, dry eye. **Body as a whole:** Infection, asthenia, chest/back pain, pain, fever/chills, increased weight. **Miscellaneous:** Tinnitus, taste perversion, SIADH, facial/peripheral edema, edema, photosensitivity, ecchymosis.

• **Zyban**

CNS: Tremors, insomnia, abnormal thinking, dizziness, insomnia, somnolence, anxiety, disturbed concentration, abnormal dreams, dysphoria, nervousness. **GI:** Dry mouth, anorexia, increased appetite, taste perversion, abdominal pain, constipation, diarrhea, dry mouth, mouth ulcer, nausea, thirst. **CV:** Hot flushes, hypertension, palpitations. **Dermatologic:** Dry skin, pruritus, rash, urticaria. **Musculoskeletal:** Arthralgia, myalgia. **Respiratory:** Bronchitis, rhinitis, increased cough, pharyngi-

---

B

tis, epistaxis, sinusitis, dyspnea. **Miscellaneous:** Allergic reaction, chest/neck pain, tinnitus, accidental injury, facial edema.

OD OVERDOSE MANAGEMENT
Symptoms: **Immediate-Release:** Seizures, hallucinations, loss of consciousness, sinus tachycardia, *multiple uncontrolled seizures*, bradycardia, fever, muscle rigidity, hypotension, rhabdomyolysis, stupor, *coma, respiratory failure, cardiac failure* and *cardiac arrest prior to death.* Consider the possibility of multiple-drug involvement. *Treatment:* Client should be hospitalized. Ensure an adequate airway, oxygenation, and ventilation. Monitor cardiac rhythm and vital signs. Monitor EEG for first 48 hr. Use general supportive and symptomatic measures. Do not induce emesis. Gastric lavage with a large-bore orogastric tube with appropriate airway protection, if needed, may be used if undertaken soon after ingestion or in symptomatic clients. Give activated charcoal. Seizures may be treated with IV benzodiazepines and other supportive procedures.

DRUG INTERACTIONS
Alcohol / ↓ Seizure threshold; may precipitate seizures
Amantadine / ↑ Risk of adverse effects, including psychotic reactions; use small initial/small gradual increases of bupropion
Antiarrhythmics, type 1C / ↑ Antiarrhythmic side effects R/T ↓ liver metabolism by CYP2D6 isoenzymes
Antipsychotics (haloperidol, risperidone, thioridazine) / ↑ Antipsychotic side effects R/T ↓ liver metabolism by CYP2D6 isoenzymes
Beta blockers / ↑ Beta blocker SE R/T ↓ liver metabolism by CYP2D6 isoenzymes
Carbamazepine / ↑ Bupropion metabolism → ↓ plasma levels
Cimetidine / Inhibits metabolism of bupropion
Clopidogrel / ↑ Bupropion AUC and peak plasma levels and ↓ bupropion clearance/AUC of hydroxyl metabolite R/T ↓ metabolism by CYP2B6 hydroxylation

Cyclosporine / ↓ Cyclosporine levels; increase dose
Fluoxetine / Panic symptoms/psychotic reactions
Levodopa / ↑ Risk of SE; use small initial/small gradual dose increases of bupropion
MAO inhibitors / ↑ Acute toxicity to bupropion, esp. with phenelzine; allow at least 14 days between discontinuation of an MAOI and initiation of bupropion
Metoprolol / ↑ Metoprolol SE R/T ↓ liver metabolism
Nicotine replacement / Possible hypertension; monitor BP
Phenobarbital / ↑ Bupropion metabolism → ↓ plasma levels
Phenytoin / ↑ Bupropion metabolism → ↓ plasma levels
Ritonavir / ↑ Risk of bupropion toxicity R/T large increases in serum bupropion; do not give together
Selective serotonin-reuptake inhibitors / ↑ SSRI SE R/T ↓ liver metabolism by CYP2D6 isoenzymes
Ticlopidine / ↑ Bupropion AUC and peak plasma levels and ↓ bupropion clearance/AUC of hydroxyl metabolite R/T ↓ metabolism by CYP2B6 hydroxylation
Tricyclic antidepressants (TCAs) / ↑ TCA SE R/T ↓ liver metabolism by CYP2D6 isoenzymes
Warfarin / Altered PT or INR with possible hemorrhagic or thrombotic complications

HOW SUPPLIED
Tablets, Extended-Release (XL-24 hr): 150 mg, 300 mg; *Tablets, Immediate-Release:* 75 mg, 100 mg; *Tablets, Sustained-Release (SR - 12 hr):* 100 mg, 150 mg, 200 mg.

DOSAGE
• **TABLETS, IMMEDIATE-RELEASE**
  Antidepressant.
Adults, initial: 100 mg in the a.m. and p.m. for the first 3 days; **then,** 100 mg 3 times per day, given in the morning, midday, and in the evening (6 hr should elapse between doses). If no response is observed after 4 weeks or more, the dose may be increased to a maximum of 450 mg/day with individual doses

---

Bold Italic = life threatening side effect   ■ = black box warning   ✦ = Available in Canada

not to exceed 150 mg. **Maintenance:** Lowest dose to control depression. Several months of treatment may be necessary. Discontinue in those who do not demonstrate an adequate response after an appropriate treatment period using 450 mg/day.

- **TABLETS, EXTENDED-RELEASE (XL)**
  Antidepressant, Seasonal affective disorder.

Initial: 150 mg/day in the morning; **maintenance:** 300 mg/day in the morning. Maintenance dose may be increased to 450 mg/day in the morning if no improvement seen after several weeks of 300 mg/day. There should be an interval of at least 24 hr between successive doses. It is not known whether the dose needed for maintenance treatment is identical to the dose needed to achieve an initial response. Periodically assess to determine the need for maintenance treatment and the appropriate dose for such treatment.

- **TABLETS, SUSTAINED-RELEASE (SR)**
  Antidepressant.

Adults, initial: 150 mg once daily in the a.m. If 150 mg is tolerated, increase to 300 mg/day given as 150 mg twice a day as early as day 4 of dosing. Allow 8 or more hr between successive doses. Do not exceed a daily dose of 400 mg given as 200 mg twice a day in clients where no clinical improvement was noted after several weeks of 300 mg/day. **Maintenance:** Periodically assess to determine the need for maintenance treatment and the appropriate dose for such treatment. It is not known whether the dose needed for maintenance treatment is identical to the dose needed to achieve an initial response.

ZYBAN
Smoking deterrent.

Initial: 150 mg/day for the first 3 days; **then,** 150 mg twice a day for 7–12 weeks (up to 6 months). Do not exceed doses of 300 mg/day. Eight hours or more should elapse between successive doses.

NURSING CONSIDERATIONS

ⓒ Do not confuse bupropion with buspirone (anti-anxiety agent) or the SR product (intended for twice-daily dosing) with the XL product (intended for once-daily dosing).

ADMINISTRATION/STORAGE

1. Administer all forms to minimize risk of seizures; do not exceed a total daily dose of 400 mg to treat depression or 300 mg as a smoking deterrent. Do not exceed a single dose of 150 mg; increase doses gradually. Discontinue and do not restart in those who experience a seizure while on the drug.

2. The risk of seizures may be minimized by using the following guidelines: For Bupropion IR: Do not exceed a total daily dose of 450 mg. The daily dose is given 3 times per day with at least 6 hr between successive doses, with each single dose not to exceed 150 mg. The rate of dose increase is very gradual. For Wellbutrin SR: Do not exceed a total daily dose of 400 mg. The daily dose is given twice daily. The rate of dose increase is gradual. No single dose should exceed 200 mg. For Bupropion XL: Do not exceed a total daily dose of 450 mg. The rate of dose increase is gradual. For Zyban: Do not exceed a total daily dose of 300 mg. The recommended daily dose for most clients is 300 mg/day given as 150 mg twice a day. No single dose should exceed 150 mg.

3. Total daily doses of the immediate- and sustained-release tablets can be converted milligram-for-milligram to a once-daily dose of the extended-release formulation.

4. Several months of therapy may be necessary to control acute depression.

5. With severe hepatic cirrhosis, do not exceed a dose of 75 mg of immediate-release product once daily; do not exceed 100 mg every day or 150 mg every other day for SR and 150 mg every other day for XL. For Zyban, give 150 mg every other day in clients with severe hepatic cirrhosis.

6. Reduce the dose and/or frequency bupropion in clients with impaired renal function.

7. Initiate Zyban treatment while client is still smoking since about 1 week of treatment is needed to reach steady-state blood levels. A 'target quit date,' usually in the second week, should be set. Continue treatment for 7 to 12 weeks. If significant progress has not been made by week 7 of treatment, it is not likely client will stop smoking during this attempt. Thus, discontinue treatment.

8. Zyban may be combined with a nicotine transdermal system for smoking cessation.

9. Store immediate-release tablets at 15–25°C (59–77°F); sustained release at 20–25°C (68–77°F); and extended-release at 15–30°C (59–86°F). Protect immediate release from light and moisture. Dispense sustained release in a tight, light-resistant container.

ASSESSMENT

1. List reasons for therapy, presenting behaviors, duration of symptoms, other agents/therapies trialed.

2. Note history of seizures, recent MI, head trauma, CNS tumor, bulimia, anorexia nervosa; precludes therapy.

3. Determine if of childbearing age or lactating.

4. Monitor lung sounds, weight, ECG, renal and LFTs; reduce dose with renal/liver dysfunction.

5. Assess mental stability and potential for compliance. Fewer side effects (no CV effects, drug interactions, sedation, and weight gain) with bupropion than other antidepressants.

6. With tobacco abuse, ensure ready to quit; note numbers of cigarettes smoked per day, nicotine content, triggers, other failures, and date desired to quit so that treatment can be started 1 week prior.

CLIENT/FAMILY TEACHING

1. Take as directed for condition treated. Do not take Zyban with Wellbutrin and do not break, crush or chew sustained release products.

2. May experience changes in taste perception; may result in appetite/weight loss. Record weights; report changes.

3. May cause menstrual irregularities and impotence. Report changes in urinary output.

4. Beneficial drug effects for depression may not be evident for 5–21 days. Continue and do not be discouraged by delayed response. Do not stop abruptly with prolonged therapy.

5. Dizziness may occur. Do not arise from lying position suddenly. If dizziness occurs during the day, sit until it subsides. May cause drowsiness, hyperactivity, GI upset, diarrhea, constipation, dry mouth. Avoid activities that require mental alertness until effects realized.

6. Report for F/U so that therapy/dosage may be evaluated/adjusted as needed.

7. Report mood swings, suicidal ideations immediately and other adverse side effects.

8. Avoid OTC agents without approval and alcohol; increases seizure risk.

9. With sustained-released formulation, for smoking cessation, will be started at a low dose for twice a day consumption. Take last dose 4 to 6 hr before bedtime to prevent insomnia. May be used with nicotine patch if needed. Start therapy while still smoking- takes about one week to achieve desired drug level; should stop smoking by week two. A formal smoking cessation program will enhance positive response rates.

OUTCOMES/EVALUATE

- Improvement in S&S of depression such as ↓ fatigue, improved eating and sleeping patterns, and ↑ socialization
- Successful nicotine/smoking cessation

Bold Italic = life threatening side effect   ■ = black box warning   ✢ = Available in Canada

Buspirone hydrochloride ⓒ
(byou-**SPYE**-rohn)

B

CLASSIFICATION(S):
Antianxiety drug, nonbenzodiazepine

PREGNANCY CATEGORY: B

Rx: BuSpar.

✤Rx: Apo-Buspirone, Gen-Buspirone, Lin-Buspirone, Novo-Buspirone, Nu-Buspirone, PMS-Buspirone, ratio-Buspirone.

USES
(1) Management of anxiety disorders. (2) Short-term relief of symptoms of anxiety. *Investigational:* Adjunct in treating withdrawal from heroin.

ACTION/KINETICS
Action
The mechanism of action is unknown. Not chemically related to the benzodiazepines; no anticonvulsant, muscle relaxant properties, or significant sedation seen. Binds to serotonin ($5\text{-}HT_{1A}$) and dopamine (D_2) receptors in the CNS; is possible that dopamine-mediated neurologic disorders may occur. These include dystonia, Parkinson-like symptoms, akathisia, and tardive dyskinesia.

Pharmacokinetics
Peak plasma levels: 1–6 ng/mL 40–90 min after a single PO dose of 20 mg. Bioavailability is increased when given with food. **$t\frac{1}{2}$:** 2–3 hr. Rapidly absorbed with extensive first-pass metabolism; active and inactive metabolites excreted in the urine and through the feces. **Plasma protein binding:** About 86%.

CONTRAINDICATIONS
Psychoses, severe liver or kidney impairment, lactation. Not usually indicated for treatment of anxiety and tension due to stress of everyday living.

SPECIAL CONCERNS
A decrease in dose may be necessary in geriatric clients due to age-related impairment of renal function.

SIDE EFFECTS
Most Common
Dizziness, drowsiness, nausea, headache, nervousness, lightheadedness, excitement.
Side effects listed have an incidence of 0.1% or more. **CNS:** Dizziness, drowsiness, headache, nervousness, insomnia, lightheadedness, decreased concentration, excitement, anger/hostility, confusion, numbness, depression, tremor, incoordination, paresthesia, dream disturbances, depersonalization, dysphoria, noise intolerance, euphoria, akathisia, fearfulness, loss of interest, dissociative reaction, hallucinations, involuntary movements, slowed reaction times, *suicidal ideation, seizures*. **GI:** N&V, dry mouth, abdominal/gastric distress, diarrhea, constipation, flatulence, anorexia, increased appetite, salivation, irritable colon, rectal bleeding. **CV:** Tachycardia/palpitations, nonspecific chest pain, syncope, hypotension, hypertension. **Dermatologic:** Skin rash, edema, pruritus, flushing, easy bruising, hair loss, dry skin, facial, edema, blisters. **GU:** Increased or decreased libido, urinary frequency, urinary hesitancy, menstrual irregularity, spotting, dysuria. **Musculoskeletal:** Aches/pains, muscle cramps, muscle spasms, rigid/stiff muscles, arthralgia. **Respiratory:** Hyperventilation, SOB, chest congestion, sore throat, nasal congestion. **Ophthalmic:** Blurred vision, redness and itching of eye, conjunctivitis. **Body as a whole:** Fatigue, weakness, sweating/clamminess, weight gain/loss, fever, malaise. **Miscellaneous:** Tinnitus, altered taste, altered smell, roaring sensation in the head.

LABORATORY TEST CONSIDERATIONS
↑ ALT, AST.

OD OVERDOSE MANAGEMENT
Symptoms: Dizziness, drowsiness, N&V, gastric distress, miosis. *Treatment:* Immediate gastric lavage; general symptomatic and supportive measures. Monitor respiration, pulse, and BP.

DRUG INTERACTIONS
Alcohol / Avoid concomitant use
Carbamazepine / ↓ Plasma buspirone levels R/T induction of metabolism by CYP3A4 liver enzymes

---

📷 = see color insert   H = Herbal   IV = Intravenous   ⓒ = sound alike drug

B

Cimetidine / ↑ Buspirone C_{max} and T_{max} but minimal effects on AUC

Clarithromycin / ↑ Plasma buspirone levels R/T inhibition of metabolism by CYP3A4 liver enzymes

Dexamethasone / ↓ Plasma buspirone levels R/T induction of metabolism by CYP3A4 liver enzymes

Diazepam / Possible dizziness, headache, and nausea

Diltiazem / ↑ Plasma buspirone levels R/T inhibition of metabolism by CYP3A4 liver enzymes

Erythromycin / ↑ Plasma buspirone levels R/T inhibition of metabolism by CYP3A4 liver enzymes

Fluoxetine / ↓ Buspirone effects

Fluvoxamine / ↑ Plasma buspirone levels R/T inhibition of metabolism by CYP3A4 liver enzymes

Grapefruit juice / ↑ Plasma levels of buspirone → excess sedation

Haloperidol / Possible ↑ haloperidol levels

Itraconazole / ↑ Plasma buspirone levels R/T inhibition of metabolism by CYP3A4 liver enzymes

Ketoconazole / ↑ Plasma buspirone levels R/T inhibition of metabolism by CYP3A4 liver enzymes

MAO inhibitors / ↑ BP; do not use together

Nefazodone / Possible lightheadedness, asthenia, dizzinesss, and somnolence; use a lower dose (2.5 mg/day) of buspirone

Phenobarbital / ↓ Plasma buspirone levels R/T induction of metabolism by CYP3A4 liver enzymes

Phenytoin / ↓ Plasma buspirone levels R/T induction of metabolism by CYP3A4 liver enzymes

Rifabutin / ↓ Plasma buspirone levels R/T induction of metabolism by CYP3A4 liver enzymes

Rifampin / ↓ Plasma buspirone levels R/T induction of metabolism by CYP3A4 liver enzymes

Ritonavir / ↑ Plasma buspirone levels R/T inhibition of metabolism by CYP3A4 liver enzymes

Verapamil / ↑ Plasma buspirone levels R/T inhibition of metabolism by CYP3A4 liver enzymes

HOW SUPPLIED
Tablets: 5 mg, 7.5 mg, 10 mg, 15 mg, 30 mg.

DOSAGE
- **TABLETS**
  Anxiety disorders, short-term relief of anxiety.
  Adults: 7.5 mg 2 times per day (i.e., 15 mg daily). May increase dose in increments of 5 mg/day q 2–3 days to achieve optimum effects; do not exceed a total daily dose of 60 mg. Divided doses of 20 to 30 mg/day have been commonly used.

NURSING CONSIDERATIONS
� Do not confuse buspirone with bupropion (antidepressant, smoking deterrent).

ADMINISTRATION/STORAGE
1. No cross-tolerance with other sedative-hypnotic drugs, including benzodiazepines.
2. Will not block the withdrawal syndrome, which may occur following cessation of sedative-hypnotics. Withdraw clients on chronic sedative-hypnotic therapy gradually prior to beginning buspirone therapy.
3. To date, no potential for abuse, tolerance, or either physical/psychologic dependence.
4. Up to 2 weeks may be required before beneficial antianxiety effects manifested.

ASSESSMENT
1. Document reasons for therapy; note pretreatment findings.
2. Determine support systems; encourage active family involvement in treatment plan.
3. Assess for recent benzodiazepine therapy; drug may be less effective.
4. Document mental status and note age; good agent to use in elderly because of less CNS suppression.
5. Determine causative factor/event that precipitated disorder.
6. Evaluate for history of drug abuse; observe for signs of misuse/abuse.

CLIENT/FAMILY TEACHING
1. Take in a consistent manner with respect to timing of dosing—either al-

---

Bold Italic = life threatening side effect   ■ = black box warning   ✤ = Available in Canada

ways with or without food; food increases bioavailability.

2. Take with food or snack to decrease nausea, a common side effect; report if persistent/severe.

3. May cause drowsiness/dizziness. Use caution when operating a motor vehicle or performing tasks that require mental alertness.

4. Avoid OTC agents and alcohol.

5. Avoid prolonged/excessive exposure to direct or artificial sunlight.

6. Do not stop suddenly; withdrawal symptoms such as N&V, dry mouth, nasal congestion, or sore throat may occur.

7. Report weakness, restlessness, nervousness, headaches, feelings of depression or lack of desired response.

8. Report involuntary, repetitive movements of the face or neck muscles, (Parkinson-like symptoms) or suicide ideations immediately.

9. Separate buspirone dosage by 6–8 hr from ingestion of grapefruit juice.

OUTCOMES/EVALUATE
Relief of agitated depressive S&S; ↓ anxiety

Busulfan

(byou-**SUL**-fan)

CLASSIFICATION(S):
Antineoplastic, alkylating
PREGNANCY CATEGORY: D
Rx: Busulfex, Myleran.

SEE ALSO *ANTINEOPLASTIC AGENTS* AND *ALKYLATING AGENTS*.

USES
Injection: With cyclophosphamide as a conditioning treatment prior to allogeneic hematopoietic progenitor cell transplantation for chronic myelogenous leukemia (CML).

Tablets: Palliative treatment of CML (granulocytic, myelocytic, myeloid). Less effective in individuals with CML who lack the Philadelphia (Ph₁) chromosome. Not effective in individuals where the disease is in the 'blastic' phase. *Investigational:* Other myeloproliferative

disorders, including severe thrombocytosis and polycythemia vera, myelofibrosis; bone marrow transplantation.

ACTION/KINETICS
Action
Is an alkylating agent. Busulfan hydrolyzes to release methylsulfonate groups that produce reactive carbonium ions; these ions can alkylate DNA. DNA damage is thought to be responsible for the cytotoxicity of busulfan. Leukocyte count drops during the second or third week; thus, weekly laboratory tests are mandatory. Resistance may develop; thought to be due to the altered transport into the cell and/or increased intracellular inactivation.

Pharmacokinetics
Rapidly and completely absorbed from the GI tract; appears in serum 0.6–2 hr after PO administration. **t½, elimination:** About 2.6 hr. Extensively metabolized by conjugation with glutathione and excreted in the urine. Clearance is more rapid in children than in adults. Increased appetite and sense of wellbeing may occur a few days after therapy is started. Sometimes administered with allopurinol to prevent symptoms of clinical gout. **Plasma protein binding:** 32% and 47% bound to plasma proteins and RBCs, respectively.

CONTRAINDICATIONS
Use of tablets unless a diagnosis of CML has been adequately established. Hypersensitivity to busulfan or any component of the product. Lactation.

SPECIAL CONCERNS
■ (1) Busulfan is a potent cytotoxic drug. Do not use unless a diagnosis of chronic myelogenous leukemia has been adequately established and the responsible healthcare provider is knowledgeable in assessing response to chemotherapy. (2) Busulfan can induce severe bone marrow hypoplasia. Reduce or discontinue the dosage immediately at the first sign of any unusual depression of bone marrow function as reflected by an abnormal decrease in any of the formed elements of the blood. Perform a bone marrow examination if the bone marrow status is uncertain. (3) Malignant tumors and acute

leukemias have been reported in clients who have received busulfan therapy, and this drug may be a human carcinogen. The World Health Organization has concluded that there is a causal relationship between busulfan exposure and the development of secondary malignancies. Four cases of acute leukemia occurred among 243 clients treated with busulfan as adjuvant chemotherapy following surgical resection of bronchogenic carcinoma. All 4 cases were from a subgroup of 19 of these 243 clients who developed pancytopenia while taking busuflan 5 to 8 years before leukemia became clinically apparent. These findings suggest that busulfan is leukemogenic, although its mode of action is uncertain.■ Avoid use of live vaccines to immunocompromised clients. Safety and efficacy of the injection have not been established in children.

SIDE EFFECTS

Most Common

Profound myelosuppression, N&V, stomatitis (mucositis), diarrhea, anorexia, abdominal pain, insomnia, anxiety, fever, headache.

Hematologic: *Pancytopenia, severe bone marrow hypoplasia,* anemia, leukopenia, thrombocytopenia, *aplastic anemia.* **GI:** N&V, stomatitis (mucositits), esophagitis, anorexia, diarrhea, abdominal pain/enlargement, ileus, dyspepsia, constipation, dry mouth, rectal disorder/discomfort, hematemesis, pancreatitis. **Hepatic:** Jaundice, hepatomegaly, *hepatotoxicity,* centrilobular sinusoidal fibrosis, hepatocellular atrophy/necrosis, *hepatic venoocclusive disease.* **CNS:** Insomnia, anxiety, dizziness, depression, confusion, lethargy, hallucinations, delirium, encephalopathy, agitation, seizures, somnolence, *cerebral hemorrhage/coma.* **Respiratory:** *Bronchopulmonary dysplasia with interstitial pulmonary fibrosis.* Rhinitis, lung disorder, cough, epistaxis, dyspnea, pharyngitis, hiccup, asthma, alveolar hemorrhage, hemoptysis, pleural effusion, sinusitis, atelectasis, hypoxia, pneumonitis. **CV:** Tachycardia, hypertension, thrombosis, vasodilation

(flushing, hot flashes) hypotension, arrhythmia, cardiomegaly, atrial fibrillation, abnormal ECG, heart block, left-sided heart failure, pericardial effusion, ventricular extrasystoles, third degree heart block, *endocardial fibrosis. Cardiac tamponade in children with thalessemia.* **Ophthalmologic:** Cataracts after prolonged use, corneal thining, lens changes. **Dermatologic:** Hyperpigmentation, especially in clients with a dark complexion. Rash, pruritus, alopecia, vesicular rash, vesiculobullous rash, maculopapular rash, acne, exfoliative dermatitis, erythema nodosum, increased local cutaneous reaction after radiotherapy. **Metabolic:** Syndrome resembling adrenal insufficiency, including symptoms of weakness, severe fatigue, weight loss, anorexia, N&V, and melanoderma (especially after prolonged use). Also, hyperuricemia/uricosuria in clients with CML. **GU:** Oliguria, hematuria, dysuria, hemorrhagic cystitis. **Miscellaneous:** Cellular dysplasia in various organs, including lymph nodes, pancreas, thyroid, adrenal glands, bone marrow, and liver. Also, fever, edema, headache, asthenia, infection, *sepsis,* chills, pain, allergic reaction, chest/back pain, myalgia, inflammation at injection site, arthralgia, pneumonia, ear disorder. Malignant tumors and acute leukemias are possible.

LABORATORY TEST CONSIDERATIONS

↑ AST, alkaline phosphatase, creatinine. Hyperbilirubinemia, hyperglycemia, hypocalcemia, hypokalemia, hypomagnesemia, hypophosphatemia, hyponatremia, hyperuricemia, hyperuricosuria.

OD OVERDOSE MANAGEMENT

Symptoms: Bone marrow toxicity, CNS stimulation with convulsions and death on the first day. Treatment: If ingestion is recent, gastric lavage or induction of vomiting followed by activated charcoal. Hematologic status must be monitored.

DRUG INTERACTIONS

Acetaminophen / ↓ Busulfan clearance
Cyclophosphamide / Cardiac tamponade in clients with thalessemia (rare), but possibly fatal in those receiving high

---

doses of both drugs
Cytotoxic drugs / Additive pulmonary toxicity
Itraconazole / ↓ Busulfan clearance up to 25%
Metronidazole / ↑ Trough plasma busulfan levels → ↑ risk of toxicity; do not use together
Myelosuppressive drugs / Additive myelosuppression
Phenytoin / ↑ Busulfan clearance by 15% or more R/T induction of glutathione-S-transferase
Thioguanine / ↑ Risk of esophageal varices with abnormal LFTs; use with caution in long-term continuous therapy

HOW SUPPLIED
Injection: 6 mg/mL; *Tablets:* 2 mg.

DOSAGE

• **TABLETS**
   CML.
Adults or children, remission induction, usual dose: 4–8 mg/day (about 60 mcg/kg or 1.8 mg/m^2 per day) until leukocyte count falls below 15,000/mcL; then, withdraw drug. **Maintenance, when leukocyte reaches about 50,000/mcL:** Resume treatment with induction dosage. When remission is less than 3 mo, consider 1–3 mg/day that may keep client under control and prevent rapid relapse.

• **IV VIA A CENTRAL VENOUS CATHETER.**
   With cyclophosphamide prior to allogeneic hematopoietic progenitor cell transplantation.
Adults: 0.8 mg/kg of IBW or actual body weight (whichever is lower) of busulfan q 6 hr for 4 days (i.e., total of 16 doses). For obese or severely obese clients, calculate the dose of busulfan based on adjusted IBW. For cyclophosphamide, 60 mg/kg given on each of 2 days as a 1-hr infusion beginning on BMT day minus 3, 6 hr following the 16th busulfan dose.

NURSING CONSIDERATIONS

⚕ Do not confuse Alkeran (melphalan), Leukeran (chlorambucil), and Myleran (busulfan), each of which is an antineoplastic.

ADMINISTRATION/STORAGE

IV 1. Do not administer without supervision and facilities for weekly CBCs.
2. Premedicate all clients with phenytoin since busulfan crosses the blood brain barrier and induces seizures.
3. Give antiemetics prior to the first dose of busulfan; continue on a fixed schedule through busulfan administration.
4. Busulfan via central catheter as a 2-hr infusion (using an infusion pump) q 6 hr for 4 consecutive days. Cyclophosphamide is given IV as a 1-hr infusion each day for 2 days beginning 6 hr following the 16th busulfan dose.
5. Dilute busulfan prior to use with either 0.9% NaCl injection or D5W. The diluent quantity should be 10 times the volume of busulfan, ensuring the final concentration is about 0.5 mg/mL or more. To prepare final solution for infusion, add 9.3 mL of busulfan to 93 mL of diluent. Always add busulfan to diluent, not diluent to busulfan. Mix thoroughly by inverting several times.
6. Diluted busulfan stable at room temperature for up to 8 hr; infusion must be completed by that time. Busulfan diluted in 0.9% NaCl is stable for up to 12 hr if refrigerated; infusion must be completed by that time.
7. Exercise caution in handling and preparing busulfan solutions as skin reactions may occur with accidental exposure. Use a vertical laminar flow safety hood; wear gloves and protective clothing.
8. Do not infuse rapidly or at the same time with any other IV solution of unknown compatibility.
9. *NOTE:* Consult the package insert for information on blood sample collection for AUC determination, instructions for drug administration and blood sample collection for therapeutic drug monitoring, and preparation for IV administration.

ASSESSMENT
1. Note history of disease, previous experience with drug therapy, any noted resistance.

B

2. Monitor renal and LFTs; CBC/platelets weekly during therapy and for 2 weeks after stopping therapy.

3. In clients with CML note presence of Philadelphia (Ph₁) chromosome. Document when disease in 'blastic' phase as drug is not effective.

4. Monitor VS and I&O. Give plenty of fluids and allopurinol to decrease uric acid levels with resultant nephropathy.

5. Assess CXR/lung sounds; may experience pulmonary fibrosis up to 4–6 months following therapy.

6. May require premedication with IV dilantin; decrease risk of seizures seen with IV infusions. Also start antiemetics before treatment on a regular schedule during IV therapy.

7. Drug may cause moderate to severe granulocyte suppression. Monitor appropriate weekly hematologic profiles. Nadir: 21 days; recovery: 42–56 days.

CLIENT/FAMILY TEACHING
1. Take at the same time each day. May take on an empty stomach if N&V occur. Extra fluid intake may be required to prevent dehydration.

2. Report early symptoms of sore throat, infection, easy bruising/bleeding; expect weekly CBC studies and keep all F/U visits.

3. Avoid vaccinations, persons infected, or those who have recently taken live virus vaccine, and all OTC agents without approval.

4. Practice reliable contraception.

5. Report skin rash immediately; may cause increased pigmentation, hair loss.

6. Allopurinol may be prescribed to decrease urate crystal formation.

7. Increased cough and visual difficulties may be S&S toxicity; report increased weight loss, fatigue, loss of appetite, blurred vision, weakness.

OUTCOMES/EVALUATE
• Maintenance of leukocytes at 20,000/mcL
• Absence of blasts on peripheral blood smear; ↓ spleen size

— **COMBINATION DRUG** —

Butalbital, Acetaminophen, and Caffeine

(byoo-**TAL**-bi-tall, ah-**SEAT**-ah-**MIN**-oh-fen, **KAF**-een)

CLASSIFICATION(S):
Barbiturate/Nonnarcotic analgesic/Stimulant combination drug
PREGNANCY CATEGORY: C
Rx: Esgic, Fioricet, Margesic, Medigesic, Repan, Triad.

SEE ALSO *ACETAMINOPHEN.*

USES
Treatment of tension headaches or mild migraine headaches.

CONTENT
Each capsule or tablet contains: Butalbital (barbiturate), 50 mg; acetaminophen (nonnarcotic analgesic), 325 mg; and, caffeine (CNS stimulant), 40 mg.

ACTION/KINETICS

Action
The role of each component in the relief of tension headaches is not completely understood.

Pharmacokinetics
Butalbital is well absorbed from the GI tract. It is excreted primarily in the urine as unchanged drug and metabolites. **t½, plasma:** About 35 hr. Acetaminophen is rapidly absorbed from the GI tract. **t½, plasma:** 1.25–3 hr (may be increased by liver damage or overdosage). Acetaminophen is metabolized by the liver and excreted in the urine as unchanged drug and metabolites. Caffeine is also rapidly absorbed. **t½, plasma:** About 3 hr. It is metabolized by the liver and excreted, mostly as metabolites, in the urine.

CONTRAINDICATIONS
Hypersensitivity to any component of the product. Porphyria. Since butalbital is habit-forming and potentially abused, extended use is not recommended.

Bold Italic = life threatening side effect   ■ = black box warning   ✦ = Available in Canada

SPECIAL CONCERNS

Use with caution in the elderly, debilitated, in those with severe renal or hepatic impairment, or acute abdominal conditions. Use during pregnancy only when clearly needed. Safety and efficacy have not been established in children 12 years of age and less.

SIDE EFFECTS

Most Common

Drowsiness, lightheadedness, dizziness, sedation, shortness of breath, N&V, abdominal pain, intoxicated feeling.

CNS: Headache, drowsiness, lightheadedness, dizziness, sedation, intoxicated feeling, shaky feeling, tingling, agitation, fainting, heavy eyelids, high energy, hot spells, numbness, sluggishness, dependence, irritability, *seizures*. Mental confusion, excitement, or depression due to intolerance (especially in the elderly or debilitated). **GI:** N&V, abdominal pain, dry mouth, difficulty swallowing, heartburn, flatulence, constipation. **CV:** Tachycardia, cardiac stimulation. **Musculoskeletal:** Leg pain, muscle fatigue. **Hematologic:** Thrombocytopenia, *agranulocytosis*. **Respiratory:** Nasal congestion, SOB. **Otic:** Earache, tinnitus. **GU:** Diuresis, nephrotoxicity. **Dermatologic:** Pruritus, rash, erythema multiforme, *toxic epidermal necrolysis*. **Body as a whole:** Hyperhidrosis, fatigue, euphoria, allergic reactions, tremor, fever. **Miscellaneous:** Hyperglycemia.

OD **OVERDOSE MANAGEMENT**

Symptoms: **Symptoms due to butalbital:** Drowsiness, confusion, coma, respiratory depression, hypotension, *hypovolemic shock*. **Symptoms due to acetaminophen:** Potentially fatal *hepatic necrosis, renal tubular necrosis, hypoglycemic coma*, thrombocytopenia, N&V, diaphoresis, general malaise. *NOTE:* Clinical and laboratory evidence of hepatic toxicity may not be apparent until 48–72 hr after ingestion. **Symptoms due to caffeine:** Insomnia, restlessness, tremor, delirium, tachycardia, extrasystoles. *Treatment:* Overdose is potentially fatal. Immediate treatment includes:

- Induction of vomiting.
- Gastric lavage. A cuffed endotracheal tube should be inserted prior to gastric lavage if the client is unconscious.
- Oral activated charcoal (1 gram/kg) should follow gastric emptying. Follow the first dose of charcoal with an appropriate cathartic. If repeated doses are needed, give consideration to giving the cathartic with alternate charcoal doses.
- Treat hypotension with fluids as it is likely due to hypovolemia. Avoid pressors.
- Maintain adequate pulmonary ventilation.
- If renal function is normal, forced diuresis may help in the elimination of butalbital.
- Alkalinization of the urine increases renal excretion of some barbiturates.
- In severe cases of intoxication, peritoneal dialysis or hemodialysis may be considered.
- If hypoprothrombinemia occurs R/T acetaminophen, give IV vitamin K.
- If the dose of acetaminophen exceeded 140 mg/kg, give acetylcysteine asap. Obtain acetaminophen serum levels, since levels four or more hours after ingestion help predict toxicity. Do not wait for acetaminophen assay results before initiating treatment. Obtain hepatic enzyme levels initially and at 24-hr intervals.
- Treat methemoglobinemia over 30% with IV methylene blue.

DRUG INTERACTIONS

See also *Acetaminophen*.

CNS depressants (other narcotic analgesics, general anesthetics, alcohol, antianxiety drug, sedative-hypnotics) / Additive CNS depression

MAO inhibitors / ↑ Butalbital effects

HOW SUPPLIED

See Content.

DOSAGE

- **TABLETS**

    Tension headache or mild migraine headache.

    Adults: 1 or 2 tablets q 4 hr, not to exceed 6 tablets a day.

B

NURSING CONSIDERATIONS

ADMINISTRATION/STORAGE

1. Since butalbital is habit-forming, it should be taken only for as long as prescribed, in the amounts prescribed, and no more frequently than prescribed.

2. Store from 15–30°C (59–86°F). Dispense in a tight, light-resistant container.

ASSESSMENT

1. Note reasons for therapy, characteristics of headaches, other agents trialed, outcome.

2. Assess renal and LFTs; avoid with porphyria, use sparingly in the elderly or debilitated and those with acute abdominal problems.

CLIENT/FAMILY TEACHING

1. Take as directed with a full glass of water.

2. Do not perform activities that require mental alertness until drug effects realized; may cause dizziness/drowsiness.

3. Avoid alcohol and CNS drugs with this therapy. Store safely away from bedside and out of reach of children to prevent OD which may be fatal.

4. May cause dependence; do not stop suddenly without provider supervision.

5. Practice reliable contraception.

6. Report adverse side effects or lack of response. Keep all F/U appointments to evaluate response to therapy.

OUTCOMES/EVALUATE

Control of headaches

Butenafine hydrochloride

(byou-**TEN**-ah-feen)

CLASSIFICATION(S):
Antifungal
PREGNANCY CATEGORY: B
OTC: Lotrimin Ultra.
Rx: Mentax.

SEE ALSO *ANTI-INFECTIVE DRUGS.*

USES

Rx: (1) Treat interdigital tinea pedis (athlete's foot), tinea corporis (ringworm), and tinea cruris (jock itch) due to *Epidermophyton floccosum*, *Trichophyton mentagrophytes*, *T. rubrum*, or *T. tonsurans*. (2) Treatment of tinea (pityriasis) versicolor due to *Malassezia fufur*.
OTC: (1) Superficial dermatophytoses. (2) Athlete's foot between toes, jock itch, ringworm and the accompanying itching, burning, cracking, and scaling that usually accompanies these conditions.

ACTION/KINETICS

Action

Acts by inhibiting epoxidation of squalene, thus blocking the synthesis of ergosterol, an essential component of fungal cell membranes. Depending on the concentration and the fungal species, the drug may be fungicidal.

Pharmacokinetics

Although applied topically, some of the drug is absorbed into the general circulation.

SPECIAL CONCERNS

Use with caution during lactation and in clients sensitive to allylamine antifungal drugs as the drugs may be cross-reactive. Safety and efficacy have not been determined in children less than 12 years of age.

SIDE EFFECTS

Most Common

Burning, stinging, itching.

Dermatologic: Contact dermatitis, burning, stinging, worsening of the condition, erythema, irritation, itching.

HOW SUPPLIED

Cream: 1%.

DOSAGE

• **CREAM (1%)**

Tinea versicolor, tinea corporis, tinea cruris.

Apply the cream to cover the affected area and immediate surrounding skin once daily for 2 weeks.

Interdigital tinea pedis.

Apply twice a day for 7 days or once daily for 4 weeks.

NURSING CONSIDERATIONS

ADMINISTRATION/STORAGE

1. For external use only; not for ophthalmic, PO, or intravaginal use.

---

2. Store the drug between 5–30°C (41–86°F).

ASSESSMENT
1. Note reasons for therapy, duration, and characteristics of symptoms.
2. Describe clinical presentation. List other agents trialed and results.

CLIENT/FAMILY TEACHING
1. Review method for site preparation and application of cream; wash hands before and after applying.
2. After bathing, dry feet thoroughly/carefully between each toe before applying; avoid occlusive dressings.
3. Avoid contact with the eyes, nose, mouth, other mucous membranes.
4. Do not stop therapy when condition shows improvement; continue for full prescribed time (usually 2–4 wk).
5. Stop therapy and report any increased swelling, itching, burning, blistering, drainage, irritation, or lack of improvement.

OUTCOMES/EVALUATE
Resolution of fungal infection

Butoconazole nitrate
(byou-toe-**KON**-ah-zohl)

CLASSIFICATION(S):
Antifungal
PREGNANCY CATEGORY: C
OTC: Femstat 3, Mycelex-3.
Rx: Gynazole-1.

USES
Vulvovaginal fungal infections caused by *Candida albicans.*

ACTION/KINETICS
Action
By permeating chitin in the fungal cell wall, butoconazole increases membrane permeability to intracellular substances, leading to reduced osmotic resistance and viability of the fungus.

Pharmacokinetics
Approximately 1.7% of drug is absorbed following vaginal administration. $t^{1/2}$: 21–24 hr.

CONTRAINDICATIONS
Use during first trimester of pregnancy.

SPECIAL CONCERNS
Pediatric dosage has not been established. Use with caution during lactation.

SIDE EFFECTS
Most Common
See below.
GU: Vaginal burning, vulvar burning or itching, discharge; soreness, swelling, and itching of the fingers.

HOW SUPPLIED
Vaginal Cream: 2%.

DOSAGE
- **VAGINAL CREAM**
  Vulvovaginal infections.
One applicatorful of Gynazole-1 intravaginally once (remains in vaginal vault for approximately four days). Or, one applicatorful a day of Mycelex-3, preferably at bedtime, for three consecutive days.

NURSING CONSIDERATIONS
ADMINISTRATION/STORAGE
1. During pregnancy, use of a vaginal applicator may be contraindicated.
2. If no response, repeat studies to confirm the diagnosis before reinstituting antifungal therapy.
3. Not to be stored above 40°C (104°F).

ASSESSMENT
1. List onset, characteristics of S&S, other contributing factors.
2. Determine if pregnant.
3. Assess vault, obtain cultures, labs as needed.

CLIENT/FAMILY TEACHING
1. Review technique; insert cream high into the vagina. S&S of vulvovaginal candidiasis usually take 3 days to resolve (6 days if pregnant).
2. Use as prescribed and continue during menstrual cycle, with OCs, and antibiotic therapy.
3. Report irritation, burning, or lack of desired response.
4. Use sanitary napkins to prevent soiling and staining of undergarments, clothing, bedding.
5. To prevent reinfection, partner should use a condom during intercourse and receive treatment if symptomatic.

---

6. If having recurrent vaginal infections, exposed to HIV, consult provider to determine the cause of symptoms. If symptoms return within 2 months, R/O pregnancy or serious underlying medical cause (e.g., diabetes, HIV infection). Keep all F/U to assess response.

OUTCOMES/EVALUATE
Eradication of fungal infection; symptomatic improvement

Butorphanol tartrate   IV Ⓒ
(byou-**TOR**-fah-nohl)

CLASSIFICATION(S):
Narcotic agonist/antagonist
PREGNANCY CATEGORY: C
Rx: Stadol, **C-IV**

SEE ALSO *NARCOTIC ANALGESICS.*

USES
Parenteral and nasal: Moderate-to-severe pain, especially after surgery. **Parenteral:** (1) Preoperative medication. (2) To supplement balanced anesthesia. (3) Pain during labor. **Nasal:** Treatment of migraine headaches.

ACTION/KINETICS

Action
Has both narcotic agonist and antagonist properties. Analgesic potency may be up to 7 times that of morphine and 30–40 times that of meperidine. Overdosage responds to naloxone. After IV use, CV effects include increased PA pressure, PCWP, LVED pressure, system arterial pressure, PVR, and increased cardiac work load.

Pharmacokinetics
Onset, IM: 10–15 min; **IV:** rapid; **nasal:** within 15 min. **Duration, IM, IV:** 3–4 hr; **nasal:** 4–5 hr. **Peak analgesia, IM, IV:** 30–60 min; **nasal:** 1–2 hr. **t½, IM:** 2.1–8.8 hr; **nasal:** 2.9–9.2 hr. The t½ is increased up to 25% in clients over 65 years of age. Metabolized in the liver and excreted by the kidney; increase the dosing interval in renal or hepatic impairment. The drug has about 1/40 the narcotic antagonist activity as na-

loxone. *NOTE:* 1 mg of tartrate salt is equal to 0.68 mg base.

CONTRAINDICATIONS
Use of the nasal form during labor or delivery. Children less than 18 years of age.

SPECIAL CONCERNS
Safe use during pregnancy, during labor for premature infants, or in children under 18 years not established. Use with extreme caution in clients with AMI, ventricular dysfunction, and coronary insufficiency (morphine or meperidine are preferred). Use with caution and in low dosage in clients with respiratory depression, severely limited respiratory reserve, bronchial asthma, obstructive respiratory conditions, or cyanosis. Use in clients physically dependent on narcotics will result in precipitation of a withdrawal syndrome. Geriatric clients may be more sensitive to side effects, especially dizziness.

SIDE EFFECTS
Most Common
After parenteral use: Somnolence, dizziness, N&V.
After nasal use: Nasal congestion, insomnia.
See *Narcotic Analgesics* for a complete list of possible side effects.

ADDITIONAL DRUG INTERACTIONS
Barbiturate anesthetics / Possible ↑ respiratory and CNS depression of butorphanol
Sumatriptan / Transient ↑ BP if used with butorphanol spray to treat migraine

HOW SUPPLIED
Injection: 1 mg/mL, 2 mg/mL; *Nasal Spray:* 10 mg/mL.

DOSAGE
• **IM**
    Analgesia.
Adults, usual: 2 mg q 3–4 hr, as necessary; **range:** 1–4 mg q 3–4 hr. Single doses should not exceed 4 mg.
    Preoperative/preanesthetic.
Adults: 2 mg 60–90 min before surgery. Individualize dosage.
    Labor.
Adults: 1–2 mg if at full term and during early labor. May be repeated after 4 hr.

- **IV**
  Analgesia.

Adults, usual: 1 mg q 3–4 hr; **range:** 0.5–2 mg q 3–4 hr. **Not recommended for use in children.**

  Balanced anesthesia.

Adults: 2 mg just before induction or 0.5–1 mg in increments during anesthesia. The increment may be up to 0.06 mg/kg, depending on drugs previously given. Total dose range: Less than 4 mg to less than 12.5 mg.

  Labor.

Adults: 1–2 mg if at full term and during early labor. May be repeated after 4 hr.

- **NASAL SPRAY**
  Analgesia.

Adults: 1 spray (1 mg) in one nostril. If pain relief is not reached within 60–90 min, an additional 1 mg may be given. The two-dose sequence may be repeated in 3–4 hr if necessary. In severe pain, 2 mg (1 spray in each nostril) may be given initially followed in 3–4 hr by additional 2-mg doses if needed. **Geriatric clients, initial:** Use one-half the usual dose at twice the usual interval. Subsequent doses and intervals are based on response.

NURSING CONSIDERATIONS

℗ Do not confuse Stadol with Haldol (antipsychotic).

ADMINISTRATION/STORAGE

1. Have naloxone for treatment of overdose.
2. Store nasal product below 30°C (86°F).
IV 3. If administered by direct IV infusion, may give undiluted at a rate of 2 mg or less over 3–5-min.

ASSESSMENT

1. Note if narcotic dependent; antagonist property of drug may precipitate acute withdrawal symptoms.
2. List reasons for therapy, characteristics of S&S; rate pain level.
3. Monitor VS, I&O, respiratory rate, CNS status during therapy.
4. With CV problems, morphine may be a preferred drug to use.
5. Give geriatric clients one-half usual dose at twice the usual interval. Have naloxone readily available.
6. With renal/hepatic impairment, increase initial dosage interval to 6–8 hr with subsequent intervals determined by client response.

CLIENT/FAMILY TEACHING

1. May cause dizziness, drowsiness, use caution with activities requiring mental alertness. Request assistance with ambulation.
2. With nasal therapy, clear nasal passages, tilt head back, shake container and insert nozzle into nostril. Administer into one nostril pointing away from the septum while holding the other nostril closed and sniff gently.
3. Cough and deep breathe every two hours following surgery to prevent atelectasis (lung collapse).
4. Drug is habit-forming when used for extended time. Withdrawal S&S may include, N&V, fever, restless/lightheadedness, loss of appetite, abdominal cramps.
5. Avoid alcohol or any CNS depressants. Report any adverse symptoms, lack of response, or allergic response.

OUTCOMES/EVALUATE

Relief of pain; termination of migraine headache

C

Calcitonin-salmon

(kal-si-**TOE**-nin)

CLASSIFICATION(S):
Calcium regulator
PREGNANCY CATEGORY: C
Rx: Fortical, Miacalcin.
❀Rx: Caltine, Miacalcin NS.

USES
Injection and nasal: Prevention of progressive loss of bone mass in postmenopausal osteoporosis in women more than 5 years postmenopause with low bone mass. Use the nasal product only in clients who cannot take estrogen.

Injection only: (1) Moderate to severe Paget's disease characterized by polyostotic involvement with elevated serum alkaline phosphatase and urinary hydroxyproline excretion. (2) Early treatment of hypercalcemic emergencies, along with other appropriate agents, when a rapid decrease in serum calcium is required (until more specific treatment can be accomplished). May be added to existing regimens for hypercalcemia.

ACTION/KINETICS
Action
Calcitonins are polypeptide hormones produced in mammals by the parafollicular cells of the thyroid gland. Calcitonin isolated from salmon has the same therapeutic effect as the human hormone, except for a greater potency per milligram and a somewhat longer duration of action. Ineffective when administered PO. Beneficial in Paget's disease of bone by reducing the rate of turnover of bone; the drug acts to block initial bone resorption, decreasing alkaline phosphatase levels in the serum, and urinary hydroxyproline excretion. Its effectiveness in treating osteoporosis or hypercalcemia is due to decreased serum calcium levels from direct inhibition of bone resorption.

Pharmacokinetics
Time to peak plasma levels, injection: 16–25 min; **nasal spray:** 31–39 min. **Duration:** 6–8 hr for hypercalcemia. **t½:** 43. Metabolized to inactive compounds in the kidneys, blood, and peripheral tissues.

CONTRAINDICATIONS
Allergy to calcitonin-salmon or its gelatin diluent.

SPECIAL CONCERNS
Circulating antibodies to calcitonin occur after 2–18 months in about one-half of Paget's disease clients. Use with caution during lactation. Safe use in children not established.

SIDE EFFECTS
Most Common
N&V, nasal symptoms after use of nasal spray (e.g., irritation, redness, sores, rhinitis), back pain, arthralgia, epistaxis, headache.

GI: N&V, anorexia, epigastric discomfort, salty taste, flatulence, increased appetite, gastritis, diarrhea, dry mouth, abdominal pain, dyspepsia, constipation. **CNS:** Dizziness, paresthesia, insomnia, anxiety, vertigo, migraine, neuralgia, agitation, depression (rare). **CV:** Hypertension, tachycardia, palpitation, bundle branch block, *MI*, *CVA*, *thrombophlebitis*, angina pectoris (rare). **Respiratory:** Sinusitis, URTI, pharyngitis, bronchitis, pneumonia, coughing, dyspnea, taste perversion, parosmia, *bronchospasm*. **Musculoskeletal:** Arthrosis, arthritis, polymyalgia rheumatica, stiffness, myalgia. **Dermatologic:** Inflammatory reactions at the injection site, flushing of face or hands, pruritus of ear lobes, edema of feet, skin rash/ulceration, eczema, alopecia, increased sweating. **Endocrine:** Goiter, hyperthyroidism. **Ophthalmic:** Abnormal lacrimation, conjunctivitis, eye pain, blurred vision, vitreous floater. **Otic:** Tinnitus, hearing loss, earache. **Hematologic:**

Lymphadenopathy, anemia, infection. **Metabolic:** Mild tetanic symptoms, asymptomatic mild hypercalcemia, cholelithiasis, thirst, hepatitis, weight increase. **Miscellaneous:** Flu-like symptoms, fatigue, nocturia, feverish sensation. Use of the nasal spray may cause rhinitis, nasal irritation/redness/sores, back pain, arthralgia, epistaxis, and headache.

LABORATORY TEST CONSIDERATIONS

↓ Alkaline phosphatase and 24-hr urinary excretion of hydroxyproline are indicative of successful therapy. Monitor urine for casts (indicative of kidney damage).

OD OVERDOSE MANAGEMENT
Symptoms: N&V.

HOW SUPPLIED

Injection: 200 international units/mL; *Nasal Spray:* 200 international units/activation.

DOSAGE

- **IM; SC**

  Paget's disease.

Adults, initial: 100 international units/day; **maintenance, usual:** 50 international units/day or every other day. Normalization of biochemical abnormalities and decreased bone pain usually seen in the first few months. Improvement of neurologic lesions requires more than 1 year.

  Hypercalcemia

Adults, initial: 4 international units/kg q 12 hr; **then,** increase the dose, if necessary after 1 or 2 days (i.e., if unsatisfactory response), to 8 international units/kg q 12 hr up to a maximum of 8 international units/kg q 6 hr. If the volume to be injected exceeds 2 mL by the SC route, give the dose IM with multiple sites used.

  Postmenopausal osteoporosis.

Adults: 100 international units/day given with calcium carbonate (1.5 grams/day) and vitamin D (400 units/day).

- **NASAL SPRAY**

  Postmenopausal (at least 5 years) osteoporosis.

200 international units (0.09 mL/activation) every day, alternating nostrils daily. Activate the pump before the first dose. Use in conjunction with calcium

supplements equivalent to at least 1,000 mg/day of elemental calcium and a vitamin D supplement of 400 international units/day.

NURSING CONSIDERATIONS

ADMINISTRATION/STORAGE

1. Check for hypersensitivity reactions. Give 1 international unit intracutaneously to inner forearm; observe for 15 min.
2. With Paget's disease, may require >1 year of therapy to treat neurologic lesions.
3. Store calcitonin-salmon injection between 2–6°C (36–43°F).
4. Store unopened nasal spray between 2–8°C. Once the pump has been activated, store at room temperature.

ASSESSMENT

1. Note hypersensitivity to drug/gelatin diluent.
2. List reasons for therapy, note baseline assessments, level of pain, age at onset, duration of disease, results of DEXA scan.
3. Review diet, intake of calcium/vitamin D; obtain levels prn.
4. Before therapy, get serum alkaline phosphatase and urinary hydroxyproline excretion. Repeat after 3 mo and q 3–6 months thereafter.

INTERVENTIONS

1. Perform test dose; note reactions at site/systemic allergic reactions.
2. Observe for hypocalcemic tetany, i.e., muscular fibrillation, twitching, tetanic spasms, convulsions. Check q 10 min for 30 min following injection; have IV calcium available.
3. Check for hypercalcemia/report, i.e., increased thirst, anorexia, polyuria, and N&V.
4. Assess for facial flushing, abdominal/epigastric distress, anorexia, diarrhea, changes in taste perception. Record weights, I&O; report if S&S persist.
5. If good clinical response initially, then relapse; check for antibody drug formation.

CLIENT/FAMILY TEACHING

1. With injection, use aseptic methods to reconstitute solution, proper injec-

C

tion technique, alternate sites. Review technique for nasal administration.

2. N&V may occur, should subside as treatment continues; report if persists, record weights.

3. With increased urine sediment, have urine tests- assess for kidney damage.

4. Continue regular exercise/activity; minimizes bone loss.

5. Take in evening to minimize flushing.

6. See dietitian for dietary adjustments.

OUTCOMES/EVALUATE

- ↓ Serum calcium, ↓ alkaline phosphatase, and ↓ 24-hr urinary excretion of hydroxyproline
- Promotion of bone formation with ↑ bone mass density
- ↓ Bone pain
- Halt in postmenopausal osteoporosis

Calcium carbonate

(**KAL**-see-um **KAR**-bon-ayt)

CLASSIFICATION(S):

Calcium salt

OTC: Capsules: Calci-Mix. **Gum:** Surpass, Surpass Extra Strength. **Tablets:** Cal-Carb Forte, Calcium-600, Caltrate 600, Nephro-Calci, Os-Cal 500, Oysco 500, Oyst-Cal 500, Oyster Shell Calcium, Trial Antacid, Tums, Tums Smooth Dissolve. **Tablets, Chewable:** Cal-Carb Forte, Cal-Gest, Calci-Chew, Calcium Antacid Extra Strength, Maalox Children's, Maalox Maximum Strength Quick Dissolve, Maalox Quick Dissolve, Mylanta Children's, Os-Cal 500, Rolaids Extra Strength Softchews, Tums Calcium for Life Bone Health, Tums Calcium for Life PMS, Tums E-X, Tums Ultra. ♣**OTC:** Apo-Cal, Calcite 500, Calcium 500, Calcium Oyster Shell.

SEE ALSO *CALCIUM SALTS.*

USES

(1) Mild hypocalcemia. (2) Antacid (including heartburn, sour stomach, and acid indigestion). (3) Antihyperphosphatemic. (4) Nutritional supplement.

SPECIAL CONCERNS

Dosage not established in children.

SIDE EFFECTS

Most Common

Constipation, headache, mild hypercalcemia (anorexia, N&V).

See *Calcium Salts* for a complete list of possible side effects.

ADDITIONAL DRUG INTERACTIONS

Omeprazole ↓ fractional calcium absorption in fasting elderly women

HOW SUPPLIED

Capsules: 125 mg, 1250 mg; *Gum:* 300 mg, 450 mg; *Gum Tablets:* 500 mg; *Lozenges:* 600 mg; *Powder:* 6,500 mg/packet; *Suspension:* 1,250 mg/5 mL; *Tablets:* 250 mg, 420 mg, 500 mg, 600 mg, 650 mg, 667 mg, 750 mg, 1,000 mg, 1,250 mg, 1,500 mg; *Tablets, Chewable:* 350 mg, 400 mg, 450 mg, 500 mg, 750 mg, 850 mg, 1,000 mg, 1,177 mg, 1,250 mg.

DOSAGE

- **LOZENGES; SUSPENSION; TABLETS; TABLETS, CHEWABLE**

    Antacid.

Adults: 0.5–1.5 grams, as needed.

- **GUM**

    Antacid

Chew 1 or 2 pieces (300–900 mg total dose) as symptoms occur. Repeat hourly if symptoms return or as directed by provider. Do not take more than 26 pieces per day of the 300 mg dosage form or more than 17 pieces per day of the 450 mg dosage form for more than 2 weeks.

- **CAPSULES; GUM TABLETS; SUSPENSION; TABLETS; TABLETS, CHEWABLE**

    Hypocalcemia, nutritional supplement.

Adults: 1.25–1.5 grams 1–3 times per day with or after meals.

    Antihyperphosphatemic.

Adults: 5–13 grams/day in divided doses with meals. *NOTE:* The preparation contains 40% elemental calcium and 400 mg elemental calcium/gram (20 mEq/gram).

NURSING CONSIDERATIONS

ASSESSMENT

1. Note reasons for therapy, age, physical condition, DEXA scan results.

---

2. Get calcium level before therapy, monitor during therapy; ensure normal renal function.

CLIENT/FAMILY TEACHING

1. Take as directed. Increase fluid intake and bulk; prevents constipation.
2. As a supplement take: 1–1½ hr after meals; as an antacid take 1 hr after meals and bedtime.
3. With gum, do not exceed 17 pieces per day of 450 mg strength or 26 pieces per day of the 300 mg strength. Do not take maximum dose for more than 2 weeks.

OUTCOMES/EVALUATE

- Desired serum calcium levels
- ↓ Gastric upset/acidity

Calcium chloride
(KAL-see-um KLOH-ryd)

CLASSIFICATION(S):
Calcium salt
PREGNANCY CATEGORY: C

SEE ALSO CALCIUM SALTS.

USES
(1) Mild hypocalcemia due to neonatal tetany, tetany due to parathyroid deficiency or vitamin D deficiency, and alkalosis. (2) Prophylaxis of hypocalcemia during exchange transfusions. (3) Intestinal malabsorption. (4) Treat effects of serious hyperkalemia as measured by ECG. (5) Cardiac resuscitation after open heart surgery when epinephrine fails to improve weak or ineffective myocardial contractions. (6) Adjunct to treat insect bites or stings to relieve muscle cramping. (7) Depression due to Mg overdosage. (8) Acute symptoms of lead colic. (9) Rickets, osteomalacia. (10) Reverse symptoms of verapamil overdosage.

CONTRAINDICATIONS
Use to treat hypocalcemia of renal insufficiency. IM or SC use.

SPECIAL CONCERNS
Use usually restricted in children due to significant irritation and possible tissue necrosis and sloughing caused by IV calcium chloride.

SIDE EFFECTS
Most Common
Peripheral vasodilation with moderate decreases in BP.
See *Calcium Salts* for a complete list of possible side effects. If given IM or SC, extravasation can cause severe necrosis, sloughing, or abscess formation.

HOW SUPPLIED
Injection: 100 mg /mL.

DOSAGE
- **IV ONLY**
  Hypocalcemia, replenish electrolytes.
  Adults: 0.5–1 gram q 1–3 days (given at a rate not to exceed 13.6–27.3 mg/min).
  Pediatric: 25 mg/kg (0.2 mL/kg up to 1–10 mL/kg) given slowly.
  Mg intoxication.
  Adults: 0.5 gram promptly; observe for recovery before other doses given.
  Cardiac resuscitation.
  Adults: 0.5–1 gram IV or 0.2–0.8 gram injected into the ventricular cavity as a single dose. **Pediatric:** 0.2 mL/kg.
  Hyperkalemia.
  Sufficient amount to return ECG to normal.
NOTE: The preparation contains 27.2% calcium and 272 mg calcium/gram (13.6 mEq/gram).

NURSING CONSIDERATIONS
ADMINISTRATION/STORAGE
1. Never administer IM or SC.
2. May give undiluted IV push.
ASSESSMENT
Note reasons for therapy, serum levels, other agents trialed.
OUTCOMES/EVALUATE
- Desired serum calcium levels
- ↓ Mg and potassium levels

Calcium gluconate
(KAL-see-um GLUE-koh-nayt)

CLASSIFICATION(S):
Calcium salt
PREGNANCY CATEGORY: C
OTC: Cal-G.
Rx: Kalcinate.

C

SEE ALSO *CALCIUM SALTS.*

USES

(1) Mild hypocalcemia due to neonatal tetany, tetany due to parathyroid deficiency or vitamin D deficiency, and alkalosis. (2) Prophylaxis of hypocalcemia during exchange transfusions. (3) Intestinal malabsorption. (4) Adjunct to treat insect bites or stings to relieve muscle cramping. (5) Depression due to Mg overdosage. (6) Acute symptoms of lead colic. (7) Rickets, osteomalacia. (8) Reverse symptoms of verapamil overdosage. (9) Decrease capillary permeability in allergic conditions, nonthrombocytopenic purpura, and exudative dermatoses (e.g., dermatitis herpetiformis). (10) Pruritus due to certain drugs. (11) Hyperkalemia to antagonize cardiac toxicity (as long as client is not receiving digitalis).

CONTRAINDICATIONS

IM, intramyocardial, or SC use due to severe tissue necrosis, sloughing, and abscess formation.

SIDE EFFECTS

Most Common

After PO use: Constipation, headache, mild hypercalcemia (anorexia, N&V).

After rapid IV use: Vasodilation, decreased BP, syncope, cardiac arrhythmias.

See *Calcium Salts* for a complete list of possible side effects.

HOW SUPPLIED

OTC: Capsules: 700 mg; **OTC: Powder for Oral Suspension**: 346.7 mg elemental calcium/15 mL; **OTC: Tablets**: 500 mg (45 mg elemental Ca), 648–650 mg (58.5–60 mg elemental Ca), 972–975 mg (87.75–90 mg elemental Ca); **Rx**: Injection 10%: 100 mg/mL.

DOSAGE

* **CAPSULES; ORAL SUSPENSION; TABLETS**
  Treatment of hypocalcemia.
Adults: 8.8–16.5 grams/day in divided doses; **Pediatric:** 0.5–0.72 gram/kg/day in divided doses.
  Nutritional supplement.
Adults: 8.8–16.5 grams/day in divided doses.
* **IV ONLY**
  Treatment of hypocalcemia.

Adults: 2.3–9.3 mEq (5–20 mL of the 10% solution) as needed (range: 4.65–70 mEq/day). **Children:** 2.3 mEq/kg/day (or 56 mEq/m^2 per day) given well diluted and slowly in divided doses. **Infants:** No more than 0.93 mEq (2 mL of the 10% solution).
Emergency elevation of serum calcium.
Adults: 7–14 mEq (15–30.1 mL). **Children:** 1–7 mEq (2.2–15 mL). **Infants:** Less than 1 mEq (2.2 mL). Depending on client response, the dose may be repeated q 1–3 days.
Hypocalcemic tetany.
Children: 0.5–0.7 mEq/kg (1.1–1.5 mL/kg) 3–4 times per day until tetany is controlled. **Infants:** 2.4 mEq/kg/day (5.2 mL/kg/day) in divided doses.
Hyperkalemia with cardiac toxicity.
2.25–14 mEq (4.8–30.1 mL) while monitoring the ECG. If needed, the dose can be repeated after 1–2 min.
Mg intoxication.
Initial: 4.5–9 mEq (9.7–19.4 mL). Subsequent dosage based on client response.
Exchange transfusion.
Adults: 1.35 mEq (2.9 mL) concurrent with each 100 mL citrated blood. **Neonates:** 0.45 mEq (1 mL)/100 mL citrated blood.
NOTE: The preparation contains 9% calcium and 90 mg calcium/gram (4.5 mEq/gram).

NURSING CONSIDERATIONS

ADMINISTRATION/STORAGE

IV 1. If precipitate noted in syringe, do not use.

2. If precipitate noted in vials or ampules, heat to 80°C (146°F) in a dry heat oven for 1 hr to dissolve. Shake vigorously and allow to cool to room temperature. Do not use if precipitate remains.

3. IV rate should not exceed 0.5–2 mL/min.

4. Give by intermittent IV infusion at a rate not exceeding 200 mg (19.5 mg calcium ion)/min. Can also be given by continuous IV infusion.

ASSESSMENT

Note therapy reasons, other agents trialed: desired levels/outcome.

Bold Italic = life threatening side effect   ■ = black box warning   ✦ = Available in Canada

CLIENT/FAMILY TEACHING
1. Take with meals to increase absorption.
2. May experience nausea or vomiting; decreased appetite, constipation, dry mouth, or increased thirst; or increased urination; report is persistent.
3. Calcium can decrease the effects of many other medicines by binding to them or by changing the acidity of the stomach or the urine. Do not take together and ensure provider aware of all drugs prescribed.

OUTCOMES/EVALUATE
- Restoration of serum calcium levels
- ↓ Mg/potassium levels

Calfactant
(kal-**FAK**-tant)

CLASSIFICATION(S):
Lung surfactant
PREGNANCY CATEGORY: C
Rx: Infasurf.

USES
Prevention and treatment of respiratory distress syndrome in premature infants.

ACTION/KINETICS
Action
Lung surfactant which contains phospholipids, neutral lipids, and hydrophobic surfactant-associated proteins B and C from calf lungs. Calfactant modifies alveolar surface tension thus stabilizing alveoli. Adsorbs rapidly to the surface of the air: liquid interface and modifies surface tension similarly to natural lung surfactant. Treatment often rapidly improves oxygenation and lung compliance.

SPECIAL CONCERNS
For endotracheal use only. Possible increased proportion of clients with both intraventricular hemorrhage and periventricular leukomalacia. These conditions were not associated with increased mortality.

SIDE EFFECTS
Most Common
Cyanosis, airway obstruction, bradycardia, reflux of surfactant into the endotracheal tube, requirement for manual ventilation.

Respiratory: Cyanosis, airway obstruction, reflux of surfactant into the endotracheal tube, requirement for manual ventilation, apnea, reintubation, periventricular leukomalacia, pulmonary air leaks, pulmonary interstitial emphysema, **pulmonary hemorrhage**. **CV:** Bradycardia, *intraventricular hemorrhage*, patent ductus arteriosus, *intracranial hemorrhage*. **GI:** *Necrotizing enterocolitis.* **Body as a whole:** Sepsis.

HOW SUPPLIED
Suspension, Intratracheal: 35 mg phospholipids/mL and 0.65 mg proteins.

DOSAGE
- **SUSPENSION, INTRATRACHEAL**
  Prophylaxis of respiratory distress syndrome at birth.
Instill 3 mL/kg of birth weight as soon as possible after birth. Give as 2 doses of 1.5 mL/kg each. Care and stabilization of the premature infant born with hypoxemia or bradycardia should precede calfactant therapy.
  Treatment of respiratory distress syndrome within 72 hr of birth.
Instill 3 mL/kg of birth weight, given as 2 doses of 1.5 mL/kg. Repeat doses of 3 mL/kg of birth weight may be given, up to a total of 3 doses 12 hr apart.

NURSING CONSIDERATIONS
ADMINISTRATION/STORAGE
1. Begin calfactant prophylaxis as soon as possible, within 30 minutes after birth.
2. Give only through an endotracheal tube. Draw dose into syringe from single-dose vial using 20-gauge or larger needle. Avoid excessive foaming. Give under supervision of clinician experienced in acute care of newborns requiring intubation.
3. Does not require reconstitution. Do not dilute, sonicate, or shake. Gently swirl/agitate vial for redispersion. Visible flecks in suspension, foaming at the surface are normal. Drug does not have to be warmed before administration.
4. Unopened, unused vials warmed to room temperature may be returned to refrigerator within 24 hr for future use.

Avoid repeated warming to room temperature.

5. Refrigerate 2–8°C (36–46°F); protect from light.

6. Vials for single use only; discard any unused drug after opening.

ASSESSMENT

1. Note condition requiring therapy, oxygen saturation, placement of ET tube.

2. Assess for reflux, airway obstruction, cyanosis, bradycardia; stop drug and take appropriate measures to alleviate. Resume dosing once infant stabilized.

3. Give only under direct supervision of one trained to use in environment with emergency equipment/personnel readily available. Instill through adaptor to ET tube during inspiration while the ventilator cycles 20–30 breaths per each dose (1.5 mL/kg x 2 doses).

4. Monitor carefully; adjust oxygen therapy and ventilatory support in response to changes in respiratory status. Reposition infant between each dose.

CLIENT/FAMILY TEACHING

1. Drug used to treat/prevent respiratory distress syndrome in newborn.

2. Reassure parents infant will be carefully monitored, breathing apparatus may be required to stay intact for the next week or more while infant continues to improve.

3. Adverse effects may occur; address as they arise. Include family in care, visits, updates, decisions.

OUTCOMES/EVALUATE

Prophylaxis/management of respiratory distress syndrome

Candesartan cilexetil

(**kan**-deh-**SAR**-tan)

CLASSIFICATION(S):

Antihypertensive, angiotensin II receptor blocker

PREGNANCY CATEGORY: C (first trimester), **D** (second and third trimesters).

Rx: Atacand.

SEE ALSO *ANGIOTENSIN II RECEPTOR ANTAGONISTS* AND *ANTIHYPERTENSIVE DRUGS.*

USES

(1) Treat hypertension alone or in combination with other antihypertensive drugs. (2) To reduce risk of death and reduce hospitalizations from heart failure (NYHA class II-IV and ejection fraction less than or equal to 40%). There is added benefit when used with an ACE inhibitor. *Investigational:* Prophylaxis of migraine headaches.

ACTION/KINETICS

Pharmacokinetics

Is about 15% bioavailable. Is rapidly and completely bioactivated to candesartan by ester hydrolysis during absorption from the GI tract. Food does not affect bioavailability. Effect somewhat less in blacks. **t½, elimination:** 9 hr. Excreted mainly unchanged in the urine (33%) and feces (67%). **Plasma protein binding:** More than 99%.

SPECIAL CONCERNS

■ When used in pregnancy during the second and third trimesters, drugs that act directly on the renin-angiotensin system may cause injury or death to the developing fetus. When pregnancy is detected, discontinue candesartan as soon as possible. Drugs that act directly on the renin-angiotensin system can cause fetal and neonatal morbidity and death when administered to pregnant women.■

SIDE EFFECTS

Most Common

URTI, dizziness, pain, rhinitis, pharyngitis.

GI: N&V, abdominal pain, diarrhea, dyspepsia, gastroenteritis. **CNS:** Headache, dizziness, paresthesia, vertigo, anxiety, depression, somnolence. **CV:** Tachycardia, palpitation; rarely, angina pectoris, *MI.* **Body as a whole:** Fatigue, asthenia, fever, peripheral edema. **Respiratory:** URTI, pharyngitis, rhinitis, bronchitis, coughing, dyspnea, sinusitis, epistaxis. **GU:** Impaired renal function, hematuria. **Dermatologic:** Rash, increased sweating. **Miscellaneous:** Back/chest pain, pain, arthralgia, myalgia, *angioedema.*

Bold Italic = life threatening side effect ■ = black box warning ♣ = Available in Canada

ADDITIONAL DRUG INTERACTIONS

When used with lithium, serum lithium levels may be increased; monitor carefully.

LABORATORY TEST CONSIDERATIONS

↑ Creatine phosphatase. Albuminuria, hyperglycemia, triglyceridemia, uricemia.

HOW SUPPLIED

Tablets: 4 mg, 8 mg, 16 mg, 32 mg.

DOSAGE

- **TABLETS**

  Hypertension, monotherapy.

Adults, usual initial: 16 mg once daily for monotherapy in those not volume depleted. Can be given once or twice daily in doses from 8 to 32 mg. If BP is not controlled, a diuretic can be added.

  Heart failure.

Adults, initial: 4 mg once daily. Target dose is 32 mg once daily; achieve by doubling the dose at approximately 2-week intervals, as tolerated.

NURSING CONSIDERATIONS

ADMINISTRATION/STORAGE

1. Most effect is noted within 2 weeks and maximum BP reduction in 4 to 6 weeks.
2. Initiate dosage with possible depletion of intravascular volume (e.g., after a diuretic) carefully; consider lower dose.
3. May give with or without food.
4. If BP not controlled by candesartan alone, may add diuretic.
5. May be given with other antihypertensive drugs.
6. No initial dosage adjustment is required for clients with mildly impaired renal or hepatic function. In moderate hepatic impairment, consider initiating at a lower dose.
7. Store from 15–30°C (59–86°F).

ASSESSMENT

1. Note disease onset/duration, other agents trialed, outcome.
2. Assess VS, electrolytes, renal and LFTs. Monitor elderly and those with renal dysfunction closely for desired response/adverse side effects.
3. With heart disease note NYHA and ejection fraction.
4. Ensure adequate hydration, especially with diuretic therapy in renal dysfunction.

CLIENT/FAMILY TEACHING

1. Take as directed with or without food; ensure adequate fluid intake.
2. Practice barrier birth control; report if pregnancy suspected.
3. With heart failure, keep daily record of weights and BP; report wt increases of >2 lb/day or 5 lb/week.
4. Continue life style modifications, i.e. diet, regular exercise, stress reduction, no smoking, moderate alcohol intake to ensure BP control. Report adverse effects.

OUTCOMES/EVALUATE

- ↓ BP ↓ hospitalizations with CHF
- Migraine prophylaxis

Capecitabine ■ ©
(cap-**SITE**-ah-bean)

CLASSIFICATION(S):
Antineoplastic, antimetabolite
PREGNANCY CATEGORY: D
Rx: Xeloda.

SEE ALSO *ANTINEOPLASTIC AGENTS.*

USES

(1) Single agent for adjuvant treatment for Duke stage C colon cancer in clients who have undergone complete resection of the primary tumor when treatment with fluoropyrimidine therapy alone is preferred. Combination chemotherapy improves disease-free survival compared with 5-fluorouracil/leucovorin. (2) First-line therapy for metastatic colorectal cancer when treatment with fluoropyrimidine therapy alone is preferred. (3) In combination with docetaxel to treat metastatic breast cancer in those for whom anthracycline therapy has failed. (4) Metastatic breast cancer in those resistant to both paclitaxel and an anthracycline-containing chemotherapy regimen or resistant to paclitaxel and for whom further anthracycline therapy is not indicated (e.g., those who have received cu-

mulative doses of 400 mg/m^2 of doxorubicin or doxorubicin equivalents). *Investigational:* Adjuvant treatment of pancreatic cancer.

ACTION/KINETICS

Action

An oral prodrug of 5′-deoxy-5-fluorouridine (5′DFUR) that is converted to 5-fluorouracil (5-FU). 5-FU is metabolized to 5-fluoro-2-deoxyuridine monophosphate (FdUMP) and 5-fluorouridine triphosphate (FUTP) which cause cell injury in two ways. First, FdUMP and the folate cofactor, N$^{5-10}$-methylenetetrahydrofolate, bind to thymidylate synthase to form a ternary complex which inhibits the formation of thymidylate from uracil. Thymidylate is essential for the synthesis of DNA so a deficiency inhibits cell division. Secondly, nuclear transcriptional enzymes can mistakenly incorporate FUTP in place of uridine triphosphate during RNA synthesis; this interferes with RNA processing and protein synthesis.

Pharmacokinetics

Readily absorbed from the GI tract. **Peak blood levels, capecitabine:** 1.5 hr; **peak blood levels, 5-FU:** 2 hr. Food reduces the rate and extent of absorption. **t½, capecitabine and 5-FU:** 45 min. Metabolites excreted in the urine. Food reduces the rate and extent of absorption; however, drug is given with food since safety and efficacy data are based on administration with food.

CONTRAINDICATIONS

Use in cancer clients with severe renal impairment (C$_{CR}$ less than 30 mL/min). Hypersensitivity to capecitabine or 5-fluorouracil. Dihydropyrimidine dehydrogenase deficiency. Lactation.

SPECIAL CONCERNS

■ Warfarin interaction. Frequently monitor the anticoagulant response (INR or PT) of clients receiving concomitant capecitabine and oral coumarin-derivative anticoagulant therapy in order to adjust the anticoagulant dose accordingly. A clinically important capecitabine-warfarin drug interaction was demonstrated in a clinical pharmacology trial. Altered coagulation parameters and/or bleeding, including death, have been reported in clients taking capecitabine concomitantly with coumarin-derivative anticoagulants such as warfarin and phenprocoumon. Postmarketing reports have shown clinically significant increases in PT and INR in clients who were stabilized on anticoagulants at the time capecitabine was introduced. These events occurred within several days and up to several months after initiating capecitabine therapy and, in a few cases, within 1 month after stopping capecitabine. These events occurred in clients with and without liver metastases. Age older than 60 years and diagnosis of cancer independently predispose clients to an increased risk of coagulopathy.■ Use with caution in impaired renal function and in the elderly. Clients 80 years of age or older may experience a greater incidence of side effects. Clients with severe diarrhea should be carefully monitored. Discontinue drug if nursing. Safety and efficacy in children less than 18 years of age have not been determined. When combined with docetaxel, more frequent side effects occur, including N&V and fatigue.

SIDE EFFECTS

Most Common

Hand-and-foot syndrome, diarrhea, N&V, stomatitis, abdominal pain, fatigue, lethargy, asthenia, dizziness, dermatitis, headache, alopecia, erythema, rash, anorexia, constipation, dysgeusia, dyspepsia, upper abdominal pain, pyrexia, conjunctivitis, peripheral sensory neuropathy.

GI: Diarrhea (may be severe), N&V, stomatitis, abdominal pain, anorexia, upper abdominal pain, constipation, dyspepsia, intestinal obstruction, rectal bleeding, GI motility disorder, ileus, oral discomfort, taste disturbance, upper GI inflammatory disorders, *GI hemorrhage*, esophagitis, gastritis, colitis, duodenitis, hematemesis, *necrotizing enterocolitis,* oral/GI/esophageal candidiasis, gastroenteritis. **CV:** Cardiotoxicity (*MI*, angina, dysrhythmias, ECG changes, *cardiogenic shock, sudden death*), angina pectoris, *cardiomyopathy,* hypo/hypertension, venous phlebi-

---

Bold Italic = life threatening side effect   ■ = black box warning   ♣ = Available in Canada

C

tis, thrombophlebitis, DVT, lymphedema, venous thrombosis, **pulmonary embolism**, **CVA**. **Hematologic:** Neutropenia (grade 3 or 4), thrombocytopenia, decreased hemoglobin, anemia (grade 3 or 4), lymphopenia, coagulation disorder, IT, pancytopenia, **sepsis**. **Dermatologic:** Hand-and-foot syndrome, alopecia, erythema, rash, dermatitis, nail disorder, increased sweating, photosensitivity, skin discoloration, radiation recall syndrome. **Neurological:** Paresthesia, fatigue, headache, dizziness, insomnia. **CNS:** Dizziness, headache, ataxia, depression, insomnia, mood alteration, encephalopathy, decreased level/loss of consciousness, confusion. **Metabolic:** Anorexia, dehydration, cachexia, hypertriglyceridemia. **Respiratory:** Dyspnea, cough, epistaxis, pharyngeal disorder, sore throat, **bronchospasm**, respiratory distress, URTI, bronchitis, pneumonia, bronchopneumonia, laryngitis. **Musculoskeletal:** Myalgia, arthralgia, back pain, pain in limb, bone pain, joint stiffness. **GU:** Nocturia, UTI. **Hepatic:** Hepatic fibrosis, cholestatic hepatitis, hepatitis. **Ophthalmic:** Conjunctivitis, eye irritation, abnormal vision. **Body as a whole:** Pyrexia, asthenia, fatigue, edema, lethargy, viral infection, dehydration. **Miscellaneous:** Hyperbilirubinemia (grade 3 or 4), chest pain, drug hypersensitivity, decreased appetite.

LABORATORY TEST CONSIDERATIONS
↑ ALT, bilirubin. ↓ Hemoglobin, lymphocytes, neutrophils, granulocytes, platelets. ↑ or ↓ Calcium.

OD **OVERDOSE MANAGEMENT**
Symptoms: N&V, diarrhea, GI irritation and bleeding, bone marrow suppression. *Treatment:* Supportive medical interventions, dose interruption, adjust dose. Dialysis may be of some benefit in removing 5′-deoxy-5-fluorouridine (a metabolite)

DRUG INTERACTIONS
Antacids / ↑ Capecitabine levels
Anticoagulants / Altered coagulation parameters and/or bleeding have been reported in clients taking coumarin-derivative anticoagulants (i.e., warfarin); monitor PT/INR closely; adjust anticoagulant dose accordingly
Leucovorin / ↑ 5-FU levels → ↑ toxicity; deaths from severe enterocolitis, diarrhea, and dehydration seen in elderly clients receiving both drugs
Phenytoin / ↑ Phenytoin levels R/T inhibition of CYP2C9; phenytoin dose may need to be ↓.

HOW SUPPLIED
Tablets: 150 mg, 500 mg.

DOSAGE
• **TABLETS**
  Colorectal cancer, Metastatic breast cancer.
For all indications: 1,250 mg/m^2 twice daily (for a total of 2,500 mg/m^2/day). Each dose should be taken about 12 hours apart at the end of a meal for 2 weeks. Follow by a 1-week rest period (i.e., give as 3-week cycles). Reduce the dose to 75% of the starting dose (i.e., 950 mg/m^2 twice daily) in clients with moderate renal impairment (C_{CR}, 30–50 mL/min). Interrupt and/or reduce dose if toxicity occurs; readjust according to adverse effects. *NOTE:* Check the package insert carefully to determine the dose reduction schedule when capecitabine is combined with docetaxel or recommended dose modification if capecitabine is used alone and there is toxicity.

NURSING CONSIDERATIONS
℘ Do not confuse Xeloda with Xenical (antiobesity drug).

ADMINISTRATION/STORAGE
1. Recommended treatment duration is six months (eight three-week cycles) when used as single-agent treatment of metastatic colorectal cancer where entire primary tumor removed and in whom fluoropyrimidine therapy alone is preferred.
2. Follow manufacturer's insert for recommended dosages R/T BSA, for dose reduction when used with docetaxel, and for adjustment of starting dose in those with impaired hepatic/renal function.
3. If dose was reduced due to toxicity, do not increase at a later time.

 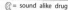

ASSESSMENT

1. Note: first line for metastatic colorectal, combo for metastatic breast cancer or resistant metastatic breast cancer, assess physical condition. List other agents/therapies trialed/failed.

2. Assess for CAD, any sensitivity to 5-FU, organ metastasis especially to liver, renal dysfuction. Monitor weights, CBC, INR/PT, renal and LFTs.

3. Give cautiously with impaired liver/renal function, for coagulation problems in elderly.

4. Monitor PT if taking both capecitabine and oral coumarin therapy; adjust anticoagulant dose accordingly-bleeding can be life threatening.

CLIENT/FAMILY TEACHING

1. Used to manage progression of cancer. Take within 30 min after meals and twice/day with water. Take for 14 days, rest for 7 days in a three week cycle. Ensure adequate fluid intake.

2. Review package for administration guidelines; expect dose adjustments during therapy.

3. May experience nausea/vomiting, diarrhea, mouth ulcers, and painful, swollen joints. Stop therapy immediately and report:

- Grade 2 diarrhea (>4–6 stools/day or at night)
- Grade 2 nausea (loss of appetite; ↓ food intake)
- Grade 2 vomiting (2–5 times per day)
- Grade 2 stomatitis (painful, red ulcers in mouth/tongue)
- Grade 2 hand-and-foot syndrome (red swollen hands/feet)
- Temperature over 100.5° For infection evidence

4. Practice reliable birth control, may harm fetus; do not breastfeed.

5. Keep all F/U appointments to evaluate response to therapy and for any adverse side effects.

OUTCOMES/EVALUATE

↓ Tumor size/spread

Capsaicin
(kap-**SAY**-ih-sin)

CLASSIFICATION(S):
Analgesic, topical
OTC: Axsain, Capsin, Capzasin-HP, Capzasin-P, Dolorac, No Pain-HP, Pain Doctor, Pain-X, R-Gel, Rid-a-Pain-HP, Zostrix, Zostrix-HP.
♣Rx: Antiphlogistine Rub A-535 Capsaicin, Capsaicin HP.

USES
(1) Temporary relief of pain due to rheumatoid arthritis and osteoarthritis. (2) Pain following herpes zoster (shingles). (3) Painful diabetic neuropathy. *Investigational:* Possible use in psoriasis, vitiligo, intractable pruritus, reflex sympathetic dystrophy, postmastectomy, vulvar vestibulitis, apocrine chromhidrosis, and postamputation and postmastectomy neuroma.

ACTION/KINETICS
Action
Derived from natural sources. May act to deplete and prevent the reaccumulation of substance P, thought to be the main mediator of pain impulses from the periphery to the CNS.

SPECIAL CONCERNS
For external use only.

SIDE EFFECTS
Most Common
Burning, stinging.
Skin: Transient burning following application, stinging, erythema. **Respiratory:** Cough, respiratory irritation.

HOW SUPPLIED
Cream: 0.025%, 0.035%, 0.075%, 0.1%, 0.25%; *Gel:* 0.025%; *Lotion:* 0.025%, 0.075%; *Roll-on:* 0.075%.

DOSAGE
- **CREAM; GEL; LOTION; ROLL-ON**
Adults and children over 2 years of age: Apply to affected area no more than 3–4 times per day.

NURSING CONSIDERATIONS
ASSESSMENT
1. Note therapy reasons, area requiring treatment, characteristics of S&S, pain level, other agents trialed, outcome.

Bold Italic = life threatening side effect   ■ = black box warning   ♣ = Available in Canada

2. Takes 1–2 weeks for arthritis pain relief, 2–4 weeks for general neuropathies, 4–6 weeks with head and neck neuralgias.

CLIENT/FAMILY TEACHING

1. Drug is for external use only. Avoid eyes and broken/irritated skin. Expect transient burning/stinging. Rub medication well into designated area until none noted on skin surface.

2. Wash hands before and immediately after application. If treatment is to hands, leave medication on for at least 30 min before washing or apply cotton gloves to protect hands from contaminating other body parts. May use a tongue blade or a small paint roller (new) to apply, or wear a glove to prevent contamination of eyes, mouth etc. Roll on is the best method of application to prevent hand contamination. Flush area with water if gets into eyes and wash with warm soapy water if contacts other sensitive body parts.

3. Do not bandage area tightly. Burning sensation increases with heat, sweating, bathing in warm water, clothing contact, and increased humidity.

4. Regular use (3–4 times per day) is required for desired response and helps decrease the intensity and frequency of burning; drug interferes with substance P (pain neurotransmitter). Must use regularly to obtain desired results.

5. Report if condition worsens, if symptoms persist >3 weeks, or if clears then recurs within a few days.

OUTCOMES/EVALUATE

Relief of pain

Captopril ■

(**KAP**-toe-prill)

CLASSIFICATION(S):

Antihypertensive, ACE inhibitor
PREGNANCY CATEGORY: C (first trimester), **D** (second and third trimesters).
Rx: Capoten.

✺**Rx:** Apo-Capto, Gen-Captopril, Novo-Captoril, Nu-Capto, PMS-Captopril, ratio-Captopril.

SEE ALSO ANGIOTENSIN-CONVERTING ENZYME (ACE) INHIBITORS.

USES

(1) Antihypertensive, alone or in combination with other antihypertensive drugs, especially thiazide diuretics. May be used as initial therapy for those with normal renal function. *NOTE:* In clients with impaired renal function, especially those with collagen vascular disease, reserve captopril for hypertensive clients who have either developed unacceptable side effects on other drugs or have failed to respond satisfactorily to drug combinations. (2) In combination with diuretics and digitalis to treat CHF. (3) To improve survival following MI in clinically stable clients with LV dysfunction manifested as an ejection fraction of 40% or less; to reduce the incidence of overt heart failure and subsequent hospitilization for CHF in these clients. (4) Treatment of diabetic nephropathy (proteinuria >500 mg/day) in those with type I insulin-dependent diabetes and retinopathy. *Investigational:* Rheumatoid arthritis, hypertensive crisis, neonatal and childhood hypertension, hypertension related to scleroderma renal crisis, diagnosis of anatomic renal artery stenosis, diagnosis of primary aldosteronism, Raynaud's syndrome, diagnosis of renovascular hypertension, enhance sensitivity and specificity of renal scintigraphy, idiopathic edema, and Bartter's syndrome.

ACTION/KINETICS

Action

Inhibits angiotensin-converting enzyme resulting in decreased plasma angiotensin II, which leads to decreased vasopressor activity and decreased aldosterone secretion.

Pharmacokinetics

Onset: 30 min or less. **Peak serum levels:** 30–90 min; presence of food decreases absorption by 30–40%. Is 75% or more bioavailable. **Time to peak effect:** 60–90 min. **Duration:** 6–10 hr (dose related). $t\frac{1}{2}$**, normal renal func-**

C

tion, elimination: 2 hr; **t½, impaired renal function:** 3.5–32 hr. More than 95% of absorbed dose excreted in urine (40–50% unchanged). **Plasma protein binding:** 25–30%.

CONTRAINDICATIONS

Use with a history of angioedema related to previous ACE inhibitor use.

SPECIAL CONCERNS

■ Can cause injury and even death in the developing fetus if used during the second and third trimesters. Discontinue as soon as possible if pregnancy is detected.■ Use with caution in cases of impaired renal function and during lactation. Use in children only if other antihypertensive therapy has proven ineffective in controlling BP. May cause a profound drop in BP following the first dose or if used with diuretics.

SIDE EFFECTS

Most Common

Rash, dysgeusia, gastric irritation, aphthous ulcers/peptic ulcer, headache, dizziness, fatigue, drowsiness, malaise, N&V, diarrhea, dry mouth.

Dermatologic: Rash (usually maculopapular) with pruritus and occasionally fever, eosinophilia, and arthralgia. Alopecia, erythema multiforme, photosensitivity, exfoliative dermatitis, **Stevens-Johnson syndrome,** reversible pemphigoid-like lesions, bullous pemphigus, onycholysis, flushing, pallor, scalded mouth sensation. **GI:** N&V, anorexia, constipation or diarrhea, gastric irritation, abdominal pain, dysgeusia, peptic/aphthous ulcers, dyspepsia, dry mouth, glossitis, pancreatitis. **Hepatic:** Jaundice, cholestasis, hepatitis. **CNS:** Headache, dizziness, insomnia, malaise, fatigue, paresthesias, confusion, depression, nervousness, ataxia, somnolence. **CV:** Hypotension, angina, **MI,** Raynaud's phenomenon, chest pain, palpitations, tachycardia, **CVA, CHF, cardiac arrest,** orthostatic hypotension, rhythm disturbances, cerebrovascular insufficiency. **Renal:** Renal insufficiency/failure, proteinuria, urinary frequency, oliguria, polyuria, nephrotic syndrome, interstitial nephritis. **Respiratory: Bronchospasm,** cough, dyspnea, asthma, **pulmonary embolism/infarction. Hemato-**

logic: Agranulocytosis, neutropenia, thrombocytopenia, pancytopenia, **aplastic/hemolytic anemia. Miscellaneous:** Decrease/loss of taste perception with weight loss (reversible), angioedema, asthenia, syncope, fever, myalgia, arthralgia, vasculitis, blurred vision, impotence, hyperkalemia, hyponatremia, myasthenia, gynecomastia, rhinitis, eosinophilic pneumonitis.

ADDITIONAL DRUG INTERACTIONS

Indomethacin / ↓ 24-hr antihypertensive effects of captopril
Iron salts / ↓ Captopril blood levels; separate administration by at least 2 hr
Probenecid / ↑ Captopril blood levels R/T ↓ renal excretion

LABORATORY TEST CONSIDERATIONS

False + test for urine acetone.

OD OVERDOSE MANAGEMENT

Symptoms: Hypotension with SBP of <80 mm Hg a possibility. *Treatment:* Volume expansion with NSS (IV) is the treatment of choice to restore BP.

HOW SUPPLIED

Tablets: 12.5 mg, 25 mg, 50 mg, 100 mg.

DOSAGE

• **TABLETS**

Hypertension.

Adults, initial: 25 mg 2–3 times per day. If unsatisfactory response after 1–2 weeks, increase to 50 mg 2–3 times per day; if still unsatisfactory after another 1–2 weeks, add a thiazide diuretic (e.g., hydrochlorothiazide, 25 mg/day). May increase dose to 100–150 mg 2–3 times per day, not to exceed 450 mg/day.

Accelerated or malignant hypertension.

Stop current medication (except for the diuretic) and initiate captopril at 25 mg 2–3 times per day. May increase dose q 24 hr until a satisfactory response is obtained or the maximum dose reached. Furosemide may be indicated.

Heart failure.

Initial: 25 mg 3 times per day; **then,** if necessary, increase dose to 50 mg 3 times per day and evaluate response. Delay further increases for at least 2 weeks to determine if a satisfactory response has been attained. **Maintenance:** 50–100 mg 3 times per day for most clients. Do not exceed 450

Bold Italic = life threatening side effect   ■ = black box warning   ✦ = Available in Canada

mg/day. *NOTE:* For adults, give an initial dose of 6.25–12.5 mg (0.15 mg/kg 3 times per day in children) 2–3 times per day to clients who are sodium- and water-depleted due to diuretics, who will continue to be on diuretic therapy, and who have renal impairment.

Left ventricular dysfunction after MI. Therapy may be started as early as 3 days after the MI. **Initial dose:** 6.25 mg; **then,** begin 12.5 mg 3 times per day and increase to 25 mg 3 times per day over the next several days. The target dose is 50 mg 3 times per day over the next several weeks. Other treatments for MI may be used concomitantly (e.g., aspirin, beta blockers, thrombolytic drugs).

Diabetic nephropathy.
25 mg 3 times per day for chronic use. Other antihypertensive drugs (e.g., beta blockers, centrally-acting drugs, diuretics, vasodilators) may be used with captopril if additional drug therapy is needed to reduce BP.

Hypertensive emergencies.
25–50 mg at 1- to 2-hr intervals.

Rheumatoid arthritis.
75–150 mg/day in divided doses.

Severe childhood hypertension.
Infants, initial: 0.15–0.3 mg/kg/dose, followed by upward titration, if needed. **Children, initial:** 0.3–0.5 mg/kg/dose q 8 hr, followed by upward titration, if needed. **Maximum dose:** 6 mg/kg/day in divided doses.

NOTE: For all uses, reduce dose in clients with renal impairment.

NURSING CONSIDERATIONS
ADMINISTRATION/STORAGE
1. Give 1 hr before meals.
2. Discontinue previous antihypertensive medication 1 week before starting captopril, if possible.
3. Tablets can be used to prepare a solution of captopril if desired.

ASSESSMENT
1. Note disease onset, other medical conditions/agents trialed, outcome.
2. Monitor VS, potassium, hematologic, renal, LFTs.

3. Note if diuretics or nitrates prescribed; may act synergistically causing more pronounced response.
4. Document ACE intolerance.
5. Assess ability to understand/comply with therapy.
6. Note ejection fraction (at or below 40%) in stable, post-MI clients.
7. Usually very effective with heart failure, diabetes, arthritis.

INTERVENTIONS
1. Observe for drop in BP within 3 hr of initial dose if on diuretic therapy and low-salt diet. If BP falls rapidly, place supine; have saline infusion available.
2. Check for proteinuria monthly for 9 months during therapy, CBC every 2 weeks for first 3 months of therapy.
3. Withhold potassium-sparing diuretics; hyperkalemia may result-may occur several months after spironolactone and captopril therapy.

CLIENT/FAMILY TEACHING
1. Take 1 hr before meals, on empty stomach; food interferes with drug absorption.
2. Report fever, skin rash, sore throat, mouth sores, fast/irregular heartbeat, chest pain, cough.
3. May develop dizziness, fainting, lightheadedness; usually disappear once body adjusts. Avoid sudden changes in posture, activities/exercise in hot weather; prevent dizziness/fainting. Consume plenty of fluids; prevent dehydration.
4. Loss of taste may be experienced first 2–3 months; report if persists/interferes with nutrition/weight.
5. Carry ID and medication list.
6. Call with questions concerning symptoms/effects of therapy; do not stop taking abruptly. Report for regular F/U, BP, electrolytes and urine protein.
7. If insulin-dependent may experience hypoglycemia; monitor FS closely.
8. Avoid OTC agents without approval.
9. Practice reliable contraception; report if pregnancy suspected.

OUTCOMES/EVALUATE
- ↓ BP
- Improved S&S CHF (↓ preload, ↓ afterload)
- Improved mortality post-MI

Carbamazepine ■Ⅳ©
(kar-bah-**MAYZ**-eh-peen)

CLASSIFICATION(S):
Anticonvulsant, miscellaneous
PREGNANCY CATEGORY: D
Rx: Carbatrol, Epitol, Equetro, Tegretol, Tegretol XR.
✿Rx: Paraplatin, Apo-Carbamazepine, Apo-Carbamazepine CR, Gen-Carbamazepine CR, Novo–Carbamaz, Nu–Carbamazepine, PMS-Carbamazepine CR, Taro-Carbamazepine.

SEE ALSO *ANTICONVULSANTS*.

USES
(1) Partial seizures with complex symptoms (psychomotor, temporal lobe). (2) Generalized tonic-clonic seizures. (3) Mixed seizure patterns that include the above, or other partial or generalized seizures. Carbamazepine is often a drug of choice. (4) Pain associated with trigeminal neuralgia and glossopharyngeal neuralgia (all products except Equetro). The drug is not a simple analgesic; do not use for relief of trivial aches or pains. (5) Acute manic and mixed episodes associated with bipolar I disorder (use Equetro only). *Investigational:* Restless leg syndrome, alternative to benzodiazepines to treat alcohol withdrawal.

ACTION/KINETICS
Action
Chemically similar to the cyclic antidepressants. Also manifests antimanic, antineuralgic, antidiuretic, anticholinergic, antiarrhythmic, and antipsychotic effects. The anticonvulsant action is not known but may involve depressing activity in the nucleus ventralis anterior of the thalamus, resulting in a reduction of polysynaptic responses and blocking posttetanic potentiation. Due to the potentially serious blood dyscrasias, undertake a benefit-to-risk evaluation before the drug is instituted.

Pharmacokinetics
Peak serum levels: 4–5 hr. **t½ (serum):** 12–17 hr with repeated doses. **Therapeutic serum levels:** 4–12 mcg/mL for both adults and children. Metabolized in the liver by the CYP3A4 isozyme to the 10,11-epoxide, which is also active. **t½, initial:** 25–65 hr but is reduced to 12–17 hr because the drug induces its own metabolism. Metabolites are excreted through the feces (28%) and urine (72%). **Plasma protein binding:** 76% bound to plasma proteins.

CONTRAINDICATIONS
History of bone marrow depression, acute intermittent porphyria. Hypersensitivity to drug or tricyclic antidepressants. Concomitant use of MAO inhibitors. Lactation. Use for relief of general aches and pains.

SPECIAL CONCERNS
■ (1) Aplastic anemia and agranulocytosis have been reported in association with the use of carbamazepine. The risk of developing these reactions is 5–8 times greater than in the general population; however, the overall risk of these reactions in the untreated general population is low, approximately 6 clients per 1 million per year for agranulocytosis and 2 clients per 1 million per year for aplastic anema. (2) Although reports of transient or persistent decreased platelet or WBC counts are not uncommon in association with the use of carbamazepine, data are not available to estimate accurately their incidence or outcome. However, the vast majority of the cases of leukopenia have not progressed to the more serious conditions of aplastic anemia or agranulocytosis. (3) Because of the very low incidence of these two conditions, the vast majority of minor hematologic changes observed in monitoring clients on carbamazepine are unlikely to signal the occurrence of either abnormality. However, obtain complete pretreatment hematological testing as a baseline. If a client exhibits low or decreased WBC or platelet counts during the course of treatment, monitor closely. Consider discontinuation of the drug if any evidence of significant bone marrow depression de-

---

Bold Italic = life threatening side effect   ■ = black box warning   ✿ = Available in Canada

velops.■ Use with caution in glaucoma and in hepatic, renal, CV disease, and a history of hematologic reaction. Use with caution in clients with mixed seizure disorder that includes atypical absence seizures (carbamazepine is not effective and may be associated with an increased frequency of generalized convulsions). Use in geriatric clients may cause an increased incidence of confusion, agitation, AV heart block, syndrome of inappropriate antidiuretic hormone, and bradycardia. In clients taking MAO inhibitors, discontinue for 14 days before taking carbamazepine. Use with caution in clients with increased intraocular pressure.

SIDE EFFECTS
Most Common
Dizziness, drowsiness, unsteadiness, headache, N&V, ataxia, somnolence, rash, diarrhea, dyspepsia, infection, pain.

GI: N&V, diarrhea, constipation, gastric distress, dyspepsia, abdominal pain, anorexia, glossitis, stomatitis, dry mouth and pharynx. **Hematologic: *Aplastic anemia***, leukopenia, eosinophilia, thrombocytopenia, *agranulocytosis*, leukocytosis, pancytopenia, *bone marrow depression*. **CNS:** Dizziness, drowsiness, unsteadiness, disturbances of coordination, somnolence, headache, fatigue, confusion, speech disturbances, visual hallucinations, depression with agitation, talkativeness, hyperacusis, abnormal involuntary movements, behavioral changes in children. **CV:** CHF, aggravation of hypertension, hypotension, syncope and collapse, edema, recurrence of or primary thrombophlebitis, aggravation of CAD, paralysis and other symptoms of cerebral arterial insufficiency, thromboembolism, *arrhythmias (including AV block)*. **GU:** Urinary frequency, acute urinary retention, oliguria with hypertension, impotence, renal failure, azotemia, albuminuria, glycosuria, increased BUN, microscopic deposits in urine. **Pulmonary:** Pulmonary hypersensitivity characterized by fever, dyspnea, pneumonitis, or pneumonia. **Dermatologic:** Pruritus, urticaria, photosensitivity, exfoliative dermatitis, erythematous rashes, alterations in pigmentation, alopecia, sweating, purpura, *toxic epidermal necrolysis* (Lyell's syndrome), *Stevens-Johnson syndrome*, aggravation of disseminated lupus erythematosus, alopecia, erythema nodosum/multiforme. **Ophthalmic:** Nystagmus, double/blurred vision, oculomotor disturbances, conjunctivitis; scattered, punctuate cortical lens opacities. **Hepatic:** Abnormal LFTs, cholestatic/hepatocellular jaundice, hepatitis, acute intermittent porphyria, *hepatic failure*. **Miscellaneous:** Peripheral neuritis, infection, pain, paresthesias, tinnitus, fever, chills, joint/muscle aches and leg cramps, adenopathy/lymphadenopathy, SIADH, frank water intoxication with hyponatremia and confusion, hypersensitivity reaction.

LABORATORY TEST CONSIDERATIONS
↓ Calcium, thyroid function tests. Interference with some pregnancy tests. Hyponatremia.

OD OVERDOSE MANAGEMENT
Symptoms: First appear after 1 to 3 hours. Neuromuscular disturbances are the most common. **Pulmonary:** Irregular breathing, *respiratory depression.* **CV:** Tachycardia, hypo- or hypertension, conduction disorders, *shock.* **CNS:** Seizures (especially in small children), impaired consciousness (deep coma possible), motor restlessness, muscle twitching or tremors, athetoid movements, ataxia, drowsiness, dizziness, nystagmus, mydriasis, psychomotor disturbances, hyperreflexia followed by hyporeflexia, opisthotonos, dysmetria, dizziness, EEG may show dysrhythmias. **GI:** N&V. **GU:** Anuria, oliguria, urinary retention. *Treatment:* Stomach should be irrigated completely even if more than 4 hr has elapsed following drug ingestion, especially if alcohol has been ingested. Activated charcoal, 50–100 grams initially, using a NGT (dose of 12.5 or more grams/hr until client is symptom free). Diazepam or phenobarbital may be used to treat seizures (although they may aggravate respiratory depression, hypotension, and coma). Respiration, ECG, BP, body temperature, pupillary reflexes, and kidney and blad-

der function should be monitored for several days. If significant bone marrow depression occurs, discontinue and determine daily CBC, platelet and reticulocyte counts. Perform bone marrow aspiration and trephine biopsy immediately and repeat often enough to monitor recovery.

DRUG INTERACTIONS

Acetaminophen / ↑ Acetaminophen breakdown → ↓ effect and ↑ risk of hepatotoxicity

Azetazolamide / ↑ Carbazepine plasma levels; adjust dose of carbamazepine as needed

Anticoagulants / Carbamazepine may ↑ metabolism of anticoagulants → ↓ hypoprothrombinemic effect; monitor PT times

Antimarlarials (e.g., chloroquine, mefloquine) / Possible antagonism of the activity of carbamazepine

Antipsychotics (e.g., aripiprazole, clozapine, olanzapine, quetiapine, risperidone, ziprasidone) / ↓ Antipychotic plasma levels

Azole, antifungal drugs (e.g., itraconazole, ketoconazole) / ↑ Plasma carbamazepine levels; closely monitor carbamazepine levels; also, possible ↓ serum itraconazole levels

Barbiturates / ↓ Plasma carbamazepine levels → ↓ effectiveness

Benzodiazepines / ↓ Effect of benzodiazepines

Bupropion / ↓ Bupropion effect R/T ↑ liver breakdown by CYP3A4 enzymes

Buspirone / ↓ Buspirone plasma levels; monitor client response

Charcoal / ↓ Carbamazepine effect R/T ↓ GI tract absorption

Cimetidine / ↑ Carbamazepine plasma levels → possible toxicity R/T ↓ liver breakdown

Cisplatin / ↓ Carbamazepine plasma levels

Clomipramine / ↑ Clomipramine plasma levels

Clozapine / ↓ Effects of clozapine

Cyclosporine / ↓ Cyclosporine effect R/T ↑ liver breakdown

Dalfopristin / ↑ Carbamazepine plasma levels → possible toxicity

Danazol / ↑ Carbamazepine effect →

possible toxicity R/T ↓ liver breakdown

Delavirdine / ↑ Carbamazepine plasma levels; possible loss of virologic response and possible resistance to delavirdine or to nonnucleoside reverse transcriptase inhibitors

Diltiazem / ↑ Carbamazepine effect → possible toxicity R/T ↓ liver breakdown

Doxorubicin / ↓ Carbamazepine plasma levels

Doxycycline / ↓ Doxycycline effect R/T ↑ liver breakdown

Erythromycin / ↑ Carbamazepine effect R/T ↓ liver breakdown

Felbamate / Possible ↓ serum levels of either drug

Felodipine / ↓ Felodipine effect

Fluoxetine / ↑ Carbamazepine levels → possible toxicity

Fluvoxamine / ↑ Carbamazepine levels → possible toxicity

Glucocorticoids (e.g., hydrocortisone) / ↓ Glucocorticoid plasma levels

Grapefruit juice / ↑ Peak levels of carbamazepine; do not give together

Haloperidol / ↓ Haloperidol effect R/T ↑ liver breakdown; also, ↑ carbamazepine effects

HMG-CoA reductase inhibitors (e.g., atorvastain, simvastatin) / ↓ Plasma levels of certain HMG-CoA reductase inhibitors → ↓ effect resulting in hypercholesterolemia; monitor closely

Hydantoins / Both ↑ and ↓ plasma hydantoin levels; also, ↓ plasma carbamazepine levels

Isoniazid / ↑ Carbamazepine effect R/T ↓ liver breakdown; also, carbamazepine may ↑ risk of drug-induced hepatotoxicity

Lamotrigine / ↓ Lamotrigine effect; also, ↑ levels of active metabolite of carbamazepine

Levetiracetam / ↑ Risk of carbamazepine toxicity

Levothyroxine / ↓ Levothyroxine plasma levels; monitor TSH

Lithium / ↑ CNS toxicity; monitor lithium serum levels

Loratidine / ↑ Carbamazepine plasma levels

Macrolide antibiotics (e.g., clarithromycin, erythromycin, troleandomycin) / ↑ Carbamazepine effect R/T ↓ liver

---

breakdown

MAO inhibitors / Do not use together; discontinue MAOI at least 14 days before giving carbamazepine

Melatonin / ↑ Melatonin bioavailability

Methadone / ↓ Methadone effects, possible ↑ methadone dose

Methylphenidate / ↓ Blood levels of methylphenidate

Mirtazapine / ↓ Mirtazapine plasma levels

Muscle relaxants, nondepolarizing / Resistance to or reversal of the neuromuscular blocking effects; ↑ muscle relaxant dose as needed

Nefazodone / ↑ Serum carbamazepine levels and ↓ nefazodone levels may result; coadministration is contraindicated

Niacin (e.g., niacinamide, niotinamide) / ↑ Carbamazepine plasma levels

Olanzapine / ↓ Plasma olanzapine levels

Oral Contraceptives / ↓ Oral contraceptive effect R/T ↑ liver breakdown

Oxcarbazepine / ↓ Oxcarbazepine plasma levels

Phenobarbital / ↓ Carbamazepine effect R/T ↑ liver breakdown

Phenytoin / ↓ Carbamazepine effect R/T ↑ liver breakdown; also, phenytoin levels may ↑ or ↓; monitor levels of both drugs

Praziquantel / ↓ Praziquantel serum levels → possible treatment failures; ↑ praziquantel dose if needed

Primidone / ↓ Carbamazepine effect R/T ↑ liver breakdown; also, either ↑ or ↓ primidone levels; monitor levels of both drugs

Probenecid / ↑ Carbamazepine metabolism by CYP3A4 and CYP2C8

Propoxyphene / ↑ Carbamazepine effect R/T ↓ liver breakdown; avoid coadministration

Protease inhibitors (e.g., amprenavir, indinavir) / ↑ Plasma carbamazepine levels → ↑ risk of toxicity; also, ↓ plasma protease inhibitor levels → treatment failure

Quinine / ↑ Carbamazepine plasma levels; monitor and adjust carbamazepine dose

Quinupristin / ↑ Carbamazepine plasma levels; monitor carbamazepine levels

Rifampin / ↓ Carbamazepine plasma levels R/T ↑ metabolism

Selective serotonin reuptake inhibitors (e.g., fluoxetine, fluvoxamine) / ↑ Carbamazepine levels → toxicity; possible ↓ plasma levels of SSRIs; closely monitor client response and adjust dose if needed

Sertraline / ↓ Sertraline effect R/T ↑ liver breakdown

Simvastatin / ↓ Simvastatin levels

Succinimides (e.g., methsuximide) / ↓ Carbamazepine and succinimide levels

Theophyllines / Either ↓ or ↑ theophylline levels; possible ↓ carbamazepine levels; monitor levels of both drugs

Thyroxine/Triiodothyronine / ↑ Elimination of thyroid hormone R/T ↑ liver breakdown

Tiagabine / ↓ Plasma tiagabine levels

Ticlopidine / ↑ Carbamazepine effect R/T ↑ liver breakdown

Topiramate / ↓ Topiramate levels → ↓ effects

Tramadol / ↓ Tramadol plasma levels

Tricyclic antidepressants (TCA) / ↓ TCA levels and TCA effects R/T ↑ liver breakdown

Valproic acid / ↓ Valproic acid effect R/T ↑ liver breakdown; ↑ carbamazepine plasma levels

Vasopressin / ↑ Vasopressin effect

Verapamil / ↑ Carbamazepine effect R/T ↓ liver breakdown; may need to ↓ carbamazepine dose by 40–50%

Voriconazole / ↓ Vorconazole levels; do not give together

Warfarin sodium / ↓ Anticoagulant effect R/T ↑ liver breakdown

Zileuton / ↑ Carbamazepine plasma levels

Ziprasidone / ↓ Plasma ziprasidone levels

Zonisamide / ↓ Zonisamide plasma levels

HOW SUPPLIED

Capsules, Extended-Release: 100 mg, 200 mg, 300 mg; *Oral Suspension:* 100 mg/5 mL; *Tablets:* 200 mg, 300 mg, 400 mg; *Tablets, Chewable:* 100 mg; *Tablets, Extended-Release:* 100 mg, 200 mg, 400 mg.

📷 = see color insert   Ⓗ = Herbal   Ⅳ = Intravenous   ⓒ = sound alike drug

DOSAGE

- **CAPSULES, EXTENDED-RELEASE; ORAL SUSPENSION; TABLETS; TABLETS, CHEWABLE; TABLETS, EXTENDED-RELEASE**

Anticonvulsant

Adults and children over 12 years old. Initial dose: 200 mg 2 times per day if using tablets or extended-release products or 100 mg (5 mL) 4 times per day of the suspension. **Titration:** For tablets or suspension, increase at weekly intervals of no more than 200 mg/day using a 3- or 4-times per day regimen. For extended-release formulations, increase at weekly intervals of no more than 200 mg/day using a 2 times per day regimen. **Maintenance:** For all formulations, adjust to minimum effective dose, usually 800–1,200 mg/day. **Maximum daily dose, all formulations:** Adults (rarely) up to 1,600 mg/day; 16 years of age and older up to 1,200 mg/day; 12 to 15 years of age up to 1,000 mg/day. **Children 6–12 years of age. Initial dose:** 100 mg 2 times per day if using tablets or extended-release formulations or 50 mg (2.5 mL) 4 times per day of the suspension. **Titration:** For tablets or suspension, increase at weekly intervals of no more than 100 mg/day using a 3- or 4-times per day regimen. For extended-release formulations, increase at weekly intervals of no more than 100 mg/day using a 2 times per day regimen. **Maintenance:** For all formulations, adjust to minimum effective dose, usually 400–800 mg/day. **Maximum daily dose:** For tablets or suspension, 1,000 mg/day; for capsules, 35 mg/kg/day. **Children younger than 6 years old, initial dose:** 10–20 mg/kg/day in 2 to 3 divided doses if using tablets and 10–20 mg/kg/day in 4 divided doses if using the suspension. **Titration:** For tablets or suspension, increase weekly to achieve optimal clinical response given 3–4 times per day. **Maintenance:** For all formulations, usually optimal responses are achieved at daily doses less than 35 mg/kg. **Maximum daily dose:** For all formulations, 35 mg/kg/day.

Anticonvulsant (Carbatrol only).

Adults and children older than 12 years of age, initial: 200 mg twice daily. Increase at weekly intervals by adding up to 200 mg/day until optimal response is reached. Dosage generally should not exceed 1,000 mg/day in children 12 to 15 years of age and 1,200 mg/day in clients older than 15 years of age. However, doses up to 1,600 mg/day have been used in adults. **Maintenance:** Usually 800–1,200 mg/day.

Children younger than 12 years of age: Optimal clinical response is reached at daily doses below 35 mg/kg. Children taking total daily doses of immediate-release carbamazepine, 400 mg or greater, may be converted to the same total daily dose of carbamazepine ER capsules, using a twice-daily regimen.

Bipolar I disorder (Equetro only).

Initial: 200 mg two times per day. **Titration:** Adjust in 200 mg daily increments to achieve optimum clinical response. **Maintenance:** Doses greater than 1,600 mg/day have not been studied.

Postherpetic neuralgia.

Initial: 100 mg at bedtime. Increase by 100 mg every 3 days until dosage is 200 mg 2 times/day, response is adequate, or blood level of the drug is 6–12 mcg/mL.

Trigeminal neuralgia.

Initial dose: 100 mg 2 times per day for tablets and extended-release tablets, 200 mg once daily for extended-release capsules, or 50 mg (2.5 mL) 4 times per day for the suspension. **Titration:** For tablets and extended-release formulations, may increase by up to 200 mg/day using 100 mg increments q 12 hr as needed. **Maintenance:** Usually 400–800 mg/day. Attempt discontinuation of drug at least 1 time every 3 months. **Maximum daily dose:** For all formulations, 1,200 mg/day. At least once every 3 months, attempts should be made to reduce the dose to the minimum effective level or even to discontinue the drug.

Trigeminal neuralgia (Carbatrol only).

Bold Italic = life threatening side effect   ■ = black box warning   ♣ = Available in Canada

Initial, Day 1: One-200 mg capsule. Daily dose may be increased by up to 200 mg/day q 12 hr only as needed to achieve freedom from pain. Do not exceed 1,200 mg/day. **Maintenance:** Usually 400–800 mg daily. Some clients require as little as 200 mg daily, while others require as much as 1,200 mg daily. At least once every 3 months, attempts should be made to reduce the dose to the minimum effective level or even to discontinue the drug.

NURSING CONSIDERATIONS

Ⓒ Do not confuse Tegretol with Tequin (an antibacterial), Toprol-XL (beta-adrenergic blocker), or Topamax (anticonvulsant/antimigraine).

ADMINISTRATION/STORAGE

1. To convert from tablets to suspension: give same number of milligrams/day in smaller, more frequent doses (e.g., tablets, 2 times per day to suspension 3 times per day).
2. Convert from conventional tablets to extended-release tablets: give same total daily milligram dose of extended-release drug.
3. When adding carbamazepine to existing anticonvulsant therapy, add gradually while other anticonvulsants maintained or gradually decreased, except phenytoin, which may have to be increased.
4. Do not administer for minimum of 2 weeks after MAO inhibitor drugs.
5. Protect tablets from moisture.
6. Start therapy gradually; use lowest dose to minimize adverse reactions. A given dose of suspension will produce higher peak levels than same dose given as the tablet; thus, start with low doses in children 6–12 y.o., increase slowly to avoid unwanted side effects.
7. If must discontinue R/T side effects, abrupt withdrawal may lead to seizures or status epilepticus.
8. Do not store chewable tablets or tablets above 30°C (86°F). Protect from light and moisture.
9. Store ER tablets from 15–30°C (59–86°F). Protect from moisture.
10. Do not store suspension above 30°C (86°F). Do not administer suspension simultaneously with other liquid medicinal agents or diluents.

ASSESSMENT

1. List reason for therapy: with seizures, describe type, onset, frequency, characteristics.
2. Assess for psychosis; may activate symptoms.
3. Do baseline CBC, renal, and LFTs; assess for dysfunction. With high doses, get weekly CBC first 3 months, then monthly: assess extent of bone marrow depression. At first sign blood dyscrasia, stop drug.
4. Obtain eye exams; assess for opacities, IOPs.
5. Obtain EEG during therapy. Use seizure precautions with quick withdrawal; may precipitate status epilepticus.
6. During dosage adjustment, monitor I&O, VS for evidence of fluid retention, renal failure, or CV complications.
7. List all drugs prescribed/consumed; ensure none interact adversely.
8. Carefully monitor high risk clients taking Equetro for bipolar disorder R/T possibility of suicide attempts.

CLIENT/FAMILY TEACHING

1. Take with meals; ↓ GI upset. Coating for extended release capsules is not absorbed; may be noticeable in stool.
2. Extended-release capsules may be opened and beads sprinkled over a teaspoon of applesauce or other similar food products. Do not crush/chew capsules or contents. May take with/without meals.
3. Withhold drug and report if any of the following symptoms occur:
- Fever, sore throat, mouth ulcers, easy bruising/bleeding (early S&S bone marrow depression).
- Urinary frequency, retention, reduced output, sexual impotence.
- Immediate attention for: CHF, fainting, collapse, swelling, blood clot, or cyanosis.
- Loss of symptom control.
4. Use caution operating car or other dangerous machinery; may interfere with vision/coordination.
5. Report skin eruptions, pigmentation changes, other adverse side effects.

C

6. Avoid excessive sunlight; wear protective clothing/sunscreen.
7. Use nonhormonal birth control; do not breast feed.
8. Avoid OTC agents, CNS depressants and alcohol.
9. Keep all F/U and labs to assesses drug response, levels and for early blood/organ dysfunction.

OUTCOMES/EVALUATE
• Control of refractory seizures
• Control of alcohol/drug withdrawal
• ↓ Pain with trigeminal neuralgia
• Therapeutic serum drug levels (4–12 mcg/mL)

Carbidopa ∎
(**KAR**-bih-doh-pah)

CLASSIFICATION(S):
Antiparkinson drug
PREGNANCY CATEGORY: C
Rx: Lodosyn.

Carbidopa/Levodopa
(**KAR**-bih-doh-pah, **LEE**-voh-doh-pah)

Rx: Parcopa, Sinemet CR, Sinemet-10/100, -25/100, or -25/250.
♣Rx: Apo-Levocarb, Novo-Levocarbidopa, Nu-Levocarb.

SEE ALSO *LEVODOPA*.

USES
(1) Parkinsonism (idiopathic, postencephalitic, following injury to the nervous system due to carbon monoxide and manganese intoxication). Not effective in drug-induced extrapyramidal symptoms. (2) Carbidopa alone is used in clients who require individual titration of carbidopa and levodopa. *Investigational:* Postanoxic intention myoclonus.
Warning: Discontinue levodopa at least 8 hr before carbidopa/levodopa therapy is initiated.

CONTENT
Carbidopa/Levodopa Orally Disintegrating Tablets: Carbidopa, 10 mg,

and levodopa, 100 mg; carbidopa, 25 mg, and levodopa, 100 mg; and carbidopa, 25 mg and levodopa, 250 mg.
Carbidopa/Levodopa Sustained-Release Tablets: Each sustained-release tablet contains: carbidopa, 25 mg, and levodopa, 100 mg or carbidopa, 50 mg, and levodopa, 200 mg. **Carbidopa/Levodopa Tablets:** Each 10/100 tablet contains: carbidopa, 10 mg, and levodopa, 100 mg. Each 25/100 tablet contains: carbidopa, 25 mg, and levodopa, 100 mg. Each 25/250 tablet contains: carbidopa, 25 mg, and levodopa, 250 mg.

ACTION/KINETICS
Action
Carbidopa inhibits peripheral, but not central, decarboxylation of levodopa because it does not cross the blood-brain barrier. Since peripheral decarboxylation is inhibited, more levodopa is available for transport to the brain, where it will be converted to dopamine, thus relieving the symptoms of parkinsonism. Carbidopa and levodopa are given together (e.g., Sinemet). However, *the dosage of levodopa must be reduced by up to 80% when combined with carbidopa.* This decreases the incidence of levodopa-induced side effects. *NOTE:* Pyridoxine will not reverse the action of carbidopa/levodopa.

Pharmacokinetics
t½, carbidopa: 1–2 hr; when given with levodopa, the t½ of levodopa increases from 1 hr to 2 hr (may be as high as 15 hr in some clients). About 30% carbidopa is excreted unchanged in the urine.

CONTRAINDICATIONS
History of melanoma. Lactation.

SPECIAL CONCERNS
∎ When carbidopa and levodopa are used together, start with no more than 20–25% of the previous daily dose of levodopa. At least 8 hr should elapse between the last dose of levodopa and the first dose of carbidopa/levodopa.∎ Use during pregnancy only if benefits outweigh risks. Safety and efficacy in children less than 18 years of age have not been determined. Lower doses may be necessary in geriatric clients due to age-related decreases in peripheral

---

Bold Italic = life threatening side effect   ∎ = black box warning   ♣ = Available in Canada dopa decarboxylase. Stop MAO inhibitors 2 weeks before therapy.

SIDE EFFECTS

Most Common

Choreiform or dystonic movements, anorexia, N&V with or without abdominal pain, dry mouth, dysphagia, dysgeusia, sialorrhea, headache, dizziness.

See *Levodopa* for a complete list of possible side effects. Because more levodopa reaches the brain, dyskinesias may occur at lower doses with carbidopa/levodopa than with levodopa alone. Clients abruptly withdrawn from levodopa may experience neuroleptic malignant-like syndrome including symptoms of muscular rigidity, hyperthermia, increased serum phosphokinase, and changes in mental status.

LABORATORY TEST CONSIDERATIONS

↓ Creatinine, BUN, and uric acid.

DRUG INTERACTIONS

Use with tricyclic antidepressants → hypertension and dyskinesia.

HOW SUPPLIED

Carbidopa: *Tablets:* 25 mg.
Carbidopa/Levodopa: *See Content.*

DOSAGE

• CARBIDOPA/LEVODOPA TABLETS, ORALLY DISINTEGRATING

Parkinsonism, clients not receiving levodopa.

Initial: 1 tablet of 10 mg carbidopa/100 mg levodopa 3–4 times per day or 25 mg carbidopa/100 mg levodopa 3 times per day; **then,** increase by 1 tablet q 1–2 days until a total of 8 tablets/day is taken. If additional levodopa is required, substitute 1 tablet of 25 mg carbidopa/250 mg levodopa 3–4 times per day.

Parkinsonism, clients receiving levodopa.

Initial: Carbidopa/levodopa dosage should be about 25% of prior levodopa dosage (levodopa dosage is discontinued 8 hr before carbidopa/levodopa is initiated); **then,** adjust dosage as required. Suggested starting dose is 1 tablet of 25 mg carbidopa/250 mg levodopa 3–4 times per day for clients taking more than 1,500 mg levodopa or 25 mg carbidopa/100 mg levodopa for clients taking less than 1,500 mg levodopa.

• TABLETS, SUSTAINED RELEASE (SINEMET CR)

Parkinsonism, clients not receiving levodopa.

1 tablet twice a day at intervals of not less than 6 hr. Depending on the response, dosage may be increased or decreased. Usual dose is 2–8 tablets per day in divided doses at intervals of 4–8 hr during waking hours (if divided doses are not equal, the smaller dose should be given at the end of the day).

Parkinsonism, clients receiving levodopa.

1 tablet twice a day. Carbidopa is available alone for clients requiring additional carbidopa (i.e., inadequate reduction in N&V); in such clients, carbidopa may be given at a dose of 25 mg with the first daily dose of carbidopa/levodopa. If necessary, additional carbidopa, at doses of 12.5 or 25 mg, may be given with each dose of carbidopa/levodopa.

• CARBIDOPA TABLETS

Clients receiving carbidopa/levodopa who require additional carbidopa.

In clients taking 10 mg carbidopa/100 mg levodopa, 25 mg carbidopa may be given with the first dose each day. Additional doses of 12.5 or 25 mg may be given during the day with each dose. If the client is taking 25 mg carbidopa/250 mg levodopa, a dose of 25 mg carbidopa may be given with any dose, as needed. The maximum daily dose of carbidopa is 200 mg.

NURSING CONSIDERATIONS

ADMINISTRATION/STORAGE

1. Individualize dosage.
2. Assess for drug interactions.
3. Do not administer carbidopa/levodopa with levodopa.
4. Giving sustained-release form of carbidopa/levodopa with food results in increased levodopa availability by 50% and increased peak levodopa levels by 25%.
5. Do not crush/chew sustained-release form of Sinemet; may administer as whole or half tablets.

C

6. Allow at least 3 days to elapse between dosage adjustments of sustained-release product.

7. When carbidopa is used as supplement to carbidopa/levodopa, 1 tablet of carbidopa may be added or omitted per day.

8. If general anesthesia necessary, continue as long as PO fluids and other medication are allowed. Resume when able to take PO medication.

ASSESSMENT

1. Note reasons for therapy. Document motor function, reflexes, gait, strength of grip, amount of tremor, agents prescribed.

2. Observe extent of tremors, noting muscle weakness, muscle rigidity, difficulty walking, or changing directions. During dosage adjustment, involuntary movement may require dosage reduction.

3. Determine usual sleep patterns; assess mental status.

4. Note CV disease, cardiac arrhythmias, COPD.

5. List drugs prescribed. Elderly may require reduced dosage. May take multivitamin with pyridoxine without losing symptom control.

6. Obtain ECG, VS, respiratory assessment; determine level of bladder function. Monitor BP supine/standing for postural hypotension.

7. Assess need for drug 'holiday' periodically based on decreased drug response. Ensure regular neurologic F/U.

CLIENT/FAMILY TEACHING

1. Food may alter availability but may take with food to lessen GI upset. Do not crush or chew sustained-release form of Sinemet. May take as whole or half tablets.

2. Use caution with activities; change positions slowly to prevent ↓ BP.

3. Report side effects as dose may need to be reduced or temporarily discontinued. May be asked to tolerate certain side effects because of overall benefits gained with therapy.

4. With improvement, may resume normal activity gradually; with increased activity, other medical conditions must be considered.

5. Do not stop abruptly. When changing medication, one drug should be withdrawn slowly and the other started in small doses under supervision. To facilitate adjustment, take last dose of levodopa at bedtime; start carbidopa/levodopa upon arising.

6. May discolor/darken urine/sweat.

7. Muscle/eyelid twitching may indicate toxicity; report immediately.

8. Keep all F/U appointments to evaluate response to therapy and adverse side effects.

OUTCOMES/EVALUATE

Control of parkinsonian symptoms (e.g., improvement in motor function, physical mobility, reflexes, gait, strength of grip, and amount of tremor)

Carboplatin
(KAR-boh-plah-tin)

CLASSIFICATION(S):
Antineoplastic, alkylating
PREGNANCY CATEGORY: D
Rx: Paraplatin.
✤**Rx:** Paraplatin-AQ.

SEE ALSO *ANTINEOPLASTIC AGENTS* AND *ALKYLATING AGENTS*.

USES
(1) Initial treatment of advanced ovarian cancer in combination with other chemotherapeutic agents. (2) Palliative treatment of recurrent ovarian cancer either initially or previously treated with chemotherapy, including cisplatin. *Investigational:* In combination with other chemotherapeutic drugs to treat small cell and non-small cell lung carcinoma; advanced or recurrent squamous cell tumors of the head and neck; seminoma of testicular cancer.

ACTION/KINETICS

Action
Related to cisplatin. Acts by producing interstrand DNA cross-links; thought to be cell-cycle nonspecific.

Pharmacokinetics
$t\frac{1}{2}$, **initial:** 1.1–2 hr; **postdistribution:** 2.6–5.9 hr. Eliminated unchanged in the urine at a rate related to C_{CR}. **Plasma**

protein binding: Not bound to plasma proteins, although platinum from carboplatin is irreversibly bound to plasma protein with a slow half-life (5 days).

ADDITIONAL CONTRAINDICATIONS

History of severe allergy to mannitol or platinum compounds (including cisplatin). Severe bone marrow depression, significant bleeding, lactation.

SPECIAL CONCERNS

■ (1) Give under the supervision of a qualified physician experienced in the use of cancer chemotherapeutic drugs. Appropriate management of therapy and complications is possible only when adequate treatment facilities are readily available. (2) Bone marrow depression is dose-related and may be severe, causing infection or bleeding. Anemia may be cumulative and require blood transfusions. (3) Vomiting is a frequent side effect due to the drug. (4) Anaphylaxis may occur within minutes of giving the drug. Symptoms may be alleviated by epinephrine, corticosteroids, and antihistamines.■ Safety and efficacy have not been detrmined in children.

SIDE EFFECTS

Most Common

Thrombocytopenia, neutropenia, anemia, central neurotoxicity, peripheral neuropathies, ototoxicity, electrolyte (magnesium, calcium, potassium, sodium) loss, N&V, alopecia, pain, asthenia, allergic reactions.

See *Antineoplastic Agents* for a complete list of possible side effects. *Bone marrow suppression may be severe.* Vomiting. **Neurologic:** Central neurotoxicity, peripheral neuropathies (more common in ages 65 and over), ototoxicity. **GU:** Nephrotoxicity (including increased BUN and serum creatinine) especially when used with aminoglycosides. **Electrolytes:** Loss of Ca, Mg, K, Na. **Allergic:** Rash, urticaria, pruritus, erythema; *bronchospasm* and hypotension (rare). **Miscellaneous:** Pain, alopecia, asthenia. CV, respiratory, mucosal side effects, *anaphylaxis*.

LABORATORY TEST CONSIDERATIONS

↑ Alkaline phosphatase, AST, total bilirubin. Abnormal LFTs.

OD OVERDOSE MANAGEMENT

Symptoms: **Bone marrow suppression, hepatic toxicity.** *Treatment:* Monitor bone marrow and LFTs. Treat symptomatically.

DRUG INTERACTIONS

Al / Precipitate formation and loss of potency R/T reaction with Al (e.g., needles, IV administration sets)

Phenytoin / ↓ Serum phenytoin levels → loss of therapeutic effect

Warfarin / ↑ Anticoagulant effect of warfarin; monitor coagulation parameters

HOW SUPPLIED

Injection: 10 mg/mL; *Powder for Injection:* 50 mg, 150 mg, 450 mg, 600 mg.

DOSAGE————

- **IV**

  Ovarian cancer, as a single agent.
  360 mg/m^2 q 4 weeks on day 1. Lower doses are recommended in clients with low C_{CR}.

  In combination with cyclophosphamide.
  Carboplatin, 300 mg/m^2 plus cyclophosphamide, 600 mg/m^2, both on day 1 q 4 weeks for 6 cycles.

NURSING CONSIDERATIONS

☺ Do not confuse carboplatin with cisplatin (also an antineoplastic drug).

ADMINISTRATION/STORAGE

1. Do not repeat single intermittent doses of carboplatin until neutrophil count is at least 2,000/mm^3 and platelet count is 100,000/mm^3.

2. May escalate dose by no more than 125% of starting dose if platelet count is greater than 100,000/mm^3 and neutrophil count is greater than 2,000/mm^3. If platelet count is less than 50,000/mm^3 and neutrophil count is less than 500/mm^3, subsequent doses should be 75% of the prior dose.

3. With impaired kidney function, adjust dose: C_{CR} of 41–59 mL/min, 250 mg/m^2 on day one; C_{CR} of 16–40 mL/min, 200 mg/m^2 on day one. No recommended dose if the C_{CR} is less than 15 mL/min.

4. Cisplatin is easily confused with carboplatin. Store separately; post signs in

---

storage areas warning of the name mixups. Do not refer to as 'platinum.'

5. Do not use with needles or IV sets containing Al.

6. Just before use, reconstitute with either sterile water, D5W, or NaCl injection to final concentration of 10 mg/mL. May further dilute to concentrations as low as 0.5 mg/mL with D5W or NaCl injection. Administered by infusion lasting 15 min or longer.

7. Reconstituted solutions stable for 8 hr at room temperature. Discard after 8 hr; no antibacterial preservative in the formulation, although vials are multidose.

8. Store unopened vials at room temperature, protected from light.

ASSESSMENT

1. List allergic reactions to mannitol or platinum compounds.

2. Note any evidence of kidney impairment.

3. Assess neurologic disorders to determine if those occurring at a later date are drug related or exacerbations of a prior condition. Monitor for ototoxicity, peripheral neuropathy, visual disturbances.

4. Check for drug-induced anemia, a frequent side effect.

5. Monitor electrolytes, C_{CR}, renal and LFTs, CBC, platelet counts before each treatment course. Platelet Nadir: day 21; back to baseline by day 28.

INTERVENTIONS

1. Premedicate with antiemetics; vomiting frequent side effect.

2. Drug dose based on CBC and C_{CR}; reduce dose with impaired liver/renal function, hold for platelet counts <100,000/mm³.

3. With kidney impairment, initially give 1–2 L of fluids slowly. Use diuretics if overhydrated.

CLIENT/FAMILY TEACHING

1. N&V may be experienced; report if pretreatment antiemetic ineffective.

2. Report hearing/vision problems, numbness, tingling, skin rash; itching, redness.

3. Maintain adequate fluid intake using fluids with electrolytes; (K^+, Ca) may be lost.

4. Report sore throat, fever, bleeding, fatigue, breathing problems, mouth sores; may indicate bone marrow depression, can be severe with therapy.

5. Avoid pregnancy; practice reliable birth control.

OUTCOMES/EVALUATE

↓ Size and spread of tumor; stabilization of malignant process

Carisoprodol
(kar-eye-so-**PROH**-dohl)

CLASSIFICATION(S):
Skeletal muscle relaxant, centrally-acting
PREGNANCY CATEGORY: C
Rx: Soma.

SEE ALSO *SKELETAL MUSCLE RELAXANTS, CENTRALLY ACTING.*

USES
As an adjunct to rest, PT, and other measures to treat skeletal muscle disorders including bursitis, low back disorders, contusions, fibrositis, spondylitis, sprains, and muscle strains.

ACTION/KINETICS

Action
Does not directly relax skeletal muscles. Sedative effects may be responsible for muscle relaxation.

Pharmacokinetics
Onset: 30 min. **Duration:** 4–6 hr. **Peak serum levels:** 4–7 mcg/mL. **t½:** 8 hr. Metabolized in the liver and excreted in urine.

CONTRAINDICATIONS
Acute intermittent porphyria. Hypersensitivity to carisoprodol or meprobamate. Not recommended for use in children under 12 years of age.

SPECIAL CONCERNS
Use with caution during lactation, in impaired liver or kidney function, in addiction-prone individuals. Idiosyncratic reactions may occur rarely within minutes or hours after the first dose. May cause GI upset and sedation in infants.

Bold Italic = life threatening side effect   ■ = black box warning   ✦ = Available in Canada

SIDE EFFECTS
Most Common
Dizziness, drowsiness, N&V, headache, tachycardia.
CNS: Ataxia, dizziness, drowsiness, excitement, tremor, syncope, vertigo, insomnia, irritability, agitation, headache, depressive reactions. **GI:** N&V, epigastric distress, hiccoughs. **CV:** Flushing of face, postural hypotension, tachycardia. **Allergic or idiosyncratic reactions (usually after the first to fourth dose):** Pruritus, skin rashes, erythema multiforme, eosinophilia, fixed drug eruptions. Symptoms of severe reactions include fever, dizziness, *angioneurotic edema*, asthmatic symptoms, 'smarting' of the eyes, weakness, hypotension, *anaphylaxis*.

OD OVERDOSE MANAGEMENT
Symptoms: Stupor, coma, *shock, respiratory depression, and rarely, death*. The effects of overdosage of carisoprodol and alcohol or other CNS depressants or psychotropic drugs can be additive even if one of the drugs has been ingested at the usual recommended dose. *Treatment:* Supportive measures. Remove any remaining drug from the stomach. Institute supportive measures. If respiration and BP become compromised, provide respiratory assistance, CNS stimulants, and pressor agents cautiously as indicated. Diuresis, osmotic diuresis, peritoneal dialysis, hemodialysis. Monitor urinary output to avoid overhydration. Observe client for possible relapse due to incomplete gastric emptying and delayed absorption.

DRUG INTERACTIONS
Alcohol / Additive CNS depressant effects
Antidepressants, tricyclic / ↑ Carisoprodol effect
Barbiturates / Possible ↑ Carisoprodol effect, followed by inhibition of carisoprodol
Chlorcyclizine / ↓ Carisoprodol effect
CNS depressants / Additive CNS depression
MAO inhibitors / ↑ Carisoprodol effect R/T ↓ liver breakdown
Phenobarbital / ↓ Carisoprodol effect R/T ↑ liver breakdown
Phenothiazines / Additive CNS depressant effects
Psychotropic drugs / Additive CNS depressant effects

HOW SUPPLIED
Tablet: 350 mg.

DOSAGE
• **TABLETS**
  Skeletal muscle disorders.
Adults: 350 mg 3–4 times per day (take last dose at bedtime).

NURSING CONSIDERATIONS

ADMINISTRATION/STORAGE
Store from 15–30°C (59–86°F). Dispense in tight, light-resistant, well-closed containers.

ASSESSMENT
1. Note sensitivity to meprobamate or carisoprodol; potential for addictive behavior-precludes therapy.
2. List reasons for therapy, onset, contributing factors, characteristics of S&S. Record extent of skeletal muscular disorders noting baseline ROM, stiffness, level of discomfort.
3. Review drugs prescribed to ensure no interactions.

CLIENT/FAMILY TEACHING
1. Take with food if GI upset. If unable to swallow tablets, mix with syrup, chocolate, or a jelly mixture.
2. Used to help relax certain muscles to relieve stiffness, pain, discomfort caused by strains, sprains, or other muscular injury. Report adverse side effects, especially gait disturbance, tremors.
3. Take last dose at bedtime. Keep F/U visits and PT referrals.
4. May cause dizziness, drowsiness, palpitations; use caution when driving or undertaking tasks requiring mental alertness. Report if severe; may necessitate drug withdrawal.
5. Avoid OTC agents and alcohol.
6. Use judiciously; psychologic dependence may occur.

OUTCOMES/EVALUATE
Improvement in skeletal muscle pain and spasticity; ↑ ROM

Carmustine (BCNU) ■ IV

(kar-**MUS**-teen)

CLASSIFICATION(S):
Antineoplastic, alkylating
PREGNANCY CATEGORY: D
Rx: BiCNU, Gliadel.

SEE ALSO *ANTINEOPLASTIC AGENTS AND ALKYLATING AGENTS.*

USES

Injection: (1) Alone or in combination with other antineoplastic agents for palliative treatment of primary (e.g., brain stem glioma, astrocytoma, glioblastoma, ependymoma, medulloblastoma) and metastatic brain tumors. (2) Multiple myeloma (in combination with prednisone). (3) Advanced Hodgkin's disease and non-Hodgkin's lymphomas (not drug of choice) in those who relapse or who fail to respond to primary therapy. *Investigational:* Malignant melanoma.

Wafer: (1) Adjunct to surgery and radiation in newly diagnosed high-grade malignant glioma. (2) To prolong survival in recurrent glioblastoma multiforme as an adjunct to surgery.

ACTION/KINETICS

Action

Alkylates DNA and RNA, as well as inhibits several enzymes by carbamoylation of amino acids in proteins. Cell-cycle nonspecific. Not cross-resistant with other alkylating agents.

Pharmacokinetics

Rapidly cleared from plasma and metabolized. Crosses blood-brain barrier (concentration in CSF at least 50% greater than in plasma). **t½:** 15–30 min. Thirty percent excreted in urine after 24 hr, 60–70% after 96 hr. Wafers are biodegradable in the brain when implanted into the cavity after tumor resection. Released carmustine diffuses into the surrounding brain tissue.

CONTRAINDICATIONS

Lactation.

SPECIAL CONCERNS

■ (1) Bone marrow depression is the major toxic side effect. Monitor CBCs weekly for at least six weeks after a dose. Do not give repeat doses more frequently than q 6 weeks. Safety and effectiveness not established in children. Bone marrow toxicity is cumulative; adjust dose based on nadir blood counts from prior dose. (2) Thrombocytopenia and leukopenia may contribute to bleeding and overwhelming infections in an already compromised client. (3) Pulmonary toxicity (can be fatal) is dose-related. Those receiving >1,400 mg/m² cumulative dose are at a higher risk. Other risk factors include history of lung disease and treatment duration. Delayed onset pulmonary fibrosis can occur years after treatment (can result in death), particularly in those treated in childhood.■

SIDE EFFECTS

Most Common

Headache, hemiplegia, convulsions, confusion, brain edema, aphasia, depression, somnolence, speech disorder, amnesia, alopecia, N&V, constipation, abnormal healing, asthenia, UTI, infection, fever, pain, rash.

See *Antineoplastic Agents* for a complete list of possible side effects. **GI:** N&V within 2 hr after administration, lasting 4–6 hr; hepatic toxicity. **CNS:** Seizures, brain edema, intracranial infection, obstructive hydrocephalus. **GU:** Renal failure, azotemia, decrease in kidney size. **Hepatic:** Reversible increases in alkaline phosphatase, bilirubin, and transaminase. **Miscellaneous:** Rapid IV administration may produce transitory intense flushing of skin and conjunctiva (onset: after 2 hr; duration: 4 hr). ***Pulmonary fibrosis,*** ocular toxicity including retinal hemorrhage. The wafer may cause healing abnormalities including wound dehiscence, delayed wound healing, cerebrospinal fluid leak, and subdural, subgaleal, or wound effusions.

DRUG INTERACTIONS

Cimetidine / Additive bone marrow suppression
Digoxin / ↓ Serum digoxin levels → ↓

Bold Italic = life threatening side effect   ■ = black box warning   ✦ = Available in Canada

effect
Mitomycin / Corneal and conjunctival epithelial damage
Phenytoin / ↓ Serum phenytoin levels → ↓ effect

HOW SUPPLIED
Powder for Injection, Lyophilized: 100 mg; *Wafer Implant:* 7.7 mg.

DOSAGE
- **IV**
  In previously untreated clients.
  150–200 mg/m² q 6 weeks as a single dose. Alternate dosing schedule: 75–100 mg/m² on 2 successive days q 6 weeks. Reduce subsequent dosage if platelet levels are less than 100,000/mm³ and leukocyte levels are less than 4,000/mm³.
- **WAFER IMPLANT**
  Recurrent glioblastoma multiforme.
  Eight wafers placed in the resection cavity if size and shape of the cavity allow. If this is not possible, use the maximum number of wafers allowed.

NURSING CONSIDERATIONS

ADMINISTRATION/STORAGE
1. Slight overlap of wafer in cavity is acceptable. May use wafer broken in half; discard wafers broken into more than two pieces.
2. To secure wafers against cavity surface, oxidized regenerated cellulose may be placed over the wafers.
3. Irrigate resection cavity after wafer placement; dura should be closed in watertight fashion.
4. Unopened foil pouches of wafers may be kept at ambient room temperature for a maximum of 6 hr. Store at or below −20°C (−4°F).
5. Discard vials in which powder has become an oily liquid.
6. Reconstitute powder with absolute ethyl alcohol (provided); then add sterile water. For injection, dilutions stable for 24 hr when stored as noted in #13 below.
7. Stock solutions diluted to 500 mL with 0.9% NaCl or D5W are stable for 48 hr when stored as noted in #13 below.
8. Administer IV over 1–2-hr; faster injection may produce intense pain and burning at injection site.

9. Check for extravasation if burning/pain at injection site; discomfort may be from alcohol diluent. If no extravasation but burning experienced, reduce rate of flow.
10. Slow rate of infusion; report intense flushing of skin, redness of conjunctiva.
11. Skin contact with reconstituted carmustine may result in hyperpigmentation (transient); wash the skin/mucosa thoroughly with soap and water.
12. *Do not use vial for multiple doses;* no preservatives.
13. Store unopened vials at 2–8°C (36–46°F); protect from light. Store diluted solutions at 4°C (39°F); protect from light.

ASSESSMENT
1. Note reasons for therapy, onset, extent of disease, other agents trialed.
2. Document/monitor pulmonary, oral, ophthalmic exams.
3. Thrombocytopenia and leukopenia may contribute to bleeding, overwhelming infections in already compromised client; monitor closely.
4. Obtain baseline renal, LFTs. Monitor uric acid, CBC up to 6 weeks after drug dose; delayed bone marrow toxicity may develop. Drug causes granulocyte and bone marrow suppression. Nadir: 21 days; recovery: 35–42 days. Do not give repeat doses more frequently than q 6 weeks. Bone marrow toxicity cumulative; adjust dose based on nadir blood counts from prior dose.

CLIENT/FAMILY TEACHING
1. Drugs (antiemetic) administered before IV therapy should help with N&V.
2. Take temperature daily. Report S&S fever/infection; increased SOB, abnormal bruising/bleeding. Consume adequate fluids; prevent dehydration.
3. Avoid vaccinations. Use soft bristled tooth brush, electric razor; avoid aspirin/NSAIDs—may cause bleeding.
4. Avoid smoking; enhances pulmonary toxicity. This can be fatal and is dose-related; may occur many years after therapy.
5. May experience hair loss. Report if mouth sores develop; a special mouthwash or anesthetic can be prescribed.

Avoid rough, hot/hard foods or citrus products to prevent oral irritation.

6. Severe flushing after IV dose should subside in 2–4 hr; may also experience N&V 2 hr after infusion.

7. Practice reliable contraception; do not breastfeed.

OUTCOMES/EVALUATE

↓ Size/spread of metastatic process

Carvedilol 📷
(kar-**VAY**-dih-lol)

CLASSIFICATION(S):
Alpha-beta adrenergic blocking agent
PREGNANCY CATEGORY: C
Rx: Coreg, Coreg CR.

SEE ALSO *ALPHA-1 AND BETA-ADRENERGIC BLOCKING AGENTS.*

USES

(1) Essential hypertension used either alone or in combination with other antihypertensive drugs, especially thiazide diuretics. (2) Mild to severe heart failure of ischemic or cardiomyopathic origin; used with diuretics, ACE inhibitors, and digitalis to increase survival and reduce risk of hospitalization. (3) Reduce CV mortality in clinically stable clients who have survived an acute MI and have a left ventricular ejection fraction of 40% or less (with or without symptomatic heart failure). *Investigational:* Chronic, stable angina pectoris; idiopathic cardiomyopathy.

ACTION/KINETICS

Action

Has both alpha- and beta-adrenergic blocking activity. Decreases cardiac output, reduces exercise- or isoproterenol-induced tachycardia, reduces reflex orthostatic hypotension, causes vasodilation, and reduces peripheral vascular resistance. BP is lowered more in the standing than in the supine position. Significantly lowers plasma renin activity when given for at least 4 weeks.

Pharmacokinetics

Significant beta-blocking activity occurs within 60 min while alpha-blocking action is observed within 30 min. Rapidly absorbed after PO administration; significant first-pass effect. **Terminal t½:** 7–10 hr. Food delays absorption rate. Plasma levels average 50% higher in geriatric compared with younger clients. Extensively metabolized in the liver mainly by CYP2D6 and CYP2C9; metabolites excreted primarily via the bile into the feces. **Plasma protein binding:** Over 98%.

CONTRAINDICATIONS

Clients with NYHA Class IV decompensated cardiac failure requiring the use of IV inotropic therapy (wean from IV therapy before starting carvedilol), bronchial asthma, or related bronchospastic conditions, second- or third-degree AV block, SSS or severe bradycardia (unless a permanent pacemaker is in place), cardiogenic shock, drug hypersensitivity. Impaired hepatic function. Lactation.

SPECIAL CONCERNS

Use with caution in hypertensive clients with CHF controlled with digitalis, diuretics, or an ACE inhibitor. Use with caution in PVD, in surgical procedures using anesthetic agents that depress myocardial function, in diabetics receiving insulin or oral hypoglycemic drugs, in those subject to spontaneous hypoglycemia, or in thyrotoxicosis. Worsening cardiac failure or fluid retention may occur during up-titration of carvedilol. Signs of hyperthyroidism or hypoglycemia, especially tachycardia, may be masked. Abrupt withdrawal may cause severe exacerbation of angina and the occurrence of MI and ventricular arrhythmias; discontinue over 1–2 weeks. Clients with a history of severe anaphylactic reaction to a variety of allergens may be more reactive to repeated challenge while taking beta blockers. Safety and efficacy have not been established in children less than 18 years of age.

SIDE EFFECTS

Most Common

Dizziness, headache, N&V, diarrhea, URTI, fatigue, pain, bradycardia, hypotension, weight increase, hyperglycemia, increased cough, SOB.

Bold Italic = life threatening side effect ■ = black box warning ✦ = Available in Canada

CV: Bradycardia, postural hypotension, AV block (may be complete), BBB, cerebrovascular disorder, extrasystoles, hyper/hypotension, palpitations, peripheral ischemia, syncope, angina, aggravated angina, *cardiac failure, CVA,* myocardial ischemia, tachycardia, CV disorder, fluid overload, peripheral vascular disorder, precipitation/worsening of symptoms of arterial insufficiency, chest pain in Prinzmetal variant angina. **CNS:** Dizziness, headache, somnolence, insomnia, ataxia, nervousness, hypesthesia, paresthesia, vertigo, depression, aggravated depression, nervousness, migraine, neuralgia, paresis, amnesia, confusion, sleep disorder, impaired concentration, abnormal thinking, paranoia, convulsions, emotional lability, hypokinesia, paroniria, *convulsions.* **Body as a Whole:** Fatigue, viral infection, rash, allergy, asthenia, malaise, pain, injury, fever, infection, flu syndrome, dependent/peripheral edema, generalized edema, somnolence, sweating, *sudden death.* **GI:** Diarrhea, abdominal/GI pain, N&V, flatulence, dry mouth, anorexia, dyspepsia, melena, periodontitis, increased hepatic enzymes, hepatotoxicity, *GI hemorrhage.* **Respiratory:** Rhinitis, pharyngitis, sinusitis, bronchitis, dyspnea, *asthma, bronchospasm,* pulmonary edema, respiratory disorder/alkalosis, dyspnea, URTI, coughing, rales, interstitial pneumonitis. **GU:** UTI, albuminuria, hematuria, frequency of micturition, abnormal renal function, impotence, renal insufficiency, kidney failure, urinary incontinence in women. **Dermatologic:** Pruritus, erythematous rash, erythema multiforme, *Stevens-Johnson syndrome, toxic epidermal necrolysis,* alopecia, maculopapular rash, psoriaform rash, photosensitivity reaction, exfoliative dermatitis, increased sweating. **Metabolic:** Hypertriglyceridemia, hypercholesterolemia, hyper/hypoglycemia, hypo/hypervolemia, hyperuricemia, weight gain/loss, gout, dehydration, glycosuria, hyponatremia, hypo/hyperkalemia, diabetes mellitus, worsening of hyperglycemia in diabetes. **Hematologic:** Thrombocytopenia, anemia, leukopenia, pancytopenia, purpura, atypical lymphocytes, *aplastic anemia (rare).* **Musculoskeletal:** Back pain, arthralgia, myalgia, arthritis, muscle cramps, hypotonia. **Otic:** Decreased hearing, tinnitus. **Miscellaneous:** Hot flushes, leg cramps, abnormal/blurred vision, decreased hearing, decreased libido in men, *anaphylactoid reaction.*

LABORATORY TEST CONSIDERATIONS

↑ ALT, AST, BUN, NPN, alkaline phosphatase, GGT, creatinine. ↓ HDL, prothrombin. Bilirubinemia.

OD OVERDOSE MANAGEMENT

Symptoms: Severe hypotension, bradycardia, cardiac insufficiency, *cardiogenic shock, cardiac arrest, generalized seizures,* respiratory problems, bronchospasms, vomiting, lapse of consciousness. *Treatment:* Place client in a supine position, monitor carefully, and treat under intensive care conditions. Continue treatment for a sufficient period consistent with the 7- to 10-hr drug half-life.

- Gastric lavage or induced emesis shortly after ingestion.
- For excessive bradycardia, atropine, 2 mg IV. If bradycardia is resistant to therapy; use pacemaker therapy.
- To support cardiovascular function, give glucagon, 5–10 mg IV rapidly over 30 sec, followed by a continuous infusion of 5 mg/hr. Sympathomimetics (dobutamine, isoproterenol, epinephrine) may be given.
- For peripheral vasodilation, give epinephrine or norepinephrine with continuous monitoring of circulatory conditions.
- For bronchospasm, give beta sympathomimetics as aerosol or IV or use aminophylline IVPB.
- With seizures, give diazepam or clonazepam slowly IV.

DRUG INTERACTIONS

Antidiabetic agents / ↑ Hypoglycemic effects R/T beta blockade

Calcium channel blocking agents (e.g., diltiazem, verapamil) / ↑ Risk of conduction disturbances (rarely with hemodynamic compromise); monitor ECG and BP

Catecholamine-depleting drugs (e.g., re-

---

serpine) / Possible hypotension/severe bradycardia

Cimetidine / ↑ Carvedilol AUC by about 30%; no change in C_{max}

Clonidine / Potentiation of BP and heart rate lowering effects; when stopping both carvedilol and clonidine, discontinue clonidine first (d/c carvedilol several days later by gradually decreasing dose)

Cyclosporine / ↑ Cyclosporine levels R/T ↓ liver breakdown; monitor cyclosporine levels closely

Digoxin / ↑ Digoxin levels by about 15%; monitor digoxin when initiating, adjusting, or d/c carvedilol

Diphenhydramine / ↑ Carvedilol plasma levels and CV effects R/T inhibition of metabolism

Disopyramide / ↓ Disopyramide clearance → sinus bradycardia and hypotension; monitor carefully

Hydroxychloroquine / ↑ Plasma and CV effects of carvedilol R/T inhibition of metabolism; monitor clients

Insulin / ↑ Glucose lowering effect of insulin; monitor blood glucose

Monoamine oxidase inhibitors / Monitor for signs of hypotension or severe bradycardia

Oral hypoglycemics / ↑ Glucose lowering effect of oral hypoglycemics; monitor blood glucose

Propafenone / ↑ Blood levels of the R(+) enantiomer of carvedilol

Quinidine / ↑ Blood levels of the R(+) enantiomer of carvedilol

Rifampin / ↓ Plasma carvedilol AUC and C_{max} by about 70%

Salicylates / ↓ BP lowering effects of carvedilol; ↓ beneficial effects of carvedilol on LVEF in those with chronic heart failure

Selective serotonin reuptake inhibitors (e.g., fluoxetine, paroxetine) / Inhibition of carvedilol metabolism → excessive bradycardia; monitor cardiac function if used together

HOW SUPPLIED

Capsules, Extended-Release: 10 mg, 20 mg, 40 mg, 80 mg (all as the phosphate); *Tablets, Immediate-Release:* 3.125 mg, 6.25 mg, 12.5 mg, 25 mg.

DOSAGE

- **TABLETS, IMMEDIATE-RELEASE**

Essential hypertension.

Initial: 6.25 mg 2 times per day. If tolerated, using standing systolic pressure measured about 1 hr after dosing, maintain dose for 7–14 days. **Then,** increase to 12.5 mg 2 times per day, if necessary, based on trough BP, using standing systolic pressure 2 hr after dosing. Maintain this dose for 7–14 days; adjust upward to 25 mg 2 times per day if necessary and tolerated. Do not exceed 50 mg/day.

Congestive heart failure.

Individualize dose and closely monitor. **Initial:** 3.125 mg 2 times per day for 2 weeks. If tolerated, increase to 6.25 mg 2 times per day. Double dose every 2 weeks to the highest tolerated level, up to a maximum of 25 mg 2 times per day in those weighing less than 85 kg and 50 mg 2 times per day in those weighing over 85 kg. Reduce dose in those experiencing bradycardia (HR <55 beats/min).

Left ventricular dysfunction following MI.

Individualize dose and monitor during up-titration. **Initial:** 6.25 mg 2 times per day; increase after 3–10 days, based on tolerability, to 12.5 mg 2 times per day. Increase again to a target dose of 25 mg 2 times per day. A lower starting dose (3.125 mg 2 times per day) may be used due to low BP, HR, or fluid retention. The dosing regimen does not need to be altered in those who received an IV or PO beta-blocker during the acute phase of the MI.

Angina pectoris.

25–50 mg 2 times per day.

Idiopathic cardiomyopathy.

6.25–25 mg 2 times per day.

- **CAPSULES, EXTENDED-RELEASE**

Essential hypertension.

Initial: 20 mg once daily. If this dose is tolerated, using standing systolic pressure measured about 1 hr after dosing, maintain this dose for 7–14 days; **then,** increase to 40 mg once daily if needed, based on trough BP; maintain this dose for 7–14 days. Dose can then be adjusted upward to 80 mg once daily if tolerated and needed. Do not exceed a total daily dose of 80 mg.

Congestive heart failure.

Initial: 10 mg once daily for 2 weeks. Those who tolerate this dose may have their dose increased to 20, 40, or 80 mg over successive intervals of at least 2 weeks. Maintain clients on lower doses if higher doses are not tolerated.

Left ventricular dysfunction following MI.

Initial: 20 mg once daily; increase after 3–10 days, based on tolerability, to 40 mg once daily and then again to the target dose of 80 mg once daily. A dose of 10 mg once daily may be used and/or the rate of up-titration may be slowed if indicated (i.e., due to low BP or HR or fluid retention). Treatment may be started as an inpatient or outpatient and should be initiated after the client is hemodynamically stable and fluid retention has been minimized. The recommended dosing regimen need not be altered in those who received treatment with an IV or PO beta-blocker during the acute phase of the MI.

NURSING CONSIDERATIONS

ADMINISTRATION/STORAGE

1. Full antihypertensive effect seen within 7–14 days.

2. Clients controlled with immediate-release (IR) carvedilol alone or in combination with other medications, can be switched to extended-release (ER) capsules based on the total daily dose as follows: If the total daily dose of IR capsules is 6.25 mg, give 10 mg once daily of the ER capsules; if the total daily dose of IR is 12.5 mg, give 20 mg once daily of the ER form; if the total daily dose if IR is 25 mg, give 40 mg once daily of the ER form; and, if the total daily dose of IR is 50 mg, give 80 mg once daily of the ER form. Individualize dosage and carefully monitor during titration.

3. Addition of a diuretic can produce additive effects and exaggerate orthostatic effect.

4. Treat fluid retention with increased dose of diuretics, whether or not heart failure symptoms have worsened.

5. Episodes of dizziness or fluid retention during initiation of therapy can usually be managed by discontinuing drug; does not preclude subsequent successful titration of or a favorable response to the drug.

6. Reduce dose if bradycardia (HR less than 55 beats/min) occurs.

7. Store both IR and ER forms from 15–30°C (59–86°F). Dispense in a tight, light-resistant container.

ASSESSMENT

1. List reasons for therapy, type/onset of symptoms, other agents trialed, outcome.

2. Note history/evidence of bronchospastic conditions, asthma, advanced AV block, severe bradycardia; drug contraindicated.

3. Do baseline VS, EKG, CBC, BNP, renal and LFTs. Assess lung sounds, check for edema. Note ejection fraction/stress test/cath results.

CLIENT/FAMILY TEACHING

1. Take as prescribed with food; slows absorption/decreases orthostatic effects. Avoid OTC agents.

2. Take the extended-release form once daily in the morning with food. Swallow as a whole capsule; do not crush, chew, or divide doses.

3. Extended-release capsules may be opened and the beads sprinkled over a spoonful of cold applesauce. Consume the mixture immediately in its entirety. Do not store applesauce-drug mixture for future use.

4. Avoid activities that require mental acuity until drug effects realized.

5. Do not stop abruptly; R/T beta-blocking activity (especially with ischemic heart disease).

6. To prevent ↓ BP, sit or lie until symptoms subside; rise slowly from a sitting or lying position. Adding a diuretic may aggravate low BP drug effects.

7. Decreased tearing may be noted by contact lens wearers.

8. Dosing adjustments made every 7–14 days based on standing SBP measured 1 hr after dosing.

9. Keep record of weight, BP, pulse for review. Report increased swelling of ex-

---

tremities, weight gain >5 lb/week, 2 lb/day.

OUTCOMES/EVALUATE
- Desired reduction of BP
- ↓ Progression of CHF
- ↓ Cardiac remodeling
- ↓ Mortality

Cefaclor
(**SEF**-ah-klor)

CLASSIFICATION(S):
Cephalosporin, second generation
PREGNANCY CATEGORY: B
Rx: Ceclor, Raniclor.
♣Rx: Apo-Cefaclor, Novo-Cefaclor, Nu-Cefaclor, PMS-Cefaclor.

SEE ALSO *ANTI-INFECTIVES* AND *CEPHALOSPORINS*.

USES
Capsules, Chewable Tablets, Oral Suspension: (1) Otitis media due to *Streptococcus pneumoniae, Hemophilus influenzae, Streptococcus pyogenes*, and staphylococci. (2) Pharyngitis and tonsillitis caused by *S. pyogenes*. (3) Lower respiratory tract infections (including pneumonia) due to *S. pneumoniae, H. influenzae*, and *S. pyogenes*. (4) UTIs (including pyelonephritis and cystitis) caused by *Escherichia coli, Proteus mirabilis, Klebsiella* species, and coagulase-negative staphylococci.

Extended-Release Tablets: (1) Uncomplicated skin and skin structure infections due to *Staphylococcus aureus* (methicillin-susceptible). (2) Pharyngitis and tonsillitis due to *S. pyogenes*. (3) Acute bacterial exacerbation of chronic bronchitis due to *H. influenzae* (non–β-lactamase-producing strains only), *Moraxella catarrhalis* (including β-lactamase-producing strains), and *S. pneumoniae*. (4) Secondary bacterial infections of acute bronchitis due to *H. influenzae* (non–β-lactamase-producing strains only), *M. catarrhalis* (including β-lactamase-producing strains), and *S. pneumoniae*.

ACTION/KINETICS
Pharmacokinetics
Peak serum levels: 5–15 mcg/mL after 1 hr. **t½: PO,** 36–54 min. Well absorbed from GI tract. From 60 to 85% excreted in urine within 8 hr.

SPECIAL CONCERNS
Safety in infants less than 1 month of age not established.

SIDE EFFECTS
Most Common
N&V, diarrhea, abdominal pain, GI upset, headache, yeast infection of the mouth or vagina.
See *Cephalosporins* for a complete list of possible side effects. Also, cholestatic jaundice, lymphocytosis.

DRUG INTERACTIONS
↓ Plasma levels of cefaclor extended-release tablets when used with antacids; take cefaclor 2 hr before or after the antacid

HOW SUPPLIED
Capsules: 250 mg, 500 mg; *Powder for Oral Suspension:* 125 mg/5 mL, 187 mg/5 mL, 250 mg/5 mL, 375 mg/5 mL; *Tablets, Chewable:* 125 mg, 187 mg, 250 mg, 375 mg; *Tablets, Extended-Release:* 250 mg.

DOSAGE
• **CAPSULES; ORAL SUSPENSION; TABLETS, CHEWABLE**
  All uses.
Adults, usual: 250 mg q 8 hr. May double dose in more severe infections or those caused by less susceptible organisms. Do not exceed 4 grams/day. **Children:** 20 mg/kg/day in divided doses q 8 hr. May double dose in more serious infections, otitis media, or for infections caused by less susceptible organisms. For otitis media and pharyngitis, the total daily dose may be divided and given q 12 hr. Do not exceed a total dose of 2 grams/day.
• **TABLETS, EXTENDED-RELEASE**
  Uncomplicated skin and skin structure infections.
Adults, 16 years of age and older: 375 mg q 12 hr for 7 to 10 days. **Total daily dose:** 750 mg.
  Pharyngitis or tonsillitis.

Adults, 16 years of age and older: 375 mg q 12 hr for 10 days. **Total daily dose:** 750 mg.

> *Acute bacterial exacerbation of chronic bronchitis or secondary bacterial infection of acute bronchitis.*

Adults, 16 years of age and older: 500 mg q 12 hr for 7 days. **Total daily dose:** 1,000 mg.

NURSING CONSIDERATIONS

ADMINISTRATION/STORAGE

1. Continue administration for a minimum of 48–72 hr after fever abates or after evidence of bacterial eradication has been obtained. For β-hemolytic streptococcal infections, continue treatment for at least 10 days as a prophylaxis for rheumatic fever or glomerulonephritis.

2. 500 mg twice a day of cefaclor extended-release tablets is clinically equivalent to 250 mg 3 times a day of cefaclor immediate-release as a capsule. 500 mg twice a day of cefaclor extended-release tablets is *not* equivalent to 500 mg 3 times a day of other cefaclor formulations.

3. Refrigerate suspension after reconstitution; discard after 2 weeks.

4. The total daily dose for otitis media and pharyngitis can be divided and given q 12 hr.

5. Store capsules, chewable tablets, and extended-release tablets from 15–30°C (59–86°F). Refrigerate suspension after reconstitution; discard after 14 days.

ASSESSMENT

1. List type, onset, characteristics of S&S, agents trialed, C&S results.

2. Note any penicillin allergy; cross-sensitivity may occur.

CLIENT/FAMILY TEACHING

1. Take as directed; do not stop when feeling better. Review how to store drug; may keep suspension refrigerated up to 14 days; shake well before using.

2. Do not cut, chew or crush tablets. Food does not affect capsule absorption. Consume adequate fluids to prevent dehydration. Take the extended-release tablets with meals (i.e., within 1 hr of eating).

3. Report any rash, adverse response, or lack of improvement after 48–72 hr.

OUTCOMES/EVALUATE

Resolution of infection; symptomatic improvement

Cefadroxil monohydrate

(sef-ah-**DROX**-ill)

CLASSIFICATION(S):

Cephalosporin, first generation

PREGNANCY CATEGORY: B

Rx: Duricef.

✲**Rx:** Apo-Cefadroxil.

SEE ALSO *ANTI-INFECTIVES* AND *CEPHALOSPORINS.*

USES

(1) UTIs caused by *Escherichia coli, Proteus mirabilis,* and *Klebsiella* species. (2) Skin and skin structure infections due to staphylococci or streptococci. (3) Pharyngitis or tonsillitis due to *Streptococcus pyogenes* (group A β-hemolytic streptococci).

ACTION/KINETICS

Pharmacokinetics

Peak serum levels: PO, 15–33 mcg/mL after 90 min. **t½: PO,** 78–96 min. 90% excreted unchanged in urine within 24 hr.

SPECIAL CONCERNS

Safe use in children not established. Determine C_{CR} in clients with renal impairment.

SIDE EFFECTS

Most Common

Diarrhea, N&V, redness/swelling of skin, skin rash/itching, vaginal inflammation, colitis.

See *Cephalosporins* for a complete list of possible side effects.

HOW SUPPLIED

Capsules: 500 mg; *Powder for Oral Suspension:* 125 mg/5 mL, 250 mg/5 mL, 500 mg/5 mL; *Tablets:* 1 gram.

DOSAGE

• **CAPSULES; ORAL SUSPENSION; TABLETS**

> *Pharyngitis, tonsillitis.*

 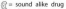

Adults: 1 gram/day in single or two divided doses for 10 days. **Children:** 30 mg/kg/day in single or two divided doses q 12 hr (for beta-hemolytic streptococcal infection, give dose for 10 or more days).

Skin and skin structure infections.
Adults: 1 gram/day in single or two divided doses. **Children:** 30 mg/kg/day in divided doses q 12 hr.

UTIs
Adults: 1 or 2 grams/day in single or two divided doses for uncomplicated lower UTI (e.g., cystitis). For all other UTIs, the usual dose is 2 grams/day in two divided doses. **Children:** 30 mg/kg/day in divided doses q 12 hr.

For clients with C_{CR} rates below 50 mL/min.
Initial: 1 gram; **maintenance,** 500 mg at following dosage intervals: q 36 hr for C_{CR} rates of 0–10 mL/min; q 24 hr for C_{CR} rates of 10–25 mL/min; q 12 hr for C_{CR} rates of 25–50 mL/min.

NURSING CONSIDERATIONS

ADMINISTRATION/STORAGE
1. Give without regard to meals. Food may decrease GI side effects.
2. Shake suspension well before using.
3. For beta-hemolytic streptococcal infections, treat for 10 days.
4. Refrigerate reconstituted suspension; discard any unused portion after 14 days.
5. Store tablets and capsules from 15–30°C (59–86°F).

ASSESSMENT
1. List reasons for therapy, type/onset of symptoms, culture results.
2. Note any penicillin allergy.

CLIENT/FAMILY TEACHING
1. Complete script as directed with/without food.
2. Refrigerate suspension, shake well before using; discard after 14 days.
3. Report any rash, adverse side effects, worsening of condition, lack of response after 72 hr.

OUTCOMES/EVALUATE
- Symptomatic improvement
- Negative culture reports

Cefdinir

(SEF-dih-near**)**

CLASSIFICATION(S):
Cephalosporin, third generation
PREGNANCY CATEGORY: B
Rx: Omnicef.

SEE ALSO *CEPHALOSPORINS.*

USES
Adults and adolescents: (1) Community-acquired pneumonia or acute exacerbations of chronic bronchitis due to *Haemophilus influenzae* (including β-lactamase producing strains), *Haemophilus parainfluenzae* (including β-lactamase producing strains), *Streptococcus pneumoniae* (penicillin-susceptible strains only), and *Moraxella catarrhalis* (including β-lactamase producing strains). (2) Acute maxillary sinusitis due to *H. influenzae* (including β-lactamase producing strains), *S. pneumoniae* (penicillin-susceptible strains only), and *M. catarrhalis* (including β-lactamase producing strains). (3) Uncomplicated skin and skin structure infections due to *Staphylococcus aureus* (including β-lactamase producing strains) and *Streptococcus pyogenes.* (4) Pharyngitis/tonsillitis due to *S. pyogenes.*
    Children (6 months through 12 years): (1) Acute bacterial otitis media due to *H. influenzae* (including β-lactamase producing strains), *S. pneumoniae* (penicillin-susceptible strains only), and *M. catarrhalis* (including β-lactamase producing strains). (2) Pharyngitis/tonsillitis due to *S. pyogenes.* Acute maxillary sinusitis. (3) Uncomplicated skin and skin structure infections due to *S. aureus* (including β-lactamase producing strains) and *S. pyogenes. NOTE:* The suspension is approved for use for all infections in children indicated above.

ACTION/KINETICS
Action
Interferes with the final step in cell wall formation (inhibition of mucopeptide biosynthesis), resulting in unstable cell membranes that undergo lysis. Also, cell division and growth are inhibited.

Bold Italic = life threatening side effect   ■ = black box warning   ✦ = Available in Canada

Pharmacokinetics
Maximum plasma levels: 2–4 hr. $t^{1}/_{2}$, **elimination:** 1.7 hr. Excreted through the urine.

CONTRAINDICATIONS
Allergy to cephalosporins.

SPECIAL CONCERNS
Reduce dose in compromised renal function. Safety and efficacy have not been determined in infants less than 6 months of age. Cefdinir has not been studied for the prevention of rheumatic fever following *S. pyrogenes* pharyngitis/tonsillitis.

SIDE EFFECTS
Most Common
Diarrhea, N&V, vaginal moniliasis/vaginitis, headache, abdominal pain, rash (children).
See *Cephalosporins* for a complete list of possible side effects.

DRUG INTERACTIONS
Antacids, Al- or Mg-containing / ↓ Cefdinir absorption → ↓ plasma levels
Probenecid / ↑ Plasma cefdinir levels → ↑ effect

HOW SUPPLIED
Capsules: 300 mg; *Oral Suspension:* 125 mg/5 mL, 250 mg/5 mL.

DOSAGE————————
- **CAPSULES**
  Community-acquired pneumonia, uncomplicated skin and skin structure infections.
Adults and adolescents age 13 and older: 300 mg q 12 hr for 10 days.
  Acute exacerbations of chronic bronchitis, acute maxillary sinusitis, or pharyngitis/tonsillitis.
Adults and adolescents age 13 and older: 300 mg q 12 hr for 5–10 days or 600 mg q 24 hr for 10 days for acute exacerbations of chronic bronchitis or pharyngitis/tonsillitis. Alternatively, 300 mg twice a day for 5 days for acute exacerbations of chronic bronchitis.
- **ORAL SUSPENSION**
  Acute bacterial otitis media or pharyngitis/tonsillitis.
Children, 6 months through 12 years: 7 mg/kg q 12 hr for 5–10 days or 14 mg/kg q 24 hr for 10 days.
  Uncomplicated skin and skin structure infections.

Children, 6 months through 12 years: 7 mg/kg q 12 hr for 10 days.
  Acute maxillary sinusitis.
Children, 6 months through 12 years: 7 mg/kg q 12 hr or 14 mg/kg q 24 hr for 10 days.

——————————————————

NURSING CONSIDERATIONS

ADMINISTRATION/STORAGE
1. For adults with C_{CR} <30 mL/min, give 300 mg once daily. For children with a C_{CR} of <30 mL/1.73 m^2, give 7 mg/kg (less than or equal to 300 mg) once daily.
2. Once daily dosing (600 mg) in adults and adolescents may be used for acute maxillary sinusitis, acute exacerbations of chronic bronchitis, or pharyngitis/tonsillitis.
3. For children, age 6 months through 12 years, the total daily dose for all infections is 14 mg/kg, up to a maximum of 600 mg/day. Except for skin infections, once-daily dosing for 10 days is as effective as twice-daily dosing.
4. The dosage of oral suspension for children is:
- **9 kg (20 lb):** 2.5 mL q 12 hr or 5 mL q 24 hr of 125 mg/5 mL formulation.
- **18 kg (40 lb):** 5 mL q 12 hr or 10 mL q 24 hr of 125 mg/5 mL formulation; or, 2.5 mL q 12 hr or 5 mL q 24 hr of 250 mg/5 mL formulation.
- **27 kg (60 lb):** 7.5 mL q 12 hr or 15 mL q 24 hr of 125 mg/5 mL formulation; or, 3.75 mL q 12 hr or 7.5 mL q 24 hr of 250 mg/5 mL formulation.
- **36 kg (80 lb):** 10 mL q 12 hr or 20 mL q 24 hr of 125 mg/5 mL formulation; or, 5 mL q 12 hr or 10 mL q 24 hr of 250 mg/5 mL formulation.
- **Greater or equal to 43 kg (95 lb):** 12 mL q 12 hr or 24 mL q 24 hr of 125 mg/5 mL formulation; or, 6 mL q 12 hr or 12 mL q 24 hr of 250 mg/5 mL formulation.
5. Hemodialysis removes cefdinir from the body. In those on chronic hemodialysis, the recommended initial dose is 300 mg or 7 mg/kg every other day. At the end of each hemodialysis session, 300 mg or 7 mg/kg should be given followed by 300 mg or 7 mg/kg every other day.

6. Store capsules/powder for suspension 15–30°C (59–86°F). After mixing, store suspension at room temperature (25°C, 77°F). Discard any unused suspension after 10 days.

ASSESSMENT
1. Check for cephalosporin/PCN allergy.
2. Note reasons for therapy, characteristics of S&S, culture results.
3. Assess CBC/liver/renal function; if C_{CR} <30 mL/min, reduce dose.

CLIENT/FAMILY TEACHING
1. Take without regard to food.
2. Iron supplements, multivitamins with iron, antacids with Mg and Al interfere with drug absorption; if needed, take either 2 hr before or 2 hr after dose.
3. Oral suspension contains 2.86 grams of sucrose per teaspoon; use capsules with diabetes. Add 38 mL water to 60 mL bottle or 63 mL water to 100 mL bottle, mix well; discard solution after 10 days. Shake well before each use.
4. May give suspension in iron fortified infant formula without losing potency.
5. Report if diarrhea persistent, exceeds 4 episodes/day, accompanied by abdominal pain. Consume adequate fluids to prevent dehydration.
6. Stools may be discolored red; should subside.
7. Report unusual side effects, worsening of condition, lack of response after 72 hr.

OUTCOMES/EVALUATE
Resolution of infection

Cefditoren pivoxil
(sef-**DIH**-tor-en)

CLASSIFICATION(S):
Cephalosporin, third generation
PREGNANCY CATEGORY: B
Rx: Spectracef.

SEE ALSO *ANTI-INFECTIVES* AND *CEPHALOSPORINS*.

USES
(1) Acute bacterial exacerbation of chronic bronchitis due to *Haemophilus influenzae* (including β-lactamase–producing strains), *Haemophilus parainfluenzae* (including β-lactamase–producing strains), *Streptococcus pneumoniae* (penicillin-susceptible strains only), and *Moraxella catarrhalis* (including β-lactamase–producing strains). (2) Pharyngitis/tonsillitis due to *Streptococcus pyogenes*. Eradicates *S. pyogenes* from the oropharynx. (3) Uncomplicated skin and skin-structure infections due to *Staphylococcus aureus* (including β-lactamase–producing strains) and *Streptococcus pyogenes*. (4) Community-acquired pneumonia due to *Haemophilus influenzae* (including β-lactamase–producing strains), *Haemophilus parainfluenzae* (including β-lactamase–producing strains), *Streptococcus pneumoniae* (penicillin-susceptible strains only), and *Moraxella catarrhalis* (including β-lactamase–producing strains).

ACTION/KINETICS
Pharmacokinetics
Absorbed from the GI tract and hydrolyzed to cefditoren by esterases. **Maximum plasma levels:** 1.5–3 hr. High fat meals increase plasma levels. **t½, terminal:** 1.6 hr. Not appreciably metabolized; mainly excreted through the urine. Clearance is decreased in renal insufficiency. **Plasma protein binding:** 88% to serum albumin.

CONTRAINDICATIONS
Use with known allergy to cephalosporin antibiotics, in those with carnitine deficiency or inborn errors of metabolism that may result in clinically significant carnitine deficiency, and in those with milk protein hypersensitivity (not lactose intolerance).

SPECIAL CONCERNS
Use with caution in clients hypersensitive to other cephalosporins, pencillins, or other drugs. Long-term use may cause carnitine deficiency or emergence and overgrowth of resistant organisms. Use with caution during lactation. Safety and efficacy have not been determined in children less than 12 years of age.

SIDE EFFECTS
Most Common
Nausea, headache, diarrhea, vaginal moniliasis.

GI: Diarrhea, N&V, abdominal pain, dyspepsia, pseudomembranous colitis, constipation, dry mouth, eructation, flatulence, gastritis, GI disorder, mouth ulceration, abnormal LFT, oral moniliasis, stomatitis, taste perversion. **CNS:** Headache, abnormal dreams, dizziness, insomnia, nervousness, somnolence. **Body as a Whole:** Asthenia, fever, fungal infection, pain, sweating, urticaria, weight loss. **Respiratory:** Pharyngitis, rhinitis, sinusitis. **GU:** Vaginal moniliasis, urinary frequency, vaginitis, hematuria. **Miscellaneous:** Allergic reaction, increased coagulation time, hyperglycemia, increased appetite, leukopenia, leukorrhea, myalgia, peripheral edema, pruritus, rash, thrombocytopenia.

LABORATORY TEST CONSIDERATIONS
Possible positive direct Coombs' test. ↑ Urine WBCs, glucose. ↓ Hematocrit.

OD OVERDOSE MANAGEMENT
Symptoms: N&V, epigastric distress, diarrhea, convulsions. *Treatment:* Hemodialysis, especially if renal function is compromised. Treat symptomatically. Institute supportive measures.

DRUG INTERACTIONS
Antacids / ↓ Cefditoren absorption
H-2 receptor antagonists / ↓ Cefditoren absorption
Probenecid / ↑ Plasma cefditoren levels

HOW SUPPLIED
Tablets: 200 mg.

DOSAGE——————————
• **TABLETS**
   Acute bacterial exacerbation of chronic bronchitis.
Adults: 400 mg twice a day for 10 days.
   Pharyngitis, tonsillitis, uncomplicated skin and skin structure infections.
Adults: 200 mg twice a day for 10 days.
   Community-acquired pneumonia.
Adults: 400 mg twice a day for 14 days.

NURSING CONSIDERATIONS

ADMINISTRATION/STORAGE
1. No dose adjustment needed with mild renal impairment (C_{CR} of 50–80 mL/min/1.73 m²). Do not give more than 200 mg 2 times per day with moderate renal impairment (C_{CR} of 30–49 mL/min/1.73 m²) and 200 mg/day with severe renal impairment (C_{CR} of <30 mL/min/1.73 m²).
2. Store 15–30°C (59–86°F). Protect from light and moisture.
3. Dispense in tight, light resistant containers.

ASSESSMENT
1. Note reasons for therapy, onset, characteristics of S&S.
2. Obtain C&S, CBC, renal and LFTs; note dysfunction- dosage may require adjustment.
3. Assess carefully for sensitivity to drug, cephalosporins, or penicillins; cross sensitivity may occur.
4. Drug not for use with carnitine deficiency/milk protein hypersensitivity.

CLIENT/FAMILY TEACHING
1. Take twice a day as directed. Take with meals; enhances absorption. Complete therapy; do not share or skip doses.
2. Do not take at same time as antacids or other drugs that decrease stomach acid (H_2antagonists). If needed take 2 hr before or after drug therapy.
3. Those with milk protein hypersensitivity (not lactose intolerance) should avoid this drug.
4. Report lack of response, worsening of symptoms, severe diarrhea, mouth pain. If rash, hives, SOB, or unusual bruising/bleeding occur, stop drug- report immediately.

OUTCOMES/EVALUATE
Resolution of infection; symptomatic improvement

Cefepime hydrochloride **IV**
(**SEF**-eh-pim)

CLASSIFICATION(S):
Cephalosporin, third generation
PREGNANCY CATEGORY: B
Rx: Maxipime.

SEE ALSO *CEPHALOSPORINS* AND *ANTI-INFECTIVES.*

USES
Adults: (1) Uncomplicated and complicated UTIs (including pyelonephritis)

---

caused by *Escherichia coli* or *Klebsiella pneumoniae;* when the infection is severe or caused by *E. coli, K. pneumoniae,* or *Proteus mirabilis;* when the infection is mild to moderate, including infections associated with concurrent bacteremia with these microorganisms. (2) Uncomplicated skin and skin structure infections caused by *Staphylococcus aureus* (methicillin-susceptible strains only) or *Streptococcus pyogenes.* (3) Moderate to severe pneumonia due to *Streptococcus pneumoniae,* including cases associated with concurrent bacteremia, *Pseudomonas aeruginosa, K. pneumoniae,* or *Enterobacter* species. (4) Monotherapy for empiric treatment of febrile neutropenia in those at high risk for infection. (5) In combination with metronidazole in complicated intra-abdominal infections due to *E. coli,* viridans group streptococci, *P. aeruginosa, K. pneumoniae, Enterobacter* species, or *Bacteroides fragilis.*

Children, 2 months to 16 years: Treatment of complicated and uncomplicated UTIs including pyelonephritis, uncomplicated skin and skin structure infections, pneumonia, and as empiric therapy for febrile neutropenic clients.

ACTION/KINETICS

Action
Antibacterial activity against both gram-negative and gram-positive pathogens, including those resistant to other β-lactam antibiotics. High affinity for the multiple penicillin-binding proteins that are essential for cell wall synthesis.

Pharmacokinetics
Peak serum levels, after IV: 78 mcg/mL. **t½, terminal:** 2 hr. About 85% of the drug is excreted unchanged in the urine.

CONTRAINDICATIONS
Use after a hypersensitivity reaction to cefepime, cephalosporins, pencillins, or any other β-lactam antibiotics.

SPECIAL CONCERNS
Increased risk of serious adverse events in clients with renal insufficiency; symptoms include encephalopathy, myoclonus, seizures, and renal failure. Use with caution during lactation. Safety and efficacy have not been determined in children <12 years old.

SIDE EFFECTS

Most Common
Rash, phlebitis, pain, inflammation at injection site, headache, nausea, dizziness, vaginal moniliasis.

See *Cephalosporins* for a complete list of possible side effects.

LABORATORY TEST CONSIDERATIONS
↑ ALT, AST, alkaline phosphatase, BUN, creatinine, potassium, total bilirubin. ↓ Hematocrit, neutrophils, platelets, WBCs. ↑ or ↓ Calcium, phosphorus. Positive Coombs' test. Abnormal PTT, PT.

DRUG INTERACTIONS
Aminoglycosides / ↑ Risk of nephrotoxicity and ototoxicity

Furosemide / ↑ Risk of nephrotoxicity

HOW SUPPLIED
Powder for Injection: 500 mg, 1 gram, 2 grams.

DOSAGE

- **IM; IV**

  Mild to moderate uncomplicated or complicated UTIs, including pyelonephritis, due to E. coli, K. pneumoniae, *or* P. mirabilis.

  Adults: 0.5–1 gram IV or IM (for *E. coli* infections) q 12 hr for 7–10 days.

  Severe uncomplicated or complicated UTIs, including pyelonephritis, due to E. coli *or* K. pneumoniae.

  Adults: 2 grams IV q 12 hr for 10 days.

  Moderate to severe pneumonia due to S. pneumoniae, P. aeruginosa, K. pneumoniae, *or* Enterobacter *species.*

  Adults: 1–2 grams IV q 12 hr for 10 days.

  Moderate to severe uncomplicated skin and skin structure infections due to S. aureus *or* S. pyogenes.

  Adults: 2 grams IV q 12 hr for 10 days.

  Febrile neutropenia.

  2 grams IV q 8 hr for 7 days, or until resolution of neutropenia.

  With metronidazole in complicated intra-abdominal infections due to E. coli, P. aeruginosa, K. pneumoniae, B. fragilis, Enterobacter *species, or viridans group streptococci.*

  Adults: 2 grams IV q 12 hr for 7–10 days

Bold Italic = life threatening side effect   ■ = black box warning   ✚ = Available in Canada

Infections in children 2 months to 16 years.

Up to 40 kg: 50 mg/kg q 12 hr (q 8 hr for febrile neutropenia) for same durations as adult dosage. Do not exceed adult dose.

NURSING CONSIDERATIONS

ADMINISTRATION/STORAGE

1. For IM use: Reconstitute with 0.9% NaCl, D5W, 0.5% or 1% lidocaine HCl, sterile water or bacteriostatic water for injection with parabens or benzyl alcohol.

2. Adjust dose/frequency (see package insert) for impaired renal function (C_{CR} <60 mL/min).

IV 3. For IV use: Reconstitute the 1 or 2 gram 100 mL bottle with 50 or 100 mL of 0.9% NaCl injection, 5% or 10% dextrose injection, M/6 sodium lactate injection, D5W/0.9% NaCl injection, D5W/RL, or Normosol-R or Normosol-M in D5W injection; administer over 30 min. Cefepime is compatible at concentrations of 1–40 mg/mL with above solutions.

4. Solutions of cefepime should not be added to ampicillin at a concentration of 40 mg/mL and should not be added to aminophylline, gentamicin, metronidazole, netilmicin sulfate, tobramycin, or vancomycin. If needed, each can be given separately.

5. Protect reconstituted drug from light; store at room temperature 20–25°C (68–77°F) for 24 hr or refrigerate at 2–8°C (36–46°F) for 7 days.

ASSESSMENT

1. Note reasons for therapy, onset, characteristics of S&S. List agents trialed; outcome.

2. Check for any sensitivity to penicillin, cephalosporins, or other antibiotics.

3. Obtain baseline cultures, CBC, renal and LFTs. Reduce dose with renal dysfunction.

4. List other agents prescribed; aminoglycosides and furosemide may increase risk of nephrotoxicity/ototoxicity.

CLIENT/FAMILY TEACHING

1. Drug administered parenterally. Must have regular dosing to maintain therapeutic blood levels.

2. May cause positive Coombs' blood test.

3. Pain and inflammation may occur at infusion site; may see rash.

4. Report adverse side effects, lack of response, prolonged/persistent diarrhea as overgrowth of colon flora may have occurred; may require additional therapy.

5. Avoid alcohol during and for 3 days following completion of therapy.

OUTCOMES/EVALUATE

Symptomatic improvement with resolution of infective organism

---

Cefixime oral
(seh-**FIX**-eem)

CLASSIFICATION(S):
Cephalosporin, third generation
PREGNANCY CATEGORY: B
Rx: Suprax.

SEE ALSO *ANTI-INFECTIVES* AND *CEPHALOSPORINS*.

USES

(1) Uncomplicated UTIs caused by *E. coli* and *P. mirabilis*. (2) Otitis media due to *H. influenzae* (beta-lactamase positive and negative strains), *Moraxella catarrhalis*, and *S. pyogenes*. (3) Pharyngitis and tonsillitis caused by *S. pyogenes*. (4) Acute bronchitis and acute exacerbations of chronic bronchitis caused by *S. pneumoniae* and *H. influenzae* (beta-lactamase positive and negative strains). (5) Uncomplicated cervical or urethral gonorrhea due to *N. gonorrhoeae* (both penicillinase- and non-penicillinase-producing strains).

ACTION/KINETICS

Pharmacokinetics

Stable in the presence of beta-lactamase enzymes. **Peak serum levels:** 2–6 hr. **$t\frac{1}{2}$:** Averages 3–4 hr. About 50% excreted unchanged in the urine and approximately 10% in the bile.

SPECIAL CONCERNS

Safe use in infants less than 6 months old not established.

SIDE EFFECTS

Most Common

N&V, diarrhea/loose stools, abdominal pain, dyspepsia, flatulence.

See *Cephalosporins* for a complete list of possible side effects. Also, **GI:** Flatulence. **Hepatic:** Elevated alkaline phosphatase levels. **Renal:** Transient increases in BUN or creatinine.

ADDITIONAL LABORATORY TEST CONSIDERATIONS

False + test for ketones using nitroprusside test.

HOW SUPPLIED

Powder for Oral Suspension: 100 mg/5 mL, 200 mg/5 mL.

DOSAGE

- **ORAL SUSPENSION**

  All uses.

Adults: Either 400 mg once daily (recommended) or 200 mg q 12 hr. **Children:** Either 8 mg/kg once daily or 4 mg/kg q 12 hr. Give the adult dose to children >50 kg or >12 years of age. *NOTE:* For clients on renal dialysis or in whom C_{CR} is 21–60 mL/min, the dose should be 75% of the standard dose (i.e., 300 mg/day). If the C_{CR} <20 mL/min or continuous ambulatory peritoneal dialysis, the dose should be 50% of the standard dose (i.e., 200 mg/day).

Uncomplicated gonorrhea.

One 400-mg tablet daily.

NURSING CONSIDERATIONS

ADMINISTRATION/STORAGE

1. Continue therapy for at least 10 days when treating *S. pyogenes*.

2. Use the following pediatric doses if using the 100 mg/5 mL suspension: **6.25 kg:** For a daily dose of 50 mg, give 2.5 mL; **12.5 kg:** For a daily dose of 100 mg, give 5 mL; **18.75 kg:** For a daily dose of 150 mg, give 7.5 mL; **25 kg:** For a daily dose of 200 mg, give 10 mL; **31.25 kg:** For a daily dose of 250 mg, give 12.5 mL; **37.5 kg:** For a daily dose of 300 mg, give 15 mL.

3. Use the following pediatric dose if using the 200 mg/5 mL suspension: **6.25 kg:** For a daily dose of 50 mg, give 1.25 mL; **12.5 kg:** For a daily dose of 100 mg, give 2.5 mL; **18.75 kg:** For a daily dose of 150 mg, give 3.75 mL; **25 kg:** For a daily dose of 200 mg, give 5 mL; **31.25 kg:** For a daily dose of 250 mg, give 6.25 mL; **37.5 kg:** For a daily dose of 300 mg, give 7.5 mL.

4. Once reconstituted, keep suspension at room temperature or under refrigeration; discard after 14 days.

5. Prior to reconstitution, store powder from 20–25°C (68–77°F).

ASSESSMENT

1. Note any prior sensitivity to cephalosporins or penicillins.

2. List onset, S&S, clinical findings, source of infection, culture results. Reduce dose with impaired renal function.

3. Use suspension in children and when treating otitis media.

CLIENT/FAMILY TEACHING

1. Take as directed; complete entire prescription. May cause GI upset; report persistent adverse side effects, esp. diarrhea. Store suspension at room temperature; discard after 14 days.

2. Once-a-day dosing should be taken at same time each day; check cost, may be prohibitive.

3. May alter results of urine glucose and ketone testing; do finger sticks for more accurate results.

4. Consult provider if condition does not improve or deteriorates after 48–72 hr. Return as scheduled for F/U.

OUTCOMES/EVALUATE

Resolution of infection; symptomatic improvement

Cefoperazone sodium

(sef-oh-**PER**-ah-zohn)

CLASSIFICATION(S):

Cephalosporin, third generation

PREGNANCY CATEGORY: B

SEE ALSO *ANTI-INFECTIVES* AND *CEPHALOSPORINS.*

USES

(1) Respiratory tract infections due to *Streptococcus pneumoniae, Haemophilus*

influenzae, Staphylococcus aureus (penicillinase/non-penicillinase producing), *S. pyogenes* (group A β–hemolytic streptococci), *Pseudomonas aeruginosa, Klebsiella pneumoniae, Escherichia coli, Proteus mirabilis,* and *Enterobacter* species. (2) Peritonitis and other intra-abdominal infections due to *E. coli, P. aeruginosa,* and anaerobic gram–negative bacilli (including *Bacteroides fragilis).* (3) Bacterial septicemia due to *S. pneumoniae, S. agalactiae, S. aureus, P. aeruginosa, E. coli, Klebsiella pneumoniae, Klebsiella* species, *Proteus* species (indole positive and indole negative), *Clostridium* species, and anaerobic gram–positive cocci. (4) Skin and skin structure infections due to *S. aureus* (penicillinase and non–penicillinase-producing species), *S. pyogenes,* and *P. aeruginosa.* (5) PID, endometritis, and other female genital tract infections due to *N. gonorrhoeae, S. epidermidis, S. agalactiae, E. coli,* and *Clostridium* species, *Bacteroides* species (including *Bacteroides fragilis,*) anaerobic gram–positive cocci. (6) UTIs due to *E. coli* and *P. aeruginosa.*

ACTION/KINETICS

Pharmacokinetics

Peak serum levels: 73–153 mcg/mL. **Steady state serum levels:** 150 mcg/mL. **t½:** 102–156 min. Approximately 30% excreted unchanged in the urine.

SPECIAL CONCERNS

Use with caution in hepatic disease or biliary obstruction. Safety and effectiveness not determined in children.

SIDE EFFECTS

Most Common

Diarrhea/loose stools, N&V, injection site reactions.

See *Cephalosporins* for a complete list of possible side effects. Also, hypoprothrombinemia resulting in bleeding and/or bruising.

ADDITIONAL DRUG INTERACTIONS

Anticoagulants / ↑ Hypoprothrombinemic effect → bleeding complications
Ethanol / Possible Antabuse-like reaction
Warfarin / ↑ Risk of bleeding

HOW SUPPLIED

Injection: 1 gram, 2, grams, 10 grams; *Powder for Injection:* 1 gram, 2 grams.

DOSAGE

- **IM; IV**
  All uses.

Adults, usual: 2–4 grams/day in equally divided doses q 12 hr (up to 6–12 grams/day divided into 2, 3, or 4 doses ranging from 1.5 to 4 grams/dose has been used in severe infections or for less sensitive organisms). Continue for at least 10 days when treating *Streptococcus pyogenes* infections.

NOTE: Significantly excreted in the bile; do not exceed 4 grams/day in hepatic disease or biliary obstruction.

NURSING CONSIDERATIONS

ADMINISTRATION/STORAGE

1. For IM: Reconstitute with 0.5% lidocaine HCl, bacteriostatic or sterile water for injection. Do not use preparations containing benzyl alcohol in infants.

2. For IM, use any of the following diluents after reconstitution: D5W, D5W/RL, D5W/0.2% or 0.9% NaCl, D10%, LR, 0.5% lidocaine HCl injection, 0.9% NaCl, D5W/Normosol M, Normosol R, bacteriostatic or sterile water for injection. If concentrations of 250 mg/mL or more are needed, prepare solutions using 0.5% lidocaine HCl injection.

[IV] 3. After reconstitution for IM or IV use, allow any foaming to dissipate; visually inspect for complete solubilization. Vigorous prolonged agitation may be necessary to solubilize concentrations of 333 mg/mL or higher.

4. For IV: Reconstitute with any of the solutions listed for IM, except 0.5% lidocaine HCl, bacteriostatic or sterile water for injection.

5. When used for intermittent infusion, further dilute reconstituted product in 20–40 mL of diluent/gram and give over 15–30 min.

6. When used IVPB for continuous infusion, dilute to a final concentration between 2 and 25 mg/mL.

7. Reconstituted drug may be frozen; however, after thawing, discard any unused portion.

[camera] = see color insert   [H] = Herbal   [IV] = Intravenous   *[@]* = sound alike drug

8. Protect unreconstituted powder from light; store in refrigerator.

9. Do not mix cefoperazone directly with an aminoglycoside. If concomitant therapy needed, use sequential intermittent IV infusion provided that separate secondary IV tubing is used and the primary IV tubing is irrigated between doses. Give prior to aminoglycoside.

ASSESSMENT

1. List reasons for therapy, onset, characteristics of S&S, culture results.

2. Note PCN/ATX sensitivity. Assess for bruising, hematuria, black stools, S&S of bleeding.

3. Obtain baseline coagulation studies and monitor; may cause hypoprothrombinemia. Assess need for prophylactic vitamin K administration (usually 10 mg/week).

4. With skin lesions, inspect closely, noting size, location, extent of involvement.

5. Assess for excessive alcohol use. Reduce dose with liver/biliary tract disease.

CLIENT/FAMILY TEACHING

1. Drug given parenterally; report unusual bruising/bleeding, diarrhea, adverse effects, or lack of response.

2. Avoid alcohol/alcohol-containing products during and for 72 hr after last dose; Antabuse-like reaction may occur.

OUTCOMES/EVALUATE

- ↓ Size and number of skin lesions; wound healing
- Resolution of infection

Cefotaxime sodium Ⅳ©

(sef-oh-**TAX**-eem)

CLASSIFICATION(S):
Cephalosporin, third generation
PREGNANCY CATEGORY: B
Rx: Claforan.

SEE ALSO *ANTI-INFECTIVES* AND *CEPHALOSPORINS*.

USES

(1) Lower respiratory tract infections, including pneumonia, due to *Streptococcus pneumoniae*, *S. pyogenes* (group A streptococci) and other streptococci (excluding enterococci), *Staphylococcus aureus* (penicillinase and nonpenicillinase producing), *Eschericia coli*, *Klepsiella* species, *Haemophilus influenzae* (including ampicillin-resistant strains), *Haemophilus parainfluenzae*, *Proteus mirabilis*, *Serratia marcescens*, *Enterobacter* species, and indole-positive *Proteus* and *Pseudomonas* species (including *P. aeruginosa*). (2) GU infections due to *Enterococcus* species, *Staphylococcus epidermidis*, *S. aureus* (penicillinase and nonpenicillinase producing), *Citrobacter* species, *Enterobacter* species, *E. coli*, *Klebsiella* species, *P. mirabilis*, *Proteus vulgaris*, *Providencia stuartii*, *Morganella morganii*, *Providencia rettgeri*, *S. marcescens*, and *Pseudomonas* species (including *P. aeruginosa*). (3) Uncomplicated gonorrhea (cervical/urethral, rectal) due to *Neisseria gonorrhoeae*, including penicillinase-producing strains. (4) Gynecologic infections, including PID, endometritis, and pelvic cellulitis due to *S. epidermidis*, *Streptococcus* species, *Enterococcus* species, *Enterobacter* species, *Klebsiella* species, *E. coli*, *P. mirabilis*, *Bacteroides* species (including *Bacteroides fragilis*), *Clostridium* species, anaerobic cocci (including *Peptostreptococcus* species and *Peptococcus* species), and *Fusobacterium* species (including *F. nucleatum*). Cefotaxime has no activity against *Chlamydia trachomatis*. (5) Bacteremia/septicemia due to *E. coli*, *Klebsiella* species, and *S. marcescens*, *S. aureus*, and *Streptococcus* species (including *S. pneumoniae*). (6) Skin and skin structure infections due to *S. aureus* (penicillinase and nonpenicillinase producing), *S. epidermidis*, *S. pyogenes* (group A streptococci) and other streptococci, *Enterococcus* species, *Acinetobacter* species, *E. coli*, *Citrobacter* species (including *C. freundii*), *Enterobacter* species, *Klebsiella* species, *P. mirabilis*, *P. vulgaris*, *M. morganii*, *P. rettgeri*, *Pseudomonas* species, *S. marcescens*, *Bacteroides* species, anaerobic cocci (includ-

---

Bold Italic = life threatening side effect ■ = black box warning ✦ = Available in Canada

ing *Peptostreptococcus* species, and *Peptococcus* species). (7) Intra-abdominal infections, including peritonitis due to *Streptococcus* species, *E. coli, Klebsiella* species, *Bacteroides* species, anaerobic cocci (including *Peptostreptococcus* species and *Peptococcus* species), *P. mirabilis,* and *Clostridium* species. (8) Bone and joint infections due to *S. aureus* (penicillinase and nonpenicillinase producing strains), *Streptococcus* species (including *S. pyogenes*), *Pseudomonas* species (including *P. aeruginosa*), and *P. mirabilis.* (9) CNS infections (e.g., meningitis, ventriculitis) due to *Neisseria meningitis, H. influenzae, S. pneumoniae, K. pneumoniae,* and *E. coli.* (10) Reduce incidence of certain infections in clients undergoing cesarean section, both intraoperatively (after clamping the umbilical cord) and postoperatively. The IV route is preferable for clients with severe or life-threatening infections; for clients after surgery; or for those manifesting malnutrition, trauma, malignancy, heart failure, or diabetes, especially if shock is present or possible. (11) Preoperatively to reduce the incidence of certain infections in clients undergoing surgical procedures (e.g., abdominal or vaginal hysterectomy, GI and GU tract surgery) that may be classified as contaminated or potentially contaminated. (12) In certain cases of confirmed or suspected gram-positive or gram-negative sepsis or in those with other serious infections in which the causative organism has not been identified; may be used together with an aminoglycoside. It is possible that nephrotoxicity may be potentiated if cefotaxime is used together with an aminoglycoside.

ACTION/KINETICS
Pharmacokinetics
$t^{1/2}$: 1 hr. **Peak serum levels after 1 gram IV:** 42–102 mcg/mL. 60% excreted unchanged in the urine.

SIDE EFFECTS
Most Common
Injection site inflammation after IV, rash, pruritus, N&V, fever, diarrhea, colitis.

See Cephalosporins for a complete list of possible side effects. Also, possibility of erythema multiforme, **Stevens-Johnson syndrome**, and **toxic epidermal necrolysis**.

HOW SUPPLIED
Injection: 1 gram, 2 grams; *Powder for Injection:* 500 mg, 1 gram, 2 grams, 10 grams.

DOSAGE
- **IM; IV**
  Uncomplicated infections.
  Adults: 1 gram q 12 hr IM or IV.
  Moderate to severe infections.
  Adults: 1–2 grams q 8 hr IM or IV.
  Septicemia and other infections requiring higher doses.
  Adults: 2 grams q 6–8 hr IV; daily dose ranges from 6–8 grams.
  Life-threatening infections.
  Adults: 2 grams q 4 hr IV, not to exceed 12 grams/day.
  Gonorrhea
  Adult males, IM: Single dose of 1 gram for rectal gonorrhea. **Adult IM:** Single dose of 0.5 gram for rectal gonorrhea in females or gonococcoal urethritis/cervicitis in males and females. For disseminated gonogoccal infections give 1 gram IV q 8 hr.
  Disseminated gonococcal infection and gonococcal scalp abscesses in newborns.
  25 mg/kg IV or IM q 12 hr for 7 days, with a duration of 10 to 14 days if meningitis is documented.
  Perioperative prophylaxis.
  Adults: 1 gram IM or IV 30–90 min prior to surgery.
  Cesarean section.
  IV: 1 gram as soon as the umbilical cord is clamped; **then,** give 1 gram IM or IV 6 and 12 hr after the first dose.
  Use in children.
  Pediatric, 0–1 week: 50 mg/kg q 12 hr IV; **1–4 weeks:** 50 mg/kg q 8 hr IV; **1 month–12 years (<50 kg):** 50–180 mg/kg/day in 4 to 6 divided doses either IM or IV. Higher doses may be used for more severe or serious infections, including meningitis. *NOTE:* Use adult dose in children 50 kg or over.
  Use in impaired renal function.
  If C_{CR} <20 mL/min/1.73 m^2, reduce dose by 50%. If only serum creatinine is avail-

C

---

able, use the following formulas to calculate C_{CR}:

- Males: Weight (kg) x (140 − age) / 72 x serum creatinine (mg/dL).
- Females: 0.85 x male value.

NURSING CONSIDERATIONS

℞ Do not confuse cefotaxime (Claforan) with cefoxitin (Mefoxin), also a cephalosporin.

ADMINISTRATION/STORAGE

1. Do not exceed a maximum daily dose of 12 grams.
2. The premixed injection is intended for IV administration after thawing. Reconstituted powder for injection may be given IM or IV.
3. Continue for a minimum of 48–72 hr after the client defervescence or after evidence of bacterial eradication has been determined. Continue therapy for a minimum of 10 days for group A β-hemolytic streptococcal infections to minimize risk of rheumatic fever/glomerulonephritis.
4. For IM: Reconstitute with sterile/bacteriostatic water for injection. Inject deeply into large muscle. Divide doses of 2 grams and administer into different sites.
IV 5. Use IV route for those with bacteremia, bacterial septicemia, peritonitis, meningitis, or other severe/life-threatening infections. Also use IV for those who may be poor risks due to lowered resistance as a result of debilitating conditions, such as malnutrition, trauma, surgery, diabetes, heart failure, or malignancy, especially if shock present/impending.
6. Cefotaxime sterile powder for injection may be reconstituted in 50 or 100 mL D5W or 0.9% NaCl in the ADD-Vantage diluent container.
7. Discontinue other IV solutions during therapy. Do not mix cefotaxime with aminoglycosides for continuous IV infusion; give each separately.
8. Cefotaxime maximally stable at pH of 5–7; do not prepare with diluents having pH >7.5 (e.g., NaHCO₃ injection).
9. Add recommended amount of diluent, shake to dissolve. Do not administer if particles are present or solution

discolored. The normal solution color ranges from light yellow to amber.
10. For intermittent IV administration, mix 1 or 2 grams cefotaxime with 10 mL sterile water for injection; administer over 3–5 min; do not give over period of less than 3 minutes. For administration by infusion, dilute in 50–100 mL of solution; infuse over 30 min.
11. After reconstitution, drug remains stable for 24 hr at room temperature, 5 days refrigerated, and 13 weeks frozen. Thaw frozen samples at room temperature before use. Do not refreeze; discard unused portions.
12. Store dry cefotaxime below 30°C (86°F); protect from excess heat/light to prevent darkening.

ASSESSMENT

1. Note reasons for therapy, onset, characteristics of S&S; assess for PCN/ATX sensitivity.
2. With joint infections, assess ROM/freedom of movement.
3. With gynecologic infections, determine extent of infection, duration, S&S.
4. Monitor labs/review culture results for organism resistance; reduce dose with renal dysfunction.

CLIENT/FAMILY TEACHING

1. Drug given parenterally. Report adverse side effects/lack of response.
2. Review appropriate technique/frequency for administration, proper storage. Inspect site for pain/redness; IM may cause thrombophlebitis.
3. Record I&O; report decrease in urinary output/persistent diarrhea.
4. Avoid alcohol in any form; an Antabuse-type reaction may occur.

OUTCOMES/EVALUATE

- Resolution of infection; symptomatic improvement
- Negative culture reports

Cefoxitin sodium **IV** ℞
(seh-**FOX**-ih-tin)

CLASSIFICATION(S):
Cephalosporin, second generation
PREGNANCY CATEGORY: B
Rx: Mefoxin.

Bold Italic = life threatening side effect   ■ = black box warning   ♣ = Available in Canada

❦**Rx:** Cefoxitin for Injection.

SEE ALSO *ANTI-INFECTIVES* AND *CEPHALOSPORINS*.

USES

(1) Lower respiratory tract infections (pneumonia and lung abscess) due to *Streptococcus pneumoniae,* other streptococci (excluding enterococci such as *S. faecalis), Staphylococcus aureus* (including penicillinase-producing strains), *Escherichia coli, Klebsiella* species, *Haemophilus influenzae,* and *Bacteroides* species. (2) UTIs due to *E. coli, Klebsiella* species, *Proteus mirabilis, Morganella morganii, Proteus vulgaris,* and *Providencia* species (including *P. rettgeri).* (3) Intra-abdominal infections (peritonitis and intra-abdominal abscess) due to *E. coli, Klebsiella* species, *Bacteroides* species (including *B. fragilis),* and *Clostridium* species. (4) Gynecological infections (endometritis, pelvic cellulitis, PID) due to *E. coli, N. gonorrhoeae* (including penicillinase-producing strains), *Bacteroides* species (including *B. fragilis* group), *Clostridium* species, *P. niger, Peptostreptococcus* species, and *Streptococcus agalactiae.* Cefoxitin has no activity against *Chlamydia trachomatis.* (5) Septicemia due to *S. pneumoniae, S. aureus* (including penicillinase-producing strains), *E. coli, Klebsiella* species, and *Bacteroides* species (including *B. fragilis).* (6) Bone/joint infections due to *S. aureus* (including penicillinase-producing strains). (7) Skin/skin structure infections due to *S. aureus* (including penicillinase-producing strains), *Staphylococcus epidermidis* (excluding enterococci, especially *S. faecalis), E. coli, P. mirabilis, Klebsiella* species, *Bacteroides* species (including the *B. fragilis* group), *Clostridium* species, *P. niger* species, and *Peptostreptococcus* species. (8) Perioperative prophylaxis, including vaginal hysterectomy, GI surgery, TURP, prosthetic arthroplasty, and C-section. (9) Infections due to *Chlamydia trachomatis.* *NOTE:* Many gram-negative infections resistant to certain cephalosporins and penicillins respond to cefoxitin.

ACTION/KINETICS

Action

Broad-spectrum cephalosporin that is penicillinase- and cephalosporinase-resistant and is stable in the presence of β-lactamases.

Pharmacokinetics

Peak serum level after 1 gram IV: 110 mcg/mL. **t½:** 40–60 min; 85% of drug excreted unchanged in urine after 6 hr.

SIDE EFFECTS

Most Common

N&V, diarrhea, thrombophlebitis.

See *Cephalosporins* for a complete list of possible side effects. Higher doses have caused increased incidence of eosinophilia and increased AST levels in children over 3 months of age.

ADDITIONAL LABORATORY TEST CONSIDERATIONS

High concentrations may interfere with the measurement of creatinine by the Jaffe method.

HOW SUPPLIED

Injection: 1 gram, 2 grams; *Powder for Injection:* 1 gram, 2 grams, 10 grams.

DOSAGE

- **IM; IV**

  Uncomplicated infections (cutaneous, pneumonia, urinary tract).

  Adults, IV: 1 gram q 6–8 hr. **Daily dosage:** 3 to 4 grams.

  Moderately severe or severe infections.

  Adults, IV: 1 gram q 4 hr or 2 grams q 6–8 hr. **Daily dosage:** 6 to 8 grams.

  Infections requiring higher dosage (e.g., gas gangrene).

  Adults, IV: 2 grams q 4 hr or 3 grams q 6 hr. **Daily dosage:** 12 grams.

  Gonorrhea

  Adults, IV: 2 grams IM with 1 gram probenecid PO.

  Prophylaxis in surgery.

  Adults, IV: 2 grams 30–60 min before surgery followed by 2 grams q 6 hr after first dose for 24 hr only (72 hr for prosthetic arthroplasty).

  Cesarean section, prophylaxis.

  IV: 2 grams as soon as the umbilical cord is clamped or a 3-dose regimen consisting of 2 grams given IV as soon as the umbilical cord is clamped followed by 2 grams 4 and 8 hr after the initial dose.

TURP, prophylaxis.
1 gram before surgery; **then,** 1 gram q 8 hr for up to 5 days.

Impaired renal function.
Adults, initial: 1–2 grams. Then, use the following as a guide: **Mild impairment (30–50 mL/min C_{CR}):** 1–2 grams q 8–12 hr. **Moderate impairment (10–29 mL/min C_{CR}):** 1–2 grams q 12–24 hr. **Severe impairment (5–9 ml/min C_{CR}):** 0.5–1 gram q 12–24 hr. **Essentially no function (<5 mL/min C_{CR}):** 0.5–1 gram q 24–48 hr.

Use in children for infections.
Children over 3 months: 80–160 mg/kg/day divided into 4 to 6 equal doses. Use the higher doses for more severe or serious infections, not to exceed 12 grams/day.

Use in children for prophylaxis.
Children over 3 months: 30–40 mg/kg q 6 hr or at the times designated for adults.

NURSING CONSIDERATIONS

℘ Do not confuse cefoxitin (Mefoxin) with cefotaxime (Claforan), also a cephalosporin.

ADMINISTRATION/STORAGE

1. Maintain therapy at least 10 days for group A beta-hemolytic streptococcal infections in order to minimize the risk of rheumatic fever or glomerulonephritis.

2. For IM injections, reconstitute each gram with 2 mL sterile water or 2 mL 0.5% lidocaine HCl (without epinephrine) to reduce pain at injection site.

3. When used for prophylactic use in surgery, give 30 to 60 minutes before the surgery. Stop prophylactic administration within 24 hr since continuing use increases the risk of side effects but, in the majority of cases, does not reduce the incidence of subsequent infection.

IV 4.   The IV route is preferable for those with bacteremia, bacterial septicemia, other severe or life-threatening infections or for those who may be poor risks because of lowered resistance resulting from debilitating conditions, including malnutrition, trauma, surgery, diabetes, heart failure, or malignancy, especially if shock is present or impending.

5. For IV: Reconstitute 1 gram with 10 or more mL of sterile water and 2 grams with 10–20 mL. The 10 gram vial may be reconstituted with 43 or 93 mL sterile water or other compatible solutions (see package insert). Do not use solutions containing benzyl alcohol in infants.

6. For intermittent IV: give 1 or 2 grams in 10 mL sterile water over 3 to 5 min. For continuous IV administration (e.g., for higher doses), add solution to 50–100 mL of D5W, NSS, D5W/0.9% NaCl, or D5W/0.02% NaHCO₃ solution and give over 15–30 min.

7. For higher doses, cefoxitin solutions may be added to an IV bottle containing D5W injection, 0.9% NaCl injection, or 5% dextrose/0.9% NaCl injection. Butterfly or scalp vein-type needles are preferred for this type of infusion.

8. Do not mix with aminoglycosides. If both needed, administer separately.

9. Store premixed products (for IV use only) at less than -20°C (-4°F). Will maintain potency after thawing for 24 hr at room temperature; 21 days if refrigerated. Discard any unused thawed solutions; do not refreeze.

10. Store dry powder below 30°C (86°F). The dry powder solutions darken depending on storage conditions; potency is unaffected.

ASSESSMENT

1. Note reasons for therapy, characteristics of S&S, culture results. Assess for PCN/ATX sensitivity.

2. Monitor I&O, renal function; reduce dose with dysfunction.

3. Assess infusion site for pain/redness; may cause thrombophlebitis.

CLIENT/FAMILY TEACHING

Drug is administered parenterally. Report any adverse effects, significant diarrhea, reduction in urinary output, rash, or lack of response.

OUTCOMES/EVALUATE

• Resolution of infection
• Surgical infection prophylaxis

Bold Italic = life threatening side effect   ■ = black box warning   ✦ = Available in Canada

Cefpodoxime proxetil
(sef-poh-**DOX**-eem)

CLASSIFICATION(S):
Cephalosporin, third generation
PREGNANCY CATEGORY: B
Rx: Vantin.

SEE ALSO *ANTI-INFECTIVES* AND
CEPHALOSPORINS.

USES
(1) Acute, community-acquired pneumonia due to *Streptococcus pneumoniae* or *Hemophilus influenzae* (including non–β-lactamase-producing strains). (2) Acute bacterial exacerbation of chronic bronchitis caused by *S. pneumoniae*, non–β-lactamase-producing *H. influenzae*, or *Moraxella catarrhalis.* (3) Acute otitis media caused by *S. pneumoniae* (excluding penicillin-resistant strains), *Streptococcus pyogenes*, *H. influenzae* (including β-lactamase-producing strains), and *M. catarrhalis* (including beta-lactamase producing strains). (4) Pharyngitis or tonsillitis due to *S. pyogenes.* (5) Acute, uncomplicated urethral and cervical gonorrhea caused by *Neisseria gonorrhoeae* (including penicillinase-producing strains). (6) Acute, uncomplicated anorectal infections in women due to *N. gonorrhoeae* (including penicillinase-producing strains). (7) Uncomplicated skin and skin structure infections due to *Staphylococcus aureus* (including penicillinase-producing strains) or *S. pyogenes.* Abscesses should be surgically drained. (8) Uncomplicated UTIs (cystitis) due to *Escherichia coli*, *Klebsiella pneumoniae*, *Proteus mirabilis*, or *Staphylococcus saprophyticus.* (9) Mild-to-moderate acute maxillary sinusitis due to *H. influenzae* (including beta-lactamase producing strains), *S. pneumoniae*, and *M. catarrhalis.*

ACTION/KINETICS
Pharmacokinetics
t½, after PO: 2–3 hr. From 29 to 33% is excreted unchanged in the urine.

SIDE EFFECTS
Most Common
N&V, diarrhea, anorexia, headache, yeast infection of the mouth or vagina. See *Cephalosporins* for a complete list of possible side effects.

DRUG INTERACTIONS
Antacids / ↓ Cefpodoxime plasma levels; take cefpodoxime 2 hr before or after the antacid
H₂ antagonists / ↓ Cefpodoxime plasma levels

HOW SUPPLIED
Granules for Oral Suspension: 50 mg/5 mL, 100 mg/5 mL; *Tablets, Film-Coated:* 100 mg, 200 mg.

DOSAGE
• **ORAL SUSPENSION; FILM-COATED TABLETS**

Acute community-acquired pneumonia.
Adults and children 12 years and over: 200 mg q 12 hr for 14 days.

Acute bacterial exacerbations of chronic bronchitis.
Adults and children 12 years and over: 200 mg q 12 hr for 10 days. Use the tablets.

Uncomplicated gonorrhea (men and women) and rectal gonococcal infections (women).
Adults and children 12 years and over: Single dose of 200 mg.

Skin and skin structure infections.
Adults and children 12 years and over: 400 mg q 12 hr for 7–14 days.

Pharyngitis, tonsillitis.
Adults and children 12 years and over: 100 mg q 12 hr for 5–10 days.
Children, 2 months through 12 years: 5 mg/kg (maximum of 100 mg/dose) q 12 hr (maximum daily dose: 200 mg) for 5–10 days.

Uncomplicated UTIs.
Adults and children 12 years and over: 100 mg q 12 hr for 7 days.

Acute otitis media.
Children, 2 months through 12 years: 5 mg/kg (maximum of 200 mg/dose) q 12 hr for 5 days.

Acute maxillary sinusitis.
Adults and children 12 years and older: 200 mg q 12 hr for 10 days. **Children, 2 months through 12 years:** 5

mg/kg (maximum of 200 mg/dose) q 12 hr for 10 days.

NURSING CONSIDERATIONS
ADMINISTRATION/STORAGE

1. In severe renal impairment (C_{CR} <30 mL/min), increase dosing interval to q 24 hr. If on hemodialysis, use dosage frequency of 3 times/week after hemodialysis. Adjustment not required with cirrhosis.
2. May use the following formula to estimate C_{CR} (mL/min): **males:** weight (kg) $\times$ (140 – age)/72 $\times$ serum creatinine (mg/dL); **females:** 0.85 $\times$ male value.
3. To prepare suspension: Add a total of 58 mL of distilled water to 50 mg/mL product or 57 mL of distilled water to the 100 mg/5 mL product. Tap bottle gently to loosen powder, then add 25 mL of water and shake vigorously for 15 sec to wet the powder. Add the remainder of the water and shake the bottle vigorously for 3 min or until all particles are suspended. Shake well before using.
4. Store tablets and unsuspended granules from 20–25°C (68–77°F).
5. After reconstitution of granules, store in refrigerator; discard after 14 days.

ASSESSMENT

1. Note any reactions to cephalosporins/penicillins; cross-sensitivity can occur.
2. List source/characteristics of infection; obtain baseline cultures.
3. Note renal dysfunction; alter dosage/frequency if evident.
4. Obtain serologic test for syphilis with gonorrhea treatment.
5. Monitor VS and I&O; evaluate persistent diarrhea for other causes, such as C. difficile.
6. Discontinue therapy/report if seizures occur.

CLIENT/FAMILY TEACHING

1. Take tablets with food to enhance absorption. Oral suspension may be given with/without food. Refrigerate suspension; discard after 14 days. Complete entire prescription.
2. Report lack of response, adverse effects, rash, persistent N&V, diarrhea; drug or dosage may require adjustment. Consume adequate fluids to prevent dehydration.
3. If receiving treatment for gonorrhea, have partner tested and treated; use barrier contraception to prevent reinfections. Drug is not effective against syphilis; all partners should be tested so that appropriate treatment may be provided.
4. Keep all F/U appointments to evaluate response to therapy.

OUTCOMES/EVALUATE
- Resolution of infection
- Symptomatic improvement

Cefprozil
(**SEF**-proh-zill)

CLASSIFICATION(S):
Cephalosporin, second generation
PREGNANCY CATEGORY: B
Rx: Cefzil.

SEE ALSO *ANTI-INFECTIVE DRUGS* AND *CEPHALOSPORINS.*

USES

(1) Pharyngitis and tonsillitis due to *Streptococcus pyogenes.* (2) Acute bacterial sinusitis due to *Streptococcus pneumoniae, Staphylococcus aureus, Haemophilus influenzae* (including β-lactamase producing strains), and *Moraxella catarrhalis* (including β-lactamase producing strains). (3) Otitis media caused by *S. pneumoniae, H. influenzae* (including β-lactamase-producing strains), and *M. catarrhalis* (including β-lactamase-producing strains). *NOTE:* Eradication rates are somewhat lower in treating otitis media due to β-lactamase-producing strains. (4) Uncomplicated skin and skin structure infections due to *S. aureus* (including penicillinase-producing strains) and *S. pyogenes.* Abscesses usually require surgical drainage. (5) Secondary bacterial infection of acute bronchitis and acute bacterial exacerbation of chronic bronchitis due to *S. pneumoniae, H. influenzae* (including β-lactamase positive and negative strains), and *M. catarrhalis* (including β-lactamase-producing strains).

ACTION/KINETICS

Pharmacokinetics

$t^{1/2}$, **after PO:** 78 min. Sixty percent is recovered in the urine unchanged.

SIDE EFFECTS

Most Common

N&V, diarrhea, abdominal pain, yeast infection of mouth or vagina.

See *Cephalosporins* for a complete list of possible side effects.

ADDITIONAL DRUG INTERACTIONS

↓ Effectiveness of oral contraceptives.

HOW SUPPLIED

Powder for Oral Suspension: 125 mg/5 mL after reconstitution, 250 mg/5 mL after reconstitution; *Tablets:* 250 mg, 500 mg.

DOSAGE

- **ORAL SUSPENSION; TABLETS**

  Pharyngitis, tonsillitis.

Adults and children over 13 years: 500 mg q 24 hr for at least 10 days (for *S. pyogenes* infections, give 10 or more days). **Children, 2–12 years:** 7.5 mg/kg q 12 hr for at least 10 days (for *S. pyogenes* infections, give 10 or more days).

  Acute sinusitis.

Adults and children over 13 years: 250 mg q 12 hr or 500 mg q 12 hr for 10 days. Use the higher dose for moderate to severe infections. **Children, 6 months–12 years:** 7.5 mg/kg q 12 hr or 15 mg/kg q 12 hr for 10 days. Use the higher dose for moderate to severe infections.

  Secondary bacterial infections of acute bronchitis and acute bacterial exacerbation of chronic bronchitis.

Adults and children over 13 years: 500 mg q 12 hr for 10 days.

  Uncomplicated skin and skin structure infections.

Adults and children over 13 years: Either 250 mg q 12 hr, 500 mg q 24 hr, or 500 mg q 12 hr (all for a duration of 10 days). **Children, 2–12 years:** 20 mg/kg q 24 hr for 10 days.

  Otitis media.

Infants and children 6 months–12 years: 15 mg/kg q 12 hr for 10 days.

NURSING CONSIDERATIONS

ADMINISTRATION/STORAGE

1. With impaired renal function (C_{CR} of 0–30 mL/min), give 50% of usual dose at standard intervals.

2. To enhance palability/adherence, a suspension is available in a bubble-gum flavor for children.

3. Store powder for oral suspension (before reconstitution) and tablets from 15–30°C (59–77°F). After reconstitution, refrigerate suspension; discard any unused portion after 14 days.

ASSESSMENT

1. Note reasons for therapy, characteristics of S&S, culture results, any PCN/ATX sensitivity.

2. Reduce dose with impaired renal function; monitor I&O and VS.

CLIENT/FAMILY TEACHING

1. Take as directed with/without food; food decreases stomach upset. Complete entire prescription, do not stop if feeling better. Refrigerate suspension and shake well before using; discard after 14 days.

2. Use nonhormonal form of contraception; may decrease OC effectiveness.

3. Report lack of response, rash, diarrhea; may occur after therapy completed. Keep all F/U to evaluate response to therapy.

OUTCOMES/EVALUATE

- Symptomatic improvement
- Resolution of infection

Ceftazidime

(sef-**TAY**-zih-deem)

CLASSIFICATION(S):

Cephalosporin, third generation

PREGNANCY CATEGORY: B

Rx: Fortaz, Tazicef, Tazidime.

SEE ALSO *ANTI-INFECTIVE DRUGS* AND *CEPHALOSPORINS*.

USES

(1) Lower respiratory tract infections (including pneumonia) due to *Pseudomonas aeruginosa* and other *Pseudomonas* species, *Haemophilus influenzae* (including ampicillin-resistant strains), *Klebsiel-*

---

la species, *Enterobacter* species, *Proteus mirabilis*, *Escherichia coli*, *Serratia* species, *Citrobacter* species, *Streptococcus pneumoniae*, *Staphylococcus aureus* (methicillin-susceptible strains). (2) Skin and skin structure infections due to *P. aeruginosa*, *Klebsiella* species, *E. coli*, *Proteus* species (including *P. mirabilis* and indole-positive *Proteus*), *Enterobacter* species, *Serratia* species, *S. aureus* (methicillin-susceptible strains), *S. pyogenes* (group A β-hemolytic streptococci). (3) UTIs, both complicated and uncomplicated, due to *P. aeruginosa*, *Enterobacter* species, *Proteus* species (including *P. mirabilis* and indole-positive *Proteus*), *Klebsiella* species, and *E. coli*. (4) Bacterial septicemia due to *P. aeruginosa*, *Klebsiella* species, *H. influenzae*, *E. coli*, *Serratia* species, *S. pneumoniae*, *S. aureus* (methicillin-susceptible strains). (5) Bone and joint infections due to *P. aeruginosa*, *Klebsiella* species, *Enterobacter* species, *S. aureus* (methicillin-susceptible strains). (6) Gynecologic infections, including endometritis, pelvic cellulitis, and other infections of the female genital tract, due to *E. coli*. (7) Intra-abdominal infections, including peritonitis, due to *E. coli*, *Klebsiella* species, *S. aureus* (methicillin-susceptible strains); polymicrobial infections due to aerobic and anaerobic organisms and *Bacteroides* species (many strains of *B. fragilis* are resistant). (8) CNS infections, including meningitis, due to *H. influenzae* and *Neisseria meningitidis* (limited effect against *P. aeruginosa* and *S. pneumoniae*). *NOTE:* May be used with aminoglycosides, vancomycin, and clindamycin in severe, life-threatening infections and in the immunocompromised client. Dosage depends on the severity of the infection and the client's condition.

ACTION/KINETICS

Pharmacokinetics

Only for IM or IV use. $t\frac{1}{2}$: 114–120 min. From 80 to 90% is excreted unchanged in the urine.

SPECIAL CONCERNS

A sodium carbonate formulation should be used if the drug is indicated for children less than 12 years of age. Possible

resistance when used to treat *Pseudomonas aeruginosa* infections.

SIDE EFFECTS

Most Common

N&V, diarrhea, yeast infection of the mouth or vagina, abdominal pain, stomach cramps, colitis, thrombophlebitis.

See *Cephalosporins* for a complete list of possible side effects. Also, hyperbilirubinemia, jaundice, renal impairment, urticaria, pain at injection site, ***anaphylaxis, severe allergic reactions (e.g., cardiopulmonary arrest)***. Myoclonia and coma in clients with renal insufficiency.

HOW SUPPLIED

Injection: 1 gram, 2 grams; *Powder for Injection:* 500 mg, 1 gram, 2 grams, 6 grams.

DOSAGE

- **IM; IV**

  Usual recommended dosage.

Adults, IM, IV: 1 gram q 8–12 hr.
  UTIs, uncomplicated.

Adults, IM, IV: 0.25 gram q 12 hr.
  UTIs, complicated.

Adults, IM, IV: 0.5 gram q 8–12 hr.
  Uncomplicated pneumonia, mild skin and skin structure infections.

Adults, IM, IV: 0.5–1 gram q 8 hr.
  Bone and joint infections.

Adults, IV: 2 grams q 12 hr.
  Serious gynecologic or intra-abdominal infections, meningitis, severe or life-threatening infections (especially in immunocompromised clients).

Adults, IV: 2 grams q 8 hr.
  Pseudomonal lung infections in cystic fibrosis clients with normal renal function.

IV: 30–50 mg/kg q 8 hr, not to exceed 6 grams/day.
  Use in neonates, infants, and children.

Neonates, 0–4 weeks, IV: 30 mg/kg q 12 hr, not to exceed the adult dose.

Infants and children, 1 month–12 years, IV: 30–50 mg/kg q 8 hr not to exceed 6 grams/day.

NURSING CONSIDERATIONS

ADMINISTRATION/STORAGE

1. Reduce dose in clients with a GFR <50 mL/min. An initial loading dose of 1

---

gram may be given. The following doses are recommended: C_{CR} 31–50 mL/min: 1 gram q 12 hr; C_{CR} 16–30 mL/min: 1 gram q 24 hr; C_{CR} 6–15 mL/min: 0.5 gram q 24 hr; C_{CR} <5 mL/min: 0.5 gram q 48 hr.

2. For dialysis clients, give a loading dose of 1 gram, followed by 1 gram after each hemodialysis period. In clients undergoing intraperitoneal dialysis and continuous ambulatory peritoneal dialysis, give loading dose of 1 gram, followed by 0.5 gram q 24 hr. In addition to IV use, ceftazidime can be incorporated in the dialysis fluid at a concentration of 250 mg for 2 L of dialysis fluid.

3. For IM: Reconstitute in sterile water or bacteriostatic water for injection, or 0.5% or 1% lidocaine HCl injection.

4. If IM, use large muscle mass and inject deeply.

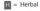 5. The IV route is preferred with bacterial septicemia, peritonitis, bacterial meningitis, or other severe/ life-threatening infections. Use IV route if poor risks R/T malnutrition, surgery, diabetes, trauma, heart failure, malignancy, or shock present/imminent.

6. For direct IV: Reconstitute 1 gram in 10 mL sterile water for injection; give over 3–5 min.

7. For intermittent administration, further dilute in 50–100 mL of solution and administer over 30–60 min. It is compatible with 0.9% NaCl, Ringer's/RL injection, D5W or D10W, M/6 sodium lactate injection, D5W and 0.225%, 0.45%, or 0.9% NaCl, 10% invert sugar in water. $NaHCO_3$ injection should not be used for reconstitution; however, a sodium carbonate formulation should be used for children <12 years old.

8. For IV infusion: The 1- or 2-gram infusion pack is reconstituted with 100 mL sterile water for injection (or a compatible IV solution).

9. Do not add ceftazidime to solutions containing aminoglycosides. Give separately.

ASSESSMENT

1. Note reasons for therapy, characteristics of S&S, culture results, any PCN/ ATX sensitivity.

2. Obtain CBC, renal function studies; reduce dose with dysfunction.

CLIENT/FAMILY TEACHING

Drug is administered parenterally. Report lack of response, adverse effects, itching, rash, SOB, or diarrhea.

OUTCOMES/EVALUATE

- Resolution of infection
- Negative culture reports

Ceftibuten   ℂ
(sef-ti-**BYOO**-tin)

CLASSIFICATION(S):
Cephalosporin, third generation
PREGNANCY CATEGORY: B
Rx: Cedax.

SEE ALSO *CEPHALOSPORINS.*

USES

(1) Acute bacterial exacerbations of chronic bronchitis due to *Haemophilus influenzae* (including β-lactamase-producing strains), *Moraxella catarrhalis* (including β-lactamase-producing strains), and penicillin-susceptible strains of *Streptococcus pneumoniae.* (2) Acute bacterial otitis media due to *H. influenzae* (including β-lactamase-producing strains), *M. catarrhalis* (including β-lactamase-producing strains), or *Staphylococcus pyogenes.* (3) Pharyngitis and tonsillitis due to *S. pyogenes.*

ACTION/KINETICS
Pharmacokinetics

Resistant to beta-lactamase. Is well absorbed from the GI tract. Food delays the time to peak serum concentration, lowers the peak concentration, and decreases the total amount of drug absorbed. **Peak serum levels:** 2 to 3 hours. **$t^{1/2}$:** 144 min. 56% excreted in the urine unchanged.

SPECIAL CONCERNS

Although ceftibuten has been approved for pharyngitis or tonsillitis, only penicillin has been shown to be effective in preventing rheumatic fever.

SIDE EFFECTS
Most Common

Diarrhea, N&V, abdominal pain, dizziness, headache.

See *Cephalosporins* for a complete list of possible side effects. Usually well tolerated.

HOW SUPPLIED

Capsules: 400 mg; *Powder for Oral Suspension:* 90 mg/5mL (after reconstitution).

DOSAGE

- **CAPSULES; ORAL SUSPENSION**
  All uses.

Adults and children over 12 years: 400 mg once daily for 10 days. The maximum daily dose is 400 mg. Adjust the dose in clients with a creatinine clearance (C_{CR}) <50 mL/min as follows. If the C_{CR} is between 30 and 49 mL/min, the recommended dose is 4.5 mg/kg or 200 mg once daily. If the C_{CR} is between 5 and 29 mL/min, the recommended dose is 2.25 mg/kg or 100 mg once daily. In clients undergoing hemodialysis 2 or 3 times/week, a single 400-mg dose of ceftibuten capsules or a single dose of 9 mg/kg (maximum of 400 mg) of PO suspension can be given at the end of each hemodialysis session.

Pharyngitis, tonsillitis, acute bacterial otitis media.

Children: 9 mg/kg, up to a maximum of 400 mg daily, for a total of 10 days. Give children over 45 kg the maximum daily dose of 400 mg.

NURSING CONSIDERATIONS

Ⓒ Do not confuse Cedax with Ceptaz or Cefzil (also cephalosporins).

ADMINISTRATION/STORAGE

1. Follow directions for mixing ceftibuten suspension carefully, depending on the final concentration and the bottle size. First, tap bottle to loosen powder; then add the appropriate amount of water in two portions. Shake well after each portion.
2. Suspension may be kept for 14 days under refrigeration. Keep container tightly closed, shake well before each use. Discard any unused drug after 14 days.
3. The dosage of the oral suspension in children is as follows:
- **10 kg (22 lb):** 5 mL daily of the 90 mg/5 mL formulation.

- **20 kg (44 lb):** 10 mL daily of the 90 mg/5 mL formulation.
- **40 kg (88 lb):** 20 mL daily of the 90 mg/5 mL formulation.

4. Store capsules and the powder for oral suspension before reconstitution from 2–25°C (36–77°F). Once reconstituted, the oral suspension is stable for 14 days from 2–8°C (36–46°F).

ASSESSMENT

1. Note reasons for therapy, characteristics of S&S; note any PCN/ATX sensitivity.
2. Monitor cultures, renal function studies; reduce dose with dysfunction.
3. Review conditions requiring treatment; drug is only approved for chronic bronchitis, bacterial otitis media, pharyngitis, tonsillitis, based on the infective organisms.

CLIENT/FAMILY TEACHING

1. Suspension must be consumed on an empty stomach, at least 2 hr before or 1 hr after a meal. Refrigerate suspension, shake well before use, and discard after 14 days.
2. Complete entire prescription; do not stop despite feeling better.
3. Report lack of response, adverse effects or persistent diarrhea. Note: suspension contains 1 gm sucrose per teaspoon.
4. Return for F/U (e.g., ear check, throat culture, x-ray).

OUTCOMES/EVALUATE

- Resolution of underlying infection
- Symptomatic improvement

Ceftizoxime sodium **Ⅳ** Ⓒ
(sef-tih-**ZOX**-eem)

CLASSIFICATION(S):
Cephalosporin, third generation
PREGNANCY CATEGORY: B
Rx: Cefizox.

SEE ALSO ANTI-INFECTIVES AND CEPHALOSPORINS.

USES

(1) Lower respiratory tract infections due to *Streptococcus* species (including

S. pneumoniae, but excluding entero-cocci), *Klebsiella* species, *Proteus mirabilis,* *Escherichia coli, Haemophilus influenzae* (including ampicillin-resistant strains), *Staphylococcus aureus* (penicillinase/nonpenicillinase-producing), *Serratia* species, *Enterobacter* species, and *Bacteroides* species. (2) UTIs due to *S. aureus* (penicillinase/nonpenicillinase-producing), *E. coli, Pseudomonas* species (including *P. aeruginosa,)* *P. mirabilis, P. vulgaris, Providencia rettgeri, Morganella morganii, Klebsiella* species, *Serratia* species (including *S. marcescens),* and *Enterobacter* species. (3) Uncomplicated cervical and urethral gonorrhea due to *N. gonorrhoeae.* (4) PID due to *N. gonorrhoeae, E. coli,* or *S. agalactiae.* Ceftizoxime has no activity against *Chlamydia trachomatis.* (5) Intra-abdominal infections due to *E. coli, S. epidermidis, Streptococcus* species (excluding enterococci), *Enterobacter* species, *Klebsiella* species, *Bacteroides* species (including *B. fragilis),* and anaerobic cocci (including *Peptococcus* and *Peptostreptococcus* species). (6) Septicemia due to *Streptococcus* species (including *S. pneumoniae,* but excluding enterococci), *S. aureus* (penicillinase/nonpenicillinease-producing), *E. coli, Bacteroides* species (including *B. fragilis), Klebsiella* species, and *Serratia* species. (7) Skin and skin structure infections due to *S. aureus* (penicillinase/nonpenicillinase-producing), *S. epidermidis, E. coli, Klebsiella* species, *Streptococcus* species (including *S. pyogenes,* but excluding enterococci), *P. mirabilis, Serratia* species, *Enterobacter* species, *Bacteroides* species (including *B. fragilis),* and anaerobic cocci (including *Peptococcus* and *Peptostreptococcus* species). (8) Bone and joint infections due to *S. aureus* penicillinase/nonpenicillinase-producing), *Streptococcus* species (excluding enterococci), *P. mirabilis, Bacteroides* species (including *B. fragilis),* and anaerobic cocci (including *Peptococcus* and *Peptostreptococcus* species). (9) Meningitis due to *H. influenzae* and limited use for *S. pneumoniae.* (10) Infections due to aerobic gram negative and by mixtures of organisms resistant to other cephalosporins, aminoglycosides, or penicillins have responded to ceftizoxime.

ACTION/KINETICS
Pharmacokinetics
$t\frac{1}{2}$: Approximately 1–2 hr. **Peak serum levels after 1 gram IV:** 60–87 mcg/mL. Approximately 80% excreted unchanged in the urine.

SIDE EFFECTS
Most Common
Rash, pruritus, fever, injection site pain/burning/cellulitis, diarrhea.

See *Cephalosporins* for a complete list of possible side effects. Also, transient increased levels of eosinophils, AST, ALT, and CPK have been seen in children over 6 months of age.

HOW SUPPLIED
Injection: 1 gram/50 mL, 2 grams/50 mL; *Powder for Injection:* 0.5 gram, 1 gram, 2 grams, 10 grams.

DOSAGE
- **IM; IV**
  Uncomplicated UTIs.
Adults: 0.5 gram IM or IV q 12 hr.
  Severe or resistant infections.
Adults: 1 gram q 8 hr or 2 grams q 8–12 hr IM or IV.
  Life-threatening infections.
Adults: 3–4 grams q 8 hr IV. Doses of 2 grams IV q 4 hr have been given.
  PID
2 grams q 8 hr IV (doses up to 2 grams q 4 hr have been used).
  Infections at other sites.
Adults: 1 gram q 8–12 hr IM or IV.
  Uncomplicated gonorrhea.
Adults: 1 gram as a single dose.
  Bacterial septicemia.
Initial: 6–12 grams/day IV in those with normal renal function; **then,** gradually reduce the dose according to clinical response and lab findings.
- **IM**
  Use in children.
Pediatric, over 6 months: 50 mg/kg q 6–8 hr up to 200 mg/kg/day (not to exceed the maximum adult dose).
  Impaired renal function.
Initial, IM, IV: 0.5–1 gram; **then,** use the following dosing schedule: **Mild impairment** (C_{CR} 50–79 mL/min): 0.5 gram q 8 hr; 0.75–1.5 grams q 8 hr for life-

 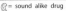

threatening infections. **Moderate to severe impairment** (C_{CR} 5–49 mL/min): 0.25–0.5 gram q 12 hr; 0.5–1 gram q 12 hr for life-threatening infections. **Dialysis clients** (C_{CR} <4 mL/min): 0.5 gram q 48 hr or 0.25 gram q 24 hr; 0.5–1 gram q 48 hr or 0.5 gram q 24 hr for life-threatening infections.

NURSING CONSIDERATIONS

℘ Do not confuse Cefizox with Ceptaz or Cedax (also cephalosporins).

ADMINISTRATION/STORAGE

1. For IM doses of 2 grams, divide dose equally; give in different large muscle masses.

IV 2. IV route may be preferred with bacterial septicemia, intra-abdominal abscess, peritonitis, other severe/life-threatening infections.

3. For direct IV: Reconstitute 1 gram in 10 mL sterile water; give slowly over 3–5 min.

4. Because UTI's R/T *P. aeruginosa* are so serious and because many strains of *Pseudomonas* are only moderately susceptible to cefitzoxime, use higher doses. Institute other therapy if response not prompt.

5. For intermittent administration/continuous infusion: Dilute reconstituted solution in 50–100 mL in one of the compatible solutions described in package insert.

6. For piggyback vials: Reconstitute with 50–100 mL of any of recommended IV solutions (see package insert). Shake well; administer as a single dose with primary IV fluids over 30 min.

7. A solution of 1 gram ceftizoxime in 13 mL sterile water for injection is isotonic.

8. Reconstituted solutions stable at room temperature for 8 hr and 48 hr if refrigerated.

9. For frozen solutions, thaw container at room temperature. After thawing, solution stable for 24 hr at room temperature or for 10 days if refrigerated. Do not refreeze or introduce additives into the solution.

10. Store unreconstituted drug, protected from excessive light, from 15–30°C (59–86°F) in the original package until used.

ASSESSMENT

Note reasons for therapy, characteristics of S&S, culture results. Assess for PCN/ATX sensitivity.

CLIENT/FAMILY TEACHING

Drug is administered parenterally. Report lack of response, adverse effects, rash, itching, or diarrhea. Consume enough fluids to prevent dehydration.

OUTCOMES/EVALUATE

- Negative culture reports
- Resolution of S&S of infection

Ceftriaxone sodium **IV**
(sef-try-**AX**-ohn)

CLASSIFICATION(S):
Cephalosporin, third generation
PREGNANCY CATEGORY: B
Rx: Rocephin.

SEE ALSO *ANTI-INFECTIVES* AND *CEPHALOSPORINS*.

USES

(1) Lower respiratory tract infections due to *Streptococcus pneumoniae, Staphylococcus aureus, Haemophilus influenzae, H. parainfluenzae, Klebsiella pneumonia, Serratia marcescens, Escherichia coli, E. aerogenes,* and *Proteus mirabilis.* (2) Skin and skin structure infections due to *S. aureus, S. epidermidis, S. pyogenes,* Viridins group streptococci, *E. coli, Enterobacter cloacae, K. oxytoca, K. pneumoniae, P. mirabilis, Pseudomonas aeruginosa, Morganella morganii, S. marcescens. Acinetobacter calcoaceticus, Bacteroides fragilis, Peptostreptococcus* species. (3) UTIs (complicated and uncomplicated) due to *E. coli, P. mirabilis, P. vulgaris, M. morganii,* and *K. pneumoniae.* (4) Uncomplicated cervical/urethral and rectal gonorrhea due to *Neisseria gonorrhoeae,* including penicillinase/non-penicillinase producing strains. Pharyngeal gonorrhea due to non-penicillinase producing strains of *N. gonorrhoeae.* (5) PID due to *N. gonorrhoeae.* Ceftriaxone has no activity against *Chlamydia trachomatis.* (6) Bac-

terial septicemia due to *S. aureus, S. pneumoniae, E. coli, H. influenzae,* and *K. pneumoniae.* (7) Bone and joint infections due to *S. aureus, S. pneumoniae, E. coli, P. mirabilis, K. pneumoniae,* and *Enterobacter* species. (8) Intra-abdominal infections due to *E. coli, K. pneumoniae, B. fragilis, Clostridium* species (most strains of *C. difficile* are resistant) and *Peptostreptococcus* species. (9) Meningitis due to *H. influenzae, N. meningitidis,* and *S. pneumoniae.* Possibly effective against *Staphylococcus epidermidis* and *E. coli.* (10) Single preoperative doses may decrease the incidence of postoperative infections following vaginal or abdominal hysterectomy or in coronary artery bypass surgery. (11) Acute bacterial otitis media due to *S. pneumoniae, H. influenzae* (including beta-lactamase-producing strains), and *Moraxella catarrhalis* (including beta-lactamase-producing strains). *Investigational:* Neurologic complications, arthritis, and carditis associated with Lyme disease in clients refractory to penicillin G.

ACTION/KINETICS

Pharmacokinetics

t½: Approximately 6–8 hr. **Serum levels after 1 gram IV:** 151 mcg/mL. One-third to two-thirds excreted unchanged in the urine. **Plasma protein binding:** Significant.

SIDE EFFECTS

Most Common

Diarrhea, rash, eosinophilia, nausea, pain/induration/tenderness/warmth at injection site

See *Cephalosporins* for a complete list of possible side effects. Also, increase in serum creatinine, presence of casts in the urine, alteration of PTs (rare).

HOW SUPPLIED

Injection: 1 gram/50 mL, 2 grams/50 mL (both strengths as base); *Powder for Injection:* 250 mg, 500 mg, 1 gram, 2 grams, 10 grams (all strengths as base).

DOSAGE——————————

- **IM; IV**

General infections.

Adults, usual: 1–2 grams/day in single or divided doses q 12 hr depending on the type and severity of infection, not to exceed 4 grams/day. Maintain therapy for 4–14 days, depending on the infection. **Pediatric, serious infections:** *Other than meningitis:* 50–75 mg/kg/day not to exceed total daily dose of 2 grams given in divided doses q 12 hr.

Meningitis

Pediatric: 100 mg/kg/day, not to exceed total daily dose of 4 grams given once daily or in equally divided doses q 12 hr for 7–14 days.

Skin and skin structure infections and serious infections other than meningitis.

Pediatric: 50–75 mg/kg once daily or in equally divided doses q 12 hr. Do not exceed a daily dose of 2 grams.

Preoperative for prophylaxis of infection in surgery.

1 gram 30–120 min prior to surgery.

Uncomplicated gonorrhea.

Adults, IM: 125 mg as a single dose plus doxycycline, 100 mg twice a day for 7 days or azithromycin, 1 gram, as a single PO dose. Or, a single dose of ceftriaxone 250 mg IM.

Disseminated gonococcal infection.

Adults: 1 gram IM or IV q 24 hr.

Gonococcal meningitis or endocarditis.

Adults: 1–2 grams IV q 12 hr for 10–14 days (meningitis) or 4 weeks (endocarditis).

Gonococcal conjunctivitis.

Adults and children over 20 kg: 1 gram given as a single IM dose.

Haemophilus ducreyi infection.

250 mg IM as a single dose.

Acute PID.

250 mg IM plus doxycycline or tetracycline.

Lyme disease in those refractory to penicillin G.

IV: 2 grams/day for 14–28 days.

Acute bacterial otitis media.

IM: Single dose of 50 mg/kg, not to exceed 1 gram.

NOTE: Dosage adjustment is not required for renal or hepatic impairment; however, monitor blood levels

NURSING CONSIDERATIONS

ADMINISTRATION/STORAGE

1. Give IM injections deep into the body of a large muscle.

IV 2. IV infusions should contain concentrations of 10–40 mg/mL. Reconstitute 500 mg in 4.8 mL of sterile water, NSS, or D5W. Then further dilute in 50–100 mL D5W or NSS and infuse over 30 min.

3. Do not mix drug with other antibiotics.

4. Stability of solutions for IM or IV use varies depending on the diluent used; check package insert carefully.

5. Maintain dosage for at least 2 days after symptoms have disappeared (usual course is 4–14 days, although complicated infections may require longer therapy).

6. Continue dosage for at least 10 days when treating *Streptococcus pyogenes* infections.

ASSESSMENT

1. Note reasons for therapy, characteristics of S&S, culture results. List any PCN/ATX sensitivity.

2. Assess for GI disease, especially colitis; use drug cautiously, report any bruising/bleeding, diarrhea.

3. Monitor renal/LFTs, coagulation studies. Use vitamin K (10 mg/week) prophylactically if bleeding occurs.

CLIENT/FAMILY TEACHING

Drug is administered parenterally. Report lack of response, injection site pain, adverse side effects.

OUTCOMES/EVALUATE

- Resolution of S&S of infection
- Negative culture reports

Cefuroxime axetil **IV** ©
(sef-your-**OX**-eem)

CLASSIFICATION(S):
Cephalosporin, second generation
PREGNANCY CATEGORY: B
Rx: Ceftin.
✦**Rx:** Apo-Cefuroxime.

Cefuroxime sodium
PREGNANCY CATEGORY: B
Rx: Zinacef.

SEE ALSO *ANTI-INFECTIVES* AND *CEPHALOSPORINS*.

USES

PO (axetil), Suspension (Children, 3 months–12 years). (1) Pharyngitis or tonsillitis due to *S. pyogenes* (group A β-hemolytic streptococci). (2) Acute bacterial otitis media due to *S. pneumoniae*, *H. influenzae* (including β-lactamase-producing strains), *M. catarrhalis* (including β-lactamase-producing strains), or *S. pyogenes*. (3) Impetigo due to *S. aureus* (including β-lactamase-producing strains) and *Streptococcus pyogenes*.

PO (axetil), Tablets. (1) Pharyngitis or tonsillitis due to *S. pyogenes* (group A β-hemolytic streptococci). (2) Acute bacterial otitis media due to *S. pneumoniae*, *H. influenzae* (including β-lactamase-producing strains), *M. catarrhalis* (including β-lactamase-producing strains), or *S. pyogenes*. (3) Acute bacterial maxillary sinusitis due to *S. pneumoniae* or *H. influenzae* (non-β-lactamase-producing strains only). (4) Acute bacterial exacerbations of chronic bronchitis and secondary bacterial infections of acute bronchitis due to *S. pneumoniae*, *H. influenzae* (β-lactamase-negative strains) or *H. parainfluenzae* (β-lactamase-negative strains). (5) Uncomplicated UTIs due to *E. coli* or *K. pneumoniae*. (6) Uncomplicated skin and skin structure infections due to *S. aureus* (including β-lactamase-producing strains) or *S. pyogenes*. (7) Uncomplicated urethral and endocervical gonorrhea due to penicillinase-producing and non-penicillinase-producing strains of *N. gonorrhoeae* and uncomplicated rectal gonorrhea in females due to non-penicillinase-producing strains of *Neisseria gonorrheae*. (8) Early Lyme disease due to *Borrelia burgdorferi*.

IM, IV (sodium). (1) Lower respiratory tract infections, including pneumonia, due to *S. pneumoniae*, *H. influenzae* (including ampicillin-resistant strains), *Klebsiella* species, *S. aureus* (penicillinase/non-penicillinase-producing), *S. pyogenes*, *E. coli*. (2) UTIs due to *E. coli* or *Klebsiella* species. (3) Skin and skin structure infections due to *S. aureus* (penicillinase/non-penicillinase-producing), *S. pyogenes, E. coli, Klebsiella* species, and *Enterobacter* species. (4) Septicemia due to *S. aureus* (penicillinase/non-penicillinase producing), *S. pneumoniae, E. coli, H. influenzae* (including ampicillin-resistant strains), and *Klebsiella* species. (5) Meningitis due to *S. pneumoniae, H. influenzae* (including ampicillin-resistant strains), *N. meningitidis* and *S. aureus* (penicillinase/non-penicillinase-producing strains). (6) Uncomplicated and disseminated gonococcal infections due to *N. gonorrhoeae* (penicillinase/non-penicillinase producing strains) in males and females. (7) Bone/joint infections due to *S. aureus* (penicillinase/non-penicillinase-producing strains). (8) Mixed skin and skin structure infections. (9) Preoperative prophylaxis in clients undergoing surgical procedures (e.g., vaginal hysterectomy) classified as clean-contaminated or potentially contaminated.

ACTION/KINETICS

Pharmacokinetics

Cefuroxime axetil is used PO, whereas cefuroxime sodium is used either IM or IV. **IM, IV: t½,** 80 min. **Peak serum levels after 1.5 grams IV:** 100 mcg/mL. 66–100% is excreted unchanged in the urine. t½ will be prolonged in clients with renal failure.

SIDE EFFECTS

Most Common

Diarrhea/loose stools, N&V, abdominal pain.

See *Cephalosporins* for a complete list of possible side effects. Also, decrease in H&H.

ADDITIONAL DRUG INTERACTIONS

↓ Effectiveness of oral contraceptives.

DRUG INTERACTIONS

H_2 antagonists ↓ cefuroxime plasma levels

ADDITIONAL LABORATORY TEST CONSIDERATIONS

False/negative reaction in the ferricyanide test for blood glucose.

HOW SUPPLIED

Cefuroxime axetil: *Powder for Oral Suspension:* 125 mg/5 mL, 250 mg/5 mL; *Tablets:* 125 mg, 250 mg, 500 mg.

Cefuroxime sodium: *Injection:* 750 mg/50 mL, 1.5 grams/50 mL; *Powder for Injection:* 750 mg, 1.5 grams, 7.5 grams.

DOSAGE

CEFUROXIME AXETIL

• **TABLETS**

Pharyngitis, tonsillitis.

Adults and children over 13 years: 250 mg q 12 hr for 10 days.

Acute bacterial exacerbations of chronic bronchitis and secondary bacterial infections of acute bronchitis, uncomplicated skin and skin structure infections.

Adults and children over 13 years: 250 or 500 mg q 12 hr for 10 days (5–10 days for secondary bacterial infections of acute bronchitis).

Uncomplicated UTIs.

Adults and children over 13 years: 250 mg q 12 hr for 7–10 days.

Acute otitis media.

Children: 250 mg twice a day for 10 days.

Uncomplicated gonorrhea.

Adults and children over 13 years: 1,000 mg as a single dose.

Early Lyme disease.

Adults and children over 13 years of age: 500 mg/day for 20 days.

Acute bacterial maxillary sinusitis.

Adults and children who can swallow tablets whole: 250 mg q 12 hr for 10 days.

• **SUSPENSION**

Pharyngitis, tonsillitis.

Children, 3 months to 12 years: 20 mg/kg/day in 2 divided doses, not to exceed 500 mg total dose/day, for 10 days.

Acute otitis media, impetigo, acute bacterial maxillary sinusitis.

Children, 3 months to 12 years: 30 mg/kg/day in 2 divided doses, not to exceed 1,000 mg total dose/day, for 10 days.

CEFUROXIME SODIUM

• **IM; IV**

Uncomplicated infections, including urinary tract, uncomplicated pneumonia, disseminated gonococcal, skin and skin structure.

Adults: 750 mg q 8 hr. **Pediatric, over 3 months:** 50–100 mg/kg/day in equally divided doses q 6–8 hr (not to exceed adult dose for severe infections).

Severe or complicated infections; bone and joint infections.

Adults: 1.5 grams q 8 hr. **Pediatric, over 3 months:** *Bone and joint infections,* **IV:** 150 mg/kg/day in equally divided doses q 8 hr (not to exceed adult dose).

Life-threatening infections or those due to less susceptible organisms.

Adults: 1.5 grams q 6 hr.

Bacterial meningitis.

Adults: Up to 3 grams q 8 hr. **Pediatric, over 3 months, initial, IV:** 200–240 mg/kg/day in divided doses q 6–8 hr; **then,** after clinical improvement, 100 mg/kg/day.

Gonorrhea (uncomplicated).

1.5 grams as a single IM dose given at two different sites together with 1 gram PO probenecid.

Prophylaxis in surgery.

Adults, IV: 1.5 grams 30–60 min before surgery; if procedure is of long duration, **IM, IV:** 0.75 gram q 8 hr.

Open heart surgery, prophylaxis.

IV: 1.5 grams when anesthesia is initiated; **then,** 1.5 grams q 12 hr for a total of 6 grams.

NOTE: Reduce the dose in impaired renal function as follows: C_{CR} over 20 mL/min: 0.75–1.5 grams q 8 hr; C_{CR} 10–20 mL/min: 0.75 gram q 12 hr; C_{CR} less than 10 mL/min: 0.75 gram q 24 hr

NURSING CONSIDERATIONS

❦ Do not confuse cefuroxime with deferoxamine (an iron chelator).

ADMINISTRATION/STORAGE

1. Cefuroxime axetil for PO use is available in tablet and suspension forms. Swallow tablets whole, do not crush; crushed tablet has a strong, bitter, persistent taste. Tablets may be taken without regard for food; however, the suspension must be taken with food. Protect tablets from excessive moisture.
2. To reconstitute suspension, loosen powder by shaking the bottle. Add appropriate amount of water (depending on bottle size). Invert bottle and shake vigorously. Shake before each use. Store reconstituted suspension either at room temperature or refrigerate. Discard any unused portion after 10 days.
3. Tablet and suspension are not bioequivalent; not substitutable on a mg-per-mg basis.
4. For IM use, constitute each 750 mg vial wit 3 mL sterile water for injection. Shake gently to disperse. Inject deep into a large muscle mass.
5. Store tablets from 15–30°C (59–86°F). Protect unit-dose packs from excessive moisture. Before reconstitution store the dry powder for the oral suspension from 2–25°C (36–77°F). After reconstitution store the suspension either in a refrigerator or at room temperature; discard after 10 days.

▐IV▌ 6. Use IV route for severe/life-threatening infections such as septicemia, or in poor-risk clients, especially in presence of shock.

7. Continue treatment for a minimum of 48 to 72 hr after client is asymptomatic or after evidence of bacterial eradication has been obtained. Treat for a minimum of 10 days for *S. pyogenes* infections in order to minimize the risk of rheumatic fever or glomerulonephritis.
8. For direct IV, reconstitute 750 mg in 8 mL sterile water; give over 3–5 min. For intermittent IV, further dilute in 100 mL of dextrose or saline solution; infuse over 30 min.
9. Constitute the 1.5 gram vial with 16 mL sterile water for injection. Withdraw completely the solution for injection. Constitute the 7.5 gram pharmacy bulk vial with 77 mL sterile water for injection; each 8 mL of the resulting solution contains 750 mg cefuroxime sodium.
10. For direct intermittent IV administration, slowly inject drug over 3 to 5 min, or give in tubing of other IV solutions. For intermittent IV infusion with a Y-type setup, may give dose in the tubing through which client is receiving other medications; however, during drug infusion, stop other solutions. For continuous IV infusion, the drug may be added to 0.9% NaCl, D5W or D10W, D5/0.45% or 0.9% NaCl, and M/6 sodium lactate injection.

11. Do not add cefuroxime sodium to solutions of aminoglycosides; if both required, give separately.

12. Prior to reconstitution, protect drug from light. The powder and reconstituted drug may darken without affecting potency.

13. Continue therapy for at least 10 days in infections due to *Streptococcus pyogenes*.

ASSESSMENT

1. Note reasons for therapy, characteristics of S&S, culture results, baseline assessments. List any PCN/ATX sensitivity.

2. Assess for anemia, renal dysfunction. Reduce dose with impaired renal function.

CLIENT/FAMILY TEACHING

1. Swallow tablets whole; do not chew or crush as crushed tablet has a strong, bitter, persistent taste. Tablets may be taken without regard for food; the suspension must be taken with food. Store suspension at room temperature or refrigerate. Discard after 10 days. Protect tablets from excessive moisture.

2. Crushed tablets have a distinctive bitter taste even when hidden in foods. If intolerable, report so alternative drug therapy may be instituted.

3. Report lack of response, persistent diarrhea or S&S of anemia (SOB, dizziness, pale skin, etc.) immediately. Keep all F/U appointments.

OUTCOMES/EVALUATE

- Resolution of S&S of infection
- Surgical infection prophylaxis

Celecoxib ■
(**sell**-ah-**KOX**-ihb)

CLASSIFICATION(S):
Nonsteroidal anti-inflammatory drug, COX-2 inhibitor
PREGNANCY CATEGORY: C
Rx: Celebrex.

SEE ALSO *NONSTEROIDAL ANTI-INFLAMMATORY DRUGS.*

USES

(1) Relief of signs and symptoms of rheumatoid arthritis and osteoarthritis in adults. (2) Acute pain in adults. (3) Relief of signs and symptoms of ankylosing spondylitis. (4) Relief of signs and symptoms of juvenile rheumatoid arthritis in clients 2 years of age and older. (5) Primary dysmenorrhea. (6) Reduce the number of adenomatous colorectal polyps in familial adenomatous polyposis, as an adjunct to usual care. Use for this purpose beyond six months has not been studied.

ACTION/KINETICS

Action

Inhibits prostaglandin synthesis, primarily by inhibiting cyclo-oxygenase-2 (COX-2), thus decreasing inflammation. does not inhibit the cyclo-oxygenase-1 (COX-1) isoenzyme. Does not affect platelet aggregation; renal effects similar to other NSAIDs. Causes fewer GI complications, such as bleeding and perforation, compared with other NSAIDs.

Pharmacokinetics

Peak plasma levels: 3 hr. $t^{1/2}$, terminal: 11 hr when fasting; low solubility prolongs absorption. Metabolized in the liver to inactive compounds; excreted in the urine (27%) and feces (57%). Blacks show a 40% increase in the total amount absorbed compared with Caucasians. **Plasma protein binding:** About 97%.

CONTRAINDICATIONS

Use in severe hepatic impairment, in those who have shown an allergic reaction to sulfonamides, or in those who have experienced asthma, urticaria, or allergic-type reactions after taking aspirin or other NSAIDs. Use in late pregnancy (may cause premature closure of ductus arteriosus). Lactation.

SPECIAL CONCERNS

■ (1) Celecoxib may cause an increased risk of serious CV thrombotic events, MI, and stroke, which can be fatal. All NSAIDs may have a similar risk. This risk may increase with duration of use. Clients with CV disease or risk factors for CV disease may be at higher risk. (2) Celecoxib is contraindicated for the treatment of perioperative pain in the setting of coronary artery bypass graft. (3) NSAIDs, including celecoxib, cause an increased risk of serious GI adverse effects, including bleeding, ulceration, and perforation of the stomach or intestines, which can be fatal. These reactions can occur at any time during use and without warning symptoms. Elderly clients are at higher risk for serious GI events.■ Use with caution in pre-existing asthma, with drugs that are known to inhibit CYP2C9 in the liver, or when initiating the drug in significant dehydration. Use with extreme caution in those with a prior history of ulcer disease or GI bleeding. Increased risk of ulceration and bleeding if used with NSAIDs. Increased risk of serious renal effects in geriatric clients. Possible serious cardiovascular side effects. Safety and efficacy have not been determined in clients less than 18 years of age.

SIDE EFFECTS

Most Common

Abdominal pain/cramps, diarrhea, nausea, dyspepsia/indigestion, URTI.

Listed are side effects with a frequency of 0.1% or greater. **GI:** Dyspepsia, diarrhea, abdominal pain, N&V, dry mouth, flatulence, constipation, GI bleeding/ulceration, **GI hemorrhage**, diverticulitis, dysphagia, eructation, esophagitis, gastritis, gastroenteritis, GERD, hemorrhoids, hiatal hernia, melena, stomatitis, tooth disorder, abnormal hepatic function. **CNS:** Headache, dizziness, insomnia, anorexia, anxiety, depression, nervousness, somnolence, hypertonia, hypoesthesia, migraine, neuropathy, paresthesia, vertigo, increased appetite. **CV:** Aggravated hypertension, angina pectoris, CAD, **MI**, palpitation, tachycardia, thrombocythemia, thrombotic events, CHF-related adverse effects. **Respiratory:** URTI, sinusitis, pharyngitis, rhinitis, bronchitis, bronchospasm, coughing, dyspnea, laryngitis, pneumonia. **Dermatologic:** Rash, ecchymosis, alopecia, dermatitis, nail disorder, photosensitivity, pruritus, erythematous/maculopapular rash, skin disorder, dry skin, increased sweating, urticaria. **Body as a Whole:** Accidental injury, back/chest pain, peripheral edema, aggravated allergy, allergic reaction, asthenia, fluid retention, generalized edema, fatigue, fever, hot flushes, flu-like symptoms, pain/peripheral pain, weight increase. **Musculoskeletal:** Arthralgia, arthrosis, bone disorder, accidental fracture, myalgia, stiff neck, synovitis, tendinitis. **Infections:** Bacterial/fungal, or viral infection; herpes simplex/ zoster, soft tissue infection, moniliasis, genital moniliasis, otitis media. **GU:** Cystitis, dysuria, frequent urination, renal calculus, urinary incontinence, UTI, breast fibroadenosis/neoplasm/pain, dysmenorrhea, menstrual disorder, vaginal hemorrhage, vaginitis, prostatic disorder. **Ophthalmic:** Glaucoma, blurred vision, cataract, conjunctivitis, eye pain. **Otic:** Deafness, ear abnormality, earache, tinnitus. **Miscellaneous:** Tenesmus, facial edema, leg cramps, diabetes mellitus, epistaxis, anemia, taste perversion.

LABORATORY TEST CONSIDERATIONS

↑ ALT, AST, BUN, CPK, NPN, creatinine, alkaline phosphatase. Hypercholesterolemia, hyperglycemia, hypokalemia, albuminuria, hematuria.

DRUG INTERACTIONS

ACE Inhibitors / ↓ Antihypertensive effect

Antacids, Al- and Mg-containing / ↓ Celecoxib absorption

Aspirin / ↑ Risk of GI ulceration

Fluconazole / ↑ Plasma celecoxib levels

Furosemide / ↓ Natriuretic drug effect

Lithium / ↑ Plasma lithium levels

Thiazide diuretics / ↓ Natriuretic drug effects

Warfarin / Possible ↑ PT with bleeding, especially in the elderly

HOW SUPPLIED

Capsules: 50 mg, 100 mg, 200 mg, 400 mg.

DOSAGE

• **CAPSULES**

Osteoarthritis.

Adults: 100 mg twice a day or 200 mg as a single dose.

Rheumatoid arthritis.

Adults: 100–200 mg twice a day.

Ankylosing spondylitis.

200 mg daily either as a single dose or divided into 2 doses. If no effect is seen after 6 weeks, a trial of 400 mg/day may be beneficial. If no effect is seen after 6 weeks on 400 mg/day, a response is not

---

Bold Italic = life threatening side effect   ■ = black box warning   ♣ = Available in Canada

likely; give consideration to alternate treatments.

Juvenile rheumatoid arthritis.
Children 2 years and older weighing 10–25 kg: 50 mg capsule twice a day. **Children 2 years of age and older weighing more than 25 kg:** 100 mg capsule twice a day.

Acute pain and primary dysmenorrhea.
Day 1, Initial: 400 mg; **then,** an additional 200 mg, if needed on Day 1. On subsequent days, 200 mg 2 times per day, as needed.

Familial adenomatous polyposis.
400 mg twice a day with food. Continue usual medical care (e.g., endoscopic surveillance, surgery).

NURSING CONSIDERATIONS

Do not confuse Celebrex with Cerebyx (an anticonvulsant) or with Celexa (an antidepressant).

ADMINISTRATION/STORAGE
1. Reduce daily dose by about 50% in clients with moderate impaired hepatic function (Child-Pugh class B).
2. For those unable to swallow capsules, the contents of a celecoxib capsule can be added to a level teaspoon of applesauce; ingest immediately with water. The applesauce-celecoxib mixture is stable for up to 6 hr when refrigerated.

ASSESSMENT
1. Note reasons for therapy, onset, characteristics of disease, ROM, deformity/loss of function, pain level, other agents trialed, outcome.
2. Determine any GI bleed/ulcer history, sulfonamide allergy, aspirin, other NSAID-induced asthma, urticaria, allergic-type reactions.
3. List drugs prescribed; ensure none interact.
4. This class of drugs has been associated with increased risk of heart attacks/stroke; monitor for S&S.
5. Assess for liver/renal dysfunction; reduce dose. Monitor CBC, electrolytes, renal, LFTs.

CLIENT/FAMILY TEACHING
1. Take with food; decreases stomach upset.
2. Avoid alcohol; may aggravate liver function.
3. Avoid prolonged exposure to direct or artificial sunlight.
4. Seek lowest effective dose. Take as directed, at same time daily. May take several days before desired effect.
5. Do not take aspirin/aspirin-containing products without consent.
6. Report unusual/persistent side effects, including dyspepsia, abdominal pain, dizziness, changes in stool/skin color.
7. Avoid during pregnancy; use reliable contraception.
8. Report weight gain, swelling of ankles, SOB, chest pain. Keep F/U appointment.

OUTCOMES/EVALUATE
- Relief of joint pain/inflammation; improved mobility
- ↓ Adenomatous colorectal polyps in familial adenomatous polyposis
- Relief of pain

Cephalexin
(sef-ah-**LEX**-in)

CLASSIFICATION(S):
Cephalosporin, first generation
PREGNANCY CATEGORY: B
Rx: Keflex.
✱**Rx:** Apo-Cephalex, Novo-Lexin, Nu-Cephalex.

SEE ALSO *ANTI-INFECTIVES* AND *CEPHALOSPORINS.*

USES
(1) Respiratory tract infections due to *Streptococcus pneumoniae* and *Streptococcus pyogenes*. (2) Otitis media due to *S. pneumoniae, Haemophilus influenzae, S. pyogenes,* and *Moraxella catarrhalis*. (3) GU infections (including acute prostatitis due to *Escherichia coli, Proteus mirabilis,* or *Klebsiella pneumoniae*). (4) Bone infections caused by *P. mirabilis* or *Staphylococcus aureus*. (5) Skin and skin structure infections due to *S. aureus* and/or *S. pyogenes*.

C

ACTION/KINETICS
Action
Interferes with the final step in cell wall formation (inhibition of mucopeptide biosynthesis), resulting in unstable cell membranes that undergo lysis. Also, cell division and growth are inhibited.

Pharmacokinetics
Peak serum levels: PO, 9–39 mcg/mL after 1 hr. **t½, PO:** 50–80 min. Absorption delayed in children. The HCl monohydrate does not require conversion in the stomach before absorption. Ninety percent of drug excreted unchanged in urine within 8 hr. **Plasma protein binding:** About 10% plasma protein bound.

SIDE EFFECTS
Most Common
Diarrhea, N&V, abdominal pain, dizziness, skin rash, fever, vaginitis.

See *Cephalosporins* for a complete list of potential side effects. Also, Nephrotoxicity, cholestatic jaundice.

HOW SUPPLIED
Cephalexin: *Capsules:* 250 mg, 333 mg, 500 mg, 750 mg; *Powder for Oral Suspension:* 125 mg/5 mL (after reconstitution), 250 mg/5 mL (after reconstitution); *Tablets:* 250 mg, 500 mg; *Tablets for Oral Suspension:* 125 mg, 250 mg.

DOSAGE
• **CAPSULES; ORAL SUSPENSION; TABLETS**
> *General infections.*

Adults, usual: 250 mg q 6 hr up to 4 grams/day in divided doses. **Pediatric:** 25–50 mg/kg/day in four equally divided doses.
> *Infections of skin and skin structures, streptococcal pharyngitis, uncomplicated cystitis, over 15 years of age.*

Adults: 500 mg q 12 hr. Large doses may be needed for severe infections or for less susceptible organisms. Continue therapy for cystitis for 7–14 days. For streptococcal pharyngitis **in children over 1 year** and for skin and skin structure infections, the total daily dose should be divided and given q 12 hr. In severe infections, the dose should be doubled.
> *Otitis media.*

Pediatric: 75–100 mg/kg/day in four divided doses.

NURSING CONSIDERATIONS
ADMINISTRATION/STORAGE
1. Refrigerate suspension after reconstitution; discard after 14 days.
2. If total daily dose is more than 4 grams, use parenteral drugs.
3. Continue for at least 10 days for β-hemolytic streptococcal infections.
4. May reduce dosage with impaired renal function; or increase for severe infections. Drug action can be prolonged by concurrent use of probenecid.
5. The tablets for oral suspension are used to prepare individual 5-mL doses.
6. Store capsules, powder for oral suspension, and tablets from 20–25°C (68–77°F).

ASSESSMENT
1. Note reasons for therapy, severity of infection, characteristics of S&S, culture results.
2. Monitor CBC, renal and LFTs; reduce dose with renal dysfunction.

CLIENT/FAMILY TEACHING
1. Take as directed/complete prescription; may take with meals for GI upset. Shake the reconstituted suspension well. Refrigerate suspension; discard after 14 days.
2. Consume 2–3 L/day of fluids to prevent dehydration.
3. Report adverse effects, rash, diarrhea, yellow discoloration of the skin/eyes, or lack of response.

OUTCOMES/EVALUATE
• Resolution of infection
• Symptomatic improvement

Cetirizine hydrochloride ©
(seh-**TIH**-rah-zeen)

CLASSIFICATION(S):
Antihistamine, second generation, piperazine
PREGNANCY CATEGORY: B
OTC: Zyrtec.
✦Rx: Apo-Cetirizine, Reactine.

SEE ALSO *ANTIHISTAMINES.*

USES

(1) Relief of symptoms associated with seasonal allergic rhinitis due to ragweed, grass, and tree pollens in adults and children over 6 years of age. Symptoms helped include sneezing, rhinorrhea, nasal pruritus, ocular pruritus, tearing, and red eyes. (2) Perennial allergic rhinitis due to allergens such as dust mites, animal dander, and molds in adults and children over 6 years of age. Symptoms helped include sneezing, rhinorrhea, postnasal discharge, nasal pruritus, ocular pruritus, and tearing. (3) Uncomplicated skin manifestations of chronic idiopathic urticaria in adults and children over 6 years of age. The drug significantly reduces the occurrence, severity, and duration of hives and significantly reduces pruritus. *Investigational:* Decrease the initial wheal response and pruritus associated with mosquito bites. Improve asthma symptom scores in clients with allergic asthma.

ACTION/KINETICS

Action

Potent H₁-receptor antagonist. Mild bronchodilator that protects against histamine-induced bronchospasm; low to negligible anticholinergic and sedative activity. No antiemetic activity.

Pharmacokinetics

Rapidly absorbed after PO administration. Food delays the time to peak serum levels but does not decrease the total amount of drug absorbed. Poorly penetrates the CNS, but high levels are distributed to the skin. **t½:** 8.3 hr (longer in elderly clients and in those with impaired liver or renal function). Excreted mostly unchanged (95%) in the urine; 10% is excreted in the feces.

CONTRAINDICATIONS

Lactation. In those hypersensitive to hydroxyzine. Use of antihistamines is not recommended in children less than 6 years of age.

SPECIAL CONCERNS

Due to the possibility of sedation, use with caution in situations requiring mental alertness. Safety and efficacy have not been determined in children less than 6 years of age.

SIDE EFFECTS

Most Common

Somnolence, dry mouth, fatigue, pharyngitis, dizziness.

See *Antihistamines* for complete list of possible side effects. Also, possible aggressive side reactions and **convulsions.**

OD OVERDOSE MANAGEMENT

Symptoms: Somnolence. *Treatment:* Symptomatic and supportive. Dialysis is not effective in removing the drug from the body.

DRUG INTERACTIONS

Ritonavir ↑ AUC, elimination t½, and volume of distribution of cetirizine

HOW SUPPLIED

Syrup: 1 mg/mL; *Tablets:* 5 mg, 10 mg; *Tablets, Chewable:* 5 mg, 10 mg.

DOSAGE

• **SYRUP; TABLETS; TABLETS, CHEWABLE**

Seasonal or perennial allergic rhinitis, chronic urticaria.

Adults and children 12 years and older, initial: Depending on the severity of the symptoms, 5 or 10 mg (most common initial dose) once daily. **Children, 6–11 years:** 5 or 10 mg once daily, depending on severity of symptoms. In clients 12 years and older with decreased renal function (C_CR 11–31 mL/min), in hemodialysis clients (C_CR <7 mL/min), and in those with impaired hepatic function, use 5 mg once daily. For the elderly, use 5 mg once a day. Do not use in children less than 6 years of age.

NURSING CONSIDERATIONS

℘ Do not confuse Zyrtec with Zyprexa (an antipsychotic).

ADMINISTRATION/STORAGE

Store syrup and tablets from 20–25°C (68–77°F). Syrup can also be refrigerated.

ASSESSMENT

1. Note onset, clinical presentation, and characteristics of allergic symptoms; note any triggers.
2. Assess for hypersensitivity to hydroxyzine. Check respiratory status; note any increase in secretions, wheezing, breathing rate.

📷 = see color insert   Ⓗ = Herbal   Ⓥ = Intravenous   ℘ = sound alike drug

3. List other drugs prescribed; drug is highly protein bound. Monitor for adverse drug interactions.

4. Assess VS, I&O, renal and LFTs; reduce dose with dysfunction.

CLIENT/FAMILY TEACHING

1. May take with or without food; can vary time of administration based on need. Food will decrease stomach upset. Syrup available for pediatric dosing.

2. Use caution when performing activities that require mental alertness until drug effects realized; may cause drowsiness/sedation.

3. May cause dry mouth, fatigue; report adverse effects that prevent taking medications. Increase fluid intake to thin secretions.

4. Avoid alcohol/CNS depressants, and other OTC antihistamines.

5. Report any behavioral changes, aggressiveness, or evidence of seizures.

6. Avoid prolonged or excessive exposure to direct or artificial sunlight.

7. Review allergens that trigger symptoms, e.g., ragweed, dust mites, molds, animal dander, etc., and how to control/avoid contact.

OUTCOMES/EVALUATE

- Symptom relief with seasonal and perennial allergic rhinitis
- ↓ Occurrence, duration, and severity of hives; ↓ pruritus with idiopathic urticaria

—— COMBINATION DRUG ——

Cetirizine hydrochloride and Pseudoephedrine hydrochloride

(seh-**TIH**-rah-zeen, soo-doh-eh-**FED**-rin)

CLASSIFICATION(S):
Antihistamine/Decongestant
PREGNANCY CATEGORY: C
OTC: Zyrtec-D 12 Hour.

SEE ALSO *CETIRIZINE HYDROCHLORIDE AND PSEUDOEPHEDRINE HYDROCHLORIDE.*

USES

Relief of nasal and non-nasal symptoms associated with seasonal or perennial allergic rhinitis in adults and children 12 years of age and older.

CONTENT

Cetirizine (antihistamine): 5 mg in an immediate-release layer and *pseudoephedrine (decongestant):* 120 mg in an extended-release layer.

ACTION/KINETICS

Action

Cetirizine, an antihistamine, selectively inhibits histamine H_1-receptors. Pseudoephedrine, a sympathomimetic amine, produces direct stimulation of both alpha- and beta-adrenergic receptors, as well as indirect stimulation through release of norepinephrine from storage sites, resulting in a decongestant effect on the nasal mucosa.

Pharmacokinetics

Mean peak plasma levels, cetirizine: 2.2 hr; **pseudoephedrine:** 4.4 hr. Food has no significant effect on amount of cetirizine absorption but T_{max} was delayed 1.8 hr and C_{max} was decreased by 30%. About 55–75% of pseudoephedrine is excreted unchanged in the urine and the remainder metabolized in the liver. Moderate renal impairment and chronic liver disease increases the $t\frac{1}{2}$ and decreases the clearance of cetirizine. The elimination $t\frac{1}{2}$ and apparent total body clearance of cetirizine may be decreased in geriatric clients.

CONTRAINDICATIONS

Due to the pseudoephedrine component, use in narrow-angle glaucoma or urinary retention and in those taking MAO inhibitor therapy or within 14 days of stopping such therapy. Also, use in severe hypertension, severe coronary artery disease, or in those who have shown hypersensitivity or idiosyncrasy to product components, to adrenergic drugs, or to other drugs of similar chemical structure. Use with alcohol or other CNS depressants due to additive decreased alertness and impaired CNS performance. Use during lactation is not recommended. Use of decongestants and antihistamines are not recommended for use in children less than 6 years of age.

SPECIAL CONCERNS

Use with caution in those with hypertension, diabetes mellitus, ischemic heart disease, increased intraocular pressure, hyperthyroidism, renal impairment, or prostatic hypertrophy. Use with caution with other sympathomimetic amines because combined CV effects may harm the client.

SIDE EFFECTS

Most Common

Insomnia, dry mouth, fatigue, somnolence, pharyngitis, epistaxis, accidental injury, dizziness.

See *Cetirizine hydrochloride* and *Pseudoephedrine hydrochloride* for the complete list of possible side effects.

DOSAGE

• **TABLETS**

Seasonal or allergic rhinitis.

Adults and children, 12 years and older: One tablet 2 times per day.

NURSING CONSIDERATIONS

ADMINISTRATION/STORAGE

Give a lower initial dose (1 tablet/day) with decreased renal function (C_CR 11–31 mL/min), those on hemodialysis (C_CR <7 mL/min), and with hepatic impairment.

ASSESSMENT

1. Note reasons for therapy, characteristics of S&S, other agents trialed, triggers/seasons if known.
2. Monitor VS, renal and LFTS; reduce dose with dysfunction.
3. List drugs prescribed to ensure none interact.
4. Assess for any CAD, HTN, BPH or other conditions that may preclude therapy.

CLIENT/FAMILY TEACHING

1. May be taken with or without food.
2. Swallow tablets whole; do not break or chew tablets.
3. Avoid alcohol and CNS depressants.
4. Do not share drugs; avoid in child <12 y.o.
5. May experience dizziness and drowsiness; do not perform activities that re-

quire mental alertness until drug effects realized.
6. Use sugarless candy or gum, ice chips or a saliva substitute for dry mouth effects.
7. Keep all F/U visits and report adverse effects or lack of response.

OUTCOMES/EVALUATE

Relief of seasonal allergy symptoms

Cetrorelix acetate
(see-**TROE**-reh-licks)

CLASSIFICATION(S):
Gonadotropin-releasing hormone antagonist
PREGNANCY CATEGORY: X
Rx: Cetrotide.

USES

Inhibition of premature LH surges in women undergoing controlled ovarian stimulation.

ACTION/KINETICS

Action

Synthetic decapeptide that competes with natural gonadotropin releasing hormone (GnRH) for binding to membrane receptors on pituitary cells, thus controlling the release of LH and FSH in a dose-dependent manner. Suppression of release of LH and FSH is maintained by continuous treatment; there is a more pronounced effect on LH than on FSH. Effects are reversible if treatment is discontinued.

Pharmacokinetics

Readily absorbed. **Onset:** About 1 hr with the 3 mg dose and 2 hr with the 0.25 mg dose. **t½:** 62.8 hr following a single 3-mg dose, 5 hr following a single 0.25-mg dose, and 20.6 hr following multiple 0.25-mg doses. **Plasma protein binding:** About 86%.

CONTRAINDICATIONS

Hypersensitivity to cetrorelix acetate, extrinsic peptide hormones, mannitol, GnRH, other GnRH analogs. Use in women with a severe allergic condition. Severe renal impairment. Clients 65 years of age and over. Known or suspected pregnancy. Lactation.

C

SPECIAL CONCERNS
Use caution in monitoring clients hypersensitive to cetrorelix as severe reactions are possible.

SIDE EFFECTS
Most Common
Ovarian hyperstimulation syndrome, nausea, headache.
GI: Nausea. **CNS:** Headache. **GU:** Ovarian hyperstimulation syndrome. **Hypersensitivity:** *Anaphylaxis*, cough, rash, hypotension. **At reaction site:** Redness, erythema, bruising, itching, swelling, pruritus.

LABORATORY TEST CONSIDERATIONS
↑ ALT, AST, GGT, alkaline phosphatase.

HOW SUPPLIED
Injection: 0.25 mg, 3 mg.

DOSAGE
- **SC**
  Inhibition of premature LH surges.

Single dose regimen: 3 mg when the serum estradiol level indicates an appropriate stimulation response (usually on stimulation day 7; range 5–9 days). If HCG has not been given within 4 days after injection of 3 mg cetrorelix, give cetrorelix, 0.25 mg once daily until the day of HCG administration. **Multiple dose regimen:** 0.25 mg cetrorelix given on either stimulation day 5 (a.m. or p.m.) or day 6 (a.m.) and continued daily until the day of HCG administration.

NURSING CONSIDERATIONS
ADMINISTRATION/STORAGE
1. Wash hands thoroughly with soap and water.
2. Flip off the plastic vial cover, wipe the Al ring and rubber stopper with alcohol swab.
3. Put injection needle with yellow mark (20 gauge) on the pre-filled syringe.
4. Push needle through the rubber vial stopper; slowly inject solvent into the vial.
5. Leave syringe on the vial and gently agitate vial until solution is clear and without residue. Avoid forming bubbles.
6. Draw the total contents of the vial into the syringe. If necessary, invert the vial and pull back the needle as far as needed to withdraw entire contents of the vial.
7. Remove the needle and replace with the injection needle (27 gauge) with grey mark.
8. Inject into lower abdomen skin at a 45 degree angle. Pull back plunger once inserted to assess for blood. If no blood evident, press plunger to administer syringe contents. If blood appears, remove the needle and discard; restart the process. Discard materials properly.

ASSESSMENT
1. Note reasons for therapy, other agents/therapies trialed for infertility, outcome.
2. Monitor VS, LFTs. Assess for hypersensitivity reactions; monitor closely after first dose for any S&S of anaphylaxis.
3. Obtain ultrasound to assess for follicle number and size, and to R/O pregnancy.

CLIENT/FAMILY TEACHING
1. If self-administering, demonstrate technique in office before leaving. Refer to administration/storage and patient leaflet for administration guidelines. Store as directed.
2. Review time commitment that therapy requires for desired outcome. Frequent monitoring, lab tests, ultrasounds are required to prevent adverse effects and to enhance desired results.
3. Drug may cause birth defects. Stop drug, report if pregnancy suspected.
4. Report any abdominal pain, cough, injection site rash, vaginal bleeding, persistent adverse effects, yellowing of eyes or skin.

OUTCOMES/EVALUATE
Desired pregnancy

Cetuximab   ■ IV
(seh-**TUX**-ih-mab)

CLASSIFICATION(S):
Antineoplastic, monoclonal antibody
PREGNANCY CATEGORY: C
Rx: Erbitux.

USES

(1) In combination with irinotecan to treat epidermal growth factor receptor (EGFR)-expressing, metastatic colorectal carcinoma in those who are refractory to irinotecan-based chemotherapy. (2) As a single agent for the treatment of EGFR-expressing, metastatic colorectal carcinoma in those who are intolerant to irinotecan-based chemotherapy. (3) In combination with radiation therapy to treat squamous cell cancer of the head and neck that cannot be removed by surgery. (4) As monotherapy to treat recurrent or metastatic squamous cell carcinoma of the head and neck when prior platinum-based chemotherapy has failed.

ACTION/KINETICS

Action

Cetuximab is a recombinant, human/mouse chimeric monoclonal antibody that binds specifically to the extracellular domain of the human epidermal growth factor receptor (EGFR) on normal and tumor cells; it competitively inhibits the binding of epidermal growth factor and other ligands (e.g., transforming growth factor-alpha). Binding of cetuximab to the EGFR blocks phosphorylation and activation of receptor-associated kinases; this results in inhibition of cell growth, induction of apoptosis, and decreased matrix metalloproteinase and vascular endothelial growth factor production. Over-expression of EGFR is noted in many human cancers, including the colon and rectum. Thus, cetuximab inhibits growth and survival of tumor cells that over-express the EGFR. Addition of irinotecan or irinotecan plus 5-fluorouracil increases the antitumor effects.

Pharmacokinetics

Steady state is reached by the third weekly infusion. **t½, terminal:** 112 hr. **Mean steady state t½:** 114 hr.

CONTRAINDICATIONS

Use during lactation and for 60 days following the last dose of cetuximab.

SPECIAL CONCERNS

■ (1) Infusion reactions. Severe infusion reactions occurred in about 3% of clients given cetuximab, rarely with fatal outcomes. About 90% of severe infusion reactions were associated with the first infusion of cetuximab. Severe infusion reactions are characterized by rapid onset of airway obstruction (e.g., bronchospasm, stridor, hoarseness), urticaria, hypotension and/or cardiac arrest. Severe infusion reactions require immediate interruption of the cetuximab infusion and permanent discontinuation from further treatment. (2) Cardiopulmonary arrest. Cardiopulmonary arrest and/or sudden death occurred in 2% of clients with squamous cell carcinoma of the head and neck treated with radiation therapy and cetuximab compared with zero clients treated with radiation therapy alone. Fatal events occurred within 1 to 43 days after the last cetuximab treatment. Use cetuximab in combination with radiation therapy with caution in head and neck cancer clients with known coronary artery disease, CHF, and arrhythmias. Although the etiology of these events is unknown, close monitoring of serum electrolytes, including serum magnesium, potassium, and calcium, during and after cetuximab therapy is recommended.■ Safety and efficacy have not been established in children. Use with caution in clients with known hypersensitivity to cetuximab, murine proteins, or any component of the product.

SIDE EFFECTS

Most Common

Acneform rash, mucositis, radiation dermatitis, abdominal pain, anorexia, xerostomia, dysphagia, asthenia, malaise, N&V, constipation, diarrhea, fever.

Side effects include those for all uses of cetuximab. **GI:** Diarrhea, N&V, xerostomia, abdominal pain, anorexia, constipation, mucositis, stomatitis, dyspepsia, dysphagia. **CV:** Cardiopulmonary arrest. **Dermatologic:** Acneform rash (including acne, dry skin, exfoliative dermatitis, maculopapular rash, pustular rash, or rash), alopecia, skin disorder, pruritus, increased hair growth, radiation dermatitis. **CNS:** Headache, insomnia, depression, confusion. **Respiratory:** Dyspnea, pharyngitis, increased cough, interstitial lung disease, SOB. **Hematologic:** Leu-

 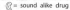

C

kopenia, anemia. **Metabolic:** Weight loss, peripheral edema, dehydration. **Infusion reaction:** Bronchospasm, stridor, hoarseness, urticaria, hypotension. **Body as a Whole:** Asthenia/malaise, chills, fever, pain, infection, hypersensitivity reactions, dehydration, peripheral edema. **Miscellaneous:** Back pain, conjunctivitis, nail disorder, infusion-related reactions.

LABORATORY TEST CONSIDERATIONS
Hypomagnesemia (may be severe).

HOW SUPPLIED
Injection: 2 mg/mL.

DOSAGE

• **IV INFUSION**
  Metastatic colorectal carcinoma.

Initial, either alone or with irinotecan: 400 mg/m^2 given as a 120-min IV infusion (maximum infusion rate, 5 mL/min). **Maintenance:** 250 mg/m^2 weekly infused over 60 minutes (maximum infusion rate, 5 mL/min).

> With radiation therapy for locally or regionally advanced squamous cell cancer of the head and neck.

Initial loading dose: 400 mg/m^2 given as a 120 min IV infusion (maximum infusion rate 5 mL/min) 1 week prior to initiation of a course of radiation therapy. **Weekly maintenance dose (all other infusions):** 250 mg/m^2 infused over 60 min (maximum infusion rate 5 mL/min) for the duration of radiation therapy (6–7 weeks).

> Monotherapy to treat recurrent or metastatic squamous cell carcinoma of the head and neck.

Initial: 400 mg/m^2 followed by 250 mg/m^2 weekly until disease progression or unacceptable toxicity.

NURSING CONSIDERATIONS
ADMINISTRATION/STORAGE
IV 1. Do not give as IV push or bolus; give as a 120-minute IV infusion using an infusion pump or syringe pump.
2. Premedicate with a H_1-histamine antagonist (e.g., 50 mg diphenhydramine IV).
3. Give using a low protein-binding 0.22 micrometer in-line filter. The solution should be clear and colorless but may contain a small amount of easily

visible, white, amorphous cetuximab particles. Do not shake or dilute.
4. If the client experiences a mild or moderate (grade 1 or 2) infusion reaction, permanently reduce the infusion rate by 50%. Immediately and permanently discontinue cetuximab in those who experience severe (grade 3 or 4) infusion reactions.
5. If a client experiences severe acneform rash, adjust treatment according to the following guidelines:

• **First occurrence of acneform rash:** Delay infusion 1–2 weeks. If improvement, continue at 250 mg/m^2; if no improvement, discontinue cetuximab.

• **Second occurrence of acneform rash:** Delay infusion 1–2 weeks. If improvement, reduce dose to 200 mg/m^2; if no improvement, discontinue cetuximab.

• **Third occurrence of acneform rash:** Delay infusion 1–2 weeks; If improvement, reduce dose to 150 mg/m^2; if no improvement, discontinue cetuximab.

• **Fourth occurrence of acneform rash:** Discontinue cetuximab.
6. Refrigerate vials from 2–8°C (36–46°F). Increased particulate formation may occur at temperatures at/below 0°C (32°F).
7. Product contains no preservatives. Preparations in infusion containers are chemically and physically stable for up to 12 hr at 2–8°C (36–46°F) and up to 8 hr from 20–25°C (68–77°F). Discard any remaining solution in the infusion container after 8 hr at controlled room temperature or after 12 hr of refrigeration. Discard any unused portion of the vial.

ASSESSMENT
1. Note disease onset, resaons for therapy: combination therapy for immunohistochemical evidence of positive EGFR expression, or irinotecan-based refractory/intolerance for EGFR expressing colorectal cancer.
2. Only to be prescribed by those experienced in this therapy. Follow guidelines for dose modifications, for infusion reactions, dermatologic and related disorder toxicities as directed.

Bold Italic = life threatening side effect   ■ = black box warning   ✦ = Available in Canada

3. Assess/monitor CBC, CXR, renal/LFTs, VS/I&O, worsening of pulmonary status, skin infections/reactions, infusion reactions. Monitor for at least 1 hr (longer in those who have experienced infusion reactions) after drug infusion.

4. Monitor periodically for hypomagnesemia that may accompany hypocalcemia and hypokalemia during and after completion of therapy.

5. After initial dose, therapy usually administered once a week. Premedicate with an H₁ antagonist (i.e., IV diphenhydramine); reduces adverse effects.

CLIENT/FAMILY TEACHING

1. Drug used to treat colorectal cancers; may cause a variety of adverse reactions. All must be reported immediately so that dosage/therapy can be adjusted/stopped.

2. Use precautions if sunlight exposed-drug may cause skin reactions; use hats, sunscreen, clothes to cover extremities.

3. Practice reliable contraception; drug is toxic to developing fetus- may cause loss of pregnancy.

4. Any unusual events should be immediately reported as therapy may be fatal. SOB, wheezing, skin reactions, rash, itching, nail disorders, diarrhea, dehydration, chest pain require immediate attention.

5. Keep all F/U appointments so that any potential problems can be addressed, labs monitored, and therapy stopped or adjusted as needed. Any severe toxicities to this therapy should render one ineligible for another course.

OUTCOMES/EVALUATE

Inhibition of metastatic colorectal carcinoma (EGFR) in those refractory to irinotecan-based chemotherapy as single agent

Chlorambucil (CHL)

(klor-**AM**-byou-sill)

CLASSIFICATION(S):

Antineoplastic, alkylating
PREGNANCY CATEGORY: D
Rx: Leukeran.

SEE ALSO ANTINEOPLASTIC AGENTS AND ALKYLATING AGENTS.

USES

Palliative treatment of chronic lymphocytic leukemia, malignant lymphomas (including lymphosarcoma), giant follicular lymphomas, and Hodgkin's disease. *Investigational:* Ovarian and testicular carcinoma, non-Hodgkin's lymphoma, Waldenstrom macroglobulinemia.

ACTION/KINETICS

Action

Cell-cycle nonspecific; cytotoxic to nonproliferating cells and has immunosuppressant activity. Forms an unstable ethylenimmonium ion which binds (alkylates) with intracellular substances such as nucleic acids. The cytotoxic effect is due to cross-linking of strands of DNA and RNA and inhibition of protein synthesis.

Pharmacokinetics

Rapidly and completely absorbed from the GI tract. **Peak plasma levels:** 1 hr. **t½, terminal:** 1.5 hr. Extensively metabolized by the liver; at least one metabolite is active. Fifteen to 60% is excreted through the urine 24 hr after drug administration; 40% is bound to tissues, including fat. **Plasma protein binding:** 99%, specifically to albumin.

CONTRAINDICATIONS

Resistance to the drug, hypersensitivity. Lactation.

SPECIAL CONCERNS

■ Can severely suppress bone marrow function. Is carcinogenic in humans and may be both mutagenic and teratogenic. Also affects fertility.■ Use during lactation only if benefits outweigh risks. Safety and efficacy have not been established in children. May be cross-hy-

 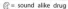

persensitivity with other alklyating agents.

SIDE EFFECTS

Most Common

Bone marrow suppression, N&V, changes in menses.

See *Antineoplastic Agents* for a complete list of possible side effects. Also, **Hepatic:** Hepatotoxicity with jaundice. **Pulmonary:** *Pulmonary fibrosis*, bronchopulmonary dysplasia. **CNS:** Children with nephrotic syndrome have an increased risk of seizures. **Miscellaneous:** Keratitis, drug fever, sterile cystitis, interstitial pneumonia, peripheral neuropathy. Cross-sensitivity (skin rashes) may occur with other alkylating agents.

LABORATORY TEST CONSIDERATIONS

↑ Uric acid levels in serum and urine.

OD OVERDOSE MANAGEMENT

Symptoms: Pancytopenia (reversible), ataxia, agitated behavior, *clonic-tonic seizures. Treatment:* General supportive measures. Monitor blood profiles carefully; blood transfusions may be required.

HOW SUPPLIED

Tablets: 2 mg.

DOSAGE

- **TABLETS**

  Leukemia, lymphomas.

  Individualized according to response of client. **Adults, children, initial and short courses:** 0.1–0.2 mg/kg (or 4–10 mg) daily in single or divided doses for 3–6 weeks; **maintenance:** 0.03–0.1 mg/kg/day (2–4 mg/day) depending on blood counts.

  Alternative for chronic lymphocytic leukemia.

  Initial: 0.4 mg/kg; **then,** repeat this dose every 2 weeks increasing by 0.1 mg/kg until either toxicity or control of condition is observed.

NURSING CONSIDERATIONS

§ Do not confuse Alkeran (melphalan), Leukeran (chlorambucil), and Myleran (busulfan), each of which is an antineoplastic.

ADMINISTRATION/STORAGE

Store at 15–25°C (59–77°F) in a dry place.

ASSESSMENT

1. List reasons for therapy, noting pretreatment lab and physical assessment findings (weight, spleen size, VS and extent of disease). List other agents trialed/outcome.

2. Monitor CXR, PFT's, CBC, liver and renal function studies, uric acid levels. Drug may cause severe granulocyte and lymphocyte suppression. Nadir: 21 days; recovery: 42–56 days.

CLIENT/FAMILY TEACHING

1. Take 1 hr before breakfast, 2 hr after the evening meal or at bedtime to reduce N&V. Take antiemetics as prescribed.

2. Consume 2–3 L/day of fluids to prevent dehydration and decrease urate crystals; may be prescribed allopurinol to control.

3. Report side effects: bruising, bleeding, stomach/joint pains, breathing difficulty, fever, sore throat, chills or S&S of infection. Skin rash may result from cross-sensitivity with other alkylating agents.

4. May lose hair; avoid vaccinations and crowds and persons with infections during therapy.

5. Drug is carcinogenic and may also be mutagenic and teratogenic; practice reliable birth control. Evalute need for sperm/egg harvesting.

OUTCOMES/EVALUATE

- Positive tumor response evidenced by ↓ tumor size/spread; suppression of malignant cell proliferation
- Immunosuppressant activity

Chloramphenicol ■ IV
(klor-am-**FEN**-ih-kohl)

CLASSIFICATION(S):
Antibiotic, chloramphenicol
PREGNANCY CATEGORY: D
Rx: Ophthalmic: Chloromycetin.
✦Rx: Capsules: Pentamycetin.

Chloramphenicol sodium succinate

Rx: Chloromycetin Sodium Succinate.

♣Rx: Chloromycetin Injection.

SEE ALSO *ANTI-INFECTIVES.*

USES

Systemic: (1) Treatment of choice for typhoid fever but not for typhoid carrier state. (2) Serious infections caused by *Salmonella, Rickettsia, Chlamydia,* and lymphogranuloma-psittacosis group. (3) Meningitis due to *Haemophilus influenzae.* (4) Brain abscesses due to *Bacteroides fragilis.* (5) Cystic fibrosis anti-infective. (6) Meningococcal or pneumococcal meningitis.

Ophthalmic: Use only in serious infections for which less potentially dangerous drugs are ineffective or contraindicated. Superficial ocular infections (involving the conjunctiva or cornea—conjunctivitis, keratitis, keratoconjunctivitis, corneal ulcers, blepharitis, blepharoconjunctivitis, acute meibomianitis, and dacrocystitis) due to *Staphylococcus aureus; Streptococcus* species, including *S. pneumoniae; Escherichia coli, H. influenzae, Klebsiella* species, *Enterobacter* species, *Moraxella lacunata, Neisseria* species. Inadequate effect against *Pseudomonas aeruginosa* and *Serratia marcescens.*

ACTION/KINETICS

Action
Interferes with or inhibits protein synthesis in bacteria by binding to 50S ribosomal subunits.

Pharmacokinetics
Therapeutic serum concentrations: **peak,** 10–20 mcg/mL; **trough:** 5–10 mcg/mL (less for neonates). **Peak serum concentration: IM,** 2 hr. **t½:** 4 hr. Metabolized in the liver; 75–90% excreted in urine within 24 hr, as parent drug (8–12%) and inactive metabolites. Mostly bacteriostatic. Well absorbed from the GI tract and distributed to all parts of the body, including CSF, pleural, and ascitic fluids; saliva; milk; and aqueous and vitreous humors.

CONTRAINDICATIONS

Hypersensitivity to chloramphenicol; pregnancy, especially near term and during labor; lactation. Avoid simultaneous administration of other drugs that may depress bone marrow. Ophthalmically in the presence of dendritic keratitis, vaccinia, varicella, mycobacterial or fungal eye infections, or following removal of a corneal foreign body.

SPECIAL CONCERNS

■ (1) Aplastic anemia, hypoplastic anemia, thrombocytopenia, and granulocytopenia may occur. Also reported is aplastic anemia terminating in leukemia. Blood dyscrasias occurred after both short-term and prolonged therapy. Do not use when less potentially dangerous drugs are effective. Not to be used for trivial infections, prophylaxis of bacterial infections, or to treat colds, flu, or throat infections. (2) Perform adequate blood studies during treatment. Such tests may detect early peripheral blood changes but they cannot be relied upon to detect bone marrow depression prior to aplastic anemia. To facilitate appropriate tests and observation, hospitalize clients. (3) When used ophthalmically, bone marrow hypoplasia including aplastic anemia and death have been reported following local application of chloramphenicol. Chloramphenicol should not be used when less potentially dangerous agents would be expected to provide effective treatment.■ Use with caution in clients with intermittent porphyria or G6PD deficiency. To avoid gray syndrome, use with caution and in reduced doses in premature and full-term infants. Ophthalmic ointments may retard corneal epithelial healing.

SIDE EFFECTS

Most Common
After systemic use: Headache, N&V, diarrhea.

Hematologic (most serious): *Aplastic anemia, hypoplastic anemia,* thrombocytopenia, granulocytopenia, *hemolytic anemia,* pancytopenia, hemoglobinuria (paroxysmal nocturnal). *Hematologic studies should be undertaken before and every 2 days during therapy.* **GI:** N&V, diarrhea, glossitis, stomatitis, unpleasant taste, enterocolitis, pruritus ani. **Allergic:** Fever, angioedema, macular and vesicular rashes, urticaria, hemorrhages of the skin, intestine, bladder, mouth,

---

anaphylaxis. **CNS:** Headache, delirium, confusion, mental depression. **Neurologic:** Optic neuritis, peripheral neuritis.

   NOTE: Neonates should be observed closely, since the drug accumulates in the bloodstream and the infant is thus subject to greater hazards of toxicity. **After Ophthalmic use:** Temporary blurring of vision, stinging, itching, burning, redness, irritation, swelling, decreased vision, persistent or worse pain.

DRUG INTERACTIONS

Acetaminophen / ↑ Chloramphenicol effect R/T ↑ serum levels
Anticoagulants, oral / ↑ Anticoagulant effect R/T ↓ liver breakdown
Antidiabetics, oral / ↑ Hypoglycemic effect R/T ↓ liver breakdown
Barbiturates / ↑ Barbiturate effect R/T ↓ liver breakdown; also, ↓ serum chloramphenicol levels
Chymotrypsin / Chloramphenicol will inhibit chymotrypsin
Cyclophosphamide / Delayed or ↓ activation of cyclophosphamide
Iron preparations / ↑ Serum levels of iron
Penicillins / Either ↑ or ↓ effect when combined to treat certain microorganisms
Phenytoin (and other hydantoins) / ↑ Phenytoin effect R/T ↓ liver breakdown; also, chloramphenicol levels may be ↑ or ↓
Rifampin / ↓ Chloramphenicol effect R/T ↑ liver breakdown
Sulfonylureas / Possible clinical manifestations of hypoglycemia
Tacrolimus / ↑ Tacrolimus blood levels R/T ↓ liver breakdown
Vitamin B_{12} / ↓ Vitamin B_{12} response when treating pernicious anemia

HOW SUPPLIED

Chloramphenicol ophthalmic: *Ointment:* 10 mg/gram; *Powder for Solution (for Reconstitution):* 25 mg/vial; *Solution:* 5 mg/mL.
Chloramphenicol sodium succinate: *Powder for Injection:* 100 mg/mL.

DOSAGE————————————

CHLORAMPHENICOL

• **Ophthalmic Ointment (10 mg/ gram)**

0.5-in. ribbon placed in lower conjunctival sac q 3–4 hr for acute infections and 2–3 times/day for mild to moderate infections.

• **Ophthalmic Solution (5 mg/mL)**

2 gtt to the affected eye(s) q 3 hr or more frequently (if deemed appropriate); continue day and night for the first 48 hr; then, increase the interval between applications. Continue for at least 48 hr after the eye appears normal.

CHLORAMPHENICOL SODIUM SUCCINATE

• **IV ONLY**

Adults: 50 mg/kg/day in four equally divided doses q 6 hr. Can be increased to 100 mg/kg/day in severe infections, but dosage should be reduced as soon as possible. **Neonates and children with immature metabolic function:** 25 mg/kg once daily in divided doses q 12 hr. **Neonates, less than 2 kg:** 25 mg/kg once daily. **Neonates, over 2 kg, over 7 days of age:** 50 mg/kg/day q 12 hr in divided doses. **Neonates, over 2 kg, from birth to 7 days of age:** 50 mg/kg once daily. **Children:** 50–75 mg/kg/day in divided doses q 6 hr (50–100 mg/kg/day in divided doses q 6 hr for meningitis). *NOTE:* Carefully follow dosage for premature and newborn infants less than 2 weeks of age because blood levels differ significantly from those of other age groups.

NURSING CONSIDERATIONS

ADMINISTRATION/STORAGE

1. Prepare the ophthalmic solution by adding sterile distilled water to the vial. To prepare a 0.16%, 0.25%, or 0.5% solution, add 15, 10, or 5 mL of sterile water to the vial, respectively.
2. Store ophthalmic products below 30°C (86°F).
IV 3. Administer IV as a 10% solution over at least a 60-sec interval by reconstituting 1 gram in 10 mL of water for injection or D5W. May further dilute in 50–100 mL of dextrose or saline solution and infuse over 30–60 min.

ASSESSMENT

1. Note hypersensitivity/previous reaction to other agents.

Bold Italic = life threatening side effect   ▆ = black box warning   ✤ = Available in Canada

2. List reasons/type of therapy, symptom characteristics, culture results, other agents prescribed. If receiving drugs that cause bone marrow depression, do not use chloramphenicol.

3. If nursing, transmission of drug to breast milk can result in infant also receiving drug; infants have underdeveloped capacity to metabolize chloramphenicol.

4. If taking oral hypoglycemic agents, may need insulin during therapy.

5. Arrange for frequent observation and hematologic studies (CBC, platelets, reticulocytes, iron q 2 days during therapy) to detect for early S&S bone marrow depression; may develop weeks to months after therapy.

6. Monitor VS, I&O, CBC, renal and LFTs; reduce dose with impaired renal function and in newborn infants.

INTERVENTIONS

1. Note drugs that enhance chloramphenicol; monitor closely for evidence of severe toxicity.

2. Avoid repeated courses of therapy; drug is highly toxic.

3. Monitor for any of the following and report:

- *Bone marrow depression* characterized by weakness, fatigue, sore throat, bleeding.
- *Optic neuritis* characterized by reduced visual acuity bilaterally.
- *Peripheral neuritis* characterized by pain/sensation disturbance.
- Development of *gray syndrome* in premature and newborn infants, characterized by rapid respiration, failure to feed, abdominal distention with/without vomiting, loose green stools, progressive cyanosis, vasomotor collapse.

4. Assess for toxic and irritative effects, such as N&V, unpleasant taste, diarrhea, perineal irritation following PO administration. Differentiation of drug-induced diarrhea from that caused by a superinfection is critical and may be accomplished by assessment and analysis of all presenting symptoms.

CLIENT/FAMILY TEACHING

1. Take 1 hr before/2 hr after meals with a full glass of water; if GI upset occurs, may be taken with food. Do not chew or crush caps.

2. Take at regularly spaced intervals *around the clock*.

3. Avoid alcohol during therapy.

4. Do not take salicylates (aspirin) or NSAIDs. Wash hands before and after instillation/application.

5. To instill in the eye, place head back and place in the lower lid (conjunctival sac); close eyes. Apply light finger pressure on the inside corner (lacrimal sac) for 1 min. to prevent systemic absorption and toxicity. Ophthalmic solutions may cause blurred vision immediately after instillation; use caution, should clear.

6. To avoid contamination, do not touch tip of eye product with any surface.

7. Do not wear contact lenses if treating bacterial conjunctivitis. If contact lenses are required, do not insert lenses for at least 15 min after using any solutions that contain benzalkonium chloride (may be absorbed by the lens).

8. During IV administration, a bitter taste may be experienced; should subside after several minutes.

9. Report adverse side effects, unusual bruising/bleeding, sore throat, fatigue or lack or response.

10. Keep all F/U appointment to evaluate response to therapy.

OUTCOMES/EVALUATE

- Resolution of infection
- Therapeutic levels (peak 10–20 mcg/mL; trough 5–10 mcg/mL)

Chlordiazepoxide [IV]

(klor-dye-**AYZ**-eh-**POX**-eyed)

CLASSIFICATION(S):
Antianxiety drug, benzodiazepine
PREGNANCY CATEGORY: D
Rx: Librium, **C-IV.**
✤Rx: Apo-Chlordiazepoxide.

SEE ALSO *TRANQUILIZERS/ ANTIMANIC DRUGS/HYPNOTICS.*

📷 = see color insert   H = Herbal   IV = Intravenous   © = sound alike drug

C

USES

PO, Parenteral: (1) Anxiety disorders or for short-term relief of anxiety symptoms. (2) Acute withdrawal symptoms in chronic alcoholics. (3) Preoperatively to reduce anxiety and apprehension.

ACTION/KINETICS

Pharmacokinetics

Onset: PO, 30–60 min; **IM,** 15–30 min (absorption may be slow and erratic); **IV,** 3–30 min. **Peak plasma levels (PO):** 0.5–4 hr. **Duration: t½:** 5–30 hr. Is metabolized to four active metabolites: desmethylchlordiazepoxide, desmethyldiazepam, oxazepam, and demoxepam. Has less anticonvulsant activity and is less potent than diazepam. About 96% protein bound.

SIDE EFFECTS

Most Common

Drowsiness, ataxia, confusion, headache, blurred vision, nausea, constipation.

See *Tranquilizers, Antimanic Drugs, Hypnotics* for a complete list of possible side effects. Also, jaundice, acute hepatic necrosis, hepatic dysfunction.

LABORATORY TEST CONSIDERATIONS

↑ 17-Hydroxycorticosteroids, 17-ketosteroids, alkaline phosphatase, bilirubin, serum transaminase, porphobilinogen. ↓ PT (clients on coumarin).

HOW SUPPLIED

Capsules: 5 mg, 10 mg, 25 mg; *Powder for Injection:* 100 mg.

DOSAGE

• CAPSULES

Mild to moderate anxiety.

Adults: 5 or 10 mg 3 to 4 times per day. **Children, initial:** 5 mg 2 to 4 times per day; may be increased in some children to 10 mg 2 to 3 times per day. Not recommended for children less than 6 years old. **Elderly clients or those with debilitating disease:** 5 mg 2 to 4 times per day.

Severe anxiety.

Adults: 20 or 25 mg 3 to 4 times per day. For elderly clients or those with debilitating disease give 5 mg 2 to 4 times per day.

Acute alcohol withdrawal.

50–100 mg; repeat as needed (up to 300 mg/day). Parenteral form usually used initially. Reduce dose to maintenance levels.

Preoperative apprehension and anxiety.

5–10 mg 3 or 4 times per day on days preceding surgery.

• IM, IV (NOT RECOMMENDED FOR CHILDREN UNDER 12 YEARS OF AGE)

Acute or severe anxiety.

Adults, initial: 50–100 mg initially; **then,** 25–50 mg 3 to 4 times per day if needed. Do not exceed 300 mg in any 24-hr period although 300 mg may be given during a 6-hr period. Use lower doses (25–50 mg initially) for elderly or debilitated clients and for children 12 years and older.

Preoperative apprehension and anxiety.

Adults: 50–100 mg IM 1 hr before surgery.

Acute alcohol withdrawal.

Adults, initial: 50–100 mg IM or IV; repeat in 2–4 hr if necessary.

NURSING CONSIDERATIONS

ADMINISTRATION/STORAGE

1. **For IM use:** Add 2 mL of special IM diluent to contents of a 5 mL ampule of chlordiazepoxide sterile powder (100 mg).
2. Avoid excessive pressure when injecting diluent because bubbles form on the surface of the solution.
3. Agitate gently until completely dissolved.
4. Do not use diluent if it is opalescent or hazy.
5. Do not give solutions made with physiological saline or sterile water for injection IM because of the pain on injection.
6. Give deep IM injection slowly into the upper outer quadrant of the gluteus muscle.
7. Do not give IV a solution made with the IM diluent because of the bubbles that form when the IM diluent is added to chlordiazepoxide powder.
8. **IV** Give IV when rapid action is mandatory.
9. **For IV use:** Prepare immediately before administration by diluting with 5 mL of sterile water for injection or sterile 0.9% NaCl solution. Agitate gently and thoroughly until dissolved.

Bold Italic = life threatening side effect   ■ = black box warning   ✦ = Available in Canada

10. Inject directly into vein over 1-min period.

11. Do not add to IV infusion because of instability of drug.

12. Do not use IV solution for IM administration.

13. Store capsules and injection from 15–30°C (59–86°F).

ASSESSMENT

1. Note reasons for therapy, pretreatment symptoms, mental status, motor responses.

2. Maintain quiet, supervised environment; keep recumbent for 3 hr following parenteral administration.

3. Assess VS, CBC, renal, and LFTs to R/O impairment.

CLIENT/FAMILY TEACHING

1. May take with food as directed; do not double doses if dose forgotten.

2. Consume extra fluids and bulk; minimizes constipating effects.

3. Use caution, may cause dizziness/drowsiness and sedation. Report unusual or persistent side effects

4. Do not stop drug suddenly after prolonged use, taper off over at least a week.

5. Avoid all OTC agents, alcohol, and any other CNS depressants.

6. Practice reliable contraception. Avoid exposure to excessive sunlight, may cause photosensitivity reaction.

OUTCOMES/EVALUATE

- ↓ Tremors; ↓ anxiety; sedation
- Termination of panic attacks
- ↓ Alcohol withdrawal symptoms

Chlorpheniramine maleate

(klor-fen-**EAR**-ah-meen)

CLASSIFICATION(S):

Antihistamine, first generation, alkylamine

PREGNANCY CATEGORY: B

OTC: Syrup: Aller-Chlor. **Tablets, Chewable:** Chlo-Amine. **Tablets:** Aller-Chlor, Allergy, Allergy Relief. **Tablets, Extended-Release:** Chlor-Trimeton Allergy 8 Hour and 12 Hour.

Rx: Capsules, Extended-Release Sustained-Release: Chlorpheniramine maleate, ODALL AR. **Caplets:** ED-CHLOR-TAN. **Oral Suspension:** Pediox—S.

♣**OTC: Repetabs Syrup Tablets:** Chlor-Tripolon.

SEE ALSO *ANTIHISTAMINES.*

USES

Allergic rhinitis, including sneezing; itchy, watery eyes; itchy throat, and runny nose due to hay fever and other upper respiratory allergies.

ACTION/KINETICS

Action

Moderate anticholinergic and low sedative activity; no antiemetic activity.

Pharmacokinetics

Onset: 15–30 min. **t½:** 21–27 hr. **Time to peak effect:** 6 hr. **Duration:** 3–6 hr.

ADDITIONAL CONTRAINDICATIONS

Use in children 5 years of age or younger.

SPECIAL CONCERNS

Geriatric clients may be more sensitive to the adult dose.

SIDE EFFECTS

Most Common

Constipation, diarrhea, dizziness, drowsiness, dry mouth/nose/throat, headache, anorexia, N&V, anxiety, insomnia, GI upset, asthenia.

See *Antihistamines* for a complete list of possible side effects.

HOW SUPPLIED

Caplets: 8 mg (as tannate); *Capsules, Extended-Release, Sustained-Release:* 8 mg, 12 mg; *Oral Suspension:* 4 mg/5 mL; *Syrup:* 2 mg/5 mL; *Tablets:* 4 mg; *Tablets, Chewable:* 2 mg; *Tablets, Extended-Release:* 8 mg, 12 mg, 16 mg.

DOSAGE

- **SYRUP; TABLETS; TABLETS, CHEWABLE**

  Allergic rhinitis.

Adults and children over 12 years: 4 mg q 4–6 hr, not to exceed 24 mg in 24 hr. **Pediatric, 6–12 years:** 2 mg (break 4-mg tablets in half) q 4–6 hr, not to exceed 12 mg in 24 hr. **2–6 years:** Not to be used.

- **CAPLETS**

  Allergic rhinitis.

 = see color insert   = Herbal   = Intravenous   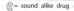 = sound alike drug

Adults and children 12 years and older: 8 mg q 12 hr, up to 16–24 mg/day. **Children, 6–12 years of age:** Consult a provider.

- **CAPSULES, EXTENDED-RELEASE; CAPSULES, SUSTAINED-RELEASE**
  Allergic rhinitis.

Adults and children over 12 years: 8 or 12 mg q 12 hr, up to 16 or 24 mg/day. **Children, 6–12 years:** 8 mg at bedtime or during the day as indicated. For ODALL AR, give 12 mg once daily, up to 24 mg in 24 hr, to those aged 12 and over.

- **ORAL SUSPENSION**
  Allergic rhinitis.

Children, 6–12 years of age: 2–4 mg (2.5–5 mL) q 12 hr; **over 12 years of age:** 4–8 mg (5–10 mL) q 12 hr.

- **TABLETS, EXTENDED-RELEASE**
  Allergic rhinitis.

Adults and children over 12 years: 8 mg q 8–12 hr or 12 mg q 12 hr, not to exceed 24 mg in 24 hr.

NURSING CONSIDERATIONS

ADMINISTRATION/STORAGE

ODALL AR contains 2 mg chlorpheniramine maleate, immediate release, and 10 mg chlorpheniramine maleate, sustained release.

ASSESSMENT

1. Note indications for therapy, other agents trialed and outcome. Attempt to identify triggers/causative agents.
2. Perform/document ENT findings; note any drainage in pharynx.

CLIENT/FAMILY TEACHING

1. Take as directed with a full glass of water. Food delays absorption.
2. Report any mental status changes, adverse effects or lack of response. May cause drowsiness; use caution.
3. Avoid alcohol in any form.
4. Anticipate dry mouth and use appropriate remedies.

OUTCOMES/EVALUATE

↓ Nasal congestion and allergic manifestations

Chlorpromazine hydrochloride
(klor-**PROH**-mah-zeen)

CLASSIFICATION(S):
Antipsychotic, phenothiazine
PREGNANCY CATEGORY: C
Rx: Thorazine.
✦Rx: Largactil.

SEE ALSO *ANTIPSYCHOTIC AGENTS, PHENOTHIAZINES*.

USES

(1) Schizophrenia. (2) Acute intermittent porphyria. (3) Preanesthetic to relieve restlessness and apprehension. (4) Adjunct to treat tetanus. (5) Intractable hiccoughs. (6) N&V. (7) Control of the manic type of manic-depressive illness. (8) Severe behavioral problems in children 1–12 years of age marked by combativeness and/or explosive hyperexcitable behavior. (9) Short-term treatment of hyperactive children who show excessive motor activity with accompanying conduct disorders with symptoms including impulsivitiy, decreased attention span, aggressiveness, mood lability, or poor frustration tolerance. *Investigational:* IM or IV to treat migraine headaches.

ACTION/KINETICS

Action

Has significant antiemetic, hypotensive, and sedative effects; moderate anticholinergic and extrapyramidal effects.

Pharmacokinetics

Is 20–40% bioavailable. **Peak plasma levels:** 2–3 hr after both PO and IM administration. $t^{1/2}$ (after IV, IM): **Initial,** 4–5 hr; **final,** 3–40 hr. Extensively metabolized in the intestinal wall and liver; certain of the metabolites are active. **Steady-state plasma levels** (in psychotics): 10–1,300 ng/mL. After 2–3 weeks of therapy, plasma levels decline, possibly because of reduction in drug absorption and/or increase in drug metabolism. **Plasma protein binding:** 92–97%.

Bold Italic = life threatening side effect   ■ = black box warning   ✦ = Available in Canada

SPECIAL CONCERNS

Use during pregnancy only if benefits outweigh risks. Safety for use during lactation has not been established. Generally, do not use chlorpromazine in children less than 6 months except where potentially life-saving; do not use for conditions for which specific children's dosages have not been established.

SIDE EFFECTS

Most Common

Constipation, drowsiness, blurred vision, decreased sweating, tremor, difficulty urinating, dark urine, dizziness, increased appetite, menstrual irregularities, swollen breasts.

See *Antipsychotic Agents, Phenothiazines* for a complete list of possible side effects.

ADDITIONAL DRUG INTERACTIONS

Epinephrine / Chlorpromazine ↓ peripheral vasoconstriction and may reverse action of epinephrine

Norepinephrine / Chlorpromazine ↓ pressor effect and eliminates bradycardia R/T norepinephrine

Smoking / ↑ Chlorpromazine hepatic metabolism and end-organ response; ↓ sedation and possible hypotension; possible ↑ dosage needed

Valproic acid / ↑ Valproic acid effect R/T ↓ clearance

LABORATORY TEST CONSIDERATIONS

Possible ↑ plasma cholesterol.

HOW SUPPLIED

Injection: 25 mg/mL; *Oral Concentrate:* 100 mg/mL; *Suppository, Rectal:* 100 mg; *Syrup:* 10 mg/5 mL; *Tablets:* 10 mg, 25 mg, 50 mg, 100 mg, 200 mg.

DOSAGE

• ORAL CONCENTRATE; SYRUP; TABLETS

Outpatients, general uses.

Adults: 10 mg 3–4 times per day or 25 mg 2–3 times per day. For more serious cases, 25 mg 3 times per day. After 1 or 2 days, increase daily dose by 20 to 50 mg semiweekly, until client becomes calm and cooperative. Maximum improvement may not be seen for weeks or months. Continue optimum dosage for 2 weeks; then, reduce gradually to maintenance levels (200 mg/day is usual). Up to 800 mg/day may be needed in discharged mental clients.

Psychotic disorders, less acutely disturbed.

Adults and adolescents: 25 mg 3 times per day; dosage may be increased by 20–50 mg/day q 3–4 days as needed, up to 400 mg/day.

Behavioral disorders/Hyperactivity in children.

Outpatients: 0.5 mg/kg (0.25 mg/lb) q 4–6 hr, as needed. **Hospitalized:** Start with low doses and increase gradually. For severe conditions: 50–100 mg/day. In older children, 200 mg or more/day may be needed. There is little evidence that improvement in severely disturbed mentally retarded clients is enhanced by doses over 500 mg/day.

Preoperative sedation.

Adults and adolescents: 25–50 mg 2–3 hr before surgery. **Pediatric:** 0.5 mg/kg (15 mg/m^2) 2–3 hr before surgery.

Intractable hiccoughs.

25–50 mg PO 3–4 times per day. If symptoms persist for 2 to 3 days, give 25–50 mg IM. Should symptoms persist, give 25–50 mg by slow IV infusion with client flat in bed. Give in 500–1,000 mL saline.

Acute intermittent porphyria in adults.

25–50 mg 3 or 4 times per day.

• IM

Acute schizophrenic or manic states in hospitalized clients.

Adults, initial: 25 mg. If necessary, give an additional 25–50 mg in 1 hr. Increase gradually over several days; up to 400 mg q 4–6 hr may be needed in severe cases. Client usually becomes quiet and cooperative within 24–48 hr. Substitute PO dosage and increase until client is calm (usually 500 mg/day, although gradual increases to 2,000 mg/day may be needed).

Prompt control of severe symptoms in outpatients.

25 mg; if needed, repeat in 1 hr. Give subsequent doses PO, 25–50 mg 3 times per day.

Intraoperative to control N&V.

Adults: 12.5 mg; repeat in 30 min if necessary and if no hypotension occurs.

Pediatric: 0.55 mg/kg (0.25 mg/lb); repeat in 30 min if necessary and if no hypotension occurs.

Preoperative sedative.

Adults: 12.5–25 mg 1–2 hr before surgery. **Pediatric:** 0.5 mg/kg (0.25 mg/lb) 1–2 hr before surgery.

Hiccoughs.

See above under PO dose.

Acute intermittent porphyria.

Adults: 25 mg q 6–8 hr until client can take PO therapy.

Tetanus.

Adults: 25–50 mg 3–4 times per day, usually with barbiturates. **Children:** 0.5 mg/kg (0.25 mg/lb) q 6–8 hr.

Behavioral disorders/Hyperactivity in children.

Outpatients: 0.5 mg/kg (0.25 mg/lb) q 6–8 hr, as needed. **Hospitalized clients, 5 years or younger or 50 lbs:** Do not exceed 40 mg/day; **5–12 years or 50–100 lbs:** Do not exceed 75 mg/day, except in unmanageable cases.

• **IV**

Intraoperative to control acute N&V.

Adults: 2 mg per fractional injection at 2-min intervals, not to exceed 25 mg (dilute with 1 mg/mL saline). **Children:** 1 mg per fractional injection at 2-min intervals, not to exceed IM dosage. Always dilute to 1 mg/mL with saline.

Tetanus.

Adults: 25–50 mg diluted to 1 mg/mL with 0.9% NaCl injection and given at a rate of 1 mg/min. **Pediatric:** 0.5 mg/kg (0.25 mg/lb) q 6–8 hr diluted to 1 mg/mL with 0.9% NaCl injection and given at a rate of 1 mg/2 min. Do not exceed 40 mg/day in children who weigh up to 23 kg (50 lb) or 75 mg/day in children who weigh 23–45 kg (50–100 lb).

• **SUPPOSITORY, RECTAL**

Behavioral disorders/Hyperactivity in children.

1 mg/kg (0.5 mg/lb) q 6–8 hr, as needed.

N&V.

Adults: 50–100 mg q 6–8 hr, as needed. **Children:** 1.1 mg/kg (0.55 mg/lb) q 6–8 hr, as needed.

NURSING CONSIDERATIONS

℮ Do not confuse chlorpromazine with chlorpropamide (an oral antidiabetic), chlorothiazide or chlorthalidone (thiazide diuretics), or with prochlorperazine or promethazine, both of which are also antipsychotics.

ADMINISTRATION/STORAGE

1. The maximum daily PO and parenteral dose for adults and adolescents should be 1 gram of the base.

2. Because of hypotensive effects, reserve IM use for bedfast clients or for acute ambulatory cases; keep client recumbent for at least 30 min after injection. If irritation is a problem, dilute injection with saline or 2% procaine; do not mix with other agents in the syringe. When administering the drug IM, select a large, well-developed muscle mass. Use the dorsogluteal site or rectus femoris in adults and the vastus lateralis in children; rotate sites.

3. Solutions may cause contact dermatitis; avoid contact with hands or clothing.

4. The oral concentrate is light sensitive; protect from light and dispense in amber glass bottle. Refrigeration is not required.

5. Slight discoloration of IM/IV or PO solutions will not affect drug action.

6. Avoid getting solution on hands or clothing due to possible contact dermatitis.

7. Protect the injection from light.

IV 8. Use IV route only for severe hiccoughs, surgery, or tetanus.

9. Discard solutions with marked discoloration; slight yellowing will not alter potency. Consult with pharmacist if unsure of drug potency.

10. A precipitate or discoloration may occur when chlorpromazine is mixed with morphine, meperidine, or other drugs preserved with creosols.

ASSESSMENT

1. Note reasons for therapy, clinical presentation, behavioral manifestations, other agents trialed.

2. After parenteral therapy, keep supine for 1 hr; advise to change positions slowly.

Bold Italic = life threatening side effect ▪ = black box warning ♣ = Available in Canada

3. List any seizure disorders; drug may be contraindicated. Diphenhydramine may help dystonic reactions.

4. Monitor VS, I&O, CBC, liver and renal function studies. Ocular exams and EEG with prolonged therapy.

5. Assess male clients for S&S of prostatic hypertrophy.

CLIENT/FAMILY TEACHING

1. Take as directed with food/milk to reduce GI upset.

2. Add needed dose of oral concentrate to 60 mL or more of tomato or fruit juice, milk, simply syrup, orange syrup, carbonated beverages, coffee, tea, water, or semisolid foods (e.g., soups, puddings).

3. Review side effects; report any extrapyramidal symptoms, especially uncontrolled twitching.

4. Urine may become discolored pinkish to brown. Report urinary retention or constipation. Protect from sun exposure; skin may develop pigmentation changes.

5. Use caution when performing activities that require mental acuity.

6. Avoid alcohol and any other CNS depressants; may potentiate drop in BP when changing positions. Support hose may help diminish problem.

7. Perform frequent toothbrushing and flossing to discourage oral fungal infections.

8. Report unusual bruising/bleeding, fever, sore throat, or malaise.

9. Avoid temperature extremes; drug may impair body's ability to regulate temperature.

10. Therapeutic psychologic effects may require 7–8 weeks of therapy.

OUTCOMES/EVALUATE

- ↓ Psychotic/manic manifestations
- Control of N&V
- Cessation of hiccoughs
- Sedation; ↓ muscular twitching

Cholestyramine resin
(koh-less-**TEER**-ah-meen)

CLASSIFICATION(S):
Antihyperlipdemic, bile acid sequestrant

PREGNANCY CATEGORY: B

Rx: Cholestyramine Light, Prevalite, Questran, Questran Light.

✦Rx: Novo-Cholamine, Novo-Cholamine Light, PMS-Cholestyramine, Questran Light.

USES

(1) Adjunct to reduce elevated serum cholesterol in primary hypercholesterolemia in those who do not respond adequately to diet. (2) Pruritus associated with partial biliary obstruction. (3) Diarrhea due to bile acids. *Investigational:* Antibiotic-induced pseudomembranous colitis (i.e., due to toxin produced by *Clostridium difficile*), digitalis toxicity, treatment of chlordecone (Kepone) poisoning, treatment of thyroid hormone overdose.

ACTION/KINETICS

Action

Binds sodium cholate (bile salts) in the intestine; thus, the principal precursor of cholesterol is not absorbed due to formation of an insoluble complex, which is excreted in the feces. Decreases cholesterol and LDL and either has no effect or increases triglycerides, VLDL, and HDL. Also, itching is relieved as a result of removing irritating bile salts. The antidiarrheal effect results from the binding and removal of bile acids.

Pharmacokinetics

Onset, to reduce plasma cholesterol: Within 24–48 hr, but levels may continue to fall for 1 yr; **to relieve pruritus:** 1–3 weeks; **relief of diarrhea associated with bile acids:** 24 hr. Cholesterol levels return to pretreatment levels 2–4 weeks after discontinuance. Fat-soluble vitamins (A, D, K) and possibly folic acid may have to be administered IM during long-term therapy because cholestyramine binds these vitamins in the intestine.

CONTRAINDICATIONS
Complete obstruction or atresia of bile duct.

SPECIAL CONCERNS
Use during pregnancy only if benefits outweigh risks. Use with caution during lactation and in children. Long-term effects and efficacy in decreasing cholesterol levels in pediatric clients are not known. Geriatric clients may be more likely to manifest GI side effects as well as adverse nutritional effects. Exercise caution in clients with phenylketonuria as Prevalite contains 14.1 mg phenylalanine per 5.5-gram dose.

SIDE EFFECTS
Most Common
Constipation (may be severe), aggravation of hemorrhoids, abdominal pain, bloating, vomiting, diarrhea, weight loss, flatulence, infection.

GI: Constipation (may be severe), N&V, diarrhea, heartburn, GI bleeding, anorexia, flatulence, belching, abdominal distention/pain or cramping, bloating, loose stools, indigestion, aggravation or bleeding of hemorrhoids, rectal bleeding or pain, black stools, bleeding duodenal ulcer, peptic ulceration, GI irritation, dysphagia, dental bleeding, hiccoughs, sour taste, pancreatitis, diverticulitis, cholecystitis, cholelithiasis. Fecal impaction in elderly clients. Large doses may cause steatorrhea. **CNS:** Migraine/sinus headaches (migraine, sinus), dizziness, anxiety, vertigo, insomnia, fatigue, lightheadedness, syncope, drowsiness, femoral nerve pain, paresthesia. **CV:** Chest pain, angina, syncope. **Hypersensitivity:** Urticaria, dermatitis, asthma, wheezing, rash. **Hematologic:** Increased PT, ecchymosis, anemia. **Musculoskeletal:** Muscle or joint pain, aches and pains in the extremities, backache, arthritis, osteoporosis. **GU:** Hematuria, dysuria, burnt odor to urine, diuresis. **Miscellaneous:** Bleeding tendencies (due to hypoprothrombinemia). Deficiencies of vitamins A and D. Uveitis, weight loss or gain, osteoporosis, swollen glands, increased libido, weakness, SOB, edema, tinnitus, tooth discoloration, swelling of hands/feet; hyperchloremic acidosis in children, rash/irritation of the skin, tongue, and perianal area.

LABORATORY TEST CONSIDERATIONS
Liver function abnormalities.

OD **OVERDOSE MANAGEMENT**
Symptoms: GI tract obstruction.

DRUG INTERACTIONS
Anticoagulants, PO / ↓ Anticoagulant effect R/T ↑ GI tract absorption
Aspirin / ↓ Aspirin absorption from GI tract
Clindamycin / ↓ Clindamycin absorption from GI tract
Clofibrate / ↓ Clofibrate absorption from GI tract
Corticosteroids / ↓ Corticosteroid serum levels R/T ↓ GI absorption
Digoxin / ↓ Digitalis effect R/T ↓ GI tract absorption
Doxepin / ↓ Doxepin serum levels R/T ↓ GI absorption
Estrogens/Progestins / ↓ Estrogen/progestin serum levels R/T ↓ GI absorption
Furosemide / ↓ Furosemide absorption from GI tract
Gemfibrozil / ↓ Gemfibrozil bioavailability
Glipizide / ↓ Serum glipizide levels
HMG-CoA reductase inhibitors / ↓ HMG-CoA reductase inhibitor serum levels R/T ↓ GI absorption
Hydrocortisone / ↓ Hydrocortisone effect R/T ↓ GI tract absorption
Imipramine / ↓ Imipramine absorption from GI tract
Iopanoic acid / Results in abnormal cholecystography
Lovastatin / Effects may be additive
Methyldopa / ↓ Methyldopa absorption from GI tract
Mycophenolate / ↓ Mycophenolate AUC by about 40%
Nicotinic acid / ↓ Nicotinic acid absorption from GI tract
NSAIDs / ↓ NSAID serum levels R/T ↓ GI absorption
Penicillin G / ↓ Penicillin G effect R/T ↓ GI tract absorption
Phenobarbital / ↓ Phenobarbital serum levels R/T ↓ GI absorption
Phenytoin / ↓ Phenytoin absorption from GI tract

Bold Italic = life threatening side effect   ■ = black box warning   ♣ = Available in Canada

Phosphate supplements / ↓ Phosphate absorption from GI tract

Piroxicam / ↑ Piroxicam elimination

Propranolol / ↓ Propranolol effect R/T ↓ GI tract absorption

Tetracyclines / ↓ Tetracycline effects R/T ↓ GI tract absorption

Thiazide diuretics / ↓ Thiazide effects R/T ↓ GI tract absorption

Thyroid hormones, Thyroxine / ↓ Thyroid effects R/T ↓ GI tract absorption

Tolbutamide / ↓ Tolbutamide absorption from GI tract

Troglitazone / ↓ Troglitazone absorption from the GI tract

Ursodiol / ↓ Ursodiol effects R/T ↓ GI tract absorption

Valproic acid / ↓ Valproic acid serum levels R/T ↓ GI absorption

Verapamil, Sustained-Release / ↓ Verapamil, Sustained-Release AUC and C_{max} by about 11% and 31% respectively

Vitamins A, D, E, K / Malabsorption of fat-soluble vitamins

Vitamin C / ↑ Vitamin C absorption

NOTE: These drug interactions may also be observed with colestipol.

HOW SUPPLIED

Powder for Suspension: 4 grams/5.5 grams powder, 4 grams/5.7 grams powder, 4 grams/6.4 grams powder, 4 grams/9 grams powder.

DOSAGE
• **POWDER**
Hypercholesterolemia, biliary obstruction.

Adults, initial: 4 grams 1–2 times per day. Dose is individualized. For Prevalite, give 1 packet or 1 level scoopful (5.5 grams Prevalite: 4 grams anhydrous cholestyramine). **Maintenance:** 2–4 packets or scoopfuls/day (8–16 grams anhydrous cholestyramine resin) mixed with 60–180 mL water or noncarbonated beverage. The recommended dosing schedule is 2 times per day but it can be given in one to six doses per day. Maximum daily dose: 6 packets or scoopfuls (equivalent to 24 grams cholestyramine). **Children, usual:** 240 mg/kg/day of anhydrous cholestyramine resin in 2–3 divided doses, normally not to exceed 8 grams/day; base dose titration on response and toler-

ance. When calculating pediatric doses, note the following content of anhydrous cholestyramine resin: 80 mg in 110 mg Prevalite, 44.4 mg in 100 mg of Questran powder, and 62.7 mg in 100 mg of Questran Light.

NURSING CONSIDERATIONS
ADMINISTRATION/STORAGE
1. Always mix powder with 60–180 mL water or noncarbonated beverage before administering; resin may cause esophageal irritation or blockage. Highly liquid soups or pulpy fruits such as applesauce or crushed pineapple may be used. Do not take in dry form.
2. After placing contents of 1 packet of resin on the surface of 4–6 oz of fluid, allow it to stand without stirring for 2 min, occasionally twirling the glass, and then stir slowly (to prevent foaming) to form a suspension.
3. Avoid inhaling powder; may be irritating to mucous membranes.
4. Cholestyramine may interfere with the absorption of other drugs taken orally; thus, take other drug(s) 1 hr before or 4–6 hr after cholestyramine dosing.
5. In clients with preexisting constipation, the initial dose should be 1 packet or 1 scoop once daily for 5–7 days, increasing to two times daily with monitoring of constipataion and of serum lipoproteins, at least twice, 4–6 weeks apart.

ASSESSMENT
1. List reasons for therapy, symptom type/onset, other agents trialed.
2. Note onset of pruritus, bile acid level with cholestasia.
3. Assess skin and eyes for evidence of jaundice or bile deposits.
4. Monitor CBC, cholesterol profile, renal and LFTs.
5. Vitamins A, D, E, K, and folic acid will need to be administered in a water-miscible form during long-term therapy. Monitor nutritional status.

CLIENT/FAMILY TEACHING
1. Other prescribed medications should be taken at least 1 hr before or 4–6 hr after taking drug. These drugs interfere with the absorption and desired effects of other medications.

2. Do not take drug in dry form; always spinkle powder on surface of liquid (preferably milk, water or juice) and let stand a few min, then stir and drink. Avoid carbonated beverages as these cause too much foaming. Add extra fluid to bottom of glass and swirl to ensure entire dose consumed. Take before meals and at bedtime.

3. Review constipating effects of drug and ways to control: daily exercise, fluid intake of 2.5–3 L/day, increased intake of citrus fruits, fruit juices, and high-fiber foods; also, a stool softener may help. If constipation persists, a change in dosage or drug may be indicated.

4. Clients with high cholesterol levels should follow dietary restrictions of fat and cholesterol as well as risk factor reduction such as smoking cessation, alcohol reduction, weight loss, and regular exercise.

5. Report tarry stools or abnormal bleeding as supplemental vitamin K (10 mg/week) may be necessary. CBC, PT, and renal function tests should be done routinely.

6. Itching (pruritus) may subside 1–3 weeks after taking the drug but may return after the medication is discontinued. Corn starch or tepid oatmeal baths may also alleviate symptoms. Report any unusual bruising/bleeding or intolerable side effects.

OUTCOMES/EVALUATE
• Control of pruritus
• ↓ Serum cholesterol levels
• ↓ Diarrheal stools
• ↓ Bile acid levels

Choriogonadotropin alfa

(**KOR**-ee-oh-goh-**nah**-dah-**troh**-pin **AL**-fah)

CLASSIFICATION(S):
Ovarian stimulant
PREGNANCY CATEGORY: X
Rx: Ovidrel.

USES
(1) Induction of final follicular maturation and early luteinization in infertile women who have undergone pituitary desensitization and who have been pretreated appropriately with FSH as part of an assisted reproductive technology program (e.g., in vitro fertilization and embryo transfer). (2) For the induction of ovulation and pregnancy in anovulatory infertile clients where the cause of infertility is functional and not due to primary ovarian failure.

ACTION/KINETICS
Action
The physicochemical, biologic, and immunologic effects of recombinant choriogonadotropin (hCG) are comparable to those of hCG derived from placental and human pregnancy urine. hCG stimulates late follicular maturation and resumption of ooctye meiosis and initiates rupture of the preovulatory ovarian follicle. Choriogonadotropin alfa binds to the LH/hCG receptor of the granulosa and theca cells of the ovary and initiates its effects in the absence of an endogenous LH surge. Choriogonadotropin alfa is given when sufficient follicular development has occurred following FSH treatment for ovulation induction.

Pharmacokinetics
Maximum serum levels: 12–24 hr. **t½, distribution, initial:** About 4.5 hr; **t½ terminal:** About 29 hr.

CONTRAINDICATIONS
Hypersensitivity to hCG products and their components; primary ovarian failure; uncontrolled thyroid or adrenal dysfunction; uncontrolled organic intracranial lesions (e.g., pituitary tumor); abnormal uterine bleeding of undetermined origin; ovarian cyst or enlargement of undetermined origin; sex hormone-dependent tumors of the reproductive tract and accessory organs; pregnancy.

SPECIAL CONCERNS
Ovarian enlargement, ovarian hyperstimulation syndrome, or multiple births may occur. Use with caution during lactation.

SIDE EFFECTS
Most Common
When used for assisted reproductive technology: Injection site pain/bruising, abdominal pain, N&V, GI system disorder, post-operative pain.
When used for induction of ovulation: Injection site pain/bruising/inflammation, ovarian cyst/hyperstimulation, abdominal pain.

Ovarian enlargement: Abdominal distention/pain. **Ovarian hyperstimulation syndrome:** Increase in vascular permeability resulting in rapid accumulation of fluid in the peritoneal cavity, thorax, and potentially the pericardium. Early warning signs include severe pelvic pain, N&V, weight gain. Symptoms include abdominal pain/distention, N&V, diarrhea, severe ovarian enlargement, weight gain, dyspnea, oliguria. Also, hypovolemia, hemoconcentration, electrolyte imbalances, ascites, hemoperitoneum, pleural effusions, hydrothorax, *acute pulmonary distress, thromboembolism*.

Side effects when used for assisted reproductive technology: GI: GI system disorder, abdominal pain, N&V, flatulence, diarrhea, hiccough. **GU:** Ectopic pregnancy, intermenstrual bleeding, breast pain, vaginal hemorrhage, cervical lesion, ovarian hyperstimulation, leukorrhea, uterine disorders, vaginitis, vaginal discomfort, UTI, urinary incontinence, dysuria, albuminuria, genital moniliasis, genital herpes, cervical carcinoma. **CNS:** Dizziness, headache, paresthesias, emotional lability, insomnia. **Respiratory:** URI, cough. **CV:** Cardiac arrhythmias, heart murmur. **At injection site:** Pain/bruising. **Miscellaneous:** Body/back pain, fever, hot flashes, malaise, leukocytosis.

Side effects when used for induction of ovulation. At injection site: Pain, bruising, inflammation. **GU:** Ovarian cyst, ovarian hyperstimulation, breast pain. **GI:** Abdominal pain, GI system disorders, flatulence, abdominal enlargement. **Respiratory:** URTI, pharyngitis. **Miscellaneous:** Hyperglycemia, pruritus.

Side effects in pregnancies resulting from HCG therapy. Spontaneous abortion, ectopic pregnancy, premature labor, postpartum fever, congenital abnormalities.

HOW SUPPLIED
Prefilled Syringes: 250 mcg/0.5 mL.

DOSAGE
• **SC**
Infertile women undergoing assisted reproductive technology; Induction of ovulation in infertile women.
250 mcg 1 day following the last dose of FSH. Do not give until adequate follicular development is confirmed by serum estradiol and vaginal ultrasonography. Withhold when there is an excessive ovarian response as indicated by clinically significant ovarian enlargement or excessive estradiol production.

NURSING CONSIDERATIONS
ADMINISTRATION/STORAGE
1. Give as single SC injection following reconstitution with 1 mL sterile water for injection. Use immediately after reconstitution.
2. Discard any unused reconstituted drug.
3. Vials for reconstitution may be stored refrigerated or at room temperature. Protect from light.
4. Store prefilled syringes at 2–8°C before dispensing to clients; syringes may then be stored at temperatures not exceeding 25°C for up to 30 days.

ASSESSMENT
1. List reasons for therapy: induction of ovulation or for in vitro fertilization program, symptom onset, clinical presentation.
2. Note any drug sensitivity. Ensure FSH treatment for ovulation induction.
3. Assess for any pituitary or sex hormone dependent tumors; uncontrolled thyroid or adrenal dysfunction or abnormal uterine bleeding as these preclude therapy.
4. Obtain estradiol levels and vaginal ultrasound to assess follicular development. If levels too high or follicles significantly enlarged hold therapy.

CLIENT/FAMILY TEACHING

1. Review reasons for therapy and anticipated results.
2. Follow self administration guideline pamphlet once initial injection done in office. May cause pain at injection site.
3. Record basal body temperature to determine if ovulation has occurred. Record daily weights. Report edema, which is common.
4. If ovulation determined (slight ↓ temperature then sharp ↑ for ovulation) attempt intercourse 3 days before and every other day until after ovulation.
5. Delayed menses, excessive menstrual bleeding, pain in the lower abdomen, weakness/fatigue are S&S of ectopic pregnancy; report immediately.
6. May experience multiple births.
7. Therapy requires long term commitment.
8. Report headache, easy fatigue, restlessness; if increasingly irritable, depressed, and changes in attention to physical appearance occur, may have to stop drug.
9. Report for lab tests/ultrasound studies as scheduled.
10. Some pregnancies may result in abortion or birth defects.

OUTCOMES/EVALUATE

Ovulation with desired pregnancy

Ciclesonide

CLASSIFICATION(S):
Glucocorticoid
PREGNANCY CATEGORY: C
Rx: Omnaris.

SEE ALSO *CORTICOSTEROIDS*.

USES
Treatment of nasal symptoms associated with seasonal and perennial allergic rhinitis in adults and adolescents, 12 years and older.

ACTION/KINETICS
Action
Precise mechanism unknown. Corticosteroids have a wide range of effects on multiple cell types and various mediators involved in allergic inflammation.

The effect on adrenal function is not known.

Pharmacokinetics
Ciclesonide is a prodrug that is enzymatically hydrolized (by esterases in the nasal mucosa) to the active metabolite, des-ciclesonide, after inhalation. A small amount is absorbed systemically. Is metabolized in the liver mainly by CYP3A4 and to a lesser extent by CYP2D6. Most excreted in the feces with small amounts excreted in the urine.

CONTRAINDICATIONS
Hypersensitivity to the drug or any component of the product.

SPECIAL CONCERNS
Use with caution during lactation. Efficacy has not been determined in children less than 12 years of age.

SIDE EFFECTS
Most Common
Headache, nasopharyngitis, epistaxis.
CNS: Headache. **Respiratory:** Nasopharyngitis, epistaxis; nasal discomfort.
Otic: Ear pain.

DRUG INTERACTIONS
Ketoconazole ↑ exposure to des-ciclesonide R/T inhibition of CYP3A4; use together with caution.

HOW SUPPLIED
Nasal Spray: 50 mcg/actuation.

DOSAGE
- **NASAL SPRAY**
  Seasonal and perennial allergic rhinitis.

Adults and adolescents, 12 years and older: Two sprays (50 mcg/spray) in each nostril once daily (i.e., total daily dose: 200 mcg). Do not exceed this dose.

NURSING CONSIDERATIONS

ADMINISTRATION/STORAGE
1. If used in geriatric clients, start at the low end of the dosing range.
2. Store from 15–30°C (59–86°F). Do not freeze.

ASSESSMENT
1. List reasons for therapy, onset, characteristics of S&S, triggers, other agents trialed, outcome.
2. Examine for evidence of nasal septal ulcers; note turbinate findings.

Bold Italic = life threatening side effect   ■ = black box warning   ♣ = Available in Canada

C

3. Assess heart and lungs. Determine if immunocompromised or actively infected. Note any recent systemic steroid therapy use and amount.

CLIENT/FAMILY TEACHING

1. Prior to initial use, gently shake the nasal spray; prime the pump by actuating 8 times. If the spray is not used for 4 consecutive days, gently shake and reprime with 1 spray or until a fine mist appears.

2. The product provides 120 metered sprays after initial priming.

3. Discard the spray bottle either after 120 sprays following initial priming or after 4 months.

4. Shake gently before each use. Do not spray in the eyes.

5. Use adequate humidity, especially during winter months when dry heat may aggravate mucosa.

6. Identify/avoid triggers that aggravate symptoms (dust, pollen, smoke, chemicals, pets).

7. Keep all F/U appointments to evaluate response to therapy.

OUTCOMES/EVALUATE

↓ Symptoms of seasonal and allergic rhinitis

Ciclopirox olamine
(sye-kloh-**PEER**-ox)

CLASSIFICATION(S):
Antifungal
PREGNANCY CATEGORY: B
Rx: Loprox, Penlac Nail Lacquer.

USES

Loprox. (1) *Cream and Suspension:* Tinea pedis, tinea cruris, and tinea corporis due to *Trichophyton rubrum, T. mentagrophytes, Epidermophyton floccosum,* and *Microsporum canis.* Candidiasis (moniliasis) due to *Candida albicans.* Tinea versicolor due to *Malassezia fufur.* (2) *Gel:* Interdigital tinea pedis and tinea corporis due to *T. rubrum, T. mentagrophytes,* or *E. floccosum.* Topical treatment of seborrheic dermatitis of the scalp. (3) *Shampoo:* Topical treatment of seborrheic dermatitis of the scalp. **Pen-**

lac Nail Lacquer: As part of total program for the topical treatment in immunocompetent clients with mild to moderate onychomycosis, due to *T. rubrum,* of the fingernails and toenails without lunula involvement. Use only on nails and immediately adjacent skin.

ACTION/KINETICS

Action

At lower concentrations the drug blocks the transport of amino acids into the cell, whereas at higher concentrations the cell membrane of the fungus is altered so that intracellular material leaks out. May also inhibit synthesis of RNA, DNA, and protein in growing fungal cells.

Pharmacokinetics

A small amount of drug is absorbed through the skin; it also penetrates to the sebaceous glands and dermis as well as into the hair.

CONTRAINDICATIONS

Ophthalmic, oral, or intravaginal use. Concomitant use of the topical solution and systemic antifungal drugs for onychomycosis.

SPECIAL CONCERNS

Use with caution during lacatation. Safety and efficacy in children under 10 years of age not established.

SIDE EFFECTS

Most Common
See individual formulations below.

- **Cream**
Pruritus at site of application, worsening of the signs and symptoms, burning.

- **Gel**
Skin burning sensation upon application, contact dermatitis, pruritus, dry skin, acne, rash, alopecia, pain upon application, eye pain, facial edema.

- **Shampoo**
Increased itching, burning, erythema, itching, seborrhea, rash, headache, ventricular tachycardia, skin disorder.

- **Topical Suspension**
Pruritus, burning.

- **Penlac Topical Solution**
Periungual erythema, erythema of the proximal nail fold, nail disorders (shape change, irritation, ingrown toenail, dis-

---

 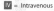

coloration), application site reactions, burning of the skin, mild rash.

HOW SUPPLIED

Cream: 0.77%; *Gel*: 0.77%; *Lotion*: 0.77%; *Shampoo*: 1%; *Penlac, Topical Solution*: 8%; *Topical Suspension*: 0.77%.

DOSAGE

- **CREAM; GEL; LOTION; TOPICAL SUSPENSION (LOPROX)**

  Dermatologic conditions.

Massage gently into the affected area and surrounding skin morning and evening. If there is no improvement after 4 weeks, reevaluate diagnosis.

- **TOPICAL SOLUTION (PENLAC)**

  Mild to moderate onychomycosis of the nails.

Apply once daily preferably at bedtime or 8 hr before washing to all affected nails using the applicator brush provided. Apply evenly over the entire nail plate and 5 mm of surrounding skin.

- **SHAMPOO (LOPROX)**

  Seborrheic dermatitis of scalp in adults.

Wet hair and apply about 5 mL to scalp; up to 10 mL can be used on long hair. Lather and leave on hair for 3 min. Rinse. Repeat twice/week for 4 weeks with a minimum of 3 days between applications.

NURSING CONSIDERATIONS

ASSESSMENT

1. List onset/characteristics of S&S, clinical presentation.
2. Describe lesion presentation, obtain scrapings; confirms diagnosis.
3. Weigh risk of removing unattached, infected nail before prescribing with insulin-dependent diabetes/diabetic neuropathy.

CLIENT/FAMILY TEACHING

1. Cleanse skin with soap/water; dry thoroughly. Apply cream with glove; wash hands before/after therapy.
2. Avoid occlusive dressings/wrappings; adult incontinence pads/diapers are occlusive.
3. Even if symptoms have improved, use for the full course.
4. Change shoes and socks at least once daily. Shoes should be well-fitted and ventilated.

5. Report any blistering, burning, itching, oozing, redness, swelling, adverse side effects.
6. When using solution, apply to nail bed, surround skin, under nail plate surface when free of nail bed. Do not remove; apply daily over the previous coat and remove with alcohol every 7 days. Up to 48 weeks may be needed, along with weekly nail trimmings and monthly professional removal of the unattached, infected nail.
7. For Penlac, avoid skin contact other than skin immediately surrounding the treated nail(s).

OUTCOMES/EVALUATE

- Resolution of fungal infection; wound healing
- Symptomatic improvement

Cidofovir

(sih-**DOF**-oh-veer)

CLASSIFICATION(S):
Antiviral
PREGNANCY CATEGORY: C
Rx: Vistide.

SEE ALSO *ANTIVIRAL DRUGS.*

USES

CMV retinitis in clients with AIDS.

ACTION/KINETICS

Action

A nucleotide analog that suppresses CMV replication by selective inhibition of viral DNA synthesis. The drug inhibits CMV DNA polymerase. Must be administered with probenecid. There may be cross resistance with ganciclovir.

CONTRAINDICATIONS

History of severe hypersensitivity to probenecid or other sulfa-containing drugs. Use by direct intraocular injection. In clients with a serum creatinine greater than 1.5 mg/dL, a calculated C_{CR} of 55 mL/min or less, or a urine protein of 100 mg/dL or more (equivalent to 2+ proteinuria or more). Use with other nephrotoxic drugs (discontinue 7 or more days prior to starting cidofovir therapy). Lactation.

Bold Italic = life threatening side effect   ■ = black box warning   ♣ = Available in Canada

SPECIAL CONCERNS

■ (1) Renal impairment is the major toxicity of cidofovir. Cases of acute renal failure resulting in dialysis or contributing to death have occurred with as few as 1 or 2 doses. To minimize possible nephrotoxicity, IV prehydration with normal saline and administration of probenecid must be used with each cidofovir infusion. Monitor renal function (serum creatinine and urine protein) within 48 hr prior to each dose of cidofovir and modify the dose or changes in renal function as appropriate. Cidofovir is contraindicated in clients who are receiving other nephrotoxic agents. (2) Neutropenia has been observed in association with cidofovir. Monitor neutrophil counts during cidofovir therapy. (3) Cidofovir is indicated only for treating CMV retinitis in clients with acquired AIDS.■ Safety and efficacy have not been determined for children or for treatment of other CMV infections, including pneumonitis, gastroenteritis, congenital or neonatal CMV disease, or CMV disease in non-HIV-infected clients. Increased risk of ocular hypotony in those with preexisting diabetes. Use caution in clients with risk factors for nephrotoxicity.

SIDE EFFECTS

Most Common

Proteinuria, N&V, fever, neutropenia, asthenia, headache, rash, infection, alopecia, diarrhea, pain, creatinine elevation, anemia, anorexia, dyspnea, chills, increased cough, oral moniliasis.

GU: Nephrotoxicity, Fanconi's syndrome and decreases in serum bicarbonate associated with renal tubular damage, hematuria, urinary incontinence, UTI, *acute renal failure*, dysuria, glycosuria, kidney stone, mastitis, metrorrhagia, nocturia, polyuria, prostatic disorder, toxic nephropathy, urethritis, urinary casts, urinary retention. **GI:** N&V, diarrhea, anorexia, abdominal pain, colitis, constipation, tongue discoloration, dyspepsia, dysphagia, flatulence, gastritis, hepatomegaly, abnormal LFTs, melena, oral candidiasis, rectal disorder, stomatitis, aphthous stomatitis, mouth ulceration, dry mouth, cholangitis, esophagitis, fecal incontinence, *GI hemorrhage*, gingivitis, hepatitis, hepatosplenomegaly, jaundice, liver damage, *liver necrosis*, pancreatitis, tooth caries. **CNS:** Headache, asthenia, amnesia, agitation, confusion, *convulsions*, depression, dizziness, abnormal gait, hallucinations, insomnia, neuropathy, paresthesia, somnolence, abnormal dreams, acute brain syndrome, agitation, ataxia, cerebrovascular disorder, delirium, dementia, drug dependence, encephalopathy, facial paralysis, hemiplegia, hyperesthesia, hypertonia, hypotony, incoordination, increased libido, myoclonus, nervousness, personality disorder, speech disorder, tremor, twitching, vertigo. **CV:** Hypotension, postural hypotension, vasodilation, pallor, syncope, tachycardia, vasodilation, *cardiomyopathy, shock*, migraine, CV disorder, hypertension, peripheral vascular disorder, phlebitis, edema. **Hematologic:** Neutropenia, thrombocytopenia, anemia, hypochromic anemia, leukocytosis, leukopenia, lymphadenopathy, lymphoma-like reaction, pancytopenia, splenic disorder, splenomegaly, thrombocytopenic purpura. **Respiratory:** Asthma, bronchitis, coughing, dyspnea, hiccup, increased sputum, lung disorder, pharyngitis, pneumonia, rhinitis, sinusitis, epistaxis, hemoptysis, hyperventilation, hypoxia, *larynx edema*, pneumothorax. **Dermatologic:** Alopecia, rash, acne, skin discoloration, dry skin, herpes simplex, pruritus, sweating, urticaria, angioedema, eczema, exfoliative dermatitis, furunculosis, nail disorder, seborrhea, skin disorder, skin hypertrophy, skin ulcer. **Musculoskeletal:** Arthralgia, myasthenia, myalgia, arthrosis, bone necrosis, bone pain, joint disorder, leg cramps, pathological fracture. **Metabolic:** Edema, dehydration, weight loss, cachexia, peripheral edema, hypoglycemic reaction, thirst. **Ophthalmic:** Ocular hypotony, amblyopia, conjunctivitis, eye disorder, iritis, retinal detachment, uveitis, decreased IOP (may cause abnormal vision), blindness, cataract, corneal lesion, corneal opacity, diplopia, dry eyes, eye pain, keratitis, miosis, refraction disorder, retinal disorder, visual

---

= see color insert   = Herbal   = Intravenous   ℛ = sound alike drug field defect. **Otic:** Ear disorder, ear pain, hearing loss, hyperacusis, otitis externa, otitis media, tinnitus. **Miscellaneous:** Allergic reactions, facial edema, malaise, back/chest/neck pain, *sarcoma, sepsis*, fever, infections, chills, taste perversion, accidental injury, adrenal cortical insufficiency, AIDS, cellulitis, cryptococcosis, cyst, *death*, flu-like syndrome, hypothermia, injection site reaction, mucous membrane disorder, photosensitivity.

LABORATORY TEST CONSIDERATIONS

↑ Creatinine, alkaline phosphatase, BUN, lactic dehydrogenase, ALT, AST. ↓ Serum bicarbonate, creatinine clearance. Proteinuria, hematuria, glycosuria, hypercalcemia, hyperglycemia, hyperkalemia, hyperlipidemia, hypocalcemia, hypoglycemia, hypokalemia, hypomagnesemia, hyponatremia, hypophosphatemia, hypoproteinemia, respiratory alkalosis.

DRUG INTERACTIONS

Amphotericin B / ↑ Risk of nephrotoxicity
Aminoglycosides / ↑ Risk of nephrotoxicity
Foscarnet / ↑ Risk of nephrotoxicity
NSAIDs / ↑ Risk of nephrotoxicity
Pentamidine, IV / ↑ Risk of nephrotoxicity
Vancomycin / ↑ Risk of nephrotoxicity
Zidovudine / ↓ Zidovudine clearance

HOW SUPPLIED

Injection: 75 mg/mL.

DOSAGE

- **IV INFUSION**
  CMV retinitis.

Induction: 5 mg/kg given once weekly for 2 consecutive weeks as an IV infusion at a constant rate over 1 hr. **Maintenance:** 5 mg/kg given once q 2 weeks as an IV infusion at a constant rate over 1 hr.

NURSING CONSIDERATIONS

ADMINISTRATION/STORAGE

1. A full course of probenecid and IV saline prehydration must be done with each dose of cidofovir. For probenecid, give 2 grams 3 hr prior to the cidofovir dose and give 1 gram at 2 hr and again at 8 hr after completion of the 1-hr cidofovir infusion (i.e., total of 4 grams probenecid). Give 1 L of 0.9% normal saline solution; infuse the saline solution over a 1- to 2-hr period immediately before cidofovir. Those who can tolerate the additional fluid load should receive a second liter. If given, start the second liter of saline at the start of the cidofovir infusion or immediately afterward; infuse over a 1- to 3-hr period.
2. Use probenecid after a meal or with an antiemetic to decrease nausea.
3. Prior to administration, dilute cidofovir in 100 mL of 0.9% NaCl solution; administer over 1 hr. If taking a nephrotoxic agent, discontinue at least 7 days before starting cidofovir.
4. If serum creatinine increases by 0.3 to 0.4 mg/dL, reduce the dose of cidofovir from 5 to 3 mg/kg. Discontinue cidofovir if the serum creatinine increases by 0.5 mg/dL or more or if there is development of 3+ or more proteinuria.
5. Store admixtures at 2–8°C (36–46°F) for no more than 24 hr. Bring to room temperature prior to use.

ASSESSMENT

1. List reasons for therapy, onset, duration, symptom characteristics.
2. Note sensitivity to probenecid or sulfa drugs; review ophthalmic exam.
3. Consider viral resistance if poor clinical response or recurrent retinitis progression during therapy.
4. Monitor CBC, renal function, and urinalysis. Identify other medical conditions/those at risk for nephrotoxicity. To minimize potential for nephrotoxicity:
- Initiate therapy only if serum creatinine is less than or equal to 1.5 mg/dL, a C_{CR} >55 mL/min, and urine protein <100 mg/mL.
- Monitor serum creatinine and urine protein within 48 hr prior to each dose; modify/discontinue dose based on renal function.
- Prehydrate with at least 1L IV of NSS and ensure adequate fluid volume status.
- Coadminister PO probenecid, 4 grams total, with each cidofovir dose.

- Avoid concomitant nephrotoxic drugs at least 7 days before initiating cidofovir.
- Neutropenia may occur. Monitor neutrophil counts during therapy.

CLIENT/FAMILY TEACHING

1. Not a cure but controls symptoms. Retinitis may progress as well as other CMV symptoms; must have regular medical/eye exams.

2. Stop zidovudine or decrease dose by 50% on cidofovir days; probenecid inhibits zidovudine clearance.

3. Report any change/decrease in urinary output; may cause renal toxicity.

4. Complete full probenecid course with each cidofovir dose; take after meals or use antiemetics to decrease nausea.

5. Women should use reliable contraception during and for 1 month following therapy. Men should practice barrier contraception during and for 3 months following therapy. Infertility may result; identify if candidate for sperm/egg harvesting.

OUTCOMES/EVALUATE

Control of symptoms of CMV retinitis with HIV

Cilostazol   ■ ©

(sih-**LESS**-tah-zohl)

CLASSIFICATION(S):
Antiplatelet drug
PREGNANCY CATEGORY: C
Rx: Pletal.

USES

Reduce symptoms of intermittent claudication, as indicated by an increased walking distance.

ACTION/KINETICS

Action

Inhibits cellular phosphodiesterase (PDE), especially PDE III. Cilostazol and several metabolites inhibit cyclic AMP PDE III. Suppression of this isoenzyme causes increased levels of cyclic AMP resulting in vasodilation and inhibition of platelet aggregation. Inhibits platelet aggregation caused by thrombin, ADP, collagen, arachidonic acid, epinephrine, and shear stress.

Pharmacokinetics

High fat meals significantly increase absorption. Extensively metabolized by the liver mainly by CYP3A4 and to a less extent by CYP2C19. Two of the metabolites are active. Primarily excreted through the urine (74%) with the rest in the feces. **t½, elimination:** 11–13 hr. **Plasma protein binding:** 95–98%.

CONTRAINDICATIONS

Use with CHF of any severity. Use in those with hemostatic disorders or active pathologic bleeding, such as bleeding peptic ulcer and intracranial bleeding. Known or suspected hypersensitivity to any component of the product. Concurrent use of grapefruit juice. Lactation.

SPECIAL CONCERNS

■ Cilostazol and several of its metabolites are phosphodiesterase III inhibitors. Such compounds have caused decreased survival in those with class III-IV CHF. Contraindicated in clients with CHF of any severity.■ Safety and efficacy have not been determined in children.

SIDE EFFECTS

Most Common

Headache, diarrhea, abnormal stools, rhinitis, infection, dizziness, peripheral edema, pharyngitis, dyspepsia, nausea, palpitations, tachycardia, vertigo, abdominal pain, flatulence, back pain, myalgia, increased cough.

GI: Abnormal stool, diarrhea, dyspepsia, flatulence, N&V, abdominal pain, anorexia, cholelithiasis, colitis, duodenal ulcer, duodenitis, *esophageal/GI hemorrhage,* esophagitis, gastritis, gastroenteritis, gum hemorrhage, hematemesis, melena, periodontal abscess, rectal hemorrhage, stomach ulcer, tongue edema. **Hepatic:** Hepatic dysfunction/abnormal liver function tests, jaundice. **CNS:** Headache, dizziness, vertigo, anxiety, insomnia, neuralgia, subdural hematoma pain, *cerebral/intracranial hemorrhage*. **CV:** Palpitation, tachycardia, hypertension, angina pectoris, atrial fibrillation/flutter, cerebral infarct/ischemia, CHF, *heart arrest,* *hemorrhage*, hypotension, MI, myocardial ischemia, nodal arrhythmia, postural hypotension, supraventricular tachycardia, syncope, varicose veins, vasodilation, ventricular extrasystole or *ventricular tachycardia,* subacute thrombosis, *CVA.* **Respiratory:** Rhinitis, pharyngitis, increased cough, dyspnea, bronchitis, asthma, epistaxis, hemoptysis, pneumonia, sinusitis, interstitial pneumonia, *pulmonary hemorrhage.* **Musculoskeletal:** Back pain, myalgia, asthenia, leg cramps, arthritis, arthralgia, bone pain, bursitis, neck rigidity. **Dermatologic:** Rash, dry skin, furunculosis, skin hypertrophy, urticaria, subcutaneous hemorrhage, pruritus, skin eruptions, extradural hematoma, *Stevens-Johnson syndrome.* **GU:** Hematuria, UTI, cystitis, urinary frequency, vaginal hemorrhage, vaginitis. **Hematologic:** Anemia, ecchymosis, iron deficiency anemia, polycythemia, purpura, agranulocytosis, granulocytopenia, leukopenia, thrombocytopenia or leukopenia progressing to agranulocytosis when cilostazol not immediately discontinued. **Ophthalmic:** Amblyopia, blindness, conjunctivitis, diplopia, eye hemorrhage, retinal hemorrhage. **Otic:** Tinnitus, ear pain. **Body as a whole:** Infection, edema, hypesthesia, paresthesia, flu syndrome, asthenia, chills, fever, hot flashes, malaise, generalized edema, diabetes mellitus, gout. **Miscellaneous:** Peripheral edema, facial edema, pelvic/chest pain, *retroperitoneal hemorrhage.*

LABORATORY TEST CONSIDERATIONS
↑ GGT, creatinine, blood glucose, uric acid, BUN, serum urea. ↓ Platelets, WBCs. Albuminuria, hyperlipemia, hyperuricemia.

OD OVERDOSE MANAGEMENT
Symptoms: Severe headache, diarrhea, hypotension, tachycardia, possible cardiac arrhythmias. *Treatment:* Observe client carefully and provide symptomatic treatment.

DRUG INTERACTIONS
Clopidogrel / Possible additive effects on bleeding time; monitor bleeding times if used together
Diltiazem / ↑ Cilostazol levels R/T inhibition of liver metabolizing enzymes; consider dose reduction of cilostazol
Erythromycin / ↑ Cilostazol levels R/T inhibition of liver metabolizing enzymes; consider dose reduction of cilostazol
Grapefruit juice / ↑ Cilostazol levels R/T inhibition of liver metabolizing enzymes
Itraconazole / ↑ Cilostazol levels R/T inhibition of liver metabolizing enzymes; consider dose reduction of cilostazol
Ketoconazole / ↑ Cilostazol levels R/T inhibition of liver metabolizing enzymes; consider dose reduction of cilostazol
Lovastatin / ↓ Cilostazol C_{max} and AUC by 15%; ↑ lovastatin AUC by about 70%
Macrolide antibiotics / ↑ Cilostazol levels R/T inhibition of liver metabolizing enzymes; consider dose reduction of cilostazol
Omeprazole / ↑ Cilostazol levels R/T inhibition of liver metabolizing enzymes; consider dose reduction of cilostazol

HOW SUPPLIED
Tablets: 50 mg, 100 mg.

DOSAGE
• **TABLETS**
Intermittent claudication.
100 mg twice a day taken 30 min or more before or 2 hr after breakfast and dinner. Consider a dose of 50 mg twice a day during coadministration of CYP3A4 inhibitors, including diltiazem, erythromycin, itraconazole, or ketoconazole and during coadministration of CYP2C19 inhibitors such as omeprazole.

NURSING CONSIDERATIONS
℀ Do not confuse Pletal with Plavix (also an antiplatelet drug).

ADMINISTRATION/STORAGE
1. Clients may respond as early as 2–4 weeks after beginning therapy but treatment for up to 12 weeks may be needed.
2. The dosage of cilostazol may be reduced or discontinued without platelet hyperaggregability.
3. Store from 15–30°C (59–86°F).

Bold Italic = life threatening side effect   ■ = black box warning   ♣ = Available in Canada

ASSESSMENT

1. Note onset/characteristics of symptoms; contributing factors. Measure distance walked before pain elicited.
2. List drugs currently prescribed to ensure none interact. Identify any CV disease or CHF.
3. Monitor CBC, and for liver/renal dysfunction. Perform/document ABIs.
4. Assess extent/amount/duration of nicotine use; nicotine constricts blood vessels.

CLIENT/FAMILY TEACHING

1. Take 30 min before or 2 hr after meals. Avoid grapefruit juice.
2. Read patient package insert carefully before starting therapy; each time renewed.
3. Use caution, may experience headaches, GI upset, dizziness, or runny nose; report if bothersome. Report any unusual bleeding, skin rash, or diarrhea.
4. Do not smoke; enroll in formal smoking cessation program.
5. Continue to walk past the point of severe pain before resting, then resume walking to improve symptoms and distance able to walk before pain recurs.
6. Beneficial effects may be seen in 2 to 4 weeks; up to 12 weeks may be needed before evident.

OUTCOMES/EVALUATE

- Increased walking distance without pain
- ↓ S&S intermittent claudication

Cimetidine

(sye-**MET**-ih-deen)

CLASSIFICATION(S):

Histamine H_2–receptor blocking drug

PREGNANCY CATEGORY: B

OTC: Acid Reducer 200, Tagamet HB 200.

Rx: Cimetidine in 0.9% Sodium Chloride, Tagamet.

✦Rx: Apo-Cimetidine, Gen-Cimetidine, Novo–Cimetine, Nu-Cimet.

SEE ALSO *HISTAMINE H₂ ANTAGONISTS.*

USES

Rx. (1) Short-term treatment and maintenance therapy for duodenal ulcers. (2) Short-term (6 weeks) treatment of benign gastric ulcers (in rare cases, healing has occurred). (3) Treatment of gastric acid hypersecretory states (Zollinger-Ellison syndrome, systemic mastocytosis). (4) GERD, including erosive esophagitis. (5) Prophylaxis of UGI bleeding in critically ill hospitalized clients (IV only). *Investigational:* As part of a multidrug regimen to eradicate *Helicobacter pylori* in the treatment of peptic ulcer; in the perioperative setting to suppress gastric acid secretion, prevent stress ulcers, and prevent aspiration pneumonitis; in combination with histamine H_1- antagonists to treat certain types of urticaria; treat cutaneous warts (conflicting data). IV only: Prevent paclitaxel hypersensitivity and reduce incidence of GI hemorrhage associated with stress-related ulcers.

OTC. (1) Relief of heartburn associated with acid indigestion and sour stomach. (2) Prevent heartburn associated with acid indigestion and sour stomach caused by certain foods and beverages.

ACTION/KINETICS

Action

Reduces postprandial daytime and nighttime gastric acid secretion by about 50–80%. May increase gastromucosal defense and healing in acid-related disorders (e.g., stress-induced ulcers) by increasing production of gastric mucus, increasing mucosal secretion of bicarbonate and gastric mucosal blood flow as well as increasing endogenous mucosal synthesis of prostaglandins. It also inhibits cytochrome P-450 and P-448, which will affect metabolism of drugs. Also possesses antiandrogenic activity and will increase prolactin levels following an IV bolus injection.

Pharmacokinetics

Well absorbed from GI tract. **Peak plasma level, PO:** 45–90 min. **Time to peak effect, after PO:** 1–2 hr. **Peak plasma levels, after PO use:** 0.7–3.2 mcg/mL (after a 300 mg dose); **after IV:** 3.5–7.5 mcg/mL. **Duration, nocturnal:** 6–8 hr;

basal: 4–5 hr. t½: 2 hr, longer in presence of renal impairment. After PO use, most metabolized in liver; after parenteral use, about 75% of drug excreted unchanged in the urine. **Plasma protein binding:** 13–25%.

CONTRAINDICATIONS

Children under 12, lactation. Cirrhosis, impaired liver and renal function.

SPECIAL CONCERNS

In geriatric clients with impaired renal or hepatic function, confusion is more likely to occur.

SIDE EFFECTS

Most Common

Headache, dizziness, diarrhea, gynecomastia, arthralgia.

GI: Diarrhea, pancreatitis (rare), hepatitis, hepatic fibrosis. **CNS:** Dizziness, sleepiness, headache, confusion, delirium, hallucinations, double vision, dysarthria, ataxia. Severely ill clients may manifest agitation, anxiety, depression, disorientation, hallucinations, mental confusion, and psychosis. **CV:** Hypotension and arrhythmias following rapid IV administration. **Hematologic:** Agranulocytosis, thrombocytopenia, *hemolytic or aplastic anemia*, granulocytopenia. **GU:** Impotence (high doses for prolonged periods of time), gynecomastia (long-term treatment). **Dermatologic:** Exfoliative dermatitis, erythroderma, erythema multiforme. **Musculoskeletal:** Arthralgia, reversible worsening of joint symptoms with preexisting arthritis (including gouty arthritis). **Miscellaneous:** Hypersensitivity reactions, pain at injection site, myalgia, rash, cutaneous vasculitis, peripheral neuropathy, galactorrhea, alopecia, bronchoconstriction.

DRUG INTERACTIONS

Antacids / ↓ Effect of cimetidine R/T ↓ GI tract absorption

Anticholinergics / ↓ Effect of cimetidine R/T ↓ GI tract absorption

Benzodiazepines / ↑ Benzodiazepine effects R/T ↓ liver breakdown

Beta-adrenergic blocking drugs / ↑ Beta-adrenergic effects R/T ↓ liver breakdown

Caffeine / ↑ Caffeine effect R/T ↓ liver breakdown

Calcium channel blockers / ↑ Calcium channel blocker effects R/T ↓ liver breakdown

Carbamazepine / ↑ Carbamazepine effect R/T ↓ liver breakdown

Carmustine / Additive bone marrow depression

Chloroquine / ↑ Chloroquine effects R/T ↓ liver breakdown

Chlorpromazine / ↓ Chlorpromazine effect R/T ↓ GI tract absorption

Cyanocobalamin / ↓ Cyanocobalamin absorption

Digoxin / ↓ Serum digoxin levels

Escitalopram / ↑ Escitalopram AUC and t½

Flecainide / ↑ Flecainide effect

Fluconazole / ↓ Fluconazole effect R/T ↓ GI tract absorption

Fluorouracil / ↑ Serum fluorouracil levels following chronic cimetidine use

Indomethacin / ↓ Indomethacin effect R/T ↓ GI tract absorption

Iron salts / ↓ Iron salt effects R/T ↓ GI tract absorption

Ketoconazole / ↓ Ketoconazole effect R/T ↓ GI tract absorption

Labetalol / ↑ Labetalol effect R/T ↓ liver breakdown

Lidocaine / ↑ Lidocaine effect R/T ↓ liver breakdown

Metoclopramide / ↓ Cimetidine effect R/T ↓ GI tract absorption

Metoprolol / ↑ Metoprolol effect R/T ↓ liver breakdown

Metronidazole / ↑ Metronidazole effect R/T ↓ liver breakdown

Moricizine / ↑ Moricizine effect R/T ↓ liver breakdown

Narcotics / Possible ↑ toxic effects (respiratory depression) of narcotics

Pentoxifylline / ↑ Pentoxifylline effect R/T ↓ liver breakdown

Phenytoin / ↑ Phenytoin effect R/T ↓ liver breakdown

Procainamide / ↑ Procainamide effect R/T ↓ kidney excretion

Propafenone / ↑ Propafenone effect R/T ↓ liver breakdown

Propranolol / ↑ Propranolol effect R/T ↓ liver breakdown

Quinidine / ↑ Quinidine effect R/T ↓ liver breakdown

Quinine / ↑ Quinine effect R/T ↓ liver

breakdown

Saquinavir / ↑ Squinavir AUC and peak plasma levels R/T inhibition of CYP3A4 liver enzymes

Sildenafil / ↑ Sildenafil effect R/T ↓ liver breakdown

Succinylcholine / ↑ Neuromuscular blockade → respiratory depression and extended apnea

Sulfonylureas / ↑ Sulfonylurea effects R/T ↓ liver breakdown

Tacrine / ↑ Tacrine effect R/T ↓ liver breakdown

Tetracyclines / ↓ Tetracycline effects R/T ↓ GI tract absorption

Theophyllines / ↑ Theophylline effects R/T ↓ liver breakdown

Tocainide / ↓ Tocainide effect

Triamterene / ↑ Triamterene effect R/T ↓ liver breakdown

Tricyclic antidepressants / ↑ TCA effects R/T ↓ liver breakdown

Valproic acid / ↑ Valproic acid effect R/T ↓ liver breakdown

Warfarin / ↑ Anticoagulant effects R/T ↓ liver breakdown

HOW SUPPLIED

Injection: 150 mg/mL; *Injection, Premixed:* 6 mg/mL; *Liquid Oral Solution:* 300 mg/5 mL; *Tablets:* 200 mg (OTC or Rx), 300 mg, 400 mg, 800 mg.

DOSAGE

- **ORAL SOLUTION; TABLETS (RX)**

  Duodenal ulcers, short-term treatment.

Adults: 800 mg at bedtime. Alternate dosage: 300 mg 4 times per day with meals and at bedtime for 4–6 weeks (administer with antacids, staggering the dose of antacids) or 400 mg 2 times per day (in the morning and evening). **Maintenance:** 400 mg at bedtime.

  Active benign gastric ulcers.

Adults: 800 mg at bedtime (preferred regimen) or 300 mg 4 times per day with meals and at bedtime for no more than 8 weeks.

  Pathologic hypersecretory conditions.

Adults: 300 mg 4 times per day with meals and at bedtime up to a maximum of 2,400 mg/day for as long as needed. Individualize dosage. If needed, give 300 mg doses more often.

  Erosive gastroesophageal reflux disease.

Adults: 800 mg 2 times per day or 400 mg 4 times per day for 12 weeks. Use beyond 12 weeks has not been determined.

  Prophylaxis of aspiration pneumonitis.

Adults: 400–600 mg 60–90 min before anesthesia.

- **TABLETS (OTC)**

  Heartburn, acid indigestion, sour stomach (OTC only).

200 mg, as symptoms present, up to 2 times per day. Take tablets with water. Do not take maximum dose for more than 2 weeks continuously unless directed by provider.

- **IM; IV; IV INFUSION**

  Hospitalized clients with pathologic hypersecretory conditions or intractable ulcers or those unable to take PO medication.

Adults: 300 mg IM or IV q 6–8 hr. If an increased dose is necessary, administer 300 mg more frequently than q 6–8 hr, not to exceed 2,400 mg per day. Give concomitant antacids as needed for pain relief.

  Prophylaxis of upper GI bleeding.

Adults: 50 mg/hr by continuous IV infusion. If C_{CR} <30 mL/min, use one-half the recommended dose. Treatment beyond 7 days has not been studied.

  Prophylaxis of aspiration pneumonitis.

Adults: 300 mg IV 60–90 min before induction of anesthetia.

NURSING CONSIDERATIONS

 Do not confuse Tagamet (Rx product) with Tagamet HB 200 (OTC product).

ADMINISTRATION/STORAGE

1. If antacids used, stagger dose with that of cimetidine; antacids (but not food) decrease absorption.
2. Administer PO medication with meals and with a snack at bedtime.
3. In renal dysfunction, a dose of 300 mg PO or IV q 12 hr may be necessary. The dose may be given, with caution, q 8 hr if needed.
4. For IM use, give undiluted.

 5. For IV injections, dilute in 0.9% NaCl (or other compatible solution) to a total volume of 20 mL. Inject over at least 2 min.

6. For intermittent IV infusion, dilute 300 mg in at least 50 mL of D5W or other compatible solution and infuse over 15–20 min.

7. For continuous IV infusion, give loading dose of 150 mg (by intermittent IV infusion); then, administer 37.5 mg/hr (900 mg/day) in 0.9% NaCl, D5W or D10W, 5% NaHCO₃ injection, RL solution, or as part of TPN. Stable for 24 hr at room temperature if mixed with these diluents.

8. May be diluted in 100–1,000 mL; if the volume for a 24-hr infusion is less than 250 mL, use a pump.

9. Do *not* introduce drugs/additives to solutions in plastic containers.

10. Not incompatible with aminophylline and barbiturates in IV solutions or in same syringe with pentobarbital sodium and a pentobarbital sodium/atropine sulfate combination.

11. Do not expose premixed single-dose product to excessive heat; store at 15–30°C (59–86°F).

ASSESSMENT

1. Note general client condition. Those receiving radiation therapy or myelosuppressive drugs may have additional side effects.

2. List drugs prescribed; ensure none interact.

3. Note reasons for therapy, type/onset of S&S, anticipated length of therapy.

4. Assess location, characteristics, extent of abdominal pain; note blood in emesis, stool, or gastric aspirate. Report loss of bowel sounds, absence of BM/gas, crampy pain or distension. Maintain gastric pH above 5 to enhance mucosal healing.

5. Monitor VS, I&O. Review radiologic/endoscopic findings; check for *H. pylori*.

6. Monitor CBC, electrolytes, B₁₂ level, renal and LFTs, esp. in elderly, severely ill, with renal impairment; most susceptible to confusion.

CLIENT/FAMILY TEACHING

1. Take with meals/snack at bedtime. Avoid antacids 1 hr before or after dose; establish regular schedule.

2. Take as prescribed even if symptoms disappear.

3. Review dietary modifications, esp. if being treated for GI problems; consult dietitian.

4. Do not perform tasks that require mental alertness until effects realized.

5. Report any breast swelling/discharge/pain or impotence.

6. Report if abdominal pain, bloody stools, or other S&S of reactivated ulcer evident.

7. Avoid alcohol, caffeine, spicy or tomato based foods, mints, NSAIDs, aspirin-containing products; may enhance GI irritation.

8. Do not smoke after the last dose of cimetidine to ensure optimal suppression of nocturnal gastric acid secretion. Attend smoking cessation program if unable to quit.

9. Report new symptoms of confusion, mood swings; more common with elderly.

10. Note increased susceptibility to infections; may develop blood problems; obtain periodic CBC.

11. Report if diarrhea develops, maintain adequate hydration, monitor frequency/severity.

12. Report skin rashes/changes, adverse effects, lack of response. May alter response to skin tests with allergenic extracts; stop drug 48–72 hr prior to testing.

OUTCOMES/EVALUATE
- ↓ Abdominal pain; ulcer healing
- Control of acid hypersecretion
- Prophylaxis of GI bleeding

Cinacalcet hydrochloride
(sin-ah-**KAL**-set)

CLASSIFICATION(S):
Calcium receptor agonist
PREGNANCY CATEGORY: C
Rx: Sensipar.

USES
(1) Hypercalcemia in clients with parathyroid carcinoma. (2) Secondary hyper-

---

parathyroidism in clients with chronic kidney disease on dialysis.

ACTION/KINETICS

Action

Secondary hyperparathyroidism (HPT) with chronic kidney disease is associated with increases in parathyroid hormone (PTH) levels and changes in calcium and phosphorus metabolism. Increased PTH stimulates osteoclastic activity, resulting in cortical bone resorption and marrow fibrosis. The goals of treatment of secondary hyperparathyroidism are to lower levels of PTH, calcium, and phosphorus in the blood to prevent progressive bone disease and the systemic consequences of disordered mineral metabolism. The calcium-sensing receptor on the surface of the chief cell of the parathyroid gland is the main regulator of parathyroid secretion. Cinacalcet directly lowers PTH levels by increasing the sensitivity of the calcium-sensing receptor to extracellular calcium. The reduction in PTH is associated with a concomitant decrease in serum calcium levels.

Pharmacokinetics

C_{max}: 2–6 hr. The C_{max} and the AUC are increased significantly when cinacalcet is given with a high fat meal. **Steady-state drug levels:** Within 7 days. Rapidly and extensively metabolized by multiple enzymes, particularly CYP3A4, CYP2D6, and CYP1A2. **t½, terminal:** 30–40 hr (prolonged in those with moderate to severe hepatic impairment). Excreted mainly through the kidney (80%) with a smaller amount (15%) in the feces. **Plasma protein binding:** About 93–97%.

CONTRAINDICATIONS

Lactation.

SPECIAL CONCERNS

Safety and efficacy have not been established in children.

SIDE EFFECTS

Most Common

N&V, anorexia, diarrhea, dizziness, myalgia, hypertension.

GI: N&V, diarrhea, anorexia. **Body as a Whole:** Myalgia, asthenia, access infection. **Miscellaneous:** Hypocalcemia, adynamic bone disease (due to suppressed PTH levels), dizziness, hypertension, noncardiac chest pain, seizures (mainly tonic-clonic).

OD OVERDOSE MANAGEMENT

Symptoms: Possible hypocalcemia. *Treatment:* Monitor for signs and symptoms of hypocalcemia; take appropriate measures to correct serum calcium levels. Hemodialysis is not an effective treatment.

DRUG INTERACTIONS

Amitriptyline / ↑ Amitriptyline and nortriptyline (active metabolite) levels by 20%

Erythromycin / ↑ Cinacalcet levels R/T inhibition of CYP3A4 enzymes; dosage adjustment may be required

Flecainide / ↑ Levels of flecainide R/T inhibition of CYP2D6 enzymes; dosage adjustment necessary

Itraconazole / ↑ Cinacalcet levels R/T inhibition of CYP3A4 enzymes; dosage adjustment may be required

Ketoconazole / ↑ Cinacalcet levels R/T inhibition of CYP3A4 enzymes; dosage adjustment may be required

Thioridazine / ↑ Levels of thioridazine R/T inhibition of CYP2D6 enzymes; dosage adjustment necessary

Tricyclic antidepressants (TCAs) / ↑ Levels of TCAs R/T inhibition of CYP2D6 enzymes; dosage adjustment necessary

Vinblastine / ↑ Levels of vinblastine R/T inhibition of CYP2D6 enzymes; dosage adjustment necessary

HOW SUPPLIED

Tablets: 30 mg, 60 mg, 90 mg.

DOSAGE

- **TABLETS**

 Parathyroid carcinoma.

Individualize dosage. **Initial:** 30 mg 2 times per day. Titrate the dose every 2 to 4 weeks through sequential doses of 30 mg 2 times per day, 60 mg 2 times per day, 90 mg 2 times per day and 90 mg 3 or 4 times per day, as needed to normalize serum calcium levels.

 Secondary hyperparathyroidism.

Initial: 30 mg once daily. Measure serum calcium and serum phosphorus within 1 week and measure intact PTH 1 to 4 weeks after initiation or dose adjustment of cinacalcet. Titrate cinacalcet no more frequently than every 2 to 4 weeks through sequential doses of 60, 90, 120, and 180 mg once daily to target PTH consistent with the National Kidney Foundation-Kidney Disease Outcomes Quality Initiative recommendation for chronic kidney disease clients on dialysis of 150 to 300 pg/mL.

NURSING CONSIDERATIONS

ADMINISTRATION/STORAGE
1. Cinacalcet can be used alone or in combination with vitamin D sterols and/or phosphate binders.
2. If PTH levels fall below recommended target range (150–300 pg/mL), reduce dose of cinacalcet and/or vitamin D sterols or stop therapy.
3. Store from 15–30°C (59–86°F).

ASSESSMENT
1. Note reasons for therapy: serum calcium reduction with parathyroid cancer or hyperparathyroidism with chronic kidney disease on dialysis. List other agents trialed/ outcome.
2. Review baseline calcium, phosphorus, PTH, CBC, alkaline phosphatase, renal and LFTs. Report if serum calcium <7.5 mg/dL or symptoms of hypocalcemia; if iPTH (intact PTH) levels below 150 pg/mL–bone turnover and fibrosis may occur. Reduce dose/stop therapy if evident.

CLIENT/FAMILY TEACHING
1. Take tablets whole; do not divide.
2. Take with food or shortly after a meal.
3. Report adverse effects or S&S of hypocalcemia: cramping, muscle pain, seizures, numbness, painful muscle spasms with convulsive movements (tetany).
4. Keep all F/U appointments to evaluate drug response, monitor labs for calcium and hyperparathyroid hormone, to determine maintenance dose.

OUTCOMES/EVALUATE
- ↓ Calcium with parathyroid carcinoma
- Reduction of PTH with chronic kidney disease

Ciprofloxacin hydrochloride   IV
(sip-row-**FLOX**-ah-sin)

CLASSIFICATION(S):
Antibiotic, fluoroquinolone
PREGNANCY CATEGORY: C
Rx: Ciloxan Ophthalmic, Cipro, Cipro I.V., Cipro XR, Proquin XR.
♣**Rx:** Cipro Oral Suspension.

SEE ALSO *FLUOROQUINOLONES*.

USES
Adults: Immediate Release (IR) Tablets and Oral Suspension. (1) Acute sinusitis due to *Haemophilus influenzae*, *Streptococcus pneumoniae*, or *Moraxella catarrhalis*. (2) Acute uncomplicated cystitis in women due to *Escherichia coli* or *Staphylococcus saprophyticus*. (3) Chronic bacterial prostatitis due to *E. coli* or *Proteus mirabilis*. (4) UTIs due to *E. coli, K. pneumoniae, E. cloacae, S. marcescens, P. mirabilis, Providencia rettgeri, M. morganii, Citrobacter diversus, C. freundii, P. aeruginosa, S. epidermidis, S. saprophysticus,* or *Enterococcus faecalis*. (5) Bone and joint infections due to *Enterobacter cloacae, Serratia marcescens,* or *Pseudomonas aeruginosa*. (6) With metronidazole for complicated intra-abdominal infections due to *E. coli, P. aeruginosa, P. mirabilis, Klebsiella pneumoniae,* or *Bacteroides fragilis*. (7) Infectious diarrhea due to *E. coli* (enterotoxigenic strains), *Campylobacter jejuni, Shigella boydii, Shigella dysenteriae, Shigella flexneri,* or *Shigella sonnei*. (8) Lower respiratory tract infections due to *E. coli, K. pneumoniae, E. cloacae, P. mirabilis, P. aeruginosa, H. influenzae, Haemophilus parainfluenzae,* or *S. pneumoniae*. Not a drug of first choice to treat presumed or confirmed pneumonia secondary to *S. pneumoniae*. (9) Acute exacerbations of chronic bronchitis due to *M. catarrhalis*. (10) Skin and skin structure infections due to *E. coli, K. pneumoniae, E. cloacae, P. mirabilis, Proteus vulgaris, Providencia stuartii, Morganella morganii, Citrobacter freundii, P. aeruginosa,*

Bold Italic = life threatening side effect   ■ = black box warning   ♣ = Available in Canada

Staphylococcus aureus (methicillin-susceptible), *Staphylococcus epidermidis,* or *Streptococcus pyogenes.* (11) Typhoid fever (enteric fever) due to *Salmonella typhi.* Efficacy in eradicating the chronic typhoid carrier state has not been demonstrated. (12) Uncomplicated cervical and urethral gonorrhea due to *Neisseria gonorrhoeae.*

Adults and Children: Immediate-Release (IR) Tablets, IV, and Oral Suspension. Reduce the incidence or progression of disease following exposure to aerosolized *Bacillus anthracis.*

Children, 1–17 years of age: Immediate-Release (IR) Tablets, IV, and Oral Suspension. Complicated UTIs and pyelonephritis due to *E. coli* (not the first drug of choice due to increased incidence of side effects).

Extended-Release (ER) Tablets Only. (1) Uncomplicated UTIs (acute cystitis) due to *E. coli, P. mirabilis, E. faecalis,* or *S. saprophyticus.* Note: Proquin XR is indicated only to treat UTIs due to *E. coli* and *K. pneumoniae.* (2) Complicated UTIs (except Proquin XR) due to *E. coli, P. aeruginosa, E. faecalis, P. mirabilis,* or *K. pneumoniae.* (3) Acute uncomplicated pyelonephritis (except Proquin XR) due to *E. coli.*

Adults: IV. (1) Acute sinusitis due to *Haemophilus influenzae, Streptococcus pneumoniae,* or *Moraxella catarrhalis.* (2) Chronic bacterial prostatitis due to *E. coli* or *P. mirabilis.* (3) UTIs due to *E. coli* (including cases with secondary bacteremia), *K. pneumoniae* (subspecies *pneumoniae*), *E. cloacae, Serratia marcescens, P. mirabilis, Providencia rettgeri, M. morganii, Citrobacter diversus, C. freundii, P. aeruginosa, S. epidermidis, Staphylococcus saprophyticus,* or *Enterococcus faecalis.* (4) Bone and joint infections due to *E. cloacae, S. marcescens,* or *P. aeruginosa.* (5) With metronidazole for complicated intra-abdominal infections due to *E. coli, P. aeruginosa, P. mirabilis, K. pneumoniae,* or *Bacteroides fragilis.* (6) Lower respiratory tract infections due to *E. coli, K. pneumoniae* (subspecies *pneumoniae*), *E. cloacae, P. mirabilis, P. aeruginosa, H. influenzae, H. parainfluenzae,* or *S. pneumoniae.* NOTE: Not the

first drug of choice to treat presumed or confirmed pneumonia secondary to *S. pneumoniae.* (6) Acute exacerbations of chronic bronchitis due to *M. catarrhalis.* (7) Nosocomial pneumonia due to *H. influenzae* or *K. pneumoniae.* (8) With piperacillin sodium as empirical therapy for febrile neutopenic clients. (9) Skin and skin structure infections due to *E. coli, K. pneumoniae* (subspecies *pneumoniae*), *E. cloacae, P. mirabilis, P. vulgaris, Providencia stuartii, Morganella morganii, Citrobacter freundii, P. aeruginosa, Staphylococcus aureus* (methicillin-susceptible), *Staphylococcus epidermidis,* or *Streptococcus pyogenes.*

Investigational: (1) Multi-drug resistant tuberculosis. (2) Alternative regimen for tularemia. (3) Alternative regimen for cutaneous and GI anthrax. (4) Alternative therapy for plague. (5) Mycobacterial diseases, including atypical mycobacterial infections when used with ciprofloxacin as combination therapy. (6) Cystic fibrosis in children (for periods of 10 days to 6 months). (7) Gastroenteritis in children.

Ocular Infections. Superficial ocular infections involving the conjunctiva or cornea, including conjunctivitis, keratitis, keratoconjunctivitis, corneal ulcers, blepharitis, blepharoconjunctivitis, acute meibomianitis, and dacryocystitis.

Ophthalmic Ointment. Bacterial conjunctivitis due to *Staphylococcus pneumoniae, Streptococcus* (viridans group), and *Haemophilus influenzae.*

Ophthalmic Solution. (1) Corneal ulcers due to *Pseudomonas aeruginosa, Serratia marcescens, Staphylococcus epidermidis, Streptococcus pneumoniae,* and *Streptococcus* (viridans group). (2) Conjunctivitis due to *Haemophilus influenzae, Staphylococcus aureus, Staphylococcus epidermidis,* and *Streptococcus pneumoniae.*

ACTION/KINETICS
Action
Interferes with DNA gyrase and topoisomerase IV. DNA gyrase is an enzyme needed for replication, transcription, and repair of bacterial DNA. Topoisomerase IV plays a key role in the partitioning of chromosomal DNA during

 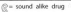

C

bacterial cell division. Effective against both gram-positive and gram-negative organisms.

Pharmacokinetics

Rapidly and well absorbed following PO administration. Food delays absorption of the drug. **Maximum serum levels:** 2–4 mcg/mL 1–2 hr after dosing. **t½:** 4 hr for PO use and 5–6 hr for IV use. Avoid peak serum levels above 5 mcg/mL. About 40–50% of a PO dose and 50–70% of an IV dose is excreted unchanged in the urine.

CONTRAINDICATIONS

Hypersensitivity to quinolones. Use in children. Lactation. Ophthalmic use in the presence of dendritic keratitis, varicella, vaccinia, and mycobacterial and fungal eye infections and after removal of foreign bodies from the cornea.

SPECIAL CONCERNS

Safety and effectiveness of ophthalmic, PO, or IV use have not been determined in children. Possible antibiotic resistance when used to treat *Pseudomonas aeruginosa* infections.

ADDITIONAL SIDE EFFECTS

Most Common

After systemic use: Headache, N&V, diarrhea, restlessness, rash.

After ophthalmic use: Irritation, burning, stinging, itching, inflammation.

See also *Side Effects* for *Fluoroquinolones.* **GI:** N&V, abdominal pain/discomfort, diarrhea, dry/painful mouth, dyspepsia, heartburn, constipation, flatulence, pseudomembranous colitis, oral candidiasis, **intestinal perforation,** anorexia, GI bleeding, bad taste in mouth. **CNS:** Headache, dizziness, fatigue, lethargy, malaise, drowsiness, restlessness, insomnia, nightmares, hallucinations, tremor, lightheadedness, irritability, confusion, ataxia, mania, weakness, psychotic reactions, depression, depersonalization, seizures. **GU:** Nephritis, hematuria, cylindruria, renal failure, urinary retention, polyuria, vaginitis, urethral bleeding, acidosis, renal calculi, interstitial nephritis, vaginal candidiasis. **Skin:** Urticaria, photosensitivity, hypersensitivity, flushing, erythema nodosum, cutaneous candidiasis, hyperpigmentation, rash, paresthesia, edema (of lips, neck, face, conjunctivae, hands), **angioedema, toxic epidermal necrolysis**, exfoliative dermatitis, **Stevens-Johnson syndrome**. **Ophthalmic:** Blurred or disturbed/double vision, eye pain, nystagmus. **CV:** Hypertension, syncope, angina pectoris, palpitations, atrial flutter, **MI, cerebral thrombosis**, ventricular ectopy, **cardiopulmonary arrest**, postural hypotension. **Respiratory:** Dyspnea, **bronchospasm, pulmonary embolism, edema of larynx or lungs**, hemoptysis, hiccoughs, epistaxis. **Hematologic:** Eosinophilia, pancytopenia, leukopenia, anemia, leukocytosis, **agranulocytosis**, bleeding diathesis. **Miscellaneous:** Superinfections; fever; chills; tinnitus; joint pain/ stiffness; back/neck/chest pain; gout flare-up; flushing; worsening of myasthenia gravis; **hepatic necrosis**; cholestatic jaundice; hearing loss, dysphasia.

• **After Ophthalmic use**

Irritation, burning, itching, **angioneurotic edema**, urticaria, maculopapular/vesicular dermatitis, crusting of lid margins, conjunctival hyperemia, bad taste in mouth, corneal staining, keratitis, keratopathy, allergic reactions, photophobia, decreased vision, tearing, lid edema. Also, a white, crystalline precipitate in the superficial part of corneal defect (onset within 1–7 days after initiating therapy; lasts about 2 weeks and does not affect continued use of the medication).

ADDITIONAL DRUG INTERACTIONS

Azlocillin / ↓ Ciprofloxacin excretion → possible ↑ effect

Caffeine / ↓ Caffeine excretion → ↑ pharmacologic effects

Calcium acetate / ↓ Relative ciprofloxacin bioavailability R/T ↓ absorption

Cyclosporine / ↑ Nephrotoxic effects

Hydantoins / ↓ Phenytoin levels

Sevelamer / ↓ Relative ciprofloxacin bioavailability R/T ↓ absorption

Tizanidine / ↑ Tizanidine AUC/peak plasma levels R/T inhibition of CYP1A2 metabolism

Theophylline / Do not take with ciprofloxacin

Bold Italic = life threatening side effect   ■ = black box warning   ✚ = Available in Canada

LABORATORY TEST CONSIDERATIONS

↑ ALT, AST, alkaline phosphatase, serum bilirubin, LDH, serum creatinine, BUN, GGT, amylase, uric acid, blood monocytes, potassium, PT, triglycerides, cholesterol. ↓ H&H. Either ↑ or ↓ blood glucose, platelets.

HOW SUPPLIED

Ophthalmic Ointment: 3.33 mg/gram (equivalent to 3 mg base); *Ophthalmic Solution:* 3.5 mg/mL; *Powder for Oral Suspension:* 250 mg/5 mL, 500 mg/5 mL; *Solution for Injection:* 200 mg, 400 mg; *Tablets:* 100 mg, 250 mg, 500 mg, 750 mg; *Tablets, Extended-Release:* 500 mg, 1,000 mg.

DOSAGE

• **ORAL SUSPENSION; TABLETS, EXTENDED-RELEASE; TABLETS, IMMEDIATE-RELEASE**

UTIs.

Adults. Acute, uncomplicated infections: 250 mg q 12 hr for 3 days or 500 mg once daily of extended-release tablets for 3 days. **Mild to moderate infections:** 250 mg q 12 hr for 7–14 days. **Severe/complicated infections:** 500 mg q 12 hr for 7–14 days or 1,000 mg once daily of extended-release tablets for 7–14 days. See *Administration/Storage* for dosing information for Proquin XR.

Pyelonephritis, acute uncomplicated.
Adults: 1,000 mg once daily of extended-release tablets for 7–14 days.

Mild to moderate chronic bacterial prostatitis.
Adults: 500 mg q 12 hr for 28 days.

Mild to moderate acute sinusitis.
Adults: 500 mg q 12 hr for 10 days.

Urethral or cervical gonococcal infections, uncomplicated.
Adults: 250 mg in a single dose.

Infectious diarrhea, mild to severe.
Adults: 500 mg q 12 hr for 5–7 days.

Skin and skin structures, lower respiratory tract, bone and joint infections.
Adults: 500 mg (mild to moderate) to 750 mg (severe or complicated) q 12 hr for 7–14 days (4–6 weeks for bone and joint infections).

Intra-abdominal infections, complicated.

Adults: 500 mg q 12 hr for 7–14 days with metronidazole.

Typhoid fever, mild to moderate.
Adults: 500 mg q 12 hr for 10 days.

Inhalational anthrax (postexposure).
Adults: 500 mg q 12 hr for 60 days. **Children:** 15 mg/kg/dose, not to exceed 500 mg/dose or 1,000 mg/day, given for 60 days.

Complicated urinary tract infections or pyelonephritis in children 1 to 17 years of age.
10–20 mg/kg q 12 hr for 10–21 days. **Maximum dose:** 750 mg/dose, not to be exceeded even in children weighing more than 51 kg.

• **IV INFUSION**
UTIs.
Adults: 200 mg (mild to moderate) to 400 mg (severe or complicated) q 12 hr for 7–14 days.

Skin and skin structures, lower respiratory tract, bone and joint infections.
Adults. Mild to moderate infections: 400 mg q 12 hr for 7–14 days. **Severe/complicated infections:** 400 mg q 8 hr for 7–14 days. Up to 4–6 weeks may be needed for bone and joint infections.

Nosocomial pneumonia, mild to severe.
Adults: 400 mg q 8 hr for 10–14 days.

Febrile neutropenic clients, empirical therapy, severe.
Adults: 400 mg q 8 hr with piperacillin, 50 mg/kg q 4 hr, not to exceed 24 grams/day, each for 7–14 days.

Acute sinusitis, mild to moderate.
Adults: 400 mg q 12 hr for 10 days.

Chronic bacterial prostatitis, mild to moderate.
Adults: 400 mg q 12 hr for 28 days.

Intra-abdominal infections, complicated.
Adults: 400 mg q 12 hr for 7–14 days.

Inhalational anthrax, postexposure.
Adults: 400 mg q 12 hr for 60 days. **Children:** 10 mg/kg q 12 hr, not to exceed 800 mg/day, for 60 days.

Disseminated gonococcal infections.
Adults: 500 mg for 24–48 hr; after improvement begins, 500 mg PO 2 times per day for 7 days.

Complicated urinary tract infections or pyelonephritis in children, 1 to 17 years of age.

6–10 mg/kg q 8 hr for 10 to 21 days. **Maximum dose:** 400 mg/dose, not to be exceeded even in children weighing more than 51 kg.

• **OPHTHALMIC OINTMENT**
Ocular infections.

Initial: Apply ½ in. ribbon to conjunctival sac 3 times per day for the first 2 days; **then,** ½ in. ribbon twice a day for the next 5 days.

• **OPHTHALMIC SOLUTION**
Corneal ulcers.

First day, initial: 2 gtt into the affected eye q 15 min for the first 6 hr; **then**, 2 gtt into the affected eye q 30 min for the remainder of the first day. **Second day:** 2 gtt into the affected eye hourly. **Third–Fourteenth day:** 2 gtt into the affected eye q 4 hr. If corneal re-epitheliazation has not occurred after 14 days, treatment may be continued.

Conjunctivitis.

Initial: 1–2 gtt into the conjunctival sac q 2 hr while awake for 2 days; **then,** 1 or 2 gtt q 4 hr while awake for the next 5 days.

NURSING CONSIDERATIONS

ADMINISTRATION/STORAGE

1. Dose must be reduced in those with a C_{CR} <50 mL/min. The dose of immediate release tablets and suspension should be 250–500 mg q 12 hr if the C_{CR} is 30–50 mL/min or 250–500 mg q 18 hr. For IV use, give 200–400 mg q 18–24 hr if the C_{CR} is 5–29 mL/min. If the client is on hemodialysis or peritoneal dialysis, the dose of immediate-release and suspension should be 250–500 mg q 24 hr after dialysis.

2. Although food delays drug absorption, it may be taken with or without meals; recommended dosing time is 2 hr after a meal.

3. Proquin XR and other PO formulations of ciprofloxacin are not interchangeable. Give Proquin XR once daily for 3 days with a main meal of the day (preferably the evening meal). Give Proquin XR at least 4 hr before or 2 hr after antacids containing magnesium or aluminum, sucralfate, Videx (didanosine) chewable/buffered tablets or pediatric powder, metal cations such as iron, and multivitamin products containing zinc. Never split, crush, or chew Proquin XR.

4. Clients on theophylline or probenecid require close observation and potential medication adjustments.

5. Do not administer to children.

6. Following instillation of ophthalmic solution, apply light finger pressure to lacrimal sac for 1 min.

7. Store immediate-release tablets below 30°C (86°F). Store extended-release tablets from 15–30°C (59–86°F). Prior to reconstitution, store oral suspension below 25 °C (77°F); after reconstitution, store below 30°C (86°F) for 14 days protected from freezing.

8. Store ophthalmic ointment from 2–25°C (36–77°F) and ophthalmic solution from 2–30°C (36–86°F). Protect from light.

IV 9. Reconstitute IV solution dose to final concentration of 1–2 mg/mL and give over 60 min. To minimize discomfort/irritation, slowly infuse dilute solution into a large vein.

10. Stable up to 14 days at refrigerated or room temperatures when diluted with 0.9% NaCl, D5W, sterile water for injection, 10% dextrose, D5W and 0.225% NaCl for injection, D5W and 0.45% NaCl, or Lactated Ringer's for injection.

11. If a Y-type IV infusion set or a piggy-back method is used, temporarily stop the administration of any other solutions during infusion.

12. If started on IV ciprofloxacin, may be switched to tablets or suspension when clinically indicated. Equivalent dosing regimens are as follows:

• 250 mg tablet q 12 hr = 200 mg IV q 12 hr.
• 500 mg tablet q 12 hr = 400 mg IV q 12 hr.
• 750 mg tablet q 12 hr = 400 mg IV q 8 hr.

13. Ciprofloxacin in admixture is incompatible with aminophylline, amoxicillin sodium, amoxicillin sodium/potassium clavulanate, clindamycin, and mezlocillin.

---

14. Store vials for IV use from 5–30°C (41–86°F). Protect from light, excessive heat, and freezing.

ASSESSMENT

1. Note reasons for therapy; onset, characteristics of S&S, culture results.
2. Not for use in children under 18 as irreversible collagen destruction has occurred.
3. Note medications currently prescribed. Fatal reactions have been reported with concurrent administration of IV ciprofloxacin and theophylline.

CLIENT/FAMILY TEACHING

1. XR tablets may be taken with meals that include milk; however, avoid with dairy products alone or with calcium-fortified products because of decreased absorption. A 2-hr window between substantial calcium intake (more than 800 mg) and dosing with XR tablets is recommended.
2. Swallow XR tablets whole; do not split, crush, or chew.
3. Take 2 hr before or 6 hr after Mg/Al antacids, sucralfate, didanosine chewable/buffered tablets, pediatric powder for oral solution, or other products containing calcium, iron, or zinc.
4. XR and IR tablets are not interchangeable.
5. Use caution- avoid sun exposure, direct or artificial sunlight may cause photosensitivity reaction.
6. Drink 2–3 L per day of fluids to keep the urine acidic and minimize risk of crystalluria.
7. Complete entire prescription to ensure desired results.
8. May cause dizziness; use caution in any activity that requires mental alertness or coordination.
9. Report any persistent joint/tendon pain (especially knee) or GI symptoms such as diarrhea, vomiting, or abdominal pain.
10. Effectiveness of oral contraceptives decreased.
11. Report adverse effects, intolerance, and lack of response.

OUTCOMES/EVALUATE

• Resolution of infection with symptomatic improvement; ↓ fever, ↓ WBCs, ↑ appetite
• Negative culture reports

Cisatracurium besylate   **IV**

(sis-ah-trah-**KYOU**-ree-um)

CLASSIFICATION(S):
Neuromuscular blocking drug
PREGNANCY CATEGORY: B
Rx: Nimbex.

SEE ALSO NEUROMUSCULAR BLOCKING AGENTS.

USES
Neuromuscular blocking agent for in- and out-patients as an adjunct to general anesthesia, to facilitate tracheal intubation, and to cause skeletal muscle relaxation during surgery or mechanical ventilation in the intensive care unit.

ACTION/KINETICS

Action
Nondepolarizing neuromuscular blocking agent that binds competitively to cholinergic receptors on the motor end-plate, resulting in antagonism of the action of acetylcholine and therefore neuromuscular blockade. The neuromuscular blocking potency of cisatracurium is about three times greater than that for atracurium.

Pharmacokinetics
Intermediate onset and duration. **Time to maximum blockade:** 2 min. **Time to recovery:** Approximately 55 min. Continuous infusion for up to 3 hr may be undertaken without tachyphylaxis or cumulative neuromuscular blockade. The time required for recovery following successive maintenance doses does not change with the number of doses given, provided that partial recovery is allowed to occur between doses. Onset, duration, and recovery are faster in children. About 95% of a dose is excreted as metabolites and unchanged drug (10%) in the urine and 4% is eliminated through the feces. Laudanosine, a major biologically active metabolite with no neuromuscular activity, may cause

transient hypotension and cerebral excitatory effects (in high doses).

CONTRAINDICATIONS

Hypersensitivity to cisatracurium or other bis-benzylisoquinolinium agents or hypersensitivity to benzyl alcohol. Use for rapid-sequence ET intubation due to its intermediate onset of action.

SPECIAL CONCERNS

Since the drug has no effect on consciousness, pain threshold, or cerebration, administration should not be undertaken before unconsciousness. May cause a profound effect in those with myasthenia gravis or the myasthenic syndrome. Burn clients may require higher doses. Onset time is faster (about 1 min) and recovery is slower (by about 1 min) in clients with impaired hepatic function. The time to maximum blockage is about 1 min slower in geriatric clients and in those with impaired renal function. Use with caution during lactation. Safety and efficacy have not been determined in children less than 2 years of age.

SIDE EFFECTS

Most Common

Bradycardia, hypotension, flushing, bronchospasm, rash.

See *Neuromuscular Blocking Agents* for a complete list of possible side effects.

OD OVERDOSE MANAGEMENT

Symptoms: Neuromuscular blockade beyond the time needed for surgery and anesthesia. *Treatment:* Maintain a patent airway and control ventilation until recovery of normal function is assured. Once recovery begins, facilitate the process by using neostigmine or edrophonium with an anticholinergic drug. Do not give these antidotes when complete blockade is evident.

DRUG INTERACTIONS

Aminoglycosides / ↑ Cisatracurium effect

Bacitracin / ↑ Cisatracurium effect

Carbamazepine / Resistance to neuromuscular blockage → slightly shorter duration.

Clindamycin / ↑ Cisatracurium effect

Colistin, sodium colistimethate / ↑ Cisatracurium effect

Enflurane/nitrous oxide/oxygen / ↑ Cisatracurium duration

Isoflurane/nitrous oxide/oxygen / ↑ Cisatracurium duration

Lincomycin / ↑ Cisatracurium effect

Lithium / ↑ Cisatracurium effect

Local anesthetics / ↑ Cisatracurium effect

Mg salts / ↑ Cisatracurium effect

Phenobarbital / Resistance to neuromuscular blockade → slightly shorter duration

Polymyxins / ↑ Cisatracurium effect

Procainamide / ↑ Cisatracurium effect

Quinidine / ↑ Cisatracurium effect

Succinylcholine / Time to onset of maximum block of cisatracurium is about 2 min faster

Tetracyclines / ↑ Cisatracurium effect

HOW SUPPLIED

Injection: 2 mg/mL, 10 mg/mL.

DOSAGE

• IV BOLUS

Neuromuscular blockade.

Adults, initial: Depending on the desired time to intubation and the anticipated length of surgery, either 0.15 or 0.2 mg/kg is used. These doses are components of a propofol/nitrous oxide/oxygen induction-intubation technique. **Maintenance during prolonged surgery:** 0.03 mg/kg given 40–50 min following an initial dose of 0.15 mg/kg and 50–60 min following an initial dose of 0.2 mg/kg.

Children, 2–12 years of age: 0.1 mg/kg over 5–10 sec during either halothane or opioid anesthesia. When given during stable opioid/nitrous oxide/oxygen anesthesia, 0.1 mg/kg produces maximum effects in about 2.8 min and a clinically effective blockade for 28 min.

• IV INFUSION

Neuromuscular blockade during extended surgery or in the ICU.

In the OR or ICU, following an initial bolus dose, a diluted solution can be given by continuous infusion to both adults and children over 2 years of age. The rate is dependent on the response of the client determined by peripheral nerve stimulation. An infusion rate of 3 mcg/kg/min can be used to counteract

---

Bold Italic = life threatening side effect   ■ = black box warning   ✦ = Available in Canada

rapid spontaneous recovery of neuromuscular blockade. Thereafter, an infusion rate of 1–2 mcg/kg/min is usually adequate to maintain blockade. Reduce infusion rate by 30–40% when given during stable isoflurane or enflurane anesthesia.

NURSING CONSIDERATIONS
ADMINISTRATION/STORAGE
IV 1. Due to slower times of onset in geriatric clients and those with impaired renal function, extend interval between drug administration and intubation.

2. Spontaneous recovery following infusion will proceed at a rate comparable to that following administration of a bolus dose.

3. Cisatracurium is acidic; thus, it may not be compatible with alkaline solutions with a pH greater than 8.5 (e.g., barbiturate solutions).

4. Drug is compatible with D5W, 0.9% NaCl, D5/0.9% NaCl, sufentanil, alfentanil HCl, fentanyl, midazolam HCl, and droperidol. Not compatible with propofol or ketorolac for Y-site administration.

5. Cisatracurium diluted in D5W, 0.9% NaCl, or D5/0.9% NaCl may be refrigerated or stored at room temperature for 24 hr without significant loss of potency. Dilutions to 0.1 or 0.2 mg/mL in DW5/RL may be refrigerated for 24 hr. Due to chemical instability, do not dilute in RL.

6. Refrigerate vials at 2–8°C (36–46°F) and protect from light. Once removed from the refrigerator, use vials within 21 days, even if rerefrigerated.

ASSESSMENT
1. List reasons for therapy, other agents trialed, anticipated duration of therapy.
2. Note hypersensitivity to benzyl alcohol.
3. Document/monitor VS, neurologic assessments, labs.

INTERVENTIONS
1. Administered only by those trained in giving neuromuscular blocking agents.
2. Client requires constant monitoring, respiratory support.

3. Medicate with analgesics for pain, agents for anxiety based on assessed need.

4. Utilize a peripheral nerve stimulator to evaluate response to therapy, to ensure partial recovery between doses.

5. Have antagonists (e.g., neostigmine) readily available. Do not use when complete blockade present.

CLIENT/FAMILY TEACHING
During drug administration you will be able to see and hear things around you but you will be completely unable to move. This will resolve once the medication is discontinued. Medications will be given for anxiety and pain as needed.

OUTCOMES/EVALUATE
- Facilitation of ET intubation
- Skeletal muscle relaxation

Cisplatin (CDDP)
(sis-**PLAH**-tin)

CLASSIFICATION(S):
Antineoplastic, alkylating
PREGNANCY CATEGORY: D
Rx: Cisplatin.

SEE ALSO *ANTINEOPLASTIC AGENTS.*

USES
Palliative therapy. (1) Combination therapy for metastatic testicular tumors or for metastatic ovarian tumors (e.g., with cyclophosphamide) in those who have received appropriate surgical or radiotherapeutic procedures. (2) Single agent in metastatic ovarian tumors as secondary therapy in those refractory to standard therapy who have not previously received cisplatin. (3) Single agent in transitional cell bladder cancer that is no longer amenable to surgery or radiotherapy. *Investigational:* Adjuvant therapy for non-small-cell lung cancer.

ACTION/KINETICS
Action
Binds to DNA and causes production of intrastrand cross-links and formation of

DNA adducts. The drug is cell-cycle nonspecific.

Pharmacokinetics

$t^{1/2}$, **plasma:** 20–30 min. **Terminal $t^{1/2}$, blood cells:** 36–47 days. Incomplete urinary excretion (only 35–51% after 5 days). Concentrates in liver, kidneys, and large and small intestines, with low penetration of CNS. About 10–40% excreted in the urine within 24 hr. **Plasma protein binding:** More than 90%.

ADDITIONAL CONTRAINDICATIONS

Lactation. Preexisting renal impairment, myelosuppression, impaired hearing, history of allergic reactions to platinum-containing compounds.

SPECIAL CONCERNS

■ (1) Administer under the supervision of a qualified physician experienced in the use of cancer chemotherapy. Appropriate management of therapy and complications is possible only when adequate diagnostic and treatment facilities are readily available. (2) Cumulative renal toxicity is severe. Other major dose-related toxicities are myelosuppression and N&V. (3) Ototoxicity, which may be more pronounced in children, is manifested by tinnitus or loss of high frequency hearing; occasionally deafness is significant. (4) Anaphylactic-type reactions have occurred. Facial edema, bronchoconstriction, tachycardia, and hypotension may occur within minutes of cisplatin administration. Epinephrine, corticosteroids, and antihistamines have been effectively used to alleviate symptoms. (5) Exercise caution to prevent inadvertent cisplatin overdose. Doses >100 mg/m^2/cycle once every 3 to 4 weeks are rarely used. Take care to avoid inadvertent cisplatin overdose due to confusion with carboplatin or prescribing practices that fail to differentiate daily doses from total dose per cycle.■ Safety and efficacy have not been determined in children. The elderly may be more susceptible to drug-related nephrotoxicity, myelosuppression, or infectious complications.

ADDITIONAL SIDE EFFECTS

Most Common

Renal toxicity, ototoxicity, myelosuppression, N&V, diarrhea.

Renal: Severe cumulative renal toxicity, including renal tubular damage and renal insufficiency. **GI:** N&V, anorexia, diarrhea, loss of taste, hiccups. **CV:** Cardiac abnormalities. **Hematologic:** Myelosuppression, including anemia and hemolytic anemia, leukopenia, thrombocytopenia. **Electrolytes:** Low levels of calcium, Mg, potassium, phosphate, and sodium. **CNS:** Seizures, peripheral neuropathies, dorsal column myelopathy, malaise, Lhermitte's sign, autonomic neuropathy. Neurotoxicity may occur 4–7 months after prolonged therapy. **Otic:** Ototoxicity characterized by tinnitus, especially in children; high frequency hearing loss, vestibular toxicity. **Ophthalmologic:** Papilledema, cerebral blindness, optic neuritis. High doses have resulted in blurred vision and altered color perception. **Body as a whole:** Asthenia, alopecia. **Metabolic:** Tetany due to hypomagnesemia and hypocalcemia. **Hypersensitivity reaction:** *Anaphylaxis*, facial edema, wheezing, tachycardia, hypotension. **Miscellaneous:** *Anaphylactic reactions*, hyperuricemia, rash, localized soft tissue toxicity, hepatotoxicity, muscle cramps, ADH syndrome, vascular toxicities (rare).

ADDITIONAL DRUG INTERACTIONS

Aminoglycosides / Cumulative nephrotoxity

Anticonvulsants / Anticonvulsant plasma levels become subtherapeutic

Loop diuretics / Additive ototoxicity

Phenytoin / ↓ Phenytoin effect R/T ↓ plasma levels

LABORATORY TEST CONSIDERATIONS

↑ Plasma iron levels, serum amylase. Nephrotoxicity results in ↑ serum uric acid, BUN, and creatinine and ↓ C$_{CR}$. Hypomagnesemia, hypocalcemia, hyponatremia, hypokalemia, hypophosphatemia.

OD OVERDOSE MANAGEMENT

Symptoms: Liver and kidney failure, deafness, ocular toxicity (including retinal detachment), significant myelosuppression, intractable N&V, neuritis, death. *Treatment:* General supportive measures

---

Bold Italic = life threatening side effect   ■ = black box warning   ♣ = Available in Canada

HOW SUPPLIED

Injection: 1 mg/mL.

DOSAGE

• IV INFUSION ONLY

Metastatic testicular tumors.

20 mg/m^2/day for 5 days per cycle in combination with other chemotherapeutic drugs.

Metastatic ovarian tumors.

Cisplatin: 75–100 mg/m^2 once every 4 weeks per cycle. Cyclophosphamide: 600 mg/m^2 once every 4 weeks on day 1. Administer cisplatin and cyclophosphamide sequentially.

Advanced bladder cancer.

50–70 mg/m^2 per cycle once q 3–4 weeks, depending on prior radiation or chemotherapy. For those heavily pretreated, give an initial dose of 50 mg/m^2/cycle repeated q 4 weeks.

NOTE: Repeat courses should not be administered until (1) serum creatinine is below 1.5 mg/dL and/or the BUN is below 25 mg/dL; (2) platelets are equal to or greater than 100,000/mm^3 and leukocyte count is equal to or greater than 4,000/mm^3; and (3) auditory activity is within the normal range

NURSING CONSIDERATIONS

🔔 Do not confuse cisplatin with carboplatin (also an antineoplastic drug).

ADMINISTRATION/STORAGE

IV 1. Add dosage recommended from vial to 2 L of D5W in one-half or one-third NSS containing 37.5 grams mannitol. Infuse over a period of 6–8 hr. Furosemide may be used instead of mannitol. Maintain adequate hydration, urinary output for 24 hr following infusion.

2. Before administration, hydrate with 1–2 L of IV fluid over a period of 8–12 hr.

3. Do *not* use any equipment with Al for preparing/administering because black precipitate will form and loss of potency will occur.

4. Platinol-AQ is a sterile, multidose vial without preservatives. Unopened containers should be stored at 15–25°C (59–77°F), protected from light. Once opened, solution is stable for 28 days protected from light, or 7 days under fluorescent lights.

5. Cisplatin has been confused with carboplatin. Place signs/label warnings to prevent name mix-ups. Do not refer to as "platinum."

6. Have emergency equipment available for anaphylactic reaction.

ASSESSMENT

1. List reasons for therapy, anticipated results. Identify previous cancer treatments (XRT, chemotherapy).

2. Obtain audiometry testing before and after therapy to ensure hearing has not been affected; an ECG during induction therapy to assess for myocarditis or focal irritability

3. Hydrate well prior to initial dose; give parenteral antiemetic at least 30 min before therapy and regularly during therapy. Hydrate to prevent urate deposits; monitor I&O during and for 24 hr after treatment.

4. *During therapy monitor for:*
- Facial edema, bronchoconstriction, tachycardia, and shock.
- Tremors that may progress to seizures due to hypomagnesemia.
- Tetany, confusion, or signs of hypocalcemia associated with hypomagnesemia; monitor Ca/Mg levels.

5. Obtain baseline CBC, uric acid, renal and LFTs. May cause severe cumulative renal toxicity; additional cisplatin doses should not be administered until renal function returned to baseline and usually not more frequently than every 3–4 weeks. Assess for mild granulocyte suppression. Nadir: 14 days; recovery: 21 days.

CLIENT/FAMILY TEACHING

1. Review reasons and frequency for therapy. Report any adverse effects, numbness, tingling, swelling, or joint pain.

2. Report ringing in ears, difficulty hearing, edema of lower extremities, decreased urination.

3. Avoid alcohol and salicylates; may increase gastric bleeding. Avoid vaccinations.

4. Use reliable birth control; may cause infertility. Identify candidates for egg/sperm harvesting.

OUTCOMES/EVALUATE
↓ Tumor size; suppression of malignant cell proliferation

Citalopram hydrobromide
(sigh-**TAL**-oh-pram)

CLASSIFICATION(S):
Antidepressant, selective serotonin reuptake inhibitor
PREGNANCY CATEGORY: C
Rx: Celexa.

SEE ALSO ANTIDEPRESSANTS.

USES
Treatment of depression in those with DSM-III and DSM III-R category of major depressive disorder. *Investigational:* Panic disorder, premenstrual dysphoric disorder (intermittent use), posttraumatic stress disorder, generalized anxiety disorder, obsessive-compulsive disorder.

ACTION/KINETICS
Action
Inhibits reuptake of serotonin into CNS neurons resulting in increased levels of serotonin in synapses. Has minimal effects on reuptake of norepinephrine and dopamine.

Pharmacokinetics
Is about 80% bioavailable. **Peak plasma levels:** 120–150 nmol/L after about 4 hr. **t½, terminal:** 35 hr. Half-life and AUC are increased in geriatric clients. **Steady state plasma levels:** About 1 week. Metabolized in the liver and excreted in the urine (20%) and feces (65%). **Plasma protein binding:** About 80%.

CONTRAINDICATIONS
Use with MAO inhibitors or with alcohol. Lactation.

SPECIAL CONCERNS
■ Antidepressants increased the risk of suicidal thinking and behavior (suicidality) in short-term studies in children and adolescents with major depressive disorder and other psychiatric disorders. Anyone considering the use of citalopram or any other antidepressant in a child or adolescent must balance this risk with the clinical need. Closely observe clients who are started on therapy for clinical worsening, suicidality, or unusual changes in behavior. Advise families and caregivers of the need for close observation and communication with the health care provider. Citalopram is not approved for use in pediatric clients. The average risk of adverse reactions representing suicidal thinking or behavior (suicidality) during the first few months of treatment in those receiving antidepressants was 4%, twice the placebo risk of 2%. No suicides occurred in these trials.■ Use with caution in severe renal impairment (dosage adjustment not necessary), a history of seizure disorders, or in diseases or conditions that produce altered metabolism or hemodynamic responses. Safety and efficacy have not been determined in children. Complications may develop in neonates exposed to citalopram; complications can develop immediately on delivery of the neonate and may require prolonged hospitalization, respiratory support, and tube feeding.

SIDE EFFECTS
Most Common
Somnolence, insomnia, nausea, excessive sweating, dry mouth, tremor, loose stools/diarrhea.

CNS: Activation of mania/hypomania, dizziness, insomnia, agitation, somnolence, anorexia, paresthesia, migraine, hyperkinesia, vertigo, hypertonia, extrapyramidal disorder, neuralgia, dystonia, abnormal gait, hypesthesia, ataxia, aggravated depression, *suicide ideation/ attempt*, confusion, aggressive reaction, drug dependence, depersonalization, hallucinations, euphoria, psychotic depression, delusions, paranoid reaction, emotional lability, panic reaction, psychosis. **GI:** N&V, dry mouth, diarrhea, dyspepsia, abdominal pain, increased salivation, flatulence, gastritis, gastroenteritis, stomatitis, eructation, hemorrhoids, dysphagia, teeth grinding, gingivitis, esophagitis. **CV:** Tachycardia, postural hypotension, hypertension, bradycardia, edema of extremities, angina pectoris, extrasystoles, *cardiac*

failure, MI, CVA, flushing, myocardial ischemia. **Musculoskeletal:** Arthralgia, myalgia, arthritis, muscle weakness, skeletal pain, leg cramps, involuntary muscle contraction. **Hematologic:** Purpura, anemia, leukocytosis, lymphadenopathy. **Metabolic/nutritional:** Decreased/increased weight, thirst. **GU:** Ejaculation disorder, impotence, dysmenorrhea, decreased/increased libido, amenorrhea, galactorrhea, breast pain/enlargement, **vaginal hemorrhage**, polyuria, frequent micturition, urinary incontinence/retention, dysuria. **Respiratory:** Coughing, epistaxis, bronchitis, dyspnea, pneumonia. **Dermatologic:** Rash, pruritus, photosensitivity reaction, urticaria, acne, skin discoloration, eczema, dermatitis, dry skin, psoriasis. **Ophthalmic:** Abnormal accommodation, conjunctivitis, eye pain. **Body as a whole:** Asthenia, fatigue, fever. **Miscellaneous:** Hyponatremia, increased sweating, yawning, hot flushes, rigors, alcohol intolerance, syncope, flu-like symptoms, taste perversion, tinnitus.

LABORATORY TEST CONSIDERATIONS
↑ Hepatic enzymes, alkaline phosphatase. Abnormal glucose tolerance.

OD **OVERDOSE MANAGEMENT**
Symptoms: Dizziness, sweating, N&V, tremor, somnolence, sinus tachycardia. Rarely, amnesia, confusion, coma, convulsions, hyperventilation, cyanosis, rhabdomyolysis, ECG changes (including QTc prolongation, nodal rhythm, ventricular arrhythmias). *Treatment:* Establish and maintain an airway. Gastric lavage with use of activated charcoal. Monitor cardiac and vital signs. General symptomatic and supportive care.

DRUG INTERACTIONS
See also *Drug Interactions* for *Selective Serotonin Reuptake Inhibitors*
Azole antifungals / ↑ Citalopram levels
Beta blockers / ↑ Beta blocker effect; reduce initial beta blocker dose
Carbamazepine / ↓ Citalopram levels; ↑ carbamazepine levels
Imipramine / ↑ Drug metabolite (desimpramine) by 50%
Lithium / Possible ↑ serotonergic citalopram effects
Macrolide antibiotics (e.g., erythromycin)/

↑ Citalopram levels
MAO inhibitors / Possible serious and sometimes fatal reactions, including hyperthermia, rigidity, myoclonus, autonomic instability, mental status changes (extreme agitation, delirium, coma)

HOW SUPPLIED
Oral Solution: 10 mg/5 mL; *Tablets:* 10 mg, 20 mg, 40 mg; *Tablets, Orally-Disintegrating:* 10 mg, 20 mg, 40 mg.

DOSAGE
- **ORAL SOLUTION; TABLETS; TABLETS, ORALLY-DISINTEGRATING**
  Depression.
Adults, initial: 20 mg once daily in a.m. or p.m. with or without food. Increase dose in increments of 20 mg at intervals of no less than 1 week. Doses greater than 40 mg/day are not recommended. For the elderly or those with hepatic impairment, 20 mg/day is recommended; titrate to 40 mg/day only for nonresponders. Initial treatment is continued for 6 or 8 weeks. **Maintenance:** Up to 24 weeks following 6 or 8 weeks of initial treatment. Periodically re-evaluate the long-term usefulness of the drug if used for extended periods.
  Panic disorder.
20–30 mg/day.

NURSING CONSIDERATIONS
℘ Do not confuse Celexa with Cerebyx (an anticonvulsant) or with Celebrex (nonsteroidal anti-inflammatory drug).

ADMINISTRATION/STORAGE
Allow at least 14 days to elapse between discontinuation of a MAOI and initiation of citalopram or vice versa.

ASSESSMENT
1. Note reasons for therapy, onset/characteristics of S&S, events that may have triggered S&S. List other agents trialed/outcome.
2. List other drugs prescribed; ensure none interact. Avoid use within 14 days before or after MAOI use.
3. Note any liver, renal dysfunction, seizure disorder; reduce dose with dysfunction.
4. If discontinued, monitor for the following symptoms: Dysphoric mood, irritability, agitation, dizziness, sensory disturbances, anxiety, confusion, head-

ache, lethargy, emotional lability, or hypomania. If intolerable symptoms occur following decrease in dose or discontinuation of the drug, consider resuming the previously prescribed dose. Subsequently the dose may be decreased but at a more gradual rate.

CLIENT/FAMILY TEACHING
1. Take as directed, once daily, with or without food.
2. Use caution operating machines or cars until drug effects known.
3. Avoid alcohol or other CNS depressants.
4. Use reliable birth control.
5. May see improvement in 1 to 4 weeks; continue therapy as prescribed. Report adverse effects; lack of response.
6. Keep all F/U appointments to evaluate response.

OUTCOMES/EVALUATE
• Relief/control of depression/panic attacks
• Control PTSD/OCD S&S

Clarithromycin
(klah-**rith**-roh-**MY**-sin)

CLASSIFICATION(S):
Antibiotic, macrolide
PREGNANCY CATEGORY: C
Rx: Biaxin, Biaxin XL.
✤Rx: Biaxin BID.

SEE ALSO *ANTI-INFECTIVES.*

USES
Oral Suspension, Tablets. Mild to moderate infections caused by susceptible strains of the following. (1) Pharyngitis/tonsillitis in adults or children due to *Streptococcus pyogenes.* Efficacy in prevention of rheumatic fever is not available. (2) Acute maxillary sinusitis in adults or children due to *Streptococcus pneumoniae, Haemophilus influenzae,* and *Moraxella catarrhalis.* The active metabolite, 14-OH clarithromycin, has significant activity (twice the parent compound) against *H. influenzae.* (3) Acute bacterial exacerbation of chronic bronchitis due to *S. pneumoniae, H. influenzae, H. parainfluenzae, M. catarrha-*

lis. (4) Community acquired pneumonia in adults or children due to *Mycoplasma pneumoniae, S. pneumoniae, Chlamydia pneumoniae* (TWAR strain), or *H. influenzae* (adults only). (5) Acute otitis media in children due to *H. influenzae, M. catarrhalis,* or *S. pneumoniae.* (6) Uncomplicated skin and skin structure infections in adults or children due to *Staphylococcus aureus* or *S. pyogenes.* (7) Disseminated mycobacterial infections in adults or children due to *Mycobacterium avium* (commonly seen in AIDS clients) and *M. intracellulare.* Prevention of disseminated *M. avium* complex in adults or children with advanced HIV. (8) In combination with other drugs (e.g., metronidazole, omeprazole or lansoprazole, amoxicillin, ranitidine bismuth citrate) for the eradication of *Helicobacter pylori* infection in clients with active duodenal ulcers associated with *H. pylori* infection.

Extended-Release Tablets. Mild to moderate infections of the following: (1) Acute maxillary sinusitis due to *H. influenzae, M. catarrhalis,* or *S. pneumoniae.* (2) Acute bacterial exacerbation of chronic bronchitis due to *H. influenzae, H. parainfluenzae, M. catarrhalis,* or *S. pneumoniae.* (3) Community-acquired pneumonia due to *H. influenzae, H. parainfluenzae, M. catarrhalis, S. pneumoniae, C. pneumoniae* (TWAR), or *M. pneumoniae.*

ACTION/KINETICS
Action
Macrolide antibiotic that acts by binding to the 50S ribosomal subunit of susceptible organisms, thus interfering with or inhibiting microbial protein synthesis.

Pharmacokinetics
Rapidly absorbed from the GI tract although food slightly delays the onset of absorption and the formation of the active metabolite but does not affect the extent of the bioavailability. **Peak serum levels:** When fasting, 2 hr for the tablet and 3 hr for the suspension. **Steady-state peak serum levels:** 1 mcg/mL within 2–3 days after 250 mg q 12 hr and 2–3 mcg/mL after 500 mg q 12 hr. Clarithromycin and 14-OH clari-

thromycin (active metabolite) are readily distributed to body tissues and fluids. **$t^1/_2$, elimination:** 3–7 hr (depending on the dose) for clarithromycin and 5–6 hr for 14-OH clarithromycin. Up to 30% of a dose is excreted unchanged in the urine.

CONTRAINDICATIONS
Hypersensitivity to clarithromycin, other macrolide antibiotics, or erythromycin. Clients taking pimozide. Use with ranitidine bismuth citrate in those with a history of acute porphyria.

SPECIAL CONCERNS
Use with caution in severe renal impairment with or without concomitant hepatic impairment and during lactation. Safety and effectiveness in children less than 6 months of age have not been determined. Safety has not been determined in MAC clients less than 20 months of age.

SIDE EFFECTS
Most Common
Diarrhea/loose stools, abdominal pain, N&V, dyspepsia, abnormal taste, headache.
GI: Diarrhea, nausea, abnormal taste, dyspepsia, abdominal discomfort/pain, pseudomembranous colitis, glossitis, stomatitis, oral moniliasis, vomiting. **CNS:** Headache, dizziness, behavioral changes, confusion, depersonalization, disorientation, hallucinations, insomnia, nightmares, vertigo. **Allergic:** Urticaria, mild skin eruptions and, rarely, ***anaphylaxis*** and ***Stevens-Johnson syndrome***. **Hepatic:** Hepatocellular cholestatic hepatitis with or without jaundice, increased liver enzymes, ***hepatic failure***. **Miscellaneous:** Hearing loss (usually reversible), alteration of sense of smell (usually with taste perversion).
In children, the most common side effects are diarrhea, vomiting, abdominal pain, rash, and headache.

LABORATORY TEST CONSIDERATIONS
↑ ALT, AST, GGT, alkaline phosphatase, LDH, total bilirubin, BUN, serum creatinine, PT. ↓ WBC count.

DRUG INTERACTIONS
See also *Drug Interactions for Erythromycins.*

Anticoagulants / ↑ Anticoagulant effects
Benzodiazepines / ↑ Plasma levels of certain benzodiazepines → ↑ and prolonged CNS effects
Buspirone / ↑ Buspirone levels → ↑ risk of side effects
Carbamazepine / ↑ Carbamazepine levels
Colchicine / Severe cholchicine intoxication R/T inhibition of metabolism by CYP3A4
Cyclosporine ↑ Cyclosporine levels → ↑ risk of nephrotoxicity and neurotoxicity
Digoxin / ↑ Digoxin levels R/T ↓ digoxin metabolism by the gut flora
Disopyramide / ↑ Plasma levels → arrhythmias and ↑ QT intervals
Ergot alkaloids / Acute drug toxicity, including severe peripheral vasospasm and dysesthesia
Fluconazole / ↑ Clarithromycin levels
HMG–CoA Reductase Inhibitors / ↑ Risk of severe myopathy or rhabdomyolysis
Lansoprazole / ↑ Lansoprazole AUC and peak plasma levels R/T inhibition of metabolism by CYP3A4
Omeprazole / ↑ Levels of omeprazole, clarithromycin, and 14-OH-clarithromycin
Pimozide / ↑ Risk of sudden death R/T cardiac effects; do not use together
Ranitidine bismuth citrate / ↑ Levels of ranitidine, bismuth citrate, and 14–OH clarithromycin
Repaglinide / ↑ Repaglinide levels likely R/T ↓ liver metabolism
Rifabutin, Rifampin / ↓ Clarithromycin effect and ↑ GI side effects
Sulfonylureas / Possible severe hypoglycemia
Tacrolimus / ↑ Tacrolimus levels → ↑ risk of toxicity (e.g., nephrotoxicity)
Theophylline / ↑ Theophylline levels
Triazolam / ↑ Risk of somnolence/confusion
Verapamil / Possible severe hypotension/bradycardia
Zidovudine (AZT) / ↓ Steady-state AZT levels in HIV-infected clients; however, peak serum AZT levels may be ↑ or ↓.

C

HOW SUPPLIED
Granules for Oral Suspension (after reconstitution): 125 mg/5 mL, 250 mg/5 mL; *Tablets:* 250 mg, 500 mg; *Tablets, Extended-Release:* 500 mg, 1,000 mg.

DOSAGE
- **ORAL SUSPENSION; TABLETS**

   Pharyngitis, tonsillitis.
Adults: 250 mg q 12 hr for 10 days.
   Acute maxillary sinusitis.
Adults: 500 mg q 12 hr for 14 days.
   Acute exacerbation of chronic bronchitis due to H. parainfluenzae *or* H. influenzae.
Adults: 500 mg q 12 hr for 7–14 days for *H. influenzae* and 7 days for *H. parainfluenzae.*
   Acute exacerbation of chronic bronchitis due to M. catarrhalis *or* S. pneumoniae.
Adults: 250 mg q 12 hr for 7–14 days.
   Community acquired pneumonia due to S. pneumoniae, M. pneumoniae, H. influenzae, *or* C. pneumoniae.
Adults: 250 mg q 12 hr for 7–14 days (7 days for *H. influenzae*).
   Uncomplicated skin and skin structure infections.
Adults: 250 mg q 12 hr for 7–14 days.
   Disseminated M. avium *complex or prophylaxis of* M. avium *complex.*
Adults: 500 mg twice a day; **children:** 7.5 mg/kg twice a day up to 500 mg twice a day.
NOTE: For all uses, the usual daily dose for children is 15 mg/kg q 12 hr for 10 days. See *Administration/Storage.*
   Active duodenal ulcers associated with H. pylori *infection.*
The following drug regimens are used:
Triple Therapy: Clarithromycin, 500 mg twice a day; amoxicillin, 1,000 mg twice a day; and *either* lansoprazole, 30 mg twice a day *or* omeprazole, 20 mg twice a day, each for 10–14 days. Take each drug with meals. In clients with an ulcer present at the time therapy begins, give omeprazole, 20 mg once daily, for an additional 18 days. **Dual Therapy:** (a) Clarithromycin, 500 mg three times per day and omeprazole, 40 mg once daily in the morning each for 14 days. Give omeprazole, 20 mg once daily, for an additional 14 days for ulcer

healing and symptom relief. (b) Clarithromycin, 500 mg either twice (q 12 hr) or three times (q 8 hr) a day and ranitidine bismuth citrate, 400 mg twice a day (q 12 hr) each for 14 days. Give ranitidine bismuth citrate twice a day for an additional 14 days for ulcer healing and symptom relief. Do not use this combination in clients with a C_{CR} <25 mL/min.
- **TABLETS, EXTENDED-RELEASE**

   Acute maxillary sinusitis.
Adults: 1,000 mg once daily for 14 days.
   Acute exacerbation of chronic bronchitis, community acquired pneumonia.
Adults: 1,000 mg once daily for 7 days.

NURSING CONSIDERATIONS
ADMINISTRATION/STORAGE
1. Usual dose for children is 15 mg/kg/day divided q 12 hr for 10 days. Use the following guidelines: **9 kg:** 62.5 mg q 12 hr; **17 kg:** 125 mg q 12 hr; **25 kg:** 187.5 mg q 12 hr; **33 kg:** 250 mg q 12 hr.
2. Tablets and granules may be given with or without food; both tablets and suspension can be given with milk. Give ER tablets with food. Food delays both the onset of absorption and the formation of 14-OH clarithromycin (the active metabolite).
3. Give without dosage adjustment in hepatic impairment if there is normal renal function. If severe renal impairment (C_{CR} <30 mL/min) with/without hepatic impairment, halve the dose or double the dosing interval.
4. Shake reconstituted suspension well before each use; use within 14 days and do not refrigerate. After mixing store at 15–30°C (59–86°F).
5. Store tablets and granules at controlled room temperature in a well-closed container. Protect 250 mg tablets from light. Store ER tablets from 20–25°C (68–77°F).

ASSESSMENT
1. Note sensitivity to erythromycin or any of the macrolide antibiotics.
2. Document onset, severity, characteristics of S&S.

Bold Italic = life threatening side effect   ■ = black box warning   ✚ = Available in Canada

3. List drugs currently prescribed to prevent any interactions.

4. Obtain baseline cultures/sensitivity, monitor CBC, renal and LFTs. Reduce dose with renal dysfunction.

5. Avoid use with pimozide and with ranitidine bismuth citrate in those with a history of acute porphyria.

CLIENT/FAMILY TEACHING

1. May take with/without meals but food may decrease chance of stomach upset; food delays onset of absorption. Drug may cause a bitter taste.

2. Take with sufficient amount of water.

3. Avoid taking with grapefruit juice.

4. Do not chew, break, or crush extended-release tablets.

5. Report any persistent diarrhea; an antibiotic-associated colitis may be precipitated by *C. difficile* and require alternative management.

6. Report adverse effects or lack of improvement after 48–72 hr.

7. Keep all F/U appointments to evaluate response to therapy.

OUTCOMES/EVALUATE

• Symptomatic improvement
• Negative follow-up cultures

Clindamycin hydrochloride   ■

(klin-dah-**MY**-sin)

CLASSIFICATION(S):
Antibiotic, lincosamide
PREGNANCY CATEGORY: B
Rx: Cleocin.
✿**Rx:** Dalacin C, ratio-Clindamycin.

Clindamycin palmitate

PREGNANCY CATEGORY: B
Rx: Cleocin Pediatric.
✿**Rx:** Dalacin C Flavored Granules.

Clindamycin phosphate

PREGNANCY CATEGORY: B
Rx: Foam, Gel, Lotion, Topical Solution: Cleocin T, ClindaMax, Clindagel, Clindets, Evoclin. **Injection:** Cleocin Phosphate. **Vaginal Cream:** Cleocin, ClindaMax, Clindesse. **Vaginal Suppositories:** Cleocin.
✿**Rx:** Dalacin C Phosphate Sterile Solution, Dalacin T Topical Solution, Dalacin Vaginal Cream.

SEE ALSO *ANTI-INFECTIVES.*

USES
Should not be used for trivial infections.

Systemic. (1) *Anareobes:* Serious respiratory tract infections (e.g., empyema, lung abscess, anaerobic pneumonitis). (2) Serious skin and soft tissue infections, septicemia, intra-abdominal infections (e.g., peritonitis, intra-abdominal abscess), infections of the female pelvis and genital tract (e.g., PID, endometritis, nongonococcal tubo-ovarian abscess, pelvic cellulitis, postsurgical vaginal cuff infection). (3) *Streptococci/ staphylococci:* Serious respiratory tract infections, serious skin and soft tissue infections, septicemia (parenteral use), acute staphylococcal hematogenous osteomyelitis (parenteral use). (4) *Pneumonococcus:* Serious respiratory tract infections. (5) Adjunct to surgery for chronic bone/joint infections. *Investigational:* Alternative to sulfonamides in combination with pyrimethamine in the acute treatment of CNS toxoplasmosis in AIDS clients. In combination with primaquine to treat *Pneumocystis carinii* pneumonia. Chlamydial infections in women. Bacterial vaginosis due to *Gardnerella vaginalis.*

Topical. (1) Inflammatory acne vulgaris. (2) Vaginally to treat bacterial vaginosis (*Haemophilus* vaginitis, *Gardnerella vaginitis*, nonspecific vaginitis, *Corynebacterium vaginitis,* or anaerobic vaginosis). Treatment of rosacea (lotion used).

ACTION/KINETICS

Action

Suppresses protein synthesis by microorganisms by binding to ribosomes (50S subunit) and preventing peptide bond formation. Is both bacteriostatic and bactericidal.

Pharmacokinetics

Does not diffuse adequately into CSF to be used to treat meningitis. Is 90% bioavailable. **Peak serum concentration: PO,** 4 mcg/mL after 300 mg; **IM,** 4.9 mcg/mL after 300 mg; **IV,** 14.7 mcg/mL after 300 mg. **t½:** 2.4–3 hr. In serious infections the rate of IV administration is adjusted to maintain appropriate serum drug concentrations: 4–6 mcg/mL. Over 90% metabolized in the liver. About 10% excreted unchanged in the urine.

CONTRAINDICATIONS

Hypersensitivity to either clindamycin or lincomycin. Use in treating viral and minor bacterial infections or in clients with a history of regional enteritis, nonbacterial infections (e.g., most URIs), ulcerative colitis, meningitis, or antibiotic-associated colitis. Lactation.

SPECIAL CONCERNS

■ (1) Systemic use may cause severe and possibly fatal colitis. Diarrhea, colitis, and pseudomembranous colitis may occur up to several weeks following cessation of therapy. Endoscopic exams may show pseudomembranous colitis. Toxin(s) produced by *Clostridia* is a primary cause of the antibiotic-associated colitis. When significant diarrhea occurs, discontinue the drug or continue only with close observation. Large bowel endoscopy is recommended. (2) Mild colitis may respond to discontinuing the drug. Promptly manage moderate-to-severe diarrhea with fluid, electrolyte, and protein supplements. Systemic corticosteroids and corticosteroid retention enemas may help. Consider other causes of colitis such as previous sensitivities to drugs or other allergens. (3) Opiates or diphenoxylate with atropine may prolong or aggravate the condition. (4) Reserve for serious infections where less toxic antibiotics are inappropriate. Do not use in clients with non-bacterial infections (e.g., most URTI).■

Use with caution in infants up to 1 month of age, in clients with GI, liver or renal disease, or a history of allergy or asthma. Use topical gel, lotion, or suspension with caution in atopic individuals. Consider if other drugs are more appropriate to treat acne due to the potential for diarrhea, bloody diarrhea, and pseudomembranous colitis. Safety and efficacy of topical products have not been established in children less than 12 years old.

SIDE EFFECTS

Most Common

After systemic use: Diarrhea, pseudomembranous colitis, tinnitis, N&V, skin rashes.

After topical use: Dry skin, burning, itching, erythema, peeling, oily skin.

GI: N&V, diarrhea, **pseudomembranous colitis** (more frequent after PO use), abdominal pain, esophagitis, unpleasant or metallic taste (after high IV doses), glossitis, stomatitis. **CV:** Hypotension; **rarely, cardiopulmonary arrest after too rapid IV use.** **Allergic:** Morbilliform rash (most common), skin rashes, urticaria, erythema multiforme, **anaphylaxis, Stevens-Johnson-like syndrome,** maculopapular rash, **angioneurotic edema. Hematologic:** Leukopenia, neutropenia, thrombocytopenia, transient eosinophilia, **agranulocytosis, aplastic anemia. Hepatic:** Jaundice, abnormal LFTs. **GU:** Renal dysfunction (azotemia, oliguria, proteinuria), vaginitis. **Miscellaneous:** Superinfection, tinnitus, polyarthritis. Also sore throat, fatigue, urinary frequency, headache.

Following IV use: Thrombophlebitis, erythema, pain, swelling.

Following IM use: Pain, induration, sterile abscesses.

Following topical use: Erythema, irritation, dryness, peeling, itching, burning, oiliness of skin, pruritus.

Following vaginal use: Cervicitis, vaginitis, vulvar irritation/moniliasis, urticaria, rash, trichomonal vaginitis, vulvovaginal disorder, vulvovaginitis, body moniliasis.

Bold Italic = life threatening side effect   ■ = black box warning   ✚ = Available in Canada

NOTE: The injection contains benzyl alcohol, which has been associated with **a fatal 'gasping syndrome'** in infants.

LABORATORY TEST CONSIDERATIONS

↓ Levels of AST, ALT, NPN, alkaline phosphatase, bilirubin, BSP retention, and ↓ platelet count.

DRUG INTERACTIONS

Antiperistaltic antidiarrheals (opiates, Lomotil) / ↑ Diarrhea R/T ↓ toxin removal from colon

Ciprofloxacin HCl / Additive antibacterial activity

Cyclosporine / ↓ Cyclosporine levels

Erythromycin / Cross-interference → ↓ effect of both drugs

Kaolin/Pectin (e.g., Kaopectate) / ↓ Effect R/T ↓ GI tract absorption

Neuromuscular blocking agents / ↑ Effect of blocking agents

HOW SUPPLIED

Clindamycin hydrochloride. *Capsules:* 75 mg, 150 mg, 300 mg.

Clindamycin palmitate. *Granules for Oral Solution:* 75 mg/5 mL.

Clindamycin phosphate *Cream:* 2%; *Foam:* 1%; *Gel:* 1%; *Injection:* 150 mg/mL; *Lotion:* 1%; *Topical Solution:* 1%; *Topical Suspension:* 1%; *Vaginal Cream:* 2%; *Vaginal Suppositories:* 100 mg (as the base).

DOSAGE

• **CAPSULES (CLINDAMYCIN HYDROCHLORIDE); ORAL SOLUTION (CLINDAMYCIN PALMITATE)**

Serious infections.

Adults: 150–300 mg q 6 hr. **Pediatric, Clindamycin hydrochloride:** 8–16 mg/kg/day divided into three or four equal doses. **Pediatric, Clindamycin palmitate hydrochloride:** 8–12 mg/kg/day divided into three or four equal doses.

More severe infections.

Adults: 300–450 mg q 6 hr. **Pediatric, Clindamycin hydrochloride:** 16–20 mg/kg/day divided into three or four equal doses. **Pediatric, Clindamycin palmitate hydrochloride:** 13–25 mg/kg/day divided into three or four equal doses. **Children less than 10 kg:** Minimum recommended dose is 37.5 mg 3 times per day.

• **IM; IV (CLINDAMYCIN PHOSPHATE)**

Serious infections due to aerobic gram-positive cocci.

Adults: 600–1,200 mg/day in two to four equal doses. **Pediatric, over 1 month to 16 years:** 350 mg/m^2/day.

More severe infections due to B. fragilis, Peptococcus, *or* Clostridium (*other than* C. perfringens).

Adults: 1,200–2,700 mg/day in two to four equal doses. May have to be increased in more serious infections. **Pediatric, over 1 month to 16 years:** 450 mg/m^2/day.

Life-threatening infections.

Adults: 4.8 grams IV. **Pediatric, 1 month to 16 years:** 20–40 mg/kg/day in three to four equal doses depending on severity of infections. **Pediatric, less than 1 month of age:** 15–20 mg/kg/day in three or four equal doses.

Acute pelvic inflammatory disease.

IV: 900 mg q 8 hr plus gentamicin loading dose of 2 mg/kg IV or IM; **then,** gentamicin, 1.5 mg/kg q 8 hr IV or IM. Therapy may be discontinued 24 hr after client improves. After discharge from the hospital, continue with doxycycline PO, 100 mg 2 times per day for 10–14 days. Alternatively, give clindamycin, PO, 450 mg 4 times per day for 14 days.

• **CREAM; LOTION; TOPICAL GEL; TOPICAL SOLUTION; TOPICAL SUSPENSION (ALL ARE CLINDAMYCIN PHOSPHATE)**

Inflammatory acne vulgaris.

Apply thin film once (Clindagel) or twice daily to affected areas. One or more pledgets may also be used.

• **VAGINAL CREAM (2%)**

Bacterial vaginosis.

One applicatorful (5 grams containing about 100 mg clindamycin phosphate), preferably at bedtime, for 3 or 7 days (nonpregnant women) or 7 (pregnant women) consecutive days. Cleocin and ClindaMax creams can be used to treat pregnant women during the second and third trimester. For Clindesse, use a single applicatorful (5 grams containing 100 mg clindamycin phosphate) given once intravaginally at anytime of the day.

- **VAGINAL SUPPOSITORIES (CLINDAMYCIN PHOSPHATE)**
  Bacterial vaginosis.

One suppository (100 mg) intravaginally/day, preferably at bedtime, for 3 days.

- **FOAM (CLINDAMYCIN PHOSPHATE)**
  Acne vulgaris.

Apply once daily to the affected area. Dispense the foam into the cap of the can or onto a cool surface; apply foam with fingertips.

NURSING CONSIDERATIONS

ADMINISTRATION/STORAGE

1. For anaerobic infections, use parenteral form initially; may be followed by PO therapy.
2. For β-hemolytic streptococci infections, continue treatment for at least 10 days.
3. Reduce dosage in severe renal impairment.
4. Single IM injections greater than 600 mg are not advisable. Inject deeply into muscle to prevent induration, pain, and sterile abscesses.
5. Do not refrigerate reconstituted solution; may become thickened and difficult to pour.
6. Shake lotion well just before using.
7. Give parenteral clindamycin only to hospitalized clients.
8. Dilute IV injections to maximum concentration of 18 mg/mL, with no more than 1,200 mg administered in 1 hr.
9. Administer IV over a period of 20–60 min, depending on dose and desired therapeutic serum concentration.
10. The phosphate is stable in NSS, D5W, and RL solution in both glass or PVC containers at concentrations of 6, 9, and 12 mg/mL for 8 weeks frozen, 32 days refrigerated, or 16 days at room temperature.

ASSESSMENT

1. List reasons for therapy, onset, characteristics of S&S; note culture results.
2. Auscultate lungs; assess extent of respiratory tract infections.
3. Describe skin/soft tissue infections; note complaints indicative of PID or intra-abdominal infections.
4. Monitor renal/LFTs; note any history of liver/renal disease, allergies, or GI problems.
5. With IV therapy, observe for hypotension; keep in bed for 30 min following infusion. Bitter taste may be evident.
6. Observe for drug interactions caused by concurrent administration of neuromuscular blocking agents. Be alert to hypotension, bronchospasms, cardiac disturbances, hyperthermia, respiratory depression.
7. Observe closely for:
- Skin rash; frequently reported
- Renal/hepatic impairment; newborns for organ dysfunction
- GI disturbances, such as abdominal pain, diarrhea, anorexia, N&V, bloody/tarry stools, excessive flatulence.

CLIENT/FAMILY TEACHING

1. Take oral medication with a full glass of water to prevent esophageal ulceration. May be taken with or without food.
2. Report side effects such as persistent vomiting, diarrhea, fever, abdominal pain, cramping.
3. Pseudomembranous colitis may occur 2–9 days or several weeks after initiation of therapy. Fluids, electrolytes, protein supplements, systemic corticosteroids, and oral antibiotics may be needed. Do not use antiperistaltic agents if diarrhea occurs; these can prolong or aggravate condition. Kaolin will reduce absorption of antibiotic; if prescribed, take 3 hr before drug.
4. The vaginal cream contains mineral oil, which may weaken latex or rubber products, such as condoms or vaginal contraceptive diaphragms; avoid for 72 hr following treatment.
5. Do not engage in intercourse when using the vaginal cream; may enhance irritation.
6. Do not use any acne or topical mercury preparations containing a peeling agent in affected area; severe irritation may occur.
7. Avoid contact of the gel, lotion, or topical suspension with the eyes; alcohol base will cause burning and irrita-

---

tion. In case of accidental contact with eyes, abraded skin, or mucous membranes, wash with copious amounts of cool tap water.

8. Apply the foam once daily to affected area(s) after washing the skin with mild soap and allowing it to dry fully. use enough to cover the entire affected area. To use the foam:

9. Do not dispense directly onto the hands or face because the foam will begin to melt on contact with warm skin.

- Remove the clear cap. Align the black mark with the nozzle of the activator.
- Hold the can at an upright angle and press firmly to dispense. Dispense enough to cover the affected area into the cap or onto a cool surface. If the can is warm or the foam is runny, run the can under cold water.
- Pick up small amounts of the foam with the fingertips and gently massage into the affected area until the foam disappears.
- Use with caution around the mouth area. 10. Keep all F/U appointments to evaluate response to therapy.

OUTCOMES/EVALUATE
- Resolution of infection
- Symptomatic improvement
- Therapeutic drug levels with IV therapy (4–6 mcg/mL)

Clobetasol propionate
(kloh-**BAY**-tah-sohl)

CLASSIFICATION(S):
Glucocorticoid
PREGNANCY CATEGORY: C
Rx: Clobevate Gel, Clobex, Cormax, Embeline, Embeline E 0.05%, Olux, Olux-E, Temovate, Temovate Emollient.
✚Rx: Dermovate, Gen-Clobetasol Cream/Ointment, Gen-Clobetasol Scalp Application, Novo-Clobetasol, ratio-Clobetasol.

SEE ALSO CORTICOSTEROIDS.

USES
(1) Relief of inflammatory and pruritic dermatoses of the skin and scalp, including eczema, atopic dermatitis, contact dermatitis, seborrhea. (2) **Foam:** Short-term treatment of inflammatory and pruritic manifestations of moderate to severe corticosteroid responsive scalp dermatoses and for short-term topical treatment of mild to moderate plaque-type psoriasis of non-scalp regions, excluding the face and intertriginous areas. (3) **Lotion:** Also used for moderate to severe plaque psoriasis if lesions occupy less than 10% of body surface area. (4) **Shampoo:** Moderate to severe scalp psoriasis in those 18 years and older. (5) **Solution:** Short-term treatment of inflammatory and pruritic manifestations of moderate to severe corticosteroid responsive scalp dermatoses. (6) **Spray:** Moderate to severe plaque psoriasis affecting up to 20% of body surface area in clients 18 years of age and older.

ACTION/KINETICS
Action
Has anti-inflammatory, antipruritic, and vasoconstrictive effects.

CONTRAINDICATIONS
Use in children less than 12 years old, use for more than 2 weeks, to treat rosacea or perioral dermatitis, and use on face, groin, axillae.

SPECIAL CONCERNS
May suppress hypothalamic-pituitary-adrenal (HPA) axis at doses as low as 2 grams/day. Use with caution during lactation.

SIDE EFFECTS
Most Common
Burning, cracking/fissuring of skin, irritation, itching, numbness of fingers, reddened skin, skin atrophy, stinging.
Dermatologic: Burning sensation, itching, stinging, irritation, dryness, pruritus, erythema, folliculitis, hypertrichosis, acneform eruptions, hypopigmentation, perioral dermatitis, allergic contact dermatitis, skin maceration, reddened skin, secondary infection, striae, millaria, cracking and fissuring of the skin, skin atrophy, numbness of fingers, telangi-

ectasia. **Miscellaneous:** Cushing's syndrome.

HOW SUPPLIED

Cream: 0.05%; *Foam:* 0.05%; *Gel:* 0.05%; *Lotion:* 0.05%; *Ointment:* 0.05%; *Shampoo:* 0.05%; *Solution for Scalp Application:* 0.05%; *Spray:* 0.05%.

DOSAGE

• **CREAM; FOAM; GEL; LOTION; OINTMENT**

Dermatoses.

Apply thin layer to affected skin or scalp twice a day, once in the morning and once in the evening. Rub in gently and completely. Use no more than 50 grams per week.

• **FOAM**

Mild to moderate plaque-type psoriasis of non-scalp regions, moderate to severe scalp dermatoses.

Apply a small amount to the affected area twice a day, morning and evening.

• **LOTION**

Plaque psoriasis.

Apply to lesions 2 times per day with no more than 50 grams given in one week. May be used for up to 4 weeks.

• **SHAMPOO**

Moderate to severe scalp psoriasis.

Apply a thin film to the affected areas of the scalp daily for no more than 4 weeks; apply to a dry scalp and leave on for 15 min before lathering and rinsing. Do not use more than 50 mL of the shampoo per week.

• **SOLUTION FOR SCALP APPLICATION**

Scalp dermatoses.

Apply to affected scalp areas twice a day, morning and evening. Do not exceed a total weekly dosage of 50 mL. Not to be used with occlusive dressings.

• **SPRAY**

Moderate to severe plaque psoriasis.

Adults 18 years and older: Up to 50 grams/week. Limit treatment beyond 2 weeks to localized moderate to severe lesions that have not improved sufficiently.

NURSING CONSIDERATIONS

ADMINISTRATION/STORAGE

1. Do not use occlusive dressings.
2. Do not refrigerate.

3. Do not use the gel on the face, groin, or axillae.

ASSESSMENT

1. Note onset, location, and characteristics of S&S (photo); note agents trialed/outcome.
2. Drug is a potent corticosteroid for short term use; assess for S&S of HPA axis suppression-may use ACTH stimulation test, a.m. cortisol, and urinary free cortisol test.

CLIENT/FAMILY TEACHING

1. Apply thin layer to affected area; gently rub in. Review type of product prescribed and use as directed- externally; avoid eye contact.
2. Wash hands before/after application. Do not cover, wrap, or bandage treatment area; may increase absorption/cause skin to shrink (atrophy).
3. Report failure to heal; may indicate contact dermatitis from agent.
4. Report any skin infections, may need antifungal/antibacterial agent.
5. Report any severe burning, stinging, swelling, numbness, lack of response. Do not use continuously for more than 2 weeks.

OUTCOMES/EVALUATE

Relief/healing of inflamed/pruritic skin manifestations

Clofarabine   IV

(klo-**FAIR**-ah-been)

CLASSIFICATION(S):

Antineoplastic, antimetabolite
PREGNANCY CATEGORY: D
Rx: Clolar.

USES

Acute lymphoblastic leukemia (ALL) in clients 1–21 years of age with relapsed or refractory ALL after at least 2 prior regimens.

ACTION/KINETICS

Action

Clofarabine is a purine nucleoside antimetabolite; it is metabolized within cells to the 5'-monophosphate metabolite by deoxycytidine kinase and mono- and di-phosphokinases to the active 5'-

triphosphate metabolite. The drug inhibits DNA synthesis by decreasing cellular deoxynucleotide triphosphate pools through inhibition of ribonucleotide reductase, and by terminating DNA chain elongation and inhibiting repair through incorporation into the DNA chain by competitive inhibition of DNA polymerases. Clofarabine 5'-triphosphate also disrupts the integrity of mitochondrial membranes resulting in release of the proapoptotic mitochondrial proteins, cytochrome C and apoptosis-inducing factor, leading to programmed cell death.

Pharmacokinetics
$t^{1/2}$, **terminal:** 5.2 hr. From 49–60% is excreted in the urine unchanged. **Plasma protein binding:** 47%, mainly albumin.

CONTRAINDICATIONS
Lactation. Use of drugs with known renal toxicity during the 5 days of clofarabine administration. Concomitant use of drugs known to induce hepatic toxicity.

SPECIAL CONCERNS
Use with caution in renal or hepatic impairment. Clients are at an increased risk for severe, opportunistic infections. Safety and efficacy have not been determined for use in adults. Use with caution, and closely monitor, clients taking drugs known to affect BP or cardiac function during administration of clofarabine.

SIDE EFFECTS
Most Common
Headache, dermatitis, pruritus, diarrhea, abdominal pain, N&V, anorexia, epistaxis, fatigue, pyrexia, rigors, flushing, hypotension, erythema, petechiae, constipation, febrile neutropenia, edema, pain in limb, cough, pain.
Hematologic: Neutropenia, anemia, leukopenia, febrile neutropenia, thrombocytopenia. **Tumor lysis syndrome/ cytokine release symptoms:** Tachycardia, tachypnea, hypotension, pulmonary edema. **Systemic inflammatory response syndrome/capillary leak syndrome:** *Respiratory distress*, hypotension, pleural and pericardial effusions, *multiple organ failure*. **GI:** N&V,

diarrhea, abdominal pain, constipation, gingival bleeding, sore throat, oral candidiasis. **CV:** Tachycardia, pericardial effusion, left ventricular systolic dysfunction, hypotension, flushing, hypertension. **CNS:** Headache, anxiety, dizziness depression, irritability, somnolence, tremor. **Dermatologic:** Pruritus, dermatitis, petechiae, erythema, palmar-plantar erythrodysesthesia syndrome, contusion, dry skin. **Hepatic:** Hepatomegaly, jaundice. **Musculoskeletal:** Pain in limb, myalgia, back pain, arthralgia. **Respiratory:** Epistaxis, cough, dyspnea, pleural effusion, pneumonia, respiratory distress. **Body as a whole:** Infections (one or more), edema, decreased weight, pyrexia, rigors, fatigue, pain, mucosal inflammation, *sepsis*, staphylococcal infection, lethargy. **Miscellaneous:** Anorexia, decreased appetite, hematuria, bacteremia, cellulitis, herpes simplex, injection site pain.

LABORATORY TEST CONSIDERATIONS
↑ ALT, AST, creatinine.

HOW SUPPLIED
Solution for Injection: 1 mg/mL.

DOSAGE
- **IV INFUSION**
  Acute lymphoblastic leukemia.
Ages, 1–21 years: 52 mg/m^2 daily infused over 2 hr for 5 consecutive days. Repeat treatment cycle following recovery or return to baseline organ function (about every 2–6 weeks).

NURSING CONSIDERATIONS
ADMINISTRATION/STORAGE
IV 1. Administer under supervision of qualified physician experienced in use of antineoplastic therapy.
2. To prevent incompatibilities, do not administer any other medication through same IV line.
3. Filter solution for injection through a sterile 0.2 micron syringe filter, and then further dilute, per package insert instructions, with D5W or 0.9% NaCl injection prior to IV infusion. Administer over 2 hours for 5 consecutive days.
4. To reduce effects of tumor lysis/other side effects, give continuous IV fluids throughout the 5 days of clofarabine administration. The use of prophylactic

---

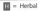 = see color insert   **H** = Herbal   **IV** = Intravenous   ℝ = sound alike drug

steroids (e.g., hydrocortisone, 100 mg/m² on days 1 through 3) may prevent S&S of systemic inflammatory response syndrome or capillary leak.

5. If the client shows early S&S of systemic inflammatory response syndrome or capillary leak, stop infusion and provide appropriate supportive measures.

6. After solution is diluted may store at room temperature for no more than 24 hr. Store vials containing undiluted clofarabine from 15–30°C (59–86°F).

ASSESSMENT

1. Used for acute lymphoblastic leukemia (ALL) in clients 1–21 years of age with relapsed or refractory ALL after at least 2 prior regimens. List other regimens trialed.

2. Dose is based on BSA, using actual height and weight before start of each treatment cycle.

3. Monitor renal and LFTs. Must be back to baseline before resuming therapy.

4. Ensure adequate hydration, give continuous IV fluids during 5 days of clofarabine.

5. Use prophylactic steroids (e.g., hydrocortisone, 100 mg/m² on days 1 through 3) to help prevent S&S of systemic inflammatory response syndrome or capillary leak (hypotension) which can be fatal. Consider allopurinol; reduces hyperuricemia from rapid cell lysis.

6. Monitor closely; report changes in VS, neurological status, renal, LFTs or CBC.

CLIENT/FAMILY TEACHING

1. Used to treat relapsed or unresponsive ALL in children. Carries high incidence of side effects; requires close/careful monitoring. Report unusual/adverse effects immediately.

2. Report any dizziness, lightheadedness, fainting reduced urine output. May experience vomiting/diarrhea; follow measures to prevent dehydration-take medications as directed.

3. If BP drops during therapy and rebounds will resume therapy but at a lower dose. If drop in BP requires medication therapy, therapy will be stopped and supportive measures continued un-

til stabilized. Labs drawn frequently to evaluate organ function and prevent adverse effects.

4. Consider egg/sperm donation in appropriate clients; fertility may be impaired. Practice reliable contraceptive measures; drug teratogenic.

OUTCOMES/EVALUATE

Inhibition of malignant cell proliferation

Clonazepam @ 📷
(kloh-**NAY**-zeh-pam)

CLASSIFICATION(S):

Anticonvulsant, miscellaneous

Rx: Klonopin, Klonopin Wafers, **C-IV**

✦Rx: Apo-Clonazepam, Clonapam, Gen-Clonazepam, Novo-Clonazepam, Nu-Clonazepam, PM-Clonazepam, Rhoxal-clonazepam, Rivotril, ratio-Clonazepam.

SEE ALSO *ANTICONVULSANTS.*

USES

(1) Alone or as an adjunct to treat absence seizures (petit mal variant) including Lennox-Gastaut syndrome. (2) Alone or as an adjunct to treat akinetic and myoclonic seizures. (3) Some effectiveness in absence seizures resistant to succinimide therapy. (4) Panic disorder with or without agoraphobia, as defined by DSM-IV. *Investigational:* Parkinsonian (hypokinetic) dysarthria, acute manic episodes of bipolar affective disorder, leg movements (periodic) during sleep, adjunct in treating schizophrenia, neuralgias (deafferentation pain syndrome), multifocal tic disorders.

ACTION/KINETICS

Action

Benzodiazepine derivative which increases presynaptic inhibition and suppresses the spread of seizure activity.

Pharmacokinetics

Peak plasma levels: 1–2 hr. **t½:** 18–50 hr. **Therapeutic serum levels:** 20–80 ng/mL. Metabolized almost completely in the liver to inactive metabolites, which are excreted in the urine. Even though a benzodiazepine, clonazepam is used mainly as an anticonvulsant.

However, contraindications, side effects, and so forth are similar to those for diazepam. **Plasma protein binding:** About 97%.

CONTRAINDICATIONS

Sensitivity to benzodiazepines. Severe liver disease, acute narrow-angle glaucoma. Pregnancy.

SPECIAL CONCERNS

Effects on lactation not known. Safety and efficacy have not been evaluated for panic disorder in clients less than 18 years of age.

SIDE EFFECTS

Most Common

Drowsiness, dizziness, fatigue, asthenia, dry mouth, diarrhea, GI upset, changes in appetite.

See *Diazepam* for a complete list of potential side effects. Also, in clients in whom different types of seizure disorders exist, clonazepam may elicit or precipitate *grand mal seizures*.

DRUG INTERACTIONS

CNS depressants / Potentiation of clonazepam CNS depressant effect
Phenobarbital / ↓ Clonazepam effect R/T ↑ liver breakdown
Phenytoin / ↓ Clonazepam effect R/T ↑ liver breakdown
Valproic acid / ↑ Chance of absence seizures

HOW SUPPLIED

Tablets: 0.5 mg, 1 mg, 2 mg; *Tablets, Oral Disintegrating (also called Wafers):* 0.125 mg, 0.25 mg, 0.5 mg, 1 mg, 2 mg.

DOSAGE——

• **TABLETS; TABLETS, ORAL DISINTEGRATING (ALSO CALLED WAFERS)**

Seizure disorders.

Adults, initial: 0.5 mg 3 times per day; do not exceed this dose. Increase by 0.5–1 mg/day q 3 days until seizures are under control or side effects become excessive; **maximum:** 20 mg/day. In those over 65 years, start on low doses and closely observe. **Pediatric up to 10 years or 30 kg:** 0.01–0.03 mg/kg/day in two to three divided doses up to a maximum of 0.05 mg/kg/day. Increase by increments of no more than 0.25–0.5 mg q 3 days until seizures are under control or maintenance of 0.1–0.2 mg/kg is attained.

Panic disorder.

Adults, initial: 0.25 mg twice a day. Can increase to the target dose by 1 mg/day after 3 days. Some may benefit from doses up to 4 mg/day (increase dose in increments of 0.125–0.25 mg twice a day every 3 days), although incidence of side effects may increase. To reduce somnolence, give 1 dose at bedtime. Discontinue treatment gradually with a decrease of 0.125 mg q 3 days until the drug is completely withdrawn.

Parkinsonian dysarthria.

Adults: 0.25–0.5 mg/day.

Acute manic episodes of bipolar affective disorder.

Adults: 0.75–16 mg/day.

Periodic leg movements during sleep.

Adults: 0.5–2 mg nightly.

Adjunct to treat schizophrenia.

Adults: 0.5–2 mg/day.

Neuralgias.

Adults: 2–4 mg/day.

Multifocal tic disorders.

Adults: 1.5–12 mg/day.

NURSING CONSIDERATIONS

ⓠ Do not confuse Klonopin with clonidine (an antihypertensive).

ADMINISTRATION/STORAGE

1. About one-third of clients show some loss of anticonvulsant activity within 3 months; dosage adjustment may reestablish effectiveness.
2. Adding clonazepam to existing anticonvulsant therapy may increase depressant effects.
3. Divide daily dose in three equal doses; if doses cannot be divided equally, give largest dose at bedtime.
4. With panic disorder, discontinue treatment gradually with a decrease of 0.125 mg twice a day every 3 days until drug is completely withdrawn. Re-evaluate long-term usefulness periodically.
5. Store from 15–30°C (59–86°F); protect from moisture.

ASSESSMENT

1. Note reasons for therapy, onset/cause of symptoms, other agents prescribed, outcome. With seizure disorder note onset, frequency, characteristics of seizures.
2. Obtain baseline CBC, renal and LFTs.

CLIENT/FAMILY TEACHING
1. Give tablets with water; swallow tablet whole.
2. Give orally disintegrating tablet with water as follows: After opening the pouch, peel back foil on the blister. Do not push tablet through foil. Immediately upon opening the blister, using dry hands, remove tablet and place in the mouth. Tablet disintegration occurs rapidly in saliva so it can be swallowed easily with or without water.
3. Take as directed; report any loss of seizure control or adverse side effects.
4. Assess drug effects before performing activities that require mental alertness.
5. Do not stop suddenly after long term use; taper to prevent seizure occurrence.
6. Avoid alcohol and any other CNS depressants. Report oversedation, lack of attentiveness or any other adverse side effects.

OUTCOMES/EVALUATE
- ↓ Number and frequency of seizures
- Therapeutic drug levels 20–80 ng/mL

Clonidine hydrochloride
(**KLOH**-nih-deen)

CLASSIFICATION(S):
Antihypertensive, centrally-acting
PREGNANCY CATEGORY: C
Rx: Catapres, Catapres-TTS-1, -2, and -3, Duraclon.
✽Rx: Apo-Clonidine, Dixarit, Novo–Clonidine, Nu-Clonidine.

SEE ALSO *ANTIHYPERTENSIVE AGENTS.*

USES
Oral, Transdermal: (1) Alone or with a diuretic or other antihypertensives to treat mild to moderate hypertension. (2) Treat spasticity. *Investigational:* Alcohol withdrawal, atrial fibrillation, attention deficit hyperactivity disorder, constitutional growth delay in children, cyclosporine-associated nephrotoxicity, diabetic diarrhea, Gilles de la Tourette's syndrome, hyperhidrosis, hypertensive emergencies, mania, menopausal flushing, opiate detoxification, diagnosis of pheochromocytoma, postherpetic neuralgia, psychosis in schizophrenia, reduce allergen-induced inflammatory reactions in extrinsic asthma, restless leg syndrome, facilitate smoking cessation, ulcerative colitis.

Epidural: With opiates for severe pain in cancer clients not relieved by opiate analgesics alone. Most effective for neuropathic pain.

ACTION/KINETICS
Action
Stimulates alpha-adrenergic receptors of the CNS, resulting in inhibition of the sympathetic vasomotor centers and decreased nerve impulses. Thus, bradycardia and a fall in both SBP and DBP occur. Plasma renin levels are decreased, while peripheral venous pressure remains unchanged. Few orthostatic effects. Although NaCl excretion is markedly decreased, potassium excretion remains unchanged. To relieve spasticity, it decreases excitatory amino acids by central presynaptic α-receptor agonism. Tolerance to the drug may develop. Epidural use causes analgesia at presynaptic and postjunctional alpha-2-adrenergic receptors in the spinal cord due to prevention of pain signal transmission to the brain.

Pharmacokinetics
Onset, PO: 30–60 min; **transdermal:** 2–3 days. **Peak plasma levels, PO:** 3–5 hr; **transdermal:** 2–3 days. **Maximum effect, PO:** 2–4 hr. **Duration, PO:** 12–24 hr; **transdermal:** 7 days (with system in place). **t½:** 12–16 hr. Approximately 50% excreted unchanged in the urine; 20% excreted through the feces. **Epidural: t½, distribution,** 19 min; **elimination:** 22 hr.

CONTRAINDICATIONS
Epidurally: Presence of an injection site infection, clients on anticoagulant therapy, in bleeding diathesis, administration above the C4 dermatome. For obstetric, postpartum, or perioperative pain.

SPECIAL CONCERNS

Use with caution during lactation and in the presence of severe coronary insufficiency, recent MI, cerebrovascular disease, or chronic renal failure. Safe use in children not established; when used for attention deficit disorder, even one extra dose can be harmful. Geriatric clients may be more sensitive to the hypotensive effects; a decreased dosage may also be necessary in these clients due to age-related decreases in renal function. For children, restrict epidural use to severe intractable pain from malignancy that is unresponsive to epidural or spinal opiates or other analgesic approaches.

SIDE EFFECTS

Most Common

Dry mouth, drowsiness, dizziness, sedation, constipation.

CNS: Drowsiness, sedation, confusion, dizziness, headache, fatigue, malaise, nightmares, nervousness, restlessness, anxiety, mental depression, increased dreaming, insomnia, hallucinations, delirium, agitation. **GI:** Dry mouth, constipation, anorexia, N&V, parotid pain, weight gain, hepatitis, parotitis, ileus, pseudo-obstruction, abdominal pain. **CV:** CHF, severe hypotension, Raynaud's phenomenon, abnormalities in ECG, palpitations, tachycardia/bradycardia, postural hypotension, conduction disturbances, sinus bradycardia, *CVA*. **Dermatologic:** Urticaria, skin rashes, sweating, *angioneurotic edema*, pruritus, thinning of hair, alopecia, skin ulcer. **GU:** Impotence, urinary retention, decreased sexual activity, loss of libido, nocturia, difficulty in urination, UTI. **Respiratory:** Hypoventilation, dyspnea. **Musculoskeletal:** Muscle/joint pain, leg cramps, weakness. **Miscellaneous:** Gynecomastia, increase in blood glucose (transient), increased sensitivity to alcohol, chest pain, tinnitus, hyperesthesia, pain, infection, thrombocytopenia, syncope, blurred vision, withdrawal syndrome, dryness of mucous membranes of nose; itching, burning, dryness of eyes; skin pallor, fever.

NOTE: When used for ADHD in children, can cause serious side effects, including bradycardia, hypotension, and respiratory depression.

Transdermal products: Localized skin reactions, pruritus, erythema, allergic contact sensitization and contact dermatitis, localized vesiculation, hyperpigmentation, edema, excoriation, burning, papules, throbbing, blanching, generalized macular rash.

NOTE: Rebound hypertension may be manifested if clonidine is withdrawn abruptly.

LABORATORY TEST CONSIDERATIONS

Transient ↑ blood glucose, serum phosphatase, and serum CPK. Weakly + Coombs' test. Electrolyte imbalance.

OD OVERDOSE MANAGEMENT

Symptoms: Hypotension, bradycardia, respiratory and CNS depression, hypoventilation, hypothermia, apnea, miosis, agitation, irritability, lethargy, *seizures, cardiac conduction defects, arrhythmias,* transient hypertension, diarrhea, vomiting. *Treatment:* Maintain respiration; perform gastric lavage followed by activated charcoal. Mg sulfate may be used to hasten the rate of transport through the GI tract. IV atropine sulfate (0.6 mg for adults; 0.01 mg/kg for children) or dopamine to treat persistent bradycardia. IV fluids and elevation of the legs are used to reverse hypotension; if unresponsive to these measures, dopamine (2–20 mcg/kg/min) may be used. To treat hypertension, diazoxide, IV furosemide, or an alpha-adrenergic blocking drug may be used.

DRUG INTERACTIONS

Alcohol / ↑ Depressant effects
Beta-adrenergic blocking agents / Paradoxical hypertension; also, ↑ severity of rebound hypertension following clonidine withdrawal
CNS depressants / ↑ CNS depressant effect
Levodopa / ↓ Levodopa effect
Local anesthetics / Epidural clonidine → prolonged duration of epidural local anesthetics
Mirtazapine / Loss of BP control → antagonism of α-2 adrenergic receptors
Prazosin / ↓ Clonidine antihypertensive effect

Narcotic analgesics / Potentiation of clonidine hypotensive effect

Tolazoline / Blocks antihypertensive effect

Tricyclic antidepressants / Blocks antihypertensive effect

Verapamil / ↑ Risk of AV block and severe hypotension

HOW SUPPLIED

Film, Extended Release, Transdermal: Catapres-TTS-1: 2.5 mg clonidine (surface area 3.5 cm^2), with 0.1 mg released daily; Catapres-TTS-2: 5 mg clonidine (surface area 7 cm^2), with 0.2 mg released daily; and Catapres-TTS-3: 7.5 mg clonidine (surface area 10.5 cm^2), with 0.3 mg released daily; *Injection:* 0.1 mg/mL, 0.5 mg/mL; *Tablets:* 0.1 mg, 0.2 mg, 0.3 mg.

DOSAGE

• TABLETS

Hypertension.

Initial: 0.1 mg twice a day; **then,** increase by 0.1–0.2 mg/day until desired response is attained; **maintenance:** 0.2–0.6 mg/day in divided doses (maximum: 2.4 mg/day). Tolerance necessitates increased dosage or concomitant administration of a diuretic. Gradual increase of dosage after initiation minimizes side effects. **Pediatric:** 0.05–0.4 mg once a day.

NOTE: In hypertensive clients unable to take PO medication, clonidine may be administered sublingually at doses of 0.2–0.4 mcg/day

Treat spasticity.

Adults and children: 0.1–0.3 mg; given in divided doses.

Alcohol withdrawal.

0.3–0.6 mg q 6 hr.

Atrial fibrillation.

0.075 mg 1–2 times per day with or without digoxin.

Attention deficit hyperactivity disorder.

0.005 mg/kg/day for 8 weeks.

Constitutional growth delay in children.

0.038–0.15 mg/m^2/day.

Diabetic diarrhea.

0.1–0.6 mg q 12 hr.

Gilles de la Tourette syndrome.

0.15–0.2 mg/day.

Hyperhidrosis.

0.25 mg 3–5 times per day.

Hypertensive urgency (diastolic >120 mm Hg).

Initial: 0.1–0.2 mg; **then,** 0.05–0.1 mg q hr to a maximum of 0.8 mg.

Menopausal flushing.

0.14–0.4 mg/day.

Withdrawal from opiate dependence.

0.015–0.016 mg/kg/day.

Diagnosis of pheochromocytoma.

0.3 mg/day.

Postherpetic neuralgia.

0.2 mg/day.

Psychosis in schizophrenia.

Less than 0.9 mg/day.

Reduce allergen-induced inflammation in extrinsic asthma.

0.15 mg for 3 days or 0.075 mg/1.5 mL saline by inhalation.

Restless leg syndrome.

0.1–0.3 mg/day, up to 0.9 mg/day.

Facilitate cessation of smoking.

0.15–0.75 mg/day for 3–10 weeks.

Ulcerative colitis.

0.3 mg 3 times per day.

• FILM, EXTENDED-RELEASE, TRANSDERMAL

Hypertension.

Initial: Use 0.1-mg system; **then,** if after 1–2 weeks adequate control has not been achieved, can use another 0.1-mg system or a larger system. The antihypertensive effect may not be seen for 2–3 days. The system should be changed q 7 days.

Treat spasticity.

Adults and children: 0.1–0.3 mg; apply patch q 7 days.

Cyclosporine-associated nephrotoxicity.

0.1–0.2 mg/day.

Diabetic diarrhea.

0.3 mg/24-hr patch (1 or 2 patches/week).

Menopausal flushing.

0.1 mg/24-hr patch.

Facilitate cessation of smoking.

0.2 mg/24-hr patch.

• EPIDURAL INFUSION

Analgesia.

Initial: 0.3 mg/hr. Dose may then be titrated up or down, depending on pain relief and side effects.

NURSING CONSIDERATIONS

℮ Do not confuse Catapres with Cataflam (a nonsteroidal anti-inflammatory drug) or with Combipres (combination antihypertensive drug). Do not confuse clonidine with Klonopin (an anticonvulsant).

ADMINISTRATION/STORAGE

1. May take 2–3 days to achieve effective blood levels using transdermal system. Therefore, reduce any prior drug dosage gradually.
2. With severe hypertension may require other antihypertensive drug therapy in addition to transdermal clonidine.
3. If drug to be discontinued, do so gradually over a period of 2–4 days.
4. Do not use preservative when given epidurally.
5. Store injection at controlled room temperature. Discard any unused portion.

ASSESSMENT

1. Identify reasons for therapy, onset, type of symptoms, and previous treatments.
2. Obtain CBC, liver and renal function studies. Promote periodic eye exams.
3. Note occupation; drug may interfere with the ability to work.
4. List drugs currently prescribed to prevent any interactions. With propranolol, observe for a paradoxical hypertensive response. With tolazoline or TCA, be aware that these may block the antihypertensive action of clonidine; clonidine dosage may need to be increased
5. Tolerance may develop with long term use; an increased dose or addition of diuretic may improve response.
6. Note evidence of alcohol, drug, or nicotine addiction. These agents usually work well in this group of clients (especially the once-a-week patch).
7. Monitor BP closely. BP decreases occur within 30–60 min after administration and may persist for 8 hr. Note any fluctuations to determine whether to use clonidine alone or concomitantly with a diuretic. A stable BP reduces orthostatic effects with postural changes.

8. Patch (transdermal) may take 2–3 days to exert effects and therefore oral therapy may be needed during this time. Assess skin sites for rash or itching and change sites weekly.

CLIENT/FAMILY TEACHING

1. With transdermal system, apply to hairless area of skin, such as upper arm or torso. Change system q 7 days; use different site with each application.
2. If taken PO, take last dose of the day at bedtime to ensure overnight control of BP. Keep a log of BP and HR.
3. Do not engage in activities that require mental alertness, such as operating machinery or driving a car; may cause drowsiness.
4. Do not change regimen or discontinue drug abruptly. Withdrawal should be gradual to prevent rebound hypertension.
5. Record weight daily, in the morning, in clothing of the same weight, to determine if there is edema caused by sodium retention. Any fluid retention should disappear after 3–4 days. Change positions slowly to prevent sudden drop in BP and associated dizziness.
6. Clonidine may reduce the effect of levodopa; report any increase in the S&S of Parkinson's disease previously controlled with levodopa.
7. Report any depression (may be precipitated by drug), especially with history of mental depression.

OUTCOMES/EVALUATE

- ↓ BP; ↓ menopausal S&S
- Control of withdrawal symptoms
- Control of neuropathic pain

Clopidogrel bisulfate

(kloh-**PID**-oh-grel)

CLASSIFICATION(S):
Antiplatelet drug
PREGNANCY CATEGORY: B
Rx: Plavix.

USES

(1) Non–ST-segment elevation acute coronary syndrome (unstable angina/non–Q-wave MI), including those who are to be managed medically and those who are to be managed with percutaneous coronary intervention (with or without stent) or coronary artery bypass graft. Clopidogrel decreases the rate of a combined end point of CV death, MI, or stroke, or refractory ischemia. (2) To reduce the rate of death from any cause and the rate of a combined end point of death, reinfarction, or stroke in those with ST-segment elevation acute MI. (3) To reduce the rate of a combined end point of new ischemic stroke (fatal or not), new MI (fatal or not), and other vascular death in those with a history of recent MI, recent stroke, or established peripheral arterial disease. *Investigational:* As a loading dose with aspirin to prevent cardiac side effects in those undergoing coronary stent implantation.

ACTION/KINETICS

Action

Inhibits platelet aggregation by inhibiting binding of adenosine diphosphate (ADP) to its platelet receptor and subsequent ADP-mediative activation of glycoprotein GPIIb/IIIa complex. Effect on receptors is irreversible; thus, platelets are affected for remainder of their lifespan. Also inhibits platelet aggregation caused by agonists other than ADP by blocking amplification of platelet activation by released ADP.

Pharmacokinetics

Rapidly absorbed from GI tract; food does not affect bioavailability. **Peak plasma levels:** About 1 hr. Extensively metabolized in liver; about 50% excreted in urine and 46% in feces. **t½, elimination:** 8 hr.

CONTRAINDICATIONS

Lactation. Active pathological bleeding such as peptic ulcer or intracranial hemorrhage.

SPECIAL CONCERNS

Use with caution in those at risk of increased bleeding from trauma, surgery, or other pathological conditions. Use with caution in severe impaired renal or hepatic function. Safety and efficacy have not been determined in children.

SIDE EFFECTS

Most Common

Skin/appendage disorders, headache, URTI, chest pain, flu-like symptoms.

CV: Edema, hyper/hypotension, syncope, palpitations, atrial fibrillation, *intracranial hemorrhage, major/life-threatening bleeding, retroperitoneal hemorrhage, hemorrhage of operative wound, cardiac failure, pulmonary hemorrhage,* ocular hemorrhage. **GI:** Abdominal pain, dyspepsia, diarrhea, constipation, N&V, taste disorders, colitis (including lymphocytic or ulcerative), pancreatitis, stomatitis, *hemorrhage,* ulcers (peptic, gastric, duodenal), GI bleeding, *perforated hemorrhagic gastritis, hemorrhagic upper GI ulcer, perforated gastric ulcer.* **Hepatic:** Infectious hepatitis, fatty liver, noninfectious hepatitis, *acute liver failure.* **CNS:** Headache, dizziness, depression, hypoesthesia, neuralgia, paresthesia, vertigo, anxiety, insomnia, confusion, hallucinations. **Body as a whole:** Chest pain, accidental injury, flu-like symptoms, pain, fatigue, asthenia, fever, allergic reactions, ischemic necrosis, generalized edema, leg cramps, gout. **Respiratory:** URTI, dyspnea, rhinitis, bronchitis, coughing, pneumonia, sinusitis, hemothorax, bronchospasm, interstitial pneumonitis. **Hematologic:** Purpura/bruises, thrombotic thrombocytopenic purpura (rare), epistaxis, hematoma, anemia, hemarthrosis, hemoptysis, thrombocytopenia, *aplastic anemia, pancytopenia,* hypochromic anemia, neutropenia, *agranulocytosis,* granulocytopenia, leukemia, leukopenia, allergic purpura. **Musculoskeletal:** Arthralgia, back pain, arthritis, arthrosis, myalgia. **Dermatologic:** Disorders of skin/appendages, rash, pruritus, eczema, skin ulceration, bullous eruption, erythematous rash, maculopapular rash, urticaria, *angioedema,* erythema multiforme, linchen planus, *Stevens-Johnson syndrome, toxic epidermal necrolysis.* **GU:** UTI, cystitis, menorrhagia, abnormal renal function, *acute renal failure,* hematuria, glomerulopathy. **Hypersensitivity:**

Bold Italic = life threatening side effect   ■ = black box warning   ♣ = Available in Canada

Angioedema, bronchospasm, *anaphylaxis*. **Ophthalmic:** Cataract, conjunctivitis; conjunctival, ocular, and retinal bleeding. **Miscellaneous:** Hernia, *anaphylactoid reactions,* hypersensitivity reactions, serum sickness, vasculitis.

LABORATORY TEST CONSIDERATIONS
Hypercholesterolemia, hematuria, bilirubinemia, hyperuricemia. ↑ Hepatic enzymes, NPN. ↓ Platelets, neutrophils. Prolonged bleeding time. Abnormal creatinine levels, abnormal LFTs.

OD **OVERDOSE MANAGEMENT**
Symptoms: Prolonged bleeding time and subsequent bleeding complications. *Treatment:* Platelet transfusion may be needed to reverse the effects of clopidogrel if a quick reversal is required.

DRUG INTERACTIONS
Aspirin / ↑ Risk of life-threatening or major bleeding events (e.g., intracranial and GI hemorrhage) in high-risk clients with recent ischemic stroke or TIAs
Atorvastatin / Inhibition of clopidogrel effects on platelet function R/T inhibition of metabolic conversion (by CYP3A4) of the prodrug clopidogrel to the active drug
Bupropion / ↑ Bupropion AUC and peak plasma levels R/T inhibition of metabolism by CYP2B6 hydroxylation of bupropion
H *Evening primrose oil* / Potential for ↑ antiplatelet effect
H *Feverfew* / Potential for ↑ antiplatelet effect
H *Garlic* / Potential for ↑ antiplatelet effect
H *Ginger* / Potential for ↑ antiplatelet effect
H *Ginkgo biloba* / Potential for ↑ antiplatelet effect
H *Grapeseed extract* / Potential for ↑ antiplatelet effect
Macrolide antibiotics (e.g., erythromycin) / Inhibition of antiplatelet effect of clopidogrel
NSAIDs (e.g., naproxen) / ↑ Risk of occult blood loss; use together with caution
Rifamycins / ↑ Clopidogrel antiplatelet effect
Simvastatin / Inhibition of clopidogrel effects on platelet function R/T inhibition of metabolic conversion (by CYP3A4) of the prodrug clopidogrel to the active drug
Statins / Possible antiplatelet drug resistance
Warfarin / Clopidogrel prolongs bleeding time → ↑ risk of major bleeding; safety of use with warfarin not established

HOW SUPPLIED
Tablets: 75 mg.

DOSAGE
• **TABLETS**
  Acute coronary syndrome, non–ST-segment elevation.
Initial: Single 300 mg loading dose; **then,** 75 mg once daily. Initiate and continue aspirin (75–325 mg once daily). Many clients also receive heparin acutely.
  Acute coronary syndrome, ST-segment elevation.
75 mg once daily, given with aspirin, with or without thrombolytics. Clopidogrel may be initiated with or without a loading dose of 300 mg.
  Recent MI, stroke, or established peripheral arterial disease.
Adults: 75 mg once daily.

NURSING CONSIDERATIONS
℘ Do not confuse Plavix with Pletal (also an antiplatelet drug) or Paxil (antidepressant).

ADMINISTRATION/STORAGE
Dosage adjustment not necessary for geriatric clients or with renal disease.

ASSESSMENT
1. Note atherosclerotic event (MI, stroke), CABG, stent (note type), or established peripheral arterial disease requiring therapy.
2. Assess for any active bleeding as with ulcers or intracranial bleeding; precludes therapy.
3. List all drugs prescribed/consumed especially OTC (i.e., NSAIDs, ASA, herbals).

CLIENT/FAMILY TEACHING
1. Take exactly as directed; may take without regard to food. Food will lessen chance of stomach upset.
2. May cause dizziness or drowsiness.

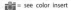

3. Avoid OTC agents especially aspirin, aspirin-containing products, or NSAIDs, unless prescribed.

4. Report any unusual bruising or bleeding; advise all providers of prescribed therapy.

5. Drug should be discontinued 7 days prior to elective surgery.

6. Keep all F/U appointments to evaluate response to therapy.

OUTCOMES/EVALUATE
- Inhibition of platelet aggregation
- Reduction of atherosclerotic events

Clorazepate dipotassium

(klor-**AYZ**-eh-payt)

CLASSIFICATION(S):
Antianxiety drug, benzodiazepine, anticonvulsant, miscellaneous

PREGNANCY CATEGORY: D

Rx: Tranxene T-tab, Tranxene-SD, Tranxene-SD Half Strength, **C-IV**
✤**Rx:** Apo-Clorazepate, Novo-Clopate.

SEE ALSO *TRANQUILIZERS/ ANTIMANIC DRUGS/HYPNOTICS.*

USES
(1) Anxiety disorders or short-term relief of symptoms of anxiety. (2) Symptomatic relief of acute alcohol withdrawal. (3) Adjunct to treat partial seizures.

ACTION/KINETICS

Pharmacokinetics
Peak plasma levels: 1–2 hr. **t½:** 40–50 hr. Hydrolyzed in the stomach to desmethyldiazepam, the active metabolite. Oxazepam is also an active metabolite. **t½, desmethyldiazepam:** 30–100 hr; **t½, oxazepam:** 5–15 hr. **Time to peak plasma levels:** 0.5–2 hr. Slowly excreted by the kidneys. **Plasma protein binding:** 97–98%.

ADDITIONAL CONTRAINDICATIONS
Depressed clients, nursing mothers.

SPECIAL CONCERNS
Use with caution with impaired renal or hepatic function.

SIDE EFFECTS

Most Common
Drowsiness, dizziness, fatigue, dry mouth, stomach upset, constipation, blurred vision, headache.

See *Tranquilizers/Antimanic Drugs/Hypnotics* for a complete list of possible side effects.

HOW SUPPLIED
Tablets, Extended-Release: 11.25 mg, 22.5 mg; *Tablets, Immediate-Release:* 3.75 mg, 7.5 mg, 15 mg.

DOSAGE

- **TABLETS, IMMEDIATE-RELEASE**
  Anxiety.
Initial: 30 mg/day in divided doses; gradually adjust dose to 15–60 mg/day. **Alternative.** Single daily dosage: **Adult, initial,** 15 mg at bedtime; subsequent dosage adjustment may be needed. **Elderly or debilitated clients, initial:** 7.5–15 mg/day.

  Acute alcohol withdrawal.
Day 1, initial: 30 mg; **then,** 30–60 mg in divided doses; **day 2:** 45–90 mg in divided doses; **day 3:** 22.5–45 mg in divided doses; **day 4:** 15–30 mg in divided doses. Thereafter, reduce to 7.5–15 mg/day and discontinue as soon as possible. Maximum daily dose: 90 mg.

  Partial seizures.
Adults and children over 12 years, initial: 7.5 mg 3 times/day; increase no more than 7.5 mg/week to maximum of 90 mg/day. **Children (9–12 years), initial, maximum:** 7.5 mg twice a day; increase by no more than 7.5 mg/week to maximum of 60 mg/day. Not recommended for children under 9 years of age.

- **TABLETS, EXTENDED-RELEASE**
  Maintenance therapy for anxiety disorders or partial seizures.
The 11.25 mg ER tablet may be given as a single dose q 24 hr as an alternate dosage form for those stabilized on a dose of 3.75 mg 3 times per day. The 22.5 mg ER tablet may be given as a single daily dose as an alternate dosage form for those stabilized on 7.5 mg 3 times per day. Do not use either strength to initiate therapy.

Bold Italic = life threatening side effect   ▮ = black box warning   ✤ = Available in Canada

NURSING CONSIDERATIONS

ADMINISTRATION/STORAGE

Store clorazepate dipotassium tablets at controlled room temperature from 15–30°C (59–86°F). Protect from moisture and light.

ASSESSMENT

1. Note reasons for therapy, symptom characteristics/behavioral manifestations; evidence of depression.
2. Monitor CBC, renal, and LFTs; assess for dysfunction especially with prolonged therapy.
3. With excessive alcohol intake, determine timing of last drink.

CLIENT/FAMILY TEACHING

1. Take as directed; do not alter prescribed dose.
2. Avoid activities requiring mental alertness until drug effects realized.
3. May use sugarless gum or candy to control dry mouth symptoms.
4. Avoid alcohol and any other CNS depressants.
5. Report increased depression or any adverse effects or lack of response.

OUTCOMES/EVALUATE

- ↓ Anxiety and tension
- ↓ S&S of alcohol withdrawal
- Control of seizures

Clotrimazole
(kloh-**TRY**-mah-zohl)

CLASSIFICATION(S):

Antifungal
PREGNANCY CATEGORY: C (systemic use), **B** (topical/vaginal use).
OTC: Lotion (1%), Solution, Topical Cream: Cruex, Desenex, Lotrimin AF. **Vaginal Cream:** Gyne-Lotrimin-3 and -7, Mycelex-7. **Vaginal Suppositories:** Gyne-Lotrimin 3. **Vaginal Cream and Vaginal Suppositories:** Gyne-Lotrimin 3, Mycelex-7.
Rx: Topical Cream, Lotion, Solution: Lotrimin. **Troche:** Mycelex.
♣**OTC:** Canesten Topical/Vaginal, Clotrimaderm.

SEE ALSO ANTI-INFECTIVES.

USES

Broad-spectrum antifungal. **Oral troche:** (1) Oropharyngeal candidiasis. (2) Reduce incidence of oropharyngeal candidiasis in clients who are immunocompromised due to chemotherapy, radiotherapy, or steroid therapy used for leukemia, solid tumors, or kidney transplant. **Topical OTC products:** Tinea pedis, tinea cruris, and tinea corporis due to *T. rubrum, T. mentagrophytes, E. floccosum,* and *M. canis.* **Topical Rx products:** Candidiasis due to *C. albicans* and tinea versicolor due to *M. furfur.* **Vaginal products:** Vulvovaginal candidiasis.

ACTION/KINETICS

Action

Depending on concentration, may be fungistatic or fungicidal. Acts by inhibiting the biosynthesis of sterols, resulting in damage to the cell wall and subsequent loss of essential intracellular elements due to altered permeability. May also inhibit oxidative and peroxidative enzyme activity and inhibit the biosynthesis of triglycerides and phospholipids by fungi. When used for *Candida albicans,* the drug inhibits transformation of blastophores into the invasive mycelial form.

Pharmacokinetics

Poorly absorbed from the GI tract and metabolized in the liver to inactive compounds that are excreted through the feces. **Duration:** Up to 3 hr.

CONTRAINDICATIONS

Hypersensitivity. First trimester of pregnancy. Topically in children less than 2 years of age. Use around the eyes.

SPECIAL CONCERNS

Use with caution during lactation. Safety and effectiveness for PO use in children age 3 or under has not been determined. For topical use, supervise children under age 12.

SIDE EFFECTS

Most Common

Topical use on skin: Irritation, rash, stinging, burning, pruritus.
Topical use in vagina: Vaginal irritation, itching, burning.
Use of troche: N&V.

Skin: Irritation including rash, stinging, pruritus, urticaria, erythema, burning, peeling, blistering, edema, general skin irritation. **Vaginal:** Lower abdominal cramps; urinary frequency; bloating; vaginal irritation, itching or burning; dyspareunia. **Hepatic:** Abnormal liver function tests. **GI:** N&V following use of troche.

HOW SUPPLIED
Oral Troche: 10 mg; *Topical Cream:* 1%; *Lotion:* 1%; *Solution:* 1%; *Vaginal Cream:* 1%, 2%; *Vaginal Suppositories:* 200 mg; *Combination/Twin Packs: Suppositories/ Cream:* 100 mg/1%, 200 mg/1%.

DOSAGE
- **TOPICAL CREAM; LOTION; SOLUTION**
  OTC for Tinea pedis/corporis.
Use daily for 4 weeks. If no improvement, consult provider.
  OTC for Tinea cruris.
Use daily for 2 weeks. If no improvement, consult provider.
  OTC cream for vaginal yeast infections.
Apply to affected areas morning and evening for 7 consecutive days or as needed.
  Rx for candidiasis and tinea versicolor.
Massage into affected skin and surrounding areas twice a day (in morning and evening). Diagnosis should be reevaluated if no improvement occurs in 4 weeks.
- **TROCHE**
  Treatment of oropharyngeal candidiasis.
One troche (10 mg) 5 times per day for 14 consecutive days.
  Prophylaxis of oropharyngeal candidiasis.
One troche 3 times per day for duration of chemotherapy or until maintenance doses of steroids are instituted.
- **VAGINAL CREAM**
  Vulvovaginal candidiasis.
Insert 1 full applicator at bedtime for 3–7 consecutive days.
- **VAGINAL SUPPOSITORIES**
  Vulvovaginal candidiasis.
Insert 1 suppository (200 mg) at bedtime for 3 consecutive days.

NURSING CONSIDERATIONS
ADMINISTRATION/STORAGE
1. Do not allow topical products to come in contact with the eyes.
2. Slowly dissolve the troche in the mouth.
3. Store Mycelex-7 vaginal cream at 2–30°C (36–86°F). Do not store Mycelex-7 100-mg vaginal troche above 35°C (95°F); store the 500-mg vaginal troche below 30°C (86°F).

ASSESSMENT
Note location, onset, and characteristics of S&S. List other agents/therapies trialed and outcome. List skin scraping/culture results.

CLIENT/FAMILY TEACHING
1. Review goals of therapy/appropriate method for administration. Wash hands before/after treatments. Unless otherwise directed, apply only after cleaning the affected area.
2. Take oral lozenge into mouth letting it dissolve over 15–30 min for best results.
3. With vaginal infections, do not engage in intercourse; or, to prevent reinfection or pain, have partner wear a condom. Avoid contact with eyes.
4. To prevent staining of clothes, use sanitary napkin with vaginal tablets or cream.
5. If exposed to HIV and recurrent vaginal yeast infections occur, seek prompt medical intervention to determine cause of symptoms.
6. Report adverse effects or lack of response.

OUTCOMES/EVALUATE
- Eradication of fungal infection
- Symptomatic improvement

Bold Italic = life threatening side effect　　■ = black box warning　　✦ = Available in Canada

—*COMBINATION DRUG*—

Clotrimazole and Betamethasone dipropionate

(kloh-**TRY**-mah-zohl,
bay-tah-**METH**-ah-zohn)

CLASSIFICATION(S):
Topical antifungal/corticosteroid
PREGNANCY CATEGORY: C
Rx: Lotrisone.

SEE ALSO *CLOTRIMAZOLE* AND
BETAMETHASONE DIPROPIONATE.

USES
Topical treatment of symptomatic inflammatory tinea pedis, tinea cruris, and tinea corporis due to *Epidermophyton floccosum, Trichophyton mentagrophytes,* and *T. rubrum.*

CONTENT
Each gram of cream or lotion contains: Clotrimazole (antifungal), 10 mg, and Betamethasone dipropionate (corticosteroid), 0.643 mg (equivalent to 0.5 mg betamethasone).

ACTION/KINETICS
Action
Clotrimazole inhibits the biosynthesis of sterols, resulting in cell wall damage and subsequent loss of essential intracellular elements due to altered permeability. May also inhibit oxidative and peroxidative enzyme activity and inhibit the biosynthesis of triglycerides and phospholipids by fungi. The anti-inflammatory effect of betamethasone results from inhibition of prostaglandin synthesis. The drug also inhibits accumulation of macrophages and leukocytes at sites of inflammation and inhibits phagocytosis and lysosomal enzyme release.

Pharmacokinetics
Skin penetration and systemic absorption of clotrimazole have not been studied. Betamethasone is absorbed after topical use, the extent of which depends on the vehicle, integrity of the epidermal barrier, and use of occlusive dressings.

CONTRAINDICATIONS
Use in clients less than 17 years of age and in those who are sensitive to clotrimazole, betamethasone, other corticosteroids or imidazoles, or to any component of the product. Use for diaper dermatitis is not recommended.

SPECIAL CONCERNS
Systemic absorption of topical corticosteroids can cause reversible hypothalamic-pituitary-adrenal axis suppression with the potential for glucocorticoid insufficiency after treatment is withdrawn. Children may be more susceptible to systemic toxicity (e.g., Cushing's syndrome, linear growth retardation, delayed weight gain, intracranial hypertension) from equivalent doses due to their large skin surface to body mass ratios. Use with caution during lactation.

SIDE EFFECTS
Most Common
Use of the Cream: Paresthesia, rash, edema, secondary infection.
Use of the Lotion: Burning/dry skin, stinging.
Dermatologic: Itching, irritation, dryness, folliculitis, hypertrichosis, acneiform eruptions, hypopigmentation, perioral dermatitis, allergic contact dermatitis, maceration of the skin, secondary infection, skin atrophy, striae, milaria, erythema, stinging, blistering, peeling, edema, pruritus, urticaria, general skin irritation, paresthesia, rash, burning or dry skin.

HOW SUPPLIED
See Content.

DOSAGE
• **CREAM; LOTION**
  Symptomatic inflammatory tinea pedis, tinea cruris, and tinea corporis.
Adults and children over 17 years of age: Gently massage sufficient cream or lotion into the affected skin areas twice a day, in the morning and evening.

NURSING CONSIDERATIONS
ADMINISTRATION/STORAGE
1. Do not use either the cream or lotion longer than 2 weeks when treating tinea corporis or tinea cruris, and amounts greater than 45 grams per

---

week of the cream or greater than 45 mL of the lotion should not be used.
2. When treating tinea corporis or tinea cruris, review the diagnosis if no improvement is seen after 1 week.
3. Do not use either the cream or lotion for longer than 4 weeks when treating tinea pedis.
4. When treating tinea pedis, review the diagnosis if no improvement is seen after 2 weeks.
5. Do not use either the cream or lotion with occlusive dressings.
6. Do not use the cream or lotion for more than 2 weeks in the groin area. Loose-fitting clothing should be worn.
7. Shake the lotion well before each use.
8. Store both the cream and lotion from 15–30°C (59–86°F).

ASSESSMENT
1. Note onset, location, and characteristics of skin lesions.
2. Describe clinical presentation and do skin scraping if lesion not definitive.

CLIENT/FAMILY TEACHING
1. Cream contains a combination of a steroid and an antifungal used to treat the inflammation and infection. Use as directed for the time directed.
2. Do not take Lotrisone cream/lotion internally and keep away from eyes. Wash hands before and after each use.
3. Wash and completely dry skin in the affected area. Gently rub the medicine into the affected and surrounding areas until evenly distributed. If in the groin area, use only for 2 weeks and apply cream sparingly; wear loose-fitting clothing.
4. Report any blistering, burning, dry skin, hives, infection, itching, peeling, reddened skin, skin eruptions and rash.
5. Avoid occlusive coverings/bandages without approval. Keep all F/U appointments to evaluate response to therapy.

OUTCOMES/EVALUATE
Healing/clearing of lesions

Clozapine
(**KLOH**-zah-peen)

CLASSIFICATION(S):
Antipsychotic
PREGNANCY CATEGORY: B
Rx: Clozaril, FazaClo.
♣Rx: Rhoxal-clozapine.

USES
(1) Severely ill schizophrenic clients who do not respond adequately to conventional antipsychotic therapy, either because of ineffectiveness or intolerable side effects from other drugs. May be effective in chronic refractory schizophrenia. (2) Recurrent suicidal behavior in schizophrenia or schizoaffective disorders in clients who are at chronic suicide risk (do not use orally disintegrating tablets for this purpose). *Investigational:* Acute manic and/or mixed episodes associated with bipolar disorder, psychosis/agitation in dementia or Alzheimer disease, psychosis in Parkinson's disease.

ACTION/KINETICS
Action
Interferes with the binding of dopamine to both D-1 and D-2 receptors; more active at limbic than at striatal dopamine receptors. Thus, is relatively free from extrapyramidal side effects and does not induce catalepsy. Also acts as an antagonist at adrenergic, cholinergic, histaminergic, and serotonergic receptors. Increases the amount of time spent in REM sleep. Causes a high incidence of sedation, anticholinergic effects, and orthostatic hypotension.

Pharmacokinetics
Is 27–47% bioavailable; food does not affect the bioavailability of clozapine. **Peak plasma levels:** 2.5 hr. **Average maximum concentration at steady state:** 122 ng/mL plasma after 100 mg twice a day. $t\frac{1}{2}$: 12 hr. Metabolized in the liver to inactive compounds and excreted through the urine (50%) and feces (30%). **Plasma protein binding:** About 97%.

CONTRAINDICATIONS

Myeloproliferative disorders. Use in those with a history of clozapine–induced agranulocytosis or severe granulocytopenia; use with other agents known to suppress bone marrow function. Use with other agents having a known potential to cause agranulocytosis or otherwise suppress bone marrow function. Severe CNS depression or coma due to any cause. Lactation. Due to the possibility of development of agranulocytosis and seizures, avoid continued use in clients failing to respond.

SPECIAL CONCERNS

■ (1) Agranulocytosis. Because of a significant risk of agranulocytosis, a potentially life-threatening adverse reaction, reserve clozapine for use in the treatment of severely ill clients with schizophrenia who fail to show an acceptable response to adequate courses of standard antipsychotic drug treatment because of insufficient efficacy or the inability to achieve an effective dose because of intolerable adverse reactions from those drugs or for reducing the risk of recurrent suicidal behavior in clients with schizophrenia or schizoaffective disorder who are judged to be at risk of reexperiencing suicidal behavior. (2) Clients being treated with clozapine must have a baseline white blood cell (WBC) count and absolute neutrophil count (ANC) before initiation of treatment as well as regular WBC counts and ANCs during treatment and for at least 4 weeks after discontinuation of treatment. (3) Clozapine is available only through a distribution system that ensures monitoring of WBC counts and ANCs. (4) Seizures have been associated with the use of clozapine. Dose appears to be an important predictor of seizure, with a greater likelihood at higher clozapine doses. Use caution when administering clozapine to clients who have a history of seizures or other predisposing factors. Advise clients not to engage in any activity in which sudden loss of consciousness could cause serious risk to themselves or others. (5) Myocarditis. Analysis of postmarketing safety databases suggest that clozapine is associated with an increased risk of fatal myocarditis, especially during, but not limited to, the first month of therapy. In clients in whom myocarditis is suspected, promptly discontinue clozapine treatment. (6) Orthostatic hypotension, with or without syncope, can occur with clozapine treatment. Rarely, collapse can be profound and be accompanied by respiratory and/or cardiac arrest. Orthostatic hypotension is more likely to occur during initial titration in association with rapid dose escalation. In clients who have had even a brief interval off clozapine (2 or more days since the last dose), start treatment with 12.5 mg once or twice daily. (7) Because collapse, respiratory arrest, and cardiac arrest during initial treatment have occurred in clients who were being administered benzodiazepines or other psychotropic drugs, caution is advised when clozapine is initiated in clients taking a benzodiazepine or any other psychotropic drug. (8) Elderly clients with dementia-related psychosis treated with atypical antipsychotic drugs are at an increased risk of death compared with placebo. Analyses revealed a risk of death in the drug-treated clients of between 1.6 and 1.7 times that seen in placebo-treated clients. Over the course of a typical 10-week controlled trial, the rate of death in drug-treated clients was about 4.5% compared with a rate of about 2.6% in the placebo group. Although the causes of death were varied, most of the deaths appeared to be either cardiovascular (e.g heart failure, sudden death) or infectious (e.g., pneumonia) in nature. Clozapine is not approved for the treatment of clients with dementia-related psychosis.■ Use with caution in clients with known CV disease, prostatic hypertrophy, narrow angle glaucoma, hepatic or renal disease. Increased incidence of cardiomyopathy.

SIDE EFFECTS

Most Common

Drowsiness, sedation/somnolence, salivation, syncope, vertigo, dizziness, constipation, dyspepsia, hypotension, tremor.

 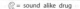

Hematologic: *Agranulocytosis*, leukopenia, neutropenia, eosinophilia. **CNS: Seizures** (appear to be dose dependent), drowsiness, sedation/somnolence, dizziness, vertigo, headache, tremor, restlessness, nightmares, hypokinesia, akinesia, agitation, akathisia, confusion, rigidity, fatigue, insomnia, hyperkinesia, weakness, lethargy, slurred speech, ataxia, depression, anxiety, epileptiform movements. **CV:** Orthostatic hypotension (especially initially) with or without syncope, tachycardia, syncope, hypertension, angina, chest pain, **cardiac abnormalities, myocarditis**, changes in ECG. **Neuroleptic malignant syndrome: Hyperpyrexia**, muscle rigidity, altered mental status, irregular pulse or BP, tachycardia, diaphoresis, cardiac dysrhythmias. **GI:** Constipation, dyspepsia, nausea, heartburn, abdominal discomfort, vomiting, diarrhea, anorexia. **GU:** Urinary abnormalities, incontinence, abnormal ejaculation, urinary frequency/urgency/ retention. **Musculoskeletal:** Muscle weakness, tremor, pain (back, legs, neck), muscle spasm/ache. **Respiratory:** Dyspnea, SOB, throat discomfort, nasal congestion. **Miscellaneous:** Salivation, sweating, visual disturbances, fever (transient), dry mouth, rash, weight gain, numb or sore tongue, increased risk of diabetes.

LABORATORY TEST CONSIDERATIONS
Hyperprolactinemia.

OD OVERDOSE MANAGEMENT
Symptoms: Drowsiness, delirium, tachycardia, **respiratory depression,** hypotension, hypersalivation, **seizures, coma.** *Treatment:* Establish airway; maintain with adequate oxygenation and ventilation. Give activated charcoal and sorbitol. Monitor cardiac status and VS. General supportive measures.

DRUG INTERACTIONS
Anticholinergic drugs / Additive anticholinergic effects
Antihypertensive drugs / Additive hypotensive effects
Benzodiazepines / Possible respiratory depression/collapse
Digoxin / ↑ Digoxin effect R/T ↓ plasma protein binding

Epinephrine / Clozapine may reverse effects when given for hypotension
Phenobarbital / ↓ Clozapine levels R/T ↑ liver breakdown
Smoking / ↓ Clozapine levels R/T ↑ hepatic metabolism by CYP1A2
H *St. John's wort* / Possible ↓ clozapine levels R/T ↑ metabolism
Warfarin / ↑ Warfarin effect R/T ↓ plasma protein binding

HOW SUPPLIED
Tablets: 12.5 mg, 25 mg, 50 mg, 100 mg, 200 mg; *Tablets, Oral Disintegrating:* 12.5 mg, 25 mg, 50 mg, 100 mg.

DOSAGE

• **TABLETS; TABLETS, ORAL DISINTEGRATING**
  Schizophrenia.

Adults, initial: 12.5 mg 1–2 times per day; **then,** if drug tolerated, the dose can be increased by 25–50 mg/day to a dose of 300–450 mg/day at the end of 2 weeks. Subsequent dosage increments should occur no more often than once or twice a week in increments not to exceed 100 mg. **Usual maintenance dose:** 300–600 mg/day (although doses up to 900 mg/day may be required in some clients). Total daily dose should not exceed 900 mg. *NOTE:* Consult manufacturer's clozapine guidelines based on WBC and ANC for treatment alterations, including reinitiation of treatment.
  Recurrent suicidal behavior.
Follow the dosage and administration recommendations for schizophrenia. **Mean daily dose:** 300 mg; **range:** 12.5–900 mg. A course of treatment for at least 2 years is recommended in order to maintain the reduction of risk for suicidal behavior. After 2 years, reassess risk of suicidal behavior. *NOTE:* Do not use orally disintegrating tablets in those with recurrent suicidal behavior.

NURSING CONSIDERATIONS

℗ Do not confuse Clozaril with Clinoril (a NSAID).

ADMINISTRATION/STORAGE
1. Clozapine is available through independent 'Clozaril treatment systems' based on a plan developed by physicians and pharmacists to ensure safe

---

Bold Italic = life threatening side effect   ■ = black box warning   ✤ = Available in Canada

use of the drug with respect to weekly CBC monitoring, data reporting, and drug dispensing. Prescriptions are limited to 1-week supplies, and drug may only be dispensed following receipt, by the pharmacist, of weekly WBC test results that fall within the established limits. All weekly blood test results must be reported by participating pharmacists to the Clozaril National Registry (1-800-448-5938).

2. If drug is effective, seek lowest maintenance doses possible to maintain remission.

3. If termination of therapy is planned, gradually reduce dose over a 1–2-week period. If cessation of therapy is abrupt due to toxicity, observe client carefully for recurrence of psychotic symptoms.

4. Clozapine therapy may be initiated immediately upon discontinuation of other antipsychotic medication; however, a 24-hr 'washout period' is desirable.

5. When restarting clients who have had even a brief interval off of clozapine (i.e., 2 days or more since the last dose), treatment should be reinitiated with 12.5 mg once or twice daily. If this dose is well tolerated, it may be possible to titrate clients back to a therapeutic dose more quickly than is recommended for initial treatment. However, any client who has previously experienced respiratory or cardiac arrest with initial dosing, but was then able to be titrated successfully to a therapeutic dose should be retitrated with extreme caution, even after 24 hr of discontinuation.

6. Clients discontinued for WBC counts below 2,000/mm³ or an ANC below 1,000/mm³ must not be restarted on clozapine.

7. Store orally disintegrating tablets, protected from moisture, from 15–30°C (59–86°F). Store tablets below 30°C (86°F).

ASSESSMENT

1. List reasons for therapy; assess behavioral manifestations. Identify other therapies trialed and outcome.

2. Note seizure disorder, enlarged prostate, CAD, or glaucoma.

3. Check baseline VS and ECG; report any irregular pulse, tachycardia, hyperpyrexia, or hypotension. Monitor S&S closely; may cause myocarditis/cardiomyopathy.

4. Obtain CBC and LFTs prior to initiating therapy. Monitor and report WBCs once weekly for the first six months of therapy, then every 2 weeks if stable.

5. Use the following therapy guidelines based on WBC and ANC:

- Do not begin treatment if WBC is <3,500/mm³ or there is a history of myelolproliferative disorder or previous clozapine-induced agranulocytosis or granulocytopenia.

- If WBC is <3,500/mm³ or >3,500/mm³ with a substantial drop from baseline, or presence of immature forms following initiation of treatment, repeat WBC and differential counts. S&S of infection include lethargy, weakness, fever, and sore throat.

- If WBC is 3,000/mm³ to 3,500/mm³ on subsequent counts and ANC is >1,500/mm³, perform twice-weekly WBC and differential counts.

- If WBC is <3,000/mm³ or ANC is <1,500/mm³, interrupt therapy and monitor for flu-like symptoms or orther symptoms of infection. Perform WBC count and differential daily. May resume therapy if no signs of infection develop, WBC count is >3,000/mm³ and ANC is >1,500/mm³. However, continue twice weekly WBC and differential counts until WBC returns to >3,500/mm³ and then monitor WBC weekly for 6 months.

- If WBC is <2,000/mm³ or ANC is <1,000/mm³, monitor WBC count and differential daily. Consider bone marrow aspiration to determine granulopoetic status. If granulopoiesis is deficient, consider protective isolation. If infection develops, perform cultures and begin antibiotics. Do not rechallenge with clozapine because agranulocytosis may develop with a shorter latency.

6. Follow manufacturer's guidelines for clients reinitiated on clozapine.

---

7. Monitor for S&S of hyperglycemia and diabetes mellitus.

8. Assess risks vs benefits of therapy with family/client. Periodically reassess to determine continued need for therapy.

CLIENT/FAMILY TEACHING

1. Do not push orally disintegrating tablet through foil. Just prior to use, peel foil from the blister and gently remove orally disintegrating tablet. Immediately place tablet in mouth, allow to disintegrate, and swallow with saliva. No water is needed. Destroy half tablets.

2. Take as directed; do not stop abruptly. Used only when conventional therapies fail due to risk of adverse side effects.

3. Report symptoms of lethargy, weakness, fever, sore throat, malaise, mucous membrane ulceration, S&S of infection or other adverse effects.

4. Rinse mouth frequently; perform regular oral care to minimize potential for candidiasis.

5. Avoid driving or other hazardous activity due to possibility of seizures.

6. Because of (orthostatic) drop in BP, use care when rising from a lying or sitting position.

7. Avoid hot showers or baths and hot weather exposure.

8. Report if pregnancy occurs or client desires to become pregnant. Do not breast feed.

9. Avoid other prescription drugs, OTC drugs, or alcohol.

10. Stress importance of weekly WBC to assess for agranulocytosis. These are reported to a national registry (Clozaril Patient Management System at 800-448-5938) and must be completed before prescriptions will be issued and filled.

OUTCOMES/EVALUATE

- Improved behavior patterns with ↓ agitation, ↓ hyperactivity, ↓ delusions, paranoia, and hallucinations
- Improved coping behaviors and thought patterns

Coagulation Factor Ⅳ VIIa (Recombinant)

CLASSIFICATION(S):
Antihemophilic agent
PREGNANCY CATEGORY: C
Rx: NovoSeven.

USES

(1) Treatment of bleeding episodes in hemophilia A or B clients with inhibitors to Factor VIII or Factor IX and in clients with acquired hemophilia. (2) Prevention of bleeding in surgical interventions or invasive procedures in hemophilia A or B clients with inhibitors to Factor VIII or Factor IX and in clients with acquired hemophilia. (3) Treatment of bleeding episodes in clients with congenital factor VII deficiency. (4) Prevention of bleeding in surgical interventions or invasive procedures in clients with congenital factor VII deficiency.

ACTION/KINETICS

Action

Structurally similar to human plasma-derived Factor VIIa. The purification process removes exogenous viruses. To eliminate the risk of human viral contamination, no human serum or other proteins are used to produce the product. Promotes hemostasis by activating the intrinsic pathway of the coagulation cascade. When complexed with tissue factor, the drug can activate coagulation Factor X to Factor Xa, as well as coagulation Factor IX to Factor IXa. Factor Xa, in complex with other factors, converts prothrombin to thrombin leading to formation of a hemostatic plug by converting fibrinogen to fibrin.

Pharmacokinetics

$t\frac{1}{2}$: 2.3 hr. **Median in vivo plasma recovery:** 44%.

CONTRAINDICATIONS

Hypersensitivity to the product, any components of the product, or to mouse, hamster, or bovine proteins. Lactation.

SPECIAL CONCERNS

Clients with DIC, advanced artherosclerotic disease, crush injury, or septicemia

---

Bold Italic = life threatening side effect   ■ = black box warning   ♣ = Available in Canada

may have an increased risk of developing thrombotic events. There is a potential increased risk of arterial thromboembolic side effects, including myocardial ischemia, MI, and cerebral ischemia and/or infarction. Use with caution for prolonged dosing.

SIDE EFFECTS

Most Common

Arthralgia, edema, headache, hemorrhage, hyper-/hypotension, injection site reactions, N&V, pain, pyrexia, rash.

CV: Hemorrhage NOS, thrombotic reactions, decreased plasma fibrinogen, hyper-/hypotension, bradycardia, coagulation disorder, *DIC*, increased fibrinolysis, decreased prothrombin, thrombosis, decreased plasma fibrinogen, thromboembolic reactions (e.g., arterial thrombosis, *cerebral infarction* and/or ischemia, *DVT*, *MI*, myocardial ischemia, *pulmonary embolism*, thrombophlebitis). **GI:** N&V. **Dermatologic:** Injection site reaction, pruritus, purpura, rash. **Musculoskeletal:** Arthralgia, arthrosis. **Hypersensitivity:** Hives, urticaria, tightness of chest, wheezing, hypotension, *anaphylaxis*. **Miscellaneous:** Fever, allergic reaction, arthrosis, hemarthrosis, edema, headache, pain, pneumonia, abnormal renal function.

DRUG INTERACTIONS

Potential interaction with activated prothrombin complex concentrates; avoid simultaneous use.

HOW SUPPLIED

Powder for Injection, Lyophilized: 1.2 mg/vial, 2.4 mg/vial, 4.8 mg/vial.

DOSAGE

• IV BOLUS ONLY

Hemophilia A or B with inhibitors.

90 mcg/kg q 2 hr until hemostasis is achieved or until treatment is deemed to be inadequate. Dosage (35–120 mcg/kg) and administration interval may be adjusted based on severity of bleeding and degree of hemostasis achieved. Clients treated for joint or muscle bleeds showed beneficial effects within 8 doses, although more doses are required for severe bleeds. The appropriate duration of post-hemostatic dosing has not been determined. For severe bleeds, continue dosing at 3–6 hr intervals after hemostasis is achieved. The biological and clinical effects of prolonged elevated levels of Factor VIIa have not been studied; thus, minimize duration of post-hemostatic dosing. Monitor clients during this time.

Surgical interventions.

Initial: 90 mcg/kg immediately before the intervention; repeat at 2-hr intervals for the duration of surgery. For minor surgery, postsurgical dosing by bolus infusion should occur at 2-hr intervals for the first 48 hr and then at 2 to 6-hr intervals until healing has occurred. For major surgery, postsurgical dosing by bolus infusion should occur at 2-hr intervals for 5 days, followed by 4-hr intervals until healing has occurred. Give additional bolus doses if needed.

Congenital factor VII deficiency.

Dose range: 15–30 mcg/kg q 4–6 hr until hemostatis is achieved. Effective treatment has been reached with doses as low as 10 mcg/kg. Adjust dose and frequency individually.

Acquired hemophilia.

Dose range: 70–90 mcg/kg repeated q 2–3 hr until hemostasis is achieved.

NURSING CONSIDERATIONS

ADMINISTRATION/STORAGE

IV 1. Use the following procedure to reconstitute:
- Bring lyophilized powder and diluent (sterile water for injection) to room temperature, but no higher than 37°C (98.6°F).
- Always use aseptic technique. Remove cap from vial to expose the central portion of the rubber stopper. Cleanse stopper with alcohol swab and allow to dry.
- Draw back plunger of sterile syringe/needle and admit air into syringe.
- Insert needle of syringe into diluent vial. Inject air into the vial and withdraw quantity required for reconstitution. For the 1.2 mg vial, add 2.2 mL of diluent; for the 4.8 mg vial add 8.5 mL of diluent.
- Insert the syringe/needle containing diluent into the vial with the powder through the center of the rubber stopper. Aim the needle against the

side so that the stream of liquid runs down the vial wall. Do not inject the diluent directly on the powder.

- Gently swirl the vial until all powder is dissolved. After reconstitution, each vial contains about 0.6 mg/mL rFVIIa. The reconstituted solution is clear and colorless (do not use if particulate matter or discoloration observed). Use within 3 hr after reconstitution.

2. Administer the reconstituted solution as follows:

- Draw back plunger of a sterile syringe/needle and admit air into the syringe.
- Insert needle into the vial of reconstituted rFVIIa and inject air into the vial. Withdraw the appropriate amount of reconstituted drug into the syringe.
- Remove and discard needle from the syringe and attach a suitable IV needle. Administer as a slow bolus injection over 2–5 min, depending on the dose.
- Discard any unused reconstituted solution after 3 hr.

3. Do not mix rFVIIa with infusion solutions (data not available).

4. Prior to reconstitution refrigerate at 2–8°C (36–46° F). Avoid exposure to direct sunlight.

5. After reconstitution, store either at room temperature or refrigerate for 3 hr or less. Do not freeze reconstituted drug or store in syringes.

ASSESSMENT

1. Note reasons for therapy i.e.; uncontrolled bleeding in hemophilia A/B clients with inhibitors to Factor VIII or IX; trauma or surgery.

2. Assess renal function, PT, PTT, and plasma FVII clotting activity. Evaluate any swelling or pain for hidden bleed.

3. Clients with DIC, advanced ASHD, crush injuries, or septicemia have increased risk of developing a thrombotic event; monitor closely.

4. Monitor VS, cardiac rhythm, neurologic findings, level of consciousness.

CLIENT/FAMILY TEACHING

1. Identify reasons for therapy, risks/benefits associated with therapy. Factor

VIIa is a man-made protein produced to replicate the naturally occurring activated factor VII (factor VIIa) in the body. Factor VIIa is used to stop bleeding of injuries for those with hemophilia by helping the blood to clot. This man-made protein, factor VIIa, is used in people who have Hemophilia A or Hemophilia B, who have also formed antibodies against other clotting proteins that help bleeding to stop.

2. The dose is based on body weight and how much, how often, and where in your body you are bleeding.

3. Report S&S of hypersensitivity i.e.; wheezing, chest tightness, itching, hives, ↓ BP, shock.

4. Avoid activities that may cause injury such as contact sports and josteling/falling activities. Report any swelling/joint pains or adverse effects.

OUTCOMES/EVALUATE

Control of bleeding episodes in hemophilia A/B clients

Codeine phosphate
(KOH-deen)

CLASSIFICATION(S):
Narcotic analgesic, C-II
PREGNANCY CATEGORY: C

Codeine sulfate

CLASSIFICATION(S):
Narcotic analgesic, C-II
PREGNANCY CATEGORY: C

SEE ALSO NARCOTIC ANALGESICS.

USES

(1) Relief of mild to moderate pain. (2) In combination with aspirin or acetaminophen to enhance analgesia. (3) Antitussive, often in combination with other respiratory drugs to treat cough.

ACTION/KINETICS

Action

Produces less respiratory depression and N&V than morphine. Moderately habit-forming and constipating. Dosages over 60 mg often cause restlessness and excitement and irritate the cough center. In lower doses it is a potent antitussive and is an ingredient in many cough syrups.

Pharmacokinetics

Onset, PO: 10–30 min; **IV:** 15 min. **Peak effect:** 30–60 min. **Duration, PO:** 4–6 hr; **IV:** 5 hr. **t½, elimination:** 2.5–3 hr. Metabolized in the liver and excreted in the urine. Codeine is two-thirds as effective PO as parenterally. Codeine phosphate may be given as an oral solution or by injection.

CONTRAINDICATIONS

Premature infants or during labor when delivery of a premature infant is expected.

SPECIAL CONCERNS

May increase the duration of labor. Use with caution and reduce the initial dose in clients with seizure disorders, acute abdominal conditions, renal or hepatic disease, fever, Addison's disease, hypothyroidism, prostatic hypertrophy, ulcerative colitis, urethral stricture, following recent GI or GU tract surgery, and in the young, geriatric, or debilitated clients. Nursing mothers who are ultrarapid metabolizers of codeine may have abnormally high levels of morphine in their breast milk that can cause serious, even fatal, side effects (increased tiredness, difficulty breathing, limpness, difficulty breast feeding) in nursing infants.

SIDE EFFECTS

Most Common

Orthostatic hypotension, tachycardia, anxiety, dizziness, lethargy, mood changes, sedation, sweating, biliary tract spasm, constipation, dry mouth, N&V, urinary hesitancy/retention, skin rash, miosis.

See *Narcotic Analgesics* for a complete list of possible side effects.

ADDITIONAL DRUG INTERACTIONS

Combination with chlordiazepoxide may induce coma.

HOW SUPPLIED

Codeine phosphate *Injection:* 15 mg/mL, 30 mg/mL; *Oral Solution:* 15 mg/5 mL.

Codeine sulfate *Tablets:* 15 mg, 30 mg, 60 mg.

DOSAGE

- **ORAL SOLUTION; TABLETS**

Analgesia.

Adults: 15–60 mg q 4–6 hr, not to exceed 360 mg/day. **Pediatric, over 1 year:** 0.5 mg/kg or 15 mg/m² q 4–6 hr.

Antitussive.

Adults: 10–20 mg q 4–6 hr, not to exceed 120 mg/day. **Pediatric, 2–6 years:** 2.5–5 mg q 4–6 hr, not to exceed 30 mg/day; **6–12 years:** 5–10 mg q 4–6 hr, not to exceed 60 mg/day.

- **INJECTION**

Analgesic.

Adults: 30 mg SC or IM q 4 hr as needed. **Usual dose range:** 15–60 mg. **Children:** 500 micrograms/kg or 15 mg/m² SC or IM q 4 hr as needed.

NURSING CONSIDERATIONS

ADMINISTRATION/STORAGE

Codeine is incompatible with soluble barbiturates.

ASSESSMENT

1. List reasons for therapy, onset, location, characteristics of S&S, other agents trialed, outcome.

2. Assess for conditions that may warrant lowered dose or cautious use. Rate pain level. Identify name, dose, form and route prescribed.

CLIENT/FAMILY TEACHING

1. Take as directed, tylenol and aspirin act synergistically with codeine and are usually given together. May take with food or milk to decrease GI upset.

2. Increase intake of fluids, fruits, and fiber to decrease constipation.

3. Use caution, may cause dizziness/drowsiness.

4. Avoid alcohol/CNS depressants. If taken with librium derivatives may cause coma.

5. Report altered mental patterns, lack of desired effect.

6. If taking codeine syrups to suppress coughs, do not overuse. If productive coughing is suppressed, may cause additional congestion.

7. Keep all F/U appointments to evaluate response.

OUTCOMES/EVALUATE

- Relief of pain

 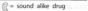

- Control of coughing with improved sleeping patterns

Colchicine
(**KOHL**-chih-seen)

CLASSIFICATION(S):
Antigout drug
PREGNANCY CATEGORY: C (oral use), **D** (parenteral use).
Rx: Colchicine Tablets.

USES
Prophylaxis and treatment of acute attacks of gout. *Investigational:* Chronic prophylactic therapy to treat familial Mediterranean fever to decrease frequency and severity of serositis attacks or as intermittent short-term therapy to abort an acute attack, primary biliary cirrhosis, hepatic cirrhosis, adjunct in the treatment of primary amyloidosis, Behçet's disease, scleroderma, Sweet's syndrome, sarcoid arthritis, acute inflammatory calcific tendonitis, arthritis associated with erythema nodosum, leukemia, adenocarcinoma of the GI tract, mycosis fungoides, intraurethral condyloma acuminata in men (topically).

ACTION/KINETICS
Action
May reduce the crystal-induced inflammation by reducing lactic acid production by leukocytes (resulting in a decreased deposition of sodium urate), by inhibiting leukocyte migration, and by reducing phagocytosis. May also inhibit the synthesis of kinins and leukotrienes. Although pain is reduced, colchicine is not an analgesic or a uricosuric.

Pharmacokinetics
$t^{1/2}$, **plasma:** 10–60 min. **Onset, IV:** 6–12 hr; **PO:** 12 hr. **Time to peak levels, PO:** 0.5–2 hr. It concentrates in leukocytes ($t^{1/2}$, about 46 hr). Metabolized in the liver and mainly excreted in the feces with 10–20% excreted unchanged through the urine.

CONTRAINDICATIONS
Blood dyscrasias. Serious GI, hepatic, cardiac, or renal disorders. Use in presence of combined renal and hepatic disease.

SPECIAL CONCERNS
Use with caution during lactation. Safety and efficacy have not been determined in children. Geriatric clients may be at greater risk of developing cumulative toxicity. Use with extreme caution for elderly, debilitated clients, especially in the presence of chronic renal, hepatic, GI, or CV disease. May impair fertility.

SIDE EFFECTS
Most Common
N&V, diarrhea (may be severe), abdominal pain/cramps, dermatoses.
The drug is toxic; thus clients must be carefully monitored. **GI:** N&V, diarrhea, abdominal cramps/pain. **Hematologic:** ***Aplastic anemia, agranulocytosis,*** or thrombocytopenia following long-term therapy. **Miscellaneous:** Peripheral neuritis, purpura, myopathy, neuropathy, alopecia, reversible azoospermia, dermatoses, hypersensitivity, thrombophlebitis at injection site (rare), liver dysfunction. If such symptoms appear, discontinue drug at once and wait at least 48 hr before reinstating drug therapy.

LABORATORY TEST CONSIDERATIONS
Alters liver function tests. ↑ Alkaline phosphatase, AST. ↓ Thrombocyte values. False + for hemoglobin or RBCs in urine.

OD OVERDOSE MANAGEMENT
Symptoms: (Acute Intoxication): Characterized at first by violent GI tract symptoms such as N&V, abdominal pain, and diarrhea. The latter may be profuse, watery, bloody, and associated with severe fluid and electrolyte loss. Also, burning of throat and skin, hematuria and oliguria, rapid and weak pulse, general exhaustion, muscular depression, and CNS involvement. ***Death is usually caused by respiratory paralysis.*** *Treatment: (Acute Poisoning):* Gastric lavage, symptomatic support, including atropine and morphine, artificial respiration, hemodialysis, peritoneal dialysis, and treatment of shock.

DRUG INTERACTIONS
Acidifying agents / Inhibit colchicine action

Bold Italic = life threatening side effect   ■ = black box warning   ✦ = Available in Canada

C

Alkalinizing agents / Potentiate colchicine action

CNS depressants / Clients may be more sensitive to CNS depressant effects

Cyclosporine / Possible severe symptoms, including GI, hepatic, renal, and neuromuscular toxicity

Macrolide antibiotics / Severe colchicine toxicity (sometimes leading to death) R/T inhibition of metabolism by CYP3A4

Sympathomimetic agents / Enhanced by colchicine

Vitamin B_{12} / Colchicine may interfere with gut absorption

HOW SUPPLIED

Injection: 0.5 mg/mL; *Tablets:* 0.6 mg.

DOSAGE

- **TABLETS**

  Acute gouty arthritis.

  Adults, usual: 1.2 mg followed by 0.6 mg q 1–2 hr until pain is relieved or nausea, vomiting, or diarrhea occurs. **Total amount required:** 4–8 mg.

  Prophylaxis during intercritical periods.

  Adults: 0.6 mg/day for 3–4 days a week if the client has less than one attack per year or 0.6 mg/day if the client has more than one attack per year.

  Prophylaxis for surgical clients.

  Adults: 0.6 mg 3 times per day for 3 days before and 3 days after surgery.

- **IV ONLY**

  Acute attack of gout.

  Adults, initial: 2 mg; **then,** 0.5 mg q 6 hr until pain is relieved; give no more than 4 mg in a 24-hr period. Some physicians recommend a single IV dose of 3 mg while others recommend no more than 1 mg for the initial dose, followed by 0.5 mg once or twice daily, if needed. If pain recurs, 1–2 mg/day may be given for several days; however, colchicine should not be given by any route for at least 7 days after a full course of IV therapy (i.e., 4 mg).

  Prophylaxis or maintenance of recurrent or chronic gouty arthritis.

  0.5–1 mg 1–2 times per day. However, PO colchicine is preferred (usually with a uricosuric drug).

NURSING CONSIDERATIONS

ADMINISTRATION/STORAGE

1. Store in tight, light-resistant containers.

2. Parenterally, give only IV; SC or IM causes severe local irritation.

IV 3. For parenteral administration, give undiluted or may dilute in 10–20 mL of NSS without a bacteriostatic agent or with sterile water. Administer over 2–5 min.

4. Avoid extravasation; may cause tissue damage with resultant nerve damage.

5. Do not use turbid solutions.

6. Not compatible with dextrose-containing solutions.

ASSESSMENT

1. List symptom onset; any other attacks, frequency, and any preventative therapy prescribed.

2. Note age and general physical condition.

3. Identify joint involvement, noting pain, swelling, and degree of mobility; may need to aspirate joint for definitive diagnosis.

4. Monitor CBC, joint x-ray, uric acid levels, and renal and LFTs.

CLIENT/FAMILY TEACHING

1. Drug seems to alter body's response to deposited uric acid crystals. This leads to less swelling and less pain. Take as prescribed; at the first sign of joint pain or other symptom of impending gout attack. The maximum dose is 10 tablets or 4–8 mg in 24 hr; do not exceed. It usually takes 12–48 hr for relief of symptoms.

2. Acute episodes may be precipitated by aspirin, alcohol, or foods high in purine; avoid.

3. Stop drug and report if N&V, or diarrhea develops; these are signs of toxicity. With severe diarrhea, medication (paregoric) may be needed.

4. Report evidence of liver dysfunction (yellow discoloration of eyes, skin, or stool). LFTs may be scheduled during long-term use.

5. Females should avoid pregnancy.

   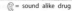

6. Drug will not prevent the progression of this disease-only controls symptoms.

7. Consume 3–3.5 L/day of fluids to enhance crystal excretion.

8. NSAIDs may help with pain and inflammation; use as prescribed. Report any unusual bruising/bleeding, weakness, numbness or tingling, fatigue, rash, sore throat or fever.

OUTCOMES/EVALUATE
- ↓ Joint pain/swelling/destruction
- Termination of acute gout attacks
- Relief of pain

Colesevelam hydrochloride
(**koh**-leh-**SEV**-eh-lam)

CLASSIFICATION(S):
Antihyperlipidemic, bile acid sequestrant

PREGNANCY CATEGORY: B

Rx: WelChol.

USES
Given alone or with an HMG-CoA reductase inhibitor, in addition to diet and exercise, to reduce elevated LDL cholesterol in those with primary hypercholesterolemia (Fredrickson Type IIa).

ACTION/KINETICS
Action
Binds bile acids, including glycocholic acid (the major bile acid in humans), in the intestine, impeding their reabsorption. As the bile acid pool becomes depleted, the hepatic enzyme, cholesterol 7-α-hydroxylase, is upregulated which increases the conversion of cholesterol to bile acids. This causes an increased demand for cholesterol in liver cells, resulting in the effects of both increasing transcription and activity of the cholesterol biosynthetic enzyme (HMG-CoA) reductase and increasing the number of hepatic LDL receptors. The result is an increased clearance of LDL cholesterol from the blood, thus lowering serum LDL cholesterol levels.

Pharmacokinetics
Is not absorbed from the GI tract. Maximum response achieved within 2 weeks.

CONTRAINDICATIONS
Use in bowel obstruction.

SPECIAL CONCERNS
Use with caution in clients with triglyceride levels greater than 300 mg/dL and in those with a susceptibility to vitamin K or fat soluble vitamin deficiencies. Safety and efficacy have not been established in children or for use in clients with dysphagia, swallowing disorders, severe GI motility disorders, or major GI tract surgery.

SIDE EFFECTS
Most Common
Flatulence, infection, headache, constipation, diarrhea, pain.

GI: Flatulence, constipation, diarrhea, nausea, dyspepsia, abdominal pain. **CNS:** Headache. **Respiratory:** Sinusitis, rhinitis, increased cough, pharyngitis. **Musculoskeletal:** Back pain, myalgia. **Body as a whole:** Infection, pain, flu syndrome, accidental injury, asthenia.

DRUG INTERACTIONS
See *Cholestyramine*. Give consideration to monitoring drug levels or effects when giving other drugs for which alterations in blood levels could have clinical significance on safety or efficacy.

HOW SUPPLIED
Tablets: 625 mg.

DOSAGE
- **TABLETS**
  Primary hypercholesterolemia.

Monotherapy, initial: Three tablets twice a day with meals or 6 tablets once per day with a meal. Can be increased to 7 tablets, depending on desired effect. **Combination therapy:** Three tablets twice a day with meals or 6 tablets once per day with a meal. Doses of 4–6 tablets per day can be taken safely with a HMG-CoA reductase inhibitor or when the 2 drugs are dosed apart.

NURSING CONSIDERATIONS
ADMINISTRATION/STORAGE
Store at room temperature and protect from moisture.

Bold Italic = life threatening side effect   ■ = black box warning   ✦ = Available in Canada

ASSESSMENT

1. Note reasons for therapy, other agents trialed, outcome.

2. Prior to starting therapy, secondary causes of hypercholesterolemia (e.g., poorly controlled diabetes, hypothyroidism, nephrotic syndrome, dysproteinemias, obstructive liver disease, other drug therapy, alcoholism) should be ruled out.

3. Obtain a 12 hr fasting lipid profile prior to therapy; assess total-C, HDL/LDL-C, and triglycerides. Avoid/monitor carefully if triglycerides are >300. Periodically assess serum cholesterol as outlined in the National Cholesterol Education Program guidelines (http://www.nhlbi.nih.gov/about/ncep/index.htm) to confirm a favorable initial and chronic response.

4. Determine any vitamin K or fat soluble vitamin deficiency, bowel, GI motility or swallowing dysfunction, or major GI tract surgery as these may preclude therapy.

CLIENT/FAMILY TEACHING

1. Take as directed with a liquid and a low fat/low cholesterol meal.

2. Continue to make lifestyle changes that lower coronary risk factors such as smoking cessation, reduction in alcohol intake, low fat/low cholesterol diet, regular daily exercise, weight loss, and reduction in stress.

3. Practice reliable birth control; stop drug and report if pregnancy suspected.

4. Consume foods high in bulk and fiber, report if constipation occurs, may require a stool softener.

5. Report any unusual bruising/bleeding or adverse effects and have labs drawn as ordered.

6. Obtain periodic labs to evaluate response and evaluate organ function.

OUTCOMES/EVALUATE

Reduced LDL cholesterol levels

Colestipol hydrochloride
(koh-**LESS**-tih-poll)

CLASSIFICATION(S):
Antihyperlipidemic, bile acid sequestrant

PREGNANCY CATEGORY: B

Rx: Colestid.

USES

As adjunctive therapy to diet to reduce elevated serum total and LDL cholesterol in those with primary hypercholesterolemia (elevated LDL, cholesterol) who do not respond adequately to diet. *Investigational:* Digitalis toxicity; hyperoxaluria; diarrhea due to bile acids; adjunctive treatment for hyperthyroidism; relief of pruritus associated with partial biliary obstruction (including primary biliary cirrhosis and various other forms of bile stasis); binds to the toxin produced by *Clostridium difficile.*

ACTION/KINETICS

Action

An anion exchange resin that binds bile acids in the intestine, forming an insoluble complex excreted in the feces. The loss of bile acids results in increased oxidation of cholesterol to bile acids and a decrease in LDL and serum cholesterol. Does not affect (or may increase) triglycerides or HDL and may increase VLDL.

Pharmacokinetics

Not absorbed from the GI tract. **Onset:** 1–2 days; **maximum effect:** 1 month. Return to pretreatment cholesterol levels after discontinuance of therapy: 1 month.

CONTRAINDICATIONS

Complete obstruction or atresia of bile duct.

SPECIAL CONCERNS

Use during pregnancy only if benefits outweigh risks. Use with caution during lactation and in children. Children may be more likely to develop hyperchloremic acidosis although dosage has not been established. Clients over 60 years of age may be at greater risk of GI side effects and adverse nutritional effects.

SIDE EFFECTS

Most Common

Constipation (may be severe), N&V, anorexia, flatulence, abdominal distention/cramping, bloating, heartburn, anorexia, headache, dizziness, drowsiness, sour taste in mouth.

GI: Constipation (may be severe and accompanied by fecal impaction), N&V, diarrhea, heartburn, GI bleeding, anorexia, flatulence, steatorrhea, abdominal distention/cramping, bloating, loose stools, indigestion, rectal bleeding/pain, black stools, hemorrhoidal bleeding, ***bleeding duodenal ulcer, peptic ulceration,*** ulcer attack, GI irritation, dysphagia, dental bleeding/caries, hiccoughs, sour taste, pancreatitis, diverticulitis, cholecystitis, cholelithiasis. **CV:** Chest pain, angina, tachycardia (rare). **CNS:** Migraine or sinus headache, anxiety, vertigo, dizziness, lightheadedness, insomnia, fatigue, tinnitus, syncope, drowsiness, femoral nerve pain, paresthesia. **Hematologic:** Ecchymosis, anemia, beeding tendencies due to hypoprothrombinemia. **Allergic:** Urticaria, dermatitis, asthma, wheezing, rash. **Musculoskeletal:** Backache, muscle/joint pain, arthritis, aches and pains in extremities. **Dermatologic:** Rash, dermatitis, urtiaria (rare). *GU:* Hematuria, burnt odor to urine, dysuria, diuresis. **Miscellaneous:** Uveitis, fatigue, weight loss or gain, increased libido, swollen glands, SOB, edema, weakness, swelling of hands/feet, osteoporosis, calcified material in biliary tree and gall bladder, hyperchloremic acidosis in children.

LABORATORY TEST CONSIDERATIONS

Transient and modest ↑ ALT, AST, alkaline phosphatase.

DRUG INTERACTIONS

See *Cholestyramine.* Also, colestipol ↓ bioavailability of diltiazem if colestipol is given with, 1 hr before, or 4 hr after diltiazem.

HOW SUPPLIED

Granules: 5 grams/7.5 grams granules; *Granules for Oral Suspension:* 5 gram packets; *Tablets:* 1 gram.

DOSAGE

• GRANULES; GRANULES FOR ORAL SUSPENSION

Antihyperlipidemic.

Adults, initial: 5 grams once or twice daily with a daily increment of 5 grams at 1- or 2-month intervals. **Range:** 5–30 grams/day (1–6 packets or level scoopfuls) given once daily or in divided doses.

• TABLETS

Antihyperlipidemic.

Adults, initial: 2 grams 1–2 times per day. Dose can be increased by 2 grams, once or twice daily, at 1–2-month intervals. **Total dose:** 2–16 grams/day given once or in divided doses.

NURSING CONSIDERATIONS

ADMINISTRATION/STORAGE

1. If compliance is good and side effects acceptable but desired effect is not obtained with 2–16 grams/day using tablets, consider combined therapy or alternative treatment.

2. In those with preexisting constipation, the starting dose of tablets should be 2 grams once daily and the starting dose of granules is 1 packet or 1 scoop once daily for 5–7 days, increasing to twice daily with monitoring of constipation and of serum lipoproteins, at least twice, 4–6 weeks apart.

3. Granules available in an orange-flavored product.

ASSESSMENT

1. Note reasons for therapy, other agents trialed, outcome.

2. Assess family history, for CAD, risk factors, dietary patterns and exercise regimes.

3. Because it sequesters bile acids, colestipol may interfere with normal fat absorption; may reduce absorption of folic acid and fat soluble vitamins such as A, D, and K.

CLIENT/FAMILY TEACHING

1. Take 30 min before meals, preferably with the evening meal, since cholesterol synthesis is increased during the evening hours. Take other drugs 1 hr before or 4 hr after to reduce interference with absorption.

Bold Italic = life threatening side effect   ■ = black box warning   ♣ = Available in Canada

2. Never take dose in dry form. Always mix granules with 90 mL or more of fruit juice, milk, water, carbonated beverages, applesauce, soup, cereal, or pulpy fruit before administering to disguise unpalatable taste and to prevent resin from causing esophageal irritation or blockage.

3. Rinse glass with a small amount of fluid and swallow to ensure the total amount of the drug is taken.

4. Tablets should be swallowed whole one at a time (i.e., they should not be cut, crushed, or chewed); may be taken with plenty of water or other fluids.

5. Consume adequate amounts of fluids, fruits, and fiber to diminish constipating drug effects. Report unusual bruising/bleeding or adverse effects and have cholesterol panel, LFTs and CBC monitored.

6. Continue to follow dietary restrictions of fat and cholesterol, regular exercise program, smoking cessation, and weight reduction in the overall goal of cholesterol reduction.

7. Serum cholesterol level will return to pretreatment levels within 1 month if drug is discontinued.

OUTCOMES/EVALUATE
↓ LDL-cholesterol levels

—— **COMBINATION DRUG** ——

Conjugated estrogens and Medroxyprogesterone acetate ■

(**KON**-jyou-**gay**-ted **ES**-troh-jens, meh-**drox**-see-proh-**JESS**-ter-ohn)

CLASSIFICATION(S):
Sex hormones
PREGNANCY CATEGORY: X
Rx: PremPro, Premphase.
✚Rx: Premplus.

SEE ALSO *ESTROGENS CONJUGATED* AND *MEDROXYPROGESTERONE ACETATE.*

USES
(1) Moderate to severe vasomotor symptoms associated with menopause in women with an intact uterus. (2) Vulvular and vaginal atrophy.

CONTENT
PremPro: Each tablet contains: Conjugated estrogens/Medroxyprogesterone, 0.3/1.5 mg, 0.45 mg/1.5 mg, 0.625 mg/2.5 mg, 0.625 mg/5 mg. *Premphase:* Two tablet types: One containing conjugated estrogens, 0.625 mg (14 tabs), and one containing conjugated estrogens, 0.625 mg, and medroxyprogesterone acetate, 5 mg (14 tabs).

ACTION/KINETICS
Action
Estrogens combine with receptors in the cytoplasm of cells, resulting in an increase in protein synthesis. During menopause, estrogens are used as replacement therapy. Medroxyprogesterone acetate reduces endometrial hyperplasia and may decrease the number of estrogen receptors.

Pharmacokinetics
Estrogens are metabolized in the liver and excreted mainly in the urine. **Medroxyprogesterone acetate, maximum levels:** 1–2 hr. **t½, after PO:** 2–3 hr for first 6 hr; then, 8–9 hr.

CONTRAINDICATIONS
Known or suspected pregnancy, including use for missed abortion or as a diagnostic test for pregnancy. Known or suspected cancer of the breast or estrogen-dependent neoplasia. Undiagnosed abnormal genital bleeding. Active or past history of thrombophlebitis, thromboembolic disease, or stroke. Liver dysfunction or disease. Lactation.

SPECIAL CONCERNS
■ Estrogens reportedly increase the risk of endometrial carcinoma in postmenopausal women. Do not use estrogens during pregnancy. Use of progestins during the first four weeks of pregnancy is not recommended.■ Use with caution in conditions aggravated by fluid retention, including asthma, epilepsy, migraine, and cardiac or renal dysfunction. Estrogens may cause significant increases in plasma triglycerides that may cause pancreatitis and other complica-

tions in clients with familial defects of lipoprotein metabolism.

SIDE EFFECTS

Most Common

Abdominal/back pain, headache, nausea, infection, depression, breast pain. See *Estrogens* and *Progesterone and Progestins* for a complete list of possible side effects.

DRUG INTERACTIONS

See individual drug entries.

HOW SUPPLIED

See Content.

DOSAGE

- **TABLETS**

  Vasomotor symptoms due to menopause, vulvar and vaginal atrophy, prevention of osteoporosis.

PremPro: One 0.625/2.5 mg tablet once daily. *Premphase:* One 0.625 mg conjugated estrogen tablet once daily on days 1 to 14 and one 0.625/5 mg tablet once daily on days 15 to 28.

NURSING CONSIDERATIONS

ADMINISTRATION/STORAGE

Prempro, 0.3 mg/1.5 mg, is approved for moderate to severe symptoms associated with menopause while the 0.45/1.5 mg product is approved for the prevention of postmenopausal osteoporosis.

ASSESSMENT

1. List reasons for therapy (hormone replacement for significant menopausal symptoms), onset, duration, and characteristics of S&S, anticipated length of therapy.

2. Note history or experience with replacement therapy. Do not give for cardiac protection; give for postmenopausal symptom control only.

3. Evaluate for active or past conditions that may preclude drug therapy: liver dysfunction, hyperlipidemia, thrombophlebitis, thromboembolic disorders, cancer of the breast or estrogen-dependent neoplasia, or any undiagnosed abnormal vaginal bleeding (AVB). Monitor closely during use.

CLIENT/FAMILY TEACHING

1. Take as directed; two cards are provided, marked cards 1 and 2.

2. Keep all follow-up exams to assess need for continued therapy. When used for treating vasomotor symptoms or vulval and vaginal atrophy, reevaluate every 3–6 months to assess treatment results.

3. Should not be used to prevent osteoporosis. Will be monitored for signs of endometrial cancer. May need to consider other available therapies such as biphosphonates if for fracture prevention. Diagnostic procedures should be undertaken to rule out malignancy in the event of persistent or recurring abnormal vaginal bleeding (AVB).

4. Report any adverse side effects/lack of desired response. Have regular pelvic exams as scheduled.

OUTCOMES/EVALUATE

Control/reduction of menopausal symptoms

Cortisone acetate

(**KOR**-tih-zohn)

CLASSIFICATION(S):

Glucocorticoid

PREGNANCY CATEGORY: D

Rx: Cortone Acetate.

SEE ALSO *CORTICOSTEROIDS*.

ADDITIONAL USES

(1) Replacement therapy in chronic cortical insufficiency. (2) Short-term (due to strong mineralocorticoid effect) for inflammatory or allergic disorders. **Sterile suspension:** Congenital adrenal hyperplasia in children.

ACTION/KINETICS

Action

Possesses both glucocorticoid and mineralocorticoid activity.

Pharmacokinetics

Short-acting. $t\frac{1}{2}$, **plasma:** 30 min; $t\frac{1}{2}$, **biologic:** 8–12 hr.

SPECIAL CONCERNS

Use during pregnancy only if benefits outweigh risks.

SIDE EFFECTS

Most Common

Insomnia, N&V, GI upset, fatigue, dizziness, muscle weakness, joint pain, in-

---

Bold Italic = life threatening side effect   ■ = black box warning   ✦ = Available in Canada

creased hunger/thirst, problems with diabetes control.

See *Corticosteroids* for a complete list of possible side effects.

HOW SUPPLIED

Injection: 50 mg/mL; *Tablets:* 5 mg, 10 mg, 25 mg.

DOSAGE

- **INJECTION; TABLETS**

  Initial or during crisis.

25–300 mg/day. Decrease gradually to lowest effective dose.

  Anti-inflammatory.

25–150 mg/day, depending on severity of the disease.

  Acute rheumatic fever.

200 mg twice a day on day 1, thereafter, 200 mg/day.

  Addison's disease.

Maintenance: 0.5–0.75 mg/kg/day.

NURSING CONSIDERATIONS

ADMINISTRATION/STORAGE

Single course of therapy should not exceed 6 weeks. Rest periods of 2–3 weeks are indicated between treatments.

ASSESSMENT

1. Note reasons for therapy: crisis or anti-inflammatory, rheumatic fever, or Addison's disease.
2. Identify levels, characteristics of S&S and previous experience with this drug.

CLIENT/FAMILY TEACHING

1. Drug reduces swelling and decreases the body's immune response. Do not take if you have serious bacterial, viral, fungal infection; reduces ability to fight infection
2. Take in the a.m. with milk or food to minimize GI upset.
3. Review correct dosage, length of therapy, rest periods, F/U labs and visit schedules. Do not stop suddenly with long term therapy; wean as directed.
4. Report any adverse effects or lack of response.
5. Do not stop suddenly if you have been taking for a few weeks. May need gradual reduction in dosage before stopping drug.

OUTCOMES/EVALUATE

- Replacement with insufficiency
- Relief of allergic manifestations

- Normal plasma cortisol levels (138–635 nmol/L at 8 a.m.)

Cromolyn sodium (Sodium cromoglycate)

(**CROH**-moh-lin)

CLASSIFICATION(S):

Antiasthmatic drug, antiallergic drug

PREGNANCY CATEGORY: B

OTC: Nasalcrom.

Rx: Crolom, Cromolyn Sodium Ophthalmic Solution, Gastrocrom, Intal.

✦Rx: Apo-Cromolyn Nasal Spray/ Sterules, Nalcrom, Nu–Cromolyn, Opticrom.

USES

Aerosol/Inhalation Solution: (1) Prophylactic and adjunct in the management of bronchial asthma in clients who have a significant bronchodilator-reversible component to their airway obstruction. (2) Prophylaxis of acute bronchospasms induced by exercise, toluene diisocyanate, known allergens, or environmental pollutants.

  Nasal, OTC: Prophylaxis and treatment of allergic rhinitis, including children 2 years and older, due to airborne pollens from trees, grasses, or ragweed and by mold, animals, and dust.

  PO: Mastocytosis (improves symptoms including diarrhea, flushing, headaches, vomiting, urticaria, nausea, abdominal pain, and itching).

  Ophthalmic: Vernal keratoconjunctivitis, vernal conjunctivitis, and vernal keratitis.

  Investigational: PO to treat food allergies and mucosal and serosal eosinophilic gastroenteritis. As alternative therapy in refractory forms of chronic urticaria/angioedema.

ACTION/KINETICS

Action

Acts locally to inhibit the degranulation of sensitized mast cells that occurs after

---

exposure to certain antigens. Prevents the release of histamine, slow-reacting substance of anaphylaxis, and other endogenous substances causing hypersensitivity reactions. When effective, reduces the number and intensity of asthmatic attacks as well as decreasing allergic reactions in the eye. No antihistaminic, anti-inflammatory, or bronchodilator effects and has no role in terminating an acute attack of asthma.

Pharmacokinetics

After inhalation, some drug is absorbed systemically. **t½:** 81 min; from lungs: 60 min. About 50% excreted unchanged through the urine and 50% through the bile. When used in the eye, approximately 0.03% is absorbed. **Onset, ophthalmic:** Several days. **Onset, nasal:** Less than 1 week. **Time to peak effect, nasal:** Up to 4 weeks.

CONTRAINDICATIONS

Hypersensitivity. Acute attacks and status asthmaticus. For mastocytosis in premature infants.

SPECIAL CONCERNS

Safety and efficacy have not been established for the aerosol in children under 5 years old, for the nebulizer in children under 2 years old, and for the ophthalmic solution in children under 4 years old. Reserve use in children under 2 years old to severe disease in which potential benefits clearly outweigh potential risks. Due to the propellants in the aerosol, use with caution in CAD or cardiac arrhythmias. Use with caution for long periods of time, in the presence of renal or hepatic disease, during pregnancy, and during lactation.

SIDE EFFECTS

Most Common

After PO/aerosol use: Bronchospasm (maybe severe), cough, nasal congestion, pharyngeal irritation, wheezing.

After ophthalmic use: Transient ocular stinging or burning after instillation

Respiratory: *Bronchospasm (may be severe and associated with a precipitous fall in pulmonary function), laryngeal edema (rare),* cough, eosinophilic pneumonia, pharyngeal irritation, nasal congestion/stinging, wheezing, or sneezing. **CNS:** Dizziness, drowsiness, headache. **Allergic:** Urticaria, rash, angioedema, serum sickness, ***anaphylaxis***. **Miscellaneous:** Nausea, urinary frequency, dysuria, joint swelling/pain, lacrimation, swollen parotid gland.

Following nebulization: Sneezing, wheezing, nasal itching, cough, nose bleeds, burning, nasal congestion, nausea, drowsiness, serum sickness, stomach ache.

Following aerosol: Lacrimation, swollen parotid gland, dysuria, urinary frequency, dizziness, headache, rash, urticaria, angioedema, joint swelling and pain, nausea, dry or irritated throat, bad taste, cough, wheezing, substernal burning, myopathy (rare).

Following nasal solution: Burning, stinging, irritation of nose; sneezing, nose bleeds, headache, bad taste in mouth, postnasal drip, rash.

Following PO use: GI: Diarrhea, taste perversion, spasm of esophagus, flatulence, dysphagia, burning of mouth and throat. **CNS:** Headache, dizziness, fatigue, migraine, paresthesia, anxiety, depression, psychosis, behavior changes, insomnia, hallucinations, lethargy, lightheadedness after eating. **Dermatologic:** Flushing, angioedema, urticaria, skin burning, skin erythema. **Musculoskeletal:** Arthralgia, stiffness and weakness in legs. **Miscellaneous:** Altered liver function test, dyspnea, dysuria, polycythemia, neutropenia.

HOW SUPPLIED

OTC. *Nasal Solution:* 5.2 mg/inh. **Rx.** *Aerosol Spray:* 800 mcg/actuation; *Ophthalmic Solution:* 4%; *Oral Concentrate:* 100 mg/5 mL; *Solution for Inhalation:* 20 mg/2 mL.

DOSAGE

• **SOLUTION FOR INHALATION**
  Prophylaxis of bronchial asthma.

Adults and children over 2 years old, initial: 20 mg inhaled 4 times per day at regular intervals.

  Prophylaxis of exercise-induced bronchospasm.

Inhale 20 mg of the nebulizer solution no more than 1 hr (the shorter the interval between the dose and exercise, the better the effect) before anticipated

---

Bold Italic = life threatening side effect   ■ = black box warning   ✤ = Available in Canada

C

exercise. Repeat as required for protection during prolonged exercise.

- **AEROSOL SPRAY**
  Management of bronchial asthma.

  Adults and children 5 years and older, initial: 2 metered sprays inhaled 4 times per day at regular intervals. Do not exceed this dose.
  Prophylaxis of acute bronchospasm.
  Inhalation of 2 metered dose sprays 10–15 min (but not more than 60 min) before exposure to precipitating factor.

- **NASAL SOLUTION (OTC)**
  Allergic rhinitis.

  Adults and children 2 years and older: 1 spray in each nostril 3–6 times per day at regular intervals q 4–6 hr. Maximum effect may not be seen for 1–2 weeks.

- **ORAL CONCENTRATE**
  Mastocytosis.

  Adults and children 13 years and older: 200 mg (i.e., 2 ampules) 4 times per day 30 min before meals and at bedtime. **Pediatric, 2–12 years:** 100 mg (i.e., 1 ampule) 4 times per day 30 min before meals and at bedtime. If relief is not seen within 2–3 weeks, dose may be increased, but should not exceed 40 mg/kg/day. **Maintenance:** Reduce dose to minimum amount to maintain client with minimum symptoms.

- **OPHTHALMIC SOLUTION**
  Vernal keratoconjunctivitis, conjunctivitis, keratitis.

  1–2 gtt in each eye 4–6 times/day at regular intervals. 1 gtt contains 1.6 mg cromolyn sodium.

NURSING CONSIDERATIONS

ADMINISTRATION/STORAGE

Continue corticosteroid dosage when initiating cromolyn therapy. If improvement occurs, taper the steroid dosage slowly. May have to reinstitute steroids if cromolyn inhalation is impaired, in times of stress, or in adrenocortical insufficiency.

ASSESSMENT

Note reasons for therapy, onset, characteristics of S&S, triggers, other agents trialed, PFTs, CXR, and pulmonary assessment findings.

CLIENT/FAMILY TEACHING

1. Institute only after acute episode is over, when airway is clear and able to inhale adequately. Acts to inhibit acute reaction by preventing histamine release.
2. Report any adverse effects or loss of response. Remember to rinse/dry all equipment thoroughly and to rinse mouth after each treatment.
3. Directions for using aerosol:
   - Remove cap from mouthpiece and shake the inhaler with canister in place for 5–10 seconds.
   - Breathe out to the end of a normal breath. Place mouthpiece into mouth, use a chamber, or position mouthpiece 2–3 finger widths from open mouth.
   - Slightly tilt head back. Breathe in through mouth slowly for 3–5 sec and press the top of the canister at the same time.
   - Remove inhaler from mouth and hold breath for about 10 sec; allow at least 1 min between inhalations.
4. Directions for using nebulizer solution:
   - Assemble the face mask or mouthpiece and connect the tubing from the port to the compressor unit.
   - Sit in an upright and comfortable position. Put the mask over your nose and mouth, making sure it fits properly to prevent mist from going into the eyes. If a mouthpiece is used, place it into your mouth.
   - Turn on compressor and take slow, deep breaths. If possible, hold breath for 10 sec before slowly exhaling. Continue until medication chamber is empty.
5. Do not swallow nebulizer solution as it is poorly absorbed.
6. When using nebulizer solution, do not mix different types of medications without provider permission.
7. Directions for using nasal spray/solution:
   - Blow nose before using spray.
   - Hold pump with thumb at bottom and nozzle between fingers. When using for the first time, prime the

 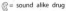

C

pump by initially spraying 5 times into the air until a fine mist appears.

- Insert nozzle into nostril, spray upward while breathing through the nose. Repeat in other nostril.
- Wipe nozzle to remove debris; cleanse.
- If the pump has not been used for 2 weeks, spray 2 times into the air before using again.
- Consult provider if used continuously for more than 12 weeks.

8. Directions for PO use:

- Take at least 30 min before meals.
- Break open ampule and squeeze contents into a glass of water. Do not mix with fruit juice, milk, or foods.
- Stir solution and drink all of the liquid.

9. Continue prescribed medications; may take up to 4 weeks for frequency of asthmatic attacks to decrease.

10. With exposure induced bronchoconstriction, use inhaler within 10–15 min prior to precipitating agent (i.e., exercise, antigen, environmental pollutants) for best results.

11. Use a peak expiratory flow meter to monitor asthma control; establish level to seek medical assistance.

12. Do not discontinue inhalation or nasal medication abruptly. Rapid withdrawal of the drug may precipitate an asthmatic attack, and concomitant corticosteroid therapy may require adjustment.

13. With eye drops, review method for instillation. Do not wear soft contact lenses during therapy; wait for several hours after therapy is discontinued. May experience slight burning or stinging upon instillation. Report any adverse side effects or lack of response.

OUTCOMES/EVALUATE

- ↓ Frequency of asthmatic attacks
- Prevention of exposure-induced bronchoconstriction
- Control of symptoms of mastocytosis (↓ diarrhea, N&V, headache, flushing, and abdominal pain)
- Relief of nasal allergic manifestations

Cyanocobalamin (Vitamin B$_{12}$)

(sye-**an**-oh-koh-**BAL**-ah-min)

CLASSIFICATION(S):
Vitamin B$_{12}$
PREGNANCY CATEGORY: A (C in doses that exceed the RDA)
OTC: Lozenges, Tablets: Big Shot B-12, Twelve Resin-K.
Rx: Nasal Gel/Spray: CaloMist, Nascobal.

Cyanocobalamin crystalline
PREGNANCY CATEGORY: C
Rx: Crystamine, Crysti 1000, Cyanoject, Cyomin, Rubesol-1000.

USES
Cyanocobalamin Nasal Gel: Nutritional Vitamin B$_{12}$ deficiency. Maintenance of hematologic status in those who are in remission following IM vitamin B$_{12}$ for the following conditions: (1) Pernicious anemia in hematologic remission with no involvement of the nervous system; (2) Dietary deficiency of vitamin B$_{12}$ in strict vegetarians; (3) Malabsorption of vitamin B$_{12}$ due to structural or functional damage to the stomach where intrinsic factor is secreted or to the ileum where intrinsic factor facilitates vitamin B$_{12}$ absorption (e.g., HIV infection, AIDS, Crohn's disease, tropical sprue, nontropical sprue); (4) Inadequate secretion of intrinsic factor due to lesions that destroy the gastric mucosa and conditions associated with a variable degree of gastric atrophy; (5) Competition for vitamin B$_{12}$ by intestinal parasites or bacteria; and, (6) Inadequate use of vitamin B$_{12}$ (i.e., if antimetabolites for the vitamin are used to treat neoplasms).

Cyanocobalamin Crystalline Parenteral: (1) Vitamin B$_{12}$ deficiency due to malabsorption syndrome as seen in pernicious anemia, GI pathology, dysfunction, or surgery. (2) Fish tapeworm infestation, malignancy of pancreas or bowel, gluten enteropathy, small bowel overgrowth of bacteria, sprue, accompanying folic acid deficiency, or total or partial gastrectomy. *NOTE:* Gel can be used in clients with HIV, AIDS, multiple sclerosis, or Crohn's disease.

Oral (OTC) Cyanocobalamin: Nutritional vitamine B12 deficiency. (These products are not treatment of pernicious anemia).

ACTION/KINETICS

Action
Required for hematopoiesis, cell reproduction, nucleoprotein and myelin synthesis. Plasma vitamin B_{12} levels: 150–750 pg/mL.

Pharmacokinetics
Rapidly absorbed following IM or SC administration. Following absorption, vitamin B_{12} is carried by plasma proteins to the liver where it is stored until required for various metabolic functions. **t½:** 6 days (400 days in the liver). **Time to peak levels, after intranasal:** 1–2 hr.

CONTRAINDICATIONS
Hypersensitivity to cobalt, Leber's disease.

SPECIAL CONCERNS
Use with caution in clients with gout. Those with severe megaloblastic anemia treated intensely with vitamin B_{12} may develop hypokalemia and sudden death. Folic acid is **not** a substitute for vitamin B_{12}.

SIDE EFFECTS

Most Common
After parenteral use: Itching, diarrhea, pain at injection site.
After intranasal use: N&V, glossitis, headache, rhinitis.

• **Following parenteral use.**
Allergic: Urticaria, itching, transitory exanthema, *anaphylaxis, shock, death.* **CV:** *Peripheral vascular thrombosis,* CHF, *pulmonary edema.* **Miscellaneous:** Polycythemia vera, optic nerve atrophy in clients with hereditary optic nerve atrophy, diarrhea, hypokalemia, body feels swollen, pain at injection site.

• **Following intranasal use.**
GI: Glossitis, N&V. **Miscellaneous:** Asthenia, headache, infection (sore throat, common cold), paresthesia, rhinitis. *NOTE:* Benzyl alcohol, which is present in certain products, may cause *fatal "gasping syndrome"* in premature infants.

LABORATORY TEST CONSIDERATIONS
Antibiotics, methotrexate, or pyrimethamine invalidate folic acid and vitamin B_{12} diagnostic blood assays.

DRUG INTERACTIONS
Alcohol / ↓ Vitamin B_{12} absorption
Aminosalicylic acid / ↓ Vitamin B_{12} effect. Also, abnormal Schilling test and symptoms of vitamin B_{12} deficiency
Chloramphenicol / ↓ Response to vitamin B_{12} in pernicious anemia
Cholestyramine / ↓ Vitamin B_{12} absorption
Cimetidine / ↓ Digestion and release of vitamin B_{12}; ↓ absorption of cyanocobalamin
Colchicine / ↓ Vitamin B_{12} absorption
Neomycin / ↓ Vitamin B_{12} absorption
Para-aminosalicylic acid / ↓ Vitamin B_{12} absorption
Potassium, timed-release / ↓ Vitamin B_{12} absorption

HOW SUPPLIED
Cyanocobalamin (OTC): *Lozenges:* 50 mcg, 100 mcg, 250 mcg, 500 mcg; *Tablets:* 100 mcg, 500 mcg, 1000 mcg, 1000 mcg (on resin), 5000 mcg.
Cyanocobalamin (Rx): *Nasal Gel/Spray:* 500 mcg/0.1 mL.
Cyanocobalamin crystalline (Rx): *Injection:* 100 mcg/mL, 1,000 mcg/mL.

DOSAGE

CYANOCOBALAMIN NASAL SPRAY
Maintenance of hematologic status in pernicious anemia, correct Vitamin B_{12} deficiencies.
500 mcg (0.1 mL of spray) once a week at least 1 hr before or after ingestion of foods or liquids.

• **LOZENGES; TABLETS (OTC)**
Vitamin B_{12} deficiency.
Dosage varies. See individual product package inserts. The RDA for adults is 2 mcg/day.

CYANOCOBALAMIN CRYSTALLINE
• **IM, SC (DEEP)**

 = see color insert   = Herbal   = Intravenous   ℚ = sound alike drug

Addisonian pernicious anemia.
Adults: 100 mcg/day for 6–7 days; **then,** if improvement noted along with a reticulocyte response, give 100 mcg every other day for seven doses and then 100 mcg q 3–4 days for 2–3 weeks. **Maintenance, IM:** 100 mcg once a month for life. Give folic acid if necessary.

Vitamin B₁₂ deficiency.
Adults: 30 mcg daily for 5–10 days; **then,** 100–200 mcg/month. Doses up to 1,000 mcg have been recommended. **Pediatric, for hematologic signs:** 10–50 mcg/day for 5–10 days followed by 100–250 mcg/dose q 2–4 weeks. **Pediatric, for neurologic signs:** 100 mcg/day for 10–15 days; **then,** 1–2 times/week for several months (can possibly be tapered to 250–1,000 mcg/month by 1 year).

Diagnosis of vitamin B₁₂ deficiency.
Adults: 1 mcg/day IM for 10 days plus low dietary folic acid and vitamin B₁₂. Loading dose for the Schilling test is 1,000 mcg given IM.

NURSING CONSIDERATIONS

ADMINISTRATION/STORAGE

1. Protect cyanocobalamin crystalline injection from light. Do not freeze.
2. With pernicious anemia, the drug cannot be administered PO.
3. Clients should be in hematologic remission before use of the nasal gel.

ASSESSMENT

1. Note reasons for therapy, onset, characteristics of S&S.
2. Check if allergic to cobalt. Obtain dietary history.
3. Note if prescribed chloramphenicol; antagonizes hematopoietic response to vitamin B₁₂.
4. Assess peripheral pulses, check for neuropathy.
5. Monitor VS, CBC, reticulocyte, potassium, folate and B₁₂ levels if being treated for megaloblastic anemia.
6. With pernicious anemia and malabsorption syndromes give parenterally and administer intrinsic factor simultaneously.

CLIENT/FAMILY TEACHING

1. With pernicious anemia, *must take* vitamin B₁₂ replacement for life. May take orally daily or parenterally monthly.
2. When repository vitamin B₁₂ used, provides drug for 4 weeks.
3. The stinging, burning sensation after injection is transitory.
4. If vitamin B₁₂ therapy is the result of dietary deficiency, identify foods (such as meats, especially liver, fermented cheeses, egg yolks, and seafood) high in B₁₂ and review diet.
5. Avoid alcohol; interferes with drug absorption.
6. Report any symptoms of urticaria, itching, and evidence of anaphylaxis immediately.
7. If diarrhea occurs, record frequency, quantity, and consistency of stools; may require a drug change.
8. When using nasal spray, prime pump before each dose.

OUTCOMES/EVALUATE

- Relief of fatigue/improved functioning level
- Plasma vitamin B₁₂ levels of 350–750 pg/mL

Cyclobenzaprine hydrochloride

(sye-kloh-**BENZ**-ah-preen)

CLASSIFICATION(S):

Skeletal muscle relaxant, centrally-acting

PREGNANCY CATEGORY: B

Rx: Amrix, Fexmid, Flexeril.

♣Rx: Apo-Cyclobenzaprine, Gen-Cyclobenzaprine, Novo–Cycloprine, Nu-Cyclobenzaprine, ratio-Cyclobenzaprine.

SEE ALSO SKELETAL MUSCLE RELAXANTS, CENTRALLY ACTING.

USES

Adjunct to rest and physical therapy for relief of muscle spasms associated with acute and/or painful musculoskeletal

---

Bold Italic = life threatening side effect   ■ = black box warning   ♣ = Available in Canada

conditions. *Investigational:* Management of fibromyalgia.

ACTION/KINETICS

Action

Thought to inhibit reflexes by reducing tonic somatic motor activity. Does not interfere with muscle function. Related to the tricyclic antidepressants; possesses both sedative and anticholinergic properties.

Pharmacokinetics

Tablets are from 33–55% bioavailable. **Onset:** 1 hr. **Time to peak plasma levels:** About 8 hr. **Therapeutic plasma levels:** 20–30 ng/mL. Food increases the C_{max} and AUC. **Duration:** 12–24 hr. **t½, elimination:** About 18 hr for tablets and 32 hr for capsules. Metabolized mainly by CYP3A4 and CYP1A2. Inactive metabolites are excreted in the urine. **Plasma protein binding:** Highly bound.

CONTRAINDICATIONS

Hypersensitivity. Arrhythmias, heart block or conduction disturbances, CHF, or during acute recovery phase of MI. Hyperthyroidism. Concomitant use of MAO inhibitors or within 14 days of their discontinuation; hyperpyretic crisis seizures and death may result if used together. Treatment of spastic diseases or cerebral palsy. Moderate to severe hepatic impairment.

SPECIAL CONCERNS

Safe use during lactation and in children under age 15 has not been established. Due to atropine-like effects, use with caution in situations where cholinergic blockade is not desired (e.g., history of urinary retention, angle-closure glaucoma, increased intraocular pressure). Geriatric clients may be more sensitive to cholinergic blockade. Use with caution in mild hepatic impairment and during lactation.

SIDE EFFECTS

Most Common

Drowsiness, dizziness, dry mouth, confusion, nausea, constipation, dyspepsia, unpleasant taste, headache, fatigue.

Since cyclobenzaprine resembles tricyclic antidepressants, side effects to these drugs should also be noted. **GI:** Dry mouth, N&V, constipation, dyspep-sia, unpleasant taste, anorexia, diarrhea, GI pain, gastritis, thirst, flatulence, ageusia, dysgeusia, paralytic ileus, discoloration of tongue, stomatitis, parotid swelling, dry throat, unpleasant taste. **Hepatic:** Abnormal liver function; rarely, cholestasis, hepatitis, jaundice. **CNS:** Drowsiness, dizziness, fatigue, asthenia, blurred vision, nervousness, headache, somnolence, insomnia, fatigue/tiredness, disturbance in attention, **convulsions**, ataxia, vertigo, dysarthria, paresthesia, hypertonia, tremors, malaise, abnormal gait, delusions, Bell's palsy, alteration in EEG patterns, extrapyramidal symptoms. Psychiatric symptoms include: Confusion, insomnia, disorientation, depressed mood, abnormal sensations, anxiety, agitation, abnormal thinking or dreaming, excitement, hallucinations, psychosis. **CV:** Tachycardia, syncope, **arrhythmias**, vasodilation, palpitations, hypotension, edema, chest pain, hypertension, MI, heart block, stroke. **GU:** Urinary frequency or retention, impaired urination, dilation of urinary tract, impotence, decreased or increased libido, testicular swelling, gynecomastia, breast enlargement, galactorrhea. **Dermatologic:** Sweating, skin rashes, urticaria, pruritus, photosensitivity, alopecia, acne. **Musculoskeletal:** Muscle twitching, weakness, myalgia. **Hematologic:** Purpura, bone marrow depression, leukopenia, eosinophilia, thrombocytopenia. **Hepatic:** Abnormal liver function, hepatitis, jaundice, cholestasis. **Ophthalmic:** Diplopia, blurred vision. **Body as a whole:** Local weakness, malaise, sweating, **anaphylaxis**, angioedema. **Miscellaneous:** Tinnitus, peripheral neuropathy, increase and decrease of blood sugar, weight gain or loss, **edema of the face and tongue**, inappropriate ADH syndrome, dyspnea.

OD OVERDOSE MANAGEMENT

Symptoms: Temporary confusion, dizziness, disturbed concentration, transient visual hallucinations, agitation, hyperactive reflexes, muscle rigidity, vomiting, **hyperpyrexia.** Also, drowsiness, hypothermia, tachycardia, hypertension, nausea, slurred speech, tremor, **cardiac arrhythmias such as bundle**

---

branch block, **ECG evidence of impaired conduction,** CHF, dilated pupils, **seizures, severe hypotension, cardiac arrest, neuroleptic malignant syndrome,** chest pain, stupor, **coma,** paradoxical diaphoresis, ECG changes. *Treatment:* In addition to the treatment outlined for skeletal muscle relaxants, physostigmine salicylate, 1–3 mg IV may be used to reverse symptoms of severe cholinergic blockade; however, profound bradycardia and asystole may occur.

DRUG INTERACTIONS
NOTE: Because of the similarity of cyclobenzaprine to tricyclic antidepressants, the drug interactions for tricyclics should also be consulted
Anticholinergics / Additive anticholinergic side effects
CNS depressants / Additive depressant effects
Guanethidine / Cyclobenzaprine may block effect of guanethidine and similar drugs
MAO inhibitors / Hyperpyretic crisis seizures and death are possible; do not use together
Tramadol / ↑ Seizure risk
Tricyclic antidepressants / Additive side effects

HOW SUPPLIED
Capsules, Extended-Release: 15 mg, 30 mg; *Tablets:* 5 mg, 7.5 mg, 10 mg.

DOSAGE
• **TABLETS**
Skeletal muscle disorders.
Adults: 5 mg 3 times/day. Depending on client response, may be increased to either 7.5 or 10 mg 3 times/day. Doses of 5 mg produce less sedation.
• **CAPSULES, EXTENDED-RELEASE**
Skeletal muscle disorders.
Adults: 15 mg once daily. Some may require 30 mg/day given once daily or 15 mg 2 times per day.

NURSING CONSIDERATIONS
℁ Do not confuse cyclobenzaprine with cyproheptadine (an antihistamine).

ADMINISTRATION/STORAGE
1. Use only for 2–3 weeks.

2. If taking an MAO inhibitor, do not administer cyclobenzaprine for at least 2 weeks after discontinuing.
3. Store from 15–30°C (59–86°F).

ASSESSMENT
1. List reasons for therapy, extent of acute or painful musculoskeletal condition, DTRs, ROM, and evidence of weakness. Review RICE (rest, ice, compression, and elevation) with acute injury to reduce swelling and recovery time.
2. Note any hypersensitivity or spastic diseases.
3. Check for evidence of cardiac arrhythmias; note history of MI. Obtain ECG, CBC, and LFTs.
4. With injury/fall, assess need for x-rays.

CLIENT/FAMILY TEACHING
1. Take as directed; take at about the same times each day. Report any adverse effects/lack of response. Moist heat, gentle stretching and PT may help during the recovery phase.
2. Report any unusual fatigue, sore throat, fever, easy bruising/bleeding; S&S of blood dyscrasia. Nausea or abdominal pain, itchy skin, or evidence of yellow sclera or skin; S&S of hepatic toxicity. Avoid alcohol during therapy. Symptoms of dry mouth, blurred vision, dizziness, tachycardia, constipation, or urinary retention should be reported.
3. Due to drug-induced drowsiness, dizziness, and/or blurred vision, observe caution if performing activities that require mental alertness.
4. Notify provider if S&S do not improve within 2–3 weeks of therapy.

OUTCOMES/EVALUATE
• ↑ ROM
• Relief of musculoskeletal spasms/pain

Cyclophosphamide **IV** ℂ (CYC)
(sye-kloh-**FOS**-fah-myd)

CLASSIFICATION(S):
Antineoplastic, alkylating
PREGNANCY CATEGORY: D
Rx: Cytoxan, Cytoxan Lyophilized, Neosar.

Bold Italic = life threatening side effect   ■ = black box warning   ✦ = Available in Canada

♣Rx: Procytox.

SEE ALSO *ANTINEOPLASTIC AGENTS* AND *ALKYLATING AGENTS*.

USES

Often used in combination with other antineoplastic drugs. (1) *Malignancies:* Malignant lymphomas (Stages III and IV, Ann Arbor Staging System), Hodgkin's disease, lymphocytic lymphoma (nodular or diffuse), mixed-cell-type lymphoma, histiocytic lymphoma, Burkitt's lymphoma, multiple myeloma, neuroblastoma (disseminated), adenocarcinoma of the ovary, retinoblastoma, carcinoma of the breast. (2) *Leukemias:* Chronic lymphocytic and granulocytic leukemia (usually ineffective in acute blastic crisis), acute myelogenous and monocytic leukemia, acute lymphoblastic leukemia in children (given during remission; cyclophosphamide is effective in prolonging remission duration). (3) *Other:* Mycosis fungoides. Nephrotic syndrome in children (not primary therapy). *Investigational:* Rheumatic diseases including rheumatoid arthritis and lupus erythematosus, Wegemer's granulomatosis, other steroid-resistant vasculitides, and in some cases of severe progressive rheumatoid arthritis and systemic lupus erythematotsus.

ACTION/KINETICS

Action

Metabolized in the liver to both active antineoplastic alkylating agents and inactive metabolites. The active metabolites alkylate nucleic acids, thus interfering with the growth of neoplastic and normal tissues. The cytotoxic action is due to cross-linking of strands of DNA and RNA and inhibition of protein synthesis. Also possesses immunosuppressive activity.

Pharmacokinetics

t½: 3–12 hr, but remnants of drug and/or metabolites detectable in serum after 72 hr; in children, the **t½** averages 4.1 hr. Metabolites are excreted through the urine with up to 25% of cyclophosphamide excreted unchanged. Cyclophosphamide is also excreted in milk.

CONTRAINDICATIONS

Lactation. Severe bone marrow depression.

SPECIAL CONCERNS

Use with caution in clients with thrombocytopenia, leukopenia, previous radiation therapy, bone marrow infiltration of tumor cells, previous therapy causing cytotoxicity, and impaired liver and kidney function. May interfere with wound healing. Increased doses may cause hepatocyte necrosis.

SIDE EFFECTS

Most Common

Alopecia, anorexia, N&V, diarrhea, mouth sores, jaundice, acne, blistering skin, weight loss, darkened/thickened skin.

See *Antineoplastic Agents* for a complete list of possible side effects. Also, acute hemorrhagic cystitis. **Bone marrow depression** appears frequently during days 9–14 of therapy. Alopecia occurs more frequently than with other drugs. **Secondary neoplasia (especially of urinary bladder), pulmonary fibrosis, cardiotoxicity**, darkening of skin or fingernails. Interference with oogenesis and spermatogenesis.

LABORATORY TEST CONSIDERATIONS

↑ Uric acid in blood and urine; false + Pap test; ↓ serum pseudocholinesterase. Suppression of certain skin tests.

OD OVERDOSE MANAGEMENT

Treatment: General supportive measures. Dialysis.

DRUG INTERACTIONS

Allopurinol / ↑ Chance of bone marrow toxicity

Anticoagulants / ↑ Anticoagulant effects

Chloramphenicol / ↓ Metabolism of cyclophosphamide to active metabolites → ↓ pharmacologic effect

Digoxin / ↓ Serum digoxin levels

Doxorubicin / ↑ Cardiotoxicity

Insulin / ↑ Hypoglycemia

Phenobarbital / ↑ Rate of metabolism of cyclophosphamide in liver

Phenytoin / Induction of metabolism of cyclophosphamide by CYP2B6 → ↑ risk of toxicity associated with cyclophosphamide active metabolite

Quinolone antibiotics / ↓ Antimicrobial effect of quinolones

Succinylcholine / ↑ Neuromuscular blockade R/T ↓ cholinesterase activity

Thiazide diuretics / ↑ Chance of leukopenia

HOW SUPPLIED

Injection, Powder for Solution: 0.5 gram, 1 gram, 2 grams; *Powder for Injection:* 100 mg cyclophosphamide/75 mg mannitol, 100 mg cyclophosphamide/82 mg sodium bicarbonate; *Tablets:* 25 mg, 50 mg.

DOSAGE

• **IV**

  Malignancies, Adults and Children.

Initial, with no hematologic deficiency, only drug used: 40–50 mg/kg in divided does over 2–5 days. **Alternative therapy:** 10–15 mg/kg q 7–10 days or 3–5 mg/kg twice weekly.

• **TABLETS**

  Malignancies.

Initial and maintenance: 1–5 mg/kg depending on client tolerance. Attempt to maintain leukocyte count at 3,000–4,000/mm³. Adjust dosage for kidney or liver disease.

  Nephrotic syndrome in children.

2.5–3 mg/kg/day for 60–90 days.

NURSING CONSIDERATIONS

◎ Do not confuse cyclophosphamide with cycloserine (an immunosupressant). Also, do not confuse Cytoxan with Cytotex (a prostaglandin derivative) or with Cytosar (an antineoplastic).

ADMINISTRATION/STORAGE

1. Prepare PO solution by dissolving injectable cyclophosphamide in aromatic elixir.

2. The initial loading dose may need to be reduced by one-third to one-half if previously received cytotoxic drugs or XRT.

IV 3. Dissolve 100 mg cyclophosphamide in appropriate amount (depending on vial strength) of sterile water for injection. Administer over 10–15 min.

4. Prepared solutions may be given IV, IM, intraperitoneally, or intrapleurally. Or, the drug may be infused IV with D5W, D5W/0.9% NaCl, D5W/Ringer's, RL, 0.45% NaCl, or 1/6M sodium lactate injection.

5. Store reconstituted solution at room temperature for 24 hr or for 6 days if refrigerated at 2–8°C (36–46°F).

ASSESSMENT

1. Note any prior radiation or chemotherapy; dose requires reduction.

2. Assess skin condition and integrity noting evidence of breakdown; may interfere with wound healing.

3. Monitor for cardiotoxicity: increased SOB, rales, increased coughing, or tachycardia. Obtain periodic CXR and PFTs.

4. Check for dysuria and hematuria; monitor urinalysis with sp.gravity to assess for SIADH.

5. Monitor uric acid, renal, LFTs, and CBC; may cause granulocyte suppression. Nadir: 14 days; recovery: 17–21 days.

CLIENT/FAMILY TEACHING

1. Take PO meds on empty stomach; may take with meals if GI upset occurs.

2. Increase fluid intake before, during, and for 24 hr after therapy.

3. Take in the a.m. so kidneys can eliminate drug before bedtime; void frequently. Stay well hydrated to prevent hemorrhagic cystitis R/T excessive urinary concentrations.

4. May discolor skin and nails.

5. Report any unusual bruising, bleeding, or fever.

6. Avoid vaccinations during therapy.

7. With alopecia, hair should grow back when drug stopped or when maintenance dosage is given.

8. Drug may cause a false positive Pap test. May also cause sterility and menstrual irregularities; identify candidates for egg/sperm harvesting.

9. Practice reliable contraception (both sexes) during therapy.

10. S&S of hypoglycemia may be precipitated by drug interactions with insulin; monitor sugars closely and consult with provider for insulin dosage adjustment.

11. Report any evidence of injury or delayed wound healing.

---

12. May suppress skin test response for *Candida,* mumps, trichophyton, and PPD.

OUTCOMES/EVALUATE
- Improved hematologic profile
- ↓ Tumor size and spread

Cyclosporine ∎ IV ©
(sye-kloh-**SPOR**-een)

CLASSIFICATION(S):
Immunosuppressant
PREGNANCY CATEGORY: C
Rx: Gengraf, Neoral, Restasis, Sandimmune.
✤Rx: Rhoxal-cyclosporine, Sandimmune I.V.

USES
(1) Prophylaxis of rejection in kidney, liver, and heart allogeneic transplants. Sandimmune is always to be taken with adrenal corticosteroids while Neoral or Gengraf have been used in combination with azathioprine and corticosteroids. (2) Sandimmune: Treatment of chronic rejection in clients previously treated with other immunosuppressants. Sandimmune has been used in children as young as 6 months with no unusual side effects. (3) Neoral or Gengraf: Severe, active rheumatoid arthritis which has not responded to methotrexate alone. Neoral and Gengraf may be used with methotrexate in RA clients who do not respond adequately to methotrexate alone. (4) Neoral or Gengraf: Adult, nonimmunocompromised clients with severe (i.e., extensive and/or disabling) recalcitrant, plaque psoriasis who have failed to respond to at least 1 systemic therapy (e.g., PUVA, retinoids, methotrexate) or in those for whom other systemic therapies are contraindicated or cannot be tolerated. (5) Restasis: Increase tear production where tear production is presumed to be suppressed due to ocular inflammation associated with keratoconjunctivitis sicca.

ACTION/KINETICS
Action
Thought to act by inhibiting the immunocompetent lymphocytes in the G_0 or G_1 phase of the cell cycle. T-lymphocytes are specifically inhibited; both the T-helper cell and the T-suppressor cell may be affected. Also inhibits interleukin 2 or T-cell growth factor production and release. Absorption from the GI tract is incomplete and variable. Children often require larger PO doses than adults, which may be due to the smaller absorptive surface area of their intestines.

Pharmacokinetics
Peak plasma levels: 3.5 hr. Food may both delay and impair drug absorption. **$t^1/2$:** Approximately 19 hr for adults and 7 hr in children. Metabolized by the liver; inactive metabolites are excreted mainly through the bile. Neoral immediately forms a microemulsion in an aqueous environment. This product has better bioequivalency; thus, Sandimmune and Neoral are not bioequivalent and cannot be used interchangeably without medical supervision. **Time to peak blood levels:** 1.5–2 hr. Food decreases the amount of drug absorbed.

CONTRAINDICATIONS
Hypersensitivity to cyclosporine or polyoxyethylated castor oil. Lactation. Use of potassium-sparing diuretics. Neoral in psoriasis or rheumatoid arthritis with abnormal renal function, uncontrolled hypertension, or malignancies. Neoral together with PUVA or UVB in psoriasis. Use in psoriasis if client is taking other immunosuppressive drugs or radiation therapy. Use of the ophthalmic emulsion with active ocular infections. Administration of the ophthalmic emulsion in those wearing contact lenses

SPECIAL CONCERNS
∎ (1) Only physicians experienced in immunosuppression therapy and management of organ transplant clients should prescribe cyclosporine. Manage clients in facilities equipped and staffed with adequate lab and supportive medical resources. The physician responsible for maintenance therapy should have complete information necessary

for client follow-up. (2) Give Sandimmune with adrenal corticosteroids but not with other immunosuppressants as there is increased susceptibility to infection and possible development of lymphoma from immunosuppression. (3) Neoral and Gengraf may increase susceptibility to infection and the development of neoplasia. In kidney, liver, and heart transplant clients, Gengraf and Neoral may be given with other immunosuppressive agents. Increased susceptibility to infection and possible development of lymphoma and other neoplasms may result from the increase in the degree of immunosuppression in transplant clients. (4) Oral absorption during chronic Sandimmune use is erratic. Monitor cyclosporine blood levels during PO therapy at repeated intervals and make dosage adjustments to avoid toxicity or possible organ rejection. This is especially important in liver transplants. (5) Sandimmune capsules and oral solution have decreased bioavailability compared with Neoral capsules, Neoral oral solution, Gengraf capsules, and Gengraf oral solution. Gengraf and Neoral are not bioequivalent to Sandimmune and cannot be used interchangeably without physician approval. For a given trough concentration, cyclosporine exposure will be greater with Neoral and Gengraf than with Sandimmune. If a client receiving exceptionally high doses of Sandimmune is converted to Neoral or Gengraf, exercise particular caution. Monitor cyclosporine blood levels in transplant and rheumatoid arthritis clients taking Gengraf and Neoral to minimize possible organ rejection due to high concentrations. Make dose adjustments in transplant clients to minimize possible organ rejection due to low concentrations. Comparison of blood concentrations in the published literature with blood concentrations obtained using current assays must be done with detailed knowledge of the assays used. (6) Psoriasis clients previously treated with PUVA and to a lesser extent, methotrexate or other immunosuppressants, UVB, coal tar, or radiation therapy are at increased risk of developing skin malignancies when taking Neoral or Gengraf. (7) In recommended doses cyclosporine can cause systemic hypertension and nephrotoxicity. Risk increases with increasing dose and duration of cyclosporine therapy. Renal dysfunction, including structural kidney damage, is a potential consequence of therapy; monitor renal function during therapy.■ Use with caution in clients with impaired renal or hepatic function. Use the ophthalmic product with caution during lactation. Safety and efficacy have not been established in children. Clients with malabsorption may not achieve therapeutic levels following PO use. Use the ophthalmic emulsion with caution during lactation.

SIDE EFFECTS
Most Common

After systemic use: Renal dysfunction, hypertension, hirsutism, tremor, gum hyperplasia, diarrhea, parestheisa, seizures, acne, N&V.

After ophthalmic use: Ocular burning

Systemic use. GI: N&V, diarrhea, gum hyperplasia, anorexia, gastritis, hiccoughs, peptic ulcer, abdominal discomfort, UGI bleeding, pancreatitis, constipation, mouth sores, swallowing difficulty. **Hematologic:** Leukopenia, lymphoma, thrombocytopenia, anemia, microangiopathic hemolytic anemia syndrome. **Allergic:** *Anaphylaxis (rare).* **CV:** Hypertension, edema, chest pain, cramps, *MI* (rare). **CNS:** Headache, tremor, confusion, fever, *seizures*, anxiety, depression, weakness, lethargy, ataxia. **GU:** Renal dysfunction, glomerular capillary thrombosis, nephrotoxicity. **Dermatologic:** Acne, hirsutism, brittle finger nails, hair breaking, pruritus. **Miscellaneous:** Hepatotoxicity, flushing, paresthesia, sinusitis, gynecomastia, conjunctivitis, hearing loss, tinnitus, muscle pain, infections (including fungal, viral), *Pneumocystis carinii* pneumonia, hematuria, blurred vision, weight loss, joint pain, night sweats, tingling, tremor, hypomagnesemia in some clients with seizures, infectious complications, increased risk of cancer. **Ophthalmic use.** Ocular burning, conjunctival hyperemia, discharge, epiphora, eye

---

Bold Italic = life threatening side effect   ■ = black box warning   ♣ = Available in Canada

pain, foreign body sensation, pruritus, stinging, visual blurring.

LABORATORY TEST CONSIDERATIONS

↑ Serum creatinine, potassium, BUN, total bilirubin, alkaline phosphatase. Possibly ↑ cholesterol, LDL, and apolipoprotein B. Hyperglycemia/-kalemia/-uricemia.

OD OVERDOSE MANAGEMENT

Symptoms: Transient hepatotoxicity and nephrotoxicity. *Treatment:* Induction of vomiting (up to 2 hr after ingestion). General supportive measures.

DRUG INTERACTIONS

Allopurinol / ↑ Cyclosporine levels

Aminoglycosides / ↑ Risk of nephrotoxicity

Amiodarone / ↑ Cyclosporine blood levels → ↑ risk of nephrotoxicity

Amphotericin B / ↑ Risk of nephrotoxicity

Androgens / ↑ Cyclosporine blood levels → possible nephrotoxicity

Azathioprine / ↑ Immunosuppression R/T suppression of lymphocytes → possible infection and malignancy

Bosentan / ↑ Bosentan trough levels → ↑ risk of toxicity; ↓ cyclosporine plasma levels

Bromocriptine / ↑ Cyclosporine plasma level R/T ↓ liver breakdown

Bupropion / Possible ↓ cyclosporine levels; ↑ cyclosporine dose

Calcium channel blockers / ↑ Cyclosporine plasma levels R/T ↓ liver breakdown; ↑ risk of toxicity

Carbamazepine / ↓ Cyclosporine plasma level R/T ↑ liver breakdown

Carvedilol / ↑ Cyclosporine blood levels → possible nephrotoxicity and neurotoxicity

Chloramphenicol / ↑ Cyclosporine blood levels in renal transplant clients

Cimetidine / ↑ Risk of nephrotoxicity

Clarithromycin / ↑ Cyclosporine plasma levels R/T ↓ liver breakdown; ↑ risk of nephro-/neurotoxicity

Clindamycin / ↓ Cyclosporine serum levels

Colchicine / Severe side effects, including GI, hepatic, renal, and neuromuscular toxicity; ↑ Risk of nephrotoxicity

Corticosteroids / ↑ Immunosuppression R/T suppression of lymphocytes → possible infection and malignancy

Cyclophosphamide / ↑ Immunosuppression R/T suppression of lymphocytes → possible infection and malignancy

Danazol / ↑ Cyclosporine plasma level R/T ↓ liver breakdown

Diclofenac / &arrowup. Risk of nephrotoxicity; also, doubling of diclofenac blood levels

Digoxin / ↑ Digoxin levels R/T ↓ clearance; also, ↓ volume of distribution of digoxin → toxicity

Diltiazem / ↑ Cyclosporine plasma level R/T ↓ liver breakdown → possible nephrotoxicity

H *Echinacea* / Do not give with cyclosporine

Erythromycin / ↑ Cyclosporine plasma level R/T ↓ liver breakdown and ↓ biliary excretion → possible nephrotoxicity

Etoposide / ↓ Etoposide renal clearance → increased toxicity

Fluconazole / ↑ Cyclosporine plasma levels R/T ↓ gut and liver metabolism → possible nephrotoxicity

Fluoroquinolones / ↑ Cyclosporine toxicity possible

Foscarnet / ↑ Risk of renal failure

Grapefruit juice / ↑ Cyclosporine blood levels due to ↓ liver breakdown

Griseofulvin / ↓ Cyclosporine levels → ↓ effect

HIV protease inhibitors / ↑ Cyclosporine plasma levels R/T ↓ liver breakdown → toxicity

Imipenem-cilastatin / ↑ CNS effects of both drugs

Isoniazid / ↓ Cyclosporine plasma level R/T ↑ liver breakdown

Itraconazole / ↑ Plasma level of cyclosporine R/T ↓ liver breakdown

Ketoconazole / ↑ Cyclosporine plasma level R/T ↓ breakdown by gut and liver metabolism → possible nephrotoxicity

Lovastatin / ↑ Risk of myopathy and rhabdomyolysis R/T ↓ cyclosporine breakdown

Melphalan / ↑ Risk of nephrotoxicity

Methotrexate / ↑ Methotrexate plasma levels and AUC perhaps R/T ↓ metabolism

Methylphenidate / Possible ↑ cyclospo-

---

rine levels; ↓ cyclosporine dose

Methylprednisolone / ↑ Cyclosporine blood levels R/T ↓ liver breakdown → toxicity

Metoclopramide / ↑ Cyclosporine plasma level R/T ↓ liver breakdown → toxicity

Micafungin / ↑ Cyclosporine single-dose whole-blood levels and ↓ cyclosporine PO clearance after single-dose and steady-state administration

Mycophenolate / Possible ↑ Mycophenolate side effects if cyclosporine discontinued

Naproxen / ↑ Risk of nephrotoxicity

Nephrotoxic drugs / Additive nephrotoxicity

Nicardipine / ↑ Cyclosporine plasma level R/T ↓ liver breakdown → possible nephrotoxicity

Nifedipine / ↑ Risk of gingival hyperplasia

Octreotide / ↓ Cyclosporine plasma level R/T ↑ liver breakdown

Oral contraceptives / ↑ Cyclosporine plasma level R/T ↓ liver breakdown; possible severe hepatotoxicity

Orlistat / Possible ↓ cyclosporine blood levels R/T ↓ absorption

Phenobarbital / ↓ Cyclosporine plasma level R/T ↑ liver breakdown

Phenytoin / ↓ Cyclosporine plasma levels R/T ↑ liver breakdown

Probucol / ↓ Cyclosporine bioavailability → ↓ clinical effect

Quercetin (in apples, berries, ginkgo, grapefruit, onions, red wine, and tea) / ↑ Cyclosporine bioavailability, AUC, and peak levels

Quinupristin/Dalfopristin / ↑ Cyclosporine blood levels

Ranitidine / ↑ Risk of nephrotoxicity

Repaglinide / ↑ Repaglinide peak serum levels R/T inhibition of hepatic metabolism

Rifabutin/Rifampin / ↓ Cyclosporine plasma level R/T ↑ liver breakdown

Saquinavir / ↑ Cyclosporine blood levels

Simvastatin / ↑ Risk of myopathy and rhabdomyolysis R/T ↓ cyclosporine breakdown

H *St. John's Wort* / Possible induction of liver enzymes → ↓ cyclosporine effect

Sulfamethoxazole and/or trimethoprim / ↑ Risk of nephrotoxicity; also, ↓ cyclosporine serum levels → possible organ rejection

Sulindac / ↑ Risk of nephrotoxicity

Tacrolimus / ↑ Risk of nephrotoxicity

Vancomycin / ↑ Risk of nephrotoxicity

Verapamil / ↑ Immunosuppression

HOW SUPPLIED

Capsules, Soft Gelatin: 25 mg, 50 mg, 100 mg; *Capsules, Soft Gelatin for Microemulsion:* 25 mg 100 mg; *Injection:* 50 mg/mL; *Ophthalmic Emulsion:* 0.05%; *Oral Solution:* 100 mg/mL.

DOSAGE

• **CAPSULES; ORAL SOLUTION**

Allogenic transplants.

Adults and children, initial: A single 15 mg/kg dose given 4–12 hr before transplantation; there is a trend to use lower initial doses of 10–14 mg/kg/day. The dose should be continued postoperatively for 1–2 weeks followed by 5% decrease in dose per week to maintenance dose of 5–10 mg/kg/day (some have used a dose of 3 mg/kg/day successfully). Compared with Sandimmune, lower maintenance doses of Neoral may be sufficient.

If converting from Sandimmune to Neoral, start with a 1:1 conversion. Then, adjust the Neoral dose to reach the pre-conversion cyclosporine blood trough levels. Until this level is reached, monitor the cyclosporine trough level q 4–7 days.

Rheumatoid arthritis (Neoral only).

Initial: 1.25 mg/kg twice a day PO. Salicylates, NSAIDs, and PO corticosteroids may be continued. If sufficient beneficial effect is not seen and the client is tolerating the medication, the dose may be increased by 0.5–0.75 mg/kg/day after 8 weeks and again after 12 weeks to a maximum dose of 4 mg/kg/day. If no benefit is seen after 16 weeks, discontinue therapy. If Neoral is combined with methotrexate, the same initial dose and dose range of Neoral can be used.

Psoriasis (Neoral only).

Initial: 1.25 mg/kg twice a day PO. Maintain this dose for 4 weeks if tolerat-

---

Bold Italic = life threatening side effect   ■ = black box warning   ♣ = Available in Canada

ed. If significant improvement is not seen, increase the dose at 2-week intervals. Based on client response, make dose increases of about 0.5 mg/kg/day to a maximum of 4 mg/kg/day. Discontinue treatment if beneficial effects can not be achieved after 6 weeks at 4 mg/kg/day. Once beneficial effects are seen, decrease the dose (doses less than 2.5 mg/kg/day may be effective). To control side effects, make dose decreases by 25% to 50% at any time.

- **IV (ONLY IN CLIENTS UNABLE TO TAKE PO MEDICATION)**
  Allogenic transplants.
  Adults: 5–6 mg/kg/day 4–12 hr prior to transplantation and postoperatively until client can be switched to PO dosage. *NOTE:* Steroid therapy must be used concomitantly.
  Investigational uses.
  Oral doses ranging from 1 to 10 mg/kg/day.
- **OPHTHALMIC SOLUTION**
  Keratoconjunctivitis sicca.
  1 gtt twice a day in each eye about 12 hr apart.

NURSING CONSIDERATIONS

℗ Do not confuse cyclosporine with cyclophosphamide (an antineoplastic) or with cycloserine (an antineoplastic).

ADMINISTRATION/STORAGE
1. Sandimmune and Neoral are not bioequivalent and should not be used interchangeably without the supervision of someone experienced in immunosuppressive therapy. Conversion from Neoral to Sandimmune using a 1:1 ratio (mg/kg/day) may result in lower cyclosporine blood levels.
2. Sandimmune capsules and oral solution are bioequivalent. Neoral capsules and oral solution are bioequivalent.
3. May dilute the PO solution with milk, chocolate milk, orange, or apple juice immediately before administering. Dilute Neoral, preferably, with orange or apple juice; grapefruit juice affects metabolism of cyclosporine and is not to be used. After removal of the protective cover, transfer the solution, using the dosing syringe supplied, to a glass of diluent. Stir well and drink at once. Do

not allow diluted solution to stand before drinking. Use a glass container (not plastic). Rinse the glass with more diluent and swallow to ensure the total dose is taken. Do not store PO solutions in the refrigerator; contents should be used within 2 months after being opened.
4. At temperatures less than 20°C (68°F), Neoral solution may gel; light flocculation or the formation of a light sediment may also occur. This will not affect product performance or dosing using the syringe provided. Allow to warm to room temperature to reverse such changes.
5. Due to variable absorption of the PO solution, monitor blood levels.
6. Clients with malabsorption from the GI tract may not achieve appropriate blood levels.
7. The ophthalmic emulsion can be used with artificial tears; allow a 15 min interval between use of products.
[IV] 8. Reserve the injection for those unable to take the soft gelatin capsules or oral solution.
9. Dilute IV concentrate 1 mL (50 mg) in 20–100 mL 0.9% NaCl or D5W injection; give infusion slowly over 2–6 hr. Do not refrigerate once cyclosporine has been added to an IV solution.
10. Following addition to an IV solution, shake vigorously to disperse the drug.
11. Protect IV solution from light.
12. The polyoxyethylated castor oil found in the concentrate for IV infusion may cause phthalate stripping from PVC.
13. Due to possibility of anaphylaxis, monitor clients receiving IV cyclosporine closely for 30 min at the start of therapy. Have epinephrine (1:1,000) for anaphylaxis.

ASSESSMENT
1. Note reasons for therapy, any previous treatments. List drugs prescribed and any potential interactions. Anticipate concomitant administration of adrenal corticosteroids.
2. Monitor VS, CBC, cyclosporine levels, liver and renal function studies. Drug

---

may increase BP, serum K, lipid, and uric acid levels.

3. Differentiate nephrotoxicity from rejection using criteria provided by the manufacturer.

CLIENT/FAMILY TEACHING

1. Review importance of following the written guidelines for medication therapy explicitly. Drug must be taken throughout one's lifetime to prevent transplant rejection.

2. Because this drug is so important in preventing rejection, a written list of all possible drug side effects and those which need to be reported will be provided.

3. Taking the drug with food may reduce nausea and GI upset. If PO form unpalatable, mix with milk or orange juice in a glass container to minimize container adherence. Measure dose accurately and take immediately after mixing.

4. Do not take with grapefruit juice due to biometabolic concerns.

5. Do not stop abruptly; must be discontinued gradually.

6. Record BP, I&O, weights daily. Report any changes or persistent diarrhea and N&V.

7. Avoid crowds and persons with infectious illnesses.

8. Practice reliable birth control.

9. Use nystatin swish and swallow to prevent development of thrush; perform oral care and routine dental exams.

10. May develop acne and hairiness; report as dermatology referral may be needed.

11. Yellow discoloration of eyes, skin, or stools; fever; other signs of hepatotoxicity require reporting.

12. Report increased fatigue, malaise, unexplained bleeding or bruising, or blood in urine.

13. If using the eye emulsion, invert the vial a few times before use to obtain a uniform, white, opaque emulsion. May be used simultaneously with artificial tears but allow 15 min between use of products.

14. If contact lenses are worn, remove them prior to using the drug. Lenses may be reinserted 15 min after using the eye emulsion.

15. Keep all F/U appointments to evaluate response and to monitor labs.

OUTCOMES/EVALUATE

- Prevention of transplant rejection; improved organ function
- Cyclosporine trough levels (100–200 ng/mL)

Cytomegalovirus Immune Globulin Intravenous, Human (CMV-IGIV) [IV]

(**sigh**-toh-**meg**-ah-lo-**VIGH**-rus im-**MYOUN GLOB**-you-lin)

CLASSIFICATION(S):
Immune globulin
PREGNANCY CATEGORY: C
Rx: CytoGam.

USES

(1) Attenuation of primary CMV disease for kidney transplant recipients who are seronegative for CMV and who receive a kidney from a CMV seropositive donor. (2) With ganciclovir to prevent CMV in clients undergoing liver, lung, pancreas, and heart transplants from CMV-seropositive donors to CMV-seronegative recipients. *NOTE:* There is a 50% decrease in primary CMV disease in renal transplant clients given this product.

ACTION/KINETICS

Action

Obtained from pooled adult human plasma that has been selected for high titers of antibody for CMV. Is purified. When reconstituted, each mL contains 50 mg of immunoglobulin that is primarily IgG with trace amounts of IgA and IgM; albumin is also present. In individuals exposed to CMV, the immune globulin can increase the relevant antibodies to levels that prevent or reduce the incidence of serious CMV disease.

CONTRAINDICATIONS

Use in clients with a history of a prior severe reaction to this product or other human immunoglobulin preparations.

SPECIAL CONCERNS

Individuals with selective immunoglobulin (Ig) A deficiency may develop antibodies to IgA and could develop anaphylactic reactions to subsequent administration of blood products that contain IgA.

SIDE EFFECTS

Most Common

During infusion: Nausea, backache, flushing.

At site of injection: Muscle stiffness, pain, tenderness. **Other side effects:** Flushing, chills, muscle cramps, fever, N&V, SOB.

Side effects often due to the rate of infusion; adhere closely to the infusion schedule. **GI:** N&V. **Body as a whole:** Flushing, chills, fever. **Respiratory:** SOB. **Musculoskeletal:** Muscle cramps, back pain, backache. **Respiratory:** Wheezing. Hypotension and allergic reactions such as *angioneurotic edema* and *anaphylactic shock* are possible but have not been observed. **Site of injection:** Muscle stiffness, pain, tenderness.

OD OVERDOSE MANAGEMENT

Symptoms: Major effects would be those related to volume overload. Also possible are anaphylaxis and a drop in BP. *Treatment:* Stop infusion immediately and have epinephrine and diphenhydramine available for treatment of acute allergic symptoms.

DRUG INTERACTIONS

The antibodies present in this product may interfere with the immune response to live virus vaccines, including measles, mumps, and rubella. Thus, such vaccinations should be deferred until at least 3 months after administration of CMV immune globulin or revaccination may be required.

HOW SUPPLIED

Injection: 50 ± 10 mg/mL.

DOSAGE

- **IV**

  Prevention of rejection of kidney transplants.

The maximum total dose/infusion is 150 mg/kg given according to the following schedule:

- Within 72 hr of transplant: 150 mg/kg.
- 2–8 weeks after transplant: 100 mg/kg.
- 12–16 weeks after transplant: 50 mg/kg.

The rate of infusion for the initial dose is 15 mg/kg/hr. If no side effects occur after 30 min, the rate may be increased to 30 mg/kg/hr. If no side effects occur after a subsequent 30-min period, the dose may be increased to 60 mg/kg/hr at a volume not to exceed 7.5 mL/hr. **This rate of infusion must not be exceeded.** For subsequent doses, the rate of infusion is 15 mg/kg/hr for 15 min. If no side effects occur, increase the rate to 30 mg/kg/hr for 15 min and then increase to a maximum rate of 60 mg/kg/hr at a volume not to exceed 7.5 mL/hr. **This rate of infusion must not be exceeded.**

NURSING CONSIDERATIONS

ADMINISTRATION/STORAGE

IV 1. The reconstituted solution should be colorless and translucent. Do not use solution if turbid.

2. After removing tab portion of the vial cap, the rubber stopper is cleaned with 70% alcohol or equivalent. Reconstitute the lyophilized powder with 50 mL of sterile water for injection using a double-ended transfer needle or large syringe. When using a double-ended transfer needle, insert one end first into the vial of water. The lyophilized powder is supplied in an evacuated vial; thus, the water should transfer by suction. To avoid foaming, do not shake vial. After water is transferred into the evacuated vial, release the residual vacuum to hasten dissolution. Rotate container gently to wet all the undissolved powder. Allow 30 min for complete dissolution of the powder.

3. This product does not contain a preservative. After reconstitution, enter vial only once; begin the infusion within 6 hr of entering vial and complete within 12 hr.

---

4. Administer drug through a separate IV line using a constant infusion pump. If not possible, the drug may be "piggy-backed" into a preexisting line that contains either NaCl or one of the following dextrose solutions (with or without NaCl added): 2.5%, 5%, 10%, or 20% dextrose in water. If used with a preexisting line, do not dilute drug more than 1:2 with any solutions. See *Dosage* for administration guidelines.

5. If minor side effects occur, slow or temporarily interrupt the infusion.

ASSESSMENT

1. List any previous experience with human immunoglobulin preparations.

2. Note any IgA deficiency; these clients may experience anaphylactic reactions with subsequent exposures to IgA products. Assess transplant before therapy.

3. Follow infusion dosing schedules carefully and assess closely during each rate change. Monitor VS continuously; if side effects develop (fever, chills, flushing, nausea, back pain), or BP drops, slow/stop infusion and report.

4. Made from human plasma (part of the blood) and may contain infectious agents (e.g., viruses) that can cause disease.

CLIENT/FAMILY TEACHING

1. Used to help prevent infection by cytomegalovirus in people who receive an organ transplant. If seronegative for CMV and receives a seropositive donor kidney, CMV disease may develop.

2. Drug has been associated with the development of kidney problems, sometimes resulting in kidney failure and/or death. Report decreased urination, sudden weight gain, fluid retention/swelling, or shortness of breath; signs of kidney problems.

3. Rarely, aseptic meningitis syndrome (AMS) has been associated with these products. Immediately report severe headache, neck stiffness, drowsiness, fever, eye sensitivity to light, painful eye movements, nausea or vomiting. Stopping therapy has resulted in resolution of AMS without any lasting problems.

4. Avoid vaccinations for at least 3 months following therapy; may require revaccination. Antibodies in suspension may interfere with immune response to live virus vaccines.

5. In order to prevent transmission of infectious agents/hepatitis virus from one client to another, sterile disposable syringes and needles should be used; do not reuse.

6. Identify support groups that may assist to cope with chronic disease condition.

OUTCOMES/EVALUATE

- CMV prophylaxis in renal transplant recipients
- Improved kidney function

Dacarbazine (DTIC, Imidazole carboxamide)
(dah-**KAR**-bah-zeen) ■ **IV**

CLASSIFICATION(S):
Antineoplastic, alkylating
PREGNANCY CATEGORY: C
Rx: DTIC-Dome.
✤Rx: DTIC.

SEE ALSO *ANTINEOPLASTIC AGENTS* AND *ALKYLATING AGENTS*.

USES
(1) Metastatic malignant melanoma. (2) Hodgkin's disease (second line therapy with other agents). *Investigational:* In combination with cyclophosphamide and vincristine for malignant pheochromocytoma. In combination with other drugs to treat advanced metastatic soft tissue sarcoma. Alone or in combination with other drugs to manage Kaposi's sarcoma.

ACTION/KINETICS

Action

Exact mechanism of action unknown. May act by three ways: (1) Alkylation by an activated carbonium ion; (2) Antimetabolite to inhibit DNA and RNA synthesis; or (3) Alkylation by combining with protein sulfhydryl groups. Is cell-cycle nonspecific.

Pharmacokinetics

$t\frac{1}{2}$, biphasic, initial: 19 min; terminal: 5 hr. The $t\frac{1}{2}$ is increased to 55 min and 7.2 hr in those with renal and hepatic dysfunction. Probably localizes in liver. Limited amounts (14% of plasma level) enter CSF. Approximately 40% of drug excreted in urine unchanged within 6 hr. Secreted through the kidney tubules rather than filtered through the glomeruli.

CONTRAINDICATIONS

Hypersensitivity to dacarbazine. Lactation.

SPECIAL CONCERNS

■ (1) Administer under the supervision of a qualified physician experienced in the use of cancer chemotherapeutic drugs. (2) Hemopoietic depression is the most common toxic effect. (3) Hepatic necrosis has been reported. (4) The drug is carcinogenic and teratogenic when used in animals. (5) In treating each client, the physician must carefully weigh the possibility of achieving therapeutic benefit against the risk of toxicity.■ Dosage not established in children.

ADDITIONAL SIDE EFFECTS

Most Common

Leukopenia, thrombocytopenia, anorexia, N&V.

Hematologic: Hemopoietic depression, especially *leukopenia and thrombocytopenia which may cause death.* **GI:** N&V (more than 90% of clients within 1 hr after initial administration, which persists for 12–48 hr), anorexia, diarrhea. **Dermatologic:** Erythematous and urticarial rashes, photosensitivity reactions, alopecia, facial flushing, paresthesia. **Miscellaneous:** Flu-like syndrome, including fever, myalgia, and malaise. Hepatotoxicity (*accompanied by hepatic vein thrombosis and hepatocellular necrosis resulting in death*), hypersensitivity, facial paresthesia, *anaphylaxis*.

LABORATORY TEST CONSIDERATIONS

↑ AST, ALT, and other enzymes.

OD OVERDOSE MANAGEMENT

Treatment: Monitor blood cell counts; supportive treatment.

HOW SUPPLIED

Powder for Injection: 100 mg, 200 mg.

DOSAGE

- **IV ONLY**

    Malignant melanoma.

2–4.5 mg/kg/day for 10 days; may be repeated at 4-week intervals; or 250 mg/m²/day for 5 days; may be repeated at 3-week intervals.

    Hodgkin's disease.

150 mg/m²/day for 5 days in combination with other drugs, and repeated q 4 weeks; or, 375 mg/m² on day 1, with other drugs and repeated q 15 days.

NURSING CONSIDERATIONS

ADMINISTRATION/STORAGE

IV 1. Avoid extravasation due to the possibility of tissue damage and severe pain.

2. Reconstitute with sterile water for injection: 9.9 mL for the 100-mg vials and 19.7 mL for the 200-mg vials for a final concentration of 10 mg/mL with a pH of 3–4. May give by IV push over 1-min period. May further dilute with 50–250 mL D5W or NaCl injection and given over 30 min.

3. Stop infusion immediately with infiltration and apply ice for 24 to 48 hr.

4. Protect dry vials from light and store at 2–8°C (36–46°F).

5. Reconstituted solutions stable for up to 72 hr at 4°C (39°F) or for 8 hr at 20°C (68°F). More dilute solutions for IV infusions are stable for 24 hr when stored at 2–8°C (36–46°F).

ASSESSMENT

1. Ascertain how fluid status is to be handled (fast for 4–6 hr before treatment to reduce emesis or have fluids up to 1 hr before administration to minimize).

2. Give antiemetic before and throughout therapy. Have phenobarbital and/or prochlorperazine available for palliation of vomiting.

 = see color insert   = Herbal   = Intravenous   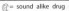 = sound alike drug

D

3. Monitor client and labs closely for bone marrow depression, liver or renal toxicity, or hypersensitivity reaction. Anticipate mild granulocyte toxicity. Nadir: 10 days; recovery: 21 days.

CLIENT/FAMILY TEACHING

1. Used to treat cancer of the lymph system, malignant melanoma (a type of skin cancer) and other types. It interferes with the growth of cancer cells, and destroys them. The growth of normal body cells may also be affected; hence other effects can occur.

2. To minimize GI effects, antiemetics, fasting, and limited fluid intake (4–6 hr preceding treatment) may be ordered. After the first 1–2 days of therapy, vomiting should cease as tolerance develops.

3. Report any unusual bruising/bleeding or flu-like symptoms (fever, aches, fatigue) that may occur. Usually occurs 1 week after treatment and may persist for 1–3 weeks. Acetaminophen may relieve symptoms. Avoid OTC agents including aspirin and NSAIDs.

4. Avoid prolonged exposure to sun or UV light and wear protective clothing; photosensitivity reaction may occur for up to two days following therapy.

5. Prepare for hair loss; report any blurred vision or numbness.

6. Practice contraception during and for several months following therapy.

7. Some effects may not occur for months or years after the medicine is used.

OUTCOMES/EVALUATE

↓ Tumor size/spread with suppression of malignant cell proliferation

---

Daclizumab   ■IV
(dah-**KLIZ**-you-mab)

CLASSIFICATION(S):
Immunosuppressant
PREGNANCY CATEGORY: C
Rx: Zenapax.

USES

Prophylaxis of acute organ rejection in renal transplants. Used with cyclosporine and corticosteroids.

ACTION/KINETICS

Action

Humanized IgG1 monoclonal antibody produced by recombinant DNA technology. As an antagonist, it binds to the alpha subunit (Tac subunit) of the human high affinity interleukin-2 (IL-2) receptor found on the surface of activated lymphocytes. This results in inhibition of IL-2 mediated activation of lymphocytes, a critical pathway in the cellular immune response involved in allograft rejection.

Pharmacokinetics

$t^{1/2}$, **terminal:** Estimated to be 20 days.

CONTRAINDICATIONS

Hypersensitivity to the drug or any component of the product. Lactation.

SPECIAL CONCERNS

■ Should be prescribed only by physicians experienced in immunosuppressive therapy and management of organ transplant clients. Prescriber should have complete information needed for follow-up of client. Should be administered by health care personnel trained in the administration of the drug who have available adequate lab and supportive medical resources.■ Avoid use during lactation. Increased risk for developing lymphoproliferative disorders and opportunistic infections. Increased risk of mortality if daclizumab is used as part of an immunosuppressive regimen with cyclosporine, mycophenolate mofetil, and corticosteroids in cardiac transplant clients. Increased risk of severe, acute hypersensitivity reactions. Use with caution in geriatric clients.

SIDE EFFECTS

Most Common

N&V, constipation, abdominal pain, dyspepsia, epigastric pain, flatulence, gastritis.

Incidence of 2% or more is reported. **GI:** Constipation, N&V, abdominal pain, pyrosis, dyspepsia, abdominal distention, epigastric pain, flatulence, gastritis, hemorrhoids. **CNS:** Tremor, headache, dizziness, insomnia, prickly sensation,

---

depression, anxiety. **CV:** Hypertension, hypotension, aggravated hypertension, tachycardia, thrombosis, bleeding. **Respiratory:** Dyspnea, pulmonary edema, coughing atelectasis, congestion, pharyngitis, rhinitis, hypoxia, rales, abnormal breathing sounds, pleural effusion. **GU:** Oliguria, dysuria, renal tubular necrosis, renal damage, hydronephrosis, urinary tract bleeding, urinary tract disorder, renal insufficiency, urinary retention. **Dermatologic:** Impaired wound healing without infection, acne, pruritus, hirsutism, rash, night sweats, increased sweating. **Musculoskeletal:** Musculoskeletal pain, back pain, arthralgia, leg cramps, myalgia. **Body as a whole:** Post-traumatic pain, chest pain, fever, pain, fatigue, insomnia, shivering, general weakness, injection site reaction, infections. **Metabolic:** Peripheral edema, edema, fluid overload, diabetes mellitus, hyperglycemia. **Hypersensitivity:** *Anaphylaxis*, hypotension, bronchospasms, wheezing, laryngeal edema, pulmonary edema, cyanosis, hypoxia, *respiratory arrest, cardiac arrhythmias, cardiac arrest*, peripheral edema, loss of consciousness, fever, rash, urticaria, diaphoresis, pruritus, injection site reactions, cytokine release syndrome. **Miscellaneous:** Blurred vision, lymphocele, increased incidence of malignancies or infectious episodes.

DRUG INTERACTIONS

 Do not give echinacea with daclizumab

HOW SUPPLIED

Injection Concentrate: 25 mg/5mL.

DOSAGE

* **IV**
  Prevent kidney transplant rejection.

Adults and children 11 months and older: 1 mg/kg q 14 days for total of five doses. Regimen also includes cyclosporine and corticosteroids.

NURSING CONSIDERATIONS

ADMINISTRATION/STORAGE

 1. Give first dose 24 hr or less before transplantation.

2. Not for direct injection. Mix calculated volume of daclizumab with 50 mL of NSS solution. Give by peripheral or central vein over 15-min period.

3. When mixing, gently invert bag to avoid foaming; do not shake.

4. Contains no preservatives or bacteriostatic agents; once prepared, give within 4 hr. If solution must be held longer, refrigerate between 2–8°C (36–46°F); discard after 24 hr. Discard any unused solution.

5. Do not add or infuse other drugs simultaneously through same IV line.

6. Have medication immediately available to treat hypersensitivity reactions.

ASSESSMENT

1. Note indications/date of kidney transplant.

2. Therapy includes cyclosporine and corticosteroids. Initiate therapy within 24 hr pretransplant and subsequent doses every 14 days for 5 total doses.

3. Monitor VS, I&O, suture line, CBC, electrolytes, liver and renal function studies.

4. Stop therapy if a severe hypersensitivity reaction occurs.

CLIENT/FAMILY TEACHING

1. Follow written guidelines for therapy explicitly. Must take exactly as prescribed to prevent transplant rejection.

2. Used to lower the body's natural immunity with kidney transplants. When one receives a transplant, the body's white blood cells will try to get rid of (reject) the transplanted kidney. Daclizumab prevents the white blood cells from getting rid of the transplanted kidney; its effect on the white blood cells may also reduce the body's ability to fight infections.

3. Review written list of all possible drug side effects and those which must be reported to transplant center.

4. Record BP, I&O, and daily weights; report sudden changes. Consume plenty of fluids and report any blood in urine, painful urination, or a reduction in urine volume.

5. Practice reliable birth control during and for 4 months following therapy.

6. May develop acne and excessive hair growth or impaired wound healing; may need dermatologic referral.

---

7. Report fever or S&S of infection, increased fatigue, malaise, breathing problems, unexplained bleeding/bruising or hematuria. Avoid vaccinations and household members should do the same until approved.

OUTCOMES/EVALUATE
Prophylaxis of acute organ rejection

Dactinomycin (Actinomycin D) ■ IV
(dack-tin-oh-**MY**-sin)

CLASSIFICATION(S):
Antineoplastic, antibiotic
PREGNANCY CATEGORY: C
Rx: Cosmegen.

SEE ALSO ANTINEOPLASTIC AGENTS.

USES
(1) In combination with vincristine, surgery, and/or irradiation for treatment of Wilms' tumor (nephroblastoma) and its metastases. (2) In combination with cyclophosphamide, doxorubicin, and vincristine to treat childhood rhabdomyosarcoma. (3) As part of combination chemotherapy and/or multimodality for treatment of metastatic nonseminomatous testicular carcinoma. (4) As part of combination chemotherapy and/or multimodality to treat Ewing's sarcoma. (5) As a single agent or part of combination chemotherapy to treat gestational trophoblastic neoplasia. (6) As a component of regional perfusion for the palliative and/or adjunctive treatment of locally recurrent or locoregional solid malignancies. *Investigational:* Ovarian cancer, Kaposi's sarcoma, osteosarcoma, malignant melanoma.

ACTION/KINETICS

Action
Acts by intercalating into the purine-pyrimidine base pair, thereby inhibiting synthesis of messenger RNA. Is cell-cycle nonspecific, although the maximum number of cells are destroyed in the G_1 phase.

Pharmacokinetics
Cleared from the blood within 2 min and concentrated in nucleated cells. **t½:** 36 hr. Does not cross the blood-brain barrier and is excreted mainly unchanged. Severity of toxicity varies and is only partly dependent on the dose.

CONTRAINDICATIONS
Concurrent infection with chickenpox or herpes zoster (death may result). Lactation. Infants less than 6–12 months of age.

SPECIAL CONCERNS
■ (1) Give under the supervision of a health care provider experienced in the use of cancer chemotherapeutic drugs. (2) Drug is highly toxic and both powder and solution must be handled and administered with care. Inhalation of dust or vapors and contact with the skin or mucous membranes, especially the eyes, must be avoided. Avoid exposure during pregnancy. Due to toxic properties (e.g., corrosivity, carcinogenicity, mutagenicity, teratogenicity), review and carefully follow special handling procedures prior to handling. (3) Drug is extremely corrosive to soft tissue. If extravasation occurs during IV use, severe damage to soft tissues will result.■ When used with x-ray therapy, erythema is seen in normal skin and on buccal and pharyngeal mucosa. Toxicity is frequent and may limit the amount that can be given. Administration to the elderly may be associated with an increased risk of myelosuppression compared with younger clients. An increased incidence of GI toxicity and bone marrow suppression may occur when combined with radiation.

SIDE EFFECTS

Most Common
N&V, diarrhea, abdominal pain, acne, rash, alopecia.

Appearance of toxic manifestations (except for N&V) may not occur for 2–4 days after a course of therapy is stopped and may not be maximal until 1–2 weeks have elapsed. **GI:** N&V, abdominal pain, anorexia, cheilitis, diarrhea, dysphagia, esophagitis, GI ulceration, hepatic veno-occlusive disease, hepatitis, hepatomegaly, liver toxicity

---

Bold Italic = life threatening side effect   ■ = black box warning   ♣ = Available in Canada

including ascites, pharyngitis, ulcerative stomatitis. **Dermatologic:** Acne, alopecia, flare-up of erythema, increased pigmentation of previously irradiated skin, skin eruptions. **Hematologic:** Agranulocytosis, anemia (even to the point of **aplastic anemia**), leukopenia, pancytopenia, reticulopenia, thrombopenia. **Miscellaneous:** **Anaphylaxis,** fatigue, fever, growth retardation, hypocalcemia, infection, lethargy, malaise, myalgia, pneumonitis, proctitis. Due to corrosiveness, extravasation causes severe damage to soft tissues. Hypocalcemia. When combined with radiation, increased severity of skin reactions, GI toxicity, and **bone marrow depression** (irreversible in clients with preexisting renal, hepatic, or bone marrow impairment).

Side effects using the perfusion technique: Hematopoietic depression, absorption of toxic products from massive destruction of neoplastic tissues, increased susceptibility to infection, impaired wound healing, superficial ulceration of the gastric mucosa, edema of the extremity involved, damage to soft tissues of the perfused area, and **potentially venous thrombosis**.

LABORATORY TEST CONSIDERATIONS
Interferes with bioassay tests used to determine antibacterial drug levels. Abnormal LFTs, bone marrow, hepatic, and renal function.

HOW SUPPLIED
Powder for Injection, Lyophilized: 0.5 mg.

DOSAGE

• **IV**

Wilms' tumor, childhood rhabdomyosarcoma, Ewing sarcoma.
15 mcg/kg daily for 5 days given in various combinations and schedules with other chemotherapeutic drugs.

Metastatic nonseminomatous testicular carcinoma.
1,000 mcg/m^2 on day 1 as part of combination regimen with cyclophosphamide, bleomycin, vinblastine, and cisplatin.

Gestational trophoblastic neoplasia.
12 mcg/kg daily for 5 days as a single agent. Alternatively, 500 mcg on days 1 and 2 as part of combination therapy

with etoposide, methotrexate, folinic acid, vincristine, cyclophosphamide, and cisplatin.

• **ISOLATION PERFUSION**

Locally recurrent and locoregional solid malignancies.
Dosage schedules and techniques vary. In general, the following doses are suggested: 50 mcg/kg for lower extremity or pelvis or 35 mcg/kg for upper extremity. Lower doses may be advisable in obese clients or when previous chemotherapy or radiation therapy have been employed.

NURSING CONSIDERATIONS
ADMINISTRATION/STORAGE
IV 1. Due to toxicity, give only in short courses. For the elderly, start at the lower end of the dosage range, depending on decreased hepatic, renal, or cardiac function and concomitant disease or other drug therapy.
2. *Drug is extremely corrosive.* Reconstitute by adding 1.1 mL sterile water for injection (without preservative). The resulting solution is a clear and gold-colored and contains about 0.5 mg/mL. Add directly to infusion solutions of D5W or NaCl injection and run over 20 to 30 min or to the tubing of a running IV infusion and give over 2–3 min.
3. Use 'two-needle technique' if given directly into the vein without use of an infusion. Reconstitute and withdraw dose from the vial with one sterile needle. Use another needle for direct injection into the vein.
4. Although stable after reconstitution, the product is preservative free. Thus, discard any unused drug.
5. Exercise extreme care in reconstituting and administering dactinomycin so that the dust or vapors are not inhaled or come in contact with skin or mucous membranes. Take special care to prevent contact with the eyes. Prepare under a laminar flow hood.
6. If any S&S of extravasation are observed, terminate the injection or infusion immediately and restart in another vein. If extravasation suspected, apply ice to the site for 15 min 4 times/ day for 3 days.

D

7. Store from 15–30°C (59–86°F). Protect from light and humidity.

ASSESSMENT

1. Note reasons for therapy, other agents trialed, outcome. Assess for any evidence of herpes zoster; check titer (VSG) if unsure of disease in youth.

2. Determine if pregnant, lactating, or infected with herpes; contraindicates therapy.

3. Interferes with bioassay test used to measure antibacterial drug levels; monitor response to antibiotic therapy carefully. Inhibits action of penicillin; do not use for infection.

4. Monitor CBC, uric acid, liver and renal function studies. Drug may cause severe granulocyte and platelet toxicity. Nadir: 10 days; recovery 21–28 days.

5. During therapy, perform leukocyte counts daily, and platelet counts q 3 days. Frequent liver and kidney function tests are recommended.

CLIENT/FAMILY TEACHING

1. Drug used to treat some kinds of cancer of the bones and soft tissue, including muscles and tendons; Wilms' tumor (a cancer of the kidney); tumors in the uterus or womb; and cancer of the testicles.

2. Report redness of the skin, which can lead to destruction and sloughing, particularly in areas previously affected by radiation. Redness may be noted in normal skin and oral and throat tissues; use topical viscous xylocaine as needed.

3. Consume 2–3 L/day of fluids to prevent dehydration and urate crystal formation; may need allopurinol therapy if inadequate fluid intake.

4. May be administered intermittently if N&V persist even when an antiemetic is given.

5. Drug is very toxic and can cause severe damage to your skin, eyes, nose, throat, or lungs. It must NOT come into contact with your skin, eyes, or any other part of your body. If receiving at home follow special handling procedures. Follow directions for protective clothing to be worn and what to do if you inhale this medicine, or if it comes into contact with your eyes or skin.

6. Report unusual bruising, bleeding, fever, oral inflammation, or persistent diarrhea.

7. Avoid vaccinations.

8. Practice contraception during and for 4 weeks following therapy. Evaluate for egg/sperm harvesting.

9. May experience hair loss 7–10 days after therapy.

10. Keep all F/U appointments to evaluate response.

OUTCOMES/EVALUATE

↓ Tumor size/spread and suppression of malignant cell proliferation

---

Dalteparin sodium ■
(**DAL**-tih-**pair**-in)

CLASSIFICATION(S):
Anticoagulant, low molecular weight heparin
PREGNANCY CATEGORY: B
Rx: Fragmin.

SEE ALSO *HEPARINS, LOW MOLECULAR WEIGHT.*

USES

(1) Prevent deep vein thrombosis (DVT) in clients undergoing hip replacement or abdominal surgery who are at risk for thromboembolic complications (i.e., pulmonary embolism). High risk includes obesity, general anesthesia more than 30 min, malignancy, history of DVT or pulmonary embolism, age 40 and over. (2) Prevent DVT in those who are at risk for thromboembolic complications (which may lead to pulmonary embolism) due to severely restricted mobility during acute illness. (3) Prevent ischemic complications due to blood clot formation in life-threatening unstable angina and non-Q-wave MI in clients coadministered aspirin. (4) Extended treatment of symptomatic venous thromboembolism (proximal deep vein thrombosis and/or pulmonary embolism) to reduce the occurrence of venous thromboembolism in clients with cancer. *Investigational:* Prophylaxis of DVT in those undergoing moderate or high risk surgery, orthopedic surgery,

---

Bold Italic = life threatening side effect   ■ = black box warning   ✦ = Available in Canada

D

hip fracture surgery, neurosurgery, in clients with ischemic stroke, in those with impaired mobility, in general medical clients (i.e., cancer, bed rest, heart failure, severe lung disease), or in pregnant clients at risk for thromboembolic complications.

ACTION/KINETICS

Pharmacokinetics
Peak plasma levels: 4 hr. **t½, SC:** 3–5 hr. t½ increased in those with chronic renal insufficiency requiring hemodialysis.

SPECIAL CONCERNS
See also *Heparins, Low Molecular Weight.* ■ (1) Spinal/epidural hematomas. When neuraxial anesthesia (spinal/epidural anesthesia) or spinal puncture is used, those who are anticoagulated or scheduled to be anticoagulated with low molecular weight heparins or heparinoids for prevention of thromboembolic complications are at risk of developing a spinal or epidural hematoma that can result in long-term or permanent paralysis. The risk is increased using indwelling epidural catheters for giving analgesics or by the concurrent use of drugs affecting hemastasis, such as NSAIDs, platelet inhibitors, or other anticoagulants. The risk also appears to increase by traumatic or repeated spinal or epidural puncture. (2) Frequently monitor clients for signs and symptoms of neurological impairment. If observed, urgent treatment is required. (3) The health care provider should consider potential benefits vs risk before neuraxial intervention in clients anticoagulated or to be anticoagulated for thromboprophylaxis.■ The multiple dose vial contains benzyl alcohol that has been associated with a fatal 'gasping syndrome' in premature infants.

SIDE EFFECTS
Most Common
Hematomas (injection site, wound), significant bleeding, pruritus/rash, hematuria, allergic reaction, fever, injection site reactions.
CV: Significant bleeding (fatal/nonfatal) from any tissue or organ, hematoma at injection site, wound hematoma, spinal or epidural hematoma, reoperation due to bleeding, postoperational transfusions. **Hematologic:** Thrombocytopenia. **Hypersensitivity:** Allergic reactions, including pruritus, rash, fever, injection site reaction, bullous eruption, skin necrosis (rare), *anaphylaxis*. **Miscellaneous:** Pain at injection site, hematuria.

HOW SUPPLIED
Injection: 2,500 international units/0.2 mL (16 mg/0.2 mL); 5,000 international units/0.2 mL (32 mg/0.2 mL); 7,500 international units/0.3 mL (48 mg/0.3 mL); 10,000 international units/0.4 mL or 1 mL (64 mg/0.4mL or 64 mg/1 mL); 12,500 units/0.5 mL (80 mg/0.5 mL); 15,000 units/0.6 mL (96 mg/0.6 mL); 18,000 units/0.72 mL (115.2 mg/0.72 mL); 95,000 units/3.8 mL (160 mg/mL); 95,000 international units/9.5 mL (64 mg/mL).

DOSAGE
- **SC ONLY**
  Prevention of DVT in abdominal surgery.
Adults: 2,500 international units each day starting 1–2 hr prior to surgery and repeated once daily for 5–10 days postoperatively. **High-risk clients:** 5,000 international units the night before surgery and repeated once daily for 5–10 days postoperatively. **In malignancy:** 2,500 international units 1–2 hr before surgery followed by 2,500 international units 12 hr later and 5,000 international units once daily for 5–10 days postoperatively.
  Prevention of DVT following hip replacement surgery.
Adults: 2,500 international units within 2 hr before surgery with a second dose of 2,500 international units in the evening on the day of surgery (six or more hr after the first dose). If surgery occurs in the evening, omit the second dose on the day of surgery. On the first postoperative day, give 5,000 international units once daily for 5–10 days. Alternatively, can give 5,000 international units the evening before surgery, followed by 5,000 international units once daily for 5–10 days, starting the evening of the day of surgery.

 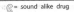

Severely restricted mobility during acute illness.

Give 5,000 international units once daily for up to 12 to 14 days.

Prevent ischemic complications in unstable angina/non-Q-wave MI.

Adults: 120 international units/kg, not to exceed 10,000 international units q 12 hr with concurrent PO aspirin (75–165 mg/day). Continue treatment until client is clinically stabilized (usually 5–8 days).

Venous thromboembolism in clients with cancer.

First 30 days of treatment: 200 units/kg total body weight once daily, not to exceed 18,000 units per day. **Months 2–6:** Approximately 150 units/kg once daily, not to exceed 18,000 units per day. Safety and efficacy beyond 6 months have not been determined.

Thrombocytopenia in clients with cancer and acute symptomatic venous thromboembolism.

Platelet counts between 50,000 and 100,000/mm³: Reduce the daily dose by 2,500 units until platelet count recovers to at least 100,000/mm³. **Platelets less than 50,000/mm³:** Discontinue dalteparin until platelet count recovers above 50,000/mm³.

NURSING CONSIDERATIONS

ADMINISTRATION/STORAGE

1. In clients in extended treatment of symptomatic venous thromboembolism and who have severe impaired renal function (C_{CR} <30 mL/min), monitor for anti-factor Xa levels. Target anti-factor Xa range is 0.5–1.5 units/mL. When monitoring anti-factor Xa in these clients, perform sampling 4–6 hr after dalteparin dosing and only after the client has received 3–4 doses.

2. Available in single-dose prefilled syringes affixed with a 27-gauge × ½-inch needle.

3. Before withdrawing drug, inspect vial for particulate matter or discoloration.

4. Do not mix with other infusions or injections unless compatibility data known.

5. To ensure delivery of full dose, do not expel air bubble from prefilled syringe before injection.

6. Store drug at controlled room temperature of 20–25°C (68–77°F). After the first penetration of rubber stopper, may store multidose vials at room temperature for up to 2 weeks. Discard any unused drug after 2 weeks.

ASSESSMENT

1. List sensitivity to heparin or pork products.

2. Note reasons for therapy, any evidence of active major bleeding, bleeding disorders, or thrombocytopenia. Monitor CBC with platelets, urinalysis, FOB during therapy.

3. Identify criteria for inclusion or if at risk for DVT (i.e., over 40, obese, prolonged general anesthesia, additional risk factors).

CLIENT/FAMILY TEACHING

1. Review reasons for therapy and administration technique. Used to prevent blood clot development after major surgery.

2. Give by deep SC injection while sitting or lying down. May give in a U-shape area around the navel, the upper outer side of the thigh, or the upper outer quadrangle of the buttock. Change/rotate the injection site daily.

3. If the area around the navel or thigh is used, a fold of skin must be lifted, using the thumb and forefinger, while giving the injection.

4. Insert the entire length of the needle at a 45–90-degree angle.

5. Avoid OTC aspirin containing products. Use electric razor and soft toothbrush to prevent tissue trauma.

6. Report any unusual bruising/bleeding or hemorrhage. Therapy may last for 5–10 days.

OUTCOMES/EVALUATE

Post-operative DVT prophylaxis

Danazol ■ ©
(**DAN**-ah-zohl)

CLASSIFICATION(S):
Androgen, synthetic
PREGNANCY CATEGORY: X
❧**Rx:** Cyclomen.

USES
(1) Endometriosis amenable to hormonal management in clients who cannot tolerate or who have not responded to other drug therapy. (2) Fibrocystic breast disease. (3) Hereditary angioedema in males and females. *Investigational:* Gynecomastia, menorrhagia, precocious puberty, idiopathic immune thrombocytopenia, lupus-associated thrombocytopenia, and autoimmune hemolytic anemia.

ACTION/KINETICS
Action
Inhibits the release of gonadotropins (FSH and LH) by the anterior pituitary; thus, inhibits synthesis of sex steroids and competitively inhibits binding of steroids to their cytoplasmic receptors in target tissues. In women this action arrests ovarian function, induces amenorrhea, and causes atrophy of normal and ectopic endometrial tissue. Has weak androgenic effects.

Pharmacokinetics
Onset, fibrocystic disease: 4 weeks. **Time to peak effect, amenorrhea and anovulation:** 6–8 weeks; **fibrocystic disease:** 2–3 months to eliminate breast pain and tenderness and 4–6 months for elimination of nodules. **t½:** 4.5 hr. **Duration:** Ovulation and cyclic bleeding usually resume 60–90 days after cessation of therapy.

CONTRAINDICATIONS
Undiagnosed genital bleeding; markedly impaired hepatic, renal, and cardiac function; porphyria; pregnancy and lactation.

SPECIAL CONCERNS
■ (1) Use contraindicated in pregnancy. A sensitive test (e.g., beta subunit test, if available) capable of determining early pregnancy is recommended immediately prior to starting therapy. Also, a nonhormonal method of contraception should be used during therapy. If the client becomes pregnant while taking danazol, discontinue the drug and advise the client of the potential risk to the fetus. (2) Thromboembolism, thrombotic and thrombophlebitic events, including sagittal sinus thrombosis and life-threatening or fatal strokes have been reported. (3) Experience with long-term danazol therapy is limited. Long-term use has resulted in peliosis hepatitis and benign adenoma; these may be silent until complicated by acute, potentially life-threatening intra-abdominal hemorrhage. Attempt to determine the lowest dose that will provide adequate protection. (4) Drug has been associated with several cases of benign intracranial hypertension. Early signs include papilledema, headache, N&V, and visual disturbances. Screen clients with these symptoms for papilledema and, if present, advise client to discontinue the drug immediately and refer to a neurologist for further diagnosis and care.■ Use with caution in children treated for hereditary angioedema due to the possibility of virilization in females and precocious sexual development in males. Use with caution in conditions aggravated by fluid retention (e.g., epilepsy, migraine, cardiac, or renal dysfunction). Geriatric clients may have an increased risk of prostatic hypertrophy or prostatic carcinoma.

SIDE EFFECTS
Most Common
Headache, dizziness, fatigue, appetite changes, GI upset, anxiety, bloating, vaginal dryness, mood changes, hot flashes.

Androgenic: Acne, edema, mild hirsutism, seborrhea, decrease in breast size, oily hair/skin, weight gain, deepening of voice and hair growth, clitoral hypertrophy, testicular atrophy. **Estrogen deficiency:** Flushing, sweating, vaginitis, vaginal dryness/irritation, decreased breast size, nervousness, changes in emotions, hot flashes. **GU:** Menstrual disturbances (e.g., spotting), alteration

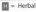

of the timing cycle, amenorrhea (may be persistent), abnormalities in semen volume, viscosity, sperm count, and motility with long-term use. **GI:** N&V, constipation, gastroenteritis, GI upset. **Hepatic:** Jaundice, dysfunction, peliosis hepatitis and benign hepatic adenoma (*intra-abdominal hemorrhage possible*) with long term use. **CV:** *Thromboembolism*, thrombotic and thrombophlebitic events including sagittal sinus thrombosis and *life-threatening or fatal strokes*. **CNS:** Fatigue, tremor, headache, dizziness, mood changes, sleep problems, paresthesia of extremities, anxiety, depression, appetite changes, pseudotumor cerebri. **Musculoskeletal:** Muscle cramps or spasms, joint swelling or lock-up, pain in back, legs, or neck. **Miscellaneous:** Allergic reactions (skin rashes and rarely nasal congestion), hematuria, increased BP, chills, pelvic pain, carpal tunnel syndrome, hair loss, change in libido.

LABORATORY TEST CONSIDERATIONS

↓ HDL and ↑ LDL (temporary but may be severe). Interference with lab determinations of testosterone, androstenedione, and dehydroepiandrosterone.

DRUG INTERACTIONS

Carbamazepine / ↑ Carbamazepine levels

Cyclosporine / ↑ Cyclosporine blood levels → possible nephrotoxicity

Insulin / ↑ Insulin requirements

Warfarin / ↑ PT in warfarin-stabilized clients

HOW SUPPLIED

Capsules: 50 mg, 100 mg, 200 mg.

DOSAGE

• **CAPSULES**

Endometriosis.

400 mg twice a day (moderate to severe) or 100–200 mg twice a day (mild) for 3–6 months (up to 9 months may be required in some clients). Begin therapy during menses, if possible, to be sure that client is not pregnant.

Fibrocystic breast disease.

50–200 mg twice a day beginning on day 2 of menses. Begin therapy during menses to ensure client is not pregnant.

Hereditary angioedema.

Initial: 200 mg 2–3 times per day; after desired response, decrease dosage by 50% (or less) at 1–3-month intervals. Treat subsequent attacks by giving up to 200 mg/day. No more than 800 mg/day should be given to adults.

NURSING CONSIDERATIONS

℘ Do not confuse danazol with Dantrium (a skeletal muscle relaxant).

ADMINISTRATION/STORAGE

Breast pain and tenderness in fibrocystic disease are usually relieved within 30 days and eliminated in 2–3 months; elimination of nodularity requires 4–6 months of uninterrupted therapy. Treatment may be reinstituted if symptoms recur (50% have recurring symptoms within 6 months).

ASSESSMENT

1. Note reasons for therapy. Assess reports of endometrial pain, breast pain, tenderness, and the presence of any nodules. Perform regular breast exams. Exclude breast carcinoma before initiating therapy for fibrocystic disease.
2. Determine any undiagnosed vaginal bleeding; note onset, frequency, extent, and precipitating factors.
3. CTS may develop due to drug-induced edema with compression of median nerve.
4. Obtain baseline CBC, renal and LFTs; determine if pregnant.
5. Identify factors that trigger angioedema (e.g., C-1 inhibitor deficiency).

CLIENT/FAMILY TEACHING

1. Take with meals to ↓ GI upset.
2. Virilization may occur with drug therapy (e.g., abnormal hair growth, acne, reduced breast size, increased skin oiliness, enlarged clitoris, voice deepening); report so dosage can be adjusted to prevent voice damage. These side effects usually disappear once drug discontinued; ovulation will resume in 60–90 days.
3. Wear cotton underwear and pay careful attention to hygiene to diminish danazol-induced vaginitis.
4. Practice non–hormonal birth control as ovulation may not be suppressed until 6–8 weeks of therapy; continue breast self-exams and report changes.

Bold Italic = life threatening side effect   ■ = black box warning   ♣ = Available in Canada

5. Clients with a history of epilepsy, migraines, and cardiac or renal dysfunction may develop fluid retention; stop drug and report.

6. With cystic breast disease, pain and discomfort usually resolve in 2–3 months while nodules take 4–6 months. Endometriosis may recur once the drug is stopped.

OUTCOMES/EVALUATE
- ↓ Endometrial pain (3–6 months)
- ↓ Breast pain (2–3 months)

Dapiprazole hydrochloride

(dah-**PIP**-rah-zol)

CLASSIFICATION(S):
Ophthalmic, alpha-adrenergic blocking drug
PREGNANCY CATEGORY: B
Rx: Rev-Eyes.

USES
Reverse diagnostic mydriasis induced by adrenergic (e.g., phenylephrine) or parasympatholytic (e.g., tropicamide) agents.

ACTION/KINETICS
Action
Produces miosis by blocking the alpha-adrenergic receptors on the dilator muscle of the iris. No significant action on ciliary muscle contraction; thus, there are no changes in the depth of the anterior chamber or the thickness of the lens. Does not alter the IOP either in normal eyes or in eyes with elevated IOP. The rate of pupillary constriction may be slightly slower in clients with brown irides than in clients with blue or green irides.

CONTRAINDICATIONS
Acute iritis or other conditions where miosis is not desirable. To reduce intraocular pressure or to treat open-angle glaucoma.

SPECIAL CONCERNS
Use with caution during lactation. Safety and effectiveness have not been determined in children. The drug may cause difficulty in adaptation to dark and may reduce the field of vision.

SIDE EFFECTS
Most Common
Conjunctival injection, burning on instillation, headaches.
Ophthalmic: Conjunctival injection lasting 20 min, burning on instillation, ptosis, lid erythema, itching, lid edema, chemosis, corneal edema, punctate keratitis, photophobia, tearing and blurring of vision, dryness of eyes. **Miscellaneous:** Headaches, brow ache.

HOW SUPPLIED
Ophthalmic Powder, Lyophilized: 20 mg (0.5% solution when reconstituted).

DOSAGE
- **OPHTHALMIC SOLUTION**
  Reverse mydriasis.
  2 gtt followed in 5 min by 2 more gtt applied to the conjunctiva of the eye after ophthalmic examination.

NURSING CONSIDERATIONS
ADMINISTRATION/STORAGE
1. Do not use more frequently than once a week.
2. To prepare solution, remove and discard Al seals and rubber plugs from drug and diluent vials. Pour diluent into drug vial; remove dropper assembly from its sterile wrapping and attach to drug vial. Shake container for several minutes to ensure adequate mixing.
3. Store reconstituted eye drops at room temperature for 21 days. Discard solution if not clear and colorless.

ASSESSMENT
1. Note any conditions that may preclude therapy or any hypersensitivity to alpha-adrenergic blocking agents.
2. List eye color. Pupillary constriction may be slightly slower in clients with brown irides as opposed to those with blue or green irides.

CLIENT/FAMILY TEACHING
1. Drops used to reverse pupil enlargement. May cause burning on instillation.
2. Use care; may impair adaptation to dark and reduce field of vision.
3. May be light sensitive after use; wear sunglasses.
4. Report any unusual adverse effects.

 = see color insert   = Herbal **IV** = Intravenous   = sound alike drug

OUTCOMES/EVALUATE
Reversal of drug-induced mydriasis (pupil dilation)

Daptomycin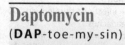
(**DAP**-toe-my-sin)

CLASSIFICATION(S):
Antibiotic, cyclic lipopeptide
PREGNANCY CATEGORY: B
Rx: Cubicin.

USES
(1) Treatment of complicated skin and skin structure infections due to the following susceptible strains of gram positive organisms: *Staphylococcus aureus* (including methicillin-resistant strains), *Streptococcus pyogenes*, *Streptococcus agalactiae*, *Streptococcus dysgalactiae* subspecies *equisimilis*, and *Enterococcus faecalis* (vancomycin-susceptible strains only). Combination therapy may be used if the documented or presumed pathogens include gram-negative or anaerobic organisms. (2) Treatment of *Staphylococcus aureus* bacteremia, including right-sided endocarditis caused by this organism that are resistant or sensitive to methicillin. Combination therapy may be used if the documented or presumed pathogens include gram-negative or anaerobic organisms.

ACTION/KINETICS
Action
Daptomycin is a cyclic lipopeptide that binds to bacterial membranes and causes a rapid depolarization of membrane potential. The loss of membrane potential leads to inhibition of protein, DNA, and RNA synthesis, leading to bacterial cell death. Daptomycin exhibits rapid, concentration-dependent bactericidal activity against gram-positive organisms.

Pharmacokinetics
Steady state levels are achieved by the third daily dose. It is reversibly bound to human plasma proteins (primarily serum albumin). **t½:** About 8 hr. Site of metabolism of the drug has not been determined. Excreted primarily by the kidney. **Plasma protein binding:** 90–93%.

CONTRAINDICATIONS
Hypersensitivity to daptomycin. Treatment of pneumonia.

SPECIAL CONCERNS
Dosage adjustment is necessary in clients with severe renal insufficiency (C_{CR} less than 30 mL/min). Safety and efficacy have not been determined in children less than 18 years of age. Use with caution during lactation. Clients older than 65 years may experience more side effects. Pseudomembranous colitis may develop; can range from mild to life-threatening. Temporarily suspend HMG-CoA reductase inhibitors in clients receiving daptomycin.

SIDE EFFECTS
Most Common
Constipation, N&V, headache, insomnia, diarrhea, rash, injection site reactions.
Side effects listed are for all uses. **GI:** Constipation, N&V, diarrhea, loose stools, dyspepsia, abdominal pain, *pseudomembranous colitis*, superinfections, abdominal distention, flatulence, stomatitis, dry mouth, epigastric discomfort, gingival pain, oral hypesthesia, jaundice, oral candidiasis, *GI hemorrhage*. **CNS:** Headache, insomnia, dizziness, anxiety, confusion, vertigo, mental status change, paresthesia, dyskinesia, hallucinations. **Dermatologic:** Rash (heat, vesicular), pruritus, eczema. **CV:** Hyper-/hypotension, *cardiac failure/arrest*, supraventricular arrhythmia, atrial fibrillation/flutter. **GU:** Renal failure (including acute), UTI, vaginal candidiasis, proteinuria, impaired renal function. **Hematologic:** Anemia, leukocytosis, thrombocytopenia, thrombocytosis, eosinophilia, lymphadenopathy. **Respiratory:** Dyspnea, cough, sore throat, pneumonia, pharyngolaryngeal pain, pleural effusion. **Musculoskeletal:** Limb/back pain, arthralgia, chest pain, myalgia, muscle cramps/pain/weakness, pain in extremity, osteomyelitis, rhabdomyolysis. **Metabolic:** Hypo-/hyperglycemia, hypokalemia, hypomagnesemia, electrolyte disturbance. **Ophthalmic:** Eye irritation, blurred vision. **Otic:** Tinnitus. **Body as a whole:** Injection

---

Bold Italic = life threatening side effect   ■ = black box warning   ✤ = Available in Canada

site reactions (including erythema), fever, edema (including peripheral edema), cellulitis, *Candida* infections, fungemia, bacteremia, **sepsis**, fatigue, weakness, asthenia, rigors, discomfort, jitteriness, flushing, hypersensitivity (including difficulty swallowing, hives, pruritus, SOB, truncal erythema), neuropathy, **anaphylaxis**. **Miscellaneous:** Decreased appetite, taste disturbance.

LABORATORY TEST CONSIDERATIONS

↑ CPK, ALT, AST, INR ratio, serum LDH, alkaline phosphatase, phosphorus, serum bicarbonate. Prolonged PT. Abnormal LFTs.

OD OVERDOSE MANAGEMENT

Treatment: Provide supportive care with maintenance of GFR. Daptomycin is slowly cleared by hemodialysis or by peritoneal dialysis. The use of high-flux dialysis membranes during 4 hr of hemodialysis may increase the percentage of dose removed compared with low-flux membranes.

DRUG INTERACTIONS

Possible rhabdomyolysis when combined with HMG-CoA reductase inhibitors.

HOW SUPPLIED

Powder for Injection, Lyophilized Cake: 500 mg.

DOSAGE

- **IV INFUSION**

    Complicated skin and skin structure infections.

Adults: 4 mg/kg given over a 30-min period by IV infusion in 0.9% NaCl injection once every 24 hr for 7–14 days. Do not dose more frequently than once a day. For clients with C_{CR} <30 mL/min (including hemodialysis or CAPD), give 4 mg/kg q 48 hr.

    Bacteremia due to Staphylococcus aureus, *including right-sided endocarditis caused by methicillin-susceptible or methicillin-resistant strains.*

Adults: 6 mg/kg in sodium chloride injection given over a 30-min period once q 24 hr for a minimum of 2–6 weeks. For clients with a C_{CR} of 30 mL/min or less, give 6 mg/kg once q 48 hr.

NURSING CONSIDERATIONS

ADMINISTRATION/STORAGE

IV 1. To reduce development of drug-resistant bacteria and maintain effectiveness of daptomycin, use drug only to treat/prevent infections that are proven/strongly suspected to be caused by susceptible organisms.

2. Reconstitute the 500 mg vial with 10 mL of 0.9% NaCl injection.

3. Further dilute reconstituted drug with 0.9% NaCl injection; give by IV infusion over a 30 min. period.

4. Product contains no preservative or bacteriostatic agent; thus, use aseptic technique in preparation of the final IV solution.

5. Reconstituted solution stable in vial for 12 hr at room temperature, up to 48 hr if refrigerated at 2–8°C (36–46°F). The diluted solution is stable in the infusion bag for 12 hr at room temperature or 48 hr if refrigerated. The combined time (vial and infusion bag) should not exceed 12 hr at room temperature and 48 hr if refrigerated.

6. Vials are for single use only.

7. Do not add additives or other medications to daptomycin single-use vials or infuse simultaneously through the same IV line. If the same IV line is used for sequential infusion of several different drugs, flush line with compatible infusion solution before and after infusion with daptomycin.

8. Daptomycin compatibile with 0.9% NaCl injection and lactated Ringer's injection. It is not compatible with dextrose-containing diluents.

9. Store original packages refrigerated at 2–8°C (36–46°F). Avoid excessive heat.

ASSESSMENT

1. Note reasons for therapy, onset, characteristics of S&S, other agents trialed, outcome.

2. Monitor CBC, CPK, cultures, renal and LFTs; reduce dose with renal dysfunction.

3. List drugs prescribed; hold statins during therapy, monitor anticoagulant activity for several days after starting daptomycin if receiving warfarin.

D

CLIENT/FAMILY TEACHING

Report immediately any muscle pain/ weakness, infusion site reactions or lack of improvement. If severe diarrhea, rash or infection evident- report.

OUTCOMES/EVALUATE

Resolution of infection; healing/clearing of skin lesions

Darbepoetin alfa ■ **IV**

(**DAR**-beh-**poh**-eh-tin **AL**-fah)

CLASSIFICATION(S):

Erythropoietin, human recombinant

PREGNANCY CATEGORY: C

Rx: Aranesp.

USES

(1) Anemia associated with chronic renal failure, including those on or not on dialysis. (2) Treat anemia in nonmyeloid malignancies in which anemia is caused by the effect of coadministered chemotherapy. *Investigational:* Anemia associated with malignancy.

ACTION/KINETICS

Action

Production of endogenous erythropoietin is decreased in those with chronic renal failure and a deficiency in erythropoietin is the causative factor. Darbepoetin alfa, produced by recombinant DNA technology, stimulates erythropoiesis-stimulating protein. Darbepoetin interacts with progenitor stem cells to increase RBC production. Usually takes 2–6 weeks to see increased hemoglobin levels.

Pharmacokinetics

Darbepoetin has about a 3-fold longer terminal t½ when given IV or SC than does epoetin alfa. **t½, after IV:** About 1.4 hr (distribution) and about 21 hr (terminal). **t½, after SC:** 49 hr (terminal). Bioavailability after SC is about 37% in adults and about 54% in children. **Peak levels after SC:** 34 hr. With once weekly dosing, steady-state serum levels are reached in 4 weeks.

CONTRAINDICATIONS

Uncontrolled hypertension. Hypersensitivity to darbepoetin alfa or any component of the product.

SPECIAL CONCERNS

■ (1) Erythropoiesis-stimulating agents: Use the lowest dose of darbepoetin alfa that will gradually increase the hemoglobin concentration to the lowest level sufficient to avoid the need for RBC transfusion. (2) Darbepoetin alfa and other erythropoiesis-stimulating agents increased the risk of death and of serious CV reactions when administered to target a hemoglobin of more than 12 grams/dL. (3) Cancer clients. Use of erythropoiesis-stimulating agents: (a) shortened the time to tumor progression in clients with advanced head and neck cancer receiving radiation therapy when administered to target a hemoglobin of more than 12 grams/dL; (b) shortened overall survival and increased deaths attributed to disease progression at 4 months in clients with metastatic breast cancer receiving chemotherapy when administered to target a hemoglobin of more than 12 grams/dL; (c) increased the risk of death when administered to target a hemoglobin of 12 grams/dL in clients with active malignant disease receiving neither chemotherapy nor radiation therapy. Erythropoiesis-stimulating agents are not indicated for this population. (4) Clients receiving erythropoiesis-stimulating agents preoperatively for reduction of allogeneic RBC transfusions. A higher incidence of DVT was documented in clients receiving epoetin alfa who were not receiving prophylactic anticoagulation. Darbepoetin alfa is not approved for this indication.■ Product is formulated with two different excipients (one containing polysorbate 80 and the other containing albumin); there is a remote risk for transmission of viral diseases with the albumin product. There is the potential for immunogenicity to develop resulting in pure red cell aplasia and severe anemia, especially in those with chronic renal failure receiving the drug SC. Use with caution during lactation. Safety and efficacy have

---

not been determined in children, in children with cancer, or in clients with underlying hematologic diseases (e.g., hemolytic anemia, sickle cell anemia, thalassemia, porphyria).

SIDE EFFECTS

Most Common

Hypertension, hypotension, cardiac arrhythmias/death, headache, fatigue, abdominal pain, diarrhea, constipation, N&V, arthralgia, limb pain, myalgia, cough, dyspnea, URTI, infection, peripheral edema, fever.

CV: Vascular access thrombosis, *access hemorrhage*, *pulmonary emboli*, *arterial and venous thromboembolic reactions*, thrombophlebitis, CHF, *cardiac arrhythmia/death*, *cardiac arrest*, *acute MI*, *stroke*, hemodialysis graft occlusion, TIA, angina pectoris, cardiac chest pain, hypertension, hypotension. **CNS:** Seizures, headache, dizziness. **GI:** Diarrhea, N&V, abdominal pain, constipation, *GI hemorrhage*. **Hematologic:** Pure red cell aplasia, severe anemia. **Body as a whole:** *Sepsis*, infection, fever, fatigue, flu-like symptoms, asthenia, dehydration, edema, *death*. **Musculoskeletal:** Myalgia, arthralgia, limb/back pain. **Dermatologic:** Pruritus. **Respiratory:** URTI, dyspnea, cough, bronchitis, pneumonia, pulmonary embolism. **Hypersensitivity reaction:** Skin rash, urticaria, *anaphylaxis*. **Miscellaneous:** Chest pain, peripheral edema, injection site pain, fluid overload, access infection, immunogenicity.

NOTE: Increasing hemoglobin levels to more than 12 grams/dL in men or women may cause increased thrombotic vascular events (e.g., pulmonary emboli, thrombophlebitis, thrombosis in cancer clients) and mortality. Further study is needed.

OD OVERDOSE MANAGEMENT

Symptoms: Increases in hemoglobin greater than about 1 gram/dL during any 2-week period may cause an increased incidence of cardiac arrest, seizures, stroke, exacerbations of hypertension, CHF, vascular thrombosis, ischemia/infarction, acute MI, and fluid overload/edema. *Treatment:* In the event of polycythemia, temporarily

withhold darbepoetin alfa. If clinically indicated, undertake phlebotomy.

HOW SUPPLIED

Solution for Injection: 25 mcg/0.42 mL, 25 mcg/1 mL, 40 mcg/0.4 mL, 40 mcg/1 mL, 60 mcg/0.3 mL, 60 mcg/1 mL, 100 mcg/0.5 mL, 100 mcg/1 mL, 150 mcg/0.3 mL, 150 mcg/1 mL, 200 mcg/0.4 mL, 200 mcg/1 mL, 300 mcg/0.6 mL, 300 mcg/1 mL, 500 mcg/1 mL.

DOSAGE

- **IV; SC**

  Anemia associated with chronic renal failure.

Initial: 0.45 mcg/kg once weekly. Titrate doses so as not to exceed a target hemoglobin concentration of 12 grams/dL. For many clients, the maintenance dose will be lower than the starting dose. Do not increase darbepoetin dose more often than once a month. If the hemoglobin is increasing and approaching 12 grams/dL, reduce dose by 25%. If hemoglobin continues to increase, withhold darbepoetin dose temporarily until the hemoglobin begins to decrease. Therapy can then be restarted at a dose of about 25% below the previous dose. Evaluate if a client fails to respond. When therapy is initiated or adjusted, follow hemoglobin levels weekly until stabilized; monitor at least monthly thereafter. IV route is recommended for those on hemodialysis. Clients with chronic renal failure not yet needing dialysis may require lower maintenance doses.

If the increase in hemoglobin is less than 1 gram/dL over 4 weeks and iron stores are adequate, the dose of darbepoetin alfa may be increased by approximately 25% of the previous dose. Further increases may be made at 4-week intervals until the specified hemoglobin level is reached.

When converting from epoetin alfa to darbepoetin alfa, estimate the starting weekly dose of darbepoetin alfa on the basis of the weekly dose of epoetin alfa at the time of substitution (see package insert). Titrate dose to maintain target hemoglobin. Due to a longer darbepoetin alfa half-life, give less frequently than epoetin alfa (e.g., give darbepoetin alfa once a week if epoetin alfa was given 2–3 times per week and give darbepoetin alfa once every 2 weeks if epoetin alfa was given once/week). Maintain the route of administration (i.e., either IV or SC).

Cancer clients receiving chemotherapy.

Initial: 2.25 mcg/kg weekly SC. The recommended starting dose given once every 3 weeks is 500 mcg as a SC injection. Adjust dose to maintain the lowest hemoglobin level sufficient to avoid the need for RBC transfusion and should not exceed 12 grams/dL. If there is less than a 1 gram/dL increase in hemoglobin after 6 weeks of therapy, increase the dose to 4.5 mcg/kg. If the hemoglobin increases by more than 1 gram/dL in a 2-week period or if the hemoglobin exceeds 11 grams/dL, reduce the dose by 40% of the previous dose. If the hemoglobin exceeds 12 grams/dL, temporarily withhold the drug until the hemoglobin falls to 11 grams/dL. Reinitiate therapy at a dose 40% below the previous dose.

NURSING CONSIDERATIONS

ADMINISTRATION/STORAGE

IV 1. For those who respond to darbepoetin with a rapid increase in hemoglobin (e.g., >1 gram/dL in any 2 week period), reduce dose due to side effects as a result of an excessive rate of rise of hemoglobin.

2. Some have been successfully treated with SC doses given every 2 weeks.

3. Check package insert carefully to determine conversion process from epoetin alfa to darbepoetin alfa.

4. When preparing injection, do not shake; vigorous shaking may denature the drug. Do not leave vials, prefilled syringes, or prefilled SureClick autoinjectors exposed to bright light. Store in their cartons until use.

5. Visually inspect vials; do not use if there is particulate matter and/or discoloration.

6. Do not dilute product and do not give with any other drug solutions.

7. Discard any unused portion; drug is packaged in single-use vials and contains no preservative. Do not pool unused portions.

8. Store at 2–8°C (36–46°F). Do not freeze; protect from light.

ASSESSMENT

1. List reasons for therapy, other agents trialed, outcome, and if epoetin alfa conversion.

2. Assess for seizure history, uncontrolled HTN, other medical conditions that may preclude therapy.

3. Obtain iron panel, H&H, and BP. Monitor weekly until stabilized or until dosage change. Add supplemental iron therapy if serum ferritin <100 mcg/L or iron saturation <20%.

4. Review product literature for administration guidelines carefully.

CLIENT/FAMILY TEACHING

1. Get instructions and review method for administration. Store safely out of reach; discard syringes as directed.

2. Drug stimulates bone marrow to produce red blood cells. Supplemental iron and vitamins may be used to enhance drug effects.

3. Administer as directed; do not increase/skip dose.

4. Do not shake vial; inactivates drug. Keep refrigerated.

5. Report as scheduled for F/U labs so drug dose can be adjusted.

6. Review list of drug side effects; report any persistent/bothersome ones, practice reliable contraception.

7. Follow prescribed dietary and dialysis recommendations; schedule activities to permit rest periods. Monitor BP and record. May experience seizures and brain dysfunction with chronic renal failure if BP not controlled.

8. Do not perform any tasks that require mental alertness until drug effects realized.

OUTCOMES/EVALUATE

↑ RBC production in anemia from CRF/chemotherapy

Darifenacin hydrobromide

(dar-ih-**FEN**-ah-sin)

CLASSIFICATION(S):
Cholinergic blocking drug
PREGNANCY CATEGORY: C
Rx: Enablex.

USES
Overactive bladder with symptoms of urge urinary incontinence, urgency, and frequency.

ACTION/KINETICS

Action
Darifenacin is a competitive muscarinic receptor antagonist. Muscarinic receptors play an important role in contractions of the urinary bladder smooth muscle and stimulation of salivary secretion. By blocking muscarinic receptors, activity of the bladder is reduced.

Pharmacokinetics
Oral bioavailability in extensive metabolizers is about 15% and 19% for the 7.5 and 15 mg tablets, respectively. **Peak plasma levels:** About 7 hr after multiple doses. **Steady-state plasma levels:** 6 days. Extensively metabolized by the liver by CYP2D6 and CYP3A4. **$t^{1}\!/_{2}$, elimination:** 13–19 hr. Excreted in both the urine (60%) and feces (40%). Clearance decreases with age. **Plasma protein binding:** About 98%.

CONTRAINDICATIONS
Use with severe hepatic impairment (Child-Pugh scores of 10–15), urinary retention, or uncontrolled narrow-angle glaucoma and in those who are at risk for these conditions. Hypersensitivity to the drug or components.

SPECIAL CONCERNS
Use with caution in clients being treated for narrow-angle glaucoma, in those with GI obstructive disorders, in those with clinically significant bladder outflow obstruction, and during lactation. Safety and efficacy have not been determined in children.

SIDE EFFECTS

Most Common
Constipation, dry mouth, dyspepsia, nausea, UTI, flu syndrome.
GI: Dry mouth, constipation, nausea, dyspepsia, abdominal pain, diarrhea. **CNS:** Headache, asthenia, dizziness. **GU:** UTI, acute urinary retention. **Miscellaneous:** Dry eyes, blurred vision, accidental injury, flu syndrome, heat prostration (when used in a hot environment).

OD OVERDOSE MANAGEMENT
Symptoms: Severe antimuscarinic effects. *Treatment:* Symptomatic and supportive. In the event of overdosage, monitor ECG.

DRUG INTERACTIONS
Anticholinergic drugs / Additive anticholinergic side effects
Clarithromycin / ↑ Darifenacin levels R/T inhibition of metabolism by CYP3A4; do not exceed 7.5 mg darifenacin/day
Desipramine / Possible ↑ desipramine C_{max} and AUC R/T ↓ metabolism by CYP2D6
Diltiazem / ↑ Darifenacin levels R/T inhibition of metabolism by CYP3A4
Erythromycin / ↑ Darifenacin levels R/T inhibition of metabolism by CYP3A4
Flecainide / Possible ↑ flecainide C_{max} and AUC R/T ↓ metabolism by CYP2D6
Fluoconazole / ↑ Darifenacin levels R/T inhibition of metabolism by CYP3A4
Imipramine / Possible ↑ imipramine C_{max} and AUC R/T ↓ metabolism by CYP2D6
Itraconazole / ↑ Darifenacin levels R/T inhibition of metabolism by CYP3A4; do not exceed 7.5 mg darifenacin/day
Ketoconazole / ↑ Darifenacin levels R/T inhibition of metabolism by CYP3A4; do not exceed 7.5 mg darifenacin/day
Nefazodone / ↑ Darifenacin levels R/T inhibition of metabolism by CYP3A4; do not exceed 7.5 mg darifenacin/day
Nelfinavir / ↑ Darifenacin levels R/T inhibition of metabolism by CYP3A4; do not exceed 7.5 mg darifenacin/day
Ritonavir / ↑ Darifenacin levels R/T inhibition of metabolism by CYP3A4; do not exceed 7.5 mg darifenacin/day

Thioridazine / Possible ↑ thioridazine C_{max} and AUC R/T ↓ metabolism by CYP2D6

Verapamil / ↑ Darifenacin levels R/T inhibition of metabolism by CYP3A4

HOW SUPPLIED

Tablets, Extended-Release: 7.5 mg, 15 mg.

DOSAGE

- **TABLETS, EXTENDED-RELEASE**
  Overactive bladder.

Initial: 7.5 mg once daily. Based on individual response, dose may be increased to 15 mg once daily as early as 2 weeks after starting therapy. For clients with moderate hepatic impairment (Child-Pugh scores of 7–9), do not exceed a daily dose of 7.5 mg.

NURSING CONSIDERATIONS

ADMINISTRATION/STORAGE

1. Do not exceed a daily dose of 7.5 mg if given with potent CYP3A4 inhibitors, such as clarithromycin, itraconazole, ketoconazole, nefazodone, nelfinavir, or ritonavir.

2. Store from 15–30°C (59–86°F); protect from light.

ASSESSMENT

1. Note reasons for therapy, onset/characteristics, other agents trialed, outcome.

2. List other drugs prescribed to ensure none interact.

3. Review voiding patterns; assess abdomen to ensure no urinary retention. Identify nonpharmacologic therapies trialed first, kugal exercises, estrogen rings, weights, etc.

4. Assess renal and LFTs; note glaucoma. Rule out UTI, obstruction, stones etc prior to starting therapy.

CLIENT/FAMILY TEACHING

1. Take with liquid, with/without food once daily.

2. Swallow whole; do not chew, divide, or crush tablets.

3. Use caution until drug effects realized; may cause dizziness or blurred vision.

4. Keep a voiding diary noting frequency and triggers; note any changes in voiding patterns after starting therapy.

5. May experience dry mouth, constipation, urinary retention. Avoid exercise in hot weather; sweating may be decreased.

6. Immediately report any adverse side effects esp. inability to pass urine.

7. Keep all F/U appointments to evaluate drug response.

OUTCOMES/EVALUATE

↓ Urinary symptoms R/T frequency, urgency and/or incontinence

Darunavir ethanolate
(dar-**UE**-na-vir)

CLASSIFICATION(S):

Antiviral drug, antiretroviral protease inhibitor

PREGNANCY CATEGORY: B

Rx: Prezista.

USES

Treatment of HIV infection, coadministered with ritonavir, 100 mg, and other antiretroviral drugs. For antiretroviral treatment-experienced adult clients, such as those with HIV-1 strains resistant to more than one protease inhibitor.

ACTION/KINETICS

Action

Inhibits HIV-1 protease. Selectively inhibits the cleavage of HIV encoded Gag-Pol polyproteins in infected cells, thus preventing the formation of mature virus particles. Darunavir is primarily metabolized by CYP3A; ritonavir is given because it inhibits CYP3A, thus increasing plasma levels of darunavir. Ritonavir, 100 mg twice daily, given with darunavir, 600 mg, results in about a 14-fold increase in systemic exposure to darunavir. The information for ritonavir should also be consulted.

Pharmacokinetics

Absolute bioavailability of darunavir, 600 mg, with ritonavir, 100 mg, is 82%. **Time to maximum levels:** 2.5–4 hr. Food increases the C_{max} and AUC of darunavir when given with ritonavir. Metabolized by CYP3A and excreted in the feces (about 80%) and urine (about

---

14%). **t½, terminal:** About 15 hr when combined with ritonavir. **Plasma protein binding:** 95%.

CONTRAINDICATIONS

Known hypersensitivity to any component of the product. Coadministration with drugs that are highly dependent on CP3A for clearance and for which increased plasma levels may result in serious and/or life-threatening events (see *Drug Interactions*). Lactation.

SPECIAL CONCERNS

Use with caution in those with a known sulfonamide allergy since darunavir contains a sulfonamide moiety. Use with caution in impaired hepatic function. During the initial phase of treatment, those responding to antiretroviral therapy may develop an inflammatory response to indolent or residual opportunistic infections (e.g., *Mycobacterium avium* complex, cytomegalovirus, *Pneumocystis jeroveci* pneumonia, tuberculosis) that may require further evaluation and treatment. Safety and efficacy have not been determined in children.

SIDE EFFECTS

Most Common

Diarrhea, headache, nasopharyngitis, N&V, abdominal pain, constipation.

GI: Abdominal pain/distension, constipation, dry mouth, dyspepsia, flatulence, N&V. **CNS:** Altered mood, anxiety, asthenia, confusion, disorientation, fatigue, headache, hypesthesia, irritability, impaired memory, nightmares, paresthesia, peripheral neuropathy, somnolence, vertigo. **CV:** Hypertension, *MI*, tachycardia, TIAs. **Dermatologic:** Allergic dermatitis, alopecia, dermatitis medicamentosa, eczema, hyperhidrosis, liopatrophy, maculopapular rash, night sweats, skin inflammation, toxic skin eruption. Severe skin rash, including erythema multiforme and ***Stevens-Johnson syndrome***. **Musculoskeletal:** Arthralgia, myalgia, osteopenia, osteoporosis, pain in extremity. **Respiratory:** Cough, dyspnea, hiccups. **GU:** Acute renal failure, gynecomastia, nephrolithiasis, polyuria, renal insufficiency. **Metabolic:** Anorexia, decreased appetite, obesity, peripheral edema, polydipsia. New onset diabetes mellitus or exacerbation of preexisting diabetes mellitus and hyperglycemia. **Hematologic:** Increased bleeding, including spontaneous skin hematomas and hemarthrosis in those with hemophilia type A and B. **Body as a whole:** Redistribution/accumulation of body fat, including central obesity, dorsocervical fat enlargement, peripheral wasting, facial wasting, breast enlargement, and 'cushingoid appearance.' **Miscellaneous:** Folliculitis, hyperthermia, pyrexia, rigors.

LABORATORY TEST CONSIDERATIONS

↑ Alanine aminotransferase, alkaline phosphatase, aspartate aminotransferase, gammaglutamyltransferase, pancreatic amylase, pancreatic lipase, PTT, plasma prothrombin. ↓ Bicarbonate, platelet count, total absolute neutrophil count, WBCs. Hyperbilirubinemia, hyper-/hypoglycemia, hyper-/hyponatremia, hyperuricemia, hypoaluminemia, hypocalcemia, hypocholesterolemia, hyperlipidemia.

DRUG INTERACTIONS

NOTE: Drug interactions are based on coadministration of darunavir and ritonavir.

Amiodarone / ↑ Amiodarone concentrations; use together with caution and monitor

Bepridil / ↑ Bepridil concentrations; use together with caution and monitor

Carbamazepine / Significant ↓ darunavir levels → loss of therapeutic effect; do not give together

Clarithromycin / ↑ Clarithromycin levels; if C_{CR} is 30–60 mL/min, decrease clarithromycin dose by 50% and if C_{CR} is <30 mL/min decrease clarithromycin dose by 75%

Cyclosporine / ↑ Cyclosporine levels; monitor levels

Dexamethasone / ↓ Darunavir levels R/T ↑ metabolism by CYP3A

Dihydroergotamine / ↑ Darunavir levels → ↑ risk of serious and/or life-threatening side effects (e.g., peripheral vasospasm, ischemia of extremities); do not use together

Efavirenz / ↓ Darunavir AUC and ↑ efavirenz AUC; use together with caution

Ergonovine / ↑ Darunavir levels → ↑

 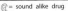

risk of serious and/or life-threatening side effects (e.g., peripheral vasospasm, ischemia of extremities); do not use together

Ergotamine / ↑ Darunavir levels → ↑ risk of serious and/or life-threatening side effects (e.g., peripheral vasospasm, ischemia of extremities); do not use together

Felodipine / ↑ Felodipine levels; use together with caution and monitor

Fluticasone / ↑ Fluticasone levels

HMG-CoA reductase inhibitors (e.g., atorvastatin, lovastatin, pravastatin, simvastatin) / ↑ Risk of myopathy (including rhabdomyolysis)

Itraconazole / ↑ Darunavir and ↑ itraconazole levels; if used together do not exceed a daily dose of itraconazole of 200 mg

Ketoconazole / ↑ Darunavir and ↑ itraconazole levels; if used together do not exceed a daily dose of ketoconazole of 200 mg

Lidocaine (systemic) / ↑ Lidocaine concentrations; use together with caution and monitor

Lopinavir/Ritonavir / ↓ Darunavir AUC by 53%

Methadone / Monitor for possible abstinence syndrome; may need to ↑ methadone dose

Methylergonovine / ↑ Darunavir levels → ↑ risk of serious and/or life-threatening side effects (e.g., peripheral vasospasm, ischemia of extremities); do not use together

Midazolam / ↑ Darunavir levels → ↑ risk of serious and/or life-threatening side effects; do not use together

Nicardipine / ↑ Nicardipine levels; use together with caution and monitor

Nifedipine / ↑ Nifedipine levels; use together with caution and monitor

Oral Contraceptives (e.g., ethinyl estradiol, norethindrone) / ↓ Ethinyl estradiol levels; use alternative or additional contraceptive measures

Phenobarbital / Significant ↓ darunavir levels → loss of therapeutic effect; do not give together

Phenytoin / Significant ↓ darunavir levels → loss of therapeutic effect; do not give together

Pimozide / ↑ Darunavir levels → ↑ risk of serious and/or life-threatening side effects (e.g., cardiac arrhythmias); do not use together

Quinidine / ↑ Quinidine concentrations; use together with caution and monitor

Rifamycins (e.g., rifabutin, rifampin) / Significant ↓ darunavir levels → loss of therapeutic effect; also, rifabutin + ritonavir → ↑ ritonavir levels. When the three drugs are used together, give rifabutin 150 mg once every other day

Saquinavir / ↓ Darunavir AUC; do not use together

Sildenafil / Use together with caution; do not exceed dose of 25 mg within 48 hr of sildenafil

Selective serotonin reuptake inhibitors / Carefully titrate SSRI dose based on antidepressant response

Sirolimus / ↑ Sirolimus levels; monitor levels

H *St. John's wort* / Significant ↓ darunavir levels → loss of therapeutic effect; do not use together

Tacrolimus / ↑ Tacrolimus levels; monitor levels

Tadalafil / Use together with caution; do not exceed dose of 10 mg within 72 hr of tadalafil

Trazodone / ↑ Trazodone levels; possible nausea, dizziness, hypotension, syncope

Triazolam / ↑ Darunavir levels → ↑ risk of serious and/or life-threatening side effects; do not use together

Vardenafil / Use together with caution; do not exceed dose of 2.5 mg within 72 hr of vardenafil

Warfarin / Warfarin levels may be affected; monitor INR frequently

HOW SUPPLIED

Tablets: 300 mg (as base).

DOSAGE

- **TABLETS**

  HIV infection.

Adults: 600 mg (two-300 mg tablets) twice daily with ritonavir, 100 mg twice daily, with food.

Bold Italic = life threatening side effect ■ = black box warning ♣ = Available in Canada

NURSING CONSIDERATIONS

ADMINISTRATION/STORAGE

1. Failure to coadminister darunavir with ritonavir and food will result in decreased darunavir plasma levels that are not high enough to achieve the desired antiviral effect.

2. Store tablets from 15–30°C (59–86°F).

ASSESSMENT

1. Note treatment history, onset, when available- genotypic or phenotypic testing results; may aid in determining darunavir susceptibility.

2. Assess for any sulfa allergy; precludes therapy.

3. List drugs prescribed/consumed to ensure none interact unfavorably.

4. Monitor renal and LFTs closely esp. with dysfunction.

5. With diabetes may aggravate control or may cause diabetes; with hemophilia may cause increased bleeding; monitor closely.

6. Drug is co-administered with 100 mg ritonavir and with other antiretroviral agents.

7. Has not been used in treatment-naive adults or pediatric clients.

CLIENT/FAMILY TEACHING

1. Drug must be co-administered with ritonavir and food to work effectively. Swallow tablets whole with water or milk.

2. Prezista is not a cure for HIV infection. May continue to develop opportunistic infections and other complications associated with HIV disease.

3. Use reliable contraception. With birth control pills, use alternate contraceptive measures during therapy because hormonal levels may decrease. Use a condom or other barrier method to lower the chance of sexual contact with any body fluids such as semen, vaginal secretions, or blood. Never reuse or share needles.

4. May experience a redistribution or accumulation of body fat in the upper back and neck, breast, and around the back, chest, and stomach area. Loss of fat from the legs, arms, and face may also occur.

5. Diarrhea, nausea, headaches, cold symptoms may occur; report if bothersome or persistent.

6. Report all drugs prescribed and avoid OTC or herbal products, including St. John's wort.

7. Drug interacts with many drugs; review pamphlet for list of drugs to avoid.

8. Store medications safely, do not share with others and keep out of the reach of children.

9. Keep all F/U appointments to evaluate response to therapy and any adverse effects.

OUTCOMES/EVALUATE

- Decreases in HIV RNA
- ↑ CD 4 cells

Dasatinib
(da-**SA**-ti-nib)

CLASSIFICATION(S):
Antineoplastic, antileukemia drug
PREGNANCY CATEGORY: D
Rx: Sprycel.

USES

(1) Treatment of adults with chronic, accelerated, or myeloid or lymphoid blast phase chronic myeloid leukemia (CML) with resistance or intolerance to prior therapy (including imatinib). (2) Treatment of adults with Philadelphia (Ph+) chromosome-positive acute lymphoblastic leukemia (ALL) with resistance or intolerance to prior therapy.

ACTION/KINETICS

Action

Dasatinib inhibits a number of kinases leading to inhibition of the growth of CML and ALL cell lines.

Pharmacokinetics

Maximum plasma levels: 0.5–6 hr. Extensively distributed to the extravascular space. Extensively metabolized, primarily by CYP3A4, to active and inactive metabolites. $t^{1/2}$, **terminal:** 3–5 hr. Eliminated mainly by the feces. **Plasma protein binding:** 96% bound to plasma proteins.

CONTRAINDICATIONS

Lactation.

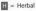

D

SPECIAL CONCERNS

Use with caution in those who have or may develop prolongation of QTc (including those with hypokalemia or hypomagnesemia, with congenital long QT syndrome, those taking antiarrhythmic medications or products that lead to QT prolongation, and cumulative high-dose anthracycline therapy). Safety and efficacy have not been determined in children less than 18 years of age.

SIDE EFFECTS

Most Common

Fluid retention, abdominal pain, diarrhea, N&V, pleural effusion, anemia, dyspnea, febrile neutropenia, GI bleeding, pneumonia, pyrexia, thrombocytopenia, cardiac failure.

GI: N&V, diarrhea, abdominal pain/distension, anorexia, constipation, mucosal inflammation (including mucositis, stomatitis), ascites, GI bleeding, dysgeusia, anal fissure, colitis, dyspepsia, dysphagia, gastritis, oral soft tissue disorder, cholecystitis, cholestasis, esophagitis, hepatitis, ileus, pancreatitis, UGI ulcer, enterocolitis infection. **CNS:** Headache, dizziness, CNS bleeding, neuropathy (including peripheral neuropathy), affect lability, anxiety, confusion, *convulsions*, depression, insomnia, somnolence, syncope, tremor, vertigo, amnesia, *CVA*, decreased libido, reversible posterior leukoencephalopathy syndrome, TIA. **CV:** *CNS hemorrhage (may be fatal),* GI hemorrhage, *other hemorrhage,* pericardial effusion, prolongation of QT interval, arrhythmia, chest pain, CHF, cardiac dysfunction, *cardiac failure, cardiomyopathy, congestive cardiomyopathy,* decreased ejection fraction, left ventricular failure, ventricular dysfunction, angina pectoris, cardiomegaly, hyper-/hypotension, *MI,* palpitations, acute coronary syndrome, livedo reticularis, myocarditis, pericarditis, ventricular tachycardia. **Hematologic:** Myelosuppression, anemia, neutropenia, thrombocytopenia, febrile neutropenia, pancytopenia, pure red cell aplasia, coagulopathy. **Respiratory:** Pulmonary edema (may be severe), pleural effusion, dry cough, dyspnea, pneumonia (bacterial, viral, fungal), pulmonary hypertension, URTI/inflammation, asthma lung infiltration, pneumonitis, a*cute respiratory distress syndrome,* bronchospasm. **Musculoskeletal:** Musculoskeletal pain, arthralgia, myalgia, muscle inflammation/weakness, musculoskeletal stiffness, rhabdomyolysis, tendonitis. **Dermatologic:** Skin rash, pruritus, flushing, acne, alopecia, dermatitis (including eczema), dry skin, hyperhidrosis, nail disorder, photosensitivity reaction, pigmentation disorder, urticaria, neutrophilic dermatosis, bullous conditions, palmar-plantar erythrodysesthesia syndrome, skin ulcer. **GU:** Gynecomastia, renal failure, urinary frequency, irregular menses, proteinuria. **Ophthalmic:** Conjunctivitis, dry eye. **Body as a whole:** Fluid retention, severe ascites, generalized/superficial edema, fatigue, asthenia, chills, pain, pyrexia, malaise, *sepsis,* infection (bacterial, viral, fungal), decreased/increased weight. **Miscellaneous:** Appetite disturbances, tinnitus, contusion, herpes virus infection, hypersensitivity, temperature intolerance, *tumor lysis syndrome.*

LABORATORY TEST CONSIDERATIONS

↑ ALT, AST, bilirubin, creatinine, CPK, troponin. Hypocalcemia, hypophosphatemia, hyperuricemia. Abnormal platelet aggregation.

DRUG INTERACTIONS

Alfentanil / Alteration of alfentanil levels R/T changes in metabolism

Antacids / ↓ Dasatinib AUC and C_{max} when given at the same time; give antacids 2 hr before or after dasatinib

Azole antifungals (itraconazole, ketoconazole) / Possible ↑ dasatinib levels R/T decreased metabolism

Carbamazepine / ↓ Dasatinib levels R/T ↑ metabolism by CYP3A4

Cyclosporine / Alteration of cyclosporine levels R/T changes in metabolism

Dexamethasone / ↓ Dasatinib levels R/T ↑ metabolism by CYP3A4

Ergot alkaloids / Alteration of ergot alkaloid levels R/T changes in metabolism

Fentanyl / Alteration of fentanyl levels R/T changes in metabolism

H_2-histamine blockers (e.g., famotidine) /

Bold Italic = life threatening side effect   ■ = black box warning   ♣ = Available in Canada

Long-term suppression of gastric acid secretion may ↓ dasatinib exposure; do not use together

Macrolide antibiotics (e.g., clarithromycin, erythromycin) / ↑ Dasatinib levels R/T ↓ metabolism; do not use together

Nefazodone / ↑ Dasatinib levels R/T ↓ metabolism; do not use together

Pemozide / Alteration of pemozide levels R/T changes in metabolism

Phenobarbital / ↓ Dasatinib levels R/T ↑ metabolism by CYP3A4

Phenytoin / ↓ Dasatinib levels R/T ↑ metabolism by CYP3A4

Protease inhibitors (e.g., atazanavir, indinavir, nelfinavir, ritonavir, saquinavir) / ↑ Dasatinib levels R/T ↓ metabolism; do not use together

Proton pump inhibitors (e.g., omeprazole) / Long-term suppression of gastric acid secretion may ↓ dasatinib exposure; to not use together

Quinidine / Alteration of quinidine levels R/T changes in metabolism

Rifampicin, rifampin / ↓ Dasatinib mean AUC and C_{max}

Simvastatin / ↑ Simvastatin AUC and C_{max}

Sirolimus / Alteration of sirolimus levels R/T changes in metabolism

 St. John's wort / ↓ Dasatinib levels; do not use together

Tacrolimus / Alteration of tacrolimus levels R/T changes in metabolism

Telithromycin / ↑ Dasatinib levels R/T ↓ metabolism; do not use together

Terfenadine / Alteration of terfenadine levels R/T changes in metabolism

HOW SUPPLIED

Tablets: 20 mg, 50 mg, 70 mg.

DOSAGE

- **TABLETS**

  Chronic myeloid leukemia, acute lymphoblastic leukemia.

Adults: 70 mg twice daily, once in the morning and once in the evening with or without a meal. Continue treatment until disease progression or until no longer tolerated by the client. Dose increase or reduction of 20 mg increments per dose is recommended based on individual safety and tolerability.

Dosage escalation to 90 mg twice daily (chronic phase of chronic myeloid leukemia) or 100 mg twice daily (advanced phase chronic myeloid leukemia or Philadelphia-chromosone positive acute lymphoblastic leukemia) was allowed in those who did not achieve a hematologic or cytogenetic response at the recommended dosage.

NURSING CONSIDERATIONS

ADMINISTRATION/STORAGE

1. The following guidelines for dose modification are used:

- Chronic phase CML (starting dose 70 mg twice daily): ANC <0.5 x 10^9/L and/or platelets, <50 x 10^9/L. (a) Stop dasatinib until ANC is >or equal to 1 x 10^9/L and platelets are >or equal to 50 x 10^9/L. (b) Resume treatment with dasatinib at original starting dose. (c) If platelets are <25 x 10^9/L and/or recurrence of ANC of 0.5 x 10^9/L for >7 days, repeat step (a) and resume dasatinib at reduced dosage of 50 mg twice daily (second episode) or 40 mg twice daily (third episode).

- Accelerated phase CML, blast phase CML, and Ph+ ALL (starting dosage 70 mg twice daily): ANC <0.5 x 10^9/L and/or platelets <10 x 10^9/L. (a) Check if cytopenia is related to leukemia (marrow aspirate or biopsy). (b) If cytopenia is unrelated to leukemia, stop dasatinib until ANC is >or equal to 1 x 10^9/L and platelets are >or equal to 20 x 10^9/L and resume at the original starting dosage. (c) If cytopenia recurs, repeat step (a) and resume dasatinib at a reduced dosage of 50 mg twice daily (second episode) or 40 mg twice daily (third episode). (d) If cytopenia is related to leukemia, consider dosage escalation to 100 mg twice daily.

2. If severe nonhematological side effects occur, withhold treatment until the event has resolved or improved. Thereafter treatment can be resumed as appropriate at a reduced dose, depending on the initial severity of the side effect.

3. Store from 15–30°C (59–86°F).

 = see color insert   = Herbal   **IV** = Intravenous   ℃ = sound alike drug

ASSESSMENT

1. Note reasons for therapy, disease onset, when imatinib was used/outcome, bone marrow results.
2. List drugs prescribed; cannot continue on H_2 blockers, PPIs and other protein bound drugs.
3. Assess physical condition, cardiac, and lung status.
4. Monitor CBC, electrolytes, Mg, renal, LFTS. Do CBC weekly for the first 2 mo then monthly thereafter.
5. Check EKG for prolonged QT, determine if lactose intolerant or pregnant; precludes drug therapy.

CLIENT/FAMILY TEACHING

1. Take with/without food. Swallow tablets whole; do not break, crush, or chew before swallowing. Take at same time each day.
2. Do not take an antacid within 2 hours before or after taking tablets.
3. May cause dizziness or drowsiness; do not perform activities that require mental alertness until drug effects realized.
4. Low blood counts (myelosuppression), may occur which can lead to bleeding, infection and fatigue. Also may experience fluid retention, headache, skin rash and nausea. Report if persistent or bothersome.
5. Practice reliable contraception. Both male and females should take precautions; pregnant females should not handle tablets. May cause fetal harm.
6. Keep all F/U appointments to evaluate LFTs, blood counts and response to therapy.

OUTCOMES/EVALUATE

- ↓ Leukemia cells in blood/bone marrow
- Restoration of normal red and white blood cell and platelet production

Daunorubicin ■ IV Ⓒ hydrochloride (DNR)
(daw-noh-**ROO**-bih-sin)

CLASSIFICATION(S):
Antineoplastic, antibiotic
PREGNANCY CATEGORY: D
Rx: Cerubidine.

Daunorubicin Citrate Liposomal

PREGNANCY CATEGORY: D
Rx: DaunoXome.

SEE ALSO *ANTINEOPLASTIC AGENTS.*

USES

Daunorubicin HCl: (1) In combination with other drugs (e.g., cytarabine) for remission induction in acute nonlymphocytic leukemia (erythroid, monocytic, myelogenous) in adults. (2) Remission induction in acute lymphocytic leukemia in children and adults (increased effectiveness when combined with prednisone and vincristine).

Daunorubicin liposomal: First-line cytotoxic therapy for advanced HIV-associated Kaposi's sarcoma. *Investigational:* Ewing's sarcoma, chronic myelocytic leukemia, neuroblastoma, non-Hodgkin's lymphomas, Wilms' tumor.

ACTION/KINETICS

Action

Anthracycline antibiotic. The liposomal product contains an aqueous solution of the citrate salt of daunorubicin encapsulated within lipid vesicles which are composed of a lipid bilayer of distearoylphosphatidylcholine and cholesterol. Most active in the S phase of cell division but is not cell-cycle specific. Inhibits synthesis of nucleic acid by inserting into the double helix of DNA. Also possesses immunosuppressive, cytotoxic, and antimitotic activity.

Pharmacokinetics

Rapidly cleared from the plasma. The liposomal preparation helps protect daunorubicin from chemical and enzy-

---

Bold Italic = life threatening side effect   ■ = black box warning   ✚ = Available in Canada matic breakdown; also, it minimizes protein binding and decreases uptake by normal tissues. Is released from the liposomal preparation over time and improves selectivity for solid tumors. Metabolized to the active daunorubinicol. **t½:** daunorubicin (nonliposomal product), 18.5 hr; daunorubinicol, 27 hr. **t½, elimination:** 4.4 hr for liposomal form. Drug rapidly taken up by heart, kidneys, lung, liver, and spleen. Chiefly excreted in bile (40%) and unchanged in urine (25%). Does not pass blood-brain barrier.

CONTRAINDICATIONS

Lactation. Hypersensitivity to previous doses. IM or SC use.

SPECIAL CONCERNS

■ (1) Give daunorubicin hydrochloride into a rapidly flowing IV infusion. Do not give IM or SC; severe local tissue necrosis will result if extravasation occurs. (2) Myocardial toxicity (e.g., fatal CHF), may occur when the total cumulative dose exceeds 400–500 mg/m^2 in adults, 300 mg/m^2 in children over 2 years of age or 10 mg/kg in children less than 2 years of age. May occur during therapy or several months or years after therapy. (3) Should be given only by physicians experienced in leukemia chemotherapy and in facilities with lab and supportive resources adequate to monitor drug tolerance and protect and maintain a client compromised by drug toxicity. (4) Both the physician and institution must be capable of responding rapidly and completely to severe hemorrhagic conditions or overwhelming infection. (5) Severe myelosuppression occurs when using therapeutic doses; may lead to infection or hemorrhage. (6) Reduce dose in clients with impaired hepatic or renal function. (7) A triad of back pain, flushing, and chest tightness has been reported in clients treated with liposomal daunorubicin. This triad usually occurs during the first 5 min of the infusion, subsides with interruption of the infusion, and generally does not recur if the infusion is then resumed at a slower rate.■ Use with caution in preexisting heart disease or bone marrow depression. Cardiotoxicity may be more frequent in children and in the elderly. Safety and efficacy have not been determined in children.

SIDE EFFECTS

Most Common

Daunorubicin hydrochloride: N&V, alopecia, mucositis, rash.

Daunorubicin citrate liposomal: N&V, fatigue, headache, fever, diarrhea, rigors, cough, dyspnea, rhinitis, neuropathy, abdominal pain, anorexia, back pain, allergic reactions.

Myocardial toxicity: Potentially fatal CHF, (especially if total dosage exceeds 400–500 mg/m^2 for adults, 300 mg/m^2 for children more than 2 years of age, and 10 mg/kg for children less than 2 years of age.) Mucositis (3–7 days after administration), red-colored urine, hyperuricemia. Severe tissue necrosis if extravasation occurs. Cross-resistance with doxorubicin (produced by similar microorganism) and vinca alkaloids. Hyperuricemia may occur due to lysis of leukemic cells; give allopurinol as a precaution, before starting antileukemic therapy.

For daunorubicin hydrochloride. GI: Acute N&V, mucositis, diarrhea, abdominal pain. **Dermatologic:** Alopecia (reversible), rash, contact drmatitis, urticaria. **At injection site due to extravasation:** Tissue necrosis, severe cellulitis, thrombophlebitis, painful induration. **Miscellaneous:** Anaphylaxis (rare), fver, chills, hyperuricemia.

For daunorubicin citrate liposomal. CNS: Fatigue, headache, neuropathy, malaise, dizziness, depression, insomnia, amnesia, anxiety, ataxia, confusion, seizures, emotional lability, abnormal gait, hallucinations, hyperkinesia, hypertonia, meningitis, somnolence, abnormal thinking, tremors. **Hematologic:** Myelosuppression, especially of the granulocytic series. Neutropenia. **CV:** Cardiomyopathy associated with a decrease in left ventricular ejection fraction (especially in clients who have received prior anthracyclines or who have preexisting cardiac disease). Also, hot flushes, hypertension, palpitation, syncope, tachycardia. **GI:** Nausea, diarrhea, anorexia, abdominal pain, vomiting,

 = see color insert H = Herbal IV = Intravenous = sound alike drug

stomatitis, constipation, increased appetite, dysphagia, **GI hemorrhage**, gastritis, gingival bleeding, hemorrhoids, hepatomegaly, melena, dry mouth, tooth caries. **Respiratory:** Cough, dyspnea, rhinitis, sinusitis, hemoptysis, hiccoughs, pulmonary infiltration, increased sputum. **Musculoskeletal:** Rigors, back pain, myalgia, arthralgia. **Dermatologic:** Alopecia, pruritus, folliculitis, seborrhea, dry skin. **GU:** Dysuria, nocturia, polyuria. **Ophthalmic:** Abnormal vision, conjunctivitis, eye pain. **Otic:** Deafness, ear pain, tinnitus. **Miscellaneous:** Fever, allergic reactions, sweating, chest pain, edema, taste perversion, tenesmus, flu-like symptoms, opportunistic infections, inflammation at injection site, lymphadenopathy, splenomegaly, dehydration, thirst. Back pain, flushing, and chest tightness have been reported within the first 5 min of the infusion.

LABORATORY TEST CONSIDERATIONS
Hyperuricemia secondary to rapid lysis of leukemic cells.

OD OVERDOSE MANAGEMENT
Symptoms: Granulocytopenia, fatigue, N&V. Also, extension of side effects. *Treatment:* Supportive care; maintain glomular filtration. Slowly cleared from the body by both hemodialysis and peritoneal dialysis.

DRUG INTERACTIONS
Cyclophosphamide / ↑ Risk of cardiotoxicity
Methotrexate / Impaired liver function → ↑ risk of toxicity
Myelosuppressive drugs / Reduce dose of daunorubicin

HOW SUPPLIED
Daunorubicin HCl. *Injection:* 5 mg/mL; *Powder for Injection, Lyophilized:* 20 mg/ 10 mL, 50 mg/20 mL.
Daunorubicin Citrate Liposomal. *Injection:* 2 mg/mL.

DOSAGE
• **IV INFUSION OF DAUNORUBICIN HCl**
  Acute nonlymphocytic leukemia.
Adults, less than 60 years old: Daunorubicin, 45 mg/m^2/day on days 1, 2, and 3 of the first course and days 1 and 2 of additional courses; cytosine arabinoside

(Ara-C), 100 mg/m^2/day, by IV infusion, for 7 days during first course and for 5 days during any additional courses of treatment. **Adults, over 60 years old:** Daunorubicin, 30 mg/m^2/day on days 1, 2, and 3 of the first course and days 1 and 2 of additional courses. Use the same dose of cytosine arabinoside as for adults less than 60 years old. Up to three courses may be required.
  Acute lymphocytic leukemia.
Adults: Daunorubicin, 45 mg/m^2, IV, on days 1, 2, and 3; vincristine, 2 mg IV, on days 1, 8, and 15; prednisone, PO, 40 mg/m^2/day for days 1–22 and then taper between days 22 and 29; and, l-asparaginase, IV, 500 international units/ kg/day on days 22–32.
  Acute lymphocytic leukemia.
Children: Daunorubicin, 25 mg/m^2, and vincristine, 1.5 mg/m^2, each IV, on day 1 every week with prednisone, 40 mg/m^2, PO, daily. Usually four courses will induce remission. *NOTE:* Calculate the dose on the basis of milligrams per kilogram if the child is less than 2 years of age or if the body surface is less than 0.5 m^2.
• **IV INFUSION OF DAUNORUBICIN CITRATE LIPOSOMAL**
  Advanced HIV-associated Kaposi's sarcoma.
40 mg/m^2 given over 1 hr. Dose is repeated q 2 weeks. This regimen is continued until there is progression of the disease or other complications of HIV disease or until other intercurrent complications preclude continued therapy. Reduce dosage for renal or hepatic disease. Recommended dose for liposomal product: three-fourths of normal dose if serum bilirubin is 1.2 to 3 mg/dL; one-half of normal dose if serum bilirubin is less than 3 mg/dL and serum creatinine is greater than 3 mg/dL.

NURSING CONSIDERATIONS
  Do not confuse daunorubicin with doxorubicin (also an antineoplastic).

ADMINISTRATION/STORAGE
IV 1. Dilute the hydrochloride in vial with 4 mL sterile water for injection USP. Agitate gently until dissolved (solution contains 5 mg daunorubicin/mL).

Bold Italic = life threatening side effect   ■ = black box warning   ✦ = Available in Canada

Withdraw desired dose into syringe containing 10–15 mL isotonic saline.

2. Inject into tubing of rapidly flowing D5W or NSS IV and administer over 3–5 min. May further dilute in 50 mL of D5W or NSS and infuse over 10–15 min (or in 100 mL of solution and infuse over 30–45 min).

3. Give into a rapidly flowing IV infusion. *Never administer IM or SC as severe local tissue necrosis will result.* Do not mix with other drugs.

4. Extravasation may cause severe local tissue necrosis.

5. Reconstituted solution stable for 24 hr at room temperature; 48 hr refrigerated. Protect from sunlight.

6. Dilute the liposomal product 1:1 with D5W dextrose injection before use. Do not use an in-line filter.

7. Refrigerate liposomal product at 2–8°C (36–46°F). Do not store the reconstituted solution for longer than 6 hr; do not freeze; protect from light.

ASSESSMENT

1. Note reasons for therapy, ensure adequate hydration; medicate 1 hr before therapy with antiemetic and again 6–8 hr after therapy to decrease N&V. Assess hydration status.

2. Assess during and following therapy for myocardial toxicity: changes in baseline ECG, edema, dyspnea, and cyanosis. A 30% decrease in QRS voltage and reduction in the systolic ejection fraction may be early signals of cardiomyopathy. Clients with a cardiac history who receive doses above 550 mg/m^2 are more susceptible to CHF.

3. Follow appropriate guidelines for dose adjustment in liver dysfunction (e.g., bilirubin 1.2–3.0 mg%, give 75% of dose; bilirubin greater than 3.0 mg%, give 50% of dose).

4. Drug may precipitate hyperuricemia; administer allopurinol.

5. Monitor VS, CBC, renal and LFTs; drug may cause severe granulocyte and platelet toxicity; allow bone marrow recovery before subsequent treatments. Nadir: 10 days; recovery: 21–28 days.

CLIENT/FAMILY TEACHING

1. Drug is used parenterally to treat leukemia and lymphoma.

2. Report S&S of cardiac toxicity (i.e., increased SOB/fatigue, and swelling of hands/feet).

3. Report adverse effects, back pain, flushing, chest pain during infusion, S&S of infection, or if mouth ulcers or pain interferes with eating. N&V usually controlled with antiemetics.

4. Urine may appear red for several days following therapy; this is not blood.

5. Consume 1.5–2 L/day of fluids. Record I&O and report alterations.

6. Avoid alcohol, NSAIDs, aspirin, and foods high in purines.

7. Practice contraception during and for at least 1 month after therapy.

8. Avoid crowds and those with active infections. Avoid vaccinations.

9. Anticipate hair loss; should grow back about 5 weeks later.

10. Report any unusual bruising/bleeding; use soft toothbrush, electric razor and avoid contact sports or excessive jostling.

OUTCOMES/EVALUATE

Suppression of malignant cell proliferation

Decitabine

(de-**SIT**-a-been)

CLASSIFICATION(S):

DNA demethylation agent
PREGNANCY CATEGORY: D
Rx: Dacogen.

USES

Treatment of myelodysplastic syndromes, including previously treated and untreated, do novo and secondary myelodysplastic syndromes.

ACTION/KINETICS

Action

Antineoplastic effects occur after phosphorylation and direct incorporation of the drug into DNA and inhibition of DNA methyltransferase, causing hypomethylation of DNA and cellular differentiation or apoptosis. In rapidly dividing cells, the cytotoxicity of decitabine may be due to the formation of covalent adducts between DNA methyltransferase and decitabine incorporated into DNA. Nonproliferating cells are relatively insensitive to the drug.

Pharmacokinetics

t½, terminal: 0.51 hr. Exact route of metabolism and excretion not known in humans. One pathway for elimination may be deamination by cytidine deaminase found in the liver (mainly), granulocytes, intestinal epithelium, and whole blood. **Plasma protein binding:** Negligible (less than 1%).

CONTRAINDICATIONS

Hypersensitivity to decitabine or any component of the product. Lactation.

SPECIAL CONCERNS

Use with caution in clients with renal or hepatic dysfunction. Safety and efficacy have not been determined in children.

SIDE EFFECTS

Most Common

Anemia, constipation, cough, diarrhea, fatigue, hyperglycemia, nausea, neutropenia, petechiae, pyrexia, thrombocytopenia.

GI: Constipation, diarrhea, N&V, abdominal pain, anorexia, decreased appetite, dyspepsia, oral mucosal petechiae, stomatitis, ascites, gingival bleeding/pain, hemorrhoids, loose stools, tongue ulceration, glossodynia, lip ulceration, oral soft tissue disorder, *UGI hemorrhage*, abdominal distension, upper abdominal pain, dysphagia, GERD, oral candidiasis, cholecystitis. **CNS:** Headache, insomnia, confusion, anxiety, hypesthesia, depression, *intracranial hemorrhage*, mental status changes. **CV:** Cardiac murmur, hypotension, atrial fibrillation, tachycardia, *cardiorespiratory arrest, intracranial hemorrhage, CHF, MI*, supraventricular tachycardia, *cardiomyopathy*. **Dermatologic:** Petechiae, pallor, ecchymosis, erythema, rash, pruritus, skin lesion, alopecia, swollen face, urticaria. **GU:** Dysuria, UTI, urinary frequency, renal failure, urethral hemorrhage. **Musculoskeletal:** Arthralgia, limb/back/chest wall pain, musculoskeletal discomfort, myalgia. **Respiratory:** Cough, pneumonia, pharyngitis, lung crackles, ↓ breath sounds, hypoxia, rales, pulmonary edema, postnasal drip, sinusitis, bronchopulmonary aspergillosis, dyspnea, hemoptysis, lung infiltration, pseudomonal lung infection, pulmonary mass, *pulmonary embolism, respiratory arrest*, RTI, URTI. **Hematologic:** Neutropenia, thrombocytopenia, febrile neutropenia, anemia, lymphadenopathy, thrombocythemia, splenomegaly. **At site of injection:** Catheter-related infection/hemorrhage, erythema, pain, swelling. **Body as a whole:** Pyrexia (including intermittent pyrexia), fatigue, rigors, asthenia, lethargy, malaise, edema, peripheral edema, dehydration, candidal infection, tenderness, pain, staphylococcal infection, *Mycobacterium avium* complex infection, fungal infection, *sepsis*. **Miscellaneous:** Blurred vision, abrasion, bacteremia, cellulitis, chest discomfort/pain, crepitations, falls, transfusion reaction, hematoma, hypersensitivity (*anaphylactic reaction*), mucosal inflammation, peridiverticular abscess, postprocedural hemorrhage/pain.

LABORATORY TEST CONSIDERATIONS

↓ ↑ AST, alkaline phosphatase, lactate dehydrogenase, urea. ↓ Albumin, chloride, total protein. ↑ or ↓ Bilirubin, blood bicarbonate. Hyperbilirubinemia, hyper-/hypokalemia, hypoalbuminemia, hyperglycemia, hypomagnesemia, hyponatremia. Abnormal LFTs.

OD **OVERDOSE MANAGEMENT**

Symptoms: Increased myelosuppression, including prolonged neutropenia and thrombocytopenia. *Treatment:* No known antidote. Provide supportive measures.

HOW SUPPLIED

Powder for Injection, Lyophilized: 50 mg.

DOSAGE

• CONTINUOUS IV INFUSION

Myelodysplastic syndromes.

First treatment cycle: 15 mg/m^2 given by continuous IV infusion over 3 hr, repeated q 8 hr for 3 days. **Subsequent treatment cycles:** Repeat the above cycle every 6 weeks. It is recommended that clients be treated for a minimum of 4 cycles; a complete or partial response may take longer than 4 cycles. Treatment may be continued as long as beneficial effects are obtained.

Bold Italic = life threatening side effect   ■ = black box warning   ✤ = Available in Canada

NURSING CONSIDERATIONS

ADMINISTRATION/STORAGE

 1. Aseptically reconstitute with 10 mL sterile water for injection; after reconstitution, product contains approximately 5 mg/mL at a pH of 6.7–7.3. Immediately after reconstitution, further dilute with 0.9% NaCl injection, D5W, or Ringer's lactate injection to a final concentration of 0.1-1 mg/mL.

2. Unless used within 15 min of reconstitution, the diluted solution must be prepared using cold (2–8°C, 36–46°F) infusion fluids and stored from 2-8°C (36-46°F) for up to a maximum of 7 hr until administration.

ASSESSMENT

1. Note onset of myelodysplastic syndrome (MDS), if previously treated (with what), or if untreated; note hematologic status (myeloblasts, plt, H/H) and physical condition of client.

2. List drugs prescribed; no data on interactions at this time.

3. Monitor VS, CBC (with platelets), renal, LFTs. Determine if pregnant-drug will cause fetal damage.

4. Assess infusion site for erythema or phlebitis. Give antiemetics before starting each infusion, after labs drawn. Cycles will be continued as long as client benefits.

CLIENT/FAMILY TEACHING

1. Drug is administered by IV infusion over 3 hr every eight hours for 3 days then every 6 weeks for at least 4 cycles.

2. Labs will be drawn before each infusion to assess for toxicity.

3. May experience fatigue, fever, nausea, cough, constipation, diarrhea, bruising, and elevated blood sugars. Will be given medication before treatments to prevent N&V; report if other S&S persistent or bothersome.

4. Practice reliable contraception. Report if pregnancy suspected. Men should not father a child while receiving decitabine treatment and for 2 months after therapy is terminated.

5. Keep all F/U appointments to assess response, evaluate labs and for toxicity.

OUTCOMES/EVALUATE

- Inhibition of MDS with <5% myeloblasts and Hb >11 g/dL
- Hematologic recovery

Delavirdine mesylate ■
(deh-lah-**VIR**-deen)

CLASSIFICATION(S):
Antiviral, non-nucleoside reverse transcriptase inhibitor
PREGNANCY CATEGORY: C
Rx: Rescriptor.

SEE ALSO *ANTIVIRAL DRUGS.*

USES
Treatment of HIV-1 infections in combination with appropriate antiretroviral agents.

ACTION/KINETICS
Action
Non-nucleoside reverse transcriptase inhibitor that binds directly to reverse transcriptase and blocks RNA-dependent and DNA-dependent DNA polymerase activities. Effect is additive if used with other antiviral drugs. Delavirdine may confer cross-resistance to other non-nucleoside reverse transcriptase inhibitors when used alone or in combination.

Pharmacokinetics
Rapidly absorbed. **Peak plasma levels:** About 1 hr. Median area under the curve is about 30% higher in females than males. Converted to inactive metabolites which are excreted in urine and feces. It inhibits its own metabolism. **$t_{1/2}$, plasma:** 2–11 hr. **Plasma protein binding:** About 98%.

CONTRAINDICATIONS
Lactation.

SPECIAL CONCERNS
■ (1) Tablets are for treatment of HIV-1 infection in combination with appropriate antiretroviral agents when therapy is warranted. (2) Resistant virus emerges rapidly when delavirdine is given as monotherapy. Always give in combination with appropriate antiretroviral therapy.■ Use with caution in impaired

---

D

hepatic function. Use with combination therapy as resistant viruses emerge with monotherapy. Safety and efficacy in combination with other antiretroviral drugs have not been determined in HIV-1-infected clients less than 16 years of age.

SIDE EFFECTS

Most Common

Rash, maculopapular rash, N&V, diarrhea, headache, fatigue, pruritus.

Body as a whole: Headache, fatigue, asthenia, allergic reaction, chest pain, chills, general or local edema, fever, flu syndrome, lethargy, malaise, neck rigidity, general or local pain, trauma. **CV:** Bradycardia, migraine, pallor, palpitation, postural hypotension, syncope, tachycardia, vasodilation. **CNS:** Headache, abnormal coordination, agitation, amnesia, anxiety, change in dreams, cognitive impairment, confusion, decreased libido, depression, disorientation, dizziness, emotional lability, hallucinations, hyperesthesia, hyperreflexia, hypesthesia, impaired coordination, insomnia, mania, nervousness, neuropathy, nightmares, paralysis, paranoia, paresthesia, restlessness, somnolence, tingling, tremor, vertigo, weakness. **GI:** N&V, diarrhea, anorexia, aphthous stomatitis, bloody stool, colitis, constipation, appetite decreased or increased, diarrhea, duodenitis, dry mouth, diverticulitis, dyspepsia, dysphagia, fecal incontinence, flatulence, enteritis, esophagitis, gastritis, gagging, gastroesophageal reflux, GI bleeding or disorder, gingivitis, gum hemorrhage, increased saliva, increased thirst, mouth ulcer, abdominal cramps/distention/pain, lip edema, hepatitis (nonspecified), pancreatitis, rectal disorder, sialadenitis, stomatitis, tongue edema, ulceration. **Dermatologic:** Skin rashes, maculopapular rash, pruritus, angioedema, dermal leukocytoblastic vasculitis, dermatitis, desquamation, diaphoresis, dry skin, erythema, erythema multiforme, folliculitis, fungal dermatitis, alopecia, nail disorder, petechial rash, seborrhea, skin disorder, skin nodule, ***Stevens-Johnson syndrome***, vesiculobullous rash, sebaceous cyst. **GU:** Breast enlargement,

kidney calculi, epididymitis, hematuria, hemospermia, impotence, kidney pain, metrorrhagia, nocturia, polyuria, proteinuria, vaginal moniliasis. **Musculoskeletal:** Back pain, neck rigidity, arthritis or arthralgia of single or multiple joints, bone disorder or pain, leg cramps, muscle weakness, myalgia, tendon disorder, tenosynovitis, tetany, muscle cramps. **Respiratory:** URTI, bronchitis, chest congestion, cough, dyspnea, epistaxis, laryngismus, pharyngitis, rhinitis, sinusitis. **Hematologic:** Anemia, bruises, ecchymosis, eosinophilia, granulocytosis, neutropenia, pancytopenia, petechiae, purpura, spleen disorder, thrombocytopenia. **Ophthalmic:** Nystagmus, blepharitis, conjunctivitis, diplopia, dry eyes, photophobia. **Miscellaneous:** Fatigue, alcohol intolerance, peripheral edema, weight increase or decrease, taste perversion, tinnitus, ear pain.

LABORATORY TEST CONSIDERATIONS

↑ ALT, AST, bilirubin, GGT, lipase, serum alkaline phosphatase, serum amylase, serum creatinine phosphatase, serum creatinine. Bilirubinemia, hyperkalemia, hyperuricemia, hypocalcemia, hyponatremia, hypophosphatemia. Prolonged PTT.

DRUG INTERACTIONS

Antacids / ↓ Delavirdine absorption; separate doses by 1 hr

Amprenavir / ↑ Amprenavir levels and AUC and ↓ amprenavir half-life; also, ↓ peak plasma level and AUC of delavirdine

Anticonvulsants (Carbamazepine, Phenobarbital, Phenytoin) / ↓ Delavirdine levels R/T ↑ hepatic metabolism

Benzodiazpines / Possible serious or life-threatening drug side effects R/T ↓ metabolism

Calcium channel blockers, dihydropyridine-type / Possible serious or life-threatening drug side effects R/T ↓ metabolism

Clarithromycin / Significant ↑ in amount absorbed of both drugs; possible serious side effects

Dapsone / Possible serious or life-threatening drug side effects of dapsone R/T ↓ metabolism

---

Bold Italic = life threatening side effect   ■ = black box warning   ✤ = Available in Canada

Didanosine / ↓ Absorption of both drugs; separate administration by at least 1 hr

Ergot derivatives / Possible serious or life-threatening ergot side effects R/T ↓ metabolism

Fluoxetine / ↑ Trough levels of delavirdine by 50%

Indinavir / ↑ Indinavir levels R/T ↓ metabolism; possible serious side effects (reduce indinavir dose to 600 mg 3 times per day)

Quinidine / Possible serious or life-threatening drug side effects R/T ↓ metabolism

Rifabutin, Rifampin / ↓ Delavirdine levels R/T ↑ hepatic metabolism; also, possible ↑ rifabutin plasma levels

H *St. John's wort* / ↓ Delavirdine levels R/T ↑ CYP3A4 metabolism

Saquinavir / ↑ Saquinavir levels R/T ↓ metabolism; possible serious side effects. Also, possible ↓ delavirdine area under the curve

Sildenafil / ↑ Sildenafil levels (do not exceed a single 25 mg dose of sildenafil in a 48-hr period)

Warfarin / ↑ Warfarin levels → possible serious or life-threatening warfarin side effects R/T ↓ metabolism

HOW SUPPLIED
Tablets: 100 mg, 200 mg.

DOSAGE

- **TABLETS**
  HIV-1 infection.
400 mg 3 times per day in combination with other antiretroviral therapy.

NURSING CONSIDERATIONS

ADMINISTRATION/STORAGE
1. Give with or without food.
2. In achlorhydria, take with an acidic beverage (e.g., cranberry or orange juice).

ASSESSMENT
1. Note disease onset/exposure times, likelihood of transmission, disease characteristics such as stage of infection, viral load.
2. List drugs prescribed.
3. Monitor CBC, LFTs, viral load, CD_4 counts.
4. Assess lifestyle and potential to resume risky behaviors.

CLIENT/FAMILY TEACHING
1. Take as directed, with or without food. Take antacids 1 hr before or 1 hr after drug ingestion.
2. Tablets may be dispersed with water prior to consumption. To prepare, add 4 tablets to at least 3 ounces of water and allow to stand for a few minutes. Stir until a uniform dispersion occurs and consume promptly. Rinse glass and swallow to ensure entire dose is taken.
3. In achlorhydria (lack of stomach acid production), take with an acidic beverage (e.g., cranberry or orange juice).
4. Drug does not cure HIV infection but only slows virus replication; may continue to have HIV related illnesses.
5. Always administer with other antiretroviral therapy.
6. Rash on upper body and arms may require interruption of therapy. Report especially if accompanied by fever, blistering, myalgia, eye or mouth lesions.
7. Avoid OTC agents without approval.
8. Continue barrier contraception; does not reduce risk of transmission.
9. If prescribed Viagra (sildenafil) do not exceed 25 mg in a 48 hr period due to risk of adverse effects such as drop in BP, vision changes and sustained painful erection (priapism).

OUTCOMES/EVALUATE
Post-exposure prophylaxis HIV; ↓ viral load

Denileukin diftitox   ■ IV

(den-ih-**LOO**-kin **DIF**-tih-tox)

CLASSIFICATION(S):
Antineoplastic, miscellaneous
PREGNANCY CATEGORY: C
Rx: Ontak.

USES
Treatment of persistent or recurrent cutaneous T-cell lymphoma whose malignant cells express the CD25 component of the IL-2 receptor.

D

ACTION/KINETICS
Action
A recombinant DNA-derived cytotoxic protein designed to direct the cytocidal action of diphtheria toxin to cells that express the IL-2 receptor. The human IL-2 receptor consists of three forms— low (CD25), intermediate (CD122/CD132), and high affinity (CD25/CD122/CD132). The high affinity form is usually found only on activated T-lymphocytes, activated B-lymphocytes, and activated macrophages. Malignant cells expressing 1 or more of the subunits of the IL-2 receptor are found in certain leukemias and lymphomas, including cutaneous T-cell lymphoma. It is believed denileukin interacts with the high affinity IL-2 receptor on the cell surface leading to inhibition of cellular protein synthesis and cell death within hours.

Pharmacokinetics
$t^{1/2}$, **distribution:** About 2–5 min; $t^{1/2}$, **terminal:** About 70–80 min. Metabolized by proteolytic degradation. Development of antibodies significantly impacts clearance rates.

CONTRAINDICATIONS
Hypersensitivity to denileukin, diphtheria toxin, interleukin-2, or excipients in the product. Lactation.

SPECIAL CONCERNS
■ Use only by those experienced with antineoplastic therapy and management of cancer clients; give in a facility equipped and staffed for CPR and where the client can be closely monitored for an appropriate time based on health status.■ Safety and efficacy have not been determined in pediatric clients or in cutaneous T-cell lymphoma whose malignant cells do *not* express the CD25 component of the IL-2 receptor. Preexisting low serum albumin levels may predict and predispose clients to the vascular leak syndrome.

SIDE EFFECTS
Most Common
Chills/fever, N&V, anorexia, rash, diarrhea, edema, dyspnea, increased cough, infection, pain, headache, chest pain, hypotension, vasodilation, tachycardia, paresthesia, nervousness, pruritus, sweating, hematuria, albuminuria, pyuria, anemia, decreased weight, myalgia, pharyngitis, rhinitis.

Up to 5% of side effects are severe or life-threatening. **Hypersensitivity:** Hypotension, back pain, dyspnea, vasodilation, rash, chest pain/tightness, tachycardia, dysphagia or laryngismus, syncope, allergic reaction, *anaphylaxis*. **Vascular leak syndrome:** Hypotension, edema, hypoalbuminemia. **GI:** N&V, anorexia, diarrhea, constipation, dyspepsia, dysphagia, pancreatitis. **CNS:** Dizziness, paresthesia, nervousness, confusion, insomnia. **CV:** Hypo-/hypertension, vasodilation, tachycardia, thrombotic events, arrhythmia. **Dermatologic:** Acute or delayed onset rash (generalized maculopapular, petechial, vesicular bullous, urticarial, or eczematous), pruritus, sweating. **GU:** Hematuria, albuminuria, pyuria, acute renal insufficiency, microscopic hematuria. **Hematologic:** Anemia, thrombocytopenia, leukopenia. **Metabolic:** Edema, weight decrease, dehydration (due to GI events). **Respiratory:** Dyspnea, increased cough, pharyngitis, rhinitis, lung disorder. **Musculoskeletal:** Myalgia, arthralgia. **Body as a whole:** Chills, fever, asthenia, infection, pain, headache, flu-like syndrome. **Miscellaneous:** Chest pain, injection site reaction, infectious complications (decreased lymphocyte counts), hyper-/hypothyroidism.

LABORATORY TEST CONSIDERATIONS
↑ Creatinine, transaminase. Hypoalbuminemia, hypocalcemia, hypokalemia.

HOW SUPPLIED
Solution for Injection, Frozen: 150 mcg/mL.

DOSAGE
• IV ONLY
   Cutaneous T-cell lymphoma.
For each treatment cycle, give 9 or 18 mcg/kg/day for 5 consecutive days q 21 days. Infuse over 15 or more min.

NURSING CONSIDERATIONS
ADMINISTRATION/STORAGE
IV 1. If side effects occur during IV infusion, stop/reduce rate, depending on reaction severity.
2. Optimal duration of therapy has not been determined.

Bold Italic = life threatening side effect   ■ = black box warning   ♣ = Available in Canada

3. Prepare and hold diluted denileukin in plastic syringes or soft plastic IV bags (adsorption will occur if glass containers are used).

4. Concentration must be 15 or more mcg/mL during all steps in the preparation of the solution for IV infusion. Ensure by withdrawing calculated dose from the vial(s) and injecting it into an empty IV infusion bag. For each 1 mL of denileukin removed from the vial(s), no more than 9 mL of sterile saline without preservative should be added to the IV bag.

5. Store frozen at −10°C (14°F) or lower. Bring to room temperature before preparing dose. May thaw vials in refrigerator for 24 hr or less or at room temperature for 1–2 hr. Do not heat. Administer prepared solutions within 6 hr. Do not refreeze.

6. Mix solution in the vial by gently swirling (do not shake vigorously). After thawing, a haze may be visible which should clear when solution reaches room temperature. Do not use unless clear, colorless, and without visible particulate matter.

7. Infuse over 15 or more min. Do not administer as a bolus injection.

8. Do not physically mix with other drugs or administer through an in-line filter.

9. Administer prepared solution within 6 hr, using a syringe pump or IV infusion bag.

10. Discard any unused portion immediately.

ASSESSMENT

1. Note disease onset, other agents trialed, outcome.

2. Assess albumin levels; delay administration until levels are >3 grams/dL. Low albumin levels may predispose to vascular leak syndrome.

3. Manage hypersensitivity reactions as follows:
- Interrupt/decrease rate of infusion, depending on severity of reaction.
- IV antihistamines, corticosteroids, and epinephrine may be required.
- Have resuscitative equipment readily available.

4. Monitor VS; observe for S&S of infection.

5. Obtain CBC, chemistry, renal and LFTs; monitor weekly.

CLIENT/FAMILY TEACHING

1. Used to treat cutaneous T-cell lymphoma, a rare type of cancer that affects certain WBCs and causes lesions to develop on the skin.

2. Monitor weight daily; report any significant gain/loss.

3. Report adverse effects, any S&S of infection, anemia, or unusual bruising/bleeding.

4. Avoid ETOH, aspirin products, or ibuprofen.

5. Practice reliable contraception during and for several months following therapy.

6. Back pain; chest pain; dizziness or faintness; difficulty swallowing; fast or irregular heartbeat; fever or chills; infection; rash; SOB; swelling of face, feet, or lower legs; warmth and flushing of skin may be experienced.

OUTCOMES/EVALUATE

Inhibition of malignant cell proliferation; ↓ tumor burden

Desipramine hydrochloride
(dess-**IP**-rah-meen)

CLASSIFICATION(S):
Antidepressant, tricyclic
PREGNANCY CATEGORY: C
Rx: Norpramin.
✤Rx: Apo-Desipramine, Novo-Desipramine, Nu-Desipramine, PMS-Desipramine, ratio-Desipramine.

SEE ALSO *ANTIDEPRESSANTS, TRICYCLIC.*

USES
Treatment of depression.

ACTION/KINETICS

Action
Slight anticholinergic, sedative, and orthostatic hypotensive effects.

Pharmacokinetics
Effective plasma levels: 125–300 ng/mL. **t½:** 12–24 hr. **Time to reach**

steady state: 2–11 days. Response usually seen within the first week.

CONTRAINDICATIONS

Use in children less than 12 years of age.

SPECIAL CONCERNS

■ (1) Antidepressants increase the risk of suicidal thinking and behavior (suicidality) in short-term studies in children and adolescents with major depressive disorders and other psychiatric disorders. Anyone considering the use of desipramine or any other antidepressant in a child or adolescent must balance this risk with the clinical need. Clients who are started on therapy should be observed closely for clinical worsening, suicidality, or unusual changes in behavior. Families and caregivers should be advised of the need for close observation and communication with the prescriber. Desipramine is not approved for use in pediatric clients. (2) Analysis of short-term (4–16 weeks) placebo-controlled trials in children and adolescents with major depressive disorder, obsessive-compulsive disorder, or other psychiatric disorders have revealed a greater risk of adverse reactions representing suicidal thinking or behavior during the first few months of treatment in those receiving antidepressants. The average risk of such reactions in such clients receiving antidepressants was 4%, twice the placebo risk of 2%. No suicides occurred in these trials.■ Safe use during pregnancy has not been established. Safety and efficacy have not been established in children.

SIDE EFFECTS

Most Common

Dizziness, drowsiness, dry mouth, taste alteration, photosensitivity, tremors, constipation, decreased libido, blurred vision.

See *Antidepressants, Tricyclic* for a complete list of possible side effects. Also, bad taste in mouth, hypertension during surgery.

HOW SUPPLIED

Tablets: 10 mg, 25 mg, 50 mg, 75 mg, 100 mg, 150 mg.

DOSAGE

- **TABLETS**

  Antidepressant.

Initial: 100–200 mg/day in single or divided doses. **Maximum daily dose:** 300 mg in severely ill clients. **Maintenance:** 50–100 mg/day. **Geriatric and adolescent clients:** 25–100 mg/day in single or divided doses up to a maximum of 150 mg/day.

NURSING CONSIDERATIONS

℮ Do not confuse desipramine with diphenhydramine (an antihistamine) or Norpramin with Normodyne (labetalol, an antihypertensive).

ADMINISTRATION/STORAGE

1. Initiate in hospital setting for those requiring 300 mg/day.
2. Give maintenance doses for at least 2 months following satisfactory response.

ASSESSMENT

Note reasons for therapy, onset, characteristics of S&S, other agents trialed, outcome.

CLIENT/FAMILY TEACHING

1. Take as directed; may take 4–6 weeks to note desired effects.
2. Take single daily dose or any dosage increases at bedtime; reduce daytime sedation. Report lack of desired response/adverse side effects.
3. Use caution; drowsiness, dizziness, or postural hypotension may occur. May require dosage reduction. Keep all F/U visits and report any adverse effects or lack of response.
4. Avoid prolonged sun exposure and use precautions when exposed.
5. Avoid alcohol and all OTC drugs without approval. Do not stop drug suddenly; with prolonged therapy may experience headaches, nausea and malaise.
6. Store safely out of child's reach. Report any increased depression or suicide ideations

OUTCOMES/EVALUATE

- ↓ Depression; ↑ self-worth
- Relief of neurogenic pain
- Therapeutic levels (125–300 ng/mL)

Bold Italic = life threatening side effect ■ = black box warning ♣ = Available in Canada

Desirudin ■
(**DEH**-sih-rue-din)

CLASSIFICATION(S):
Antithrombin drug
PREGNANCY CATEGORY: C
Rx: Iprivask.

USES
Prophylaxis of DVT that may lead to pulmonary embolism in clients undergoing elective hip replacement surgery.

ACTION/KINETICS
Action
A specific inhibitor of free-circulating and clot-bound human thrombin. Desirudin prolongs the clotting time of human plasma by increasing aPTT. One molecule of desirudin binds to 1 molecule of thrombin, thereby blocking the thrombogenic activity of thrombin. As a result, all thrombin-dependent coagulation assays are affected. Thrombin time may exceed 200 seconds, even at low plasma desirudin levels; thus, this test is unsuitable for routine monitoring of desirudin therapy. At therapeutic serum levels, the drug has no effect on factors IXa, Xa, kallikrein, plasmin, tissue plasminogen activator, or activated protein.

Pharmacokinetics
Maximum plasma levels: 1–3 hr. Primarily metabolized and eliminated by the kidney with about 40–50% excreted unchanged. $t^{1/2}$, **elimination:** 2–3 hr after SC use.

CONTRAINDICATIONS
IM use. Known hypersensitivity to natural or recombinant hirudins and in those with active bleeding and/or irreversible coagulation disorders.

SPECIAL CONCERNS
■ (1) When neuraxial anesthesia (epidural/spinal anesthesia) or spinal puncture is employed, clients anticoagulated or scheduled to be anticoagulated with selective thrombin inhibitors, such as desirudin, may be at risk of developing an epidural or spinal hematoma which can result in long-term or permanent paralysis. (2) The risk of the above events may be increased by the use of indwelling spinal catheters for administration of analgesia or by the concomitant use of drugs affecting hemostasis, such as NSAIDs, platelet inhibitors, or other anticoagulants. The risk appears to be increased by traumatic or repeated epidural or spinal puncture. (3) Frequently monitor clients for signs and symptoms of neurological impairment. If neurological compromise is noted, urgent treatment is required. (4) The physician should consider the potential benefit versus risk before neuraxial intervention, in clients anticoagulated or to be anticoagulated for thromboprophylaxis.■ Use with caution in clients with increased risks of hemorrhage, including those with recent major surgery, organ biopsy, or puncture of a non-compressible vessel within the last month; also, a history of hemorrhagic stroke, intracranial or intraocular bleeding including diabetic retinopathy, recent ischemic stroke, severe uncontrolled hypertension, bacterial endocarditis, congenital or acquired hemostatic disorder (e.g., hemophilia, liver disease), or a history of GI or pulmonary bleeding within the past 3 months. Use with caution in clients with renal impairment, especially in those with moderate and severe renal impairment (C_{CR} less than 60 mL/min/1.74 m^2 body surface area) and in those with impaired liver function. Risk of side effects may be greater in elderly clients.

SIDE EFFECTS
Most Common
Hemorrhage, injection site mass, wound secretion, anemia, deep thrombophlebitis, nausea.

Hemorrhagic events: Hematomas; hemorrhages, including retroperitoneal, intracranial, intraocular, intraspinal, or in a major prosthetic joint. **CV:** Deep thrombophlebitis, thrombosis, hypotension, CV disorder. **GI:** N&V. **Body as a whole:** Wound secretion, fever, impaired healing. **Miscellaneous:** Injection site mass, anemia, leg edema, decreased hemoglobin, hematuria, dizziness, epistaxis, leg pain, hematemesis, hypersensitivity reactions, including ***anaphylaxis***.

 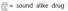

D

OD OVERDOSE MANAGEMENT

Symptoms: Hemorrhagic complications, excessively high aPTT values. *Treatment:* Discontinue desirudin therapy. Effects of desirudin are partially reversed by using thrombin-rich plasma concentrates. aPTT levels can be decreased by IV administration of 0.3 mcg/kg of desmopressin. Institute emergency procedures as appropriate.

DRUG INTERACTIONS

Abciximab / Use with caution with desirudin

Alteplase / ↑ Risk of bleeding

Anticoagulants (heparin, low molecular weight heparins) / Prolongation of aPTT; do not use together

Aspirin / Use with caution with desirudin

Clopidogrel / Use with caution with desirudin

Dextran / ↑ Risk of bleeding

Dipyridamole / Use with caution with desirudin

Glucocorticoids / ↑ Risk of bleeding

Ketorolac / Use with caution with desirudin

NSAIDs / Use with caution with desirudin

Salicylates / Use with caution with desirudin

Streptokinase / ↑ Risk of bleeding

Sulfinpyrazone / Use with caution with desirudin

Ticlopidine / Use with caution with desirudin

HOW SUPPLIED

Powder for Injection, Lyophilized: 15 mg.

DOSAGE

• **SC**

  Prophylaxis of DVT during hip replacement surgery.

15 mg q 12 hr with the initial dose given up to 5–15 min before surgery, but after induction of regional block anesthesia (if used). May be given up to 12 days (average is 9–12 days).

NURSING CONSIDERATIONS

ADMINISTRATION/STORAGE

1. Reduce dosage with renal insufficiency as follows:

• If C_{CR} is between 31 and 60 mL/min/1.73 m², begin therapy at 5 mg SC q 12 hr. Monitor aPTT and serum creatinine at least daily. If aPTT exceeds 2 times control, interrupt therapy until the value returns to <2 times control and resume therapy at a reduced dose guided by the initial degree of aPTT abnormality.

• If C_{CR} <31 mL/min/1.73 m², begin therapy at 1.7 mg SC q 12 hr. Monitor aPTT and serum creatinine at least daily. If aPTT exceeds 2 times control, interrupt therapy until the value returns to <2 times control and consider further dose reductions guided by the initial degree of aPTT abnormality.

2. Reconstitute under sterile conditions; each vial with 0.5 mL of provided diluent (mannitol, 3%, in water for injection). Shake gently until drug is fully reconstituted.

3. Once reconstituted, each 0.5 mL contains 15.75 mg of desirudin.

4. Use the reconstituted solution immediately, although stable for up to 24 hr when stored at room temperature and protected from light. Discard any unused solution. Do not mix with other injections, solvents, or infusions.

5. To administer SC, use a 26- or 27-gauge ½-in needle. Withdraw the entire reconstituted solution (15.75 mg/0.5 mL) into the syringe and inject the total volume (will deliver 15 mg).

6. Desirudin can not be used interchangeably with other hirudins as they differ in their manufacturing process and specific biological activity.

7. Do not use any vial that is discolored or that has particles in it.

8. Protect from light. Store unopened vials from 15–30°C (59–86°F).

ASSESSMENT

1. With elective THR, administer initial dose 5–15 min before surgery but after induction of regional block anesthesia if used. Given every 12 hr SC for 9–12 days following surgery. If epidural/spinal anesthesia or spinal puncture employed assess carefully for epidural or spinal hematoma which can result in long-term or permanent paralysis.

Bold Italic = life threatening side effect   ■ = black box warning   ♣ = Available in Canada

2. Monitor CBC, renal and LFTs. Decrease dosage with impaired renal function.

3. Assess for any recent surgery or bleeding episodes, bleeding or coagulation disorders or other conditions that may preclude therapy.

CLIENT/FAMILY TEACHING

1. Drug is used to prevent the development of blood clots in the legs or lungs after elective hip replacement surgery.

2. To administer, lie down and grasp a fold of skin on the abdomen between the thumb and forefinger. Insert the entire length of the needle straight in; use a 25- to 26-gauge needle to minimize tissue trauma. Hold the skin fold throughout the injection; do not rub or massage area after administration; rotate sites with each injection.

3. Alternate administration between the left and right anterolateral and posterolateral abdominal walls.

4. Avoid OTC aspirin containing products. Use electric razor, soft bristled toothbrush to prevent tissue trauma.

5. Report any unusual chest pain, SOB, bruising/bleeding, acute SOB, itching, rash or swelling of extremities.

OUTCOMES/EVALUATE

Post-operative DVT prophylaxis

Desloratadine

(**des**-lor-**AT**-ah-deen)

CLASSIFICATION(S):
Antihistamine, second generation, piperidine
PREGNANCY CATEGORY: C
Rx: Clarinex, Clarinex Reditabs.

SEE ALSO ANTIHISTAMINES (H₁ BLOCKERS).

USES

(1) Relief of nasal and nonnasal symptoms of seasonal allergic rhinitis in adults and children 6 years and older. (2) Relief of nasal and nonnasal symptoms of perennial allergic rhinitis in adults and children 6 years and older. (3) Symptomatic relief of chronic idiopathic pruritus and reduction in the number and size of hives in adults and children 6 years and older.

ACTION/KINETICS

Action

Desloratadine, a major metabolite of loratadine, is a long-acting selective histamine H₁-receptor antagonist. Low to no anticholinergic or sedative activity.

Pharmacokinetics

Maximum plasma levels: About 3 hr. Neither food nor grapefruit juice affect bioavailability. Metabolized to 3-hydroxydesloratadine which is also active. There are both slow and normal metabolizers of desloratadine; people of African descent have a higher frequency of slow metabolism. **t½, elimination:** 27 hr. Reduce dose in clients with renal or hepatic impairment.

CONTRAINDICATIONS

Lactation. Antihistamines are not recommended for use in children less than 6 years of age.

SPECIAL CONCERNS

Use with caution in elderly clients.

SIDE EFFECTS

Most Common

Dizziness, drowsiness/somnolence, headache, fatigue, pharyngitis, myalgia, dry mouth/nose/throat.

See also *Antihistamines* (H₁-Blockers) for a complete list of possible side effects. **CNS:** Fatigue, drowsiness/somnolence, headache, dizziness. **GI:** Dry mouth, nausea, dyspepsia. **Miscellaneous:** Pharyngitis, myalgia, dysmenorrhea, tachycardia, dry nose/throat, rarely hypersensitivity reactions (e.g., rash, pruritus, urticaria, edema, dyspnea, **anaphylaxis**).

LABORATORY TEST CONSIDERATIONS

↑ Liver enzymes, bilirubin.

HOW SUPPLIED

Syrup: 2.5 mg/5 mL; *Tablets:* 5 mg; *Tablets, Rapidly Disintegrating:* 2.5 mg, 5 mg.

DOSAGE

• SYRUP; TABLETS; TABLETS, RAPIDLY DISINTEGRATING

Chronic idiopathic urticaria, perennial/seasonal allergic rhinitis.

Adults and children over 12 years: 5 mg once daily (10 mL of the syrup). **Children, 6–11 years:** 2.5 mg once dai-

---

ly (5 mL of the syrup). In adults with liver or renal impairment, start with 5 mg every other day.

NURSING CONSIDERATIONS

ADMINISTRATION/STORAGE

1. Protect syrup from light.
2. Protect tablets from excessive moisture.
3. Store tablets, syrup and disintegrating tablets from 15–30°C (59–86°F).

ASSESSMENT

1. Note reasons for therapy, onset, characteristics of S&S, time of year, triggers if know. List other agents trialed/outcome.
2. Assess liver and renal function, reduce dose/frequency of dosing with dysfunction.

CLIENT/FAMILY TEACHING

1. May be taken without regard to meals.
2. With dry hands, place the rapidly disintegrating tablet on the tongue immediately after opening the blister. Do not push the tablet through the foil backing. Peel back the foil backing and remove the tablet (disintegrates rapidly); give with or without water.
3. Do not increase dose or dosing frequency as effectiveness is not increased and sleepiness may occur.
4. Avoid activities that require mental alertness until drug effects realized.
5. Keep a diary and attempt to identify triggers.
6. Report unusual side effects, lack of response, or worsening of symptoms.

OUTCOMES/EVALUATE

- Control of S&S of seasonal/allergic rhinitis
- Relief from idiopathic urticaria

Desmopressin acetate [IV]

(des-moh-**PRESS**-in)

CLASSIFICATION(S):

Antidiuretic hormone, synthetic
PREGNANCY CATEGORY: B
Rx: DDAVP, Minirin, Stimate.

♣Rx: Apo-Desmopressin, DDAVP Injection/Spray/Tablets, DDAVP Rhinyle Nasal Solution, Minirin, Octostim Injection/Spray.

USES

DDAVP: (1) Primary noctural enuresis (intranasal). (2) Central cranial diabetes insipidus (DI) (intranasal, oral, parenteral). (3) Hemophilia A with factor VIII levels greater than 5% (intranasal, parenteral). (4) von Willebrand's disease (type I) with factor VIII levels greater than 5% (intranasal, parenteral). **Stimate, DDAVP:** (1) Hemophilia A with factor VIII levels greater than 5%. (2) von Willebrand's disease with factor VIII levels greater than 5%. *Investigational:* Chronic autonomic failure (nocturnal polyuria, overnight weight loss, morning postural hypotension).

ACTION/KINETICS

Action

A synthetic analog of arginine vasopressin which possesses antidiuretic activity but is devoid of vasopressor and oxytocic effects. Acts to increase absorption of water in the kidney by increasing permeability of cells in the collecting ducts.

Pharmacokinetics

Onset: 1 hr. **Peak, intranasal:** 1–5 hr.; **peak, PO:** 4–7 hr. **Duration:** 8–20 hr. **t½:** initial, 8 min; final: 75 min. Effect ceases abruptly. It also increases factor VIII levels (**onset:** 30 min; **peak:** 1.5–2 hr) and von Willebrand's factor activity. **Time to reach maximum plasma levels, after PO or intranasal:** 0.9–1.5 hr.

CONTRAINDICATIONS

Hypersensitivity to drug. Use for treatment of hemophilia A with factor VIII levels less than or equal to 5%, treatment of hemophilia B or in clients who have factor VIII antibodies. Treatment of severe classic von Willebrand's disease (type I) and when an abnormal molecular form of factor VIII antigen is present. Use for type IIB von Willebrand's disease. Parenteral administration for DI in infants under 3 months and intranasal administration in infants less than 11 months. Nephrogenic DI, polyuria due to psychogenic DI, renal disease, hypercalcemia, hyperkalemia, or administration of demeclocycline or lithium.

SPECIAL CONCERNS

Safety for use during lactation not established. Use with caution and with restricted fluid intake in infants due to an increased risk of hyponatremia and water intoxication. Geriatric clients may have a greater risk of developing hyponatremia and water intoxication. Use with caution in clients with coronary artery insufficiency and/or hypertensive CV disease. Use cautiously with other pressor agents. Safety and efficacy have not been determined in children less than 12 years of age (parenteral) or less than 2 months of age (intranasal) with DI.

SIDE EFFECTS

Most Common

See below.

• **Intranasal DDAVP**

Respiratory: Nasal congestion, rhinitis, cough, epistaxis, nostril pain, sore throat, nose bleed, URTI. **GI:** Abdominal pain (mild), nausea, GI disorder. **CNS:** Headache (transient), dizziness. **Ophthalmic:** Conjunctivitis, eye edema, lacrimation disorder. **Miscellaneous:** Facial flushing, asthenia, chills.

• **Intranasal Stimate**

GI: Dyspepsia, vomiting. **CNS:** Agitation, insomnia, dizziness, somnolence. **CV:** Palpitations, tachycardia. **Ophthalmic:** Itchy or light sensitive eyes, balanitis. **Miscellaneous:** Chest pain, chills, edema, pain, warm feeling.

• **Parenteral DDAVP**

GI: Abdominal pain (mild), nausea. **CNS:** Headache (transient). **CV:** BP changes. **Miscellaneous:** Facial flushing, burning pain, edema, erythema (local), vulval pain, anaphylaxis.

OD OVERDOSE MANAGEMENT

Symptoms: Headache, abdominal cramps, facial flushing, dyspnea, fluid retention, mucous membrane irritation. *Treatment:* Reduce dose, decrease frequency of administration, or withdraw the drug depending on the severity of the condition.

DRUG INTERACTIONS

Carbamazepine / Possible potentiation of desmopressin effects

Chlorpropamide / Possible potentiation of desmopressin effects

Pressor drugs / Use large nasal or parenteral doses (0.3 mcg/kg) of desmopressin with caution with other pressor drugs

HOW SUPPLIED

Injection: 4 mcg/mL; *Nasal Solution:* 0.1 mg/mL, 1.5 mg/mL; *Nasal Spray:* 0.1 mg; *Tablets:* 0.1 mg, 0.2 mg.

DOSAGE

• **DIRECT IV, SC**

Neurogenic DI.

Adults: 0.5–1 mL/day in two divided doses, adjusted separately for an adequate diurnal rhythm of water turnover. If switching from intranasal to IV, the comparable IV antidiuretic dose is about ¹⁄₁₀ the intranasal dose.

Hemophilia A, von Willebrand's disease (type I).

Adults: 0.3 mcg/kg diluted in 50 mL 0.9% NaCl injection infused IV over 15–30 min; dose may be repeated, if necessary. **Pediatric, 3 months or older, weighing 10 kg or less, IV:** 0.3 mcg/kg diluted in 10 mL of 0.9% NaCl injection and given over 15–30 min; repeat if necessary. **Pediatric, 3 months or older, weighing 10 kg or more, IV:** 0.3 mcg/kg diluted in 50 mL of 0.9% NaCl injection and given over 15–30 min; repeat if necessary.

• **INTRANASAL (SOLUTION, SPRAY)**

Neurogenic DI.

Adults: 0.1–0.4 mL/day, either as a single dose or divided into two to three doses (usual: 0.2 mL/day in two divided doses). Adjust morning and evening doses separately for an adequate diurnal rhythm of water turnover. **Children, 3 months to 12 years:** 0.05–0.3 mL/day, either as a single dose or two divided doses.

Nocturnal enuresis.

Age 6 years and older, initial: 20 mcg (0.2 mL) at bedtime with one-half the dose in each nostril; if no response, the dose may be increased to 40 mcg.

Hemophilia A and type I von Willebrand's disease.

In clients weighing 50 kg or more: One spray per nostril (total dose of 300 mcg). **In clients weighing less than 50**

 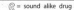

kg: Given as a single spray of 150 mcg. The drug may be given 2 hr prior to minor surgery in the same doses as described above.

Renal concentration capacity test.

Adults: 40 mcg (20 mcg in each nostril) given any time during the day. **Children, 3–12 years:** 20 mcg given in the morning.

• **TABLETS**

Central cranial DI.

Adults, initial: 0.05 mg twice a day; adjust individually to optimum therapeutic dose and adjust each dose for an adequate diurnal rhythm of water turnover. Total daily dose should be increased or decreased (range 0.1–1.2 mg divided 2–3 times per day) as needed to obtain adequate antidiuresis. **Children, initial:** 0.05 mg. Careful restriction of fluid intake in children is required to prevent hyponatremia and water intoxication.

Primary nocturnal enuresis.

Age 6 years and older, initial: 0.2 mg at bedtime. May be increased to 0.6 mg, depending on client response.

NURSING CONSIDERATIONS

ADMINISTRATION/STORAGE

1. Measure the dosage exactly because the drug is potent.

2. Note the three graduation marks on the soft flexible plastic nasal tube: 0.2, 0.1, and 0.05 mL. The 0.05-level is not designated by number. Cleanse and dry tube appropriately.

3. Stimate nasal spray pump can only deliver 0.1 mL (150 mcg). The pump must be primed prior to the first use by pressing down four times. Discard the bottle after 25 (150 mcg per dose) doses since the amount delivered thereafter may be much less than 150 mcg.

4. Refrigerate nasal solution at 2–8°C (36–46° F) although the product will be stable for up to 3 weeks when stored at room temperature. Refrigerate the injection at the same temperature as the nasal spray.

5. If used for hemophilia A or von Willebrand's disease, do not use it more often than q 2 days as tachyphylaxis may occur.

6. To determine the renal concentration capacity in adults, the urine voided within 1 hr after drug administration is discarded; the two subsequent urines collected within 8 hr are saved and tested for osmolality. In children, osmolality is measured on urine voided during 3–5 hr after drug administration. Advise to drink only small amounts of fluid during the test day.

IV 7. For direct IV administration (with neurogenic DI) give each dose over 1 min. With hemophilia, may dilute drug in 50 mL of NSS and infuse over 15–30 min.

8. Refrigerate the solution and injection at 4°C (39.2°F).

ASSESSMENT

1. Note reasons for therapy and clinical presentation. Monitor BP, CBC, calcium, blood sugar, electrolytes, and factor levels.

2. Observe for early S&S of water intoxication (drowsiness, headache, and vomiting, excessive fluid consumption, weight gain, and/or seizures). Adjust fluid intake to avoid water intoxication and hyponatremia; excessive retention, may be treated with a diuretic.

3. With hemophilia, monitor BP and HR closely during IV therapy.

4. With neurogenic DI, monitor urine osmolarity and volume; weigh daily; assess for edema/dehydration.

5. With enuresis monitor duration of sleep. The amount of sleep, together with the client's daily I&O, provide parameters to estimate the clinical response to drug therapy.

CLIENT/FAMILY TEACHING

1. Drug is a synthetic analogue of vasopressin and an antidiuretic hormone. It may be used to maintain bleeding or for antidiuretic replacement therapy in the management of central (cranial) diabetes insipidus and for the management of the temporary polyuria and polydipsia following head trauma or surgery in the pituitary region.

2. If spray is prescribed, administer after instruction using the special catheter provided. Insert tip of catheter into

---

nose and blow on the other end of the catheter to deliver the medication deep into the nasal cavity. (A syringe filled with air may be used in children and comatose persons; rinse after use.)

3. Review recommendations concerning fluid intake. Measure I&O and keep an accurate record of fluid status. Report any symptoms of water intoxication and swelling.

4. Notify provider at the earliest signs of trouble, such as ↓ urinary output, headaches, or severe nasal congestion which may be mistaken for a URI.

5. Avoid alcohol in any form.

6. Tolerance may develop over time and response may be diminished.

OUTCOMES/EVALUATE

• Prevention of hemorrhage
• Control of nocturnal enuresis
• Desired antidiuretic effects (↓ urine volume, ↑ urine osmolarity, and relief of polydipsia) with DI

Dexamethasone acetate

CLASSIFICATION(S):
Glucocorticoid

Rx: Cortastat LA, Dalalone D.P., Dalalone L.A., Decaject-L.A., Dexasone L.A.

SEE ALSO CORTICOSTEROIDS.

ACTION/KINETICS

Action

Practically insoluble; provides the prolonged activity suitable for repository injections, although it has a prompt onset of action. Not for IV use.

SPECIAL CONCERNS

Use during pregnancy only if benefits outweigh risks.

SIDE EFFECTS

Most Common

Increased appetite, irritability, insomnia, fluid retention, heartburn, muscle weakness, impaired wound healing, hyperglycemia.

See Corticosteroids for a complete list of possible side effects.

HOW SUPPLIED

Injection: 8 mg/mL, 16 mg/mL.

DOSAGE

• IM REPOSITORY INJECTION

8–16 mg q 1–3 weeks, if necessary.

• INTRALESIONAL

0.8–1.6 mg.

• INJECTION, SOFT TISSUE; INTRA-ARTICULAR

4–16 mg repeated at 1–3-week intervals.

NURSING CONSIDERATIONS

ASSESSMENT

1. Note reasons for therapy, onset/duration, characteristics of S&S, events surrounding injury, other agents/treatments trialed, outcome.

2. Review ROM, x-rays, bone density, labs.

CLIENT/FAMILY TEACHING

1. Drug is a steroid; reduces swelling and decreases the body's immune response.

2. Do not overuse joint/limb as futher injury may occur. Use support/aids and exercise as directed.

3. Report adverse effects, lack of response, worsening of symptoms.

OUTCOMES/EVALUATE

• ↓ Inflammation
• Symptomatic improvement

Dexamethasone sodium phosphate [IV]

CLASSIFICATION(S):
Glucocorticoid

PREGNANCY CATEGORY: C

Rx: Ophthalmic/Topical: Decadron Phosphate. Injection: Cortastat, Dalalone, Decadron Phosphate, Decaject, Dexasone, Hexadrol Phosphate.

✤Rx: PMS-Dexamethasone Injection.

SEE ALSO CORTICOSTEROIDS.

ADDITIONAL USES

Systemic: For IV or IM use in emergency situations when dexamethasone cannot be given PO.

Intranasal: Nasal polyps, allergic or inflammatory nasal conditions.

Ophthalmic: Ophthalmic inflammatory conditions (See Dexamethasone).

Otic: Inflammatory conditions of the external auditory meatus, such as allergic otitis externa and selected purulent and nonpurulent infective otitis external when the risks of steroid use are accepted to obtain decreased edema and inflammation.

ACTION/KINETICS
Pharmacokinetics
Rapid onset and short duration of action.

CONTRAINDICATIONS
Acute infections, persistent positive sputum cultures of *Candida albicans*. Lactation.

SPECIAL CONCERNS
Use during pregnancy only if benefits outweigh risks. Safety and efficacy of the otic solution has not been determined in children.

SIDE EFFECTS
Most Common
Following ophthalmic use: Increased intraocular pressure, eye pain, blurred vision, dry eye, eye inflammation, abnormal sensation in eye, glaucoma, tearing, conjunctival hemorrhage, cataracts.
Following otic use: Rarely, stinging and burning.
Following topical use: Burning, itching, irritation, erythema, dryness.
See *Corticosteroids* for a complete list of possible side effects.

HOW SUPPLIED
Cream: 0.1%; *Injection:* 4 mg/mL, 10 mg/mL, 20 mg/mL, 24 mg/mL; *Ophthalmic Ointment:* 0.05%; *Ophthalmic Solution:* 0.1%; *Otic Solution:* 0.1% (as phosphate).

DOSAGE
• **IM; IV**
Most uses.
Range: 0.5–9 mg/day (⅓ to ½ the PO dose q 12 hr).
Cerebral edema.
Adults, initial: 10 mg IV; **then,** 4 mg IM q 6 hr until maximum effect is obtained (usually within 12–24 hr). Switch to PO therapy (1–3 mg 3 times/day) as soon as feasible and then slowly withdraw over 5–7 days.
Shock, unresponsive.

Initial: Either 1–6 mg/kg IV or 40 mg IV; **then,** repeat IV dose q 2–6 hr as long as necessary.
• **INTRA-ARTICULAR; INTRALESIONAL; SOFT TISSUE INJECTIONS**
0.4–6 mg, depending on the site (e.g., small joints: 0.8–1 mg; large joints: 2–4 mg; soft tissue infiltration: 2–6 mg; ganglia: 1–2 mg; bursae: 2–3 mg; tendon sheaths: 0.4–1 mg).
• **OPHTHALMIC OINTMENT**
Instill a small amount of the ointment into the conjunctival sac 3–4 times per day. As response is obtained, reduce the number of applications.
• **OPHTHALMIC SOLUTION**
Initial: Instill 1–2 gtt into the conjunctival sac q hr during day and q 2 hr at night until response is obtained. After favorable response, reduce to 1 gtt q 4 hr and later 1 gtt 3–4 times per day.
• **OTIC SOLUTION**
Otic inflammatory conditions.
Initial: 3 or 4 gtt 2 or 3 times daily directly into the aural canal. Reduce dose when a favorable response is obtained. Duration of treatment may extend from a few days to several weeks. Relapses usually respond to retreatment.
• **TOPICAL CREAM**
Apply sparingly to affected areas and rub in.

NURSING CONSIDERATIONS
ADMINISTRATION/STORAGE
1. The ophthalmic ointment is useful when an eye pad is used and for situations when prolonged contact of dexamethasone with ocular tissues is required.
2. If preferred, the aural canal may be packed with a gauze wick saturated with the solution. Keep the wick moist with the solution and remove from the ear after 12–24 hr. Repeat treatment as often as needed.
IV 3. For IV administration may give undiluted over 1 min. Do not use preparation containing lidocaine IV.

ASSESSMENT
Note reasons for therapy, clinical presentation, onset, characteristics of S&S,

---

Bold Italic = life threatening side effect   ■ = black box warning   ♣ = Available in Canada

any triggers, other agents trialed, outcome.

CLIENT/FAMILY TEACHING
1. Review appropriate method/frequency for administration and use as directed.
2. Report any loss of response, adverse side effects, or worsening of symptoms.

OUTCOMES/EVALUATE
- Improved airway exchange
- Relief of allergic manifestations
- Suppression of inflammatory response; enhanced tissue perfusion

Dexmedetomidine hydrochloride **IV**

(dex-**med**-ih-**TOM**-ih-deen)

CLASSIFICATION(S):
Sedative-hypnotic, nonbenzodiazepine
PREGNANCY CATEGORY: C
Rx: Precedex.

USES
For sedation in initially intubated and mechanically ventilated clients for treatment in an intensive care setting. *Investigational:* Treat shivering. Adjunct to regional or general anesthesia. As a bridge to ICU sedation and analgesia. As a supplement to regional block in those undergoing carotid endarterectomy or during awake craniotomy. In certain clients with CHF. Control agitation while receiving noninvasive ventilatory support, such as mask continuous or bilevel positive airway pressure. Minimize withdrawal symptoms in critically ill clients who have received long-term benzodiazepines and opiates during hospitalization.

ACTION/KINETICS
Action
An alpha$_2$-adrenoceptor agonist with sedative effects. No evidence of respiratory depression when given at recommended doses.

Pharmacokinetics
Rapidly distributed; **t$\frac{1}{2}$:** About 6 min. Almost completely metabolized in the liver; excreted in the urine and feces. **t$\frac{1}{2}$, terminal:** About 2 hr. Possibility of accumulation of metabolites with long-term infusions in clients with impaired renal function.

CONTRAINDICATIONS
Use for infusions lasting over 24 hr, during labor and delivery, or in pediatric patients under 18 years of age.

SPECIAL CONCERNS
A higher incidence of hypotension and bradycardia is seen in geriatric and hypovolemic clients; consider a dose reduction. Use with caution in advanced heart block or during lactation. If chronically given and then abruptly discontinued, withdrawal symptoms (e.g., nervousness, agitation, headaches, increase in BP) may occur.

SIDE EFFECTS
Most Common
Somnolence, N&V, constipation, skin rashes, angioedema, apnea, hypoventilation, bradycardia, hypotension, syncope.
CV: Bradycardia, sinus arrest, hypotension, syncope, atrial fibrillation, BP fluctuation, heart disorder, aggravated hypertension, arrhythmia, ventricular arrhythmia, AV block, *cardiac arrest, ventricular tachycardia*, extrasystoles, heart block, T-wave inversion, tachycardia, supraventricular tachycardia. **GI:** N&V, constipation, abdominal pain, diarrhea, dry mouth. **CNS:** Dizziness, headache, neuralgia, neuritis, speech disorder, agitation, confusion, delirium, hallucinations, illusions, somnolence. **Respiratory:** Hypoxia, pleural effusion, pulmonary edema, apnea, bronchospasm, dyspnea, hypercapnia, hypoventilation, pulmonary congestion. **Body as a whole:** Thirst, skin rashes, angioedema, anemia, pain, infection, leukocytosis, fever, hyperpyrexia, rigors, increased sweating, *hemorrhage*, acidosis, hyperglycemia. **Miscellaneous:** Oliguria, hypovolemia, photopsia, abnormal vision.

LABORATORY TEST CONSIDERATIONS

↑ AST, ALT, SGGT, alkaline phosphatase. Acidosis, respiratory acidosis, hyperkalemia.

DRUG INTERACTIONS

Possible enhanced CNS depression when given with anesthetics, hypnotics, narcotics, or sedatives. Consider dosage reduction.

HOW SUPPLIED

Injection: 100 mcg/mL.

DOSAGE

- **IV INFUSION**

  Sedation in intensive care setting.

Adults: Loading infusion of 1 mcg/kg over 10 min, followed by a maintenance infusion of 0.2–0.7 mcg/kg/hr. Adjust rate to achieve desired level of sedation. Reduce dosage in impaired hepatic function.

NURSING CONSIDERATIONS

ADMINISTRATION/STORAGE

IV 1. Administer using a controlled infusion device.

2. To prepare the infusion, withdraw 2 mL and add to 48 mL of 0.9% NaCl injection (i.e., total of 50 mL). Shake gently to mix. Ampules and vials are intended for single use only.

3. Dexmedetomidine is compatible with lactated Ringer's, D5W, 0.9% NaCl in water, 20% mannitol, thiopental sodium, etomidate, vecuronium bromide, pancuronium bromide, succinylcholine, atracurium besylate, mivicurium chloride, glycopyrrolate bromide, phenylephrine HCl, atropine sulfate, midazolam, morphine sulfate, fentanyl citrate, and plasma substitute.

4. May adsorb to some types of natural rubber; use administration components made with synthetic or coated natural rubber gaskets.

5. Store at controlled room temperature of 25°C (77°F).

ASSESSMENT

1. Note reasons for and goals of therapy, intended length of use.

2. Give in a continuously monitored environment. Client may develop cardiac arrhythmias, heart block, GI upset, respiratory distress.

3. With chronic use, taper dosage to prevent withdrawal symptoms.

4. Monitor VS, renal and LFTs, reduce dose with dysfunction, assess HTN during infusion, in older clients.

CLIENT/FAMILY TEACHING

1. Drug is used to sedate before surgery and during procedures. Do not attempt to get up or walk without assistance.

2. May awaken when stimulated; may experience atrial fibrillation, burning at injection site, change in mental status, and respiratory suppression. Therefore drug is only administered in a carefully monitored environment by trained personnel where client can be closely attended.

OUTCOMES/EVALUATE

Desired sedation; control of intubated clients being mechanically ventilated

Dexmethylphenidate ■ hydrochloride

(dex-**meth**-il-**FEN**-ah-dayt)

CLASSIFICATION(S):
CNS stimulant
PREGNANCY CATEGORY: C
Rx: Focalin, Focalin XR, **C-II**

USES

As part of a total program to treat attention deficit hyperactivity disorder in children 6 years of age and older. Effectiveness of use for more than 6 weeks using tablets or for more than 7 weeks using extended-release capsules has not been studied.

ACTION/KINETICS

Action

Precise mechanism to treat attention deficit disorder is not known. Drug is thought to block reuptake of norepinephrine and dopamine into the pre-synaptic neuron and increase the release of these neurotransmitters into the extraneuronal space.

Bold Italic = life threatening side effect   ■ = black box warning   ♣ = Available in Canada

Pharmacokinetics

Immediate-release tablets: Rapidly absorbed; **maximum levels:** 1–1.5 hr. Food delays the time to maximum levels. Metabolized in the liver; 90% excreted through the urine. **t½, elimination:** About 2.2 hr. **Extended-release capsules:** Produce a bimodal concentration-time profile about 4 hr apart. The initial release is similar to immediate-release tablets. High fat meals cause a longer lag time until absorption begins and variable delays until the first peak concentration, the time until the interpeak minimum, and the time until the second peak. The drug is metabolized in the liver and excreted mainly in the urine.

CONTRAINDICATIONS

Clients with marked anxiety, tension, and agitation. Those with glaucoma, motor tics, or with a family history of Tourette's syndrome, during treatment with MAO inhibitors or within a minimum of 14 days following discontinuation of a MAO inhibitor (hypertensive crisis may result). Use to treat severe depression or to prevent or treat normal fatigue states.

SPECIAL CONCERNS

■ (1) Use with caution in those with a history of drug dependence or alcoholism. (2) Chronic, abusive use may lead to marked tolerance and psychological dependence with abnormal behavior. (3) Parenteral abuse may result in frank psychotic episodes. (4) Careful supervision is needed during drug withdrawal from abusive use because severe depression may occur. (5) Withdrawal following chronic therapy may unmask symptoms of the underlying disorder that may require follow-up.■ In psychotic children, worsening of symptoms of behavior disturbance and thought disorder may occur. Use with caution during lactation and in medical conditions that might be compromised by increases in BP or HR (e.g., preexisting hypertension, heart failure, recent MI, hyperthyroidism). Safety and efficacy have not been determined in children less than 6 years of age.

SIDE EFFECTS

Most Common

Immediate-Release: Abdominal pain, nausea, anorexia, fever, nervousness, anxiety, irritability, insomnia, weight loss, tachycardia, motor/vocal tics.

Extended-Release: Headache, dyspepsia, decreased appetite, anxiety, dry mouth, pharyngolaryngeal pain, feeling jittery, dizziness.

CNS: Nervousness, insomnia, dizziness, drowsiness, anxiety, irritability, dyskinesia, headache, motor/vocal tics, feeling jittery, Tourette's syndrome (rare), toxic psychosis (rare), transient depressed mood, lowering of seizure threshold in those with a history of seizures or with prior EEG abnormalities, treatment emergent psychotic or manic symptoms, aggressive behavior or hostility. **GI:** Abdominal pain, anorexia, nausea, dyspepsia, dry mouth. **CV:** Tachycardia, angina, arrhythmia, palpitations, increased or decreased pulse/BP, cerebral arteritis or occlusion, *sudden death in those with structural cardiac abnormalities or other serious heart problems.* **Dermatologic:** Skin rash, urticaria, exfoliative dermatitis, erythema multiforme with findings of necrotizing vasculitis, thrombocytopenia purpura. **Hematologic:** Leukopenia, anemia. **Ophthalmic:** Difficulties with accommodation and blurring of vision. **Miscellaneous:** Weight loss, scalp hair loss, temporary slowing of growth rate in consistently medicated children, pharyngolaryngeal pain, *neuroleptic malignant syndrome* (rare).

LABORATORY TEST CONSIDERATIONS

↑ Urinary excretion of epinephrine. Abnormal liver function (ranging from ↑ transaminase levels to hepatic coma).

OD OVERDOSE MANAGEMENT

Symptoms: Agitation, cardiac arrhythmias, confusion, convulsions (may be followed by coma), delirium, dry mucous membranes, euphoria, flushing, hallucinations, headache, hyperpyrexia, hyperreflexia, hypertension, muscle twitching, mydriasis, palpitations, sweating, tachycardia, tremors, vomiting. *Treatment:* Appropriate supportive measures. Protect against self-injury and external stimuli. Gastric lavage (control agitation and seizures before gastric lavage). Administration of activated charcoal and a cathartic. Maintain adequate circulation and respiratory exchange. External cooling procedures to treat hyperpyrexia.

DRUG INTERACTIONS

Antacids / Possible alteration of the release of dexmethylphenidate

Antihypertensives / ↓ Effect of antihypertensives

Clonidine / Possible serious side effects

Gastric acid suppressants / Possible alteration of the release of dexmethylphenidate

MAO inhibitors / Possible hypertensive crisis, hyperthermia, convulsions, coma; do not use together or within 14 days following discontinuation of MAO therapy

Phenobarbital / ↑ Effect of phenobarbital R/T ↓ metabolism

Phenytoin / ↑ Effect of phenytoin R/T ↓ metabolism

Pressor drugs (dopamine, epinephrine, phenylephrine) / Due to possible effects on BP, use cautiously with pressor drugs

Primidone / ↑ Effect of primidone R/T ↓ metabolism

Selective serotonin reuptake inhibitors / ↑ Effect of SSRIs R/T ↓ metabolism

Tricyclic antidepressants / ↑ TCA effect R/T ↓ metabolism

Warfarin / ↓ Metabolism of warfarin; monitor coagulation times when starting or stopping therapy with possible dosage adjustment

HOW SUPPLIED

Capsules, Extended-Release: 5 mg, 10 mg, 15 mg, 20 mg; *Tablets:* 2.5 mg, 5 mg, 10 mg.

DOSAGE

• TABLETS

Attention deficit hyperactivity disorder.

Clients new to methylphenidate: Initially, 2.5 mg twice a day of dexmethylphenidate. May adjust dose in 2.5–5 mg increments up to a maximum of 20 mg/day (10 mg twice a day). Dosage adjustments may be made at weekly intervals. **Those currently taking methylphenidate:** Start dexmethylphenidate at one-half the dose of racemic methylphenidate being used. Maximum recommended dose is 20 mg/day (10 mg twice a day). Clients currently using immediate-release dexmethylphenidate tablets may be switched to the same dose of extended-release dexmethylphenidate capsules.

• CAPSULES, EXTENDED-RELEASE

Attention deficit hyperactivity disorder.

Clients new to methylphenidate: 10 mg/day for adults and 5 mg/day for children given once daily. Adjust dose, if needed, in 5 mg increments to a maximum of 20 mg/day for children and in 10 mg/day increments to a maximum of 20 mg/day for adults. Observe the client for a sufficient period of time at a given dose to ensure that a maximum benefit has been reached before a dose increase is considered. Periodically assess need for the drug.

NURSING CONSIDERATIONS

ADMINISTRATION/STORAGE

1. Give twice a day at least 4 hr apart, with/without food.

2. If extended treatment deemed necessary, evaluate long-term usefulness with periods off drug to assess ability to function without medication.

3. If paradoxical aggravation of symptoms or other side effects occur, decrease/discontinue drug.

4. Discontinue drug if improvement is not seen after appropriate dosage adjustment over a 1-month period.

5. Withdrawal after use may cause severe depression.

6. Withdrawal from chronic therapeutic use may unmask symptoms of underlying disorder.

7. Store from 15–30°C (59–86°F). Protect from light and moisture.

ASSESSMENT

1. Note reasons for therapy, symptom characteristics, other agents trialed, outcome. List other drugs prescribed that may interact unfavorably.

2. Assess for family history of Tourette's syndrome, evidence of glaucoma, tics, or depression; may preclude therapy.

3. Ensure psychologic evaluations show no evidence of psychotic disorder or severe stress/anxiety reaction.

4. Obtain baseline VS, LFTs, CBC, CNS evaluation, ECG and monitor.

5. Assess for possible growth suppression. Monitor height and weight especially with long-term therapy and provide periodic 'drug holiday' to determine need for continued therapy.

CLIENT/FAMILY TEACHING

1. Drug thought to work by restoring the balance of certain natural substances (neurotransmitters) in the brain. It helps increase ability to pay attention, stay focused on an activity, and control behavior problems. It may also help improve listening skills, help stop fidgeting, and allow you to organize your tasks better.

2. Take before/with breakfast and lunch to avoid interference with sleep. For immediate-release tablets take twice daily at least 4 hr apart, with or without food. Take extended-release capsules once daily in the morning.

3. Take extended-release capsules whole or by sprinkling the contents on a small amount of applesauce. Do not crush, chew, or divide capsules. Consume the mixture with applesauce immediately; to not store for future use.

4. Store safely out of reach, may cause tolerance and psychological dependence.

5. Do NOT stop suddenly with long-term therapy, reduce dose with supervised direction.

6. Use caution when driving or operating hazardous machinery; may mask fatigue and/or cause physical incoordination, dizziness, drowsiness.

7. Record weight twice a week; weight loss may occur.

8. Report any overt changes in client mood or attention span.

9. Any adverse S&S as well as skin rashes, fever, or joint pains should be reported immediately.

10. Therapy may be interrupted periodically ('drug holiday') to determine if it is still necessary in those responsive to therapy and in some to permit normal growth.

OUTCOMES/EVALUATE
Ability to sit quietly and concentrate

Dextroamphetamine ■ sulfate

(dex-troh-am-**FET**-ah-meen)

CLASSIFICATION(S):
CNS stimulant

PREGNANCY CATEGORY: C

Rx: Dexedrine, Dexedrine Spansules, Dextrostat, **C-II**

SEE ALSO *AMPHETAMINES AND DERIVATIVES.*

USES

(1) As part of a total treatment program for attention deficit disorders with hyperactivity in children 3 to 16 years of age. (2) Narcolepsy.

ACTION/KINETICS

Action

Stronger CNS effects and weaker peripheral action than amphetamine; thus, dextroamphetamine manifests fewer undesirable CV effects.

Pharmacokinetics

After PO, completely absorbed in 3 hr. **Duration: PO,** 4–24 hr; **t½, adults:** 10–12 hr; **children:** 6–8 hr. Excreted in urine. Acidification will increase excretion, while alkalinization will decrease it.

ADDITIONAL CONTRAINDICATIONS

Lactation. Use for obesity. Not recommended for use in children less than 3 years of age.

SPECIAL CONCERNS

■ High potential for abuse. Use for prolonged periods may lead to drug dependence and must be avoided. Particular attention should be paid to the possibility of subjects obtaining amphetamines for nontherapeutic use or distribution to others, and the drugs should be prescribed or dispensed sparingly.■ Higher rates of serious CV events and sudden death are seen with amphetamine compared with methylphenidate in both children and adults, with more events seen in adults rather than children. Use of extended-release capsules for attention deficit disorders in children less than 6 years of age and the tablets for attention deficit disorders in children less than 3 years of age is not recommended. Dosage for narcolepsy has not been determined in children less than 6 years of age.

SIDE EFFECTS

Most Common

Nausea, GI upset, cramps, anorexia, diarrhea, constipation, dry mouth, headache, nervousness, dizziness, insomnia, irritability, restlessness.

See *Amphetamines and Derivatives* for a complete list of possible side effects.

HOW SUPPLIED

Capsules, Sustained-Release: 5 mg, 10 mg, 15 mg; *Tablets:* 5 mg, 10 mg.

DOSAGE

• **CAPSULES, SUSTAINED-RELEASE; TABLETS**

Attention deficit disorders in children.
Children, 3–5 years: 2.5 mg/day initially; increase in increments of 2.5 mg/day at weekly intervals until optimum response reached. **Children, 6 years and older:** 5 mg once or twice daily initially; increase in increments of 5 mg/day at weekly intervals until optimum response reached. Dosage will rarely exceed 40 mg/day. When appropriate, use the sustained-release capsules for once daily dosing.

Narcolepsy.
Adults and children over 12 years: Initial: 10 mg/day; increase dose in increments of 10 mg/day at weekly intervals. Reduce dose if side effects occur. **Children, 6–12 years: Initial:** 5 mg/day; increase in increments of 5 mg at weekly intervals until optimum effect is reached, up to a maximum of 60 mg/day.

NURSING CONSIDERATIONS

ADMINISTRATION/STORAGE

1. Use the lowest effective dose; adjust dosage individually.
2. Avoid late evening doses, especially with sustained-release capsules due to the possibility of insomnia.
3. Sustained-release capsules may be used for once-a-day dosing in attention deficit disorders and narcolepsy.

4. When tablets are used for ADD or narcolepsy, give first dose upon awakening with one or two additional doses given at intervals of 4–6 hr. Give the last dose 6 hr before bedtime.
5. If receiving an MAO inhibitor, wait 14 days after stopping before initiating dextroamphetamine.
6. Where possible interrupt drug administration occasionally to determine the need for continued therapy.
7. Store from 15–30°C (59–86°F); dispense in a tight, light- and child-resistant container.

ASSESSMENT

1. Note reasons for therapy, characteristics of S&S, testing results, other agents trialed, outcome.
2. Obtain baseline labs, EKG, vital signs, ht and wt; monitor during therapy.
3. Products contain FD&C Yellow No. 5 (tartrazine).

CLIENT/FAMILY TEACHING

1. Do not crush or chew SR tablets.
2. With tablets, give the first dose upon awakening; give additional doses (1 or 2) at intervals of 4 to 6 hr. Take last dose at least 6 hr before bedtime to ensure adequate rest.
3. Avoid activities that require alertness until drug effects realized. May exerience fatigue as drug starts to wear off.
4. Check weight weekly to ensure no significant loss. In children check height and growth rate. Eat regular meals with snacks to prevent weight loss. Avoid caffeine or caffeinated drinks.
5. Do not stop suddenly after prolonged use; drug may cause psychological dependence. Reduce dose gradually to prevent acute withdrawal effects or severe depression. Keep all F/U appointments to evaluate drug response.

OUTCOMES/EVALUATE

• Improved attention span and concentration levels
• ↓ Daytime sleeping

Dextromethorphan hydrobromide

(dex-troh-meth-**OR**-fan)

D

CLASSIFICATION(S):
Antitussive, nonnarcotic

PREGNANCY CATEGORY: C

OTC: Freezer Pops: PediaCare Children's Long-Acting Cough. **Gelcaps:** DexAlone, Robitussin CoughGels. **Liquid/Oral Solution:** Children's Pedia Care Long-Acting Cough, Creo-Terpin, Robitussin Maximum Strength Cough, Simply Cough, Vicks 44 Cough Relief. **Lozenges:** Hold DM, Scot-Tussin DM Cough Chasers, Trocal. **Oral Suspension, Extended-Release:** Delsym. **Strips, Orally Disintegrating:** TheraFlu Thin Strips Long-Acting Cough, Triaminic Thin Strips Long Acting Cough. **Syrup:** Creomulsion Adult Formula, Creomulsion for Children, ElixSure Children's Cough, Robitussin Pediatric Cough, Silphen DM.
Rx: Suspension: AeroTuss 12.
♣**OTC:** Balminil DM Children, Koffex DM Children, Koffex DM Syrup, Novahistex DM, Novahistine DM, Robitussin Honey Cough DM.

USES
Symptomatic relief of nonproductive cough due to colds or inhaled irritants.

ACTION/KINETICS
Action
Selectively depresses the cough center in the medulla. Dextromethorphan 15–30 mg is equal to 8–15 mg codeine as an antitussive. Does not produce physical dependence or respiratory depression.

Pharmacokinetics
Well absorbed from GI tract. **Onset:** 15–30 min. **Duration:** 3–6 hr. The sustained liquid contains dextromethorphan plistirex equivalent to 30 mg dextromethorphan hydrobromide per 5 mL.

CONTRAINDICATIONS
Persistent or chronic cough or when cough is accompanied by excessive secretions. Use during first trimester of pregnancy unless directed otherwise by physician. Use in children less than 6 years of age.

SPECIAL CONCERNS
Use with caution in clients with nausea, vomiting, high fever, rash, or persistent headache. Dextromethorphan abuse can lead to brain damage, seizures, loss of consciousness, irregular heartbeat, and death.

SIDE EFFECTS
Most Common
Dizziness, drowsiness, GI disturbances.
CNS: Dizziness, drowsiness. **GI:** N&V, stomach pain.

OD **OVERDOSE MANAGEMENT**
Symptoms: **Adults:** Dysphoria, slurred speech, ataxia, altered sensory perception. **Children:** Ataxia, ***convulsions, respiratory depression.*** *Treatment:* Treat symptoms and provide support.

DRUG INTERACTIONS
Grapefruit juice / ↑ Bioavailability of dextromethorphan
MAO inhibitors / May cause hyperpyrexia, abnormal muscle movement, hypotension, coma, and death; avoid concomitant use for 2 weeks after stopping MAOI.
Quinidine / ↑ Plasma dextromethorphan levels R/T ↓ liver metabolism
Silbutramine / Accumulation of brain serotonin → serotonin syndrome (myoclonus, hyperreflexia, confusion, disorientation, agitation, hypomania, rigidity, tremor, sweating, shivering, seizures, coma, hypertension)

HOW SUPPLIED
Freezer pops: 7.5 mg/25 mL (per pop); *Gelcaps:* 15 mg, 30 mg; *Liquid:* 5 mg/5 mL, 7.5 mg/5 mL, 10 mg/5 mL, 15 mg/5 mL, 30 mg/5 mL; *Lozenges:* 5 mg, 7.5 mg; *Oral Suspension, Extended-Release:* 30 mg/5 mL; *Strips, Orally Disintegrating:* 7.5 mg, 12.5 mg, 15 mg; *Suspension:* 30 mg/5 mL; *Syrup:* 5 mg/5 mL, 7.5 mg/5 mL, 10 mg/5 mL, 20 mg/15 mL.

DOSAGE
• **FREEZER POPS**
Antitussive.

Children, 6 to <12 years old: 2 freezer pops (50 mL), if needed, q 6–8 hr, up to 8 freezer pops (200 mL)/day.
• **GELCAPS**

Antitussive.

Adults and children 12 years and older: 30 mg q 6–8 hr, not to exceed 120 mg/24 hr. Do not use in children less than 12 years old.

- **LOZENGES**

Antitussive.

Adults and children 12 years and older: 5–15 mg q 1–4 hr, up to 120 mg/day. **Children, 6–12 years of age:** 5–10 mg q 1–4 hr, not to exceed 60 mg/day. Do not give to children under 6 years of age unless directed by provider.

- **LIQUID; ORAL SOLUTION; SYRUP**

Antitussive.

Adults and children 12 years and older: 10–20 mg q 4 hr or 30 mg q 6–8 hr, not to exceed 120 mg/day. **Children, 6–12 years of age:** 10 mg q 4 hr or 15 mg q 6–8 hr, up to 60 mg/day.

- **ORAL SUSPENSION, EXTENDED-RELEASE**

Antitussive.

Adults and children 12 years and older: 60 mg q 12 hr, up to 120 mg/day. **Children, 6–12 years of age:** 30 mg q 12 hr, up to 60 mg/day.

NURSING CONSIDERATIONS

ADMINISTRATION/STORAGE

1. Increasing the dose of dextromethorphan will not increase its effectiveness but will increase the duration of action.

2. Do not give lozenges to children under 6 years of age.

ASSESSMENT

1. List sputum characteristics, C&S results. Note duration of cough, if persists beyond several weeks, stop drug and reassess cause. List drugs prescribed to ensure none interact.

2. Determine presence of nausea, vomiting, persistent headaches, or a high fever.

3. If pregnant, determine trimester; contraindicated in first trimester.

4. Assess VS, ENT, lung sounds; determine need for CXR/sinus films.

CLIENT/FAMILY TEACHING

1. Take exactly as directed and do not exceed dosing schedule.

2. Avoid tasks that require mental alertness until drug effects realized.

3. Avoid alcohol in any form.

4. Add humidity to environment.

5. Increase fluids to decrease thickness of secretions.

6. Cigarette smoke, dust, and chemical fumes are irritants that may aggravate condition.

7. Symptoms that persist for more than a week require medical intervention; record/report onset, triggers, characteristics of secretions, medications, and response to therapy.

OUTCOMES/EVALUATE

Control of cough with improved sleep patterns

Diazepam [IV]

(dye-**AYZ**-eh-pam)

CLASSIFICATION(S):

Antianxiety drug, benzodiazepine
PREGNANCY CATEGORY: D
Rx: Diastat AcuDial, Diazepam Intensol, Valium, **C-IV**
✦Rx: Apo-Diazepam, Diazemuls, Valium Roche.

SEE ALSO *TRANQUILIZERS/ ANTIMANIC DRUGS/HYPNOTICS.*

USES

PO: (1) Management of anxiety disorders or for short-term relief of symptoms of anxiety. (2) Adjunct therapy in convulsive disorders; effectiveness as sole therapy has not been proven. (3) Adjunct for relief of skeletal muscle spasm caused by reflex spasm to local pathology (e.g., inflammation of muscles or joints or secondary to trauma). Also, spasticity due to upper motor neuron disorders (e.g., cerebral palsy, paraplegia). Athetosis, stiff-man syndrome. (4) Acute alcohol withdrawal for symptomatic relief of acute agitation, tremor, impending or acute delirium tremens, and hallucinosis.

Parenteral: (1) Adjunct therapy in status epilepticus and severe recurrent convulsive seizures. (2) IV prior to cardioversion for relief of anxiety and tension and to decrease client's recall. (3)

Relief of anxiety and tension in those undergoing surgical procedures. As an adjunct prior to endoscopic or surgical procedures if apprehension, anxiety, or acute stress reactions are present; also, to diminish client recall of the procedures. (4) Treatment of tetanus. (5) Adjunct for the relief of skeletal muscle spasm due to reflex spasm caused by local pathology (e.g., inflammation of muscles or joints, secondary to trauma). Also, spasticity due to upper motor neuron disorders (e.g., cerebral palsy, paraplegia); athetosis; stiff-man syndrome. (6) Symptomatic relief of acute agitation, tremor, impending or acute delirium tremens, and hallucinosis.

Rectal gel: Management of selective refractory clients with epilepsy who are stable on regimens of anticonvulsant drugs who require intermittent diazepam to control increased seizure activity.

ACTION/KINETICS
Action
Reduces anxiety by increasing or facilitating the inhibitory neurotransmitter activity of GABA. The skeletal muscle relaxant effect may be due to enhancement of GABA-mediated presynaptic inhibition at the spinal level as well as in the brain stem reticular formation.

Pharmacokinetics
Onset: PO, 30–60 min; **IM,** 15–30 min; **IV,** more rapid. **Peak plasma levels: PO,** 0.5–2 hr; **IM,** 0.5–1.5; **IV,** 0.25 hr. **Duration:** 3 hr. **t½:** 20–50 hr. Metabolized in the liver to the active metabolites desmethyldiazepam, oxazepam, and temazepam. Diazepam and metabolites are excreted through the urine. **Plasma protein binding:** 97–99%.

ADDITIONAL CONTRAINDICATIONS
Narrow-angle glaucoma, children under 6 months, lactation, and parenterally in children under 12 years.

SPECIAL CONCERNS
When used as an adjunct for seizure disorders, diazepam may increase the frequency or severity of clonic-tonic seizures, for which an increase in the dose of anticonvulsant medication is necessary. Safety and efficacy of parenteral diazepam have not been determined in neonates less than 30 days of age. Prolonged CNS depression has been observed in neonates, probably due to inability to biotransform diazepam into inactive metabolites. Use IV diazepam with extreme caution in the elderly, in very ill clients, and in those with limited pulmonary reserve as apnea or cardiac arrest may occur. Tonic status epilepticus may be precipitated in those treated with IV diazepam for petit mal status or petit mal variant status.

SIDE EFFECTS
Most Common
Drowsiness (transient), ataxia, confusion.

See *Tranquilizers/Antimanic Drugs/Hypnotics* for a complete list of possible side effects.

ADDITIONAL DRUG INTERACTIONS
1. Diazepam potentiates antihypertensive effects of thiazides and other diuretics.
2. Diazepam potentiates muscle relaxant effects of *d*-tubocurarine and gallamine.

Fluoxetine / ↑ Diazepam half-life
Isoniazid / ↑ Diazepam half-life
Ranitidine / ↓ GI absorption of diazepam
Smoking / Possible ↑ Diazepam hepatic metabolism → ↓ response

HOW SUPPLIED
Injection: 5 mg/mL; *Oral Solution:* 1 mg/mL; *Rectal Gel:* 2.5 mg, 10 mg, 20 mg; *Solution, Intensol:* 5 mg/mL; *Tablets:* 2 mg, 5 mg, 10 mg.

DOSAGE
• **ORAL SOLUTION; SOLUTION, INTENSOL; TABLETS**

Management and relief of anxiety disorders.

Adults: 2–10 mg 2 to 4 times per day. **Children, initial:** 1–2.5 mg 3–4 times per day; **then,** increase gradually as needed and tolerated. Not to be used in children less than 6 months of age. **Elderly clients or in presence of debilitating disease, initial:** 2–2.5 mg 1 or 2 times per day; **then,** increase gradually as needed and tolerated.

Acute alcohol withdrawal.

---

10 mg 3 or 4 times per day during the first 24 hr; reduce to 5 mg 3 or 4 times per day, as needed.

Adjunct in skeletal muscle spasms.

Adults: 2–10 mg 3 or 4 times per day. **Children:** 0.12–0.8 mg/kg/24 hr divided 3 to 4 times per day.

Adjunct in convulsive disorders.

Adults: 2–10 mg 2–4 times per day. **Elderly or debilitated clients, initial:** 2–2.5 mg 1 or 2 times per day; **then,** increase dose gradually as needed and tolerated. Limit dose to the smallest effective amount to preclude development of ataxia or oversedation. **Children at least 6 months of age, initial:** 1–2.5 mg 3 or 4 times per day; **then,** increase dose gradually as needed and tolerated.

• **IM; IV**

Moderate anxiety disorders and symptoms of anxiety.

Adults: 2–5 mg IM or IV. Repeat in 3–4 hr if needed.

Severe anxiety disorders and symptoms of anxiety.

Adults: 5–10 mg IM or IV. Repeat in 3–4 hr if needed.

Acute alcohol withdrawal.

Adults, initial: 10 mg IM or IV; **then,** 5–10 mg in 3–4 hr if needed.

Endoscopic procedures.

Adults, IV: Titrate dosage to desired sedative response (e.g., slurring of speech). Give slowly and just prior to procedure. Reduce narcotic dosage by at least one-third; in some cases, narcotics may be omitted. **Usual:** 10 mg or less; up to 20 mg may be used, especially when concomitant narcotics are omitted. **Adults, IM:** 5–10 mg 30 min prior to procedure if IV route cannot be used.

Muscle spasms.

Adults, initial: 5–10 mg IM or IV; **then,** 5–10 mg in 3–4 hr if needed. Tetanus may require larger doses.

Sedation or muscle relaxation in children.

0.04–0.2 mg/kg/dose q 2–4 hr up to a maximum of 0.6 mg/kg within an 8-hr period.

Tetanus.

Children, 5 years and older: 5–10 mg given q 3–4 hr, if needed. **Infants older than 30 days of age:** 1–2 mg IM or slowly IV given q 3–4 hr as needed.

Preoperative medication.

Adults: 10 mg IM before surgery. If atropine, scopolamine, or other premedications are desired, use separate syringes.

Cardioversion.

Adults: 5–15 mg IV, 5–10 min prior to procedure.

Status epilepticus or severe recurrent convulsive seizures.

Adults, initial: 5–10 mg IV (preferred); **then,** may be repeated at 10–15 min intervals up to a maximum of 30 mg, if needed. May repeat therapy in 2–4 hr. Use with extreme caution in chronic lung disease or unstable cardiovascular status. **Children, at least 5 years of age:** 1 mg q 2–5 min IV (preferred) up to a maximum of 10 mg. Repeat in 2–4 hr if needed. **Infants older than 30 days of age and younger than 5 years of age:** 0.2–0.5 mg by slow IV q 2–5 min up to a maximum of 5 mg. May be repeated in 2–4 hr if needed.

• **RECTAL GEL**

Convulsive disorders.

Depending on age dose ranges from 0.2–0.5 mg/kg; calculate the recommended dose by rounding up to the next available unit dose. If needed, a second dose may be given 4–12 hr after the first dose. Do not treat more than 5 episodes/month or more than 1 episode q 5 days. **Adults and children 12 years and older:** 0.2 mg/kg. In the elderly or debilitated, adjust dose downward to reduce ataxia or oversedation. **Children, 6–11 years of age:** 0.3 mg/kg; **children, 2–5 years of age:** 0.5 mg/kg.

NURSING CONSIDERATIONS

ADMINISTRATION/STORAGE

1. Mix Intensol solution with beverages such as water, soda, and juices or soft foods such as applesauce or puddings. Use only the calibrated dropper provided to withdraw drug; once withdrawn and mixed, use immediately.

Bold Italic = life threatening side effect   ■ = black box warning   ✦ = Available in Canada

2. Except for the deltoid muscle, absorption from IM sites is slow, erratic and painful and not generally recommended.

3. The rectal delivery system includes a plastic applicator with a flexible, molded tip available in two lengths. The Diastat AcuDial 2.5 mg and 10 mg syringes are available with a 4.4 cm tip and the Diastat AcuDial 20 mg syringe is available with a 6 cm tip.

4. Store the rectal gel from 15–30°C (59–86°F).

 5. IV route is preferred in the convulsing client; EEG monitoring of seizure may be helpful.

6. IV diazepam will control seizures promptly; however, many clients experience a return to seizure activity (probably due to the short duration of IV diazepam). Be prepared to readminister.

7. Diazepam is not recommended for maintenance of seizure control. Consider other agents for long-term control.

8. In children, EEG monitoring of seizures may be helpful.

9. Parenteral administration may cause bradycardia, respiratory/cardiac arrest; have emergency equipment/drugs available.

10. Diazepam interacts with plastic; putting into plastic containers or administration sets will decrease drug availability.

11. To reduce IV site reactions, give diazepam slowly (5 mg/min); avoid small veins or intra-arterial administration. For pediatric use, give IV solution slowly over a 3-min period.

12. Due to the possibility of precipitation and instability, do not infuse diazepam. Do not mix or dilute with other solutions or drugs in the syringe or infusion container.

13. Store injection at room temperature protected from light. Do not use if solution is darker than slightly yellow or contains a precipitate.

ASSESSMENT

1. Identify reasons for therapy, onset, characteristics of S&S, other agents prescribed/trialed.

2. Assess emotional status; note depression or drug abuse. Avoid simultaneous use of CNS depressants. Reduce drug gradually to avoid withdrawal symptoms such as anxiety, tremors, anorexia, insomnia, weakness, headache, and N&V.

3. Monitor VS, CBC, renal, and LFTs. Do not use with glaucoma (narrow angle).

4. Review anxiety level; identify contributing factors.

5. Elderly clients, very ill clients, those with limited pulmonary reserve may experience adverse reactions more quickly than others; use a lower dose in these groups.

CLIENT/FAMILY TEACHING

1. Drug acts by slowing down the nervous system. Review why prescribed, dose, form, frequency and desired outcome.

2. May cause dizziness/drowsiness; avoid activities that require mental alertness until drug effects realized.

3. Avoid alcohol and other CNS depressants.

4. Smoking may increase drug metabolism; thus requiring higher dose than nonsmoker. Do not stop drug abruptly.

5. Report if pregnancy suspected. adverse side effects, lack of response. Prolonged use may cause dependence.

6. Inspect the prefilled syringes of the rectal gel for cracks frequently; cracks can cause leakage of the drug so client may not get sufficient medication to control seizures. Review administration procedure prior to use.

7. Keep all F/U appointments to evaluate response to therapy.

OUTCOMES/EVALUATE

- ↓ Anxiety/tension episodes
- Control alcohol withdrawal
- Control of status epilepticus
- Relief of muscle spasms
- Effective sedation

Diazoxide IV
(dye-az-**OX**-eyed)

CLASSIFICATION(S):
Antihypertensive, direct-acting
PREGNANCY CATEGORY: C
Rx: Hyperstat IV.

SEE ALSO *ANTIHYPERTENSIVE AGENTS* AND *DIAZOXIDE ORAL*.

USES

May be the drug of choice for hypertensive crisis (malignant and nonmalignant hypertension) in hospitalized adults and children. Often given concomitantly with a diuretic. Especially suitable for clients with impaired renal function, hypertensive encephalopathy, hypertension complicated by LV failure, and eclampsia. Ineffective for hypertension due to pheochromocytoma.

ACTION/KINETICS

Action

Exerts a direct action on vascular smooth muscle to cause arteriolar vasodilation and decreased peripheral resistance.

Pharmacokinetics

Onset: 1–5 min. **Time to peak effect:** 2–5 min. **Duration** (variable): Usual, 3–12 hr. Excreted through the kidney (50% unchanged).

CONTRAINDICATIONS

Hypersensitivity to drug or thiazide diuretics. Treatment of compensatory hypertension due to aortic coarctation or AV shunt. Dissecting aortic aneurysm.

SPECIAL CONCERNS

A decrease in dose may be necessary in geriatric clients due to age-related decreases in renal function. If given prior to delivery, fetal or neonatal hyperbilirubinemia, thrombocytopenia, or altered carbohydrate metabolism may result. Use with caution during lactation and in clients with impaired cerebral or cardiac circulation.

SIDE EFFECTS

Most Common

Hypotension, N&V, dizziness, weakness.

CV: Hypotension (may be severe enough to cause shock), sodium and water retention, especially in clients with impaired cardiac reserve, *atrial or ventricular arrhythmias*, *cerebral or myocardial ischemia*, marked ECG changes with possibility of *MI*, palpitations, bradycardia, SVT, chest discomfort or nonanginal chest tightness. **CNS:** Cerebral ischemia manifested by unconsciousness, *seizures*, paralysis, confusion, numbness of the hands. Headache, dizziness, weakness, drowsiness, lightheadedness, somnolence, lethargy, euphoria, weakness of short duration, apprehension, anxiety, malaise, blurred vision. **Respiratory:** Tightness in chest, cough, dyspnea, choking sensation. **GI:** N&V, diarrhea, anorexia, parotid swelling, change in taste sense, salivation, dry mouth, ileus, constipation, acute pancreatitis (rare). **Miscellaneous:** Hyperglycemia (may be serious enough to require treatment), sweating, flushing, sensation of warmth, transient neurologic findings due to alteration in regional blood flow to the brain, hyperosmolar coma in infants, tinnitus, hearing loss, retention of nitrogenous wastes, acute pancreatitis, back pain, increased nocturia, lacrimation, hypersensitivity reactions, papilledema, hirsutism, decreased libido. Pain, cellulitis without sloughing, warmth or pain along injected vein, phlebitis at injection site, extravasation.

LABORATORY TEST CONSIDERATIONS

False + or ↑ uric acid.

OD **OVERDOSE MANAGEMENT**

Symptoms: Hypotension, excessive hyperglycemia. *Treatment:* Use the Trendelenburg position to reverse hypotension.

DRUG INTERACTIONS

Anticoagulants, oral / ↑ Anticoagulant effect R/T ↓ plasma protein binding
Nitrites / ↑ Hypotensive effect
Phenytoin / ↓ Anticonvulsant effect of phenytoin
Sulfonylureas / Destablization of the client → hyperglycemia
Thiazide diuretics / ↑ Hyperglycemic, hyperuricemic, and antihypertensive diazoxide effect
Vasodilators, peripheral / ↑ Hypotensive effect

HOW SUPPLIED

Injection: 15 mg/mL.

DOSAGE

- **IV PUSH (30 SEC OR LESS)**

    Hypertensive crisis.

Adults: 1–3 mg/kg up to a maximum of 150 mg; may be repeated at 5–15-min intervals until adequate BP response obtained. Drug may then be repeated at 4–24-hr intervals for 4–5 days or until

---

Bold Italic = life threatening side effect   ■ = black box warning   ✦ = Available in Canada

oral antihypertensive therapy can be initiated. **Pediatric:** 1–3 mg/kg (30–90 mg/m²) using the same dosing intervals as adults.

Repeated use can result in sodium and water retention; therefore, a diuretic may be needed to avoid CHF and for maximum reduction of BP.

NURSING CONSIDERATIONS

ADMINISTRATION/STORAGE
IV 1. Do not administer IM or SC. Medication is highly alkaline.

2. Ensure patency; inject rapidly (30 sec) undiluted into a peripheral vein to maximize response.

3. Assess site for signs of irritation/extravasation. If extravasation occurs, apply ice packs.

4. Protect from light, heat, freezing.

5. Have norepinephrine (sympathomimetic drug), available to treat severe hypotension should it occur.

6. Protect ampules from light; store between 2–30°C (36–86°F).

ASSESSMENT
1. Note sensitivity to thiazide diuretics, sulfa drugs, diazoxide.

2. Can cause serious elevations in blood sugar levels. Note complaints of sweating, flushing, evidence of hyperosmolar NKDM or hyperglycemia in diabetics.

3. Obtain uric acid level; assess for hyperuricemia.

4. Monitor VS/BP frequently until stabilized, then hourly until crisis resolved. Obtain final BP upon arising, prior to ambulation. Keep recumbent during and for 30 min after injection to avoid orthostatic hypotension; for 8–10 hr if furosemide is also administered. Assess for CHF, peripheral edema, monitor electrolytes.

CLIENT/FAMILY TEACHING
Drug is injected IV to rapidly lower BP in a monitored environment when other measures fail or a rapid reduction is needed. Must remain flat for 30 min after injection. Do not change positions suddenly; may experience adverse side effects of sudden drop in BP (postural hypotension).

OUTCOMES/EVALUATE
Reduction in BP during hypertensive crisis

Diclofenac epolamine ■ ©
(dye-**KLOH**-fen-ack)

CLASSIFICATION(S):
Nonsteroidal anti-inflammatory drug
PREGNANCY CATEGORY: B
Rx: Flector.

Diclofenac potassium
PREGNANCY CATEGORY: B
Rx: Cataflam.
✦**Rx:** Apo-Diclo Rapide, Voltaren Rapide.

Diclofenac sodium
PREGNANCY CATEGORY: B
Rx: Gel: Solaraze. **Ophthalmic:** Voltaren. **Tablets:** Voltaren, Voltaren-XR.
✦**Rx:** Apo-Diclo, Apo-Diclo SR, Novo-Difenac, Novo-Difenac SR, Novo-Difenac-K, Nu-Diclo, Nu-Diclo-SR, PMS-Diclofenac SR, Voltaren Ophtha.

SEE ALSO *NONSTEROIDAL ANTI-INFLAMMATORY DRUGS.*

USES
PO, Immediate-release (Diclofenac potassium): (1) Acute and chronic treatment of signs and symptoms of rheumatoid arthritis and osteoarthritis. (2) Ankylosing spondylitis. (3) Mild-t-moderate pain. (4) Primary dysmenorrhea. Use immediate-release when prompt relief is desired. **PO, Delayed-Release or Extended-Release (Diclofenac sodium):** (1) Signs and symptoms of rheumatoid arthritis and osteoarthritis. (2) Acute or long-term use for ankylosing spondylitis (Delayed-Release). *Investigational:* Mild-to-moderate

D

 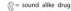

pain, juvenile rheumatoid arthritis, acute painful shoulder, sunburn.

Transdermal Patch (Diclofenac epolamine): Topical treatment of acute pain due to minor strains, sprains, and contusions.

Ophthalmic: (1) Postoperative inflammation following cataract removal. (2) Temporary relief of pain and photophobia following corneal refractive surgery.

Topical Gel: Actinic keratoses.

ACTION/KINETICS

Action

Anti-inflammatory effect is due to inhibition of the enzyme cyclo-oxygenase. Inhibition of cyclo-oxygenase results in decreased prostaglandin synthesis. Prostaglandin will cause inflammation. Effective in reducing joint swelling, pain, and morning stiffness and increases mobility in those with inflammatory disease.

Pharmacokinetics

Available as both the potassium (immediate-release) and sodium (delayed-release) salts. *Immediate-release product.* Is 50–60% bioavailable. **Onset:** 30 min. **Peak plasma levels:** 1 hr. **Duration:** 8 hr. *Delayed-release product.* **Peak plasma levels:** 2–3 hr. **t½:** 1–2 hr. For all dosage forms, food will affect the rate, but not the amount, absorbed from the GI tract. Metabolized in the liver and excreted by the kidneys. **Plasma protein binding:** Greater than 99% bound to plasma proteins.

CONTRAINDICATIONS

Use to treat perioperative pain following coronary artery bypass graft surgery. Wearers of soft contact lenses. Use of the gel in those with hypersensitivity to benzyl alcohol, polyethylene glycol monomethyl ether 350, or hyaluronate sodium. Use of the gel during lactation or in children.

SPECIAL CONCERNS

■ (1) NSAIDs may cause an increased risk of serious CV thrombotic events, MI, and stroke, which can be fatal. This risk may increase with duration of use. Clients with CV disease or risk factors for CV disease may be at greater risk. (2) Diclofenac epolamine, potassium, or sodium are contraindicated to treat perioperative pain in the setting of coronary artery bypass graft surgery. (3) NSAIDs cause an increased risk of serious GI side effects including inflammation, bleeding, ulceration, and perforation of the stomach or intestines, which can be fatal. These events can occur at any time during use and without warning symptoms. Elderly clients are at greater risk for serious GI events.■ Starting therapy with maximum doses in those at increased risk due to renal or hepatic disease, low body weight (less than 60 kg), advanced age, a known ulcer diathesis, or known hypersensitivity to NSAID effects is likely to increase the frequency of side effects. Use with caution during lactation. Safety and effectiveness have not been determined in children. When used ophthalmically, may cause increased bleeding of ocular tissues in conjunction with ocular surgery. Healing may be slowed or delayed.

SIDE EFFECTS

Most Common

After PO use: Headache, dizzness, abdominal pain/cramps, nausea, diarrhea, constipation, dyspepsia/indigestion.

See *Nonsteroidal Anti-Inflammatory Drugs* for a complete list of possible side effects.

Following ophthalmic use: Keratitis, increased IOP, ocular allergy, N&V, anterior chamber reaction, viral infections, transient burning/stinging on administration. When used with soft contact lenses, may cause ocular irritation, including redness/burning.

HOW SUPPLIED

Diclofenac epolamine. *Transdermal patch:* 180 mg.

Diclofenac potassium. *Tablets, Immediate-Release:* 50 mg.

Diclofenac sodium *Gel:* 3%; *Ophthalmic Solution:* 0.1%; *Tablets, Delayed-Release:* 25 mg, 50 mg, 75 mg; *Tablets, Extended-Release:* 100 mg.

DOSAGE

DICLOFENAC POTASSIUM

• **TABLETS, IMMEDIATE-RELEASE**
  Analgesia, primary dysmenorrhea.

Adults, initial: 50 mg 3 times per day of immediate-release tablets. In some, an initial dose of 100 mg followed by 50-mg doses may achieve better results. After the first day, the total daily dose should not exceed 150 mg.

Rheumatoid arthritis.
Adults: 150–200 mg/day in divided doses (e.g., 50 mg 3 or 4 times per day). Do not exceed 225 mg/day.

Osteoarthritis.
Adults: 100–150 mg/day in divided doses (e.g., 50 mg 2 or 3 times per day). Doses greater than 200 mg/day have not been evaluated.

Ankylosing spondylitis.
Adults: 50 mg 2 times per day; **range:** 100–125 mg/day. Doses greater than 125 mg/day have not been evaluated.

DICLOFENAC SODIUM
• **DELAYED-RELEASE TABLETS**
Ankylosing spondylitis.
100–125 mg/day, given as 25 mg 4 times per day, with an extra 25 mg at bedtime, if necessary.

Osteoarthritis.
100–150 mg/day (e.g., 50 mg 2 or 3 times per day or 75 mg 2 times per day).

Rheumatoid arthritis.
150–200 mg/day in divided doses (50 mg 3 or 4 times per day or 75 mg 2 times per day).

• **EXTENDED-RELEASE TABLETS**
Osteoarthritis.
100 mg/day.

Rheumatoid arthritis.
100 mg/day. If this dose is not satisfactory, dose may be increased to 100 mg 2 times per day if the benefits outweigh the risk of increased side effects.

• **OPHTHALMIC SOLUTION, 0.1%**
Following cataract surgery.
1 gtt in the affected eye 4 times per day beginning 24 hr after cataract surgery and for 2 weeks thereafter.

Corneal refractive surgery.
1–2 gtt within 1 hr prior to surgery; then, apply 1–2 gtt within 15 min of surgery and continue 4 times per day for up to 3 days.

• **TOPICAL GEL, 3%**
Actinic keratoses.

Apply gel 2 times per day to lesion areas for 60–90 days.

DICLOFENAC EPOLAMINE
• **TRANSDERMAL PATCH**
Acute pain due to minor strains, sprains, contusions.
Apply 1 patch to the most painful area twice a day. Change patch once every 12 hr. Remove patch if irritation occurs.

NURSING CONSIDERATIONS

🅒 Do not confuse Cataflam with Catapres (an antihypertensive).

ADMINISTRATION/STORAGE

1. The lowest dose should be sought for each client.

2. In those weighing less than 60 kg (132 lbs) or where the severity of the disease, concomitant medications, or other diseases warrant, reduce the maximum recommended total dose of diclofenac potassium.

3. The various dosage forms are not necessarily bioequivalent even if the milligram strength is the same.

4. Up to 3 weeks may be required for beneficial effects to be realized when used for rheumatoid arthritis or osteoarthritis.

5. Do not store diclofenac potassium or sodium above 30°C (86°F); protect from moisture.

6. Store ophthalmic solution from 15–30°C (59–86° F).

7. Protect ophthalmic solution from light; dispense in original, unopened container.

8. Store the patch from 15–30°C (59–86°F). Keep the envelopes sealed at all times when not in use. Discard unused patches 3 months after opening the envelope.

ASSESSMENT

1. Note reasons for therapy, symptom characteristics, other agents trialed/failed.

2. Assess for redness, infection, pain, vision changes with eye therapy.

3. With arthritis, assess joints for inflammation, deformity, erosion, ROM, loss of function; rate pain level.

4. Monitor VS, CBC, renal and LFTs; perform FOB with long-term therapy.

 = see color insert   = Herbal   = Intravenous   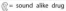 = sound alike drug

5. Ensure drug administered in high enough doses for anti-inflammatory effect when needed and in low doses for an analgesic effect.

CLIENT/FAMILY TEACHING

1. Take with meals, a full glass of water or milk if GI upset occurs; remain upright for 30 min after taking drug to reduce esophageal irritation.

2. Do not crush or chew delayed-release tablets.

3. Do not apply the patch to damaged or nonintact skin; do not apply when bathing or showering.

4. Wash hands after applying, handling, or removing the patch. Avoid eye contact.

5. When disposing of the patch, fold so that the adhesive side sticks to itself. Safely discard where children and pets cannot access.

6. Limit intake of sodium, monitor weights, report any swelling or unusual weight gain.

7. Clients with diabetes should monitor BS levels closely; may alter response to antidiabetic agents.

8. Avoid alcohol, OTC products, and prolonged sun exposure without protection.

9. Do not wear contacts when using eye therapy.

10. Maintain fluid intake of 2 L/day.

11. Report adverse effects, changes in stools, ringing in ears, stomach pain, unusual bruising/bleeding, lack of response.

OUTCOMES/EVALUATE

- Relief of joint pain/inflammation with improved mobility
- ↓ Eye inflammation

Dicyclomine hydrochloride ©

(dye-**SYE**-kloh-meen)

CLASSIFICATION(S):
Cholinergic blocking drug
PREGNANCY CATEGORY: C
Rx: Antispas, Bentyl, Byclomine, Di-Spaz, Dibent, Dilomine, Or-Tyl.

✢**Rx:** Bentylol, Lomine.

SEE ALSO *CHOLINERGIC BLOCKING AGENTS.*

USES
Hypermotility and spasms of GI tract associated with irritable colon and spastic colitis, mucous colitis.

ACTION/KINETICS
Action Prevents acetylcholine from combining with postganglionic parasympathetic nerve receptors (muscarinic) resulting in decreased vagal impulses to the GI tract. Results in a decrease in GI motility.

Pharmacokinetics
t½, initial: 1.8 hr; **secondary:** 9–10 hr.

ADDITIONAL CONTRAINDICATIONS
Use for peptic ulcer.

SPECIAL CONCERNS
Lower doses may be needed in elderly clients due to confusion, agitation, excitement, or drowsiness.

SIDE EFFECTS
Most Common
Dry mouth, N&V, constipation, urinary hesitancy/retention, headache, blurred vision.

See *Cholinergic Blocking Agents* for a complete list of possible side effects. Also, brief euphoria, slight dizziness, feeling of abdominal distention. **Use of the syrup in infants less than 3 months of age:** *Seizures,* syncope, respiratory symptoms, fluctuations in pulse rate, *asphyxia,* muscular hypotonia, *coma.*

HOW SUPPLIED
Capsules: 10 mg; *Injection:* 10 mg/mL; *Syrup:* 10 mg/5 mL; *Tablets:* 20 mg.

DOSAGE
- **CAPSULES; SYRUP; TABLETS**
  Hypermotility and spasms of GI tract.
Adults, initial: 10–20 mg 3–4 times per day; **then,** may increase to total daily dose of 160 mg if side effects do not limit this dosage. **Pediatric, 6 months–2 years, syrup:** 5–10 mg 3–4 times per day; **2 years and older:** 10 mg 3–4 times per day. The dose should be adjusted to need and incidence of side effects.
- **IM ONLY**
  Hypermotility and spasms of GI tract.

Bold Italic = life threatening side effect   ■ = black box warning   ✢ = Available in Canada

Adults: 20 mg q 4–6 hr. **Not for IV use.**

NURSING CONSIDERATIONS

🕮 Do not confuse dicyclomine with doxycycline (an antibiotic); do not confuse Bentyl with Benadryl (an antihistamine) or Aventyl (an antidepressant).

ADMINISTRATION/STORAGE
Can be administered to clients with glaucoma with caution.

ASSESSMENT
1. List reasons for therapy, symptom characteristics, any triggers, other agents trialed, outcome.
2. Determine presence/history PUD; assess abdomen, review UGI, endoscopy/colonoscopy findings.

CLIENT/FAMILY TEACHING
1. Take 30 min before meals and at bedtime, report lack of response, rash, skin eruption, or adverse effects.
2. Use caution with activities requiring mental alertness; may cause drowsiness, blurred vision.
3. Consume adequate fluids to prevent dehydration/constipation; may use sugarless candy/gum for dry mouth. Avoid strenuous activity during hot conditions; heatstroke may occur.

OUTCOMES/EVALUATE
Restoration of normal bowel function/GI motility; Relief of GI spasms/pain.

Didanosine (ddI, dideoxyinosine) ■
(die-**DAN**-oh-seen)

CLASSIFICATION(S):
Antiviral, nucleoside reverse transcriptase inhibitor
PREGNANCY CATEGORY: B
Rx: Videx, Videx EC.

SEE ALSO *ANTIVIRAL AGENTS.*
USES
Videx: In combination with other antiretroviral drugs to treat HIV-1 infections. May be used in children over 2 weeks of age.

Videx EC: In combination with other antiretroviral drugs to treat HIV-1 infection in adults where treatment requires once-daily treatment of didanosine or an alternative didanosine formulation.

ACTION/KINETICS

Action
A nucleoside analog of deoxyadenosine. After entering the cell, it is converted to the active dideoxyadenosine triphosphate (ddATP) by cellular enzymes. Due to the chemical structure of ddATP, its incorporation into viral DNA leads to chain termination and therefore inhibition of viral replication. ddATP also inhibits viral replication by interfering with the HIV–RNA-dependent DNA polymerase by competing with the natural nucleoside triphosphate for binding to the active site of the enzyme. Didanosine has shown in vitro antiviral activity in a variety of HIV-infected T-cell and monocyte/macrophage cell cultures.

Pharmacokinetics
Is broken down quickly at acidic pH; therefore, PO products contain buffering agents to increase the pH of the stomach. Food decreases the rate of absorption. Oral availability differs between adults (about 42%) and children (about 25%). $t^{1}\!/_{2}$, **elimination:** 1.5 hr for adults and 0.8 hr for children. Metabolized in the liver and excreted mainly through the urine.

CONTRAINDICATIONS
Lactation.

SPECIAL CONCERNS
■ (1) Fatal and nonfatal pancreatitis has occurred with didanosine alone or in combination regimens in treatment-naive and treatment-experienced clients, regardless of the degree of immunosuppression. Suspend didanosine in those suspected of pancreatitis and discontinue in those with confirmed pancreatitis. (2) Lactic acidosis and severe hepatomegaly with steatosis, including death, may occur with use of nucleoside analogs alone or in combination, including didanosine and other antiretrovirals. (3) Fatal lactic acidosis has been reported in pregnant women who received the combination of didanosine and stavudine with other antiretroviral drugs. Use the combination of didanosine and stavudine with caution during

D

pregnancy; use only if the potential benefit clearly outweighs the potential risk.■ Use with caution in renal and hepatic impairment and in those on sodium-restricted diets. Use the combination of didanosine and ribavirin with caution due to increased exposure to the active metabolite of didanosine that may cause fatal hepatic failure, peripheral neuropathy, pancreatitis, and symptomatic hyperlactatemia or lactic acidosis. Opportunistic infections and other complications of HIV infection may continue to develop; thus, keep clients under close observation. High rate of virologic failure and emergence of nucleoside reverse transcriptase inhibitor resistance-associated mutations.

SIDE EFFECTS

Most Common

Diarrhea, N&V, headache, peripheral neurologic symptoms/neuropathy, abdominal pain, rash, pruritus, pancreatitis.

Commonly pancreatitis (fatal or nonfatal) and peripheral neuropathy (manifested by distal numbness, tingling, or pain in the feet or hands). Lactic acidosis (may be fatal), including pregnant women also receiving stavudine along with other antiretroviral drugs. Hepatotoxicity (may be fatal) used alone or in combination. Neuropathy occurs more frequently in clients with a history of neuropathy or neurotoxic drug therapy.

In adults. GI: Diarrhea, abdominal pain, N&V, anorexia, dyspepsia, dry mouth, ileus, colitis, constipation, eructation, flatulence, gastroenteritis, *GI hemorrhage,* severe hepatomegaly with steatosis, *liver failure*, oral moniliasis, stomatitis, mouth sores, sialadenitis, *stomach ulcer hemorrhage*, melena, oral thrush, liver abnormalities, parotid gland enlargement, *pancreatitis*. **CNS:** Headache, *tonic-clonic seizures*, abnormal thinking, anxiety, nervousness, twitching, confusion, depression, acute brain syndrome, amnesia, aphasia, ataxia, dizziness, hyperesthesia, hypertonia, incoordination, *intracranial hemorrhage*, paralysis, paranoid reaction, psychosis, insomnia, sleep disorders, speech disorders, tremor. **Hema-**

tologic: Leukopenia, granulocytopenia, thrombocytopenia, microcytic anemia, *hemorrhage*, ecchymosis, petechiae. **Dermatologic:** Rash, pruritus, herpes simplex, skin disorder, sweating, eczema, impetigo, excoriation, erythema. **Musculoskeletal:** Asthenia, myopathy, arthralgia, myopathy, arthritis, myalgia (with or without increases in creatine phosphokinse), muscle atrophy, decreased strength, hemiparesis, neck rigidity, joint disorder, leg cramps, *rhabdomyolysis, including acute renal failure*. **CV:** Chest pain, hypertension, hypotension, migraine, palpitation, peripheral vascular disorder, syncope, vasodilation, arrhythmias. **Body as a whole:** Chills, fever, asthenia, pain, infection, allergic reaction, pain, abscess, cellulitis, cyst, dehydration, malaise, flu syndrome, numbness of hands and feet, weight loss, alopecia, *anaphylaxis*. **Metabolic:** Diabetes mellitus, hypo—/hyperglycemia, *lactic acidosis*. **Respiratory:** Pneumonia, dyspnea, asthma, bronchitis, increased cough, rhinitis, rhinorrhea, epistaxis, laryngitis, decreased lung function, pharyngitis, hypoventilation, sinusitis, rhonchi, rales, congestion, interstitial pneumonia, respiratory disorders. **Ophthalmic:** Blurred vision, conjunctivitis, diplopia, dry eye, glaucoma, retinitis, photophobia, strabismus, optic neuritis, retinal depigmentation. **Otic:** Ear disorder, otitis (externa and media), ear pain. **GU:** Impotency, kidney calculus, kidney failure, abnormal kidney function, nocturia, urinary frequency, vaginal hemorrhage. **Miscellaneous:** Peripheral edema, sarcoma, hernia, hypokalemia, lymphoma-like reaction.

In children. GI: Diarrhea, N&V, liver abnormalities, abdominal pain, stomatitis, mouth sores, pancreatitis, anorexia, increase in appetite, constipation, oral thrush, melena, dry mouth, *pancreatitis*. **CNS:** Headache, nervousness, insomnia, dizziness, poor coordination, lethargy, neurologic symptoms, *seizures*. **Hematologic:** Ecchymosis, *hemorrhage*, petechiae, leukopenia, granulocytopenia, thrombocytopenia, anemia. **Dermatologic:** Rash, pruritus, skin disorder, eczema, sweat-

---

Bold Italic = life threatening side effect   ■ = black box warning   ✤ = Available in Canada

ing, impetigo, excoriation, erythema. **Musculoskeletal:** Arthritis, myalgia, muscle atrophy, decreased strength. **Body as a whole:** Chills, fever, asthenia, pain, malaise, failure to thrive, weight loss, flu syndrome, alopecia, dehydration, lactic acidosis. **CV:** Vasodilation, arrhythmia. **Respiratory:** Cough, rhinitis, dyspnea, asthma, rhinorrhea, epistaxis, pharyngitis, hypoventilation, sinusitis, rhonchi, rales, congestion, pneumonia. **Ophthalmic:** Photophobia, strabismus, visual impairment, optic neuritis, retinal changes. **Otic:** Ear pain, otitis. **Miscellaneous:** Urinary frequency, diabetes mellitus, diabetes insipidus, liver abnormalities.

LABORATORY TEST CONSIDERATIONS
↑ AST, ALT, alkaline phosphatase, bilirubin, uric acid, amylase, lipase.

OD **OVERDOSE MANAGEMENT**
Symptoms: Pancreatitis, peripheral neuropathy, diarrhea, hyperuricemia, hepatic dysfunction. *Treatment:* There are no antidotes; treatment should be symptomatic.

DRUG INTERACTIONS
Allopurinol / ↑ Didanosine levels
Antacids, Mg- or Al-containing / ↑ Risk of side effects R/T antacid components
Antifungal drugs (azoles) / ↓ Absorption of azole antifungals
Antiretroviral drugs (delavirdine, indinavir) / Significantly ↓ levels of antiretroviral drugs
Ganciclovir / ↑ Didanosine levels; ↓ ganciclovir levels
Itraconazole / ↓ Itraconazole effect; give 2 or more hr before didanosine
Ketoconazole / ↓ Ketoconazole absorption R/T gastric pH change caused by buffering agents in didanosine
Methadone / ↓ Didanosine levels
Pentamidine (IV) / ↑ Risk of pancreatitis
Quinolone antibiotics / ↓ Quinolone levels R/T ↓ absorption
Ranitidine / ↓ Ranitidine absorption R/T gastric pH change caused by buffering agents in didanosine
Ribavirin / ↑ Risk of fatal hepatic failure, peripheral neuropathy, pancreatitis, symptomatic hyperlactatemia, or lactic acidosis

Stavudine / ↑ Risk of fatal lactic acidosis in pregnant women, especially when combined with other drugs
Tenofovir / ↑ Didanosine toxicity (lactic acidosis, pancreatitis, peripheral neuropathy) and poor therapeutic outcomes (↓ virologic response, ↓ CD4+ T-cell counts); adjust dosage
Tetracyclines / ↓ Tetracycline absorption R/T gastric pH changes caused by buffering agents in didanosine

HOW SUPPLIED
Didanosine: *Powder for Oral Solution, Buffered:* 100 mg, 250 mg; *Powder for Pediatric Oral Solution:* 2 grams, 4 grams; *Tablets, Buffered (Chewable/Dispersible):* 25 mg, 50 mg, 100 mg, 200 mg.
Didanosine Enteric Coated: *Capsule, Enteric-Coated:* 125 mg, 200 mg, 250 mg, 400 mg.
Didanosine Delayed-Release: *Capsules, Delayed-Release (with enteric-coated beads):* 200 mg, 250 mg, 400 mg.

DOSAGE
• **CAPSULE, ENTERIC-COATED; POWDER FOR ORAL SOLUTION, BUFFERED; POWDER FOR PEDIATRIC ORAL SOLUTION; TABLETS, BUFFERED (CHEWABLE/DISPERSIBLE)**
Adults, initial, over 60 kg: 200 mg q 12 hr (or 400 mg/day) for tablets; 250 mg 2 times/day for buffered oral solution; or, 400 mg/day for enteric-coated capsules. **Adults, less than 60 kg:** 125 mg q 12 hr (or 250 mg/day) for tablets; 167 mg 2 times/day for buffered oral solution; or, 250 mg/day for enteric-coated capsules. **Pediatric:** 120 mg/m^2 2 times per day. Once-daily dosing may lower the virologic response; twice-daily dosing is preferred.
For adults with impaired renal function, the following dosage regimens are used: (1) **C_{CR} 60 mL or more per min:** See above. (2) **C_{CR} 30–59 mL/min, 60 kg or more:** 200 mg daily or 100 mg twice a day for tablets; or, 100 mg daily for buffered oral solution; or 200 mg per day for enteric-coated capsules. (3) **C_{CR} 30–59 mL/min, <60 kg:** 150 mg daily or 75 mg twice a day for tablets; or, 100 mg twice a day for buffered oral solution; or 125 mg daily for enteric-

coated capsules. (4) **C$_{CR}$ 10–29 mL/min, 60 kg or more:** 150 mg daily for tablets; or 167 mg per day for buffered oral solution; or, 125 mg/day for enteric-coated capsules. (5) **C$_{CR}$ 10–29 mL/min, <60 kg:** 100 mg daily for tablets; or, 100 mg daily for buffered oral solution; or 125 mg daily for enteric-coated capsules. (6) **C$_{CR}$ <10 mL/min, 60 kg or more:** 100 mg daily for tablets; or 100 mg buffered oral solution; or 125 mg daily for enteric-coated capsules. (7) **C$_{CR}$ <10 mL/min, <60 kg:** 75 mg daily for tablets or 100 mg daily for buffered oral solution (do not use enteric-coated capsules in these clients). *NOTE:* For clients requiring continuous ambulatory peritoneal dialysis or hemodialysis, give ¼ of the total daily dose once daily. For clients with a C$_{CR}$ <10 mL/min, do not give a supplemental dose of didanosine following hemodialysis.

NURSING CONSIDERATIONS
ADMINISTRATION/STORAGE
1. Twice-daily dosing may be more effective than once-daily dosing.
2. Administer all formulations 30 min before or 1 hr after meals. Didanosine EC should be given on an empty stomach and swallowed intact. Didanosine EC has not been studied in children.
3. For either once- or twice-daily dosing, clients must take at least 2 of the appropriate strength tablets at each dose to provide adequate buffering and to prevent gastric acid degradation of didanosine.
4. When taken with tenofovir, reduce dose of didanosine as follows: For adults weighing at least 60 kg with a C$_{CR}$ of >60 mL/min, reduce didanosine dose to 250 mg once daily; for adults weighing less than 60 kg with a C$_{CR}$ <60 mL/min, reduce the didanosine dose to 200 mg.
5. To reduce GI side effects, do not give more than 4 tablets at each dose.
6. To disperse tablets, add 2 tablets (for adults) to about 1 oz of water. Stir until a uniform dispersion forms; drink entire dispersion immediately. The dispersion may be diluted with 1 oz of clear apple juice. Pediatric dispersion is prepared similarly.
7. To prepare the buffered powder for PO solution for adults, mix with 4 oz of drinking water; do not mix powder with fruit juice or other acid-containing beverages. Stir mixture until the powder dissolves completely (about 2–3 min). Consume the entire solution immediately.
8. To prepare powder for pediatric oral solution, mix the dry powder with purified water to an initial concentration of 20 mg/mL. The resulting solution is then mixed with antacid (e.g., Mylanta Double Strength Liquid, Extra Strength Maalox Plus Suspension, or Maalox TC Suspension) to a final concentration of 10 mg/mL. Shake this admixture thoroughly prior to use. May be stored in a tightly closed container, in the refrigerator for up to 30 days.

ASSESSMENT
1. Note all experiences with zidovudine therapy; list reasons for transfer to didanosine. List drugs prescribed to ensure none interact.
2. Monitor CBC, CD$_4$ counts/viral load, renal and LFTs.
3. Reduce dose with liver and renal impairment. Note baseline VS and weight. Monitor for S&S pancreatitis.

CLIENT/FAMILY TEACHING
1. Used with other drugs to treat HIV infections. Follow dosing guidelines carefully; review drug administration insert. Food decreases the rate of drug absorption by 50%; take 30 min before or 2 hr after meals.
2. Do not swallow tablets whole. Tablets may be chewed or crushed thoroughly before taking or dispersed in at least 1 oz of drinking water (stir thoroughly and drink immediately).
3. Report any symptoms of neuropathy (numbness, burning, or tingling in the hands or feet); drug should be discontinued until symptoms subside. May tolerate a reduced dose once these S&S are resolved.
4. Report any abdominal pain and N&V immediately; may be clinical signs of pancreatitis. Stop drug and report; re-

---

Bold Italic = life threatening side effect   ■ = black box warning   ✦ = Available in Canada

sume only after pancreatitis has been ruled out.

5. With salt-restricted diets, sodium content is higher in the single-dose packet than the two-tablet dose. Each single-dose packet of buffered powder for oral solution contains 1,380 mg sodium and each 2 tablet dose contains 529 mg sodium.

6. Chewable/dispersible buffered tablets contain 73 mg phenylalanine per 2-tablet dose.

7. Increase fluid intake; report S&S of diarrhea or hyperuricemia (joint pains).

8. Any changes in vision should be evaluated by an ophthalmologist. Get retinal exams every 6 months to rule out depigmentation with children.

9. Avoid alcohol and any other drugs that may exacerbate toxicity of didanosine.

10. Drug is not a cure, but alleviates the symptoms of HIV infections; may continue to acquire opportunistic infections.

11. *Does not* reduce the risk of transmission of HIV to others through sexual contact or blood contamination; use appropriate precautions/protection.

12. Identify local support groups that may assist client/family to understand and cope with disease.

OUTCOMES/EVALUATE

- Control of symptoms of AIDS, ARC, and Opportunistic Infections in clients with HIV who are intolerant or have clinically deteriorated during Zidovudine therapy.
- ↓ HIV RNA Replication

Diflunisal ∎
(dye-**FLEW**-nih-sal)

CLASSIFICATION(S):
Nonsteroidal anti-inflammatory drug
PREGNANCY CATEGORY: C
✤**Rx:** Apo-Diflunisal, Novo-Diflunisal, Nu-Diflunisal.

USES
(1) Acute or long-term use for mild to moderate pain. (2) Acute or long-term use for symptomatic treatment of rheumatoid arthritis or osteoarthritis.
ACTION/KINETICS
Action
Has analgesic, anti-inflammatory, and antipyretic effects. Salicylic acid derivative, although not metabolized to salicylic acid. Mechanism not known; may be an inhibitor of prostaglandin synthetase.
Pharmacokinetics
Rapidly and completely absorbed. **Onset:** 20 min (analgesic, antipyretic). **Peak plasma levels:** 2–3 hr. **Peak effect:** 2–3 hr. **Duration:** 4–6 hr $t\frac{1}{2}$: 8–12 hr. Metabolites excreted in urine. **Plasma protein binding:** 99%.
CONTRAINDICATIONS
Hypersensitivity to diflunisal, aspirin, or other anti-inflammatory drugs. Acute asthmatic attacks, urticaria, or rhinitis precipitated by aspirin. Advanced renal disease. During lactation and in children less than 12 years of age.
SPECIAL CONCERNS
∎ (1) Cardiovascular risk. NSAIDs may cause an increased risk of serious CV thrombotic reactions, MI, and stroke, which can be fatal. This risk may increase with duration of use. Clients with CV disease or risk factors for CV disease may be at greater risk. (2) Diflunisal is contraindicated for the treatment of perioperative pain in the setting of coronary artery bypass graft surgery. (3) GI risk. NSAIDs cause an increased risk of serious GI adverse reactions, including bleeding, ulceration, and perforation of the stomach or intestines, which can be fatal. These reactions can occur at any time during use and without warning symptoms. Elderly clients are at greater risk for serious GI reactions.∎ Use with extreme caution in presence of ulcers or in clients with a history thereof, GI bleeding, in clients with hypertension, compromised cardiac function, or in conditions leading to fluid retention. Use with caution in only first two trimesters of pregnancy. Geriatric clients may be at greater risk of GI toxicity. It is

possible diflunisal may be associated with Reye syndrome.

SIDE EFFECTS
Most Common
Headache, rash, nausea, dyspepsia, GI pain, diarrhea, fatigue, tiredness, tinnitus.

GI: N&V, dyspepsia, GI pain and bleeding, diarrhea, constipation, flatulence, peptic ulcer, eructation, anorexia, gastritis, GI inflammation, ulceration, stomatitis, ***perforation of the stomach/small intestine/large intestine.*** **Hepatic:** Cholestasis, hepatitis, jaundice. **CNS:** Headache, fatigue, fever, malaise, tiredness, dizziness, somnolence, insomnia, nervousness, confusion, depression, disorientation, vertigo, hallucinations, light-headedness, nervousness, paresthesias. **Dermatologic:** Rashes, pruritus, sweating, ***Stevens-Johnson syndrome, toxic epidermal necrolysis,*** exfoliative dermatitis, dry mucous membranes, erythema multiforme, photosensitivity, urticaria. **CV:** Palpitations, syncope, edema, hypertension (new or worsening of existing), ***serious thrombotic events, MI, stroke***. **GU:** Dysuria, hematuria, interstitial nephritis, proteinuria, impaired renal function including renal failure, nephrotic syndrome (rare), renal papillary necrosis. **Hematologic:** Agranulocytosis, hemolytic anemia, thrombocytopenia, anemia. **Hypersensitivity:** ***Acute anaphylaxis with bronchospasm,*** angioedema, flushing, hypersensitivity syndrome, hypersensitivity vasculitis. **Ophthalmic:** Transient visual disturbances including blurred vision. **Otic:** Tinnitus, hearing loss (rare). **Miscellaneous:** Asthenia, chest pain, ***anaphylaxis***, dyspnea, muscle cramps, fluid retention, edema, ***fulminant necrotizing fasciitis.***

LABORATORY TEST CONSIDERATIONS
↑ ALT, AST. Abnormal LFTs.

OD OVERDOSE MANAGEMENT
Symptoms: Drowsiness, N&V, diarrhea, tachycardia, sweating, tinnitus, hyperventilation, stupor, disorientation, diminished urine output, ***coma, cardiorespiratory arrest.*** *Treatment:* Supportive measures to treat symptoms. To empty the stomach perform gastric lavage. Hemodialysis may not be effective since the drug is significantly bound to plasma protein.

DRUG INTERACTIONS
Acetaminophen / ↑ Acetaminophen levels
ACE Inhibitors / ↓ Antihypertensive effect; in those with renal dysfunction → further renal function deterioration
Angiotensin II antagonists / ↓ Antihypertensive effect; in those with renal dysfunction → further renal function deterioration
Antacids / ↓ Diflunisal levels
Anticoagulants / ↑ PT
Aspirin / Potential for ↑ side effects R/T ↓ diflunisal plasma protein binding
Cyclosporine / ↑ Cyclosporine toxicity possibly R/T ↓ synthesis of renal prostacyclin; use together with caution
Furosemide / ↓ Furosemide hyperuricemic effect
Hydrochlorothiazide / ↑ Hydrochlorothiazide levels and ↓ hyperuricemic effect
Indomethacin / ↓ Indomethacin renal clearance → ↑ plasma levels
Lithium / ↑ Lithium levels; monitor for lithium toxicity
Methotrexate / ↑ Methotrexate toxicity
Naproxen / ↓ Urinary naproxen and metabolite excretion
NSAIDs / ↑ Chance of GI toxicity with little or no ↑ efficacy
Probenecid / ↑ Probenecid pharmacologic and toxic effects
Sulindac / ↓ Plasma levels of the active sulindac metabolite by one-third
Thiazide diuretics / ↓ Natriuertic and hyperuricemic effects

HOW SUPPLIED
Tablets: 500 mg.

DOSAGE
* **TABLETS**
  Mild to moderate pain.
Adults, initial: 1,000 mg; **then,** 500 mg q 12 hr. Some may require 500 mg q 8 hr. A lower dosage may be appropriate for some (e.g., 500 mg initially followed by 250 mg q 8 hr).
  Rheumatoid arthritis, osteoarthritis.
Adults: 250–1,000 mg/day in 2 divided doses. Dose may be increased or decreased depending on client response.

Bold Italic = life threatening side effect   ■ = black box warning   ✢ = Available in Canada

Maintenance doses greater than 1,500 mg/day are not recommended.

NURSING CONSIDERATIONS

ADMINISTRATION/STORAGE
1. Maximum relief occurs in 2–3 weeks when used for pain/swelling of arthritis. Serum salicylate levels are not used as guide to dosage or toxicity; drug is not hydrolyzed to salicylic acid.
2. Store from 20–25°C (68–77°F).

ASSESSMENT
1. Note reasons for therapy, characteristics of S&S. Assess for hypersensitivity to salicylates, other NSAIDs.
2. With arthritis, assess joints for inflammation, deformity, erosion, ROM, loss of function. Rate pain levels.
3. Determine PUD, HTN, cardiac dysfunction. List drugs prescribed to ensure none interact.
4. Check for pregnancy; avoid drug/use with extreme caution during first two trimesters.
5. Give in high enough doses for anti-inflammatory effects when needed; use lower dose for analgesic effects. Reduce dose by half in those over 65 years old.
6. With long-term therapy, monitor CBC, renal. LFTs; reduce dose with renal dysfunction.

CLIENT/FAMILY TEACHING
1. May give with water, milk, or meals to reduce gastric irritation. Do not crush or chew tablets.
2. Report adverse effects, unusual bruising/bleeding, or lack of response; may inhibit platelets which is reversible with drug discontinuation. Do not give with acetaminophen or aspirin.
3. May cause dizziness or drowsiness; use care when operating machinery or driving.
4. Report stool color changes or diarrhea; can cause electrolyte imbalance or GI bleed.
5. Must take on a regular basis to sustain anti-inflammatory effect.
6. Report for medical follow-up; drug needs to be adjusted according to age, condition, and changes in disease activity.

OUTCOMES/EVALUATE
- ↓ Pain/inflammation; ↑ joint mobility
- Prevention of vascular headaches

Digoxin
(dih-**JOX**-in)

D

CLASSIFICATION(S):
Cardiac glycoside
PREGNANCY CATEGORY: A
Rx: Digitek, Digoxin Injection Pediatric, Lanoxicaps, Lanoxin.
✤Rx: Digoxin Injection C.S.D., Digoxin Pediatric Injection C.S.D.

USES
(1) CHF, including that due to venous congestion, edema, dyspnea, orthopnea, and cardiac arrhythmia. May be drug of choice for CHF because of rapid onset, relatively short duration, and ability to be administered PO or IV. (2) Control of rapid ventricular contraction rate in clients with atrial fibrillation or flutter. (3) Slow HR in sinus tachycardia due to CHF. (4) SVT. (5) Prophylaxis and treatment of recurrent paroxysmal atrial tachycardia with paroxysmal AV junctional rhythm. (6) Cardiogenic shock (value not established).

ACTION/KINETICS
Action
Increases the force and velocity of myocardial contraction (positive inotropic effect) by increasing the refractory period of the AV node and increasing total peripheral resistance. This effect is due to inhibition of sodium/potassium–ATPase in the sarcolemmal membrane, which alters excitation-contraction coupling. Inhibiting sodium/potassium–ATPase results in increased calcium influx and increased release of free calcium ions within the myocardial cells, which then potentiate the contractility of cardiac muscle fibers. Digoxin also decreases HR, decreases the rate of conduction and increases the refractory period of the AV node due to an increase in parasympathetic tone and a decrease in sympathetic tone. Clinical

D

effects are not seen until steady-state plasma levels are reached. The initial dose of digoxin is larger (loading dose) and is traditionally referred to as the *digitalizing dose;* subsequent doses are referred to as *maintenance doses.*

Pharmacokinetics

Onset: PO, 0.5–2 hr; **time to peak effect:** 2–6 hr. **Duration:** Over 24 hr. **Onset, IV:** 5–30 min; **time to peak effect:** 1–4 hr. **Duration:** 6 days. **t½:** 30–40 hr. **Therapeutic serum level:** 0.5–2.0 ng/mL. Serum levels above 2.5 ng/mL indicate toxicity. Fifty percent to 70% is excreted unchanged by the kidneys. Bioavailability depends on the dosage form: Tablets (60–80%), capsules (90–100%), and elixir (70–85%). Thus, changing dosage forms may require dosage adjustments. **Plasma protein binding:** 20–25%.

CONTRAINDICATIONS

Ventricular fibrillation or tachycardia (unless congestive failure supervenes after protracted episode not due to digitalis), in presence of digoxin toxicity, hypersensitivity to cardiac glycosides, beriberi heart disease, certain cases of hypersensitive carotid sinus syndrome.

SPECIAL CONCERNS

Use with caution in clients with ischemic heart disease, acute myocarditis, hypertrophic subaortic stenosis, hypoxic or myxedemic states, Adams-Stokes or carotid sinus syndromes, cardiac amyloidosis, or cyanotic heart and lung disease, including emphysema and partial heart block. Those with carditis associated with rheumatic fever or viral myocarditis are especially sensitive to digoxin-induced disturbances in rhythm. Electric pacemakers may sensitize the myocardium to cardiac glycosides. Also use with caution and at reduced dosage in elderly, debilitated clients, pregnant women and nursing mothers, and newborn, term, or premature infants who have immature renal and hepatic function and in reduced renal and/or hepatic function.

The half-life of digoxin is prolonged in the elderly; anticipate smaller drug doses. Be especially alert to cardiac arrhythmias in children. This sign of toxicity occurs more frequently in children than in adults.

SIDE EFFECTS

Most Common

Tachycardia, headache, dizziness, mental disturbances, N&V, diarrhea, anorexia, blurred or yellow vision.

Digoxin is extremely toxic and has caused *death* even in clients who have received the drug for long periods of time. There is a narrow margin of safety between an effective therapeutic dose and a toxic dose. Overdosage caused by the cumulative effects of the drug is a constant danger in therapy. Digoxin toxicity is characterized by a wide variety of symptoms, which are hard to differentiate from those of the cardiac disease itself. One of the most serious side effects of digoxin is hypokalemia. This may lead to cardiac arrhythmias, muscle weakness, hypotension, and respiratory distress. Other agents causing hypokalemia reinforce this effect and increase the chance of digitalis toxicity. Such reactions may occur in clients who have been on digoxin maintenance for a long time. **CV:** Changes in the rate, rhythm, and irritability of the heart and the mechanism of the heartbeat. Extrasystoles, bigeminal pulse, coupled rhythm, ectopic beat, and other forms of arrhythmias have been noted. ***Death most often results from ventricular fibrillation.*** Discontinue digoxin in adults when pulse rate falls below 60 beats/min. All cardiac changes are best detected by the ECG, which is also most useful in clients suffering from intoxication. ***Acute hemorrhage.*** **GI:** Anorexia, N&V, excessive salivation, epigastric distress, abdominal pain, diarrhea, bowel necrosis. Clients on digoxin therapy may experience two vomiting stages. The first is an early sign of toxicity and is a direct effect of digoxin on the GI tract. Late vomiting indicates stimulation of the vomiting center of the brain, which occurs after the heart muscle has been saturated with digoxin. **CNS:** Headaches, fatigue, lassitude, irritability, malaise, muscle weakness, insomnia, stupor. Psychotomimetic effects (especially in elderly or arteriosclerotic clients

---

Bold Italic = life threatening side effect   ■ = black box warning   ✦ = Available in Canada

or neonates) including disorientation, confusion, depression, aphasia, delirium, hallucinations, and, rarely, **convulsions**. **Neuromuscular:** Neurologic pain involving the lower third of the face and lumbar areas, paresthesia. **Visual disturbances:** Blurred vision, flickering dots, white halos, borders around dark objects, diplopia, amblyopia, color perception changes. **Hypersensitivity: (5–7 days after starting therapy):** Skin reactions (urticaria, fever, pruritus, facial and **angioneurotic edema**). **Miscellaneous:** Chest pain, coldness of extremities.

LABORATORY TEST CONSIDERATIONS
May ↓ PT. Alters tests for 17-ketosteroids and 17-hydroxycorticosteroids.

OD **OVERDOSE MANAGEMENT**
Symptoms: The relationship of digoxin levels to symptoms of toxicity varies significantly from client to client; thus, it is not possible to identify digoxin levels that would define toxicity accurately. **Toxicity: GI:** Anorexia, N&V, diarrhea, abdominal discomfort, or pain. **CNS:** Blurred, yellow, or green vision and halo effect; headache, weakness, drowsiness, mental depression, apathy, restlessness, disorientation, confusion, **seizures,** EEG abnormalities, delirium, hallucinations, neuralgia, psychosis. **CV:** VT, unifocal or **multiform PVCs** (especially in bigeminal or trigeminal patterns), paroxysmal/nonparoxysmal nodal rhythms, AV dissociation, accelerated junctional rhythm, excessive slowing of the pulse, **AV block (may proceed to complete block),** atrial fibrillation, **ventricular fibrillation (most common cause of death).** **Children:** Visual disturbances, headache, weakness, apathy, and psychosis occur but may be difficult to recognize. **CV:** Conduction disturbances, supraventricular tachyarrhythmias (e.g., **AV block**), atrial tachycardia with or without block, nodal tachycardia, unifocal or multiform ventricular premature contractions, **ventricular tachycardia**, sinus bradycardia (especially in infants).
Treatment in Adults:
- Discontinue drug, admit to ICU for continuous ECG monitoring.
- If serum potassium is below normal, KCl should be administered in divided PO doses totaling 3–6 grams (40–80 mEq). Potassium should not be used when severe or complete heart block is due to digoxin and not related to tachycardia.
- *Atropine:* A dose of 0.01 mg/kg IV to treat severe sinus bradycardia or slow ventricular rate due to secondary AV block.
- *Cholestyramine, colestipol, activated charcoal:* To bind digitalis in the intestine, thus preventing enterohepatic recirculation.
- *Digoxin immune FAB:* See drug entry. Given in approximate equimolar quantities as digoxin, it reverses S&S of toxicity, often with improvement within 30 min.
- *Lidocaine:* A dose of 1 mg/kg given over 5 min followed by an infusion of 15–50 mcg/kg/min to maintain normal cardiac rhythm.
- *Phenytoin:* For atrial or ventricular arrhythmias unresponsive to potassium, can give a dose of 0.5 mg/kg at a rate not exceeding 50 mg/min (given at 1–2 hr intervals). The maximum dose should not exceed 10 mg/kg/day.
- *Countershock:* A direct-current countershock can be used *only as a last resort.* If required, initiate at low voltage levels.
Treatment in Children: Give potassium in divided doses totaling 1–1.5 mEq/kg (if correction of arrhythmia is urgent, a dose of 0.5 mEq/kg/hr can be used) with careful monitoring of the ECG. The potassium IV solution should be dilute to avoid local irritation although IV fluid overload must be avoided. *Treatment:* Digoxin immune FAB may also be used.

Digoxin is not removed effectively by dialysis, by exchange transfusion, or during cardiopulmonary bypass as most of the drug is found in tissues rather than the circulating blood.

DRUG INTERACTIONS
The following drugs increase serum digoxin levels, leading to possible toxicity: Aminoglycosides, amiodarone, anticholinergics, atorvastatin, benzodiaze-

D

pines, captopril, diltiazem, dipyridamole, erythromycin, esmolol, flecainide, hydroxychloroquine, ibuprofen, indomethacin, itraconazole, nifedipine, quinidine, quinine, telmisartan, tetracyclines, tolbutamide, verapamil.

Albuterol / ↑ Digoxin binding to skeletal muscle

H *Aloe* / Potential for ↑ digoxin effect R/T aloe-induced hypokalemia

Amiloride / ↓ Digoxin inotropic effects

Aminoglycosides / ↓ Digoxin effect R/T ↓ GI tract absorption

Aminosalicylic acid / ↓ Digoxin effect R/T ↓ GI tract absorption

Amphotericin B / ↑ K depletion caused by digoxin; ↑ risk of digitalis toxicity

Antacids / ↓ Digoxin effect R/T ↓ GI tract absorption

Beta blockers / Complete heart block possible

H *Buckthorn bark/berry* / Potential for ↑ digoxin effect R/T to buckthorn-induced hypokalemia

Calcium preparations / Cardiac arrhythmias following parenteral calcium

H *Cascara sagrada bark* / Potential for ↑ digoxin effect R/T to cascara-induced hypokalemia

Chlorthalidone / ↑ K and Mg loss with ↑ chance of digitalis toxicity

Cholestyramine / Binds digoxin in the intestine and ↓ its absorption

Colestipol / Binds digoxin in the intestine and ↓ its absorption

Disopyramide / May alter effect of digoxin

H *Ephedra* / ↑ Chance of cardiac arrhythmias

Ephedrine / ↑ Chance of cardiac arrhythmias

Epinephrine / ↑ Chance of cardiac arrhythmias

Ethacrynic acid / ↑ K and Mg loss with ↑ chance of digitalis toxicity

Fluoxetine / Possible ↑ serum digoxin levels

Furosemide / ↑ K and Mg loss with ↑ chance of digoxin toxicity

H *German chamomile flower* / Potential for ↑ digoxin effect R/T to chamomile-induced hypokalemia

H *Ginseng* / ↑ Digoxin levels

Glucose infusions / Large infusions of glucose may cause ↓ K and ↑ chance of digoxin toxicity

Grapefruit juice / ↑ Digoxin bioavailability; do not take digoxin with grapefruit juice

H *Hawthorn* / Potentiation of digoxin effect

Hypoglycemic drugs / ↓ Effect of digitalis glycosides R/T ↑ liver breakdown

H *Iceland moss* / Potential for ↑ digoxin effect R/T to iceland moss-induced hypokalemia

H *Indian snakeroot* / ↑ Risk of bradycardia

H *Ivy leaf* / Potential for ↑ digoxin effect R/T to ivy leaf-induced hypokalemia

Levothyroxine / ↓ Serum levels and therapeutic digoxin effect

H *Licorice* / Potential for ↑ digoxin effect R/T to licorice-induced hypokalemia

H *Marshmallow root* / Potential for ↑ digoxin effect R/T to marshmallow root-induced hypokalemia

Methimazole / ↑ Chance of toxic effects of digitalis

Metoclopramide / ↓ Digoxin effect R/T ↓ GI tract absorption

Muscle relaxants, nondepolarizing / ↑ Risk of cardiac arrhythmias

Penicillamine / ↓ Serum digoxin levels

Propranolol / Potentiates digitalis-induced bradycardia

H *Rhubarb root* / Potential for ↑ digoxin effect R/T to rhubarb root-induced hypokalemia

H *St. John's wort* / ↓ Digoxin plasma levels R/T ↑ renal excretion

H *Sarsaparilla root* / Potential for ↑ absorption of digoxin

H *Senna pod/leaf* / Potential for ↑ digoxin effect R/T to senna-induced hypokalemia

Spironolactone / Either ↑ or ↓ toxic effects of digoxin

Succinylcholine / ↑ Chance of cardiac arrhythmias

Sulfasalazine / ↓ Digoxin effect R/T ↓ GI tract absorption

Sympathomimetics / ↑ Chance of cardiac arrhythmias

Bold Italic = life threatening side effect   ■ = black box warning   ✤ = Available in Canada

Thiazides / ↑ K and Mg loss with ↑ chance of digoxin toxicity

Thioamines / ↑ Effect and toxicity of digoxin

Thyroid / ↓ Digoxin effect

Triamterene / ↑ Digoxin effects

HOW SUPPLIED

Capsules: 0.05 mg, 0.1 mg, 0.2 mg; *Elixir, Pediatric:* 0.05 mg/mL; *Injection:* 0.1 mg/mL, 0.25 mg/mL; *Tablets:* 0.125 mg, 0.25 mg.

DOSAGE

• **CAPSULES**

Digitalization: Rapid.

Adults: 0.4–0.6 mg initially followed by 0.1–0.3 mg q 6–8 hr until desired effect achieved.

Digitalization: Slow.

Adults: A total of 0.05–0.35 mg/day divided in two doses for a period of 7–22 days to reach steady-state serum levels. **Pediatric.** Digitalizing dosage is divided into three or more doses with the initial dose being about one-half the total dose; doses are given q 4–8 hr. **Children, 10 years and older:** 0.008–0.012 mg/kg. **5–10 years:** 0.015–0.03 mg/kg. **2–5 years:** 0.025–0.035 mg/kg. **1 month–2 years:** 0.03–0.05 mg/kg. **Neonates, full-term:** 0.02–0.03 mg/kg. **Neonates, premature:** 0.015–0.025 mg/kg.

Maintenance.

Adults: 0.05–0.35 mg once or twice daily. **Premature neonates:** 20–30% of total digitalizing dose divided and given in two to three daily doses. **Neonates to 10 years:** 25–35% of the total digitalizing dose divided and given in two to three daily doses.

• **ELIXIR; TABLETS**

Digitalization: Rapid.

Adults: A total of 0.75–1.25 mg divided into two or more doses each given at 6–8-hr intervals.

Digitalization: Slow.

Adults: 0.125–0.5 mg/day for 7 days. **Pediatric.** (Digitalizing dose is divided into two or more doses and given at 6–8-hr intervals.) **Children, 10 years and older, rapid or slow:** Same as adult dose. **5–10 years:** 0.02–0.035 mg/kg. **2–5 years:** 0.03–0.05 mg/kg. **1 month–2 years:** 0.035–0.06 mg/kg.

Premature and newborn infants to 1 month: 0.02–0.035 mg/kg.

Maintenance.

Adults: 0.125–0.5 mg/day. **Pediatric:** One-fifth to one-third the total digitalizing dose daily. *NOTE:* An alternate regimen (referred to as the "small-dose" method) is 0.017 mg/kg/day. This dose causes less toxicity.

• **IV**

Digitalization.

Adults: Same as tablets. **Maintenance:** 0.125–0.5 mg/day in divided doses or as a single dose. **Pediatric:** Same as tablets.

D

NURSING CONSIDERATIONS

ADMINISTRATION/STORAGE

1. Measure liquids precisely using calibrated dropper/syringe.

2. Obtain written parameters for high/low pulse rates, at which cardiac glycosides are to be held; changes in rate or rhythm may indicate toxicity.

3. Lanoxicaps gelatin capsules are more bioavailable than tablets. Thus, the 0.05-mg capsule is equivalent to the 0.0625-mg tablet; the 0.1-mg capsule is equivalent to the 0.125-mg tablet, and the 0.2-mg capsule is equivalent to the 0.25-mg tablet.

4. Differences in bioavailability have been noted between products; monitor when changing from one product to another.

5. If switching from tablets or elixir to liquid-filled capsules or parenteral route, expect reduction in dosage; absorption is much higher with capsules and parenteral form.

6. Protect from light.

IV 7. Give IV injections over 5 min (or longer) either undiluted or diluted fourfold or greater with sterile water for injection, 0.9% NaCl, RL injection, or D5W.

ASSESSMENT

For clients starting on a digitalizing dose:

1. List type, onset, characteristics of S&S. If administered for heart failure, note causes; ensure failure not solely related to diastolic dysfunction- drug's positive inotropic effect may increase

---

 = see color insert   = Herbal   = Intravenous   = sound alike drug cardiac outflow obstruction with hypertrophic cardiomyopathy.

2. Note any drugs prescribed that would adversely interact with digoxin and monitor; diuretics may increase toxicity.

3. Assess for hyper/hypothyroidism; hypothyroid clients sensitive to glycosides while hyperthyroid clients may require a higher dose of drug.

4. Monitor CBC, serum electrolytes, calcium, Mg, BNP, renal and LFTs. Reduce dose with renal dysfunction. Monitor digoxin levels.

5. Obtain ECG; note rhythm/rate.

6. Document cardiopulmonary findings; note presence of S3, JVD, HJR, displaced PMI, HR above 100 bpm, rales, peripheral edema, DOE, PND, echo, MUGA, and/or cardiac catheterization findings. Note NYHA Classification.

7. Observe elderly clients for early S&S of toxicity (N&V, anorexia, confusion, visual disturbances); their rate of drug elimination is slower.

INTERVENTIONS

For clients being digitalized and for clients on maintenance dose digoxin:

1. With digitalization, monitor closely.

2. Observe and monitor for bradycardia/arrhythmias, count apical rate for at least 1 min before administering drug. Obtain written parameters (e.g., HR >60 bpm) for drug administration.

- Document adult HR below 50 bpm; hold drug. Report if arrhythmia (irregular pulse) or any sudden increase/decrease in pulse rate, pulse deficit, changes in rhythm occurs.
- If child's HR is 90–110 bpm or if arrhythmia present; withhold drug and report.

3. Anticipate more than once-daily dosing in most children (up to age 10) R/T higher metabolic activity.

4. With coworker simultaneously take apical and radial pulse for 1 min; report pulse deficit (e.g., the wrist rate is less than the apical rate); may indicate adverse drug reaction.

5. Monitor weights and I&O. Weight gain may indicate edema. Adequate intake will help prevent cumulative toxic drug effects.

6. If taking non-potassium-sparing diuretics as well as digoxin, will need potassium supplements. Provide the most palatable preparation available. (Liquid potassium preparations are usually bitter.)

7. If gastric distress experienced, use antacid. Antacids containing Al or Mg and kaolin/pectin mixtures should be given 6 hr before or 6 hr after dose of cardiac glycoside to prevent decreased therapeutic effects.

8. When given to newborns, use cardiac monitor to identify early evidence of toxicity: excessive slowing of sinus rate, sinoatrial arrest, prolonged PR interval.

9. Monitor digoxin levels periodically, assess for symptoms of toxicity; draw specimen more than 6 hr after last dose. Have digoxin antidote available (digoxin immune FAB) for severe toxicity.

10. Use caution; digoxin withdrawal may worsen heart failure.

CLIENT/FAMILY TEACHING

1. Take after meals to lessen gastric irritation.

2. Do not take with grapefruit juice.

3. Maintain written record of pulse rates and weights; review guidelines for withholding medication and reporting abnormal pulse rates. Report wt gains of >2 lb/day or >5 lb/week.

4. Do not change brands; different preparations have variations in bioavailability and may cause toxicity or loss of effect.

5. Follow directions carefully for taking medication. If one dose is accidentally missed, do not double up on the next dose.

6. Report adverse effects or toxic drug symptoms: Anorexia, N&V, abdominal pain and diarrhea are often early symptoms due to the toxic effects on the GI tract and CTZ stimulation. Disorientation, agitation, visual disturbances, changes in color perception, irregular heartbeat, and hallucinations may also occur.

7. Maintain a sodium-restricted diet. Read labels and review foods low in sodium; consult dietitian for assistance in

---

Bold Italic = life threatening side effect   ■ = black box warning   ♣ = Available in Canada

food selection, meal planning, and preparation.

8. Consult provider before taking any other medications, whether prescribed or OTC, because drug interactions occur frequently with cardiac glycosides.

9. Report persistent cough, difficulty breathing, or swelling (S&S of CHF).

10. Identify community health agencies to assist in maintaining health.

11. Return for scheduled follow-up visits, EKG, and lab tests.

OUTCOMES/EVALUATE

- Stable cardiac rate and rhythm, ↓ severity of S&S of CHF, improved CO, improved activity tolerance
- Serum drug levels within therapeutic range (e.g., digoxin 0.5–2.0 ng/mL)

Digoxin Immune Fab (Ovine) **IV**

CLASSIFICATION(S):
Antidote for digoxin poisoning
PREGNANCY CATEGORY: C
Rx: DigiFab, Digibind.

USES
Life-threatening digoxin toxicity or overdosage. Symptoms of toxicity include severe sinus bradycardia, second- or third-degree heart block which does not respond to atropine, ventricular tachycardia, and ventricular fibrillation.

NOTE: Cardiac arrest can be expected if a healthy adult ingests more than 10 mg digoxin or a healthy child ingests more than 4 mg. Also, steady-state serum concentrations of digoxin greater than 10 ng/mL or potassium concentrations greater than 5 mEq/L as a result of digoxin therapy require use of digoxin immune Fab.

ACTION/KINETICS

Action
Digoxin immune Fab are antibodies that bind to digoxin making them unavailable to bind at their site of action. In cases of digoxin toxicity, the antibodies bind to digoxin and the complex is excreted through the kidneys. As serum levels of digoxin decrease, digoxin

bound to tissue is released into the serum to maintain equilibrium and this is then bound and excreted. The net result is a decrease in both tissue and serum digoxin.

Pharmacokinetics
Onset: Less than 1 min. Improvement in signs of toxicity occurs within 30 min. **t½:** 15–20 hr (after IV administration). Each vial contains either 38 mg or 40 mg of pure digoxin immune Fab, which will bind approximately 0.5 mg digoxin.

SPECIAL CONCERNS
Use with caution during lactation. Use in infants only if benefits outweigh risks. Clients sensitive to products of sheep origin may also be sensitive to digoxin immune Fab. Skin testing may be appropriate for high-risk clients.

SIDE EFFECTS

Most Common
Hypokalemia.

CV: Worsening of CHF or low CO, atrial fibrillation (all due to withdrawal of the effects of digoxin). **Miscellaneous:** Hypokalemia. Rarely, hypersensitivity reactions occur, including fever and *anaphylaxis*.

HOW SUPPLIED
Digibind: *Injection:* 38 mg/vial.
DigiFab: *Injection:* 40 mg/vial.

DOSAGE——————
- IV

Dosage depends on the serum digoxin concentration. A large dose has a faster onset but there is an increased risk of allergic or febrile reactions. The package insert should be carefully consulted.

Acute ingestion of an unknown amount of digoxin.
Adults and children: Twenty vials (760 mg Digibind or 800 mg DigiFab). In small children, monitor the amount of overload.

Toxicity during chronic therapy.
Adults: Six vials (228 mg of Digibind or 240 mg DigiFab) is usually enough to reverse most cases of toxicity. **Children, <20 kg:** A single vial (38 mg Digibind or 40 mg DigiFab) should be sufficient.

NURSING CONSIDERATIONS

ADMINISTRATION/STORAGE

IV 1. Dose of antidote estimated based on ingested digoxin differs significantly from that calculated based on the serum digoxin levels. Errors in amount of antidote required may result from inaccurate estimates of amount of digoxin ingested or absorbed from non-steady-state serum digoxin concentrations. Also, inaccurate serum digoxin level measurements are a possible source of error.

2. To calculate dose (in number of vials) of antidote for acute ingestion of a known amount of digitalis, divide the total digitalis body load (in mg) by 0.5 (i.e., amount of digitalis bound/vial). The total body load (mg) will be about equal to the amount ingested in mg for digoxin capsules.

3. To estimate number of vials for adults when a steady-state serum digoxin level is known, multiply the serum digoxin concentration in ng/mL times the weight in kg and divide by 100.

4. Reconstitute lyophilized material with 4 mL of sterile water for injection to give a concentration of 10 mg/mL (DigiFab) or 9.5 mg/mL (Digibind). If small doses required (e.g., in infants), Digibind or DigiFab can be further diluted (34 mL sterile isotonic saline when using Digibind or 36 mL sterile isotonic saline for DigiFab) for concentration of 1 mg/mL.

5. Administer over a 30-min period through a 0.22-μm membrane filter; may use bolus injection if immediate danger of cardiac arrest.

6. Use reconstituted antibody immediately. May store up to 4 hr at 2–8°C (36–46°F). Unreconstituted vials of Digibind can be stored up to 30°C (86°F) for a total of 30 days. Do not freeze Digi-Fab.

7. If acute digoxin ingestion results in severe symptoms and serum concentration is not known, 800 mg (20 vials) of digoxin immune Fab may be given. Monitor for volume overload in small children.

8. Administer to infants with a tuberculin syringe.

ASSESSMENT

1. List amount, time of drug ingestion, serum digoxin level.

2. If previous reaction suspected or high-risk client, perform skin testing: Prepare a 10-mL solution (0.1 mL of drug in 9.9 mL NSS). Administer 0.1 mL intradermally or perform a scratch test by placing 1 drop of solution on the skin and making a scratch through the drop with a sterile needle; assess site in 20 min. **Do not** use if reaction is positive: urticarial wheal with erythematous surrounding skin.

3. **Do not** administer with known allergy to sheep proteins.

4. Monitor VS/cardiac rhythm. Assess for electrolyte imbalance; note hypokalemia. evidence of CHF.

5. Wait several days for redigitalization to ensure complete elimination of Digibind. Levels will take 5–7 days to stabilize following treatment, although improvement in S&S of toxicity should be evident in 30 min.

CLIENT/FAMILY TEACHING

Drug is used to reverse the effects of too high a concentration of digoxin in the body. Should take effect in a couple of hours but digoxin levels will not show changes until about 2 days later. Report any chest pain, dizziness, or breathing difficulty.

OUTCOMES/EVALUATE

- Resolution of digoxin toxicity
- Controlled cardiac rhythm

Diltiazem hydrochloride **IV**

(dill-**TIE**-ah-zem)

CLASSIFICATION(S):

Calcium channel blocker

PREGNANCY CATEGORY: C

Rx: Capsule, Extended-Release: Cardizem CD, CartiaXT, Dilacor XR, Dilt-CD, Dilt-XR, Diltia XT, Diltiazem

HCl Extended Release, Taztia XT, Tiazac. **Injection:** Cardizem. **Tablets, Immediate-Release:** Cardizem. **Tablets, Extended-Release:** Cardizem LA.

✤Rx: Apo-Diltiaz CD, Apo-Diltiaz Injectable, Apo-Diltiaz SR, Gen-Diltiazem, Novo-Diltazem SR, Novo-Diltiazem, Novo-Diltiazem CD, Nu-Diltiaz, Nu-Diltiaz-CD, Rhoxal-Diltiazem CD, ratio-Diltiazem CD.

SEE ALSO *CALCIUM CHANNEL BLOCKING AGENTS.*

USES
PO: (1) Angina pectoris due to coronary artery spasm. (2) Chronic stable angina (classic effort-associated angina). (3) Hypertension (extended- or sustained-release only). **Parenteral:** (1) Temporary control of rapid ventricular rate in atrial fibrillation or flutter. (2) Rapid conversion of paroxysmal SVT to sinus rhythm (including AV nodal re-entrant tachycardias and reciprocating tachycardias associated with an extranodal accessory pathway such as Wolff-Parkinson-White syndrome or short PR syndrome). *Investigational:* Prophylaxis of reinfarction of non–Q-wave MI; tardive dyskinesia, Raynaud's syndrome.

ACTION/KINETICS
Action
Inhibits influx of calcium through the cell membrane, resulting in a depression of automaticity and conduction velocity in cardiac muscle. Decreases SA and AV conduction and prolongs AV node effective and functional refractory periods. Also decreases myocardial contractility and peripheral vascular resistance. Slight decrease in HR.

Pharmacokinetics
Tablets, Immediate Release: Onset, 30–60 min; **time to peak plasma levels:** 2–4 hr; **$t^{1/2}$, elimination:** about 3–4.5 hr (5–8 hr with high and repetitive doses); **duration:** 4–8 hr. **Extended-Release Capsules/Tablets: Onset,** 2–3 hr; **time to peak plasma levels:** 10–14 hr; **$t^{1/2}$, elimination:** 4–9.5 hr; **duration:** 12 hr. **IV, $t^{1/2}$, elimination:** About 3.4 hr. **Therapeutic serum levels:** 0.05–0.2 mcg/mL. Metabolized in the liver to desacetyldiltiazem, which

manifests 25–50% of the activity of diltiazem. Excreted through both the bile and urine. **Plasma protein binding:** 70–80%.

CONTRAINDICATIONS
Hypotension or cardiogenic shock. Second- or third-degree AV block and sick sinus syndrome except in presence of a functioning ventricular pacemaker. Acute MI, pulmonary congestion. IV diltiazem with IV beta-blockers. Atrial fibrillation or atrial flutter associated with an accessory bypass tract (e.g., as in W-P-W syndrome or PR syndrome). Ventricular tachycardia. Use of Cardizem LyoJect Syringe in newborns (due to presence of benzyl alcohol). Lactation.

SPECIAL CONCERNS
Safety and effectiveness in children have not been determined. The half-life may be increased in geriatric clients. Use with caution in hepatic disease and in CHF. Abrupt withdrawal may cause an increase in the frequency and duration of chest pain. Use with beta blockers or digitalis is usually well tolerated, although the effects of coadministration cannot be predicted (especially in clients with left ventricular dysfunction or cardiac conduction abnormalities).

SIDE EFFECTS
Most Common
AV block, bradycardia, edema, dizziness/lightheadedness, headache, pain, dyspnea, rhinitis, infection.
CV: AV block, bradycardia, CHF, hypotension, syncope, palpitations, peripheral edema, *arrhythmias*, angina, tachycardia, *abnormal ECG*, *ventricular extrasystoles*. **GI:** N&V, diarrhea, constipation, anorexia, abdominal discomfort, cramps, dry mouth, dysgeusia. **CNS:** Weakness, nervousness, dizziness, lightheadedness, headache, depression, psychoses, hallucinations, disturbances in sleep, somnolence, insomnia, amnesia, abnormal dreams. **Dermatologic:** Rashes, dermatitis, pruritus, urticaria, erythema multiforme, *Stevens-Johnson syndrome*. **Miscellaneous:** Photosensitivity, joint pain/stiffness, flushing, nasal/chest congestion, dyspnea, SOB, nocturia/polyuria, sexual difficulties, weight gain, paresthesia, tinnitus, trem-

or, asthenia, gynecomastia, gingival hyperplasia, petechiae, ecchymosis, purpura, bruising, hematoma, leukopenia, double vision, epistaxis, eye irritation, thirst, alopecia, abnormal gait, hyperglycemia. ***bundle branch block***,

ADDITIONAL DRUG INTERACTIONS

Amiodarone / Possible cardiotoxicity with bradycardia and ↓ CO
Amlodipine / ↑ Amlodipine levels possibly R/T ↓ liver metabolism
Anesthetics / ↑ Risk of depression of cardiac contractility, conductivity, and automaticity as well as vascular dilation
Buspirone / ↑ Buspirone effects
Carbamazepine / ↑ Diltiazem effect R/T ↓ liver breakdown
Cimetidine / ↑ Diltiazem bioavailability
Colestipol / ↓ Diltiazem bioavailability when colestipol given 1 hr before or 4 hr after diltiazem R/T ↓ diltiazem absorption
Cyclosporine / ↑ Cyclosporine effect → possible renal toxicity
Digoxin / Possible ↑ digoxin levels
HMG-CoA reductase inhibitors / ↑ HMG-CoA reductase inhibitors levels
Imipramine / ↑ Serum levels
Indinavir + Ritonavir / ↑ Diltiazem AUC R/T ↓ CYP 3A metabolism of diltiazem
Lithium / ↑ Risk of neurotoxicity
Methylprednisolone / ↑ Pharmacologic and toxicologic effects of methylprednisolone
Moricizine / ↑ Moricine levels and ↓ diltiazem levels
Quinidine / ↑ Therapeutic and toxic effects of quinidine
Ranitidine / ↑ Diltiazem bioavailability
Sirolimus / ↑ Sirolimus levels
Tacrolimus / ↑ Tacrolimus levels → ↑ toxicity
Theophyllines / ↑ Risk of pharmacologic and toxicologic theophylline effects

LABORATORY TEST CONSIDERATIONS
↑ Alkaline phosphatase, CPK, LDH, AST, ALT.

HOW SUPPLIED
Capsules, Extended-Release: 60 mg, 90 mg, 120 mg, 180 mg, 240 mg, 300 mg, 360 mg, 420 mg; *Injection:* 5 mg/mL; *Powder for Injection:* 25 mg; *Tablets, Extended-Release:* 120 mg, 180 mg, 240 mg, 300 mg, 360 mg, 420 mg; *Tablets,* *Immediate-Release:* 30 mg, 60 mg, 90 mg, 120 mg.

DOSAGE
- **TABLETS, IMMEDIATE-RELEASE**
  Angina.
Individualize dose. **Adults, initial:** 30 mg 4 times/day before meals and at bedtime; **then,** increase gradually to total daily dose of 180–360 mg (given in three to four divided doses). Increments may be made q 1–2 days until the optimum response is attained.
- **TABLETS, EXTENDED-RELEASE**
  Hypertension.
Individualize dose. **Adults, initial, monotherapy:** 180–240 mg once daily; some may respond to lower doses. May be titrated to a maximum dose of 540 mg/day. Schedule dosage adjustments accordingly as maximum effect usually seen within 14 days.
  Angina.
Individualize dose. **Adults, initial:** 180 mg; **then,** may increase dose at intervals of 7–14 days if adequate response not obtained. Doses above 360 mg appear not to have any additional benefit.
- **CAPSULES, EXTENDED-RELEASE**
  Angina.
Cardizem CD and Cartia XT: Adults, initial: 120 or 180 mg once daily. Up to 480 mg/day may be required. Dosage adjustments should be carried out over a 7–14-day period.
Dilacor XR and Diltia XT: Adults, initial: 120 mg once daily; **then,** dose may be titrated, depending on the needs of the client, up to 480 mg once daily. Titration may be carried out over a 7–14-day period.
Tiazac: Adults, initial: 120–180 once daily. Some may respond to higher doses up to 540 mg once daily. When necessary, carry out titration over 7–14 days.
  Hypertension.
Cardizem CD and Cartia XT: Adults, initial: 180–240 mg once daily. Some respond to lower doses. Maximum antihypertensive effect usually reached within 14 days. Usual range is 240–360 mg once daily.
Dilacor XR and Diltia XT: Adults, initial: 180–240 mg once daily. Clients 60

years and older may respond to a lower dose of 120 mg. Usual range is 180–480 mg once daily. The dose may be increased to 540 mg/day with little or no increased risk of side effects. May be used alone or in combination with other antihypertensive drugs, such as diuretics

Tiazac: Adults, initial: 120–240 mg once daily. Maximum effect usually reached by 14 days of therapy; thus, schedule dosage adjustments accordingly. Usual range is 120–540 mg once daily. May be used alone or with other antihypertensive drugs.

- **IV BOLUS**
  Atrial fibrillation/flutter; paroxysmal SVT.

Adults, initial: 0.25 mg/kg (average 20 mg) given over 2 min; **then,** if response is inadequate, a second dose may be given after 15 min. The second bolus dose is 0.35 mg/kg (average 25 mg) given over 2 min. Subsequent doses should be individualized. Some clients may respond to an initial dose of 0.15 mg/kg (duration of action may be shorter).

- **IV, CONTINUOUS INFUSION**
  Atrial fibrillation/flutter.

Adults, initial: For continuous reduction of HR (up to 24 hr) for those with atrial fibrillation/flutter, begin an IV infusion immediately after the IV bolus dose. Initial infusion rate is 10 mg/hr; may be increased in 5 mg increments to 15 mg/hr. Infusion longer than 24 hr at a dose of 15 mg/hr is not recommended.

NURSING CONSIDERATIONS

ℭ Do not confuse Cardizem with Cardene (also a calcium channel blocker). Do not confuse Cartia-XT with Cartia (an enteric-coated aspirin tablet).

ADMINISTRATION/STORAGE

1. Sublingual nitroglycerin may be taken concomitantly for acute angina. Diltiazem may also be taken together with long-acting nitrates.
2. Clients treated with diltiazem alone or in combination with other medications may be switched safely to once daily extended-release diltiazem capsules or tablets at the nearest equivalent total daily dose. However, subsequent titration to a higher or lower dose may be necessary and should be initiated if needed.
3. Use with beta blockers or digitalis is usually well tolerated, but the combined effects cannot be predicted, especially with cardiac conduction abnormalities or LV dysfunction.

IV 4. May administer direct IV over 2 min or as infusion (see *Dosage*). For IV infusion, may mix drug with NSS, D5W, or D5/0.45% NaCl.
5. Do not mix Cardizem LyoJect or Cardizem Monovial with any other drugs in the same container.
6. Do not give diltiazem injection, Cardizem LyoJect, and Cardizem Monovial in the same IV line.
7. Infusion may be maintained for up to 24 hr; beyond 24 hr is not recommended.
8. Refrigerate the injection at 2–8°C (36–46°F). May be stored at room temperature for 1 month; then, discard remaining solution.
9. Store Cardizem LyoJect and Cardizem Monovial at room temperature (15–20°C; 59–86°F). Do not freeze. Reconstituted drug is stable for 24 hr at controlled room temperature. Discard any unused portion of Cardizem LyoJect.

ASSESSMENT

1. List reasons for therapy, onset, S&S, other drugs trialed.
2. Assess for edema or CHF; review ECG for AV block.
3. Monitor VS, renal and LFTs; reduce dose with impaired function.
4. Drug half-life may be prolonged in elderly; monitor closely.

CLIENT/FAMILY TEACHING

1. Take extended-release capsules on an empty stomach. Do not open, chew, or crush; swallow whole.
2. Use caution; may cause drowsiness/dizziness. Record BP for review.
3. Rise slowly from a lying to a sitting and standing position; may cause ↓ BP.
4. Report persistent/bothersome side effects including headaches, constipation, unusual tiredness, or weakness.

5. Continue carrying short-acting nitrites (nitroglycerin) at all times; use as directed. Avoid prolonged sun exposure; use precaution if exposed to prevent photosensitivity reaction.

6. Continue diet (low fat/low Na), regular exercise, and decreased caffeine; stop tobacco and alcohol. Reduce fluid and salt intake to control swelling.

OUTCOMES/EVALUATE
- ↓ Frequency and intensity of vasospastic anginal attacks
- ↓ BP; stable cardiac rhythm

Dimenhydrinate IV ⓒ
(dye-men-**HY**-drih-nayt)

CLASSIFICATION(S):
Cholinergic blocking drug, antiemetic

PREGNANCY CATEGORY: B
OTC: Liquid: Children's Dramamine, Dramamine, Triptone. **Tablets:** Calm-X, Dramamine, Triptone. **Tablets, Chewable:** Dramamine.
Rx: Injection: Dinate, Dramanate, Dymenate. **Liquid:** Dramamine.
✿**Rx: Tablets, Chewable:** Apo-Dimenhydrinate, Gravol.

SEE ALSO ANTIHISTAMINES AND ANTIEMETICS.

USES
(1) Motion sickness, especially to relieve nausea, vomiting, or dizziness. (2) Vertigo.

ACTION/KINETICS
Action
Contains both diphenhydramine and chlorotheophylline. Antiemetic mechanism not known, but it does depress labyrinthine and vestibular function. May mask ototoxicity due to aminoglycosides. Possesses anticholinergic activity.

Pharmacokinetics
Duration: 3–6 hr.

SPECIAL CONCERNS
Use of the injectable form is not recommended in neonates. Geriatric clients may be more sensitive to the usual adult dose.

SIDE EFFECTS
Most Common
Drowsiness, confusion (especially in children), headache, dizziness, blurred/double vision.
See *Antihistamines* for a complete list of possible side effects.

HOW SUPPLIED
OTC. *Liquid:* 12.5 mg/4 mL, 12.5 mg/5 mL; *Tablets:* 50 mg; *Tablets, Chewable:* 50 mg.
Rx. *Injection:* 50 mg/mL; *Liquid:* 15.62 mg/5 mL.

DOSAGE
- **LIQUID; TABLETS; TABLETS, CHEWABLE**
  Motion sickness.
  Adults: 50–100 mg q 4 hr, not to exceed 400 mg/day. **Pediatric, 6–12 years:** 25–50 mg q 6–8 hr, not to exceed 150 mg/day; **2–6 years:** 12.5–25 mg q 6–8 hr, not to exceed 75 mg/day.
- **IM; IV**
  Adults: 50 mg as required. **Pediatric, over 2 years:** 1.25 mg/kg (37.5 mg/m^2) 4 times/day, not to exceed 300 mg/day.
- **IV**
  Adults: 50 mg in 10 mL sodium chloride injection given over 2 min; may be repeated q 4 hr as needed. **Pediatric:** 1.25 mg/kg (37.5 mg/m^2) in 10 mL of 0.9% sodium chloride given slowly over 2 min; may be repeated q 6 hr, not to exceed 300 mg/day.

NURSING CONSIDERATIONS
ⓒ Do not confuse dimenhydrinate with diphenhydramine (also an antihistamine).

ADMINISTRATION/STORAGE
IV 1. Dilute 50 mg in 10 mL of NSS and administer slowly over 2 min.
2. Adjust pediatric dosage per BSA.

ASSESSMENT
1. List reasons for therapy and symptom onset.
2. Assess for vestibular damage when administered with antihistamines.
3. Note other agents trialed and outcome.
4. Evaluate need for further neurologic workup.

Bold Italic = life threatening side effect   ■ = black box warning   ✿ = Available in Canada

CLIENT/FAMILY TEACHING
1. Take at least 30 min before departure; may repeat before meals and upon retiring for motion sickness prevention.
2. Avoid activities that require mental alertness until effects realized. Avoid alcohol and any other CNS depressants.
3. May alter skin testing results; wait 72 hr after use.
4. Report adverse effects or lack of response.

OUTCOMES/EVALUATE
Prevention of N&V; control of vertigo

Dinoprostone (PGE$_2$)
(**die**-noh-**PROS**-tohn)

CLASSIFICATION(S):
Abortifacient
PREGNANCY CATEGORY: C
Rx: Cervidil, Prepidil Gel, Prostin E$_2$.
✦**Rx:** Prostin E$_2$ Vaginal Gel.

USES
(1) Ripening of an unfavorable cervix in pregnant women at or near term with a medical or obstetric need for induction of labor. (2) Evacuation of uterus in the management of missed abortion or intrauterine fetal death up to 28 weeks gestational age. (3) Management of nonmetastatic gestational trophoblastic disease (benign hydatidiform mole). (4) Termination of pregnancy from 12–20 weeks calculated from the first day of the last normal menstrual period.

ACTION/KINETICS
Action
Interacts with prostaglandin receptor to produce changes in the consistency, dilation, and effacement of the cervix. May also stimulate the smooth muscle of the GI tract, causing vomiting and diarrhea.

Pharmacokinetics
Extensively metabolized in the lungs on first pass through the pulmonary circulation. Metabolites are excreted through the kidneys. **t½:** 2.5–5 min.

CONTRAINDICATIONS
Use when oxytocic drugs are contraindicated or when prolonged uterine contractions are inappropriate (e.g., history of cesarean section or major uterine surgery), presence of cephalopelvic disproportion, history of difficult labor and/or traumatic delivery, grand multiparae with six or more previous term pregnancies, non-vertex presentation, hyperactive or hypertonic uterine patterns, fetal distress where delivery is not imminent, obstetric emergencies when surgical intervention may be favored. Also, use is contraindicated in ruptured membranes, hypersensitivity to prostaglandins or constituents of the gel, placenta previa or unexplained vaginal bleeding during current pregnancy, or when vaginal delivery is contraindicated (e.g., vasa previa or active herpes genitalis). Use in conjunction with oxytocic agents.

SPECIAL CONCERNS
Uterine rupture is possible when high-tone uterine contractions are sustained. Use with caution in clients with asthma or a history thereof; hypotension or hypertension; cardiovascular, renal, or hepatic disease; anemia; jaundice; diabetes; epilepsy; a compromised (scarred) uterus; glaucoma or increased intraocular pressure. Use dinoprostone suppositories with caution in presence of cervicitis, infected endocervical lesions, or acute vaginitis.

SIDE EFFECTS
Most Common
N&V, diarrhea, headache, chills/shivering.

GI: N&V, diarrhea. **CV:** Arrhythmias, chest pain/tightness, **MI** (in those with a history of CV disease), transient diastolic BP decreases of >20 mm Hg. **CNS:** Headache, flushing, anxiety, tension, hot flashes, paresthesia, syncope, dizziness, weakness. **GU:** Endometritis, uterine rupture, uterine/vaginal pain, vaginitis, vulvitis, vaginismus, breast tenderness, urine retention. **Respiratory:** Coughing, dyspnea, wheezing, pharyngitis, laryngitis. **Musculoskeletal:** Joint inflammation, arthralgia, myalgia, stiff neck, back ache, muscle

---

cramp/pain, leg cramps. **Dermatologic:** Skin discoloration, rash. **Ophthalmic:** Eye pain, blurred vision. **Body as a whole:** Chills, shivering, tremor, dehydration, diaphoresis, fever. **Miscellaneous:** Hearing impairment.

OD OVERDOSE MANAGEMENT

Symptoms: Uterine hypercontractility, uterine hypertonus. *Treatment:* Symptoms may be relieved by changing maternal position, giving oxygen to the mother, or the use of beta-adrenergic drugs to treat hyperstimulation.

DRUG INTERACTIONS

Dinoprostone may ↑ action of other oxytocics.

HOW SUPPLIED

Vaginal Gel/Jelly: 0.5 mg/3 grams; *Vaginal Insert, Controlled-Release:* 10 mg (releases 0.3 mg/hr); *Vaginal Suppositories:* 20 mg.

DOSAGE

• **GEL**

Initial: 0.5 mg. If there is no cervical/uterine response, repeat doses of 0.5 mg may be given q 6 hr. The maximum cumulative dose for 24 hr is 1.5 mg dinoprostone.

• **VAGINAL INSERT**

One insert (10 mg), designed to release approximately 0.3 mg dinoprostone/hr over a 12-hr period. The insert should be removed upon onset of active labor or 12 hr after insertion.

• **VAGINAL SUPPOSITORIES**

20 mg repeated every 3–5 hr; dose adjusted according to client response.

NURSING CONSIDERATIONS

ADMINISTRATION/STORAGE

1. Bring gel to room temperature just prior to administration.
2. Avoid contact with the skin; wash hands thoroughly with soap and water after administration.
3. Gel is intended for endocervical placement; do not administer above level of the internal os. The degree of cervical effacement will regulate shielded catheter size to be used (20-mm catheter for no effacement and 10-mm catheter for 50% effacement).

4. Administer gel by sterile technique; introduce just below level of the internal os.
5. Keep supine for at least 15–30 min after administration.
6. If desired response obtained from the initial dose, the recommended interval before giving oxytocin is 6–12 hr. A dosing interval of at least 30 min is recommended following removal of vaginal insert.
7. The insert is placed transversely in the posterior fornix of the vagina immediately after removal from the foil package. Insertion does not require sterile conditions. Do not use insert without its retrieval system.
8. Insert may be placed in the vagina with a minimal amount of water-miscible lubricant. Prevent excess contact or coating with the lubricant, thus preventing optimal swelling and release of the drug.
9. The gel has a shelf life of 24 months when stored under refrigeration at 2–8°C (36–46°F). Store the insert in a freezer between −20 to −10°C (−4 to −14°F). When stored in a freezer, the insert is stable for up to 3 years.

ASSESSMENT

1. Note reasons for therapy and maternal condition. List calculated and ultrasound-derived due date; note fetopelvic relationships.
2. Check cervix for degree of effacement (shortening of cervical canal) to determine size of shielded endocervical catheter needed.
3. Note system used, time of insertion, and dosing intervals. Insert must be removed with retrieval system after 12 hr or onset of labor.
4. Monitor uterine contractions, fetal heart tones, cervical dilation and effacement by visual assessment, auscultation, and electronic fetal monitor.
5. Continuous monitoring of uterine activity and fetal status should be undertaken esp. with history of hypertonic uterine contractility or tetanic uterine contractions. Monitor for uterine rupture with sustained high-tone myometrial contractions.

Bold Italic = life threatening side effect   ■ = black box warning   ♣ = Available in Canada

CLIENT/FAMILY TEACHING

1. Review reasons for therapy and anticipated outcome.
2. Gel may produce increased vaginal warmth.
3. Must remain supine for 30 min after gel insertion.
4. Avoid douches, tampons, intercourse, and tub baths for at least 2 weeks.
5. Monitor temperature (late afternoon) for a few days after discharge; report any new onset fever, bleeding, cramps/pain or foul-smelling discharge.
6. Pretreatment or concurrent use of antiemetic and antidiarrheal drugs help decrease the incidence of GI effects.

OUTCOMES/EVALUATE

- Desired cervical presentation to facilitate induction of labor
- Evacuation of uterus

Diphenhydramine hydrochloride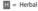

(dye-fen-**HY**-drah-meen)

CLASSIFICATION(S):

Antihistamine, second generation, ethanolamine

PREGNANCY CATEGORY: B

**OTC: Anti-Allergy/Anti-Cough.
Capsules or Capsules, Soft Gel:** Banophen, Benadryl Allergy Kapseals, Benadryl Dye-Free Allergy Liqui Gels, Diphenhist, Genahist.**Elixir:** Banophen Allergy, Siladryl. **Liquid:** Allermax, Altaryl Children's Allergy, Benadryl Children's Allergy, Benadryl Children's Dye-Free Allergy, Diphen AF, Genahist, Scot-Tussin Allergy Relief Formula Clear. **Oral Solution:** Children's Pedia Care Nighttime Cough, Diphenhist. **Strips, Oral Disintegrating:** Benadryl Allergy Quick Dissolve Strips, TheraFlu Thin Strips Multi-Symptom, Triaminic Thin Strips Cough & Runny Nose, Triaminic Thin Strips Multi-Symptoms. **Syrup:** Hydramine Cough, Silphen Cough. **Tablets:** AllerMax Caplets Maximum Strength, Banophen Caplets, Benadryl Allergy Ultratabs, Diphenist Captabs, Genahist. **Tablets,**

Chewable: Benadryl Allergy. **Tablets, Oral Disintegrating:** Children's Benadryl Allergy Fastmelt. **Sleep Aids. Capsules:** Compoz Gel Caps, Dormin, Maximum Strength Sleepinal Capsules and Soft Gels, Maximum Strength Unisom SleepGels. **Tablets:** 40 Winks, Dormin, Maximum Strength Nytol, Midol PM, Miles Nervine, Nighttime Sleep Aid, Nytol, Simply Sleep, Sleep-eze 3, Sleepwell 2-nite, Snooze Fast, Sominex, Twilite. **Rx: Injection:** Benadryl. **Syrup:** Tusstat.

SEE ALSO *ANTIHISTAMINES, ANTIEMETICS, AND ANTIPARKINSON AGENTS.*

USES

(1) Hypersensitivity reactions (type I), including perennial and seasonal allergic rhinitis, vasomotor rhinitis and sneezing caused by the common cold, allergic conjunctivitis caused by inhalant allergens and foods, mild uncomplicated allergic skin manifestations of urticaria and angioedema, amerlioration of allergic reactions to blood or plasma, dermatographism, adjunctive anaphylactic therapy, uncomplicated allergic conditions of the immediated type. (2) Motion sickness (injection only). (3) Parkinsonism (postencephalitic, arteriosclerotic, idiopathic, drug/chemical induced). (4) Nighttime sleep aid. (5) Antitussive (syrup only).

ACTION/KINETICS

Action

High sedative, anticholinergic, and antiemetic effects.

CONTRAINDICATIONS

Use in children 5 years of age and younger. Use of oral OTC diphenhydramine products with other products containing diphenhydramine, including topical products.

SPECIAL CONCERNS

Increased risk of cognitive decline in the elderly.

SIDE EFFECTS

Most Common

Drowsiness, constipation, diarrhea, dizziness, dry mouth/nose/throat, headache, anorexia, N&V, anxiety, GI upset, asthenia.

See *Antihistamines* for a complete list of possible side effects.

ADDITIONAL DRUG INTERACTIONS

Diphenhydramine ↑ effects of metoprolol.

HOW SUPPLIED

OTC. *Capsules:* 25 mg, 50 mg; *Capsules, Soft Gel:* 25 mg; *Elixir:* 12.5 mg/5 mL; *Liquid:* 12.5 mg/5 mL; *Oral Solution:* 12.5 mg/5 mL; *Strips, Orally Disintegrating:* 12.5 mg, 25 mg; *Syrup:* 12.5 mg/5 mL; *Tablets:* 25 mg, 50 mg; *Tablets, Chewable:* 12.5 mg; *Tablets, Oral Disintegrating:* 12.5 mg.

Rx. *Injection:* 50 mg/mL; *Syrup:* 12.5 mg/5 mL.

DOSAGE

● **CAPSULES; CAPSULES, SOFT GEL; ELIXIR; LIQUID; ORAL SOLUTION; SYRUP; TABLETS; TABLETS, CHEWABLE; TABLETS, ORAL DISINTEGRATING**

Hypersensitivity reactions, motion sickness, parkinsonism.

Adults: 25–50 mg PO 3–4 times per day, not to exceed 300 mg/day; **pediatric, 6–12 years:** 12.5–25 mg PO 3–4 times per day, not to exceed 150 mg/day.

Sleep aid.

Adults and children over 12 years: 50 mg at bedtime.

● **LIQUID**

Antitussive.

Adults and children 12 years of age and older: 25–50 mg q 4 hr, not to exceed 300 mg in 24 hr. **Children, 6–12 years of age:** 12.5–25 mg q 4 hr, not to exceed 150 mg in 24 hr. **Children, 6 years and younger:** Do not use.

● **ORAL SOLUTION**

Antitussive.

Children, 6 to <12 years of age: 12.5 mg (5 mL) q 4 hr, up to 75 mg (30 mL)/day. **Children, less than 6 years of age:** Do not use.

● **STRIPS, ORALLY DISINTEGRATING**

Antiallergic.

Adults: Take one q 4 to 6 hr, up to 6 doses/day.

● **SYRUP**

Antitussive.

Adults: 25 mg q 4 hr, not to exceed 150 mg/day; **pediatric, 6–12 years:** 12.5

mg q 4 hr, not to exceed 75 mg/day; **pediatric, 2–6 years:** do not use.

● **IM (DEEP); IV**

Hypersensitivity reactions, motion sickness, parkinsonism.

Adults: 10–50 mg up to 100 mg if needed (not to exceed 400 mg/day); **pediatric, 6 years and older:** 1.25 mg/kg (or 37.5 mg/m²) 4 times per day, not to exceed a total of 300 mg/day divided into 4 doses given IV at a rate not exceeding 25 mg/min or deep IM.

NURSING CONSIDERATIONS

Do not confuse diphenhydramine with desipramine (an antidepressant) or with dimenhydrinate (also an antihistamine).

ADMINISTRATION/STORAGE

1. With motion sickness, give full prophylactic dose 30 min prior to travel and 1–2 hr before exposures that precipitate sickness.

2. Take similar doses with meals and at bedtime.

3. Do not use more than 2 weeks to treat insomnia.

4. Store liquid and syrup from 15–30°C (59–86°F).

IV 5. For IV, may give undiluted.

6. For adults or children, do not exceed an IV rate of 25 mg/min.

7. Protect the injection from freezing and light.

ASSESSMENT

Note reasons for therapy, onset, S&S of characteristics, other agents trialed, triggers, outcome.

CLIENT/FAMILY TEACHING

1. May cause drowsiness; use caution until drug effects realized.

2. Take 30 minutes before travel to prevent motion sickness.

3. Use sun protection; may cause photosensitivity reaction.

4. Use sugarless gum/candy to diminish dry mouth effects.

5. Avoid alcohol and any other CNS depressants unless prescribed.

6. Stop therapy 72 to 96 hr before skin testing performed.

7. Report adverse side effects or lack of response. May require different antihistamine to offset tolerance if it occurs.

Bold Italic = life threatening side effect　　■ = black box warning　　✦ = Available in Canada

OUTCOMES/EVALUATE

- ↓ Allergic manifestations
- Relief of nausea/insomnia
- Relief of dyskinesias/extrapyramidal symptoms with parkinsonism

—**COMBINATION DRUG**—

Diphenoxylate hydrochloride with Atropine sulfate

(dye-fen-**OX**-ih-layt, **AH**-troh-peen)

CLASSIFICATION(S):
Antidiarrheal
PREGNANCY CATEGORY: C
Rx: Logen, Lomanate, Lomotil, Lonox, **C-V**

SEE ALSO CHOLINERGIC BLOCKING AGENTS.

USES

(1) Symptomatic treatment of chronic and functional diarrhea. (2) Diarrhea associated with gastroenteritis, irritable bowel, regional enteritis, malabsorption syndrome, ulcerative colitis, acute infections, food poisoning, postgastrectomy, and drug-induced. Therapeutic results for control of acute diarrhea are inconsistent. (3) Control of intestinal passage time in clients with ileostomies and colostomies.

CONTENT

Each tablet or 5 mL of liquid contains: *Antidiarrheal:* Diphenoxylate HCl, 2.5 mg. *Anticholinergic:* Atropine sulfate, 0.025 mg.

ACTION/KINETICS

Action

Chemically related to the narcotic analgesic drug meperidine but without the analgesic properties. Inhibits GI motility and has a constipating effect. May aggravate diarrhea due to organisms that penetrate the intestinal mucosa (e.g., *Escherichia coli, Salmonella, Shigella*) or in antibiotic-induced pseudomembranous colitis. High doses over prolonged periods may cause euphoria and physical dependence. The product also contains small amounts of atropine sulfate which will prevent abuse by deliberate overdosage.

Pharmacokinetics

Onset: 45–60 min. **t½, diphenoxylate:** 2.5 hr; **diphenoxylic acid:** 12–24 hr. **Duration:** 2–4 hr. Metabolized in the liver to the active diphenoxylic acid and excreted through the urine.

CONTRAINDICATIONS

Obstructive jaundice, liver disease, diarrhea associated with pseudomembranous enterocolitis after antibiotic therapy or enterotoxin-producing bacteria, children under the age of 2.

SPECIAL CONCERNS

Use with caution during lactation, when anticholinergics may be contraindicated, and in advanced hepatic-renal disease or abnormal renal functions. Children (especially those with Down syndrome) are susceptible to atropine toxicity. Children and geriatric clients may be more sensitive to the respiratory depressant effects of diphenoxylate. Dehydration, especially in young children, may cause a delayed diphenoxylate toxicity.

SIDE EFFECTS

Most Common
Dizziness, drowsiness, dry mouth, bloating, anorexia.

GI: N&V, dry mouth, anorexia, abdominal discomfort, bloating, paralytic ileus, megacolon. **Allergic:** Pruritus, *angioneurotic edema*, swelling of gums. **CNS:** Dizziness, drowsiness, malaise, restlessness, headache, depression, numbness of extremities, *respiratory depression, coma*. **Dermatologic:** Dry skin and mucous membranes, flushing. **Miscellaneous:** Anorexia, tachycardia, urinary retention, hyperthermia.

OD **OVERDOSE MANAGEMENT**
Symptoms: Dry skin and mucous membranes, flushing, *hyperthermia*, mydriasis, restlessness, tachycardia followed by miosis, lethargy, hypotonic reflexes, nystagmus, *coma, severe (and possibly fatal) respiratory depression*. *Treatment:* Gastric lavage, induce vomiting, establish a patent airway, and assist respiration. Activated charcoal (100 grams) given as a slurry. IV administration of a

narcotic antagonist. Administration may be repeated after 10–15 min. Observe client and readminister antagonist if respiratory depression returns.

DRUG INTERACTIONS

Alcohol / Additive CNS depression
Antianxiety agents / Additive CNS depression
Barbiturates / Additive CNS depression
MAO inhibitors / ↑ Chance of hypertensive crisis
Narcotics / ↑ Effect of narcotics

HOW SUPPLIED

See Content.

DOSAGE

DIPHENOXYLATE

• **ORAL SOLUTION; TABLETS**

Adults, initial: 2.5–5 mg (of diphenoxylate) 3–4 times per day; **maintenance:** 2.5 mg 2–3 times per day. **Pediatric, 2–3 years:** 0.75–1.5 mg 4 times per day; **3–4 years:** 1–1.5 mg 4 times per day; **4–5 years:** 1–2 mg 4 times per day; **5–6 years:** 1.25–2.25 mg 4 times per day; **6–9 years;** 1.25–2.5 mg 4 times per day; **9–12 years:** 1.75–2.5 mg 4 times per day. Maintain dosage at initial levels until symptoms are under control; then reduce to maintenance levels.

NURSING CONSIDERATIONS

ADMINISTRATION/STORAGE

1. For liquid preparations, use only plastic dropper supplied by manufacturer to measure dosage.
2. If clinical improvement not evident after 10 days with a maximum dose of 20 mg/day, further use will not likely control symptoms.

ASSESSMENT

1. List reasons for therapy, onset/frequency of stools, unusual foods/exposures and other agents trialed.
2. Note fluid & electrolyte status. Dehydration occurs rapidly in young children: may cause delayed toxicity. Correct before therapy.
3. Review culture reports to determine if drug is appropriate if not effective after 24–36 hr.
4. Note mental status, any hepatic or renal dysfunction.
5. Assess GI function, for abdominal distension and toxic megacolon.

CLIENT/FAMILY TEACHING

1. Used to control diarrhea. Take as prescribed; do not exceed dosage.
2. May cause drowsiness; use caution.
3. Report lack of response or adverse effects
4. Keep all F/U appointments to evaluate response to therapy.

OUTCOMES/EVALUATE

Relief of diarrhea

Dipyridamole

(dye-peer-**ID**-ah-mohl)

CLASSIFICATION(S):

Anticoagulant, platelet adhesion inhibitor

PREGNANCY CATEGORY: B

Rx: Persantine.

✤Rx: Apo-Dipyridamole FC, Dipyridamole for Injection, Novo-Dipiradol.

USES

As an adjunct to coumarin anticoagulants in preventing post-operative thromboembolic complications of cardiac valve replacement. *Investigational:* Use with aspirin to prevent myocardial reinfarction and reduction of post-MI mortality (combination therapy does not appear to be any more beneficial than use of aspirin alone).

ACTION/KINETICS

Action

In higher doses may act by several mechanisms, including inhibition of red blood cell uptake of adenosine, itself an inhibitor of platelet reactivity; inhibition of platelet phosphodiesterase, which leads to accumulation of cAMP within platelets; direct stimulation of release of prostacyclin or prostaglandin D_2; and/or inhibition of thromboxane A_2 formation. Dipyridamole prolongs platelet survival time in clients with valvular heart disease and has maintained platelet count in open heart surgery. Also causes coronary vasodilation which may be due to inhibition of adenosine deaminase in the blood, thus allowing accumulation of adenosine which is a potent vasodilator. Vasodilation may also be caused by delaying the hydrolysis of cyclic 3′,5′-adenosine monophosphate as a result of inhibition of the enzyme phosphodiesterase.

Pharmacokinetics
Incompletely absorbed from the GI tract. **Peak plasma levels, after PO:** 75 min. **$t^{1}/_{2}$, after PO: initial,** 40 min; **terminal,** 10–12 hr. Metabolized in the liver and mainly excreted in the bile. **Plasma protein binding:** Significant.

SPECIAL CONCERNS
Use with caution in hypotension (can cause peripheral vasodilation) and during lactation. Safety and efficacy have not been determined in children less than 12 years of age.

SIDE EFFECTS
Most Common
Dizziness, abdominal distress, headache, rash.
GI: Abdominal distress, diarrhea, vomiting, liver dysfunction (rare). **CNS:** Dizziness, headache. **CV:** Angina pectoris. **Dermatologic:** Rash, flushing, pruritus.

OD OVERDOSE MANAGEMENT
Symptoms: Hypotension of short duration. *Treatment:* Use of a vasopressor may be beneficial. Due to the high percentage of protein binding of dipyridamole, dialysis is not likely to be beneficial.

DRUG INTERACTIONS
Digoxin / ↑ Digoxin bioavailability
H *Evening primrose oil* / Potential for ↑ antiplatelet effect
H *Feverfew* / Potential for ↑ antiplatelet effect
H *Garlic* / Potential for ↑ antiplatelet effect
H *Ginger* / Potential for ↑ antiplatelet effect
H *Ginkgo biloba* / Potential for ↑ antiplatelet effect
H *Ginseng* / Potential for ↑ antiplatelet effect
H *Grapeseed extract* / Potential for ↑ antiplatelet effect
Warfarin / ↑ Risk of major bleeding

HOW SUPPLIED
Tablets: 25 mg, 50 mg, 75 mg.

DOSAGE
• **TABLETS**

Adjunct in prophylaxis of thromboembolism after cardiac valve replacement.
Adults: 75–100 mg 4 times per day as an adjunct to warfarin therapy. Do not give aspirin concomitantly.

NURSING CONSIDERATIONS
ASSESSMENT
1. Note reasons for therapy, type, onset, characteristics of S&S.
2. List drugs currently prescribed to ensure none interact unfavorably.
3. Assess mental status, skin color, cardiopulmonary findings.
4. Monitor VS, ECG, CBC, PT, PTT, INR.

CLIENT/FAMILY TEACHING
1. Drug helps prevent clots by inhibiting platelet stickiness; may also decrease frequency of chest pain and increase exercise tolerance. May take several months of therapy before effects evident.
2. Avoid alcohol and tobacco due to hypotensive vasoconstrictive effects; avoid use of any unprescribed drugs including aspirin without approval.
3. May cause dizziness and lightheadedness; use caution and change positions slowly to minimize ↓ BP.
4. Try small frequent meals if nausea or gastric distress experienced.
5. Report any increased chest pain, rash, fainting or severe headaches.

OUTCOMES/EVALUATE
• CAD evaluation with imaging
• Prevention of thromboembolism

Dirithromycin
(die-**rih**-throw-**MY**-sin)

CLASSIFICATION(S):
Antibiotic, macrolide
PREGNANCY CATEGORY: C
Rx: Dynabac, Dynabac D5-Pak.

USES
(1) Acute bacterial exacerbations of chronic bronchitis due to *Haemophilus influenzae, Moraxella catarrhalis* or *Streptococcus pneumoniae.* (2) Secondary bacterial infections of acute bron-

   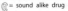

D

chitis due to *M. catarrhalis* or *S. pneumoniae*. (3) Community-acquired pneumonia due to *Legionella pneumophila*, *Mycoplasma pneumoniae*, or *S. pneumoniae*. (4) Pharyngitis or tonsillitis due to *Streptococcus pyogenes*. (5) Uncomplicated infections of the skin and skin structures due to *Staphylococcus aureus* (methicillin-susceptible strains) or *S. pyogenes*.

ACTION/KINETICS
Action
Erythromycylamine, the active metabolite, acts by binding to the 50S ribosomal subunits of microorganisms, resulting in inhibition of protein synthesis.

Pharmacokinetics
Rapidly absorbed and converted during intestinal absorption to the active erythromycylamine. Distributed throughout the body, including the lungs, GI tract, skin, soft tissues, and GU tract. **t½:** 2–36 hr. From 81 to 97% of erythromycylamine is excreted in the feces via the bile.

CONTRAINDICATIONS
Hypersensitivity to erythromycin or any other macrolide antibiotic. Use in children less than 12 years of age. Use in clients with known, suspected, or potential bacteremias since serum levels of the drug are not high enough in the serum to be effective. Use for the empiric treatment of acute bacterial exacerbations of chronic or secondary bacterial infections of acute bronchitis or for empiric treatment of uncomplicated skin and skin structure infections.

SPECIAL CONCERNS
Although dirithromycin eradicates *S. pyogenes* from the nasopharynx, data are lacking as to its effectiveness in preventing rheumatic fever. Use with caution during lactation. Safety and efficacy have not been determined in children less than 12 years of age.

SIDE EFFECTS
Most Common
Abdominal pain/discomfort, headache, N&V, diarrhea/loose stools, dyspepsia, dizziness, asthenia, non-specific pain.

GI: ***Pseudomembranous colitis***, abdominal pain/discomfort, nausea, diarrhea/loose stools, vomiting, dyspep-

sia, GI disorder, flatulence, abnormal stools, constipation, dry mouth, gastritis, gastroenteritis, mouth ulceration, taste perversion, thirst, dysphagia. **CNS:** Headache, dizziness, vertigo, insomnia, anxiety, depression, nervousness, paresthesia, somnolence. **CV:** Palpitation, vasodilation, syncope. **GU:** Dysmenorrhea, urinary frequency, vaginal moniliasis, vaginitis. **Dermatologic:** Rash, pruritus, urticaria, sweating. **Respiratory:** Increased cough, dyspnea, hyperventilation. **Miscellaneous:** Nonspecific pain, asthenia, anorexia, dehydration, edema, epistaxis, eye disorder, fever, flu syndrome, hemoptysis, malaise, peripheral edema, ***allergic reaction***, amblyopia, myalgia, neck pain, tinnitus, tremor, thirst.

LABORATORY TEST CONSIDERATIONS
↑ ALT, AST, alkaline phosphatase, potassium, serum CPK, bands, segs, basophils, eosinophils, platelet count, total bilirubin, creatinine, GGT, leukocyte count, lymphocytes, monocytes, phosphorus, uric acid, Ca, hematocrit, hemoglobin. ↓ Platelet count, albumin, chloride, hematocrit, hemoglobin, lymphocytes, segmented neutrophils, phosphorus, serum alkaline phosphatase, serum uric acid, total protein.

OD **OVERDOSE MANAGEMENT**
Symptoms: N&V, epigastric distress, diarrhea. *Treatment:* Treat symptoms.

DRUG INTERACTIONS
Antacids / Slightly ↑ absorption of dirithromycin
H₂-Antagonists / Slightly ↑ absorption of dirithromycin
Pimozide / Not to be used together due to possible sudden death

HOW SUPPLIED
Tablets, Delayed-Release: 250 mg.

DOSAGE
- **TABLETS, DELAYED-RELEASE**
  Acute bacterial exacerbations of chronic bronchitis.
Adults and children over 12 years of age: 500 mg once a day for 5–7 days.
  Secondary bacterial infection of acute bronchitis.
500 mg once a day for 7 days.
  Community-acquired pneumonia.

Bold Italic = life threatening side effect   ■ = black box warning   ♣ = Available in Canada

Adults and children over 12 years of age: 500 mg once a day for 14 days.
Pharyngitis or tonsillitis.

Adults and children over 12 years of age: 500 mg once a day for 10 days.
Uncomplicated skin and skin structure infections.

Adults and children over 12 years of age: 500 mg once a day for 5–7 days.

NURSING CONSIDERATIONS

ASSESSMENT

1. List reasons for therapy, onset, symptom characteristics. Assess for allergies/macrolide sensitivity.
2. Obtain VS, renal, LFTs and culture results; assess for superinfections.
3. Does not appear to cause CV problems. Note other drugs prescribed, may increase theophylline blood levels.

CLIENT/FAMILY TEACHING

1. Take as prescribed with food or within 1 hr of eating.
2. Do not crush, cut, or chew enteric-coated tablets.
3. Report worsening of S&S or new onset diarrhea; drug alters normal colon flora, permitting clostridia overgrowth; requires drug withdrawal and symptom management. Consume 2 L/day of fluids with diarrhea.

OUTCOMES/EVALUATE

- Resolution of infection
- Negative culture reports

Disulfiram ■
(dye-**SUL**-fih-ram)

CLASSIFICATION(S):
Treatment of alcoholism
PREGNANCY CATEGORY: C
Rx: Antabuse.

USES

To prevent further ingestion of alcohol in chronic alcoholics. Should be given only to cooperating clients fully aware of the consequences of alcohol ingestion.

ACTION/KINETICS

Action

Produces severe hypersensitivity to alcohol. Inhibits liver enzymes that participate in the normal degradation of alcohol. This results in accumulation of acetaldehyde in the blood. High levels of acetaldehyde produce a series of symptoms referred to as the disulfiram-alcohol reaction or syndrome. The specific symptoms are listed under *Side Effects..*

Pharmacokinetics

The symptoms vary individually, are dose-dependent with respect to both alcohol and disulfiram, and persist for periods ranging from 30 min to several hours. A single dose of disulfiram may be effective for 1–2 weeks. **Onset:** May be delayed up to 12 hr because disulfiram is initially localized in fat stores.

CONTRAINDICATIONS

Alcohol intoxication. Severe myocardial or occlusive coronary disease, psychoses, hypersensitivity to disulfiram or other thiuram derivatives used in pesticides and rubber vulcanization, clients receiving or who have recently received metronidazole, paraldehyde, alcohol, or alcohol-containing preparations (e.g., cough syrups, tonics). If client is exposed to ethylene dibromide. Lactation.

SPECIAL CONCERNS

■ Never give to anyone in a state of alcohol intoxication or without the client's full knowledge. Instruct the clients family accordingly.■ Use in pregnancy only if benefits outweigh risks. Use with caution in narcotic addicts or clients with diabetes, goiter, epilepsy, psychosis, hypothyroidism, hepatic cirrhosis, or nephritis. Do not expose clients to ethylene dibromide or its vapors; a toxic interaction may occur. Safety and efficacy have not been determined in children.

SIDE EFFECTS

Most Common

See below for use in absence of or in presence of alcohol.

In the absence of alcohol. CNS: Drowsiness, fatigue, headache, psychotic reactions. **Neurologic:** Peripheral neuropathy, peripheral neuritis, polyneuritis, optic neuritis. **GI:** Metallic or garlic-like aftertaste (usually during the first 2 weeks of therapy), hepatotoxicity, cholestatic and fulminant hepatitis, *hepatic failure*. **Dermatologic:** Skin eruptions (occasional), acneform eruptions, allergic dermatitis. **Miscellaneous:** Impotence.

In the presence of alcohol. CV: Flushing, chest pain, palpitations, tachycardia, hypotension, syncope, arrhythmias, *CV collapse, MI, acute CHF*. **CNS:** Throbbing headaches, vertigo, weakness, uneasiness, confusion, unconsciousness, *seizures, death*. **GI:** Nausea, severe vomiting, thirst. **Respiratory:** Respiratory difficulties, dyspnea, hyperventilation, *respiratory depression*. **Miscellaneous:** Throbbing in head and neck, sweating. In the event of an Antabuse-alcohol interaction, measures should be undertaken to maintain BP and treat shock. Oxygen, antihistamines, ephedrine, and/or vitamin C may also be used.

DRUG INTERACTIONS

Alcohol / Severe alcohol intolerance reactions (e.g., flushing, increased respiration, pulse rate, and CO); avoid alcohol in all forms
Anticoagulants, oral / ↑ Anticoagulant effects by ↑ hypoprothrombinemia
Barbiturates / ↑ Barbiturate effects R/T ↓ liver breakdown
Caffeine / ↑ CV and CNS stimulant effects of caffeine
Chlordiazepoxide, diazepam / ↑ Chlordiazepoxide/diazepam effects R/T ↓ plasma clearance
Chlorzoxazone / Inhibition of chlorzoxazone metabolism; ↓ chlorzoxazone dose
Cocaine / ↑ CV side effects of cocaine
Hydantoins / ↑ Serum hydantoin levels → ↑ pharmacologic and toxic effects
Isoniazid / ↑ Isoniazid side effects (especially CNS)
Metronidazole / Acute toxic psychosis or confusional state
Paraldehyde / Antabuse-like effects
Phenytoin / ↑ Phenytoin effects R/T ↓ liver breakdown
Theophyllines / ↓ Theophylline metabolism → toxic effects

Tricyclic antidepressants / ↑ Risk of acute organic brain syndrome
Warfarin / ↑ Anticoagulant effect of warfarin

HOW SUPPLIED

Tablets: 250 mg.

DOSAGE

- **TABLETS**

  Prevent further ingestion of alcohol in chronic alcoholics.

Adults, initial (after alcohol-free interval of 12–48 hr): 500 mg/day for 1–2 weeks; **maintenance: usual,** 250 mg/day (range: 120–500 mg/day). Do not exceed 500 mg/day. Maintenance may be needed for months or years.

NURSING CONSIDERATIONS

ASSESSMENT

1. Note reasons for therapy, other agents/therapies trialed, living situation, client's mental status/level of understanding. Identify length of time with disease.
2. Perform baseline and follow-up LFTs (10–14 days) to detect hepatic dysfunction. Perform CBC and serum chemistries.

CLIENT/FAMILY TEACHING

1. May crush tablets or mix with liquid.
2. Never give without client's knowledge. Ingesting 30 mL of 100-proof alcohol (e.g., one shot) may cause severe symptoms (within 15 min; lasting several hours) and possibly death. Avoid alcohol in any form, in foods, sauces, or other medications, such as cough syrups or tonics; avoid vinegar, paregoric, skin products, linaments, or lotions containing alcohol. Read all labels before consuming.
3. CNS side effects should lessen with continued therapy.
4. May feel tired, experience drowsiness, headaches, and develop a metallic or garlic-like taste; should subside after 2 weeks of therapy.
5. May have occasional impotence, usually transient; report.
6. Report if skin eruptions occur; an antihistamine may be prescribed.
7. Carry card stating 'taking disulfiram' and describing symptoms and treatment if a disulfiram reaction occurs. In-

clude provider/contact person, and phone number.

8. Attend local support group meetings, e.g., Alcoholics Anonymous and Al-Anon, to gain the support, structure, referral, and encouragement to obtain an alcohol-free life.

OUTCOMES/EVALUATE
Freedom from alcohol and its effects; sobriety

Divalproex sodium
(dye-**VAL**-proh-ex)

PREGNANCY CATEGORY: D
Rx: Depakote.
♣Rx: Apo-Divalproex, Epival, Epival ER, Novo-Divalproex, Nu-Divalproex.

SEE ALSO SEE *VALPROIC ACID.*

ADDITIONAL USES
Extended-Release Tablets: Treatment of acute manic or mixed episodes associated with bipolar disorder, with or without psychotic features.

LABORATORY TEST CONSIDERATIONS
False + for ketonuria. Altered thyroid function tests.

HOW SUPPLIED
Capsules, Enteric-Coated: 125 mg; *Tablets, Enteric-Coated:* 125 mg, 250 mg, 500 mg; *Tablets, Extended-Release:* 500 mg.

Dobutamine hydrochloride   IV Ⓒ
(doh-**BYOU**-tah-meen)

CLASSIFICATION(S):
Sympathomimetic, direct-acting
PREGNANCY CATEGORY: B
Rx: Dobutamine hydrochloride.

SEE ALSO *SYMPATHOMIMETIC DRUGS.*

USES
When parenteral therapy is needed for inotropic support in the short-term treatment of cardiac decompensation in adults secondary due to depressed contractility resulting from organic heart disease or cardiac surgical procedures. Experience does not extend beyond 48 hr of use. *Investigational:* Congenital heart disease in children undergoing diagnostic cardiac catheterization.

ACTION/KINETICS
Action
Directly stimulates beta-1 receptors (in the heart), increasing cardiac function, CO, and SV, with minor effects on HR. Decreases afterload reduction although SBP and pulse pressure may remain unchanged or increase (due to increased CO). Also decreases elevated ventricular filling pressure and helps AV node conduction. It does not cause the release of norepinephrine.

Pharmacokinetics
Onset: 1–2 min. **Peak effect:** 10 min. **t½:** 2 min. **Therapeutic plasma levels:** 40–190 ng/mL. Metabolized by the liver and excreted in urine.

CONTRAINDICATIONS
Idiopathic hypertrophic subaortic stenosis. Previous hypersensitivity to dobutamine.

SPECIAL CONCERNS
Safe use after AMI not established. Dobutamine is less effective than dopamine in premature neonates in raising systemic BP without causing undue tachycardia.

SIDE EFFECTS
Most Common
Marked increase in HR, BP, ventricular ectopic activity; premature ventricular beats, hypotension, nausea, headache, SOB.
CV: Marked increase in HR, BP, and ***ventricular ectopic activity***, precipitous drop in BP, premature ventricular beats, anginal and nonspecific chest pain, palpitations. **Hypersensitivity:** Skin rash, pruritus of the scalp, fever, eosinophilia, ***bronchospasm.*** **Infusion site reactions:** Inadvertent infiltration, cutaneous necrosis, local inflammation. **Miscellaneous:** Nausea, headache, SOB, fever, phlebitis, and local inflammatory changes at the injection site.

📷 = see color insert   H = Herbal   IV = Intravenous   Ⓒ = sound alike drug

LABORATORY TEST CONSIDERATIONS
Thrombocytopenia. Mild ↓ serum potassium.

OD OVERDOSE MANAGEMENT
Symptoms: Excessive alteration of BP, anorexia N&V, tremor, anxiety, palpitations, headache, SOB, anginal and nonspecific chest pain, hypertension, hypotension, tachyarrhythmias, *myocardial ischemia, ventricular fibrillation or tachycardia. Treatment:* Reduce the rate of administration or discontinue temporarily until the condition stabilizes. Establish an airway, ensuring oxygenation and ventilation. Initiate resuscitative measures immediately. Treat severe ventricular tachyarrhythmias with propranolol or lidocaine.

DRUG INTERACTIONS
Bretylium / Possible potentiation of vasopressor action → arrhythmias
Guanethidine / Possible ↑ pressor response → severe hypertension
Halogenated hydrocarbon anesthetics / Possible sensitization of the myocardium → serious arrhythmias; use together with extreme caution
Nitroprusside / ↑CO and ↓ PAWP
Oxytocics / Possible severe persistent hypertension
Tricyclic antidepressants / Possible potentiation of the pressor response

HOW SUPPLIED
Injection: 12.5 mg/mL.

DOSAGE
• **IV INFUSION**
Treatment of cardiac decompensation.
Adults, individualized, usual: 2.5–10 mcg/kg/min (up to 40 mcg/kg/min). Rate of administration and duration of therapy depend on response of client, as determined by HR, presence of ectopic activity, BP, and urine flow.
Children with congenital heart disease undergoing diagnostic cardiac catheterization.
Children: 2 and 7.75 mcg/kg/min infused for 10 min. *NOTE:* This dosage is investigational.

NURSING CONSIDERATIONS

☙ Do not confuse dobutamine with dopamine (also a sympathomimetic).

ADMINISTRATION/STORAGE
IV 1. Reconstitute according to manufacturer directions; takes place in two stages.
2. Before administration, solution is diluted further according to client fluid needs. Use this more dilute solution within 24 hr. Solutions that can be used for further dilution include D5W, D5W/0.45% NaCl injection, D5W/0.9% NaCl injection, D10W, Isolyte M with D5W injection, RL injection, D5W/RL, Normosol-M in D5W, 20% Osmitrol in water for injection, 0.9% NaCl injection, and sodium lactate injection.
3. May refrigerate the more concentrated solution for 48 hr or store at room temperature for 6 hr. After dilution (in glass or Viaflex containers), solution is stable for 24 hr at room temperature. Dilute solutions may darken; does not affect potency when used within designated time spans.
4. Drug is incompatible with alkaline solutions. Do not give with agents or diluents containing both sodium bisulfite and ethanol. Physically incompatible with hydrocortisone sodium succinate, cefazolin, cefamandole, neutral cephalothin, penicillin, sodium ethacrynate, and heparin sodium.
5. Compatible when given through same tubing with dopamine, lidocaine, tobramycin, verapamil, nitroprusside, KCl, and protamine sulfate.
6. Give using electronic infusion device. Carefully reconstitute and calculate dosage according to weight and desired response.
7. Contains sodium bisulfite that may cause allergic reactions, including anaphylaxis and life-threatening or less severe asthmatic episodes.
8. Store from 15–30°C (59–86°F).

ASSESSMENT
Note reasons for therapy; ensure hydrated prior to infusion. Administered in a monitored environment; assess for increased ectopy with dose titration.

INTERVENTIONS
1. During acute use: Monitor CVP to assess vascular volume and cardiac pumping efficiency. Normal range 5–10 cm water (1–7 mm Hg). Elevated CVP

may indicate disruption of CO, as in pump failure or pulmonary edema; low CVP may indicate hypovolemia.

2. Monitor PAWP to assess the pressures in the left atrium and ventricle and to measure the efficiency of CO; usual range is 6–12 mm Hg.

3. Assess ECG and BP continuously during drug administration; review written parameters for SBP and titrate infusion. Drug increases AV node conduction causing those with AFib to develop rapid ventricular rate; have digoxin available to give in this event.

4. Record I&O.

5. Monitor glucose in diabetics; more insulin may be needed.

CLIENT/FAMILY TEACHING

Drug is administered IV to improve cardiac function thus increasing BP and improving urine output. Report any chest pain, increased SOB, headaches, or IV site pain.

OUTCOMES/EVALUATE

- ↑ CO; ↑ urine output
- SBP >90 mm Hg

Docetaxel
(doh-seh-**TAX**-ell)

CLASSIFICATION(S):
Antineoplastic, miscellaneous
PREGNANCY CATEGORY: D
Rx: Taxotere.

SEE ALSO *ANTINEOPLASTIC AGENTS.*

USES

(1) Locally advanced or metastatic breast cancer after failure of prior chemotherapy. (2) In combination with doxorubicin and cyclophosphamide for the adjuvant treatment of operable node-positive breast cancer. (3) As a single agent to treat locally advanced or metastatic non-small cell lung cancer after failure of prior platinum-based chemotherapy. (4) With cisplatin for first-line treatment of unresectable locally advanced or metastatic non-small cell lung cancer in clients who have not received prior chemotherapy. (5) With prednisone to treat androgen-independent (hormone-refactory) advanced metastatic prostate cancer. (6) With cisplatin and 5-fluorouracil to treat advanced gastric adenocarcinoma, including adenocarcinoma of the gastro-esophageal junction, in those who have not previously received chemotherapy for advanced disease. (7) With cisplatin and fluorouracil for induction of treatment of inoperable locally advanced squamous cell carcinoma of the head and neck. *Investigational:* Ovarian cancer, urothelial cancer, small cell lung cancer, esophageal cancer.

ACTION/KINETICS

Action

Effect is due to disruption of the microtubular network in cells that is required for mitotic and interphase cellular functions. Thus, mitosis is inhibited.

Pharmacokinetics

t^{1}_{2}, **3 phases:** 4 min, 36 min, and 11.1 hr. Metabolized in the liver, and metabolites and small amounts of unchanged drug are excreted through both the feces (75%) and urine (6%). **Plasma protein binding:** About 94%.

CONTRAINDICATIONS

Severe hypersensitivity to docetaxel or to other drugs formulated with polysorbate 80. Use in those with neutrophil counts less than 1,500 cells/mm^3, in those with bilirubin greater than the upper limit of normal (ULN), or in those with AST or ALT greater than 1.5 times the ULN. Lactation.

SPECIAL CONCERNS

■ (1) Give docetaxel under the supervision of a qualified health care provider experienced in the use of antineoplastic drugs. Appropriate management of complications is possible only when adequate diagnostic and treatment facilities are readily available. (2) The incidence of treatment-related mortality is increased in clients with abnormal liver function, in those receiving higher doses, and in clients with non-small cell lung cancer and a history of prior treatment with platinum-based chemotherapy who receive docetaxel as a single agent at a dose of 100 mg/m^2. (3) Hepatic function impairment. In general, do not give to clients with bilirubin greater than the upper limit of normal (ULN) or to those with AST and/or ALT over 1.5 x ULN concomitant with alkaline phosphatase over 2.5 x ULN. Those with elevations of bilirubin or abnormalities of transaminase concurrent with alkaline phosphatase are at increased risk for developing grade 4 neutropenia, febrile neutropenia, infections, severe thrombocytopenia, severe stomatitis, severe skin toxicity, and toxic death. Those with isolated elevations of transaminases greater than 1.5 x ULN also had a higher rate of febrile neutropenia grade 4 but did not have an increased incidence of toxic death. Obtain and review bilirubin, AST or ALT, and alkaline phosphatase values before each cycle of docetaxel therapy. (4) Neutropenia. Do not give to those with a neutrophil count less than 1,500 cells/mm^3. In order to monitor the occurrence of neutropenia, which may be severe and result in infection, perform frequent blood cell counts on all clients receiving docetaxel. (5) Hypersensitivity. Severe hypersensitivity reactions, characterized by general rash/erythema, hypotension and/or bronchospasm or, very rarely, fatal anaphylaxis, have been reported in clients who received the recommended 3-day dexamethasone premedication. Hypersensitivity reactions require immediate discontinuation of the docetaxel infusion and administration of appropriate therapy. Do not give docetaxel to clients who have a history of severe hypersensitivity reactions to docetaxel or other drugs formulated with polysorbate 80. (6) Fluid retention. Severe fluid retention is a possibility despite use of 3-day dexamethasone premedication regimen. Fluid retention was characterized by one or more of the following reactions: Poorly tolerated peripheral edema, generalized edema, pleural effusion requiring urgent drainage, dyspnea at rest, cardiac tamponade, or pronounced abdominal distention (due to ascites).■ The incidence of treatment-related mortality is increased in clients with abnormal liver function and in those re-

ceiving higher doses. Select doses carefully in the elderly as side effects may be more common. Safety and efficacy have not been determined in children less than 16 years of age.

SIDE EFFECTS

Most Common

Neutropenia, leukopenia, asthenia, fatigue, neurosensory effects, alopecia, nail changes, N&V, diarrhea, stomatitis, anemia, hypersensitivity reactions, fluid retention, myalgia, fever, infections, skin toxicity, constipation.

Hematologic: Neutropenia (virtually in 100% of clients given 100 mg/m^2). Leukopenia, thrombocytopenia, anemia, febrile neutropenia, acute myeloid leukemia. **GI:** N&V, diarrhea (may be severe), stomatitis (may be severe), pharyngitis, anorexia (may be severe/life-threatening), abdominal pain, colitis, constipation, ulcer, esophagitis, dysphagia, odynophagia, GI pain/cramps, heartburn, ***GI perforation, GI hemorrhage/bleeding***, intestinal obstruction, ileus, ischemic colitis, neutropenic enterocolitis, taste perversion, duodenal ulcer, impaired hepatic function, ***hepatitis***. **CNS:** Confusion, dizziness, lethargy, loss of consciousness (rare), ***seizures*** (rare). **CV:** Fluid retention (even with premedication), hypotension, atrial fibrillation, ***DVT***, ECG abnormalities, cardiac arrhythmias, thrombophlebitis, CHF, ***pulmonary embolism, heart failure***, syncope, tachycardia, sinus tachycardia, atrial flutter, dysrhythmia, unstable angina, vasodilation, pulmonary edema, myocardial ischemia, ***MI***, cardiac left ventricular function, hypertension (rare). **Respiratory:** Dyspnea, cough, epistaxis, pleural effusion, interstitial pneumonia, ***acute pulmonary edema, ARDS***, pulmonary fibrosis. **Dermatologic:** Reversible cutaneous reactions characterized by a rash, including localized eruptions on the hands, feet, arms, face, or thorax, and usually associated with pruritus. Localized erythema of the extremities with edema followed by desquamation. Nail changes, alopecia, itching, dry skin, cutaneous lupus erythematosus (rare), bullous eruption (e.g., erythema multiforme), ***Stevens-John-***

Bold Italic = life threatening side effect   ■ = black box warning   ✦ = Available in Canada

son syndrome, toxic epidermal necro-lysis. **Hypersensitivity:** Flushing, local-ized skin reactions, back pain, chest tightness, chills, drug fever, dyspnea, rash (with or without pruritus). Severe hypersensitivity reactions characterized by hypotension, bronchospasm, or gen-eralized rash/erythema, **anaphylactic shock**. **Musculoskeletal:** Myalgia, ar-thralgia. **GU:** Amenorrhea, impaired re-nal function. **Neurologic:** Paresthesia, dysesthesia, pain in those with anthra-cycline-resistant breast cancer, pares-thesia, dysestheisa, pain. Distal extremi-ty weakness. **Reactions at infusion site:** Hyperpigmentation, inflammation, redness or dryness of the skin, phlebitis, extravasation, mild swelling of the vein. **Ophthalmic:** Conjunctivitis, lacrimation disorder (tearing), flashes, flashing lights, scotomata. **Otic:** Altered hearing, hearing loss. **Body as a whole:** Infec-tions, fluid retention, asthenia, fatigue, lymphedema, peripheral edema, weight gain/loss, dehydration (due to GI reac-tions), bleeding episodes. **Miscellane-ous:** *Septic/nonseptic death, treat-ment-related death*, fever (including in absence of infections), diffuse pain, chest pain, renal insufficiency, syncope, allergy, cancer pain.

LABORATORY TEST CONSIDERATIONS
↑ ALT, AST, alkaline phosphatase.

OD OVERDOSE MANAGEMENT
Symptoms: Bone marrow suppression, peripheral neurotoxicity, mucositis. *Treatment:* No known antidote. Keep client in a specialized unit to monitor vital functions. Give therapeutic G-CSF as soon as possible after overdose dis-covered. Treat symptomatically.

DRUG INTERACTIONS
Clarithromycin / Substantial ↑ docetax-el levels
Itraconazole / ↑ Docetaxel levels → ↑ risk of toxicity (e.g., neutropenia); coad-minister with caution and ↓ dose as needed
Ketoconazole / ↑ Docetaxel levels → ↑ risk of toxicity (e.g., neutropenia); coad-minister with caution and ↓ dose as needed
Nefazodone / Substantial ↑ docetaxel levels

Nelfinavir / Substantial ↑ docetaxel lev-els

HOW SUPPLIED
Injection: 20 mg/0.5 mL, 80 mg/2 mL.

DOSAGE
- **IV**
  Breast cancer.
60–100 mg/m² given IV over 1 hr q 3 weeks. Reduce the dose to 75 mg/m² or discontinue therapy in those who are dosed initially at 100 mg/m² and who experience febrile neutropenia, neutro-phils less than 500/mm³ for more than 1 week, severe or cumulative cutaneous reactions, or severe peripheral neuropa-thy. If these reactions continue, either decrease the dosage from 75 to 55 mg/m² or discontinue treatment. Those who are dosed at 60 mg/m² and do not experience these symptoms may toler-ate higher doses. Discontinue treat-ment in those who develop greater than grade 3 peripheral neuropathy.

  Combination therapy with doxorubicin and cyclophosphamide for breast can-cer.
Docetaxel, 75 mg/m² given as a 1hr IV infusion after doxorubicin, 50 mg/m², and cyclophosphamide, 500 mg/m², ev-ery 3 weeks for 6 treatment cycles. Give when the neutrophil count is 1,500 cells/mm³ or more. Prophylactic granu-locyte colony-stimulating factor may be given to reduce the risk of hematologi-cal toxicities. Those who experience fe-brile neutropenia should receive granu-locyte colony-stimulating factor in all subsequent cycles. Clients who con-tinue to experience febrile neutropenia should remain on granulocyte colony-stimulating factor and have their doce-taxel dose decreased to 60 mg/m². Those who experience grade 3 or 4 sto-matitis, severe or cumulative cutaneous reactions, or moderate neurosensory signs and/or symptoms should have their docetaxel dose reduced to 60 mg/m². If the client continues to experience these reactions at 60 mg/m², discontin-ue treatment.

  Non-small cell lung cancer, after fail-ure of prior platinum-based chemo-therapy.

75 mg/m^2 IV over 1 hr q 3 weeks. Withhold treatment until toxicity is resolved for those who experience either febrile neutropenia, neutrophils less than 500/mm^3 for more than 1 week, severe or cumulative cutaneous reactions, or severe peripheral neuropathy. Resume at 55 mg/m^2. Discontinue entirely if clients develop grade 3 or greater peripheral neuropathy.

Non-small cell lung cancer, chemotherapy naive clients.

75 mg/m^2 IV over 1 hr immediately followed by cisplatin, 75 mg/m^2 over 30–60 min q 3 weeks. In those whose nadir of platelet count during the previous course of therapy is less than 25,000 cells/mm^3, in those who experience febrile neutropenia, and in clients with serious nonhematologic toxicities, reduce the docetaxel dosage in subsequent cycles to 65 mg/m^2. If the client requires a further dose reduction, a dose of 50 mg/m^2 is recommended.

Metastatic prostate cancer.

75 mg/m^2 by IV infusion over 1 hr q 3 weeks with PO prednisone, 5 mg, twice a day continuously. For androgen-dependent metastatic prostate cancer, give dexamethasone 8 mg PO at 12 hr, 3 hr, and 1 hr before the docetaxel infusion. Reduce the dose of docetaxel from 75 mg/m^2 to 60 mg/m^2 if febrile neutropenia, neutrophils less than 500/mm^3 for more than 1 week, severe or cumulative cutaneous reactions, or moderate neurosensory signs and/or symptoms occur during docetaxel therapy. If the client continues to experience these reactions at 60 mg/m^2, discontinue the drug.

Head and neck cancer.

75 mg/m^2 as a 1-hr IV infusion, followed by cisplatin, 75 mg/m^2 IV over 1 hour both on day 1; follow with fluorouracil, 750 mg/m^2 as a continuous IV infusion for 5 days. Give this regimen q 3 weeks for 4 cycles. Following chemotherapy, clients should receive radiotherapy. Clients must receive premedication with antiemetics and appropriate hydration (prior to and after cisplatin administration). Prophylactic antibiotics are also often given.

Granulocyte colony-stimulating factor has been given during the second and/or subsequent cycles in the event of febrile neutropenia, documented infection with neutropenia, or neutropenia lasting longer than 7 days. If these symptoms occur despite granulocyte colony-stimulating factor use, reduce the dose of docetaxel to 60 mg/m^2. If subsequent episodes of complicated neutropenia occur, reduce the docetaxel dose to 45 mg/m^2.

In cases of grade 4 thrombocytopenia, reduce the docetaxel dose to 60 mg/m^2. Do not retreat clients with subsequent cycles of docetaxel until neutrophils recover to a level more than 1,500 cells/mm^3 and platelets recover to a level of more than 100,000/mm^3. Discontinue treatment if these toxicities persist.

The recommended dose modifications for diarrhea, stomatitis, and/or mucositis are as follows: (1) Diarrhea grade 3: Reduce the fluorouracil dose by 20% after the first episode. Reduce the docetaxel dose by 20% after the second episode. (2) Diarrhea, grade 4: Reduce the docetaxel and fluorouracil doses by 20% after the first episode. Discontinue treatment after the second episode. (3) Stomatitis/mucositis, grade 3: Reduce the fluorouracil dose by 20% after the first episode. For the second episode, discontinue fluorouracil only, at all subsequent cycles. For the third episode, reduce the docetaxel dose by 20%. (4) Stomatitis/mucositis, grade 4: Discontinue fluorouracil only, at all subsequent cycles, at the first episode. Reduce the docetaxel dose by 20% at the second episode.

Gastric adenocarcinoma.

75 mg/m^2 as a 1-hr IV infusion, followed by cisplatin, 75 mg/m^2, as a 1- to 3-hr IV infusion (both on day 1), followed by fluorouracil, 750 mg/m^2/day given as a 24-hr continuous IV infusion for 5 days (start at the end of the cisplatin infusion). Repeat treatment q 3 weeks. Clients must receive premedication with antiemetics and appropriate hydration for cisplatin administration. *NOTE:* See information under *Head and*

Bold Italic = life threatening side effect   ■ = black box warning   ✦ = Available in Canada

Neck Cancer above for dose reduction guidelines in the event of toxicities.

NURSING CONSIDERATIONS

ℂ Do not confuse Taxotere with Taxol (also an antineoplastic).

ADMINISTRATION/STORAGE

IV 1. Premedicate clients with oral corticosteroids, such as dexamethasone, 16 mg/day (e.g., 8 mg twice a day) for 3 days starting 1 day prior to docetaxel in order to reduce the incidence and severity of fluid retention and hypersensitivity reactions

2. Check package insert for cisplatin and fluorouracil dose modifications and delays.

3. Allow vials to stand at room temperature for about 5 min before using. Both injection concentrate and the diluent vials contain an overfill. The 20-mg vial contains 23.6 mg and the 80-mg vial contains 94.4 mg of the drug. Only the final concentration of 10 mg/mL, prepared with the supplied diluent, should be used for preparing doses. Using the entire vial content for each 20- or 80-mg dose may result in a significant overdose when using multiple vials.

4. Diluted concentrate of 10 mg/mL is then used to prepare the solution for infusion. Withdraw the required amount of docetaxel using a calibrated syringe. Inject into a 250-mL infusion bag or bottle of either 0.9% NaCl injection or D5W to produce a final concentration of 0.3–0.9 mg/mL; administer as a 1-hr infusion. If doses greater than 240 mg are required, use more solution so that the concentration to be infused does not exceed 0.9 mg/mL.

5. Protect drug from light; refrigerate at 2–8°C (36–46°F). The premixed solution is stable for 8 hr. Do not store in PVC bags.

ASSESSMENT

1. List reasons for therapy, disease onset, previous agents used, outcome.

2. Note previous experience with this drug. If previous hypersensitivity, do not rechallenge. Premedication helps prevent hypersensitivity reactions and reduce adverse side effects.

3. List other drugs prescribed; ensure none interact.

4. Monitor CBC, LFTs. Drug causes bone marrow suppression. Do not give if AST or ALT above 1.5 ULN, alkaline phosphatase above 2.5 ULN or neutrophil count <1,500/mm³; Nadir: 8 days.

CLIENT/FAMILY TEACHING

1. Used to treat resistant cancers and can cause a drop in WBCs and altered liver function which must be monitored closely to prevent any severe reactions.

2. May experience a rash 1 week after treatment; should subside.

3. Prepare for hair loss.

4. Report adverse effects including infection, fever, sore throat, unusual bruising/bleeding, fluid retention, illness. Avoid crowds and people with contagious diseases.

OUTCOMES/EVALUATE

Control of metastatic process

Docusate calcium (Dioctyl calcium sulfosuccinate)

(**DOCK**-you-sayt)

CLASSIFICATION(S):

Laxative, emollient

PREGNANCY CATEGORY: C

OTC: DC Softgels, Pro-Cal-Sof, Sulfolax Calcium, Surfak Liquigels.

♣**OTC:** ratio-Docusate Calcium.

Docusate sodium (Dioctyl sodium sulfosuccinate)

PREGNANCY CATEGORY: C

OTC: Colace, D-S-S, D.O.S., Dioctyn Softgels, Docu, Dulcolax Stool Softener, Ex-Lax Stool Softener, Gena Soft, Non-Habit Forming Stool Softener, Phillips Liqui-Gels, Regulex SS, Silace Stool Softener, Soflax.

♣**OTC:** Selax, Soflax, ratio-Docusate Sodium.

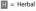

SEE ALSO *LAXATIVES.*

USES

(1) To lessen strain of defecation in persons with hernia or CV diseases or other diseases in which straining at stool should be avoided. (2) Megacolon or bedridden clients. (3) Constipation associated with dry, hard stools. *NOTE:* The microemulsion formulation is indicated for relief of occasional constipation in children over the age of 3 years.

ACTION/KINETICS

Action

Acts by lowering the surface tension of the feces and promoting penetration by water and fat, thus increasing the softness of the fecal mass. Not absorbed systemically and does not seem to interfere with the absorption of nutrients.

Pharmacokinetics

A microenema formulation is available for clients aged 3 and older. **Onset:** 12–72 hr.

CONTRAINDICATIONS

Nausea, vomiting, abdominal pain, and intestinal obstruction.

SIDE EFFECTS

Most Common

Diarrhea, N&V, perianal irritation, flatulence, cramps.

See *Laxatives* for a complete list of possible side effects.

DRUG INTERACTIONS

Docusate may ↑ absorption of mineral oil from the GI tract

HOW SUPPLIED

Docusate calcium. *Capsules:* 50 mg, 240 mg.

Docusate sodium. *Capsules:* 50 mg, 100 mg, 250 mg; *Capsules, Soft Gel:* 50 mg, 100 mg, 250 mg; *Oral Liquid:* 10 mg/mL; *Syrup:* 20 mg/5 mL, 50 mg/15 mL, 60 mg/15 mL, 100 mg/30 mL; *Tablets:* 100 mg.

DOSAGE

Docusate Calcium

- **CAPSULES**

  Laxative.

Adults: 240 mg/day until bowel movements are normal; **pediatric, over 6 years:** 50–150 mg/day.

Docusate Sodium

- **CAPSULES; CAPSULES, SOFT GEL; ORAL LIQUID; SYRUP; TABLETS**

  Laxative.

Adults and children over 12 years: 50–500 mg, depending on the product; **6–12 years:** 40–120 mg, depending on the product; **3–6 years:** 20–60 mg; **pediatric, under 3 years:** 10–40 mg.

NURSING CONSIDERATIONS

ASSESSMENT

1. Note reasons for therapy, onset, causes, other agents prescribed.
2. Assess activity levels, diet, water intake, exercise routines. Have client identify habits and BM frequency.
3. When used in enemas, add 50–100 mg (5–10 mL) to a retention or flushing enema.

CLIENT/FAMILY TEACHING

1. May give oral solutions with milk or juices to help mask bitter taste.
2. Drink a glass of water with each dose.
3. Because docusate salts are minimally absorbed, it may require 1–3 days to soften fecal matter.

OUTCOMES/EVALUATE

Elimination of a soft, formed stool; ↓ straining

Dofetilide   ■

(doh-**FET**-ih-lyd)

CLASSIFICATION(S):

Antiarrhythmic

PREGNANCY CATEGORY: C

Rx: Tikosyn.

SEE ALSO *ANTIARRHYTHMIC DRUGS.*

USES

(1) Conversion of atrial fibrillation or atrial flutter to normal sinus rhythm. (2) Maintenance of normal sinus rhythm in clients witih atrial fibrillation/atrial flutter of more than 1 week duration and who have been converted to normal sinus rhythm. Reserve for those in whom atrial fibrillation/atrial flutter is highly symptomatic due to life-threatening ventricular arrhythmias. *NOTE:* Available only to hospitals and prescrib-

---

ers who receive dosing and treatment initiation education through the *Tikosyn in Pharmacy System* (phone: 1-877-845-6796 or www.tikosyn.com/TIPS_info.asp.

ACTION/KINETICS
Action
Acts by blocking the cardiac ion channel carrying the rapid component of the delayed rectifier potassium currents. Blocks only I_{Kr} with no significant block of other repolarizing potassium currents (e.g., I_{Ks}, I_{K1}). No effect on sodium channels or adrenergic receptors. Dofetilide increases the monophasic action potential duration due to delayed repolarization.

Pharmacokinetics
Maximum plasma levels: 2–3 hr during fasting. Steady state plasma levels reached in 2–3 days. Metabolized in the liver and excreted in the urine. **t½, terminal:** About 10 hr. Women have lower oral clearances than men.

CONTRAINDICATIONS
Congenital or acquired long QT syndromes, in those with a baseline QT interval greater than 440 msec (500 msec in clients with ventricular conduction abnormalities), severe renal impairment (C_{CR} less than 20 mL/min). Concomitant use of verapamil, cimetidine, trimethoprim (alone or with sulfamethoxazole), ketoconazole, prochlorperazine, megestrol. Lactation.

SPECIAL CONCERNS
■ (1) To minimize risk of induced arrhythmia, place clients started or restarted on dofetilide in a facility that can determine creatinine clearance and provide continuous ECG monitoring and cardiac resuscitation for a minimum of 3 days. (2) Drug is available only to hospitals and prescribers who have received appropriate dofetilide dosing and treatment initiation education.■ There is a greater risk of dofetilide-induced TdP (type of ventricular tachycardia) in female clients than in male clients. Use with caution in severe hepatic impairment. Use with drugs that prolong the QT interval has not been studied with dofetilide use; therefore, do not use bepridil, certain macrolide antibiotics, phenothiazines, or TCAs with dofetilide. Safety and efficacy have not been determined in children less than 18 years of age.

SIDE EFFECTS
Most Common
Headache, chest pain, dizziness, ventricular tachycardia/arrhythmias, respiratory tract infection, dyspnea, nausea, flu syndrome, insomnia.

CV: Ventricular arrhythmias (especially TdP type ventricular tachycardia, *torsades de pointes*, angina pectoris, atrial fibrillation, hypertension, palpitation, supraventricular tachycardia, ventricular tachycardia, bradycardia, cerebral ischemia, *CVA, MI, heart arrest, ventricular fibrillation*, AV block, bundle branch block, heart block. **CNS:** Headache, dizziness, insomnia, anxiety, paresthesia. **GI:** Nausea, diarrhea, abdominal pain. **Respiratory:** Respiratory tract infection, dyspnea, increased cough. **Miscellaneous:** Chest pain, flu syndrome, accidental injury, back pain, rash, arthralgia, asthenia, pain, peripheral edema, sweating, UTI, angioedema, edema, facial paralysis, flaccid paralysis, liver damage, paralysis, *sudden death*, syncope.

OD OVERDOSE MANAGEMENT
Symptoms: Excessive prolongation of QT interval. *Treatment:* Symptomatic and supportive. Initiate cardiac monitoring. Can use charcoal slur but is effective only when given within 15 min of dofetilide. To treat TdP or overdose, may give isoproterenol infusion, with or without cardiac pacing. IV Mg sulfate may be useful to manage TdP. Monitor until QT interval returns to normal.

DRUG INTERACTIONS
Amiloride / Possible ↑ dofetilide levels
Amiodarone / Possible ↑ dofetilide levels
Cannabinoids / Possible ↑ dofetilide levels
Cimetidine / ↑ Risk of arrhythmia (TdP) R/T ↓ liver metabolism of dofetilide
Digoxin / ↑ Risk of torsades de pointes
Diltiazem / Possible ↑ dofetilide levels
Grapefruit juice / Possible ↑ dofetilide levels

 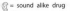

D

Ketoconazole / ↑ Risk of arrhythmia (TdP) R/T ↓ liver metabolism of dofetilide

Macrolide antibiotics / Possible ↑ dofetilide levels

Megestrol / Possible ↑ dofetilide levels → arrhythmias

Metformin / Possible ↑ dofetilide levels

Nefazadone / Possible ↑ dofetilide levels

Norfloxacin / Possible ↑ dofetilide levels

Potassium-depleting diuretics / Hypokalemia or hypomagnesemia may occur, → ↑ potential for torsades de pointes

Prochlorperazine / Possible ↑ dofetilide levels → arrhythmias

Quinine / Possible ↑ dofetilide levels

Triamterene / Possible ↑ dofetilide levels

Trimethoprim or Trimethoprim/Sulfamethoxazole / ↑ Risk of arrhythmia (TdP) R/T ↓ liver metabolism of dofetilide

Verapamil / Possible ↑ dofetilide levels → arrhythmias

Zafirlukast / Possible ↑ dofetilide levels

HOW SUPPLIED

Capsules: 125 mcg, 250 mcg, 500 mcg.

DOSAGE

- **CAPSULES**

  Conversion of atrial fibrillation/flutter; maintenance of normal sinus rhythm.

The dosing for dofetilide must be undertaken using the following steps:

1. Before giving the first dose, determine the QTc using an average of 5–10 beats. If the QTc is greater than 440 msec (500 msec in those with ventricular conduction abnormalities), dofetilide is contraindicated. Also, do not use if the heart rate <60 bpm.

2. Before giving the first dose, calculate the C_{CR} using the following formulas: *Males:* (Weight [kg] x [140–age])/(72 x serum creatinine [mg/dL]) *Females:* 0.84 x male value

3. Determine starting dose of dofetilide as follows: **C_{CR} >60 mL/min:** 500 mcg 2 times/day; **C_{CR} 40–60 mL/min:** 250 mcg 2 times/day; **C_{CR} 20 to <40 mL/min:** 125 mcg 2 times/day; **C_{CR} <20 mL/min:** DO NOT USE DOFETILIDE; CONTRAINDICATED IN THESE CLIENTS. The maximum daily dose is 500 mcg 2 times/day.

4. Give adjusted dose based on C_{CR} and begin continuous ECG monitoring.

5. At 2–3 hr after giving the first dofetilide dose, determine the QTc. If the QTc has increased by >15% compared with the baseline established in Step 1 or if the QTc is 500 msec (550 msec in those with ventricular conduction abnormalities), adjust subsequent dosing as follows: If the starting dose based on C_{CR} is 500 mcg 2 times/day, the adjusted dose (for QTc prolongation) is 250 mcg twice/day. If the starting dose is 250 mcg twice a day, the adjusted dose (for QTc prolongation) is 125 mcg 2 times/day. If the starting dose is 125 mcg twice a day, the adjusted dose (for QTc prolongation) is 125 mcg once daily.

6. At 2–3 hr after each subsequent dose of dofetilide, determine QTc for in-hospital doses 2 through 5. No further down titration of dofetilide based on QTc is recommended. Discontinue if at any time after the second dose of dofetilide, the QTc is greater than 500 msec (550 msec in those with ventricular conduction abnormalities).

7. Continuously monitor by ECG for a minimum of 3 days or for a minimum of 12 hr after electrical or pharmacologic conversion to normal sinus rhythm, whichever time is greater.

NURSING CONSIDERATIONS

ADMINISTRATION/STORAGE

1. Therapy must be started (and, if necessary, reinitiated) in a setting where continuous ECG monitoring and personnel trained in the management of serious ventricular arrhthymias are available for a minimum of 3 days.

2. Do not discharge clients within 12 hr of electrical or pharmacologic conversion to normal sinus rhythm.

3. Prior to electrical or pharmacologic cardioversion, anticoagulate clients with atrial fibrillation according to usual medical practices. Anticoagulants may be continued after cardioversion. Correct hypokalemia before starting dofetilide therapy.

4. Re-evaluate renal function q 3 months or as warranted. Discontinue dofetilide if the QTc is >500 msec (550

msec in those with ventricular conduction abnormalities) and monitor carefully until QTc returns to baseline levels. If renal function decreases, adjust dose as directed under *Dosage*.

5. The highest dose of 500 mcg twice a day is the most effective. However, the risk of torsades de pointes (TdP) is increased. Thus, a lower dose may be used. If at any time the lower dose is increased, the client must be hospitalized for 3 days. Previous tolerance of higher doses does not eliminate the need for hospitalization.

6. Do not consider electrical conversion if the client does not convert to normal sinus rhythm within 24 hr after starting dofetilide.

7. Withdraw previous antiarrhythmic drug therapy before starting dofetilide therapy; during withdrawal, carefully monitor for a minimum of 3 plasma half-lives. Do not initiate dofetilide following amiodarone therapy until amiodarone plasma levels are less than 0.3 mcg/mL or until amiodarone has been withdrawn for 3 or more months.

8. Protect capsules from moisture and humidity. Dispense in tight containers.

ASSESSMENT

1. Identify arrhythmia and duration. Note S&S associated with arrhythmia. Monitor ECG rhythm continuously for at least three days after starting therapy for evidence of prolonged QT interval; requires reduction in dose or stopping therapy.

2. Note drugs prescribed; ensure none interact. Do not give within 3 mo of amiodarone therapy unless level below 0.3 mcg/mL. Avoid use of drugs that prolong QT interval.

3. Monitor electrolytes, renal and LFTs; avoid use with dysfunction. Low K and Mg can increase risk of torsades de pointes.

4. Drug is available only through the Tikosyn Dosing Program with provider education.

CLIENT/FAMILY TEACHING

1. Take exactly as prescribed without regard to food or meals; avoid grapefruit juice.

2. Do not double the next dose if dose missed. Take next dose at usual time.

3. Report any change in prescriptions or OTC/supplement use. Inform all providers if hospitalized or prescribed a new medication for any condition. Do not take any interacting drugs for at least two days after stopping dofetilide; allow drug to get out of system.

4. **Do not** use OTC Tagamet, **may use** Zantac, Pepcid, Axid and Prevacid for acid indigestion or ulcer therapy.

5. Report adverse effects including diarrhea, sweating, vomiting, loss of thirst/appetite to provider immediately.

6. Read the package insert prior to use. Drug adherence is imperative with this therapy. Must report as scheduled for ECG evaluation and report any adverse effects to ensure no serious drug-related complications.

OUTCOMES/EVALUATE

- Conversion of atrial fibrillation/flutter to NSR
- Maintenance of NSR once converted

Dolasetron mesylate
(dohl-**AH**-seh-tron)

CLASSIFICATION(S):
Antinauseant, serotonin 5-HT$_3$ antagonist
PREGNANCY CATEGORY: B
Rx: Anzemet.

USES
(1) Prevention of N&V associated with emetogenic cancer chemotherapy (initially and repeat courses). (2) Prevention of postoperative N&V. (3) Treatment of postoperative N&V (IV use). *Investigational:* Radiotherapy-induced N&V.

ACTION/KINETICS
Action
Selective serotonin 5-HT$_3$ antagonist that prevents N&V by inhibiting released serotonin from combining with receptors on vagal efferents that initiate vomiting reflex. May also cause acute,

usually reversible, PR and QTc prolongation and QRS widening, perhaps due to blockade of sodium channels by active metabolite of dolasetron.

Pharmacokinetics

Well absorbed from GI tract. Metabolized to active hydrodolasetron. **Peak plasma levels:** 1 hr; **$t^{1/2}$:** 8.1 hr. Food does not affect bioavailability. Hydrodolasetron is excreted through urine and feces. Is eliminated more quickly in children than in adults.

SPECIAL CONCERNS

Use with caution during lactation and in those who have or may develop prolongation of cardiac conduction intervals, including QTc. These include clients with hypokalemia or hypomagnesemia, those taking diuretics with potential for electrolyte abnormalities, in congenital QT syndrome, those taking anti-arrhythmic drugs or other drugs which lead to QT prolongation, and cumulative high dose anthracycline therapy. Safety and efficacy in children less than 2 years of age have not been determined.

SIDE EFFECTS

Most Common

Headache, diarrhea, fatigue, drowsiness, dizziness, bradycardia, hypotension, hypertension, abdominal pain, fever, pain.

Chemotherapy clients. Headache, fatigue, diarrhea, bradycardia, dizziness, pain, tachycardia, dyspepsia, chills, shivering. **Postoperative clients.** Headache, hypotension, dizziness, fever, pruritus, oliguria, hypertension, tachycardia. **Chemotherapy or postoperative clients. CV:** Hypotension, edema, peripheral edema, peripheral ischemia, thrombophlebitis, phlebitis. **GI:** Constipation, dyspepsia, abdominal pain, anorexia, pancreatitis, taste perversion. **CNS:** Flushing, vertigo, paresthesia, tremor, ataxia, twitching, agitation, sleep disorder, depersonalization, confusion, anxiety, abnormal dreaming. **Dermatologic:** Rash, increased sweating. **Hematologic:** Hematuria, epistaxis, anemia, purpura, hematoma, thrombocytopenia. **Hypersensitivity:** Rarely, *anaphylaxis*, facial edema, urticaria.

Musculoskeletal: Myalgia, arthralgia. **Respiratory:** Dyspnea, bronchospasm. **GU:** Dysuria, polyuria, acute renal failure. **Ophthalmic:** Abnormal vision, photophobia. **Miscellaneous:** Tinnitus.

LABORATORY TEST CONSIDERATIONS

↑ PTT, AST, ALT, alkaline phosphatase. Prolonged prothrombin time.

DRUG INTERACTIONS

Atenolol / ↓ Hydrodolasetron clearance (by about 27%) when dolasetron given IV
Cimetidine / ↑ Hydrodolasetron levels after given with cimetidine for 7 days
Rifamycins / ↓ Dolasetron levels
Ziprasidone / ↑ Risk of life-threatening cardiac arrhythmias, including torsade de pointes; do not give together

HOW SUPPLIED

Injection: 20 mg/mL; *Tablets:* 50 mg, 100 mg.

DOSAGE

- **TABLETS**

  Prevention of cancer chemotherapy-induced N&V.

  Adults: 100 mg within 1 hr before chemotherapy. **Children, 2 to 16 years:** 1.8 mg/kg within 1 hr before chemotherapy, up to a maximum of 100 mg.

  Prevention of postoperative N&V.

  Adults: 100 mg within 2 hr before surgery. **Children, 2 to 16 years:** 1.2 mg/kg within 2 hr before surgery, up to a maximum of 100 mg.

- **IV**

  Prevention of cancer chemotherapy-induced N&V.

  Adults: 1.8 mg/kg as a single dose about 30 min before chemotherapy. Alternatively, a fixed dose of 100 mg can be given over 30 seconds. **Children, 2 to 16 years:** 1.8 mg/kg as a single dose about 30 min before chemotherapy, up to a maximum of 100 mg.

  Prevention or treatment of postoperative N&V.

  Adults: 12.5 mg given as a single dose. **Children, 2 to 16 years:** 0.35 mg/kg, up to a maximum of 12.5 mg. For adults and children, give about 15 min before cessation of anesthesia or as soon as nausea and vomiting presents.

Bold Italic = life threatening side effect   ■ = black box warning   ✦ = Available in Canada

NOTE: For children, injection may be mixed with apple or apple-grape juice and used for oral dosing. When injection is used PO, recommended dose for prevention of cancer chemotherapy N&V is 1.8 mg/kg (up to a maximum of 100 mg) and dose for prevention of postoperative N&V is 1.2 mg/kg (up to a maximum of 100 mg). Diluted injection may be kept up to 2 hr at room temperature before use.

NURSING CONSIDERATIONS

 Do not confuse Anzemet with Avandamet (combination drug oral hypoglycemic).

ADMINISTRATION/STORAGE

[IV] 1. Injection can be safely infused as rapidly as 100 mg/30 seconds. May also be diluted to 50 mL with 0.9% NaCl, D5W, D5/0.45% NaCl, D5/RL, RL, and 10% mannitol injection. Dilutions are given over 15 min. Diluted product is stable for 24 hr (48 hr if refrigerated).
2. Do not mix with any other drugs.
3. Flush infusion line before and after administration of dolasetron.
4. Inspect visually for particulate matter and discoloration before using.
5. Store injection at controlled room temperature protected from light.

ASSESSMENT

1. Note reasons for therapy: N&V R/T chemotherapy or postoperatively.
2. List drugs prescribed; ensure none interact.
3. Monitor CBC, electrolytes, Mg, ECG and fluid status. Assess for prolonged conduction intervals (QT).
4. Give 1 hr before chemotherapy or 2 hr before surgery to gain desired effect. May experience headache.
5. With children, calculate appropriate dose (cancer chemotherapy or postop N&V); may administer orally with apple or apple-grape juice.

CLIENT/FAMILY TEACHING

1. Drug is given parenterally to prevent N&V with chemo/surgery.
2. May mix injection in apple juice for oral administration just before dosing. Discard mixture after 2 hours.
3. Report any adverse effects or lack of response.

OUTCOMES/EVALUATE

Inhibition of chemotherapy induced/ postop N&V

Donepezil hydrochloride
(dohn-**EP**-eh-zil)

D

CLASSIFICATION(S):
Treatment of Alzheimer's disease
PREGNANCY CATEGORY: C
Rx: Aricept, Aricept ODT.

USES

Treatment of mild to severe dementia of the Alzheimer's type. Is combined with memantine (Namenda) to lower the decline of mental and physical function in Alzheimer's disease. *Investigational:* Vascular dementia; improve memory in multiple sclerosis clients; post-stroke aphasia.

ACTION/KINETICS

Action

A decrease in cholinergic function may be the cause of Alzheimer's disease. Donepezil, a cholinesterase inhibitor, exerts its effect by enhancing cholinergic function by increasing levels of acetylcholine through reversible inhibition of acetylcholinesterase. No evidence that the drug alters the course of the underlying dementing process.

Pharmacokinetics

Well absorbed from the GI tract; is 100% bioavailable. **Peak plasma levels:** 3–4 hr; steady state reached in 15 days. Food does not affect the rate or extent of absorption. **t½, elimination:** 70 hr. Metabolized in the liver, and both unchanged drug and metabolites are excreted in the urine and feces. **Plasma protein binding:** 96%.

CONTRAINDICATIONS

Hypersensitivity to piperidine derivatives.

SPECIAL CONCERNS

Use with caution in clients with a history of asthma or obstructive pulmonary disease. Safety and efficacy have not been determined for use in children.

D

SIDE EFFECTS
Most Common
Anorexia, diarrhea, fatigue, insomnia, muscle cramps, N&V, dizziness, headache, ecchymosis.
NOTE: Side effects with an incidence of 1% or greater are listed. **GI:** N&V, diarrhea, anorexia, fecal incontinence, GI bleeding (especially those at risk of developing ulcers), bloating, epigastric pain, abdominal pain, constipation, dyspepsia, gastroenteritis. **CNS:** Insomnia, dizziness, depression, confusion, abnormal dreams, somnolence, abnormal crying, aggression/hostility, aphasia, ataxia, delusions, increased libido, irritability, nervousness, paresthesia, restlessness, tremor, ataxia, emotional lability, hallucinations, personality disorder, abnormal gait, anxiety, *seizures*. **CV:** Hypertension, vasodilation, atrial fibrillation, hot flashes, hypotension, heart block, bradycardia, *hemorrhage*, syncope, ecchymosis, ECG abnormalities, *heart failure*. **Body as a whole:** Headache, pain (in various locations), fever, asthenia, infection, accident, fatigue, influenza, fungal infection, chest/back pain, edema, peripheral edema, toothache. **Hematologic:** Anemia. **Musculoskeletal:** Muscle cramps, arthritis, bone fracture. **Dermatologic:** Diaphoresis, urticaria, pruritus, eczema, rash, skin ulcer. **GU:** Urinary incontinence, nocturia, frequent urination, cystitis, hematuria, UTI. **Respiratory:** Dyspnea, sore throat, bronchitis, increased cough, pharyngitis, pneumonia. **Ophthalmic:** Cataract, eye irritation, blurred vision. **Miscellaneous:** Dehydration, ecchymosis, weight loss.

LABORATORY TEST CONSIDERATIONS
↑ Creatine phosphokinase, alkaline phosphatase, ALT, AST, lactic dehydrogenase. Hyperlipemia, glycosuria.

OD OVERDOSE MANAGEMENT
Symptoms: Cholinergic crisis characterized by severe N&V, salivation, sweating, bradycardia, hypotension, respiratory depression, collapse, convulsions, increased muscle weakness (may cause death if respiratory muscles are involved). *Treatment:* Atropine sulfate at an initial dose of 1–2 mg IV with subsequent doses based on the response. General supportive measures.

DRUG INTERACTIONS
Anticholinergic drugs / The cholinesterase inhibitor activity of donepezil interferes with the activity of anticholinergics
Bethanechol / Synergistic effect
Carbamazepine / ↑ Donepezil elimination R/T induction of CYP3A4 and CYP2D6
Dexamethasone / ↑ Donepezil elimination R/T induction of CYP3A4 and CYP2D6
Ketoconazole / ↑ Peak plasma levels of donepezil R/T ↓ breakdown by liver
NSAIDs / ↑ Gastric acid secretion due to donepezil → ↑ risk of active or occult GI bleeding
Phenobarbital / ↑ Donepezil elimination R/T induction of CYP3A4 and CYP2D6
Quinidine / ↑ Peak plasma levels of donepezil R/T ↓ breakdown by liver
Rifampin / ↑ Donepezil elimination R/T induction of CYP3A4 and CYP2D6
Succinylcholine / ↑ Muscle relaxant effect

HOW SUPPLIED
Oral Solution: 1 mg/mL; *Tablets:* 5 mg, 10 mg; *Tablets, Oral Disintegrating:* 5 mg, 10 mg.

DOSAGE
• **ORAL SOLUTION; TABLETS; TABLETS, ORAL DISINTEGRATING**
Mild to moderate Alzheimer's disease.
Initial: 5 or 10 mg once daily. Use of a 10-mg dose did not provide a clinical effect greater than the 5-mg dose; however, in some clients, 10 mg daily may be superior. Do not increase the dose to 10 mg until clients have been on a daily dose of 5 mg for 4 to 6 weeks.
Severe Alzheimer's disease.
10 mg given once daily. Do not achieve a dose of 10 mg until clients have been on a daily dose of 5 mg for 4–6 weeks.

NURSING CONSIDERATIONS
© Do not confuse Aricept with Aciphex (a proton pump inhibitor).

ADMINISTRATION/STORAGE
1. Donepezil orally disintegrating tablets are bioequivalent to donepezil tab-

---

Bold Italic = life threatening side effect   ■ = black box warning   ♣ = Available in Canada

lets. Donepezil oral solution is bioequivalent to donepezil tablets.

2. Store at controlled room temperatures from 15–30°C (59–86°F).

ASSESSMENT

1. Document onset/duration, other agents trialed, outcome.

2. Describe clinical presentation. Note MME (mini mental exam) scores.

3. Note history of asthma or COPD.

4. Monitor for symptoms of active or occult GI bleeding.

5. Assess ECG and labs.

CLIENT/FAMILY TEACHING

1. Take in the evening, just prior to bedtime. May take with or without food.

2. Place the oral disintegrating tablet on the tongue; after the tablet dissolves, drink water.

3. Drug does not cure disease but helps alleviate symptoms or slow physical and mental progression of disease, especially when used with memantine.

4. Report adverse effects including irregular pulse or dizzy spells, lack of response, worsening of symptoms.

5. Ensure caregiver is aware of outside programs available to these clients for socialization and activity. Advise all providers that drug is prescribed; especially before anesthesia use.

OUTCOMES/EVALUATE

Improved cognitive functioning with Alzheimer's-type dementia.

Dopamine hydrochloride ■ IV ⓒ

(**DOH**-pah-meen)

CLASSIFICATION(S):

Sympathomimetic, direct-acting and indirect-acting

PREGNANCY CATEGORY: C

Rx: Dopamine hydrochloride.

SEE ALSO *SYMPATHOMIMETIC DRUGS.*

USES

(1) Correction of hemodynamic imbalances present in the shock syndrome due to MI, trauma, endotoxic septicemia, open heart surgery, renal failure, and chronic cardiac decompensation in CHF. (2) Poor perfusion of vial organs, including the kidney. Concurrent administration of dopamine and diuretics may produce an additive or potentiating effect. (3) Increase cardiac output. (4) Hypotension due to inadequate cardiac output. Dopamine has little effect on systemic vascular resistance. *Investigational:* Chronic obstructive pulmonary disease, CHF, respiratory distress syndrome in infants.

ACTION/KINETICS

Action

Dopamine is the immediate precursor of epinephrine in the body. Exogenously administered, it produces direct stimulation of beta-1 receptors and variable (dose-dependent) stimulation of alpha receptors (peripheral vasoconstriction). Will cause a release of norepinephrine from its storage sites. These actions result in increased myocardial contraction, CO, and SV, as well as increased renal blood flow and sodium excretion. Exerts little effect on DBP and induces fewer arrhythmias than are seen with isoproterenol.

Pharmacokinetics

Onset: 5 min after IV. **Duration:** <10 min (MAO inhibitors increase duration to 1 hr). **t½, plasma:** 2 min. Does not cross the blood-brain barrier. Metabolized in liver and 80% excreted in urine. About 25% is taken up into adrenergic nerve terminals where it is hydroxylated to form norepinephrine.

ADDITIONAL CONTRAINDICATIONS

Pheochromocytoma, uncorrected tachycardia, ventricular fibrillation, or arrhythmias. Pediatric clients.

SPECIAL CONCERNS

■ Antidote for peripheral ischemia: To prevent sloughing and necrosis in ischemic areas, the area should be infiltrated as soon as possible with 10 to 15 mL of saline solution containing 5 to 10 mg of phentolamine, an adrenergic blocking agent. A syringe with a fine hypodermic needle should be used, and the solution liberally infiltrated throughout the ischemic area. Sympathetic blockade with phentolamine causes immedi-

---

ate and conspicuous local hyperemic changes if the area is infiltrated within 12 hours. Therefore, phentolamine should be given as soon as possible after the extravasation is noted.■ Use with caution during lactation. Safety and efficacy have not been established in children. Dosage may have to be adjusted in clients with a history of occlusive vascular disease.

SIDE EFFECTS

Most Common

Tachycardia, anginal pain, palpitations, dyspnea, N&V, headache, anxiety, hypertension, hypotension.

CV: Ectopic heartbeats, tachycardia, anginal pain, palpitations, vasoconstriction, hypo-/hypertension. Infrequently: Aberrant conduction, bradycardia, widened QRS complex. **CNS:** Headache, anxiety. **GI:** N&V. **Dermatologic:** Piloerection. **Respiratory:** Dyspnea. **Metabolic:** Azotemia. **Miscellaneous:** Gangrene of the extremities, especially if given for long periods or in those with occlusive vascular disease; peripheral cyanosis. Extravasation may result in necrosis and sloughing of surrounding tissue.

ADDITIONAL DRUG INTERACTIONS

Alpha- or beta-adrenergic blocking drugs / Antagonism of dopamine effects
Anesthetics, halogenated hydrocarbon / Sensitization of myocardium to dopamine → serious arrhythmias
Diuretics / Additive or potentiating effect
Ergonovine / Possible severe hypertension
Guanethidine / Partial or total reversal of antihypertensive effect of guanethidine
Haloperidol / Suppression of dopaminergic renal and mesenteric vasodilation induced with low dose dopamine infusion
MAO inhibitors / ↑ Pressor response to dopamine by 6 to 20 fold → hypertension; avoid concomitant use
Oxytocic drugs / Possible severe persistent hypertension
Phenothiazines / Suppression of dopaminergic renal and mesenteric vasodilation induced with low dose dopamine infusion

Phenytoin / Possible seizures, severe hypotension, and bradycardia
Propranolol / ↓ Effect of dopamine
Tricyclic antidepressants / Possible ↓ dopamine pressor effect

OD **OVERDOSE MANAGEMENT**

Symptoms: Extravasation. Overdose may cause excessive BP elevation. *Treatment:* To prevent sloughing and necrosis if extravasation occurs, infiltrate as soon as possible with 10–15 mL of 0.9% NaCl solution containing 5–10 mg phentolamine using a syringe with a fine needle. Infiltrate liberally throughout the ischemic area. For overdosage, reduce the rate of administration or discontinue temporarily until condition has stablilized.

HOW SUPPLIED

Injection: 40 mg/mL, 80 mg/mL, 160 mg/mL; *Injection in 5% Dextrose:* 80 mg/100 mL (0.8 mg/mL), 160 mg/100 mL (1.6 mg/mL), 320 mg/100 mL (3.2 mg/mL).

DOSAGE

• IV INFUSION

Shock.

Initial: 2–5 mcg/kg/min; **then,** increase in increments of 1–4 mcg/kg/min at 10–30-min intervals until desired response is obtained.

Severely ill clients.

Initial: 5 mcg/kg/min; **then,** increase rate in increments of 5–10 mcg/kg/min up to 20–50 mcg/kg/min as needed. *NOTE:* Dopamine is a potent drug. Be sure to dilute the drug before administration. The drug should not be given as a bolus dose.

NURSING CONSIDERATIONS

℘ Do not confuse dopamine with dobutamine (also a sympathomimetic).

ADMINISTRATION/STORAGE

IV 1. Dopamine is a potent drug. It must be diluted before use—see package insert.
2. For reconstitution use dextrose or saline solutions: 200 mg/250 mL for a concentration of 0.8 mg/mL or 800 mcg/mL; 400 mg/250 mL for a concentration of 1.6 mg/mL or 1,600 mcg/mL. Alkaline solutions such as 5% NaHCO₃,

---

Bold Italic = life threatening side effect   ■ = black box warning   ♣ = Available in Canada

oxidizing agents, or iron salts will inactivate drug.

3. Infuse into a large vein (e.g., veins of the antecubital fossa) when possible to prevent possibility of extravasation into adjacent tissue. Extravasation may cause necrosis and tissue sloughing.

4. Avoid mixing dopamine with alteplase in the same container as a visible particulate matter has been observed.

5. Do not mix, add dopamine to amphotericin B solutions as amphotericin B is physically unstable in dopamine solutions.

6. Dilute just prior to administration, solution stable for 24 hr at room temperature; protect from light.

7. To prevent fluid overload, may use more concentrated solutions with higher doses.

8. Hypoxia, hypercapnia, and acidosis may reduce the effectiveness and/or increase the incidence of side effects of dopamine. Correct these conditions prior to or concurrently with dopamine administration.

9. If hypotension occurs during administration, rapidly increase infusion rate until adequate BP is reached. If hypotension persists, discontinue dopamine and use a more potent vasoconstrictor (e.g., norepinephrine).

10. Reduce dose if an increased number of ectopic beats are observed.

11. Administer using an electronic infusion device. Carefully reconstitute and calculate dosage.

12. When discontinuing, gradually decrease dose; sudden cessation may cause marked hypotension.

13. Some products contain sodium metabisulfite that may cause allergic reactions, including anaphylaxis and life-threatening or less severe asthmatic symptoms in susceptible people.

ASSESSMENT

Note reasons for therapy; ensure adequate hydration prior to infusion. List drugs prescribed to ensure none interact.

INTERVENTIONS

1. Monitor VS, I&O, and ECG; titrate infusion to maintain SBP as ordered.

2. Be prepared to monitor CVP and PAWP. Report ectopy, palpitations, anginal pain, or vasoconstriction.

CLIENT/FAMILY TEACHING

Drug is administered IV to improve cardiac function thus increasing BP and improving urine output. Report any chest pain, increased SOB, headaches, or IV site pain.

OUTCOMES/EVALUATE

- SBP >90; ↑ urine output
- Improved organ perfusion

Dornase alfa recombinant
(**DOR**-nace **AL**-fah)

CLASSIFICATION(S):
Treatment of cystic fibrosis
PREGNANCY CATEGORY: B
Rx: Pulmozyme.

USES

In cystic fibrosis (CF) clients in conjunction with standard therapy to decrease the frequency of respiratory infections that require parenteral antibiotics and to improve pulmonary function.

ACTION/KINETICS

Action

This drug is a highly purified solution of genetically engineered recombinant human deoxyribonuclease I (rhDNase), an enzyme that selectively cleaves DNA. The amino acid sequence is identical to that of the native human enzyme. Cystic fibrosis (CF) clients have viscous purulent secretions in the airways that contribute to reduced pulmonary function and worsening of infection. These secretions contain high concentrations of extracellular DNA released by degenerating leukocytes that accumulate as a result of infection. Dornase alfa hydrolyzes the DNA in sputum of CF clients, thereby reducing sputum viscoelasticity and reducing infections.

CONTRAINDICATIONS

Known sensitivity to dornase alfa or products from Chinese hamster ovary cells.

SPECIAL CONCERNS

Safety and effectiveness of daily use have not been demonstrated in clients with forced vital capacity (FVC) of less than 40% of predicted, or for longer than 12 months. Use with caution during lactation.

SIDE EFFECTS

Most Common

Pharyngitis, chest pain, rash, voice alteration, conjunctivitis, laryngitis.

Respiratory: Pharyngitis, voice alteration, laryngitis, *apnea*, bronchiectasis, bronchitis, change in sputum, cough increase, dyspnea, hemoptysis, lung function decrease, nasal polyps, pneumonia, pneumothorax, rhinitis, sinusitis, sputum increase, wheezing. **Body as a whole:** Abdominal pain, asthenia, fever, flu syndrome, malaise, sepsis, weight loss. **GI:** Intestinal obstruction, gall bladder disease, liver disease, pancreatic disease. **Miscellaneous:** Rash, urticaria, chest pain, conjunctivitis, diabetes mellitus, hypoxia.

HOW SUPPLIED

Solution for Inhalation: 1 mg/mL.

DOSAGE

- **SOLUTION FOR INHALATION**
  Cystic fibrosis.

One 2.5-mg (2.5 mL) single-dose ampule inhaled once daily using a recommended nebulizer (see *Administration/Storage*). Older clients and clients with baseline FVC above 85% may benefit from twice-daily dosing.

NURSING CONSIDERATIONS

ADMINISTRATION/STORAGE

1. Approved nebulizers include the disposable jet nebulizer Hudson T U-draft II, disposable jet nebulizer Marquest Acorn II in conjunction with a Pulmo-Aide compressor, and the reusable PARI LC Jet+ nebulizer in conjunction with the PARI PRONEB compressor. Safety and efficacy have been demonstrated with these only.
2. Do not dilute or mix with other drugs in nebulizer. Mixing could lead to adverse physicochemical or functional changes in dornase alfa.
3. Must be stored in the refrigerator at 2–8°C (36–46°F) in the protective foil pouch and protected from strong light.
4. Refrigerate when transported and do not expose to room temperature for more than 24 hr.
5. Discard if cloudy or discolored.
6. Product does not contain a preservative; thus, once opened, entire ampule must be used or discarded.

ASSESSMENT

1. Note age of CF symptom onset, therapies trialed, and outcome.
2. Drug is produced by genetically engineered Chinese hamster ovary cells; assess for sensitivity.
3. Monitor VS, PFTs, respiratory patterns and lung sounds.

CLIENT/FAMILY TEACHING

1. Drug is administered by inhalation of an aerosol mist generated by a compressed air-driven nebulizer system; review dose, frequency, and method for inhalation. Ensure familiarity with use, care, and storage of equipment and drug. Rinse equipment and mouth after each use.
2. Must be performed on a daily schedule to obtain full benefits. Must continue standard therapies for CF, e.g., chest PT, antibiotics, bronchodilators, oral and inhaled corticosteroids, enzyme supplements, vitamins, and analgesics during therapy.
3. Report symptoms that require immediate medical intervention: Severe rashes, itching, respiratory distress, fever. Have family members learn CPR.
4. Identify support groups that may assist to cope with this disease.

OUTCOMES/EVALUATE

- ↓ Respiratory tract infectious exacerbations; ↓ sputum viscosity
- Improved PFTs

Dorzolamide hydrochloride ophthalmic solution

(dor-**ZOH**-lah-myd)

CLASSIFICATION(S):
Antiglaucoma drug
PREGNANCY CATEGORY: C
Rx: Trusopt.

USES
Elevated intraocular pressure (IOP) in adults and children with ocular hypertension or open-angle glaucoma.

ACTION/KINETICS
Action
Decreases aqueous humor secretion in the ciliary processes of the eye by inhibiting carbonic anhydrase. Occurs by decreasing the formation of bicarbonate ions with a reduction in sodium and fluid transport and a subsequent decrease in intraocular pressure.

Pharmacokinetics
The drug may reach the systemic circulation, where it and the metabolite are excreted through the urine. The drug and metabolite also accumulate in RBCs.

CONTRAINDICATIONS
Use with severe renal impairment (C_{CR} <30 mL/min) or in soft contact lens wearers as the preservative (benzalkonium chloride) may be absorbed by the lenses. Lactation.

SPECIAL CONCERNS
Dorzolamide is a sulfonamide and, as such, may cause similar systemic reactions, including side effects and allergic reactions, as sulfonamides. Use with caution in hepatic impairment. Due to additive effects, concurrent use of dorzolamide with systemic carbonic anhydrase inhibitors is not recommended. Safety and efficacy have not been determined in children. It is possible geriatric clients may show greater sensitivity to the drug.

SIDE EFFECTS
Most Common
Ocular burning, stinging/discomfort immediately following administration, bitter taste, superficial punctate keratitis, ocular allergic reaction.

Ophthalmic: Conjunctivitis, lid reactions, bacterial keratitis (due to contamination by concurrent corneal disease). Ocular burning, stinging, or discomfort immediately following administration. Also, superficial punctate keratitis, ocular allergic reaction, blurred vision, tearing, dryness, photophobia, iridocyclitis (rare). **Miscellaneous:** Acid-base and electrolyte disturbances (i.e., similar to systemic use of carbonic anhydrase inhibitors). Also, bitter taste following instillation, headache, nausea, asthenia, fatigue. Rarely, skin rashes, urolithiasis, iridocyclitis.

HOW SUPPLIED
Ophthalmic Solution: 2%.

DOSAGE
- **OPHTHALMIC SOLUTION**
  Increased intraocular pressure.
  1 gtt in the affected eye(s) 3 times per day.

NURSING CONSIDERATIONS
ADMINISTRATION/STORAGE
Protect from light and store at 15–30°C (59–86°F).

ASSESSMENT
Document visual symptoms and baseline IOP. Note sensitivity to sulfonamides or impaired renal function.

CLIENT/FAMILY TEACHING
1. Review instillation procedure. Do not let dispenser tip come in contact with eye or surrounding structures; contamination may result. Apply light pressure to tear duct to prevent systemic drug absorption. Wash hands before and after administration.
2. Use only as prescribed. Report evidence of conjunctivitis, eye or lid reaction and stop therapy. Burning or stinging may accompany administration. A bitter taste may also be noted.
3. May be used with other topical ophthalmic drugs. If using more than one, give them at least 10 min apart.

 = see color insert   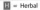 = Herbal   IV = Intravenous   = sound alike drug

4. Do not administer drops while wearing contact lenses; may absorb solution preservative. Remove, administer, and reinsert 15 min after administration.

OUTCOMES/EVALUATE

↓ IOP

Doxazosin mesylate ©
(dox-**AYZ**-oh-sin)

CLASSIFICATION(S):
Antihypertensive, peripherally-acting

PREGNANCY CATEGORY: B

Rx: Cardura, Cardura XL.

✚Rx: Apo-Doxazosin, Cardura-1, -2, -4, Gen-Doxazosin, Novo-Doxazosin, ratio-Doxazosin.

USES
(1) Hypertension, alone or in combination with diuretics, calcium channel blockers, ACE inhibitors, or beta blockers. (2) BPH, both urinary outflow obstruction and obstructive and irritative symptoms. May be used in BPH clients whether hypertensive or normotensive. Cardura XL is used only for BPH.

ACTION/KINETICS
Action
Blocks the alpha-1 (postjunctional) adrenergic receptors resulting in a decrease in systemic vascular resistance and a corresponding decrease in BP.

Pharmacokinetics
Peak plasma levels: 2–3 hr. **Peak effect:** 2–6 hr. Metabolized in the liver to active and inactive metabolites, which are excreted through the feces and urine. **t½:** 22 hr. **Plasma protein binding:** 98%.

CONTRAINDICATIONS
Clients allergic to prazosin or terazosin.

SPECIAL CONCERNS
Use with caution during lactation, in impaired hepatic function, or in those taking drugs known to influence hepatic metabolism. Safety and effectiveness have not been demonstrated in children. Due to the possibility of severe hypotension, do not use the 2-, 4-, and 8-mg tablets for initial therapy.

SIDE EFFECTS
Most Common
Dizziness, somnolence, headache, edema, fatigue/malaise, N&V, asthenia.

CV: Dizziness, syncope, vertigo, light-headedness, edema, palpitation, arrhythmia, postural hypotension, tachycardia, peripheral ischemia. **CNS:** Fatigue, headache, paresthesia, kinetic disorders, ataxia, somnolence, nervousness, depression, insomnia. **Musculoskeletal:** Arthralgia, arthritis, muscle weakness/cramps, myalgia, hypertonia. **GU:** Polyuria, sexual dysfunction, urinary incontinence/frequency. **GI:** Nausea, diarrhea, dry mouth, constipation, dyspepsia, flatulence, abdominal pain, vomiting. **Respiratory:** Rhinitis, epistaxis, dyspnea. **Miscellaneous:** Fatigue or malaise, rash, pruritus, flushing, urticaria, abnormal vision, conjunctivitis, eye pain, tinnitus, chest pain, asthenia, facial edema, generalized pain, slight weight gain.

OD OVERDOSE MANAGEMENT
Symptoms: Hypotension. *Treatment:* IV fluids.

HOW SUPPLIED
Tablets: 1 mg, 2 mg, 4 mg, 8 mg; *Tablets, Extended-Release:* 4 mg, 8 mg.

DOSAGE
• **TABLETS**
Hypertension.
Adults: initial, 1 mg once daily at bedtime; **then,** depending on the response (client's standing BP both 2–6 hr and 24 hr after a dose), the dose may be increased to 2 mg/day, and then 4 mg, 8 mg, and 16 mg (maximum), if needed to control BP.
Benign prostatic hyperplasia.
Initial: 1 mg once daily in the morning or evening. **Maintenance:** Depending on the urodynamics and symptoms, dose may be increased to 2 mg daily and then 4 or 8 mg once daily (maximum recommended dose). The recommended titration interval is 1–2 weeks.

• **TABLETS, EXTENDED-RELEASE**
Benign prostatic hyperplasia.
Initial: 4 mg once daily with breakfast. Depending on the response and tolerability, the dose may be increased to 8 mg, the maximum recommended dose.

Bold Italic = life threatening side effect   ■ = black box warning   ✚ = Available in Canada

Titrate at intervals of 3–4 weeks. If administration is discontinued for several days, restart therapy using the 4 mg daily dose.

NURSING CONSIDERATIONS

@ Do not confuse Cardura with Ridaura (gold-containing anti-inflammatory).

ADMINISTRATION/STORAGE

1. To minimize the possibility of severe hypotension, limit initial dosage to 1 mg/day.

2. Increasing the dose higher than 4 mg/day increases the possibility of severe syncope, postural dizziness, vertigo, and postural hypotension.

3. If switching from immediate-release to extended-release tablets, start therapy with 4 mg once daily. Before starting therapy with extended-release tablets, the final evening dose of the immediate-release tablets should not be taken.

4. Store from 15–30°C (59–86°F).

ASSESSMENT

1. Note reasons for therapy, other agents trialed. Explore experience with, any allergy to prazosin or terazosin; a quinazoline derivative.

2. Assess supine and standing BP at 2 to 6 hr and 24 hr after dosing. Check ECG for arrhythmia.

3. With BPH, score severity.

CLIENT/FAMILY TEACHING

1. Take once daily; do not stop abruptly. May take first dose at bedtime to minimize side effects.

2. Record BP and weight; note swelling of hands/feet. Dosage may be increased every 2 weeks for high BP and every 1 to 2 weeks for prostate enlargement.

3. Rise slowly to a sitting position before attempting to stand to prevent ↓ BP. This may occur 2–6 hr after a dose.

4. Driving and hazardous tasks should be avoided for 24 hr after first dose until effects are evident; may experience dizziness and fainting. Use care.

5. Report adverse effects or if S&S do not improve after several weeks of therapy as drug dosage may need adjustment.

OUTCOMES/EVALUATE

• ↓ BP

• ↓ S&S of BPH/nocturia

Doxepin hydrochloride ■ @

(**DOX**-eh-pin)

CLASSIFICATION(S):
Antidepressant, tricyclic
PREGNANCY CATEGORY: C
Rx: Prudoxin Cream 5%, Sinequan, Zonalon.
✦Rx: Apo-Doxepin, Novo-Doxepin.

SEE ALSO *ANTIDEPRESSANTS, TRICYCLIC*.

USES

Systemic. (1) Psychoneurotic clients with depression or anxiety. (2) Depression or anxiety due to alcoholism (do not give concomitantly with alcohol). (3) Psychotic depressive disorders with associated anxiety, including involutional depression and manic-depressive disorders. (4) Depression or anxiety associated with organic disease. *NOTE:* The symptoms of psychoneurosis that are most responsive include anxiety, tension, depression, somatic symptoms and concerns, sleep disturbances, guilt, lack of energy, fear, apprehension, and worry.

Topical. Dermatologic disorders including chronic urticaria, angioedema, atopic dermatitis, lichen simplex chronicus in adults, and nocturnal pruritus due to atopic eczema.

ACTION/KINETICS

Action

Metabolized to the active metabolite, desmethyldoxepin. Moderate anticholinergic effects and orthostatic hypotension; high sedative effects.

Pharmacokinetics

Therapeutic plasma levels of both doxepin and desmethyldoxepin: 100–200 ng/mL. **Time to reach steady state:** 2–8 days. **t½:** 8–24 hr.

CONTRAINDICATIONS

Use in children less than 12 years of age. Glaucoma or a tendency for urinary retention.

 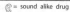

D

SPECIAL CONCERNS

■ Antidepressants increase the risk of suicidal thinking and behavior (suicidality) in short-term studies in children and adolescents with major depressive disorders and other psychiatric disorders. Anyone considering the use of doxepin or any other antidepressant in a child or adolescent must balance this risk with the clinical need. Clients who are started on therapy should be observed closely for clinical worsening, suicidality, or unusual changes in behavior. Families and caregivers should be advised of the need for close observation and communication with the prescriber. Doxepine is not approved for use in pediatric clients. Analysis of short-term (4–16 weeks) placebo-controlled trials in children and adolescents with major depressive disorder, obsessive-compulsive disorder, or other psychiatric disorders have revealed a greater risk of adverse reactions representing suicidal thinking or behavior during the first few months of treatment in those receiving antidepressants. The average risk of such reactions in such clients receiving antidepressants was 4%, twice the placebo risk of 2%. No suicides occurred in these trials.■ Safety has not been determined in pregnancy.

SIDE EFFECTS

Most Common

Drowsiness, dry mouth, blurred vision, constipation, urinary retention, sweating, tachycardia, weight gain/loss, orthostatic hypotension.

See also *Antidepressants, Tricyclic* for a complete list of possible side effects.

• **After systemic use**
Sedation, decreased libido, extrapyramidal symptoms, dermatitis, pruritus, fatigue, weight gain, edema, paresthesia, breast engorgement, insomnia, tremor, chills, tinnitus, and photophobia.

• **After topical use**
Burning, stinging, drowsiness, dry mouth.

HOW SUPPLIED

Capsules: 10 mg, 25 mg, 50 mg, 75 mg, 100 mg, 150 mg; *Cream:* 5%; *Oral Concentrate:* 10 mg/mL.

DOSAGE

• **CAPSULES; ORAL CONCENTRATE**
Antidepressant, mild to moderate anxiety or depression.

Adults, initial: 25 mg 3 times per day (up to 150 mg can be given at bedtime); **then,** adjust dosage to individual response (usual optimum dosage: 75–150 mg/day). **Geriatric clients, initially:** 25–50 mg/day; dose can be increased as needed and tolerated.

Severe symptoms.
Initial: 50 mg 3 times per day; **then,** gradually increase to 300 mg/day, if needed. Additional effects rarely obtained using doses over 300 mg/day.

Emotional symptoms with organic disease.
25–50 mg/day.

Antipruritic.
10–30 mg at bedtime.

• **CREAM, 5%**
Apply thin film 4 times per day with at least a 3–4 hr interval between applications.

NURSING CONSIDERATIONS

⍟ Do not confuse doxepin with Doxapram (an analeptic) or doxazosin (antidrenergic drug). Do not confuse Sinequan with saquinavir (antiviral) or with Singulair (an antiasthmatic).

ADMINISTRATION/STORAGE

1. Dilute oral concentrate with 4 oz water, milk, or orange, grapefruit, tomato, prune, or pineapple juice just before ingestion. Do not mix concentrate with carbonated beverages or grape juice.
2. For clients on methadone maintenance, concentrate can be mixed with methadone syrup and lemonade, orange juice, water, or sugar water (but not with grape juice).
3. Do not prepare or store bulk dilutions.
4. The antianxiety effect is manifested rapidly; however, it may take 2 to 3 weeks to observe optimum antidepressant effect.

ASSESSMENT

1. Note type, onset, characteristics of S&S. List other therapy trialed, outcome.
2. Assess depression/anxiety and identify any contributing factors. List all

---

Bold Italic = life threatening side effect   ■ = black box warning   ✦ = Available in Canada

drugs prescribed to ensure none interact.

CLIENT/FAMILY TEACHING
1. Take at bedtime to minimize sedative effects. Beneficial antidepressant effects may take up to 3 weeks, whereas antianxiety effects occur rapidly.
2. Do not perform activities that require mental alertness until drug effects realized; may experience drowsiness/dizziness (should subside after several weeks of therapy). Change positions slowly to prevent sudden drop in BP.
3. Avoid alcohol and any other CNS depressants. Do not stop drug abruptly.
4. Report adverse effects and lack of response; keep all followup visits.

OUTCOMES/EVALUATE
- ↓ S&S of anxiety/depression
- Improved sleeping patterns
- Control of neurogenic pain
- Relief of nocturnal pruritus

Doxorubicin hydrochloride, conventional (ADR)
(dox-oh-**ROO**-bih-sin)

CLASSIFICATION(S):
Antineoplastic, antibiotic
PREGNANCY CATEGORY: D
Rx: Adriamycin PFS, Adriamycin RDF.

Doxorubicin hydrochloride liposomal
PREGNANCY CATEGORY: D
Rx: Doxil.
✤Rx: Caelyx.

SEE ALSO ANTINEOPLASTIC AGENTS.

USES
Conventional doxorubicin: (1) To produce regression in the following disseminated cancers: Acute lymphoblastic leukemia, acute myeloblastic leukemia, Wilms' tumor, soft tissue and osteogenic sarcomas, neuroblastoma; cancer of the breast, ovaries, lungs, bladder, and thyroid; lymphomas (Hodgkin's and non-Hodgkin's), bronchogenic carcinoma (especially small cell histologic type) and gastric carcinoma. (2) With cyclophosphamide as a part of adjuvant therapy where there is evidence of axillary node tumor involvement following resection of primary breast cancer. *Investigational:* Cancer of the head and neck, cervix, liver, pancreas, prostate, testes, and endometrium.

Liposomal doxorubicin: (1) AIDS-related Kaposi's sarcoma in clients where the disease has progressed on prior combination therapy or in those who are intolerant of such therapy. (2) Metastatic ovarian cancer in women who have failed or relapsed after cisplatin- or paclitaxel-based chemotherapy.

ACTION/KINETICS
Action
Cell-cycle specific for the S phase of cell division. Antineoplastic activity may be due to binding to DNA by intercalating between base pairs resulting in inhibition of synthesis of DNA and RNA by template disordering and steric obstruction. The liposomal product is produced with surface-bound methoxypolyethylene in order to protect liposomes from detection by mononuclear phagocytes and to increase blood circulation time. It is believed the liposomes are able to penetrate altered and often compromised vasculature of tumors.

Pharmacokinetics
Conventional product is rapidly distributed to body tissues. Conventional doxorubicin is significantly bound to tissue and plasma proteins whereas the liposomal product is confined mostly to the vascular fluid and does not bind to plasma proteins. Metabolized in the liver to the active doxorubicinol as well as inactive metabolites, which are excreted mainly through the bile. **t½, doxorubicin, conventional: triphasic:** 12 min, 3.3 hr, and about 30–40 hr. **t½, liposomal:** About 55 hr. **Plasma protein binding:** About 75%.

D

CONTRAINDICATIONS

History of hypersensitivity to conventional or liposomal doxorubicin or their components. Malignant melanoma, cancer of the kidney, large bowel carcinoma, brain tumors and metastases to the CNS (not responsive to doxorubicin therapy). Initiation of therapy in those with marked myelosuppression induced by previous treatment with other drugs or with radiotherapy. Use in preexisting heart disease. Previous treatment with complete cumulative doses of doxorubicin, daunorubicin, idarubicin, or other anthracyclines and anthracenes. Lactation. Depressed bone marrow or cardiac disease. IM or SC use.

SPECIAL CONCERNS

■ Doxorubicin, Conventional. (1) Extravasation will cause severe local tissue necrosis. Do not give IM or SC. (2) Myocardial toxicity, with potential fatal CHF, may occur either during therapy or months to years after termination of therapy. The risk of CHF increases rapidly with increasing total cumulative doses of doxorubicin in excess of 450 mg/m^2. This toxicity may occur at lower cumulative doses in those with prior mediastinal irradiation or on concurrent cyclophosphamide therapy or with preexisting heart disease. Pediatric clients are at increased risk for developing delayed cardiotoxicity. (3) Reduce the dose in those with impaired renal function. (4) Severe myelosuppression may occur. (5) Give only under the supervision of a physician experienced in the use of cancer chemotherapeutic drugs.

Doxorubicin, Liposomal. (1) Myocardial damage may lead to CHF and may be encountered as the total cumulative dose of doxorubin approaches 550 mg/m^2. The use of liposomal doxorubin may lead to cardiac toxicity. Include prior use of other anthracyclines or anthracenediones in calculations of total cumulative dosage. Cardiac toxicity may also occur at lower cumulative doses in clients with prior mediastinal irradiation or who are receiving concurrrent cyclophosphamide therapy. (2) Acute infusion-related reactions, including, but not limited to, flushing, shortness of breath, facial swelling, headache, chills, back pain, tightness in the chest or throat, and/or hypotension have occurred in up to 10% of clients treated with liposomal doxorubicin. In most clients, these reactions resolve over the course of several hours or a day once the infusion is terminated. In some clients, the reaction has resolved with slowing of the infusion rate. Serious and sometimes life-threatening or fatal allergic/anaphylactoid-like infusion reactions have been reported. Medications to treat such reactions, as well as emergency equipment, should be available for immediate use. Administer liposomal doxorubicin at an initial rate of 1 mg/min to minimize the risk of infusion reactions. (3) Severe myelosuppresion may occur. (4) Reduce the dose in those with impaired hepatic function. (5) Accidental substitution of liposomal doxorubicin for conventional doxorubicin has resulted in severe side effects. Do not substitute liposomal doxorubicin for conventional doxorubicin on a mg-per-mg basis. (6) Liposomal doxorubicin should be given only under the supervision of a health care provider experienced in the use of cancer chemotherapeutic agents.■ Use with caution in necrotizing colitis.

SIDE EFFECTS

Most Common

Conventional: N&V, diarrhea, anorexia, alopecia, rash, hoarseness, red color to urine/sweat/tears, opportunistic infections (candidiasis, cytomegalovirus, herpes simplex, *Pneumocystis carinii* pneumonia, mycobacterium avium).

Liposomal: Palmar-plantar skin eruptions, myelosuppression, asthenia, alopecia, rash, abdominal pain, anorexia, N&V, constipation, diarrhea, dyspepsia, stomatitis, dyspnea, pharyngitis, fever, mucous membrane disorder, pain/back pain, infection.

See also *Antineoplastic Agents* for a complete list of potential side effects.

Myocardial toxicity: Potentially fatal ***CHF, including acute left ventricular failure.*** **Infusion reactions** (liposomal product): Flushing, fever, SOB, facial

---

swelling, headache, chills, chest/back pain, tightness in chest and throat, hypotension, tachycardia, pruritus, rash, cyanosis, syncope, **bronchospasm, asthma, apnea, anaphylaxis. GI:** N&V, mucositis (stomatitis, esophagitis), anorexia, diarrhea. **Ulceration and necrosis of the colon. Dermatologic:** Reversible complete alopecia, hyperpigmentation of nail beds and dermal creases (especially in children), onycholysis, recall of skin reaction to prior radiotherapy, palmar-plantar erythrodysesthesia (swelling, pain, erythema, and desquamation of the skin on the hands and feet). **Local:** Severe cellulitis, vesication, and tissue necrosis if the drug is extravasated. Erythematous streaking along the vein next to injection site. **Hypersensitivity:** Fever, chills, urticaria, crosssensitivity with lincomycin, **anaphylaxis. Hematologic:** Myelosuppression, neutropenia. **Ophthalmic:** Conjunctivitis, lacrimation.

OD OVERDOSE MANAGEMENT
Symptoms: Mucositis, leukopenia, thrombocytopenia, pancytopenia. Increased risk of **cardiomyopathy** and subsequent **CHF** with chronic overdosage. *Treatment:* If the client is myelosuppressed, antibiotics and platelet and granulocyte transfusions may be necessary. Treat symptoms of mucositis. Treat CHF with digitalis preparations and diuretics as well as peripheral vasodilators.

DRUG INTERACTIONS
Actinomycin-D / Acute 'recall' pneumonitis in pediatric clients
Ciprofloxacin/other quinolones / Liposomal doxorubicin ↓ effect of quinolones
Cyclophosphamide / ↑ Risk of hemorrhagic cystitis
Cyclosporine / ↑ Doxorubicin levels R/T ↓ metabolism → more profound and prolonged hematologic toxicity
Digoxin / ↓ Digoxin plasma levels
6-Mercaptopurine / ↑ Risk of hemorrhagic cystitis
Paclitaxel / ↓ Doxorubicin clearance → more profound neutropenic and stomatitis episodes
Phenobarbital / ↑ Elimination of doxorubicin

Phenytoin / Possible ↓ phenytoin levels
Progesterone / More pronounced doxorubicin-induced neutropenia and thrombocytopenia
Radiation / ↑ Radiation-induced toxicity to the myocardium, mucosa, skin, and liver
Streptozocin / Possible inhibition of doxorubicin hepatic metabolism

HOW SUPPLIED
Conventional. *Aqueous Injection:* 2 mg/mL; *Injection:* 2 mg/mL; *Powder for Injection, Lyophilized:* 10 mg, 20 mg, 50 mg, 150 mg.
Liposomal. *Solution for Injection:* 20 mg, 50 mg.

DOSAGE
CONVENTIONAL DOXORUBICIN
• **IV ONLY**
Various cancers (see Uses).
Adults, highly individualized: 60–75 mg/m^2 as a single injection q 21 days. Use the lower dose for clients with inadequate marrow reserves due to old age, prior therapy, or neoplastic marrow infiltration. Use reduced dosage in clients with hepatic dysfunction, depending on serum bilirubin level. If bilirubin is 1.2–3 mg/100 mL, give 50% of usual dose; if it is greater than 3 mg/100 mL, give 25% of usual dose.
LIPOSOMAL DOXORUBICIN
• **IV ONLY**
AIDS-related Kaposi's sarcoma.
Adults: 20 mg/m^2 over 30 min once q 3 weeks, as long as the client responds satisfactorily and tolerates the drug. Use an initial rate of 1 mg/min to minimize the risk of infusion-related reactions. For clients with hepatic dysfunction, use the same dosing schedule as conventional doxorubicin.
Metastatic ovarian carcinoma.
50 mg/m^2 at an initial rate of 1 mg/min. If no adverse effects occur, increase the rate of infusion to complete administration in 1 hr. Give q 4 weeks.

NURSING CONSIDERATIONS
Do not confuse doxorubicin with daunorubicin (also an antineoplastic). Also, do not confuse Adriamycin with Aredia (bone growth regulator).

ADMINISTRATION/STORAGE

IV 1. Initiate while hospitalized. Give by slow IV into the tubing of a running NaCl or D5W infusion attached to a butterfly needle inserted into a large vein. Avoid veins over joints or in extremities with compromised venous or lymphatic drainage. Although infusion rate depends on vein size, do not administer in less than 3 to 5 min.

2. Reconstitute conventional drug with saline to give a final concentration of 2 mg/mL (e.g., dilute 10-mg vial with 5 mL, 20-mg vial with 10 mL, the 50-mg vial with 25 mL, and the 150-mg vial with 75 mL of 0.9% NaCl) and administer over 3–5 min. The reconstituted solution is stable for 24 hr at room temperature and 48 hr if stored at 2–8°C (36–46°F). The liposomal product is diluted, up to 90 mg, in 250 mL of D5W prior to administration. Do not use inline filters. Refrigerate diluted liposomal doxorubicin at 2–8°C (36–46°F). Short-term freezing (less than 1 month) should not affect liposomal product.

3. If the powder or solution comes in contact with the skin or mucous membranes, wash with soap and water thoroughly.

4. **Do not** administer SC or IM because severe necrosis of tissue may result. To minimize danger of extravasation, inject as directed. Monitor carefully; stinging, burning, or edema may indicate extravasation. Stop infusion and change sites to avoid tissue necrosis.

5. Be prepared with an injectable corticosteroid for local infiltration and flood site with NSS. Examine area frequently for ulceration which may necessitate early wide excision followed by plastic surgery.

6. Do not give liposomal product as a bolus injection or as undiluted solution. Rapid infusion may increase risk of infusion-related events. Have emergency equipment and medication available for immediate use in the event of serious, life-threatening symptoms.

7. Do not mix conventional doxorubicin with heparin, dexamethasone sodium phosphate, or cephalothin; a precipitate may form. Mixing with aminophylline or 5-FU will result in a change from red to blue-purple indicating decomposition. Do not mix liposomal doxorubicin with other drugs and do not use with any diluent other than D5W. Liposomal doxorubicin is a translucent, red liposomal dispersion.

8. Check package insert carefully for alternate dosing regimens for liposomal doxorubicin in clients with palmar-plantar erythrodysesthesia, hematologic toxicity, or stomatitis.

ASSESSMENT

1. Note resaons for therapy, onset, characteristics of S&S; list other agents/therapies trialed.

2. Observe for cardiac arrhythmias, ST segment depression, sinus tachycardia, and/or respiratory difficulties indicative of cardiac toxicity. Have dexrazoxane available to prevent drug-induced cardiomyopathy. Monitor for late-onset (up to 6 mo) CHF.

3. Administer antiemetics 30–45 min before therapy and ATC as needed.

4. Monitor VS and I&O; encourage fluid intake of 2–3 L/day. Anticipate allopurinol administration and alkalinization of urine to decrease urate stone formation.

5. Monitor CBC, uric acid, renal, LFTs; drug may cause granulocyte toxicity. Nadir: 10–14 days; recovery: 21 days.

CLIENT/FAMILY TEACHING

1. If medication reactivates previous radiotherapy damage, such as erythema, edema, and desquamation; should resolve after 7 days.

2. Consume 2–3 L/day of fluids.

3. Avoid foods with citric acid, hot or rough textures.

4. Report mouth ulcers; inflammation may occur 5–10 days after dose and last for 3–7 days. A special mouth rinse may help control symptoms.

5. May experience increased tearing; avoid rubbing eyes.

6. Urine will turn red-brown for 1–2 days; this is not blood.

7. Nail beds may become discolored.

8. Any hair loss should grow back 2–3 months after therapy.

9. Report any flu-like symptoms; causes severe myelosuppression.

Bold Italic = life threatening side effect   ▬ = black box warning   ♣ = Available in Canada

10. Avoid vaccinations.
11. Practice contraception during and for 4 mo after therapy.

OUTCOMES/EVALUATE
Inhibition of malignant cell proliferation

Doxycycline anhydrous
IV @

(dox-ih-**SYE**-kleen)

CLASSIFICATION(S):
Antibiotic, tetracycline
PREGNANCY CATEGORY: D
Rx: Oracea.

Doxycycline calcium
PREGNANCY CATEGORY: D
Rx: Vibramycin.

Doxycycline hyclate
PREGNANCY CATEGORY: D
Rx: Atridox, Doryx, Doxy 100 and 200, Periostat, Vibra-Tabs, Vibramycin.
✤Rx: Apo-Doxy, Apo-Doxy-Tabs, Doxycin, Novo-Doxylin, Nu-Doxycycline, ratio-Doxycycline.

Doxycycline monohydrate
PREGNANCY CATEGORY: D
Rx: Adoxa, Monodox, Vibramycin.

SEE ALSO *ANTI-INFECTIVES* AND *TETRACYCLINES*.

USES
Doxycycline calcium, doxycycline hyclate, and doxycycline monohydrate. (1) Gram-negative organisms, including *Haemophilus ducreyi* (chancroid), *Francisella tularensis* (tularemia), *Yersenia pestis* (plague), *Bartonella bacilliformis* (bartonellosis), *Campylobacter fetus* (fetus infections), *Vibrio cholerae* (cholera), *Brucella* species (with streptomycin) to treat brucellosis, *Calymmatobacterium granulomatis* (granuloma inguinale). (2) *Rickettsiae* (e.g., Rocky Mountain spotted fever, typhus fever and the typhus group, Q fever, rickettsialpox, tick fevers). (3) *Mycoplasma pneumoniae* (e.g., respiratory tract infections). (4) *Chlamydia trachomatis* (e.g., lymphogranuloma venereum, trachoma, inclusion conjunctivitis, uncomplicated urethral, endocervical, or rectal infections). (5) *Chlamydia psittaci* (psittacosis). (6) *Borellia recurrentis* (e.g., relapsing fever). (7) *Ureaplasma urealyticum* (e.g., nongonococcal urethritis). (8) For the following infections following susceptibility testing as resistance has been documented: *Escherichia coli*, *Enterobacter aerogenes*, *Acinetobacter* species, *Haemophilus influenzae* (e.g., respiratory tract infections), *Klebsiella* species (e.g., respiratory and urinary tract infections), *Streptococcus pneumoniae* (e.g., upper respiratory tract infections), and *Shigella* species. (9) Alternative therapy for the following infections when penicillin is contraindicated: Uncomplicated gonorrhrea due to *Neisseria gonorrhoeae*, syphilis due to *Treponema pallidum*, yaws due to *Treponema pertenue*, listeriosis due to *Listeria monocytogenes*, Vincent's infection due to *Fusobacterium fusiforme*, actinomycosis due to *Actinomyces israelii*, and infections due to *Clostridium* species. (10) Adjunct to amebicides for acute intestinal amebiasis. (11) Adjunctive therapy for severe acne. (12) Reduce incidence or progression of anthrax (including inhalational anthrax) following exposure to aerosolized *Bacillus anthracis*. (13) Prophylaxis of malaria due to *Plasmodium falciparum* in short-term travelers (less than 4 months) to areas with chloroquine and/or pyrimethamine-sulfadoxine resistant strains. *Investigational:* Lyme disease, syphilis, pelvic inflammatory disease, epididymitis due to gonococcal or chlamydial infection, sexual assault prophylaxis.

Doxycycline hyclate. (1) Trachoma (infectious agent not always eliminated). (2) Inclusion conjunctivitis (may also be combined with topical drugs). (3) Acute epididymo-orchitis due to *Chlamydia trachomatis*.

Doxycycline monohydrate. Treatment of only inflammatory lesions (papules and pustules) or rosacea in adults.

Dental: (1) Atridox injection for chronic adult periodontitis for a gain in clinical attachment, reduction in probing depth, and reduction in bleeding on probing. (2) Periostat as an adjunct to scaling and root planing to promote attachment level gain and reduce pocket depth in adult periodontitis.

NOTE: Do not use for streptococcal disease unless organism is susceptible. Tetracyclines are not the drugs of choice to treat any type of staphylococcal infection.

ACTION/KINETICS

Action
Inhibits protein synthesis by binding to the ribosomal 30S subunit. Blocks binding of aminoacyl transfer RNA to the messenger RNA complex. Cell wall synthesis is not inhibited.

Pharmacokinetics
More slowly absorbed, and thus more persistent, than other tetracyclines. Preferred for clients with impaired renal function for treating infections outside the urinary tract. **t½:** 15–25 hr; 30–42% excreted unchanged in urine. High lipid solubility. **Plasma protein binding:** From 80–95%.

CONTRAINDICATIONS
Prophylaxis of malaria in pregnant individuals and in children less than 8 years old. Use during pregnancy (may stunt fetal growth) and in children up to 8 years of age (tetracycline may cause permanent discoloration of the teeth). Lactation.

SPECIAL CONCERNS
Safety for IV use in children less than 8 years of age has not been established.

SIDE EFFECTS

Most Common
Anorexia, N&V, diarrhea, dizziness, headache, rashes.

See *Tetracyclines* for complete listing of possible side effects.

ADDITIONAL DRUG INTERACTIONS
Barbiturates, carbamazepine, phenytoin / ↓ Doxycycline effect by ↑ liver breakdown

Methotrexate / Possible GI and hematologic toxicity after high doses of methotrexate

HOW SUPPLIED
Doxycycline anhydrous. *Capsules:* 40 mg (30 mg immediate-release and 10 mg delayed-release).

Doxycycline calcium. *Syrup:* 50 mg/5 mL.

Doxycycline hyclate. *Capsules:* 50 mg, 100 mg; *Capsules, Coated Pellets:* 75 mg, 100 mg; *Gel:* 10%; *Powder for Injection, Lyophilized:* 100 mg, 200 mg; *Tablets:* 20 mg, 100 mg; *Tablets, Delayed-Release:* 75 mg, 100 mg.

Doxycycline monohydrate. *Capsules:* 50 mg, 100 mg; *Powder for Oral Suspension:* 25 mg/5 mL (after reconstitution); *Tablets:* 50 mg, 75 mg, 100 mg, 150 mg.

DOSAGE
- **CAPSULES; CAPSULE, ENTERIC-COATED; IV; ORAL SUSPENSION; SYRUP; TABLETS; TABLETS, DELAYED-RELEASE**

Infections.
Adult: First day, 100 mg q 12 hr; **maintenance:** 100 mg/day. For more severe infections (e.g., chronic UTIs), give 100 mg q 12 hr. **Children, over 8 years (45 kg or less): First day,** 4.4 mg/kg in 2 doses; **then,** 2.2–4.4 mg/kg/day in divided doses depending on severity of infection. Children over 45 kg should receive the adult dose.

Uncomplicated gonorrhea in adults (except anorectal infections in men).
Adults: 100 mg twice a day for at least 7 days. Alternatively, 300 mg immediately followed in 1 hr with 300 mg. Give with plenty of water.

Nongonococcal urethritis due to C. trachomatis or U. urealyticum.
100 mg PO twice a day for 7 days.

Syphilis, early.
100 mg PO twice a day for 2 weeks (except Doryx). When using Doryx: Give 300 mg/day in divided PO doses for 10 days.

Syphilis, more than 1 year duration.
100 mg PO 2 times/day for 4 weeks (except Adoxa, Doryx, Monodox).

Uncomplicated urethral, endocervical or rectal infections in adults due to C. trachomatis.

Bold Italic = life threatening side effect   ■ = black box warning   ✦ = Available in Canada

100 mg PO twice a day for at least 7 days.

Acute epididymo-orchitis due to N. gonorrhoeae or C. trachomatis.

100 mg PO twice a day for at least 10 days.

Pelvic inflammatory disease.

100 mg PO or IV q 12 hr *plus* cefotetan, 2 grams IV, q 12 hr *or* cefoxitin, 2 grams IV, q 6 hr. May discontinue parenteral therapy after 24 hr; continue PO therapy with doxycycline for 14 days.

Epididymitis likely due to gonococcal or chlamydial infection.

100 mg twice a day for 10 days *plus* a single dose of ceftriaxone, 250 mg IM.

Sexual assault prophylaxis.

100 mg twice a day for 7 days plus ceftriaxone and metronidazole.

Prophylaxis of malaria.

Adults: 100 mg PO once daily (except Doryx); **children, over 8 years of age:** 2 mg/kg/day up to 100 mg/day. Begin 1–2 days before travel to endemic area and continue during travel and for 4 weeks after returning.

Anthrax, inhalation, post-exposure.

Adults and children weighing 45 kg or more: 100 mg q 12 hr for 60 days. **Children, less than 45 kg:** 2.2 mg/kg q 12 hr for 60 days.

Lyme disease.

Tick bite from endemic area: 200 mg once. **Early Lyme disease:** 100 mg twice a day for 14–21 days. **Carditis (first degree AV block):** 100 mg twice a day for 14–21 days. **Facial nerve paralysis:** 100 mg twice a day for 14–21 days. **Arthritis:** 100 mg twice a day for 30–60 days.

ORACEA

- **TABLETS**

  Inflammatory lesions of rosacea.

40 mg once daily in the morning on an empty stomach, preferably at least 1 hr before or 2 hr after meals. Oracea contains 30 mg immediate release and 10 mg delayed release anhydrous doxycycline.

PERIOSTAT

- **TABLETS**

  Adjunct to promote attachment and level gain and to reduce pocket depth in adult periodontitis.

20 mg twice a day following scaling and planing. May be used for up to 9 months. Do not exceed recommended dose.

ATRIDOX

- **INJECTION**

  Chronic adult periodontitis.

After preparing the injection (see package insert), keeping the tip near the base of the pocket, express the drug into the pocket until the formulation reaches the top of the gingival margin. Cover the pocket containing doxycycline with either Coe-Pak periodontal dressing or Octyldent dental adhesive.

- **IV INFUSION ONLY**

  Infections.

Adults: 200 mg IV on day 1 given in 1 or 2 infusions; **then,** 100–200 mg, depending on severity of condition (give 200 mg in 1 or 2 infusions). **Children, over 8 years of age, up to 45 kg:** 4.4 mg/kg on day 1 in 1 or 2 infusions; **then,** 2.2–4.4 mg/kg given as 1 or 2 infusions, depending on severity of the infection. **Children, over 45 kg:** Use adult dose.

- **GEL, 10%**

  Reduce bacteria due to periodontal disease.

Apply to affected area; gel conforms to shape of the periodontal pocket and solidifies. It releases doxycycline for about 7 days.

NURSING CONSIDERATIONS

© Do not confuse Doxycycline with Dicyclomine (an anticholinergic/antispasmodic).

ADMINISTRATION/STORAGE

1. When used for streptococcal infections, continue therapy for 10 days.

2. Malaria prophylaxis can begin 1–2 days before travel begins, during travel, and for 4 weeks after leaving the malarial area.

3. The powder for suspension expires 12 months from date of issue.

4. Reconstituted PO solution is stable for 2 weeks when refrigerated.

IV 5. Avoid rapid administration. Duration of IV infusion may vary with the dose; usually from 1–4 hr. A recommended minimum infusion time for 100

---

mg of a 0.5 mg/mL solution is 1 hr. Switch to oral therapy as soon as possible.

6. Continue therapy for at least 24–48 hr after symptoms and fever have subsided.

7. Follow directions on vial for dilution. Concentrations should be no lower than 0.1 mg/mL and no higher than 1.0 mg/mL.

8. During infusion protect solution from light.

9. When diluted with NaCl injection, D5W, Ringer's injection, 10% invert sugar in water, Normosol-M in D5W, Normosol-R in D5W, Plasma-Lyte 56 in D5W, or Plasma-Lyte 148 in D5W, infusion of the solution (about 1 mg/mL) or lower concentrations (not less than 0.1 mg/mL) must be completed within 12 hr after reconstitution to ensure adequate stability.

10. Administer solutions diluted with RL or D5/RL within 6 hr.

11. Reconstituted solutions (0.1–1 mg/mL) may be stored up to 72 hr prior to start of the infusion, if refrigerated and protected from sun or artificial light.

ASSESSMENT

1. Note reasons for therapy, onset, and characteristics of S&S.

2. Obtain cultures when indicated.

3. Check for any allergic/hypersensitivity reactions; note expiration date as expired tetracycline products are nephrotoxic.

CLIENT/FAMILY TEACHING

1. May take with food; take caps with a full glass of water to prevent esophageal ulceration and remain upright for 45 min.

2. Avoid direct exposure to sunlight and wear protective clothing and sunscreens when exposed.

3. With STDs advise that partner be tested and treated. Use condoms until medically cleared.

4. Take entire prescription; do not stop if symptoms subside. Report adverse effects or lack of response.

OUTCOMES/EVALUATE

- Resolution of infection
- Symptomatic improvement

Drotrecogin alfa (Activated)   IV

(droh-treh-**KOH**-jin **AL**-fah)

CLASSIFICATION(S):
Sepsis drug
PREGNANCY CATEGORY: C
Rx: Xigris.

USES

Reduce mortality in adults with sepsis associated with acute organ dysfunction who have a high risk of death. Safety and efficacy have not been determined in clients with severe sepsis and a lower risk of death or in children with severe sepsis.

ACTION/KINETICS

Action

Drotrecogin alfa is a recombinant human activated Protein C. Activated Protein C exerts an antithrombotic effect by inhibiting Factors Va and VIIIa. Activated Protein C has indirect profibrolytic activity by inhibiting plasminogen activator inhibitor-1 and limiting generation of activated thrombin-activatable-fibrinolysis-inhibitor. Activated Protein C may also exert an anti-inflammatory effect by inhibiting tumor necrosis factor production by monocytes, by blocking leukocyte adhesion to selectins, and by limiting the thrombin-induced inflammatory responses within the microvascular endothelium. Activated Protein C levels in those with severe sepsis are below detectable levels.

Pharmacokinetics

Infusion of drotrecogin alfa rapidly produces steady-state levels that are proportional to infusion rates. In most clients, plasma levels of drotrecogin alfa fall below detectable levels within 2 hr after stopping infusion. Inactivated by endogenous plasma protease inhibitors. Plasma clearance in those with severe sepsis is about 50% higher than in healthy subjects.

Bold Italic = life threatening side effect   ■ = black box warning   ✦ = Available in Canada

CONTRAINDICATIONS

Due to increased risk of bleeding, use in active internal bleeding, within 3 months of hemorrhagic stroke, within 2 months of intracranial or intraspinal surgery or severe head trauma, trauma with an increased risk of life-threatening bleeding, presence of an epidural catheter, and intracranial neoplasm or mass lesion with evidence of cerebral herniation. Hypersensitivity to the drug or any component of the product. Lactation.

SPECIAL CONCERNS

Use with caution with other drugs that affect hemostasis. For the following conditions, carefully consider the increased risk of bleeding if drotrecogin alfa is used:

- Concurrent therapeutic dosing of heparin to treat active thrombotic or embolic event (low doses of heparin do not affect safety)
- Platelet count less than 30,000 x 10^6/L (even if platelet count is increased after transfusions)
- Prothrombin time (INR) greater than 3
- Within 6 weeks of GI bleeding
- Within 3 days of thrombolytic therapy
- Within 7 days of PO anticoagulants or glycoprotein IIb/IIIa inhibitors
- Within 3 months of ischemic stroke
- Intracranial arteriovenous malformation or aneurysm
- Known bleeding diathesis
- Chronic severe hepatic disease
- Any other condition in which bleeding constitutes a significant hazard or would be particularly difficult to treat due to its location.

Carefully consider the risk vs benefits in those with single organ dysfunction after recent surgery as these clients may be at high risk of death. Safety and efficacy have not been determined in children from newborns to 18 years of age.

SIDE EFFECTS

Most Common

Bleeding.

Hematologic: Bleeding (most common side effect), including the following sites of hemorrhage: *Intracranial, GI, intra-abdominal, intrathoracic, retroperitoneal, GU, skin/soft tissue.* Possibility of immunogenicity.

LABORATORY TEST CONSIDERATIONS

Prolongation of aPTT. Interference with factor VIII, IX, and XI assays (values obtained that are lower than the true concentrations).

OD OVERDOSE MANAGEMENT

Symptoms: Bleeding. *Treatment:* No known antidote. Immediately stop the infusion and monitor closely for hemorrhagic complications.

DRUG INTERACTIONS

Use with caution if used with other drugs that affect hemostasis → increased risk of bleeding

HOW SUPPLIED

Powder for Injection, Lyophilized: 5 mg, 20 mg.

DOSAGE

- **IV**
  Sepsis.

IV, at an infusion rate of 24 mcg/kg/hr for a total duration of 96 hr. Do **not** adjust dose based on clinical or lab parameters. If infusion is interrupted, restart at the 24 mcg/kg/hr infusion rate.

NURSING CONSIDERATIONS

ADMINISTRATION/STORAGE

IV 1. Do not escalate dose or give by bolus injection.

2. To minimize risk of higher than prescribed infusion rates, carefully check package insert for calculating final concentration of infusion solution, the duration of the infusion, and the actual infusion rate of the diluted drug solution.

3. Stop infusion immediately if clinically significant bleeding occurs.

4. Discontinue 2 hr before undergoing invasive surgical procedure or procedures with an inherent risk of bleeding. Once adequate hemostasis has been achieved, drotrecogin alfa may be reconsidered 12 hr after any major invasive procedure or surgery and may be restarted immediately after uncomplicated less invasive procedures.

5. The drug has not been readministered to clients with severe sepsis.

ASSESSMENT

1. Note reasons for therapy, characteristics of S&S, other agents trialed, organ function/failure status.

2. Evaluate carefully and weigh anticipated benefits versus potential risks of therapy. Certain conditions are likely to increase the risk of bleeding. In clients with 1 or more of the following conditions, use drotrecogin alfa therapy cautiously:

- Concurrent therapeutic heparin (15 or more units/kg/hr)
- Platelet count <30,000 x 10⁶/L, even if platelet count is elevated after transfusions
- Prothrombin time-(INR) >3
- Within 6 weeks of GI bleeding
- Within 3 days of thrombolytic therapy
- Within 7 days of oral anticoagulants or glycoprotein IIb/IIIa inhibitors
- Within 7 days of aspirin, >650 mg/day or other platelet inhibitors
- Within 3 months of ischemic stroke
- Intracranial arteriovenous malformation or aneurysm
- Known bleeding diathesis
- Chronic severe hepatic disease
- Any other condition in which bleeding constitutes a significant hazard or would be difficult to manage because of its location

3. Place in a carefully monitored environment which permits continuous assessment for any evidence of significant active bleeding. If evident- stop infusion; report.

4. Monitor VS, cultures, CBC, PT/INR, renal and LFTs. Sepsis predisposes client to a coagulopathy associated with prolongation of PTT/PT. Drotrecogin alfa may alter the PTT thus making it an unreliable test to assess coagulopathy status.

CLIENT/FAMILY TEACHING

Those with severe sepsis (infection in blood) and organ failure may experience many adverse events that are life-threatening, which predisposes this population to a high risk of death. The benefits must far outweigh the risks when this therapy is selected. Report any adverse effects and evidence of bleeding. Bleeding may occur for up to 28 days after treatment.

OUTCOMES/EVALUATE

Improved mortality with severe sepsis

Duloxetine hydrochloride
(doo-**LOX**-eh-teen)

CLASSIFICATION(S):

Antidepressant, selective serotonin and norepinephrine reuptake inhibitor

PREGNANCY CATEGORY: C

Rx: Cymbalta.

USES

(1) Treatment of major depressive disorder as defined in the DSM-IV. (2) Management of neuropathic pain associated with diabetic peripheral neuropathy. (3) Treatment of generalized anxiety disorder. *Investigational:* Fibromyalgia; stress urinary incontinence.

ACTION/KINETICS

Action

Mechanism is unknown. Antidepressant and pain inhibitory effect believed to be related to potentiation of serotonergic and noradrenergic activity in the CNS. Potent inhibitor of neuronal reuptake of serotonin and norepinephrine.

Pharmacokinetics

Well absorbed after PO administration. **Maximum plasma levels:** 6 hr (there is a 2-hr lag until absorption begins). Food delays the time to peak levels from 6 to 10 hr. There is a 3-hr delay in absorption and a one-third increase in apparent clearance after an evening dose compared with a morning dose. Undergoes extensive metabolism by the liver isoenzymes, CYP2D6 and CYP1A2. **t½, elimination:** 8–17 hr. Excreted in both the urine (70%) and feces (20%). **Plasma protein binding:** More than 90%.

CONTRAINDICATIONS

Use in end-stage renal disease or severe renal impairment (C_{CR} less than 30

---

mL/min), any hepatic insufficiency, chronic liver disease, substantial alcohol use, uncontrolled narrow-angle glaucoma, or concomitant use in those taking MAO inhibitors. Lactation.

SPECIAL CONCERNS

■ (1) Antidepressants increase the risk of suicidal thinking and behavior (suicidality) in children and adolescents with major depressive disorder and other psychiatric disorders. Anyone considering the use of duloxetine or other antidepressants in a child or adolescent must balance this risk with the clinical need. Closely observe clients for clinical worsening, suicidality, or unusual changes in behavior. Advise families and caregivers of the need for close observation and communication with the prescriber. Duloxetine is not approved for use in children. (2) Short-term (4 to 6 weeks) placebo-controlled trials of 9 antidepressant drugs (SSRIs and others) in children and adolescents with major depressive disorder, OCD, or other psychiatric disorders have revealed a greater risk of side effects representing suicidality during the first few months of treatment in those receiving antidepressants. The average risk of such reactions in those receiving antidepressants was 4%, twice the placebo risk of 2%. No suicides occurred in these trials.■ Both adults and children with major depressive disorder may experience worsening of their depression and/or suicidal ideation and behavior, whether or not they are taking antidepressant medication. Use with caution in clients with a history of mania, seizure disorder, with controlled narrow-angle glaucoma, in the elderly, and with conditions that may slow gastric emptying. Safety and efficacy have not been determined in children. Use during labor and delivery only if the potential benefit justifies the potential risk to the fetus.

SIDE EFFECTS

Most Common

N&V, somnolence, dizziness, headache, constipation, dry mouth, fatigue, insomnia, decreased appetite, increased sweating.

Side effects with an incidence of 1% or greater are listed. **CNS:** Insomnia, dizziness, somnolence, tremor, anxiety, agitation, decreased libido, headache, hypoesthesia, paresthesia, irritability, lethargy, nervousness, nightmares/abnormal dreams, restlessness, sleep disorder, *completed suicide*, mania, mood swings, pressure of speech, sluggishness, suicide attempt, activation of mania/hypomania, *seizures*. **Serotonin syndrome:** Agitation, coma, hallucinations, hyperthermia, labile BP, tachycardia, hyperreflexia, incoordination, diarrhea, N&V. **GI:** N&V, dry mouth, constipation, diarrhea, dyspepsia, loose stools, gastritis, blood in stool, colitis, dysphagia, dysgeusia, acquired esophageal stenosis, gastric ulcer, gingivitis, irritable bowel syndrome, abdominal pain, flatulence, hepatitis, cholestatic jaundice. **GU:** Erectile dysfunction, delayed ejaculation, dysuria, ejaculatory dysfunction, abnormal orgasm, dysuria, micturition urgency, urinary hesitation/incontinence/retention, decreased urine flow, pollakiuria. **CV:** Peripheral edema, phlebitis, ECG changes, small increase in BP and HR, orthostatic hypotension, syncope, palpitations. **Dermatologic:** Night sweats, pruritus, rash, hyperhidrosis, acne, alopecia, skin ulcer, cold sweat, ecchymosis, eczema, erythema, face edema, increased tendency to bruise, photosensitivity reaction. **Hematologic:** Anemia, leukopenia, lymphadenopathy, thrombocytopenia. **Musculoskeletal:** Muscle cramps, myalgia, musculoskeletal pain. **Respiratory:** Cough, pharyngolaryngeal pain, nasopharyngitis. **Ophthalmic:** Blurred vision, mydriasis. **Body as a whole:** Decreased appetite, decreased/increased weight, anorexia, fatigue, hot flushes, asthenia, pyrexia, chills, rigors. **Miscellaneous:** Decreased glycemic control in diabetics, yawning, vertigo.

LABORATORY TEST CONSIDERATIONS

Slight ↑ AST, ALT, CPK, alkaline phosphatase. ↑ WBCs. Hyponatremia.

OD OVERDOSE MANAGEMENT

Symptoms: Serotonin syndrome, somnolence, *seizures*, vomiting, *death* (rare and usually with mixed drugs). *Treat-*

 = see color insert   = Herbal   IV = Intravenous   = sound alike drug *ment:* Treat serotonin syndrome with cyproheptadine and/or temperature control. Ensure an adequate airway, oxygenation and ventilation; monitor cardiac rhythm and vital signs. Do not induce vomiting. Gastric lavage with a large-bore orogastric tube with appropriate airway protection, if needed, may be performed soon after ingestion or in symptomatic clients. Activated charcoal may limit duloxetine absorption from the GI tract. Consider the possibility of multiple drug involvement.

DRUG INTERACTIONS

Alcohol / Liver injury manifested by ↑ ALT and total bilirubin

Almotriptan / ↑ Risk of serotonin syndrome

Cimetidine / ↑ Duloxetine AUC, C_{max}, and $t\frac{1}{2}$ R/T inhibition of the CYP1A2 isoenzyme

CNS drugs / Use together with caution

Eletriptan / ↑ Risk of serotonin syndrome

Flecainide / Both are metabolized by CYP2D6 → ↑ levels of flecainide; approach coadministration with caution

Fluvoxamine / ↑ Duloxetine AUC, C_{max}, and $t\frac{1}{2}$ R/T inhibition of the CYP1A2 isoenzyme

Fluoxetine / ↑ Duloxetine levels R/T inhibition of CYP2D6 isoenzyme

Lithium / ↑ Risk of serotonin syndrome

MAO Inhibitors / ↑ Risk of serious side effects, including hyperthermia, rigidity, myoclonus, autonomic instability, mental status changes, and death, R/T ↑ levels of serotonin and norepinephrine. Do not use with an MAOI or within at least 14 days of discontinuing an MAOI; allow 5 days after stopping duloxetine before starting an MAOI

Naratriptan / ↑ Risk of serotonin syndrome

Paroxetine / ↑ Duloxetine levels R/T inhibition of CYP2D6 isoenzyme

Phenothiazines / Both are metabolized by CYP2D6 → ↑ levels of phenothiazine; approach coadministration with caution

Propafenone / Both are metabolized by CYP2D6 → ↑ levels of propafenone; approach coadministration with caution

Quinidine / ↑ Duloxetine levels R/T inhibition of CYP2D6 isoenzyme

Quinolone antibiotics / ↑ Duloxetine AUC, C_{max}, and $t\frac{1}{2}$ R/T inhibition of the CYP1A2 isoenzyme

Selective serotonin reuptake inhibitors / ↑ Risk of serotonin syndrome

Sumatriptan / ↑ Risk of serotonin syndrome

Thioridazine / Both are metabolized by CYP2D6 → ↑ Risk of serious arrhythmias and sudden death; do not use together

Tramadol / ↑ Risk of serotonin syndrome

Tryptophan / ↑ Risk of serotonin syndrome

Tricyclic antidepressants / Both are metabolized by CYP2D6 → ↑ levels of tricyclic antidepressant; approach coadministration with caution

Warfarin / ↑ Free levels of warfarin due to displacement from plasma protein binding sites by duloxetine

HOW SUPPLIED

Capsules, Delayed-Release: 20 mg, 30 mg, 60 mg.

DOSAGE

• CAPSULES, DELAYED-RELEASE

Major depressive disorder.

Adults, initial: 20 mg twice a day to 60 mg/day (given either once a day or 30 mg twice a day) without regard to meals. There is no evidence that doses greater than 60 mg/day confer additional benefits. Periodically evaluate to determine need for maintenance treatment.

Diabetic peripheral neuropathic pain.

Adults, initial: 60 mg/day given once a day without regard to meals. Periodically evaluate to determine need for maintenance treatment; efficacy beyond 12 weeks has not been evaluated.

Generalized anxiety disorder.

Initial: 60 mg once daily without regard to meals. For some, it may be beneficial to start at 30 mg once daily for 1 week to allow adjustment to the drug before increasing to 60 mg once daily. There is no evidence that doses higher than 60 mg daily confer additional benefit. If doses greater than 60 mg are used, increase doses in increments of 30 mg

---

Bold Italic = life threatening side effect   ■ = black box warning   ✦ = Available in Canada

once daily up to a maximum of 120 mg once daily. Efficacy of duloxetine for more than 10 weeks has not been evaluated. Periodically evaluate the long-term usefulness of the drug.

Fibromyalgia.
60 mg twice a day in those with and without depression.

NURSING CONSIDERATIONS

Do not confuse duloxetine with fluoxetine (also a selective serotonin reuptake inhibitor).

ADMINISTRATION/STORAGE

1. Before beginning therapy with duloxetine, screen clients with depressive symptoms carefully to determine if they are at risk for bipolar disorder.
2. Treatment for several months or longer may be needed for acute episodes of major depression. Periodically reassess clients to determine need for and appropriate dose for maintenance therapy.
3. Abrupt discontinuation may cause dizziness, N&V, headache, paresthesia, irritability, and nightmares. Reduce dose gradually rather than abruptly discontinuing the drug.
4. If intolerable symptoms occur following a decrease in dose or upon discontinuing the drug, resume the previously prescribed dose. The provider may continue decreasing the dose but at a more gradual rate.
5. Wait at least 14 days between discontinuing a MAO inhibitor and initiating duloxetine. Also, at least 5 days should elapse after stopping duloxetine and starting a MAO inhibitor.
6. Store at 25°C (77°F); permitted range is 15–30°C (59–86°F).

ASSESSMENT

1. List reasons for therapy, characteristics of S&S, contributing factors, other agents trialed, outcome.
2. Monitor BP, renal and LFTs; avoid use with ESRD and hepatic insufficiency. May cause elevation of liver enzymes; avoid in those that have substantial alcohol use.
3. Assess history and use cautiously with seizures, controlled narrow angle glaucoma, history of mania, or drug abuse/dependence, and conditions that may slow gastric emptying.
4. Note EMG results, extent of neuropathy and any contributing factors.

CLIENT/FAMILY TEACHING

1. Take as directed without regard to meals. Do not chew, crush, or sprinkle contents, or mix with liquids; swallow whole to protect enteric coating.
2. Avoid activities that require mental alertness until drug effects realized.
3. May experience dizziness, N&V, headache, paresthesia, irritability, and nightmares. Do not stop suddenly; reduce dose gradually. Report adverse new onset side effects, especially worsening of depression, inability to sleep, suicide thoughts, anxiety, agitation, hostility, and impulsiveness.
4. Avoid heavy alcohol use, may cause severe liver injury.
5. Practice reliable contraception; report if pregnant, desire to become pregnant, or if breastfeeding.
6. Keep all F/U appointments and counselling sessions. May take up to 4 weeks before improvement noted.

OUTCOMES/EVALUATE

- Relief of depression/anxiety
- Control of neuropathic pain R/T diabetic peripheral neuropathy

Dutasteride
(dew-**TAS**-teer-ide)

CLASSIFICATION(S):
Androgen hormone inhibitor
PREGNANCY CATEGORY: X
Rx: Avodart.

USES

Symptomatic benign prostatic hypertrophy in men with enlarged prostate to improve symptoms, decrease risk of acute urinary retention, and decrease risk/need for surgery.

ACTION/KINETICS

Action

Competitively inhibits conversion of testosterone to the active 5α-dihydrotestosterone (DHT) by

5α-reductase. DHT develops and enlarges the prostate gland.

Pharmacokinetics
Time to peak serum levels: 2–3 hr. Metabolized by the CYP3A4 isoenzyme. Excreted mainly in the feces. **t½, terminal:** About 5 weeks at steady state. **Steady-state serum level after 0.5 mg for 1 year:** 40 ng/mL. **Plasma protein binding:** Over 99%.

CONTRAINDICATIONS
Use in women and children. Known hypersensitivity to dutasteride or other 5α-reductase inhibitors.

SPECIAL CONCERNS
Use with caution in liver disease.

SIDE EFFECTS
Most Common
GU: Impotence, decreased libido, ejaculation disorder, gynecomastia (both breast enlargement and tenderness).

LABORATORY TEST CONSIDERATIONS
↓ PSA levels.

DRUG INTERACTIONS
Dutasteride may ↑ levels of CYP3A4 inhibitors, including cimetidine, ciprofloxacin, diltiazem, ketoconazole, ritonavir, and verapamil.

HOW SUPPLIED
Capsules: 0.5 mg.

DOSAGE
- **CAPSULES**
  Benign prostatic hypertrophy.
0.5 mg/day with or without food.

NURSING CONSIDERATIONS
ADMINISTRATION/STORAGE
1. Swallow capsules whole.
2. Store between 15–30°C (59–77°F).

ASSESSMENT
1. Note characteristics of S&S, other agents trialed/outcome.

2. List other drugs prescribed to ensure none interact.
3. Assess urinary tract symptoms to R/O other urological diseases; assess for obstructive uropathy with reduced flow or increased residuals. Note prostate exam findings.
4. Obtain baseline/monitor PSA, DRE, and LFTs; assess for liver dysfunction.

CLIENT/FAMILY TEACHING
1. Take as directed once daily. May take with or without food but swallow capsule whole. Review printed drug guide for updates.
2. Drug causes the prostate to decrease in size and thus decreases urination complaints.
3. Ejaculation volume may decrease; this does not appear to affect normal sexual function. Drug related side effects (impotence, ↓ libido, and ejaculation disorder) may decrease with continued therapy.
4. May experience breast enlargement/tenderness; report if persistent.
5. Women should use caution when handling dutasteride capsules; if contact is made with leaking capsules, wash contact area immediately with soap and water.
6. Women who are pregnant or who may be pregnant should not handle dutasteride capsules due to the possibility of absorption and potential risk to a male fetus.
7. Men treated with dutasteride should not give blood until at least 6 months have passed since the last dose.

OUTCOMES/EVALUATE
Control of S&S of BPH: ↓ nocturia ↑ urinary stream

Bold Italic = life threatening side effect   ■ = black box warning   ✤ = Available in Canada

E

Efalizumab

(eh-fah-**LIH**-zyoo-mab)

CLASSIFICATION(S):
Immunosuppressant
PREGNANCY CATEGORY: C
Rx: Raptiva.

USES

Treat adults (18 years and older) with chronic moderate to severe plaque psoriasis who are candidates for systemic therapy or phototherapy.

ACTION/KINETICS

Action

Lymphocyte activation and trafficking to skin play a role in the pathophysiology of chronic plaque psoriasis. It is believed efalizumab affects the activation, adhesion, migration, and numbers of cells other than T lymphocytes. Efalizumab binds to CD11a, the α subunit of leukocyte function antigen–1 (LFA-1) that is expressed on all leukocytes, and decreases cell surface expression of CD11a. Efalizumab inhibits binding of LFA-1 to intercellular adhesion molecule–1 (ICAM-1), thus inhibiting the adhesion of leukocytes to other cell types. Interaction between LFA-1 and ICAM-1 contributes to the initiation and maintenance of multiple processes, including activation of T lymphocytes, adhesion of T lymphocytes to endothelial cells, and migration of T lymphocytes to sites of inflammation, including psoriatic skin. The drug also causes an increase in WBC count, a doubling of mean lymphocyte counts, and an increase of eosinophil counts.

Pharmacokinetics

Serum steady state levels: 4 weeks.

CONTRAINDICATIONS

Lactation. Use with other immunosuppressive drugs. Administration of acellular, live, and live-attenuated vaccines during efalizumab treatment.

SPECIAL CONCERNS

Safety and efficacy have not been established beyond 1 year. Clients who become pregnant while taking efalizumab should be enrolled in the efalizumab pregnancy registry. Use with caution in the elderly. Safety and efficacy have not been determined in children.

SIDE EFFECTS

Most Common

Headache, infection, chills, nausea, pain, myalgia, flu syndrome, fever, back pain, acne. The most serious side effects include serious infections, malignancies, thrombocytopenia, and psoriasis.

First dose reaction complex: Headache, chills, fever, nausea, myalgia within 2 days following the first 2 injections. **Body as a whole:** Infection (including URI), chills, nausea, pain, myalgia, flu syndrome, fever, asthenia, arthralgia, psoriasis, inflammatory/immune-mediated reactions (including hemolytic anemia), low titer antibodies to efalizumab or other protein components of the drug product. **Serious infections:** Cellulitis, pneumonia, abscess, sepsis, sinusitis, bronchitis, gastroenteritis, aseptic meningitis, Legionnaire's disease, septic arthritis, vertebral osteomyelitis, necrotizing fasciitis, tuberculosis pneumonia, bacterial sepsis. **Malignancies:** Nonmelanoma skin cancer, noncutaneous solid tumors, Hodgkin and non-Hodgkin lymphoma, malignant melanoma. **Hypersensitivity:** Laryngospasm, angioedema, erythema multiforme, asthma, allergic drug eruption. **Miscellaneous:** Headache, acne, peripheral edema, thrombocytopenia.

LABORATORY TEST CONSIDERATIONS

↑ Leukocyte counts.

HOW SUPPLIED

Powder for Injection, Lyophilized: 150 mg (to deliver 125 mg/1.25 mL).

DOSAGE

- **SC**

  Plaque psoriasis.

Single 0.7 mg/kg conditioning dose SC followed by weekly SC doses of 1 mg/kg, with a single dose not to exceed a total of 200 mg.

NURSING CONSIDERATIONS

ADMINISTRATION/STORAGE

1. Discontinue drug if hemolytic anemia occurs.

2. Prepare efalizumab solution as follows:

- Slowly inject 1.3 mL of sterile water for injection into efalizumab vial using provided prefilled diluent syringe.
- Swirl vial with a gentle rotary motion to dissolve drug. Do not shake; shaking causes foaming. Dissolution takes less than 5 min.

3. Reconstitute immediately before use; use only once. Product provided as a single-use vial and contains no antibacterial preservatives. Discard any unused reconstituted solution.

4. If reconstituted solution not used immediately, store vial at room temperature; use within 8 hr.

5. Do not add other medications to solutions containing efalizumab; do not reconstitute with any other diluent.

6. Injection sites include the abdomen, thigh, buttocks, or upper arm; rotate sites.

7. If appropriate, clients may self-inject efalizumab after proper training in the preparation and injection technique, and with medical follow-up.

8. Refrigerate at 2–8°C (36–46°F) until addition of diluent. Protect from exposure to light. Store in original carton until time of use.

ASSESSMENT

1. Note clinical presentation, extent of involvement, other agents trialed, outcome.

2. Monitor CBC with platelet count during therapy; then monitor every 3 months for evidence of thrombocytopenia.

CLIENT/FAMILY TEACHING

1. Drug used to decrease inflammation of psoriatic skin when other therapies have failed. It is administered SC once a week by injection.

2. After instruction and return demonstration, client may administer at home. Follow reconstitution guidelines, prepare just before use and do not shake vial. Do not use if solution contains particles or is discolored. If not able to use immediately, may store at room temperature for 8 hr and then discard if not used. Rotate injection sites using the abdomen, thigh, buttocks, or upper arm and report adverse effects or site reactions.

3. Report immediately any unusual bruising/bleeding, infections, weight changes, worsening of psoriasis, sudden illness, or newly diagnosed malignancy.

4. Practice reliable contraception; stop drug and report if pregnancy suspected.

5. Avoid vaccines during therapy; may be immunocompromised. Keep all F/U appointments to evaluate response to therapy and to monitor platelet counts.

OUTCOMES/EVALUATE

↓ Inflammation and clearing of plaque psoriasis

Efavirenz

(eh-**FAH**-vih-rehnz)

CLASSIFICATION(S):

Antiviral, non-nucleoside reverse transcriptase inhibitor

PREGNANCY CATEGORY: D

Rx: Sustiva.

SEE ALSO *ANTIVIRAL AGENTS.*

USES

In combination with other antiretroviral drugs to treat HIV-1 infection.

ACTION/KINETICS

Action

A nonnucleoside reverse transcriptase inhibitor of HIV-1 that acts mainly by noncompetitive inhibition of HIV-1.

Pharmacokinetics

Peak plasma levels: 3–5 hr. **Steady-state plasma levels:** 6–10 days. Metabolized by the cytochrome P450 system to inactive metabolites which are excreted in the urine and feces. Will induce its own metabolism. **t¹⁄₂, terminal:** 52–76 hr after a single dose and 40–55 hr after multiple doses. **Plasma protein binding:** 99.5–99.75%.

CONTRAINDICATIONS

Use as a single agent to treat HIV (resistant virus emerges rapidly) or added on as a sole agent to a failing regimen. High-fat meals (increase absorption). Use with cisapride, ergot derivatives, midazolam, or triazolam. Pregnancy or in those of childbearing age due to increased risk of birth defects. Lactation (to prevent postnatal transmission of HIV infection).

SPECIAL CONCERNS

Use with caution in impaired hepatic function.

SIDE EFFECTS

Most Common

Adults: Rash, N&V, dizziness, headache, insomnia, diarrhea, impaired concentration, dyspepsia, fatigue, abnormal dreams, somnolence, depression, nervousness.

Children: Rash, diarrhea/loose stools, fever, cough, dizziness, lightheadedness, fainting, ache/pain/discomfort, N&V, headache.

CNS: Delusions, inappropriate behavior (especially in those with a history of mental illness or substance abuse), severe acute depression with **suicidal ideation/attempts**, dizziness, lightheadedness, fainting, impaired concentration, somnolence, abnormal dreams, insomnia, fatigue, headache, hypoesthesia, depression, anorexia, nervousness, ataxia, confusion, **convulsions**, impaired coordination, migraine headaches, neuralgia, paresthesia, peripheral neuropathy, speech disorder, tremor, vertigo, aggravated depression, agitation, amnesia, anxiety, apathy, emotional lability, euphoria, hallucinations, psychosis, aggressive reactions, agitation, delusions, emotional lability, mania, neurosis, paranoia, **suicide**. **Dermatologic:** Skin rash, including moist or dry desquamation, ulceration, erythema, pruritus, diffuse maculopapular rash, vesiculation, erythema multiforme. Increased sweating, alopecia, eczema, folliculitis, urticaria, nail disorders, skin discoloration. Rarely, **Stevens-Johnson syndrome, toxic epidermal necrolysis**, necrosis requiring surgery, exfoliative dermatitis. **GI:** N&V, diarrhea, dyspepsia, abdominal pain, flatulence, dry mouth, pancreatitis, hepatitis, constipation, malabsorption, hepatic failure. **CV:** Flushing, palpitations, tachycardia, thrombophlebitis. **Respiratory:** Dyspnea, cough. **GU:** Hematuria, renal calculus. **Musculoskeletal:** Arthralgia, myalgia, myopathy, aches/pains. **Ophthalmic:** Abnormal vision, diplopia. **Miscellaneous:** Parosmia, taste perversion, alcohol intolerance, allergic reaction, asthenia, fever, hot flushes, malaise, pain, peripheral edema, syncope, tinnitus, asthma, redistribution/accumulation of body fat, gynecomastia, dyspnea.

LABORATORY TEST CONSIDERATIONS

↑ AST, ALT, total cholesterol, serum amylase, serum triglycerides. False + urine cannabinoid tests using the CEDIA DAU Multi-Level THC assay.

OD OVERDOSE MANAGEMENT

Symptoms: Increased nervous system symptoms. *Treatment:* General supportive measures, including monitoring of vital signs. Activated charcoal may be used to aid removal of unabsorbed drug.

DRUG INTERACTIONS

Amprenavir / ↓ Serum amprenavir levels

Carbamazepine / ↓ Levels of both drugs; monitor carbamazepine levels

Clarithromycin / ↓ Clarithromycin levels and ↑ levels of metabolite; use alternative therapy such as azithromycin

CNS depressants / Additive CNS depression

Ergot derivatives / Inhibition of ergot metabolism → possible cardiac arrhythmias, prolonged sedation, or respiratory depression

Indinavir / ↓ Indinavir levels R/T enzyme induction; ↑ indinavir dose

Methadone / ↑ Risk of methadone withdrawal symptoms R/T ↑ liver breakdown

Midazolam / Inhibition of midazolam metabolism → possible cardiac arrhythmias, prolonged sedation, or respiratory depression

Phenobarbital / ↓ Levels of both drugs; monitor phenobarbital levels

Phenytoin / ↓ Levels of both drugs; monitor levels

Rifabutin / Possible ↓ rifabutin levels and ↑ clearance of efavirenz

Rifampin / ↓ Efavirenz levels

Ritonavir / ↑ Levels of both drugs; higher frequency of dizziness, nausea, paresthesia, and elevated liver enzymes

Saquinavir / ↓ Saquinavir AUC and C_{max}

H *St. John's wort* / Possible significant ↓ efavirenz levels R/T ↑ hepatic metabolism by CYP3A4 isoenzymes

Triazolam / Inhibition of triazolam metabolism → possible cardiac arrhythmias, prolonged sedation, or respiratory depression

Warfarin / Possible ↑ or ↓ levels of warfarin

HOW SUPPLIED
Capsules: 50 mg, 100 mg, 200 mg; *Tablets:* 300 mg, 600 mg.

DOSAGE
- **CAPSULES; TABLETS**
  HIV-1 infections.
Adults: 600 mg once daily in combination with a protease inhibitor or nucleoside analog reverse transcriptase inhibitors. **Children, 3 years and older, 10 to <15 kg:** 200 mg once daily; **15 to <20 kg:** 250 mg once daily; **20 to <25 kg:** 300 mg once daily; **25 to <32.5 kg:** 350 mg once daily; **32.5 to <40 kg:** 400 mg once daily; **40 kg or more:** 600 mg once daily.

NURSING CONSIDERATIONS

ADMINISTRATION/STORAGE
1. Always initiate therapy with 1 or more other new antiretroviral drugs to which client has not been previously exposed.
2. May be taken with or without food; high-fat meals may increase absorption and are to be avoided.
3. Use bedtime dosing during first 2 to 4 weeks to improve tolerability of nervous system side effects.

ASSESSMENT
1. Note reasons for therapy, other agents trialed. Monitor lipid profile, LFTs.
2. May cause false-positive cannabinoid urine test.

CLIENT/FAMILY TEACHING
1. Take as directed and with other antiretroviral agents.
2. May take with food but avoid high-fat meals; may increase drug absorption.
3. May cause dizziness, drowsiness, delusions, and impaired concentration. Take at bedtime to increase tolerability; avoid tasks requiring concentration/dexterity until effects realized.
4. Drug does not cure disease but works to reduce viral load.
5. Practice reliable barrier contraception with additional form of birth control; do not breast feed.
6. Most clients will experience a rash. This should resolve after several weeks; report if persistent or extensive.
7. Avoid alcohol and any OTC agents.

OUTCOMES/EVALUATE
↓ HIV-RNA levels; ↑ CD_4 cell counts

Eletriptan hydrobromide
(**EH**-leh-trip-tan)

CLASSIFICATION(S):
Antimigraine drug
PREGNANCY CATEGORY: C
Rx: Relpax.

SEE ALSO *SEROTONIN 5-HT₁ RECEPTOR AGONISTS (ANTIMIGRAINE DRUGS).*

USES
Treatment of migraine with or without aura.

ACTION/KINETICS
Action
Binds with high affinity to $5\text{-}HT_{1B}$, $5\text{-}HT_{1D}$, and $5\text{-}HT_{1F}$ receptors. It is believed activation of these receptors located on intracranial blood vessels leads to vasoconstriction, which causes relief of migraine headache. The drug may also ac-

---

Bold Italic = life threatening side effect   ■ = black box warning   ♣ = Available in Canada

tivate 5-HT$_1$ receptors on sensory nerve endings in the trigeminal system resulting in inhibition of pro-inflammatory neuropeptide release.

Pharmacokinetics
Well absorbed; **peak plasma levels:** About 1.5 hr. Is approximately 50% bioavailable. A high-fat meal increases AUC and C$_{max}$ by 20–30%. Is metabolized by the CYP3A4 enzyme. The N-demethylated metabolite is active and contributes significantly to the overall effect of eletriptan. t$\frac{1}{2}$, **terminal:** 4 hr. The half-life is increased in the elderly. **Plasma protein binding:** About 85%.

CONTRAINDICATIONS
Use for prophylaxis of migraine or use in the management of hemiplegic or basilar migraine. Use in clients with the following: Ischemic heart disease (e.g., angina pectoris, history of MI, documented silent ischemia) or in those who have symptoms or findings consistent with ischemic heart disease, coronary artery vasospasm (including Prinzmetal's variant angina), or other significant underlying CV disease. Use in clients with cerebrovascular syndromes (including, but not limited to, strokes of any type as well as transient ischemic attacks), in peripheral vascular disease (including, but not limited to, ischemic bowel disease), in those with uncontrolled hypertension, within 24 hr of treatment with another 5-HT$_1$ agonist (e.g., dihydroergotamine, methysergide), or in those with severe hepatic impairment.

SPECIAL CONCERNS
Safety and efficacy have not been determined for cluster headache. Use with caution during lactation.

SIDE EFFECTS
Most Common
Asthenia, dizziness, nausea, paresthesia, somnolence, headache, chest tightness/pressure/heaviness, dry mouth.
See *Serotonin 5-HT$_1$ Receptor Agonists (Antimigraine Drugs)* for a complete list of possible side effects. **GI:** Nausea, dry mouth, dyspepsia, dysphagia. **CNS:** Somnolence, dizziness, headache. **Body as a whole:** Paresthesia, flushing/feeling of warmth, asthenia. **Miscellane-**

ous: Chest tightness, pain or pressure; abdominal pain, discomfort; stomach pain; cramps/pressure.

DRUG INTERACTIONS
Ergot-containing drugs (e.g., dihydroergotamine) / Prolonged vasospastic reactions; do not use within 24 hr of each other
Erythromycin / ↑ Eletriptan C$_{max}$ and AUC R/T ↓ metabolism
Fluoconazole / ↑ Eletriptan C$_{max}$ and AUC R/T ↓ metabolism
Ketoconazole / ↑ Eletriptan C$_{max}$ and AUC R/T ↓ metabolism
SSRIs / Possible weakness, hyperreflexia, and incoordination
Verapamil / ↑ Eletriptan C$_{max}$ and AUC R/T ↓ metabolism

HOW SUPPLIED
Tablets: 24.2 mg eletriptan hydrobromide (equivalent to 20 mg of the base), 48.5 mg eletriptan hydrobromide (equivalent to 40 mg of the base).

DOSAGE
● **TABLETS**
  Migraine with or without aura.
Adults: Individualize dose. Usually a single 20-mg or 40-mg dose (greater chance of a response). Maximum single dose: 40 mg; maximum daily dose: 80 mg. If after the initial dose the headache improves and then returns, a repeat dose may be beneficial. If a second dose is required, take at least 2 hr after the initial dose. If the initial dose is ineffective, a second dose may not be beneficial either.

NURSING CONSIDERATIONS
ADMINISTRATION/STORAGE
1. Do not use within 72 hr of treatment with clarithromycin, ketoconazole, itraconazole, nefazodone, nelfinavir, ritonavir, and troleandomycin.
2. Safety of treating an average of >3 headaches in a 30-day period has not been determined.
ASSESSMENT
1. Note reasons for therapy, neurologic evaluations, S&S, other agents trialed.
2. Assess for CHD, uncontrolled BP, CVA, severe liver problems; precludes drug therapy.

📷 = see color insert　　H = Herbal　　IV = Intravenous　　ℭ = sound alike drug

3. Note any evidence of increased cholesterol, obesity, smoking, or menopause.

CLIENT/FAMILY TEACHING

1. Take as directed; do not exceed prescribed dosage. Read info sheet accompanying product; do not share medications. Take at first sign of migraine; if headache returns, may take a second dose after 2 hr.

2. Drug works by reducing swollen blood vessels around the brain and reducing release of nerve substances that cause migraine headache symptoms.

3. Use caution, may experience nausea, dizziness, tiredness, or weakness, as well as pain or pressure in chest/throat. Report any increased SOB, pains, heaviness, or tightness in chest, jaw, or neck. Report adverse effects, or lack of response.

4. Do not take if you have used any other type of special headache medicines within 24 hr of clarithromycin, itraconazole, ketoconazole, nefazodone, nelfinavir, ritonavir, or troleandomycin. Do not use within 72 hr with drugs that have demonstrated potent CYP3A4 inhibition. Contact provider if unsure; avoid all OTC agents without approval.

OUTCOMES/EVALUATE

Relief of migraine headaches

Emtricitabine ∎
(em-trih-**SIGH**-tah-been)

CLASSIFICATION(S):
Antiretroviral drug, nucleoside reverse transcriptase inhibitor
PREGNANCY CATEGORY: C
Rx: Emtriva.

USES

In combination with other antiretroviral drugs for HIV-1 infection in clients older than 3 months of age. In antiretroviral treatment-experienced clients, emtricitabine may be considered for those with HIV strains that are expected to be susceptible to emtricitabine as assessed by genotypic or phenotypic testing. *In-*

vestigational: Hepatitis B virus (HBV) treatment.

ACTION/KINETICS

Action

Emtricitabine is phosphorylated by cellular enzymes to form emtricitabine 5′-triphosphate which then inhibits the activity of the HIV-1 reverse transcriptase by competing with the natural substrate deoxycytidine 5′-triphosphate. It is also incorporated into nascent viral DNA, which results in chain termination.

Pharmacokinetics

Pharmacokinetic data for children from birth to 3 months of age is similar to those of older infants, children, and adolescents. Rapidly and extensively absorbed; **peak plasma levels:** 1–2 hr. May be taken with or without food. Metabolized in the liver and excreted in both the feces (14%) and urine (86%). $t^1/_2$, **plasma:** About 10 hr. $t^1/_2$, **terminal, children:** About 8.9 hr. Is eliminated in the urine by both glomerular filtration and active tubular secretion; thus, there may be competition for elimination with other drugs/compounds that are also renally eliminated.

CONTRAINDICATIONS

Hypersensitivity to the drug or any components of the product. Lactation.

SPECIAL CONCERNS

∎ (1) Lactic acidosis and severe hepatomegaly with steatosis, including fatal cases, have been reported with the use of nucleoside analogs alone or in combination with other antiretroviral drugs. (2) Emtricitabine is not indicated for the treatment of chronic hepatitis B virus (HBV) infection, and the safety and efficacy of emtricitabine have not been established in clients coinfected with HBV and HIV. Severe acute exacerbations of hepatitis B have been reported in clients after the discontinuation of emtricitabine. Closely monitor hepatic function with clinical and laboratory follow-up for at least several months in clients who discontinue emtricitabine and are coinfected with HIV and HBV. If appropriate, initiation of anti-HBV therapy may be warranted.∎ Use with caution in the elderly. Safety and efficacy

---

Bold Italic = life threatening side effect   ∎ = black box warning   ♣ = Available in Canada have not been determined in children less than 3 months of age.

SIDE EFFECTS

Most Common

Headache, diarrhea, nausea, rash, asthenia, increased cough, rhinitis.

CNS: Headache, insomnia, depressive disorders, paresthesia, dizziness, neuropathy/peripheral neuritis, abnormal dreams. **GI:** Diarrhea, N&V, abdominal pain, dyspepsia. **Metabolic:** Redistribution or accumulation of body fat, including central obesity, dorsocervical fat enlargement (buffalo hump), peripheral/facial wasting, breast enlargement, and 'cushingoid' appearance. **Musculo-skeletal:** Myalgia, arthralgia. **Respiratory:** Rhinitis, increased cough. **Dermatologic:** Rash, pruritus, urticaria maculopapular/vesiculobullous/pustular rash, skin discoloration (hyperpigmentation on the palms and/or soles). **Miscellaneous:** Asthenia, immune reconstitution syndrome (inflammatory response to indolent or residual opportunistic infections, including *Mycobacterium avium*, cytomegalovirus, *Pneumocystis jirovecii*, pneumonia, tuberculosis), *allergic reactions.*

LABORATORY TEST CONSIDERATIONS

↑ ALT, AST, bilirubin, creatine kinase, pancreatic amylase, serum lipase, triglycerides. ↓ Neutrophils. ↑ or ↓ Serum glucose.

OD OVERDOSE MANAGEMENT

Symptoms: If overdose occurs, monitor for signs of toxicity and begin standard supportive care. There is no known antidote. Hemodialysis removes about 30% of an emtricitabine dose over a 3-hr period. *Treatment:* There is no known antidote. Hemodialysis removes about 30% of an emtricitabine dose over a 3-hr period.

HOW SUPPLIED

Capsules: 200 mg; *Oral Solution:* 10 mg/mL.

DOSAGE

- **CAPSULES; ORAL SOLUTION**
  HIV-1 infection in adults and children, 3 months and older.

Adults, 18 years and older: 200 mg of the capsules or 240 mg (24 mL) of the oral solution once daily with or without food. **Children, 3 months through 17 years:** For children weighing more than 33 kg who can swallow an intact capsule, one 200 mg capsule once daily. For the oral solution, 6 mg/kg, up to a maximum of 240 mg (24 mL) once daily. See *Administration/Storage* for the dosing interval in clients with baseline C_{CR} <50 mL/min.

NURSING CONSIDERATIONS

ADMINISTRATION/STORAGE

1. Adjust the dose as follows in clients with impaired renal function:
- $C_{CR,}$ 50 mL/min and greater: 200 mg q 24 hr of the capsule or 240 mg (24 mL) q 24 hr of the oral solution.
- C_{CR} 30–49 mL/min: 200 mg q 48 hr of the capsule or 120 mg (12 mL) q 24 hr of the oral solution.
- $C_{CR,}$ 15–20 mL/min: 200 mg q 72 hr of the capsule or 80 mg (8 mL) q 24 hr of the oral solution.
- $C_{CR,}$ <15 mL/min and those clients requiring hemodialysis: 200 mg q 96 hr of the capsule and 60 mg (6 mL) of the oral solution q 24 hr.

2. Store capsules from 15–30°C (59–86°F) and the oral solution refrigerated from 2–8°C (36–46°F). Use the oral solution within three months if stored from 15–30°C (59–86°F).

ASSESSMENT

1. Note disease onset, characteristics of S&S, other agents trialed, outcome. List drugs prescribed to ensure none interact.

2. Monitor HIV RNA, renal and LFTs; reduce dose with renal dysfunction based on C_{CR}.

CLIENT/FAMILY TEACHING

1. Take as directed with other antiretroviral therapy; always used in combination therapy. Must take for life.

2. Do not take any unprescribed/OTC medications/herbals without provider consent.

3. Drug may cause a redistribution of body fat. Does not prevent disease transmission or STDs; practice safe sex and use protection. Practice reliable birth control and report immediately if pregnancy suspected.

4. May continue to experience opportunistic infections. Long-term drug effects are unknown. May cause liver toxicity, and lactic acidosis; keep all F/U appointments/lab visits and report adverse side effects.

OUTCOMES/EVALUATE
↓ HIV RNA

Enalapril maleate
(en-**AL**-ah-prill)

CLASSIFICATION(S):
Antihypertensive, ACE inhibitor
PREGNANCY CATEGORY: D
Rx: Enalaprilat, Vasotec.

SEE ALSO ANGIOTENSIN-CONVERTING ENZYME INHIBITORS.
USES
PO: (1) Alone or in combination with other antihypertensives (especially thiazide diuretics) for the treatment of hypertension. Hypertension in children. (2) In combination with digitalis and diuretic in acute and chronic CHF. (3) Asymptomatic left ventricular dysfunction in clinically stable asymptomatic clients.

IV: Treatment of hypertension when PO is not practical.

Investigational: Hypertension related to scleroderma renal crisis. Treatment of diabetic nephropathy in normotensive clients. Enalaprilat may be used for hypertensive emergencies (effect is variable).

ACTION/KINETICS
Action
Enalapril (and its active metabolite enalaprilat) inhibit angiotensin-converting enzyme resulting in decreased plasma angiotensin II, which leads to decreased vasopressor activity and decreased aldosterone secretion. The parenteral product is enalaprilat injection.

Pharmacokinetics
About 60% bioavailable after PO. **Onset, PO:** 1 hr; **IV:** 15 min. **Time to peak action, PO:** 4–6 hr; **IV:** 1–4 hr. **Duration, PO:** 24 hr or more; **IV:** About 6 hr.

t½, enalapril, PO: 1.3 hr; **IV:** 15 min. **t½, enalaprilat, PO:** 11 hr. Excreted through the urine (half unchanged) and feces; over 90% of enalaprilat is excreted through the urine. **Plasma protein binding:** Approximately 50–60%.

SPECIAL CONCERNS
■ When used during the second and third trimesters of pregnancy, injury and even death can result in the developing fetus. When pregnancy is detected, discontinue as soon as possible.■ Use with caution during lactation. Safety and effectiveness have not been determined in children.

SIDE EFFECTS
Most Common
Dizziness, headache, hypotension, syncope, chest pain, fatigue, diarrhea, cough.

CV: Palpitations, hypotension, chest pain, angina, *CVA, MI*, orthostatic hypotension/effects, disturbances in rhythm, tachycardia, *cardiac arrest*, atrial fibrillation, tachycardia, bradycardia, Raynaud's phenomenon. **GI:** N&V, diarrhea, abdominal pain, alterations in taste, anorexia, dry mouth, constipation, dyspepsia, glossitis, ileus, melena, stomatitis. **CNS:** Insomnia, headache, fatigue, dizziness, paresthesias, nervousness, sleepiness, ataxia, confusion, depression, vertigo, abnormal dreams. **Hepatic:** Hepatitis, hepatocellular or cholestatic jaundice, pancreatitis, elevated liver enzymes, hepatic failure. **Respiratory:** Bronchitis, cough, dyspnea, bronchospasm, URI, pneumonia, pulmonary infiltrates, asthma, *pulmonary embolism and infarction, pulmonary edema*. **Renal:** Renal dysfunction, oliguria, UTI, transient increases in creatinine and BUN. **Hematologic:** Rarely, neutropenia, thrombocytopenia, bone marrow depression, decreased H&H in hypertensive or CHF clients. Hemolytic anemia, including hemolysis, in clients with G6PD deficiency. **Dermatologic:** Rash, pruritus, alopecia, flushing, erythema multiforme, exfoliative dermatitis, photosensitivity, urticaria, increased sweating, pemphigus, *Stevens-Johnson syndrome*, herpes zoster, *toxic epidermal necrolysis*. **Miscellaneous:** *Angi-*

Bold Italic = life threatening side effect   ■ = black box warning   ✦ = Available in Canada

oedema, asthenia, impotence, blurred vision, fever, arthralgia, arthritis, vasculitis, eosinophilia, tinnitus, syncope, myalgia, muscle cramps, rhinorrhea, sore throat, hoarseness, conjunctivitis, tearing, dry eyes, loss of sense of smell, hearing loss, peripheral neuropathy, anosmia, myositis, flank pain, gynecomastia.

ADDITIONAL DRUG INTERACTIONS

Rifampin may ↓ the effects of enalapril. Do not discontinue without first reporting to the provider.

HOW SUPPLIED

Injection: 1.25 mg/mL (as enalaprilat); *Tablets:* 2.5 mg, 5 mg, 10 mg, 20 mg.

DOSAGE

ENALAPRIL

- **TABLETS**

  Antihypertensive in clients not taking diuretics.

Initial: 5 mg/day; **then,** adjust dosage according to response (range: 10–40 mg/day in one to two doses). In some clients treated once daily, the antihypertensive effect may decrease toward the end of the dosing interval; if this occurs, consider an increase in dosage or twice-daily administration.

  Antihypertensive in clients taking diuretics.

Initial: 2.5 mg. Since hypotension may occur following the initiation of enalapril, the diuretic should be discontinued, if possible, for 2–3 days before initiating enalapril. If BP is not maintained with enalapril alone, diuretic therapy may be resumed.

  Hypertension in children.

Initial: 0.08 mg/kg, up to 5 mg, once daily. Adjust dose depending on response. Do not give to neonates and children with a GFR <30 mL/min/1.73 m^2

  Adjunct with diuretics and digitalis in heart failure.

Initial: 2.5 mg 1–2 times per day; **then,** depending on the response, 2.5–20 mg/day in two divided doses. Dose should not exceed 40 mg/day. Dosage must be adjusted in clients with renal impairment or hyponatremia.

  In clients with impaired renal function.

Initial: 5 mg/day if C_{CR} ranges between 30 and 80 mL/min and serum creatinine is less than 3 mg/dL; 2.5 mg/day if C_{CR} is less than 30 mL/min and serum creatinine is more than 3 mg/dL and in dialysis clients on dialysis days.

  Renal impairment or hyponatremia.

Initial: 2.5 mg/day if serum sodium is less than 130 mEq/L and serum creatinine is more than 1.6 mg/dL. The dose may be increased to 2.5 mg twice a day and then 5 mg twice a day or higher if required; dose is given at intervals of 4 or more days. Maximum daily dose is 40 mg.

  Asymptomatic LV dysfunction following MI.

2.5 mg twice a day, titrated as tolerated to the daily dose of 20 mg in divided doses.

ENALAPRILAT

- **IV**

  Hypertension.

1.25 mg over a 5-min period; repeat q 6 hr.

  Antihypertensive in clients taking diuretics.

Initial: 0.625 mg over 5 min; if an adequate response is seen after 1 hr, administer another 0.625-mg dose. Thereafter, 1.25 mg q 6 hr. In those taking diuretics, start with 0.625 mg enalaprilat over 5 min; if there is an inadequate effect after 1 hr, repeat the 0.625 mg dose. Give additional doses of 1.25 mg q 6 hr.

  Clients with impaired renal function.

Give enalaprilat, 1.25 mg q 6 hr for clients with a C_{CR} more than 30 mL/min and an initial dose of 0.625 mg for clients with a C_{CR} less than 30 mL/min. If there is an adequate response, an additional 0.625 mg may be given after 1 hr; thereafter, additional 1.25-mg doses can be given q 6 hr. For dialysis clients, the initial dose is 0.625 mg q 6 hr.

  Hypertensive emergency.

1.25 mg IV over 5 min q 6 hr; titrate by 1.25 mg increments up to a maximum dose of 5 mg.

NURSING CONSIDERATIONS

℞ Do not confuse enalapril with Anafranil (an antidepressant) or with Eldepryl (an antiparkinson drug).

📷 = see color insert   H = Herbal   IV = Intravenous   ℞ = sound alike drug

ADMINISTRATION/STORAGE

1. To convert from IV to PO therapy in clients on a diuretic, begin with 2.5 mg/day for clients responding to a 0.625-mg IV dose. Thereafter, 2.5 mg/day may be given.

2. Use lower dose if receiving diuretics or impaired renal function.

3. A 1 mg/mL suspension may be prepared for use in children (see instructions in the labeling).

4. Carefully select dosage of all enalapril products in the geriatric client R/T decreased renal function with advancing age.

IV 5. To convert from PO to IV therapy in clients not on a diuretic, use the recommended IV dose (i.e., 1.25 mg every 6 hr). To convert from IV to PO therapy, begin with 5 mg/day.

6. Following IV administration, first dose peak effect may take 4 hr (whether or not on a diuretic). For subsequent doses, the peak effect is usually within 15 min.

7. Give enalaprilat as a slow IV infusion (over 5 min) either alone or diluted up to 50 mL with an appropriate diluent. Any of the following can be used: D5W, D5/RL, McGaw Isolyte E, 0.9% NaCl, D5/0.9% NaCl.

8. When used initially for heart failure, observe for at least 2 hr after initial dose and until BP has stabilized for an additional hour. If possible, reduce dose of diuretic.

9. Store below 30°C (86°F).

ASSESSMENT

1. Note reasons for therapy, presenting symptoms, other agents trialed, outcome.

2. Record ECG, VS, and weight.

3. Monitor CBC, electrolytes, renal and LFTs. Reduce dose with impaired renal function/hyponatremia.

CLIENT/FAMILY TEACHING

1. For BP lowering. Use caution, may cause low BP effects and dizziness.

2. Maintain healthy diet; limit intake of caffeine; avoid alcohol, salt substitutes, or high Na and high K foods.

3. Report any weight loss that may result from the loss of taste; or rapid weight gain that may result from fluid overload.

4. Any persistent dry cough, flu-like symptoms, rash, or unusual side effects should be reported immediately. Keep record of home BP readings for provider review.

OUTCOMES/EVALUATE

- ↓ BP
- ↓ Preload and afterload with CHF

Enfuvirtide
(en-**FYOU**-vir-tide)

CLASSIFICATION(S):
Antiretroviral drug, fusion inhibitor
PREGNANCY CATEGORY: B
Rx: Fuzeon.

USES

In combination with other antiretroviral drugs to treat HIV-1 infection in treatment-experienced clients with evidence of HIV-1 replication despite ongoing antiretroviral therapy.

ACTION/KINETICS

Action

Enfuvirtide is an inhibitor of the fusion of HIV-1 with CD4+ cells. The drug interferes with the entry of HIV-1 into cells by inhibiting the fusion of the viral and cellular membranes.

Pharmacokinetics

Time to peak levels: 3–12 hr. Is about 84% bioavailable. Since the drug is a peptide, it is expected to undergo catabolism into its constituent amino acids with subsequent recycling of the amino acids in the body pool. **t½:** 3.8 hr. Clearance is 20% lower in women than men; no dosage adjustment is necessary, however. Clearance decreases with decreased body weight; no dosage adjustment is necessary. **Plasma protein binding:** About 92% in HIV-infected plasma.

CONTRAINDICATIONS

Hypersensitivity to the drug or any component of the product. Lactation.

SPECIAL CONCERNS

Theoretically, enfuvirtide use may cause production of antienfuvirtide antibod-

---

Bold Italic = life threatening side effect   ■ = black box warning   ✤ = Available in Canada

ies that cross-react with HIV gp41. This could result in a false-positive HIV test with an ELISA assay; a confirmatory Western blot test would be expected to be negative. SC injections with the needle-free Biojector 2000 has been associated with neuralgia and/or paresthesia lasting up to 6 months when used at sites where large nerves course close to the skin (e.g., elbow, knee, groin, medial sections of the buttocks). Safety and efficacy have not been determined in children less than 6 years of age.

SIDE EFFECTS

Most Common

Injection site reaction (pain/discomfort, induration, erythema, nodules/cysts, pruritus, ecchymosis), diarrhea, nausea, fatigue, weight loss, sinusitis, abdominal pain, cough, herpes simplex.

Local injection site reactions: Pain, discomfort, induration, erythema, nodules and cysts, pruritus, ecchymosis. **Hypersensitivity:** Rash, fever, N&V, chills, rigors, hypotension, elevated serum liver transaminases, primary immune complex reaction, respiratory distress, glomerulonephritis, Guillain-Barre syndrome. **CNS:** Insomnia, peripheral neuropathy, depression, anxiety, taste disturbance, sixth nerve palsy. **GI:** Diarrhea, nausea, decreased appetite, constipation, anorexia, pancreatitis, upper abdominal pain. **Hematologic:** Thrombocytopenia, neutropenia, fever. **Infections:** Increased rate of bacterial pneumonia, herpes simplex, sinusitis, herpes simplex, skin papilloma, influenza. **GU:** Glomerulonephritis, renal failure. **Body as a whole:** Fatigue, decreased weight, asthenia, pruritus. **Miscellaneous:** Cough, myalgia, sinusitis, lymphadenopathy, conjunctivitis, hyperglycemia.

LABORATORY TEST CONSIDERATIONS

↑ Amylase, lipase, ALT, AST, creatine phosphokinase, GGT, triglycerides. ↓ Hemoglobin. Eosinophilia.

HOW SUPPLIED

Powder for Injection, Lyophilized: 108 mg (about 90 mg/mL when reconstituted).

DOSAGE

• **SC**

HIV-1 infection.

Adults: 90 mg (1 mL) twice a day SC into the upper arm, anterior thigh, or abdomen. **Children, 6–16 years:** 2 mg/kg twice a day, up to a maximum of 90 mg twice a day SC into the upper arm, anterior thigh, or abdomen. (See *Administration/Storage* for specific pediatric dosing guidelines.)

NURSING CONSIDERATIONS

ADMINISTRATION/STORAGE

1. Pediatric dosing guidelines for enfuvirtide using the 90 mg/mL reconstituted solution are: **11–15.5 kg:** 27 mg/dose (0.3 mL); **15.6–20 kg:** 36 mg/dose (0.4 mL); **20.1–24.5 kg:** 45 mg/dose (0.5 mL); **24.6–29 kg:** 54 mg/dose (0.6 mL); **29.1–33.5 kg:** 63 mg/dose (0.7 mL); **33.6–38 kg:** 72 mg/dose (0.8 mL); **38.1–42.5 kg:** 81 mg/dose (0.9 mL); **42.6 kg or greater:** 90 mg/dose (1 mL).

2. Reconstitute only with 1.1 mL of sterile water for injection.

3. Enfuvirtide contains no preservatives. Once reconstituted, inject immediately or keep refrigerated in original vial; use within 24 hr. Bring refrigerated reconstituted solution to room temperature before injection. Visually inspect vial to ensure that the contents are fully dissolved in solution and solution is clear, colorless, and without bubbles or particulate matter.

4. Product is for single use only; discard unused portions.

5. Give each injection at a different site from preceding injection site and only where there is no current injection site reaction from an earlier dose.

6. Do not inject enfuvirtide directly over a blood vessel or into moles, scar tissue, bruises, tatoos, burn sites, near the navel, or where there is an injection site reaction.

7. Store lyophilized powder for injection from 15–30°C (59–86°F). Store reconstituted solution under refrigeration at 2–8°C (36–46°F); use within 24 hr.

ASSESSMENT

1. Note disease onset, characteristics of S&S, other agents trialed, outcome.

2. List drugs prescribed to ensure none interact.

3. Note Western blot results as HIV test with an ELISA assay may be false positive.

CLIENT/FAMILY TEACHING

1. Drug is given subcutaneously by injection twice a day. Injections with the needle-free Biojector 2000 has been associated with neuralgia and/or paresthesia lasting up to 6 months when used near elbow, knee, groin, medial sections of the buttocks. It is taken with other antiretroviral drugs.

2. If given sc may experience pain and inflammation at injection site. Review how to prepare and inject medication, dispose of needles, rotate sites and notify provider if redness and swelling at site do not resolve.

3. Do not perform activities that require mental alertness until drug effects realized; may experience dizziness.

4. Report fever, ↑ SOB, cough, and labored breathing, as pneumonia has been reported. Clients developing S&S of hypersensitivity reaction (rash, N&V, fever, chills) should discontinue drug and seek medical evaluation immediately. Do not restart therapy.

5. Practice safe sex and reliable contraception; report if pregnant or plan to become pregnant. Alert provider if planning to breastfeed. Drug is not a cure for HIV, may continue to experience opportunistic infections.

6. Clients may have medication dispensed by their own pharmacist at the pharmacy of their choice (no longer available only through Chronimed, Inc.). May call 1-877-438-9366 or 1-877-4fuzeon Mon-Fri 8am-8pm or go to www.fuzeon.com for more information on self-administration/drug therapy or the FUZEON as soon as possible program (FUZEON Accelerated Simultaneous Access Program).

7. A 'FUZEON Travel Card' is also available at www.fuzeon.com. This card, with a healthcare provider's signature, is required for those who plan to travel by air with the syringes required for FUZEON administration.

OUTCOMES/EVALUATE

↓ HIV RNA

Enoxaparin   ■ IV
(ee-**nox**-ah-**PAIR**-in)

CLASSIFICATION(S):
Anticoagulant, low molecular weight heparin
PREGNANCY CATEGORY: B
Rx: Lovenox.
✦**Rx:** Lovenox HP.

SEE ALSO *HEPARINS, LOW MOLECULAR WEIGHT.*

USES

(1) Acute (in the hospital) and extended (at home for up to three weeks) prophylaxis of DVT, which may lead to pulmonary embolism, after hip or knee replacement surgery or abdominal surgery in those at risk for thromboembolic complications, including severely restricted mobility due to acute illness. (2) With warfarin for inpatient treatment of DVT with and without pulmonary embolism; with warfarin for outpatient treatment of DVT without pulmonary embolism. (3) With aspirin to prevent ischemic complications of unstable angina and non-Q-wave MI. Can be used in geriatric clients. (4) Acute ST-segment elevation myocardial infarction in those receiving thrombolysis and being managed medically or with percutaneous coronary intervention.

ACTION/KINETICS

Pharmacokinetics

t½, elimination: 4.5 hr after SC use. Elimination may be delayed in the elderly. **Duration:** 12 hr following a 40-mg dose. Excreted mainly through the urine.

CONTRAINDICATIONS

IM use. Use with prosthetic heart valves due to possible valve thrombosis, especially in pregnant women. Hypersensitivity to enoxaparin, heparin, pork products and in those with active major bleeding.

SPECIAL CONCERNS

■ (1) Spinal/Epidural hematomas. When neuraxial anesthesia (epidural/spinal anesthesia) or spinal puncture is used,

---

Bold Italic = life threatening side effect   ■ = black box warning   ✦ = Available in Canada

those anticoagulated or scheduled to be anticoagulated with low molecular weight heparins or heparinoids to prevent thromboembolic complications are at risk of developing a spinal or epidural hematoma that can result in long-term or permanent paralysis. Risk is increased using indwelling epidural catheters for giving analgesics or by the concomitant use of drugs affecting hemostasis, such as NSAIDs, platelet inhibitors, or other anticoagulants. The risk also appears to increase by traumatic or repeated spinal or epidural puncture. (2) Frequently monitor for signs and symptoms of neurological impairment. If observed, urgent treatment is required. (3) The health care provider should consider potential benefits vs. risk before neuraxial intervention in clients anticoagulated or to be anticoagulated for thromboprophylaxis.■

Use with caution during pregnancy.

SIDE EFFECTS
Most Common
Anemia, dyspnea, edema, fever, peripheral edema, confusion, pruritus/rash, nausea, diarrhea, thrombocytopenia, injection site reactions including hemorrhage.

Hematologic: Thrombocytopenia, thrombocythemia, thrombocytosis, hematoma, *hemorrhage*, hypochromic anemia, ecchymosis, epidural/spinal hematoma when used with spinal/epidural anesthesia or spinal puncture. **Injection site:** Mild local irritation, pain, hematoma, erythema, hemorrhage, inflammation, nodules, skin necrosis, oozing. **GI:** Nausea, diarrhea. **CNS:** Confusion. **CV:** Atrial fibrillation, *heart failure*. **Dermatologic:** Pruritus, rash, cutaneous vasculitis, purpura. **GU:** Hematuria. **Respiratory:** Dyspnea, lung edema, pneumonia. **Miscellaneous:** Fever, pain, edema, peripheral edema, hypersensitivity.

LABORATORY TEST CONSIDERATIONS
Hyperlipidemia (rare).

HOW SUPPLIED
Injection: 30 mg/0.3 mL, 40 mg/0.4 mL, 60 mg/0.6 mL, 80 mg/0.8 mL, 100 mg/1 mL, 120 mg/0.8 mL, 150 mg/1 mL, 300 mg/3 mL.

DOSAGE
• **SC ONLY**
Prophylaxis of DVT in hip or knee replacement.
Adults: 30 mg q 12 hr with the initial dose given within 12–24 hr after surgery (providing hemostasis has been established) for 7–10 days (usually), up to 14 days. For hip replacement, a dose of 40 mg once daily may be considered; give 9–15 hr before surgery and continue for 3 weeks.
Prophylaxis of DVT in abdominal surgery.
Adults: 40 mg once daily, with the initial dose given 2 hr prior to surgery. Give for 7–10 days, up to 12 days.
Prophylaxis of DVT for medical clients during acute illness.
40 mg once daily for 6–11 days (up to 14 days has been well tolerated).
Treatment of DVT with or without pulmonary embolism for outpatients.
1 mg/kg SC q 12 hr.
Treatment of DVT without pulmonary embolism in outpatients.
1 mg/kg q 12 hr SC.
Treatment of DVT with or without pulmonary embolism for inpatients.
1 mg/kg SC q 12 hr or 1.5 mg/kg SC once daily at the same time each day. *NOTE:* For both in- and outpatients, initiate warfarin within 72 hr of enoxaparin. Continue enoxaparin for a minimum of 5 days and until an INR of 2–3 is reached (average duration is 7 days; up to 17 days has been well tolerated).
Acute ST-segment elevation myocardial infarction.
Single IV bolus of 30 mg plus a 1 mg/kg SC dose followed by 1 mg/kg given SC q 12 hr (maximum of 100 mg for the first 2 doses only, followed by 1 mg/kg dosing for the remaining doses). Adjust dosage in those over 75 years of age.

When given with a thrombolytic (fibrin-specific or nonfibrin-specific), give enoxaparin between 15 minutes before and 30 minutes after the start of fibrolytic therapy. All clients should receive aspirin as soon after acute ST-segment elevation MI has been diagnosed and maintained with 75–325 mg aspirin once daily unless contraindicated.

For clients managed with percutaneous coronary intervention, no additional dosing is needed if the last SC injection was given less than 8 hr before balloon inflation. If the last SC injection was given more than 8 hr before balloon inflation, give an IV bolus of enoxaparin of 0.3 mg/kg.

Acute ST-segment elevation MI in those 75 years of age and older.

Initial: 0.75 mg/kg SC q 12 hr (maximum of 75 mg for the first 2 doses only) followed by 0.75 mg/kg for the remaining doses. **Do not use an initial IV bolus.**

Unstable angina/Non-Q-wave MI.

1 mg/kg q 12 hr with PO aspirin (100–325 mg once/day). Use for a minimum of 2 days; usual duration for enoxaparin is 2–8 days, up to 12.5 days.

NOTE: For clients with a C_{CR} less than 30 mL/min, the dose is 30 mg once daily for DVT prophylaxis in abdominal surgery, hip or knee replacement surgery, or medical clients during acute illness. The dose is 1 mg/kg once daily for prophylaxis of ischemic complications of unstable angina and non-Q-wave MI (when used with aspirin), inpatient treatment of acute DVT with or without pulmonary embolism (when used with warfarin), or outpatient treatment of acute DVT without pulmonary embolism (when given with warfarin). For treatment of acute ST-segment elevation MI in clients less than 75 years of age, the dose is 30 mg as a single IV bolus plus a 1 mg/kg SC dose followed by 1 mg/kg given SC once a day. For treatment of acute ST-segment elevation MI in clients over 75 years of age, give 1 mg/kg SC once daily (no initial bolus).

NURSING CONSIDERATIONS

ADMINISTRATION/STORAGE

1. Consider adjusting dose for low weight (<45 kg) clients and those with a C_{CR} <30 mL/min.
2. Use tuberculin syringe or equivalent to ensure withdrawal of appropriate drug volume.
3. Give only by deep SC while lying down; do *not* give IM.

4. Continue treatment throughout postsurgical period until risk of DVT decreased.
5. Do not mix with other injections/infusions.
6. Discard any unused solution.
7. Do *not* interchange (unit for unit) with unfractionated heparin or other low molecular weight heparins as they differ in their manufacturing process, molecular weight distribution, anti-Xa and anti-IIa activities, units, and dosage.
8. Injection is clear and colorless to pale yellow; store at 15–30°C (59–86°F). Do not freeze.
9. Do not store the multidose vial for more than 28 days after the first use.
IV 10.   For IV injection use the multidose vial. Give through an IV line.
11. May be safely given with normal saline solution or D5W.
12. Do not mix or coadminister with other drug.
13. To avoid possible mixture of enoxaparin with other drugs, flush the IV access with a sufficient amount of saline or dextrose solution prior to and following IV bolus administration to clear the port of the drugs.

ASSESSMENT

1. Note reasons for therapy, clinical presentation, S&S of pulmonary embolism or DVT.
2. Assess for a bleeding disorder before giving enoxaparin, unless the drug is urgently needed.
3. Assess for heparin or pork product sensitivity; disorders that may preclude drug therapy.
4. List baseline hematologic parameters, liver function, and coagulation studies. If normal coagulation, monitor platelet counts. Drug may cause significant, nonsymptomatic increases in SGOT and SGPT.
5. Monitor VS; observe for early S&S of bleeding. Any unexplained fall in hematocrit or BP should lead to a search for a bleeding site. Those with spinal or epidural anesthesia should have neuro assessments regularly.
6. Assess clients with renal dysfunction, the elderly closely. Drug is extremely

---

expensive order in small lots. Report any evidence of thromboembolic event.

CLIENT/FAMILY TEACHING

1. May self-inject once provider determines appropriate and with medical follow-up. Lie down during self-administration; use prefilled syringes and administer at the same time each day.

2. Alternate administration between the left and right anterolateral and posterolateral abdominal wall.

3. Introduce the entire length of the needle into a skin fold held between the thumb and forefinger; hold throughout the injection. To minimize bruising, do not rub site.

4. May experience mild discomfort, irritation, hematoma at injection site. Report unusual bruising, bleeding or weakness. Practice reliable contraception.

5. Avoid OTC agents that contain aspirin; use electric razor to shave, a soft toothbrush, and a nightlight to prevent falls and potential bleeding.

OUTCOMES/EVALUATE

• DVT prophylaxis post-surgery

• Thromboembolic occurrence/recurrence prophylaxis

Entacapone
(en-**TAH**-kah-pohn)

CLASSIFICATION(S):
Antiparkinson drug
PREGNANCY CATEGORY: C
Rx: Comtan.

USES

As an adjunct with levodopa/carbidopa to treat idiopathic parkinsonism clients who experience signs and symptoms of end-of-dose 'wearing off.'

ACTION/KINETICS

Action

A selective and reversible catechol-O-methyltransferase (COMT) inhibitor. COMT eliminates catechols (e.g., dopa, dopamine, norepinephrine, epinephrine) and in the presence of a decarboxylase inhibitor (e.g., carbidopa), COMT becomes the major metabolizing enzyme for dopa. Thus, in the presence of a COMT inhibitor, levels of dopa and dopamine increase. When entacapone is given with levodopa and carbidopa, plasma levels of levodopa are greater and more sustained than after levodopa/carbidopa alone. This leads to more constant dopaminergic stimulation in the brain resulting in improvement of the signs and symptoms of Parkinson's disease.

Pharmacokinetics

Rapidly absorbed. Almost completely metabolized in the liver with most excreted in the feces. **t½, elimination:** Biphasic 0.4–0.7 hr and 2.4 hr. **Plasma protein binding:** 98%.

CONTRAINDICATIONS

Concomitant use with a nonselective MAO inhibitor (e.g., phenelzine, tranylcypromine).

SPECIAL CONCERNS

Use with caution during lactation and in clients with biliary obstruction. At present, there is no potential use in children. Use with caution with drugs known to be metabolized by COMT (e.g., apomorphine, bitolterol, dobutamine, dopamine, epinephrine, isoetharine, isoproterenol, methyldopa, norepinephrine) due to the possibility of increased HR, arrhythmias, and excessive changes in BP.

SIDE EFFECTS

Most Common

Dyskinesia, nausea, hyperkinesia, diarrhea, urine discoloration, hypokinesia, dizziness, abdominal pain, constipation, fatigue.

CNS: Dyskinesia, hyper/hypokinesia, dizziness, anxiety, somnolence (may be sudden and uncontrolled), agitation, hallucinations. **GI:** Nausea, diarrhea, abdominal pain, constipation, vomiting, dry mouth, dyspepsia, flatulence, gastritis, GI disorder. **Body as a whole:** Fatigue, asthenia, increased sweating, bacterial infection. **Miscellaneous:** Urine discoloration, back pain, dyspnea, purpura, taste perversion, rhabdomyolysis.

OD OVERDOSE MANAGEMENT

Symptoms: Abdominal pain, loose stools. *Treatment:* Symptomatic with

---

supportive care. Consider hospitalization. Monitor respiratory and circulatory systems. Review for possible drug interactions.

DRUG INTERACTIONS

Ampicillin / ↓ Entacapone biliary excretion

Apomorphine / Possible ↑ HR, arrhythmias, and excessive BP changes

Bitolterol / Possible ↑ HR, arrhythmias, and excessive BP changes

Chloramphenicol / ↓ Entacapone biliary excretion

Cholestyramine / ↓ Entacapone biliary excretion

Dobutamine / Possible ↑ HR, arrhythmias, and excessive BP changes

Dopamine / Possible ↑ HR, arrhythmias, and excessive BP changes

Epinephrine / Possible ↑ HR, arrhythmias, and excessive BP changes

Erythromycin / ↓ Entacapone biliary excretion

Isoetharine / Possible ↑ HR, arrhythmias, and excessive BP changes

Isoproterenol / Possible ↑ HR, arrhythmias, and excessive BP changes

MAO inhibitors (phenelzine, tranylcypromine) / Significant ↑ levels of catecholamines

Methyldopa / Possible ↑ HR, arrhythmias, and excessive BP changes

Norepinephrine / Possible ↑ HR, arrhythmias, and excessive BP changes

Probenecid / ↓ Entacapone biliary excretion

Rifampicin / ↓ Entacapone biliary excretion

HOW SUPPLIED

Tablets: 200 mg.

DOSAGE

• **TABLETS**

Parkinsonism.

200 mg given concomitantly with each levodopa/carbidopa dose up to a maximum of 8 times per day (i.e., 1,600 mg/day).

NURSING CONSIDERATIONS

ADMINISTRATION/STORAGE

1. Always give in combination with levodopa/carbidopa; entacapone has no antiparkinson effect by itself.

2. Most clients required a decreased daily levodopa dose (about 25%) if their daily levodopa dose was 800 mg or more, or if they had moderate or severe dyskinesias prior to entacapone treatment.

3. Entacapone can be given with immediate- or sustained-release levodopa/carbidopa formulations.

4. Rapid withdrawal or abrupt reduction in entacapone dose can lead to emergence of S&S of parkinsonism and could lead to a complex resembling neuroleptic malignant syndrome (hyperpyrexia and confusion).

5. If necessary to discontinue treatment, withdraw clients slowly from entacapone.

ASSESSMENT

1. Note onset of Parkinson's disease, levodopa/carbidopa dosage, and when symptoms occur in dosage cycle. Assess mental status, mood, and involuntary movement/occurrence.

2. Determine any evidence of liver or biliary dysfunction. Monitor LFTs, H&H and ferritin levels with prolonged therapy.

3. List drugs prescribed to ensure none interact.

CLIENT/FAMILY TEACHING

1. Take as directed with levodopa/carbidopa with or without food. Do not crush or chew tablets.

2. Drug is used to prevent end-of-dose 'wearing off' effects of Sinemet; alone it has no antiparkinson effect.

3. Never stop abruptly! Report any high fever or rigidity immediately.

4. Do not perform activities that require mental or physical alertness until drug effects realized.

5. May experience loss of consciousness, nausea, diarrhea, hallucinations, increase in involuntary movements, altered pulmonary or kidney function. Report if evident.

6. Urine may appear brownish-orange in color.

7. Rise slowly from a sitting or lying position to prevent sudden drop in BP or dizziness.

8. Avoid alcohol during therapy.

Bold Italic = life threatening side effect   ■ = black box warning   ✦ = Available in Canada

9. Drug is not for use during pregnancy or breastfeeding. Report if pregnancy suspected or desired.

OUTCOMES/EVALUATE
Improved control of Parkinson's disease; (↓ (dyskinesia): stiffness, tremor and shuffling; ↑ coordination)

Ephedrine sulfate [IV]
(eh-**FED**-rin)

E

CLASSIFICATION(S):
Sympathomimetic, direct- and indirect-acting
PREGNANCY CATEGORY: C
OTC: Capsules: Ephedrine Sulfate.
Rx: Injection: Ephedrine Sulfate.

SEE ALSO *SYMPATHOMIMETIC DRUGS.*

USES
PO: Temporary relief of shortness of breath, tightness of chest, and wheezing due to bronchial asthma or bronchospasm.
   Parenteral: (1) Allergic disorders, including bronchial asthma. (2) Pressor agent, especially during spinal anesthesia when hypotension occurs frequently. (3) Stokes-Adams syndrome with complete heart block. (4) Myasthenia gravis. (5) CNS stimulant in narcolepsy.
   Investigational: Depression (to enhance physical and mental energy).

ACTION/KINETICS
Action
Releases norepinephrine from synaptic storage sites. Has direct effects on alpha, beta-1, and beta-2 receptors, causing increased BP due to arteriolar constriction and cardiac stimulation, bronchodilation, relaxation of GI tract smooth muscle, nasal decongestion, mydriasis, and increased tone of the bladder trigone and vesicle sphincter. It may also increase skeletal muscle strength, especially in myasthenia clients. Significant CNS effects include stimulation of the cerebral cortex and subcortical centers. Hepatic glycogenolysis is increased, but not as much as

with epinephrine. More stable and longer-lasting than epinephrine.

Pharmacokinetics
Rapidly and completely absorbed following parenteral use. **Onset, IM:** 10–20 min; **PO:** 15–60 min; **SC:** >20 min. **Duration, IM, SC:** 30–60 min; **PO:** 3–5 hr. t$^{1/2}$, **elimination:** About 3 hr when urine is at a pH of 5 and about 6 hr when urinary pH is 6.3. Excreted mostly unchanged through the urine (rate dependent on urinary pH-increased in acid urine).

ADDITIONAL CONTRAINDICATIONS
Angle closure glaucoma, anesthesia with cyclopropane or halothane, thyrotoxicosis, diabetes, obstetrics where maternal BP is greater than 130/80. Lactation.

SPECIAL CONCERNS
Geriatric clients may be at higher risk to develop prostatic hypertrophy. May cause hypertension resulting in intracranial hemorrhage or anginal pain in clients with coronary insufficiency or ischemic heart disease. Use with special caution in those with heart disease, angina pectoris, diabetes, hyperthyroidism, prostatic hypertrophy, hypertension, and in those taking digitalis.

SIDE EFFECTS
Most Common
Palpitations, tachycardia, PVCs, dizziness/vertigo, nervousness, headache, insomnia, N&V, sweating, anorexia.
See *Sympathomimetics* for a complete list of possible side effects. **CNS:** Nervousness, shakiness, confusion, delirium, insomnia, vertigo, headache, hallucinations. Anxiety and nervousness following prolonged use. **GI:** N&V, anorexia. **CV:** Precordial pain, tachycardia, palpitations, cardiac arrhythmias, **excessive doses may cause hypertension sufficient to result in cerebral hemorrhage.** **GU:** Difficult and painful urination, urinary retention in males with prostatism, decrease in urine formation. **Miscellaneous:** Pallor, sweating, respiratory difficulty, hypersensitivity reactions. **Abuse:** Prolonged abuse can cause an anxiety state, including symptoms of paranoid schizophrenia, tachy-

---

cardia, poor nutrition and hygiene, dilated pupils, cold sweat, and fever.

ADDITIONAL DRUG INTERACTIONS

Alpha-adrenergic blockers / Antagonism of vasoconstricting and hypertensive effects of ephedrine

Dexamethasone / ↓ Dexamethasone effect

Digitalis / Possible cardiac arrhythmias R/T sensitization of the myocardium

Diuretics / Diuretics ↓ response to sympathomimetics

Furazolidone / ↑ Pressor effect → possible hypertensive crisis and intracranial hemorrhage

Guanethidine / ↓ Guanethidine effect by displacement from its action site

Halothane / Serious arrhythmias R/T sensitization of myocardium to sympathomimetics by halothane

MAO Inhibitors / ↑ Pressor effect → possible hypertensive crisis and intracranial hemorrhage; do not give ephedrine during or within 14 days following administration of MAO inhibitors

Methyldopa / Effect of ephedrine ↓ in methyldopa-treated clients

Oxytocic drugs / Severe persistent hypertension

OD OVERDOSE MANAGEMENT

Symptoms: **Acute poisoning: Convulsions,** N&V, chills, cyanosis, irritability, nervousness, fever, suicidal behavior, tachycardia, dilated pupils, blurred vision, opisthotonos, spasms, pulmonary edema, gasping respirations, **coma, respiratory failure,** hypertension followed by hypotension accompanied by anuria. *Treatment:* Artificial respiration if breathing is shallow or cyanosis is present. Maintain BP but do not give vasopressors. For hypertension, can use phentolamine mesylate diluted in saline IV or 100 mg PO. Control convulsions by diazepam. Cool applications and dexamethasone, 1 mg/kg, given slowly IV, may control pyrexia.

HOW SUPPLIED

Capsules: 25 mg; *Injection:* 50 mg/mL.

DOSAGE

• CAPSULES

Bronchial asthma.

Adults and children over 12 years of age: 12.5–25 mg q 4 hr, not to exceed 150 mg in 24 hr. **Children, less than 12 years:** Consult a provider.

• IM; SC; SLOW IV

Allergic disorders, including bronchial asthma.

Adults: 25–50 mg SC or IM; or, 5–25 mg by slow IV repeated q 5–10 min, if needed. **Children, usual:** 0.5 mg/kg (16.7–25 mg/m²) SC, IM q 4–6 hr.

Vasopressor.

Adults: 25–50 mg (IM or SC) or 5–25 mg (by slow IV push) repeated at 5- to 10-min intervals, if necessary. Absorption following IM is more rapid than following SC use. **Pediatric (IM):** 16.7 mg/m² q 4–6 hr.

NURSING CONSIDERATIONS

ADMINISTRATION/STORAGE

1. Tolerance may develop; temporary cessation of therapy restores original drug response.

IV 2. May administer 10 mg IV undiluted over at least 1 min.

3. Use only clear solutions; discard any unused solution. Protect against exposure to light; drug is subject to oxidation.

ASSESSMENT

1. Note reasons for therapy; symptom characteristics.

2. Assess mental status, pulmonary function; monitor ECG and VS. If administered for hypotension, monitor BP until stabilized.

3. If used for prolonged periods, assess for drug resistance. Rest without medication for 3–4 days, then resume to regain response.

CLIENT/FAMILY TEACHING

1. Report if SOB unrelieved by medication and accompanied by chest pain, dizziness, or palpitations; any elevated or irregular pulse.

2. Review proper method for nasal instillation.

3. Avoid activities that require mental alertness until drug effects realized. Do not take within 2 hr of bedtime; may cause insomnia.

4. With males, report difficulty or pain with voiding; may be drug-induced urinary retention.

Bold Italic = life threatening side effect   ■ = black box warning   ♣ = Available in Canada

E

5. Report any depression, lack of interest in personal appearance, complaints of insomnia, anorexia or decreased effectiveness. Tolerance may occur within 1–2 months.

6. Avoid OTC drugs and alcohol. Keep F/U appointments.

OUTCOMES/EVALUATE

- Relief of SOB, chest tightness and wheezing with asthma
- ↓ Nasal congestion/mucus
- ↑ BP
- Control of narcolepsy

Epinephrine   **IV**
(ep-ih-**NEF**-rin)

CLASSIFICATION(S):
Sympathomimetic, direct-acting
PREGNANCY CATEGORY: C
OTC: Aerosol (OTC): Epinephrine Mist, Primatene Mist.
Rx: Injection: EpiPen, EpiPen Jr.

Epinephrine hydrochloride
PREGNANCY CATEGORY: C
OTC: Inhalation Solution (as Racenephrine hydrochloride): AsthmaNefrin, MicroNefrin, Nephron, S-2 Inhalant.
Rx: Inhalation Solution: Adrenalin Chloride. **Injection:** Adrenalin Chloride.
✦**Rx:** Vaponefrin.

SEE ALSO *SYMPATHOMIMETIC DRUGS.*

USES
Inhalation (Rx and OTC): Temporary relief of shortness of breath, tightness of chest, and wheezing due to bronchial asthma.
    Injection, 1:1,000 product: (1) Relieve respiratory distress due to bronchospasms. (2) Rapid relief of hypersensitivity reactions to drugs and other allergens. (3) Prolong the action of anesthetics used in local and regional anesthesia. (4) Restore cardiac rhythm in cardiac arrest due to various causes, al-

though it is not used in cardiac failure or in hemorrhagic, traumatic, or cardiogenic shock.
    Injection, 1:1,000 (autoinjector) and 1:2,000 (autoinjector): Emergency treatment of allergic reactions (anaphylaxis) to insect stings or bites, foods, drugs, and other allergens, as well as idiopathic or exercise-induced anaphylaxis. Autoinjectors are for emergency supportive therapy only and are not replacements or substitutes for immediate medical or hospital care.
    Injection, 1:10,000 (IV use): (1) Acute hypersensitivity (anaphylactoid reactions) to drugs, animal serums, and other allergens. (2) Acute asthmatic attacks to relieve bronchospasms not controlled by inhalation or SC administration of other solutions of the drug. (3) Prophylaxis of cardiac arrest and attacks of transitory AV heart block with syncopal seizures (Stokes-Adams syndrome). (4) Acute attacks of ventricular standstill, use physical measures first. When external cardiac compression and attempts to restore circulation by electrical defibrillation or use of a pacemaker fail, intracardiac puncture, and intramyocardial injection of epinephrine may be effective.
    Investigational: Endoscopic injection to manage acute lower GI bleeding.

ACTION/KINETICS
Action
Causes marked stimulation of alpha, beta-1, and beta-2 receptors, causing sympathomimetic stimulation, pressor effects, cardiac stimulation, bronchodilation, and decongestion. It crosses the placenta but not the blood-brain barrier. **Extreme caution must be taken never to inject 1:100 solution intended for inhalation–injection of this concentration has caused death.**
Pharmacokinetics
SC: Onset, 5–10 min; **duration:** 4–6 hr. **Inhalation: Onset,** 1–5 min; **duration:** 1–3 hr. **IM, Onset:** variable; duration: 1–4 hr. Ineffective when given PO.
ADDITIONAL CONTRAINDICATIONS
Unless directed by a provider use if the client has heart disease, hypertension, thyroid disease, difficulty in urination

due to enlarged prostate gland. Use if taking a MAOI for four weeks after stopping the MAOI. Inhalation if the client has ever been hospitalized for asthma or if the client is taking prescription medication for asthma. Seek medical advice before using during pregnancy or lactation.

SPECIAL CONCERNS

May cause anoxia in the fetus. Administer parenteral epinephrine to children with caution. Syncope may occur if epinephrine is given to asthmatic children. Administration of the SC injection by the IV route may cause severe or fatal hypertension or cerebrovascular hemorrhage. Epinephrine may temporarily increase the rigidity and tremor of parkinsonism. Use with caution and in small quantities in the toes, fingers, nose, ears, and genitals or in the presence of peripheral vascular disease as vasoconstriction-induced tissue sloughing may occur. Use the injection with caution in geriatric clients and in those with CV disease, hypertension, diabetes, hyperthyroidism, psychoneurotic clients, and during pregnancy. Epinephrine may cause potentially serious cardiac arrhythmias in clients not suffering from heart disease and in those with organic heart disease or who are receiving drugs that sensitize the myocardium.

SIDE EFFECTS

Most Common
When used for bronchodilation: Palpitations, tachycardia, PVCs, dizziness/vertigo, nervousness, headache, insomnia, N&V, sweating, anorexia.
When used to treat shock: Anginal pain, tachycardia, palpitations, restlessness, headache, tremor, dizziness, N&V, sweating, anxiety.
Use of autoinjectors: Palpitations, tachycardia, sweating, N&V, respiratory difficulty, pallor dizziness, weakness, tremor, headache, apprehension, nervousness, anxiety.
See *Sympathomimetic Drugs* for a complete list of possible side effects. **CV:** *Fatal ventricular fibrillation, cerebral or subarachnoid hemorrhage*, obstruction of central retinal artery. *A rapid*

and large increase in BP may cause aortic rupture, cerebral hemorrhage, or angina pectoris. **GU:** Decreased urine formation, urinary retention, painful urination. **CNS:** Anxiety, fear, pallor. Parenteral use may cause or aggravate disorientation, memory impairment, psychomotor agitation, panic, hallucinations, *suicidal or homicidal tendencies*, schizophrenic-type behavior. **Miscellaneous:** Prolonged use or overdose may cause elevated serum lactic acid with severe metabolic acidosis. **At injection site:** Bleeding, urticaria, wheal formation, pain. Repeated injections at the same site may cause necrosis from vascular constriction.

ADDITIONAL DRUG INTERACTIONS

Alpha-adrenergic blocking agents / Antagonism of vasoconstrictor and hypertensive effects
Antihistamines / Epinephrine effects potentiated
Beta-adrenergic blocking agents / Possible hypertension and reflex bradycardia R/T predominance of alpha-receptor effects
Cardiac glycosides / Possible sensitization of the myocardium to actions of epinephrine
Chlorpromazine / Possible reversal of epinephrine effects
Diuretics / ↓ Vascular response
Ergot alkaloids / Reversal of epinephrine pressor effects
General anesthetics (halothane, cyclopropane) / ↑ Sensitivity of myocardium to epinephrine → arrhythmias
Levothyroxine / Potentiation of epinephrine effects
Nitrites / Reversal of epinephrine pressor effects
Phenothiazines / Reversal of epinephrine pressor effects
Sympathomimetic drugs / Possible additive effects and ↑ toxicity (e.g., serious cardiac arrhythmias) when used with other sympathomimetic drugs; do not use together

OD OVERDOSE MANAGEMENT

Symptoms: From overdosage or inadvertent IV administration: Precordial distress, vomiting, headache, dyspnea, elevated BP. Also, angina pectoris, aortic

---

Bold Italic = life threatening side effect   ■ = black box warning   ♣ = Available in Canada

rupture, or cerebral rupture due to the sharp increase in BP. Pulmonary edema (may be fatal) due to peripheral vascular constriction together with cardiac stimulation. *Treatment:* Injection of an alpha- and a beta-adrenergic blocker. If there is a sharp increase in BP, use rapid-acting vasodilators such as nitrites or an alpha-adrenergic blocker.

HOW SUPPLIED

Epinephrine: *Aerosol (OTC):* 0.2 mg/inh; *Autoinjector (Rx):* 0.5 mg/mL, 1 mg/mL; *Solution for Injection (Rx):* 1:1,000 (1 mg/mL), 1:2,000 (0.5 mg/mL), 1:10,000 (0.1 mg/mL).

Epinephrine hydrochloride: *Injection (Rx):* 1:1,000 (1 mg/mL); *Solution for Inhalation (Rx):* 1:100 (10 mg/mL); *Solution for Inhalation (Racenephrine HCl) (OTC):* 2.25% (1.125% epinephrine base).

DOSAGE

EPINEPHRINE/EPINEPHRINE HYDROCHLORIDE

• **INHALATION AEROSOL**
Bronchodilation.

Adults and children 4 years and older, initial: 1 inhalation; **then,** wait 1 min or more—if no relief, use once more. Do not reuse for 3 or more hr. **Children less than 4 years of age:** Consult a provider.

• **NEBULIZATION**
Bronchodilation.

Adults and children 4 years and older (for AsthmaNefrin, 12 years and older). *Hand pump nebulizer:* place 0.5 mL (about 8–10 drops) of racemic epinephrine into the reservoir. Place the nebulizer nozzle into the partially opened mouth and squeeze the bulb 1–3 times. Inhale deeply. Give 2–3 additional inhalations if relief does not occur within 2–3 min. Can use 4–6 times/day but no more often than q 3 hr. *Aerosol nebulizer:* Add 0.5 mL (about 10 drops) of racemic epinephrine to 3 mL of diluent or 0.2–0.4 mL (about 4–8 drops) of Micro-Nefrin to 4.6–4.8 mL water. Give for 15 min q 3–4 hr. **Children younger than 4 years of age:** Consult a provider.

• **IM; SC**
Bronchodilation.

Adults, initial: 0.2–1 mL (0.2–1 mg) of the 1:1000 solution SC (preferred) or IM q 4 hr. Start with a small dose and in-crease if necessary. **Children:** 0.01 mL/kg or 0.3 mL/m² (0.1 mg/kg or 0.3 mg/m²) SC. Do not exceed 0.5 mL (0.5 mg) in a single pediatric dose. Can repeat q 4 hr, if necessary. **Neonates:** 0.01 mg/kg; for an infant, 0.05 mg is an adequate initial dose; may be repeated at 20–30 min intervals in the management of asthma attacks. *NOTE:* For bronchial asthma and certain allergic symptoms (e.g., angioedema, urticaria, serum sickness, anaphylactic shock), use epinephrine SC.

• **IV**
Bronchodilation, hypersensitivity reactions.

Adults: 0.1-0.25 mg (1–2.5 mL) of the 1:10,000 solution injected slowly. **Infants, initial:** 0.05 mg; may be repeated at 20–30 min intervals to manage asthma attacks. **Neonates:** 0.01 mg/kg. *NOTE:* If the client is intubated, the IV dose of epinephrine can be given via the endotracheal tube directly into the bronchial tree as it is rapidly absorbed through the lung capillary bed.

• **AUTOINJECTOR (1:200), IM**
Anaphylaxis.

Given IM into the anterolateral aspect of the thigh, through clothing if necessary. **Adults:** 0.3 mg. **Children:** 0.15 mg or 0.3 mg, depending on body weight; **recommended dose:** 0.01 mg/kg. The autoinjectors deliver a single dose. Epi-Pen Jr. provides a dosage of 0.15 mg which may be more appropriate for clients weighing less than 30 kg. EpiPen provides 0.3 mg of epinephrine for those weighing more than 30 kg. In cases of a severe reaction, repeat injections may be necessary.

• **INTRACARDIAC, IV**
Cardiac arrest.

Adults, intracardiac or IV: 0.5 mg *(0.5 mL of 1:1,000 solution)* diluted to 10 mL with NaCl injection or 0.5–1 mg *(5–10 mL of 1:10,000 solution).* During a resuscitation effort, give 0.5 mg (5 mL of 1:10,000 solution) IV q 5 min. Intracardiac dose usually ranges from 0.3 to 0.5 mg (3 to 5 mL of 1:10,000 solution). Follow intracardiac administration with external cardiac massage to permit the drug to enter the coronary circulation.

Alternatively, if the client has been intubated, epinephrine can be injected via the endotracheal tube directly into the bronchial tree at the same dosage as for IV injection. **Do not confuse the 1:1,000 solution with the 1:10,000 solution.** *NOTE:* Intracardiac injection should be given by personnel well trained in the technique. External cardiac massage should follow intracardiac administration to permit the drug to enter the coronary circulation. Use intracardiac administration secondarily to unsuccessful attempts with physical or electromechanical methods.

Use with local anesthetics.
Epinephrine, 1:100,000 (0.01 mg/mL) to 1:20,000 (0.05 mg/mL) is the usual concentration used with local anesthetics.
• REGIONAL OR INTRASPINAL
  Regional anesthesia; Intraspinal use.
Regional anesthesia. A final concentration of 1:200,000 is recommended for infiltration injection, nerve block, caudal, or other epidural blocks. From 0.3–0.4 mg epinephrine (0.3–0.4 mL of 1:1,000 solution) may be mixed with spinal anesthetic agents.
Intraspinal use. Usual dose is 0.2–0.4 mL added to the anesthetic spinal fluid mixture (may prolong anesthetic action by limiting absorption). Epinephrine 1:100,000 to 1:20,000 is the usual concentration used with local anesthetics.

NURSING CONSIDERATIONS
ADMINISTRATION/STORAGE
1. The 1:1,000 solution may be given IM or SC (preferred). The 1:10,000 solution is given by IV injection or, in cardiac arrest, by intracardiac injection into the left ventricular chamber or via endotracheal tube directly into the bronchial tree.
2. The 1:100 epinephrine solution is intended only for PO (not nasal) use. Because of the higher concentration of the 1:100 solution, it is not suitable for parenteral use.
3. Seek medical attention immediately if symptoms are not relieved within 20 min or if they become worse.

4. Excessive use may cause nervousness and rapid heart beat and possibly adverse cardiac effects.
5. Briskly massage site of SC or IM injection to hasten drug action. Do not expose drug to heat, light, or air, as this causes deterioration.
6. Discard solution if reddish brown and after expiration date. Protect from light.
7. Accidental injection of the autoinjector into the hands or feet may result in loss of blood flow to the area and should be avoided.
8. Store autoinjectors in the tube provided from 15–30°C (59–86°F); do not refrigerate. Autoinjectors do not contain latex.
9. **Never administer** 1:100 solution IV; use the 1:1,000 solution.
10. Use a tuberculin syringe to measure. Parenteral doses are small and drug is potent, thus errors in measurement may be disastrous.
11. For direct IV administration to adults, the drug must be well diluted as a 1:1,000 solution; inject quantities of 0.05–0.1 mL of solution cautiously taking about 1 min for each injection; note response (BP and pulse). Dose may be repeated several times if necessary. May be further diluted in D5W or NSS.
ASSESSMENT
1. List reasons for therapy; describe type/onset of symptoms and anticipated results.
2. Assess for sulfite sensitivity. Note cardiopulmonary function.
3. During IV therapy, continuously monitor ECG, BP, and pulse until desired effect achieved. Take VS every 2–5 min until stabilized; once stable, monitor BP q 15–30 min.
4. Note any symptoms of shock such as cold, clammy skin, cyanosis, and loss of consciousness.
CLIENT/FAMILY TEACHING
1. Take as directed. Review method for administration carefully. When prescribed for anaphylaxis, administer autoinjector immediately and seek medical care. Check expiration dates.
2. Report any increased restlessness, chest pain, heart fluttering, SOB, lack of

---

Bold Italic = life threatening side effect   ■ = black box warning   ✦ = Available in Canada

response, adverse effects, or insomnia as dosage adjustment may be necessary. May elevate blood sugar.

3. Limit intake of caffeine (colas, coffee, tea, and chocolate); avoid OTC drugs without approval.

4. Rinse mouth and inhaler after use. If also prescribed steroid inhaler take bronchodilator first and wait at least 5 min before administering steroid inhaler so air passages are open and receptive.

5. Nasal application may sting slightly. Nasal OTC products may work initially but with prolonged use exacerbate symptoms.

6. Ophthalmic solution may burn initially and a brow headache may occur; this should subside. Remove contact lenses; may stain lens.

7. Use caution when performing activities that require careful vision; ophthalmic solution may diminish visual fields, cause double vision, and alter night vision.

8. Discard any discolored or precipitated solutions.

OUTCOMES/EVALUATE

- Restoration of cardiac activity
- Improved CO with EC bypass
- ↓ IOP
- Reversal of S&S of anaphylaxis
- Improved airway exchange
- Hemostasis with ocular surgery

Epirubicin hydrochloride ■ IV

(ep-ee-**ROO**-bih-sin)

CLASSIFICATION(S):

Antineoplastic, antibiotic
PREGNANCY CATEGORY: D
Rx: Ellence.
♣Rx: Pharmorubicin PFS.

SEE ALSO *ANTINEOPLASTIC AGENTS.*

USES

Adjunct to treat breast cancer in clients with evidence of axillary node tumor involvement after resection of primary breast cancer. *Investigational:* In combination with cisplatin and 5-fluorouracil to treat advanced esophageal cancer.

ACTION/KINETICS

Action

Cell cycle phase nonspecific anthracycline; has maximum cytotoxic effects on the S and G_2 phases. Precise mechanism of action is not known. It does form a complex with DNA by intercalation of its planar rings between nucleotide base pairs resulting in inhibition of DNA and RNA synthesis. Intercalation triggers DNA cleavage by topoisomerase II, resulting in cell death. The drug also inhibits DNA helicase activity which prevents enzymatic separation of double-stranded DNA and interferes with replication and transcription. The drug is also involved in oxidation-reduction reactions by generating cytotoxic free radicals.

Pharmacokinetics

Following IV, it is rapidly and widely distributed; appears to concentrate in RBCs. Extensively and rapidly metabolized by the liver and RBCs. Parent drug and metabolites are excreted through both the feces and urine. **t½:** Triphasic with half-lives of about 3 min, 2.5 hr, and 33 hr. **Plasma protein binding:** About 77%.

CONTRAINDICATIONS

Severe hepatic dysfunction; previous anthracycline treatment up to the maximum cumulative dose; severe myocardial insufficiency or recent MI; severe arrhythmias; hypersensitivity to epirubicin, other anthracyclines, or anthracenediones; baseline neutrophil count <1500 cells/mm^3. Lactation.

SPECIAL CONCERNS

■ (1) Severe local tissue necrosis will occur if extravasation occurs during administration. Do not give IM or SC. (2) Myocardial toxicity, including fatal CHF, may occur either during therapy or months to years after termination of therapy. The risk of developing CHF increases rapidly with increasing total cumulative doses in excess of 900 mg/m^2; exceed this cumulative dose only with extreme caution. (3) Active or dormant CV disease, prior or concomitant radiotherapy to the mediastinal/pericardial area, previous therapy with other anthracyclines or anthracenediones, or concomitant use of other cardiotoxic drugs may increase the risk of cardiac toxicity. Cardiac toxicity may occur at lower cumulative doses whether or not cardiac risk factors are present. (4) Secondary acute myelogenous leukemia may occur with epirubicin use. Is more common when given in combination with DNA-damaging antineoplastic agents, when clients have been heavily pretreated with cytotoxic drugs, or when doses of anthracyclines have been escalated. (5) Reduce dosage in clients with impaired hepatic function. (6) Severe myelosuppression may occur. (7) Give only under the supervision of a physician experienced in use of cancer chemotherapeutic agents.■ Use of epirubicin after previous radiation therapy may cause an inflammatory recall reaction at the site of irradiation. When used in combination with other cytotoxic drugs, additive hematologic and GI toxicity may occur. Safety and efficacy have not been determined in pediatric clients.

SIDE EFFECTS
Most Common
Leukopenia, neutropenia, anemia, thrombocytopenia, amenorrhea, lethargy, N&V, mucositis, alopecia, hot flashes.

GI: N&V, mucositis (oral stomatitis, esophagitis), diarrhea, anorexia. **CV:** CHF, sinus tachycardia, nonspecific ST-T wave changes, PVCs, *ventricular tachycardia*, bradycardia, AV and bundle branch block. **Dermatologic:** Alopecia, local toxicity, rash, itch, skin changes, flushes, skin and nail hyperpigmentation, photosensitivity, hypersensitivity to irradiated skin, urticaria, *anaphylaxis*. **Hematologic:** Leukopenia, neutropenia, anemia, thrombocytopenia, secondary acute myelogenous leukemia, acute lymphoid leukemia. **Endocrine:** Amenorrhea, hot flashes. **Miscellaneous:** Lethargy, infection, febrile neutropenia, fever, conjunctivitis/keratitis, tumor lysis syndrome, injection site reactions (venous sclerosis, local pain,

severe tissue lesions, necrosis), hypersensitivity (urticaria, *anaphylaxis*).

DRUG INTERACTIONS
Cardioactive drugs (e.g., calcium channel blockers) / Possible heart failure
Cimetidine / ↑ Epirubicin blood levels by 50%; stop cimetidine therapy during use of epirubicin

HOW SUPPLIED
Injection: 2 mg/mL; *Powder for Injection, Lyophilized:* 2 mg/mL.

DOSAGE
- **IV INFUSION**
  Breast cancer with evidence of axillary node tumor.

The following regimens are recommended: (1) epirubicin, 100 mg/m^2; 5-fluorouracil, 500 mg/m^2; and cyclophosphamide, 500 mg/m^2. All drugs are given on day 1 and repeated q 21 days for 6 cycles. Clients given epirubicin, 120 mg/m^2 are also given prophylactic antibiotic therapy with trimethoprim-sulfamethoxazole or a fluoroquinolone. (2) epirubicin, 60 mg/m^2 on days 1 and 8; 5-fluorouracil, 500 mg/m^2 on days 1 and 8; and cyclophosphamide, 75 mg/m^2 PO on days 1 to 14. The regimen is repeated q 28 days for 6 cycles.

NURSING CONSIDERATIONS
ADMINISTRATION/STORAGE
IV 1. Make dosage adjustments after the first treatment cycle based on hematologic and nonhematologic toxicity:
- Reduce day 1 dose in subsequent cycles to 75% of the day 1 dose given in the current cycle in clients experiencing cycle nadir platelet counts <50,000/mm^3, absolute neutrophil counts (ANC) <250/mm^3, neutropenic fever, or Grades 3/4 nonhematologic toxicity. Delay day 1 chemotherapy in subsequent courses of treatment until platelet counts are 100,000/mm^3 or more, ANC is 1,500/mm^3 or more, and nonhematologic toxicities have recovered to Grade 1 or less.
- For clients receiving a divided dose of epirubicin on days 1 and 8, reduce the day 8 dose to 75% of day 1 if platelet counts are 75,000–100,000/mm^3 and ANC is 1,000–1,499/mm^3.

Bold Italic = life threatening side effect   ■ = black box warning   ♣ = Available in Canada

Omit the day 8 dose, if day 8 platelet counts are <75,000/mm^3, ANC is <1,000/mm^3, or Grade 3/4 nonhematologic toxicity has occurred.

2. Consider a lower starting dose (75–90 mg/m^2) for heavily pretreated clients, those with preexisting bone marrow depression, or in the presence of neoplastic bone marrow infiltration.

3. With elevated serum AST or serum total bilirubin levels, consider the following doses of epirubicin:

- Bilirubin, 1.2–3 mg/dL, or AST, 2–4 times ULN, give one-half the recommended starting dose.
- Bilirubin >3 mg/dL or AST >4 times ULN, give one-fourth the recommended starting dose.

4. Consider lower doses of epirubicin with severe renal impairment (serum creatinine >5 mg/dL).

5. Clients given 120 mg/m^2 of epirubicin as part of combination therapy should receive prophylactic antibiotic therapy with a fluoroquinolone or trimethoprim-sulfamethoxazole.

6. Consider prophylactic use of antiemetics to reduce N&V, esp. if epirubicin given with other emetogenic drugs.

7. Do not mix epirubicin with heparin or fluorouracil due to chemical incompatibility that may cause precipitation.

8. Avoid prolonged contact with any alkaline solution; hydrolysis of the drug will occur.

9. The solution is manufactured preservative-free and as a ready-to-use solution. Give over a 3–5 min period into the tubing of a freely flowing IV infusion (0.9% NaCl or D5W). Do not use a direct push injection due to the possibility of extravasation.

10. Wear protective clothing when handling drug and do not handle if pregnant. Use within 24 hr of first penetration of the rubber stopper.

ASSESSMENT

1. Note disease onset, symptom characteristics, staging, other medical conditions, other agents trialed.

2. Obtain baseline CBC, renal, LFTs, ECG, and LVEF; monitor for anthracycline-induced cardiomyopathy by ECHO or MUGA determination of LVEF during therapy. Note any rhythm changes, S$_3$, SOB, edema; may experience delayed cardiac toxicity 2–3 mo to years after completing therapy. Do not exceed 900 mg/m^2 cumulative dose. May cause inflammatory reaction at previous XRT sites.

3. Assess IV site carefully; drug is a vesicant. Venous sclerosis at injection site or extravasation may occur; may cause pain and tissue necrosis. Give slowly over 3–5 min to prevent facial flushing or erythematous streaking along vein.

4. Give antiemetics 30–60 min before therapy to diminish N&V. Ensure adequate hydration, alkalinization of urine, treatment for tumor lysis syndrome (allopurinol).

5. With 120 mg/m^2 regimen in combination therapy, also give ATX prophylaxis with trimethoprim-sulfamethoxazole or fluoroquinolone.

6. Lower dose with hematologic, renal or liver dysfunction. Follow dosing guidelines carefully.

CLIENT/FAMILY TEACHING

1. Therapy usually given once every three weeks for 6 cycles for node positive resectable primary breast cancer.

2. May experience N&V, diarrhea, hair loss, inflammation or sores in the oral mucosa; report side effects or complaints.

3. There is a risk of irreversible myocardial damage and treatment-related leukemia; need frequent studies (ECHO or MUGA scans) and blood work.

4. Report increased SOB, chest pains, lower extremity swelling, vomiting, dehydration, fever, infection or injection site pain after therapy.

5. Urine may be red for several days after therapy; not worrisome.

6. If platelet counts, white count, or nonhematologic toxicities occur, dosage will be reduced with next dose or discontinued if prolonged.

7. Use reliable birth control; men may experience chromosomal sperm damage and women may develop premature menopause or irreversible amenorrhea. Determine if sperm/egg harvesting indicated.

8. Avoid cimetidine during therapy. Keep all F/U appointments.

9. Avoid crowds and persons with known infections; vaccinations during therapy.

OUTCOMES/EVALUATE
Control of malignant cell proliferation in breast cancer

Eplerenone
(eh-**PLEH**-reh-none)

CLASSIFICATION(S):
Aldosterone receptor antagonist
PREGNANCY CATEGORY: B
Rx: Inspra.

USES
(1) Hypertension, alone or in combination with other antihypertensive drugs. (2) Improve survival of stable clients with left ventricular systolic dysfunction (ejection fraction of 40% or less) and clinical evidence of CHF after an acute MI. *Investigational:* Alone or in combination with an angiotensin-converting enzyme inhibitor for reducing left ventricular hypertrophy. As adjunctive therapy in diabetic hypertension with microalbuminuria.

ACTION/KINETICS
Action
Binds to the mineralocorticoid receptor and blocks binding of aldosterone. Aldosterone increases BP through induction of sodium reabsorption and other mechanisms. Thus, by blocking aldosterone binding, sodium is not reabsorbed and BP decreases.

Pharmacokinetics
Peak plasma levels: About 1.5 hr. **Steady state:** Reached in 2 days. Absorption not affected by food. Metabolized primarily via CYP3A4 in the liver. About two-thirds excreted in the urine and one-third in the feces. $t^{1/2}$, **terminal:** 4–6 hr. **Plasma protein binding:** About 50%.

CONTRAINDICATIONS
Serum potassium greater than 5.5 mEq/L at initiation, type 2 diabetes with microalbuminuria, serum creatinine greater than 2 mg/dL in males or greater than 1.8 mg/dL in females, C_{CR} less than 30 mL/min. Also, clients concurrently taking potassium supplements, potassium-sparing diuretics (e.g., amiloride, spironolactone, triamterene), or strong inhibitors of CYP3A4 drugs (clarithromycin, ketoconazole, itraconazole, nefazodone, nelfinavir, ritonavir, troleandomycin). Lactation.

SPECIAL CONCERNS
Safety and efficacy have not been determined in children.

SIDE EFFECTS
Most Common
Hyperkalemia, diarrhea, abdominal pain, dizziness, coughing, fatigue, flu-like symptoms.

Hyperkalemia is the primary risk; can result in decreased renal function and serious, sometimes *fatal arrhythmias.* **GI:** Diarrhea, abdominal pain. **GU:** Mastodynia in males, abnormal vaginal bleeding, gynecomastia (males). **Miscellaneous:** Dizziness, coughing, fatigue, flu-like symptoms.

LABORATORY TEST CONSIDERATIONS
↑ ALT, BUN, uric acid, serum creatinine. Hyponatremia, hypercholesterolemia, albuminuria, hypertriglyceridemia, hyperkalemia.

DRUG INTERACTIONS
ACE inhibitors / ↑ Risk of hyperkalemia
Angiotensin II antagonists / ↑ Risk of hyperkalemia
CYP3A4 inhibitors (itraconazole, ketoconazole) / Up to a 5-fold increase in eplerenone exposure
Lithium / Potential lithium toxicity; monitor serum lithium levels
NSAIDs / Potential ↓ antihypertensive effect and severe hyperkalemia
H *St. John's wort* / About a 30% ↓ in eplerenone AUC

HOW SUPPLIED
Tablets: 25 mg, 50 mg.

DOSAGE
- **TABLETS**
  Hypertension.
Initial: 50 mg once daily. If inadequate response, increase dose to 50 mg twice a day. Higher doses are not recommended as no greater effect is noted and there is an increased risk of hyper-

---

Bold Italic = life threatening side effect ■ = black box warning ✦ = Available in Canada

kalemia. For clients taking weak CYP3A4 inhibitors (erythromycin, fluconazole, saquinavir, verapamil), reduce starting dose to 25 mg once daily.

CHF post-MI.

Initial: 25 mg once daily; titrate to target dose of 50 mg once daily, preferably within 4 weeks, as tolerated. Adjust dose as follows based on serum potassium. **Less than 5 mEq/L potassium:** Increase dose from 25 mg every other day to 25 mg daily to 50 mg daily; **Serum potassium from 5–5.4 mEq/L:** Maintain dosage; no adjustment; **Serum potassium, 5.5–5.9 mEq/L:** Decrease dose from 50 mg daily to 25 mg daily to 25 mg every other day to withholding the drug; **Serum potassium, 6 mEq/L or greater:** Withhold drug.

NURSING CONSIDERATIONS

ADMINISTRATION/STORAGE
Store from 15–30°C (59–86°F).

ASSESSMENT
1. Note reasons for therapy, symptom characteristics, other agents trialed.
2. List drugs prescribed to ensure none interact.
3. Assess BP, serum K+, renal, and LFTs. With post-MI heart failure, note LV ejection fraction and systolic dysfunction.

CLIENT/FAMILY TEACHING
1. Take as directed with or without food. Do not take with grapefruit juice; avoid all supplements containing potassium.
2. Keep log of BP and HR for provider review.
3. Avoid activities that require mental alertness until drug effects realized.
4. Report as scheduled for F/U. Continue lifestyle changes that help control BP, i.e., weight loss, regular daily exercise, tobacco/alcohol cessation, stress/salt reduction.
5. Avoid OTC meds and ETOH.

OUTCOMES/EVALUATE
↓ BP ↓ Mortality post-MI with CHF

Epoetin alfa recombinant ■ IV
(ee-**POH**-ee-tin)

E

CLASSIFICATION(S):
Erythropoietin, human recombinant
PREGNANCY CATEGORY: C
Rx: Epogen, Procrit.
✦Rx: Eprex.

USES
(1) Treatment of anemia associated with chronic renal failure in adults and children, including clients on dialysis (end-stage renal disease) or adults not on dialysis. Not intended for those who require immediate correction of severe anemia; epoetin alfa may decrease the need for maintenance transfusions but is not a substitute for emergency transfusion. (2) Zidovudine-induced anemia in HIV-infected clients to decrease the need for transfusions. (3) Treatment of anemia in clients with nonmyeloid malignancies in which anemia is due to the effect of coadministered chemotherapy. Epoetin alfa decreases the need for transfusions in those who will be receiving concomitant chemotherapy for a minimum of 2 months. (4) Treatment of anemic clients (hemoglobin more than 10 to less than 13 grams/dL) to reduce allogeneic blood transfusions in clients scheduled to undergo elective, noncardiac, nonvascular surgery. *Investigational:* Anemia associated with critically ill clients, CHF, chronic disease (e.g., rheumatoid arthritis), postpartum anemia, sickle cell disease, thalassemia, multiple myeloma, Jehovah's witnesses, radiation treatment, epidermolysis bullosa, porphyria. For athletic enhancement, sexual dysfunction, and transfusional iron overload.

ACTION/KINETICS
Action
Made by recombinant DNA technology; it has the identical amino acid sequence and same biologic effects as endogenous erythropoietin (which is normally synthesized in the kidney and

 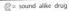

stimulates RBC production). Epoetin alfa will stimulate RBC production and thus elevate or maintain the RBC level, decreasing the need for blood transfusions.

Pharmacokinetics

t½: 4–13 hr in clients with chronic renal failure, but is about 20% longer in those with chronic renal failure compared with healthy subjects. **Peak serum levels after SC:** 5–24 hr.

CONTRAINDICATIONS

Uncontrolled hypertension. Hypersensitivity to mammalian cell-derived products or to human albumin. Use in chronic renal failure clients who need severe anemia corrected. To treat anemia in HIV-infected or cancer clients due to factors such as iron or folate deficiencies, hemolysis, or GI bleeding. Anemic clients willing to donate autologous blood.

SPECIAL CONCERNS

■ (1) Erythropoiesis-stimulating agents. Use the lowest dose of epoetin alfa that will gradually increase the hemoglobin concentration to the lowest level sufficient to avoid the need for red blood cell transfusion. (2) Epoetin alfa and other erythropoiesis-stimulating agents increased the risk of death and serious CV reactions when administered to target a hemoglobin of more than 12 grams/dL. (3) Cancer clients: Use of erythropoiesis-stimulating agents: (a) shortened the time to tumor progression in clients with advanced head and neck cancer receiving radiation therapy when administered to target a hemoglobin of more than 12 grams/dL; (b) shortened overall survival and increased deaths attributed to disease progression at 4 months in clients with metastatic breast cancer receiving chemotherapy when administered to target a hemoglobin of more than 12 grams/dL; (c) increased the risk of death when administered to target a hemoglobin of 12 grams/dL in clients with active malignant disease receiving neither chemotherapy nor radiation therapy. Erythropoiesis-stimulating agents are not indicated for this population. (4) Clients receiving erythropoiesis-stimulating agents preoperatively for reduction of allogeneic RBC transfusions: A higher incidence of deep vein thrombosis was documented in clients receiving epoetin alfa who were not receiving prophylactic anticoagulation. Strongly consider antithrombotic prophylaxis when epoetin alfa is used to reduce allogeneic RBC transfusions.■ Safety and efficacy have not been established in children less than 1 month of age or in clients with a history of seizures or underlying hematologic disease (e.g., hypercoagulable disorders, myelodysplastic syndromes, sickle cell anemia). Use with caution in clients with porphyria, during lactation, and preexisting vascular disease. Increased anticoagulation with heparin may be required in clients on epoetin alfa undergoing hemodialysis. Since epoetin alfa contains albumin, there is a remote risk for transmission of viral diseases.

SIDE EFFECTS

Most Common

Hypertension, headache, fatigue, N&V, diarrhea, edema, asthenia, respiratory congestion, cough, pyrexia, rash, SOB, insomnia, pruritus, DVT (in surgery clients).

In Chronic Renal Failure Clients (symptoms may be due to the disease): CV: Hypertension (including hypertensive encephalopathy), tachycardia, edema, *MI*, CVA, TIA, clotted vascular access. Rarely, thromboembolic reactions, including microvascular thrombosis, migratory thrombophlebitis, pulmonary embolus, and thrombosis of the retinal artery and temporal and renal veins. **CNS:** Headache, fatigue, dizziness, *seizures*. **GI:** N&V, diarrhea, worsening of porphyria. **Allergic reactions:** Skin rashes, urticaria, circumoral edema, *anaphylaxis*. **Hematologic:** Pure red cell aplasia, severe anemia (with or without cytopenias). **Miscellaneous:** SOB, hyperkalemia, arthralgias, myalgia, chest pain, skin reaction at administration site, asthenia, injection site stinging in dialysis clients. *NOTE:* In children on dialysis, the pattern of most side effects was similar to adults. The following additional side effects were observed: Abdominal pain, constipation, cough, dialysis access complications (e.g., infections, peritonitis), fever, pharyngitis, URTI.

In Zidovudine-Treated HIV-Infected Clients: CNS: Pyrexia, fatigue, headache, dizziness, *seizures*. **Respiratory:** Cough, respiratory congestion, SOB. **GI:** Diarrhea, nausea. **Miscellaneous:** Rash, asthenia, reaction at injection site, *allergic reactions*.

In Cancer Clients: CNS: Pyrexia, fatigue, dizziness. **GI:** Diarrhea, N&V. **Musculoskeletal:** Asthenia, paresthesia, trunk pain. **Respiratory:** SOB, URTI. **Miscellaneous:** Edema, asthenia, *increased mortality* and tumor progression.

In Surgery Clients: CNS: Pyrexia, insomnia, headache, dizziness, anxiety. **GI:** N&V, constipation, diarrhea, dyspepsia. **CV:** Hypertension, DVT, edema. **Dermatologic:** Pruritus, reaction at injection site, skin pain. *GU:* UTI.

NOTE: For all uses, epoetin alfa increases the risk for death and serious CV events when given to target a hemoglobin of more than 12 grams/dL. There is an increased risk of serious arterial and venous thromboembolic reactions, include MI, stroke, CHF, and hemodialysis graft occlusion.

LABORATORY TEST CONSIDERATIONS Hyperkalemia.

OD OVERDOSE MANAGEMENT
Symptoms: Polycythemia. *Treatment:* Withhold drug until hematocrit returns to the target range. Phlebotomy may be used to decrease hemoglobin.

HOW SUPPLIED
Injection Solution: 2,000 units/mL, 3,000 units/mL, 4,000 units/mL, 10,000 units/mL, 20,000 units/mL, 40,000 units/mL.

DOSAGE————————————
• **IV; SC**
  Chronic renal failure.
IV, initial (dialysis or nondialysis clients), SC (nondialysis clients), adults: 50–100 units/kg 3 times per week. The rate of increase of hematocrit depends on both dosage and client variation. **Maintenance, nondialysis clients:** Individualize; 75–150 units/kg/week have maintained hematocrits of

36–38% for up to 6 months; **hemodialysis clients:** 12.5–525 units/kg 3 times per week (median dose is 75 units/kg 3 times per week). **Maintenance, peritoneal dialysis clients:** 24–323 units/kg/week given in divided doses 2–3 times per week. Median dosage is 76 units/kg/week in divided doses.

Children on dialysis: 50 units/kg 3 times per week IV or SC; **maintenance, median dose:** 167 units/kg/week; range: 49–477 units/kg/week in divided doses 2–3 times per week. **Children, 3 months–20 years, not requiring dialysis:** 50–250 units/kg weekly to 3 times per week SC or IV.

NOTE: Reduce dose by about 25% if hemoglobin approaches 12 grams/dL or if hemoglobin increases by more than 1 gram/dL in any 2-week period. If hemoglobin continues to increase, temporarily withhold epoetin alfa until hemoglobin begins to decrease at which point reinitiate therapy at a dose about 25% below the previous dose.

Increase dose if hemoglobin does not increase by 2 grams/dL after 8 weeks of therapy and hemoglobin remains at a level not sufficient to avoid the need for RBC transfusion. Do not increase the dose more frequently than once per month. If the increase in hemoglobin is less than 1 gram/dL over 4 weeks and iron stores are adequate, the dose of epoetin alfa may be increased by about 25% of the previous dose. Further increases may be made at 4-week intervals until the specified hemoglobin is obtained.

Zidovudine-treated, HIV infections.
Adults, initial, IV, SC: 100 units/kg 3 times per week for 8 weeks (in clients with serum erythropoietin levels less than or equal to 500 milliunits/mL who are receiving less than or equal to 4,200 mg/week of zidovudine). If a satisfactory response is obtained, the dose can be increased by 50–100 units/kg 3 times per week. Evaluate the response q 4–8 weeks thereafter with dosage adjusted by 50–100 units/kg increments 3 times per week. If clients have not responded to 300 units/kg 3 times per week, it is not likely they will respond to

E

higher doses. If the hemoglobin exceeds 12 grams/dL, discontinue the dose until the hemoglobin drops below 11 grams/dL. Reduce the dose by 25% when treatment is resumed and then titrate to maintain the desired hemoglobin.

Children, 8 months–17 years: 50–400 units/kg 2 to 3 times per week.

Cancer clients on chemotherapy.

Adults, initial, SC: 150 units/kg three times per week. **Children, initial, IV:** 600 units/kg (maximum of 40,000 units) once a week. Treatment of clients with highly elevated erythropoetin levels (>200 milliunits/mL) is not recommended. Target hemoglobin range: 10-12 grams/dL.

Dosage adjustment, 3 times per week dosing:

- Increase the dosage to 300 units/kg 3 times per week if response is not satisfactory (i.e., no reduction in transfusion requirements or rise in hemoglobin) after 8 weeks. Goal is to achieve and maintain the lowest hemoglobin level sufficient to avoid the need for RBC transfusion, not to exceed 12 grams/dL.
- Reduce the dose by 25% when hemoglobin approaches 12 grams/dL or increases by more than 1 gram/dL in any two week period.
- Withhold the dose if hemoglobin exceeds 12 grams/dL, until hemoglobin falls below 11 grams/dL; restart the dose at 25% below the previous dose.

Dosage adjustment, weekly dosing:

- Increase the dose to 60,000 units SC weekly for adults and 900 units/kg IV (maximum 60,000 units) in children if response is not satisfactory (see above).
- Reduce the dose by 25% when hemoglobin approaches 12 grams/dL or increases by more than 1 gram/dL in any two week period.
- Withhold the dose if hemoglobin exceeds 12 grams/dL, until the hemoglobin falls below 11 grams/dL; restart the dose at 25% below the previous dose.

Surgery to reduce allogeneic blood transfusions.

SC: 300 units/kg/day for 10 days before surgery, on the day of surgery, and for 4 days after surgery. Alternative: 600 units/kg SC once a week 21, 14, and 7 days before surgery plus a fourth dose on the day of surgery. Iron supplementation is required at the time of epoetin therapy and continuing throughout the course of therapy.

NURSING CONSIDERATIONS

ADMINISTRATION/STORAGE

1. *Do not* give with any other drug solutions. At time of SC administration, the drug may be admixed in a syringe with bacteriostatic 0.9% NaCl injection with benzyl alcohol, 0.9%, at a 1:1 ratio. The benzyl alcohol acts as a local anesthetic that may reduce discomfort at the SC injection site.

2. If a client with chronic renal failure fails to respond or maintain a response, undertake a cause. If the transferrin saturation is less than 20%, give supplemental iron.

3. A hemoglobin rise of more than 1 gram/dL over 2 weeks may contribute to increased mortality, serious CV and thromboembolic events.

4. Absolute or functional iron deficiency may develop.

5. Using aseptic technique, attach a sterile needle to a sterile syringe. Remove the flip top from the vial containing epoetin alfa and wipe the septum with a disinfectant. Insert the needle into the vial and withdraw into the syringe an appropriate volume of solution.

6. Do not dilute or give in conjunction with other drug solutions. At the time of SC administration, however, preservative-free epoetin alfa from single-use vials may be mixed in a syringe with bacteriostatic sodium chloride (0.9% injection with benzyl alcohol 0.9%) at a 1:1 ration using aseptic technique. Admixing is not necessary when using multidose vials as these contain benzyl alcohol.

IV 7. IV usually given as a bolus 3 times/week. May be given into venous

---

line at end of dialysis procedure to obviate need for additional venous access.

8. During hemodialysis, may require increased anticoagulation with heparin to prevent clotting of artificial kidney.

9. Determine hematocrit twice weekly until stabilized in the target range and the maintenance dose of epoetin alfa has been determined. Do not adjust more often than once a month, unless clinically indicated. After any dosage adjustment, monitor hematocrit twice a week for 2–6 weeks.

10. If hematocrit approaches 36%, decrease dose to maintain suggested target hematocrit range. If dose decrease does not stop the rise in hematocrit and it exceeds 35%, temporarily withhold doses until hematocrit begins to decrease; then, restart therapy at a lower dose. Determine maintenance doses individually.

11. Individualize hemoglobin target level. If rate of rise of hemoglobin exceeds 1 gram/dL over a 2-week period, interrupt dose and modify rate of rise of hemoglobin. Target hemoglobin with cancer should not exceed 12 grams/dL in men and women. Withhold dose if hemoglobin is 13 grams/dL or above. This applies whether drug is given 3 times weekly or once weekly.

12. If the hematocrit does not increase by 5–6 points after 8 weeks of therapy and iron stores are adequate, increase dose incrementally. Further increases may be made at 4–6-week intervals until a desired response observed.

13. Do **not** shake; shaking will denature the glycoprotein, making it biologically inactive.

14. Do not use vials showing particulate matter or discoloration.

15. The 1 mL single-dose vial contains no preservative; use only one dose/vial. Do not reenter the vial; discard unused portions.

16. The multidose 1 and 2 mL vials contain preservative. Store from 2–8°C (36–46°F) after initial entry and between doses. Discard 21 days after initial entry.

17. Store at 2–8°C (36–46°F). Do not freeze or shake.

ASSESSMENT

1. Note sensitivity to mammalian cell-derived products or human albumin.

2. List reasons for therapy, conditions requiring therapy, goal Hct, expected duration of therapy. Follow dosing guidelines carefully; initially monitor Hct 2 times weekly.

3. Determine CBC and iron stores. Transferrin saturation should be at least 20% and serum ferritin should be at least 200 ng/mL. Provide supplemental iron to increase or maintain transferrin to levels required to support stimulation of erythropoiesis by epoetin alfa.

4. With HIV, note when zidovudine therapy was instituted, and anemia cause.

5. Assess BP; control hypertension.

6. Monitor CBC, renal function studies, I&O, electrolytes, phosphorus and uric acid levels; especially with CRF.

7. Assess for seizures if hematocrit increases by 4 points in 2 weeks.

CLIENT/FAMILY TEACHING

1. Do not shake vial; inactivates drug. Keep refrigerated.

2. Over 95% of clients with CRF manifested significant increases in hematocrit and nearly all were transfusion-independent within 2 months after beginning therapy; drug does not cure renal disease and desired drug response may take up to 6 weeks.

3. Supplemental iron and vitamins are administered to enhance drug effects; take as directed.

4. Report as scheduled for lab studies so dose can be adjusted.

5. Review list of drug side effects; report persistent/bothersome ones. Practice contraception during therapy.

6. Must continue to follow prescribed dietary and dialysis recommendations; schedule activities to permit rest periods. Monitor BP and keep record.

7. Do not perform tasks that require mental alertness until drug effects realized (especially during the first 3 months of therapy).

OUTCOMES/EVALUATE

- ↑ Hematocrit
- Relief of symptoms of anemia

- ↓ Need for allogeneic blood transfusions

Epoprostenol sodium

(eh-poh-**PROST**-en-ohl)   **IV**

CLASSIFICATION(S):
Vasodilator, peripheral
PREGNANCY CATEGORY: B
Rx: Flolan.

SEE ALSO *ANTIHYPERTENSIVE AGENTS.*

USES
Long-term IV treatment of primary pulmonary hypertension and pulmonary hypertension associated with scleroderma spectrum of the disease in NYHA Class III and Class IV clients who do not respond adequately to conventional therapy. *NOTE:* Should be used only by practitioners experienced in the diagnosis and treatment of pulmonary hypertension.

ACTION/KINETICS
Action
Acts by direct vasodilation of pulmonary and systemic arterial vascular beds and by inhibition of platelet aggregation. IV infusion in clients with pulmonary hypertension results in increases in cardiac index and SV and decreases in pulmonary vascular resistance, total pulmonary resistance, and mean systemic arterial pressure.

Pharmacokinetics
Is rapidly hydrolyzed at the neutral pH of the blood as well as by enzymatic degradation. Steady state plasma levels reached within 15 min and are proportional to infusion rates. Metabolites are less active than the parent compound. $t\frac{1}{2}$: 6 min. Most excreted in the urine with a small amount in the feces.

CONTRAINDICATIONS
Known hypersensitivity to the drug or structurally related compounds. Chronic use in those with CHF due to severe LV systolic dysfunction and in those who develop pulmonary edema during dosing.

SPECIAL CONCERNS
Abrupt withdrawal or sudden large decreases in the dose may cause rebound pulmonary hypertension (symptoms include dizziness, asthenia, and dyspnea). Use caution in dose selection in the elderly due to the greater frequency of decreased hepatic, renal, or cardiac function, as well as concomitant disease or other drug therapy. Use with caution during lactation. Safety and efficacy not determined in children.

SIDE EFFECTS
Most Common
Flushing, headache, N&V, hypotension, anxiety/nervousness, agitation, chest pain, dizziness, bradycardia, abdominal pain, musculoskeletal pain, dyspnea, back pain, tachycardia.

Those occurring during acute dosing and escalation of dose. CV: Flushing, hypotension, bradycardia, tachycardia. **GI:** N&V, abdominal pain, dyspepsia. **CNS:** Headache, anxiety, nervousness, agitation, dizziness, hypesthesia, paresthesia. **Miscellaneous:** Chest/ back/ musculoskeletal pain, dyspnea, sweating.

Those occurring as a result of the drug delivery system. Due to the chronic indwelling catheter: Local infection, pain at the injection site, sepsis, infections, injection site hemorrhage.

Those occurring during chronic dosing. CV: Flushing, tachycardia. **GI:** N&V, diarrhea. **CNS:** Headache, anxiety, nervousness, tremor, dizziness, hypesthesia, hyperesthesia, paresthesia. **Musculoskeletal:** Jaw pain, myalgia, nonspecific musculoskeletal pain. **Miscellaneous:** Flu-like symptoms, chills, fever, sepsis.

Side effects regardless of attribution. CV: Palpitation, flushing, cyanosis, arrhythmia, hypotension, pallor, angina pectoris, *hemorrhage*, rectal hemorrhage, bradycardia, supraventricular tachycardia, *CVA*, myocardial ischemia, syncope, heart failure, right heart failure, vascular disorder, peripheral vascular disorder, *shock*. **CNS:** Depression, headache, confusion, *convulsion*, insomnia, dizziness, anxiety, hyperkinesia, nervousness, tremor, depression, hyperesthesia, hypesthesia, paresthesia, somnolence. **GI:** Abdominal pain, anorexia, diarrhea, N&V, ascites, constipation, esophageal reflux/gastritis, enlarged abdomen, flatulence. **Dermatologic:** Sweating, rash, pruritus, eczema, urticaria, skin ulcer, collagen disease. **Musculoskeletal:** Chest/back pain, arthralgia, jaw/neck pain, pain, arthritis, leg cramps. **Respiratory:** Dyspnea, increased cough, epistaxis, pleural effusion, pharyngitis, pneumonia, pneumothorax, pulmonary edema, respiratory disorder, sinusitis, rhinitis. **GU:** Hematuria, UTI. **Hematologic:** Thrombocytopenia, anemia, hypersplenism, pancytopenia, splenomegaly. **Metabolic:** Edema, peripheral/genital edema, weight reduction/gain, hypo-/hyperkalemia, hypercalcemia, hypoxia. **Ophthalmic:** Amblyopia, abnormal vision. **Miscellaneous:** Asthenia, chills, fever, *sepsis*, flu-like symptoms, infection, hyperthyroidism.

OD OVERDOSE MANAGEMENT
Symptoms: Flushing, headache, hypotension, tachycardia, nausea, vomiting, diarrhea, hypoxemia, *respiratory arrest*. *Treatment:* Reduce dose of epoprostenol.

DRUG INTERACTIONS
Anticoagulants / Possible ↑ risk of bleeding
Antiplatelet drugs / Possible ↑ risk of bleeding
Diuretics / Additional ↓ in BP
Vasodilators / Additional ↓ in BP

HOW SUPPLIED
Powder for Reconstitution: 0.5 mg, 1.5 mg.

DOSAGE
• **CHRONIC IV INFUSION**
Pulmonary hypertension.
Acute dosing: Initial: 2 ng (nanograms)/kg/min. Increase in increments of 2 ng/kg/min every 15 min or longer until dose-limiting pharmacologic effects are observed or until a tolerance limit to the drug is established and further increases in the infusion rate are not clinically warranted. If the initial infusion rate of 2 ng/kg/min is not tolerated, identify a lower dose that is tolerated. **Dosage adjustments:** Changes in

the chronic infusion rate are based on persistence, recurrence, or worsening of the symptoms of primary pulmonary hypertension. Consider increments in dose if symptoms of pulmonary hypertension persist or recur after improving. Increase the infusion by 1 to 2 ng/kg/min increments at intervals sufficient to allow assessment of response. These intervals should be at least 15 min. Following establishment of a new chronic infusion rate, observe the client and monitor standing and supine BP and HR for several hours to ensure that the new dose is tolerated. If a decrease in infusion rate is necessary, gradually make 2 ng/kg/min decrements every 15 min or longer until the dose-limiting effects resolve. Avoid abrupt withdrawal or sudden large reductions in infusion rates.

NURSING CONSIDERATIONS
ADMINISTRATION/STORAGE
IV 1. Initiate dosage in a setting with adequate personnel and equipment for physiologic monitoring and emergency care.
2. Chronic administration delivered continuously by a permanent indwelling central venous catheter and an ambulatory infusion pump (see package insert for requirements for the infusion pump). Unless contraindicated, give therapy to decrease the risk of pulmonary thromboembolism or systemic embolism.
3. Follow package instructions for reconstitution and dilution.
4. Do not dilute reconstituted solutions or administer with other parenteral solutions or medications.
5. Check package insert carefully to make 100 mL of a solution with the appropriate final concentration of drug and for infusion delivery rates for doses equal to or less than 16 ng/kg/min based on client weight, drug delivery rate, and concentration of solution to be used.
6. Protect unopened vials from light; store at 15–25°C (59–77°F). Protect reconstituted solutions from light; refrigerate at 2–8°C (36–46°F) for no more than 40 hr.

---

7. Do not freeze reconstituted solutions; discard any solution refrigerated for >48 hr.

8. A single reservoir of reconstituted solution can be given at room temperature for 8 hr; alternatively, it can be used with a cold pouch and given for up to 24 hr. Do not expose solution to sunlight.

ASSESSMENT

1. Perform full cardiopulmonary assessment. Based on symptoms, determine NYHA functional class (III or IV). List other agents used, outcome.

2. Note clinical presentation, fatigability, ability to ambulate, to perform ADLs, need for continuous oxygen, oxygen saturation levels.

3. Assess mental status, ability to handle medication preparation, IV administration; or identify someone that can and is willing to perform this function on a regular basis. Get home infusion referral for supplies.

4. Ensure that permanent indwelling central venous catheter is available for continuous ambulatory delivery once dosing completed.

5. Assess central venous access site for any evidence of infection, discharge, odor, erythema, or swelling and review with client/significant other.

6. Consult manufacturer's guidelines for dosage and delivery rate based on client weight for acute dosing.

7. Monitor cardiopulmonary response during therapy. Drug helps reduce RV and LV afterload and increases CO and SV.

CLIENT/FAMILY TEACHING

1. Drug helps reduce work of the heart thus improving symptoms of SOB, fatigue, and exercise intolerance.

2. Administered continuously through an indwelling catheter to the heart by a portable external infusion pump; may be needed for years to help control symptoms.

3. Proper site care, pump maintenance (troubleshooting and care) and accurate reconstitution for prescribed drug concentration; proper storage, light protection, pouch filling, pump settings, and port care are imperative to

safe therapy. Review written guidelines for all the above regularly. Call with questions or problems.

4. When drug is reconstituted and administered at room temperature, the pump must be programmed to administer pouch contents in 8 hr, whereas if drug is reconstituted and refrigerated at 2–8°C (36–46°F) may be administered in cold pouch over 24 hr.

5. Side effects that indicate excessive dosing and require a reduction in dosage and reporting include fast heart rate, headache, N&V, diarrhea, hypotension.

6. Brief interruptions in therapy may cause rapid deterioration in condition. Report loss of effect, worsening of condition or any S&S of infusion site infection. Do not run out of medication, call infusion team in a timely manner to ensure continuous availability.

OUTCOMES/EVALUATE

- Improvement in exercise capacity
- ↓ Dyspnea and fatigue with pulmonary hypertension

Eprosartan mesylate ■

(eh-proh-**SAR**-tan)

CLASSIFICATION(S):

Antihypertensive, angiotensin II receptor blocker

PREGNANCY CATEGORY: C (first trimester), **D** (second and third trimesters).

Rx: Teveten.

USES

Hypertension, alone or with other antihypertensives (diuretics, calcium channel blockers).

ACTION/KINETICS

Action

Acts by blocking the vasoconstrictor and aldosterone-secreting effects of angiotensin II by blocking selectively the binding of angiotensin II to angiotensin II receptors located in the vascular smooth muscle and adrenal gland. BP is thus reduced.

Bold Italic = life threatening side effect   ■ = black box warning   ✦ = Available in Canada

Pharmacokinetics

About 13% bioavailable. **Peak plasma levels:** 1–2 hr. Food delays absorption. **t½, terminal:** 5–9 hr. Excreted mostly unchanged in both the feces (about 90%) and urine (about 7%). **Plasma protein binding:** About 98%.

SPECIAL CONCERNS

■ When used during the second and third trimesters of pregnancy, drugs that act directly on the renin-angiotensin system can cause injury and even death to the developing fetus. When pregnancy is detected, discontinue use of eprosartan as soon as possible.■ Symptomatic hypotension may be seen in clients who are volume- and/or salt-depleted (e.g., those taking diuretics). Safety and efficacy have not been determined in children.

SIDE EFFECTS

Most Common

URTI, cough, pharyngitis, rhinitis, UTI, viral infection, arthralgia, abdominal pain, fatigue.

GI: Abdominal pain, diarrhea, dyspepsia, anorexia, constipation, dry mouth, esophagitis, flatulence, gastritis, gastroenteritis, gingivitis, nausea, periodontitis, toothache, vomiting. **CNS:** Depression, headache, dizziness, anxiety, ataxia, insomnia, migraine, neuritis, nervousness, paresthesia, somnolence, tremor, vertigo. **CV:** Angina pectoris, bradycardia, abnormal ECG, extrasystoles, atrial fibrillation, hypotension, tachycardia, palpitations, peripheral ischemia. **Respiratory:** URTI, sinusitis, bronchitis, chest pain, rhinitis, pharyngitis, cough, asthma, epistaxis. **Musculoskeletal:** Arthralgia, myalgia, arthritis, aggravated arthritis, arthrosis, skeletal/back pain, tendonitis. **GU:** UTI, albuminuria, cystitis, hematuria, frequent micturition, polyuria, renal calculus, urinary incontinence. **Metabolic:** Diabetes mellitus, gout. **Body as a whole:** Viral infection, injury, fatigue, alcohol intolerance, asthenia, substernal chest pain, peripheral edema, dependent edema, fatigue, fever, hot flushes, flu-like symptoms, malaise, rigors, pain, leg cramps, herpes simplex. **Hematologic:** Anemia, purpura, leukopenia, neutropenia, thrombocytopenia. **Dermatologic:** Eczema, furunculosis, pruritus, rash, maculopapular rash, increased sweating. **Ophthalmic:** Conjunctivitis, abnormal vision, xerophthalmia. **Otic:** Otitis external, otitis media, tinnitus.

LABORATORY TEST CONSIDERATIONS

↑ ALT, AST, creatine phosphokinase, BUN, creatinine, alkaline phosphatase. ↓ Hemoglobin. Glycosuria, hypercholesterolemia, hyperglycemia, hyper-/hypokalemia, hyponatremia.

HOW SUPPLIED

Tablets: 600 mg.

DOSAGE

- **TABLETS**
  Hypertension.

Adults, initial: 600 mg once daily as monotherapy in clients who are not volume-depleted. Can be given once or twice daily with total daily doses ranging from 400–800 mg.

NURSING CONSIDERATIONS

ADMINISTRATION/STORAGE

1. If antihypertensive effect using once-daily dosing is inadequate, a twice-a-day regimen at the same total daily dose or an increase in dose may be more effective.
2. Maximum BP reduction may not occur for 2–3 weeks.
3. May be used in combination with thiazide diuretics or calcium channel blockers if additional BP lowering effect is needed.
4. Discontinuing treatment does not lead to a rapid rebound increase in BP.
5. No initial dosage adjustment is needed for the elderly or those with hepatic or renal impairment (maximum dose: 600 mg/day).
6. Store from 20–25°C (68–77°F).

ASSESSMENT

1. Note onset, symptoms, other agents trialed.
2. Correct volume depletion. Monitor BP, CBC, K⁺, sodium, microalbumin, renal, and LFTs.

CLIENT/FAMILY TEACHING

1. Take as directed once or twice daily with or without food.
2. Continue lifestyle modifications, i.e., regular exercise, weight loss, smoking/

E

alcohol cessation, low fat/salt diet for BP control.

3. Practice reliable birth control. Report if pregnant.

4. Immediately report any lip, tongue or facial swelling as well as any fever or sore throat. Report any persistent dry cough.

5. Keep a record of BP readings and bring for provider review.

OUTCOMES/EVALUATE

↓ BP; control of HTN

Eptifibatide   IV
(**ep**-tih-**FY**-beh-tide)

CLASSIFICATION(S):
Antiplatelet drug, glycoprotein IIb/IIIa inhibitor
PREGNANCY CATEGORY: B
Rx: Integrilin.

USES
(1) Treatment of acute coronary syndrome (unstable angina or non-Q-wave MI), including those to be managed medically and those undergoing percutaneous coronary intervention. (2) Treatment of those undergoing percutaneous coronary intervention, including those undergoing intracoronary stenting.

ACTION/KINETICS
Action
Reversibly inhibits platelet aggregation by preventing the binding of fibrinogen, von Willebrand factor, and other adhesive ligands to GP IIb/IIIa.
Pharmacokinetics
Immediately effective after IV use. **t½, elimination:** 2.5 hr. Drug and metabolites are excreted through kidneys.

CONTRAINDICATIONS
History of bleeding diathesis or evidence of active abnormal bleeding within the past 30 days. Severe hypertension (systolic BP >200 mm Hg or diastolic BP >110 mm Hg) inadequately controlled. Major surgery within the past 6 weeks, history of stroke within 30 days or any history of hemorrhagic stroke, current or planned use of another parenteral GP IIb/IIIa inhibitor, platelet count less than 100,000/mm³, dependency on renal dialysis. Serum creatinine of 2.0 mg/dL or more (for the 180 mcg/kg bolus and the 2 mcg/kg/min infusion) or 4.0 mg/dL or more (for the 135 mcg/kg bolus and the 0.5 mcg/kg/min infusion). Lactation.

SPECIAL CONCERNS
Bleeding is the most common complication; there is a greater risk in older clients. Use with caution when used with other drugs that affect hemostasis, including thrombolytics, oral anticoagulants, NSAIDs, dipyridamole, ticlopidine, and clopidogrel. Use with caution during lactation. Safety and efficacy have not been determined in children.

SIDE EFFECTS
Most Common
Bleeding, hypotension.
CV: Major bleeding, including ***intracranial hemorrhage***, bleeding from the femoral artery access site, and bleeding that leads to decreases in hemoglobin greater than 5 grams/dL. Minor bleeding, including spontaneous gross hematuria, spontaneous hematemesis, or blood loss with a hemoglobin decrease of more than 3 grams/dL. Oropharyngeal (especially gingival), genitourinary, GI, and retroperitoneal bleeding. Hypotension. **Hypersensitivity/allergy: *Anaphylaxis*,** other allergic S&S.

DRUG INTERACTIONS
Possible additive effects when used with thrombolytics, anticoagulants, or other antiplatelet drugs.
H *Evening primrose oil* / Potential for ↑ antiplatelet effect
H *Feverfew* / Potential for ↑ antiplatelet effect
H *Garlic* / Potential for ↑ antiplatelet effect
H *Ginger* / Potential for ↑ antiplatelet effect
H *Ginkgo biloba* / Potential for ↑ antiplatelet effect
H *Ginseng* / Potential for ↑ antiplatelet effect
H *Grapeseed extract* / Potential for ↑ antiplatelet effect

HOW SUPPLIED
Injection: 0.75 mg/mL, 2 mg/mL.

Bold Italic = life threatening side effect   ■ = black box warning   ♣ = Available in Canada

DOSAGE

- **IV**

Acute coronary syndrome.

Adults, initial: IV bolus of 180 mcg/kg as soon as possible following diagnosis, followed by a continuous infusion of 2 mcg/kg/min until hospital discharge or initiation of coronary artery bypass surgery, up to 72 hr. If the client is to undergo a PCI while receiving eptifibatide, continue the infusion up to hospital discharge, or for up to 18 to 24 hr after the procedure, whichever comes first, allowing up to 96 hr of therapy.

The recommended adult dosage in clients with acute coronary syndrome with an estimated C_{CR} <50 mL/min or a serum creatinine >2 mg/dL (if C_{CR} is not available) is an IV bolus of 180 mcg/kg as soon as possible following diagnosis, immediately followed by a continuous infusion of 1 mcg/kg/min.

Percutaneous coronary intervention.

Adults with normal renal function: IV bolus of 180 mcg/kg given immediately before initiation of PCI followed by a continuous infusion of 2 mcg/kg/min and a second bolus dose of 180 mcg/kg 10 min after the first bolus. This is followed by a continuous infusion until hospital discharge or for up to 18–24 hr, whichever comes first. A minimum of 12 hr of infusion is recommended. Give those weighing more than 121 kg a maximum of 22.6 mg/bolus followed by a maximum infusion rate of 7.5 mg/hr. **Adults, in those with a C_{CR} <50 mL/min or creatinine >2 mg/dL:** IV bolus of 180 mcg/kg given immediately before initiation of PCI, immediately followed by a continuous infusion of 1 mcg/kg/min and a second 180 mcg/kg bolus given 10 min after the first. Give those weighing more than 121 kg a maximum of 22.6 mg/bolus followed by a maximum infusion rate of 7.5 mg/hr.

NURSING CONSIDERATIONS

ADMINISTRATION/STORAGE

IV 1. If undergoing CABG surgery, discontinue prior to surgery.

2. Aspirin has been used with eptifibatide with the following possible doses: In acute coronary syndrome, aspirin, 160–325 mg initially and daily thereafter; in PCI, aspirin, 160–325 mg 1–24 hr prior to intervention and daily thereafter.

3. The following aspirin and heparin doses are recommended:

- **Acute coronary syndrome:** Aspirin, 160–325 mg PO initially and daily thereafter. For heparin, achieve a target aPTT of 50–70 sec during medical management of the following: If weight is 70 or more kg, give a 5,000 units heparin bolus followed by infusion of 1,000 units/hr. If the weight is <70 kg, give a 60 units/kg bolus followed by infusion of 12 units/kg/hr. If heparin is initiated prior to PCI, additional boluses during PCI to maintain an ACT target of 200 to 300 seconds. Heparin infusion after the PCI is discouraged.

- **PCI:** Aspirin, 160–325 mg PO 1 to 24 hr prior to PCI and daily thereafter. For heparin, achieve a target ACT of 200–300 seconds for the following: Heparin, 60 units/kg, as a bolus initially in those not treated with heparin within 6 hr prior to PCI. Give additional boluses during PCI to maintain ACT within target. Do not give heparin infusion after the PCI.

4. Inspect vial for particulate matter or discoloration before use.

5. May be given in the same IV line as alteplase, atropine, dobutamine, heparin, lidocaine, meperidine, metoprolol, midazolam, morphine, nitroglycerin, or verapamil; do not give in same line as furosemide.

6. May be given in the same IV line with 0.9% NaCl or D5W/NSS; may also contain up to 60 mEq/L of KCl.

7. Withdraw bolus dose from the 10-mL vial and give by IV push over 1–2 min. Immediately following the bolus dose, start continuous infusion. If using an infusion pump, give undiluted directly from the 100-mL vial by spiking the 100-mL vial with a vented infusion set. Center spike within the circle on the stopper top.

8. Store vials at 2–8°C (36–46°F). Protect from light until use. Discard any portion left in the vial.

 = see color insert   **H** = Herbal   **IV** = Intravenous   ℞ = sound alike drug

ASSESSMENT

1. Note onset, duration, characteristics of S&S.
2. Note conditions that preclude therapy: recent CVA or surgery, platelets <100,000/mm³, uncontrolled BP, abnormal bleeding or history of bleeding diathesis, hemorrhagic stroke, renal failure, or dialysis.
3. Monitor VS, ECG, bleeding times, renal and LFTs.
4. Stop drug prior to CABG surgery.
5. Used in conjunction with aspirin and heparin; review dosing guidelines.
6. Assess femoral artery access site for evidence of bleeding. Stop heparin and eptifibatide therapy if unable to stop bleeding with pressure.

CLIENT/FAMILY TEACHING

1. Review risks associated with therapy. Drug is a blood thinner used to prevent clot formation with unstable angina and non-Q-wave MI.
2. Bleeding is most common side effect of therapy; usually occurs at graft site but may also occur as GU, GI, oropharyngeal, or retroperitoneal bleeding. Report any unusual bleeding, change in mental status, sudden drop in BP, or other adverse side effects.
3. Encourage family to learn CPR.

OUTCOMES/EVALUATE

- Inhibition of platelet aggregation
- ↓ Death/MI with acute coronary syndrome

Erlotinib
(er-**LOE**-tye-nib)

CLASSIFICATION(S):

Epidermal growth factor receptor inhibitor
PREGNANCY CATEGORY: D
Rx: Tarceva.

USES

(1) Non-small cell lung cancer (locally advanced or metastatic) after failure of at last 1 prior chemotherapy regimen. (2) With gemcitabine for first-line treatment of locally advanced, unresectable, or metastatic pancreatic cancer. *Investi-*
gational: Squamous cell head and neck cancer.

ACTION/KINETICS

Action

Erlotinib inhibits the intracellular phosphorylation of tyrosine kinase associated with the epidermal growth factor receptor. Epidermal growth factor receptors are expressed on the cell surface of both normal and cancer cells. Precise mechanism is not known.

Pharmacokinetics

Bioavailability is about 60%; food increases bioavailability to almost 100%. **Peak plasma levels:** 4 hr. $t^{1/2}$: 36 hr. Metabolized predominately by CYP3A4 and to a lesser extent by CYP1A2. Excreted mainly through the feces (83%).

CONTRAINDICATIONS

Lactation.

SPECIAL CONCERNS

Use with caution in impaired hepatic function. Safety and efficacy have not been determined in children.

SIDE EFFECTS

Most Common

When used to treat non-small cell lung cancer: Rash, diarrhea, anorexia, N&V, cough, dyspnea, fatigue, infection. **When used to treat pancreatic cancer (with gemcitabine):** Rash, diarrhea, fatigue, N&V, anorexia, abdominal pain, constipation, weight loss, infection, pyrexia, edema.

When used to treat non-small cell lung cancer. Respiratory: Dyspnea, cough, fever, epistaxis, *interstitial lung disease*. **CV:** *MI*, ischemia, *CVA*. **GI:** Diarrhea, GI bleeding, anorexia, N&V, stomatitis, abdominal pain, gastritis, gastroduodenal ulcers, hematemesis, hematochezia, melena, hemorrhage from possible colitis. **Hematologic:** Microangiopathic hemolytic anemia with thrombocytopenia (when used for pancreatic cancer). **Dermatologic:** Rash, dry skin, pruritus. **Ophthalmic:** Conjunctivitis, keratoconjunctivitis sicca. **Miscellaneous:** Fatigue, infection.

When used with gemcitabine to treat pancreatic cancer. GI: N&V, diarrhea, anorexia, abdominal pain, constipation, stomatitis, dyspepsia, flatulence, ileus, pancreatitis, GI bleeding, gastritis,

---

gastroduodenal ulcers, hematemesis, hematochezia, melena, hemorrhage from possible colitis. **CNS:** Depression, dizziness, headache, insomnia, anxiety, neuropathy, rigors. **CV:** Syncope, arrhythmias, DVT, *MI*/ischemia, *CVA (including cerebral hemorrhage)*. **Dermatologic:** Rash, alopecia. **Musculoskeletal:** Bone pain, myalgia. **Respiratory:** Dyspnea, cough, epistaxis. **Hematologic:** Hemolytic anemia (including microangiopathic hemolytic anemia with thrombocytopenia). **Ophthalmic:** Conjunctivitis, keratitis. **Body as a whole:** Fatigue, weight loss, edema, infection, pyrexia. **Miscellaneous:** Renal insufficiency.

LABORATORY TEST CONSIDERATIONS
↑ INR, ALT, AST, bilirubin.

OD **OVERDOSE MANAGEMENT**
Symptoms: Doses of 400 mg daily may cause diarrhea, rash, and elevated liver transaminases. *Treatment:* Withhold erlotinib and begin symptomatic treatment.

DRUG INTERACTIONS
Coumarin derivatives / ↑ Risk of bleeding episodes
CYP3A4 inducers (e.g., carbamazepine, phenobarbital, phenytoin, rifabutin, rifapentine, St. John's wort) / Potential ↓ erlotinib AUC R/T ↑ metabolism
CYP3A4 inhibitors (e.g., atazanavir, clarithromycin, indinavir, itraconazole, ketoconazole, nefazodone, nelfinavir, ritonavir, saquinavir, telithromycin, troleandomycin, voriconazole) / ↓ Erlotinib dosage if side effects occur
NSAIDs / ↑ Risk of bleeding episodes
Rifampin / ↓ Erlotinib AUC by about two-thirds R/T induction of CYP3A4; consider alternate treatment with drug lacking CYP3A4 inducing activity
Warfarin / ↑ Risk of bleeding episodes

HOW SUPPLIED
Tablets: 25 mg, 100 mg, 150 mg.

DOSAGE
• TABLETS
Non-small cell lung cancer.
150 mg once daily taken at least 1 hr before or 2 hr after ingestion of food. Continue treatment until disease progresses or unacceptable toxicity occurs.

When reduction of dose is necessary, reduce in 50 mg decrements.

Pancreatic cancer.
100 mg per day taken at least 1 hr before or 2 hr after ingestion of food. Taken in combination with gemcitabine. Continue treatment until disease progresses or unacceptable toxicity occurs. When dose reduction is needed, reduce the erlotinib dose in 50 mg decrements.

E

NURSING CONSIDERATIONS
ADMINISTRATION/STORAGE
1. In those who develop an acute onset of new or progressive pulmonary symptoms (e.g., dyspnea, cough, or fever), interrupt treatment pending diagnostic evaluation. If interstitial lung disease diagnosed, discontinue and institute appropriate treatment.
2. Diarrhea can usually be managed by loperamide. Severe diarrhea unresponsive to loperamide or in those who become dehydrated may require dose reduction or temporary interruption of therapy.
3. Those with severe skin reactions may require dose reduction or temporary interruption of therapy.
4. Store from 15–30°C (59–86°F).

ASSESSMENT
1. Note reasons for therapy, disease onset, other chemotherapy regimen trialed/failed. List drugs prescribed to ensure none interact.
2. Assess/monitor pulmonary condition; include PFTs, CXR and CT/MRI findings, bronchocospy biopsy results.
3. Monitor CBC, renal and LFTs; may need to reduce dose or stop therapy with dysfunction.

CLIENT/FAMILY TEACHING
1. Drug is used to treat non-small cell lung cancer after at least one other therapy trialed/failed. Take one hour before or two hours after food.
2. May cause worsening of lung condition; report any increased SOB, coughing, fever, or sudden change in breathing condition.
3. Report inability to eat, severe diarrhea or vomiting, eye irritation, onset/worsening of SOB or cough.

📷 = see color insert   **H** = Herbal   **IV** = Intravenous   ⓒ = sound alike drug

4. Diarrhea is managed with loperamide. In those with severe diarrhea who are unresponsive to loperamide or who become dehydrated, dose will be reduced or therapy temporarily interrupted until resolved.

5. Practice reliable contraception during and for 2 weeks after completing therapy.

OUTCOMES/EVALUATE
Inhibition of malignant cell proliferation with non-small cell lung cancer or pancreatic cancer

---

Erythromycin base ©
(eh-**rih**-throw-**MY**-sin)

CLASSIFICATION(S):
Antibiotic, macrolide
PREGNANCY CATEGORY: B (A/T/S, Erymax, Staticin, and T-Stat are C)
Rx: Capsules, Delayed-Release; Tablets, Delayed-Release; Tablets, Film-Coated; Tablets, Polymer Coated Particles: Ery-Tab, Eryc, Erythromycin Film-Tabs, PCE Dispertab. **Gel, Topical:** A/T/S, Emgel. **Ointment, Topical:** Akne-Mycin. **Ophthalmic Ointment:** Ilotycin Ophthalmic. **Pledgets, Topical:** Ery Pads. **Solution, Topical:** A/T/S, Eryderm 2%.
♣**Rx: Capsules: Tablets:** Apo-Erythro Base, Apo-Erythro E-C, Erybid, PCE, PMS-Erythromycin.

SEE ALSO *ANTI-INFECTIVE AGENTS.*
USES
(1) Mild to moderate upper respiratory tract infections due to *Streptococcus pyogenes* (group A beta-hemolytic streptococci), *Streptococcus pneumoniae,* and *Haemophilus influenzae* (combined with sulfonamides). (2) Mild-to-moderate lower respiratory tract infections due to *S. pyogenes* (group A beta-hemolytic streptococci) and *S. pneumoniae.* Respiratory tract infections due to *Mycoplasma pneumoniae.* (3) Pertussis (whooping cough) caused by *Bordetella pertussis;* may also be used as prophylaxis of pertussis in exposed individuals. (4) Mild-to-moderate skin and skin structure infections due to *S. pyogenes* and *Staphylococcus aureus* (resistant staphylococci may emerge during treatment). Topically for acne vulgaris. (5) As an adjunct to antitoxin in diphtheria (caused by *Corynebacterium diphtheriae),* to prevent carriers, and to eradicate the organism in carriers. (6) Intestinal amebiasis due to *Entamoeba histolytica* (PO erythromycin only). (7) As an alternative to penicillin to treat acute pelvic inflammatory disease due to *Neisseria gonorrhoeae* (erythromycin lactobionate IV followed by PO erythromycin). (8) Erythrasma due to *Corynebacterium minutissimum.* (9) *Chlamydia trachomatis* infections causing urogenital infections during pregnancy, conjunctivitis in the newborn, or pneumonia during infancy. Also, uncomplicated chlamydial infections of the urethra, endocervix, or rectum in adults (when tetracyclines are contraindicated or not tolerated). (10) Nongonococcal urethritis caused by *Ureaplasma urealyticum* when tetracyclines are contraindicated or not tolerated (PO erythromycin only). (11) Legionnaires' disease due to *Legionella pneumophilia.* (12) PO as an alternative to penicillin (in penicillin-allergic clients) to treat primary syphilis caused by *Treponema pallidum.* (13) Prophylaxis of initial or recurrent attacks of rheumatic fever in clients allergic to penicillin or sulfonamides. (14) Infections due to *Listeria monocytogenes.* (15) Bacterial endocarditis due to alpha-hemolytic streptococci, Viridans group, in clients allergic to penicillins.

Investigational: (1) Acne vulgaris to decrease population of lipophilic bacteria. (2) Bacilly angiomatosis in immunocompromised clients due to *Bartonella henselae* or *B. quintana.* (3) Enteritis due to *Campylobacter jejuni.* (4) As an alternative to treat erysipelas cellulitis of the extremities not associated with venous catheter or diabetes. (5) Chancroid due to *Haemophilus ducreyi.* (6) As an alternative to doxycycline or trimethoprim to treat Granuloma inguinale due to *Calymmatobacterium granulomatis.* (7) As an alternative to treat nonbullous lesions of ecthyma impetigo. (8) Inclusion

---

Bold Italic = life threatening side effect   ■ = black box warning   ♣ = Available in Canada

conjunctivitis in adults due to *C. trachomatis*. (9) As an alternative to treat mild to moderate, uncomplicated, infected wounds of the extremities. (10) Moderate to severe leptospirosis due to *Leptospira* species. (11) As an alternative to treat early Lyme disease due *Borrelia burgorferi*. (12) As an alternative to doxycycline to treat *Lymphogranuloma venereum*. (13) Tick-borne relapsing fever and louse-borne relapsing fever. (14) As an alternative to treat tetanus due to *Clostridium tetani*.

Ophthalmic ointment: (1) Treatment of superficial ocular infections involving the conjunctiva and cornea (e.g., conjunctivitis, keratitis, keratoconjunctivitis, corneal ulcers, blepharitis, blepharoconjunctivitis, acute meibomianitis, and dacryocystitis) due to *Streptococcus pneumoniae, Staphylococcus aureus, S. pyogenes, Corynebacterium* species, *Haemophilus influenzae*, and *Bacteroides* infections. (2) Prophylaxis of ophthalmia neonatorum due to *Neisseria gonorrhoeae* and *Chlamydia trachomatis*. The efficacy in preventing ophthalmia caused by penicillinase-producing *N. gonorrhoeae* is not established.

Topical solution: Acne vulgaris.

Topical ointment: (1) Prophylaxis of infection in minor skin abrasions; treatment of superficial infections of the skin. (2) Acne vulgaris.

ACTION/KINETICS

Action

Erythromycins are macrolide antibiotics. They inhibit protein synthesis of microorganisms by binding reversibly to a ribosomal subunit (50S), thus interfering with the transmission of genetic information and inhibiting protein synthesis. The drugs are effective only against rapidly multiplying organisms.

Pharmacokinetics

Absorbed from the upper part of the small intestine. Those for PO use are manufactured in enteric-coated or film-coated forms to prevent destruction by gastric acid. Achieves concentrations in body tissues about 40% of those in the plasma. Diffuses into body tissues: Peritoneal, pleural, ascitic, and amniotic fluids; saliva; through the placental circulation; and across the mucous membrane of the tracheobronchial tree. Diffuses poorly into spinal fluid, although penetration is increased in meningitis. Alkalinization of the urine (to pH 8.5) increases the gram-negative antibacterial action. **Peak serum levels: PO,** 1–4 hr. **t½:** 1.5–2 hr, *but prolonged in clients with renal impairment*. Partially metabolized by the liver and primarily excreted in bile. Also excreted in breast milk. **Plasma protein binding:** Approximately 70%.

CONTRAINDICATIONS

Hypersensitivity to erythromycin; *in utero* syphilis. Use of topical preparations in the eye or near the nose, mouth, or any mucous membrane. Ophthalmic use in dendritic keratitis, vaccinia, varicella, myobacterial infections of the eye, fungal diseases of the eye. Use with steroid combinations following uncomplicated removal of a corneal foreign body.

SPECIAL CONCERNS

Use with caution in liver disease and during lactation. Use may result in bacterial and fungal overgrowth (i.e., superinfection). Use of other drugs for acne may result in a cumulative irritant effect. Although still recommended, use to treat whooping cough in newborns may cause pyloric stenosis. Use with certain CYP3A inhibitors, such as certain calcium-channel blockers, certain antifungal drugs, and some antidepressants, causes a greater risk of sudden death from cardiac causes.

SIDE EFFECTS

Most Common

After systemic use: Abdominal pain/ discomfort, headache, diarrhea/loose stools, increased cough, dyspepsia, N&V, dizziness, rash.

GI: Abdominal discomfort or pain, anorexia, diarrhea or loose stools, dyspepsia, flatulence, GI disorder, N&V, pseudomembranous colitis, hepatotoxicity. Possibility of hypertrophic pyloric stenosis in infants. **CV:** Ventricular arrhythmias, including *ventricular tachycardia and torsades de pointes in clients with prolonged QT intervals*. After IV, in-

crease in heart rate and prolongation of QT interval. **Dermatologic:** Pruritus, rash, urticaria, bullous eruptions, eczema, erythema multiforme, ***Stevens-Johnson syndrome, toxic epidermal necrolysis.*** **CNS:** Dizziness, headache, insomnia. **Miscellaneous:** Asthenia, dyspnea, increased cough, non-specific pain, vaginitis, allergic reaction, ***anaphylaxis.*** Reversible hearing loss in those with renal or hepatic insufficiency, in the elderly, and after doses greater than 4 grams/day.
Following IV use: Venous irritation, thrombophlebitis.
Following IM use: Pain at the injection site, with development of necrosis or sterile abscesses.
Following topical use: Erythema, desquamation, burning sensation, eye irritation, tenderness, dryness, pruritus, oily skin, peeling, itching, contact sensitization, generalized urticaria.

LABORATORY TEST CONSIDERATIONS
Interference with fluorometric assay for urinary catecholamines. ↑ Bicarbonate, eosinophils, platelet count, segmented neutrophils, serum CPK.

OD OVERDOSE MANAGEMENT
Symptoms: N&V, diarrhea, epigastric distress, acute pancreatitis (mild), hearing loss (with or without tinnitus and vertigo). *Treatment:* Induce vomiting. General supportive measures. Allergic reactions should be controlled with conventional therapy.

DRUG INTERACTIONS
Alfentanil / ↓ Alfentanil excretion → ↑ effect
Antacids / Slight ↓ in elimination rate of erythromycin
Anticoagulants / ↑ Anticoagulant effects → possible hemorrhage
Benzodiazepines (alprazolam, diazepam, midazolam, triazolam) / ↑ Benzodiazepine levels → ↑ CNS depressant effects
Bromocriptine / ↑ Bromocriptine levels → ↑ pharmacologic and toxic effects
Buspirone / ↑ Buspirone levels → ↑ pharmacologic and toxic effects
Carbamazepine / ↑ Carbamazepine effect (and toxicity requiring hospitalization and resuscitation) R/T ↓ liver breakdown

Clindamycin / Antagonism of effect if used together topically
Colchicine / Possible severe colchicine toxicity (may cause death) R/T inhibition of CYP3A4 metabolism of colchicine
Cyclosporine / ↑ Cyclosporine effect R/T ↓ excretion (possibly with renal toxicity)
Digoxin / ↑ Digoxin levels R/T effect on gut flora
Diltiazem / Possible sudden death due to cardiac causes R/T inhibition of CYP3A metabolism
Disopyramide / ↑ Disopyramide levels → arrhythmias and ↑ QTc intervals
Ergot alkaloids / Acute ergotism manifested by peripheral ischemia and dysesthesia
Felodipine / ↑ Felodipine drug levels → ↑ pharmacologic and toxic effects
Fluvoxamine (PO)/Lidocaine (IV) / Combination of the three drugs → ↓ lidocaine elimination R/T inhibition of CYP1A2 metabolism of lidocaine by fluvoxamine
Grapefruit juice / ↑ Erythromycin levels and AUC R/T ↓ metabolism in the small intestine
Grepafloxacin / ↑ Risk of life-threatening cardiac arrhythmias, including torsades de pointes
HMG-CoA reductase inhibitors / ↑ Risk of myopathy or rhabdomyolysis; also ↑ levels of atorvastatin, lovastatin, or simvastatin R/T ↓ liver breakdown
Methylprednisolone / ↑ Methylprednisolone effect R/T ↓ liver breakdown
Penicillin / Either ↓ or ↑ effect of penicillins
Pimozide / Possibility of sudden death; do not use together
Quetiapine / ↑ Quetiapine AUC, peak plasma levels, and $t\frac{1}{2}$ R/T inhibition of metabolism by CYP3A4
Rifabutin, rifampin / ↓ Erythromycin effect; ↑ risk of GI side effects
Sildenafil / ↑ AUC and peak sildenafil levels R/T inhibition of sildenafil first pass metabolism
Sodium bicarbonate / ↑ Erythromycin effect in urine R/T alkalinization

---

Bold Italic = life threatening side effect　　■ = black box warning　　✦ = Available in Canada

Sparfloxacin / ↑ Risk of life-threatening cardiac arrhythmias, including torsades de pointes

Tacrolimus / ↑ Tacrolimus levels → ↑ risk of nephrotoxicity

Theophyllines / ↑ Theophylline effects R/T ↓ liver breakdown; ↓ erythromycin levels may also occur

Verapamil / Possible sudden death due to cardiac causes R/T inhibition of CYP3A metabolism

Vinblastine / ↑ Risk of vinblastine toxicity (constipation, myalgia, neutropenia)

HOW SUPPLIED

Capsules, Delayed-Release: 250 mg; *Gel, Topical:* 2%; *Ointment, Topical:* 2%; *Ophthalmic Ointment:* 0.5%; *Pledgets, Topical:* 2%; *Solution, Topical:* 2%; *Tablets, Delayed-Release:* 250 mg, 333 mg, 500 mg; *Tablets, Film-Coated:* 250 mg, 500 mg; *Tablets, Polymer Coated Particles:* 333 mg, 500 mg.

DOSAGE

NOTE: Doses are listed as erythromycin base.

• **CAPSULES, DELAYED-RELEASE; TABLETS, DELAYED-RELEASE; TABLETS, FILM-COATED; TABLETS, POLYMER COATED PARTICLES**

Respiratory tract infections due to My-coplasma pneumoniae.

Adults: 500 mg q 6 hr for 14–21 days (for severe infections). **Children:** 20–50 mg/kg/day in 3 or 4 divided doses for 14–21 days.

Upper respiratory tract infections (mild to moderate) due to S. pyogenes or S. pneumoniae.

Adults: 250 mg q 6 hr, or 333 mg q 8 hr, or 500 mg q 12 hr for 10 days or longer, up to a maximum of 4 grams/day. **Children:** 20–50 mg/kg/day in divided doses, not to exceed the adult dose, for 10 days or longer.

URTIs due to H. influenzae.

Erythromycin ethylsuccinate, 50 mg/kg/day for children, plus sulfisoxazole, 150 mg/kg/day, given together for 10 days.

Lower UTRIs (mild to moderate) due to S. pyogenes or S. pneumoniae.

250–500 mg 4 times per day (or 20–50 mg/kg/day in divided doses) for 10 days.

Intestinal amebiasis due to Entamoeba histolytica.

Adults: 250 mg of the base (or 400 mg of ethylsuccinate) 4 times per day or 333 mg of the base q 8 hr or 500 mg q 12 hr for 10–14 days; **pediatric:** 30–50 mg/kg/day in divided doses for 10 -14 days.

Legionnaires' disease.

1–4 grams/day in divided doses for 10–14 days.

Bordetella pertussis.

500 mg 4 times per day for 10 days (or for children, 40–50 mg/kg/day in divided doses for 5–14 days).

Infections due to Corynebacterium diphtheriae.

500 mg q 6 hr for 14 days (7 days for cutaneous diphtheria and carriers).

Primary syphilis.

30–40 grams (or 48–64 grams of ethylsuccinate) in divided doses over 10–15 days.

Conjunctivitis of the newborn, pneumonia of infancy, urogenital infections during pregnancy due to Chlamydia trachomatis.

Infants: 50 mg/kg/day in four divided doses for 14 (conjunctivitis) to 21 (pneumonia) days or longer. **Adults:** 500 mg 4 times per day or 666 mg q 8 hr for urogenital infections during pregnancy. For women unable to tolerate the above regimen, give 250 mg q 6 hr or 333 mg q 8 hr, or 500 mg q 12 hr for 14 days or longer.

Mild to moderate skin and skin structure infections due to S. pyogenes or S. aureus.

250–500 mg q 6 hr (or 20–50 mg/kg/day for children, in divided doses—to a maximum of 4 grams/day) for 10 days.

Listeria monocytogenes infections.

Adults: 500 mg q 12 hr (or 250 mg q 6 hr), up to a maximum of 4 grams/day.

Pelvic inflammatory disease, acute due to N. gonorrhoeae.

Erythromycin lactobionate, 500 mg IV q 6 hr for 3 days; **then,** erythromycin base, 250 mg PO q 6 hr or 333 mg q 8 hr for 7 days.

Prevention of initial rheumatic fever attack; Prophylaxis of recurrent attacks of rheumatic fever.

Prevention of initial attack: 400 mg q 6 hr for 10 days. Prevention of recurrent attacks: 250 mg twice a day of the base or 400 mg of ethylsuccinate given continuously.

Bacterial endocarditis due to alpha-hemolytic streptococcus.

Adults: 1 gram 1–2 hr prior to the procedure; **then,** 500 mg 6 hr after the initial dose. **Pediatric,** 20 mg/kg 2 hr prior to the procedure; **then,** 10 mg/kg 6 hr after the initial dose.

Uncomplicated urethral, endocervical, or rectal infections due to C. trachomatis.

500 mg 4 times per day for 7 days (or 250 mg 4 times per day for 14 days).

Nongonococcal urethritis due to Ureaplasma urealyticum.

Adults: 500 mg 4 times per day, or 666 mg q 8 hr, or 800 mg (as ethylsuccinate) 4 times per day for 7 days or longer. **Children, 45 kg or less:** 50 mg/kg/day in 4 divided doses for 14 days.

Erythrasma due to Corynebacterium minutissimum.

250 mg q 6 hr for 14 days.

• **OPHTHALMIC OINTMENT (0.5%)**
Ophthalmic infections.

Approximately 1 cm of ointment applied directly to the eye(s) up to 6 times/day, depending on the severity of the infection.

Prophylaxis of neonatal gonococcal or chlamydial conjunctivitis.

Approximately 1 cm of ointment instilled into each lower conjunctival sac. Do not flush the ointment from the eye after instillation.

• **TOPICAL GEL (2%); TOPICAL OINTMENT (2%); TOPICAL PLEDGETS (2%); TOPICAL SOLUTION (2%)**
Acne vulgaris.

Clean the affected area thoroughly and pat dry. **Gel:** Apply sparingly and lightly as a thin film to affected area(s) once or twice a day. If there is no improvement after 6–8 weeks, or if the condition gets worse, discontinue treatment. **Ointment:** Apply to affected area in the morning and evening. **Pledgets:** Rub the pad over the affected area(s) twice a day. Use each pledget once and discard. **Solution:** Apply to the affected area(s) in the morning and evening. Use enough solution to thoroughly wet the affected area(s).

• **INVESTIGATIONAL USES**
Diarrhea due to Campylobacter enteritis or enterocolitis. Chancroid due to Haemophilus ducreyi.

500 mg 4 times per day for 7 days.

Genital, inguinal, or anorectal infections due to Lymphogranuloma venereum. Early syphilis due to Treponema pallidum.

500 mg 4 times per day for 14 days.

Tetanus due to Clostridium tetani.

500 mg q 6 hr for 10 days.

Granuloma inguinale due to Calymmatobacterium granulomatis.

500 mg PO 4 times per day for 21 or more days.

NURSING CONSIDERATIONS

�911 Do not confuse Eryc with Ery-Tab, both of which are trade names for erythromycin base.

ADMINISTRATION/STORAGE

Prepare topical gel by adding 3 mL of ethyl alcohol to the vial and immediately shaking to dissolve erythromycin. This solution is added to the gel and stirred until it appears homogenous (1–1.5 min). Refrigerate gel.

ASSESSMENT

1. List type, onset, characteristics of S&S, other agents used, outcome.
2. Note allergy to any antibiotics; assess for sensitivity reactions.
3. Obtain cultures, LFTs, CBC, wound documentation, appropriate diagnostic studies.
4. Avoid if also prescribed digoxin and theophyllines; erythromycins can inhibit cytochrome P-450 and enhance effects of these drugs or cause lethal arrhythmias. Assess for hepatotoxicity and ototoxicity.

CLIENT/FAMILY TEACHING

1. Take on an empty stomach; delayed-release forms of base can be taken without regard for meals. Do not administer with or immediately prior to ingestion of fruit juice or other acidic

drinks; acidity may decrease drug activity. Consume up to 8 oz of water with each dose and ensure a fluid intake of 2.5 L/day.

2. May take with food to diminish GI upset; food decreases absorption of most erythromycins. Take as directed and complete entire prescription despite feeling better.

3. If tablets are not coated, take 2 hr after meals. Stomach acid destroys erythromycin base; must be administered with enteric coating.

4. Evenly space doses over 24 hr. Report any unusual/intolerable side effects or lack of response.

5. If nausea intolerable, report so prescription can be changed to coated tablets; can be taken with meals.

6. Report symptoms of superinfection, i.e., furry tongue, vaginal itching, rectal itching, or diarrhea. Also rash, yellow discoloration of skin or eyes, or irritation of the mouth or tongue should be reported.

7. Drug may increase GI motility with diabetic gastric paresis.

8. With topical use, clean affected area before applying ointment; wash hands before and after therapy. If no improvement in 6–8 weeks or if condition worsens, consult provider.

9. A sterile bandage may be used with the topical ointment. Drying and peeling following topical use may be controlled by reducing the frequency of applications.

10. Report any hearing loss; usually temporary.

11. Do not wash ophthalmic ointment from the eyes. Topical and ophthalmic products are for external use only.

12. Keep all F/U appointments to evaluate response to therapy.

OUTCOMES/EVALUATE

- Resolution of infection (negative culture reports, ↓ temperature, ↑ wound healing, ↓ WBCs)
- Desired infection prophylaxis

Erythromycin estolate ■

CLASSIFICATION(S):
Antibiotic, macrolide
PREGNANCY CATEGORY: B

SEE ALSO *ERYTHROMYCIN BASE.*

USES
See *Erythromycin Base.*

ACTION/KINETICS

Pharmacokinetics
Most active form of erythromycin, with relatively long-lasting activity.

ADDITIONAL CONTRAINDICATIONS
Cholestatic jaundice or preexisting liver dysfunction. Treatment of chronic disorders such as acne, furunculosis, or prophylaxis of rheumatic fever.

SPECIAL CONCERNS

■ Hepatic dysfunction, with or without jaundice, has occurred, mainly in adults. It may be accompanied by malaise, N&V, abdominal colic, and fever. In some cases, severe abdominal pain may stimulate an abdominal surgical emergency. If any of the above occurs, discontinue erythromycin estolate oral suspension promptly. Erythromycin estolate oral suspension is contraindicated for clients with a known history of sensitivity to the drug and for those with pre-existing liver disease.■

HOW SUPPLIED
Suspension: 125 mg (as the base)/5 mL, 250 mg (as the base)/5 mL.

DOSAGE

- **SUSPENSION**

  See *Erythromycin base.* Similar blood levels are achieved using erythromycin base, estolate, or stearate.

NURSING CONSIDERATIONS

ASSESSMENT

1. Note reasons for therapy, onset, symptom characteristics.

2. Assess clinical presentation, C&S results, CBC and LFTs. Drug may cause significant hepatoxicity; monitor LFTs.

CLIENT/FAMILY TEACHING

1. Take without regard to meals. Chew or crush chewable tablets.

2. Shake suspension well before using; do not store for more than 2 weeks at room temperature.

3. Report lack of response, adverse drug effects; esp. change in skin/eye color, abdominal pain, stool color change, N&V, and fever.

4. Keep all F/U appointments to evaluate response to therapy.

OUTCOMES/EVALUATE
Resolution of infection

Erythromycin ethylsuccinate

CLASSIFICATION(S):
Antibiotic, macrolide
PREGNANCY CATEGORY: B
Rx: E.E.S. 200 and 400, E.E.S. Granules, EryPed 200, EryPed 400, EryPed Drops.
♣Rx: Apo-Erythro-ES, EES 600.

SEE ALSO ERYTHROMYCIN BASE.
USES
See *Erythromycin Base.*
ADDITIONAL CONTRAINDICATIONS
Preexisting liver disease.
HOW SUPPLIED
Powder for Oral Suspension: 200 mg (of the base)/5 mL (when reconstituted), 400 mg (of the base)/5 mL (when reconstituted); *Suspension:* 100 mg (as the base)/2.5 mL, 200 mg (as the base)/5 mL, 400 mg (as the base)/5 mL; *Tablets:* 400 mg.
DOSAGE
• **ORAL SUSPENSION; TABLETS**
See Erythromycin base. NOTE: 400 mg of erythromycin ethylsuccinate will achieve the same blood levels of erythromycin as 250 mg of the base, estolate, or stearate forms.
Hemophilus influenzae infections.
Erythromycin ethylsuccinate, 50 mg/kg/day with sulfisoxazole, 150 mg/kg/day, both for a total of 10 days.

NURSING CONSIDERATIONS
ASSESSMENT
List reasons for therapy, onset/characteristics of S&S, culture results. Monitor CBC, renal and LFTs.

CLIENT/FAMILY TEACHING
1. Take without regard to meals. Complete entire prescription.
2. May chew or crush chewable tablets.
3. Refrigerate oral suspension; store for 1 week maximum.
4. Report lack of response or adverse drug effects. Keep all F/U appointments to evaluate response to therapy.

OUTCOMES/EVALUATE
Resolution of infection

Erythromycin lactobionate   IV

CLASSIFICATION(S):
Antibiotic, macrolide
PREGNANCY CATEGORY: B

SEE ALSO ERYTHROMYCIN BASE.
USES
See *Erythromycin Base.*
ADDITIONAL DRUG INTERACTIONS
Do not add drugs to IV solutions of erythromycin lactobionate.
HOW SUPPLIED
Powder for Injection, Lyophilized: 500 mg, 1 gram.
DOSAGE
• **IV**
Severe infections.
Adults and children: 15–20 mg/kg/day up to 4 grams/day in severe infections.
Acute pelvic inflammatory disease caused by gonorrhea.
500 mg q 6 hr for 3 days followed by 250 mg erythromycin stearate, **PO,** q 6 hr for 7 days.
Legionnaire's disease.
1–4 grams/day in divided doses. Change to PO therapy as soon as possible.

NURSING CONSIDERATIONS
ADMINISTRATION/STORAGE
IV 1. Sterile water for injection is preferred diluent. D5W or D5/RL may also be used if buffered with 4% NaHCO₃ injection.
2. For intermittent IV administration: Further dilute in 100 to 250 mL of D5W or NSS and infused over 20–60 min.

Bold Italic = life threatening side effect   ■ = black box warning   ♣ = Available in Canada

3. The initial reconstituted solution is stable for 2 weeks refrigerated or for 24 hr at room temperature if final diluted solution is used within 8 hr. Use the reconstituted piggyback vial within 24 hr if refrigerated or 8 hr if stored at room temperature.

4. If reconstituted solution is frozen, may be stored for 30 days. Once thawed, use within 8 hr. Do not refreeze thawed solutions.

ASSESSMENT

1. Note reasons for therapy, onset, characteristics of S&S. Obtain CBC, cultures.

2. Assess for hearing deficits. Monitor renal and LFTs.

CLIENT/FAMILY TEACHING

Drug is administered by injection. Report any rash, fever, nausea, abdominal pain, or lack of response.

OUTCOMES/EVALUATE

Resolution of infection; negative C&S

Erythromycin stearate

CLASSIFICATION(S):
Antibiotic, macrolide
PREGNANCY CATEGORY: B
Rx: Erythrocin Stearate.
✦Rx: Apo-Erythro-S, Nu-Erythromycin-S.

SEE ALSO *ERYTHROMYCIN BASE.*

USES
See *Erythromycin Base.*

ADDITIONAL SIDE EFFECTS
Causes more allergic reactions (e.g., skin rash and urticaria) than other erythromycins.

HOW SUPPLIED
Tablets, Film-Coated: 250 mg, 500 mg.

DOSAGE

- **TABLETS, FILM-COATED**
  See Erythromycin base. Similar blood levels are achieved using erythromycin base, estolate, or stearate forms.

NURSING CONSIDERATIONS

ASSESSMENT
List reasons for therapy, characteristics of S&S, culture results, CBC, renal and LFTs.

CLIENT/FAMILY TEACHING

1. Take on an empty stomach; food decreases absorption.

2. Report lack of effect or evidence of allergic reaction, i.e., rash or itching. Keep all F/U appointments to evaluate response to therapy.

OUTCOMES/EVALUATE
Resolution of infection

Escitalopram oxalate
(eh-sye-**TAL**-oh-pram)

CLASSIFICATION(S):
Antidepressant, selective serotonin reuptake inhibitor
PREGNANCY CATEGORY: C
Rx: Lexapro.

SEE ALSO *SELECTIVE SEROTONIN REUPTAKE INHIBITORS.*

USES
(1) Major depressive disorder, including maintenance, as defined in the DSM-IV-TR category. (2) Generalized anxiety disorder. *Investigational:* Panic disorder.

ACTION/KINETICS

Action
Inhibits CNS neuronal reuptake of serotonin. Minimal effects on norepinephrine and dopamine reuptake.

Pharmacokinetics
80% is bioavailable. **Peak plasma levels:** About 5 hr. Absorption is not affected by food. **Steady state:** About 1 week following once-daily dosing. Metabolized in the liver by the CYP3A4 and CYP2C19 isoenzymes. **$t^{1}/_{2}$, terminal:** 27–32 hr. About 7% excreted in the urine. **Plasma protein binding:** About 56%.

CONTRAINDICATIONS
Clients taking monoamine oxidase inhibitors or citalopram (Celexa). Hyper-

sensitivity to the drug or any component of the product. Alcohol use.

SPECIAL CONCERNS

■ Antidepressants increased the risk of suicidal thinking and behavior (suicidality) in short-term studies in children and adolescents with major depressive disorder and other psychiatric disorders. Anyone considering the use of citalopram or any other antidepressant in a child or adolescent must balance this risk with the clinical need. Closely observe clients who are started on therapy for clinical worsening, suicidality, or unusual changes in behavior. Advise families and caregivers of the need for close observation and communication with the health care provider. Citalopram is not approved for use in pediatric clients. The average risk of adverse reactions representing suicidal thinking or behavior (suicidality) during the first few months of treatment in those receiving antidepressants was 4%, twice the placebo risk of 2%. No suicides occurred in these trials.■ To prevent serious reactions, do not use escitalopram in combination with a MAOI, within 14 days of discontinuing treatment with a MAOI, or within 14 days after discontinuing escitalopram before starting a MAOI. There is some risk of developing a serotonin syndrome. Use with caution in seizure disorders, in clients with diseases or conditions that produce altered metabolism or hemodynamic responses, in impaired hepatic function, severe renal impairment, and in those taking CNS drugs. Use with caution during lactation. There is a risk of clinical worsening and suicidal ideation and behavior, especially at the beginning of drug therapy and during dosage adjustments. Safety and efficacy have not been determined in children. There may be a need for prolonged hospitalization, respiratory support, and tube feeding in neonates exposed to escitalopram late in the third trimester.

SIDE EFFECTS

Most Common

Nausea, dry mouth, increased sweating, dizziness, diarrhea, flu-like symptoms, fatigue, insomnia, somnolence, rhinitis, ejaculation disorder.

CNS: Insomnia, somnolence, dizziness, decreased appetite, activation of mania/hypomania, *suicide attempts*, paresthesia, light-headedness, migraine, tremor, vertigo, abnormal dreaming, yawning, irritability, impaired concentration, seizures. **GI:** N&V, dry mouth, diarrhea, constipation, indigestion, abdominal pain, flatulence, heartburn, toothache, gastroenteritis, abdominal cramps, gastroesophageal reflux. **CV:** Palpitation, hypertension. **GU:** Ejaculatory delay, decreased libido, impotence, anorgasmia (females), menstrual cramps, UTI, urinary frequency. **Respiratory:** Rhinitis, sinusitis, bronchitis, sinus headache/congestion, coughing, nasal congestion. **Musculoskeletal:** Arthralgia, neck/shoulder pain, muscle cramps, myalgia. **Dermatologic:** Increased sweating. **Body as a whole:** Fatigue, flu-like symptoms, allergy, hot flushes, fever, increased/decreased weight, lethargy. **Miscellaneous:** Pain in limb, chest pain, blurred vision, earache, tinnitus.

DRUG INTERACTIONS

Cimetidine / ↑ Escitalopram AUC and $t\frac{1}{2}$ R/T possible inhibition of metabolism

MAO inhibitors / Serious (may be fatal) reactions, including hyperthermia, rigidity, myoclonus, autonomic instability, mental status changes (extreme agitation, delirium, coma)

Metoprolol / ↑ Metoprolol C_{max} and AUC

Omeprazole / ↑ Escitalopram AUC and $t\frac{1}{2}$ R/T possible inhibition of metabolism

Sumatriptan / Potential for weakness, hyperreflexia, incoordination

HOW SUPPLIED

Oral Solution: 5 mg (as base)/5 mL; *Tablets:* 5 mg (as base), 10 mg (as base), 20 mg (as base).

DOSAGE

- **ORAL SOLUTION; TABLETS**
  Major depressive illness.
Initial: 10 mg once daily, including the elderly or those with hepatic impairment. Increase dose to 20 mg, if neces-

---

Bold Italic = life threatening side effect   ■ = black box warning   ♣ = Available in Canada

sary, after a minimum of 1 week. **Maintenance therapy:** 10 or 20 mg/day for up to 36 weeks after an initial 8 weeks of treatment.

Generalized anxiety disorder.

Initial: 10 mg once daily. Dose may be increased to 20 mg once daily after a minimum of one week. Efficacy after eight weeks of treatment has not been determined.

NURSING CONSIDERATIONS
ADMINISTRATION/STORAGE
1. Give once daily in the morning or evening with or without food.
2. Discontinuing escitalopram may cause symptoms, including dysphoric mood, irritability, agitation, dizziness, sensory disturbances, anxiety, confusion, headache, lethargy, emotional lability, hypomania, or insomnia. A gradual reduction in dose, rather than abrupt cessation, is recommended whenever possible.
3. Store from 15–30°C (59–86°F).

ASSESSMENT
1. Note reasons for therapy, onset/characteristics of symptoms, clinical presentation. List other agents trialed, outcome.
2. Note other drugs prescribed; ensure none interact. Avoid use within 14 days before/after MAOI use.
3. Determine liver, renal dysfunction or seizure disorder. Review history for metabolic disorders; diseases that preclude therapy.
4. Monitor EKG, electrolytes, renal, and LFTs.

CLIENT/FAMILY TEACHING
1. Take as directed, once daily, with or without food.
2. Drug is an isomer of Celexa and should not be taken with Celexa.
3. Use caution operating machines or cars until drug effects known. May experience insomnia, fatigue, nausea, sweating and ejaculation disorders.
4. Avoid alcohol, OTC agents, or CNS depressants.
5. Use reliable birth control; report if pregnancy suspected.
6. May see improvement in 1 to 4 weeks; continue as prescribed.
7. Report lack of response or adverse side effects. Keep F/U appointments.

OUTCOMES/EVALUATE
Relief/control of depression/anxiety

Esmolol hydrochloride [IV]
(**EZ**-moh-lohl)

E

CLASSIFICATION(S):
Beta-adrenergic blocking agent
PREGNANCY CATEGORY: C
Rx: Brevibloc, Brevibloc Double Strength.

SEE ALSO *BETA-ADRENERGIC BLOCKING AGENTS.*

USES
(1) Supraventricular tachycardia in those with atrial fibrillation or atrial flutter in perioperative, postoperative, or other emergent situations when short-term control is needed. (2) Noncompensatory sinus tachycardia when rapid heart rate requires intervention. (3) Tachycardia and hypertension during induction and tracheal intubation, during surgery, on emergence from anesthesia, and postoperatively.

ACTION/KINETICS
Action
Preferentially inhibits beta-1 receptors. Has no membrane-stabilizing or intrinsic sympathomimetic activity. Decreases HR and AV nodal conduction velocity and increases AV refractory period.

Pharmacokinetics
Rapid onset (<5 min) and a short duration of action. Low lipid solubility. $t\frac{1}{2}$: 9 min. Rapidly metabolized by esterases in RBCs.

SPECIAL CONCERNS
Dosage has not been established in children.

SIDE EFFECTS
Most Common
N&V, dizziness, sweating, pain/redness at injection site, headache, confusion, fatigue, hypotension, somnolence, local thrombophlebitis, rash, itchy skin.

See *Beta-Adrenergic Blocking Agents* for a complete list of possible side effects. **Dermatologic:** Inflammation at site of infusion, flushing, pallor, induration, erythema, burning, skin discoloration, edema. **Miscellaneous:** Urinary retention, midscapular pain, asthenia, changes in taste.

ADDITIONAL DRUG INTERACTIONS

Digoxin / ↑ Digoxin levels
Morphine / ↑ Esmolol levels

HOW SUPPLIED

Injection: 10 mg/mL, 20 mg/mL, 250 mg/mL.

DOSAGE

- **IV INFUSION**
  SVT.

Initial: 500 mcg/kg/min for 1 min; **then,** 50 mcg/kg/min for 4 min. If after 5 min an adequate effect is not achieved, repeat the loading dose followed by a maintenance infusion of 100 mcg/kg/min for 4 min. This procedure may be repeated, increasing the maintenance infusion by 50 mcg/kg/min increments (for 4 min) until the desired HR or lowered BP is approached. **Then,** omit the loading infusion and reduce incremental infusion rate from 50 to 25 mcg/kg/min or less. The interval between titrations may be increased from 5 to 10 min.

Once the HR has been controlled, the client may be transferred to another antiarrhythmic agent. Reduce the infusion rate of esmolol by 50% 30 min after the first dose of the alternative antiarrhythmic agent. If satisfactory control is observed for 1 hr after the second dose of the alternative agent, the esmolol infusion may be stopped.

Intraoperative and postoperative tachycardia and hypertension.

Immediate control: 80 mg (about 1 mg/kg) bolus dose over 30 sec followed by 150 mcg/kg/min for 1 min followed by a 4-min maintenance infusion of 50 mcg/kg/min. If an adequate effect is not seen in 5 min, repeat the same loading dose and follow with a maintenance infusion of 100 mcg/kg/min. **Gradual control:** Dosing schedule is the same as for supraventricular tachycardia (SVT).

NURSING CONSIDERATIONS

ADMINISTRATION/STORAGE

IV 1. Infusions may be necessary for 24–48 hr.
2. Not for direct IV push administration.
3. Do not dilute concentrate with sodium bicarbonate.
4. To minimize irritation and thrombophlebitis, do not infuse concentrations greater than 10 mg/mL.
5. Diluted esmolol (concentration of 10 mg/mL) is compatible with D5W, D5W/RL, D5W/Ringer's injection, D5W/0.9% NaCl, D5W/0.45% NaCl, 0.45% NaCl, RL, KCl (40 mEq/L) in D5W, and 0.9% NaCl.

ASSESSMENT

1. Note reasons for therapy, type, onset, characteristics of S&S.
2. List CP assessments, ECG, VS. Assess for hypotension, bradycardia.
3. Administer in a monitored environment; wean using guidelines.

CLIENT/FAMILY TEACHING

Drug is administered IV to control cardiac arrhythmias.

OUTCOMES/EVALUATE

- Suppression of SVT
- Restoration of stable rhythm

Esomeprazole Magnesium **IV** 📷
(**es**-oh-**MEP**-rah-zole)

CLASSIFICATION(S):

Proton pump inhibitor
PREGNANCY CATEGORY: B
Rx: Nexium.

USES

PO only: (1) Short-term treatment (4–8 weeks) in the healing and symptomatic resolution of diagnostically confirmed erosive esophagitis. An additional 4- to 8-week course may be instituted for those who have not healed. (2) To maintain symptom resolution and healing of erosive esophagitis. (3) Treatment of heartburn and other symptoms associated with GERD in adults. (4) Reduce occurrence of gastric ulcers associated with continuous NSAID therapy

---

Bold Italic = life threatening side effect   ■ = black box warning   ♣ = Available in Canada

in those at risk for developing gastric ulcers (those 60 years and older and/or documented history of gastric ulcers). (5) In combination with amoxicillin and clarithromycin to treat and eradicate *H. pylori* infection and duodenal ulcer disease (active or history in the past 5 years). (6) Long-term treatment of pathological hypersecretory conditions, including Zollinger-Ellison syndrome. *Investigational:* Non–GERD dyspepsia, Barrett esophagus, stress ulcer prophylaxis.

IV only: Short-term treatment (up to 10 days) of GERD clients with a history of erosive esophagitis as an alternative to PO therapy when therapy with capsules is not possible or appropriate. *Investigational:* Stress ulcer prophylaxis.

ACTION/KINETICS
Action
Suppresses the final step in gastric acid production by inhibiting the H^+/K^+-ATPase in the gastric parietal cells. This decreases gastric acid secretion.

Pharmacokinetics
About 90% bioavailable after multiple doses. **Peak plasma levels:** 1.5 hr. Absorption is decreased by food. Extensively metabolized in the liver by the cytochrome P450 enzyme system. **$t\frac{1}{2}$, elimination:** 1–1.5 hr. About 80% excreted as inactive metabolites in the urine with 20% excreted in the feces. **Plasma protein binding:** 97%.

CONTRAINDICATIONS
Known hypersensitivity to any component of the formulation or to any macrolide antibiotic. Lactation.

SPECIAL CONCERNS
Symptomatic response does not preclude the presence of gastric malignancy. Safety and efficacy have not been determined in children.

SIDE EFFECTS
Most Common
Headache, diarrhea, nausea, stomach pain, constipation, dry mouth.
GI: Diarrhea, nausea, flatulence, abdominal/stomach/epigastric pain, constipation, dry mouth, bowel irregularity, dyspepsia, dysphagia, GI dysplasia, eructation, esophageal disorder, frequent stools, gastroenteritis, *GI hemorrhage*, hiccough, melena, mouth/pharynx/rec-

tal/tongue disorder, tongue edema, ulcerative stomatitis, vomiting. **CNS:** Headache, anorexia, apathy, increased appetite, confusion, aggravated depression, dizziness, hypertonia, nervousness, hypoesthesia, impotence, insomnia, migraine, paresthesia, sleep disorder, somnolence, tremor, vertigo. **CV:** Hypertension, tachycardia. **Hematologic:** Anemia, hypochromic anemia, cervical lymphoadenopathy, leukocytosis, leukopenia, thrombocytopenia. **Respiratory:** Aggravated asthma, cough, dyspnea, epistaxis, *laryngeal edema*, pharyngitis, rhinitis, sinusitis. **Dermatologic:** Acne, *angioedema*, dermatitis, flushing, pruritus, pruritus ani, rash, erythematous/maculopapular rash, skin inflammation, increased sweating, urticaria. **Otic:** Earache, tinnitus, otitis media. **Ophthalmic:** Conjunctivitis, abnormal vision, visual field defect. **Musculoskeletal :** Arthralgia, aggravated arthritis, arthropathy, cramps, fibromyalgia syndrome, hernia, polymyalgia rheumatica. **GU:** Dysmenorrhea, menstrual disorder, vaginitis, abnormal urine, cystitis, dysuria, fungal infection, hematuria, frequent micturition, moniliasis, genital moniliasis, polyuria. **Body as a whole:** Enlarged abdomen, *allergic reaction*, *anaphylaxis*, asthenia, back/chest/substernal chest pain, facial/peripheral/leg edema, hot flushes, fatigue, fever, flu-like symptoms, generalized edema, malaise, pain, rigors. **Miscellaneous:** Goiter, abnormal hepatic function, thirst, increased/decreased weight, vitamin B_{12} deficiency, parosmia, taste loss/perversion.

LABORATORY TEST CONSIDERATIONS
↑ AST, ALT, GGT, alkaline phosphatase, bilirubin, serum creatinine, serum gastrin, uric acid, TSH, hemoglobin, platelets, WBC count, potassium, sodium, thyroxine. Glycosuria, hyponatremia, hypoglycemia. Bilirubinemia, hyperuricemia, albuminuria.

DRUG INTERACTIONS
Esomeprazole may interfere with the absorption of drugs where gastric pH is an important factor in bioavailability (e.g., digoxin, iron salts, ketoconazole).

E

HOW SUPPLIED

Capsules, Delayed-Release: 20 mg (as base), 40 mg (as base); *Powder for Injection, Freeze-Dried:* 20 mg, 40 mg; *Powder for Suspension, Delayed-Release:* 20 mg, 40 mg.

DOSAGE

- **CAPSULES, DELAYED-RELEASE; SUSPENSION, DELAYED-RELEASE**

Healing of erosive esophagitis.

20 or 40 mg once daily for 4–8 weeks. For those who do not heal within 4–8 weeks, consider an additional 4–8 weeks of therapy.

Maintenance of healing of erosive esophagitis.

20 mg once daily, for up to 6 months.

Symptomatic GERD.

20 mg once daily for 4 weeks. If symptoms do not resolve completely, consider an additional 4 weeks of therapy.

Eradication of H. pylori to reduce risk of duodenal ulcer recurrence.

Use the following triple therapy. Esomeprazole, 40 mg once daily for 10 days; amoxicillin, 1,000 mg twice a day for 10 days; and, clarithromycin, 500 mg twice a day for 10 days.

Reduce risk of NSAID-associated gastric ulcers.

20 or 40 mg once daily for up to 6 months.

Short-term treatment of GERD in children, 12–17 years of age.

20 or 40 mg once daily for up to 8 weeks.

Pathological hypersecretory conditions, including Zollinger-Ellison syndrome.

40 mg twice daily; adjust dose to needs of client.

- **IV**

GERD with history of erosive esophagitis.

20 or 40 mg given once daily by IV injection (no less than 3 minutes) or by IV infusion over 10–30 minutes.

NURSING CONSIDERATIONS

ADMINISTRATION/STORAGE

1. Do not exceed a dose of 20 mg daily in clients with severe hepatic dysfunction.

2. For clients unable to swallow capsules, add one tablespoon of applesauce to an empty bowl. Carefully empty the pellets from the capsule onto the applesauce. Mix the pellets with the applesauce and swallow immediately. Do not use hot applesauce and do not chew or crush the pellets. Do not store the pellet/applesauce mixture for future use.

3. For clients with a nasogastric tube in place, open the capsules and empty the intact granules into a 60 mL syringe. Mix with 50 mL of water. Replace the plunger and shake the syringe vigorously for 15 seconds. Hold the syringe with the tip up and check for granules remaining in the tip. Attach the syringe to the NG tube and deliver the contents through the NG tube into the stomach. Flush the NG tube with additional water.

4. Store between 15–30°C (59–86°F) with container tightly closed.

IV 5. Discontinue treatment as soon as the client is able to resume treatment with the delayed-release capsule.

6. Safety and efficacy of esomeprazole IV for use for more than 10 days in GERD clients with a history of erosive esophagitis has not been demonstrated.

7. In clients with severe impaired liver function (Child-Pugh class C), do not exceed a dose of 20 mg.

8. Reconstitute with 5 mL of 0.9% NaCl injection. Withdraw 5 mL of the reconstituted solution and give IV over no less than 3 minutes.

9. For use by IV infusion over 10–30 minutes, reconstitute the contents of 1 vial with 5 mL of 0.9% NaCl, lactated Ringer's injection, or D5W; further dilute to a final volume of 50 mL. Give the final diluted solution as an IV infusion over 10–30 min.

10. Store the admixture at room temperature up to 30°C (86°F) and give as follows: Give within 12 hr if diluted with 0.9% NaCl or lactated Ringer's injection and within 6 hr if diluted with D5W.

11. Do not give esomeprazole IV with any other medication through the same IV site and/or tubing. Always flush the

---

Bold Italic = life threatening side effect   ■ = black box warning   ✦ = Available in Canada

IV line with the diluent both prior to and after administration of the drug.

ASSESSMENT

1. List reasons for therapy, type, onset, and characteristics of symptoms. List other agents prescribed; ensure no interaction.

2. Determine if pregnant.

3. Record abdominal assessments, radiographic/endoscopic and *H. pylori* findings.

4. Monitor CBC and LFTs; note any liver dysfunction.

CLIENT/FAMILY TEACHING

1. Take the delayed-release capsules whole at least 1 hr before meals. If unable to swallow whole may empty capsule onto one tablespoon of applesauce in a cup. Mix pellets into applesauce and swallow immediately, taking care not to chew pellets. The capsule may also be opened and the intact granules emptied into a syringe and delivered through a nasogastric tube.

2. Mix the contents of the packet of delayed-release powder for suspension with 15 mL of water; leave 2–3 min to thicken; stir and drink within 30 min. The suspension may also be administered via a nasogastric or gastric tube. To do so, add 15 mL water to a syringe and add contents of the packet. Shake the syringe; leave 2–3 min to thicken. Shake the syringe and inject through the nasogastric or gastric tube within 30 min.

3. May take antacids.

4. Avoid alcohol and OTC products unless approved.

5. Drug is for short-term use only; it inhibits gastric acid secretion. Side effects of prolonged therapy and suppression of acid secretion alter bacterial colonization and lead to hypochlorhydria and hypergastrinemia, which may lead to an increased risk for gastric tumors.

OUTCOMES/EVALUATE

- Promotion of ulcer healing; relief of pain; ↓ gastric acid production.
- Eradication of *H. pylori* with designated ATXs.

Esterified estrogens ■
(es-**TER**-ih-fyd **ES**-troh-jens)

CLASSIFICATION(S):
Estrogen, natural
PREGNANCY CATEGORY: X
Rx: Menest.

E

SEE ALSO *ESTROGENS.*

USES

(1) Moderate to severe vasomotor symptoms associated with menopause. (2) Atrophic vaginitis and kraurosis vulvae due to menopause. (3) Female hypogonadism. (4) Female castration and primary ovarian failure. (5) Inoperable, progressing breast cancer (palliation only) in selected women and men with metastatic disease. (6) Inoperable, progressing, prostate cancer (palliation only).

ACTION/KINETICS

Pharmacokinetics

This product is a mixture of sodium salts of sulfate esters of natural estrogenic substances: 75–85% estrone sodium sulfate and 6–15% equilin sulfate in such proportion that the total of the components is not less than 90% of the total esterified estrogens content. Less potent than estrone.

ADDITIONAL CONTRAINDICATIONS

Pregnancy as use may cause severe harm to the fetus.

SPECIAL CONCERNS

■ See Estrogens in Chapter 2 for Black Box Warnings.■

SIDE EFFECTS

Most Common

N&V, breakthrough bleeding/spotting, loss of menses or excessively long menses, breast pain, breast enlargement, edema, increased/decreased libido.

See *Estrogens* for a complete list of possible side effects.

HOW SUPPLIED

Tablets: 0.3 mg, 0.625 mg, 1.25 mg, 2.5 mg.

DOSAGE
- **TABLETS**

E

Moderate to severe vasomotor symptoms.

1.25 mg/day given cyclically (3 weeks on and then 1 week off).

Atrophic vaginitis, kraurosis vulvae.

0.3–1.25 mg or more daily depending on the individual tissue response. Short-term use only. Give cyclically. Re-evaluate at 3- to 6- month intervals for tapering or terminating therapy.

Female hypogonadism.

2.5–7.5 mg daily in divided doses for 20 days followed by a 10-day rest period. If bleeding does not occur by the end of this period, repeat the same dosage schedule. The number of courses of therapy to produce bleeding depends on the endometrial responsiveness. If bleeding occurs before the end of the 10-day period, begin with an estrogen-progestin cyclic regimen of 2.5–7.5 mg daily of estrogen in divided doses for 20 days. During the last 5 days of estrogen therapy give a PO progestin. If bleeding occurs before the end of this regimen, discontinue therapy and resume on the 5th day of bleeding.

Female castration, primary ovarian failure.

1.25 mg/day; give cyclically. Adjust dose up or down according to severity of symptoms and client response. For maintenance, adjust dose to lowest level that will provide effective control.

Prostatic cancer, inoperable, progressing.

1.25–2.5 mg 3 times per day given chronically. Judge effectiveness of therapy by symptomatic improvement and phosphatase determinations.

Breast cancer, inoperable, progressing in selected men and women.

10 mg 3 times per day for at least 3 months.

NURSING CONSIDERATIONS

ADMINISTRATION/STORAGE

1. When used for moderate to severe vasomotor symptoms: If client has not menstruated within the last 2 months or more, cyclic administration is started arbitrarily. If the client is menstruating, start cyclic use on day 5 of bleeding. For short-term use only. Use the lowest dose to control symptoms and discontinue as soon as possible. Re-evaluate at 3–6 month intervals for tapering or discontinuation of therapy.

2. When used for atrophic vaginitis, kraurosis vulvae: For short-term use only. Discontinue as soon as possible. Re-evaluate at 3–6 month intervals for tapering or stopping therapy.

3. When estrogen is used for a post-menopausal woman with an intact uterus, monitor closely for signs of endometrial cancer; undertake appropriate diagnostic measures to rule out malignancy in the event of persistent or recurring abnormal vaginal bleeding.

ASSESSMENT

1. Note reasons for therapy, type, onset, characteristics of S&S.

2. Review associated hazards of prolonged therapy.

CLIENT/FAMILY TEACHING

1. May take oral tablets at bedtime or mealtime to minimize GI upset or nausea.

2. Report abdominal pain, severe headaches, SOB, chest pain, visual changes, vaginal bleeding /discharge, breast lumps, yellow skin or eyes, dark urine, light-colored stools or swelling of hands and feet.

3. Stop therapy 1 month before planned procedure that may result in prolonged imbolization to reduce risk of blood clot formation.

4. Keep all F/U appointments and yearly exams. Will need lipid and liver panel, BP, and body weight monitored; perform BSE regularly. Report unusual side effects or lack of desired response.

5. Smoking significantly increases risk of blood clots; so stop.

OUTCOMES/EVALUATE

- Stimulation of menses
- Relief of postmenopausal S&S
- Suppression of tumor growth/spread

Estradiol gel ■

(ess-trah-**DYE**-ohl)

CLASSIFICATION(S):
Estrogen, semisynthetic
PREGNANCY CATEGORY: X
Rx: Divigel, Elestrin, Estrogel.

SEE ALSO *ESTROGENS.*

USES

(1) Moderate to severe vasomotor symptoms associated with menopause. (2) Moderate to severe symptoms of vulvar and vaginal atrophy associated with menopause (Estrogel only).

SPECIAL CONCERNS

■ (1) Endometrial cancer. Close clinical surveillance of all women taking estrogen is important. Adequate diagnostic measures, including endometrial sampling when indicated, should be undertaken to rule out malignancy in all cases of undiagnosed persistent or recurring abnormal vaginal bleeding. There is no evidence that the use of 'natural' estrogens results in a different endometrial risk profile than synthetic estrogens at equivalent estrogenic doses. (2) CV and other risks. Estrogens with or without progestins should not be used for the prevention of CV disease or dementia. The Women's Health Initiative (WHI) estrogen alone substudy reported increased risk of stroke and deep vein thrombosis (DVT) in postmenopausal women (50 to 79 years of age) during 6.8 and 7.1 years, respectively of treatment with daily oral conjugated estrogens, 0.625 mg, relative to placebo. (3) The estrogen and progestin WHI substudy reported increased risks of MI, stroke, invasive breast cancer, pulmonary emboli, and DVT in postmenopausal women (50 to 79 years of age) during 5.6 years of treatment with daily oral conjugated estrogens, 0.625 mg, combined with medroxyprogesterone acetate, 2.5 mg relative to placebo. (4) The WHI Memory Study, a substudy of the WHI, reported an increased risk of developing probable dementia in postmenopausal women 65 years of age and older during 5.2 years of treatment with daily conjugated estrogen, 0.625 mg alone and during 4 years of treatment with daily conjugated estrogens, 0.625 mg combined with medroxyprogesterone acetate, 2.5 mg, relative to placebo. It is unknown whether this finding applies to younger postmenopausal women. (5) Other doses of conjugated estrogens and medroxyprogesterone acetate, and other combinations of estrogens and progestins, were not studied in the WHI and, in the absence of comparable data, these risks should be assumed to be similar. Because of these risks, estrogens with or without progestins should be prescibed at the lowest effective doses and for the shortest duration consistent with treatment goals and risks for the individual woman.■

SIDE EFFECTS

Most Common

Dizziness, lightheadedness, headache, N&V, GI upset, bloating, weight changes, increased/decreased libido, breast tenderness, edema, redness/irritation at application site.

See *Estrogens* for a complete list of possible side effects.

HOW SUPPLIED

Gel: **Divigel:** 0.25, 0.5, or 1 gram per single-dose foil packet. **Elestrin:** 0.52 mg/0.87 gram unit dose (0.06%). **Estrogel:** 0.75 mg/1.25 gram unit dose (0.06%).

DOSAGE————————

• **DIVIGEL**

  Moderate to severe vasomotor symptoms associated with menopause.

Initial, usual: 0.25 gram. Adjust subsequent doses based on individual client response. Doses of 0.25 gram, 0.5 gram, and 1 gram/day may be used. Periodically assess.

• **ELESTRIN**

  Moderate to severe vasomotor symptoms associated with menopause.

Apply 1 pump per day (0.87 gram/day containing 0.52 mg estradiol) to the upper arm. Adjust subsequent doses based on client response.

• **ESTROGEL**

E

E

Moderate to severe vasomotor symptoms and/or moderate to severe symptoms of vulvar and vaginal atrophy associated with menopause.
1.25 grams (containing 0.75 mg estradiol). The lowest effective dose has not been determined.

NURSING CONSIDERATIONS
ADMINISTRATION/STORAGE
Store at 20–25°C (68–77°F).
ASSESSMENT
Note reasons for therapy, age at menopause onset, other therapies trialed, GYN findings.
CLIENT/FAMILY TEACHING
1. Before using pump for the first time, it must be primed. Remove the large pump cover and fully depress pump twice. After priming, the pump is ready to use. Discard unused gel by thoroughly rinsing down the sink or placing it in the household trash in a manner that prevents accidental exposure or ingestion by household members or pets.
2. *Estrogel:*
- Estrogel pump contains enough drug to allow for initial priming of the pump twice and to deliver 64 daily doses. Discard the pump after priming twice and after 64 doses have been used.
- Apply the gel at the same time each day. Apply daily dose of gel to clean, dry, unbroken skin. Apply after bath, shower, or sauna. Be sure skin is completely dry before applying the gel.
- Leave as much time as possible between applying the gel and going swimming.
- To obtain gel from the pump, collect gel into the palm of the hand by pressing the pump firmly and fully with 1 fluid motion without hesitation.
- Apply the gel to one arm using the hand. Spread the gel as thinly as possible over the entire area on the inside and outside of the arm from wrist to shoulder to cover 750 cm^2 of skin.
- Always place the cap back on the tip of the pump and the large pump

cover over the top of the pump after each use.
- To reduce the chance that the estradiol will spread to other people, wash hands with soap and water after applying the gel.
- It is not necessary to massage or rub in the gel. Allow the gel to dry for up to 5 min before dressing.
3. *Divigel:*
- Apply once daily on the skin of either the right or left upper thigh. The application surface area should be about 5 by 7 inches (about the size of 2 palm prints).
- The entire contents of a unit dose packet should be applied each day.
- To avoid potential skin irritation, apply to the right or left upper thigh on alternating days.
- Do not apply to the face, breasts, or irritated skin, or in or around the vagina.
- After application, allow the gel to dry before dressing.
- Do not wash the application site within 1 hr after applying Divigel.
- Avoid contact of the gel with eyes.
- Wash hands after each application.
4. Alcohol-based gels are flammable. Avoid fire, flame, or smoking until the gel has dried.
5. When using the tube, apply the gel to one arm using the applicator. Be sure to transfer all of the gel from the applicator to the arm.
6. Keep all regular visits for F/U and lab evaluation. Review associated adverse effects of estrogen. Report any rash, adverse side effects, or lack of response.
OUTCOMES/EVALUATE
Relief of menopausal symptoms

Estradiol hemihydrate
(ess-trah-**DYE**-ohl)

CLASSIFICATION(S):
Estrogen, semisynthetic
PREGNANCY CATEGORY: X
Rx: Vagifem.

⚘Rx: Oesclim.

SEE ALSO *ESTROGENS*.

USES

Atrophic vaginitis.

SPECIAL CONCERNS

■ See Estrogens in Chapter 2 for Black Box Warnings.■

SIDE EFFECTS

Most Common

Breakthrough bleeding/spotting, dizziness, lightheadedness, headache, GI upset, bloating, N&V, weight changes, increased/decreased libido, breast tenderness, edema.

See *Estrogens* for a complete list of possible side effects.

HOW SUPPLIED

Vaginal Tablets: 25 mcg.

DOSAGE

• **VAGINAL TABLETS**
  Atrophic vaginitis.

Initial: 1 tablet, inserted vaginally, once daily for 2 weeks; **maintenance:** 1 tablet, inserted vaginally, twice a week.

NURSING CONSIDERATIONS

ADMINISTRATION/STORAGE

Attempt to discontinue or taper the drug at 3- to 6-month intervals.

ASSESSMENT

Note reasons for therapy, age at menopause onset, characteristics of S&S. Review associated hazards of therapy and alternative treatments available.

CLIENT/FAMILY TEACHING

1. Gently insert the vaginal tablet into the vagina as far as it can comfortably go without force. Use the supplied applicator.

2. Insert the tablet at the same time each day.

3. Report any pain, odor, increased discharge.

OUTCOMES/EVALUATE

Relief of S&S of atrophic vaginitis

Estradiol topical ■ emulsion

(ess-trah-**DYE**-ohl)

CLASSIFICATION(S):

Estrogen, semisynthetic

PREGNANCY CATEGORY: X

Rx: Estrasorb.

E

SEE ALSO *ESTROGENS*.

USES

Moderate to severe vasomotor symptoms associated with menopause.

SPECIAL CONCERNS

■ See Estrogens in Chapter 2 for Black Box Warnings.■

SIDE EFFECTS

Most Common

Dizziness, lightheadedness, headache, N&V, GI upset, bloating, weight changes, increased/decreased libido, breast tenderness, edema, redness/irritation at application site.

See *Estrogens* for a complete list of possible side effects.

HOW SUPPLIED

Topical Emulsion: 2.5 mg estradiol hemihydrate/gram.

DOSAGE

• **TOPICAL EMULSION**
  Moderate to severe vasomotor symptoms.

The single approved dose is 3.48 grams/day (of the product). The lowest effective dose has not been determined. Use the lowest effective dose and for the shortest period of time determined by goals of treatment and risks involved. Periodically re-evaluate (e.g., at 3- and 6-months) to determine need for continued treatment.

NURSING CONSIDERATIONS

ADMINISTRATION/STORAGE

1. When estrogen is prescribed for a women with a uterus, also initiate a progestin to reduce the risk of endometrial cancer. When indicated, rule out malignancy in cases of undiagnosed persistent or recurring abnormal vaginal bleeding.

2. Store at 15–30°C (59–86°F).

ASSESSMENT

1. List reasons for therapy, age at onset, other agents trialed, outcome. Review potential hazards of therapy.

2. Determine if client has undergone GYN exam, understands risks associated with and is a candidate for therapy.

3. Monitor VS, weight, blood sugar, liver and lipid panels. Therapy may increase risk of thromboembolism especially with smoking.

4. Review potential risks R/T to prolonged therapy in postmenopausal women. Progestin helps to minimize risk of endometrial hyperplasia.

CLIENT/FAMILY TEACHING

1. Drug is administered topically to relieve S&S of post menopausal symptoms.

2. The following procedure for application of two-1.74 grams foil-laminated pouches should be followed:

- Open each pouch individually and apply in a comfortable sitting position to clean, dry skin on both legs each morning.
- Cut or tear the first pouch at the notches indicated near the top of the pouch.
- Apply the emulsion in the pouch to the top of the left thigh; push the entire contents from the bottom through the neck of the pouch.
- Using one or both hands, rub the emulsion into the entire left thigh and left calf for 3 minutes until thoroughly absorbed. Rub any excess estradiol remaining on both hands on the buttocks.
- Cut or tear the second pouch at the notches indicated near the top of the pouch. Apply the emulsion in the pouch to the top of the right thigh; push the entire contents from the bottom through the neck of the pouch.
- Using one or both hands, rub the emulsion into the entire right thigh and right calf for 3 minutes until thoroughly absorbed. Rub any excess estradiol remaining on both hands on the buttocks.
- To avoid transfer to other persons, allow the application to dry completely before covering with clothing.
- When application is completed, wash both hands with soap and water to remove any residual estradiol.

3. Report any rash, irritation or skin discoloration at application sites. Do not smoke.

4. Any sudden pain in chest or calves, severe headaches, dizziness, swelling of hands or feet, speech or vision changes, SOB, changes in mental status or abnormal vaginal bleeding, yellow skin or other adverse side effects should be reported immediately.

OUTCOMES/EVALUATE

Relief/control of post menopausal vasomotor symptoms

Estradiol transdermal system ■

CLASSIFICATION(S):
Estrogen, semisynthetic

PREGNANCY CATEGORY: X

Rx: Alora, Climara, Esclim, Estraderm, Estradiol Transdermal System, Menostar, Vivelle, Vivelle-Dot.

SEE ALSO *ESTROGENS.*

USES

(1) Vasomotor symptoms (moderate to severe) associated with menopause (except Menostar). (2) Hypoestrogenism due to hypogonadism, castration, or primary ovarian failure (except Menostar). (3) Vulvar and vaginal atrophy associated with menopause (except Menostar). When prescribing solely for vulvar and vaginal atrophy, consider topical vaginal products. (4) Prevention of postmenopausal osteoporosis. Consider this therapy only for women at significant risk of osteoporosis; carefully consider nonestrogen medications.

ACTION/KINETICS

Action

This transdermal system allows a constant low dose of estradiol to directly reach the systemic circulation. The system overcomes certain problems associated with PO use, including first-pass hepatic metabolism, GI upset, and induction of liver enzymes.

Pharmacokinetics

The system is available in various surface areas, release rates, and total estradiol content (the package insert should be carefully consulted). The patches are made either with a reservoir and a rate-controlling membrane or using a matrix where estradiol is embedded in the adhesive, allowing for a translucent, small, thin patch.

ADDITIONAL CONTRAINDICATIONS

Use with liver dysfunction or disease.

SPECIAL CONCERNS

■ (1) Endometrial cancer. Close clinical surveillance of all women taking estrogen is important. Adequate diagnostic measures, including endometrial sampling when indicated, should be undertaken to rule out malignancy in all cases of undiagnosed persistent or recurring abnormal vaginal bleeding. There is no evidence that the use of 'natural' estrogens results in a different endometrial risk profile than synthetic estrogens at equivalent estrogenic doses. (2) CV and other risks. Estrogens with or without progestins should not be used for the prevention of CV disease or dementia. The Women's Health Initiative (WHI) estrogen alone substudy reported increased risk of stroke and deep vein thrombosis (DVT) in postmenopausal women (50 to 79 years of age) during 6.8 and 7.1 years, respectively of treatment with daily oral conjugated estrogens, 0.625 mg, relative to placebo. (3) The estrogen and progestin WHI substudy reported increased risks of MI, stroke, invasive breast cancer, pulmonary emboli, and DVT in postmenopausal women (50 to 79 years of age) during 5.6 years of treatment with daily oral conjugated estrogens, 0.625 mg, combined with medroxyprogesterone acetate, 2.5 mg relative to placebo. (4) The WHI Memory Study, a substudy of the WHI, reorted an increased risk of developing probable dementia in postmenopausal women 65 years of age and older during 5.2 years of treatment with daily conjugated estrogen, 0.625 mg alone and during 4 years of treatment with daily conjugated estrogens, 0.625 mg combined with medroxyprogesterone acetate, 2.5 mg, relative to placebo. It is unknown whether this finding applies to younger postmenopausal women. (5) Other doses of conjugated estrogens and medroxyprogesterone acetate, and other combinations of estrogens and progestins, were not studied in the WHI and, in the absence of comparable data, these risks should be assumed to be similar. Because of these risks, estrogens with or without progestins should be presbiced at the lowest effective doses and for the shortest duration consistent with treatment goals and risks for the individual woman.■

SIDE EFFECTS

Most Common

Breakthrough bleeding/spotting, dizziness, lightheadedness, headache, GI upset, bloating, N&V, weight changes, increased/decreased libido, breast tenderness, edema, redness/irritation at site of application.

See *Estrogens* for a complete list of possible side effects.

HOW SUPPLIED

Transdermal System: Release rate: 0.014 mg/24 hr, 0.025 mg/24 hr, 0.0375 mg/24 hr, 0.05 mg/24 hr, 0.06 mg/24 hr, 0.075 mg/24 hr, 0.1 mg/24 hr.

DOSAGE

• **TRANSDERMAL SYSTEM**

Menopausal symptoms.

Initial: To treat vasomotor symptoms, use a system that delivers 0.025 mg estradiol/day. To treat moderate to severe vasomotor symptoms, vulvar and vaginal atrophy associated with menopause, hypoestrogenism caused by hypogonadism, castration, or primary ovarian failure, use a system that delivers 0.025–0.05 mg estradiol/day. Depending on the system selected, apply to the skin once or twice weekly. Do not make dosage adjustments until after the first month of therapy. Try to taper or discontinue at 3- to 6-month intervals but try to discontinue as soon as possible.

Prevention of postmenopausal osteoporosis.

Initial: 0.05 mg/day is the minimum established dosage; initiate as soon as possible after menopause. Adjust dosage to control concurrent menopausal symptoms. In women who are not taking oral estrogens or in women switching from another estradiol transdermal product, start treatment immediately. In women who are currently taking oral estrogens, start treatment 1 week after withdrawal of oral therapy or sooner if symptoms reappear in less than 1 week.

NURSING CONSIDERATIONS

ADMINISTRATION/STORAGE

1. Therapy may be given continuously to those who do not have an intact uterus. For clients with an intact uterus, give cyclically (3 weeks on, 1 week off). Vivelle may be given continuously or on a cyclic schedule with a progestin.

2. A progestin is given to postmenopausal women with an intact uterus to reduce the risk of endometrial cancer. A woman without a uterus does not require a progestin. Menostar may be used in women both with and without a uterus.

3. Alora, Estraderm, Esclim, Vivelle, and Vivelle-Dot are applied twice a week. Climara and Menostar are applied once a week.

4. Menostar should only be prescribed to postmenopausal women who are at significant risk of osteoporosis. Carefully consider nonestrogen approaches. It is recommended that women who have a uterus and are to be treated with Menostar receive a progestin for 14 days q 6 to 12 months, as well as undergo an endometrial biopsy at yearly intervals or as clinically indicated.

5. Store at 25°C (77°F). Do not store above 30°C (86°F). Do not store unpouched. Apply immediately upon removal from the protective pouch.

ASSESSMENT

1. Note reasons for therapy, age, other agents trialed, outcome. Review potential hazards of therapy.

2. Ensure client has undergone GYN exam, understands the risks associated with contraception and is a candidate for therapy.

3. Therapy may increase risk of thromboembolism especially with smoking, CVA, and ↑ BP readings. Monitor VS, blood sugar and lipid panel.

CLIENT/FAMILY TEACHING

1. If taking oral estrogens, stop pills and wait 1 week before applying the system.

2. Without a hysterectomy, the system is usually used for 3 weeks, followed by 1 week of rest. May be used continuously in those without an intact uterus.

3. Place system on a clean, dry area of the skin on the trunk of the body (preferably the abdomen). Avoid using areas with excessive amounts of hair. Also may use on the hip or buttock. Do not apply to the breasts or the waistline.

4. Rotate application site; date patch. Allow 1 week intervals between reapplication to same site. Wear only 1 patch at a time.

5. Apply system immediately after the pouch is opened and the protective liner is removed. Firmly press in place with the palm for approximately 10 sec. Ensure good contact, especially around the edges. If system falls off, reapply the same system (except Climara or Menostar) or place a new one and follow the same schedule. If Climara or Menostar falls off, apply a new system for the remainder of the 7-day dosing interval. Continue the original treatment schedule.

6. If the client forgets to apply a patch, apply a new one as soon as possible on the original treatment schedule. Interruption of treatment may increase the likelihood of breakthrough bleeding, spotting, and recurrence of symptoms.

7. Swimming, bathing, or using a sauna while the patch is in place may decrease adhesion of the patch and thus delivery of estradiol.

8. To avoid irritation, slowly and carefully remove the system. If any adhesive remains on the skin after removal of the system, allow the area to dry for 15 min. Then, gently rub the area with an oil-based cream or lotion to remove the adhesive residue.

9. Used patches still contain estradiol. Thus, carefully fold each patch in half so

---

Bold Italic = life threatening side effect   ▇ = black box warning   ✦ = Available in Canada that it sticks to itself before discarding. Discard in household trash such that accidental application or ingestion by children, pets, or others is prevented.

10. Weight gain may occur; report if marked or if extremity swelling noted.

11. Stop smoking; smoking increases risk of blood clots.

12. Addition of a progestin for 7 or more days may reduce the incidence of endometrial hyperplasia.

13. Report adverse side effects, sudden pain in chest or calves, headaches, speech or vision changes, SOB, changes in mental status or abnormal vaginal bleeding.

OUTCOMES/EVALUATE
- Relief of menopausal symptoms
- Therapeutic estrogen levels

Estrogens conjugated, oral (conjugated estrogenic substances)

(**ES**-troh-jens)

CLASSIFICATION(S):
Estrogen, natural and synthetic
PREGNANCY CATEGORY: X
Rx: Premarin.
✤**Rx:** C.E.S., Congest, Conjugated Estrogens C.S.D., PMS-Conjugated Estrogens.

Estrogens conjugated, parenteral

PREGNANCY CATEGORY: X
Rx: Premarin Intravenous.

Estrogens conjugated, synthetic (A & B)

PREGNANCY CATEGORY: X
Rx: Cenestin, Enjuvia.

Estrogens conjugated, vaginal

PREGNANCY CATEGORY: X
Rx: Premarin Vaginal Cream.

SEE ALSO *ESTROGENS* AND *ESTERIFIED ESTROGENS.*

USES
Conjugated Estrogens, PO: (1) Moderate to severe vasomotor symptoms due to menopause. (2) Moderate to severe symptoms of vulvar and vaginal atrophy associated with menopause. (3) Prophylaxis of postmenopausal osteoporosis. (4) Hypoestrogenism due to hypogonadism, castration, or primary ovarian failure. (5) Palliation of breast cancer in selected women and men with metastatic disease. (6) Palliation only of advanced androgen-dependent prostatic carcinoma.

Conjugated Estrogens, Synthetic, A & B, PO: (1) Moderate to severe vasomotor symptoms associated with menopause. (2) Vulvar and vaginal atrophy (Synthetic Conjugated Estrogens A).

Conjugated Estrogens, Parenteral: Abnormal bleeding due to imbalance of hormones and in the absence of disease.

Conjugated Estrogens, Vaginal: Atrophic vaginitis and kraurosis vulvae associated with menopause.

ACTION/KINETICS
Action
Estrogens combine with receptors in the cytoplasm of cells, resulting in an increase in protein synthesis. During menopause, estrogens are used as replacement therapy. These products contain a blend of various estrogenic substances.

Pharmacokinetics
Metabolized in the liver and excreted mainly in the urine.

CONTRAINDICATIONS
Use for prevention of CV disease due to increased risk of MI, stroke, invasive breast cancer, and venous thromboembolism.

SPECIAL CONCERNS
■ See Estrogens in Chapter 2 for Black Box Warnings. Also, due to the in-

creased risk of MI, stroke, invasive breast cancer, and venous thromboembolism, give for the shortest amount of time consistent with treatment goals.■

Use of estrogen replacement therapy for prolonged periods of time may increase the risk of fatal ovarian cancer and an increased risk of endometrial cancer.

SIDE EFFECTS

Most Common

After PO Use: Abdominal/back pain, asthenia, breast pain, headache, infection, dyspepsia, nausea, arthralgia, pharyngitis, URTI.

See *Estrogens* for a complete list of possible side effects.

HOW SUPPLIED

Estrogens conjugated, oral. *Tablets:* 0.3 mg, 0.45 mg, 0.625 mg, 0.9 mg, 1.25 mg.

Estrogens conjugated, parenteral. *Injection:* 25 mg.

Estrogens conjugated, synthetic A. *Tablets:* 0.3 mg, 0.45 mg, 0.625 mg, 0.9 mg, 1.25 mg.

Estrogens conjugated, synthetic B. *Tablets:* 0.3 mg, 0.45 mg, 0.625 mg, 1.25 mg.

Estrogens conjugated, vaginal. *Cream:* 0.625 mg/gram.

DOSAGE

ESTROGENS CONJUGATED, ORAL (PREMARIN)

- **TABLETS**

  Moderate to severe vasomotor symptoms due to menopause, moderate to severe symptoms of vulvar and vaginal atrophy associated with menopause.

Start with the lowest dose: 1.25 mg/day given cyclically. If the client has not menstruated in 2 or more months, begin therapy on any day; if, however, the client is menstruating, begin therapy on day 5 of bleeding.

  Primary ovarian failure, female castration.

1.25 mg/day given cyclically (3 weeks on, 1 week off). Adjust dose to lowest effective level.

  Hypogonadism in females.

0.3–0.625 mg/day given cyclically (3 weeks on, 1 week off). Adjust dose depending on severity of symptoms and

responsiveness of the endometrium. Dose may be gradually titrated upward at 6–12 month intervals as needed to achieve appropriate bone age advancement and eventual epiphyseal closure. Chronic dosing with 0.625 mg is sufficient to induce artificial cyclical menses with sequential progestin administration and to maintain bone density after skeletal maturity has been achieved.

  Palliation of mammary carcinoma in men or postmenopausal women.

10 mg 3 times/day for at least 90 days.

  Palliation of prostatic carcinoma.

1.25–2.5 mg 3 times per day. Effectiveness can be measured by phosphatase determinations and symptomatic improvement.

  Prophylaxis of osteoporosis.

0.625 mg/day continuously or cyclically (such as 25 days on, 5 days off). Mainstays of therapy include calcium; exercise and nutrition may be important adjuncts.

ESTROGENS CONJUGATED, SYNTHETIC A (CENESTIN)

- **TABLETS**

  Moderate-to-severe vasomotor symptoms due to menopause.

Initial: 0.45 mg daily; **then,** adjust dose based on individual client response. Discontinue as soon as possible. Attempt to discontinue or taper dosage at 3- to 6-month intervals.

  Vulvar and vaginal atrophy.

0.3 mg/day.

ESTROGENS CONJUGATED, SYNTHETIC B (ENJUVIA)

- **TABLETS**

  Moderate-to-severe vasomotor symptoms due to menopause.

Initial: 0.3 mg daily. Adjust dosage based on individual client response. Periodically reassess dosage.

ESTROGENS CONJUGATED, PARENTERAL (PREMARIN INTRAVENOUS)

- **IM; IV**

  Abnormal bleeding.

25 mg; repeat after 6–12 hr if necessary.

ESTROGENS CONJUGATED, VAGINAL (PREMARIN VAGINAL CREAM)

- **VAGINAL CREAM**

  Atrophic vaginitis and kraurosis vulvae associated with menopause.

Bold Italic = life threatening side effect   ■ = black box warning   ✤ = Available in Canada

½–2 grams daily for 3 weeks on and 1 week off. Repeat as needed. Attempt to taper the dose or discontinue the medication at 3- to 6-month intervals.

NURSING CONSIDERATIONS

ADMINISTRATION/STORAGE

1. For all uses, except palliation of mammary and prostatic carcinoma, oral conjugated estrogens are best administered cyclically—3 weeks on and 1 week off.

2. When used vaginally, insert the cream high into the vagina (two-thirds the length of the applicator).

3. When estrogen is used for a postmenopausal woman with a uterus, also initiate a progestin to reduce the risk of endometrial cancer. Those without a uterus do not require a progestin.

4. For women who have a uterus, undertake adequate diagnostic measures, such as endometrial sampling, when indicated to rule out malignancy in cases of undiagnosed persistent or recurring abnormal vaginal bleeding.

IV 5. Administer IV Premarin slowly to prevent flushing.

6. Parenteral solutions of conjugated estrogens are compatible with NSS, invert sugar solutions, and dextrose solutions.

7. Parenteral solutions are incompatible with acid solutions, ascorbic acid solutions, and protein hydrolysates.

8. Use reconstituted parenteral solutions within a few hours after mixing if kept at room temperature. Note date and time of reconstitution on the label. If refrigerated, the reconstituted solution is stable for 60 days. Do not use if solution is dark or has a precipitate.

9. IV use is preferred over IM as it induces a more rapid response.

ASSESSMENT

1. Indicate reasons for therapy, age, characteristics of S&S, other agents trialed.

2. Review potential risks R/T the development of breast and fatal ovarian cancers with prolonged therapy.

3. Monitor serum phosphatase levels with prostatic cancer.

CLIENT/FAMILY TEACHING

1. Take tablets cyclically as directed, i.e., 3 weeks on, 1 week off.

2. May take with food to decrease GI upset.

3. Cenestin is the only plant derived form of estrogen.

4. Review potential risks of prolonged therapy, i.e., endometrial cancer, abnormal blood clotting, gallbladder disease, and breast cancer.

5. Review how to use esp with cream and/or rings.

6. If no hysterectomy has been performed remember to add a progestin to help prevent cancer. Review hazards related to hormone replacement therapy.

OUTCOMES/EVALUATE

- Control of abnormal uterine bleeding
- Relief of menopausal symptoms
- Treatment of urogenital S&S R/T postmenopausal atrophy of vagina and lower urinary tract

Estropipate ■ (Piperazine estrone sulfate)
(es-troh-**PIE**-payt)

CLASSIFICATION(S):
Estrogen, semisynthetic
PREGNANCY CATEGORY: X
Rx: Ogen, Ogen Vaginal Cream, Ortho-Est.

SEE ALSO *ESTROGENS.*

USES

PO: (1) Moderate to severe vasomotor symptoms associated with menopause. (2) Vulval and vaginal atrophy. (3) Hypoestrogenism due to primary ovarian failure, castration, or hypogonadism. (4) Prevention of osteoporosis.

Vaginal: Atrophic vaginitis and kraurosis vulvae associated with menopause.

ACTION/KINETICS

Action

Contains solubilized crystalline estrone stabilized with piperazine.

E

CONTRAINDICATIONS
Use during pregnancy. Use to treat nervous symptoms or depression that might occur during menopause.

SPECIAL CONCERNS
■ See Estrogens in Chapter 2 for Black Box Warnings.■

SIDE EFFECTS
Most Common
Anorexia, N&V, swollen/tender breasts, acne, decreased libido, dizziness, edema, changes in menstrual cycle, breakthrough bleeding, depression.
See *Estrogens* for a complete list of possible side effects.

HOW SUPPLIED
Tablets (equivalent to estropipate): 0.75 mg, 1.5 mg, 3 mg, 6 mg; *Vaginal Cream*: 1.5 mg/gram.

DOSAGE
• **TABLETS**
Moderate to severe vasomotor symptoms; atrophic vaginitis or kraurosis vulvae due to menopause.
0.75–6 mg/day for short-term therapy (give cyclically). May also be used continuously. The lowest dose that will control symptoms should be selected. Attempt to discontinue or taper the dose at 3- to 6-month intervals.
Hypogonadism, primary ovarian failure, castration.
Initial, 1.5–9 mg/day (calculated as 0.625 to 5 mg estrone sulfate) for first 3 weeks; **then,** rest period of 8–10 days. PO progestin can be given during the third week if withdrawal bleeding does not occur.
Prevention of osteoporosis.
0.75 mg estropipate/day for 25 days of a 31-day cycle per month. Mainstay of therapy includes calcium; exercise and nutrition may be important adjuncts.
• **VAGINAL CREAM**
Atrophic vaginitis and kraurosis vulvae associated with menopause.
2–4 grams (containing 3–6 mg estropipate) daily for 3 weeks followed by a 1-week rest period. Attempt to taper the dose or discontinue the medication at 3- to 6-month intervals.

NURSING CONSIDERATIONS
ADMINISTRATION/STORAGE
1. Administration should be cyclic—3 weeks on and 1 week off medication.
2. When used to relieve vasomotor symptoms, cyclic administration is initiated on day 5 of bleeding if menstruating. If the client has not menstruated within the last 2 months (or more), cyclic administration may be initiated at any time.
3. When estrogen is used for a postmenopausal woman with a uterus, also initiate a progestin to reduce the risk of endometrial cancer. A woman without a uterus does not require a progestin.
4. Store tablets from 15–30°C (59–86°F).

ASSESSMENT
1. Note reasons for therapy, characteristics of S&S, other agents trialed. Ensure regular physical and GYN exams.
2. Monitor VS, weight, liver and lipid panels.
3. Review potential risks R/T to prolonged therapy in postmenopausal women. Cyclic therapy using lowest doses reduces risk of endometrial cancer. Progestin helps to minimize risk of endometrial hyperplasia with intact uterus.

CLIENT/FAMILY TEACHING
1. Take medications at the same time each day.
2. Relieve nausea during PO therapy by consuming solid foods.
3. Report any evidence of thromboembolic S&S (headache, blurred vision, pain, swelling or tenderness in the extremities); fluid retention (weight gain, swelling of extremities); hepatic dysfunction (yellowing of skin or eyes, itching, dark urine, clay-colored stools); changes in mental status or unusual bleeding.
4. With vaginal preparations, administer at bedtime, remain supine for 30 min; protect clothing and bed linens by using a sanitary pad. Avoid tampons during therapy. Wash vaginal area with soap and water prior to application. To deliver cream, the end of the applicator (after the appropriate amount is intro-

---

Bold Italic = life threatening side effect   ■ = black box warning   ✤ = Available in Canada

duced) should be inserted high into the vagina and the plunger pushed all the way down. Between uses remove the plunger and wash in warm, soapy water. Avoid hot or boiling water.

5. Report any chest pressure, SOB, severe headaches, abdominal pain, blurred vision, breast lumps, vaginal bleeding, changes in skin or urine darkening immediately

6. Drug may cause increased skin pigmentation. Wear protective clothing and sunscreen; avoid prolonged sun exposure.

7. Stop drug and report if pregnant. Do not smoke.

OUTCOMES/EVALUATE
- Relief of menopausal symptoms
- Stimulation of menses
- Restoration of hormonal balance

Eszopiclone
(ess-**ZOP**-eye-klone)

CLASSIFICATION(S):
Sedative-hypnotic, nonbenzodiazepine

PREGNANCY CATEGORY: C

Rx: Lunesta.

USES
Treatment of insomnia.

ACTION/KINETICS

Action
Precise mechanism is unknown but may interfere with GABA-receptor complexes at binding domains located close to or allosterically coupled to benzodiazepine receptors.

Pharmacokinetics
Rapidly absorbed; **peak plasma levels:** 1 hr. Extensively metabolized by CYP3A4 and CYP2E1 enzymes; one of the metabolites has hypnotic activity. **t½:** About 6 hr. Excreted in the urine (75%); less than 10% is excreted as the parent drug.

SPECIAL CONCERNS
Use with caution in those with diseases that could affect metabolism or hemodynamic responses, in those with compromised respiratory function, in those

with signs and symptoms of depression, and during lactation. Safety and efficacy have not been demonstrated in children less than 18 years of age.

SIDE EFFECTS

Most Common
Unpleasant taste, headache, dizziness, diarrhea, dry mouth, dyspepsia, nervousness, somnolence.

CNS: Headache, somnolence, nervousness, dizziness, depression, anxiety, confusion, hallucinations, abnormal dreams, neuralgia, decreased libido, agitation, apathy, ataxia, emotional lability, hostility, hypertonia, hypesthesia, incoordination, insomnia, impaired memory, neurosis, nystamus, paresthesia, decreased reflexes, difficulty concentrating. **GI:** N&V, dry mouth, unpleasant taste, dyspepsia, anorexia, cholelithiasis, increased appetite, melena, mouth ulceration, thirst, ulcerative stomatitis, halitosis. **GU:** Dysmenorrhea, gynecomastia (in men), UTI, amenorrhea, breast engorgement/enlargement/pain, breast neoplasm, cystitis, dysuria, female lactation, hematuria, kidney calculus/pain, mastitis, menorrhagia, metrorrhagia, urinary frequency/incontinence, ***uterine/vaginal hemorrhage***, vaginitis. **Dermatologic:** Rash, pruritus, acne, alopecia, contact dermatitis, dry skin, eczema, skin discoloration, sweating, urticaria. **Musculoskeletal:** Arthrits, bursitis, joint disorder (pain, stiffness, swelling) leg cramps, myasthenia, twitching. **Respiratory:** Asthma, bronchitis, dyspnea, epistaxis, hiccup, laryngitis. **Hematologic:** Anemia lymphadenopathy. **Ophthalmic:** Conjunctivitis, dry eyes. **Otic:** Ear pain, otitis externa, otitis media, tinnitus, vestibular disorder. **Body as a whole:** Allergic reaction, cellulitis, fever, heat stroke, malaise, photosensitivity, accidental injury, pain. **Miscellaneous:** Infection, viral infection, migraine, hypertension, peripheral edema, hypercholesteremia, weight gain/loss, chest pain, facial edema, hernia, neck rigidity.

OD OVERDOSE MANAGEMENT
Symptoms: Exaggeration of the pharmacologic effects, including impairment of consciousness ranging from somno-

lence to coma. *Treatment:* General symptomatic and supportive care. Immediate gastric lavage, if appropriate. Give IV fluids as needed. Flumazenil may be useful. Monitor respiration, pulse, BP, hypotension, and CNS depression. The value of dialysis has not been determined.

DRUG INTERACTIONS

Clarithromycin / ↑ Eszoplicone levels, C_{max}, and t½ R/T ↓ metabolism by CYP3A4

CNS depressants, including anticonvulsants, antihistamines / Additive CNS depressant effects

Ethanol / Do not use together

Ketoconazole / ↑ Eszoplicone levels, C_{max}, and t½ R/T ↓ metabolism by CYP3A4

Nefazodone / ↑ Eszoplicone levels, C_{max}, and t½ R/T ↓ metabolism by CYP3A4

Olanzapine / ↓ Psychomotor function

Rifampin / ↓ Eszoplicone levels R/T ↑ metabolism by CYP3A4

Ritonovir / ↑ Eszoplicone levels, C_{max}, and t½ R/T ↓ metabolism by CYP3A4

HOW SUPPLIED

Tablets: 1 mg, 2 mg, 3 mg.

DOSAGE

• **TABLETS**

Insomnia.

Adults, initial: 2 mg immediately before bedtime for most nonelderly clients. May be initiated at or raised to 3 mg if indicated, as 3 mg is more effective for sleep maintenance. The recommended starting dose for the elderly is 1 mg immediately before bedtime; dose may be increased to 2 mg if indicated. For the elderly who have difficulty staying asleep, give 2 mg immediately before bedtime. Use a starting dose of 1 mg in severe hepatic impairment.

NURSING CONSIDERATIONS

ADMINISTRATION/STORAGE

1. Absorption is slowed if taken with or immediately after a heavy, high-fat meal; this results in a reduced effect on sleep latency.

2. Do not exceed a starting dose of 1 mg in clients coadministered eszopiclone with potent CYP3A4 inhibitors.

3. Store from 15–30°C (59–86°F).

ASSESSMENT

1. List reasons for therapy, other agents trialed, outcome. List drugs prescribed to ensure none interact.

2. Indentify triggers (i.e., napping during daytime, high caffeine intake, depression, or pain).

3. Monitor renal and LFTs. Anticipate reduced dosage with the elderly and those with impaired liver function.

4. Assess for depression, memory problems, and any dependent behaviors.

CLIENT/FAMILY TEACHING

1. Take as directed just before bedtime as drug acts quickly. Do not crush or break tablets and ensure at least 8 hours before required to be up and active.

2. Use caution, do not perform activities that require mental alertness until drug effects are realized. May experience unpleasant taste, dizziness, drowsiness, lightheadedness, and impaired coordination.

3. Avoid alcohol and OTC meds without provider approval.

4. Report any unusual or disturbing thoughts or behavior or other adverse side effects or lack of response immediately.

5. May experience more sleeping problems after stopping drug for the first one or two nights. With prolonged therapy may experience mild withdrawal symptoms.

6. Do not share medications. Store safely out of reach of children.

7. Do not use if nursing or pregnant.

OUTCOMES/EVALUATE

Relief of insomnia

Etanercept

(eh-**TAN**-er-sept)

CLASSIFICATION(S):
Immunomodulator
PREGNANCY CATEGORY: B
Rx: Enbrel.

USES
(1) Reduce S&S, delays structural damage, and improves physical function in moderate to severe active rheumatoid arthritis in adults who have had an inadequate response to one or more antirheumatic drugs. May be used in combination with methotrexate, in those who do not respond adequately to methotrexate alone. Used to induce a major clinical response lasting 6 months. (2) Reduce signs and symptoms of active ankylosing spondylitis. (3) Reduce signs and symptoms of moderate to severe active polyarticular-course juvenile rheumatoid arthritis in those who have had an inadequate response to one or more disease-modifying antirheumatic drugs. (4) Reduce signs and symptoms, inhibiting the progression of structural damage of active arthritis, and improving physical function in those with psoriatic arthritis. Can be used in combination with methotrexate in those who do not respond adequately to methotrexate alone. (5) Chronic, moderate to severe plaque psoriasis in adults 18 years of age and older who are candidates for systemic therapy or phototherapy. *Investigational:* Wegener granulomatosis.

ACTION/KINETICS
Action
Binds specifically to tumor necrosis factor (TNF) and blocks its interaction with cell surface TNF receptors. TNF is a cytokine that is involved in normal inflammatory and immune responses. Thus, the drug renders TNF biologically inactive. It is possible for etanercept to affect host defenses against infections and malignancies since TNF mediates inflammation and modulates cellular immune responses. It may also reverse CHF by decreasing inflammation in the heart.

Pharmacokinetics
t½: About 102 hr. Individual clients may undergo a two- to five-fold increase in serum levels with repeated dosing.

CONTRAINDICATIONS
Sepsis. Use in any chronic or localized active infection. Concurrent administration of live vaccines. Lactation.

SPECIAL CONCERNS
Use with caution in the elderly and in those with a history of recurring infections or with a condition that predisposes to infections (e.g., advanced or poorly controlled diabetes). Use with caution in those with preexisting or recent-onset CNS-demyelinating disorders. Safety and efficacy have not been determined in those with immunosuppression, chronic infections, in children with plaque psoriasis, or in children less than 4 years of age. Serious infections and sepsis, including fatalities, are possible.

SIDE EFFECTS
Most Common
URTI, non-URTI, injection site reaction, infection, headache, nausea, dizziness, rash, abdominal pain, cough, pharyngitis, asthenia, peripheral edema.

Injection site reactions: Erythema, itching, pain, swelling. **GI:** Abdominal pain, N&V, diarrhea, altered taste sense, mouth ulcer, dyspepsia, dry mouth, cholecystitis, pancreatitis, appendicitis, cholecystitis, GI bleeding, *GI hemorrhage, intestinal perforation.* **CNS:** Headache, dizziness, depression, *stroke, seizures,* paresthesias, normal pressure hydrocephalous, *seizure, CVA.* Rarely, demyelinating disorders (multiple sclerosis, transverse myelitis, optic neuritis). **CV:** *Heart failure,* chest pain, flushing, *MI,* myocardial ischemia, cerebral ischemia, deep vein thrombosis, thrombophlebitis, coagulopathy, cutaneous vasculitis, hypertension, hypotension, vasodilation, cutaneous vasculitis, CHF (either new or worsening of existing). **Hematologic:** *Pancytopenia, including aplastic anemia*; adenopathy, anemia, leukopenia, neutropenia, thrombocytopenia, lymphadenopathy. **Respiratory:** URTI, non-URTI, sinusitis, rhinitis, pharyngitis, cough, pneumonitis, respiratory disorder, dyspnea, interstitial lung disease, worsening of prior lung disorder, pulmonary disease, sarcoidosis, *pulmonary embolism.* **Ophthalmic:** Ocular inflammation, dry eyes, optic neuritis. **Dermatologic:** Urticaria, pruritus, rash, alopecia, cutaneous vasculitis, subcutaneous nodules, worsening psoriasis. **GU:** Membranous glomerulonephropathy, UTI, kidney calculus. **Musculoskeletal:** Bursitis, polymyositis, joint pain, urticaria, SC nodules, transverse myelitis, lupus-like syndrome (including rash consistent with subacute or discoid lupus). **Body as a whole:** Formation of autoimmune antibodies, malignancies (including lymphoma), asthenia, *serious infections and sepsis*, *hypersensitivity reactions (including angioedema)*, generalized pain, fatigue, abscess with bacteremia, fever, flu-like symptoms, tuberculosis arthritis. **Miscellaneous:** Peripheral edema, anorexia, weight gain, chest pain.

Side effects noted in juveniles. GI: N&V, gastroenteritis, abdominal pain, esophagitis, gastritis. **CNS:** Depression, headache, personality disorder, *seizures*. **CV:** Cutaneous vasculitis. **Hematologic:** Coagulopathy, pancytopenia. **GU:** UTI. **Ophthalmic:** Optic neuritis. **Body as a whole:** Group A streptococcal septic shock, type 1 diabetes mellitus, soft tissue and postoperative wound infection, infections, abscess with bacteremia. **Miscellaneous:** Varicella, tuberculosis arthritis, ↑ transaminases.

DRUG INTERACTIONS
Anakinra / ↑ Incidence of serious infections compared with use of etanercept alone.
Sulfasalazine / Mild ↓ in mean neutrophil counts

HOW SUPPLIED
Injection: 50 mg/mL; *Powder for Injection, Lyophilized:* 25 mg.

DOSAGE————————————
• **SC**

Moderate to severe active rheumatoid arthritis; psoriatic arthritis; ankylosing spondylitis.

Adults: 50 mg per week given as one SC injection using a 50 mg/mL single-use prefilled syringe, or as two-25 mg injections given either on the same day or 3 or 4 days apart. Doses greater than 50 mg per week are not recommended. Methotrexate, glucocorticoids, salicylates, NSAIDs, or analgesics may be used during treatment.

Children with active polyarticular-course juvenile rheumatoid arthritis.

Children, 4–17 years: 0.8 mg/kg/week (up to a maximum of 50 mg/week). Maximum dose at a single injection site: 25 mg. For children weighing from 31–62 kg, give the total weekly dose as 2 SC injections, either on the same day or 3 or 4 days apart using the multiple-use vial. Give the dose for children weighing less than 31 kg as a single SC injection once weekly using the correct volume from the multiple-use vial. Glucocorticoids, NSAIDs, or analgesics may be continued during treatment. Concurrent use of methotrexate and higher doses of etanercept have not been studied in children.

Plaque psoriasis in adults.

Adults, initial: 50 mg given twice weekly (3 or 4 days apart) for 3 months; **then,** reduce dose to 50 mg/week. Starting doses of 25 mg or 50 mg per week were also shown to be effective.

NURSING CONSIDERATIONS
ADMINISTRATION/STORAGE
1. Clients must enroll with the makers of etanercept so that pharmacies can obtain the product.
2. Reconstitute multiple-use vial aseptically with 1 mL of the supplied sterile bacteriostatic water for injection to yield a solution containing 25 mg/mL. During reconstitution, inject the diluent slowly into the vial. Some foaming will occur. To avoid excessive foaming, do not shake or vigorously agitate. Swirl the contents slowly during dissolution which takes less than 10 minutes. The reconstituted solution should be clear and colorless. Withdraw only the dose to be given from the vial into the syringe. Some foam or bubbles may remain in the vial. Do not filter the reconstituted solution during preparation or administration.
3. Allow the single-use prefilled syringe to come to room temperature (about 15–30 min) before using. Do not remove the needle shield while allowing the prefilled syringe to reach room temperature.

Bold Italic = life threatening side effect   ■ = black box warning   ✤ = Available in Canada

4. Methotrexate, glucocorticoids, salicylates, NSAIDs, or analgesics may be continued during therapy for rheumatoid arthritis.

5. Glucocorticoids, NSAIDs, or analgesics may be continued during treatment for polyarticular juvenile rheumatoid arthritis.

6. Some clients treated, without interruption, for 3 years may be able to reduce the dose or stop concomitant therapy with methotrexate or corticosteroids.

7. The needle cover of the diluent syringe contains latex; do not handle if sensitive to latex.

8. Before administration, visually inspect for particulate matter and discoloration. Do not use if discolored, cloudy, or if particulate matter remains after reconstitution.

9. Do not add other medications to solutions containing etanercept and do not reconstitute with other diluents.

10. Do not filter reconstituted solution during preparation/administration.

11. Give a 50 mg dose as 1 SC injection using a 50 mg/mL single-use prefilled syringe or as two 25 mg SC injections using the multiple-use vial. Give the two 35 mg injections either on the same day or 3 or 4 days apart.

12. Store the sterile powder at 2–8°C (36–46°F). Refrigerate etanercept sterile powder (do not freeze). Solutions reconstituted with the diluent provided may be stored for up to 14 days if refrigerated. Do not freeze.

13. Keep single-use prefilled syringes refrigerated at 2–8°C (36–46°F). Do not freeze. Keep prefilled syringes in the original carton to protect from light until the time of use. Do not shake.

ASSESSMENT

1. Note reasons for therapy, joints affected, presenting characteristics, other agents/therapies trialed/failed. Assess baseline functionality; monitor.

2. Observe as client performs first injection after instruction.

3. Monitor closely if a new infection occurs during treatment. Discontinue if serious infection develops.

4. Certain joints may require individual steroid injections during flares to control pain and enhance mobility.

5. Ensure juvenile clients brought up to date with all immunizations prior to starting etanercept therapy.

6. A pregnancy register is available to monitor outcomes of pregnant women exposed to etanercept. Health care providers should register clients by calling 1-877-311-8972.

CLIENT/FAMILY TEACHING

1. Drug consists of a protein injected under the skin. Each tray contains all materials needed for administration. Follow written guidelines for mixing and administering explicitly. May request prefilled syringes and autoinjector to facilitate administration.

2. Review procedures for storage, reconstitution, inspection, withdraw, administration, site rotation, and disposal of syringes.

3. If self-administering etanercept, the first injection will be performed by the client under the supervision of a qualified health care professional.

4. Always rotate sites for self-injection which include the thigh, abdomen, or upper arm. Give new injections at least 1 inch from the old site and never into areas where the skin is tender, bruised, red, or hard.

5. Report any abdominal pain, S&S of infection, dizziness, SOB, chest pain, rash, other adverse side effects.

6. If traveling must keep refrigerated or carry in cooler.

7. Avoid immunizations with live vaccines.

8. Practice reliable contraception. Do not use if breast-feeding.

9. The manufacturer maintains and active web site www.enbrel.com with patient support services and information. Additionally may call 1-888-4ENBREL (1-888-436-2735) with questions and nurse support.

OUTCOMES/EVALUATE

• ↓ Joint pain/swelling
• Improved ROM
• Delayed structural damage with RA

Ethacrynate sodium ■ IV

(eth-ah-**KRIH**-nayt)

CLASSIFICATION(S):
Diuretic, loop
PREGNANCY CATEGORY: B

Ethacrynic acid

(eth-ah-**KRIH**-nik)

PREGNANCY CATEGORY: B
Rx: Edecrin.

SEE ALSO *DIURETICS, LOOP.*

USES
Of value with resistance to less potent diuretics. (1) CHF, acute pulmonary edema, edema associated with nephrotic syndrome, ascites due to idiopathic edema, lymphedema, malignancy. (2) Short-term use for ascites as a result of malignancy, lymphedema, or idiopathic edema. (3) Short-term use in pediatric clients (except infants) with congenital heart disease. *Investigational:* **Ethacrynic acid:** Single injection into the eye to treat glaucoma (effective for a week or more). **Ethacrynate sodium:** Hypercalcemia, bromide intoxication, and with mannitol in ethylene glycol poisoning.

ACTION/KINETICS
Action
Inhibits the reabsorption of sodium and chloride in the loop of Henle; it also decreases reabsorption of sodium and chloride and increases potassium excretion in the distal tubule. Also acts directly on the proximal tubule to enhance excretion of electrolytes. Large quantities of sodium and chloride and smaller amounts of potassium and bicarbonate ion are excreted during diuresis.

Pharmacokinetics
Onset, PO: 30 min; **IV:** Within 5 min. **Peak, PO:** 2 hr; **IV:** 15–30 min. **Duration, PO:** 6–8 hr. **IV:** 2 hr. **t½, after PO:** 60 min. Metabolites are excreted through the urine. Diuresis and electro-lyte loss are more pronounced with ethacrynic acid than with thiazide diuretics. Is often effective in clients refractory to other diuretics. Careful monitoring of the diuretic effects is necessary.

CONTRAINDICATIONS
Pregnancy (usually), lactation, use in neonates. Anuria and severe renal damage.

SPECIAL CONCERNS
■ Potent diuretic; excess amounts can lead to a profound diuresis with water and electrolyte depletion. Careful medical supervision is required; individualize dosage.■ Geriatric clients may be more sensitive to the usual adult dose. Use with caution in diabetics and in those with hepatic cirrhosis (who are particularly susceptible to electrolyte imbalance). Monitor gout clients carefully. Safety and efficacy of oral use in infants and IV use in children have not been established.

SIDE EFFECTS
Most Common
Dizziness, lightheadedness, blurred vision, anorexia, itching, GI upset, headache, weakness, muscle cramps, N&V, hearing difficulty, pain.

Electrolyte imbalance: Hypokalemia, hyponatremia, hypochloremic alkalosis, hypomagnesemia, hypocalcemia. **GI:** Anorexia, N&V, diarrhea (may be sudden, watery, profuse diarrhea), acute pancreatitis, abdominal discomfort/pain, jaundice, *GI bleeding or hemorrhage*, dysphagia. **Hematologic:** Severe neutropenia, thrombocytopenia, *agranulocytosis*, rarely Henoch-Schoenlein purpura in clients with rheumatic heart disease. **CNS:** Apprehension, confusion, dizziness, lightheadedness, vertigo, headache. **Body as a whole:** Fever, chills, fatigue, malaise, weakness, muscle cramps. **Otic:** Sense of fullness in the ears, tinnitus, irreversible hearing loss. **Miscellaneous:** Hematuria, acute gout, abnormal LFTs in seriously ill clients on multiple drug therapy including ethacrynic acid, blurred vision, rash, local irritation and pain following parenteral use, hyperuricemia/glycemia.
Ethacrynic acid may cause death in critically ill clients refractory to other

---

Bold Italic = life threatening side effect   ■ = black box warning   ✦ = Available in Canada

diuretics. These include (a) clients with severe myocardial disease who also received digitalis and who developed acute hypokalemia with fatal arrhythmias and (b) those with severely decompensated hepatic cirrhosis with ascites, with or without encephalopathy, who had electrolyte imbalances. *Death is due to intensification of the electrolyte effect.*

OD OVERDOSE MANAGEMENT
Symptoms: Profound water loss, electrolyte depletion (causes dizziness, weakness, mental confusion, vomiting, anorexia, lethargy, cramps), dehydration, reduction of blood volume, *circulatory collapse (possibility of vascular thrombosis and embolism).* *Treatment:* Replace electrolytes and fluid and monitor urine output and serum electrolyte levels. Induce emesis or perform gastric lavage. Artificial respiration and oxygen may be needed. Treat other symptoms.

HOW SUPPLIED
Ethacrynate Sodium: *Powder for Injection:* 50 mg/vial.
Ethacrynic Acid: *Tablets:* 25 mg, 50 mg.

DOSAGE
ETHACRYNATE SODIUM
• IV
  Diuresis.
Adults: 50 mg (base) (or 0.5–1 mg/kg); may be repeated in 2–4 hr, although only one dose is usually needed. A single 100-mg dose IV has also been used.
ETHACRYNIC ACID
• TABLETS
  Diuresis.
Adults, initial: 50–200 mg/day in single or divided doses to produce a gradual weight loss of 1–2 lb/day. The dose can be increased by 25–50 mg/day if needed. **Maintenance:** Usually 50–200 mg (up to a maximum of 400 mg) daily may be required in severe, refractory edema. If used with other diuretics, the initial dose should be 25 mg with increments of 25 mg. **Pediatric, initial:** 25 mg/day; can increase by 25 mg/day if needed. **Maintenance:** Adjust dose to needs of client. Dosage for infants has not been determined.

NURSING CONSIDERATIONS
ADMINISTRATION/STORAGE
1. Due to local pain and irritation, do not give SC or IM.
2. Ammonium chloride or arginine chloride may be prescribed for those at a higher risk of developing metabolic acidosis.
IV 3. Reconstitute by adding 50 mL of D5W or NaCl injection to powder.
4. Administer intermittent IV slowly over a 30-min period, given either directly or through IV tubing. For direct IV, may give at a rate of 10 mg/min.
5. When reconstituted with D5W injection, if the resulting solution is hazy or opalescent; do not use. Do not mix solution with whole blood or its derivatives.
6. If a second IV injection is necessary, use a different site to prevent thrombophlebitis.
7. Use reconstituted solutions within 24 hr; discard any unused solution.

ASSESSMENT
1. Note reasons for therapy, other agents trialed, outcome.
2. Assess for diabetes or cirrhosis; ensure not anuric.
3. Drug acts on the ascending loop of Henle and the proximal and distal tubules. Urinary output usually dose dependent and R/T fluid accumulation. Water and electrolyte excretion may be several times that with thiazide diuretics, since drug inhibits reabsorption
4. Monitor electrolytes, CBC, renal and LFTs; avoid with severe liver/renal failure. With prolonged therapy, obtain hearing test.

INTERVENTIONS
1. Monitor VS, I&O, and weight. Note excessive diuresis or weight loss; electrolyte imbalance may occur quickly.
2. With rapid excessive diuresis, assess for pain in calves, pelvic area, or the chest; rapid hemoconcentration may cause thromboembolic effects.
3. Drug should be withdrawn if severe, watery diarrhea presents. Test for occult blood in urine and stools.
4. Observe for vestibular disturbances. Do not administer concomitantly with

E

any other ototoxic agent. Hearing loss is most common following high or rapid IV dosing.

5. Monitor serum K$^+$ levels; assess need for supplemental potassium.

6. Since drug has such a profound effect on sodium excretion, dietary salt restriction is not necessary; if sodium is restricted, hyponatremia may result.

CLIENT/FAMILY TEACHING

1. Take tablets after meals and early in the day to ensure sleep is not interrupted due to voiding.

2. Change positions slowly to prevent any sudden drop in BP and associated dizziness. Avoid activities that require mental alertness until drug effects realized.

3. Monitor weight, I&O, and BP; report any excessive weight gain, SOB, swelling of hands or feet, adverse effects, or lack of response.

4. Keep all F/U appointments to evaluate response to therapy.

OUTCOMES/EVALUATE

• Enhanced diuresis
• ↓ Edema (↑ weight loss)
• ↓ Abdominal girth R/T ascites

Ethosuximide
(eth-oh-**SUCKS**-ih-myd)

CLASSIFICATION(S):
Anticonvulsant, succinimide
PREGNANCY CATEGORY: C
Rx: Zarontin.

SEE ALSO *ANTICONVULSANTS.*

USES

Absence (petit mal) seizures. May be given concomitantly with other anticonvulsants if other types of epilepsy are manifested with absence seizures.

ACTION/KINETICS

Action

Suppresses the paroxysmal 3-cycle/sec spike and wave activity that is associated with lapses of consciousness seen in absence seizures. Act by depressing the motor cortex and by raising the threshold of the CNS to convulsive stimuli.

Pharmacokinetics

Rapidly absorbed from the GI tract. **Peak serum levels:** 3–7 hr. t½, **adults:** 40–60 hr; t½, **children:** 30 hr. Steady serum levels reached in 7–10 days. **Therapeutic serum levels:** 40–100 mcg/mL. Metabolized in the liver. Both inactive metabolites and unchanged drug are excreted in the urine. Not bound to plasma protein.

CONTRAINDICATIONS

Hypersensitivity to succinimides.

SPECIAL CONCERNS

Safe use during pregnancy has not been established. Use with caution in clients with abnormal liver and kidney function.

SIDE EFFECTS

Most Common

Drowsiness, dizziness, blurred vision, GI upset, anorexia, headache, hiccoughs.

CNS: Drowsiness, ataxia, dizziness, headaches, euphoria, lethargy, fatigue, insomnia, irritability, nervousness, dream-like state, hyperactivity. Psychiatric or psychologic aberrations such as mental slowing, hypochondriasis, sleep disturbances, inability to concentrate, depression, night terrors, instability, confusion, aggressiveness. Rarely, auditory hallucinations, paranoid psychosis, increased libido, suicidal behavior. **GI:** N&V, hiccoughs, anorexia, diarrhea, GI upset, weight loss, abdominal/epigastric pain, cramps, constipation. **Hematologic:** Leukopenia, granulocytopenia, eosinophilia, *agranulocytosis,* pancytopenia with or without bone marrow suppression, monocytosis. **Dermatologic:** Pruritus, urticaria, erythema multiforme, lupus erythematosus, *Stevens-Johnson syndrome,* pruritic erythematous rashes, skin eruptions, alopecia, hirsutism, photophobia. **GU:** Urinary frequency, vaginal bleeding, renal damage, microscopic hematuria. **Miscellaneous:** Blurred vision, muscle weakness, hyperemia, hypertrophy of gums, swollen tongue, myopia, periorbital edema.

OD OVERDOSE MANAGEMENT

Symptoms: **Acute Overdose:** Confusion, sleepiness, slow shallow respiration, N&V, *CNS depression with coma and*

---

respiratory depression, hypotension, cyanosis, hyper/hypothermia, absence of reflexes, unsteadiness, flaccid muscles.
Chronic Overdose: Ataxia, dizziness, drowsiness, confusion, depression, proteinuria, skin rashes, hangover, irritability, poor judgment, N&V, muscle weakness, periorbital edema, hepatic dysfunction, **fatal bone marrow aplasia, delayed onset of coma,** nephrosis, hematuria, casts.
Treatment: General supportive measures. Charcoal hemoperfusion may be helpful.

DRUG INTERACTIONS
Estrogens, Progestins / ↓ Plasma hormone levels → ↓ effect
Hydantoins / ↑ Hydantoin effect R/T ↓ breakdown by the liver
Isoniazid / ↑ Ethosuximide effects
Valproic acid / ↑ Ethosuximide effects

HOW SUPPLIED
Capsules: 250 mg; *Syrup:* 250 mg/5 mL.

DOSAGE
- **CAPSULES; SYRUP**
  Absence seizures.
Adults and children over 6 years, initial: 250 mg twice a day; the dose may be increased by 250 mg/day at 4–7-day intervals until seizures are controlled or until total daily dose reaches 1.5 grams.
Children under 6 years, initial: 250 mg/day; dosage may be increased by 250 mg/day every 4–7 days until control is established or total daily dose reaches 1 gram.

NURSING CONSIDERATIONS
ADMINISTRATION/STORAGE
May be given with other anticonvulsants when other forms of epilepsy are present.
ASSESSMENT
1. Note reasons for therapy, onset, characteristics of seizures, other agents trialed, outcome. List any predisposing factors (e.g., SAH, head trauma, etc.).
2. Monitor EKG, CBC, renal, LFTs. Assess clinical presentation, mental/emotional status; ensure not pregnant.
3. Any S&S of infection (e.g., sore throat, fever) warrant blood counts.

There have been several cases of lupus associated with drug therapy.
CLIENT/FAMILY TEACHING
1. Take with meals to minimize GI upset. Do not stop abruptly; may increase severity and frequency of seizures. Report any increase in frequency of seizures or unusual side effects.
2. Avoid hazardous activities while on drug therapy. May experience dizziness, drowsiness, confusion, headaches, and blurred vision.
3. Any persistent fever, swollen glands, and bleeding gums may signal a blood dyscrasia and require reporting. Report significant weight loss, rash, joint pain, fever.
4. Need lab studies q 3 mo to assess uric acid levels, hematologic values, liver and renal function.
5. Avoid alcohol and CNS depressants during therapy.
6. Alert family to the possibility of transient personality changes, hypochondriacal behavior, and aggressiveness, which should be reported. Keep all F/U appointments to evaluate response to therapy.

OUTCOMES/EVALUATE
- ↓ Frequency; ↑ control of seizures
- Therapeutic serum drug levels (40–100 mcg/mL)

Etidronate disodium
(eh-tih-**DROH**-nayt)

CLASSIFICATION(S):
Bone growth regulator, bisphosphonate
PREGNANCY CATEGORY: B
Rx: Didronel.

USES
PO: (1) Paget's disease (osteitis deformans), especially of the polyostotic type accompanied by pain and increased urine levels of hydroxyproline and serum alkaline phosphatase. (2) Prevention and treatment of heterotopic ossification due to spinal cord injury or total hip replacement. *Investigational:* Pre-

vention and treatment of corticosteroid-induced osteoporosis.

ACTION/KINETICS

Action
Slows bone metabolism, thereby decreasing bone resorption, bone turnover, and new bone formation; it also reduces bone vascularization. Renal tubular reabsorption of calcium is not affected.

Pharmacokinetics
Absorption: Dose-dependent; after 24 hr, one-half of absorbed drug is excreted unchanged. Absorption is affected by food or preparations containing divalent ions. **Onset:** 1 month for Paget's disease and within 24 hr for hypercalcemia. The drug remaining in the body is adsorbed to bone, where therapeutic effects for Paget's disease persist 3–12 months after discontinuation of the drug. **Plasma t½:** 6 hr; **bone t½:** Over 90 days. Approximately 50% excreted unchanged in the urine; unabsorbed drug is excreted through the feces.

CONTRAINDICATIONS
Enterocolitis, fracture of long bones, hypercalcemia of hyperparathyroidism. Serum creatinine greater than 5 mg/dL.

SPECIAL CONCERNS
Use with caution in the presence of renal dysfunction, in active UGI problems, and during lactation. Safety and efficacy have not been established in children.

SIDE EFFECTS
Most Common
After PO use: Diarrhea, nausea, increased or recurrent bone pain at pagetic sites, onset of pain at previously asymptomatic sites.
GI: Nausea, diarrhea, constipation, ulcerative stomatitis, altered taste, loss of taste. **Bones:** Increased incidence of bone fractures and increased or recurrent bone pain. Drug should be discontinued if fracture occurs and not restarted until healing takes place. Onset of pain at previously asymptomatic sites. Osteonecrosis, primarily in the jaw, especially with cancers of the oral cavity. **Allergy:** Angioedema, rash, pruritus, urticaria. **Electrolytes:** Hypophosphatemia, hypomagnesemia. **Miscellaneous:** Metallic taste, chest pain, abnormal hepatic function, fever, fluid overload, dyspnea, convulsions. Symptoms of rachitic syndrome have been reported in children receiving 10 mg or more/kg daily for long periods (up to 1 year) to treat heterotopic ossification or soft tissue calcification.

LABORATORY TEST CONSIDERATIONS
Hypomagnesemia, hypophosphatemia.

OD OVERDOSE MANAGEMENT
Symptoms: Following PO ingestion, hypocalcemia may occur. Rapid IV administration may cause renal insufficiency. *Treatment:* Gastric lavage following PO ingestion. Treat hypocalcemia by giving calcium IV.

DRUG INTERACTIONS
Products containing calcium or other multivalent cations ↓ absorption of etidronate

HOW SUPPLIED
Tablets: 200 mg, 400 mg.

DOSAGE
• TABLETS
Paget's disease.
Adults, initial: 5–10 mg/kg/day for 6 months or less; or, 11–20 mg/kg for a maximum of 3 months. Reserve doses above 10 mg/kg when lower doses are ineffective, when there is a need for suppression of increased bone turnover, or when a prompt decrease in cardiac output is needed. Do not exceed doses of 20 mg/kg/day. Another course of therapy may be instituted after a rest period of 3 months if there is evidence of active disease process. Monitor every 3 to 6 months.

Heterotopic ossification due to spinal cord injury.
Adults: 20 mg/kg/day for 2 weeks; **then** 10 mg/kg/day for 10 weeks. Treatment should be initiated as soon as possible after the injury, preferably before evidence of heterotopic ossification.

Heterotopic ossification due to total hip replacement.
Initial: 20 mg/kg/day for 1 month preoperatively; **then,** 20 mg/kg/day for 3 months postoperatively for a total treatment duration of 4 months.

NURSING CONSIDERATIONS

ADMINISTRATION/STORAGE

1. Administer PO as a single dose (if GI upset occurs, divide dose) with juice or water 2 hr before meals.

2. There are no indications to date that etidronate will affect mature heterotopic bone.

3. Avoid excessive heat (over 104°F) for tablets.

ASSESSMENT

1. Note reasons for therapy, other agents trialed, clinical presentation; rate pain level.

2. Assess for evidence of renal dysfunction. Monitor uric acid, alkaline phosphatase, urinary hydroxyproline excretion, electrolytes, Mg, phosphate, calcium, PTH, and renal function studies.

3. Determine if pregnant.

4. Review x-rays/bone density for evidence of bone loss/fracture or pagetic lesions.

CLIENT/FAMILY TEACHING

1. Drug slows accelerated bone turnover (resorption and accretion) in pagetic lesions and, to a lesser extent, in normal bone.

2. Maintain a well-balanced diet with adequate intake of calcium and vitamin D; see dietitian p.r.n.

3. Take with a full glass of water. Do not eat for 2 hr after taking medication. Foods high in calcium (e.g., milk, milk products) and vitamins with mineral supplements (e.g., Al, calcium, iron, or Mg) may decrease absorption. If GI upset with single dose, may divide dose.

4. Report any unusual pain, muscle twitching/spasms, diarrhea, headaches, restricted mobility or pain/heat over bone site, and S&S of hypercalcemia, i.e., lethargy, N&V, anorexia, tremors, and pain.

5. Obtain lab studies as scheduled: with Paget's disease, reduced levels of urinary hydroxyproline excretion and serum alkaline phosphatase indicate a beneficial therapeutic response. Levels usually decrease 1–3 months after initiation of therapy.

6. With hypercalcemia, serum calcium levels show drug response and need for continued therapy. Reduction usually occurs in 2–8 days in hypercalcemia R/T bone metastasis. Therapy may be repeated only after 7 days of rest; risk for hypocalcemia greatest 3 days after IV therapy.

OUTCOMES/EVALUATE

- Suppression of bone resorption
- ↓ Serum calcium levels; ↓ fractures
- Reductions in serum alkaline phosphatase and urinary hydroxyproline levels
- ↓ Bone pain with Paget's disease

Etodolac
(ee-toh-**DOH**-lack)

CLASSIFICATION(S):
Nonsteroidal anti-inflammatory drug
PREGNANCY CATEGORY: C
✤Rx: Apo-Etodolac, Ultradol.

SEE ALSO *NONSTEROIDAL ANTI-INFLAMMATORY DRUGS.*

USES

(1) Relief of signs and symptoms of osteoarthritis, rheumatoid arthritis, and juvenile rheumatoid arthritis. (2) Mild to moderate pain.

ACTION/KINETICS

Action

Etodolac is an NSAID in a class called the pyranocarboxylic acids. Anti-inflammatory effect likely due to inhibition of cyclo-oxygenase which results in decreased prostaglandin synthesis. Effective in reducing joint swelling, pain, and morning stiffness in those with inflammatory disease.

Pharmacokinetics

Over 80% bioavailable. **Time to peak levels:** 1–2 hr. **Onset of analgesic action:** 30 min; **duration:** 4–12 hr. t½: 7.3 hr. The drug is metabolized by the liver and metabolites are excreted through the kidneys (72%) and feces (16%). **Plasma protein binding:** More than 99%.

CONTRAINDICATIONS

Clients in whom etodolac, aspirin, or other NSAIDs have caused asthma, rhinitis, urticaria, or other allergic reactions. Use during lactation, during labor and delivery, and in children.

SPECIAL CONCERNS
Use with caution in impaired renal or hepatic function, heart failure, those on diuretics, and in geriatric clients. Safety and effectiveness have not been determined in children.

ADDITIONAL SIDE EFFECTS
Most Common
Dizziness, asthenia/malaise, abdominal pain/cramps, diarrhea, nausea, flatulence.
See *Nonsteroidal Anti-Inflammatory Drugs* for a complete listing of side effects. **GI:** Diarrhea, gastritis, thirst, ulcerative stomatitis, anorexia. **CNS:** Nervousness, depression. **CV:** Syncope. **Respiratory:** Asthma. **Dermatologic:** *Angioedema*, vesiculobullous rash, cutaneous vasculitis with purpura, hyperpigmentation. **Miscellaneous:** Jaundice, hepatitis.

ADDITIONAL DRUG INTERACTIONS
Cyclosporine / ↑ Cyclosporine levels R/T ↓ renal excretion; ↑ risk of cyclosporine-induced nephrotoxicity
Digoxin / ↑ Digoxin levels R/T ↓ renal excretion
Lithium / ↑ Lithium levels R/T ↓ renal excretion
Methotrexate / ↑ Methotrexate levels R/T ↓ renal excretion

LABORATORY TEST CONSIDERATIONS
False + reaction for urinary bilirubin and for urinary ketones (using the dip-stick method). ↑ Liver enzymes, serum creatinine. ↑ Bleeding time.

OD OVERDOSE MANAGEMENT
Symptoms: N&V, drowsiness, lethargy, epigastric pain, **anaphylaxis.** Rarely, hypertension, acute renal failure, respiratory depression. *Treatment:* Since there are no antidotes, treatment is supportive and symptomatic. If discovered within 4 hr, emesis followed by activated charcoal and an osmotic cathartic may be tried.

HOW SUPPLIED
Capsules: 200 mg, 300 mg; *Tablets:* 400 mg, 500 mg; *Tablets, Extended-Release:* 400 mg, 500 mg, 600 mg.

DOSAGE
• CAPSULES; TABLETS; TABLETS, EXTENDED-RELEASE
Osteoarthritis, rheumatoid arthritis.
Adults, initial: 300 mg 2–3 times per day, 400 mg 2 times/day, or 500 mg 2 times per day using capsules or tablets. Dose may be adjusted up or down during long-term use, depending on the clinical response. A dose of 600 mg may suffice for chronic administration. In clients who tolerate 1,000 mg/day, the dose may be increased to 1,200 mg/day if a higher level of activity is needed. *Tablets, Extended-Release:* 400–1,000 mg given once daily. Doses above 1,200 mg/day have not been evaluated adequately, although the dose may be increased to 1,200 mg/day if needed.
Acute pain.
Adults: 200–400 mg q 6–8 hr, up to 1,000 mg/day. In some, the dose may be increased to 1,200 mg/day. Use capsules or tablets.
NOTE: Do not exceed 20 mg/kg in clients weighing 60 kg or less.
Juvenile rheumatoid arthritis (use Extended-Release Tablets).
Children, 6–16 years of age based on body weight. 20–30 kg: 1–400 mg tablet once daily. **31–45 kg:** 1–600 mg tablet once daily. **46–60 kg:** 2–400 mg tablets once daily. **>60 kg:** 2–500 mg tablets once daily.

NURSING CONSIDERATIONS
ADMINISTRATION/STORAGE
1. Seek the lowest dose and longest dosing interval for each client.
2. Dosage adjustment is usually not required in clients with mild-to-moderate renal impairment.
3. In chronic conditions, a therapeutic response with extended-release tablets may be seen within 1 week, but most often is seen by 2 weeks.
4. Store capsules and tablets from 15–30°C (59–86° F). Store extended-release tablets from 20–25°C (68–77° F).
5. Protect from excessive heat and humidity; store in tight, light-resistant containers.

Bold Italic = life threatening side effect   ■ = black box warning   ♣ = Available in Canada

ASSESSMENT
1. Note any previous experience with NSAIDs or acetylsalicylic acid and results.
2. List reasons for therapy (i.e., analgesic or anti-inflammatory), include onset, characteristics of symptoms, status of ROM; rate pain level.
3. With long-term therapy, monitor CBC, chemistry, renal and LFTs.
4. Determine history of ulcers, heart disease, or cardiac failure.
5. Note age and weight; if currently prescribed diuretics.

CLIENT/FAMILY TEACHING
1. Drug works by reducing hormones that cause inflammation and pain in the body
2. Take with milk or food to decrease GI upset.
3. May cause dizziness or drowsiness, avoid activities requiring alertness until drug effects realized.
4. Report any unusual bruising/bleeding, rash, yellow skin discoloration, dark/tarry stools, or lack of response.
5. Stop drug and report, sudden weight gain, loss of BP control, swelling in extremities, blood in stools or urine.
6. Avoid alcohol, aspirin, and other NSAIDs.
7. Use protection if exposed and avoid prolonged sun exposure.
8. Practice reliable contraception during therapy.

OUTCOMES/EVALUATE
Control of pain and inflammation with improved joint mobility

——COMBINATION DRUG——

Etonogestrel/ Ethinyl estradiol vaginal ring ■

CLASSIFICATION(S):
Contraceptive
PREGNANCY CATEGORY: X
Rx: NuvaRing.

SEE ALSO *ESTROGENS* AND *ORAL CONTRACEPTIVES: ESTROGEN-PROGESTERONE COMBINATIONS*

USES
Prevention of pregnancy.

CONTENT
In each ring: 11.7 mg etonogestrel and 2.7 mg ethinyl estradiol.

ACTION/KINETICS
Action
The product is a nonbiodegradable, flexible, transparent, colorless to almost colorless contraceptive vaginal ring containing a progestin (etonogestrel) and an estrogen (ethinyl estradiol). In the vagina, each ring releases an average of 0.12 mg/day of etonogestrel and 0.015 mg/day of ethinyl estradiol over a 3-week period of use. The primary action is inhibition of ovulation although changes in the cervical mucus (decreasing sperm motility) and the endometrium (reducing possibility of implantation) add to the contraceptive effectiveness.

Pharmacokinetics
Both hormones are rapidly absorbed into the systemic circulation and are metabolized by the liver cytochrome CYP3A4 isoenzyme. Both hormones are excreted in the urine, bile, and feces.

CONTRAINDICATIONS
See *Estrogens* and *Oral Contraceptives: Estrogen-Progesterone Combinations.*

SPECIAL CONCERNS
See *Estrogens* and *Oral Contraceptives: Estrogen-Progesterone Combinations..*
■ See Estrogens in Chapter 2 for Black Box Warnings.■

SIDE EFFECTS
Most Common
Vaginitis, headache, URTI, leukorrhea, sinusitis, weight gain, nausea.
See *Estrogens* and *Oral Contraceptives: Estrogen-Progesterone Combinations* for a complete list of possible side effects. **Device-related events:** Foreign body sensation, coital problems, device expulsion, vaginal discomfort, vaginitis, leukorrhea, headache, emotional lability, weight gain. **Serious: *Thrombophlebitis, venous thrombosis with or without embolism, arterial thromboembolism, pulmonary embolism, MI, cerebral hemorrhage, cerebral thrombosis, hepatic adenomas,*** hypertension, gall bladder disease, benign liver

E

tumors, mesenteric thrombosis, retinal thrombosis. **GI:** Cholestatic jaundice, abdominal cramps, bloating, N&V. **GU:** Amenorrhea, breakthrough bleeding, breast tenderness/enlargement/secretion, change in cervical erosion and secretion, change in menstrual flow, decrease in lactation when given immediately postpartum, spotting, temporary infertility after discontinuing treatment, vaginal candidiasis. **Miscellaneous:** Increase or decrease in weight, steepening of corneal curvature, edema, intolerance to contact lenses, melasma, mental depression, migraine, allergic rash, decreased tolerance to carbohydrates.

DRUG INTERACTIONS
See *Estrogens* and *Oral Contraceptives: Estrogen-Progesterone Combinations*

HOW SUPPLIED
See *Content*.

DOSAGE

• **VAGINAL RING**
Prevention of pregnancy.
One vaginal ring is inserted by the woman in the vagina. Ring remains in place for 3 weeks and is removed for a 1-week break. A new ring is inserted 1 week after the last ring was removed on the same day of the week as it was inserted in the previous cycle.

NURSING CONSIDERATIONS
ADMINISTRATION/STORAGE
1. If switching from a progestin-only method, insert the first vaginal ring as follows:

• Any day of the month when switching from a progestin-only tablet; do not skip any days between the last tablet and the first day of vaginal ring use.

• On the same day as the contraceptive implant removal.

• On the same day as removal of a progestin-containing IUD.

• On the day when the next contraceptive injection would be due. In all of these situations, advise use of an additional method of contraception for the first 7 days after ring insertion.

2. The client may start using the vaginal ring within the first 5 days following a complete first trimester abortion. No additional method of contraception is required. If the vaginal ring is not inserted within 5 days and no preceding hormonal contraceptive was used in the past month, count the first day of menses as day 1 and insert the vaginal ring on or prior to day 5 of the cycle, even if menses has not finished.

3. Following delivery or a second-trimester abortion, insert the vaginal ring 4 weeks postpartum in women who are not breast-feeding. A woman who is breast-feeding should not use the vaginal ring until the child is weaned. Initiate use of the vaginal ring 4 weeks after a second-trimester abortion. However, there is an increased risk of thromboembolic disease. If a woman begins using the vaginal ring postpartum and has not yet had a period, it is possible that ovulation and conception has occurred prior to the insertion of the vaginal ring.

4. If the client has not adhered to the prescribed regimen, consider the possibility of pregnancy at the time of the first missed period. Discontinue the use of the vaginal ring if pregnancy is confirmed. Rule out pregnancy if the client has adhered to the regimen and misses 2 consecutive periods.

5. Once dispensed to the user, the vaginal rings can be stored for up to 4 months at 15–30°C (59–86°F). Avoid storing in direct sunlight. When dispensed to the user, place an expiration date on the label. The date should not be more than 4 months from the date of dispensing or the expiration date, whichever comes first.

ASSESSMENT
1. Ensure client has undergone gyn exam and understands contraception and ring use and is a candidate for therapy.

2. Therapy may increase risk of thromboembolism especially with smoking, CVA, and BP readings. Monitor VS, blood sugar and lipid panel.

CLIENT/FAMILY TEACHING
1. The flexible ring is placed in the vagina to prevent pregnancy. It is inserted and left in place for 3 weeks.

Bold Italic = life threatening side effect   ■ = black box warning   ♣ = Available in Canada

2. Wash and dry your hands.

3. Remove one contraceptive ring from its foil pouch, but do not throw away the pouch. Save the pouch so you can use it to discard the old contraceptive ring after you remove it.

4. May select the insertion position that is most comfortable (e.g., standing with one leg up, squatting, or lying down). Compress the ring and insert into the vagina. The exact position of the ring inside the vagina is not critical for activity.

5. Remove the vaginal ring after three weeks in place by hooking the index finger under the forward rim or by grasping the rim between the index and middle finger and pulling it out. Place the used ring in the foil pouch and discard in a waste receptacle out of the reach of children and pets. Do not flush in the toilet.

6. Withdrawal bleeding usually starts on day 2 to 3 after removal but may not have finished before the next ring is inserted. However, it is imperative that the new ring must be inserted 1 week after the previous one was removed in order to maintain contraceptive efficacy.

7. It is possible that ovulation and conception may occur before the first use of the vaginal ring. During the first cycle, an additional method of contraception should be used until after the first 7 days of ring use.

8. If no preceding hormonal contraceptive was used in the past month, count the first day of menses as day 1 and insert the vaginal ring on or prior to day 5 of the cycle, even if menses has not finished.

9. If switching from a combination oral contraceptive to the vaginal ring, insert the vaginal ring anytime within 7 days after the last combination oral contraceptive tablet and no later than the day that a new cycle of tablets would have started. No backup method of contraception is required.

10. If there has been inadvertent removal, expulsion, or prolonged ring-free intervals during the 3-week use period, rinse the ring with cool to lukewarm (not hot) water and reinsert as soon as possible, at the latest within 3 hours. Contraceptive effectiveness is reduced if the ring has been out of the vagina for more than 3 hours. Thus, use an additional form of contraception until the ring has been used continuously for 7 days. Consider the possibility of pregnancy if the ring-free interval has been extended beyond 1 week.

11. If the vaginal ring has been left in place for up to 1 extra week, remove it and insert a new ring after a 1-week ring-free interval. Rule out pregnancy if the vaginal ring has been left in place for more than 4 weeks.

12. Ring does not prevent the spread of HIV or other sexually transmitted diseases.

13. Store away from light/heat.

14. Report any problems related to usage or adverse side effects or suspected pregnancy.

OUTCOMES/EVALUATE
Desired contraception

Etoposide ■ IV
(VP-16–213)
(eh-**TOH**-poh-syd)

CLASSIFICATION(S):
Antineoplastic, miscellaneous
PREGNANCY CATEGORY: D
Rx: Etopophos, Toposar, VePesid.

SEE ALSO ANTINEOPLASTIC AGENTS.

USES
With combination therapy to treat refractory testicular tumors and small cell lung cancer. *Investigational:* Alone or in combination to treat acute monocytic leukemia, non-Hodgkin's lymphoma, Hodgkin's disease, AIDS-associated Kaposi's sarcoma, Ewing's sarcoma. Also, choriocarcinoma; hepatocellular carcinoma; non-small cell lung, breast, endometrial, and gastric cancers; acute lymphocytic leukemia; soft tissue carcinoma; rhabdomyosarcoma.

ACTION/KINETICS

Action

Acts as a mitotic inhibitor at the G_2 portion of the cell cycle to inhibit DNA synthesis. At high doses, cells entering mitosis are lysed, whereas at low doses, cells will not enter prophase.

Pharmacokinetics

$t\frac{1}{2}$: **biphasic, initial,** 1.5 hr; **final,** 4–11 hr. **Effective plasma levels:** 0.3–10 mcg/mL. Poor CNS penetration. Eliminated through both the urine and bile unchanged and as liver metabolites. Is water soluble.

CONTRAINDICATIONS

Lactation.

SPECIAL CONCERNS

■ Severe myelosuppression with resulting infection or bleeding may occur.■ Safety and efficacy in children have not been established.

SIDE EFFECTS

Most Common

Alopecia (reversible), leukopenia, anorexia, N&V, diarrhea, stomatitis, neutropenia, anemia, thrombocytopenia, dysphagia, abdominal pain.

See *Antineoplastic Agents* for a complete list of possible side effects. ***Anaphylactic-type reactions***, hypotension, peripheral neuropathy, somnolence.

ADDITIONAL DRUG INTERACTIONS

Atovaquone / ↑ Risk of etoposide-related secondary acute myeloid leukemia
Grapefruit juice / ↓ Etoposide AUC and absolute bioavailability

HOW SUPPLIED

Capsules: 50 mg; *Injection:* 20 mg/mL; *Powder for Injection, Lyophilized:* 100 mg.

DOSAGE

• **IV**

Testicular carcinoma.

50–100 mg/m²/day on days 1–5 or 100 mg/m²/day on days 1, 3, and 5 q 3–4 weeks (i.e., after recovery from toxic effects). Used in combination with other agents.

Small cell lung carcinoma.

35 mg/m²/day for 4 days to 50 mg/m²/day for 5 days, repeated q 3–4 weeks.

• **CAPSULES**

Small cell lung carcinoma.

70 mg/m² (rounded to the nearest 50 mg) daily for 4 days to 100 mg/m² (rounded to the nearest 50 mg) daily for 5 days; repeat q 3–4 weeks. *NOTE:* Etopophos is given in higher concentrations than VePesid. Doses above are for VePesid.

NURSING CONSIDERATIONS

ADMINISTRATION/STORAGE

1. Store capsules at 2–8°C (36–46°F); do not freeze.

IV 2. For IV use, dilute drug with either D5W or 0.9% NaCl for final concentration of 0.2 or 0.4 mg/mL (5-mL vial in 250 or 500 mL of IV solution).

3. A slow infusion over 30–60 min will decrease chance of hypotension. Do not give by rapid IV push; may give over a period of 5 min.

4. Wear gloves when preparing; if drug comes in contact with the skin or mucosa, wash immediately and thoroughly with soap and water.

5. Diluted solutions with a final concentration of 0.2 mg/mL are stable for 96 hr at room temperature; final concentrations of 0.4 mg/mL are stable for 48 hr at room temperature.

ASSESSMENT

1. Note condition being treated, other agents trialed, outcome. Assess nutritional status. Pretreat with antiemetic; drug may cause N&V.

2. Determine if pregnant. Monitor CBC, renal and LFTs; may cause increased uric acid levels and granulocyte and platelet suppression. Nadir: 14 days; recovery: 21 days.

3. Assess for signs of infection and bleeding; occurs more often with this drug than with most antineoplastic agents. Be prepared to treat anaphylactic reactions.

4. With infusions, stress bed rest and supervise ambulation as orthostatic hypotension may occur. Record BP during infusions and at least twice a day with PO therapy; note any decreases.

CLIENT/FAMILY TEACHING

1. Take as directed; store capsules in the refrigerator.

Bold Italic = life threatening side effect   ■ = black box warning   ♣ = Available in Canada

2. Report any flu-like symptoms; drug combination therapy may cause severe bone marrow suppression.

3. Consume 2–3 L/day of fluids to prevent kidney damage.

4. May experience sudden drop in BP; change positions slowly. May also cause marked hair loss and blood cell abnormalities.

5. Report sores in mouth so treatment may be initiated. Avoid irritants such as tobacco, alcohol, and hot spicy foods.

6. May feel fatigued and sleepy during/after drug administration; schedule activities to ensure adequate rest.

7. Report any tingling sensations or numbness (S&S of peripheral neuropathy). Report weight loss or if N&V impairs food/fluid intake.

8. Practice reliable contraception.

OUTCOMES/EVALUATE
• ↓ Malignant cell proliferation
• Improved hematologic parameters with leukemia

Etravirine
(ee-tra-**VIR**-een)

CLASSIFICATION(S):
Antiviral, non-nucleoside reverse transcriptase inhibitor
PREGNANCY CATEGORY: B
Rx: Intelence.

USES
In combination with other antiretroviral drugs to treat HIV-1 infection in antiretroviral treatment-experienced clients who have evidence of viral replication and HIV-1 strains resistant to nonnucleoside reverse transcriptase inhibitors and other antiretroviral drugs.

ACTION/KINETICS
Action
Entravirine binds directly to reverse transcriptase and blocks the RNA- and DNA-dependent DNA polymerase activities by causing a disruption of the enzyme's catalytic site. The drug does not inhibit the human DNA polymerases alpha, beta, or gamma.

Pharmacokinetics
Time to maximum plasma levels: About 2.5–4 hr. Absorption is not affected by drugs that increase gastric pH (e.g., omeprazole, ranitidine). The AUC is decreased by about 50% under fasting conditions; thus, always take etravirine following a meal. Metabolized primarily by CYP3A4, CYP2C9, and CYP2C19. Nearly 94% is excreted in the feces. $t^{1/2}$, **terminal elimination:** About 41 hr. **Plasma protein binding:** About 99.9%.

CONTRAINDICATIONS
Lactation.

SPECIAL CONCERNS
Use caution when selecting the dose for geriatric clients. Safety and efficacy have not been determined in children.

SIDE EFFECTS
Most Common
Rash (any type), N&V, diarrhea, fatigue, abdominal pain, hypertension, peripheral neuropathy, headache.

GI: Diarrhea, N&V, abdominal pain/distension, anorexia, constipation, dry mouth, flatulence, gastritis, GERD, hematemesis, *pancreatitis*, retching, stomatitis. **Hepatic:** Cytolytic hepatitis, hepatic steatosis, hepatitis, hepatomegaly. **CNS:** Peripheral neuropathy, headache, abnormal dreams, amnesia, anxiety, confused state, *convulsion*, disorientation, hypersomnia, hypesthesia, insomnia, nervousness, nightmares, paresthesia, sleep disorders, sluggishness, somnolence, syncope, tremor. **CV:** Hypertension, angina pectoris, atrial fibrillation, *MI, hemorrhagic stroke*. **Dermatologic:** Mild to moderate rash, dry skin, hyperhidrosis, lipohypertrophy, night sweats, pruritus, swelling face, *Stevens-Johnson syndrome, hypersensitivity reaction, erythema multiforme*. **Respiratory:** *Bronchospasm*, exertional dyspnea. **GU:** Gynecomastia, renal failure. **Hematologic:** Anemia, hemolytic anemia. **Metabolic:** Diabetes mellitus, dyslipidemia. **Body as a whole:** Fatigue, redistribution/accumulation of body fat (including central obesity, dorsocervial fat enlargement, peripheral wasting, facial wasting, breast enlargement, cushingoid appear-

E

---

ance), immune reconstitution syndrome (i.e., inflammatory response to indolent or residual opportunistic infections, such as *Mycobacterium avium* complex, cytomegalovirus, *Pneumocystis jiroveci*, pneumonia, tuberculosis), **angioneurotic edema. Miscellaneous:** Blurred vision, vertigo, drug hypersensitivity, acquired lipodystrophy.

LABORATORY TEST CONSIDERATIONS

↑ Pancreatic amylase, lipase, creatinine, neutrophils, platelets, total cholesterol, LDL, triglycerides, glucose, ALT, AST. ↓ Hemoglobin. *NOTE:* ALT and AST abnormalities occur more frequently in clients with hepatitis B and/or hepatitis C.

OD OVERDOSE MANAGEMENT

Symptoms: Extension of side effects. *Treatment:* General supportive measures, including monitoring of vital signs and observation of the clinical status. Eliminate unabsorbed drug by gastric lavage and/or administration of activated charcoal. Because etravirine is highly bound to plasma proteins, it is unlikely hemodialysis or peritoneal dialysis will remove significant quantities of the drug.

DRUG INTERACTIONS

Because etravirine is a substrate of CYP3A4, CYP2C9, and CYP2C19, coadministration with drugs that induce or inhibit these enzymes may alter the therapeutic effect or side effects of etravirine. Also, etravirine is an inducer of CYP3A4 and inhibitor of CYP2C9 and CYP2C19; thus, coadministration of drugs that are substrates of these enzymes with etravirine may alter the therapeutic effect or side effects of the coadministered drug(s).

Antiarrhythmic drugs (e.g., amiodarone, bepridil, disopyramide, flecainide, systemic lidocaine, mexiletine, propafenone, quinidine) / ↓ Concentrations of antiarrhythmic drugs; use together with caution

Anticonvulsants (e.g., carbamazepine, phenobarbital, phenytoin) / Significant ↓ in etravirine levels → loss of therapeutic effect R/T induction of CYP450 enzymes

Atazanavir/Ritonavir / Etravirine AUC 100% higher; also, possible significant ↓ in atazanavir minimum plasma levels → loss of atazanavir therapeutic effect

Clarithromycin / ↓ Clarithromycin levels but ↑ of the active 14-hydroxyclarithromycin; consider using azithromycin

Darunavir/Ritonavir / Etravirine AUC ↓ by about 37%; no dosage adjustments needed

Delavirdine / ↑ Etravirine levels; do not use together

Dexamethasone (systemic) / ↓ Etravirine levels → loss of therapeutic effect; consider an alternative corticosteroid, especially if used long-term

Diazepam / ↑ Diazepam levels; possibly ↓ diazepam dose

Fluconazole / ↑ Etravirine levels

Fosamprenavir/Ritonavir / Significant ↑ amprenavir levels; do not use together

HMG-CoA reductase inhibitors (e.g., atorvastatin, fluvastatin, lovastatin, simvastatin) / ↓ Lovastatin and simvastatin levels and ↑ fluvastatin levels; possibly adjust dosage levels

Immunosuppressants (cyclosporine, sirolimus, tacrolimus) / Use together with caution R/T plasma levels of immunosuppressant may be affected

Itraconazole / ↑ Etravirine levels; ↓ itraconazole levels; dosage adjustment may be needed

Ketoconazole / ↑ Etravirine levels; ↓ ketoconazole levels; dosage adjustment may be needed

Lopinavir/Ritonavir / Etravirine AUC 85% higher; coadminister with caution

Methadone / Methadone maintenance therapy may have to be adjusted in some clients

Non-nucleoside reverse transcriptase inhibitors (e.g., efavirenz, nevirapine) / Significant ↓ etravirine levels → loss of therapeutic effect; avoid coadministration

PDE-5 inhibitors (e.g., sildenafil, tadalafil, vardenafil) / Dose of sildenafil may need adjustment depending on clinical effect

Posaconazole / ↑ Etravirine levels

Protease inhibitors (atazanavir, fosamprenavir, indinavir, nelfinavir) / Possible significant alteration (↑ or ↓) of plasma levels of protease inhibitor if taken without low-dose ritonavir; do not give

---

Bold Italic = life threatening side effect   ■ = black box warning   ✦ = Available in Canada

etravirine with protease inhibitors without low-dose ritonavir

Rifampin or Rifapentine / Significant ↓ etravirine levels → loss of therapeutic effect; do not use together

Ritonavir / Significant ↓ etravirine levels if used with ritonavir, 600 mg twice a day → loss of therapeutic effect

Saquinavir/Ritonavir / Etravirine AUC ↓ 33%; no dosage adjustment needed

H *St. John's wort* / Significant ↓ etravirine levels → loss of therapeutic effect; do not use together

Tipranavir/Ritonavir / Significant ↓ etravirine levels → loss of therapeutic effect; do not use together

Voriconazole / ↑ Plasma levels of both drugs; dosage adjustment may be needed

Warfarin / Possible ↑ warfarin levels; monitor INR

HOW SUPPLIED

Tablets: 100 mg.

DOSAGE

- **TABLETS**
  HIV-1 infection.
200 mg (2 x 100 mg tablets) twice a day following a meal. The type of food does not affect exposure to the drug.

NURSING CONSIDERATIONS

ADMINISTRATION/STORAGE

1. To monitor maternal-fetal outcomes of pregnant women exposed to etravirine, health care providers are encouraged to register clients by calling 1-800-258-4263.

2. Store from 15-30°C (59-86°F) in the original bottle. Protect from moisture. Do not remove the desiccant pouches.

ASSESSMENT

1. Note disease onset, disease characteristics such as stage of infection, viral load and other therapies trialed/failed.

2. List all drugs prescribed to prevent interactions.

3. Identify if also infected with hepatitis virus.

4. Monitor CBC, LFTs, viral load, CD_4 counts. Determine if pregnant.

5. Assess lifestyle and potential to resume risky behaviors.

CLIENT/FAMILY TEACHING

1. Take as prescribed following a meal twice daily. Swallow tablets whole with water.

2. If unable to swallow tablets may place the tablets in a glass of water. Once dispersed, stir contents well and drink immediately. Rinse glass with water several times; completely swallow each rinse to ensure the entire dose is taken.

3. If a dose is missed within 6 hours of the time it is usually taken, then may take following a meal as soon as possible, and then take the next dose at the regularly scheduled time. If dose is missed by more than 6 hours of when usually taken, do not take the missed dose just resume the usual dosing schedule. Take only the dose prescribed do not increase of decrease dose or stop therapy without provider approval.

4. Drug is not a cure for HIV infection; may continue to develop opportunistic infections and other complications associated with HIV disease. Drug is always used in combination with other antiretroviral drugs.

5. Does not reduce risk of transmitting HIV through sexual contact, sharing needles, or being exposed to blood. Must continue to practice safe sex and use latex or polyurethane condoms to reduce chance of sexual contact with any body fluids such as semen, vaginal secretions or blood. Never re-use or share needles.

6. Sustained decreases in viral levels have been associated with a reduced risk of progression to AIDS and death.

7. Avoid other prescription or OTC agents; interacts with many other drugs. Herbal products, including St. John's wort has caused severe and potentially life-threatening rash. Stop therapy if severe rash develops.

8. A redistribution or accumulation of body fat may occur in those receiving antiretroviral therapy; cause and long-term health effects of this are unknown at this time.

9. Practice reliable contraception as drug effects on fetus may be harmful;

E

monitoring by drug company is requested.

10. Keep all F/U appointments and labs to evaluate response to therapy and for adverse side effects.

OUTCOMES/EVALUATE
- ↓ HIV RNA
- Improved survival rates in those with HIV resistant to nonnucleoside reverse transcriptase inhibitors (NNRTI) and other antiretroviral drugs

Exemestane
(ex-eh-**MESS**-tayn)

CLASSIFICATION(S):
Antineoplastic, hormone
PREGNANCY CATEGORY: D
Rx: Aromasin.

USES
(1) Treatment of advanced breast cancer in postmenopausal women where the disease has progressed following tamoxifen therapy. (2) Adjuvant therapy in menopausal women whose estrogen receptor-positive early breast cancer has progressed despite two or three years of tamoxifen therapy. Exemestane therapy is intended to complete a total of five consecutive years of adjuvant hormonal therapy. *Investigational:* Prevention of prostate cancer.

ACTION/KINETICS
Action
Irreversible, steroidal aromatase inactivator. Acts as a false substrate for the aromatase enzyme, which is the principal enzyme that converts androgens to estrogens. Drug is processed to an intermediate form that binds irreversibly to the active enzyme site causing its inhibition (called 'suicide inhibition'). Significantly lowers circulating estrogen levels in postmenopausal women; has no detectable effect on adrenal biosynthesis of corticosteroids or aldosterone.

Pharmacokinetics
Rapidly absorbed. **t½, terminal:** About 24 hr. Metabolized in the liver and metabolites (some are active) excreted in both the urine and feces in equal amounts.

CONTRAINDICATIONS
Premenopausal women.

SPECIAL CONCERNS
Safety and efficacy have not been established in children.

SIDE EFFECTS
Most Common
Hot flashes, fatigue, pain, N&V, depression, insomnia, anxiety, edema, abdominal pain, anorexia, flu-like symptoms, increased sweating.

GI: N&V, abdominal pain, anorexia, GI upset, constipation, diarrhea, increased appetite, dyspepsia. **CNS:** Depression, insomnia, anxiety, dizziness, headache, hypoesthesia, confusion. **Respiratory:** Dyspnea, coughing, bronchitis, sinusitis, chest pain, URTI, pharyngitis, rhinitis. **Body as a whole:** Fatigue, edema, fever, generalized weakness, paresthesia, asthenia, peripheal edema, leg edema, flu-like symptoms, increased sweating, rash, itching, infection. **Miscellaneous:** Hypertension, hot flashes, pain, pathological fracture, UTI, lymphedema, pain at tumor site, arthralgia, skeletal back pain, alopecia, lymphocytopenia.

LABORATORY TEST CONSIDERATIONS
↑ AST, ALT, alkaline phosphatase, gamma glutamyl transferase. Slight ↑ serum LH and FSH. ↓ Sex hormone binding globulin.

HOW SUPPLIED
Tablets: 25 mg.

DOSAGE
- **TABLETS**
  Breast cancer.
  25 mg once daily after a meal.

NURSING CONSIDERATIONS
ADMINISTRATION/STORAGE
Glucocorticoid and mineralocorticoid replacement therapy is not necessary.

ASSESSMENT
1. Note reasons for therapy, disease onset, other therapies trialed; tamoxifen failure.
2. Drug is not for use in premenopausal women.
3. Treatment should continue until tumor progression is evident.

Bold Italic = life threatening side effect   ■ = black box warning   ♣ = Available in Canada

4. List drugs prescribed; if a potent CYP3A4 inducer such as rifampicin or phenytoin, the recommended dose requires adjustment to 50 mg from 25 mg daily.

5. Monitor VS, CBC, chemistry, renal and LFTs.

6. Continue mammograms/CT to follow disease progression.

CLIENT/FAMILY TEACHING

1. Used for the treatment of advanced breast cancer in postmenopausal women whose disease has progressed following tamoxifen therapy.

2. Take once daily after a meal. Consume adequate fluids to prevent dehydration.

3. Drug will lower estrogen levels; anticipate therapy may be for prolonged period of time.

4. Report if GI upset, headaches, depression, fatigue or edema become intolerable. Keep regularly scheduled F/U appointments.

OUTCOMES/EVALUATE

- Treatment of progressive breast cancer in postmenopausal women
- Prevention of prostate cancer

Exenatide

(ex-**EN**-a-tide)

CLASSIFICATION(S):
Antidiabetic, incretin mimetic
PREGNANCY CATEGORY: C
Rx: Byetta.

USES

Adjunct therapy to improve glycemic control in type 2 diabetics who are taking a thiazolidinedione alone or in combination with metformin but have not achieved adequate glycemic control.

ACTION/KINETICS

Action

Exenatide enhances glucose-dependent insulin secretion by pancreatic beta-cells, suppresses inappropriately elevated glucagon secretion, and slows gastric emptying. Exenatide is an incretin (glucagon-like peptide-1) mimetic agent that mimics the enhancement of glucose-depenent insulin secretion, as well as several other antihyperglycemic actions of incretins. The drug binds and activates known human glucagon-like peptide-1 receptors, leading to an increase in both glucagon-dependent synthesis of insulin and secretion of insulin from pancreatic beta cells in the presence of elevated glucose concentrations. Glycemic control is improved by reducing fasting and postprandial glucose levels.

Pharmacokinetics

Peak plasma levels: 2.1 hr. Eliminated mainly by glomerular filtration and subsequent proteolytic degradation. **$t\frac{1}{2}$, terminal:** 2.4 hr.

CONTRAINDICATIONS

Hypersensitivity to the product or any of its components. Use with type-1 diabetes or to treat diabetic ketoacidosis. Use in end-stage renal disease or severe renal impairment (C_{CR} <30 mL/min) or in severe GI disease.

SPECIAL CONCERNS

It is possible clients may develop anti-exenatide antibodies; antibody titers diminish with time. It is possible that exenatide, by slowing gastric emptying time, may reduce the rate and extent of absorption of oral drugs; thus, use with caution in those receiving oral medications that require rapid GI absorption. Use with caution during lactation. Safety and efficacy have not been determined in children.

SIDE EFFECTS

Most Common

N&V, dizziness, headache, jittery feeling, diarrhea, dyspepsia.

Metabolic: Hypoglycemia (mild to moderate usually). **GI:** N&V, diarrhea, dyspepsia, decreased appetite, gastroesophageal reflux disease. **CNS:** Dizziness, jittery feeling, headache. **Body as a whole:** Asthenia, hyperhidrosis, development of anti-exenatide antibodies.

OD OVERDOSE MANAGEMENT

Symptoms: Hypoglycemia (may be a rapid fall in BG), severe N&V. *Treatment:* Treat hypoglycemia with PO carbohydrate. Initiate appropriate supportive treatment according to the client's clinical signs and symptoms.

DRUG INTERACTIONS

Acetaminophen / ↓ Acetaminophen AUC and C_{max} and ↑ acetaminophen T_{max}; give acetaminophen 1 hr before exenatide

Antibiotics / Possible ↓ absorption of antibiotics; take the antibiotic at least 1 hr before exenatide injection

Digoxin / ↓ Exenatide C_{max} and delayed T_{max} by about 2.5 hr

Lisinopril / Lisinopril steady-state T_{max} delayed 2 hr

Lovastatin / ↓ Lovastatin AUC and C_{max}; T_{max} delayed about 4 hr

Oral contraceptives / Possible ↓ absorption of contraceptive; take oral contraceptives at least 1 hr before exenatide injection

Sulfonylureas / ↑ Risk of hypoglycemia; consider reducing the dose of the sulfonylurea

Warfarin / ↑ Effect of warfarin; T_{max} of warfarin delayed by a mean of 2 hr when given 30 min after exenatide; possible ↑ INR

HOW SUPPLIED

SC Injection: 5 mcg/dose, 10 mcg/dose.

DOSAGE

• **SC**

Diabetes mellitus, type 2

Initial: 5 mcg/dose given 2 times per day at any time within the 60-minute period before the morning and evening meals. Do not give after a meal. Dose can be increased to 10 mcg after 1 month.

NURSING CONSIDERATIONS

ADMINISTRATION/STORAGE

1. Give the dose in the thigh, abdomen, or upper arm.

2. When exenatide is added to metformin therapy, the current dose of metformin can be continued as it is unlikely the hypoglycemia will require dosage adjustment.

3. Refrigerate from 2–8°C (36–46°F). Do not freeze; do not use if the drug has been frozen. Protect from light. Discard the pen 30 days after first use, even if some drug remains in the pen.

ASSESSMENT

1. Note reasons for therapy, age of disease onset, other agents trialed, outcome. List drugs prescribed to ensure none interact unfavorably.

2. Monitor VS, weight, HbA1c, renal and LFTs.

3. Assess for gastroparesis; drug slows stomach emptying so food passes more slowly through stomach. Determine if timing of other prescribed medications i.e., birth control pills, antibiotics should be changed to accommodate these effects.

CLIENT/FAMILY TEACHING

1. Drug is used to help control blood sugars in adults with type 2 diabetes. It is injected twice a day one hour before breakfast and dinner by a pen. Review patient information pamphlet.

2. It is generally used with metformin or a sulfonylurea. The drug is injected under the skin in client's upper leg, stomach, or upper arm. The first dose should be given in the provider's office so technique can be observed.

3. The drug comes in a prefilled pen with 60 doses to allow 30 days of therapy. Pen needles are ordered separately and are to be discarded after each injection.

4. Read the instructions for use prior to using pen. Must follow directions in the 'New pen setup' section for each new pen before its first use.

5. Store pen in original carton and refrigerate once activated. Thirty days after activating, discard Byetta pen even if not completely empty. Mark with date when pen first used.

6. Liquid in the pen cartridge should be clear, colorless, and free of particles. Report any damaged or broken pens at 800-868-1190.

7. Keep out of reach of children.

8. Report any adverse side effects including injection site reactions, persistently low blood sugars, dizziness, N&V.

9. Practice reliable contraceptive measures. Do not use if breast feeding.

10. Keep all visits so dosage adjustment can be performed as needed.

OUTCOMES/EVALUATE

Control of blood sugars; HbA1c <7

Ezetimibe
(eh-**ZET**-eh-myb)

CLASSIFICATION(S):
Antihyperlipidemic drug
PREGNANCY CATEGORY: C
Rx: Zetia.

USES
(1) Primary hypercholesterolemia, either as monotherapy or combination therapy with HMG-CoA reductase inhibitors to reduce elevated total cholesterol, LDL-C, and apo B. (2) With atorvastatin or simvastatin for homozygous familial hypercholesterolemia as an adjunct to other lipid-lowering treatments. (3) As adjunctive therapy to diet for homozygous sitosterolemia. (4) With fenofibrate as adjunctive therapy to diet to reduce total cholesterol, LDL-C, apo B, and non–high-density lipoprotein cholesterol in clients with mixed hyperlipidemia.

ACTION/KINETICS
Action
Acts by inhibiting the absorption of cholesterol from the small intestine, leading to a decrease in the delivery of cholesterol to the liver. This complements the mechanism of action of HMG-CoA reductase inhibitors. Reduces total cholesterol, LDL cholesterol, Apo B, and triglycerides as well as increases HDL cholesterol. Has no effect on the fat-soluble vitamins A, D, and E.

Pharmacokinetics
Peak plasma ezetimibe levels: 4–12 hr. **t½, parent drug and active metabolite:** 22 hr. After PO administration, is rapidly conjugated to the active phenolic glucuronide in the small intestine and liver. Mainly excreted through the feces with smaller amounts through the urine. **Plasma protein binding:** More than 90% (ezetimibe-glucuronide).

CONTRAINDICATIONS
Use with HMG-CoA reductase inhibitors in pregnant or nursing women and in active liver disease or unexplained persistent elevations in serum transaminases. As monotherapy in moderate to severe hepatic insufficiency and during lactation. Use in children under 10 years old.

SPECIAL CONCERNS
If used with HMG-CoA reductase inhibitors, be aware of contraindications, special concerns, and side effects of these drugs as well.

SIDE EFFECTS
Most Common
Back/abdominal pain, diarrhea, arthralgia, sinusitis, coughing, pharyngitis.
GI: Diarrhea, nausea, abdominal pain, cholelithiasis, hepatitis, cholecystitis, ***pancreatitis***. **CNS:** Headache, dizziness. **Hematologic:** Thrombocytopenia. **Musculoskeletal:** Myalgia, back pain, arthralgia, possible myopathy or rhabdomyolysis. **Respiratory:** URTI, sinusitis, pharyngitis, coughing. **Miscellaneous:** Chest pain, fatigue, viral infection; hypersensitivity reactions including ***anaphylaxis***, angioedema, rash, urticaria.

LABORATORY TEST CONSIDERATIONS
↑ Liver enzymes greater than or equal to 3 times ULN, CPK.

DRUG INTERACTIONS
Antacids / ↓ Ezetimibe C_{max} after both Mg- and Ca-containing antacids; no effect on AUC
Cholestyramine / ↓ Ezetimibe AUC probably R/T ↓ absorption
Cyclosporine / ↑ Total ezetimibe levels; monitor carefully; possibly ↑ cyclosporine AUC
Fenofibrate/Gemfibrozil / ↑ Total ezetimibe levels

HOW SUPPLIED
Tablets: 10 mg.

DOSAGE
- **TABLETS**
  Primary hypercholesterolemia, homozygous familial hypercholesterolemia, homozygous sitosterolemia, with fenofibrate in mixed hyperlipidemia.
  10 mg once daily with or without food.

NURSING CONSIDERATIONS
ADMINISTRATION/STORAGE
1. Place client on a standard cholesterol-lowering diet before therapy and for duration of treatment.
2. May be given with a HMG-CoA reductase inhibitor for an incremental ef-

fect. Dose of both drugs can be given at the same time.

3. Give at least 2 hr before or at least 4 hr after giving a bile sequestrant.

4. Before initiating therapy exclude or, if appropriate, treat secondary causes for dyslipidemia (e.g., diabetes, hypothyroidism, obstructive liver disease, chronic renal failure, drugs that increase LDL-C and decrease HDL-C.

5. Store from 15–30°C (59–86°F) protected from moisture.

ASSESSMENT

1. Note reasons for therapy: plaque stability or elevated TG/LDL cholesterol in CAD. List other agents trialed, outcome.

2. Monitor CBC, lipid panel, renal and LFTs. Schedule LFTs at the beginning of therapy (6 weeks) and if stable, semiannually for the first year of therapy. Special attention should be paid to elevated serum transaminase levels.

3. List all drugs prescribed; ensure none interact unfavorably. Identify cardiac risk factors.

4. Assess level of adherence to weight reduction, exercise, cholesterol-lowering diet, and BP or BS control. Note any alcohol abuse or liver dysfunction.

CLIENT/FAMILY TEACHING

1. Take daily as directed with or without food. Avoid taking with antacids; reduces drug effect.

2. A low-cholesterol diet must be followed during drug therapy. Consult dietitian for assistance in meal planning and food preparation.

3. Report any S&S of infections, unexplained muscle pain, tenderness/weakness (especially if accompanied by fever or malaise), surgery, trauma, or metabolic disorders. Report as scheduled for lab tests, eye exam, and F/U.

4. Review importance of following a low-cholesterol diet, regular exercise, low alcohol consumption, and not smoking in the overall plan to reduce serum cholesterol levels and inhibit progression of CAD.

5. Not for use during pregnancy; use barrier contraception.

6. Drug acts by inhibiting cholesterol absorption in the small intestine. May

experience GI upset and muscle and back pains; report if persistent.

OUTCOMES/EVALUATE

↓ Total cholesterol, LDL cholesterol, and triglycerides; ↑ HDL cholesterol

—— COMBINATION DRUG ——

Ezetimibe and Simvastatin

(eh-**ZET**-eh-myb, **sim**-vah-**STAH**-tin)

CLASSIFICATION(S):
Combination antihyperlipidemic drugs

PREGNANCY CATEGORY: X

Rx: Vytorin 10/10, 10/20, 10/40, or 10/80.

SEE ALSO *EZETIMIBE* **AND** *SIMVASTATIN.*

USES

(1) Adjunctive therapy to diet to reduce elevated total-C, LDL-C, Apo B, triglycerides, and non-HDL-C and to increase HDL-C in clients with primary (heterozygous familial or non-familial) hypercholesterolemia or mixed hyperlipidemia. (2) Reduction of elevated total-C and LDL-C in clients with homozygous familial hypercholesterolemia, as an adjunct to other lipid-lowering treatments (or if such treatments are not available).

CONTENT

All strengths contain ezetimibe, 10 mg with either 10 mg, 20 mg, 40 mg, or 80 mg simvastatin.

ACTION/KINETICS

Action

Ezetimibe reduces blood cholesterol by inhibiting absorption of cholesterol by the small intestine, leading to a decrease of hepatic cholesterol stores and an increased clearance of cholesterol from the blood. Simvastatin decreases cholesterol by inhibiting conversion of HMG-CoA to mevalonate, an early step in the biosynthesis of cholesterol. Also, simvastatin reduces VLDL and triglycerides and increases HDL-C.

Pharmacokinetics

Ezetimibe is absorbed and converted to the active exetimibe-glucuronide. High fat or non-fat meals have no effect on the extent of absorption. Ezetimibe is metabolized in the small intestine and liver by glucuroide conjugation and excreted in both the feces and urine. Simvastatin undergoes extensive first-pass liver metabolism and is mainly excreted in the bile.

CONTRAINDICATIONS

Use not recommended with moderate or severe hepatic insufficiency. Lactation.

SPECIAL CONCERNS

Give to women of childbearing age only when such clients are highly unlikely to conceive. Use with caution with niacin. Safety and efficacy for use in children have not been sufficiently evaluated.

SIDE EFFECTS

Most Common

Headache, myalgia, URTI, influenza, abdominal pain, diarrhea, arthralgia, back pain, sinusitis, chest pain.

See *Ezetimibe* and *Simvastatin* for a complete list of possible side effects.

LABORATORY TEST CONSIDERATIONS

↑ Serum transaminases (>3 x ULN).

DRUG INTERACTIONS

Amiodarone / ↑ Risk of myopathy/rhabdomyolysis; do not use more than Vytorin, 10/20 mg daily

Clarithromycin / ↑ Risk of myopathy/rhabdomyolysis; do not use together

Cyclosporine / ↑ Risk of myopathy/rhabdomyolysis; do not use more than Vytorin, 10/10 mg daily

Danazol / ↑ Risk of myopathy/rhabdomyolysis; do not use more than Vytorin, 10/10 mg daily

Erythromycin / ↑ Risk of myopathy/rhabdomyolysis; do not use together

Gemfibrozil / ↑ Risk of myopathy/rhabdomyolysis; do not use Vytorin more than 10/10 mg daily

Grapefruit juice (>1 qt daily) / ↑ Risk of myopathy/rhabdomyolysis; do not use together

HIV Protease Inhibitors / ↑ Risk of myopathy/rhabdomyolysis; do not use together

Itraconazole / ↑ Risk of myopathy/rhabdomyolysis; do not use together

Ketoconazole / ↑ Risk of myopathy/rhabdomyolysis; do not use together

Nefazodone / ↑ Risk of myopathy/rhabdomyolysis; do not use together

Telithromycin / ↑ Risk of myopathy/rhabdomyolysis; do not use together

Verapamil / ↑ Risk of myopathy/rhabdomyolysis; do not use more than Vytorin, 10/20 mg daily

HOW SUPPLIED

See Content.

DOSAGE

• **TABLETS**

Primary hypercholesterolemia.

Usual, initial: 10/20 mg/day. Beginning with 10/10 mg/day may be considered for those requiring less aggressive LDL-C reductions. Those requiring a larger LDL-C reduction (>55%) may be started on 10/40 mg/day. After initiation or titration of Vytorin, lipid levels may be analyzed after 2 or more weeks; adjust dosage, if necessary. **Dose range:** 10/10 mg/day through 10/80 mg/day.

Homozygous familial hypercholesterolemia.

10/40 mg/day or 10/80 mg/day, with other lipid-lowering treatments (e.g., LDL apheresis).

NURSING CONSIDERATIONS

ADMINISTRATION/STORAGE

1. Prior to beginning therapy with Vytorin, secondary causes for dyslipidemia (i.e., diabetes, hypothyroidism, obstructive liver disease, chronic renal failure, and drugs that increase LDL-C and decrease HDL-C) should be excluded or, if appropriate, treated.

2. Place client on a standard cholesterol-lowering diet before giving Vytorn; continue the diet during Vytorin treatment.

3. Individualize Vytorin dose according to baseline LDL-C, recommended goal of therapy, and client's response.

4. No dosage adjustment is needed with mild hepatic insufficiency or mild to moderate renal insufficiency. In severe renal insufficiency, do not begin Vytorin unless client has tolerated treatment with simvastatin, at a dose of 5

mg or higher. Use caution when using Vytorin in these clients; monitor closely.

5. If given with bile acid sequestrants, give Vytorin either 2 hr or more before or 4 hr or more after giving the bile acid sequestrant.

6. Store from 20–25°C (68–77°F). Store in original container until time of use.

ASSESSMENT

1. Note reasons for therapy, family history, risk factors, other agents trialed, outcome. List drugs prescribed to ensure none interact.

2. Monitor VS, lipid panel, renal, LFTs; reduce with dysfunction. Identify any metabolic, endocrine or electrolyte disorders.

3. Assess for seizure history and any muscle problems/disease.

4. Check adherence to cholesterol lowering diet, weight control and regular daily exercise.

CLIENT/FAMILY TEACHING

1. Take as a single dose in the evening, with or without food. If also prescribed bile acid sequestrant (eg, cholestyramine, colestipol, colesevelam), take Vytorin at least 2 hours before or at least 4 hours after bile acid sequestrant.

2. May cause visual changes or drowsiness; avoid activities that require mental alertness until drug effects realized.

3. Avoid grapefruit and grapefruit juice; may increase drug concentrations and adverse effects.

4. Report any new onset muscle pain, weakness, tenderness or fever.

5. Use reliable contraception; do not take if pregnancy suspected.

6. Continue to follow low fat low cholesterol diet, regular daily exercise, weight control, smoking cessation in overall goal of cholesterol control.

7. Avoid alcohol: may increase risk of liver problems.

8. Keep all F/U appointments for lab and to evaluate drug response.

OUTCOMES/EVALUATE

↓ Total and LDL cholesterol

Factor IX Concentrates, Human

IV

(**FAK**-tor 9)

CLASSIFICATION(S):
Hemostatic, systemic
PREGNANCY CATEGORY: C
Rx: AlphaNine SD, Bebulin VH, BeneFIX, Mononine, Profilnine SD, Proplex T.
♣Rx: Immunine VH.

USES

(1) To prevent or control bleeding in clients with factor IX deficiency, especially hemophilia B (Christmas disease).
(2) Hemarthroses in hemophiliacs when inhibitors to Factor VII can not be resolved by administration of factor IX complex and in other types of bleeding episodes in factor VII-inhibitor clients (Proplex T only).

ACTION/KINETICS

Action

Causes an increase in factor IX levels, thus minimizing hemorrhage in those with factor IX deficiency. Factors II, VII, and X may also be increased following administration of Bebulin VH and Proplex T.

Pharmacokinetics

t^{1}_{2}: 22 hr. The mean increase in circulating factor IX after IV infusion is 0.67–1.15 international units/dL rise per international units/kg body weight. One unit is the activity present in 1 mL of pooled normal fresh plasma.

CONTRAINDICATIONS

Factor VII deficiency, except for Proplex T. Use in mild Factor IX deficiency when fresh frozen plasma is effective. Liver disease with suspected intravascular

---

Bold Italic = life threatening side effect   ■ = black box warning   ♣ = Available in Canada

coagulation or fibrinolysis. Hypersensitivity to mouse (Mononine) or hamster (BeneFIX) proteins.

SPECIAL CONCERNS

Assess benefit versus risk prior to use in liver disease or elective surgery. Factor IX products may be derived from pooled units of human plasma; although precautions are taken, the risk of viral infections from such products can not be eliminated completely. Safety and efficacy have not been determined in children less than 6 years of age (except for Mononine).

SIDE EFFECTS

Most Common

Nausea, discomfort at IV site, altered taste, burning sensation in the jaw and skull, allergic rhinitis, lightheadedness, headache.

CV: *DIC, thrombosis. High doses may cause MI, venous or pulmonary thrombosis,* hypotension, thrombosis. **Symptoms due to rapid infusion:** N&V, headache, fever, chills, tingling, flushing, urticaria, and changes in BP or pulse rate. Most of these side effects disappear when rate of administration is slowed. **Hypersensitivity:** Hives, generalized urticaria, angioedema, chest tightness, dyspnea, wheezing, faintness, hypotension, tachycardia, *anaphylaxis*. **GI:** Nausea, altered taste. **CNS:** Lightheadedness, headache, dizziness, drowsiness. **Respiratory:** Dry cough/sneeze, tight chest, dyspnea, *laryngeal edema*. **Miscellaneous:** Chills, fever, cyanosis, nephrotic syndrome, discomfort at IV site, burning sensation in jaw and skull, allergic rhinitis, rash, phlebitis/cellulitis at IV site.

NOTE: The preparation also contains trace amounts of blood groups A and B and isohemagglutinins, which may cause intravascular hemolysis when administered in large amounts to clients with blood groups A, B, and AB. Although careful screening is undertaken, both hepatitis and AIDS may be transmitted using factor IX concentrates since it is derived from pooled human plasma.

DRUG INTERACTIONS

↑ Risk of thrombosis if administered with aminocaproic acid

HOW SUPPLIED

Injection, Powder for Solution: Most products are 250, 500, or 1,000 international units/single dose vials.

DOSAGE

- **IV**

  Factor IX deficiency (hemophilia B [Christmas disease]).

  Individualized, depending on severity of bleeding, degree of deficiency, body weight, and level of factor required. As a guide in determining the units required to raise blood level percentages of factor IX, use the following formulas. **For human-derived factor IX:** 1 international unit/kg × body weight (kg) × desired increase (% of normal). **For recombinant factor IX:** 1.2 international units/kg × body weight (kg) × desired increase (% of normal).

  As a general rule, 1 unit of human-derived factor IX activity/kg will increase the circulating level of factor IX by 1% of normal and 1 unit of recombinant factor IX/kg will increase the circulating activity of factor IX by 0.8 units/dL. If inhibitors to factor IX are present, use sufficient additional dosage to overcome the inhibitors. **For minor hemorrhage:** Uncomplicated hemarthroses, superficial muscle, or soft tissue, 20–30 units/dL of circulating factor IX are required. Give q 12–24 hr for 1–2 days. **For moderate hemorrhage:** Intramuscular or soft tissue with disconnection, mucous membranes, dental extractions, or hematuria, 25–50 units/dL of circulating factor IX are required. Give q 12–24 hr and treat until bleeding stops and healing begins (about 2–7 days). **For major hemorrhage:** Pharynx, retropharynx, retroperitoneum, CNS, surgery, 50–100 units/dL of circulating factor IX are required. Give q 12–24 hr for 7–10 days.

  Factor VII deficiency (Proplex T only). To determine the units needed to raise blood level percentages, use the following: 0.5 unit/kg × body weight (kg) × desired increase (% of normal). The dose may be repeated q 4–6 hr as needed. In preparation for and following surgery, maintain levels more than 25% for at least 1 week. To maintain levels more than 25% for a reasonable time, calculate each dose to raise levels to 40-60% of normal.

Factor VIII inhibitor (Proplex T only). Use dosage levels approximating 75 international units/kg.

NURSING CONSIDERATIONS

ADMINISTRATION/STORAGE

IV 1. Rate of administration varies with the product. As a general guideline, infuse about 100–200 international units/min at a rate of 2–3 mL/min, do not exceed 3 mL/min. If headache, flushing, or changes in pulse rate or BP occur, stop the infusion until symptoms subside; then resume at a slower rate. Use the factor IX assay for precise monitoring.

2. Before reconstitution, warm diluent to room temperature but not above 40°C (104°F).

3. Agitate solution gently until powder dissolved.

4. Administer within 3 hr of reconstitution; avoid incubation in case contamination occurred during preparation. Do not refrigerate after reconstitution; active ingredient may precipitate out.

5. Use the following guidelines for administration of BeneFIX:

- Use the following equation to calculate the factor IX BeneFIX dose: number of factor IX units required = body weight (kg) x desired factor IX increase (% or units/dL) x reciprocal of observed recovery (units/kg per units/dL).

- Administer using the infusion set provided in the kit and the prefilled syringe provided or a single sterile disposable syringe. Withdraw the solution from the vial using the vial adapter.

- Agglutination of RBCs in the tubing/syringe has occurred. To minimize this possibility, limit the amount of blood entering the tubing. Blood should not enter the syringe. If RBC agglutination is observed in the tub-

ing or syringe, discard all material (i.e., tubing, syringe, BeneFIX solution) and resume administration with a new package.

- Reconstitute lyophilized BeneFIX powder for injection with the diluent supplied (0.234% NaCl solution) from the prefilled syringe provided. Following injection of the diluent into the vial, gently rotate the vial until all powder is dissolved.

- After reconstitution, the solution is drawn back into the syringe. The solution should be clear and colorless. Discard the solution if visible particulate matter or discoloration is observed.

- Administer within 3 hr of reconstitution. The reconstituted solution may be stored at room temperature until given.

- Reconstituted BeneFIX contains polysorbate 80 which increases the rate of extraction of di-(2-ethylhexyl)phthalate (DEHP) from polyvinyl chloride (PVC). Consider this in the storage time when using a PVC container.

- Store the BeneFIX product as packaged for sale from 2-8°C (36-46°F). Prior to the expiration date the product may also be stored at room temperature (not to exceed 25°C (77°F) for up to 6 months. Avoid freezing to prevent damage to the diluent syringe.

6. Store products from 2–8°C (36–46°F). Do not freeze provided diluent.

7. Discard 2 years after date of manufacture or as directed.

ASSESSMENT

1. List any previous experience/treatment with factor replacement and outcome.

2. Obtain weight, height, and blood type. Dose must be individualized based on weight, degree of deficiency, and severity of bleed. Maintain plasma level at least 20% of normal until hemostasis achieved.

3. Note any S&S of liver disease (i.e., urticaria, fever, pruritus, anorexia, N&V); monitor LFTs, VS, CBC, coagulation, and factor assay levels.

4. Assess carefully for abnormal bruising/bleeding, i.e., enlarged joints, restricted joint movement, oral mucosa for gingival bleeding, drop in H&H, increased menses etc.

INTERVENTIONS

1. Monitor BP and pulse q 30 min during infusion.

2. Report increased bleeding and joint swelling; use rest, ice, and elevation with affected joints.

3. Reduce flow rate and report if a tingling sensation, headache, chills, or fever occur.

4. Avoid aminocaproic acid administration; may cause clot formation.

5. Assess for DIC if factor IX level is increased above 50% of normal. At 50% or greater, there is an increased risk for the development of a thromboembolic event and/or DIC.

6. Make sure client has received hepatitis A and B vaccines.

7. Monitor I&O; test urine for occult blood. Hemolytic reactions are more pronounced in clients with A, B, and AB type blood.

CLIENT/FAMILY TEACHING

1. This drug is a type of protein that is normally produced in your body that helps your blood to form clots to prevent you from bleeding out.

2. Product is prepared from human plasma, has been treated but may carry risks (i.e., hepatitis, AIDS). The man made product does not have these viruses.

3. Avoid contact sports and any activities that may lead to injury or excessive jostling.

4. Use soft bristled tooth brush and electric razor to prevent unnecessary bleeding.

5. Report any uncontrolled bleeding, joint pain, swelling. May note changes in skin coloring, sob, chest pains; report all side effects.

6. Ensure family members are screened and genetically counselled; disease is hereditary.

7. Avoid OTCs and aspirin-containing products.

8. Identify local support groups that may assist to cope with this disease.

OUTCOMES/EVALUATE

- Prevention of hemorrhage
- Factor levels within desired range

Famciclovir

(fam-**SY**-kloh-veer)

CLASSIFICATION(S):

Antiviral

PREGNANCY CATEGORY: B

Rx: Famvir.

SEE ALSO *ANTIVIRAL AGENTS.*

USES

(1) Treatment of acute herpes zoster (shingles). (2) Treatment or suppression of recurrent episodes of genital herpes in immunocompetent clients. (3) Treatment of recurrent mucocutaneous herpes simplex infections in HIV-infected clients. (4) Treatment of recurrent herpes labialis (cold sores) in immunocompetent clients. *Investigational:* Management of initial episodes of herpes genitalis. *NOTE:* The efficacy of famciclovir has not been determined for initial episode genital herpes infection, ophthalmic zoster, disseminated zoster, or in immunocompromised clients with herpes zoster.

ACTION/KINETICS

Action

Undergoes rapid biotransformation to the active compound penciclovir. Inhibits viral DNA synthesis and therefore replication in HSV types 1 (HSV-1) and 2 (HSV-2) and varicella-zoster virus.

Pharmacokinetics

Absolute bioavailability is 77%. **Time to C_{max}:** 0.9 hr after PO use. Food decreased C_{max}; but not AUC. **$t\frac{1}{2}$, plasma:** 2.3 hr following PO use of famciclovir. Penciclovir, the active metabolite, is further metabolized to inactive compounds that are excreted through the urine. Half-life increased in renal insufficiency.

CONTRAINDICATIONS

Use during lactation. Hypersensitivity to famciclovir, its components, or penciclovir cream. Those with galactose intolerance, a severe lactose deficiency, or glucose-galactose malabsorption.

SPECIAL CONCERNS

Safety and efficacy have not been determined in children less than 18 years of age.

SIDE EFFECTS

Most Common

Headache, N&V, diarrhea, paresthesia, fatigue, flatulence, pruritus, abdominal pain.

GI: N&V, diarrhea, constipation, anorexia, abdominal pain, dyspepsia, flatulence, jaundice. **CNS:** Headache, dizziness, paresthesia, migraine, somnolence, insomnia, confusion (especially in the elderly), hallucinations. **Body as a whole:** Fatigue, fever, pain, rigors, injury. **Musculoskeletal:** Back pain, arthralgia. **Respiratory:** Pharyngitis, sinusitis, URI. **Hematologic:** Anemia, leukopenia, neutropenia, thrombocytopenia. **Dermatologic:** Pruritus, rash, urticaria, signs/symptoms/complications of zoster and genital herpes, erythema multiforme. **Miscellaneous:** Dysmenorrhea.

LABORATORY TEST CONSIDERATIONS

↑ AST, ALT, total bilirubin, serum creatinine, amylase, lipase.

DRUG INTERACTIONS

Digoxin / ↑ Digoxin levels
Probenecid / ↑ Penciclovir levels
Theophylline / ↑ Penciclovir levels

HOW SUPPLIED

Tablets: 125 mg, 250 mg, 500 mg.

DOSAGE

- **TABLETS**

  Herpes zoster infections.

500 mg q 8 hr for 7 days. Initiate as soon as herpes zoster is diagnosed. Dosage reduction is recommended in clients with impaired renal function: For C_{CR} of 40–59 mL/min: 500 mg q 12 hr; C_{CR} of 20–39 mL/min: 500 mg q 24 hr; C_{CR} <20 mL/min: 250 mg q 48 hr. For hemodialysis clients: 250 mg given after each dialysis treatment.

  Recurrent genital herpes.

1,000 mg q 12 hr for 1 day. Should be taken at the first sign or symptom. Dosage reduction is as follows for those with impaired renal function: For C_{CR} of 40 to 59 mL/min: 500 mg q 12 hr for 1 day; C_{CR} of 20–39 mL/min: A single dose

of 500 mg; C_{CR} <20 mL/min: A single dose of 250 mg. Hemodialysis clients: A single dose of 250 mg after each dialysis treatment.

  Suppression of recurrent genital herpes.

250 mg q 12 hr for up to 1 year (safety and efficacy beyond one year have not been established). Dosage reduction is as follows for those with impaired renal function: C_{CR}, over 20–39 mL/min: 125 mg q 12 hr hr; C_{CR} <20 mL/min: 125 mg q 24 hr. Hemodialysis clients: 125 mg after each dialysis treatment.

  Recurrent orolabial or genital herpes infection in HIV-infected clients.

500 mg twice a day for 7 days. Dosage reduction is as follows for those with impaired renal function: C_{CR} of 40 mL/min or greater: 500 mg q 12 hr; C_{CR} of 20–39 mL/min: 500 mg q 24 hr; C_{CR} <20 mL/min: 250 mg q 24 hr. Hemodialysis clients: 250 mg after each dialysis treatment.

  Recurrent herpes labialis (cold sores).

1,500 mg as a single dose. Initiate therapy at the earliest sign or symptom of a cold sore. Dosage reduction is as follows for those with impaired renal function: C_{CR}, 40–59 mL/min: 750 mg as a single dose; C_{CR}, 20–39 mL/min: 500 mg as a single dose; C_{CR}, <20 mL/min: 250 mg as a single dose. Hemodialysis clients: 250 mg as a single dose following dialysis.

  Management of initial episodes of herpes genitalis.

250 mg 3 times per day for 5 days.

NURSING CONSIDERATIONS

ADMINISTRATION/STORAGE

1. Initiate therapy as soon as herpes zoster is diagnosed and at the first symptoms of genital herpes.
2. Therapy is most useful if started within first 48 hr of rash appearance.
3. Effect is greatest in those over 50 years of age.

ASSESSMENT

1. Note onset of symptoms, location, extent of lesions; duration/frequency of recurrence.
2. Initiate as soon as diagnosis is confirmed.

Bold Italic = life threatening side effect   ▪ = black box warning   ♣ = Available in Canada

3. Monitor CBC and renal function studies. Anticipate reduced dosage with renal dysfunction; follow dosing guidelines.

4. To monitor maternal fetal outcomes of pregnant women exposed to famciclovir, Novartis Pharmaceutical Corporation, the manufacturer, maintains a famciclovir pregnancy registry. Register clients by calling 1-888-669-6682.

CLIENT/FAMILY TEACHING

1. Drug is an antiviral that slows spread and growth of virus so body can fight off infections.

2. May be taken without regard to meals.

3. Review frequency, amount of drug to consume, and duration of therapy.

4. Side effects often associated with therapy include diarrhea, nausea, headaches, and fatigue; report if intolerable.

5. When lesions are open and draining, carrier is extremely contagious and should avoid any exposure or outside contact unless confirmed that the person(s) have had the chickenpox and are not pregnant.

6. Wear condoms to prevent spreading to others. Women should have yearly Pap smears as cervical cancer is an increased risk.

7. Report adverse side effects, lack of response or any evidence of infection. Keep all F/U appointments.

OUTCOMES/EVALUATE

- Resolution of herpetic lesions
- ↓ Duration of neuralgia

Famotidine   IV

(fah-**MOH**-tih-deen)

CLASSIFICATION(S):
Histamine H_2 receptor blocking drug

PREGNANCY CATEGORY: B

OTC: Pepcid AC, Pepcid AC Maximum Strength.

Rx: Pepcid, Pepcid RPD.

✤Rx: Apo-Famotidine, Gen-Famotidine, Novo-Famotidine, Nu-Famotidine, Pepcid Tablets, Rhoxal-famotidine, ratio-Famotidine.

SEE ALSO *HISTAMINE H_2 ANTAGONISTS.*

USES

PO/Injection, Rx: (1) Treatment, up to 8 weeks, of active duodenal ulcers. Maintenance therapy for duodenal ulcer after active ulcer has healed. (2) Pathologic hypersecretory conditions such as Zollinger-Ellison syndrome or multiple endocrine adenomas. (3) Treatment, up to 6 weeks, of GERD, including ulcerative disease diagnosed by endoscopy or erosive esophagitis. (4) Treatment, up to 8 weeks, of active, benign gastric ulcer. *Investigational:* Prevent aspiration pneumonitis; for prophylaxis of stress ulcers; perioperatively to suppress gastric acid secretion; in combination with histamine H-1 antagonists to treat certain types of urticaria; as part of multidrug therapy to eradicate *Helicobacter pylori.*

PO, OTC: (1) Relief of heartburn associated with indigestion and sour stomach. (2) Prevent heartburn associated with acid indigestion and sour stomach due to certain foods and beverages.

IV: (1) Some hospitalized clients with pathological hypersecretory conditions or intractable ulcers. (2) Alternative to PO dosage forms for short-term use in those who are unable to take PO medication. *Investigational:* Prevent paclitaxel hypersensitivity; prevent recurrent bleeding after successful endoscopic treatment of bleeding peptic ulcer; reduce incidence of GI hemorrhage associated with stress-related ulcers.

ACTION/KINETICS

Action

Competitive inhibitor of histamine H_2 receptors leading to inhibition of gastric acid secretion. Both basal and nocturnal gastric acid secretion stimulated by food or pentagastrin are inhibited.

Pharmacokinetics

Bioavailability after PO use is 40–45%. **Peak plasma levels:** 1–3 hr. **$t^1/_2$:** 2.5–3.5 hr. **Onset:** 1 hr. **Duration:** 10–12 hr. Does not inhibit the cytochrome P450 system in the liver; thus, drug interactions due to inhibition of liver metabolism are not expected to occur. From 25 to 30% of a PO dose is eliminated through the kidney unchanged; from 65 to 70% of an IV dose is excreted through the kidney unchanged. **Plasma protein binding:** From 15–20% bound to plasma proteins.

CONTRAINDICATIONS

Cirrhosis of the liver, impaired renal or hepatic function, lactation.

SPECIAL CONCERNS

CNS side effects are possible in those with moderate to severe renal insufficiency. Use of IV famotidine in children younger than 1 year has not been adequately studied. Do not give the OTC product to children younger than 12 years unless otherwise directed.

SIDE EFFECTS

Most Common

Headache, dizziness, diarrhea, constipation, N&V, anxiety, confusion.

GI: Constipation, diarrhea, N&V, anorexia, dry mouth, abdominal discomfort. **CNS:** Dizziness, headache, paresthesias, depression, anxiety, confusion, hallucinations, insomnia, fatigue, sleepiness, agitation, **grand mal seizure**, psychic disturbances. **Skin:** Rash, acne, pruritus, alopecia, urticaria, dry skin, flushing. **CV:** Palpitations. **Musculoskeletal:** Arthralgia, asthenia, musculoskeletal pain. **Hematologic:** Thrombocytopenia. **Miscellaneous:** Fever, orbital edema, conjunctival injection, bronchospasm, tinnitus, taste disorders, decreased libido, impotence, pain at injection site (transient).

DRUG INTERACTIONS

Antacids / ↓ Famotidine absorption from the GI tract
Diazepam / ↓ Diazepam absorption from the GI tract

HOW SUPPLIED

OTC. *Gelcaps:* 10 mg; *Tablets:* 10 mg, 20 mg; *Tablets, Chewable:* 10 mg.
Rx. *Injection:* 10 mg/mL; *Injection (Premix):* 20 mg/50 mL; *Powder for Oral Suspension:* 40 mg/5 mL (when reconstituted); *Tablets:* 20 mg, 40 mg; *Tablets, Oral Disintegrating:* 20 mg, 40 mg.

DOSAGE

• **RX: ORAL SUSPENSION; TABLETS; TABLETS, ORAL DISINTEGRATING**
Duodenal ulcer, acute therapy.

Adults: 40 mg once daily at bedtime or 20 mg twice a day. Most ulcers heal within 4 weeks and it is rarely necessary to use the full dosage for 6–8 weeks.
Duodenal ulcer, maintenance therapy.
Adults: 20 mg once daily at bedtime.
Benign gastric ulcers, acute therapy.
Adults: 40 mg once daily at bedtime.
Children: Peptic ulcers.
Children, 1–16 years of age: 0.5 mg/kg/day at bedtime or divided twice a day up to 40 mg/day. Individualize dose based on clinical response and/or gastric/esophageal pH and endoscopy.
Pathological hypersecretory conditions.
Adults, individualized, initial: 20 mg q 6 hr; **then,** adjust dose to response, although doses of up to 160 mg q 6 hr may be required for severe cases of Zollinger-Ellison syndrome. Continue as long as clinically indicated.
Adults: Gastroesophageal reflux disease.
Adults: 20 mg twice a day for 6 weeks. For esophagitis with erosions and ulcerations, give 20 or 40 mg twice a day for up to 12 weeks.
Children: GERD with or without esophagitis, including erosions and ulcerations.
Children, 1–16 years of age: 1 mg/kg/day PO divided twice daily, up to 40 mg twice daily.
Infants: GERD.
Children, less than 1 year of age, initial: 0.5 mg/kg/dose of the oral suspension for up to 8 weeks. Give once daily (i.e., 0.5 mg/kg) in children younger than 3 months of age and twice daily (i.e., 0.5 mg/kg twice daily) to children from 3 months to younger than 1 year.
Prophylaxis of upper GI bleeding.
Adults: 20 mg twice a day.
Prophylaxis of stress ulcers.
Adults: 40 mg/day.
• **IV; IV INFUSION**
Hospitalized clients with hypersecretory conditions, duodenal ulcers, gastric ulcers; unable to take PO medication.
Adults: 20 mg IV q 12 hr. **Children, 1–16 years of age:** Individualize. **Initial:** 0.25 mg/kg given over 2 or more minutes or as a 15-min infusion q 12 hr

---

Bold Italic = life threatening side effect   ■ = black box warning   ♣ = Available in Canada

up to 40 mg/day. **Initial, infants less than one year of age:** 0.5 mg/kg/dose once daily, for up to 8 weeks in infants younger than 3 months of age and 0.5 mg/kg/dose twice daily, for up to 8 weeks in infants 3 months to younger than 1 year of age. These clients should also receive conservative measures (e.g., thickened feedings).

• **OTC: GELCAPS ; TABLETS ; TABLETS, CHEWABLE**

Relief and prevention of heartburn, acid indigestion, and sour stomach.

Adults and children over 12 years of age, for prevention: 10 or 20 mg 15–60 min before eating food or drinking a beverage expected to cause symptoms. **Relief (acute therapy):** 10 mg or 20 mg with water. **Maximum dose:** 20 mg/24 hr. Not to be used continuously for more than 2 weeks unless medically prescribed. Do not give OTC product to children less than 12 years of age unless otherwise directed.

NURSING CONSIDERATIONS

ADMINISTRATION/STORAGE

1. Use antacids concomitantly if needed.

2. The oral suspension may be substituted for tablets for any use.

3. To prepare the oral suspension, slowly add 46 mL of purified water. Shake vigorously for 5–10 seconds immediately after adding the water and immediately before use.

4. Reduce dose in moderate to severe renal impairment (C_{CR} mL/min) to half the usual dose at the usual dosage interval or the usual dose every 36–48 hr.

5. Store PO Rx forms from 15–30°C (59–86°F). Protect suspension from freezing; discard any unused suspension after 30 days. Store OTC forms from 20–30°C (68–86°F); protect from moisture.

IV 6. For IV, dilute 2 mL (containing 10 mg/mL) with 0.9% NaCl or other compatible IV solution to a total volume of 5–10 mL; give over at least a 2-min period.

7. For IV infusion, dilute 2 mL (20 mg) with 100 mL of D5W or other compatible IV solution and infuse over 15–30 min. Infuse the premixed solution over 15–30 min.

8. A solution is stable for 7 days at room temperature when added to or diluted with water for injection, 0.9% NaCl, D5W or D10W, RL injection, or 5% NaHCO₃ injection.

9. Stable when mixed with various TPN solutions. Length of stability depends on the solution.

10. Store non-premixed injection at 2–8°C (36–46°F). Avoid exposure of premixed injection to excessive heat. If the solution freezes, bring to room temperature, allowing sufficient time to solubilize all the components.

ASSESSMENT

1. List reasons for therapy, type, onset, characteristics of S&S.

2. Note location, extent, and type of abdominal pain.

3. Review UGI/endoscopic findings; note modifications trialed with GERD (i.e. staying upright for 3 hr after eating, elevating head of bed on 5 inch blocks, avoiding food triggers).

4. Check for occult blood in stools/GI secretions; note presence of *H. pylori* antibodies.

5. Assess mental status; history of seizures.

6. If pregnant, list benefits versus risks.

7. Note hepatic/renal dysfunction and need for dose reduction; review CBC, assess for bleeding.

CLIENT/FAMILY TEACHING

1. Take with food at night, do not smoke after last dose (increases acid production) or if more than one dose daily, take last dose at bedtime.

2. Drug is used to help heal ulcers or control acid reflux S&S by reducing the amount of stomach acid produced. May take with antacids for pain relief. Drug may cause dizziness, headaches, and anxiety; use caution with activities requiring mental alertness and report if symptoms persist.

3. Report any increasing lack of concern for personal appearance, depression, or sleeplessness, diarrhea, constipation, appetite loss, easy bruising, or fatigue. Increase fluids and bulk in diet to prevent constipation.

4. Avoid alcohol, aspirin-containing products, OTC cough and cold products, smoking, and foods that increase GI irritation (i.e., citrus, carbonated drinks, caffeine, black pepper, harsh spices). Smoking causes increased secretion of gastric acid and may aggravate problems.

5. Report a reduction in urinary output, adverse side effects or lack of response; may need dosage changed. Keep all F/U appointments.

OUTCOMES/EVALUATE

- ↓ Abdominal pain
- Prophylaxis of stress ulcers
- Control of hypersecretion of acid
- Duodenal ulcer healing
- Control of symptoms of GERD

Felbamate ■
(**FELL**-bah-mayt)

CLASSIFICATION(S):
Anticonvulsant, miscellaneous
PREGNANCY CATEGORY: C
Rx: Felbatol.

SEE ALSO *ANTICONVULSANTS*.

USES
(1) Alone or as part of adjunctive therapy for the treatment of partial seizures with and without generalization in adults with epilepsy. (2) Adjunct in the treatment of partial and generalized seizures associated with Lennox-Gastaut syndrome in children. Used only as second-line therapy.

ACTION/KINETICS

Action
Mechanism not known. Felbamate may reduce seizure spread and increase seizure threshold. Has weak inhibitory effects on both GABA and benzodiazepine receptor binding.

Pharmacokinetics
Well absorbed after PO use. **Terminal t½:** 20–23 hr. Trough blood levels are dose dependent. From 40–50% excreted unchanged in the urine.

CONTRAINDICATIONS
History of hepatic dysfunction or blood dyscrasia. Hypersensitivity to carbamates.

SPECIAL CONCERNS
■ (1) Use is associated with a marked increase in the incidence of aplastic anemia. Use only in those whose epilepsy is so severe that the risk of aplastic anemia is deemed acceptable in view of the benefits from its use. Clients should not be placed on or continued on felbamate without consideration of appropriate expert hematologic consultation. (2) Clinical manifestations of aplastic anemia may not be seen until after a client has been on the drug for several months (5–30 weeks); however, the injury to bone marrow stem cells may occur weeks to months earlier, placing clients at risk for developing anemia for a variable and unknown period after drug discontinuation. (3) It is not known whether or not the risk of developing aplastic anemia changes with the duration of exposure, dose, or concomitant use of antiepileptic drugs or other drugs. (4) Aplastic anemia typically develops without premonitory clinical or laboratory signs. The full-blown syndrome presents with signs of infection, bleeding, or anemia. Thus, routine blood testing cannot be reliably used to reduce the incidence of aplastic anemia. It will, in some cases, allow the detection of the hematologic changes before the syndrome is seen clinically. Discontinue felbamate if any evidence of bone marrow depression occurs. (5) Hepatic failure resulting in death has been reported with a marked increase in frequency in those taking felbamate. Thus, only use felbamate in those whose epilepsy is so severe that potential benefits of seizure control outweigh the risk of liver failure. Reliable estimates cannot be made of the incidence of hepatic failure or to identify the factors, if any, that might be used to predict which client is at greater risk. (6) It is not known whether the risk of developing hepatic failure changes with duration of exposure, dosage, or concomitant use of other antiepileptic drugs or

---

other drugs. (7) Avoid use in those with a history of hepatic dysfunction. (8) Clients prescribed felbamate should have liver function tests (AST, ALT, bilirubin) performed before starting therapy and at 1- to 2-week intervals while treatment continues. A client who develops abnormal liver function tests should be immediately withdrawn from the drug.■ Use with caution during lactation. Safety and efficacy have not been established in children other than those with Lennox-Gastaut syndrome.

SIDE EFFECTS
Most Common
When used as adjunctive therapy: Headache, N&V, somnolence, anorexia, dizziness, fatigue, dyspepsia, constipation.
When used for Lennox-Gastaut in children: Anorexia, URTI, somnolence, vomiting, fever, insomnia, nervousness, constipation, purpura.

CNS: Insomnia, headache, anxiety, somnolence, dizziness, nervousness, tremor, abnormal gait, depression, paresthesia, ataxia, stupor, abnormal thinking, emotional lability, agitation, psychologic disturbance, aggressive reaction, hallucinations, euphoria, *suicide attempt*, migraine. **GI:** Dyspepsia, N&V, constipation, diarrhea, dry mouth, nausea, anorexia, abdominal pain, hiccoughs, esophagitis, increased appetite. **Respiratory:** URTI, rhinitis, sinusitis, pharyngitis, coughing. **CV:** Palpitation, tachycardia, SVT. **Body as a whole:** Fatigue, weight decrease or increase, facial edema, fever, chest pain, pain, asthenia, malaise, flu-like symptoms, *anaphylaxis*. **Ophthalmologic:** Miosis, diplopia, abnormal vision. **GU:** Urinary incontinence, intramenstrual bleeding, UTI. **Hematologic:** *Aplastic anemia*, purpura, leukopenia, lymphadenopathy, leukocytosis, thrombocytopenia, granulocytopenia, positive antinuclear factor test, *agranulocytosis*, qualitative platelet disorder. **Dermatologic:** Acne, rash, pruritus, urticaria, bullous eruption, buccal mucous membrane swelling, *Stevens-Johnson syndrome*. **Miscellaneous:** Otitis media, *acute liver failure*, taste perversion, myalgia, photosensitivity, substernal chest pain, dystonia, allergic reaction.

NOTE: Side effects may differ depending on whether the drug is used as monotherapy or adjunctive therapy in adults or for Lennox-Gastaut syndrome in children.

LABORATORY TEST CONSIDERATIONS
↑ ALT, AST, GGT, LDH, alkaline phosphatase, CPK. Hypophosphatemia, hypokalemia, hyponatremia.

DRUG INTERACTIONS
Carbamazepine / ↓ Carbamazepine steady-state levels and ↑ steady-state carbamazepine epoxide (metabolite) levels. Also, drug → 50% ↑ in felbamate clearance
Methsuximide / ↑ Normethsuxmide levels; decrease methsuximide dose
Phenobarbital / ↑ Phenobarbital levels and ↓ in felbamate levels
Phenytoin / ↑ Phenytoin steady-state drug levels necessitating a 40% decrease in drug dose. Also, drug ↑ felbamate clearance
Valproic acid / ↑ Steady-state valproic acid levels

HOW SUPPLIED
Oral Suspension: 600 mg/5 mL; *Tablets:* 400 mg, 600 mg.

DOSAGE
• **TABLETS**
Monotherapy, initial therapy.
Adults over 14 years of age, initial: 1,200 mg per day in divided doses 3–4 times per day. The dose may be increased in 600-mg increments q 2 weeks to 2,400 mg/day based on clinical response and thereafter to 3,600 mg/day, if needed.
Conversion to monotherapy.
Adults: Initiate at 1,200 mg/day in divided doses 3–4 times per day. Reduce dose of concomitant antiepileptic drugs by one-third at initiation of felbamate therapy. At week 2, the felbamate dose should be increased to 2,400 mg/day while reducing the dose of other antiepileptic drugs up to another one-third of the original dose. At week 3, increase the felbamate dose to 3,600 mg/day and continue to decrease the dose of other antiepileptic drugs as indicated by response.

Adjunctive therapy.
Add felbamate at a dose of 1,200 mg/day in divided doses 3–4 times per day while reducing current antiepileptic drugs by 20%. Further decreases of concomitant antiepileptic drugs may be needed to minimize side effects due to drug interactions. The dose of felbamate can be increased by 1,200-mg/day increments at weekly intervals to 3,600 mg/day.

Lennox-Gastaut syndrome in children, aged 2–14 years.
As an adjunct, add felbamate at a dose of 15 mg/kg/day in divided doses 3–4 times per day while decreasing present antiepileptic drugs by 20%. Further decreases in antiepileptic drug dosage may be needed to minimize side effects due to drug interactions. The dose of felbamate may be increased by 15 mg/kg/day increments at weekly intervals to 45 mg/kg/day.

NURSING CONSIDERATIONS

ADMINISTRATION/STORAGE
1. Shake suspension well before use.
2. Store in a tightly closed container at room temperature away from heat, direct sunlight, or moisture. Keep away from children.
3. Most side effects seen during adjunctive therapy resolve as the dose of concomitant antiepileptic drugs is decreased.
4. For geriatric clients, start at the low end of the dosage range.

ASSESSMENT
1. Note type, location, duration, characteristics of seizures, other agents trialed.
2. Check if monotherapy or adjunctive therapy needed.
3. List drugs prescribed to ensure none interact; assess need for dosage change.
4. Inform of potentially lethal side effects R/T aplastic anemia. Provide written explanation of risks and have consent form signed.
5. Monitor CBC, renal, LFTs and seizure occurrence.

CLIENT/FAMILY TEACHING
1. Take only as prescribed; store appropriately to prevent loss of effectiveness (away from sunlight, heat and moisture)
2. Shake bottle well before measuring prescribed dosage.
3. Avoid activities that require mental alertness until drug effects realized.
4. Side effects include anorexia, vomiting, insomnia, nausea, and headaches; report if persistent. May take with food if GI upset.
5. Report any changes in mental status or loss of seizure control; clinical response determines dosage.
6. Do not stop taking; may increase seizure frequency.
7. Seizure control benefit should far outweigh the potential for development of aplastic anemia; assess risk.

OUTCOMES/EVALUATE
Control of seizures

Felodipine
(feh-**LOHD**-ih-peen)

CLASSIFICATION(S):
Calcium channel blocker
PREGNANCY CATEGORY: C
Rx: Plendil.
✤**Rx:** Renedil.

SEE ALSO *CALCIUM CHANNEL BLOCKING AGENTS.*

USES
Hypertension, alone or with other antihypertensives. *Investigational:* Raynaud's syndrome, CHF.

ACTION/KINETICS
Action
Moderate increase in HR and moderate decrease in peripheral resistance. No effect on the QRS complex, PR interval, or QT interval with no effect to a slight decrease on myocardial contractility.

Pharmacokinetics
Onset after PO: 120–300 min. **Peak plasma levels:** 2.5–5 hr. **t½, elimination:** 11–16 hr. Metabolized in the liver with 70% excreted in the urine and 10% excreted in the feces. **Plasma protein binding:** Over 99%.

Bold Italic = life threatening side effect   ■ = black box warning   ✤ = Available in Canada

CONTRAINDICATIONS
Lactation.
SPECIAL CONCERNS
Use with caution in clients with CHF or compromised ventricular function, especially in combination with a beta-adrenergic blocking agent. Use with caution in impaired hepatic function or reduced hepatic blood flow. May cause a greater hypotensive effect in geriatric clients. Safety and effectiveness have not been determined in children.
SIDE EFFECTS
Most Common
Peripheral edema, asthenia, dizziness, lightheadedness, headache, dyspepsia, constipation, cough, URTI, flushing.
CV: Significant hypotension, syncope, angina pectoris, peripheral edema, palpitations, AV block, *MI*, **arrhythmias**, tachycardia. **CNS:** Dizziness, lightheadedness, headache, nervousness, sleepiness, irritability, anxiety, insomnia, paresthesia, depression, amnesia, paranoia, psychosis, hallucinations. **Body as a whole:** Asthenia, flushing, muscle cramps, pain, inflammation, warm feeling, influenza. **GI:** Nausea, abdominal discomfort, cramps, dyspepsia, diarrhea, constipation, vomiting, dry mouth, flatulence. **Dermatologic:** Rash, flushing, dermatitis, urticaria, pruritus. **Respiratory:** Rhinitis, URTI, rhinorrhea, pharyngitis, sinusitis, nasal and chest congestion, SOB, wheezing, dyspnea, cough, bronchitis, sneezing, respiratory infection. **Miscellaneous:** Anemia, gingival hyperplasia, sexual difficulties, epistaxis, back pain, facial edema, erythema, urinary frequency or urgency, dysuria.
ADDITIONAL DRUG INTERACTIONS
Barbiturates / ↓ Effect of felodipine
Carbamazepine / ↓ Felodipine effects
Cimetidine / ↑ Bioavailability of felodipine
Cyclosporine / ↑ Pharmacologic and toxic effects of felodipine; ↑ cyclosporine levels and toxicity
Digoxin / ↑ Peak plasma levels of digoxin
Erythromycins / ↑ Erythromycin effects; monitor CV status closely
Fentanyl / Possible severe hypotension or ↑ fluid volume

Grapefruit juice / ↑ Plasma levels of felodipine R/T ↓ liver breakdown
Itraconazole / ↑ Felodipine serum levels
Nelfinavir / Possible leg edema and orthostatic hypotension
Oxcarbazepine / ↓ Felodipine effects
Phenytoin / ↓ Effects of felodipine
Ranitidine / ↑ Bioavailability of felodipine
HOW SUPPLIED
Tablets, Extended-Release: 2.5 mg, 5 mg, 10 mg.
DOSAGE————————
• **TABLETS, EXTENDED-RELEASE**
  Hypertension
Initial: 5 mg once daily (2.5 mg in clients over 65 years of age and in those with impaired liver function); **then:** adjust dose according to response, usually at 2-week intervals with the usual dosage range being 2.5–10 mg once daily. Doses greater than 10 mg increase the rate of peripheral edema and other vasodilatory side effects.

NURSING CONSIDERATIONS
ADMINISTRATION/STORAGE
Bioavailability is not affected by food. It is increased more than twofold when taken with doubly concentrated grapefruit juice as compared with water or orange juice.
ASSESSMENT
1. Note disease onset, other agents used, outcome. Check for history of heart failure or compromised ventricular function. Assess EKG, or for evidence of disease associated organ damage.
2. List drugs currently prescribed to ensure no interactions.
3. During dosage adjustments, monitor BP closely in clients over 65 or with impaired hepatic function.
CLIENT/FAMILY TEACHING
1. Swallow tablets whole; do not chew or crush. Avoid taking with grapefruit juice.
2. Do not stop abruptly; abrupt withdrawal may increase frequency and duration of chest pain.
3. Avoid activities that require mental alertness until effects are realized.

4. Rise slowly from a lying position and dangle feet before standing to minimize low BP effects.

5. Report any headaches, flushing or extremity swelling. Keep written record of BP and HR for review.

6. Practice frequent oral hygiene to minimize incidence and severity of drug-induced gingival hyperplasia.

OUTCOMES/EVALUATE

Control of hypertension

Fenofibrate 📷

(**fee**-noh-**FY**-brayt)

CLASSIFICATION(S):

Antihyperlipidemic

PREGNANCY CATEGORY: C

Rx: Antara, Lipofen, Lofibra, Tricor, Triglide.

✦**Rx: Fenofibrate:** Apo-Feno-Micro, Apo-Fenofibrate, Nu-Fenofibrate. **Fenofibrate Microcoated:** Lipidil Supra. **Fenofibrate Micronized:** Gen-Fenofibrate Micro, Lipidil Micro, Novo-Fenofibrate Micronized, PMS-Fenofibrate Micro.

USES

(1) Adjunctive therapy to diet to reduce elevated LDL-C, total-C, triglycerides, and Apo B and to increase HDL-C in adults with primary hypercholesterolemia or mixed dyslipidemia (Fredrickson Types IIa and II b). (2) Adjunctive therapy to diet to treat adults with hypertriglyceridemia (Fredrickson Types IV and V hyperlipidemia). *Investigational:* Hyperuricemia.

ACTION/KINETICS

Action

Is converted to the active fenofibric acid, which lowers plasma triglycerides. Probable mechanism is to inhibit triglyceride synthesis, resulting in a reduction of cholesterol, triglycerides, apolipoprotein B, and VLDL and by stimulating catabolism of triglyceride-rich lipoprotein. Increases urinary excretion of uric acid.

Pharmacokinetics

Well absorbed; absorption is increased when given with food. **Peak plasma levels:** 4–8 hr, depending on the product; **steady-state plasma levels:** within 5–7 days. **t½:** 20–23 hr with once daily dosing. Fenofibric acid and an inactive metabolite are excreted through the urine (60%) and feces (25%). **Plasma protein binding:** 99%.

CONTRAINDICATIONS

Hepatic or severe renal dysfunction (including primary biliary cirrhosis), those with unexplained, persistent abnormal liver function, and preexisting gallbladder disease. Lactation.

SPECIAL CONCERNS

Due to similarity to clofibrate and gemfibrozil, side effects, including death, are possible. Select dosage carefully in the elderly. Safety and efficacy have not been determined in children.

SIDE EFFECTS

Most Common

Abnormal LFTs, respiratory disorder, abdominal/back pain, headache, nausea, diarrhea, rhinitis.

GI: *Pancreatitis,* cholelithiasis, dyspepsia, N&V, diarrhea, abdominal pain, dry mouth, constipation, flatulence, eructation, hepatitis, cholecystitis, hepatomegaly, gastroenteritis, rectal disorder, esophagitis, gastritis, colitis, tooth disorder, anorexia, GI disorder, duodenal/peptic ulcer, *rectal hemorrhage*, fatty liver deposit. **CNS:** Decreased libido, dizziness, increased appetite, insomnia, paresthesia, depression, vertigo, anxiety, hypertonia, nervousness, neuralgia, somnolence. **CV:** Angina pectoris, hyper/hypotension, vasodilation, coronary artery disorder, abnormal ECG, ventricular extrasystoles, *MI*, peripheral vascular disorder, migraine, varicose vein, palpitation, CV/vascular disorder, arrhythmia, phlebitis, tachycardia, atrial fibrillation. **Dermatologic:** Rash, pruritus, eczema, herpes simplex/zoster, urticaria, acne, sweating, contact/fungal dermatitis, alopecia, maculopapular rash, nail/skin disorder, skin ulcer. **Respiratory:** Rhinitis, respiratory disorder, increased cough, sinusitis, allergic pulmonary alveolitis, pharyngitis, bronchitis, dyspnea, asthma, pneumonia, laryngitis. **GU:** Polyuria, vaginitis, prostatic disorder, dysuria, abnormal kidney function, urolithiasis, gynecomastia, unintended pregnancy, vaginal moniliasis, cystitis, urinary frequency. **Hematologic:** Anemia, leukopenia, ecchymosis, eosinophilia, lymphadenopathy, thrombocytopenia. **Musculoskeletal:** Myopathy, myositis, arthralgia, myalgia, myasthenia, rhabdomyolysis, arthritis, tenosynovitis, joint disorder, arthrosis, leg cramps, bursitis. **Hypersensitivity:** Severe skin rashes, urticaria; rarely, *Stevens-Johnson syndrome and toxic epidermal necrolysis.* **Ophthalmic:** Eye irritation, blurred/abnormal vision, conjunctivitis, eye floaters, eye disorder, amblyopia, cataract, refraction disorder. **Otic:** Ear pain, otitis media. **Body as a whole:** Infections, pain, headache, asthenia, fatigue, flu syndrome, photosensitivity, malaise, allergic reaction, fever, weight gain/loss. **Miscellaneous:** Back/chest pain, cyst, hernia, accidental injury, diabetes mellitus, gout, edema, peripheral edema, increased appetite.

LABORATORY TEST CONSIDERATIONS
↑ AST, ALT, CPK, creatinine, blood urea. Initial ↓ hemoglobin, hematocrit, WBCs. Hypoglycemia, hyperuricemia. Abnormal LFTs.

DRUG INTERACTIONS
Anticoagulants, oral / Potentiation of coumarin anticoagulants (prolongation of PT/INR); determine PT/INR frequently and dose reduction is advisable
Bile acid sequestrants / ↓ Absorption of fenofibrate R/T binding; give fenofibrate at least 1 hr before to 4–6 hr after a bile acid binding resin
Cyclosporine / ↑ Risk of nephrotoxicity; use lowest effective dose
HMG-CoA reductase inhibitors / ↑ Possibility of rhabdomyolysis, ↑ creatine kinase, and myloglobinuria → acute renal failure; avoid concomitant use unless benefits outweigh risks

HOW SUPPLIED
Capsules: 50 mg, 100 mg, 150 mg; *Capsules, Micronized (Antara, Lofibra):* 43 mg, 67 mg, 130 mg, 134 mg, 200 mg; *Tablets (Lofibra, Triglide, Tricor):* 48 mg, 50 mg, 54 mg, 145 mg, 160 mg.

DOSAGE
• **CAPSULES; TABLETS**

Primary hypertriglyceridemia., mixed hyperlipidemia.
Individualize dose depending on client response; adjust, if necessary, following repeat lipid determinations at 4- to 8-week intervals. **Antara, initial:** 130 mg/day with meals; for renal function impairment or the elderly, give 43 mg/day initially. **Lipofen, initial:** 150 mg/day. In the elderly and in impaired renal function, start with 50 mg/day. **Lofibra capsules, initial:** 200 mg/day with meals; for renal function impairment or the elderly, give 67 mg/day. **Lofibra, tablets, initial:** 160 mg/day with meals; for renal function impairment or the elderly, give 54 mg/day. **Tricor, initial:** 145 mg/day; for renal function impairment or the elderly, give 48 mg/day initially. **Triglide, initial:** 160 mg/day with food; for renal function impairment or the elderly, give 50 mg/day.

Hypertriglyceridemia.
Individualize dosage according to client response and adjust if necessary following repeat lipid determinations at 4- to 8-week intervals. **Antara, initial:** 43–130 mg/day without regard to meals; maximum dosage: 130 mg/day. **Lipofen, initial:** 50–150 mg/day. **Lofibra capsules, initial:** 67–200 mg/day with meals; maximum dosage: 200 mg/day. **Lofibra tablets, initial:** 54–160 mg/day; maximum dosage: 160 mg/day. **Tricor, initial:** 48–145 mg/day; maximum dosage: 145 mg/day. **Triglide, initial:** 50–160 mg/day; maximum dosage: 160 mg/day.

NURSING CONSIDERATIONS
ADMINISTRATION/STORAGE
1. Place clients on an appropriate triglyceride-lowering diet before starting fenofibrate and continue during treatment.
2. Give capsules and tablets with food to optimize bioavailability. Antara and Tricor can be given without regard to meals.
3. Reduce dosage in clients who have C_{CR} <50 mL/min.
4. Store from 15–30°C (59–86°F); protect from moisture.

ASSESSMENT
1. Note reasons for therapy, other agents trialed, cardiac risk factors.
2. Control BP, BS and assess renal and LFTs regularly; avoid drug with severe dysfunction.
3. Monitor lipids, CBC, renal and LFTs; if ALT or AST >3 times normal, discontinue therapy. Reduce dosage with C_{CR} <50 mL/min.

CLIENT/FAMILY TEACHING
1. Take as directed with/without meals; except take triglide tablets with food.
2. Follow prescribed diet for triglyceride reduction as well as regular exercise program, smoking cessation, alcohol and salt reduction.
3. Report skin rash, GI upset, persistent abdominal pain, muscle pain, tenderness, fatigue, GU dysfunction or weakness.
4. Avoid therapy with pregnancy and breastfeeding.
5. Report as scheduled for regular liver tests and triglyceride levels. Drug therapy should be reevaluated after 2 months if desired lipid reduction is not evident with maximum dose therapy.
6. Advise to take 1 or more before or 4–6 hr after a bile acid binding resin to avoid decreased absorption. Keep all F/U appointment to evaluate response to therapy.

OUTCOMES/EVALUATE
↓ Triglyceride levels ↓ ASHD events

Fenoldopam mesylate   Ⅳ
(feh-**NOL**-doh-pam)

CLASSIFICATION(S):
Treatment of hypertensive emergency
PREGNANCY CATEGORY: B
Rx: Corlopam.

USES
Adults: In-hospital, short-term (up to 48 hr) management of severe hypertension when rapid, quickly reversible, emergency reduction of BP is needed (including malignant hypertension with deteriorating end-organ function). **Children:** In-hospital, short-term (up to 48 hr) reduction of BP.

ACTION/KINETICS
Action
Rapid-acting vasodilator that is an agonist for D_1-like dopamine receptors and α_2-adrenoreceptors. Causes vasodilation in coronary, renal, mesenteric, and peripheral arteries; vascular beds do not respond uniformly.

Pharmacokinetics
Steady-state levels: About 20 min. **$t\frac{1}{2}$, elimination:** About 5 min in mild to moderate hypertensives. Metabolized in liver; 90% is excreted in urine and 10% in the feces.

CONTRAINDICATIONS
Use with beta-blockers or in those with sulfite sensitivity.

SPECIAL CONCERNS
Use with caution during lactation and in those with glaucoma or intraocular hypertension. Effects have been studied in children less than 1 month of age (at least 2 kg or full term) to 12 years of age; use caution in selecting dosage for 12–16-year-old clients.

SIDE EFFECTS
Most Common
In adults: Headache, dizziness, N&V, hypotension, back pain, sweating.
In children: Hypotension, tachycardia.
CV: Tachycardia, hypotension, flushing, ST-T abnormalities, postural hypotension, extrasystoles, palpitations, bradycardia, *heart failure, ischemic heart disease, MI*, angina pectoris. **Body as a whole:** Headache, sweating, back pain, non-specific chest pain, pyrexia, limb cramp. **CNS:** Nervousness, anxiety, insomnia, dizziness. **GI:** N&V, abdominal pain or fullness, constipation, diarrhea. **Respiratory:** Nasal congestion, dyspnea, upper respiratory disorder. **Hematologic:** Leukocytosis, bleeding. **Miscellaneous:** Reaction at injection site, UTI, oliguria. ocular hypertension.

LABORATORY TEST CONSIDERATIONS
↑ Creatinine, BUN, serum glucose, transaminase, LDH. Hypokalemia.

Bold Italic = life threatening side effect   ■ = black box warning   ✤ = Available in Canada

OD **OVERDOSE MANAGEMENT**
Symptoms: Excessive hypotension.
Treatment: Discontinue the drug. Provide supportive treatment.

HOW SUPPLIED
Injection: 10 mg/mL; *Injection Concentrate:* 10 mg/mL.

DOSAGE

• **IV, CONTINUOUS INFUSION**
Hypertensive emergency.

Adults: Rate of infusion is individualized according to body weight and to desired speed and extent of effect. See package insert for table of infusion rates. Doses range from 0.01 mcg/kg/min–0.3 mcg/kg/min. Titrate the initial dose upward or downward, no more frequently than every 15 min. The recommended increments for titration are 0.05–0.1 mcg/kg/min. **Children, usual initial:** 0.2 mcg/kg/min. Increased doses of up to 0.3-0.5 mcg/kg/min every 20–30 min are generally well tolerated.

NURSING CONSIDERATIONS

ADMINISTRATION/STORAGE

IV 1. Do not use a bolus dose.
2. Most of the effect of a given infusion is reached in 15 min.
3. Initial dose is titrated up or down no more often than every 15 min, and less frequently as desired BP is approached. Recommended increments for titration are 0.05–0.1 mcg/kg/min.
4. Initial doses of 0.03–0.1 mcg/kg/min have been associated with less reflex tachycardia than higher doses (>0.3 mcg/kg/min).
5. Administer using a calibrated mechanical infusion pump that can deliver desired infusion rate accurately.
6. Infusion may be discontinued abruptly or tapered gradually prior to discontinuation.
7. Transition to PO therapy can be started any time after BP is stabilized during infusion.
8. Dilute ampule concentrate in 0.9% NaCl or D5W injection for a final concentration of 40 mcg/mL (i.e., add 4 mL of the concentrate to 1,000 mL; 2 mL of the concentrate to 500 mL; or, 1 mL of the concentrate to 250 mL). Each mL of

concentrate contains 10 mg of drug. Each ampule is for single use only.
9. Store ampules at 2–30°C (36–86°F).
10. Diluted solution is stable under normal light and temperature for 24 hr or less. Discard any diluted solution that is not used within 24 hr.

ASSESSMENT

1. Note clinical presentation, onset, characteristics of S&S, evidence of neurologic involvement/changes.
2. Assess for glaucoma, sulfite sensitivity, or intraocular hypertension. List drugs prescribed to ensure none interact unfavorably; avoid use with beta-blockers.
3. Monitor VS, ECG, electrolytes, renal and LFTs; obtain weight.
4. Assess for physical conditions that may have precipitated event; evaluate life-style changes needed; continue meds to control BP.

CLIENT/FAMILY TEACHING

Drug is administered by IV infusion to help lower very high blood pressure readings quickly.

OUTCOMES/EVALUATE

Reduction in BP with hypertensive crisis

Fenoprofen calcium
(fen-oh-**PROH**-fen) ■ ℘

CLASSIFICATION(S):
Nonsteroidal anti-inflammatory drug
PREGNANCY CATEGORY: B
Rx: Nalfon.

SEE ALSO *NONSTEROIDAL ANTI-INFLAMMATORY DRUGS.*

USES

(1) Relief of S&S of rheumatoid arthritis and osteoarthritis. Is used for treatment of acute flare-ups and exacerbations and for long-term management of these diseases. (2) Mild to moderate pain. *Investigational:* Juvenile rheumatoid arthritis, prophylaxis of migraine, migraine due to menses, sunburn.

ACTION/KINETICS

Pharmacokinetics

Peak serum levels: 1–2 hr. **Peak effect:** 2 hr. **Duration:** 4–6 hr. **t½:** 2–3 hr. **Onset, as antiarthritic:** Within 2 days; **maximum effect:** 2–3 weeks. Food (but not antacids) delays absorption and decreases the total amount absorbed. 99% eliminated through the kidneys. **Plasma protein binding:** 99%.

CONTRAINDICATIONS

Use in pregnancy and children less than 12 years of age. Renal dysfunction.

SPECIAL CONCERNS

■ (1) Cardiovascular risk. NSAIDs may cause an increased risk of serious CV thrombotic events, MI, and stroke, which can be fatal. This risk may increase with duration of use. Clients with CV disease or risk factors for CV disease may be at greater risk. (2) Fenoprofen is contraindicated for treatment of perioperative pain in the setting of coronary artery bypass graft surgery. (3) GI risk. NSAIDs cause an increased risk of serious GI adverse events, including bleeding, ulceration, and perforation of the stomach or intestines, which can be fatal. These events can occur at any time during use and without warning symptoms. Elderly clients are at greater risk for serious GI events.■ Safety and efficacy in children have not been established.

SIDE EFFECTS

Most Common

Headache, dizziness, asthenia/malaise, nervousness, somnolence, nausea, constipation, dyspepsia/indigestion, peripheral edema.

See *Nonsteroidal Anti-Inflammatory Drugs* for a complete list of possible side effects. Also, **GU:** Dysuria, hematuria, cystitis, interstitial nephritis, nephrotic syndrome. Overdosage has caused tachycardia and hypotension.

HOW SUPPLIED

Capsules: 200 mg, 300 mg; *Tablets:* 600 mg.

DOSAGE

• **CAPSULES; TABLETS**

Rheumatoid and osteoarthritis.

Adults: 300–600 mg 3–4 times per day, not to exceed a total daily dose of 3,200 mg. Adjust dose according to response of client. 2–3 weeks may be needed for improvement. Those with rheumatoid arthritis seem to require larger doses than do those with osteoarthritis.

Mild to moderate pain.

200 mg q 4–6 hr, as needed, up to a total daily dose of 3,200 mg.

NURSING CONSIDERATIONS

℀ Do not confuse fenoprofen with flurbiprofen (also a NSAID).

ADMINISTRATION/STORAGE

1. Those over 70 years of age generally require half the usual adult dose.
2. Store from 15–30°C (59–86°F).

ASSESSMENT

1. List reasons for therapy, symptom characteristics, other agents trialed, outcome.
2. Assess joints for inflammation, swelling, deformities, mobility; rate pain levels.
3. Obtain periodic ophthalmic, auditory tests with chronic therapy.
4. Monitor BP, CBC, PT/PTT, renal and LFTs with chronic therapy; avoid with renal dysfunction.
5. Assess for CAD; an increased risk of thrombotic events, MI and stroke may occur.

CLIENT/FAMILY TEACHING

1. Take 30 min before or 2 hr after meals; peak blood levels are delayed or diminished if taken with food but the total amount absorbed is not affected. If GI upset occurs, may be taken with meals or milk.
2. With swallowing problems, tablets can be crushed and contents mixed with applesauce or other similar foods.
3. Report any unusual bruising/bleeding, blood oozing from gums/nose, sore throat, fever, extremity swelling, sob, or wt gain. May elevate BP.
4. Avoid aspirin, alcohol, and OTC agents.
5. Report evidence of liver toxicity, such as jaundice, RUQ pain, or a change in the color/consistency of stools.
6. If vomiting or diarrhea occurs, monitor appetite, and weight; report if persistent.

Bold Italic = life threatening side effect   ■ = black box warning   ♣ = Available in Canada

7. Report increased headaches, sleepiness, dizziness, nervousness, weakness, or fatigue. Report lack of response, adverse side effects, or severe GI upset.

OUTCOMES/EVALUATE

↓ Joint pain and inflammation with ↑ mobility

Fentanyl citrate ■Ⅳ
(FEN-tah-nil)

CLASSIFICATION(S):
Narcotic analgesic
PREGNANCY CATEGORY: C
Rx: Injection: Sublimaze, **C-II Lozenge on a Stick:** Actiq, Fentanyl Citrate Transmucosal. **Tablets, Buccal:** Fentora.

SEE ALSO *NARCOTIC ANALGESICS.*

USES
Parenteral: (1) Preanesthetic medication. (2) Induction and maintenance of anesthesia of short duration and immediate postoperative period. (3) Opioid analgesic supplement in general or regional anesthesia. (4) Combined with droperidol for preanesthetic medication, induction of anesthesia, or as adjunct in maintenance of general or regional anesthesia. (5) Combined with oxygen for anesthesia in high-risk clients undergoing open heart surgery, orthopedic procedures, or complicated neurologic procedures.

Oral (transmucosal-lozenge and buccal tablet): Management of breakthrough cancer pain in those with cancer who are already receiving and are tolerate of opioid therapy for their underlying persistent cancer pain.

Investigational: (1) Pain and anxiety management in pediatric burn clients undergoing dressing change and tubbing. (2) Reduce postoperative anxiety and excitement in ambulatory children.

ACTION/KINETICS
Action
Effects similar to those of morphine and meperidine. May have profound effects on respiration.

Pharmacokinetics
IV, onset: Immediate; **IM, onset:** 7–8 min. **Peak effect:** Approximately 30 min for the injection and 20–30 min for transmucosal product. **Duration:** 30–60 min after IV and 1–2 hr after IM. **t½:** 3.65 hr for the injection and 7 hr for transmucosal. When the oral lozenge (transmucosal administration) is sucked, fentanyl citrate is absorbed through the mucosal tissues of the mouth and GI tract. Actiq resembles a lollipop; sucking provides a rapid onset of action. Faster-acting and shorter duration than morphine or meperidine. Metabolized by CYP3A4 enzymes in the liver and excreted in the urine.

CONTRAINDICATIONS
The transmucosal form is contraindicated in children who weigh less than 10 kg, for the treatment of acute or chronic pain (safety for this use not established), and for doses in excess of 15 mcg/kg in children and in excess of 5 mcg/kg (maximum of 400 mcg) in adults. Use outside the hospital setting is contraindicated. Myasthenia gravis and other conditions in which muscle relaxants should not be used. Clients particularly sensitive to respiratory depression. Use during labor. Lactation.

SPECIAL CONCERNS
■ (1) Fentanyl is an opioid agonist and a Schedule II controlled substance with an abuse liability similar to other opioid analgesics. Fentanyl can be abused in a manner similar to other opioid agonists, legal or illicit. This should be considered when prescribing or dispensing fentanyl in situations in which the health care provider or pharmacist is concerned about an increased risk of misuse, abuse, or diversion. (2) Schedule II opioid substances, which include morphine, oxycodone, hydromorphone, oxymorphone, and methadone, have the highest abuse potential for abuse and risk of fatal overdose due to respiratory depression. (3) The fentanyl lozenge and buccal tablet are indicated only for the management of breakthrough cancer pain in clients with cancer already receiving and tolerant to opioid therapy for their underlying per-

sistent cancer pain. Clients considered opioid-tolerant are those who are taking oral morphine 60 mg/day or more, transdermal fentanyl 25 mcg/hr, oxycodone 20 mg/day, oral hydromorphone 8 mg/day, or an equianalgesic dose of another opioid for a week or longer. (4) Because life-threatening respiratory depression could occur at any dose in clients not taking chronic opiates, it is contraindicated in the management of acute or postoperative pain. This product is not indicated for use in opioid-nontolerant clients. (5) Instruct clients and their caregivers that this drug contains a medicine in an amount that can be fatal to a child. Keep all units out of the reach of children, and discard opened units properly. (6) This medicine should be used only in the care of cancer clients and only by health care providers who are knowledgeable of and skilled in the use of Schedule II opioids to treat cancer pain. (7) *Tablet:* Because of the higher bioavailability of fentanyl in the buccal tablet, when converting clients from other oral fentanyl products (including fentanyl lozenge) to the buccal tablet, do not substitute the buccal tablet on a mcg per mcg basis. Adjust dosage as appropriate.■ Safety and efficacy have not been determined in children less than 2 years of age. Use with caution and at reduced dosage in poor-risk clients, children, the elderly, and when other CNS depressants are used. Use of the transmucosal form carries a risk of hypoventilation that may result in death. The respiratory depressant effect of fentanyl may last longer than the analgesic effect.

SIDE EFFECTS
Most Common
Injection: Bradycardia, circulatory depression, hypotension, dizziness, sweating, N&V, chest wall/muscle rigidity, respiratory depression, blurred vision.
Transmucosal: N&V, anxiety, asthenia, confusion, depression, headache, insomnia, sedation/somnolence, itching, rash, constipation.
See *Narcotic Analgesics* for a complete list of possible side effects. Also, skeletal and thoracic muscle rigidity, especially after rapid IV administration. Bradycardia, *seizures*, diaphoresis. Transmucosal form may cause *life-threatening hypoventilation.*

ADDITIONAL DRUG INTERACTIONS
Diazepam / ↑ Risk of CV depression
Droperidol / Hypotension and ↓ pulmonary arterial pressure
Nitrous oxide / ↑ Risk of CV depression
Protease inhibitors / ↑ CNS and respiratory depression
Ritonavir / ↑ Fentanyl effect R/T ↓ liver metabolism

HOW SUPPLIED
Fentanyl Citrate: *Injection:* 50 mcg/mL; *Lozenge on a Stick:* 200 mcg, 400 mcg, 600 mcg, 800 mcg, 1,200 mcg, 1,600 mcg (all as the base); *Tablets, Buccal:* 100 mcg, 200 mcg, 400 mcg, 600 mcg, 800 mcg.

DOSAGE
● **IM; IV**
Preoperative medication.
Adults: 50–100 mcg IM 30–60 min before surgery.
Adjunct to general anesthesia.
Adults, total low dose: 2 mcg/kg IV for minor, painful surgical procedures and postsurgical relief; **maintenance low dose:** 2 mcg/kg (additional doses are infrequently needed in minor procedures). **Adults, total moderate dose:** 2–20 mcg/kg IV, depending on length and depth of anesthesia desired; **maintenance moderate dose:** 2–20 mcg/kg when indicated. Use 25–200 mcg total IV or IM when movement and/or changes in vital signs indicate surgical stress or lightening of anesthesia. **Adults, total high dose:** 20–50 mcg/kg for 'stress free' anesthesia. Use this dose during open heart surgery and complicated neurosurgical and orthopedic procedures where surgery is prolonged and stress response is detrimental. Use with nitrous oxide/oxygen to reduce the stress response. Postoperative ventilation and observation are required. **Maintenance, high dose:** 20–50 mcg/kg (range: 25 to half the initial loading dose). Individualize dose; administer when vital signs indicate surgical stress and lightening of anesthesia.

Bold Italic = life threatening side effect   ■ = black box warning   ✦ = Available in Canada

Adjunct to regional anesthesia.
Adults: 50–100 mcg IM or slowly IV over 1–2 min as required.
Postoperatively, recovery room.
Adults: 50–100 mcg IM q 1–2 hr for control of pain, tachypnea, and emergence delirium.
As general anesthetic with oxygen and a muscle relaxant.
50–100 mcg/kg (up to 150 mcg/kg may be required) with oxygen and a muscle relaxant when attenuation of the responses to surgical stress is very important; used for open heart surgery and other major surgical procedures to protect the myocardium from excess oxygen demand and for complicated neurological and orthopedic procedures.
Children, induction and maintenance of anesthesia.
Pediatric, 2–12 years: 2–3 mcg/kg. Safety and efficacy have not been determined in children less than 2 years of age.

• **TRANSMUCOSAL (ORAL LOZENGE)**
Breakthrough cancer pain.
Individualize according to weight, age, physical status, general condition and medical status, underlying pathology, use of other drugs, type of anesthetic to be used, and the type and length of the surgical procedure. **Initial:** 200 mcg. Until the appropriate dose is determined, it may be necessary to use an additional unit during a single episode. Redosing may start 15 min after the previous unit has been completed (30 min after the start of the previous unit). Do not give more than 2 units for each individual breakthrough cancer pain episode while clients are in the titration phase and consuming units that individually may be subtherapeutic. If treatment of several consecutive breakthrough cancer episodes requires more than 1 fentanyl lozenge per episode, consider an increase in dose to the next higher available strength. At each new dose during titration, 6 units of the titration dose should be prescribed. Evaluate each new dose in the titration period of several episodes of breakthrough cancer pain (usually 1–2 days) to determine whether the dose is adequate with acceptable side effects. Once a successful dose has been determined (i.e., an average episode is treated with a single unit), clients should limit consumption to 4 units/day or less. If consumption increases to more than 4 units/day, reevaluate the dose of the long-acting opioid for persistent cancer pain.

Dosage adjustment of the lozenge and the maintenance (around-the-clock) opioid analgesic may be needed in some clients to provide adequate relief of breakthrough cancer pain.

Gradually titrate downward for discontinuation as it is not known at what dose level the opioid may be discontinued without producing the signs and symptoms of abrupt withdrawal.

• **TABLETS, BUCCAL**
Breakthrough cancer pain.
Titrate to a dose of the buccal tablet that provides adequate analgesia with tolerable side effects. **Initial:** 100 mcg. Initiate titration using multiples of the fentanyl, 100 mcg buccal tablet. Those needing to titrate above 100 mcg can be instructed to use two 100 mcg tablets (one on each side of the mouth). Once a successful dose has been established, more than 4 breakthrough pain episodes per day, re-evaluate the dose of the maintenance (around-the-clock) opioid used for persistent pain.

Dosing may be repeated once during a single episode of breakthrough pain if pain is not adequately relieved by one buccal tablet. Redosing may occur over 20 min after the start of administration of the buccal tablet; use the same dosage strength.

For clients switching from oral transmucosal fentanyl to the buccal tablet, use the following conversion:
• Current PO dose of transmucosal fentanyl: 200 mcg or 400 mcg; the initial buccal tablet dose is 100 mcg.
• Current PO dose of transmucosal fentanyl: 600 mcg or 800 mcg; the initial buccal tablet dose is 200 mcg.
• Current PO dose of transmucosal fentanyl: 1,200 mcg or 1,600 mcg; the initial buccal tablet dose is 400 mcg.

NURSING CONSIDERATIONS

ADMINISTRATION/STORAGE

1. Other opioids should be used with fentanyl in reduced initial doses of one-fourth to one-third of recommended doses.

2. Reduce dose of injection in elderly and debilitated clients and those with renal or hepatic dysfunction.

3. Protect injection from light; store from 15–25°C (59–77°F). Protect transmucosal and buccal tablet products from freezing and moisture, Store the lozenge and buccal tablets from 15–30°C (59–86°F).

4. Consider lower doses of the transmucosal form with head injury, CV, pulmonary/hepatic disease or liver dysfunction.

5. When using transmucosal form, monitor at all times by an individual skilled in airway management and resuscitative techniques. Have naloxone available in event of overdose.

6. When discontinuing transmucosal fentanyl, titrate downward gradually; not known at what dose level opioid may be discontinued without causing S&S of withdrawal.

IV 7. Direct IV infusions may be given, undiluted, over a period of 1–3 min.

ASSESSMENT

1. List reasons for therapy, anticipated time frame, any previous use. Have opioid antagonist (naloxone) available to reverse drug effects.

2. Monitor VS; assess for skeletal, thoracic muscle rigidity and weakness. Respiratory depression may persist.

3. Note any neurovascular or pulmonary disease. Instruct in C&DB exercises before therapy to ensure compliance.

CLIENT/FAMILY TEACHING

1. Actiq and Fentora are only for opiod tolerant persons; generally used with cancer pain.

2. If prescribed buccal tabs do not open Fentora blister pack until ready to administer and do not store tablet once it has been removed from the blister package.

3. Fentora tablets should not be sucked, chewed, or swallowed. Place tablets between the cheek and gum and leave until disintegrated, which usually takes 14 to 25 min. If any remains after 30 min, may be swallowed with a glass of water.

4. Use caution, Actiq contains approximately 2 g of sugar/unit; dry mouth associated with fentanyl use may increase risk of dental decay.

5. Place the Actiq unit between the cheek and lower gum. The unit should not be sucked or chewed

6. Reinforce with child that transmucosal agent is not candy; it is a very potent medication that may be fatal and should not be chewed or swallowed. Place in mouth in between cheek and lower gum and ensure that the lozenge is sucked.

7. Dispose of units remaining from a prescription as soon as they are no longer needed. Drug can cause dependence and has the potential for abuse. Store appropriately. Partially consumed units are a special risk because they are no longer protected by a child-resistant pouch, yet may contain enough drug to be fatal to a child. Use temporary storage bottle provided in the event that a partially consumed unit cannot be disposed of promptly.

8. Rise slowly; may experience orthostatic hypotension (sudden drop in BP). Drug causes dizziness and drowsiness; use caution.

9. Avoid alcohol and CNS depressants for at least 24 hr.

10. Recall or memory may be suppressed; may not fully recall events surrounding procedure. Advise that procedure was done, answer any questions; reassure that this is normal and provide written guidelines for F/U for client/family to review.

OUTCOMES/EVALUATE

• Desired analgesia/relaxation
• Conscious sedation
• Control of pain

Fentanyl Transdermal System

(**FEN**-tah-nil)

CLASSIFICATION(S):
Narcotic analgesic
PREGNANCY CATEGORY: C
Rx: Duragesic-12, -25, -50, -75, and -100, Ionsys.

SEE ALSO *NARCOTIC ANALGESICS* AND *FENTANYL CITRATE.*

USES

(1) **Duragesic:** Restrict use for the management of moderate to severe chronic pain that requires continuous around-the-clock opioid administration for an extended period of time and cannot be managed by other means, such as opioid combinations, nonsteroidal analgesics, immediate-release opioids, acetaminophen-opioid combinations, or as-needed dosing with short-acting opioids. Use only in clients who are already receiving opioid therapy, who have demonstrated opioid tolerance, and who require a total daily dose at least equivalent to fentanyl transdermal system, 25 mcg/hr. Clients who are opioid tolerant are those who have been taking, for a week or longer, morphine, 60 mg/day or more; oral oxycodone, 30 mg/day or more; oral hydromorphone, 8 mg/day or more; or, an equianalgesic dose of another opioid. Can be used in opioid-tolerant pediatric clients 2 years of age and older. (2) **Ionsys:** Short-term management of acute postoperative pain in adults needing opioid analgesia while hospitalized. Not intended for home use.

ACTION/KINETICS

Action

The system provides continuous delivery of fentanyl for up to 72 hr. The amount of fentanyl released from each system each hour depends on the surface area (25 mcg/hr is released from each 10 cm^2). Each system also contains 0.1 mL of alcohol/10 cm^2; the alcohol enhances the rate of drug flux through the copolymer membrane and also increases the permeability of the skin to fentanyl.

Ionsys delivers up to 80 40-mcg doses of fentanyl in 24 hr. Each unit is powdered by a 3-volt lithium battery.

Pharmacokinetics

Following application of the system, the skin under the system absorbs fentanyl, resulting in a depot of the drug in the upper skin layers, which is then available to the general circulation. After the system is removed, the residual drug in the skin continues to be absorbed so that serum levels fall 50% in about 17 hr. Metabolized in the liver and excreted mainly in the urine.

CONTRAINDICATIONS

Use for acute or postoperative pain (including outpatient surgeries). To manage mild or intermittent pain that can be managed by acetaminophen-opioid combinations, NSAIDs, or short-acting opioids. Hypersensitivity to fentanyl or adhesives. ICP, impaired consciousness, coma, medical conditions causing hypoventilation. Use during labor and delivery. Use of initial doses exceeding 25 mcg per hr, use in children less than 2 years of age. Lactation.

SPECIAL CONCERNS

■ **Transdermal System.** (1) Fentanyl transdermal systems contain a high concentration of the potent schedule II opioid agonist, fentanyl. Schedule II drugs, which include fentanyl, hydromorphone, methadone, morphine, oxycodone, and oxymorphone, have the highest potential for abuse and associated risk of fatal overdose due to respiratory depression. Fentanyl can be abused and is subject to criminal diversion. The high content of fentanyl in the patches may be a particular target for abuse and diversion. (2) Fentanyl transdermal system is indicated for the management of persistent, moderate to severe chronic pain (such as that of malignancy) that requires continuous round-the-clock opioid administration for an extended period of time and cannot be managed by other means such as acetaminophen-opioid combinations, nonsteroidal analgesics, opioid combination products, or immediate-release

F

opioids. (3) Only use the 50, 75, and 100 mcg/hr dosages in clients who are already on and tolerant of opioid therapy. (4) Only use fentanyl transdermal system in clients who are already receiving opioid therapy, who have demonstrated opioid tolerance, and who require a total daily dose at least equivalent to fentanyl transdermal system, 25 mcg/hr transdermal system. Those who are considered opioid tolerant are those who have been taking, for a week or longer, morphine 60 mg/day or more, or oral oxycodone 30 mg/day or more, or oral hydromorphone 8 mg/day or more, or an equianalgesic dose of another opioid. (5) Because serious or life-threatening hypoventilation can occur, the transdermal product is contraindicated as follows: In those who are not opioid tolerant, in the management of acute pain or in those who require opioid analgesia for a short period of time; in the management of acute or postoperative pain, including use after outpatient or day surgeries (e.g., tonsillectomies); in the management of mild pain; in the management of intermittent pain responsive to as-needed therapy or nonopioid therapy; or, in doses exceeding 25 mcg/hr at the initiation of opioid therapy. (6) Because the peak fentanyl levels occur between 24 and 72 hr after treatment, be aware that serious or life-threatening hypoventilation may occur, even in opioid-tolerant clients, during the initial application period. (7) The concomitant use of fentanyl transdermal system with potent CYP3A4 inhibitors (e.g., clarithromycin, itraconazole, ketoconazole, nefazodone, nelfinavir, ritonavir, troleandomycin) may result in an increase in fentanyl plasma levels, which could increase or prolong adverse drug effects and may cause potentially fatal respiratory depression. Carefully monitor clients receiving fentanyl transdermal system and potent CYP3A4 inhibitors for an extended period of time and adjust dosage if warranted. (8) The safety of fentanyl has not been established in children younger than 2 years of age. Only administer to children if they are opioid tolerant and 2 years of age or older. (9) Fentanyl transdermal system is only for use in those who are already tolerant to opioid therapy of comparable potency. Use in nonopioid-tolerant clients may lead to fatal respiratory depression. Overestimating the fentanyl transdermal system dose when converting clients from another opioid medication can result in fatal overdose with the first dose. Because of the 17-hour mean elimination half-life of fentanyl transdermal system, those who are thought to have had a serious adverse event, including overdose, will require monitoring and treatment for at least 24 hr. (10) Fentanyl transdermal system can be abused in a manner similar to other opioid agonists, legal or illict. Consider this risk when giving, prescribing, or dispensing in situations where there is concern about increased risk of misuse, abuse, or diversion. (11) Persons at increased risk for opioid abuse include those with a personal or family history of substance abuse (including drug or alcohol abuse or addiction) or mental illness (e.g., major depression). Assess clients for their clinical risks for opioid abuse or addiction prior to prescribing opioids. Routinely monitor all clients receiving opioids for signs of misuse, abuse, and addiction. Clients at increased risk of opioid abuse may still be appropriately be treated with modified-release opioid formulations; however, these clients will require intensive monitoring for signs of misuse, abuse, or addiction. (12) Fentanyl transdermal patches are for transdermal use on intact skin only. Using damaged or cut fentanyl transdermal patches can lead to rapid release of the contents of the patch and absorption of a potentially fatal dose of fentanyl.

Iontophoretic Transdermal System. (1) This system is only for the treatment of hospitalized clients. Discontinue treatment with the fentanyl iontophoretic transdermal system before clients are discharged from the hospital. (2) Treatment with fentanyl may result in potentially life-threatening respiratory depression and death. To avoid potential overdosing, only the client should activate the fentanyl iontophoretic transdermal system dosing. (3) Inappropriate use of the iontophoretic transdermal system leading to ingestion, contact with mucous membranes, or unintended exposure to fentanyl hydrogel could lead to the absorption of a potentially fatal dose of fentanyl. Therefore, the hydrogels should not come into contact with the fingers or the mouth. (4) Fentanyl is a potent opioid agonist and Schedule II controlled substance with high potential for abuse similar to hydromorphone, methadone, morphine, and oxycodone. Fentanyl can be abused in a manner similar to other opioid agonists, legal or illicit. Consider this when prescribing or dispensing the iontophoretic transdermal system in situations in which there is concern about an increased risk of misuse, abuse, or diversion. After the maximum dosage administration, a significant amount of fentanyl remains in the device. (5). Keep the iontophoretic transdermal system out of the reach of children.■ Use with caution in clients with brain tumors and bradyarrhythmias, as well as in elderly, cachectic, or debilitated individuals.

SIDE EFFECTS

Most Common

N&V, anxiety, asthenia, confusion, depression, dizziness, euphoria, hallucinations, headache, nervousness, sedation/somnolence, itching/pruritus, abdominal pain, anorexia, constipation, dry mouth, diarrhea, dyspepsia, urinary retention.

See *Narcotic Analgesics* for a complete list of possible side effects. Also, sustained hypoventilation.

HOW SUPPLIED

Iontophoretic Transdermal System: 10.8 mg (to deliver eighty 40 mcg doses in 24 hr); *Transdermal Film, Extended-Release:* 12.5 mcg/hr, 25 mcg/hr, 50 mcg/hr, 75 mcg/hr, 100 mcg/hr.

DOSAGE

• **TRANSDERMAL SYSTEM**
  Analgesia.

Individualize dose. Adults, usual initial: 25 mcg per hr unless the client is tolerant to opioids (Duragesic-50, -75,

and -100 are intended for use only in clients tolerant to opioids). Initial dose should be based on (1) the daily dose, potency, and characteristics (i.e., pure agonist, mixed agonist/antagonist) of the drug the client has been taking; (2) the reliability of the relative potency estimates used to calculate the dose as estimates vary depending on the route of administration; (3) the degree, if any, of tolerance to narcotics; and (4) the general condition and status of the client.

To convert clients from PO or parenteral opioids to the transdermal system, the following method should be used: (1) the previous 24-hr analgesic requirement should be calculated; (2) convert this amount to the equianalgesic PO morphine dose; (3) find the calculated 24-hr morphine dose and the corresponding transdermal fentanyl dose using the table provided with the product; and (4) initiate treatment using the recommended fentanyl dose.

The dose may be increased no more frequently than 3 days after the initial dose or q 6 days thereafter. The ratio of 90 mg per 24 hr of PO morphine to 25 mcg per hr increase in transdermal fentanyl dose should be used to base appropriate dosage increments on the daily dose of supplementary opioids. If the dose of the fentanyl transdermal system exceeds 300 mcg per hr, it may be necessary to change clients to another narcotic analgesic. In such cases, the transdermal system should be removed and treatment initiated with one-half the equianalgesic dose of the new opioid 12–18 hr later. The dose of the new analgesic should be titrated based on the level of pain reported by the client.

• **IONTOPHORETIC TRANSDERMAL SYSTEM**
  Short-term management of pain after surgery in hospitalized adults.

Adults: Apply one unit q 24 hr to intact skin on the chest or upper outer arm (for up to 72 hr). Clients should already be receiving an acceptable level of analgesia from other products. Activation

F

of the dosing button initiates delivery of 40 mcg of fentanyl over 10 min.

NURSING CONSIDERATIONS

ADMINISTRATION/STORAGE

Transdermal System:

1. Elderly, cachetic, or debilitated clients should not be started on fentanyl transdermal system doses higher than 25 mcg/hr unless they are already tolerating an around-the-clock opioid at a dose and potency comparable with fentanyl transdermal system, 25 mcg/hr.

2. Multiple systems may be used if the delivery rate needs to exceed 100 mcg/hr.

3. Do not undertake initial evaluation of the maximum analgesic effect until 24 hr after system applied.

4. If required, a short-acting analgesic may be used for the first 24 hr (i.e., until analgesic efficacy reached with transdermal system).

5. Clients may continue to require periodic supplemental doses of a short-acting analgesic to treat breakthrough pain.

6. Upon removal of the system, it takes 17 hr or more for the seum levels of fentanyl to fall by 50%. Titrate the dose of new analgesic based on client report of pain until adequate analgesia has been reached.

7. If opioid therapy is to be discontinued, a gradual decrease in dose is recommended to minimize S&S of abrupt narcotic withdrawal.

8. Do not store the system above 25°C (77°F).

Fentanyl Iontophoretic Transdermal System:

1. Test each iontophoretic transdermal system before dispensing to a client. Consult the package insert for testing procedures. Functionality test should be performed by the pharmacist or pharmacy technician with the system still in its sealed pouch.

2. Apply to intact, nonirritated, and nonirradiated skin on the chest or upper outer arm. Do not place on scars, burns, or tattoos. Clip (not shave) any excessive hair at the administration site.

Wipe the application site with a standard alcohol swab and allow the skin to dry completely before applying the system. Do not use any soaps, oils, lotions, or any other agent that might irritate the skin or alter the absorption characteristics of the system.

3. Consult the package insert for specific instructions on the application procedure.

4. Clients must have access to supplemental analgesia during treatment with the iontophoretic transdermal system.

5. Only the client should administer doses from the iontophoretic transdermal system. To activate, press the button firmly twice within 3 seconds; an audible tone indicates the start of delivery of each dose; the red light remains on throughout the 10-minute dosing period. The red light turns off after the 10-minute dosing period.

6. A maximum of six doses/hr can be given by this system. The maximum amount fentanyl that can be administered from a single system over 24 hr is 3.2 mg (i.e., eighty 40 mcg doses). Each iontophoretic transdermal system operates for 24 hr or until 80 doses have been given, whichever comes first.

7. Between doses, a red light will flash in 1-second pulses to indicate the approximate number of doses that have been given up to the present time. Each 1-second flash of light indicates administration of up to 5 doses. The system may also be queried during delivery of an on-demand dose by a single press of the button.

8. Up to 3 consecutive iontophoretic transdermal systems can be used sequentially, each applied to a different skin site for a maximum of 72 hr of therapy for short-term postoperative pain.

9. The iontophoretic transdermal system may be removed at any time. Once a system has been removed, the same system should *not* be reapplied. At the end of 24 hours of use, or after 80 doses have been delivered, the system will deactivate and should be removed from the skin of the client.

Bold Italic = life threatening side effect   ■ = black box warning   ✦ = Available in Canada

10. When removing the system, use gloves. Ensure both hydrogels remain with the removed system. If the hydrogel becomes separated from the system during removal, use gloves or tweezers to remove the hydrogel from the skin.

11. If the hydrogel drug reservoir is touched accidentally, rinse the area thoroughly with water; do not use soap.

12. Accidental ingestion of the fentanyl hydrogel or contact of the hydrogel with mucous membranes could lead to absorption of a potentially fatal dose of fentanyl.

13. Properly dispose of the hydrogel in accordance with state and federal regulations for controlled substances.

14. If the client requires additional analgesia, a new system can be applied to a new skin site on the upper outer arm or chest.

15. Clients on chronic opioid therapy or with a history of opioid abuse may require higher analgesic doses in the postoperative period. Frequently evaluate these clients to ensure they are receiving adequate analgesia.

16. To convert clients to another opioid or other analgesic, remove the transdermal system and titrate the dose of the new analgesic based on the client's report of pain until adequate analgesia has been obtained. Use caution since serum fentanyl levels will decrease slowly following removal of the system.

17. Store the iontophoretic transdermal system from 15–30°C (59–86°F). Apply to the skin immediately after removal from the individually sealed package.

ASSESSMENT

1. List reasons for therapy, previous agents used, outcome. Note all drugs prescribed to ensure none compete/interact.

2. Rate pain level at various times throughout the day to ensure adequate dosing. Determine that dose required is based on conversion guidelines provided by manufacturer.

3. It takes 17 or more hr for fentanyl serum levels to fall by 50% after system removal. Titrate dose of new analgesic based on client's report of pain until adequate analgesia reached. If opioids are to be discontinued, titrate downward gradually since it is not known at what dose level the opioid may be discontinued without causing S&S of abrupt withdrawal.

4. Note ↑ ICP or brain tumors; precludes drug therapy.

5. Assess for any history of illicit drug use; monitor for compliance and level of pain control.

Fentanyl Iontophoretic Transdermal System:

1. Ionsys should only be used during hospitalization. Treatment should be discontinued before hospital discharge.

2. Titrate clients to an acceptable level of analgesia before initiating treatment with Ionsys.

3. Check for any hypersensitivity to fentanyl, cetylpyridinium chloride (e.g. Cepacol) or any components of the Ionsys system.

4. Apply system to intact, non-irritated, and non-irradiated skin on the chest or upper outer arm. Avoid exposing Ionsys to water as this could cause the system to fall off or stop working. If system loosens, a non-allergenic tape may be used to be sure all of the system's edges make complete contact with the skin. Take care not to tape over the button or the red light.

5. Only those who are able to understand and follow the instructions for operation should use the system.

6. System contains metal parts and should be removed before an MRI procedure, cardioversion, or defibrillation to avoid damage to the system from the strong electromagnetic fields set up by these procedures.

7. The error detection circuitry uses a series of audible signals to alert when a dose is not being delivered in response to the clients attempt to activate a dose. Use with caution in those who have high frequency hearing impairment.

8. System provides a 40 mcg dose. Each on-demand dose is delivered over a 10-minute period. To initiate administration of a fentanyl dose, the client must press the button twice firmly within 3 seconds. An audible tone

F

(beep) indicates the start of delivery of each dose; the red light remains on throughout the 10-minute dosing period.

9. A maximum of six 40-mcg doses per hour can be administered by Ionsys. The maximum amount of fentanyl that can be administered from a single Ionsys system over 24 hours is 3.2 mg (eighty 40-mcg doses). Each system operates for 24 hours or until 80 doses have been administered, whichever occurs first.

CLIENT/FAMILY TEACHING

Fentanyl Transdermal System:

1. Apply system to a nonirritated and nonirradiated fatty, flat surface of the skin, preferably on the upper torso. May clip hair (not shave) from site prior to application.

2. Use only clear water, if needed, to cleanse the site prior to application. Do not use soaps, oils, lotions, alcohol, or other agents that might irritate the skin. Allow skin to dry completely prior to applying the system. If liquid comes in contact with the skin, use clear water only to remove.

3. Remove system from sealed package and apply immediately by pressing firmly in place (for 10–20 sec) with the palm of the hand. *Never cut or open the system.* Ensure complete contact of system, especially around the edges. Date and time patches and tape securely to avoid confusion or dislodgement.

4. Keep each system in place for 72 hr; if additional analgesia is required, use breakthrough analgesic and record. A new system can be applied to a different skin site after removal of the previous system.

5. Fold system removed from a skin site so that the adhesive side adheres to itself; flush down the toilet immediately after removal. Keep systems out of reach of children.

6. Dispose of any unused systems as soon as they are no longer needed by removing them from their package and flushing or double bagging.

7. Note time and frequency of short-acting analgesic use for breakthrough pain. Report if use exceeds expected needs; transdermal dosage may require adjustment.

8. Use only as prescribed; do not stop suddenly. Directions for use of fentanyl transdermal must be followed exactly to prevent death or serious side effects associated with overdose.

9. Avoid activities that require mental alertness. Excessive heat may increase absorption and excessive perspiration may alter adhesive stickiness.

Fentanyl Iontophoretic Transdermal System:

1. System is only used in the hospital for acute pain.

2. The system is composed of a plastic top housing that contains the battery and mechanics, and a red plastic bottom housing containing two hydrogel reservoirs and a skin adhesive.

3. A clear plastic release liner covers the hydrogels and must be removed and discarded prior to contact with the skin. The system is powered by a 3-volt lithium battery.

4. The bottom housing has a red tab that is used only for system removal from the skin and during disposal. The hydrogels should not come into contact with fingers or mouth.

5. When you trigger a dose, an electrical current is activated, which moves a dose of fentanyl from the drug-containing reservoir through the skin and into the systemic circulation.

6. System should be applied on the upper outer arm or the chest. Do not touch the sticky side of the system and do not touch the gels. Fentanyl is rapidly absorbed by the eyes and mouth, and could be harmful or fatal if absorbed this way.

7. Do not allow anyone else to activate the dosing button on the Ionsys system since only the patient knows how much pain they are experiencing. Could lead to fatal overdose.

OUTCOMES/EVALUATE

Patch: Desired pain control with chronic conditions. **Ionsys System:** Short-term management of acute postoperative pain in adults

Ferrous sulfate ■
(**FAIR**-us **SUL**-fayt)

CLASSIFICATION(S):
Antianemic, iron
PREGNANCY CATEGORY: A
OTC: Feosol, Fer-Gen-Sol, Fer-in-Sol, FeroSul.
✿OTC: Apo-Ferrous Sulfate, Ferrodan.

Ferrous sulfate, dried

OTC: Feosol, Feratab, Slow FE, Slow Release Iron.

USES
(1) Prophylaxis and treatment of iron deficiency and iron-deficiency anemias. (2) Dietary supplement for iron. Optimum therapeutic responses are usually noted within 2–4 weeks. *Investigational:* Clients receiving epoetin therapy (failure to give iron supplements either IV or PO can impair the hematologic response to epoetin).

ACTION/KINETICS
Action
The normal daily iron intake for males is 12–20 mg and for females is 8–15 mg, although only about 10% (1–2 mg) of this iron is absorbed. Iron is absorbed from the duodenum and upper jejunum by an active mechanism through the mucosal cells where it combines with the protein transferrin. Iron is stored in the body as hemosiderin or aggregated ferritin which is found in reticuloendothelial cells of the liver, spleen, and bone marrow. About two-thirds of total body iron is in the circulating RBCs in hemoglobin.

Pharmacokinetics
Absorption of iron is enhanced when stored iron is depleted or when erythropoiesis occurs at an increased rate. Food decreases iron absorption by up to two-thirds. The daily loss of iron through urine, sweat, and sloughing of intestinal mucosal cells is 0.5–1 mg in healthy men; in menstruating women, 1–2 mg is the normal daily loss. Least expensive, most effective iron salt for PO therapy. Ferrous sulfate products contain 20% elemental iron, whereas ferrous sulfate dried products contain 30% elemental iron. The exsiccated form is more stable in air.

CONTRAINDICATIONS
Hemosiderosis, hemochromatosis, peptic ulcer, regional enteritis, and ulcerative colitis. Hemolytic anemia, pyridoxine-responsive anemia, and cirrhosis of the liver. Use in those with normal iron balance.

SPECIAL CONCERNS
■ Accidental overdose of iron-containing products is a leading cause of fatal poisoning in children younger than 6 years of age. Keep products out of the reach of children. In case of accidental overdose, call a doctor or poison control center immediately.■ Allergic reactions may result due to certain products containing tartrazine and some products containing sulfites.

SIDE EFFECTS
Most Common
Constipation, gastric irritation, nausea, abdominal cramps, anorexia, diarrhea, dark-colored stools.
GI: Constipation, gastric irritation, N&V, abdominal cramps, anorexia, diarrhea, dark-colored stools. These effects may be minimized by administering preparations as a coated tablet. Soluble iron preparations may stain the teeth.

LABORATORY TEST CONSIDERATIONS
Iron may affect electrolyte balance determinations.

OD OVERDOSE MANAGEMENT
Symptoms: Symptoms may occur when at least 20 mg/kg is ingested. Acute poisoning will produce symptoms in the following 4 stages:
1. Within 6 hours: Abdominal pain, coma, diminished tissue perfusion, dyspnea, fever, hyperglycemia, hypotension, lethargy, leukocytosis, metabolic acidosis, N&V, tarry stools, weak-rapid pulse.
2. If not immediately fatal, symptoms may subside within 12–24 hr.

---

3. Symptoms return 12–48 hr after ingestion and may include: Anuria, **convulsions, death**, **diffuse vascular congestion**, hyperthermia, metabolic acidosis, pulmonary edema, **shock.**
4. If client survives, in 2–6 weeks after ingestion, pyloric or antral stenosis, hepatic cirrhosis, and CNS damage may occur.

Treatment: Maintain a proper airway, respiration, and circulation. Perform gastric lavage in those who are candidates for GI decontamination. Systemic chelation with deferoxamine may be recommended for those with serum iron levels greater than 350–500 mcg/dL or in those with symptoms of iron toxicity. IM deferoxamine therapy may suffice, but severe poisoning (e.g., shock, coma) may require IV deferoxamine therapy. Specific treatment for shock, convulsions, acidosis, and renal failure may be necessary. Treatment includes usual supportive measures.

DRUG INTERACTIONS
Antacids, oral / ↓ Iron absorption from GI tract
Ascorbic acid / Ascorbic acid, 200 mg or more, ↑ iron absorption
Calcium salts / ↓ GI absorption of iron; separate administration times
Captopril / Concomitant use within 2 hr may promote formation of inactive captopril disulfide dimer
Cefdinir / ↓ GI cefdinir absorption by up to 80%; give cefdinir 2 hr before or after iron supplements
Chloramphenicol / ↑ Serum iron levels
Cholestyramine / ↓ Iron absorption from GI tract
Cimetidine / ↓ Iron absorption from GI tract
Digestive enzymes / Serum iron response to PO iron may be ↓ by pancreatic extracts
Fluoroquinolones / ↓ Fluoroquinolone absorption from GI tract R/T formation of a ferric ion-quinolone complex; do not use together
Histamine H-2 receptor antagonists / ↓ GI iron absorption
Levodopa / ↓ Levodopa absorption R/T formation of chelates with iron salts

Levothyroxine / ↓ Levothyroxine efficacy R/T ↓ absorption
Methyldopa / ↓ Methyldopa absorption from GI tract
Mycophenolate mofetil / ↓ GI absorption of mycophenolate R/T formation of a drug-iron complex in the GI tract
Pancreatic extracts / ↓ Iron absorption from GI tract
Penicillamine / ↓ Penicillamine absorption from GI tract due to chelation
Proton pump inhibitors / ↓ GI absorption of iron
H *St. John's wort /* May ↓ absorption of iron
Tetracyclines / ↓ Absorption of both tetracyclines and iron from GI tract
Thyroid hormone / ↓ Thyroid absorption; do not use together
Trientine / The two drugs inhibit absorption of each other; give at least 2 hr apart
Vitamin E / ↓ Response to iron therapy

HOW SUPPLIED
Ferrous sulfate. *Drops:* 75 mg/0.6 mL; *Elixir:* 220 mg/5 mL; *Liquid:* 300 mg/5 mL; *Tablets:* 325 mg.
Ferrous sulfate, dried. *Tablets:* 200 mg, 300 mg; *Tablets, Slow-Release:* 160 mg.

DOSAGE

FERROUS SULFATE
• **DROPS; ELIXIR; LIQUID; TABLETS**
  Prophylaxis of anemia.
Adults: 300 mg/day. **Pediatric:** 5 mg/kg/day.
  Anemia.
Adults: 300 mg twice a day increased to 300 mg 4 times per day as needed/tolerated. If using the liquid, give 5 mL three times per day. **Pediatric:** 10 mg/kg 3 times per day. Consult a provider if the liquid is being considered for a child. The enteric-coated tablets are not recommended for use in children.

FERROUS SULFATE, DRIED
• **TABLETS**
  Prophylaxis of anemia.
Adults: 200 mg/day. **Pediatric:** 5 mg/kg/day.
  Anemia.
Adults: 200 mg 3 times per day up to 200 mg 4 times per day as needed and

tolerated. **Pediatric:** 10 mg/kg 3 times per day.
- **TABLETS, SLOW-RELEASE**
  Anemia.

Adults: 160 mg 1–2 times per day. This dosage form is not recommended for use in children.

NURSING CONSIDERATIONS
ADMINISTRATION/STORAGE
1. Substitution of one iron salt for another without proper adjustment may result in serious over or under dosing.
2. For infants and young children, administer liquid preparations with a dropper. Deposit liquid well back against the cheek.
3. Eggs, milk, coffee, or tea consumed with a meal or 1 hr after may significantly inhibit absorption of dietary iron.
4. Ingestion of calcium and iron supplements with food can decrease iron absorption by one-third; iron absorption is not decreased if calcium carbonate is used and taken between meals.
5. Do not crush or chew sustained-release products.

ASSESSMENT
1. Take a drug history, including:
- Antacid use; any drugs used that may interact
- OTC drugs, i.e., iron compounds or vitamin E use
- Recent abdominal surgery; currently prescribed drugs
- Allergy to sulfites or tartrazines (may be present in some products)
2. Note any GI bleeding; tarry stools or bright blood in stool or vomitus.
3. Assess for thalassemia (mediterranean descent); obtain hemoglobin electrophoresis, as iron administration could be lethal.
4. Note any complaints of fatigue, pallor, poor skin turgor, or change in mental status, especially in the elderly.
5. Assess nutritional status and diet history through questioning and intake if possible.
6. Review pregnancies and menstruation history; note frequency, amounts, and heavy or abnormal bleeding. Pregnancy is an indication for iron prophylactically.

7. Monitor VS, CBC, chemistry profile, stool for occult blood, reticulocytes, serum transferrin, and iron panel results. Discontinue if 500 mg of iron daily does not cause a 1-gram rise of hemoglobin in 1 mo. Note cause (i.e., iron-deficient or megaloblastic anemia) or if further workup is needed.

CLIENT/FAMILY TEACHING
1. Adhere to prescribed regimen; report any problems immediately. Coated tablets may diminish GI effects such as nausea, constipation or diarrhea, gastric irritation, and abdominal cramps.
2. Review form of iron prescribed (bi- or trivalent), frequency of administration.
3. Take with meals to reduce gastric irritation. Taking with citrus juices enhances iron absorption. Milk products, eggs, and antacids inhibit absorption so avoid unless taking ferrous lactate. Coffee and tea consumed within 1 hr of meals may inhibit absorption of dietary iron.
4. May cause indigestion, change in stool color (black and tarry or dark green), abdominal cramps, diarrhea, or constipation; may be relieved by changing the medication, dosage, or time of administration.
5. Increase intake of fruit, fiber, and fluids to minimize constipating effects. Eat a well-balanced diet with foods high in iron (i.e., meat proteins, dried fruits) and affordable foods (i.e., raisins, dark green leafy vegetables, and liver versus apricots or prunes).
6. Will reduce tetracycline absorption. If to receive both, allow at least 2 hr to elapse between doses.
7. Store out of reach of children; overdosage can be fatal.
8. Dilute liquid preparations well with water or fruit juice and use a straw to minimize teeth staining.
9. Pregnant women need an iron-rich diet. The American Academy of Pediatrics recommends an iron supplement for infants during their first year of life.
10. Follow administration guidelines for each product to minimize side effects. Do not self-medicate with vitamin, mineral, and iron supplements.

OUTCOMES/EVALUATE

- Resolution of S&S of anemia; if hemoglobin has not increased 1 gram in 4 weeks, then reconfirm diagnosis
- Restoration of serum iron levels
- Improvement in exercise tolerance and level of fatigue
- Improvement in skin pallor, color of nail beds, Hb and iron levels

Fexofenadine hydrochloride

(fex-oh-**FEN**-ah-deen)

CLASSIFICATION(S):

Antihistamine, second generation, piperidine

PREGNANCY CATEGORY: C

Rx: Allegra, Allegra ODT.

♣Rx: Allegra 12 Hour, Allegra 24 Hour.

SEE ALSO ANTIHISTAMINES.

USES

(1) Seasonal allergic rhinitis, including sneezing; rhinorrhea; itchy nose, throat, or palate; and itchy, watery, and red eyes in adults and children 6 years of age and older. (2) Uncomplicated skin manifestations of chronic idiopathic urticaria in adults and children 6 years of age and older. Significantly reduces pruritus and number of wheals.

ACTION/KINETICS

Action

Fexofenadine, a metabolite of terfenadine, is an H_1-histamine receptor blocker. Low to no sedative or anticholinergic effects.

Pharmacokinetics

Onset: Rapid. **Peak plasma levels:** 2.6 hr. **t½, terminal:** 14.4 hr. Approximately 90% of the drug is excreted through the feces (80%) and urine (10%) unchanged.

CONTRAINDICATIONS

Antihistamines are not recommended for use in children less than 6 years of age.

SPECIAL CONCERNS

Use with care during lactation. Safety and efficacy have not been determined in children under 12 years of age; use is not recommended in children less than 6 years of age.

SIDE EFFECTS

Most Common

Headache, dyspepsia, coughing, URTI, viral infection, back pain.

CNS: Drowsiness, fatigue, headache, dizziness. **GI:** Nausea, dyspepsia. **Respiratory:** Coughing, URTI, nasopharyngitis. **Musculoskeletal:** Back pain, myalgia. **Miscellaneous:** Viral infection (flu, colds), dysmenorrhea, back pain, accidental injury, fever, pain, otitis media, pain in extremity.

DRUG INTERACTIONS

NOTE: No differences in side effects or the QTc interval were observed when fexofenadine was given with either *erythromycin* or *ketoconazole.*

Grapefruit juice / ↓ Fexofenadine absorption from GI tract

Probenecid / ↑ Fexofenadine AUC R/T ↓ renal clearance

Verapamil / ↑ Fexofenadine peak plasma level and AUC R/T inhibiting P-glycoprotein transport

HOW SUPPLIED

Oral Suspension: 6 mg/mL; *Tablets:* 30 mg, 60 mg, 180 mg; *Tablets, Oral Disintegrating:* 30 mg.

DOSAGE

- **ORAL SUSPENSION; TABLETS; TABLETS, ORAL DISINTEGRATING**

> *Seasonal allergic rhinitis; chronic idiopathic urticaria.*

Adults and children over 12 years: 60 mg twice a day or 180 mg once daily. **Children, 6–11 years:** 30 mg twice a day. *NOTE:* **Adults and children over 12 years with decreased renal function, initial:** 60 mg once daily. **Children 6–11 years with decreased renal function, initial:** 30 mg once daily.

NURSING CONSIDERATIONS

ADMINISTRATION/STORAGE

Store oral suspension and tablets from 20–25°C (68–77°F); protect tablets from excessive moisture.

ASSESSMENT

1. Note onset, characteristics of S&S; identify triggers/time of year.

---

2. List other agents trialed, length of use, outcome.

3. Assess for renal dysfunction; reduce dose.

CLIENT/FAMILY TEACHING

1. Take as directed; do not crush, break or chew sustained release tabs.

2. May take with food to decrease stomach upset. Avoid taking with grapefruit juice.

3. Shake oral suspension well before each use.

4. Do not take closely within 15 min of aluminum- or magnesium-containing antacids.

5. May experience headaches, sore throat, nausea, and dysmenorrhea.

6. Avoid alcohol and CNS depressants. Avoid activities that require mental alertness until drug effects realized.

7. Evade prolonged or excessive exposure to direct or artificial sunlight.

8. Report if symptoms intensify; don't improve after 48 hr.

9. Identify and avoid triggers.

10. Protect from excessive moisture.

OUTCOMES/EVALUATE

- Control of symptoms of seasonal allergic rhinitis i.e. ↓ sneezing, pruritus, nasal congestion, watery/red eyes, itchy eyes/nose
- Relief of itching

—— *COMBINATION DRUG* ——

Fexofenadine hydrochloride and Pseudoephedrine hydrochloride

(fex-oh-**FEN**-ah-deen, soo-doh-eh-**FED**-rin)

CLASSIFICATION(S):
Antihistamine/Decongestant Combination

PREGNANCY CATEGORY: C

Rx: Allegra-D 12 Hour, Allegra-D 24 Hour.

SEE ALSO *FEXOFENADINE HYDROCHLORIDE AND PSEUDOEPHEDRINE HYDROCHLORIDE.*

USES

Relief of symptoms associated with seasonal allergic rhinitis in adults and children, 12 years and older. Symptoms relieved include sneezing, rhinorrhea, itchy nose/palate, itchy throat, itchy/watery/red eyes, nasal congestion.

CONTENT

Each Allegra-D 12 Hour tablet contains: Fexofenadine hydrochloride (*antihistamine*), 60 mg for immediate release and Pseudoephedrine hydrochloride (*decongestant*), 120 mg for extended release.

Each Allegra-D 24 Hour tablet contains: Fexofenadine hydrochloride, 180 mg for immediate release and Pseudoephedrine hydrochloride, 240 mg for extended release.

ACTION/KINETICS

Action

Fexofenadine is an antihistamine with selective histamine H_1-receptor antagonist activity. No sedative or other CNS effects are observed. Pseudoephedrine is a sympathomimetic amine that has decongestant activity on the nasal mucosa. CNS effects are similar to, but less intense than, amphetamines. At recommended PO doses, it has little or no pressor activity in normotensive adults.

Pharmacokinetics

Fexofenadine . Rapidly absorbed. **Peak plasma levels:** 2 hr. High fat meals decrease bioavailability by 50%. About 5% eliminated by hepatic metabolism. $t\frac{1}{2}$, **elimination:** 14.4 hr. Excreted mainly in the feces (80%). **Pseudoephedrine. Peak plasma levels:** 6 hr. Food does not affect extent of absorption. Less than 1% is eliminated by hepatic metabolism. $t\frac{1}{2}$, **elimination:** 4–6 hr (dependent on urine pH); mainly excreted unchanged in the urine. **Plasma protein binding:** From 60–70% of fexofenadine bound to plasma proteins. Protein binding of pseudoephedrine is unknown.

CONTRAINDICATIONS

Known hypersensitivity to any of the product components. Use with narrow-angle glaucoma or urinary retention, in those receiving MAO inhibitor therapy or within 14 days of stopping such treatment, with severe hypertension, or severe coronary artery disease. Antihistamines and decongestants are not recommended for use in children less than 6 years of age.

SPECIAL CONCERNS
Use with caution in those with hypertension, diabetes mellitus, ischemic heart disease, increased intraocular pressure, hyperthyroidism, renal impairment, or prostatic hypertrophy. Elderly clients are more likely to have side effects due to sympathomimetic amines. Use during pregnancy only if benefit justifies the potential risk to the fetus. Use with caution during lactation. Safety and efficacy with the 12 Hour product have not been determined below the age of 12 years.

SIDE EFFECTS
Most Common
Headache, insomnia, nausea, dry mouth, dyspepsia, throat irritation, URTI.
See *Fexofenadine hydrochloride* and *Pseudoephedrine hydrochloride* for a complete list of possible side effects. Also, *seizures or CV collapse* with accompanying hypotension may occur.

DRUG INTERACTIONS
Antacids (Al- and Mg-containing) / ↓ Fexofenadine AUC and C_{max}
Erythromycin / ↑ Fexofenadine levels R/T enhanced GI absorption
Ketoconazole / ↑ Fexofenadine levels R/T enhanced GI absorption
MAO inhibitors / Significant ↑ BP
Sympathomimetic amines / ↑ Risk of CNS stimulation with seizures or CV collapse with accompanying hypotension

HOW SUPPLIED
See Content.

DOSAGE
- **TABLETS, EXTENDED-RELEASE 12 HOUR**
  Seasonal allergic rhinitis.

Adults and children over 12 years:
One tablet twice daily given on an empty stomach with water. In clients with decreased renal function, initial dose is one tablet once daily.

- **TABLETS, EXTENDED-RELEASE 24 HOUR**
  Seasonal allergic rhinitis.

Adults and children over 12 years:
One tablet once daily given on an empty stomach with water. Avoid use of the 24 Hour product in clients with renal insufficiency.

NURSING CONSIDERATIONS

ADMINISTRATION/STORAGE
Store from 20–25°C (68–77°F).

ASSESSMENT
1. List reasons for therapy, clinical presentation/symptoms, triggers, other agents trialed.
2. Assess HEENT, note findings. List drugs prescribed to ensure none interact.
3. Reduce dose with renal dysfunction.
4. Determine any narrow-angle glaucoma, urinary retention, (MAOI) therapy, severe CAD/hypertension; precludes drug therapy.

CLIENT/FAMILY TEACHING
1. Drug prescribed for the relief of symptoms of seasonal allergic rhinitis.
2. Take on an empty stomach with water. Swallow tablet whole; do not break or chew tablet.
3. Something that resembles the tablet may occasionally be eliminated in the feces; this is the inactive ingredients.
4. If nervousness, dizziness, or sleeplessness occur, stop drug and report.
5. Do not take within 30 min of aluminum and magnesium-containing antacids.
6. Practice reliable contraception.
7. Keep all F/U appointments to evaluate response to therapy and symptom control.

OUTCOMES/EVALUATE
Prevention of sneezing; runny nose; itching, watery eyes; and other allergic symptoms

---

Bold Italic = life threatening side effect   ■ = black box warning   ✦ = Available in Canada

Filgrastim   IV

(fill-**GRASS**-tim)

CLASSIFICATION(S):
Granulocyte colony-stimulating factor, human
PREGNANCY CATEGORY: C
Rx: Neupogen.

USES

(1) Decrease the incidence of infection, as manifested by febrile neutropenia, in clients with nonmyeloid malignancies who are receiving myelosuppressive anticancer drugs that are associated with severe neutropenia with fever. (2) Reduce the duration of neutropenia in clients with nonmyeloid malignancies undergoing myeloablative chemotherapy followed by bone marrow transplantation. (3) Reduce infection in severe chronic neutropenia (e.g., congenital, cyclical, or idiopathic neutropenia) after other diseases have been ruled out. (4) Mobilization of hematopoietic progenitor cells into the peripheral blood for leukapheresis collection. (5) Reduce the time to neutrophil recovery and the duration of fever in clients being treated for acute myelogenous leukemia. *Investigational:* Use in AIDS, aplastic anemia, hairy cell leukemia, myelodysplasia, drug-induced and congenital agranulocytosis, and alloimmune neonatal neutropenia.

ACTION/KINETICS

Action

Is a human granulocyte colony stimulating factor (G-CSF) produced by recombinant DNA technology by *Escherichia coli* that has been inserted with the human G-CSF gene. Endogenous G-CSF is a glycoprotein that is produced by monocytes, fibroblasts, and other endothelial cells; it regulates the production of neutrophils in the bone marrow. Has minimal effects, either *in vivo* or *in vitro*, on the production of other hematopoietic cell types. Filgrastim has an amino acid sequence that is identical to the natural sequence predicted from human DNA sequence analysis except there is an N-terminal methionine that is required for expression in *E. coli*.

Pharmacokinetics

IV infusion of 20 mcg/kg over 24 hr resulted in a mean serum level of 48 ng/mL, whereas SC administration of 11.5 mcg/kg resulted in a maximum serum level of 49 ng/mL within 2–8 hr. **t½, elimination:** 3.5 hr.

CONTRAINDICATIONS

Hypersensitivity to proteins derived from *E. coli*. The safety and effectiveness of filgrastim given simultaneously with cytotoxic chemotherapy has not been determined; thus, filgrastim should not be given 24 hr before to 24 hr after cytotoxic chemotherapy.

SPECIAL CONCERNS

Use with caution during lactation. Use with caution in any malignancy with myeloid characteristics since the drug may act as a growth factor for any tumor type. Filgrastim does not cause any greater incidence of toxicity in children than in adults. Safety and efficacy have not been determined in neonates and clients with autoimmune neutropenia of infancy. The safety and effectiveness of chronic filgrastim therapy have not been determined. Hypersensitivity reactions usually occur within 30 min after administration and are more frequent in clients receiving the drug IV.

SIDE EFFECTS

Most Common
N&V, skeletal pain, alopecia, diarrhea, neutropenic fever, mucositis, fever, fatigue, anorexia, dyspnea, headache.
When used for myelosuppressive therapy: Musculoskeletal: Medullary bone pain, skeletal pain. **GI:** N&V, diarrhea, anorexia, stomatitis, constipation, peritonitis, splenic rupture. **Hypersensitivity:** Skin rash, facial edema, wheezing, dyspnea, hypotension, tachycardia. **Hematologic:** Leukocytosis; greater risk of thrombocytopenia and anemia. **Respiratory:** Dyspnea, cough, chest pain, sore throat. **Body as a whole:** Alopecia, neutropenic fever, fever, fatigue, headache, skin rash, mucositis, generalized weakness, unspecified pain. **CV:** Decreased BP (transient), cutaneous vasculitis, hypertension, *arrhythmias, MI.*

When used for severe chronic neutropenia: Musculoskeletal: Mild to moderate bone pain, abdominal/flank pain, arthralgia, osteoporosis. **Hematologic:** Thrombocytopenia, epistaxis (associated with thrombocytopenia), anemia, myelodysplasia or myeloid leukemia. **Dermatologic:** Exacerbation of certain skin conditions (e.g., psoriasis), rash, alopecia. **Miscellaneous:** Palpable splenomegaly, hepatomegaly, monosomy, reaction at injection site, cutaneous vasculitis, hematuria, proteinuria.

When used for bone marrow transplantation. GI: N&V, stomatitis, peritonitis. **CV:** Hypertension, capillary leak syndrome (rare). **Hematologic:** Decreased platelet counts, anemia, increase in neutrophil count, WBC count greater than 100,000/mm^3. **Miscellaneous:** Rash, renal insufficiency, erythema nodosum. When used for peripheral blood progenitor cell collection.

LABORATORY TEST CONSIDERATIONS
↑ Uric acid, LDH, alkaline phosphatase.

HOW SUPPLIED
Injection: 300 mcg/0.5 mL, 300 mcg/mL, 600 mcg/mL.

DOSAGE
• **IV; SC**
Myelosuppressive chemotherapy.

Initial: 5 mcg/kg/day as a single injection, either as a SC bolus, by short IV infusion (15–30 min), or by continuous SC or IV infusion (over a 24-hr period). The dose may be increased in increments of 5 mcg/kg for each chemotherapy cycle depending on the duration and severity of the absolute neutrophil count (ANC) nadir. The dose should be given daily for up to 2 weeks, until ANC has reached 10,000/mm^3 following the expected chemotherapy-induced neutrophil nadir.

Severe chronic neutropenia.
5 mcg/kg/day SC for idiopathic and cyclic disease; 6 mcg/kg/day SC for congenital disease.

Bone marrow transplantation.
10 mcg/kg/day given as an IV infusion of 4 or 24 hr or as a continuous 24-hr SC infusion.
NOTE: During the period of neutrophil recovery, the daily dose should be titrated against the neutrophil response as follows:

• When ANC is greater than 1,000/mm^3 for 3 consecutive days, reduce the dose of filgrastim to 5 mcg/kg/day. If ANC decreases to less than 1,000/mm^3 at any time during the 5-mcg/kg/day dosage, increase filgrastim to 10 mcg/kg/day.

• If ANC remains greater than 1,000/mm^3 for 3 more consecutive days, discontinue filgrastim.

• If ANC decreases to less than 1,000/mm^3, resume filgrastim at 5 mcg/kg/day.

Peripheral blood progenitor cell collection.
10 mcg/kg/day SC, either as a bolus or a continuous infusion. Filgrastim should be given at least 4 days before the first leukapheresis procedure and continued until the last leukapheresis.

NURSING CONSIDERATIONS

ADMINISTRATION/STORAGE

1. Discontinue therapy if ANC is greater than 10,000/mm^3 after chemotherapy-induced neutrophil nadir.

2. For myelosuppressive therapy or bone marrow transplantation, do not give filgrastim 24 hr before to 24 hr after administration of chemotherapy.

3. Discontinuing therapy usually results in a 50% decrease in circulating neutrophils within 1–2 days and return to pretreatment levels in 1–7 days.

4. Do not freeze; store in the refrigerator at 2–8°C (36–46°F). Prior to use, can be at room temperature for a maximum of 24 hr. Discard if left at room temperature more than 24 hr.

5. Solution should be clear and colorless.

6. Do not shake. Use only one dose from each vial; do not reenter the vial.

7. Compatible with glass, PVC, or plastic syringes.

IV 8. May be diluted in D5W. When diluted to concentrations between 5 and 15 mcg/mL, protect from adsorption to plastic materials by adding human albumin to a final concentration of 2 mg/mL.

Bold Italic = life threatening side effect   ■ = black box warning   ✦ = Available in Canada

9. The following drugs are incompatible as an admixture with filgrastim: Amphotericin B, cefonicid, cefoperazone, cefotaxime, cefoxitin, ceftizoxime, ceftriaxone, cefuroxime, clindamycin, dactinomycin, etoposide, fluorouracil, furosemide, heparin, mannitol, metronidazole, methylprednisolone, mezlocillin, mitomycin, prochlorperazine, piperacillin, and thiotepa.

ASSESSMENT

1. Note experience/sensitivity to *E. coli*-derived products.
2. List reasons for therapy (i.e., chemotherapy-induced neutropenia, myelopsuppressive therapy for bone marrow transplantation, leukapheresis), expected time frame.
3. Monitor CBC with platelet counts twice weekly during therapy.
4. Clients reporting left upper abdominal and/or shoulder tip pain should be evaluated for an enlarged spleen or splenic rupture.
5. Note last dose of cytotoxic agent and determine ANC nadir. Do not administer from 24 hr before to 24 hr after cytotoxic chemotherapy.

CLIENT/FAMILY TEACHING

1. Drug helps bone marrow make new white blood cells to protect you from infection.
2. Show appropriate technique for administering. Review written guidelines concerning dose, administration, drug storage/handling, and discarding syringes.
3. Do not shake container; only enter the vial once, then discard.
4. 'Flu-like' symptoms (N&V and aching; bone pain) may be side effects of drug therapy. Take at bedtime, with prescribed analgesics.
5. Record temperatures; report bone pain, unusual bruising/bleeding or infection.
6. Avoid crowds and persons with infectious diseases.
7. Keep F/U lab appointments to evaluate response to therapy.

OUTCOMES/EVALUATE

- Prevention of infection
- ↓ Duration of neutropenia
- Improved neutrophil counts
- Mobilization of progenitor cells into peripheral blood

Finasteride
(fin-**AS**-teh-ride)

CLASSIFICATION(S):
Androgen hormone inhibitor
PREGNANCY CATEGORY: X
Rx: Propecia, Proscar.

F

USES

(1) Improve symptoms of benign prostatic hyperplasia to reduce risk of acute urinary infection and reduce risk for surgery and prostatectomy (Proscar only). (2) In combination with doxazosin to decrease risk of benign prostatic hypertrophy symptoms from progressing over time. (3) Male pattern baldness (vertex and anterior midscalp) in clients between 18 and 41 years of age (Proscar only). *Investigational:* Prostate cancer; hirsutism (use with caution, if at all, in women of childbearing age), male chronic pelvic pain syndrome (chronic nonbacterial prostatitis).

ACTION/KINETICS

Action
Is a specific inhibitor of 5-α-reductase, the enzyme that converts testosterone to the active 5-α-dihydrotestosterone (DHT). Thus, there are significant decreases in serum and tissue DHT levels, resulting in rapid regression of prostate tissue and an increase in urine flow and symptomatic improvement. Also a decrease in scalp DHT levels.

Pharmacokinetics
Well absorbed after PO administration with a bioavailability of 63–65%. **Elimination $t^{1}/_{2}$:** 6 hr in clients 45–60 years of age and 8 hr in clients over 70 years of age. Slow accumulation after multiple dosing. Metabolized in the liver and excreted through both the urine and feces.

CONTRAINDICATIONS

Hypersensitivity to finasteride or any excipient in the product. Use in women and in children. Handling of crushed or broken tablets in women who may potentially be pregnant. Lactation.

SPECIAL CONCERNS

Use with caution in clients with impaired liver function.

SIDE EFFECTS

Most Common

Impotence, decreased libido, postural hypotension, dizziness, asthenia, headache, ejaculation disorder.

GU: Impotence, decreased libido, decreased volume of ejaculate, ejaculation disorder. **CNS:** Dizziness, somnolence, headache. **CV:** Postural hypotension, hypotension. **Respiratory:** Rhinitis, dyspnea. **Miscellaneous:** Breast tenderness and enlargement (Propecia only), hypersensitivity reactions (including pruritus, urticaria, skin rash and lip swelling), breast cancer in men, testicular pain, gynecomastia, asthenia, peripheral edema.

LABORATORY TEST CONSIDERATIONS

↓ Serum PSA levels.

DRUG INTERACTIONS

Significant ↑ plasma levels of finasteride when used with terazosin

HOW SUPPLIED

Tablets: 1 mg, 5 mg.

DOSAGE————————

- **TABLETS**

  Benign prostatic hyperplasia.

  5 mg per day, with or without meals.

  Androgenetic alopecia.

  Males: 1 mg once a day with or without meals.

NURSING CONSIDERATIONS

ADMINISTRATION/STORAGE

1. At least 6–12 months of therapy may be required to determine whether a beneficial response has been achieved for BPH.

2. Daily use for three months or longer is necessary to observe beneficial effects for androgenetic alopecia.

3. Continued use is required to sustain beneficial effects for hair growth. Withdrawal leads to reversal of effects within 12 months.

4. Women who are pregnant or may become pregnant should not handle crushed finasteride tablets as there is potential for drug absorption and sub-

sequent potential risk to the male fetus. When the male's sexual partner is or may become pregnant, exposure of semen to his partner should be avoided or drug use discontinued.

5. Do not adjust dosage in the elderly or in those with impaired renal function.

ASSESSMENT

1. Note reasons for therapy, onset, characteristics of S&S, associated family history.

2. Review urologic exam to rule out other conditions similar to BPH (e.g., prostate cancer, infection, stricture, hypotonic bladder, neurogenic disorders).

3. Monitor LFTs and PSA. May cause a decrease in PSA levels (prostate-specific antigen: a blood screening study to detect prostate cancer) even in the presence of prostate cancer. Schedule regular digital rectal exams to assess prostate gland. With liver impairment, monitor closely.

4. Not all clients show a response to finasteride. With a large residual urinary volume or severely diminished urinary flow, assess for obstructive uropathy; may not be finasteride candidate.

5. Complete history/physical exam. Not for use in females. May obtain pre-treatment scalp photos with hair loss to assess/gauge response.

CLIENT/FAMILY TEACHING

1. The following symptoms of BPH should show improvement with continued drug therapy: hesitancy, feelings of incomplete bladder emptying, interruption of urinary stream, impairment of size and force of urinary stream, and terminal urinary dribbling. May take 6–12 months of continued therapy before a beneficial effect is evident.

2. May lower PSA levels (prostate-specific antigen: a blood screening study to detect prostate cancer) even in the presence of prostate cancer.

3. Use barrier contraception. If partner is pregnant or may become pregnant, avoid exposure to semen. Drug may cause damage to male fetus; stop drug or use a condom. Women who are pregnant or desire to become pregnant

---

should not handle crushed or broken tablets due to potential for fetal harm.

4. Take once a day with/without meals. More than prescribed dose will not increase hair growth but may cause adverse symptoms. May take 3 mg or more before any response noted and up to 3 months of therapy.

5. Decreased volume of ejaculate may occur but does not interfere with sexual function. Impotence and decreased libido may occur.

6. Keep F/U lab, checkups, and prostate exams; report side effects. Do not donate blood for up to 1 month after therapy completed/stopped.

7. Interruption of therapy will reverse effects within 12 months and BPH symptoms will return as well as hair loss.

OUTCOMES/EVALUATE

- ↓ Size of enlarged prostate gland
- Symptomatic improvement
- Regrowth of hair in male pattern baldness

Flecainide acetate ■ ©
(fleh-**KAY**-nyd)

CLASSIFICATION(S):
Antiarrhythmic, Class IC
PREGNANCY CATEGORY: C
Rx: Tambocor.

SEE ALSO *ANTIARRHYTHMIC DRUGS.*

USES
(1) Life-threatening arrhythmias manifested as sustained ventricular tachycardia. (2) Prevention of paroxysmal atrial fibrillation associated with disabling symptoms and paroxysmal supraventricular tachycardias (PSVT), including atrioventricular nodal reentrant tachycardia, atrioventricular reentrant tachycardia, and other supraventricular tachycardias of unspecified mechanism associated with disabling symptoms in those without structural heart disease.

NOTE: Not recommended in those with less severe ventricular arrhythmias even if clients are symptomatic.

ACTION/KINETICS
Action
The antiarrhythmic effect is due to a local anesthetic action, especially on the His-Purkinje system in the ventricle. Drug decreases single and multiple PVCs and reduces the incidence of ventricular tachycardia.
Pharmacokinetics
Peak plasma levels: 3 hr; **steady state levels:** 3–5 days. **Effective plasma levels:** 0.2–1 mcg/mL (trough levels). **t½:** 20 hr (12–27 hr). Approximately 30% is excreted in urine unchanged. Metabolized by the CYP2D6 isoenzyme system. Impaired renal function decreases rate of elimination of unchanged drug and prolongs the half-life. Food or antacids do not affect absorption. **Plasma protein binding:** 40%.

CONTRAINDICATIONS
Cardiogenic shock, preexisting second- or third-degree AV block, RBBB when associated with bifascicular block (unless pacemaker is present to maintain cardiac rhythm). Recent MI. Chronic atrial fibrillation. Frequent PVCs and symptomatic nonsustained ventricular arrhythmias. Lactation.

SPECIAL CONCERNS
■ (1) Flecainide was included in the National Heart Lung and Blood Institutes Cardiac Arrhythmia Suppression Trial. An excessive mortality or non-fatal cardiac arrest rate was seen in those treated with flecainide compared with that seen in those assigned to a carefully matched placebo-control group. The average duration of treatment with felcainide in the study was 10 months. (2) The applicability of this study to other populations is uncertain. However, it is advisable to consider the risks of Class IC agents (including flecainide), coupled with the lack of any evidence of improved survival, generally unacceptable in those without life-threatening ventricular arrhythmias, even if the clients are experiencing unpleasant, but not life-threatening, symptoms or signs. (3) Ventricular tachycardia was noted (0.4%) in clients treated with PO flecainide for paroxysmal atrial fibrillation. Flecainide is not recommended for use in

F

those with chronic atrial fibrillation. Case reports of ventricular proarrhythmic effects in those treated with flecainide for atrial fibrillation/flutter have included increased PVCs, ventricular tachycardia, ventricular fibrillation, and death. (4) As with other Class I drugs, those treated with flecainide for atrial flutter have been reported with a 1:1 atrioventricular conduction due to slowing the atrial rate. A paradoxical increase in the ventricular rate may also occur in those with atrial fibrillation who receive flecainide. Concomitant negative chronotropic therapy, such as digoxin or beta-blockers, may lower the risk of this complication.■ Use with caution in SSS, in clients with a history of CHF or MI, in disturbances of potassium levels, in clients with permanent pacemakers or temporary pacing electrodes, renal and liver impairment. Safety and efficacy in children less than 18 years of age are not established. The incidence of proarrhythmic effects may be increased in geriatric clients.

SIDE EFFECTS
Most Common
Dizziness, lightheadedness, faintness, unsteadiness and near syncope, dyspnea, headache, nausea, fatigue, palpitation, chest pain, asthenia, tremor, constipation, edema, abdominal pain.

CV: *New or worsened ventricular arrhythmias, increased risk of death in clients with non-life-threatening cardiac arrhythmias,* new or worsened CHF, palpitations, chest pain, sinus bradycardia, sinus pause, sinus arrest, *ventricular fibrillation, ventricular tachycardia that cannot be resuscitated,* second- or third-degree AV block, nonfatal cardiac arrest, tachycardia, hypertension, hypotension, bradycardia, angina pectoris. **CNS:** Dizziness, faintness, syncope, lightheadedness, neuropathy, unsteadiness and near synocope, headache, fatigue, paresthesia, paresis, hypoesthesia, insomnia, anxiety, twitching, weakness, neuropathy, malaise, vertigo, depression, *seizures,* euphoria, confusion, depersonalization, apathy, morbid dreams, speech disorders, stupor, amnesia, weakness, somnolence. **GI:** Nausea, constipation, abdominal pain, vomiting, anorexia, dyspepsia, dry mouth, diarrhea, flatulence, change in taste. **Ophthalmic:** Blurred vision, difficulty in focusing, spots before eyes, diplopia, photophobia, eye pain, nystagmus, eye irritation, photophobia. **Hematologic:** Leukopenia, thrombocytopenia. **GU:** Decreased libido, impotence, urinary retention, polyuria. **Musculoskeletal:** Asthenia, tremor, ataxia, arthralgia, myalgia. **Dermatologic:** Skin rashes, urticaria, exfoliative dermatitis, pruritus, alopecia. **Miscellaneous:** Edema, dyspnea, fever, fatigue, *bronchospasm,* flushing, increased sweating, tinnitus, swollen mouth, lips, and tongue.

OD OVERDOSE MANAGEMENT
Symptoms: Lengthening of PR interval; increase in QRS duration, QT interval, and amplitude of T wave; decrease in HR and contractility; conduction disturbances; hypotension; *respiratory failure* or *asystole. Treatment:* Charcoal will remove unabsorbed drug up to 90 min after drug ingestion. Administration of dopamine, dobutamine, or isoproterenol. Artificial respiration. Intraaortic balloon pumping, transvenous pacing (to correct conduction block). Acidification of the urine may be beneficial, especially in those with an alkaline urine. Due to the long duration of action of the drug, treatment measures may have to be continued for a prolonged period of time.

DRUG INTERACTIONS
Acidifying agents / ↑ Renal excretion of flecainide → ↓ bioavailability
Alkalinizing agents / ↓ Renal excretion of flecainide → ↑ bioavailability
Amiodarone / ↑ Flecainide levels
Cimetidine / ↑ Flecainide levels and half-life
Digoxin / ↑ Digoxin levels
Disopyramide / Additive negative inotropic effects; do not use together unless benefits outweigh risks
Propranolol / Additive negative inotropic effects; also, ↑ levels of both drugs
Ritonavir / Significant ↑ flecainide levels; do not use together
Smoking (Tobacco) / ↑ Plasma clearance of flecainide; dose of flecainide

---

may need to be ↑
Verapamil / Additive negative inotropic effects

HOW SUPPLIED
Tablets: 50 mg, 100 mg, 150 mg.

DOSAGE

- **TABLETS**
  Sustained ventricular tachycardia.
Initial: 100 mg q 12 hr; **then,** increase by 50 mg twice/day q 4 days until effective dose reached. **Usual effective dose:** 150 mg q 12 hr, not to exceed 400 mg/day.
  PSVT, PAF.
Initial: 50 mg q 12 hr; **then,** dose may be increased in increments of 50 mg twice/day q 4 days until effective dose reached. Maximum recommended dose for those with paroxysmal supraventricular arrhythmias: 300 mg/day.
  NOTE: For PAF clients, increasing the dose from 50 to 100 mg twice a day may increase efficacy without a significant increase in side effects. For clients with a C_{CR} <35 mL/min/1.73m^2, the starting dose is 100 mg once daily (or 50 mg twice a day). For less severe renal disease, the initial dose may be 100 mg q 12 hr.

NURSING CONSIDERATIONS

℞ Do not confuse Tambocor with Pamelor (a tricyclic antidepressant).

ADMINISTRATION/STORAGE
1. For most situations, start in a hospital setting (especially in clients with symptomatic CHF, sustained ventricular arrhythmias, compensated clients with significant myocardial dysfunction, or sinus node dysfunction).
2. In renal impairment, increase dose at intervals greater than 4 days. Monitor for adverse toxic effects.
3. Most treated successfully had trough plasma levels between 0.2 and 1 mcg/mL. The chance of toxic effects increases if the trough plasma levels exceed 1 mcg/mL.
4. If being transferred to flecainide from another antiarrhythmic, allow at least two to four plasma half-lives to elapse for the drug being discontinued before initiating flecainide therapy.

5. Dosing at 8-hr intervals may benefit some.
6. If given with amiodarone, reduce flecainide dose by 50% and monitor closely for side effects.
7. To minimize toxicity, reduce dose once arrhythmia controlled.

ASSESSMENT
1. Note physical assessment findings i.e., heart, lungs, JVD, weight. Review history, echocardiograms, ECGs for evidence of CHF, ventricular arrhythmias, sinus node dysfunction, abnormal EF.
2. Monitor VS, ECG, CXR, electrolytes, renal and LFTs. Assess ECG for increased arrhythmias, RBBB with LAH, or AV block. Preexisting hypo/hyperkalemia may alter drug effects; correct. Monitor for labile BP.
3. Concomitant administration with disopyramide, propranolol, or verapamil will promote negative inotropic (depressant) effects.
4. Check pacing thresholds with pacemakers; adjust before and 1 week following drug therapy.
5. Obtain urinary pH to detect alkalinity or acidity. Alkalinity decreases renal excretion and acidity increases renal excretion, affecting rate of drug elimination.

CLIENT/FAMILY TEACHING
1. Take at dose and frequency prescribed. Report changes in elimination.
2. Report bruising or increased bleeding tendencies, dyspnea, edema, chest pain.
3. Keep appointments; drug effectiveness must be monitored carefully.
4. Report adverse CNS effects, such as dizziness, visual disturbances, headaches, nausea, depression.
5. Change positions slowly from lying to standing to prevent drop in BP. Avoid hazardous activities until drug effects realized.

OUTCOMES/EVALUATE
- Termination of lethal ventricular arrhythmias; stable cardiac rhythm
- Therapeutic serum (trough) drug levels (0.2–1.0 mcg/mL)

📷 = see color insert   H = Herbal   IV = Intravenous   ℞ = sound alike drug

Floxuridine ■
(flox-**YOUR**-ih-deen)

CLASSIFICATION(S):
Antineoplastic, antimetabolite
PREGNANCY CATEGORY: D
Rx: FUDR.

SEE ALSO *ANTINEOPLASTIC AGENTS.*

USES
Intra-arterially as palliative treatment of GI adenocarcinoma metastatic to the liver (especially in clients incurable by surgery or other treatment). Used in clients with disease limited to an area capable of infusion by a single artery. *Investigational:* Tumors of the liver, ovaries, or kidneys.

ACTION/KINETICS
Action
Cell-cycle specific for the S phase of cell division. Rapidly metabolized to fluorouracil. The drug inhibits DNA and RNA synthesis. Crosses blood-brain barrier.

Pharmacokinetics
t½: 5–20 min. From 60 to 80% of fluorouracil is excreted as respiratory CO_2 (8–12 hr); small amount (15%) excreted in urine (1–6 hr).

CONTRAINDICATIONS
If client is at poor risk, including depressed bone marrow function, nutritionally poor, or potentially serious infections. Lactation. Do not use during pregnancy unless benefits clearly outweigh risks.

SPECIAL CONCERNS
■ (1) It is recommended that floxuridine be given only by or under the supervision of a qualified physician who is experienced in cancer chemotherapy and intraarterial drug therapy and is well versed in the use of potent antimetabolites. (2) Because of the possibility of severe toxic reactions, all clients should be hospitalized for initiation of the first course of therapy.■

SIDE EFFECTS
Most Common
N&V, diarrhea, enteritis, stomatitis, localized erythema, anemia, leukopenia, thrombocytopenia.
CNS: Lethargy, malaise, weakness, acute cerebellar syndrome (my persist after treatment discontinued), headache, disorientation, confusion, euphoria. **GI:** Stomatitis/esophagopharyngitis (may lead to sloughing/ulceration), diarrhea, anorexia, N&V, enteritis, cramps, duodenal ulcer, watery stools, duodenitis, gastritis, glossitis, pharyngitis, intra-/extrahepatic biliary sclerosis, acalculus cholecystitis, GI ulceration/bleeding. **CV:** Myocardial ischemia, angina. **Dermatologic:** Alopecia, dermatitis (often as pruritic maculopapular rash on extremities or trunk), nonspecific skin toxicity, photosensitivity (erythema, increased skin pigmentation), nail changes (e.g., loss of nails), dry skin, fissuring, vein pigmentation. **Hematologic:** Leukopenia, thrombocytopenia, pancytopenia, agranulocytosis, anemia, thrombophlebitis. **Hypersensitivity:** Generalized allergic reactions, anaphylaxis. **Ophthalmic:** Photophobia, lacrimation, decreased vision, nystagmus, diplopia, lacrimal duct stenosis, visual changes. **At catheter site:** Bleeding, occluded/displaced/leaking catheters, embolism, fibromyositis, infection, thrombophlebitis. **Miscellaneous:** Complications of intra-arterial administration are arterial aneurysm, arterial ischemia, arterial thrombosis. Fever, epistaxis.

LABORATORY TEST CONSIDERATIONS
↑ Excretion of 5-hydroxyindoleacetic acid. ↑ Serum transaminase and bilirubin, LDH, alkaline phosphatase. ↓ Plasma albumin.

HOW SUPPLIED
Powder for Injection, Lyophilized: 0.5 gram.

DOSAGE
• **INTRA-ARTERIAL INFUSION ONLY**
   Palliation of GI adenocarcinoma metastatic to the liver.
0.1–0.6 mg/kg/day by continuous infusion over 24 hr. Infusion is continued as long as a response continues.

NURSING CONSIDERATIONS
ADMINISTRATION/STORAGE
1. Higher doses (0.4–0.6 mg) are best given by hepatic artery infusion; liver metabolizes drug, reducing possibility of systemic toxicity.
2. Give until adverse effects manifested; resume therapy after effects have subsided. Maintain therapy as long as the response to floxuridine continues.
3. Use infusion pump to overcome pressure in large arteries and to assure a uniform infusion rate.
4. Reconstitute each vial with 5 mL sterile water to yield a 100 mg/mL concentration. This may be further reconstituted in D5W or NSS and infused intra-arterially.
5. Store reconstituted vials in the refrigerator at 2–8°C (36–46°F) for no longer than 2 weeks.

ASSESSMENT
1. Note reasons for therapy; CT/MRI confirmation of metastasis; monitor CBC, uric acid, creatinine and LFTs. WBC nadir: 1 week; Platelet nadir: 10 days.
2. Assess carefully for bleeding at catheter site, S&S of infection, catheter displacement. Should be inserted under fluoroscopy by trained individual.

CLIENT/FAMILY TEACHING
1. Drug is administered under pressure into an artery. Any dislodgement may cause significant bleeding; report immediately.
2. May cause temporary thinning of hair.
3. Report any mouth lesions, diarrhea, intractable vomiting or infections.
4. Will be premedicated for N&V, report recurrence so that therapy may be re-administered.

OUTCOMES/EVALUATE
Suppression of metastatic processes

Fluconazole   IV
(flew-**KON**-ah-zohl)

CLASSIFICATION(S):
Antifungal
PREGNANCY CATEGORY: C
Rx: Diflucan.

♣**Rx:** Apo-Fluconazole, Apo-Fluconazole-150, Diflucan-150.

USES
(1) Oropharyngeal and esophageal candidiasis. (2) Serious systemic candidal infection (including UTIs, peritonitis, candidemia, disseminated candidiasis, and pneumonia). (3) Cryptococcal meningitis. (4) Vaginal candidiasis and infections due to *Candida*. (5) Decrease the incidence of candidiasis in clients undergoing a bone marrow transplant who receive cytotoxic chemotherapy or radiation therapy. (6) Cryptococcal meningitis and candidal infections in children.

ACTION/KINETICS
Action
Is a highly selective inhibitor of fungal cytochrome P450 and sterol C-14 alpha-demethylation. The loss of normal sterols correlates with accumulation of 14-alpha-methyl sterols in fungi and may be responsible for the fungistatic activity. There is a decrease in cell wall integrity and extrusion of intracellular material, leading to death.

Pharmacokinetics
Bioavailability is 90% after PO use. Apparently does not affect the cytochrome P-450 enzyme in animals or humans. **Peak plasma levels:** 1–2 hr. **Steady-state levels:** 5–10 days after 50–400 mg given once a day. **t½:** 30 hr, which allows for once daily dosing. Penetrates all body fluids at steady state. Not affected by agents that increase gastric pH. Eighty percent of the drug is excreted unchanged by the kidneys. **Plasma protein binding:** 11–12%.

CONTRAINDICATIONS
Hypersensitivity to fluconazole. Lactation.

SPECIAL CONCERNS
Use with caution if client shows hypersensitivity to other azoles. Use with extreme caution in renal impairment. Efficacy has not been determined in children less than 6 months of age.

SIDE EFFECTS
Most Common
Following single doses: Headache, nausea, abdominal pain, diarrhea.
Following multiple doses: Nausea, headache, skin rash, vomiting, abdominal pain.

Following single doses: GI: Nausea, abdominal pain, diarrhea, dyspepsia, taste perversion. **CNS:** Headache, dizziness. **Miscellaneous: *Angioedema, anaphylaxis (rare).***

Following multiple doses: Side effects are more frequently reported in HIV-infected clients than in non-HIV-infected clients. **GI:** N&V, abdominal pain, diarrhea, ***serious hepatic reactions*.** **CNS:** Headache, ***seizures*.** **Dermatologic:** Skin rash, exfoliative skin disorders (including ***Stevens-Johnson syndrome*,** and ***toxic epidermal necrolysis*),** alopecia. **Hematologic:** Leukopenia, thrombocytopenia. **Miscellaneous:** Hypercholesterolemia/triglyceridemia, hypokalemia.

LABORATORY TEST CONSIDERATIONS
↑ AST, serum transaminase (especially if used with isoniazid, oral hypoglycemic agents, phenytoin, rifampin, valproic acid).

DRUG INTERACTIONS
Alfentanil / ↑ Pharmacologic and side effects R/T ↓ liver metabolism by CYP3A4
Benzodiazepines / ↑ And prolonged serum levels → CNS depression and psychomotor impairment
Buspirone / ↑ Buspirone levels R/T ↓ metabolism
Carbamazepine / ↑ Carbamazepine levels R/T ↓ metabolism by CYP3A4
Cimetidine / ↓ Fluconazole AUC and C_{max}
Corticosteroids / ↑ Corticosteroid effects and toxicity R/T ↓ metabolism
Cyclosporine / ↑ Cyclosporine levels in renal transplant clients with or without impaired renal function
Glipizide / ↑ Glipizide levels R/T ↓ liver breakdown
Glyburide / ↑ Glyburide levels R/T ↓ liver breakdown
Haloperidol / ↑ Haloperidol levels → ↑ risk of side effects

HMG-CoA reductase inhibitors / ↑ HMG-CoA reductase inhibitor levels → possible rhabdomyolysis
Hydrochlorothiazide / ↑ Fluconazole levels R/T ↓ renal clearance
Losartan / ↑ Losartan antihypertensive and toxicity R/T ↓ metabolism by CYP2D9
Nateglinide / ↑ Nateglinide levels R/T ↓ metabolism by CYP2C9
Nisoldipine / ↑ Effects/toxicity of nisoldipine levels R/T ↓ metabolism by CYP3A4
Oral contraceptives / Possible ↑ or ↓ ethinyl estradiol and levonorgestrel levels
Phenytoin / ↑ Phenytoin levels
Protease inhibitors / Possible ↑ protease inhibitor levels with possible ↑ toxicity
Rifabutin, Rifampin / ↓ Fluconazole levels R/T ↑ liver breakdown; possible uveitis if rifabutin/fluconazole given together
Sirolimus / ↑ Sirolimus levels R/T ↓ gut metabolism
Sulfonamides / ↑ Sulfonamide levels
Sulfonylureas / ↓ Sulfonylurea metabolism → ↑ plasma levels
Tacrolimus / ↑ Tacrolimus levels R/T ↓ gut metabolism; possible nephrotoxicity
Theophylline / ↑ Theophylline levels
Tolbutamide / ↑ Tolbutamide levels R/T ↓ liver breakdown
Tolterodine / ↑ Tolterodine levels; do not give more than 1 mg twice daily of tolterodine when given with azole antifungals
Tricyclic antidepressants / ↑ TCA effects/toxicity R/T ↓ metabolism by CYP2C9
Vinca alkaloids / ↑ Risk of vinca toxicity (constipation, myalgia, neutropenia)
Warfarin / ↑ Warfarin effect → ↑ PT
Zidovudine / ↑ Zidovudine levels
Zolpidem / ↑ Zolpidem effects; possible toxicity

HOW SUPPLIED
Injection: 2 mg/mL; *Powder for Oral Suspension:* 10 mg/mL, 40 mg/mL; *Tablets:* 50 mg, 100 mg, 150 mg, 200 mg.

DOSAGE
• IV; ORAL SUSPENSION; TABLETS

Bold Italic = life threatening side effect   ■ = black box warning   ✦ = Available in Canada

Vaginal candidiasis.
150 mg as a single oral dose.
Oropharyngeal or esophageal candidiasis.
Adults, first day: 200 mg; **then,** 100 mg/day for a minimum of 14 days (for oropharyngeal candidiasis) or 21 days (for esophageal candidiasis). Up to 400 mg/day may be required for esophageal candidiasis. **Children, first day:** 6 mg/kg; **then,** 3 mg/kg once daily for a minimum of 14 days (for oropharyngeal candidiasis) or 21 days (for esophageal candidiasis).
Candidal UTI and peritonitis.
50–200 mg/day.
Systemic candidiasis (e.g., candidemia, disseminated candidiasis, and pneumonia).
Optimal dosage and duration in adults have not been determined although doses up to 400 mg/day have been used. **Children:** 6–12 mg/kg/day.
Acute cryptococcal meningitis.
Adults, first day: 400 mg; **then,** 200 mg/day (up to 400 mg may be required) for 10 to 12 weeks after CSF culture is negative. **Children, first day:** 12 mg/kg; **then,** 6 mg/kg once daily for 10 to 12 weeks after CSF culture is negative.
Maintenance to prevent relapse of cryptococcal meningitis in AIDS clients.
Adults: 200 mg once daily. **Pediatric:** 6 mg/kg once daily.
Prevention of candidiasis in bone marrow transplant.
400 mg once daily. In clients expected to have severe granulocytopenia (less than 500 neutrophils/mm³), start fluconazole several days before the anticipated onset of neutropenia and continue for 7 days after the neutrophil count rises above 1,000 cells/mm³. In clients with renal impairment, an initial loading dose of 50–400 mg can be given; then daily dose is based on C_{CR}.

NURSING CONSIDERATIONS
ADMINISTRATION/STORAGE
1. Daily dose is same for PO and IV administration. Store tablets below 30°C (86°F).

2. A loading dose of twice the daily dose is recommended for the first day of therapy in order to obtain plasma levels close to the steady state by the second day of therapy.
3. Due to a long half-life, once daily dosing (either IV or PO) is possible.
4. To prevent relapse, maintenance therapy usually required in clients with AIDS, cryptococcal meningitis, or recurrent oropharyngeal candidiasis.
5. Do not give more than 1 mg of tolterodine twice a day when given with azole antifungals
6. To reconstitute the oral suspension, add 24 mL distilled water or purified water; shake vigorously to suspend powder. Shake oral suspension well before using. Store reconstituted suspension at 5–30°C (41–86°F). Discard any unused drug after 2 weeks. Do not freeze suspension.
7. Store glass bottles from 5–30°C (41–86°F); protect from freezing.
IV 8. Do not use IV solution if cloudy, precipitated, or if seal not intact.
9. Do not exceed continuous IV infusion rate of 200 mg/hr. Check site frequently for extravasation/necrosis.
10. Do not add supplementary medication to IV bag.
11. For IV use of Viaflex Plus plastic containers, do not remove unit from overwrap until ready for use. The overwrap is a moisture barrier and the inner bag maintains sterility. Do not use plastic containers in series connections as such use can cause an air embolism.

ASSESSMENT
1. Describe clinical presentation of fungal infection; culture reports. Note sensitivity to azoles or similar drugs.
2. List drugs prescribed to ensure no interactions/dosage adjustments.
3. If HIV infected may increase risk for side effects and relapse; may need maintenance therapy.
4. Obtain baseline cultures, renal and LFTs. Monitor hematologic, renal, and hepatic status. If abnormal LFTs, monitor closely for development of more serious liver toxicity. Reduce dose with renal dysfunction using guidelines.

CLIENT/FAMILY TEACHING

1. Review goals of therapy, appropriate method and schedule for administration. Take as directed; complete entire script even if infection has cleared.
2. Report rash, N&V, diarrhea, yellowing of skin, clay-colored stools, dark urine, lack of response, or persistent side effects; may need to be discontinued.
3. Avoid prolonged or excessive exposure to direct or artificial sunlight.
4. Keep all F/U and lab appointments to ensure desired response. Consume fluids to ensure hydration.

OUTCOMES/EVALUATE

- Elimination of pathogenic fungi (candida, cryptococcal meningitis)
- Candida prophylaxis in transplant recipients

Fludarabine phosphate ■ IV
(floo-**DAIR**-ah-bean)

CLASSIFICATION(S):
Antineoplastic, antimetabolite
PREGNANCY CATEGORY: D
Rx: Fludara.

SEE ALSO *ANTINEOPLASTIC AGENTS.*

USES

Chronic lymphocytic leukemia in individuals who have not responded to at least one standard alkylating agent-containing regimen. *Investigational:* Non-Hodgkin's lymphoma. In combination therapy to treat primary resistant or relapsing acute myelogenous leukemia, acute lymphoblastic leukemia, and secondary acute myelogenous leukemia.

ACTION/KINETICS

Action

Rapidly dephosphorylated to 2-fluoro-ara-A and then phosphorylated within the cell by the enzyme deoxycytidine kinase by the active 2-fluoro-ara-ATP. This compound inhibits DNA polymerase alpha, ribonucleotide reductase, and DNA primase, resulting in inhibition of DNA synthesis.

Pharmacokinetics

$t\frac{1}{2}$, **2-fluoro-ara-A:** About 20 hr. Approximately 23% of a dose of fludarabine is excreted in the urine as unchanged 2-fluoro-ara-A.

CONTRAINDICATIONS

Lactation.

SPECIAL CONCERNS

■ (1) Give under the supervision of a qualified physician experienced in the use of antineoplastic therapy. Can severely depress bone marrow function. (2) High doses in those with acute leukemia were associated with severe neurologic effects, including blindness, coma, and death. This severe CNS toxicity occurred in 36% of clients treated with doses about four times higher (96 mg/m²/day for 5–7 days) than the recommended dose. Rarely, similar severe CNS toxicity has occurred in clients treated at doses in the range of the dose recommended for chronic lymphocytic leukemia. (3) Instances of life-threatening and sometimes fatal autoimmune hemolytic anemia have been reported after 1 or more cycles of fludarabine treatment. Evaluate and closely monitor for hemolysis. (4) There was an unacceptably high incidence of fatal pulmonary toxicity when using fludarabine with pentostatin for the treatment of refractory chronic lymphocytic leukemia. Do not use together.■ Use with caution in clients with renal insufficiency. The safety and effectiveness of fludarabine in children and in previously untreated or nonrefractory chronic lymphocytic leukemia clients have not been established. An increased risk of toxicity is possible in geriatric clients, in renal insufficiency, and in bone marrow impairment.

SIDE EFFECTS

Most Common

Fever, N&V, diarrhea, infection, pain, chills, cough, pneumonia, dyspnea, sinusitis, malaise, weakness, anorexia, stomatitis, rash, edema, paresthesia.

Hematologic: Neutropenia, thrombocytopenia, anemia, *pancytopenia after trilineage bone marrow hypoplasia or aplasia.* **Tumor lysis syndrome:** Hyperuricemia, hyperphosphatemia, hypo-

---

Bold Italic = life threatening side effect   ■ = black box warning   ✦ = Available in Canada

calcemia, hyperkalemia, hematuria, metabolic acidosis, urate crystalluria, renal failure. Flank pain and hematuria may signal the onset of the syndrome. **GI:** N&V, diarrhea, anorexia, stomatitis, GI bleeding, esophagitis, mucositis, constipation, dysphagia, liver failure, cholelithiasis. **CNS:** Malaise, fatigue, weakness, headache, cerebellar syndrome, sleep disorder, impaired mentation, depression, agitation, confusion, coma. **CV:** Edema, angina, arrhythmia, CHF, ***CVA, MI***, DVT, phlebitis, supraventricular tachycardia, transient TIA. **Neuromuscular:** Peripheral neuropathy, paresthesia, myalgia, osteoporosis, arthralgia. **Respiratory:** Pneumonia, dyspnea, cough, interstitial pulmonary infiltrate, sinusitis, URTI, bronchitis, epistaxis, hemoptysis, hypoxia, pharyngitis, allergic pneumonitis, pulmonary toxicity (including ***ARDS, respiratory distress, pulmonary hemorrhage, pulmonary fibrosis, and respiratory failure***). **GU:** Dysuria, urinary infection, hematuria, urinary hesitancy, renal failure, hemorrhagic cystitis (rare). **Miscellaneous:** Skin rashes, fever, chills, ***serious opportunistic infections***, pain, visual disturbances, hearing loss, ***hemorrhage***, dehydration, diaphoresis, infection.

LABORATORY TEST CONSIDERATIONS
Abnormal renal function test. Proteinuria, hyperglycemia.

OD OVERDOSE MANAGEMENT
Symptoms: Irreversible CNS toxicity including delayed blindness, ***coma, and death.*** Severe thrombocytopenia and neutropenia. *Treatment:* Discontinue the drug and treat symptoms. Monitor the hematologic profile.

DRUG INTERACTIONS
Fludarabine combined with pentostatin ↑ risk of severe pulmonary toxicity

HOW SUPPLIED
Injection: 25 mg/mL; *Powder for Reconstitution, Lyophilized:* 50 mg.

DOSAGE
• **IV**
Chronic lymphocytic leukemia.
Adults, usual: 25 mg/m^2 given over a period of 30 min for 5 consecutive days. Initiate a 5-day course of therapy every 28 days. Reduce the dose by 20% in clients with a C_{CR} of <30 mL/min/1.73m^2.

NURSING CONSIDERATIONS

ADMINISTRATION/STORAGE
IV 1. Dose may be decreased or delayed based on presence of hematologic or neurotoxicity.

2. After maximal response, give three additional cycles, then discontinue.

3. Reconstitute lyophilized product with 2 mL of sterile water for injection, USP. Each mL of the resulting solution will contain 25 mg fludarabine (final pH range: 7.2 to 8.2). This may then be diluted in 100 or 125 mL of D5W, or 0.9% NaCl, and given over 30 min.

4. Use reconstituted drug within 8 hr; contains no preservatives.

5. If solution comes in contact with the skin or mucous membranes, wash thoroughly with soap and water. Rinse eyes thoroughly with plain water. Record exposure.

6. Store the product under refrigeration at 2–8°C (36–46°F).

ASSESSMENT
1. Note reasons for therapy, onset, previous agents used, outcome.

2. List baseline CNS assessment, bone marrow impairment, and renal dysfunction; high doses may precipitate toxicity.

3. Monitor hematologic, renal and LFTs; Reduce dose with renal impairment. Causes severe bone marrow suppression; Nadir: 5–25 days.

CLIENT/FAMILY TEACHING
1. Report flank pain or blood in urine; may precede a tumor lysis syndrome.

2. Practice barrier contraception. May interfere with menstrual cycle in women and may stop sperm production in men.

3. Report any evidence of infection (sore throat, fever), abnormal bruising or bleeding, tingling of the hands or feet, mental confusion, or loss of coordination.

4. Avoid vaccinations during therapy.

OUTCOMES/EVALUATE
• Hematologic improvement
• Control of malignant process

Flumazenil   IV
(floo-**MAZ**-eh-nill)

CLASSIFICATION(S):
Benzodiazepine receptor antagonist
PREGNANCY CATEGORY: C
Rx: Romazicon.
♣**Rx:** Anexate.

F

USES
Complete or partial reversal of benzodiazepine-induced depression of the ventilatory responses to hypercapnia and hypoxia. Situations include cases where general anesthesia has been induced or maintained by benzodiazepines, where sedation has been produced by benzodiazepines for diagnostic and therapeutic procedures, and for the management of benzodiazepine overdosage.

ACTION/KINETICS
Action
Antagonizes the effects of benzodiazepines on the CNS by competitively inhibiting their action at the benzodiazepine recognition site on the GABA/benzodiazepine receptor complex. Does not antagonize the CNS effects of ethanol, general anesthetics, barbiturates, or opiates. Depending on the dose, there will be partial or complete antagonism of sedation, impaired recall, and psychomotor impairment.

Pharmacokinetics
Onset of reversal: 1–2 min. **Peak effect:** 6–10 min. The duration of reversal is related to the plasma levels of the benzodiazepine and the dose of flumazenil. **Distribution t½, initial:** 7–15 min; **terminal t½:** 41–79 min. Metabolized in the liver with 90–95% excreted through the urine and 5–10% excreted in the feces. Hepatic impairment prolongs the half-life of the drug. Ingestion of food results in a 50% increase in clearance of flumazenil.

CONTRAINDICATIONS
Use in clients given a benzodiazepine for control of intracranial pressure or status epilepticus. In clients manifesting signs of serious cyclic antidepressant overdose. Use during labor and delivery or in children as the risks and benefits are not known. To treat benzodiazepine dependence or for the management of protracted benzodiazepine abstinence syndrome. Use until the effects of neuromuscular blockade have been fully reversed.

SPECIAL CONCERNS
The reversal of benzodiazepine effects may be associated with the onset of seizures in certain high-risk clients (e.g., concurrent major sedative-hypnotic drug withdrawal, recent therapy with repeated doses of parenteral benzodiazepines, myoclonic jerking or seizure activity prior to administration of flumazenil in cases of overdose, and concurrent cyclic antidepressant overdosage). Use with caution in clients with head injury as the drug may precipitate seizures or alter cerebral blood flow in clients receiving benzodiazepines. Use with caution in clients with alcoholism and other drug dependencies due to the increased frequency of benzodiazepine tolerance and dependence. Use with caution during lactation.

Flumazenil may precipitate a withdrawal syndrome if the client is dependent on benzodiazepines. May cause panic attacks in clients with a history of panic disorder.

Use with caution in mixed-drug overdosage as toxic effects (e.g., cardiac dysrhythmias, convulsions) may occur (especially with cyclic antidepressants).

SIDE EFFECTS
Most Common
Sweating, flushing, hot flashes, dizziness, agitation, dry mouth, tremors, palpitations, insomnia, dyspnea, hyperventilation, N&V, abnormal vision, blurred vision, headache, injection site pain.

Deaths have occurred in clients receiving flumazenil, especially in those with serious underlying disease or in those who have ingested large amounts of nonbenzodiazepine drugs (usually cyclic antidepressants) as part of an overdose. Seizures are the most common serious side effect noted. **CNS:** Dizziness, vertigo, ataxia, anxiety, nervousness, tremor, palpitations, insom-

---

Bold Italic = life threatening side effect   ■ = black box warning   ♣ = Available in Canada

nia, dyspnea, hyperventilation, abnormal crying, depersonalization, euphoria, increased tears, depression, dysphoria, paranoia, delirium, difficulty concentrating, **seizures**, somnolence, stupor, speech disorder. **GI:** N&V, hiccoughs, dry mouth. **CV:** Sweating, flushing, hot flushes, **arrhythmias (atrial, nodal, ventricular extrasystoles)**, bradycardia, tachycardia, hypertension, chest pain. **At injection site:** Pain, thrombophlebitis, rash, skin abnormality. **Body as a whole:** Headache, increased sweating, asthenia, malaise, rigors, shivering, paresthesia. **Ophthalmologic:** Abnormal vision including visual field defect and diplopia; blurred vision. **Otic:** Transient hearing impairment, tinnitus, hyperacusis.

HOW SUPPLIED

Injection: 0.1 mg/mL.

DOSAGE

- **IV ONLY**

  To reverse sedation from benzodiazepines.

Adults, initial: 0.2 mg (2 mL) given IV over 15 sec. If the desired level of consciousness is not reached after waiting an additional 45 sec, a second dose of 0.2 mg (2 mL) can be given and repeated at 60-sec intervals, up to a maximum total dose of 1 mg (10 mL). Most clients will respond to doses of 0.6–1 mg. To treat resedation, repeat doses may be given at 20-min intervals; give no more than 1 mg (given as 0.2 mg/min) at any one time and give no more than 3 mg in any 1 hr.

Management of suspected benzodiazepine overdose.

Adults, initial: 0.2 mg (2 mL) given IV over 30 sec; a second dose of 0.3 mg (3 mL) can be given over another 30 sec. Further doses of 0.5 mg (5 mL) can be given over 30 sec at 1-min intervals up to a total dose of 3 mg (although some clients may require up to 5 mg given slowly as described). If the client has not responded 5 min after receiving a cumulative dose of 5 mg, the major cause of sedation is probably not due to benzodiazepines and additional doses of flumazenil are likely to have no effect. For resedation, repeated doses may be given at 20-min intervals; no more than 1 mg (given as 0.5 mg/min) at any one time and no more than 3 mg in any 1 hr should be administered.

NURSING CONSIDERATIONS

ADMINISTRATION/STORAGE

IV 1. Must individualize dosage. Give only smallest amount effective. The 1-min wait between individual doses in dose-titration recommended for general uses may be too short for high-risk clients as it takes 6–10 min for any single dose of flumazenil to reach full effects. Slow rate of administration in high-risk clients.

2. Major risk is resedation; duration of effect of a long-acting or a large dose of a short-acting benzodiazepine may exceed that of flumazenil. With resedation, give repeated doses at 20-min intervals as needed.

3. Best given as a series of small injections to allow provider to control reversal of sedation to desired end point and to decrease possibility of side effects.

4. Reduce dose to 40–60% of normal with severe hepatic dysfunction.

5. Give through freely running IV infusion into a large vein to minimize pain at injection site.

6. Doses larger than a total of 3 mg do not reliably produce additional effects.

7. Compatible with D5W, RL, and NSS solutions. If drawn into a syringe or mixed with any of these solutions, discard after 24 hr.

8. For optimum sterility, keep in the vial until just before use.

9. Before administering, have a secure airway and IV access; awaken clients gradually.

ASSESSMENT

1. Note history of seizure disorder or panic attacks. Drug may cause seizures and respiratory impairment.

2. List type/time and amount of drug ingested; note any TCA or mixed-drug overdose.

3. Check for liver dysfunction; subsequent doses require adjustment.

4. Assess for evidence of head injury or increased ICP.

---

5. Note evidence of sedative or benzodiazepine dependence, alcohol abuse, or any recent use; may precipitate withdrawal symptoms.

INTERVENTIONS

1. The effects of flumazenil usually wear off before the effects of many benzodiazepines. Observe closely for resedation, depressed respirations, or other benzodiazepine effects up to 2 hr after administration.

2. Intended as an adjunct to, not a substitute for, proper management of the airway, assisted breathing, circulatory access and support, use of lavage and charcoal, and adequate clinical evaluation. Prior to giving flumazenil, proper measures should be undertaken to secure an airway for ventilation and IV access. Be prepared for clients attempting to withdraw ET tubes or IV lines due to confusion and agitation following awakening; awakening should be gradual. Drug should be used with caution in the ICU due to increased risk of unrecognized benzodiazepine dependence; may produce convulsions. Drug is not intended to be used to diagnose benzodiazepine-induced sedation in the ICU. Failure to respond may be masked by metabolic disorders, traumatic injury, or drugs.

3. Use seizure precautions; increased risk for seizures with large overdoses of cyclic antidepressants and with longterm benzodiazepine sedation. Drug-associated convulsions may be treated with benzodiazepines, phenytoin, or barbiturates. (Higher doses of benzodiazepines may be needed.)

4. Do not use until the effects of neuromuscular blockade have been fully reversed.

5. Flumazenil does not consistently reverse amnesia. Therefore, clients may not remember instructions during the postprocedure period; provide written instructions.

CLIENT/FAMILY TEACHING

1. Do not undertake activities requiring complete alertness; do not operate hazardous machinery or motor vehicle until at least 18–24 hr after discharge and until determined that no residual sedative effects of benzodiazepines remain. Memory and judgment may be impaired.

2. Avoid alcohol or nonprescription drugs for 18–24 hr after administration of flumazenil or if the effects of the benzodiazepines persist.

OUTCOMES/EVALUATE

Reversal of benzodiazepine sedative/psychomotor effects

Flunisolide ∎
(flew-**NISS**-oh-lyd)

CLASSIFICATION(S):
Glucocorticoid
PREGNANCY CATEGORY: C
Rx: Inhalation Aerosol: AeroBid, AeroBid-M. **Intranasal:** Nasarel.
✤**Rx:** Apo-Flunisolide, ratio-Flunisolide.

Flunisolide Hemihydrate
CLASSIFICATION(S):
Glucocorticoid
PREGNANCY CATEGORY: C
Rx: AeroSpan.

SEE ALSO *CORTICOSTEROIDS.*

USES

AeroBid, AeroBid-M, AeroSpan: (1) Maintenance treatment of asthma as prophylactic therapy in adults and children, 6 years and older. (2) For those who require systemic corticosteroids where adding flunisolide may reduce or eliminate the need for PO corticosteroids. **Nasarel:** Relief and management of nasal symptoms of seasonal and perennial allergic rhinitis.

ACTION/KINETICS

Action

Minimal systemic effects with intranasal use.

Pharmacokinetics

Significant first-pass after inhalation; rapidly metabolized by the liver. Several days may be required for full beneficial effects. 50% bioavailable. $t^{1/2}$: 1–2 hr.

Metabolized in the liver and excreted by the feces (50%) and urine (50%).

CONTRAINDICATIONS

Active or quiescent TB, especially of the respiratory tract. Untreated fungal, bacterial, systemic viral infections. Ocular herpes simplex. Use until healing occurs following recent ulceration of nasal septum, nasal surgery, or trauma. Lactation.

SPECIAL CONCERNS

■ (1) Use care when transferring from systemic corticosteroids to flunisolide inhaler due to possibility of death because of adrenal insufficiency. Several months may be needed to restore hypothalamic-pituitary-adrenal function. During this period, clients may exhibit signs and symptoms of adrenal insufficiency when exposed to trauma, surgery, or infections (especially gastroenteritis). (2) Although flunisolide inhaler may provide control of asthmatic symptoms during these episodes, it does not provide the systemic steroid needed for coping with these emergencies. During periods of stress or a severe asthmatic attack, instruct clients who have been withdrawn from systemic steroids to resume systemic steroids (in large doses) immediately and to contact their provider for further instructions. (3) Instruct clients to carry a warning card indicating they may need supplementary systemic steroids during periods of stress or a severe asthmatic attack. (4) To assess the risk of adrenal insufficiency in emergency situations, perform routine tests of adrenal cortical function periodically, including measurement of early morning resting cortisol levels. An early morning resting cortisol level may be accepted as normal if it falls at or near the normal mean level.■ Safety and efficacy in children less than 6 years of age have not been determined.

SIDE EFFECTS

Most Common

After use of the aerosol: N&V, diarrhea, flu, sore throat, headache, cold symptoms, nasal congestion, URTI, unpleasant taste.

After use of the solution/spray: Burning, dryness, nasal irritation, sneezing, throat irritation/itching.

See *Corticosteroids* for a complete list of possible side effects. Also, **Respiratory:** Hoarseness, coughing, throat irritation; *Candida* infections of nose, larynx, and pharynx.

• **Intranasal use**

Nasopharyngeal irritation, stinging, burning, dryness, headache.

GI: Dry mouth. Systemic corticosteroid effects, especially if recommended dose is exceeded.

HOW SUPPLIED

Flunisolide. *Aerosol:* About 250 mcg/actuation; *Solution/Spray:* 25 mcg/inh.

Flunisolide Hemihydrate. *Aerosol:* About 80 mcg flunisolide hemihydrate (78 mcg flunisolide)/actuation.

DOSAGE

FLUNISOLIDE

• **AEROSOL (AEROBID, AEROBID-M)**
  Chronic asthma.

Adults: 2 inhalations twice daily, morning and evening, for a total daily dose of 1 mg. Do not exceed a maximum daily dose of 4 inhalations twice/day (i.e., total of 2 mg/day). **Children and adolescents, 5–15 years of age:** 2 inhalations twice daily for a total daily dose of 1 mg. *NOTE:* Insufficient information available for use in children <6 years old.

• **SOLUTION/SPRAY (NASAREL)**
  Allergic rhinitis.

Adults: 2 sprays in each nostril twice a day. Dose may be increased to 2 sprays in each nostril 3 times per day. **Maximum dose:** 8 sprays in each nostril daily. **Children, 6–14 years:** 1 spray in each nostril 3 times per day or 2 sprays in each nostril twice a day. **Maximum dose:** 4 sprays in each nostril daily. **Maintenance, adults, children:** Smallest dose necessary to control symptoms. Some clients (approximately 15%) are controlled on 1 spray in each nostril daily.

FLUNISOLIDE HEMIHYDRATE

• **AEROSOL (AEROSPAN)**
  Chronic asthma.

Adults, 12 years of age and older, initial: 160 mcg twice daily, not to exceed 320 mcg twice daily. **Children, 6–11 years of age, initial:** 80 mcg twice daily, not to exceed 160 mcg twice daily.

NURSING CONSIDERATIONS

ADMINISTRATION/STORAGE

1. When initiating in those receiving systemic corticosteroids, use aerosol concomitantly with the systemic steroid for 1 week. Then, slowly withdraw the systemic corticosteroid over several weeks.

2. The recommended dosage of flunisolide hemihydrate relative to flunisolide is lower due to differences in delivery characteristics between the products. Any client switched from flunisolide to flunisolide hemihydrate should be dosed appropriately, taking into account the recommended dosage; monitor to ensure that the dose of the hemihydate is safe and effective.

3. When flunisolide is used chronically at 2 mg/day for asthma, periodically monitor for effects on the hypothalamic-pituitary-adrenal axis.

4. If nasal congestion is present, use a decongestant before administration to ensure drug reaches site of action.

5. If beneficial effects do not occur within 3 weeks, discontinue therapy. Improvement of symptoms usually is evident within a few days, but may take up to 2 weeks for allergic rhinitis and 1–4 weeks for chronic asthma.

6. Store products from 15–30°C (59–86°F).

ASSESSMENT

1. Note onset, symptoms and triggers as well as assessment.

2. When used chronically, monitor children for growth and effects on the HPA axis.

CLIENT/FAMILY TEACHING

1. Before use, prime the nasal spray by pushing down on the pump 5 or 6 times until a fine mist appears. If the pump has not been used for 5 days or more, the spray must be primed again.

2. Use a demonstrator and instruct client and family how to administer nasal spray or inhalant. If prescribed a bronchodilator, instruct to use that first so steroid can better penetrate mucosa.

3. Clear nasal passages before using nasal spray. Gargle and rinse mouth with water after inhalation to prevent alterations in taste and to maintain adequate oral hygiene. Report any symptoms of irritation or fungal infections.

4. Mild nasal bleeding may occur; this is usually transient.

5. Do not puncture the aerosol, store or administer near heat or open flame, or throw container into a fire or incinerator. Report lack of response or worsening of condition.

OUTCOMES/EVALUATE

- Improved airway exchange
- ↓ Allergic manifestations

Fluorouracil ■ IV (5-Fluorouracil, 5-FU)

(flew-roh-**YOUR**-ah-sill)

CLASSIFICATION(S):
Antineoplastic, antimetabolite
PREGNANCY CATEGORY: X
Rx: Adrucil, Carac, Efudex, Fluoroplex.

SEE ALSO *ANTINEOPLASTIC AGENTS.*

USES

Systemic: (1) Palliative management of certain cancers of the rectum, stomach, colon, pancreas, and breast. (2) In combination with levamisole for Dukes' stage C colon cancer after surgical resection. (3) In combination with leucovorin for metastatic colorectal cancer. *Investigational:* Cancer of the bladder, ovaries, prostate, cervix, endometrium, lung, liver, head, and neck. Also, malignant pleural, peritoneal, and pericardial effusions.

Topical (as solution or cream): (1) Multiple actinic or solar keratoses. (2) Superficial basal cell carcinoma (5% strength). *Investigational:* Condylomata acuminata (1% solution in 70% ethanol or the 5% cream).

ACTION/KINETICS

Action

Pyrimidine antagonist that inhibits the methylation reaction of deoxyuridylic acid to thymidylic acid. Thus, synthesis of DNA and, to a lesser extent, RNA is inhibited. Cell-cycle specific for the S phase of cell division. When used topically, the following response occurs:

- Early inflammation: Erythema for several days (minimal reaction)
- Severe inflammation: Burning, stinging, vesiculation
- Disintegration: Erosion, ulceration, necrosis, pain, crusting, reepithelialization
- Healing: Within 1–2 weeks with some residual erythema and temporary hyperpigmentation

Pharmacokinetics
t½, **initial:** 5–20 min; **final:** 20 hr. From 60 to 80% eliminated as respiratory CO_2 (8–12 hr); small amount (15%) excreted unchanged in urine (1–6 hr). Highly toxic; initiate use in hospital.

ADDITIONAL CONTRAINDICATIONS

Systemic: Clients in poor nutritional state, with severe bone marrow depression, severe infection, or recent (4-week-old) surgical intervention. Pregnancy or lactation. **Topical:** Use in women who are pregnant or who may become pregnant. Use of Carac in dihydropyrimidine dehydrogenase enzyme deficiency. Application to mucous membranes due to possible local inflammation and ulceration and miscarriage/birth defects when applied during pregnancy.

SPECIAL CONCERNS

■ It is recommended that fluorouracil injection be given only by or under the supervision of a qualified physician who is experienced in cancer chemotherapy and who is well versed in the use of potent antimetabolites. Because of the possibility of severe toxic reactions, it is recommended that clients be hospitalized at least during the initial course of therapy.■ Safety and efficacy of topical products have not been established in children. Occlusive dressings may result in increased inflammation in adjacent normal skin when topical products are used. To be used with caution in clients with hepatic or liver dysfunction.

SIDE EFFECTS
Most Common
After systemic use: Diarrhea, heartburn, sores in mouth and on lips, anorexia, N&V, skin rash, itching, weakness, alopecia.
After topical use: Rash, skin irritation, burning, inflammation, itching, pain, tenderness, changes in skin color at application site.

Systemic use. GI: Stomatitis, sores in mouth and on lips, esophagopharyngitis (may lead to sloughing and ulceration), diarrhea, anorexia, N&V, enteritis, cramps, duodenal ulcer, watery stools, duodenitis, gastritis, glossitis, pharyngitis, intra- and extrahepatic biliary schleroris, acalculus cholecystitis, GI ulceration, bleeding. **CNS:** Lethargy, malaise, weakness, acute cerebellar syndrome (may persist after discontinuation of treatment), headache, disorientation, confusion, euphoria. **CV:** Myocardial ischemia, angina. **Dermatologic:** Alopecia, dermatitis (often as a pruritis maculopapular rash on the extremities or trunk), nonspecific skin toxicity, itching, photosensitivity (erythema, increased skin pigmentation), nail changes (including nail loss), dry skin, fissuring, vein pigmentation. **Hematologic:** Leukopenia, thrombocytopenia, pancytopenia, *agranulocytosis*, anemia, thrombophlebitis, low WBC counts. **Ophthalmic:** Photophobia, lacrimation, decreased vision, nystagmus, diplopia, lacrimal duct stenosis, visual changes. **Regional arterial infusion complications:** *Arterial aneurysm*, arterial ischemia, arterial thrombosis, bleeding at catheter site, catheter blocked/displaced/leaking, *embolism*, fibromyositis, abscesses, infection at catheter site, thrombophlebitis. **Hypersensitivity:** *Anaphylaxis*, generalized allergic reactions. **Miscellaneous:** Fever, epistaxis.
Topical Use. Dermatologic: Local pain, pruritus, itching, hyperpigmentation, irritation, inflammation, burning at site of application, allergic contact dermatitis, scarring, soreness, tenderness, suppuration, scaling, swelling, change in skin color at application site. **Miscellaneous:** Alopecia, insomnia, irritability,

F

stomatitis, medicinal taste, photosensitivity, lacrimation, telangiectasia, uticara, toxic gramulation.

NOTE: The following side effects are possible when using Carac: **Dermatologic:** Application site reaction, burning, dryness, edema, erosion, erythema, irritation, pain. **Miscellaneous:** Eye irritation, sinusitis, common cold, headache, allergy.

LABORATORY TEST CONSIDERATIONS
↑ Alkaline phosphatase, LDH, serum bilirubin, and serum transaminase. Abnormal lab tests: BSP, prothrombin, total proteins, sed rate, thrombocytopenia.

OD OVERDOSE MANAGEMENT
Symptoms: N&V, diarrhea, GI ulceration, GI bleeding, thrombocytopenia, *agranulocytosis,* leukopenia. *Treatment:* Monitor hematologically for at least 4 weeks.

DRUG INTERACTIONS
Leucovorin calcium ↑ toxicity of fluorouracil.

HOW SUPPLIED
Cream: 0.5%, 1%, 5%; *Injection:* 50 mg/mL; *Topical Solution:* 2%, 5%.

DOSAGE
• **IV**
Palliative management of selected carcinomas.
Individualize dosage. Initial: 12 mg/kg/day for 4 days, not to exceed 800 mg/day. If no toxicity seen, administer 6 mg/kg on days 6, 8, 10, and 12. Discontinue therapy on day 12 even if there are no toxic symptoms. **Maintenance:** Repeat dose of first course q 30 days or when toxicity from initial course of therapy is gone; or, give 10–15 mg/kg/week as a single dose. Do not exceed 1 gram/week. **If client is debilitated or is a poor risk:** 6 mg/kg/day for 3 days; if no toxicity, give 3 mg/kg on days 5, 7, and 9 (daily dose should not exceed 400 mg).

Metastatic colorectal cancer.
Leucovorin, **IV,** 200 mg/m²/day for 5 days followed by fluorouracil, **IV,** 370 mg/m²/day for 5 days. Repeat q 28 days to maximize response and to prolong survival.
• **CREAM; TOPICAL SOLUTION**

Multiple actinic or solar keratoses.
Apply to cover lesion 1–2 times per day for 2–6 weeks.
Superficial basal cell carcinoma.
Apply 5% cream or solution to cover lesion twice a day for 3–6 weeks (up to 10–12 weeks may be required).

NURSING CONSIDERATIONS
ADMINISTRATION/STORAGE
1. Apply cream or solution with fingertips, nonmetallic applicator, or rubber gloves. Wash hands immediately thereafter.
2. Avoid contact with eyes, nose, and mouth.
3. Limit occlusive dressings to lesions; causes inflammatory reactions in normal skin. Increased absorption is possible through ulcerated or inflamed skin.
4. Complete healing of keratoses may require 2 months.
IV 5. Further dilution not needed; solution may be injected directly into the vein with a 25-gauge needle over 1–2 min.
6. Drug can be diluted in D5W or NSS and administered by IV infusion for periods of 30 min–8 hr. This method produces less systemic toxicity than rapid injection.
7. Do not mix with other drugs or IV additives.
8. If precipitate forms, resolubilize by heating to 60°C (140°F) with vigorous shaking. Allow to return to room temperature, allow air to settle out before withdrawing and administering medication.
9. Solution may discolor slightly during storage; potency and safety not affected.
10. Store in a cool place (10–27°C, or 50–80°F). Do not freeze. Excessively low temperature causes precipitation. Do not expose the solution to light.
ASSESSMENT
1. List reasons for therapy, onset, area requiring treatment, clinical presentation, other agents trialed.
2. Observe for intractable vomiting, stomatitis, diarrhea; early signs of toxicity requiring immediate withdrawal of drug.

3. Hydrate well before and after therapy. Give antiemetics 1 hr before therapy.

4. Protect and supervise ambulation if symptoms of cerebellar dysfunction occur (altered balance, dizziness, or weakness).

5. Prevent exposure to strong sunlight and other ultraviolet rays; these intensify skin reactions.

6. Hair loss and mouth lesions may occur but are usually transient.

7. Use precautions and strict asepsis when WBC count is below 2,000/mm³.

8. Discontinue if WBC and platelet counts are depressed below 3,500/mm³ and 100,000/mm³, respectively. Nadir: 10–20 days; recovery: 30 days.

CLIENT/FAMILY TEACHING

1. Review method for topical application. Do not wear plastic eyeglass frames during treatment. Contact may cause severe skin burns. Apply at night when glasses may be removed.

2. To apply Carac, use the following procedure:
- Apply once a day using fingertips; cover lesions with a thin film.
- Do not apply near eyes, nostrils, or mouth. Apply 10 min after thoroughly washing, rinsing, and drying the entire area.
- Wash hands thoroughly immediately after application.
- Continued treatment up to 4 weeks results in greater lesion reduction. Local irritation is not significantly increased by extending treatment from 2 to 4 weeks; irritation is generally resolved within 2 weeks after stopping treatment.

3. Affected area may appear much worse before healing takes place in 1–2 months. Expect severe red skin areas and then scaling and peeling of area. If dressing is needed, use only porous gauze; avoid occlusive dressings. May apply moisturizer and sunscreen two hours after application.

4. Drink plenty of fluids (2–3 L/day) during therapy.

5. Practice barrier contraception during systemic therapy.

6. Avoid exposure to sunlight. If exposed, wear protective clothing, sunglasses, and sunscreen.

7. Hair loss and mouth sores may occur but are usually transient with parenteral therapy.

8. Avoid contact with people who have colds, the flu, or other contagious illnesses; do not receive vaccines that contain live strains of a virus (e.g., live oral polio vaccine) during treatment. Avoid contact with individuals who have recently been vaccinated with a live vaccine.

OUTCOMES/EVALUATE
- Control of malignant process
- Reepithelialization of skin lesion

Fluoxetine hydrochloride ■ⓒ
(flew-**OX**-eh-teen)

CLASSIFICATION(S):
Antidepressant, selective serotonin reuptake inhibitor

PREGNANCY CATEGORY: B

Rx: Prozac, Prozac Pulvules, Prozac Weekly, Sarafem Pulvules.

✦Rx: Apo-Fluoxetine, CO Fluoxetine, Gen-Fluoxetine, Novo-Fluoxetine, Nu-Fluoxetine, PMS-Fluoxetine, Rhoxal-fluoxetine, ratio-Fluoxetine.

SEE ALSO *SELECTIVE SEROTONIN REUPTAKE INHIBITORS*.

USES

Prozac: (1) Major depressive disorder as defined in the DSM-IV in children (8–18 years) and adults. (2) Obsessive-compulsive disorders (OCD; as defined in the DSM-III-R) in children (8–18 years) and adults. (3) Long-term treatment of moderate to severe bulimia nervosa. (4) Panic disorder with or without agoraphobia as defined in DSM-IV. **Serafem:** Premenstrual dysphoric disorder. *Investigational:* Posttraumatic stress disorder, Raynaud phenomenon, generalized anxiety disorder, hot flashes, prophylaxis of migraine (second-line treatment).

ACTION/KINETICS

Action

Antidepressant effect likely due to inhibition of CNS neuronal uptake of serotonin and to a less extent norepinephrine and dopamine. Results in increased levels of serotonin in synapses.

Pharmacokinetics

Metabolized in the liver to norfluoxetine, a metabolite with equal potency to fluoxetine. Norfluoxetine is further metabolized by the liver to inactive metabolites that are excreted by the kidneys. **Time to peak plasma levels:** 6–8 hr. **Peak plasma concentrations:** 15–55 ng/mL. $t^{1/2}$, **fluoxetine:** 1–6 days; $t^{1/2}$, **norfluoxetine:** 4–16 days. **Time to steady state:** About 4 weeks. Active drug maintained in the body for weeks after withdrawal. Impaired hepatic function increases the half-life. **Plasma protein binding:** About 94.5%.

CONTRAINDICATIONS

Use of thioridazine with fluoxetine or within a minimum of 5 weeks after fluoxetine has been discontinued.

SPECIAL CONCERNS

■ (1) Antidepressants increased the risk of suicidal thinking and behavior (suicidality) in short-term studies in children and adolescents with major depressive disorder and other psychiatric disorders. Anyone considering the use of fluoxetine or any other antidepressant in a child or adolescent must balance this risk with the clinical need. Clients who are started on therapy should be observed closely for clinical worsening, suicidality, or unusual changes in behavior. Families and caregivers should be advised of the need for close observation and communication with the prescriber. Fluoxetine is approved for use in pediatric clients with major depressive disorder and obsessive-compulsive disorder. (2) Short-term placebo-controlled trials of 9 antidepressant drugs in children and adolescents with major depressive disorder, obsessive-compulsive disorder, or other psychiatric disorders revealed a greater risk of adverse reactions during the first few months of treatment. The average risk of such reactions in clients receiving antidepressants was 4%, twice the placebo risk of 2%. No suicides occurred in these trials.■ A lower dose or less frequent dosing should be considered for those with impaired hepatic function, elderly clients, those with concurrent diseases, or those who are taking multiple medications. Use in hospitalized clients, use for longer than 5–6 weeks for depression, or use for more than 13 weeks for obsessive-compulsive disorder has not been studied adequately.

SIDE EFFECTS

Most Common

Insomnia, nausea, somnolence, nervousness, anxiety, tremor, diarrhea/loose stools, anorexia, dry mouth.

A large number of side effects have been reported for this drug. Listed are those with a reported frequency of greater than 1%. **CNS:** Headache, activation of mania or hypomania, insomnia, anxiety, nervousness, dizziness, fatigue, sedation, decreased libido, drowsiness, somnolence, lightheadedness, decreased ability to concentrate, tremor, disturbances in sensation, agitation, abnormal dreams. Although less frequent than 1%, *some clients may experience seizures or attempt suicide.* **GI:** Nausea, diarrhea/loose stools, vomiting, constipation, dry mouth, dyspepsia, anorexia, abdominal pain, flatulence, alteration in taste, gastroenteritis, increased appetite. **CV:** Hot flashes, palpitations. **GU:** Sexual dysfunction, impotence, anorgasmia, frequent urination, UTI, dysmenorrhea. **Respiratory:** URTI, pharyngitis, cough, dyspnea, rhinitis, bronchitis, nasal congestion, sinusitis, sinus headache, yawn. **Skin:** Rash, pruritus, excessive sweating. **Musculoskeletal:** Muscle, joint, limb or back pain. **Miscellaneous:** Flu-like symptoms, asthenia, fever, chest pain, allergy, visual disturbances, blurred vision, weight loss, bacterial or viral infection, chills.

ADDITIONAL DRUG INTERACTIONS

Alprazolam / ↑ Alprazolam levels and ↓ psychomotor performance

Buspirone / ↓ Buspirone effects; worsening of OCD

Bold Italic = life threatening side effect   ■ = black box warning   ♣ = Available in Canada

Carbamazepine / ↑ Carbamazepine levels → toxicity
Clozapine / ↑ Clozapine levels
Cyproheptadine / ↓ or Reversal of fluoxetine effect
Dextromethorphan / Possibility of hallucinations
Diazepam / ↑ Diazepam half-life → excessive sedation or impaired psychomotor skills
Digoxin / ↓ AUC of digoxin; use together with caution
Haloperidol / ↑ Haloperidol levels
Lithium / ↑ Lithium levels → possible neurotoxicity
Olanzapine / ↑ Olanzapine peak levels
Phenytoin / ↑ Phenytoin levels

HOW SUPPLIED

Capsules: 10 mg, 20 mg, 40 mg; *Capsules, Delayed-Release:* 90 mg; *Oral Solution:* 20 mg/5 mL; *Tablets:* 10 mg, 15 mg, 20 mg.

DOSAGE

PROZAC

• **CAPSULES; CAPSULES, DELAYED RELEASE; ORAL SOLUTION; TABLETS**

Major depressive disorder.

Adults, initial: 20 mg/day in the morning. If clinical improvement is not observed after several weeks, the dose may be increased to a maximum of 80 mg/day in two equally divided doses. For weekly dosing for stabilized clients requiring maintenance therapy, can use Prozac Weekly (90 mg delayed release capsule), given 7 days after the last 20 mg dose. If satisfactory response is not maintained, reestablish a daily dosing regimen. **Children, 8–18 years of age, initial:** 10 or 20 mg/day. After 1 week at 10 mg/day increase the dose to 20 mg/day.

OCD.

Initial: 20 mg/day in the morning. If improvement is not significant after several weeks, the dose may be increased. Full effect may be delayed until 5 weeks of treatment or longer. **Usual dosage range:** 20–60 mg/day; the total daily dosage should not exceed 80 mg. Adjust dose to maintain client on lowest effective dosage. **Children, 8–18 years of age, initial:** 10 mg/day. After 2 weeks, increase the dose to 20 mg/day;

additional dose increases may be considered after several more weeks if clinical improvement is insufficient. Recommended dose range: 20–60 mg/day. A dose range of 20–30 mg/day is recommended for lower weight children. **Maintenance, adults and children:** Clients have been continued on therapy for an additional 6 months after an initial 13 weeks of treatment, without loss of efficacy. Adjust dose to maintain on lowest effective dose; periodically reassess to determine need for continued treatment.

Bulimia nervosa.

Initial: 60 mg/day given in the morning. May be necessary to titrate up to this dose over several days. **Maintenance:** Therapy has been continued for an additional 52 weeks beyond the initial 8 weeks.

Panic disorder.

Initial: 10 mg/day. After 1 week, increase the dose to 20 mg/day. A dose increase may be considered after several weeks if no improvement is noted. Doses above 60 mg/day have not been evaluated in panic disorders.

Migraine, prophylaxis (second-line).

10–40 mg/day.

PTSD.

10–80 mg/day.

Generalized anxiety disorder.

20 mg/day.

Raynaud phenomenon.

20–60 mg/day.

Hot flashes.

20 mg/day.

SERAFEM

• **CAPSULES**

Premenstrual dysphoric disorder.

Initial: 20 mg/day (not to exceed 80 mg/day) given every day of the menstrual cycle or intermittently (starting a daily dose 14 days before anticipated menses onset through the first full day of menses; repeat with each new cycle). Efficacy has been maintained for up to 6 months at doses of 20 mg/day given continuously and up to 3 months at a dose of 20 mg/day given intermittently. Reassess clients to determine continued need for the drug.

F

NURSING CONSIDERATIONS

✪ Do not confuse fluoxetine with duloxetine (another selective serotonin reuptake inhibitor).

ADMINISTRATION/STORAGE

1. Divide doses greater than 20 mg/day and give in the a.m. and at noon.

2. If doses lower than 20 mg are necessary, the drug may be emptied from the capsule into cranberry, orange, or apple juice; this should not be refrigerated (is stable for 2 weeks). *NOTE:* A liquid preparation (20 mg/5 mL) is also available.

3. The maximum therapeutic effect may not be observed until 4–5 weeks after beginning therapy.

4. Elderly clients, clients taking multiple medications, and those with liver or kidney dysfunction should take lower or less frequent doses.

5. When used for obsessive-compulsive disorders and therapy has been continued for over 6 months, reassess periodically to determine if continued drug therapy is needed.

6. When given with tricyclic antidepressants or if fluoxetine has been recently discontinued, the dose of TCA may need to be reduced and plasma levels monitored temporarily.

7. Allow 14 days to elapse between discontinuing a MAOI and starting fluoxetine therapy; also, allow 5 weeks or more to elapse between stopping fluoxetine and starting a MAOI.

8. Do not give thioridazine with fluoxetine or within a minimum of 5 weeks after fluoxetine has been discontinued.

9. Store drug at controlled room temperature protected from light.

ASSESSMENT

1. Note reasons for therapy, onset, characteristics of S&S, other agents trialed, outcome.

2. Review drugs currently prescribed to ensure that none interact.

3. Determine if pregnant or lactating.

4. Obtain renal and LFTs; reduce dose with elderly or debilitated, hepatic/renal dysfunction.

5. Periodically reassess to determine need for continued therapy.

6. Drug has long half-life up to 3 days and its metabolite 16 days.

CLIENT/FAMILY TEACHING

1. Take at the designated times; nervousness and insomnia may occur.

2. May be taken with food to decrease chance of stomach upset.

3. Use caution when driving or performing tasks that require mental alertness; may cause drowsiness/dizziness. Change positions slowly to avoid drop in BP.

4. Report side effects, especially rashes, hives, increased anxiety, loss of appetite or lack of response. Use reliable birth control during therapy.

5. Usually takes 1 month to note any significant benefits from therapy. Do not become discouraged and discontinue before benefits attained.

6. Avoid alcohol; do not take any OTC agents without approval. Use sunscreen and avoid prolonged sun exposure.

7. Keep all F/U appointments. Any thoughts of suicide or evidence of increased suicide ideations should be reported immediately. Parents should monitor children carefully for any indications of suicide ideations.

OUTCOMES/EVALUATE

- ↓ Symptoms of depression, as evidenced by improved sleeping and eating patterns, ↓ fatigue, and ↑ social involvement and activity
- Control of repetitive behavioral manifestations (OCD), bulimia nervosa, panic disorder

Fluphenazine decanoate
(flew-**FEN**-ah-zeen)

CLASSIFICATION(S):
Antipsychotic, phenothiazine
PREGNANCY CATEGORY: C

♣**Rx:** Apo-Fluphenazine Decanoate Injection, Fluphenazine Omega, Modecate Concentrate, Modecate Decanoate, PMS-Fluphenazine Decanoate.

Bold Italic = life threatening side effect   ▬ = black box warning   ♣ = Available in Canada

Fluphenazine hydrochloride

PREGNANCY CATEGORY: C

✦**Rx:** Apo-Fluphenazine, Moditen HCl.

SEE ALSO *ANTIPSYCHOTIC AGENTS, PHENOTHIAZINES.*

USES

(1) Psychotic disorders. (2) Schizophrenia. (3) Decanoate for prolonged and parenteral neuroleptic therapy (e.g., chronic schizophrenics).

NOTE: For severely agitated clients, treat initially with the hydrochloride; after acute symptoms improve, can give the decanoate and adjust dose as required.

ACTION/KINETICS

Action

High incidence of extrapyramidal symptoms and a low incidence of sedation, anticholinergic effects, antiemetic effects, and orthostatic hypotension.

Pharmacokinetics

Only 2.7% bioavailable when given PO and 3.4% bioavailable when given IM or SC. The decanoate ester dramatically increases the duration of action. *Decanoate:* **Onset,** 24–72 hr; **peak plasma levels,** 24–48 hr; **t½** (approximate), 21 days; **duration,** 4 or more weeks. *Hydrochloride:* **Peak plasma levels:** 2.8 hr; **t½:** About 18 hr. Fluphenazine hydrochloride can be cautiously administered to clients with known hypersensitivity to other phenothiazines.

SPECIAL CONCERNS

In those with phenothiazine sensitivity or with disorders that may cause undue reactions, begin therapy cautiously with the hydrochloride. May then follow with the decanoate.

SIDE EFFECTS

Most Common

After PO use: Drowsiness, dizziness, agitation, dry mouth, anorexia, nausea, constipation, headache, changes in vision.

After parenteral use: Drowsiness, dizziness, lethargy, nausea, anorexia, blurred vision, dry mouth, constipation, extrapyramidal symptoms.

See *Antipsychotic Agents, Phenothiazines* for a complete list of possible side effects.

HOW SUPPLIED

Fluphenazine decanoate: *Injection:* 25 mg/mL.

Fluphenazine hydrochloride: *Elixir:* 2.5 mg/5 mL; *Injection:* 2.5 mg/mL; *Oral Solution, Concentrate:* 5 mg/mL; *Tablets:* 1 mg, 2.5 mg, 5 mg, 10 mg.

DOSAGE

HYDROCHLORIDE

• **ELIXIR; ORAL SOLUTION CONCENTRATE; TABLETS**

Psychotic disorders.

Adults initial: 2.5–10 mg/day in divided doses q 6–8 hr; **then,** reduce gradually to maintenance dose of 1 or 5 mg/day (usually given as a single dose, not to exceed 20 mg/day). **Geriatric, emaciated, debilitated clients, initial:** 1–2.5 mg/day; **then,** dosage determined by response.

HYDROCHLORIDE

• **IM**

Psychotic disorders.

Adults, initial: 1.25 mg (0.5 mL); **initial daily dose:** 2.5–10 mg; divide and give q 6–8 hr. Use doses greater than 10 mg/day with caution. When symptoms are controlled, switch to PO therapy often with single daily doses.

DECANOATE

• **IM; SC**

Chronic schizophrenia.

Adults, initial: 12.5–25 mg (0.5–1 mL); **then,** the dose may be repeated or increased q 1–3 weeks. The usual maintenance dose is 50 mg/1–4 weeks. Maximum adult dose: 100 mg/dose. If doses greater than 50 mg are needed, increase succeeding doses cautiously in 12.5 mg increments.

NURSING CONSIDERATIONS

ADMINISTRATION/STORAGE

1. In poor risk clients (i.e., phenothiazine hypersensitivity or with disorders that predispose to untoward reactions), start PO or parenteral drug cautiously.

2. Store at room temperature and avoid freezing the elixir.

3. Color of parenteral solution may vary from colorless to light amber. Do not

use solutions that are darker than light amber.

4. Do not mix the hydrochloride concentrate with any beverage containing caffeine, tannates (e.g., tea), or pectins (e.g., apple juice) due to a physical incompatibility.

5. Give the hydrochloride form when beginning phenothiazine therapy. Consider the decanoate form after the response to the drug has been evaluated and for those who demonstrate compliance problems.

6. An approximate conversion is 20 mg of the hydrochloride to 25 mg of the decanoate.

7. Store tablets, elixir, and injection at room temperature of 15–30°C (59–86°F). Avoid excessive heat and protect from light. Do not freeze elixir or injection.

ASSESSMENT

1. List reasons for therapy, onset and characteristics of S&S, other therapies trialed, outcome; note clinical presentation.

2. Obtain labs and monitor periodically during prolonged therapy: LFTs, CBC, and eye exams.

3. Note age, mental status, physical condition. Elderly and debilitated clients are increased risk for acute extrapyramidal symptoms.

CLIENT/FAMILY TEACHING

1. Review administration times; determine if able to assume responsibility for self-medication. Many long term clients do better on monthly injection.

2. Avoid activities that require mental alertness until drug effects realized.

3. Review written guidelines concerning side effects that should be reported and when to return for follow-up. Stress importance of regular psychotherapy.

4. Avoid hot tubs, hot shower and tub baths as low BP may occur; in hot weather, avoid strenous activity, keep cool as heat stroke may occur.

5. Do not stop abruptly. Change positions slowly to avoid low BP effects.

6. Report jaw, neck, and back muscle spasms, slow or difficult speech, shuffling walk, persistent fine tremor or inability to sit still, fever, chills, sore throat, or flu-like symptoms, mouth sores, unusual fatigue, difficulty breathing or swallowing, severe skin rash, yellowing of the skin or eyes, irregular heartbeat. May need labs and drug withdrawn.

7. Wear sunscreen to prevent sunburns, increase fluids to prevent constipation and for dry mouth effects. Urine may turn pink-reddish brown.

8. Avoid alcohol, CNS depressants, and OTC drugs or cough remedies. Report any unusual or intolerable side effects. Cigarette smoking may decrease drug effectiveness.

OUTCOMES/EVALUATE

• Improved behavior patterns with ↓ agitation, ↓ paranoia and withdrawal

• Control of tics

Flurbiprofen ■ ©
(flur-BIH-proh-fen)

CLASSIFICATION(S):
Nonsteroidal anti-inflammatory drug
PREGNANCY CATEGORY: C
Rx: Ansaid.
♣Rx: Apo-Flurbiprofen, Froben, Froben SR, Novo-Flurprofen, Nu-Flurbiprofen, ratio-Flurbiprofen.

Flurbiprofen sodium
PREGNANCY CATEGORY: C
Rx: Flurbiprofen Sodium Ophthalmic, Ocufen.

SEE ALSO *NONSTEROIDAL ANTI-INFLAMMATORY DRUGS.*

USES
Ophthalmic: Prevention of intraoperative miosis.

PO: Relief of signs and symptoms of rheumatoid arthritis and osteoarthritis. *Investigational:* Inflammation following cataract surgery, uveitis syndromes. Topically to treat cystoid macular edema. Primary dysmenorrhea, sunburn, mild to moderate pain.

ACTION/KINETICS

Action
By inhibiting prostaglandin synthesis, when used ophthalmically flurbiprofen reverses prostaglandin-induced vasodilation, leukocytosis, increased vascular permeability, and increased intraocular pressure. Also inhibits miosis occurring during cataract surgery.

Pharmacokinetics
PO form, time to peak levels: 1.5 hr; **t½:** 5.7 hr. Over 70% excreted in the urine. Limited if any absorption after ophthalmic use. **Plasma protein binding:** More than 99%.

CONTRAINDICATIONS
Dendritic keratitis.

SPECIAL CONCERNS
■ (1) Cardiovascular risk. NSAIDs may cause an increased risk of serious CV thrombotic events, MI, and stroke, which can be fatal. This risk may increase with duration of use. Clients with CV disease or risk factors for CV disease may be at greater risk. (2) Flurbiprofen is contraindicated for treatment of perioperative pain in the setting of coronary artery bypass graft surgery. (3) GI risk. NSAIDs cause an increased risk of serious GI adverse eevents, including bleeding, ulceration, and perforation of the stomach or intestines, which can be fatal. These events can occur at any time during use and without warning symptoms. Elderly clients are at greater risk for serious GI events.■ Use with caution in clients hypersensitive to aspirin or other NSAIDs and during lactation. Wound healing may be delayed with use of the ophthalmic product. Acetylcholine chloride and carbachol may be ineffective when used with ophthalmic flurbiprofen. Safety and efficacy in children have not been established.

SIDE EFFECTS

Most Common
After PO use: Headache, abdominal pain/cramps, diarrhea, nausea. dyspepsia/indigestion, UTI/symptoms, edema.
After ophthalmic use: Ocular irritation, transient stinging or burning.

See **Nonsteroidal Anti-Inflammatory Drugs** for a complete list of possible side effects.
Ophthalmic: Ocular irritation, transient stinging or burning following use, delay in wound healing. Increased bleeding of ocular tissues in conjunction with ocular surgery.

HOW SUPPLIED
Flurbiprofen: *Tablets:* 50 mg, 100 mg.
Flurbiprofen sodium: *Ophthalmic Solution:* 0.03%.

DOSAGE
- **OPHTHALMIC SOLUTION**
  Inhibit intraoperative miosis.
Beginning 2 hr before surgery, instill 1 gtt q 30 min (i.e., total of 4 gtt of 0.03% solution).
- **TABLETS**
  Rheumatoid arthritis, osteoarthritis.
Adults, initial: 200–300 mg/day in divided doses 2, 3, or 4 times per day; **then,** adjust dose to client response. The largest recommended single dose in a multiple-dose daily regimen is 100 mg. Doses greater than 300 mg/day are not recommended.
  Dysmenorrhea.
50 mg 4 times/day.

NURSING CONSIDERATIONS
℅ Do not confuse flurbiprofen with fenoprofen (also a NSAID). Also, do not confuse Ocufen with Ocuflox (a fluoroquinolone antibiotic).

ADMINISTRATION/STORAGE
1. Use a dose of 300 mg only for initiating therapy or for treating acute exacerbations of the disease.
2. Seek the lowest dose for each client.
3. Store ophthalmic solution from 15–25°C (59–79°F) and tablets from 20–25°C (68–77°F).

ASSESSMENT
1. Rate pain level; note reasons for therapy, onset, location, characteristics.
2. Assess ROM of involved extremity, noting any discoloration, swelling, crepitus, deformity, or warmth.
3. Note any heart disease, heart attack, stroke, if smoker, have high cholesterol, high blood pressure, or diabetes.
4. Prior to eye surgery, carefully follow the prescribed dosing intervals. Use

F

care not to touch eye surface with dropper. Report any post-op tearing, dry eye, pain, light sensitivity.

CLIENT/FAMILY TEACHING

1. May take tablets with food to decrease GI upset. Do not cut or chew tablets.

2. Review appropriate method of administering eye medication. Wash hands before administering. Do not allow dropper to come in contact with any skin surfaces, avoid rubbing eyes after instilled. Report stinging, burning, or irritation immediately.

3. Report delays in wound healing, unusual bruising/bleeding, lack of response.

4. Perform muscle-strengthening (weight-bearing) exercises daily.

5. Avoid alcohol and aspirin as they may increase GI upset.

6. Review risks of having a heart attack or a stroke with continued NSAID use.

OUTCOMES/EVALUATE

- ↓ Pain and inflammation with ↑ joint mobility
- ↓ Optic inflammation
- ↓ Abnormal pupillary contractions

Flutamide ■ⓒ
(**FLOO**-tah-myd)

CLASSIFICATION(S):
Antineoplastic, hormone

PREGNANCY CATEGORY: D

Rx: Eulexin.

✤**Rx:** Apo-Flutamide, Euflex, Novo-Flutamide, PMS-Flutamide.

SEE ALSO ANTINEOPLASTIC AGENTS.

USES

(1) In combination with leuprolide acetate (i.e., a LHRH agonist) to treat stage D$_2$ metastatic prostatic carcinoma as well as locally confined stage B$_2$-C prostate cancer. (2) In combination with goserelin acetate depots (Zoladex) to treat locally confined early stage B$_2$-C prostate cancer before and during radiation therapy. *Investigational:* Treat hirsutism in women.

ACTION/KINETICS

Action

Acts either to inhibit uptake of androgen or to inhibit nuclear binding of androgen in target tissues. Thus, the effect of androgen is decreased in androgen-sensitive tissues.

Pharmacokinetics

Rapidly metabolized to active (α-hydroxylated derivative) and inactive metabolites in the liver and mainly excreted in the urine. **t½ of active metabolite:** 6 hr (8 hr in geriatric clients). **Plasma protein binding:** 94–96%.

CONTRAINDICATIONS

Use during pregnancy or severe hepatic impairment (if baseline serum ALT values exceed twice ULN).

SPECIAL CONCERNS

 (1) There have been postmarketing reports of hospitalization and rarely death from liver failure. Evidence of hepatic injury included elevated serum transaminase levels, jaundice, hepatic encephalopathy, and death related to hepatic failure. Hepatic injury was reversible after discontinuing therapy in some clients. About half of the reported cases occurred within the initial 3 months of treatment. (2) Measure serum transaminase levels before starting treatment. Flutamide is not recommended in clients whose ALT values exceed twice ULN. Serum transaminase levels should then be measured monthly for the first 4 months of therapy, and periodically thereafter. Also obtain LFTs at the first signs and symptoms suggestive of liver dysfunction (e.g., N&V, abdominal pain, fatigue, anorexia, flu-like symptoms, hyperbilirubinemia, jaundice, right upper quadrant tenderness). If at any time a client has jaundice or their ALT rises greater than twice ULN, discontinue flutamide immediately, with close follow-up of LFTs until resolution. ■

SIDE EFFECTS

Most Common

Hot flashes, loss of libido, impotence, diarrhea, N&V, anorexia, gynecomastia, anemia, edema.

Side effects are listed for treatment with flutamide and LHRH agonist. **GU:** Loss

---

of libido, impotence. **CV:** Hot flashes, hypertension. **GI:** N&V, diarrhea, GI disturbances, anorexia. **CNS:** Confusion, depression, drowsiness, anxiety, nervousness. **Hematologic:** Anemia, leukopenia, thrombocytopenia, *hemolytic anemia*, macrocytic anemia, methemoglobinemia, sulfhemoglobinemia. **Hepatic:** Hepatitis, cholestatic jaundice, hepatic encephalopathy, jaundice, *hepatic necrosis, liver failure*. **Dermatologic:** Rash, injection site irritation, erythema, ulceration, bullous eruptions, photosensitivity, *epidermal necrolysis*. **Miscellaneous:** Gynecomastia, edema, neuromuscular symptoms, pulmonary symptoms, GU symptoms, malignant breast tumors.

LABORATORY TEST CONSIDERATIONS

↑ AST, ALT, serum creatinine, SGGT, BUN, bilirubin. Urine may be colored amber or yellow-green due to the drug or its metabolites.

OD OVERDOSE MANAGEMENT

Symptoms: Breast tenderness, gynecomastia, increases in AST. Also possible are ataxia, anorexia, vomiting, decreased respiration, lacrimation, sedation, hypoactivity, and piloerection. *Treatment:* Induce vomiting if client is alert. Frequently monitor VS and observe closely.

HOW SUPPLIED

Capsules: 125 mg.

DOSAGE

• **CAPSULES**

  Locally confined stage B_2-C and stage D_2 metastatic cancer of the prostate.
250 mg (2 capsules) 3 times/day q 8 hr for a total daily dose of 750 mg.

  Hirsutism in women.
250 mg/day.

NURSING CONSIDERATIONS

℘ Do not confuse flutamide with remantadine (an antiviral). Also, do not confuse Eulexin with Edecrin (a diuretic).

ADMINISTRATION/STORAGE

1. For stage B_2-C prostatic cancer, start flutamide and the LHRH agonist 8 weeks prior to initiating and continue during radiation therapy.

2. For maximum benefit in stage D_2 metastatic prostatic cancer, start flutamide and the LHRH agonist together and continue until disease progression.

ASSESSMENT

1. Note reasons for therapy, agents previously used, outcome.

2. Administer with an LHRH agonist (such as leuprolide acetate).

3. Monitor CBC and LFTs; check liver function prior to therapy, monthly for the first 4 months, and periodically thereafter. Stop therapy (or do not start therapy) if ALT exceeds 2X ULN or if jaundice develops.

4. Monitor methemoglobinemia in those susceptible to aniline toxicity (i.e., G-6-P dehydrogenase deficiency, hemoglobin M disease, smokers).

CLIENT/FAMILY TEACHING

1. Used to treat cancer of the prostate gland; blocks the effect of the male hormone testosterone in the body. Take flutamide and the LHRH agonist (leuprolide) at the same time which works to lower levels of testosterone produced by the testicles.

2. Drug therapy should not be interrupted or discontinued without consulting provider.

3. Hot flashes, impotence, and diarrhea are all potential side effects of drug therapy; report if persistent or bothersome. Compliance may be a problem if diarrhea experienced. Manage diarrhea by cutting down on dairy products, drinking plenty of fluids, not using laxatives, using antidiarrheal products, and eating smaller, more frequent meals high in dietary fibers.

4. Report any N&V, abdominal pain, nausea, vomiting, fatigue, anorexia, flu-like symptoms, right upper quadrant pain/tenderness, loss of appetite, dark yellow or brown urine, and yellowing of the skin or eyes.

5. Sexual problems may be drug induced (impotence, decreased libido, gynecomastia). Counseling may be indicated. Keep all F/U visits.

OUTCOMES/EVALUATE

• ↓ Production of testosterone
• ↓ Prostatic tumor size
• Control of metastatic processes

F

Fluticasone furoate ■
(flu-**TIH**-kah-sohn)

CLASSIFICATION(S):
Glucocorticoid
PREGNANCY CATEGORY: C
Rx: Veramyst.

Fluticasone propionate

CLASSIFICATION(S):
Glucocorticoid
PREGNANCY CATEGORY: C
Rx: Cream, Lotion, Ointment: Cutivate. **Aerosol:** Flovent. **Powder for Inhalation:** Flovent Rotadisk. **Spray:** Flonase.
♣Rx: Flovent HFA.

SEE ALSO *CORTICOSTEROIDS*.

USES
Fluticasone furoate. Intranasal: Symptoms of seasonal and perennial allergic rhinitis in clients 2 years of age and older.

Fluticasone propionate. Respiratory Inhalation: Maintenance treatment of asthma as prophylactic therapy in clients 4 years of age and older (Flovent HFA, Flovent Rotadisk, and Flovent Diskus). **Intranasal:** As needed to manage nasal symptoms of seasonal and perennial allergic and nonallergic rhinitis in adults and children over 4 years of age (Flonase). **Topical:** (1) Relief of inflammatory and pruritic corticosteroid-responsive dermatoses in adults. (2) Atopic dermatitis in clients as young as 3 months.

ACTION/KINETICS
Action
Anti-inflammatory due to ability to inhibit prostaglandin synthesis. Also inhibits accumulation of macrophages and leukocytes at sites of inflammation as well as to inhibit phagocytosis and lysosomal enzyme release.

Pharmacokinetics
Following intranasal use, a small amount is absorbed into the general circulation. Bioavailability is less than 2%. **Onset:** Approximately 12 hr. **Maximum effect:** May take several days. **t½:** About 3.1 hr. Absorbed drug is metabolized in the liver by CYP3A4 and excreted in the feces (>95%) and urine (<5%). **Plasma protein binding:** About 91%.

CONTRAINDICATIONS
Use for relief of acute bronchospasm. Use following nasal septal ulcers, nasal surgery, or nasal trauma until healing has occurred. Use of Flovent Rotadisk in those with hypersensitivity to any ingredient, including lactose.

SPECIAL CONCERNS
■ (1) Use care when transferring from systemic corticosteroids to fluticasone propionate because deaths due to adrenal insufficiency have occurred in those with asthma during and after transfer from systemic corticosteroids to less systemically available inhaled corticosteroids. After withdrawal from systemic corticosteroids, a number of months are required for recovery of hypothalamic-pituitary-adrenal (HPA) function. (2) Clients who have been previously maintained on 20 mg/day or more of prednisone (or its equivalent) may be most susceptible, particularly when their systemic corticosteroids have been almost completely withdrawn. During this period of HPA suppression, clients may exhibit signs and symptoms of adrenal insufficiency when exposed to trauma, surgery, or infections (particularly gastroenteritis) or other conditions associated with severe electrolyte loss. Although fluticasone propionate inhalation may provide control of asthma symptoms during these episodes, in recommended doses it supplies less than normal physiological amounts of glucocorticoid systemically and does not provide the mineralocorticoid activity that is necessary for coping with these emergencies. (3) During periods of stress or severe asthma attack, clients who have been withdrawn from systemic corticosteroids should be instructed to resume oral corticosteroids (in large doses) immediately and to contact their providers for further instruction. These clients should also be

F

instructed to carry a warning card indicating that they may need supplementary systemic corticosteroids during periods of stress or a severe asthma attack.■ Clients on immunosuppressant drugs, such as corticosteroids, are more susceptible to infections. Use with caution, if at all, in active or quiescent tuberculosis infections; untreated fungal, bacterial, or systemic viral infections. or ocular herpes simplex. Use with caution during lactation.

SIDE EFFECTS

Most Common

Use of Flonase: Headache, pharyngitis, epistaxis, nasal burning/irritation, N&V, asthma symptoms, cough.

Use of Flovent: Throat irritation, URTI, sinusitis/sinus infection, oral candidiasis, headache, fever.

Allergic: Rarely, immediate hypersensitivity reactions or contact dermatitis. Rotadisk blisters contain lactose; *anaphylaxis* may occur in those allergic to milk protein. **Respiratory:** Epistaxis, URTI, nasal burning/ulcer, blood in nasal mucus, pharyngitis, cough, asthma symptoms, irritation of nasal mucous membranes, sneezing, runny nose, sinusitis/sinus infection, nasal congestion/dryness, bronchitis, nasal septum excoriation, *possible severe fatal asthma*. **CNS:** Headache, dizziness. **Ophthalmic:** Eye disorder, cataracts, glaucoma, increased intraocular pressure. **GI:** N&V, xerostomia, oral candidiasis. **Miscellaneous:** Unpleasant taste, fever, urticaria. High doses have resulted in hypercorticism and adrenal suppression.

DRUG INTERACTIONS

Cimetidine / ↑ Fluticasone plasma levels R/T ↓ liver breakdown by CYP3A4
Clarithromycin / ↑ Fluticasone levels R/T ↓ liver breakdown by CYP3A4
Erythromycin / ↑ Fluticasone levels R/T ↓ liver breakdown by CYP3A4
Itraconazole / ↑ Fluticasone levels R/T ↓ liver breakdown by CYP3A4
Ketoconazole / ↑ Fluticasone levels R/T ↓ liver breakdown by CYP3A4
Ritonavir / ↑ Fluticasone levels R/T ↓ liver breakdown by CYP3A4

HOW SUPPLIED

Fluticasone furoate: *Intranasal suspension spray:* 27.5 mcg/spray.
Fluticasone propionate: *Aerosol (Flovent HFA):* 44 mcg/inh, 110 mcg/inh, 220 mcg/inh; *Cream:* 0.05%; *Lotion:* 0.05%; *Nasal Spray (Flonase):* 50 mcg/inh; *Ointment:* 0.005%; *Powder for Inhalation (Flovent Rotadisk):* 50 mcg/inh, 100 mcg/inh, 250 mcg/inh.

DOSAGE

FLUTICASONE PROPIONATE
FLOVENT HFA
• **AEROSOL**
Asthma.

Adults and children over 4 years of age, initial: 88 mcg twice a day (maximum: 440 mcg twice a day) if previous therapy was bronchodilators alone; 88–220 mcg twice a day (maximum: 440 mcg twice a day) if previous therapy was inhaled corticosteroids; and, 440 mcg twice a day (maximum: 880 mcg twice a day) if previous therapy was oral corticosteroids. Starting doses more than 88 mcg twice daily may be considered for those with poor asthma control or those who have previously required doses of inhaled corticosteroids that are in the higher range for that specific agent.

FLOVENT ROTADISK
• **POWDER FOR INHALATION**
Prevention of asthma.

Adults and children, 12 years and older: 100 mcg twice a day (maximum: 500 mcg twice a day) if previous therapy was bronchodilators alone; 100–250 mcg twice a day (maximum: 500 mcg twice a day) if previous therapy was inhaled corticosteroids; and, 500 (using the Diskus) to 1,000 mcg twice a day (maximum: 1,000 mcg twice a day) if previous therapy was oral corticosteroids. **Children, 4–11 years:** 50 mcg twice a day (maximum: 100 mcg twice a day) if previous therapy was bronchodilators alone or inhaled corticosteroids.

FLONASE
• **NASAL SPRAY**
Allergic rhinitis.

Adults, initial: Two sprays (50 mcg each) per nostril once daily (total daily dose: 200 mcg). Or, 100 mcg given twice a day (e.g., 8 a.m. and 8 p.m.) Maximum dose is two sprays (200 mcg) in each nostril once a day. After a few days, may reduce dose to 100 mcg (1 spray/nostril) once daily for maintenance. **Adolescents and children 4 years and older, initial:** 100 mcg (1 spray/nostril once a day). If no response to 100 mcg, may use 200 mcg/day (2 sprays/nostril). Once control achieved, decrease dose to 100 mcg (1 spray/nostril) daily. Do not exceed a dose of 200 mcg/day. The spray is not recommended for children under 4 years of age.

• **CREAM; LOTION; OINTMENT**
   Dermatoses in adults, atopic dermatitis.

Apply sparingly to affected area 2–4 times daily. For Cutivate Cream, apply a thin film to the affected areas once daily. For Cutivate Lotion, apply a thin film to the affected areas once daily.

FLUTICASONE FUROATE

• **SPRAY, INTRANASAL SUSPENSION**
   Seasonal and perennial allergic rhinitis.

Adults and children 12 years and older, initial: 110 mcg once daily given as 2 sprays (27.5 mcg/spray) in each nostril. Titrate to the minimum effective dose to reduce the possibility of side effects. When the maximum benefit has been reached, reduce the dose to 55 mcg (1 spray in each nostril) once daily. **Children, 2–11 years of age, initial:** 55 mcg once daily given as 1 spray (27.5 mcg/spray) in each nostril. Children not responding adequately to the 55 mcg dose may use 110 mcg (2 sprays/nostril) once daily. Once symptoms have been controlled, decrease the dose to 55 mcg daily.

NURSING CONSIDERATIONS

ADMINISTRATION/STORAGE

1. Effectiveness depends on regular use. Individuals will vary with respect to time to onset and degree of relief. Improvement may occur within 24 hr while maximum benefits may not occur for 1–2 weeks or longer.
2. If taking chronic oral steroids, reduce prednisone no faster than 2.5 mg/day

on a weekly basis, beginning after 1 or more weeks of aerosol therapy. After prednisone reduction is complete, decrease fluticasone dosage to the lowest effective dose.
3. Store nasal spray (Flonase) at 4–30°C (39–86°F). Store aerosol between 2–30°C (36–86°F) and the powder at 20–25°C (68–77°F) in a dry place. Store the intranasal suspension spray (Veramyst) upright from 15–30°C (59–86°F); do not freeze or refrigerate.
4. Store aerosol canister with nozzle end down; protect from freezing and direct sunlight. For best results, the aerosol cansister should be at room temperature before use.
5. Use Rotadisk blisters within 2 months of opening the moisture-protective foil.
6. For Flonase, initially prime the pump with 6 actuations before use or after a period of non-use of 1 week or more.
7. Before use of Flonase, shake gently. Discard the Flonase bottle when the labeled number of actuations has been used.

ASSESSMENT

1. List reasons for therapy, onset, characteristics of S&S, other agents trialed, outcome.
2. Examine for evidence of nasal septal ulcers; note turbinate findings.
3. Determine if immunocompromised or actively infected. Note recent systemic steroid therapy use and amount.
4. Assess heart and lungs; note PFTs and CXR findings.

CLIENT/FAMILY TEACHING

1. Review technique for administration. With nasal spray (Flonase), clear nasal passages before using. Shake inhalation and nasal product well. With inhalers, if others prescribed, use the bronchodilator first so steroid better permeates mucosa. Rinse mouth and inhaler with water after use to prevent infections.
2. With the intranasal suspension spray (Veramyst), prime before using for the first time by shaking the container well and releasing 6 test sprays into the air away from the face. When the drug has not been used for more than 2 weeks or if the cap has been left off the bottle for

---

5 days or more, prime the pump again until a fine mist appears. Store upright, shake well before each use. Discard after 120 sprays have been used, even though the bottle is not completely empty.

3. Use Rotadisk blisters within 2 months of opening the moisture-protective foil.

4. Do not exceed prescribed dose, it may take several days to achieve full benefits. Take at regular intervals to ensure effectiveness.

5. Do not interrupt therapy if side effects evident; notify provider as drug may require slow withdrawal. The dosage should also be slowly reduced if S&S of hypercorticism or adrenal suppression occur such as depression, lassitude, joint and muscle pain; report if evident, especially when replacing systemic corticosteroids with topical.

6. Use adequate humidity, especially during winter months when dry heat may aggravate mucosa.

7. Avoid persons with active infections. Report exposure to chicken pox or measles. (If not immunized or previously infected with the disease, Varicella or Immune Globulin prophylaxis may be given to high-risk clients on long-term therapy).

8. Height and weight will be monitored periodically in adolescents to detect any growth suppression.

9. Identify/avoid triggers that aggravate asthma (dust, pollen, smoke, chemicals, pets). Use peak flow meter to help manage asthma.

10. During high stress or acute asthma attack, if previously on systemic corticosteroids, resume oral corticosteroids (in large doses) immediately and contact provider for further instruction. Carry an alert indicating they may need supplementary systemic corticosteroids during periods of stress or a severe asthma attack.

11. With topical products report evidence of infection lack of healing or lack of response; do not cover with occlusive dressing. Do not apply to face, underarms, or groin areas unless specifically directed.

12. Keep all F/U appointments to evaluate response to therapy and adjust dosage as needed.

OUTCOMES/EVALUATE
- Control of asthma
- ↓ Symptoms of allergic rhinitis
- Relief of inflammatory and pruritic corticosteroid-responsive dermatoses in adults/atopic dermatitis as young as 3 mo.

─── *COMBINATION DRUG* ───

Fluticasone propionate and Salmeterol xinafoate
(flu-**TIH**-kah-sohn, sal-**MET**-er-ole)

CLASSIFICATION(S):
Anti-asthmatic combination drug.
PREGNANCY CATEGORY: C
Rx: Advair Diskus, Advair HFA.

SEE ALSO *FLUTICASONE PROPIONATE* AND *SALMETEROL XINAFOATE.*

USES
(1) Long-term, twice-daily maintenance treatment of asthma in clients 4 years of age and older (Advair Diskus) or in clients 12 years of age and older (Advair HFA). (2) Twice-daily maintenance treatment of airflow obstruction in clients with COPD associated with chronic bronchitis (use only Advair Diskus: Fluticasone 250 mcg/Salmeterol 50 mcg). Do not use higher doses of fluticasone.

CONTENT
Advair Diskus 100/50 Inhalation Powder: Fluticasone propionate (corticosteroid), 100 mcg and Salmeterol (beta-2 adrenergic agonist), 50 mcg. *Advair Diskus 250/50 Inhalation Powder:* Fluticasone propionate, 250 mcg and Salmeterol, 50 mcg. *Advair Diskus 500/50 Inhalation Powder:* Fluticasone propionate, 500 mcg and Salmeterol, 50 mcg.
Advair HFA Inhalation Aerosol Spray: Fluticasone propionate (corticosteroid), 45 mcg and Salmeterol (beta-2 adrenergic agonist), 21 mcg; Fluticasone propio-

F

nate, 115 mcg and Salmeterol, 21 mcg; Fluticasone propionate, 230 mcg and Salmeterol, 21 mcg.

ACTION/KINETICS

Action

Fluticasone is an anti-inflammatory corticosteroid. The precise mechanism is unknown but corticosteroids inhibit multiple cell types (e.g., mast cells, eosinophils, lymphocytes, macrophages, and neutrophils) and mediator production or secretion (e.g., histamine, eicosanoids, leukotriens, cytokines) involved in the asthmatic response. Salmeterol is a long-acting beta$_2$-adrenergic agonist that catalyzes the conversion of ATP to cyclic-AMP. Increased cyclic-AMP levels cause relaxation of bronchial smooth muscle and inhibition of release of mediators of immediate hypersensitivity, especially from mast cells.

Pharmacokinetics

Onset: 30–60 min; **maximum improvement in forced expiratory volume in 1 second (FEV$_1$):** Within 3 hr; **duration:** 12 hr.

Fluticasone propionate. Peak plasma levels: 1–2 hr. **t½, elimination:** 7.8 hr. Metabolized by CYP3A4 in the liver. Excreted in the feces as parent drug and metabolites.

Salmeterol xinafoate. Peak plasma levels: About 5 min but plasma levels are low. Extensively metabolized; eliminated mostly in the feces. **Plasma protein binding:** About 91% of fluticasone and 96% of salmeterol are bound to plasma proteins.

CONTRAINDICATIONS

Hypersensitivity to any component of the product. Primary treatment of status epilepticus or other acute episodes of asthma where intensive measures are needed. Use to relieve acute bronchospasm. Do not use Advair Diskus for transferring clients from systemic corticosteroid therapy due to the possibility of deaths due to adrenal insufficiency.

SPECIAL CONCERNS

■ Long-acting beta$_2$ adrenergic agonists, such as salmeterol, one of the active ingredients in fluticasone/salmeterol, may increase the risk of asthma-related death. Therefore, when treating clients with asthma, only prescribe fluticasone/salmeterol for clients not adequately controlled on other asthma-controller medications (e.g., low- to medium-dose inhaled corticosteroids) or whose disease severity clearly warrants initiation of treatment with two maintenance therapies. Data from a large placebo-controlled study showed an increase in asthma-related deaths in clients receiving salmeterol.■ Use with caution in hepatic disease. Use with caution in CV disorders, especially coronary insufficiency, cardiac arrhythmias, and hypertension. Use with caution, if at all, with active quiescent tuberculosis infections of the respiratory tract; untreated systemic fungal, bacterial, viral, or parasitic infections; or, ocular herpes simplex. Use with caution during lactation. Restrict use during labor to those in whom the benefits clearly outweigh the risks. Safety and efficacy have not been shown in children less than 12 years of age.

SIDE EFFECTS

Most Common

URTI, pharyngitis, headache, URT inflammation, cough, hoarseness/dysphonia, bronchitis, N&V.

See *Fluticasone propionate* and *Salmeterol xinafoate* for a complete list of possible side effects. Also, **Respiratory: *Paradoxical bronchospasm, laryngeal spasm,*** irritation, swelling of upper airway, stridor, ***choking.* Immediate Hypersensitivity:** Urticaria, *angioedema,* rash, ***bronchospasm.* CV:** Changes in BP and pulse rate. **Hematologic:** Systemic eosinophilia, vasculitis consistent with Churg-Strauss syndrome. **Miscellaneous:** Immunosuppression.

OD OVERDOSE MANAGEMENT

Symptoms: **Salmeterol:** Excessive beta-adrenergic stimulation and/or occurrence or exaggeration of side effects, including ***seizures,*** angina, hypertension/hypotension, tachycardia (rates up to 200 beats/min); arrhythmias, nervousness, headache, tremor, muscle cramps, dry mouth, palpitation, nausea, dizziness, fatigue, malaise, insomnia, hypokalemia, hyperglycemia. Also, pro-

---

Bold Italic = life threatening side effect   ■ = black box warning   ✦ = Available in Canada

longation of the QTc interval which can produce **arrhythmias.** *Treatment:* **Salmeterol:** Discontinue salmeterol. Institute appropriate supportive therapy based on symptoms. Use a cardioselective beta-receptor blocker but such drugs can cause bronchospasm. Cardiac monitoring is recommended.

DRUG INTERACTIONS

Beta-adrenergic blockers / Block pulmonary effects of salmeterol; also may produce severe bronchospasms

Diuretics (loop or thiazide) / ECG change and/or hypokalemia may be worsened

Ketoconazole / ↑ Fluticasone levels R/T inhibition of metabolism by CYP3A4

MAO inhibitors / Action of salmeterol may be potentiated; administer with extreme caution or within 2 weeks of discontinuation of MAOIs

Ritonavir / ↑ Fluticasone levels R/T inhibition of metabolism by CYP3A4

Tricyclic antidepressants / Action of salmeterol may be potentiated; administer with extreme caution or within 2 weeks of discontinuation of TCAs

HOW SUPPLIED

See Content.

DOSAGE

- **INHALATION AEROSOL (ADVAIR HFA)**

Asthma.

Adults and children over 12 years of age: Two inhalations twice a day (morning and evening) every day. For those who do not respond adequately to the initial dose after 2 weeks of therapy, replace the current strength of Advair HFA with a higher strength. **Maximum dosage:** Two inhalations of Advair HFA 230/21 twice a day.

- **INHALATION POWDER (ADVAIR DISKUS)**

Asthma.

Adults and children 12 years and older: 1 inhalation twice daily (morning and evening) about 12 hours apart. Recommended starting doses depend on clients' current asthma therapy. Clients not currently on inhaled corticosteroid, whose disease severity warrants treatment with two maintenance therapies, including those on non-corticosteroid maintenance therapy, start with Advair Diskus 100/50 twice daily. For clients on inhaled corticosteroid, dosage depends on the steroid being used but the recommended Advair Diskus dosage is 500/50 twice daily. **Children, 4–11 years of age:** 1 Inhalation of fluticasone 100 mcg/salmeterol 50 mcg Diskus twice daily (morning and evening), approximately 12 hr apart.

COPD associated with chronic bronchitis.

Adults: 1 Inhalation of fluticasone 250 mcg/ salmeterol 50 mcg twice daily (morning and evening) about 12 hr apart. The 250 mcg/50 mcg product is the only strength approved for COPD with chronic bronchitis. If shortness of breath occurs in the period between doses, an inhaled short–acting beta$_2$ agonist (e.g., formoterol) should be taken for immediate relief.

NURSING CONSIDERATIONS

ADMINISTRATION/STORAGE

1. Do not use inhaled, long-acting beta$_2$-agonists in conjunction with Advair Diskus.

2. Titrate to the lowest effective strength after adequate asthma stability is achieved.

3. More frequent administration than twice daily is not recommended. If symptoms arise between doses, an inhaled, short-acting beta$_2$-agonist should be used for immediate relief.

4. Improvement in asthma control can occur within 30 min but maximum benefits may not be reached for 1 week or longer after beginning treatment.

5. For those who do not respond adequately to the initial dose after 2 weeks of therapy, replacing the current strength of Advair Diskus with a higher strength may provide additional asthma control.

6. If a previously effective dosage regimen fails to provide adequate asthma control, reevaluate the therapeutic regimen and consider additional therapeutic options, including replacing the current strength with a higher strength, adding additional inhaled corticosteroid, or initiating oral corticosteroids.

7. The Diskus inhalation device is not reusable. Discard 1 month after removal from the moisture-protective foil overwrap pouch or after every blister has been used (i.e., when the dosage indicator reads '0').

8. Store from 20–25°C (68–77°F) in a dry place away from direct heat or sunlight.

ASSESSMENT

1. List reasons for therapy, characteristics of S&S, other agents trialed/outcome.

2. Assess/monitor for conditions that may preclude drug therapy; i.e., seizure disorder, glaucoma, TB, osteoporosis, CV disease, uncontrolled HTN, thyroid disorder or renal/liver disorder.

3. Determine that CXR, PFTs completed. Note pulmonary and cardiac findings.

4. Monitor VS, lung sounds, peak flow, renal and LFTs.

CLIENT/FAMILY TEACHING

1. Administer Advair Diskus by the orally inhaled route only. After inhalation, rinse the mouth with water without swallowing.

2. Prime Advair HFA before using for the first time by releasing 4 test sprays into the air, away from the face. Shake well for 5 seconds before each spray. If the inhaler has not been used for more than 4 weeks or when it has been dropped, prime the inhaler again by shaking well before each spray and releasing 2 test sprays into the air, away from the face. Do not use the purple actuator supplied with Advair HFA with any other product canisters; also, do not use actuators from other canisters with the Advair HFA canister.

3. The correct amount of medication in each inhalation of Advair HFA cannot be ensured after 120 inhalations, even though the canister is not completely empty and will continue to operate. Discard the inhaler when 120 actuations have been used.

4. Inhaler improves lung function and makes breathing easier by reducing airway swelling and irritation and by causing muscle relaxation; combination of steroid and bronchodilator.

5. Drug will not treat an asthma attack that has already begun. Not for use with acute breathing problems.

6. Monitor peak flow readings and identify when to seek additional medical care.

7. Do not give to child under 12 years; can affect growth in children. Keep F/U to assess growth rate of child if using this medication.

8. Long-term use of steroids may lead to bone loss (osteoporosis), especially in smoker, if no regular exercise, if vitamin D or calcium deficient in diet, or if family history of osteoporosis.

9. Can lower the blood cells that help your body fight infections. This can make it easier to get sick. Avoid being near people who are sick or have infections.

10. Keep all F/U appointments to evaluate response to therapy; report any adverse side effects or lack or response.

OUTCOMES/EVALUATE

- Improved breathing patterns and air exchange
- Asthma control

Fluvastatin sodium
(flu-vah-**STAH**-tin)

CLASSIFICATION(S):
Antihyperlipidemic, HMG-CoA reductase inhibitor

PREGNANCY CATEGORY: X

Rx: Lescol, Lescol XL.

SEE ALSO ANTIHYPERLIPIDEMIC AGENTS— HMG-COA REDUCTASE INHIBITORS.

USES

(1) Reduce elevated total and LDL cholesterol, apo-B, and triglyceride levels and to increase HDL cholesterol in clients with primary hypercholesterolemia (heterozygous familial and nonfamilial) and mixed dyslipidemia (Fredrickson type IIa and IIb) whose response to diet and other nondrug measures has been inadequate. The lipid-lowering effects of fluvastatin are enhanced when it is combined with a

bile-acid binding resin or with niacin. (2) Adjunct to diet to reduce total and LDL cholesterol and apo-B levels in adolescent boys and girls 10 to 16 years of age who are at least 1 year postmenarche, with heterozygous familial hypercholesterolemia whose response to dietary restriction has not been adequate and the following are present: (a) LDL-C remains at 190 mg/dL or more or (b) LDL-C remains at 160 mg/dL or more and there is a positive family history of premature CV disease or 2 or more other CV disease risk factors present. (3) To slow the progression of coronary atherosclerosis in coronary heart disease as part of a treatment plan to lower total and LDL cholesterol to target levels. (4) Reduce the risk of undergoing coronary revascularization procedures in those with coronary heart disease.

ACTION/KINETICS

Action

Decreases cholesterol, triglycerides, VLDL, and HDL and increases HDL.

Pharmacokinetics

98% absorbed. **Absolute bioavailability:** 24%. Undergoes extensive first-pass metabolism by CYP2C9. Metabolized in the liver with 90% excreted through the feces and 5% through the urine. $t^{1/2}$: Less than 3 hr for immediate-release and about 9 hr for extended release. **Plasma protein binding:** More than 98%.

SPECIAL CONCERNS

Use with caution in clients with severe renal impairment, a history of liver disease, or heavy alcohol consumption.

SIDE EFFECTS

Most Common

UTRI, dysgeusia, diarrhea, abdominal pain/cramps, N&V, constipation, myalgia, back pain, arthralgia, rhinitis, pharyngitis, influenza, accidental trauma.

See *Antihyperlipidemic Agents–HMG-CoA Reducase* Inhibitors for a complete list of possible side effects. Also, **GI:** N&V, diarrhea, dysgeusia, abdominal pain/cramps, constipation, flatulence, dyspepsia, tooth disorder. **Musculoskeletal:** Myalgia, back pain, arthralgia, arthritis. **CNS:** Headache, dizziness, insomnia. **Respiratory:** URTI, rhinitis, cough, pharyngitis, sinusitis. **Miscellaneous:** Rash, pruritus, fatigue, influenza, allergy, accidental trauma.

ADDITIONAL DRUG INTERACTIONS

Alcohol / ↑ Fluvastatin absorbed

Cimetidine / Significant ↑ in fluvastatin C_{max} and AUC

Diclofenac / ↑ Mean diclofenac C_{max} and AUC

Digoxin / ↑ Digoxin C_{max} and slight ↑ digoxin urinary clearance

Glyburide / ↑ Glyburide C_{max}, AUC, and $t^{1/2}$ and ↑ fluvastatin C_{max} and AUC

HMG—CoA Redutase Inhibitors / Concomitant use not recommended

Omeprazole / Significant ↑ in fluvastatin C_{max} and AUC

Phenytoin / ↑ Fluvastatin C_{max} and AUC; minimal ↑ phenytoin C_{max} and AUC

Ranitidine / Significant ↑ in fluvastatin C_{max} and AUC

Rifampin / ↑ Fluvastatin C_{max} and AUC and ↑ plasma clearance

Warfarin / ↑ INR

LABORATORY TEST CONSIDERATIONS

↑ Serum transaminases.

HOW SUPPLIED

Capsules (Lescol): 20 mg (as base), 40 mg (as base); *Tablets, Extended-Release (Lescol XL):* 80 mg (as base).

DOSAGE

• **CAPSULES; TABLETS, EXTENDED-RELEASE**

Hypercholesterolemia and mixed dyslipidemia. Antihyperlipidemic to slow progression of coronary atherosclerosis. Secondary prevention of coronary events.

For those requiring LDL cholesterol reduction to 25% or more, **Adults, initial:** 40 mg as one capsule in the evening or 80 mg as one tablet any time of day. Or, 80 mg in divided doses using the 40 mg capsule twice a day. For those requiring LDL cholesterol reduction to less than 25%, **Adults, initial:** 20 mg. **Dose range:** 20–80 mg/day. **Children:** 1–20 mg capsule. Adjust dosage at 6-week intervals, up to a maximum daily dose of 40 mg capsules twice a day or 1–80 mg extended-release tablet once a day.

Slow progression of coronary athero-sclerosis in coronary heart disease.
40 mg twice a day, initiated shortly after a first percutaneous coronary intervention procedure.

NURSING CONSIDERATIONS
ADMINISTRATION/STORAGE
1. Place on standard cholesterol-lowering diet before receiving fluvastatin; continue diet during therapy.
2. Lipid lowering effects on total cholesterol and LDL cholesterol are additive when immediate-release fluvastatin is combined with a bile-acid-binding resin or niacin. Maximum reductions of LDL cholesterol are usually seen within 4 weeks; order periodic lipid determinations during this time, with dosage adjusted accordingly.
3. To avoid fluvastatin binding to a bile-acid binding resin (if given together), give the fluvastatin at bedtime and the resin at least 2 hr before.
4. Store from 15–30°C (59–86°F). Dispense in tight containers and protect from light.

ASSESSMENT
1. Identify risk factors. Attempt to change/modify as many as possible. Note lipid profile.
2. Monitor LFTs prior to starting treatment, 6–8 weeks into therapy, 3 months later, then yearly if stable; 12 weeks after a dose increase.
3. Evaluate on a standard cholesterol-lowering diet before giving fluvastatin unless client has metabolic syndrome, increased risk factors, HTN with microalbuminuria or diabetes. Continue diet during treatment.

CLIENT/FAMILY TEACHING
1. May be taken with /without food; usually consumed with the evening meal.
2. Used to lower blood cholesterol and fat levels, which have been proven to promote CAD.
3. Practice reliable contraception; report if pregnancy suspected or desired.
4. Must continue risk factor reduction, dietary restrictions of saturated fat and cholesterol, and regular exercise programs in addition to drug therapy in

the overall goal of lowering cholesterol levels and CHD risk.
5. Report muscle pain or weakness, especially with fever or severe fatigue, or other adverse effects. Keep scheduled lab visits.
6. Avoid alcohol consumption.

OUTCOMES/EVALUATE
↓ Triglycerides, LDL, and total cholesterol levels

Fluvoxamine maleate ■
(flu-**VOX**-ah-meen)

CLASSIFICATION(S):
Antidepressant, selective serotonin reuptake inhibitor
PREGNANCY CATEGORY: C
✤**Rx:** Apo-Fluvoxamine, Novo-Fluvoxamine, Nu-Fluvoxamine, PMS-Fluvoxamine, ratio-Fluvoxamine.

SEE ALSO *SELECTIVE SEROTONIN REUPTAKE INHIBITORS.*
USES
Obsessive-compulsive disorder (as defined in DSM-III-R) for adults, adolescents, and children. *Investigational:* Depression, panic disorder, bulimia nervosa, social anxiety disorder.

ACTION/KINETICS
Action
Minimal to no anticholinergic or sedative effects; no orthostatic hypotension.
Pharmacokinetics
About 53% is bioavailable. **Maximum plasma levels:** 3–8 hr. t½: 13.6–15.6 hr. **Peak plasma concentration:** 88–546 ng/mL. **Time to reach steady state:** About 7 days. Elderly clients manifest higher mean plasma levels and a decreased clearance. Metabolized in the liver and about 94% excreted through the urine. **Plasma protein binding:** About 80%.

ADDITIONAL CONTRAINDICATIONS
Alcohol ingestion. Use with alosetron, pimozide, thioridazine, or tizanidine.
SPECIAL CONCERNS
■ (1) Suicidality in children and adolescent. Antidepressants increased the risk

of suicidal thinking and behavior (suicidality) in short-term studies in children and adolescents with major depressive disorder and other psychiatric disorders. Anyone considering the use of fluvoxamine or any other antidepressant in a child or adolescent must balance this risk with the clinical need. Clients who are started on therapy should be observed closely for clinical worsening, suicidality, or unusual changes in behavior. Families and caregivers should be advised of the need for close observation and communication with the prescriber. Fluvoxamine is not approved for use in pediatric clients with major depressive disorder and obsessive-compulsive disorder. (2) Short-term placebo-controlled trials of 9 antidepressant drugs in children and adolescents with major depressive disorder, obsessive-compulsive disorder, or other psychiatric disorders revealed a greater risk of adverse reactions during the first few months of treatment. The average risk of such reactions in clients receiving antidepressants was 4%, twice the placebo risk of 2%. No suicides occurred in these trials.■ Use with caution in clients with a history of mania, seizure disorders, and liver dysfunction and in those with diseases that could affect hemodynamic responses or metabolism.

SIDE EFFECTS

Most Common

Nausea, insomnia, somnolence, headache, nervousness, asthenia, dizziness, diarrhea/loose stools, dyspepsia, dry mouth, constipation, URTI.

Side effects listed occur at an incidence of 0.1% or greater. **CNS:** Somnolence, insomnia, nervousness, dizziness, tremor, anxiety, hypertonia, agitation, decreased libido, depression, CNS stimulation, amnesia, apathy, hyperkinesia, hypokinesia, manic reaction, myoclonus, psychoses, fatigue, malaise, agoraphobia, akathisia, ataxia, **convulsion**, delirium, delusion, depersonalization, drug dependence, dyskinesia, dystonia, emotional lability, euphoria, extrapyramidal syndrome, unsteady gait, hallucinations, hemiplegia, hostility, hypersomnia, hypochondriasis, hypotonia, hysteria, incoordination, increased libido, neuralgia, paralysis, paranoia, phobia, sleep disorders, stupor, twitching, vertigo, activation of mania/hypomania, seizures. **GI:** Nausea, dry mouth, diarrhea/loose stools, constipation, dyspepsia, anorexia, vomiting, flatulence, toothache, tooth caries, dysphagia, colitis, eructation, esophagitis, gastritis, gastroenteritis, **GI hemorrhage**, GI ulcer, gingivitis, glossitis, hemorrhoids, melena, rectal hemorrhage, stomatitis. **CV:** Palpitations, hypertension, postural hypotension, vasodilation, syncope, tachycardia, angina pectoris, bradycardia, **cardiomyopathy**, CV disease, cold extremities, conduction delay, **heart failure, MI,** pallor, irregular pulse, ST segment changes. **Respiratory:** URTI, dyspnea, yawn, increased cough, sinusitis, asthma, bronchitis, epistaxis, hoarseness, hyperventilation. **Body as a whole:** Headache, asthenia, flu syndrome, chills, malaise, edema, weight gain or loss, dehydration, hypercholesterolemia, allergic reaction, neck pain, neck rigidity, photosensitivity, **suicide attempt. Dermatologic:** Excessive sweating, acne, alopecia, dry skin, eczema, exfoliative dermatitis, furunculosis, seborrhea, skin discoloration, urticaria. **Musculoskeletal:** Arthralgia, arthritis, bursitis, generalized muscle spasm, myasthenia, tendinous contracture, tenosynovitis. **GU:** Delayed ejaculation, urinary frequency, impotence, anorgasmia, urinary retention, anuria, breast pain, cystitis, delayed menstruation, dysuria, female lactation, hematuria, menopause, menorrhagia, metrorrhagia, nocturia, polyuria, PMS, urinary incontinence, UTI, urinary urgency, impaired urination, **vaginal hemorrhage**, vaginitis. **Hematologic:** Anemia, ecchymosis, leukocytosis, lymphadenopathy, thrombocytopenia. **Ophthalmic:** Amblyopia, abnormal accommodation, conjunctivitis, diplopia, dry eyes, eye pain, mydriasis, photophobia, visual field defect. **Otic:** Deafness, ear pain, otitis media. **Miscellaneous:** Taste perversion or loss, parosmia, hypothyroidism, hypercholesterolemia, dehydration.

ADDITIONAL DRUG INTERACTIONS

Beta-adrenergic blockers / Possible ↑ effects on BP and HR

Buspirone / ↓ Buspirone effects

Carbamazepine / ↑ Risk of carbamazepine toxicity

Clozapine / ↑ Risk of orthostatic hypotension and seizures

Diazepam / ↑ Diazepam effect R/T ↓ clearance

Diltiazem / ↑ Risk of bradycardia

Grapefruit juice / ↑ Fluvoxamine mean AUC and C_{max}

Haloperidol / ↑ Haloperidol levels

Lansoprazole / ↑ Lansoprazole AUC and prolongation of $t\frac{1}{2}$ in homozygous and heterozygeous extensive metabolizers R/T inhibition of CYP2C19 metabolism

Lidocaine (IV) / ↓ Lidocaine elimination R/T inhibition of metabolism by CYP1A2; adding erythromycin further ↓ lidocaine elimination R/T inhibition of metabolism by CYP3A4

Lithium / ↑ Risk of seizures

H *Melatonin* / ↑ Plasma melatonin levels

Methadone / ↑ Risk of methadone toxicity

Mexiletine / ↓ Mexiletine clearance R/T ↓ metabolism

Midazolam / ↑ Midazolam effect R/T ↓ clearance

Nitroprusside / ↑ Nitroprusside-induced venodilation

Olanzapine / ↑ Olanzapine levels R/T ↓ liver metabolism

Sildenafil / ↑ Sildenafil exposure and $t\frac{1}{2}$

Smoking / ↓ Fluvoxamine plasma levels R/T ↑ metabolism by CYP1A2; smokers may need to ↑ dose

Sumatriptan / ↑ Risk of weakness, hyperreflexia, incoordination

Theophylline / ↑ Risk of theophylline toxicity (decrease dose by one-third the usual daily maintenance dose)

Thioridazine / ↑ Thioridazine levels

Tizanidine / ↑ Tizanidine intensity and duration of effects R/T ↓ metabolism by CYP1A2 enzymes

Tolbutamide / ↓ Tolbutamide clearance R/T ↓ metabolism

Triazolam / ↑ Triazolam effect R/T ↓ clearance

OD OVERDOSE MANAGEMENT

Treatment: Establish an airway and maintain respiration as needed. Monitor VS and ECG. Activated charcoal may be as effective as emesis or lavage in removing drug from the GI tract. Since absorption in overdose may be delayed, measures to reduce absorption may be required for up to 24 hr.

HOW SUPPLIED

Tablets: 25 mg, 50 mg, 100 mg.

DOSAGE

• **TABLETS**

  Obsessive-compulsive disorder.

Adults, initial: 50 mg at bedtime; **then,** increase the dose in 50 mg increments q 4–7 days, as tolerated, until a maximum benefit is reached, not to exceed 300 mg/day. Give total daily doses greater than 100 mg in 2 divided doses; if doses are unequal, give the larger dose at bedtime. **Children and adolescents, 8 to 17 years, initial:** 25 mg as a single daily dose at bedtime; **then,** increase the dose in 25 mg increments q 4–7 days until a maximum benefit is reached, not to exceed 200 mg/day up to 11 years of age and 300 mg/day up to 17 years of age. Divide total daily doses more than 50 mg into 2 doses; if the 2 divided doses are not equal, give the larger dose at bedtime. The therapeutic effect may be reached in female children with lower doses. **Maintenance:** Although efficacy has not been documented beyond 10 weeks, consider continuation in a responding client since OCD is a chronic condition. Adjust dose to maintain the lowest effective dosage; periodically reasses to determine need for continued treatment.

NURSING CONSIDERATIONS

ADMINISTRATION/STORAGE

1. If total daily dose exceeds 100 mg for adults or 50 mg in children, give in two divided doses. If the doses are unequal, give the larger dose at bedtime.

2. Initial and incremental doses may need to be lower in geriatric clients and with impaired hepatic function.

3. Store from 15–30°C (59–86°F); protect from high humidity.

Bold Italic = life threatening side effect   ■ = black box warning   ✣ = Available in Canada

ASSESSMENT

1. Note reasons for therapy, presenting/reported behavioral manifestations, other agents trialed, outcome.
2. List agents currently prescribed to ensure none interact.
3. Note history of mania, seizure disorders, liver dysfunction.
4. Monitor ECG, CBC, renal and LFTs; reduce dose with dysfunction.

CLIENT/FAMILY TEACHING

1. Take only as directed, usually at bedtime, do not exceed dosage. May initially experience N&V; should subside.
2. May cause dizziness and drowsiness. Do not perform activities that require mental or physical alertness until drug effects realized.
3. Report any rash, hives, or unusual itching or bleeding; increased depression or suicide ideations
4. Avoid alcohol and other drugs or herbals without approval. Smoking may reduce drug effectiveness.
5. Practice reliable birth control.
6. Report for scheduled appointments so response to therapy, dosage, and need for continued therapy can be determined.

OUTCOMES/EVALUATE

- Reduction in excessive, repetitive behaviors
- ↓ Depression

Folic acid

(FOH-lik AH-sid)

CLASSIFICATION(S):
Vitamin B complex
PREGNANCY CATEGORY: A
Rx: Deplin, Folvite.
❋Rx: Apo-Folic.

USES

Treatment of megaloblastic anemias due to folic acid deficiency (e.g., tropical and nontropical sprue, pregnancy, infancy or childhood, nutritional causes). Diagnosis of folate deficiency.

ACTION/KINETICS

Action

Folic acid (which is converted to tetra-hydrofolic acid) is necessary for normal production of RBCs and for synthesis of nucleoproteins. Tetrahydrofolic acid is a cofactor in the biosynthesis of purines and thymidylates of nucleic acids. Megaloblastic and macrocytic anemias in folic acid deficiency are believed to be due to impairment of thymidylate synthesis. Natural sources of folic acid include liver, dried beans, peas, lentils, whole-wheat products, asparagus, beets, broccoli, brussels sprouts, spinach, and oranges.

Pharmacokinetics

Synthetic folic acid is absorbed from the GI tract even if the client suffers from malabsorption syndrome. **Peak plasma levels after an oral dose:** 1 hr. It is stored in the liver.

CONTRAINDICATIONS

Use in aplastic, normocytic, or pernicious anemias (is ineffective). Folic acid injection that contains benzyl alcohol should not be used in neonates or immature infants.

SPECIAL CONCERNS

Daily folic acid doses of 0.1 mg or greater may obscure pernicious anemia. Prolonged folic acid therapy may cause decreased vitamin B_{12} levels.

SIDE EFFECTS

Most Common
Folic acid is relatively nontoxic in humans.
Allergic: Skin rash, itching, erythema, general malaise, respiratory difficulty due to **bronchospasm**. **GI:** Nausea, anorexia, abdominal distention, flatulence, bitter or bad taste (in those taking 15 mg/day for 1 month). **CNS:** In doses of 15 mg daily, altered sleep patterns, irritability, excitement, difficulty in concentration, overactivity, depression, impaired judgment, confusion.

DRUG INTERACTIONS

Aminosalicylic acid / ↓ Serum folate levels
Corticosteroids (chronic use) / ↑ Folic acid requirements
Methotrexate / Folic acid antagonist

Oral contraceptives / ↑ Risk of folate deficiency
Phenytoin / ↑ Seizure frequency; ↓ folic acid levels
Pyrimethamine / ↓ Pyrimethamine effect in toxoplasmosis; also, a folic acid antagonist
Sulfonamides / ↓ Absorption of folic acid
Triamterene / ↓ Utilization of folic acid; folic acid antagonist
Trimethoprim / ↓ Utilization of folic acid; folic acid antagonist

HOW SUPPLIED
Injection: 5,000 mcg/mL; *Tablets:* 400 mcg, 800 mcg, 1,000 mcg; 7.5 mg (as L-methylfolate).

DOSAGE—————————
- **TABLETS**
  Dietary supplement.
Adults and children: 100 mcg/day (up to 1 mg in pregnancy); may be increased to 500–1,000 mcg if requirements increase.
  Treatment of deficiency.
Adults, initial: 250–1,000 mcg/day until a hematologic response occurs; **maintenance:** 400 mcg/day (800 mcg during pregnancy and lactation). **Pediatric, initial:** 250–1,000 mcg/day until a hematologic response occurs. **Maintenance, infants:** 100 mcg/day; **children up to 4 years:** 300 mcg/day; **children 4 years and older:** 400 mcg/day.
- **DEEP SC; IM; IV**
  Treatment of deficiency.
Adults and children: 250–1,000 mcg/day until a hematologic response occurs.
  Diagnosis of folate deficiency.
Adults, IM: 100–200 mcg/day for 10 days plus low dietary folic acid and vitamin B_{12}.

NURSING CONSIDERATIONS
ℂ Do not confuse folic acid with folinic acid (leucovorin calcium).

ADMINISTRATION/STORAGE
1. Given PO; if there is severe malabsorption, give either IV or SC.
2. Regardless of age, dosage should never be less than 0.1 mg/day.
IV 3. Folic acid will remain stable in solution if the pH is kept above 5.

4. May be administered IM, by direct IV push or added to infusions. When given IV, do not exceed 5 mcg/min.
5. When parenteral forms are used, have drugs and equipment available to treat anaphylactic reactions.

ASSESSMENT
1. Note reasons for therapy; monitor CBC, reticulocytes, MCV, serum folate and B_{12} levels. Assess for pernicious anemia with Shilling test; serum B_{12} levels to prevent permanent neurologic damage.
2. Review drugs prescribed; oral contraceptives, trimethoprim, hydantoins, and alcohol may cause increased body loss of folic acid.

CLIENT/FAMILY TEACHING
1. Take only as directed. Avoid alcohol.
2. Dietary sources of folic acid include dark green leafy vegetables, beans, fortified breads, and cereals. Prolonged cooking destroys folate in vegetables.
3. Drug may discolor urine a deep yellow.
4. U.S. Public Health Service recommends that all women of childbearing age consume 0.4 mg of folic acid to reduce the risk of neural tube birth defects. Folic acid may prevent the development of spinal canal or brain defects, which occur during the first month of pregnancy.

OUTCOMES/EVALUATE
- Desired hematologic response (↑ retic count in 5 days)
- Reversal of symptoms of folic acid deficiency and megaloblastic anemia
- Prophylaxis of newborn neural tube defects

Follitropin alfa
(fol-ih-**TROH**-pin **AL**-fah)

CLASSIFICATION(S):
Ovarian stimulant, gonadotropin
PREGNANCY CATEGORY: X
Rx: Gonal-f, Gonal-f RFF Pen.

Bold Italic = life threatening side effect   ■ = black box warning   ✤ = Available in Canada

Follitropin beta
(fol-ih-**TROH**-pin **BAY**-tah)

PREGNANCY CATEGORY: X
Rx: Folistem AQ Cartridge/Folistim Pen, Follistim.
♣Rx: Puregon.

USES
Follitropin alfa: (1) Induction of ovulation and pregnancy in anovulatory infertile clients where cause of infertility is functional and not primary ovarian failure. (2) Stimulate development of multiple follicles in ovulatory clients undergoing in-vitro fertilization. (3) Induce spermatogenesis in men with primary and secondary hypogonadotropic hypogonadism where failure is not due to primary testicular failure.

Follitropin beta: (1) Development of multiple follicles in ovulatory clients participating in an assisted reproductive technology program.(2) Induction of ovulation and pregnancy in anovulatory infertile clients in whom the cause of infertility is functional and not due to primary ovarian failure.

ACTION/KINETICS
Action
Both products are human FSH prepared by recombinant DNA technology. When given with hCG, products stimulate ovarian follicular growth in women who do not have primary ovarian failure. Increased risk of multiple births.

Pharmacokinetics
Steady state plasma levels reached within 4 to 5 days. Increased body weight or body mass index (BMI) results in a decrease in rate of absorption.

CONTRAINDICATIONS
Use in primary ovarian failure; uncontrolled thyroid or adrenal dysfunction; in presence of any cause of infertility other than anovulation; tumor of ovary, breast, uterus, hypothalamus, or pituitary gland; abnormal vaginal bleeding of undetermined origin; ovarian cysts or enlargement not due to polycystic ovary syndrome; pregnancy; use in children; hypersensitivity to products.

SPECIAL CONCERNS
Use with caution during lactation.

SIDE EFFECTS
Most Common
Headache, nausea, flatulence, intermenstrual bleeding, abdominal/pelvic pain, URTI, increased weight, vaginal hemorrhage.

CV: Intravascular thrombosis and embolism causing venous thrombophlebitis, **pulmonary embolism**, pulmonary infarction, **stroke,** arterial occlusion (leading to loss of limb). **Pulmonary:** Atelectasis, ARDS, exacerbation of asthma. **Ovarian hyperstimulation syndrome:** Ovarian enlargement, abdominal pain/distention, N&V, diarrhea, dyspnea, oliguria, ascites, pleural effusion, hypovolemia, electrolyte imbalance, hemoperitoneum, thromboembolic events. **Hypersensitivity:** Febrile reaction, chills, musculoskeletal aches, joint pains, malaise, headache, fatigue. **GI:** N&V, diarrhea, abdominal cramps, bloating. **Dermatologic:** Dry skin, body rash, hair loss, hives. **Miscellaneous:** Ovarian cysts, pain, swelling, headache, irritation at site of injection, breast tenderness.

HOW SUPPLIED
Follitropin alfa: *Injection: FSH activity:* 415 units or more/0.5 mL (to deliver 300 units or more/0.5 mL), 568 units or more/0.75 mL (to deliver 450 units or more/0.75 mL), 1,026 units or more/1.5 mL (to deliver 900 units or more/1.5 mL); *Powder for Injection, Lyophilized: FSH activity:* 82 units (to deliver 75 units), 600 units (to deliver 450 units), 1,200 units (to deliver 1,050 units).

Follitropin beta: *Injection:* 75 units/0.5 mL, 150 units/0.5 mL; *Injection Cartridge for use with Follistim Pen:* 175 units/0.21 mL, 350 units/0.42 mL, 650 units/0.78 mL, 975 units/1.17 mL.

DOSAGE
FOLLITROPIN ALFA
• **SC**
Ovulation induction.

Initial, first cycle: 75 units/day. An incremental adjustment up to 37.5 units may be considered after 14 days; further increases can be made, if needed, every 7 days. To complete follicular development and effect ovulation in absence of an endogenous LH surge, give 5,000 units of hCG 1 day after last dose of follitropin alfa. Withhold hCG if serum estradiol is greater than 2,000 pg/mL. Base initial dose in subsequent cycles on response in the preceding cycle. Doses greater than 300 units/day are not recommended routinely. As in initial cycle, hCG at a dose of 5,000 is given 1 day after last dose of follitropin alfa.

Multifollicular development during assisted reproductive technology.

Initiate on day 2 or 3 of the follicular phase at a dose of 150 units/day, until sufficient follicular development is achieved. Usually, therapy does not exceed 10 days. In those undergoing in vitro fertilization whose endogenous gonadotropin levels are suppressed, initiate follitropin alfa at a dose of 225 units/day. Consider dosage adjustments after 5 days based on client response; adjust subsequent dosage every 3 to 4 days and by no more than 75 to 150 units additional drug at each adjustment, not to exceed 450 international units/day. Once follicular development is achieved, give hCG, 5,000–10,000 units, to cause final follicular maturation in preparation for oocyte retrieval.

Male infertility.

Individualize dose. Give in conjunction with hCG. Prior to therapy with follitropin alfa and hCG, pretreat with hCG alone (1,000–2,250 units 2–3 times per week). Continue treatment until serum testosterone levels are within the normal range (may require 3–6 months); dose of hCG may need to be increased to achieve normal testosterone levels. After normal testosterone levels are reached, give follitropin alfa, 150 units SC 3 times per week with hCG, 1,000 units 3 times per week. Use the lowest dose of follitropin alfa that induces spermatogenesis. If azoospermia persists, may increase dose of follitropin alfa to 300 units 3 times per week; may

need to administer for up to 18 months to achieve adequate spermatogenesis.

FOLLITROPIN BETA

• **IM; SC**

Ovulation induction.

Use stepwise, gradually increasing dosage regimen. **Initial:** 75 international units per day for up to 14 days; increase by 37.5 international units at weekly intervals until follicular growth or serum estradiol levels indicate response. Maximum daily dose: 300 international units. Treat until ultrasonic visualization or serum estradiol levels indicate preovulatory conditions greater than or equal to normal values. Then, give hCG 5,000–10,000 international units.

Multifollicular development during assisted reproductive technology.

Initial: 150–225 international units for first 4 days of treatment. Dose may be adjusted based on ovarian response. Daily maintenance doses from 75–300 international units (however, doses from 375–600 international units have been used) for 6 to 12 days are usually sufficient. Maximum daily dose: 600 international units. When sufficient number of follicles of adequate size are present, induce final maturation by giving hCG, 5,000–10,000 international units. Oocyte retrieval is undertaken 34–36 hr later.

• **INJECTION CARTRIDGE FOR USE WITH FOLLISTIM PEN**

Assisted reproductive technology.

Initial: 150–225 units for the first 5 days; **then**, adjust dose based on response, up to a maximum daily dose of 450 units. *NOTE:* If the health care provider generally uses a starting dose from 150–225 units, a lower starting dose should be considered if using Follistim Pen (See *Administration/Storage*). Also, consider lower maintenance doses. When sufficient numbers of follicles are present, give human chorionic gonadotropin (hCG) at a dose of 5,000–10,000 units for final maturation. If the ovaries are abnormally enlarged on the last day of treatment, withhold hCG.

Ovulation induction.

Initial: 75 units/day for up to 7 days; **then,** increase the dose by 25 or 50 units at weekly intervals until follicular growth and/or serum estradiol levels indicate an adequate ovarian response. **Maximum daily dose:** 175 units. *NOTE:* If a health care provder generally uses a starting dose of 75 units/day, consideration should be given to use a lower starting dose when using cartridges (see *Administration/Storage*). When preovulatory conditions are satisfactory, give hCG, 5,000 to 10,000 units. If the ovaries are abnormally enlarged on the last day of treatment, withhold hCG.

Using Conventional Syringe:	Using Follistim Pen:
75 units	50 units
150 units	125 units
225 units	175 units
300 units	250 units
375 units	300 units
450 units	375 units

NURSING CONSIDERATIONS

ADMINISTRATION/STORAGE

1. For follitropin alfa or beta:
- Store vials in refrigerator or at room temperature and protect from light.
- Use immediately after reconstitution; discard unused drug.

2. For follitropin alfa single-dose ampules, dissolve powder from one or more vials in 0.5–1 mL of sterile water for injection. Concentration should not exceed 225 international units/0.5 mL. For multiple-dose vials, dissolve contents of 1 multi-dose vial (1,200 units) with the contents of 1 prefilled syringe (2 mL) containing bacteriostatic water for injection. Resulting concentration will be 600 units/mL. Product will deliver about 1,050 units of FSH. Clients should use the accompanying syringes callibrated in FSH units (International Units FSH) for administration.

3. For follitropin beta, consider a lower starting dose for gonadotropin stimulation when converting for administration with the Follistim Pen. The difference is due to more accurate dosing possible with the Follistim Pen. Use the following conversion:

4. For follitropin beta, inject 1 mL of 0.45% NaCl injection into the vial. Do not shake but gently swirl until the solution is clear. It usually dissolves immediately.

5. When using either drug, if ovaries are abnormally enlarged on last day of therapy, withhold hCG to reduce risk of ovarian hyperstimulation syndrome.

6. Gonal-f RFF Pen is used to make several days worth of the formulation at one time.

7. Store Gonal-f RFF or Folistim AQ Cartridge from 2–8°C. Clients may keep the pens at 20–25°C for up to one month or from 2–8°C or 20–25°C for up to 28 days after the first injection.

ASSESSMENT

1. Note reasons for therapy, history including GYN (hysterosalpingogram) and endocrine evaluation, indications for therapy, other agents/therapies trialed.

2. Obtain serum hormonal levels, gonadotropin levels, pregnancy test, CBC, electrolytes, thyroid adrenal function studies; document neurovascular assessments, peripheral pulses.

INTERVENTIONS

1. Obtain urinary estrogen excretion levels daily. If >100 mcg or if daily estriol excretion exceeds 50 mcg, *withhold* hCG; signals impending hypersti-mulation syndrome.

2. If hospitalized for hyperstimulation, perform the following:
- Place client on bed rest.
- Monitor I&O; weigh daily.
- Monitor urine specific gravity, serum and urine electrolytes.
- Assess for hemoconcentration. May need heparin to prevent hypercoagulability.

- Increase fluid intake; replace electrolytes.
- Provide analgesics for comfort.

3. Monitor for respiratory distress or exacerbation of asthma. Report unexplained fever, ovarian enlargement, or complaints of abdominal pain.

CLIENT/FAMILY TEACHING

1. Helps to develop eggs in the ovaries in women and produce more sperm in men with a low sperm count. Dose is individualized. Alfa is given SC in the abdomen or upper thigh at 45° angle; beta is given SC or IM with IM administered in upper outer buttocks muscle at 90° angle.

2. May become dizzy. Report pain, coolness, or pale bluish color of an extremity (signs of arterial bloodclot).

3. Fever or development of lower abdominal pain may be result of overstimulation of ovaries that has caused cysts to form, loss of fluid into peritoneum, or bleeding; report immediately. Need exam for this at least every other day during drug therapy and for 2 weeks thereafter; hospitalize if evident.

4. Record temperatures. Signs that indicate ovulation include increase in basal body temperature, and increase in appearance and volume of cervical mucus.

5. Engage in daily intercourse from day before hCG is administered until ovulation occurs.

6. If symptoms indicate overstimulation of ovaries, significant ovarian enlargement may have occurred. Report and abstain from intercourse; ↑ risk of ovarian cyst rupture.

7. Ultrasound is used to monitor for follicular maturation and serum estradiol levels.

8. Pregnancy usually occurs 4–6 weeks after completion of therapy. Multiple births may occur.

OUTCOMES/EVALUATE

- Induction of ovulation
- Pregnancy
- Spermatogenesis

Fondaparinux sodium ■
(**fon**-dah-**PAIR**-in-uks)

CLASSIFICATION(S):
Anticoagulant, antithrombin
PREGNANCY CATEGORY: B
Rx: Arixtra.

USES

(1) Prophylaxis of deep vein thrombosis, which may lead to pulmonary embolism, in clients undergoing hip fracture surgery (including extended prophylaxis), hip replacement surgery, knee replacement surgery, or abdominal surgery in those at risk for thromboembolic complications. May be used for up to 60 days in clients undergoing hip fracture surgery. (2) With warfarin to treat acute DVT. (3) With warfarin to treat acute pulmonary embolism when initial therapy is started in the hospital.

ACTION/KINETICS

Action

Antithrombotic action is due to antithrombin III (ATIII)-mediated selective inhibition of Factor Xa. By selectively binding to ATIII, fondaparinux potentiates the innate neutralization of Factor Xa by ATIII. Neutralization of Factor Xa interrupts the blood coagulation cascade and thus inhibits thrombin formation and thrombus development. Does not inactivate thrombin (activated Factor II), has no known effect on platelet function, and does not affect fibrinolytic activity or bleeding time.

Pharmacokinetics

Rapidly and completely absorbed following SC administration; 100% bioavailable. **Maximum levels:** 2 hr. Excreted unchanged in the urine. **t½, elimination:** 17–21 hr. Elimination is prolonged in the elderly, in those with renal impairment, and in those weighing less than 50 kg. Anticoagulant effect may last for 2–4 days after discontinuation in clients with normal renal function and even longer in those with renal impairment. **Plasma protein binding:** Does not significantly bind to plasma proteins or RBCs.

CONTRAINDICATIONS

IM use. In those with severe renal impairment (C_{CR} <30 mL/min) or with body weight <50 kg needing prophylactic therapy and undergoing hip-fracture or knee-replacement surgery (due to increased risk for major bleeding episodes). In those with active major bleeding, bacterial endocarditis, thrombocytopenia associated with a positive *in vitro* test for antiplatelet antibody in the presence of fondaparinux, or with known sensitivity to fondaparinux.

SPECIAL CONCERNS

■ (1) When epidural/spinal anesthesia is used, clients anticoagulated or scheduled to be anticoagulated with low molecular weight heparins, heparinoids, or fondaparinux for prevention of thromboembolic complications are at risk of developing an epidural or spinal hematoma that can cause long-term or permanent paralysis. The risk of such events is increased by the use of indwelling epidural catheters for administration of analgesia or by the concomitant use of drugs affecting hemostasis, such as NSAIDs, platelet inhibitors, or other anticoagulants. The risk also seems to be increased by traumatic or repeated epidural or spinal puncture. (2) Frequently monitor clients for signs and symptoms of neurologic impairment. If neurologic compromise is noted, urgent treatment is necessary. (3) Consider the potential benefit vs risk before neuraxial intervention in clients anticoagulated or to be anticoagulated for thromboprophylaxis. (4) Fondaparinux, like other anticoagulants should be used with extreme caution in conditions with increased risk of hemorrhage, such as congenital or acquired bleeding disorders, active ulcerative and angiodysplastic GI disease, hemorrhagic stroke, or shortly after brain, spinal, or ophthalmological surgery, or in those treated concomitantly with platelet inhibitors.■ The risk of hemorrhage increases with increasing renal impairment. Use with caution during lactation, in moderate renal impairment (C_{CR} 30–50 mL/min), in the elderly, in those with a history of heparin-induced thrombocytopenia, in those with a bleeding diathesis, uncontrolled arterial hypertension, history of recent GI ulceration, diabetic retinopathy, and hemorrhage. Use with extreme caution in conditions with increased risk of hemorrhage, including congenital or acquired bleeding disorders, active ulcerative and angiodysplastic GI disease, hemorrhagic stroke, in those treated concomitantly with platelet inhibitors, or shortly after brain, spinal, or ophthalmologic surgery. Safety and efficacy have not been determined in children.

SIDE EFFECTS

Most Common

Bleeding complications (see below), hypotension, confusion, dizziness, insomnia, constipation, headache, N&V, UTI, anemia, purpura, rash, edema, fever. The most common side effect is **bleeding complications (hemorrhage)** which include intracranial, cerebral, retroperitoneal, intra-ocular, pericardial, or spinal bleeding, bleeding in the adrenal gland, or reoperation due to bleeding. **CV:** Edema, hypotension. **GI:** N&V, constipation, diarrhea, dyspepsia, abdominal pain. **CNS:** Insomnia, dizziness, confusion, headache, anxiety. **GU:** UTI, urinary retention. **Dermatologic:** Rash, bullous eruption, pruritus, bruising. **Respiratory:** Coughing, epistaxis. **Hematologic:** Anemia, hematoma, purpura, *postoperative hemorrhage*. **Miscellaneous:** Thrombocytopenia, injection site bleeding, anemia, fever, increased wound drainage, pain, back/chest/leg pain, abnormal hepatic function.

LABORATORY TEST CONSIDERATIONS

↑ AST, ALT, hepatic enzymes. ↓ Prothrombin. Hypokalemia.

OD **OVERDOSE MANAGEMENT**

Symptoms: Hemorrhagic complications. *Treatment:* Discontinue treatment. There is no known antidote. Initiate appropriate therapy. Clearance can increase by 20% during hemodialysis.

DRUG INTERACTIONS

Increased risk of hemorrhage if used with agents that enhance the risk of hemorrhage; discontinue such agents or if co-administration is essential, monitor closely.

HOW SUPPLIED

Injection: 2.5 mg/0.5 mL, 5 mg/0.4 mL, 7.5 mg/0.6 mL, 10 mg/0.8 mL.

DOSAGE

- **SC**

Prophylaxis of DVT in hip fracture, hip or knee replacement surgery.

Adults, initial: 2.5 mg given 6–8 hr after surgery. Administration before 6 hr after surgery has been associated with an increased risk of major bleeding. **Duration:** Give 2.5 mg once daily for 5–9 days (up to 11 days has been tolerated).

Treatment of acute DVT without pulmonary embolism; acute pulmonary embolism.

Adults: 5 mg/day for clients weighing less than 50 kg, 7.5 mg for those weighing 50–100 kg, and 10 mg for those over 100 kg. Continue therapy for at least 5 days and until an INR of 2.0–3.0 is achieved with warfarin sodium.

Abdominal surgery in those at risk for thromboembolic complications.

Adults: 2.5 mg once daily for 5–9 days, with the first dose given 6–8 hr after surgery, once hemostasis has been established. Can be given for up to 10 days.

NURSING CONSIDERATIONS

ADMINISTRATION/STORAGE

1. Stop therapy if major bleeding occurs or coagulation indicators change unexpectedly.

2. Drug provided in single dose, prefilled syringe affixed with an automatic needle protection system.

3. Can not be used interchangeably (unit for unit) with heparin, low molecular weight heparins, or heparinoids; products differ in manufacturing process, anti-Xa and anti-IIa activity, units, and dosage.

4. To avoid loss of drug with the prefilled syringe, do not expel the air bubble from the syringe before injection.

5. Do not mix with other injections or infusions.

6. Give in the fatty tissue, alternating injection sites (i.e., between the left and right anterolateral or the left and right posterolateral abdominal wall).

7. Store between 15–30°C (59–86°F). Keep out of the reach of children.

ASSESSMENT

1. Note condition(s) requiring therapy, onset, estimated duration of therapy.

2. Assess for conditions that may affect therapy (i.e. age, weight, history of GI ulcerations, diabetic retinopathy, uncontrolled HTN, bleeding diathesis/disorders, hemorrhage, hemorrhagic stroke, or shortly after brain, spinal or eye surgery or in those treated concomitantly with platelet inhibitors. Risk of hemorrhage increases with increasing renal impairment or heparin induced thrombocytopenia.

3. Monitor all sites, incisions, orifices for bleeding. Assess mobility and adherence to exercise program.

4. Assess carefully for S&S of neurologic impairment; anticoagulated clients undergoing epidural/spinal anesthesia may sustain a spinal/epidural hematoma which could result in paralysis.

5. Monitor CBC, creatinine, K$^+$, renal, LFTs and stool for occult blood.

CLIENT/FAMILY TEACHING

1. Drug is used to prevent the formation of blood clots in those extremities that have compromised functioning due to a surgical procedure. Clots may enter the circulation and be transported to the lung causing a pulmonary embolus which can be lethal.

2. Review guidelines for SC administration and demonstrate. Start with proper skin prep, pinching and holding a fold of skin for the injection, injecting the solution, removing the syringe, and discarding into a designated container. The syringe has a retractable needle to prevent punctures. Rotate sites to prevent hardening of the tissues between the right and left anterolateral/posterolateral abdominal wall).

3. Store prefilled syringes and used syringes safely out of reach and dispose of properly.

4. Report adverse effects as well as extremity pain, chest pain, SOB, bleeding, or other unusual symptoms.

Bold Italic = life threatening side effect   ■ = black box warning   ♣ = Available in Canada

5. Avoid OTC agents including aspirin, NSAIDs and other agents without provider approval. Keep all F/U visits to evaluate incision site, response to therapy, recovery, and labs.

OUTCOMES/EVALUATE

DVT(blood clot) prevention in those undergoing hip fracture repair or hip/knee replacements or abdominal surgery where mobility is impaired

Formoterol fumarate ■

(for-**MOH**-tur-all)

CLASSIFICATION(S):
Sympathomimetic, direct-acting
PREGNANCY CATEGORY: C
Rx: Foradil Aerolizer, Perforomist.

SEE ALSO *SYMPATHOMIMETICS.*

USES

Inhalation Powder in Capsules: (1) Long-term maintenance treatment of asthma and to prevent bronchospasms in adults and children 5 years of age and older who have reversible obstructive airway disease, including nocturnal asthma, who require regular treatment with inhaled, short-acting, beta$_2$-agonists. Not to be used in those whose asthma can be managed successfully by inhaled corticosteroids or other medications along with occasional use of inhaled, short-acting beta$_2$-agonists. (2) Acute prevention of exercise-induced bronchospasm in adults and children 5 years of age and older. Used on an occasional, as needed, basis.

Inhalation Powder or Solution: Long-term use in the maintenance treatment of bronchoconstriction in those with COPD, including chronic bronchitis and emphysema.

ACTION/KINETICS

Action

Long-acting selective beta$_2$-agonist. Acts locally in the lung as a bronchodilator. Acts in part by increasing cyclic AMP levels causing relaxation of bronchial smooth muscle and inhibition of release of mediators of immediate hypersensitivity, especially from mast cells.

Pharmacokinetics

When inhaled, is rapidly absorbed into the plasma reaching maximum plasma levels within 5 min. Metabolized in the liver to inactive metabolites. Excreted in the urine and feces. **t½ terminal:** 10 hr. **Plasma protein binding:** 61–64%.

CONTRAINDICATIONS

Use for those whose asthma can be controlled by occasional use of inhaled, short-acting, beta$_2$-agonists. Use to treat acute symptoms of asthma.

SPECIAL CONCERNS

■ Long-acting beta$_2$-adrenergic agonists may increase the risk of asthma-related death. Therefore, when treating clients with asthma, only use formoterol as additional therapy for clients not adequately controlled on other asthma-controller medications (e.g., low-to-medium dose inhaled corticosteroids) or whose disease severity clearly warrants initiation of treatment with two maintenance therapies, including formoterol. Data from studies that compared the safety of another long-acting beta$_2$-adrenergic agonist (salmeterol) or placebo added to usual asthma therapy showed an increased in asthma-related deaths in clients receiving salmeterol. This finding with salmeterol may apply to formoterol (a long-acting beta$_2$-adrenergic agonist).■ May cause life-threatening, paradoxical bronchospasms. Use with extreme caution in clients treated with MAO inhibitors, tricyclic antidepressants, or drugs known to prolong the QTc interval (effect of adrenergic agonists may be prolonged). Use with caution during the co-administration of beta-agonists with nonpotassium-sparing diuretics (loop or thiazide diuretics) since ECG changes and/or hypokalemia can be acutely worsened by beta-agonists. Use with caution in CV disorders (especially coronary insufficiency, cardiac arrhythmias, and hypertension), in convulsive disorders, in thyrotoxicosis, in those unusually responsive to sympathomimetics, and during lactation.

F

SIDE EFFECTS

Most Common

Viral infection, bronchitis, chest infection/pain, dyspnea, tremor, dizziness, dry mouth, insomnia.

See also *Sympathomimetics* for a complete list of possible side effects. Also, **CV:** Increased pulse rate and BP, ECG changes (e.g., flattening of T wave, prolongation of QTc interval, and ST segment depression). **Body as a whole:** Immediate hypersensitivity reactions, including severe hypotension, *anaphylaxis*, and angioedema. Viral infection, fever, trauma. **Respiratory:** Worsening of asthma, bronchitis, chest infection, dyspnea, chest pain, tonsilitis, URTI, pharyngitis, sinusitis, increased sputum. **CNS:** Dizziness, insomnia, anxiety. **Musculoskeletal:** Back pain, leg/muscle cramps. **Miscellaneous:** Tremor, rash, dysphonia, pruritis, dry mouth.

LABORATORY TEST CONSIDERATIONS

Hypokalemia (transient and usually does not require supplementation).

HOW SUPPLIED

Foradil: Powder in Capsules for use in Aerolizer: 12 mcg; **Perforomist:** Inhalation Solution: 20 mcg/2 mL.

DOSAGE

Foradil Aerolizer

• **CAPSULES FOR USE IN AEROLIZER**
  Maintenance treatment of asthma and to prevent bronchospasm.

Adults and children over 5 years: Inhale contents of one 12 mcg-capsule q 12 hr (morning and evening) using the Aerolizer inhaler. Do not exceed 24 mcg/day. If symptoms appear between doses, use an inhaled short-acting beta$_2$-agonist for immediate relief.
  Prevention of exercise-induced bronchospasm.

Adults and adolescents 12 years and older: Inhale contents of one 12-mcg capsule at least 15 min before exercise. Give on an occasional, as needed, basis. When used for prevention, protection may last up to 12 hr; do not use additional doses for 12 hr.
  Maintenance treatment of COPD.

Inhale contents of one 12-mcg capsule q 12 hr (morning and evening) using the Aerolizer inhaler. Do not exceed 24 mcg/day.

Perforomist Inhalation Solution

• **INHALATION SOLUTION**
  Maintenance treatment of COPD, including chronic bronchitis and emphysema.

20 mcg given twice daily (morning and evening) by nebulization, not to exceed 40 mcg/day.

NURSING CONSIDERATIONS

ADMINISTRATION/STORAGE

1. Use only with Aerolizer inhaler, do not take orally.

2. Can be used together with short-acting beta$_2$-agonists, inhaled or systemic corticosteroids, and theophylline.

3. If asthma symptoms arise between doses, an inhaled short-acting, beta$_2$-agonist may be used for immediate relief.

4. If a previously used dose for asthma or COPD does not result in the usual response, seek medical advice immediately; this is often a sign of deteriorating asthma or COPD. Re-evaluate therapeutic regimen and consider additional options such as systemic corticosteroids.

5. If taking formoterol in twice-daily doses for asthma, do not take additional doses for exercise-induced bronchospasms.

6. A satisfactory response to formoterol does not eliminate the need for continued treatment with an anti-inflammatory drug.

7. Do not start formoterol therapy in clients with significantly worsening or acutely deteriorating asthma, which may be a life-threatening condition.

8. Formoterol is not a substitute for inhaled or oral corticosteroids.

9. When starting formoterol therapy, instruct clients who have been taking inhaled, short-acting beta$_2$-agonists on a regular basis (4 times/day) to discontinue the regular use of these drugs and use only for symptomatic relief of acute asthma symptoms.

10. Do not swallow orally. Store in the blister and remove immediately before use.

Bold Italic = life threatening side effect   ■ = black box warning   ♣ = Available in Canada

11. Before dispensing, store at 2–8°C (36–46°F). After dispensing, store at 20–25°C (68–77°F). Protect from heat and moisture.

ASSESSMENT

1. List reasons for therapy, symptom characteristics, PFT results, other agents trialed, outcome.
2. Assess for CAD, seizures, and HTN.
3. Monitor VS, electrolytes, PFTs, CXR, and lung sounds.

CLIENT/FAMILY TEACHING

1. Use only as directed, do not take orally. Demonstrate appropriate method for administration and storage. Review *Patient Use Instructions*.
2. Use the capsules only with the Aerolizer inhaler provided. Do not use Aerolizer inhaler with any other capsules. Do not exceed dosage of 2 capsules per day. Capsules must be punctured by Aerolizer inhaler in order to release powder. Always store capsules in the blister package and remove from the blister immediately before use.
3. Administer the inhalation solution by the orally inhaled route via a standard jet nebulizer connected to an air compressor.
4. If symptoms of asthma arise between doses, an inhaled short-acting, beta$_2$-agonist may be used for immediate relief.
5. If a previously used dose for asthma or COPD does not result in the usual response, seek medical advice immediately as this is often a sign of deteriorating asthma or COPD. Use incentive spirometer to monitor breathing status. Not for use with marked reduction in spirometry readings or acute worsening of asthma condition.
6. Clients taking formoterol in twice-daily doses for asthma should not take additional doses for exercise-induced bronchospasms.
7. With exercise-induced asthma, use 15 min before exercise.
8. Do not expose capsules to moisture; handle with dry hands. Do not wet or wash the Aerolizer inhaler; keep dry. Always use the new Aerolizer inhaler with each refill.

9. Do not use Aerolizer inhaler with a spacer and never exhale into the Aerolizer inhaler.
10. Store capsules as directed and only pierce once. If gelatin capsule breaks, the screen in the Aerolizer inhaler should retain it. Be aware that it may escape into the mouth or throat after inhalation.
11. Practice reliable contraception, report if pregnancy suspected.
12. Report any unusual side effects, loss of control of breathing patterns or intolerance to therapy. Keep F/U appointments to evaluate drug effects and prevent deterioration of lung function.
13. Store the inhalation solution in the foil pouch and only remove immediately before use. Discard the contents of any partially used container.

OUTCOMES/EVALUATE

Improved breathing patterns, ↓ bronchospasms

Fosamprenavir calcium

(fos-am-**PREN**-ah-veer)

CLASSIFICATION(S):

Antiretroviral agent, protease inhibitor

PREGNANCY CATEGORY: C

Rx: Lexiva.

USES

In combination with other antiretroviral drugs to treat HIV infection in adults.

ACTION/KINETICS

Action

Fosamprenavir is a prodrug of amprenavir which is a HIV-1 protease inhibitor. Fosamprenavir is rapidly converted to amprenavir and inorganic phosphate by cellular phosphatases in the gut epithelium. Amprenavir binds to the active site of HIV-1 protease, thus preventing the processing of viral Gag and Gag-Pol polyprotein precursors; this results in formation of immature noninfectious viral particles.

Pharmacokinetics
Time to peak amprenavir levels:
1.5–4 hr. Food does not affect the C_{max}, T_{max}, or AUC of the tablets. However there is a reduction in the C_{max}, T_{max}, and AUC if the oral suspension is taken with a high-fat meal. Amprenavir is rapidly and almost completely metabolized in the liver by the CYP3A4 enzyme system. Metabolites are excreted in both the urine (14%) and feces (75%). **Plasma $t\frac{1}{2}$, elimination of amprenavir:** About 7.7 hr. **Plasma protein binding:** About 90%.

CONTRAINDICATIONS
Hypersensitivity to the drug or any component of the product or to amprenavir. Coadministration with dihydroergotamine, ergotamine, ergonovine, methylergonovine, midazolam, pimozide, or triazolam. Fosamprenavir with ritonavir coadministered with either flecainide or propafenone. Lactation.

SPECIAL CONCERNS
Select doses carefully in geriatric clients. Use with caution in those with impaired hepatic function and in those with known sulfonoamide allergy (due to possible cross-sensitivity). If used with ritonavir at doses higher than recommended, elevations in serum transaminase may occur. Safety and efficacy have not been determined in children less than 2 years of age.

SIDE EFFECTS
Most Common
N&V, diarrhea, abdominal pain, headache, fatigue, redistribution of body fat, symptoms of hyperglycemia.
GI: Diarrhea, N&V, abdominal pain. Worsening of transaminase elevations if those with hepatitis B or C. **CNS:** Headache, fatigue, depressive mood disorders, oral paresthesia. **Hematologic:** *Acute hemolytic anemia*, neutropenia, spontaneous bleeding in hemophilia A and B clients treated with protease inhibitors. **Dermatologic:** Severe or *life-threatening skin reactions*, including mild or moderate maculopapular rashes, some with pruritus, and ***Stevens-Johnson syndrome***. **Metabolic:** New-onset diabetes mellitus, exacerbation of preexisting diabetes mellitus, di-

abetic ketoacidosis, hyperglycemia. Redistribution of body fat, including central obesity, dorsocervical fat enlargement (buffalo hump), peripheral/facial wasting, breast enlargement, and 'cushingoid' appearance. **Miscellaneous:** Development of opportunistic infections including those due to *Mycobacterium avium* complex, cytomegalovirus, *Pneumocystis carinii*, and tuberculosis. Immune reconstitution syndrome.

LABORATORY TEST CONSIDERATIONS
↑ Triglycerides, serum lipase, ALT, AST. ↓ Neutrophils. Hyperglycemia.

DRUG INTERACTIONS
Amprenavir, the active form of fosamprenavir, is metabolized by CYP3A4 enzyme system and is an inhibitor (and possible inducer) of CYP3A4. Coadministration of fosamprenavir and drugs that induce CYP3A4 may decrease amprenavir levels and decrease efficacy. Coadministration of amprenavir and drugs that inhibit CYP3A4 may increase amprenavir levels and increase the incidence of side effects. Also, the potential for drug interactions changes when fosamprenavir is given with ritonavir, a potent CYP3A4 inhibitor. Because ritonavir is also a CYP2D6 inhibitor, significant interactions may occur when fosamprenavir plus ritonavir are given with drugs metabolized by CYP2D6.
Amiodarone / Possible serious/life-threatening reactions (e.g., cardiac arrhythmias); give together with caution
Amiodarine plus ritonavir / Possible ↑ amiodarone plasma levels → serious and/or life-threatening reactions, including cardiac arrhythmias when the three are given together
Amitriptyline / Monitor therapeutic levels of amitriptyline
Antacids / ↓ Amprenavir C_{max} and AUC
Benzodiazepines (alprazolam, clorazepate, diazepam, flurazepam, midazolam, triazolam) / Do not use together R/T possible serious/life-threatening reactions, such as prolonged or increased sedation/respiratory depression
Bepridil plus ritonavir / Possible ↑ bepridil plasma levels → serious and/or life-threatening reactions, including cardiac arrhythmias when the three are

---

Bold Italic = life threatening side effect ■ = black box warning ✤ = Available in Canada

given together

Calcium channel blockers (e.g., amlodipine, diltiazem, felodipine, nifedipine, verapamil) / Possible ↑ levels of CCBs; use together with caution and monitor

Carbamazepine / ↑ Carbamazepine levels → ↑ risk of toxicity

Corticosteroids (e.g., nasal fluticasone, oral prednisone) / Possible inhibition of corticosteroid metabolism by CYP3A4 → ↑ risk of toxicity; do not give fluticasone together with fosamprenavir and ritonavir unless benefits outweigh risks

Cyclosporine / Monitor therapeutic levels of cyclosporine as toxicity may occur

CYP4503A4 inhibitors (e.g., clarithromycin) / Possible ↑ amprenavir plasma levels; use together with caution

Delavirdine / Possible loss of virologic response and resistance to fosamprenavir/other protease inhibitors

Dexamethasone / Possible loss of virologic response and resistance to fosamprenavir/other protease inhibitors

Efavirenz / ↓ Fosamprenavir levels if given with/without ritonavir

Efavirenz plus ritonavir / ↑ Amprenavir C_{max} and AUC if fosamprenavir is also given with ritonavir; give an additional 100 mg/day of ritonavir

Ergot derivatives (e.g., dihydroergotamine, ergonovine, ergotamine, methylergonovine) / Do not use together R/T potential for serious/life-threatening reactions, such as acute ergot toxicity (peripheral vasospasm, ischemia of the extremities)

Esomeprazole / Possible ↑ esomeprazole plasma levels

Flecainide plus ritonavir / Possible ↑ plasma levels of flecainide if given with fosamprenavir and ritonavir → serious and/or life-threatening cardiac arrhythmias

Fluconazole / Possible ↑ fluconazole side effects; dosage may need to be reduced

Histamine H_2-receptor antagonists / Possible decreased virologic response and resistance to fosamprenavir/other protease inhibitors

HMG-CoA reductase inhibitors / Possible ↑ serum levels of HMG-CoA reductase inhibitors → ↑ toxicity, including myopathy and rhabdomyolysis; also ↓ amprenavir C_{max} and AUC

Imipramine / Monitor therapeutic levels of imipramine

Indinavir / ↑ Amprenavir levels; possible ↓ indinavir levels

Itraconazole / Possible ↑ itraconazole side effects; dosage reduction may be needed; possible ↑ amprenavir plasma levels → ↑ risk of toxicity

Ketoconazole / Possible ↑ ketoconazole side effects; may require dosage reduction; possible ↑ amprenavir plasma levels → ↑ risk of toxicity

Lidocaine (systemic) / Possible serious/life-threatening reactions (e.g., cardiac arrhythmias); give together with caution

Lidocaine plus ritonavir / Possible ↑ lidocaine plasma levels → serious and/or life-threatening reactions, including cardiac arrhythmias when the three are given together

Lopinavir plus ritonavir / ↓ Amprenavir C_{max} and AUC if also given with ritonavir; ↑ lopinavir C_{max} and AUC

Methadone / Possible need to ↑ methadone dose; also, ↓ amprenavir C_{max}, AUC, and C_{min}; may need to ↑ methadone dosage

Narcotic analgesics (e.g., alfentanil, buprenorphine, fentanyl sufentanil)/ Possible ↑ narcotic analgesic plasma levels and $t^{1}/_{2}$ → ↑ risk of toxicity

Nelfinavir / ↑ Amprenavir levels

Nevirapine / ↓ Amprenavir levels; possible ↑ nevirapine plasma levels; do not give nevirapine and fosamprenavir without ritonavir

Oral contraceptives (ethinyl estradiol, norethindrone) / Possible alteration of hormonal levels; use nonhormonal contraceptive methods; also, possible ↓ amprenavir AUC and ↑ transaminase elevations

Paroxetine / Significant ↓ paroxetine plasma levels when given with fosamprenavir and ritonavir

Phenobarbital / Possible loss of virologic response and resistance to fosamprenavir and/or other protease inhibitors R/T ↓ amprenavir plasma levels

Phenytoin / Possible loss of virologic response and resistance to fosamprenavir/other protease inhibitors R/T ↓ amprenavir plasma levels

Pimozide / Do not use together; possible serious and/or life-threatening reactions, including cardiac arrhythmias

Propafenone plus ritonavir / Possible ↑ propafenone plasma levels → serious and/or life-threatening reactions, including cardiac arrhythmias when the three are given together

Proton pump inhibitors / Possible loss of virologic response and resistance to fosamprenavir/other protease inhibitors

Quinidine plus ritonavir / Possible serious/life-threatening reactions (e.g., cardiac arrhythmias) when the three are given together

Ranitidine / ↓ Amprenavir C_{max} and AUC

Ranolazine / Possible ↑ Ranolazine plasma levels → ↑ risk of dose-related prolongation of the QTc interval, torsades de pointes-type arrhythmias and sudden death

Rifabutin / Monitor weekly for neutropenia; reduce dose by at least one-half when given with fosamprenavir or three-fourths if given with both fosamprenavir and ritonavir

Rifampin / Possible loss of virologic response and resistance to fosamprenavir/other protease inhibitors

Saquinavir / ↓ Amprenavir levels

Sildenafil / ↑ Sildenafil plasma levels → ↑ risk of side effects; ↓ sildenafil dose to 25 mg q 48 hr and monitor for side effects

H   *St. John's wort* / Possible loss of virologic response and resistance R/T ↑ fosamprenavir hepatic metabolism by CYP3A4 enzymes

Tacrolimus / Monitor therapeutic levels of tacrolimus as toxicity may occur

Tadalafil / ↑ Tadalafil plasma levels → ↑ side effects; ↓ tadalafil dose to no more than 10 mg q 72 hr

Trazodone / ↑ Trazodone plasma levels → ↑ pharmacologic and side effects when given with fosamprenavir alone or with fosamprenavir and ritonavir; decrease trazodone dose

Tricyclic antidepressants (e.g., amitriptyline, imipramine) / Serious and/or life-threatening reactions possible; monitor TCA plasma levels

Vardenafil / ↑ Vardenafil plasma levels → ↑ side effects; ↓ vardenafil dose to 2.5 mg q 24 hr; if given with fosamprenavir and ritonavir, ↓ vardenafil dose to no more than 2.5 mg q 72 hr

Warfarin / Levels of warfarin may be affected; monitor INR

Zidovudine / Possible ↑ in levels of both amprenavir and zidovudine

HOW SUPPLIED

Oral Suspension: 50 mg/mL (equivalent to 43 mg amprenavir); *Tablets:* 700 mg (equivalent to 600 mg amprenavir).

DOSAGE

• ORAL SUSPENSION; TABLETS

HIV infections, therapy-naive clients.

Adults: Fosamprenavir, 1,400 mg twice a day (without ritonavir); or, fosamprenavir, 1,400 mg once daily plus ritonavir, 200 mg once daily; or, fosamprenavir, 700 mg twice a day plus ritonavir, 100 mg once a day; or, fosamprenavir, 700 mg twice daily plus ritonavir, 100 mg twice daily.

HIV infections, protease inhibitor-experienced clients.

Adults: Fosamprenavir, 700 mg twice a day plus ritonavir, 100 mg twice a day. Once daily fosamprenavir and ritonavir is not recommended.

HIV infections, concomitant therapy with efavirenz.

Adults: An additional 100 mg/day (i.e., 300 mg total) of ritonavir is recommended when efavirenz is given with fosamprenavir plus ritonavir once daily.

HIV infections, children, 2 to 18 years of age.

Children, 2–5 years of age, therapy-naive: 30 mg/kg of the PO suspension twice daily, not to exceed the adult dose of 1,400 mg twice daily.

Children, 6 years and older, therapy-naive: 30 mg/kg of the PO suspension twice daily, not to exceed the adult dose of 1,400 mg twice daily; or, 18 mg/kg of the PO suspension plus ritonavir, 3 mg/kg twice daily, not to exceed the adult dose of 700 mg plus ritonavir, 100 mg twice daily.

Children, 2–5 years of age, therapy-experienced: Data are insufficient to recommend any dosing regimen.

Bold Italic = life threatening side effect   ■ = black box warning   ✤ = Available in Canada

Children, 6 years and older, therapy-experienced: 18 mg/kg of the PO suspension plus ritonavir, 3 mg/kg twice daily, not to exceed the adult dose of fosamprenavir, 700 mg twice daily plus ritonavir, 100 mg twice daily. When given without ritonavir, the adult regimen of the tablets, 1,400 mg twice daily may be used for children weighing at least 47 kg. When given with ritonavir, the tablets may be used for children weighing at least 39 kg; ritonavir capsules may be used for children weighing at least 33 kg.

NURSING CONSIDERATIONS
ADMINISTRATION/STORAGE
1. Use the following guidelines for use of fosamprenavir in clients with hepatic impairment:
- **For mild hepatic impairment (Child-Pugh score from 5 to 6):** Reduce dosage of fosamprenavir to 700 mg twice daily without ritonavir or 700 mg twice daily plus ritonavir, 100 mg once daily in therapy-naive or protease inhibitor-experienced clients.
- **For moderate hepatic impairment (Child-Pugh score from 7 to 9):** Reduce dosage of fosamprenavir to 700 mg twice daily without ritonavir or 450 mg twice daily plus ritonavir, 100 mg once daily in therapy-naive or protease inhibitor-experienced clients.
- **For severe hepatic impairment (Child-Pugh score from 10 to 12):** Reduce dosage of fosamprenavir to 350 mg twice daily without ritonavir. There are no data on the use of fosamprenavir in combination with ritonavir in those with severe hepatic impairment.
2. Store tablets from 15–30°C (59–86°F) and the oral suspension from 5–30°C (40–86°F).
ASSESSMENT
1. Note disease onset, characteristics of S&S, other agents trialed, outcome. List drugs prescribed to ensure none interact.
2. List sulfa allergy; precludes drug therapy.

3. Monitor HIV RNA, renal and LFTs; reduce dose with liver dysfunction.
CLIENT/FAMILY TEACHING
1. Works by blocking protease, a protein that HIV needs to make more copies of itself.
2. Take tablets as directed with or without food and with other antiretroviral therapy; always used in combination therapy. Do not double or change dose; if dose missed take when remembered. Adults should take the oral suspension should be taken without food while children should take the oral suspension with food. If emesis occurs within 30 min after dosing, redose the fosamprenavir oral suspension.
3. Do not take any unprescribed or OTC medications/herbals without approval due to potential for adverse interactions.
4. May experience a change in body fat distribution/accumulation, high cholesterol, increased bleeding in those with hemophilia, high blood sugar levels, and onset or worsening of diabetes.
5. Use nonhormonal contraception; drug may alter hormone levels. Does not prevent disease transmission or STDs; practice safe sex.
6. Report any unusual rash or side effects. May continue to experience opportunistic infections. Long term drug effects are unknown.
OUTCOMES/EVALUATE
↓ HIV RNA

Foscarnet sodium ■ IV
(fos-**KAR**-net)

CLASSIFICATION(S):
Antiviral
PREGNANCY CATEGORY: C
Rx: Foscavir.

SEE ALSO *ANTIVIRAL AGENTS.*

USES
(1) Treatment of CMV retinitis in clients with AIDS. (2) Treatment of acyclovir-resistant HSV infections in immunocompromised clients. (3) With ganciclovir in

those who have relapsed after monotherapy with either drug.

ACTION/KINETICS

Action

Inhibits replication of all known herpes viruses by selective inhibition at the pyrophosphate binding site on virus-specific DNA polymerases and reverse transcriptases at levels that do not affect cellular DNA polymerases. Active against herpes simplex virus mutants deficient in thymidine kinase. CMV strains resistant to ganciclovir may be sensitive to foscarnet; viral reactivation of CMV occurs after termination of foscarnet therapy. The latent state of any of the human herpes viruses is not sensitive to foscarnet.

Pharmacokinetics

Believed to accumulate in human bone and has variable penetration into the CSF. **t½, plasma:** About 3 hr. Approximately 80–90% of IV foscarnet is excreted unchanged through the urine.

SPECIAL CONCERNS

■ (1) Renal impairment is the major toxicity. Continually assess client risk, frequently monitor serum creatinine with dose adjustment for changes in renal function. Ensure adequate hydration when drug is administered. (2) Seizures, related to alterations in plasma minerals and electrolytes, have been associated with foscarnet. Carefully monitor clients for such changes and their potential sequelae. Mineral and electrolyte supplementation may be required. (3) Foscarnet is indicated only for use in immunocompromised clients with CMV retinitis and mucocutaneous acyclovir-resistant HSV infections. ■ Use with caution during lactation and in clients with impaired renal function (the effects of the drug have not been determined in clients with a C_{CR} <50 mL/min or serum creatinine >2.8 mg/dL). Use with caution with drugs that alter serum calcium levels as foscarnet decreases serum levels of ionized calcium. Safety and effectiveness have not been determined in children, for the treatment of other CMV infections such as pneumonitis or gastroenteritis, for congenital or neonatal CMV disease, and in nonimmuno-

compromised clients. Transient changes in electrolytes may increase the risk of cardiac disturbances and seizures. Side effects such as renal impairment, electrolyte abnormalities, and seizures may contribute to client death. The drug is not a cure for HSV infections and relapse occurs in most clients. Repeated treatment has led to the development of viral resistance.

SIDE EFFECTS

Most Common

Fever, N&V, anemia, diarrhea, abnormal renal function, headache, seizures.

GU: Renal impairment (most common), albuminuria, dysuria, polyuria, urinary retention, urethral disorder, UTIs, *acute renal failure*, nocturia, hematuria, glomerulonephritis, urinary frequency, toxic nephropathy, nephrosis, urinary incontinence, pyelonephritis, renal tubular disorders, urethral irritation, uremia, perineal pain in women, penile inflammation. **Metabolic/Electrolyte:** Hypocalcemia, hypokalemia, hypomagnesemia, hypophosphatemia, hyponatremia, hyperphosphatemia, hypercalcemia, acidosis, thirst, decreased weight, dehydration, glycosuria, diabetes mellitus, abnormal glucose tolerance, hypochloremia, hypervolemia, hypoproteinemia. **Hematologic:** Anemia (one-third of clients), granulocytopenia, neutropenia, leukopenia, thrombocytopenia, platelet abnormalities, thrombosis, WBC abnormalities, lymphadenopathy, coagulation disorders, decreased coagulation factors, decreased prothrombin, hypochromic anemia, pancytopenia, hemolysis, leukocytosis, cervical lymphadenopathy, lymphopenia. **Body as a whole:** Fever, fatigue, asthenia, pain, infection, rigors, malaise, sepsis, death, back or chest pain, cachexia, flu-like symptoms, edema, bacterial or fungal infections, abscess, moniliasis, leg edema, peripheral edema, hypothermia, syncope, substernal chest pain, ascites, *malignant hyperpyrexia*, herpes simplex, viral infections, toxoplasmosis. **CNS:** Headache, dizziness, *seizures (including tonic-clonic)*, tremor, ataxia, dementia, stupor, meningitis, aphasia, abnormal coordination, EEG abnormali-

---

Bold Italic = life threatening side effect   ■ = black box warning   ✦ = Available in Canada

ties, vertigo, coma, encephalopathy, dyskinesia, extrapyramidal disorders, hemiparesis, paraplegia, speech disorders, tetany, cerebral edema, depression, confusion, anxiety, insomnia, somnolence, amnesia, aggressive reaction, nervousness, agitation, hallucinations, impaired concentration, emotional lability, psychosis, *suicide attempt*, delirium, sleep disorders, personality disorders. **Peripheral nervous system:** Hypesthesia, neuropathy, sensory disturbances, generalized spasms, abnormal gait, hyperesthesia, hypertonia, hyperkinesia, vocal cord paralysis, hyporeflexia, hyperreflexia, neuralgia, neuritis, peripheral neuropathy. **Musculoskeletal:** Arthralgia, myalgia, involuntary muscle contractions, leg cramps, arthrosis, synovitis, torticollis. **GI:** N&V, diarrhea, anorexia, abdominal pain, dry mouth, dysphagia, dyspepsia, rectal hemorrhage, constipation, melena, flatulence, pancreatitis, ulcerative stomatitis, enteritis, glossitis, enterocolitis, proctitis, stomatitis, tenesmus, pseudomembranous colitis, gastroenteritis, oral leukoplakia, oral hemorrhage, rectal disorders, colitis, duodenal ulcer, hematemesis, paralytic ileus, ulcerative proctitis, tongue ulceration, esophageal ulceration. **Hepatic:** Abnormal hepatic function, cholecystitis, cholelithiasis, hepatitis, hepatosplenomegaly, cholestatic hepatitis, jaundice. **CV:** Hypertension, palpitations, sinus tachycardia, first degree AV block, nonspecific ST-T segment changes, hypotension, flushing, cerebrovascular disorder, *cardiomyopathy, cardiac failure, cardiac arrest*, bradycardia, arrhythmias, extrasystole, atrial fibrillation, phlebitis, superficial thrombophlebitis of arm, mesenteric vein thrombophlebitis. **Respiratory:** Cough, dyspnea, pneumonia, sinusitis, rhinitis, pharyngitis, respiratory insufficiency, pulmonary infiltration, *pulmonary embolism*, pneumothorax, hemoptysis, stridor, bronchospasm, laryngitis, bronchitis, respiratory depression, pleural effusion, *pulmonary hemorrhage*, pneumonitis. **Ophthalmic:** Visual field defects, nystagmus, periorbital edema, eye pain, conjunctivitis, diplopia, blindness, retinal detachment, mydriasis, photophobia. **Otic:** Deafness, earache, tinnitus, otitis. **Dermatologic:** Increased sweating, rash, skin ulceration, pruritus, seborrhea, erythematous rash, maculopapular rash, facial edema, skin discoloration, acne, alopecia, dermatitis, anal pruritus, genital pruritus, aggravated psoriasis, psoriaform rash, skin disorders, dry skin, urticaria, skin hypertrophy, verruca. **Miscellaneous:** Epistaxis, taste perversions, pain or inflammation at injection site, lymphoma-like disorder, sarcoma, *malignant lymphoma*, ADH disorders, decreased gonadotropins, gynecomastia.

LABORATORY TEST CONSIDERATIONS
↑ Alkaline phosphatase, AST, ALT, LDH, BUN, CPK, serum creatinine. ↓ C_{CR}. Abnormal x-ray. Abnormal A-G ratio.

OD OVERDOSE MANAGEMENT
Symptoms: Extensions of the preceding side effects. Of most concern are development of *seizures,* renal function impairment, paresthesias in limbs or periorally, and electrolyte disturbances especially involving calcium and phosphate. *Treatment:* Monitor the client for S&S of electrolyte imbalance and renal impairment. Symptomatic treatment. Hemodialysis and hydration may be of some benefit.

DRUG INTERACTIONS
Aminoglycosides / ↓ Elimination of foscarnet → ↑ risk of renal impairment
Amphotericin B / ↓ Elimination of foscarnet → ↑ risk of renal impairment
Didanosine / ↓ Elimination of foscarnet → ↑ risk of renal impairment
Pentamidine, IV / ↓ Elimination of foscarnet → ↑ risk of renal impairment; also, pentamidine causes hypocalcemia
Zidovudine / ↑ Risk of anemia

HOW SUPPLIED
Injection: 24 mg/mL.

DOSAGE
• **IV INFUSION**
  CMV retinitis in AIDS.
Individualized, initial, normal renal function: Either 60 mg/kg over a minimum of 1 hr q 8 hr or 90 mg/kg q 12 hr for 2–3 weeks, depending on the response. **Maintenance:** 90–120 mg/kg/day (depending on renal func-

---

tion) given as an IV infusion over 2 hr. Start most clients on the 90 mg/kg/day dose; however, consider increasing the dose to 120 mg/kg/day due to progression of retinitis.

Acyclovir-resistant HSV infections in immunocompromised clients.

Initial: 40 mg/kg for clients with normal renal function given IV at a constant rate over a minimum of 1 hr q 8 or 12 hr for 2 to 3 weeks or until lesions are healed. **Maintenance:** See dose for CMV retinitis.

NURSING CONSIDERATIONS

ADMINISTRATION/STORAGE

IV 1. To avoid local irritation, infuse only into veins with adequate blood flow to allow rapid dilution and distribution.

2. Rate of infusion must be no more than 1 mg/kg/min using controlled IV infusion either by a central venous line or a peripheral vein. Do not give by rapid or bolus IV injection.

3. If using a central venous catheter for infusion, the standard 24 mg/mL solution may be used without dilution. If peripheral vein catheter used, dilute the 24 mg/mL solution to 12 mg/mL with D5W or NSS to avoid vein irritation. Use diluted solutions within 24 hr of first entry into sealed bottle.

4. To minimize potential for renal impairment, hydrate during drug administration; establish and maintain diuresis.

5. Adjust dose in renal impairment; use dosing guide.

6. Do not give any other drug or supplement through the same catheter. Foscarnet is incompatible with 30% dextrose, amphotericin B, and calcium-containing solutions (e.g., RL and TPN). Other incompatibilities include acyclovir sodium, diazepam, digoxin, diphenhydramine, dobutamine, droperidol, ganciclovir, gentamicin, haloperidol, isoethionate, leucovorin, midazolam, morphine sulfate, pentamidine, phenytoin, prochlorperazine, trimethoprim/sulfamethoxazole, trimetrexate, and vancomycin. A precipitate can result if foscarnet is given at the same time as divalent cations.

7. Store drug at room temperature of 15–30°C (59–86°F). Do not freeze. Concentrations of 12 mg/mL in NSS are stable for 30 days at 5°C (41°F).

ASSESSMENT

1. List reasons for therapy.

2. Confirm CMV retinitis by indirect ophthalmoscopy reports.

3. Note history of cardiac or neurologic dysfunction.

4. Monitor CBC, electrolytes, calcium, phosphorus, Mg, renal and LFTs.

INTERVENTIONS

1. Hydrate to minimize potential for renal impairment; establish and maintain diuresis. Determine C_{CR} 2–3 times per week during induction therapy, and at least once every 1–2 weeks during maintenance therapy, especially in geriatric clients who commonly have decreased GFRs.

2. Observe for possibility of chelation of divalent metal ions, which will alter serum levels of electrolytes.

3. Observe for any seizure activity; use seizure precautions.

4. Follow dilution and administration guidelines carefully. Ideally, product should be prepared daily, under a biologic hood, by the pharmacist. Refer to home infusion program for home therapy.

CLIENT/FAMILY TEACHING

1. Foscarnet is not a cure for CMV retinitis; may continue to experience progression of condition during or following treatment.

2. Report if sore throat, swollen lymph nodes, fatigue, fever and other S&S of infection occur.

3. Keep scheduled eye exams.

4. Report any evidence of numbness of the extremities, loss of sensation, or oral tingling as these are symptoms of hypocalcemia. Stop infusion and notify provider to correct imbalance before resuming the infusion.

OUTCOMES/EVALUATE

Ophthalmic evidence of successful treatment of CMV retinitis

Bold Italic = life threatening side effect   ■ = black box warning   ✦ = Available in Canada

Fosinopril sodium ■©
(foh-**SIN**-oh-prill)

CLASSIFICATION(S):
Antihypertensive, ACE inhibitor
PREGNANCY CATEGORY: D
Rx: Monopril.

SEE ALSO ANGIOTENSIN-CONVERTING ENZYME INHIBITORS.

USES
(1) Alone or in combination with other antihypertensive agents (especially thiazide diuretics) to treat hypertension. Diabetic hypertensive clients show a reduction in major CV events. (2) Treat CHF as adjunctive therapy when added to conventional therapy, including diuretics with or without digoxin.

ACTION/KINETICS
Action
Fosinopril inhibits angiotensin-converting enzyme resulting in decreased plasma angiotensin II, which leads to decreased vasopressor activity and decreased aldosterone secretion.

Pharmacokinetics
About 36% bioavailable. **Onset:** 1 hr. **Time to peak serum levels:** About 3 hr. Metabolized in the liver to the active fosinoprilat. **Peak effect:** 2–6 hr. **t½:** 12 hr for fosinoprilat (prolonged in impaired renal function) following IV administration. **Duration:** 24 hr. Approximately 50% excreted through the urine and 50% in the feces. Food decreases the rate, but not the extent, of absorption of fosinopril. **Plasma protein binding:** More than 99%.

CONTRAINDICATIONS
Use during lactation.

SPECIAL CONCERNS
■ When used during the second and third trimesters of pregnancy, injury and even death can result in the developing fetus. When pregnancy is detected, discontinue as soon as possible.■

SIDE EFFECTS
Most Common
Dizziness, headache, hypotension, chest pain, fatigue, diarrhea, URTI.

CV: Orthostatic hypotension, chest pain, hyper/hypotension, palpitations, angina pectoris, *CVA, MI*, rhythm disturbances, TIA, tachycardia, *hypertensive crisis*, claudication, bradycardia, conduction disorder, *sudden death, cardiorespiratory arrest, shock.* **CNS:** Headache, dizziness, fatigue, confusion, memory/sleep disturbances, depression, behavior change, tremors, drowsiness, mood change, insomnia, vertigo. **GI:** N&V, diarrhea, constipation, dry mouth, dysphagia, taste disturbance, abdominal distention/pain, flatulence, heartburn, appetite/weight changes. **Hepatic:** Hepatitis, *pancreatitis*, hepatomegaly, *hepatic failure.* **Respiratory:** Cough, sinusitis, dyspnea, URTI, *bronchospasm*, asthma, pharyngitis, laryngitis, tracheobronchitis, abnormal breathing, sinus abnormalities. **Hematologic:** Leukopenia, eosinophilia, decreases in hemoglobin (mean of 0.1 gram/dL) or hematocrit, neutropenia. **Dermatologic:** Diaphoresis, photosensitivity, flushing, exfoliative dermatitis, pruritus, rash, urticaria. **Body as a whole:** *Angioedema*, muscle cramps, fever, syncope, influenza, cold sensation, pain, myalgia, arthralgia, arthritis, edema, weakness, musculoskeletal pain. **GU:** Decreased libido, sexual dysfunction, renal insufficiency, urinary frequency, abnormal urination, kidney pain. **Miscellaneous:** Paresthesias, tinnitus, gout, lymphadenopathy, rhinitis, epistaxis, vision disturbances, eye irritation, swelling/weakness of extremities, abnormal vocalization, pneumonia, muscle ache.

LABORATORY TEST CONSIDERATIONS
↑ Serum potassium. Transient ↓ H&H. False low measurement of serum digoxin levels with DigiTab RIA Kit for Digoxin.

HOW SUPPLIED
Tablets: 10 mg, 20 mg, 40 mg.
DOSAGE
• **TABLETS**
Hypertension.
Initial: 10 mg once daily; **then,** adjust dose depending on BP response at peak (2–6 hr after dosing) and trough (24 hr after dosing) blood levels. **Main-**

© = see color insert   **H** = Herbal   **IV** = Intravenous   © = sound alike drug

tenance: Usually 20–40 mg/day, although some clients manifest beneficial effects at doses up to 80 mg.

In clients taking diuretics.

Symptomatic hypotension may occur following the initial dose. To reduce this possibility, discontinue diuretic 2–3 days before starting fosinopril. If diuretic cannot be discontinued, use an initial dose of 10 mg fosinopril.

Congestive heart failure.

Initial: 10 mg once daily; **then,** following initial dose, observe the client for at least 2 hr for the presence of hypotension or orthostasis (if either is present, monitor until BP stabilizes). An initial dose of 5 mg is recommended in heart failure with moderate to severe renal failure or in those who have had significant diuresis. Increase the dose over several weeks, not to exceed a maximum of 40 mg daily (usual effective range is 20–40 mg once daily).

NURSING CONSIDERATIONS

℮ Do not confuse Monopril with minoxidil (an antihypertensive).

ADMINISTRATION/STORAGE

1. If antihypertensive effect decreases at end of dosing interval with once-daily dosing, consider twice a day administration.

2. If also taking a diuretic, discontinue diuretic 2–3 days prior to beginning fosinopril therapy. If BP not controlled, restart diuretic. If the diuretic cannot be discontinued, give an initial dose of 10 mg fosinopril.

3. Do not adjust the dose of fosinopril in renal insufficiency except as noted in *Dosage*.

4. Store from 15–30°C (59–86°F). Protect from moisture by keeping bottle tightly closed.

ASSESSMENT

1. Note disease onset, other agents trialed, outcome.

2. Monitor BP, CBC, BNP, electrolytes, microalbumin, renal and LFTs.

CLIENT/FAMILY TEACHING

1. Take as directed with or without food. BP control does not exceed 24 hr; take at same time(s) each day.

2. May initially cause dizziness and light-headedness; use care. Avoid dehydration, use caution in hot weather and with increased exercise. Record BP at different times during the day.

3. Avoid OTC agents without provider approval; salt substitutes containing potassium should be avoided.

4. Change positions slowly to avoid sudden drop in BP.

5. Use reliable contraception. Stop drug and report if pregnancy suspected.

6. Report adverse side effects especially S&S infection, sore throat, swelling of hands and feet, chest pain, SOB, mouth sores, unusual bruising/bleeding, or irregular heart beat.

7. Continue life style changes aimed at controlling BP: salt/fat restriction, regular exercise, weight reduction, and smoking/alcohol cessation.

8. Keep all F/U appointments to evaluate response to therapy.

OUTCOMES/EVALUATE

Control of BP/CHF

Fosphenytoin sodium

(**FOS**-fen-ih-toyn)

CLASSIFICATION(S):
Anticonvulsant, hydantoin
PREGNANCY CATEGORY: D
Rx: Cerebyx.

SEE ALSO *ANTICONVULSANTS AND PHENYTOIN.*

USES

Short-term parenteral use for the control of generalized convulsive status epilepticus and prophylaxis and treatment of seizures occurring during neurosurgery. It can be substituted, short term, for PO phenytoin when PO administration is not possible.

ACTION/KINETICS

Action

Fosphenytoin is a prodrug of phenytoin; thus, its anticonvulsant effects are due to phenytoin. For every millimole of fosphenytoin administered, 1 mmol of phenytoin is produced. Fosphenytoin is better tolerated at the infusion site than is phenytoin (i.e., pain and burning associated with IV phenytoin is decreased).

Pharmacokinetics

$t\frac{1}{2}$, fosphenytoin: 15 min after IV infusion. **Peak plasma levels, after IM:** 30 min. Fosphenytoin displaces phenytoin from plasma protein binding sites. The IV infusion rate for fosphenytoin is three times faster than for IV phenytoin. IM use results in systemic phenytoin concentrations that are similar to PO phenytoin, thus allowing interchangeable use. Phenytoin derived from fosphenytoin is extensively metabolized in the liver and excreted in the urine. **Plasma protein binding:** 95–99%.

CONTRAINDICATIONS

Hypersensitivity to fosphenytoin, phenytoin, or other hydantoins. Use in clients with sinus bradycardia, SA block, second- and third-degree AV block, and Adams-Stokes syndrome. Use to treat absence seizures. Use during lactation.

SPECIAL CONCERNS

The safety and efficacy of fosphenytoin have not been determined for longer than 5 days. Safety has not been determined in pediatric clients. After administration of fosphenytoin to those with renal and/or hepatic dysfunction or in those with hypoalbuminemia, fosphenytoin clearance to phenytoin may be increased without a similar increase in phenytoin clearance, thus increasing the potential for serious side effects.

SIDE EFFECTS

Most Common

Ataxia, dizziness, headache, nystagmus, paresthesia, pruritus, and somnolence. See *Phenytoin* for a complete list of possible side effects.

LABORATORY TEST CONSIDERATIONS

See *Phenytoin*. Alters LFTs, ↑ blood glucose values, and ↓ PBI values. ↑ Gamma globulins. Phenytoin ↓ immunoglobulins A and G. False + Coombs' test.

OD OVERDOSE MANAGEMENT

Symptoms: N&V, **cardiac dysrhythmia or arrest,** hypotension, syncope, hypocalcemia, metabolic acidosis, **death.** *Treatment:* See Phenytoin.

DRUG INTERACTIONS

See *Phenytoin*

HOW SUPPLIED

NOTE: Doses of fosphenytoin are expressed as phenytoin sodium equivalents (PE = phenytoin sodium equivalent) to avoid the need to perform molecular weight adjustments when converting between fosphenytoin and phenytoin sodium doses. *Injection:* 75 mg/mL.

DOSAGE

- **IV**

   Status epilepticus.

Loading dose: 15–20 mg PE/kg given at a rate of 100–150 mg PE/min. The loading dose is followed by maintenance doses of either fosphenytoin or phenytoin, either PO or parenterally.

- **IM; IV**

   Nonemergency loading and maintenance dosing.

Loading dose: 10–20 mg PE/kg given at a rate of 100–150 mg PE/min. **Maintenance:** 4–6 mg PE/kg/day.

   Temporary substitution for PO phenytoin.

Use the same daily PO dose of phenytoin in milligrams given at a rate not to exceed 150 mg PE/min.

NURSING CONSIDERATIONS

Ⓒ Do not confuse Cerebyx with Celebrex (nonsteroidal antiinflammatory drug) or with Celexa (an antidepressant).

ADMINISTRATION/STORAGE

1. Fosphenytoin can be substituted for PO phenytoin sodium therapy at the same total daily dose.

2. Phenytoin capsules as Dilantin are approximately 90% bioavailable by the PO route and fosphenytoin (available as Cerebyx) is 100% bioavailable by both the IM and IV routes. Plasma phenytoin may increase modestly when IM or IV fosphenytoin (as Cerebyx) is substituted for PO phenytoin sodium therapy.

3. Do not use IM fosphenytoin to treat status epilepticus because therapeutic phenytoin concentrations may not be reached as quickly as with IV administration.

---

4. Do not use vials that develop particulate matter.

5. Do not store at room temperature for more than 48 hr. Store under refrigeration at 2–8°C (36–46°F).

IV 6. Prior to IV infusion fosphenytoin must be diluted in D5W or NSS solution to obtain a concentration ranging from 1.5 to 25 mg/PE (phenytoin sodium equivalents)/mL.

7. Due to risk of hypotension, do not administer at a rate greater than 150 PE/min.

8. Because the full antiepileptic effect of phenytoin (given as either fosphenytoin or parenteral phenytoin) is not known immediately, other measures to control status epilepticus (e.g., use of an IV benzodiazepine) will be necessary.

ASSESSMENT

1. Note type, onset, characteristics of seizures; list other agents trialed, outcome.

2. Fosphenytoin converts to phenytoin and may be administered IV or IM; prescribed and dispensed in PE units.

3. Monitor ECG, albumin, CBC, renal and LFTs. During IV administration, continuously monitor ECG, BP, and respirations.

4. Do not use with bradycardia or heart block; may cause atrial and ventricular conduction depression.

5. The waiting period before ordering laboratory tests for phenytoin plasma levels is 2 hr following IV infusion and 4 hr following IM injection.

CLIENT/FAMILY TEACHING

1. Review goals of therapy; drug is for short-term use of seizure control.

2. Report fever, sore throat, bruising/bleeding, rash, jaundice, slurred speech, joint pain, N&V, severe headaches, swollen lymph glands.

3. Use caution with activities that require alertness; may experience dizziness and drowsiness, itching, tingling of groin and face. Presence of REMs, gait and speech impairment may indicate toxicity.

4. If rash appears, stop therapy and report. If mild, therapy may resume once rash has cleared. If rash recurs, do not reuse this class of drugs.

5. Practice reliable contraception. Keep all check up visits.

OUTCOMES/EVALUATE

- Control of seizures
- Seizure prophylaxis with surgery
- Short-term substitution for PO phenytoin

Frovatriptan succinate

(**froh**-vah-**TRIP**-tan)

CLASSIFICATION(S):
Antimigraine drug
PREGNANCY CATEGORY: C
Rx: Frova.

USES
Acute treatment of migraine, with or without aura, in adults. Use only where a clear diagnosis of migraine has been established.

ACTION/KINETICS

Action
Frovatriptan is a selective $5\text{-HT}_{1B/1D}$ receptor agonist which binds with high affinity to 5-HT_{1B} and 5-HT_{1D} receptors. Believed to act on extracerebral, intracranial arteries to cause constriction and to inhibit excessive dilation of these vessels in migraine.

Pharmacokinetics
From 29.6% (2.5 mg PO) to 17.5% (40 mg PO) bioavailable. **Maximum blood levels:** 2–4 hr. **Time to onset of action:** 2–3 hr. **Time to peak effect:** 2–4 hr. Food has no significant effect on bioavailability but delays the maximum levels by 1 hr. Metabolized in the liver with about one third unchanged drug and metabolites excreted in the urine and two-thirds in the feces. **t½, mean terminal:** 25.7–29.7 hr, depending on the dose. **Plasma protein binding:** About 15%.

CONTRAINDICATIONS
Use for prophylaxis of migraine or use in management of hemiplegic or basilar migraine. Use in those with ischemic heart disease (e.g., angina pectoris, history of MI, documented silent ischemia)

---

or in those who have symptoms or findings consistent with ischemic heart disease, coronary artery vasospasm (including Prinzmetal's variant angina), or other significant underlying CV disease. Use in those with CV syndromes, including (but not limited to) strokes of any type as well as TIAs. Use in those with peripheral vascular disease (including, but not limited to ischemic bowel disease), uncontrolled hypertension, use within 24 hr of treatment with another 5-HT$_1$ agonist or an ergotamine-containing or ergot-type medication (e.g., dihydroergotamine, methysergide), or in those hypersensitive to frovatriptan or any ingredients of the product. Use in those with documented ischemic or vasospastic CAD or in whom unrecognized CAD is predicted by the presence of risk factors (e.g., hypertension, hypercholesterolemia, smoking, obesity, diabetes, strong history of CAD, females with surgical or physiological menopause, or males over 40 years of age) unless a CV evaluation provides evidence that the client is reasonably free of CAD and ischemic myocardial disease. Use in children less than 18 years of age.

SPECIAL CONCERNS
Use with caution during lactation. Safety and efficacy have not been established for use in children less than 18 years of age or for cluster headaches (present in an older, predominantly male population).

SIDE EFFECTS
Most Common
Palpitations, dysesthesia, hypesthesia, insomnia, anxiety, increased sweating, N&V, abdominal pain, diarrhea, sinusitis, rhinitis, abnormal vision, tinnitus, pain.
GI: Dry mouth, dyspepsia, vomiting, abdominal pain, diarrhea, dysphagia, flatulence, constipation, anorexia, esophagospasm, increased salivation. **CNS:** Dizziness, paresthesia, headache, dysesthesia, hypoesthesia, tremor, hyperesthesia, aggravated migraine, vertigo, ataxia, abnormal gait, speech disorder, insomnia, anxiety, confusion, nervousness, agitation, euphoria, impaired concentration, depression, emotional lability, amnesia, abnormal thinking, depersonalization. **CV:** *Acute MI, life-threatening disturbances of cardiac rhythm, death, cerebral hemorrhage, subarachnoid hemorrhage, stroke, ventricular fibrillation,* coronary artery vasospasm, transient myocardial ischemia, ventricular tachycardia, peripheral vascular ischemia, colonic ischemia (with abdominal pain and bloody diarrhea), hypertension, palpitations, tachycardia, abnormal ECG. **Body as a whole:** Fatigue, flushing, hot or cold sensation, pain, asthenia, rigors, fever, hot flashes, malaise, dehydration, syncope. **Musculoskeletal:** Skeletal pain, involuntary muscle contraction, myalgia, back pain, arthralgia, arthrosis, leg cramps, muscle weakness. **Respiratory:** Sinusitis, rhinitis, pharyngitis, dyspnea, hyperventilation, laryngitis, epistaxis. **Dermatologic:** Increased sweating, pruritis, bullous eruption. **GU:** Frequent micturition, polyuria. **Ophthalmic:** Abnormal vision, eye pain, conjunctivitis, abnormal lacrimation. **Otic:** Tinnitus, earache, hyperacusis. **Miscellaneous:** Chest pain, thirst, taste perversion. Sensations of pain, tightness, pressure, and heaviness in the chest, throat, neck, and jaw.

DRUG INTERACTIONS
Dihydroergotamine / Prolonged vasospastic reaction; do not use within 24 hr of each other
Ergotamine / Frovatriptan maximum levels and AUC ↓ 25%
Methysergide / Prolonged vasospastic reaction; do not use within 24 hr of each other
Oral contraceptives / Frovatriptan maximum levels and AUC ↑ 30%
Propranolol / ↑ Frovatriptan maximum levels and AUC
Selective serotonin reuptake inhibitors / Possible weakness, hyperreflexia, incoordination

HOW SUPPLIED
Tablets: 2.5 mg (as base).

DOSAGE
• **TABLETS**
  Migraine headache.
Adults: Single dose of 2.5 mg taken with fluids. If the headache recurs after

initial relief, a second tablet (2.5 mg) may be taken provided there is an interval of at least 2 hr between doses. Do not exceed a total daily dose of 3 tablets (7.5 mg).

NURSING CONSIDERATIONS

ADMINISTRATION/STORAGE

1. If first dose does not produce response, reconsider diagnosis of migraine before giving a second dose. There is no evidence that a second dose is effective in clients who do not respond to a first dose.
2. The safety of treating an average of 4 migraine attacks in a 30-day period has not been determined.
3. Store at controlled room temperature of 15–30°C (59–86°F). Protect from moisture and light.

ASSESSMENT

1. Note reasons for therapy, onset, family history, characteristics of symptoms, other agents trialed, outcome. Ensure not hemiplegic or basilar type of migraine headaches. Review neurologist reports/findings.
2. List drugs currently prescribed to ensure none interact.
3. Assess for CAD, uncontrolled HTN, circulation problems, IBD, or history of CVA/TIAs. With increased CAD risk factors, get EKG, give first dose in the office and assess client for adverse effects.
4. Determine renal and LFT's; evaluate for dysfunction.

CLIENT/FAMILY TEACHING

1. Take as directed for migraine headaches; do not use for other types of headaches. Never share medications with others no matter what the symptoms.
2. If headache returns may repeat dose in 2 hours; do not exceed 7.5 mg in 24 hr.
3. Use caution if driving or performing activities that require mental alertness; may cause dizziness, fatigue, or drowsiness.
4. Store in a safe place and away from heat, light, and moisture. Do not take within 24 hr of taking any other ergotamine or serotonin receptor agonist type headache medicine.

5. Drug acts to shrink swollen blood vessels surrounding the brain that cause migraine headaches. Keep a headache diary and identify factors/foods/events that surround migraine headaches.
6. Avoid known triggers, i.e., chocolate, cheese, citrus fruit, caffeine, alcohol, missing sleep/meals etc.
7. Report any chest pain, SOB, palpitations, rash/itching, or unusual side effects, intolerance, or lack of response.

OUTCOMES/EVALUATE

Resolution of acute migraine attack

Fulvestrant
(**FULL**-veh-strant)

CLASSIFICATION(S):
Antiestrogen
PREGNANCY CATEGORY: D
Rx: Faslodex.

USES

Hormone receptor-positive metastatic breast cancer in postmenopausal women with disease progression following antiestrogen therapy.

ACTION/KINETICS

Action

Is an estrogen receptor antagonist. Competitively binds to the estrogen receptor and down regulates the estrogen receptor protein in human breast cancer cells.

Pharmacokinetics

Peak plasma levels, IM: 7 days. **t½:** 40 days. After 250 mg IM every month, plasma levels reach steady state after 3 to 6 doses. Metabolized in the liver by CYP3A4. About 90% excreted in the feces with negligible (less than 1%) excreted in the urine. **Plasma protein binding:** About 99%.

CONTRAINDICATIONS

Pregnancy, lactation. Hypersensitivity to the drug or any of its components.

SPECIAL CONCERNS

Safety and efficacy have not been determined in children or in moderate to severe hepatic impairment.

Bold Italic = life threatening side effect   ■ = black box warning   ✦ = Available in Canada

SIDE EFFECTS
Most Common
Headache, N&V, constipation, diarrhea, abdominal pain, bone pain, pharyngitis, dyspnea, increased cough, asthenia, pain, vasodilation (hot flushes), back pain, injection site pain/inflammation.
GI: N&V, constipation, diarrhea, abdominal pain, anorexia. **CNS:** Headache, dizziness, insomnia, paresthesia, depression, anxiety, vertigo. **Dermatologic:** Rash, sweating. **Musculoskeletal:** Bone pain, arthritis, myalgia. **Respiratory:** Pharyngitis, dyspnea, increased cough. **At injection site:** Mild transient pain, inflammation. **Body as a whole:** Asthenia, pain, vasodilation (hot flushes), peripheral edema, flu syndrome, fever, accidental injury, anemia. **Miscellaneous:** Back/pelvic/chest pain, UTI, thromboembolic phenomenon, leukopenia, vaginal bleeding mainly during the first 6 weeks of therapy.

HOW SUPPLIED
Injection: 50 mg/mL.

DOSAGE
- **IM**
  Metastatic breast cancer.
Adults: 250 mg IM (give slowly) into the buttock as a single 5-mL injection at 1-month intervals. Alternatively, 2 concurrent 2.5-mL injections can be given.

NURSING CONSIDERATIONS
ADMINISTRATION/STORAGE
Store in a refrigerator at 2–8°C (36–46°F) in the original container.
ASSESSMENT
1. Note disease onset, other therapies/surgeries trialed and outcome.
2. Ensure client is not pregnant.
3. Monitor CBC and injection site for adverse reactions.
CLIENT/FAMILY TEACHING
1. Blocks the effects of the estrogen hormone in the body. Therefore, the amount of estrogen that the tumor is exposed to is reduced, limiting the growth of the tumor.
2. Drug is administered slowly, once monthly IM, as one 5 mL injection or two 2.5 mL injections to control progression of breast cancer.
3. May experience GI upset, headaches, back pain, sore throat and hot flashes; report any persistent or intolerable side effects. Report swelling of face, arms, hands, lower legs, or feet; rapid weight gain; tingling of hands or feet; unusual weight gain or loss.
4. Practice reliable contraception; report if pregnancy suspected as drug may cause fetal damage. Keep all F/U appointments.
OUTCOMES/EVALUATE
Control of hormone receptor– positive metastatic breast cancer progression

Furosemide
(fur-**OH**-seh-myd)

CLASSIFICATION(S):
Diuretic, loop
PREGNANCY CATEGORY: C
Rx: Lasix.
♣Rx: Apo-Furosemide, Lasix Special.

SEE ALSO *DIURETICS, LOOP.*
USES
(1) Edema associated with CHF, nephrotic syndrome, hepatic cirrhosis, and ascites. (2) IV for acute pulmonary edema. (3) PO to treat hypertension in conjunction with spironolactone, triamterene, and other diuretics *except* ethacrynic acid. *Investigational:* Hypercalcemia. As an antihypertensive in postpartum clients with severe preeclampsia.
ACTION/KINETICS
Action
Inhibits the reabsorption of sodium and chloride in the proximal and distal tubules as well as the ascending loop of Henle; this results in the excretion of sodium, chloride, and, to a lesser degree, potassium and bicarbonate ions. The resulting urine is more acid. Diuretic action is independent of changes in clients' acid-base balance. Has a slight antihypertensive effect.
Pharmacokinetics
Onset: PO, IM: 30–60 min; **IV:** 5 min.
Peak: PO, IM: 1–2 hr; **IV:** 20–60 min. **t½:**

F

About 2 hr after PO use. **Duration: PO, IM:** 6–8 hr; **IV:** 2 hr. Metabolized in the liver and excreted through the urine. May be effective for clients resistant to thiazides and for those with reduced GFRs.

CONTRAINDICATIONS

Never use with ethacrynic acid. Anuria, hypersensitivity to drug, severe renal disease associated with azotemia and oliguria, hepatic coma associated with electrolyte depletion. Lactation.

SPECIAL CONCERNS

■ Furosemide is a potent diuretic. Excess amounts can lead to profound diuresis with water and electrolyte depletion. Careful medical attention is needed; individualize dosage.■ Use with caution in premature infants and neonates due to prolonged half-life in these clients (dosing interval must be extended). Geriatric clients may be more sensitive to the usual adult dose. Allergic reactions may be seen in clients who show hypersensitivity to sulfonamides.

SIDE EFFECTS

Most Common

Jaundice, tinnitus, hearing impairment, hypotension, water/electrolyte depletion, pancreatitis, abdominal pain, dizziness, anemia.

Electrolyte and fluid effects: Fluid and electrolyte depletion leading to dehydration, hypovolemia, thromboembolism. Hypokalemia and hypochloremia may cause metabolic alkalosis. Hyperuricemia, azotemia, hyponatremia. **GI:** Nausea, oral and gastric irritation, abdominal pain, vomiting, anorexia, diarrhea (especially in children) or constipation, cramps, pancreatitis, jaundice, ischemic hepatitis. **Otic:** Tinnitus, hearing impairment (may be reversible or permanent), reversible deafness (usually following rapid IV or IM administration of high doses). **CNS:** Vertigo, headache, dizziness, blurred vision, restlessness, paresthesias, xanthopsia. **CV:** Orthostatic hypotension, thrombophlebitis, chronic aortitis. **Hematologic:** Anemia, thrombocytopenia, neutropenia, leukopenia, *agranulocytosis*, purpura. *Rarely, aplastic anemia.* **Allergic:**

Rashes, pruritus, urticaria, photosensitivity, exfoliative dermatitis, vasculitis, erythema multiforme. **Miscellaneous:** Interstitial nephritis, fever, weakness, hyperglycemia, glycosuria, exacerbation/aggravation/worsening of SLE, increased perspiration, muscle spasms, urinary bladder spasm, urinary frequency.

Following IV use: Thrombophlebitis, *cardiac arrest*.

Following IM use: Pain and irritation at injection site, *cardiac arrest*. Because this drug is resistant to the effects of pressor amines and potentiates the effects of muscle relaxants, it is recommended that the PO drug be discontinued 1 week before surgery and the IV drug 2 days before surgery.

ADDITIONAL DRUG INTERACTIONS

Charcoal / ↓ Absorption of furosemide from GI tract
Clofibrate / Enhanced diuretic effect
Hydantoins / ↓ Diuretic effect of furosemide
Propranolol / ↑ Plasma propranolol levels

OD **OVERDOSE MANAGEMENT**

Symptoms: Profound water loss, electrolyte depletion (manifested by weakness, anorexia, vomiting, lethargy, cramps, mental confusion, dizziness), decreased blood volume, *circulatory collapse (possibly vascular thrombosis and embolism).* *Treatment:* Replace fluid and electrolytes. Monitor urine electrolyte output and serum electrolytes. Induce emesis or perform gastric lavage. Oxygen or artificial respiration may be needed. Treat symptoms.

HOW SUPPLIED

Injection: 10 mg /mL; *Oral Solution:* 10 mg/mL, 40 mg/5 mL; *Tablets:* 20 mg, 40 mg, 80 mg.

DOSAGE————

• **ORAL SOLUTION; TABLETS**
Edema.

Adults, initial: 20–80 mg/day as a single dose. For resistant cases, dosage can be increased by 20–40 mg q 6–8 hr until desired diuretic response is attained. Maximum daily dose should not exceed 600 mg. **Pediatric, initial:** 2 mg/kg as a single dose; **then,** dose can

---

Bold Italic = life threatening side effect   ■ = black box warning   ✦ = Available in Canada

be increased by 1–2 mg/kg q 6–8 hr until desired response is attained (up to 5 mg/kg may be required in children with nephrotic syndrome; maximum dose should not exceed 6 mg/kg). A dose range of 0.5–2 mg/kg twice a day has also been recommended.

Hypertension.
Adults, initial: 40 mg twice a day. Adjust dosage depending on response.

CHF and chronic renal failure.
Adults: 2–2.5 grams/day.

Antihypercalcemic.
Adults: 120 mg/day in one to three doses.

• **IM; IV**
Edema.
Adults, initial: 20–40 mg; if response inadequate after 2 hr, increase dose in 20-mg increments. **Pediatric, initial:** 1 mg/kg given slowly; if response inadequate after 2 hr, increase dose by 1 mg/kg. Doses greater than 6 mg/kg should not be given.

Antihypercalcemic.
Adults: 80–100 mg for severe cases; dose may be repeated q 1–2 hr if needed.

• **IV**
Acute pulmonary edema.
Adults: 40 mg slowly over 1–2 min; if response inadequate after 1 hr, give 80 mg slowly over 1–2 min. Concomitant oxygen and digitalis may be used.

CHF, chronic renal failure.
Adults: 2–2.5 grams/day. For IV bolus injections, the maximum should not exceed 1 gram/day given over 30 min.

Hypertensive crisis, normal renal function.
40–80 mg.

Hypertensive crisis with pulmonary edema or acute renal failure.
100–200 mg.

NURSING CONSIDERATIONS

℞ Do not confuse Lasix with Lanoxin (a cardiac glycoside).

ADMINISTRATION/STORAGE
1. Give 2–4 days per week.
2. Food decreases bioavailability of furosemide and ultimately the degree of diuresis.
3. Slight discoloration resulting from light does not affect potency. However, do not dispense discolored tablets or injection.
4. If used with other antihypertensives, reduce dose of other agents by at least 50% when furosemide is added in order to prevent an excessive drop in BP.
5. Store in light-resistant containers at room temperature (15–30°C, or 59–86°F).
6. In CHF or chronic renal failure, oral and parenteral doses of 2–2.5 grams/day (or higher) are well tolerated.
IV 7. Give IV injections slowly over 1–2 min.
8. Do not mix with solutions with a pH below 5.5. After pH adjustment, furosemide can be mixed with NaCl injection, RL injection, and D5W and infused at a rate not to exceed 4 mg/min, to prevent ototoxicity.
9. A precipitate may form if mixed with gentamicin, netilmicin, or milrinone in either D5W or NSS.

ASSESSMENT
1. Note reasons for therapy, clinical presentation, other agents trialed, outcome. When more than 40 mg/day is required, give in divided doses, i.e., 40 mg PO twice a day (7 a.m. and 3 p.m.)
2. With renal impairment or if receiving other ototoxic drugs, observe for ototoxicity.
3. Assess closely for signs of vascular thrombosis and embolism, particularly in the elderly. With history of gout, monitor uric acid levels.
4. Monitor BP, weight, edema, breath sounds, I&O, electrolytes; observe for S&S of hypokalemia.
5. With rapid diuresis, observe for dehydration and circulatory collapse; monitor BP and pulse.
6. With chronic use, assess for thiamine deficiency; if used with zaroxlyn assess for low phosphate levels.

CLIENT/FAMILY TEACHING
1. Take in the morning on an empty stomach to enhance absorption and avoid interruption of sleep. May take with food or milk if GI upset. Time administration to participate in social activities.

2. Immediately report any muscle weakness/cramps, dizziness, ringing in the ears, sore throat, fever, severe abdominal pain, numbness, or tingling.

3. Drug may cause BP drop. Change positions from lying to standing slowly. Avoid alcohol and do not exercise heavily in hot weather.

4. Refrigerate solution. Sorbitol in the solution may result in diarrhea, especially in children.

5. Consult provider before taking excessive aspirin for any reason. Salicylate intoxication occurs at lower levels than normal because of competition at the renal excretory sites.

6. Use sunscreens and protective clothing when sun exposed to minimize the effects of drug-induced photosensitivity.

7. Management of end stage heart disease requires diligent monitoring, management, and titration on provider and client part; keep all visits and report any changes or adverse effects.

8. Record BP and weights; report any gains of >2 lb per day or >5 lb per week.

9. Supplement diet with vegetables and fruits that are high in potassium (bananas, oranges, peaches, dried dates) if oral supplements are not prescribed. Those on a salt-restricted diet should not increase salt intake; NSAIDs and alpha blockers may also cause sodium retention.

10. Keep all F/U appointments to evaluate response to therapy.

OUTCOMES/EVALUATE
- Enhanced diuresis; ↓ BP
- Resolution of pulmonary edema
- ↓ Dependent edema

G

Gabapentin
(**gab**-ah-**PEN**-tin)

CLASSIFICATION(S):
Anticonvulsant, miscellaneous
PREGNANCY CATEGORY: C
Rx: Gabarone, Neurontin.
❋Rx: Apo-Gabapentin, Novo-Gabapentin, PMS-Gabapentin.

SEE ALSO *ANTICONVULSANTS.*

USES
(1) Treatment of partial seizures with and without secondary generalization in clients 12 years and older. (2) Adjunct to treat partial seizures in children 3–12 years of age. (3) In adults, management of post-herpetic neuralgia or pain in the area affected by herpes zoster after treating the disease. *Investigational:* Neuropathic pain, bipolar disorder, prevent migraine, tremors associated with MS. With morphine to treat diabetic neuropathy or postherpetic neuralgia.

ACTION/KINETICS
Action
Anticonvulsant and analgesic mechanisms are not known. Is related chemically to GABA but does not interact with GABA receptors.

Pharmacokinetics
Food has no effect on the rate and extent of absorption; however, as the dose increases, the bioavailability decreases. **t½:** 5–7 hr. Excreted unchanged through the urine. Adjust dosage in those with impaired renal function.

SPECIAL CONCERNS
Use during lactation only if benefits outweigh risks. Plasma clearance is reduced in geriatric clients and in those with impaired renal function. Use in children 3–12 years of age is associated with various neuropsychiatric side effects (e.g., emotional lability, hostility including aggression, thought disorder including concentration problems and change in school performance, hyperkinesia). Safety and efficacy have not

---

Bold Italic = life threatening side effect   ■ = black box warning   ❋ = Available in Canada been determined in children less than 3 years of age.

SIDE EFFECTS

Most Common

Dizziness, somnolence, peripheral edema, ataxia, nystagmus, tremor.

Side effects listed are those with an incidence of 0.1% or greater. **CNS:** Most common: Somnolence, ataxia, dizziness, and fatigue. Also, nystagmus, tremor, nervousness, dysarthria, amnesia, depression, abnormal thinking/coordination, twitching, headache, *convulsions (including the possibility of precipitation of status epilepticus)*, confusion, insomnia, emotional lability, vertigo, hyperkinesia, paresthesia, decreased/increased/absent reflexes, anxiety, hostility, CNS tumors, syncope, abnormal dreaming, aphasia, hypesthesia, *intracranial hemorrhage*, hypo/dystonia, dysesthesia, paresis, hemiplegia, facial paralysis, stupor, cerebellar dysfunction, positive Babinski sign, decreased position sense, subdural hematoma, apathy, hallucinations, decreased or loss of libido, agitation depersonalization, euphoria, 'doped-up' sensation, *suicidal tendencies, sudden unexplained deaths*, psychoses. **Neuropsychiatric effects in children:** Emotional lability (behavioral problems), hostility (aggressive behavior), thought disorder (concentration problems and change in school performance), restlessness, hyperactivity. **GI:** Most common is: N&V. Also, dyspepsia, dry mouth and throat, constipation, dental abnormalities, increased appetite, abdominal pain, diarrhea, anorexia, flatulence, gingivitis, glossitis, *gum hemorrhage,* thirst, stomatitis, taste loss, unusual taste, increased salivation, gastroenteritis, hemorrhoids, bloody stools, fecal incontinence, hepatomegaly. **CV:** Hyper/hypotension, vasodilation, angina pectoris, peripheral vascular disorder, palpitation, tachycardia, migraine, murmur. **Musculoskeletal:** Myalgia, fracture, tendinitis, arthritis, joint stiffness/swelling, positive Romberg test. **Respiratory:** Rhinitis, pharyngitis, coughing, pneumonia, epistaxis, dyspnea, apnea. **Dermatologic:** Pruritus, abrasion, rash, acne, alopecia, eczema, dry skin, increased sweating, urticaria, hirsutism, seborrhea, cyst, herpes simplex. **Body as a whole:** Back pain, weight increase/decrease, peripheral edema, asthenia, facial edema, allergy, chills. **GU:** Hematuria, dysuria, frequent urination, cystitis, urinary retention/incontinence, *vaginal hemorrhage*, amenorrhea, dysmenorrhea, menorrhagia, breast cancer, inability to climax, abnormal ejaculation, impotence. **Hematologic:** Leukopenia, decreased WBCs, purpura, anemia, thrombocytopenia, lymphadenopathy. **Ophthalmic:** Diplopia, amblyopia, abnormal vision, cataract, conjunctivitis, dry eyes, visual field defect, photophobia, bilateral/unilateral ptosis, eye twitching/pain/hemorrhage, hordeolum. **Otic:** Hearing loss, earache, tinnitus, inner ear infection, otitis, ear fullness.

LABORATORY TEST CONSIDERATIONS

False + reading with Ames N-Multistix SG dipstick test for urinary protein.

OD OVERDOSE MANAGEMENT

Symptoms: Double vision, slurred speech, drowsiness, lethargy, diarrhea. *Treatment:* Hemodialysis.

DRUG INTERACTIONS

Alcohol / Intensifies effects of gabapentin

Antacids / ↓ Bioavailability of gabapentin

Cimetidine / ↓ Renal excretion of gabapentin

Hydrocodone / ↑ Gabapentin AUC values and ↓ hydrocodone C_{max} and AUC

Morphine / ↑ Morphine AUC by 44%

HOW SUPPLIED

Capsules: 100 mg, 300 mg, 400 mg; *Oral Solution:* 250 mg/5 mL; *Tablets:* 100 mg, 300 mg, 400 mg, 600 mg, 800 mg.

DOSAGE

• CAPSULES; ORAL SOLUTION; TABLETS

Partial seizures with and without secondary generalization.

Clients 12 years and older: Dose range of 900–1,800 mg/day in three divided doses using 300 or 400 mg capsules or 600 or 800 mg tablets. **Initial dose:** 300 mg 3 times per day; dose may be increased, as needed, up to 1,800 mg/day. Doses up to 2,400 and

3,600 mg/day have been well tolerated for short periods. In clients with a C_{CR} of 30–60 mL/min, the dose is 300 mg twice a day; if the C_{CR} is 15–30 mL/min, the dose is 300 mg/day; if the C_{CR} <15 mL/min, the dose is 300 mg every other day.

Adjunctive therapy for partial seizures in children.

Ages 3–12 years, initial: 10–15 mg/kg/day in 3 divided doses. Attain effective dose by titration over 3 days. Effective dose in clients 5 years and older is 25–35 mg/kg/day and in clients 3 and 4 years of age is 40 mg/kg/day; give in divided doses 3 times per day. May use capsules, oral solution or tablets.

Postherpetic neuralgia.

Adults, initial: Single 300 mg dose on day 1; 600 mg/day on day 2 (divided twice daily); and, 900 mg/day on day 3 (divided 3 times daily). Then, titrate dose up as needed for pain relief to a daily dose of 1,800 mg (divided 3 times daily). Beneficial effects of dose greater than 1,800 mg/day not determined.

NURSING CONSIDERATIONS

℗ Do not confuse Neurontin with Noroxin (a fluoroquinolone antibiotic).

ADMINISTRATION/STORAGE

1. Do not allow 12 hr to pass between any 2 doses using the 3 times per day daily regimen.
2. If gabapentin discontinued or alternate anticonvulsant added to regimen, do gradually over a 1-week period.
3. The first dose on day 1 may be taken at bedtime to minimize somnolence, dizziness, fatigue, and ataxia.

ASSESSMENT

1. Note reasons for therapy, onset, frequency, characteristics of seizures/symptoms, other agents prescribed, outcome. With chronic pain/neuralgia, rate pain level.
2. List other drugs prescribed to ensure none interact.
3. Monitor renal and LFTs; reduce dose in elderly and with impaired renal function.

4. When drug therapy is discontinued or supplemental therapy added, do so gradually over at least 1 week.

CLIENT/FAMILY TEACHING

1. May be taken with or without food. Do not chew or crush; use half tablets within several days of breaking the scored tablet. May take first dose at bedtime to decrease sedative effects.
2. Do not take antacids at any time while taking gabapentin or at least stagger 2 hr apart; decreases drug absorption.
3. If trouble swallowing, may open capsule and mix with applesauce or juice. Mix only one dose at a time just before taking it.
4. May cause dizziness, fatigue, drowsiness, incoordination, and eye twitching. Do not perform any activities that require mental alertness until full drug effects realized.
5. Report any seizures, visual changes, unusual bruising/bleeding, loss of effect, new/unusual side effects. Do not stop suddenly with prolonged therapy.
6. Avoid alcohol, CNS depressants; do not take any OTC agents without approval.
7. Keep all F/U appointments to evaluate labs and response to therapy.

OUTCOMES/EVALUATE

- Control of seizure activity
- Chronic pain control
- Relief postherpetic neuralgia/diabetic neuropathy

Galantamine hydrobromide ℗
(gah-**LAN**-tah-meen)

CLASSIFICATION(S):
Treatment of Alzheimer's disease
PREGNANCY CATEGORY: B
Rx: Razadyne, Razadyne ER.

USES
Treatment of mild to moderate dementia of the Alzheimer's type. *Investigational:* Vascular dementia.

ACTION/KINETICS

Action

The drug is a competitive and reversible inhibitor of acetylcholinesterase. It is believed the drug enhances cholinergic function, which is believed to be impaired in Alzheimer's disease. The drug's effect may lessen as the disease process advances and as fewer cholinergic neurons remain functionally intact. There is no evidence the drug alters the course of the underlying dementing process.

Pharmacokinetics

Well absorbed; absolute bioavailability: 90%. **Time to peak levels, immediate-release:** About 1 hr; **time to peak levels, delayed-release:** 4.5–5 hr. Food does not affect the amount absorbed but does delay the maximum time by 1.5 hr. Metabolized by CYP2D6 and CYP3A4. **t½, terminal:** 7 hr. Mainly excreted in the urine.

CONTRAINDICATIONS

Hypersensitivity to galantamine or any components of the product. Use in those with severe hepatic impairment (Child-Pugh class 10–15) or severe renal impairment or C_{CR} less than 9 mL/min. Lactation, use in children.

SPECIAL CONCERNS

Use with caution in those with severe asthma, obstructive pulmonary disease, or moderately impaired renal function. Possible increase in mortality in clients with mild cognitive impairment due to various vascular causes (e.g., MI, stroke, and sudden death).

SIDE EFFECTS

Most Common

Dry mouth, headache, depression, dizziness, insomnia, N&V, fever, malaise, anorexia, diarrhea, weight decrease, dyspepsia, urinary incontinence, UTI, fatigue/lethargy.

GI: N&V, anorexia, diarrhea, abdominal pain, dyspepsia, constipation, active/occult GI bleeding, PUD, flatulence, gastritis, melena, dysphagia, *rectal hemorrhage*, dry mouth, increased salivation, diverticulitis, gastroenteritis, hiccough, esophageal perforation (rare), upper and lower GI bleeding. **CNS:** Dizziness, headache, tremor, depression, insomnia, somnolence, agitation, confusion, anxiety, hallucination, vertigo, hypertonia, aggression, *convulsions,* paresthesia, ataxia, hypo-/hyperkinesia, apraxia, aphasia, apathy, paroniria, paranoid reaction, increased libido, delirium, suicidal ideation (rare), *suicide* (very rare). **CV:** Bradycardia (rarely severe), AV block, syncope, hyper-/hypotension, chest pain, postural hypotension, *cardiac failure*, palpitation, atrial fibrillation, prolonged QT, BBB, SVT, VT-wave inversion, *myocardial ischemia or infarction*, purpura, TIA, *CVA.* **GU:** UTI, hematuria, urinary retention/hesitancy/difficulty, urinary incontinence, frequent micturition, cystitis, nocturia, renal calculi. **Respiratory:** Rhinitis, URTI, bronchitis, coughing, epistaxis. **Musculoskeletal:** Leg cramps, involuntary muscle contractions. **Hematologic:** Purpura, thrombocytopenia. **Body as a whole:** Weight decrease, fever, malaise, fatigue/lethargy, anemia, peripheral/dependent edema, asthenia, dehydration. **Miscellaneous:** Injury, back/chest pain, fall, injury, tinnitus.

LABORATORY TEST CONSIDERATIONS

↑ Alkaline phosphatase. Hyperglycemia, hypokalemia.

OD OVERDOSE MANAGEMENT

Symptoms: Severe N&V, GI cramping, salivation, lacrimation, urination, defecation, sweating, bradycardia, hypotension, respiratory depression, *collapse, convulsions.* Also, *increasing muscle weakness which may result in death* if respiratory muscles are involved. *Treatment:* IV atropine sulfate at an initial dose of 0.5–1 mg with subsequent doses based on clinical response.

DRUG INTERACTIONS

Amitriptyline / ↓ Galantamine clearance R/T ↓ liver metabolism
Anticholinergic drugs / Possible interference with activity of anticholinergics
Bethanecol / Synergistic effects
Cimetidine / ↑ Galantamine bioavailability
Cholinesterase inhibitors / Synergistic effect
CYP 2D6 or CYP3A4 inhibitors / Possible ↑ galantamine AUC
Erythromycin / ↑ Galantamine AUC R/T

↓ liver metabolism
Fluoxetine / ↓ Galantamine clearance R/T ↓ liver metabolism
Fluvoxamine / ↓ Galantamine clearance R/T ↓ liver metabolism
Ketoconazole / ↑ Galantamine AUC R/T ↓ liver metabolism
Neuromuscular blocking drugs / Possible exaggeration of neuromuscular blockade
Nonsteroidal anti-inflammatory drugs / Galantamine ↑ gastric secretion; monitor for symptoms of active or occult GI bleeding
Paroxetine / ↑ Galantamine bioavailability R/T ↓ liver metabolism
Quinidine / ↓ Galantamine clearance R/T ↓ liver metabolism
Succinylcholine-type drugs / Exaggeration of neuromuscular blocking effects

HOW SUPPLIED

Capsules, Extended-Release: 8 mg, 16 mg, 24 mg; *Oral Solution:* 4 mg/mL; *Tablets:* 4 mg, 8 mg, 12 mg.

DOSAGE

- **CAPSULES, EXTENDED-RELEASE**
  Dementia of the Alzheimer type.
Initial: 8 mg/day; increase the dose to the initial maintenance dose of 16 mg/day after a minimum of 4 weeks. Attempt a further increase to 24 mg/day after a minimum of 4 weeks at 16 mg/day. **Dose range:** 16–24 mg/day.
- **ORAL SOLUTION; TABLETS**
  Dementia of the Alzheimer's type.
Initial: 4 mg twice a day. After a minimum of 4 weeks if this dose is well tolerated, increase to 8 mg twice a day. Attempt a further increase to 12 mg twice a day only after a minimum of 4 weeks. Although a dosage range of 16–32 mg/day given as twice daily dosing is possible, due to side effects the recommended dose range is 16–24 mg/day given as twice a day dosing.

NURSING CONSIDERATIONS

℃ Due to errors confusing Reminyl with Amaryl (glimerpiride: an oral hypoglycemic), the manufacturer has chanced the name from Reminyl to Razadyne.

ADMINISTRATION/STORAGE

1. Do not exceed a dose of 16 mg/day in those with moderately impaired hepatic function (Child-Pugh class 7–9) or in those with moderate renal function impairment.
2. Store all dosage forms from 15–30°C (59–86°F). do not freeze the oral solution.

ASSESSMENT

1. Identify onset/duration of behavioral changes, family history, other agents trialed, outcome.
2. Note cognitive functioning, MMSE/ Alzheimer's Disease Assessment Scale (ADAS-cog), ability to perform ADLs, clinical presentation, family reports.
3. List history of GI bleed, asthma, CAD, COPD, BPH, liver/renal dysfunction; reduce dose with liver/renal dysfunction.
4. Monitor ECG, VS, labs, for GI bleeding; may cause ↑ gastric acid secretion and vagotonic effects.

CLIENT/FAMILY TEACHING

1. Take oral solution or tablets twice daily, with morning and evening meals; take extended-release capsules once in the morning with food.
2. Most side effects occur during periods of increasing dosage. Make dose adjustments no more often than every 4 weeks. Take with food, use prescribed anti-emetics, ensure adequate fluid intake to reduce impact of side effects especially N&V.
3. If therapy interrupted for several days or longer, must restart at the lowest dose and increase back up to the current dose.
4. Report any irregular, slow pulse, dizzy spells, ↑ abdominal pain, urinary difficulty, lack of response, worsening of symptoms. Keep all F/U appointments.

OUTCOMES/EVALUATE

Improved cognitive functioning with Alzheimer's disease

Ganciclovir sodium (DHPG) ■ IV ℃
(gan-**SYE**-kloh-veer)

CLASSIFICATION(S):
Antiviral
PREGNANCY CATEGORY: C
Rx: Cytovene, Vitrasert.

USES

IV: (1) Treatment of CMV retinitis in immunocompromised clients, including those with AIDS. Diagnosis may be confirmed by culture of CMV from the blood, urine, or throat; note that a negative CMV culture does not rule out CMV retinitis. (2) Prevention of CMV disease in transplant clients at risk; duration of treatment depends on duration and degree of immunosuppression.

PO: (1) Alternative to IV for maintenance treatment of CMV retinitis in immunocompromised (including AIDS) clients. (2) Prevention of CMV disease in solid organ transplant clients and in those with advanced HIV infection at risk for developing CMV pneumonitis. *Investigational:* CMV pneumonia in organ transplants, CMV gastroenteritis in those with irritable bowel disease, and CMV pneumonitis.

Intraocular implant: CMV retinitis in those with AIDS.

ACTION/KINETICS

Action

Upon entry into viral cells infected by CMV, ganciclovir is converted to ganciclovir triphosphate by the CMV. Ganciclovir triphosphate inhibits viral DNA synthesis by competitive inhibition of viral DNA polymerases and direct incorporation into viral DNA; this results in eventual termination of viral DNA elongation. Ganciclovir is active against CMV, herpes simplex virus-1 and -2, Epstein-Barr virus, and varicella zoster virus. Use of the intraocular implant causes a significantly slower disease progression than did the use of IV ganciclovir.

Pharmacokinetics

$t\frac{1}{2}$: Approximately 2.9 hr. Believed to cross the blood-brain barrier. Most excreted unchanged through the urine. Renal impairment increases the $t\frac{1}{2}$ of the drug; make dosage adjustments based on C_{CR}.

CONTRAINDICATIONS

Hypersensitivity to acyclovir or ganciclovir. Lactation. Use when the absolute neutrophil count is less than 500/mm³

or the platelet count is less than 25,000/mm³.

SPECIAL CONCERNS

■ (1) Clinical toxicity includes granulocytopenia, anemia, and thrombocytopenia. In animal studies, the drug was carcinogenic, teratogenic, and caused aspermatogenesis. (2) IV ganciclovir is indicated only to treat cytomegalovirus retinitis in immunocompromised clients and for the prevention of CMV disease in transplant clients at risk for CMV disease. (3) The capsules are indicated only for prevention of CMV disease in clients with advanced HIV infection at risk for CMV disease, for maintenance treatment of CMV retinitis in immunocompromised clients, and for prevention of CMV disease in solid organ transplant recipients. (4) Oral ganciclovir is associated with a risk of more rapid rate of CMV retinitis progression; thus, use as maintenance treatment only in those clients for whom this risk is balanced by the benefit associated with avoiding daily IV infusions.■ Safety and effectiveness of ganciclovir have not been established for nonimmunocompromised clients, treatment of other CMV infections such as pneumonitis or colitis, or congenital or neonatal CMV disease. Use with caution in impaired renal function, in elderly clients, or with preexisting cytopenias or with a history of cytopenic reactions to other drugs, chemicals, or irradiation. Use in children only if potential benefits outweigh potential risks, including carcinogenicity and reproductive toxicity. Not a cure for CMV retinitis and progression of the disease may continue in immunocompromised clients. Treatment with zidovudine and ganciclovir (e.g., in AIDS clients) will likely not be tolerated and lead to severe granulocytopenia.

SIDE EFFECTS

Most Common

Diarrhea, fever, rash, leukopenia, anemia, anorexia, vomiting, sweating, infection, neuropathy, chills, sweating, puritus, thrombocyopenia.

Hematologic: Granulocytopenia, thrombocytopenia, neutropenia (may be irreversible), eosinophilia, leukopenia, anemia, hypochromic anemia, bone marrow depression, pancytopenia, **leukemia, lymphoma**. **CNS:** Ataxia, **coma**, neuropathy, confusion, abnormal dreams or thoughts, dizziness, headache, paresthesia, psychosis, nervousness, somnolence, tremor, agitation, amnesia, anxiety, depression, euphoria, hypertonia, hypesthesia, insomnia, manic reaction, **seizures**, trismus, emotional lability. **GI:** N&V, aphthous stomatitis, diarrhea, anorexia, dry mouth, **GI hemorrhage, pancreatitis**, abdominal pain, flatulence, dyspepsia, constipation, dysphagia, esophagitis, eructation, fecal incontinence, melena, mouth ulceration, tongue disorder, hepatitis, weight loss. **CV:** Hypertension or hypotension, arrhythmias, phlebitis, deep thrombophlebitis, **cardiac arrest, intracranial hypertension, MI, stroke**, pericarditis, vasodilation, migraine. **Body as a whole:** Fever, chills, edema, infections, malaise, neuropathy, **sepsis, multiple organ failure**, asthenia, enlarged abdomen, abscess, back pain, cellulitis, chest pain, facial edema, neck pain or rigidity. **Dermatologic:** Rash, sweating, alopecia, pruritus, urticaria, sweating, acne, dry skin, fixed eruption, herpes simplex, maculopapular rash, skin discoloration, vesiculobullous rash, photosensitivity, phototoxicity. **GU:** Hematuria, breast pain, kidney failure, abnormal kidney function, urinary frequency, UTI. **At injection site:** Catheter infection, catheter sepsis, inflammation or pain, abscess, edema, hemorrhage, phlebitis. **Musculoskeletal:** Arthralgia, bone pain, leg cramps, myalgia, myasthenia. **Ophthalmologic:** Abnormal vision, amblyopia, blindness, conjunctivitis, eye pain, glaucoma, retinitis, photophobia, cataracts, vitreous disorder. **Respiratory:** Dyspnea, increased cough, pneumonia. **Hepatic:** Cholestasis, cholangitis. **Miscellaneous:** Abnormal gait, decreased libido, deafness, **anaphylaxis,** taste perversion, tinnitus, acidosis, congenital anomaly, encephalopathy, impotence, transverse myelitis, infertility, splenomegaly, **Stevens-Johnson syndrome, unexplained death**, retinal detachment in CMV retinitis clients.

LABORATORY TEST CONSIDERATIONS
↑ Serum creatinine, BUN, alkaline phosphatase, CPK, LDH, AST, ALT. ↓

Blood glucose. Abnormal LFT. Hypokalemia, hyponatremia.

OD OVERDOSE MANAGEMENT
Symptoms: Neutropenia. Possibility of hypersalivation, anorexia, vomiting, bloody diarrhea, inactivity, cytopenia, testicular atrophy, increased BUN and LFT results. *Treatment:* Hydration, hemodialysis.

DRUG INTERACTIONS
Adriamycin / Additive cytotoxicity in rapidly dividing cells
Amphotericin B / Additive cytotoxicity in rapidly dividing cells; also, ↑ serum creatinine levels
Cyclosporine / ↑ Serum creatinine levels
Cytotoxic drugs / Additive cytotoxicity
Didanosine / ↑ Didanosine AUC
Flucytosine / Additive cytotoxicity in rapidly dividing cells
Imipenem/Cilastatin combination / Possibility of seizures
Nephrotoxicity / ↑ Serum creatinine
Pentamidine / Additive cytotoxicity in rapidly dividing cells
Probenecid / ↑ Effect of ganciclovir R/T ↓ renal excretion
Sulfamethoxazole/Trimethoprim combinations / Additive cytotoxicity in rapidly dividing cells
Vinblastine / Additive cytotoxicity in rapidly dividing cells
Vincristine / Additive cytotoxicity in rapidly dividing cells
Zidovudine / ↑ Risk of neutropenia and anemia

HOW SUPPLIED
Capsules: 250 mg, 500 mg; *Ocular Implant:* 4.5 mg; *Powder for Injection:* 500 mg/vial.

DOSAGE

• **CAPSULES; IV INFUSION**
CMV retinitis.
Induction treatment: 5 mg/kg IV over 1 hr q 12 hr for 14–21 days in clients with normal renal function. Do not use PO treatment for induction. **Maintenance, IV:** 5 mg/kg by IV infusion daily for 7 days or 6 mg/kg/day for 5 days each week. Dosage must be reduced in clients with renal impairment. **Maintenance, PO:** 1,000 mg 3 times per day with food. Or, 500 mg 6 times

---

per day q 3 hr with food during waking hours.

Prevention of CMV retinitis in those with advanced HIV infection and normal renal function.

1,000 mg 3 times/day with food.

Prophylaxis of CMV disease in transplant clients

Initial dose, IV: 5 mg/kg over 1 hr q 12 hr for 7–14 days in those with normal renal function. **Maintenance:** 5 mg/kg/day on 7 days each week (or 6 mg/kg/day on 5 days each week). The PO prophylactic dose is 1,000 mg 3 times per day with food.

In renal impairment, the following dosages are recommended. **IV. C_{CR} 50–69 mL/min:** Induction dose of 2.5 mg/kg q 12 hr and maintenance dose of 2.5 mg/kg q 24 hr; **C_{CR} 25–49 mL/min:** Induction dose of 2.5 mg/kg q 24 hr and maintenance dose of 1.25 mg/kg q 24 hr; **C_{CR} 10–24 mL/min:** Induction dose of 1.25 mg/kg q 24 hr and maintenance dose of 0.625 mg/kg q 24 hr; **C_{CR} <10 mL/min:** Induction dose of 1.25 mg/kg 3 times/week following hemodialysis and maintenance dose of 0.625 mg/kg 3 times/week following hemodialysis. **PO. C_{CR} 50–69 mL/min:** 1,500 mg once daily or 500 mg 3 times/day; **C_{CR} 25–49 mL/min:** 1,000 mg once daily or 500 mg twice a day; **C_{CR} 10–24 mL/min:** 500 mg once daily; **C_{CR} <10 mL/min:** 500 mg 3 times/week after hemodialysis.

• **OCULAR IMPLANT**

CMV retinitis.

The 4.5 mg implant releases the drug over a 5- to 8-month period. Following depletion of the ganciclovir from the implant, it may be removed and replaced.

NURSING CONSIDERATIONS

🕲 Do not confuse Cytovene with Cytosar (an antineoplastic) or Cytotec.

ADMINISTRATION/STORAGE

1. Use capsules only where risk of more rapid progression of the disease is offset by the benefit of avoiding daily IV infusions.

IV 2. Reconstitute by injecting 10 mL sterile water for injection followed by shaking. Discard if particulate matter or discoloration is noted.

3. Parabens is incompatible with ganciclovir; do not use bacteriostatic water for injection for reconstitution.

4. IV infusion concentrations greater than 10 mg/mL are not recommended. Further reconstitute ganciclovir with 100 mL of any of the following solutions: D5W, RL or Ringer's solution, 0.9% NaCl. Infuse over 1 hr. Doses greater than 6 mg/kg infused over 1 hr may result in increased toxicity.

5. Due to high pH (9–11) of reconstituted ganciclovir, do not give IM or SC. Do not give by IV bolus or rapid IV injection.

6. To minimize phlebitis/pain at injection site, give into veins with an adequate blood flow to allow rapid dilution and distribution.

7. Do not exceed 1.25 mg/kg/day in clients undergoing hemodialysis.

8. Reconstituted solution stable for 12 hr at room temperature.

9. Follow guidelines for handling and disposal of cytotoxic drugs. Avoid inhalation and contact with skin. Wear latex gloves and safety glasses and mix under a biologic hood.

ASSESSMENT

1. Note disease onset, other medical conditions, characteristics of S&S, therapies trialed.

2. Confirm CMV retinitis by indirect ophthalmoscopy reports.

3. Assess orientation and mentation levels.

4. Monitor CBC, CD4+ cell count, renal function studies; reduce dose with impaired renal function. Granulocytopenia and thrombocytopenia are side effects of drug therapy; do not administer if neutrophil count drops below 500 cells/mm^3 or plt. count falls below 25,000/mm^3. Concomitant therapy with zidovudine may increase neutropenia.

5. Monitor I&O. Ensure adequate hydration before/during IV therapy.

6. May experience pain/phlebitis at infusion site because pH of *diluted* solution is high (pH 9–11). Follow administration guidelines carefully. Avoid contact with drug.

7. List drugs prescribed and review list of drug interactions; some may induce renal failure, have additive toxicity if given during ganciclovir therapy.

CLIENT/FAMILY TEACHING

1. Not a cure; used to control symptoms. Take tablets with food to increase bioavailability. Ensure adequate hydration

2. Do not interrupt drug therapy, unless by provider; a relapse may occur.

3. Report dizziness, S&S of infection, confusion, bleeding, seizures immediately.

4. Use protection (sunglasses, clothing/hat, sunscreen) with sun exposure to prevent photosensitivity reaction.

5. Have regular eye exams because retinitis may progress to blindness (retinal detachment). Following surgical insertion of the ocular implant, may experience blurred vision in the eye, which clears within two to four weeks. Implant can be removed when depleted of drug, usually within five to eight months, and a new Vitrasert Implant can be inserted. Effect is only on eye and not elsewhere in the body.

6. May impair fertility; determine if candidate for sperm/egg harvesting. During and for 90 days following drug therapy, women of childbearing age should use safe contraception and men should practice barrier contraception; inhibits sperm production.

7. Avoid crowds and persons with known infections. Report any unusual behavior or altered thought processes.

8. Report for scheduled labs; may require dose adjustment or stoppage of therapy.

OUTCOMES/EVALUATE

- ↓ Progression of CMV retinitis
- CMV prophylaxis in transplant and at-risk clients
- Prevention of CMV retinitis in those with advanced HIV infection

Ganirelix acetate
(**gan**-ih-**REL**-icks)

CLASSIFICATION(S):
Gonadotropin-releasing hormone antagonist
PREGNANCY CATEGORY: X
Rx: Antagon.
✤Rx: Orgalutran.

USES
Infertility treatment to inhibit premature LH surges in women undergoing controlled ovarian stimulation.

ACTION/KINETICS
Action
Synthetic decapeptide that antagonizes gonadotropin-releasing hormone (GnRH). Acts by competitively blocking GnRH receptors in the pituitary gland leading to a rapid, reversible suppression of gonadotropin secretion. When discontinued, pituitary LH and FSH levels fully recover within 48 hr.

Pharmacokinetics
Steady state: Within 3 days. Metabolized to peptides. Excreted in both the feces and urine. **t½, elimination:** 16.2 hr after multiple doses.

CONTRAINDICATIONS
Hypersensitivity to ganirelix or any of its components, hypersensitivity to GnRH or GnRH analogs, known or suspected pregnancy. Lactation.

SPECIAL CONCERNS
Use with caution in hypersensitivity to GnRH. Packaging of the product contains natural rubber latex, which may cause allergic reactions.

SIDE EFFECTS
Most Common
Abdominal pain (gynecologic or GI), headache, ovarian hyperstimulation syndrome, vaginal bleeding.

GU: Abdominal pain (gynecologic), **fetal death,** ovarian hyperstimulation syndrome, vaginal bleeding. **CNS:** Headache. **GI:** Nausea, abdominal pain. **Miscellaneous:** Injection site reaction.

LABORATORY TEST CONSIDERATIONS
↑ Neutrophils. ↓ Hematocrit, total bilirubin.

Bold Italic = life threatening side effect   ■ = black box warning   ✤ = Available in Canada

DRUG INTERACTIONS

Because ganirelix suppresses secretion of pituitary gonadotropins, dosage adjustments of exogenous gonadotropins may be necessary when used during controlled ovarian hyperstimulation.

HOW SUPPLIED

Injection: 250 mcg/0.5 mL.

DOSAGE

- **SC ONLY**
  Infertility treatment.

Initiate FSH therapy on day 2 or 3 of the cycle (may reduce exogenous FSH requirement). Give ganirelix, 250 mcg, SC once daily during the early to mid follicular phase. Continue ganirelix treatment daily until the day of chorionic gonadotropion (hCG) treatment. When a sufficient number of follicles of adequate size are present (assess by ultrasound), give hCG to finalize maturation of follicles.

NURSING CONSIDERATIONS

ADMINISTRATION/STORAGE

1. Most convenient sites for SC administration are upper thigh or abdomen around the navel.
2. Swab injection site with disinfectant. Clean about 2 inches around the point where the needle will be inserted. Let the disinfectant dry a minute or more before proceeding.
3. Pinch up a large area of skin between the finger and thumb. Insert the needle at the base of the pinched-up skin at a 45–90° angle to the skin surface.
4. When the needle is positioned correctly, it will be difficult to draw back on the plunger. If the needle tip penetrates a vein (if blood is drawn into the syringe), withdraw the needle slightly and reposition without removing it from the skin. Alternatively, remove the needle and use a new, sterile, prefilled syringe.
5. Once needle is positioned correctly, depress the plunger slowly and steadily so solution is correctly injected and skin is not damaged.
6. Pull the syringe out quickly and apply pressure to site with a swab containing disinfectant. The site should stop bleeding within 1 or 2 min.

7. Use the sterile, prefilled syringe only once and dispose of correctly.
8. Store the syringes at 25°C (77°F). Protect from light.

ASSESSMENT

1. Note reasons for therapy, other medical conditions, duration of infertility, history.
2. Use cautiously in gonadotropin-releasing hormone (GnRH) hypersensitivity.
3. Ensure not pregnant.
4. Product packaging contains latex.

CLIENT/FAMILY TEACHING

1. Drug keeps woman from ovulating too soon when undergoing infertility treatment.
2. Therapy requires SC administration daily during early to mid follicular phases after initial FSH therapy on day 2 or 3 of cycle. It must be continued until day of hCG administration.
3. Will be shown how to administer drug under the skin and the body areas where to inject. Review package insert for proper administration procedure. Rotate sites using the abdomen or upper thigh for injection. Store drug at room temperature away from heat, light, and children. Keep track of where you give each shot to make sure you rotate body areas. Use a new needle and syringe for each administration.
4. An ultrasound is used to check for sufficient number and size of follicles.
5. May experience abdominal pain, fetal death, headache, ovarian hyperstimulation syndrome, unusual vaginal bleeding, nausea, injection site pain/swelling/redness. Report rapid weight gain or bloating, severe/ongoing nausea, vomiting, diarrhea, severe stomach or pelvic pain. Not for use in pregnancy; may cause fetal loss.
6. Therapy requires a long term commitment for administration and F/U and medical visits from user.

OUTCOMES/EVALUATE

Inhibition of premature LH surges during controlled ovarian stimulation

Gatifloxacin

(**gat**-ih-**FLOX**-ah-sin)

CLASSIFICATION(S):
Antibiotic, quinolone
PREGNANCY CATEGORY: C
Rx: Zymar.

SEE ALSO *ANTI-INFECTIVE DRUGS.*

USES

Ophthalmic. Bacterial conjunctivitis due to susceptible strains of *Corynebacterium propinguum, S. aureus, S. epidermidis, Streptococcus mitis, S. pneumoniae,* or *Haemophilis influenzae.*

ACTION/KINETICS

Pharmacokinetics
Used only ophthalmically.

CONTRAINDICATIONS

Hypersensitivity to any component of the product. Use with epithelial herpes, dendritic keratitis, vaccinia, varicella, mycobacterial infections of the eye, or fungal disease of the ocular structure.

SPECIAL CONCERNS

Systemic use may prolong the QTc interval.

SIDE EFFECTS

Most Common
After ophthalmic use: Transient irritation, burning, stinging, itching, inflammation.

Transient irritation, burning, stinging, itching, inflammation, angioneurotic edema, urticaria, vesicular and maculopapular dermatitis.

HOW SUPPLIED

Ophthalmic Solution: 0.3%.

DOSAGE

- **OPHTHALMIC SOLUTION**
  Bacterial conjunctivitis.

Days 1 and 2: 1 gtt in affected eye(s) q 2 hr while awake, up to 8 times per day.
Days 3 through 7: 1 gtt up to 4 times per day while awake.

NURSING CONSIDERATIONS

Ⓒ Do not confuse gatifloxacin with gemifloxacin (also a fluoroquinolone antibiotic).

ADMINISTRATION/STORAGE

Store ophthalmic solution from 15–25°C (59–77°F). Protect from freezing.

ASSESSMENT

Assess for quinolone sensitivity or diabetes; precludes drug therapy.

CLIENT/FAMILY TEACHING

1. Protect the ophthalmic solution from freezing.
2. When instilling eye drops: wash hands; do not allow dropper to touch eye. Tilt head back and look up; pull lower eyelid down; instill prescribed number of drops. Close eye for 1 to 2 min and apply gentle pressure to bridge of nose. Do not rub eye.
3. If more than 1 topical eye drug is being used, administer the drugs at least 5 min apart.
4. Avoid wearing contacts with bacterial conjunctivitis.

OUTCOMES/EVALUATE

Resolution of infection; symptomatic improvement

Gefitinib

(geh-**FIH**-tih-nib)

CLASSIFICATION(S):
Antineoplastic, epidermal growth factor receptor inhibitor
PREGNANCY CATEGORY: D
Rx: Iressa.

USES

Monotherapy for locally advanced or metastatic non-small cell lung cancer after failure of platinum-based and docetaxel chemotherapies. *NOTE:* The drug should be used only in cancer clients who have already taken the drug; new clients should not be started on the medication as it does not improve survival.

ACTION/KINETICS

Action
Mechanism not fully characterized. Gefitinib inhibits intracellular phosphorylation of numerous tyrosine kinases associated with transmembrane cell surface receptors, including the tyrosine

---

Bold Italic = life threatening side effect   ■ = black box warning   ✦ = Available in Canada

kinases associated with epidermal growth factor receptor. Epidermal growth factor receptor is expressed on the cell surface of many normal and cancer cells.

Pharmacokinetics

Slowly absorbed; **peak plasma levels:** 3–7 hr. About 60% bioavailable. Undergoes extensive hepatic metabolism, predominantly by CYP3A4. Cleared mainly by the liver; t½, **terminal:** 48 hr after IV administration. Excreted mainly by the feces (86%) with a small amount (4%) through the urine. **Plasma protein binding:** 90%.

CONTRAINDICATIONS

Severe hypersensitivity to gefitinib or any component of the product. Lactation.

SPECIAL CONCERNS

Pulmonary toxicity (can be fatal) may occur. Has the potential to inhibit the cardiac action potential repolarization (i.e., QT interval); clinical relevance is not known at the present time. Use with caution in impaired renal and hepatic function. Safety and efficacy have not been determined in children.

SIDE EFFECTS

Most Common

Diarrhea, rash, acne, dry skin N&V, pruritus, anorexia, asthenia, weight loss.

Pulmonary: Interstitial lung disease, including interstitial pneumonia, pneumonitis, alveolitis, acute onset dyspnea (sometimes associated with cough or low-grade fever). **GI:** Diarrhea, N&V, anorexia, mouth ulceration, pancreatitis (rare). **Body as a whole:** Rash, pruritus, asthenia, weight loss, **hemorrhage** (including epistaxis and hematuria). **Dermatologic:** Acne, dry skin, vesiculobullous rash; rarely, toxic epidermal necrolysis, erythema multiforme. **Ophthalmic:** Amblyopia, conjunctivitis, eye pain, corneal erosion/ulcer (sometimes with aberrant eyelash growth); very rarely corneal membrane sloughing, ocular ischemia/hemorrhage. **Miscellaneous:** Peripheral edema. Rarely, allergic reactions, including angioedema and urticaria.

DRUG INTERACTIONS

Cimetidine / ↓ Gefitinib levels R/T ↓ GI absorption

CYP3A4 inducers (e.g., phenytoin, rifampin) / ↓ Gefitinib levels R/T ↑ liver metabolism; consider a dosage increase

CYP3A4 inhibitors (e.g., itraconazole, ketoconazole) / ↑ Gefitinib levels R/T ↓ liver metabolism; use together with caution

H₂ histamine antagonists (e.g., cimetidine, ranitidine) / ↓ Gefitinib levels R/T ↑ gastric pH → ↓ efficacy

Metoprolol / ↑ Metoprolol levels

Sodium bicarbonate / ↓ Gefitinib levels R/T ↑ gastric pH → ↓ efficacy

Vinorelbine / Exacerbation of neutropenic effect of vinorelbine

Warfarin / ↑ INR and bleeding events; monitor PT or INR regularly

HOW SUPPLIED

Tablets: 250 mg.

DOSAGE

- **TABLETS**

  Non-small cell lung cancer.

  250 mg/day with or without food. Higher doses do not give a better response and may increase toxicity.

NURSING CONSIDERATIONS

ADMINISTRATION/STORAGE

1. Clients with poorly tolerated diarrhea (possibly with dehydration) or skin toxicity may be successfully managed by up to a 14-day drug free period followed by reinstatement of the 250 mg/day dose.

2. If acute onset or worsening of pulmonary symptoms (e.g., dyspnea, cough, fever) occur, stop gefitinib therapy, evaluate promptly, and begin appropriate treatment. If interstitial lung disease is confirmed, stop therapy and treat appropriately.

3. If new eye symptoms develop (e.g., pain), evaluate and manage appropriately, including stopping gefitinib therapy and removing an aberrant eyelash if present. After symptoms and eye changes resolve, decide on reinitiating the 250 mg/day dose.

4. In those receiving a potent CYP3A4 inducer (e.g., phenytoin or rifampin), consider increasing dose to 500

mg/day, provided there are no severe side effects; carefully monitor response and toxicity.

5. Store tablets at room temperature (20–25°C, 68–77°F).

ASSESSMENT

1. Note reasons for therapy, other agents trialed, outcome. Should only be used in cancer clients who have already taken the drug; new clients should not be started on this drug as it does not improve survival.

2. Monitor CBC, renal and LFTs; reduce dose with dysfunction. List drugs prescribed to ensure none interact.

3. Assess eye findings, lungs sounds, CXR and EKG.

CLIENT/FAMILY TEACHING

1. Take exactly as directed with or without food.

2. Stop drug and report any persistent diarrhea, increased SOB, N&V, eye problems, or rash.

3. Consume adequate fluids to prevent dehydration.

4. Practice reliable contraception. Avoid pregnancy; may harm fetus.

5. Review side effects related to pulmonary toxicity which may be lethal. Keep all F/U appointments and evaluations.

OUTCOMES/EVALUATE

Inhibition of malignant cell proliferation

Gemcitabine hydrochloride [IV]

(jem-**SIGHT**-ah-been)

CLASSIFICATION(S):
Antineoplastic, miscellaneous
PREGNANCY CATEGORY: D
Rx: Gemzar.

SEE ALSO *ANTINEOPLASTIC AGENTS.*

USES

(1) In combination with paclitaxel as first-line treatment of metastatic breast cancer after failure of prior anthracycline-containing adjuvant chemotherapy, unless anthracyclines were contraindicated. (2) In combination with cisplatin as first-line treatment of inoperable, locally advanced (stage IIIA or IIIB) or metastatic (stage IV) non-small cell lung cancer. (3) In combination with carboplatin for advanced ovarian cancer that has relapsed at least 6 months after completion of platinum-based therapy. (4) As first-line treatment of locally advanced (nonresectable stage II or stage III) or metastatic (stage IV) adenocarcinoma of the pancreas. Indicated for those previously treated with 5-fluorouracil. *Investigational:* Biliary cancer, bladder cancer, relapsed or refractory testicular cancer, squamous cell carcinoma of the head and neck.

ACTION/KINETICS

Action

A nucleoside analog that kills cells undergoing DNA synthesis (S-phase) and by blocking the progression of cells through the G1/S-phase boundary. Metabolized within cells by nucleoside kinases to the active gemcitabine diphosphate and triphosphate nucleosides. The diphosphate inhibits ribonucleotide reductase, which is responsible for catalyzing reactions that generate the deoxynucleoside triphosphate for DNA synthesis. Inhibition of the reductase enzyme causes a decrease in the levels of deoxynucleotides. The triphosphate competes with triphosphate nucleosides for incorporation into DNA, resulting in inhibition of DNA synthesis. DNA polymerase is not able to remove the gemcitabine nucleoside and repair the growing DNA strands.

Pharmacokinetics

The metabolite of gemcitabine nucleoside is excreted through the urine. $t\frac{1}{2}$, **short infusions:** 42-94 min; $t\frac{1}{2}$, **long infusions:** 245-638 min (depends on age and gender). Higher levels are found in women and the elderly due to lower clearance.

CONTRAINDICATIONS

Lactation.

SPECIAL CONCERNS

Use with caution in those with preexisting renal impairment or hepatic insufficiency. Safety and efficacy have not been determined in children.

SIDE EFFECTS

Most Common

N&V, anemia, leukopenia, neutropenia, pain, fever, dyspnea, thrombocytopenia, constipation, diarrhea, hemorrhage, infection, alopecia.

Side effects include those observed with combination therapy. **GI:** N&V, diarrhea, constipation, stomatitis, anorexia, pharyngitis. **CNS:** Somnolence, mild to severe paresthesias, insomnia, neuropathy (motor and sensory). **CV:** Arrhythmia, hypotension, hypertension, CHF, *MI*, *CVA*, gangrene, vasculitis. **Hematologic:** Anemia, leukopenia, neutropenia, thrombocytopenia, platelet transfusions. **Respiratory:** Dyspnea, bronchospasm, cough, rhinitis, rarely parenchymal lung toxicity, including adult respiratory distress syndrome, interstitial pneumonitis, pulmonary edema, and pulmonary fibrosis, *respiratory failure, death* (rare). **Muscluoskeletal:** Myalgia, arthralgia, bone pain. **Dermatologic:** Alopecia, rash, desquamation, macular or finely granular maculopapular pruritic eruptions, pruritus, hair loss (minimal), cellulitis, injection site reactions, bullous skin eruptions. **GU:** Renal failure, hemolytic uremic syndrome. **Body as a whole:** Pain, fever, fatigue, peripheral edema; flu syndrome (including fever), asthenia, chills, sweating, malaise. **Miscellaneous:** *Hemorrhage, sepsis,* infections, petechiae, anaphylaxis (rare).

LABORATORY TEST CONSIDERATIONS

↑ ALT, AST, alkaline phosphatase, bilirubin, BUN, creatinine, GGT. Proteinuria, hematuria, hyperglycemia, hypocalcemia, hypomagnesemia.

OD OVERDOSE MANAGEMENT

Symptoms: Myelosuppression, paresthesias, severe rash. *Treatment:* Monitor with appropriate blood counts. Supportive therapy as needed.

DRUG INTERACTIONS

↓ Clearance and ↑ gemcitabine levels when given with paclitaxel.

HOW SUPPLIED

Powder for Injection, Lyophilized: 200 mg, 1 gram.

DOSAGE

- **IV ONLY**

Metastatic breast cancer not responding to anthracycline-containing adjuvant chemotherapy.

Gemcitabine, 1,250 mg/m^2 by IV infusion over 30 min on days 1 and 8 of each 21-day cycle and paclitaxel, 175 mg/m^2 by IV infusion over 3 hr before the administration of gemcitabine on day 1.

Adjust the gemcitabine dosage as follows for hematological toxicity based on granulocyte and platelet counts taken on day 8 of therapy: (a) If the absolute granulocyte count is greater than or equal to 1,200 x 10^6/L and the platelet count is greater than 75,000 x 10^6/L, give 100% of the full dose. (b) If the absolute granulocyte count is between 1,000 and 1,199 x 10^6/L or the platelet count is between 50,000 and 75,000 x 10^6/L, give 75% of the full dose. (c) If the absolute granulocyte count is between 700 and 999 x 10^6/L and the platelet count is greater than or equal to 50,000 x 10^6/L, give 50% of the full dose. (d) If the absolute granulocyte count is less than 700 x 10^6/L or the platelet count is less than 50,000 x 10^6/L, withhold the dose.

Non-small cell lung cancer.

Two schedules are used. (1) Four-week schedule: Gemcitabine, 1,000 mg/m^2 over 30 min on days 1, 8, and 15 of each 28-day cycle. Give cisplatin, IV, 100 mg/m^2 on day 1 after gemcitabine. (2) Three-week schedule: Gemcitabine, 1,250 mg/m^2 over 30 min on days 1 and 8 of each 21-day cycle. Give cisplatin, IV, 100 mg/m^2 after gemcitabine on day 1. Dosage modifications may be required for hematological toxicity.

Ovarian cancer.

Adults: Gemcitabine 1,000 mg/m^2 over 30 min on days 1 and 8 of each 21-day cycle plus carboplatin AUC 4 should be given IV on day 1 after gemcitabine administration. Monitor clients prior to each dose; clients should have an absolute granulocyte count of 1,500 x 10^6/L or greater and a platelet count of 100,000 x 10^6/L or greater prior to each cycle.

If marrow suppression is observed on day 8 of therapy within a treatment cycle, use the following dosage modifications: (a) If the absolute granulocyte count is 1,500 x 10^6/L or greater and the platelet count is 100,000 x 10^6/L or greater, give 100% of the full dose; (b) If the absolute granulocyte count is between 1,000 and 1,499 x 10^6/L and/or the platelet count is between 75,000 and 99,999 x 10^6/L, give 50% of the dose. (c) If the absolute granulocyte count is less than 1,000 x 10^6/L and/or the platelet count is less than 75,000 x 10^6/L, withhold the dose.

The dose of gemcitabine should be reduced to 800 mg/m^2 on days 1 and 8 in case of any of the following hematologic toxicities: (a) Absolute granulocyte count less than 500 x 10^6/L for more than 5 days; (b) absolute granulocyte count less than 100 x 10^6/L for more than 3 days; (c) febrile neutropenia; (d) platelets less than 25,000 x 10^6/L; (e) cycle delay of more than 1 week because of toxicity.

Adenocarcinoma of the pancreas.
Adults: 1,000 mg/m^2 given over 30 min once a week for up to 7 weeks (or until toxicity necessitates reducing or holding a dose). This is followed by a 1-week rest period. Subsequent cycles should consist of infusions once a week for 3 consecutive weeks out of 4. Those who complete the entire 7 weeks of initial therapy or a subsequent 3-week cycle at the 1,000-mg/m^2 dose may have the dose for subsequent cycles increased by 25% to 1,250 mg/m^2 provided that the absolute neutrophil count nadir exceeds 1,500 × 10^6/L and the platelet nadir exceeds 100,000 × 10^6/L and if nonhematologic toxicity has not been greater than World Health Organization Grade 1. If clients tolerate a dose of 1,250 mg/m^2 once weekly, the dose for the next cycle can be increased to 1,500 mg/m^2 provided the absolute neutrophil count and platelet nadirs are as defined above.
The dose should be reduced to 75% of the full dose if the absolute granulocyte count is 500–999 × 10^6/L and the platelet count is 50,000–99,000 × 10^6/L. The dose should be held if the absolute granulocyte count falls below 500 × 10^6/L and the platelet count falls below 50,000 × 10^6/L.

NURSING CONSIDERATIONS
ADMINISTRATION/STORAGE
IV 1. To reconstitute drug, use 0.9% NaCl injection without preservatives. The maximum concentration upon reconstitution is 40 mg/mL; greater concentrations may cause incomplete dissolution.

2. Give over 30 min; prolonging infusion time beyond 60 min and more frequent administration than once weekly increases toxicity.

3. To reconstitute, add 5 mL of 0.9% NaCl to the 200-mg vial or 25 mL to the 1-gram vial. Shake to dissolve. This results in a concentration of 40 mg/mL which may be further diluted, if needed, with 0.9% NaCl to concentrations as low as 0.1 mg/mL.

4. Do not refrigerate reconstituted drug as crystallization may occur. Store diluted product at controlled room temperatures of 20–25°C (68–77°F). Reconstituted solutions are stable at these temperatures for 24 hr.

ASSESSMENT
1. Note disease stage, onset, symptoms, organ(s) involved, and other therapies trialed.

2. Monitor CBC prior to each dose; check liver and renal function tests periodically; causes thrombocytopenia and myelosuppression. Nadir: 1 week.

CLIENT/FAMILY TEACHING
1. Anticipate IV therapy once weekly over 30 min for up to 7 weeks; then weekly for 3 out of every 4 weeks.

2. May experience fever and flu-like symptoms as well as a rash involving trunk and extremities.

3. Report any evidence of blood or pain with voiding.

4. Use reliable birth control during and for several months following therapy; can cause fetal harm.

OUTCOMES/EVALUATE
Suppression of malignant cell proliferation

Bold Italic = life threatening side effect   ■ = black box warning   ✚ = Available in Canada

Gemfibrozil ©

(jem-**FIH**-broh-zill)

CLASSIFICATION(S):
Antihyperlipidemic, fibric acid derivative

PREGNANCY CATEGORY: C

Rx: Lopid.

❀**Rx:** Apo-Gemfibrozil, Gen-Gemfibrozil, Novo-Gemfibrozil, Nu-Gemfibrozil, PMS-Gemfibrozil.

USES

(1) Hypertriglyceridemia (type IV and type V hyperlipidemia) unresponsive to dietary control or in clients who are at risk of pancreatitis and abdominal pain. (2) Reduce risk of coronary heart disease in clients with type IIb hyperlipidemia who have not responded to diet, weight loss, exercise, and other drug therapy.

ACTION/KINETICS

Action

Gemfibrozil, a fibric acid derivative, decreases triglycerides, cholesterol, and VLDL and increases HDL; LDL levels either decrease or do not change. Also, decreases hepatic triglyceride production by inhibiting peripheral lipolysis and decreasing extraction of free fatty acids by the liver. Also, gemfibrozil decreases VLDL synthesis by inhibiting synthesis of VLDL carrier apolipoprotein B, as well as inhibits peripheral lipolysis and decreases hepatic extraction of free fatty acids (thus decreasing hepatic triglyceride production). May be beneficial in inhibiting development of atherosclerosis.

Pharmacokinetics

Onset: 2–5 days. **Peak plasma levels:** 1–2 hr; **t½:** 1.5 hr. Metabolized in the liver with nearly 70% excreted in the urine.

CONTRAINDICATIONS

Gallbladder disease, primary biliary cirrhosis, hepatic or renal dysfunction. Lactation.

SPECIAL CONCERNS

Safety and efficacy have not been established in children. The dose may have to be reduced in geriatric clients due to age-related decreases in renal function.

SIDE EFFECTS

Most Common

Fatigue, vertigo, dyspepsia, eczema, rash, abdominal pain, diarrhea, N&V.

GI: Cholelithiasis, abdominal/epigastric pain, N&V, diarrhea, dyspepsia, constipation, acute appendicitis, colitis, **pancreatitis**, cholestatic jaundice, hepatoma. **CNS:** Dizziness, headache, fatigue, vertigo, somnolence, paresthesia, hypesthesia, depression, confusion, syncope, peripheral neuritis, **seizures**. **CV:** Atrial fibrillation, extrasystoles, peripheral vascular disease, **intracerebral hemorrhage**. **Hematopoietic:** Anemia, leukopenia, eosinophilia, thrombocytopenia, bone marrow hypoplasia. **Musculoskeletal:** Painful extremities, arthralgia, myalgia, myopathy, myositis, myasthenia, rhabdomyolysis, synovitis. **Allergic:** Urticaria, lupus-like syndrome, **angioedema**, **laryngeal edema**, vasculitis, **anaphylaxis**. **Dermatologic:** Eczema, dermatitis, pruritus, skin rashes, exfoliative dermatitis, alopecia. **GU:** Impotence, decreased libido/male fertility, impaired renal function, UTI. **Ophthalmic:** Blurred vision, retinal edema, cataracts. **Miscellaneous:** Increased chance of viral and bacterial infections, taste perversion, weight loss.

LABORATORY TEST CONSIDERATIONS

↑ AST, ALT, LDH, CPK, alkaline phosphatase, bilirubin. Hypokalemia, hyperglycemia. Positive antinuclear antibody. ↓ Hemoglobin, WBCs, hematocrit.

OD **OVERDOSE MANAGEMENT**

Symptoms: Abdominal cramping, N&V, diarrhea, abnormal LFTs, ↑ Serum creatine phosphokinase, joint and muscle pain.

DRUG INTERACTIONS

Anticoagulants, oral / ↑ Anticoagulant effects; adjust dosage

Cyclosporine / ↓ Cyclosporine effect

Lovastatin / Possible rhabdomyolysis

Pioglitazone / ↑ Pioglitazone AUC R/T inhibition of the CYP2C8 isoenzyme

Repaglinide / Significant ↑ repaglinide levels R/T ↓ metabolism by CYP2C8

Rosiglitazone / ↑ Rosiglitazone AUC R/T

inhibition of the CYP2C8 isoenzyme
Rosuvastatin / Two-fold ↑ Rosuvastatin levels
Simvastatin / Possible rhabdomyolysis
Sulfonylureas / ↑ Hypoglycemic effect

HOW SUPPLIED
Tablets: 600 mg.

DOSAGE

- **TABLETS**
  Hypertriglyceridemia, hyperlipidemia.
Adults: 600 mg twice a day 30 min before the morning and evening meal. Dosage has not been established in children. Discontinue if significant improvement not observed within 3 months.

NURSING CONSIDERATIONS

ℂ Do not confuse gemfibrozil with gemifloxacin (a fluoroquinolone antibiotic) or Lopid with Lorabid (a beta-lactam antibiotic).

ASSESSMENT

1. Note reasons for therapy, other agents trialed, outcome, serum HDL and TG levels.
2. Monitor CBC, blood sugars, (HbA1c), CPK, LFTs; identify risk factors. Assess for gall bladder disease, liver/renal dysfunction.
3. Assess compliance with therapeutic regimens/life-style changes i.e., restriction of fat in diet, blood sugar control, weight reduction, regular exercise, avoidance of alcohol.

CLIENT/FAMILY TEACHING

1. Take 30 min before meals as directed-pill is rather large so use care when swallowing; continue to follow prescribed dietary guidelines restricting sugar and CHO, and regular exercise program to reduce risk factors.
2. Use caution when driving/performing dangerous tasks until drug effects realized; may experience dizziness, blurred vision.
3. Report unusual bruising/bleeding. If also on anticoagulant therapy, a reduction in anticoagulant may be necessary.
4. Limit intake of alcohol. Report any muscle pain/cramps, RUQ abdominal pain or change in stool color or consistency.
5. Report any S&S of gallstones, such as abdominal pain and vomiting.
6. Keep all F/U appointments to evaluate liver and renal function, cholesterol panel, adverse side effects, and response to therapy.

OUTCOMES/EVALUATE

↓ Cholesterol and triglyceride levels ↑ HDL

Gemifloxacin mesylate
(gem-ih-**FLOCK**-sah-sin)

CLASSIFICATION(S):
Antibiotic, fluoroquinolone
PREGNANCY CATEGORY: C
Rx: Factive.

SEE ALSO *FLUOROQUINOLONES.*

USES

(1) Acute bacterial exacerbation of chronic bronchitis due to *Streptococcus pneumoniae, Haemophilus influenzae, H. parainfluenzae,* or *Moraxella catarrhalis.* (2) Community-acquired pneumonia (mild to moderate) due to *S. pneumoniae* (including multi-drug resistant strains), *H. influenzae, M. catarrhalis, Mycoplasma pneumoniae, Chlamydia pneumoniae,* or *Klebsiella pneumoniae.*

NOTE: To prevent development of drug-resistant bacteria and maintain efficacy, use only to treat infections proven or strongly suspected to be caused by susceptible bacteria.

ACTION/KINETICS

Pharmacokinetics

Rapidly absorbed from the GI tract. **Peak plasma levels:** 0.5–2 hr. About 71% of the drug is bioavailable. Food does not affect absorption. Widely distributed throughout the body after PO administration. A small percentage is metabolized in the liver. Unchanged drug and metabolites are excreted in the feces (about 61%) and urine (about 36%). **t½, elimination:** About 7 hr.

CONTRAINDICATIONS

Hypersensitivity to gemifloxacin, fluoroquinolone antibiotics, or any component of the product. Use in clients with a history of prolongation of the QTc interval, those with uncorrected electrolyte disorders (hypokalemia, hypomagnesemia), in clients taking class IA (e.g., quinidine, procainamide) or class III (e.g., amiodarone, sotalol) antiarrhythmic drugs. Lactation.

SPECIAL CONCERNS

Use reduced dosage in clients with a C_{CR} <40 mL/min. Safety and efficacy have not been determined in children <18 years old, in pregnancy, or during lactation. Use with caution when given with erythromycin, antipsychotics, and tricyclic antidepressants and in clients with ongoing proarrhythmic conditions (clinically significant bradycardia, acute myocardial ischemia) due to possible prolongation of QTc interval. Possibility of prolongation of the QTc interval increases with increasing doses.

SIDE EFFECTS

Most Common

Nausea, GI upset, anorexia, diarrhea, drowsiness, dizziness, headache, dry mouth, altered taste, constipation, insomnia.

GI: N&V, diarrhea, GI upset, abdominal pain, taste perversion, anorexia, constipation, dry mouth, dyspepsia, flatulence, gastritis, gastroenteritis, nonspecified GI disorder. **CNS:** Headache, dizziness, insomnia, somnolence/drowsiness, nervousness, vertigo. **Dermatologic:** Rash, dermatitis, pruritus, urticaria, eczema, flushing. **CV:** Prolongation of QT interval. **Hypersensitivity: Anaphylaxis, CV collapse, hypotension/shock, acute respiratory distress, seizures,** loss of consciousness, tingling, angioedema, bronchospasm, shortness of breath, dyspnea, urticaria, itching, serious skin reactions. **Hematologic:** Leukopenia, thrombocythemia, anemia, eosinophilia, granulocytopenia, thrombocytopenia. **Musculoskeletal:** Back pain, leg cramps, myalgia. **Respiratory:** Dyspnea, pharyngitis, pneumonia. **GU:** Genital moniliasis, vaginitis, abnormal urine. **Body as a whole:** Arthralgia, fatigue, fungal infection, moniliasis, asthenia, pain, tremor. **Miscellaneous:** Hot flashes, vision abnormality.

LABORATORY TEST CONSIDERATIONS

↑ ALT, AST, creatine phosphokinase, GGT, potassium, alkaline phosphatase, total bilirubin, BUN, serum creatinine, calcium. ↓ Sodium, albumin, total protein. Hyperglycemia, bilirubinemia.

DRUG INTERACTIONS

Antacids, Al- or Mg-containing / ↓ Absorption of gemifloxacin from the GI tract

Didanosine (chewable/buffered tablets, pediatric powder for PO solution) / ↓ Absorption of gemifloxacin from the GI tract

Ferrous sulfate or iron-containing products / ↓ Absorption of gemifloxacin from the GI tract

Probenecid / Significant ↑ in gemifloxacin AUC and prolongation of half-life

Sucralfate / ↓ Absorption of gemifloxacin from the GI tract

HOW SUPPLIED

Tablets: 320 mg.

DOSAGE

- **TABLETS**

  Acute bacterial exacerbation of chronic bronchitis

  One 320 mg tablet daily for 5 days.

  Mild to moderate community-acquired pneumonia.

  One 320 mg tablet daily for 7 days.

  NOTE: For both uses, a dose of 160 mg q 24 hr should be used in those with C_{CR} of 40 mL/min or less and in those requiring routine hemodialysis or continuous ambulatory peritoneal dialysis.

NURSING CONSIDERATIONS

🕮 Do not confuse gemifloxacin with gatifloxacin (also a fluoroquinolone antibiotic).

ADMINISTRATION/STORAGE

Store from 15–30°C (59–86°F) protected from light.

ASSESSMENT

1. Note reasons for therapy, characteristics of S&S, other agents trialed/outcome, culture results. Review family history for QT prolongation.
2. Determine sensitivity reactions. Assess for CNS effects such as anxiety, tremors.

3. Monitor EKG, CBC, LFTs; liver enzymes may become elevated during therapy but should resolve.

CLIENT/FAMILY TEACHING

1. May take without regard to meals. Swallow tablets whole with a liberal amount of liquid.

2. Complete entire therapy even if feeling better to prevent resistance to antibiotic.

3. Allow 3 hr before or 2 hr after dosing if using calcium, iron, sucrafatre, multivits with zinc, or antacids.

4. Avoid activities that require mental alertness until drug effects realized. May experience tremors and anxiety; report.

5. Use protection when exposed; avoid excessive exposure to sunlight.

6. Report persistent diarrhea. Consume adequate fluids to prevent dehydration.

7. Stop drug and report any pain, inflammation, or tendon rupture. Avoid OTC agents without provider approval. Report adverse side effects or lack of response.

8. Women on hormone therapy may experience rash as well as clients under age 40; stop drug if evident and report.

OUTCOMES/EVALUATE

Resolution of infection

Gemtuzumab ozogamicin ■ IV

(gem-**TOO**-zeh-mab oh-zoh-**GAM**-ih-sin)

CLASSIFICATION(S):

Antineoplastic, monoclonal antibody

PREGNANCY CATEGORY: D

Rx: Mylotarg.

USES

Treatment of CD33 positive acute myeloid leukemia in first relapse in those 60 years or older who are not candidates for other cytotoxic chemotherapy.

ACTION/KINETICS

Action

Composed of a recombinant humanized IgG$_4$ kappa antibody conjugated with a cytotoxic antitumor antibiotic (calicheamicin). Binding of the anti-CD33 antigen forms a complex that is internalized. Upon internalization, the calicheamicin derivative is released inside the lysosomes of the myeloid cell. The released calicheamicin derivative binds to DNA in the minor groove resulting in DNA double strand breaks and cell death. The drug is cytotoxic to the CD33 positive HL-60 human leukemia cell line. There is significant myelosuppression but this is reversible because pluripotent hematopoietic stem cells are spared.

Pharmacokinetics

$t\frac{1}{2}$, **elimination, after first dose:** About 45 hr for total and 100 hr for unconjugated calicheamicin. $t\frac{1}{2}$, **elimination, after second dose:** About 60 hr for total calicheamicin, while $t\frac{1}{2}$ for unconjugated calicheamicin did not change from the first dose. Appears to be metabolized by liver microsomes.

CONTRAINDICATIONS

Hypersensitivity to gemtuzumab ozogamicin or any of its components: Anti-CD33 antibody, calicheamicin derivatives, or inactive ingredients. Lactation.

SPECIAL CONCERNS

■ (1) Give under the supervision of a health care provider experienced in the treatment of acute leukemia and in facilities equipped to monitor and treat leukemia clients. (2) There are no controlled trials demonstrating efficacy and safety using gemtuzumab in combination with other chemotherapeutic agents. Therefore, use gemtuzumab only as a single agent chemotherapy and not in combination chemotherapy regimens outside clinical trials. (3) Severe myelosuppression occurs when gemtuzumab is used at recommended doses. (4) Gemtuzumab administration can result in severe hypersensitivity reactions (including anaphylaxis) and other infusion-related reactions that may include severe pulmonary events. Infrequently, hypersensitivity reactions and pulmonary events have been fatal. In most cases, infusion-related symptoms occurred during the infusion or within

24 hr of administration of gemtuzumab and resolved. Interrupt gemtuzumab infusion for clients experiencing dyspnea or clinically significant hypotension. Monitor clients until signs and symptoms completely resolve. Strongly consider discontinuation of treatment for clients who develop anaphylaxis, pulmonary edema, or acute respiratory distress syndrome. Because clients with high peripheral blast counts may be at greater risk for pulmonary events and tumor lysis syndrome, consider leukoreduction with hydroxyurea or leukapheresis to reduce the peripheral white count to below 30,000/mcL before administration of gemtuzumab. (5) Hepatotoxicity, including severe hepatic venoocclusive disease, has been reported in association with the use of gemtuzumab as a single agent, as part of a combination chemotherapy regimen, and in clients without a history of liver disease or hematopoietic stem-cell transplant. Clients who receive gemtuzumab either before or after hematopoietic stem-cell transplant, clients with underlying hepatic disease or abnormal liver function, and clients receiving gemtuzumab in combination with other chemotherapy are at increased risk for developing venoocclusive disease, including severe venoocclusive disease. Death from liver failure and from venoocclusive disease has been reported in clients who received gemtuzumab. Monitor clients carefully for symptoms of hepatotoxicity, particularly venoocclusive disease. These symptoms can include rapid weight gain, right upper quadrant pain, hepatomegaly, ascites, and elevations in bilirubin and/or liver enzymes. However, careful monitoring may not identify all clients at risk or prevent the complications of hepatotoxicity.■ Use with caution in hepatic impairment. Safety and efficacy have not been determined in children.

SIDE EFFECTS

Most Common

N&V, fever, chills, thrombocytopenia, leukopenia, headache, diarrhea, abdominal pain, anorexia, constipation, stomatitis, mucositis, anemia, hypokalemia, dyspnea, epsitaxis, asthenia. sepsis.

Myelosuppression: Grade 3 or 4 neutropenia, anemia, and/or thrombocytopenia. **GI:** Mucositis, abdominal pain, stomatitis, hepatotoxicity, N&V, diarrhea, anorexia, constipation, gum hemorrhage, dyspepsia, *venoocclusive disease*. **CV:** Bleeding, including epistaxis; *hemorrhage*, hyper-/hypotension, tachycardia. **CNS:** Depression, dizziness, anxiety, headache, insomnia. **Respiratory:** Dyspnea, epistaxis, hypoxia, increased cough, pharyngitis, pneumonia, rales, rhonchi, change in breath sounds, rhinitis. **Dermatologic:** Herpes simplex, rash, local reaction, peripheral edema, ecchymosis, pruritus, petechiae. **Musculoskeletal:** Back pain, myalgia. **GU:** Hematuria, metrorrhagia, *vaginal hemorrhage.* **Infusion reactions:** *Severe hypersensitivity, anaphylaxis, fatal pulmonary events*, tumor lysis syndrome. **Body as a whole:** Infections (grade 3 or 4), including opportunistic infections; arthralgia, asthenia, chills, fever, neutropenic fever, pain, *sepsis.* **Miscellaneous:** Enlarged abdomen, abdominal pain, back pain, peripheral edema.

LABORATORY TEST CONSIDERATIONS

↑ ALT, AST, alkaline phosphatase, bilirubin, LDH, creatinine. Hypokalemia, hypomagnesemia, hyper-/hypoglycemia, hypocalcemia, hypophosphatemia. Changes in hemoglobin, total absolute neutrophils, WBCs, lymphocytes, platelet count, PT/PTT.

HOW SUPPLIED

Powder for Injection, Lyophilized: 5 mg.

DOSAGE

• **IV**

   Acute myeloid leukemia.

Adults: 9 mg/m^2 as a 2-hr infusion. Give the following prophylactic medications 1 hr before gemtuzumab: Diphenhydramine, 50 mg PO and acetaminophen, 650–1,000 mg PO. Thereafter, 2 additional doses of acetaminophen, 650–1,000 mg PO q 4 hr as needed. The recommended treatment course for gemtuzumab is a total of 2 doses, 14 days apart. *NOTE:* Consider leukoreduction with hydroxyurea or leukapheresis to reduce the peripheal WBC count to below 30,000/mcL before giving gemtuzumab.

NURSING CONSIDERATIONS

ADMINISTRATION/STORAGE

IV 1. Methylprednisolone given before gemtuzumab may reduce infusion-related symptoms.

2. Full recovery from hematologic toxicity is not a requirement for administration of a second dose of gemtuzumab.

3. Protect from direct and indirect sunlight and unshielded fluorescent light during preparation and administration of the infusion.

4. Prepare in a biologic safety hood with the fluorescent light off.

5. Prior to reconstitution, allow drug vials to come to room temperature.

6. Reconstitute each vial with 5-mL sterile water for injection, using sterile syringes. Gently swirl each vial. The final concentration is 1 mg/mL.

7. Inspect visually for particulate matter and discoloration following reconstitution and prior to administration.

8. Withdraw desired volume from each vial and inject into a 100-mL IV bag of 0.9% NaCl injection. Place the 100-mL bag into a UV protectant bag. Use the resulting drug solution in the IV bag immediately.

9. Do not give as an IV push or bolus.

10. Give over 2 hr. Use a separate IV line equipped with a low protein-binding 1.2-micron terminal filter. May be given peripherally or through a central line.

11. Only dilute with 0.9% NaCl solution; do not dilute with any other electrolyte solution or D5W; do not mix with other drugs and do not coadminister other drugs through the same infusion line.

12. To reduce the risk of a severe pulmonary event, consider reducing the peripheral WBC count with hydroxyurea therapy or leukapheresis before giving gemtuzumab.

13. Store refrigerated at 2–8°C (36–46°F) and protect from light. While in the vial, the reconstituted drug may be stored refrigerated and protected from light for 8 hr or less.

ASSESSMENT

1. Note indications for therapy, CD33 receptor determined before treatment started, date of first treatment for CD33 AML, why client not candidate for cytotoxic chemotherapy.

2. Premedicate with diphenhydramine and acetaminophen/steroids to help control side effects.

3. Monitor CBC, electrolytes, uric acid, and LFTs; use cautiously with any liver impairment. Stop if hepatomegaly, ascites, elevation in LFTS or bilirubin.

4. Ensure adequate hydration and medication (allopurinol) to prevent hyperuricemia.

5. Assess for myelosuppression and thrombocytopenia; nadir: days 35–45.

CLIENT/FAMILY TEACHING

1. This antibody attaches to the CD33 receptor and is taken into the cell, along with the chemotherapy. This kills the leukemic cell. 80% of AML clients have this receptor.

2. Report any fever, sore throat, or S&S of infections. May experience a post infusion reaction during the first 24 hr after administration; use acetaminophen every 4 hr prn to control.

3. Avoid hazardous activities, contact sports, or other situations and tasks; may experience dizziness and confusion. Protect from injury/infection during bone marrow suppression.

4. Report any unusual bruising or bleeding or dark tarry stools.

5. Do not touch your eyes or the inside of your nose unless you have just washed your hands and have not touched anything else.

6. Report any S&S of liver toxicity or venoocclusive disease i.e., RUQ pain, rapid wt gain, ascites, yellow skin/eye discoloration.

7. Avoid immunizations during therapy as drug lowers body resistance. Avoid persons with infections and those who have recently received live virus vaccines (polio).

8. Keep all F/U appointments and report all adverse effects.

OUTCOMES/EVALUATE

Hematologic improvement/recovery with AML

Bold Italic = life threatening side effect   ■ = black box warning   ♣ = Available in Canada

Gentamicin sulfate

■ IV

(jen-tah-**MY**-sin)

CLASSIFICATION(S):
Antibiotic, aminoglycoside
PREGNANCY CATEGORY: C
Rx: Injection: Pediatric Gentamicin Sulfate. **Ophthalmic Ointment:** Garamycin, Genoptic S.O.P., Gentak. **Ophthalmic Solution:** Garamycin, Genoptic, Gentacidin.
✦Rx: Alcomicin, Minims Gentamicin, ratio-Gentamicin.

SEE ALSO *AMINOGLYCOSIDES.*

USES
Injection: (1) Serious infections of the conjunctiva or cornea caused by *Pseudomonas aeruginosa, Proteus, Klebsiella, Enterobacter, Serratia, Citrobacter,* and *Staphylococcus.* Infections include bacterial neonatal sepsis, bacterial septicemia, and serious infections of the skin, bone, soft tissue (including burns), urinary tract, GI tract (including peritonitis), and CNS (including meningitis). Should be considered as initial therapy in suspected or confirmed gram-negative infections. (2) In combination with carbenicillin for treating life-threatening infections due to *P. aeruginosa.* (3) In combination with penicillin for treating endocarditis caused by group D streptococci. (4) In combination with penicillin for treating suspected bacterial sepsis or staphylococcal pneumonia in the neonate. (5) Intrathecal administration is used in combination with systemic gentamicin for treating meningitis, ventriculitis, or other serious CNS infections due to *Pseudomonas. Investigational:* Pelvic inflammatory disease.

Ophthalmic: Ophthalmic bacterial infections, including conjunctivitis, keratitis, keratoconjunctivitis, corneal ulcers, blepharitis, blepharoconjunctivitis, acute meibomianitis, and dacryocystitis infections due to *Staphylococcus epidermidis, Streptococcus pyogenes, Streptococcus pneumoniae, Enterobacter aerogenes, E. coli, Haemophilus influenzae,* *Klebsiella pneumoniae, Neisseria gonorrhoeae, Pseudomonas aeruginosa, Serratia marcescens.*

Topical: (1) Primary skin infections, including impetigo contagiosa, superficial folliculitis, ecthyma, furunculosis, sycosis barbae, and pyoderma gangrenosum. (2) Secondary skin infections, including infectious eczematoid dermatitis, pustular acne, pustular psoriasis, infected seborrheic dermatitis, infected contact dermatitis (including poison ivy), infected excoriations, and bacterial superinfections of fungal or viral infections. (3) Infected skin cysts and certain other skin abscesses when preceded by incision and drainage to permit adequate contact between the antibiotic and the causative bacteria. (4) Other infections, including infected stasis and other skin ulcers, superficial burns, paronychia, infected insect bites and stings, lacerations and abrasions, and wounds from minor surgery.

ACTION/KINETICS
Pharmacokinetics
Therapeutic serum levels: IM, 4–8 mcg/mL. **Toxic serum levels:** >12 mcg/mL (peak) and >2 mcg/mL (trough). Prolonged serum levels above 12 mcg/mL should be avoided. **t½:** 2 hr. Can be used with carbenicillin to treat serious *Pseudomonas* infections; do not mix these drugs in the same flask as carbenicillin will inactivate gentamicin.

CONTRAINDICATIONS
Ophthalmic use to treat dendritic keratitis, vaccinia, varicella, mycobacterial infections of the eye, fungal diseases of the eye, use with steroids after uncomplicated removal of a corneal foreign body. Concurrent use with nephrotoxic drugs or diuretics. Lactation.

SPECIAL CONCERNS
■ See Aminoglycosides in Chapter 2.■
Use with caution in premature infants and neonates. Ophthalmic ointments may retard corneal epithelial healing.

SIDE EFFECTS
Most Common
After parenteral use: GI upset, diarrhea, anorexia, N&V, tinnitus, dizziness.

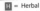 = see color insert   H = Herbal   IV = Intravenous   = sound alike drug

After ophthalmic use: Transient irritation, burning, stinging, itching, inflammation, mydriasis, lid itching/swelling.
After topical use: Erythema, pruritus. See *Aminoglycosides* for a complete list of possible side effects. Also, Muscle twitching, numbness, *seizures*, increased BP, alopecia, purpura, pseudotumor cerebri. Photosensitivity when used topically.
After ophthalmic use: Transient irritation, burning, stinging, itching, inflammation, angioneurotic edema, urticaria, vesicular and maculopapular dermatitis, mydriasis, conjunctival paresthesia, conjunctival hyperemia, nonspecific conjunctivitis, conjunctival epithelial defects, lid itching/swelling, bacterial/fungal corneal ulcers.
After topical use: Erythema, pruritus, photosensitivity; overgrowth of nonsusceptible organisms (superinfection), including fungi.

ADDITIONAL DRUG INTERACTIONS
Carbenicillin / ↑ Effect when used for *Pseudomonas* infections
Diuretics / ↑ Risk of ototoxicity
Nephrotoxic drugs / ↑ Risk of toxicity
Ticarcillin / ↑ Effect when used for *Pseudomonas* infections

HOW SUPPLIED
Injection: 10 mg/mL, 40 mg/mL; *Ophthalmic Ointment:* 3 mg/gram; *Ophthalmic Solution:* 3 mg/mL; *Topical Cream:* 0.1% (as base); *Topical Ointment:* 0.1%.

DOSAGE
• **IM (USUAL); IV**
Infections.
Adults with normal renal function: 1 mg/kg q 8 hr, up to 5 mg/kg/day in life-threatening infections; **children:** 2–2.5 mg/kg q 8 hr; **infants and neonates:** 2.5 mg/kg q 8 hr; **premature infants or neonates less than 1 week of age:** 2.5 mg/kg q 12 hr. Therapy may be required for 7–10 days.
Prevention of bacterial endocarditis, dental or respiratory tract procedures.
Adults: 1.5 mg/kg gentamicin (not to exceed 80 mg) plus 1 gram ampicillin, each IM or IV, 30–60 min before the procedure; one additional dose of each can be given 8 hr later (alternative: Pen-

icillin V, 1 gram PO, 6 hr after initial dose).
Prophylaxis of bacterial endocarditis in GI or GU tract procedures or surgery.
Adults: 1.5 mg/kg gentamicin (not to exceed 80 mg) plus 2 grams ampicillin, each IM or IV, 30–60 min before procedure; dose should be repeated 8 hr later. **Children:** 2 mg/kg gentamicin plus penicillin G, 30,000 units/kg, or ampicillin, 50 mg/kg in same dosage interval as for adults. Pediatric dosage should not exceed single or 24-hr adult doses. *NOTE:* In clients allergic to penicillin, vancomycin, 1 gram IV given slowly over 1 hr, may be substituted; the dose of vancomycin should be repeated 8–12 hr later. **Adults with impaired renal function:** To calculate interval (hr) between doses, multiply serum creatinine (mg/100 mL) by 8.
• **IV**
Septicemia.
Initially: 1–2 mg/kg infused over 30–60 min; **then,** maintenance doses may be administered.
• **INTRATHECAL**
Meningitis.
Use only the intrathecal preparation. Adults, usual: 4–8 mg/day; **children and infants 3 months and older:** 1–2 mg/day
Pelvic inflammatory disease.
Initial: 2 mg/kg IV; **then,** 1.5 mg/kg 3 times per day plus clindamycin, 500 mg IV 4 times per day. Continue for at least 4 days and at least 48 hr after client improves. Continue clindamycin, 450 mg PO 4 times per day for 10–14 days.
• **OPHTHALMIC SOLUTION (3 MG/ML)**
Ophthalmic bacterial infections.
Initially: 1–2 gtt in conjunctival sac q 4 hr. For severe infections, dose may be increased to 2 gtt once every hour.
• **OPHTHALMIC OINTMENT (3 MG/GRAM)**
Ophthalmic bacterial infections.
Apply a small amount (about ½ inch) to the affected eye 2–3 times a day.
• **TOPICAL CREAM/OINTMENT (0.1%)**
All uses.
Apply 3–4 times per day to affected area. The area may be covered with a sterile bandage.

NURSING CONSIDERATIONS

ADMINISTRATION/STORAGE

1. When used intrathecally, the usual site is the lumbar area.

2. Store ophthalmic ointment and solution from 2–30°C (36–86°F).

IV 3. For intermittent IV administration, dilute adult dose in 50–200 mL of NSS or D5W and administer over a 30–120-min period; use less volume for infants and children.

4. Do not mix with other drugs for parenteral use.

5. For parenteral use, the duration of treatment is 7–10 days; a longer course may be required for severe or complicated infections.

ASSESSMENT

1. Note type, onset and characteristics of S&S.

2. Obtain renal function studies, CBC, and appropriate specimens for culture.

3. With eye disorders, note baseline ophthalmologic examinations.

4. Assess for tinnitus, vertigo, or hearing losses during therapy. Persistently increased gentamicin levels have been associated with 8th CN dysfunction. Monitor levels and ensure adequate hydration.

CLIENT/FAMILY TEACHING

1. Review appropriate method and frequency for administration. Wash hands before and after treatment; prepare site and apply as directed.

2. With topical administration:

- Remove crusts (of impetigo contagiosa) before applying cream/ointment to permit maximum contact between antibiotic and infection.

- Wash affected area with soap and water, rinse, and dry thoroughly.

- Apply cream or ointment gently and cover with gauze dressing if ordered.

- Avoid direct exposure to sunlight; photosensitivity reaction may occur.

- Avoid further contamination of infected skin.

3. Identify symptoms and wound changes that require medical attention; i.e., pain, redness, swelling, increased drainage or odor.

4. With eye therapy, apply pressure to the inner eye for 1 min after instilling and keep eyes closed for 1–2 min to ensure dosage. May experience blurred vision for several min following therapy.

5. Report any visual impairment, vertigo, dizziness, hearing impairment/changes, or worsening of S&S

6. Consume adequate fluids to prevent dehydration.

7. Avoid vaccinations during treatment. Keep all F/U appointments to assess response to therapy.

OUTCOMES/EVALUATE

- Resolution of infection
- Therapeutic serum drug levels 4–8 mcg/mL; (peak: 4–8 mcg/mL; trough: 2 mcg/mL)

G

Glatiramer acetate
(glah-**TER**-ah-mer)

CLASSIFICATION(S):
Immunosuppressant
PREGNANCY CATEGORY: B
Rx: Copaxone.

USES
Reduce frequency of relapsing-remitting multiple sclerosis.

ACTION/KINETICS

Action
May act by modifying immune processes responsible for pathology of multiple sclerosis. Some of the drug enters the lymphatic circulation reaching regional lymph nodes. MRI gadolinium-enhanced lesions are reduced following treatment.

CONTRAINDICATIONS
Hypersensitivity to glatiramer or mannitol.

SPECIAL CONCERNS
Use with caution during lactation. Safety and efficacy have not been determined in children less than 18 years of age. May interfere with useful immune function.

SIDE EFFECTS

Most Common
Pain, erythema, inflammation, infection, pruritus, vasodilation, anxiety, hyperto-

---

nia, pain, arthralgia, chest pain, flu syndrome, nausea.

Side effects listed are those with incidence of 1% or more. **Immediate-post injection reaction:** Flushing, chest pain, palpitations, anxiety, dyspnea, laryngeal constriction, urticaria. **CNS:** Anxiety, hypertonia, tremor, vertigo, agitation, foot drop, nervousness, nystagmus, speech disorder, confusion, abnormal dreams, emotional lability, stupor, migraine. **GI:** Nausea, diarrhea, anorexia, vomiting, GI disorder, abdominal pain, gastroenteritis, bowel urgency, oral moniliasis, salivary gland enlargement, tooth caries, ulcerative stomatitis. **CV:** Vasodilation, palpitations, tachycardia, syncope, hypertension. **Body as a whole:** Infection, asthenia, pain, arthritis, transient chest pain, flu syndrome, back pain, fever, neck pain, face edema, bacterial infection, chills, cyst, headache, injection site ecchymosis, accidental injury, neck rigidity, malaise, injection site edema or atrophy, abscess, peripheral edema, edema, weight gain. **Dermatologic:** Rash, pruritus, sweating, herpes simplex, erythema, urticaria, skin nodule, eczema, herpes zoster, pustular rash, skin atrophy and warts. **GU:** Urinary urgency, vaginal moniliasis, dysmenorrhea, amenorrhea, hematuria, impotence, menorrhagia, suspicious Pap smear, *vaginal hemorrhage.* **Hematologic:** Ecchymosis, lymphadenopathy. **Respiratory:** Dyspnea, allergic rhinitis, bronchitis, laryngismus, hyperventilation. **At injection site:** Pain, erythema, inflammation, pruritus, mass, induration, welt, hemorrhage, urticaria. **Miscellaneous:** Ear pain, eye disorder, arthralgia.

DRUG INTERACTIONS

H Do not give echinacea with glatiramer.

HOW SUPPLIED

Injection, Premixed: 20 mg; *Powder for Injection:* 20 mg.

DOSAGE

- **SC**
  Multiple sclerosis.
  Adults: 20 mg/day.

NURSING CONSIDERATIONS

ADMINISTRATION/STORAGE

1. SC sites include arms, abdomen, hips, and thighs.

2. Reconstitute with diluent provided (sterile water for injection). Gently swirl vial after diluent is added. Let stand at room temperature until solid material is dissolved.

3. Use reconstituted drug immediately; contains no preservative. Before reconstitution store at 2–8°C (36–46°F).

ASSESSMENT

1. Note age at onset, frequency of exacerbations, degree of physical disability, other therapies trialed.

2. RRMS is characterized by recurrent attacks of neurologic dysfunction followed by complete or incomplete recovery; assess frequency.

CLIENT/FAMILY TEACHING

1. Use exactly as directed; do not stop without consulting provider.

2. Reconstitute with diluent provided and gently swirl vial. Let stand at room temperature until solid material is dissolved. Administer SC into arms, abdomen, hips, or thighs, rotating sites.

3. Patient information booklet is enclosed with drug for review of self–injection procedure.

4. Drug is used to slow accumulation of physical disability and to decrease frequency of clinical exacerbations with MS. Continue to use aids, i.e., cane, brace, walker, etc. for ambulation.

5. May experience pain, itching, swelling, and hardening of skin at injection site. Report adverse effects.

6. Chest tightness, flushing, SOB, and anxiety may occur within minutes of injection and last up to 30 min. Keep regular F/U appointments and lab tests as ordered.

7. Practice reliable contraception.

OUTCOMES/EVALUATE

↓ Frequency and severity of MS exacerbations

Bold Italic = life threatening side effect   ■ = black box warning   ✦ = Available in Canada

Glimepiride @ 📷
(GLYE-meh-pye-ride)

CLASSIFICATION(S):
Antidiabetic, oral; second generation sulfonylurea
PREGNANCY CATEGORY: C
Rx: Amaryl.

SEE ALSO *ANTIDIABETIC AGENTS: HYPOGLYCEMIC AGENTS.*

USES
(1) As an adjunct to diet and exercise to lower blood glucose in non-insulin-dependent diabetes mellitus (type 2 diabetes mellitus) whose hyperglycemia can not be controlled by diet and exercise alone. (2) In combination with insulin to decrease blood glucose in those whose hyperglycemia cannot be controlled by diet and exercise in combination with an oral hypoglycemic drug. (3) In combination with metformin (Glucophage) if control is not reached with diet, exercise, and either hypoglycemic alone.

ACTION/KINETICS
Action
Lowers blood glucose by stimulating the release of insulin from functioning pancreatic beta cells and by increasing the sensitivity of peripheral tissues to insulin.
Pharmacokinetics
Completely absorbed from the GI tract within 1 hr. **Onset:** 2–3 hr. **t½, serum:** About 9 hr. **Duration:** 24 hr. Completely metabolized in the liver and metabolites are excreted through both the urine and feces.

CONTRAINDICATIONS
Diabetic ketoacidosis with or without coma. Use during lactation.

SPECIAL CONCERNS
The use of oral hypoglycemic drugs has been associated with increased CV mortality compared with treatment with diet alone or diet plus insulin. Safety and efficacy have not been determined in children.

SIDE EFFECTS
Most Common
Hypoglycemia, dizziness, weakness, headache, blurred vision, N&V, stomach pain, photosensitivity.
GI: N&V, GI pain, diarrhea, stomach pain, cholestatic jaundice (rare). **CNS:** Dizziness, headache. **Dermatologic:** Pruritus, erythema, urticaria, morbilliform or maculopapular eruptions, photosensitivity. **Hematologic:** Leukopenia, agranulocytosis, thrombocytopenia, hemolytic anemia, *aplastic anemia,* pancytopenia. **Body as a Whole:** Hypoglycemia, weakness. **Miscellaneous:** Hyponatremia, increased release of ADH, changes in accommodation and/or blurred vision.

DRUG INTERACTIONS
See *Antidiabetic Agents: Hypoglycemic Agents.*

HOW SUPPLIED
Tablets: 1 mg, 2 mg, 4 mg.

DOSAGE
- **TABLETS**
  Non-insulin-dependent diabetes mellitus (Type 2 diabetes).
Adults, initial: 1–2 mg once daily, given with breakfast or the first main meal. The initial dose should be 1 mg in those sensitive to hypoglycemic drugs, in those with impaired renal or hepatic function, and in elderly, debilitated, or malnourished clients. The maximum initial dose is 2 mg or less daily. **Maintenance:** 1–4 mg once daily up to a maximum of 8 mg once daily. After a dose of 2 mg is reached, increase the dose in increments of 2 mg or less at 1- to 2-week intervals (determined by the blood glucose response). **When combined with insulin therapy:** 8 mg once daily with the first main meal with low-dose insulin. The fasting glucose level for beginning combination therapy is greater than 150 mg/dL glucose in the plasma or serum. After starting with low-dose insulin, upward adjustments of insulin can be done about weekly as determined by frequent fasting blood glucose determinations.
Type 2 diabetes—transfer from other hypoglycemic agents.

G

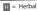

When transferring clients to glimepiride, no transition period is required. However, observe clients closely for 1 to 2 weeks for hypoglycemia when being transferred from longer half-life sulfonylureas (e.g., chlorpropamide) to glimepiride.

NURSING CONSIDERATIONS

€ Do not confuse Amaryl with Reminyl (an anti-Alzheimer's drug). NOTE: The manufacturer has changed the trade name of Reminyl to Razadyne.

ADMINISTRATION/STORAGE
1. Dispense tablets in well-closed containers with safety caps.
2. Store tablets at 15–30°C (59–86°F).

ASSESSMENT
1. Note reasons for therapy, if newly diagnosed or transferred therapy, glycemic control, disease characteristics, family hx.
2. List other agents trialed, drugs currently taking to ensure none interact.
3. Assess lifestyle and diet, identify risk factors and changes needed.
4. Monitor electrolytes, BS, HbA1c, Ca, Mg, microalbumin, and LFTs.

CLIENT/FAMILY TEACHING
1. Drug helps insulin get into the cells where it can work properly to lower blood sugar and help restore the way you use food to make energy.
2. Review dose, frequency for administration. Usually once a day with first main meal of day.
3. Record finger sticks, include 1 or 2 hr post meal FS.
4. Continue regular exercise and dietary restrictions, BP and cholesterol control in addition to drug therapy.
5. Avoid alcohol and direct or artificial sun exposure. Report any adverse effects.
6. Report as scheduled for teaching reinforcement, follow-up labs, BP, eye/foot exams, and medication response.

OUTCOMES/EVALUATE
FBS <100 and HbA1c <7

Glipizide €
(**GLIP**-ih-zyd)

CLASSIFICATION(S):
Antidiabetic, oral; second generation sulfonylurea

PREGNANCY CATEGORY: C
Rx: Glipizide Extended-Release, Glucotrol, Glucotrol XL.

SEE ALSO *ANTIDIABETIC AGENTS: HYPOGLYCEMIC AGENTS.*

USES
Adjunct to diet for control of hyperglycemia in clients with type 2 diabetes. Begin therapy when diet alone has been unsuccessful in controlling hyperglycemia.

ACTION/KINETICS

Action
Lowers blood glucose by stimulating the release of insulin from functioning pancreatic beta cells and by increasing the sensitivity of peripheral tissues to insulin. Also has mild diuretic effects.

Pharmacokinetics
Onset: 1–3 hr. **t½:** 2–4 hr. **Duration:** 10–24 hr. Metabolized in liver to inactive metabolites, which are excreted through the kidneys.

SIDE EFFECTS

Most Common
Hypoglycemia, headache, dizziness, hives, skin rash, jaundice.

See *Antidiabetic Agents: Hypoglycemic Agents* for a complete list of possible side effects.

ADDITIONAL DRUG INTERACTIONS
Cimetidine may ↑ glipizide effect R/T ↓ liver breakdown.

HOW SUPPLIED
Tablets, Extended-Release: 2.5 mg, 5 mg, 10 mg; *Tablets, Immediate-Release:* 5 mg, 10 mg.

DOSAGE
• **TABLETS, IMMEDIATE-RELEASE**
Type 2 diabetes.
Adults, initial: 5 mg 30 min before breakfast; **then,** adjust dosage by 2.5–5 mg every few days, depending on the blood glucose response, until adequate control is achieved. **Maintenance:**

15–40 mg/day; divide total daily doses over 15 mg/day. Older clients or those with liver disease should begin with 2.5 mg.

- **TABLETS, EXTENDED-RELEASE**
  Type 2 diabetes.
  Adults (including geriatric clients), initial: 5 mg with breakfast. Monitor response to therapy by measuring HbA1c at 3-month intervals. Dose can be increased to 10 mg if response is inadequate. **Maintenance:** 5 or 10 mg once daily; some may require 20 mg/day (maximum).

NURSING CONSIDERATIONS

Ⓖ Do not confuse glipizide with glyburide (another oral hypoglycemic drug).

ADMINISTRATION/STORAGE

1. Some are better controlled on once daily dosing while others are better controlled with divided dosing.
2. Divide maintenance doses greater than 15 mg/day; give before the morning and evening meals. Total daily doses of 30 mg or more may be given safely on twice daily dosing.
3. If on immediate-release glipizide, can be safely switched to extended-release tablets once a day at the nearest equivalent total daily dose. Can also be titrated to the appropriate dose of extended-release tablets starting with 5 mg once daily.
4. No transition period needed when transferring to extended-release tablets from other oral antidiabetic drugs. Observe for 1–2 weeks if transferred from long half-life sulfonylureas (e.g., chlorpropamide) to extended-release glipizide due to overlapping effects.
5. When transferring from insulin dose of <20 units/day, insulin may be discontinued abruptly. When transferring from an insulin dose of >20 units/day, reduce insulin dose by 50%; further reduce depending on response. The initial glipizide dose when transferring from insulin is 5 mg/day.
6. Assess lifestyle to ensure that maximal changes in the areas of diet and exercise have been taken before increasing dosage. Once maximum dosage is attained, if renal function is normal, consider adding metformin, pioglitazone, or rosiglitazone for better control.
7. Store immediate-release tablets below 30°C (86°F) and extended-release tablets, protected from moisture and humidity, from 15–30°C (59–86°F).

ASSESSMENT

1. List reasons for therapy, if newly diagnosed or transferred therapy; glycemic control, disease characteristics, family hx.
2. List other agents trialed, drugs currently taking to ensure none interact.
3. Assess lifestyle and diet, identify changes needed, identify risk factors.
4. Monitor BP, Wt. electrolytes, BS, HbA1c, Ca, Mg, U/A, microalbumin, renal and LFTs.

CLIENT/FAMILY TEACHING

1. Helps insulin get into cells where it can work properly to lower blood sugar and help restore the way you use food to make energy.
2. Take 30 min before or with meals (to lessen chance of stomach upset). Do not chew or crush extended release form (i.e., Glucotrol XL).
3. Report CNS side effects: drowsiness, headache; check fingerstick.
4. May have anorexia, constipation, diarrhea, vomiting, stomach pain. Report if severe, record weight, I&O.
5. Report if skin reactions occur. Avoid exposure to direct/artificial light; use sunscreen, sunglasses, protective clothing when out doors.
6. Assess lifestyle and diet, identify changes needed. Practice barrier contraception
7. Avoid alcohol; OTC agents without approval.
8. Continue prescribed diet, weight loss, and regular exercise program. Record FS, also obtain FS 1–2 hr after eating. Report as scheduled for teaching reinforcement, F/U labs, BP, eye/foot exams, and medication review.

OUTCOMES/EVALUATE

FBS <100; HbA1c <7

G

Glyburide Ⓒ

(**GLYE**-byou-ryd)

CLASSIFICATION(S):

Antidiabetic, oral; second generation sulfonylurea

PREGNANCY CATEGORY: B

Rx: Diaβeta, Glynase PresTab, Micronase.

✦Rx: Apo-Glyburide, Euglucon, Gen-Glybe, Novo-Glyburide, Nu-Glyburide, PMS-Glyburide, ratio-Glyburide.

SEE ALSO ANTIDIABETIC AGENTS: HYPOGLYCEMIC AGENTS.

USES

Type 2 diabetes whose hyperglycemia cannot be controlled by diet alone. May be used with metformin when diet and glyburide or diet and metformin alone do not provide adequate control.

ACTION/KINETICS

Action

Lowers blood glucose by stimulating the release of insulin from functioning pancreatic beta cells and by increasing the sensitivity of peripheral tissues to insulin. Has a mild diuretic effect.

Pharmacokinetics

Onset, nonmicronized: 2–4 hr; **micronized:** 1 hr. **t½, nonmicronized:** 10 hr; **micronized:** Approximately 4 hr. **Time to peak levels:** 4 hr. **Duration, nonmicronized:** 16–24 hr; **micronized:** 12–24 hr. Metabolized in liver to weakly active metabolites. Excreted in bile (50%) and through the kidneys (50%). Micronized glyburide (3 mg tablets) produces serum levels that are not bioequivalent to those from nonmicronized glyburide (5 mg tablets).

SIDE EFFECTS

Most Common

Hypoglycemia, nausea, epigastric distress, heartburn, allergic skin reactions, blurred vision.

See *Antidiabetic Agents: Hypoglycemic Agents* for a complete list of possible side effects.

ADDITIONAL DRUG INTERACTIONS

Anticoagulants / Either ↑ or ↓ anticoagulant effect

Ciprofloxacin / Potentiation of hypoglycemic effect

HOW SUPPLIED

Tablets, Micronized: 1.5 mg, 3 mg, 4.5 mg, 6 mg; *Tablets, Nonmicronized:* 1.25 mg, 2.5 mg, 5 mg.

DOSAGE

DIAβETA/MICRONASE

• **TABLETS, NONMICRONIZED**
  Type 2 diabetes.

Adults, initial: 2.5–5 mg/day given with breakfast (or the first main meal); **then,** increase by 2.5 mg at weekly intervals to achieve the desired response. **Maintenance:** 1.25–20 (maximum) mg/day. Clients sensitive to sulfonylureas should start with 1.25 mg/day.

GLYNASE PRESTAB

• **TABLETS, MICRONIZED**
  Type 2 diabetes.

Adults, initial: 1.5–3 mg/day given with breakfast (or the first main meal). Those sensitive to sulfonylureas should start with 0.75 mg/day. Increase by no more than 1.5 mg at weekly intervals to achieve the desired response. **Maintenance:** 0.75–12 (maximum) mg/day.

NURSING CONSIDERATIONS

Ⓒ Do not confuse glyburide with glipizide (also an oral hypoglycemic) or glyburide with Glucotrol (also an oral hypoglycemic). Do not confuse Diaβeta with Zebeta (a beta-adrenergic blocker).

ADMINISTRATION/STORAGE

1. For best results, administer 30 min prior to meals.

2. To avoid hypoglycemic reactions, the initial and maintenance doses should be conservative in the elderly, the debilitated, or in those with impaired hepatic or renal function.

3. Do not exceed 20 mg/day of the nonmicronized product and 12 mg/day of the micronized product.

4. If daily dosage of the nonmicronized product exceeds 15 mg or the micronized product exceeds 6 mg, dividing the dose and giving before the morning and evening meals may be more effective.

5. When transferring from oral hypoglycemics, other than chlorpropamide, no transition and no initial priming

---

dose are required. When transferring from chlorpropamide, use caution for the first 2 weeks due to the long duration of action of chlorpropamide and possible overlapping drug effects.

6. A maintenance dose of 5 mg nonmicronized glyburide or 3 mg of micronized glyburide tablets provides about the same degree of blood glucose control as 250–375 mg chlorpropamide, 250–375 mg tolazamide, 500–750 mg acetohexamide, or 1,000–1,500 mg tolbutamide.

7. Add glyburide tablets gradually to the dosing regimen of those who have not responded to the maximum dose of metformin monotherapy after 4 weeks. Attempt to find the optimal dose of each drug needed to achieve blood glucose control.

8. Use the following guidelines when transferring from insulin to glyburide:

• Insulin dose <20 units/day, start with 1.5–3 mg/day micronized or 2.5–5 mg/day nonmicronized glyburide. Insulin may be discontinued abruptly.

• Insulin dose from 20–40 units/day, start with 3 mg/day micronized or 5 mg/day nonmicronized glyburide. Insulin may be discontinued abruptly.

• Insulin dose >40 units/day, start with 3 mg/day micronized or 5 mg/day nonmicronized glyburide. Reduce insulin dose by 50%; reduce further as determined by response. Consider hospitalization during the transition.

9. Store from 15–30°C (59–86°F).

ASSESSMENT

1. Note reasons for therapy, if newly diagnosed or transferred therapy; glycemic control, disease characteristics, family Hx.

2. List other agents trialed, drugs currently taking to ensure none interact.

3. Assess BMI, lifestyle, diet, identify risk factors and changes needed.

4. Monitor BP, electrolytes, BS, HbA1c, Ca, Mg, U/A, microalbumin, lipid panel, renal and LFTs.

CLIENT/FAMILY TEACHING

1. Works by causing your pancreas to release more insulin into the blood stream, helps insulin get into the cells to lower blood sugar and help restore the way you use food to make energy. Take as directed with meals.

2. Record finger sticks at various times (i.e., fasting, 1 or 2 hr after meal, bedtime).

3. Continue regular daily exercise, lifestyle changes, BP control, Wt loss, and dietary restrictions to control cholesterol and glucose.

4. Avoid alcohol, OTC agents without approval. Practice reliable contraception.

5. Report as scheduled for teaching reinforcement, F/U labs, foot/eye exams, and medication response.

OUTCOMES/EVALUATE

FBS <100; HbA1c <7

──── *COMBINATION DRUG* ────

Glyburide and Metformin hydrochloride ■
(**GLYE**-byou-ryd, met-**FOR**-min)

CLASSIFICATION(S):

Antidiabetic, oral

PREGNANCY CATEGORY: B

Rx: Glucovance.

SEE ALSO *GLYBURIDE, METFORMIN, AND ANTIDIABETIC AGENTS: HYPOGLYCEMIC AGENTS.*

USES

(1) As an adjunct to diet and exercise, and as initial therapy, to improve glycemic control in type 2 diabetes in those who can not be controlled satisfactorily with diet and exercise alone. (2) Second-line therapy when diet, exercise, and initial therapy with a sulfonylurea or metformin do not provide adequate control in those with type 2 diabetes. If additional control is needed, a thiazolidinedione may be added to Glucovance therapy.

CONTENT

Each tablet, 1.25 mg/250 mg, contains glyburide, 1.25 mg and metformin, 250 mg. Each tablet, 2.5 mg/500 mg, contains glyburide, 2.5 mg and metformin, 500 mg. Each tablet, 5 mg/500 mg, contains gluburide, 5 mg and metformin, 500 mg.

ACTION/KINETICS

Action

Glyburide stimulates release of insulin from the pancreas, which is dependent upon functioning pancreatic beta islets. Extrapancreatic effects may also be involved in the long-term effectiveness of glyburide. Metformin decreases hepatic glucose production, decreases intestinal absorption of glucose, and improves insulin sensitivity by increasing peripheral glucose uptake and utilization. Thus the mechanisms are complementary.

Pharmacokinetics

Glyburide is rapidly absorbed; **peak levels:** 4 hr. Food decreases the extent and slightly delays the absorption of metformin. Glyburide is significantly bound to plasma proteins while metformin is negligibly bound. Steady state metformin levels are reached within 24–48 hr. **Glyburide, $t_{1/2}$, terminal:** About 10 hr; excreted as metabolites in the bile and urine (about 50% by each route). Metformin is excreted unchanged in the urine; $t_{1/2}$, **elimination:** About 17.6 hr.

CONTRAINDICATIONS

Use in renal disease or renal dysfunction (including that due to shock, acute MI, septicemia), CHF requiring pharmacologic treatment, acute or chronic metabolic acidosis (including diabetic ketoacidosis, with or without coma), and known hypersensitivity to glyburide or metformin. Not recommended for use during pregnancy.

SPECIAL CONCERNS

■ (1) Lactic acidosis is a rare, but serious, metabolic complication that can occur due to metformin accumulation during treatment with Glucovance. When it occurs, it is fatal in approximately 50% of cases. Lactic acidosis may also occur in association with a number of pathophysiologic conditions, including diabetes mellitus, and whenever there is significant tissue hypoperfusion and hypoxemia. (2) Lactic acidosis is characterized by elevated blood lactate levels (>5 mmol/L), decreased blood pH, electrolyte disturbances with an increased anion gap, and an increased lactate/pyruvate ratio. When metformin is implicated as the cause of lactic acidosis, metformin plasma levels >5 μgrams/mL are generally found. (3) The incidence of lactic acidosis in those receiving metformin is approximately 0.03 case/1,000 client years, with approximately 0.015 fatal cases/1,000 client years. Reported cases have occurred primarily in diabetic clients with significant renal insufficiency, including both intrinsic renal disease and renal hypoperfusion, often in the setting of multiple concomitant medical/surgical problems and multiple concomitant medications. (4) Clients with CHF requiring pharmacologic management, in particular those with unstable or acute CHF who are at risk of hypoperfusion and hypoxemia, are at increased risk of lactic acidosis. The risk of lactic acidosis increases with the degree of renal dysfunction and the client's age. The risk of lactic acidosis, therefore, may be significantly decreased by regular monitoring of renal function in clients taking metformin and by use of the minimum effective dose of metformin. (5) In particular, treatment of the elderly should be accompanied by careful monitoring of renal function. Glucovance treatment should not be initiated in clients >80 years of age unless measurement of creatinine clearance demonstrates that renal function is not reduced, as these clients are more susceptible to developing lactic acidosis. (6) Glucovance should be promptly withheld in the presence of any condition associated with hypoxemia, dehydration, or sepsis. (7) Because impaired hepatic function may significantly limit the ability to clear lactate, Glucovance should generally be avoided in clients with clinical or laboratory evidence of hepatic disease. (8) Clients should be cautioned against excessive alcohol intake, either acute or chronic, when taking Glucovance, since alcohol potentiates the effects of metformin on lactate metabolism. (9) In addition, Glucovance should be temporarily discontinued prior to any intravascular radiocontrast study and for any surgical procedure. (10) The onset of lactic acidosis often is subtle, and accompanied only by nonspecific symptoms such as malaise, myalgias, respiratory distress, increasing somnolence, and nonspecific abdominal distress. There may be associated hypothermia, hypotension, and resistant bradyarrhythmias with more marked acidosis. The client and the client's provider must be aware of the possible importance of such symptoms and the client should be instructed to notify the provider immediately if they occur. Glucovance should be withdrawn until the situation is clarified. (11) Serum electrolytes, ketones, blood glucose, and if indicated, blood pH, lactate levels, and even blood metformin, are unlikely to be drug related. (12) Later occurrence of GI symptoms could be due to lactic acidosis or other serious disease. (13) Levels of fasting venous plasma lactate above the upper limit of normal but less than 5 mmol/L in clients taking Glucovance do not necessarily indicate impending lactic acidosis and may be explainable by other mechanisms, such as poorly controlled diabetes or obesity, vigorous physical activity, or technical problems in sample handling. (14) Lactic acidosis should be suspected in any diabetic client with metabolic acidosis lacking evidence of ketoacidosis (ketonuria and ketonemia). (15) Lactic acidosis is a medical emergency that must be treated in a hospital setting. In a client with lactic acidosis taking Glucovance, the drug should be discontinued immediately and general supportive measures promptly instituted. Because metformin is dialyzable (with a clearance of up to 170 mL/min under good hemodynamic conditions), prompt hemodialysis is recommended to correct the acidosis and remove the accumulated metformin. Such management often results in prompt reversal of symptoms and recovery.■ To avoid the risk of hypoglycemia, generally do not titrate the eld-

erly, debilitated, or malnourished clients to the maximum dose of Glucovance.

SIDE EFFECTS
Most Common
URTI, diarrhea, hypoglycemia, headache, N&V, abdominal pain, dizziness. See *Glyburide, Metformin,* and *Antidiabetic Agents: Hypoglycemic Agents* for a complete list of possible side effects.

DRUG INTERACTIONS
See *Glyburide, Metformin,* and *Antidiabetic Agents; Hypoglycemic Agents* for a complete list of possible drug interactions.

HOW SUPPLIED
See Content.

DOSAGE
- **TABLETS**
  Type 2 diabetes, initial therapy.
Initial: 1.25 mg/250 mg once a day with a meal. In those with baseline HbA1c >9% or an FPG >200 mg/dL, give an initial dose of 1.25 mg/250 mg twice a day with the morning and evening meals. Do not use Glucovance, 5 mg/500 mg, as initial therapy due to the increased risk of hypoglycemia. Make dosage increases in increments of 1.25 mg/250 mg per day every two weeks up to the minimum effective dose needed to control blood glucose, not to exceed 20 mg glyburide/2,000 mg metformin daily.
  Type 2 diabetes, in previously treated clients (second-line therapy).
Initial: Either 2.5 mg/500 mg or 5 mg/500 mg twice a day with the morning and evening meals. Titrate the daily dose in increments of no more than 5 mg/500 mg, up to the minimum effective dose to achieve adequate blood glucose control or a maximum dose of 20 mg/2,000 mg daily.

NURSING CONSIDERATIONS
℘ Do not confuse Glucovance with Glucophage (metformin only).

ADMINISTRATION/STORAGE
1. For those previously treated with combination therapy or glyburide (or another sulfonylurea) plus metformin, if switched to Glucovance, do not exceed the daily dose of glyburide (or

G

equivalent dose of another sulfonyl-urea) and metformin already being tak-en. Monitor closely for S&S of hypogly-cemia.

2. For clients not adequately controlled on Glucovance, a thiazolidinedione can be added to therapy. When a thiazolidi-nedione is added, the current dose of Glucovance can be continued and the thiazolidinedione added at its recom-mended starting dose. If additional gly-cemic control is needed, the dose of the thiazolidinedione can be increased based on its recommended titration schedule. However, the risk of hypogly-cemia increases. If hypoglycemia oc-curs, reduce dose of the glyburide com-ponent of Glucovance.

3. Temporarily discontinue Glucovance in those undergoing radiologic studies involving intravascular administration of iodinated contrast materials; use of such products may result in acute alter-ation of renal function.

ASSESSMENT

1. Note reasons for therapy, disease on-set, characteristics of S&S, other agents trialed, outcome.

2. List agents prescribed to ensure none interact.

3. Monitor renal and LFTs; avoid use in elderly, debilitated clients. Stop therapy if creatinine >1.5 males or >1.4 females to prevent acidosis.

4. Assess for alcohol use; this potenti-ates the effects of metformin on lactate metabolism.

5. Determine any heart disease, history of MI, stroke, or liver disease.

CLIENT/FAMILY TEACHING

1. Drug is a combination of two oral hypoglycemic agents (glyburide and metformin) to help control blood sugar.

2. Take with meals as directed. Do not take if meal skipped.

3. May cause drowsiness, dizziness, blurred vision; avoid activities that re-quire mental alertness until drug effects realized.

4. Monitor FS to ensure glucose con-trol. Follow prescribed diabetic diet, ex-ercise, and weight control program.

5. Report symptoms of lactic acidosis: weakness, increasing sleepiness, slow heart rate, cold feeling, muscle pain, shortness of breath, stomach pain, feel-ing light-headed, fainting.

6. Avoid alcohol - lowers blood sugar and may predispose one to lactic acido-sis.

7. May cause photosensitivity; avoid prolonged sun exposure and use pro-tection if exposed.

8. Any procedure scheduled (x-ray or CT scan) using dye which is injected into veins, client should temporarily stop taking drug to prevent renal fail-ure.

9. Keep all F/U labs and appointments to check drug response.

OUTCOMES/EVALUATE
HbA1c <7

Goserelin acetate
(**GO**-seh-rel-in)

CLASSIFICATION(S):
Antineoplastic, hormone
PREGNANCY CATEGORY: X (when used for endometriosis), **D** (when used for breast cancer).
Rx: Zoladex.
♣Rx: Zoladex LA.

SEE ALSO ANTINEOPLASTIC AGENTS.

USES
Implant, 3.6 mg or 10.8 mg: Palliative treatment of advanced prostatic carci-noma as an alternative to orchiectomy or estrogen administration when these are either unacceptable to the client or not indicated. **Implant, 3.6 mg only:** (1) Endometriosis, including pain relief and reduction of endometriotic lesions. Use limited to women 18 years and old-er who have been treated for 6 months. (2) Palliative treatment of advanced breast cancer in pre- and postmeno-pausal women. (3) For endometrial thinning prior to ablation for dysfunc-tional uterine bleeding. **Implant, 10.8 mg only:** In combination with flutam-ide to manage locally confined T2b-T4 (Stage B2 to C) cancer of the prostate. Begin treatment 8 weeks prior to begin-

---

Bold Italic = life threatening side effect   ■ = black box warning   ♣ = Available in Canada

ning radiation therapy and continue during radiation therapy.

ACTION/KINETICS

Action

Synthetic decapeptide analog of LHRH (or GnRH) which is a potent inhibitor of gonadotropin secretion from the pituitary gland. Initially, there is actually an increase in serum luteinizing hormone and FSH. This is followed by a long-term suppression of pituitary gonadotropins with serum levels of testosterone decreasing to those seen in surgically castrated males. When used for endometriosis, the drug controls the secretion of hormones required for the ovary to synthesize estrogen resulting in plasma estrogen levels seen in menopause.

Pharmacokinetics

Peak serum levels after SC implantation of 3.6 mg: 12–15 days in males and 8–22 days in females. **Mean peak serum levels:** Approximately 2.5 ng/mL. Available as an implant in a preloaded syringe. For the first 8 days of the treatment cycle, the rate of absorption of the 3.6 mg implant is slower than for the remainder of the period. For the 10.8 mg implant, mean levels increase to a peak within the first 24 hr and then decline rapidly until day 4; thereafter, mean levels remain constant until the end of the treatment period. **t½, elimination:** 4.2 hr in males and 2.3 hr in females with normal renal function and 12.1 hr for C_{CR} less than 20 mL/min. Rapidly cleared by a combination of hepatic metabolism and urinary excretion.

CONTRAINDICATIONS

Pregnancy, lactation, nondiagnosed vaginal bleeding, hypersensitivity to LHRH or LHRH agonist analogs. Use of the 10.8-mg implant in women.

SPECIAL CONCERNS

Safety and effectiveness have not been determined in clients less than 18 years of age. May be initial worsening of the symptoms or occurrence of additional symptoms of prostate or breast cancer. Use with caution in males who are at particular risk of developing ureteral obstruction or spinal cord compression.

SIDE EFFECTS

Most Common

Hot flashes, headache, vaginitis, emotional lability, decreased libido, depression, sweating, acne, breast atrophy, vasodilation, peripheral edema, seborrhea.

In males. GU: Sexual dysfunction, decreased erections, lower urinary tract symptoms, gynecomastia, renal insufficiency, urinary obstruction, UTI, bladder neoplasm, hematuria, impotence, urinary frequency, incontinence, urinary tract disorder, impaired urination. **CV:** CHF, **CVA, MI, heart failure, pulmonary embolus**, arrhythmia, hypertension, peripheral vascular disorder, chest pain, angina pectoris, cerebral ischemia, varicose veins. **CNS:** Lethargy, dizziness, insomnia, asthenia, anxiety, depression, headache, paresthesia. **GI:** N&V, diarrhea, constipation, ulcer, anorexia, hematemesis. **Respiratory:** URTI, COPD, increased cough, dyspnea, pneumonia. **Metabolic:** Gout, hypercalcemia, weight increase, diabetes mellitus. **Miscellaneous:** Pelvic or bone pain, anemia, chills, fever, breast pain, breast swelling or tenderness, abdominal or back pain, flu syndrome, sepsis, aggravation reaction, herpes simplex, pruritus, peripheral edema, injection site reaction, hot flashes, rash, sweating, complications of surgery, hypersensitivity, pain, edema.

In females. GU: Vaginitis, decreased or increased libido, pelvic symptoms, dyspareunia, dysmenorrhea, urinary frequency, UTI, vaginal bleeding (during the first 2 months) of varying duration and intensity. **CV:** **Hemorrhage**, hypertension, palpitations, migraine, tachycardia. **CNS:** Emotional lability, depression, headache, insomnia, dizziness, nervousness, anxiety, paresthesia, somnolence, abnormal thinking, malaise, fatigue, lethargy. **GI:** N&V, abdominal pain, increased appetite, anorexia, constipation, diarrhea, dry mouth, dyspepsia, flatulence. **Musculoskeletal:** Asthenia, back pain, myalgia, hypertonia, arthralgia, joint disorder, decrease of vertebral trabecular bone mineral density. **Dermatologic:** Sweating, acne, sebor-

G

rhea, hirsutism, pruritus, alopecia, dry skin, ecchymosis, rash, skin discoloration, hair disorders. **Respiratory:** Pharyngitis, bronchitis, increased cough, epistaxis, rhinitis, sinusitis. **Ophthalmic:** Amblyopia, dry eyes. **Miscellaneous:** Hot flashes, breast atrophy or enlargement, breast pain, tumor flare, pain, infection, application site reaction, flu syndrome, voice alterations, weight gain, allergic reaction, chest pain, fever, peripheral edema, hypercalcemia, osteoporosis, hypersensitivity.

LABORATORY TEST CONSIDERATIONS
↑ LDL and HDL cholesterol, triglycerides, AST, ALT. Misleading results of pituitary-gonadotropic and gonadal function tests conducted during treatment.

HOW SUPPLIED
Implant: 3.6 mg, 10.8 mg.

DOSAGE

- **SC IMPLANT, 3.6 MG**
  Endometriosis, advanced breast cancer.

3.6 mg q 28 days into the upper abdominal wall using sterile technique under the direction of the provider.

  Thinning prior to endometrial ablation for dysfunctional uterine bleeding.

1 or 2 depots (each depot given 4 weeks apart).

- **SC IMPLANT, 10.8 MG**
  Advanced prostatic carcinoma.

10.8 mg q 12 weeks into the upper abdominal wall using sterile technique under the direction of the provider.

  With flutamide to treat Stage B2-C prostatic carcinoma.

One goserelin 3.6 mg implant followed in 28 days by one 10.8 mg implant. Alternatively, 4 injections of the 3.6 mg depot can be given at 28-day intervals, 2 depots preceding and 2 during radiotherapy.

NURSING CONSIDERATIONS

ADMINISTRATION/STORAGE

1. Do not remove sterile syringe containing the drug until immediately before use. Examine syringe for damage and to ensure drug is visible in the translucent chamber.

2. Administer drug under physician supervision/orders.

3. Clean the area with an alcohol swab; a topical (i.e., ethyl chloride) or a local anesthetic may be used prior to the injection.

4. To administer, stretch the skin with one hand and grip the needle with the fingers around the barrel of the syringe. Insert needle into the SC fat; do not aspirate. If a large vessel is penetrated, blood will be seen immediately in the syringe; withdraw needle and make injection elsewhere with a new syringe.

5. The direction of the needle is changed so it parallels the abdominal wall. The needle is then pushed in until the barrel hub touches the skin. The plunger is depressed to deliver the drug. The needle is then withdrawn and the area bandaged.

6. To confirm the drug has been delivered, ensure that the tip of the plunger is visible within the tip of the needle.

7. If there is need to remove goserelin surgically, it can be located by ultrasound.

8. Adhere to the 28-day and 12-week schedules as closely as possible.

9. Store at room temperatures not exceeding 25°C (77°F).

10. There is no evidence the drug accumulates with either hepatic and/or renal dysfunction.

11. Duration of treatment for endometriosis is 6 months.

12. Males with ureteral obstruction or spinal cord compression should have appropriate treatment prior to initiating goserelin therapy.

ASSESSMENT

1. Note reasons for therapy, clinical presentation, other agents trialed, outcome.

2. List PSA and testosterone levels with prostate cancer; pain with endometriosis.

CLIENT/FAMILY TEACHING

1. Drug will be implanted into abdomen with a syringe every 28 days to 3 mo as prescribed. Be sure not to miss scheduled administration days.

2. The most common side effects (e.g.; hot flashes, decreased erections, and sexual dysfunction) R/T ↓ testosterone levels.

Bold Italic = life threatening side effect   ■ = black box warning   ✦ = Available in Canada

3. Symptoms may grow worse initially as a result of transient increases of testosterone.

4. May experience increased bone pain and develop spinal cord compression or ureteral obstruction; usually only temporary but must be reported promptly so that appropriate treatment may be initiated. Report all unusual/adverse side effects.

5. Not for use in women who are likely to become pregnant or who are pregnant. Drug may harm fetus and may impair fertility; identify for sperm or egg harvesting.

6. Clients with prostate cancer who decide against surgery (orchiectomy), for medication therapy, must come in regularly for abdominal implants for the rest of their lives.

7. Identify appropriate resources and support groups.

OUTCOMES/EVALUATE

- Symptom control; ↑ comfort
- ↓ Tumor size and spread
- ↓ Testosterone levels

Granisetron hydrochloride   Ⅳ

(gran-**ISS**-eh-tron)

CLASSIFICATION(S):
Antiemetic, 5-HT$_3$ receptor antagonist

PREGNANCY CATEGORY: B

Rx: Kytril.

USES
(1) Prevention of N&V associated with initial/repeat cancer chemotherapy, including high-dose cisplatin (IV and PO). (2) Prevention of N&V associated with radiation, including total body irradiation/fractionated abdominal radiation (PO only). (3) Prevention/treatment of postoperative nausea and vomiting (IV only).

ACTION/KINETICS

Action
Selective 5-HT$_3$ (serotonin) receptor antagonist with little or no affinity for other 5-HT, beta-adrenergic, dopamine, or histamine receptors. During chemotherapy-induced vomiting, mucosal enterochromaffin cells release serotonin, which stimulates 5-HT$_3$ receptors. The stimulation of 5-HT$_3$ receptors by serotonin causes vagal discharge resulting in vomiting. Granisetron blocks serotonin stimulation and subsequent vomiting.

Pharmacokinetics
In adult cancer clients undergoing chemotherapy, infusion of a single 40-mcg/kg dose over 5 min produced the following data. **Peak plasma level:** 63.8 ng/mL. **Plasma t½, terminal:** 5–9 hr, depending on age and disease state. Metabolized in the liver with unchanged drug (12%) and metabolites excreted through both the urine and feces.

CONTRAINDICATIONS
Known hypersensitivity to the drug.

SPECIAL CONCERNS
Use with caution during lactation. Safety and efficacy in children less than 2 years of age have not been established.

SIDE EFFECTS

Most Common

After parenteral use: Headache, asthenia, constipation, pain, fever, anemia, abdominal pain, constipation, dizziness, bradycardia, somnolence, diarrhea.

After PO use: Headache, constipation, asthenia, diarrhea, abdominal pain, dyspepsia, dizziness, insomnia, N&V, leukopenia, anorexia, fever, anemia.

After IV use. CNS: Headache, somnolence, dizziness, agitation, anxiety, CNS stimulation, insomnia, extrapyramidal syndrome. **GI:** Diarrhea, constipation, taste disorder, abdominal pain. **CV:** Hyper-/hypotension, arrhythmias (e.g., sinus bradycardia, atrial fibrillation, *AV block*, ventricular ectopy including nonsustained tachycardia, ECG abnormalities). **Allergic:** *Hypersensitivity reactions (anaphylaxis)*, skin rashes. **Hematologic:** Anemia. **Miscellaneous:** Asthenia, fever, pain.

After PO use. CNS: Headache, dizziness, insomnia, anxiety, somnolence. **GI:** N&V, diarrhea, constipation, abdominal pain, dyspepsia. **CV:** Hyper-/hypo-

---

G

tension, angina, atrial fibrillation, syncope (rare). **Hypersensitivity:** Rarely, hypersensitivity reactions; *severe anaphylaxis*, shortness of breath, urticaria. **Miscellaneous:** Fever, asthenia, leukopenia, decreased appetite, anemia, alopecia, thrombocytopenia.

LABORATORY TEST CONSIDERATIONS
↑ AST, ALT.

DRUG INTERACTIONS
Because granisetron is metabolized by hepatic cytochrome P-450 drug-metabolizing enzymes, agents that induce or inhibit these enzymes may alter the clearance (and thus the half-life) of granisetron.

HOW SUPPLIED
Injection: 1 mg/mL; *Oral Solution:* 1 mg/ 5 mL; *Tablets:* 1 mg.

DOSAGE
• **IV**
Antiemetic during cancer chemotherapy.
Adults and children over 2 years of age: 10 mcg/kg within 30 min before initiation of chemotherapy given either undiluted over 30 seconds, or diluted and infused over 5 min.
Prevention and treatment of postoperative nausea and vomiting.
Adults: 1 mg, undiluted, given over 30 seconds, before induction of anesthesia or immediately before reversal of anesthesia. Treatment of nausea and/or vomiting after surgery is 1 mg, undiluted, given over 30 seconds. Safety and efficacy have not been established in children.
• **ORAL SOLUTION; TABLETS**
Protection from chemotherapy-induced N&V.
Adults: 2 mg (two-1 mg tablets or 10 mL of oral solution) once daily or 1 mg (one-1 mg tablet or 5 mL of oral solution) twice daily. In the 2 mg once daily regime, two 1 mg tablets are given up to 1 hr before chemotherapy. In the 1 mg twice a day regime, the first 1 mg tablet is given up to 1 hr before chemotherapy and the second tablet is given 12 hr after the first. Either regimen is administered only on the day(s) chemotherapy is given. Data are not available for PO use in children.

Protection from radiation-induced N&V.
Adults: 2 mg (two-1 mg tablets or 10 mL of oral solution) once daily taken within 1 hr of radiation.

NURSING CONSIDERATIONS

ADMINISTRATION/STORAGE
1. Give drug only on the day chemotherapy is given.
2. Dosage adjustment not necessary for geriatric clients or with impaired renal/hepatic function.
3. Store oral solution and tablets from 15–30°C (59–86°F) protected from light.
IV 4. Administer either undiluted over 30 seconds or diluted with NSS or D5W to a total volume of 20 to 50 mL; infuse over 5 minutes. Drug is stable for at least 24 hr when diluted in NSS or D5W and stored at room temperature under normal lighting.
5. Do not mix in solution with other drugs.
6. Do not freeze vial; protect from light.
7. Once multidose vial is penetrated, use within 30 days.
8. Store single- and multi-use vials from 15–30°C (59–86°F).

ASSESSMENT
1. Note reasons for therapy: XRT/chemo/postoperative N&V.
2. Give drug 30 min before the start of emetogenic cancer chemotherapy.
3. Monitor LFTs, frequency/severity of vomiting, and fluid balance.

CLIENT/FAMILY TEACHING
1. Review the appropriate method/frequency of dosing.
2. May be given IV/orally to ↓ chemotherapy-induced N&V.
3. Report constipation/diarrhea/rashes/adverse effects. May experience headaches; usually relieved with acetaminophen. Drug may mask an ileus and/or gastric distention.

OUTCOMES/EVALUATE
• Prevention of N&V
• Protection from XRT/chemotherapy-induced N&V

Guaifenesin ©

(gwye-**FEN**-eh-sin)

CLASSIFICATION(S):
Expectorant

PREGNANCY CATEGORY: C

OTC: Oral Liquid: Mucinex Children's, Naldecon Senior EX, Robitussin, Scot-Tussin Expectorant, Siltussin SA. **Syrup:** Altarussin, Guiatuss. **Tablets, Extended-Release:** Humabid Maximum Strength, Mucinex. **Granules:** Mucinex Mini-Melts Children's, Mucinex Mini-Melts Junior Strength.

Rx: Oral Liquid: Diabetic Tussin, Organidin NR. **Tablets:** Liquidbid, Organidin NR.

♣OTC: Balminil Expectorant, Benylin-E Extra Strength.

USES

(1) Dry, nonproductive cough due to colds and minor upper respiratory tract infections when there is mucus in the respiratory tract. (2) To loosen phlegm and thin bronchial secretions.

ACTION/KINETICS

Action

May increase the output of fluid from the respiratory tract by reducing the viscosity and surface tension of respiratory secretions, thereby removing accumulated secretions from the upper and lower airway.

Pharmacokinetics

Readily absorbed from the GI tract. Rapidly metabolized and excreted in the urine. **t½:** 1 hr.

CONTRAINDICATIONS

Chronic cough (e.g., due to smoking, asthma, or emphysema), cough accompanied by excess secretions. Use in children under age 6. Lactation.

SPECIAL CONCERNS

Persistent cough may indicate a serious infection; thus, the provider should be consulted if cough lasts for more than 1 week, is recurring, or is accompanied by high fever, rash, or persistent headache. Taking large quantities of guaifenesin products may increase the risk of drug-induced kidney stones.

SIDE EFFECTS

Most Common

N&V, GI discomfort.

GI: N&V, GI upset/discomfort. **CNS:** Dizziness, headache. **Dermatologic:** Rash, urticaria.

LABORATORY TEST CONSIDERATIONS

↑ Renal urate clearance and thus ↓ serum uric acid levels. ↑ Urinary 5-hydroxyindoleacetic acid and falsely ↑ vanillylmandelic acid test for catechols.

OD **OVERDOSE MANAGEMENT**

Symptoms: N&V. *Treatment:* Treat symptomatically.

DRUG INTERACTIONS

Inhibition of platelet adhesiveness by guaifenesin may result in bleeding tendencies.

HOW SUPPLIED

Granules: 50 mg/packet, 100 mg/packet; *Oral Liquid:* 100 mg/5 mL, 200 mg/5 mL; *Syrup:* 100 mg/5 mL; *Tablets:* 200 mg, 400 mg; *Tablets, Extended-Release:* 600 mg, 1,200 mg.

DOSAGE

- **GRANULES**
  Expectorant.

Children, 12 years and older: 200–400 mg (2 to 4 of the 100 mg/packet strength) q 4 hr, up to 6 doses/day. **Children, 6 to <12 years of age:** 100–200 mg (1 to 2 of the 100 mg/packet strength or 2 to 4 of the 50 mg/packet strength) q 4 hr, up to 6 doses/day.

- **ORAL LIQUID; SYRUP; TABLETS**
  Expectorant.

Adults and children 12 years and older: 200–400 mg q 4 hr, not to exceed 2,400 mg/day; **pediatric, 6–11 years:** 100–200 mg q 4 hr, not to exceed 1,200 mg/day; **pediatric, less than 6 years of age: Do not use.**

- **TABLETS, EXTENDED-RELEASE**
  Expectorant.

Adults and children 12 years and over: 600–1,200 mg q 12 hr, not to exceed 2,400 mg/day.

NOTE: The liquid dosage forms may be more suitable for children from 6–12 years of age.

NURSING CONSIDERATIONS

Ⓒ Do not confuse Mucinex with Mucomyst (a mucolytic).

ADMINISTRATION/STORAGE

Naldecon Senior EX and Mucinex are not recommended for children less than 12 years of age.

ASSESSMENT

1. Note type, frequency, duration, and characteristics of cough and sputum production.

2. List pulmonary assessment findings, CXR.

3. Assess for tobacco/nasal drug use, fever/chills, loss of appetite, or increased fatigue.

CLIENT/FAMILY TEACHING

1. Take only as directed and do not exceed prescribed dose. Take tablets with a full glass of water.

2. If symptoms persist more than 1 week, recur, or are accompanied by a persistent headache, fever, or rash, notify provider.

3. Report any evidence of increased bruising/bleeding, fever, change in secretions, or lack of response.

4. Do not perform activities that require mental alertness; drug may cause drowsiness.

5. Increase fluids to 2.5 L/day to decrease secretion viscosity.

6. Avoid triggers: dust, chemicals, cleansers, cigarette smoke, environmental pollutants, and perfumes.

OUTCOMES/EVALUATE

- Control of coughing episodes
- Mobilization of mucus

Guanfacine hydrochloride

(**GWON**-fah-seen)

CLASSIFICATION(S):

Antihypertensive, centrally-acting
PREGNANCY CATEGORY: B
Rx: Tenex.

SEE ALSO ANTIHYPERTENSIVE AGENTS.

USES

Hypertension alone or with a thiazide diuretic. *Investigational:* Withdrawal from heroin use, to reduce the frequency of migraine headaches.

ACTION/KINETICS

Action

Thought to act by central stimulation of alpha-2 receptors. Causes a decrease in peripheral sympathetic output and HR resulting in a decrease in BP. May also manifest a direct peripheral alpha-2 receptor stimulant action.

Pharmacokinetics

Onset: 2 hr. **Peak plasma levels:** 1–4 hr. **Peak effect:** 6–12 hr. **t½:** 12–23 hr. **Duration:** 24 hr. Approximately 50% excreted through the kidneys unchanged.

CONTRAINDICATIONS

Hypersensitivity to guanfacine. Acute hypertension associated with toxemia. Children less than 12 years of age.

SPECIAL CONCERNS

Use with caution during lactation and in clients with recent MI, cerebrovascular disease, chronic renal or hepatic failure, or severe coronary insufficiency. Geriatric clients may be more sensitive to the hypotensive and sedative effects. Safety and efficacy in children less than 12 years of age have not been determined.

SIDE EFFECTS

Most Common

Dry mouth, somnolence, dizziness, constipation, fatigue, headache, insomnia.

GI: Dry mouth, constipation, nausea, abdominal pain, diarrhea, dyspepsia, dysphagia, taste perversion or alterations in taste. **CNS:** Sedation/somnolence, weakness, dizziness, headache, fatigue, insomnia, amnesia, confusion, depression, vertigo, agitation, anxiety, malaise, nervousness, tremor. **CV:** Bradycardia, substernal pain, palpitations, syncope, chest pain, tachycardia, cardiac fibrillation, CHF, heart block, MI (rare), cardiovascular accident (rare). **Ophthalmic:** Visual disturbances, conjunctivitis, iritis, blurred vision. **Dermatologic:** Pruritus, dermatitis, purpura, sweating, skin rash with exfoliation, alopecia, rash. **GU:** Decreased libido, impo-

---

Bold Italic = life threatening side effect　　■ = black box warning　　♣ = Available in Canada

tence, urinary incontinence or frequency, testicular disorder, nocturia, acute renal failure. **Musculoskeletal:** Leg cramps, hypokinesia, arthralgia, leg pain, myalgia. **Miscellaneous:** Rhinitis, tinnitus, dyspnea, paresthesias, paresis, asthenia, edema, abnormal LFTs.

OD OVERDOSE MANAGEMENT
Symptoms: Drowsiness, bradycardia, lethargy, hypotension. *Treatment:* Gastric lavage. Supportive therapy, as needed. The drug is not dialyzable.

DRUG INTERACTIONS
Additive sedative effects when used concomitantly with CNS depressants.

HOW SUPPLIED
Tablets: 1 mg, 2 mg.

DOSAGE

- **TABLETS**
  Hypertension.
Initial: 1 mg/day alone or with other antihypertensives; if satisfactory results are not obtained in 3–4 weeks, dosage may be increased by 1 mg at 1–2-week intervals up to a maximum of 3 mg/day in one to two divided doses.
  Heroin withdrawal.
0.03–1.5 mg/day.
  Reduce frequency of migraine headaches.
1 mg/day for 12 weeks.

NURSING CONSIDERATIONS

ADMINISTRATION/STORAGE
1. Divide the daily dose if a decrease in BP is not maintained for over 24 hr; however, the incidence of side effects increases.

2. Adverse effects increase significantly when dose exceeds 3 mg/day.
3. Initiate antihypertensive therapy in clients already taking a thiazide diuretic.
4. Abrupt cessation may result in increases in plasma and urinary catecholamines, symptoms of nervousness and anxiety, and BPs greater than those prior to therapy.

ASSESSMENT
1. Note reasons for therapy, onset, S&S, any previous agents used, outcome.
2. Determine evidence of CAD, and renal or liver dysfunction.

CLIENT/FAMILY TEACHING
1. To minimize daytime drowsiness, take at bedtime. Do not perform activities that require mental alertness until drug effects realized.
2. Do not stop drug abruptly; may experience rebound effect. Continue life style changes to ensure BP control, i.e., salt restriction, lipid control, absence of proteinuria, tobacco and alcohol cessation, regular daily exercise and weight control.
3. Avoid alcohol. Use sugarless gum, ice chips, or sips of water for dry mouth.
4. May cause constipation or skin rash; report if persistent or severe.
5. Avoid OTC cough/cold remedies. Keep record of BP for provider review at F/U visits.

OUTCOMES/EVALUATE
- ↓ BP
- ↓ S&S of heroin withdrawal
- ↓ Migraine headaches

G

Haloperidol ©
(hah-low-**PAIR**-ih-dohl)

CLASSIFICATION(S):
Antipsychotic
PREGNANCY CATEGORY: C
♣**Rx:** Apo-Haloperidol,
Novo–Peridol, ratio-Haloperidol.

Haloperidol decanoate

PREGNANCY CATEGORY: C
Rx: Haldol Decanoate 50 and 100.
♣**Rx:** Apo-Haloperidol Decanoate
Injection, Haloperidol LA, Haloperidol Long Acting, Haloperidol-LA
Omega, PMS Haloperidol-LA.

Haloperidol lactate

PREGNANCY CATEGORY: C

USES
(1) Psychotic disorders including schizophrenia. (The decanoate is used for prolonged therapy in chronic schizophrenia). (2) Severe behavior problems in children (those with combative, explosive hyperexcitability not accounted for by immediate provocation). Use reserved only after failure to respond to psychotherapy or drugs other than antipsychotics. (3) Short-term treatment of hyperactive children who show excessive motor activity with accompanying conduct consisting of impulsivity, poor attention, aggression, mood lability, or poor frustration tolerance. (4) Control of tics and vocal utterances associated with Tourette's syndrome in adults and children. *Investigational:* Intractable hiccoughs, N&V.

ACTION/KINETICS
Action
Precise mechanism not known. Competitively blocks dopamine receptors in the tuberoinfundibular system to cause sedation. Also causes alpha-adrenergic blockade, decreases release of growth hormone, and increases prolactin release by the pituitary. Causes significant extrapyramidal effects, as well as a low incidence of sedation, anticholinergic effects, and orthostatic hypotension. Narrow margin between the therapeutically effective dose and that causing extrapyramidal symptoms. Also has antiemetic effects.

Pharmacokinetics
Is 60–65% bioavailable after PO administration. **Peak plasma levels, PO:** 3–5 hr; **IM:** 20 min; **IM, decanoate:** approximately 6 days. **Therapeutic serum levels:** 3–10 ng/mL. **t½, PO:** About 18 hr; **IM:** 13–36 hr; **IM, decanoate:** 3 weeks; **IV:** approximately 14 hr. Metabolized in liver, slowly excreted in urine and feces. **Plasma protein binding:** 92%.

CONTRAINDICATIONS
Use with extreme caution, or not at all, in clients with parkinsonism. Lactation.

SPECIAL CONCERNS
PO dosage has not been determined in children less than 3 years of age; IM dosage is not recommended in children. Geriatric clients are more likely to exhibit orthostatic hypotension, anticholinergic effects, sedation, and extrapyramidal side effects (such as parkinsonism and tardive dyskinesia).

SIDE EFFECTS
Most Common
Extrapyramidal symptoms, drowsiness, dizziness, blurred vision, GI upset, anorexia, headache, salivation, dry mouth, sweating, sleep disturbances, restlessness, constipation.
CNS: Agitation, akathisia, anxiety, catatonic-like states, confusion, *seizures*, depression, drowsiness, dizziness, sleep disturbances, sedation, somnolence, dystonia, extrapyramidal symptoms, hallucinations, headache, insomnia, lightheadedness, neuroleptic malignant syndrome, pseudoparkinsonism, psy-

---

Bold Italic = life threatening side effect   ■ = black box warning   ♣ = Available in Canada

chosis, restlessness, tardive dyskinesia, tardive dystonia, vertigo. **GI:** Anorexia, constipation, diarrhea, dry mouth, GI upset, dyspepsia, N&V, salivation. **Hepatic:** Jaundice impaired liver function. **CV:** Hypo-/hypertension, ECG changes, prolonged QTc interval, tachycardia. **Dermatologic:** Acne, alopecia, maculo-papular skin reactions, photosensitivity, diaphoresis/sweating. **GU:** Breast engorgement, galactorrhea, gynecomastia, impotence, menstrual irregularities, priapism, urinary retention. **Hematologic:** Anemia, agranulocytosis (rare), leukocytosis, leukopenia. **Ophthalmic:** Cataracts, oculogyric crisis, blurred vision, visual disturbances. **Miscellaneous:** Opisthotonos, hyperpyrexia/hyperthermia, *sudden death*, withdrawal syndrome.

LABORATORY TEST CONSIDERATIONS
↑ Alkaline phosphatase, bilirubin, serum transaminase; ↓ PT (clients on coumarin), serum cholesterol.

OD **OVERDOSE MANAGEMENT**
Symptoms: CNS depression, hyper-/hypotension, extrapyramidal symptoms (may be severe), agitation, restlessness, fever, hypo-/hyperthermia, *seizures, cardiac arrhythmias,* changes in the ECG, autonomic reactions, *coma.* *Treatment:* Treat symptomatically. Antiparkinson drugs, diphenhydramine, or barbiturates can be used to treat extrapyramidal symptoms. Fluid replacement and vasoconstrictors (either norepinephrine or phenylephrine) can be used to treat hypotension. Ventricular arrhythmias can be treated with phenytoin. To treat seizures, use pentobarbital or diazepam. A saline cathartic can be used to hasten the excretion of sustained-release products.

DRUG INTERACTIONS
Amphetamine / ↓ Amphetamine effect by ↓ uptake of drug at its site of action
Anticholinergics / ↓ Haloperidol effect
Antidepressants, tricyclic / ↑ TCA effects R/T ↓ liver breakdown
Barbiturates / ↓ Effect of haloperidol R/T ↑ liver breakdown
H *Ginkgo biloba* / Increased beneficial effect and decreased extrapyramidal symptoms when used to treat schizo-phrenia
Guanethidine / ↓ Guanethidine effect by ↓ uptake of drug at site of action
Lithium / ↑ Toxicity of haloperidol
Methyldopa / ↑ Toxicity of haloperidol
Phenytoin / ↓ Effect of haloperidol R/T ↑ liver breakdown
Smoking / ↑ Haloperidol clearance → ↓ serum levels

HOW SUPPLIED
Haloperidol: *Tablets:* 0.5 mg, 1 mg, 2 mg, 5 mg, 10 mg, 20 mg.
Haloperidol decanoate: *Injection:* 50 mg/mL, 100 mg/mL.
Haloperidol lactate: *Injection:* 5 mg/mL; *Oral Concentrate:* 2 mg/mL.

DOSAGE
HALOPERIDOL, HALOPERIDOL LACTATE
• **ORAL CONCENTRATE; TABLETS**
  Psychoses.
Adults: 0.5–2 mg 2–3 times per day up to 3–5 mg 2–3 times per day for severe symptoms; **maintenance:** reduce dosage to lowest effective level. Up to 100 mg/day may be required in some. **Geriatric or debilitated clients:** 0.5–2 mg 2–3 times per day. **Pediatric, 3–12 years or 15–40 kg:** 0.5 mg/day (25–50 mcg/kg/day) in two to three divided doses; if necessary the daily dose may be increased by 0.5-mg increments q 5–7 days for a total of 0.15 mg/kg/day for psychotic disorders
  Tourette's syndrome.
Adults, initial: 0.5–1.5 mg 3 times per day, up to 10 mg daily. Adjust dose carefully to obtain the optimum response. **Children, 3 to 12 years or 15–40 kg:** 0.05–0.075 mg/kg/day. Higher doses may be needed for those severely disturbed.
  Behavioral disorders/hyperactivity in children.
Children, 3 to 12 years or 15–40 kg: 0.05–0.075 mg/kg/day. Higher doses may be needed for those severely disturbed.
  Intractable hiccoughs (investigational).
1.5 mg 3 times per day.
  Infantile autism (investigational).
0.5–4 mg/day.
HALOPERIDOL LACTATE
• **IM**
  Acute psychoses.

Adults and adolescents, initial: 2–5 mg to control acute agitation; may be repeated if necessary q 4–8 hr to a total of 100 mg/day. Switch to **PO** therapy as soon as possible.

HALOPERIDOL DECANOATE

• IM

Chronic therapy.

Adults, initial dose, first month: 10–15 times the daily PO dose for those stabilized on low daily PO doses (10 mg/day or less) and in the elderly or debilitated. **then, monthly maintenance:** 10–15 times the previous daily PO dose (decanoate is not to be given IV). For clients stabilized on higher doses with risk of relapse or those tolerant to oral haloperidol, give 20 times the daily PO dose the first month followed by monthly maintenance doses of 10–15 times the previous daily PO dose. For elderly or debilitated clients, give lower initial doses and more gradual adjustments. *NOTE:* The initial dose should not exceed 100 mg, regardless of the previous oral antipsychotic dose. If the conversion requires more than 100 mg haloperidol decanoate as an initial dose, give that dose in 2 injections (maximum of 100 mg initially followed by the balance in 3–7 days).

NURSING CONSIDERATIONS

℗ Do not confuse Haldol with Medrol (a corticosteroid).

ADMINISTRATION/STORAGE

1. Give the decanoate by deep IM injection using a 21-gauge needle. Do not exceed a volume of 3 mL/site.

2. Do not give decanoate IV.

3. Replace injectable with PO form asap. For an approximation of the total daily dose needed, determine parenteral dose given during the preceding 24 hr; carefully monitor for the first several days. Give the first PO dose within 12–24 hr after the last parenteral dose.

4. Store tablets from 15–30°C (59–86°F). Store injection from 15–30°C (59–86°F) protected from light.

ASSESSMENT

1. Note behavior, appearance, response to environment, characteristics of symptoms; note any of parkinsonism and tardive dyskinesias. Monitor for relapse of psychotic symptoms.

2. Use with caution in the elderly; they tend to exhibit toxicity more frequently and S&S that may not be resolvable; may also benefit from a periodic 'drug holiday.'

3. List onset extrapyramidal symptoms; may be drug induced.

4. Assess CBC, electrolytes, liver, and renal function.

CLIENT/FAMILY TEACHING

1. Take exactly as prescribed. Do not stop abruptly with long-term therapy.

2. Avoid activities that require mental alertness until drug effects realized.

3. Avoid alcohol. May use sugarless gum, ice chips, or sips of water for dry mouth effects.

4. Report muscle weakness/stiffness. Change position slowly to avoid sudden drop in BP.

5. May take up to 6 weeks for full benefits to occur.

6. Immediately report any new onset involuntary, dyskinetic movements, temperature elevation, muscle rigidity, altered mental status; stop drug.

7. Keep all F/U appointments to assess response to therapy and need for continued therapy.

OUTCOMES/EVALUATE

• Improved behavior patterns: ↓ Agitation, hostility, psychosis, delusions

• Control of tics/vocal utterances, intractable hiccoughs

• ↓ Hyperactive behaviors

Heparin sodium lock flush solution (**HEP**-ah-rin) ⅣV ℗

CLASSIFICATION(S):

Anticoagulant, heparin

PREGNANCY CATEGORY: C

Rx: Hep-Flush 10, Hep-Lock, Hep-Lock U/P, Heparin I.V. Flush Syringe, Heparin Lock Flush.

Bold Italic = life threatening side effect   ■ = black box warning   ✤ = Available in Canada

Heparin sodium and sodium chloride

PREGNANCY CATEGORY: C

Rx: Heparin Sodium and 0.45% Sodium Chloride, Heparin Sodium and 0.9% Sodium Chloride.

Heparin sodium injection

PREGNANCY CATEGORY: C

♣Rx: Hepalean, Hepalean-Lok, Heparin Leo.

USES

(1) Prophylaxis and treatment of venous thrombosis and its extension; pulmonary embolism; peripheral arterial embolism; atrial fibrillation with embolization. (2) Diagnosis and treatment of acute and chronic consumption coagulopathies (disseminated intravascular coagulation). (3) Low-dose regimen for the prevention of post-operative deep venous thrombosis and pulmonary embolism in those undergoing major abdominothoracic surgery or who are at risk of developing thromboembolic disease. (4) Prevention of clotting in arterial and heart surgery, blood transfusions, extracorporeal circulation, dialysis procedures, and blood samples. *Investigational:* (1) Prophylaxis of left ventricular thrombi and cerebrovascular accidents after MI. (2) Continuous infusion for treating MI in unstable angina refractory to conventional treatment. Heparin decreases the number of anginal attacks and silent ischemic episodes and reduces the daily duration of ischemia. (3) Prevention of cerebral thrombosis in the evolving stroke. (4) Adjunct in treating coronary occlusion with acute MI.

Heparin lock flush solution: Dilute solutions are used to maintain patency of indwelling catheters used for IV therapy or blood sampling. Not to be used therapeutically.

ACTION/KINETICS

Action

Anticoagulants do not dissolve previously formed clots, but they do forestall their enlargement and prevent new clots from forming. Heparin potentiates the inhibitory action of antithrombin III on various coagulation factors including factors IIa, IXa, Xa, XIa, and XIIa. This occurs due to the formation of a complex with antithrombin III and causing a conformational change in the antithrombin III molecule. Inhibition of factor Xa results in interference with thrombin generation; thus, the action of thrombin in coagulation is inhibited. Heparin also increases the rate of formation of antithrombin III–thrombin complex causing inactivation of thrombin and preventing the conversion of fibrinogen to fibrin. By inhibiting the activation of fibrin-stabilizing factor by thrombin, heparin also prevents formation of a stable fibrin clot. Therapeutic doses of heparin prolong thrombin time, whole blood clotting time, activated clotting time, and PTT. Heparin also decreases the levels of triglycerides by releasing lipoprotein lipase from tissues; the resultant hydrolysis of triglycerides causes increased blood levels of free fatty acids.

Pharmacokinetics

Onset: IV, immediate; **deep SC:** 20–60 min. **Peak plasma levels, after SC:** 2–4 hr. **t½:** 30–180 min in healthy persons. t½ increases with dose, severe renal disease, and cirrhosis and in anephric clients and decreases with pulmonary embolism and liver impairment other than cirrhosis. **Metabolism:** Probably by reticuloendothelial system, although up to 50% is excreted unchanged in the urine. Clotting time returns to normal within 2–6 hr.

CONTRAINDICATIONS

Active bleeding, blood dyscrasias (or other disorders characterized by bleeding tendencies such as hemophilia), clients with frail or weakened blood vessels, purpura, thrombocytopenia, liver disease with hypoprothrombinemia, suspected intracranial hemorrhage, suppurative thrombophlebitis, inaccessible ulcerative lesions (especially of the GI tract), open wounds, extensive denudation of the skin, and increased capillary permeability (as in ascorbic acid deficiency). IM use.

Do not administer during surgery of the eye, brain, or spinal cord or during continuous tube drainage of the stomach or small intestine. Use is also contraindicated in subacute endocarditis, shock, threatened abortion, severe hypertension, diverticulitis, colitis, SBE, or hypersensitivity to drug. Premature neonates due to the possibility of a fatal 'gasping syndrome.' Also, regional anesthesia and lumbar block, vitamin K deficiency, leukemia with bleeding tendencies, open wounds or ulcerations, acute nephritis, or impaired hepatic or renal function. In the presence of drainage tubes in any orifice. Alcoholism.

SPECIAL CONCERNS

Use with caution in menstruation, in pregnant women (heparin may cause hypoprothrombinemia in the infant), during lactation, during the postpartum period, and following cerebrovascular accidents. Geriatric clients may be more susceptible to developing bleeding complications, unusual hair loss, and itching.

SIDE EFFECTS

Most Common

Hemorrhage (see below), chills, fever, urticaria, local irritation, erythema, mild pain, hematoma.

CV: *Hemorrhage ranging from minor local ecchymoses to major hemorrhagic complications from any organ or tissue.* Higher incidence is seen in women over 60 years of age. Hemorrhagic reactions are more likely to occur in prophylactic administration during surgery than in the treatment of thromboembolic disease. White clot syndrome. **Hematologic:** Heparin-induced thrombocytopenia (both early and delayed). **Hypersensitivity:** Chills, fever, urticaria are the most common. Rarely, asthma, lacrimation, headache, N&V, rhinitis, *shock, anaphylaxis.* Allergic vasospastic reaction within 6–10 days after initiation of therapy (lasts 4–6 hr) including painful, ischemic, cyanotic limbs. Use a test dose of 1,000 units in clients with a history of asthma or allergic disease. **Miscellaneous:** Hyperkale-

mia, cutaneous necrosis, osteoporosis (after long-term high doses), delayed transient alopecia, priapism, suppressed aldosterone synthesis. Discontinuance of heparin has resulted in rebound hyperlipemia.

Following IM (usual), SC: Local irritation, erythema, mild pain, ulceration, hematoma, and tissue sloughing.

LABORATORY TEST CONSIDERATIONS

↑ AST and ALT.

OD OVERDOSE MANAGEMENT

Symptoms: Nosebleeds, hematuria, tarry stools, petechiae, and easy bruising may be the first signs. *Treatment:* Drug withdrawal is usually sufficient to correct heparin overdosage. Protamine sulfate (1%) solution; each mg of protamine neutralizes about 100 USP heparin units.

DRUG INTERACTIONS

Alteplase, recombinant / ↑ Risk of bleeding, especially at arterial puncture sites

Anticoagulants, oral / Additive ↑ PT

Antihistamines / ↓ Effect of heparin

Aspirin / Additive ↑ PT

H *Bromelain* / ↑ Tendency for bleeding

Cephalosporins / ↑ Risk of bleeding R/T additive effect

H *Cinchona bark* / ↑ Anticoagulant effect

Dextran / Additive ↑ PT

Digitalis / ↓ Effect of heparin

Dipyridamole / Additive ↑ PT

H *Feverfew* / Possible additive antiplatelet effect

H *Ginger* / Possible additive antiplatelet effects

H *Ginkgo biloba* / ↑ Effect on blood coagulation

H *Ginseng* / Potential for ↓ effect on platelet aggregation

H *Goldenseal* / Antagonizes action of heparin

Hydroxychloroquine / Additive ↑ PT

Ibuprofen / Additive ↑ PT

Indomethacin / Additive ↑ PT

Insulin / Heparin antagonizes insulin effect

Nicotine / ↓ Effect of heparin

Nitroglycerin / ↓ Effect of heparin

NSAIDs / Additive ↑ PT

Penicillins / ↑ Risk of bleeding R/T possible additive effects

Salicylates / ↑ Risk of bleeding

Smoking / Possible ↑ heparin elimination, ↓ t½; dosage may need to be ↑

Streptokinase / Relative resistance to effects of heparin

Tetracyclines / ↓ Effect of heparin

Ticlopidine / Additive ↑ PT

HOW SUPPLIED

Heparin sodium injection: *Injection:* 1,000 units/mL, 2,000 units/mL, 2,500 units/mL, 5,000 units/mL, 7,500 units/mL, 10,000 units/mL, 20,000 units/mL, 40,000 units/mL.

Heparin sodium and sodium chloride: *Injection:* 200 units/100 mL-0.9% NaCl; 5,000 units/100 mL-0.45% NaCl; 10,000 units/100 mL-0.45% NaCl.

Heparin sodium lock flush solution: *:* 1 unit/mL, 10 units/mL, 100 units/mL.

DOSAGE

NOTE: Adjusted for each client on the basis of laboratory tests. Dosage is adequate when whole blood clotting time is about 2.5 to 3 times control value, or when aPTT is 1.5 to 2 times normal.

• **DEEP SC**

General heparin dosage.

Initial loading dose: 10,000–20,000 units; **maintenance:** 8,000–10,000 units q 8 hr or 15,000–20,000 units q 12 hr. Use concentrated solution.

Prophylaxis of postoperative thromboembolism.

5,000 units of concentrated solution 2 hr before surgery and 5,000 units q 8–12 hr thereafter for 7 days or until client is ambulatory whichever is longer.

• **IV, INTERMITTENT**

General heparin dosage.

Initial loading dose: 10,000 units undiluted or in 50–100 mL saline; **then,** 5,000–10,000 units q 4–6 hr undiluted or in 50–100 mL saline.

• **IV, CONTINUOUS INFUSION**

General heparin dosage.

Initial loading dose: 20,000–40,000 units/day in 1,000 mL saline (preceded initially by 5,000 units IV).

• **SPECIAL USES**

Use in children.

Use the following as a guideline. **Initial:** 50 units/kg IV bolus. **Maintenance:** 100 units/kg/dose IV drip q 4 hr or 20,000 units/m²/24 hr continuous IV infusion.

Deep venous thrombosis.

If the PTT is <45 seconds give 5,000 units as a bolus and increase by 250 units/hr. If the PTT is from 45-54 seconds, increase by 150 units/hr. If the PTT is from 55-85 seconds, do not change dosage. If the PTT is 85-110 seconds, stop the infusion for 1 hr and decrease by 150 units/hr. If the PTT is >110 seconds, stop the infusion for 1 hr and decrease by 250 units/hr.

Surgery of heart and blood vessels.

Initial, 150–400 units/kg to clients undergoing total body perfusion for open heart surgery. *NOTE:* 300 units/kg may be used for procedures less than 60 min while 400 units/kg is used for procedures lasting more than 60 min. To prevent clotting in the tube system, add heparin to fluids in pump oxygenator.

Extracorporeal renal dialysis.

See instructions on equipment.

Blood transfusion.

400–600 units/100 mL whole blood. 7,500 units should be added to 100 mL 0.9% sodium chloride injection; from this dilution, add 6–8 mL/100 mL whole blood.

Laboratory samples.

70–150 units/10- to 20-mL sample to prevent coagulation.

Heparin lock sets.

To prevent clot formation in a heparin lock set, inject 10–100 units/mL heparin solution through the injection hub in a sufficient quantity to fill the entire set to the needle tip.

NURSING CONSIDERATIONS

℘ Do not confuse heparin with low molecular weight heparins (LMWH)

ADMINISTRATION/STORAGE

1. May be given by intermittent IV injection, continuous IV infusion, or deep SC injection. Continuous IV infusion is generally preferred due to the higher chance of bleeding complications with other routes. Do *not* administer IM.

2. Administer by deep SC injection to minimize local irritation, hematoma, and tissue sloughing and to prolong drug action.

- Z-track method: Use any fat roll, but abdominal fat rolls are preferred. Use a ½-in. or ⅝-in. 25- or 27-gauge needle. Grasp skin layer of the fat roll and lift up. Insert needle at about a 45° angle to the skin's fat layer and then administer the medication. Not necessary to aspirate to check if needle is in a blood vessel. Rapidly withdraw the needle while releasing the skin.
- 'Bunch technique' method: Grasp tissue around injection site, creating a tissue roll of about ½ in. in diameter. Insert needle into tissue roll at a 90° angle to the skin surface and inject medication. Not necessary to aspirate. Withdraw needle rapidly when skin is released.
- Do not administer within 2 in. of umbilicus (R/T increased vascularity of area).

3. Do not massage site. Rotate sites of administration.

4. Slight discoloration does not affect potency.

IV 5. Hospitalize for IV therapy.

6. May be diluted in dextrose, NSS, or Ringer's solution and administered over 4–24 hr with an infusion pump.

7. Protect solutions from freezing.

8. Have protamine sulfate, a heparin antagonist, available should excessive bleeding occur.

9. NaCl, 0.9%, is effective in maintaining patency of peripheral (noncentral) intermittent infusion devices and in reducing medical costs. The following procedure is recommended:

- Determine patency by aspirating lock.
- Flush with 2 mL NSS.
- Administer medication therapy (flush between drugs).
- Flush with 2 mL NSS.
- Frequency of flushing to maintain patency when not actively in use varies from every 8 hr to every 24–48 hr.
- This does NOT apply to any central venous access devices. Must use heparin.

ASSESSMENT

1. When given by continuous IV infusion, perform coagulation tests every 4 hr in the early stages. When given by intermittent IV infusion, perform coagulation tests before each dose during early stages and at appropriate intervals thereafter. After deep SC injection, perform coagulation tests 4-6 hr after the injections.

2. Note reasons for therapy. Identify any bleeding incidents, i.e., bleeding tendencies, family history, or any other incidents of unexplained or active bleeding.

3. Perform test dose (1,000 units SC) on clients with multiple allergies or asthma history.

4. Review drug profile to ensure none interact unfavorably; otherwise, anticipate heparin dosage adjustment.

5. Assess for defects in clotting mechanism or any capillary fragility; obtain baseline coagulation values. PTT values 1½ to 2 times control indicates anticoagulation.

6. Note time frame for therapy (i.e., DVT [initial] 6 months; certain valve replacements—lifetime), and desired INR, PT/PTT, and record.

7. Review PMH for conditions that may preclude therapy: alcoholic, chronic GI tract ulcerations, severe renal or liver dysfunction, infections of the endocardium, or PUD which may be a potential site of bleeding. Note any evidence of intracranial hemorrhage.

8. Monitor CBC with platelets, PT, PTT, renal, and LFTs. Note bleeding precautions at bedside.

INTERVENTIONS

1. Post/advise at bedside 'client receiving anticoagulant therapy.'

2. Monitor CBC and PTT closely.

3. Question about bleeding (gums, urine, stools, vomit, bruises). If urine discolored, determine cause, i.e., from drug therapy or hematuria. Indanedione-type anticoagulants turn alkaline urine a red-orange color; acidify urine or test for occult blood.

4. Sudden lumbar pain may indicate retroperitoneal hemorrhage.

5. GI dysfunction may indicate intestinal hemorrhage. Test for blood in urine and feces; check H&H to assess for bleeding.

Bold Italic = life threatening side effect   ■ = black box warning   ♣ = Available in Canada

6. Have protamine sulfate for heparin overdose available (generally for every 100 units of heparin administer 1 mg protamine sulfate IV).

7. Apply pressure to all venipuncture and injection sites to prevent bleeding and hematoma formation.

8. In heparin lock devices, the presence of heparin or NSS may cause lab test interferences.

- To clear flush solution: aspirate and discard 1 mL of fluid from device before withdrawing blood sample.
- Inject 1 mL of flush solution into lock after blood samples are drawn.
- With excessively abnormal results, obtain a repeat sample from another site before altering treatment.

9. With SC administration, do not aspirate or massage; administer in lower abdomen and rotate sites.

For Heparin Lock Flush Solution:

1. Aspirate lock to determine patency. Maintain patency: inject 1 mL of flush solution into device diaphragm after each use (maintains catheter patency for up to 24 hr).

2. If administering a drug incompatible with heparin, flush with 0.9% NaCl solution or sterile water for injection before and immediately after incompatible drug administered. Inject another dose of heparin lock flush solution after the final flush.

3. Observe coagulation times carefully with underlying bleeding disorders; ↑ risk for hemorrhage.

4. The presence of heparin or NSS may cause lab test interferences. To clear flush solution:

- Aspirate and discard 1 mL of fluid from device before withdrawing blood sample.
- Inject 1 mL of flush solution into lock after blood samples are drawn.
- With excessively abnormal results, obtain a repeat sample from another site before initiating treatment.

5. Monitor for allergic reactions due to various biologic sources of heparin.

CLIENT/FAMILY TEACHING

1. Review administration technique. Can only be given parenterally. For SC administration inject in lower abdomen.

Do not massage after injection. Rotate sites with each dose.

2. Report signs of active bleeding or any excessive menstrual flow; may need to withhold/reduce dosage.

3. Report alterations in urine function, urine color, or any injury.

4. Use an electric razor for shaving and a soft-bristle toothbrush to decrease gum irritation. Hair loss is generally temporary.

5. Arrange furniture to allow open space for unimpeded ambulation and to diminish chances of bumping into objects that may cause bruising/bleeding. Use a night light to illuminate trips to the bathroom. Always wear shoes or slippers.

6. Avoid contact sports and any activities where excessive bumping, bruising or injury may occur.

7. Eat potassium-rich foods (e.g., baked potato, orange juice, bananas, beef, flounder, haddock, sweet potato, turkey, raw tomato). Avoid eating large amounts of vitamin K food (yellow and dark green vegetables).

8. Report increased bruising, bleeding of nose, mouth, gums, mucus or oral secretions, tarry stools, GI upset, SOB, chest pain or difficulty breathing.

9. Avoid alcohol, aspirin, tobacco, and NSAIDs due to increased anticoagulant response.

10. Alert all providers of therapy and wear/carry drug identification.

OUTCOMES/EVALUATE

- PTT: 2–2.5 times the control/normal
- Prevention of thrombus formation
- Clot prophylaxis/treatment
- Indwelling catheter patency

Hyaluronic acid derivatives, dermal

(hie-loo-**RON**-ik)

CLASSIFICATION(S):
Physical adjunct
PREGNANCY CATEGORY: C
Rx: Hylaform, Juvederm 24 HV, 30, and 30 HV, Restylane.

 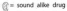

USES
Mid-to-deep dermal implantation for the correction of moderate to severe facial wrinkles and folds, such as nasolabial folds.

ACTION/KINETICS
Action
Hyaluronic acid is generated by *Streptococcus* species of bacteria. It is a clear, colorless gel without particulates.

CONTRAINDICATIONS
Severe allergies manifested by a history of anaphylaxis or history or presence of multiple severe allergies. Use in those with a history of allergies to proteins found in gram-positive bacteria (the product contains trace amounts of gram-positive bacterial proteins). Use in breast augmentation and for implantation into bone, tendon, ligament, muscle, or blood vessels. Implantation into blood vessels (implantation into dermal vessels may cause vascular occlusion, infarction, or embolic phenomena). Use in those with known hypersensitivity to keloid formation or hypertrophic scarring. Use in sites in which an active inflammatory process or infection is present (e.g., cysts, pimples, rash, hives); defer treatment until the inflammation has been controlled. Long-term safety and efficacy have not been determined for use beyond 1 year.

SPECIAL CONCERNS
Use with caution in clients on immuo-suppressive therapy. Safety and efficacy have not been established to treat anatomic regions other than nasolabial folds, or for use in pregnancy, during lactation, and in children under 18 years of age.

SIDE EFFECTS
Most Common
Bruising, itching, pain, redness, swelling, tenderness, URTI, acne.

Dermatologic: Bruising, itching, pain, redness, swelling, tenderness, acne, contact dermatitis, localized superficial necrosis, inflammatory reaction at injection site (including swelling, redness, tenderness, induration, and rarely acneiform papules at the injection site); inflammation at the implant site if laser treatment, chemical peeling, or any other procedure is undertaken. **Hypersensitivity:** Swelling, redness, tenderness, induration, acneiform papules (rare). **CNS:** Depression, headache, migraine, aggravation of depression. **Respiratory:** URTI, sinusitis, bronchitis, pneumonia. **Miscellaneous:** Inflicted injury, tooth disorder, back pain, allergic reaction, arthralgia, herpes simplex, osteoporosis, urinary incontinence, bacterial infection, hypercholesterolemia, necrosis.

DRUG INTERACTIONS
Possible increased bleeding or bruising if used with aspirin or NSAIDs.

HOW SUPPLIED
Gel for Injection: 5.5 mg/mL (as hylan B), 20 mg/mL, 24 mg/mL.

DOSAGE
- **GEL FOR INJECTION**
  Facial wrinkles and folds.
Usual: Limit to 1.5 mL per treatment site.

NURSING CONSIDERATIONS
ADMINISTRATION/STORAGE
1. Hyaluronic acid is supplied in a syringe ready for use; never mix with other products prior to injection of the device.
2. If the content of a syringe shows signs of separation and/or appears cloudy, do not use.
3. Do not resterilize hyaluronic acid as this may damage or alter the product.
4. Hyaluronic acid is packaged for single-client use.
5. Use the following administration procedure:
- Counsel the client and discuss the indication, risks, benefits, and expected responses to treatment. Advise of necessary precautions before beginning the procedure.
- Assess the need of the client for pain management.
- Clean the area to be treated with alcohol or other suitable antiseptic solution.
- Before injecting, press the rod carefully until a small droplet is visible at the tip of the needle.

Bold Italic = life threatening side effect   ■ = black box warning   ✤ = Available in Canada

- Inject, applying even pressure on the plunger rod while slowly pulling the needle backwards.
- The wrinkle should be lifted and eliminated by the end of the injection.
- Stop the injection just before the needle is pulled out of the skin to prevent material from leaking out or ending up too superficially in the skin.
- Only correct to 100% of the dermal volume effect; do not overcorrect.
- With cutaneous contour deformities, the best results are seen if the defect can be manually stretched to the point where it is eliminated.
- When the injection is completed, gently massage the treated site so that it conforms to the contour of the surrounding tissue. If an overcorrection has occurred, massage the area firmly between the fingers or against the underlying superficial bone to obtain optimal results.

6. Administer using a thin gauge needle (30 gauge x $\frac{1}{2}$ in.) The needle is inserted at an approximate angle of 30° parallel to the length of the wrinkle or fold. The bevel of the needle should face upwards and the drug injected into the middle of the dermis. For mid-dermis placement, the contour of the needle should be visible but not the color of it.

7. If the product is injected too deep or IM, the duration of action will be shorter. If the product is injected too superficially, visible lumps and/or grayish discoloration may result.

8. If 'blanching' is observed (i.e., the overlying skin turns a whitish color), stop the injection immediately and massage the area until it returns to a normal color.

9. The degree and duration of correction depend on the character of the defect treated, the tissue stress at the implant site, the depth of the implant in the tissue, and the injection technique. Markedly indurated defects may be difficult to correct.

10. If further treatment is needed, repeat the same procedure with several punctures of the skin until a satisfactory result is obtained. Additional treatment may be needed to achieve the desired correction. With clients who have localized swelling, the degree of correction is sometimes difficult to judge at the time of treatment. In such cases, a touch-up session may be needed after 1 or 2 weeks.

11. Defer use at specific sites in which an active inflammatory process (e.g., skin eruptions such as cysts, pimples, rashes, or hives) or infection are present until the inflammation has been controlled.

12. Must be used prior to expiration date. Do not freeze and protect from sunlight. Store at a temperature up to 25°C (77°F); refrigeration is not needed.

ASSESSMENT

1. Obtain pre-treatment photos to document extent of wrinkles and folds.
2. Ensure no history of multiple allergies or keloid formation.
3. Assess emotional status and ensure ready for procedure; review potential adverse reactions.

CLIENT/FAMILY TEACHING

1. Drug has been approved only for injection into nasolabial folds to decrease folds and wrinkling.
2. To be administered only by those trained to use this therapy.
3. May experience bruising, itching, pain, redness, swelling, and acne at treatment site.
4. Report any adverse effects, including infection, elevated cholesterol levels, or deformity, and keep all F/U appointments.
5. Minimize exposure of the treated area to excessive sun, UV lamps, and extreme cold weather until any initial swelling and redness have resolved.

OUTCOMES/EVALUATE

Correction of nasolabial wrinkles and folds

Hydrochlorothiazide

(**hy**-droh-klor-oh-**THIGH**-ah-zyd)

CLASSIFICATION(S):
Diuretic, thiazide
PREGNANCY CATEGORY: B
Rx: Ezide, Hydro-Par, HydroDIURIL, Microzide Capsules.
♣Rx: Apo-Hydro.

SEE ALSO DIURETICS, THIAZIDE.

USES

(1) Hypertension. Hydrochlorothiazide is a component of a large number of combination drugs used to treat hypertension. (2) Diuretic to treat edema due to CHF, nephrosis, nephritis, renal failure, PMS, hepatic cirrhosis, corticosteroid or estrogen therapy. (3) Microzide is available for once-daily, low-dose treatment for hypertension.

ACTION/KINETICS

Action
Promote the excretion of sodium and chloride, and thus water, by the distal renal tubule. Also increases excretion of potassium and to a lesser extent bicarbonate. The antihypertensive activity is thought to be due to direct dilation of the arterioles, as well as to a reduction in the total fluid volume of the body and altered sodium balance.

Pharmacokinetics
Onset: 2 hr. **Peak effect:** 4–6 hr. **Duration:** 6–12 hr. **t½:** 5.6–14.8 hr. Hydrochlorothiazide is not metabolized but is eliminated rapidly by the kidney.

SPECIAL CONCERNS

Geriatric clients may be more sensitive to the usual adult dose.

SIDE EFFECTS

Most Common
Orthostatic hypotension, hypokalemia, weakness, headache, diarrhea, dizziness, gastric upset/irritation/cramping.
See also *Diuretics, Thiazides* for a complete list of possible side effects. Also, **CV:** Allergic myocarditis, hypotension. **Dermatologic:** Alopecia, exfoliative dermatitis, **toxic epidermal necrolysis,** erythema multiforme, **Stevens-Johnson syndrome. Miscellaneous: Anaphylactic reactions, respiratory distress including pneumonitis and pulmonary edema,** cognitive and neurologic impairment.

HOW SUPPLIED

Capsules: 12.5 mg; *Oral Solution:* 50 mg/5 mL; *Tablets:* 25 mg, 50 mg, 100 mg.

DOSAGE

• **CAPSULES; ORAL SOLUTION; TABLETS**
Diuretic.
Adults, initial: 25–200 mg/day for several days until dry weight is reached; **then,** 25–100 mg/day or intermittently. Some clients may require up to 200 mg/day.
Antihypertensive.
Adults, initial: 25 mg/day as a single dose. The dose may be increased to 50 mg/day in one to two daily doses. Doses greater than 50 mg may cause significant reductions in serum potassium. **Pediatric, under 6 months:** 3.3 mg/kg/day in two doses; **up to 2 years of age:** 12.5–37.5 mg/day in two doses; **2–12 years of age:** 37.5–100 mg/day in two doses

NURSING CONSIDERATIONS

ADMINISTRATION/STORAGE

1. Divide daily doses in excess of 100 mg.
2. Give twice a day at 6–12-hr intervals.
3. When used with other antihypertensives, hydrochlorothiazide dose is usually not more than 50 mg.

ASSESSMENT

1. Note reasons for therapy, disease onset, other agents trialed, outcome.
2. Assess for glucose intolerance.
3. Monitor BP, weight, uric acid, renal function, microalbumin, and electrolytes; replace potassium as needed.

CLIENT/FAMILY TEACHING

1. Take in the a.m. to prevent nighttime urinary frequency with a glass of orange juice. May take with food if GI upset. Report side effects or lack of response.
2. May cause dizziness; change positions slowly and avoid activities that re-

---

Bold Italic = life threatening side effect   ■ = black box warning   ♣ = Available in Canada

quire mental alertness until drug effects realized.

3. Report swelling of extremities or weight gain of >2 lb/day.

4. Avoid alcohol, OTC drugs and prolonged sun exposure; may cause delayed (10–14 day) photosensitivity reaction.

5. With diabetes, monitor BS and potassium closely, may cause glucose intolerance.

6. Keep a log of BP recordings to share with provider.

OUTCOMES/EVALUATE

- ↓ BP
- ↑ Urine output; ↓ edema

— **COMBINATION DRUG** —

Hydrocodone bitartrate and Acetaminophen

(**high**-droh-**KOH**-dohn, ah-**seat**-ah-**MIN**-oh-fen)

CLASSIFICATION(S):

Analgesic

PREGNANCY CATEGORY: C

Rx: Anexia 10/660, Anexia 5/325, Anexia 5/500, Anexia 7.5/325, Anexia 7.5/650, Bancap HC, Ceta-Plus, Co-Gesic, Dolacet, Duocet, Hy-Phen, Hycet, Hydrocet, Hydrogesic, Liquicet, Lorcet Plus, Lorcet-10/650, Lorcet-HD, Lortab 10/500, Lortab 5/500, Lortab 7.5/500, Margesic H, Maxidone, Norco, Norco 5/325, Norco 7.5/325, Panacet 5/500, Stagesic, T-Gesic, Vicodin, Vicodin ES, Vicodin HP, Xodol, Zydone, **C-III**

SEE ALSO *NARCOTIC ANALGESICS* AND *ACETAMINOPHEN*.

USES

Relief of moderate to moderately severe pain.

CONTENT

Capsules/Tablets: Several possible combinations of hydrocodone bitartrate (*narcotic analgesic*) and acetaminophen (*nonnarcotic analgesic*)— amount of hydrocodone listed first: 2.5 mg/108 mg, 2.5 mg/325 mg, 2.5 mg/ 500 mg, 5 mg/300 mg, 5 mg/325 mg, 7.5 mg/325 mg, 10 mg/325 mg, 5 mg/ 500 mg, 7.5 mg/325 mg, 7.5 mg/400 mg, 7.5 mg/500 mg, 7.5 mg/650 mg, 7.5 mg/750 mg, 10 mg/325 mg, 10 mg/400 mg, 10 mg/500 mg, 10 mg/650 mg, 10 mg/660 mg, 10 mg/750 mg.

Elixir/Oral Solution: Hydrocodone bitartrate, 2.5 mg and acetaminophen, 108 mg/5 mL (oral solution); hydrocodone bitartrate, 2.5 mg and acetaminophen, 167 mg/5 mL (elixir); hydrocodone bitartrate, 10 mg and acetaminophen, 500 mg/15 mL.

ACTION/KINETICS

Action

Hydrocodone produces its analgesic activity by an action on the CNS via opiate receptors. The analgesic action of acetaminophen is produced by both peripheral and central mechanisms.

Pharmacokinetics

Hydrocodone, maximum serum levels: About 1.3 hr. **Acetaminophen, $t^{1/2}$:** 1.25–3 hr. Both hydrocodone and acetaminophen are metabolized in the liver and excreted through the urine.

CONTRAINDICATIONS

Hypersensitivity to acetaminophen or hydrocodone. Lactation.

SPECIAL CONCERNS

Use with caution, if at all, in clients with head injuries as the CSF pressure may be increased further. Use with caution in geriatric or debilitated clients; in those with impaired hepatic or renal function; in hypothyroidism, Addison's disease, prostatic hypertrophy, or urethral stricture; and in clients with pulmonary disease. Use shortly before delivery may cause respiratory depression in the newborn. Safety and efficacy have not been determined in children.

SIDE EFFECTS

Most Common

N&V, urinary retention, lightheadedness, dizziness, sedation, mental clouding.

CNS: Lightheadedness, dizziness, sedation, drowsiness, mental clouding, lethargy, impaired mental and physical performance, anxiety, fear, dysphoria, psychologic dependence, mood changes.

GI: N&V. **Respiratory:** Respiratory depression (dose-related), irregular and periodic breathing. **GU:** Ureteral spasm, spasm of vesical sphincters, urinary retention.

OD OVERDOSE MANAGEMENT
Symptoms: ***Acetaminophen overdose may result in potentially fatal hepatic necrosis.*** Also, renal tubular necrosis, hypoglycemic coma, and thrombocytopenia. Symptoms of hepatotoxic overdose include N&V, diaphoresis, and malaise. Symptoms of hydrocodone overdose include respiratory depression, somnolence progressing to stupor or ***coma***, skeletal muscle flaccidity, cold and clammy skin, bradycardia, and hypotension. ***Severe overdose may cause apnea, circulatory collapse, cardiac arrest, and death.***
Treatment: **Acetaminophen:**
- Empty stomach promptly by lavage or induction of emesis.
- Serum acetaminophen levels should be determined as early as possible but no sooner than 4 hr after ingestion.
- Determine liver function initially and at 24-hr intervals.
- The antidote, *N-* acetylcysteine, should be given within 16 hr of overdose for optimal results.

Hydrocodone:
- Re-establish adequate respiratory exchange with a patent airway and assisted or controlled ventilation.
- Respiratory depression can be reversed by giving naloxone IV.
- Oxygen, IV fluids, vasopressors, and other supportive measures may be instituted as required.

DRUG INTERACTIONS
Anticholinergics / ↑ Risk of paralytic ileus
CNS depressants, including other narcotic analgesics, antianxiety agents, antipsychotics, alcohol / Additive CNS depression
MAO inhibitors / ↑ Effect of either the narcotic or the antidepressant
Tricyclic antidepressants / ↑ Effect of either the narcotic or the antidepressant

HOW SUPPLIED
See Content.

DOSAGE
- **CAPSULES; TABLETS**
  Analgesia.
For 2.5/500 product: 1 or 2 q 4 hr, up to 8 per day. **For 5/500 products:** 1 or 2 q 4–6 hr, up to 8 per day. **For 5/300, 5/325, 7.5/325, 10/325, and 7.5/400 products:** 1 q 4–6 hr, up to 6 or 8 per day, depending on the product. **For 7.5/500 and 7.5/650 products:** 1 q 4–6 hr. **For the 7.5/750 product:** 1 q 4–6 hr, up to 5 per day. **For 10/325, 10/400, 10/500, and 10/650 products:** 1 q 4–6 hr, up to 6 per day. **For 10/650, 10/660, and 10/750 products:** 1 q 4–6 hr, up to 5 per day.
- **ORAL SOLUTION**
  Analgesia.
Children, 14 years and older: 15 mL q 4–6 hr, up to 120 mL/day; **10–13 years:** 10 mL q 4–6 hr, up to 60 mL/day; **7–9 years:** 7.5 mL q 4–6 hr, up to 45 mL/day; **4–6 years:** 5 mL q 4–6 hr, up to 30 mL/day; **2–3 years:** 3.75 mL q 4–6 hr, up to 22.5 mL/day. *NOTE:* **Dosages are based on a concentration of 2.5 mg hydrocodone bitartrate and 108 mg acetaminophen/5 mL.**

NURSING CONSIDERATIONS
ASSESSMENT
1. Note onset, location, and characteristics of S&S, other agents prescribed, outcome, if pain acute or chronic; rate pain level.
2. Assess for head injury, hypothyroidism, BPH, urethral stricture, Addison's disease, severe pulmonary disease; precludes therapy.
3. Monitor renal and LFTs avoid with dysfunction.

CLIENT/FAMILY TEACHING
1. Take as directed. May take with food/milk to decrease GI upset.
2. Do not perform activities that require mental alertness; causes dizziness, lethargy, and impaired physical and mental performance.
3. Report evidence of abnormal bruising/bleeding, breathing problems, N&V, constipation, urinary difficulty, excessive sedation or lack of desired pain control.

Bold Italic = life threatening side effect   ■ = black box warning   ✚ = Available in Canada

4. Avoid alcohol and OTC agents or CNS depressants.

5. Store appropriately, away from the bedside and safely out of the reach of children.

6. Drug is for short term use; may be habit forming.

OUTCOMES/EVALUATE
Desired pain control

Hydrocortisone (Cortisol)   IV ©

(hy-droh-**KOR**-tih-zohn)

CLASSIFICATION(S):
Glucocorticoid
PREGNANCY CATEGORY: C
OTC: Roll-on Applicator: Maximum Strength Cortaid Faststick. **Topical Cream:** Allercort, Bactine, Cortizone-10 External Anal Itch, Cortizone-10 Plus, Dermolate Anti-Itch, Dermtex HC, Hydro-Tex, HydroSkin. **Topical Gel:** Alcortin, Extra Strength CortaGel. **Topical Liquid:** Scalpicin, T/Scalp. **Topical Lotion:** Dermolate Scalp-Itch, HydroSkin. **Topical Ointment:** HydroSkin. **Topical Spray:** Cortaid, Cortizone-10 Quickshot, Dermolate Anti-Itch, Maximum Strength Cortaid, Pro-cort.

Rx: Parenteral: Sterile Hydrocortisone Suspension. **Rectal Cream/Gel:** Dermolate Anal-Itch, Procto-Cream-HC 2.5%, Proctocort. **Retention Enema (Suspension):** Colocort. **Roll-on:** Cortaid FastStick. **Tablets:** Cortef, Hydrocortone. **Topical Cream:** Ala-Cort, Alphaderm, Cort-Dome, Cortifair, Dermacort, DermiCort, H_2Cort, Hi-Cor 1.0 and 2.5, Hytone, Nutracort, Penecort, Synacort. **Topical Gel:** Alcortin. **Topical Lotion:** Acticort 100, Ala-Cort, Ala-Scalp, Allercort, Cetacort, Cort-Dome, Delacort, Dermacort, Gly-Cort, Hytone, LactiCare-HC, Lemoderm, Lexocort Forte, My Cort, Nutracort, Pentacort, Rederm, S-T Cort. **Topical Ointment:** Allercort, Cortril, Hytone, Lemoderm, Penecort. **Topical Solution:** Emo-Cort Scalp Solution, Penecort, Texacort, Texacort Scalp Solution.

✤**Rx: Rectal Gel:** Cortenema, Rectocort. **Retention Enema:** Hycort, Rectocort. **Topical Lotion:** Aquacort, Cortate, Emo-Cort, Sarna HC. **Topical Cream:** Cortate, Emo-cort Prevex HC. **Topical Ointment:** Cortoderm.

Hydrocortisone acetate

PREGNANCY CATEGORY: C (topical and dental products)
OTC: Topical Cream: Cortaid, Cortef Feminine Itch, Corticaine, FoilleCort, Gynecort Female Cream, Lanacort 10, Lanacort 5, Maximum Strength Cortaid, Rhulicort. **Topical Lotion:** Cortaid, Rhulicort. **Topical Ointment:** Cortef Acetate, Hydrocortisone Acetate Maximum Strength, Lanacort, Lanacort 5, Maximum Strength Cortaid.

Rx: Intrarectal Foam: Cortifoam. **Parenteral:** Hydrocortone Acetate. **Paste:** Orabase-HCA. **Rectal Gel:** Cort-Dome High Potency, Cortenema, Corticaine, Cortifoam. **Topical Cream/Topical Ointment:** Maximum Strength Hydrocortisone Acetate, U-cort. **Topical Cream:** Calde-CORT Light, Carmol-HC, Gynecort, Lanacort, Pharma-Cort. **Topical Gel:** Novacort. **Topical Ointment:** Nov-Hydrocort.

✤**Rx: Ophthalmic:** Cortamed. **Suppositories:** Cortiment, Rectocort. **Topical Cream:** Corticreme, Hyderm. **Topical Ointment:** DermaPlex HC1%.

Hydrocortisone butyrate

PREGNANCY CATEGORY: C (topical products)
Rx: Topical Cream, Lotion, Ointment, Solution: Locoid, Locoid Lipocream.

Hydrocortisone cypionate

PREGNANCY CATEGORY: C
Rx: Oral Suspension: Cortef.

H

Hydrocortisone probutate

PREGNANCY CATEGORY: C

Rx: Topical Cream: Pandel.

Hydrocortisone sodium phosphate

PREGNANCY CATEGORY: C

Rx: Parenteral: Hydrocortone Phosphate.

Hydrocortisone sodium succinate

PREGNANCY CATEGORY: C

Rx: Parenteral: A-Hydrocort, Solu-Cortef.

SEE ALSO *CORTICOSTEROIDS*.

USES

See *Corticosteroids*.

ACTION/KINETICS

Pharmacokinetics

Short-acting. t½: 80–118 min. Topical products are available without a prescription in strengths of 0.5% and 1%.

SIDE EFFECTS

See *Corticosteroids*.

HOW SUPPLIED

Hydrocortisone (Cortisol): *Cream:* 0.5%, 1%, 2.5%; *Enema (Suspension):* 100 mg/60 mL; *Gel:* 1%, 2%; *Liquid:* 1%; *Lotion:* 0.25%, 0.5%, 1%, 2%, 2.5%; *Ointment:* 0.5%, 1%, 2.5%; *Pad:* 0.5%, 1%; *Rectal Cream:* 2.5%; *Solution:* 1%, 2.5%; *Spray:* 1%; *Spray Pump:* 1%; *Stick, Roll-On:* 1%; *Tablets:* 5 mg, 10 mg, 20 mg. **Hydrocortisone acetate:** *Cream:* 0.5%, 1%; *Foam:* 10%; *Gel:* 2%; *Injection:* 25 mg/mL, 50 mg/mL; *Ointment:* 0.5%, 1%; *Suppositories:* 10 mg, 25 mg, 30 mg. **Hydrocortisone butyrate:** *Cream:* 0.1%; *Lotion:* 0.1%; *Ointment:* 0.1%; *Solution:* 0.1%. **Hydrocortisone cypionate:** *Suspension:* 10 mg/5 mL. **Hydrocortisone probutate:** *Cream:* 0.1%, 1%. **Hydrocortisone sodium phosphate:** *Injection:* 50 mg/mL.

Hydrocortisone sodium succinate: *Powder for Injection:* 100 mg, 250 mg, 500 mg, 1 gram. **Hydrocortisone valerate:** *Cream:* 0.2%; *Ointment:* 0.2%.

DOSAGE

HYDROCORTISONE

• **TABLETS**

20–240 mg/day, depending on disease.

• **ENEMA**

100 mg in retention enema nightly for 21 days (up to 2 months of therapy may be needed; discontinue gradually if therapy exceeds 3 weeks).

• **CREAM; GEL; LOTION; SOLUTION; SPRAY; TOPICAL OINTMENT**

Apply sparingly to affected area and rub in lightly 3–4 times per day.

HYDROCORTISONE ACETATE

• **INTRA-ARTICULAR; INTRALESIONAL; SOFT TISSUE**

Large joints: 25 mg (occasionally, 37.5 mg). **Small joints:** 10–25 mg. **Tendon sheaths:** 5–12.5 mg. **Soft tissue infiltration:** 25–50 mg (occasionally 75 mg). **Bursae:** 25–37.5 mg. **Ganglia:** 12.5–25 mg.

• **INTRARECTAL FOAM**

1 applicatorful (90 mg) 1–2 times per day for 2–3 weeks; **then** every second day.

• **TOPICAL**

See *Hydrocortisone*.

HYDROCORTISONE BUTYRATE

• **OINTMENT; SOLUTION; TOPICAL CREAM**

Apply a thin film to the affected area 2–3 times per day.

HYDROCORTISONE CYPIONATE

• **SUSPENSION**

20–240 mg/day, depending on the severity of the disease.

HYDROCORTISONE PROBUTATE

• **TOPICAL CREAM**

Apply a thin film to the affected area 1–2 times per day.

HYDROCORTISONE SODIUM PHOSPHATE

• **IM; IV; SC**

General uses.

Initial: 15–240 mg/day depending on use and on severity of the disease. Usually, one-half to one-third of the PO dose is given q 12 hr.

Adrenal insufficiency, acute.

Adults, initial: 100 mg IV; **then,** 100 mg q 8 hr in an IV fluid; **older children, initial:** 1–2 mg/kg by IV bolus; **then,** 150–250 mg/kg/day **IV** in divided doses; **infants, initial:** 1–2 mg/kg by IV bolus; **then,** 25–150 mg/kg/day in divided doses.

HYDROCORTISONE SODIUM SUCCINATE
• **IM; IV**
Initial: 100–500 mg; **then,** may be repeated at 2-, 4-, and 6-hr intervals depending on response and severity of condition.

HYDROCORTISONE VALERATE
• **OINTMENT; TOPICAL CREAM**
See *Hydrocortisone.*

NURSING CONSIDERATIONS

ⓒ Do not confuse hydrocortisone with hydrocodone (a narcotic analgesic). Also, do not confuse Hytone with Vytone (also a topical corticosteroid). Do not confuse HCTZ (hydrochlorothiazide) with HCT (hydrocortisone); spell out all drug names to prevent error and confusion.

ADMINISTRATION/STORAGE
Ⅳ 1. Check label of parenteral hydrocortisone because IM and IV preparations are not necessarily interchangeable.
2. Give reconstituted direct IV solution at a rate of 100 mg over 30 sec. Doses larger than 500 mg should be infused over 10 min. Drug may be further diluted in 50–100 mL of dextrose or saline solutions and administered as ordered within 24 hr.

ASSESSMENT
1. Note reasons for therapy, type, location, onset, characteristics of S&S. List other agents used and the outcome.
2. Describe clinical presentation; use photographs to document as indicated.
3. Identify any medical conditions that may preclude therapy.
4. Assess weight, VS, CBC, BS, chemistry profile, renal and LFTs. Note findings of x-ray, TB skin test, EKG.

CLIENT/FAMILY TEACHING
1. When using topical products, wash area prior to application or shower/bathe first, to increase drug penetration. Use only a small amount and rub into area thoroughly. Do not allow topical product to come in contact with the eyes.
2. Avoid prolonged use of topical products near the genital/rectal areas and eyes, on the face, and in creases of the skin.
3. For the butyrate topical products, use an occlusive dressing only on advice of the provider if used to treat psoriasis or other deep-seated dermatoses.
4. Do not use probutate products in the diaper area. With the probutate products, do not use tight-fitting diapers or plastic pants (occlusive).
5. No part of the intrarectal foam aerosol container should be inserted into the anus. With the suspension, shake well. Lie on left side with left leg extended and the right leg forward and flexed. Insert applicator tip of the suspension into the rectum pointed towards the navel and slowly instill medication as directed.
6. Report worsening of condition or lack of improvement; may need dosage adjustment. Report any fever, sore throat, muscle aches, slow healing, sudden weight gain, or swelling of extremities.
7. With prolonged use of oral products, do not stop suddenly. Drug must be weaned/tapered down to prevent adrenal crisis. Cushingoid S&S of adrenal insufficiency include fatigue, dizziness, nausea, lack of appetite, weakness, SOB, joint pain.
8. Avoid alcohol, caffeine, and all OTC agents without approval.
9. Use appropriate prescribed form only as directed; call with questions or problems.

OUTCOMES/EVALUATE
• Replacement of adrenocortical deficiency
• Restoration of skin integrity
• Relief of allergic manifestations
• ↓ Inflammation

Hydromorphone ■Ⅳ ⓒ
hydrochloride

CLASSIFICATION(S):
Narcotic analgesic

PREGNANCY CATEGORY: C

Rx: Dilaudid, Dilaudid-HP, Hydromorphone HP 10, 20, and 50, Palladone, **C-II**

✦Rx: Dilaudid Sterile Powder, Dilaudid-HP-Plus, Dilaudid-XP, Hydromorphone HP Forte, PMS-Hydromorphone.

SEE ALSO *NARCOTIC ANALGESICS.*

USES
Moderate to severe pain (e.g., surgery, cancer, biliary colic, burns, renal colic, MI, bone or soft tissue trauma). Dilaudid-HP is a concentrated solution intended for those tolerant to narcotics. *NOTE:* The ER Capsules have been removed from the market based on a potential fatal interaction with alcohol.

ACTION/KINETICS

Action
Hydromorphone is 7–10 times more analgesic than morphine, with a shorter duration of action. It manifests less sedation, less vomiting, and less nausea than morphine, although it induces pronounced respiratory depression.

Pharmacokinetics
Onset: 15 min (IM, SC); 30 min (PO). **Peak effect:** 30–60 min. **Duration:** 4–5 hr (immediate release) and 4–5 hr (IM, SC). **t½, elimination:** 2.3 hr (immediate release) and 2.6 hr (IM, SC). Metabolized in the liver and excreted in the urine. Give rectally for prolonged activity. **Plasma protein binding:** 60–80%.

ADDITIONAL CONTRAINDICATIONS
Migraine headaches. Use in children or during labor. Status asthmaticus, obstetrics, respiratory depression in absence of resuscitative equipment. Lactation.

SPECIAL CONCERNS
■ (1) HP injection is a highly concentrated solution of hydromorphone intended for use in opioid-tolerant clients. Do not confuse HP injection with standard parenteral formulations of injection or other opioids. Overdose and death could result. (2) Schedule II opioid agonists (e.g., hydromorphone, fentanyl, methadone, morphine, oxycodone, oxymorphone) have the highest risk of fatal overdoses because of respiratory depression, as well as the highest potential for abuse. ER capsules can be abused in a manner similar to other opioid agonists, legal or illict. Consider these risks when administering, prescribing, or dispensing ER capsules in situations where there is concern about increased risk of misuse, abuse, or diversion. (3) People at increased risk for opioid abuse include those with a personal or family history of substance abuse (including drug or alcohol abuse or addiction) or mental illness (e.g., major depression). Assess clients for clinical risks of opoid abuse or addiction prior to prescribing opioids. Routinely monitor all clients receiving opioids for signs of misuse, abuse, and addiction. Clients at increased risk of opioid abuse may still be appropriately treated with modified-release opioid formulations; however, these clients will require intensive monitoring for signs of misuse, abuse, or addiction.■ Use Dilaudid-HP with caution in clients with circulatory shock.

SIDE EFFECTS

Most Common

Constipation, N&V, asthenia, headache, sleepiness/sedation/somnolence, itching/pruritus.

See *Narcotic Analgesics* for a complete list of potential side effects. Also, nystagmus.

ADDITIONAL DRUG INTERACTIONS
↑ CNS and respiratory depression when used with protease inhibitors.

HOW SUPPLIED
Capsules, Extended-Release: 12 mg, 16 mg, 24 mg, 32 mg; *Injection:* 1 mg/mL, 2 mg/mL, 4 mg/mL, 10 mg/mL; *Liquid, Oral:* 1 mg/mL; *Powder for Injection, Lyophilized:* 250 mg/vial (10 mg/mL after reconstitution); *Suppositories:* 3 mg; *Tablets:* 2 mg, 4 mg, 8 mg.

DOSAGE

• CAPSULES, EXTENDED-RELEASE
Analgesia.

To be used only in clients who are opioid-dependent and who require a total daily dose of analgesic equivalent to PO hydromorphone of 12 mg. To calculate the dose of the extended-release capsules, calculate the total daily (24-hour) dose of the client's previous opioid. Using standard conversion ratio estimates, multiply the milligrams per day of the previous opioids by the appropriate conversion factors to obtain the equivalent total daily dose of PO hydromorphone. If necessary, modify the dose. Round off to a dose that is appropriate for the available capsule strengths (i.e., 12, 16, 24, 32, mg). Discontinue all other around-the-clock opioid analgesics when beginning the extended-release capsules

- **ORAL LIQUID**
  Analgesia.
  Initial: 2.5-10 mg q 3-6 hr.
- **SUPPOSITORIES**
  Analgesia.
  Adults: 3 mg q 6–8 hr or as directed by provider.
- **TABLETS**
  Analgesia.
  Adults, initial: 2–4 mg q 4–6 hr; for more severe pain, 4 or more mg q 4–6 hr. A gradual increase may be needed if the pain increases in severity, analgesia is not adequate, or tolerance occurs.
- **IM; IV; SC**
  Analgesia.
  Adults, initial: 1–2 mg IM or SC q 4–6 hr as needed. For severe pain, 3–4 mg q 4–6 hr. May be given by slow IV over 2–3 min.

NURSING CONSIDERATIONS

 Do not confuse hydromorphone with morphine (also a narcotic analgesic).

ADMINISTRATION/STORAGE

1. Most clients given around-the-clock therapy with controlled-release opioids may require immediate-release medication for worsening of pain or to treat or prevent pain that occurs predictably during certain client activities (incident pain). Refrigerate suppositories.

2. Reconstitute the lyophilized sterile powder for injection immediately prior to use with 25 mL sterile water for injection to provide a sterile solution containing 10 mg/mL.

[IV] 3. May be given by slow IV injection. Administer slowly to minimize hypoten-

sive effects and respiratory depression. Administer at a rate of 2 mg over 5 min.

ASSESSMENT

1. Note type, location, onset, and characteristics of symptoms. Use a rating scale to rate pain.

2. Assess for respiratory depression; more profound with hydromorphone than with other narcotic analgesics. Encourage to turn, cough, deep breathe or use incentive spirometry every 2 hr to prevent atelectasis.

3. List drugs prescribed to ensure none interact unfavorably. Avoid use with migraine headaches, during labor, or with status asthmaticus.

4. Drug may mask symptoms of acute pathology; assess abdomen carefully.

CLIENT/FAMILY TEACHING

1. Use exactly as directed at the onset of pain and in the dose prescribed. Report any unusual or intolerable side effects, difficulty breathing, or loss of pain control.

2. May be given as Dilaudid brand cough syrup. Be alert to an allergic response in those sensitive to yellow dye number 5.

3. Store away from bedside.

4. Increase intake of fluids and fiber to offset constipating effects; request therapy when needed.

5. Do not perform activities that require mental alertness or coordination. Change positions slowly to avoid dizziness.

6. Do not stop suddenly with long term use; drug dependence occurs.

7. Avoid alcohol and any other CNS depressants without approval.

OUTCOMES/EVALUATE

Relief of pain; control of cough

Hydroxyurea (Abbreviation: HYD)
(hy-**DROX**-ee-you-**ree**-ah)

CLASSIFICATION(S):
Antineoplastic, antimetabolite
PREGNANCY CATEGORY: D
Rx: Droxia, Hydrea.
♣**Rx:** Gen-Hydroxyurea.

 = see color insert   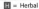 = Herbal   [IV] = Intravenous   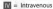 = sound alike drug

SEE ALSO *ANTINEOPLASTIC AGENTS.*

USES

(1) Chronic, resistant, myelocytic leukemia. (2) Carcinoma of the ovary (recurrent, inoperable, or metastatic). (3) Melanoma. (4) With irradiation to treat primary squamous cell carcinoma of the head and neck (but not the lip). (5) **Droxia:** Reduce frequency of painful crises and reduce need for blood transfusions in adults with sickle cell anemia. *Investigational:* Thrombocythemia, HIV, refractory psoriasis.

ACTION/KINETICS

Action

Inhibits DNA synthesis but not synthesis of RNA or protein. As an antimetabolite, it interferes with the conversion of ribonucleotides to deoxyribonucleotides due to blockade of the ribonucleotide reductase system. May also inhibit incorporation of thymidine into DNA. Effectiveness in sickle cell anemia may be due to increases in hemoglobin F levels in RBCs, decrease in neutrophils, increases in the water content of RBCs, increases in the deformability of sickled cells, and altered adhesion of RBCs to the endothelium.

Pharmacokinetics

Rapidly absorbed from GI tract. **Peak serum concentration:** 1–2 hr. **t½:** 3–4 hr. Crosses the blood-brain barrier. Degraded in liver. 80% excreted through the urine with 50% unchanged; also excreted as respiratory CO_2.

CONTRAINDICATIONS

Leukocyte count less than 2,500/mm³ or thrombocyte count less than 100,000/mm³. Severe anemia.

SPECIAL CONCERNS

■ (1) Use of hydroxyurea capsules may result in severe, sometimes life-threatening side effects. Administer under the supervision of a physician experienced in the use of this drug for the treatment of sickle cell anemia. (2) Hydroxyurea is mutagenic and clastogenic and causes cellular transformation to a tumorigenic phenotype. Thus, it is genotoxic and a presumed transspecies carcinogen that implies a carcinogenic risk to humans. In clients receiving long-term hydroxyurea for myelosuppressive diseases, such as polycythemia vera and thrombocythemia, secondary leukemias have been reported. It is unknown whether this leukemogenic effect is secondary to hydroxyurea or is associated with the client's underlying disease. The physician and client must carefully consider the benefits versus risks of developing secondary malignancies.■ Use during pregnancy only if benefits clearly outweigh risks. Give with caution to clients with marked renal dysfunction. Geriatric clients may be more sensitive to the effects of hydroxyurea necessitating a lower dose. Clients who have received prior irradiation therapy may have worsening of postirradiation erythema. Possible cutaneous vasculitic toxicity may occur in those with myeloproliferative disorders (especially in those with a history of, or currently receiving, interferon therapy). Dosage has not been established in children.

SIDE EFFECTS

Most Common

Stomatitis, N&V, diarrhea, anorexia, headache, dizziness, rash, fever, chills, malaise.

GI: Stomatitis, anorexia, N&V, diarrhea, constipation. **CNS:** Headache, dizziness, disorientation, hallucinations, seizures (rare), moderate drowsiness with large doses. **Dermatologic:** Maculopapular rash, skin ulceration, facial erythema, alopecia (rare). **Respiratory:** Acute pulmonary reactions, including diffuse pulmonary infiltrates, fever, dyspnea. **Body as a whole:** Mucositis, fever, chills, malaise. **Miscellaneous:** Renal toxicity/impairment, dysuria, erythrocyte abnormalities including megaloblastic erythropoiesis.

LABORATORY TEST CONSIDERATIONS

↑ Serum uric acid, BUN, and creatinine.

HOW SUPPLIED

Droxia: *Capsules:* 200 mg, 300 mg, 400 mg.
Hydrea: *Capsules:* 500 mg.

DOSAGE

- **CAPSULES**

  Solid tumors, intermittent therapy or when used together with irradiation.

Dose individualized. Usual: 80 mg/kg as a single dose every third day. Intermittent dosage offers advantage of reduced toxicity. If effective, maintain client on drug indefinitely unless toxic effects preclude such a regimen.

Solid tumors, continuous therapy.
20–30 mg/kg/day as a single dose.

Resistant chronic myelocytic leukemia.
20–30 mg/kg/day in a single dose or two divided daily doses.

Concomitant therapy with irradiation for carcinoma of the head and neck.
80 mg/kg as a single dose every third day.

Reduce platelet count and prevent thrombosis in essential thrombocytopenia.
About 15 mg/kg/day.

Refractory psoriasis.
0.5–1.5 grams/day.

Sickle cell anemia (Use Droxia).
Base dose on the smaller of ideal or actual body weight. **Initial:** 15 mg/kg/day as a single dose. If blood counts are acceptable, may increase dose by 5 mg/kg/day q 12 weeks until a maximum tolerated dose (highest dose that does not produce toxic blood counts over 24 consecutive weeks) or 35 mg/kg/day is reached.

NURSING CONSIDERATIONS

ADMINISTRATION/STORAGE
1. Calculate dosage based on actual or ideal weight (whichever is less).
2. Start hydroxyurea at least 7 days before initiation of irradiation; continue through irradiation and indefinitely afterward as long as the client can tolerate dose. The dosage of radiation is not usually adjusted with concomitant usage of hydroxyurea.
3. Do not store in excessive heat.

ASSESSMENT
1. Note reasons for therapy, onset, characteristics of disease. Assess for exacerbation of postirradiation erythema.
2. Monitor uric acid, renal and LFTs. With sickle cell anemia, monitor blood count q 2 weeks; adjust dosage to keep neutrophil, platelet, hemoglobin, and reticulocyte counts within acceptable ranges.
3. Initially, obtain hematologic profiles weekly. Drug may cause severe granulocyte and platelet suppression. Nadir: 7 days; recovery: 14 days.

CLIENT/FAMILY TEACHING
1. Take as directed; continue for at least 6 weeks before efficacy is assessed.
2. If unable to swallow capsule, contents may be given in glass of water and drunk immediately; some material may not dissolve and may float on top of water.
3. Consume 8–10 glasses of fluids per day.
4. Monitor temperatures. Report any S&S of infection: fever, chills, sore throat, flu-like symptoms, N&V, loss of appetite, unusual bruising or bleeding, or sores in the mouth.
5. Drug is a carcinogenic risk to humans; may develop secondary malignancies.
6. Use during pregnancy only if benefits clearly outweigh risks. Practice reliable contraception.
7. Keep all F/U appointments to evaluate response to therapy and labs to assess for toxicity.

OUTCOMES/EVALUATE
- Suppression of malignant process
- ↓ Tumor size and spread
- ↓ Occurrence of sickle cell crisis

Hydroxyzine hydrochloride
(hy-**DROX**-ih-zeen)

CLASSIFICATION(S):
Antianxiety drug, nonbenzodiazepine
PREGNANCY CATEGORY: C
✽**Rx:** Apo-Hydroxyzine, Novo-Hydroxyzide, PMS Hydroxyzine.

Hydroxyzine pamoate
PREGNANCY CATEGORY: C
Rx: Vistaril.

 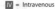

USES
(1) Sedation when used as premedication and following general anesthesia. (2) Anxiety and tension associated with psychoneurosis and as an adjunct in organic diseases in which anxiety is manifested. (3) Pruritus due to allergic conditions such as chronic urticaria or atopic or contact dermatoses; also, histamine-mediated pruritus.

ACTION/KINETICS
Action
Action may be due to a suppression of activity in selected key regions of the subcortical areas of the CNS. Manifests anticholinergic, antiemetic, antispasmodic, local anesthetic, antihistaminic, and skeletal relaxant effects. Has mild antiarrhythmic activity and mild analgesic effects. Significant sedative and antiemetic effects and moderate anticholinergic activity.

Pharmacokinetics
Rapidly absorbed. **Onset:** 15–30 min. **t½:** 3 hr. **Duration:** 4–6 hr. Metabolized by the liver and excreted through the urine. The pamoate salt is believed to be converted to the hydrochloride in the stomach.

CONTRAINDICATIONS
Hypersensitivity to hydroxyzine or cetirizine. Pregnancy (especially early) or lactation. Treatment of morning sickness during pregnancy or as sole agent for treatment of psychoses or depression. Use in porphyria. IV, SC, or intra-arterial use.

SPECIAL CONCERNS
Possible increased anticholinergic and sedative effects in geriatric clients.

SIDE EFFECTS
Most Common
Sedation, drowsiness, tiredness, dizziness, disturbed coordination, drying/thickening of oral and other respiratory secretions, stomach upset.

Low incidence at recommended dosages. **CNS:** Drowsiness, dizziness, sedation, tiredness, sleepiness, confusion, nervousness, irritability, tremor. **GI:** Stomach upset, loss of appetite, nausea, dry mouth. **Respiratory:** Drying and thickening of oral and other respiratory secretions. **Dermatologic:** Urticaria, skin reactions. **Ophthalmic:** Blurred vision, double vision. **Miscellaneous:** Disturbed coordination, involuntary motor activity, hypersensitivity, worsening of porphyria, ECG abnormalities (e.g., alterations in T-waves). Marked discomfort, induration, and even gangrene at site of IM injection.

OD OVERDOSE MANAGEMENT
Symptoms: Oversedation. *Treatment:* Immediate gastric lavage. General supportive care with monitoring of VS. Control hypotension with IV fluids and either levarterenol, norepinephrine, or metaraminol (do not use epinephrine).

DRUG INTERACTIONS
See *Drug Interactions* for *Tranquilizers.* Additive effects when used with other CNS depressants, including narcotics, nonnarcotic analgesics, and barbiturates.

HOW SUPPLIED
Hydroxyzine hydrochloride: *Injection:* 25 mg/mL, 50 mg/mL; *Syrup:* 10 mg/5 mL; *Tablets:* 10 mg, 25 mg, 50 mg. **Hydroxyzine pamoate:** *Capsules:* 25 mg, 50 mg, 100 mg; *Oral Suspension:* 25 mg/5 mL.

DOSAGE
HYDROXYZINE HYDROCHLORIDE AND HYDROXYZINE PAMOATE
- **CAPSULES; ORAL SUSPENSION; SYRUP; TABLETS**
  Sedation.
Adults: 50–100 mg as premedication or following general anesthesia. **Children:** 0.6 mg/kg.
  Anxiety and tension.
Adults: 50—100 mg 4 times per day. **Children over 6 years old:** 50—100 mg/day in divided doses. **Children less than 6 years old:** 50 mg/day in divided doses.
  Pruritus.
Adults: 25 mg 3–4 times per day. **Children, over 6 years old:** 50–100 mg/day in divided doses. **Children, <6 years old:** 50 mg/day in divided doses.
HYDROXYZINE HYDROCHLORIDE
- **IM**
  Sedation.
Adults: 50—100 mg as premedication or following general anesthesia. **Children:** 0.6 mg/kg.

Anxiety and tension.
Adults: 50–100 mg 4 times per day.
Pruritus.
Adults only: 25 mg 3–4 times/day.

NURSING CONSIDERATIONS

ℂ Do not confuse Atarax with Ativan (lorazepam), each of which is an anti-anxiety drug. Do not confuse hydroxy-zine with hydralazine (an antihyperten-sive).

ADMINISTRATION/STORAGE
1. Start geriatric clients on low doses and observe closely.
2. Inject IM only. Make injection into the upper, outer quadrant of the but-tocks or the midlateral muscles of the thigh. In children, inject into the midla-teral muscles of the thigh. In infants and small children, to minimize sciatic nerve damage, use the periphery of the upper outer quadrant of the gluteal re-gion only when necessary (e.g., burn clients). Do not make IM injections into the lower and mid—third of the upper arm.
3. Shake suspension vigorously until completely resuspended.
4. Store PO dosage forms from 15–30°C (59–86°F).
5. Dispense in tight, light-resistant con-tainers.
6. Store injection below 30°C (86°F); protect from freezing.

ASSESSMENT
1. List reasons for therapy, type, onset, and characteristics of S&S; identify trig-gers.
2. Note any associated contributing factors (i.e., dehydration, sweating, hives, asthma, urticaria, areas of pruritus and any potential contact).

CLIENT/FAMILY TEACHING
1. Take only as directed, do not exceed dosing guidelines.
2. Careful mouth care with frequent rinsing, sucking hard candy, chewing sugarless gum, and increased fluid in-take may relieve S&S of dry mouth.
3. Wait and evaluate sedative effects of drug before performing tasks that re-quire mental alertness.
4. Avoid alcohol, CNS depressants, or OTC agents.

5. Drug is for short-term use; keep F/U appointment to evaluate response to therapy and adverse effects.

OUTCOMES/EVALUATE
- ↓ Anxiety and agitation
- Relief of itching/allergic S&S
- Control of N&V/chronic urticaria

Hyoscyamine sulfate
(high-oh-**SIGH**-ah-meen)

CLASSIFICATION(S):
Cholinergic blocking drug
PREGNANCY CATEGORY: C
Rx: Anaspaz, Cystospaz, ED-SPAZ, IB-Stat, Levbid, Levsin, Levsin Drops, Levsin/SL, Levsinex Time-caps, Mar-Spas, Neosol, NuLev, Sy-max Duotab, Symax FasTab, Sy-max-SL, Symax-SR.

SEE ALSO *CHOLINERGIC BLOCKING AGENTS.*

USES
(1) To control gastric secretion, visceral spasm, and hypermotility in spastic coli-tis, spastic bladder, cystitis, pyloros-pasm, and associated abdominal cramps. (2) Relieve symptoms in func-tional intestinal disorders (e.g., mild dy-senteries and diverticulitis), infant colic, biliary colic. (3) Adjunct to treat peptic ulcer. (4) Irritable bowel syndrome (e.g., irritable colon, spastic colon, mucous colitis, acute enterocolitis, functional GI disorders). (5) Neurogenic bowel distur-bances, including splenic flexure syn-drome and neurogenic colon. (6) Re-duce pain and hypersecretion in pan-creatitis. (7) As a drying agent to relieve symptoms of acute rhinitis. (8) In Par-kinsonism to reduce rigidity and trem-ors and to control associated sialorrhea and hyperhidrosis. (9) Treat poisoning by anticholinesterase agents. (10) Treat cystitis or renal colic. (11) Certain cases of partial heart block associated with vagal activity. (12) Preoperative medica-tion to reduce salivary, tracheobronchi-al, and pharyngeal secretions. (13) Par-

---

enterally to reduce duoendal motility to facilitate the diagnostic radiologic procedure, hypotonic duodenography. May also improve radiologic visibility of the kidneys.

ACTION/KINETICS

Action

One of the belladonna alkaloids; acts by blocking the action of acetylcholine at the postganglionic nerve endings of the parasympathetic nervous system.

Pharmacokinetics

$t^{1}\!/_{2}$: 3.5 hr for tablets, 7 hr for extended-release capsules, and 9 hr for extended-release tablets. Majority of the drug is excreted in the urine unchanged.

SPECIAL CONCERNS

Heat prostration may occur if the drug is taken in the presence of high environmental temperatures. Use with caution during lactation.

SIDE EFFECTS

Most Common

Dry mouth, drowsiness, flushing of face, headache, blurred vision, photosensitivity, constipation, decreased sweating, thirst.

See *Cholinergic Blocking Agents* for a complete list of possible side effects.

HOW SUPPLIED

Capsules, Extended-Release: 0.375 mg; *Capsules, Timed-Release:* 0.375 mg; *Drops:* 0.125 mg/mL; *Elixir:* 0.125 mg/5 mL; *Injection:* 0.5 mg/mL; *Oral Spray:* 0.125 mg/mL; *Tablets:* 0.125 mg, 0.15 mg; *Tablets, Extended-Release / Tablets, Sustained-Release:* 0.375 mg (includes Duotab containing 0.125 mg immediate-release and 0.5 mg extended-release); *Tablets, Oral Disintegrating:* 0.125 mg; *Tablets, Sublingual:* 0.125 mg, 0.25 mg.

DOSAGE

- **CAPSULES, EXTENDED-RELEASE; TABLETS, EXTENDED-RELEASE; TABLETS, TIMED-RELEASE**

Adults and children over 12 years of age: 0.375–0.750 mg q 12 hr, not to exceed 1.5 mg in 24 hr.

- **TABLETS; TABLETS, SUBLINGUAL**

Adults and children over 12 years of age: 0.125–0.25 mg q 4 hr or as needed, not to exceed 1.5 mg in 24 hr.

- **TABLETS, ORAL DISINTEGRATING**

0.125 mg: Adults and children over 12 years: 1 or 2 tablets q 4 hr, up to 12/day or 2 tablets 4 times per day. **Children, 2 to less than 12 years:** ½–1 tablet q 4 hr, up to 6 per day.

0.25 mg: Adults and children over 12 years: ½–1 tablet 3–4 times per day, 30 min to 1 hr before meals and at bedtime. This dosage form is not recommended for children under 12 years old.

- **ELIXIR**

Adults and children over 12 years of age: 0.125 mg–0.25 mg (5–10 mL) q 4 hr, not to exceed 1.5 mg (60 mL) in 24 hr. **Children, 2 to 12 years of age: 10 kg:** 1.25 mL (0.031 mg) q 4 hr; **20 kg:** 2.5 mL (0.062 mg) q 4 hr; **40 kg:** 3.75 mL (0.093 mg) q 4 hr; **50 kg:** 5 mL (0.125 mg) q 4 hr.

- **DROPS**

Adults and children over 12 years of age: 0.125–0.25 mg (5–10 mL) q 4 hr, not to exceed 1.5 mg (12 mL) in 24 hr. **Children, 2 to 12 years of age:** 0.031–0.125 mg (0.22–1 mL) q 4 hr or as needed, not to exceed 0.75 mg (6 mL) in 24 hr. **Children, under 2 years of age: 3.4 kg:** 4 drops q 4 hr, not to exceed 24 drops in 24 hr; **5 kg:** 5 drops q 4 hr, not to exceed 30 drops in 24 hr; **7 kg:** 6 drops q 4 hr, not to exceed 36 drops in 24 hr; **10 kg:** 8 drops q 4 hr, not to exceed 48 drops in 24 hr.

- **ORAL SPRAY**

Children, 12 years and younger: 1–2 mL (1 or 2 sprays) q 4 hr as needed, up to 12 mL/day (12 sprays/day).

- **INJECTION**

GI disorders.

Adults: 0.25–0.5 mg (0.5–1 mL). Some clients need only one dose while others require doses 2, 3, or 4 times per day at 4 hr intervals.

Diagnostic procedures.

Adults: 0.25–0.5 mg (0.5–1 mL) given IV 5 to 10 min prior to the procedure.

Preanesthetic medication.

Adults and children over 2 years of age: 0.005 mg/kg 30–60 min prior to the time of induction of anesthesia. May also be given at the time the preanesthetic sedative or narcotic is given.

Bold Italic = life threatening side effect　　■ = black box warning　　✦ = Available in Canada

During surgery to reduce drug-induced bradycardia.

Adults and children over 2 years of age: Increments of 0.125 mg (0.25 mL) IV repeated as needed.

Reverse neuromuscular blockade.

Adults and children over 2 years of age: 0.2 mg (0.4 mL) for every 1 mg neostigmine or equivalent dose of physostigmine or pyridostigmine.

NURSING CONSIDERATIONS

℞ Do not confuse Levbid or Levsin with Lithobid (lithium), Lopid (an antihyperlipidemic), or Lorabid (a beta-lactam antibiotic).

ADMINISTRATION/STORAGE
1. May take hyoscyamine SL tablets sublingually, PO, or chewed. May take hyoscyamine tablets PO or SL.
2. Depending on the use, may give injection SC, IM, or IV.
IV 3. Visually inspect the injectable form for particulate matter/discoloration.

ASSESSMENT
1. Note reasons for therapy, type, onset, characteristics of S&S.
2. List other agents trialed, outcome. Reduce dose in elderly.
3. Determine evidence of glaucoma, bladder neck or GI tract obstruction.

4. Assess elimination/output, abdomen, UGI, CT/US abdomen to R/O pathology.

CLIENT/FAMILY TEACHING
1. Take as prescribed; avoid antacids within 1 hr of taking drug (decreases effectiveness).
2. Do not perform activities that require mental alertness until drug effects realized; dizziness, drowsiness, and blurred vision may occur.
3. Report any loss of symptom control so provider can adjust dose and frequency of administration. Report diarrhea as it may be symptom of intestinal obstruction, especially with a colostomy or ileostomy.
4. Avoid excessive temperatures and activity; drug impairs heat regulation and may decrease perspiration, which may cause fever, heat prostration, or stroke.
5. Males with enlarged prostrate may experience urinary retention/hesitancy; report if persistent or bothersome.
6. Stop drug and report any mental confusion, impaired gait, disorientation, or hallucinations.
7. Avoid alcohol and CNS depressants. Use dark glasses when outside to prevent blurred vision. Keep all F/U visits.

OUTCOMES/EVALUATE
- ↓ GI motility
- Control of epigastric pain/spasm

Ibandronate sodium **IV** 📷
(eye-**BAN**-droh-nayt)

CLASSIFICATION(S):
Bone growth regulator, bisphosphonate
PREGNANCY CATEGORY: C
Rx: Boniva.

USES
Tablets: Prophylaxis of postmenopausal osteoporosis in women who are at risk of developing osteoporosis and for whom the desired clinical outcome is to maintain bone mass and reduce the risk of fracture.

Injection/Tablets: Treatment of postmenopausal osteoporosis to increase bone mineral density and reduce the incidence of vertebral fractures.

Investigational: Prevention and treatment of complications of metastatic bone disease in breast cancer.

ACTION/KINETICS

Action

A bisphosphonate that inhibits osteoclast activity and reduces bone resorption and turnover. In postmenopausal women, the drug reduces the elevated rate of bone turnover, leading to a net gain in bone mass.

Pharmacokinetics

Time to maximum plasma levels, after PO: 0.5–2 hr. Absorption is impaired by food or beverages (other than plain water). After absorption, ibandronate either binds rapidly to bone or is excreted in the urine. Drug not bound to bone is excreted unchanged by the kidney (about 50–60% of the absorbed dose). Unabsorbed drug is excreted unchanged in the feces. **$t\frac{1}{2}$, terminal, after PO:** 10–60 hr. **Plasma protein binding:** 90.9–99.5%.

CONTRAINDICATIONS

Hypersensitivity to the drug or any component of the product. Uncorrected hypocalcemia. Inability to stand or sit upright for at least 60 min. Severe renal impairment (C_{CR} less than 30 mL/min).

SPECIAL CONCERNS

Use with caution with aspirin or NSAIDs and during lactation. Safety and efficacy have not been determined in children. Greater sensitivity can not be ruled out in some geriatric clients.

SIDE EFFECTS

Most Common

Back/arm/leg pain, diarrhea, dyspepsia, abdominal pain, constipation, pain/difficulty swallowing, headache, nausea, rash.

GI: UGI disorders, including dysphagia, esophagitis, esophageal or gastric ulcer. Dyspepsia, diarrhea, constipation, abdominal pain, pain/difficulty swallowing, tooth disorder, N&V, gastritis. **CNS:** Headache, dizziness, vertigo, nerve root lesion. **Musculoskeletal:** Myalgia, back/arm/leg pain, joint disorder, arthritis, osteonecrosis of jaw. **Respiratory:** URTI, bronchitis, pneumonia, pharyngitis. **Ophthalmic:** Ocular inflammation, including uveitis and scleritis. **Body as a whole:** Infection, asthenia, rash, allergic reaction. **Miscellaneous:** UTI, hypercholesterolemia.

LABORATORY TEST CONSIDERATIONS

↓ Alkaline phosphatase.

OD OVERDOSE MANAGEMENT

Symptoms: Hypocalcemia/phosphatemia, UGI side effects, including upset stomach, dyspepsia, esophagitis, gastritis, ulcer. *Treatment:* Milk or antacids to bind the drug. Do not induce vomiting due to the risk of esophageal irritation. Keep client fully upright

DRUG INTERACTIONS

Antacids containing Ca, Al, Mg / ↓ Ibandronate absorption from GI tract

Foods containing Ca / ↓ Ibandronate absorption from GI tract

Iron-containing products / ↓ Ibandronate absorption from GI tract

HOW SUPPLIED

Injection: 1 mg/mL (as base); *Tablets:* 2.5 mg (as base), 150 mg (as base).

DOSAGE

- **IV ONLY**

  Postmenopausal osteoporosis.

  3 mg q 3 months given over 15–30 seconds.

- **TABLETS**

  Treat or prevent postmenopausal osteoporosis.

  Adults: 2.5 mg once daily or one 150 mg tablet taken once monthly on the same date each month.

NURSING CONSIDERATIONS

ADMINISTRATION/STORAGE

1. Therapy must include calcium and vitamin D supplements.

2. No dosage adjustment needed with mild or moderate renal impairment (where C_{CR} is equal to or greater than 30 mL/min).

3. Store tablets between 15–30°C (59–86°F).

IV 4. Do not administer intra-arterially or paravenously due to possible tissue damage.

5. Use the needle provided; prefilled syringes are for single use only. Discard any unused portion.

6. Do not mix the injection with calcium-containing solutions or other IV administered drugs.

Bold Italic = life threatening side effect   ■ = black box warning   ✤ = Available in Canada

7. If the IV dose is missed, administer as soon as it can be rescheduled. Thereafter, schedule injections every 3 months from the date of the last injection. Do not give more frequently than every three months.

8. Store from 15–30°C (59–86°F). Discard any unused portion.

ASSESSMENT

1. Note reasons for therapy, risk factors, BMD. List drugs prescribed to ensure none interact.

2. Assess renal function, electrolytes; ensure calcium and vitamin D WNL. May cause elevated cholesterol and reduced total alkaline phosphatase.

CLIENT/FAMILY TEACHING

1. Take as directed once daily at least 60 min before the first food or drink (other than water) of the day and before any PO medications containing Al, calcium, or Mg, including supplements and vitamins.

2. If once-monthly dose is missed, and the next scheduled ibandronate day is more than 7 days away, take one 150 mg tablet in the morning of the date that it is remembered. Return taking the one 150 mg tablet every month in the morning of the chosen day, according to the original schedule.

3. Do not take two 150 mg tablets during the same week. If the next scheduled ibandronate tablet is only 1–7 days away, wait until the next scheduled ibandronate day to take the tablet. Return to taking one 150 mg tablet every month in the morning of the chosen day, according to the original schedule.

4. Swallow tablets whole with a full glass of plain water (6–8 oz) while standing or sitting in an upright position. Do not lie down for 60 min after taking the drug. Do not double up or take dose later in the day.

5. Plain water is the only liquid that should be taken with ibandronate. Some mineral waters contain a higher concentration of calcium and thus should not be used.

6. Do not chew or suck the tablet due to the possibility of throat ulceration.

7. Review drug insert with each refill. May experience heartburn, swallowing problems, diarrhea, bone pain, ulcers, or chest pain. Report adverse effects to provider.

8. Eat well balanced meals, perform regular daily exercise, stop smoking, avoid alcohol consumption; behaviors that add to osteoporosis risk.

9. Do not take any OTC medications, vitamins or supplements without approval; may inhibit drug action. Should be prescribed supplemental calcium and vitamin D.

10. Practice reliable contraception; report if pregnancy suspected or if planning to breastfeed. Keep all F/U appointments to evaluate response.

OUTCOMES/EVALUATE

↑ Bone mineral density in post menopausal women; ↓ vertebral fractures

Ibritumomab tiuxetan ■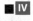

(ib-rih-**TOO**-moh-mab)

CLASSIFICATION(S):
Antineoplastic Agent
PREGNANCY CATEGORY: D
Rx: Zevalin.

SEE ALSO *ANTINEOPLASTIC AGENTS*

USES

Relapsed or refractory low-grade, follicular, or transformed B-cell non-Hodgkin's lymphoma, including rituximab-refractory follicular non-Hodgkin's lymphoma. Ibritumomab tiuxetan is part of a therapeutic regimen that first includes an infusion of rituximab followed by an injection of ibritumomab tiuxetan. This same regimen is repeated 7–9 days after the first course of therapy.

ACTION/KINETICS

Action

Drug is the immunoconjugate from a stable thiourea covalent bond between the monoclonal antibody, ibritumomab, and the linker-chelator, tiuxetan. The linker-chelator provides a high affinity, conformationally restricted chelation site for either Indium-111 or Yttrium-90. The ibritumomab antibody acts against the CD20 antigen, which is found on the surface of normal and malignant B lymphocytes. The chelate, tiuxetan, which tightly binds In-111 or Y-90 is covalently linked to the amino groups of exposed lysines and arginines contained within the antibody. The beta emission from Y-90 causes cellular damage by forming free radicals in the target and neighboring cells. Administration of ibritumomab tiuxetan results in sustained depletion of B cells. Median serum levels of IgG and IgA remain within the normal range through the period of B-cell depletion. However, median IgM levels drop below normal after treatment but recover to normal values within 6 months after therapy.

Pharmacokinetics

t½ of Y-90: 30 hr.

CONTRAINDICATIONS

Type I hypersensitivity or anaphylactic reactions to murine proteins or any component of the product, including rituximab, yttrium chloride, or indium chloride. Administration of Y-90 ibritumomab tiuxetan to those with altered biodistribution as determined by imaging with In-111 ibritumomab tiuxetan. Lactation.

Use in clients with 25% or more lymphoma marrow involvement or impaired bone marrow reserve; platelet count <100,000 cells/mm³; neutrophil count <1,500 cells/mm³; hypocellular bone marrow (less than or equal to 15% cellularity or marked reduction in bone marrow precursors); or a history of failed stem cell collection.

Receipt of growth factor for 2 weeks prior to ibritumomab tiuxetan therapy and for 2 weeks following completion of the regimen.

SPECIAL CONCERNS

■ (1) Fatal infusion reactions. Deaths have occurred within 24 hr of rituximab infusion. Deaths were associated with an infusion reaction, including symptoms of hypoxia, pulmonary infiltrates, acute respiratory distress syndrome, MI, ventricular fibrillation, or cardiogenic shock. About 80% of such fatalities occurred in association with the first infusion. Discontinue rituximab, In-111 ibri-

tumomab tiuxetan, and Y-90 ibritumomab tiuxetan infusions in clients who develop severe infusion reactions; give medical treatment. (2) Prolonged and severe cytopenias. Y-90 ibritumomab tiuxetan administration results in severe and prolonged cytopenias in most clients. Do not give the ibritumomab tiuxetan administration regimen to clients with 25% or more lymphoma marrow involvement or impaired bone marrow reserve. (3) Severe cutaneous and mucocutaneous reactions. Severe cutaneous and mucocutaneous reactions, some with fatal outcome, have been reported in association with ibritumomab tiuxetan therapeutic regimen. Do not administer any further component of the ibritumomab tiuxetan therapeutic regimen to clients experiencing a severe cutaneous or mucocutaneous reaction; those clients should seek prompt medical evaluation. (4) Dosing. (a) The prescribed, measured, and administered dose of Y-90 ibritumomab tiuxetan should not exceed the absolute maximum allowable dose of 32 mCi (1184 MBq). (b) Do not adminster Y90 ibritumomab tiuxetan to clients with altered biodistribution as determined by imaging with IN-111 ibritumomab tiuxetan. (5) In-111 ibritumomab tiuxetan and Y-90 ibritumomab tiuxetan are radiopharmaceuticals and should be used only by physicians and other professionals qualified by training and experience in the safe use and handling of radionuclides. ■ Use with caution with drugs that interfere with platelet function or coagulation after the ibritumomab tiuxetan therapeutic regimen; monitor clients carefully who receive such drugs. Safety and efficacy have not been determined in children.

SIDE EFFECTS

Most Common

Anemia, anorexia, anxiety, arthralgia, dizziness, dyspnea, ecchymosis, abdominal pain, diarrhea, N&V, increased cough, neutropenia, thrombocytopenia, chills, infection, pain, fever.

Severe infusion reactions: Hypotension, angioedema, hypoxia, bronchospasms, pulmonary infiltrate, *ARDS, MI,*

Bold Italic = life threatening side effect   ■ = black box warning   ✦ = Available in Canada

ventricular fibrillation, cardiogenic shock, death. **Hematologic:** Prolonged and severe cytopenias, including thrombocytopenia (most common) and neutropenia; anemia, ecchymosis, pancytopenia. **CV:** *Hemorrhage (while thrombocytopenic), including fatal cerebral hemorrhage and severe infections,* hypotension, tachycardia. **GI:** N&V, abdominal pain/enlargement, diarrhea, throat irritation, constipation, dyspepsia, melena, *GI hemorrhage,* hematemesis. **CNS:** Dizziness, anorexia, anxiety, headache, insomnia, encephalopathy, *subdural hematoma.* **Respiratory:** Increased cough, dyspnea, rhinitis, bronchospasm, epistaxis, *apnea,* lung edema, *pulmonary embolus.* **Musculoskeletal:** Arthralgia, myalgia, arthritis. **Dermatologic:** Urticaria, sweats, petechia, pruritus, rash, flushing, erythema multiforme, *Stevens-Johnson syndrome, toxic epidermal necrolysis,* bullous dermatitis, exfoliative dermatitis. **Infections:** UTI, febrile neutropenia, sepsis, pneumonia, cellulitis, colitis, diarrhea, osteomyelitis, URTI. Serious infections (primarily bacterial), including *sepsis,* empyema, pneumonia, febrile neutropenia, biliary stent-associated colangitis. Serious infections from 3 months to 4 years after start of treatment, including UTI, bacterial or viral pneumonia, febrile neutropenia, perihilar infiltrate, pericarditis, IV drug-associated viral hepatitis, respiratory disease, *sepsis.* **Body as a whole:** Development of secondary malignancies (myeloid, dysplasias), possible immunogenicity, allergic reactions (*bronchospasm, angioedema*), peripheral edema, asthenia, infection, chills, fever, pain, back/tumor pain, *vaginal hemorrhage.*

DRUG INTERACTIONS
Possible ↑ risk of bleeding and hemorrhage if client receives drugs that interfere with platelet function or coagulation

HOW SUPPLIED
Injection: 3.2 mg.

DOSAGE
• **IV**
Non-Hodgkin's lymphoma.

Step 1: Give rituximab, 250 mg/m² IV at an initial rate of 50 mg/hr. Do not mix or dilute rituximab with other drugs. If hypersensitivity or infusion-related events do not occur, escalate the infusion rate in 50 mg/hr increments every 30 min to a maximum of 400 mg/hr. If hypersensitivity or an infusion-related event occurs, temporarily slow or interrupt the infusion; the infusion can continue at 50% of the previous rate upon improvement of client symptoms. **Then,** within 4 hr following completion of the rituximab dose, inject 5 mCi (1.6 mg total antibody dose) of In-111 ibritumomab tiuxetan over a 10-min period. Assess biodistribution as follows: First image, 2–24 hr after In-111 ibritumomab tiuxetan; second image, 48–72 hr after In-111 ibritumomab tiuxetan. An optional third image may be taken 90–120 hr after In-111 ibritumomab tiuxetan. If biodistribution is not acceptable, do not proceed.

Step 2: Initiate Step 2, 7 to 9 days following Step 1. Give rituximab, 250 mg/m² IV at an initial rate of 100 mg/hr (50 mg/hr if infusion-related events were documented during Step 1). Increase by 100 mg/hr increments at 30-min intervals to a maximum of 400 mg/hr, as tolerated. **Then,** within 4 hr after completion of the rituximab dose, inject IV, Y-90 ibritumomab tiuxetan, over a period of 10 min, 0.4 mCi/kg (14.8 MBq/kg) actual body weight for clients with a platelet count greater than 150,000 cells/mm³ and 0.3 mCi/kg (11.1 MBq/kg) actual body weight for clients with a platelet count of 100,000 to 149,000 cells/mm³. The prescribed, measured, and administered dose of Y-90 ibritumomab tiuxetan must not exceed the maximum allowable dose of 32 mCi (1,184 MBq) regardless of the client's weight.

NURSING CONSIDERATIONS
ADMINISTRATION/STORAGE
IV 1. Establish free-flowing IV line prior to Y-90 ibritumomab tiuxetan injection. Monitor carefully for extravasation when giving drug. If any signs of extrav-

asation occur, immediately terminate the infusion and restart in another vein.

2. Do not give Y-90 ibritumomab tiuxetan to clients with a platelet count less than 100,000/mm³.

3. For product preparation, see manufacturer's product labeling.

4. Two separate kits (distinctly labeled) are to be ordered for the preparation of a single dose each of In-111 ibritumomab tiuxetan and Y-90 ibritumomab tiuxetan. Note that these are both radiopharmaceuticals and must be used only by physicians and other professionals qualified by training in the safe use and handling of such agents.

5. Changing the ratio of any of the reactants in the radiolabeling process may adversely impact results.

6. Do not use either In-111 ibritumomab tiuxetan or Y-90 ibritumomab tiuxetan in the absence of the rituximab predose.

ASSESSMENT

1. Note reasons for therapy, other agents trialed, outcome.

2. Infusion reactions (ARDS, hypoxia, pulmonary infiltrates, MI, VF, or cardiogenic shock) may occur. Monitor closely and stop infusion as reactions fatal. Must only be administered by qualified trained individuals.

3. Avoid drugs that interfere with platelet function or bleeding times; monitor CBC, platelets weekly until recovered.

4. Monitor carefully for infections, allergic reactions, and hemorrhage. Drug is radiopharmaceutical; utilize radionuclide precautions (minimize exposure to client and medical staff).

CLIENT/FAMILY TEACHING

1. Used to treat relapsed or refractory non-Hodgkin's lymphoma; consists of two infusions approximately one week apart.

2. Elderly may show greater sensitivity to the regimen.

3. Use effective contraception during treatment and for 12 months following regimen.

4. Ensure client/family aware of risks: that myeloid malignancies have oc-

curred with therapy and that infusion reactions may be fatal.

OUTCOMES/EVALUATE

Inhibition of malignant cell proliferation

Ibuprofen ■ IV
(eye-byou-**PROH**-fen)

CLASSIFICATION(S):
Nonsteroidal anti-inflammatory drug

PREGNANCY CATEGORY: B (first two trimesters), **D** (third trimester).

OTC: Capsules: Advil Liqui-Gels, Advil Migraine. **Gelcaps**: Ibutab, Midol Maximum Strength Cramp Formula, Motrin IB. **Oral Drops**: Infants' Motrin, PediaCare Fever. **Suspension**: Children's Advil, Children's Motrin, PediaCare Fever, Pediatric Advil Drops. **Tablets**: Advil, Junior Strength Motrin, Menadol, Motrin IB, Motrin Migraine Pain. **Tablets, Chewable**: Children's Advil, Children's Motrin, Junior Strength Advil, Junior Strength Motrin.

Rx: Tablets: Motrin.

✷**Rx:** Apo-Ibuprofen, Novo-Profen, Nu-Ibuprofen.

Ibuprofen lysine
Rx: NeoProfen.

SEE ALSO NONSTEROIDAL ANTI-INFLAMMATORY DRUGS.

USES

Ibuprofen. Rx: (1) Analgesic for mild to moderate pain. (2) Primary dysmenorrhea. (3) Relief of signs and symptoms of rheumatoid arthritis or osteoarthritis. *Investigational:* Resistant acne vulgaris (with tetracyclines); inflammation due to ultraviolet-B exposure (sunburn), juvenile rheumatoid arthritis. High doses to treat progressive lung deterioration in cystic fibrosis. Prophylactically to lower the risk of Alzheimer's disease.

OTC. Liquid-Filled Capsules, Adults: Migraine headaches. **Gelcaps and Tablets, Adults:** (1) Temporary relief of minor aches and pains due to the common cold, headache, toothache, muscular aches, backache, minor pain of arthritis, menstrual cramps. (2) Reduce fever. **Chewable Tablets, Junor Strength Tablets, Oral Suspension, Oral Drops, Children:** (1) Temporary reduction of fever. (2) Relief of minor aches and pains due to colds, flu, sore throat, headaches, and toothaches.

Ibuprofen lysine. Rx (IV): To close clinically significant patent ductus arteriosus in infants whose gestational age is 32 weeks or less, weight is 500–1,500 grams, and the condition cannot be managed through usual therapy (e.g., diuretics, fluid restriction, respiratory support).

ACTION/KINETICS

Action

Anti-inflammatory effect is likely due to inhibition of cyclo-oxygenase. Inhibition of cyclo-oxygenase results in decreased prostaglandin synthesis. Effective in reducing joint swelling, pain, and morning stiffness, as well as to increase mobility in those with inflammatory disease. Ibuprofen does not alter the course of the disease, however. The antipyretic action occurs by decreasing prostaglandin synthesis in the hypothalamus resulting in an increase in peripheral blood flow and heat loss, as well as promoting sweating. The mechanism to close patent ductus arteriosus is not known.

Pharmacokinetics

Greater than 80% bioavailable after PO. **Time to peak levels:** 1–2 hr. **Onset:** 30 min for analgesia and approximately 1 week for anti-inflammatory effect. **Peak serum levels:** 1–2 hr. **Duration:** 4–6 hr for analgesia and 1–2 weeks for anti-inflammatory effect. Food delays absorption rate but not total amount of drug absorbed. $t\frac{1}{2}$: 1.8–2 hr. 45–79% excreted in the urine. **Plasma protein binding:** 99%.

CONTRAINDICATIONS

Pregnancy, especially during the last trimester. Use in clients with the aspirin triad (bronchial asthma, rhinitis, aspirin intolerance). Use to treat perioperative pain in the setting of coronary artery bypass graft surgery. Ibuprofen lysine is contraindicated in preterm infants with a proven or suspected infection not receiving treatment; congenital heart disease needing a patent ductus arteriosus to acheive satisfactory pulmonary or systemic blood flow; thrombocytopenia; in those who are bleeding (especially those with active intracranial hemorrhage or GI bleeding); a coagulation defect, proven or suspected necrotizing enterocolitis, or significant impaired renal function.

SPECIAL CONCERNS

■ (1) NSAIDs may cause an increased risk of serious CV thrombotic events, MI, and stroke, which can be fatal. This risk may increase with duration of use. Clients with CV disease or risk factors for CV disease may be at a greater risk. (2) Ibuprofen is contraindicated for treatment of perioperative pain in the setting of coronary artery bypass graft surgery. (3) NSAIDs cause an increased risk of serious GI adverse events including bleeding, ulceration, and perforation of the stomach or intestines, which can be fatal. These events can occur at any time during use and without warning symptoms. Elderly clients are at greater risk for serious GI events.■ Individualize dosage by body weight for children less than 12 years of age as safety and effectiveness have not been established. May cause stomach bleeding in individuals who consume large amounts of alcohol regularly. Blocks the heart-protecting effects of aspirin. Ibuprofen chewable tablets may cause stomach bleeding if more than the recommended dose is taken.

Ibuprofen lysine may alter the usual signs of infection. Use the drug with extra care in the presence of controlled infection and in infants at risk of infection. Use with caution in infants with elevated total bilirubin.

SIDE EFFECTS

Most Common

Ibuprofen: Dizziness, rash, nausea, epigastric/GI pain, heartburn.

Ibuprofen lysine: Skin lesion/irritation, **sepsis**, GI disorders, anemia, **intraventricular hemorrhage**, impaired renal function, **apnea**, respiratory failure, RTI.

 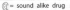

See also *Nonsteroidal Anti-Inflammatory Drugs* for a complete list of possible side effects.

Ibuprofen: Also, dermatitis (maculopapular type), rash. Hypersensitivity reaction consisting of abdominal pain, fever, headache, *meningitis*, N&V, abnormal platelet function (returns to normal within 24 hr), signs of liver damage; especially seen in clients with SLE.

Ibuprofen lysine: GI: GI disorders, including non-necrotizing enterocolitis, abdominal distention, gastritis, gastroesophageal reflux, ileus, cholestasis, jaundice. **CNS: *Convulsions*. CV: *Cardiac failure,*** hypotension, tachycardia. **GU:** UTI, reduced urine output, inguinal hernia. **Hematologic:** Anemia, *intraventricular hemorrhage* (all grades), other bleeding disorders, neutropenia, thrombocytopenia. **Metabolic:** Hypernatremia, hypocalcemia, hypo/hyperglycemia. **GU:** Renal failure, impaired renal function, decreased urine output. **Respiratory:** Apnea, *respiratory failure*, atelectasis, RTI. **Dermatologic:** Skin lesions/irritation. **Miscellaneous: *Sepsis*,** edema, adrenal insufficiency, injection site reactions, feeding problems, various infections.

ADDITIONAL DRUG INTERACTIONS

Aspirin / Ibuprofen may ↓ or negate the cardioprotective effects of low-dose aspirin

Furosemide / ↓ Diuretic effect R/T ↓ renal prostaglandin synthesis

H *Ginkgo biloba* / Possible (rare) intracerebral mass bleeding

Lithium / ↑ Plasma lithium levels

Thiazide diuretics / See furosemide

LABORATORY TEST CONSIDERATIONS

Ibuprofen lysine: ↑ Blood urea, blood urea increased with hematuria, blood creatinine.

HOW SUPPLIED

Ibuprofen: OTC: Capsules: 200 mg; *Oral Drops:* 40 mg/mL; *Suspension:* 100 mg/2.5 mL, 100 mg/5 mL; *Tablets:* 100 mg, 200 mg.; *Tablets, Chewable:* 50 mg, 100 mg; **Rx:** Tablets: 400 mg, 600 mg, 800 mg.

Ibuprofen lysine: Injection: 17.1 mg/mL (equivalent to 10 mg/mL ibuprofen).

DOSAGE
IBUPROFEN
• **RX: TABLETS**

Rheumatoid arthritis and osteoarthritis, including flareups of chronic disease.

Either 300 mg 4 times per day or 400, 600, or 800 mg 3–4 times per day; adjust dosage according to client response. Individual clients may show a better response to 3,200 mg daily compared with 2,400 mg. However, evaluate the increased clinical benefits of the higher dose to potential increased risk. Full therapeutic response may not be noted for 2 or more weeks.

Mild to moderate pain.

Adults: 400 mg q 4–6 hr, as needed. Doses greater than 400 mg are no more effective than the 400 mg dose.

Primary dysmenorrhea.

Adults: 400 mg q 4 hr, as needed, for the relief of pain. Begin treatment with the earliest onset of pain.

• **OTC: ORAL DROPS**

Antipyretic.

Children, 6–11 months (12–17 pounds): 50 mg (1.25 mL) q 6–8 hr, up to 4 times per day. **Children, 12–23 months (18–23 pounds):** 75 mg (1.875 mL) q 6–8 hr, up to 4 times per day.

• **OTC: GELCAPS AND TABLETS**

Mild to moderate pain, antipyretic, dysmenorrhea.

Adults: 200 mg q 4–6 hr while symptoms persist. If pain or fever does not respond to 1 gelcap or tablet, 2 gelcaps or tablets (i.e., 400 mg) may be taken, but do not exceed 6 gelcaps or tablets (i.e., 1,200 mg) in 24 hr unless directed by provider. For capsules, do not take more than 2 capsules in 24 hr.

• **OTC: ORAL SUSPENSION**

Pain, fever.

Usual dose: 7.5 mg/kg. **Children, 2–3 years of age (24–35 pounds):** 100 mg (5 mL) q 6–8 hr, up to 4 times per day. **Children, 4–5 years of age (36–47 pounds):** 150 mg (7.5 mL) q 6–8 hr, up to 4 times per day. **Children, 6–8 years of age (48–59 pounds):** 200 mg (10 mL) q 6–8 hr, up to 4 times per day. **Children, 9–10 years of age (60–71 pounds):** 250 mg (12.5 mL) q 6–8 hr, up

---

Bold Italic = life threatening side effect   ■ = black box warning   ✦ = Available in Canada

to 4 times per day. **Children, 11 years of age (72–95 pounds):** 300 mg (15 mL) q 6–8 hr, up to 4 times per day.

• **OTC: CHEWABLE TABLETS (50 MG)**

Pain, fever.

Children, 4–5 years of age (36–47 pounds): 150 mg (3 tablets) q 6–8 hr, up to 4 times per day. **Children, 6–8 years of age (48–59 pounds):** 4 tablets (200 mg) q 6–8 hr, up to 4 times per day. **Children, 9–10 years of age (60–71 pounds):** 250 mg (5 tablets) q 6–8 hr, up to 4 times per day. **Children, 11 years of age (72–95 pounds):** 300 mg (6 tablets) q 6–8 hr, up to 4 times per day. Usually use weight to dose; otherwise, use age.

• **OTC: JUNIOR STRENGTH CHEWABLE TABLETS (100 MG)**

Pain, fever.

Children, 6–8 years of age (48–59 pounds): 200 mg (2 tablets) q 6–8 hr, up to 4 times per day. **Children, 9–10 years of age (60–71 pounds):** 250 mg (2.5 tablets) q 6–8 hr, up to 4 times per day. **Children, 11 years of age (72–95 pounds):** 300 mg (3 tablets) q 6–8 hr, up to 4 times per day. Use weight to dose; otherwise use age.

IBUPROFEN LYSINE

• **IV INFUSION**

Patent ductus arteriosus.

10 mg/kg by IV infusion over 15 min for one dose and then 5 mg/kg 24 and 48 hr later, with all doses based on birth weight. Administration of the second or third dose to an infant with urinary output <0.6 mL/kg/hr should be delayed until renal function returns to normal.

NURSING CONSIDERATIONS

ADMINISTRATION/STORAGE

1. Do not use OTC ibuprofen as an antipyretic for more than 3 days or as an analgesic for more than 10 days, unless medically prescribed.

2. Children's Chewable Tablets are for children, 4–11 years of age; Junior Strength Tablets are for children, 6–11 years of age; Oral Suspension is for children 2–11 years of age; and, Oral Drops are for children 6 months–3 years of age.

3. Do not take more than 3.2 grams/day of prescription products.

4. If GI distress occurs with any product, take with meals or milk.

5. Oral Drops: Consult a provider before giving to children who are less than 6 months of age or weigh less than 24 pounds.

6. Oral Suspension: Consult a provider before giving to children who are less than 2 years of age or weigh less than 24 pounds.

7. Chewable Tablets (50 mg): Consult a provider before giving to children who are less than 4 years of age or weigh less than 36 pounds.

8. Chewable Tablets (100 mg): Consult a provider before giving to children who are less than 6 years of age or weigh less than 48 pounds.

9. Store Capsules, Gelcaps, and Tablets from 20–25°C (68–77°F). Avoid excessive heat greater than 40°C (104°F). Store Oral Suspension and Oral Drops from 15–30°C (59–86°F).

IV 10. If the ductus arteriosus closes or is significantly reduced in size after completion of the first course of ibuprofen lysine, no further doses are necessary. If during continued treatment the ductus arteriosus fails to close or re-opens, then a second course of ibuprofen, alternative pharmacologic therapy, or surgery may be necessary.

11. Dilute the solution for injection to an appropriate volume with dextrose or saline. Prepare for infusion and administer within 30 min of preparation.

12. Infuse continuously over a period of 15 min.

13. Administer through the IV port that is nearest the insertion site.

14. After the first withdrawal from the vial, discard any remaining solution because ibuprofen lysine contains no preservative.

15. Administer carefully to avoid extravasation as the product is irritating to tissues.

16. Do not administer ibuprofen lysine simultaneously in the same IV line with TPN. If necessary, interrupt TPN for 15 min prior to and after drug administration.

17. Maintain line patency using dextrose or saline.

18. Store the injection from 15–30°C (59–86°F) protected from light. Store vials in the carton until used.

ASSESSMENT

1. Note reasons for therapy, onset, location, characteristics of S&S. With pain, rate level; evaluate for effectiveness.

2. Review history for any conditions that may preclude drug therapy, i.e., PUD, lupus, ASA intolerance, heavy alcohol intake.

3. Obtain/monitor VS, CBC, renal and LFTs, x-rays, eye exam prior to initiating long-term therapy.

4. Observe preterm infants for signs of bleeding.

CLIENT/FAMILY TEACHING

1. Take with a snack, milk, antacid, or meals to decrease GI upset. Report N&V, diarrhea, or constipation.

2. Take the dosage prescribed for best results; report lack of response.

3. May cause dizziness/drowsiness. Perform activities that require mental alertness once evaluated.

4. With history of CHF or compromised cardiac function, keep weight records, and report weight gain/swelling (drug causes sodium retention).

5. Report ringing in ears, blurred vision; obtain periodic eye exams with chronic therapy.

6. Avoid prolonged sun exposure; use protection when exposed.

7. Avoid alcohol, NSAIDS, corticosteroids, and ASA; bleeding may occur.

8. Report as scheduled for follow-up evaluations: ROM, CBC, renal function, x-rays, and stool for blood.

OUTCOMES/EVALUATE

- ↓ Joint pain and ↑ mobility
- ↓ Fever, ↓ Inflammation
- ↓ Dysmenorrhea

Ibutilide fumarate ■ IV
(ih-**BYOU**-tih-lyd)

CLASSIFICATION(S):
Antiarrhythmic
PREGNANCY CATEGORY: C
Rx: Corvert.

USES

Rapid conversion of atrial fibrillation or atrial flutter of recent onset to sinus rhythm. Base determination of clients to receive ibutilide on expected benefits of maintaining sinus rhythm and whether this outweighs both the risks of the drug and of maintenance therapy. Used in post-cardiac surgery clients.

ACTION/KINETICS

Action

Class III antiarrhythmic agent. Delays repolarization by activation of a slow, inward current (mostly sodium), rather than by blocking outward potassium currents (the way other class III antiarrhythmics act). This results in prolongation in the duration of the atrial and ventricular action potential and refractoriness. Also a dose-related prolongation of the QT interval.

Pharmacokinetics

High systemic plasma clearance that approximates liver blood flow. $t^{1}/_{2}$, **terminal:** 6 hr. Over 80% is excreted in the urine (with 7% excreted unchanged) and approximately 20% is excreted through the feces. **Plasma protein binding:** Less than 40%.

CONTRAINDICATIONS

Use of certain class Ia antiarrhythmic drugs (e.g., disopyramide, quinidine, procainamide) and certain class III drugs (e.g., amiodarone and sotalol) concomitantly with ibutilide or within 4 hr of postinfusion.

SPECIAL CONCERNS

■ (1) May cause potentially fatal arrhythmias, especially sustained polymorphic ventricular tachycardia, usually in association with QT prolongation (torsades de pointes). Arrhythmias can be reversed if treated promptly. (2) It is

---

essential that ibutilide be given in a setting of continuous ECG monitoring and by personnel trained in identification and treatment of acute ventricular arrhythmias, especially polymorphic ventricular tachycardia. (3) Clients with atrial fibrillation of more than 2 to 3 days duration must be adequately anticoagulated, usually for at least 2 weeks. (4) Clients with chronic atrial fibrillation have a strong tendency to revert after conversion to sinus rhythm; treatments to maintain sinus rhythm carry risks. Thus, select clients carefully to be treated with ibutilide, so that the expected benefits of maintaining sinus rhythm outweigh the immediate risks and the risks of maintenance therapy are likely to offer an advantage compared with alternative management.■ Effectiveness has not been determined in clients with arrhythmias of more than 90 days duration. Breast feeding should be discouraged during therapy. Safety and efficacy have not been determined in children less than 18 years of age.

SIDE EFFECTS

Most Common

Sustained/nonsustained polymorphic ventricular tachycardia, nonsustained monomorphic ventricular extrasystoles, sinus tachycardia, headache, hypotension, bundle branch block.

CV: *Life-threatening arrhythmias, either sustained or nonsustained polymorphic ventricular tachycardia (torsades de pointes).* Induction/worsening of ventricular arrhythmias. Nonsustained monomorphic ventricular extrasystoles/*ventricular tachycardia,* sinus tachycardia, SVT, hypo-/hypertension, postural hypotension, BBB, AV block, bradycardia, QT-segment prolongation, palpitation, supraventricular extrasystoles, nodal arrhythmia, CHF, *idioventricular rhythm, sustained monomorphic VT.* **Miscellaneous:** Headache, nausea, syncope, renal failure.

OD OVERDOSE MANAGEMENT

Symptoms: Increased ventricular ectopy, monomorphic ventricular tachycardia, AV block, nonsustained polymorphic VT. *Treatment:* Treat symptoms.

DRUG INTERACTIONS

Amiodarone / ↑ Risk of prolonged refractoriness

Antidepressants, tricyclic and tetracyclic / ↑ Risk of proarrhythmias

Digoxin / Supraventricular arrhythmias; ibutilide, may mask cardiotoxicity R/T high digoxin levels

Disopyramide / ↑ Risk of prolonged refractoriness

Histamine H₁ receptor antagonists / ↑ Risk of proarrhythmias

Phenothiazines / ↑ Risk of proarrhythmias

Procainamide / ↑ Risk of prolonged refractoriness

Quinidine / ↑ Risk of prolonged refractoriness

Sotalol / ↑ Risk of prolonged refractoriness

HOW SUPPLIED

IV Solution: Injection 5 mg, 10 mg, 20 mg.

DOSAGE

- **IV INFUSION**

  Atrial fibrillation or atrial flutter of recent onset.

Clients weighing 60 kg or more, initial: 1 mg (one vial) infused over 10 min. **Clients weighing less than 60 kg, initial:** 0.01 mg/kg infused over 10 min. If the arrhythmia does not terminate within 10 min after the end of the initial infusion (regardless of the body weight), a second 10-min infusion of equal strength may be given 10 min after completion of the first infusion.

NURSING CONSIDERATIONS

ADMINISTRATION/STORAGE

IV 1. Anticoagulate clients with atrial fibrillation (>2–3 days duration) for at least 2 weeks.

2. May give undiluted or diluted in 50 mL of 0.9% NaCl or D5W. One vial (1 mg) mixed with 50 mL of diluent forms an admixture of approximately 0.017 mg/mL of ibutilide; administer infusion over 10 min.

3. Either PVC or polyolefin bags are compatible with drug admixtures.

4. Admixtures with approved diluents are chemically and physically stable for

I

---

24 hr at room temperature and for 48 hr if refrigerated.

ASSESSMENT

1. Note onset of arrhythmia, associated symptoms. Those with AF >2–3 days require anticoagulation for at least 2 weeks prior to ibutilide therapy.
2. List drugs prescribed to ensure none interact.
3. Monitor VS, I&O, Mg, electrolytes, ECG.
4. Must be given in a setting with continuous ECG monitoring and by those trained in the identification/treatment of acute ventricular arrhythmias, especially polymorphic VT.
5. Document conversion to NSR (usually within 30–90 min). Stop infusion when arrhythmia terminated or in the event of sustained/nonsustained VT or marked prolongation of QT interval.
6. Observe for at least 4 hr following infusion or until QT interval has returned to baseline. Monitor longer if arrhythmic activity observed.

CLIENT/FAMILY TEACHING

1. Understand reasons for dosing and why new-onset atrial fibrillation should be terminated (to prevent embolus formation).
2. Review benefits and possible adverse side effects. Drug can only be given IV, may experience rapid irregular heart beat, headache, and other arrhythmias. Report any chest pain, SOB, numbness or tingling in extremities.
3. Requires close medical follow-up to determine stability of rhythm.

OUTCOMES/EVALUATE

Conversion of atrial fibrillation to sinus rhythm

Idarubicin hydrochloride

(eye-dah-**ROOB**-ih-sin)

CLASSIFICATION(S):
Antineoplastic, antibiotic
PREGNANCY CATEGORY: D
Rx: Idamycin PFS.

♣Rx: Idamycin.

SEE ALSO *ANTINEOPLASTIC AGENTS.*

USES

In combination with other drugs (often cytarabine) to treat AML in adults, including French-American-British classifications M1–M7. Compared with daunorubicin, idarubicin is more effective in inducing complete remissions in clients with AML.

ACTION/KINETICS

Action

Inhibits nucleic acid synthesis and interacts with the enzyme topoisomerase II. Rapidly taken up into cells due to significant lipid solubility.

Pharmacokinetics

t½ terminal: 22 hr when used alone and 20 hr when used with cytarabine. Metabolized in the liver to the active idarubicinol, which is excreted through both the bile and urine. **Plasma protein binding:** Idarubicin: 97%; Idarubicinol: 94%.

CONTRAINDICATIONS

Lactation. Preexisting bone marrow suppression induced by previous drug therapy or radiotherapy (unless benefit outweighs risk). Administration by the IM or SC routes.

SPECIAL CONCERNS

■ (1) Give idarubicin slowly into a freely flowing IV infusion; never give IM or SC. Severe local tissue necrosis can occur if there is extravasation during administration. (2) Can cause myocardial toxicity leading to CHF. Cardiac toxicity is more common in those who have received prior anthracyclines or who have preexisting heart disease. (3) Severe myelosuppression occurs at therapeutic doses. (4) Give only under the supervision of a physician experienced in leukemia chemotherapy and in facilities with lab and supportive resources adequate to monitor drug tolerance; protect and maintain a client compromised by drug toxicity. The physician and institution must be capable of responding rapidly and completely to severe hemorrhagic conditions or overwhelming infections. (5) Reduce dosage in clients with impaired hepatic or renal function.■ Safety and efficacy have not been demonstrated in children. Skin reactions may occur if the powder is not handled properly. Clients over 60 years of age experienced CHF, serious arrhythmias, chest pain, MI, and asymptomatic declines in LVEF more frequently than younger clients.

SIDE EFFECTS
Most Common
Infection, alopecia, abdominal cramps, diarrhea, hemorrhage, mucositis, changes in mental status, fever, headache.

GI: N&V, mucositis, diarrhea, abdominal pain/cramps, *hemorrhage*. **Hematologic:** *Severe myelosuppression, hemorrhage.* **Dermatologic:** Alopecia, generalized rash, urticaria, bullous erythrodermatous rash of the palms/soles, hives at injection site. **CNS:** Headache, *seizures,* altered mental status. **CV:** CHF, *serious arrhythmias including AF, chest pain, MI, cardiomyopathies,* decreased LV ejection fraction. *NOTE:* Cardiac toxicity more common in clients who received anthracycline drugs previously or who have preexisting cardiac disease. **Miscellaneous:** Altered hepatic/renal function tests, infection (95% of clients), fever, pulmonary allergy, neurologic changes in peripheral nerves, infection, alopecia.

LABORATORY TEST CONSIDERATIONS
Changes in hepatic/renal function tests (usually transient and occurred in those with sepsis and who were receiving potentially hepatotoxic and nephrotoxic antibiotics and antifungal drugs).

OD OVERDOSE MANAGEMENT
Symptoms: Severe GI toxicity, myelosuppression. *Treatment:* Supportive treatment including antibiotics and platelet transfusions. Treat mucositis.

HOW SUPPLIED
Injection: 1 mg/mL.

DOSAGE
• IV
Induction therapy in adults with AML.
12 mg/m²/day for 3 days by slow (10–15 min) IV injection in combination with cytarabine, 100 mg/m²/day given by continuous infusion for 7 days or as a 25-mg/m² IV bolus followed by 200 mg/m²/day for 5 days by continuous infusion. A second course may be given if there is evidence of leukemia after the first course. Delay the second course in those with severe mucositis until recovery occurs; a dosage reduction of 25% is recommended. Consider a dosage reduction in clients with impaired hepatic or renal function; do not give if the bilirubin level is greater than 5 mg/dL.

NURSING CONSIDERATIONS
℘ Do not confuse Idamycin (Idarubicin) with Adriamycin (Doxorubicin HCl)

ADMINISTRATION/STORAGE
IV 1. Reconstitute the 5-, 10-, and 20-mg vials with 5, 10, and 20 mL, respectively, of 0.9% NaCl injection to give a final concentration of 1 mg/mL. Do not use diluents containing bacteriostatic agents.

2. Vial contents under negative pressure. To minimize aerosol formation during reconstitution use care when needle is inserted. Avoid inhalation of any aerosol formed.

3. Give slowly into a freely flowing IV infusion of 0.9% NaCl injection or D5W over 10–15 min. Attach tubing to a butterfly needle or other suitable device and insert into a large vein.

4. If extravasation suspected/evident terminate injection or infusion immediately and restart in another vein. Keep extremity elevated and apply intermittent ice packs over area (immediately for ½ hr, then 4 times per day at one-half hr intervals for 3 days).

5. Do not mix IV solution with any other drugs.

6. Reconstituted solutions are stable for 7 days if refrigerated and 3 days at room temperature. Discard unused solution.

7. If drug comes in contact with skin, wash area thoroughly with soap and water. Use goggles, gloves, and protective gowns to prepare/administer.

ASSESSMENT
1. Note disease onset, other agents trialed, outcome. Drug is given in com-

bination with other drugs (often cytarabine) to treat AML in adults.

2. List any preexisting cardiac disease; assess cardiac status closely.

3. Note previous radiation therapy or treatment with anthracyclines. Assess infusion site carefully.

4. Monitor CBC, platelets, uric acid, renal and LFTs. Reduce dose with impaired hepatic or renal function; hold if bilirubin levels >5 mg/dL.

CLIENT/FAMILY TEACHING

1. Nausea and diarrhea are frequent side effects of therapy; take antiemetic 1 hr before therapy.

2. Hair loss may occur. Urine may become orange-red.

3. Report any SOB or chest pain; may cause myocardial toxicity.

4. Report S&S of anemia, i.e., dyspnea, fatigue, or faintness. Severe myelosuppression may occur; report any abnormal bruising/bleeding or infection.

5. Severe abdominal pains should be reported.

6. Use reliable contraception before, during, and for several months after therapy.

7. Avoid all OTC products without provider approval; avoid vaccinia, crowds and those with infections.

8. Consume high fluid intake; keep urine slightly alkaline to prevent the formation of uric acid stones. Those with gout may require therapy.

OUTCOMES/EVALUATE

- Presence of leukemia cells (second course of therapy may be indicated after hematologic recovery)
- Complete remission; improved hematologic parameters

Ifosfamide ■ IV
(eye-**FOS**-fah-myd)

CLASSIFICATION(S):
Antineoplastic, alkylating
PREGNANCY CATEGORY: D
Rx: Ifex.

SEE ALSO *ANTINEOPLASTIC AGENTS AND ALKYLATING AGENTS.*

USES
As third-line therapy, in combination with other antineoplastic drugs, for germ cell testicular cancer. *Always give with mesna to prevent ifosfamide-induced hemorrhagic cystitis. Investigational:* Cancer of the breast, lung, pancreas, ovary, and stomach. Also for sarcomas, acute leukemias (except AML), malignant lymphomas.

ACTION/KINETICS
Action
Synthetic analog of cyclophosphamide that must be converted in the liver to active metabolites. The alkylated metabolites of ifosfamide then interact with DNA.

Pharmacokinetics
$t\frac{1}{2}$, **elimination:** 7 hr. Excreted in the urine both as unchanged drug and metabolites.

CONTRAINDICATIONS
Severe bone marrow depression. Hypersensitivity to ifosfamide. Lactation.

SPECIAL CONCERNS
■ (1) Urotoxic side effects (especially hemorrhagic cystitis) and CNS toxicities (e.g., confusion and coma) have been associated with ifosfamide. When they occur, cessation of ifosfamide therapy may be required. (2) Severe myelosuppression has occurred.■ Use with caution in clients with compromised bone marrow reserve, impaired renal function, and during lactation. Safety and efficacy have not been established in children. May interfere with wound healing.

SIDE EFFECTS
Most Common
Hematuria, alopecia, myelosuppression, hemorrhagic cystitis, dysuria, urinary frequency, metabolic acidosis, somnolence, confusion, depressive psychosis, hallucinations.

See *Antineoplastic Agents* for a complete list of possible side effects. Also, **GU:** *Hemorrhagic cystitis*, hematuria, dysuria, urinary frequency. **CNS:** Confusion, depressive psychosis, somnolence, hallucinations. Less frequently: Dizziness, disorientation, cranial nerve dysfunction, *seizures, coma.* **GI:** Salivation, stomatitis. **Miscellaneous:** Myelosuppression (especially when given with other chemotherapeutic drugs), metabolic acidosis, alopecia, infection, liver dysfunction, phlebitis, fever of unknown origin, dermatitis, fatigue, hyper-/hypotension, polyneuropathy, pulmonary symptoms, *cardiotoxicity*, interference with normal wound healing.

LABORATORY TEST CONSIDERATIONS
↑ Liver enzymes, bilirubin, BUN, serum creatinine.

OD OVERDOSE MANAGEMENT
Symptoms: See *Side Effects. Treatment:* General supportive measures.

HOW SUPPLIED
Powder for Injection: 1 gram/single-dose vial, 3 grams/single-dose vial.

DOSAGE
• **IV**
  Testicular cancer.
1.2 grams/m^2/day for 5 consecutive days. Treatment may be repeated q 3 weeks or after recovery, if platelet counts are at least 100,000/mm^3 and WBCs are at least 4,000/mm^3.

NURSING CONSIDERATIONS

ADMINISTRATION/STORAGE
IV 1. To prevent bladder toxicity, give with at least 2 L/day of PO or IV fluid as well as with mesna.
2. To reconstitute, add either sterile or bacteriostatic water for injection for a final concentration of 50 mg/mL. Solutions may be further diluted to achieve concentrations from 0.6 to 20 mg/mL by adding D5W, 0.9% NaCl, RL, or sterile water for injection. Infuse slowly over 30 min.
3. Reconstituted solutions (50 mg/mL) are stable for 1 week at 30°C (86°F) or 3 weeks at 5°C (41°F).
4. Refrigerate dilutions of ifosfamide not prepared with bacteriostatic water for injection; use within 6 hr.

ASSESSMENT
1. Note reasons for therapy, other agents/therapies trialed. Anticipate concomitant administration with mesna to minimize hemorrhagic cystitis.
2. Send urine for analysis prior to each dose of ifosfamide. If hematuria occurs (>10 RBCs per HPF) hold therapy until it

clears and adjust dose of mesna as needed.
3. Document neurologic status; assess for hallucinations, agitation, confusion or unusual fatigue; stop infusion if evident.
4. Monitor renal, LFTs, CBC; immunosuppression may activate latent infections such as herpes.

CLIENT/FAMILY TEACHING
1. Antiemetic may be given before therapy to decrease nausea. Give mesna with or before drug therapy to prevent hemorrhagic cystitis.
2. Consume adequate fluids to prevent dehydration and reduce bladder irritation.
3. Hair loss and N&V are frequent side effects of drug therapy.
4. Hyperpigmentation of skin and mucous membranes may occur; report any injury or interference with normal wound healing.
5. Report confusion, hallucinations, or marked drowsiness as dosage may require reduction.
6. Females should practice contraceptive measures during and for at least 4 months following treatments. Infertility may result if treatment lasts 6 months.
7. Report presence of frothy dark urine, jaundice, or light-colored stools; S&S of hepatotoxicity requiring dosage adjustments. Consume 2–3 L/day of fluids and void frequently to lessen irritation.
8. Joint or flank pain may be caused by the increase in uric acid that results from the rapid cytolysis of tumor and RBCs.
9. Report symptoms of neurotoxicity (numbness, tingling). Assess for evidence of infection. Monitor and record temperature daily. Elicit family support in making observations/evaluations and recording.
10. Do not take salicylates or alcohol.
11. Avoid crowds, vaccinations, and persons with known infections.

OUTCOMES/EVALUATE
• ↓ Tumor size and spread
• Desired hematologic parameters

📷 = see color insert   **H** = Herbal   **IV** = Intravenous   @ = sound alike drug

Iloprost inhalational
(**EYE**-loe-prost)

CLASSIFICATION(S):
Vasodilator, prostacyclin analog
PREGNANCY CATEGORY: C
Rx: Ventavis.

USES
Pulmonary arterial hypertension (WHO group I) in those with NYHA class III or IV symptoms. *Investigational:* IV to treat severe Raynaud phenomenon associated with systemic sclerosis.

ACTION/KINETICS
Action
Iloprost is a synthetic analog of prostacyclin PGI$_2$. It dilates systemic and pulmonary arterial beds; it also affects platelet aggregation (relevance to use is unknown).

Pharmacokinetics
Absolute bioavailability of inhaled iloprost is not known. Following inhalation of 5 mcg of iloprost, peak serum levels reached 150 pg/mL. Iloprost is not detectable in plasma 30–60 min after inhalation. **t½:** 20–30 min. Metabolized mainly by beta-oxidation. Excreted in the urine (68%) and feces (12%). **Plasma protein binding:** About 60%.

CONTRAINDICATIONS
Lactation.

SPECIAL CONCERNS
Use caution in selecting the dose for elderly clients; start at the low end of the dosing range due to the greater frequency of decreased hepatic, renal, and cardiac function and other concomitant diseases or drug therapy. Iloprost has not been studied in clients with COPD, severe asthma, or acute pulmonary infections. Use with caution in clients on dialysis and in those with at least Child-Pugh class B hepatic impairment. Safety and efficacy have not been determined in children.

SIDE EFFECTS
Most Common
Flushing, headache, N&V, increased cough, flu syndrome, trismus, syncope, hypotension.

CV: Vasodilation (flushing), hypotension, syncope, palpitations, chest pain/tightness/discomfort, ***CHF,*** supraventricular tachycardia. **CNS:** Headache, insomnia, dizziness (high doses). **GI:** N&V. **Respiratory:** Increased cough, hemoptysis, pneumonia, dyspnea, pulmonary edema. **Miscellaneous:** Flu syndrome, trismus, back/chest pain, muscle cramps, tongue pain, kidney failure, peripheral edema.

LABORATORY TEST CONSIDERATIONS
↑ Alkaline phosphatase, GGT.

OD **OVERDOSE MANAGEMENT**
Symptoms: Extensions of the pharmacologic effects, including diarrhea, flushing, headache, hypotension, N&V. *Treatment:* Interruption of the inhalation session, monitoring, and symptomatic treatment.

DRUG INTERACTIONS
Anticoagulants / Potential for ↑ bleeding R/T inhibition of platelet function by iloprost
Antihypertensive drugs / Potential to ↑ hypotensive effect
Vasodilators / Potential to ↑ hypotensive effect

HOW SUPPLIED
Solution for Inhalation: 10 mcg/mL.

DOSAGE
• **SOLUTION FOR INHALATION**
  Pulmonary arterial hypertension.
First inhaled dose: 2.5 mcg (delivered at the mouthpiece). If this dose is well tolerated, increase the dose to 5 mcg and maintain this dose. The drug is taken 6–9 times per day (no more than q 2 hr) during waking hours, depending on individual need and tolerability. **Maximum daily dose evaluated:** 45 mcg (5 mcg 9 times per day). *NOTE:* If signs of pulmonary edema occur, stop treatment immediately as this may be a sign of pulmonary venous hypotension.

NURSING CONSIDERATIONS
ADMINISTRATION/STORAGE
1. Iloprost is intended for inhalation using only the Prodose AAD system, a pulmonary drug delivery device. To avoid potential interruptions in drug delivery due to equipment failure, client

---

should have easy access to a backup Prodose AAD system.

2. Each inhalation treatment requires 1single-use ampule. Each ampule delivers 20 mcg/2 mL to the medication chamber of the Prodose AAD system and delivers a nominal dose of either 2.5 or 5 mcg to the mouthpiece.

3. For each inhalation session, transfer the entire contents of one opened ampule into the Prodose AAD system medication chamber just before use. After each inhalation session, discard any remaining solution. Using any remaining solution will result in unpredictable dosing. Clean the Prodose AAD system after each dose administration; follow manufacturer's directions for cleaning.

4. Mixing of iloprost with other medications has not been evaluated.

5. Use of iloprost with other treatments for pulmonary hypertension has not been studied. If clients deteriorate while on iloprost, consider alternative treatments (e.g., some clients were helped taking IV epoprostenol).

6. Do not allow iloprost solution to come into contact with skin or eyes; avoid oral ingestion.

7. Store from 15–30°C (59–86°F).

ASSESSMENT

1. Note reasons for therapy, NYHA class, clinical S&S, other agents trialed, outcome.

2. List drugs prescribed to ensure none interact; vasodilators and antihypertensives may increase hypotensive drug effects.

3. Monitor VS, oxygen sats, renal, LFTs. Do not administer if systolic BP <85 mm Hg. Adjust dose as directed for hepatic/renal dysfunction.

CLIENT/FAMILY TEACHING

1. Drug used with the special Prodose AAD system and administered by inhalation. Follow prescribed dose and frequency using the following preparation directions: (a) With one hand, hold the bottom of the ampule with the blue dot facing away from the body. (b) With the other hand, wrap the included rubber pad around the entire ampule. (c) Using thumbs, break open the neck of the ampule by snapping the top away from

the body. (d) Transfer the entire contents of the ampule into the medication chamber of the Prodose AAD system. (e) Safely dispose of the open ampule, out of the reach of children, as instructed by provider. (f) Follow manufacturer's instructions for administration of iloprost dose and maintenance of the system.

2. Inhale drug at intervals of not less than 2 hrs; the acute benefits may not last 2 hrs. Always keep a back up Prodose AAD system in the event of malfunctions.

3. Keep log of BP recordings. Do not administer if systolic BP <85 mm Hg. May experience a fall in BP and become dizzy or faint. Stand up slowly when getting out of bed or chair to prevent these symptoms. If symptoms worsen, alert provider.

4. Avoid skin contact with solution or oral ingestion.

5. Use only the prescribed material in the Prodose AAD system; do not add any other medications to this medication system.

6. May experience facial flushing (due to the dilation of blood vessels), increased cough, headache, nausea, drop in BP, fainting, and spasm of the jaw muscles (may impair opening of mouth); report if persistent or worsen. Any SOB, chest pain, palpitations, change in urinary output or other adverse side effects should be reported immediately.

7. Practice reliable contraception.

8. Keep all F/U appointments to evaluate response to therapy.

OUTCOMES/EVALUATE

- Improved exercise tolerance
- Inhibition of clinical deterioration with pulmonary artery hypertension

Imatinib mesylate
(eh-**MAT**-eh-nib)

CLASSIFICATION(S):
Antineoplastic, miscellaneous
PREGNANCY CATEGORY: D
Rx: Gleevec.

USES

(1) Treatment of adults with relapsed or refractory Philadelphia chromosome-positive (Ph+) acute lymphoblastic leukemia. (2) Treatment of adults with aggressive systemic mastocytosis without the D816V c-Kit mutation or with c-Kit mutation status unknown. (3) Treatment of newly diagnosed adults and children with Ph+ chronic myeloid leukemia (CML) in chronic phase; for the treatment of PH+ CML in blast crisis, accelerated phase, or in chronic phase after failure of interferon alpha therapy; for the treatment of children with Ph+ chronic phase CML whose disease has recurred after stem-cell transplant or who are resistant to interferon alpha therapy. (4) Treatment of adults with unresectable, recurrent, and/or metastatic dermatofibrosarcoma protuberans. (5) Treatment of Kit (CD117) positive unresectable and/or metastatic malignant GI stromal tumors. (6) Treatment of adults with hypereosinophilic syndrome and/or chronic eosinophilic leukemia who have the FIP1L1-platelet derived growth factor receptor (PDGFR)α fusion kinase and for those with hypereosinophilic syndrome and/or chronic eosinophilic leukemia who are FIP1L1-PDGFRα fusion kinase negative or unknown. (7) Treatment of adults with myelodysplastic/myeloproliferative diseases associated with PDGFR gene rearrangements.

ACTION/KINETICS

Action

Imatinib is a protein-tyrosine kinase inhibitor that inhibits the Bcr-Abl tyrosine kinase which is the abnormal form of tyrosine kinase created by the Philadelphia chromosome abnormality in chronic myeloid leukemia (CML). Imatinib inhibits proliferation and causes apoptosis in Bcr-Abl positive cell lines, as well as fresh leukemic cells from Philadelphia chromosome positive CML. The drug may also inhibit receptor tyrosine kinases for platelet-derived growth factor and stem cell factor, c-Kit; inhibits platelet-derived growth factor and stem cell factor cellular events.

Pharmacokinetics

Well absorbed after PO administration; mean absolute bioavailability is 98%. **Maximum levels: 2–4 hr. t½, terminal, imatinib and N-desmethyl derivative (active metabolite):** About 18 and 40 hr, respectively. Metabolized in the liver by the CYP3A4 enzyme with 68% excreted in the feces and 18% in the urine.

CONTRAINDICATIONS

Hypersensitivity to any component of the product. Lactation.

SPECIAL CONCERNS

Safety and efficacy have been determined only in children with Ph+ chronic phase CML with recurrence after stem cell transplantation or resistance to interferon-alfa therapy. There are no data in children younger than 2 years.

SIDE EFFECTS

Most Common

N&V, fluid retention, superficial edema, hemorrhage, pyrexia, diarrhea, musculoskeletal pain, abdominal pain, fatigue, arthralgia, myalgia, joint pain, muscle cramps.

Side effects listed are either those with a frequency of 0.1% or more or those that are potentially serious. **GI:** N&V, diarrhea, GI irritation, *GI/tumor hemorrhage*, dyspepsia, abdominal pain/distention, constipation, taste disturbance, flatulence, hepatotoxicity (may be severe), hepatitis, gastroesophageal reflux, mouth ulceration, gastric ulcer, gastritis, gastroenteritis, loose stools. **CNS:** Headache, dizziness, insomnia, anxiety, *CNS hemorrhage, cerebral edema, increased intracranial pressure*, paresthesia, depression, impaired memory, migraine, peripheral neuropathy, somnolence, syncope. **CV:** Pericardial effusion, *grade 3/4 hemorrhage (tumor, cerebral, GI tract), cardiac failure*, CHF, left ventricular dysfunction, flushing, hyper-/hypotension, peripheral coldness, tachycardia, hypereosinophilic cardiac toxicity. **Musculoskeletal:** Musculoskeletal/back pain, muscle cramps, arthralgia, myalgia, joint pain/swelling, joint/muscle stiffness, sciatica. **Dermatologic:** Skin rash, pruritus, night sweats, petechiae, ecchymosis, alopecia, dry skin, bullous eruption, exfoliative dermatitis, nail disorder, photosensitivity reaction, psoriasis, purpura, skin pigmentaion changes, erythema multiforme, **Stevens-Johnson syndrome**. **Respiratory:** Cough, dyspnea, pneumonia, epistaxis, nasopharyngitis, pharyngitis, sinusitis, URTI, sore throat, chest pain, pleural effusion, pulmonary edema, pharynlaryngeal pain. **Hematologic:** Neutropenia, thrombocytopenia, anemia, pancytopenia. **GU:** Breast enlargement, hematuria, menorrhagia, sexual dysfunction, urinary frequency, renal failure. **Ophthalmic:** Increased lacrimation, edema of the optic disk, conjunctivitis, blurred vision, conjunctival hemorrhage, dry eye, periorbital edema. **Body as a whole:** Edema, dehydration, gout, decreased/increased weight, fluid retention, superficial edema, ascites, fatigue, asthenia, influenza, rigors, pyrexia, weakness, rapid weight gain with or without superficial edema, ascites, facial edema, **sepsis**. **Miscellaneous:** Anasarca, anorexia, appetite disturbances, tinnitus, vertigo, herpes simplex/zoster, hypokalema.

LABORATORY TEST CONSIDERATIONS
↑ AST, ALT, bilirubin, creatinine, alkaline phosphatase, blood creatine phosphokinase, blood lactate dehydrogenase, albumin. Hypophosphatemia.

DRUG INTERACTIONS
Acetaminophen / ↑ Risk of hepatotoxicity

Benzodiazepines (certain ones) / ↑ Benzodiazepine levels R/T ↓ metabolism by CYP3A4

Calcium channel blockers (dihydropyridine-type) / ↑ CCB levels R/T ↓ metabolism by CYP3A4

Carbamazepine / ↓ Imatinib levels R/T ↑ metabolism by CYP3A4

Clarithromycin / ↑ Imatinib levels R/T ↓ metabolism by CYP3A4

Cyclosporine / Use with caution with CYP3A4 substrates that have a narrow therapeutic margin

Dexamethasone / ↓ Imatinib levels R/T ↑ metabolism by CYP3A4

Dihydropyridine / ↑ Dihydropyridine levels R/T ↓ metabolism by CYP3A4

Erythromycin / ↑ Imatinib levels R/T ↓ metabolism by CYP3A4

Erythromycin / ↑ Imatinib levels R/T ↓ metabolism by CYP3A4

Ethinyl estradiol / ↑ Ethinyl estradiol levels R/T ↓ metabolism by CYP3A4

Itraconazole / ↑ Imatinib levels R/T ↓ metabolism by CYP3A4

Ketoconazole / ↑ Imatinib levels R/T ↓ metabolism by CYP3A4

Levothyroxine / Symptoms of hypothyroidism and ↑ TSH levels after undergoing thyroidectomy; ↑ levothyroxine dose

Oral contraceptives / ↑ OC levels R/T ↓ metabolism by CYP3A4

Phenobarbital / ↓ Imatinib levels R/T ↑ metabolism by CYP3A4

Phenytoin / ↓ Imatinib levels R/T ↑ metabolism by CYP3A4

Pimozide / Use with caution with CYP3A4 substrates that have a narrow therapeutic margin

Rifampicin / ↓ Imatinib levels R/T ↑ metabolism

Rifampin / ↓ Imatinib peak levels and AUC R/T ↑ metabolism by CYP3A4

Simvastastin / ↑ Simvastatin AUC and maximum concentration R/T ↓ metabolism by CYP3A4

H *St. John's wort* / ↓ Imatinib levels R/T ↑ metabolism by CYP3A4

Triazolobenzodiazepines / ↑ Triazolobenzodiazepine levels

Warfarin / Possible ↑ warfarin effect R/T ↓ metabolism by CYP2C9 and CYP3A4; use low molecular weight heparins or standard heparin

HOW SUPPLIED
Tablets: 100 mg (as base), 400 mg (as base).

DOSAGE
• **TABLETS**

Chronic myeloid leukemia in adults. 400 mg/day for those in chronic phase of CML and 600 mg/day for those in accelerated phase or blast crisis. Increases in dose from 400 mg to 600 mg may be considered in those with chronic phase disease or from 600 mg to 800 mg (400 mg twice a day) in those with accelerated phase or blast crisis if there are no severe side effects, severe non-leukemia-related neutropenia, or thrombocytopenia in the following situ-

---

ations: Disease progression, failure to achieve a satisfactory hematologic response after 3 or more months of treatment, or loss of a previously achieved hematologic response.

CML in chronic phase in children.

Children, newly diagnosed Ph+ CML: 340 mg/m^2/day (not to exceed 600 mg). **Children with Ph+ chronic phase CML recurrent after stem-cell transplant or resistant to interferon alpha:** 260 mg/m^2/day given either once daily or split into two daily doses.

Gastrointestinal stromal tumors.

Adults: 400 or 600 mg/day.

Acute lymphoblastic leukemia.

Adults: 600 mg/day in those with relapsed/refractory Ph+ acute lymphoblastic leukemia.

Aggressive systemic mastocytosis.

Adults: 400 mg/day in those without the D816V c-kit mutation. For those with aggressive systemic mastocytosis associated with eosinophilia, begin with 100 mg/day. May increase the dose from 100 to 400 mg/day in the absence of adverse side effects if assessment shows an insufficient response to therapy.

Dermatofibrosarcoma protuberans.

Adults: 800 mg/day.

Hypereosinophilic syndrome and/or chronic eosinophilic leukemia.

Adults: 400 mg/day. In those with demonstrated FIP1L1-PDGFRα fusion kinase, give a starting dose of 100 mg/day. Dose may be increased from 100 mg/day to 400 mg/day in the absence of side effects if assessments show an insufficient response to therapy.

Myelodysplastic/myeloproliferative diseases.

Adults: 400 mg/day.

NURSING CONSIDERATIONS

ADMINISTRATION/STORAGE

1. Therapy should be initiated by a health care provider experienced in the treatment of those with hematological malignancies or malignant sarcomas.
2. Start with a dose of 400 mg/day in those with mild to moderate impaired hepatic function. Start with a dose of 300 mg/day in those with severe hepatic impairment.
3. Increase imatinib dose by at least 50% and monitor carefully in clients receiving imatinib with a potent CYP3A4 inducer (e.g., phenytoin, rifampin).
4. For daily dosing of 800 mg or more, use the 400 mg tablet to reduce exposure to iron.
5. If severe hepatotoxicity or fluid retention occurs, withhold imatinib until event resolved. Treatment can be resumed depending on the initial severity of the event.
6. If elevations in bilirubin >3 times IULN or in liver transaminases >5 IULN occur, withhold imatinib until bilirubin levels have returned to <1.5 times IULN and transaminase levels to <2.5 times IULN. Treatment with imatinib may be continued at a reduced daily dose (400 mg reduced to 300 mg or 600 mg reduced to 400 mg).
7. Use the following guidelines to adjust dose for neutropenia and thrombocytopenia:

- **For chronic phase CML (starting dose 400 mg), myelodysplastic/myeloproliferative diseases (starting dose 400 mg), or GI stromal tumors (starting dose either 400 or 600 mg):** If ANC is <1 x 10^9/L and/or platelets are <50 x 10^9/L, stop imatinib until ANC is 1.5 or more x 10^9/L and platelets are 75 or more x 10^9/L. Resume treatment at the original starting dose of 400 mg or 600 mg. If recurrence of ANC and/or platelets occur at levels indicated above, withhold until levels return to those indicated above and resume at reduced dose (300 mg if the starting dose was 400 mg and 400 mg if the starting dose was 600 mg)

- **For accelerated phase of CML and blast crisis (starting dose 600 mg) and relapsed or refractory Philadelphia chromosome-positive acute ALL (starting dose 600 mg):** If ANC is <0.5 x 10^9/L and/or platelets are <10 x 10^9/L, check if cytopenia is related to leukemia. If cytopenia unrelated to leukemia, reduce dose of imatinib to 400 mg. If cytopenia persists 2 weeks, reduce further to 300 mg. If cytopenia persists 4 weeks and is still unrelated to leukemia, stop imatinib until ANC is 1 or more x 10^9/L and platelets are 20 or more x 10^9/L and resume treatment at 300 mg.

- **Aggressive systemic mastocytosis associated with eosinophilia (starting dose 100 mg):** If ANC is <1 x 10^9/L and/or platelets <50 x 10^9/L, stop imatinib until ANC is 1.5 x 10^9/L or more and platelets are 75 x 10^9/L or more. Resume treatment with imatinib at previous dose (i.e., before severe side effects).

- **Hypereosinophilic syndrome with FIP1L1-PDGFRα fusion kinase (starting dose 100 mg):** If ANC is <1 x 10^9/L and/or platelets <50 x 10^9/L, stop imatinib until ANC is 1.5 x 10^9/L or more and platelets are 75 x 10^9/L or more. Resume treatment with imatinib at previous dose (i.e., before severe side effects).

- **Dermatofibrosarcoma protuberans (starting dose 800 mg):** If ANC is <1 x 10^9/L or platelets <50 x 10^9/L, stop imatinib until ANC is 1.5 x 10^9/L or more and platelets are 75 x 10^9/L or more. Resume treatment with imatinib at 600 mg. In the event of recurrence of ANC <1 x 10^9/L and/or platelets <50 x 10^9/L, repeat the previous step and resume imatinib at reduced dose of 400 mg.

- **Newly diagnosed pediatric chronic CML (start at dose 340 mg/m²):** If ANC is <1 x 10^9/L and/or platelets <50 x 10^9/L, stop imatinib until ANC is 1.5 x 10^9/L or more and platelets are 75 x 10^9/L or more. Resume treatment with imatinib at previous dose (i.e., before serious side effects). In the event of recurrence of ANC <1 x 10^9/L and/or platelets <50 x 10^9/L, repeat the previous step and resume imatinib at reduced dose of 250 mg/m².

- **Children with chronic phase CML recurring after transplant or resistant to interferon (start at dose 260 mg/m²):** If ANC is <1 x 10^9/L and/or platelets <50 x 10^9/L, stop im-

atinib until ANC is 1.5 x 10^9/L or more and platelets are 75 x 10^9/L or more. Resume treatment with imatinib at previous dose (i.e., before severe side effects). In the event of recurrence of ANC <1 x 10^9/L and/or platelets <50 x 10^9/L, repeat the previous step and resume imatinib at reduced dose of 200 mg/m².

ASSESSMENT

1. Note reasons for therapy, disease onset, phase of disease, other therapies trialed/failed, last interferon-alpha therapy.

2. List drugs prescribed to ensure none interact unfavorably.

3. Closely monitor those with hepatic impairment; exposure to imatinib may increase liver dysfunction.

4. Monitor VS, weight, CBC, renal and LFTs.

5. Follow administration guidelines carefully; dose is adjusted for various phases of disease, types of disease, as well as altered renal/liver function, neutropenia/thrombocytopenia.

CLIENT/FAMILY TEACHING

1. Take with food and a large glass of water to minimize GI irritation.

2. Drug is given once daily initially; may be increased to twice daily.

3. Monitor weight; report any significant increases/decreases.

4. Avoid OTC agents especially with acetaminophen unless provider approved.

5. Women of childbearing age should avoid pregnancy during therapy.

6. May experience N&V, diarrhea, swelling of extremities/around the eyes, skin rash, muscle cramps. May also experience increased SOB, changes in urinary output, ↑ bruising/bleeding, and ↓ exercise intolerance. Report any of these symptoms.

7. Keep all F/U visits so drug may be adjusted as needed and labs monitored for neutropenia/thrombocytopenia or liver/renal toxicity.

OUTCOMES/EVALUATE

- Hematologic stabilization of CML
- Control of malignant cell proliferation with metastatic GI stromal tumors

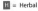

——COMBINATION DRUG——

Imipenem-Cilastatin IV sodium

(em-ee-**PEN**-em, sigh-lah-**STAT**-in)

CLASSIFICATION(S):
Antibiotic, carbapenem
PREGNANCY CATEGORY: C
Rx: Primaxin I.M., Primaxin I.V.

SEE ALSO *ANTI-INFECTIVE DRUGS*.

USES

IV: (1) Lower respiratory tract infections due to *Staphylococcus aureus* (penicillinase-producing), *Escherichia coli*, *Klebsiella* sp., *Enterobacter* sp., *Haemophilus influenzae*, *Haemophilus parainfluenzae*, *Acinetobacter* sp., and *Serratia marcescens*. (2) Urinary tract infections (complicated and uncomplicated) due to *Enterococcus faecalis*, *S. aureus* (penicillinase-producing), *E. coli*, *Klebsiella* sp., *Enterobacter* sp., *Proteus vulgaris*, *Providencia rettgeri*, *M. morganii*, and *P. aeruginosa*. (3) Intra-abdominal infections due to *E. faecalis*, *S. aureus* (penicillinase-producing), *Staphylococcus epidermidis*, *E. coli*, *Klebsiella* sp., *Enterobacter* sp., *Proteus* sp., *Morganella morganii*, *P. aeruginosa*, *Citrobacter* sp., *Clostridium* sp., *Bacteroides* sp., including *B. fragilis*, *Fusobacterium* sp., *Peptococcus* sp., *Peptostreptococcus* sp., *Eubacterium* sp., *Propionibacterium* sp., and *Bifidobacterium* sp. (4) Gynecologic infections due to *E. faecalis*, *S. aureus* (penicillinase-producing), *S. epidermidis*, *Streptococcus agalactiae* (group B streptococcus), *E. coli*, *Klebsiella* sp., *Proteus* sp., *Enterobacter* sp., *Bifidobacterium* sp., *Bacteroides* sp., including *B. fragilis*, *Gardnerella vaginalis*, *Peptococcus* sp., *Peptostreptococcus* sp., *Propionibacterium* sp. (5) Bacterial septicemia due to *E. faecalis*, *S. aureus* (penicillinase-producing), *E. coli*, *Klebsiella* sp., *P. aeruginosa*, *Serratia* sp., *Enterobacter* sp., *Bacteroides* sp. (6) Bone and joint infections due to *E. faecalis*, *S. aureus* (penicillinase-producing), *S. epidermidis*, *Enterobacter* sp., *P. aeruginosa*.

(7) Skin and skin structure infections due to *E. faecalis*, *S. aureus* (penicillinase-producing), *S. epidermidis*, *E. coli*, *Klebsiella* sp., *Enterobacter* sp., *P. vulgaris*, *P. rettgeri*, *M. morganii*, *P. aeruginosa*, *Serratia* sp., *Citrobacter* sp., *Acinetobacter* sp., *Bacteroides* sp., *Fusobacterium* sp., *Peptococcus* sp., and *Peptostreptococcus* sp. (8) Endocarditis due to *S. aureus* (penicillinase-producing). (9) Polymicrobic infections, including those in which *S. pneumoniae* (pneumonia, septicemia), *S. pyogenes* (skin and skin structure), or nonpenicillinase-producing *S. aureus* is one of the causative organisms.

IM: (1) Lower respiratory tract infections, including pneumonia and bronchitis as an exacerbation of COPD due to *S. pneumoniae* and *H. influenzae*. (2) Intra-abdominal infections including acute gangrenous or perforated appendicitis and appendicitis with peritonitis that are caused by group *Streptococcus*, including *E. faecalis*, streptococcus (viridans group), *E. coli*, *Klebsiella pneumoniae*, *P. aeruginosa*, *Bacteroides* sp., including *B. fragilis*, *B. distasonis*, *B. intermedius*, *B. thetaiotaomicron*, *Fusobacterium* sp., and *Peptostreptococcus* sp. (3) Skin and skin structure infections, including abscesses, cellulitis, infected skin ulcers, and wound infections due to *S. aureus* (including penicillinase-producing strains), *Streptococcus pyogenes*, group D streptococcus including *E. faecalis*, *Acinetobacter* sp., including *A. calcoaceticus*, *Citrobacter* sp., *E. coli*, *Enterobacter cloacae*, *K. pneumoniae*, *P. aeruginosa*, *Bacteroides* sp., including *B. fragilis*. (4) Gynecologic infections, including postpartum endomyometritis due to group D streptococcus such as *E. faecalis*, *E. coli.*, *K. pneumoniae*, *B. intermedius*, and *Peptostreptococcus* sp. NOTE: IM use is not intended for severe or life-threatening infections, including bacterial sepsis or endocarditis, or in major physiological impairments (e.g., shock).

CONTENT

The powder for IM injection contains: Imipenem, 500 mg, and cilastatin, 500 mg, or imipenem, 750 mg, and cilastatin, 750 mg. The powder for IV injection

---

contains: Imipenem, 250 mg, and cilastatin, 250 mg, or imipenem, 500 mg, and cilastatin, 500 mg.

ACTION/KINETICS

Action

Inhibits cell wall synthesis. Is bactericidal against a wide range of gram-positive and gram-negative organisms. Stable in the presence of beta-lactamases. Addition of cilastatin prevents the metabolism of imipenem in the kidneys by dehydropeptidase I, thus ensuring high levels of the imipenem in the urinary tract.

Pharmacokinetics

$t\frac{1}{2}$, **after IV:** 1 hr for each component. **Peak plasma levels of imipenem, after 20 min IV infusion:** 14–24 mcg/mL for the 250-mg dose, 21–58 mcg/mL for the 500-mg dose, and 41–83 mcg/mL for the 1-gram dose. **Peak plasma levels, after IM:** 10–12 mcg/mL within 2 hr. Compared with IV administration, imipenem is approximately 75% bioavailable after IM use with cilastatin being 95% bioavailable. $t\frac{1}{2}$, **imipenem:** 2–3 hr. About 70% of imipenem and cilastatin is recovered in the urine within 10 hr of administration.

CONTRAINDICATIONS

IM use in clients allergic to local anesthetics of the amide type and use in clients with heart block (due to use of lidocaine HCl diluent) or severe shock. Use in clients with a C_{CR} of less than or equal to 5 mL/min/1.73 m^2, unless hemodialysis is begun within 48 hr. IV use in children with CNS infections due to the risk of seizures and in children less than 30 kg with impaired renal function.

SPECIAL CONCERNS

Use with caution in pregnancy and lactation. Due to cross sensitivity, use with caution in clients with penicillin allergy. Safety and effectiveness have not been determined for IM use in children less than 12 years of age.

SIDE EFFECTS

Most Common

After IM use: Pain at injection site, nausea, diarrhea, rash, vomiting.
After IV use: Hypotension, phlebitis/thrombophlebitis, pain, erythema at injection site, N&V, diarrhea, fever, seizures, dizziness, rash, pruritus.

GI: Pseudomembranous colitis, nausea, diarrhea, vomiting, abdominal pain, heartburn, increased salivation, *hemorrhagic colitis*, gastroenteritis, glossitis, pharyngeal pain, tongue papillar hypertrophy, hepatitis, jaundice, staining of the teeth or tongue. **CNS:** Fever, confusion, *seizures*, dizziness, sleepiness, myoclonus, headache, vertigo, paresthesia, encephalopathy, tremor, psychic disturbances (including hallucinations). **CV:** Hypotension, tachycardia, palpitations. **Dermatologic:** Rash, urticaria, pruritus, flushing, cyanosis, facial edema, erythema multiforme, skin texture changes, hyperhidrosis, angioneurotic edema, *toxic epidermal necrolysis, Stevens-Johnson syndrome*. **CV:** Hypotension, palpitations, tachycardia. **Respiratory:** Chest discomfort, dyspnea, hyperventilation. **GU:** Pruritus vulvae, anuria/oliguria, acute renal failure, polyuria, urine discoloration. **Hematologic:** Pancytopenia, bone marrow depression, thrombocytopenia, neutropenia, leukopenia, hemolytic anemia. **Miscellaneous:** Candidiasis, superinfection, tinnitus, polyarthralgia, asthenia, muscle weakness, transient hearing loss in clients with existing hearing impairment, taste perversion, thoracic spine pain. **Children, 3 months and older:** Diarrhea, rash, phlebitis, gastroenteritis, vomiting, IV site irritation, urine discoloration. **Children, newborn to 3 months:** Convulsions, diarrhea, oliguria, anuria, oral candidiasis, rash, tachycardia. **The following side effects may occur at the injection site:** Thrombophlebitis, phlebitis, pain, erythema, vein induration, infused vein infection.

LABORATORY TEST CONSIDERATIONS

IV: ↑ AST, ALT, alkaline phosphatase, bilirubin, LDH, BUN, creatinine, eosinophils, monocytes, lymphocytes, basophils, potassium, chloride. ↓ Neutrophils, hemoglobin, hematocrit. ↑ or ↓ WBCs, platelets. Positive Coombs' test and abnormal PT. Presence of protein, RBCs, WBCs, casts, bilirubin, or urobilinogen in the urine.

IM: ↑ AST, ALT, alkaline phosphatase, bilirubin, BUN, creatinine, PT. ↓ Hemoglobin, hematocrit, erythrocytes. ↑ or ↓ WBCs and platelets. Presence of RBCs, WBCs, casts, and bacteria in urine.

DRUG INTERACTIONS

Cyclosporine / ↑ CNS side effects of both drugs
Ganciclovir / ↑ Risk of generalized seizures
Probenecid / ↑ Imipenem levels and half-life; do not use together

HOW SUPPLIED

See Content.

DOSAGE

- **IV**

  Fully susceptible gram-positive organisms, gram-negative organisms, anaerobes.

Mild: 250 mg q 6 hr (total daily dose: 1 gram); **moderate:** 500 mg q 6 hr or q 8 hr (total daily dose: 1.5 or 2 grams); **severe/life-threatening:** 500 mg q 6 hr (total daily dose: 2 grams).

  Urinary tract infections due to fully susceptible organisms.

Uncomplicated: 250 mg q 6 hr (total daily dose: 1 gram); **complicated:** 500 mg q 6 hr (total daily dose: 2 grams).

  Moderately susceptible organisms (especially some strains of P. aeruginosa).

Mild: 500 mg q 6 hr (total daily dose: 2 grams); **moderate,** 500 mg q 6 hr to 1 gram q 6 hr (total daily dose: 2 or 3 grams); **severe/life-threatening,** 1 gram q 6 or 8 hr (total daily dose: 3 or 4 grams).

  Urinary tract infections due to moderately susceptible organisms.

Uncomplicated: 250 mg q 6 hr (total daily dose: 1 gram); **complicated:** 500 mg q 6 hr (total daily dose: 2 grams).

  Pediatric, non-CNS infections.

Children, 3 months of age or older: 15–25 mg/kg/dose q 6 hr, up to a maximum dose of 2 grams/day for treating infections with fully susceptible organisms and up to a maximum of 4 grams/day for infections with moderately susceptible organisms. Doses as high as 90 mg/kg/day have been used in older children with cystic fibrosis. **Children, three months of age or less (weighing 1,500 grams or more):** Less than 1 week of age, 25 mg/kg q 12 hr; 1–4 weeks of age, 25 mg/kg q 8 hr; 4 weeks to 3 months of age, 25 mg/kg q 6 hr. Give doses less than or equal to 500 mg by IV infusion over 15 to 20 min; give doses greater than 500 mg by IV infusion over 40 to 60 min. *NOTE:* IV use is not recommended for children with CNS infections due to the risk of seizures and in children <30 kg with impaired renal function as no data are available.

- **IM**

  Mild to moderate lower respiratory tract, skin and skin structure, or gynecologic infections.

500 or 750 mg q 12 hr depending on severity.

  Mild to moderate intra-abdominal infections.

Adults: 750 mg q 12 hr. The total daily dose should not exceed 1.5 grams. **Children:** 10–15 mg/kg q 6 hr for all uses.

NURSING CONSIDERATIONS

ADMINISTRATION/STORAGE

1. When used IM, give in large muscle mass (e.g., gluteal muscles or lateral part of the thigh) with a 21-gauge 2-in. needle.
2. Total daily IM doses >1,500 mg/day are not recommended.
3. For IM use, prepare with 1% lidocaine HCl solution without epinephrine. Prepare the 500 mg vial with 2 mL and the 750 mg vial with 3 mL of lidocaine HCl. Use reconstituted IM solutions within 1 hr of preparation.
4. Continue IM use for at least 2 days after S&S of infection are absent. Safety and effectiveness have not been established for use more than 14 days.
5. Reduce dosage with a C_{CR} of 70 mL/min/1.73 m² or less. Check package insert for dosage information.
6. Reconstitute for IV use by mixing with 100 mL of diluent.
7. Base initial dose on the type and severity of infection. Give doses of 125 mg, 250 mg, and 500 mg by IV infusion over 20–30 min. Give doses of 750 mg or 1 gram by IV infusion over 40–60

min. If nausea develops, decrease infusion rate. Do not exceed more than 50 mg/kg/day or 4 grams/day, whichever is lower as there is no evidence higher doses provide greater efficacy.

8. The following solutions can be used as diluents: 0.9% NaCl, D5/W or D10/W, D5/0.9% NaCl, D5W% with either 0.225% or 0.45% saline solution, D5/W with 0.15% KCl solution, or mannitol (2.5%, 5%, or 10%).

9. Reconstituted IV solutions vary from colorless to yellow while reconstituted IM solutions vary from white to light tan in color. Color variations do not affect potency.

10. Do not mix with other antibiotics; however, may be administered with other antibiotics, if necessary.

11. Most reconstituted IV solutions can be stored at room temperature for 4 hr and, if refrigerated, for 24 hr. The exception is imipenem-cilastatin reconstituted with 0.9% NaCl solution, which is stable at room temperature for 10 hr and, if refrigerated, for 48 hr.

ASSESSMENT

1. Note reasons for therapy, onset, duration, characteristics of S&S. Check CBC, cultures.

2. Do not use in clients allergic to local anesthetics of the amide type or with heart block (due to the use of lidocaine HCl diluent) or severe shock. Use cautiously with penicillin, beta-lactams or cephalosporin allergy. Assess for seizure history. The cilastatin component prevents renal metabolism of imipenem.

3. Monitor renal function; avoid if C_{CR} is less than or equal to 5 mL/min/1.73 m^2, unless hemodialysis is begun within 48 hr. See administration guidelines.

4. Avoid IV use in children with CNS infections R/T risk of seizures and in children <30 kg with impaired renal function.

5. Assess IV site for phlebitis, pain, erythema.

CLIENT/FAMILY TEACHING

1. Drug is used to kill organisms that cause infection. May experience pain at injection site.

2. Report any unusual or persistent adverse side effects or lack of response.

OUTCOMES/EVALUATE

- Resolution of infection
- Symptomatic improvement

Imipramine hydrochloride ■ ⓒ

(im-**IHP**-rah-meen)

CLASSIFICATION(S):
Antidepressant, tricyclic
PREGNANCY CATEGORY: B
Rx: Tofranil.
✤Rx: Apo-Imipramine.

Imipramine pamoate
PREGNANCY CATEGORY: B
Rx: Tofranil-PM.

SEE ALSO *ANTIDEPRESSANTS, TRICYCLIC*.

USES
(1) Symptoms of depression; endogenous depression is more likely to be helped. (2) Enuresis in children 6 years or older.

ACTION/KINETICS

Action
Moderate anticholinergic and sedative effects; high orthostatic hypotensive effects. Biotransformed into its active metabolite, desmethylimipramine (desipramine).

Pharmacokinetics
Effective plasma level of imipramine and desmethylimipramine: 200–350 ng/mL. t½: 11–25 hr. **Time to reach steady state:** 2–5 days.

SPECIAL CONCERNS
■ (1) Antidepressants increase the risk of suicidal thinking and behavior (suicidality) in short-term studies in children and adolescents with major depressive disorders and other psychiatric disorders. Anyone considering the use of imipramine or any other antidepressant in a child or adolescent must balance this risk with the clinical need. Clients who are started on therapy should be observed closely for clinical worsening, suicidality, or unusual changes in be-

havior. Families and caregivers should be advised of the need for close observation and communication with the prescriber. Imipramine and imipramine pamoate are not approved for use in pediatric clients. (2) Analysis of short-term (4–16 weeks) placebo-controlled trials in children and adolescents with major depressive disorder, obsessive-compulsive disorder, or other psychiatric disorders have revealed a greater risk of adverse reactions representing suicidal thinking or behavior during the first few months of treatment in those receiving antidepressants. The average risk of such reactions in such clients receiving antidepressants was 4%, twice the placebo risk of 2%. No suicides occurred in these trials.■ Elderly and adolescent clients may have low tolerance to the drug.

SIDE EFFECTS
Most Common

Dry mouth, blurred vision, headache, drowsiness, dizziness, constipation, N&V, anorexia, diarrhea, stomach cramps, weight gain/loss, increased sweating.

See *Antidepressants, Tricyclic* for a complete list of possible side effects. Also, increased frequency of *seizures* in epileptics and *seizures* in nonepileptics following high doses.

ADDITIONAL DRUG INTERACTIONS

Smoking / ↓ Imipramine levels R/T ↑ hepatic metabolism

H St. John's wort / Possible ↓ imipramine levels R/T ↑ metabolism

LABORATORY TEST CONSIDERATIONS

↑ Metanephrine (Pisano test); ↓ urinary 5-HIAA.

HOW SUPPLIED

Imipramine hydrochloride: *Tablets:* 10 mg, 25 mg, 50 mg.
Imipramine pamoate: *Capsules:* 75 mg, 100 mg, 125 mg, 150 mg.

DOSAGE
- **CAPSULES; TABLETS**
  Depression.

Hospitalized clients, initial: 100–150 mg/day; may be increased to 200 mg/day. Can be increased by 25 mg every few days up to 200 mg/day. After 2 weeks, dosage may be increased gradually to maximum of 250–300 mg/day at bedtime. **Outpatients, initial:** 75 mg/day, increased to 150 mg/day. Maximum dose for outpatients is 200 mg/day. Decrease when feasible to maintenance dosage: 75–150 mg/day at bedtime. **Adolescent and geriatric clients, initial:** 25–50 mg/day up to maximum of 100 mg/day. Use the pamoate capsules when the total daily dose is established at 75 mg or more. The total daily maintenance dose may be given on a once-a-day basis, preferably at bedtime.
  Childhood enuresis.

Age 6 years and over: 25 mg/day 1 hr before bedtime. If satisfactory effect is not seen in 1 week, increase dose to 50 mg/day up to 12 years of age and to 75 mg/day in children over 12 years of age. Dose should not exceed 2.5 mg/kg/day. *NOTE:* Use tablets for treating childhood enuresis.

NURSING CONSIDERATIONS

Ⓒ Do not confuse Imipramine with Desipramine (Norpramin) also an antidepressant.

ADMINISTRATION/STORAGE

1. Total daily dose can be given once daily at bedtime.
2. In early night bed wetters, the drug may be more effective if given in doses of 25 mg in midafternoon and 25 mg at bedtime.
3. Children who relapse after discontinuing the drug may not respond to a subsequent course. Gradually tapering the dose may decrease tendency to relapse.

ASSESSMENT

1. Note reasons for therapy, behavioral presentation, characteristics of S&S, other agents trialed.
2. Obtain baseline EKG; monitor during therapy. May cause prolonged PR and Q-T intervals.
3. Monitor VS, CBC, renal and LFTs.

CLIENT/FAMILY TEACHING

1. Review appropriate times and methods for administration depending on condition being treated.
2. May take with food or milk if GI upset.

3. Take dose at bedtime to prevent daytime sedation. May experience drop in BP upon arising; use caution.

4. Report any increase in frequency of seizures in epileptics; any occurrence of seizures in nonepileptics.

5. Children may experience mild N&V, unusual tiredness, nervousness, or insomnia; report if pronounced.

6. Avoid prolonged exposure to sunlight; wear protective clothing if exposed; may cause photosensitivity reaction.

7. Avoid alcohol, smoking, and OTC meds during therapy without approval.

8. Do not perform activities that require mental alertness until drug effects realized; may cause sedation.

9. With enuresis, refer parents to regional centers with incontinence programs if bed-wetting persists.

OUTCOMES/EVALUATE

- Improved S&S of depression
- Control of bed-wetting/severe neurogenic pain
- Therapeutic serum drug levels (200–350 ng/mL)

Immune globulin IV (Human) ■ IV

(im-**MYOUN GLOH**-byou-lin)

CLASSIFICATION(S):

Immune globulin

PREGNANCY CATEGORY: C

Rx: Carimune NF, Flebogamma 5%, Gammagard 10%, Gammagard Liquid 10%, Gamunex, Octagam, Polygam S/D, Privigen.

✤**Rx:** Iveegam Immuno.

USES

All products: Severe combined immunodeficiency and primary immunoglobulin deficiency syndromes, including congenital agammaglobulinemia, X-linked agammaglobulinemia with or without hyper IgM, severe combined immunodeficiency, and Wiskott-Aldrich syndrome. **Carimune NF:** Maintenance treatment of primary immunodeficiencies, including common variable immunodeficiency, X-linked aggamglobulinemia, or severe combined immunodeficiency. **Flebogamma:** Primary (inherited) humoral immunodeficiency disorders, including common variable immunodeficiency, X-linked agammaglobulinemia, severe combined immunodeficiency, and Wisksott-Aldrich syndrome. Especially useful when rapid IgG replacement or attainment of high IgG serum levels are desired. **Octagam:** Primary immune deficient diseases, including congenital aggamglobulinemia and hypogammaglobulinemia, common variable immunodeficiency, Wiskott-Aldrich syndrome, and severe combined immunodeficiencies. **Polygam S/D:** (1) Idiopathic thrombocytopenic purpura (ITP) in children and adults. (2) B-cell CLL in those with hypogammaglobulinemia or recurrent associated bacterial infections. (3) To prevent coronary artery aneurysms associated with Kawasaki disease (given with high-dose aspirin).

ACTION/KINETICS

Action

Derived from a human volunteer pool. Contains the various IgG antibodies normally occurring in humans. The products may also contain traces of IgA and IgM. Plasma in the manufacturing pool has been found nonreactive for hepatitis B antigen. No documented cases of viral transmission. Antibodies present in the products will cause both opsonization and neutralization of microbes and toxins. Reconstituted products may contain sucrose, maltose, protein, and/or small amounts of sodium chloride. Immune globulin IV provides immediate antibody levels.

Pharmacokinetics

The percentage of IgG in the products is over 90%. **t½:** Gamimune N and Sandoglobulin, 3 weeks; Venoglobulin-I, 29 days.

CONTRAINDICATIONS

Clients with selective IgA deficiency who have antibodies to IgA (the products contain IgA). Sensitivity to human immune globulin.

SPECIAL CONCERNS

■ These products have been associated with renal dysfunction, acute renal failure, osmotic nephrosis, and death. Clients predisposed to acute renal failure include those with any degree of pre-existing renal insufficiency, diabetes mellitus, those over 65 years of age, volume depletion, sepsis, paraproteinemia, or those receiving known nephrotoxic drugs. IGIV should be given in such clients at the minimum concentration available and the minimum rate of infusion practical. While reports of renal dysfunction and acute renal failure have been associated with many of the IGIV products, those containing sucrose as a stabilizer account for a disproportionate share of the total number.■ The various products are used for different conditions and at different doses; thus, check information carefully. Possible thrombotic events, especially following rapid infusion or high doses.

SIDE EFFECTS

Most Common

Back ache, chills, dizziness, fever, flushing, headache, increased sweating, leg cramps, muscle aches/pains, N&V, malaise, pain/tenderness at injection site.
CNS: Headache, malaise, feeling of faintness, dizziness. Aseptic meningitis syndrome, including symptoms of severe headache, nuchal rigidity, drowsiness, fever, photophobia, painful eye movements. **Allergic:** Hypersensitivity or *anaphylactic reactions*. **Body as a whole:** Fever, chills, flushing, increased sweating. **GI:** N&V. **At injection site:** Pain, tenderness. **Miscellaneous:** Chest tightness, dyspnea; chest, back, or hip pain; leg cramps, mild erythema following infiltration; burning sensation in the head; tachycardia, renal insufficiency and acute renal failure. Agammaglobulinemic and hypogammaglobulinemic clients never having received immunoglobulin therapy or where the time from the last treatment is more than 8 weeks may manifest side effects if the infusion rate exceeds 1 mL/min. Symptoms include flushing of the face, hypotension, tightness in chest, chills, fever, dizziness, diaphoresis, and nausea.

HOW SUPPLIED

Injection: 5% (50 mg/mL), 10% (100 mg/mL); *Liquid:* 10% (100 mg protein/mL); *Powder for Injection:* 5%, 10%; *Powder for Injection, Freeze-Dried:* 50 mg/mL; *Powder for Injection, lyophilized:* 5%, 1 grams, 3 grams, 6 grams, 12 grams.

DOSAGE

NOTE: Due to differences in products, dosage must be listed separately for each product.

FLEBOGAMMA, OCTAGAM

- **IV ONLY**
  Primary humoral immunodeficiency disorders.

300–600 mg/kg q 3–4 weeks. Dose may be adjusted over time to achieve the desired trough IgG levels and clinical response.

GAMUNEX

- **IV ONLY**
  Primary humoral Immunodeficiency.

Individualize dose. **Dose range:** 300–600 mg/kg q 3–4 weeks.
  ITP.

Total dose of 2 grams/kg divided in two doses of 1 gram/kg given on two consecutive days or into five doses of 0.4 mg/kg given on five consecutive days. If after giving the first of two daily 1 gram/kg doses, an adequate increase in the platelet count is seen at 24 hr, the second dose of 1 gram/kg may be withheld.

CARIMUNE NF

- **IV ONLY**
  Immunodeficiency syndrome.

0.2 gram/kg given once a month by IV infusion. If clinical response is inadequate, the dose may be increased to 0.3 gram/kg or the infusion may be repeated more frequently than once a month. The first infusion in previously untreated agammaglobulinemic or hypogammaglobulinemic clients must be given as a 3% immunoglobulin solution. Start with a flow rate of 10–20 gtt (0.5–1 mL/min). After 15–30 min, the rate of infusion may be further increased to 30–50 gtt (1.5–2.5 mL/min). After the first bottle of 3% solution is given and the client shows good tolerance, subsequent infusions may be given at a high-

---

Bold Italic = life threatening side effect   ■ = black box warning   ✦ = Available in Canada

er rate or concentration. Make such increases gradually allowing 15–30 min before each increment.

POLYGAM S/D
• IV ONLY
Immunodeficiency syndrome.
Initial: 200–400 mg/kg may be given; **then,** 100 mg/kg/month. Rate of administration for all uses: Initially, 0.5 mL/kg/hr. If there is no distress, the rate can be gradually increased, not to exceed 4 mL/kg/hr. Those who tolerate the 5% solution at a rate of 4 mL/kg/hr can receive the 10% solution starting at 0.5 mL/kg/hr. If the rate causes the client no distress, it may be increased, not to exceed 8 mL/kg/hr.
B-cell CLL.
400 mg/kg q 3 to 4 weeks.
ITP.
1 gram/kg. Depending on response, additional doses can be given—three separate doses on alternate days can be given, if needed. For all uses: In clients at risk of developing renal dysfunction, it may be wise to reduce the amount of product infused per unit time by infusing IGIV at a rate <13.3 mg/kg/min (<0.27 mL/kg/min of 5% or <0.13 mL/kg/min of 10%).

GAMMAGARD LIQUID (10%)
• IV
Immunodeficiency disease.
Usual: 300–600 mg/kg q 3–4 weeks, with the first dose given at an initial rate of 0.5 mL/kg/hr and increased gradually q 30 min to the level the client can tolerate but no more than 5 mL/kg/hr. In clients at risk of renal dysfunction or thrombotic complications, the recommended rate of administration is <2 mL/kg/hr.

NURSING CONSIDERATIONS

ADMINISTRATION/STORAGE

[IV] 1. Store Polygam S/D <25°C (77°F). Avoid freezing. Begin infusion of Polygam S/D 2 hr or less after reconstitution; discard any unused solution.
2. Store Carimune NF at room temperature, not exceeding 30°C (86°F). Do not use after expiration date.
3. Octagam may be stored for 24 months at 2–8°C (36–46°F) or may be stored at temperatures not to exceed 25°C (77°F) for up to 18 months from the date of manufacture. Do not use after expiration date.
4. Store Flebogamma from 2–25°C (36–77°F); do not freeze. Discard after expiration date.
5. Store Gammagard Liquid at 25°C (77°F) for up to 9 months after manufacture or from 2–8°C (36–46°F) for up to 36 months.
6. Follow administration guidelines explicitly and the manufacturer's directions carefully for reconstitution of either the 5% or 10% solution.
7. In agamma- or hypogammaglobulinemic clients, use the 3% solution. Initially, administer at a rate of 10–20 gtt/min (0.5–1 mL/min). After 15–30 min the rate may be increased to 30–50 gtt/min (1.5–2.5 mL/min). Subsequent infusions may be given at a rate of 40–50 gtt/min (2–2.5 mL/min). If the first bottle of the 3% solution is given with good tolerance, subsequent infusions may be given using the 6% solution.
8. Infuse only if the solution is clear and at room temperature. Do not shake the solutions because excessive foaming will occur.
9. Give only IV using a pump to administer; the IM or SC routes have not been evaluated.
10. Give by a separate IV line; do not mix with other fluids or medications.
11. A rapid decrease in serum IgG level in the first week postinfusion will be observed; this is expected and due to the equilibration of IgG between the plasma and extravascular space.
12. Have epinephrine readily available in the event of an acute anaphylactic reaction.

ASSESSMENT

1. List reasons for therapy; for passive immunization note date and type of exposure; assess closely for anaphylaxis.
2. Give within 2 weeks of exposure to hepatitis A, within 6 days after measles exposure, and within 7 days after hepatitis B exposure.
3. Any history of ITP warrants close hematologic monitoring. Monitor CBC, de-

termine if pregnant; requires close observation/management.

4. Monitor VS; if hypotension occurs, decrease/interrupt infusion rate until hypotension subsides.

5. Administer in a closely monitored environment away from persons with active infections if immunocompromised.

6. Monitor LFTs, hematologic parameters, IgG levels, and appropriate blood/urine chemistries.

7. To reduce the risk of IGIV-associated acute renal failure:

- Ensure client adequately hydrated before infusing IGIV.
- Be especially cautious when giving IGIV to those at increased risk for acute renal failure (renal insufficiency, diabetes mellitus, those over 65 years of age, volume depletion, sepsis, paraproteinemia, or clients taking nephrotoxic drugs).
- Do not exceed the recommended dose. For those at risk of acute renal failure, dilute or reconstitute the product so the IGIV concentration is as low and the infusion rate as slow as is practical. Do not exceed infusion rate of 3 mg/kg/min.
- Assess renal function before infusing IGIV and at regular intervals.

CLIENT/FAMILY TEACHING

1. Immunoglobulin helps to prevent and/or reduce intensity of various infectious diseases. With thrombocytopenia, expect increased platelets and enhanced clotting.

2. Once-monthly therapy is needed to maintain IgG serum levels.

3. Drug may cause N&V, fever, chills, flushing, lightheadedness, respiratory difficulty, and tightness in the chest; report immediately, may be dosage and rate related.

4. Close observation and frequent labs are essential with pregnancy to improve chances of a healthy baby and to ensure maternal safety.

5. Warm soaks to injection site and PO acetaminophen may relieve discomfort.

6. Drug is derived from human plasma (except for those engineered genetically); be aware of potential risks.

OUTCOMES/EVALUATE

- IgG levels within normal range
- ↑ Antibody titer; passive immunity
- ↑ Platelets; ↓ hemorrhaging

Inamrinone lactate

(in-**AM**-rih-nohn)

CLASSIFICATION(S):
Inotropic drug
PREGNANCY CATEGORY: C
Rx: Inamrinone lactate.

USES
Congestive heart failure (short-term therapy in clients unresponsive to digitalis, diuretics, and/or vasodilators). Can be used in digitalized clients.

ACTION/KINETICS

Action
Causes an increase in CO by increasing the force of contraction of the heart, probably by inhibiting cyclic AMP phosphodiesterase, thereby increasing cellular levels of c-AMP. It reduces afterload and preload by directly relaxing vascular smooth muscle.

Pharmacokinetics
Time to peak effect: 10 min. **t½, elimination, after rapid IV:** 3.6 hr; **after IV infusion:** 5.8 hr. **Steady-state plasma levels:** 2.4 mcg/mL by maintaining an infusion of 5–10 mcg/kg/min. **Duration:** 30 min–2 hr, depending on the dose. Excreted primarily in the urine both unchanged and as metabolites. Children have a larger volume of distribution and a decreased elimination half-life. *NOTE:* Due to medication errors and confusion with amiodarone, the generic name for amrinone was changed to inamrinone.

CONTRAINDICATIONS
Hypersensitivity to inamrinone or bisulfites. Severe aortic or pulmonary valvular disease in lieu of surgery. Acute MI.

SPECIAL CONCERNS
Safety and efficacy have not been established in children. Use with caution during lactation.

SIDE EFFECTS

Most Common

Arrhythmias, hypotension, N&V, thrombocytopenia, fever, anorexia.

GI: N&V, abdominal pain, anorexia. **CV:** Hypotension, *supraventricular and ventricular arrhythmias*. **Allergic:** Pericarditis, pleuritis, ascites, allergic reaction to sodium bisulfite present in the product, vasculitis with nodular pulmonary densities, hypoxemia, jaundice. **Miscellaneous:** Thrombocytopenia, *hepatotoxicity*, fever, chest pain, burning at site of injection.

OD **OVERDOSE MANAGEMENT**

Symptoms: Hypotension. *Treatment:* Reduce or discontinue drug administration and begin general supportive measures.

DRUG INTERACTIONS

Excessive hypotension when used with disopyramide

HOW SUPPLIED

Injection: 5 mg/mL.

DOSAGE

- **IV**

    CHF.

Initial: 0.75 mg/kg as a bolus given slowly over 2–3 min; may be repeated after 30 min if necessary. **Maintenance, IV infusion:** 5–10 mcg/kg/min. Do not exceed a daily dose of 10 mg/kg, although up to 18 mg/kg/day has been used in some clients for short periods.

NURSING CONSIDERATIONS

© Do not confuse inamrinone with amiodarone (an antiarrhythmic).

ADMINISTRATION/STORAGE

IV 1. Administer undiluted or diluted in 0.9% or 0.45% saline to a concentration of 1–3 mg/mL. Use diluted solutions within 24 hr.

2. Do not dilute with solutions containing dextrose (glucose) prior to injection. However, the drug may be injected into running dextrose (glucose) infusions through a Y connector or directly into the tubing.

3. Administer loading dose over 2–3 min; may be repeated in 30 min.

4. Solutions should be clear yellow.

5. Do not administer with furosemide; precipitate will form.

6. Protect from light and store at room temperature.

ASSESSMENT

1. Note reasons for therapy, other agents trialed, outcome.

2. Obtain baseline VS, CXR, and ECG. Assess electrolytes, BNP, and CBC. Document ejection fraction and pulmonary assessments, noting any new onset S_3, JVD, crackles, or edema.

3. Monitor VS, I&O, weights, urine output. Document CVP, CO, and PA pressures.

4. Assess for any hypersensitivity reactions, including pericarditis, pleuritis, or ascites.

CLIENT/FAMILY TEACHING

1. Drug is used IV for congestive heart failure in those who have not responded to the normal treatment with digoxin, diuretics, or vasodilators.

2. Expect frequent monitoring of ECG, BP and heart rate as well as weights. Drug may cause more frequent voiding.

3. Report any increased dizziness, weakness, fatigue, numbness, tingling or swelling of extremities, or pain at IV site. Keep all F/U appointments.

OUTCOMES/EVALUATE

- ↓ Preload and afterload; ↑ CO, EF
- Improvement in S&S of CHF.

Indapamide

(in-**DAP**-ah-myd)

CLASSIFICATION(S):

Diuretic, thiazide

PREGNANCY CATEGORY: B

Rx: Lozol.

✦**Rx:** Apo-Indapamide, Novo-Indapamide, PMS-Indapamide.

Indapamide hemihydrate

PREGNANCY CATEGORY: B

✦**Rx:** Gen-Indapamide, Lozide, Nu-Indapamide.

SEE ALSO *DIURETICS, THIAZIDES.*

USES
(1) Alone or in combination with other drugs for treatment of hypertension. (2) Edema in CHF.

ACTION/KINETICS
Pharmacokinetics
Onset: 1–2 weeks after multiple doses. **Peak levels:** 2 hr. **Duration:** Up to 8 weeks with multiple doses. **t½:** 14 hr. Nearly 100% is absorbed from the GI tract. Excreted through the kidneys (70% with 7% unchanged) and the GI tract (23%).

SPECIAL CONCERNS
Dosage has not been established in children. Geriatric clients may be more sensitive to the hypotensive and electrolyte effects.

SIDE EFFECTS
Most Common
Dizziness/lightheadedness, headache, weakness, fatigue/malaise, anxiety, nervousness, muscle cramps/spasms.

See *Diuretics, Thiazides* for a complete list of possible side effects.

HOW SUPPLIED
Tablets: 1.25 mg, 2.5 mg.

DOSAGE
• **TABLETS**
Edema of CHF.
Adults: 2.5 mg as a single dose in the morning. If necessary, may be increased to 5 mg/day after 1 week
Hypertension.
Adults: 1.25 mg as a single dose in the morning. If the response is not satisfactory after 4 weeks, the dose may be increased to 2.5 mg taken once daily. If the response to 2.5 mg is not satisfactory after 4 weeks, the dose may be increased to 5 mg taken once daily (however, consideration should be given to adding another antihypertensive).

NURSING CONSIDERATIONS
ADMINISTRATION/STORAGE
1. May be combined with other antihypertensive agents if response inadequate. Initially, reduce the dose of other agents by 50%.
2. Doses greater than 5 mg/day do not increase effectiveness but may increase hypokalemia.

ASSESSMENT
1. Note reasons for therapy, type, onset, characteristics of S&S, other agents trialed; outcome.
2. List drugs prescribed to ensure none interact unfavorably.
3. Monitor VS, weight, I&O, edema, renal function, electrolytes, uric acid levels.

CLIENT/FAMILY TEACHING
1. Drug is used to remove fluids and lower BP. Take in the morning upon awakening to prevent frequent nighttime voiding.
2. Change positions slowly to prevent sudden drop in BP and dizziness.
3. Follow low sodium diet; choose foods high in potassium (cantalope, broccoli, oranges, grapefruit, bananas, dried fruits, etc). Continue healthy life style by exercising regularly, stop smoking, limit alcohol consumption and strive for weight reduction.
4. Monitor BP and weight; report any gain of more than 2 lbs per day or 10 lbs per week.
5. Avoid prolonged sun exposure and use protection if exposed. Keep all F/U appointments for labs and evaluation.

OUTCOMES/EVALUATE
• ↓ BP
• ↑ Urinary output with ↓ edema

Indinavir sulfate
(in-**DIN**-ah-veer)

CLASSIFICATION(S):
Antiviral, protease inhibitor
PREGNANCY CATEGORY: C
Rx: Crixivan.

SEE ALSO *ANITIVIRAL DRUGS.*

USES
Treatment of HIV infection in adults in combination with other antiretroviral drugs.

ACTION/KINETICS
Action
Binds to active sites on the HIV protease enzyme resulting in inhibition of enzyme activity. Inhibition prevents cleavage of the viral polyproteins resulting in the formation of immature noninfec-

---

Bold Italic = life threatening side effect   ■ = black box warning   ✚ = Available in Canada

tious viral particles. Varying degrees of cross resistance have been noted between indinavir and other HIV-protease inhibitors.

Pharmacokinetics
Rapidly absorbed in fasting clients; **time to peak plasma levels:** Approximately 0.8 hr. Administration with a meal high in calories, fat, and protein results in a significant decrease in the amount absorbed and in the peak plasma concentration. **t½:** 1.8 hr. Metabolized in the liver with both parent drug and metabolites excreted through the feces (over 80%) and the urine (20% unchanged). **Plasma protein binding:** Approximately 60%.

CONTRAINDICATIONS
Lactation. Use with amiodarone, dihydroergotamine, ergonovine, ergotamine, methylergonovine, midazolam, pimozide, rifampin, terfenadine, and triazolam. Mild to moderate liver or kidney disease. Use in HIV-infected pregnant women.

SPECIAL CONCERNS
Not a cure for HIV infections; clients may continue to develop opportunistic infections and other complications of HIV disease. Not been shown to reduce the risk of transmission of HIV through sexual contact or blood contamination. No data on the effect of indinavir therapy on clinical progression of HIV infection, including survival or the incidence of opportunistic infections. Hemophiliacs treated for HIV infections with protease inhibitors may manifest spontaneous bleeding episodes. Drug resistance and cross resistance with other HIV protease inhibitors have been noted. Optimal dosing regimens have not been determined in children.

SIDE EFFECTS
Most Common:
Nephrolithiasis/urolithiasis, abdominal pain, N&V, back pain, headache, pruritus, dizziness, diarrhea.
NOTE: Many side effects are the result of combination therapy with other antiretroviral drugs. **GI:** N&V, diarrhea, abdominal pain/distention, acid regurgitation, anorexia, dry mouth, aphthous stomatitis, cheilitis, cholecystitis, cholestasis, constipation, dyspepsia, eructation, flatulence, gastritis, gingivitis, glossodynia, gingival hemorrhage, increased appetite, infectious gastroenteritis, jaundice, hepatitis, *pancreatitis, hepatic failure, impaired liver function, liver cirrhosis.* **CNS:** Headache, insomnia, dizziness, somnolence, agitation, anxiety, bruxism, decreased mental acuity, depression, dream abnormality, dysesthesia, excitement, fasciculation, hypesthesia, nervousness, neuralgia, neurotic disorder, oral paresthesia, peripheral neuropathy, sleep disorder, tremor, vertigo. **CV:** CV disorder, palpitation, *MI*, angina pectoris, vasculitis. **Musculoskeletal:** Back/leg pain, arthralgia, myalgia, muscle cramps/weakness, musculoskeletal pain, shoulder pain, stiffness. **Body as a whole:** Asthenia, fatigue, malaise, chest/flank pain, chills, fever, flu-like illness, fungal infection, pain, syncope. **Hematologic:** Anemia, lymphadenopathy, spleen disorder, *acute hemolytic anemia*, spontaneous bleeding in hemophilia A and B. **Respiratory:** Cough, dyspnea, halitosis, SOB, difficulty breathing, pharyngeal hyperemia, pharyngitis, pneumonia, rales, rhonchi, *respiratory failure*, sinus disorder, sinusitis, URTI. **Dermatologic:** Body odor, pruritus, rash, contact dermatitis, dermatitis, dry skin, flushing, folliculitis, herpes simplex/zoster, night sweats, pruritus, seborrhea, alopecia, hyperpigmentation, ingrown toenails, skin disorder/infection, sweating, urticaria, erythema multiforme, *Stevens-Johnson syndrome.* **GU:** Nephrolithiasis, urolithiasis, dysuria, hematuria, hydronephrosis, nocturia, PMS, proteinuria, renal colic, urinary frequency/abnormality, UTI, urine sediment abnormality, tubulointerstitial nephritis, crystalluria, dysuria, interstitial nephritis, leukocyturia, acute renal failure, pyelonephritis with or without bacteremia. **Ophthalmic:** Accommodation disorder, blurred vision, eye pain/swelling, orbital edema. **Body as a whole:** Asthenia, fatigue, fever, malaise, vasculitis, *anaphylaxis.* **Miscellaneous:** Asymptomatic hyperbilirubinemia, asthenia, fatigue, food allergy, taste disorder, increased

appetite, new-onset diabetes mellitus, exacerbation of pre-existing diabetes mellitus, hyperglycemia, immune reconstitution syndrome (when given with other antiretroviral drugs). Redistribution of body fat including central obesity, dorsocervical fat enlargement ('buffalo hump'), peripheral wasting, breast enlargement, and 'cushingoid appearance.'

LABORATORY TEST CONSIDERATIONS
↑ Serum transaminases (ALT, AST), total serum bilirubin, serum amylase, glucose, creatinine, serum cholesterol, serum triglycerides. ↓ Hemoglobin, platelet count, neutrophils. Hyperbilirubinemia.

OD OVERDOSE MANAGEMENT
Symptoms: Nephrolithiasis, urolithiasis, flank pain, hematuria, N&V, diarrhea. *Treatment:* It is not known if indinavir is dialyzable by peritoneal or hemodialysis.

DRUG INTERACTIONS
Aldesleukin / ↑ Plasma indinavir levels R/T ↓ liver metabolism
Amiodarone / Possible ↑ amiodarone levels R/T ↓ liver metabolism; do not use together
Amlodipine / ↑ Amlodipine AUC when given with indinavir and ritonavir R/T ↓ CYP3A metabolism of amlodipine
Atazanavir / Both drugs associated with indirect (unconjugated) hyperbilirubinemia; do not use together
Atorvastatin / ↑ Atorvastatin levels → ↑ risk of myopathy (including rhabdomyolysis); use lowest possible dose of atorvastatin
Azole antifungal drugs / ↑ Indinavir levels
Benzodiazepines / Possible severe sedation and respiratory depression
Bepridil / Use together with caution; monitor therapeutic levels
Calcium channel blockers (dihydropyridine-type: felodipine, nicardipine, nifedipine) / Use with caution together; monitor
Carbamazepine / ↓ Indinavir levels → ↓ effectiveness
Clarithromycin / ↑ Levels of both indinavir and clarithromycin → ↑ pharmacologic and toxic effects

Delavirdine / ↑ Indinavir levels; reduce indinavir dose to 600 mg q 8 hr when given with delavirdine, 400 mg 3 times/day
Didanosine / pH Dependent ↓ in absorption; give at least 1 hr apart on an empty stomach
Diltizaem / ↑ Amlodipine AUC when given with indinavir and ritonavir R/T ↓ CYP3A metabolism of amlodipine
Efavirenz / ↓ Indinavir levels R/T ↑ metabolism
Ergot derivatives (dihydroergotamine, ergonovine, ergotamine, methylergonovine) / ↑ Risk of ergot toxicity (peripheral vasospasm, ischemia of the extremities); do not give together
Fentanyl / ↑ Fentanyl levels → possible toxicity (respiratory depression)
Fluconazole / ↓ Levels of indinavir
Grapefruit juice / Slight delay in absorption of indinavir; no effect on bioavailability
Interleukins / ↑ Indinaviar levels → ↑ risk of toxicity
Isoniazid / ↑ Isoniazid levels
Itraconazole / ↑ Indinavir levels; reduce indinavir dose to 600 mg q 8 hr when giving itraconazole, 200 mg 2 times/day
Ketoconazole / ↑ Levels of indinavir; reduce indinavir dose to 600 mg q 8 hr
Lidocaine (systemic) / Use together with caution; monitor therapeutic levels
Lovastatin / ↑ Lovastatin levels → ↑ risk of myopathy (including rhabdomyolysis); do not use together
Midazolam / ↓ Midazolam metabolism → possibility of cardiac arrhythmias and prolonged sedation; do not use together
Nevirapine / ↓ Indinavir levels; monitor levels and adjust dose appropriately
Oral contraceptives / ↑ Levels of both estrogen and progestin components of product
Phenobarbital / ↓ Indinavir levels → ↓ effectiveness
Phenytoin / ↓ Indinavir levels → ↓ effectiveness
Quinidine / ↑ Indinavir levels; use together with caution; monitor therapeutic levels
Rifabutin / ↑ Rifabutin levels; ↓ rifabutin dose by 50% and increase indinavir

---

dose to 1,000 mg q 8 hr

Rifampin / ↓ Levels of indinavir; use together is not recommended

Rifapentine / ↓ Indinavir levels; use together with extreme caution, if at all

Ritonavir / ↑ Ritonavir levels → possible toxicity

H *St. John's wort* / Significant ↓ indinavir levels R/T ↑ liver metabolism

Saquinavir / ↑ Saquinavir levels → ↑ pharmacologic and toxic effects

Sildenafil / ↑ Sildenafil levels → severe and potentially fatal hypotension, visual changes, and priapism; do not exceed a sildenafil dose of 25 mg in a 48-hr period

Simvastatin / ↑ Simvastatin levels → ↑ risk of myopathy (including rhabdomyolysis); do not use together

Sirolimus / ↑ Sirolimus levels

Stavudine / ↑ Stavudine levels

Tacrolimus / ↑ Tacrolimus levels

Tadalafil / ↑ Tadalafil levels → severe and potentially fatal hypotension, visual changes, and priapism; do not exceed a tadalafil dose of 10 mg in a 72-hr period

Trazodone / ↑ Trazodone levels → ↑ pharmacologic and toxic effects; monitor and adjust dosage if necessary

Triazolam / ↓ Triazolam metabolism → possibility of cardiac arrhythmias and prolonged sedation; do not use together

Trimethoprim/Sulfamethoxazole / ↑ Levels of trimethoprim (no change in sulfamethoxazole levels)

Vardenafil / ↑ Vardenafil levels → severe and potentially fatal hypotension, visual changes, and priapism; do not exceed a vardenafil dose of 2.5 mg in a 24-hr period

Vitamin C (high doses) / ↓ Indinavir peak levels and AUC R/T induction of CYP3A4

Zidovudine / ↑ Levels of both indinavir and zidovudine

HOW SUPPLIED

Capsules: 100 mg, 200 mg, 333 mg, 400 mg.

DOSAGE————

• **CAPSULES**

HIV infections.

Adults: 800 mg (two 400-mg capsules) q 8 hr ATC. The dosage is the same whether the drug is used alone or in combination with other retroviral agents (except when noted below). Although optimal dosing regimens have not been determined in children, a dose of 500 mg/m^2 q 8 hr has been studied.

NURSING CONSIDERATIONS

ADMINISTRATION/STORAGE

1. Capsules are moisture sensitive. Store in original container; keep desiccant in the bottle. Keep tightly closed, protected from moisture and at a room temperature of 15–30°C (59–86°F).

2. Modify dosage or dosage schedule when indinivir is taken with the following drugs:

- Consider reducing dose of indinivir to 600 mg q 8 hr when given with delavirdine, 400 mg 3 times/day.
- If indinavir and didanosine are given together, give at least 1 hr apart on an empty stomach.
- Increase dose of indinavir to 1,000 mg q 8 hr when taken with efavirenz.
- Reduce dose of indinavir to 600 mg q 8 hr when taken with itraconazole, 200 mg twice a day.
- Reduce dose of indinavir to 600 mg q 8 hr when taken with ketoconazole.
- When taken with rifabutin, reduce the dose of rifabutin to one-half the standard dose and increase the indinavir dose to 1,000 mg (3 x 333 mg capsules) q 8 hr.

3. In mild to moderate hepatic insufficiency due to cirrhosis, reduce indinavir dosage to 600 mg q 8 hr.

4. In those with nephrolithiasis or urolithiasis, therapy may have to be interrupted temporarily (1–3 days) or discontinued even with adequate hydration.

5. Store from 15–30°C (59–86°F).

ASSESSMENT

1. Note symptom onset, confirmation of HIV, other agents trialed, outcome.

2. Monitor CD4 cell count, CBC, viral load, LFTs. Anticipate reduced dosage with impaired liver function; drug is hepatically metabolized.

3. Review list of drugs currently prescribed to ensure none interact.

CLIENT/FAMILY TEACHING

1. Take as prescribed at 8-hr intervals ATC with water 1 hr before or 2 hr after meals for optimal absorption. May be taken with other liquids, such as skim milk, juice, coffee, or tea, or with a light meal (e.g., dry toast with jelly, juice, and coffee with skim milk and sugar; or corn flakes, skim milk, and sugar). Avoid grapefruit juice, foods high in calories, fat, or protein.

2. If a dose is missed by more than 2 hr, wait and take the next dose at the regularly scheduled time. If a dose is missed by less than 2 hr, take immediately.

3. May cause dizziness or drowsiness; avoid activities that require mental alertness until drug effects realized.

4. To ensure adequate hydration, drink at least 1.5 L of liquids during a 24-hr period.

5. Report any symptoms of kidney stones (e.g., flank pain with or without hematuria, including microscopic hematuria); therapy should be interrupted for 1–3 days.

6. Drug is not a cure for HIV; continue to take precautions with disease transmission; opportunistic infections may occur.

7. Use reliable birth control and barrier protection; drug does not decrease the risk of transmitting disease through sexual contact or blood contamination. Do not breastfeed. If using viagra may experience adverse side effects: drop in BP, visual changes, and prolonged erection requiring medical attention; do not exceed 25 mg in 48 hr.

8. Report severe N&V, diarrhea, fever, chills, personality changes or changes in the color of urine or stool.

9. If also taking didanosine, must take on an empty stomach 1 hr apart.

10. The original desiccant must be dispensed with the medication. Counsel to store the drug in original container at room temperature away from moisture.

OUTCOMES/EVALUATE

Interference with progression of HIV infection

Indomethacin ■ IV ©
(in-doh-**METH**-ah-sin)

CLASSIFICATION(S):
Nonsteroidal anti-inflammatory drug

PREGNANCY CATEGORY: C (do not use late in pregnancy due to possible premature closure of ductus arteriosus),

Rx: Indocin, Indocin SR, Indomethacin Extended-Release, Indomethacin SR.

✦Rx: Apo-Indomethacin, Indocid, Novo–Methacin, Nu-Indo, Rhodacine, ratio-Indomethacin.

Indomethacin sodium trihydrate
(in-doh-**METH**-ah-sin)

Rx: Indocin I.V.
✦Rx: Indocid P.D.A.

SEE ALSO NONSTEROIDAL ANTI-INFLAMMATORY DRUGS.

USES

Not a simple analgesic; use only for the conditions listed.

PO: (1) Moderate to severe rheumatoid arthritis (including acute flares of chronic disease). (2) Moderate-to-severe osteoarthritis. (3) Moderate-to-severe ankylosing spondylitis. (4) Acute painful shoulder (tendinitis, bursitis). (5) Acute gouty arthritis (Capsules and Oral Suspension only).

Rectal: (1) Moderate to severe rheumatoid arthritis, including acute flares of chronic disease. (2) Moderate to severe osteoarthritis. (3) Acute gouty arthritis. (4) Moderate to severe ankylosing spondylitis. (5) Acute painful shoulder (bursitis, tendinitis).

IV: To close hemodynamically significant patent ductus arteriosus in premature infants weighing between 500 and 1750 grams if, after 48 hr, usual medical management is ineffective.

Bold Italic = life threatening side effect   ■ = black box warning   ✦ = Available in Canada

ACTION/KINETICS

Action

Anti-inflammatory effect is likely due to inhibition of cyclo-oxygenase. Inhibition of cyclo-oxygenase results in decreased prostaglandin synthesis. Effective in reducing joint swelling, pain, and morning stiffness, as well as to increase mobility in those with inflammatory disease. Indomethacin does not alter the course of the disease, however.

Pharmacokinetics

PO. Onset: 30 min for analgesia and up to 1 week for anti-inflammatory effect. Is 98% bioavailable. **Peak plasma levels:** 1–2 hr (2–4 hr for sustained-release). **Peak action for gout:** 24–36 hr; swelling gradually disappears in 3–5 days. **Peak activity for antirheumatic effect:** About 4 weeks. **Duration:** 4–6 hr for analgesia and 1–2 weeks for anti-inflammatory effect. **Therapeutic plasma levels:** 10–18 mcg/mL. **t½:** Approximately 5 hr (up to 6 hr for sustained-release). Metabolized in the liver and excreted in both urine and feces. **Plasma protein binding:** Approximately 90%.

ADDITIONAL CONTRAINDICATIONS

Pregnancy and lactation. PO indomethacin in children under 14 years of age. GI lesions or history of recurrent GI lesions. **IV use:** GI or intracranial bleeding, thrombocytopenia, renal disease, defects of coagulation, necrotizing enterocolitis. **Suppositories:** Recent rectal bleeding, history of proctitis.

SPECIAL CONCERNS

■ (1) NSAIDs may cause an increased risk of serious CV thrombotic events, MI, and stroke, which can be fatal. This risk may increase with duration of use. Clients with CV disease or risk factors for CV disease may be at a greater risk. (2) Indomethacin is contraindicated for treatment of perioperative pain in the setting of coronary artery bypass graft surgery. (3) NSAIDs cause an increased risk of serious GI adverse events including bleeding, ulceration, and perforation of the stomach or intestines, which can be fatal. These events can occur at any time during use and without warning symptoms. Elderly clients are at greater risk for serious GI events.■ Restrict use in children to those unresponsive to or intolerant of other anti-inflammatory agents; efficacy has not been determined in children less than 14 years of age. Geriatric clients are at greater risk of developing CNS side effects, especially confusion. Use with caution in clients with history of epilepsy, psychiatric illness, or parkinsonism and in the elderly. Use with extreme caution in the presence of existing, controlled infections.

ADDITIONAL SIDE EFFECTS

Most Common

After PO: Headache, dizziness, N&V, diarrhea, constipation, dyspepsia/indigestion, GI distress, tinnitus.

After IV: Renal dysfunction in infants, GI bleeding, elevated serum potassium, fluid retention, hyponatremia, intracranial bleeding, retrolental fibroplasia.

See also *Nonsteroidal Anti-Inflammatory Drugs* for a complete list of possible side effects. Also, reactivation of latent infections may mask signs of infection. More marked CNS manifestations than for other drugs of this group. Aggravation of depression or other psychiatric problems, epilepsy, and parkinsonism.

ADDITIONAL DRUG INTERACTIONS

Captopril / ↓ Captopril effect, probably R/T prostaglandin synthesis inhibition
Diflunisal / ↑ Plasma levels of indomethacin; also, possible fatal GI hemorrhage
Digitalis / Digitalis t½ maybe further prolonged in premature infants
Diuretics (loop, potassium-sparing, thiazide) / May reduce antihypertensive and natriuretic action of diuretics
Furosemide / Indomethacin may blunt natriuretic effect of furosemide
Lisinopril / Possible ↓ lisinopril effect
Losartan / ↓ Antihypertensive effect of losartan
Prazosin / ↓ Antihypertensive drug effects

HOW SUPPLIED

Indomethacin: *Capsules:* 25 mg, 50 mg; *Capsules, Sustained-Release:* 75 mg; *Oral Suspension:* 25 mg/5 mL; *Suppositories:* 50 mg.

Indomethacin sodium trihydrate:
Powder for Injection: 1 mg.

DOSAGE

INDOMETHACIN

- **CAPSULES; ORAL SUSPENSION; SUPPOSITORIES**

    Moderate to severe rheumatoid arthritis (including acute flares), osteoarthritis, or ankylosing spondylitis.

Adults, initial: 25 mg 2–3 times per day; may be increased by 25–50 mg at weekly intervals, according to condition and if tolerated until satisfactory response is obtained. With persistent night pain or morning stiffness, a maximum of 100 mg of the total daily dose can be given at bedtime either PO or rectally. **Maximum daily dosage:** 150–200 mg. In acute flares of chronic rheumatoid arthritis, the dose may need to be increased by 25–50 mg/day until the acute phase is under control.

    Acute gouty arthritis.

Adults, initial: 50 mg 3 times per day until pain is tolerable; **then,** reduce dosage rapidly until drug is withdrawn. Pain relief usually occurs within 2–4 hr, tenderness and heat subside in 24–36 hr, and swelling disappears in 3–4 days. Use only Capsules, Oral Suspension, or Suppositories.

    Acute painful shoulder (bursitis/tendinitis).

Adults: 75–150 mg/day in three to four divided doses for 1–2 weeks. Discontinue after signs and symptoms of inflammation have been controlled for several days. Usual course of therapy: 7 to 14 days.

- **CAPSULES, EXTENDED-RELEASE**

    Antirheumatic, anti-inflammatory.

Adults: 75 mg, of which 25 mg is released immediately, 1–2 times per day.

    Acute painful shoulder (bursitis, tendinitis).

75 mg two times per day. Discontinue after signs and symptoms of inflammation have been controlled for several days. Usual course of therapy: 7 to 14 days.

INDOMETHACIN SODIUM TRIHYDRATE

- **IV**

    Closure of patent ductus arteriosus.

A course of therapy is defined as 3 IV doses given 12–24 hr apart. Dose according to age as follows:

Age at first dose, <48 hr: First dose is 0.2 mg/kg; doses two and three are 0.1 mg/kg. **Age at first dose, 2–7 days:** All three doses are 0.2 mg/kg. **Age at first dose, >7 days:** First dose is 0.2 mg/kg; doses two and three are 0.25 mg/kg.

NURSING CONSIDERATIONS

ℭ Do not confuse Indocin with Minocin (an antibiotic).

ADMINISTRATION/STORAGE

1. If indomethacin is used for pediatric clients 2 years of age or older, monitor closely, including periodic assessment of liver function. If indomethacin is initiated, a suggested starting dose is 2 mg/kg/day, in divided doses. Maximum daily dose should not exceed 4 mg/kg/day or 150–200 mg/day, which is less. As symptoms subside, reduce the dose to the lowest level needed to control symptoms, or discontinue the drug.

2. The ER capsules can be given once a day and can be substituted for the 25 mg capsules 3 times per day. However, significant differences will be noted between the 2 dosage regimens in indomethacin blood levels, especially after 12 hours. The ER capsules can also be substituted for the 50 mg capsules 3 times a day.

3. Do not crush sustained-release form; do not use sustained-release form for acute gouty arthritis.

4. With dysphagia, the capsule contents may be emptied into applesauce, food, or liquid to ensure that client receives the prescribed dose.

5. Use smallest effective dose, based on individual need. Adverse reactions are dose related.

6. Do not use in conjunction with aspirin or other salicylates as such a combination does not produce any greater therapeutic effect and the incidence of GI side effects significantly increases.

7. Capsules: Store from 15–30°C (59–86°F). Protect from light. Dispense in a tight, light-resistant container using a child-resistant container.

Bold Italic = life threatening side effect   ■ = black box warning   ✤ = Available in Canada

8. Extended-Release Capsules: Store from 15–30°C (59–86°F). Potect from moisture.

9. Oral Suspension: Store below 30°C (86°F). Avoid temperatures above 50°C (122°F). Protect from freezing.

IV 10. If the ductus arteriosus closes or is significantly reduced in size after 48 hr or more from completion of the first course, no further doses are needed. If the ductus arteriosus reopens, a second course of 1 to 3 doses may be given; separate each dose by 12 to 24 hr.

11. Prepare the IV solution with 1–2 mL of sodium chloride 0.9% or water for injection. All diluents should be preservative free.

ASSESSMENT

1. List reasons for therapy, onset, characteristics of S&S, other agents prescribed.

2. Assess involved joint(s), including goniometric measurements, ROM, functional ability, swelling, erosion, erythema, pain level; note x-ray/CT/MRI findings.

3. Note U/A, CBC, renal, uric acid, and LFTs; avoid with severe renal impairment.

4. Monitor heart sounds, US, and respiratory status throughout therapy with patent ductus arteriosus.

CLIENT/FAMILY TEACHING

1. Take with food or milk to decrease GI upset. Do not crush or break capsules; may sprinkle capsule contents on food if unable to swallow.

2. Use caution when operating potentially hazardous equipment; may cause lightheadedness and decreased alertness.

3. In the event of lack of response or adverse side effects, withhold drug and report, since many may be serious enough to stop therapy.

4. Avoid prolonged sun exposure during therapy, may cause photosensitivity reaction.

5. Record weights, especially if N/V occur; report any abdominal pain or diarrhea.

6. Indomethacin masks infections; report any S&S of infection or fever.

7. Avoid alcohol and OTC agents without approval.

8. Return for scheduled eye exams and lab studies.

9. It will take from 2 to 4 days with gout flare and 2 to 4 weeks with arthritic conditions before significant improvement is evident. Follow prescribed dosing regimen carefully and refrain from becoming discouraged.

OUTCOMES/EVALUATE

- ↓ Pain and inflammation; ↑ joint mobility
- Relief from gout flare
- Closure of patent ductus arteriosus
- Therapeutic serum drug levels (10–18 mcg/mL)

Infliximab ■ **IV**
(in-**FLIX**-ih-mab)

CLASSIFICATION(S):
Treatment of Crohn's disease
PREGNANCY CATEGORY: B
Rx: Remicade.

USES

(1) In adults and children to reduce S&S and inducing and maintaining clinical remission of moderate to severe Crohn's disease unresponsive to conventional therapy. (2) Long-term use in adults to reduce the number of draining enterocutaneous fistulas in fistulizing Crohn's disease. (3) With methotrexate for inhibition of structural damage progression in those with moderate-to-severe rheumatoid arthritis who do not respond adequately to methotrexate alone. (4) Reduce S&S in active anklyosing spondylitis. (5) Reduce signs and symptoms of active arthritis in those with psoriatic arthritis to inhibit the progression of structural damage and improve physical function. (6) Reduce signs and symptoms, achieve clinical remission and mucosal healing, and eliminate corticosteroid use in those with moderately to severely active ulcerative colitis who have had an inadqequate response to conventional therapy. (7) Treat adults with chronic, severe,

plaque psoriasis who are candidates for systemic therapy and when other systemic therapies are less appropriate. Only administer to those who will be monitored closely and have regular follow-up visits to their healthcare provider. *Investigational:* Juvenile idiopathic arthritis associated with uveitis.

ACTION/KINETICS

Action

Chimeric $IgG1_K$ monoclonal antibody produced by a recombinant cell line. Acts by neutralizing the biological activity of TNF-α by high–affinity binding to its soluble and transmembrane forms and inhibits TNF-α receptor binding. In rheumatoid arthritis, infliximab reduces infiltration of inflammatory cells in inflamed areas of the joint as well as expression of molecules mediating cellular adhesion. In Crohn's disease, infliximab reduces infiltration of inflammatory cells and TNF-α production in inflamed areas of the intestine and reduces the proportion of mononuclear cells from the lamina propria able to express TNF-α and interferon.

Pharmacokinetics

$t\frac{1}{2}$, **terminal:** 7.7–9.5 days. No systemic accumulation of drug occurs. Development of antibodies increases infliximab clearance.

CONTRAINDICATIONS

Hypersensitivity to any component of the product or to murine proteins. Lactation. Administration of doses greater than 5 mg/kg to those with moderate to severe heart failure (NYHA Class III/IV). CHF or in those with a clinically important, active infection. Readministration to those who have experienced a severe hypersensitivity reaction to the drug. Concurrent use with live vaccines (e.g., measles, mumps, oral polio) as vaccinations may be less effective.

SPECIAL CONCERNS

■ (1) Risk of infections. Clients treated with infliximab are at increased risk for infections, including progression to serious infections leading to hospitalization or death. These infections have included bacterial sepsis, tuberculosis (TB), and invasive fungal, and other opportunistic infections. Educate clients about the symptoms of infection, and closely monitor for signs and symptoms of infection during and after treatment with infliximab; clients should have access to appropriate medical care. Evaluate clients who develop an infection for appropriate antimicrobial therapy and discontinue for serious infections. (2) Tuberculosis (frequently disseminated or extrapulmonary), has been observed in clients receiving inflixmab. Evalute clients for TB risk factors and test for latent TB infection prior to initiating infliximab and during therapy. Initiate treatment of latent TB infection prior to therapy with infliximab. Treatment of latent TB in clients with a reactive tuberculin test reduces the risk of TB reactivation in those receiving infliximab. Some clients who tested negative for latent TB prior to receiving infliximab have developed active TB. Monitor clients receiving infliximab for signs and symptoms of active TB, including those who tested negative for latent TB infections. (3) Hepatosplenic T-cell lymphomas. Rare postmarketing cases of hepatosplenic T-cell lymphoma have been reported in adolescent and young adult clients with Crohn disease treated with infliximab. This rare type of T-cell lymphoma has a very aggressive disease course and is usually fatal. All of these hepatosplenic T-cell lymphomas with infliximab have occurred in clients on concomitant treatment with azathioprine or 6-mercaptopurine.■ Use with caution in the elderly and in, or pre-existing or recent-onset CNS demyelinating or seizure disorders. Serious infections, including sepsis and death, have occurred in those treated with TNF-blocking agents. Thus, use with caution in clients with a chronic infection or a history of recurrent infection, or in mild heart failure. May worsen CHF. Those with Crohn's disease or rheumatoid arthritis, especially those with highly active disease or chronic exposure to immunosuppressant therapies, may be at a higher risk for the development of lymphoma. Safety and efficacy have not been determined for use in children less than 6 years of age with Crohn dis-

---

Bold Italic = life threatening side effect   ■ = black box warning   ✦ = Available in Canada

ease; also, safety and efficacy have not been determined in children with juvenile rheumatoid arthritis, ulcerative colitis, or plaque psoriasis.

SIDE EFFECTS

Most Common

URTI, nausea, headache, diarrhea, abdominal pain, pharyngitis, sinusitis, coughing, bronchitis, pain, fatigue, rash, dyspepsia, UTI, arthralgia.

Infusion-related (during infusion or within 2 hr post-infusion): Flu-like symptoms, headache, dyspnea, hypotension, transient fever, chills, GI symptoms, skin rashes, anaphylaxis (may occur anytime during infusion). **Hypersensitivity:** Urticaria, dyspnea, hypotension, *layrngeal/pharyngeal edema, severe bronchospasms, anaphylaxis (including laryngeal/pharyngeal edema, severe bronchospasm, seizures).* **Infections:** Pneumonia, cellulitis, infection at CNS venous catheter, sepsis, cholecystitis, endophthalmitis, furunculosis, histoplasmosis, listeriosis, pneumocytosis, tuberculosis (disseminated or extrapulmonary), invasive fungal infections, other opportunistic infections. **GI:** N&V, diarrhea, abdominal pain, constipation, dyspepsia, flatulence, intestinal obstruction, oral pain, ulcerative stomatitis, toothache, *GI hemorrhage,* ileus, *intestinal perforation,* intestinal stenosis, pancreatitis, peritonitis, proctaliga. **Hepatic:** *Acute liver failure,* jaundice, hepatitis, cholestasis, biliary pain, cholecystitis, cholelithiasis, hepatotoxicity, hepatitis B reactivation. **CNS:** Headache, fatigue, dizziness, paresthesia, vertigo, anxiety, depression, insomnia, optic neuritis, *seizures,* multiple sclerosis, CNS manifestations of systemic vasculitis, confusion, meningitis, neuritis, peripheral neuropathy, *suicide attempt.* **Neurolorlgic:** Optic neuritis, seizures, new onset or worsening of CNS demyelinating disorders as multiple sclerosis, neuropathies, Guillain-Barré syndrome. **CV:** Hypotension, hypertension, tachycardia, *worsening heart failure (may be fatal),* arrhythmia, bradycardia, brain infarction, *cardiac arrest, circulatory failure, MI, pulmonary embolism,* syncope, thrombophlebitis, systemic and cutaneous vasculitis, thrombotic thrombocytopenic purpura, *pericardial effusion.* **Dermatologic:** Rash, pruritus, acne, alopecia, fungal dermatitis, eczema, erythema, erythematous/maculopapular rash, papular rash, dry skin, increased sweating, ulceration, urticaria, ecchymoses, flushing, hematoma, erythema multiforme, *Stevens-Johnson syndrome,* toxic epidermal necrolysis. **Hematologic:** Leukopenia, neutropenia, thrombocytopenia, anemia, idiopathic thrombocytopenic purpura, lymphadenopathy, *hepatosplenic T-cell lymphomas, hemolytic anemia, pancytopenia.* **GU:** Dysuria, micturition frequency, UTIs, menstrual irregularity, renal calculus, renal failure, moniliasis. **Musculoskeletal:** Myalgia, back pain, arthralgia, arthritis, intervertebral disk herniation, tendon disorder, transverse myelitis. **Respiratory:** Dyspnea, URTI, pharyngitis, bronchitis, rhinitis, coughing, sinusitis, laryngitis, respiratory tract allergic reaction, ARDS, lower RTI (including pneumonia), pleural effusion, pleurisy, pulmonary edema, respiratory insufficiency, interstitial pneumonitis/fibrosis. **Miscellaneous:** Fatigue, fever, pain, moniliasis, chest pain, chills, peripheral edema, fall, hot flashes, malaise, anemia, abscess, flu syndrome, conjunctivitis, malignancies (basal cell and breast), cellulitis, *sepsis,* serum sickness, dehydration, diaphragmatic hernia, lymphoproliferative disorders (including lymphoma), lymphoadenopathy, lupus-like syndrome, infections (bacterial, fungal, protozoal, viral), opportunistic infections and TB in children.

NOTE: Possible formation of autoimmune antibodies (anti–dsDNA antibodies); development of lupus–like syndrome. Retreatment after an extended treatment-free period may cause delayed, potentially serious side effects. Symptoms include fever, myalgia, polyarthralgia, pruritus, rash and, less frequently, facial or hand edema, dysphagia, urticaria, sore throat, and headache. Use of acetaminophen, antihistamines, corticosteroids, or epinephrine helps the symptoms.

DRUG INTERACTIONS

Anakinra / Possible ↑ risk of neutropenia and serious infections

Etanercept / ↑ Risk of neutropenia

Immunosuppressants / Fewer infusion reactions compared with those taking no immunosuppressants

HOW SUPPLIED

Injection, Lyophilized Powder for Solution: 100 mg.

DOSAGE

• **IV**

Moderate to severe Crohn's disease or fistulizing Crohn's disease.

Adults, induction: 5 mg/kg IV at 0, 2, and 6 weeks followed by maintenance of 5 mg/kg q 8 weeks thereafter. If response is lost, consider 10 mg/kg. Those who do not respond by week 14 are not likely to respond with continued dosing; consider discontinuing infliximab. **Children:** 5 mg/kg IV at 0, 2, and 6 weeks followed by a maintenance regimen of 5 mg/kg q 8 weeks.

With methotrexate to treat rheumatoid arthritis.

Infliximab, 3 mg/kg at 2 and 6 weeks; then, q 8 weeks thereafter. If response is incomplete, may adjust the dose up to 10 mg/kg or treat as often as q 4 weeks. *NOTE:* The risk of serious infections is increased at higher doses.

Ankylosing spondylitis.

5 mg/kg by IV infusion, followed by additional similar doses at 2 and 6 weeks after the first infusion. Then, give every 6 weeks thereafter.

Psoriatic arthritis.

Initial: 5 mg/kg by IV infusion, followed by additional similar doses 2 and 6 weeks after the first infusion, and every 8 weeks thereafter. Can be used with or without methotrexate.

Ulcerative colitis, moderate to severe.

Initial, induction: 5 mg/kg at 0, 2, and 6 weeks, followed by a maintenance regimen of 5 mg/kg q 8 weeks thereafter.

Plaque psoriasis.

5 mg/kg as an IV infusion followed by additional doses at 2 and 6 weeks after the first infusion; then, q 8 weeks thereafter.

NURSING CONSIDERATIONS

ADMINISTRATION/STORAGE

IV 1. TO prevent and minimize infusion reactions, premedicate with antihistamines (H_1-antihistamines with or without H_2-antihistamines), acetaminophen, and/or corticosteroids. Discontinue treatment in those who experience severe infusion-related reactions.

2. Shortening the dosing interval may work as well (or better) than increasing the dose in those who do not respond to the dosage regimen of 3 mg/kg q 8 weeks for treating arthritis.

3. Do not give more than 5 mg/kg to clients with CHF.

4. Use vials immediately after reconstitution as there is no preservative. Do not reuse or store any unused portion of the infusion solution.

5. Infliximab solution is incompatible with PVC equipment or devices. Prepare only in glass infusion bottles or polypropylene or polyolefin infusion bags. Infuse through polyethylene-lined infusion sets.

6. Calculate total amount of reconstituted solution required. Reconstitute each vial with 10 mL sterile water for injection using a syringe equipped with a 21-gauge or smaller needle. Direct stream of water to the glass wall of the vial. Gently swirl solution by rotating the vial to dissolve contents. Do not shake; some foaming is usual. Allow reconstituted solution to stand for 5 min. The solution should be colorless to light yellow and opalescent; a few translucent particles (protein) may develop. Inspect for particulate matter and discoloration prior to administration. If there are visible opaque particles, discoloration, or other foreign particulates, do not use solution.

7. Dilute reconstituted infliximab dose to a total of 250 mL with 0.9% NaCl injection. Slowly add reconstituted solution to the 250 mL infusion bag/bottle. Mix gently.

8. Administer for 2 or more hours using an in-line, sterile, nonpyrogenic, low protein-binding filter (1.2 μm or less pore size).

Bold Italic = life threatening side effect   ■ = black box warning   ✦ = Available in Canada

9. Do not infuse concomitantly in the same IV line with other agents.

10. Store the lyophilized product at 2–8°C (36–46°F). Do not freeze.

ASSESSMENT

1. Note disease onset, surgeries, previous treatments trialed. List medical conditions that may preclude therapy. In those with worsening CHF, stop infliximab.

2. List stool frequency and consistency with Crohn's disease. Assess abdomen; note pain levels, mucus production. With fistulas, assess number, size, amount, type of drainage.

3. With arthritis, assess characteristics of involved joint(s), including goniometric measurements, ROM, functional ability, swelling, erythema. Rate pain levels.

4. Evaluate for latent tuberculosis; drug quadruples risk of TB so test prior to starting therapy.

5. Update immunizations prior to starting infliximab therapy.

6. Consider cessation of therapy when significant hematologic or CNS side effects occur.

7. Evaluate liver enzyme levels in those seropositive for hepatitis B surface antigen before beginning infliximab therapy and during treatment.

CLIENT/FAMILY TEACHING

1. Drug is for short term therapy. Infusion-related symptoms, i.e. headache, fever, itching, nausea, and pain may be managed with antihistamines, acetaminophen, corticosteroids and/or epinephrine.

2. With prolonged symptoms and diffuse disease in ulcerative colitis, surgical intervention may improve quality of life and prevent increased mortality.

3. Infliximab may cause dizziness; use caution while driving or performing other tasks requiring alertness, coordination, or physical dexterity. Keep all F/U visits.

OUTCOMES/EVALUATE

- ↓ Number of draining enterocutaneous fistulas in fistulizing Crohn's disease
- Control of arthritis pain with improved mobility

Insulin aspart
(**IN**-sue-lin **AS**-part)

CLASSIFICATION(S):
Insulin, rDNA origin
PREGNANCY CATEGORY: C
Rx: NovoLog, Novolog Mix 70/30.
✤**Rx:** NovoRapid.

SEE ALSO *ANTIDIABETIC AGENTS: INSULINS.*

USES
Treat diabetes mellitus in adults and children (ages 2–18 years). Due to the short duration of action, use with an intermediate or long-acting insulin. *NOTE:* Insulin aspart is the only insulin analog approved for use in external pump systems for continuous SC insulin infusion.

ACTION/KINETICS

Action
Rapid-acting. Is homologous with regular human insulin except for a single substitution of the amino acid proline by aspartic acid in position B28. This reduces the tendency of the molecule to form hexamers as with regular human insulin.

Pharmacokinetics
Has a faster absorption, faster onset, and shorter duration than regular human insulin after SC use. **Onset:** 15 min. **Peak:** 1–3 hr. **Duration:** 3–5 hr. **t½:** 90 min (compared with 141 min for regular human insulin). *NOTE:* Novolog Mix 70/30 contains 70% insulin aspart protamine suspension and 30% insulin aspart. **Onset:** 15–20 min. **Peak:** 1–4 hr. **Duration:** 1–24 hr.

SPECIAL CONCERNS
Use with caution during lactation.

SIDE EFFECTS

Most Common
Hypoglycemia, hypokalemia, injection site reaction, lipodystrophy, pruritus, rash.

See *Antidiabetic Agents: Insulins* for a complete list of possible side effects.

LABORATORY TEST CONSIDERATIONS
Small, but persistent ↑ in alkaline phosphatase.

DRUG INTERACTIONS

ACE inhibitors / ↑ Blood glucose lowering effect and susceptibility to hypoglycemia

Clonidine / Either potentiate or weaken blood-glucose lowering effect of insulin

Danazol / ↓ Blood glucose lowering effect

Disopyramide / ↑ Blood glucose lowering effect and susceptibility to hypoglycemia

Diuretics / ↓ Blood glucose lowering effect

Fluoxetine / ↑ Blood glucose lowering effect and susceptibility to hypoglycemia

Isoniazid / ↓ Blood glucose lowering effect

Lithium salts / Either potentiate or weaken blood-glucose lowering effect of insulin

MAO inhibitors / ↑ Blood glucose lowering effect and susceptibility to hypoglycemia

Niacin / ↓ Blood glucose lowering effect

Octreotide / ↑ Blood glucose lowering effect and susceptibility to hypoglycemia

Propoxyphene / ↑ Blood glucose lowering effect and susceptibility to hypoglycemia

Salicylates / ↑ Blood glucose lowering effect and susceptibility to hypoglycemia

Somatropin / ↓ Blood glucose lowering effect

Sulfonamides / ↑ Blood glucose lowering effect and susceptibility to hypoglycemia

HOW SUPPLIED

Injection: 100 units/mL.

DOSAGE

- **SC ONLY**

  Diabetes mellitus.

Individualized. The total daily individual insulin dosage requirement is usually between 0.5–1 unit/kg/day. About 50–70% may be provided by insulin aspart and the rest by an intermediate- or long-acting insulin. Clients may require more basal insulin and more total insulin when using insulin aspart compared with regular insulin; additional basal insulin injections may be required. *NOTE:* Start the meal within 5 to 10 min after injection.

NURSING CONSIDERATIONS

ADMINISTRATION/STORAGE

1. Addition of color branding has occurred with insulin products to prevent errors when using or dispensing Novolog and Novolog Mix 70/30.

2. If used with NPH human insulin immediately before injection, there is some attenuation in the peak level of insulin aspart but the time to peak and the total bioavailability are not affected significantly.

3. If insulin aspart is mixed with NPH human insulin, draw insulin aspart into the syringe first. Make the injection immediately upon mixing.

4. Do not mix insulin aspart with crystalline zinc insulin products.

5. IV use is possible under medical supervision with close monitoring of blood glucose and potassium levels to avoid hypoglycemia and hypokalemia. For IV, use concentrations from 0.05 to 1 unit/mL in infusion systems with infusion fluids (0.9% NaCl, D5W, or 10% dextrose with KCl (40 mml/L) using polypropylene infusion bags.

6. May be infused SC by external infusion pumps. Do not mix with any other insulins or diluent.

7. Visually inspect. Never use if the product contains particulate matter or has become viscous or cloudy. Do not use after the expiration date.

8. Store between 2–8°C (36–46°F). Do not freeze and do not use if the product has been frozen. Vials may be kept at room temperature below 30°C (86°F) for up to 28 days but should never be exposed to excessive heat or sunlight.

ASSESSMENT

1. Note onset of diabetes, level of control, other agents used, outcome.

2. Monitor VS, BS, electrolytes, HbA1c, U/A, microalbumin, renal and LFTs. Adjust dosage with impaired hepatic/renal function.

CLIENT/FAMILY TEACHING

1. This insulin is of rapid onset (1–3 hr) and short duration (3–5 hr) and may

---

also be used with an intermediate- or long- acting insulin to maintain glucose control.

2. Due to the fast onset of action, immediately follow the insulin aspart injection by a meal within 5–10 min.

3. Monitor BS; adjust dosage with any change in physical activity or usual meal plan. Illness, emotional disturbances, and stress may alter insulin requirements.

4. Continue diet, exercise, and life style changes necessary to enhance blood sugar control.

5. May initially experience local itching, swelling or redness; report if persistent. SOB, wheezing, diffuse rash, ↑ heart rate, and ↓ BP are S&S of shock.

6. Avoid pregnancy; if desired notify provider.

7. Keep all F/U appointments for evaluation of diabetes control, BP control, LDL levels, foot and eye exams.

OUTCOMES/EVALUATE
Glycemic control; HbA1c <7

Insulin detemir (rDNA origin) injection

(**IN**-sue-lin **DE**-te-meer)

CLASSIFICATION(S):
Insulin, rDNA origin
PREGNANCY CATEGORY: C
Rx: Levemir.

SEE ALSO *ANTIDIABETIC AGENTS: INSULINS*

USES
Once- or twice-daily treatment of adult and pediatric clients with type 1 diabetes mellitus or adult clients with type 2 diabetes mellitus who require long-acting insulin to control hyperglycemia.

ACTION/KINETICS
Action
Binds to insulin receptors and lowers blood glucose by facilitating uptake of glucose into skeletal muscle and fat cells and by inhibiting the output of glucose from the liver. Insulin inhibits lipolysis in the adipocyte, inhibits proteolysis, and enhances protein synthesis.

Pharmacokinetics
Slower, more prolonged, absorption over 24 hr compared with NPH human insulin. Absolute bioavailability: 60%. **Maximum serum levels:** 6–8 hr. **t½, terminal:** 5–7 hr, depending on the dose. **Plasma protein binding:** 98% bound to albumin.

SIDE EFFECTS
Most Common
Hypoglycemia, hypokalemia, injection site reaction, lipodystrophy, pruritus, rash.

See *Antidiabetic Agents: Insulins* for a complete list of possible side effects.

HOW SUPPLIED
Injection: 100 units/mL.

DOSAGE
- **SC**
  Type 1 diabetes mellitus in adults and children; Type 2 diabetes mellitus in adults.

Once or twice daily. Determine dose according to blood glucose levels. Individualize according to needs of the client.

NURSING CONSIDERATIONS
ADMINISTRATION/STORAGE
1. For clients treated once daily, give dose with the evening meal or at bedtime. For clients who require twice-daily dosing, the evening dose can be given with the evening meal, at bedtime, or 12 hr after the morning dose.

2. Administer by SC injection in the thigh, abdominal wall, or upper arm. Rotate injection sites within the same region.

3. Duration of action varies according to the dose, injection site, blood flow, temperature, and level of physical activity.

4. For those with type 1 or type 2 diabetes who are on basal-bolus treatment, changing the basal insulin to insulin detemir can be undertaken on a unit-to-unit basis. Adjust dose of insulin detemir to achieve glycemic targets. In some clients with type 2 diabetes, more insulin detemir may be needed than neutral protamine (NPH) insulin.

5. For clients receiving only basal insulin, changing the basal insulin to insulin detemir can be undertaken on a unit-to-unit basis.

6. For insulin-naive clients with type 2 diabetes who are not controlled on oral hypoglycemic drugs, start insulin detemir at a dose of 0.1–0.2 units/kg once daily in the evening or 10 units once or twice daily. Adjust dose to achieve glycemic targets.

7. Store unused insulin detemir from 2–8°C (36–46°F). Do not freeze. Do not use insulin detemir if it has been frozen.

8. After initial use, store vials in a refrigerator (never a freezer). If refrigeration is not possible, the in-use vial can be kept at room temperature, below 30°C (86°F) for up to 42 days, as long as kept as cool as possible and away from direct heat and light.

9. After initial use, a cartridge or prefilled syringe cartridge may be used for up to 42 days if kept at room temperature, below 30°C (86°F). Do not store in-use cartridges and prefilled syringes in a refrigerator or with the needle in place. Keep away from direct heat and sunlight.

ASSESSMENT

1. Note reasons for therapy, age at onset, Ht and WT, HbA1c, other agents trialed and outcome.

2. List medications prescribed to ensure none interact.

3. Monitor VS, BUN, creatinine, lytes, HbA1c, lytes, EKG, and blood sugar.

CLIENT/FAMILY TEACHING

1. Use exactly as directed. Return demonstrate appropriate use of cartridge or syringe. Store syringes/cartridges in a safe container until destroyed.

2. May cause drowsiness, dizziness, blurred vision, or lightheadedness. Do not drive, operate machinery, or perform any activities that require mental alertness. Using Insulin Detemir Cartridges alone, with certain other medicines, or with alcohol may lessen your ability to drive or perform other potentially dangerous tasks. Do not drink alcohol without approval; may increase risk of high/low blood sugar.

3. Illness, especially N&V, emotional problems, stress, or changes in diet or activity level may cause insulin requirements to change. Even if you are not eating, you still require insulin. Identify a sick day plan to use in case of illness. When you are sick, test your blood/urine frequently and call provider as needed. If traveling across time zones, ask provider about adjustments to your insulin schedule.

4. Proper diet, regular exercise, and regular testing of blood sugar are important for best results when using Insulin Detemir Cartridges. If blood sugar level is higher than it should be and you are taking Insulin Detemir Cartridges according to the directions, check with your provider.

5. Carry ID card at all times that says you have diabetes.

6. Do not exceed the recommended dose, use Insulin Detemir Cartridges more often than prescribed, or change type or dose of insulin you're taking without first discussing with provider.

7. An insulin reaction resulting from low blood sugar levels (hypoglycemia) may occur if you take too much insulin, skip a meal, or exercise too much. Signs of hypoglycemia include ↑ heartbeat, headache, chills, sweating, tremor, increased hunger, changes in vision, nervousness, weakness, dizziness, drowsiness, or fainting. Carry glucose tablets or gel to treat low blood sugar. If you do not have a reliable source of glucose available, eat a quick source of sugar such as table sugar, honey, or candy, or drink a glass of orange juice or non-diet soda to quickly raise your blood sugar level; advise provider.

8. Developing a fever or infection, eating significantly more than usual, or missing your dose of insulin may cause high blood sugar (hyperglycemia). Symptoms of hyperglycemia include thirst, increased urination, confusion, drowsiness, flushing, rapid breathing, and fruity breath odor. If these S&S occur, report immediately. If not treated, loss of consciousness, coma, or death may occur.

Bold Italic = life threatening side effect   ■ = black box warning   ✤ = Available in Canada

9. Use with caution in the elderly; may be more sensitive to its effects, especially low blood sugar. Use Cartridges with extreme caution in those under 6 years old.

10. Practice reliable contraception; report if pregnancy occurs. Do not breastfeed.

11. Skin depression, enlargement or thickening; redness, swelling, mild pain, or itching at the injection site may occur. Seek medical attention if any severe side effects occur i.e., severe allergic reactions (rash; hives; difficulty breathing; tightness in the chest; swelling of the mouth, face, lips, or tongue); changes in vision; chills; dizziness; drowsiness; fainting; fast heartbeat; fast, shallow breathing; headache; hoarseness; increased hunger, thirst, or urination; loss of consciousness; nervousness; seizures; slurred speech; stomach pain; sweating; sweet or fruity breath; swelling of arms or legs; tremor; weakness.

12. Lab tests, such as fasting blood glucose levels or glycosylated hemoglobin levels, may be performed to monitor progress or to check for side effects. Keep all provider and lab appointments.

OUTCOMES/EVALUATE
- HbA1c <7
- Desired control of blood sugar

Insulin glargine ©
(**IN**-sue-lin **GLAR**-jeen)

CLASSIFICATION(S):
Insulin, rDNA origin
PREGNANCY CATEGORY: C
Rx: Lantus.

SEE ALSO *ANTIDIABETIC AGENTS: INSULINS.*

USES
Once daily treatment of adult and pediatric clients (6 years and older) with type 1 diabetes mellitus or adults with type 2 diabetes mellitus who require long-acting insulin to control hyperglycemia. Not the insulin of choice for treatment of diabetic acidosis.

ACTION/KINETICS
Action
Long-acting recombinant human insulin analog. Differs from human insulin in that the amino acid asparagine at position A21 is replaced by glycine and two arginines are added to the C-terminus of the B-chain. Is designed to have low aqueous solubility at neutral pH; at pH 4, it is completely soluble. After injection into SC tissue, the acidic solution is neutralized, leading to formation of microprecipitates from which small amounts of insulin glargine are slowly released. This allows a relatively constant concentration/time profile over 24 hr with no pronounced peak.

Pharmacokinetics
Onset: 1.1 hr. **Peak:** No pronounced peak; small amounts are released slowly resulting in relatively constant levels over 24 hr. **Duration:** Prolonged (greater than 24 hr) when compared with NPH human insulin (about 14.5 hr). Metabolized in the liver. Dosage adjustment may be necessary in impaired renal or hepatic function.

CONTRAINDICATIONS
IV use.

SPECIAL CONCERNS
The long duration of insulin glargine may delay recovery from hypoglycemia. Use with caution during lactation. Not the drug of choice for diabetic ketoacidosis (use a short-acting IV insulin). Safety and efficacy have not been determined in children under 6 years old.

ADDITIONAL SIDE EFFECTS
Most Common
Hypoglycemia, hypokalemia, injection site reaction, lipodystrophy, pruritus, rash, allergic reactions.

See *Antidiabetic Agents: Insulins* for a complete list of potential side effects. Also, higher incidence of treatment-emergent injection site pain compared with NPH insulin-treated clients.

DRUG INTERACTIONS
ACE inhibitors / ↑ Blood glucose lowering effect and susceptibility to hypoglycemia

---

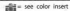

Clonidine / Either potentiates or weakens blood-glucose lowering effect of insulin

Danazol / ↓ Blood glucose lowering effect

Disopyramide / ↑ Blood glucose lowering effect and susceptibility to hypoglycemia

Diuretics / ↓ Blood glucose lowering effect

Fluoxetine / ↑ Blood glucose lowering effect and susceptibility to hypoglycemia

Isoniazid / ↓ Blood glucose lowering effect

Lithium salts / Either potentiate or weaken blood-glucose lowering effect of insulin

MAO inhibitors / ↑ Blood glucose lowering effect and susceptibility to hypoglycemia

Niacin / ↓ Blood glucose lowering effect

Octreotide / ↑ Blood glucose lowering effect and susceptibility to hypoglycemia

Propoxyphene / ↑ Blood glucose lowering effect and susceptibility to hypoglycemia

Salicylates / ↑ Blood glucose lowering effect and susceptibility to hypoglycemia

Somatropin / ↓ Blood glucose lowering effect

Sulfonamides / ↑ Blood glucose lowering effect and susceptibility to hypoglycemia

HOW SUPPLIED
Injection: 100 units/mL.

DOSAGE
- **SC**
  Diabetes mellitus.
  Dose individualized. Give once daily at bedtime. **Initial:** Average of 10 units once daily at the same time each day; **then,** adjust according to client need to a total daily dose ranging from 2–100 units.

NURSING CONSIDERATIONS

℗ Do not confuse insulin glargine with insulin glulisine. Do not confuse Lantus with Lente insulin (insulin zinc suspension).

ADMINISTRATION/STORAGE
1. Do not dilute or mix with any other insulin or solution as the mixture may become cloudy and the properties of either insulin glargine or other insulins may be altered.
2. Use only if the solution is clear and colorless with no visible particles.
3. Syringes must not contain any other medicinal product or residue.
4. If changing from an intermediate- or long-acting insulin to insulin glargine, the amount and timing of the short-acting insulin or fast-acting insulin analog may need to be adjusted.
5. Store unopened product in a refrigerator at 2–8°C (36–46°F). Do not store in the freezer and do not allow product to freeze. If refrigeration is not possible, 10 mL vials/cartridges can be kept unrefrigerated for up to 28 days and 5 mL vials/cartridges can be kept unrefrigerated for up to 14 days, away from direct heat and light, as long as the temperature does not exceed 30°C (86°F).
6. Once the cartridge is placed in an OptiPen One, do not put in the refrigerator.

ASSESSMENT
1. Note disease onset, level of control, other agents trialed, outcome.
2. Monitor VS, BS, electrolytes, HbA1c, U/A, microalbumin, renal and LFTs. List drugs prescribed.
3. Adjust dosage with hepatic/renal dysfunction.

CLIENT/FAMILY TEACHING
1. Insulin glargine is usually given once daily at anytime of the day for continual blood sugar control. Rotate sites.
2. Do not dilute or mix with any other insulin solution. Carry oral glucose tablets in event of hypoglycemia (low blood sugar).
3. Monitor/record FS and assess for hypo/hyperglycemia S&S.
4. Report any systemic rash, cough, or dizziness.
5. Continue lifestyle changes and diabetic diet necessary to control blood sugar.
6. Avoid pregnancy; consult provider if desired.

Bold Italic = life threatening side effect   ■ = black box warning   ♣ = Available in Canada

7. Attend diabetes education classes with spouse and keep all F/U visits to evaluate BS/BP control, eye/foot exams, ↓ LDL, and associated symptoms.

8. Store in refrigerator. If not available can keep unrefrigerated away from direct heat or light <86°F (30°C) and use within 28 days. Once placed in OptiPen One, do not refrigerate.

OUTCOMES/EVALUATE

Glycemic control; HbA1c <7

Insulin glulisine ©
(**IN**-sue-lin glue-**LIH**-seen)

CLASSIFICATION(S):
Insulin product, rDNA origin
PREGNANCY CATEGORY: C
Rx: Apidra.

USES

Control of hyperglycemia in adults with diabetes mellitus. Usually used in regimens that include a longer-acting insulin or basal insulin analog. May also be infused SC by external insulin infusion pumps.

ACTION/KINETICS

Action

A recombinant insulin analog equipotent to human insulin.

Pharmacokinetics

After SC administration, it has a more rapid onset of action and a shorter duration of action than regular human insulin. **Onset:** 15 min. **Peak:** 30–90 min. **Duration:** 1–2.5 hr. **t½:** 0.7 hr. One unit of insulin glulisine has the same glucose-lowering effect as one unit of regular human insulin.

SIDE EFFECTS

Most Common

Hypoglycemia, hypokalemia, injection site reaction, lipodystrophy, pruritus, rash.

See *Antidiabetic Agents:* Insulins for a complete list of possible side effects.

HOW SUPPLIED

Injection: 100 units per mL.

DOSAGE

• **SC**

Diabetes mellitus in adults.

Individualize dosage based on needs of client.

NURSING CONSIDERATIONS

© Do not confuse insulin glulisine with insulin glargine.

ADMINISTRATION/STORAGE

1. Give SC in the abdominal wall, thigh, or deltoid, or by continuous SC infusion in the abdominal wall.

2. Rotate injection sites and infusion sites within an injection area (e.g., abdomen, thigh, deltoid) from one injection to the next.

3. Use only if solution is clear and colorless with no particles visible.

4. When used in a pump, do not mix insulin glulisine with other insulins or with a diluent.

5. If glulisine is mixed with NPH human insulin, draw the glulisine into the syringe first. Make injection immediately after mixing. Do not mix glulisine with insulin products other than NPH.

6. Store unopened glulisine vials in the refrigerator at 2–8°C (36–46°F). Protect from light. Do not store in the freezer or allow to freeze. Discard vial if frozen.

7. Opened vials, whether or not refrigerated, must be used within 28 days. Discard if not used within 28 days. If refrigeration is not possible, the open vial may be kept unrefrigerated for up to 28 days away from direct heat and light as long as the temperature does not exceed 25°C (77°F).

8. Discard infusion sets (e.g., reservoirs, tubing, catheters) and insulin glulisine in the reservoir after no more than 48 hours of use or after exposure to temperatures that exceed 37°C (98.6°F).

CLIENT/FAMILY TEACHING

1. Drug onset of action is quicker than regular human insulin. Take within 15 min before a meal or within 20 min after starting a meal.

2. Administer subcutaneously into the abdomen, thigh or arm. Rotate injection sites and monitor finger sticks regularly.

3. May also be administered via pump into the abdomen as directed.

© = see color insert   H = Herbal   IV = Intravenous   © = sound alike drug

4. Continue diet, exercise and weight control along with insulin to control blood sugar and prevent organ damage. Ensure BP and LDL cholesterol well controlled and keep all F/U appointments for labs and medical evaluation.

OUTCOMES/EVALUATE
Control of diabetes; HbA1c <7

Insulin injection (Regular insulin) [IV]

(**IN**-sue-lin)

CLASSIFICATION(S):
Insulin product
OTC: Human Insulin: Humulin R, Novolin R, Novolin R PenFill, Novolin R Prefilled. **Pork Insulin:** Regular Iletin II.
✤**Rx: Human Insulin:** Novolin ge Toronto. **Pork Insulin:** Iletin II Pork Regular.

SEE ALSO *ANTIDIABETIC AGENTS: INSULINS.*

USES
Suitable for treatment of diabetic coma, diabetic acidosis, or other emergency situations. Especially suitable for the client suffering from labile diabetes. During acute phase of diabetic acidosis or for the client in diabetic crisis, client is monitored by serum glucose and serum ketone levels.

ACTION/KINETICS
Action
Rarely administered as the sole agent due to its short duration of action. Injections of 100 units/mL are clear; cloudy, colored solutions should not be used. Regular insulin is the only preparation suitable for IV administration. Available only as 100 units/mL.
Pharmacokinetics
Onset, SC: 30–60 min; **IV:** 10–30 min. **Peak, SC:** 2–5 hr; **IV:** 15–30 min. **Duration, SC:** 8–12 hr; **IV:** 30–60 min. Is compatible with all other insulins.

SIDE EFFECTS
Most Common
Hypoglycemia, hypokalemia, injection site reaction, lipodystrophy, pruritus, rash.

See *Antidiabetic Agents:* Insulins for a complete list of possible side effects.

HOW SUPPLIED
Injection: 100 units/mL.

DOSAGE
• **SC**
Diabetes.
Adults, individualized, usual, initial: 5–10 units; **pediatric:** 2–4 units. Injection is given 15–30 min before meals and at bedtime.
Diabetic ketoacidosis.
Adults: 0.1 unit/kg/hr given by continuous IV infusion.

NURSING CONSIDERATIONS
ASSESSMENT
1. Note disease onset, level of control/ understanding of disease, previous agents trialed, outcome.
2. Monitor VS, CBC, HbA1c, U/A: microalbumin, renal and LFTs.
CLIENT/FAMILY TEACHING
1. Use as directed.
2. Report adverse effects or lack of sugar control. Continue diet, exercise and weight control.
3. Record FS and keep all F/U appointments for evaluation of diabetes control, BP control, LDL levels, foot and eye exams.
OUTCOMES/EVALUATE
Control of hyperglycemia; A1C <7

Insulin injection, concentrated

CLASSIFICATION(S):
Insulin product
PREGNANCY CATEGORY: C
Rx: Humulin R Regular U-500 (Concentrated).

SEE ALSO *ANTIDIABETIC AGENTS: INSULINS.*

USES
Insulin resistance requiring more than 200 units insulin/day (a large dose may be given SC in a reasonable volume).
ACTION/KINETICS
Action
Concentrated insulin injection (500 units/mL) is a recombinant DNA product. Response varies among clients. In-

sulin resistance is frequently self-limiting; responsiveness to insulin may be regained after several weeks or months necessitating dosage reduction. Only given SC.

Pharmacokinetics
Has a duration similar to repository insulin; a single dose lasts for 24 hr.

CONTRAINDICATIONS
IV or IM use due to possible inadvertent overdosage.

SPECIAL CONCERNS
Use with caution during lactation.

ADDITIONAL SIDE EFFECTS
Most Common
Hypoglycemia, hypokalemia, injection site reaction, lipodystrophy, pruritus, rash.

See *Antidiabetic Agents: Insulins* for a complete list of possible side effects. Also, deep secondary hypoglycemia 18–24 hr after administration; hypoglycemia may be prolonged and severe.

DRUG INTERACTIONS
Do not use together with PO hypoglycemic agents.

HOW SUPPLIED
Injection: 500 units/mL.

DOSAGE ─────────────
• **SC ONLY**
Individualized, depending on severity of condition. Clients must be kept under close observation until dosage is established. Some clients may require only 1 dose/day while others may require 2 or 3 injections/day.

NURSING CONSIDERATIONS
ADMINISTRATION/STORAGE
1. Administer only water/clear solutions. Discoloration, turbidity, or unusual viscosity means deterioration or contamination.
2. Use a tuberculin or insulin syringe for accuracy of measurement.
3. Deep secondary hypoglycemia may occur 18–24 hr after administration; monitor closely and have 10–20% dextrose solution available.
4. Some clients who have experienced hypoglycemic reactions after transfer from animal-source insulin to human insulin have reported that the early warning symptoms of hypoglycemia

were less pronounced or different from those experienced with their previous insulin.
5. Keep in a cold location, preferably a refrigerator. Do not freeze.

ASSESSMENT
1. Observe closely for S&S of hyper- or hypoglycemia until dosage established. Counsel that this insulin is very concentrated and not to share or use without monitoring FS.
2. Monitor BP, BS, LDL cholesterol, and HbA1c. Keep all scheduled appointments, especially eye exams and foot exams.

CLIENT/FAMILY TEACHING
1. Review technique for self-administration.
2. Be alert for signs of hypoglycemia, which may indicate that responsiveness to insulin has been regained and that a reduction in dosage is warranted.
3. Record FS especially 2 hr PP to assess response. Keep all F/U visits and lab exams.
4. Continue BP/weight control, diet, and exercise to achieve glycemic control and to prevent complications.

OUTCOMES/EVALUATE
• BS and HbA1c within desired range
• Prevention of MI and organ damage

Insulin lispro injection
(**IN**-sue-lin **LYE**-sproh)

CLASSIFICATION(S):
Insulin, rDNA origin
PREGNANCY CATEGORY: B
Rx: Humalog, Humalog Mix 75/25.

SEE ALSO ANTIDIABETIC AGENTS: INSULINS.

USES
(1) Type 1 diabetes mellitus. In combination with sulfonylureas to treat high blood glucose in children over 3 years of age and adults over 65 years of age. (2) In combination with sulfonylureas in type 2 diabetes. Do not use a long-acting insulin when combined with sulfonylureas.

ACTION/KINETICS

Action

Is a rapid-acting human insulin analog created when the amino acids at positions 28 and 29 on the insulin B-chain are reversed. Absorbed faster than regular human insulin. Compared to regular insulin, has a more rapid onset of glucose-lowering activity, an earlier peak for glucose lowering, and a shorter duration of glucose-lowering activity. However, is equipotent to human regular insulin (i.e., one unit of insulin lispro has the same glucose-lowering capacity as one unit of regular insulin). May lower the risk of nocturnal hypoglycemia in clients with type 1 diabetes.

Pharmacokinetics

Onset: 15 min. **Peak effect:** 30–90 min. **t½:** 1 hr. **Duration:** 2–5 hr. *NOTE:* Humalog Mix 75/25 is a mixture of insulin lispro protamine suspension (75%) and insulin lispro injection (25%). It has glucose-lowering effects similar to Humulin 70/30 on a unit for unit basis. **Onset:** 5 min. **Peak:** 7–12 hr. **Duration:** 1–24 hr.

CONTRAINDICATIONS

Use during episodes of hypoglycemia. Hypersensitivity to insulin lispro.

SPECIAL CONCERNS

Since insulin lispro has a more rapid onset and shorter duration of action than regular insulin, clients with type 1 diabetes also require a longer acting insulin to maintain glucose control. Requirements may be decreased in impaired renal or hepatic function. Use with caution during lactation. Safety and efficacy of Humalog have not been determined in children less than 12 years of age. For Humalog Mix 75/25, safety and efficacy have not been determined in children less than 18 years of age.

SIDE EFFECTS

Most Common

Hypoglycemia, hypokalemia, injection site reaction, lipodystrophy, pruritus, rash, allergic reactions.

See *Antidiabetic Agents: Insulins* for a complete list of possible side effects.

DRUG INTERACTIONS

See *Antidiabetic Agents: Insulins*

HOW SUPPLIED

Injection: 100 units/mL. Humalog Mix 75/25 contains 75% insulin lispro protamine suspension and 25% insulin lispro injection.

DOSAGE

- **SC**

  Diabetes.

Individualized, depending on severity of the condition.

NURSING CONSIDERATIONS

℘ Do not confuse Humalog with Humulin (another insulin product).

ADMINISTRATION/STORAGE

1. When used as a mealtime insulin, give within 15 min before a meal or 15 min of finishing a meal, as compared with human regular insulin, which is best given 30–60 min before a meal.

2. May be mixed with Humalog, Humulin N, Humulin 50/50, Humulin 70/30, and NPH Iletin to a concentration of 1:10 or 1:2.

3. Mixing with Humulin N or Humulin U does not decrease the rate of absorption or the total bioavailability of insulin lispro.

4. Given alone or with Humulin N, insulin lispro causes a more rapid absorption and glucose-lowering effect than human regular insulin.

5. If Humalog is mixed with a longer-acting insulin (e.g., Humulin N or Humulin U), draw Humalog into the syringe first to prevent clouding of the Humalog by the longer-acting insulin.

6. After abdominal administration, insulin lispro levels are higher than those following deltoid or thigh injections. Also, the duration of action following abdominal injection is slighter shorter than deltoid or femoral injection.

7. Do not give mixtures IV.

8. May be given by an external insulin pump. The reservoir syringe, tubing, catheter, cartridge adapter, and insulin should be replaced every 48 hr or sooner. Also, a new infusion site should be selected. If an insulin cartridge is used, discard after 7 days. Do not expose the insulin in the external pump to a temperature above 37°C.

Bold Italic = life threatening side effect   ■ = black box warning   ✚ = Available in Canada

9. Store in the refrigerator at 2–8°C (36–46°F). Do not freeze. If refrigeration not possible, can store unrefrigerated for up to 28 days, provided it is kept as cool as possible and away from direct heat and light. Do not use if the product has been frozen.

10. Diluted insulin lispro may be used for 28 days when stored at 5°C (41°F) and for 14 days when stored at 30°C (86°F).

11. Do not use if the product is cloudy, contains particulate matter, is thickened, or discolored.

ASSESSMENT

1. Note disease onset, level of control, previous agents trialed, outcome.

2. Monitor VS, CBC, HbA1c, U/A: microalbumin, renal and LFTs.

CLIENT/FAMILY TEACHING

1. Review method for preparation, storage, and administration; rotate sites.

2. Prime the disposable insulin-delivery device before each injection.

3. Drug has a more rapid onset of action and a shorter duration of action than regular insulin.

4. Take within 15 min of meals and immediately after mixing, with combined therapy.

5. Monitor/record FS, especially 2 hr PP until response evident. Review S&S of hypoglycemia and appropriate management. Continue BP control, diet, and exercise for disease control.

6. Clients with type 1 diabetes also require a longer-acting insulin preparation for adequate glucose control.

7. Report for F/U labs, reinforcement of teaching, and evaluation of drug response. Bring Glucometer to all appointments.

OUTCOMES/EVALUATE

HbA1c <7; Prevention of MI and end organ disease

Insulin zinc suspension (Lente) (IN-sue-lin)

CLASSIFICATION(S):
Insulin product
PREGNANCY CATEGORY: B
OTC: Pork Insulin: Lente Iletin II.
♣OTC: Human Insulin: Novolin ge Lente. **Pork Insulin**: Iletin II.

SEE ALSO *ANTIDIABETIC AGENTS: INSULINS.*

USES

Allergy to other types of insulin and in clients disposed to thrombotic phenomena in which protamine may be a factor. Not a replacement for regular insulin and is not suitable for emergency use.

ACTION/KINETICS

Action

Contains 70% crystalline and 30% amorphous insulin suspension. Principal advantage is the absence of a sensitizing agent such as protamine.

Pharmacokinetics

Considered intermediate-acting. **Onset:** 1–2.5 hr. **Peak:** 7–15 hr. **Duration:** 24 hr.

SIDE EFFECTS

Most Common

Hypoglycemia, hypokalemia, injection site reaction, lipodystrophy, pruritus, rash.

See *Antidiabetic Agents: Insulins* for a complete list of possible side effects.

HOW SUPPLIED

Injection: 100 units/mL.

DOSAGE

• **SC**

Diabetes.

Adults, initial: 7–26 units 30–60 min before breakfast. Dosage is then increased by daily or weekly increments of 2–10 units until satisfactory readjustment is established. A second smaller dose may be given prior to the evening meal or at bedtime. Clients on NPH can be transferred to insulin zinc suspension on a unit-for-unit basis. Clients being transferred from regular insulin should begin zinc insulin at two-thirds to three-fourths the regular insulin dosage. If the client is being transferred from protamine zinc insulin, the dose of zinc insulin should be about 50% of that required for protamine zinc insulin.

NURSING CONSIDERATIONS

℗ Do not confuse Lente insulin with Lantus Insulin (insulin glargine).

ADMINISTRATION/STORAGE
Can be mixed with regular or semilente insulins.

ASSESSMENT
1. Note disease onset, level of control, previous agents trialed, outcome.
2. Monitor VS, CBC, HbA1c, U/A: microalbumin, renal, LFTs.

CLIENT/FAMILY TEACHING
1. Review technique for self-administration.
2. Be alert for S&S of hypoglycemia; may indicate responsiveness to insulin has been regained and a reduction in dosage is warranted.
3. Record FS especially 2 hr PP to assess response. Keep all F/U visits and lab exams.
4. Continue BP control, diet, and exercise to achieve glycemic control and to prevent disease complications.

OUTCOMES/EVALUATE
Normalization of BS; HbA1c <7

Interferon alfa-2a ■ recombinant (rIFN-A; IFLrA)

(in-ter-**FEER**-on **AL**-fah)

CLASSIFICATION(S):
Antineoplastic, miscellaneous
PREGNANCY CATEGORY: C
Rx: Roferon-A.

USES
(1) Hairy cell leukemia in select clients over age 18. Can be used in splenectomized and nonsplenectomized clients. (2) AIDS-related Kaposi's sarcoma in select clients over age 18. (3) In chronic phase, Philadelphia chromosome (Ph)-positive chronic myelogenous leukemia, in those minimally pretreated (within 1 year of diagnosis). (4) Chronic hepatitis C in select clients over age 18. *Investigational:* Bladder tumors, mycosis fungoides, essential thrombocythemia, non-Hodgkin's lymphoma, ovarian and cervical cancer, renal cell carcinoma, melanoma.

ACTION/KINETICS
Action
Recombinant DNA product whose activity is expressed as International Units, which are determined by comparing the antiviral activity of recombinant interferons with the activity of the international reference standard of human leukocyte interferon. Interferons bind to specific receptors on the cell surface, resulting in inhibition of virus replication in virus-infected cells, suppression of cell proliferation, increase in the phagocytic activity of macrophages, and enhancement of the toxic effects of leukocytes for target cells.

Pharmacokinetics
Peak serum levels: 3.8–7.3 hr. **t½, elimination:** 3.7–8.5 hr. Metabolized by the kidney.

CONTRAINDICATIONS
Lactation. Use in clients with a history of autoimmune hepatitis, history of autoimmune disease, or immunosuppressed transplant clients. Use to treat visceral AIDS-related Kaposi's sarcoma associated with rapid progressive or life-threatening disease.

SPECIAL CONCERNS
■ Causes or aggravates fatal or life-threatening neuropsychiatric, autoimmune, ischemic, and infectious disorders. Closely monitor clients with periodic clinical and lab evaluations. Withdraw clients with persistently severe or worsening signs or symptoms of these conditions due to therapy. In many, but not all cases, these conditions resolve after terminating interferon alfa-2a therapy.■ Use with caution in clients with a history of unstable angina, uncontrolled CHF, COPD, diabetes mellitus prone to ketoacidosis, thrombophlebitis, pulmonary embolism, seizure disorders, severe renal and hepatic disease, compro-

---

Bold Italic = life threatening side effect　　■ = black box warning　　♣ = Available in Canada

mised CNS function, and severe myelosuppression. Possible development or aggravation of vision loss or decrease, retinopathy, retinal hemorrhage, cotton-wool spots, optic neuritis, papilledema. Safety and efficacy in individuals less than 18 years of age have not been established.

SIDE EFFECTS

Most Common

Fatigue, myalgia/arthralgia/bone pain, flu-like symptoms, fever, chills, headache, dizziness, asthenia/fatigue, N&V, diarrhea, abdominal pain, anorexia, coughing, depression, irritability, injection site reaction, alopecia, insomnia.

When used to treat hairy cell leukemia. CNS: Depression, paresthesia, numbness, sleep disturbance, decreased mental status, anxiety, lethargy, visual disturbances, confusion, nervousness, vertigo. **GI:** Anorexia, N&V, abdominal pain, diarrhea, throat irritation, bleeding gums. **CV:** Chest pain, edema, hyper-/hypotension, cardiac murmur, thrombophlebitis. **Musculoskeletal:** Joint/bone pain, arthritis/polyarthritis. **Dermatologic:** Skin rash, diaphoresis, partial alopecia, dry skin, pruritus, ecchymosis, urticaria, petechiae. **Respiratory:** Cough, dyspnea, rhinorrhea, pneumonia, sinusitis, epistaxis. **Flu-like syndrome:** Fever, fatigue, myalgias, headache, chills, weight loss, dizziness. **Miscellaneous:** Pain, generalized pain, gait disturbance, inflammation at injection site, syncope. **When used to treat AIDS-related Kaposi's sarcoma. CNS:** Dizziness, decreased mental status, depression, paresthesia, confusion, sleep disturbance, visual disturbance, numbness, anxiety, nervousness, emotional lability, vertigo, forgetfulness, ataxia, seizures, neuropathy, aphasia, aphonia, dysarthria, amnesia. **GI:** Anorexia, nausea, diarrhea, emesis, abdominal pain, constipation, flatulence, gastric distress. **CV:** Cardiac palpitations, hypotension, arrhythmia, cardiomyopathy. **Respiratory:** Cough, dryness/inflammation of oropharynx, dyspnea, chest pain/congestion, rhinorrhea, sinusitis, pneumonia, bronchospasm, rhinitis. **Dermatologic:** Partial alopecia, rash, dry skin, pruritus, cyanosis, flushing of skin, night sweats, urticaria. **Musculoskeletal:** Poor coordination, muscle contractions, dysarthria. **Flu-like symptoms:** Fatigue, fever, myalgia, headache, chills, arthralgia. **Miscellaneous:** Weight loss, taste perversion, edema, poor coordination, pain at injection site, earache, eye irritation, lethargy, tremor, involuntary movements, syncope, weakness. **When used to treat CML. CNS:** Headache, depression, decreased mental status, dizziness, sleep disturbances, paresthesia, involuntary movements, visual disturbances, confusion, seizures, memory loss. **GI:** Anorexia, N&V, diarrhea. **Dermatologic:** Hair changes (e.g., alopecia), skin rash, sweating, dry skin, pruritus. **Hematologic:** Coombs' positive hemolytic anemia, *aplastic anemia*. **CV:** Syncope, hypotension, coagulopathy, cardiomyopathy. **Flu-like symptoms:** Fever, asthenia, fatigue, myalgia, chills, arthralgia, bone pain, headache. **Miscellaneous:** Chest pain, impotence, taste/hearing alteration, disturbances of libido, bruising, hypothyroidism, hypertriglyceridemia, bronchospasm. NOTE: For all uses, can cause leukopenia, neutropenia, thrombocytopenia, severe anemia, severe cytopenias. Also, although rare, severe or *fatal GI hemorrhage*.

LABORATORY TEST CONSIDERATIONS

↑ AST, ALT, LDH, BUN, serum creatinine, alkaline phosphatase, bilirubin, uric acid, serum glucose, serum phosphorus. ↓ H&H. Hypocalcemia, proteinuria, hyperglycemia. Leukopenia, neutropenia, thrombocytopenia, anemia.

DRUG INTERACTIONS

Cardiotoxic drugs / ↑ Effect of cardiotoxic drug
Hematotoxic drugs / ↑ Effects of hematotoxic drug
Interleukin-2 / ↑ Risk of renal failure
Neurotoxic drugs / ↑ Effects of neurotoxic drug
Theophylline / ↓ Theophylline clearance

HOW SUPPLIED

Prefilled Syringes: 3 million international units/syringe, 6 million international units/syringe, 9 million international units/syringe.

DOSAGE

- **IM; SC**

Hairy cell leukemia.

Induction: 3 million international units/day for 16–24 weeks; **maintenance,** 3 million international units 3 times per week. Reduce dose by 50% or withhold individual doses when severe side effects occur. Doses higher than 3 million international units are not recommended. Some clients have been treated for up to 24 consecutive months; the optimal duration of treatment has not been determined.

AIDS-related Kaposi's sarcoma.

Induction: 36 million international units/day for 10–12 weeks; or, 3 million international units/day on days 1–3; 9 million international units/day on days 4–6; and 18 million international units/day on days 7–9 followed by 36 million international units/day for the remainder of the 10 to 12-week induction period. **Maintenance:** 36 million international units 3 times per week. If severe side effects occur, the dose can be withheld or reduced by one-half.

Chronic myelogenous leukemia, chronic phase Ph-positive.

Induction: 9 million international units/day. The dose can be graded during the first week of therapy to improve short-term tolerance by giving 3 million international units/day for 3 days to 6 million international units/day for 3 days then to target dose of 9 million international units/day. **Maintenance:** Optimal dose and duration of therapy have not been determined. Continue regimen until the disease progresses. Limited data are available on the use in children with chronic myelogenous leukemia.

Chronic hepatitis C.

3 million international units, SC or IM, 3 times per week for 12 mo. **Alternative dose:** Induction dose of 6 million international units 3 times per week for the first 12 weeks followed by 3 million international units 3 times per week for 36 weeks. Reduce the dose by 50% in those who do not tolerate the prescribed dose. If side effects resolve, reinstitute the original prescribed dose. For those who cannot tolerate the reduced dose, temporarily cease therapy. Those who relapse following discontinuation of the drug may be retreated with either 3 million international units 3 times per week or with 6 million international units 3 times per week for 6-12 months.

NURSING CONSIDERATIONS

ADMINISTRATION/STORAGE

1. Stop treatment if leukemia does not respond within 6 months.

2. If severe reactions occur, reduce dose of drug by one-half or withhold individual doses. Assess effect on bone marrow of previous radiation or chemotherapy.

3. Although optimal treatment duration has not been established, clients have been treated for up to 20 consecutive months. Consider SC route with platelet count <50,000/mm^3.

4. Although not approved by the FDA, interferon alfa-2a has been given by continuous or intermittent IV infusion as well as ophthalmically and intravaginally.

5. The reconstituted solution is stable for 30 days when stored at 2–8°C (36–46°F) and for 24 hr when stored at room temperature. The undiluted drug is not stable in syringes R/T adhesion to syringe surfaces.

ASSESSMENT

1. Note reasons for therapy, other agents trialed, disease onset, baseline labs.

2. Perform eye examination initially and on those with a preexisting eye disorder periodically during therapy. Terminate therapy if an eye condition develops or worsens.

3. Prior to therapy, premedicate with acetaminophen to decrease flu like side effects. Ensure adequate hydration.

4. Ensure clients aware drug can cause blood cell abnormalities such as leukopenia, neutropenia, thrombocytopenia, severe anemia/cytopenias. Monitor CBC; Nadir: leukocytes, 20–40 days; platelets, 15–20 days.

Bold Italic = life threatening side effect   ■ = black box warning   ✦ = Available in Canada

CLIENT/FAMILY TEACHING

1. Review appropriate method for administration, care, and safe storage of drug and equipment.

2. Most common side effects are flu-like symptoms, such as fever, fatigue, headache, chills, nausea, and loss of appetite; may be minimized by taking at bedtime.

3. Flu-like symptoms usually diminish in severity as treatment continues. Acetaminophen may be used for fever and headache. Drink 2–3 L/day of fluids.

4. Use caution: low BP may occur up to 2 days following drug therapy; sit before standing and rise slowly to offset effects.

5. Do not change brands of interferon without approval; changes in dosage may occur with different brands.

6. Report for CBC, electrolytes, and LFTs as scheduled.

7. Practice safe sex and birth control.

8. Report any adverse effects and evidence of neurologic or psychologic disturbances.

9. Avoid alcohol and any other unprescribed CNS depressants. Hair loss may occur.

OUTCOMES/EVALUATE

- ↓ Tumor size and spread
- Inhibition of viral replication
- ↓ Lesions with Kaposi's sarcoma

Interferon alfa-2b ■IV recombinant (rIFN-α2; α-2-interferon; IFN-alpha)

(in-ter-**FEER**-on **AL**-fah)

CLASSIFICATION(S):
Antineoplastic, miscellaneous
PREGNANCY CATEGORY: C
Rx: Intron A.

USES

NOTE: Not all dosage forms and strengths are appropriate for some indications. (1) Hairy cell leukemia in clients over age 18 (in both splenectomized and nonsplenectomized clients). (2) Intralesional use for external genital or perianal warts (*Condylomata acuminata*) in clients 18 years and older. (3) AIDS-related Kaposi's sarcoma in clients over age 18. (4) Chronic hepatitis C in clients at least 18 years of age with compensated liver disease and a history of blood or blood product exposure or who are HCV antibody positive. (5) Chronic hepatitis B in clients 1 year of age and older with compensated liver disease and HBV replication (clients must be serum HBsAg positive for at least 6 months and have HBV replication with elevated serum ALT). (6) Adjunct therapy for malignant melanoma in those who are 18 years of age or older who are free of the disease but at a high risk for recurrence within 56 days of surgery. (7) With an anthracycline drug for the initial treatment of clinically aggressive non-Hodgkin's lymphoma in clients 18 years and older. *Investigational:* The drug has been used for a large number of conditions. Significant activity has been noted against the following neoplastic diseases: Locally for superficial bladder tumors, carcinoid tumor, chronic myelogenous leukemia, cutaneous T-cell lymphoma, essential thrombocythemia, low-grade non-Hodgkin's lymphoma, and chronic granulocytic leukemia. Limited activity has been noted in acute leukemias, cervical carcinoma, chronic lymphocytic leukemia, Hodgkin's disease, malignant gliomas, melanoma, multiple myeloma, nasopharyngeal carcinoma, osteosarcoma, ovarian carcinoma, renal carcinoma, and chronic granulomatous disease.

Interferon alfa-2b has also been used to treat the following viral infections: Significant activity has been seen against cutaneous warts, CMVs, herpes keratoconjunctivitis, and herpes simplex. Limited activity has been noted against papillomaviruses, rhinoviruses, vaccinia virus, varicella zoster, and HIV (used with foscarnet/zidovudine). It has also been used to treat multiple sclerosis.

ACTION/KINETICS

Action

Recombinant product whose activity is expressed as International Units, which are determined by comparing the antiviral activity of the recombinant interferon with the activity of the international reference standard of human leukocyte interferon. Interferons bind to specific receptors on the cell surface, resulting in inhibition of virus replication in virus-infected cells, suppression of cell proliferation, increase in the phagocytic activity of macrophages, and enhancement of the toxic effects of leukocytes for target cells.

Pharmacokinetics

Peak serum levels after IM, SC: 18–116 international units/mL after 3–12 hr. **t½, IM, SC:** 2–3 hr. **Peak serum levels after IV infusion:** 135–270 international units/mL at the end of the infusion. **t½, IV:** 2 hr. The main site of metabolism may be the kidney.

CONTRAINDICATIONS

Lactation. Use to treat rapidly progressive visceral disease in AIDS-related Kaposi's sarcoma. Use in clients with decompensated liver disease, autoimmune hepatitis, history of autoimmune disease, or immunosuppressed transplant clients. Use of interferon alfa-2b and ribavirin by women who are pregnant, by men whose female partners are pregnant, or in those with autoimmune hepatitis.

SPECIAL CONCERNS

■ Alpha interferons, including interferon alfa-2b, recombinant, cause or aggravate fatal or life-threatening neuropsychiatric, autoimmune, ischemic, and infectious disorders. Closely monitor clients with periodic clinical and lab evaluations. Terminate therapy in clients with persistently severe or worsening S&S of these conditions R/T therapy. In many, but not all, these conditions resolve after terminating therapy.■ Use with caution in clients with a history of unstable angina, uncontrolled CHF, COPD, diabetes mellitus prone to ketoacidosis, thrombophlebitis, pulmonary embolism, seizure disorders, severe renal and hepatic disease, compromised CNS function, and severe myelosuppression. Safety and efficacy in individuals less than age 18 have not been established.

SIDE EFFECTS

Most Common

Musculoskeletal pain/weakness, confusion, depression, dizziness, paresthesia, alopecia, rash, pruritus, back pain, chills, dry mouth, fatigue, fever, flu-like symptoms, headache, myalgia, N&V, anorexia, diarrhea, taste alteration, coughing, asthenia, increased sweating, rigors.

Flu-like symptoms: Fever, headache, fatigue, myalgia, chills. **CV:** Hypo-/hypertension, *arrhythmias,* tachycardia, syncope, coagulation disorders, chest pain, palpitations, flushing, atrial fibrillation, bradycardia, *cardiac failure, cardiomyopathy*, extrasystoles, postural hypotension. **CNS:** Depression, confusion, somnolence, migraine, dizziness, ataxia, insomnia, irritability, paresthesia, anxiety, nervousness, emotional lability, amnesia, impaired concentration, weakness, tremor, syncope, abnormal coordination, hypesthesia, aggravated depression, aggressive reaction, hypertonia, impaired consciousness, neuropathy, agitation, apathy, aphasia, dysphonia, extrapyramidal disorder, hot flashes, hyper-/hypoesthesia, hypo-/hyperkinesia, neurosis, paresis, paronria, parosmia, personality disorder, *seizures, coma*, polyneuropathy, *suicide attempt.* **GI:** N&V, diarrhea, stomatitis, weight loss, anorexia, flatulence, thirst, dehydration, constipation, eructation, loose stools, abdominal distention/pain, dysphagia, esophagitis, gastric ulcer, *GI hemorrhage*, GI mucosal discoloration, gum hyperplasia, gingival bleeding, gingivitis, increased saliva/appetite, melena, oral leukoplakia, rectal bleeding after stool, *rectal hemorrhage*, ulcerative stomatitis, ascites, gallstones, gastroenteritis, halitosis. **Hematologic:** Thrombocytopenia, granulocytopenia, anemia, *hemolytic anemia*, leukopenia. **Musculoskeletal:** Arthralgia, leg cramps, asthenia, arthrosis, arthritis, muscle pain/weakness, back/bone pain, rigors, CTS. **Respiratory:** Pharyngitis, coughing, dyspnea, sinusitis, rhinitis, epistaxis, nasal congestion, dry mouth, **bronchospasm**, pleural pain, pneumonia, rhinorrhea, sneezing, wheezing, bronchitis, cyanosis, lung fibrosis. **EENT:** Alteration/loss of taste, tinnitus, hearing/vision disorders, conjunctivitis, photophobia, eye pain, diplopia, dry eyes, earache, lacrimal gland/speech disorder, periorbital edema, vertigo. **Dermatologic:** Rash, pruritus, alopecia, urticaria, dry skin, dermatitis, purpura, photosensitivity, acne, nail disorder, facial edema, moniliasis, reaction at injection site, abnormal hair texture, cold/clammy skin, cyanosis of the hand, epidermal necrolysis, dermatitis lichenoides, furunculosis, increased hair growth, erythema, melanosis, nonherpetic cold sores, peripheral ischemia, skin depigmentation/discoloration, vitiligo, folliculitis, lipoma, psoriasis. **GU:** Amenorrhea, hematuria, impotence, leukorrhea, menorrhagia, urinary frequency, nocturia, polyuria, uterine bleeding, increased BUN, incontinence, pelvic pain. **Endocrine:** Gynecomastia, thyroid disorder, aggravation of diabetes mellitus, virilism. **Hepatic:** Jaundice, RUQ pain, *hepatic encephalopathy/failure*. **Miscellaneous:** Pain, increased sweating, malaise, decreased libido, herpes zoster/simplex, lymphadenopathy, chest pain, abscess, cachexia, hypercalcemia, peripheral edema, stye, substernal chest pain, weakness, sepsis, dehydration, fungal/viral infection, trichomoniasis.

LABORATORY TEST CONSIDERATIONS

↑ AST, ALT, LDH, BUN, serum creatinine, alkaline phosphatase. ↓ H&H. Abnormal LFT, bilirubinemia.

DRUG INTERACTIONS

Theophyllines / ↓ Theophylline clearance R/T ↓ liver breakdown

Zidovudine / ↑ Risk of neutropenia

HOW SUPPLIED

Injection: 3 million international units/dose, 5 million international units/dose, 10 million international units/dose; *Powder for Injection:* 5 million international units/vial, 10 million international units/vial, 18 million international units/vial, 25 million international units/vial, 50 million international units/vial; *Solution for Injection:* 3 million international units/vial, 5 million international units/vial, 10 million international units/vial, 18 million international units/vial, 25 million international units/vial.

DOSAGE

- **IM; SC**

  Hairy cell leukemia.

  2 million international units/m^2 3 times per week. Higher doses are not recommended. May require 6 or more months of therapy for improvement. Do not use the 50 million-international unit strength of the powder for injection for treating hairy cell leukemia. If severe side effects occur, reduce the dose by 50% or temporarily discontinue the drug until side effects abate. Discontinue if intolerance persists or recurs following adequate dosage adjustment, or if disease progresses.

  AIDS-related Kaposi's sarcoma

  30 million international units/m^2 3 times per week SC or IM using only the 50 million international unit vial. Do not use the 18 and 25 million international unit multidose strengths for treatment of AIDS-related Kaposi's sarcoma as concentrations are inappropriate. Using this dose, clients should tolerate an average dose of 110 million international units/week at the end of 12 weeks of therapy and 75 million international units/week at the end of 24 weeks of therapy.

  Chronic hepatitis C.

  3 million international units 3 times per week for 16 weeks. At 16 weeks, extend treatment to 18 to 24 months at 3 million international units 3 times per week to improve the sustained response of normalization of ALT. Discontinue therapy if there is no response after 16 weeks.

  Chronic hepatitis B.

  30–35 million international units/week SC or IM, given as either 5 million international units/day or 10 million international units 3 times per week for 16 weeks. If serious side effects occur, the dose may be decreased by 50%. **Children:** 3 million international units/m^2 3 times per week for the first week followed by dose escalation to 6 million international units/m^2 3 times per week (maximum of 10 million international units 3 times per week) for a total of 16–24 weeks.

• **IV**

Malignant melanoma.

20 million international units/m² IV on 5 consecutive days per week for 4 weeks. **Maintenance:** 10 million international units/m² SC 3 times per week for 48 weeks. The Solution for Injection is not recommended for this use. If side effects develop, especially if granulocytes decrease to <500/mm³ or ALT/AST rises to more than 5 times ULN, temporarily discontinue the drug until side effects abate. Restart at 50% of the previous dose. If intolerance persists, granulocytes decrease to less than 250/mm³, or ALT/AST increases to more than 10 times ULN, discontinue the drug.

Follicular lymphoma.

5 million international units SC 3 times per week for up to 18 months in conjunction with an anthracycline-containing chemotherapy regimen. Consider withdrawing therapy temporarily if neutrophil count is less than 1,000/mm³ or platelet count is less than 50,000/mm³; reduce the dose by 50% to 2.5 million international units 3 times per week for a neutrophil count of >1,000/mm³ but <1,500/mm³. Reinstitution of the initial dose of 5 million international 3 times/week may be tolerated after resolution of hematologic toxicity. Discontinue therapy if AST exceeds more than 5 times ULN or serum creatinine is more than 2 mg/dL.

• **INTRALESIONAL**

Condylomata acuminata (genital or venereal warts).

1 million international units (either 0.1 mL of reconstituted 10 million international units or 0.1 mL of the 5 million international units, the 10 million international units, or the 25 million international units strengths of solution for injection, each having a final concentration of 10 million international units/mL) 3 times per week for 3 weeks. To reduce side effects, give in the evening with acetaminophen. Maximum response usually occurs within 4–8 weeks.

If results are unsatisfactory after 12–16 weeks, a second course may be started.

NURSING CONSIDERATIONS

ADMINISTRATION/STORAGE

1. Prior to administration, reconstitute drug with provided bacteriostatic water for injection. Consult chart with product package to prepare powder for injection based on use. Client may self-administer dose at bedtime.

2. If severe side effects occur, dose may be reduced as much as 50% or therapy can be discontinued until side effects subside, i.e., if the granulocyte count is <750/mm³ and the platelet count is <50,000/mm³, reduce dose by 50%; if the granulocyte count is <500/mm³ and the platelet count <30,000/mm³, interrupt drug therapy until counts return to normal or baseline levels. Nadir: 3–5 days.

3. Discontinue treatment for leukemia if no response within 6 months.

4. When used for venereal or genital warts, direct needle at the center of the base of the wart and at an angle almost parallel to the plane of the skin. Maximum response usually occurs 4–8 weeks after therapy is initiated. If results not satisfactory after 12–16 weeks, a second course of therapy may be undertaken.

5. Although the optimal duration of treatment has not been established, clients have been treated for up to 20 consecutive months.

6. If platelet count is <50,000/mm³, give SC rather than IM.

7. Use a tuberculin-type syringe with a 25- to 30-gauge needle for intralesion administration. Do not give beneath the lesion too deeply or inject too superficially. As many as five lesions can be treated at one time.

8. Store powder from 2–8°C (36–46°F). The reconstituted solution is stable for 30 days when stored from 2–8°C (36–46°F). The solution for injection is stable at 35°C (95°F) for up to 7 days and at 30°C (86°F) for up to 14 days. The undiluted drug is not stable in syringes due to adhesion to syringe surfaces.

Bold Italic = life threatening side effect   ■ = black box warning   ✦ = Available in Canada

IV 9. Although not approved by the FDA, interferon alfa-2b has been given by continuous or intermittent IV infusion as well as ophthalmically and intravaginally.

10. For infusion solutions, after reconstitution, withdraw appropriate dose and inject into a 100-mL bag of 0.9% NaCl solution. The final concentration should be 10 million international units/10 mL or more. Infuse over a 20-min period. Prepare solution immediately prior to use.

ASSESSMENT

1. Note reasons for therapy, other agents trialed. outcome.

2. Monitor labs, VS, and lesions/viral loads as indicated.

CLIENT/FAMILY TEACHING

1. Flu-like symptoms may be minimized by administering drug at bedtime. Check temperatures; use acetaminophen for fever and headache.

2. Consume 2–3 L/day of fluids.

3. May cause dizziness/confusion or low BP; avoid hazardous tasks until drug effects realized.

4. Fatigue may be experienced. Report if depression, hallucinations, or suicide ideations occur.

5. Report for labs and bone marrow (hairy cell) determinations as ordered. Report any adverse or intolerable side effects.

OUTCOMES/EVALUATE

- Improved hematologic response
- ↓ Size/number of genital/venereal warts
- ↓ Viral load

Interferon alfa-n3
(in-ter-**FEER**-on **AL**-fah)

CLASSIFICATION(S):
Antineoplastic
PREGNANCY CATEGORY: C
Rx: Alferon N.

USES

Intralesional treatment of refractory or recurring external condylomata acuminata (genital or venereal warts) in clients 18 years of age or older. *Investigational:* Alpha interferons are being tested for use in a large number of neoplastic diseases and viral infections.

ACTION/KINETICS

Action

Is a sterile, aqueous formulation of purified, natural, human interferon alpha proteins. Binds to receptors on cell surfaces leading to a sequence of events including inhibition of virus replication and suppression of cell proliferation. Also, causes immunomodulation characterized by enhanced phagocytosis by macrophages, augmentation of the cytotoxicity of lymphocytes, and enhancement of human leukocyte antigen expression.

Pharmacokinetics

Intralesional use of interferon alfa-n3 does not result in detectable plasma levels of the drug.

CONTRAINDICATIONS

Hypersensitivity to human interferon alpha; clients who are allergic to mouse immunoglobulin (IgG), egg protein, or neomycin (the production process involves a nutrient medium containing neomycin although it has not been detected in the final product). Lactation. Use in clients less than 18 years of age.

SPECIAL CONCERNS

Due to fever and flu-like symptoms with use of interferon alfa-n3, use with caution in clients with debilitating diseases, including unstable angina, uncontrolled CHF, COPD, diabetes mellitus with ketoacidosis, thrombophlebitis, pulmonary embolism, hemophilia, severe myelosuppression, or seizure disorders. Use with caution in fertile men. Since the drug is made from human blood, it may carry a risk of transmitting infections. Safety and effectiveness have not been determined in children less than 18 years of age.

SIDE EFFECTS

Most Common

Myalgias, fever, headache, fatigue, chills, malaise, dizziness, nausea, arthralgia, back pain.

Flu-like symptoms: Commonly, fever, headache, myalgias which decrease with repeated doses. Also, chills, fatigue, malaise. **Hypersensitivity reaction:** Urticaria, angioedema, bronchoconstriction, *anaphylaxis*. **CNS:** Dizziness, headache, lightheadedness, insomnia, depression, nervousness, decreased ability to concentrate. **GI:** N&V, heartburn, dyspepsia, diarrhea, tongue hyperesthesia, thirst, altered taste, increased salivation. **Musculoskeletal/Skin:** Arthralgia, myalgia, back pain, hot sensation at bottom of feet, tingling of legs/feet, muscle cramps. **Respiratory:** Nose or sinus drainage, nose bleed, throat tightness, pharyngitis. **Miscellaneous:** Pruritus, swollen lymph nodes, heat intolerance, visual disturbances, sensitivity to allergens, papular rash on neck, hot flashes, herpes labialis, dysuria, photosensitivity, sweating, vasovagal reaction.

NOTE: When used for treatment of cancer, the incidence of many of the preceding side effects was increased. Additional side effects were noted including: **GI:** Constipation, anorexia, stomatitis, dry mouth, mucositis, sore mouth. **Miscellaneous:** Insomnia, blurred vision, ocular rotation pain, sore injection site, chest pains, low BP.

LABORATORY TEST CONSIDERATIONS
↓ WBC. The following may be affected in cancer clients: Hemoglobin levels, WBC and platelet count, GGT, AST, alkaline phosphatase, and total bilirubin.

HOW SUPPLIED
Injection: 5 million international units/mL.

DOSAGE

Condylomata acuminata.
0.05 mL (250,000 international units)/wart twice a week for up to 8 weeks. The maximum recommended dose per treatment session is 0.5 mL (2.5 million international units). The safety and effectiveness of a second course of treatment have not been determined.

NURSING CONSIDERATIONS
ADMINISTRATION/STORAGE
1. Inject drug into base of the wart using a 30-gauge needle.
2. For large warts, inject at several points around the wart periphery using a total of 0.05 mL/wart.

3. Do not give further drug or conventional therapy for 3 mo after the initial 8-week course of treatment unless the warts enlarge or new warts appear.
4. Store drug at 2–8°C (36–46°F). Do not freeze or shake.

ASSESSMENT
1. Note reasons for therapy, assess for allergy to egg protein or neomycin; may have increased sensitivity to drug.
2. List any preexisting debilitating diseases; note functional level.
3. For condylomata therapy, measure and document size and number of lesions.

CLIENT/FAMILY TEACHING
1. Intralesional treatment should be continued for 8 weeks.
2. Genital warts may disappear both during and after treatment has been completed. When this occurs, unless new warts appear or warts become enlarged, there should be a 3-month waiting period after the first 8-week course of therapy.
3. Do not change brands without approval; manufacturing process, strength, and type of interferon may vary.
4. Practice reliable contraception. Consider egg/sperm harvesting if pregnancy desired.
5. Report early signs of hypersensitivity reactions (e.g., hives, chest tightness, generalized urticaria, hypotension, wheezing, anaphylaxis).
6. Keep F/U appointment for labs and response to therapy.

OUTCOMES/EVALUATE
• ↓ Pain, number of genital warts
• Suppression of malignant cell proliferation

Interferon alfacon-1 ■

(in-ter-**FEER**-on **AL**-fah-kon)

CLASSIFICATION(S):
Immunomodulator
PREGNANCY CATEGORY: C
Rx: Infergen.

Bold Italic = life threatening side effect   ■ = black box warning   ✦ = Available in Canada

SEE ALSO *INTERFERON ALFA-2A* AND *INTERFERON ALFA-2B*.

USES

Chronic hepatitis C infections in those 18 years of age or older with compensated liver disease who have anti-HCV (hepatitis C virus) serum antibodies or the presence of HCV RNA. *Investigational:* With G-CSF therapy to treat hairy-cell leukemia.

ACTION/KINETICS

Action

Prepared by recombinant technology. Has antiviral, antiproliferative, and immunomodulatory effects, regulation of cell surface major histocompatibility antigen expression, and regulation of cytokine expression.

Pharmacokinetics

Plasma levels are too low to measure.

CONTRAINDICATIONS

Hypersensitivity to alpha interferons or to products derived from *E. coli*. Use in autoimmune hepatitis or in decompensated hepatic disease.

SPECIAL CONCERNS

■ Causes or aggravates fatal or life-threatening neuropsychiatric, autoimmune, ischemic, and infectious disorders. Closely monitor clients with periodic clinical and lab evaluations. Terminate therapy in clients with persistently severe or worsening signs or symptoms of these conditions due to therapy. In many, but not all, these conditions resolve after terminating therapy.■ Use with caution during lactation and in preexisting cardiac disease, in depression, in those with abnormally low peripheral blood cell counts, in those receiving myelosuppressive agents, in the elderly, and in autoimmune disorder. Safety and efficacy have not been determined in children less than 18 years of age.

SIDE EFFECTS

Most Common

Headache, fatigue, fever, myalgia, rigors, arthralgia, body pain, abdominal pain, nausea, back pain, insomnia, nervousness, pharyngitis, URTI, dizziness, diarrhea, anorexia, dyspepsia, injection site erythema, limb pain, depression, cough.

Flu-like symptoms: Headache, fatigue, fever, myalgia, rigors, arthralgia, increased sweating. **Body as a whole:** Body pain, access pain, non-cardiac chest pain, hot flushes, malaise, asthenia, peripheral edema, allergic reactions, weight loss, infection, exacerbation of autoimmune disease. **Hypersensitivity:** Urticaria, angioedema, bronchoconstriction, *anaphylaxis*. **CNS:** Insomnia, dizziness, paresthesia, amnesia, hypoesthesia, hypertonia, nervousness, depression, anxiety, emotional lability, abnormal thinking, agitation, decreased libido, apathy, confusion, hyperesthesia, somnolence, *suicidal ideation, suicide*. **GI:** Abdominal pain, N&V, diarrhea, anorexia, dyspepsia, constipation, flatulence, toothache, hemorrhoids, decreased saliva, gingivitis, ulcerative stomatitis, taste perversion, hepatomegaly, tender liver. **CV:** Hypertension, palpitation. **Hematologic:** Granulocytopenia, thrombocytopenia, leukopenia, ecchymosis, lymphadenopathy, lymphocytosis, anemia. **Respiratory:** Pharyngitis, URI, cough, sinusitis, rhinitis, respiratory tract/URT congestion, epistaxis, dyspnea, bronchitis. **Dermatologic:** Alopecia, pruritus, rash, erythema, dry skin, wound. **Musculoskeletal:** Back/limb/neck/skeletal pain, musculoskeletal disorder. **GU:** Dysmenorrhea, vaginitis, menstrual disorder, menorrhagia, genital moniliasis. **Ophthalmic:** Conjunctivitis, eye pain, decrease or loss of vision, macular edema, retinal artery or vein thrombosis, retinal hemorrhages, cotton wool spots, optic neuritis, papilledema. **Otic:** Tinnitus, earache, otitis. **At injection site:** Erythema, pain, ecchymosis.

LABORATORY TEST CONSIDERATIONS

↑ TSH, triglycerides. ↓ H&H. Abnormal thyroid tests.

DRUG INTERACTIONS

Drugs metabolized by cytochrome P450 / Possible changes in therapeutic and/or toxic levels of these drugs
Myelosuppressive drugs / Use caution when given with such drugs

HOW SUPPLIED

Injection: 9 mcg, 15 mcg; *Prefilled Syringes:* 9 mcg, 15 mcg.

DOSAGE

- **SC INJECTION**

Chronic hepatitis C infection.

Adults over 18 years of age: 9 mcg SC as a single injection 3 times per week for 24 weeks. At least 48 hr should elapse between doses. Those who tolerate therapy but did not respond or relapsed following discontinuation may be subsequently treated with 15 mcg 3 times per week for 6 months.

NURSING CONSIDERATIONS

ADMINISTRATION/STORAGE

1. Withhold dose temporarily if severe side effects experienced. If side effects do not become tolerable, discontinue therapy.
2. Reduction of dose to 7.5 mcg may be necessary following an intolerable side effect. If side effects continue to occur at reduced dosage, discontinue treatment or reduce dosage further. Decreased efficacy may result from continued treatment at doses less than 7.5 mcg.
3. Do not give 15 mcg 3 times per week if client has not received or tolerated an initial course of therapy.
4. Store refrigerated but do not freeze. Avoid vigorous shaking.

ASSESSMENT

1. Note reasons for therapy, other therapies trialed/outcome, disease characteristics.
2. Note any cardiac disease, hypertension, severe psychiatric disorders; these preclude drug therapy.
3. Monitor CBC, TSH, HCV RNA, renal. LFTs.

CLIENT/FAMILY TEACHING

1. Review dose and method of administration (SC); usually administered 3 times per week with 48 hr between doses.
2. May experience flu-like symptoms, including headache, fatigue, fever, muscle/joint pain, rigors, increased sweating.
3. Stop drug, report any S&S of depression, suicide thoughts/attempt.
4. Report as scheduled for F/U labs, evaluations. Do not change brands of interferon without provider approval.

OUTCOMES/EVALUATE

Improvement in LFTs; ↓ viral load

Interferon beta-1a
Interferon beta-1b
(r1FN-B)

(in-ter-**FEER**-on **BAY**-tah)

CLASSIFICATION(S):

Immunomodulator
PREGNANCY CATEGORY: C
Rx: Interferon beta-1a: Avonex, Rebif, **Interferon beta-1b**: Betaseron.

USES

Interferon beta-1a: Treatment of relapsing forms of MS to slow the appearance of physical disability (and possibly mental decline) and decrease the frequency of clinical exacerbations. Safety and efficacy have not been established in those with chronic progressive MS.
Interferon beta-1b: Treatment of relapsing forms of MS to reduce the frequency of clinical exacerbations. Those in whom efficacy has been shown include clients who have experienced a first clinical episode and have magnetic resonance imaging features consistent with MS. Evidence of efficacy beyond 2 years is not known. Safety and efficacy in chronic progressive MS have not been studied. *Investigational:* Treatment of AIDS, AIDS-related Kaposi's sarcoma, metastatic renal cell carcinoma, herpes of the lips or genitals, malignant melanoma, cutaneous T-cell lymphoma, and acute non-A/non-B hepatitis.

ACTION/KINETICS

Action

Interferon beta-1a is produced by mammalian cells into which the human interferon beta gene has been introduced. Interferon beta-1b is a genetically engineered plasmid containing the gene for human interferon beta$_{ser17}$. Interferon betas have antiviral, antiproliferative, and immunoregulatory effects. Mechanism for the beneficial effect in

---

MS is unknown, although the effects are mediated through combination with specific cell receptors located on the cell membrane. The receptor-drug complex induces the expression of a number of interferon-induced gene products that are thought to be the mediators of the biologic effects of interferon beta-1a and beta-1b.

Pharmacokinetics
t½, interferon beta-1a: 10 hr. Kinetic information is not available for interferon beta-1b since serum levels are low or not detectable following SC administration to MS clients. **Peak serum levels of beta-1b:** Within 1–8 hr with a mean serum concentration of 40 international units/mL. Mean terminal half-lives ranged from 8 min to 4.3 hr.

CONTRAINDICATIONS
Hypersensitivity to natural or recombinant interferon beta or human albumin. Use of Avonex with other hepatotoxic drugs. Lactation.

SPECIAL CONCERNS
The safety and efficacy for use in chronic progressive MS and in children less than 18 years of age have not been studied. Use with caution in clients with depression and other severe psychiatric symptoms as depression, attempted suicide, and suicide have occurred. Potential to be an abortifacient. Use with caution in those with preexisting seizure disorder.

SIDE EFFECTS
Most Common
Interferon beta-1a: Headache, flu-like symptoms, nausea, myalgia, URTI, fever, pain, asthenia, chills, infection, sleep difficulty, dizziness, diarrhea, sinusitis.
Interferon beta-1b: Injection site reaction, headache, fever, flu-like symptoms, pain, asthenia, chills, abdominal pain, mental symptoms, hypertonia, dizziness, diarrhea, constipation, vomiting, myalgia, sinusitis.

• Interferon beta-1a and -1b
Body as a whole: Headache, fever, pain, asthenia, chills, reaction at injection site (including necrosis/inflammation/pain), malaise. **Flu-like symptoms:** Muscle aches, fever, chills, asthenia, headache, pain, nausea, diarrhea, infec-

tion, sleep difficulty, dizziness. **GI:** Abdominal pain, diarrhea, dry mouth, **GI hemorrhage**, gingivitis, hepatomegaly, intestinal obstruction, periodontal abscess, proctitis. **CV:** Arrhythmia, hypotension, postural hypotension. **CNS:** Dizziness, depression, speech disorder, convulsion, **suicide attempt**, abnormal gait, depersonalization, facial paralysis, hyperesthesia, neurosis, psychosis. **Respiratory:** Sinusitis, dyspnea, hemoptysis, hyperventilation. **Musculoskeletal:** Myalgia, arthritis, arthralgia, back pain, myasthenia, skeletal pain. **Dermatologic:** Contact dermatitis, furunculosis, seborrhea, skin ulcer, photosensitivity. **GU:** Epididymitis, gynecomastia, hematuria, kidney calculus, nocturia, **vaginal hemorrhage**, ovarian cyst. **Miscellaneous:** Abscess, ascites, cellulitis, hernia, chest pain, hypothyroidism, **sepsis**, hiccoughs, thirst, leukorrhea.

• Interferon beta-1a
Body as a whole: Infection, neutralizing antibodies (significance unknown). **GI:** Nausea, dyspepsia, anorexia, blood in stool, colitis, constipation, diverticulitis, gall bladder disorder, gastritis, gum hemorrhage, hepatoma, increased appetite, **intestinal perforation**, periodontitis, tongue disorder. **Hepatic:** Autoimmune hepatitis. Avonex may cause hepatic injury (including hepatic failure), elevated serum LFTs (asymptomatic), and hepatitis. **CV:** Syncope, vasodilation, arteritis, **heart arrest, hemorrhage, pulmonary embolus, CHF, cardiomyopathy, cardiomyopathy with CHF**, palpitation, pericarditis, peripheral ischemia, peripheral vascular disorder, spider angioma, telangiectasia. **CNS:** Sleep difficulty, muscle spasm, ataxia, amnesia, Bell's palsy, clumsiness, drug dependence, increased libido, new or worsening psychiatric disorders, **seizures**. **Respiratory:** URTI, emphysema, laryngitis, pharyngeal edema, pneumonia. **Musculoskeletal:** Arthralgia, bone pain, myasthenia, osteonecrosis, synovitis. **Dermatologic:** Urticaria, alopecia, nevus, herpes zoster/simplex, basal cell carcinoma, blisters, cold clammy skin, erythema, genital pruritus, skin discoloration. **GU:** Vaginitis, fibroids, kidney

---

pain, breast fibroadenosis/pain, dysuria, fibrocystic change of the breast, menopause, PID, penis disorder, Peyronie's disease, polyuria, postmenopausal hemorrhage, testis/prostatic disorder, pyelonephritis, urethral pain, urinary urgency/retention/incontinence, menorrhagia, metrorrhagia. **Hematologic:** Anemia, ecchymosis at injection site, eosinophils >10%, hematocrit <37%, increased coagulation time, ecchymosis, lymphadenopathy, petechia, rarely pancytopenia or thrombocytopenia, idiopathic thrombocytopenia, ***pancytopenia*** (rare). **Metabolic:** Dehydration, hypoglycemia/magnesemia/-kalemia, hypo-/hyperthyroidism. **Ophthalmic:** Abnormal vision, conjunctivitis, eye pain, vitreous floaters. **Miscellaneous:** Otitis media, decreased hearing, facial edema, fibrosis/ hypersensitivity at injection site, rarely ***anaphylaxis, allergic reactions***, lipoma, neoplasm, photosensitivity, toothache, sinus headache, chest pain.

• **Interferon beta-1b**
Body as a whole: Generalized edema, hypothermia, ***anaphylaxis, shock***, adenoma, sarcoma. **GI:** Constipation, vomiting, GI disorder, aphthous stomatitis, cardiospasm, cheilitis, cholecystitis, cholelithiasis, duodenal ulcer, enteritis, esophagitis, fecal impaction or incontinence, flatulence, gastritis, glossitis, hematemesis, ileus, increased salivation, melena, nausea, oral leukoplakia/ moniliasis, ***pancreatitis, rectal hemorrhage***, salivary gland enlargement, stomach ulcer, peritonitis, tenesmus. **Hepatic:** Autoimmune hepatitis, severe liver damage leading to hepatic failure and transplant, hepatic neoplasia, hepatitis. **CV:** Migraine, palpitation, hypertension, tachycardia, peripheral vascular disorder, ***hemorrhage***, angina pectoris, atrial fibrillation, cardiomegaly, ***cardiac arrest, cerebral hemorrhage, heart failure, MI, pulmonary embolus, ventricular fibrillation, cardiomyopathy, DVT***, cerebral ischemia, endocarditis, pericardial effusion, spider angioma, subarachnoid hemorrhage, syncope, thrombophlebitis, thrombosis, varicose veins, vasospasm, venous pressure increase,

ventricular extrasystoles. **CNS:** Mental symptoms, hypertonia, somnolence, hyperkinesia, acute/chronic brain syndrome, agitation, apathy, aphasia, ataxia, confusion, depersonalization, emotional lability, paresthesia, ***seizures***, brain edema, ***coma***, delirium, delusions, dementia, dystonia, encephalopathy, euphoria, hallucinations, hemiplegia, hypalgesia, incoordination, intracranial hypertension, decreased libido, manic reaction, meningitis, neuralgia, neuropathy, paralysis, paranoid reaction, decreased reflexes, stupor, subdural hematoma, torticollis, tremor. **Respiratory:** Laryngitis, apnea, asthma, atelectasis, lung carcinoma, hypoventilation, interstitial pneumonia, ***bronchospasm***, lung edema, pleural effusion, pneumothorax. **Musculoskeletal:** Myasthenia, arthrosis, bursitis, leg cramps, muscle atrophy, myopathy, myositis, ptosis, tenosynovitis. **Dermatologic:** Sweating, alopecia, erythema nodosum, pruritus, skin discoloration, exfoliative dermatitis, hirsutism, leukoderma, lichenoid dermatitis, maculopapular rash, photosensitivity, psoriasis, benign skin neoplasm, urticaria, skin hypertrophy/necrosis/carcinoma, vesiculobullous rash. **GU:** Dysmenorrhea, menstrual disorder, metrorrhagia, cystitis, breast pain, menorrhagia, urinary urgency, fibrocystic breast, breast neoplasm, urinary retention, anuria, balanitis, breast engorgement, cervicitis, impotence, kidney failure, tubular disorder, nephritis, oliguria, polyuria, UTI, urosepsis, salpingitis, urethritis, urinary incontinence, enlarged uterine fibroids, uterine neoplasm. **Hematologic:** Lymphocytes <1,500/mm^3, active neutrophil count <1,500/mm^3, WBCs <3,000/mm^3, lymphadenopathy, CLL, petechia, hemoglobin <9.4 g/dL, platelets <75,000/mm^3, splenomegaly, anemia, thrombocytopenia. **Metabolic:** Weight gain/loss, goiter, glucose <55 mg/dL or >160 mg/dL, AST or ALT >5 times baseline, total bilirubin >2.5 times baseline, urine protein >1+, alkaline phosphatase >5 times baseline, BUN >40 mg/dL, calcium >11.5 mg/dL, increased GGT, hypocalcemia, hyperuricemia, increased triglycerides, cyanosis,

---

Bold Italic = life threatening side effect   ■ = black box warning   ✤ = Available in Canada

edema, glycosuria, hypoglycemic reaction, hypoxia, ketosis. **Endodrine:** Hypo-/hyperthroidism, thyroid dysfunction. **Ophthalmic:** Conjunctivitis, abnormal vision, diplopia, nystagmus, oculogyric crisis, papilledema, blepharitis, blindness, dry eyes, iritis, keratoconjunctivitis, mydriasis, photophobia, retinitis, visual field defect. **Hematologic:** Anemia, thrombocytopenia. **Miscellaneous:** Pelvic pain, hydrocephalus, alcohol intolerance, otitis/externa/media, parosmia, taste loss/perversion, *fatal capillary leak syndrome*.

LABORATORY TEST CONSIDERATIONS
↑ ALT, total bilirubin, AST, BUN, urine protein. Hypoglycemia or hyperglycemia. Ketosis.
Interferon beta-1b: ↑ GGT, triglycerides. Hypocalcemia, hyperuricemia.

HOW SUPPLIED
Interferon Beta-1a: *Injection (Rebif):* 8.8 mcg/0.2 mL, 22 mcg/0.5 mL, 44 mcg/0.5 mL.; *Powder for Injection, Lyophilized (Avonex):* 33 mcg (6.6 million international units when reconstituted); *Prefilled Syringes (Avonex):* 30 mcg/0.5 mL.
Interferon Beta-1b: *Powder for Injection, Lyophilized (Betaseron):* 0.3 mg.

DOSAGE
INTERFERON BETA-1A

• **IM; SC**
Relapsing forms of MS.
Avonex: 30 mcg IM once a week. Sites include the thigh or upper arm.
Rebif: Usually start with 20% of the prescribed dose 3 times per week and increase over a 4-week period to the targeted dose, either 22 mcg or 44 mcg three times per week. For a prescribed dose of 44 mcg, give 8.8 mcg three times per week for weeks 1 and 2 and 22 mcg three times per week for weeks 3 and 4. For a prescribed dose of 22 mcg, give 4.4 mcg three times per week for weeks 1 and 2 and 11 mcg three times per week for weeks 3 and 4. Give the full prescribed dose beginning week 5. Give, if possible, at the same time (preferably late afternoon or evening) on the same days each week, at least 48 hr apart (e.g., Monday, Wednesday, Friday). Rotate injection sites.
INTEFERON BETA-1B

• **SC**
Relapsing-remitting MS.
Goal: 0.25 mg SC every other day. Sites include arms, abdomen, hips, and thigh. Generally start clients at 0.0625 mg (0.25 mL) SC every other day for weeks 1 and 2; then, for weeks 3 and 4, give 0.125 mg (0.5 mL) every other day; for weeks 5 and 6, give 0.1875 mg (0.75 mL) every other day; and, beginning week 7, give 0.25 mg (1 mL) every other day.

NURSING CONSIDERATIONS
ADMINISTRATION/STORAGE
1. Avonex and Rebif are intended for use under the direction of a physician. Clients may self-inject only if the physician determines it is appropriate and with medical follow-up, as needed, after proper training in IM (for Avonex) or SC (for Rebif) injection technique.
2. To reconstitute and use Avonex (interferon beta-1a) use the following process:
• Use a sterile syringe and *Micro Pin* to inject 1.1 mL of the supplied diluent, sterile water for injection, into the vial and swirl gently to dissolve. Do not shake.
• The reconstituted solution should be clear to slightly yellow without particles. Discard if the product contains particulate matter or is discolored.
• Each vial contains 30 mcg/mL of drug
• Withdraw 1 mL of reconstituted solution into a sterile syringe. Replace the cover on the *Micro Pin* and attach the sterile 23-gauge 1.25 inch needle and inject IM.
• Vials must be stored in a refrigerator at 2–8°C (36–46°F).
• Following reconstitution, use within 6 hr; store at same temperatures as unreconstituted drug.
3. If using Avonex prefilled syringes, hold the prefilled syringe upright (rubber cap facing up). Remove the protective cover by turning and gently pulling the rubber cap in a clockwise motion. Attach the 23-gauge, 1.25 inch needle, and inject IM. The prefilled syringe is for single use only.

---

4. When using Rebif, rotate injection sites.

5. Store Rebif from 2–8°C (36–46°F). Do not freeze. If refrigeration is not available, store Rebif at or below 25°C (77°F) for up to 30 days away from heat and light.

6. Concurrent use of analgesics or antipyretics may help decrease flu-like symptoms on Rebif treatment days.

7. To reconstitute and use Betaseron (interferon beta-1b), use the following process:

- Using the sterile single-use syringe and needle, slowly inject 1.2 mL of diluent provided (0.54% NaCl) into the vial. Swirl gently to dissolve the drug completely. Do not shake.
- Visually inspect reconstituted product; discard if it contains particulate matter or is discolored.
- Withdraw 1 mL of the reconstituted solution from the vial into a sterile syringe fitted with a 27-gauge needle and inject SC. Injection sites include the arms, abdomen, hips, and thighs.
- Since the reconstituted product contains no preservative, discard any unused portions after one use.
- Before reconstitution, store from 2–8°C (36–46°F). After reconstitution, if not used immediately, refrigerate and use within 3 hr. Do not freeze. If refrigeration is not possible, keep vials and diluent as cool as possible below 30°C (86°F), away from heat and light; use within 7 days.

ASSESSMENT

1. List age at diagnosis, frequency of exacerbations, other therapies prescribed, outcome.

2. Note any hypersensitivity to human albumin or interferon beta. Assess psychological status noting depression or suicidal ideations; use with extreme caution.

3. Check for pregnancy; drug has abortifacient properties.

4. Monitor hematologic profile and hepatic enzyme levels q 3 months.

5. Conduct LFTs 1, 3, and 6 months after beginning interferon beta-1b ther-

apy and then periodically thereafter in the absence of clinical symptoms.

CLIENT/FAMILY TEACHING

1. Review guidelines for drug reconstitution, proper dose, administration, and care and disposal of equipment. Do not change dose or administration schedule without approval.

2. If possible, give Rebif at the same time, preferably in the late afternoon or evening on the same 3 days (e.g., Monday, Wednesday, Friday) at least 48 hr apart each week.

3. For Rebif, a starter kit is available to titrate the dose during the first 4 weeks of therapy. Following the administration of each dose, discard any unused product in the syringe.

4. Use Rebif only under the guidance and supervision of provider. Review the proper technique to self-administer SC using the prefilled syringes; rotate injection sites.

5. Flu-like symptoms are common; analgesics or antipyretics may help.

6. Report any mental status changes, depression, suicide thoughts.

7. Practice reliable birth control; drug may harm fetus.

8. May cause photosensitivity reactions; wear protective clothing, sunscreen, sun glasses, and a hat when sun exposed.

9. Avoid alcohol in any form.

10. With diabetes, monitor FS and report any overt changes.

11. Identify support groups that may assist to cope with chronic disease.

OUTCOMES/EVALUATE

↓ Frequency and severity of MS exacerbations

Interferon gamma-1b **IV**

(in-ter-**FEER**-on **GAM**-uh)

CLASSIFICATION(S):
Immunomodulator
PREGNANCY CATEGORY: C
Rx: Actimmune.

USES

(1) Decrease the frequency and severity of serious infections associated with chronic granulomatous disease. (2) Delay time to disease progression in severe, malignant osteoporosis.

ACTION/KINETICS

Action

Manifests potent phagocyte-activating effects including generation of toxic oxygen metabolites within phagocytes. Such metabolites result in the death of microorganisms such as *Staphylococcus aureus, Toxoplasma gondii, Leishmania donovani, Listeria monocytogenes,* and *Mycobacterium avium intracellulare.* Since interferon gamma regulates activity of immune cells, it is characterized as a lymphokine of the interleukin type. Interferon gamma interacts functionally with other interleukin molecules (e.g., interleukin-2) and all interleukins form part of a complex, lymphokine regulatory network. As an example, interferon gamma and interleukin-4 may interact reciprocally to regulate murine IgE levels; interferon gamma can suppress IgE levels and inhibit the production of collagen at the transcription level in humans.

Pharmacokinetics

Slowly absorbed after SC injection. $t\frac{1}{2}$, **elimination: SC,** 5.9 hr. **Peak plasma levels:** 7 hr after SC.

CONTRAINDICATIONS

Hypersensitivity to interferon gamma or *E. coli*-derived products. Lactation.

SPECIAL CONCERNS

Safety and effectiveness have not been determined in children less than 1 year of age. Use with caution in clients with preexisting cardiac disease, including symptoms of ischemia, arrhythmia, or CHF, and in clients with myelosuppression or taking other potentially myelosuppressive drugs, seizure disorders, or compromised CNS function.

SIDE EFFECTS

Most Common

Fever, headache, rash, chills, injection site erythema/tenderness, fatigue, diarrhea, N&V, abdominal pain, myalgia.
The following side effects were noted in clients with chronic granulomatous dis-

ease or severe, malignant osteoporosis receiving the drug SC. **GI:** Diarrhea, N&V, abdominal pain, anorexia. **CNS:** Fever (over 50%), headache, fatigue, depression. **Miscellaneous:** Rash, chills, erythema or tenderness/pain at injection site, weight loss, myalgia, arthralgia, back pain, myelosuppression, hypersensitivity reactions. When used in clients other than those with chronic granulomatous disease, in addition to the preceding, the following side effects were reported. **GI:** *GI bleeding,* pancreatitis, hepatic insufficiency. **CV:** Hypotension, heart block, *heart failure,* syncope, *tachyarrhythmia, MI.* **CNS:** Confusion, disorientation, symptoms of parkinsonism, gait disturbance, *seizures,* hallucinations, TIAs. **Hematologic:** *DVT, pulmonary embolism.* **Respiratory:** *Bronchospasm,* tachypnea, interstitial pneumonitis. **Metabolic:** Hyperglycemia, hyponatremia. **Miscellaneous:** Reversible renal insufficiency, worsening of dermatomyositis.

HOW SUPPLIED

Injection: 2 million international units/ 0.5 mL, 3 million international units/0.5 mL.

DOSAGE

- **SC**

Chronic granulomatous disease. Severe, malignant osteoporosis.
50 mcg/m^2 (1 million units/m^2) for clients whose body surface is greater than 0.5 m^2. If the body surface is less than 0.5 m^2, the dose of interferon gamma should be 1.5 mcg/kg/dose. The drug is given 3 times per week (e.g., Monday, Wednesday, Friday).

NURSING CONSIDERATIONS

ADMINISTRATION/STORAGE

1. Preferred injection sites: right and left deltoid; anterior thigh.
2. Does not contain a preservative. Use the vial only for a single dose and discard any unused portion.
3. Safety and effectiveness have not been determined for doses greater or less than 50 mcg/m^2.
4. If severe side effects occur, dose can be reduced by 50% or therapy can be discontinued until these subside.

5. May be administered using either sterilized glass or plastic disposable syringes.

6. Do not shake the vial; avoid vigorous agitation.

7. Vials must be stored at 2–8°C (36–46°F) to assure optimal retention of activity. Do not freeze vial.

8. Discard vials stored at room temperature for more than 12 hr.

9. Do not store undiluted drug in syringes due to syringe adhesion.

IV 10. Although not FDA approved, the drug has been given by continuous (10 days to 8 weeks) or intermittent (at 1, 6, or 24 hr) IV infusion as well as by IM injection.

ASSESSMENT

1. List age at onset, any treatments used in the past to reduce frequency/severity of infections, DEXA bone scan results.

2. Note history of CAD or CNS disorders; assess for symptoms or seizure history.

3. Monitor urinalysis, CBC, renal, LFTs q 3 months.

CLIENT/FAMILY TEACHING

1. Review reconstitution, method for administration, storage (keep vial refrigerated), and disposal of drug/equipment.

2. Keep drug in the refrigerator; do *not* shake container.

3. Take at bedtime with acetaminophen to minimize flu-like symptoms (fever and headaches).

4. Consume 2–3 L/day of fluids.

5. Avoid alcohol and any other CNS depressants.

6. Avoid activities that require mental alertness until drug effects realized.

7. Close medical supervision is imperative with this disease and genetically engineered drug therapy as dosage may require frequent adjustments. Report concerns and adverse effects.

OUTCOMES/EVALUATE

- Suppression of infective organisms associated with chronic granulomatous disease

- Control of malignant osteoporosis progression

Ipratropium bromide

(eye-prah-**TROH**-pee-um)

CLASSIFICATION(S):
Cholinergic blocking drug

PREGNANCY CATEGORY: B

Rx: Atrovent, Atrovent HFA.

✿**Rx:** Apo-Ipravent, Gen-Ipratropium, Novo-Ipramide, Nu-Ipratropium, PMS-Ipratropium, ratio-Ipratropium, ratio-Ipratropium UDV.

SEE ALSO *CHOLINERGIC BLOCKING AGENTS.*

USES

Aerosol or solution for inhalation: Alone or with other bronchodilators, especially beta-adrenergics, as a bronchodilator for maintenance treatment of bronchospasm associated with COPD, including chronic bronchitis and emphysema.

Nasal spray: (1) Symptomatic relief (using 0.03%) of rhinorrhea associated with allergic and nonallergic perennial rhinitis in clients over 6 years of age. (2) Symptomatic relief (using 0.06%) of rhinorrhea associated with the common cold in those aged 5 and older. It does not relieve nasal congestion or sneezing associated with the common cold or seasonal allergic rhinits. *NOTE:* The use of ipratropium with sympathomimetic bronchodilators, methylxanthines, steroids, or cromolyn sodium (all of which are used in treating COPD) are without side effects.

ACTION/KINETICS

Action

Chemically related to atropine. Antagonizes the action of acetylcholine. Prevents the increase in intracellular levels of cyclic guanosine monophosphate, which is caused by the interaction of acetylcholine with muscarinic receptors in bronchial smooth muscle; this leads to bronchodilation which is primarily a local, site-specific effect.

Pharmacokinetics

Poorly absorbed into the systemic cir-

Bold Italic = life threatening side effect   ◼ = black box warning   ✿ = Available in Canada culation (about 7%). About 50% of unchanged drug excreted through the urine. t½, **elimination:** 2 hr after use of the inhalation aerosol and 1.6 hr after use of the nasal spray.

CONTRAINDICATIONS

Hypersensitivity to atropine, ipratropium, or derivatives. Hypersensitivity to soy lecithin or related food products, including soybean or peanut (inhalation aerosol). Use for initial treatment of acute bronchospasms.

SPECIAL CONCERNS

Use with caution in clients with narrow-angle glaucoma, prostatic hypertrophy, or bladder neck obstruction and during lactation. Use of ipratropium as a single agent for the relief of bronchospasm in acute COPD has not been studied adequately. Safety and efficacy of the aerosol has not been derermined in children; of the solution in children less than 12 years of age; of the nasal spray, 0.03%, in children less than 6 years of age; and of the nasal spray, 0.06%, in children less than 5 years of age.

SIDE EFFECTS

Most Common

Use of inhalation aerosol: Headache, dizziness, chest pain, URTI, nausea, bronchitis, coughing, dyspnea, pharyngitis, pain.

Use of nasal spray: Headache, pharyngitis, URTI, epistaxis, nasal dryness, nausea, nasal irritation. dry mouth/throat, taste perversion.

Inhalation aerosol. CNS: Cough, nervousness, dizziness, headache, fatigue, insomnia, drowsiness, difficulty in coordination, tremor. **GI:** Dryness of oropharynx, GI distress, dry mouth, nausea, constipation. **CV:** Palpitations, tachycardia, flushing. **Dermatologic:** Itching, hives, alopecia. **Miscellaneous:** Irritation from aerosol, worsening of symptoms, rash, hoarseness, blurred vision, difficulty in accommodation, drying of secretions, urinary difficulty, paresthesias, mucosal ulcers. **Inhalation solution. CNS:** Dizziness, insomnia, nervousness, tremor, headache. **GI:** Dry mouth, nausea, constipation.
CV: Hypertension, aggravation of hypertension, tachycardia, palpitations.

Respiratory: Worsening of COPD symptoms, URTI, coughing, dyspnea, bronchitis, **bronchospasm**, increased sputum, URI, pharyngitis, rhinitis, sinusitis. **Miscellaneous:** Urinary retention, UTIs, urticaria, pain, flu-like symptoms, back/chest pain, arthritis. **Nasal spray. CNS:** Headache, dizziness. **GI:** Nausea, dry mouth, taste perversion. **CV:** Palpitation, tachycardia. **Respiratory:** URTI, epistaxis, pharyngitis, nasal dryness, miscellaneous nasal symptoms, nasal irritation, blood-tinged mucus, dry throat, cough, nasal congestion/burning, coughing. **Ophthalmic:** Ocular irritation, blurred vision, conjunctivitis. **Miscellaneous:** Hoarseness, thirst, tinnitis, urinary retention. **All products. Allergic:** Skin rash, angioedema of the tongue, throat, lips, and face; urticaria, **laryngospasm**, oropharyngeal edema, **bronchospasm, anaphylaxis. Anticholinergic reactions:** Precipitation or worsening of narrow angle glaucoma, prostatic disorders, tachycardia, urinary retention, constipation, bowel obstruction, blurred vision, difficulty in accommodation. *NOTE:* Rarely, immediate hypersensitivity reactions may occur. Symptoms include urticaria, angioedema, rash, **bronchospasm, anaphylaxis, and oropharyngeal edema.**

DRUG INTERACTIONS

Potential additive interaction when used concomitantly with other anticholinergics

HOW SUPPLIED

Inhalation Aerosol: 17 mcg/inh (HFA aerosol), 18 mcg/inh; *Nasal Spray:* 0.03% (21 mcg/spray), 0.06% (42 mcg/spray); *Solution for Inhalation:* 0.02% (500 mcg/vial).

DOSAGE

• **INHALATION AEROSOL (HFA)**
  Treat bronchospasms.
Adults: 2 inhalations (34 mcg) 4 times per day. Additional inhalations may be required but should not exceed 12 inhalations/day.

• **SOLUTION FOR INHALATION**
  Treat bronchospasms.
Adults: 500 mcg (1-unit-dose vial) given 3–4 times per day by oral nebulization with doses 6–8 hr apart. Can be

---

mixed in the nebulizer with albuterol or metaproterenol if used within 1 hr.

- **NASAL SPRAY, 0.03%**
  Perennial rhinitis.

Adults and children, 6 years and older: 2 sprays (42 mcg) per nostril 2–3 times per day for a total daily dose of 168–252 mcg/day. Optimum dose varies.

- **NASAL SPRAY, 0.06%**
  Rhinitis due to the common cold.

Adults and children, 12 years and older: 2 sprays (84 mcg) per nostril 3–4 times per day for a total daily dose of 504–672 mcg/day. **Children, 5–11 years:** 2 sprays (84 mcg) per nostril 3 times per day (total dose of 504 mcg/day). Safety and efficacy for use for the common cold for more than 4 days have not been determined.

Rhinorrhea associated with seasonal allergic rhinitis.

Adults and children, 5 years and older: 2 sprays (84 mcg) per nostril 4 times per day (total of 672 mcg/day). Safety and efficacy for use beyond 3 weeks have not been determined.

NURSING CONSIDERATIONS

⚸ Do not confuse Atrovent with Alupent (a sympathomimetic).

ADMINISTRATION/STORAGE

1. Use of a nebulizer with mouthpiece rather than a face mask may be preferable to reduce the chance of the nebulizer solution reaching the eyes.
2. Store the aerosol between 15–30°C (59–86°F); avoid excessive humidity.
3. Store solution between 15–30°C (59–86°F); protect from light. Store unused vials in the foil pouch.
4. Store nasal spray tightly closed between 15–30°C (59–86°F). Avoid freezing.

ASSESSMENT

1. List type, onset, characteristics of S&S, other agents used, outcome.
2. Perform full pulmonary assessment; monitor PFTs and x-rays.
3. Note any prostate gland enlargement, difficulty urinating; may aggravate.

CLIENT/FAMILY TEACHING

1. Take only as directed; shake well before using. Review administration technique. Rinse mouth and equipment after use. With inhalers do not exceed 12 inhalations in 24 hr; with nasal spray do not exceed 8 sprays in each nostril in 24 hr.
2. Prime or actuate the HFA inhalation aerosol before using for the first time by releasing 2 test sprays into the air away from the face. In cases where the inhaler has not been used for more than 3 days, prime the inhaler again by releasing 2 sprays into the air away from the face.
3. If using more than one inhalation per dose, wait 3 min before administering the second inhalation. If also prescribed steroid inhaler use ipratropium and then wait 5 min before using the steroid inhaler.
4. Drug is not for use in terminating an acute attack; effects take up to 15 min. Have another prescribed agent readily available in this event.
5. Avoid contact with the eyes. A spacer may be useful with the inhaler and a mouthpiece with the nebulizer to help prevent solution (mist) contact with the eyes; also enhances lung dispersion.
6. May experience a bitter taste and dry mouth; use frequent mouth rinses and hard candy to relieve.
7. Transient dizziness, insomnia, blurred vision, or excessive weakness may occur, use caution.
8. Stop smoking now to preserve current level of lung function and to prevent further damage; utilize smoking cessation program.
9. Keep all F/U appointments to evaluate response to therapy.

OUTCOMES/EVALUATE

- Improved airway exchange and breathing patterns
- ↓ Wheezing, dyspnea
- Relief of rhinorrhea

—COMBINATION DRUG—

Ipratropium bromide and Albuterol sulfate

(eye-prah-**TROH**-pee-um, al-**BYOU**-ter-ohl)

CLASSIFICATION(S):
Cholinergic blocking drug and sympathomimetic

PREGNANCY CATEGORY: C

Rx: Combivent, DuoNeb.

SEE ALSO *IPRATROPIUM BROMIDE AND ALBUTEROL SULFATE.*

USES
Treatment of COPD (including bronchospasms) in those who are on regular aerosol bronchodilator therapy and who require a second bronchodilator.

CONTENT
Combivent: Each actuation of the Aerosol delivers: Ipratropium bromide (*cholinergic blocking drug*), 18 mcg; and Albuterol sulfate (*sympathomimetic*), 103 mcg. **DuoNeb:** Inhalation Solution contains: Ipratropium bromide (*cholinergic blocking drug*), 0.5 mg and Albuterol sulfate (*sympathomimetic*), 3 mg (equivalent to 2.5 mg albuterol base).

ACTION/KINETICS
Action
Ipratropium is an anticholinergic drug that acts to inhibit the effect of acetylcholine following vagal nerve stimulation. This results in bronchodilation which is primarily a local, site-specific effect. Albuterol is a beta$_2$-adrenergic agonist that also causes bronchodilation.

Pharmacokinetics
Ipratropium is poorly absorbed into the systemic circulation. About 50% of unchanged drug excreted in the urine. **t½, elimination:** 2 hr after inhalation. After inhalation, the onset for albuterol is within 5 min; peak effect occurs within 60–90 min and duration is 3–6 hr. Albuterol and metabolites are excreted in the urine and feces.

CONTRAINDICATIONS
History of hypersensitivity to soy lecithin or related food products, such as soybean and peanuts. Lactation.

SPECIAL CONCERNS
Use with caution in CV disorders, especially coronary insufficiency, cardiac arrhythmias, and hypertension. Use with caution in narrow-angle glaucoma, prostatic hypertrophy, bladder-neck obstruction, convulsive disorders, hyperthyroidism, diabetes mellitus, in those unusually responsive to sympathomimetic amines, and renal or hepatic disease. Safety and efficacy have not been determined in children.

SIDE EFFECTS
Most Common
Bronchitis, URTI, headache, pain, dyspnea, coughing, nausea, pharyngitis, sinusitis.

Respiratory: *Paradoxical bronchospasm*, bronchitis, dyspnea, coughing, respiratory disorders, pneumonia, URTI, pharyngitis, sinusitis, rhinitis. **CV:** ECG changes including flattening of T wave, prolongation of QTc interval, and ST segment depression. Also, arrhythmias, palpitation, tachycardia, angina, hypertension. **Hypersensitivity, immediate:** Urticaria, *angioedema, bronchospasm, anaphylaxis, oropharyngeal edema.* **Body as a whole:** Headache, pain, flu, chest pain, edema, fatigue. **GI:** N&V, dry mouth, diarrhea, dyspepsia. **CNS:** Dizziness, nervousness, headache, paresthesia, tremor, dysphonia, insomnia. **Miscellaneous:** Arthralgia, increased sputum, taste perversion, UTI, dysuria, pain.

DRUG INTERACTIONS
See individual drugs.

HOW SUPPLIED
See Content.

DOSAGE
- **AEROSOL (COMBIVENT)**
  COPD.
  2 inhalations q 6 hr not to exceed 12 inhalations/24-hr.
- **INHALATION SOLUTION (DUONEB)**
  COPD.
  One 3-mL vial given 4 times per day via nebulization with up to 2 additional 3-mL doses daily, if needed.

NURSING CONSIDERATIONS

Ⓒ Do not confuse Combivent with Combivir (combination antiviral drug to treat AIDS).

ADMINISTRATION/STORAGE
1. Aerosol canister provides sufficient medication for 200 inhalations.
2. Discard canister after labeled number of inhalations used.
3. Give DuoNeb via a jet nebulizer connected to an air compressor with an adequate air flow, equipped with mouthpiece or suitable face mask.
4. Store Combivent between 15–30°C (59–86°F). Avoid excessive humidity. Canister should be at room temperature before use.
5. Store DuoNeb between 2–25°C (36–77°F). Protect from light.

ASSESSMENT
1. Assess for soybean or peanut allergy.
2. Note reasons for therapy, characteristics/frequency of symptoms/sputum production, other agents trialed, outcome.
3. Assess breath sounds, triggers; monitor CXR, symptoms, and PFTs.

CLIENT/FAMILY TEACHING
1. Use as directed; do not increase dose or frequency of administration unless specifically directed.
2. Avoid excessive humidity. For best results, have canister at room temperature before use.
3. Shake canister well before using. Review administration guidelines and rinse mouth and equipment after each use. Use a spacer to facilitate dispersion.
4. Test canister spray 3 times before first use and again if the canister has not been used for 24 hr.
5. Report any loss of effectiveness, change in symptoms early to prevent exacerbation and resultant hospitalization. If steroid inhaler also prescribed, use combivent first and wait 5 min before using the steroid to ensure better lung penetration.
6. Avoid eye contact; report any visual disturbances or eye irritation.
7. Drug is not for use in terminating an acute attack; effects take up to 15 min.

Have another prescribed agent readily available.
8. Stop smoking to preserve current level of lung function and to prevent further damage; utilize smoking cessation program.

OUTCOMES/EVALUATE
Improved airway exchange with ↓ cough/SOB/sputum production

Irbesartan ■ 📷
(ihr-beh-**SAR**-tan)

CLASSIFICATION(S):
Antihypertensive, angiotensin II receptor blocker
PREGNANCY CATEGORY: C (first trimester), **D** (second and third trimesters).
Rx: Avapro.

SEE ALSO *ANGIOTENSIN II RECEPTOR ANTAGONISTS AND ANTIHYPERTENSIVE DRUGS.*

USES
(1) Hypertension, alone or in combination with other antihypertensives. (2) Nephropathy in type 2 diabetics with an elevated serum creatinine and proteinuria (greater than 300 mg/day). Will reduce rate of progression of renal disease. *Investigational:* Heart failure.

ACTION/KINETICS

Action
Competitively blocks the angiotensin AT_1 receptor located in vascular smooth muscle and the adrenal glands, thus blocking the vasoconstrictor and aldosterone-secreting effects of angiotensin II (a potent vasoconstrictor). Thus, BP is reduced.

Pharmacokinetics
Rapid absorption after PO use. **Peak plasma levels:** 1.5–2 hr. Is 60–80% bioavailable; food does not affect bioavailability. Effect somewhat less in Blacks. t_{max}: 1.5–2 hr. $t\frac{1}{2}$, **terminal elimination:** 11–15 hr. Metabolized in liver by CYP2C9 and both unchanged drug and metabolites excreted through urine (20%) and feces (80%). **Plasma protein binding:** More than 90%.

Bold Italic = life threatening side effect   ■ = black box warning   ✦ = Available in Canada

SPECIAL CONCERNS

■ When used during the second and third trimester of pregnancy, drugs that act directly on the renin-angiotensin system can cause injury and even death to the fetus. When pregnancy is detected, discontinue as soon as possible.■ Safety and efficacy have not been determined in children less than 6 years of age.

SIDE EFFECTS

Most Common

URTI, cough, fatigue, dyspepsia/heartburn, diarrhea.

GI: Diarrhea, dyspepsia, heartburn, abdominal distension/pain, N&V, constipation, oral lesion, gastroenteritis, flatulence. **CV:** Tachycardia, syncope, orthostatic hypo/hypertension, hypotension (especially in volume- or salt-depletion), flushing, cardiac murmur, *MI, cardiorespiratory arrest, heart failure, hypertensive crisis, CVA*, angina pectoris, arrhythmias, conduction disorder, TIA. **CNS:** Sleep disturbance, fatigue, anxiety, nervousness, dizziness, numbness, somnolence, emotional disturbance, depression, paresthesia, tremor. **Musculoskeletal:** Extremity swelling, muscle cramp/ache/weakness, arthritis, musculoskeletal pain, musculoskeletal chest pain, joint stiffness, bursitis. **Respiratory:** Cough, epistaxis, tracheobronchitis, congestion, pulmonary congestion, dyspnea, wheezing, URTI, rhinitis, pharyngitis, sinus abnormality. **GU:** Abnormal urination, prostate disorder, UTI, sexual dysfunction, libido change. **Dermatologic:** Pruritus, dermatitis, ecchymosis, facial erythema, urticaria. **Ophthalmic:** Vision disturbance, conjunctivitis, eyelid abnormality. **Otic:** Hearing abnormality, ear infection/pain/abnormality. **Miscellaneous:** Gout, fever, fatigue, chills, facial edema, upper extremity edema, headache, influenza, rash, chest pain.

LABORATORY TEST CONSIDERATIONS

↑ BUN (minor), serum creatinine. ↓ Hemoglobin. Neutropenia.

HOW SUPPLIED

Tablets: 75 mg, 150 mg, 300 mg.

DOSAGE

• **TABLETS**

Hypertension.

150 mg once daily with or without food, up to 300 mg once daily. Lower initial dose of 75 mg is recommended for clients with depleted intravascular volume or salt. If BP is not controlled by irbesartan alone, hydrochlorothiazide may have an additive effect. Clients not adequately treated by 300 mg irbesartan are unlikely to get benefit from higher dose or twice a day dosing. **Children, 6–12 years, initial:** 75 mg once daily. Titrate those requiring further reduction in BP to 150 mg once daily. **Children, 13–16 years, initial:** 150 mg once daily. Titrate those requiring further reduction in BP to 300 mg once daily.

Nephropathy in type 2 diabetics.

Adults: Target dose is 300 mg once daily. **Adolescents, 13–16 years of age, initial:** 150 mg once daily. Titrate those requiring further reduction in BP to 300 mg once daily. **Children, 6–12 years of age, initial:** 75 mg once daily. Titrate those requiring further reduction in BP to 150 mg once daily.

NURSING CONSIDERATIONS

ADMINISTRATION/STORAGE

1. Dose adjustment is not required in geriatric clients or in hepatic or renal impairment.
2. May be given with other antihypertensive drugs.
3. Store between 15–30°C (59–86°F).

ASSESSMENT

1. Note reasons for therapy, onset, duration, characteristics of symptoms, other agents trialed.
2. If pregnancy detected, stop drug as soon as possible.
3. Observe infants exposed to angiotensin II inhibitor in utero for hypotension, oliguria, and ↑ K.
4. Monitor VS, electrolytes, U/A, microalbumin, renal and LFTs.

CLIENT/FAMILY TEACHING

1. Take only as directed. May take with or without food.
2. Avoid tasks that require mental alertness until drug effects realized; may cause dizziness or drowsiness; change

positions slowly to prevent sudden drop in BP.

3. Continue low-fat, low-cholesterol diet, regular exercise, tobacco cessation, salt restriction, and lifestyle changes necessary to maintain lowered BP.

4. Practice reliable contraception. Stop drug and report if pregnancy suspected.

5. Record BP for provider review; report muscle/joint pains, anxiety, nervousness, cold symptoms, diarrhea, headaches, unusual tiredness, heartburn, stomach discomfort.

OUTCOMES/EVALUATE
↓ BP; Renal protection in DM.

—COMBINATION DRUG—

Irbesartan and Hydrochlorothiazide ■ 📷

(ihr-beh-**SAR**-tan, hy-droh-klor-oh-**THIGH**-ah-zyd)

CLASSIFICATION(S):
Antihypertensive (combination drug)
PREGNANCY CATEGORY: C (first trimester), **D** (second and third trimesters).
Rx: Avalide.

SEE ALSO *IRBESARTAN* AND *HYDROCHLOROTHIAZIDE*.

USES
Treatment of hypertension. Not indicated for initial therapy.

CONTENT
Avalide 150/12.5: Irbesartan (*angiotensin II receptor blocker*), 150 mg and hydrochlorothiazide (*thiazide diuretic*), 12.5 mg. *Avalide 300/12.5:* Irbesartan, 300 mg and hydrochlorothiazide, 12.5 mg. *Avalide 300/25:* Irbesartan, 300 mg and hydrochlorothiazide, 25 mg.

ACTION/KINETICS
Action
Irbesartan competitively blocks the angiotensin AT_1 receptor located in vascular smooth muscle and the adrenal glands, thus blocking the vasoconstric-

tor and aldosterone-secreting effects of angiotensin II (a potent vasoconstrictor). Thus, BP is reduced. The antihypertensive activity of hydrochlorothiazide is thought to be due to direct dilation of the arterioles, as well as to a reduction in the total fluid volume of the body and altered sodium balance.

Pharmacokinetics
Irbesartan is rapidly absorbed; absolute bioavailability is 60–80%. **Irbesartan, peak plasma levels:** 1.5–2 hr. **Maximum effect:** 4 hr; **duration:** 24 hr. Food does not affect bioavailability. **t½, terminal, irbesartan:** 11–15 hr. Irbesartan is mainly excreted unchanged (>80%) through the urine and feces. **Hydrochlorothiazide, onset:** 2 hr; **peak effect:** 4–6 hr; **duration:** 6–12 hr. **t½:** 5.6–14.8 hr. Hydrochlorothiazide is not metabolized but is eliminated rapidly by the kidney; about 61% excreted unchanged within 24 hr. **Plasma protein binding:** Irbesartan is 90% bound to plasma proteins.

CONTRAINDICATIONS
Hypersensitivity to any component of the product. In clients with anuria or hypersensitivity to sulfonamide-derived drugs. Use of lithium with diuretics reduces renal clearance of lithium and adds a high risk of lithium toxicity. Lactation.

SPECIAL CONCERNS
■ When used in pregnancy during the second and third trimesters, drugs that act directly on the renin-angiotensin system can cause injury and even death to the developing fetus. When pregnancy is detected, discontinue Avalide as soon as possible.■ Use with caution in impaired hepatic function or progressive liver disease since minor alterations of fluid and electrolyte imbalance can cause hepatic coma. Safety and efficacy have not been determined in children less than 18 years of age.

SIDE EFFECTS
Most Common
Hypokalemia, lightheadedness, musculoskeletal pain, fatigue, dizziness, edema, N&V.

See *Irbesartan* and *Hydrochlorothiazide* for a list of possible side effects. Also,

---

Bold Italic = life threatening side effect   ■ = black box warning   ✦ = Available in Canada

hypersensitivity reactions (with or without a history of allergy or bronchial asthma). Exacerbation or activation of systemic lupus erythematosus. Postmarketing side effects: Urticaria, **angioedema** (including swelling of the face, lips, pharynx, and/or tongue), hepatitis, jaundice (rare), **rhabdomyolysis** (rare).

LABORATORY TEST CONSIDERATIONS
Slight ↑ serum creatinine, BUN. Rarely, ↑ liver enzymes and/or serum bilirubin.

HOW SUPPLIED
See Content.

DOSAGE

- **TABLETS**
  Hypertension.
  Adults, usual: One tablet daily (i.e., 150 or 300 mg irbesartan and 12.5–25 mg hydrochlorothiazide). A lower initial dose of irbesartan (75 mg) is recommended in clients with depletion of intravascular volume.

NURSING CONSIDERATIONS

ADMINISTRATION/STORAGE
1. No dosage adjustment is needed in mild to severe renal impairment (unless the client is also volume depleted) or in hepatic insufficiency.
2. Clients not responding adequately to 300 mg irbesartan once daily are not likely to derive additional benefit from a higher dose or twice-daily dosing.
3. It is usually appropriate to begin combination therapy only after monotherapy has failed.
4. Avalide may be given with other antihypertensive drugs.
5. Store from 25–30°C (59–86°F).

ASSESSMENT
1. Note reasons for therapy, disease onset, other therapies trialed, outcome. Ensure adequately hydrated.
2. List agents prescribed to ensure none interact. Assess for sulfonamide allergy.
3. Monitor BP, electrolytes, renal, LFTs; determine if pregnant.

CLIENT/FAMILY TEACHING
1. May take with or without food with a full glass of water. Do not skip doses or double up if dose missed.
2. Take early in the day to prevent nighttime awakening to urinate.
3. May experience dizziness or drowsiness; avoid activities that require mental alertness until drug effects realized.
4. If lightheadedness or fainting occur, may be aggravated if diarrhea, vomiting, excessive sweating, poor fluid intake, or if on a low-salt diet.
5. Avoid alcohol or prolonged activities in hot weather; may cause dehydration and increased lightheadedness. Change positions slowly to prevent sudden drop in BP.
6. With diabetes may have elevated blood sugar; monitor finger sticks closely and adjust dosage of meds as needed.
7. Wear sunscreen and protective clothing if sun exposed; may cause photosensitivity reaction.
8. Practice reliable contraception; stop drug if pregnancy suspected.
9. Keep all F/U appointments for labs and drug response. Bring BP log for provider review. Report any adverse effects or lack of response.

OUTCOMES/EVALUATE
Desired BP control

Irinotecan hydrochloride ∎ IV
(**eye**-rih-noh-**TEE**-kan)

CLASSIFICATION(S):
Antineoplastic, hormone
PREGNANCY CATEGORY: D
Rx: Camptosar.

SEE ALSO *ANTINEOPLASTIC AGENTS.*

USES
(1) First-line therapy with 5-fluorouracil and leucovorin for metastatic colon or rectal carcinomas. (2) Metastatic carcinoma of the colon or rectum in those whose disease has recurred or progressed following 5-fluorouracil therapy.

ACTION/KINETICS

Action

The cytotoxic effect is due to double-strand DNA damage produced during DNA synthesis when replication enzymes interact with the ternary complex formed by topoisomerase I, DNA, and either irinotecan or SN-38 (its active metabolite). Conversion of irinotecan to SN-38 occurs in the liver.

Pharmacokinetics

$t^{1/2}$, terminal, irinotecan: About 6 hr; $t^{1/2}$, terminal, SN-38: About 10 hr. Plasma protein binding: SN-38: 95%.

CONTRAINDICATIONS

Use with the Mayo Clinic regimen of 5-FU/LV (i.e., administration for 4 to 5 days q 4 weeks) due to increased toxicity, including deaths. Lactation.

SPECIAL CONCERNS

■ (1) Give under the supervision of a physician experienced in the use of cancer chemotherapeutic drugs. Appropriate management of complications is possible only when adequate diagnostic and treatment facilities are readily available. (2) Irinotecan can cause both early and late forms of diarrhea that are mediated by different mechanisms. Both forms may be severe. Early diarrhea may be accompanied by cholinergic symptoms, including rhinitis, increased salivation, miosis, lacrimation, diaphoresis, flushing, and intestinal hyperperistalsis that may cause abdominal cramping. This type of diarrhea may be treated with atropine. Late diarrhea (occurring more than 24 hr after giving the drug) may be life-threatening because it may be prolonged and lead to dehydration, electrolyte imbalance, or sepsis. Treat late diarrhea promptly with loperamide. Monitor clients with diarrhea carefully and give fluid and electrolyte replacement if dehydration occurs, or give antibiotics if clients develop ileus, fever, or severe neutropenia. Stop irinotecan therapy and reduce subsequent dosage if severe diarrhea occurs. (3) Severe myelosuppression may occur.■ Clients who have previously received pelvic or abdominal irradiation are at an increased risk for severe myelosuppression when treated with irinotecan. Safety and efficacy have not been determined in children.

SIDE EFFECTS

Most Common

Neutropenia, anemia, leukopenia, thrombocytopenia, diarrhea, N&V, abdominal pain/cramping, anorexia, constipation, mucositis, dyspnea, cough, asthenia, pain, fever, infection, cholinergic syndrome.

NOTE: Side effects listed include symptoms of combination therapy with 5-FU and leucovorin. GI: Diarrhea (both early and late; may be life-threatening), cholinergic syndrome, N&V, anorexia, abdominal cramping or pain, constipation, flatulence, stomatitis, mucositis, dyspepsia, colitis, ileus. Hematologic: Severe myelosuppression, including leukopenia, anemia, neutropenia (including neutropenic fever/infection), serious thrombocytopenia (rare). CNS: Insomnia, dizziness, somnolence, confusion. Respiratory: Dyspnea, increased coughing, pneumonia, rhinitis, severe pulmonary events (rare). CV: Vasodilation, flushing, thromboembolism, orthostatic hypotension. Body as a whole: Asthenia, fever, pain, headache, back pain, chills, minor infections (usually UTI), edema, abdominal enlargement. Dermatologic: Alopecia, sweating, rashes, exfoliative dermatitis, hand and foot syndrome. Metabolic/nutritional: Decreased body weight, dehydration, hypersensitivity reactions, including *anaphylaxis*.

LABORATORY TEST CONSIDERATIONS

↑ AST, alkaline phosphatase, bilirubin.

OD OVERDOSE MANAGEMENT

Symptoms: Extension of side effects. Treatment: Maximum supportive care to prevent dehydration due to diarrhea. Treat any infections.

DRUG INTERACTIONS

Antineoplastic agents / ↑ Risk of myelosuppression and diarrhea

Dexamethasone / ↑ Risk of lymphocytopenia and hyperglycemia

Diuretics / ↑ Risk of dehydration secondary to diarrhea and vomiting

Phenytoin / ↓ AUC and ↑ irinotecan clearance

Prochlorperazine / ↑ Risk of akathisia

HOW SUPPLIED
Injection: 20 mg/mL.

DOSAGE

- **IV INFUSION**
  Metastatic carcinoma of the colon or rectum.

Combination agent dosage regimen 1: *Irinotecan:* 125 mg/m^2 given as an IV infusion over 90 min on days 1, 8, 15, and 22, followed by a 2-week rest period. *5-Fluorouracil:* 500 mg/m^2 by IV bolus on days 1, 8, 15, and 22 followed by a 2-week rest period. *Leucovorin:* 20 mg/m^2 by IV bolus on days 1, 8, 15, and 22, followed by a 2-week rest period. Next course begins on day 43.

Combination agent dosage regimen 2: *Irinotecan:* 180 mg/m^2 by IV infusion over 90 min on days 1, 15, and 29. *5-Fluorouracil:* 400 mg/m^2 by IV bolus on days 1, 2, 15, 16, 29, and 30. This is followed by an IV infusion over 22 hr of 600 mg/m^2 on days 1, 2, 15, 16, 29, and 30. *Leucovorin:* 200 mg/m^2 IV over 2 hr on days 1, 2, 15, 16, 29, and 30. Next course begins on day 43. *NOTE:* Modifications of the dosage are based on the degree of neutropenia, neutropenic fever, diarrhea, and other toxicities. Consult the package insert for specific dosage modifications.

Single-agent dosage schedule regimen 1, initial: 125 mg/m^2 IV over 90 min on days 1, 8, 15, and 22, followed by a 2-week rest period. Subsequent doses may be adjusted as high as 150 mg/m^2 or as low as 50 mg/m^2 in 25-50 mg/m^2 decrements depending on toxicity. If intolerable toxicity does not occur, courses of treatment may be continued indefinitely, as long as beneficial effects are noted.

Single-agent dosage schedule regimen 2: 350 mg/m^2 given IV over 90 min once every three weeks. Subsequent doses may be adjusted as low as 200 mg/m^2 in 50 mg/m^2 decrements, depending on toxicity.

NURSING CONSIDERATIONS

ADMINISTRATION/STORAGE

[IV] 1. Avoid extravasation. If extravasation occurs, flush site with sterile water and apply ice.

2. Causes vomiting; give antiemetic therapy; this includes dexamethasone, 10 mg, and a 5-HT$_3$ blocker such as granisetron or ondansetron; give 30 min before giving irinotecan.

3. Prepare infusion solution by diluting in D5W (preferred) or 0.9% NaCl to a final concentration of 0.12-1.1 mg/mL; administer over 90 min.

4. Solutions diluted in D5W, stored in the refrigerator, and protected from light are stable for 48 hr. However, due to possible microbial contamination during dilution, use refrigerated admixtures within 24 hr or, if kept at room temperature, use within 6 hr. Do not refrigerate admixtures containing 0.9% NaCl. Freezing irinotecan or admixtures may cause drug precipitation.

ASSESSMENT

1. Note reasons for therapy; assess for any history of pelvic/abdominal irradiation and last 5-FU therapy.

2. List all drugs currently prescribed to ensure none exacerbate side effects.

3. Drug is emetogenic; administer antiemetics 30 min prior to therapy.

4. May need IV atropine for those who experience early-onset abdominal cramps, diarrhea, or diaphoresis.

5. Assess infusion site carefully; flush site with sterile water and apply ice with extravasation.

6. Obtain CBC before each treatment. Hold if ANC below 500/mm^3 or neutropenic fever occurs. Any significant reduction in WBC (<2,000/mm^3), neutrophil count (<1,000/mm^3), or platelet count (<100,000/mm^3) warrants dose reduction.

CLIENT/FAMILY TEACHING

1. Drug is administered IV usually weekly but depends on condition and reasons for treatment.

2. Diarrhea may occur within 24 hr of therapy; is cholinergic in nature and usually transient.

3. Report if temperature is over 101°F or diarrhea, vomiting, or dehydration develop.

4. With late-onset diarrhea (usually 10 days after therapy) take 4 mg of loperamide, followed by 2 mg q 2 h for 12 hr until diarrhea free (or other antidiar-

---

rheal prescribed). After the first treatment, delay weekly chemotherapy in clients with diarrhea until bowel function returns to pretreatment status. Consume extra fluids to prevent dehydration. Report if persistent or unresponsive to therapy.

5. Avoid laxatives unless approved. Keep all F/U appointments for labs and evaluation.

6. Practice birth control during and for several months following therapy.

7. Avoid crowds, those with active infections, and immunizations during drug therapy. Report any unusual bruising/bleeding. Avoid alcohol and OTC agents without approval.

OUTCOMES/EVALUATE
Inhibition of malignant cell proliferation

Iron dextran parenteral ■ IV

CLASSIFICATION(S):
Antianemic, iron
PREGNANCY CATEGORY: C
Rx: DexFerrum, InFeD.
♣Rx: Dexiron, Infufur.

USES
IV or IM treatment of documented iron deficiency where oral use is unsatisfactory or impossible. *Investigational:* Iron supplementation in clients receiving epoetin therapy.

ACTION/KINETICS
Action
A complex of ferric hydroxide and dextran that is removed from the plasma by the reticuloendothelial system which splits the complex into iron and dextran. The iron is bound to protein to form hemosiderin or ferritin, which replenishes hemoglobin and depleted iron stores.

Pharmacokinetics
After IM, most absorbed within 72 hr and the rest over 3–4 weeks. $t\frac{1}{2}$: From 5 hr (circulating iron dextran) to more than 20 hr (total iron, both circulating and bound). Negligible amounts of iron in iron dextran are lost via the urine and feces.

CONTRAINDICATIONS
All anemias not associated with iron deficiency. Acute phase of infectious kidney disease. Use in infants less than 4 months of age.

SPECIAL CONCERNS
■ Parenteral complexes of iron and carbohydrates may cause anaphylactic reactions. Deaths have been reported; thus, use iron dextran injection only in those clients in whom the indications have been clearly established and laboratory tests confirm an iron-deficient acute state not amenable to oral iron therapy. Because fatal anaphylactic reactions have been reported after administration of iron dextran injection, give the drug only when resuscitation techniques and treatment of anaphylactic and anaphylactoid shock are readily available.■ Use with extreme caution in seriously impaired liver function. Use with caution during lactation and in clients with a history of significant allergies/asthma. Rheumatoid arthritis clients may have an acute exacerbation of joint pain and swelling after iron dextran. Side effects may exacerbate CV complications in clients with preexisting CV disease. Unwarranted therapy will cause excess storage of iron with the possibility of exogenous hemosiderosis.

Large IV or IM doses may cause arthralgia, backache, chills, dizziness, moderate to high fever, headache, malaise, myalgia, N&V (onset is 24–48 hr; symptoms usually subside within 3–4 days after IV and within 3–7 days after IM).

SIDE EFFECTS
Most Common
Flushing, headache, dizziness, tingling of hands/feet, N&V, diarrhea, shivering, injection site reaction, metallic taste.

Delayed reactions (1–2 days): Arthralgia, backache, chills, dizziness, moderate to high fever, headache, malaise, myalgia, N&V. **Hypersensitivity:** *Anaphylaxis.* **GI:** Abdominal pain, N&V, diarrhea. **CNS:** Convulsions, syncope, headache, weakness, unresponsiveness, paresthesia, febrile episodes, dizziness, disorientation, numbness, uncon-

---

sciousness. **CV:** Chest pain, chest tightness, shock, *cardiac arrest*, hypotension, hypertension, tachycardia, bradycardia, flushing, arrhythmias. Also, flushing and hypotension from too rapid IV injection. **Respiratory:** Dyspnea, bronchospasm, wheezing, *respiratory arrest*. **Musculoskeletal:** Arthralgia, tingling of hands/feet, arthritis (including reactivation), myalgia, backache, sterile abscess, atrophy/fibrosis (at IM injection site), soreness or pain at or near IM injection site, cellulitis, swelling, inflammation, local phlebitis at or near IV injection site, brown skin or underlying tissue discoloration. **Hematologic:** Leukocytosis, lymphadenopathy. **Dermatologic:** Urticaria, pruritus, purpura, rash, cyanosis. **Miscellaneous:** Hematuria, sweating, shivering, chills, malaise, altered taste (metallic), carcinogenesis after IM injection. *Note:* Unwarranted therapy with parenteral iron will cause excess storage of iron with possible exogenous hemosiderosis, especially in those with hemoglobinopathies and other refractory anemias that might be erroneously diagnosed as iron deficiency anemia.

OD OVERDOSE MANAGEMENT
Symptoms: Hemosiderosis. Probably no acute manifestations. *Treatment:* Monitor serum ferritin levels periodically to determine a deleterious progressive accumulation of iron resulting from impaired uptake of iron from the reticuloendothelial system in concurrent medical conditions, such as chronic renal failure, Hodgkin's disease, and rheumatoid arthritis.

DRUG INTERACTIONS
If taken with chloramphenicol, may see ↑ serum iron levels R/T ↓ iron clearance and erythropoiesis R/T direct bone marrow toxicity.

HOW SUPPLIED
Injection: 50 mg iron/mL (as dextran).

DOSAGE
- **IM, IV**
  Iron deficiency.
Dosage is based on results of hematology data. The table in the package insert must be used to estimate the total iron required to restore hemoglobin to normal or near normal levels plus an additional allowance to replenish iron stores. The information in the table is to be used only in clients with iron deficiency anemia; it is not to be used to determine dosage in those needing iron replacement for blood loss.

IV injection. Prior to the first therapeutic dose, give an IV test dose of 0.5 mL slowly (over 30 seconds for InFeD or 5 minutes or more for DexFerrum). To ensure the client does not experience an anaphylactic reaction, allow 1 hr or more to elapse before the remainder of the initial therapeutic dose is given. Individual doses of 2 mL or less may be given daily until the calculated total amount of iron required has been administered. Give undiluted and slowly 50 mg or less/min (1 mL or less/min).

IM injection. As with IV administration, give a 0.5 mL test dose as described above. If no side effects occur, give injections as follows until the calculated total amount of iron has been administered. Do not exceed a daily dose of 25 mg iron (i.e., 0.5 mL) for infants less than 5 kg, 50 mg iron (i.e., 1 mL) for children less than 10 kg, and 100 mg iron (i.e., 2 mL) for all others.

NURSING CONSIDERATIONS
ADMINISTRATION/STORAGE
1. For IM, inject into the upper outer quadrant of the buttock; never inject into the arm or other exposed areas. Inject deeply with a 2 or 3 inch 19- or 20-gauge needle.
2. If client is standing, have client bear weight on the leg opposite the injection site. If in bed, have client lie in a lateral position with injection site uppermost.
3. To avoid leakage or injection into SC tissue, use a Z-track technique.
IV 4. Do not mix iron dextran with other drugs or add to parenteral nutrition solutions for IV infusion.
5. No more than 2 mL should be given daily.
ASSESSMENT
1. Note reasons for therapy (ensure iron deficieny anemia), onset, reason

oral replacement not used, previous therapies trialed.

2. Assess for CAD, significant allergies, asthma.

3. With rheumatoid arthritis may experience acute exacerbation of joint swelling and pain after dosing.

4. Ensure test dose performed as directed (0.5 mL given over 5 min before first IM or IV dose to assess response to drug; allow 1 hr to elapse before therapy). Delayed reactions may occur manifested by N&V, chills, fever, arthralgia, backache, malaise, myalgia.

5. Assess H&H and reticulocyte count. Serum iron levels not useful until 3 weeks, ferritin peaks in 7–9 days and reliable at 3 weeks.

6. May alter bone scans and discolor blood brown in samples drawn 4 hr after treatment.

7. May falsely elevate bilirubin and decrease calcium. Keep this in mind when monitoring lab values.

CLIENT/FAMILY TEACHING

1. Iron is essential for red cell synthesis so is replaced when iron stores depleted.

2. May notice pain and brown staining at injection site. Stools usually appear black to dark green in color during therapy.

3. Do not consume oral iron or vitamins when receiving injections. Iron poisoning may occur if intake is excessive.

4. Report any bleeding sources, unusual or adverse side effects. Therapy may end once anemia is corrected.

OUTCOMES/EVALUATE

Iron replacement with iron deficiency anemia

Isoniazid (INH, Isonicotinic acid hydrazide) ■
(eye-so-**NYE**-ah-zid)

CLASSIFICATION(S):
Antitubercular drug
PREGNANCY CATEGORY: C
Rx: Nydrazid Injection.
✤Rx: Isotamine, PMS-Isoniazid.

USES

(1) Tuberculosis caused by human, bovine, and BCG strains of *Mycobacterium tuberculosis*. Not to be used as the sole tuberculostatic agent. (2) Prophylaxis of tuberculosis in the following: HIV, close contacts with those newly diagnosed with infectious tuberculosis, recent converters, abnormal chest radiographs, IV drug users, those with increased risk of tuberculosis, those less than 35 years of age with tuberculin skin test reaction 10 mm or greater, and children less than 4 years of age if they have greater than 10 mm induration from a purified protein derivative Mantoux tuberculin skin test. *Investigational:* To improve severe tremor in clients with multiple sclerosis.

ACTION/KINETICS

Action

The most effective tuberculostatic agent. Probably interferes with lipid and nucleic acid metabolism of growing bacteria, resulting in alteration of the bacterial wall. Is tuberculostatic.

Pharmacokinetics

Readily absorbed after PO and parenteral (IM) administration and widely distributed in body tissues, including cerebrospinal, pleural, and ascitic fluids. **Peak plasma concentration: PO,** 1–2 hr. **$t^{1/2}$, fast acetylators:** 0.5–6 hr; **$t^{1/2}$, slow acetylators:** 2–5 hr. Liver and kidney impairment increase these values. Metabolized in liver and excreted primarily in urine. The metabolism of isoniazid is genetically determined. Clients fall into two groups, depending on the rapidity with which they metabolize isoniazid. As a rule, 50% of Whites and Blacks inactivate the drug slowly, whereas the majority of American Indians, Eskimos, Japanese, and Chinese are rapid acetylators (inactivators).

1. **Slow acetylators:** These clients show earlier, favorable response but have more toxic reactions (e.g., neuropathies because of higher blood levels of drug).

2. **Rapid acetylators:** These clients have possible poor clinical response due to rapid inactivation, which is 5–6 times faster than slow acetylators. This group requires an increased daily dose of the drug. They are more likely to develop hepatitis.

CONTRAINDICATIONS
Severe hypersensitivity to isoniazid or in clients with previous isoniazid-associated hepatic injury or side effects. Active liver disease.

SPECIAL CONCERNS
■ (1) Severe and sometimes fatal hepatitis may occur even after several months of therapy; incidence is age-related. Daily alcohol use increases the risk. (2) Carefully monitor and interview clients at monthly intervals. For people over 25 years, in addition to monthly interviews, measure AST and ALT prior to starting isoniazid therapy and periodically during therapy. Isoniazid-induced hepatitis usually occurs during the first three months of treatment. Enzyme levels generally return to normal even if continuing drug therapy; in some cases, however, progressive liver dysfunction occurs. (3) Other factors associated with an increased risk of hepatitis include daily use of alcohol, chronic liver disease, and injection drug use. There is an increased risk of fatal hepatitis in minority women, especially Blacks and Hispanics, as well as postpartum. Consider more careful monitoring in these groups. If abnormal liver function 3 to 5 times ULN occurs, consider discontinuing isoniazid. (4) Liver function tests are not a substitute for clinical evaluation at monthly intervals or for the prompt assessment of signs or symptoms of side effects occurring during regularly scheduled evaluations. Instruct clients to report immediately signs and symptoms consistent with liver damage or other side effects. These include: Unexplained anorexia, N&V, dark urine, icterus, rash, persistent paresthesias of the hands and feet, persistent fatigue, weakness or fever more than 3 days duration, or abdominal tenderness (especially right upper quadrant discomfort). If these symptoms appear or signs suggestive of hepatic damage are detected, discontinue isoniazid promptly as continued use may cause a more severe form of liver damage. (5) Treat clients with tuberculosis who have hepatitis due to isoniazid with appropriate alternative drugs. Reinstitute isoniazid after symptoms and lab abnormalities have become normal. Restart the drug in small doses; gradually increase doses and withdraw immediately if there is any indication of recurrent liver involvement. (6) Defer preventive treatment in those with acute hepatic diseases.■ Extreme caution should be exercised in clients with convulsive disorders, in whom the drug should be administered only when the client is adequately controlled by anticonvulsant medication. Also, use with caution for the treatment of renal tuberculosis and, in the lowest dose possible, in clients with impaired renal function and in alcoholics.

SIDE EFFECTS
Most Common
Peripheral neuropathy, N&V, heartburn, dizziness, optic neuritis, hepatitis.

Neurologic: Peripheral neuropathy characterized by symmetrical numbness and tingling of extremities (dose-related). Rarely, toxic encephalopathy, optic neuritis, optic atrophy, *seizures*, impaired memory, toxic psychosis. **GI:** N&V, epigastric distress, heartburn, xerostomia, hepatitis. **Hypersensitivity:** Fever, skin rashes and eruptions, vasculitis, lymphadenopathy. **Hepatic:** Liver dysfunction, jaundice, bilirubinemia, bilirubinuria, *serious and sometimes fatal hepatitis (even many months after treatment)* especially in clients over 50 years of age. Increases in serum AST and ALT. **Hematologic:**

Agranulocytosis, eosinophilia, thrombocytopenia, *hemolytic, sideroblastic, or aplastic anemia.* **Metabolic/Endocrine:** Metabolic acidosis, pyridoxine deficiency, pellagra, hyperglycemia, gynecomastia. **Miscellaneous:** Tinnitus, dizziness, urinary retention, rheumatic syndrome, lupus-like syndrome, arthralgia. *NOTE:* Pyridoxine, 10–50 mg/day, may be given concomitantly with isoniazid to decrease CNS side effects. Ophthalmologic and liver function tests are recommended periodically.

OD OVERDOSE MANAGEMENT
Symptoms: N&V, dizziness, blurred vision, slurred speech, visual hallucinations within 30–180 min. Severe overdosage may cause respiratory distress, *CNS depression (coma can occur), severe seizures,* metabolic acidosis, acetonuria, hyperglycemia. *Treatment:* Maintain respiration and undertake gastric lavage (within first 2–3 hr providing seizures are not present). To control seizures, give diazepam or a short-acting IV barbiturate followed by pyridoxine (1 mg IV/1 mg isoniazid ingested). Sodium bicarbonate IV to correct metabolic acidosis. Forced osmotic diuresis; monitor fluid I&O. For severe cases, consider hemodialysis or peritoneal dialysis.

DRUG INTERACTIONS
Al salts / ↓ Effect of isoniazid R/T ↓ GI tract absorption
Aminosalicylate / ↑ Effect of isoniazid by ↑ blood levels
Anticoagulants, oral / ↓ Anticoagulant effect
Atropine / ↑ Side effects of isoniazid
Benzodiazepines / ↑ Effect of benzodiazepines that undergo oxidative metabolism (e.g., diazepam, triazolam)
Carbamazepine / ↑ Risk of carbamazepine and isoniazid toxicity
Chlorzoxazone / ↑ Chlorzoxazone peak levels and plasma elimination t½ R/T ↓ liver metabolism
Cycloserine / ↑ Risk of cycloserine CNS side effects
Disulfiram / ↑ Risk of acute behavioral and coordination changes
Enflurane / May → high levels of hydrazine → ↑ defluorination of enflurane

Ethanol / ↑ Chance of isoniazid-induced hepatitis
Halothane / ↑ Risk of hepatotoxicity and hepatic encephalopathy
Hydantoins (phenytoin) / ↑ Hydantoins effect R/T ↓ liver breakdown
Ketoconazole / ↓ Serum ketoconazole levels → ↓ effect
Meperidine / ↑ Risk of hypotension or CNS depression
Niacin / Possible ↑ of niacin requirements
Pyridoxine / Possible ↑ of pyridoxine requirements
Rifampin / Additive liver toxicity

HOW SUPPLIED
Injection: 100 mg/mL; *Syrup:* 50 mg/5 mL; *Tablets:* 50 mg, 100 mg, 300 mg.

DOSAGE
• **SYRUP; TABLETS**
  Active tuberculosis.
Adults: 5 mg/kg/day (up to 300 mg/day) as a single dose; **children and infants:** 10–20 mg/kg/day (up to 300 mg total) in a single dose.
  Prophylaxis of tuberculosis.
Adults: 300 mg/day in a single dose; **children and infants:** 10 mg/kg/day (up to 300 mg total) in a single dose.
• **IM**
  Active tuberculosis.
Adults: 5 mg/kg (up to 300 mg) once daily. **Pediatric:** 10–20 mg/kg (up to 300 mg) once daily.
  Prophylaxis of tuberculosis.
Adults/adolescents: 300 mg/day. **Pediatric:** 10 mg/kg/day.
  NOTE: Pyridoxine, 10–50 mg/day, is recommended in the malnourished and those prone to neuropathy (e.g., alcoholics, diabetics).

NURSING CONSIDERATIONS
ADMINISTRATION/STORAGE
1. Store in dark, tightly closed containers.
2. Solutions for IM injection may crystallize at low temperature; warm to room temperature if precipitation evident.
3. Anticipate slight local irritation at injection site. Rotate and document injection sites.

Bold Italic = life threatening side effect   ■ = black box warning   ♣ = Available in Canada

4. Administer with pyridoxine, 10–50 mg/day, in malnourished, alcoholic, or diabetic clients to prevent symptoms of peripheral neuropathy.

ASSESSMENT

1. Note reasons for therapy, type/onset of symptoms; note birth origin, travel outside of country. List other therapies used, outcome.

2. Obtain baseline labs, CXR, and AFB sputums; note date of PPD conversion if positive. Monitor renal and LFTs; reduce dose with dysfunction.

3. New PPD converters without symptoms still require treatment and then yearly CXR. +AFB clients require treatment and isolation initially and tracking/treatment of contacts if +AFB or PPD converters.

4. Perform pulmonary assessment; note cough/sputum characteristics.

CLIENT/FAMILY TEACHING

1. Take on an empty stomach 1 hr before or 2 hr after meals.

2. Consume 2–3 L/day of fluids to ensure adequate hydration.

3. Pyridoxine is given to prevent neurotoxic drug effects (peripheral neuritis). Report any numbness or tingling of hands or feet.

4. Avoid alcohol to prevent hepatic toxicity. May be advised to avoid certain foods (tyramine-containing) during therapy.

5. Withhold drug and report fatigue, weakness, malaise, yellow eyes/skin, dark urine, and loss of appetite (S&S of liver problems).

6. Report any visual disturbances; may precede optic neuritis.

7. With diabetes, monitor FS closely.

8. Take drugs as ordered, missing doses may require retreatment; therapy may take 6 months to a year. Report for periodic lab, provider visits, and eye exams.

OUTCOMES/EVALUATE

- Negative sputum cultures for AFB
- ↓ Neurotoxic drug effects
- Symptomatic improvement (↓ fever, ↓ secretions, ↑ appetite)

Isophane insulin suspension (NPH)
(**EYE**-so-fayn **IN**-sue-lin)

CLASSIFICATION(S):
Insulin product
PREGNANCY CATEGORY: B
OTC: Human: Humulin N, Novolin N, Novolin N PenFill, Novolin N Prefilled.
✚Rx: Iletin II Pork NPH. **Human:** Novolin ge NPH.

SEE ALSO *ANTIDIABETIC AGENTS: INSULINS*.

ACTION/KINETICS

Action

Contains zinc insulin crystals modified by protamine, appearing as a cloudy or milky suspension. Not recommended for emergency use. Not suitable for IV administration or in the presence of ketosis.

Pharmacokinetics

Onset: 1–1.5 hr. **Peak:** 4–12 hr. **Duration:** 24 hr. May be mixed with regular insulin.

SIDE EFFECTS

Most Common

Hypoglycemia, hypokalemia, injection site reaction, lipodystrophy, pruritus, rash, allergic reactions.

See *Hypoglycemic Agents: Insulins* for a complete list of possible side effects.

HOW SUPPLIED

Injection: 100 units/mL.

DOSAGE

- **SC**

  Diabetes.

Adult, individualized, usual, initial: 7–26 units as a single dose 30–60 min before breakfast. A second smaller dose may be given, if needed, prior to the evening meal or at bedtime. If necessary, the daily dose may be increased in increments of 2–10 units at daily or weekly intervals until desired control is achieved. Clients on insulin zinc may be transferred directly to isophane insulin on a unit-for-unit basis. If client is being transferred from regular insulin, the initial dose of isophane should be from two-thirds to three-fourths the dose of regular insulin.

NURSING CONSIDERATIONS
ASSESSMENT
1. Note reasons for therapy, age at onset, other therapies trialed, outcome.
2. Monitor BP, Wt, HbA1c, renal and LFTs, lipid panel, and microalbumin.

CLIENT/FAMILY TEACHING
1. Review technique for self-administration. Keep current with regular diabetes education class attendance.
2. Be alert for signs of hypoglycemia, loss of glucose control, kidney, eye or foot problems and report promptly.
3. Record FS at different times during the day/night to assess response. Keep all F/U visits and lab exams.
4. Continue BP control, diet, and exercise to achieve glycemic control and to prevent complications.

OUTCOMES/EVALUATE
- Control of BS; HbA1c <7
- Prevention of target organ damage

—— *COMBINATION DRUG* ——

Isophane insulin suspension and Insulin injection

CLASSIFICATION(S):
Insulin product
PREGNANCY CATEGORY: B
OTC: Human Insulin: Humulin 50/50, Humulin 70/30, Novolin 70/30, Novolin 70/30 PenFill, Novolin 70/30 Prefilled.
♣OTC: Humulin (20/80 and 30/70), Novolin ge (10/90, 20/80, 30/70, 40/60, and 50/50).

SEE ALSO ANTIDIABETIC AGENTS: INSULINS.

CONTENT
Humulin 50/50: Contains 50% isophane insulin and 50% regular insulin injection. **Humulin 70/30 and Novolin 70/30:** Contain 70% isophane insulin and 30% regular insulin injection. *NOTE:* Canadian products contain amounts of isophane and regular insulins that are different.

ACTION/KINETICS
Pharmacokinetics
Onset: 45 min. **Peak effect:** 7–12 hr. **Duration:** 16–24 hr. Insulin injection provides for a rapid onset while the long duration is due to isophane insulin.

SIDE EFFECTS
Most Common
Hypoglycemia, hypokalemia, injection site reaction, lipodystrophy, pruritus, rash.

See *Antidiabetic Agents: Insulins* for a complete list of possible side effects.

HOW SUPPLIED
See Content.

DOSAGE
- **SC**
  Diabetes.
Adults: Individualized and given once daily 15–30 min before breakfast, or as directed. **Children:** Individualized according to client size.

NURSING CONSIDERATIONS
ASSESSMENT
1. Note reasons for therapy, age at disease onset, other agents trialed, outcome.
2. Monitor BP, Wt, HbA1c, renal panel, LDL, and microalbumin.
3. Education related to diet, medication, exercise, weight, life style changes, disease should be initiated and reinforced.

CLIENT/FAMILY TEACHING
1. Review technique for self-administration. Keep current with regular diabetes education class attendance.
2. Be alert for signs of hypoglycemia, loss of glucose control, kidney, eye or foot problems and report promptly.
3. Record FS at different times during the day/night to assess response. Keep all F/U visits and lab exams.
4. Continue BP control, diet, and exercise to achieve glycemic control and to prevent complications.

OUTCOMES/EVALUATE
Control of BS; HbA1c <7

Isoproterenol hydrochloride   IV

(eye-so-proe-**TER**-e-nole)

CLASSIFICATION(S):
Sympathomimetic
PREGNANCY CATEGORY: C
Rx: Isuprel, Isuprel Mistometer.

SEE ALSO *SYMPATHOMIMETIC DRUGS.*

USES

Inhalation: Relief of bronchospasms associated with acute and chronic asthma, chronic bronchitis, or emphysema.
Injection: (1) Bronchospasm during anesthesia. (2) As an adjunct to fluid and electrolyte replacement therapy to treat hypovolemic and septic shock, low cardiac output states, CHF, and cardiogenic shock. (3) Mild or transient heart block that does not require electric shock or pacemaker therapy. (4) For serious episodes of heart block and Adams-Stokes attacks, except when caused by ventricular tachycardia or fibrillation. (5) Cardiac arrest until electric shock or pacemaker therapy (treatments of choice) is available. *NOTE:* May produce beneficial hemodynamic and metabolic effects when a low arterial pressure has been elevated by other means.

ACTION/KINETICS

Action

Produces pronounced stimulation of both beta-1 and beta-2 receptors of the heart, bronchi, skeletal muscle vasculature, and the GI tract. Has both positive inotropic and chronotropic activity resulting in increased CO; systolic BP may increase while diastolic BP may decrease. Thus, mean arterial BP may not change or may be decreased. Causes less hyperglycemia than epinephrine, but produces bronchodilation and the same degree of CNS excitation.

Pharmacokinetics

Readily absorbed after aerosol use. **Inhalation: Onset,** 2–5 min; **peak effect:** 3–5 min; **duration:** 1–3 hr. **IV: Onset,** immediate; **duration:** less than 1 hr. Metabolized by COMT but is a poor substrate for MAO; excreted in urine.

CONTRAINDICATIONS

Tachyarrhythmias, tachycardia, or heart block caused by digitalis intoxication, ventricular arrhythmias that require inotropic therapy, and angina pectoris.

SPECIAL CONCERNS

May have a harmful effect on the failing or injured heart; not recommended for use as the initial drug in treating cardiogenic shock following MI. Use with caution during lactation and in the presence of tuberculosis. Use special caution if given to those with coronary artery disease, coronary insufficiency, diabetes, hyperthyroidism, and sensitivity to sympathomimetic amines. Safety and effectiveness have not been determined in children under age 12.

SIDE EFFECTS

Most Common

Nausea, warmth, diaphoresis, dizziness, pallor, visual blurring, shakiness, weakness, headache, dyspnea.

See *Sympathomimetic Drugs* for a complete list of possible side effects. Also, **CV: *Cardiac arrest*,** Adams-Stokes attack, hypo-/hypertension, precordial pain or distress, tachycardia, palpitations, angina, ***Adams-Stokes attacks***, ventricular arrhythmias, tachyarrhythmias, ***cardiac dysrhythmias myocardial necrosis*. CNS:** Hyperactivity, hyperkinesia, nervousness, dizziness, shakiness, headache, mild tremors. **Respiratory:** Wheezing, bronchitis, dyspnea, increase in sputum, ***pulmonary/bronchial edema and inflammation, paradoxical airway resistance*.** Excessive inhalation causes refractory bronchial obstruction. **Dermatologic:** Flushing, warmth, diaphoresis, pallor. **Miscellaneous:** Visual blurring, weakness, swelling of the parotid gland. Sublingual administration may cause buccal ulceration. Side effects of drug are less severe after inhalation.

DRUG INTERACTIONS

Aminophylline & Corticosteroids / Possible additive cardiotoxic effects → myocardial necrosis and death

---

Bretylium / Possibility of arrhythmias

Epinephrine / Do not give together; possible serious arrhythmias; may be given alternately if proper interval between doses

Guanethidine / ↑ Pressor response of isoproterenol → severe hypertension

Halogenated hydrocarbon anesthetics / Sensitization of the heart to catecholamines → serious arrhythmias; use together with caution

Oxytocic drugs / Possibility of severe, persistent hypertension

Tricyclic antidepressants / Potentiation of pressor effect; use together with caution

HOW SUPPLIED

Isoproterenol Hydrochloride. *Injection:* 0.02 mg/mL (1:50,000), 0.2 mg/mL (1:5,000); *Metered Dose Inhaler:* (Aerosol) 103 mcg/inh; *Solution for Inhalation:* 0.5% (1:200), 1% (1:100).

DOSAGE

ISOPROTERENOL HYDROCHLORIDE

• **INHALATION**

Acute bronchial asthma.

Hand bulb nebulizer. **Adults and children:** Give 5–15 deep inhalations of the 1:200 solution. Alternatively, in adults, give 3–7 deep inhalations of the 1:100 solution. If no relief occurs after 5–10 min, repeat doses once more. If acute attack recurs, can repeat treatment up to 5 times per day, if necessary. *Metered dose inhaler (aerosol).* One inhalation (103 mcg). Wait 1 min to determine effect before considering a second inhalation. Repeat up to 5 times per day, if necessary.

Bronchospasm in COPD.

Hand bulb nebulizer. Give 5–15 deep inhalations using the 1:200 solution. Severe attacks may require 3–7 inhalations using the 1:100 solution. Wait at least 3–4 hr between doses. *Nebulization by compressed air or oxygen.* Dilute 0.5 mL of the 1:200 solution to 2–2.5 mL with appropriate diluent for a concentration of 1:800 to 1:1,000. Deliver the solution over 10–20 min. May repeat up to 5 times per day. *Intermittent positive pressure breathing.* Dilute 0.5 mL of the 1:200 solution to 2–2.5 mL with water or isotonic saline. Deliver over 15–20

min. May repeat up to 5 times per day. *Metered dose inhaler (aerosol).* 1 or 2 inhalations repeated at no less than 3–4 hr intervals (6–8 times per day). **Children:** For acute bronchospasms, use the 1:200 solution. Do not use more than 0.25 mL of the 1:200 solution for each 10–15 min programmed treatment.

• **IV**

Bronchospasms during anesthesia.

Bolus IV injection: Dilute 1 mL (0.2 mg) of the 1:5,000 solution to 10 mL with NaCl injection or D5W. **Initial dose:** 0.01–0.02 mg (0.5–1 mL of diluted solution). Repeat when necessary or use a 1:50,000 solution undiluted and give as an initial dose of 0.01–0.02 mg (0.5–1 mL).

Hypovolemic and septic shock.

IV infusion: Dilute 5 mL (1 mg) of the 1:5,000 solution in 500 mL D5W. **Infusion rate:** 0.5—5 mcg/min (0.25—2.5 mL of diluted solution/minute). Adjust the rate of infusion based on HR, central venous pressure, systemic BP, and urine flow. If the HR exceeds 110 beats/min, it may be advisable to decrease or temporarily discontinue the infusion.

Heart block, Adams-Stokes attacks, cardiac arrest.

Bolus IV injection. Dilute 1 mL of the 1:5,000 solution (0.2 mg) to 10 mL with NaCl or D5W or use the 1:50,000 solution undiluted. **Initial dose:** 0.02–0.06 mg (1–3 mL of diluted solution or of the 1:50,000 solution); **then,** 0.01–0.2 mg (0.5–10 mL of diluted solution). *IV infusion.* Dilute 10 mL of the 1:5,000 solution (2 mg) in 500 mL of D5W or dilute 5 mL of the 1:5,000 solution (1 mg) in 250 mL of D5W. **Initial dose:** 5 mcg/min (1.25 mL/min of diluted solution).

NURSING CONSIDERATIONS

ADMINISTRATION/STORAGE

1. Administration to children, except where noted, is the same as that for adults; their smaller ventilatory exchange capacity will permit a proportionally smaller aerosol intake. For their acute bronchospasms, use 1:200 solution.

Bold Italic = life threatening side effect   ■ = black box warning   ✦ = Available in Canada

2. In children, no more than 0.25 mL of the 1:200 solution should be used for each 10–15 min of programmed treatment.

3. Elderly clients usually receive a lower dose.

IV 4. The injection should be initiated at the lowest recommended dose and the rate of administration increased gradually, if needed, while carefully monitoring the client.

5. Isoproterenol injection, 1:50,000 is given IV. The 1:5,000 injection is suitable only for addition to a large volume IV solution single-dose container to prepare a dilute concentration for slow IV infusion.

6. The initial IV dose of isoproterenol in children (7 to 19 years of age) ranges between 0.05–0.17 mcg/kg/min, which is increased gradually by 0.1 to 0.2 mcg/kg/min at intervals of 15 to 20 min, titrated to clinical response. The maximum dose range used is 1.3–2.7 mcg/kg/min. General postoperative pediatric cardiac clients with bradycardia require lower doses (0.029 ± 0.002 mcg/kg/min) of IV isoproterenol than do asthma clients (0.5 ± 0.21 mcg/kg/min).

7. Administer IV in a continuously monitored environment.

8. Do not use the injection if it is pinkish to brownish in color. Protect from light and store at 15–30°C (59–86°F).

ASSESSMENT

1. Note reasons for therapy, triggers, characteristics of S&S.

2. Perform pulmonary assessment; note PFTs, CXRs. Report respiratory problems that worsen after administration; refractory reactions may necessitate drug withdrawal.

3. Obtain EKG. Identify arrhythmias (especially ventricular) and angina; may preclude drug therapy.

CLIENT/FAMILY TEACHING

1. Review method for inhaler use; a spacer enhances dispersion.

2. Rinse mouth and equipment with water; removes drug residue and minimizes dryness after inhalation.

3. Maintain fluid intake of 2–3 L/day to help liquefy secretions. Reduce intake of caffeine during therapy.

4. Sputum and saliva may appear pink after inhalation therapy; do not become alarmed.

5. With more than one inhalation therapy prescribed, wait 2 min before second inhalation. When also taking inhalant glucocorticoids, take isoproterenol first and wait 5 min before using the next inhaler.

6. Do not use more often than prescribed; overuse can cause severe cardiac and respiratory problems. Report any chest pain/tightness or increased SOB.

7. Identify parotid gland; withhold drug and report if enlarged.

8. Stop smoking to preserve current level of lung function; enroll in smoking cessation program.

9. Keep all F/U appointments to evaluate response to therapy.

OUTCOMES/EVALUATE

• Improved airway exchange
• ↓ Bronchoconstriction/spasms
• Stable cardiac rhythm

Isosorbide dinitrate ©
(eye-so-**SOR**-byd)

CLASSIFICATION(S):
Coronary vasodilator

PREGNANCY CATEGORY: C

Rx: Capsules, Sustained-Release: Dilatrate-SR. **Tablets**: Isordil Titradose. **Tablets, Extended-Release**: Isochron. **Tablets, Sublingual**: Isosorbide dinitrate.

♣Rx: Apo-ISDN.

SEE ALSO ANTIANGINAL DRUGS- NITRATES/NITRITES.

USES

(1) Treatment of angina pectoris (sublingual tablets only). (2) Prevention of angina pectoris caused by coronary artery disease. The onset is not sufficiently rapid for this product to be used to abort an acute anginal attack. *Investigational:* With hydralazine to increase survival among black clients with advanced heart failure; treat acute angle-

closure glaucoma in emergency situations (not for long-term management); achalasia.

ACTION/KINETICS
Action
Relaxes vascular smooth muscle by stimulating production of intracellular cyclic guanosine monophosphate. Dilation of postcapillary vessels decreases venous return to the heart due to pooling of blood; thus, LV end-diastolic pressure (preload) is reduced. Relaxation of arterioles results in a decreased systemic vascular resistance and arterial pressure (afterload).

Pharmacokinetics
Sublingual chewable. Onset: 2–5 min; **duration:** 1–3 hr. **Oral Capsules/Tablets. Onset:** 20–40 min; **duration:** 4–6 hr. **Extended-Release. Onset:** up to 4 hr; **duration:** 6–8 hr.

ADDITIONAL CONTRAINDICATIONS
Use to abort acute anginal attacks.

SPECIAL CONCERNS
Use with caution during lactation. Safety and efficacy have not been established in children.

SIDE EFFECTS
Most Common
Headache, vascular headache, lightheadedness, hypotension.

See *Antianginal Drugs–Nitrates/Nitrites* for a complete list of possible side effects. Vascular headaches occur especially frequently.

ADDITIONAL DRUG INTERACTIONS
Acetylcholine / Acetylcholine effect antagonized
Norepinephrine / Norepinephrine effect antagonized

HOW SUPPLIED
Capsules, Sustained-Release: 40 mg; *Tablets:* 5 mg, 10 mg, 20 mg, 30 mg, 40 mg; *Tablets, Extended-Release:* 40 mg; *Tablets, Sublingual:* 2.5 mg, 5 mg.

DOSAGE
• TABLETS
Antianginal.

Initial: 5–20 mg 2–3 times per day; **maintenance:** 10–40 mg 2–3 times per day. To minimize tolerance, a daily dose-free interval of at least 14 hr is recommended.

• TABLETS, SUBLINGUAL
Antianginal, acute attack.

Initial: 2.5–5 mg. The dose can be titrated upward until angina is relieved or side effects occur. To minimize development of tolerance, a daily dose-free interval must be longer than 14 hr.

Prophylaxis of angina.

2.5–5 mg about 15 min before activity that is likely to cause angina. Sublingual tablets may be used to abort an acute anginal episode, but use is recommended only in those who fail to respond to sublingual nitroglycerin.

• CAPSULES, SUSTAINED-RELEASE; TABLETS, EXTENDED-RELEASE
Antianginal.

Initial: 40 mg; **maintenance:** 40–80 mg q 8–12 hr. Tolerance may occur to these agents. Consider giving the short-acting products 2 or 3 times daily (last dose no later than 7 p.m.) and the sustained-release products once daily or twice daily at 8 a.m. and 2 p.m.

NURSING CONSIDERATIONS
Ⓖ Do not confuse Isordil with Isuprel (a beta-adrenergic agonist) or Inderal (a beta-adrenergic blocker).

ADMINISTRATION/STORAGE
1. Capsules, Sustained-Release: Store from 15–30°C (59–86°F) in a dry location.
2. Tablets: Store at room temperature protected from light. Keep bottles tightly closed. Dispense in a light-resistant, tight container.
3. Tablets, Extended-Release: Store from 15–30°C (59–86°F). Dispense in a well-closed container.
4. Tablets, Sublingual: Store from 15–30°C (59–86°F) protected from light and moisture. Dispense in a tight, light-resistant container.

ASSESSMENT
1. Note reasons for therapy; include onset, location, characteristics of chest pain; rate pain levels.
2. Assess VS and ECG; note stress thallium, catheterization, or IVUS findings as well as CAD history/interventions.

CLIENT/FAMILY TEACHING
1. Take tablets with meals to eliminate/reduce headaches; otherwise, take on an empty stomach to facilitate absorp-

tion. Leave product in original container.

2. Tolerance may develop (stay nitrate free for 8–14 hr, usually at night, to prevent tolerance). Short-acting products can be given 2–3 times per day with the last dose no later than 7:00 p.m. The extended-release products can be given once or twice daily at 8:00 a.m. and 2:00 p.m. or as prescribed

3. Review method for administration; do not chew sublingual tablets. May take SL tablets at first symptom of chest pain. None of the products should be crushed or chewed, unless ordered. Do not stop abruptly; may cause heart spasms.

4. Hold chewable tablets in the mouth for 1–2 min; allows absorption through cheek membranes.

5. Take before any stressful activity (sexual activity, exercise).

6. Change positions slowly to avoid sudden drop in BP. Avoid hazardous activities if dizziness occurs.

7. Acetaminophen (tylenol) may assist to relieve drug-induced headaches.

8. Avoid alcohol and any OTC agents without approval.

9. Report if symptoms not controlled or intolerable side effects occur with therapy.

OUTCOMES/EVALUATE

- ↓ Frequency/severity of anginal attacks
- ↑ CO/Exercise tolerance

Isosorbide mononitrate ©

(eye-so-**SOR**-byd)

CLASSIFICATION(S):
Coronary vasodilator
PREGNANCY CATEGORY: C
Rx: Tablets: ISMO, Monoket. **Tablets, Extended-Release**: Imdur.

SEE ALSO *ANTIANGINAL DRUGS-NITRATES/NITRITES* AND *ISOSORBIDE DINITRATE.*

USES
(1) Treatment of angina pectoris (Monoket only). (2) Prophylaxis of angina pectoris caused by coronary artery disease. The onset of action of the mononitrate is not sufficiently rapid to be used in aborting an acute angina attach. *Investigational:* With nadolol to prevent recurrent variceal bleeding.

ACTION/KINETICS
Action
Isosorbide mononitrate is the major metabolite of isosorbide dinitrate. The mononitrate is not subject to first-pass metabolism. Relaxes vascular smooth muscle by stimulating production of intracellular cyclic guanosine monophosphate. Dilation of postcapillary vessels decreases venous return to the heart due to pooling of blood; thus, LV end-diastolic pressure (preload) is reduced. Relaxation of arterioles results in a decreased systemic vascular resistance and arterial pressure (afterload).

Pharmacokinetics
Bioavailability is nearly 100%. **Onset:** 30–60 min. t_{max}, **tablets:** 0.6–0.7 hr; t_{max}, **ER tablets:** 2.9–4.5 hr. $t^{1}\!/_{2}$, **tablets:** About 5 hr; $t^{1}\!/_{2}$, **ER tablets:** 6.2 hr.

CONTRAINDICATIONS
To abort acute anginal attacks. Use in acute MI or CHF.

SPECIAL CONCERNS
Use with caution during lactation and in clients who may be volume depleted or who are already hypotensive. Safety and effectiveness have not been determined in children. The benefits have not been established in acute MI or CHF.

SIDE EFFECTS
Most Common
Dizziness, headache, hypotension, N&V, increased cough, allergic reaction.
CV: Hypotension (may be accompanied by paradoxical bradycardia and increased angina pectoris), CV disorder, chest pain. **CNS:** Headache, lightheadedness, dizziness, fatigue, emotional lability. **GI:** N&V, diarrhea, abdominal pain. **Dermatologic:** Pruritus, rash. **Respiratory:** Increased cough, URTI. **Miscellaneous:** Possibility of methemoglobinemia, allergic reactions, flushing, pain.

📷 = see color insert   H = Herbal   IV = Intravenous   © = sound alike drug

OD OVERDOSE MANAGEMENT

Symptoms: Increased intracranial pressure manifested by throbbing headache, confusion, moderate fever. Also, vertigo, palpitations, visual disturbances, N&V, syncope, air hunger, dyspnea (followed by reduced ventilatory effort), diaphoresis, skin either flushed or cold and clammy, heart block, bradycardia, paralysis, ***coma, seizures, death.*** *Treatment:* Direct therapy toward an increase in central fluid volume. Do *not* use vasoconstrictors.

DRUG INTERACTIONS

Ethanol / Additive vasodilation
Calcium channel blockers / Severe orthostatic hypotension
Organic nitrates / Severe orthostatic hypotension

HOW SUPPLIED

Tablets: 10 mg, 20 mg; *Tablets, Extended-Release:* 30 mg, 60 mg, 120 mg.

DOSAGE

• TABLETS

Prophylaxis of angina.

20 mg twice a day with the two doses given 7 hr apart, with the first dose upon awakening. A starting dose of 5 mg (one-half of the 10 mg tablet) may be appropriate for clients of particularly small stature; however, increase to at least 10 mg by the second or third day. This dosing regimen provides a daily nitrate-free interval to minimize tolerance development.

• TABLETS, EXTENDED-RELEASE

Prophylaxis of angina.

Initial: 30 mg or 60 mg once daily; **then,** after several days dosage may be increased to 120 mg (given as a single 120 mg tablet or as two-60 mg tablets). Rarely, 240 mg daily may be needed. The suggested regimen is to give the dose in the a.m. on arising.

NURSING CONSIDERATIONS

�θ Do not confuse Imdur with Imuran (an immunosuppressant) or Inderal (a beta-adrenergic blocker).

ADMINISTRATION/STORAGE

1. The treatment regimen minimizes the development of refractory tolerance.

2. Tablets: Store from 15–30°C (59–86°F). Keep tightly closed.
3. Protect from excessive moisture.

ASSESSMENT

1. Note reasons for therapy, cardiac history, onset/frequency of angina, triggers.
2. Monitor VS, EKG, cardiac status, family history, risk factors, and electrolytes.
3. List drugs prescribed to ensure none interact. Do not use if taking any drug for erectile dysfunction of phosphodiesterase type 5 inhibitors (eg, sildenafil, tadalafil, vardenafil) because the risk of severe low BP is inherent.

CLIENT/FAMILY TEACHING

1. Consume 1–2 L/day of fluids to ensure adequate hydration. Do not stop abruptly
2. Take the extended-release tablet in the morning upon arising as directed. Do not crush or chew; take with a half glass of water.
3. May cause dizziness or lightheadedness. Alcohol, hot weather, exercise, and fever can increase these effects. Use caution performing activities that require mental alertness until drug effects realized. Change positions slowly to prevent dizziness.
4. Not to be used to stop an attack of angina; intended only for prevention of an attack.
5. Avoid alcohol. Report if chest pain persists/recurs and adverse effects. Keep all F/U appointments, labs, and EKGs to assess response to therapy.

OUTCOMES/EVALUATE

Angina prophylaxis

Isotretinoin ■ ℂ

(eye-so-**TRET**-ih-noyn)

CLASSIFICATION(S):

Retinoid

PREGNANCY CATEGORY: X

Rx: Accutane, Amnesteem, Claravis, Sotret.

✚Rx: Accutane, Isotrex, Roche.

USES

Severe recalcitrant nodular acne unresponsive to standard therapies. Severe refers to many nodules that are inflam-

---

Bold Italic = life threatening side effect   ■ = black box warning   ✚ = Available in Canada

matory with a diameter of 5 mm or more. *NOTE:* To decrease further the chances of pregnancy during therapy, pharmacies, wholesalers, and clients must register with the SMART Program to obtain and distribute isotretinoin. *Investigational:* Treat premalignant lesions and reduce incidence of second primary tumors in clients with prior head and neck, lung, or liver cancers.

ACTION/KINETICS

Action

Reduces sebaceous gland size, decreases sebum secretion, and inhibits abnormal keratinization.

Pharmacokinetics

Approximately 25% of the PO dosage form is bioavailable. **Peak plasma levels:** 3 hr. **Steady-state blood levels following 80 mg/day:** 160 ng/mL. **t½, terminal** to Metabolized in the liver to 4-oxo-isotretinoin, which is also active. **t½, terminal of 4-oxo-isotretinoin:** 17–50 hr. Approximately equal amounts are excreted through the urine and in the feces. **Plasma protein binding:** Nearly 100%.

CONTRAINDICATIONS

Due to the possibility of fetal abnormalities or spontaneous abortion at any dose, women who are pregnant or intend to become pregnant should not use the drug. Certain conditions for use should be met in women with childbearing potential (see package insert). Hypersensitivity to parabens (in the product).

SPECIAL CONCERNS

■ (1) Must not be used by females who are pregnant. There is an extremely high risk that a deformed infant can result if pregnancy occurs while taking isotretinoin in any amount, even for short periods of time. There are no accurate means of determining, after isotretinoin exposure, which fetus has been affected and which fetus has not been affected. (2) There is an increased risk of spontaneous abortion; also, premature births have been reported. (3) Documented external abnormalities include: Skull abnormality; ear abnormalities, including anotia, micropinna, small or absent external auditory canals; eye abnormalities, including microphthalmia; facial dysmorphia; cleft palate. Documented internal abnormalities include cerebral abnormalities, cerebellar malformation, hydrocephalus, microcephaly, cranial nerve deficit; CV abnormalities; thymus gland abnormality; parathyroid hormone deficiency. In some cases death has occurred with certain of the previously listed abnormalities. Cases of IQ scores less than 85 with or without obvious CNS abnormalities have also been reported. (4) Is contraindicated in women of childbearing age unless they meet the following criteria: Must not be pregnant or breast feeding; must be capable of complying with mandatory contraceptive measures and understand behaviors associated with an increased risk of pregnancy; and must be reliable in understanding and carrying out instructions. (5) Accutane must be prescribed under the 'System to Manage Accutane-Related Teratogenicity (SMART).' Check this process carefully. (6) For a female client, the yellow self-adhesive Accutane Qualification Sticker signifies she understands a number of things including two negative urine or serum pregnancy tests; must have selected and committed to using 2 forms of effective contraception simultaneously; must have signed a patient information/consent form that contains warnings about the risk of potential birth defects if the fetus is exposed to isotretinoin; and, must have been informed of the purpose and importance of participating in the Accutane survey and given the opportunity to enroll. (7) The yellow qualification sticker documents that the woman is qualified and includes the date of qualification, client gender, cut-off date for filling the prescription, and up to a 30-day supply limit with no refills. (8) If pregnancy does occur during isotretinoin therapy, the desirability of continuing the pregnancy should be addressed. Prescribers are encouraged to report to the company all cases of pregnancy. (9) Isotretinoin should be prescribed only by those who have demonstrated special competence in the diagnosis and treatment of severe recalcitrant nodular acne; are experienced in the use of systemic retinoids; have read the SMART Guide to Best Practices; signed and returned the completed SMART letter of understanding; and, obtained yellow self-adhesive Accutane Qualification Stickers. Do not prescribe or dispense Accutane without a yellow self-adhesive Accutane Qualification Sticker. (10) The yellow self-adhesive Accutane Qualification Stickers should also be used for male clients. (11) Isotretinoin may only be dispensed in no more than a 30-day supply; only on presentation of an Accutane prescription with a yellow self-adhesive Accutane Qualification Sticker; prescription written within the previous 7 days; refills require a new prescription with a yellow self-adhesive Accutane Qualification Sticker; and, no telephone or computerized prescriptions are permitted. (12) An Accutane medication guide must be given to the client each time the drug is dispensed, as required by law. This guide is an important part of the risk management program for the client. (13) Studies have not ruled out the possibility that isotretinoion decreases the effectiveness of hormonal contraceptives.■ Intolerance to contact lenses may develop. Increased risks for birth defects, aggressive and/or violent behavior, psychiatric disorders (including suicidal tendencies). Give for no longer than the recommended duration. Avoid use during lactation. Check lipids before therapy, and then at intervals until response established (within 4 weeks). Monitor LFTs before therapy, weekly or biweekly until response established. Avoid prolonged UV rays or sunlight, and donating blood up to 1 month after discontinuing therapy. Use with caution with genetic predisposition for age-related osteoporosis, history of childhood osteoporosis, osteomalacia, other bone metabolism disorders (i.e., anorexia nervosa). Use with caution with drugs that cause drug-induced osteoporosis/osteomalacia and affect vitamin D metabolism disorders (i.e., corticosteroids, phenytoin).

SIDE EFFECTS

Most Common

Dry skin, itching, dry nose, epistaxis, chelitis, dry mouth, conjunctivitis, joint aches, depression, hallucinations, suicidal behavior, increase blood glucose and triglycerides.

Skin: Cheilitis, itching, skin fragility, pruritus, dry skin, desquamation of facial skin, drying of mucous membranes, brittle nails, photosensitivity, rash (including facial erythema, seborrhea, and eczema), hypo- or hyperpigmentation, urticaria, erythema nodosum, hirsutism, excess granulation of tissues as a result of healing, petechiae, peeling of palms and soles, skin infections (including disseminated herpes simplex), paronychia, thinning of hair, nail dystrophy, pyogenic granuloma, bruising, acne fulminans, alopecia, eruptive xanthomas, sweating, increased susceptibility to sunburn. **CNS:** Headache, fatigue, pseudotumor cerebri (i.e., headaches, papilledema, disturbances in vision, dizziness), depression, psychosis, hallucinations, suicidal ideation, *suicide attempts, suicide,* drowsiness, insomnia, lethargy, malaise, nervousness, paresthesias, *seizures, stroke,* syncope, weakness, emotional instability. Aggressive and/or violent behaviors. **Hematologic:** Neutropenia, thrombocytopenia, anemia, *agranulocytosis (rare).* **Ocular/Ophthalmic:** Conjunctivitis, optic neuritis, corneal opacities, dry eyes, decrease in acuity of night vision, photophobia, eyelid inflammation, cataracts, visual disturbances, color vision disorder, keratitis. **GI:** Dry mouth, N&V, abdominal pain, nonspecific GI symptoms, hepatitis, hepatotoxicity, inflammatory bowel disease (including regional enteritis), anorexia, weight loss, *acute pancreatitis,* inflammation and bleeding of gums, colitis, ileitis. **Neuromuscular:** Arthralgia; muscle, bone and joint pain and stiffness; skeletal hyperostosis, calcification of tendons and ligaments, premature epiphyseal closure, arthritis, tendonitis, back pain, rhabdomyolysis (rare). Reports of osteoporosis, osteopenia, bone fractures, and delayed healing of bone fractures. Decrease in

---

Bold Italic = life threatening side effect   ■ = black box warning   ✦ = Available in Canada

lumbar spine bone mineral density. **CV:** Flushing, palpitation, tachycardia, vascular thrombotic disease. **GU:** White cells in urine, proteinuria, nonspecific urogenital findings, microscopic or gross hematuria, abnormal menses, glomerular nephritis. **Respiratory:** Bronchospasms with or without history of asthma, respiratory infections, voice alterations, epistaxis, dry nose. **Ophthalmic:** Decreased night vision (may persist), corneal opacities, conjunctivitis, optic neuritis, photophobia, eyelid inflammation, cataracts, color vision disorder, visual disturbances, keratitis, dry eyes. **Otic:** Impaired hearing, tinnitus. **Miscellaneous:** Dry mouth, disseminated herpes simplex, edema, transient chest pain, development of diabetes, vasculitis (including Wegener's granulomatosis), lymphadenopathy, flushing, severe allergic reactions (including ***anaphylaxis***, cutaneous allergic reactions, allergic vasculitis, purpura).

LABORATORY TEST CONSIDERATIONS
↑ Plasma triglycerides, sedimentation rate, platelet counts, alkaline phosphatase, AST, ALT, GGTP, LDH, fasting blood glucose, uric acid in blood, serum cholesterol, CPK levels in clients who exercise vigorously. ↓ HDL, RBC parameters, WBC counts. Hypertriglyceridemia.

OD OVERDOSE MANAGEMENT
Symptoms: Abdominal pain, ataxia, cheilosis, dizziness, facial flushing, headache, vomiting. Symptoms are transient. *Treatment:* Symptoms are quickly resolved with drug cessation or decrease in dose.

DRUG INTERACTIONS
Alcohol / Potentiation of ↑ serum triglycerides
Minocycline / ↑ Risk of developing pseudotumor cerebri or papilledema
Oral contraceptives and injectable/implantable contraceptives, microdose progesterone products / Possible inadequate pregnancy protection
H *St. John's wort* / May cause breakthrough bleeding with oral contraceptives
Tetracycline / ↑ Risk of developing pseudotumor cerebri or papilledema
Vitamin A / ↑ Risk of toxicity

HOW SUPPLIED
Capsules: 10 mg, 20 mg, 30 mg, 40 mg.

DOSAGE
• **CAPSULES**
Recalcitrant cystic acne.
Adults and children 12 years and older, individualized, initial: 0.5–1 mg/kg/day (range: 0.5–2 mg/kg/day) divided in two doses for 15–20 weeks. Adjust dose based on toxicity and clinical response; if cyst count decreases by 70% or more, drug may be discontinued. If necessary, a second course of therapy may be instituted after a rest period of 2 months. Doses of 0.05–0.5 mg/kg/day are effective but result in higher frequency of relapses.
Investigational: Keratinization disorders.
Doses up to 4 mg/kg/day have been used.
Prevent second tumors in squamous-cell carcinoma of the head and neck. 50–100 mg/m^2.

NURSING CONSIDERATIONS
℗ Do not confuse Accutane with Accupril (ACE inhibitor).

ADMINISTRATION/STORAGE
1. Requirements for dispensing isotretinoin are:
• Prescription must bear a yellow self-adhesive Accutane Qualification Sticker completely and correctly filled out by the prescriber.
• Telephone, fax, or computer-generated orders are not acceptable.
• No more than a 30-day supply may be dispensed and there are no refills.
• Prescriptions for females must be filled within 7 days of the qualification date on the sticker. Prescriptions presented later are to be considered expired.
• A medication guide must be dispensed to every client with an Accutane prescription.
2. A rest period of 2 months is recommended if a second course of therapy is needed.

ASSESSMENT
1. Note clinical presentation, other agents/therapies trialed, outcome; use photos to document.

---

2. Perform pregnancy test on all females of child bearing age.

3. Monitor serum glucose levels, chemistry, CBC, urinalysis, LFTs, lipoprotein, cholesterol, and triglycerides.

CLIENT/FAMILY TEACHING

1. Isotretinoin is available only through a restricted-access program. Before receiving isotretinoin, clients must sign an informed consent form that details the risks associated with isotretinoin use. Clients will also receive a medication guide and must have watched the videotape that gives information about contraceptive methods. Females must confirm they have a negative result for the second urine pregnancy request, conducted on the second day of the next menstrual period or 11 days or more after the last unprotected act of sexual intercourse, whichever is later.

2. Do not crush capsules. Food or milk will increase the absorption of isotretinoin.

3. Avoid donating blood for 30 days after discontinuing drug therapy.

4. Drug is teratogenic; perform monthly pregnancy test. Females of childbearing age should practice 2 reliable forms of birth control 1 month before, during, and 1 month following therapy; severe fetal damage may occur.

5. A 30-day prescription will be dispensed with no refills to ensure compliance. It must be filled within 7 days of order date and prescription must have yellow qualification sticker.

6. Report if persistent headache, N&V, or visual disturbances occur. Avoid abrasive skin cleaners, medicated soaps, topical acne preparations/alcohol based products and peeling agents. Lubricants may help diminish symptoms of dry, chapped skin and lips.

7. Contact lens wearers may develop sensitivity to contacts during and after therapy. Excessively dry eyes may require an eye lubricant.

8. Condition may become worse before healing starts. Report any muscle, joint, or bone pains.

9. Avoid OTC medications, especially vitamin A, without consent.

10. Eliminate or markedly reduce consumption of alcohol; may increase triglyceride levels.

11. Avoid prolonged sunlight exposure; may cause photosensitivity. Wear protective clothing, sunscreen, and sunglasses when exposed.

12. Keep all F/U appointments to assess response to therapy and eval any adverse effects.

OUTCOMES/EVALUATE

↓ Number/size and severity of cystic acne lesions; Healing/clearing and restoration of skin integrity

Isradipine
(iss-**RAD**-ih-peen)

CLASSIFICATION(S):
Antihypertensive, calcium channel blocking drug
PREGNANCY CATEGORY: C
Rx: DynaCirc, DynaCirc CR.

SEE ALSO CALCIUM CHANNEL BLOCKING AGENTS.

USES
Essential hypertension, alone or with thiazide diuretics. *Investigational:* Raynaud's phenomenon.

ACTION/KINETICS

Action
Binds to calcium channels resulting in the inhibition of calcium influx into cardiac and smooth muscle and subsequent arteriolar vasodilation. Reduced systemic resistance leads to a decrease in BP with a small increase in resting HR. In clients with normal ventricular function, the drug reduces afterload leading to some increase in CO. Causes a slight increase in QT interval and CO and a slight decrease in myocardial contractility.

Pharmacokinetics
Well absorbed from the GI tract, although it undergoes significant first-pass metabolism. Bioavailability increases in those over 65 years of age, those with impaired hepatic function, and those with mild impaired renal function. **Peak plasma levels:** 1 ng/mL

Bold Italic = life threatening side effect   ■ = black box warning   ✦ = Available in Canada

after 1.5 hr. **Onset:** 2–3 hr. Food increases the time to peak effect by about 1 hr, although the total bioavailability does not change. For the capsules, the antihypertensive effect usually occurs within 2–3 hr with maximal response in 2–4 wk. For the controlled-release tablets, the antihypertensive response occurs within 2 hr with the peak response in 8–10 hr with BP reduction maintained for 24 hr. **t½, initial:** 1.5–2 hr; **terminal,** 8 hr. Completely metabolized in the liver with 60–65% excreted through the kidneys and 25–30% through the feces. Maximum effect may not be observed for 2–4 weeks. **Plasma protein binding:** 95%.

CONTRAINDICATIONS
Lactation.

SPECIAL CONCERNS
Safety and effectiveness have not been determined in children. Use with caution in clients with CHF, especially those taking a beta-adrenergic blocking agent.

SIDE EFFECTS
Most Common
Edema, tachycardia, dizziness/lightheadedness, fatigue/lethargy, headache, abdominal discomfort, constipation, diarrhea, nausea, polyuria, dyspnea, flushing.
CV: Palpitations, edema, flushing, tachycardia, SOB, hypotension, transient ischemic attack, *stroke*, atrial fibrillation, *ventricular fibrillation, MI,* CHF, angina. **CNS:** Headache, dizziness/lightheadedness, fatigue, drowsiness, insomnia, lethargy, nervousness, depression, syncope, amnesia, psychosis, hallucinations, weakness, jitteriness, paresthesia. **GI:** Nausea, abdominal discomfort, diarrhea, vomiting, constipation, dry mouth. **Respiratory:** Dyspnea, cough. **Dermatologic:** Pruritus, urticaria. **Miscellaneous:** Chest pain, rash, pollakiuria, cramps of the legs and feet, nocturia, polyuria, hyperhidrosis, visual disturbances, numbness, throat discomfort, leukopenia, sexual difficulties.

LABORATORY TEST CONSIDERATIONS
↑ LFTs.

DRUG INTERACTIONS
Azole antifungals / ↑ Isradipine levels
Beta-blockers / Possible additive or synergistic effects; isradipine may ↓ metabolism of certain beta-blockers
Cimetidine / Possible ↑ Isradipine levels
Fentanyl / Severe hypotension with a beta-blocker and isradipine
Lovastatin / ↓ Lovastatin levels
Rifampin / ↓ Isradipine effect

HOW SUPPLIED
Capsules: 2.5 mg, 5 mg; *Tablets, Controlled-Release:* 5 mg, 10 mg.

DOSAGE
DYNACIRC
● **CAPSULES**
   Hypertension.
Adults, initial: 2.5 mg twice a day alone or in combination with a thiazide diuretic. If BP is not decreased satisfactorily after 2–4 weeks, the dose may be increased in increments of 5 mg/day at 2 to 4-week intervals up to a maximum of 20 mg/day. Adverse effects increase at doses above 10 mg/day.
DYNACIRC CR
● **TABLETS, CONTROLLED-RELEASE**
   Hypertension.
Adults: 5 mg once daily alone or with a thiazide diuretic. If needed, dose can be increased in increments of 5 mg at 2 to 4-week intervals up to a maximum of 20 mg/day. *NOTE:* For clients over 65 years of age, those with impaired hepatic function, and those with mild renal impairment, the initial dose should be 2.5 mg twice a day for capsules and 5 mg once daily for tablets.

NURSING CONSIDERATIONS
ADMINISTRATION/STORAGE
Store below 30°C (86°F) in a tight container protected from light, moisture, and humidity.
ASSESSMENT
1. Note reasons for therapy, disease onset, other therapies trialed, outcome. With angina, assess characteristics; list other drugs prescribed to ensure none interact unfavorably.
2. Monitor VS, EKG, I&O, weight, CXR, lung sounds, renal, LFTs.
CLIENT/FAMILY TEACHING
1. Take as directed with or without food. Swallow controlled-release tablets whole; do not bite or divide.

---

2. Use caution, may cause dizziness and confusion; assess drug effects. Change positions slowly to prevent rapid drop in BP.

3. Report any SOB, swelling of extremities, irregular heart beat, or prolonged dizziness.

4. Report any increased frequency of anginal attacks.

5. Avoid alcohol and OTC meds without approval.

6. Keep log of BP recordings for provider review.

7. Report for scheduled lab tests: liver and renal function studies every 3–6 months.

OUTCOMES/EVALUATE
Control of HTN

Itraconazole ■ IV
(**ih**-trah-**KON**-ah-zohl)

CLASSIFICATION(S):
Antifungal
PREGNANCY CATEGORY: C
Rx: Sporanox.

USES
Capsules and Injection: (1) Pulmonary and extrapulmonary aspergillosis in nonimmunocompromised or immunocompromised clients who are intolerant of or refractory to amphotericin B therapy. (2) Pulmonary and extrapulmonary blastomycosis in nonimmunocompromised or immunocompromised clients. (3) Histoplasmosis, including chronic cavitary pulmonary disease and disseminated, nonmeningeal histoplasmosis in nonimmunocompromised or immunocompromised clients.

Capsules only: Onychomycosis of the toenail with or without fingernail involvement and onychomycosis of the fingernail because of dermatophytes (*Tinea unguium*) in nonimmunocompromised clients.

Oral Solution: Oropharyngeal and esophageal candidiasis. NOTE: If clients with cystic fibrosis do not respond to the PO solution, consider switching to alternative therapy.

Oral Solution and Injection: For empiric therapy of febrile neutropenic clients with suspected fungal infections.

Investigational: (1) Solution (200 mg/day) as an alternative to fluconazole as secondary prevention of oropharyngeal, vaginal, or esophageal candidiasis in HIV-infected clients who have severe or frequent recurrences. (2) Capsules (200 mg/day) as an alternative to fluconazole for primary prevention of cryptococcosis in adults with advanced HIV disease (CD4 counts less than 50 cells/mcL). (3) Capsules as an alternative to fluconazole for lifelong secondary prevention of cryptococcal disease in HIV-infected adults. (4) Capsules (200 mg/day) as first-line therapy in the primary prevention of histoplasmosis in adults with advanced HIV disease (CD4 counts less than 100 cells/mcL) and live in endemic areas (rate greater than or equal to 10 cases/100 patient-years). Also as first-line drug (200 mg/day) for lifelong secondary prophylaxis. (5) Capsules (200 mg/day) as an alternate drug to fluconazole for lifelong secondary prevention of coccidioidomycosis in HIV-infected adults. (6) Oral products for secondary prevention of histoplasmosis (first line: 2–5 mg/kg q 12–48 hr), cryptococcal disease (alternative therapy: 2–5 mg/kg q 12–24 hr), and coccidioidomycosis (alternative therapy: 2–5 mg/kg q 12–48 hr) in children with HIV. (7) Oral products (2–5 mg/kg q 12–24 hr) for primary prevention of histoplasmosis (first-line drug) and cryptococcal disease (alternative drug) in children with HIV, severe immunosuppression, and live in endemic histoplasmosis areas.

ACTION/KINETICS
Action
Believed to inhibit cytochrome P-450-dependent synthesis of ergosterol, a necessary component of fungal cell membranes.

Pharmacokinetics
Oral bioavailability is maximum when capsules are taken with a full meal. Absorption was increased under fasting conditions in those with AIDS when taken with a cola beverage. Absorption is

---

decreased in the presence of decreased gastric acidity. Concentrates in fatty tissues, omentum, liver, kidney, and skin. T_{max}, **capsules, steady-state:** 4.6 hr. **$t^{1/2}$ for capsules at steady-state:** 64 hr. Extensively metabolized in the liver by CYP3A4; the major metabolite is hydroxyitraconazole, which also has antifungal activity. Metabolites are excreted in both the urine and feces. **Plasma protein binding:** Itraconazole and hydroxyitraconazole: More than 99%.

CONTRAINDICATIONS

Concomitant use of dofetilide, pimozide, quinidine, triazolam, or oral midazolam due to possible serious CV events. Hypersensitivity to the drug or its excipients. Lactation. Use for the treatment of onychomycosis in pregnant women or in women wishing to become pregnant. Use with severe renal dysfunction (C_{CR} less than 30 mL/min). Use of capsules in clients with a history of cardiac dysfunction (e.g., CHF or a history of CHF) or other ventricular dysfunction. Use with HMG-CoA reductase inhibitors (e.g., lovastatin, simvastatin) or ergot alkaloids (e.g., dihydroergotamine, ergotamine, ergonovine, methylergonovine) metabolized by the CYP3A4 enzyme system. Initiation of therapy in clients with elevated or abnormal liver enzyme levels, active liver disease, or a previous incident of hepatotoxicity during therapy with any drug.

SPECIAL CONCERNS

■ (1) Do not give itraconazole to treat onychomycosis or dermatomycoses in clients with evidence of cardiac dysfunction, such as CHF or a history of CHF. Discontinue if S&S of CHF occur during treatment. If S&S of CHF occur during treatment for more serious fungal infections involving other parts of the body, continued use of itraconazole should be reassessed. Possible negative inotropic effects may occur. (2) Coadministration with dofetilide, pimozide, or quinidine is contraindicated. Itraconazole is a potent inhibitor of the CYP3A4 isoenzyme system and may raise plasma concentrations of drugs metabolized by this pathway. Serious CV events, including QT prolongation, torsade de pointes, ventricular tachycardia, cardiac arrest, or sudden death have occurred in those taking itraconazole with these drugs, which are inhibitors of the CYP3A4 system.■ Use with caution in clients with hypersensitivity to other azoles. Safety and efficacy have not been determined in children 3–16 years of age although pediatric clients have been treated for systemic fungal infections. Liver enzymes may be elevated more than twice that of normal.

SIDE EFFECTS

Most Common

N&V, rash, asthenia, headache, abdominal pain, diarrhea, dyspepsia, flatulence, rhinitis, sinusitis, URTI, coughing, fever.

GI: N&V, diarrhea, abdominal pain, anorexia, taste perversion, flatulence, general GI disorders, constipation, dyspepsia, gingivitis, ulcerative stomatitis, gastritis, gastroenteritis, increased appetite, dyspepsia, dysphagia, hemorrhoids, abnormal hepatic function, hepatitis, *serious hepatotoxicity, liver failure*, jaundice. **CNS:** Headache, anxiety, depression, vertigo, dizziness, somnolence, decreased libido, abnormal dreaming, insomnia. **CV:** Hypertension, hypotension, orthostatic hypotension, vasculitis, *CHF*, tachycardia, vein disorder. **Respiratory:** URTI, rhinitis, sinusitis, pharyngitis, coughing, dyspnea, pneumonia, increased sputum, pulmonary edema/infiltration. **Dermatologic:** Increased sweating, skin disorders, hot flushes, rash, pruritus, alopecia, erythematous rash, skin disorder, *Stevens-Johnson syndrome*. **GU:** UTI, impotence, cystitis, menstrual disorders, abnormal renal function, gynecomastia, hematuria. **Allergic:** Rash, pruritus, urticaria, angioedema, *anaphylaxis* (rare). **Body as a whole:** Edema, fatigue, pain, fever, malaise, myalgia, rigors, asthenia, tremor, dehydration, infection, jaundice, fluid overload. **Miscellaneous:** Bursitis, injury, herpes zoster, neutropenia, chest pain, *Pneumocystis carinii* infection, reaction at injection/application site, adrenal insufficiency, back pain, male breast pain, tinnitus, abnormal vision, weight loss, peripheral edema, peripheral neuropathy.

LABORATORY TEST CONSIDERATIONS

↑ ALT, AST, alkaline phosphatase, BUN, serum creatinine, LDH, GGT. Hypertriglyceridemia, hypokalemia, hypocalcemia, hypomagnesemia, hypophosphatemia, albuminuria, bilirubinemia. Abnormal hepatic function.

OD OVERDOSE MANAGEMENT

Symptoms: Extension of side effects. *Treatment:* Use supportive measures, including gastric lavage and sodium bicarbonate. Dialysis will not remove itraconazole.

DRUG INTERACTIONS

Alfentanil / ↑ Alfentanil effect and toxicity R/T inhibition of metabolism

Almotriptan / ↑ Almotriptan levels→ ↑ pharmacologic and side effects; do not take almotriptan within 7 days of itraconazole

Alprazolam / ↑ And prolonged alprazolam levels → ↑ CNS depression and psychomotor impairment

Amphotericin B / ↓ Activity of amphotericin B

Antacids / ↓ Itraconazole absorption R/T ↓ gastric acidity; give antacid at least 1 hr before or 2 hr after itraconazole capsules

Aripiprazole / ↑ Aripiprazole levels → ↑ pharmacologic and side effects; reduce aripiprazole dose by 50% if given with itraconazole

Buspirone / ↑ Buspirone levels → ↑ effects and toxicity

Busulfan / ↑ Busulfan levels → ↑ risk of toxicity (e.g., pancytopenia)

Calcium channel blockers / Inhibition of metabolism of felodipine, nifedipine, nisoldipine, and verapamil; also ↑ negative inotropic effects and possible edema

Carbamazepine / ↑ Carbamazepine levels → ↑ clinical and adverse effects; also, possible ↓ itraconazole levels

Cilostazol / ↑ Cilostazol levels → ↑ pharmacologic and side effects

Clarithromycin / ↑ Itraconazole levels R/T inhibition of metabolism by CYP3A4

Corticosteroids (budesonide, dexamethasone, methylprednisolone) / ↓ Corticosteroid metabolism → ↑ corticosteroid pharmacologic and toxic effects

Cyclosporine / ↑ Cyclosporine levels (dose of cyclosporine should be ↓ by 50% if itraconazole doses are much greater than 100 mg/day)

Diazepam / ↑ And prolonged diazepam levels → ↑ CNS depression and psychomotor impairment

Didanosine (buffered formulation) / ↓ Itraconazole effects; give itraconazole 2 hr or more before didanosine chewable tablets

Digoxin / ↑ Digoxin levels → ↑ pharmacologic and toxic effects

Disopyramide / ↑ Disopyramide levels; potential to ↑ QT interval

Docetaxel / Inhibition of docetaxel metabolism

Dofetilide / ↑ Dofetilide levels → possible serious CV events, including QT prolongation, torsades de pointes, ventricular tachycardia, cardiac arrest, or sudden death; do not use together

Eletriptan / ↑ Eletriptan levels→ ↑ pharmacologic and side effects; do not take eletriptan within 72 hr of itrconazole

Eplerenone / ↑ Eplerenone levels → ↑ risk of hyperkalemia and associated serious arrhythmias; do not use together

Ergot alkaloids (dihydroergotamine, ergonovine, ergotamine, methylergonovine) / ↑ Risk of ergot toxicity (i.e., peripheral vasospasm, ischemia of the extremities, and/or cerebral ischemia

Erythromycin / ↑ Itraconazole levels R/T inhibition of metabolism by CYP3A4

Felodipine / ↑ Felodipine levels (possible edema)

Grapefruit juice / ↓ Itraconazole bioavailability R/T inhibition of absorption

Haloperidol / ↑ Haloperidol levels → ↑ risk of side effects

H$_2$ Antagonists / ↓ Itraconazole absorption R/T ↓ gastric acidity; give itraconazole with a cola beverage

HMG-CoA Reductase Inhibitors (atorvastatin, lovastatin, simvastatin) / ↑ Plasma levels and side effects of reductase inhibitors; possibility of rhabdomyolysis; do not use lovastatin or simvastatin with itraconazole

Indinavir / ↑ Indinavir levels R/T inhibition of metabolism by CYP3A4 → ↑ risk of toxicity; also, possible ↑ itraconazole levels

---

Isoniazid / ↓ Plasma itraconazole levels

Losartan / ↑ Losartan antihypertensive effect

Lovastatin / ↑ Lovastatin levels → possible rhabdomyolysis; do not use together

Methylprednisolone / Inhibition of methylprednisolone metabolism

Midazolam, oral / ↑ Prolonged levels of oral midazolam → ↑ CNS depression and psychomotor impairment

Neviripine / ↓ Itraconazole levels

Nisoldipine / ↑ Nisoldipine levels

Oral Contraceptives / ↓ Oral contraceptive effect

Oral Hypoglycemics / Possible severe hypoglycemia; monitor blood glucose

Phenobarbital / ↓ Itraconazole levels

Phenytoin / ↓ Effect of itraconazole and ↑ effect of phenytoin; do not use together

Pimozide / Possible serious CV events, including QT prolongation, torsade de pointes, ventricular tachycardia, cardiac arrest/sudden death; do not use together

Proton pump inhibitors / ↓ Itraconazole absorption R/T ↓ gastric acidity

Quinidine / Possible serious CV events, including QT prolongation, torsade de pointes, ventricular tachycardia, cardiac arrest and/or sudden death; do not use together

Rifampin, Rifabutin, Rifapentine / ↓ Itraconazole levels; possible ↑ rifabutin levels; do not use together

Ritonavir / ↑ Ritonavir levels R/T inhibition of metabolism by CYP3A4 → ↑ risk of toxicity; also, possible ↑ itraconazole levels

Sildenafil / ↑ Sildenafil levels → ↑ risk of side effects; give sildenafil with caution and in reduced doses

Simvastatin / ↑ Simvastatin levels → possible rhabdomyolysis; do not use together

Sirolimus / Possible ↑ sirolimus levels; monitor for sirolimus toxicity

Sulfonylureas / ↑ Hypoglycemia risk

Tacrolimus / ↑ Tacrolimus levels → ↑ toxicity

Tadalafil / ↑ Tadalafil levels → ↑ risk of side effects; give tadalafil with caution and in reduced doses

Tolterodine / ↑ Tolterodine levels; do not give more than 1 mg tolterodine twice a day

Triazolam / ↑ & Prolonged triazolam levels → ↑ CNS depression and psychomotor impairment

Trimetrexate / Inhibition of trimetrexate metabolism

Vardenafil / ↑ Vardenafil levels → ↑ risk of side effects; give vardenafil with caution and in reduced doses

Vinca alkaloids / ↑ Risk of vinca alkaloid toxicity (e.g., constipation, myalgia, neutropenia) R/T inhibition of metabolism; do not use together

Warfarin / ↑ Anticoagulant effect; monitor PT and INR values q 2 days when adding or discontinuing an azole antifungal

Zolpidem / ↑ Zolpidem effects R/T inhibition of metabolism

HOW SUPPLIED

Capsules: 100 mg; Injection: 10 mg/mL; Oral Solution: 10 mg/mL.

DOSAGE

- **CAPSULES**

    Blastomycosis or chronic pulmonary histoplasmosis.

Adults: 200 mg once daily. If there is no improvement or the disease is progressive, the dose may be increased in 100-mg increments to a maximum of 400 mg/day. Give doses greater than 200 mg/day in 2 divided doses. For life-threatening situations, a loading dose of 200 mg 3 times per day may be given for the first 3 days of treatment.

    Aspergillosis.

200–400 mg daily.

    Onychomycosis, fingernails only.

Two treatment pulses, each consisting of 200 mg twice a day for 1 week. Pulses are separated by a 3-week period without the drug.

    Onychomycosis, toenails with or without fingernail involvement.

200 mg/day for 12 weeks.

    Life-threatening situations.

Loading dose: 200 mg 3 times/day for the first 3 days of treatment; continue treatment for a minimum of 3 months and until clinical parameters and lab tests indicate the active fungal infection has subsided.

- **ORAL SOLUTION**

Esophageal candidiasis.

100 mg/day (10 mL) for a minimum of 3 weeks. Continue treatment for 2 weeks following resolution of symptoms. Doses of 200 mg/day may be used based on medical judgment of response.

Empiric therapy of febrile neutropenia with suspected funal infections.

After about 14 days of IV therapy, continue treatment with PO solution, 200 mg (20 mL) twice a day, until resolution of clinically significant neutropenia. Safety and efficacy for more than 28 days are not known.

Oropharyngeal candidiasis.

200 mg/day (20 mL) for 1–2 weeks. For those unresponsive or refractory to treatment with fluconazole tablets, the recommended dose of itraconazole is 100 mg twice a day. A response should occur within 2–4 weeks. Clients may relapse shortly after discontinuing therapy. Data on use for more than 6 months is lacking.

- **IV**

Blastomycosis, histoplasmosis, aspergillosis.

200 mg twice a day for 4 doses, followed by 200 mg/day. Infuse each IV dose over 1 hr. The safety and efficacy of IV use for more than 14 days is not known. Continue total itraconazole therapy (injection followed by capsules) for a minimum of 3 months and until clinical parameters and lab tests indicate the active fungal infection has subsided. Do not use in clients with a C_{CR} <30 mL/min.

Empiric therapy of febrile neutropenia with suspected fungal infections.

200 mg twice a day for 4 doses, followed by 200 mg once daily for up to 14 days. Infuse each IV dose over 1 hr. Continue treatment with itraconazole PO solution, 200 mg (20 mL) twice a day until resolution of clinically significant neutropenia. The safety and efficacy of itraconazole use exceeding 28 days for this condition is not known.

NURSING CONSIDERATIONS

ADMINISTRATION/STORAGE

1. Take capsules, but not oral solution, after a full meal to ensure maximal absorption. Swallow capsules whole. Swish solution in oral cavity and swallow; do not rinse after swallowing. Do not use capsules and oral solution interchangeably.

2. Give daily doses greater than 200 mg in two divided doses.

3. Continue treatment for a minimum of 3 months until symptoms and lab tests indicate the active fungal infection has subsided. Recurrence of active infection may occur with inadequate treatment period.

4. Absorption from capsules is impaired when gastric acidity is decreased (e.g., use of antacids, proton pump inhibitors, H_2-histamine blockers). Thus, give such drugs at least 2 hr after itraconazole.

5. Give with a cola beverage when co-administering with H_2-antagonists or other gastric acid suppressors

6. Plasma levels using capsules are lower in neutropenic and AIDS clients than in healthy subjects due to hypochlorhydria. However, the bioavailability of the oral solution in AIDS clients is not different from healthy subjects.

7. Protect capsules from light and moisture. Do not freeze the oral solution; discard any unused oral solution 3 months after opening.

IV 8. To prepare, add the full contents (25 mL) of the ampule into the infusion bag provided (contains 50 mL of 0.9% NaCl injection). Mix gently. Do not dilute with D5W or lactated Ringer's.

9. Using a flow control device, infuse 60 mL of the dilute solution (which contains 3.33 mg/mL; therefore total dose will be 200 mg) over 60 min, using an extension line and the infusion set provided. After administration, flush infusion set with 15–20 mL of 0.9% NaCl injection over 0.5–15 min via the 2-way stopcock. Discard the entire infusion line.

10. Do not introduce any other medication through the same bag or same

line. Other drugs may be given after flushing the line/catheter with 0.9% NaCl injection, and removing and replacing the entire infusion line.

11. Do not use IV if C_{CR} is less than 30 mL/min.

12. Store the injection at 25°C (77°F) or less and protect from light and freezing after reconstitution. Refrigerate the diluted drug at 2–8°C (36–46°F) or store at room temperature from 15–25°C (59–77°F) for up to 48 hr. Protect from direct light.

ASSESSMENT

1. Note reasons for therapy, location, onset, characteristics of S&S, other agents prescribed, noting compliance/outcome. Drug is extremely expensive and should not be used as first-line therapy with typical fungal infections.

2. Due to possibility of liver failure, confirm diagnosis of onychomycosis through scrapings/lab tests. If symptoms of CHF develop, stop drug.

3. List drugs currently prescribed to prevent any unfavorable effects. Note any previous liver dysfunction with any other therapy; precludes drug therapy.

4. Monitor CBC, electrolytes, fungal cultures/scrapings, renal and LFTs. Stop therapy if S&S of hepatotoxicity occur; do not reinstitute therapy. Drug is not intended for pregnant or nursing mothers.

5. The response rate of histoplasmosis in HIV-infected clients is similar to non-HIV-infected clients, although the clinical course in HIV-infected clients is more severe and usually requires maintenance therapy to prevent relapse.

6. Absorption may be decreased in HIV-infected clients with hypochlorhydria.

CLIENT/FAMILY TEACHING

1. Take capsules with food to enhance absorption and only as directed (usually for 3 months). Do not take the oral solution with food. Swish oral solution in mouth vigorously for 10 seconds and then swallow. Noncompliance or inadequate treatment period may lead to recurrence of active infection.

2. Practice reliable hygiene measures to prevent spread of infection and reinfection.

3. Avoid activities requiring mental alertness until drug effects realized; may cause drowsiness.

4. Report S&S suggesting liver dysfunction; appetite loss, unusual fatigue, N&V, diarrhea, yellow skin/eyes, or dark urine. Avoid alcohol during therapy.

5. Report symptoms that may indicate reactivation of histoplasmosis, such as weight loss, chest pain, SOB, fever, crackles, and pain.

6. S&S of blastomycosis include SOB, rales, hemoptysis, chest pain, fever, cough, skin lesions, rashes, and weight loss; requires immediate attention.

7. Avoid alcohol and OTC agents without provider approval. Keep F/U appointment to evaluate response to therapy and any adverse side effects.

OUTCOMES/EVALUATE

Eradication of infecting organisms; subjective improvement

Ixabepilone

(ix-ab-**EP**-i-lone)

CLASSIFICATION(S):

Antineoplastic agent, antimitotic (epothilone)

PREGNANCY CATEGORY: D

Rx: Ixempra.

USES

(1) In combination with capecitabine to treat metastatic or locally advanced breast cancer resistant to treatment with an anthracycline or a taxane, or in those whose cancer is taxane-resistant and for whom further anthracycline therapy is contraindicated. (2) As monotherapy to treat metastatic or locally advanced breast cancer in clients whose tumors are resistant or refractory to anthracyclines, taxanes, and capecitabine.

ACTION/KINETICS

Action Ixabepilone binds directly to β-tubulin subunits on microtubules, leading to suppression of microtubule dynamics. The drug blocks cells in the mitotic phase of the cell division cycle, leading to cell death.

Pharmacokinetics

Maximum plasma levels: 3 hr. Extensively metabolized in the liver by CYP3A4. Eliminated primarily as metabolites in the feces (65%) and urine (21%). **t½, elimination:** 52 hr.

CONTRAINDICATIONS

In those with a history of severe (CTC grade 3/4) hypersensitivity reaction to drugs containing polyoxyethylated castor oil. Clients who have neutrophil counts less than 1,500 cells/mm^3 or a platelet count less than 100,000 cells/mm^3. In combination with capecitabine in those with AST or ALT greater than 2.5 times ULN or bilirubin greater than 1 times ULN. Lactation.

SPECIAL CONCERNS

■ Ixabepilone in combination with capecitabine is contraindicated in clients with AST or ALT greater than 2.5 times ULN or bilirubin greater than 1 times ULN because of an increased risk of toxicity and neutropenia-related death.■ Use with caution in those with a history of cardiac disease. Incidence of toxicity is higher in the elderly. Safety and efficacy have not been determined in children.

SIDE EFFECTS

Most Common

Alopecia, diarrhea, fatigue/asthenia, musculoskeletal pain, myalgia, arthralgia, peripheral neuropathy, stomatitis, mucositis, N&V, palmar-plantar erythrodysesthesia syndrome, nail disorder, hematologic abnormalities.

Side effects listed are for monotherapy as well as therapy combined with capecitabine. **GI:** Diarrhea, stomatitis, anorexia, mucositis, N&V, abdominal pain, constipation, GERD, taste disorder, colitis, dysphagia, enterocolitis, esophagitis, gastritis, *GI hemorrhage*, ileus, impaired gastric emptying. **Hepatic:** *Acute hepatic failure*, jaundice. **CNS:** Neuropathy (burning sensation, hyper-/hypoesthesia, paresthesia, discomfort, neuropathic pain), motor neuropathy, insomnia, dizziness, headache, abnormal coordination, *cerebral hemor-*

rhage, cognitive disorder, lethargy, syncope. **Dermatologic:** Palmar-plantar erythrodysesthesia syndrome, alopecia, nail disorder, skin hyperpigmentation, skin exfoliation, pruritus, erythema multiforme. **Hematologic:** Anemia, leukopenia, thrombocytopenia, neutropenia, febrile neutropenia, coagulopathy, lymphopenia, neutropenic infection. **CV:** Hot flush, angina pectoris, atrial flutter, *cardiomyopathy, embolism, hemorrhage,* hypotension, hypovolemic shock, left ventricular dysfunction, *MI,* myocardial ischemia, supraventricular tachycardia, *thrombosis,* vasculitis. **Musculoskeletal:** Myalgia, arthralgia, musculoskeletal pain, chest pain, muscle spasms, muscle weakness, trismus. **Respiratory:** Dyspnea, cough, URTI, acute pulmonary edema, dysphonia, hypoxia, laryngitis, lower RTI, pharyngolaryngeal pain, pneumonia, pneumonitis, *respiratory failure.* **GU:** UTI, nephrolithiasis, renal failure. **Metabolic/Nutritional:** Decreased weight, dehydration. **Ophthalmic:** Increased lacrimation. **Body as a whole:** Fatigue, asthenia, edema, hypersensitivity reactions, pain, pyrexia, bacterial infection, chills, infection, *sepsis*.

LABORATORY TEST CONSIDERATIONS

↑ Blood alkaline phosphatase, GGT, ALT, AST. Hypokalemia, hyponatremia, hypovolemia, metabolic acidosis.

DRUG INTERACTIONS

Azole antifungals (e.g., fluconazole, itraconazole, ketoconazole, voriconazole) / ↑ Ixabepilone levels R/T inhibition of CYP3A4; if alternative treatment not possible, consider dosage adjustment

Carbamazepine / ↓ Ixabepilone levels R/T induction of CYP3A4 → subtherapeutic levels

Delavirdine / ↑ Ixabepilone levels R/T inhibition of CYP3A4; avoid coadministration

Dexamethasone / ↓ Ixabepilone levels R/T induction of CYP3A4 → subtherapeutic levels

Grapefruit juice / ↑ Ixabepilone plasma levels; do not use together

Macrolide antibiotics (e.g., clarithromycin, erythromycin) / ↑ Ixabepilone levels R/T inhibition of CYP3A4; avoid co-

---

Bold Italic = life threatening side effect   ■ = black box warning   ✦ = Available in Canada

administration

Nefazodone / ↑ Ixabepilone levels R/T inhibition of CYP3A4; avoid coadministration

Phenobarbital / ↓ Ixabepilone levels R/T induction of CYP3A4 → subtherapeutic levels

Phenytoin / ↓ Ixabepilone levels R/T induction of CYP3A4 → subtherapeutic levels

Protease inhibitors (e.g., amprenavir, atazanavir, indinavir, nelfinavir, ritonavir, saquinavir) / ↑ Ixabepilone levels R/T inhibition of CYP3A4; avoid coadministration

Rifamycins (e.g., rifabutin, rifamycin, rifampin) / ↓ Ixabepilone levels R/T induction of CYP3A4 → subtherapeutic levels

H *St. John's wort* / ↓ Ixabepilone levels unpredictably; avoid concomitant use

Telithromycin / ↑ Ixabepilone levels R/T inhibition of CYP3A4; avoid coadministration

Verapamil / ↑ Ixabepilone levels R/T inhibition of CYP3A4; use together with caution and monitor closely for toxicity

HOW SUPPLIED

Injection, Lyophilized Powder for Injection, Concentrate: 15 mg, 45 mg.

DOSAGE

- **IV ONLY**

    Breast cancer.

40 mg/m^2 given over 3 hr q 3 weeks. Doses for those with body surface area greater than 2.2 m^2 should be calculated based on 2.2 m^2.

NURSING CONSIDERATIONS

ADMINISTRATION/STORAGE

1. Premedicate clients with both an H$_1$- and H$_2$- antagonist about 1 hr before ixabepilone infusion and observe for hypersensitivity reactions. In cases of severe hypersensitivity reactions, stop the infusion and begin aggressive supportive treatment (e.g., epinephrine, corticosteroids).
2. The ixabepilone kit contains 2 vials—one labeled ixabepilone for injection that contains the drug and the other containing the diluent (use only this diluent to reconstitute). Before re-constituting, allow the kit to stand at room temperature for about 30 min.
3. To allow for withdrawal losses, the vial labeled 15 mg for injection contains 16 mg and the vial labeled 45 mg for injection contains 47 mg.
4. To reconstitute, aseptically withdraw the diluent with a suitable syringe and slowly inject it into the ixabepilone for injection vial. The 15 mg kit contains 8 mL of the diluent and the 45 mg kit contains 23.5 mL of the diluent. Gently swirl and invert the vial until the powder is completely dissolved. After reconstituting with the diluent, the concentration of ixabepilone is 2 mg/mL.
5. Before administration, the reconstituted solution must be further diluted only with Ringer's lactate injection, supplied in di-(2-ethylhexyl)phthalate-free bags. For most doses, a 250 mL bag of Ringer's lactate is sufficient. The final concentration of the diluted solution for infusion must be between 0.2 and 0.6 mg/mL. To calculate the final infusion concentration, use the following formulas:

- Total infusion volume = mL of reconstituted solution + mL of Ringer's lactate injection

6. Administer the infusion solution through an appropriate inline filter with a microporous membrane of 0.2-1.3 microns. Discard any remaining solution. Administration of diluted ixabepilone must be completed within 6 hr.
7. To minimize the risk of dermal exposure, wear impervious gloves when handling vials containing ixabepilone.
8. Evaluate all clients receiving ixabepilone for toxicity and delay treatment to allow recovery. The following are dosage adjustments for monotherapy and combination therapy:

- Decrease the dose by 20% in the event of grade 2 neuropathy (moderate) lasting 7 or more days.
- Decrease the dose by 20% in the event of grade 2 neuropathy (severe) lasting less than 7 days.
- Discontinue treatment in the event of grade 2 neuropathy (severe) lasting 7 or more days or disabling neuropathy.

- Decrease dose by 20% for any grade 3 toxicity (severe) other than neuropathy.
- No change in the dose of ixabepilone is needed in the event of transient grade 3 arthralgia/myalgia or fatigue or for grade 3 hand-foot syndrome (palmar-plantar erythrodysesthesia).
- Discontinue treatment for any grade 4 toxicity (disabling).
- Decrease the dose by 20% if neutrophils are <500 cells/mm^3 for 7 or more days.
- Decrease the dose by 20% in the event of febrile neutropenia.
- Decrease the dose by 20% if platelets are <25,000/mm^3 or platelets are <50,000/mm^3 with bleeding.
- NOTE: If toxicities recur, reduce the dose by an additional 20%.

9. Dosage adjustment for capecitabine when used in combination with ixabepilone.

- For nonhematologic toxicity, follow the guidelines on the capecitabone label.
- If platelets are <25,000/mm^3 or <50,000/mm^3 with bleeding, hold for concurrent diarrhea or stomatitis until platelet count is >50,000/mm^3; then continue at the same dose.
- If neutrophils are <500 cells/mm^3 for 7 days or longer or if febrile neutropenia, hold for concurrent diarrhea or stomatitis until neutrophil count is >1,000 cells/mm^3; then continue at the same dose.

10. Clients should not begin a new cycle of treatment unless the neutrophil count is at least 1,500 cells/mm^3, the platelet count is at least 100,000 cells/mm^3, and nonhematologic toxicities have improved to grade 1 (mild) or resolved.

11. All clients must be premedicated with a H-1 antagonist (e.g., diphenhydramine, 50 mg PO or equivalent) and a H-2 antagonist (e.g., ranitidine, 150-300 mg PO or equivalent) about 1 hr before the ixabepilone infusion begins. Those who experienced a hypersensitivity reaction required premedication with corticosteroids (e.g., dexamethasone, 20 mg IV 30 min before the infusion or PO 60 min before the infusion) in addition to pretreatment with H-1 and H-2 antagonists.

12. If a strong CYP3A4 inhibitor (see *Drug Interactions*) is required, reduce the dose of ixabepilone by 20 mg/m^2. If the strong inhibitor is discontinued, allow a washout period of about 1 week before the ixabepilone dose is adjusted upward to the indicated dose.

13. Store the ixabepilone kit from 2-8°C (36-46°F) in the original package to protect from light.

ASSESSMENT

1. Note reasons for therapy, clinical presentation, therapies trialed.

2. List all drugs prescribed to ensure none interact.

3. Perform clinical examination and identify findings. Obtain baseline CBC, renal, LFTs; monitor during therapy. If abnormal– adjust dosage as outlined in administration.

4. Identify any liver or heart disease; precludes therapy.

5. Assess for any allergy to taxol or castor oil.

CLIENT/FAMILY TEACHING

1. Drug is generally given IV over 3 hrs every 3 weeks along with the medicine capecitabine. Will be medicated 1 hr before infusion with benadryl and zantac to help prevent allergic reactions.

2. Infusion contains alcohol. Avoid activities that require mental alertness i.e., driving or operating machinery as dizziness or drowsiness may occur.

3. Do not drink grapefruit juice while receiving Ixempra; may cause increased blood levels of Ixempra and increase adverse side effects.

4. Report any numbness and tingling of extremities, fever over 100.5° F or chills, cough, burning or pain on urination. If itching, rash, flushing, swelling, SOB, chest tightness or other allergic reactions occur report immediately.

5. Use reliable contraception to prevent pregnancy and avoid nursing.

6. Any pain, difficulty breathing, palpitations or unusual weight gain should be evaluated.

Bold Italic = life threatening side effect   ■ = black box warning   ✤ = Available in Canada

7. Keep all F/U appointments for lab studies and to evaluate response to therapy.

OUTCOMES/EVALUATE
Tumor regression with metastatic breast cancer

Ketoconazole ■

(kee-toe-**KON**-ah-zohl)

CLASSIFICATION(S):
Antifungal
PREGNANCY CATEGORY: C
OTC: Nizoral, Nizoral A-D.
Rx: Extina; Ketoconazole Cream, Shampoo, and Tablets; Xolegel.
✦Rx: Apo-Ketoconazole, Ketoderm, Novo-Ketoconazole.

SEE ALSO *ANTI-INFECTIVE DRUGS.*

USES
PO: (1) Candidiasis, chronic mucocutaneous candidiasis, candiduria, histoplasmosis, chromomycosis, oral thrush, blastomycosis, coccidioidomycosis, paracoccidioidomycosis. (2) Recalcitrant cutaneous dermatophyte infections not responding to other therapy. *Investigational:* Onychomycosis due to *Trichophyton* and *Candida*. CNS fungal infections (high doses). Cushing's syndrome.

   Cream: (1) Tinea pedis, tinea corporis, and tinea cruris due to *Trichophyton rubrum, T. mentagrophytes,* and *Epidermophyton floccosum.* (2) Tinea versicolor caused by *Microsporum furfur.* (3) Cutaneous candidiasis caused by *Candida* sp. (4) Seborrheic dermatitis.

   Foam/Gel: Seborrheic dermatitis in immunocompetent adults and children 12 years and older. Safety and efficacy to treat fungal infections have not been established.

   Shampoo: Reduce scaling, flaking, and itching due to dandruff.

ACTION/KINETICS
Action
Inhibits synthesis of ergosterol (the main sterol of fungal cell membranes), damaging the cell membrane and resulting in loss of essential intracellular material. Also inhibits biosynthesis of triglycerides and phospholipids and inhibits oxidative and peroxidative enzyme activity. When used to treat *Candida albicans,* it inhibits transformation of blastospores into the invasive mycelial form. Inhibits growth of *Pityrosporum ovale* when used to treat dandruff. Use in Cushing's syndrome is due to its ability to inhibit adrenal steroidogenesis.

Pharmacokinetics
Peak plasma levels: 3.5 mcg/mL after 1–2 hr after a 200-mg dose. **t½, biphasic:** first, 2 hr; second, 8 hr. Requires acidity for dissolution. Metabolized in liver to inactive metabolites and most excreted through feces.

CONTRAINDICATIONS
Hypersensitivity, fungal meningitis. Topical products not for ophthalmic use. Use during lactation.

SPECIAL CONCERNS
■ PO ketoconazole has been associated with hepatic toxicity, including some fatalities. Closely monitor clients and inform them of the risk.■ Use tablets with caution in children less than 2 years of age. The safety and effectiveness of topical products have not been determined in children. Use with caution during lactation.

SIDE EFFECTS
Most Common
Systemic use: N&V, abdominal pain, pruritus.
Topical use: Stinging, irritation, pruritus.
TABLETS. GI: N&V, abdominal pain, diarrhea, hepatotoxicity (including fatalities). **CNS:** Headache, dizziness, somnolence, fever, chills, suicidal tendencies, depression (rare). **Hematologic:** Thrombocytopenia, leukopenia, *hemolytic*

anemia. **Miscellaneous:** Hepatotoxicity, photophobia, pruritus, gynecomastia, impotence, bulging fontanelles, urticaria, decreased serum testosterone levels, anaphylaxis (rare).

TOPICAL CREAM. Stinging, irritation (may be severe), pruritus.

SHAMPOO. Increased hair loss; irritation; abnormal hair texture; itching; oiliness or dryness of the scalp and hair; scalp pustules.

LABORATORY TEST CONSIDERATIONS

Transient ↑ serum liver enzymes. ↓ Serum testosterone.

DRUG INTERACTIONS

Almotriptan / ↑ AUC and plasma levels of almotriptan R/T ketoconazole inhibition of gut wall and hepatic first-pass metabolism of almotriptan

Antacids / ↓ Absorption of ketoconazole R/T ↑ pH

Anticoagulants / ↑ Anticoagulant effect

Benzodiazepines / Prolonged levels → ↑ CNS depression and psychomotor impairment

Buspirone / ↑ Buspirone levels

Carbamazepine / ↑ Carbamazepine levels

Corticosteroids / ↑ Risk of drug toxicity R/T ↑ bioavailability

Cyclosporine / ↑ Cyclosporine levels (ketaconazole may be used therapeutically to decrease cyclosporine dose) R/T inhibition of metabolism

Didanosinse / ↓ Ketoconazole effect R/T ↓ absorption

Docetaxel / ↓ Docetaxel clearance R/T ↓ metabolism by CYP3A4

Donepezil / ↑ Levels of donepezil R/T ↓ liver metabolism

Histamine H₂ antagonists / ↓ Ketoconazole absorption R/T ↑ gastric pH

Imatinib / ↑ Imatinib AUC and peak levels and ↓ AUC and peak level of imatinib R/T inhibition of CYP3A4 metabolism

Isoniazid / ↓ Bioavailability of ketoconazole

Nisoldipine / ↑ Nisoldipine levels R/T ↓ liver metabolism

Oral Contraceptives / Possible ↓ effect of contraceptive

Protease inhibitors (Indinavir, Ritonavir, Saquinavir) / ↑ Levels of protease inhibitor

Proton pump inhibitors / ↓ Ketoconazole effect R/T ↓ bioavailability

Quinidine / ↑ Quinidine levels

Rifampin / ↓ Levels of either drug

Rosiglitazone / ↑ Rosiglitazone AUC and peak plasma levels and prolonged t½ R/T inhibition of CYP2C8 and CYP2C9

Sucralfate / ↓ Ketoconazole effect R/T ↓ bioavailability

Sulfonylureas / ↑ Hypoglycemic effect R/T ↑ serum levels

Theophyllines / ↓ Serum theophylline levels R/T ↓ absorption

Tolterodine / ↑ Tolterodine t½ and AUC in those deficient in CYP2D6 enzymes

Tricyclic antidepressants / ↑ TCA levels

Vinca alkaloids / ↑ Risk of vinca toxicity R/T inhibition of metabolism

Zolpidem / ↑ Half-life of zolpidem R/T ↓ liver metabolism

HOW SUPPLIED

Cream, Topical (Rx): 2%; *Foam, Topical (Rx):* 2%; *Gel, Topical (Rx):* 2%; *Shampoo:* 1% (OTC), 2% (Rx); *Tablets (Rx):* 200 mg.

DOSAGE

• **TABLETS**

Fungal infections.

Adults: 200 mg once daily; in serious infections or if response is not sufficient, increase to 400 mg once daily. **Pediatric, over 2 years:** 3.3–6.6 mg/kg once daily. Dosage has not been established for children less than 2 years of age.

CNS fungal infections.

Adults: 800–1,200 mg/day.

Cushing's syndrome.

800–1,200 mg/day.

• **CREAM, TOPICAL**

Tinea corporis, tinea cruris, tinea versicolor, tinea pedis, cutaneous candidiasis.

Cover the affected and immediate surrounding areas once daily (twice daily for more resistant cases). Duration of treatment is usually 2 weeks for tinea versicolor and 6 weeks for tinea pedis.

Seborrheic dermatitis.

Apply to affected area once a day for 2 weeks.

• **FOAM**

Seborrheic dermatitis.
Apply to the affected area twice daily for 4 weeks.
- **GEL, TOPICAL**
  Seborrheic dermatitis.
  Apply once daily to affected area for 2 weeks.
- **SHAMPOO**
  Reduction of scaling due to dandruff.
  Apply sufficient shampoo to produce enough lather to wash scalp and hair and gently massage it over the entire scalp area for about 1 minute. Rinse hair thoroughly with warm water and repeat leaving shampoo on the scalp for an additional 3 minutes. Shampoo twice a week for 4 weeks with at least 3 days between each shampooing. Then, use intermittently as needed.

NURSING CONSIDERATIONS
ADMINISTRATION/STORAGE
1. Give a minimum of 2 hr before administration of drugs that increase gastric pH (such as antacids, anticholinergics, or H_2 blockers).
2. The minimum treatment for candidiasis (using tablets) is 1–2 weeks; for other systemic mycoses 6 months. The minimum treatment for recalcitrant dermatophyte infections is 4 weeks in cases involving glabrous skin; palmar and plantar infections may respond more slowly.
ASSESSMENT
1. Note reasons for therapy, clinical presentation, other agents trialed, outcome.
2. Monitor LFTs before/during therapy.
3. List all drugs/agents prescribed to ensure none interact.
CLIENT/FAMILY TEACHING
1. Take tablets with food to decrease GI upset. Take 2 hr before drugs (antacids) that change gastric pH. Water, fruit juice, coffee, or tea provides an acid medium for dissolution and absorption.
2. Apply shampoo to wet hair in sufficient quantities to cover the entire scalp for 1 min. Rinse with warm water; repeat, leaving shampoo on the scalp for 3 min. After the second washing, rinse thoroughly and dry hair with towel or warm air flow. Use twice a week

for 4 weeks with at least 3 days between treatments.
3. Report persistent fever, pain, rash, severe N&V, unusual bruising/bleeding, yellow skin or eyes, dark urine, pale stools, or diarrhea.
4. With lack of stomach acid, may dissolve each tablet in 4 mL aqueous solution of 0.2 N HCl; use a straw to avoid contact with teeth. Follow by drinking a full glass of water.
5. Use caution when driving or performing hazardous tasks; tablets may cause headaches, dizziness, and drowsiness. Avoid all forms of alcohol. Report adverse effects or lack of response.
6. Wear sunglasses, sunscreen, and protective clothing to prevent photosensitivity reactions.
7. Complete the full course of therapy. Long-term therapy is needed and beneficial effects may not be evident for several weeks. Interruption of therapy may cause recurrence of infection.

OUTCOMES/EVALUATE
- Eradication of fungal infections
- Clearing of skin lesions
- Control of dandruff with ↓ scaling

Ketoprofen
(kee-toe-**PROH**-fen)

CLASSIFICATION(S):
Nonsteroidal anti-inflammatory drug
PREGNANCY CATEGORY: B
♣Rx: Apo-Keto, Apo-Keto-E, Apo-Keto-SR, Novo-Keto, Novo-Keto-EC, Nu-Ketoprofen, Nu-Ketoprofen-SR, Orudis-SR, Rhodis, Rhodis SR, Rhodis-EC, Rhovail.

SEE ALSO NONSTEROIDAL ANTI-INFLAMMATORY DRUGS.
USES
Rx: (1) Acute or chronic rheumatoid arthritis and osteoarthritis (both immediate-release and sustained-release capsules). (2) Primary dysmenorrhea (immediate-release capsules only). (3) Analgesic for mild to moderate pain (immediate-release capsule only).

OTC: Temporary relief of aches and pains associated with the common cold, toothache, headache, muscle aches, backache, menstrual cramps, reduction of fever, and minor arthritic pain.

ACTION/KINETICS

Action

Possesses anti-inflammatory, antipyretic, and analgesic properties. Known to inhibit both prostaglandin and leukotriene synthesis, to have antibradykinin activity, and to stabilize lysosomal membranes.

Pharmacokinetics

Onset: 15–30 min. **Peak plasma levels:** 0.5–2 hr. **Duration:** 4–6 hr. $t\frac{1}{2}$: 2–4 hr. $t\frac{1}{2}$, **geriatrics:** Approximately 5 hr. For Ketoprofen ER: **Peak:** 6–7 hr; $t\frac{1}{2}$: 5.4 hr. Food does not alter the bioavailability; however, the rate of absorption is reduced. **Plasma protein binding:** 99%.

CONTRAINDICATIONS

Use during late pregnancy, in children, and during lactation. Use of the extended-release product for acute pain in any client or for initial therapy in clients who are small, elderly, or who have renal or hepatic impairment.

SPECIAL CONCERNS

Safety and effectiveness have not been established in children. Geriatric clients may manifest increased and prolonged serum levels due to decreased protein binding and clearance. Use with caution in clients with a history of GI tract disorders, in fluid retention, hypertension, and heart failure.

SIDE EFFECTS

Most Common

Abdominal pain/cramps, diarrhea, N&V, constipation, flatulence, dyspepsia/indigestion, headache, CNS depression or excitation, impaired renal function, edema.

See *Nonsteroidal Anti-Inflammatory Drugs* for a complete list of possible side effect. Also, **GI:** Peptic ulcer, *GI bleeding,* dyspepsia, nausea, diarrhea, constipation, abdominal pain, flatulence, anorexia, vomiting, stomatitis. **CNS:** Headache. **CV:** Peripheral edema, fluid retention.

ADDITIONAL DRUG INTERACTIONS

Acetylsalicylic acid / ↑ Plasma ketoprofen levels R/T ↓ plasma protein binding

Hydrochlorothiazide / ↓ Chloride and potassium excretion

Methotrexate / Concomitant use → toxic plasma levels of methotrexate

Probenecid / ↓ Plasma clearance of ketoprofen and ↓ plasma protein binding

Warfarin / Additive effect to cause bleeding

HOW SUPPLIED

Capsules, Extended-Release: 100 mg, 150 mg, 200 mg; *Capsules, Intermediate-Release:* 50 mg, 75 mg; *Tablets:* 12.5 mg (OTC).

DOSAGE

- **CAPSULES, EXTENDED-RELEASE; CAPSULES, IMMEDIATE-RELEASE**

  Rheumatoid arthritis, osteoarthritis.

  Adults, initial: 75 mg 3 times per day or 50 mg 4 times per day for immediate release; for extended-release, 200 mg once a day. Doses above 300 mg/day for the immediate-release or 200 mg/day for the extended-release are not recommended. Decrease dose by one-half to one-third in clients with impaired renal function or in elderly.

- **CAPSULES, IMMEDIATE-RELEASE ONLY**

  Mild to moderate pain, dysmenorrhea.

  Adults: 25–50 mg q 6–8 hr as required, not to exceed 300 mg/day. Reduce dose in smaller or geriatric clients and in those with liver or renal dysfunction. Doses greater than 75 mg do not provide any added therapeutic effect.

- **TABLETS (OTC)**

  Adults, over 16 years, of age: 12.5 mg with a full glass of liquid every 4 to 6 hr. If pain or fever persists after 1 hr follow with an additional 12.5 mg. Experience may determine that an initial dose of 25 mg gives a better effect. Do not exceed a dose of 25 mg in a 4- to 6-hr period or 75 mg in a 24-hr period.

NURSING CONSIDERATIONS

ADMINISTRATION/STORAGE

1. The maximum recommended daily dose in those with mild renal impair-

ment is 150 mg. In those with a more severe renal impairment (C_{CR} <25 mL/min/1.73 m^2 or end-stage renal impairment) the maximum recommended daily dose is 100 mg.

2. Reduce initial dose of both immediate-release and extended-release capsules in elderly clients (>75 years old).

3. The maximum daily dose should be 100 mg in clients with impaired liver function and serum albumin levels <3.5 grams/L. If good tolerance is demonstrated, the dose may be increased to the recommended dosage for the general population.

4. Store from 15–30°C (59–86°F). Protect from direct light and excessive heat and humidity.

ASSESSMENT

1. List reasons for therapy, type, onset, location, ADL/pain level, symptom characteristics.

2. Note history of GI disorders/bleeding, cardiac failure, hypertension, or edema.

3. With cardiac disease determine risk factors; advise increased risk of thrombotic events, MI, and stroke, which can be fatal with prolonged use.

4. Determine if pregnant. Not for children under age 12.

5. Monitor CBC, renal and LFTs. In high doses, may prolong bleeding times by decreasing platelet aggregation. Reduce dose/stop with increased renal dysfunction/GI bleeding; consider adding H2 blocker.

CLIENT/FAMILY TEACHING

1. GI side effects may be minimized by taking with antacids, milk, or food.

2. Use caution; may cause dizziness and drowsiness. Review risks of prolonged therapy.

3. Avoid alcohol; may increase risk for GI bleed. Report adverse effects or lack of response.

4. Do not take any OTC agents or aspirin products unless specifically prescribed/approved.

5. Report any new symptoms such as rash, headaches, black stools, disturbances in vision, unexplained bruising, or bleeding from the gums or nose.

6. Report any S&S of liver dysfunction such as fatigue, upper right quadrant pain, clay-colored stools, or yellowing of the skin and eyes.

7. Avoid prolonged sun exposure; use protection if exposed.

8. Keep all F/U appointments to evaluate CBC, renal and LFTS and response to therapy.

OUTCOMES/EVALUATE
- ↓ Joint pain/swelling; ↑ mobility
- ↓ Uterine cramping

Ketorolac tromethamine

■ IV

(kee-toh-**ROH**-lack)

K

CLASSIFICATION(S):
Nonsteroidal anti-inflammatory drug

PREGNANCY CATEGORY: C

Rx: Acular, Acular LS, Acular PF.

✿**Rx:** Apo-Ketorolac, Apo-Ketorolac Injectable, Novo-Ketorolac, Toradol IM.

SEE ALSO *NONSTEROIDAL ANTI-INFLAMMATORY DRUGS.*

USES

PO: Short-term (up to 5 days) management of severe, acute pain in adults that requires analgesia at the opiate level, usually in a postoperative setting. Always initiate therapy with IV or IM followed by PO only as continuation treatment, if necessary. The combination of ketorolac tromethamine IV/IM and ketorolac tromethamine oral is not to exceed 5 days due to the potential of increased frequency and severity of side effects. Switch clients to alternative analgesics as soon as possible.

IM/IV: As a single or multiple dose regimen on a regular or as needed schedule for the management of moderately severe acute pain that requires analgesia at the opioid level, usually in a postoperative setting. Switch to alternative analgesics as soon as possible, but no later than after 5 days.

Ophthalmic, Acular (0.5%): (1) Relieve itching caused by seasonal allergic conjunctivitis. (2) Postoperative inflammation following cataract surgery.

Ophthalmic, Acular LS (0.4%): Reduce ocular pain, burning, and stinging after corneal refractive surgery.

Ophthalmic, Acular PF (0.5%): Reduction of ocular pain and photophobia following incisional refractive surgery. Is a preservative-free product.

ACTION/KINETICS
Action
Possesses anti-inflammatory, analgesic, and antipyretic effects.

Pharmacokinetics
Completely absorbed following IM use. **Onset:** Within 30 min. **Maximum effect:** 1–2 hr after IV or IM dosing. **Duration:** 4–6 hr. **Peak plasma levels:** 2.2–3.0 mcg/mL 50 min after a dose of 30 mg. **$t^{1/2}$, terminal:** 3.8–6.3 hr in young adults and 4.7–8.6 hr in geriatric clients. Metabolized in the liver with over 90% excreted in the urine and the remainder excreted in the feces. **Plasma protein binding:** More than 99%.

CONTRAINDICATIONS
Hypersensitivity to the drug or allergic symptoms (angioedema, bronchospasm) to aspirin or other NSAIDs. Active peptic ulcer disease, recent GI bleeding or perforation, history of peptic ulcer disease or GI bleeding. Advanced renal impairment and in those at risk for renal failure due to volume depletion. Suspected or confirmed cerebrovascular bleeding, hemorrhagic diathesis, or incomplete hemostasis and in those with a high risk of bleeding. As prophylactic analgesic before any major surgery or intraoperatively when hemostasis is critical (due to increased risk of bleeding). Intrathecal or epidural administration (due to alcohol content of product). Use of injection/tablets in labor, delivery, or during lactation. Use with aspirin or other NSAIDs. Use of the ophthalmic solution in clients wearing soft contact lenses.

SPECIAL CONCERNS
■ (1) Indicated for the short-term (up to 5 days) management of moderately severe acute pain that requires analgesia at the opioid level in adults. Not to be used for minor or chronic painful conditions. Is a potent NSAID analgesic; its use carries many risks. Side effects can be serious in certain clients for whom ketorolac is indicated, especially when used inappropriately. Increasing the dose beyond the label recommendations will not provide better efficacy but will result in increased risk of developing serious side effects. (2) GI effects. Ketorolac tromethamine can cause peptic ulcers, GI bleeding, or perforation. Therefore, it is contraindicated in clients with active peptic ulcer disease, in clients with recent GI bleeding or perforation, and in those with a history of peptic ulcer disease or GI bleeding. (3) Renal effects. Ketorolac tromethamine is contraindicated in those with advanced renal impairment and in clients at risk for renal failure due to volume depletion. (4) Risk of bleeding. Ketorolac tromethamine inhibits platelet function and is, therefore, contraindicated in clients with suspected or confirmed cerebrovascular bleeding, hemorrhagic diathesis, incomplete hemostasis, and in those at high risk of bleeding. It is also contraindicated as a prophylactic analgesic before any major surgery and is contraindicated intraoperatively when hemostasis is critical because of the increased risk of bleeding. (5) Hypersensitivity. Hypersensitivity reactions ranging from bronchospasm to anaphylactic shock have occurred and appropriate counteractive measures must be available when administering the first dose of ketorolac tromethamine IV/IM. Ketorolac is contraindicated in those who have previously demonstrated hypersensitivity to ketorolac or allergic manifestations to aspirin or other NSAIDs. (6) Intrathecal or epidural administration. Ketorolac tromethamine is contraindicated for neuraxial (epidural or intrathecal) administration due to its alcohol content. (7) Labor, delivery, and nursing. Ketorolac tromethamine is contraindicated in labor and delivery because it may adversely affect fetal circulation and inhibit uterine contractions. The use is contraindicated in nursing mothers because of the potential adverse effects of prostaglandin-inhibiting

drugs on neonates. (8) Concomitant use with NSAIDs. Ketorolac tromethamine is contraindicated in clients currently receiving aspirin or NSAIDs because of the cumulative risks of inducing serious NSAID-related adverse effects. (9) Ketorolac tromethamine oral is indicated only as continuation therapy to ketorolac tromethamine IV/IM, and the combined duration of use of ketorolac tromethamine IV/IM and ketorolac tromethamine oral is not to exceed 5 days because of the increased risk of serious adverse effects. The recommended total daily dose of ketorolac tromethamine oral (maximum 40 mg) is significantly lower than that for ketorolac tromethamine IV/IM (maximum 120 mg). (10) Special populations. Dosage should be adjusted for clients greater than or equal to 65 years of age, for clients less than 50 kg (110 lbs) of body weight, and for clients with moderately elevated serum creatine. Doses of ketorolac IV/IM are not to exceed 60 mg (total dose per day) in these clients. Ketorolac is indicated as a single dose therapy in pediatric clients; not to exceed 30 mg for IM administration and 15 mg for IV administration.■ The age of the client, dosage, and duration of therapy should receive special consideration when using this drug. Use of ophthalmic products in clients with complicated ocular surgeries, corneal denervation, corneal epithelial defects, diabetes mellitus, ocular surface diseases, rheumatoid arthritis, or repeat ocular surgeries within a short period of time may be at increased risk for corneal side effects that may be sight-threatening. Safety and effectiveness of the systemic products have not been determined in children less than 2 years of age and of the ophthalmic product in children less than 3 years of age. Use ophthalmic products with caution during lactation.

SIDE EFFECTS

Most Common

Systemic use: Headache, dizziness, drowsiness, diarrhea, nausea, dyspepsia/indigestion, epigastric/GI pain, edema.

Ophthalmic use: Transient burning/stinging upon administration, ocular irritation.

See *Nonsteroidal Anti-Inflammatory Drugs* for a complete set of possible side effects, as well as information under *Special Concerns*. Also, **CV:** Vasodilation, pallor. **GI:** GI pain, peptic ulcers, nausea, dyspepsia, flatulence, GI fullness, stomatitis, excessive thirst, GI bleeding (higher risk in geriatric clients), **perforation**. **CNS:** Headache, nervousness, abnormal thinking, depression, euphoria. **Hypersensitivity: *Bronchospasm, anaphylaxis*. Miscellaneous:** Purpura, asthma, abnormal vision, abnormal liver function. **Ophthalmic Solution.** Transient stinging and burning following instillation, ocular irritation, allergic reactions, superficial ocular infections, superficial keratitis.

DRUG INTERACTIONS

Ketorolac may ↑ plasma levels of salicylates due to ↓ plasma protein binding.

HOW SUPPLIED

Injection: 15 mg/mL, 30 mg/mL; *Ophthalmic Solution:* 0.4%, 0.5%; *Tablets:* 10 mg.

DOSAGE

- **IM**

   Analgesic, single dose.

Adults, less than 65 years of age: One 60-mg dose. **Adults, over 65 years of age, in renal impairment, or weight less than 50 kg:** One 30-mg dose. **Children, 2–16 years of age:** One dose of 1 mg/kg, up to a maximum of 30 mg.

- **IV**

   Analgesic, single dose.

Adults, less than 65 years of age: One 30-mg dose. **Adults, over 65 years of age, in renal impairment, or weight less than 50 kg (110 lbs):** One 15-mg dose. **Children, 2–16 years of age:** One dose of 0.5 mg/kg, up to a maximum of 15 mg.

- **IM; IV**

   Analgesic, multiple dose.

Adults, less than 65 years of age: 30 mg q 6 hr, not to exceed 120 mg daily. **Adults, over 65 years of age, in renal impairment, or weight less than 50 kg (110 lbs):** 15 mg q 6 hr, not to exceed 60 mg daily. For breakthrough pain, do not increase the dose or the frequency of ketorolac tromethamine; consider supplementing with low doses of opioids as needed, unless otherwise contraindicated.

- **TABLETS**
  Transition from IV/IM to PO.

Adults less than 65 years of age: 20 mg as a first PO dose for clients who received 60 mg IM single dose, 30 mg IV single dose, or 30 mg multiple dose IV/IM; **then,** 10 mg q 4–6 hr, not to exceed 40 mg PO in a 24-hr period. **Adults, over 65 years of age, in renal impairment, or weight less than 50 kg:** 10 mg as a first PO dose for those who received a 30-mg IM single dose, a 15-mg IV single dose, or a 15-mg multiple dose IV/IM; **then,** 10 mg q 4–6 hr, not to exceed 40 mg PO in a 24-hr period.

- **OPHTHALMIC SOLUTION, 0.5%**
  Ocular itching.

Acular: 1 gtt (0.25 mg) 4 times per day.
Following catract extraction.

Acular: 1 gtt to the affected eye(s) 4 times per day beginning 24 hr after cataract surgery and continuing through the first 2 weeks of the postoperative period. **Acular PF:** 1 gtt 4 times per day in the operated eye, as needed for pain and photophobia for up to 3 days after incisional refractive surgery.

- **OPHTHALMIC SOLUTION, 0.4%**
  Following cataract extraction.

Acular LS: 1 gtt 4 times per day in the operated eye, as needed for pain and burning/stinging for up to 4 days following corneal refractive surgery.

NURSING CONSIDERATIONS

ADMINISTRATION/STORAGE

1. Use as part of a regular analgesic schedule rather than on an as-needed basis.

2. If given on p.r.n. basis, base size of a repeat dose on the duration of pain relief from the previous dose. If pain returns within 3–5 hr, the next dose can be increased by up to 50% (as long as the total daily dose is not exceeded). If pain does not return for 8–12 hr, the next dose can be decreased by as much

as 50% or the dosing interval can be increased to q 8–12 hr.

3. Shortening the dosing intervals recommended will lead to an increased frequency and duration of side effects.

4. Correct hypovolemia prior to administering.

5. Store Acular and Acular PF from 15–30°C (59–86°F) protected from light. Store Acular LS from 15–25°C (59–77°F).

6. Store tablets from 15–30°C (59–86°F).

IV 7. Do not mix IV/IM ketorolac in a small volume (i.e., a syringe) with morphine sulfate, meperidine HCl, promethazine HCl, or hydroxyzine HCl; will precipitate from solution.

8. The IV bolus must be given over no less than 15 sec. Give IM slowly and deeply into the muscle.

9. Protect the injection from light.

ASSESSMENT

1. Identify reasons for therapy, onset, location, pain intensity/level, characteristics of S&S.

2. Note any previous experience with NSAIDs and results.

3. Assess for any asthma, aspirin-induced allergy, PUD/recent GI bleed or nasal polyps.

4. Check for liver or renal dysfunction; assess hydration status.

5. List drugs prescribed; note if any are ace inhibitors, anticonvulsants or antidepressants—may cause adverse effects with prolonged therapy.

CLIENT/FAMILY TEACHING

1. Take only as directed; do not exceed prescribed dosage. May take with food/milk if GI upset occurs. Report if symptoms unrelieved.

2. Drug may cause drowsiness and dizziness; avoid activities that require mental alertness until drug effects realized.

3. Avoid alcohol, aspirin, and all OTC agents without approval.

4. Report any unusual bruising/bleeding, weight gain, swelling of feet/ankles, increased joint pain, change in urine patterns or lack of response.

5. With eye drops, transient stinging or burning may occur. Do not wear soft contact lens. Report eye reactions that do not subside with therapy.

Bold Italic = life threatening side effect   ■ = black box warning   ✚ = Available in Canada

6. Drug is for short-term use only, review adverse effects R/T prolonged therapy and with other conditions.

OUTCOMES/EVALUATE
• Effective pain control
• ↓ Ocular allergic manifestations
• ↓ Ocular pain/photophobia

Ketotifen fumarate
(kee-**TOHT**-ih-fen)

CLASSIFICATION(S):
Ophthalmic decongestant
PREGNANCY CATEGORY: C
OTC: Alaway.
Rx: Zaditor.
✤**Rx:** Apo-Ketotifen, Novo-Ketotifen, Zaditen.

USES
Temporary prophylaxis of itching of the eye due to allergic conjunctivitis, including that due to pollen, ragweed, grass, animal hair, and dander.

ACTION/KINETICS
Action
Selective, non-competitive histamine H_1 receptor antagonist and mast cell stabilizer. Inhibits release of mediators from cells involved in hypersensitivity reactions. Decreased chemotaxis and activation of eosinophils.
Pharmacokinetics
Rapid acting; effect seen within minutes of administration.

CONTRAINDICATIONS
Use orally or by injection. Use to treat contact-lens-related irritation.

SPECIAL CONCERNS
Use with caution during lactation. Safety and efficacy have not been determined in children less than 3 years of age.

SIDE EFFECTS
Most Common
Conjunctival injection, headache, rhinitis, burning, stinging.
Ophthalmic: Burning, stinging, conjunctivitis, conjunctival injection, discharge, dry eyes, eye pain, eyelid disorder, itching, keratitis, lacrimation disorder, mydriasis, photophobia. **Miscella-**

neous: Headache, rhinitis, allergic reactions, rash, flu syndrome, pharyngitis.

HOW SUPPLIED
Ophthalmic Solution: 0.025%.

DOSAGE
• **OPHTHALMIC SOLUTION**
  Allergic conjunctivitis.
1 gtt in the affected eye(s) q 8–12 hr.

NURSING CONSIDERATIONS
ASSESSMENT
1. Note reasons for therapy, onset, characteristics of S&S.
2. Assist to identify triggers; teach avoidance.

CLIENT/FAMILY TEACHING
1. Use as directed. To prevent contaminating the dropper tip and solution, do not touch the eyelids or surrounding areas with the dropper tip.
2. For eye (topical) use only. Keep bottle tightly closed when not in use.
3. Benzalkonium chloride, the preservative in the product, may be absorbed by soft contact lenses. For those who wear soft contact lenses and whose eyes are not red, wait 10 min or longer after instilling ketotifen before inserting contact lenses. Not for use with contact lens or related irritation; do not wear contact lenses if eyes are red/irritated.
4. May experience burning, stinging and inflammation with instillation; notify provider if persistent. Report adverse side effects or lack of desired response.

OUTCOMES/EVALUATE
Relief of S&S of allergic conjunctivitis

K

Kunecatechins (Topical)

CLASSIFICATION(S):
Catechins.
PREGNANCY CATEGORY: C
Rx: Veregen.

USES
Topical treatment of external genital and perianal warts (due to *Condyloma acuminatum*) in immunocompetent clients 18 years and older.

ACTION/KINETICS
Action
Action in treating genital and perianal warts is unknown.

CONTRAINDICATIONS
Hypersensitivity to any components of the product. Avoid use on open wounds.

SPECIAL CONCERNS
Safety and efficacy have not been determined in immunosuppressed clients or in children. It is not known whether topically applied kunecatechins are excreted in breast milk.

SIDE EFFECTS
Most Common
Burning, erythema, erosion/ulceration, pruritus, edema, pain/discomfort, induration.
Dermatologic: Pruritus, burning, erythema, erosion/ulceration, vescular rash, desquamation, discharge, regional lymphadenitis, bleeding, irritation, rash, scars, discoloration, dryness, eczema, hyperesthesia, necrosis, papules, perianal infection, pigmentation changes, pyodermatitis, superinfection of warts and ulcers. **GU:** Urethritis, phimosis, dysuria, urethral meatus erosions, genital herpes simplex, inguinal lymphadenitis, urethral meatus stenosis, vulvitis. **Miscellaneous:** Pain/discomfort, edema, induration, hypersensitivity reactions.

HOW SUPPLIED
Ointment: 15%.

DOSAGE
• **OINTMENT**
  External genital and perianal warts.
Adults: Apply 3 times per day to all external genital and perianal warts. Apply about 0.5 cm strand of ointment to each wart using the fingers, ensuring complete coverage.

NURSING CONSIDERATIONS
ADMINISTRATION/STORAGE
1. Safety and efficacy have not been determined in the treatment of warts beyond 16 weeks or for multiple treatment courses.
2. Continue treatment until complete clearance of all warts, but no longer than 16 weeks.
3. Local skin reactions (e.g., erythema) are frequent; however, continue treatment when the severity of the local skin reaction is acceptable.
4. Store refrigerated prior to dispensing. After dispensing, store refrigerated (2–8°C, 36–46°F) or at a temperature up to 25°C (77°F). Do not freeze.

ASSESSMENT
Note onset, location, number/extent of genital/perianal warts, other agents trialed.

CLIENT/FAMILY TEACHING
1. Administered topically to infected area as directed. Apply a 0.5 cm strand externally in a thin layer over all genital and perianal warts, three times a day.
2. Wash hands before/after application. Not necessary to wash off the ointment from the treated area prior to the next application.
3. The mechanism of catechins is unknown; they are powerful anti-oxidants and are linked to evidence of fighting tumors as well as enhancing immune system function.
4. Avoid exposure of the genital and perianal area to sunlight and UV light during treatment.
5. May experience itching, burning, pain/discomfort, redness, swelling, ulceration or rash at site; report if bothersome or progresses.
6. Keep all F/U appointments to evaluate response to therapy and for adverse drug effects. Not for use >16 weeks.
7. Use barrier contraception to prevent transmission to partner.

OUTCOMES/EVALUATE
Resolution of perianal/genital warts

L

Labetalol hydrochloride

IV ©

(lah-**BET**-ah-lohl)

CLASSIFICATION(S):
Alpha-beta adrenergic blocking agent
PREGNANCY CATEGORY: C
Rx: Normodyne, Trandate.
✦Rx: Apo-Labetalol.

SEE ALSO *BETA-ADRENERGIC BLOCKING AGENTS* AND *ANTIHYPERTENSIVE AGENTS*.

USES
PO: Hypertension, alone or in combination with other drugs (especially thiazide and loop diuretics).
IV: Severe hypertension.
Investigational: Pheochromocytoma, clonidine withdrawal hypertension.

ACTION/KINETICS
Action
Decreases BP by blocking both alpha- and beta-adrenergic receptors. Standing BP is lowered more than supine. Significant reflex tachycardia and bradycardia do not occur, although AV conduction may be prolonged.

Pharmacokinetics
Completely absorbed after PO. Food increases bioavailability of the drug. **Onset, PO:** 2–4 hr; **IV:** 5 min. **Peak plasma levels, PO:** 1–2 hr. **Peak effects, PO:** 2–4 hr. **Duration, PO:** 8–12 hr. **t½, PO:** 6–8 hr; **IV:** 5.5 hr. Significant first-pass effect; metabolized in liver. Excreted in the urine and feces.

CONTRAINDICATIONS
Cardiogenic shock, overt cardiac failure, bronchial asthma, severe bradycardia, greater than first-degree heart block.

SPECIAL CONCERNS
Use with caution during lactation, in impaired renal and hepatic function, in chronic bronchitis and emphysema, in those with a history of heart failure who are well compensated, and in diabetes (may prevent premonitory signs of acute hypoglycemia). Elderly clients may experience orthostatic hypotension, dizziness, and lightheadedness. Safety and efficacy in children have not been established.

SIDE EFFECTS
Most Common
Headache, nausea, dizziness, impotence, tingling scalp, fatigue, dry itchy skin, insomnia, anxiety/nervousness.
See also *Beta-Adrenergic Blocking Agents.*
After PO Use. GI: Nausea, diarrhea, cholestasis with or without jaundice. **CNS:** Fatigue, dizziness, drowsiness, paresthesias, headache, anxiety/nervousness, insomnia, syncope (rare). **GU:** Impotence, priapism, ejaculation failure, difficulty in micturition, Peyronie's disease, acute urinary bladder retention. **Respiratory:** Dyspnea, nasal stuffiness, *bronchospasm*. **Musculoskeletal:** Muscle cramps, asthenia, toxic myopathy. **Dermatologic:** Dry itchy skin, generalized maculopapular, lichenoid, or urticarial rashes; bullous lichen planus, psoriasis, facial erythema, reversible alopecia. **Ophthalmic:** Abnormal vision, dry eyes. **Miscellaneous:** SLE, + antinuclear factor, antimitochondrial antibodies, fever, edema.

After parenteral use. CV: Ventricular arrhythmias. **CNS:** Numbness, somnolence, yawning, hypesthesia. **Renal:** Transient increases in BUN and serum creatinine associated with drops in BP usually in those with prior renal insufficiency. **Miscellaneous:** Pruritus, flushing, wheezing.

After PO or parenteral use. CV: Depression of myocardial contractility causing more heart failure, postural hypotension. **GI:** N&V, dyspepsia, taste distortion, jaundice or hepatic dysfunction (rare). **CNS:** Dizziness, tingling of skin or scalp, vertigo. **Miscellaneous:**

📷 = see color insert   H = Herbal   IV = Intravenous   © = sound alike drug

Postural hypotension, increased sweating, hypersensitivity reactions.

LABORATORY TEST CONSIDERATIONS
False + increase in urinary catecholamines or for amphetamine when screening urine for drugs. Transient ↑ serum transaminases, BUN, serum creatinine.

OD OVERDOSE MANAGEMENT
Symptoms: Excessive hypotension and bradycardia. *Treatment:* Induce vomiting or perform gastric lavage. Place clients in a supine position with legs elevated. If required, the following treatment can be used:

- Epinephrine or a beta₂-agonist (aerosol) to treat bronchospasm.
- Atropine or epinephrine to treat bradycardia.
- Digitalis glycoside and a diuretic for cardiac failure; dopamine or dobutamine may also be used.
- Diazepam to treat seizures.
- Norepinephrine (or another vasopressor) to treat hypotension.
- Administration of glucagon (5–10 mg rapidly over 30 sec), followed by continuous infusion of 5 mg/hr, may be effective in treating severe hypotension and bradycardia.

DRUG INTERACTIONS
Beta-adrenergic bronchodilators / ↓ Bronchodilator drug effects; ↑ dose of bronchodilator may be required
Calcium channel blockers (e.g., verapamil) / Use together with caution
Cimetidine / ↑ Bioavailability of PO labetalol
Glutethimide / ↓ Labetalol effects R/T ↑ liver breakdown
Halothane / ↑ Risk of severe myocardial depression → hypotension; do not use together
Nitroglycerin / Additive hypotension; labetalol blunts reflex tachycardia due to nitroglycerin without preventing hypotension
Tricyclic antidepressants / ↑ Risk of tremors

HOW SUPPLIED
Injection: 5 mg/mL; *Tablets:* 100 mg, 200 mg, 300 mg.

DOSAGE
- **TABLETS**

Hypertension.
Individualize. Initial: 100 mg twice a day alone or with a diuretic. After 2 or 3 days, using BP as a guide, titrate dosage in increments of 100 mg twice a day, q 2–3 days. **Maintenance:** 200–400 mg twice a day up to 1,200–2,400 mg/day for severe cases. Geriatric clients will generally require lower maintenance doses.

- **IV**
  Hypertension.
Individualize. Initial: 20 mg slowly over 2 min; **then,** 40–80 mg q 10 min until desired effect occurs or a total of 300 mg has been given.

- **IV INFUSION**
  Hypertension.
Initial: 2 mg/min; **then,** adjust rate according to response. **Usual dose range:** 50–300 mg.
  Transfer from IV to PO therapy.
Initial: 200 mg; **then,** 200–400 mg 6–12 hr later, depending on response. Thereafter, dosage based on response.

NURSING CONSIDERATIONS
Ⓒ Do not confuse Normodyne with Norpramine (an antidepressant).

ADMINISTRATION/STORAGE
1. When transferring to PO labetalol from other antihypertensive therapy, slowly reduce dosage of current therapy.
2. Full antihypertensive effect is usually seen within the first 1–3 hr after the initial dose or dose increment.
IV 3. To transfer from IV to PO therapy in hospitalized clients, begin when supine BP begins to increase.
4. Not compatible with 5% sodium bicarbonate injection, furosemide, or other alkaline products.
5. May give IV undiluted (20 mg over 2 min) or reconstituted with dextrose or saline solutions (infuse at a rate of 2 mg/min). When given by IV infusion, use an infusion control device.
6. Labetalol, at a final concentration of 1.25–3.75 mg/mL is compatible and stable for 24 hr with: Ringer's, Lactated Ringer's, D5W and Ringer's, LR and D5W, D5W, 0.9% NaCl, D5W and 0.2% NaCl, 2.5% Dextrose and 0.45% NaCl,

---
Bold Italic = life threatening side effect   ■ = black box warning   ♣ = Available in Canada

D5W and 0.9% NaCl, and D5W and 0.33% NaCl.

ASSESSMENT

1. Note reasons for therapy, other agents trialed, outcome. List any conditions that may preclude therapy.

2. Assess effect of labetalol tablets on standing BP before hospital discharge. Obtain standing BP at different times (in left and right arm) during day to assess full effects.

3. To reduce chance of orthostatic hypotension, keep supine for 3 hr after receiving parenteral labetalol.

CLIENT/FAMILY TEACHING

1. Take as directed with meals. Do not stop taking abruptly; may cause chest pain.

2. Use caution and change positions slowly; may precipitate sudden drop in BP and cause dizziness. Report any low heart rate, confusion, fever, swelling of extremities, difficulty breathing, night cough, or persistent dizziness. Record heart rate, weight, and BP for provider review.

3. May cause increased sensitivity to cold; dress appropriately.

4. Avoid alcohol, OTC products (especially cold remedies), high sodium intake, and tobacco.

5. Keep all F/U appointments to evaluate response to therapy and adverse side effects.

OUTCOMES/EVALUATE

↓ BP

Lamivudine (3TC) ■
(lah-**MIH**-vyou-deen)

CLASSIFICATION(S):
Antiviral, nucleoside reverse transcriptase inhibitor
PREGNANCY CATEGORY: C
Rx: Epivir, Epivir-HBV.
✦Rx: 3TC, Heptovir.

SEE ALSO *ANTIVIRAL DRUGS*.

USES

Epivir. In combination with other antiretroviral drugs for the treatment of HIV infection. **Epivir-HBV.** (1) Chronic hepatitis B associated with evidence of hepatitis B replication and active liver inflammation. (2) Hepatitis B in children 2–17 years of age.

ACTION/KINETICS

Action

Synthetic nucleoside analog effective against HIV. Converted to active 5'-triphosphate (L-TP) metabolite which inhibits HIV reverse transcription via viral DNA chain termination. L-TP also inhibits the RNA- and DNA-dependent DNA polymerase activities of reverse transcriptase. Lamivudine-resistant HIV-1 mutants are cross-resistant to didanosine and zalcitabine.

Pharmacokinetics

Rapidly absorbed after PO administration; absolute bioavailability is about 86%. Most eliminated unchanged through the urine.

CONTRAINDICATIONS

Lactation. Use of Epivir-HBV tablets or oral solution to treat HIV infections (due to the lower amount of lamivudine compared with Epivir).

SPECIAL CONCERNS

■ (1) Lactic acidosis and severe hepatomegaly with steatosis, including death, may occur with the use of nucleoside analogs alone or in combination with lamivudine and other antiretroviral agents. A majority of these cases have been in women. Obesity and prolonged nucleoside exposure may be risk factors. Most of these reports have described clients receiving nucleoside analogs for treatment of HIV infection, but there have been reports of lactic acidosis in those receiving lamivudine for hepatitis B virus (HBV). (2) Exercise particular caution when administering lamivudine to any clients with known risk factors for liver disease; however, cases have also been reported in clients with no known risk factors. Suspend treatment with lamivudine in any client who develops clinical or laboratory findings suggestive of lactic acidosis or pronounced heptotoxicity (which may include hepatomegaly and steatosis, even in the absence of marked transaminase elevations). (3) Lamivudine tablets and oral solution (used to treat HIV infection) contain a higher dose of the active ingredient (lamivudine) than lamivudine-HBV tablets and oral solution (used to treat chronic hepatitis B). Clients with HIV infection should receive only dosing forms appropriate for treatment of HIV. The formulation and dosage of lamivudine-HBV are not appropriate for those dually infected with HBV and HIV. (4) Offer HIV counseling and testing to all clients before beginning Epivir HBV and periodically during treatment because Epivir-HBV tablets and oral solution contain a lower dose of lamivudine as do Epivir tablets and oral solution used to treat HIV infection. If treatment with Epivir-HBV is prescribed for chronic hepatitis B for a client with unrecognized or untreated HIV infection, rapid emergence of HIV resistance is likely due to the subtherapeutic dose and inappropriate monotherapy. (5) Severe acute exacerbations of hepatitis B have been reported in clients who have discontinued anti-hepatitis B therapy (including lamivudine-HBV) or are coinfected with HBV and HIV and have discontinued lamivudine. Monitor hepatic function closely with both clinical and laboratory follow-up for at least several months in those who discontinue anti-hepatitis B therapy or who discontinue lamivudine and are coinfected with HIV and HBV. If appropriate, initiation of anti-hepatitis B therapy may be warranted.■ Clients taking lamivudine and zidovudine may continue to develop opportunistic infections and other complications of HIV infection. Use with caution and at a reduced dose in those with impaired renal function. Use lamivudine with caution in pediatric clients with a history of prior antiretroviral nucleoside exposure, a history of pancreatitis, or other significant risk factors for the development of pancreatitis. Data on the use of lamivudine and zidovudine in pediatric clients are lacking; however, use the combination with extreme caution in children with pancreatitis. Safety and efficacy of Epivir-HBV have not been determined in those with decompensated liver disease or organ transplants, in children

under age 2, or in clients dually infected with HBV and HIV, hepatitis delta, or HIV. Possible virologic failure and emergence of nucleoside reverse transcriptase–associated mutations with a regimen consisting of didanosine enteric-coated beadlets, lamivudine, and tenofovir disoproxil fumarate.

SIDE EFFECTS
Most Common
When used for HIV treatment: Headache, nausea, nasal signs/symptoms, cough, malaise, fatigue, diarrhea, fever.
When used for chronic hepatitis B: Ear/nose/throat infections, malaise, fatigue, headache, N&V, abdominal discomfort/pain.

Side effects include those when lamivudine is taken alone or with other antiretroviral drugs.

When used to treat HIV. Adults: CNS: Headache, neuropathy, insomnia and other sleep disorders, dizziness, depression, dreams. **GI:** N&V, diarrhea, anorexia, abdominal pain/cramps, dyspepsia, *severe hepatomegaly with steatosis, pancreatitis*, posttreatment worsening of hepatitis B. **Dermatologic:** Skin rashes. **Musculoskeletal:** Musculoskeletal pain, myalgia, arthralgia. **Respiratory:** Nasal signs/symptoms, cough. **Hematologic:** Anemia, neutropenia. **GU:** UTI. **Body as a whole:** Malaise, fatigue, fever, chills. **Children: CNS:** Paresthesias, peripheral neuropathies. **GI:** Hepatomegaly, diarrhea, N&V, stomatitis, splenomegaly, *pancreatitis*. **Dermatologic:** Skin rashes. **Respiratory:** Cough, nasal discharge or congestion, abnormal breath sounds/wheezing. **Otic:** Pain, discharge, erythema, or swelling of an ear. **Body as a whole:** Fever, lymphadenopathy.

When used for chronic hepatitis B: Adults and children: CNS: Headache, paresthesia, peripheral neuropathy. **GI:** Abdominal discomfort/pain, N&V, diarrhea, stomatitis, severe *hepatomegaly with steatosis, pancreatitis*. **Dermatologic:** Skin rashes, alopecia, pruritus, rash, urticaria. **Musculoskeletal:** Myalgia, arthralgia, rhabdomyolysis, muscle weakness. **Respiratory:** Sore throat, ear/nose/throat infections; cough, bron-

L

Bold Italic = life threatening side effect   ■ = black box warning   ♣ = Available in Canada

chitis, viral respiratory tract infections in children; abnormal breath sounds, wheezing. **Hematologic:** Anemia (including pure red cell aplasia and severe anemias), lymphadenopathy, splenomegaly. **Body as a whole:** Fever, chills, fatigue, malaise, lactic acidosis, hyperglycemia, redistribution/accumulation of body fat, weakness. **Miscellaneous:** *Anaphylaxis,* posttreatment worsening of hepatitis B. *NOTE:* Pediatric clients have an increased risk to develop *pancreatitis.*

LABORATORY TEST CONSIDERATIONS
↑ ALT, AST, amylase, bilirubin, serum lipase, CPK. ↓ Hemoglobin, ANC, platelets, neutrophils.

DRUG INTERACTIONS
Interferon alfa / May cause hepatic decompensation (some fatal)
Ribavirin / Possible ↓ phosphorylation of lamivudine
Trimethoprim-Sulfamethoxazole / Significant ↑ (44%) in lamivudine levels
Zalcitabine / Inhibition of the intracellular phosphorylation of one another; do not use together
Zidovudine / ↑ (about 39%) C_{max} of zidovudine

HOW SUPPLIED
Epivir. *Oral Solution:* 10 mg/mL; *Tablets:* 150 mg, 300 mg.
Epivir-HBV. *Oral Solution:* 5 mg/mL; *Tablets:* 100 mg.

DOSAGE
EPIVIR
• **ORAL SOLUTION; TABLETS**
  HIV infection.
Adults: 150 mg twice a day or 300 mg once daily in combination with other antiretroviral drugs. For adults with low body weight (<50 kg), recommended dose is 2 mg/kg twice a day in combination with other antiretroviral drugs. **Children, 3 months to 16 years old:** 4 mg/kg twice a day (up to a maximum of 150 mg twice a day) in combination with other antiretroviral drugs.

In clients over age 16, adjust dose as follows in impaired renal function: C_{CR} 50 mL/min or more: 150 mg twice a day or 300 mg once daily; C_{CR} 30–49 mL/min: 150 mg once daily; C_{CR} 15–29 mL/min: 150 mg for the first dose fol-

lowed by 100 mg once daily; C_{CR} 5–14 mL/min: 150 mg for the first dose followed by 50 mg once daily; C_{CR} <5 mL/min: 50 mg for the first dose followed by 25 mg once daily.
EPIVIR HBV
• **ORAL SOLUTION; TABLETS**
  Chronic hepatitis B.
Adults: 100 mg once daily. **Children, 2–17 years:** 3 mg/kg once daily, not to exceed 100 mg daily. Safety and efficacy beyond 1 year in adults and children have not been determined.

Adjust dose in adults as follows in impaired renal function: C_{CR} 50 mL/min or more: 100 mg once daily; C_{CR} 30–49 mL/min: 100 mg for the first dose followed by 50 mg once daily; C_{CR} 15–29 mL/min: 100 mg for the first dose followed by 25 mg once daily; C_{CR} 5–14 mL/min: 35 mg for the first dose followed by 15 mg once daily; C_{CR} <5 mL/min: 35 mg for the first dose followed by 10 mg once daily.

NURSING CONSIDERATIONS
ADMINISTRATION/STORAGE
1. Consult zidovudine or other antiviral drug prescribing information before using with lamivudine.
2. Safety and efficacy of twice-daily lamivudine in combination with other antiretroviral drugs have been established in children over 3 months of age.
3. Store Epivir Solution at 2–25°C (36–77°F). Store Epivir and Epivir-HBV Tablets from 15–30°C (59–86°F). Store Epivir-HBV Solution from 20–25°C (68–77°F).

ASSESSMENT
1. Note disease onset/confirmation, other agents trialed, outcome.
2. Monitor child for clinical symptoms of pancreatitis.
3. Assess for HIV, HCV, hepatitis delta when treating hepatitis B.
4. Monitor liver, renal, and hematologic parameters, including CD_4 and viral load. Adjust dose with impaired renal function.

CLIENT/FAMILY TEACHING
1. Take as prescribed with other antiretroviral drug(s) twice a day. Drug works by blocking the growth of HIV.

---

2. May take without regard to food. Report any adverse side effects. Drug is not a cure; may continue to experience illnesses and opportunistic infections associated with HIV.

3. Use barrier protection with sexual partners to prevent HIV transmission. Review transmission of HIV and hepatitis.

4. May experience fainting or dizziness; GI upset, and insomnia may resolve after 3–4 weeks of therapy; use caution with activities that require mental alertness.

5. With children, report symptoms of pancreatitis (i.e., abdominal pain, N&V, fever, loss of appetite, yellow skin discoloration).

6. Keep all F/U appointments to assess response to therapy and to monitor labs.

OUTCOMES/EVALUATE

- Control of HIV disease progression with other antiretroviral.
- Stabilization of hepatitis B disease

—— *COMBINATION DRUG* ——

Lamivudine/ Zidovudine   ■ ©

(lah-**MIH**-vyou-deen, zye-**DOH**-vyou-deen)

CLASSIFICATION(S):
Antiviral, nucleoside reverse transcriptase inhibitors
PREGNANCY CATEGORY: C
Rx: Combivir.

SEE ALSO *LAMIVUDINE, ZIDOVUDINE, AND ANTIVIRAL DRUGS.*

USES
Treatment of HIV-1 infection in combination with other antiretrovirals.

CONTENT
Each Combivir tablet contains: *Antiviral:* Lamivudine, 150 mg and *Antiviral:* Zidovudine, 300 mg.

ACTION/KINETICS
Action
Both drugs are reverse transcriptase inhibitors with activity against HIV. Combination results in synergistic antiretroviral effect.

Pharmacokinetics
Each drug is rapidly absorbed. **t½, lamivudine:** 5–7 hr; **t½, zidovudine:** 0.5–3 hr. Most lamivudine is excreted unchanged in the urine. Zidovudine is metabolized by the liver and unchanged drug and metabolites are excreted in the urine. **Plasma protein binding:** Less than 36% of lamivudine and less than 38% of zidovudine are bound to plasma proteins.

CONTRAINDICATIONS
Use in clients requiring dosage reduction of lamivudine/zidovudine (product is a fixed-dose combination), children <12 years old, C_{CR} <50 mL/min, body weight <50 kg, and in those experiencing dose-limiting side effects. Lactation.

SPECIAL CONCERNS
■ (1) Zidovudine has been associated with hematologic toxicity, including neutropenia and severe anemia, particularly in clients with advanced HIV disease. Prolonged use of zidovudine has been associated with symptomatic myopathy. (2) Lactic acidosis and severe hepatomegaly with steatosis, including deaths, have been reported with use of nucleoside analogs alone or in combination, including lamivudine, zidovudine, and other antiretrovirals. (3) Severe acute exacerbations of hepatitis B have been reported in clients who are coinfected with hepatitis B virus (HBV) and HIV and have discontinued lamivudine. Monitor hepatic function closely with both clinical and laboratory follow-up for at least several months in those who discontinue lamivudine/zidovudine and are coinfected with HIV and HBV. If appropriate, initiation of hepatitis B therapy may be warranted.■ Use with caution in clients with bone marrow compromise as evidenced by granulocyte count <1,000 cells/mm³ or hemoglobin <9.5 grams/dL.

SIDE EFFECTS
Most Common
Headache, N&V, ear/nose/throat infections, malaise/fatigue, diarrhea, anorexia, dizziness, myalgia, musculoskeletal pain, neuropathy, cough, fever, chills.

Bold Italic = life threatening side effect   ■ = black box warning   ✦ = Available in Canada

See *Lamivudine* and *Zidovudine* for a complete list of possible side effects. Note especially, possibility of hematologic toxicity, lactic acidosis, myopathy and myositis, and severe hepatomegaly with steatosis. Hepatic decompensation (some fatal) has occurred in HIV/HCV coinfected clients receiving combination antiretroviral therapy for HIV and interferon alfa and ribavirin. Immune reconstitution syndrome is possible. Redistribution/accumulation of body fat, including central obesity, dorsocervical fat enlargement, peripheral wasting, facial wasting, breast enlargement, and cushingoid appearance are possible.

ADDITIONAL DRUG INTERACTIONS

See *Lamivudine* and *Zidovudine* for a complete list of possible side effects. Trimethoprim, Trimethoprim/Sulfamethoxazole / ↑ Lamivudine plasma levels R/T inhibition of lamivudine renal secretion; also, ↑ serum levels of zidovudine and its metabolite especially in those with impaired hepatic glucuronidation

HOW SUPPLIED

See Content

DOSAGE

- **TABLETS**
  HIV infection.

Adults and children over 12 years of age: One combination tablet—150 mg lamivudine/300 mg zidovudine—twice a day.

NURSING CONSIDERATIONS

⟨ Do not confuse Combivir with Combivent (combination drug for COPD).

ADMINISTRATION/STORAGE

1. May be taken without regard to food.
2. Since Combivir is a fixed-dose combination, do not use for those requiring dosage adjustment, such as with reduced renal function (C_{CR} <50 mL/min) or those experiencing dose-limiting side effects.
3. A decrease in dosage may be needed in those with mild to moderate impaired hepatic function or liver cirrhosis. Since Combivir is a fixed-dose combination, do not use in clients with impaired hepatic function.
4. Store between 2–30°C (36–86°F).

ASSESSMENT

1. Note disease onset, clinical characteristics, other agents trialed, outcome.
2. Weigh client; not for use in those with low body weight or C_{CR} <50 mL/min.
3. Monitor liver, renal, and hematologic parameters, including CD_4 and viral load; report dysfunction.
4. Assess for hepatomegaly and lactic acidosis (pH <7.35 or serum lactate >5–6 mEq/L).

CLIENT/FAMILY TEACHING

1. Take as directed, with or without food, twice daily.
2. Report adverse effects including severe abdominal pain, fatigue, SOB, dizziness, or muscle pain/weakness; drug may cause low white count and anemia.
3. Drug is not a cure; may experience opportunistic infections. May cause lactic acidosis and liver swelling/toxicity.
4. Practice barrier contraception; drug does not prevent disease transmission. Do not breastfeed.
5. Keep all F/U appointments to evaluate response to therapy and adverse side effects.

OUTCOMES/EVALUATE

Control of HIV; ↓ HIVRNA (viral load)

Lamotrigine
(lah-**MOH**-trih-jeen)

CLASSIFICATION(S):

Anticonvulsant, miscellaneous
PREGNANCY CATEGORY: C

Rx: Lamictal, Lamictal Chewable Dispersible Tablets.

SEE ALSO *ANTICONVULSANTS*.

USES

(1) Adjunct in treatment of partial seizures in adults and children 2 years and older. (2) Adjunct in treating seizures in adults and children 2 years and older with Lennox-Gastaut syndrome. (3) Adjunct to treat primary generalized tonic-clonic seizures in adults and children 2 years of age and older. (4) Conversion to monotherapy in adults with partial

seizures who are receiving carbamaze-pine, phenytoin, phenobarbital, primidone, or valproate as the single antiepileptic drug. Safety and efficacy of lamotrigine have not been determined as initial monotherapy. (5) Long-term maintenance of bipolar I disorder to delay occurrence of mood episodes in those treated for acute mood episodes (depression, mania, hypomania, mixed episodes) with standard therapy. The efficacy in the acute treatment of mood episodes has not been determined. *Investigational:* Children with absence seizures; juvenile myoclonic epilepsy; and temporal lobe seizures.

ACTION/KINETICS

Action

Mechanism of anticonvulsant action not known. May act to inhibit voltage-sensitive sodium channels. This effect stabilizes neuronal membranes and modulates presynaptic transmitter release of excitatory amino acids such as glutamate and aspartate. The mechanism for efficacy in biopolar disorder has not been determined.

Pharmacokinetics

Rapidly and completely absorbed after PO use with negligible first-pass metabolism; absolute bioavailability is 98% and is not affected by food. **Peak plasma levels:** 1.4–4.8 hr. **t½, after repeated doses:** Depends on whether taken alone or with other anticonvulsant drugs; ranges from about 12 to 70 hr in adults. The chewable/dispersible tablets are equivalent in terms of rate and extent of absorption whether they are given as dispersed in water, chewed and swallowed, or swallowed whole as compared with compressed tablets. Metabolized by the liver with metabolites and unchanged drug excreted mainly through the urine (94%). Lamotrigine induces its own metabolism following multiple doses. Eliminated more rapidly in clients who have been taking antiepileptic drugs that induce liver enzymes. However, valproic acid decreases the clearance of lamotrigine. **Plasma protein binding:** About 55% (does not displace other antiepileptic drugs from protein-binding sites).

CONTRAINDICATIONS

Hypersensitivity to the drug or any component of the product. Lactation. Children less than 16 years of age, other than as adjunctive therapy for generalized seizures of Lennox-Gastaut syndrome or for generalized tonic-clonic seizures in children older than 2 years.

SPECIAL CONCERNS

■ (1) Serious rashes requiring hospitalization and discontinuation of treatment have been reported in association with the use of lamotrigine. The incidence of these rashes, which have included Stevens-Johnson syndrome, is approximately 0.8% in pediatric clients (younger than 16 years of age) receiving lamotrigine as adjunctive therapy for epilepsy and 0.3% in adults on adjunctive therapy for epilepsy. In clinical trials of bipolar and other mood disorders, the rate of serious rash was 0.08% in adult clients receiving lamotrigine as initial monotherapy and 0.13% in adult clients receiving lamotrigine as adjunctive therapy. In a prospectively followed cohort of 1,983 pediatric clients with epilepsy taking adjunctive lamotrigine, there was one rash-related death. In worldwide postmarketing experience, rare cases of toxic epidermal necrolysis or rash-related death have been reported in adult and pediatric clients, but those numbers are too few to permit a precise estimate of the rate. (2) Other than age, no factors have been identified that are known to predict the risk of occurrence or the severity of rash associated with lamotrigine. It is suggested, although not yet proven, that the risk of rash may also be increased by coadministration of lamotrigine with valproate (includes valproic acid and divalproex sodium), exceeding the recommended initial dose of lamotrigine, or exceeding the recommended dose escalation for lamotrigine. (3) Nearly all cases of life-threatening rashes associated with lamotrigine have occurred within 2 to 8 weeks of treatment initiation. However, isolated cases have been reported after prolonged treatment (e.g., 6 months). Accordingly, duration of therapy cannot be relied upon as a

---

Bold Italic = life threatening side effect   ■ = black box warning   ✦ = Available in Canada

means to predict the potential risk heralded by the first appearance of a rash. (4) Although benign rashes also occur with lamotrigine, it is not possible to predict reliably which rashes will prove to be serious or life-threatening. Accordingly, lamotrigine should ordinarily be discontinued at the first sign of rash, unless the rash is clearly not drug related. Discontinuation of treatment may not prevent a rash from becoming life-threatening or permanently disabling or disfiguring.■ Use with caution in clients with diseases or conditions that could affect metabolism or elimination of the drug, such as in impaired renal, hepatic, or cardiac function. Sudden unexplained death has occurred, rarely. Use caution in dose selection in the elderly due to greater frequency of decreased hepatic, renal, or cardiac function and greater incidence of concomitant diseases. Abrupt withdrawal may increase seizure frequency. Safety and efficacy for use in bipolar disorder have not been determined in children less than 18 years of age.

SIDE EFFECTS

Most Common

When used as adjunctive therapy: Dizziness, ataxia, somnolence, headache, diplopia, blurred vision, N&V, rash. **When used as monotherapy:** N&V, abnormal coordination, dyspepsia, dizziness, rhinitis, anxiety, insomnia, infection, pain, weight decrease, chest pain, dysmenorrhea.

When used for bipolar disorder: Dizziness, rash, diarrhea, dream abnormality, headache, pruritus, insomnia, nausea, somnolence.

When used during conversion to monotherapy (add-on) period: Dizziness, headache, N&V, asthenia, abnormal coordination, rash, somnolence, diplopia, ataxia, accidental injury, tremor, blurred vision, insomnia, nystagmus, diarrhea, lymphadenopathy, pruritus, sinusitis.

Side effects listed are for all uses and with an incidence of 0.1% or greater or a more serious side effect. **CNS:** Dizziness, headache, ataxia, anxiety, somnolence, incoordination, insomnia, depression, tremor, vertigo, mania, speech disorder, irritability, agitation, **convulsions**, disturbed concentration, seizure exacerbation, amnesia, decreased or increased reflexes, dream abnormality, increased/decreased libido, hypesthesia, emotional lability, dyspraxia, nervousness, abnormal thinking, confusion, paresthesia, akathisia, apathy, aphasia, depersonalization, dysarthria, dyskinesia, euphoria, hallucinations, hostility, hyperkinesia, hypoesthesia, hypertonia, decreased memory, mind racing, movement disorder, myoclonus, panic attack, paranoid reaction, personality disorder, psychosis, sleep disorder, tics, stupor, gait abnormality, mania/hypomania/ mixed mood episodes (when used for bipolar I disorder), **suicidal ideation. GI:** N&V, diarrhea, abdominal pain, dry mouth, dyspepsia, constipation, tooth disorder, anorexia, flatulence, peptic ulcer, dysphagia, eructation, gastritis, gingivitis, increased appetite, increased salivation, mouth ulceration, esophagitis, pancreatitis, **rectal hemorrhage. CV:** Migraine, flushing, hot flashes, hypertension, palpitations, postural hypotension, syncope, tachycardia, vasodilation, vasculitis, **hemorrhage** (in children). **Dermatologic:** Rash, pruritus, contact dermatitis, dry skin, sweating, eczema, acne, alopecia, hirsutism, maculopapular rash, skin discoloration, urticaria, **Stevens—Johnson syndrome, toxic epidermal necrolysis. Musculoskeletal:** Arthralgia, myalgia, gait abnormality, arthritis, leg cramps, myasthenia, twitching, rhabdomyolysis (in those experiencing hypersensitivity reactions). **Respiratory:** Rhinitis, pharyngitis, sinusitis, increased cough, respiratory disorder, bronchitis, **bronchospasm**, dyspnea, epistaxis, yawn, apnea. **Hematologic:** Lymphadenopathy, ecchymosis, anemia, thrombocytopenia, leukopenia, agranulocytosis, **aplastic anemia, disseminated intravascular coagulation,** hemolytic anemia, neutropenia, pancytopenia, red pure cell aplasia. **GU:** Amenorrhea, dysmenorrhea, vaginitis, menstrual disorder, UTI, penis disorder, urinary frequency, abnormal ejaculation, breast pain, hema-

L

---

turia, impotence, menorrhagia, polyuria, urinary abnormality, urinary incontinence. **Ophthalmic:** Diplopia, blurred vision, abnormal vision, nystagmus, amblyopia, abnormal accommodation, conjunctivitis, dry eye. **Otic:** Ear disorder, ear pain, tinnitus. **Body as a whole:** Fever, flu syndrome, asthenia, fatigue, paresthesia, infection, weight gain/decrease, edema, accidental injury, pain, photosensitivity, allergic reaction, chills, malaise, hypersensitivity reaction. **Miscellaneous:** Neck/back/chest pain, peripheral/facial edema, halitosis, taste perversion, worsening of Parkinsonism in those with preexisting Parkinson's disease, lupus-like reaction, ***multiorgan failure***, progressive immunosuppression.

OD OVERDOSE MANAGEMENT
Symptoms: Ataxia, nystagmus, increased seizures, decreased level of consciousness, coma, intraventricular conduction delay. *Treatment:* There is no specific antidote. Use the following general guidelines:
- Hospitalization with general supportive care.
- Frequent monitoring of vital signs and close observation.
- Perform gastric lavage.
- Protect the airway.
- Hemodialysis may or may not be effective.

DRUG INTERACTIONS
Acetaminophen / ↓ Serum lamotrigine levels; lamotrigine dosage adjustment may be required
Carbamazepine / 40% ↓ in lamotrigine levels; possible ↑ in carbamazepine levels
Folate inhibitors / Lamotrigine inhibits dihydrofolate reductase
Oral contraceptives / ↓ Lamotrigene levels R/T ↑ lamotrigine clearance → ↓ seizure control; maintenance dose of lamotrigine may need to be ↑ by as much as 2-fold over the recommended target dose; during hormone free weeks, plasma lamotrigine levels may ↑ leading to side effects (ataxia, diplopia, dizziness)
Oxcarbazepine / ↓ Lamotrigine levels by 29% R/T ↑ liver metabolism; adjust

lamotrigine dose as needed
Phenobarbital / 40% ↓ in lamotrigine levels
Phenytoin / 40% ↓ in lamotrigine levels
Primidone / 40% ↓ in lamotrigine levels
Progestins / ↓ Lamotrigene levels → ↓ seizure control
Rifamycins (e.g., Rifampin) / ↓ Lamotrigine levels R/T ↑ liver metabolism; adjust lamotrigine dose as needed
Succinimides (e.g., ethosuximide) / ↓ Lamotrigine levels → ↓ therapeutic effects; adjust dosage as needed
Topiramate / 15% ↑ in topiramate levels
Valproic acid / Twofold ↑ in lamotrigine levels; 25% ↓ in valproic acid levels; ↓ lamotrigine dose to less than ½
NOTE: Lamotrigine is a dihydrofolate reductase inhibitor; use caution when prescribing other drugs that inhibit folate metabolism.

HOW SUPPLIED
Tablets: 25 mg, 100 mg, 150 mg, 200 mg; *Tablets, Chewable Dispersible:* 2 mg, 5 mg, 25 mg.

DOSAGE
• **TABLETS; TABLETS, CHEWABLE DISPERSIBLE**
Partial seizures, lamotrigine added to valproic acid.
Adults and children over 12 years of age: Weeks 1 and 2, 25 mg q other day. **Weeks 3 and 4,** 25 mg every day. **Week 5 onwards to maintenance:** Increase by 25–50 mg/day q 1 to 2 weeks. **Maintenance, usual:** 100–400 mg/day in 1 or 2 divided doses (100–200 mg/day with valproate alone). **Children, 2–12 years: Weeks 1 and 2,** 0.15 mg/kg/day in 1 or 2 divided doses, rounded down to the nearest whole tablet. **Weeks 3 and 4,** 0.3 mg/kg/day in 1 or 2 divided doses; round down to the nearest whole tablet. **Week 5 onwards to maintenance:** Increase dose q 1 to 2 weeks as follows: Calculate 0.3 mg/kg/day; round this amount down to the nearest whole tablet and add this amount to the previously administered daily dose. **Maintenance, usual:** 1–5 mg/kg/day in 1 or 2 divided doses, not to exceed 200 mg/day. Maintenance doses in children weighing less than 30

L

kg may need to be increased by as much as 50%, based on clinical response.

If dosage is calculated on a weight basis in children 2–12 years of age, use the following guide: 6.7 to <14 kg: Weeks 1 and 2: 2 mg every other day; weeks 3 and 4: 2 mg per day. **14.1 to <27 kg:** Weeks 1 and 2: 2 mg per day; weeks 3 and 4: 4 mg per day. **27.1 to <34 kg:** Weeks 1 and 2: 4 mg per day; weeks 3 and 4: 8 mg per day; **34.1 to <40 kg:** Weeks 1 and 2: 5 mg per day; weeks 3 and 4: 10 mg per day. Give daily doses using the most appropriate combination of 2 mg and 5 mg tablets. **Maintenance:** 1–3 mg/kg/day (see above).

Partial seizures, clients taking enzyme-inducing antiepileptic drugs (e.g., carbamazepine, phenobarbital, phenytoin, primidone) without valproic acid.
Adults and children over 12 years: Weeks 1 and 2, 50 mg/day. **Weeks 3 and 4,** 100 mg/day in 2 divided doses. **Week 5 onwards to maintenance:** Increase by 100 mg/day q 1–2 weeks. **Maintenance, usual:** 300–500 mg/day in 2 divided doses. **Children, 2–12 years: Weeks 1 and 2,** 0.6 mg/kg/day in 2 divided doses, rounded down to the nearest whole tablet. **Weeks 3 and 4,** 1.2 mg/kg/day in 2 divided doses, rounded down to the nearest whole tablet. **Week 5 onwards to maintenance:** Increase the dose as follows q 1–2 weeks: Calculate 1.2 mg/kg/day and round down to the nearest whole tablet; add this amount to the previously administered daily dose. **Maintenance, usual:** 5–15 mg/kg/day, to a maximum of 400 mg/day in 2 divided doses. Doses for those weighing less than 30 kg may need to be increased by as much as 50%, based on clinical response.

Partial seizures, clients taking antiepileptic drugs other than carbamazepine, phenobarbital, phenytoin, primidone, or valproate.
Adults and children older than 12 years of age: Weeks 1 and 2: 25 mg/day; **weeks 3 and 4:** 50 mg/day; **weeks 5 onwards to maintenance:** Increase by 50 mg/day q 1–2 weeks; **maintenance, usual:** 225–375 mg/day in 2 divided doses.
Children, 2–12 years of age: Weeks 1 and 2: 0.3 mg/kg/day in 1 or 2 divided doses, rounded down to the nearest whole tablet; **Weeks 3 and 4:** 0.6 mg/kg/day in 2 divided doses, rounded down to the nearest whole tablet; **Week 5 onward to maintenance:** Dose should be increased every 1–2 weeks as follows: Calculate 0.6 mg/kg/day and round this amount down to the nearest whole tablet, and add this amount to the previously administered daily dose; **maintenance, usual:** 4.5–7.5 mg/kg/day, up to a maximum of 300 mg/day in 2 divided doses. Maintenance doses in children weighing less than 30 kg may need to be increased by as much as 50%, based on clinical response.

Conversion from adjunctive therapy with carbamazepine, phenytoin, phenobarbital, primidone, or valproate as the single antiepileptic drug to monotherapy with lamotrigene in clients 16 years and older with epilepsy.
Clients 16 years and older: 500 mg/day (maintenance dose) in 2 divided doses. To convert, titrate lamotrigine to 500 mg/day in 2 divided doses while maintaining the dose of the enzyme-inducing drug at a fixed level. Withdraw the enzyme-inducing drug by 20% decrements each week over a 4-week period.

Conversion from adjunctive therapy with valproate to monotherapy with lamotrigine.
The conversion requires four steps. **Step 1:** Achieve a dosage of 200 mg/day lamotrigine (see above where lamotrigine is added to an antiepileptic drug regimen containing valproate in clients 12 years and older, if not already on 200 mg/day). Maintain previous stable valproate dose. **Step 2:** Maintain lamotrigine at 200 mg/day. Decrease valproate dosage to 500 mg/day by decrements no greater than 500 mg/day per week and then maintain the dose of 500 mg/day for one week.

L

Step 3: Increase the lamotrigine dose to 300 mg/day and maintain for one week. Simultaneously decrease the valproate dose to 250 mg/day and maintain for one week. **Step 4:** Increase the lamotrigine dose by 100 mg/day every week to achieve a maintenance dose of 500 mg/day. Discontinue valproate.

Bipolar disorder, escalation regimen for lamotrigine.

For clients not taking carbamazepine, phenytoin, phenobarbital, primidone, or rifampin and not taking valproate: Weeks 1 and 2: 25 mg/day; **weeks 3 and 4:** 50 mg/day; **week 5:** 100 mg/day; **weeks 6 and 7:** 200 mg/day.

For clients taking carbamazepine, phenytoin, phenobarbital, primidone, or rifampin and not taking valproate: Weeks 1 and 2: 50 mg/day; **weeks 3 and 4:** 100 mg/day in divided doses; **week 5:** 200 mg/day in divided doses; **week 6:** 300 mg/day in divided doses; **week 7:** Up to 400 mg/day in divided doses.

For clients taking valproate: Weeks 1 and 2: 25 mg every other day; **weeks 3 and 4:** 25 mg/day; **week 5:** 50 mg/day; **weeks 6 and 7:** 100 mg/day.

Bipolar disorder, adjustments to lamotrigine dosing following discontinuation of psychotropic medications.

Discontinuing of psychotropic drugs (excluding valproate, carbamazepine, phenytoin, phenobarbital, primidone, rifampin). Weeks 1, 2, and 3 and beyond: Maintain current lamotrigine dosage.

After discontinuation of carbamazepine, phenytoin, phenobarbital, primidone, or rifampin (current lamotrigine dose of 400 mg/day). Week 1: 400 mg/day; **week 2:** 300 mg/day; **week 3 and beyond:** 200 mg/day.

After discontinuation of valproate (current lamotrigine dose of 100 mg/day). Week 1: 150 mg/day; **week 2:** 200 mg/day; **week 3 and beyond:** 200 mg/day.

NURSING CONSIDERATIONS

℀ Do not confuse Lamictal with Lamisil (an antifungal) or with Lomotil (an antidiarrheal).

ADMINISTRATION/STORAGE

1. Dose based on the therapeutic response since a therapeutic plasma level has not been determined.
2. Use caution in selecting doses for geriatric clients.
3. It is recommended that lamotrigine not be restarted in those who discontinue due to rash associated with prior treatment unless potential benefits clearly outweigh risks. The greater the interval of time since the previous dose, the greater consideration that should be given to restarting with the initial dosing regimen.
4. If the calculated dose can not be achieved using whole tablets, round the dose down to the nearest whole tablet.
5. If a change in seizure control or worsening of side effects is noted in clients on lamotrigine in combination with other antiepileptics, reevaluate all drugs in the regimen.
6. Discontinuing an enzyme-inducing antiepileptic drug should prolong the drug half-life, whereas discontinuing valproic acid should shorten the half-life of lamotrigine.
7. If decided to discontinue lamotrigine therapy, a stepwise reduction of dose over 2 weeks (about 50% per week) is recommended unless safety concerns mandate a more rapid withdrawal.
8. Initial, escalation, and maintenance doses should generally be reduced by 50% in clients with moderate (Child-Pugh grade B) and 75% in clients with severe (Child-Pugh grade C) hepatic impairment.
9. Store all tablets from 15–30°C (59–86°F).

ASSESSMENT

1. Note type, onset, characteristics of seizures, previous agents used, outcome.
2. If also prescribed other anticonvulsant agents (i.e., valproate, carbamazepine), monitor closely for adverse ef-

fects. List drugs prescribed to ensure none interact.

3. With bipolar disorder assess clinical behavioral presentation including mood, mania, and ideation; monitor for suicide behaviors.

4. With renal or liver dysfunction, or hypersensitivity reaction, monitor CBC, renal and LFTs.

5. Discontinue drug at first sign of rash.

CLIENT/FAMILY TEACHING

1. Swallow chewable dispersible tablets whole, chewed, or dispersed in water or diluted fruit juice. If chewed, drink a small amount of water or diluted fruit juice to help in swallowing. To disperse chewable tablets, add the tablets to 5 mL (or enough to cover the drug) of liquid. About 1 min later, when tablets are completely dispersed, swirl the solution and consume the entire amount immediately. Do not take partial amounts of dispersed tablets.

2. Do not stop abruptly; may cause increased seizure frequency. Drug should be gradually decreased over at least 2 weeks unless safety concerns require rapid withdrawal.

3. Do not perform activities that require mental alertness and/or coordination until drug effects realized; may cause dizziness, sleepiness, walking problems, headache, and blurred vision.

4. Immediately report loss of seizure control or occurrence of a rash.

5. Avoid alcohol and CNS depressants.

6. Do not start or stop using birth control pills or other female hormonal products during therapy. Report unusual changes in menstrual cycle (i.e., break-through bleeding).

7. Keep all F/U appointments to ensure desired response and to monitor labs.

OUTCOMES/EVALUATE

- Control of seizures
- Mood swing stabilization with bipolar disorder

Lansoprazole IV ℂ 📷
(lan-**SAHP**-rah-zohl)

CLASSIFICATION(S):
Proton pump inhibitor
PREGNANCY CATEGORY: B
Rx: Prevacid, Prevacid IV.

USES

PO. (1) Short-term treatment (up to 4 weeks) for healing and symptomatic relief of active duodenal ulcer (PO only). (2) Maintain healing of duodenal ulcer (PO only). (3) With clarithromycin and/or amoxicillin to eradicate *Helicobacter pylori* infection in active or recurrent duodenal ulcers (PO only). (4) Short-term treatment (up to 8 weeks) for healing and symptomatic relief of active benign gastric ulcer. (5) Treatment of NSAID-associated gastric ulcer in those who continue NSAID use. (6) Reduce the risk of NSAID-associated gastric ulcer in those with a history of documented gastric ulcer who required an NSAID (PO only). (7) Short-term treatment (up to 8 weeks) for healing and symptomatic relief of all grades of erosive esophagitis. Maintain healing of erosive esophagitis. (8) Long-term treatment of pathologic hypersecretory conditions, including Zollinger-Ellison syndrome (PO only). (9) Heartburn and other symptoms of GERD. (10) Short-term treatment of symptomatic GERD and erosive esophagitis including in children, aged 1 to 17 years (PO only).

IV. Short-term (up to 7 days) treatment of all grades of erosive esophagitis. Then, switch to PO lansoprazole formulations.

Investigational: Treat GERD in infants and children. With amoxicillin/clarithromycin for eradication of *H. pylori* in children with *H. pylori*-induced gastritis. Improve pancreatic enzyme absorption in cystic fibrosis clients with intestinal malabsorption.

ACTION/KINETICS

Action

Drug is a gastric acid (proton) pump inhibitor in that it blocks the final step of acid production. Suppresses gastric acid secretion by inhibition of the (H^+, K^+)-ATPase system located at the secretory surface of the parietal cells in the stomach. Both basal and stimulated gastric acid secretion are inhibited, regardless of the stimulus. May have antimicrobial activity against *H. pylori*.

Pharmacokinetics
Absorption begins only after lansoprazole granules leave the stomach, but absorption is rapid. Bioavailability is greater than 80%. **Peak plasma levels:** 1.7 hr. **Mean plasma t½, PO:** 1.5 hr; **IV,** 1.3 hr. **Onset:** 1–3 hr. **Duration:** Over 24 hr. Food does not appear to affect the rate of absorption, if given before meals. Metabolized in the liver with metabolites excreted through both the urine (33%) and feces (66%). **Plasma protein binding:** More than 97%.

CONTRAINDICATIONS
Lactation. Use with rabeprazole.

SPECIAL CONCERNS
Reduce dosage in impaired hepatic function. Symptomatic relief does not preclude the presence of gastric malignancy. Safety and efficacy have not been determined in children less than 18 years of age.

SIDE EFFECTS
Most Common
Diarrhea, headache, N&V, constipation, rash.

GI: Diarrhea, abdominal pain, N&V, melena, anorexia, bezoar, cardiospasm, cholelithiasis, constipation, dry mouth, thirst, dyspepsia, dysphagia, eructation, esophageal stenosis/ulcer, esophagitis, fecal discoloration, flatulence, gastric nodules, fundic gland polyps, gastroenteritis, *GI hemorrhage, rectal hemorrhage, pancreatitis,* hematemesis, increased appetite/salivation, stomatitis, tenesmus, vomiting, ulcerative colitis, hepatotoxicity. **CV:** Angina, hyper/hypotension, *CVA, MI, shock,* palpitations, vasodilation. **CNS:** Headache, agitation, amnesia, anxiety, apathy, confusion, depression, syncope, dizziness, hallucinations, hemiplegia, aggravated hostility, decreased libido, nervousness, paresthesia, abnormal thinking, speech disorder. **GU:** Abnormal menses, breast en-

largement/tenderness/pain, dysmenorrhea, dysuria, gynecomastia, hematuria, albuminuria, glycosuria, impotence, kidney calculus/pain, leukorrhea, menorrhagia, menstrual disorder, polyuria, penis/testis disorder, urethral pain, urinary frequency/urgency/retention, UTI, impaired urination, vaginitis. **Respiratory:** Asthma, bronchitis, increased cough, dyspnea, epistaxis, hemoptysis, hiccoughs, laryngeal neoplasia, pharyngitis, pleural/respiratory disorder, pneumonia, rhinitis, sinusitis, stridor, URTI/inflammation. **Endocrine:** Diabetes mellitus, goiter, hypo/hyperglycemia, hypothyroidism. **Hematologic:** Anemia, eosinophilia, hemolysis, lymphadenopathy, leukopenia, neutropenia, *pancytopenia,* agranulocytosis, *aplastic anemia,* hemolytic anemia. **Musculoskeletal:** Arthritis, arthralgia, bone/joint disorder, leg cramps, musculoskeletal pain, myalgia, myasthenia, synovitis. **Dermatologic:** Acne, alopecia, pruritus, rash, urticaria; severe dermatological reactions, including erythema multiforme, *Stevens-Johnson syndrome, toxic epidermal necrolysis,* thrombocytopenia, thrombotic thrombocytopenic purpura. **Ophthalmic:** Amblyopia, abnormal/blurred vision, eye pain, visual field defect, conjunctivitis, dry eyes, photophobia, retinal degeneration. **Otic:** Deafness, otitis media, tinnitus, ear disorder. **Body as a whole:** Dehydration, edema, gout, peripheral edema, weight loss/gain, asthenia, candidiasis, chills, fever, flu syndrome, infection, malaise, *carcinoma, allergic reaction, anaphylactoid-like reaction.* **Miscellaneous:** Taste loss/perversion, chest/back/neck/pelvic pain, neck rigidity, fever, halitosis, parosmia.

LABORATORY TEST CONSIDERATIONS
Abnormal LFTs. ↑ AST, ALT, creatinine, alkaline phosphatase, globulins, GGTP, glucocorticoids, LDH, gastrin. ↑,↓ or abnormal WBC and platelets. Abnormal AG ratio, RBC. Bilirubinemia, hyperlipemia. ↑ or ↓ Electrolytes or cholesterol.

DRUG INTERACTIONS
Ampicillin / ↓ Ampicillin effect R/T ↓ absorption

Clarithromycin / ↑ Lansoprazole AUC and peak plasma levels R/T inhibition of metabolism by CYP2C19

Digoxin / ↓ Digoxin effect R/T ↓ absorption

Fluvoxamine / ↑ Lansoprazole AUC and prolonged elimination $t\frac{1}{2}$ R/T inhibition of metabolism by CYP2C19

Iron salts / ↓ Effect of iron salts R/T ↓ absorption

Ketoconazole / ↓ Ketoconazole effect R/T ↓ absorption

Sucralfate / Delayed absorption of lansoprazole

HOW SUPPLIED

Capsules, Delayed-Release: 15 mg, 30 mg; Granules for Oral Suspension, Delayed-Release: 15 mg, 30 mg; Powder for Injection, Lyophilized: 30 mg/vial; Tablets, Orally Disintegrating, Delayed-Release: 15 mg, 30 mg.

DOSAGE

• **CAPSULES, DELAYED-RELEASE; ORAL SUSPENSION, DELAYED-RELEASE; TABLETS, ORALLY DISINTEGRATING, DELAYED-RELEASE**

Treatment of duodenal ulcer.

Adults, short-term treatment: 15 mg once daily before breakfast for 4 weeks.

Maintenance of healed duodenal ulcer.

Adults: 15 mg once daily.

Duodenal ulcer associated with H. pylori infections.

The following regimens may be used: (1) Triple therapy. Lansoprazole, 30 mg, plus clarithromycin, 500 mg, plus amoxicillin, 1 gram, each taken twice a day (q 12 hr) for 10 or 14 days. (2) Dual Therapy. Lansoprazole, 30 mg plus amoxicillin, 1 gram each taken 3 times/day (q 8 hr) for 14 days (for clients intolerant or resistant to clarithromycin).

Treatment of gastric ulcer.

30 mg once daily for up to 8 weeks.

Reduce risk of NSAID-associated gastric ulcer.

15 mg once daily for up to 12 weeks.

Treatment of NSAID-associated gastric ulcer.

30 mg once daily for 8 weeks.

GERD.

Adults and children, 12–17 years: 15 mg once daily for up to 8 weeks. **Chil-**

dren, 1–11 years of age, 30 kg or less: 15 mg/day for up to 12 weeks; if symptoms remain after 2 or more weeks, can increase the dose to 30 mg twice a day. **Children, 1–11 years of age, over 30 kg:** 30 mg/day for up to 12 weeks; if symptoms remain after 2 or more weeks, can increase the dose to 30 mg twice a day.

Erosive esophagitis.

Adults, and children 12–17 years, short-term treatment: 30 mg once daily before meals for up to 8 weeks. For adults who do not heal in 8 weeks, an additional 8 weeks of therapy may be given. If there is a recurrence, an additional 8-week course may be considered. **Adults, maintenance:** 15 mg once daily. **Children, 1–11 years of age, short-term treatment, 30 kg or less:** 15 mg/day for up to 12 weeks; if symptoms remain after 2 or more weeks, can increase the dose to 30 mg twice a day. **Children, 1–11 years, short-term treatment, over 30 kg:** 30 mg/day for up to 12 weeks; if symptoms remain after 2 or more weeks, can increase the dose to 30 mg twice a day.

Pathologic hypersecretory conditions (including Zollinger-Ellison syndrome).

Individualize dose. **Initial:** 60 mg once daily. Adjust the dose to client need. Dosage may be continued as long as necessary. Doses up to 90 or 120 mg (in divided doses) have been given. Some clients have been treated for longer than 4 years.

• **IV**

Erosive esophagitis.

Adults: 30 mg/day given over 30 min for up to 7 days. When able to take PO medication, switch to PO Prevacid and continue for up to 6–8 weeks.

NURSING CONSIDERATIONS

ℹ Do not confuse lansoprazole with aripiprazole (an antipsychotic). Also, do not confuse Prevacid with Pravachol (an antihyperlipidemic).

ADMINISTRATION/STORAGE

1. Consider dosage reduction in those with severe liver disease.

2. Do not crush or chew any lansoprazole PO product.

L

3. For those unable to swallow capsules, open delayed-release capsule and sprinkle contents on a tablespoon of applesauce, *Ensure,* pudding, cottage cheese, yogurt, or strained pears and swallow immediately. Alternatively, contents of the capsule can be mixed with about 2 oz of either apple, orange or tomato juice, mixed briefly, and swallowed immediately. To ensure complete delivery of the medication, rinse the glass with 2 or more volumes of juice and swallow contents immediately. Do not chew or crush the granules.

4. To give capsules with an NG tube in place, open capsule and mix intact granules with 40 mL of apple juice; do not use other liquids. Instill through NG tube into the stomach, flushing with additional apple juice to clear the tube.

5. The delayed-release, orally disintegrating tablets may be given with an oral syringe or NG tube. To give via syringe or NG tube, dissolve a 15 mg tablet in 4 mL water or a 30 mg tablet in 10 mL water; shake gently and give within 15 min. Refill the syringe with approximately 5 mL of water, shake gently, and flush the NG tube.

6. Store in a tight container protected from moisture. Store between 15–30°C (59–86°F).

IV 7. Store powder for injection from 15–30°C (59–86°F) protected from light. To reconstitute in the vial, inject 5 mL of only Sterile Water for Injection into a 30 mg vial of lansoprazole IV. The resulting solution will contain lansoprazole, 6 mg/mL. Mix gently until the powder is dissolved. The reconstituted solution can be held for 1 hr when stored at 25°C (77°F).

8. The reconstituted solution must be further diluted before administration and given over 30 min. After dilution, store the admixture at 25°C (77°F) and give within the following time periods: 24 hr if diluted with 0.9% NaCl injection (pH about 10.2) or lactated Ringer's injection (pH about 10) and within 12 hr if mixed with D5W (pH about 9.5).

9. Give lansoprazole admixtures IV using the in-line filter provided. The filter removes precipitate that may form when the reconstituted drug product is mixed with IV solutions. Follow directions carefully for priming and using the filter.

ASSESSMENT

1. List reasons for therapy, onset, duration, characteristics of S&S, other agents trialed, triggers.

2. Note findings of abdominal assessment, US, UGI, barium swallow, endoscopy. Check *H. pylori* results.

3. Monitor CBC, electrolytes, triglycerides, renal and LFTs; reduce dose with severe liver disease.

CLIENT/FAMILY TEACHING

1. Acts by decreasing the amount of acid produced in the stomach. Take as prescribed (usually 30 min before meals); do not exceed dose or share medications. Place orally disintegrating tablets on the tongue and allow to dissolve and then swallow small particles.

2. Swallow capsules whole; do not open, chew, or crush. Those who have difficulty swallowing capsules may open capsule and sprinkle the contents onto applesauce, *Ensure,* yogurt, cottage cheese, strained pears, or juices.

3. To prepare the oral suspension, empty packet contents into 30 mL water (do not use other liquids or food). Stir well and drink immediately. Do not crush/chew the granules. If any material remains after drinking, add more water, stir, and drink immediately.

4. Follow prescribed diet and activities to control S&S of GERD. Drug should be withdrawn once condition resolved; avoid triggers.

5. Keep scheduled appointments. Drug is generally for short-term use and stopped once condition is healed. Long-term effects are not known; users should be assessed periodically for gastric malignancy.

6. May have to stop drug if reports of any severe headaches, worsening of symptoms, fever, chills, or diarrhea.

7. Avoid hazardous activities until drug effects realized; dizziness many occur.

8. Avoid alcohol, aspirin, NSAIDs, and OTC agents unless prescribed; may increase GI irritation.

Bold Italic = life threatening side effect   ■ = black box warning   ✤ = Available in Canada

OUTCOMES/EVALUATE
- Suppression of acid secretion
- Healing of ulcer/erosive esophagitis
- ↓ Pain; relief of heartburn

Lanthanum carbonate
(**LAN**-tha-num)

CLASSIFICATION(S):
Phosphate binder
PREGNANCY CATEGORY: C
Rx: Fosrenol.

USES
Reduce serum phosphate in clients with end-stage renal disease (ESRD).

ACTION/KINETICS
Action
In the acid environment of the upper GI tract, lanthanum dissociates to release lanthanum ions. Lanthanum ions then bind dietary phosphate released from food during digestion. The absorption of phosphate is inhibited R/T the formation of highly insoluble lanthanum phosphate complexes, thus reducing serum phosphate and calcium phosphate.
Pharmacokinetics
Lanthanum is not metabolized. **t½, elimination:** 53 hr.

CONTRAINDICATIONS
Use in children is not recommended.

SPECIAL CONCERNS
Use with caution during lactation.

SIDE EFFECTS
Most Common
N&V, abdominal pain, dialysis graft occlusion, headache, diarrhea.
GI: N&V, diarrhea, abdominal pain, constipation. **CV:** Hypotension. **CNS:** Headache. **Respiratory:** Bronchitis, rhinitis. **Miscellaneous:** Dialysis graft occlusion/complication.

LABORATORY TEST CONSIDERATIONS
Hypercalcemia.

DRUG INTERACTIONS
Do not take drugs known to interact with antacids within 2 hr of dosing with lanthanum.

HOW SUPPLIED
Tablets, Chewable: 250 mg, 500 mg, 750 mg, 1,000 mg.

DOSAGE
- **TABLETS, CHEWABLE**
  Reduce serum phosphate in end-stage renal disease.
Initial, total daily dose: 750–1,500 mg. Divide the total daily dose and take with meals. Titrate the dose every 2–3 weeks until an acceptable serum phosphate level is reached.

NURSING CONSIDERATIONS
ADMINISTRATION/STORAGE
Store from 15–30°C (59–86°F); protect from moisture.

ASSESSMENT
Note onset and reasons for therapy, factors R/T ESRD, other agents trialed. outcome. Monitor BP, dietary habits, serum calcium, lytes, bun, creatinine, phosphate levels.

CLIENT/FAMILY TEACHING
1. Drug is used to lower serum phosphate levels in those with end stage renal disease (ESRD). Chew tablets completely before swallowing; do not swallow intact tablets.
2. Divide total daily prescribed dose in thirds and take with or immediately after each meal.
3. Avoid agents known to interact with antacids for at least 2 hrs of drug administration; consult with provider if unsure.
4. Report any persistent N&V, stomach pain, or diarrhea. Keep all F/U visits to evaluate labs and dialysis graft patency if applicable.
5. Practice reliable contraception. Keep out of reach of children. Reports as scheduled for labs and evaluation of condition.

OUTCOMES/EVALUATE
↓ Serum phosphate with ESRD

Lapatinib

(la-**PA**-ti-nib)

CLASSIFICATION(S):
Protein tyrosine kinase inhibitor
PREGNANCY CATEGORY: D
Rx: Tykerb.

USES
In combination with capecitabine to treat advanced or metastatic breast cancer whose tumors overexpress human epidermal receptor type 2 (HER2) and who have received prior therapy, including an anthracycline, a taxane, and trastuzumab.

ACTION/KINETICS

Action
Inhibits intracellular tyrosine kinase domains of both epidermal growth factor receptor and human epidermal receptor type 2. Thus, proliferation of breast cancer cells is inhibited.

Pharmacokinetics
Absorption is incomplete and variable. **Peak plasma levels:** About 4 hr. Steady state reached in 6-7 days. Systemic levels are increased by food. Undergoes extensive metabolism primarily by CYP3A4 and CYP3A5. **t½, terminal:** 14.2 hr. Mainly excreted in the feces. **Plasma protein binding:** More than 99%.

CONTRAINDICATIONS
Avoid concomitant use of strong CYP3A4 *inhibitors* (e.g., atazanavir, clarithromycin, indinavir, itraconazole, ketoconazole, nefazodone, nelfinavir, ritonavir, saquinavir, telithromycin, and voriconazole). Avoid concomitant use of strong CYP3A4 *inducers* (e.g., carbamazepine, dexamethasone, phenobarbital, phenytoin, rifampin, rifabutin, rifapentin, St. John's wort). Lactation.

SPECIAL CONCERNS
Use with caution in those who have or may develop prolongation of QTc (e.g., hypokalemia, hypomagnesemia, congenital long QT syndrome, antiarrhythmic drugs, cumulative high-dose anthracycline therapy). Safety and efficacy have not been determined in children.

SIDE EFFECTS

Most Common
Diarrhea, N&V, palmar-plantar erythrodysesthesia, rash, fatigue.

GI: Diarrhea, N&V, stomatitis, dyspepsia. **CNS:** Insomnia. **CV:** Decrease in left ventricular cardiac ejection fraction, prolongation of QT. **Dermatologic:** Palmar-plantar erythrodysesthesia, rash, dry skin. **Musculoskeletal:** Pain in extremity, back pain. **Respiratory:** Dyspnea. **Miscellaneous:** Fatigue, mucosal inflammation.

LABORATORY TEST CONSIDERATIONS
↑ ALT, AST, total bilirubin. ↓ Hemoglobin, neutrophils, platelets.

OD OVERDOSE MANAGEMENT
Symptoms: Diarrhea, vomiting, nausea. *Treatment:* Interrupt treatment. Institute IV hydration. Hemodialysis is not expected to be effective.

DRUG INTERACTIONS
Azole antifungals (itraconazole, ketoconazole, voriconazole) / ↑ Lapatinib levels R/T inhibition of CYP3A4; do not use together

Carbamazepine / ↓ Lapatinib levels R/T induction of CYP3A4; do not use together

Clarithromycin / ↑ Lapatinib levels R/T inhibition of CYP3A4; do not use together

Dexamethasone / ↓ Lapatinib levels R/T induction of CYP3A4; do not use together

Digitoxin / Avoid concomitant use; if use can not be avoided, consider dose ↓ of digitoxin

Grapefruit juice / ↑ Lapatinib plasma levels; do not use together

Hydantoins (e.g., fosphenytoin, phenytoin) / ↓ Lapatinib levels R/T induction of CYP3A4; do not use together

Nefazodone / ↑ Lapatinib levels R/T inhibition of CYP3A4; do not use together

Phenobarbital / ↓ Lapatinib levels R/T induction of CYP3A4; do not use together

Protease inhibitors (e.g., atazanavir, indinavir, nelfinavir, ritonavir, saquinavir) / ↑ Lapatinib levels R/T inhibition of CYP3A4; do not use together

Rifamycins (e.g., rifabutin, rifampin, rifa-

L

pentin) / ↓ Lapatinib levels R/T induction of CYP3A4; do not use together

H *St. John's wort* / ↓ Lapatinib levels R/T induction of CYP3A4; do not use together

Telithromycin / ↑ Lapatinib levels R/T inhibition of CYP3A4; do not use together

Theophylline / Avoid concomitant use; if use can not be avoided, consider dose ↓ of theophylline

Warfarin / Avoid concomitant use; if use can not be avoided, consider dose ↓ of warfarin

HOW SUPPLIED

Tablets: 250 mg.

DOSAGE

- **TABLETS**

  Breast cancer.

1,250 mg (5 tablets) PO once daily on days 1 to 21 continuously in combination with capacitabine, 2,000 mg/m²/day (given PO in 2 doses approximately 12 hr apart) on days 1 to 14 in a repeating 21-day cycle.

NURSING CONSIDERATIONS

ADMINISTRATION/STORAGE

1. Correct hypokalemia or hypomagnesemia prior to lapatinib administration.

2. If a dose is missed, do not double the dose the next day.

3. Continue treatment until disease progression or unacceptable toxicity occurs.

4. Discontinue in clients with a decreased left ventricular ejection fraction (LVEF) that is grade 2 or more by the National Cancer Institute Common Terminology Criteria for Adverse Events. Also discontinue in those with a LVEF that drops below the institution's lower limit of normal. Lapatinib may be restarted at a reduced dose (1,000 mg/day) after a minimum of 2 weeks if the LVEF recovers to normal and the client is asymptomatic.

5. Reduce the initial dose of lapatinib to 750 mg/day in clients with Child-Pugh class C impaired hepatic function.

6. Discontinue or interrupt dosing in clients who develop NCI-CTC toxicity of grade 2 or more. The drug can be restarted at 1,250 mg/day when the toxicity improves to grade 1 or less. If the toxicity recurs, restart lapatinib at a lower dose of 1,000 mg/day.

7. If strong CYP3A4 inhibitors (see *Contraindications* and *Drug Interactions*) must be used concomitantly with lapatinib, reduce the dose of lapatinib to 500 mg/day. If the strong inhibitor is discontinued, a washout period of about 1 week should be allowed before the lapatinib dose is adjusted upward to the indicated dose.

8. If strong CYP3A4 inducers (see *Contraindications* and *Drug Interactions*) must be used concomitantly with lapatinib, titrate the dose of lapatinib gradually from 1,250 mg/day up to 4,500 mg/day, based on tolerability. If the strong inducer is discontinued, reduce the lapatinib dose to the indicated dose.

9. Store from 15–30°C (59–86°F).

ASSESSMENT

1. Note reasons for therapy, prior therapy with an anthracycline, a taxane, and trastuzumab and when, outcome. List drugs prescribed to ensure none interact.

2. Assess clinical condition and for any CAD, prolonged Q-T syndrome, renal or liver disease.

3. Monitor EKG, Mg, lytes, CBC, renal and LFTs. Obtain MUGA to assess EF if impairment likely.

CLIENT/FAMILY TEACHING

1. Take lapatinib at least 1 hr before or 1 hr after a meal. Take capecitabine with food or within 30 min after food.

2. Lapatinib is given once daily for 21 consecutive days, and capecitabine is given twice daily for the first 14 days. This 21-day cycle is then repeated, unless your condition gets worse or have serious side effects.

3. The usual dose of lapatinib is equal to 5 tablets. May swallow each tablet individually, but take entire dose at the same time each day.

4. Do not eat grapefruit or drink grapefruit juice while taking Lapatinib.

5. Practice reliable contraception during therapy, do not nurse.

6. Report any adverse side effects including chest pain, palpitations, sob,

L

---

redness or swelling of extremities, severe stomach pain or diarrhea, severe tiredness or weakness, unusual bruising or bleeding; yellowing of the eyes or skin.

7. Keep all F/U appointments to evaluate labs and response to therapy.

OUTCOMES/EVALUATE
Inhibits epidermal growth factor receptor and (HER) human epidermal receptor 2–driven tumor cell growth with metastatic breast cancer

Latanoprost
(lah-**TAH**-noh-prost)

CLASSIFICATION(S):
Prostaglandin agonist
PREGNANCY CATEGORY: C
Rx: Xalatan.

USES
Reduce intraocular pressure in open-angle glaucoma and ocular hypertension in clients who are intolerant of other intraocular pressure lowering medications or who failed to achieve target IOP over time.

ACTION/KINETICS
Action
A prostaglandin $F^2\alpha$ analog that decreases intraocular pressure by increasing the outflow of aqueous humor. Absorbed through the cornea where it is hydrolyzed by esterases to the active acid.

Pharmacokinetics
Peak levels in aqueous humor: 2 hr. **Onset:** 3–4 hr. **Maximum effect:** 8–12 hr. The active acid is metabolized in the liver and excreted in the urine. **t½, elimination:** 17 min.

CONTRAINDICATIONS
Hypersensitivity to latanoprost or benzalkonium chloride. Use while wearing contact lenses or in active intraocular inflammation.

SPECIAL CONCERNS
May gradually change eye color by increasing the amount of brown pigment in the iris; the resultant color changes may be permanent. Use with caution during lactation and in those with a history of intraocular inflammation (i.e., iritis/uveitis). The drug product contains benzalkonium chloride, which may be absorbed by contact lenses. Safety and efficacy have not been determined in children.

SIDE EFFECTS
Most Common
Blurred vision, burning, stinging, conjunctival hyperemia, foreign body sensation, itching, increased pigmentation of the iris, punctate epithelial keratopathy.

Ophthalmic: Blurred vision, burning, stinging, conjunctival hyperemia, foreign body sensation, itching, increased pigmentation of the iris, punctate epithelial keratopathy, dry eye, excessive tearing, eye pain, lid crusting/edema/erythema, lid discomfort/pain, photophobia, conjunctivitis, diplopia, discharge from the eye, retinal artery embolus, retinal detachment, macular edema, bacterial keratitis (i.e., from contaminated multidose containers), vitreous hemorrhage from diabetic retinopathy (rare). **Systemic:** URTI (e.g., cold, flu), pain in muscles/joints/back, chest pain/angina pectoris, rash, allergic skin reactions.

DRUG INTERACTIONS
A precipitate may form if latanoprost is used with eyedrops containing thimerosal; if such drugs are used, give with an interval of at least 5 min between applications.

HOW SUPPLIED
Ophthalmic Solution: 0.005%.

DOSAGE
- **SOLUTION, 0.005%**
  Elevated intraocular pressure.
1 gtt (1.5 mcg) in the affected eye(s) once daily in the evening. More frequent use may decrease the intraocular pressure lowering effect.

NURSING CONSIDERATIONS
ADMINISTRATION/STORAGE
1. May be used concomitantly with other topical ophthalmic drugs to lower IOP. If more than one drug is used, give at least 5 min apart.

Bold Italic = life threatening side effect   ■ = black box warning   ✤ = Available in Canada

2. Protect from light. Refrigerate unopened bottles. Once opened, may store container at room temperature (up to 25°C; 77°F) for 6 weeks.

ASSESSMENT

Note eye exam findings, pressures, and client ability to comply with therapy and F/U appointments.

CLIENT/FAMILY TEACHING

1. Drug reduces pressure in the eye by increasing the amount of fluid that drains from the eye.

2. Wash hands before and after use. Avoid touching any part of the eye with the container tip to prevent contamination and eye infections. Contaminated solutions may cause eye damage and loss of vision.

3. Use once daily, in the evening. Report any lid or eye reactions, especially redness.

4. At least 5 min should elapse between administration of latanoprost and other eye drops, especially drops containing thimerosal.

5. Prior to administration, remove contact lenses and do not reinsert for at least 15 min.

6. Iris color changes may occur due to an increase of brown pigment in the iris; this may be permanent. Occurs primarily in people with blue or green eyes and only in the eye being treated.

OUTCOMES/EVALUATE

↓ IOP

Leflunomide ■
(leh-**FLOON**-oh-myd)

CLASSIFICATION(S):
Antiarthritic drug
PREGNANCY CATEGORY: X
Rx: Arava.

USES

(1) Treatment of active rheumatoid arthritis in adults, including to retard structural damage. (2) Improvement of physical function in adults with active rheumatoid arthritis.

ACTION/KINETICS

Action

Inhibits dihydroorotate dehydrogenase, an enzyme involved in de novo pyrimidine synthesis; has antiproliferative activity and anti-inflammatory and uricosuric effects.

Pharmacokinetics

After PO, is metabolized to an active metabolite (M1). **Peak levels, M1:** 6–12 hr. **t½, M1:** About 2 weeks. M1 is extensively bound to albumin. M1 is further metabolized and excreted through the kidney (more significant over the first 96 hr) and bile.

CONTRAINDICATIONS

Use in pregnancy, lactation, in children less than 18 years of age, in hepatic insufficiency, or positive hepatitis B or C. Also, use in those with severe immunodeficiency, bone marrow dysplasia, severe uncontrolled infections, or vaccination with live vaccines.

SPECIAL CONCERNS

■ Before starting treatment, exclude pregnancy. Contraindicated in women, or women of childbearing age, who are not using reliable contraception. Pregnancy must be avoided during leflunomide treatment or prior to the completion of the drug elimination procedure after treatment.■ Use with caution in those with renal insufficiency. Rare, serious hepatic injury (may be fatal) can occur within 6 months of therapy in clients with multiple risk factors for hepatotoxicity. Clients have died from interstitial lung disease that developed during therapy; onset or worsening of cough or dyspnea may require further evaluation; the drug elimination process may be required (See *Administration/Storage*).

SIDE EFFECTS

Most Common

Diarrhea, respiratory infection, hypertension, alopecia, rash, headache, nausea, bronchitis, dyspepsia, GI/abdominal pain, back pain, UTI.

GI: Diarrhea, N&V, dyspepsia, abnormal liver enzymes, GI/abdominal pain, anorexia, dry mouth, gastroenteritis, mouth ulcer, cholelithiasis, colitis, constipation, esophagitis, flatulence, gastritis, gingivitis, melena, oral moniliasis, pharyngitis, enlarged salivary gland, stomatitis or aphthous stomatitis, tooth disorder, acute hepatotoxicity with **hepatic necrosis, serious hepatic injury. CNS:** Headache, dizziness, paresthesia, anxiety, depression, insomnia, neuralgia, neuritis, sleep disorder, sweat, vertigo. **CV:** Hypertension (as preexisting condition was over represented in drug treatment groups), chest pain, angina pectoris, migraine, palpitation, tachycardia, vasculitis, vasodilation, varicose vein. **Dermatologic:** Alopecia, rash, pruritus, eczema, dry skin, acne, contact/fungal dermatitis, hair discoloration, hematoma, herpes simplex/zoster, nail disorder, subcutaneous nodule, maculopapular rash, skin disorder/discoloration/ulcer/nodule. **Musculoskeletal:** Back pain, joint disorder, tenosynovitis, synovitis, arthralgia, leg/muscle cramps, arthrosis, bursitis, myalgia, bone pain/necrosis, tendon rupture. **Respiratory:** Respiratory infection, bronchitis, increased cough, pharyngitis, pneumonia, rhinitis, sinusitis, asthma, dyspnea, epistaxis, lung disorder. **GU:** Albuminuria, cystitis, dysuria, hematuria, menstrual disorder, vaginal moniliasis, prostate disorder, urinary frequency, UTI. **Hematologic:** Anemia, including iron deficiency anemia; ecchymosis. **Metabolic:** Weight loss, hypokalemia, peripheral edema, hyperglycemia, hyperlipidemia. **Ophthalmic:** Blurred vision, cataract, conjunctivitis, eye disorder. **Miscellaneous:** Diabetes mellitus, hyperthyroidism, taste perversion, injury accident, infection, asthenia, allergic reaction, flu syndrome, pain, abscess, cyst, fever, hernia, malaise, neck/pelvic pain.

LABORATORY TEST CONSIDERATIONS
↑ ALT, AST, CPK. Uricosuric effect, hypophosphatemia.

OD OVERDOSE MANAGEMENT
Symptoms: See *Side Effects. Treatment:* Give cholestyramine or charcoal. Dose of cholestyramine is 8 grams 3 times per day PO for 24 hr. Dose of charcoal is 50 grams made into a suspension for PO or NGT given q 6 hr for 24 hr.

DRUG INTERACTIONS
Charcoal / Rapid and significant ↓ in leflunomide active M1 metabolite
Cholestyramine / Rapid and significant ↓ in leflunomide active M1 metabolite
Hepatotoxic drugs / ↑ Side effects
Rifampin / ↑ M1 peak levels

HOW SUPPLIED
Tablets: 10 mg, 20 mg, 100 mg.

DOSAGE
- **TABLETS**
  Rheumatoid arthritis.
  Loading dose: 100 mg/day PO for 3 days. **Maintenance:** 20 mg/day; if this dose is not well tolerated, decrease to 10 mg/day. Doses greater than 20 mg/day are not recommended due to increased risk of side effects.

NURSING CONSIDERATIONS
ADMINISTRATION/STORAGE
1. Aspirin, NSAIDs, or low-dose corticosteroids may be continued during leflunomide therapy.
2. Use the drug elimination procedure to achieve nondetectable plasma levels (<0.02 mcg/mL) after stopping treatment: Give cholestyramine, 8 grams 3 times/day for 11 days (no need to be consecutive unless need to lower plasma levels rapidly). Verify plasma levels by 2 separate tests at least 14 days apart. Without the drug elimination procedure, it may take 2 years or less to reach plasma M1 levels of 0.02 mcg/mL due to variations in drug clearance.

ASSESSMENT
1. Note reasons for therapy, pain level, functional limitations, quality of life, joint(s) characteristics, other agents trialed.
2. Assess for liver dysfunction, hepatitis B or C; precludes therapy.
3. Obtain negative pregnancy test.
4. Monitor SGPT (ALT) and SGOT (AST) monthly; adjust dosage with elevations. If elevations persist 2–3x ULN and continued therapy is desired, consider liver biopsy.
5. Drug metabolite M1 has an extremely long half-life (up to 2 years). Cholestyramine may accelerate drug elimination. Women of childbearing age desiring pregnancy should undergo the

---

Bold Italic = life threatening side effect   ■ = black box warning   ♣ = Available in Canada

drug elimination procedure to prevent fetal death or damage.

CLIENT/FAMILY TEACHING

1. Therapy consists of a 3-day loading dose and then a daily maintenance dose.

2. May take with or without food; takes up to 8 weeks for desired effects.

3. Drug will cause fetal damage. Practice reliable birth control. If pregnancy desired or suspected in females, or males wish to father a child, start drug elimination procedure. Do not breastfeed during therapy.

4. Avoid live vaccines during therapy.

5. May experience dizziness, diarrhea, nausea, GI upset, URI, headache, and rash; report if persistent or intolerable.

6. Report as scheduled for monthly liver function studies to prevent possibility of fatal liver damage.

OUTCOMES/EVALUATE

- ↓ Bone erosion/joint narrowing
- Slowed RA disease progression
- Improved functioning level/quality of life

Lenalidomide ■
(le-na-**LID**-oh-mide)

CLASSIFICATION(S):
Immunomodulator
PREGNANCY CATEGORY: X
Rx: Revlimid.

USES
(1) Treatment of transfusion-dependent anemia due to low- or intermediate-1 risk myelodysplastic syndrome associated with a deletion 5q cytogenetic abnormality with or without additional cytogenetic abnormalities. (2) In combination with dexamethasone to treat multiple myeloma in those who have received at least one prior therapy.

ACTION/KINETICS

Action
The mechanism of action is not fully understood; the drug possesses antineoplastic, immunomodulatory, and antiangiogenic properties. It is known to inhibit proinflammatory cytokines and increase the secretion of anti-inflammatory cytokines from peripheral blood mononuclear cells.

Pharmacokinetics
Rapidly absorbed. **Maximum plasma levels:** 0.63–1.5 hr. Food does not affect the AUC but does decrease C_{max}. About two-thirds excreted unchanged in the urine. $t\frac{1}{2}$, **elimination:** About 3 hr. **Plasma protein binding:** About 30%.

CONTRAINDICATIONS
Hypersensitivity to the drug or any component of the product. Pregnancy and women of childbearing potential since lenalidomide is structurally similar to thalidomide. Lactation.

SPECIAL CONCERNS
■ Warnings. (1) Potential for human birth defects. Lenalidomide is an analog of thalidomide. Thalidomide is a known human teratogen that causes severe, life-threatening human birth defects. If lenalidomide is taken during pregnancy, it may cause birth defects or death to a fetus. Advise women to avoid pregnancy while taking lenalidomide. Because of this potential toxicity and to avoid fetal exposure to lenalidomide, the drug is only available under a special restricted distribution program, RevAssist. Under this program, only health care providers and pharmacists registered with the program are able to prescribe and dispense the products. In addition, lenalidomide is only dispensed to clients who are registered and meet all the conditions of the RevAssist program. **Consult the package insert for a detailed description of Celgene's RevAssist Program, and especially use in women of childbearing age.** (2) Hematologic toxicity (neutropenia and thrombocytopenia). Lenalidomide is associated with significant neutropenia and thrombocytopenia. Eighty percent of clients had to have a dose delay/reduction during the major study. Thirty-four percent of clients had to have a second dose delay/reduction. Grade 3 or 4 hematologic toxicity was seen in 80% of clients enrolled in the study. Clients on therapy for deletion 5q myelodysplastic syndrome should have their complete blood count moni-

L

tored weekly for the first 8 weeks of therapy and at least monthly thereafter. Clients may require dose interruption and/or reduction. Clients may require use of blood product support and/or growth factors. (3) Deep vein thrombosis (DVT) and pulmonary embolism (PE). Use of lenalidomide has demonstrated a significantly increased risk of DVT and PE in those with multiple myeloma who were treated with lenalidomide combination therapy. Clients and health care providers are advised to be observant for the signs and symptoms of thromboembolism. Instruct clients to seek medical care if they develop symptoms such as shortness of breath, chest pain, or arm or leg swelling. It is not known whether prophylactic anticoagulation or antiplatelet therapy prescribed in conjunction with lenalidomde may lessen the potential for venous thromboembolic events. The decision to take prophylactic measures should be done carefully after an assessment of an individual client's underlying risk factors. (4) Information about lenalidomide and the RevAssist program can be obtained at http://www.revlimid.com or by calling the manufacturer's toll-free number 1-888-423-5436.■ Use with caution in impaired renal function and in the elderly (more likely to experience diarrhea, fatigue, pulmonary embolism, and syncope). Safety and efficacy have not been determined in children less than 18 years of age.

SIDE EFFECTS
Most Common
Thrombocytopenia, neutropenia, diarrhea, pruritus, rash, fatigue, dizziness, headache, dry skin, constipation, N&V, arthralgia, back pain, muscle cramps, myalgia, cough, dyspnea, nasopharyngitis, URTI, asthenia, peripheral edema, pyrexia.

Side effects listed are for all uses. **GI:** Abdominal pain, upper abdominal pain, anorexia, constipation, diarrhea, dry mouth, dysgeusia, loose stools, N&V, pseudomembranous colitis, ischemic colitis, colonic polyp, diverticulitis, dysphagia, gastritis, gastroenteritis, GERD, *GI hemorrhage*, *intestinal perforation*,

IBS, melena, obstructive inguinal hernia, *pancreatitis* (including that due to biliary obstruction), perirectal abscess, *rectal hemorrhage*, small intestinal obstruction, *peptic ulcer hemorrhage, UGI hemorrhage*. **Hepatic:** Cholecystitis (including acute), *hepatic failure*, hyperbilirubinemia, toxic hepatitis. **CV:** Hyper-/hypotension, orthostatic hypotension, palpitations, pulmonary hypertension, *pulmonary embolism,* angina pectoris, aortic disorder, atrial fibrillation (including aggravated), bradycardia, *cardiac arrest/failure,* CHF, *cardiorespiratory arrest, cardiogenic shock, cardiomyopathy, DVT*, ischemia, *MI*, myocardial/cerebral/peripheral ischemia, pulmonary edema, supraventricular arrhythmia, tachyarrhythmia, superficial thrombophlebitis, thrombosis, ventricular dysfunction, *subarachnoid hemorrhage*, TIA, postprocedural hemorrhage, *cerebellar/cerebral infarction, CVA, postprocedural hemorrhage, intracranial venous sinus thrombosis* (when used with dexamethasone), atrial flutter, circulatory collapse, phlebitis, subacute endocarditis, limb venous thrombosis, *intracranial hemorrhage*. **CNS:** Depression, dizziness, fatigue, headache, hypesthesia, insomnia, peripheral neuropathy, rigors, syncope, aphasia, confusion, decreased level of consciousness, dysarthria, falls, abnormal gait, vertigo, migraine, spinal cord compression, paresthesia, tremor, delirium, delusion, encephalitis, leukoencephalopathy, impaired memory, changes in mental status, decreased performance status, psychotic disorder, somnolence. **Dermatologic:** Dry skin, ecchymosis, erythema, pruritus, night sweats, rash, increased sweating, acute febrile neutrophilic dermatosis, skin desquamation. **GU:** Dysuria, UTI, azotemia, ureteric calculus, hematuria, kidney infection, renal failure (including acute), renal mass, pelvic pain, metastatic prostate cancer, acquired Fanconi syndrome, renal tubular necrosis, urinary retention. **Hematologic:** Anemia, febrile neutropenia, leukopenia, lymphopenia, neutropenia, thrombocytopenia, granulocytopenia, *pancytope-*

Bold Italic = life threatening side effect   ■ = black box warning   ✦ = Available in Canada

nia, acute leukemia, acute myeloid leukemia, bone marrow depression, coagulopathy, hemolysis, hemolytic anemia, lymphoma, refractory anemia, splenic infarction, warm type hemolytic anemia, *neutropenic sepsis.* **Musculoskeletal:** Arthralgia, back pain, muscle cramps/weakness, myalgia, limb pain, arthritis, aggravated arthritis, chondrocalcinosis pyrophosphate, gouty arthritis, neck pain, cervical vertebral fracture, femoral neck fracture, femur/pelvis/hip/rib fracture, pelvic pain, spinal compression fracture, cerebral vertebral fracture, myopathy (including that due to steroids). **Respiratory:** Bronchitis, cough, dyspnea, exertional dyspnea, epistaxis, hypoxia, nasopharyngitis, pharyngitis, pneumonia, rhinitis, sinusitis (including acute), URTI, respiratory tract infection, hypoxia, pleural effusion, pneumonia, pneumonitis, respiratory distress, exaggerated chronic obstructive airway disease, exacerbated dyspnea, interstitial lung disease, lobar pneumonia, lung infiltration, pulmonary edema, *respiratory failure,* wheezing, bronchopneumonia, bronchopneumopathy, bronchoalveolar carcinoma, metastatic lung cancer. **Infections:** Bacteremia, central line infection, clostridial infection, ear infection, *Enterobacter* sepsis or bacteremia, fungal infection, herpes viral infection, influenza, kidney infection, *Klebsiella* sepsis, localized infection, oral infection, GI infection, *Pseudomonas* infection, *Staphylococcal* infection (including pneumonia), ***Streptococcal sepsis,*** urosepsis, lung infection, *Escherichia* sepsis, *Pneumocystis carnii* pneumonia, bacterial pneumonia, cytomegaloviral pneumonia, pneumococcal pneumonia, primary atypical pneumonia, infective bursitis, herpes zoster, ***sepsis, septic shock.*** **Ophthalmic:** Blurred vision, blindness, ophthalmic herpes zoster. **Otic:** Ear infection. **Body as a whole:** Asthenia, cellulitis, edema, peripheral edema, pain, peripheral swelling, pyrexia (including intermittent), dehydration, rigors, hypersensitivity, increased/decreased weight, diabetes mellitus, diabetes with hyperosmolarity, diabetic ketoacidosis. **Miscel-**

laneous: Acquired hypothyroidism, adrenal insufficiency, chest pain, ear infection, contusion, gout, ***multi-organ failure,*** Basedow disease, nodule, cellulitis (including staphylococcal), transfusion reaction, ***sudden death.***

LABORATORY TEST CONSIDERATIONS

↑ AST, blood creatinine, troponin I, C-reactive protein, INR. ↓ Hemoglobin, WBC. Abnormal LFTs. Hypokalemia, hypomagnesemia, hypernatremia, hypo-/hyperglycemia, hypocalcemia.

DRUG INTERACTIONS

Digoxin / ↑ Digoxin C_{max} (AUC did not change)

HOW SUPPLIED

Capsules: 5 mg, 10 mg, 15 mg, 25 mg.

DOSAGE

• **CAPSULES**

Myelodysplastic syndrome with transfusion-dependent anemia.

Initial: 10 mg daily with water. See *Administration/Storage* for dosage information for clients who experience thrombocytopenia or neutropenia.

Multiple myeloma.

Lenalidomide, 25 mg/day with water given as a single 25 mg capsule on days 1 through 21 of repeated 28-day cycles. The dose of dexamethasone is 40 mg/day PO on days 1 through 4, 9 through 12, and 17 through 20 of each 28-day cycle for the first 4 cycles of therapy; then, 40 mg/day PO on days 1 through 4 every 28 days. Dosing is continued or modified based on clinical and lab findings.

NURSING CONSIDERATIONS

ADMINISTRATION/STORAGE

1. The following dosage schedule is used for those who are dosed initially at 10 mg/day lenalidomide for myelodysplastic syndrome and who experience thrombocytopenia *within* 4 weeks of starting treatment:

• Interrupt lenalidomide treatment when platelets fall to fewer than 50,000/mcL. Resume lenalidomide at 5 mg/day when platelets return to 50,000/mcL or greater.

• Interrupt lenalidomide treatment when platelets fall to 50% of baseline value. Resume lenalidomide at 5

L

mg/day if baseline is 60,000/mcL or greater and returns to 50,000/mcL or greater.

- Interrupt lenalidomide treatment when platelets fall to 50% of baseline value. Resume lenalidomide at 5 mg/day if baseline is <60,000/ mcL and returns to 30,000/mcL or more.

2. The following dosage schedule is used for those who are dosed initially at 10 mg/day lenalidomide for myelodysplastic syndrome and who experience thrombocytopenia *after* 4 weeks of starting treatment:

- Interrupt lenalidomide treatment when platelets are <30,000/mcL or <50,000 mcL and platelet transfusions. Resume lenalidomide at 5 mg/day when platelets return to 30,000/mcL or more (without hemostatic failure).

3. The following dosage schedule is used for those who experience thrombocytopenia at 5 mg/day when used for myelodysplastic syndrome:

- Interrupt lenalidomide treatment when platelets are 30,000/mcL or less or 50,000/mcL or less and platelet transfusions. Resume lenalidomate at 5 mg every other day when platelets return to 30,000/mcL or more (without hemostatic failure).

4. The following dosage schedule is used for those who are dosed initially at 10 mg/day for myelodysplastic syndrome and experience neutropenia *within* 4 weeks of starting treatment:

- If baseline ANC is 1,000/mcL or greater, interrupt lenalidomnide treatment when neutrophils fall to <750/mcL. Resume lenalidomide at 5 mg/day when neutrophils return to 1,000/mcL or greater.
- If baseline ANC is <1,000/mcL, interrupt lenalidomide treatment when neutrophils fall to <500/mcL. Resume lenalidomide at 5 mg/day when neutrophils return to 500/mcL or greater.

5. The following dosage schedule is used for those who are dosed initially at 10 mg/day for myelodysplastic syndrome and experience neutropenia *after* 4 weeks of starting treatment:

- Interrupt lenalidomide treatment when neutrophils are <500/mcL for 7 days or more or neutrophils are <500/mcL associated with fever (38.5°C/101°F) or greater. Resume lenalidomide at 5 mg/day when neutrophils return to 500/mcL or more.

6. The following dosage schedule is used for those who experience neutropenia at 5 mg/day when used for myelodysplastic syndrome:

- Interrupt lenalidomide treatment when neutrophils are <500/mcL for 7 days or more or neutrophils are <500/mcL associated with fever (38.5°C/101°F). Resume lenalidomide at 5 mg every other day when neutrophils return to 500 mcL or more.

7. When used to treat multiple myeloma, use the following dosage adjustments due to thrombocytopenia or neutropenia:

- Interrupt lenalidomide treatment and follow CBC weekly when platelets fall to <30,000/mcL. Resume lenalidomde at 15 mg/day when platelets return to >30,000/mcL or more. For each subsequent platelet count drop to <30,000/mcL, interrupt lenalidomide therapy. When platelet counts return to 30,000/mcL or more after subsequent drops, resume treatment at 5 mg less than the previous dose; do not dose below 5 mg/day.
- Interrupt lenalidomide treatment, add granulocyte colony-stimulating factor, and follow CBC weekly when neutrophils fall to <1,000/mcL. Resume lenalidomide at 25 mg/day when neutrophils return to 1,000/ mcL or more and neutropenia is the only toxicity. When neutrophils return to >1,000/mcL and there is other toxicity, resume lenalidomide at 15 mg/day. Interrupt lenalidomide for each subsequent neutrophil count drop to <1,000/mcL. When neutrophils return to >1,000/mcL or more, resume lenalidomide at 5 mg less than the previous dose; do not dose below 5 mg/day.

8. For other grade 3/4 toxicities that are related to lenalidomide, hold treat-

ment and restart at the next lower dose level when toxicity has resolved to grade 2 or less.

9. Store from 15-30°C (59-86°F).

ASSESSMENT

1. Note reasons for therapy, MDS/MM, other agents trialed, outcome.

2. List all drugs/agents consumed to ensure none interact. Identify all other medical conditions; assess renal function.

3. Obtain CBC weekly during first 8 weeks of therapy and then monthly thereafter with 5q MDS and q 2 weeks x 12 weeks then monthly with MM. Follow dosing guidelines carefully under administration/storage based on blood count results.

4. Ensure negative pregnancy test drug teratogenic and a derivative of thalidomide.

5. For uninsured or underinsured, drug company participates in Patient Support Solutions; provider may call for new case application forms at 1-888-423-5436.

6. Chromosonal abnormality involving 5q evident in 20-30% of all MDS clients.

CLIENT/FAMILY TEACHING

1. Myelodysplastic syndrome (5q MDS) have low red blood cell counts that require treatment with blood transfusions. This is caused by bone marrow that does not produce enough mature blood cells.

2. Take capsules whole with water daily. Do not break, chew or open capsules. Do not double up on dose. No more than a 28 day supply will be dispensed at one time.

3. All providers, dispensing pharmacies, and clients must enroll in the RevAssist program and follow all of the guidelines/requirements and sign the Patient-Physician Agreement form in order to get Revlimid.

4. Do not donate blood during and for 4 weeks following drug therapy.

5. Females that can become pregnant will get regular pregnancy testing weekly for 4 weeks and must agree to use 2 separate forms of birth control at the same time: 4 weeks before, during and 4 weeks after stopping drug.

6. Males, even those that have had a vasectomy, must agree to use a latex condom during sexual contact with a female that can become or is pregnant. Do not donate sperm during and for 4 weeks following therapy.

7. May experience diarrhea, rash, fatigue, itching. Other adverse effects include birth defects, low white blood cells and platelets, blood clots in the veins and the lungs. Report immediately any SOB, chest pain or sudden swelling in hands and/or feet.

8. With MDS, your blood counts are checked weekly for 8 weeks then monthly thereafter; with multiple myeloma, drug is administered with dexamethasone; blood counts should be checked every two weeks for the first 12 weeks and then at least monthly after that.

9. Keep all F/U appointments for labs and evaluation of therapy.

OUTCOMES/EVALUATE

Restoration of blood cells without blood transfusion with MDS

Lepirudin   IV

(leh-**PEER**-you-din)

CLASSIFICATION(S):
Anticoagulant, thrombin inhibitor
PREGNANCY CATEGORY: B
Rx: Refludan.

SEE ALSO ANTICOAGULANTS.

USES

Anticoagulation in heparin-induced thrombocytopenia (HIT) and associated thromboembolic disease to prevent further complications. *Investigational:* Adjunct to treat unstable angina, acute MI without ST elevation, prevent deep vein thrombosis, and in those undergoing percutaneous coronary intervention.

ACTION/KINETICS

Action

Lepirudin is a highly specific direct inhibitor of thrombin. One antithrombin unit (ATU) is the amount of lepirudin that neutralizes one unit of World Health Organization preparation 89/588 of thrombin. One molecule of lepirudin binds to one molecule of thrombin, blocking the thrombogenic activity of thrombin. Thus, all thrombin-dependent assays are affected (i.e., activated partial thromboplastin time [aPTT], resulting in an increase in aPTT.

Pharmacokinetics

t½, distribution: About 10 min; **t½, elimination:** About 1.3 hr. Systemic clearance is dependent on glomerular filtration rate. About half is excreted in the urine as unchanged drug and other fragments. Thought to be metabolized by release of amino acids via catabolic hydrolysis of the parent drug. The systemic clearance in women is about 25% lower than in men and clearance in the elderly is 20% less than in younger clients. Dose must be adjusted based on C_{CR} as elimination half-lives are prolonged up to 2 days.

CONTRAINDICATIONS

Hypersensitivity to hirudins. Lactation.

SPECIAL CONCERNS

Assess risk of therapy in those with an increased risk of bleeding, including recent puncture of large vessels or organ biopsy; anomaly of vessels or organs; recent CVA, stroke, intracerebral surgery or other neuraxial procedures; severe uncontrolled hypertension; bacterial endocarditis; advanced renal impairment; hemorrhagic diathesis; recent major surgery; recent intracranial, GI, intraocular, or pulmonary major bleeding; recent active peptic ulcer. Formation of antihirudin antibodies or serious hepatic injury may increase the anticoagulant effect. Increased risk of allergic reactions in those also receiving thrombolytic therapy (e.g., streptokinase) for acute MI or contrast media for coronary angiography. Intracranial bleeding following concomitant thrombolytic therapy with alteplase or streptokinase may be life-threatening. Safety and efficacy have not been determined in children.

SIDE EFFECTS

Most Common

Bleeding from puncture sites/wounds, anemia, hematuria, GI/rectal bleeding, fever, abnormal liver function, pneumonia.

Hemorrhagic events: Bleeding from puncture sites and wounds, anemia or isolated drop in hemoglobin, hematoma, hematuria, GI/rectal bleeding, epistaxis, hemothorax, intracranial bleeding, hemoperitoneum, hemoptysis, liver/vaginal/lung/mouth/retroperitoneal bleeding. CV: *Heart failure, pericardial effusion, ventricular fibrillation.* **Allergic reactions:** Cough, *bronchospasms,* stridor, dyspnea, pruritus, urticaria, rash, flushes, chills, *anaphylaxis,* angioedema, *facial/tongue/larynx edema.* **Miscellaneous:** Fever, pneumonia, anemia, sepsis, allergic skin reactions, abnormal kidney/liver function, unspecified infections, *multiorgan failure.*

OD OVERDOSE MANAGEMENT

Symptoms: Bleeding. *Treatment:* Immediately stop administration. Determine aPTT and other coagulation levels as appropriate. Determine hemoglobin and prepare for blood transfusion. Follow guidelines for treatment of shock. Hemofiltration or hemodialysis may be helpful.

DRUG INTERACTIONS

Coumarin derivatives / ↑ Risk of bleeding

Thrombolytics (streptokinase, TPA) / ↑ Risk of bleeding complications and ↑ effect on aPTT prolongation

HOW SUPPLIED

Powder for Injection: 50 mg.

DOSAGE————————

- **IV**

  Heparin-induced thrombocytopenia and associated thromboembolic disease.

Adults, initial: 0.4 mg/kg given slowly over 15–20 seconds as a bolus dose followed by 0.15 mg/kg/hr as a continuous IV infusion for 2–10 days or longer if needed. Normally the initial dose is based on body weight; this is valid for clients up to 110 kg; for those over 110 kg, do not increase the initial dosage beyond the 110 kg body weight dose (the maximum bolus dose is 44 mg and the maximal initial infusion dose is 16.5 mg/hr). Adjust dose according to the aPTT ratio (client aPTT at a given time over an aPTT reference value, usually median of the lab normal range for aPTT). The target range for aPTT is 1.5 to 2.5. To avoid initial overdosing, do not start therapy in clients with a baseline aPTT ratio of 2.5 or more. The bolus and infusion doses must be reduced in known or suspected renal insufficiency (C_{CR} <60 mL/min or serum creatinine >1.5 mg/dL).

Concomitant use with thrombolytics.
Initial IV bolus: 0.2 mg/kg; **continuous IV infusion:** 0.1 mg/kg/hr.

NURSING CONSIDERATIONS

ADMINISTRATION/STORAGE

[IV] 1. If client is to receive coumarin derivatives for PO anticoagulation after lepirudin, gradually reduce lepirudin dose to reach an aPTT ratio just above 1.5 before initiating PO anticoagulation. As soon as an INR of 2 is reached, stop drug.

2. Do not mix with other drugs except water for injection, 0.9% NaCl, or D5W injection.

3. Reconstitution and further dilution are to be done under sterile conditions as follows:

- Use D5W or water for injection for reconstitution
- For further dilution, 0.9% NaCl injection or D5W injection is suitable.
- For rapid, complete reconstitution, inject 1 mL of diluent into the vial and shake gently. A clear, colorless solution is usually obtained in a few seconds, but <3 min.
- Do not use solutions that are cloudy or contain particles.
- Use reconstituted solution immediately; it is stable for 24 hr or less at room temperature (i.e., during infusion).
- Warm product to room temperature before administration.
- Discard any unused solution.

4. For the initial IV bolus, use a 5 mg/mL solution. Prepare as follows:

- Reconstitute one vial (50 mg) with 1 mL of 0.9% NaCl or water for injection.
- To obtain a final concentration of 5 mg/mL, transfer contents of the vial into a sterile, single-use syringe (10 mL or greater capacity); dilute solu-

tion to a total volume of 10 mL using water for injection, 0.9% NaCl, or D5W.

5. For continuous IV infusion, use a concentration of 0.2 or 0.4 mg/mL. Prepare as follows:

- Reconstitute two vials (50 mg each) with 1 mL each using either 0.9% NaCl or water for injection.
- To obtain a final concentration of 0.2 or 0.4 mg/mL, transfer contents of both vials into an infusion bag containing 500 or 250 mL of 0.9% NaCl or D5W.
- The infusion rate (mL/hr) is determined according to body weight).

ASSESSMENT

1. Assess for conditions that preclude therapy: recent surgery, bleed, ulcers etc. Note allergic reactions with thrombolytic therapy.

2. Monitor LFTs, CBC, bleeding parameters, renal function studies; reduce dose with dysfunction.

3. If weight is more than 110 kg, do not increase dosage beyond that weight dose.

4. Monitor carefully at all sites for evidence of excessive bleeding. Have RBCs available for transfusion.

5. Get aPTT 4 hr after first dose and at least daily during therapy (more frequently with liver/renal impairment). If aPTT ratio >2.5 stop infusion (for at least 2 hr) report.

CLIENT/FAMILY TEACHING

1. Drug is used to thin the blood and prevent blood clots in those with low platelets caused by heparin.

2. Report any evidence of bleeding or oozing from catheter sites, under skin or gums, in urine or stools or adverse effects.

3. Use soft-bristled toothbrush, electric razor, night-light, and slippers to prevent injury; avoid contact sports or aggressive hugging, juggling, or wrestling.

4. May experience redness or pain at injection site. Keep all F/U appointments to evaluate response to therapy and for any adverse effects.

OUTCOMES/EVALUATE

- Inhibition of thromboembolic complications
- PTT ratio 1.5 to 2.5

L

Letrozole ©

(**LET**-roh-zohl)

CLASSIFICATION(S):
Antineoplastic, hormone
PREGNANCY CATEGORY: D
Rx: Femara.

SEE ALSO *ANTINEOPLASTIC AGENTS.*

USES

(1) First-line treatment of advanced or metastatic breast cancer in postmenopausal women who have hormone-receptor positive disease or hormone-receptor unknown disease and where there is progression following antiestrogen therapy. (2) Extended adjuvant treatment of early breast cancer in postmenopausal women who have received 5 years of adjuvant tamoxifen therapy. (3) First-line treatment of postmenopausal women with hormone receptor-positive or hormone receptor-unknown locally advanced or metastatic breast cancer with disease progression following antiestrogen therapy. *Investigational:* Stimulation of ovulation to improve chances of pregnancy.

ACTION/KINETICS

Action

A nonsteroidal competitive inhibitor of aromatase, resulting in inhibition of conversion of androgens to estrogens. It acts by competitively binding to heme of the cytochrome P450 subunit of aromatase, leading to decreased biosynthesis of estrogen in all tissues. Does not cause an increase in serum FSH and does not affect synthesis of adrenocorticosteroids, aldosterone, or thyroid hormones.

Pharmacokinetics

Rapidly and completely absorbed. $t\frac{1}{2}$, **terminal elimination:** About 2 days. Steady state plasma levels after daily doses of 2.5 mg reached in 2 to 6 weeks. Slowly broken down in the liver to inactive metabolites that are excreted in urine.

CONTRAINDICATIONS

Hypersensitivity to any component of the product.

SPECIAL CONCERNS

Use with caution during lactation and in those with severely impaired hepatic function. Safety and efficacy have not been determined in children.

SIDE EFFECTS

Most Common
Bone pain, hot flashes, flushing, back pain, nausea, arthralgia/arthritis, dyspnea, fatigue/lethargy/asthenia, headache, weight increase, increased sweating, edema.

CNS: Headache, somnolence, insomnia, dizziness, vertigo, depression, anxiety, hemiparesis. **GI:** N&V, constipation, diarrhea, abdominal pain, anorexia, dyspepsia. **CV:** Hypertension, angina, coronary heart disease, thrombophlebitis, *MI, pulmonary embolism, thrombotic or hemorrhagic strokes,* myocardial ischemia, portal vein thrombosis, TIAs, venous thrombosis. **GU:** Renal disorders, vaginal hemorrhage, vulvovaginal dryness, breast pain, UTIs. **Body as a whole:** Fatigue, lethargy, malaise, increased sweating, viral infections, infections and infestations, peripheral edema (including lower leg), asthenia, weakness, influenza, increased or decreased weight, nonspecific pain. **Dermatologic:** Hot flashes, flushing, rash (erythematous, maculopapular, psoriaform, vesicular), pruritus, alopecia, increased sweating. **Respiratory:** Dyspnea, coughing, pleural effusion. **Musculoskeletal:** Bone/back/limb pain, arthralgia, arthritis, myalgia, fracture. **Miscellaneous:** Chest wall pain, chest pain, peripheral edema, hypercholesterolemia, hypercalcemia, postmastectomy lymphedema.

LABORATORY TEST CONSIDERATIONS

↑ AST, ALT, GGT. ↓ Lymphocyte counts. Hypercholesterolemia, hypercalcemia.

DRUG INTERACTIONS

Tamoxifen may ↓ letrozole plasma levels by about 37%; clinical significance not known

HOW SUPPLIED

Tablets: 2.5 mg.

DOSAGE

• TABLETS

All uses.

Adults and elderly: 2.5 mg once per day without regard to meals. Continue until tumor progression is evident; discontinue treatment at relapse. Dosage adjustment is not needed in renal impairment if C_{CR} is greater than or equal to 10 mL/min. **Severe hepatic impairment or cirrhosis:** 2.5 mg every other day (i.e., decrease dose by 50%).

NURSING CONSIDERATIONS

@ Do not confuse Femara with Femhrt (an estrogen-progestin combination).

ADMINISTRATION/STORAGE

ASSESSMENT

1. Note disease onset, clinical findings, previous antiestrogen therapy, and response.
2. Monitor bone mineral density, CBC, calcium, renal and LFTs; reduce dose with liver dysfunction. Stop drug if tumor progression evident.

CLIENT/FAMILY TEACHING

1. Take as directed; may take without regard to meals.
2. Report any severe rash, chills, fever, diarrhea, pain, severe depression, changes in color of urine/stool or skin/sclera, SOB, or chest pain. May experience hot flashes, headaches, light-headedness, and nausea; report if persistent.
3. May experience drowsiness/dizziness; use caution with activities requiring mental alertness. Avoid alcohol and OTC agents without approval.
4. Practice reliable contraception; may cause serious fetal harm.

OUTCOMES/EVALUATE

↓ Tumor mass; ↓ malignant cell proliferation

Leucovorin calcium (Citrovorum factor, Folinic acid)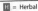

(loo-koh-**VOR**-in)

CLASSIFICATION(S):
Folic acid derivative
PREGNANCY CATEGORY: C
Rx: Leucovorin calcium.

USES

PO and parenteral: (1) Prophylaxis and treatment of toxicity due to methotrexate and folic acid antagonists (e.g., pyrimethamine and trimethoprim). (2) Leucovorin rescue following high doses of methotrexate for osteosarcoma.

Parenteral: (1) Megaloblastic anemias due to nutritional deficiency, sprue, pregnancy, and infancy when oral folic acid is not appropriate. (2) Adjunct with 5-FU to prolong survival in the palliative treatment of metastatic colorectal carcinoma. *NOTE:* It is recommended for megaloblastic anemia caused by pregnancy even though the drug is pregnancy category C.

ACTION/KINETICS

Action

Is a mixture of the diastereoisomers of the 5-formyl derivative of tetrahydrofolic acid. Does not require reduction by dihydrofolate reductase to be active in intracellular metabolism; thus, it is not affected by dihydrofolate inhibitors. Quickly metabolized to 1,5-methyltetrahydrofolate, which is then metabolized by other pathways back to 5,10-methylene-tetrahydrofolate and then converted to 5-methyltetrahydrofolate using the cofactors $FADH_2$ and NADPH. Leucovorin can counteract the therapeutic and toxic effects of methotrexate (acts by inhibiting dihydrofolate reductase) but can enhance the effects of 5-fluorouracil (5-FU).

Pharmacokinetics

Rapidly absorbed following PO administration. Is rapidly absorbed. **Peak serum levels, PO:** Approximately 2.3 hr; **after IM:** 52 min; **after IV:** 10 min. Onset, PO: 20–30 min; IM: 10–20 min; IV: <5 min. **Terminal t½:** 5.7 hr (PO), 6.2 hr (IM and IV). **Duration:** 3–6 hr. Excreted by the kidney.

CONTRAINDICATIONS

Pernicious anemia or megaloblastic anemia due to vitamin B_{12} deficiency.

SPECIAL CONCERNS

Use with caution during lactation. May increase the frequency of seizures in susceptible children. When leucovorin is used with 5-FU for advanced colorectal cancer, the dosage of 5-FU must be lower than usual as leucovorin enhances the toxicity of 5-FU. The benzyl alcohol in the parenteral form may cause a fatal gasping syndrome in premature infants.

SIDE EFFECTS

Most Common

Urticaria, anaphylaxis (no other side effects attributed to leucovorin alone).
Leucovorin alone. Allergic reactions, including urticaria and ***anaphylaxis.***
Leucovorin and 5-FU. GI: N&V, diarrhea, stomatitis, constipation, anorexia. **Hematologic:** Leukopenia, thrombocytopenia. **CNS:** Fatigue, lethargy, malaise. **Miscellaneous:** Infection, alopecia, dermatitis.

DRUG INTERACTIONS

5-FU / ↑ 5-FU toxicity
Methotrexate / High doses ↓ effect of intrathecal methotrexate
PAS / ↓ Folate levels → folic acid deficiency
Phenobarbital / ↓ Phenobarbital effect → ↑ seizure frequency, especially in children
Phenytoin / ↓ Phenytoin effect R/T ↑ rate of liver breakdown; also, drug may ↓ folate levels
Primidone / ↓ Primidone effect → ↑ seizure frequency, especially in children
Sulfasalazine / ↓ Folate levels → folic acid deficiency

HOW SUPPLIED

Injection: 3 mg/mL, 10 mg/mL; *Powder for Injection:* 50 mg, 100 mg, 350 mg; *Tablets:* 5 mg, 15 mg, 25 mg.

DOSAGE

• **IM; IV; TABLETS**

Advanced colorectal cancer.

Either leucovorin, 200 mg/m^2 by slow IV over a minimum of 3 min followed by 5-FU, 370 mg/m^2 IV **or** leucovorin 20 mg/m^2 IV followed by 5-FU, 425 mg/m^2 IV. Treatment is repeated daily for 5 days with the 5-day treatment course repeated at 28-day intervals for two courses and then repeated at 4- to 5-week intervals as long as the client has recovered from the toxic effects.

Leucovorin rescue after high-dose methotrexate therapy.

The dose of leucovorin is based on a methotrexate dose of 12–15 mg/m^2 given by IV infusion over 4 hr. The dose of leucovorin is 15 mg (10 mg/m^2) PO, IM, or IV q 6 hr for 10 doses starting 24 hr after the start of the methotrexate infusion. Give leucovorin parenterally if there is nausea, vomiting, or GI toxicity. If serum methotrexate levels are greater than 0.2 μM at 72 hr and greater than 0.05 μM at 96 hr after administration, leucovorin should be continued at a dose of 15 mg PO, IM, or IV q 6 hr until methotrexate levels are less than 0.05 μM. If serum methotrexate levels are equal to or greater than 50 μM at 24 hr, or equal to or greater than 5 μM at 48 hr after administration, or if there is a 100% or greater increase in serum creatinine levels at 24 hr after methotrexate administration, the dose of leucovorin should be 150 mg IV q 3 hr until methotrexate levels are less than 1 μM; **then,** give leucovorin, 15 mg IV q 3 hr until methotrexate levels are less than 0.05 μM. If significant clinical toxicity is seen following methotrexate, leucovorin rescue should total 14 doses over 84 hr in subsequent courses of methotrexate therapy.

Impaired methotrexate elimination or accidental overdose.

Start leucovorin rescue as soon as the overdose is discovered and within 24 hr of methotrexate administration when excretion is impaired. Give leucovorin, 10 mg/m^2 PO, IM, or IV q 6 hr until serum methotrexate levels are less than 10^{-8} M. If the 24-hr serum creatinine has increased 50% over baseline or if the 24- or 48-hr methotrexate level is more than 5×10^{-6} M or greater than 9×10^{-7}

Bold Italic = life threatening side effect   ■ = black box warning   ✦ = Available in Canada

M, respectively, the dose of leucovorin should be increased to 100 mg/m^2 IV q 3 hr until the methotrexate level is less than 10^{-8} M. Urinary alkalinization with sodium bicarbonate solution (to maintain urine pH at 7 or greater) and hydration with 3 L/day should be undertaken at the same time.

Overdosage of folic acid antagonists.
5–15 mg/day

Megaloblastic anemia due to folic acid deficiency.

Adults and children: Up to 1 mg/day.

NURSING CONSIDERATIONS

🕮 Do not confuse folinic acid with folic acid (Vitamin B complex).

ADMINISTRATION/STORAGE

1. Oral solution stable for 14 days refrigerated or 7 days stored at room temperature.

2. If used for methotrexate (MTX) rescue, hydrate well and alkalinize urine to reduce nephrotoxicity.

IV 3. Dilute with 5 mL bacteriostatic water for injection and use within 1 week. If sterile water for injection is added, use the solution immediately.

4. Give doses higher than 25 mg parenterally because PO absorption is saturated.

5. Do not use leucovorin calcium injection containing benzyl alcohol in doses greater than 10 mg/m^2.

6. Parenteral use is preferred if there is a possibility client may vomit or not absorb leucovorin.

7. In treating overdosage due to folic acid antagonists, give as soon as possible. As the time interval between the overdosage and administration of leucovorin increases, the effectiveness of leucovorin decreases.

8. Protect from light.

ASSESSMENT

1. Note reasons for therapy: replacement or rescue. If for rescue therapy, administer promptly (first dose within 1 hr) following a high dose of folic acid antagonists; follow dosage exactly to be effective.

2. Note history of B$_{12}$ deficiency that has resulted in pernicious or megaloblastic anemia. Leucovorin may obscure the diagnosis of pernicious anemia if previously undiagnosed.

3. Determine any history of seizure disorders; assess for recurrence.

4. Monitor renal, B$_{12}$, folic acid, MTX, and hematologic values. Creatinine increases of 50% over pretreatment levels indicate severe renal toxicity.

5. Urine pH should be >7.0; monitor q 6 hr during therapy. Urine alkalinization with NaHCO$_3$ or acetazolamide may be necessary to prevent nephrotoxic effects.

CLIENT/FAMILY TEACHING

1. This drug is used to save or 'rescue' normal cells from the damaging effects of chemotherapy, allowing them to survive while the cancer cells die.

2. Report immediately any skin rash, itching, uneasiness, or difficulty breathing.

3. IV therapy is used following chemotherapy; N&V may prevent oral absorption.

4. When high-dose therapy is used, be alert for mental confusion and impaired judgment. Safety measures and supervision help ensure safety and protection.

5. Consume at least 3 L/day of fluids with rescue therapy.

OUTCOMES/EVALUATE

- Symptom improvement (↓ fatigue, ↑ weight, improved mentation)
- ↑ Normoblasts (with anemia)
- MTX level <5 x 10^{-8}M
- Prevention/reversal of GI, renal, and bone marrow toxicity in MTX therapy or during overdosage of folic acid antagonists

Leuprolide acetate
(loo-**PROH**-lyd)

CLASSIFICATION(S):
Antineoplastic, hormone
PREGNANCY CATEGORY: X

Rx: Eligard, Lupron, Lupron Depot, Lupron Depot-3 Month, Lupron Depot-4 Month, Lupron Depot-Ped, Lupron for Pediatric Use, Viadur.

📷 = see color insert   H = Herbal   IV = Intravenous   🕮 = sound alike drug

♣**Rx:** Lupron Depot 3.75 mg/ 11.25 mg, Lupron/Lupron Depot 3.75 mg/7.5 mg, Lupron/Lupron Depot 7.5 mg/22.5 mg/30 mg.

SEE ALSO *ANTINEOPLASTIC AGENTS.*

USES
(1) Palliative treatment in advanced prostatic cancer when orchiectomy or estrogen treatment are not appropriate (use injection, implant, or depot 7.5, 22.5, 30 mg, or 45 mg). (2) Viadur is used as a once yearly implant for advanced prostate cancer. (3) Endometriosis (use depot 3.75 or 11.25 mg). (4) Central precocious puberty (use pediatric injection or Lupron Depot-Ped). (5) In combination with iron supplements for the presurgical treatment of anemia caused by uterine leiomyomata (use depot form, 3.75 or 11.25 mg). *Investigational:* With flutamide for metastatic prostatic cancer.

ACTION/KINETICS
Action
Related to the naturally occurring GnRH. By desensitizing GnRH receptors, gonadotropin secretion is inhibited. Initially, however, LH and FSH levels increase, leading to increases of sex hormones; decreases in these hormones will be observed within 2–4 weeks. Levels of serum testosterone and prostate-specific antigen in men with advanced prostate cancer are decreased to castrate levels.

Pharmacokinetics
Peak plasma levels: 4 hr for various doses. $t\frac{1}{2}$: 3 hr. Chronic use results in a measurable increase in body length, return to prepubertal state of reproductive organs, and cessation of menses (if present). A miniature titanium implant is available which releases leuprolide over one year and provides an alternative to frequent injections. **Plasma protein binding:** From 43–49%.

CONTRAINDICATIONS
Pregnancy, in women who may become pregnant while receiving the drug, and during lactation. Sensitivity to benzyl alcohol (found in leuprolide injection). Undiagnosed abnormal vaginal bleeding. Hypersensitivity to GnRH or GnRH agonist analogs. Use of the 7.5 mg (monthly), 22.4 mg (3-month), and 30 mg (4-month) injections in women and children. Lactation.

SPECIAL CONCERNS
Safety and efficacy have not been determined in children (except Lupron Depot-PED). May cause increased bone pain and difficulty in urination during the first few weeks of therapy for prostatic cancer. An increase in signs and symptoms of central precocious puberty, endometriosis/uterine leiomyomata, and advanced prostate cancer may be noted at the beginning of therapy.

SIDE EFFECTS
Most Common
Injection site reactions, peripheral edema, general pain, hot flashes/sweats, asthenia, malaise/fatigue, decreased bone density, GI disorders, edema, testicular atrophy, skin reactions, headache, depression/emotional lability, dizziness/vertigo, N&V, headache/migraine, vaginitis.

When used for central precocious puberty. Dermatologic: Acne, seborrhea, injection site reactions (including induration, abscess), rash (including erythema multiforme), alopecia, skin striae, rash, urticaria, photosensitivity reactions, hair growth. **GI:** Dysphagia, gingivitis, N&V, hepatic dysfunction. **CNS:** Emotional lability, nervousness, personality disorder, somnolence, peripheral neuropathy, spinal fracture/paralysis. **CV:** Syncope, vasodilation, hypotension, *pulmonary embolism*. **Respiratory:** Epistaxis, respiratory disorders. **Musculoskeletal:** Tenosynovitis-like symptoms, fibromyalgia, decreased bone density. **GU:** Vaginitis/bleeding/discharge, cervix disorder, gynecomastia, breast disorders, urinary incontinence, prostate pain. **Body as a whole:** Body odor, fever, headache, infection. **Miscellaneous:** General pain, accelerated sexual maturity, peripheral edema, weight gain, decreased WBCs, hearing disorder, hard nodule in throat, weight gain, increased uric acid.

When used for advanced prostate cancer (all dosage forms). CNS: Dizziness, lightheadedness, general pain,

---

headache, insomnia/sleep disorders, anxiety, agitation, lethargy, memory disorder mood swings, nervousness, numbness, paresthesia, peripheral neuropathy, syncope/blackouts, depression, spinal fracture/paralysis, disturbance of smell/taste, vertigo, delusions, hypesthesia, abnormal thinking, amnesia, confusion, **convulsions**, dementia. **GI:** Anorexia, constipation, flatulence, N&V, diarrhea, dysphagia, GI bleeding, dyspepsia, GI disturbance, duodenal/peptic ulcer, rectal polyps, hepatic dysfunction, gastroenteritis, colitis, eructation, thirst/dry mouth, increased appetite, **GI hemorrhage,** gingivitis, gum hemorrhage, hepatomegaly, intestinal obstruction, periodontal abscess. **CV:** CHF, EEG changes, ischemia, high BP, heart murmur, peripheral edema, phlebitis, thrombosis, hypo-/hypertension, TIA, angina, CHF, arrhythmia, bradycardia, varicose vein, atrial fibrillation, deep thrombophlebitis, **heart failure, stroke, pulmonary embolism**. **Dermatologic:** Dermatitis, carcinoma of skin/ear, dry skin, ecchymosis, hair loss/growth, alopecia, itching, local skin reactions, pigmentation, skin lesions, erythema, transient burning/stinging, pain, mild bruising, pruritus, induration/abscess at injection site, ulceration, hot flashes, sweating, night sweats, clamminess, herpes zoster, melanosis. **Musculoskeletal:** Bone/joint/neck pain, myalgia, ankylosing spondylosis, pelvic fibrosis, backache, tremor, changes in bone density, arthralgia, limb pain/cramps, muscle atrophy, fibromyalgia, tenosynovitis-like syndrome, pathological fracture. **Respiratory:** Dyspnea, sinus congestion, cough, pleural rub, pneumonia, pulmonary fibrosis, pulmonary infiltrate, respiratory disorders, emphysema, hemoptysis, increased sputum, lung edema, epistaxis, pharyngitis, pleural effusion, hypoxia, asthma, bronchitis, lung disorder, sinusitis, voice alteration, hiccup. **Endocrine:** Impotence, decreased/increased libido, thyroid enlargement. **GU:** Gynecomastia, breast enlargement, breast tenderness/pain/soreness, urinary frequency/urgency, urinary difficulty, hematuria, decreased testicular size/testicular atrophy, UTI, bladder spasms, dysuria, incontinence, testicular/prostate pain, urinary obstruction, scanty urination, penile swelling, nocturia, erectile dysfunction, reduced penis size, balanitis, prostate pain, impotence, bladder carcinoma, epididymitis. **Hematologic:** Anemia, decreased WBCs/RBCs, hemoptysis, decreased H&H, lymphedema, lymphadenopathy. **Ophthalmic:** Blurred vision, temporal bone swelling, abnormal vision, amblyopia, dry eyes, ptosis. **Otic:** Hearing disorder, tinnitus. **Hypersensitivity:** Rash, urticaria, photosensitivity, **anaphylaxis**. **At site of injection:** Induration, abscess. **Body as a whole:** Asthenia, diabetes, fatigue, malaise, chills, fever, lethargy, weakness, rigors, generalized edema, dehydration, general pain, infection, cellulitis, flu syndrome. **Miscellaneous:** Taste disorder, infection, inflammation, hard nodule in throat, weight gain/loss, increased uric acid, enlarged abdomen, neoplasm, abnormal healing, abscess, accidental injury, allergic reaction, cyst, hernia.

When used for endometriosis (all dosage forms). GI: Appetite changes, dry mouth, GI disturbances, N&V, thirst, altered bowel function. **CV:** Hot flashes/sweats, palpitations, syncope, tachycardia. **CNS:** Anxiety, depression, headache/migraine, emotional lability, dizziness/vertigo, insomnia, sleep disorder, changes in libido, memory disorder, nervousness, delusions, memory disorder, personality disorder. **Musculoskeletal:** Neuromuscular disorders. **Dermatologic:** Alopecia, ecchymosis, hair disorder, skin/mucous membrane reaction. **GU:** Dysuria, lactation, breast pain/tenderness, menstrual disorders, vaginitis. **Body as a whole:** Asthenia, pain. **Miscellaneous:** Lymphadenopathy, ophthalmologic disorders, edema, weight changes, injection site reaction.

When used for uterine leiomyomata (all dosage forms). CV: Hot flashes, sweats, tachycardia. **GI:** Appetite changes, dry mouth, GI disturbances, N&V. **CNS:** Depression, emotional lability, headache/migraine, anxiety, decreased libido, dizziness, insomnia, nervousness, paresthesias. **Respiratory:** Rhinitis. **Dermatologic:** Androgen-like effects, nail disorder, skin reactions. **GU:** Vaginitis, breast changes, menstrual disorders. **Musculoskeletal:** Joint disorder, neuromuscular disorders, changes in bone density. **Body as a whole:** Asthenia, general pain, body odor, flu syndrome. **Miscellaneous:** Edema, weight changes, conjunctivitis, taste perversion, injection site reactions.

When used for endometriosis or uterine leiomyomata (all dosage forms). **CNS:** Mood swings including depression, peripheral neuropathy, spinal fracture/paralysis, decreased libido, dizziness/vertigo, nervousness, paresthesias, headache, anxiety, delusions, insomnia/sleep disorders, memory disorder, personality disorder, hypesthesia, agitation, *suicidal ideation/attempt*. **GI:** N&V, GI disturbances, appetite changes, dry mouth, thirst, glossitis, altered bowel function. **CV:** Hypotension, hot flashes, sweats, palpitations, syncope, tachycardia, *pulmonary embolism*. **Musculoskeletal:** Fibromyalgia, tenosynovitis-like symptoms, neuromuscular disorders, joint disorder, myalgia. **Dermatologic:** Skin reactions, acne, hirsutism, alopecia, hair/nail disorder. **Respiratory:** Rhinitis, laryngitis. **GU:** Prostate pain, breast changes/tenderness/pain, vaginitis, dysuria, lactation, menstrual disorders, pyelonephritis, urinary disorders, lactation. **Hematologic:** Decreased WBCs, ecchymosis, lymphadenopathy. **Ophthalmic:** Conjunctivitis, ophthalmologic disorders. **At injection site:** Induration, abscess. **Hypersensitivity:** Rash, urticaria, photosensitivity reactions, asthma-like symptoms, *anaphylaxis*. **Body as a whole:** Asthenia, general pain, body odor, flu syndrome. **Miscellaneous:** Edema, weight gain/loss, androgen-like effects, taste perversion, facial edema, ear pain.

LABORATORY TEST CONSIDERATIONS
Injection and Depot. ↑ Calcium. ↓ WBC. Hypoproteinemia. **Injection:** ↑ BUN, creatinine. **Depot:** ↑ LDH, alkaline phosphatase, AST, uric acid, cholesterol, LDL, triglycerides, PT, PTT, glucose, WBC. ↓ Platelets, potassium. Hyperphosphatemia, abnormal LFTs. Misleading results from tests of pituitary gonadotropic and gonadal function up to 4–8 weeks after discontinuing depot therapy.

HOW SUPPLIED
Implant (Viadur): 72 mg; *Injection (Lupron):* 5 mg/mL; *Injection, Depot (Eligard):* 22.5 mg (3-month), 30 mg (4-month), 45 mg (6-month); *Microspheres for Injection, Lyophilized (Lupron Depot, Lupron Depot-Ped, Lupron Depot-3 Month, Lupron Depot-4 Month):* 3.75 mg, 7.5 mg. 11.25 mg, 15 mg, 22.5 mg, 30 mg; *Powder for Injection, Lyophilized (Eligard):* 7.5 mg.

DOSAGE
• **INJECTION; DEPOT INJECTION; IMPLANT**

Advanced prostatic cancer.
Injection (SC): 1 mg/day using the syringes provided. **Depot (IM):** 7.5 mg monthly, 22.5 mg q 3 months, 30 mg q 4 months, or 45 mg q 6 months. **Implant:** One implant q 12 months. The implant delivers 120 mcg/day.

Central precocious puberty.
Individualize, based on a mg/kg ratio of drug to body weight. Younger children require higher doses on a mg/kg ratio. **Injection, initial:** 50 mcg/kg/day SC as a single dose. If down regulation is not achieved, titrate dose upward by 10 mcg/kg/day, which is the maintenance dose. **Lupron Depot-Ped, initial:** 0.3 mg/kg/4 weeks (minimum 7.5 mg) as a single IM dose. Determine the starting dose as follows: If weight is 25 kg or less, give 7.5 mg; if weight is 25–37.5 kg, give 11.25 mg; if weight is >37.5 kg, give 15 mg. If total down regulation is not reached, titrate upward in 3.75 mg increments q 4 weeks (which will be the maintenance dose). *NOTE:* The first dose to cause an adequate down regulation can probably be maintained for duration of therapy in most children.

Endometriosis.
Depot only: 3.75 mg IM once a month or 11.25 mg IM q 3 months for at least 6 months for endometriosis. If further treatment is contemplated, assess bone density prior to beginning therapy.

Uterine leiomyomata.

Use 3.75 mg of the depot only IM monthly or one 11.25 mg IM injection for three months with concomitant iron therapy. The 11.25 mg depot is for women for whom 3 months of hormonal suppression is needed. Duration of therapy is 3 months or less. If further treatment is contemplated, assess bone density prior to beginning therapy.

NURSING CONSIDERATIONS

ADMINISTRATION/STORAGE

1. Follow manufacturer's guidelines carefully to prepare the depot form. Reconstitute only with the diluent provided; after reconstitution, the preparation is stable for 24 hr. There is no preservative so discard if not used immediately.

2. Due to different release properties, a fractional dose of the 3-month and 4-month depot formulations is not equivalent to the same dose of the monthly product; thus, do not interchange.

3. When injecting depot form, do not use needles smaller than 22 gauge.

4. Give the injection using only the syringes provided. If alternate syringes are needed, use insulin syringes.

5. For a single IM injection, reconstitute the lyophilized microspheres with the diluent provided. Withdraw the appropriate amount of diluent from the ampule (1 or 1.5 mL) using a 22-gauge needle and inject into the vial. Shake well to obtain uniform suspension which will appear milky. Withdraw entire contents into the syringe and inject immediately.

6. If using the prefilled dual-chamber syringe, the suspension will be milky. If the microspheres adhere to the stopper, tap the syringe against a finger. Remove the needle guard and advance the plunger to expel air from the syringe. Inject the entire contents of the syringe IM (Lupron) or SC (Eligard). Mix and use immediately as the suspension settles quickly following reconstitution. Reshake suspension if settling occurs.

7. Titanium implant is placed under the skin in the inner aspects of the arm.

8. Injection: Store below room temperature at 25°C (77°F) or less. Avoid freezing and protect from light. Store vial in carton until use.

9. Depot: Store Lupron from 15–30°C (59–86°F). The product does not contain a preservative; thus, discard if not used immediately. Store Eligard from 2–8°C (35–46°F); once mixed, must be given within 30 min.

ASSESSMENT

1. Note reasons for therapy, onset/characteristics of S&S, other agents trialed, outcome.

2. After 1–2 months of initiating therapy or changing doses, monitor with a GnRH stimulation test, sex steroids, and Tanner staging to confirm down regulation.

3. Monitor measurements of bone age for advancement every 6–12 months.

CLIENT/FAMILY TEACHING

1. With prostate cancer drug is used as an alternative to orchiectomy but must be administered for lifetime. With central precocious puberty, drug is given continuously until before girl reaches age 11 and before boy reaches age 12. Undergo careful instruction before assuming responsibility to administer drug therapy.

2. Hot flashes may occur with drug therapy.

3. Record weight; report gains of more than 2 lb/day or 10 lbs per week.

4. Immediately report any weakness, numbness, respiratory difficulty, or impaired urination.

5. Altered sexual effects (impotence, decreased testes size) may occur; identify appropriate resources for counseling and support.

6. Women should expect menstrual irregularities; practice nonhormonal form of contraception.

7. Increased bone pain may be evident at the start of therapy; analgesics may be used for pain control.

OUTCOMES/EVALUATE

- ↓ Tumor size and spread
- Improved symptoms with endometriosis

Levetiracetam [IV] [C]

(**lehv**-ah-ter-**ASS**-ah-tam)

CLASSIFICATION(S):
Anticonvulsant, miscellaneous
PREGNANCY CATEGORY: C
Rx: Keppra.

USES

PO. (1) Adjunctive treatment of partial onset seizures in adults and children 4 years and older with epilepsy. (2) Adjunctive treatment of myoclonic seizures in adults and adolescents, 12 years and older, with juvenile myoclonic epilepsy. (3) Adjunctive treatment of primary generalized tonic-clonic seizures in adults and children 6 years and older with idiopathic generalized seizures. *Investigational:* Treatment of migraines; as adjunctive therapy for bipolar disorder; as monotherapy in new-onset pediatric epilepsy.

IV. Adjunctive treatment of partial-onset seizures in adults with epilepsy and as an alternative for clients when PO administration is temporarily not feasible.

ACTION/KINETICS

Action

Precise mechanism unknown. May act in synaptic plasma membranes in the CNS to inhibit burst firing without affecting normal neuronal excitability. Thus, it may selectively prevent hypersynchronization of epileptiform burst firing and propagation of seizure activity.

Pharmacokinetics

Rapidly and almost completely absorbed; oral bioavailability is 100%. Food does not affect the extent of absorption but it decreases C_{max} and delays time to T_{max}. **Peak plasma levels:** 1 hr during fasting. **Steady state:** Within 2 days of twice a day dosing. Not extensively metabolized in the liver. $t\frac{1}{2}$: 7 hr. Excreted through the urine as metabolites and unchanged (66%) drug. Half-life is longer (by 2.5 hr) in elderly clients. Total body clearance is reduced in those with impaired renal function.

CONTRAINDICATIONS

Lactation.

SPECIAL CONCERNS

Reduce dosage in clients with impaired renal function. Clearance is increased in children. Use care in dose selection in the elderly due to possible decreased renal function. Safety and efficacy have not been determined in children less than 4 years of age for PO products and in children younger than 16 years of age for IV use.

SIDE EFFECTS

Most Common

Somnolence, asthenia, headache, infection, dizziness, pain, pharyngitis, neck pain, pharyngitis.

Adults: CNS: Somnolence, headache, dizziness, depression, nervousness, ataxia, vertigo, amnesia, anxiety, hostility, paresthesia, emotional lability, confusion, insomnia, abnormal thinking, psychotic symptoms, ***convulsion, generalized tonic-clonic convulsions,*** withdrawal seizures, coordination difficulties, abnormal thinking, confusion, tremor, ***suicidal behavior*** (including completed suicide). **Respiratory:** Pharyngitis, rhinitis, sinusitis, increased cough, bronchitis, influenza. **GI:** Abdominal pain, constipation, diarrhea, dyspepsia, gastroenteritis, gingivitis, N&V, dyspepsia, ***pancreatitis.*** **Hepatic:** Abnormal liver function, hepatic failure, hepatitis. **Hematologic:** Leukopenia, neutropenia, pancytopenia, thrombocytopenia. **Musculoskeletal:** Pain, arthralgia, back pain, chest pain. **Dermatologic:** Rash, ecchymosis, alopecia. **Hematologic:** Leukopenia, neutropenia, ***pancytopenia*** (with bone marrow suppression), thrombocytopenia. **Ophthalmic:** Diplopia, amblyopia, **Body as a whole:** Asthenia, infection, fever, flu syndrome, weight gain/loss. **Miscellaneous:** Anorexia, coordination difficulties, accidental injury, fungal infection, otitis media, UTI.

Children: CNS: Somnolence, hostility, nervousness, personality disorder, dizziness, agitation, emotional lability, depression, vertigo, confusion, increased reflexes, abnormal thinking, ataxia, ***convulsion***, headache, hyper-

---

Bold Italic = life threatening side effect   ■ = black box warning   ✦ = Available in Canada

kinesia, insomnia, *status epilepticus*, tremor, irritability, mood swings, hypersomnia. Behavioral symptoms in children, including agitation, anxiety, apathy, depersonalization, depression, emotional lability, hostility, hyperkinesia, nervousness, neurosis, personality disorder. **GI:** Vomiting, anorexia, diarrhea, gastroenteritis, constipation, abdominal pain, nausea. **Respiratory:** Rhinitis, increased cough, pharyngitis, nasopharyngitis, asthma, epistaxis, sinusitis. **Dermatologic:** Pruritus, skin discoloration, vesiculobullous rash, ecchymosis, rash. **GU:** Urine abnormality/incontinence. **Ophthalmic:** Conjunctivitis, amblyopia, diplopia. **Body as a whole:** Asthenia, dehydration, facial edema, flu syndrome, pain, viral infection, allergic reaction, infection, fatigue. **Miscellaneous:** Accidental injury, pain, ear pain, ecchymosis, otitis media.

LABORATORY TEST CONSIDERATIONS
Infrequent abnormalities in hematologic parameters (significant ↓ in total mean RBC count, mean hemoglobin, and mean hematocrit) and LFTs.

OD OVERDOSE MANAGEMENT
Symptoms: Drowsiness (most common), aggression, agitation, coma, depressed level of consciousness, respiratory depression, somnolence. *Treatment:* Emesis or gastric lavage; maintain airway. General supportive care. Monitor VS. Hemodialysis may be beneficial.

DRUG INTERACTIONS
Carbamazepine / ↑ Risk of carbamazepine toxicity
Probenecid / Doubling of the maximum steady-state plasma level of the levetiracetam metabolite

HOW SUPPLIED
Oral Solution: 100 mg/mL; *Solution for Injection:* 100 mg/mL; *Tablets:* 250 mg, 500 mg, 750 mg, 1,000 mg.

DOSAGE

• **ORAL SOLUTION; TABLETS**
  Partial onset seizures in adults and children 4 to younger than 16 years.
Adults, 16 years and older, initial: 500 mg twice a day. Can increase dose by 1,000 mg/day q 2 weeks up to a maximum daily dose of 3,000 mg. There is no evidence that doses above 3,000 mg/day confer additional benefits. For impaired renal function, use the following doses: C_{CR}, **50–80 mL/min:** 500–1,000 mg q 12 hr; C_{CR}, **30–50 mL/min:** 250–750 mg q 12 hr; C_{CR}, **less than 30 mL/min:** 250–500 mg q 12 hr. **ESRD clients using dialysis:** 500–1,000 mg q 24 hr; following dialysis, a 250–500 mg supplemental dose is recommended.

Children, 4 to younger than 16 years of age, initial: 20 mg/kg in 2 divided dose (i.e.,10 mg/kg twice a day). Increase the daily dose q 2 weeks by increments of 20 mg/kg to a recommended daily dose of 60 mg/kg (30 mg/kg twice a day). If the client cannot tolerate a dose of 60 mg/kg, the daily dose can be reduced. Use the oral solution in those with a body weight of 20 kg or less.

  Myoclonic seizures, 12 years and older.
Initial: 500 mg twice a day. Increase the daily dose by 1,000 mg/day q 2 weeks to the recommended daily dose of 3,000 mg.

  Primary generalized tonic-clonic seizures.
Adults, 16 years and older, initial: 500 mg twice a day. Increase the daily dose by 1,000 mg/day q 2 weeks to the recommended daily dose of 3,000 mg.
Children, 6 years to younger than 16 years, initial: 10 mg/kg twice a day. Increase the daily dose q 2 weeks by increments of 20 mg/kg to the recommended daily dose of 60 mg/kg (i.e., 30 mg/kg twice a day). Use the oral solution in those with a body weight less than 20 kg.

• **IV ONLY**
  Adjunct to treat partial onset seizures in adults.
Adults, initial: 500 mg twice a day. Dose may be increased by 1,000 mg/day every 2 weeks to a maximum of 3,000 mg/day. There is no evidence that doses greater than 3,000 mg/day provide additional benefit. *NOTE:* See above under dosage for partial-seizures for doses to be used in the event of impaired renal function.

L

NURSING CONSIDERATIONS

℮ Do not confuse Keppra with Kaletra (combination antiretroviral drug containing ritonavir and lopinavir).

ADMINISTRATION/STORAGE

1. Withdraw levetiracetam slowly to minimize the potential of increased seizure frequency.

2. The manufacturer has established the levetiracetam pregnancy registry. Either the client or health care provider can initiate enrollment by calling 1-888-537-7734. Clients may also enroll in the North American Antiepileptic Drug Pregnancy Registry by calling 1-888-233-2334.

IV 3. For IV use, dilute in 100 mL of 0.9% NaCl injection, lactated Ringer's injection, or D5W injection prior to administration.

4. Give as a 15-minute IV infusion.

5. Levetiracetam is compatible with lorazepam, diazepam, and valproate sodium.

6. When switching from PO levetiracetam, the initial total daily IV dose should be equivalent to the total daily dosage and frequency of PO levetiracetam. At the end of the IV treatment period, the client may be switched to PO levetiracetam at the equivalent daily dosage and frequency of the IV administration.

7. Do not use if the product shows particulate matter or discoloration.

8. Store the IV product from 15–30°C (59–86°F).

ASSESSMENT

1. List history and characteristics of seizures. Note drugs currently prescribed.

2. Monitor CBC, renal, LFTs; with impaired renal function, drug dose based on C_{CR}.

3. Clients weighing <20 kg should receive the PO solution, not the tablets. Use the weight-based guide for determining dosage in children weighing >20 kg and the equation provided for calculating the volume of the PO solution to be given to lighter-weight children.

CLIENT/FAMILY TEACHING

1. Take exactly as directed. May take with food to ↓ GI upset. Take with other prescribed seizure medications.

2. May cause dizziness and sleepiness. Do not engage in activities that require mental alertness until drug effects realized. Rise slowly from a sitting or lying position.

3. Use reliable birth control. Notify provider if pregnant or planning to become pregnant.

4. Report any unusual side effects or loss of seizure control. Do not stop suddenly.

OUTCOMES/EVALUATE

Control of seizures

Levobetaxolol hydrochloride

(**lee**-voh-bay-**TAX**-oh-lohl)

CLASSIFICATION(S):
Beta-adrenergic blocking agent
PREGNANCY CATEGORY: C
Rx: Betaxon.

USES

Decrease IOP in chronic open-angle glaucoma or ocular hypertension.

ACTION/KINETICS

Action

A cardioselective (beta-1-adrenergic) receptor blocking agent. No significant membrane-stabilizing (i.e., local anesthetic) activity and is devoid of sympathomimetic activity. Reduces IOP probably by decreasing aqueous humor production.

Pharmacokinetics

Onset: 30 min. **Maximum effect:** 2 hr. **Duration:** 12 hr.

CONTRAINDICATIONS

Use with sinus bradycardia, greater than first-degree AV block, cardiogenic shock, or overt cardiac failure.

SPECIAL CONCERNS

May be absorbed systemically leading to respiratory and cardiac effects. Use with caution in those with a history of

---

Bold Italic = life threatening side effect   ■ = black box warning   ✦ = Available in Canada

cardiac failure or heart block; in those subject to spontaneous hypoglycemia, or in diabetics receiving insulin or oral hypoglycemic drugs; in those with excessive restriction of pulmonary function; and during lactation. Safety and efficacy have not been determined in children.

SIDE EFFECTS

Most Common

Transient ocular discomfort and eye pain upon instillation, blurred vision.

Ophthalmic: Transient blurred vision, transient ocular discomfort and eye pain upon instillation, cataracts, vitreous disorders. **CV:** Bradycardia, heart block, hypertension, hypotension, tachycardia, vascular anomaly. **CNS:** Anxiety, dizziness, hypertonia, vertigo. **GI:** Constipation, dyspepsia. **Musculoskeletal:** Arthritis, tendinitis. **Respiratory:** Bronchitis, dyspnea, pharyngitis, pneumonia, rhinitis, sinusitis. **Metabolic/Endocrine:** Gout, hypercholesterolemia, hyperlipidemia, diabetes, hypothyroidism. **Dermatologic:** Alopecia, dermatitis, psoriasis. **GU:** Breast abscess, cystitis. **Miscellaneous:** Accidental injury, headache, infection.

HOW SUPPLIED

Ophthalmic Suspension: 0.5% (as base).

DOSAGE

- **OPHTHALMIC SUSPENSION**
  Lower IOP.

1 gtt in affected eye(s) twice a day. In some, a few weeks may be needed to stabilize.

NURSING CONSIDERATIONS

ADMINISTRATION/STORAGE

1. The use of two topical beta-adrenergic agents is not recommended.
2. Protect from light.
3. Shake well before using.

ASSESSMENT

1. Note disease onset, ocular findings, pressures, other agents prescribed.
2. Assess for any restrictive airway disease, diabetes, or severe CAD.
3. Monitor EKG and VS; periodically assess lipid panel, TSH, glucose.

CLIENT/FAMILY TEACHING

1. Use drops as directed; do not skip therapy.

2. Drug is used to lower pressures in the eye with ocular hypertension or chronic open-angle glaucoma to help prevent optic nerve damage and visual field loss.
3. When instilling, wash hands, do not touch dropper tip to any surface, as this may result in contamination.
4. Do not use with contact lenses in the eyes.
5. Report any increased SOB, edema, or eye irritation, pain, swelling, or itching.

OUTCOMES/EVALUATE

↓ IOP

Levobunolol hydrochloride

(lee-voh-**BYOU**-no-lohl)

CLASSIFICATION(S):

Beta-adrenergic blocking agent

PREGNANCY CATEGORY: C

Rx: AKBeta, Betagan Liquifilm.

✤Rx: Apo-Levobunolol, Novo-Levobunolol, PMS-Levobunolol, ratio-Levobunolol.

SEE ALSO *BETA-ADRENERGIC BLOCKING AGENTS.*

USES

To decrease intraocular pressure in chronic open-angle glaucoma or ocular hypertension.

ACTION/KINETICS

Action

Both beta-1- and beta-2-adrenergic receptor agonist. May act by decreasing the formation of aqueous humor.

Pharmacokinetics

Onset: <60 min. **Peak effect:** 2–6 hr. **Duration:** 24 hr.

CONTRAINDICATIONS

Use of 2 or more topical ophthalmic beta-adrenergic blocking agents simultaneously.

SPECIAL CONCERNS

Safety and effectiveness have not been determined in children. Significant absorption in geriatric clients may result in myocardial depression. Also, use with caution in angle-closure glaucoma (use with a miotic), in clients with muscle weaknesses, and in those with decreased pulmonary function.

SIDE EFFECTS

Most Common

Transient burning/stinging, blepharoconjunctivitis.

Ophthalmic: Stinging and burning (transient), decreased corneal sensitivity, blepharoconjunctivitis, iridocyclitis. **CNS:** Ataxia, dizziness, headache, lethargy. **Dermatologic:** Urticaria, pruritus. **CV:** Bradycardia, arrhythmia, hypotension, syncope.

HOW SUPPLIED

Ophthalmic Solution: 0.25%, 0.5%.

DOSAGE

• OPHTHALMIC SOLUTION

Decrease IOP.

Adults, usual: 1–2 gtt of 0.25% solution in affected eye(s) twice a day or 1–2 gtt of 0.5% solution in affected eye(s) once a day (use twice a day in more severe or uncontrolled glaucoma).

NURSING CONSIDERATIONS

ADMINISTRATION/STORAGE

1. If IOP is not decreased sufficiently, pilocarpine, epinephrine, or systemic carbonic anhydrase inhibitors may be used.
2. Due to diurnal IOP variations, a satisfactory response to twice-daily therapy is best determined by measuring IOP at different times during the day.
3. Do not give two or more ophthalmic beta-adrenergic blocking agents simultaneously.

ASSESSMENT

1. Note reasons for therapy, disease onset, other agents trialed, pressures.
2. List other drops prescribed to ensure not beta blockers.
3. Assess for angle-closure glaucoma, clients with muscle weaknesses, decreased pulmonary function, geriatric clients; use cautiously.

CLIENT/FAMILY TEACHING

1. Used to lower pressures in the eye and to prevent vision loss.
2. Wash hands. Apply gentle pressure to the inside corner of the eye for approximately 60 sec following instillation.
3. When instilling, do not touch dropper tip to any surface, as this may result in contamination.
4. Wait at least 5 min before instilling other eyedrops.
5. Do not close the eyes tightly or blink more frequently than usual after instillation of the drug.
6. May experience transient burning, stinging, itching; report if persistent.
7. Return for evaluation of intraocular pressure and drug's effectiveness.

OUTCOMES/EVALUATE

↓ IOP

Levocetirizine

(lee-voe-se-**TIR**-i-zeen)

CLASSIFICATION(S):

Antihistamine, second generation, piperazine

PREGNANCY CATEGORY: B

Rx: Xyzal.

SEE ALSO *ANTIHISTAMINES (H₁ BLOCKERS)*.

USES

(1) Symptomatic relief of allergic rhinitis (seasonal and perennial) in adults and children 6 years and older. (2) Uncomplicated skin manifestations of chronic idiopathic urticaria in adults and children 6 years and older.

ACTION/KINETICS

Action

Levocetirizine is metabolized to the active cetirizine which is an antagonist at the H-1 histamine receptor. Not expected to have QT/QTc effects.

Pharmacokinetics

Rapidly and extensively absorbed. **Peak plasma levels, adults:** 0.9 hr. **Steady state:** 2 days. A high fat meal delays T_{max} and decreases C_{max} but not significantly. Metabolized in part by CYP3A4. Excreted in the urine (about 85%) and feces (about 13%). **$t\frac{1}{2}$, plasma, adults:** 8 hr. **Plasma protein binding:** 91-92%.

CONTRAINDICATIONS

Hypersensitivity to levocetirizine or any component of the product. End-stage renal disease (C_{CR} <10 mL/min or those

---

Bold Italic = life threatening side effect   ■ = black box warning   ♣ = Available in Canada

on hemodialysis). Children, 6-11 years of age with impaired renal function. Use during lactation is not recommended.

SPECIAL CONCERNS
Use caution in dose selection in the elderly. Safety and efficacy have not been determined in children less than 6 years of age.

SIDE EFFECTS
Most Common
Adults: Somnolence, fatigue, asthenia, pharyngitis, nasopharyngitis, dry mouth.
Children, 6-12 years: Pyrexia, cough, somnolence, epistaxis
See *Antihistamines (H₁-Blockers)* for a complete list of potential side effects. Also, **CNS:** Somnolence, *convulsion*, aggression, agitation, hallucinations, suicidal ideation. **GI:** Dry mouth, nausea, hepatitis, cholestasis. **CV:** Syncope, palpitations, hypotension. **Dermatologic:** Pruritus, rash, urticaria. **Respiratory:** Pharyngitis, nasopharyngitis, epistaxis, cough, dyspnea. **Musculoskeletal:** Myalgia, orofacial dyskinesia. **Body as a whole:** Asthenia, fatigue, pyrexia, *anaphylaxis,* hypersensitivity, *angioneurotic edema*, fixed drug eruption, weight gain. **Miscellaneous:** Visual disturbances, glomerulonephritis, *still birth.*

LABORATORY TEST CONSIDERATIONS
↑ Blood bilirubin, transaminases.

OD **OVERDOSE MANAGEMENT**
Symptoms: Drowsiness in adults and agitation and restlessness in children followed by drowsiness. *Treatment:* Symptomatic and supportive treatment. There is no specific antidote. The drug is not effectively removed by dialysis.

DRUG INTERACTIONS
Ritonavir / ↑ Cetirizine (active metabolite) AUC and t½; ↓ cetirizine clearance
Theophylline / Small (16%) ↓ clearance of cetirizine (active metabolite)

HOW SUPPLIED
Tablets: 5 mg.

DOSAGE
• **TABLETS**
Allergic rhinitis, chronic idiopathic urticaria.

Adults and children, 12 years and older: 5 mg once daily in the evening. Some may be controlled adequately by 2.5 mg once daily in the evening. **Children, 6–11 years of age:** 2.5 mg (half of a tablet) once daily in the evening; do not exceed this dose.

NURSING CONSIDERATIONS

ADMINISTRATION/STORAGE
1. For mild impaired renal function (C_CR 50–80 mL/min), use a dose of 2.5 mg once daily. For moderate impaired renal function (C_CR 50–80 mL/min), use a dose of 2.5 mg every other day. For severe impaired renal function (C_CR 10–30 mL/min), use a dose of 2.5 mg given twice a week (once q 3–4 days). Do not use in clients with end-stage renal disease (C_CR <10 mL/min) or in hemodialysis clients.
2. No dosage adjustment is needed in those with only impaired hepatic function. Adjust the dose as recommended above in clients with both hepatic and renal function impairment.,
3. Store from 15–30°C (59–86°F).

ASSESSMENT
1. Note onset, characteristics of S&S; identify triggers/time of year.
2. List other agents trialed, length of use, outcome.
3. Assess renal and liver function; adjust dose with renal dysfunction.

CLIENT/FAMILY TEACHING
1. May take with or without food; take only prescribed dose as increased dose will increase risk of somnolence
2. Use caution when performing activities that require mental alertness; may cause drowsiness/sedation.
3. May cause dry mouth, fatigue; report adverse effects that prevent taking medications. May increase fluid intake to thin secretions.
4. Avoid alcohol/CNS depressants, and other OTC antihistamines; increases sedative effects.
5. Report any behavioral changes, aggressiveness, or evidence of seizures.
6. Practice reliable contraception; may cause still birth.
7. Review allergens that trigger symptoms, e.g., ragweed, dust mites, molds,

animal dander, etc., and how to control/avoid contact.

OUTCOMES/EVALUATE

• Control of symptoms of seasonal allergic rhinitis i.e. ↓ sneezing, pruritus, nasal congestion, watery/red eyes, itchy eyes/nose
• ↓ Pruritus with idiopathic urticaria

Levodopa
(lee-voh-**DOH**-pah)

CLASSIFICATION(S):
Antiparkinson drug
Rx: Dopar, L-Dopa, Larodopa.

USES

Idiopathic, arteriosclerotic, or postencephalitic parkinsonism due to carbon monoxide or manganese intoxication and in the elderly associated with cerebral arteriosclerosis. Not effective in drug-induced extrapyramidal symptoms. Levodopa only provides symptomatic relief and does not alter the course of the disease. When effective, it relieves rigidity, bradykinesia, tremors, dysphagia, seborrhea, sialorrhea, and postural instability. NOTE: Often used in combination with carbidopa. See *Carbidopa/Levodopa*. *Investigational:* Pain from herpes zoster; restless legs syndrome.

ACTION/KINETICS

Action
Depletion of dopamine in the striatum of the brain is thought to cause the symptoms of Parkinson's disease. Levodopa, a dopamine precursor, is able to cross the blood-brain barrier to enter the CNS. It is decarboxylated to dopamine in the basal ganglia, thus replenishing depleted dopamine stores.

Pharmacokinetics
Peak plasma levels: 0.5–2 hr (may be delayed if ingested with food). **t½, plasma:** 1–3 hr. **Onset:** 2–3 weeks, although some clients may require up to 6 months. Extensively metabolized (>95%) both in the periphery and the liver; metabolites are excreted in the urine.

CONTRAINDICATIONS

Concomitant use with MAO inhibitors, except MAO-B inhibitors (e.g., selegiline). History of melanoma or in clients with undiagnosed skin lesions. Lactation. Hypersensitivity to drug, narrow-angle glaucoma, blood dyscrasias, hypertension, coronary sclerosis.

SPECIAL CONCERNS

Use with extreme caution in clients with history of MIs, convulsions, arrhythmias, bronchial asthma, emphysema, active peptic ulcer, psychosis or neurosis, wide-angle glaucoma, and renal, hepatic, or endocrine diseases. Use during pregnancy only if benefits clearly outweigh risks. Safety has not been established in children less than 12 years of age. Geriatric clients may require a lower dose as they have a reduced tolerance for the drug and its side effects (including cardiac effects). Clients may experience an "on-off" phenomenon in which they experience an improved clinical status followed by loss of therapeutic effect.

SIDE EFFECTS

Most Common
Choreiform and/or dystonic movements, anorexia, N&V, abdominal pain, dry mouth, dysphagia, dysgeusia, headache, dizziness, sialorrhea, malaise, fatigue, euphoria.

The side effects of levodopa are numerous and usually dose related. Some may abate with usage. **CNS:** Choreiform and/or dystonic movements, sudden sleep attacks, paranoid ideation, psychotic episodes, depression (with possibility of suicidal tendencies), dementia, *seizures* (rare), dizziness, headache, faintness, confusion, insomnia, nightmares, hallucinations, delusions, agitation, anxiety, malaise, fatigue, euphoria. **GI:** N&V, anorexia, abdominal pain, dry mouth, sialorrhea, dysphagia, dysgeusia, hiccups, diarrhea, constipation, burning sensation of tongue, bitter taste, flatulence, weight gain/loss, *upper GI hemorrhage* (in clients with a history of peptic ulcer), *GI bleeding* (rare), *duodenal ulcer* (rare). **CV:** Cardiac irregularities, palpitations, orthostatic hypotension, hypertension, phlebitis,

---

Bold Italic = life threatening side effect   ■ = black box warning   ♣ = Available in Canada

hot flashes. **Ophthalmic:** Diplopia, dilated pupils, blurred vision, development of Horner's syndrome, oculogyric crisis. **Hematologic:** *Hemolytic anemia, agranulocytosis,* leukopenia. **Musculoskeletal:** Muscle twitching (early sign of overdose), tonic contraction of the muscles of mastication, increased hand tremor, ataxia. **Miscellaneous:** Blepharospasm (early sign of overdose), urinary retention/incontinence, increased sweating, unusual breathing patterns, weakness, numbness, bruxism, alopecia, priapism, hoarseness, edema, dark sweat/urine, flushing, skin rash, sense of stimulation. Levodopa interacts with many other drugs (see below) and must be administered cautiously.

LABORATORY TEST CONSIDERATIONS
↑ BUN, AST, LDH, ALT, bilirubin, alkaline phosphatase, protein-bound iodine, uric acid (with colorimetric test). ↓ H&H, WBCs. False + Coombs' test. Interference with tests for urinary glucose and ketones.

OD OVERDOSE MANAGEMENT
Symptoms: Muscle twitching, blepharospasm. Also see *Side Effects. Treatment:* Immediate gastric lavage for acute overdose. Maintain airway and give IV fluids carefully. General supportive measures.

DRUG INTERACTIONS
Antacids / ↑ Effect of levodopa R/T ↑ absorption from GI tract
Anticholinergic drugs / Possible ↓ levodopa effect R/T ↑ levodopa breakdown in stomach (R/T delayed gastric emptying time)
Antidepressants, tricyclic / ↓ Levodopa effect R/T ↓ GI tract absorption; also, ↑ risk of hypertension
Benzodiazepines / ↓ Levodopa effect
Clonidine / ↓ Levodopa effect
Digoxin / ↓ Digoxin effect
Furazolidone / ↑ Levodopa effect R/T ↓ liver breakdown
Guanethidine / ↑ Hypotensive drug effect
Hypoglycemic drugs / Levodopa upsets diabetic control with hypoglycemic agents

H *Indian snakeroot* / ↓ Effect of levodopa but ↑ extrapyramidal symptoms
MAO inhibitors / Concomitant administration may result in hypertension, light-headedness, and flushing R/T ↓ breakdown of dopamine and norepinephrine formed from levodopa
Methionine / ↓ Levodopa effect
Methyldopa / Additive effects including hypotension
Metoclopramide / ↑ Bioavailability of levodopa; ↓ metoclopramide effect
Papaverine / ↓ Levodopa effect
Phenothiazines / ↓ Levodopa effect R/T ↓ neuronal uptake of dopamine
Phenytoin / Antagonizes levodopa effect
Propranolol / May antagonize the hypotensive and positive inotropic effect of levodopa
Pyridoxine / Reverses levodopa-induced improvement in Parkinson's disease
Thioxanthines / ↓ Levodopa effect in Parkinson clients
Tricyclic antidepressants / ↓ Levodopa absorption and bioavailability → ↓ effect

HOW SUPPLIED
Capsules: 100 mg, 250 mg, 500 mg; *Tablets:* 100 mg, 250 mg, 500 mg.

DOSAGE
• **CAPSULES; TABLETS**
  Parkinsonism.
Adults, initial: 250 mg 2–4 times per day taken with food; **then,** increase total daily dose by no more than 750 mg/day q 3–7 days until optimum dosage reached (should not exceed 8 grams/day). Up to 6 mo may be required to achieve a significant therapeutic effect.

NURSING CONSIDERATIONS
ADMINISTRATION/STORAGE
1. If unable to swallow tablets or capsules, crush tablets or empty the capsule into a small amount of fruit juice at the time of administration.
2. Often administered together with an anticholinergic agent.

ASSESSMENT
1. Assess condition and document baseline rigidity, tremors, motor func-

tion, and involuntary movements r/t Parkinson's disease. Note mental status.
2. Review medical history for any contraindications to therapy. Stop drug 24 hr before surgery and note when drug is to be restarted.
3. Identify adverse effects that may require ↓ drug dose or 'drug holiday.' Very low dose therapy used with RLS.
4. Monitor VS, ECG, CBC, liver/renal function studies, PBI tests.

CLIENT/FAMILY TEACHING
1. Take exactly as prescribed; may take with food to decrease GI upset.
2. Report headaches; may indicate drug-induced glaucoma. Twitching or eye spasms may indicate toxicity.
3. Dosage should not exceed 8 grams/day; do not stop abruptly.
4. Avoid fortified cereals and taking multivitamin preparations containing 10–25 mg of B_6 as they may reverse the antiparkinson effect. *Larobec* is a form of multivitamin that does not contain pyridoxine.
5. Significant results may take up to 6 mo to be realized.
6. May cause dizziness or drowsiness. Do not perform tasks that require mental alertness until drug effects realized. Change from a sitting or lying position slowly, and wear elastic hose to decrease dizziness.
7. Sweat and urine may appear dark; this is not harmful.
8. If sustained erection occurs; report immediately.
9. Report any evidence of depression or psychosis, other unusual mental or behavioral changes.
10. Report for all scheduled visits so that drug effectiveness can be evaluated and dosage adjusted as needed.
11. Identify local support groups/services.

OUTCOMES/EVALUATE
- Improvement in motor function, reflexes, gait, strength of grip, amount of tremor, and quality of life
- Relief of S&S of RLS (restless leg syndrome)

Levofloxacin 〖IV〗📷
(**lee**-voh-**FLOX**-ah-sin)

CLASSIFICATION(S):
Antibiotic, fluoroquinolone
PREGNANCY CATEGORY: C
Rx: Levaquin, Quixin.

SEE ALSO FLUOROQUINOLONES.

USES
Systemic. (1) Acute maxillary sinusitis due to *Streptococcus pneumoniae, Haemophilus influenzae,* or *Moraxella catarrhalis.* (2) Acute bacterial exacerbation of chronic bronchitis due to *Staphylococcus aureus, S. pneumoniae, H. influenzae, Haemophilus parainfluenzae,* or *M. catarrhalis.* (3) Community acquired pneumonia due to *S. aureus, S. pneumoniae* (including multidrug resistant *S. pneumoniae*), *H. influenzae, H. parainfluenzae, Klebsiella pneumoniae, M. catarrhalis, Chlamydia pneumoniae, Legionella pneumophila* or *Mycoplasma pneumoniae.* (4) Nosocomial (hospital acquired) pneumonia due to methicillin-susceptible *S. aureus, Pseudomonas aeruginosa, Serratia marcescens, E. coli, Klebsiella pneumoniae, H. influenzae,* or *S. pneumoniae.* When *P. aeruginosa* is documented or presumed to be the pathogen, also use an antipseudomonal beta-lactam. (5) Uncomplicated mild to moderate infections of the skin and skin structures, including abscesses, cellulitis, furuncles, impetigo, pyoderma, and wound infections due to *S. aureus* or *Streptococcus pyogenes.* (6) Complicated skin and skin structure infections, including surgical incisions, infected bites and lacerations, major abscesses, and infected ulcers due to methicillin-sensitive *S. aureus, Enterococcus faecalis, S. pyogenes,* or *Proteus mirabilis.* (7) Mild to moderate complicated UTIs due to *Enterococcus faecalis, Enterobacter cloacae, Escherichia coli, Klebsiella pneumoniae, P. mirabilis,* or *Pseudomonas aeruginosa.* (8) Uncomplicated UTIs (mild to moderate) due to *E. coli, K. pneumoniae,* or *Staphylococcus saprophyticus.* (9) Acute mild to moderate pyelonephritis

---

Bold Italic = life threatening side effect   ■ = black box warning   ✤ = Available in Canada

due to *E. coli.* (10) Chronic bacterial prostatitis due to *E. coli, Enterococcus faecalis,* or *Staphylococcus epidermidis.* (11) Prevent the development of inhalational anthrax following exposure to *Bacillus anthracis. Investigational:* (1) Epididymitis (alternative regimen). (2) Disseminated gonococcal infections (alternative regimen). (3) Uncomplicated gonococcal infections of the cervix, urethra, and rectum. (4) Nongonococcal urethritis (alternative regimen). (5) Pelvic inflammatory disease (alternative regimen).

Ophthalmic. (1) Bacterial conjunctivitis caused by *Staphylococcus aureus* (methicillin-susceptible strains only), *Corynebacterium* species, *Staphylococcus epidermidis* (methicillin-susceptible strains only), *Streptococcus pneumoniae, Streptococcus* (Groups C/F and G), Viridans Group streptococci, *Acinetobacter lwoffi, Haemophilus influenzae, Serratia marcescens.* (2) Corneal ulcers caused by *S. aureus, S. epidermidis, S. pneumoniae, P. aeruginosa, S. marcescens.*

ACTION/KINETICS

Action

Interferes with DNA gyrase and topoisomerase IV. DNA gyrase is an enzyme needed for replication, transcription, and repair of bacterial DNA. Topoisomerase IV plays a key role in the partitioning of chromosomal DNA during bacterial cell division. Effective against both gram-positive and gram-negative organisms.

Pharmacokinetics

About 99% bioavailable. **t½, after multiple doses:** 7–8.8 hr. About 87% excreted unchanged in the urine after PO use.

CONTRAINDICATIONS

Lactation. IM, intrathecal, intraperitoneal, or SC administration.

SPECIAL CONCERNS

The dose must be reduced with impaired renal function. (See *Administration/Storage.*) Safety and efficacy have not been determined in those less than 18 years of age.

SIDE EFFECTS

Most Common

Headache, dizziness, insomnia, N&V, diarrhea, dyspepsia/heartburn, constipation.

See *Fluoroquinolones* for a complete list of possible side effects.

ADDITIONAL DRUG INTERACTIONS

↑ Risk of tendon rupture, especially in the elderly, if taken with corticosteroids

HOW SUPPLIED

Injection Concentrate: 500 mg (25 mg/mL), 750 mg (25 mg/mL); *Injection (Premix):* 250 mg (5 mg/mL), 500 mg (5 mg/mL), 750 mg (5 mg/mL); *Ophthalmic Solution:* 0.5%, 1.5%; *Oral Solution:* 25 mg/mL; *Tablets:* 250 mg, 500 mg, 750 mg.

DOSAGE

- **SLOW IV INFUSION; ORAL SOLUTION; TABLETS**

  Acute maxillary (bacterial) sinusitis.
  500 mg q 24 hr for 10–14 days or 750 mg q 24 hr for 5 days.

  Acute bacterial exacerbation of chronic bronchitis.
  500 mg once daily for 7 days.

  Community-acquired pneumonia.
  500 mg once daily for 7–14 days. Or, 750 mg once daily for 5 days to treat infections due to *S. pneumoniae* (except MDRSP), *H. influenzae, H. parainfluenzae, M. pneumoniae,* and *C. pneumoniae.*

  Inhalation anthrax (postexposure).
  Adults: 500 mg q 24 hr for 60 days. Begin therapy as soon as possible after suspected or confirmed exposure to aerosolized *B. anthracis.* Safety beyond use for 28 days has not been studied; only use prolonged therapy in adults when the benefit outweighs the risk.

  Nosocomial pneumonia.
  750 mg q 24 hr for 7–14 days.

  Uncomplicated skin and skin structure infections.
  500 mg once daily for 7–10 days.

  Complicated skin and skin structure infections.
  750 mg once daily for 7–14 days.

  Complicated UTIs.
  250 mg once daily for 10 days.

  Uncomplicated UTIs.
  250 mg once daily for 3 days.

  Acute pyelonephritis.

250 mg once daily for 10 days.

Chronic bacterial prostatitis.

500 mg q 24 hr for 28 days.

Epididymitis.

500 mg/day PO for 10 days.

Disseminated gonococcal infections.

250 mg once daily IV for 24–48 hr (after improvement begins); then, 500 mg/day PO for 7 days.

Uncomplicated gonococcal infections of the cervix, urethra, rectum.

250 mg PO in a single dose plus 1 gram azithromycin as a single oral dose or 100 mg doxycycline PO 2 times per day for 7 days if chlamydial infection is not ruled out.

Nongonococcal urethritis.

500 mg/day for 7 days.

Pelvic inflammatory disease.

500 mg/day PO for 14 days.

* **OPHTHALMIC SOLUTION**

Bacterial conjunctivitis.

Days 1 and 2: 1–2 gtt in affected eye(s) q 2 hr while awake, up to 8 times per day; **Days 3 through 7:** 1–2 gtt in affected eye(s) q 4 hr while awake, up to 4 times per day.

Bacterial corneal ulcer.

Days 1 and 2: 1–2 gtt in the affected eye(s) q 30 min while awake. Awaken at about 4 and 6 hr after retiring and instill 1–2 gtt. **Days 3 through 7 to 9:** Instill 1–2 gtt hourly while awake. **Days 7 to 9 to treatment completion:** 1–2 gtt 4 times per day.

Corneal ulcer.

Days 1 through 3: 1–2 gtt in the affected eye(s) q 30 min to 2 hr while awake and about every 4–6 hr after retiring; **Days 4 through treatment completion:** 1–2 gtt in the affected eye(s) q 1 to 4 hr while awake.

NURSING CONSIDERATIONS

ADMINISTRATION/STORAGE

1. For PO or IV dosing, reduce dose with impaired renal function as follows when used for *acute maxillary sinusitis, acute bacterial exacerbation of chronic bronchitis, community-acquired pneumonia, uncomplicated skin and skin structure infections, chronic bacterial prostatitis, and inhalational anthrax postexposure (IV):* If C_{CR} is between 20 and 49 mL/min, the initial dose is 500 mg and subsequent doses are 250 mg q 24 hr. If C_{CR} is between 10 and 19 mL/min, the initial dose is 500 mg and subsequent doses are 250 mg q 48 hr. If on hemodialysis or chronic ambulatory peritoneal dialysis, initial dose is 500 mg and subsequent doses are 250 mg q 48 hr.

2. For PO or IV dosing, reduce dose, as follows, with impaired renal function when used for *complicated UTI* or *acute pyelonephritis:* If C_{CR} is 20 mL/min or more, no dosage adjustment is needed. If the C_{CR} is between 10 and 19 mL/min, the initial dose is 250 mg and subsequent doses are 250 mg q 48 hr. For uncomplicated UTIs, no dosage adjustment is needed.

3. For PO and IV dosing, reduce dose, as follows, with impaired renal function when used for *complicated skin and skin structure infections, community-acquired pneumonia, nosocomial pneumonia, and bacterial sinusitis (IV dosing):* If C_{CR} is from 20–49 mL/min, the initial dose is 750 mg and subsequent doses are 750 mg q 48 hr; if C_{CR} is from 10–19 mL/min, the initial dose is 750 mg and subsequent doses are 500 mg q 48 hr. If on hemodialysis or chronic ambulatory peritoneal dialysis, initial dose is 750 mg and subsequent doses are 500 mg q 48 hr.

4. Oral doses are given at least 2 hr before or 2 hr after antacids containing Mg or Al, as well as sucralfate, iron products, multivitamin preparations containing zinc, and didanosine (chewable/buffered tablets or pediatric powder for PO solution).

5. Store tablets in a tight container at 15–30°C (59–85°F).

IV 6. Injectable form may be mixed with 0.9% NaCl, D5W, D5/0.9% NaCl, D5/RL, Plasma-Lyte 56/5% dextrose, D5/0.45% NaCl, 0.15% KCl injection, or M/6 sodium lactate injection.

7. Administer doses of 250 or 500 mg by slow infusion over 60 min q 24 hr or 750 mg given by slow infusion over 90 min q 24 hr. Avoid rapid or bolus IV infusion.

Bold Italic = life threatening side effect   ■ = black box warning   ✦ = Available in Canada

8. Diluted solutions for IV use are stable for 72 hr up to a concentration of 5 mg/mL when stored in IV containers at 25°C or less (77°F or less). Such solutions are stable for 14 days when stored under refrigeration at 5°C (41°F). Diluted solutions that are frozen in glass bottles or plastic IV containers are stable for 6 months when stored at -20°C (-4°F).

9. Thaw frozen solutions at room temperature or in refrigerator. Do not thaw in a microwave or by bath immersion. After initial thawing, do not refreeze.

ASSESSMENT

1. Note reasons for therapy, onset, characteristics of S&S. List drugs trialed/outcome.

2. Assess for seizure history or CNS disorders; may preclude therapy. If also prescribed corticosteroids, may precipitate tendon rupture esp in elderly.

3. Obtain baseline cultures, CBC, BS, renal and LFTs. Follow guidelines for reducing dosage with renal impairment based on C_{CR}.

CLIENT/FAMILY TEACHING

1. Tablets can be taken without regard to food. Consume plenty of fluids to prevent urinary crystal formation.

2. Take the oral solution 1 hr before or 2 hr after eating.

3. Avoid multivitamins with zinc, iron products, sucralfate, and Mg- or Al-containing antacids 4 hr before and after dose.

4. Practice reliable birth control. Avoid prolonged exposure to sunlight or UV light. Advise diabetics to monitor BS closely and report if hypoglycemia occurs.

5. Use caution until drug effects realized; may experience dizziness, drowsiness or visual changes. May also experience N&V, abdominal pain, diarrhea/constipation, and photosensitivity.

6. Report pain or inflammation in tendon of foot, rash, or if S&S do not improve or worsen after 72 hr of therapy.

7. Keep all F/U appointments to evaluate response and monitor labs.

OUTCOMES/EVALUATE

- Symptomatic improvement
- Resolution of infection

Levothyroxine sodium (T₄) ■ IV
(lee-voh-thigh-**ROX**-een)

CLASSIFICATION(S):
Thyroid product
PREGNANCY CATEGORY: A
Rx: Levothroid, Levoxyl, Synthroid, Thyro-Tabs, Tirosint, Unithroid.
✦**Rx:** Synthroid.

SEE ALSO *THYROID DRUGS*.

USES
(1) Replacement or supplemental therapy for congenital or acquired hypothyroidism of any etiology, except transient hypothyroidism during the recovery phase of subacute thyroiditis. (2) Treatment or prevention of various types of euthyroid goiters, including thyroid nodules, subacute or chronic lymphocytic thyroiditis, and multinodular goiter. (3) Adjunct to surgery and radioiodine therapy to manage thyrotropin-dependent well-differentiated thyroid cancer.

ACTION/KINETICS

Action
Levothyroxine is the synthetic sodium salt of the levoisomer of T_4 (tetraiodothyronine). Levothyroxine, 0.05–0.6, mg equals approximately 60 mg (1 grain) of thyroid.

Pharmacokinetics
Absorption from the GI tract is incomplete and variable, especially when taken with food. Has a slower onset but a longer duration than sodium liothyronine. More active on a weight basis than thyroid. Is usually the drug of choice. Effect is predictable as thyroid content is standard. **Time to peak therapeutic effect:** 3–4 weeks. t½: 6–7 days in a euthyroid person, 9–10 days in a hypothyroid client, and 3–4 days in a hyperthyroid client. **Duration:** 1–3 weeks after withdrawal of chronic therapy. *NOTE:* All levothyroxine products are not bioequivalent; thus, changing

 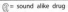

brands is not recommended. **Plasma protein binding:** 99%.

SPECIAL CONCERNS

■ Drugs with thyroid hormone activity, alone or with other drugs, have been used to treat obesity. In euthyroid clients, doses within the range of daily hormonal requirements are ineffective for weight reduction. Larger doses may produce serious or even life-threatening manifestations of toxicity, especially when given with sympathomimetic amines such as those used for their anorectic effects.■ Use with caution in those with underlying CV disease, in the elderly, and in those with concomitant adrenal insufficiency. Errors have occurred when prescribers have ordered 0.25 mg (250 mcg) instead of the correct dose of 0.025 mg (25 mcg). Be careful with decimal point placements and when converting a dose from micrograms to milligrams.

SIDE EFFECTS

Most Common

Symptoms of hyperthyroidism.

See *Thyroid Drugs* for a complete list of possible side effects.

DRUG INTERACTIONS

Al hydroxide / Adsorption of levothyroxine to the Al and increased fecal elimination of levothyroxine

Carbamazepine / ↑ Levothyroxine elimination R/T ↑ liver metabolism

Cholestyramine / ↓ Absorption of thyroxine R/T binding to cholestyramine in the GI tract

Digoxin / ↓ Digoxin levels and therapeutic effect

Imitinib / Hypothyroidism and ↑ TSH levels in those receiving levothyroxine after thyroidectomy

Iron salts / ↓ Absorption of levothyroxine R/T complex formation with iron in the GI tract

Raloxifene / ↓ Levothyroxine absorption

Sucralfate / ↓ Absorption of thyroxine R/T binding to cholestyramine in the GI tract

Theophylline / ↓ Theophylline effect R/T ↑ elimination

Warfarin / ↑ Risk of bleeding

HOW SUPPLIED

Capsules: 12.5 mcg, 25 mcg, 50 mcg, 75 mcg, 100 mcg, 125 mcg, 150 mcg; *Powder for Injection, Lyophilized*: 200 mcg, 500 mcg; *Tablets*: 25 mcg, 50 mcg, 75 mcg, 88 mcg, 100 mcg, 112 mcg, 125 mcg, 137 mcg, 150 mcg, 175 mcg, 200 mcg, 300 mcg.

DOSAGE

• **CAPSULES; TABLETS**

Mild hypothyroidism.

Adults, initial: 50 mcg once daily; **then,** increase by 25–50 mcg q 2–3 weeks until desired clinical response is attained; **maintenance, usual:** 75–125 mcg/day (although doses up to 200 mcg/day may be required in some clients).

Severe hypothyroidism.

Adults, initial: 12.5–25 mcg once daily; **then,** increase dose, as necessary, in increments of 25 mcg at 2- to 3-week intervals.

Congenital hypothyroidism.

Pediatric, 12 years and older: 2–3 mcg/kg once daily until the adult daily dose (usually 150 mcg) is reached. **6–12 years of age:** 4–5 mcg/kg/day or 100–150 mcg once daily. **1–5 years of age:** 5–6 mcg/kg/day or 75–100 mcg once daily. **6–12 months of age:** 6–8 mcg/kg/day or 50–75 mcg once daily. **Less than 6 months of age:** 8–10 mcg/kg/day or 25–50 mcg once daily.

• **IM; IV**

Myxedematous coma.

Adults, initial: 400 mcg by rapid IV injection, even in geriatric clients; **then,** 100–200 mcg/day, IV. **Maintenance:** 100–200 mcg/day, IV. Smaller daily doses should be given until client can tolerate PO medication.

Hypothyroidism.

Adults: 50–100 mcg once daily; **pediatric, IV, IM:** A dose of 75% of the usual PO pediatric dose should be given.

TSH suppression in well-differentiated thyroid cancer or thyroid nodules.

Individualize dose. **Usual dose:** 2 mcg/kg/day.

NURSING CONSIDERATIONS

ADMINISTRATION/STORAGE

1. Take with a full glass of water to prevent choking, gagging, dysphagia, or getting tablets stuck in the throat.

Bold Italic = life threatening side effect   ■ = black box warning   ✦ = Available in Canada

2. In infants with congenital or acquired hypothyroidism, institute therapy with full doses as soon as the diagnosis is made.

3. In infants and children who cannot swallow tablets, the correct dosage tablet may be crushed and suspended in a small amount of formula or water and given by dropper or spoon. The crushed tablet may also be sprinkled over cooked cereal or applesauce.

4. Transfer from liothyronine to levothyroxine: Administer replacement drug for several days before discontinuing liothyronine. Transfer from levothyroxine to liothyronine: Discontinue levothyroxine before starting low daily dose of liothyronine.

IV 5. Prepare solution for injection immediately before administration. Reconstitute by adding 5 mL of 0.9% NaCl or bacteriostatic NaCl injection and shake vial to ensure complete mixing. Give IV push.

6. Discard any unused portion of the IV medication.

7. Do not mix with other IV infusion solutions.

ASSESSMENT

1. With thyroid disease, elderly clients are likely to have undetected cardiac problems. Obtain ECG prior to initiating therapy; monitor VS and symptoms. Adjust dose based on thyroid panels.

2. If pregnant, must continue taking thyroid preparations throughout the pregnancy.

3. Note height, weight, and psychomotor development in child.

4. List drugs currently consumed to ensure none interact.

5. Errors have occurred when prescribers have ordered 0.25 mg (250 mcg) instead of the correct dose of 0.025 mg (25 mcg). Review orders carefully and question if unsure.

CLIENT/FAMILY TEACHING

1. Used to replace a hormone that is low in the body causing hypothyroidism. Drug is not a cure for hypothyroidism; must be taken for life to control symptoms.

2. Take at the same time each day on an empty stomach 1 hr before or 2–3 hr after a meal. Take in the morning to prevent insomnia. Do not take with food unless specifically instructed; may interfere with absorption. Avoid iodine-rich foods.

3. Do not switch brands; bioavailability may change.

4. Report severe headache, palpitations, chest pain, diarrhea, irritability, excitability, insomnia, intolerance to heat, significant weight loss, and/or excessive sweating.

5. Avoid OTC medications unless approved. Report as scheduled for evaluation of response, VS, and labs.

6. Child may experience hair loss; should regrow. Return for evaluation of bone age, growth, labs, and psychomotor functioning.

7. If taking raloxifene, take levothyroxine at least 12 hr earlier in the day.

OUTCOMES/EVALUATE

- Promotion of normal metabolism
- ↑ Levels of T_3 and T_4, ↓ TSH

Lidocaine hydrochloride   **IV**
(**LYE**-doh-kayn)

CLASSIFICATION(S):
Antiarrhythmic, Class IB
PREGNANCY CATEGORY: B
Rx: IM: LidoPen Auto-Injector. **Direct IV, IV Admixtures:** Lidocaine HCl for Cardiac Arrhythmias, Xylocaine HCl IV for Cardiac Arrhythmias. **IV Infusion:** Lidocaine HCl in 5% Dextrose.
✦Rx: Xylocard.

SEE ALSO ANTIARRHYTHMIC AGENTS.

USES

IV: Acute ventricular arrhythmias (i.e., following MIs or occurring during surgery). Ineffective against atrial arrhythmias. *Investigational:* IV in children who develop ventricular couplets or frequent premature ventricular beats.

IM: Single doses in certain emergency situations (e.g., ECG equipment not available; by the client in the prehospital phase of suspected acute MI, directed by qualified medical personnel viewing the transmitted ECG).

ACTION/KINETICS

Action

Shortens the refractory period and suppresses the automaticity of ectopic foci without affecting conduction of impulses through cardiac tissue. Increases the electrical stimulation threshold of the ventricle during diastole. It does not affect BP, CO, or myocardial contractility. Since lidocaine has little effect on conduction at normal antiarrhythmic doses, use in acute situations (instead of procainamide) in instances in which heart block might occur.

Pharmacokinetics

IV, Onset: 45–90 sec; **duration:** 10–20 min. **IM, Onset:** 5–15 min; **duration:** 60–90 min. **t½:** 1–2 hr. **Therapeutic serum levels:** 1.5–6 mcg/mL. **Time to steady-state plasma levels:** 3–4 hr (8–10 hr in clients with AMI). Ninety percent is rapidly metabolized in the liver to active metabolites. **Plasma protein binding:** 40–80%.

CONTRAINDICATIONS

Hypersensitivity to amide-type local anesthetics, Stokes-Adams syndrome, Wolff-Parkinson-White syndrome, severe SA, AV, or intraventricular block (when no pacemaker is present). Use of the IM autoinjector for children.

SPECIAL CONCERNS

Use with caution during labor and delivery, during lactation, and in the presence of liver or severe kidney disease, CHF, marked hypoxia, digitalis toxicity with AV block, reduced cardiac output, severe respiratory depression, or shock. In geriatric clients, the rate and dose for IV infusion should be decreased by one-half and slowly adjusted. Accelerated ventricular rate may occur when given to clients with atrial flutter or fibrillation. Safety and efficacy have not been determined in children.

SIDE EFFECTS

Most Common

N&V, nervousness, anxiety, dizziness, drowsiness, sensation of heat or cold, numbness, injection site pain.

Body as a whole: Malignant hyperthermia characterized by tachycardia, tachypnea, labile BP, metabolic acidosis, temperature elevation. **GI:** N&V. **CV:** Precipitation or aggravation of arrhythmias (following IV use), hypotension, bradycardia *(with possible cardiac arrest), CV collapse.* **CNS:** Dizziness, apprehension, euphoria, light-headedness, nervousness, anxiety, drowsiness, confusion, changes in mood, hallucinations, twitching, 'doom anxiety,' *convulsions,* unconsciousness. **Respiratory:** Difficulties in breathing or swallowing, *respiratory depression or arrest.* **Allergic:** Rash, cutaneous lesions, urticaria, edema, *anaphylaxis.* **Miscellaneous:** Tinnitus, blurred/double vision, vomiting, numbness, sensation of heat or cold, twitching, tremors, soreness at IM injection site, fever, *venous thrombosis or phlebitis (extending from site of injection),* extravasation. *NOTE:* During anesthesia, CV depression may be the first sign of lidocaine toxicity. During other usage, convulsions are the first sign of lidocaine toxicity.

LABORATORY TEST CONSIDERATIONS

↑ CPK following IM use.

OD OVERDOSE MANAGEMENT

Symptoms: Dependent on plasma levels. If plasma levels range from 4 to 6 mcg/mL, mild CNS effects are observed. Levels of 6 to 8 mcg/mL may result in significant CNS and CV depression while levels greater than 8 mcg/mL cause hypotension, decreased CO, respiratory depression, obtundation, *seizures, and coma. Treatment:* Discontinue the drug and begin emergency resuscitative procedures. Seizures can be treated with diazepam, thiopental, or thiamylal. Succinylcholine, IV, may be used if the client is anesthetized. IV fluids, vasopressors, and CPR are used to correct circulatory depression.

DRUG INTERACTIONS

Aminoglycosides / ↑ Neuromuscular blockade
Beta-adrenergic blockers / ↑ Lidocaine levels with possible toxicity
Cimetidine / ↓ Clearance of lidocaine → possible toxicity
Fluvoxamine / ↓ Lidocaine elimination;

Bold Italic = life threatening side effect   ■ = black box warning   ✦ = Available in Canada

adding PO erythromycin further ↓ lidocaine elimination; R/T inhibition of lidocaine metabolism by CYP3A4

Phenytoin / IV phenytoin → excessive cardiac depression

Procainamide / Additive cardiodepressant effects

Smoking / ↑ Hepatic metabolism of lidocaine

Succinylcholine / ↑ Succinylcholine action by ↓ plasma protein binding

Tocainide / ↑ Risk of side effects

Tubocurarine / ↑ Neuromuscular blockade

HOW SUPPLIED

Direct IV Injection: 1% (10 mg/mL), 2% (20 mg/mL); *IM Injection:* 10% (300 mg/ 3 mL); *IV Admixtures:* 4% (40 mg/mL), 10% (100 mg/mL), 20% (200 mg/mL); *IV Infusion:* 0.2% (2 mg/mL), 0.4% (4 mg/mL), 0.8% (8 mg/mL).

DOSAGE

- **IV BOLUS**
  Antiarrhythmic.

Adults: 50–100 mg at a rate of 25–50 mg/min. Bolus is used to establish rapid therapeutic plasma levels. Repeat if necessary after 5 min interval. Onset of action is 10 sec. **Maximum dose/hour:** 200–300 mg. Reduce the dose in those with CHF or reduced cardiac output and in the elderly; some recommended, however, that the usual loading dose be given and only the maintenance dose be reduced.

- **IV INFUSION**
  Antiarrhythmic.

20–50 mcg/kg at a rate of 1–4 mg/min. No more than 200–300 mg/hr should be given. Reduce maintenance doses in those with heart failure or liver disease or who are also receiving other drugs known to decrease lidocaine clearance or liver blood flow, and in clients over 70 years of age. **Pediatric, bolus dose:** 1 mg/kg IV or intrathecally q 5–10 min until desired effect reached (maximum total dose: 5 mg/kg); **maintenance:** 20–50 mcg/kg/min.

- **IM**
  Antiarrhythmic.

Adults: 4.5 mg/kg (approximately 300 mg for a 70-kg adult). Switch to IV lidocaine or oral antiarrhythmics as soon as possible although an additional IM dose may be given after 60–90 min.

NURSING CONSIDERATIONS

ADMINISTRATION/STORAGE

1. For IM use, the deltoid muscle is preferred. Use only the 10% solution for IM injection.

IV 2. *Do not add lidocaine to blood transfusion assembly.*

3. Do not use lidocaine solutions that contain epinephrine to treat arrhythmias. Make certain that vial states, "For Cardiac Arrhythmias." Check prefilled syringes closely to ensure appropriate dose has been obtained. (Lidocaine prefilled syringes come in both milligrams and grams.)

4. Use D5W to prepare solution; this is stable for 24 hr. Administer with an electronic infusion device.

5. Reduce IV bolus dosage in clients over 70 years old, with CHF or liver disease, and if taking cimetidine or propranolol (i.e., where metabolism of lidocaine is reduced).

ASSESSMENT

1. List reasons for therapy; any hypersensitivity to amide-type local anesthetics.

2. Those with hepatic or renal disease or who weigh less than 45.5 kg will need to be watched closely for adverse side effects; adjust dosage as directed.

3. Note CNS status. Report sudden changes in mental status, dizziness, visual disturbances, twitching, tremors; may precede convulsions. Review pulmonary findings; assess for respiratory depression. Monitor renal, LFTs, electrolytes, VS, ECG; assess for hypotension, cardiac collapse.

4. View monitor strips for myocardial depression, variations of rhythm, aggravation of arrhythmia during infusion.

5. IM use may increase CPK levels.

CLIENT/FAMILY TEACHING

1. Drug is used to eradicate ventricular arrhythmias. It is generally administered IV in a continuously monitored environment.

2. Report any evidence of dizziness or altered mentation; may be S&S of toxicity and progress to seizures and coma.

L

3. Smoking is not permitted during drug therapy. Refer to smoking cessation for alternative therapy.

OUTCOMES/EVALUATE

- Control of ventricular arrhythmias
- Therapeutic serum drug levels (1.5–6 mcg/mL)

Liothyronine sodium (T₃)

(lye-oh-**THIGH**-roh-neen)

CLASSIFICATION(S):
Thyroid product
PREGNANCY CATEGORY: A
Rx: Cytomel, Sodium-L-Triiodothyronine, Triostat.

SEE ALSO *THYROID DRUGS.*

USES

(1) Replacement or supplemental therapy for congenital or acquired hypothyroidism of any etiology, except transient hypothyroidism during the recovery phase of subacute thyroiditis. (2) Treatment or prevention of various types of euthyroid goiters, including thyroid nodules, subacute or chronic lymphocytic thyroiditis, and multinodular goiter. (3) Adjunct to surgery and radioiodine therapy to manage thyrotropin-dependent well-differentiated thyroid cancer. (4) Diagnostic agent in suppression tests to differentiate suspected mild hypothyroidism or thyroid gland autonomy.

ACTION/KINETICS

Action

Synthetic sodium salt of the levoisomer of T₃. Has more predictable effects due to standard hormone content. From 15 to 37.5 mcg is equivalent to about 60 mg of desiccated thyroid. May be preferred when a rapid effect or rapidly reversible effect is required. Has a rapid onset, which may result in difficulty in controlling the dosage as well as the possibility of cardiac side effects and changes in metabolic demands. However, its short duration allows quick adjustment of dosage and helps control overdosage.

Pharmacokinetics

t½: 24 hr for euthyroid clients, approximately 34 hr in hypothyroid clients, and approximately 14 hr in hyperthyroid clients. **Duration:** Up to 72 hr. **Plasma protein binding:** 99%.

ADDITIONAL CONTRAINDICATIONS

Use in children with cretinism because there is some question about whether the hormone crosses the blood-brain barrier.

SPECIAL CONCERNS

■ Drugs with thyroid hormone activity, alone or with other drugs, have been used to treat obesity. In euthyroid clients, doses within the range of daily hormonal requirements are ineffective for weight reduction. Larger doses may produce serious or even life-threatening manifestations of toxicity, especially when given with sympathomimetic amines such as those used for their anorectic effects.■

SIDE EFFECTS

Most Common

Symptoms of hyperthyroidism.

See *Thyroid Drugs* for a complete list of possible side effects.

HOW SUPPLIED

Injection: 10 mcg/mL; *Tablets:* 5 mcg, 25 mcg, 50 mcg.

DOSAGE————————

- **TABLETS**

    Mild hypothyroidism.

Adults, individualized, initial: 25 mcg/day. Increase by 12.5–25 mcg q 1–2 weeks until satisfactory response has been obtained. **Usual maintenance:** 25–75 mcg/day (100 mcg may be required in some clients). Use lower initial dosage (5 mcg/day) for the elderly, children, and clients with CV disease. Increase only by 5 mcg increments.

    Myxedema.

Adults, initial: 5 mcg/day increased by 5–10 mcg/day q 1–2 weeks until 25 mcg/day is reached; **then,** increase q 1–2 weeks by 12.5–50 mcg. **Usual maintenance:** 50–100 mcg/day.

    Simple (nontoxic) goiter.

Adults, initial: 5 mcg/day; **then,** increase q 1–2 weeks by 5–10 mcg until

L

25 mcg/day is reached; **then,** dose can be increased by 12.5–25 mcg/week until the maintenance dose of 50–100 mcg/day is reached (usual is 75 mcg/day).

T₃ suppression test.

75–100 mcg/day for 7 days followed by a repeat of the I¹³¹ thyroid uptake test (a 50% or greater suppression of uptake indicates a normal thyroid-pituitary axis).

Congenital hypothyroidism.

Adults and children, initial: 5 mcg/day; **then,** increase by 5 mcg/day q 3–4 days until the desired effect is achieved. Approximately 20 mcg/day may be sufficient for infants a few months of age while children 1 year of age may require 50 mcg/day. Children above 3 years may require the full adult dose.

• **IV ONLY**

Myxedema coma, precoma.

Adults, initial: 25–50 mcg. Base subsequent doses on continuous monitoring of client's clinical status and response. Doses should be given at least 4 hr, and no more than 12 hr, apart. Total daily doses of 65 mcg in initial days of therapy are associated with a lower incidence of mortality. In cases of known CV disease, give an initial dose of 10–20 mcg.

NURSING CONSIDERATIONS

ⓒ Do not confuse Liothyronine with Liotrix or Levothyroxine (both thyroid products). Do not confuse Cytomel with Cytotec (a prostaglandin).

ADMINISTRATION/STORAGE

1. *Transfer from other thyroid preparations to liothyronine:* Discontinue old preparation before starting on low daily dose of liothyronine. *Transfer from liothyronine to another thyroid preparation:* Start therapy with replacement drug several days prior to complete withdrawal of sodium liothyronine.

2. If symptoms of hyperthyroidism noted, the drug can be withdrawn for 2–3 days and can be reinstituted at a lower dose.

Ⅳ 3. A *Cytomel* injection kit is available for the emergency treatment of myxedema coma.

ASSESSMENT

1. Note reasons for therapy, other agents trialed, outcome. List drugs prescribed to ensure none interact.

2. Stress importance of adherence to therapy and not to change brands once dosage stabilized.

3. Monitor VS, EKG, thyroid function tests and those with CAD for evidence of insufficiency.

CLIENT/FAMILY TEACHING

1. Take once a day at the same time, preferably before breakfast to prevent insomnia.

2. This drug is used to control symptoms of hypothyroidism; require replacement for life.

3. Report any chest pain, palpitations, fever, insomnia, irritability, unusual sweating, bruising/bleeding, heat intolerance, diarrhea, weight loss, and headaches.

4. Report as scheduled for physical exams and blood work.

OUTCOMES/EVALUATE

Desired thyroid hormone replacement

Liotrix ∎
(**LYE**-oh-trix)

CLASSIFICATION(S):
Thyroid product
PREGNANCY CATEGORY: A
Rx: Thyrolar.

*SEE ALSO **THYROID DRUGS.***

USES

(1) Replacement or supplemental therapy for congenital or acquired hypothyroidism of any etiology, except transient hypothyroidism during the recovery phase of subacute thyroiditis. (2) Treatment or prevention of various types of euthyroid goiters, including thyroid nodules, subacute or chronic lymphocytic thyroiditis, and multinodular goiter. (3) Adjunct to surgery and radioiodine therapy to manage thyrotropin-dependent   well-differentiated

thyroid cancer. (4) Diagnostic agent in suppression tests to differentiate suspected mild hypothyroidism or thyroid gland autonomy.

ACTION/KINETICS

Action

Mixture of synthetic levothyroxine sodium (T_4) and liothyronine (T_3) in a 4:1 ratio by weight and in a 1:1 ratio by biologic activity.

SPECIAL CONCERNS

■ Drugs with thyroid hormone activity, alone or with other drugs, have been used to treat obesity. In euthyroid clients, doses within the range of daily hormonal requirements are ineffective for weight reduction. Larger doses may produce serious or even life-threatening manifestations of toxicity, especially when given with sympathomimetic amines such as those used for their anorectic effects.■

SIDE EFFECTS

Most Common

Symptoms of hyperthyroidism.

See *Thyroid Drugs* for a complete list of possible side effects.

HOW SUPPLIED

Tablets: T_3/T_4: 3.1 mcg/12.5 mcg; 6.25 mcg/25 mcg; 12.5 mcg/50 mcg; 25 mcg/100 mcg; 37.5 mcg/150 mcg.

DOSAGE

• **TABLETS**

Hypothyroidism.

Adults and children, initial: 50 mcg levothyroxine and 12.5 mcg liothyronine (Thyrolar); **then,** at monthly intervals, increments of like amounts can be made until the desired effect is achieved. **Usual maintenance:** 50–100 mcg of levothyroxine and 12.5–25 mcg liothyronine daily.

Congenital hypothyroidism.

Children, 0–6 months: 3.1 mcg/12.5 (T_3/T_4) to 6.25 mcg/25 mcg (T_3/T_4); **6–12 months:** 6.25 mcg/25 mcg (T_3/T_4) to 9.35 mcg/37.5 mcg (T_3/T_4); **1–5 years:** 9.35 mcg/37.5 mcg (T_3/T_4) to 12.5 mcg/ 50 mcg (T_3/T_4); **6–12 years:** 12.5 mcg/ 50 mcg (T_3/T_4) to 18.75 mcg/75 mcg (T_3/T_4); **over 12 years:** more than 18.75 mcg/75 mcg (T_3/T_4).

NURSING CONSIDERATIONS

ADMINISTRATION/STORAGE

1. In infants with congenital hypothyroidism, begin therapy with full doses as soon as the diagnosis is made.
2. In children, make dosing increments q 2 weeks until desired response attained.
3. Protect tablets from light, heat, and moisture.

ASSESSMENT

1. Note onset of disease, any S&S, TFTs, dose at start of therapy.
2. Always do thyroid function tests before initiating dosage changes.

CLIENT/FAMILY TEACHING

1. Take once a day as a single dose before breakfast. May split dose if nausea and diarrhea persist.
2. Drug used to control symptoms of hypothyroidism; requires replacement for life. Do not stop suddenly.
3. Report any chest pain, palpitations, fever, insomnia, irritability, unusual sweating, heat intolerance, diarrhea, weight loss, and headaches.
4. Report as scheduled for physical exam and blood work.

OUTCOMES/EVALUATE

Thyroid hormone replacement

Lisdexamfetamine dimesylate ■
(lis-**DEX**-am-**FET**-a-meen)

CLASSIFICATION(S):
CNS stimulant
PREGNANCY CATEGORY: C
Rx: Vyvanse.

SEE ALSO *AMPHETAMINES AND DERIVATIVES.*

USES

Treatment of attention-deficit/hyperactivity disorder (ADHD).

ACTION/KINETICS

Action

Lisdexamfetamine is a prodrug and is converted to dextroamphetamine, the active moiety. The mechanism of action for ADHD is not known. However, amphetamines are thought to block the reuptake of norepinephrine and dopamine into presynaptic neurons and increase the release of monoamines into the extraneuronal space leading to CNS effects.

Pharmacokinetics
Rapidly absorbed; T_{max}: 3.5 after a single dose. Food does not affect the AUC or C_{max} but prolongs the T_{max} by about 1 hr. Dextroamphetamine and metabolites (98%) are excreted in the urine. **t½, plasma elimination:** Less than 1 hr.

CONTRAINDICATIONS
Advanced arteriosclerosis, symptomatic CV disease (structural cardiac abnormalities, cardiomyopathy, serious heart rhythm abnormalities), recent MI, moderate to severe hypertension, hyperthyroidism, hypersensitivity or idiosyncrasy to sympathomimetics, glaucoma, agitated states, history of drug abuse, during or within 14 days following administration of MAO inhibitors (hypertensive crisis may occur). Use not recommended during lactation and in children less than 3 years of age.

SPECIAL CONCERNS
■ Amphetamines have a high potential for abuse. Administration of amphetamines for prolonged periods of time may lead to drug dependence. Particular attention should be paid to the possibility of subjects obtaining amphetamines for non-therapeutic use or distribution to others and the drugs should be prescribed or dispensed sparingly. Misuse of amphetamine may cause sudden death and serious cardiovascular adverse events.■ Worsening of symptoms of behavior disturbance and thought disorder may occur in those with pre-existing psychotic disorder. Possible lowering of the threshold in clients with prior history of seizures, in those without a history of seizures, and no prior EEG evidence of seizures. Use with caution with concomitant use of other sympathomimetic drugs. Tolerance, significant psychological dependence, and severe social disability have occurred with amphetamine use/abuse. Safety and efficacy have not been de-

termined in children less than 3 years of age or over 12 years of age.

SIDE EFFECTS
Most Common
Decreased appetite, insomnia, upper abdominal pain, headache, irritability, decreased weight, N&V, dry mouth, dizziness.
CNS: Insomnia, headache, irritability, dizziness, somnolence, affect lability, tic, initial insomnia, psychomotor hyperactivity, treatment emergent psychotic or manic symptoms (e.g., hallucinations, delusional thinking, mania), overstimulation, restlessness, euphoria, dyskinesia, dysphoria, depression, tremor, aggressive behavior/hostility, worsening of motor and phonic tics and Tourette's syndrome, **seizures**. **GI:** Decreased appetite, upper abdominal pain, N&V, dry mouth, diarrhea, constipation, unpleasant taste. **CV:** ↑ BP/HR, palpitations, tachycardia, **cardiomyopathy** with chronic use, **CVA, MI. Dermatologic:** Rash. **Allergic:** Urticaria, **angioedema, anaphylaxis,** serious skin rashes including **Stevens-Johnson syndrome** and **toxic epidermal necrolysis. Ophthalmic:** Accommodation difficulty, blurred vision. **Body as a whole:** Decreased weight, pyrexia, long-term suppression of growth. **Miscellaneous:** Impotence, changes in libido, **sudden death**.

LABORATORY TEST CONSIDERATIONS
↑ Plasma corticosteroid levels. Interference with urinary steroid determinations.

OD OVERDOSE MANAGEMENT
SEE ALSO *AMPHETAMINES AND DERIVATIVES*.

DRUG INTERACTIONS
Adrenergic blockers / ↓ Effect of adrenergic blockers
Antihistamines / Amphetamines may counteract the sedative effects of antihistamines
Antihypertensives / Amphetamines may antagonize the hypotensive effect of antihypertensives
Chlorpromazine / Inhibition of CNS stimulant effect of amphetamines R/T blockade of dopamine and norepinephrine receptors
Ethosuximide / Possible delayed absorp-

L

tion of ethosuximide

Haloperidol / ↓ Amphetamine effect R/T blockade of dopamine receptors

Lithium carbonate / ↓ Anorectic and stimulatory effect of amphetamine

MAO Inhibitors / ↓ Amphetamine metabolism → ↑ effect of amphetamine, including headaches and other signs of hypertensive crisis, malignant hyperpyrexia, **death**

Meperidine / Potentiation of meperidine's analgesic effect

Methenamine / ↓ Amphetamine effect R/T ↑ urinary excretion

Norepinephrine / ↑ Adrenergic effects of norepinephrine

Phenobarbital / Delayed phenobarbital absorption; also, synergistic anticonvulsant action

Phenytoin / Delayed phenytoin absorption; also, synergistic anticonvulsant action

Propoxyphene / In event of propoxyphene overdosage, amphetamine CNS stimulation is potentiated; **fatal convulsions possible**

Sympathomimetics / ↑ Effect of sympathomimetics

Tricyclic antidepressants / ↑ Effect of TCAs; also, significant ↑ amphetamine brain levels → potentiation of cardiac effects

Urinary acidifiers (e.g., ammonium chloride, sodium acid phosphate) / ↓ Amphetamine blood levels R/T ↑ urinary excretion → ↓ efficacy

HOW SUPPLIED

Capsules: 20 mg, 30 mg, 40 mg, 50 mg, 60 mg, 70 mg.

DOSAGE

• **CAPSULES**

Attention deficit-hyperactivity disorder.
Individualize. **Children, 6–12 years of age, initial:** 30 mg once daily in the morning. If a dosage increase is needed, adjust in increments of 10 mg or 20 mg at approximately weekly intervals. **Maximum daily dose:** 70 mg. A dose of 20 mg/day may be started in some children.

NURSING CONSIDERATIONS

ADMINISTRATION/STORAGE

1. The least amount of the drug should be prescribed or dispensed at one time in order to minimize possible overdosage.

2. When possible interrupt the drug occasionally to determine if there is a recurrence of behavioral symptoms to warrant continued use of the drug.

3. The efficacy for use longer than 4 weeks has not been determined.

4. Store from 15–30°C (59–86°F) in tight, light-resistant containers.

ASSESSMENT

1. Note reasons for therapy, onset/characteristics of S&S, other drugs trialed/outcome and those currently prescribed that may interact unfavorably.

2. Assess for conditions that may preclude therapy: advanced/ symptomatic CV disease (structural cardiac abnormalities, cardiomyopathy, serious heart rhythm abnormalities), recent MI, moderate to severe hypertension, hyperthyroidism, hypersensitivity or idiosyncrasy to sympathomimetics, glaucoma, agitated states, history of drug abuse, during or within 14 days following administration of MAO inhibitors

3. Ensure psychologic evaluations show no evidence of psychotic disorder, excessive stimulation, or severe stress. Obtain/monitor VS, CBC, CNS status, ECG.

4. Assess growth (ht and wt); provide periodic 'drug holiday' to determine need for continued therapy.

5. Monitor scripts and evaluate for any drug overuse/abuse.

CLIENT/FAMILY TEACHING

1. May be taken whole with or without food. The capsule may be opened and the entire contents dissolved in a glass of water. Consume the solution immediately. Rinse to ensure that entire contents consumed.

2. Take in the morning to ensure ability to sleep at bedtime. Avoid afternoon doses to minimize insomnia.

3. Use caution when driving or operating hazardous machinery; drug may mask fatigue and/or cause physical in-

---

Bold Italic = life threatening side effect   ■ = black box warning   ✦ = Available in Canada

coordination, dizziness, blurred vision, drowsiness.

4. Record BP, HR, and weight 2 times per week; report any significant wt loss or changes.

5. Report changes in mood, attention span; seizure disorder.

6. Skin rashes, fever, or joint pains should be reported immediately.

7. Therapy may be interrupted every few months ('drug holiday') to determine if still needed in those responsive to therapy.

8. May require more rest as drug effects fade.

9. Chronic use may lead to psychic dependence and marked tolerance. Scripts will be carefully monitored to prevent overdose and overuse.

10. Keep all F/U appointments to evaluate response to therapy and for any adverse side effects.

OUTCOMES/EVALUATE

↑ Ability to sit quietly/focus/concentrate in those with ADHD

Lisinopril
(lie-**SIN**-oh-prill)

CLASSIFICATION(S):
Antihypertensive, ACE inhibitor
PREGNANCY CATEGORY: C
Rx: Prinivil, Zestril.
✚Rx: Apo-Lisinopril.

SEE ALSO *ANGIOTENSIN-CONVERTING ENZYME INHIBITORS.*

USES

(1) Alone or in combination with a diuretic (usually a thiazide) to treat hypertension. (2) Hypertension in children, aged 6–16 years. (3) In combination with digitalis and a diuretic for treating CHF not responding to other therapy. (4) Use within 24 hr of acute MI to improve survival in hemodynamically stable clients (clients should receive the standard treatment, including thrombolytics, aspirin, and beta blockers). *Investigational:* Prophylactic treatment of migraine.

ACTION/KINETICS

Action

Inhibits angiotensin-converting enzyme resulting in decreased plasma angiotensin II, which leads to decreased vasopressor activity and decreased aldosterone secretion. Both supine and standing BPs are reduced, although the drug is less effective in African Americans than in Caucasians.

Pharmacokinetics

Although food does not alter the bioavailability of lisinopril, only 25% of a PO dose is absorbed. **Onset:** 1 hr. **Peak serum levels:** 7 hr. **Duration:** 24 hr. **t½:** 12 hr. 100% of the drug is excreted unchanged in the urine.

CONTRAINDICATIONS

Use in children less than 6 years of age or in children with a GFR less than 30 mL/min/1.73 m².

SPECIAL CONCERNS

■ When used during the second and third trimesters of pregnancy, injury and even death can result in the developing fetus. When pregnancy is detected, discontinue as soon as possible.■ Use with caution during lactation. Safety and efficacy have not been established in children. Geriatric clients may manifest higher blood levels. Reduce the dosage in clients with impaired renal function.

SIDE EFFECTS

Most Common

Chest pain, dizziness, headache, hypotension, fatigue, diarrhea, URTI.

CV: Hypotension, orthostatic hypotension, angina, tachycardia, palpitations, rhythm disturbances, ***stroke,*** chest pain, orthostatic effects, peripheral edema, *MI, CVA,* worsening of heart failure, chest sound abnormalities, PVCs, TIAs, atrial fibrillation. **CNS:** Dizziness, headache, fatigue, vertigo, insomnia, depression, sleepiness, paresthesias, malaise, nervousness, confusion, ataxia, impaired memory, tremor, irritability, hypersomnia, peripheral neuropathy, spasm. **GI:** Diarrhea, N&V, dyspepsia, anorexia, constipation, dysgeusia, dry mouth, abdominal pain, flatulence, gastritis, heartburn, GI cramps, weight loss/gain, taste alterations, increased salivation. **Respiratory:** URTI, cough, dyspnea, bronchitis, upper respiratory symptoms, nasal congestion, sinusitis, pharyngeal pain, **bronchospasm**, asthma, pulmonary edema infiltrates, **pulmonary embolism/infarction,** PND, chest discomfort, common cold, pleural effusion, wheezing, painful respiration, epistaxis, laryngitis, pharyngitis, rhinitis, rhinorrhea, orthopnea. **Musculoskeletal:** Asthenia, muscle cramps, pain (neck, hip, leg, knee, arm, joint, shoulder, back, pelvic, flank), myalgia, arthralgia, arthritis, lumbago. **Hepatic:** Hepatitis, hepatocellular/cholestatic jaundice, pancreatitis, hepatomegaly. **Dermatologic:** Rash, pruritus, flushing, increased sweating, urticaria, alopecia, erythema multiforme, photophobia. **GU:** Impotence, oliguria, progressive azotemia, acute renal failure, UTI, anuria, uremia, renal dysfunction, pyelonephritis, dysuria. **Ophthalmic:** Blurred vision, visual loss, diplopia. **Miscellaneous:** *Angioedema (may be fatal if laryngeal edema occurs),* hyperkalemia, neutropenia, anemia, *bone marrow depression,* decreased libido, fever, syncope, vasculitis of the legs, gout, eosinophilia, fluid overload, dehydration, diabetes mellitus, chills, virus infection, edema, *anaphylactoid reaction, malignant lung neoplasms,* hemoptysis, breast pain.

LABORATORY TEST CONSIDERATIONS
↑ Serum potassium, BUN, serum creatinine. ↓ H&H.

OD OVERDOSE MANAGEMENT
Symptoms: Hypotension. *Treatment:* Supportive. To correct hypotension, IV normal saline is treatment of choice. Lisinopril may be removed by hemodialysis.

DRUG INTERACTIONS
Diuretics / Excess ↓ BP
Indomethacin / Possible ↓ lisinopril effect
Potassium-sparing diuretics / Significant ↑ serum potassium

HOW SUPPLIED
Tablets: 2.5 mg, 5 mg, 10 mg, 20 mg, 30 mg, 40 mg.

DOSAGE
• **TABLETS**

Essential hypertension, used alone.
Adults, Initial: 10 mg once daily. Adjust dosage depending on response (range: 20–40 mg/day given as a single dose). Doses greater than 80 mg/day do not give a greater effect. **Children over 6 years of age, initial:** 0.07 mg/kg once daily up to 5 mg total). Adjust dose according to BP response; doses above 0.61 mg/kg (or in excess of 40 mg) have not been studied in children.
Essential hypertension in combination with a diuretic.
Initial: 5 mg. The BP-lowering effects of the combination are additive. Reduce dosage in renal impairment as follows: C_{CR}, 10–30 mL/min: Give an initial dose of 5 mg/day for hypertension. C_{CR}, less than 10 mL/min: Give an initial dose of 2.5 mg/day and adjust dose depending on BP response.
CHF.
Initial: 5 mg once daily (2.5 mg/day in clients with hyponatremia) in combination with diuretics and digitalis. **Dosage range:** 5–20 mg/day as a single dose.
Acute MI to improve survival.
First dose: 5 mg within 24 hr of the onset of symptoms; **then,** 5 mg after 24 hr, 10 mg after 48 hr, and then 10 mg daily. Continue dosing for 6 weeks. In clients with a systolic pressure less than 120 mm Hg when treatment is started or within 3 days after the infarct should be given 2.5 mg. If hypotension occurs (systolic BP less than 100 mm Hg), the dose may be temporarily reduced to 2.5 mg. If prolonged hypotension occurs, withdraw the drug.

NURSING CONSIDERATIONS
Ⓒ Do not confuse lisinopril with Lioresal (a muscle relaxant). Also, do not confuse Prinivil with Prilosec (a proton pump inhibitor) or Proventil (a sympathomimetic).

ADMINISTRATION/STORAGE
1. To prepare a suspension (200 mL) of a 1 mg/mL concentration, add 10 mL purified water to a polyethylene terephthalate bottle containing ten 20 mg tablets of lisinopril. Shake for at least 1 min. Add 30 mL Bicitra diluent and 160 mL of Ora-Sweet SF to the concentrate

in the bottle; shake gently for several seconds to disperse the ingredients. Store the suspension at or below 25°C (77°F) for up to 4 weeks. Shake the suspension before each use.

2. When considering use of lisinopril in a client taking diuretics, discontinue the diuretic, if possible, 2–3 days before beginning lisinopril therapy. If diuretic cannot be discontinued, the initial dose of lisinopril should be 5 mg; observe closely for at least 2 hr.

3. Maximum antihypertensive effects may not be observed for 2–4 weeks.

4. When starting treatment for CHF, give under medical supervision, especially if SBP <100 mm Hg.

5. With clients whose BP is controlled with lisinopril, 20 mg, plus hydrochlorothiazide 25 mg, given separately may trial Prinzide 12.5 mg or Zestoretic 20–12.5 mg before Prinzide 25 mg or Zestoretic 20–25 mg is used.

6. The maximum recommended daily dose of lisinopril is 80 mg in a single daily dose. Clients usually do not require hydrochlorothiazide in doses exceeding 50 mg/day, especially if combined with other antihypertensives.

7. Use of potassium supplements, potassium-sparing diuretics, or potassium salt substitutes with Prinzide or Zestoretic may lead to increases in serum potassium.

8. Prinzide or Zestoretic is recommended for those with C_{CR} >30 mL/min.

9. Anticipate reduced dosage with renal insufficiency—initial dose of 10 mg/day if C_{CR} >30 mL/min, 5 mg/day if C_{CR} is between 10 and 30 mL/min, and 2.5 mg/day in dialysis clients (i.e., C_{CR} <10 mL/min).

10. Store tablets from 15–30°C (59–86°F); protect from moisture.

ASSESSMENT

1. Note reasons for therapy, agents trialed and outcome.

2. Perform physical exam noting cardiopulmonary status, review history for any existing conditions, and labs for any organ dysfunction.

3. Obtain ECG, VS, CXR, and baseline labs. Reduce dose with renal dysfunction.

4. Identify risk factors and those that are modifiable to reduce CHD progression.

5. Start within 24 hr of AMI in addition to ASA, beta blockers, statins, and thrombolytics to reduce mortality.

CLIENT/FAMILY TEACHING

1. Must be taken as directed at least once a day to control BP.

2. Avoid symptoms of low BP (i.e., rise slowly from sitting or lying position and wait until symptoms subside).

3. Avoid all potassium supplements as well as foods high in potassium, unless otherwise directed.

4. Review drug side effects; record BP.

5. Report new or unusual side effects or aggravation of existing conditions, as well as sore throat, hoarseness, cough, chest pain, difficulty breathing, or swelling of hands, feet, or face.

6. Avoid OTC agents without approval; may affect drug action.

7. Keep all F/U appointments to evaluate response to therapy, EKG and labs.

OUTCOMES/EVALUATE

- ↓ BP
- Improved survival with acute MI

—— COMBINATION DRUG ——

Lisinopril and Hydrochlorothiazide

(lie-**SIN**-oh-prill, **hy**-droh-klor-oh-**THIGH**-ah-zyd)

CLASSIFICATION(S):

Antihypertensive (combination ACE inhibitor and thiazide diuretic)

PREGNANCY CATEGORY: C (first trimester), **D** (second and third trimesters).

Rx: Prinzide, Zestoretic.

SEE ALSO *LISINOPRIL* AND *HYDROCHLOROTHIAZIDE*.

USES

Hypertension (not indicated for initial therapy).

CONTENT

Prinzide or Zestoretic: 10–12.5 (10 mg lisinopril, *an ACE inhibitor*, and 12.5 mg hydrochlorothiazide, *a thiazide diuretic*); 20–12.5 (20 mg lisinopril and 12.5 mg hydrochlorothiazide; 20–25 (20 mg lisinopril and 25 mg hydrochlorothiazide).

ACTION/KINETICS

Action

Lisinopril inhibits angiotensin-converting enzyme resulting in decreased plasma angiotensin II, which leads to decreased vasopressor activity and decreased aldosterone secretion. Hydrochlorothiazide promotes the excretion of sodium and chloride, and thus water, by the distal renal tubule. Also increases excretion of potassium and to a lesser extent bicarbonate. The antihypertensive activity is thought to be due to direct dilation of the arterioles, as well as to a reduction in the total fluid volume of the body and altered sodium balance.

Pharmacokinetics

Lisinopril, about 25% absorbed; peak serum levels: About 7 hr. Lisinopril absorption not affected by food. Hydrochlorothiazide: **Onset, 2 hr; peak effect:** 4 hr; **duration:** 6–12 hr. **t½, lisinopril:** 12 hr; hydrochlorothiazide, 5.6–14.8 hr. Lisinopril and hydrochlorothiazide are excreted unchanged in the urine.

CONTRAINDICATIONS

Use in clients hypersensitive to any components of the product, a history of angioedema related to previous treatment with ACE inhibitors, hereditary or idiopathic angioedema, anuria, or hypersensitivity to other sulfonamide-derived drugs. Lactation.

SPECIAL CONCERNS

Angioedema and anaphylactoid reactions are possible with ACE inhibitors. Black clients receiving ACE inhibitors have a higher incidence of angioedema compared with non-Blacks. Use thiazides with caution in severe renal disease, impaired hepatic function, or progressive liver disease. Use lisinopril with caution in aortic stenosis or hypertrophic cardiomyopathy. Safety and efficacy have not been determined in children.

SIDE EFFECTS

Most Common

Dizziness, headache, cough, fatigue, orthostatic hypotension, hypokalemia.

See *Angiotensin-Converting Enzyme Inhibitors* and *Diuretics, Thiazides* for a complete list of possible side effects.

DRUG INTERACTIONS

See *Angiotensin-Converting Enzyme Inhibitors* and *Diuretics, Thiazides*.

HOW SUPPLIED

See Content.

DOSAGE

• TABLETS

Hypertension.

Individualized, usual: 1 or 2 tablets daily of one of the strengths (depending on response). For geriatric clients, begin therapy at the low end of the dosage range.

NURSING CONSIDERATIONS

ADMINISTRATION/STORAGE

1. To minimize dose-independent side effects, in general, use combination therapy only after a client has failed to achieve the desired effect with monotherapy.

2. Clients whose BP is controlled adequately with 25 mg/day of hydrochlorothiazide, but who experience significant hypokalemia, may achieve similar or greater BP control with less potassium loss if they are switched to the 10/12.5 mg product

3. Dosages higher than lisinopril, 80 mg, and hydrochlorothiazide, 50 mg, should not be used.

4. The usual dosage does not require adjustment if the client's C_{CR} is >30 mL/min/1.73 m². In those with more severe renal impairment, do not use thiazides.

5. Store from 15–30°C (59–86°F). Protect from excessive light and humidity.

ASSESSMENT

1. Note disease onset, other drugs trialed/outcome, age, other co-morbidities.

2. Monitor VS, CBC, lytes, renal and LFTs; reduce dose with dysfunction. Use cautiously with aortic stenosis or hypertrophic cardiomyopathy.

3. Assess for sulfa based allergies; precludes therapy.

Bold Italic = life threatening side effect　　■ = black box warning　　✤ = Available in Canada

CLIENT/FAMILY TEACHING
1. Take as directed with a full glass of water; do not skip or forget doses.
2. May cause dizziness/drowsiness use caution until drug effects realized.
3. Report any swelling of face, extremities, or difficulty swallowing.
4. Record BP to share at all F/U visits.
5. Avoid activities that cause excessive overheating; may become dehydrated.
6. Do not use salt substitutes with potassium.
7. Use reliable contraception; harmful to fetus in 2nd and 3rd trimester.

OUTCOMES/EVALUATE
BP <140/85 or <130/80 with diabetes, renal disease

Lithium carbonate ■ ©
(**LITH**-ee-um)

CLASSIFICATION(S):
Antimanic
PREGNANCY CATEGORY: D
Rx: Eskalith CR, Lithobid, Lithonate, Lithotabs.
♣Rx: Apo-Lithium Carbonate, Carbolith, Duralith, Lithane, PMS-Lithium Carbonate.

Lithium citrate
PREGNANCY CATEGORY: D
♣Rx: PMS-Lithium Citrate.

USES
Control of mania in manic-depressive clients. *Investigational:* To reverse neutropenia induced by cancer chemotherapy, in children with chronic neutropenia, and in AIDS clients receiving zidovudine. Prophylaxis of cluster headaches. Also for premenstrual tension, alcoholism accompanied by depression, tardive dyskinesia, bulimia, hyperthyroidism, excess ADH secretion, postpartum affective psychosis, corticosteroid-induced psychosis.

ACTION/KINETICS
Action
Mechanism for the antimanic effect of lithium is unknown. Various hypotheses include: (a) a decrease in catecholamine neurotransmitter levels caused by lithium's effect on Na^+–K^+ ATPase to improve transneuronal membrane transport of sodium ion; (b) a decrease in cyclic AMP levels caused by lithium which decreases sensitivity of hormonal-sensitive adenyl cyclase receptors; or (c) interference by lithium with lipid inositol metabolism ultimately leading to insensitivity of cells in the CNS to stimulation by inositol. Affects the distribution of calcium, Mg, and sodium ions and affects glucose metabolism.

Pharmacokinetics
Peak serum levels (regular release): 1–4 hr; (slow-release): 4–6 hr. **Onset:** 5–14 days. **Therapeutic serum levels:** 0.4–1.0 mEq/L (must be carefully monitored because toxic effects may occur at these levels and significant toxic reactions occur at serum lithium levels of 2 mEq/L). **$t\frac{1}{2}$, plasma:** 24 hr (longer in presence of renal impairment and in the elderly). Lithium and sodium are excreted by the same mechanism in the proximal tubule. Thus, to reduce the danger of lithium intoxication, sodium intake must remain at normal levels.

CONTRAINDICATIONS
Cardiovascular or renal disease. Brain damage. Dehydration, sodium depletion, clients receiving diuretics. Lactation.

SPECIAL CONCERNS
■ Toxicity is closely related to serum lithium levels and can occur at therapeutic doses. Facilities to monitor serum lithium are required.■ Safety and efficacy have not been established for children less than 12 years of age. Use with caution in geriatric clients because lithium is more toxic to the CNS in these clients; also, geriatric clients are more likely to develop lithium-induced goiter and clinical hypothyroidism and are more likely to manifest excessive thirst and larger volumes of urine.

SIDE EFFECTS
Most Common
Due to initial therapy: Fine hand tremor, polyuria, thirst, transient and mild nausea, general discomfort.

The following side effects are dependent on the serum level of lithium. **CV:** Arrhythmia, hypotension, *peripheral circulatory collapse,* bradycardia, sinus node dysfunction with *severe bradycardia causing syncope*; reversible flattening, isoelectricity, or inversion of T waves. **CNS:** Blackout spells, epileptiform seizures, slurred speech, dizziness, vertigo, somnolence, psychomotor retardation, restlessness, sleepiness, confusion, stupor, *coma,* acute dystonia, startled response, hypertonicity, slowed intellectual functioning, hallucinations, poor memory, tics, cog wheel rigidity, tongue movements. Pseudotumor cerebri leading to increased intracranial pressure and papilledema; if undetected may cause enlargement of the blind spot, constriction of visual fields, and eventual blindness. Diffuse slowing of EEG; widening of frequency spectrum of EEG; disorganization of background rhythm of EEG. **GI:** Anorexia, N&V, diarrhea, dry mouth, gastritis, salivary gland swelling, abdominal pain, excessive salivation, flatulence, indigestion, incontinence of urine or feces, dysgeusia/taste distortion, salty taste, swollen lips, dental caries. **Dermatologic:** Drying and thinning of hair, anesthesia of skin, chronic folliculitis, xerosis cutis, alopecia, exacerbation of psoriasis, acne, angioedema. **Neuromuscular:** Tremor, muscle hyperirritability (fasciculations, twitching, clonic movements), ataxia, choreo-athetotic movements, hyperactive DTRs, polyarthralgia. **GU:** Albuminuria, oliguria, polyuria, glycosuria, decreased C_{CR}, symptoms of nephrogenic diabetes, impotence/sexual dysfunction. **Thyroid:** Euthyroid goiter or hypothyroidism, including myxedema, accompanied by lower T_3 and T_4. **Miscellaneous:** Fatigue, lethargy, dehydration, weight loss, transient scotomata, tightness in chest, hypercalcemia, hyperparathyroidism, thirst, swollen painful joints, fever.

The following symptoms are unrelated to lithium dosage. Transient EEG and ECG changes, leukocytosis, headache, diffuse nontoxic goiter with or without hypothyroidism, transient hyperglycemia, generalized pruritus with or without rash, cutaneous ulcers, albuminuria, worsening of organic brain syndrome, excessive weight gain, edematous swelling of ankles or wrists, thirst or polyuria (may resemble diabetes mellitus), metallic taste, symptoms similar to Raynaud's phenomenon.

LABORATORY TEST CONSIDERATIONS
False + urinary glucose test (Benedict's). ↑ Serum glucose, CK. False − or ↓ serum PBI, uric acid; ↑ TSH, I^{131} uptake; ↓ T_3, T_4.

OD OVERDOSE MANAGEMENT
Symptoms: Symptoms dependent on serum lithium levels.
Levels less than 2 mEq/L: N&V, diarrhea, muscle weakness, drowsiness, loss of coordination.
Levels of 2–3 mEq/L: Agitation, ataxia, blackouts, blurred vision, choreoathetoid movements, confusion, dysarthria, fasciculations, giddiness, hyperreflexia, hypertonia, agitation or manic-like behavior, myoclonic twitching or movement of entire limbs, slurred speech, tinnitus, urinary or fecal incontinence, vertigo.
Levels over 3 mEq/L: Complex clinical picture involving multiple organs and organ systems. *Arrhythmias, coma,* hypotension, *peripheral vascular collapse, seizures (focal and generalized)*, spasticity, stupor, twitching of muscle groups. *Treatment:* Early symptoms are treated by decreasing the dose or stopping treatment for 24–48 hr. In severe cases, first eliminate lithium from the body.
- Use gastric lavage.
- Restore fluid and electrolyte balance (can use saline).
- Regulate and maintain kidney function.
- Increase lithium excretion by giving aminophylline, mannitol, or urea.
- Prevent infection. Maintain adequate respiration.
- Chest x-rays
- Monitor thyroid function.
- Institute hemodialysis, especially if lithium levels are >3.5 to 4 mEq/L.

DRUG INTERACTIONS

Acetazolamide / ↓ Lithium effect by ↑ renal excretion

Bumetanide / ↑ Lithium toxicity R/T ↓ renal clearance

Carbamazepine / ↑ Risk of lithium toxicity

Diazepam / ↑ Risk of hypothermia

Ethacrynic acid / ↑ Lithium toxicity R/T ↓ renal clearance

Fluoxetine / ↑ Serum lithium levels

Furosemide / ↑ Lithium toxicity R/T ↓ renal clearance

Haloperidol / ↑ Risk of neurologic toxicity

Iodide salts / Additive effect to cause hypothyroidism

Mannitol / ↓ Lithium effect by ↑ renal excretion

Mazindol / ↑ Chance of lithium toxicity R/T ↑ serum levels

Methyldopa / ↑ Chance of neurotoxic effects with or without ↑ lithium serum levels

Neuromuscular blocking agents / Lithium ↑ neuromuscular blockade → severe respiratory depression/apnea

NSAIDs / ↓ Lithium renal clearance, possibly R/T inhibition of renal prostaglandin synthesis

Phenothiazines / ↓ Phenothiazine levels or ↑ lithium levels

Phenytoin / ↑ Risk of lithium toxicity

Probenecid / ↑ Risk of lithium toxicity R/T ↑ serum levels

Sibutramine / Additive serotonergic effects → possible serotonin syndrome

Sodium chloride / Excretion of lithium is proportional to amount of sodium chloride ingested; if client is on salt-free diet, may develop lithium toxicity since less lithium excreted

Sympathomimetics / ↓ Drug pressor effects

Theophyllines, including aminophylline / ↓ Lithium effect R/T ↑ renal excretion

Thiazide diuretics, triamterene / ↑ Risk of lithium toxicity R/T ↓ renal clearance

Tricyclic antidepressants / ↑ TCA effects

Urea / ↓ Lithium effect by ↑ renal excretion

Urinary alkalinizers / ↓ Lithium effect by ↑ renal excretion

Verapamil / ↓ Lithium levels and toxicity

HOW SUPPLIED

Lithium carbonate: *Capsules:* 150 mg, 300 mg, 600 mg; *Oral Solution:* 8 mEq lithium/5 mL (equivalent to 300 mg lithium carbonate); *Tablets:* 300 mg; *Tablets, Extended-Release:* 300 mg, 450 mg.
Lithium citrate: *Syrup:* 300 mg/5 mL.

DOSAGE

• **CAPSULES; ORAL SOLUTION; SYRUP; TABLETS; TABLETS, EXTENDED-RELEASE**

Acute mania.

Adults: Individualized and according to lithium serum level (not to exceed 1.4 mEq/L) and clinical response. **Usual initial:** 300–600 mg 3 times/day or 600–900 mg twice per day of slow-release form; **elderly and debilitated clients:** 0.6–1.2 grams/day in three divided doses. **Maintenance:** 300 mg 3–4 times/day. Administration of drug is discontinued when lithium serum level exceeds 1.2 mEq/L and resumed 24 hr after it has fallen below that level.

To reverse neutropenia.

300–1,000 mg/day (to achieve serum levels of 0.5–1.0 mEq/L) for 7–10 days.

Prophylaxis of cluster headaches.

600–900 mg/day.

NURSING CONSIDERATIONS

ⓒ Do not confuse Lithonate, Lithobid, and Lithotabs (all trade names for lithium carbonate).

ADMINISTRATION/STORAGE

1. To prevent toxic serum levels, determine blood levels 1–2 times per week during initiation of therapy, and monthly thereafter, on blood drawn 8–12 hr after dosage.

2. Full beneficial drug effects may not be noted for 6–10 days.

ASSESSMENT

1. Note reasons for therapy, other agents trialed, characteristics of S&S, behavioral presentation. Conduct a drug history; determine if taking other medications likely to interact, i.e., thiazide diuretics which may induce dehydration.

2. With arthritic conditions, document anti-inflammatory agent(s) used.

 = see color insert   = Herbal   = Intravenous   ⓒ = sound alike drug

3. Monitor lithium levels, kidney and thyroid function studies; assess for decreased function.

4. Assess mental status, CV function, VS, chemistry, thyroid function, urinalysis, weight, and ECG.

CLIENT/FAMILY TEACHING

1. Take with food or immediately after meals. Avoid any caffeinated beverages/foods; may aggravate mania.

2. Report persistent diarrhea; may need supplemental fluids or salt.

3. Maintain a constant level of salt intake to avoid fluctuations in lithium activity. Weight gain and swelling may be related to sodium retention; report if excessive.

4. Drink 10–12 glasses of water each day; avoid dehydration (e.g., vigorous exercise, sunbathing, sauna) to prevent increased concentrations of lithium in urine.

5. Review goals of therapy, drug interactions/side effects. Report diarrhea, vomiting, drowsiness, muscular weakness, or lack of coordination.

6. Do not engage in physical activities that require alertness or physical coordination until drug effects realized; may cause drowsiness.

7. Will take several weeks to realize a behavioral benefit from therapy.

8. Do not change brands of drug. Avoid all OTC agents.

9. Lithium works well in the manic phase; concomitant antidepressant use may be necessary during depressive phases.

10. Transient acneiform eruptions, folliculitis, altered sexual function in men may occur.

11. Carry name and telephone number of persons to contact if needed or if family members note behavioral/physical changes contrary to expectations. Carry ID, noting diagnosis and prescribed medications.

12. Keep all F/U appointments to evaluate response to therapy, adverse side effects and drug levels.

OUTCOMES/EVALUATE

• Stabilization of mood swings

• ↓ Symptoms of mania (↓ hyperactivity, ↓ sleeplessness; improved judgment)

• Therapeutic serum drug levels (0.4–1.0 mEq/L)

Lomefloxacin hydrochloride
(**Ioh**-meh-**FLOX**-ah-sin)

CLASSIFICATION(S):
Antibiotic, fluoroquinolone
PREGNANCY CATEGORY: C
Rx: Maxaquin.

SEE ALSO *FLUOROQUINOLONES.*

USES

(1) Acute bacterial exacerbation of chronic bronchitis caused by *Haemophilus influenzae* or *Moraxella catarrhalis.* (Not to be used for empiric treatment of acute bacterial exacerbation of chronic bronchitis due to *Streptococcus pneumoniae*). (2) Uncomplicated UTIs (cystitis) due to *Escherichia coli, Klebsiella pneumoniae, Proteus mirabilis,* or *Staphylococcus saprophyticus.* (3) Complicated UTIs due to *E. coli, K. pneumoniae, P. mirabilis, Pseudomonas aeruginosa, Citrobacter diversus,* or *Enterobacter cloacae.* Safety and efficacy in treating pseudomonas bacteremia has not been determined. (4) Reduce the incidence of UTIs in the early postoperative period (3–5 days postsurgery) after transurethral surgical procedures. Do not use for simple cystoscopy or retrograde pyelography. (5) Reduce incidence of UTIs in transrectal prostate biopsy in the early (3–5 days) and late (3–4 weeks) postoperative periods.

ACTION/KINETICS

Pharmacokinetics

Mean peak plasma levels: 4.2 mcg/mL after a 400-mg dose. The rate and extent of absorption are decreased if taken with food. $t\frac{1}{2}$: 8 hr. Metabolized in the liver with 65% excreted unchanged through the urine and 10% excreted unchanged in the feces.

Bold Italic = life threatening side effect   ■ = black box warning   ✦ = Available in Canada

CONTRAINDICATIONS

Use in minor urologic procedures for which prophylaxis is not indicated (e.g., simply cystoscopy, retrograde pyelography). Use for the empiric treatment of acute bacterial exacerbation of chronic bronchitis due to *Streptococcus pneumoniae*. Lactation.

SPECIAL CONCERNS

Plasma clearance is reduced in the elderly. Safety and efficacy have not been determined in children less than 18 years of age. Serious hypersensitivity reactions that are occasionally fatal have occurred, even with the first dose. No dosage adjustment is needed for elderly clients with normal renal function. Not efficiently removed from the body by hemodialysis or peritoneal dialysis.

SIDE EFFECTS

Most Common

Headache, dizziness, photosensitivity, N&V, abdominal pain/discomfort/cramping.

See *Fluoroquinolones* for a complete list of possible side effects. **CNS:** Confusion, tremor, vertigo, nervousness, anxiety, hyperkinesia, anorexia, agitation, increased appetite, depersonalization, paranoia, *coma.* **GI:** GI inflammation or bleeding, dysphagia, tongue discoloration, bad taste in mouth. **GU:** Dysuria, hematuria, micturition disorder, anuria, leukorrhea, intermenstrual bleeding, perineal pain, vaginal moniliasis, orchitis, epididymitis, proteinuria, albuminuria. **Hypersensitivity Reactions:** Urticaria, itching, pharyngeal or facial edema, *CV collapse,* tingling, loss of consciousness, dyspnea. **CV:** Hypotension, tachycardia, bradycardia, extrasystoles, cyanosis, *arrhythmia, cardiac failure,* angina pectoris, *MI, pulmonary embolism, cardiomyopathy,* phlebitis, cerebrovascular disorder. **Respiratory:** Dyspnea, respiratory infection, epistaxis, *bronchospasm,* cough, increased sputum, respiratory disorder, stridor. **Hematologic:** Eosinophilia, leukopenia, increase or decrease in platelets, increase in ESR, lymphocytopenia, decreased hemoglobin, anemia, bleeding, increased PT, increase in monocytes. **Dermatologic:** Urticaria, eczema, skin exfoliation, skin disorder. **Ophthalmic:** Conjunctivitis, eye pain. **Otic:** Earache, tinnitus. **Musculoskeletal:** Back or chest pain, asthenia, leg cramps, arthralgia, myalgia. **Miscellaneous:** Increase or decrease in blood glucose, flushing, increased sweating, facial edema, influenza-like symptoms, decreased heat tolerance, purpura, lymphadenopathy, increased fibrinolysis, thirst, gout, hypoglycemia, phototoxicity, peripheral neuropathy (including paresthesias, hypesthesias, dysesthesias, and weakness).

LABORATORY TEST CONSIDERATIONS

↑ ALT, AST, alkaline phosphatase, bilirubin, BUN, GGT. ↑ or ↓ Potassium. Abnormalities of urine specific gravity or serum electrolytes.

HOW SUPPLIED

Tablets: 400 mg.

DOSAGE

• TABLETS

Acute bacterial exacerbation of chronic bronchitis. Uncomplicated cystitis due to K. pneumoniae, P. mirabilis, or S. saprophyticus.

Adults: 400 mg once daily for 10 days.

Complicated UTIs.

Adults: 400 mg once daily for 14 days.

Uncomplicated cystitis in females due to E. coli.

400 mg once daily for 3 days.

Prophylaxis of infection before surgery for transurethral procedures.

Single 400-mg dose 2–6 hr before surgery.

Transrectal prostate biopsy.

Single 400 mg dose 1–6 hr prior to the procedure.

NURSING CONSIDERATIONS

ADMINISTRATION/STORAGE

1. Dosage modification is required for C_{CR} <40 mL/min/1.73 m^2 and >10 mL/min/1.73 m^2. Following an initial loading dose of 400 mg, give daily maintenance doses of 200 mg for the duration of treatment. Assess lomefloxacin levels to determine any need to alter dosing interval. Follow this same regimen for clients on hemodialysis.

2. Hemodialysis clients should receive an initial loading dose of 400 mg fol-

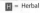

lowed by maintenance doses of 200 mg (½ tablet) once daily for the duration of treatment.

3. Store tablets from 15–25°C (59–77°F).

ASSESSMENT

1. Note reasons for therapy, onset, characteristics of S&S.

2. Obtain cultures, renal function studies; modify dosage with dysfunction.

CLIENT/FAMILY TEACHING

1. May take without regard to food. Increase fluid intake to 2 L/day and complete entire prescription.

2. Avoid antacids for 2 hr surrounding drug dose.

3. May experience dizziness and lightheadedness; use caution until drug effects realized.

4. Avoid prolonged sunlight exposure; may experience photosensitivity. Photosensitivity may be reduced by taking the drug at least 12 hr before exposure to the sun (e.g., in the evening).

5. Report lack of response or any rash, severe GI upset, diarrhea, weakness, tremors, visual changes or seizures. Discontinue if symptoms of neuropathy occur (e.g., burning, pain, tingling, numbness, and/or weakness or deficits in light touch, pain, temperature, position sense, vibratory sense, or motor strength).

OUTCOMES/EVALUATE

• Prostate/bladder/urinary infection prophylaxis

• Resolution of infective organism

Lomustine ■
(loh-**MUS**-teen)

CLASSIFICATION(S):
Antineoplastic, alkylating
PREGNANCY CATEGORY: D
Rx: CeeNu (Abbreviation: CCNU).

SEE ALSO *ANTINEOPLASTIC AGENTS* AND *ALKYLATING AGENTS*.

USES

(1) Used alone or in combination to treat primary and metastatic brain tumors. (2) Secondary therapy in Hodg-

kin's disease (in combination with other antineoplastics).

ACTION/KINETICS

Action

Alkylating agent that inhibits DNA and RNA synthesis through DNA alkylation. It also affects other cellular processes, including RNA, protein synthesis and the processing of ribosomal and nucleoplasmic messenger RNA; DNA base component structure; the rate of DNA synthesis and DNA polymerase activity. Is cell cycle nonspecific.

Pharmacokinetics

Rapidly absorbed from the GI tract; crosses the blood-brain barrier resulting in concentrations higher than in plasma. **Peak plasma level:** 1–6 hr; **t½:** biphasic; **initial,** 6 hr; **postdistribution:** 1–2 days. From 15 to 20% of drug remains in body after 5 days. Fifty percent of drug excreted within 12 hr through the kidney, 75% within 4 days. Small amounts are excreted through the lungs and feces. Metabolites present in milk.

CONTRAINDICATIONS

Lactation.

SPECIAL CONCERNS

■ (1) Bone marrow suppression, especially thrombocytopenia and leukopenia, which may contribute to bleeding and overwhelming infections in an already compromised client, is the most common and severe toxic effect. (2) Because the major toxicity is delayed bone marrow suppression, monitor blood counts weekly for 6 or more weeks after a dose. Do not give courses of lomustine more frequently than every 6 weeks at the recommended dose. (3) Bone marrow toxicity is cumulative. Consider dosage adjustments on the basis of nadir blood counts from prior dosage.■

SIDE EFFECTS

Most Common

N&V, sore mouth/lips/throat, alopecia, lethargy, ataxia, disorientation, bone marrow suppression.

See *Antineoplastic Agents* for a complete list of possible side effects. Also, High incidence of N&V 3–6 hr after administration and lasting for 24 hr. Renal

---

and pulmonary toxicity. Dysarthria. Delayed bone marrow suppression may occur due to cumulative bone marrow toxicity. **Thrombocytopenia and leukopenia may lead to bleeding and overwhelming infections.** Secondary malignancies.

LABORATORY TEST CONSIDERATIONS
↑ LFTs (reversible).

HOW SUPPLIED
Capsules: 10 mg, 40 mg, 100 mg; *Dose Pack:* 2–100 mg capsules, 2–40 mg capsules, and 2–10 mg capsules.

DOSAGE
• **CAPSULES**
Metastatic brain tumors; secondary therapy in Hodgkin's disease.
Adults and children, initial: 130 mg/m^2 as a single dose q 6 weeks. If bone marrow function is reduced, decrease dose to 100 mg/m^2 q 6 weeks. Subsequent dosage based on blood counts of clients (platelet count above 100,000/mm^3 and leukocyte count above 4,000/mm^3). Undertake weekly blood tests and do not repeat therapy before 6 weeks.

NURSING CONSIDERATIONS

ADMINISTRATION/STORAGE
1. Store below 40°C (104°F).
2. Given alone or in combination with other drugs, surgery, or XRT.

ASSESSMENT
1. Note reasons for therapy, onset, other agents/therapies trialed, outcome.
2. Monitor CBC; causes platelet and leukocyte suppression. Nadir: 3–7 weeks.

CLIENT/FAMILY TEACHING
1. Medication comes in capsules of three strengths and a combination of capsules will make up the correct dose in the dose pack; take all at one time.
2. May have N&V up to 36 hr after treatment; may be followed by 2–3 days of anorexia. Take antiemetics as prescribed. GI distress may be reduced by taking antiemetics before drug therapy or by taking the drug after fasting.
3. Report feelings of depression caused by prolonged N&V so that various antiemetics can be tried and to ensure that psychological support is available as needed.
4. Report abnormal bruising or bleeding, sore throat, or S&S of flu.
5. Avoid all OTC agents.
6. Six-week intervals are needed between doses for optimum effect with minimal toxicity; hematologic profiles should be assessed weekly.

OUTCOMES/EVALUATE
Control/remission of metastatic processes

Loperamide hydrochloride
(loh-**PER**-ah-myd)

CLASSIFICATION(S):
Antidiarrheal
PREGNANCY CATEGORY: B
OTC: Diar-aid Caplets, Imodium, Imodium A-D Caplets, K-Pek II, Kaopectate II Caplets, Maalox Anti-Diarrheal Caplets, Neo-Diaral, Pepto Diarrhea Control.
Rx: Imodium.
✦**OTC:** Apo-Loperamide, Novo-Loperamide, PMS-Loperamide Hydrochloride, Rhoxal-Loperamide, Riva-Loperamide.

USES
Rx: (1) Symptomatic relief of acute non-specific diarrhea and of chronic diarrhea associated with inflammatory bowel disease. (2) Decrease the volume of discharge from ileostomies.
OTC: Control symptoms of diarrhea, including traveler's diarrhea. *Investigational:* With trimethoprim-sulfamethoxazole to treat traveler's diarrhea.

ACTION/KINETICS
Action
Slows intestinal motility by acting on the nerve endings and/or intramural ganglia embedded in the intestinal wall. The prolonged retention of the feces in the intestine results in reducing the volume of the stools, increasing viscosity, and decreasing fluid and electrolyte loss. Reportedly more effective than diphenoxylate.

Pharmacokinetics

Time to peak effect, capsules: 5 hr;
PO solution: 2.5 hr. **t½:** 9.1–14.4 hr.
Twenty-five percent excreted unchanged in the feces.

CONTRAINDICATIONS

In clients in whom constipation should be avoided. OTC if body temperature is over 38°C (101°F) and in presence of bloody diarrhea. Use in acute diarrhea associated with organisms that penetrate the intestinal mucosa, such as *E. coli*, *Salmonella*, and *Shigella*.

SPECIAL CONCERNS

Safe use in children under age 2 and during lactation has not been established. Fluid and electrolyte depletion may occur in clients with diarrhea. Children under age 3 are more sensitive to the narcotic effects of loperamide.

SIDE EFFECTS

Most Common

Abdominal pain/distention/discomfort, constipation, dry mouth, N&V, epigastric distress, dizziness, drowsiness.

GI: Abdominal pain, distention, or discomfort. Constipation, dry mouth, N&V, epigastric distress. Toxic megacolon in clients with acute colitis. **CNS:** Drowsiness, dizziness, fatigue. **Miscellaneous:** Allergic skin rashes.

OD **OVERDOSE MANAGEMENT**

Symptoms: Constipation, CNS depression, GI irritation. *Treatment:* Give activated charcoal (it will reduce absorption up to ninefold). If vomiting has not occurred, perform gastric lavage followed by activated charcoal, 100 grams, through a gastric tube. Give naloxone for respiratory depression.

DRUG INTERACTIONS

Ritonavir / ↑ Loperamide AUC and peak plasma levels
Saquinavir / ↑ Loperamide levels and ↓ saquinavir levels perhaps R/T ↓ saquinavir absorption

HOW SUPPLIED

Capsules: 2 mg; *Liquid:* 1 mg/1 mL, 1 mg/5 mL, 1 mg/7.5 mL; *Tablets:* 2 mg.

DOSAGE

• **RX: CAPSULES**

Acute diarrhea.

Adults, initial: 4 mg, followed by 2 mg after each unformed stool, up to maximum of 16 mg/day. **Pediatric:** *Day 1 doses:* **8–12 years:** 2 mg 3 times per day; **6–8 years:** 2 mg twice a day; **2–5 years:** 1 mg 3 times per day using only the liquid. *After day 1:* 1 mg/10 kg after a loose stool (total daily dosage should not exceed day 1 recommended doses).

Chronic diarrhea.

Adults: 4–8 mg/day as a single or divided dose. Dosage not established for chronic diarrhea in children.

• **OTC: CAPSULES, LIQUID, TABLETS**

Acute diarrhea.

Adults: 4 mg after the first loose bowel movement (LBM) followed by 2 mg after each subsequent bowel movement to a maximum of 8 mg/day for no more than 2 days. **Pediatric, 9–11 years:** 2 mg after the first LBM followed by 1 mg after each subsequent LBM, not to exceed 6 mg/day for no more than 2 days. **Pediatric, 6–8 years:** 1 mg after the first bowel movement followed by 1 mg after each subsequent LBM, not to exceed 4 mg/day for no more than 2 days.

NURSING CONSIDERATIONS

ASSESSMENT

1. Note reasons for therapy, onset, frequency, characteristics of stools. Identify any contributing/causative factors, i.e., travel, drinking untreated water.
2. Note any experience with this drug or any allergy to piperidine derivatives.
3. Stop drug promptly and report if abdominal distention develops in clients with acute ulcerative colitis.
4. Ensure colonoscopy completed for chronic diarrhea to note etiology.

CLIENT/FAMILY TEACHING

1. May cause a dry mouth; try ice, sugarless gum, and candy to alleviate.
2. Use caution while driving or performing tasks requiring alertness; may cause dizziness/drowsiness.
3. OTC products are not intended for use in children less than 6 years of age unless provider prescribed.
4. Record the number, frequency, and consistency of stools per day and the amount of drug consumed. Report if diarrhea lasts up to 5 days without relief.

Bold Italic = life threatening side effect   ■ = black box warning   ✦ = Available in Canada

5. In *acute diarrhea*, discontinue after 48 hr and report if ineffective.

6. If no improvement within 10 days after using up to 16 mg/day for *chronic diarrhea*, symptoms are not likely to improve with further use. Seek medical intervention.

7. Report if fever, nausea, abdominal pain/distention occurs; may require dosage adjustment.

8. In children, dietary treatment of diarrhea is preferred. Avoid apple juices, formulas, and high fat or spicy foods.

OUTCOMES/EVALUATE
Reduction/Control of diarrhea

Loratidine
(loh-**RAH**-tih-deen)

CLASSIFICATION(S):
Antihistamine, second generation, piperidine

PREGNANCY CATEGORY: B

OTC: Oral Solution: Claritin Allergy Children's, Clear-Atadine Children's. **Syrup:** Alavert Children's, Children's Loratidine Syrup, Claritin, Dimetapp Children's ND Non-Drowsy Allergy, Non-Drowsy Allergy Relief for Kids. **Tablets:** Claritin 24-Hour Allergy, Claritin Hives Relief, Clear-Atadine, Tavist ND. **Tablets, Chewable:** Claritin Children's Allergy. **Tablets, Orally Disintegrating:** Alavert, Claritin RediTabs, Dimetapp Children's ND Non-Drowsy Allergy, Non-Drowsy Allergy Relief, Triaminic Allerchews.

❧**Rx:** Apo-Loratidine, Claritin Kids.

SEE ALSO *ANTIHISTAMINES.*

USES
(1) Relief of nasal and nonnasal symptoms of seasonal allergic rhinitis, including runny nose, itchy and watery eyes, itchy palate, and sneezing. (2) Relief of itching due to hives in adults and children 6 years and older.

ACTION/KINETICS

Action
Metabolized in the liver to active metabolite descarboethoxyloratidine. Low to no sedative and anticholinergic effects; no antiemetic effect. Does not alter cardiac repolarization and has not been linked to development of torsades de pointes as seen with astemizole and terfenadine.

Pharmacokinetics
Onset: 1–3 hr. **Maximum effect:** 8–12 hr. Food delays absorption. $t^{1/2}$, **loratidine:** 8.4 hr; $t^{1/2}$, **descarboethoxyloratidine:** 28 hr. **Duration:** 24 hr. Excreted through both the urine and feces.

CONTRAINDICATIONS
Use in children less than 6 years of age.

SPECIAL CONCERNS
Use with caution, if at all, during lactation. Give a lower initial dose in liver impairment.

SIDE EFFECTS
Most Common
Headache, somnolence, fatigue, dry mouth.

GI: Altered salivation, dry mouth, gastritis, dyspepsia, stomatitis, toothache, thirst, altered taste, flatulence. **CNS:** Headache, somnolence, hypoesthesia, hyperkinesia, migraine, anxiety, depression, agitation, paroniria, amnesia, impaired concentration. **Ophthalmic:** Altered lacrimation, conjunctivitis, blurred vision, eye pain, blepharospasm. **Respiratory:** URTI, epistaxis, pharyngitis, dyspnea, coughing, rhinitis, sinusitis, sneezing, bronchitis, *bronchospasm,* hemoptysis, laryngitis. **Body as a whole:** Fatigue, asthenia, increased sweating, flushing, malaise, rigors, fever, dry skin, aggravated allergy, pruritus, purpura. **Musculoskeletal:** Back/chest pain, leg cramps, arthralgia, myalgia. **GU:** Breast pain, menorrhagia, dysmenorrhea, vaginitis. **Miscellaneous:** Earache, dysphonia, dry hair, urinary discoloration.

HOW SUPPLIED
Oral Solution: 5 mg/5 mL; *Syrup:* 5 mg/5 mL; *Tablets:* 10 mg; *Tablets, Chewable:* 5 mg; *Tablets, Orally Disintegrating:* 5 mg, 10 mg.

DOSAGE
• **ORAL SOLUTION; SYRUP; TABLETS; TABLETS, ORAL DISINTEGRATING; TABLETS, RAPIDLY DISINTEGRATING**
Allergic rhinitis, chronic idiopathic urticaria.

L

Adults and children, 6 and older: 10 mg once daily. *In clients with impaired kidney function (GFR <30 mL/min):* **Adults and children 6 years and older:** 10 mg every other day initially.

NURSING CONSIDERATIONS

ADMINISTRATION/STORAGE

1. Use the syrup or chewable/orally disintegrating tablets for children ages 6 to 11.
2. Use caution. The concentration of the syrup is 5 mg/5 mL.
3. Protect unit dose packs, unit-of-use packs, and rapidly disintegrating tablets from excessive moisture.
4. Store tablets from 2–30°C (36–86°F). Store syrup and rapidly disintegrating tablets from 2–25°C (36–77°F).

ASSESSMENT

1. List reasons for therapy, type, onset, characteristics of S&S. List other agents trialed; outcome.
2. Monitor LFTs; reduce dose with dysfunction. Assess elderly and clients with hepatic and renal impairment for increasing somnolence.
3. Note pulmonary findings; assess throat, cervical nodes, turbinates, skin testing when necessary.
4. Identify triggers contributing to allergic S&S. Advise to remove carpet, enclose mattress and pillows in plastic, control dust, vacuum regularly, remove pets and plants from sleeping area.
5. Review drug profile. Cautiously coadminister with drugs that inhibit hepatic metabolism (i.e., macrolide antibiotics, cimetidine, ranitidine, ketoconazole, or theophylline).

CLIENT/FAMILY TEACHING

1. Take on an empty stomach; food may delay absorption. If stomach upset occurs, can take with food.
2. If using rapidly disintegrating tablets, place under the tongue. Disintegration occurs within seconds, after which the tablet contents may be swallowed with or without water.
3. Use rapidly disintegrating tablets within 6 months of opening the foil pouch and immediately after opening the individual tablet blister.

4. Do not perform activities that require mental alertness until drug effects realized; should not cause drowsiness.
5. Avoid prolonged or excessive exposure to direct or artificial sunlight.
6. Identify triggers, i.e., foods, detergents, or materials that may have induced allergic/itching response. Keep all F/U appointments.

OUTCOMES/EVALUATE

- Relief of nasal congestion and seasonal allergic manifestations
- Control of skin eruption R/T antigenic offender

Lorazepam   IV ©
(lor-**AYZ**-eh-pam)

CLASSIFICATION(S):
Antianxiety drug, benzodiazepine
PREGNANCY CATEGORY: D
Rx: Ativan, Lorazepam Intensol, **C-IV**
🍁**Rx:** Apo-Lorazepam, Novo-Lorazem, Nu-Loraz.

SEE ALSO *TRANQUILIZERS/ ANTIMANIC DRUGS/HYPNOTICS.*

USES

PO: Short-term relief of anxiety disorders or symptoms of anxiety with depression. *Investigational:* Short-term improvement of chronic insomnia.
    Parenteral: (1) Preanesthetic medication to produce sedation, relief of anxiety, and a decreased ability to recall events related to surgery. (2) Status epilepticus.

ACTION/KINETICS

Action

Reduces anxiety by increasing or facilitating the inhibitory neurotransmitter activity of GABA.

Pharmacokinetics

Absorbed and eliminated faster than other benzodiazepines. **Peak plasma levels, PO:** 1–6 hr; **IM:** 1–1.5 hr. **t½:** 10–20 hr. Metabolized to inactive compounds, which are excreted through the kidneys.

ADDITIONAL CONTRAINDICATIONS

Narrow-angle glaucoma. Parenterally in children less than 18 years.

Bold Italic = life threatening side effect   ■ = black box warning   🍁 = Available in Canada

SPECIAL CONCERNS

PO dosage has not been established in children less than 12 years of age and IV dosage has not been established in children less than 18 years of age. Use cautiously in presence of renal and hepatic disease.

SIDE EFFECTS

Most Common

Drowsiness (transient), ataxia, confusion.

See *Tranquilizers/Antimanic Drugs/Hynpotics* for a complete list of possible side effects.

ADDITIONAL DRUG INTERACTIONS

With parenteral lorazepam, scopolamine → sedation, hallucinations, and behavioral abnormalities

HOW SUPPLIED

Injection: 2 mg/mL, 4 mg/mL; *Oral Solution, Concentrated:* 2 mg/mL; *Tablets:* 0.5 mg, 1 mg, 2 mg.

DOSAGE

- **ORAL CONCENTRATE; TABLETS**
  Anxiety.

Adults, initial: 2–3 mg/day given 2 or 3 times per day. Dose range varies from 1 to 10 mg/day given in divided doses.

Insomnia due to anxiety or transient situational stress.
Single dose of 2–4 mg at bedtime.

- **IM**
  Preanesthetic.

0.05 mg/kg, up to a maximum of 4 mg. For optimum effect, give at least 2 hr before surgical procedure. Administer narcotic analgesics at their usual preoperative time.

- **IV**
  Status epilepticus.

Adults, 18 years and older, usual: 4 mg given slowly (2 mg/min). If seizures continue or recur after a 10–15-min period, an additional 4 mg IV may be given slowly.

Preanesthetic.
Initial: 2 mg total or 0.044 mg/kg (whichever is smaller). This will sedate most adults. Do not exceed dose in clients over 50 years of age. Doses as high as 0.05 mg/kg (up to a total of 4 mg) may be given if a greater lack of recall is desired. For optimum effect, give 15–20 min prior to procedure.

NURSING CONSIDERATIONS

ⓖ Do not confuse lorazepam (Ativan) with alprazolam (Xanax) or with hydroxyzine (Atarax), each of which is an antianxiety agent.

ADMINISTRATION/STORAGE

1. Individualize dosage. If higher doses required, increase evening dose before the daytime doses. Increase gradually to minimize side effects.

2. For the elderly or debilitated, start with 1–2 mg/day of tablet or solution in divided doses. Adjust dose as needed and tolerated. When higher doses are needed, increase the evening dose before the daytime dose.

3. Intensol product is a concentrated PO solution. Mix with liquid or semi-solid foods such as water, juices, soda or soda-like beverages, applesauce, or puddings.

4. Use only the calibrated dropper provided with the Intensol solution. Draw prescribed amount into the dropper; squeeze contents onto the liquid or semi-solid food and stir gently for a few seconds. Consume entire amount of the mixture immediately. Do not store for future use.

5. For IM, inject deep into muscle mass.

6. IM administration is not recommended for status epilepticus as therapeutic levels may not be reached as quickly as with IV. IM can be used when an IV port is not available.

7. Reduce dose of lorazepam by 50% when given with probenecid or valproate.

8. It may be necessary to increase dose of lorazepam in females who are also taking oral contraceptives.

9. Refrigerate injection and oral solution from 2–8°C (36–46°F). Protect from light.

10. Store tablets at controlled room temperature from 15–30°C (59–86°F). Protect from moisture.

ⅣⅤ 11. For IV use, dilute just before use with equal amounts of either sterile water, NaCl, or 5% dextrose injection. Do not shake vigorously; will result in air entrapment.

📷 = see color insert   H = Herbal   ⅣⅤ = Intravenous   ⓖ = sound alike drug

12. Inject directly into tubing of an existing IV infusion.

13. Do not exceed 2 mg/min IV. Have available equipment to maintain a patent airway.

14. Do not use if solution is discolored or contains a precipitate.

ASSESSMENT

1. Note reasons for therapy, onset, characteristics of S&S. Assess mental status; describe anxiety symptoms, any associated factors/triggers.

2. List other agents trialed, outcome. Monitor CBC, renal and LFTs.

3. Determine if psychological evaluation/counselling has been initiated.

4. Check for sleep apnea, severe respiratory conditions that may preclude therapy. Avoid with narrow angle glaucoma.

CLIENT/FAMILY TEACHING

1. Take as directed; report loss of effectiveness. Do not share meds.

2. May cause dizziness, drowsiness, loss of recall; use with caution until drug effects realized.

3. Report increased depression or suicidal ideations.

4. Avoid alcohol and CNS depressants.

5. With long-term therapy, do not stop suddenly; must be tapered to prevent withdrawal symptoms. Keep all F/U appointments to evaluate response and need to continue.

OUTCOMES/EVALUATE

- ↓ Anxiety ↓ Insomnia
- Termination of seizures
- Control of alcohol withdrawal
- Muscle relaxation/amnesia

Losartan potassium

(loh-**SAR**-tan)

CLASSIFICATION(S):

Antihypertensive, angiotensin II receptor blocker

PREGNANCY CATEGORY: C (first trimester), **D** (second and third trimesters).

Rx: Cozaar.

SEE ALSO *ANGIOTENSIN II RECEPTOR ANTAGONISTS* AND *ANTIHYPERTENSIVE AGENTS*.

USES

(1) Antihypertensive, alone or in combination with other antihypertensive drugs (including diuretics). (2) Reduce risk of stroke in clients with hypertension and left ventricular hypertrophy. Is evidence this use does not apply to African American clients. (3) Nephropathy in type 2 diabetics.

ACTION/KINETICS

Action

Competitively blocks the angiotensin AT_1 receptor located in vascular smooth muscle and the adrenal glands, thus blocking the vasoconstrictor and aldosterone-secreting effects of angiotensin II (a potent vasoconstrictor). Thus, BP is reduced.

Pharmacokinetics

Undergoes significant first-pass metabolism (by CYP2C9 and CYP3A4) in the liver, where it is converted to an active carboxylic acid metabolite that is responsible for most of the angiotensin receptor blockade. About 33% is bioavailable. Rapidly absorbed after PO administration, although food slows absorption. **Peak plasma levels of losartan and metabolite:** 1 hr and 3–4 hr, respectively. When used alone, decrease in BP in African Americans was less than in Non-African Americans. **$t\frac{1}{2}$, losartan:** 2 hr; **$t\frac{1}{2}$, metabolite:** 6–9 hr. **Maximum effects:** 1 week (3 to 6 weeks in some clients). Drug and metabolites are excreted through both the urine (35%) and feces (60%). **Plasma protein binding:** 98.7% of the drug and 99.8% of the metabolite.

CONTRAINDICATIONS

Use during second and third trimesters of pregnancy due to possible injury and death to developing fetus. Use in children less than 6 years of age or in children with a GFR <30 mL/min/1.73m².

SPECIAL CONCERNS

■ When used during the second and third trimester of pregnancy, drugs that act directly on the renin-angiotensin system can cause injury and even death to the developing fetus. When pregnan-

---

Bold Italic = life threatening side effect   ■ = black box warning   ✤ = Available in Canada

cy is detected, discontinue as soon as possible.■ In severe CHF there is a risk of oliguria and/or progressive azotemia with acute renal failure and/or death (which are rare). In those with unilateral or bilateral renal artery stenosis, there is a risk of increased serum creatinine or BUN. Lower doses are recommended in those with hepatic insufficiency.

SIDE EFFECTS

Most Common

URTI, dizziness, cough, diarrhea, sinus disorder, nasal congestion, dyspepsia/heartburn, pain.

GI: Diarrhea, dyspepsia, anorexia, constipation, dental pain, dry mouth, flatulence, gastritis, vomiting, taste perversion. **CV:** Angina pectoris, second-degree AV block, vasculitis, ***CVA, MI, ventricular tachycardia, ventricular fibrillation,*** hypotension, palpitation, sinus bradycardia, tachycardia, orthostatic effects. **CNS:** Dizziness, insomnia, anxiety, anxiety disorder, ataxia, confusion, depression, abnormal dreams, hypesthesia, decreased libido, impaired memory, migraine, nervousness, paresthesia, peripheral neuropathy, panic disorder, sleep disorder, somnolence, tremor, vertigo. **Respiratory:** URTI, cough, nasal congestion, sinus disorder, sinusitis, dyspnea, bronchitis, pharyngeal discomfort, epistaxis, rhinitis, respiratory congestion. **Musculoskeletal:** Muscle cramps, myalgia, joint swelling, musculoskeletal pain, stiffness, arthralgia, arthritis, fibromyalgia, muscle weakness; pain in the back, legs, arms, hips, knees, shoulders. **Dermatologic:** Alopecia, dermatitis, dry skin, ecchymosis, erythema, flushing, photosensitivity, pruritus, rash, sweating, urticaria. **GU:** Impotence, nocturia, urinary frequency, UTI. **Ophthalmic:** Blurred vision, burning/stinging in the eye, conjunctivitis, decrease in visual acuity. **Miscellaneous:** Gout, anemia, tinnitus, facial edema, fever, syncope, pain.

LABORATORY TEST CONSIDERATIONS

Minor ↑ BUN, serum creatinine. Occasional ↑ liver enzymes and/or serum bilirubin. Small ↓ H&H.

OD OVERDOSE MANAGEMENT

Symptoms: Hypotension, tachycardia, bradycardia (due to vagal stimulation). *Treatment:* Supportive treatment. Hemodialysis is not indicated.

DRUG INTERACTIONS

Grapefruit juice / ↓ Liver metabolism of losartan to its active form
Indomethacin / ↓ Antihypertensive effect of losartan
Phenobarbital / ↓ Plasma losartan levels (20%)

HOW SUPPLIED

Tablets: 25 mg, 50 mg, 100 mg.

DOSAGE

- **TABLETS**

Hypertension.

Adults: 50 mg once daily with or without food. Total daily doses range from 25 to 100 mg. In those with possible depletion of intravascular volume (e.g., clients treated with a diuretic), use 25 mg once daily. If the antihypertensive effect (measured at trough) is inadequate, a twice-a-day regimen, using the same dose, may be tried; or an increase in dose may give a more satisfactory result. Range of total daily dose: 25–100 mg. If BP is not controlled by losartan alone, a diuretic (e.g., hydrochlorothiazide, 12.5 mg with losartan, 50 mg once daily) may be added.

Hypertensives with left ventricular hypertrophy.

Initial: 50 mg once daily. Add hydrochlorothiazide, 12.5 mg/day, and/or increase the dose of losartan to 100 mg once daily followed by an increase in hydrochlorothiazide to 25 mg once daily based on BP response.

Nephropathy in type 2 diabetics.

Initial: 50 mg once daily. Increase to 100 mg once daily based on BP response. May be given with insulin and other hypoglycemic drugs.

Pediatric hypertension (age 6 years and older).

Initial: 0.7 mg/kg once daily (up to 50 mg total) given as a tablet or suspension. Adjust dose according to BP response. Doses above 1.4 mg/kg (or in excess of 100 mg) daily have not been evaluated in children.

L

NURSING CONSIDERATIONS

⊕ Do not confuse Cozaar with Zocor (an antihyperlipidemic) or with Hyzaar (combination of losartan potassium and hydrochlorothiazide).

ADMINISTRATION/STORAGE

1. No initial dosage adjustment is needed for the elderly or for those with renal impairment, including those on dialysis.

2. To prepare 200 mL of a 2.5 mg/mL suspension, add 10 mL of purified water to a 240 mL (8 oz) amber polyethylene terephthalate bottle containing ten 50 mg losartan tablets. Immediately shake for at least 2 min. Let the concentrate stand for 1 hr and then shake for 1 min to disperse the tablet contents. Separately prepare a 50/50 volumetric mixture of Ora-Plus and Ora-Sweet SF. Add 190 mL of the 50/50 Ora-Plus/Ora-Sweet SF mixture to the tablet and water slurry and shake for 1 min to disperse the ingredients. Refrigerate the suspension; can be stored for up to 4 weeks. Shake the suspension prior to each use and return promptly to the refrigerator.

3. Store from 15–30°C (59–86°F) and protect from light. Keep container tightly closed.

ASSESSMENT

1. List reasons for therapy, onset, other agents used, other related conditions (diabetes, low EF), outcome.

2. Monitor CBC, microalbumin, renal and LFTs. Correct any volume depletion prior to using to prevent sympathomimetic hypotension. Reduce starting dose with volume depletion or renal/hepatic impairment. Observe for S&S of fluid or electrolyte imbalance.

3. When pregnancy is detected, discontinue as soon as possible.

CLIENT/FAMILY TEACHING

1. Take as directed with or without food. Do not take with grapefruit juice. Avoid any OTC agents unless directed.

2. Regular exercise, proper low-salt diet, and lifestyle changes (i.e., no smoking, low alcohol, low-fat diet, low stress, adequate rest) may also contribute to enhanced BP control. Avoid salt substitutes containing potassium; may cause high potassium levels with this drug.

3. Do not change positions suddenly, dangle legs before rising, and rest until symptoms subside to prevent low BP and dizziness.

4. May cause photosensitivity reaction; avoid prolonged sun exposure and use precautions.

5. Use effective contraception; report immediately if pregnancy is suspected because drug use during second and third trimesters is associated with fetal injury and morbidity. Keep all F/U appointments to evaluate response to therapy and labs.

OUTCOMES/EVALUATE

BP control; Cardiac/renal protection

—— COMBINATION DRUG ——

Losartan potassium and Hydrochlorothiazide
(loh-**SAR**-tan, **hy**-droh-klor-oh-**THIGH**-ah-zyd)

CLASSIFICATION(S):

Antihypertensive (combination of angiotensin II receptor blocker and thiazide diuretic)

PREGNANCY CATEGORY: C (first trimester), **D** (second and third trimesters).

Rx: Hyzaar.

SEE ALSO *LOSARTAN POTASSIUM AND HYDROCHLOROTHIAZIDE*

USES

(1) Hypertension. Not indicated for initial therapy, except when hypertension is severe enough that the value of achieving prompt BP control exceeds the risk of initiating combination therapy. (2) Reduce risk of stroke in those with hypertension and left ventricular hypertrophy. Is evidence this benefit does not apply to Black clients.

CONTENT

Hyzaar 50–12.5 contains losartan (*antiotensin II receptor blocker*), 50 mg, and

---

Bold Italic = life threatening side effect   ■ = black box warning   ✤ = Available in Canada

hydrochlorothiazide (*thiazide diuretic*), 12.5 mg. Hyzaar 100–12.5 contains losartan, 100 mg, and hydrochlorothiazide, 12.5 mg. Hyzaar 100–25 contains losartan, 100 mg, and hydrochlorothiazide, 25 mg.

ACTION/KINETICS

Action

Losartan competitively blocks the angiotensin AT_1 receptor located in vascular smooth muscle and the adrenal glands, thus blocking the vasoconstrictor and aldosterone-secreting effects of angiotensin II (a potent vasoconstrictor). Thus, BP is reduced. Hydrochlorothiazide promotes the excretion of sodium and chloride, and thus water, by the distal renal tubule. Also increases excretion of potassium and to a lesser extent bicarbonate. The antihypertensive activity is thought to be due to direct dilation of the arterioles, as well as to a reduction in the total fluid volume of the body and altered sodium balance.

Pharmacokinetics

Losartan undergoes significant first-pass metabolism (by CYP2C9 and CYP3A4) in the liver, where it is converted to an active carboxylic acid metabolite that is responsible for most of the angiotensin receptor blockade. About 33% is bioavailable. Rapidly absorbed after PO administration, although food slows absorption. **Peak plasma levels of losartan and metabolite:** 1 hr and 3–4 hr, respectively. **t½, losartan:** 2 hr; **t½, metabolite:** 6–9 hr. **Maximum effects:** 1 week (3 to 6 weeks in some clients). Drug and metabolites are excreted through both the urine (35%) and feces (60%). Hydrochlorothiazide, **onset:** 2 hr; **peak effect:** 4–6 hr; **duration:** 6–12 hr. **t½:** 5.6–14.8 hr. Hydrochlorothiazide is not metabolized but is eliminated rapidly by the kidney.

CONTRAINDICATIONS

Hypersensitivity to any components of the product. In those with anuria or hypersensitivity to other sulfonamide-derived drugs. Not recommended for use during pregnancy or lactation. Not recommended for use in those with hepatic impairment who require titration with losartan (the lower starting dose of losartan recommended for use in such clients can not be given using Hyzaar). Use with lithium.

SPECIAL CONCERNS

■ When used during the second and third trimester of pregnancy, drugs that act directly on the renin-angiotensin system can cause injury and even death to the developing fetus. When pregnancy is detected, discontinue as soon as possible.■ Use with caution in impaired hepatic function or progressive liver disease (minor alterations of fluid and electrolyte balance may precipitate hepatic coma). Hypersensitivity reactions to hydrochlorothiazide may occur in those with or without a history of allergy or bronchial asthma (are more likely in clients with such a history). Thiazide diuretics may cause exacerbation or activation of systemic lupus erythematosus. Safety and efficacy have not been determined in children.

SIDE EFFECTS

Most Common

Hypokalemia, dizziness, URTI, cough, back pain, rash, edema/swelling, palpitation.

See *Losartan potassium* and *Hydrochlorothiazide* for a complete list of possible side effects.

OD OVERDOSE MANAGEMENT

Symptoms: **Due to losartan:** Hypotension and tachycardia. Possible bradycardia due to parasympathetic stimulation. **Due to hydrochlorothiazide:** Hypokalemia, hypochloremia, hyponatremia, dehydration. *Treatment:* Supportive treatment. Hemodialysis does not remove losartan.

DRUG INTERACTIONS

See *Losartan potassium* and *Hydrochlorothiazide* for lists of possible drug interactions.

HOW SUPPLIED

See Content.

DOSAGE

- **TABLETS**

  Hypertension.

Individualize. Usual, initial: Losartan, 50 mg once daily (25 mg for those with intravascular volume depletion and in those with a history of hepatic impairment). **Losartan, range:** 25–100 mg

 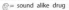

once or twice a day. **Hydrochlorothiazide, usual:** 12.5–50 mg once daily and can be given at doses of 12.5–25 mg as Hyzaar. The usual dose of Hyzaar is one tablet of Hyzaar, 50–12.5 once daily. More than 2 tablets of Hyzaar, 50–12.5 once daily or more than 1 tablet of Hyzaar, 100–25 once daily is not recommended.

Severe hypertension.

Initial: 1 Hyzaar, 50–12.5 tablet once daily. For those who do not respond adequately to the 50–12.5 dose after 2–4 weeks of therapy, the dosage may be increased to Hyzaar, 100–25 once daily (maximum recommended dose).

Hypertension with left ventricular hypertrophy.

Initial: Losartan alone, 50 mg once daily. Add hydrochlorothiazide, 12.5 mg or Hyzaar 50–12.5 if further BP reduction is needed. If additional BP reduction is needed, Hyzaar 100–12.5 may be substituted followed by Hyzaar, 100–25. For further BP reduction, add other antihypertensives.

NURSING CONSIDERATIONS

ℂ Do not confuse Hyzaar with Cozaar (contains only losartan potassium).

ADMINISTRATION/STORAGE

1. In clients who are intravascularly volume-depleted (e.g., those treated with diuretics), symptomatic hypotension may result after initiation of Hyzaar therapy. Correct this condition before administering Hyzaar.

2. To minimize dose-dependent side effects, begin combination therapy only after the client has failed to achieve the desired effect with monotherapy.

3. The maximal antihypertensive effect is reached about 3 weeks after beginning therapy.

4. The usual dosage regimen of Hyzaar may be followed as long as the client's C_{CR} is >30 mL/min. In clients with more severe renal impairment, loop diuretics are preferred to thiazides. Thus, Hyzaar is not recommended for these clients.

ASSESSMENT

1. Note disease onset, other agents trialed/outcome, all co-morbidities, (diabetes, low EF).

2. Monitor VS, EKG, electrolyes, microalbumin, renal and LFTs.

3. Correct any volume depletion prior to using to prevent sympathomimetic hypotension. Reduce starting dose with volume depletion or renal/hepatic impairment. Observe for S&S of fluid or electrolyte imbalance.

4. When pregnancy is detected, discontinue as soon as possible.

CLIENT/FAMILY TEACHING

1. Take as directed once daily with a full glass of water.

2. Avoid activities that may require mental alertness until drug effects realized; may cause dizziness/drowsiness.

3. Ensure adequate hydration; avoid excessive overheating/perspiration.

4. Keep record of BP for provider review. Report unusual or adverse effects.

5. Avoid potassium replacements and high salt diet.

6. Practice reliable contraception; do not use if pregnant.

OUTCOMES/EVALUATE

• Desired BP control
• ↓ Incidence of stroke with LVH

Loteprednol etabonate
(**loh**-teh-**PRED**-nohl)

CLASSIFICATION(S):
Glucocorticoid
PREGNANCY CATEGORY: C
Rx: Alrex, Lotemax.

SEE ALSO CORTICOSTEROIDS.

USES

Alrex (0.2% Suspension): Temporary relief of seasonal allergic conjunctivitis.

Lotemax (0.5% Suspension): (1) Steroid-responsive inflammatory conditions of the palpebral and bulbar conjunctiva, cornea, and anterior segment of the globe (e.g., allergic conjunctivitis, superficial punctuate keratitis, herpes zoster keratitis, acne rosacea, iritis, cyclitis, certain infective conjunctivitis). (2) Treatment of postoperative inflammation after ocular surgery.

Bold Italic = life threatening side effect   ■ = black box warning   ✦ = Available in Canada

ACTION/KINETICS
Action
Rapidly metabolized to inactive compounds by eye esterases. After ocular use, minimal amounts are absorbed.

CONTRAINDICATIONS
Bacterial, fungal, or viral eye infections.

SPECIAL CONCERNS
Use with caution with cataracts, diabetes mellitus, glaucoma, intraocular hypertension, use beyond 10 days. Safety and efficacy have not been determined in children.

SIDE EFFECTS
Most Common
Blurred vision, discharge, burning on instillation, dry eyes.
Ophthalmic: Increased IOP, thinning of sclera or cornea, blurred vision, discharge, dry eyes, burning on instillation.

HOW SUPPLIED
Ophthalmic Suspension: 0.2%, 0.5%.

DOSAGE
- **ALREX OPHTHALMIC SUSPENSION, 0.2%**
  Seasonal allergic conjunctivitis.
1 gtt in the affected eye(s) 4 times per day.
- **LOTEMAX OPHTHALMIC SUSPENSION, 0.5%**
  Steroid-responsive disease.
1–2 gtt into the conjunctival sac of the affected eye 4 times per day. For the first week, dose may be increased to 1 gtt every hour. Do not discontinue prematurely. Re-evaluate if client does not improve after 2 days.
  Postoperative inflammation.
1–2 gtt into the conjunctival sac of the operated eye(s) 4 times per day beginning 24 hr after surgery and continuing for 2 weeks.

NURSING CONSIDERATIONS
ADMINISTRATION/STORAGE
Store upright from 15–25°C (59–77°F). Do not freeze.

ASSESSMENT
Note indications for therapy, symptoms, and related factors (triggers).

CLIENT/FAMILY TEACHING
1. Shake well before use. Instill as directed. Avoid contact of the container tip with the eye or surrounding tissues to prevent infection.
2. Contact lenses may continue to be worn if the drug is used to treat lens-associated giant papillary conjunctivitis. Remove lens prior to each instillation; reinsert 10–15 min later.
3. Report if symptoms do not improve or worsen after 2 days of treatment.
4. When used for steroid responsive disease, do *not* discontinue therapy prematurely.

OUTCOMES/EVALUATE
↓ Eye irritation, inflammation, and allergic S&S

Lovastatin (Mevinolin)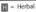
(**LOW**-vah-**STAT**-in, me-**VIN**-oh-lin)

CLASSIFICATION(S):
Antihyperlipidemic, HMG-CoA reductase inhibitor
PREGNANCY CATEGORY: X
Rx: Altoprev, Mevacor.
✤Rx: Apo-Lovastatin, Gen-Lovastatin, ratio-Lovastatin.

SEE ALSO *ANTIHYPERLIPIDEMIC AGENTS— HMG-COA REDUCTASE INHIBITORS.*
USES
Immediate-Release Only: (1) As an adjunct to diet to reduce elevated total and LDL cholesterol in primary hypercholesterolemia (types IIa and IIb) when the response to diet restricted in saturated fat and cholesterol and to other nonpharmacological regimens has been inadequate. (2) As an adjunct to diet to reduce total and LDL cholesterol and apolipoprotein B levels in adolescent boys and girls (who are at least 1 yr postmenarche) and 10–17 years old, with heterozygous familial hypercholesterolemia. Used in those after an adequate trial of diet, the LDL cholesterol remains higher than 189 mg/dL or if LDL cholesterol remains higher than 160 gm/dL *and* there is a positive family

history of premature CV disease or 2 or more CV disease risk factors present.

Extended-Release Only: Adjunct to diet to decrease elevated total and LDL cholesterol, apolipoprotein B, and triglycerides and to increase HDL cholesterol in those with primary hypercholesterolemia (heterozygous familial and nonfamilial and mixed dyslipidemia Fredrickson types IIa and IIb) when response to diet restricted in saturated fat and cholesterol and other nonpharmacological measures have been inadequate.

Immediate-Release or Extended-Release: (1) To slow the progression of coronary atherosclerosis in clients with CAD in order to lower total and LDL cholesterol levels to target levels. (2) Primary prevention of coronary heart disease in those without symptomatic CV disease, average to moderately elevated total cholesterol and LDL cholesterol, and below average HDL cholesterol. Used to reduce risk of MI, unstable angina, and coronary revascularization procedures.

Investigational: Diabetic dyslipidemia, nephrotic hyperlipidemia, familial dysbetalipoproteinemia, and familial combined hyperlipidemia.

ACTION/KINETICS
Action
Competitively inhibits HMG-CoA reductase; this enzyme catalyzes the early rate-limiting step in the synthesis of cholesterol. Thus, cholesterol synthesis is inhibited/decreased. Decreases total cholesterol, triglycerides, LDL, and VLDL and increases HDL.

Pharmacokinetics
Approximately 35% of a dose is absorbed. Extensive first-pass metabolism (by CYP2C9); less than 5% reaches the general circulation. Absorption is decreased by about one-third if the drug is given on an empty stomach rather than with food. **Onset:** Within 2 weeks using multiple doses. **Time to peak plasma levels:** 2–4 hr. **Time to peak effect:** 4–6 weeks using multiple doses. **t½:** 3–4 hr for immediate-release. **Duration:** 4–6 weeks after termination of therapy. Metabolized in the liver (its

main site of action) to active metabolites. Severe renal impairment increases plasma levels. Over 80% of a PO dose is excreted in the feces, via the bile, and approximately 10% is excreted through the urine. **Plasma protein binding:** Over 95%.

ADDITIONAL CONTRAINDICATIONS
Use with mibefradil (Posicor).

SPECIAL CONCERNS
Carefully monitor clients with impaired renal function.

SIDE EFFECTS
Most Common
Headache, diarrhea, flatulence, N&V, abdominal pain/cramps, constipation, dyspepsia, myalgia, back pain, rash/pruritus, flu syndrome, infection, pain.
See *Antihyperlipidemic Agents—HMG-CoA Reductase Inhibitors* for a complete list of side effects. **CNS:** Headache, dizziness, paresthesia, insomnia. **GI:** Flatus (most common), abdominal pain, cramps, diarrhea, constipation, dyspepsia, N&V, heartburn, dysgeusia, acid regurgitation, dry mouth. **Musculoskeletal:** Myalgia, muscle cramps, arthralgia, leg/shoulder pain, localized pain. **Miscellaneous:** Blurred vision, eye irritation, rash, pruritus, chest pain, alopecia.

LABORATORY TEST CONSIDERATIONS
↑ Risk of elevated serum transaminases in clients with homozygous familial hypercholesterolemia.

DRUG INTERACTIONS
Clarithromycin / ↑ Risk of myopathy or rhabdomyolysis R/T ↓ lovastatin elimination R/T inhibition of CYP3A4
Cyclosporine / ↑ Risk of myopathy or rhabdomyolysis, especially if given with higher doses of lovastatin
Danazol / ↑ Risk of myopathy or rhabdomyolysis especially, if given with higher doses of lovastatin
Erythromycin / ↑ Risk of myopathy or rhabdomyolysis R/T ↓ lovastatin elimination R/T inhibition of CYP3A4
Fibrates / ↑ Risk of myopathy
Gemfibrozil / ↑ Risk of myopathy
Grapefruit juice (>1 qt daily) / ↑ Risk of myopathy or rhabdomyolysis R/T ↓ lovastatin elimination R/T inhibition of CYP3A4

HIV protease inhibitors / ↑ Risk of myopathy or rhabdomyolysis R/T ↓ lovastatin elimination R/T inhibition of CYP3A4

Isradipine / ↑ Clearance of lovastatin

Itraconazole / ↑ Risk of myopathy or rhabdomyolysis R/T ↓ lovastatin elimination R/T inhibition of CYP3A4

Ketoconaozle / ↑ Risk of myopathy or rhabdomyolysis R/T ↓ lovastatin elimination R/T inhibition of CYP3A4

Nefazodone / ↑ Risk of myopathy or rhabdomyolysis R/T ↓ lovastatin elimination R/T inhibition of CYP3A4

Niacin/Nicotinic acid / ↑ Risk of myopathy

Telithromycin / ↑ Risk of myopathy or rhabdomyolysis R/T ↓ lovastatin elimination R/T inhibition of CYP3A4

HOW SUPPLIED

Tablets, Extended-Release: 10 mg, 20 mg, 40 mg, 60 mg; *Tablets, Immediate-Release:* 10 mg, 20 mg, 40 mg.

DOSAGE

- **TABLETS, EXTENDED-RELEASE**

  Hyperlipidemia, coronary heart disease, primary prevention of coronary heart disease.

Initial: 20, 40, or 60 mg once a day at bedtime; **range:** 10–60 mg/day in single doses. Start with 10 mg once a day for those requiring small reductions in lipid levels. Adjust dose at intervals of 4 weeks or more.

- **TABLETS, IMMEDIATE-RELEASE**

  Hypercholesterolemia, coronary heart disease, primary prevention of coronary heart disease.

Adults/adolescents, initial: 20 mg once daily with the evening meal. Initiate at 10 mg/day in clients who require smaller reductions. Initiate at 20 mg/day in those requiring reductions in LDL-C of 20% or more. **Dose range:** 10–80 mg (maximum)/day in single or two divided doses. Adjust dose at intervals of every 4 weeks, if necessary. If C_{CR} is less than 30 mL/min, use doses greater than 20 mg/day with caution.

  Adolescents, age 10–17 years, with heterozygous familial hypercholesterolemia.

Dose range: 10–40 mg/day (maximum). Individualize dose depending on goal of therapy. Start clients with 20 mg/day who require decreases in LDL cholesterol of 20% or more to achieve their goal. For those requiring smaller reductions, start with 10 mg/day. Adjust dose at intervals of 4 weeks or more.

NURSING CONSIDERATIONS

ⓒ Do not confuse lovastatin with Lotensin (an ACE inhibitor).

ADMINISTRATION/STORAGE

1. Immediate-release is effective alone or when used together with bile acid sequestrants. Avoid use of extended-release with fibrates or niacin; if such combinations are used, do not exceed a dose of 20 mg/day of lovastatin

2. If lovastatin is used with gemfibrozil, other fibrates, or lipid-lowering doses of niacin (1 gram or more), do not exceed a dose of 20 mg/day of lovastatin R/T increased risk of myopathy.

3. Do not exceed dose of 40 mg/day of lovastatin if taking amiodarone or verapamil. Do not exceed a dose of 20 mg/day of lovastatin if taking cyclosporine R/T increased risk of myopathy.

4. Store immediate-release tablets between 5–30°C (41–86°F) protected from light in a well-closed, light-resistant container. Store extended-release tablets at controlled room temperature of 20–25°C (68–77°F); avoid excess heat and humidity.

ASSESSMENT

1. Note lipid profile, cardiac risk factors, family history, other therapies trialed, outcome.

2. Assess for hepatic disease, heavy alcohol consumption.

3. Determine if pregnant.

4. Request recent eye exam; slight changes have been noted in the lenses of some clients.

5. Assess LFTs q 4–6 weeks for the first 12 mo of therapy. A threefold increase in serum transaminase or new-onset abnormal LFTs is an indication to stop therapy as well as severe myalgia.

6. Assess lifestyle, including weight, diet (intake of fats, CHOs, and proteins), activity (regular exercise), alcohol consumption, smoking history. Identify ar-

eas that may contribute to increased cholesterol levels.

CLIENT/FAMILY TEACHING
1. Take with meals. Avoid coadministration with grapefruit juice due to increased serum levels of lovastatin. Continue cholesterol-lowering diet and exercise program. Cholesterol production by the liver is highest in the evening; usually taken with the evening meal.
2. Follow a standard cholesterol-lowering diet before starting lovastatin and continue during therapy. Adhere to dietary restrictions, daily exercise, and weight loss in the overall management and control of hypercholesterolemia/hyperlipidemia.
3. Practice reliable birth control; drug is pregnancy category X.
4. Report malaise, myalgia, muscle spasms, or fever. These may be mistaken for the flu, but could be serious side effects of drug therapy.
5. Keep all F/U appointments for labs and to evaluate response to therapy.
6. Any RUQ abdominal pain or yellowing of eyes, skin, stools should be reported.
7. Periodic LFTs and eye exams are mandatory; report early visual disturbances.

OUTCOMES/EVALUATE
• ↓ LDL and total cholesterol levels
• ↓ Progression of coronary atherosclerosis

Lubiprostone
(loo-bi-**PROS**-tone)

CLASSIFICATION(S):
Drug for chronic idiopathic constipation.
PREGNANCY CATEGORY: C
Rx: Amitiza, **C-IV**

USES
Treatment of chronic idiopathic constipation in adults.
ACTION/KINETICS
Action
Lubiprostone is a locally acting chloride channel activator that enhances a chloride-rich intestinal fluid secretion without changing sodium and potassium serum levels. By increasing intestinal fluid secretion the drug increases intestinal motility, thereby increasing the passage of stool and alleviating symptoms associated with chronic idiopathic constipation. The main site of action appears to be the luminal portion of the GI epithelium.
Pharmacokinetics
Low systemic availability prevents determination of plasma levels. Rapidly and extensively metabolized in the liver by carbonyl reductase. Excreted in the urine (60%) and feces (30%). **t½:** 0.9–1.4 hr. **Plasma protein binding:** About 94% bound to plasma proteins.
CONTRAINDICATIONS
Hypersensitivity to any component of the product. Use in those with a history of mechanical GI obstruction. Decide whether to discontinue breast-feeding or the drug, taking into account the importance of the drug to the mother.
SPECIAL CONCERNS
Lubiprostone has not been studied in children.
SIDE EFFECTS
Most Common
Fatigue, dizziness, headache, hypesthesia, abdominal discomfort/pain, diarrhea, flatulence, N&V, UTI, back pain, retching, dyspnea, sinusitis, URTI, chest discomfort, peripheral edema.
GI: Abdominal discomfort/distension/pain, lower/upper abdominal pain, constipation, diarrhea, dry mouth, dyspepsia, flatulence, viral gastroenteritis, GERD, loose stools, N&V, stomach discomfort, abnormal bowel sounds, dysgeusia, fecal incontinence, frequent bowel movements, retching, watery stools. **CNS:** Anxiety, depression, dizziness, fatigue, headache, hypesthesia, insomnia, nervousness, paresthesia, syncope, tremor, vertigo. **CV:** Hypertension, flushing, palpitations, vasovagal episode. **GU:** UTI. **Musculoskeletal:** Arthralgia, back pain, muscle cramps, pain in extremities. **Respiratory:** Bronchitis, cough, dyspnea, nasopharyngitis, pharyngolaryngeal pain, sinusitis, URTI, asthma, painful respiration, throat tightness.

Body as a whole: Peripheral edema, influenza, pyrexia, viral infection, asthenia, malaise, pain, rigors, flushing/hot flashes, pallor, hyperhidrosis. **Miscellaneous:** Chest discomfort/pain, decreased appetite/anorexia, skin irritation.

HOW SUPPLIED
Capsules: 24 mcg.

DOSAGE
- **CAPSULES**
  Chronic idiopathic constipation.

Adults: 24 mcg twice a day with food. Periodically assess the need for continued therapy.

NURSING CONSIDERATIONS
ASSESSMENT
1. Note onset, duration, reasons for therapy, other agents trialed.
2. List drugs prescribed/consumed including herbals to ensure none interact.
3. Assess for bowel obstruction/blockage history, diarrhea, pregnancy, breast feeding, renal or liver dysfunction; precludes drug therapy.
4. Check for bowel sounds and palpate abdomen. Note bowel patterns, fluid intake, diet, and activity levels.

CLIENT/FAMILY TEACHING
1. Take as directed with food; do not double up if dose missed.
2. Drug works by increasing fluid secretion in the intestine, which increases intestinal muscle movement and helps the stool to pass.
3. May cause dizziness. Do not drive or perform activities that require mental alertness until drug effects realized. Using Lubiprostone alone, with certain other medicines, or with alcohol may lessen your ability to drive or perform other potentially dangerous tasks.
4. Back pain, diarrhea, dizziness, gas, heartburn, headache, N &/or V, stomach pain/upset, bloating or tiredness may occur; report if bothersome.
5. Practice reliable contraception; stop drug and report if pregnancy suspected-may cause fetal harm.
6. Review importance of diet, fluid intake, and regular daily exercise.

OUTCOMES/EVALUATE
Relief of chronic constipation

Lutropin alfa
(**LOO**-troe-pin alfa)

CLASSIFICATION(S):
Gonadotropin
PREGNANCY CATEGORY: X
Rx: Luveris.

USES
Given with follitropin alfa for stimulation of follicular development in infertile, hypogonadotropic, hypogonadal women with profound luteinizing hormone deficiency (<1.2 units/mL).

ACTION/KINETICS
Action
The physicochemical, immunological, and biological activities of lutropin alfa are comparable with those of human pituitary LH. During the follicular phase in the ovaries, LH stimulates theca cells to secrete androgens that will be used as the substrate by granulosa cell aromatase enzyme to synthesize estradiol (that supports FSH-induced follicular development). Lutropin alfa is given with follitropin alfa to stimulate development of a potentially competent follicle and to prepare, indirectly, the reproductive tract for implantation and pregnancy.

Pharmacokinetics
Peak serum levels after SC: 4–16 hr. **$t^{1}/_{2}$, terminal, after SC:** About 18 hr.

CONTRAINDICATIONS
Contraindicated in women who manifest the following; (1) Prior hypersensitivity to hLH preparations or their excipients. (2) Primary ovarian failure. (3) Uncontrolled thyroid or adrenal dysfunction. (4) Uncontrolled organic intracranial lesion, such as pituitary tumor. (5) Abnormal uterine bleeding of undetermined origin. (6) Ovarian cyst or enlargement of undetermined origin. (7) Sex-hormone dependent tumors of the reproductive tract and accessory organs. (8) Pregnancy. Not indicated for use in children; safety and efficacy have not been determined in children.

L

SPECIAL CONCERNS

The safety and efficacy of concomitant administration of lutropin alfa with any other preparation of recombinant human FSH or urinary human FSH is unknown. There is the potential risk of multiple births. Use with caution during lactation.

SIDE EFFECTS

Most Common

Abdominal pain, breast pain (females), ovarian cyst, headache, flatulence, injection site reaction, URTI, pain, diarrhea, dysmenorrhea, ovarian hyperstimulation.

GI: Abdominal pain, flatulence, diarrhea, nausea, constipation. **Miscellaneous:** Headache, injection site reaction, pain, fatigue, URTI. **GU:** Ovarian cyst, ovarian disorder, dysmenorrhea, breast pain, spontaneous abortion, ectopic pregnancy, premature labor, postpartum fever, congenital abnormalities. Overstimulation of the ovary resulting in mild to moderate uncomplicated ovarian enlargement which may be accompanied by abdominal distention/pain. **Ovarian hyperstimulation syndrome:** Increase (dramatic) in vascular permeability with rapid accumulation of fluid in the peritoneal cavity, thorax, and potentially the pericardium. Early warning signs include: Severe pelvic pain, N&V, weight gain. Symptoms of syndrome: Abdominal pain/distension, N&V, diarrhea, severe ovarian enlargement, weight gain, dyspnea, oliguria. Also, hypovolemia, hemoconcentration, electrolyte imbalances, ascites, hemoperitoneum, pleural effusions, hydothorax, *acute pulmonary distress, thromboembolic events*. **From menotropins:** Adnexal torsion, pulmonary and vascular complications, congenital abnormalities, mild to moderate ovarian enlargement.

HOW SUPPLIED

Powder for Injection, Lyophilized: 82.5 units/vial.

DOSAGE

• **SC**

Follicle stimulation.

Initial treatment cycle: Lutropion alfa, 75 units, given with follitropin alfa (Go-nal-F), 75–150 units, as 2 separate injections. Administer both drugs daily until adequate follicular development is indicated by ovary ultrasonography and serum estradiol. Duration of treatment: Do not exceed 14 days unless signs of imminent follicular development are present. To complete follicular development and effect ovulation in the absence of an endogenous LH surge, give human chorionic gonadotropin 1 day after the last dose of lutropin alfa and follitropin alfa.

Individualize doses given in subsequent cycles for each client based on the response in the preceding cycle. Doses of follitropin alfa greater than 225 units/day are not routinely recommended. As in the initial cycle, hCG must be given to complete follicular development and induce ovulation.

NURSING CONSIDERATIONS

ADMINISTRATION/STORAGE

1. Withhold hCG treatment if the ovaries are abnormally enlarged or if excessive estradiol production has occurred. If the ovaries are abnormally enlarged or abdominal pain occurs, discontinue treatment with lutropin alfa and follitropin alfa and do not give hCG. Advise the couple not to have intercourse as this may reduce the chances of developing ovarian hyperstimulation syndrome and, should spontaneous ovulation occur, reduce the chances of multiple gestation.

2. To prepare the product for use, dissolve the contents of 1 vial of lutropoin alfa in 1 mL sterile water for injection. Mix gently; do not shake. Give the entire contents of each vial SC as separate injections.

3. For single use. Use immediately after reconstitution; discard unused material.

4. Vials may be refrigerated or stored at room temperature (2–25°C; 36–77°F). Protect from light. Store in original package.

ASSESSMENT

1. Note reasons for therapy, other agents trialed, outcome.

2. Ensure drug is monitored and administered through an approved infer-

---

Bold Italic = life threatening side effect   ■ = black box warning   ✦ = Available in Canada

tility clinic/specialist so that all labs and monitoring requirements are performed.

3. Assess for any conditions that may preclude therapy: primary ovarian failure, uncontrolled thyroid/adrenal dysfunction, prior hypersensitivity to hLH preparation or excepients, sex hormone dependent tumors of reproductive tract or accessory organs, abnormal uterine bleeding of unknown origin, uncontrolled organic intracranial lesions such as pituitary tumor, and pregnancy.

4. Dosage will be individualized based on client response to preceding cycle.

5. Assess for abnormally enlarged ovaries if abdominal pain reported (US), and hyperstimulation syndrome and ovulation during the luteal phase.

6. Monitor serum estradiol levels, weight, temperature, BP, CBC, LFTs, electrolytes and fluid status regularly.

CLIENT/FAMILY TEACHING

1. Drug is given with follitropin alfa for stimulation of follicular development in infertile (hypogonadotropic, hypogonadal women with profound luteinizing hormone deficiency) women by several injections daily.

2. Therapy requires a commitment to long-term therapy and frequent lab tests and ultrasounds to monitor condition and progress.

3. Expect to have intercourse daily, beginning on day prior to hCG administration until ovulation confirmed by provider (rise in basal body temperature, increase in serum progesterone, menstruation after a shift in body temperature, or sonographic evidence of ovulation).

4. Record basal body temperatures; report a sudden rise (may indicate ovulation).

5. Immediately report any sudden accumulation of fluid in the belly, chest/pelvic pain, N&V diarrhea, weight gain, SOB, or other unusual effects; requires careful monitoring.

6. May experience ovarian hyperstimulation syndrome, ectopic pregnancy, spontaneous abortion, congenital abnormalities, postpartum fever, premature labor, pulmonary and vascular complications and multiple births. Keep all F/U visits for evaluation of drug response.

OUTCOMES/EVALUATE

Follicular development and ovulation to achieve desired conception

Lymphocyte immune globulin, anti-thymocyte globulin sterile solution (equine) ■ IV

(**LIM**-foh-sight im-**MYOUN GLOH**-byou-lin, an-tih-**THIGH**-moh-sight **GLOH**-byou-lin **EE**-kwine)

CLASSIFICATION(S):
Immunosuppressant
PREGNANCY CATEGORY: C
Rx: Atgam.

USES

(1) Management of allograft rejection in renal transplant clients, given either at the time of rejection or as an adjunct with other immunosuppressants to delay onset of the first rejection episode. (2) Treatment of moderate to severe aplastic anemia in those who are unsuitable for bone marrow transplantation. *Investigational:* As an immunosuppressant in liver, bone marrow, heart, or other organ transplants. Treatment of multiple sclerosis, pure red-cell aplasia, and scleroderma. NOTE: Only physicians with experience in immunosuppressive therapy in treating renal transplant or aplastic anemia should use this drug.

ACTION/KINETICS

Action

Obtained from hyperimmune serum of horses immunized with human thymus lymphocytes. Reduces the number of circulating, thymus-dependent lymphocytes that form rosettes from sheep erythrocytes. Antilymphocytic effect may be due to alteration of the function of T-lymphocytes, which are responsible, in part, for cell-mediated immunity.

Pharmacokinetics

t½, serum: 5.7 days when the drug is given with other immunosuppressants and measured as horse IgG.

CONTRAINDICATIONS

In those who have demonstrated a severe systemic reaction during prior administration of the drug or any other equine gamma globulin preparation.

SPECIAL CONCERNS

■ (1) Only physicians experienced in immunosuppressive therapy in the treatment of renal transplant or aplastic anemia clients should use this drug. (2) Treat clients receiving this drug in facilities equipped and staffed with adequate lab and supportive medical resources.■ A systemic reaction, such as a generalized rash, tachycardia, dyspnea, hypotension, or anaphylaxis, precludes any further administration of the drug. Potency may vary from lot to lot. The possibility of transmission of infectious agents exists. Use with caution during lactation.

SIDE EFFECTS

Most Common

When used for renal transplantation: Fever, chills, leukopenia, rash, pruritus, urticaria, wheal, flare, thrombocytopenia.

When used for aplastic anemia: Chills, arthralgia, headache, myalgia, nausea, chest pain, phlebitis.

General side effects. Whole Body: Fever, chills, systemic or localized infection, malaise, serum sickness, edema, sweating. **GI:** N&V, diarrhea, *GI bleeding or perforation,* sore mouth or throat, epigastric or stomach pain, abdominal pain. **CNS:** Headache, *seizures,* confusion, disorientation, dizziness, faintness, paresthesias. **CV:** Hypertension or hypotension, tachycardia, DVT, thrombophlebitis, CHF, vasculitis, renal artery thrombosis. **Hematologic:** Thrombocytopenia, leukopenia, eosinophilia, neutropenia, granulocytopenia, anemia, lymphadenopathy, aplasia, pancytopenia, hemolysis, hemolytic anemia. **Dermatologic:** Rashes. **Respi-**

ratory: Dyspnea, apnea, cough, *pulmonary edema,* nosebleed. **Musculoskeletal:** Chest/back/flank pain; arthralgia, myalgias, abnormal involuntary movement or tremor, rigidity. **Miscellaneous:** Herpes simplex infection, swelling or redness at infusion site, *anaphylaxis, laryngospasm/edema,* hyperglycemia, *acute renal failure,* viral hepatitis, enlarged or ruptured kidney.

When used for renal transplantation with other immunosuppressants. Whole Body: Fever, chills, weakness or faintness. **CNS:** Headache, dizziness, paresthesia, *seizures.* **GI:** Diarrhea, nausea/vomiting, stomatitis, hiccoughs, epigastric pain, malaise. **Hematologic:** Leukopenia, thrombocytopenia. **Dermatologic:** Rash, pruritus, urticaria, wheal, flare. **CV:** Hypotension, peripheral thrombophlebitis, edema, hypertension, renal artery stenosis, tachycardia. **Musculoskeletal:** Arthralgia, chest or back pain (or both), myalgia. **Respiratory:** Dyspnea, laryngospasm, pulmonary edema. **Miscellaneous:** Clotted AV fistula, pain at infusion site, night sweats, *anaphylaxis,* herpes simplex reactivation, hyperglycemia, iliac vein obstruction, localized infection, lymphadenopathy, serum sickness, systemic infection, *toxic epidermal necrosis,* wound dehiscence.

When used for aplastic anemia with support therapy. Whole Body: Fever, chills, diaphoresis, aches. **GI:** N&V, diarrhea. **CNS:** Headache, agitation, lethargy, listlessness, light-headedness, *seizures,* encephalitis or postviral encephalopathy. **CV:** Chest pain, phlebitis, bradycardia, myocarditis, cardiac irregularity, hypotension, CHF, hypertension. **Hematologic:** Lymphadenopathy, postcervical lymphadenopathy, tender lymph nodes. **Respiratory:** Bilateral pleural effusion, respiratory distress. **Musculoskeletal:** Arthralgia, myalgia, joint stiffness, muscle aches. **Miscellaneous:** Periorbital edema, edema, hepatosplenomegaly, burning soles/palms, foot sole pain, proteinuria, *anaphylaxis.*

Bold Italic = life threatening side effect   ■ = black box warning   ♣ = Available in Canada

LABORATORY TEST CONSIDERATIONS
↑ ALT, AST, alkaline phosphatase, serum creatinine.

DRUG INTERACTIONS
Previously masked reactions to Atgam may appear when the drug is given concomitantly with corticosteroids or other immunosuppressants.

HOW SUPPLIED
Injection: 50 mg horse gamma globulin/mL.

DOSAGE
- **IV ONLY**
  Renal allograft recipients.

Adults: 10–30 mg/kg daily. **Children:** 5–25 mg/kg daily. Usually used concomitantly with azathioprine and corticosteroids. When used to delay the onset of allograft rejection, a fixed dose of 15 mg/kg for 14 days is used; then, the dose is given every other day for 14 days for a total of 21 doses in 28 days. Give the first dose within 24 hr before or after the transplant. When used to treat allograft rejection, the first dose can be delayed until the first rejection episode is diagnosed. **Recommended dose:** 10–15 mg/kg daily for 14 days; additional alternate day therapy can be given for a total of 21 doses.

  Aplastic anemia.
10–20 mg/kg daily for 8–14 days; additional alternate day therapy may be given for a total of 21 doses. Thrombocytopenia can be associated with Atgam use; thus, clients may need prophylactic platelet transfusions to maintain platelets at an acceptable level.

NURSING CONSIDERATIONS
ADMINISTRATION/STORAGE
IV 1. Recommended that clients be skin tested with an intradermal injection of 0.1 mL of a 1:1,000 dilution (5 mcg horse IgG) of Atgam in NaCl and a contralateral NaCl injection. Observe every 15–20 min the first hour after intradermal injection. A local reaction of 10 mm or greater with a wheal or erythema (or both) with or without pseudopod formation and itching or a marked local swelling should be considered a positive test. A systemic reaction such as a generalized rash, tachycardia, dyspnea, hypotension, or anaphylaixs precludes any additional administration.
NOTE: Allergic reactions and anaphylaxis have occurred following negative skin tests.

2. Dilution of Atgam with dextrose injection is not recommended, as low sugar concentrations may cause precipitation.

3. Avoid highly acidic infusion solutions due to the possibility of physical instability over time.

4. The product can be transparent to slightly opalescent, colorless to faintly pink or brown. A slight granular or flaky deposit may form during storage.

5. To avoid excessive foaming and/or denaturation of protein, do not shake either diluted or undiluted Atgam.

6. For IV infusion, dilute in an inverted bottle of sterile vehicle so the undiluted drug does not come in contact with the air inside. Do not exceed a 4 mg/mL concentration; gently rotate or swirl the diluted solution so it is thoroughly mixed. Allow diluted drug to come to room temperature before administration.

7. Administer drug into a vascular shunt, arterial venous fistula, or a high-flow central vein through an in-line filter with a pore size of 0.2–1.0 micron. The filter prevents administration of any insoluble material that may develop during product storage. Use of high-flow veins will minimize development of phlebitis and thrombosis.

8. Do not administer in less than 4 hr.

9. Diluted Atgam is stable for up to 24 hr at concentrations up to 4 mg/mL in 0.9% NaCl, D5W/0.25% NaCl, and D5W/0.45% NaCl. Store diluted solution in the refrigerator. Do not keep diluted form for more than 24 hr (including actual infusion time).

10. Store refrigerated from 2–8°C (36–46°F). Do not freeze; discard if frozen.

ASSESSMENT
1. List type of symptoms, date of transplant, hematologic profile.
2. Administer concomitantly with corticosteroids, antihistamines, and antipy-

retics to help control drug-induced side effects.

3. With repeated treatments, exclude those exhibiting any evidence of a systemic reaction.

4. Monitor ECG, electrolytes, hematologic profile, renal, LFTs.

5. Assess for S&S of infection, and pregnancy. Ensure skin testing has been completed prior to treatment.

INTERVENTIONS

1. Only those experienced with immunosuppressive therapy in treating clients with aplastic anemia or renal transplant should use the drug. Ensure intradermal skin test performed 1 hr before first dose. Observe for evidence of wheal >10 mm; indicates potential for severe systemic reactions. Some clients with negative skin test results have also experienced anaphylaxis.

2. Discontinue if any of the following occurs: (a) symptoms of anaphylaxis, (b) severe and unremitting thrombocytopenia or leukopenia.

3. Observe for evidence of concurrent infection, thrombocytopenia, or leukopenia.

4. Continuously observe for possible allergic reactions. Respiratory distress and pain in the chest, back, or flank may indicate anaphylactoid reaction; stop drug and report.

5. Clients with aplastic anemia may require platelet transfusions during therapy to maintain acceptable platelet levels.

CLIENT/FAMILY TEACHING

1. Drug is used to prevent transplant rejection; close follow-up is required.

2. Report any fever, chills, fatigue, sore throat, chest/flank/back pain, night sweats or adverse side effects.

3. Use effective contraception during treatment and for 12 weeks after completing therapy.

4. Keep all F/U appointments to assess response to therapy and for any adverse effects.

OUTCOMES/EVALUATE

- Interruption of cell-mediated renal allograft rejection
- ↓ Rejection and graft loss
- Hematologic remission

Magnesium sulfate IV

(mag-**NEE**-see-um **SUL**-fayt)

CLASSIFICATION(S):
Anticonvulsant, miscellaneous; and laxative, saline
PREGNANCY CATEGORY: A
Rx: Epsom Salts.

SEE ALSO ANTICONVULSANTS AND LAXATIVES.

USES

Parenteral. (1) Prevention and treatment of seizures in severe pre-eclampsia or eclampsia without producing deleterious CNS depression in mother or infant. (2) To control hypertension, encephalopathy, and convulsions associated with acute nephritis in children. (3) Replacement therapy in Mg deficiency, especially in acute hypomagnesemia accompanied by signs of tetany similar to those seen in hypocalcemia. (4) Added to total parenteral nutrition therapy to correct or prevent hypomagnesemia that may occur during the course of therapy. *Investigational:* (1) As a tocolytic agent to manage premature labor (not a first-line agent). (2) IV use as an adjunct to treat acute exacerbations of moderate to severe asthma in clients who respond poorly to beta agonists. (3) In adults to prevent recurrences of torsades de pointes by suppressing early-after depolarizations.

Oral. Laxative.

ACTION/KINETICS
Action
Magnesium (Mg) is an essential element for muscle contraction, certain

enzyme systems, and nerve transmission. Extracellular fluid levels: 1.5–2.5 mEq/L. Mg depresses the CNS and controls convulsions by blocking release of acetylcholine at the myoneural junction. Also, Mg decreases the sensitivity of the motor end plate to acetylcholine and decreases the excitability of the motor membrane. As a laxative, it acts in the small and large intestine to attract and retain water in the intestinal lumen, increasing intraluminal pressure; also releases cholecystokinin.

Pharmacokinetics
Therapeutic anticonvulsant serum levels: 2.5 or 3–7.5 mEq/L (normal Mg levels: 1.5–2.5 mEq/L). **Onset, IM:** 1 hr; **IV:** immediate. **Duration, IM:** 3–4 hr; **IV:** 30 min. Excreted by the kidneys at a rate proportional to the serum concentration and GFR. **Plasma protein binding:** 30% bound to albumin.

CONTRAINDICATIONS
In the presence of heart block or myocardial damage. In toxemia of pregnancy during the 2 hr prior to delivery.

SPECIAL CONCERNS
Use with caution in clients with renal disease because Mg is removed from the body solely by the kidneys; use in renal disease may cause magnesium intoxication. The elderly may require reduced dosage due to impaired renal function. Magnesium sulfate is compatible with breast feeding.

SIDE EFFECTS
Most Common
Magnesium intoxication when used parenterally (see below for symptoms).
Magnesium intoxication: Cardiac and CNS depression preceding respiratory paralysis, circulatory collapse, depressed reflexes, flaccid paralysis, flushing, hypotension, hypothermia, sweating. **CNS:** Depression. **CV:** Flushing, hypotension, *circulatory collapse, depression of the myocardium*. **Miscellaneous:** Sweating, hypothermia, muscle/flaccid paralysis, CNS depression, *respiratory paralysis*. Suppression of knee jerk reflex can be used to determine toxicity. *Respiratory failure may occur if given after knee jerk reflex disappears*. Hypocalcemia with signs of tetany secondary to Mg sulfate when used for eclampsia.

NOTE: Magnesium toxicity may occur in the newborn especially if the mother has received an IV infusion for more than 24 hr prior to delivery. Elevated Mg levels may persist for up to 7 days in the newborn.

OD **OVERDOSE MANAGEMENT**
Symptoms: Sharp drop in BP and respiratory paralysis. Disappearance of patellar reflex indicates onset of magnesium toxicity. ECG changes include increased PR interval, increased QRS complex, and prolonged QT interval. Heart block and asystole may occur. Other symptoms depend on serum levels with respiratory arrest, asystole, and death possible if serum levels exceed 14 mEq/L. Hypermagnesemia in the newborn, including neuromuscular or respiratory depression. *Treatment:* Artificial respiration and IV calcium salt to antagonize the effects of magnesium. A dose of 5–10 mEq calcium gluconate will usually reverse respiratory depression and heart block. In extreme cases, may need peritoneal dialysis or hemodialysis. Hypermagnesemia in the newborn may require resuscitation and assisted ventilation via endotracheal intubation or intermittent positive pressure ventilation, as well as IV calcium.

DRUG INTERACTIONS
CNS depressants (general anesthetics, sedative-hypnotics, narcotics) / Additive CNS depression
Neuromuscular blocking agents / Possible potentiation of neuromuscular blockade
Streptomycin / ↓ Streptomycin antibiotic activity
Tetracycline / ↓ Tetracycline antibiotic activity
Tobramycin / ↓ Tobramycin antibiotic activity

HOW SUPPLIED
Oral Solutions; Injection: 4% (0.325 mEq/mL), 8% (0.65 mEq/mL), 12.5% (1 mEq/mL), 50% (4 mEq/mL).

DOSAGE
• **IM**
Acute nephritis in children.

20–40 mg/kg as needed to control seizures. Dilute the 50% concentration to a 20% solution and give 0.1–0.2 mL/kg of the 20% solution.

Mild magnesium deficiency.

Adults: 1 g (8.12 mEq; 2 mL of a 50% solution) IM q 6 hr for 4 doses (total of 32.5 mEq/24 hr).

Severe hypomagnesemia.

As much as 3 mEq/kg (0.5 mL of a 50% solution) within 4 hr, if necessary.

• **IV/IM**

Seizures associated with eclampsia.

Initial: 10–14 grams. To initiate therapy, 4 grams Mg sulfate in water for injection or 4–5 grams in 250 mL of D5W or 0.9% NaCl may be given IV. Simultaneously, 4–5 grams may be given IM into each buttock using undiluted 50% Mg sulfate. Alternatively, the initial IV dose of 4 grams may be given by diluting the 50% solution to a 10% or 20% concentration; the diluted solution (40 mL of a 10% solution or 20 mL of a 20% solution) may be given IV over a period of 3–4 hr. After the initial IV dose, 1–2 grams/hr may be given by IV infusion. Subsequent IM doses of 4–5 grams may be injected into alternate buttocks q 4 hr, depending on the presence of the patellar reflex, adequate respiratory function, and absences of signs of Mg toxicity. A serum level of 3–6 mg/dL (2.5–5 mEq/L) is considered optimal for seizure control; do not exceed a total daily dose of 20–40 grams of magnesium sulfate. Continue therapy until paroxysms cease.

• **IV INFUSION**

Hypomagnesemia, severe.

Adults: 5 grams (40 mEq)/L of D5W injection or sodium chloride injection by **slow** infusion over period of 3 hr. Use caution to prevent exceeding renal excretory capacity.

Hyperalimentation.

Adults: 8–24 mEq/day; **infants:** 2–10 mEq/day.

• **ORAL SOLUTION**

Laxative.

Adults and children 12 years and older: 5–10 mL in one-half glass of water. **Children, 6–12 years:** 2.5–5 mL in one-half glass of water.

NURSING CONSIDERATIONS

ADMINISTRATION/STORAGE

1. When used as laxative, dissolve in a glassful of ice water or other chilled fluid to lessen the disagreeable taste.
2. Dilutions for IM: Deep injection of 50% concentrate for adults. Use a 20% solution for children.

[IV] 3. Reserve IV use in eclampsia for immediate control of life-threatening convulsions. Give slowly to avoid producing hypermagnesemia. When given by continuous IV infusion to toxemic mothers, the newborn may show signs of magnesium toxicity. Hypermagnesemia in the newborn may require resuscitation and assisted ventilation via endotracheal intubation, as well as IV calcium.

4. For IV infusion, dilute to a concentration of 20% or less. Generally do not exceed an IV rate of 1.5 mL of a 10% concentration (or its equivalent) per min (150 mg/min), except in severe eclampsia with seizures.

5. Mg sulfate in solution may cause a precipitate when mixed with solutions containing the following: High concentrations of alcohol, alkali carbonates and bicarbonates, alkali hydroxides, arsenates, barium, calcium, clindamycin phosphate, heavy metals, hydrocortisone sodium succinate, phosphates, polymyxin B sulfate, procaine HCl, salicylates, strontium, and tartrates.

ASSESSMENT

1. List reasons for therapy, onset, characteristics of S&S.
2. Evaluate cardiac status, respirations, ECG. Monitor I&O.
3. Note any kidney disease. Assess Mg levels (S&S of toxicity begin at 4 mEq/L) and renal function.
4. With premature labor, continually assess fetal heart rate, intensity and timing of contractions.

INTERVENTIONS

1. Before administering IV check for the following conditions:
• Absent patellar reflexes
• Respirations below 16/min
• Urine output <100 mL in past 4 hr

- Early signs of hypermagnesemia: flushing, sweating, hypotension, or hypothermia
- Past history of heart block or myocardial damage; prolonged PR and widened QRS intervals
2. Adjust dose of CNS depressants.
3. Digitalis toxicity treated with calcium is extremely dangerous and may result in heart block.
4. Do not administer for 2 hr preceding delivery. If mother received continuous IV Mg therapy 24 hr prior to delivery, assess newborn constantly for neurologic and respiratory depression.

CLIENT/FAMILY TEACHING
1. Do not exceed prescribed dose.
2. Ensure well-balanced diet, with increased bulk, increased water intake, and regular daily exercise to promote bowel motility.
3. Report adverse side effects or lack of response.

OUTCOMES/EVALUATE
- Control of seizures
- Mg levels (1.8–3 mEq/L)
- Successful evacuation of stool

Mannitol **IV**
(MAN-nih-tol)

CLASSIFICATION(S):
Diuretic, osmotic
PREGNANCY CATEGORY: C
Rx: Osmitrol, Resectisol.

USES
(1) Diuretic to prevent or treat the oliguric phase of acute renal failure before irreversible renal failure occurs. (2) Decrease ICP and cerebral edema by decreasing brain mass. (3) Decrease elevated intraocular pressure when the pressure cannot be lowered by other means. (4) To promote urinary excretion of toxic substances. (5) As a urinary irrigant to prevent hemolysis and hemoglobin buildup during transurethral prostatic resection or other transurethral surgical procedures. *Investigational:* Prevent hemolysis during cardiopulmonary bypass surgery.

ACTION/KINETICS
Action
Increases the osmolarity of the glomerular filtrate, which decreases the reabsorption of water and increases excretion of sodium and chloride. It also increases the osmolarity of the plasma, which causes enhanced flow of water from tissues into the interstitial fluid and plasma. Thus, cerebral edema, increased ICP, and CSF volume and pressure are decreased.

Pharmacokinetics
Onset, IV: 30–60 min for diuresis and within 15 min for reduction of cerebrospinal and intraocular pressures. **Peak:** 30–60 min. **Duration:** 6–8 hr for diuresis and 4–8 hr for reduction of intraocular pressure. $t^{1/2}$: 15–100 min. Over 90% excreted through the urine unchanged. A test dose is given in clients with impaired renal function or oliguria.

CONTRAINDICATIONS
Anuria, pulmonary edema, severe dehydration, active intracranial bleeding except during craniotomy, progressive heart failure or pulmonary congestion after mannitol therapy, progressive renal damage following mannitol therapy.

SPECIAL CONCERNS
Use with caution during lactation. If blood is given simultaneously with mannitol, add at least 20 mEq of sodium chloride to each liter of mannitol solution to avoid pseudoagglutination. Sudden expansion of the extracellular volume that occurs after rapid IV mannitol may lead to fulminating CHF. Mannitol may obscure and intensify inadequate hydration or hypovolemia.

SIDE EFFECTS
Most Common
Headache, N&V, diarrhea, dry mouth, irritation/pain/swelling at injection site.
Electrolyte: Fluid and electrolyte imbalance, acidosis, loss of electrolytes, dehydration. **GI:** N &/or V, dry mouth, thirst, diarrhea. **CV:** Edema, hypo-/hypertension, increased heart rate, angina-like chest pain, CHF, thrombophlebitis. **At injection site:** Irritation, pain, swelling. **CNS:** Dizziness, headaches, blurred vision, *seizures*. **Miscellaneous:** Pulmo-

nary congestion, marked diuresis, rhinitis, chills, fever, urticaria, pain in arms, skin necrosis.

LABORATORY TEST CONSIDERATIONS
↑ or ↓ Inorganic phosphorus. ↑ Ethylene glycol values because mannitol is oxidized to an aldehyde during test.

OD OVERDOSE MANAGEMENT
Symptoms: Increased electrolyte excretion, especially sodium, chloride, and potassium. Sodium depletion results in orthostatic tachycardia or hypotension and decreased CVP. Potassium loss can impair neuromuscular function and cause intestinal dilation and ileus. If urine flow is inadequate, pulmonary edema or water intoxication may occur. Other symptoms include hypotension, polyuria that rapidly becomes oliguria, stupor, *seizures,* hyperosmolality, and hyponatremia. *Treatment:* Discontinue the infusion immediately and begin supportive measures to correct fluid and electrolyte imbalances. Hemodialysis is effective.

DRUG INTERACTIONS
May cause deafness when used in combination with kanamycin

HOW SUPPLIED
Injection: 5%, 10%, 15%, 20%, 25%; *Irrigation Solution:* 5%.

DOSAGE
• **IV INFUSION ONLY**
 Test dose (oliguria or reduced renal function).
Either 50 mL of a 25% solution, 75 mL of a 20% solution, or 100 mL of a 15% solution infused over 3–5 min. If urine flow is 30–50 mL/hr, therapeutic dose can be given. If urine flow does not increase, give a second test dose; if still no response, client must be reevaluated.
 Prevention of acute renal failure (oliguria).
Adults: 50–100 grams, as a 5–25% solution, given at a rate to maintain urine flow of at least 30–50 mL/hr.
 Treatment of oliguria.
Adults: 50–100 grams of a 15–25% solution.
 Reduction of intracranial pressure and brain mass.

Adults: 1.5–2 grams/kg as a 15–25% solution, infused over 30–60 min.
 Reduction of intraocular pressure.
Adults: 1.5–2 grams/kg as a 20% solution (7.5–10 mL/kg) or as a 15% solution (10–13 mL/kg) given over 30–60 min. When used preoperatively, the dose should be given 1–1.5 hr before surgery to maintain the maximum effect.
 Antidote to remove toxic substances.
Adults: Dose depends on the fluid requirement and urinary output. IV fluids and electrolytes are given to replace losses. If a beneficial effect is not seen after 200 grams mannitol, the infusion should be discontinued.
• **IRRIGATION SOLUTION**
 Urologic irrigation.
Adults: Use as a 2.5% irrigating solution for the bladder (this concentration minimizes the hemolytic effect of water alone).

NURSING CONSIDERATIONS

ADMINISTRATION/STORAGE
IV 1. Use a filter with concentrated mannitol (15%, 20%, and 25%).
2. Concentrations >15% may crystallize. To redissolve, warm bottle in a hot water bath or autoclave; cool to body temperature before administering.
3. Do not add to other IV solutions or mix with other medications.
4. If blood is administered concurrently, add 20 mEq of NaCl to each liter of mannitol to prevent pseudoagglutination.

ASSESSMENT
1. Note reasons for therapy, type/onset/characteristics S&S, underlying cause.
2. List other medications prescribed to ensure none alter drug effects.
3. Note neurologic findings.
4. When used to reduce ICP and brain mass, evaluate circulatory and renal reserve, fluid/electrolyte balance, body weight, total I&O before/after infusion.
5. Assess for S&S of electrolyte imbalances and dehydration; replace as needed. If renal failure or oliguria present, ensure test dose performed (under dosage).

---

6. Monitor VS, I&O. Report S&S of pulmonary edema manifested by dyspnea, cyanosis, rales, frothy sputum or any other adverse event.

CLIENT/FAMILY TEACHING

1. Drug is administered IV to increase water excretion or to decrease intracranial or intraocular (eye) pressures.

2. May experience increased thirst or dry mouth; do not exceed amount of fluid provided.

3. Increased SOB or pain in chest, back, or legs should be reported immediately.

OUTCOMES/EVALUATE

• Desired diuresis with ↓ edema
• ↓ ICP, intraocular pressures

Maraviroc ■

(mare-ah-**VYE**-rock)

CLASSIFICATION(S):
Cellular chemokine receptor antagonist

PREGNANCY CATEGORY: B

Rx: Selzentry.

USES

In combination with other antiretroviral agents to treat adult clients infected only with chemokine receptor 5-tropic HIV-1 detectable, who have evidence of viral replication and HIV-1 strains resistant to multiple antiretroviral agents.

ACTION/KINETICS

Action

Maraviroc selectively binds to the human chemokine receptor CCR5 present on the cell membrane, thus preventing the interaction of HIV-1 gp120 and CCR5 which is necessary for CCR5-tropic HIV-1 to enter cells.

Pharmacokinetics

Peak plasma levels: 0.5-4 hr, depending on the dose. Absolute bioavailability is about 33%. A high fat meal will decrease C_{max} and AUC, although it can be taken with or without food. Plasma levels may be higher in those with impaired hepatic function. Metabolized in the liver by CYP3A. **t½, terminal:** 14-18 hr. Excreted in the feces (76%) and urine (20%). **Plasma protein binding:** About 76%.

CONTRAINDICATIONS

Lactation.

SPECIAL CONCERNS

■ Hepatotoxicity has been reported with maraviroc use. Evidence of a systemic allergic reaction (e.g., eosinophilia or elevated immunoglobulin E, pruritic rash) prior to development of hepatotoxicity may occur. Immediately evaluate clients with signs or symptoms of hepatitis or allergic reactions following use of maraviroc.■ Cross resistance is possible. Use with caution in the elderly, in those with preexisting impaired hepatic or renal function, in those who are coinfected with hepatitis B or C, and in those with a history of postural hypotension or on concomitant antihypertensive medications. The safety, efficacy, and pharmacokinetics have not been determined in children less than 16 years of age; do not use marviroc in this population.

SIDE EFFECTS

Most Common

Abdominal pain, cough, dizziness, postural dizziness, musculoskeletal symptoms, pyrexia, rash, URTI.

CNS: Dizziness/postural dizziness, disturbances in initiating and maintaining sleep, paresthesias, dysesthesias, depressive disorders, disturbances in consciousness, sensory abnormalities, peripheral neuropathies. **GI:** GI and abdominal pains, constipation, dyspeptic signs/symptoms, stomatitis (ulceration). **Hepatic:** Hepatotoxicity with allergic features, cholestatic jaundice, hepatic cirrhosis, *hepatic failure*. **CV:** Vascular hypertensive disorders, *CVA, acute cardiac failure,* coronary artery disease/occlusion, *MI*, myocardial ischemia, unstable angina. **Dermatologic:** Rash, apocrine/eccrine gland disorders, pruritus, folliculitis, dermatitis/eczema, lipodystrophies, benign skin neoplasms. **GU:** Bladder/urethral symptoms, Condyloma acuminatum. **Musculoskeletal:** Musculoskeletal and connective tissue S&S, joint-related S&S, muscle pains, myositis, osteonecrosis, rhabdomyolysis. **Respiratory:** URTI, coughing, sinusitis, bronchitis, breathing abnormalities, bronchospasm and obstruction, paranasal sinus disorders, pneumonia, respiratory tract disorders, influenza. **Body as a whole:** Pain/discomfort, pyrexia, *septic shock*. **Miscellaneous:** Immune reconstitution syndrome, increased risk of infections, appetite disorders, herpes infection, *Clostridium difficle* colitis, viral meningitis; benign/malignant/unspecified neoplasms.

LABORATORY TEST CONSIDERATIONS
↑ ALT, AST, total bilirubin, amylase, lipase, blood creatine kinase. ↓ Absolute neutrophil count.

OD OVERDOSE MANAGEMENT
Symptoms: Postural hypotension. *Treatment:* Institute general supportive measures. Keep client in a supine position. Assess vital signs, BP, and ECG. Gastric lavage and activated charcoal can be used to aid in removal of the drug. Dialysis may also be beneficial.

DRUG INTERACTIONS
Atazanavir / ↑ Maraviroc C_{max}, C_{min}, and AUC R/T inhibition of CYP3A4
Atazanavir/Ritonavir / ↑ Maraviroc C_{max}, C_{min}, and AUC R/T inhibition of CYP3A4
Efavirenz / ↓ Maraviroc C_{max}, C_{min}, and AUC R/T induction of CYP3A4
Ketoconazole / ↑ Maraviroc C_{max}, C_{min}, and AUC R/T inhibition of CYP3A4
Lopinavir/Ritonavir / ↑ Maraviroc C_{max}, C_{min}, and AUC R/T inhibition of CYP3A4
Rifampicin / ↓ Maraviroc C_{max}, C_{min}, and AUC R/T induction of CYP3A4
Ritonavir / ↑ Maraviroc C_{max}, C_{min}, and AUC R/T inhibition of CYP3A4
Saquinavir/Ritonavir / ↑ Maraviroc C_{max}, C_{min}, and AUC R/T inhibition of CYP3A4
H *St. John's wort* / ↓ Maraviroc levels → suboptimal maraviroc levels and loss of virologic response and possible resistance; do not use together

HOW SUPPLIED
Tablets: 150 mg, 300 mg.

DOSAGE
• **TABLETS**
HIV infection.
As a result of drug interactions, the recommended dose of maraviroc differs based on use of concomitant drugs. The dose of maraviroc is 150 mg twice a day if given with protease inhibitors (except tipranavir/ritonavir), delavirdine, ketoconazole, itraconazole, clarithromycin, or other strong CYP3A inhibitors (e.g., nefazodone, telithromycin).

The dose of maraviroc is 300 mg twice a day if given with tipranavir/ritonavir, nevirapine, all nucleoside reverse transcriptase inhibitors, and enfuvirtide.

The dose of maraviroc is 600 mg twice a day if given with CYP3A inducers, including carbamazepine, phenobarbital, phenytoin, efavirenz, or rifampin.

NURSING CONSIDERATIONS
ADMINISTRATION/STORAGE
1. Maraviroc must be given in combination with other antiretroviral drugs.
2. May be taken with or without food.
3. Store from 15-30°C (59-86°F).

ASSESSMENT
1. Note CCR5-tropic HIV-1 detectable disease. It is used along with other HIV medicines to prevent virus from entering the cells.
2. List all drugs prescribed to ensure none interact.
3. Assess for history of liver problems, hepatitis B or C, heart or kidney problems.
4. Monitor CBC, renal, and LFTs.

CLIENT/FAMILY TEACHING
1. May take with or without food. Swallow whole; do not break, crush, or chew before swallowing.
2. Take even if feeling well; do not miss/skip any doses. Do not stop taking Maraviroc, even for a short period of time. The virus may grow resistant to the medicine and become harder to treat.
3. Avoid activities that require mental alertness until drug effects realized; may cause dizziness
4. Report any sore throat, weakness, cough, or evidence of infection. Avoid those with known infections.
5. Report any difficulty breathing, chest tightness/pain, swelling of the mouth, face, lips, or tongue, rash, bloody diarrhea, or confusion.
6. Drug does not prevent spread of HIV to others through blood or sexual con-

---

tact; practice barrier protection. Do not share needles, injection supplies, toothbrushes or razors.

7. To monitor maternal-fetal outcomes of pregnant women exposed to maraviroc and other antiretroviral drugs, an antiretroviral registry has been established. Health care providers are encouraged to register clients by calling 1-800-258-4263.

8. Keep all F/U appointments to evaluate labs and response to therapy.

OUTCOMES/EVALUATE

- ↓ HIV RNA
- Inhibition of HIV viral replication

Mebendazole
(meh-**BEN**-dah-zohl)

CLASSIFICATION(S):
Anthelmintic
PREGNANCY CATEGORY: C
Rx: Vermox.

USES
Single or mixed infections of whipworm, pinworm, roundworm, and common and American hookworm. Not effective for hydatid disease.

ACTION/KINETICS
Action
Anthelmintic effect occurs by blocking the glucose uptake of the organisms, thereby reducing their energy until death results. It also inhibits the formation of microtubules in the helminth.
Pharmacokinetics
Peak plasma levels: 2–4 hr. Poorly absorbed from the GI tract. Excreted in feces as unchanged drug or metabolites.

CONTRAINDICATIONS
Hypersensitivity to mebendazole.

SPECIAL CONCERNS
Use with caution in children under 2 years of age and during lactation.

SIDE EFFECTS
Most Common
Transient abdominal pain, diarrhea.
GI: Transient abdominal pain and diarrhea. **Hematologic:** Reversible neutropenia. **Miscellaneous:** Fever.

DRUG INTERACTIONS
Carbamazepine and hydantoin may ↓ effect due to ↓ plasma levels of mebendazole.

HOW SUPPLIED
Tablets, Chewable: 100 mg.

DOSAGE
- **TABLETS, CHEWABLE**
  Whipworm, roundworm, and hookworm.

Adults and children: 1 tablet morning and evening on 3 consecutive days.
  Pinworms.

1 tablet, one time. All treatments can be repeated after 3 weeks if the client is not cured.

NURSING CONSIDERATIONS
ASSESSMENT
Note clinical confirmation of organism, onset and characteristics of S&S, and any other contributory factors. Identify all persons in contact and potentially infected.

CLIENT/FAMILY TEACHING
1. Tablets may be chewed, swallowed, or crushed and mixed with food. Fasting or purging are not required.
2. Pinworms may be highly contagious. To prevent reinfection:
- Carefully wash hands with soap and water frequently during the day and especially before and after eating and toileting; clean nails and keep out of mouth.
- Advise school nurse of treatment.
- Do not scratch the infected area or place your fingers in your mouth.
- Do not share washcloths and towels. Wear tight underpants day and night; change daily. Sleep alone; wear shoes during waking hours.
- Do not shake clothing/linens before washing. Change and wash daily-underwear, bed linens, towels, clothes, and pajamas in hot water.
- Clean toilet and seats with disinfectant daily; vacuum or wet-mop bedroom floors daily during treatment and for several days after treatment. Avoid dry sweeping; stirs up dust.
- All family members should be treated simultaneously

 = see color insert   = Herbal   = Intravenous   ⓒ = sound alike drug

M

3. Wash all fruits and vegetables. Thoroughly cook all meats and vegetables.
4. Immobilization followed by death of parasites is slow. Complete clearance from the GI tract may take up to 3 days after initiation of treatment.
5. Report if S&S do not improve or worsen after three weeks.

OUTCOMES/EVALUATE
- Three consecutive negative stool and/or perianal swabs
- Organism expulsion/destruction

Mecasermin (rDNA origin) Injection
(meh-kah-**SIR**-min)

CLASSIFICATION(S):
Insulin-like Growth Factor
PREGNANCY CATEGORY: C
Rx: Increlex.

Mecasermin rinfabate (rDNA origin) Injection
Rx: Iplex.

USES
Long-term treatment of growth failure in children with severe primary insulin-like growth factor-1 deficiency or with growth hormone gene deletion who have developed neutralizing antibodies to growth hormone. *NOTE:* Mecasermin is not a substitute for growth hormone treatment.

ACTION/KINETICS
Action
Insulin-like growth factor-1 (IGF-1) is the principal hormonal mediator of statural growth. Under normal conditions, growth hormone binds to its receptor in the liver and other tissues and stimulates the synthesis and secretion of IGF-1. In target tissues, the type 1 IGF-1 receptor is activated by IGF-1, leading to intracellular signaling, which stimulates multiple processes leading to statural growth. The metabolic actions of IGF-1 are, in part, directed at stimulating the uptake of glucose, fatty acids, and amino acids so that metabolism supports growing tissues. IGF-1 suppresses hepatic glucose production and stimulates peripheral utilization of glucose; thus, the drug may cause hypoglycemia. IGF-1 also inhibits insulin secretion.

Pharmacokinetics
Bioavailability after SC administration is thought to be close to 100%. Both the liver and kidney metabolize IGF-1. **t½, terminal:** 5.8 hr. **Plasma protein binding:** >80% bound to IGF binding protein 3.

CONTRAINDICATIONS
Use to treat secondary forms of insulin-like growth factor-1 deficiency, such as growth hormone deficiency, malnutrition, hypothyroidism, or chronic treatment with pharmacologic doses of anti-inflammatory steroids. Use for growth promotion in clients with closed epiphyses, in the presence of active or suspected neoplasia, IV administration, and in those allergic to IGF-1 or any ingredients in the product.

SPECIAL CONCERNS
Use with caution during lactation. Safety and efficacy have not been evaluated in adults over 65 years of age or in adults or children <3 years old with primary insulin-like growth factor deficiency.

SIDE EFFECTS
Most Common
Hypoglycemia, tonsillar hypertrophy, bruising, otitis media, snoring, headache, dizziness, vomiting, injection site reactions, muscular atrophy, pain in extremity.

Metabolic: Hypoglycemia. **Hematologic:** Thymus hypertrophy, iron-deficiency anemia, lymphadenopathy. Lymphoid tissue (e.g., tonsillar and adenoidal) hypertrophy associated with complications, such as snoring, sleep apnea, and chronic middle-ear effusions. **GI:** Vomiting. **CNS:** *Convulsions,* dizziness, headache. Intracranial hypertension with papilledema (visual changes, headache, N&V), visual changes, headache, N &/or V. **CV:** Cardiac murmur, valvulopathy. **Musculoskeletal:** Arthralgia, pain in ex-

---

Bold Italic = life threatening side effect   ■ = black box warning   ✦ = Available in Canada

tremities, bone pain, muscular atrophy. **GU:** Hematuria, increase in kidney size. **Injection site reactions:** Erythema, hair growth at injection site, lipohypertrophy. **Otic:** Abnormal tympanometry, ear pain, ear tube insertion, fluid in middle ear, hypoacusis, otitis media, serous otitis media. **Body as a whole:** Hypersensitivity reactions (local or systemic), development of antibodies to mecasermin. Bruising. **Miscellaneous:** Thickening of soft tissues of the face, thyromegaly, development of antibodies to the protein complex.

LABORATORY TEST CONSIDERATIONS
↑ ALT, AST, LDH, cholesterol, triglycerides.

OD OVERDOSE MANAGEMENT
Symptoms: Hypoglycemia. Long-term overdosage may cause S&S of acromegaly. *Treatment:* Use methods to reverse hypoglycemia (e.g., consume PO glucose and food). If an overdose causes loss of consciousness, IV glucose or parenteral glucagon may be needed to reverse the hypoglycemia.

HOW SUPPLIED
Mecasermin (Increlex): *Injection:* 10 mg/mL.
Mecasermin rinfabate (Iplex): *Injection:* 36 mg/0.6 mL.

DOSAGE
MECASERMIN
- **SC**
    Growth failure in children with insulin-like growth factor-1 deficiency.
Individualize dosage. **Initial:** 0.04–0.08 mg/kg (40–80 mcg/kg) twice daily. If well tolerated for at least 1 week, the dose may be increased by 0.04 mg/kg/dose to the maximum dose of 0.12 mg/kg given twice daily. Doses greater than 0.12 mg/kg may cause hypoglycemia.
MECASERMIN RINFABATE
- **SC**
    Growth failure in children with insulin-like growth factor-1 deficiency.
Individualize dosage. **Initial:** 0.5 mg/kg; increase to the therapeutic dosage range of 1–2 mg/kg, given once daily. A maximum of 2 mg/kg/day can be given based on measurement of IGF-1 levels 8–18 hr after the previous dose. Can be

given in the morning or evening but at about the same time each day.

NURSING CONSIDERATIONS
ADMINISTRATION/STORAGE
1. Give shortly before or after (about 20 min) a meal or snack. If client is unable to eat shortly before or after dose, withhold dose of mecasermin. Subsequent doses should never be increased to make up for 1 or more omitted doses.
2. If severe or persistent hypoglycemia occurs during treatment despite adequate food intake, consider dose reduction.
3. Rotate injection sites to a different site with each injection.
4. Give using sterile disposable syringes and needles. The syringes should be of small enough volume so that the correct dose can be withdrawn from the vial with reasonable accuracy.
5. Product contains benzyl alcohol as a preservative; has been associated with neurologic toxicity in neonates.
6. Do not use if solution is cloudy or contains particulate matter. Discard any remaining unused drug after 30 days following initial vial entry.
7. Discontinue therapy if evidence of neoplasia develops.
8. **For mecasermin:** Before opening, store vials from 2–8°C (35–46°F); do not freeze vials. Protect from direct light.
9. **For mecasermin:** After opening, vials are stable for 30 days after initial vial entry when stored from 2–8°C (35–46°F); do not freeze vials. Protect from direct light.
10. **For mecasermin rinfabate:** Must be kept frozen while transferring it to a home freezer (-20°C, -4°F). Can be stored frozen up to 2 months in the freezer. For use, remove from freezer and thaw at room temperature (20–25°C, 68–77°F) for 45 min prior to use. Do not use if it thaws during transfer or storage as stability may be affected.
11. **For mecasermin rinfabate:** After thawing at room temperature for 45 min, swirl vial gently in a rotary motion to ensure a uniform content. Do not shake. Inspect visually for particulate

M

matter and discoloration; discard if particulate matter noted or solution is cloudy or discolored. If solution is cloudy, may indicate drug was thawed previously or exposed to extreme temperatures. Use within 1 hr of reaching room temperature; do not use if at room temperature for more than 2 hr. Discard any unused portion.

ASSESSMENT

1. Drug is used for growth failure in children with IGF-1 deficiency (primary IGFD) or growth homone gene deletion; note reasons.

2. Severe primary IGFD is defined by: (a) height standard deviation score less than or equal to -3.0; (b) basal IGF-1 standard deviation score less than or equal to -3.0; and (c) normal or elevated GH. Note findings. Obtain baseline measurements; monitor during therapy.

3. Assess for evidence of malnutrition, hypothyroidism or chronic therapy with anti-inflammatory steroids. Must correct thyroid and nutritional deficiencies before starting Mecasermin therapy.

4. Drug suppresses hepatic glucose production and stimulates peripheral glucose use; increased incidence of hypoglycemia. Check preprandial glucose when starting treatment and until established well tolerated dose reached.

5. Do not use dug for growth promotion in those with closed epiphyses; skeletal growth occurs at the cartilage growth plates of the epiphyses.

6. Assess for thickening of the soft tissues of the face. Evaluate lymphhoid tissue (tonsillar) for atrophy and associated symptoms such as snoring, sleep apnea or middle ear-effusions. Refer for fundoscopic exam with complaints of headaches, N&V or visual changes and periodically during therapy.

7. Monitor for slipped capital femoral epiphysis and scoliosis with rapid growth.

CLIENT/FAMILY TEACHING

1. Review/demonstrate correct method for subcutaneous administration. Ensure that sites are rotated with each injection and that a new needle and syringe are used for each injection. Inject mecasermin rinfabate just below the skin in child's upper arm, upper thigh, stomach area, or buttocks.

2. Give shortly before or after (about 20 min) a meal or snack. If unable to eat shortly before or after a dose, withhold the dose of mecasermin. Subsequent doses should never be increased to make up for 1 or more omitted doses.

3. Dosage will be started low and gradually increased to ensure no adverse side effects.

4. Avoid activities that require alertness (driving, machine operation) within 2–3 hr of dosing esp when starting therapy (and for 3–5 days thereafter) and until a well-tolerated dose established.

5. Do not use if solution is cloudy or contains particulate matter. Discard any remaining unused drug after 30 days following initial vial entry.

6. Parents must pay careful attention to small children whose oral intake may not be consistent. Ensure mecasermin administered just before or after a meal or snack.

7. Report any S&S of low blood sugar: weakness, drowsiness, dizziness, confusion, shaky, cold, clammy, sweaty, headaches. May use food or oral glucose to relieve.

8. Keep all scheduled follow up visits and labs to ensure proper dosing and desired results.

9. Report any unusual or adverse side effects. Keep out of reach of children and dispose of syringes in a puncture-resistant container. Store according to instructions and review patient education pamphlet.

OUTCOMES/EVALUATE

Desired growth of bones and muscles with IGF-1 deficiency

Mechlorethamine hydrochloride (Nitrogen mustard) ■ Ⅳ

(meh-klor-**ETH**-ah-meen)

CLASSIFICATION(S):
Antineoplastic, alkylating
PREGNANCY CATEGORY: D
Rx: Mustargen.

SEE ALSO *ANTINEOPLASTIC AGENTS* AND *ALKYLATING AGENTS*.

USES

IV: (1) Palliative treatment of bronchogenic carcinoma. (2) Palliative treatment of CLL and CML. (3) Palliative treatment of stages III and IV of Hodgkin's disease. (4) Palliative treatment of polycythemia vera. (5) Palliative treatment of mycosis fungoides. (6) Palliative treatment of lymphosarcoma.

Intracavity (Intrapericardial, intraperitoneal, or intrapleural): Metastatic carcinoma resulting in effusion. *NOTE:* Tumors of the bone and nervous tissue respond poorly to this drug.

Investigational: **Topical:** Cutaneous mycosis fungoides.

ACTION/KINETICS

Action

Cell-cycle nonspecific. Forms an unstable ethylenimmonium ion, which then alkylates or binds with various compounds, including nucleic acids. Cytotoxic activity is due to cross-linking of DNA and RNA strands and protein synthesis. When used for intracavitary tumors, exerts both an inflammatory reaction and sclerosis on serous membranes, which causes adherence of the drug to serosal surfaces.

Pharmacokinetics

Reacts rapidly with tissues and within minutes after administration the active drug is no longer present. Metabolites are excreted through the urine.

CONTRAINDICATIONS

Lactation. During infectious disease.

SPECIAL CONCERNS

■ (1) Administer only under the supervision of a physician experienced in the use of cancer chemotherapeutic drugs. (2) This drug is highly toxic and the powder and solution must be handled and administered with care. Inhalation of dust or vapors and contact with skin or mucous membranes, especially those of the eyes, must be avoided. Avoid exposure during pregnancy. Because of the toxic properties of the drug (e.g., corrosive, carcinogenic, mutagenic, teratogenic), review special handling procedures prior to handling and follow diligently. (3) Extravasation into SC areas causes painful inflammation. The area usually becomes indurated; sloughing may occur. If leakage of drug is obvious, promptly infiltrate the area with sterile isotonic sodium thiosulfate (1/6 molar), and apply an ice compress for 6–12 hr. For a 1/6 molar solution of sodium thiosulfate, use 4.14 grams sodium thiosulfate per 100 mL sterile water for injection or 2.64 grams anhydrous sodium thiosulfate per 100 mL, or dilute 4 mL sodium thiosulfate injection (10%) with 6 mL sterile water for injection.■ Use in children has been limited although the drug has been used in MOPP (mechlorethamine, Oncovin, procarbazine, prednisone) therapy.

SIDE EFFECTS

Most Common
N&V, diarrhea, headache, anorexia, confusion, drowsiness, metallic taste, weakness, alopecia.

See *Antineoplastic Agents* for a complete list of possible side effects. High incidence of N&V. Amyloidosis, hyperuricemia, petechiae, SC hemorrhages, tinnitus, deafness, herpes zoster, or temporary amenorrhea, hypersensitivity reactions. Extravasation into SC tissue causes painful inflammation.

OD OVERDOSE MANAGEMENT

Symptoms: Severe leukopenia, anemia, thrombocytopenia, and hemorrhagic diathesis with subsequent delayed bleeding. Death may follow. *Treatment:* The only treatment is repeated blood product transfusions, antibiotic treatment of complicating infections, and general supportive measures.

DRUG INTERACTIONS

Amphotericin B / Combination ↑ possibility of blood dyscrasias

HOW SUPPLIED

Powder for Injection: 10 mg.

DOSAGE

- **IV**

  All uses.

Adults, children: A total dose of 0.4 mg/kg per course of therapy given as a single dose or in two to four divided doses of 0.1–0.2 mg/kg over 2–4 days. Depending on blood cell count, a second course may be given after 3 weeks.

- **INTRAPERITONEAL, INTRAPERICARDIAL; INTRAPLEURAL INJECTION**

0.4 mg/kg (0.2 mg/kg or 10–20 mg has been used intrapericardially).

NURSING CONSIDERATIONS

ADMINISTRATION/STORAGE

1. For intracavitary administration, may be further diluted in 100 mL of NSS; turn client every 60 sec for 5 min to the following positions: prone, supine, right side, left side, and knee-chest. Lack of effect often results from failure to move client often enough. Remaining fluid may be removed after 24–36 hr.

IV 2. Drug is highly irritating; avoid skin contact. Wear gloves during preparation. Should accidental eye contact occur, immediately begin copious irrigation with water, normal saline, or balanced salt ophthalmic irrigating solution for at least 15 min. Follow with prompt ophthalmologic consultation. Should accidental contact with the skin occur, irrigate the affected part immediately with copious amounts of water for 15 min while removing contaminated clothing and shoes. Follow by 2% sodium thiosulfate solution. Seek medical attention immediately. Destroy contaminated clothing.

3. Best administered through tubing of a rapidly flowing IV saline infusion.

4. Prepare solution immediately before administration because it decomposes on standing.

5. Drug is available in a rubber-stoppered vial to which 10 mL of either NaCl

or sterile water for injection is added to give a concentration of 1 mg/mL; administer over 3–5 min.

6. Insert the needle and keep it inserted until the medication is dissolved and the required dose withdrawn. Carefully discard the vial with the remaining solution so that no one will come in contact with it.

7. Use aqueous solution of equal parts 5% sodium thiosulfate and 5% $NaHCO_3$ to clean glassware, tubings, and other articles after drug administration. Soak for 45 min.

8. Monitor IV closely because extravasation causes swelling, erythema, induration, and sloughing. In case of extravasation, remove IV, infuse area with 1/6 molar isotonic sodium thiosulfate, and apply cold compresses. If sodium thiosulfate is not available, use isotonic NaCl solution or 1% lidocaine. Apply ice for 6–12 hr (on for 10 min, off for 30 min).

9. N&V usually begin 1–3 hr after administration. Vomiting may disappear in the first 8 hr; nausea may persist for 24 hr. N&V may be so severe as to cause vascular accidents in those with a hemorrhagic tendency. Premedication with antiemetics and sedatives may be beneficial.

ASSESSMENT

1. Note reasons for therapy, route of administration any agents used previously.

2. Monitor I&O, uric acid, renal and hematologic function. Assess for dehydration, anemia, infection, and gout (allopurinol may help lower uric acid levels).

3. Drug causes granulocyte and platelet suppression. Nadir: 7–14 days; recovery 21 days.

INTERVENTIONS

1. Ensure phenothiazine and/or sedative ordered (30–45 min prior to medication and RTC as needed) to control severe N&V that usu. occurs 1–3 hr after administration.

2. Give late afternoon or early evening; follow with a sedative (sleeping pill) to control adverse S&S and induce sleep.

3. If drug comes in contact with the eye, irrigate with copious amounts of

---

Bold Italic = life threatening side effect　　　■ = black box warning　　　✣ = Available in Canada saline solution and consult opthalmologist. Irrigate skin with water for 15 min and then with 2% sodium thiosulfate solution in the event of accidental contact. Destroy contaminated clothing.

CLIENT/FAMILY TEACHING

1. Drug may be administered either IV or directly into a body cavity.
2. Medications will be given to control N&V and to help you relax and sleep.
3. Hair loss may occur.
4. Avoid vaccinia and exposure to infections or infected persons.
5. Drug may cause irreversible gonadal suppression; identify if candidate for sperm/egg harvesting.
6. Practice birth control during and for 4 months following therapy.
7. Consume increased fluid volume. Report any unusual bruising or bleeding, a rash consistent with herpes zoster, S&S of infection, or hearing loss.

OUTCOMES/EVALUATE

- ↓ Tumor size/spread
- Improved hematologic profile
- Resolution of effusion

Meclizine hydrochloride

(**MEK**-lih-zeen)

CLASSIFICATION(S):

Antiemetic

PREGNANCY CATEGORY: B

OTC: Dramamine Less Drowsy Formula.

Rx: Antivert, Antivert/25 and /50, Antrizine, Meni-D.

✤**OTC:** Bonamine.

SEE ALSO *ANTIHISTAMINES* AND *ANTIEMETICS.*

USES

(1) Prevention and treatment of nausea, vomiting, and dizziness of motion sickness. (2) Possibly effective for vertigo associated with diseases of the vestibular system.

ACTION/KINETICS

Action

Meclizine has antiemetic, anticholinergic, and antihistaminic effects. Mechanism for the antiemetic effect may be due to a central anticholinergic effect to decrease vestibular stimulation and depress labyrinthine activity. May also act on the CTZ to decrease vomiting.

Pharmacokinetics

Onset: 30–60 min; **Duration:** 8–24 hr. t½: 6 hr.

SPECIAL CONCERNS

Safety for use during lactation and in children less than 12 years of age has not been determined. Use with caution in glaucoma, obstructive disease of the GI or GU tract, and in prostatic hypertrophy. Pediatric and geriatric clients may be more sensitive to the anticholinergic effects of meclizine.

SIDE EFFECTS

Most Common

Drowsiness, dry mouth, nervousness, insomnia, constipation.

CNS: Drowsiness, excitation, nervousness, restlessness, insomnia, euphoria, vertigo, auditory or visual hallucinations (especially when doses recommended are exceeded). **GI:** N&V, diarrhea, constipation, dry mouth, anorexia. **GU:** Urinary frequency or retention; difficulty in urination. **CV:** Hypotension, tachycardia, palpitations. **Dermatologic:** Rash, urticaria. **Miscellaneous:** Dry nose and throat, blurred or double vision, tinnitus.

OD **OVERDOSE MANAGEMENT**

Symptoms: Hyperexcitability alternating with drowsiness. Massive overdosage may cause **convulsions**, hallucinations, and **respiratory paryalysis**. *Treatment:* Appropriate supportive and symptomatic treatment. Do **not** use morphine or other respiratory depressants.

HOW SUPPLIED

Capsules: 25 mg; *Tablets:* 12.5 mg, 25 mg, 50 mg; *Tablets, Chewable:* 25 mg.

DOSAGE

- **CAPSULES; TABLETS; TABLETS, CHEWABLE**

Motion sickness.

Adults: 25–50 mg 1 hr before travel; may be repeated q 24 hr during travel.

Vertigo.

Adults: 25–100 mg/day in divided doses.

M

NURSING CONSIDERATIONS

ASSESSMENT

1. Note onset, duration, characteristics of symptoms. Identify triggers if known, any recent cold or URI, fever.

2. Assess for adverse symptoms; drug may mask signs of drug overdose or pathology such as increased ICP or intestinal obstruction.

3. Determine any asthma, emphysema, enlarged prostate, glaucoma, intestinal or urinary tract blockage; precludes drug therapy.

CLIENT/FAMILY TEACHING

1. Take as directed; report if condition does not improve or worsens

2. Antiemetics tend to cause drowsiness and dizziness. Do not drive or perform other hazardous tasks until drug response evident.

3. For dryness of the mouth may get some relief with sugarless candy or gum, melting ice chips in your mouth, or using a saliva substitute

4. With motion sickness, take 1 hr before departure to ensure best results.

5. Avoid alcohol; markedly increases sedative effects.

OUTCOMES/EVALUATE

- Prevention of motion sickness
- Control of vertigo

Medroxy-progesterone acetate ■ ©

(meh-**drox**-see-proh-**JESS**-ter-ohn)

CLASSIFICATION(S):

Progestin

PREGNANCY CATEGORY: X

Rx: Amen, Depo-Provera, Depo-Provera C-150, Depo-Sub Q Provera 104, Provera.

♣Rx: Gen-Medroxy, Novo-Medrone, ratio-MPA.

SEE ALSO PROGESTERONE AND PROGESTINS AND ANTINEOPLASTIC AGENTS.

USES

(1) Secondary amenorrhea. (2) Abnormal uterine bleeding due to hormonal imbalance (no organic pathology). (3) Adjunct in palliative treatment of inoperable, recurrent, or metastatic endometrial or renal carcinoma. (4) Long-acting contraceptive (injectable form given q 3 months). (5) Reduce endometrial hyperplasia in postmenopausal women receiving 0.625 mg conjugated estrogen for 12 to 14 days/month; can begin on the 1st or 16th day of the cycle. (6) Depo-Sub Q Provera 104 to manage pain associated with endometriosis in women. *Investigational:* Polycystic ovary syndrome, precocious puberty. With estrogen to treat menopausal symptoms and hypermenorrhea. To stimulate respiration in obesity-hypoventilation syndrome (oral). Treatment of advanced breast cancer.

ACTION/KINETICS

Action

Synthetic progestin devoid of estrogenic and androgenic activity. Prevents stimulation of endometrium by pituitary gonadotropins. Priming with estrogen is necessary before response is noted.

Pharmacokinetics

Rapidly absorbed from GI tract. **Maximum levels:** 1–2 hr. **t½, after PO:** 2–3 hr for first 6 hr; then, 8–9 hr. **t½, long-acting forms IM:** About 10 weeks with maximum levels within 24 hr.

CONTRAINDICATIONS

Clients with CV disease or a history of thrombophlebitis, thromboembolic disease, cerebral apoplexy. Liver dysfunction. Known or suspected malignancy of the breasts or genital organs. Missed abortion; as a diagnostic for pregnancy. Undiagnosed vaginal bleeding. Use during the first 4 months of pregnancy.

SPECIAL CONCERNS

■ (1) The use of progestins during the first four months of pregnancy is not recommended. There is the possibility that intrauterine exposure to progestational drugs in the first trimester of pregnancy may cause genital abnormalities in female and male fetuses. If the client is exposed to progestational drugs during the first 4 months of pregnancy or if the woman becomes pregnant while taking a progestational drug, apprise her of the potential risks to the fetus. (2) Significant bone mineral density loss has been associated with the use of the drug; loss may be greater with increased duration of use. Bone loss may not be completely reversible. (3) Use is not recommended for long-term birth control (longer than 2 years) unless other methods are inadequate.■ The overall risk of breast, liver, ovarian, endometrial, and cervical cancer is not thought to increase with use of the injectable long-acting contraceptive preparation. Possibility of ectopic pregnancy. Use with caution with a history of depression. Due to the possibility of fluid retention, use with caution in clients with epilepsy, migraine, asthma, or cardiac or renal dysfunction.

SIDE EFFECTS

Most Common

Breast tenderness, breakthrough bleeding, spotting, change in menstrual flow, urticaria/pruritus, acne, generalized rash.

GU: Amenorrhea or infertility for up to 18 months, breast tenderness, breakthrough bleeding, spotting, change in menstrual flow. **CV:** Thrombophlebitis, **pulmonary embolism. GI:** Nausea (rare), jaundice. **CNS:** Nervousness, drowsiness, insomnia, fatigue, dizziness, headache (rare). **Dermatologic:** Pruritus, urticaria, rash, acne, hirsutism, alopecia, angioneurotic edema. **Miscellaneous: Hyperpyrexia, anaphylaxis,** decrease in glucose tolerance, weight gain, fluid retention.

DRUG INTERACTIONS

Aminoglutethimide may ↑ metabolism of medroxyprogesterone → ↓ effect

HOW SUPPLIED

Injection: 104 mg/0.65 mL, 150 mg/mL, 400 mg/mL; Tablets: 2.5 mg, 5 mg, 10 mg.

DOSAGE
• **IM**

Endometrial or renal carcinoma.

Initial: 400–1,000 mg/week; **then,** if improvement noted, 400 mg/month. Medroxyprogesterone is not intended to be the primary therapy.

Long-acting contraceptive.

150 mg of depot form q 3 months by deep IM injection given only during the first 5 days after the onset of a normal menstrual period, within 5 days postpartum if not breastfeeding, or 6 weeks postpartum if breastfeeding.

Pain associated with endometriosis.

On injection (104 mg) q 3 months.
• **TABLETS**

Secondary amenorrhea.

5–10 mg/day for 5–10 days, with therapy beginning at any time during the menstrual cycle. If endometrium has been estrogen primed: 10 mg medroxyprogesterone/day for 10 days beginning any time. Bleeding usually begins within 3–7 days.

Abnormal uterine bleeding with no pathology.

5 or 10 mg/day for 5–10 days, with therapy beginning on day 16 or 21 of the menstrual cycle. If endometrium has been estrogen primed: 10 mg/day for 10 days, beginning on day 16 of the menstrual cycle. Bleeding usually begins within 3–7 days.

Endometrial hyperplasia.

5 or 10 mg/day for 12–14 consecutive days per month, beginning either on the 1st day of the cycle or the 16th day of the cycle.

NURSING CONSIDERATIONS

ⓒ Do not confuse Amen with Ambien (sedative-hypnotic). Also, do not confuse Provera with Premarin (an estrogen).

ASSESSMENT

1. Note reasons for therapy, type, onset, and characteristics of S&S.
2. List any thromboembolic disease, liver dysfunction, malignancy of the breasts or genital organs; precludes therapy.
3. Monitor BMD, calcium levels, and LFTs. With severe hypercalcemia, have IV fluids, diuretics, corticosteroids, and phosphate supplements available; monitor closely once corrected.

CLIENT/FAMILY TEACHING

1. With oral administration may take with food to ↓ GI upset; mark calendar to ensure dosing. IM injection may be painful. After repeated injections, infer-

tility and amenorrhea may last as long as 18 mo.

2. With cancer therapy, the combined effect of the drug and osteolytic metastases may result in hypercalcemia. Report insomnia, lethargy, anorexia, and N&V. Increase fluids to minimize hypercalcemia.

3. Keep scheduled appointments for contraceptive evaluation and regular GYN exams. Additional barrier protection is necessary to prevent STDs and HIV transmission. Practice regular breast exams. May induce mild masculinization of the external genitalia of the female fetus, as well as hypospadias in the male fetus; avoid use during the first 4 mo of pregnancy.

4. Report pain/swelling in calves, sudden chest pain, shortness of breath as well as any other unusual side effects. Keep all follow up visits.

OUTCOMES/EVALUATE

- Prevention of pregnancy
- Control of tumor size and spread
- Regular menses; normal hormone levels
- ↓ Endometrial hyperplasia in postmenopausal women receiving estrogen

Mefloquine hydrochloride

(meh-**FLOH**-kwin)

CLASSIFICATION(S):
Antimalarial
PREGNANCY CATEGORY: C
Rx: Lariam.

USES

(1) Mild to moderate acute malaria caused by mefloquine-susceptible strains of *Plasmodium falciparum* (both chloroquine susceptible and resistant strains) or *P. vivax*. Data are not available regarding effectiveness in treating *P. ovale* or *P. malariae*. (2) Prophylaxis of *P. falciparum* and *P. vivax* infections, including prophylaxis of chloroquine-resistant strains of *P. falciparum*. NOTE:

Clients with acute *P. vivax* malaria are at a high risk for relapse as mefloquine does not eliminate the exoerythrocytic (hepatic) parasites. Thus, these clients should also be treated with primaquine. Strains of *P. falciparum* are reported to be resistant to mefloquine.

ACTION/KINETICS

Action

Related chemically to quinine and acts as a blood schizonticide. It may increase intravesicular pH in acid vesicles of parasite. It shows myocardial depressant activity with about 20% of the antifibrillatory activity of quinidine and 50% of the increase in the PR interval noted with quinine.

Pharmacokinetics

Mefloquine is a mixture of enantiomeric molecules that results in differences in the rates of release, absorption, distribution, metabolism, elimination, and activity of the drug. $t\frac{1}{2}$: 13–24 days (average 3 weeks). Is concentrated in blood erythrocytes (i.e., the target cells in treatment of malaria). **Plasma protein binding:** 98%.

CONTRAINDICATIONS

Hypersensitivity to mefloquine or related compounds (e.g., quinine, quinidine). Use as prophylaxis with active or recent history of depression, anxiety, generalized anxiety disorder, psychosis or schizophrenia, or other major psychiatric disorder, or with a history of convulsions. Lactation.

SPECIAL CONCERNS

In long-term therapy >1 year, monitor LFTs and perform ophthalmic exams. Use with extreme caution with cardiovascular disease. Use with caution with hepatic dysfunction and epilepsy (may increase risk of seizures). If used in clients with *P. vivax*, there is high risk of relapse as mefloquine does not eliminate the exoerythrocytic phase of the parasite.

SIDE EFFECTS

Most Common

N&V, diarrhea/loose stools, abdominal pain, dizziness, vertigo, loss of balance, headache, somnolence, insomnia, abnormal dreams.

Bold Italic = life threatening side effect   ■ = black box warning   ♣ = Available in Canada

NOTE: At the doses used, it is difficult to distinguish side effects due to the drug from symptoms attributable to the disease itself.

When used for treatment of acute malaria. GI: N&V, diarrhea, abdominal pain, loss of appetite. **CNS:** Dizziness, fever, headache, fatigue, emotional problems, *seizures.* **Miscellaneous:** Myalgia, loss of balance, chills, skin rash, tinnitus, bradycardia, hair loss, pruritus, asthenia.

When used for prophylaxis of malaria. CNS: Dizziness, syncope, encephalopathy of unknown etiology. **Miscellaneous:** Vomiting, extrasystoles. *Post-marketing surveillance.* **CNS:** Vertigo, psychoses, confusion, anxiety, depression, *seizures*, hallucinations, insomnia, abnormal dreams, forgetfulness, motor and sensory neuropathy, psychiatric events. **CV:** Hypertension, hypotension, tachycardia, palpitations, chest pain, bradycardia, irregular pulse, extrasystoles, AV block, other transient cardiac conduction alterations (rare). **Dermatologic:** Flushing, urticaria, erythema multiforme, *Stevens-Johnson syndrome*, rash, exanthema, erythema, pruritus, edema, hair loss. **Musculoskeletal:** Muscle weakness, muscle cramps, myalgia, arthralgia (rare). **Miscellaneous:** Visual disturbances, vestibular disorders (including tinnitus, hearing impairment), dyspnea, asthenia, malaise, fatigue, fever, sweating, chills, dyspepsia, loss of appetite (rare).

LABORATORY TEST CONSIDERATIONS
When used for prophylaxis: Transient ↑ transaminases, leukocytosis, thrombocytopenia. **When used for treatment of acute malaria:** ↓ Hematocrit, transient ↑ transaminases, leukocytosis, thrombocytopenia.

OD OVERDOSE MANAGEMENT
Symptoms: Cardiotoxic effects, vomiting, diarrhea. *Treatment:* Induce vomiting and administer fluid therapy to treat vomiting and diarrhea.

DRUG INTERACTIONS
Anticonvulsants / Loss of seizure control R/T ↓ anticonvulsant blood levels
Drugs known to alter cardiac conduction (i.e., anti-arrhythmic or beta-adrenergic blocking agents, calcium channel blockers, H₁ antihistamines, tricyclic antidepressants and phenothiazines) / May contribute to a prolongation of the QTc interval
Chloroquine / ↑ Risk of seizures
Quinidine / ↑ Risk of ECG abnormalities or cardiac arrest
Quinine / ↑ Risk of seizures, ECG abnormalities, or cardiac arrest
Halofantrine / May prolong QTc interval; avoid use

HOW SUPPLIED
Tablets: 250 mg.

DOSAGE
• **TABLETS**
  Mild to moderate malaria caused by susceptible strains of P. falciparum *or* P. vivax.

Adults: 1,250 mg (5 tablets) as a single dose with at least 8 oz of water (not to be taken on an empty stomach). Take with food and 8 oz of water. **Children, 6 months and older:** 20–25 mg/kg, split in 2 doses. Take 6–8 hrs apart. If vomiting occurs <30 minutes after dose, give a second full dose. If vomiting occurs 30–60 minutes after dose, give additional half-dose.
  Prophylaxis of malaria.

Adults: 250 mg/week. Start 1 week before departure to endemic area and continue weekly while in area. Continue for 4 weeks after leaving the area. Take with food and 8 oz of water. **Children, 3 months and older:** 3–5 mg/kg/week. **>45 kg:** 250 mg/week. **31–45 kg:** ¾ tab/week. **21–30 kg:** ½ tab/week. **5–20 kg:** ¼ tab/week. Take with food and water. May crush and mix with water.

M

NURSING CONSIDERATIONS
ADMINISTRATION/STORAGE
1. Vaccinations with attenuated live bacteria (e.g., typhoid vaccine) should be completed at least 3 days before the first dose of mefloquine.
2. Store tablets at 15–30°C (59–86°F).
ASSESSMENT
1. Note if for prophylaxis or treatment; dosages differ. List travel location and time of visit.
2. Country-specific information on malaria can be obtained from the CDC.

3. Obtain laboratory confirmation of causative organism; monitor CBC/LFTs.

4. Note any psychiatric disturbances or severe emotional lability, assess for anxiety, depression, restlessness, or confusion. With seizure disorder, monitor anticonvulsant blood levels.

5. With life-threatening *P. falciparum* infection, treat with an IV antimalarial and follow with mefloquine to complete therapy.

6. To reduce cardiotoxic effects, induce vomiting with overdose.

CLIENT/FAMILY TEACHING

1. Do not take on an empty stomach; take with at least 8 oz of water. May be crushed and put in water, milk, or juice if necessary.

2. Avoid activities that require mental alertness until drug effects realized.

3. Report any unusual side effects, S&S of infection, mental status changes, visual disturbances; obtain periodic eye exams.

4. For prophylaxis, the CDC recommends a single dose taken weekly starting 1 week before travel, continued weekly during travel, and for 4 weeks after leaving malarious areas.

5. Report if fever or "flu-like" S&S occur during your travels or within 2 to 3 months after you leave the area.

OUTCOMES/EVALUATE

Treatment/prophylaxis of malaria (with drug-sensitive malarial parasites)

Megestrol acetate ■
(meh-**JESS**-trohl)

CLASSIFICATION(S):
Progestin
PREGNANCY CATEGORY: D
Rx: Megace, Megace ES.
♣Rx: Apo-Megestrol, Lin-Megestrol, Megace OS, Nu-Megestrol.

SEE ALSO *PROGESTERONE AND PROGESTINS* AND *ANTINEOPLASTIC AGENTS*.

USES
Tablets: Palliative treatment of advanced endometrial or breast cancer –

recurrent, inoperable, or metastatic disease. Do not use in place of chemotherapy, radiation, or surgery.

Oral suspension: Treatment of anorexia, cachexia, or an unexplained, significant weight loss in clients with a diagnosis of AIDS. *Investigational:* Appetite stimulant for cachexia in advanced cancer. Treatment of hot flashes.

ACTION/KINETICS
Action
Antineoplastic activity is due to suppression of gonadotropins (antiluteinizing effect). Has appetite-enhancing properties (mechanism unknown). Contains tartrazine, which can cause allergic-type reactions, including asthma, often occurring in aspirin sensitivity.

CONTRAINDICATIONS
Use as a diagnostic aid test for pregnancy, in known or suspected pregnancy, or for prophylaxis to avoid weight loss. Use during the first 4 months of pregnancy. Use for other types of neoplasms.

SPECIAL CONCERNS
■ The use of progestins during the first four months of pregnancy is not recommended. There is the possibility that intrauterine exposure to progestational drugs in the first trimester of pregnancy may cause genital abnormalities in female and male fetuses. If the client is exposed to progestational drugs during the first 4 months of pregnancy or if the woman becomes pregnant while taking a progestational drug, apprise her of the potential risks to the fetus.■ Use with caution in clients with a history of thromboembolic disease. Use in HIV-infected women with endometrial or breast cancer has not been widely studied. Long-term use may increase the risk of respiratory infections and may cause secondary adrenal suppression. Safety and efficacy in children have not been determined.

SIDE EFFECTS
Most Common
Diarrhea, impotence, rash, flatulence, hypertension, asthenia, insomnia, nausea, anemia, fever, headache.

GI: Diarrhea, flatulence, nausea, dyspepsia, vomiting, constipation, dry

---

Bold Italic = life threatening side effect   ■ = black box warning   ♣ = Available in Canada

mouth, hepatomegaly, increased salivation, abdominal pain, oral moniliasis. **CV:** Hypertension, *cardiomyopathy*, palpitation. **CNS:** Insomnia, headache, paresthesia, confusion, *seizures*, depression, neuropathy, hypesthesia, abnormal thought process. **Respiratory:** Pneumonia, dyspnea, cough, pharyngitis, chest pain, lung disorder, increased risk of respiratory infection with chronic use. **Dermatologic:** Rash, alopecia, herpes, pruritus, vesiculobullous rash, sweating, skin disorder. **GU:** Impotence, decreased libido, urinary frequency, albuminuria, urinary incontinence, UTI, gynecomastia. **Body as a whole:** Asthenia, anemia, fever, pain, moniliasis, infection, sarcoma. **Miscellaneous:** Leukopenia, edema, peripheral edema, amblyopia.

LABORATORY TEST CONSIDERATIONS
Hyperglycemia, ↑ LDH.

HOW SUPPLIED
Oral Suspension: 40 mg/mL, 125 mg/mL; *Tablets:* 20 mg, 40 mg.

DOSAGE
- **ORAL SUSPENSION**
  Appetite stimulant in AIDS clients.
Adults, initial: 800 mg/day (20 mL/day of the 40 mg/mL oral suspension). The dose should be adjusted to 400 mg/day (10 mL/day of the 40 mg/mL oral suspension) after 1 month. **Extra strength oral suspension:** 625 mg/day (5 mL/day). Can be taken without regard to meals.
- **TABLETS**
  Breast cancer.
40 mg 4 times per day.
  Endometrial cancer.
40–320 mg/day in divided doses. To determine efficacy, treatment should be continued for at least 2 months.

NURSING CONSIDERATIONS

ADMINISTRATION/STORAGE
1. The oral suspension is available in a lemon-lime flavor that contains 40 mg of micronized megestrol acetate/mL; shake well before using.
2. Store suspension from 15–25°C (59–77°F); dispense in a tight container. Protect from heat.
3. Store tablets from 15–30°C (59–86°F). Protect from temperatures above 40°C (104°F).

ASSESSMENT
1. Note reasons for therapy, other agents trialed, symptom onset, weight history.
2. List any sensitivity to tartrazines or thromboembolic disease.
3. Determine if pregnant; avoid.
4. With long-term therapy, assess for respiratory infections and adrenal suppression.

CLIENT/FAMILY TEACHING
1. Take exactly as prescribed; do not skip or double up doses. May take with meals if GI upset occurs. Consume plenty of fluids to prevent dehydration.
2. Report vaginal bleeding, headaches, breast tenderness, back/abdominal pain or pain/weakness in hands (CTS).
3. Practice reliable birth control. Do not breastfeed during therapy.
4. Report any pain, swelling or warmth in calves (S&S of DVT); as well as any other unusual side effects.
5. Monitor weights when used to stimulate appetite.
6. Keep all scheduled F/U appointments; with cancer therapy may take two months to determine effectiveness.

OUTCOMES/EVALUATE
- ↓ Tumor size and spread
- ↑ Appetite and weight gain especially in HIV-related cachexia

Meloxicam
(meh-**LOX**-ih-kam)

CLASSIFICATION(S):
Nonsteroidal anti-inflammatory drug
PREGNANCY CATEGORY: C
Rx: Mobic.
✤**Rx:** Mobicox.

SEE ALSO *NONSTEROIDAL ANTI-INFLAMMATORY DRUGS*

USES
(1) Signs and symptoms of osteoarthritis. (2) Signs and symptoms of rheumatoid arthritis in adults. (3) Relief of signs

and symptoms of pauciarticular or poly-articular course juvenile rheumatoid arthritis in clients 2 years of age and older. *Investigational:* Treatment of ankylosing spondylitis and acute shoulder pain.

ACTION/KINETICS
Action
Anti-inflammatory effect is likely due to inhibition of cyclo-oxygenase. Inhibition of cyclo-oxygenase results in decreased prostaglandin synthesis. Effective in reducing joint swelling, pain, and morning stiffness, as well as to increase mobility in those with inflammatory disease. Does not alter the course of the disease, however.

Pharmacokinetics
Prolonged drug absorption. 89% is bioavailable. Steady state reached in 5 days. Metabolized in the liver by P450-mediated metabolism. **Peak:** 4–5 hr. **t½, elimination:** 15–20 hr. Excreted in about equal amounts in the urine and feces. **Plasma protein binding:** More than 99%.

CONTRAINDICATIONS
Use in those who have exhibited asthma, urticaria, or allergic-type reactions after taking aspirin or other NSAIDs (anaphylaxis is possible). Use for treatment of perioperative pain in the setting of coronary artery bypass graft surgery. Use in advanced renal disease or late pregnancy (may cause premature closure of the ductus arteriosus). Lactation.

SPECIAL CONCERNS
■ (1) NSAIDs may cause an increased risk of serious CV thrombotic events, MI, and stroke, which can be fatal. The risk may increase with duration of use. Clients with CV disease or risk factors for CV disease may be at higher risk. (2) Meloxicam is contraindicated for the treatment of peri-operative pain in the setting of coronary artery bypass graft surgery. (3) NSAIDs cause an increased risk of serious GI adverse reactions, including bleeding, ulceration, and perforation of the stomach or intestines, which can be fatal. These reactions can occur at any time during use and without warning symptoms. Elderly clients are at higher risk for serious GI reactions.■ Use in clients with severe hepatic or renal failure has not been studied. Use with caution in those 65 years of age and older. Safety and efficacy have not been determined in children less than 18 years of age.

SIDE EFFECTS
Most Common
Headache, dizziness, insomnia, rash, abdominal pain/cramps, diarrhea, N&V, constipation, flatulence, dyspepsia/indigestion, UTI, edema, URTI, pharyngitis.

See also *Nonsteroidal Anti-Inflammatory Drugs* for a complete list of possible side effects. Side effects listed are those with an incidence of 2% or greater. **GI:** Abdominal pain, cramps, diarrhea, dyspepsia, indigestion, constipation, flatulence, N&V. **CNS:** Dizziness, headache, insomnia. **Respiratory:** Pharyngitis, URTI, coughing. **GU:** Renal papillary necrosis, micturition frequency, UTI. **Hematologic:** Anemia. **Musculoskeletal:** Arthralgia, back pain. **Dermatologic:** Pruritus, rash. **Body as a whole:** Fluid retention, edema, pain, flu-like symptoms, accidents.

LABORATORY TEST CONSIDERATIONS
Elevation of LFTs.

DRUG INTERACTIONS
ACE Inhibitors / ↓ Antihypertensive effect of ACE inhibitors
Aspirin / ↑ Risk of GI side effects, including GI ulceration or other complications
Cholestyramine / ↑ Meloxicam clearance
Lithium / ↑ Plasma lithium levels
Warfarin / ↑ Risk of bleeding

HOW SUPPLIED
Oral Suspension: 7.5 mg/5 mL; *Tablets:* 7.5 mg, 15 mg.

DOSAGE
- **ORAL SUSPENSION; TABLETS**
  Osteoarthritis, rheumatoid arthritis.
Initial and maintenance: 7.5 mg once daily. Some may gain additional benefit from 15 mg once daily. Maximum recommended daily dose: 15 mg.
  Pauciarticular/polyarticular course juvenile rheumatoid arthritis.
Recommended PO dose: 0.125 mg/kg once daily, up to a maximum of 7.5 mg

---

Bold Italic = life threatening side effect   ■ = black box warning   ♣ = Available in Canada

daily. The following dosage recommendations are based on weight using the oral suspension (1.5 mg/mL): **12 kg (26 lbs):** 1 mL (1.5 mg); **24 kg (54 lbs):** 2 mL (3 mg); **36 kg (80 lbs):** 3 mL (4.5 mg); **48 kg (106 lbs):** 4 mL (6 mg); **greater or equal to 60 kg (132 lbs):** 5 mL (7.5 mg).

NURSING CONSIDERATIONS

ADMINISTRATION/STORAGE

1. Consider the potential benefits and risks before deciding to use meloxicam.
2. Use the lowest dose for the shortest duration consistent with individual client treatment goals. Adjust dose to suit the individual client's needs.
3. The oral suspension, 7.5 mg/5 mL or 15 mg/10 mL, may be substituted for meloxicam tablets, 7.5 or 15 mg respectively.
4. The maximum recommended daily dose is 15 mg, regardless of the formulation.
5. May be taken without regard to meals.
6. Store at 15–30°C (59–86°F). Keep in a dry place in a tight container.

ASSESSMENT

1. Identify reasons for therapy, onset, characteristics of disease, ROM, deformity/loss of function, level of pain, other agents trialed, outcome. List drugs prescribed to ensure none interact.
2. Check for any GI bleed or ulcer history, aspirin or other NSAID-induced asthma, urticaria, or allergic-type reactions.
3. Monitor CBC, electrolytes, renal and LFTs within 3 months of starting therapy and then q 6 months. Avoid with severe liver/renal dysfunction, perioperative CABG pain, pregnancy.

CLIENT/FAMILY TEACHING

1. Take as directed at the same time each day. May take with or without food. Shake the oral suspension gently before using.
2. The lowest dose for symptom control will be used. Class of drugs may cause serious CV side effects, such as MI or stroke.
3. Avoid activities that require mental alertness until drug effects realized; may cause dizziness or drowsiness.

4. Report unusual or persistent side effects including dyspepsia, abdominal pain, dizziness, and changes in stool or skin color. Alcohol and tobacco may aggravate GI S&S.
5. Avoid therapy during pregnancy; may cause premature closure of baby's heart duct.
6. Report weight gain, skin rash, swelling of ankles, chest pain, SOB, or lack of effect.

OUTCOMES/EVALUATE

• Relief of joint pain and inflammation with improved mobility

Melphalan (L-PAM, L-Phenylalanine mustard, L-Sarcolysin, MPL)

(**MEL**-fah-lan)

CLASSIFICATION(S):

Antineoplastic, alkylating
PREGNANCY CATEGORY: D
Rx: Alkeran.

SEE ALSO *ANTINEOPLASTIC AGENTS* AND *ALKYLATING AGENTS*.

USES

(1) Palliative treatment of multiple myeloma. Use IV only when PO therapy is not appropriate. (2) Palliative treatment of nonresectable epithelial carcinoma of ovary (tablets only). *Investigational:* Cancer of the breast and testes. Bone marrow transplantation.

ACTION/KINETICS

Action

A bifunctional alkylating agent that forms an unstable ethylenimmonium ion that binds to or alkylates various intracellular substances including nucleic acids. It produces a cytotoxic effect by cross-linking of DNA and RNA strands as well as inhibition of protein synthesis.

Pharmacokinetics

Absorption from GI tract is variable and incomplete. $t\frac{1}{2}$ **after PO:** 90 min. Inacti-

---

vated in tissues and body fluids although it will remain active in the blood for approximately 6 hr. Within 24 hr, 10% is excreted unchanged in the urine.

CONTRAINDICATIONS
Lactation. Hypersensitivity to the drug. Known resistance to drug.

SPECIAL CONCERNS
■ (1) Administer under the supervision of a qualified physician experienced in the use of cancer chemotherapeutic drugs. (2) Severe bone marrow depression with resulting infection or bleeding may occur. More myelosuppression occurs with IV use than with PO use. (3) Hypersensitivity reactions, including anaphylaxis, have occurred in about 2% of clients who received the IV product. (4) Melphalan is leukemogenic in humans. It produces chromosomal aberrations in vitro and in vivo; thus, it is potentially mutagenic to humans.■ Safety and efficacy have not been determined in children less than 12 years of age. Use with extreme caution in those with compromised bone marrow function due to prior chemotherapy or radiation. Use caution in dose selection in the elderly. Reduce IV dosage in impaired renal function.

SIDE EFFECTS
Most Common
N&V, diarrhea, stomatitis, rash, amenorrhea, alopecia, leukopenia, thrombocytopenia.
See *Antineoplastic Agents* for a complete list of possible side effects. **Severe bone marrow depression (especially after IV use,** chromosomal aberrations (may be mutagenic), **leukemia (acute, nonlymphatic) in clients with multiple myeloma.** Also, hypersensitivity reactions including **anaphylaxis, pulmonary fibrosis,** interstitial pneumonia, vasculitis, **hemolytic anemia,** hepatitis, jaundice.

LABORATORY TEST CONSIDERATIONS
↑ Uric acid and urinary 5-HIAA levels. Abnormal LFTs.

OD OVERDOSE MANAGEMENT
Symptoms: Severe N&V, decreased consciousness, **seizures,** muscle paralysis, cholinomimetic symptoms, diarrhea, severe mucositis, stomatitis, colitis, **hemorrhage of GI tract, bone marrow toxicity.** *Treatment:* General supportive treatment, blood transfusions, antibiotics. Monitor hematology for up to 6 weeks. Use of filgrastim or sargramostim may decrease the period of pancytopenia.

DRUG INTERACTIONS
Carmustine / ↑ Risk of lung toxicity
Cisplatin / Drug-induced renal dysfunction → ↓ melphalan excretion
Cyclosporine / ↑ Risk of nephrotoxicity
Interferon alfa / ↓ Levels of melphalan
Nalidixic acid / ↑ Risk of severe hemorrhagic necrotic enterocolitis in pediatric clients

HOW SUPPLIED
Powder for Injection, Lyophilized: 50 mg; *Tablets:* 2 mg.

DOSAGE
• **TABLETS**
  Multiple myeloma.
One of the following regimens may be used. (1) 6 mg given once daily for 2–3 weeks (adjust dose based on weekly blood counts). Drug is then discontinued for up to 4 weeks with blood count being monitored. When WBC and platelet counts are increasing, a maintenance dose of 2 mg/day can be started. (2) 10 mg/day for 7–10 days. Maximum leukocyte and platelet suppression occurs within 3–5 weeks with recovery within 4–8 weeks. When the WBC exceeds 4,000/mm^3 and the platelet count is greater than 100,000/mm^3, a maintenance dose of 2 mg/day can be started. Dose is then adjusted to 1–3 mg/day, depending on the hematologic response. Keep leukocytes in the range of 3,000–3,500 cells/mm^3. (3) 0.15 mg/kg/day for 7 days followed by a rest period of at least 2 weeks (up to 5 weeks may be needed). During the rest period, the leukocyte count will decrease; when WBC and platelet counts are increasing, a maintenance dose of 0.05 mg/kg/day may be given. (4) 0.25 mg/kg/day for 4 consecutive days (or 0.2 mg/kg/day for 5 consecutive days) for a total dose of 1 mg/kg/course of therapy. The 4 to 5 day courses can be repeated q 4–6 weeks if the granulo-

M

cyte and platelet counts have returned to normal.

Epithelial ovarian cancer.

0.2 mg/kg/day for 5 days repeated q 4–5 weeks (as long as blood counts return to normal).

- **IV**

Multiple myeloma.

Adults, usual: 16 mg/m² as a single infusion over 15–20 min. Give this dose at 2 week intervals for a total of four doses; then, after adequate recovery from toxicity, at 4-week intervals. Reduce the dose up to 50% in clients with a BUN less than or equal to 30 mg/dL.

NURSING CONSIDERATIONS

Ⓒ Do not confuse Alkeran (melphalan), Leukeran (chlorambucil), and Myleran (busulfan), each of which is an antineoplastic.

ADMINISTRATION/STORAGE

1. Store tablets in a refrigerator between 2–8°C (36–46°F). Protect from light. Dispense in glass.

IV 2. About one-third to one-half of clients with multiple myeloma show a favorable response to IV melphalan.

3. For IV use, reconstitute powder with 10 mL of the supplied diluent for a concentration of 5 mg/mL. Then shake vial vigorously until a clear solution is obtained. Immediately dilute the dose to be given with 0.9% NaCl injection to a concentration of less than or equal to 0.45 mg/mL. Administer diluted infusion over 15 min.

4. Complete administration within 60 min after reconstitution. After dilution, about 1% label strength of melphalan hydrolyzes every 10 min.

5. Protect from light and dispense in glass.

6. Store IV product at 15–30°C (59–86°F). Protect from light. A precipitate will form if the reconstituted solution is stored at 5°C (41°F). Do not refrigerate the reconstituted product.

ASSESSMENT

1. Note reasons for therapy, other agents trialed, outcome.

2. Identify previous radiation or chemotherapy treatments. Do not give full dosage until 4 weeks after chemo or XRT due to risk of severe bone marrow depression; give under direction of oncologist.

3. Monitor CBC, uric acid, renal, LFTs–reduce dose with dysfunction. Drug causes granulocyte and platelet suppression. Nadir: 14 days; recovery: 28–40 days.

CLIENT/FAMILY TEACHING

1. Take once a day as directed on an empty stomach. May divide dose if N&V severe. Usually given by injection in providers office.

2. Use reliable birth control; may cause severe birth defects.

3. Increase fluid intake to protect against ↑ uric acid levels. Avoid crowds and those with active infections. Ask provider before accepting vaccinations.

4. Report any unusual bruising, bleeding, fever, chills, SOB, sore throat, stomach/flank/joint pains, or black tarry stools. Expect hair loss; will regrow.

OUTCOMES/EVALUATE

- ↓ Malignant cell proliferation
- Improved hematologic profile

Memantine hydrochloride Ⓒ 📷

(meh-**MAN**-teen)

CLASSIFICATION(S):

Drug for Alzheimer's disease

PREGNANCY CATEGORY: B

Rx: Namenda.

USES

Moderate to severe dementia of the Alzheimers type. When combined with donepezil (Aricept), the decline of mental and physical function may be less. *Investigational:* Treatment of vascular dementia.

ACTION/KINETICS

Action

It is believed that activation of N-methyl-D-aspartate (NMDA) receptors in the brain by glutamate, an excitatory amino acid, contributes to the symptomatology of Alzheimer's disease. Memantine is believed to have low to moderate affinity as an antagonist for open-channel NMDA receptors thus preventing activation by glutamate. The drug does not prevent or slow neurodegeneration in Alzheimer's disease. The drug also shows antagonistic effects at the 5HT₃ receptor and for nicotinic acetylcholine receptors.

Pharmacokinetics
Well absorbed after PO administration; **peak levels:** 3–7 hr. Food has no effect on the absorption. Excreted mainly unchanged in the urine. $t^1/_2$, **terminal:** 60–80 hr. **Plasma protein binding:** 45%.

CONTRAINDICATIONS
Known hypersensitivity to memantine or any excipients in the formulation, including lactose monohydrate. Conditions that raise urine pH may decrease the urinary elimination of memantine resulting in increased plasma levels. Severe renal impairment.

SPECIAL CONCERNS
It is likely that clients with moderate to severe renal impairment will have higher levels of the drug; dose reduction should be considered. Use with caution in renal tubular acidosis, severe UTIs, and during lactation. Safety and efficacy have not been determined in children.

SIDE EFFECTS
Most Common
Fatigue, pain, increased BP, dizziness, headache, constipation, vomiting, back pain, confusion, somnolence, hallucinations, coughing, dyspnea.

GI: Constipation, vomiting. Infrequently, gastroenteritis, diverticulitis, *GI hemorrhage*, melena, esophageal ulceration. **CNS:** Dizziness, headache, vertigo, ataxia, hypokinesia, confusion, somnolence, hallucinations, aggressive reaction. Infrequently, paresthesia, *convulsions*, extrapyramidal disorder, hypertonia, tremor, aphasia, hypoesthesia, abnormal coordination, hemiplegia, hyperkinesia, stupor, *cerebral hemorrhage*, neuralgia, neuropathy, delusions, personality disorder, emotional lability, nervousness, sleep disorder, increased libido, psychosis, amnesia, apathy, paranoid reaction, abnormal thinking, abnormal crying, paroniria, deliri-

um, depersonalization, neurosis, *suicide attempt*. **CV:** Hypertension, TIA, syncope, *CVA, cardiac failure*. Infrequently, angina pectoris, bradycardia, *MI, cardiac arrest*, *pulmonary embolism*, thrombophlebitis, atrial fibrillation, hypotension, postural hypotension, pulmonary edema. **Respiratory:** Coughing, difficulty breathing, dypsnea, pneumonia. Infrequently, *apnea*, asthma, hemoptysis. **Dermatologic:** Rash. Infrequently, skin ulceration, pruritus, cellulitis, eczema, dermatitis, erythematous rash, alopecia, urticaria. **GU:** Frequent micturition. Infrequently, dysuria, hematuria, urinary retention. **Ophthalmic:** Cataract, conjunctivitis. Infrequently, macula lutea degeneration, ptosis, decreased visual acuity, blepharitis, blurred vision, corneal opacity, glaucoma, conjunctival hemorrhage, eye pain, retinal hemorrhage, xerophthalmia, diplopia, abnormal lacrimation, myopia, retinal detachment. **Body as a whole:** Fatigue, pain, syncope. Infrequently, hypothermia, allergic reaction, dehydration, aggravated diabetes mellitus, involuntary muscle contractions. **Miscellaneous:** Increased appetite, back pain, anemia, leukopenia (infrequent), decreased hearing, tinnitus, decreased weight.

LABORATORY TEST CONSIDERATIONS
↑ Alkaline phosphatase. Hyponatremia.

OD OVERDOSE MANAGEMENT
Symptoms: See *Side Effects. Treatment:* Use general supportive measures; treat symptoms. Can enhance elimination by acidification of the urine.

DRUG INTERACTIONS
Amantadine / Use with memantine with caution as amantadine is also a NMDA antagonist
Carbonic anhydrase inhibitors / Accumulation of memantine → ↑ side effects
Cimetidine / Possible altered plasma levels of both drugs
Dextromethorphan / Use with memantine with caution as dextromethorphan is also a NMDA antagonist
Hydrochlorothiazide / Possible altered plasma levels of both drugs

---

Bold Italic = life threatening side effect   ■ = black box warning   ✦ = Available in Canada

Ketamine / Use with memantadine with caution as ketamine is also a NMDA antagonist
Nicotine / Possible altered plasma levels of both drugs
Quinidine / Possible altered plasma levels of both drugs
Ranitidine / Possible altered plasma levels of both drugs
Sodium bicarbonate / Accumulation of memantine → ↑ side effects
Triamterene / Possible altered plasma levels of both drugs

HOW SUPPLIED
Oral Solution: 2 mg/mL; *Tablets:* 5 mg, 10 mg.

DOSAGE
• **ORAL SOLUTION; TABLETS**
  Alzheimer's disease.
Initial: 5 mg/day. Dose should be increased in 5 mg increments to 10 mg/day (5 mg twice a day), then 15 mg/day (5 mg and 10 mg as separate doses), and finally 20 mg/day (10 mg twice a day). The minimum recommended interval between dose increases is one week. Reduce the dose in clients with moderate renal impairment.

NURSING CONSIDERATIONS
⏚ Do not confuse memantine with amantadine (antiviral and antiparkinson drug).

ADMINISTRATION/STORAGE
Store from 15–30°C (59–86°F).

ASSESSMENT
1. Note reasons for therapy, when diagnosed with Alzheimers disease and when treatment began.
2. Assess for other medical conditions that require careful monitoring, i.e., seizure disorder, liver or renal dysfunction. Monitor weight, VS, renal and LFTs.
3. List all drugs prescribed to ensure none interact. Review MMSE score before therapy and then several months after to determine effectiveness.

CLIENT/FAMILY TEACHING
1. May take with or without food; with food if GI upset.
2. Drug is used in Alzheimers disease to improve level of cognitive functioning,

does not cure disease but assists with symptoms.
3. Avoid alcohol and any OTC products or herbals without provider approval to prevent interactions. May cause dizziness, constipation, headache, pain.
4. Report any adverse side effects and ensure caregiver keeps all follow up appointments to evaluate drug response and assess renal and liver function.

OUTCOMES/EVALUATE
Improved cognitive functioning and ↓ confusion.

Meperidine hydrochloride (Pethidine hydrochloride) IV
(meh-**PER**-ih-deen)

CLASSIFICATION(S):
Narcotic analgesic
PREGNANCY CATEGORY: C
Rx: Demerol Hydrochloride, **C-II**

SEE ALSO *NARCOTIC ANALGESICS.*

USES
PO, Parenteral: Analgesic for moderate-to-severe pain. **Parenteral:** (1) Preoperative medication. (2) Adjunct to support anesthesia. (3) Obstetrical analgesia (except 10 mg/mL).

ACTION/KINETICS
Action
One-tenth as potent an analgesic as morphine. Its analgesic effect is only one-half when given PO rather than parenterally. Has no antitussive effects and does not produce miosis. Less smooth muscle spasm, constipation, and antitussive effect than equianalgesic doses of morphine. Produces both psychologic and physical dependence; overdosage causes severe respiratory depression (see *Narcotic Overdose*).

Pharmacokinetics
Onset: 10–45 min. **Peak effect:** 30–60 min. **Duration:** 2–4 hr (duration is less than that of most opiates; keep in mind when establishing a dosing schedule).

t½: 3–6 hr for meperidine and <20 hr for normeperidine (active metabolite).

ADDITIONAL CONTRAINDICATIONS

Hypersensitivity to drug, convulsive states as in epilepsy, tetanus, and strychnine poisoning, children under 6 months, diabetic acidosis, head injuries, shock, liver disease, respiratory depression, increased intracranial pressure, and before labor during pregnancy. Use with sibutramine.

SPECIAL CONCERNS

Use with caution during lactation, in older, or debilitated clients. Use with extreme caution in clients with asthma. Atropine-like effects may aggravate glaucoma, especially when given with other drugs used with caution in glaucoma.

SIDE EFFECTS

Most Common

Constipation, dry mouth, N&V, anorexia, dizziness, fatigue, lightheadedness, muscle twitches, sweating, itching, decreased urination, decreased libido.

See *Narcotic Analgesics* for a complete list of possible side effects. Also, transient hallucinations, transient hypotension (high doses), visual disturbances. Active metabolite may accumulate in renal dysfunction, leading to an increased risk of CNS toxicity.

ADDITIONAL DRUG INTERACTIONS

Antidepressants, tricyclic / Additive anticholinergic side effects

Cimetidine / ↑ Respiratory and CNS depression

Hydantoins / ↓ Meperidine effect R/T ↑ liver breakdown

MAO inhibitors / ↑ Risk of severe symptoms including hyperpyrexia, restlessness, hyper- or hypotension, convulsions, or coma

Protease inhibitors / Avoid combination

Sibutramine / Possibility of life-threatening serotonin syndrome

Smoking / ↓ Analgesia R/T ↑ hepatic metabolism; takes several weeks to occur

OD OVERDOSE MANAGEMENT

Symptoms: Severe respiratory depression. See *Narcotic Analgesics*. *Treatment:* Naloxone 0.4 mg IV is effective in the treatment of acute overdosage. In PO overdose, gastric lavage and induced emesis are indicated. Treatment, however, is aimed at combating the progressive respiratory depression usually through artificial ventilation.

HOW SUPPLIED

Injection: 25 mg/mL, 50 mg/mL, 75 mg/mL, 100 mg/mL; *Oral Solution:* 50 mg/5 mL; *Syrup:* 50 mg/5 mL; *Tablets:* 50 mg, 100 mg.

DOSAGE

- **ORAL SOLUTION; SYRUP; TABLETS**
  Analgesic.
Adults: 50–100 mg q 3–4 hr as needed; **pediatric:** 1.1–1.75 mg/kg, up to adult dosage, q 3–4 hr as needed.
- **IM, SC**
  Analgesic.
Adults: 50–150 mg q 3–4 hr, as needed. For elderly clients, use the lower end of the dosage range and observe closely. **Children:** 1.1–1.75 mg/kg, up to the adult dose, q 3–4 hr, as needed.
  Preoperatively.
Adults: 50–100 mg 30–90 min before beginning anesthesia. Use the lower end of the dosage range for elderly clients and observe closely. **Children:** 1.1–2.2 mg/kg, up to the adult dose, 30–90 min before beginning anesthesia.
  Obstetrical analgesia.
Adults: 50–100 mg when the pain becomes regular; may repeat at 1 to 3 hr intervals.
- **IV**
  Analgesia.
Adults: 15–35 mg/hr by continuous infusion.
  Analgesic using a compatible Hospira infusion device.
Adults, initial: 10 mg using the 10 mg/mL strength; **range:** 1–5 mg/incremental dose. The recommended lockout interval is 6–10 min with the minimum recommended lockout interval of 5 min. Dose may be adjusted upward or downward or the lockout interval may be increased or decreased, depending on client response.
  Support of anesthesia.
Continuous IV infusion: 1 mg/mL or **slow IV injection:** 10 mg/mL until client needs met.

Bold Italic = life threatening side effect   ■ = black box warning   ♣ = Available in Canada

NURSING CONSIDERATIONS

ADMINISTRATION/STORAGE

1. Adjust the dose depending on the severity of the pain and the client response.

2. For repeated doses, IM administration is preferred over SC use.

3. More effective when given parenterally than when given PO.

4. Take the syrup with half a glass of water to minimize anesthetic effect on mucous membranes.

5. If used concomitantly with phenothiazines or antianxiety agents, reduce the PO or parenteral dose by 25–50%.

6. Adjust parenteral doses according to the severity of pain and client response. Reduce the dose in poor-risk clients, in the very young or very old, in those with impaired renal or hepatic function, and in clients receiving other CNS depressants.

7. For surgical clients, adjust parenteral doses based on response of the client, other premedications and concomitant medications, the anesthetic being used, and the nature and duration of the surgery.

IV 8. IV doses should be decreased and the injection given very slowly, preferably using a diluted solution (e.g., 10 mg/mL). Rapid injection increases the incidence of side effects.

9. When given parenterally, especially IV, the client should be lying down.

10. Meperidine for IV use is incompatible with the following drugs: Aminophylline, barbiturates, heparin, iodide, methicillin, morphine sulfate, phenytoin, sodium bicarbonate, sulfadiazine, and sulfisoxazole.

11. The following IV solutions are compatible with meperidine: D5/RL, dextrose-saline combinations, dextrose (2.5%, 5%, 10%) in water; Ringer's, LR, 0.45% or 0.5% NaCl; or ⅙ M sodium lactate.

12. Store PO forms from 15–30°C (59–86°F). Store parenteral forms (except the 10 mg/mL) at room temperature (up to 25°C, 77°F). Store the 10 mg/mL injection from 20–25 °C (68–77°F).

ASSESSMENT

1. Note reasons for therapy, with pain - location, onset, characteristics of pain; rate pain level. List drugs prescribed to ensure none interact unfavorably.

2. List any head injury, seizure disorder, glaucoma, asthma, or conditions that may compromise respirations.

3. Monitor renal and LFTs; note dysfunction.

CLIENT/FAMILY TEACHING

1. Take drug within ordered intervals to prevent pain recurring; report pain levels and lack of effectiveness.

2. Drug causes dizziness and drowsiness; do not engage in activities that require mental alertness.

3. Due to low BP effects, rise slowly and do not change positions abruptly.

4. Increase fluid intake and bulk; report constipation if evident.

5. Avoid alcohol and other CNS depressants.

6. Store safely away from bedside; record dose and time of administration. Drug causes dependence.

OUTCOMES/EVALUATE

Desired level of analgesia/pain control

Mercaptopurine (6-Mercaptopurine, 6-MP) ©

(mer-kap-toe-**PYOUR**-een)

CLASSIFICATION(S):
Antineoplastic, antimetabolite
PREGNANCY CATEGORY: D
Rx: Purinethol.

SEE ALSO *ANTINEOPLASTIC AGENTS.*

USES

(1) Acute lymphocytic or myelocytic leukemia. Use combination therapy. (2) Lymphoblastic leukemia, especially in children. (3) Acute myelogenous and myelomonocytic leukemia. Use combination therapy. Effectiveness varies depending on use. Not effective for leukemia of the CNS, solid tumors, lympho-

M

mas, or chronic lymphocytic leukemia. *Investigational:* Inflammatory bowel disease, chronic myelocytic leukemia, polycythemia vera, non-Hodgkin's lymphoma, psoriatic arthritis.

ACTION/KINETICS

Action

Cell-cycle specific for the S phase of cell division. Converted to thioinosinic acid by the enzyme hypoxanthine-guanine phosphoribosyltransferase. Thioinosinic acid then inhibits reactions involving inosinic acid. Also, both thioinosinic acid and 6-methylthioinosinate (also formed from mercaptopurine) inhibit RNA synthesis.

Pharmacokinetics

Absorption is incomplete and variable, averaging about 50%. **Plasma t½:** 47 min in adults and 21 min in children. Metabolites are excreted in urine with up to 39% excreted unchanged. Cross-resistance with thioguanine has been observed. **Plasma protein binding:** About 19%.

CONTRAINDICATIONS

Use in resistance to mercaptopurine or thioguanine. Prophylaxis or treatment of CNS leukemia, CLL, lymphomas (including Hodgkin's disease), solid tumors. Lactation.

SPECIAL CONCERNS

Use with caution in clients with impaired renal function. Use during lactation only if benefits clearly outweigh risks. Severe bone marrow depression (anemia, leukopenia, thrombocytopenia) may occur. There is an increased risk of pancreatitis when used for inflammatory bowel disease.

SIDE EFFECTS

Most Common

Myelosuppression (anemia, leukopenia, thrombocytopenia), alopecia, skin rash, hyperpigmentation, fatigue, weakness, yellow eyes/skin, N&V, anorexia, abdominal pain.

See *Antineoplastic Agents* for a complete list of possible side effects. Also, **hepatotoxicity**, oral lesions, drug fever, hyperuricemia. Produces less GI toxicity than folic acid antagonists. Side effects are less frequent in children than in adults. Pancreatitis (when used for in-

flammatory bowel disease). Alopecia, oligospermia.

OD OVERDOSE MANAGEMENT

Symptoms: Immediate symptoms include N&V, diarrhea, and anorexia while delayed symptoms include myelosuppression, gastroenteritis, and liver dysfunction. *Treatment:* Induction of emesis if detected soon after ingestion. Supportive measures.

DRUG INTERACTIONS

Allopurinol / ↑ Methotrexate effect R/T ↓ liver breakdown (reduce methotrexate dose from 25–33%)

Balsalazide / Possible leukopenia and ↑ in whole blood 6-thioguanine nucleotide levels in clients with Crohn's disease

Mesalamine / Possible leukopenia and ↑ in whole blood 6-thioguanine in clients with Crohn's disease

Sulfasalazine / Possible leukopenia and ↑ in whole blood 6-thioguanine nucleotide levels in clients with Crohn's disease

Trimethoprim–Sulfamethoxazole / ↑ Risk of bone marrow suppression

HOW SUPPLIED

Tablets: 50 mg.

DOSAGE

- **TABLETS**

   Leukemias.

Highly individualized. **Induction therapy:** 2.5 mg/kg/day (**Adults, usual:** 100–200 mg; **pediatric:** 50 mg.) Calculate the dose to the closest multiple of 25 mg. Dose may be given all at once. Dosage may be increased to 5 mg/kg/day after 4 weeks if beneficial effects are not noted. Dosage is increased until symptoms of toxicity appear. **Maintenance after remission:** 1.5–2.5 mg/kg/day but varies from client to client.

NURSING CONSIDERATIONS

⊗ Do not confuse Purinethol (mercaptopurine) with propylthiouracil (antithyroid drug).

ADMINISTRATION/STORAGE

1. Start with lower doses in clients with impaired renal function.
2. When used for acute lymphocytic leukemia, combine with vincristine,

---

prednisone, and L-asparaginase which induces complete remission more frequently than mercaptopurine alone. Remission is brief without use of maintenance therapy; although mercaptopurine alone can prolong complete remission, combination therapy has proven more effective.

3. In children with acute lymphoblastic leukemia, there is lowered risk of relapse if drug is given in the evening rather than morning.

4. Since maximum effect on blood count may be delayed and the count may drop for several days after drug has been discontinued, stop therapy at first sign of abnormally large drop in leukocyte count. Nadir: 14 days.

ASSESSMENT

1. Note reasons for therapy, characteristics of S&S, other agents trialed, outcome.

2. Obtain CBC, uric acid, renal, LFTs. Drug causes granulocyte and platelet suppression. Nadir: 10–14 days; recovery: 21–28 days.

CLIENT/FAMILY TEACHING

1. Take as directed with or without food.

2. Drink 8–10 glasses of water/fluids each day. Avoid alcoholic beverages.

3. Report any S&S of infection, dizziness, SOB, mouth sores, fever, chills, unusual bruising/bleeding, or pain.

4. Avoid persons with infections; avoid activities that may cause bruising or injury.

5. Practice reliable contraception.

OUTCOMES/EVALUATE

- Improved hematologic profile
- ↓ Malignant cell proliferation
- Disease remission

Mesalamine (5-Aminosalicylic acid)
(mes-**AL**-ah-meen)

CLASSIFICATION(S):
Anti-inflammatory drug
PREGNANCY CATEGORY: B
Rx: Asacol, Canasa, Lialda, Pentasa, Rowasa.
❦Rx: Mesasal, Novo-5 ASA, Pentasa, Salofalk.

USES
PO: Maintain remission and treatment of mild to moderate active ulcerative colitis.
   Rectal: Treatment of active mild to moderate distal ulcerative colitis, proctosigmoiditis, or proctitis.

ACTION/KINETICS
Action
Chemically related to acetylsalicylic acid. Acts locally in the colon to inhibit cyclo-oxygenase and therefore prostaglandin synthesis, resulting in a reduction of inflammation of colitis.

Pharmacokinetics
Following PR administration, between 10% and 30% is absorbed and is excreted in the urine as the N-acetyl-5-aminosalicylic acid metabolite; the remainder is excreted in the feces. PO tablets are coated with an acrylic-based resin that prevents release of mesalamine until it reaches the terminal ileum and beyond. Approximately 28% of the drug found in tablets is absorbed with the remaining drug available for action in the colon. Capsules are methylcellulose coated, controlled release designed to release the drug throughout the GI tract; from 20–30% is absorbed. **t½, mesalamine:** 0.5–1.5 hr; **t½, N-acetyl mesalamine:** 5–10 hr. **Time to reach maximum plasma levels:** 4–12 hr for both mesalamine and metabolite. Excreted mainly through the kidneys.

CONTRAINDICATIONS
Hypersensitivity to salicylates.

M

SPECIAL CONCERNS

Use with caution in clients with sulfasalazine sensitivity, in those with impaired renal function, and during lactation. Safety and efficacy have not been established in children. Pyloric stenosis may delay the drug in reaching the colon.

SIDE EFFECTS

Most Common

After use of capsules: Headache, rash/spots, abdominal pain/cramps, diarrhea, N&V.

After use of rectal suppositories/suspension: Dizziness, fever, headache, malaise/fatigue, itching, rash/spots, abdominal pain/cramps, diarrhea, flatulence, nausea, cold/sore throat, flu syndrome.

After use of tablets: Asthenia, chills, dizziness, fever, headache, rash/spots, abdominal pain/cramps, diarrhea, constipation, dyspepsia, eructation, nausea, arthralgia, back pain, hypertonia, pharyngitis, pain.

Sulfite sensitivity: Hives, wheezing, itching, *anaphylaxis*. **Intolerance syndrome:** Acute abdominal pain, cramping, bloody diarrhea, rash, fever, headache. **GI:** Abdominal pain or discomfort, flatulence, cramps, dyspepsia, nausea, diarrhea, hemorrhoids, rectal pain/burning/urgency, constipation, bloating, worsening of colitis, eructation, pain following insertion of enema, vomiting (after PO use). **CNS:** Headache, dizziness, insomnia, fatigue, malaise, chills, fever, asthenia. **Respiratory:** Cold, sore throat; increased cough, pharyngitis, rhinitis following PO use. **Dermatologic:** Acne, pruritus, itching, rash. **Musculoskeletal:** Back pain, hypertonia, arthralgia, myalgia, leg/joint pain, arthritis. **Miscellaneous:** Flu-like symptoms, hair loss, anorexia, peripheral edema, urinary burning, sweating, pain, chest pain, conjunctivitis, dysmenorrhea, pancreatitis. In addition to the preceding, PO use may result in the following side effects. **GI:** Anorexia, gastritis, gastroenteritis, cholecystitis, dry mouth, increased appetite, oral ulcers, tenesmus, perforated peptic ulcer, bloody diarrhea, duodenal ulcer, dysphagia, esophageal ulcer, fecal incontinence, GI bleeding, oral moniliasis, rectal bleeding, abnormal stool color and texture. **CNS:** Anxiety, depression, hyperesthesia, nervousness, confusion, peripheral neuropathy, somnolence, emotional lability, vertigo, paresthesia, migraine, tremor, transverse myelitis, Guillain-Barré syndrome. **Dermatologic:** Dry skin, psoriasis, pyoderma gangrenosum, urticaria, erythema nodosum, eczema, photosensitivity, lichen planus, nail disorder. **CV:** Pericarditis, myocarditis, vasodilation, palpitations, *fatal myocarditis*, chest pain, T-wave abnormalities. **GU:** Nephropathy, interstitial nephritis, urinary urgency, dysuria, hematuria, menorrhagia, epididymitis, amenorrhea, hypomenorrhea, metrorrhagia, nephrotic syndrome, urinary frequency, albuminuria, nephrotoxicity. **Hematologic:** *Agranulocytosis*, anemia, eosinophilia, leukopenia, thrombocytopenia, lymphadenopathy, thrombocythemia, ecchymosis. **Respiratory:** Worsening of asthma, sinusitis, interstitial pneumonitis, pulmonary infiltrates, fibrosing alveolitis. **Ophthalmic:** Eye pain, blurred vision. **Miscellaneous:** Ear pain, tinnitus, taste perversion, neck pain, enlargement of abdomen, facial edema, gout, hypersensitivity pneumonitis, breast pain, Kawasaki-like syndrome.

LABORATORY TEST CONSIDERATIONS

↑ AST, ALT, BUN, LDH, alkaline phosphatase, serum creatinine, amylase, lipase, GTTP.

OD OVERDOSE MANAGEMENT

Symptoms: Salicylate toxicity manifested by tinnitus, vertigo, headache, confusion, drowsiness, sweating, hyperventilation, vomiting, and diarrhea. Severe toxicity results in disruption of electrolyte balance and blood pH, *hyperthermia,* and *dehydration. Treatment:* Therapy to treat salicylate toxicity, including emesis, gastric lavage, fluid and electrolyte replacement (if necessary), maintenance of adequate renal function.

DRUG INTERACTIONS

When used with azathioprine or mercaptopurine, possible leukopenia and ↑ in whole blood 6-thioguanine nucleotide levels in Crohn's disease clients.

HOW SUPPLIED

Capsules, Controlled-Release: 250 mg, 500 mg; *Rectal Suspension Enema:* 4 grams/60 mL; *Suppositories, Rectal:* 500 mg, 1,000 mg; *Tablets, Delayed-Release:* 400 mg, 1.2 grams.

DOSAGE

- **SUPPOSITORIES, RECTAL**
  Mild to moderate distal ulcerative colitis, proctosigmoiditis, proctitis.
  One suppository (500 mg) twice a day
- **RECTAL SUSPENSION ENEMA**
  Mild to moderate distal ulcerative colitis, proctosigmoiditis, proctitis.
  4 grams in 60 mL once daily for 3–6 weeks, usually given at bedtime; retain for 8 hr. For maintenance, the drug can be given every other day or every third day at doses of 1–2 grams.
- **CAPSULES, CONTROLLED-RELEASE**
  Mild to moderate active ulcerative colitis.
  1 gram (4 capsules) 4 times per day for a total daily dose of 4 grams for up to 8 weeks.
- **TABLETS, DELAYED-RELEASE**
  Mild to moderate active ulcerative colitis.
  800 mg 3 times per day for a total dose of 2.4 grams/day for 6 weeks. Or, 2.4 grams once daily (of Lialda) with meals.

NURSING CONSIDERATIONS

◊ Do not confuse Asacol with Avelox (fluoroquinolone antibiotic).

ADMINISTRATION/STORAGE

1. Shake bottle well to ensure suspension is homogeneous.
2. Beneficial effects using the suppository or enema may occur within 3–21 days, with a full course of therapy lasting up to 6 weeks.

ASSESSMENT

1. Note onset, character/frequency of stools. Assess abdomen for bowel sounds, distension, pain/tenderness.
2. Check for sulfite sensitivity
3. Monitor lytes, renal, LFTs, U/A; abdominal films.

CLIENT/FAMILY TEACHING

1. Do not chew; take tablets whole, being careful not to break the outer coating.
2. Review technique for enema/suppository administration.
- Prior to use, shake bottle until all contents are thoroughly mixed.
- Lie on the left side with the lower leg extended and the upper right leg flexed forward. The knee-chest position may also be used for suppository administration.
- Remove cap, insert tip into rectum, and squeeze steadily to completely discharge contents.
- Retain the enema for 8 hr to ensure proper absorption; may best be accomplished by administering at bedtime, after BM; retain throughout the sleep cycle.
- Remove foil wrapper from suppository; avoid excess handling as the suppository will melt at body temperature.
- Insert the pointed end first into the rectum.
- For maximal effect, retain suppository for 1–3 hr or more.
- Protect bed linens with towels or rubber pads.
3. Hold drug and report severe abdominal pain, cramping, bloody diarrhea, rash, fever, or headache.
4. Avoid smoking and cold foods; increases bowel motility.
5. The therapy may last 3–6 weeks; follow as prescribed. Report lack of response.

OUTCOMES/EVALUATE

- Relief of pain and diarrhea
- Normalization of bowel patterns

Mesna   [IV]
(MEZ-nah)

CLASSIFICATION(S):
Antidote for ifosfamide toxicity
PREGNANCY CATEGORY: B
Rx: Mesnex.
❦**Rx:** Uromitexan.

USES

Prophylactically to reduce the incidence of hemorrhagic cystitis caused by ifosfamide. *Investigational:* Reduce incidence of hemorrhagic cystitis in bone marrow transplantation in those receiving high-dose cyclophosphamide. As a uroprotective drug in those receiving antimetabolite regimens containing high-dose cyclophosphamide and in a limited number of clients receiving cyclophosphamide for immunologically mediated disorders (e.g., systemic lupus erythematosus, polyarteritis, Wegener's granulomatosis, dermatomyositis).

ACTION/KINETICS
Action
Ifosfamide is metabolized to products that cause hemorrhagic cystitis. In the kidney, mesna disulfide is reduced to the free thiol compound, mesna, which reacts chemically with the urotoxic ifosfamide metabolites resulting in their detoxification.

Pharmacokinetics
Following IV use, mesna is rapidly oxidized to mesna disulfide (dimesna), which is eliminated by the kidneys. **$t^{1/2}$ in blood, mesna:** 0.36 hr; **dimesna:** 1.17 hr. **$t^{1/2}$, terminal:** 7 hr.

CONTRAINDICATIONS
Hypersensitivity to thiol compounds. Lactation.

SPECIAL CONCERNS
This product contains benzyl alcohol, which may cause a fatal 'gasping syndrome' in infants. Safety and efficacy have not been determined in children.

SIDE EFFECTS
Most Common
N&V, constipation, fatigue, fever, anorexia, abdominal pain, leukopenia, thrombocytopenia, anemia, granulocytopenia, alopecia, asthenia.
Since mesna is used with ifosfamide and other antineoplastic agents, it is difficult to identify those side effects that are due to mesna. The following symptoms are believed possible. **GI:** N&V, constipation, anorexia, abdominal pain, diarrhea, dyspepsia. **CNS:** Dizziness, headache, somnolence, anxiety, confusion, insomnia, hyperesthesia. **CV:** Chest pain, hypotension, hypertension, tachycardia, ST-segment elevation. **Hematologic:** Leukopenia, thrombocytopenia, anemia, granulocytopenia, decreased platelet counts (associated with

allergic reactions). **Dermatologic:** Alopecia, injection site reaction (including pain and erythema), pallor, flushing. **Respiratory:** Dyspnea, pharyngitis, pneumonia, coughing, tachypnea. **Body as a whole:** Fatigue, fever, asthenia, malaise, hypokalemia, pain, increased sweating, peripheral edema, edema, dehydration, flu-like symptoms, allergic/hypersensitivity reactions (including ***anaphylaxis).*** **Miscellaneous:** Back pain, facial edema, limb pain, myalgia, hematuria.

LABORATORY TEST CONSIDERATIONS
False + test for urinary ketones. ↑ Liver enzymes.

HOW SUPPLIED
Injection: 100 mg/mL; *Tablets:* 400 mg.

DOSAGE
• **IV BOLUS**
  Prophylaxis of ifosfamide-induced hemorrhagic cystitis.
Dosage of mesna equal to 20% of the ifosfamide dose given at the same time as ifosfamide and at 4 and 8 hr after each dose of ifosfamide. Thus, the total daily dose of mesna is 60% of the ifosfamide dose (e.g., an ifosfamide dose of 1.2 grams/m^2 would mean doses of mesna would be 240 mg/m^2 at the time the ifosfamide dose was given, 240 mg/m^2 after 4 hr, and 240 mg/m^2 after 8 hr). This dosage should be given on each day that ifosfamide is administered.

• **TABLETS**
  Prophylaxis of ifosfamide-induced hemorrhagic cystitis.
Initial: IV mesna equal to 20% of the ifosfamide dose, given at the time of ifosfamide, followed 2 and 6 hr later by PO doses of mesna equal to 40% of the ifosfamide dose. The total daily dose of mesna is 100% of the ifosfamide dose. Give a repeat PO mesna dose if client vomits within 2 hr of ingesting mesna. Or, a replacement IV dose may be given. PO mesna therapy has not been thoroughly evaluated for ifosfamide doses greater than 2 grams/m^2.

NURSING CONSIDERATIONS
ADMINISTRATION/STORAGE
IV 1. If the dosage of ifosfamide is increased or decreased, adjust mesna dosage accordingly.

Bold Italic = life threatening side effect   ■ = black box warning   ♣ = Available in Canada

2. Reconstitute to a final concentration of 20 mg mesna/mL fluid by adding D5W, D5W/0.2% NaCl, D5W/0.33% NaCl, D5W/0.45% NaCl, 0.9% NaCl, or RL injection.

3. Mesna and ifosfamide are compatible in the same infusion fluid.

4. Mesna is not compatible with cisplatin or carboplatin.

5. Diluted solutions are stable for 24 hr at 25°C (77°F). When mesna is exposed to oxygen, dimesna is formed; use a new ampule for each administration.

6. Mesna multidose vials may be stored and used for up to 8 days.

ASSESSMENT

1. Drug must be administered with each dose of ifosfamide and at 4 and 8 hr intervals following the initial dose to be effective against drug-induced hemorrhagic cystitis.

2. Analyze morning urine specimen each day before ifosfamide therapy for hematuria.

3. Note age and any sensitivity to benzyl alcohol. May alter tests for ketones in urine.

CLIENT/FAMILY TEACHING

1. Drug is used to prevent ifosofamide-induced hemorrhagic cystitis; will not prevent any other drug-associated adverse reactions or toxicities.

2. May experience a bad taste in the mouth during drug therapy; use hard candy to mask taste.

3. N&V and diarrhea are frequent side effects of drug therapy; report those and headaches if persistent or bothersome. If vomiting occurs within 2 hrs of oral administration report as dose may need to be repeated or given IV.

OUTCOMES/EVALUATE

Prevention of ifosfamide-induced hemorrhagic cystitis

Metaproterenol sulfate (Orciprenaline sulfate) @

(met-ah-proh-**TER**-ih-nohl)

CLASSIFICATION(S):
Sympathomimetic, direct-acting
PREGNANCY CATEGORY: C
Rx: Alupent.
✿Rx: Apo-Orciprenaline, ratio-Orciprenaline.

SEE ALSO *SYMPATHOMIMETIC DRUGS.*

USES

Inhalation: (1) Asthma and bronchitis or emphysema when a reversible component is present in adults. (2) Acute asthmatic attacks in children 6 years of age and older. **Oral:** Bronchial asthma and for reversible bronchospasm that may occur in association with bronchitis and emphysema.

ACTION/KINETICS

Action

Markedly stimulates beta-2 receptors, resulting in relaxation of smooth muscles of the bronchial tree, as well as peripheral vasodilation. Minimal effects on beta-1 receptors. Similar to isoproterenol but with a longer duration of action and fewer side effects.

Pharmacokinetics

Onset, aerosol, hand bulb nebulizer or IPPB: 5–30 min; **duration:** 1–6 or more hr after repeated doses. **PO: Onset,** 15–30 min; **peak effect:** 1 hr. **Duration:** 4 hr. Marked first-pass effect after PO use. Metabolized in the liver and excreted through the kidney.

ADDITIONAL CONTRAINDICATIONS

PO in children less than 6 years old.

SPECIAL CONCERNS

Dosage of syrup or tablets not determined in children less than 6 years of age.

SIDE EFFECTS

Most Common

Tachycardia, tremor, nervousness/tension, N&V, palpitations, dizziness/vertigo, weakness, headache, insomnia, GI distress, cough, dry throat/irritation/pharyngitis.

See *Sympathomimetic Drugs* for a complete list of possible side effects. Also, **GI:** Diarrhea, bad taste or taste changes. **Respiratory:** Worsening of asthma, nasal congestion, hoarseness. **Miscellaneous:** Hypersensitivity reactions, rash, fatigue, backache, skin reactions.

DRUG INTERACTIONS
Possible potentiation of adrenergic effects if used before or after other sympathomimetic bronchodilators

HOW SUPPLIED
Aerosol: 0.65 mg/actuation; *Solution for Inhalation:* 0.4%, 0.6%, 5%; *Syrup:* 10 mg/5 mL; *Tablets:* 10 mg, 20 mg.

DOSAGE

• **INHALATION OF 5% SOLUTION USING HAND-BULB NEBULIZER**
  Bronchodilation.
Adults and children 12 years and older: 10 inhalations (range: 5–15 inhalations) of undiluted solution.

• **NEBULIZER USING 5% SOLUTION**
  Bronchodilation.
Adults and children 12 years and older: 0.3 mL (range: 0.2–0.3 mL) of 5% solution diluted approximately 2.5 mL in saline solution or other diluent. **Children, 6–12 years:** 0.1 mL (0.1–0.2 mL) of 5% solution diluted in saline to 3 mL.

• **IPPB USING 5% SOLUTION**
  Bronchodilation.
Adults and children 12 years and older: 0.3 mL (range: 0.2–0.3 mL) of 5% solution diluted to 2.5 mL saline or other diluent.

• **SOLUTION FOR INHALATION, 0.4% AND 0.6%**
  Bronchodilation.
Give the unit-dose vial as follows: **Adults:** 1 vial/nebulization treatment given by IPPB. Each 0.4% vial is equal to 0.2 mL of the 5% solution diluted to 2.5 mL with normal saline. Each 0.6% vial is equal to 0.3 mL of the 5% solution diluted to 2.5 mL with normal saline.

• **MDI (AEROSOL)**
  Bronchodilation.
Usual: 2–3 inhalations (1.30–2.25 mg) q 3–4 hr. Do not exceed a total daily dose

of 12 inhalations (9 mg). Not for use in children less than 12 years of age.

• **SYRUP; TABLETS**
  Bronchodilation.
Adults: 20 mg 3 or 4 times per day. **Children, over 9 years old and >60 lb:** 20 mg 3 or 4 times per day; **children, 6–9 years old and <60 lb:** 10 mg 3 or 4 times per day; **children less than 6 years of age:** 1.3–2.6 mg/kg of the syrup (limited clinical trials). Tablets are not recommended for children less than 6 years of age.

NURSING CONSIDERATIONS
⚐ Do not confuse Alupent with Atrovent (cholinergic blocking agent). Do not confuse Metaproterenol with Metoprolol or Metipranolol (both are adrenergic blocking agents).

ADMINISTRATION/STORAGE
1. Store inhalant solution at less than 25°C (77°F) and protect from light.
2. Do not use solution if darker than slightly yellow, pinkish, or if it contains a precipitate.
3. Protect tablets from moisture.
4. Store syrup and tablets from 15–30°C (59–86°F).

ASSESSMENT
1. Note reasons for therapy, characteristics of S&S, onset, duration, frequency, any precipitating factors.
2. Assess PFTs, CXR, environmental/home triggers, tobacco use/exposure, lung sounds. Note any anxiety; may contribute to air hunger.
3. Monitor pulmonary status (i.e., breath sounds, VS, peak flow, ABGs) for effects of the therapy.

CLIENT/FAMILY TEACHING
1. Review method for administration. Shake container well before each use.
2. Report loss of effectiveness with prescribed dosage and frequency.
3. Store inhalant solution at room temperature; avoid excessive heat and light.
4. Do not use solution if it is brown or shows a precipitate.
5. Do not use inhalant solutions more often than every 4 hr to relieve acute bronchospasms. In chronic bronchospastic disease, the dose can be given

3–4 times per day. A single dose of nebulized drug may not completely abort acute asthma attack. Allow 2 or more minutes between inhalations; rinse equipment and mouth with water after each use.

6. If also using steroid inhaler use bronchodilator first, wait 5 minutes before administering corticosteroid. Monitor peak flow to assess need for additional therapy/hospitalization.

7. Report lack/loss of response, infections, or drop in readings. Stop smoking to help preserve lung function. Avoid triggers.

OUTCOMES/EVALUATE

- Improved airway exchange; ↑ oxygen saturation levels
- Relief of respiratory distress

Metformin hydrochloride
(met-**FOR**-min)

CLASSIFICATION(S):

Antidiabetic, oral; biguanide

PREGNANCY CATEGORY: B

Rx: Fortamet, Glucophage, Glucophage XR, Glumetza, Riomet.

♣Rx: Apo-Metformin, Gen-Metformin, Novo-Metformin, Nu-Metformin, PMS-Metformin, Rhoxal-metformin, Rhoxal-metformin FC, ratio-Metformin.

USES

(1) As monotherapy, as an adjunct to diet and exercise, to improve glycemic control in clients with type 2 diabetes. The immediate-release tablets and PO solution can be used in clients 10 years of age and older. (2) Extended-release form used to treat type 2 diabetes as initial therapy or in combination with a sulfonylurea or insulin in clients aged 17 years and older. *Investigational:* Polycystic ovary syndrome to improve rate of ovulation, cervical scores, and pregnancy rates. Treat antipsychotic-induced weight gain.

ACTION/KINETICS

Action

Decreases hepatic glucose production, decreases intestinal absorption of glucose, and increases peripheral uptake and utilization of glucose. Does not cause hypoglycemia in either diabetic or nondiabetic clients, and it does not cause hyperinsulinemia. Insulin secretion remains unchanged, while fasting insulin levels and day-long plasma insulin response may decrease. In contrast to sulfonylureas, the body weight of clients treated with metformin remains stable or may decrease somewhat.

Pharmacokinetics

Bioavailability of immediate-release tablets is 50–60%. Food decreases and slightly delays the absorption of metformin. Steady-state plasma levels (less than 1 mcg/mL) are reached within 24–48 hr. Excreted unchanged in the urine; no biliary excretion. **t½, plasma elimination:** 6.2 hr. The plasma and blood half-lives are prolonged with decreased renal function and in the elderly. **Plasma protein binding:** Negligible.

CONTRAINDICATIONS

Renal disease or dysfunction (serum creatinine levels greater than 1.5 mg/dL in males and greater than 1.4 mg/dL in females) or abnormal C_{CR} due to cardiovascular collapse, acute MI, or septicemia. In CHF requiring pharmacologic intervention. In clients undergoing radiologic studies using iodinated contrast media, because use of such products may cause alteration of renal function, leading to acute renal failure and lactic acidosis. Acute or chronic metabolic acidosis, including diabetic ketoacidosis, with or without coma. Abnormal hepatic function. Acute hemodynamic compromise of hypoxic states. Dehydration. Lactation.

SPECIAL CONCERNS

■ (1) Lactic acidosis is a rare, but serious, metabolic complication that can occur due to metformin accumulation during treatment with metformin. When it occurs, it is fatal in approximately 50% of cases. Lactic acidosis may also occur in association with a number of pathophysiologic conditions, including diabetes mellitus, and whenever there is significant tissue hypoperfusion and hypoxemia. (2) Lactic acidosis is characterized by elevated blood lactate levels (>5 mmol/L), decreased blood pH, electrolyte disturbances with an increased anion gap, and an increased lactate/pyruvate ratio. When metformin is implicated as the cause of lactic acidosis, metformin plasma levels >5 µg/mL are generally found. (3) The incidence of lactic acidosis in those receiving metformin is approximately 0.03 cases/1,000 client years, with approximately 0.015 fatal cases/1,000 client years. Reported cases have occurred primarily in diabetic clients with significant renal insufficiency, including both intrinsic renal disease and renal hypoperfusion, often in the setting of multiple concomitant medical/surgical problems and multiple concomitant medications. (4) Clients with CHF requiring pharmacologic management, in particular those with unstable or acute CHF who are at risk of hypoperfusion and hypoxemia, are at increased risk of lactic acidosis. The risk of lactic acidosis increases with the degree of renal dysfunction and the client's age. The risk of lactic acidosis, therefore, may be significantly decreased by regular monitoring of renal function in clients taking metformin and by use of the minimum effective dose of metformin. (5) In particular, treatment of the elderly should be accompanied by careful monitoring of renal function. Metformin treatment should not be initiated in clients >80 years of age unless measurement of creatinine clearance demonstrates that renal function is not reduced, as these clients are more susceptible to developing lactic acidosis. (6) Metformin should be promptly withheld in the presence of any condition associated with hypoexmia, dehydration, or sepsis. (7) Because impaired hepatic function may significantly limit the ability to clear lactate, metformin should generally be avoided in clients with clinical or laboratory evidence of hepatic disease. (8) Clients should be cautioned against excessive alcohol intake, either acute or chronic, when taking metformin, since alcohol potentiates the effects of metformin on lactate metabolism. (9) In addition, metformin should be temporarily discontinued prior to any intravascular radiocontrast study and for any surgical procedure. (10) The onset of lactic acidosis often is subtle, and accompanied only by nonspecific symptoms such as malaise, myalgias, respiratory distress, increasing somnolence, and nonspecific abdominal distress. There may be associated hypothermia, hypotension, and resistant bradyarrhythmias with more marked acidosis. The client and the client's provider must be aware of the possible importance of such symptoms and the client should be instructed to notify the provider immediately if they occur. Metformin should be withdrawn until the situation is clarified. (11) Serum electrolytes, ketones, blood glucose, and if indicated, blood pH, lactate levels, and even blood metformin, are unlikely to be drug related. (12) Later occurrence of GI symptoms could be due to lactic acidosis or other serious disease. (13) Levels of fasting venous plasma lactate above the upper limit of normal but less than 5 mmol/L in clients taking metformin do not necessarily indicate impending lactic acidosis and may be explained by other mechanisms, such as poorly controlled diabetes or obesity, vigorous physical activity, or technical problems in sample handling. (14) Lactic acidosis should be suspected in any diabetic client with metabolic acidosis lacking evidence of ketoacidosis (ketonuria and ketonemia). (15) Lactic acidosis is a medical emergency that must be treated in a hospital setting. In a client with lactic acidosis taking metformin, the drug should be discontinued immediately and general supportive measures promptly instituted. Because metformin is dialyzable (with a clearance of up to 170 mL/min under good hemodynamic conditions), prompt hemodialysis is recommended to correct the acidosis and remove the accumulated metformin. Such management often results in prompt reversal of symptoms and recovery.■ Use of oral hypoglycemic agents may increase the risk of *cardiovascular mortality.* Although hypoglycemia does not usually occur with metformin, it may result with deficient caloric intake, with strenuous exercise not supplemented by increased intake of calories, or when metformin is taken with sulfonylureas or alcohol. Because of age-related decreases in renal function, use with caution as age increases. Safety and efficacy of the extended-release tablet have not been determined in children.

SIDE EFFECTS

Most Common
Hypoglycemia, diarrhea, N&V, asthenia, flatulence, headache, abdominal pain/discomfort.

Metabolic: *Lactic acidosis* (fatal in approximately 50% of cases). **GI:** Diarrhea, N&V, abdominal bloating/pain/discomfort, flatulence, anorexia, unpleasant or metallic taste, abnormal stools, taste disorder. **CNS:** Light-headedness, headache. **Hematologic:** Asymptomatic subnormal serum vitamin B_{12} levels. **Body as a whole:** Asthenia, rash, chills, flu syndrome, flushing, increased sweating. **Miscellaneous:** Hypoglycemia, myalgia, dyspnea, nail disorder, chest discomfort, palpitation. *NOTE:* Common side effects for metformin, extended-release, include N&V, diarrhea, constipation, abdominal distention/pain, dyspepsia, heartburn, flatulence, dizziness, headache, URTI, taste disturbance.

OD **OVERDOSE MANAGEMENT**
Symptoms: Lactic acidosis, hypoglycemia. *Treatment:* Hemodialysis since metformin is dialyzable with a clearance up to 170 mL/min.

DRUG INTERACTIONS
Alcohol / ↑ Metformin effect on lactate metabolism
Cimetidine / ↑ (by 60%) Peak metformin plasma and whole blood levels and a 40% ↑ in AUC
Furosemide / ↑ Metformin plasma and blood levels; also, metformin ↓ the half-life of furosemide
Iodinated contrast media / ↑ Risk of acute renal failure and lactic acidosis

Nifedipine / ↑ Absorption of metformin, leading to ↑ plasma metformin levels
Propantheline / ↑ Absorption of metformin R/T slowed GI motility

HOW SUPPLIED
Oral Solution: 500 mg/5 mL; *Tablets:* 500 mg, 850 mg, 1,000 mg; *Tablets, Extended-Release:* 500 mg, 750 mg, 1,000 mg.

DOSAGE
● **ORAL SOLUTION**
  Type 2 diabetes.
Individualize dosage. **Adults and adolescents over 16 years of age:** Up to 2,550 mg/day; **Children, 10–16 years of age:** up to 2,000 mg/day.
● **TABLETS; TABLETS, EXTENDED-RELEASE**
  Type 2 diabetes.
Individualize dosage regimen. Adults, using 500-mg immediate-release tablet: Starting dose is one 500-mg tablet twice a day given with the morning and evening meals. Dosage increases may be made in increments of 500 mg every week, given in divided doses, up to a maximum of 2,500 mg/day. If a 2,500-mg daily dose is required, it may be better tolerated when given in divided doses 3 times/day with meals. The extended-release tablet is given once daily. **Adults, using 850-mg immediate-release tablet:** Starting dose is 850 mg once daily given with the morning meal. Dosage increases may be made in increments of 850 mg every other week, given in divided doses, up to a maximum of 2,550 mg/day. **Usual maintenance dose:** 850 mg twice a day with the morning and evening meals. However, some may require 850 mg 3 times per day with meals. **Adults, using 500-mg extended-release tablet: Initial:** 500 mg once daily with the evening meal. Adjust dose, if needed, in increments of 500 mg/week, up to a maximum of 2,000 mg once daily with the evening meal. If glycemic control is not achieved on 2,000 mg once daily, consider 1,000 mg twice a day. If higher doses are needed, use total daily dose up to 2,550 mg given in divided doses. **Adults using 1,000-mg extended-release tab-**

M

let: Initial: 1,000 mg once daily with the evening meal. Dosage may be increased weekly in 500 mg increments, based on efficacy and tolerance, but must not exceed 2,500 mg/day. *NOTE:* Initial dose of metformin immediate release in children is 500 mg twice a day given with meals. Increase dose, if necessary, in increments of 500 mg/week, up to a maximum of 2,000 mg daily given in divided doses. Safety and efficacy of metformin extended-release have not been determined in children.

NURSING CONSIDERATIONS

Do not confuse Glucophage with Glucovance (combination antidiabetic product containing metformin and glyburide).

ADMINISTRATION/STORAGE

1. Individualize dosage based on tolerance and effectiveness.
2. Give with meals starting at a low dose with gradual escalation. This will reduce GI side effects and allow determination of the minimal dose necessary for adequate BS control.
3. May safely switch from metformin to metformin extended-release (ER) once daily at the same total daily dose, up to 2,000 mg once daily. Once switched, closely monitor glycemic control and make dosage adjustments as needed.
4. No transition period required when transferring from standard oral hypoglycemic drugs (other than chlorpropamide) to metformin. When transferring from chlorpropamide, exercise caution during first 2 weeks R/T chlorpropamide's long duration of action.
5. Glumetza, 500 mg, is an extended-release tablet with a novel drug-delivery system that provides controlled and prolonged release of metformin. Can be used alone or as combination therapy (e.g., sulfonylurea or insulin).
6. If maximum dose of metformin for 4 weeks does not provide adequate control of blood glucose, gradual addition of an oral sulfonylurea (data are available for glyburide, chlorpropamide, tolbutamide, and glipizide) may be considered, while maintaining maximum dose of metformin. Desired control of

blood glucose may be attained by adjusting the dose of each drug.
7. If initiating metformin or metformin ER, continue current insulin dose. Start metformin or metformin ER at 500 mg once daily. For those not responding, increase metformin or metformin ER dose by 500 mg after about 1 week and by 500 mg every week thereafter until adequate control reached. Maximum recommended daily dose is 2,500 mg for metformin and 2,000 mg for metformin ER. Decrease insulin dose by 10–25% when fasting glucose levels decrease to less than 120 mg/dL in those receiving both metformin/metformin extended-release and insulin.
8. Be conservative with initial and maintenance doses in the elderly because of possible decreased renal function. Generally, do not titrate geriatric clients to the maximum dose. Do not start metformin or metformin ER in clients 80 years and older unless tests show renal function is not decreased.
9. If no response to 1–3 months of concomitant metformin and oral sulfonylurea therapy, consider initiating insulin therapy and discontinuing oral agents.
10. If exposed to stress (e.g., fever, trauma, infection, surgery) may experience loss of glycemic control. May be necessary to withhold metformin and administer insulin temporarily.
11. Temporarily suspend metformin for dye and surgical procedures (unless minor and not associated with restricted intake of food and fluids). Do not restart until oral intake has resumed and renal function is normal.
12. Store tablets and oral solution from 15–30°C (59–86°F).

ASSESSMENT

1. Note age at diabetes onset, BMI, family Hx, previous therapies utilized, outcome.
2. Monitor BP, CBC, BS, electrolytes, HbA1c, urinalysis, microalbumin, renal, LFTs. Assess for liver/renal failure; may precipitate lactic acidosis (i.e., serum lactate levels greater than 5 mmol/L, decreased blood pH, increased anion gap).

3. Withhold for surgery and iodinated procedures (usually 48 hr before and 48 hr after). May administer when normal diet resumed or the day after the procedure.

4. If anemia develops, exclude vitamin B_{12} deficiency; may interfere with B_{12} absorption.

5. A small dose with insulin therapy may enhance glucose control.

6. Avoid with CHF, may alter furosemide effects. During times of acute stress, monitor carefully, may require insulin therapy.

CLIENT/FAMILY TEACHING

1. Take with food to ↓ GI upset. Do not crush or chew extended-release tablets.

2. May cause a metallic taste; should subside.

3. The inactive components in the extended-release tablets may pass into the feces and appear as a soft, hydrated mass.

4. Regular exercise, decreased caloric intake, and weight loss are required to reduce blood glucose levels; medication neither replaces nor excuses compliance with these modalities.

5. Inadequate caloric intake or strenuous exercise without caloric replacement may precipitate hypoglycemia.

6. Do regular blood sugar monitoring (fingersticks), especially 1–2 hr after meals, if symptomatic, and maintain record for provider review.

7. Avoid alcohol and situations that may precipitate dehydration.

8. Consume plenty of fluids; report when illnesses with fever, vomiting, and diarrhea are persistent/severe.

9. Stop drug and immediately report any symptoms of difficulty breathing, severe weakness, muscle pain, increased sleepiness, dizziness, palpitation, or sudden increased abdominal distress.

OUTCOMES/EVALUATE

- Control of BS; prevention of microvascular complications
- HbA1c <7%

Methadone hydrochloride ■
(METH-ah-dohn)

CLASSIFICATION(S):
Narcotic analgesic
PREGNANCY CATEGORY: C
Rx: Dolophine Hydrochloride, Methadone HCl Diskets, Methadose, **C-II**
✚**Rx:** Metadol.

SEE ALSO *NARCOTIC ANALGESICS.*

USES
(1) Severe pain. (2) Detoxification and temporary maintenance of narcotic dependence (except dispersible tablets and certain oral concentrates). *NOTE:* If used to treat heroin dependence for longer than 3 weeks, the procedure goes from treatment of acute withdrawal syndrome to maintenance therapy. Maintenance may be undertaken only by approved methadone programs. (3) Detoxification treatment of opioid addiction (heroin or other morphine-type drugs (use Diskets). (4) For maintenance treatment of opioid addiction (heroin and other morphine-type drugs) in conjunction with appropriate social and medical services.

ACTION/KINETICS
Action
Produces only mild euphoria, which is the reason it is used as a heroin withdrawal substitute and for maintenance programs. Produces physical dependence; withdrawal symptoms develop more slowly and are less intense but more prolonged than those associated with morphine. Does not produce sedation or narcosis. Not effective for preoperative or obstetric anesthesia. Only one-half as potent PO as when given parenterally.

Pharmacokinetics
PO administration results in a delay of onset, lower peak, and an increased duration of analgesic effect. **Onset, PO:** 30–60 min; **parenteral**: 10–20 min. **Peak effects:** 30–60 min. **Duration:** 4–6 hr. **t½, elimination:** 8–59 hr. Both the

M

duration and half-life increase with repeated use due to cumulative effects. Metabolized in the liver primarily by CYP3A4 and to a lesser extent by CYP2D6. Excreted in the urine and feces.

ADDITIONAL CONTRAINDICATIONS

IV use, liver disease, during pregnancy, in children, or in obstetrics (due to long duration of action and chance of respiratory depression in the neonate). Use to relieve general anxiety.

SPECIAL CONCERNS

■ (1) To treat narcotic addiction in detoxification or maintenance programs, methadone should be dispensed only by hospitals, community pharmacies, and maintenance programs approved by the FDA and designated state authorities. Approved maintenance programs shall dispense and use methadone in oral form only and according to treatment requirements stipulated in Federal Methadone Opioid Treatment Standards. Failure to abide by the requirements in these regulations may result in criminal prosecution, seizure of drug supply, revocation of program approval, and injunction precluding program operation. (2) Regulatory exceptions to the general requirement for certification to provide opioid agonist treatment: (a) During inpatient care, when the client was admitted for any condition other than concurrent opioid addiction to facilitate the treatment of the primary admitting diagnosis and (b) during an emergency period of no longer than 3 days while definitive care for the addiction is being sought in an appropriately licensed facility. (3) Methadone, used as an analgesic, may be dispensed in any licensed pharmacy. (4) Methadone dispersible tablets are for PO administration only. This preparation contains insoluble excipients and therefore must not be injected. It is recommended that methadone dispersible tablets, if dispensed, be packaged in child-resistant containers and kept out of the reach of children to prevent accidental ingestion. (5) Deaths have been reported during initiation of methadone treatment for opioid dependence. In some cases, drug interactions with other drugs, both licit and illicit, have been suspected. However, in other cases, deaths appear to have occurred because of the respiratory or cardiac effects of methadone and too-rapid titration without appreciation for the accumulation of methadone over time. It is critical to understand the pharmacokinetics of methadone and to exercise vigilance during treatment initiation and dose titration. Clients must also be strongly cautioned against self-medicating with CNS depressants during initiation of methadone treatment. (6) Respiratory depression is the chief hazard associated with methadone administration. Methadone's peak respiratory depressant effects typically occur later and persist longer than its peak analgesic effects, particularly in the early dosing period. These characteristics can contribute to the cases of iatrogenic overdose, particularly during treatment initiation and dose titration. (7) Cardiac conduction effects. Laboratory studies have demonstrated that methadone inhibits cardiac potassium channels and prolongs the QT interval. Cases of QT interval prolongation and serious arrhythmia (torsades de pointes) have been observed during treatment with methadone. These cases appear to be more commonly associated with, but not limited to, higher dose treatment (greater than 200 mg/day). Most cases involve clients being treated for pain with large, multiple daily doses of methadone, although cases have been reported in clients receiving doses commonly used for maintenance treatment of opioid addiction.■ Use with caution during lactation. Methadone can build up in the body to toxic levels if it is taken too often, if the amount taken is too high, or if it is take with other drugs or supplements.

SIDE EFFECTS

Most Common

Insomnia, dizziness, anxiety, nervousness, weakness, drowsiness, N&V, diarrhea, anorexia, constipation, dry mouth, impotence, decreased libido.

Bold Italic = life threatening side effect   ■ = black box warning   ♣ = Available in Canada

See *Narcotic Analgesics* for a complete list of possible side effects. Also, marked constipation, excessive sweating, pulmonary edema, choreic movements. Possible **torsade de pointes** during high-dose methadone treatment, especially in those with predisposing factors.

ADDITIONAL DRUG INTERACTIONS

Cimetidine / ↑ Respiratory and CNS depression

Desipramine / ↑ Desipramine blood levels

Nelfinavir / ↓ Methadone plasma levels

Phenytoin / ↓ Methadone effect R/T ↑ liver metabolism

Protease inhibitors / ↑ Respiratory and CNS depression

Ritonavir / ↓ Methadone plasma levels

Rifampin / ↓ Methadone effect R/T ↑ liver metabolism; may precipitate withdrawal

LABORATORY TEST CONSIDERATIONS

↑ Immunoglobulin G.

HOW SUPPLIED

Injection: 10 mg/mL; *Oral Concentrate:* 10 mg/mL; *Oral Solution:* 5 mg/5 mL, 10 mg/5 mL; *Tablets:* 5 mg, 10 mg; *Tablets, Dispersable:* 40 mg.

DOSAGE————————

• **INJECTION; ORAL CONCENTRATE; ORAL SOLUTION; TABLETS; TABLETS, DISPERSABLE**

Analgesia.

Adults, individualized: 2.5–10 mg q 3–4 hr, although higher doses may be necessary for severe pain or due to development of tolerance.

Narcotic withdrawal.

Initial: 15–20 mg/day PO (some may require 40 mg/day); **then,** depending on need, slowly decrease dosage.

Maintenance following narcotic withdrawal.

Adults, individualized, initial: 20–40 mg PO 4–8 hr after heroin is stopped; **then,** adjust dosage as required up to 120 mg/day.

• **DISKETS**

Detoxification treatment of opioid addiction (e.g., heroin or other morphine-type drugs).

The initial methadone should be given under supervision when there are no signs of sedation or intoxication and the client shows symptoms of withdrawal. **Initial:** Single dose of 20-30 mg; do not exceed 30 mg. An additional 5-10 mg may be given if withdrawal symptoms have not been suppressed or if symptoms reappear. **Total first day dose:** Do not exceed 40 mg. Make dosage adjustments over the first week based on control of withdrawal symptoms at the time of expected peak methadone activity (i.e., 2-4 hr after dosing). *NOTE:* Diskets can only be given in 10 mg increments and thus may not be appropriate for initial dosing in many clients. A methadone dose will hold for a longer period of time as tissue stores of methadone accumulate.

NURSING CONSIDERATIONS

ADMINISTRATION/STORAGE

1. Dilute solution in at least 90 mL of water prior to administration.

2. If taking dispersible tablets, dilute in 120 mL of water, orange juice, citrus-flavored drink, or other acidic fruit drink. Allow at least 1 min for complete drug dispersion.

3. For repeated analgesic doses, IM administration is preferred over SC administration due to local irritation. Inspect sites for signs of irritation.

4. Duration of treatment for detoxification purposes is no longer than 21 days. Do not repeat treatment for 4 weeks.

ASSESSMENT

1. Note reasons for therapy: opioid withdrawal or chronic pain control, other therapies/agents trialed, outcome.

2. With long-term therapy, assess EKG and monitor for QT prolongation.

CLIENT/FAMILY TEACHING

1. Take as prescribed for pain control.

2. If ambulatory and not suffering acute pain, side effects may be more pronounced.

3. Avoid activities that require mental alertness until drug effects realized, causes sedation, drowsiness, impaired vision.

4. Avoid alcohol. Report N&V; a lower drug dose may relieve symptoms. Practice reliable contraception.

M

---

5. To minimize constipation, exercise regularly, increase intake of fluids, fruit, and bulk, and use stool softener.

6. May adversely affect employment R/T type of drug consumed and drug association. Drug causes tolerance and dependence with long-term use. Do not stop drug suddenly, it must be weaned slowly.

7. For clients on narcotic withdrawal therapy, store drug out of the reach of children. Continue to attend group therapy such as Narcotics Anonymous. Identify social service groups for assistance in child care, food and living arrangements, and expenses.

OUTCOMES/EVALUATE
- Control of severe/chronic pain
- Detoxification and maintenance in narcotic-dependent individual

---

Methocarbamol
(meth-oh-**KAR**-bah-mohl)

CLASSIFICATION(S):
Skeletal muscle relaxant, centrally-acting
PREGNANCY CATEGORY: C
Rx: Robaxin, Robaxin-750.

SEE ALSO SKELETAL MUSCLE RELAXANTS, CENTRALLY ACTING.

USES
(1) Adjunct to rest, physical therapy, and other measures for the relief of acute, painful musculoskeletal conditions (e.g., sprains, strains). (2) Adjunct to treat neuromuscular symptoms of tetanus. Methocarbamol does not replace the usual treatment of debridement, tetanus antitoxin, penicillin, tracheotomy, appropriate fluid balance, and supportive care.

ACTION/KINETICS
Action
Beneficial effect may be related to the sedative properties of the drug. Has no direct effect on the contractile mechanism of striated muscle, the motor endplate, or the nerve fiber, and it does not directly relax tense skeletal muscles.

Pharmacokinetics
Onset: 30 min. **Peak plasma levels:** 2 hr after 2 grams. **$t\frac{1}{2}$:** 1–2 hr. Inactive metabolites are excreted in the urine with small amounts in the feces.

CONTRAINDICATIONS
Hypersensitivity, when muscle spasticity is required to maintain upright position, seizure disorders, pregnancy, lactation, children under 12 years. Renal disease (parenteral dosage form only since it contains polyethylene glycol 300). SC use.

SPECIAL CONCERNS
Use the PO and injectable forms with caution in suspected or known epileptics.

SIDE EFFECTS
Most Common
Drowsiness, dizziness, GI upset/nausea, blurred vision, fever.

After PO Use. CNS: Lightheadedness, dizziness, drowsiness, headache. **GI:** Nausea. **Dermatologic:** Urticaria, pruritus, rash. **Ophthalmic:** Conjunctivitis with nasal congestion, blurred vision. **Miscellaneous:** Fever.

After IV Use. CNS: Dizziness, lightheadedness, vertigo, headache, drowsiness, fainting, *seizures* in epileptics. **CV:** Syncope, hypotension, bradycardia. **GI:** GI upset, metallic taste. **Dermatologic:** Urticaria, pruritus, rash, flushing. **Ophthalmic:** Blurred vision, conjunctivitis with nasal congestion, nystagmus, diplopia. **Miscellaneous:** Sloughing or pain at the injection site, thrombophlebitis, *anaphylaxis*, fever.

LABORATORY TEST CONSIDERATIONS
Color interference in certain screening tests for 5-HIAA and VMA.

OD **OVERDOSE MANAGEMENT**
Symptoms: CNS depression, including coma, is often seen when methocarbamol is used with alcohol or other CNS depressants. *Treatment:* Supportive, depending on the symptoms.

DRUG INTERACTIONS
CNS depressants (including alcohol) may ↑ the effect of methocarbamol.

HOW SUPPLIED
Tablets: 500 mg, 750 mg.

DOSAGE
- **TABLETS**

Bold Italic = life threatening side effect   ■ = black box warning   ♣ = Available in Canada

Skeletal muscle disorders.
Adults, initial: 1.5 grams 4 times/day, for the first 2–3 days (for severe conditions, 8 grams/day may be given); **maintenance:** 1 gram 4 times/day, 0.75 gram q 4 hr, or 1.5 grams 3 times/day.

NURSING CONSIDERATIONS

ASSESSMENT

1. Note reasons for therapy, onset, characteristics of S&S, associated factors, other agents trialed, outcome.
2. Rate pain level, assess range of motion, stiffness, x-ray if indicated, note assessment findings and renal function.

INTERVENTIONS

1. Monitor VS. Observe seizure precautions.
2. Keep side rails up, supervise ambulation of elderly or those who have been immobilized prior to drug therapy.

CLIENT/FAMILY TEACHING

1. Take as directed with meals or milk. Do not exceed dosage parameters; usually tapered off over 1–2 weeks with extended use.
2. Causes drowsiness; do not operate dangerous machinery or drive a car.
3. Rise slowly from a recumbent position and dangle legs before standing up to minimize low BP effects.
4. Double/blurred vision, and involuntary eye movement may occur; report if persistent.
5. Report skin eruptions/rash or itching (allergic responses which may require drug withdrawal).
6. Nausea, anorexia, metallic taste may occur; report if severe or interferes with nutrition.
7. Avoid alcohol/CNS depressants.
8. Urine may turn black, brown, or green (upon standing); will resolve once drug stopped.
9. Drug for short-term use during acute sprain/strain. Use as needed and perform exercises/stretching, PT/exercises as directed.

OUTCOMES/EVALUATE

- Improvement in muscle spasticity, pain, and mobility
- Control of tetanus-induced neuromuscular manifestations

Methotrexate, ■ Ⅳ ©
Methotrexate sodium
(Amethopterin, MTX)
(meth-oh-**TREKS**-ayt)

CLASSIFICATION(S):
Antineoplastic, antimetabolite; Antipsoriasis drug
PREGNANCY CATEGORY: X
Rx: Methotrexate LPF Sodium, Rheumatrex, Rheumatrex Dose Pack, Trexall.
✤Rx: ratio-Methotrexate.

SEE ALSO *ANTINEOPLASTIC AGENTS.*

USES

(1) Certain carcinomas including uterine choriocarcinoma (curative), chorioadenoma destruens, hydatidiform mole, acute lymphocytic and lymphoblastic leukemia, lymphosarcoma, and other disseminated neoplasms in children. (2) Meningeal leukemia. (3) Some beneficial effect in regional chemotherapy of head and neck tumors, breast tumors, and lung cancer. (4) In combination for advanced stage non-Hodgkin's lymphoma. (5) Advanced mycosis fungoides. (6) High doses followed by leucovorin rescue in combination with other drugs for prolonging relapse-free survival in nonmetastatic osteosarcoma in individuals who have had surgical resection or amputation for the primary tumor. (7) Severe, recalcitrant, disabling psoriasis not responsive to other therapy. Use only when diagnosis has been established by biopsy or after dermatologic consultation. (8) Rheumatoid arthritis (severe, active, classical, or definite) in clients who have had inadequate response to NSAIDs at least one or more antirheumatic drugs (disease modifying). *Investigational:* Severe corticosteroid-dependent asthma to reduce corticosteroid dosage; adjunct to treat osteosarcoma. Psoriatic arthritis and Reiter's disease.

M

ACTION/KINETICS

Action

Cell-cycle specific for the S phase of cell division. Acts by inhibiting dihydrofolate reductase, which prevents reduction of dihydrofolate to tetrahydrofolate; this results in decreased synthesis of purines and consequently DNA. The most sensitive cells are bone marrow, fetal cells, dermal epithelium, urinary bladder, buccal mucosa, intestinal mucosa, and malignant cells. When used for rheumatoid arthritis it may affect immune function. In psoriasis, the rate of production of epithelial cells in the skin is greater than normal skin; methotrexate interferes with DNA synthesis, repair, and cellular replication, especially in actively proliferating tissues.

Pharmacokinetics

Variable absorption from GI tract. Food may delay the absorption and reduce peak levels. **Peak serum levels, IM:** 30–60 min; **PO:** 1–2 hr. **t½:** initial, 1 hr; intermediate, 2–3 hr; final, 8–12 hr. May accumulate in the body. Excreted by kidney (55–92% in 24 hr).

CONTRAINDICATIONS

Clients with psoriasis or rheumatoid arthritis (1) with alcoholism, alcoholic liver disease, or other chronic liver disease; (2) who have overt or lab evidence of immunodeficiency syndromes; or (3) who have pre-existing blood dyscrasias (e.g., bone marrow hypoplasia, leukopenia, thrombocytopenia, significant anemia). Pregnancy and lactation.

SPECIAL CONCERNS

■ (1) The high doses required for treating osteosarcoma require meticulous care. (2) Use only in life-threatening, neoplastic diseases, or in those with psoriasis Pneumocystis carinii pneumonia or rheumatoid arthritis (RA) with severe, recalcitrant, disabling disease that is not adequately responsive to other types of therapy. Deaths have occurred with the use of methotrexate in malignancy, psoriasis, and RA. Closely monitor clients for bone marrow, liver, lung, and kidney toxicities. (3) Marked bone marrow depression may occur with resultant anemia, leukopenia, or thrombocytopenia. (4) Unexpected severe (sometimes fatal) bone marrow suppression, aplastic anemia, and GI toxicity have occurred with coadministration of methotrexate (usually high doses) with some NSAIDs. (5) Monitor periodically for toxicity, including CBC with differential and platelet counts; liver and renal function testing is mandatory. Periodic liver biopsies may be necessary in some situations. Monitor those at increased risk for impaired methotrexate elimination (e.g., renal dysfunction, pleural effusion, ascites) more frequently. (6) Causes hepatotoxicity, fibrosis, and cirrhosis, usually only after prolonged use. Acutely, liver enzyme elevations are frequent but are usually transient and asymptomatic; they do not seem predictive of subsequent liver disease. Liver biopsy after sustained use often shows histologic changes, and fibrosis and cirrhosis have occurred; these latter lesions are not preceded by symptoms of abnormal LFTs. Thus, periodic liver biopsies are usually recommended for those who are treated long-term. Persistent abnormalities in LFTs may precede appearance of fibrosis or cirrhosis in those with RA. (7) Methotrexate-induced lung disease is a potentially dangerous lesion that may occur acutely at any time during therapy; has occurred at doses as low as 7.5 mg/week. Is not always fully reversible. Pulmonary symptoms (especially a dry, nonproductive cough) may require interruption of treatment and careful investigation. (8) Fetal death and/or congenital anomalies have occurred; do not use in women of childbearing age unless benefits outweigh possible risks. Pregnant women with psoriasis or RA should not receive methotrexate. (9) Use with extreme caution in clients with impaired renal function and at reduced dosage because renal dysfunction will prolong elimination. (10) Diarrhea and ulcerative stomatitis require interruption of therapy. Hemorrhagic enteritis and death from intestinal perforation may occur. (11) Do not use methotrexate formulations and diluents containing preservatives for intrathecal or experimental high dose methotrexate therapy. (12)

Bold Italic = life threatening side effect   ■ = black box warning   ✚ = Available in Canada

Malignant lymphomas, which may regress following withdrawal of methotrexate, may occur in those receiving low-dose methotrexate; they may not require cytotoxic treatment. Discontinue methotrexate first and, if the lymphoma does not regress, start appropriate treatment. (13) Methotrexate may induce tumor lysis syndrome in clients with rapidly growing tumors. (14) Severe, occasionally fatal skin reactions have been reported following single or multiple doses of methotrexate. Reactions have occurred within days of PO, IM, IV, or intrathecal administration. Recovery occurs with discontinuation of therapy. (15) Potentially fatal opportunistic infections, especially *Pneumocystis carinii pneumonia*, may occur with methotrexate therapy. (16) May increase the risk of soft tissue necrosis and osteonecrosis when given concomitantly with radiotherapy. (17) Because of the possibility of severe toxic reactions (that may be fatal), inform clients fully of the risks involved and assure constant supervision.■ Use with caution in impaired renal function and elderly clients. Use with extreme caution in the presence of active infection and in debilitated clients. Safety and efficacy have not been established for children other than in cancer chemotherapy and in polyarticular-course juvenile rheumatoid arthritis. Read prescription order carefully; do not give daily when the order reads weekly dosing.

SIDE EFFECTS

Most Common

Ulcerative stomatitis, leukopenia, nausea, abdominal distress, malaise, fatigue, chills, fever, dizziness, decreased resistance to infection.

GI: Gingivitis, stomatitis, anorexia, N&V, diarrhea, hematemesis, melena, GI ulceration/perforation, GI bleeding, *enteritis (including hemorrhagic), pancreatitis*. **CNS:** Headache, drowsiness, aphasia, dizziness, hemiparesis, paresis, *convulsions,* speech impairment (including dysarthria). Following low doses: Transient subtle cognitive dysfunction, mood alteration, unusual cranial sensations, leukoencephalopathy, encephalopathy. **CV:** Pericarditis, *pericardial effusion*, hypotension, thromboembolic events (including, arterial thrombosis, *cerebral thrombosis*, DVT, retinal vein thrombosis, thrombophlebitis, vasculitis, *pulmonary embolism)*. **Pulmonary:** Chronic interstitial pulmonary disease, *respiratory fibrosis, respiratory failure*, interstitial pneumonitis, URTI, cough, epistaxis. **Dermatologic:** Erythematous rashes, pruritus, urticaria, photosensitivity, pigmentary changes, sweating, alopecia, ecchymosis, telangiectasia, acne, furunculosis, erythema multiforme, *toxic epidermal necrolysis, Stevens-Johnson syndrome,* skin necrosis, skin ulceration, exfoliative dermatitis, 'burning skin' lesions, plaque erosions (rare). **Hematologic:** Bone marrow depression, leukopenia, thrombocytopenia, suppressed hematopoiesis causing anemia, *aplastic anemia*, pancytopenia, neutropenia, decreased hematocrit, lymphadenopathy, lymphoproliferative disorders, hypogammaglobulinemia (rare). **GU:** Renal failure (acute), cystitis, hematuria, severe nephropathy, defective oogenesis or spermatogenesis, transient oligospermia, menstrual dysfunction, vaginal discharge, infertility, *abortion*, fetal defects, gynecomastia, dysuria. **Hepatic:** Hepatotoxicity, acute hepatitis, chronic fibrosis, cirrhosis. **Musculoskeletal:** Stress fractures, arthralgia, myalgia, chest pain, osteoporosis (rare). **Ophthalmic:** Blurred vision, transient blindness, conjunctivitis, serious visual changes of unknown etiology, eye discomfort. **Body as a whole:** Malaise, fatigue, chills, fever, decreased resistance to infection, soft tissue necrosis, osteonecrosis. **Miscellaneous:** Diabetes, *sudden death, anaphylaxis*, nodulosis, loss of libido/impotence, reversible lymphomas, *tumor lysis syndrome*, opportunistic infections, including *Pneumocystis carinii* (some may be fatal). **Following intrathecal use.** Acute chemical arachnoiditis (headache, back pain, nuchal rigidity, fever). Subacute myelopathy (paraparesis/paraplegia with involvement of spinal nerve roots). Chronic leukoencephalopathy (confusion, irrita-

M

bility, somnolence, ataxia, dementia, **seizures, coma**).

LABORATORY TEST CONSIDERATIONS

Azotemia. ↑ Liver enzymes. ↓ Serum albumin.

OD OVERDOSE MANAGEMENT

Symptoms: See *Antineoplastic Agents.* *Treatment:* Leucovorin, given as soon as possible, may decrease toxic effects. The dose used is 10 mg/m² PO or parenterally followed by 10 mg/m² PO q 6 hr for 72 hr. In massive overdosage, routine hemodialysis and hemoperfusion are ineffective. Hydration and urinary alkalinization are needed to prevent precipitation of methotrexate and metabolites in the renal tubules.

DRUG INTERACTIONS

Alcohol, ethyl / Additive hepatotoxicity; combination can → coma
Aminoglycosides, oral / ↓ Absorption of PO methotrexate
Anticoagulants, oral / Additive hypoprothrombinemia
Azathioprine / ↑ Risk of hepatotoxicity; monitor closely
Caffeine / Ingestion of more than 180 mg/day of caffeine may ↓ effect of methotrexate compared with ingestion of less than 120 mg/day
Charcoal / ↓ Methotrexate absorption and ↑ removal from systemic circulation
Chloramphenicol, oral / ↓ Methotrexate intestinal absorption or interference with enterohepatic circulation by inhibiting bowel flora and suppressing metabolism of the drug by bacteria
Cyclosporine / ↑ Methotrexate peak plasma levels and AUC and ↓ AUC and urinary excretion of the 7-hydroxy-methotrexate metabolite
Digoxin / ↓ Serum digoxin levels
Doxycycline / GI and hematologic toxicity after high-dose methotrexate
Etretinate / Possible hepatotoxicity if used together for psoriasis; monitor closely
Folic acid–containing vitamin preparations / ↓ Methotrexate systemic response
Ibuprofen / ↑ Methotrexate effect by ↓ renal secretion

NSAIDs / Possible fatal interaction R/T ↑ and prolongation of serum methotrexate levels
PABA / ↑ Methotrexate effect by ↓ plasma protein binding
Penicillins / ↑ Serum methotrexate levels → toxicity
Phenytoin / ↓ Serum phenytoin levels → ↓ therapeutic effect
Probenecid / ↑ Methotrexate effect by ↓ renal clearance
Procarbazine / Possible ↑ nephrotoxicity
Pyrimethamine / ↑ Methotrexate toxicity
Salicylates (aspirin) / ↑ Methotrexate effect by ↓ tubular secretion of methotrexate; also, salicylates ↓ methotrexate renal excretion
Smallpox vaccination / Methotrexate impairs immunologic response to smallpox vaccine
Sulfasalazine / ↑ Risk of hepatotoxicity; monitor closely
Sulfonamides / ↑ Risk of methotrexate-induced bone marrow suppression
Tetracyclines / ↑ Methotrexate effect by ↓ plasma protein binding
Theophylline / ↓ Theophylline clearance
Thiopurines (e.g., azathioprine) / ↑ Plasma drug levels
Trimethoprim / ↑ Risk of methotrexate-induced bone marrow suppression and megaloblastic anemia
Vancomycin / ↑ Methotrexate serum levels and markedly delayed methotrexate excretion

HOW SUPPLIED

Methotrexate: *Tablets:* 2.5 mg, 5 mg, 7.5 mg, 10 mg, 15 mg.
Methotrexate Sodium: *Injection:* 25 mg/mL (as base); *Powder for Injection, Lyophilized:* 20 mg/vial (as base-preservative free), 1 gram/vial (as base-preservative free).

DOSAGE

• **IA; IM; INTRATHECAL; IV; TABLETS**
Choriocarcinoma and similar trophoblastic diseases.
Dose individualized. PO, IM, 15–30 mg/day for 5 days. May be repeated 3–5 times with 1-week rest period between courses.

Bold Italic = life threatening side effect   ■ = black box warning   ✦ = Available in Canada

Acute lymphatic (lymphoblastic) leukemia.

Initial: 3.3 mg/m^2 (with 60 mg/m^2 prednisone daily); **maintenance: PO, IM,** 30 mg/m^2 2 times per week or **IV,** 2.5 mg/kg q 14 days.

Meningeal leukemia.

Intrathecal: 12 mg/m^2 q 2–5 days until cell count returns to normal.

Lymphomas.

PO: 10–25 mg/day for 4–8 days for several courses of treatment with 7- to 10-day rest periods between courses.

Mycosis fungoides.

PO: 2.5–10 mg/day for several weeks or months; **alternatively, IM:** 50 mg once weekly or 25 mg twice weekly.

Lymphosarcoma.

0.625–2.5 mg/kg/day in combination with other drugs.

Osteosarcoma.

Used in combination with other drugs, including doxorubicin, cisplatin, bleomycin, cyclophosphamide, and dactinomycin. **Usual IV starting dose for methotrexate:** 12 grams/m^2; dose may be increased to 15 grams/m^2 to achieve a peak serum level of 10^{-3} mol/L at the end of the methotrexate infusion.

Psoriasis.

Adults, usual: PO, IM, IV: 10–25 mg/week, continued until beneficial response observed. Weekly dose should not exceed 30 mg. **Alternate regimens:** PO, 2.5 mg q 12 hr for three doses or q 8 hr for four doses each week (not to exceed 30 mg/week). Once beneficial effects are noted, reduce dose to lowest possible level with longest rest periods between doses.

Rheumatoid arthritis.

Initial: Single PO doses of 7.5 mg/week or divided PO doses of 2.5 mg at 12-hr intervals for three doses given once a week; **then,** adjust dosage to achieve optimum response, not to exceed a total weekly dose of 20 mg. Once response has been reached, reduce the dose to the lowest possible effective dose.

NURSING CONSIDERATIONS

Ⓒ Do not confuse methotrexate with metolazone (a thiazide diuretic).

ADMINISTRATION/STORAGE

1. Use only sterile, preservative-free NaCl injection to reconstitute powder for intrathecal administration.

2. Prevent inhalation of drug particles and skin exposure.

3. When used for rheumatoid arthritis, improvement is thought to be maintained for up to 2 years with continuous therapy. When discontinued, arthritis usually worsens within 3–6 weeks.

IV 4. Six hours prior to initiation of a methotrexate infusion, hydrate with 1 L/m^2 of IV fluid. Continue hydration at 125 mL/m^2/hr during methotrexate infusion and for 2 days after infusion completed.

5. Alkalinize urine (see *Sodium Bicarbonate*) to a pH >7 during infusion.

6. Follow guidelines provided for leucovorin rescue schedule following high doses of methotrexate.

ASSESSMENT

1. Note reasons for therapy, onset, characteristics of S&S. With arthritis, note joint findings, ROM, pain level, other agents trialed, outcome.

2. List drugs prescribed. Identify if receiving other organic acids, such as aspirin, phenylbutazone, probenecid, and/or sulfa drugs; these affect renal clearance of methotrexate and increase thrombocytopenia and GI side effects. Note any acute infections.

3. Renal function tests are recommended before initiation of therapy; perform daily leukocyte counts during therapy.

4. Monitor CBC, uric acid, renal and LFTs; report oliguria. Drug causes granulocyte and platelet suppression. Nadir: 10 days; recovery: 14 days.

5. Have calcium leucovorin—a potent antidote for folic acid antagonists—readily available in case of overdosage. Antidotes are ineffective if not administered within 4 hr of overdosage; may give corticosteroids concomitantly with initial dose of methotrexate. Allow maximum rest between doses.

CLIENT/FAMILY TEACHING

1. Take at bedtime with an antacid to minimize GI upset. Prepare calendar to ensure correct dosage days. Do not consume OTC vitamins.

M

2. Avoid salicylates and alcohol as liver toxicity/bleeding may result. Avoid contact sports.

3. Report oral ulcerations, one of the first signs of toxicity.

4. May experience hair loss; should regrow with stoppage of therapy.

5. Avoid crowds, those with infections, vaccinations (esp. smallpox); impaired immunologic response may result in vaccinia.

6. Consume 2–3 L/day of fluids to prevent renal damage and facilitate drug excretion.

7. Test urine pH, report if less than 6.5; bicarbonate tablets may be prescribed to assist in alkalinizing urine.

8. Drug may precipitate gouty arthritis; allopurinol may be added to reduce uric acid levels.

9. Avoid sun exposure, use sunscreens, sunglasses, and appropriate clothing when necessary. Report if psoriasis worsens.

10. Practice reliable contraception during and for at least 8 weeks following therapy.

OUTCOMES/EVALUATE
- Suppression of malignant cell proliferation, ↓ tumor size/spread
- Improvement in skin lesions
- ↓ Joint swelling/pain; ↑ mobility

Methyldopa
(meth-ill-**DOH**-pah)

CLASSIFICATION(S):
Antihypertensive, centrally-acting
PREGNANCY CATEGORY: B (PO), **C** (IV).
♣Rx: Apo-Methyldopa, Nu-Medopa.

Methyldopate hydrochloride
PREGNANCY CATEGORY: B (PO), **C** (IV).
Rx: Aldomet Hydrochloride.

SEE ALSO *ANTIHYPERTENSIVE AGENTS.*

USES
PO: Moderate to severe hypertension. Particularly useful for clients with impaired renal function, renal hypertension, resistant cases of hypertension complicated by stroke, CAD, or nitrogen retention. **IV:** Hypertensive crisis. *Investigational:* Hypertension in pregnancy.

ACTION/KINETICS
Action
The active metabolite, alpha-methyl-norepinephrine, lowers BP by stimulating central inhibitory alpha-adrenergic receptors, false neurotransmission, and/or reduction of plasma renin. Little change in CO.

Pharmacokinetics
PO, Onset: 7–12 hr. **Duration:** 12–24 hr. All effects terminated within 48 hr. Absorption is variable. **IV, Onset:** 4–6 hr. **Duration:** 10–16 hr. Seventy percent of drug excreted in urine. **Full therapeutic effect:** 1–4 days. $t\frac{1}{2}$: 1.7 hr. Metabolites excreted in the urine.

CONTRAINDICATIONS
Sensitivity to drug (including sulfites), labile and mild hypertension, pregnancy, active hepatic disease (e.g., acute hepatitis, active cirrhosis), use with MAO inhibitors, or pheochromocytoma. Use if previous methyldopa therapy has been associated with liver disorders.

SPECIAL CONCERNS
Use with caution in clients with a history of liver or kidney disease. A decrease in dose in geriatric clients may prevent syncope.

SIDE EFFECTS
Most Common
Dizziness, drowsiness, headache, flatulence, dry mouth, N&V, fatigue, stomach upset, menstrual irregularities, rash, impotence.

CNS: Sedation (transient), drowsiness, weakness, headache, asthenia, dizziness, paresthesias, Parkinson-like symptoms, psychic disturbances, symptoms of CV impairment, choreoathetotic movements, Bell's palsy, decreased mental acuity, verbal memory impairment. **CV:** Bradycardia, orthostatic hypotension, hypersensitivity of carotid sinus, worsening of angina, paradoxical hypertensive response (after IV), myo-

---

carditis, CHF, pericarditis, vasculitis. **GI:** N&V, stomach upset, abdominal distention, diarrhea or constipation, flatus, colitis, dry mouth, sore or 'black tongue,' pancreatitis, sialoadenitis, hepatotoxicity, jaundice. **Hematologic: *Hemolytic anemia*,** leukopenia, granulocytopenia, thrombocytopenia, ***bone marrow depression*. Endocrine:** Gynecomastia, amenorrhea, galactorrhea, lactation, hyperprolactinemia. **GU:** Impotence, menstrual irregularities, failure to ejaculate, decreased libido. **Dermatologic:** Rash, ***toxic epidermal necrolysis*. Hepatic:** Jaundice, hepatitis, liver disorders, abnormal LFTs. **Miscellaneous:** Edema, weight gain, fever, lupus-like symptoms, nasal stuffiness, arthralgia, myalgia, ***septic shock-like syndrome*.**

LABORATORY TEST CONSIDERATIONS Positive Coombs' test. Hepatotoxicity may cause ↑ alkaline phosphatase, AST, ALT, bilirubin, and prothrombin time; also, eosinophilia. Interference with urinary uric acid by phosphotungstate method; serum creatinine by the alkaline picrate method; AST by colorimetric methods.

OD OVERDOSE MANAGEMENT
Symptoms: CNS, GI, and CV effects, including sedation, weakness, light-headedness, dizziness, coma, bradycardia, acute hypotension, impairment of AV conduction, constipation, diarrhea, distention, flatus, N&V. *Treatment:* Induction of vomiting or gastric lavage if detected early. General supportive treatment with special attention to HR, CO, blood volume, urinary function, electrolyte imbalance, paralytic ileus, and CNS activity. In severe cases, hemodialysis is effective.

DRUG INTERACTIONS
Anesthetics, general / Additive hypotension
Antidepressants, tricyclic / May block methyldopa hypotensive effects
Ferrous gluconate or sulfate / ↓ Bioavailability of methyldopa
Haloperidol / ↑ Haloperidol toxic effects
Levodopa / ↑ Effect of both drugs
Lithium / ↑ Possibility of lithium toxicity

MAO inhibitors / Accumulation of methyldopa metabolites may → excessive sympathetic stimulation
Methotrimeprazine / Additive hypotensive effect
Phenothiazines / Possible ↑ BP
Propranolol / Paradoxical hypertensive crisis
Sympathomimetics / Potentiation of pressor effects → hypertension
Thiazide diuretics / Additive hypotensive effect
Thioxanthenes / Additive hypotensive effect
Tolbutamide / ↑ Hypoglycemia R/T ↓ liver breakdown
Tricyclic antidepressants / ↓ Methyldopa effect
Vasodilator drugs / Additive hypotensive effect
Verapamil / ↑ Methyldopa effect

HOW SUPPLIED
Methyldopa: *Tablets:* 250 mg, 500 mg. **Methyldopate hydrochloride:** *Injection:* 50 mg/mL.

DOSAGE
METHYLDOPA
• **TABLETS**
Hypertension.
Initial: 250 mg 2–3 times per day for 2 days. Adjust dose q 2 days. If dose increased, start with evening dose. **Usual maintenance:** 0.5–2.0 grams/day in two to four divided doses; **maximum:** 3 grams/day. Gradually transfer to and from other antihypertensive agents, with initial dose of methyldopa not exceeding 500 mg. *NOTE:* Do not use combination medication to initiate therapy. **Pediatric, initial:** 10 mg/kg/day in 2–4 divided doses, adjusting maintenance to a maximum of 65 mg/kg/day (or 3 grams/day, whichever is less).

METHYLDOPATE HCL
• **IV INFUSION**
Hypertensive crisis.
Adults: 250–500 mg q 6 hr; **maximum:** 1 gram q 6 hr for hypertensive crisis. Switch to PO methyldopa, at same dosage level, when BP is brought under control. **Pediatric:** 20–40 mg/kg/day in divided doses q 6 hr; **maximum:** 65

mg/kg/day (or 3 grams/day, whichever is less).

NURSING CONSIDERATIONS

⚕ Do not confuse Aldomet with Aldoril (also an antihypertensive).

ADMINISTRATION/STORAGE

1. Tolerance may occur following 2–3 months of therapy. Increasing the dose or adding a diuretic often restores effect on BP.

IV 2. For IV, mix with 100 mL of D5W or administer in D5W at a concentration of 10 mg/mL. Infuse over 30–60 min.

ASSESSMENT

1. Note reasons for therapy, onset/characteristics of S&S, other agents trialed, outcome.

2. Monitor BP, CBC, renal, LFTs. If blood transfusion required, check direct and indirect Coombs' tests; if positive, consult hematologist.

3. Avoid during pregnancy. Note if jaundiced; avoid with active hepatic disease.

4. Assess for depression, drug tolerance; may occur during the second or third month of therapy.

CLIENT/FAMILY TEACHING

1. To prevent dizziness and fainting, rise slowly to a sitting position and dangle legs over the bed edge. Use caution, sedation may occur initially; should disappear once maintenance dose established.

2. In rare cases, may darken or turn urine blue; not harmful.

3. Withhold and report any of the following symptoms: tiredness, fever, depression, or yellowing of eyes/skin.

4. Continue to follow prescribed diet and exercise program in the overall goal of BP control. Keep log of BP recordings and weight for provider review.

5. Do not take any other medications or remedies unless approved.

6. Report any S&S of infection such as fever, or sore throat. May use ice chips or sugarless gums/candy to relieve dry mouth.

OUTCOMES/EVALUATE

BP control

Methylergonovine maleate   **IV**

(meth-ill-er-**GON**-oh-veen)

CLASSIFICATION(S):
Oxytocic drug
PREGNANCY CATEGORY: C
Rx: Methergine.

USES

(1) Management and prevention of postpartum and postabortal hemorrhage by producing firm uterine contractions and decreasing uterine bleeding. (2) During the second stage of labor following delivery of the anterior shoulder, but only under full obstetric supervision. *Investigational:* Ergonovine has been used to diagnose Prinzmetal's angina (variant angina).

ACTION/KINETICS

Action

Synthetic drug related to ergonovine. Acts directly on the uterine smooth muscle to stimulate the rate, tone, and amplitude of uterine contractions. It induces a rapid, sustained tetanic uterotonic effect that shortens the third stage of labor and reduces blood loss. The uterus becomes more sensitive to the drug toward the end of pregnancy.

Pharmacokinetics

Decrease in bioavailability after PO use probably due to first-pass metabolism in the liver. **Onset** (uterine contractions), **PO:** 5–10 min; **IM:** 2–5 min; **IV:** immediate. $t\frac{1}{2}$, **IV:** 2–3 min (initial) and 20–30 min (final). **Duration, PO, IM:** 3 hr; **IV:** 45 min. $t\frac{1}{2}$, **elimination:** 3.4 hr.

CONTRAINDICATIONS

Pregnancy, toxemia, hypertension. Ergot hypersensitivity. To induce labor or threatened spontaneous abortions. Administration before delivery of the placenta. Use with CYP3A4 inhibitors (e.g., protease inhibitors, macrolide antibiotics, azole antifungal drugs).

SPECIAL CONCERNS

Use with caution in sepsis, obliterative vascular disease, impaired renal or hepatic function, during the second stage of labor, and during lactation. Do not routinely use IV due to possible induction of sudden hypertension and CVA.

SIDE EFFECTS

Most Common
Hypertension associated with seizure or headache.

CV: Hypertension that may be associated with seizure or headache; hypotension, *acute MI*, thrombophlebitis, palpitation, transient chest pains. **GI:** N&V, diarrhea, foul taste. **CNS:** Dizziness, headache, tinnitus, hallucinations, seizures. **Miscellaneous:** Sweating, dyspnea, hematuria, water intoxication, leg cramps, nasal congestion.

NOTE: *Use of methylergonovine during labor may result in uterine tetany with rupture, cervical and perineal lacerations, embolism of amniotic fluid as well as hypoxia and intracranial hemorrhage in the infant.*

OD OVERDOSE MANAGEMENT
Symptoms: Initially, N&V, abdominal pain, increase in BP, tingling of extremities, numbness. Symptoms of severe overdose include hypotension, hypothermia, *respiratory depression, seizures, coma*. Treatment: Induce vomiting or perform gastric lavage. Administer a cathartic; institute diuresis. Maintain respiration, especially if seizures or coma occur. Treat seizures with anticonvulsant drugs. Warm extremities to control peripheral vasospasm.

DRUG INTERACTIONS
Azole antifungals (itraconazole, ketoconazole, voriconazole) / ↑ Risk of vasospasm leading to cerebral ischemia and/or ischemia of the extremities; do not use together
Clarithromycin / ↑ Risk of vasospasm leading to cerebral ischemia and/or ischemia of the extremities; do not use together
Erythromycin / ↑ Risk of vasospasm leading to cerebral ischemia and/or ischemia of the extremities; do not use together
Protease inhibitors / ↑ Risk of vasospasm leading to cerebral ischemia and/or ischemia of the extremities; do not use together

Reverse transcriptase inhibitors / ↑ Risk of vasospasm leading to cerebral ischemia and/or ischemia of the extremities; do not use together
Sympathomimetics / Hypertension R/T additive vasoconstriction
Troleoandomycin / ↑ Risk of vasospasm leading to cerebral ischemia and/or ischemia of the extremities; do not use together

HOW SUPPLIED
Injection: 0.2 mg/mL; Tablets: 0.2 mg.

DOSAGE

- **IM; IV (EMERGENCIES ONLY)**
  Prevention and treatment of postpartum and postabortal hemorrhage; during second stage of labor following delivery of anterior shoulder.
  0.2 mg q 2–4 hr following delivery of placenta, of the anterior shoulder, or during the puerperium.
- **TABLETS**
  Prevention and treatment of postpartum and postabortal hemorrhage.
  0.2 mg 3–4 times per day in the puerperium for a maximum of 1 week.

NURSING CONSIDERATIONS

ADMINISTRATION/STORAGE
1. Store tablets below 25°C (77°F) in tight, light-resistant containers.
IV 2. Administer slowly over 1 min; check VS for evidence of shock or hypertension after IV administration. Have emergency drugs available.
3. Give only if solution is clear and colorless; discard ampules if discolored.
4. Store ampules from 2–8°C (36–46°F). Protect from light.

ASSESSMENT
1. Note reasons for therapy, onset, characteristics of S&S. Avoid with liver or renal dysfunction. List drugs prescribed to ensure none interact.
2. Assess fundal tone and nonphasic contractures; massage to check for relaxation or severe cramping.
3. Monitor baseline calcium; correct if low to improve drug effectiveness. Monitor prolactin levels; assess for decreased milk production.
4. With postpartum bleeding, report frequency, amount, color, and any associated S&S.

CLIENT/FAMILY TEACHING

1. Take only as directed; do not exceed dosage.

2. Avoid smoking; nicotine constricts blood vessels.

3. Report any S&S of ergotism (cold/numb fingers/toes, N&V, headache, muscle or chest pain, weakness) or infection.

4. Abdominal cramps may be experienced; report any severe cramping, increased bleeding, or other adverse effects. F/U with provider to ensure no complications.

OUTCOMES/EVALUATE

Improved uterine tone; control of postpartum hemorrhage

Methylphenidate hydrochloride ■

(meth-ill-**FEN**-ih-dayt)

CLASSIFICATION(S):

CNS stimulant

PREGNANCY CATEGORY: C

Rx: Capsules, Extended-Release: Metadate CD, Ritalin LA. **Oral Solution**: Methylin. **Tablets**: Methylin, Ritalin. **Tablets, Chewable**: Methylin. **Tablets, Extended-Release**: Concerta, Metadate ER, Methylin ER, Ritalin-SR. **Transdermal Patch**: Daytrana, **C-II**

♣Rx: PMS-Methylphenidate, ratio-Methylphenidate.

USES

(1) Attention-deficit disorders (ADD) and attention-deficit hyperactivity disorders (ADHD) in children as part of overall treatment regimen. Syndrome characterized by moderate to severe distractibility, short attention span, hyperactivity, emotional lability, and impulsivity. Transdermal patch used only for ADHD. (2) Narcolepsy (Concerta, Metadate CD, Ritalin LA only). *Investigational:* Depression in medically ill (including stroke) elderly clients. Alleviation of neurobehavioral symptoms after traumatic brain injury. Improvement in

pain control, sedation, or both in those receiving opiates.

ACTION/KINETICS

Action

Mechanism unknown; may activate the brain stem arousal system and cortex to produce stimulation. In children with attention-deficit disorders, methylphenidate causes decreases in motor restlessness with an increased attention span. In narcolepsy the drug acts on the cerebral cortex and subcortical structures (e.g., thalamus) to increase motor activity and mental alertness and decrease fatigue.

Pharmacokinetics

Rapidly and well absorbed from the GI tract. Food delays peak levels of the chewable tablets by about 1 hr. **Peak blood levels, children:** 1.9 hr for tablets; 1–2 hr for chewable tablets; and, 4.7 hr for extended-release tablets. **Duration:** 4–6 hr. **t½ tablets, chewable tablets, Concerta tablets:** 1–3.5 hr; **t½,** Metatate CD: 6.8 hr. Metabolized by the liver and excreted by the kidney. *NOTE:* The various methylphenidate products have different pharmacokinetic properties. For example, the extended-release capsules (Ritalin LA) are taken once/day to eliminate the need for dosing during school hours. Drug is released in two parts—the second dose 4 hr after the first dose. Ritalin-SR is also for once daily dosing but provides continuous release over 8 hr.

CONTRAINDICATIONS

Marked anxiety, tension and agitation, glaucoma. Severe depression (either endogenous or exogenous), to prevent or treat normal fatigue, diagnosis or family history of Tourette's syndrome, motor tics. In children who manifest symptoms of primary psychiatric disorders (psychoses) or acute stress. Concurrent treatment of Concerta, Metadate CD, Ritalin, Ritalin LA, and Ritalin-SR with monoamine oxidase inhibitors and within a minimum of 14 days after stopping MAOI therapy (hypertensive crisis may occur). Use in children less than 6 years of age.

Bold Italic = life threatening side effect   ■ = black box warning   ♣ = Available in Canada

SPECIAL CONCERNS

■ (1) Give cautiously to emotionally unstable clients, such as those with a history of drug dependence or alcoholism, because such clients may increase dosage on their own initiative. (2) Chronic abuse can lead to marked tolerance and psychic dependence with varying degrees of abnormal behavior. Frank psychotic episodes can occur, especially after parenteral abuse. (3) Careful supervision is required during drug withdrawal because severe depression, as well as the effects of chronic overactivity, can be unmasked. (4) Long-term follow-up may be required due to the client's basic personality disturbances. (5) There is an increased risk of serious CV events and sudden death with CNS stimulants of this class.■ Use with caution during lactation. Use with great caution in clients with history of hypertension or convulsive disease or to emotionally unstable clients (e.g., those with history of drug dependence or alcoholism). Lowers seizure threshold in those with a history of seizures or with prior EEG abnormalities in the absence of seizures. May worsen symptoms of behavior disturbances and thought disorder. Safety and efficacy in children less than 6 years of age have not been established.

SIDE EFFECTS

Most Common

Headache, URTI, abdominal pain, anorexia, insomnia, vomiting, accidental injury, nervousness, anxiety/irritability.
CNS: Nervousness, insomnia, headaches, dizziness, drowsiness, chorea, depressed mood (transient). Toxic psychosis, dyskinesia, Tourette's syndrome, neuroleptic malignant syndrome (rare). Psychologic dependence. **CV:** Palpitations, tachycardia, angina, arrhythmias, hyper/hypotension, cerebral arteritis and/or occlusion. **GI:** N&V, anorexia, abdominal pain, weight loss (chronic use). GI obstruction (Concerta only as it is nondeformable and does not change shape appreciably in the GI tract.) **Respiratory:** URTI, increased cough, pharyngitis, sinusitis. **Allergic:** Skin rashes, fever, urticaria, arthralgia, exfoliative dermatitis, erythema multiforme with necrotizing vasculitis, erythema. **Hematologic:** Thrombocytopenic purpura, leukopenia, anemia. **Ophthalmic:** Accommodation difficulty, blurred vision. **Miscellaneous:** Scalp hair loss, accidental injury, abnormal liver function (including transaminase elevation to *hepatic coma*). **In children, in addition to the above, the following side effects are common:** Loss of appetite, abdominal pain, weight loss during chronic use, insomnia, tachycardia, dysmenorrhea, rhinitis, fever.

OD OVERDOSE MANAGEMENT

Symptoms: Characterized by CNS overstimulation and excessive sympathomimetic effects including: Vomiting, agitation, tremors, hyperreflexia, muscle twitching, **convulsions (may be followed by coma), hyperpyrexia,** euphoria, confusion, hallucinations, delirium, sweating, flushing, headache, tachycardia, palpitations, cardiac arrhythmias, hypertension, mydriasis, dry mucous membranes. *Treatment:* Symptomatic. Treat excess CNS stimulation by keeping the client in quiet, dim surroundings to reduce external stimuli. Protect the client from self-injury. A short-acting barbiturate may be used. Undertake emesis or gastric lavage if the client is conscious. Adequate circulatory and respiratory function must be maintained. Hyperpyrexia may be treated by cooling the client (e.g., cool bath, hypothermia blanket).

DRUG INTERACTIONS

Anticoagulants, oral (coumarin) / ↑ Anticoagulant effect R/T ↓ liver breakdown
Anticonvulsants (phenobarbital, phenytoin, primidone) / ↑ Anticonvulsant effect and ↑ toxic effects R/T ↓ liver breakdown
Carbamazepine / ↓ Methylphenidate levels
Clonidine / Possible serious side effects
Guanethidine / ↓ Guanethidine effect by displacement from its action site
MAO inhibitors / Possibility of hypertensive crisis, hyperthermia, convulsions, coma; do not use with Concerta, Metadate CD, Ritalin, Ritalin LA, Ritalin SR

Selective serotonin reuptake inhibitors / ↑ Serum levels of SSRIs

Tricyclic antidepressants / ↑ Plasma levels and TCA effect R/T ↓ liver breakdown

HOW SUPPLIED

Capsules, Extended-Release: 10 mg, 20 mg, 30 mg, 40 mg, 50 mg, 60 mg; Oral Solution: 5 mg/5 mL, 10 mg/5 mL; Tablets, Immediate-Release: 5 mg, 10 mg, 20 mg; Tablets, Chewable: 2.5 mg, 5 mg, 10 mg; Tablets, Extended-Release: 10 mg, 18 mg, 20 mg, 27 mg, 36 mg, 54 mg; Tablets, Sustained-Release: 20 mg; Transdermal Patch: 10 mg, 15 mg, 20 mg, 30 mg (each strength is the amount delivered over 9 hr).

DOSAGE

- **CAPSULES, EXTENDED-RELEASE; ORAL SOLUTION; TABLETS, CHEWABLE; TABLETS, IMMEDIATE-RELEASE; TABLETS, EXTENDED-RELEASE**

    Narcolepsy.

Adults, average dose: 20–30 mg/day in 2 to 3 divided doses (range: 10–15 to 40–60 mg/day), preferably 30–45 min before meals. For those unable to sleep if the medication is given late in the day, take the last dose before 6 p.m.

    Attention-deficit/hyperactivity disorder.

Individualize dose. Children, 6 years and older, initial: 5 mg twice a day before breakfast and lunch; **then,** increase gradually by 5–10 mg/week to a maximum of 60 mg/day. If no improvement is noted after a 1-month period, discontinue the drug. NOTE: See Administration/Storage for additional dosing information.

- **TRANSDERMAL PATCH**

    Attention-deficit/hyperactivity disorder.

Children, 6–12 years of age, initial: 10 mg over 9 hr for the first week with the patch applied to the client's hip 2 hr before an effect is needed; remove after 9 hr. **Week 2:** 15 mg over 9 hr; **week 3:** 20 mg over 9 hr; **week 4 and thereafter:** 30 mg over 9 hr.

NURSING CONSIDERATIONS

ADMINISTRATION/STORAGE

1. Discontinue periodically to assess condition as drug therapy is not indefinite; discontinue at puberty.
2. Sustained-release (SR) and Methylin ER tablets are effective for 8 hr and may be substituted for regular-release tablets if the 8-hr dosage of the sustained-release tablets is the same as the titrated 8-hr dosage of regular tablets. ER tablets must be swallowed whole, never crushed or chewed.
3. If paradoxical aggravation of symptoms or other side effects occur, reduce dose or discontinue drug.
4. Give Concerta once daily in the a.m. with or without food. Swallow tablets whole with liquids; do not chew, divide, or crush.
5. The recommended starting dose for Concerta is 18 mg/day for those not currently taking methylphenidate or if on stimulants other than methylphenidate. Dose may be adjusted in 18 mg increments at weekly intervals up to a maximum of 54 mg/day taken once in the a.m. For adolescents, aged 13–17 years, maximum dose may be 72 mg/day, but not more than 2 mg/kg/day, taken once in the morning.
6. The recommended dose for Concerta for clients currently taking methylphenidate 2 or 3 times per day, or SR at doses from 10–60 mg/day:
- 18 mg every a.m. if previously taking methylphenidate 5 mg 2 or 3 times per day or methylphenidate-SR, 20 mg/day.
- 36 mg every a.m. if previously taking methylphenidate 10 mg 2 or 3 times per day or methylphenidate-SR, 40 mg/day.
- 54 mg every a.m. if previously taking methylphenidate 15 mg 2 or 3 times per day or methylphenidate-SR, 60 mg/day.
7. For Metadate CD form, give once daily in the a.m. before breakfast. Swallow capsules whole with liquids; do not chew, divide, or crush. May also be given by sprinkle administration (e.g., on applesauce).

Bold Italic = life threatening side effect   ■ = black box warning   ✦ = Available in Canada

8. If Metadate CD is to be sprinkled onto soft food, the entire capsule contents must be used as a single 20-mg dose. Dose cannot be split because the immediate-release and continuous-release beads cannot be physically distinguished from one another. Give dose immediately after sprinkling; do not store for future use. The beads must not be crushed or chewed.

9. For Metadate CD, the dose is 20 mg once daily. Thirty percent is rapidly released and remaining 70% is released continuously permitting once daily dosage. Adjust dose in weekly 20 mg increments up to maximum of 60 mg/day taken once daily in a.m.

10. For Ritalin LA, start with 20 mg q day. Adjust dose, if needed, in 10 mg increments weekly up to a maximum of 60 mg/day taken once daily in the a.m. If a lower initial dose is appropriate, begin with an immediate-release methylphenidate. After titration to 10 mg twice a day, switch to Ritalin LA according to the following guidelines:

- If previous methylphenidate dose was 10 mg twice a day or 20 mg methylphenidate SR, give 20 mg Ritalin LA once daily.
- If previous methylphenidate dose was 15 mg twice a day, give 30 mg Ritalin LA once daily.
- If previous methylphenidate dose was 20 mg twice a day or 40 mg methylphenidate SR, give 40 mg Ritalin LA once daily.
- If previous methylphenidate dose was 30 mg twice a day or 60 mg methylphenidate SR, give 60 mg Ritalin LA once daily.

11. Each methylphenidate chewable tablet, 2.5 mg, contains phenylalanine, 0.42 mg; each 5 mg chewable tablet contains phenylalanine, 0.84 mg; and, each 10 mg chewable tablet contains phenylalanine, 1.68 mg.

12. Do not store Ritalin above 30°C (86°F). Protect from light, dispense in tight, light-resistant container.

13. Store Concerta, Metadate CD, and Ritalin LA from 25–30°C (59–86°F). Protect from humidity; store in a tight container.

14. Store Metadate ER, Methylin, and Methylin ER from 15–30°C (59–86°F). Protect from moisture and light. Dispense in a tight, light-resistant container.

ASSESSMENT

1. Note reasons for therapy, onset/characteristics of S&S, other drugs prescribed that may interact unfavorably.

2. Ensure psychologic evaluations show no evidence of psychotic disorder, excessive stimulation, or severe stress. Obtain/monitor VS, CBC, CNS status, ECG.

3. Assess growth (ht and wt); provide periodic 'drug holiday' to determine need for continued therapy.

4. May cause Tourette syndrome in child; monitor effects carefully.

CLIENT/FAMILY TEACHING

1. With ADD, take before breakfast and lunch to avoid interference with sleep. Take Ritalin SR and Concerta tablets whole; do not chew or crush. May swallow whole or sprinkle contents of Metadate CD onto a small amount of applesauce and take immediately. May notice the shell of the Concerta tablet in the stool.

2. Use caution when driving or operating hazardous machinery; drug may mask fatigue and/or cause physical incoordination, dizziness, blurred vision, drowsiness.

3. Record weight 2 times per week; report any significant loss as this may occur.

4. Report changes in mood, attention span; seizure disorder.

5. Skin rashes, fever, or joint pains should be reported immediately.

6. Therapy may be interrupted every few months ('drug holiday') to determine if still needed in those responsive to therapy.

7. Avoid caffeine in any form. May require more rest as drug effects fade.

8. Both adults and children should take the chewable tablets with at least 8 ounces of water or other fluid. Failure to do so may cause choking.

9. Chronic use may lead to psychic dependence and marked tolerance. Scripts will be carefully monitored.

OUTCOMES/EVALUATE
- ↑ Ability to sit quietly/concentrate
- ↓ Daytime sleeping

Methylprednisolone
(meth-ill-pred-**NISS**-oh-lohn)

CLASSIFICATION(S):
Glucocorticoid
PREGNANCY CATEGORY: C
Rx: Tablets: Medrol.

Methylprednisolone acetate
PREGNANCY CATEGORY: C
Rx: Parenteral: Depo-Medrol, dep-Medalone-40 and -80.

Methylprednisolone sodium succinate
PREGNANCY CATEGORY: C
Rx: A-methaPred, Solu-Medrol.

SEE ALSO CORTICOSTEROIDS.

ADDITIONAL USES
(1) Severe hepatitis due to alcoholism.
(2) Within 8 hr of severe spinal cord injury (to improve neurologic function).
(3) Septic shock (controversial).

ACTION/KINETICS

Action
The anti-inflammatory effect is due to inhibition of prostaglandin synthesis. The drug also inhibits accumulation of macrophages and leukocytes at sites of inflammation and inhibits phagocytosis and lysosomal enzyme release. Low incidence of increased appetite, peptic ulcer, psychic stimulation, and sodium and water retention. May mask negative nitrogen balance.

Pharmacokinetics
Onset: Slow, 12–24 hr. **t½, plasma:** 78–188 min. **Duration:** Long, up to 1 week. Rapid onset of sodium succinate by both IV and IM routes. Long duration of action of the acetate.

SPECIAL CONCERNS
Use during pregnancy only if benefits outweigh risks.

SIDE EFFECTS

Most Common
After PO use: GI upset, headache, dizziness, changes in menstrual cycle, insomnia, weight gain.
After parenteral use: Nausea, increased appetite, indigestion, dizziness, weight gain, weakness, sleep disturbances.

See *Corticosteroids* for a complete list of possible side effects.

ADDITIONAL DRUG INTERACTIONS
Aprepitant / ↑ Methylprednisolone AUC, peak levels, and t½ R/T ↓ metabolism by CYP3A4
Erythromycin / ↑ Methylprednisolone effect R/T ↓ liver metabolism
Grapefruit juice / ↑ AUC, peak levels, and t½ of methylprednisolone R/T ↓ liver metabolism
Nefazodone / ↑ Methylprednisolone AUC and prolonged t½ R/T ↓ metabolism
Troleandomycin / ↑ Methylprednisolone effect R/T ↓ liver metabolism

LABORATORY TEST CONSIDERATIONS
↓ Immunoglobulins A, G, M.

HOW SUPPLIED
Methylprednisolone: *Tablets:* 2 mg, 4 mg, 8 mg, 16 mg, 24 mg, 32 mg.
Methylprednisolone acetate: *Injection:* 20 mg/mL, 40 mg/mL, 80 mg/mL.
Methylprednisolone sodium succinate: *Powder for Injection:* 40 mg, 125 mg, 500 mg, 1 gram, 2 grams.

DOSAGE

METHYLPREDNISOLONE
- **TABLETS**

  Rheumatoid arthritis.
Adults: 6–16 mg/day. Decrease gradually when condition is under control.
Pediatric: 6–10 mg/day.

  SLE.
Adults, acute: 20–96 mg/day; **maintenance:** 8–20 mg/day.

  Acute rheumatic fever.
1 mg/kg body weight daily. Drug is always given in four equally divided doses after meals and at bedtime.

METHYLPREDNISOLONE ACETATE
- **IM**

M

Adrenogenital syndrome.
40 mg q 2 weeks.
Rheumatoid arthritis.
40–120 mg/week.
Dermatologic lesions, dermatitis.
40–120 mg/week for 1–4 weeks; for severe cases, a single dose of 80–120 mg should provide relief.
Seborrheic dermatitis.
80 mg/week.
Asthma, rhinitis.
80–120 mg.

• **INJECTION, SOFT TISSUE; INTRA-ARTICULAR INJECTION; INTRALESIONAL**
4–80 mg, depending on site.
METHYLPREDNISOLONE SODIUM SUCCINATE

• **IM; IV**
Most conditions.
Adults, initial: 10–40 mg, depending on the disease; **then,** adjust dose depending on response, with subsequent doses given either **IM, IV.**
Severe conditions.
Adults: 30 mg/kg infused IV over 10–20 min; may be repeated q 4–6 hr for 2–3 days only. **Pediatric:** Not less than 0.5 mg/kg/day.

NURSING CONSIDERATIONS

@ Do not confuse Medrol with Haldol (an antipsychotic). Do not confuse Solu-Medrol with Solu-Cortef (a hydrocortisone product). Do not confuse methylprednisolone with medroxyprogesterone (a progestin).

ADMINISTRATION/STORAGE
1. Dosage must be individualized.
2. Methylprednisolone acetate is not for IV use.
3. Use sodium succinate solutions within 48 hr after preparation.
4. For alternate day therapy, twice the usual PO dose is given every other morning (client receives beneficial effect while minimizing side effects).

ASSESSMENT
1. List reasons for treatment, onset, characteristics of S&S; describe clinical presentation.
2. Note any aspirin allergy; the 24 mg tablets distributed as Medrol contain tartrazine which may cause allergic reaction.

3. Monitor VS, weight, CBC, HbA1c, glucose, renal/LFTs, TFTs, cholesterol, and electrolytes with prolonged therapy.

CLIENT/FAMILY TEACHING
1. Take as directed; may take with food or milk to diminish GI upset. Do not ↑, ↓, or stop taking suddenly after prolonged use without provider consent; may cause rebound symptoms/adrenal crisis. Usually if administered before 9 a.m. may mimic normal peak body corticosteroid levels and prevent insomnia.
2. Report unusual weight gain, extremity swelling (cushingoid symptoms), fatigue, nausea, anorexia, joint pain, muscle weakness, dizziness, fever (adrenal insufficiency), black or tarry stools, prolonged sore throat/colds, infections, or worsening of problem.
3. Avoid live vaccines and persons with infections or diseases.
4. Severe stress or trauma may require increased dosage.
5. Prolonged use may cause glucose intolerance requiring treatment with insulin or oral agents.
6. Do not stop suddenly with prolonged use; must be tapered off to prevent adverse SE. Report any unusual SE or lack of response.

OUTCOMES/EVALUATE
• Relief of allergic manifestations
• ↓ Pain/inflammation; ↑ mobility
• ↓ Nerve fiber destruction in spinal cord injury (SCI)

Metipranolol hydrochloride
(met-ih-**PRAN**-oh-lohl)

CLASSIFICATION(S):
Beta-adrenergic blocking agent
PREGNANCY CATEGORY: C
Rx: OptiPranolol.

SEE ALSO *BETA-ADRENERGIC BLOCKING AGENTS.*

USES
Reduce IOP in ocular hypertension or chronic open-angle glaucoma.

M

ACTION/KINETICS

Action

Blocks both beta-1- and beta-2-adrenergic receptors. Reduction in intraocular pressure may be related to a decrease in production of aqueous humor and a slight increase in the outflow of aqueous humor. A decrease from 20–26% in intraocular pressure may be seen if the intraocular pressure is greater than 24 mm Hg at baseline. When used topically, has no local anesthetic effect and exerts no action on pupil size or accommodation.

Pharmacokinetics

May be absorbed and exert systemic effects. **Onset:** 30 min. **Maximum effect:** 1–2 hr. **Duration:** 12–24 hr.

SPECIAL CONCERNS

Use with caution during lactation. Safety and effectiveness have not been determined in children.

SIDE EFFECTS

Most Common

Transient local discomfort, conjunctivitis, blurred vision, browache, tearing, headache, dizziness, photophobia.

Ophthalmic: Transient local discomfort, dermatitis of the eyelid, blepharitis, conjunctivitis, browache, tearing, blurred/abnormal vision, photophobia, edema. Due to absorption, the following systemic side effects have been reported. **CV:** Hypertension, *MI*, atrial fibrillation, angina, bradycardia, palpitation. **CNS:** Headache, dizziness, anxiety, depression, somnolence, nervousness. **Respiratory:** Dyspnea, rhinitis, bronchitis, coughing. **Miscellaneous:** Allergic reaction, asthenia, nausea, epistaxis, arthritis, myalgia, rash.

HOW SUPPLIED

Ophthalmic Solution: 0.3%.

DOSAGE

- **OPHTHALMIC SOLUTION, 0.3%**
  Reduce IOP in ocular hypertension or chronic open-angle glaucoma.

Adults: 1 gtt in the affected eye(s) twice a day. Increasing the dose or more frequent administration does not increase the beneficial effect.

NURSING CONSIDERATIONS

ADMINISTRATION/STORAGE

1. May be used concomitantly with other drugs to lower IOP.
2. Due to diurnal variation in response, measure IOP at different times during the day.

ASSESSMENT

1. Note ocular condition, onset, pretreatment pressures.
2. Document clinical presentation, baseline ECG, acuity level, VS.

CLIENT/FAMILY TEACHING

1. Transient burning or stinging is common during administration; report if severe.
2. To prevent contamination/infection wash hands before and after instillation and do not permit dropper to come in contact with eye.
3. Take only as directed; report any persistent bothersome side effects or symptoms of intolerance.
4. Report for follow up visits to assess for systemic effects, measure intraocular pressures, and access effectiveness.

OUTCOMES/EVALUATE

↓ IOP

Metoclopramide IV ©
(meh-toe-kloh-**PRAH**-myd)

CLASSIFICATION(S):

Gastrointestinal stimulant
PREGNANCY CATEGORY: B
Rx: Maxolon, Octamide PFS, Reglan.
♣Rx: Apo-Metoclop, Metoclopramide Omega, Nu-Metoclopramide.

USES

PO: (1) Short-term (4 to 12 weeks) therapy for adults with symptomatic documented gastroesophageal reflux who fail to respond to conventional treatment. (2) Symptomatic relief of acute and recurrent diabetic gastroparesis. Relief of vomiting and anorexia may precede the relief of abdominal fullness by 1 week or more.

Bold Italic = life threatening side effect   ■ = black box warning   ♣ = Available in Canada

Parenteral: (1) Prevention of N&V associated with emetogenic cancer chemotherapy. (2) Prevention of postoperative N&V when nasogastric suction is undesirable. (3) Facilitate small bowel intubation when the tube does not pass the pylorus with conventional methods (use single doses). (4) Stimulate gastric emptying and intestinal transit of barium in clients where delayed emptying interferes with radiological examination of the stomach or small intestine. (5) Symptomatic relief of diabetic gastroparesis.

Investigational: To improve lactation. N&V due to various causes, including vomiting during pregnancy and labor, gastric ulcer, anorexia nervosa. Improve client response to ergotamine, analgesics, and sedatives when used to treat migraine (may increase absorption). Postoperative gastric bezoars. Atonic bladder. Esophageal variceal bleeding.

ACTION/KINETICS

Action

Dopamine antagonist that acts by increasing sensitivity to acetylcholine; results in increased motility of the upper GI tract and relaxation of the pyloric sphincter and duodenal bulb. Gastric emptying time and GI transit time are shortened. No effect on gastric, biliary, or pancreatic secretions. Facilitates intubation of the small bowel and speeds transit of a barium meal. Produces sedation, induces release of prolactin, increases circulating aldosterone levels (is transient), and is an antiemetic.

Pharmacokinetics

Onset, IV: 1–3 min; **IM:** 10–15 min; **PO:** 30–60 min. **Duration:** 1–2 hr. **t½:** 5–6 hr. Significant first-pass effect following PO use; unchanged drug and metabolites excreted in urine. Renal impairment decreases clearance of the drug.

CONTRAINDICATIONS

Gastrointestinal hemorrhage, obstruction, or perforation; epilepsy; clients taking drugs likely to cause extrapyramidal symptoms, such as phenothiazines. Pheochromocytoma.

SPECIAL CONCERNS

Use with caution during lactation and in hypertension. Extrapyramidal effects are more likely to occur in children and geriatric clients.

SIDE EFFECTS

Most Common

Extrapyramidal symptoms, restlessness, drowsiness, fatigue, lassitude, akathisia, dizziness, nausea, diarrhea.

CNS: Restlessness, drowsiness, fatigue, lassitude, akathisia, anxiety, insomnia, confusion. Headaches, dizziness, extrapyramidal symptoms (especially acute dystonic reactions), Parkinson-like symptoms (including cogwheel rigidity, mask-like facies, bradykinesia, tremor), dystonia, myoclonus, *depression (with suicidal ideation)*, tardive dyskinesia (including involuntary movements of the tongue, face, mouth, or jaw), *seizures*, hallucinations. **GI:** Nausea, bowel disturbances (usually diarrhea). **CV:** Hypertension (transient), hypotension, SVT, bradycardia. **Hematologic:** *Agranulocytosis*, leukopenia, neutropenia. Methemoglobinemia in premature and full-term infants at doses of 1–4 mg/kg/day IM, IV, or PO for 1–3 or more days. **Endocrine:** Galactorrhea, amenorrhea, gynecomastia, impotence (due to hyperprolactinemia), fluid retention (due to transient elevation of aldosterone). **Neuroleptic malignant syndrome: Hyperthermia,** altered consciousness, autonomic dysfunction, muscle rigidity, *death*. **Miscellaneous:** Incontinence, urinary frequency, porphyria, visual disturbances, flushing of the face and upper body, hepatotoxicity.

OD OVERDOSE MANAGEMENT

Symptoms: Agitation, irritability, hypertonia of muscles, drowsiness, disorientation, EPS. *Treatment:* Treat extrapyramidal effects by giving anticholinergic drugs, antiparkinson drugs, or antihistamines with anticholinergic effects. General supportive treatment. Reverse methemoglobinemia by giving methylene blue.

DRUG INTERACTIONS

Acetaminophen / ↑ Acetaminophen absorption
Anticholinergics / ↓ Metoclopramide effect

Cimetidine / ↓ Cimetidine effect R/T ↓ GI tract absorption

CNS depressants / Additive sedative effects

Cyclosporine / ↑ Cyclosporine absorption → ↑ immunosuppressive and toxic effects

Digoxin / ↓ Digoxin effect R/T ↓ GI tract absorption

Ethanol / ↑ Ethanol GI absorption

Levodopa / ↑ Levodopa GI absorption and ↓ metoclopramide effects on gastric emptying and lower esophageal pressure

MAO inhibitors / ↑ Release of catecholamines → toxicity

Narcotic analgesics / ↓ Metoclopramide effect

Sertraline / Possible serotonin syndrome with EPS

Succinylcholine / ↑ Succinylcholine effect R/T plasma cholinesterase inhibition

Tetracyclines / ↑ Tetracycline GI absorption

Venlafaxine / Possible serotonin syndrome with EPS

HOW SUPPLIED

Injection: 5 mg/mL; *Syrup:* 5 mg/5 mL; *Tablets:* 5 mg, 10 mg.

DOSAGE

- **SYRUP; TABLETS**

Diabetic gastroparesis.

Adults: 10 mg 30 min before meals and at bedtime for 2–8 weeks (therapy should be reinstituted if symptoms recur).

Gastroesophageal reflux.

Adults: 10–15 mg 4 times per day, 30 min before meals and at bedtime. If symptoms occur only intermittently, single doses up to 20 mg prior to the provoking situation may be used.

Enhance lactation.

Adults: 30–45 mg/day.

Postoperative gastric bezoars.

10 mg 3–4 times per day.

- **IM; IV**

Diabetic gastroparesis.

10 mg 30 min before each meal and at bedtime for 2–8 weeks. May take up to 10 days for symptoms subside; then, begin PO therapy. Reinstitute therapy at the earliest manifestation.

Prophylaxis of vomiting due to chemotherapy.

Initial: 2 mg/kg IV (1 mg/kg may be adequate for less emetogenic regimens) q 2 hr for two doses, with the first dose 30 min before chemotherapy; **then,** 10 mg or more q 3 hr for three doses. Inject slowly IV over 15 min.

Prophylaxis of postoperative N&V.

Adults: 10–20 mg IM near the end of surgery.

Facilitate small bowel intubation.

IV. Adults: 10 mg; **pediatric, 6–14 years:** 2.5–5 mg; **pediatric, less than 6 years:** 0.1 mg/kg. Give a single undiluted dose slowly IV over 1–2 min.

Radiologic examinations to increase intestinal transit time.

Adults: 10 mg as a single dose given IV over 1–2 min.

NURSING CONSIDERATIONS

℮ Do not confuse metoclopramide with metoprolol (a beta-adrenergic blocker) or with metolazone (a thiazide diuretic).

ADMINISTRATION/STORAGE

1. Determine route of administration to treat diabetic gastroparesis by the severity of symptoms. With only the earliest symptoms, begin PO therapy. If symptoms are severe, begin with parenteral therapy. Administer 10 mg over 1–2 min.

2. If C_{CR} is <40 mL/min, begin therapy at approximately one-half the recommended dosage. Depending on efficacy and safety, the dose may be increased or decreased as needed.

3. After PO use, absorption of certain drugs from the GI tract may be affected (see *Drug Interactions*).

4. For outpatient treatment when PO dosing is not possible, suppositories containing 25 mg metoclopramide have been made extemporaneously. Give 1 suppository 30–60 min before each meal and at bedtime.

IV 5. Inject slowly IV over 1–2 min to prevent transient feelings of anxiety/restlessness.

6. Metoclopramide is physically/chemically incompatible with a number of drugs; check package insert if drug is to be admixed.

Bold Italic = life threatening side effect   ■ = black box warning   ✦ = Available in Canada

7. For IV, dilute doses greater than 10 mg in 50 mL of D5W, D5/0.45% NaCl, RL, Ringer's injection, or NaCl; infuse over 15 min.

ASSESSMENT
1. Note reasons for therapy, type, onset, characteristics of S&S. List drugs prescribed, ensuring none interact.
2. Assess abdomen for bowel sounds, distention, N&V.

CLIENT/FAMILY TEACHING
1. Take as directed; may dilute syrup in water, juice or carbonated beverage just before taking.
2. Drug increases the movements or contractions of the stomach and intestines.
3. Do not operate a car or hazardous machinery until drug effects realized; drug has a sedative effect up to 2 hr after dosing.
4. Report lack of response, persistent side effects so they can be properly evaluated and counteracted.
5. Avoid alcohol and CNS depressants.
6. Extrapyramidal effects (trembling hands, facial grimacing) should be reported; may be treated with parenteral diphenhydramine.

OUTCOMES/EVALUATE
- Prevention of N&V
- Enhanced gastric motility
- Promotion of gastric emptying
- Prophylaxis of gastric bezoars

Metolazone @

(meh-**TOH**-lah-zohn)

CLASSIFICATION(S):
Diuretic, thiazide
PREGNANCY CATEGORY: B
Rx: Mykrox, Zaroxolyn.

SEE ALSO DIURETICS, THIAZIDE.

USES
Slow availability tablets: (1) Edema accompanying CHF; edema accompanying renal diseases, including nephrotic syndrome and conditions of reduced renal function. (2) Alone or in combination with other drugs for the treatment of hypertension.

Rapid availability tablets: Treatment of newly diagnosed mild to moderate hypertension alone or in combination with other drugs. The rapid availability tablets are not to be used to produce diuresis.
Investigational: Alone or as an adjunct to treat calcium nephrolithiasis, premanagement of menstrual syndrome, and adjunct treatment of renal failure.

ACTION/KINETICS
Pharmacokinetics Onset: 1 hr. **Peak blood levels, rapid availability tablets:** 2–4 hr; **t½, elimination:** About 14 hr. **Peak blood levels, slow availability tablets:** 8 hr. **Duration, rapid or slow availablity tablets:** 24 hr or more. Most excreted unchanged through the urine.

CONTRAINDICATIONS
Anuria, prehepatic and hepatic coma, allergy or hypersensitivity to metolazone. Routine use during pregnancy. Lactation.

SPECIAL CONCERNS
Use with caution in those with severely impaired renal function and in the elderly. Safety and effectiveness have not been determined in children.

SIDE EFFECTS
Most Common
Dizziness, headache, muscle cramps, malaise, lethargy, lassitude, joint pain/swelling, chest pain.
See *Diuretics, Thiazide* for a complete list of possible side effects. Also, ***toxic epidermal necrolysis and Stevens-Johnson syndrome.***

ADDITIONAL DRUG INTERACTIONS
Alcohol / ↑ Hypotensive effect
Barbiturates / ↑ Hypotensive effect
Narcotics / ↑ Hypotensive effect
NSAIDs / ↓ Hypotensive effect of metolazone
Salicylates / ↓ Hypotensive effect of metolazone

HOW SUPPLIED
Tablets: 0.5 mg, 2.5 mg, 5 mg, 10 mg.

DOSAGE
ZAROXOLYN
- **SLOW AVAILABLE TABLETS**
  Edema due to cardiac failure or renal disease.

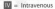

M

Adults: 5–20 mg once daily. For those who experience paroxysmal nocturnal dyspnea, a larger dose may be required to ensure prolonged diuresis and saluresis for a 24-hr period.

Mild to moderate essential hypertension.

Adults: 2.5–5 mg once daily.

MYKROX

• **RAPID AVAILABILITY TABLETS**

Mild to moderate essential hypertension.

Adults, initial: 0.5 mg once daily, usually in the morning. If inadequately controlled, the dose may be increased to 1 mg once a day. Increasing the dose higher than 1 mg does not increase the effect.

NURSING CONSIDERATIONS

℣ Do not confuse metolazone with methotrexate (an antineoplastic) or with metoclopramide (a GI stimulant).

ADMINISTRATION/STORAGE

1. Formulations of slow availability tablets should not be interchanged with formulations of rapid availability tablets as they are not therapeutically equivalent.

2. The antihypertensive effect may be observed from 3 to 4 days to 3 to 6 weeks.

3. If BP is not controlled with 1 mg of the rapid availability tablets, add another antihypertensive drug, with a different mechanism of action, to the therapy.

4. Store tablets at room temperature in a tight, light-resistant container.

ASSESSMENT

1. Note reasons for therapy, onset, duration, clinical characteristics; has synergistic effect with furosemide.

2. Monitor weight, BP, ECG, CBC, electrolytes, uric acid, renal, LFTs; assess for S&S of electrolyte imbalance (i.e., ↓ Na/K/Mg/P and hypochloremic alkalosis).

CLIENT/FAMILY TEACHING

1. Take with/without food exactly as directed; early in the day to prevent nighttime awakening for urination.

2. May cause sudden drop in BP and syncope; use caution and change positions slowly. Avoid alcohol during therapy.

3. Check weight regularly; report increases of more than 3 lb/day or 5 lb/week or lack of response to extremity swelling.

4. Avoid exposure to sun or bright lights; may cause photosensitivity.

5. May cause potassium depletion; eat a K-rich diet (whole grain cereals, legumes, meat, bananas, apricots, orange juice, potatoes, raisins); keep all follow up appointments for labs and evaluation.

6. Report any muscle weakness/cramps, fatigue, nausea, dizziness, or adverse effects.

OUTCOMES/EVALUATE

↓ Edema; ↓ BP

Metoprolol succinate

(me-toe-**PROH**-lohl)

CLASSIFICATION(S):
Beta-adrenergic blocking agent
PREGNANCY CATEGORY: C
Rx: Toprol XL.

Metoprolol tartrate

PREGNANCY CATEGORY: B
Rx: Lopressor.
✤**Rx:** Apo-Metoprolol, Apo-Metoprolol (Type L), Betaloc, Betaloc Durules, Gen-Metoprolol, Gen-Metoprolol (Type L), Novo-Metoprol, Nu-Metop, PMS-Metoprolol-B, PMS-Metoprolol-L.

SEE ALSO *BETA-ADRENERGIC BLOCKING AGENTS.*

USES

Metoprolol Succinate: (1) Alone or with other drugs to treat hypertension. (2) Chronic management of angina pectoris. (3) Treatment of stable, symptomatic (NYHA Class II or III) heart failure of ischemic, hypertensive, or cardiomyopathic origin.

   Metoprolol Tartrate: (1) Hypertension (either alone or with other antihypertensive agents, such as thiazide diuretics). (2) Acute MI in hemodynamically stable clients. (3) Angina pectoris. *Investigational:* IV to suppress atrial ectopy in COPD, aggressive behavior, prophylaxis of migraine, ventricular arrhythmias, enhancement of cognitive performance in geriatric clients, essential tremors.

ACTION/KINETICS
Action
Combines reversibly mainly with $beta_1$-adrenergic receptors to block the response to sympathetic nerve impulses, circulating catecholamines, or adrenergic drugs. Blockade of $beta_1$-receptors decreases HR, myocardial contractility, and CO and slows AV conduction, all of which lead to a decrease in BP. $Beta_2$-receptors are blocked at high doses. Has no membrane-stabilizing or intrinsic sympathomimetic effects.

Pharmacokinetics
Moderate lipid solubility. **Onset:** 15 min. **Peak plasma levels:** 90 min. **t½:** 3–7 hr. Effect of drug is cumulative. Food increases bioavailability. Exhibits significant first-pass effect. Metabolized in liver and excreted in urine.

ADDITIONAL CONTRAINDICATIONS
Myocardial infarction in clients with a HR of less than 45 bpm, in second- or third-degree heart block, or if SBP is less than 100 mm Hg. Moderate to severe cardiac failure.

SPECIAL CONCERNS
Safety and effectiveness have not been established in children. Use with caution in impaired hepatic function and during lactation.

SIDE EFFECTS
Most Common
Fatigue, dizziness, depression, shortness of breath, bradycardia, diarrhea.
See *Beta-Adrenergic Blocking* Agents for a complete list of possible side effects.

ADDITIONAL DRUG INTERACTIONS
Cimetidine / May ↑ plasma metoprolol levels
Contraceptives, oral / May ↑ metoprolol effects
Diphenhydramine / ↓ Metoprolol clearance → prolonged negative chronotropic and inotropic effects in extensive metabolizers
Hydroxychloroquine / ↑ Bioavailability of metoprolol in homozygous extensive metabolizers
Methimazole / May ↓ metoprolol effects
Phenobarbital / ↓ Metoprolol effect R/T ↑ liver metabolism
Propylthiouracil / May ↓ metoprolol effects
Quinidine / May ↑ metoprolol effects
Rifampin / ↓ Metoprolol effect R/T ↑ liver metabolism

LABORATORY TEST CONSIDERATIONS
↑ Serum transaminase, LDH, alkaline phosphatase.

HOW SUPPLIED
Metoprolol succinate: *Tablets, Extended-Release:* 25 mg, 50 mg, 100 mg, 200 mg (all are equivalent to metoprolol tartrate).
Metoprolol tartrate: *Injection:* 1 mg/mL; *Tablets:* 2 mg, 50 mg, 100 mg.

DOSAGE
METOPROLOL SUCCINATE
• **TABLETS, EXTENDED-RELEASE**
Angina pectoris.
Individualized, Initial: 100 mg/day in a single dose. Dose may be increased slowly, at weekly intervals, until optimum effect is reached or there is a pronounced slowing of HR. Doses above 400 mg/day have not been studied.
Hypertension.
Initial: 25–100 mg/day in a single dose with or without a diuretic. Dosage may be increased in weekly intervals until maximum effect is reached. Doses above 400 mg/day have not been studied.
CHF.
Individualize dose. **Initial:** 25 mg once daily for 2 weeks in clients with NYHA Class II heart failure and 12.5 mg once daily in those with more severe heart failure. Double the dose q 2 weeks to the highest dose level tolerated or up to 200 mg.
METOPROLOL TARTRATE
• **TABLETS**
Hypertension.
Initial: 100 mg/day in single or divided doses; **then,** dose may be increased

weekly to maintenance level of 100–450 mg/day. A diuretic may also be used.

Angina pectoris.
Initial: 100 mg/day in 2 divided doses. Dose may be increased gradually at weekly intervals until optimum response is obtained or a pronounced slowing of HR occurs. Effective dose range: 100–400 mg/day. If treatment is to be discontinued, reduce dose gradually over 1–2 weeks.

Aggressive behavior.
200–300 mg/day.

Essential tremors.
50–300 mg/day.

Prophylaxis of migraine.
50–100 mg twice a day.

Ventricular arrhythmias.
200 mg/day.

• **INJECTION (IV); TABLETS**
Early treatment of MI.

Three IV bolus injections of 5 mg each at approximately 2-min intervals. If clients tolerate the full IV dose, give 50 mg q 6 hr PO beginning 15 min after the last IV dose (or as soon as client's condition allows). This dose is continued for 48 hr followed by **late treatment:** 100 mg twice a day as soon as feasible; continue for 1–3 months (although data suggest treatment should be continued for 1–3 years). In clients who do not tolerate the full IV dose, begin with 25–50 mg q 6 hr PO beginning 15 min after the last IV dose or as soon as client's condition allows.

NURSING CONSIDERATIONS

Ⓒ Do not confuse metoprolol with metoclopramide (GI stimulant), metaproterenol (bronchodilator), or with misoprostol (prostaglandin derivative). Also, do not confuse Toprol-XL with Topamax (an antiepileptic, antimigraine drug) or Tegretol and Tegretol-XR (an antiepileptic).

ADMINISTRATION/STORAGE
1. If transient worsening of heart failure occurs; treat with increased doses of diuretics. May need to lower dose of metoprolol or temporarily discontinue.
2. For CHF, do not increase dose until symptoms of worsening CHF have been

stabilized. Initial difficulty with titration should not preclude attempts later to use metoprolol.
3. If CHF clients experience symptomatic bradycardia, reduce dose.

ASSESSMENT
1. Note reasons for therapy: CAD, recent MI, NYHA class.
2. Monitor VS, EF, CXR, CBC, liver/renal function studies, ECG, echocardiogram.
3. Assess for asthma, emphysema, depression, myasthenia gravis, circulation problems, chf, or heartblock, thyroid, liver or kidney disorders; may preclude drug therapy.

CLIENT/FAMILY TEACHING
1. Take at same time each day; do not stop suddenly.
2. Take with food. Do not crush or chew the extended-release products; swallow tablets whole.
3. Avoid activities that require mental alertness until drug effects realized. Alcohol may intensify these effects.
4. Before taking any OTC agents, obtain medical advice; some may affect action of metoprolol.
5. Continue with diet, regular exercise, and weight loss in the overall plan to control BP.
6. Report any symptoms of fluid overload such as sudden weight gain, SOB, or swelling of extremities. Avoid salt.
7. Dress appropriately; may cause an increased sensitivity to cold. Do not smoke.
8. Keep a log of symptoms, Wt, BP, and HR readings; report if heart rate <50 or irregular.

OUTCOMES/EVALUATE
• ↓ BP; ↓ anginal attacks
• Prevention of myocardial reinfarction and associated mortality

Metronidazole   ■ Ⅳ
(meh-troh-**NYE**-dah-zohl)

CLASSIFICATION(S):
Trichomonacide, amebicide
PREGNANCY CATEGORY: B
Rx: Injection: Flagyl I.V., Flagyl I.V.

RTU. **PO:** Flagyl, Flagyl 375, Flagyl ER, Metric 21, Protostat. **Topical:** MetroCream, MetroGel, MetroLotion, Noritate. **Vaginal Gel/Jelly:** MetroGel Vaginal, Vandazole.

✤**Rx:** Apo-Metronidazole, Metro-Cream, NidaGel, Novo–Nidazol.

SEE ALSO *ANTI-INFECTIVE DRUGS.*

USES
Systemic: (1) Serious infections due to susceptible anaerobic bacteria, including *Bacteroides fragilis* resistant to clindamycin, chloramphenicol, and penicillin. (2) Peritonitis, intra-abdominal abscess and liver abscess due to *B. fragilis*, *B. distasonis, B. ovatus, B. thetaiotaomicron, B. vulgatus, Clostridium* species, *Eubacterium* species, *Peptostreptococcus* species, and *Peptococcus niger.* (3) Skin and skin structure infections due to *Bacteroides* species including *B. fragilis* group, *Clostridium* species, *Peptostreptococcus* species, *Fusobacterium* species, and *Peptococcus niger.* (4) Endometritis, endomyometritis, tubo-ovarian abscess, and postsurgical vaginal cuff infection due to *Bacteroides* species including the *B. fragilis* group, *Clostridium* species, *Peptococcus* species, and *Peptostreptococcus* species. Bacterial vaginosis (use Flagyl ER only). Symptomatic trichomoniasis in males and females (endocervicitis, cervicitis, cervical erosion). (5) Bacterial septicemia due to *Bacteroides* species including the *B. fragilis* group and *Clostridium* species. (6) Adjunct therapy to treat bone and joint infections due to *Bacteroides* species including the *B. fragilis* group. (7) Meningitis and brain abscess due to *Bacteroides* species including the *B. fragilis* group. (8) Pneumonia, empyema, and lung abscess due to *Bacteroides* species including the *B. fragilis* group. (9) Endocarditis due to *Bacteroides* species including the *B. fragilis* group. (10) Amebiasis. Symptomatic and asymptomatic trichomoniasis; to treat asymptomatic partner. (11) To reduce postoperative anaerobic infection following colorectal surgery, elective hysterectomy, and emergency appendectomy. (12) As part of combination therapy to eradicate *Helicobacter pylori* infections. (13) Hepatic encephalopathy. (14) Crohn's disease. (15) Diarrhea associated with *Clostridium difficile.* (16) Recurrent and persistent urethritis. (17) Pelvic inflammatory disease as an alternative parenteral regimen. (18) Prophylaxis after sexual assault. (19) Bacterial vaginosis. *Investigational:* Giardiasis, *Gardnerella vaginalis.*

Topical: Inflammatory papules, pustules, and erythema of rosacea. *Investigational:* Infected decubitus ulcers (use gel or 1% solution or suspension).

Vaginal: Bacterial vaginosis.

ACTION/KINETICS
Action
Effective against anaerobic bacteria and protozoa. Specifically inhibits growth of trichomonae and amoebae by binding to DNA, resulting in loss of helical structure, strand breakage, inhibition of nucleic acid synthesis, and cell death. The mechanism for its effectiveness in reducing the inflammatory lesions of acne rosacea is not known.

Pharmacokinetics
Well absorbed from GI tract and widely distributed in body tissues. Rate of absorption of extended-release tablet is increased in the fed state resulting in alteration of the extended-release characteristics. **Peak serum concentration, PO:** 6–40 mcg/mL, depending on the dose, after 1–2 hr. **t½, PO:** 6–12 hr; average: 8 hr. t½ is inversely related to gestational age in newborns. Eliminated primarily in urine (20% unchanged), which may be red-brown in color following either PO or IV use.

CONTRAINDICATIONS
Blood dyscrasias, active organic disease of the CNS, trichomoniasis during the first trimester of pregnancy, lactation. Is carcinogenic in rodents; avoid unnecessary use. Topical use if hypersensitive to parabens or other ingredients of the formulation. Consumption of alcohol during use. For the vaginal gel, hypersensitivity to the drug, parabens, or other.

SPECIAL CONCERNS
■ Metronidazole is carcinogenic in rats; avoid unnecessary use.■ Use with caution in those with evidence or history of blood dyscrasias or in those with im-

paired hepatic function. Safety and efficacy have not been established in children except for treating amebiasis. Those with candidiasis may show more pronounced symptoms during metronidazole therapy; treat with a candicidal drug.

SIDE EFFECTS

Most Common

Following systemic use: Headache, vaginitis, nausea, metallic taste, genital pruritus, bacterial infection, flu-like symptoms.

Systemic Use. GI: Nausea, dry mouth, metallic taste, vomiting, diarrhea, abdominal discomfort, constipation, epigastric distress, abdominal cramping/pain, proctitis. **CNS:** Headache, dizziness, vertigo, incoordination, ataxia, confusion, irritability, depression, weakness, insomnia, syncope, *seizures*, peripheral neuropathy including paresthesias. **Hematologic:** Leukopenia (reversible), thrombocytopenia (reversible), *bone marrow aplasia*. **CV:** Flattening of the T-wave in ECG tracings, thrombophlebitis after IV infusion. **GU:** Vaginitis, genital pruritus, dysmenorrhea, UTI, burning, dysuria, cystitis, polyuria, incontinence, sense of pelvic pressure, proliferation of *Candida* in the vagina, dryness of vagina or vulva, dyspareunia, dark brown color to urine, decreased libido. **Respiratory:** URTI, rhinitis, sinusitis, pharyngitis. **Allergic:** Urticaria, pruritus, erythematous rash, flushing, nasal congestion, fever, joint pain. **Miscellaneous:** Furry tongue, glossitis, stomatitis (all due to overgrowth of *Candida*), fleeting joint pain sometimes resembling serum sickness, bacterial infection, flu-like symptoms, moniliasis. **Topical Use.** Watery eyes if gel applied too closely to this area. Acne, burning/stinging, contact dermatitis, dryness, erythema, local allergic reaction, metallic taste, nausea, pruritus, skin irritation, tingling/numbness of extremities, transient redness, worsening of rosacea. **Vaginal Use.** Symptomatic *Candida vaginitis*, N&V.

LABORATORY TEST CONSIDERATIONS

May interfere with chemical analyses for AST, ALT, LDH, triglycerides, and glucose hexokinase; zero values may result.

OD OVERDOSE MANAGEMENT

Symptoms: Ataxia, N&V, peripheral neuropathy, *seizures* up to 5–7 days. *Treatment:* Supportive treatment.

DRUG INTERACTIONS

Barbiturates / Possible therapeutic failure of metronidazole R/T ↑ elimination

Busulfan / ↑ Busulfan trough plasma levels; ↑ risk of toxicity

Cimetidine / ↑ Serum metronidazole levels R/T ↓ clearance

Disulfiram / Concurrent use may cause confusion or acute psychosis; do not give metronidazole to clients who have taken disulfiram within the past 2 weeks

Ethanol / Possible disulfiram-like reaction, including flushing, palpitations, tachycardia, and N&V

Hydantoins / ↑ Hydantoins effect R/T ↓ clearance

Lithium / ↑ Lithium levels and toxicity

Phenytoin / Possible therapeutic failure of metronidazole R/T ↑ elimination

Warfarin / ↑ Anticoagulant effect → prolonged prothrombin time

HOW SUPPLIED

Capsules: 375 mg; *Cream:* 0.75%, 1%; *Gel (Topical):* 0.75%, 1%; *Injection:* 5 mg/1 mL (ready-to-use); *Injection, Lyophilized:* 500 mg; *Lotion:* 0.75%; *Tablets:* 250 mg, 500 mg; *Tablets, Extended-Release:* 750 mg; *Vaginal Gel/Jelly:* 0.75%.

DOSAGE

• **CAPSULES; TABLETS**

Amebiasis: Acute amebic dysentery or amebic liver abscess.

Adult: 500–750 mg 3 times per day for 5–10 days; **pediatric:** 35–50 mg/kg/day in three divided doses for 10 days.

Trichomoniasis, female.

Female: 250 mg if using tablets 3 times per day for 7 days, 2 grams given on 1 day in single or divided doses, or 375 mg if using capsules twice a day for 7 days. **Pediatric:** 5 mg/kg 3 times per day for 7 days. An interval of 4–6 weeks should elapse between courses of therapy. *NOTE:* Do not treat pregnant women during the first trimester. **Male:** Individualize dosage; usual, 250 mg 3 times per day for 7 days.

Treat Helicobacter pylori *infections.*

One of the following regimens may be used: (1) Metronidazole, 500 mg twice a day; clarithromycin, 500 mg twice a day; and, either lansoprazole, 30 mg a day or omeprazole, 20 mg twice a day. All drugs given with meals for 2 weeks. (2) Metronidazole, 500 mg twice a day for 2 weeks, or amoxicillin, 1 gram twice a day for 2 weeks, or tetracycline, 500 mg twice a day for 2 weeks; plus, clarithromycin, 500 mg twice a day for 2 weeks and ranitidine bismuth citrate, 400 mg twice a day for 2 weeks. (3) Tetracycline, 500 mg 4 times per day; metronidazole, 500 mg 3 times per day for 2 weeks with meals and at bedtime; bismuth subsalicylate, 525 mg 4 times per day with meals and at bedtime for 2 weeks; and, either lansoprazole, 30 mg once daily for 2 weeks or omeprazole, 20 mg once daily for 2 weeks. (4) Tetracycline, 500 mg 4 times per day for 2 weeks; metronidazole, 250 mg 4 times per day with meals and at bedtime for 1 week; bismuth subsalicylate, 525 mg 4 times per day with meals and at bedtime for 2 weeks; and, a H_2-receptor antagonist as directed for 2 or more weeks. (5) Amoxicillin, 1 gram twice a day with meals; metronidazole, 500 mg twice a day with meals; and, omeprazole, 20 mg twice a day before meals. Each drug is given for 2 weeks.

Giardiasis.

250 mg 3 times per day for 7 days.

G. vaginalis.

500 mg twice a day for 7 days.

- **TABLETS, EXTENDED-RELEASE**
  Bacterial vaginosis.

One 750-mg tablet per day for 7 days.

- **IV**
  Anaerobic bacterial infections.

Adults, initially: 15 mg/kg infused over 1 hr; **then,** after 6 hr, 7.5 mg/kg q 6 hr for 7–10 days (daily dose should not exceed 4 grams). Treatment may be necessary for 2–3 weeks, although PO therapy should be initiated as soon as possible.

Prophylaxis of anaerobic infection during surgery.

Adults: 15 mg/kg given over a 30- to 60-min period, with completion 1 hr prior to surgery and 7.5 mg/kg infused over 30–60 min 6 and 12 hr after the initial dose.

- **TOPICAL CREAM; TOPICAL GEL; TOPICAL LOTION**
  Rosacea.

After washing, apply a thin film and rub in well either once daily or twice a day in the morning and evening for 4–9 weeks.

- **VAGINAL GEL (0.75%)**
  Bacterial vaginosis.

One applicatorful (5 grams which contains 37.5 mg metronidazole) once or twice daily for 5 days. Metro-Gel Vaginal allows for once-daily dosing at bedtime.

NURSING CONSIDERATIONS

ADMINISTRATION/STORAGE

1. Reduce dose in those with hepatic disease. Dosage reduction may be necessary in geriatric clients.

2. For topical use, therapeutic results should be seen within 3 weeks with continuing improvement through 9 weeks of therapy.

3. Metronidazole used vaginally may be absorbed in sufficient quantities to produce systemic effects.

4. Cosmetics may be used after application of topical metronidazole.

IV 5. Do not give by IV bolus. Administer each single dose over 1 hr.

6. Do not use syringes with Al needles or hubs.

7. Discontinue primary IV infusion during infusion of metronidazole.

8. The order of mixing to prepare powder for injection is important:
- Reconstitute.
- Dilute in IV solutions in glass or plastic containers.
- Neutralize pH with $NaHCO_3$ solution. Do not refrigerate neutralized solutions.

9. Premixed, ready-to-use Flagyl comes as 5 mg/mL (500 mg metronidazole in 100 mL of solution) in plastic bags; administer over 1 hr.

10. Drug has a high sodium content.

ASSESSMENT

1. Note reasons for therapy and symptom characteristics.

2. Monitor CBC, LFTs, and cultures. Reduce dose with liver dysfunction.

3. With amebiasis, monitor stool number/characteristics. With IV therapy assess for sodium retention. With pregnancy use the 7-day regimen for trichomoniasis. Use only after *T. vaginalis* or *E. histolytica* has been confirmed by wet smear/culture/identification process.

CLIENT/FAMILY TEACHING

1. Take with food or milk to reduce GI upset; may cause a metallic taste. Take ER tablets at least 1 hr before or 2 hr after meals.

2. Report lack of response, any symptoms of CNS toxicity, i.e., uncoordinated movements/tremors, numbness, seizures, any unusual bruising/bleeding.

3. Do not perform tasks that require mental alertness until drug effects are realized; dizziness may occur.

4. During treatment for trichomoniasis, treat partner also since organisms may be in the male urogenital tract and reinfect partner. Use condom to prevent re-infections.

5. Do not engage in intercourse while using the vaginal gel.

6. With topical preparation, cleanse area then apply a thin film onto affected area. Avoid eye contact. May apply cosmetics after application and after ensuring that the area is dry.

7. Drug may turn urine brown; do not be alarmed.

8. No alcohol until at least 48 hr after therapy completed; a disulfiram-like reaction may occur. Symptoms include abdominal cramps, vomiting, flushing, and headache.

OUTCOMES/EVALUATE

- Symptomatic improvement
- Negative culture reports

Mexiletine hydrochloride ■

(mex-**ILL**-eh-teen)

CLASSIFICATION(S):
Antiarrhythmic, Class IB
PREGNANCY CATEGORY: C
Rx: Mexitil.
✦**Rx:** Novo-Mexiletine.

SEE ALSO *ANTIARRHYTHMIC DRUGS*.

USES

Documented life-threatening ventricular arrhythmias (such as ventricular tachycardia). *Investigational:* Prophylactically to decrease the incidence of ventricular tachycardia and other ventricular arrhythmias in the acute phase of MI. To reduce pain, dysesthesia, and paresthesia associated with diabetic neuropathy.

ACTION/KINETICS

Action

Similar to lidocaine but is effective PO. Inhibits the flow of sodium into the cell, thereby reducing the rate of rise of the action potential. The drug decreases the effective refractory period in Purkinje fibers. BP and pulse rate are not affected following use, but there may be a small decrease in CO and an increase in peripheral vascular resistance. Also has both local anesthetic and anticonvulsant effects.

Pharmacokinetics

Bioavailability: About 90%. **Onset:** 30–120 min. **Peak blood levels:** 2–3 hr. **Therapeutic plasma levels:** 0.5–2 mcg/mL. **Plasma t½:** 10–12 hr. Metabolized in the liver mainly by CYP2D6. Approximately 10% excreted unchanged in the urine; acidification of the urine enhances excretion, whereas alkalinization decreases excretion.

CONTRAINDICATIONS

Cardiogenic shock, preexisting second- or third-degree AV block (if no pacemaker is present). Use with lesser arrhythmias. Lactation.

Bold Italic = life threatening side effect   ■ = black box warning   ✦ = Available in Canada

SPECIAL CONCERNS

■ Clients with asymptomatic, non life-threatening ventricular arrhythmias who had an MI more than 6 days but less than 2 years previously may show an excessive mortality or nonfatal cardiac arrest. Use of mexilitene should be reserved for those with life-threatening ventricular arrhythmias.■ Use with caution in hypotension, severe CHF, or known seizure disorders. Safety and efficacy have not been determined in children.

SIDE EFFECTS

Most Common

Upper GI distress, tremor, lightheadedness, dizziness, coordination difficulties, nervousness, headache, blurred vision, paresthesias, N&V, heartburn, fatigue, constipation.

CV: *Worsening of arrhythmias*, palpitations, chest pain, increased ventricular arrhythmias (PVCs), CHF, angina or angina-like pain, hypotension, bradycardia, syncope, ***AV block or conduction disturbances***, atrial arrhythmias, hypertension, ***cardiogenic shock***, hot flashes, edema, worsening of CHF in those with pre-existing compromised ventricular function. **GI:** High incidence of UGI distress, N&V, heartburn. Also, diarrhea/constipation, changes in appetite, dry mouth, abdominal cramps/pain/discomfort, salivary changes, dysphagia, altered taste, pharyngitis, changes in oral mucous membranes, UGI bleeding, peptic ulcer, esophageal ulceration, dyspepsia, pancreatitis (rare). **CNS:** High incidence of lightheadedness, dizziness, tremor, coordination difficulties, and nervousness. Also, changes in sleep habits, headache, fatigue, weakness, tinnitus, paresthesias, numbness, depression, confusion, difficulty with speech, short-term memory loss, hallucinations, malaise, psychosis, drowsiness, ataxia, ***seizures***, loss of consciousness. **Hematologic:** Leukopenia, neutropenia, agranulocytosis, thrombocytopenia. **GU:** Decreased libido, impotence, urinary hesitancy/retention. **Dermatologic:** Rash, dry skin. Rarely, exfoliative dermatitis, and ***Stevens-Johnson syndrome***. **Pulmonary:** Dyspnea, laryn-geal or pharyngeal changes, pulmonary fibrosis, pulmonary infilatration. **Ophthalmic:** Blurred vision, visual disturbances, nystamus. **Miscellaneous:** Arthralgia, fever, diaphoresis, loss of hair, hiccoughs, syndrome of SLE, myelofibrosis, hypersensitivity reaction.

LABORATORY TEST CONSIDERATIONS

↑ AST. Positive ANA. Abnormal LFTs.

`OD` OVERDOSE MANAGEMENT

Symptoms: Nausea. CNS symptoms (dizziness, drowsiness, confusion, paresthesias, seizures) usually precede CV symptoms (hypotension, sinus bradycardia, intermittent LBBB, ***temporary asystole, AV heart block, ventricular tachyarrhythmias, CV collapse). Massive overdoses cause coma and respiratory arrest.*** *Treatment:* General supportive treatment. Give atropine to treat hypotension or bradycardia. Give anticonvulsants for seizures. Transvenous cardiac pacing may be helpful. Acidification of the urine may increase rate of excretion.

DRUG INTERACTIONS

Al hydroxide / ↓ Mexiletine absorption
Atropine / ↓ Mexiletine absorption
Caffeine / ↓ Drug clearance (50%)
Cimetidine / ↑ or ↓ Plasma mexiletine levels
Fluvoxamine / ↓ Oral clearance and ↑ in AUC and peak serum levels of mexiletine R/T ↓ liver metabolism by CYP1A2
Mg hydroxide / ↓ Mexiletine absorption
Metoclopramide / ↑ Mexiletine absorption
Narcotics / ↓ Mexiletine absorption
Phenobarbital / ↓ Plasma mexiletine levels
Phenytoin / ↑ Mexiletine clearance → ↓ plasma mexiletine levels
Propafenone / ↓ Metabolic clearance of mexiletine in extensive metabolizers → no differences between extensive and poor metabolizers
Rifampin / ↑ Clearance → ↓ plasma mexiletine levels
Smoking / ↑ Mexiletine clearance → ↓ t$\frac{1}{2}$
Theophylline / ↑ Drug effect R/T ↑ serum levels
Urinary acidifiers / ↑ Rate of mexiletine

excretion

Urinary alkalinizers / ↓ Rate of mexiletine excretion

HOW SUPPLIED

Capsules: 150 mg, 200 mg, 250 mg.

DOSAGE

- **CAPSULES**

Antiarrhythmic.

Adults, individualized, initial: 200 mg q 8 hr if rapid control of arrhythmia not required; dosage adjustment may be made in 50- or 100-mg increments q 2–3 days, if required. **Maintenance:** 200–300 mg q 8 hr, depending on response and tolerance of client. If adequate response is not achieved with 300 mg or less q 8 hr, 400 mg q 8 hr may be tried although the incidence of CNS side effects increases. If the drug is effective at doses of 300 mg or less q 8 hr, the same total daily dose may be given in divided doses q 12 hr (e.g., 450 mg q 12 hr). Maximum total daily dose: 1,200 mg.

Rapid control of arrhythmias.

Initial loading dose: 400 mg followed by a 200-mg dose in 8 hr.

Diabetic neuropathy.

Initial: 150 mg/day for 3 days; **then,** 300 mg/day for 3 days. **Maintenance:** 10 mg/kg/day.

NURSING CONSIDERATIONS

ADMINISTRATION/STORAGE

1. If transferring to mexiletine from other class I antiarrhythmics, initiate mexiletine at a dose of 200 mg and then titrate according to the response at the following times: 6–12 hr after the last dose of quinidine sulfate, 3–6 hr after the last dose of procainamide, 6–12 hr after the last dose of disopyramide, or 8–12 hr after the last dose of tocainide.

2. Hospitalize client when transferring to mexiletine if there is a chance that withdrawal of the previous antiarrhythmic may produce life-threatening arrhythmias.

3. When transferring from lidocaine to mexiletine, stop the lidocaine infusion when the first PO dose of mexiletine is given. Maintain the IV line until suppression of the arrhythmia appears satisfactory.

4. Avoid concurrent drugs or diets which may markedly affect urinary pH.

ASSESSMENT

1. List reasons for therapy, other agents trialed, outcome.

2. Note evidence of CHF; assess ECG for AV block.

3. Assess pulmonary status; note SaO$_2$/PO$_2$.

4. Monitor ECG, CXR, CBC, lytes, renal, LFTs.

5. Reduce dose with severe liver disease, marked right-sided CHF.

6. Check urinary pH; alkalinity decreases/acidity increases renal drug excretion.

CLIENT/FAMILY TEACHING

1. Take with food or an antacid to ↓ GI upset.

2. Do not stop drug suddenly; maintain acidity level in urine by not changing dietary patterns.

3. Report any bruising, bleeding, fevers, or sore throat or adverse CNS effects such as dizziness, tremor, impaired coordination, N&V.

4. Immediately report any increase in heart palpitations, irregularity, or rate less than 50 bpm.

5. Do not perform tasks that require mental alertness until drug effects are realized.

6. Carry identification that lists drugs currently prescribed. Keep regularly scheduled F/U appointments.

OUTCOMES/EVALUATE

- Control of ventricular arrhythmias
- Therapeutic drug levels (0.5–2 mcg/mL)
- ↓ S&S of diabetic neuropathy

Micafungin sodium ℞

(me-ka-**FUN**-jin)

CLASSIFICATION(S):
Antifungal
PREGNANCY CATEGORY: C
Rx: Mycamine.

USES

(1) Treatment of esophageal candidiasis. (2) Prophylaxis of Candida infections in clients undergoing hematopoietic stem cell transplantation.

ACTION/KINETICS

Action

Micafungin, a semisynthetic lipopeptide, inhibits the synthesis of 1,3-β-D-glucan, an essential component of fungal cell walls; it is not present in mammalian cells.

Pharmacokinetics

t½: 14–17.2 hr, depending on the use and dose. Metabolized to M-1 (catechol form) and subsequently to M-2 (methoxy form). Excreted mainly through the feces. **Plasma protein binding:** >99% mainly to albumin.

SPECIAL CONCERNS

Use with caution during lactation.

SIDE EFFECTS

Most Common

Headache, N&V, phlebitis, rash, diarrhea, leukopenia, neutropenia, pyrexia, rigors.

Histamine-mediated symptoms: Rash, pruritus, facial swelling, vasodilation. **Injection site reactions:** Phlebitis, thrombophlebitis, thrombosis. **GI:** N&V, diarrhea, dysgeusia, dyspepsia, constipation, hiccups, abdominal pain, upper abdominal pain. **Hepatic:** Significant hepatic dysfunction, hepatitis, hepatomegaly, jaundice, *hepatic failure*. **CNS:** Headache, delirium, dizziness, somnolence, convulsions, encephalopathy, *intracranial hemorrhage*. **CV:** Hyper-/hypotension, flushing, arrhythmia, *cardiac arrest*, cyanosis, *DVT, MI,* tachycardia. **Dermatologic:** Rash, pruritus, erythema multiforme, skin necrosis, urticaria. **GU:** Significant renal dysfunction, acute renal failure, anuria, renal tubular necrosis, oliguria. **Respiratory:** Apnea, dyspnea, hypoxia, pneumonia, *pulmonary embolism*. **Hematologic:** Leukopenia, anemia, neutropenia, thrombocytopenia, lymphopenia, febrile neutropenia, coagulopathy, hemolysis, pancytopenia, thrombotic thrombocytopenic purpura; *acute intravascular hemolysis* and hemoglobinuria when used with PO prednisolone. Also hemolysis and *hemolytic anemia* when used alone. Hypersensitivity reactions, including *shock*. **Body as a whole:** Rigors, pyrexia, decreased appetite, acidosis, arthralgia, infection, *sepsis*. **Miscellaneous:** Mucosal inflammation.

LABORATORY TEST CONSIDERATIONS

↑ ALT, AST, BUN, creatinine, blood alkaline phosphatase/LDH. Hypomagnesemia, hyperbilirubinemia, hypocalcemia, hypokalemia, hyponatremia, hemoglobinuria. Abnormal LFTs.

DRUG INTERACTIONS

Cyclosporine / ↑ Cyclosporine PO clearance and ↑ single-dose cyclosporine whole blood levels R/T inhibition of CYP3A metabolism
Nifedipine / ↑ Nifedipine AUC and C_{max}
Sirolimus / ↑ Sirolimus AUC

HOW SUPPLIED

Powder for Injection: 50 mg, 100 mg.

DOSAGE

• **IV INFUSION**

Esophageal candidiasis.

150 mg/day.

Prophylaxis of Candida *infections in hematopoietic stem cell transplantation.*

50 mg/day.

NURSING CONSIDERATIONS

ADMINISTRATION/STORAGE

IV 1. Give over a period of 1 hr. More rapid infusion may cause more frequent histamine-mediated reactions.

2. Flush existing IV line with 0.9% NaCl injection prior to infusing micafungin.

3. Do not mix or coinfuse micafungin with other drugs. Micafungin will precipitate when mixed directly with a number of other commonly used drugs.

4. Solutions for infusion are prepared as follows:

• Aseptically add 5 mL of 0.9% NaCl injection (without a bacteriostatic agent) to each 50 mg vial to yield a preparation containing about 10 mg/mL micafungin.

• To minimize excess foaming, gently dissolve the micafungin powder by swirling the vial. Do not shake vigorously. Visually inspect the vial for particulate matter.

📷 = see color insert　　H = Herbal　　IV = Intravenous　　ⓒ = sound alike drug

- Protect the diluted solution from light, although it is not necessary to cover the infusion drip chamber or the tubing.

5. For prophylaxis of Candida infections, add 50 mg of reconstituted micafungin in 5 mL NaCl injection into 100 mL of 0.9% NaCl; infuse over 1 hr.

6. For treatment of esophageal candidiasis, add micafungin, 150 mg (i.e., from 3–50 mg vials) reconstituted in 15 mL NaCl injection into 100 mL of 0.9% NaCl injection; infuse over 1 hr.

7. Since micafungin is preservative free, discard partially used vials.

8. The reconstituted drug may be stored in the original vial for up to 24 hr at room temperature. Protect the diluted infusion solution from light; it may be stored for up to 24 hr at room temperature.

ASSESSMENT

1. Note reasons for therapy: treatment or prophylaxis, schedule for hematopoietic stem cell transplantation (HSCT), or cause of infection, other agents trialed and those currently prescribed.

2. Monitor during infusion for S&S of hypersensitivity reaction.

3. Assess cultures, K+, Ca, Mg, CBC, renal and LFTs. If any dysfunction occurs stop drug, report. Drug is highly protein bound and not dialyzable.

CLIENT/FAMILY TEACHING

1. Drug is administered intravenously to treat or prevent a type of fungal infection. Therapy usually is any where from 7–21 days.

2. Report any headaches, skin rashes, N&V, diarrhea, pain at injection site, swelling of extremities, unusual bruising/bleedings, itching, cough, fever or chills.

OUTCOMES/EVALUATE

- Resolution of esophageal candidiasis
- Prophylaxis of Candida infections in HSCT recipients

Miconazole nitrate
(my-**KON**-ah-zohl)

CLASSIFICATION(S):
Antifungal
PREGNANCY CATEGORY: C
OTC: Topical: Fungoid Tincture, Lotrimin AF, Micatin, Neosporin AF, Prescription Strength Desenex, Tetterine, Ting, Zeasorb-AF. **Vaginal:** Femizol-M, M-Zole 7 Dual Pack, Monistat 7, Monistat 7 Combination Pack, Vagistat-3 Combination Pack.
Rx: Topical: Monistat-Derm. **Vaginal:** M-Zole 3 Combination Pack, Monistat 1 Combination Pack, Monistat 3, Monistat 3 Combination Pack, Monistat Dual-Pak.
✚**Rx:** Micozole, Monazole 7.

SEE ALSO *ANTI-INFECTIVE DRUGS.*
USES
Topical: Tinea pedis (athlete's foot), tinea cruris (jock itch), tinea corporis (ringworm) caused by *Trichophyton rubrum, T. mentagrophytes,* and *Epidermophyton floccosum* (both OTC and Rx).
   Vaginal: Vulvovaginal candidiasis (suppositories). Relief of external vulvar itching and irritation associated with a yeast infection (cream).
ACTION/KINETICS
Action
Broad-spectrum fungicide that alters the permeability of the fungal membrane by inhibiting synthesis of sterols; thus, essential intracellular materials are lost. The drug also inhibits biosynthesis of triglycerides and phospholipids and also inhibits oxidative and peroxidative enzyme activity. May be fungistatic or fungicidal, depending on the concentration.

CONTRAINDICATIONS
Hypersensitivity. Use of topical products in or around the eyes. Use of topical products in children less than 2 years of age unless directed by a physician.

SPECIAL CONCERNS
Safe use in children less than 1 year of age has not been established.

SIDE EFFECTS

Most Common

Following topical use: Irritation, burning, maceration, allergic contact dermatitis.

Following vaginal use: Irritation, sensitization, vulvovaginal burning.

At vaginal administration site: Burning, irritation, sensitization, vulvovaginal burning, pruritus, discharge, edema, pain. **Miscellaneous:** GI cramping, nausea, headache, genital erythema, vaginal tenderness, dysuria, allergic reaction, dry mouth, flatulence, perianal burning, pelvic cramping, rash, urticaria, skin irritation, periorbital edema, conjunctival pruritus.

HOW SUPPLIED

Topical: *Cream:* 2%; *Gel:* 2%; *Ointment:* 2%; *Powder:* 2%; *Solution:* 2%; *Spray Powder:* 2%; *Spray Liquid:* 2%.

Vaginal: *Cream:* 2%; *Suppositories and Topical Cream:* Dual-Pak or Combination Pack: Suppository, 100 mg and Topical Cream, 2%; Suppository, 200 mg and Topical Cream, 2%; Suppository, 1,200 mg, and Topical Cream, 2%; *Suppositories:* 100 mg, 200 mg.

DOSAGE

- **TOPICAL GEL; POWDER; SOLUTION; SPRAY LIQUID/POWDER; CREAM; OINTMENT; SOLUTION**

Apply to cover affected areas in morning and evening (once daily for tinea versicolor) for 2 weeks for tinea cruris and for 4 weeks for tinea pedis and tinea corporis.

- **VAGINAL CREAM; VAGINAL SUPPOSITORIES**

Suppositories: One suppository daily at bedtime for 7 days (100-mg suppositories), 3 consecutive days (200-mg suppositories), or 1 day (1,200 mg). **Cream:** 1 applicator-full intravaginally once daily at bedtime for 3–7 days. For topical use, apply cream to affected areas twice a day (morning and evening) for up to 7 days or as needed. Repeat course, if needed, after ruling out other pathogens.

NURSING CONSIDERATIONS

ADMINISTRATION/STORAGE

1. The lotion is preferred for intertriginous areas.

2. Store topical products from 15-30°C (59–86°F). Refrigerate vaginal products below 15–30°C (59–86°F).

ASSESSMENT

1. Note clinical presentation, size/number/extent of lesions. List any previous experience/sensitivity with this drug; response obtained.

2. Monitor cultures/skin scraping, CBC, lytes, LFTs and healing/clearing progress.

CLIENT/FAMILY TEACHING

1. Review administration technique; use only as directed. Complete full course of therapy despite symptom improvement. To ensure success, tinea cruris, tinea corporis, and candida should be treated for 2 weeks; tinea pedis should be treated for 1 month.

2. When used for vaginal infections, refrain from intercourse or use a condom to prevent reinfection. Use sanitary pads to protect clothing and linens when using cream or suppositories. When used vaginally, continue treatment during menses.

3. If pregnant or breastfeeding, ask a health care professional before use.

4. Report if exposed to HIV and recurrent vaginal infections occur.

5. Report lack of response, persistent N&V, diarrhea, dizziness, itching, or other adverse SE.

OUTCOMES/EVALUATE

- Negative culture reports
- Clearing of fungal infection
- Resolution of vaginitis evidenced by ↓ itching/burning; ↓ discharge
- ↓ Size and number of lesions

M

Midazolam hydrochloride

■ ▣Ⅳ ©

(my-**DAYZ**-oh-lam)

CLASSIFICATION(S):

Benzodiazepine, adjunct to general anesthesia

PREGNANCY CATEGORY: D

Rx: Midazolam hydrochloride, **C-IV**
❧Rx: Apo-Midazolam.

SEE ALSO *TRANQUILIZERS/ ANTIMANIC DRUGS/HYPNOTICS.*

USES

IV, IM: Preoperative sedation, anxiolysis, and amnesia. **IV:** (1) Sedation, anxiolysis, and amnesia prior to or during short diagnostic, therapeutic, or endoscopic procedures (either alone or with other CNS depressants). (2) Induction of general anesthesia before administration of other anesthetics. (3) Supplement to nitrous oxide and oxygen in balanced anesthesia. (4) Sedation of intubated and mechanically ventilated clients as a component of anesthesia or during treatment in a critical care setting. **Syrup:** Preprocedural sedation and anxiolysis in children. *Investigational:* Treat epileptic seizures. Alternative to terminate refractory status epilepticus.

ACTION/KINETICS

Action

Short-acting benzodiazepine with sedative–general anesthetic properties. Depresses the response of the respiratory system to carbon dioxide stimulation, which is more pronounced in clients with COPD. Possible mild to moderate decreases in CO, mean arterial BP, SV, and systemic vascular resistance. HR may rise somewhat in those with slow HRs (<65 bpm) and decrease in others (especially those with HRs >85 bpm).

Pharmacokinetics

Onset, IM: 15 min; **IV:** 2–2.5 min for induction (if combined with a preanesthetic narcotic, induction is about 1.5 min). If preanesthetic medication (morphine) is given, the **Peak plasma levels, IM:** 45 min. **Maximum effect:** 30–60 min. **Time to recovery:** Usually within 2 hr, although up to 6 hr may be required. **t½, elimination:** 1.2–12.3 hr. Rapidly metabolized in the liver to inactive compounds; excreted through the urine. **Plasma protein binding:** About 97%.

CONTRAINDICATIONS

Hypersensitivity to benzodiazepines. Acute narrow-angle glaucoma. Use in obstetrics, coma, shock, or acute alcohol intoxication where VS are depressed. IA injection.

SPECIAL CONCERNS

■ (1) IV midazolam has been associated with respiratory depression and respiratory arrest. In some cases, when not recognized and treated effectively, death or hypoxic encephalopathy resulted. (2) Use IV midazolam in a hospital or ambulatory care setting, including physicians' offices, that provide for continuous monitoring of respiratory and cardiac function. Ensure immediate availability of resuscitative drugs and equipment and personnel trained in their use. (3) The initial IV dose for conscious sedation may be as little as 1 mg, and should not exceed 2.5 mg in a normal healthy adult. Lower doses are necessary for older (over 60 years) or debilitated clients and in clients receiving concomitant narcotics or other CNS depressants. (4) Never give the initial dose and all subsequent doses as a bolus; rather, give over at least 2 min and allow an additional 2 or more min to evaluate fully the sedative effect. Use of a 1 mg/mL formulation or dilution of 1 mg/mL or 5 mg/mL formulation is recommended to facilitate slower injection.■ Use with caution during lactation. Pediatric clients may require higher doses than adults. Severe hypotension and seizures are possible in neonates after rapid IV injection, especially with concurrent fentanyl; do not give by rapid IV injection in this group. Hypotension may be more common in conscious sedated clients who have received a preanesthetic narcotic. Geriatric and debilitated clients require lower doses to induce anesthesia and they are more prone to side effects. Use IV with

---

M

---

extreme caution in severe fluid or electrolyte disturbances.

SIDE EFFECTS

Most Common

Following IM or IV use: Fluctuations in VS, including decreased respiratory rate and tidal volume; apnea.

Following IM use: Headache, pain at injection site, muscle stiffness, induration, redness.

Following IV use: Coughing, oversedation, headache, drowsiness, bronchospasm.

Fluctuations in VS, including decreased respiratory rate and tidal volume, apnea, variations in BP and pulse rate are common. The following are general side effects regardless of the route of administration. **CV:** Hypotension, *cardiac arrest*. **CNS:** Oversedation, headache, drowsiness, grogginess, confusion, retrograde amnesia, euphoria, nervousness, agitation, anxiety, argumentativeness, restlessness, emergence delirium, increased time for emergence, dreaming during emergence, nightmares, insomnia, tonic-clonic movements, ataxia, muscle tremor, involuntary or athetoid movements, dizziness, dysphoria, dysphonia, slurred speech, paresthesia. **GI:** Hiccoughs, N&V, acid taste, retching, excessive salivation. **Ophthalmic:** Double/blurred vision, nystagmus, pinpoint pupils, visual disturbances, cyclic eyelid movements, difficulty in focusing. **Dermatologic:** Hives, swelling or feeling of burning, warmth or cold feeling at injection site, hive-like wheal at injection site, pruritus, rash. **Miscellaneous:** Blocked ears, loss of balance, chills, weakness, faint feeling, lethargy, yawning, toothache, hematoma. **More common following IM use:** Pain at injection site, headache, induration and redness, muscle stiffness. **More common following IV use:** **Respiratory:** *Bronchospasm*, coughing, dyspnea, *laryngospasm*, hyperventilation, shallow respirations, tachypnea, *airway obstruction*, wheezing, respiratory depression and *respiratory arrest* when used for conscious sedation. **CV:** PVCs, bigeminy, bradycardia, tachycardia, vasovagal episode, nodal rhythm. **At injection site:** Tenderness, pain, redness, induration, phlebitis.

DRUG INTERACTIONS

Alcohol / ↑ Risk of apnea, airway obstruction, desaturation, or hypoventilation

Anesthetics, inhalation / ↓ Dose if midazolam used as an induction agent

Antifungals, azole / ↑ Effect of midazolam R/T ↓ liver metabolism

Aprepitant / ↑ Midazolam AUC, peak, plasma levels, and t½ R/T inhibition of metabolism by CYP3A4

Cimetidine / ↑ Sedation

Clarithromycin / ↑ Effect of midazolam R/T ↓ liver metabolism

CNS depressants / ↑ Risk of apnea, airway obstruction, desaturation, or hypoventilation

Contraceptives, oral / Prolongation of midazolam half-life

Droperidol / ↑ Hypnotic effect of midazolam when used as a premedication

Erythromycin / ↑ Effect of midazolam R/T ↓ liver metabolism

Fentanyl / ↑ Hypnotic effect of midazolam when used as a premedication

Fluvoxamine / ↑ Serum midazolam levels, reduced clearance, and prolonged half-life

Indinavir / Possible prolonged sedation and respiratory depression

Meperidine / See *Narcotics;* also, ↑ risk of hypotension

Narcotics / ↑ Hypnotic effect of midazolam when used as premedication

Propofol / ↑ Effect of propofol

Protease inhibitors / ↑ Effect of midazolam R/T ↓ liver metabolism

Rifamycins / Possible pharmacokinetic changes of midazolam

Ritonavir / Possible prolonged sedation and respiratory depression

Selective serotonin reuptake inhibitors / ↑ Effect of midazolam R/T ↓ liver metabolism

Theophyllines / Antagonism of midazolam's sedative effects

Thiopental / ↓ Dose if midazolam used as an induction agent

Valproic acid / Possible ↓ liver metabolism of midazolam

Verapamil / Possible ↑ CNS depression and prolonged midazolam effects

HOW SUPPLIED

Injection: 1 mg/mL, 5 mg/mL; *Syrup:* 2 mg/mL.

DOSAGE

- **IM**

  Preoperative sedation, anxiolysis, amnesia.

Adults: 0.07–0.08 mg/kg IM (average: 5 mg) 1 hr before surgery. **Children:** 0.1–0.15 mg/kg (up to 0.5 mg/kg may be needed for more anxious clients).

- **IV**

  Conscious sedation, anxiolysis, amnesia for endoscopic or CV procedures in healthy adults under age 60.

Using the 1 mg/mL (can be diluted with 0.9% sodium chloride or D5W) product, titrate slowly to the desired effect (usually slurred speech); initial dose should be no higher than 2.5 mg IV (may be as low as 1 mg IV) within a 2-min period; wait an additional 2 min to evaluate the sedative effect. If additional sedation is necessary, give small increments waiting an additional 2 min or more after each increment to evaluate the effect. Total doses greater than 5 mg are usually not required. **Children:** Dosage must be individualized by the physician.

Conscious sedation for endoscopic or CV procedures in debilitated or chronically ill clients or clients aged 60 or over.

Slowly titrate to the desired effect using no more than 1.5 mg initially IV (may be as little as 1 mg IV) given over a 2-min period; wait an additional 2 min or more to evaluate the effect. If additional sedation is needed, no more than 1 mg should be given over 2 min; wait an additional 2 min or more after each increment in dose. Total doses greater than 3.5 mg are usually not needed.

Induction of general anesthesia, before use of other general anesthetics, in unmedicated clients.

Adults, unmedicated clients up to 55 years of age, IV, initial: 0.3–0.35 mg/kg given over 20–30 sec, waiting 2 min for effects to occur. If needed, increments of about 25% of the initial

dose can be used to complete induction; or, induction can be completed using a volatile liquid anesthetic. Up to 0.6 mg/kg may be used but recovery will be prolonged. **Adults, unmedicated clients over 55 years of age who are good risk surgical clients, initial IV:** 0.15–0.3 mg/kg given over 20–30 sec. **Adults, unmedicated clients over 55 years of age with severe systemic disease or debilitation, initial IV:** 0.15–0.25 mg/kg given over 20–30 sec. **Pediatric:** 0.05–0.2 mg/kg IV.

Induction of general anesthesia, before use of other general anesthetics, in medicated clients.

Adults, premedicated clients up to 55 years of age, IV, initial: 0.15–0.35 mg/kg. If less than 55 years of age, 0.25 mg/kg may be given over 20–30 sec, allowing 2 min for effect. **Adults, premedicated clients over 55 years of age who are good risk surgical clients, initial, IV:** 0.2 mg/kg. **Adults, premedicated clients over 55 years of age with severe systemic disease or debilitation, initial, IV:** 0.15 mg/kg may be sufficient.

Maintenance of balanced anesthesia for short surgical procedures.

IV: Incremental injections about 25% of the dose used for induction when signs indicate anesthesia is lightening. *NOTE:* Narcotic preanesthetic medication may include fentanyl, 1.5–2 mcg/kg IV 5 min before induction; morphine, up to 0.15 mg/kg IM; meperidine, up to 1 mg/kg IM; or, Innovar, 0.02 mL/kg IM. Sedative preanesthetic medication may include secobarbital sodium, 200 mg PO or hydroxyzine pamoate, 100 mg PO. Except for fentanyl, give all preanesthetic medications 1 hr prior to midazolam. Always individualize doses.

- **SYRUP**

  Preprocedural sedation and anxiolysis in children.

Children: 0.25–1 mg/kg, not to exceed 20 mg.

NURSING CONSIDERATIONS

℘ Do not confuse Versed with Vistaril (an antianxiety drug) or with VePesid (an antineoplastic).

Bold Italic = life threatening side effect   ■ = black box warning   ♣ = Available in Canada

ADMINISTRATION/STORAGE

1. When used for procedures via the mouth, use a topical anesthetic.

2. Give IM doses in a large muscle mass.

 3. When used for conscious sedation, do not give by rapid or single bolus IV; may cause respiratory depression.

4. When used for induction of general anesthesia, give the initial dose over 20–30 sec.

5. If preanesthetic medications with a depressant component are given (e.g., narcotic analgesics or CNS depressants), reduce the midazolam dosage by 50% compared with healthy, young unmedicated clients.

6. Give maintenance doses to all clients in increments of 25% of the dose first required to achieve the sedative endpoint.

7. Give a narcotic preanesthetic for bronchoscopic procedures.

8. Carefully monitor all IV doses with the immediate availability of oxygen, resuscitative equipment, and personnel who are skilled in maintaining a patent airway and ventilation support; continue monitoring during recovery period.

9. May be mixed in the same syringe with atropine, meperidine, morphine, or scopolamine

10. At a concentration of 0.5 mg/mL midazolam is compatible with D5W and 0.9% NaCl for up to 24 hr and with RL solution for up to 4 hr.

ASSESSMENT

1. Note reasons for therapy, general client condition, VS, airway integrity, oxygen saturation during procedure.

2. Have oxygen and resuscitative equipment readily available in the event of respiratory depression.

CLIENT/FAMILY TEACHING

1. Drug may cause dizziness and drowsiness. Avoid alcohol, CNS depressants, and activities that require mental alertness for 24–48 hr following drug administration.

2. Repeat post-procedure instructions and obtain in writing, as may not fully recall instructions; transient amnesia is normal and memory of procedure may be minimal.

OUTCOMES/EVALUATE

Desired level of sedation and amnesia; ↓ anxiety

Mifepristone ■ ⓒ
(mih-feh-**PRIS**-tohn)

CLASSIFICATION(S):
Abortifacient
PREGNANCY CATEGORY: X
Rx: Mifeprex.

USES

Medical termination of intrauterine pregnancy through day 49 of pregnancy. Pregnancy is dated from the first day of the last menstrual period in a presumed 28-day cycle with ovulation occurring at mid-cycle. When mifepristone and misoprostol fail to cause termination of intrauterine pregnancy, pregnancy termination by surgery is recommended. Not effective to treat ectopic pregnancy. *Investigational:* Emergency contraception, uterine leiomyomata.

ACTION/KINETICS

Action

Competes with progesterone at progesterone-receptor sites, thus inhibiting the activity of endogenous or exogenous progesterone. During pregnancy, the drug sensitizes the myometrium to the contraction-inducing activity of prostaglandins. Termination of pregnancy results. Also exhibits antiglucocorticoid and weak antiandrogenic activity.

Pharmacokinetics

Rapidly absorbed. **Peak plasma levels:** 1.98 mg/L after 90 min. Absolute bioavailability is 69%. **t½, elimination:** 50% eliminated between 12 and 72 hr followed by a more rapid phase with a terminal **t½** of 18 hr. Metabolized in the liver by CYP3A4 with most eliminated in the feces. **Plasma protein binding:** 98%.

CONTRAINDICATIONS

Use for termination of pregnancy in any one of the following conditions: Confirmed or suspected ectopic pregnancy or undiagnosed adnexal mass; IUD in place; chronic adrenal failure; concurrent long-term corticosteroid therapy; history of allergy to mifepristone, misoprostol, or other prostaglandins; hemorrhagic disorders or concurrent anticoagulant therapy; pregnancy termination >49 days; inherited porphyrias. Use if client does not have adequate access to medical facilities equipped to provide emergency treatment of incomplete abortion, blood transfusions, and emergency resuscitation during the period from the first visit until discharged by the administering physician. Use in those who cannot understand the effects of the treatment procedure or comply with its regimen.

SPECIAL CONCERNS

■ (1) Serious and sometimes fatal infections and bleeding occur very rarely following spontaneous, surgical, and medical abortions, including following mifepristone use. Before prescribing mifepristone, inform the client about the risk of these serious events and discuss the Medication Guide and the Patient Agreement. Ensure that the client knows whom to call and what to do, including going to an emergency room, if none of the provided contacts are reachable, or if she experiences sustained fever, severe abdominal pain, prolonged heavy bleeding, or syncope. (2) Clients with serious bacterial infections and sepsis can present without fever, bacteremia, or significant findings on pelvic examination following an abortion. No causal relationship between the use of mifepristone and misoprostol and these events has been established. A high index of suspicion is needed to rule out sepsis. (3) Prolonged heavy bleeding may be a sign of incomplete abortion or other complications, and prompt medical or surgical intervention may be needed. Advise clients to seek immediate medical attention if they experience prolonged heavy vaginal bleeding. (4) Advise clients to take their Medication Guide with them if they visit an emergency room or another health care provider who did not prescribe mifepristone, so that provider will be aware that the client is undergoing a medical abortion.■ Clients should expect vaginal bleeding or spotting for an average of 9–16 days. Safety and efficacy have not been determined for use in cardiovascular, hypertensive, hepatic, respiratory, or renal disease; IDDM; severe anemia; heavy smoking; or, pediatric clients. Use with caution during lactation; decision may be made to discard breast milk for a few days following use.

SIDE EFFECTS

Most Common

Bleeding, uterine cramping, abdominal pain/cramping, N&V, diarrhea, headache, back pain, fatigue, dizziness.

NOTE: Bleeding and cramping are expected results of therapy. **GI:** N&V, diarrhea, abdominal pain, dyspepsia. **GU:** Uterine cramping/bleeding/hemorrhage, vaginitis, leukorrhea, pelvic pain, endometritis, salpingitis, pelvic inflammatory disease, postabortal infection, *ruptured ectopic pregnancy*. **CV:** Hypotension (including orthostatic), shortness of breath, tachycardia (including racing pulse, heart palpitations, heart pounding). **CNS:** Headache, dizziness, insomnia, anxiety, syncope, lightheadedness, loss of consciousness. **Hematologic:** Anemia, decreased hemoglobin. **Body as a whole:** Asthenia, fatigue, fever, viral infection, chills/shaking, allergic reaction (including rash, hives, itching). **Miscellaneous:** Fainting, pelvic/back/leg pain, sinusitis, serious infection (including *septic shock*), *MI*.

LABORATORY TEST CONSIDERATIONS

Rarely, ↑ AST, ALT, alkaline phosphatase, GGT. ↓ H & H, RBCs in women who bleed heavily.

DRUG INTERACTIONS

Carbamazepine / Possible ↓ mifepristone levels R/T ↑ liver metabolism
Dexamethasone / Possible ↓ mifepristone levels R/T ↑ liver metabolism
Erythromycin / Possible ↑ mifepristone levels R/T ↓ liver metabolism
Grapefruit juice / Possible ↑ mifepristone levels R/T ↓ liver metabolism

---

Itraconazole / Possible ↑ mifepristone serum levels R/T ↓ liver metabolism
Ketoconazole / Possible ↑ mifepristone levels R/T ↓ liver metabolism
Misoprostol ↑ Risk of bacterial infection and sepsis with possible death
Phenobarbital / Possible ↓ mifepristone levels R/T ↑ liver metabolism
Phenytoin / Possible ↓ mifepristone serum levels R/T ↑ liver metabolism
Rifampin / Possible ↓ mifepristone serum levels R/T ↑ liver metabolism
H *St. John's wort* / Possible ↓ mifepristone levels R/T ↑ liver metabolism
NOTE: When used with mifepristone, possible increase in serum levels of drugs that are CYP3A4 substrates. Use with caution with such drugs that have a narrow therapeutic range (e.g., some agents used during general anesthesia).

HOW SUPPLIED
Tablets: 200 mg.

DOSAGE

- **TABLETS**
  Termination of intrauterine pregnancy.
  Treatment includes both mifepristone and misoprostol and requires three office visits. **Day 1:** Three-200 mg tablets (600 mg) of mifepristone taken as a single dose. **Day 3:** Unless abortion has occurred and has been confirmed by clinical examination or ultrasonographic scan, clients must take misoprostol, 400 mcg (2–200 mcg tablets) PO. **Day 14:** Client returns for follow-up visit to confirm by clinical examination or ultrasonographic scan that complete termination of pregnancy has occurred.

NURSING CONSIDERATIONS

ⓒ Do not confuse mifepristone with misoprostol (prostaglandin used with mifepristone to terminate pregnancy).

ADMINISTRATION/STORAGE
1. The drug is supplied only to licensed physicians who sign and return a Prescriber's Agreement. It is not available to the public through licensed pharmacies.
2. Remove any IUD before beginning mifepristone treatment.
3. Available only in single-dose packaging.

4. Administration must be under the supervision of a qualified provider.
5. Clients must read the Medication Guide and read and sign the Patient Agreement before mifepristone is given.
6. Mifepristone may be less effective if misoprostol is given more than 2 days after mifepristone use.

ASSESSMENT
1. The duration of pregnancy can be determined from menstrual history and clinical examination. Use an ultrasonographic scan if the duration of pregnancy is uncertain or if ectopic pregnancy is suspected.
2. Ensure client fully understands the results of treatment and is in concurrence. Provide a copy of the Medication Guide and the Patient Agreement. May obtain by contacting Danco-Laboratories.
3. List drugs prescribed to ensure none interact unfavorably (CYP3A4 metabolism).
4. Obtain history to assess for CAD, HTN, IDDM, smoking, hepatic/respiratory/renal disease, or severe anemia as drug has not been studied in these groups.

CLIENT/FAMILY TEACHING
1. Review Medication Guide and Patient Agreement to understand the treatment procedure and its effects. Request clarification or pose questions as needed and sign agreement.
2. The treatment consists of three visits to the provider. On day one a dose of mifepristone (600 mg) PO is administered. Return on day 3 to determine if abortion has occurred by clinical exam or by ultrasound. If not, misoprostol 400 mcg will be administered orally. Finally, must return on day 14–16 to confirm termination of pregnancy.
3. Onset of action usually occurs between 2 and 24 hr of initial treatment. Menses should begin within 5 days of treatments and will last 1–2 weeks.
4. May experience vaginal bleeding and uterine cramping, nausea, vomiting, diarrhea, and headache.
5. Prolonged, heavy bleeding does not confirm a complete expulsion. With

treatment failure, there is an increased risk of fetal malformation.

6. If medical treatment fails, these cases are managed by surgical termination (D&C).

7. Contraception must be initiated as soon as the termination of pregnancy has been confirmed or before sexual intercourse is resumed as pregnancy can occur before resumption of normal menses.

8. In addition to uterine bleeding and cramping, may experience N&V, pelvic pain, diarrhea, fainting, headaches, and dizziness. Bleeding and spotting may occur for over 2 weeks after treatment. Report immediately if persistent or significant side effects.

OUTCOMES/EVALUATE
Termination of pregnancy

Miglitol
(MIG-lih-tohl)

CLASSIFICATION(S):
Antidiabetic, oral; alpha-glucosidase inhibitor
PREGNANCY CATEGORY: B
Rx: Glyset.

SEE ALSO *ANTIDIABETIC AGENTS: HYPOGLYCEMIC AGENTS.*

USES
(1) Alone as adjunct to diet to treat non-insulin-dependent diabetes when hyperglycemia cannot be managed with diet alone. (2) With a sulfonylurea when diet plus either miglitol or a sulfonylurea alone do not result in adequate control (effects of sulfonylurea and miglitol are additive).

ACTION/KINETICS
Action
Acts by delaying digestion of ingested carbohydrates resulting in smaller rise in blood glucose levels after meals. Effect is due to reversible inhibition of membrane-bound intestinal glucoside hydrolase enzymes which hydrolyze oligosaccharides and disaccharides to glucose and other monosaccharides. Reduces levels of glycosylated hemoglobin in type 2 diabetes. Does not enhance insulin secretion or increase insulin sensitivity. Does not cause hypoglycemia when given in fasted state. **Pharmacokinetics** Absorption is saturable at high doses (i.e., only 50 to 70% of 100 mg dose is absorbed while 25 mg dose is 100% absorbed). **Peak levels:** 2–3 hr. Drug is not metabolized and is eliminated unchanged in urine. Reduce dose in impaired renal function.

CONTRAINDICATIONS
Lactation, diabetic ketoacidosis, IBD, colonic ulceration, partial intestinal obstruction, those predisposed to intestinal obstruction, chronic intestinal diseases associated with marked disorders of digestion or absorption, conditions that may deteriorate due to increased gas formation in the intestine, hypersensitivity to drug.

SPECIAL CONCERNS
When given with sulfonylurea or insulin, miglitol causes further decrease in blood sugar and increased risk of hypoglycemia. Safety and efficacy have not been determined in children.

SIDE EFFECTS
Most Common
Flatulence, diarrhea, abdominal pain.
GI: Flatulence, diarrhea, abdominal pain/discomfort, soft stools. **Dermatologic:** Skin rash (transient). **Miscellaneous:** Low serum iron.

DRUG INTERACTIONS
Amylase / ↓ Miglitol effect
Charcoal / ↓ Miglitol effect; do not take together
Digestive enzymes / ↓ Miglitol absorption
Digoxin / May ↓ digoxin levels
Pancreatin / ↓ Miglitol effect
Propranolol / Significant ↓ in propranolol bioavailability
Ranitidine / Significant ↓ in ranitidine bioavailability

HOW SUPPLIED
Tablets: 25 mg, 50 mg, 100 mg.

DOSAGE
• **TABLETS**
Type 2 diabetes.
Individualize dosage. **Initial:** 25 mg 3 times per day with first bite of each main meal (some may benefit from

---

starting with 25 mg once daily to minimize GI side effects). After 4 to 8 weeks of 25 mg 3 times per day dose, increase dosage to 50 mg 3 times per day for about 3 months. Measure glycosylated hemoglobin; if not satisfactory, increase dose to 100 mg 3 times per day. **Maintenance:** 50 mg 3 times per day, up to 100 mg 3 times per day (maximum).

NURSING CONSIDERATIONS
ASSESSMENT
1. Note age, onset, characteristics of disease, other agents trialed, outcome.
2. List any IBD, colonic ulceration, intestinal obstruction, severe digestion/absorption problems from colonoscopy.
3. Monitor BS, HbA1c, renal function; reduce dose with impaired function; avoid if creatinine >2 mg/dL.

CLIENT/FAMILY TEACHING
1. Take with first bite of each meal, 3 times per day as directed.
2. Attend diabetic education program to enhance understanding of disease, dietary control, weight loss, foot/eye care, BP, and exercise as it relates to overall health.
3. May experience abdominal pain and diarrhea which should diminish with continued treatment.
4. Any stress, fever, trauma, infection, or surgery may alter glucose control; monitor/record FS regularly.
5. Drug inhibits breakdown of table sugar; have glucose available for episodes of marked hypoglycemia.
6. Continue prescribed diet and regular exercise. Report for labs and follow up as ordered.

OUTCOMES/EVALUATE
↓ BS; HbA1c <7

Milrinone Lactate

(**MILL**-rih-nohn)

CLASSIFICATION(S):
Inotropic drug
PREGNANCY CATEGORY: C
Rx: Primacor.

USES
Short-term IV treatment of CHF, usually in clients receiving digoxin and diuretics.

ACTION/KINETICS
Action
Selective inhibitor of peak III cyclic AMP phosphodiesterase isozyme in cardiac and vascular muscle, resulting in a direct inotropic effect and a direct arterial vasodilator activity. Also improves diastolic function as manifested by improvements in LV diastolic relaxation. In clients with depressed myocardial function, produces a prompt increase in CO and a decrease in pulmonary wedge pressure and vascular resistance, without a significant increase in HR or myocardial oxygen consumption. Causes an inotropic effect in clients who are fully digitalized without causing signs of glycoside toxicity. Also, LV function has improved in clients with ischemic heart disease.

Pharmacokinetics
Therapeutic plasma levels: 150–250 ng/mL. $t^{1/2}$: 2.3 hr following doses of 12.5–125 mcg/kg to clients with CHF. Metabolized in the liver and excreted primarily through the urine.

CONTRAINDICATIONS
Hypersensitivity to the drug. Use in severe obstructive aortic or pulmonary valvular disease in lieu of surgical relief of the obstruction.

SPECIAL CONCERNS
Use with caution during lactation. Safety and efficacy have not been determined in children.

SIDE EFFECTS
Most Common
Ventricular arrhythmias (see below), hypotension, angina/chest pain, headaches.
CV: *Ventricular and supraventricular arrhythmias, including ventricular ectopic activity, nonsustained ventricular tachycardia, sustained ventricular tachycardia, and ventricular fibrillation.* Infrequently, *life-threatening arrhythmias associated with preexisting arrhythmias*, metabolic abnormalities, abnormal digoxin levels, and catheter insertion. Also, hypotension, angina,

chest pain. **Miscellaneous:** Mild to moderately severe headaches, hypokalemia, tremor, thrombocytopenia, bronchospasm (rare).

OD OVERDOSE MANAGEMENT

Symptoms: Hypotension. *Treatment:* If hypotension occurs, reduce or temporarily discontinue administration of milrinone until the condition of the client stabilizes. Use general measures to support circulation.

HOW SUPPLIED

Injection, premixed: 200 mcg/mL in D5W.

DOSAGE

- **IV INFUSION**

  CHF in clients receiving digoxin and diuretics.

Adults, loading dose: 50 mcg/kg administered slowly over 10 min. **Maintenance, minimum:** 0.59 mg/kg/24 hr (infused at a rate of 0.375 mcg/kg/min); **maintenance, standard:** 0.77 mg/kg/24 hr (infused at a rate of 0.5 mcg/kg/min); **maintenance, maximum:** 1.13 mg/kg/24 hr (infused at a rate of 0.75 mcg/kg/min).

NURSING CONSIDERATIONS

℆ Do not confuse milrinone with inamrinone (an inotropic drug).

ADMINISTRATION/STORAGE

IV 1. Give IV infusions at rates described in the package insert.
2. Adjust rate depending on the hemodynamic and clinical response.
3. Prepare dilutions using 0.45% or 0.9% NaCl or 5% dextrose injection.
4. Reduce rate in renal impairment (see package insert for chart).
5. Do not give furosemide in IV lines containing milrinone as a precipitate will form.
6. Store at room temperatures of 15–30°C (59–86°F).

ASSESSMENT

1. Note onset, characteristics of S&S. Identify NYHA class, other therapies used, outcome.
2. Monitor CBC, electrolytes, renal, LFTs. Document ECG, CO, CVP, and PAWP; rule out acute MI.

INTERVENTIONS

1. Monitor I&O, electrolyte levels, and renal function. Potassium loss due to excessive diuresis may cause arrhythmias in digitalized clients; correct hypokalemia.
2. Monitor VS; review parameters for interruption of infusion (e.g., SBP <80; HR <50).
3. Observe EKG for increased supraventricular and ventricular arrhythmias on monitor.

CLIENT/FAMILY TEACHING

May experience headaches; report as mild analgesics may alleviate i.e. acetaminophen.

OUTCOMES/EVALUATE

- ↑ CO and ↓ PACWP
- Resolution of S&S of CHF
- Therapeutic drug levels (150–250 ng/mL)

Minocycline hydrochloride IV

(mih-no-**SYE**-kleen)

CLASSIFICATION(S):

Antibiotic, tetracycline

PREGNANCY CATEGORY: D

Rx: Arestin, Cleeravue-M, Dynacin, Minocin, Myrac, Solodyn.

✤**Rx:** Apo-Minocycline, Gen-Minocycline, Novo-Minocycline, Rhoxal-minocycline, ratio-Minocycline.

SEE ALSO *ANTI-INFECTIVE DRUGS AND TETRACYCLINES.*

USES

PO. (1) Gram-negative infections due to *Haemophilis ducreyi* (chancroid); *Francisella tularensis* (tularemia); *Yersinia pestis* (plague); *Bartonella bacilliformis* (bartonellosis); *Campylobacter fetus; Vibrio cholerae* (cholera); *Brucella* species (used with streptomycin); *Neisseria gonorrhoeae* (uncomplicated urethritis in men). Do not use extended-release products for these infections. (2) Infections caused by the following miscellaneous organisms: *Rickettsiae* (Rocky Mountain spotted fever, typhus fever and the typhus group; Q fever; rickettsiapox; tick fevers); *Mycoplasma pneumoniae* (respiratory tract infections); *Chlamydia trachomatis* (lymphogranuloma venereum; trachoma, inclusive conjunctivitis), *Chlamydia psittaci* (psittacosis); *Borellia recurrentis* (relapsing fever); *Ureaplasma urealyticum* (nongonococcal urethritis). Do not use extended-release products for these infections. (3) Following susceptibility testing (resistance has been shown): *Eschericia coli; Enterobacter aerogenes; Acinetobacter* and *Shigella* species; *Haemophilus influenzae* (respiratory tract infections); *Klebsiella* species (respiratory and urinary tract infections); *Streptococcus pneumoniae* (upper respiratory infections); *Staphylococcus aureus* (skin and skin structure infections). (4) Alternative therapy for the following infections when penicillin is contraindicated: *Neisseria gonorrhoeae* infections; syphilis due to *Treponema pallidum;* yaws due to *Treponema pertenue;* listeriosis due to *Listeria monocytogenes;* anthrax due to *Bacillus anthracis;* Vincent's infections due to *Fusobacterium fusiforme;* actinomycosis due to *Actinomyces israelii;* infections due to *Clostridium* species. Do not use extended-release products for these infections. (5) As an adjunct to amebicides to treat acute intestinal amebiasis. Do not use extended-release products for these infections. (6) As an adjunct to treat severe acne. (7) Treat asymptomatic meningococcal carriers due to *N. meningitidis.* Do not use extended-release products for this infection. (8) Adjunctive treatment to scaling and root planing procedures to reduce pocket depth adult periodontitis (Arestin). (9) Inflammatory lesions of moderate to severe acne vulgaris without nodules in clients age 12 years and older. *Investigational:* Early rheumatoid arthritis; gallbladder infections due to *E. coli;* alternative drug for nocardiosis in those who cannot take sulfa drugs; chronic malignant pleural effusion.

Injection. (1) Infections due to the following susceptible strains: Rocky Mountain spotted fever; typhus fever and the typhus group; Q fever; rickettsial pox and tick fevers caused by rickettsia; respiratory tract infections due to *Mycoplasma pneumoniae;* lymphogranuloma venereum due to *Chlamydia trachomatis;* psittacosis (ornithosis) due to *Chlamydia psittaci;* trachoma due to *C. trachomatis* (infection not always eliminated); inclusion conjunctivitis due to *C. trachomatis;* nongonococcal urethritis, endocervical, or rectal infections in adults due to *Ureaplasma urea lyticum* or *C. trachomatis;* relapsing fever due to *Borrelia recurrentis;* chancroid due to *Haemophilus ducreyi;* plague due to *Yersinia pestis;* tularemia due to *Francisella tularensis;* cholera due to *Vibrio cholerae; Campylobacter fetus* infections due to *C. fetus;* brucellosis due to *Brucella* species (in conjunction with streptomycin); bartonellosis due to *Bartonella bacilliformis;* granuloma inguinale due to *Calymmatobacterium granulomatis.* (2) Infections due to the following gram-negative microorganisms susceptible to the drug: *E. coli; Enterobacter aerogenes; Shigella* species; *Acinetobacter* species; respiratory tract infections due to *Haemophilus influenzae;* respiratory tract and urinary tract infections due to *Klebsiella* species. (3) Infections due to the following gram-positive microorganisms susceptible to the drug: Upper respiratory tract infections due to *Streptococcus pneumoniae;* skin and skin structure infections due to *Staphylococcus aureus* (minocycline is not the drug of choice). (4) As an alternative drug for the following infections when penicillin is contraindicated: Uncomplicated urethritis in men due to *Neisseria gonorrhoeae* and to treat other gonococcal infections; infections in women due to *N. gonorrhoeae;* meningitis due to *Neisseria meningitidis;* syphilis due to *Treponema pallidum* subspecies *pallidum;* yaws due to *T. pallidum* subspecies *pertenue;* listeriosis due to *Listeria monocytogenes;* anthrax due to *Bacillus anthracis;* Vincent infection due to *Fusobacterium fusiforme;* actinomycosis due to *Actinomyces israelii;* infections due to *Clostridum* species. (5) Adjunct to amebicides to treat acute intestinal amebiasis. (6) Adjunct therapy to treat severe acne.

NOTE: Do not use tetracyclines for streptococci infections unless the organism has been shown to be susceptible. Tetracyclines are not the drugs of choice to treat any type of staphylococcal infection.

ACTION/KINETICS

Action

Inhibits protein synthesis by binding to the ribsomal 30S subunit, thereby interfering with protein synthesis. Blocks the binding of aminoacyl transfer RNA to the messenger RNA complex. Cell wall synthesis is not inhibited.

Pharmacokinetics

In fasting adults, 90–100% of an oral dose is absorbed. **Peak plasma levels:** 1–4 hr. Absorption is less affected by milk or food than for other tetracyclines. **$t\frac{1}{2}$, elimination:** 11–26 hr after PO use and 15–23 hr after IV use. Metabolized in the liver. 5–10% excreted in the urine.

SPECIAL CONCERNS

Use the dental product (Arestin) with caution in clients with a history of predisposition to oral candidiasis.

SIDE EFFECTS

Most Common

Diarrhea, dizziness, unsteadiness, drowsiness, headache, vomiting.

See *Tetracyclines* for a complete list of possible side effects. Also, blue-gray pigmentation areas of cutaneous inflammation, vertigo, ataxia, drowsiness, Stevens-Johnson syndrome (rare).

When used for adult periodontitis: Tooth discoloration, periodontitis, tooth disorder, tooth caries, dental pain, stomatitis, infection, headache, gingivitis, flu syndrome, pharyngitis, dental infection, pain, mucous membrane disorder, dyspepsia, mouth ulceration. Also, overgrowth of nonsusceptible microorganisms, including fungi. Stevens-Johnson syndrome (rare).

HOW SUPPLIED

Capsules: 50 mg, 75 mg, 100 mg; *Capsules, Pellet-Filled:* 50 mg, 100 mg; *Oral Suspension:* 50 mg/5 mL; *Powder for Injection, Cryodesiccated:* 100 mg/vial; *Powder, Extended-Release, Dental:* 1 mg; *Tablets:* 50 mg, 75 mg, 100 mg; *Tablets,*

Extended-Release: 45 mg, 90 mg, 135 mg.

DOSAGE

- **CAPSULES; CAPSULES, PELLET-FILLED; INJECTION; ORAL SUSPENSION**

Infections against which effective.

Adults, initial: 200 mg; **then,** 100 mg q 12 hr. An alternative regimen is 100–200 mg initially followed by 50 mg q 6 hr. **Children over 8 years of age, initial:** 4 mg/kg; **then,** 2 mg/kg q 12 hr. When used parenterally do not exceed 400 mg per day in adults; for children, do not exceed the adult dose.

Uncomplicated urethral infections in adults due to C. trachomatis or Ureaplasma urealyticum.

Adults: 100 mg q 12 hr for at least 7 days.

Uncomplicated gonococcal urethritis in men.

100 mg q 12 hr for 5 days.

Uncomplicated gonococcal infections except urethritis and anorectal infections in men.

Initial: 200 mg; **then,** 100 mg q 12 hr for at least 4 days, with posttherapy cultures within 2–3 days.

Meningococcal carrier state.

100 mg q 12 hr for 5 days.

Mycobacterium marinum infections.

Usual: 100 mg q 12 hr for 6–8 weeks.

- **MICROSPHERES, SUSTAINED-RELEASE**

Adult periodontitis.

Amount given depends on the size, shape, and number of pockets being treated. The unit-dose cartridge is inserted into a cartridge handle in order to administer.

- **TABLETS, EXTENDED-RELEASE**

Moderate-to-severe acne vulgaris without nodules.

91–136 kg (200–300 lbs): 0.99–1.48 mg/kg (use 135 mg strength); **60–90 kg (132–100 lbs):** 1–1.5 mg/kg (use 90 mg strength); **45–59 kg (99–131 lbs):** 0.76–1 mg/kg (use 45 mg strength).

NURSING CONSIDERATIONS

Do not confuse Minocin with Indocin (NSAID).

Bold Italic = life threatening side effect ■ = black box warning ✚ = Available in Canada

ADMINISTRATION/STORAGE

1. Minocycline microspheres (Arestin) are delivered directly into the infected periodontal pocket after scaling and root planing. No refrigeration or mixing is needed and the product does not require removal.

2. Decrease the recommended dose and/or increase the dosing intervals in clients with renal impairment. Do not exceed a dose of 200 mg/day of Minocin (whether using PO or injection) in these clients.

3. When used for syphilis, give usual dose over a period of 10–15 days. Close follow-up, including lab tests, is recommended.

4. Store capsules, suspension, and microspheres from 15–30°C (59–86°F). Do not freeze. Protect from light, moisture and excessive heat.

IV 5. Do not dissolve in solutions containing calcium; forms a precipitate.

6. Reconstitute the cryodesiccated powder with 5 mL sterile water for injection; immediately dilute further to 500–1,000 mL with sodium chloride injection, dextrose injection, dextrose and sodium chloride injection, Ringer's injection, or Ringer's lactate injection. When diluted in 500 to 1,000 mL the pH usually ranges from 2.5 to 4, except when using Ringer's lactate where the pH ranges from 4.5 to 6.

7. Administer immediately although reconstituted solutions may be stored at room temperature up to 24 hr. Discard any unused portions after 24 hr at room temperature.

8. Store the Powder for Injection from 20–25°C (68–77°F). Protect from light, moisture, and excessive heat.

ASSESSMENT

1. List reasons for therapy, onset, location, characteristics of S&S, cultures, other agents trialed/outcome.

2. Monitor C&S, renal, LFTs, CBC; identify contacts when treating contagious diseases; get infectious disease referral.

3. Reduce dose/dosing intervals with renal dysfunction.

CLIENT/FAMILY TEACHING

1. Take with or without food, with a full glass of water and at least 1 hr prior to bedtime to prevent esophageal irritation. Check expiration date; discard outdated products to prevent adverse effects.

2. Avoid activities that require mental alertness until drug effects realized.

3. With STDs, use condoms during therapy to prevent reinfections and obtain periodic cultures.

4. Avoid in children under 8 years old during tooth development; may stain teeth.

5. Practice reliable non-hormonal birth control; drug may cause fetal harm.

6. Avoid prolonged sunlight exposure; may cause photosensitivity reaction.

7. Report any dizziness, unusual bruising/bleeding, severe rash or diarrhea, difficulty breathing, dark urine or stools, severe cramps, and lack of improvement after 72 hr.

8. Keep all follow up appointments to evaluate response to therapy and dose adequacy.

OUTCOMES/EVALUATE

Symptomatic improvement; resolution of infection

Minoxidil, oral
(mih-**NOX**-ih-dil)

CLASSIFICATION(S):

Antihypertensive, peripheral vasodilator

PREGNANCY CATEGORY: C

SEE ALSO *ANTIHYPERTENSIVE AGENTS*.

USES

Severe hypertension not controllable by the use of a diuretic plus two other antihypertensive drugs. Usually taken with at least two other antihypertensive drugs (a diuretic and a drug to minimize tachycardia such as a beta-adrenergic blocking agent). Can produce severe side effects; reserve for resistant cases of hypertension. Close medical supervision required, including possible hospitalization during initial administration.

ACTION/KINETICS

Action

Decreases elevated BP by decreasing peripheral resistance by a direct effect. Causes increase in renin secretion, increase in cardiac rate and output, and salt/water retention. Does not cause orthostatic hypotension.

Pharmacokinetics

Onset: 30 min. **Peak plasma levels:** Reached within 60 min; **plasma t½:** 4.2 hr. **Duration:** 24–48 hr. Ninety percent absorbed from GI tract; excretion: renal (90% metabolites). The time needed to reach the maximum effect is inversely related to the dose.

CONTRAINDICATIONS

Pheochromocytoma. Within 1 month after a MI. Dissecting aortic aneurysm. Use in milder forms of hypertension.

SPECIAL CONCERNS

 (1) May produce serious side effects. Can cause pericardial effusion, occasionally progressing to tamponade. Can also worsen angina pectoris. Reserve for hypertensive clients who do not respond adequately to maximum therapeutic doses of a diuretic and two other antihypertensive agents. (2) In experimental animals, minoxidil caused several kinds of myocardial lesions and other adverse cardiac effects. (3) Give under close supervision, usually together with a beta-adrenergic blocking agent, to prevent tachycardia and increased myocardial workload. Usually must be given with a diuretic, frequently one acting in the ascending limb of the loop of Henle, to prevent serious fluid accumulation. (4) When first given, hospitalize and monitor clients with malignant hypertension and those already receiving guanethidine to avoid too rapid or large orthostatic decreases in BP.■ Safe use during lactation not established. Use with caution and at reduced dosage in impaired renal function. Geriatric clients may be more sensitive to the hypotensive and hypothermic effects of minoxidil; also, may be necessary to decrease the dose due to age-related decreases in renal function. BP controlled too rapidly may cause syncope, stroke, MI, and ischemia of affected organs. Experience with use in children is limited.

SIDE EFFECTS

Most Common

Edema (temporary), change in direction and magnitude of T waves; enhanced hair growth, pigmentation and thickening of fine body hair; malaise, dizziness, drowsiness, headache.

CV: Edema (temporary), ***pericardial effusion that may progress to tamponade*** (acute compression of heart caused by fluid or blood in pericardium), CHF, angina pectoris, changes in direction and magnitude of T waves, increased HR. In children, rebound hypertension following slow withdrawal. **GI:** N&V. **CNS:** Headache, fatigue, dizziness, drowsiness. **Hypersensitivity:** Rashes, including bullous eruptions and ***Stevens-Johnson syndrome***. **Hematologic:** Initially, decrease in hematocrit, hemoglobin, and erythrocyte count but all return to normal. Rarely, thrombocytopenia and leukopenia. **Miscellaneous:** Hypertrichosis (enhanced hair growth, pigmentation and thickening of fine body hair 3–6 weeks after initiation of therapy), breast tenderness, darkening of skin.

LABORATORY TEST CONSIDERATIONS

Nonspecific changes in ECG. ↑ Alkaline phosphatase, serum creatinine, and BUN.

OD OVERDOSE MANAGEMENT

Symptoms: Excessive hypotension. *Treatment:* Give NSS IV (to maintain BP and urine output). Vasopressors, such as phenylephrine and dopamine, can be used but only in underperfusion of a vital organ.

DRUG INTERACTIONS

Concomitant use with guanethidine may result in severe hypotension

HOW SUPPLIED

Tablets: 2.5 mg, 10 mg.

DOSAGE

• TABLETS

Hypertension.

Adults and children over 12 years: Initial: 5 mg/day. For optimum control, dose can be increased to 10, 20, and then 40 mg in single or divided doses/day. Do not exceed 100 mg/day. **Chil-**

Bold Italic = life threatening side effect   ■ = black box warning   ♣ = Available in Canada

dren under 12 years: Initial, 0.2 mg/kg/day. Effective dose range: 0.25–1.0 mg/kg/day. Dosage must be titrated to individual response. Do not exceed 50 mg/day. *NOTE:* Clients with renal failure or undergoing dialysis may require smaller doses.

NURSING CONSIDERATIONS

◉ Do not confuse minoxidil with Monopril (an ACE inhibitor).

ADMINISTRATION/STORAGE

1. Give once daily if supine DBP has been reduced less than 30 mm Hg and twice daily (in two equal doses) if it has been reduced more than 30 mm Hg.
2. Wait at least 3 days between dosage adjustments as the full response is not obtained until then. However, if more rapid control is required, may adjust q 6 hr but with careful monitoring.

ASSESSMENT

1. Note reasons for therapy, other agents trialed, outcome. Be sure diuretic is prescribed to relieve fluid accumulation and beta blocker to control tachycardia.
2. Assess cardiopulmonary status; may cause pericardial effusion which may progress to tamponade. Also, may worsen angina pectoris.
3. Monitor VS, (anticipate BP decreases within 30 min), CBC, glucose, electrolytes, and renal function studies; adjust dose with dysfunction. Give after dialysis as drug removed by hemodialysis.

CLIENT/FAMILY TEACHING

1. Can be taken with fluids and without regard to meals.
2. Record BP, HR, and weight daily for provider; report any S&S of fluid overload (gain of 6 lb/week; swelling of extremities, face, abdomen; or ↑ SOB).
3. Report any symptoms of chest pain, fainting, dizziness, or ↑ SOB that occurs, especially when lying down.
4. Drug may cause elongation, thickening, and increased pigmentation of body hair; should resolve once discontinued.
5. Keep all follow up appointments to evaluate response.

OUTCOMES/EVALUATE

↓ BP; control of hypertension

Minoxidil, topical solution

(mih-**NOX**-ih-dil)

CLASSIFICATION(S):
Hair growth stimulant
PREGNANCY CATEGORY: C
OTC: Minoxidil Extra Strength for Men, Minoxidil Topical Solution 2% for Men, Minoxidil Topical Solution 2% for Women, Rogaine Extra Strength for Men, Rogaine Men's Extra Strength, Rogaine for Men Solution, Rogaine for Women Solution.
✦**OTC:** Apo-Gain.

USES

To treat male and female pattern baldness (alopecia androgenetica). Extra Strength (5%) is only for treatment of hereditary male pattern baldness. *Investigational:* Alopecia areata.

ACTION/KINETICS

Action

The topical solution stimulates vertex hair growth in clients with male pattern baldness or in women with androgenetic alopecia. Mechanism may be related to dilation of arterioles and stimulation of resting hair follicles into active growth. Following topical administration, approximately 1.4% is absorbed into the systemic circulation.

Pharmacokinetics

Onset: 4 months but is variable. **Duration:** New hair growth may be lost 3–4 months after withdrawal of therapy. Minoxidil and its inactive metabolites are excreted in the urine. Also, see *Minoxidil, oral.*

CONTRAINDICATIONS

Lactation. Use of 5% solution in women.

SPECIAL CONCERNS

Use with caution in clients with hypertension, coronary heart disease, or predisposition to heart failure. Safety and efficacy in clients under 18 years of age have not been determined. Increased systemic absorption may occur if the scalp is irritated or there are abrasions.

M

M

SIDE EFFECTS

Most Common

Allergic contact dermatitis, irritant dermatitis, diarrhea, N&V, headache, dizziness, lightheadedness, faintness.

Dermatologic: Allergic contact dermatitis, irritant dermatitis, pruritus, dry skin, flaking of scalp, alopecia, hypertrichosis, erythema, eczema, worsening of hair loss. **Allergic:** Hives, facial swelling, allergic rhinitis, nonspecific allergic reactions. **GI:** N&V, diarrhea. **CNS:** Dizziness, lightheadedness, headache, faintness, anxiety, depression, fatigue. **CV:** Edema, chest pain, BP increase or decrease, palpitations, increase/decrease in pulse rate. **Respiratory:** Sinusitis, bronchitis, URTI. **Endocrine:** Menstrual changes, breast symptoms. **GU:** UTI, renal calculi, urethritis, prostatitis, epididymitis, vaginitis, vulvitis, vaginal discharge, itching. **Hematologic:** Lymphadenopathy, thrombocytopenia, anemia. **Musculoskeletal:** Fractures, back pain, tendonitis, aches and pains. **Ophthalmic:** Conjunctivitis, visual disturbances, decreased visual acuity. **Miscellaneous:** Vertigo, ear infections, edema, weight gain. *NOTE:* The incidence of side effects due to placebos is often similar to the incidence of side effects R/T the drug itself.

DRUG INTERACTIONS

Corticosteroids, topical / Enhances absorption of topical minoxidil
Guanethidine / Possible ↑ risk of orthostatic hypotension
Petrolatum / Enhances absorption of topical minoxidil
Retinoids / Enhances absorption of topical minoxidil

HOW SUPPLIED

Aerosol Foam, Topical: 5%; *Solution, Topical:* 2%, 5%.

DOSAGE

- **AEROSOL FOAM, TOPICAL**
  Stimulate hair growth.
  Apply ½ capful two times per day.
- **TOPICAL SOLUTION: 2%, 5%**
  Stimulate hair growth.

Adults: Apply 1 mL twice a day directly onto the scalp in the hair loss area. 5% solution not to be used on women.

NURSING CONSIDERATIONS

ADMINISTRATION/STORAGE

1. Use only in clients with normal, healthy scalps. Dermatitis, scalp abrasions, scalp psoriasis, or severe sunburn may increase the absorption of topical minoxidil and lead to systemic side effects (See *Minoxidil, oral*).

2. Hair may be shampooed before treatment, but dry the hair and scalp prior to topical application.

3. The product comes with a metered spray attachment (for application to large areas of the scalp), extender spray attachment (for application to small scalp areas or under the hair), and a rub-on applicator tip (to spread the solution on the scalp). Follow directions on the package insert carefully for each of these methods of application. Warn not to inhale the spray mist.

4. If the fingertips are used to apply the drug, wash hands thoroughly after application.

5. At least 4 months of continuous therapy is necessary before evidence of hair growth can be expected. Further hair growth continues through 1 year of treatment.

6. The alcohol base in topical minoxidil will cause irritation and burning of the eyes, abraded skin, or mucous membranes. If contact with any of these areas, wash site with copious amounts of water.

7. Avoid inhaling the spray mist.

CLIENT/FAMILY TEACHING

1. Review method and frequency for application. Solution may dry and leave a residue on the hair; this is harmless.

2. May permanently discolor linens, hats and pillows with prolonged use/contact.

3. More frequent than prescribed applications will not enhance hair growth but will increase systemic side effects. Review info booklet.

4. New hair growth will be soft and hard to see and is not permanent. Drug is a treatment, not a cure; stopping therapy will lead to hair loss within a few months. Topical minoxidil must be used indefinitely to sustain the effect.

Bold Italic = life threatening side effect ■ = black box warning ✤ = Available in Canada

5. Treatment has positive benefits for only approximately one-half the population. May take up to 4 months of continuous therapy before any response is noted.

6. Report any evidence of irritation or rash.

7. Do not apply any other topical products to the scalp without approval.

8. Consult provider before using if no family history of gradual hair loss, if hair loss is sudden or patchy, if hair loss is accompanied by other symptoms, or if the reasons for hair loss are not clear.

OUTCOMES/EVALUATE
Stimulation of hair growth

Mirtazapine ■
(mir-**TAZ**-ah-peen)

CLASSIFICATION(S):
Antidepressant, tetracyclic
PREGNANCY CATEGORY: C
Rx: Remeron, Remeron SolTab.

USES
Treatment of major depressive disorder.

ACTION/KINETICS

Action
Enhances central noradrenergic and serotonergic activity, perhaps by antagonism at central presynaptic alpha$_2$-adrenergic inhibitory autoreceptors and heteroreceptors. Also a potent antagonist of 5-HT$_2$, 5-HT$_3$, and histamine H$_1$ receptors. Moderate antagonist of peripheral alpha$_1$-adrenergic receptors and muscarinic receptors.

Pharmacokinetics
Rapidly and completely absorbed from the GI tract. **Peak plasma levels:** Within 2 hr. **t½, elimination:** 20–40 hr. Extensively metabolized in the liver and excreted in both the urine (75%) and feces (15%). Females exhibit significantly longer elimination half-lives than males.

CONTRAINDICATIONS
Use in combination with an MAO inhibitor or within 14 days of initiating or discontinuing therapy with a MAO in-hibitor. Known or suspected seizure disorders. During acute phase of MI.

SPECIAL CONCERNS
■ (1) Antidepressants increased the risk of suicidal thinking and behavior (suicidality) in short-term studies in children and adolescents with major depressive disorder and other psychiatric disorders. Anyone considering the use of mirtazapine or any other antidepressant in a child or adolescent must balance this risk with the clinical need. Clients who are started on therapy should be observed closely for clinical worsening, suicidality, or unusual changes in behavior. Families and caregivers should be advised of the need for close observation and communication with the prescriber. Mirtazapine is not approved for use in pediatric clients with major depressive disorder and obsessive-compulsive disorder. (2) Short-term placebo-controlled trials of 9 antidepressant drugs in children and adolescents with major depressive disorder, obsessive-compulsive disorder, or other psychiatric disorders revealed a greater risk of adverse reactions during the first few months of treatment. The average risk of such reactions in clients receiving antidepressants was 4%, twice the placebo risk of 2%. No suicides occurred in these trials.■ Use with caution in those with impaired renal or hepatic disease, in geriatric clients, during lactation, in CV or cerebrovascular disease that can be exacerbated by hypotension (e.g., history of MI, angina, ischemic stroke), and in conditions that would predispose to hypotension (e.g., dehydration, hypovolemia, treatment with antihypertensive medications). The effect of mirtazapine for longer than 6 weeks has not been evaluated, although treatment is indicated for 6 months or longer. Safety and efficacy have not been determined in children. Suicide attempts and suicidal thinking have occurred in pediatric clients taking antidepressant drugs for major depressive disorder.

SIDE EFFECTS

Most Common

Somnolence, dry mouth, constipation, increased appetite, dizziness, weight gain, asthenia, abnormal dreams.

Side effects with an incidence of 0.1% or greater are listed. **CNS:** Somnolence, dizziness, activation of mania or hypomania, **suicidal ideation**, sedation, drowsiness, abnormal dreams, abnormal thinking, tremor, confusion, hypesthesia, apathy, depression, hypokinesia, vertigo, twitching, agitation, anxiety, amnesia, hyperkinesia, paresthesia, ataxia, delirium, delusions, depersonalization, EPS, increased libido, abnormal coordination, dysarthria, hallucinations, neurosis, dystonia, hostility, increased reflexes, emotional lability, euphoria, paranoid reaction. **GI:** N&V, anorexia, dry mouth, constipation, ulcer, eructation, glossitis, cholecystitis, gum hemorrhage, stomatitis, colitis, abnormal LFTs. **CV:** Hypertension, vasodilation, angina pectoris, **MI**, bradycardia, ventricular extrasystoles, syncope, migraine, orthostatic hypotension. **Hematologic:** Agranulocytosis. **Body as a whole:** Asthenia, flu syndrome, back pain, malaise, abdominal pain, acute abdominal syndrome, chills, fever, facial edema, photosensitivity reaction, neck rigidity, neck pain, enlarged abdomen. **Respiratory:** Dyspnea, increased cough, sinusitis, epistaxis, bronchitis, asthma, pneumonia. **GU:** Urinary frequency, UTI, kidney calculus, cystitis, dysuria, urinary incontinence, urinary retention, vaginitis, hematuria, breast pain, amenorrhea, dysmenorrhea, leukorrhea, impotence. **Musculoskeletal:** Myalgia, myasthenia, arthralgia, arthritis, tenosynovitis. **Dermatologic:** Pruritus, rash, acne, exfoliative dermatitis, dry skin, herpes simplex, alopecia. **Metabolic/nutritional:** Increased appetite, weight gain, peripheral edema, edema, thirst, dehydration, weight loss. **Ophthalmic:** Eye pain, abnormal accommodation, conjunctivitis, keratoconjunctivitis, lacrimation disorder, glaucoma. **Miscellaneous:** Deafness, hyperacusis, ear pain.

LABORATORY TEST CONSIDERATIONS

↑ ALT and nonfasting cholesterol and triglycerides.

OD **OVERDOSE MANAGEMENT**

Symptoms: Disorientation, drowsiness, impaired memory, tachycardia. *Treatment:* General supportive measures. If the client is unconscious, establish and maintain an airway. Consider induction of emesis or gastric lavage and administration of activated charcoal. Monitor cardiac and vital signs.

DRUG INTERACTIONS

Clonidine / Possible ↓ clonidine's hypertensive effect

CNS depressants / Enhanced CNS depressant effect

Diazepam / Additive impairment of motor skills

Fluvoxamine / Possible ↑ mirtazapine serum levels

Phenytoin / ↓ Plasma mirtazapine levels R/T ↑ liver metabolism

HOW SUPPLIED

Tablets: 7.5 mg, 15 mg, 30 mg, 45 mg; *Tablets, Oral Disintegrating:* 15 mg, 30 mg, 45 mg.

DOSAGE

• **TABLETS; TABLETS, ORAL DISINTEGRATING**

Treatment of depression.

Initial: 15 mg/day given as a single dose, preferably in the evening before sleep. Those not responding to the 15-mg dose may respond to doses up to a maximum of 45 mg/day. Do not make dose changes at intervals of less than 1 to 2 weeks. Consider treatment for up to 6 months.

NURSING CONSIDERATIONS

ADMINISTRATION/STORAGE

1. The oral disintegrating tablet (Sol-Tab) can be swallowed with or without water, chewed, or allowed to disintegrate.

2. Clearance is decreased in the elderly and in clients with moderate to severe renal or hepatic impairment.

3. At least 2 weeks should elapse between discontinuing an MAOI and starting mirtazapine therapy. Also, 14 or more days should elapse after stopping mirtazapine and starting an MAOI.

Bold Italic = life threatening side effect   ■ = black box warning   ♣ = Available in Canada

4. Store from 15–30°C (59–86°F). Protect from light and moisture.

ASSESSMENT

1. Note reasons for therapy, onset, triggers, behavioral manifestations. Identify events that may be R/T to depression, i.e., death, divorce, illness, or job loss.
2. List drugs prescribed; ensure no MAOI use within past 2 weeks.
3. Monitor mental status, ECG, CBC, LFTs, cholesterol, and triglyceride levels.

CLIENT/FAMILY TEACHING

1. Take as directed; do not exceed prescribed dosing schedule.
2. For the orally disintegrating tablet, open tablet blister pack with dry hands and place tablet on tongue; it will disintegrate within 30 seconds and can be swallowed with saliva or chewed. Do not split the tablet and do not open the blister pack until just before use.
3. Report any S&S of infection or flu (fever, sore throat, stomatitis, etc.); drug may cause (↓ WBCs) agranulocytosis.
4. Do not engage in activities that require mental alertness until drug effects realized; dizziness and drowsiness may occur.
5. Avoid alcohol and OTC agents; may potentiate drug's cognitive and motor skill impairment.
6. Report as scheduled for F/U labs, counselling, and evaluation of clinical response to drug therapy.
7. Parents should consult medication guide and think about four important things when their child is prescribed an antidepressant: (1) Risk of suicidal thoughts or actions; (2) How to try to prevent suicidal thoughts or actions in your child; (3) watch for certain signs if your child is taking an antidepressant; and (4) There are benefits and risks when using antidepressants. These are all delineated in the guide and should be.

OUTCOMES/EVALUATE

Improved sleeping and eating patterns; improved mood, ↑ interest in social activities, ↓ depression

Misoprostol
(my-soh-**PROST**-ohl)

CLASSIFICATION(S):
Prostaglandin
PREGNANCY CATEGORY: X
Rx: Cytotec.
✦Rx: Apo-Misoprostol, Novo-Misoprostol.

USES

(1) Prevention of aspirin and other nonsteroidal anti-inflammatory-induced gastric ulcers in clients with a high risk of gastric ulcer complications (e.g., geriatric clients with debilitating disease) or in those with a history of ulcer. (2) In combination with mifepristone to terminate pregnancy. *Investigational:* Vaginally to produce cervical ripening and induction of labor and to treat serious postpartum hemorrhage in the presence of uterine atony. Chronic, idiopathic constipation.

ACTION/KINETICS

Action

Synthetic prostaglandin E_1 analog that inhibits gastric acid secretion, protects the gastric mucosa by increasing bicarbonate and mucus production, and decreases pepsin levels during basal conditions. May also stimulate uterine contractions that may endanger pregnancy.

Pharmacokinetics

Extensively absorbed and rapidly converted to the active misoprostol acid. **Time for peak levels of misoprostol acid:** 12 min. $t\frac{1}{2}$, **misoprostol acid:** 20–40 min. Excreted in the urine.

NOTE: Misoprostol does not prevent development of duodenal ulcers in clients on NSAIDs. **Plasma protein binding:** Less than 90%.

CONTRAINDICATIONS

Allergy to prostaglandins, during lactation (may cause diarrhea in nursing infants). Use in pregnancy to reduce risk of ulcers induced by NSAIDs.

SPECIAL CONCERNS

■ (1) If given to pregnant women, can cause abortion, premature birth, or

M

birth defects. Uterine rupture has been reported if given to pregnant women to induce labor or to induce abortion beyond week 8 of pregnancy. (2) Not to be taken by pregnant women to reduce risk of ulcers induced by NSAIDs. (3) Advise clients of the abortifacient property and warn them not to give the drug to others. (4) Should not be used to reduce risk of NSAID-induced ulcers in women of childbearing age unless the client is at high risk of developing complications from gastric ulcers associated with NSAID use, or is at high risk of developing gastric ulceration. In such clients, misoprostol may be prescribed if the client:

• Has had a negative serum pregnancy test within 2 weeks prior to beginning therapy.

• Is capable of complying with effective contraceptive measures.

• Has received both oral and written warnings of the hazards of misoprostol, the risk of possible contraception failure, and the danger to other women of childbearing age should the drug be taken by mistake.

• Will begin misoprostol only on the second or third day of the next normal menstrual period.■

SIDE EFFECTS
Most Common
Diarrhea, abdominal pain, N&V, flatulence, dyspepsia, headache, uterine cramping.

GI: Diarrhea (may be severe, but is usually self-limiting), abdominal pain, nausea, dyspepsia, flatulence, vomiting, constipation. **GU:** Spotting, cramps, dysmenorrhea, hypermenorrhea, menstrual disorders, postmenopausal vaginal bleeding. **Miscellaneous:** Headache.

OD OVERDOSE MANAGEMENT
Symptoms: Abdominal pain, diarrhea, dyspnea, sedation, tremor, fever, palpitations, bradycardia, hypotension, *seizures.* *Treatment:* Use supportive therapy.

HOW SUPPLIED
Tablets: 100 mcg, 200 mcg.

DOSAGE
• **TABLETS**

Reduce risk of NSAID-induced gastric ulcers.

Adults: 200 mcg 4 times per day with food for the duration of NSAID therapy. Dose can be reduced to 100 mcg if the larger dose cannot be tolerated. In renal impairment, the 200 mcg dose can be reduced if necessary.

With mifepristone to terminate pregnancy.

Treatment includes both mifepristone and misoprostol and requires three office visits. **Day 1:** Three-200 mg tablets (600 mg) of mifepristone taken as a single dose. **Day 3:** Unless abortion has occurred and has been confirmed by clinical examination or ultrasonographic scan, clients must take misoprostol, 400 mcg (two-200 mcg tablets) PO. **Day 14:** Client returns for follow-up visit to confirm by clinical examination or ultrasonographic scan that complete termination of pregnancy has occurred.

NURSING CONSIDERATIONS
℮ Do not confuse misoprostol with mifepristone (an abortifacient) or with metoprolol (a beta-adrenergic blocker). Also, do not confuse Cytotec with Cytoxan (an antineoplastic) or with Cytosar (an antineoplastic).

ADMINISTRATION/STORAGE
1. Reduce diarrhea by giving after meals and at bedtime; avoid Mg-containing antacids. Diarrhea is usually self-limiting.
2. Maximum plasma levels are decreased if drug is taken with food.
3. Take for the duration of NSAID therapy.
4. Drug may increase gastric bicarbonate and mucus production.

ASSESSMENT
1. Note any ulcer disease; assess GI S&S, clinical presentation, other agents trialed.
2. Obtain a negative pregnancy test unless being used with methotrexate to induce abortion.

CLIENT/FAMILY TEACHING
1. Drug reduces stomach acid and protects stomach.

Bold Italic = life threatening side effect   ■ = black box warning   ♣ = Available in Canada

2. Avoid foods/spices that may aggravate condition: caffeine, alcohol, and black pepper.

3. Take exactly as prescribed for the duration of aspirin or NSAID therapy to prevent ulcer formation.

4. May experience abdominal discomfort, diarrhea; take misoprostol after meals and at bedtime to minimize these side effects. Avoid Mg-containing antacids.

5. Report persistent diarrhea, postmenopausal bleeding, or increased menstrual bleeding.

6. All women of childbearing age must practice effective contraceptive measures; drug has abortifacient properties. Never share medications.

7. With abortion, report any increased bleeding, pain, or fever.

OUTCOMES/EVALUATE

Prevention of drug-induced gastric ulcers

Mitomycin (MTC) ■ IV
(my-toe-**MY**-sin)

CLASSIFICATION(S):
Antineoplastic, antibiotic
PREGNANCY CATEGORY: X
Rx: MitoExtra, Mutamycin.

SEE ALSO *ANTINEOPLASTIC AGENTS.*

USES
Palliative treatment and adjunct to surgical or radiologic treatment of disseminated adenocarcinoma of the stomach and pancreas when other treatment fails. Used in combination with other agents (not recommended as a single agent for primary treatment or in place of surgery and/or radiotherapy). *Investigational:* Superficial bladder cancer (by the intravesical route). As an ophthalmic solution as an adjunct to surgical excision in primary or recurrent pterygia.

ACTION/KINETICS
Action
Antibiotic produced by *Streptomyces caespitosus* that inhibits DNA synthesis.

The guanine and cytosine content correlates with the degree of mitomycin-induced cross-linking. At high doses both RNA and protein synthesis are inhibited. Most active during late G_1 and early S stages.

Pharmacokinetics
Rapidly cleared from the serum. $t\frac{1}{2}$, **initial:** 17 min after a 30 mg bolus injection; **final:** 50 min. Metabolized in liver; 10% excreted unchanged in urine, more when dose is increased.

CONTRAINDICATIONS
Primary therapy as a single agent. Use to replace surgery or radiotherapy. Hypersensitivity or idiosyncratic reaction to mitomycin. Pregnancy and lactation. Thrombocytopenia, coagulation disorders, increase in bleeding tendency due to other causes. In clients with a serum creatinine level greater than 1.7 mg/dL.

SPECIAL CONCERNS
■ (1) Bone marrow suppression, especially thrombocytopenia and leukopenia, which may contribute to overwhelming infection in an already compromised client, is the most common and severe toxic effect. (2) Hemolytic uremic syndrome, a serious syndrome of microangiopathic hemolytic anemia, thrombocytopenia, and irreversible renal failure has occurred.■ Use with extreme caution in presence of impaired renal function.

SIDE EFFECTS
Most Common
Thrombocytopenia, leukopenia, cellulitis at injection site, stomatitis, alopecia, fever, anorexia, N&V.

See *Antineoplastic Agents* for a complete list of possible side effects. Also, severe bone marrow depression, especially leukopenia and thrombocytopenia. Pulmonary toxicity including dyspnea with nonproductive cough. **Microangiopathic hemolytic anemia with renal failure and hypertension (hemolytic uremic syndrome),** especially when used long-term in combination with fluorouracil. Cellulitis. Extravasation causes severe necrosis of surrounding tissue. **Acute respiratory distress syndrome in adults,** especially when used with other chemotherapy.

M

DRUG INTERACTIONS
Severe bronchospasm and SOB when used with vinca alkaloids

HOW SUPPLIED
Powder for Injection: 5 mg, 20 mg, 40 mg.

DOSAGE

- **IV ONLY**

  Adenocarcinoma of the stomach and pancreas.

After hematological recovery from previous chemotherapy, give 20 mg/m^2 as a single dose via infusion q 6–8 wk. Subsequent courses of treatment are based on hematologic response; do not repeat until leukocyte count is at least 4,000/mm^3 and platelet count is at least 100,000/mm^3. Adjust the dose as follows depending on the nadir after prior dose/mm^3: If leukocytes are between 3,000 and 3,999 and platelets are between 75,000 and 99,999, give 100% of the prior dose; if leukocytes are between 2,000 and 2,999 and platelets are between 25,000 and 74,999, give 70% of the prior dose; if leukocytes are less than 2,000 and platelets are less than 25,000, give 50% of the prior dose.

NURSING CONSIDERATIONS

ADMINISTRATION/STORAGE

IV 1. Drug is toxic; avoid extravasation. Observe infusion site closely for evidence of erythema or complaints of discomfort. Apply ice and use thiosulfate for infiltrate.

2. Reconstitute 5-, 20-, or 40-mg vial with 10, 40, or 80 mL sterile water for injection, respectively, as indicated and administer over 5–10 min; will dissolve if allowed to remain at room temperature.

3. Drug concentration of 0.5 mg/mL is stable for 14 days under refrigeration or 7 days at room temperature.

4. Diluted concentrations of 20–40 mcg/mL, are stable for 3 hr in D5W, for 12 hr in isotonic saline, and for 24 hr in sodium lactate injection.

5. Mitomycin (5–15 mg) and heparin (1,000–10,000 units) in 30 mL of isotonic saline are stable for 48 hr at room temperature.

ASSESSMENT

1. Note reasons for therapy, other agents trialed/failed, anticipated length of therapy.

2. List pulmonary function. Obtain CXR; pulmonary infiltrates and fibrosis can occur with cumulative doses. Observe closely for early evidence of pulmonary complications, such as dyspnea, nonproductive cough, and abnormal ABGs/lung sounds.

3. Obtain baseline CBC, PT, PTT, and renal function; do not initiate if serum creatinine level is >1.7 mg/dL. Drug may cause platelet and granulocyte suppression. Nadir: 28 days; recovery: 40–55 days. Follow dosing schedule based on platelets and leukocytes.

CLIENT/FAMILY TEACHING

1. Drug is used with other agents to treat disseminated adenocarcinoma of stomach and pancreas.

2. Report any adverse side effects, S&S of cold/flu or respiratory distress. May lose hair; should regrow.

3. Avoid vaccinations during active therapy. Mitomycin may lower your body's resistance and there is a chance you might get the infection the immunization is meant to prevent. In addition, other persons living in your household should not take oral polio vaccine since there is a chance they could pass the polio virus on to you. Also, avoid persons who have taken oral polio vaccine. Do not get close to them, and do not stay in the same room with them for very long. If you cannot take these precautions, you should consider wearing a protective face mask that covers the nose and mouth.

4. Mitomycin can temporarily lower the number of WBCs in your blood, increasing chances of getting an infection. It can also lower the number of platelets, which are necessary for proper blood clotting. If this occurs, there are certain precautions you can take, esp when your blood count is low, to reduce the risk of infection or bleeding:

- Avoid people with infections. Report immediately: fever or chills, cough or hoarseness, lower back or side pain, or painful or difficult urination.

- Any unusual bleeding or bruising; black, tarry stools; blood in urine or stools; or pinpoint red spots on your skin.
- Be careful when using a regular toothbrush, dental floss, or toothpick. Use a soft bristled tooth brush and waxed dental floss. Check before having any dental work done.
- Do not touch your eyes or the inside of your nose unless you have just washed your hands and have not touched anything else in the meantime.
- Be careful not to cut yourself when using sharp objects such as a safety razor or fingernail or toenail cutters.
- Avoid contact sports or other situations where bruising or injury could occur.

5. If mitomycin accidentally seeps out of the vein into which it is injected, it may damage the skin and cause scarring. In some, this may occur weeks or even months after this medicine is given. Report if you notice redness, pain, or swelling at the place of injection or anywhere else on your skin.

6. Practice reliable contraception throughout therapy.

OUTCOMES/EVALUATE
↓ Tumor size/spread

Mitoxantrone hydrochloride ■ IV
(my-toe-**ZAN**-trohn)

CLASSIFICATION(S):
Antineoplastic, antibiotic
PREGNANCY CATEGORY: D
Rx: Novantrone.

SEE ALSO *ANTINEOPLASTIC AGENTS.*

USES
(1) In combination with other drugs, for the initial treatment of acute nonlymphocytic leukemias, including monocytic, promyelocytic, myelocytic, and acute erythroid leukemias. (2) In combination with corticosteroids as initial chemotherapy to treat pain from advanced hormone-refractory prostate cancer. (3) Reduce neurologic disability and/or the frequency of clinical relapses in those with secondary (chronic) progressive, progressive relapsing, or worsening relapsing-remitting MS. Not indicated to treat those with primary progressive MS. *Investigational:* Treat breast cancer; non-Hodgkin's lymphomas, and autologous bone marrow transplantation.

ACTION/KINETICS
Action
A synthetic antineoplastic anthracenedione. Is a DNA-reactive drug that intercalates into DNA through hydrogen bonding, causes cross-links and strand breaks. It also interferes with RNA and is a potent inhibitor of topoisomerase II (enzyme responsible for uncoiling and repairing damaged DNA). The drug has a cytocidal effect and is considered not to be cell-cycle specific. Low distribution to the brain, spinal cord, spinal fluid, and eyes.

Pharmacokinetics
$t^{1/2}$, **alpha:** 6–12 min; $t^{1/2}$, **beta:** 1.1–3.1 hr; $t^{1/2}$, **terminal:** about 75 hr. Excreted through both the feces (via the bile) and the urine (up to 65% unchanged). **Plasma protein binding:** 75%.

CONTRAINDICATIONS
Preexisting myelosuppression (unless benefits outweigh risks). Use with baseline neutrophil counts less than 1,500 cells/mm^3 (except for treatment of acute nonlymphocytic leukemia). To treat primary progressive multiple sclerosis. In MS clients who have received a cumulative lifetime dose of 140 mg/m^2 or more, in those with hepatic impairment, in those with either a left ventricular ejection fraction of less than 50%, or a clinically significant reduction in LVEF. Lactation. Intrathecal, SC, IM, or intra-arterial use.

SPECIAL CONCERNS
■ (1) Administer under the supervision of a physician experienced in the use of cytotoxic chemotherapeutic drugs. (2) Give slowly into a freely flowing IV infusion. Never give SC, IM, or intra-arterially. Severe local tissue damage may occur if there is extravasation during administration. (3) Do not use intrathecal-

M

ly; severe injury with permanent sequelae may result if given intrathecally. (4) Except to treat nonlymphocytic leukemia, mitoxantrone generally should not be given to clients with baseline neutrophil counts less than 1,500 cells/mm^3. In order to monitor the occurrence of bone marrow suppression, primarily neutropenia, which may be severe and result in infection, perform frequent peripheral cell counts in all clients receiving mitoxantrone. (5) Use of mitoxantrone has been associated with cardiotoxicity. Cardiotoxicity can occur at any time during therapy, and the risk increases with cumulative doses. CHF, potentially fatal, may occur either during therapy with mitoxantrone or months to years after termination of therapy. All clients should be carefully assessed for cardiac signs and symptoms by history and physical examination prior to the start of mitoxantrone therapy. Baseline physical evaluation of left ventricular ejection fraction (LVEF) by echocardiogram or multi-gated radionuclide angiography (MUGA) should be performed. Multiple sclerosis (MS) clients with baseline LVEF less than 50% should not be treated with mitoxantrone. LVEF should be reevaluated by echocardiogram or MUGA prior to each dose administration to those with MS. Additional doses of mitoxantrone should not be administered to MS clients who have experienced either a drop in LVEF to below 50% or a clinically significant reduction in LVEF during mitoxantrone therapy. Clients with MS should not receive a cumulative dose greater than 140 mg/m^2. In cancer clients the risk of symptomatic CHF was estimated to be 2.6% for those receiving up to a cumulative dose of 140 mg/m^2. Presence or history of cardiovascular disease, prior or concomitant radiotherapy to the mediastinal/pericardial area, previous therapy with other anthracyclines or anthracenediones, or concomitant use of other cardiotoxic drugs may increase the risk of cardiac toxicity. Cardiac toxicity with mitoxantrone may occur whether or not cardiac risk factors are present. (6) Secondary acute myelogenous leukemia has been reported in MS and cancer clients treated with mitoxantrone. Mitoxantrone is an anthracenedione, a related drug. The occurrence of refractory secondary leukemia is more common when anthracyclines are given in combination with DNA-damaging antineoplastic drugs, when clients have been heavily pretreated with cytotoxic drugs, or when doses of anthracyclines have been escalated. Secondary leukemias have been reported in cancer clients treated with mitoxantrone in combination with other cytotoxic agents, or when doses of anthracyclines have been escalated.■ Older clients may be more sensitive to the drug. Safety and efficacy have not been established in children. May be mutagenic.

SIDE EFFECTS
Most Common
URTI, alopecia, N&V, diarrhea, menstrual disorder, UTI, amenorrhea, pharyngitis, asthenia, bleeding, headache, GI mucositis/stomatitis, fever, infections, sepsis, decreased LVEF, fatigue, anorexia, constipation, edema.

Hematologic: Severe myelosuppression, ecchymosis, bleeding, petechiae, secondary acute myelogenous leukemia, acute leukemia, myelodysplasia, leukopenia, granulocytopenia, anemia. **GI:** N&V, diarrhea, stomatitis, mucositis, abdominal pain, dyspepsia, gastralgia, stomach burn, epigastric pain, aphthosis, constipation, jaundice, GI bleeding/***hemorrhage***. **CNS:** Headache, seizures, anxiety, depression, malaise, fatigue. **CV: *CHF (potentially fatal),*** decreases in LV ejection fraction, arrhythmias, tachycardia, chest pain, hypotension, abnormal ECG, cardiac dysrhythmia, cardiac ischemia, hypertension. **Respiratory:** Cough, dyspnea, URTI (increased risk of pneumonia), pharyngitis, throat infection, rhinitis, sinusitis, interstitial pneumonitis. **GU:** Menstrual disorder, amenorrhea, menorrhagia, UTI, abnormal urine, renal failure, hematuria, impotence, sterility. **Dermatologic:** Alopecia, skin infection, nail bed changes, cutaneous mycosis. **Body as a whole:** Rashes, edema, urticaria, alope-

---

cia, fever, asthenia, jaundice, infections, fungal infections, weight gain/loss, myalgia, arthralgia, **sepsis**. **Hypersensitivity:** Hypotension, urticaria, dyspnea, rashes, **anaphylaxis** (rare). **Ophthalmic:** Conjunctivitis, blurred vision. **Miscellaneous:** Anorexia, hyperuricemia, back pain, extravasation at injection site (tissue necrosis, phlebitis, erythema, swelling, pain, burning and/or blue skin discoloration).

LABORATORY TEST CONSIDERATIONS
↑ AST, ALT, gamma-GT, BUN, alkaline phosphatase, creatinine, glucose. Leukopenia, granulocytopenia, anemia. ↓ WBC, ANC, lymphocytes, hemoglobin, platelets, potassium. Hematuria, proteinuria. Hyperglycemia, hypocalcemia, hypokalemia, hyponatremia.

OD **OVERDOSE MANAGEMENT**
Symptoms: Severe leukopenia with infection. *Treatment:* Antibiotic therapy. Monitor hematology.

HOW SUPPLIED
Injection: 2 mg (base)/mL.

DOSAGE
- **IV INFUSION**
  Initial therapy for acute nonlymphocytic leukemia, induction.
Mitoxantrone, 12 mg/m^2/day on days 1–3 combined with cytarabine, 100 mg/m^2 as a continuous 24-hr infusion on days 1–7. If the response is incomplete, a second induction course may be given using the same daily dosage, but giving mitoxantrone for 2 days and cytosine arabinoside for 5 days. *Consolidation therapy, approximately 6 weeks after final induction therapy.* Mitoxantrone, 12 mg/m^2/day on days 1 and 2 combined with cytosine arabinoside, 100 mg/m^2 as a continuous 24-hr infusion on days 1–5. A second consolidation course of therapy may be given 4 weeks after the first.
  Secondary progressive multiple sclerosis.
12 mg/m^2 over 5–15 min q 3 months. Due to the risk of cardiotoxicity, no more than 8–12 doses can be given over 2–3 years (i.e., a cumulative lifetime dose of 140 mg/m^2).
  Hormone-refractory prostate cancer.

12–14 mg/m^2 as a short IV infusion q 21 days.

NURSING CONSIDERATIONS
ADMINISTRATION/STORAGE
IV 1. Do not mix in the same infusion with other drugs.
2. Must be diluted prior to use with at least 50 mL of either D5W or 0.9% NaCl injection.
3. Give diluted solution into a freely running IV infusion of either D5W or 0.9% NaCl slowly over at least 3 min.
4. Avoid extravasation at the injection site. Do not allow contact with the eyes, mucous membranes, or skin.
5. Do not freeze.
6. Closely follow hospital procedures for the handling and disposal of antineoplastic drugs.

ASSESSMENT
1. Note reasons for therapy, other agents trialed, any cardiac disease. Perform baseline ECG; assess for S&S of cardiotoxicity. Evaluate LVEF by echocardiogram or MUGA prior to therapy.
2. Anticipate N&V, mucositis/stomatitis; initiate appropriate protocol. Assess need for allopurinol therapy with rapid tumor lysis.
3. Monitor VS, CBC, uric acid, renal and LFTs. Drug may cause granulocyte and platelet suppression. Nadir: 10–14 days; recovery: 21 days.
4. Do not use in MS clients with an LVEF <50%, in those with a clinically significant reduction in LVEF, or to those who have received a cumulative lifetime dose of >140 mg/m^2.
5. Systemic infections should be treated concomitantly with or just prior to initiating therapy.

CLIENT/FAMILY TEACHING
1. Drug is usually given for 3 days IV with cytosine or other drug therapy; frequent lab tests will be done to evaluate drug effects.
2. May temporarily discolor urine/whites of eyes a greenish blue for 24 hr after therapy. Report any persistent diarrhea, sores in mouth, N&V, abnormal bruising/bleeding, sore throat, severe SOB, swelling of extremities, severe joint pain, or any S&S of infection.

M

---

3. Consume 2–3 L per day of fluids to prevent ↑ uric acid levels.

4. Avoid vaccinia, persons with infections, and crowds, especially during flu season.

5. Practice reliable contraception.

6. May experience hair loss; should regrow.

7. Keep all F/U appointments to evaluate labs, cardiac function and response to therapy.

OUTCOMES/EVALUATE

• Improved hematologic parameters

• Suppression of malignant cell proliferation

Mometasone furoate monohyrate

(moh-**MET**-ah-sohn)

CLASSIFICATION(S):
Glucocorticoid
PREGNANCY CATEGORY: C
Rx: Nasonex.

Mometasone furoate

Rx: Cream, Lotion, Ointment: Elocon. **Powder for Inhalation**: Asmanex Twisthaler.

SEE ALSO *CORTICOSTEROIDS*.

USES

Mometasone furoate monohydrate. Spray: (1) Treatment of the nasal symptoms of seasonal allergic rhinitis and perennial allergic rhinitis in adults and children 2 years and older. (2) Prophylaxis of nasal symptoms of seasonal or perennial allergic rhinitis in adults and adolescents 12 years and older. (3) Treatment of nasal polyps in clients 18 years and older.

Mometasone furoate. Cream, Lotion, Ointment, Topical Solution: Dermatoses. **Powder for Inhalation:** (1) Maintenance treatment of chronic asthma in clients 12 years and older. (2) For asthma clients who require PO corticosteroid therapy, where adding mometasone may reduce or eliminate the need for PO corticosteroids.

ACTION/KINETICS

Action

Anti-inflammatory due to ability to inhibit prostaglandin synthesis. Also inhibits accumulation of macrophages and leukocytes at sites of inflammation as well as to inhibit phagocytosis and lysosomal enzyme release.

Pharmacokinetics

Undetected in plasma although some may be swallowed after use. No effect on adrenal function. Metabolized in the liver by CYP3A4 enzymes. **t½:** 5.8 hr. Excreted in the feces and urine. **Plasma protein binding:** 98–99%.

CONTRAINDICATIONS

Use in those with recent nasal septum ulcers, nasal surgery, or nasal trauma until healing has occurred. Not indicated to relieve acute bronchospasms.

SPECIAL CONCERNS

Use with caution, if at all, in those with active or quiescent tuberculosis infection of the respiratory tract, or in untreated fungal, bacterial, systemic viral infections, or ocular herpes simplex. Use with caution during lactation. Safety and efficacy of Nasonex has not been determined in children less than 2 years of age for use in allergic rhinitis and in children less than 18 years of age to treat nasal polyps.

SIDE EFFECTS

Most Common

For Asmanex: Dry/irritated throat, hoarseness, cough, dry mouth, taste alteration.

For Nasonex: Headache, pharyngitis, epistaxis, nasal burning/irritation.

Respiratory: Pharyngitis, epistaxis, nasal burning/irritation/ulceration, dry/irritated throat, hoarseness, blood-tinged mucus, coughing, URI, sinusitis, rhinitis, asthma, bronchitis. Rarely, nasal ulcers and nasal and oral candidiasis. **GI:** Diarrhea, dyspepsia, nausea, dry mouth, taste alteration. **Miscellaneous:** Headache, viral infection, dysmenorrhea, musculoskeletal pain, arthralgia, chest pain, conjunctivitis, earache, flu-like symptoms, myalgia, increased IOP.

HOW SUPPLIED

Mometasone furoate: *Cream, Lotion, Ointment, Topical Solution:* Each is 0.1%;

Bold Italic = life threatening side effect   ■ = black box warning   ✦ = Available in Canada

Powder for Inhalation: 220 mcg (delivers 200 mcg/actuation of mometasone furoate).

Mometasone furoate monohydrate: *Nasal Spray:* 0.05% (50 mcg/actuation).

DOSAGE

MOMETASONE FUROATE MONOHYDRATE
- **NASAL SPRAY**
  Prophylaxis and treatment of seasonal/perennial allergic rhinitis.

Adults and children over 12 years: 2 sprays (50 mcg in each spray) in each nostril once daily (i.e., total daily dose: 200 mcg). In those with a known seasonal allergen that precipitates seasonal allergic rhinitis, give prophylactically, 200 mcg/day, 2 to 4 weeks prior to the anticipated start of the pollen season.

Children 2–11 years of age: One spray (50 mcg) in each nostril once daily (total daily dose: 100 mcg).

Treatment of nasal polyps.

Adults 18 years and older: 2 sprays (100 mcg) into each nostril twice a day (i.e., total daily dose of 400 mcg). In some, a dose of 2 sprays once daily in each nostril (i.e., total daily dose of 200 mcg) may be effective.

MOMETASONE FUROATE
- **CREAM, LOTION, OINTMENT**
  Dermatoses.

Apply sparingly to affected area(s) 2–4 times per day.

- **TOPICAL SOLUTION**
  Dermatoses.

Apply a few drops to the affected skin once a day; massage lightly until solution disappears.

- **POWDER FOR INHALATION**
  Chronic asthma.

Recommended starting dose, previous therapy of bronchodilators alone or inhaled corticosteroids: 220 mcg once daily in the evening; **highest recommended daily dose:** 440 mcg. **Recommended starting dose, previous therapy of oral corticosteroids:** 440 mcg twice daily; **highest recommended daily dose:** 880 mcg.

NURSING CONSIDERATIONS

ADMINISTRATION/STORAGE

1. Improvement is usually seen within 11 hours to 2 days after the first dose. Maximum benefit: Within 1 to 2 weeks.

2. Giving mometasone by the orally inhaled route will result in a variable time to onset and degree of symptom relief.

3. Store nasal spray from 2–25°C (36–77°F) protected from light. Avoid prolonged exposure to direct light when removed from cardboard container.

4. Store inhaler in a dry place from 15–30°C (59–86°F).

ASSESSMENT

1. Note onset, duration, and characteristics of S&S. Assess EENT and describe clinical presentation.

2. Attempt to identify triggers with seasonal allergy and asthma.

CLIENT/FAMILY TEACHING

1. Shake nasal spray well before using. Review enclosed instructions for proper use.

2. Prior to initial use, prime the pump by actuating ten times or until a fine spray appears.

3. The pump may be stored, unused, for up to 1 week without repriming. If more than one week has elapsed between use, reprime by actuating 2 times, or until a fine spray appears.

4. Use regularly as directed. Do not increase dose/frequency; does not increase effectiveness. A spacer facilitates oral inhaler administration.

5. Protect nasal spray from sunlight.

6. Discard oral inhaler 45 days after opening the foil pouch or when the dose counter reads '00,' whichever comes first.

7. When using oral inhaler, inhale deeply and rapidly and hold breath for about 10 seconds, or as long as possible. Do not breathe out through the inhaler. Rinse mouth/equipment after inhalation use.

8. Do not spray into the eyes or directly onto the nasal septum. If on immunosuppressant doses of corticosteroids, avoid exposure to chickenpox or measles, and report if exposed.

9. Identify triggers and practice avoidance. Report if condition does not improve or worsens after 3–5 days of therapy.

OUTCOMES/EVALUATE

- Prophylaxis/relief of allergic rhinitis

M

- Control of asthma S&S
- Clearing of skin lesions

Montelukast sodium ©

(mon-teh-**LOO**-kast)

CLASSIFICATION(S):
Antiasthmatic, leukotriene receptor antagonist
PREGNANCY CATEGORY: B
Rx: Singulair.

USES
(1) Prophylaxis and chronic treatment of asthma in adults and children 12 months of age and older. (2) Relief of symptoms of seasonal allergic rhinitis in adults and children 2 years of age and older. (3) Relief of symptoms of perennial allergic rhinitis in adults and children 6 months of age and older. (4) Prevention of exercise-induced bronchoconstriction in clients 15 years of age and older. *Investigational:* Chronic urticaria. Atopic dermatitis.

ACTION/KINETICS
Action
Cysteinyl leukotrienes and leukotriene receptor occupation are associated with symptoms of asthma, including airway edema, smooth muscle contraction, and inflammation. Montelukast binds with cysteinyl leukotriene receptors thus preventing the action of cysteinyl leukotrienes.

Pharmacokinetics
Rapidly absorbed after PO use. **Time to peak levels:** 3–4 hr for 10 mg tablet, 2–2.5 hr for 5 mg tablet, and 2 hr for the 4 mg chewable tablet. The 4 mg oral granule formulation is bioequivalent to the 4 mg chewable tablet. Metabolized extensively in the liver by cytochromes CYP3A4 and CYP2C9; mainly excreted in feces. **t½:** 2.7–5.5 hr for healthy, young adults. **Plasma protein binding:** More than 99%.

CONTRAINDICATIONS
Use to reverse bronchospasm in acute asthma attacks, including status asthmaticus. Use to abruptly substitute for inhaled or oral corticosteroids. Use as monotherapy to treat and manage exercise-induced bronchospasm. Use with known aspirin or NSAID sensitivity.

SPECIAL CONCERNS
Use with caution during lactation. Safety and efficacy in children less than 12 months of age with asthma, 2 years of age and younger with seasonal allergic rhinitis, 6 months of age with perennial allergic rhinitis, or 15 years of age and younger with exercise-induced bronchoconstriction have not been determined.

SIDE EFFECTS
Most Common
Adults and adolescents 15 years and older: Headache, cough, abdominal pain, influenza, dyspepsia, dizziness, asthenia/fatigue, dental pain.
Adolescents and adults aged 15 and older: GI: Dyspepsia, infectious gastroenteritis, abdominal pain, dental pain. **CNS:** Headache, dizziness, somnolence. **Body as a whole:** Asthenia, fatigue, fever, trauma. **Respiratory:** Influenza, cough, nasal congestion, URTI, epistaxis, sinus headache, sinusitis. **Dermatologic:** Rash. **Miscellaneous:** Pyuria.
Children, aged 6 to 14 years: GI: Nausea, diarrhea, dyspepsia, gastroenteritis, tooth infection. **CNS:** Headache. **Otic:** Otitis media. **Respiratory:** Pharyngitis, laryngitis, sinusitis, infective rhinitis, acute bronchitis, URTI. **Dermatologic:** Atopic dermatitis, skin infection, varicella. **Miscellaneous:** Viral infection, influenza, fever, myopia, eosinophilic conditions consistent with Churg-Strauss syndrome.
Children, aged 2 to 5 years: Respiratory: Rhinorrhea, cough, sinusitis, pneumonia, pharyngitis, URTI. **GI:** Abdominal pain, diarrhea, gastroenteritis. **CNS:** Headache. **Dermatologic:** Rash, urticaria, eczema, varicella, dermatitis. **Otic:** Otitis media, ear pain. **Miscellaneous:** Fever, influenza, conjunctivitis.
Children, aged 12 to 23 months: Respiratory: URTI, wheezing, pharyngitis, tonsillitis, rhinitis, cough. **Otic:** Otitis media.

Bold Italic = life threatening side effect   ■ = black box warning   ♣ = Available in Canada

Postmarketing side effects: CNS: Dream abnormalities, hallucinations, drowsiness, irritability, agitation (including aggressive behavior and tremor), restlessness, insomnia, *seizures (very rare)*, paresthesia, hypesthesia. **GI:** N&V, dyspepsia, diarrhea, *pancreatitis (very rare)*. **Hepatic:** Cholestatic jaundice, hepatocellular liver injury, mixed-pattern liver injury. **Hypersensitivity:** Urticaria, pruritus, angioedema, *anaphylaxis*, hepatic eosinophilic infiltration (very rare). **Musculoskeletal:** Arthralgia; myalgia, including muscle cramps. **Miscellaneous:** Increased bleeding tendency, systemic eosinophilia, vasculitis (consistent with Churg-Strauss syndrome), palpitations, edema, bruising.

LABORATORY TEST CONSIDERATIONS
↑ ALT, AST.

OD OVERDOSE MANAGEMENT
Symptoms: In children, symptoms include thirst, somnolence, mydriasis, hyperkinesia, abdominal pain. *Treatment:* Usual supportive measures, including removing unabsorbed drug from GI tract and clinical monitoring.

DRUG INTERACTIONS
Phenobarbital / ↓ Montelukast plasma levels → ↓ effect
Prednisone / ↑ Prednisone adverse effects (e.g., edema)
Rifampin / ↓ Montelukast plasma levels → ↓ effect

HOW SUPPLIED
Granules, Oral: 4 mg/packet; *Tablets:* 10 mg; *Tablets, Chewable:* 4 mg, 5 mg.

DOSAGE
- **TABLETS**
  Asthma, Seasonal/perennial allergic rhinitis, Prophylaxis of exercise-induced bronchoconstriction.

Adolescents and adults age 15 years and older: One 10 mg tablet once daily (in the evening for asthma; anytime for allergic rhinits). To prevent exercise-induced bronchoconstriction, take at least 2 hr before exercise. An additional dose is not to be taken within 24 hr of a previous dose.
- **GRANULES; TABLETS, CHEWABLE**
  Asthma, Seasonal/perennial allergic rhinitis.

Pediatric clients aged 6 to 14 years: One 5 mg chewable tablet once daily (in the evening for asthma; anytime for allergic rhinitis). **Pediatric clients aged 2 to 5 years:** One 4 mg chewable tablet or one 4 mg oral granule packet taken once daily (in the evening for asthma; anytime for allergic rhinitis).
- **GRANULES**
  Asthma.

Children 12–23 months of age: One packet of 4 mg granules once daily in the evening.
  Perennial allergic rhinits.
Children, 6–23 months of age: 1 packet of 4 mg daily.

NURSING CONSIDERATIONS
℞ Do not confuse Singulair with Sinequan (doxepin, a tricyclic antidepressant).

ADMINISTRATION/STORAGE
1. Take daily as prescribed, even when symptom free. Contact provider if asthma is not well controlled.
2. The 4 and 5 mg chewable tablets contain phenylalanine (a component of aspartame).
3. Do not abruptly substitute montelukast for inhaled or oral corticosteroids.
4. Store all tablets at room temperature; protect from moisture and light.

ASSESSMENT
1. List reasons for therapy, onset, triggers, characteristics of disease, assess EENT and note findings. List other agents trialed, outcome.
2. Review other agents prescribed for asthma; identify which should be continued.
3. Do not use with aspirin or NSAID allergy.
4. Document LFTs, lung assessments, PFTs, and x-rays.
5. Chewable 5 mg tablet contains 0.842 mg of phenylalanine and 4 mg tablet contains 0.674 mg phenylalanine; not to be used with phenylketonurics.
6. Assist to identify and eliminate/minimize triggers.

CLIENT/FAMILY TEACHING
1. Take once daily in evening for asthma; for seasonal allergic rhinitis, the time of administration can be individu-

M

alized. For those with combined asthma and seasonal allergic rhinitis, give one tablet daily in the evening. Granules can be given directly in the mouth or mixed with a spoonful of cold or room-temperature food such as applesauce, carrots, rice, or ice cream. Do not open packet until ready to use. The full dose must be given within 15 min. Do not store drug mixed with food. Oral granules are not intended to be dissolved in liquid. Granules can be given without regard to meals; may take with food to decrease stomach upset.

2. Those taking montelukast, 1 tablet daily, for another indication (including chronic asthma) should not take an additional dose to prevent exercise-induced bronchoconstriction. Have a short-acting beta agonist available for rescue.

3. Continue drug during acute attacks as well as during symptom free periods.

4. Use short-acting prescribed β-agonist inhalers to treat acute asthma attacks. Report if increased use/frequency of inhalers needed for symptom control.

5. Continue other prescribed antiasthma medications during this therapy.

6. With exercise-induced asthma, continue to use prescribed inhaler for prophylaxis.

7. Report unusual side effects, changes in disease, or significant drop in peak flow readings.

8. Notify provider if pregnancy suspected or planned.

9. Ensure that environment assessed for triggers and that appropriate steps taken to minimize or avoid exposures.

10. Inform parents of phenylketonuric clients that both the 4 and 5 mg chewable tablets contain phenylalanine.

11. Keep all follow up appointments to evaluate respiratory status and response to therapy.

OUTCOMES/EVALUATE

- Asthma prophylaxis; ↑ FEV_1
- Control of seasonal allergies

Moricizine hydrochloride
(mor-**IS**-ih-zeen)

CLASSIFICATION(S):
Antiarrhythmic, Class IA
PREGNANCY CATEGORY: B
Rx: Ethmozine.

SEE ALSO ANTIARRHYTHMIC DRUGS.

USES

Documented life-threatening ventricular arrhythmias (e.g., sustained VT) where benefits of the drug are determined to outweigh the risks. *Investigational:* Ventricular premature contractions, couplets, and nonsustained VT.

ACTION/KINETICS

Action

Causes a stabilizing effect on the myocardial membranes as well as local anesthetic activity. Shortens phase II and III repolarization leading to a decreased duration of the action potential and an effective refractory period. Also, there is a decrease in the maximum rate of phase O depolarization and a prolongation of AV conduction in clients with ventricular tachycardia. Whether the client is at rest or is exercising, has minimal effects on cardiac index, stroke volume, systemic or pulmonary vascular resistance or ejection fraction, and pulmonary capillary wedge pressure. There is a small increase in resting BP and HR. The time, course, and intensity of antiarrhythmic and electrophysiologic effects are not related to plasma levels of the drug.

Pharmacokinetics

Onset: 2 hr. **Peak plasma levels:** 30–120 min. $t\frac{1}{2}$: 1.5–3.5 hr (reduced after multiple dosing). **Duration:** 10–24 hr. Significant first-pass effect. Metabolized almost completely by the liver with metabolites excreted through both the urine and feces; the drug induces its own metabolism. Food delays the rate of absorption resulting in lower peak plasma levels; however, the total amount absorbed is not changed. **Plasma protein binding: 95%.**

CONTRAINDICATIONS

Preexisting second- or third-degree block, right bundle branch block when associated with bifascicular block (unless the client has a pacemaker), cardiogenic shock. Lactation.

SPECIAL CONCERNS

There is the possibility of increased risk of death when used in clients with non-life-threatening cardiac arrhythmias. Safety and effectiveness in children less than 18 years of age have not been determined. Geriatric clients have a higher rate of side effects. Increased survival rates following use of antiarrhythmic drugs have not been proven in clients with ventricular arrhythmias. Use with caution in clients with sick sinus syndrome due to the possibility of sinus bradycardia, sinus pause, or sinus arrest. Use with caution in clients with CHF.

SIDE EFFECTS

Most Common

Palpitations, dizziness, headache, fatigue, nausea, dyspnea.

CV: *Proarrhythmias, including new rhythm disturbances or worsening of existing arrhythmias*; ECG abnormalities, including conduction defects, sinus pause, junctional rhythm, AV block; palpitations, *sustained VT*, cardiac chest pain, CHF, *cardiac death*, hypotension, hypertension, atrial fibrillation, atrial flutter, syncope, bradycardia, *cardiac arrest, MI, pulmonary embolism*, vasodilation, thrombophlebitis, *cerebrovascular events*. **CNS:** Dizziness, anxiety, headache, fatigue, nervousness, paresthesias, sleep disorders, tremor, hypoesthesias, depression, euphoria, somnolence, agitation, confusion, *seizures*, hallucinations, loss of memory, vertigo, coma. **GI:** Nausea, dry mouth, abdominal pain, vomiting, diarrhea, dyspepsia, anorexia, ileus, flatulence, dysphagia, bitter taste. **Musculoskeletal:** Asthenia, abnormal gait, akathisia, ataxia, abnormal coordination, dyskinesia, pain. **GU:** Urinary retention, dysuria, urinary incontinence, urinary frequency, impotence, kidney pain, decreased libido.

Respiratory: Dyspnea, apnea, asthma, hyperventilation, pharyngitis, cough, sinusitis. **Ophthalmic:** Nystagmus, diplopia, blurred vision, eye pain, periorbital edema. **Dermatologic:** Rash, pruritus, dry skin, urticaria. **Miscellaneous:** Sweating, drug fever, hypothermia, temperature intolerance, swelling of the lips and tongue, speech disorder, tinnitus, jaundice.

LABORATORY TEST CONSIDERATIONS

↑ Bilirubin and liver transaminases.

OD OVERDOSE MANAGEMENT

Symptoms: Vomiting, hypotension, lethargy, worsening of CHF, *MI, conduction disturbances, arrhythmias (e.g., junctional bradycardia, VT, ventricular fibrillation, asystole), sinus arrest, respiratory failure.* *Treatment:* In acute overdose, induce vomiting, taking care to prevent aspiration. Hospitalize and closely monitor for cardiac, respiratory, and CNS changes. Provide life support, including an intracardiac pacing catheter, if necessary.

DRUG INTERACTIONS

Cimetidine / ↑ Plasma moricizine levels R/T ↓ excretion
Digoxin / Additive prolongation of the PR interval (but no significant increase in the rate of second- or third-degree AV block)
Propranolol / Additive prolongation of the PR interval
Theophylline / ↓ Plasma theophylline levels R/T ↑ rate of clearance

HOW SUPPLIED

Tablets: 200 mg, 250 mg, 300 mg.

DOSAGE

- **TABLETS**
  Antiarrhythmic.

Adults: 600–900 mg/day in equally divided doses q 8 hr. If needed, the dose can be increased in increments of 150 mg/day at 3-day intervals until the desired effect is obtained. In clients with hepatic or renal impairment, the initial dose should be 600 mg or less with close monitoring and dosage adjustment.

M

NURSING CONSIDERATIONS

ADMINISTRATION/STORAGE

1. When transferring clients from other antiarrhythmics to moricizine, withdraw the previous drug for one to two plasma half-lives before starting moricizine. For example, when transferring from quinidine or disopyramide, moricizine can be started 6–12 hr after the last dose; when transferring from procainamide, moricizine can be initiated 3–6 hr after the last dose; when transferring from mexiletine, propafenone, or tocainide, start 8–12 hr after the last dose; and, when transferring from flecainide, start moricizine 12–24 hr after the last dose.

2. If clients are well controlled on an 8-hr regimen, they might be given the same total daily dose q 12 hr to increase compliance.

ASSESSMENT

1. Note cardiac history, preexisting conditions, ECG abnormalities requiring treatment.

2. Monitor VS (report any persistent temp elevations) ECG, lytes, CXR, PFTs, renal and LFTs; correct any electrolyte disturbances, reduce dose with liver/renal dysfunction.

3. Monitor cardiac rhythm closely for drug-induced rhythm disturbances.

4. Antiarrhythmic response may be determined by ECG, exercise testing, or programmed electrical stimulation testing and used as a guide to dosage adjustment. Assess pacing parameters with pacemakers.

CLIENT/FAMILY TEACHING

1. Drug is used to terminate life-threatening ventricular arrhythmias.

2. Take before meals; food delays rate of absorption.

3. Drug may cause dizziness. Use care when rising from a lying or sitting position. Report any unusual or adverse effects.

4. Advise family member or significant other to learn CPR.

OUTCOMES/EVALUATE

Termination of life-threatening ventricular arrhythmias

Morphine sulfate

(**MOR**-feen **SUL**-fayt)

CLASSIFICATION(S):

Narcotic analgesic

PREGNANCY CATEGORY: C

Rx: Capsules, Extended-Release Pellets: Avinza, Kadian. **Injection**: Astramorph PF, Duramorph, Infumorph 200 and 500, Morphine Sulfate in 5% Dextrose. **Injection, Extended-Release Liposomal**: DepoDur. **Oral Solution**: MSIR, Roxanol, Roxanol 100, Roxanol T. **Rectal Suppository**: RMS. **Tablets, Controlled-Release**: MS Contin, Oramorph SR, **C-II**

♣**Rx:** M-Eslon, M.O.S.-Sulfate, Morphine HP, Morphine LP Epidural, Statex, ratio-Morphine SR.

SEE ALSO *NARCOTIC ANALGESICS.*

USES

Oral: (1) Immediate-Release (IR) tablets/solution: Relief of moderate to severe pain. (2) Controlled-/Extended-/Sustained-Release Tablets: Relief of moderate to severe pain in those requiring continuous, around-the-clock opioid therapy for an extended period of time. Not indicated for use as an as-needed analgesic.

IV: (1) Relief of severe pain (MI, severe injuries, severe chronic pain associated with terminal cancer after all non-narcotic analgesics have failed). (2) Preoperatively for sedation and to reduce apprehension. (3) Facilitate induction of anesthesia and reduce anesthetic dose. (4) Control postoperative pain. (5) Relieve anxiety and reduce left ventricular work by reducing preload pressure. (6) Treat dyspnea associated with acute left ventricular failure and pulmonary edema. (7) Anesthesia for open-heart surgery.

SC, IM: (1) Relief of moderate to severe pain. (2) Reduce preoperative apprehension and produce sedation. (3) Control postoperative pain. (4) Supplement to anesthesia. (5) Analgesia dur-

Color Photo Quick Reference Guide

This color photo quick reference guide provides rapid identification of 74 most commonly prescribed drugs. Actual-sized tablets and capsules, with their strength, are organized alphabetically by generic name and include appropriate trade name and manufacturer.

ALENDRONATE SODIUM
Fosamax
MERCK

10 mg

Rx

AMLODIPINE
Norvasc
PFIZER

10 mg

Rx

AMLODIPINE BESYLATE AND BENAZEPRIL HYDROCHLORIDE
Lotrel
NOVARTIS

2.5 mg/10 mg

5 mg/10 mg

Rx

AMPHETAMINE MIXTURES
Adderall
SHIRE

10 mg

Rx   C-II

Adderall XR
SHIRE

5 mg

10 mg

20 mg

Rx   C-II

ARIPIPRAZOLE
Abilify
BRISTOL-MYERS SQUIBB

30 mg

Rx

ATORVASTATIN CALCIUM
Lipitor
PFIZER

10 mg

20 mg

40 mg

Rx

BUPROPION HYDROCHLORIDE
Wellbutrin XL
GLAXOSMITHKLINE

300 mg

Rx

BUTALBITAL, ACETAMINOPHEN AND CAFFEINE
Fioricet
WATSON

50 mg/325 mg/40 mg

Rx

CANDESARTAN CILEXETIL
Atacand
ASTRAZENECA LP

16 mg

32 mg

Rx

CARVEDILOL
Coreg
GLAXOSMITHKLINE

25 mg

Rx

CEFDINIR
Omnicef
ABBOTT

300 mg

Rx

CELECOXIB
Celebrex
PFIZER

100 mg

200 mg

Rx

CITALOPRAM HYDROBROMIDE
Celexa
FOREST

40 mg

Rx

CLONAZEPAM
Klonopin
ROCHE

1 mg

Rx   C-IV

CLOPIDOGREL BISULFATE
Plavix
BRISTOL-MYERS SQUIBB

75 mg

Rx

CYCLOBENZAPRINE HYDROCHLORIDE
Flexeril
ORTHO-MCNEIL

5 mg

Rx

DESLORATADINE
Clarinex
SCHERING-PLOUGH

5 mg

Rx

DIGOXIN
Lanoxin
GLAXOSMITHKLINE

0.125 mg

Rx

DULOXETINE HYDROCHLORIDE
Cymbalta
ELI LILLY

20 mg

60 mg

Rx

ESCITALOPRAM OXALATE
Lexapro
FOREST

10 mg

20 mg

Rx

ESOMEPRAZOLE MAGNESIUM
Nexium
ASTRAZENECA LP

40 mg

Rx

ESTROGENS, CONJUGATED
Premarin
WYETH

0.625 mg

Rx

EZETIMIBE
Zetia
MERCK/SCHERING-PLOUGH

10 mg

Rx

EZETIMIBE AND SIMVASTATIN
Vytorin
MERCK/SCHERING-PLOUGH

10 mg/20 mg

10 mg/40 mg

10 mg/80 mg

Rx

FENOFIBRATE
Tricor
ABBOTT LABORATORIES

145 mg

Rx

FEXOFENADINE HYDROCHLORIDE AND PSEUDOEPHEDRINE HYDROCHLORIDE
Allegra D
SANOFI-AVENTIS

60 mg/120 mg

308
AV

180 mg/240 mg

Rx

FUROSEMIDE
Lasix
SANOFI-AVENTIS

40 mg

Rx

GABAPENTIN
Neurontin
PFIZER

300 mg

Rx

GLIMEPIRIDE
Amaryl
SANOFI-AVENTIS

2 mg

Rx

IBANDRONATE SODIUM
Boniva
ROCHE

150 mg

Rx

IRBESARTAN
Avapro
BRISTOL-MYERS SQUIBB

150 mg

Rx

IRBESARTAN AND HYDROCHLOROTHIAZIDE
Avalide
BRISTOL-MYERS SQUIBB

150 mg/12.5 mg

Rx

LAMOTRIGINE
Lamictal
GLAXOSMITHKLINE

100 mg

150 mg

200 mg

Rx

LANSOPRAZOLE
Prevacid
TAP

30 mg

Rx

LEVOFLOXACIN
Levaquin
ORTHO MCNEIL

250 mg

500 mg

750 mg

Rx

LOSARTAN POTASSIUM
Cozaar
MERCK

50 mg

Rx

LOSARTAN POTASSIUM AND HYDROCHLOROTHIAZIDE
Hyzaar
MERCK

50 mg/12.5 mg

100 mg/25 mg

Rx

MELOXICAM
Mobic
BOEHRINGER INGELHEIM

7.5 mg

Rx

MEMANTINE HYDROCHLORIDE
Namenda
FOREST

10 mg

Rx

METFORMIN HYDROCHLORIDE
Glucophage
BRISTOL-MYERS SQUIBB

1000 mg

Rx

MOXIFLOXACIN HYDROCHLORIDE
Avelox
SCHERING

400 mg

Rx

NIFEDIPINE
Procardia XL
PFIZER

30 mg

60 mg

Rx

OLANZAPINE
Zyprexa
ELI LILLY

5 mg

10 mg

15 mg

Rx

OLMESARTAN MEDOXOMIL
Benicar
DAIICHI-SANYKO

20 mg

Rx

OLMESARTAN MEDOXOMIL AND HYDROCHLOROTHIAZIDE
Benicar HCT
DAIICHI-SANYKO

20 mg/12.5 mg

Rx

OMEPRAZOLE
Prilosec
ASTRAZENECA LP

40 mg

Rx

OXCARBAZEPINE
Trileptal
NOVARTIS

600 mg

Rx

PANTOPRAZOLE SODIUM
Protonix
WYETH

40 mg

Rx

PAROXETINE HYDROCHLORIDE
Paxil CR
GLAXOSMITHKLINE

25 mg

37.5 mg

Rx

PIOGLITAZONE HYDROCHLORIDE
Actos
TAKEDA

15 mg

30 mg

45 mg

Rx

PRAVASTATIN SODIUM
Pravachol
BRISTOL-MYERS SQUIBB

40 mg

80 mg

Rx

PREGABALIN
Lyrica
PFIZER

75 mg

100 mg

Rx   C-V

QUETIAPINE FUMARATE
Seroquel
ASTRAZENECA LP

200 mg

Rx

RABEPRAZOLE SODIUM
Aciphex
EISAI

20 mg

Rx

RALOXIFENE HYDROCHLORIDE
Evista
ELI LILLY

60 mg

Rx

RAMIPRIL
Altace
KING

5 mg

Rx

RISPERIDONE
Risperdal
JANSSEN L.P.

3 mg

4 mg

Rx

ROPINIROLE HYDROCHLORIDE
Requip
GLAXOSMITHKLINE

1 mg

2 mg

3 mg

Rx

ROSIGLITAZONE MALEATE
Avandia
GLAXOSMITHKLINE

2 mg

Rx

ROSUVASTATIN CALCIUM
Crestor
ASTRAZENECA LP

10 mg

20 mg

Rx

SERTRALINE HYDROCHLORIDE
Zoloft
PFIZER

25 mg

50 mg

Rx

SILDENAFIL CITRATE
Viagra
PFIZER

50 mg

100 mg

Rx

TADALAFIL
Cialis
ELI LILLY

10 mg

20 mg

Rx

TAMSULOSIN HYDROCHLORIDE
Flomax
BOEHRINGER INGELHEIM

0.4 mg

Rx

TOLTERODINE TARTRATE
Detrol LA
PHARMACIA/UPJOHN

4 mg

Rx

TOPIRAMATE
Topomax
ORTHO-MCNEIL

100 mg

Rx

TRAMADOL HYDROCHLORIDE
Ultram
ORTHO-MCNEIL

50 mg

Rx

TRAMADOL HYDROCHLORIDE AND ACETAMINOPHEN
Ultracet
ORTHO-MCNEIL

37.5 mg/325 mg

Rx

VALACYCLOVIR HYDROCHLORIDE
Valtrex
GLAXOSMITHKLINE

500 mg

1 gram

Rx

VALSARTAN
Diovan
NOVARTIS

80 mg

Rx

VALSARTAN AND HYDROCHLOROTHIAZIDE
Diovan HCT
NOVARTIS

160 mg/25 mg

160 mg/12.5 mg

Rx

VARDENAFIL HYDROCHLORIDE
Levitra
SCHERING

20 mg

Rx

VENLAFAXINE HYDROCHLORIDE
Effexor XR
WYETH

37.5 mg

75 mg

150 mg

Rx

ZOLPIDEM TARTRATE
Ambien
SANOFI-AVENTIS

10 mg

Rx   C-IV

Ambien CR
SANOFI-AVENTIS

6.25 mg

12.5 mg

Rx   C-IV

ing labor. (6) Acute pulmonary edema. (7) Allay anxiety.

Epidural, Intrathecal: (1) Management of pain not responsive to nonnarcotic analgesics. (2) Treat intractable chronic pain (Infumorph only).

ER Epidural: Treatment of pain following major surgery. Is a liposomal preparation for single-dose administration by the epidural route, at the lumbar level. Is given prior to surgery or after clamping the umbilical cord during cesarean section.

Rectal: Severe acute and chronic pain.

Investigational: Combined with gabapentin to treat diabetic neuropathy or postherpetic neuralgia.

ACTION/KINETICS

Action

Morphine is the prototype for opiate analgesics. Morphine combines with specific receptors located in the CNS to produce various effects. The mechanism is believed to involve decreased permeability of the cell membrane to sodium, which results in diminished transmission of pain impulses and therefore analgesia.

Pharmacokinetics

Onset, IM/SC:10–30 min. **Peak effect, PO:** 60 min; **epidural:** 10–15 min. **Duration, SC:** 4–5 hr. **t½, elimination:** 1.5–2 hr. Oral morphine is only one-third to one-sixth as effective as parenteral products. Metabolized in the liver by glucuronidation. Excreted in the urine.

ADDITIONAL CONTRAINDICATIONS

Epidural or intrathecal morphine: If infection is present at injection site; with anticoagulant therapy; bleeding diathesis; if client has received parenteral corticosteroids within the past 2 weeks. **Morphine injection:** Heart failure secondary to chronic lung disease, cardiac arrhythmias, brain tumor, acute alcoholism, delirium tremens, convulsive states. **Immediate-release oral solution of morphine:** Respiratory insufficiency, severe CNS depression, heart failure secondary to chronic lung disease, cardiac arrhythmias, increased intracranial or CSF pressure, head injuries, brain tumor, acute alcoholism, de-

lirium tremens, after biliary tract surgery, suspected surgical abdomen, convulsive disorders, surgical anastomosis, with MAO inhibitors or within 14 days of these drugs.

SPECIAL CONCERNS

■ (1) Avinza: These capsules are a modified-release formulation of morphine indicated for once daily administration for relief of moderate to severe pain requiring continuous, around-the-clock opioid therapy for an extended period of time. Avinza capsules are to be swallowed whole or the contents of the capsules sprinkled on applesauce. The capsule beads are not to be chewed, crushed, or dissolved because of the risk of rapid release and absorption of a potentially fatal dose of morphine. (2) Morphine release is increased when Avinza capsules are exposed to ethanol. Clients must not use prescription or nonprescription medications containing alcohol while on Avinza therapy. Consumption of alcohol while taking Avinza may result in the rapid release and absorption of a potentially fatal dose of morphine. (3) Kadian. Morphine has an abuse liability similar to other opioid analgesics. Morphine can be abused in a manner similar to other opioid agonists, legal or illicit. Consider this when prescribing or dispensing Kadian in situations in which the health care provider or pharmacist is concerned about an increased risk of misuse, abuse, or diversion. (4) Kadian capsules are an extended-release oral formulation of morphine indicated for the management of moderate to severe pain requiring a continuous, around-the-clock opioid analgesic for an extended period of time. (5) Kadian capsules are NOT for use as an as-needed analgesic. Kadian 100 and 200 mg capsules are for use in opioid-tolerant clients only. Ingestion of these capsules or of the pellets within the capsules may cause fatal respiratory depression when administered to clients not already tolerant to high doses of opioids. Kadian capsules are to be swallowed whole or the contents of the capsules sprinkled on applesauce. The pellets in the capsules are not to be chewed, crushed, or dissolved because of the risk of rapid release and absorption of a potentially fatal dose of morphine. (6) Astromorph PF, Duramorph, Infumorph: Because of the risk of severe adverse effects when the epidural or intrathecal route of administration is employed, clients must be observed in a fully equipped and staffed environment for at least 24 hr after the initial dose. (7) Infumorph: Is not recommended for single-dose IV, IM, or SC administration because of the very large amount of morphine in the ampule and the associated risk of overdosage.■ May increase the length of labor. Clients with known seizure disorders may be at greater risk for morphine-induced seizure activity. Respiratory depression may be delayed up to 24 hr after epidural or intrathecal use. Use with extreme caution in aged or debilitated clients; lower doses are usually satisfactory.

SIDE EFFECTS

Most Common

N&V, constipation, somnolence, headache.

See *Narcotic Analgesics* for a complete list of possible side effects.

ADDITIONAL DRUG INTERACTIONS

Amitriptyline / ↑ CNS and respiratory depression

Cimetidine / ↑ CNS and respiratory depression

Clomipramine / ↑ CNS and respiratory depression

Nortriptyline / ↑ CNS and respiratory depression

Smoking / ↓ Analgesia R/T ↑ hepatic metabolism; takes several weeks to occur

Warfarin / ↑ Warfarin anticoagulant effect

HOW SUPPLIED

Capsules, Extended-Release Pellets: 10 mg, 20 mg, 30 mg, 50 mg, 60 mg, 80 mg, 90 mg, 100 mg, 120 mg, 200 mg; *Injection:* 0.5 mg/mL, 1 mg/mL, 2 mg/mL, 4 mg/mL, 5 mg/mL, 8 mg/mL, 10 mg/mL, 15 mg/mL, 25 mg/mL, 50 mg/mL; 1 mg/mL in 5% Dextrose; *Injection, Extended-Release Liposomal:* 10 mg/mL; *Oral Solution:* 10 mg/5 mL, 20 mg/mL (concentrate), 20 mg/5 mL, 100 mg/5 mL (concentrate); *Suppository, Rectal:* 5 mg, 10 mg, 20 mg, 30 mg; *Tablets:* 15 mg, 30 mg; *Tablets for Injection, Soluble:* 10 mg, 15 mg, 30 mg; *Tablets, Controlled-Release:* 15 mg, 30 mg, 60 mg, 100 mg, 200 mg; *Tablets, Extended-Release:* 15 mg, 30 mg, 60 mg, 100 mg, 200 mg.

DOSAGE

• **ORAL SOLUTION; TABLETS; TABLETS, SOLUBLE**

Analgesia.

5–30 mg (solution or tablets) on a regularly scheduled basis q 4 hr at the lowest dosage level that will achieve adequate analgesia.

• **CAPSULES, EXTENDED-RELEASE PELLETS**

Analgesia.

Avinza. Initial, no proven opioid tolerance: 30 mg once daily (at 24-hour intervals). Increase the dose conservatively in these clients; adjust the dose in increments not greater than 30 mg q 4 days. Some degree of tolerance may develop requiring a dosage adjustment until a balance is reached between analgesia and opioid side effects. If necessary, increase the total daily dose until pain relief is reached or clinically significant opioid-related side effects occur. If breakthrough pain occurs, Avinza may be supplemented with a small dose (5–15% of the total daily dose of morphine) of a short-acting analgesic.

Limit the daily dose of Avinza to a maximum of 1,600 mg; doses over 1,600 mg/day contain an amount of fumaric acid that has not been shown to be safe and may cause serious renal toxicity. The 60, 90, and 120 mg capsules are for use only in opioid-tolerant clients. All doses are intended to be given once daily.

Kadian. Initial: 20 mg daily in clients who do not have a proven tolerance to opioids. The first dose may be taken with the last dose of any immediate-release morphine product because of the long delay until the peak effect occurs with Kadian. Increase the dose at a rate of up to 20 mg every other day. Individualize dosage. The 100 mg and 200 mg

---

capsules are for use only in opioid-tolerant clients.

Give one-half of the estimated daily PO morphine dose q 12 hr (twice a day) or give the total daily PO morphine dose q 24 hr (once a day). To avoid accumulation, do not reduce the dosing interval below 12 hr. Titrate the dose no more frequently than every other day to allow clients to stabilize before escalating the dose. If breakthrough pain occurs, the dose of Kadian may be supplemented with a small dose (less than 20% of the total daily dose) of a short-acting analgesic.

Clients who are excessively sedated after a once-daily dose of Kadian or who regularly experience inadequate analgesia before the next dose should be switched to a twice-daily dose. Most clients will rapidly develop some degree of tolerance, requiring adjustment of dosage until a balance between baseline analgesia and opioid side effects have occurred. Increase the total daily dose of Kadian until the desired therapeutic end point is reached or clinically significant opioid-related side effects occur.

- **TABLETS, CONTROLLED-RELEASE; TABLETS, EXTENDED-RELEASE**
  Analgesia.

Titrate first to analgesia using an immediate-release product dosing q 4–6 hr. Transfer to a long-acting controlled- or extended-release product in either of 2 ways. (1) Give one-half the total 24-hr PO morphine dose as MS Contin or Oramorph SR q 12 hr or (2) Give one-third of the client's 24-hr requirement using MS Contin on an every 8-hr schedule. Use the 15 mg extended-release MS Contin tablet for initial conversion if the client's total daily requirement is expected to be less than 60 mg. The 30 mg extended-release product of Oramorph SR is recommended for those with a daily morphine requirement of 60 to 120 mg. When the total daily dose is expected to be greater than 120 mg, the appropriate tablet strength should be used. The MS Contin 200 mg tablet is only for narcotic-tolerant clients requiring daily morphine equivalent doses of 400 mg or more.

- **IM; SC**
  Analgesia.

Adults: 10 mg (range: 5–20 mg)/70 kg q 4 hr as needed. **Pediatric:** 0.1–0.2 mg/kg q 4 hr, up to a maximum of 15 mg/dose. For analgesia during labor, 10 mg is the usual dose. If using soluble tablets, prepare in sterile water and filter through a 0.22 micron membrane filter. For analgesia: **Adults:** 10 mg/70 kg body weight (range, 5–20 mg); **children:** 0.1–0.2 mg/kg (maximum dose: 15 mg). For preanesthetic medication: **Adults:** 10 mg (range: 5–20 mg)/70 kg body weight; **children, 1 year of age and older:** 0.1 mg/kg, up to a maximum dose of 10 mg.

- **IV**
  Analgesia.

Adults: 2–10 mg/70 kg. A strength of 2.5–15 mg can be used in 4–5 mL of water for injection (administer slowly over 4–5 min).

Relief of pain and as a preanesthetic.

Adult, usual: 10 mg q 4 hr, depending on the severity of the condition and the client response. Individual dose range: 5–15 mg; usual daily dose range: 12–120 mg. **Children (as an analgesic):** 50–100 micrograms/kg (0.05—0.1 mg/kg) given very slowly, not exceed 10 mg/dose.

Chronic severe pain associated with terminal cancer.

Initial: Loading dose of 15 mg or more of morphine by IV push followed by the infusion of 0.2–1 mg/mL. Infusion amount may range from 0.8–80 mg/hr, up to 144 mg/hr. Thus, for the 1 mg/mL solution, the infusion may be run from 0.8–80 mL/hr and for the 0.5 mg/mL solution, the infusion may be run from 1.6–160 mL/hr. A constant infusion rate must be maintained with an infusion pump in order to assure proper control of dosage. Avoid overdosage (respiratory depression) or abrupt cessation of therapy, which may cause withdrawal symptoms.

Open-heart surgery.

0.5–3 mg/kg (large doses) as the sole anesthetic or with a suitable anesthetic.

Give oxygen and adequate ventilation to maintain CV function.

MI pain.

8–15 mg. For very severe pain, additional smaller doses may be given q 3–4 hr, as needed.

- **INTRATHECAL**

  Pain not responsive to nonnarcotic analgesics.

Adults: 0.2–1 mg as a single daily injection; may provide relief for up to 24 hr. NOTE: The dose is only 0.4–2 mL of the 0.5 mg/mL potency or 0.2–1 mL of the 1 mg/mL product. Do not inject intrathecally more than 2 mL of the 0.5 mg/mL potency or 1 mL of the 1 mg/mL potency product. Use in lumbar area only. Repeated intrathecal injections are not recommended. A constant IV infusion of naloxone, 0.6 mg/hr, for 24 hr after intrathecal injection may reduce the incidence of potential side effects. Continue client monitoring for at least 24 hr after each dose due to the possibility of delayed respiratory depression. *NOTE:* The intrathecal dose is usually one tenth the epidural dose.

- **EPIDURAL**

  Pain not responsive to nonnarcotic analgesics.

Initial: 5 mg/day in the lumbar region may provide pain relief for up to 24 hr; if analgesia is not manifested in 1 hr, increasing doses of 1–2 mg can be given, not to exceed 10 mg/day. Thoracic use has been shown to dramatically increase the incidence of early and late respiratory depression even at doses of 1 to 2 mg. Administer with extreme caution to aged or debilitated clients; doses less than 5 mg may provide satisfactory analgesia for up to 24 hr. For continuous infusion, 2–4 mg/day with additional doses of 1–2 mg if analgesia is not satisfactory. Usual starting dose of Infumorph for those not tolerant to opiates ranges from 2.5–7.5 mg/day whereas the usual starting dose for continuous epidural infusion in those who have some degree of opiate tolerance is 4.5–10 mg/day. Dose requirements may increase significantly (i.e., up to 20–30 mg/day) during treatment.

- **INJECTION, EXTENDED-RELEASE LIPOSOMAL (DEPO-DUR)**

  Pain resulting from major surgery.

One-time dose of DepoDur: 15 mg for major orthopedic surgery of the lower extremity, 10–15 mg for lower abdominal or pelvic surgery, and 10 mg for cesarean section. DepoDur is not intended for intrathecal, IV, or IM use. Give via needle or catheter at the lumbar level. May be given undiluted or diluted up to 5 mL total volume with preservative-free 0.9% NaCl. Do not use an in-line filter during administration of DepoDur. *NOTE:* Use in clients 65 years and older only after careful evaluation of their underlying medication condition and the risks associated with use. The dose for such clients should be at the low end of the dose range.

- **RECTAL SUPPOSITORY**

  Severe chronic and acute pain.

Adults, usual: 10–20 mg q 4 hr or as directed by prescriber. Give on a regular schedule and at the lowest dose that will achieve adequate analgesia. During the first 2 to 3 days of effective pain relief, the client may sleep for many hours. This may be misinterpreted as an excessive analgesic dose rather than the first sign of relief of a pain-exhausted client. Therefore, maintain dosage for at least 3 days before reduction. Following successful relief of severe pain, periodic attempts to reduce dose of narcotic should be made as lower doses may be feasible due to a physiologic change or improved mental status of the client.

NURSING CONSIDERATIONS

 (1) Do not confuse morphine with hydromorphone (also a narcotic analgesic). (2) Do not confuse Avinza (extended-release morphine sulfate) with Evista (raloxifene-used to treat and prevent osteoporosis in postmenopausal women). (3) Do not confuse Roxanol with Uroxatral (drug for benign prostatic hypertrophy) or Oxytrol (drug for overactive bladder).

ADMINISTRATION/STORAGE

1. Begin therapy using an immediate-release morphine product as it may be

more difficult to titrate a client to adequate analgesia using a controlled- or extended-release product.

2. During the first 2 to 3 days of immediate-release morphine therapy, the client may sleep for many hours. This may be the first sign of relief in a pain-exhausted client rather than the effect of excessive dosing. Thus, if respiratory activity and other vital signs are adequate, maintain the dose for at least 3 days before reduction. Following successful relief of severe pain, reduce the narcotic dose periodically. Smaller doses or complete discontinuation of the narcotic may be feasible due to a physiologic change or the improved mental state of the client.

3. If signs of excessive opioid effects are seen early in the dosing interval when using controlled-/extended-release products, the next dose should be decreased. If this dosage reduction leads to breakthrough pain late in the dosing interval, the dosing interval may be shortened. If breakthrough pain occurs when Kadian is given on an every 24-hr dosing regimen, consider dosing q 12 hr. Alternatively, a supplemental dose of a short-acting analgesic may be given.

4. The MS Contin 200 mg tablet is for use only in opioid-tolerant clients requiring daily morphine-equivalent doses of 400 mg or more. Reserve this strength for those who have already been titrated to a stable analgesic regimen using lower strengths of MS Contin or other opioids.

5. The contents of the immediate-release capsule may be delivered through an NG or a gastric tube.

6. Conversion from parenteral morphine or parenteral or PO other opioids to controlled-/extended-release PO morphine: Initial dosing regimens should be conservative since there is intersubject variation in relative estimates of opioid potency and cross-tolerance (i.e., an underestimation of the 24-hr PO morphine requirement is preferred to an overestimate). In clients whose daily PO requirements are expected to be no more than 120 mg, the

30 mg tablet is recommended for the initial titration period. Once a stable dose regimen is reached the client can be converted to the 60 or 100 mg tablet or appropriate combination of tablet strengths.

7. From 2 to 6 mg of PO morphine may be required to provide analgesia equivalent to 1 mg of parenteral morphine. A dose of PO morphine 3 times the daily parenteral morphine requirement may be sufficient for chronic use. A reasonable initial dose of Avinza would be about 3 times the previous daily parenteral morphine requirement.

8. Conversion from controlled-/extended-release PO morphine to parenteral opioids: Assume that the parenteral-to-PO potency is high. To estimate the required 24-hr dose of morphine for IM use, a conversion of 1 mg morphine IM for every 6 mg morphine as a controlled-release tablet can be used. The IM 24-hr dose is divided by six (6) and given on an every 4-hr regimen. This approach is least likely to cause an overdose.

9. When converting from Avinza or Kadian to parenteral opioids, calculate an equivalent parenteral dose and then begin treatment at one-half of this calculated value. For example, an estimated 24-hr parenteral morphine requirement of a client receiving Avinza or Kadian is one-third of the dose of Avinza or Kadian. This estimated dose should then be divided in half and this last calculated dose is the total daily dose. This value should be further divided by six (6) if the desire is to dose with parenteral morphine every 4 hr. This approach may require a dosage increase in the first 24 hr for many clients. However, this method is less likely to result in overdose. *Example:* A client takes 360 mg of Avinza or Kadian per day. The estimated total 24-hr parenteral morphine requirement would be one-third of 360 mg (i.e., 120 mg). Dividing by two (2) gives the total daily dose of 60 mg. If parenteral morphine is to be given at 4-hr intervals, 10 mg (60 mg divided by 6) would be given q 4 hr.

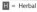 = see color insert   **H** = Herbal   **IV** = Intravenous   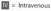 = sound alike drug

10. Conversion of extended-release morphine (Avinza or Kadian) to other controlled-/extended-release PO morphine products: Kadian is *not* equivalent to other extended-release morphine products. For a given dose, the same total amount of morphine is available from Avinza or Kadian as from PO morphine solution or controlled-/extended-release morphine tablets. However, the slower release of Kadian results in reduced maximum and increased minimum plasma levels than with shorter-acting morphine products. Conversion from Kadian or Avinza to the same total daily dose of another controlled-/extended-release morphine formulation may lead to either excessive sedation at peak or inadequate analgesia at trough. Close observation and appropriate dosing adjustments are recommended. *NOTE:* Persistence of Avinza-derived plasma morphine levels may be in excess of 36 hr when making a conversion to other pain control therapies.

11. For intrathecal use, do not give more than 2 mL of the 0.5-mg/mL preparation or 1 mL of the 1-mg/mL product.

12. Give intrathecally only in the lumbar region; repeated injections are not recommended.

13. To reduce chance of side effects with intrathecal administration, a constant IV infusion of naloxone (0.6 mg/hr for 24 hr after intrathecal injection) is recommended.

14. For Infumorph, Duramorph, and Astromorph PF use epidural doses of 20 mg or more with caution R/T the increased possibility of serious side effects.

15. In certain circumstances (e.g., tolerance, severe pain), provider may prescribe doses higher than those listed under *Dosage.*

16. Dose may be lower in geriatric clients or those with respiratory disease.

17. Intraventricular administration may be effective in select clients with a short life expectancy and recalcitrant pain due to head and neck malignancies and tumors and breast cancer that affect the brachial plexus. Only 1–2 doses/day are usually needed.

18. Use caution interpreting dosage, especially for concentrated morphine sulfate oral solutions. **Do not interchange milligrams for milliliters.** Prescription should contain concentration of morphine oral solution to be dispensed and intended dose of morphine in milligrams with the corresponding volume in milliliters written out in the directions. As an example, a prescription should look as follows: 'Roxanol Concentrated Oral Solution, 20 mg/mL' at a dose of '15 mg (0.75 mL) q 4 hr as needed.'

19. Store PO solution, soluble tablets for injection, and capsules at controlled room temperature of 15–30°C (59–86°F) protected from light and moisture. Solutions made from soluble tablets for injection may darken with age; do not use if solution is darker than pale yellow, discolored in any way, or contains a precipitate.

20.

IV listFor IV use, dilute 2–10 mg with at least 5 mL sterile water or NSS and administer over 4–5 min. For continous infusions, reconstitute to concentration of 0.1–1 mg/mL and administer as prescribed to control symptoms.

21. Rapid IV administration increases risk of adverse effects; do not give IV unless a narcotic antagonist (e.g., naloxone) immediately available.

22. When the client no longer requires therapy, taper doses gradually to prevent signs and symptoms of withdrawal in the physically-dependent client.

23. Store injections at controlled room temperature; do not use if injection is darker than pale yellow, discolored in any way, or contains a precipitate.

24. Store Infumorph, Duramorph, or Astromorph PF injections from 15–30°C (59–86°F) protected from light; do not freeze. Discard any unused portion as products contain no preservative or antioxidant. Do not heat sterilize.

25. Store DepoDur in the refrigerator at 2–8°C (36–46°F). May be held at 15–30°C (59–86°F) for up to 7 days in sealed, intact (unopened) vials. Product

---

is sterile but does not contain bacteriostatic agents; thus, give within 4 hr after withdrawal from vial. Do not heat or gas sterilize. Protect from freezing; do not give if suspected that the vial has been frozen.

ASSESSMENT

1. Identify reasons for therapy, onset, location and characteristics of pain. Rate pain level using a pain-rating scale.
2. List other agents prescribed, outcome.
3. Note any seizure disorder or head trauma. Monitor VS and respiratory status.
4. With continous IV drips follow established protocols for infusion (i.e. Resp Rate >10).

CLIENT/FAMILY TEACHING

1. May take with food to diminish GI upset. Do not crush or chew controlled- or extended-release capsules or tablets as this will lead to the rapid release and absorption of a potentially fatal dose of morphine.
2. Avinza or Kadian beads sprinkled over applesauce are bioequivalent to Avinza or Kadian capsules swallowed whole under fasting conditions. Capsules may be opened and the entire bead contents sprinkled on a small amount of applesauce immediately prior to ingestion. The applesauce should be at room temperature or cooler. Clients should ingest the mixture immediately without chewing or crushing the beads; clients should then rinse their mouths and swallow to ensure all beads have been ingested. Do not divide the applesauce into separate doses.
3. The entire capsule contents of Kadian may also be administered through a 16-French gastrostomy tube. Flush the tube with water to ensure that it is wet. Sprinkle the Kadian pellets into 10 mL of water. Using a swirling motion pour the pellets and water into the gastrostomy tube through a funnel. Rinse the beaker with a further 10 mL of water and pour this into the funnel. Repeat rinsing until no pellets remain in the beaker. Do not administer Kadian pellets through a nasogastric tube.

4. Immediate-release capsules may be swallowed intact or the contents of the capsule may be sprinkled on food or stirred in juice to avoid the bitter taste.
5. Drug may cause dizziness and drowsiness; avoid activities that require mental alertness.
6. Practice cough and deep-breathing exercises and incentive spirometry to decrease risk of atelectasis.
7. Record drug use for breakthrough pain when SR therapy prescribed, to ensure adequate dosage.
8. Avoid alcohol/CNS depressants and OTC agents. Keep out of reach of children and away from bedside.
9. Report adverse side effects or lack of desired response.

OUTCOMES/EVALUATE

- ↓ Pain rating/ ↑ pain control
- Control of respirations during mechanical ventilation

Moxifloxacin hydrochloride 🔳Ⓒ📷
(**mox**-ee-**FLOX**-ah-sin)

CLASSIFICATION(S):
Antibiotic, fluoroquinolone
PREGNANCY CATEGORY: C
Rx: Avelox, Avelox I.V., Vigamox.

SEE ALSO *FLUOROQUINOLONES.*

USES

Systemic. All uses are for adults at least 18 years of age. (1) Acute bacterial sinusitis due to *Streptococcus pneumoniae, Haemophilus influenzae,* or *Moraxella catarrhalis.* (2) Acute bacterial exacerbation of chronic bronchitis due to *S. pneumoniae, H. influenzae, Haemophilus parainfluenzae, Klebsiella pneumoniae, Staphylococcus aureus* (methicillin-susceptible), or *M. catarrhalis.* (3) Community-acquired pneumonia due to *S. pneumoniae* (including penicillin-resistant strains, MIC penicillin 2 mcg/mL or above), *H. influenzae, Mycoplasma pneumoniae, Chlamydia pneumoniae, M. catarrhalis* (methicillin-susceptible), *K. pneumoniae,* or *S. aureus.* (4) Uncompli-

M

cated skin and skin structure infections due to *S. aureus* or *Streptococcus pyogenes*. (5) Methicillin-susceptible complicated skin and skin structure infections due to *S. aureus, E. coli, K. pneumoniae,* or *Enterobacter cloacae* in adults. (6) Complicated intra-abdominal infections, including polymicrobial infection such as abscess due to *E. coli, Bacteroides fragilis, Streptococcus anginosus, Streptococcus constellatus, Enterococcus faecali, Proteus mirabilis, Clostridium perfringens, Bacteroides thetaiotaomicron,* or *Peptostreptococcus* species.

Ophthalmic. Bacterial conjunctivitis due to *Corynebacterium* species, *Micrococcus luteus, S. aureus, S. epidermidis, S. haemolyticus, S. hominis, S. warneri, S. pneumoniae, Streptococcus viridans* group, *Acinetobacter lwoffi, H. influenzae, H. parainfluenzae,* and *Chlamydia trachomatis.*

ACTION/KINETICS
Action
Interferes with DNA gyrase and topoisomerase IV. DNA gyrase is an enzyme needed for replication, transcription, and repair of bacterial DNA. Topoisomerase IV plays a key role in the partitioning of chromosomal DNA during bacterial cell division. Effective against both gram-positive and gram-negative organisms.

Pharmacokinetics
Well absorbed from the GI tract (about 90% bioavailable). A high-fat meal does not affect absorption. **$t_{1/2}$, elimination:** About 12 hr. Steady state is reached in 3 days (400 mg/day). Widely distributed in the body. Metabolized in the liver; metabolites and unchanged drug are excreted in the feces and urine.

CONTRAINDICATIONS
Hypersensitivity to moxifloxacin or any quinolone antibiotic. Use with moderate to severe hepatic insufficiency. Use in clients with known prolongation of the QT interval (the drug prolongs the QT interval in some), with uncorrected hypokalemia, and in those receiving class IA (e.g., quinidine, procainamide) or Class III (e.g., amiodarone, sotalol) antiarrhythmic drugs. IM, intrathecal, IP, or SC use. Lactation.

SPECIAL CONCERNS
Use with caution in those with clinically significant bradycardia or acute myocardial ischemia, in clients with known or suspected CNS disorders (e.g., severe cerebral arteriosclerosis, epilepsy), or in the presence of risk factors that predispose to seizures or lower the seizure threshold. Safety and efficacy have not been determined in children, adolescents less than 18 years of age, in pregnancy, and during lactation.

SIDE EFFECTS
Most Common
N&V, diarrhea, dizziness, headache, dyspepsia/heartburn.

Hypersensitivity: *Anaphylaxis after the first dose, CV collapse,* loss of consciousness, tingling, pharyngeal or facial edema, dyspnea, urticaria, itching. **CNS:** Dizziness, headache, convulsions, confusion, tremors, hallucinations, depression, insomnia, nervousness, anxiety, depersonalization, hypertonia, incoordination, somnolence, vertigo, paresthesia, psychotic reaction, syncope, suicidal thoughts/acts (rare). **GI:** N&V, diarrhea, abdominal pain, taste perversion, dyspepsia, heartburn, dry mouth, constipation, oral moniliasis, anorexia, stomatitis, gastritis, glossitis, GI disorder, pseudomembranous colitis, cholestatic jaundice, hepatitis. **CV:** Palpitation, vasodilatation, tachycardia, hypertension, peripheral edema, hypotension. **Body as a whole:** Asthenia, moniliasis, pain, malaise, allergic reaction, leg/pelvic/back/chest/hand pain, chills, infection. **Hematologic:** Thrombocytopenia, thrombocythemia, eosinophilia, leukopenia. **Respiratory:** Asthma, dyspnea, increased cough, pneumonia, pharyngitis, rhinitis, sinusitis. **Musculoskeletal:** Arthralgia, myalgia, tendon ruptures. **Dermatologic:** Rash, pruritus, sweating, urticaria, dry skin, *Stevens-Johnson syndrome.* **GU:** Vaginal moniliasis, vaginitis, cystitis. **Miscellaneous:** Tinnitus, amblyopia.

LABORATORY TEST CONSIDERATIONS
↑ GGTP, LDH, MCH, WBCs, PT ratio, ionized calcium, chloride, albumin, globulin, bilirubin. ↓ Hemoglobin, RBCs, eosinophils, basophils, glucose,

---

pO$_2$. Either ↑ or ↓ Amylase, PT, bilirubin, neutrophils. Hyperglycemia, hyperlipidemia. Abnormal LFTs and kidney function.

DRUG INTERACTIONS

Antacids / Significant ↓ bioavailability of moxifloxacin
Antidepressants, tricyclic / Potential to add to the QTc prolonging effect of moxifloxacin
Antipsychotics / Potential to add to the QTc prolonging effect of moxifloxacin
Didanosine / ↓ Absorption of moxifloxacin
Erythromycin / Potential to add to the QTc prolonging effect of moxifloxacin
Iron products / Significant ↓ bioavailability of moxifloxaicn
NSAIDs / ↑ Risk of CNS stimulation and convulsions
Sucralfate / ↓ Absorption of moxifloxacin
Warfarin / ↑ Anticoagulant effect of warfarin

HOW SUPPLIED

Injection (Premix): 400 mg; *Ophthalmic Solution:* 0.5%; *Tablets:* 400 mg.

DOSAGE

• **IV; TABLETS**
Acute bacterial sinusitis.
Adults 18 years and older: 400 mg q 24 hr for 10 days.
Acute bacterial exacerbation of chronic bronchitis.
Adults 18 years and older: 400 mg q 24 hr for 5 days.
Community-acquired pneumonia.
Adults 18 years and older: 400 mg q 24 hr for 7–14 days.
Uncomplicated skin and skin structure infections.
Adults 18 years and older: 400 mg q 24 hr for 7 days.
Complicated skin and skin structure infections.
Adults 18 years and older: 400 mg q 24 hr for 7–21 days.
Complicated intra-abdominal infections.
Adults 18 years and older: 400 mg q 24 hr for 5–14 days. Begin therapy with the IV formulation.

• **OPHTHALMIC SOLUTION**
Bacterial conjunctivitis.

Adults and children at least 1 year of age: 1 gtt in affected eye 3 times per day for 7 days.

NURSING CONSIDERATIONS

ⓒ Do not confuse Avelox with Asacol (an anti-inflammatory drug).

ADMINISTRATION/STORAGE

1. Avoid high humidity when storing tablets. Not for IM, SC, intrathecal, or intraperitoneal use.
IV 2. No dosage adjustment needed when switching from IV to PO dosing.
3. Give only by IV infusion over 60 min through a Y-type IV infusion set. Avoid rapid or bolus IV infusion. Do not add additives or other medications to IV moxifloxacin or infuse at the same time through the same IV line. If the same IV line is used for sequential infusion of other drugs, flush line before and after moxifloxacin infusion with a compatible solution.
4. Moxifloxacin IV is compatible with the following IV solutions at ratios from 1:10 to 10:1: 0.9% NaCl injection, 1 M NaCl injection, D5W, sterile water for injection, 10% dextrose for injection, or lactated Ringer's for injection.
5. If Y-type or piggyback method used, temporarily discontinue administration of other solutions during moxifloxacin IV administration.
6. The premix containers are for single use only; discard any unused portion.
7. Store IV solution and tablets from 15–30°C (59–86°F). Do not refrigerate IV solution.

ASSESSMENT

1. Note onset, location, characteristics of S&S and cultures. List drugs prescribed to ensure none interact.
2. Avoid with uncorrected hypokalemia, prolonged QT intervals, if receiving class 1A or III antiarrhythmic agents, or seizure disorder.
3. Monitor cultures, electrolytes, CBC, renal and LFTs; avoid with moderate to severe liver dysfunction.

CLIENT/FAMILY TEACHING

1. Take once daily at the same time, as directed. May take with/without meals. Drink fluids liberally.

2. Take at least 4 hr before or 8 hr after multivitamins containing iron, zinc, antacids containing Mg/calcium/Al, sucralfate, or didanosine (chewable/buffered tablets or the pediatric powder for PO solution).

3. Do not perform activities that require mental alertness until drug effects realized.

4. May cause GI upset, dizziness, and headaches. Report pain or inflammation in a tendon, muscle weakness, paralysis, pain or numbness, a burning sensation, or a 'pins and needles' sensation if experienced.

5. Avoid excess sunlight and tanning beds and low potassium levels.

6. Stop drug and report skin rash immediately. Report adverse effects, lack of effectiveness, or worsening of condition.

OUTCOMES/EVALUATE
Resolution of infection; symptomatic improvement

Mupirocin ©

(myou-**PEER**-oh-sin)

CLASSIFICATION(S):
Antibiotic, topical
PREGNANCY CATEGORY: B
Rx: Bactroban Nasal, Bactroban Ointment, Centany Ointment.

Mupirocin calcium

PREGNANCY CATEGORY: B
Rx: Bactroban Cream, Bactroban Nasal, Centany.

USES

Nasal Ointment: Eradication of nasal colonization with methicillin-resistant *S. aureus* in adult clients and health care workers as part of a comprehensive infection control program to reduce risk of infection among clients at high risk of methicillin-resistant *S. aureus* infection during institutional outbreaks of infections. **Topical Cream:** Secondarily infected traumatic skin lesions (up to 10 cm in length or 100 cm²) due to suscep-

tible strains of *Staphylococcus aureus* and *Streptococcus pyogenes*. **Topical Ointment:** Impetigo due to *Staphylococcus aureus*, *Streptococcus pyogenes*, and beta-hemolytic streptococcus. *Investigational:* Topical products to treat diaper dermatitis due to *Candida*.

ACTION/KINETICS

Action

Binds to bacterial isoleucyl transfer RNA synthetase, which results in inhibition of protein synthesis by the organism. Not absorbed into the systemic circulation. Serum present in exudative wounds decreases the antibacterial activity. No cross resistance with other antibiotics such as chloramphenicol, erythromycin, gentamicin, lincomycin, methicillin, neomycin, novobiocin, penicillin, streptomycin, or tetracyclines.

Pharmacokinetics

Metabolized to the inactive monic acid in the skin which is removed by normal skin desquamation.

CONTRAINDICATIONS

Hypersensitivity to any component of the product. Ophthalmic use. Use if absorption of large quantities of polyethylene glycol is possible (i.e., large, open wounds). Use with other nasal products.

SPECIAL CONCERNS

Superinfection may result from chronic use. Use with caution during lactation. Safety and efficacy have not been established in children less than 12 years for mupirocin nasal; safety and efficacy of the cream and ointment have not been established in children 2 months to 16 years of age.

SIDE EFFECTS

Most Common

Use of nasal ointment: Headache, rhinitis, upper respiratory tract congestion, pharyngitis, taste perversion, burning/stinging, cough.

Use of topical cream: Headache, rash, nausea.

Use of topical ointment: Burning, stinging, pain, itching.

● **TOPICAL CREAM**
Headache, rash, nausea, abdominal pain, burning at application site, cellulitis, dermatitis, dizziness, pruritus, secon-

---

dary wound infection, ulcerative stomatitis.

- **TOPICAL OINTMENT**

Burning, stinging or pain, itching, rash, nausea, erythema, dry skin, tenderness, swelling contact dermatitis, increased exudate.

- **NASAL USE**

Headache, rhinitis, respiratory disorder (including upper respiratory tract congestion), pharyngitis, taste perversion, burning, stinging, cough, pruritus, blepharitis, diarrhea, dry mouth, ear pain, epistaxis, nausea, rash.

HOW SUPPLIED

Nasal Ointment: 2%; *Topical Ointment:* 2%; *Topical Cream:* 2%.

DOSAGE

- **NASAL OINTMENT**

Eradication of nasal colonization with methicillin-resistant S. aureus.

Adults and adolescents 12 years and older: Divide about one-half of the ointment from the single-use tube between the nostrils and apply in the morning and evening for 5 days. The single-use tube will deliver about 0.25 gram/nostril.

- **TOPICAL CREAM**

Traumatic skin lesions due to S. aureus *or* S. pyogenes.

Apply to affected area 3 times per day for 10 days. May be covered with a gauze dressing. If no response in 3–5 days, re-evaluate.

- **TOPICAL OINTMENT**

Impetigo due to S. aureus, S. pyogenes, *or beta-hemolytic streptococcus.*

A small amount of ointment is applied to the affected area 3 times per day. Area may be covered with a gauze dressing. If no response in 3–5 days, re-evaluate.

NURSING CONSIDERATIONS

℘ Do not confuse Bactroban with bacitracin (also a topical antibacterial agent).

ADMINISTRATION/STORAGE

1. After application of the nasal product, close the nostrils by pressing them together for about 1 min.

2. Store the topical ointment between 15–30°C (59–86°F); store the topical cream or nasal ointment below 25°C (77°F).

ASSESSMENT

1. Note reasons for therapy, onset, duration, characteristics of S&S.

2. Assess labs and culture results.

CLIENT/FAMILY TEACHING

1. Review technique for administering topical and/or nasal medications; use aseptic measures and hand washing before and after therapy to prevent contamination. For external use only.

2. Report any symptoms of chemical irritation or hypersensitivity such as increased rash, itching, pain at site, or lack of healing.

3. Clear nasal passages and do not use other nasal products during nasal therapy.

4. Report if no improvement in skin infection after 3–5 days of therapy.

5. Notify school nurse to ensure appropriate screening is performed when treating school-aged children with impetigo.

OUTCOMES/EVALUATE

- Healing of lesions; symptomatic improvement
- Eradication of nasal colonization MRSA

Muromonab-CD3 ∎
(myour-oh-**MON**-ab)

CLASSIFICATION(S):
Immunosuppressant
PREGNANCY CATEGORY: C
Rx: Orthoclone OKT 3.

USES

(1) Reverse acute allograft rejection in kidney transplant clients; used in combination with azathioprine, cyclosporine, corticosteroids. (2) Steroid-resistant acute allograft rejection in cardiac and hepatic transplant clients.

ACTION/KINETICS

Action

A murine monoclonal antibody that is a purified IgG$_{2a}$ immunoglobulin. Acts to prevent rejection of transplanted kidney tissue by blocking the action of T cells, which play a significant role in acute rejection. Specifically, the CD3 molecule in the membrane of T cells is blocked; this molecule is necessary for signal transduction. Does not cause myelosuppression. Antibodies to muromonab-CD3 have been observed after approximately 20 days.

Pharmacokinetics
Average serum levels after 3 days: 0.9 mcg/mL. **Time to steady-state trough levels:** 3 days. **Duration:** 1 week for return of circulating CD3 positive T cells to pretreatment levels.

CONTRAINDICATIONS
Hypersensitivity to drug (or any product of murine origin), clients with antimouse titers greater than or equal to 1:1,000. Clients with fluid overload or uncompensated CHF as confirmed by CXR or more than a 3% weight gain within the week prior to treatment. History of seizures or predisposition to seizures. Use during pregnancy (IgG antibody potentially hazardous to the fetus) and lactation.

SPECIAL CONCERNS
■ (1) Should be used only by providers experienced in immunosuppressive therapy and management of renal transplant clients. (2) Anaphylactic or anaphylactoid reactions may occur following administration of any dose or course of muromonab-CD3. Serious and occasionally life-threatening systemic, CV, and CNS reactions have been reported. These have included pulmonary edema (especially in those with volume overload), shock, CV collapse, cardiac or respiratory arrest, seizures, and coma. Thus, those treated with muromonab-CD3 must be managed in a facility equipped and staffed for cardiopulmonary resuscitation.■ Although used in children, safety and effectiveness have not been assessed. Following the first two to three doses, a cytokine release syndrome (CRS) due to the release of cytokines by activated lymphocytes or monocytes may occur. Clients at greatest risk for CRS are those with unstable angina, recent MI, symptomatic ischemic heart disease, heart failure, pulmonary edema, COPD, intravascular volume overload or depletion, cerebrovascular disease, advanced symptomatic vascular disease or neuropathy, history of seizures, or septic shock.

SIDE EFFECTS
Most Common
Infections (herpes simplex, CMV, fungal), pyrexia, dyspnea, N&V, chest pain, diarrhea, tremor, wheezing, headache, tachycardia, rigors, hypertension (most of these symptoms due to cytokine release syndrome).

Cytokine release syndrome (CRS). Flu-like symptoms, such as pyrexia, chills, dyspnea, N&V, chest pain, diarrhea, tremor, wheezing, headache, tachycardia, rigor, and hypertension. *Rarely, severe, life-threatening shock-like syndrome including serious CV and CNS effects.*

Within the first 45 days of therapy for renal transplants. *Infections (which may be life-threatening)* due to CMV, HSV, *Staphylococcus epidermidis, Pneumocystis carinii, Legionella, Cryptococcus, Serratia,* and other gram-negative bacteria.

Within the first 45 days of therapy for liver transplants. *CMV, fungal infections, HSV, Legionella,* and other severe, life-threatening gram-positive, gram-negative, and viral infections.

Within the first 45 days of therapy for heart transplants. Most commonly herpes simplex, fungal, and CMV infections. **Hypersensitivity reactions:** *Cardiovascular collapse, cardiorespiratory arrest, shock,* loss of consciousness, hypotension, tachycardia, tingling, angioedema, *airway obstruction, bronchospasm,* dyspnea, urticaria, pruritus. **Neuropsychiatric:** *Seizures,* encephalopathy, cerebral edema, *aseptic meningitis,* headaches. **CV:** *Cardiac arrest, shock, heart failure, CV collapse, MI,* hypotension, angina, tachycardia, bradycardia, hemodynamic instability, hypertension, LV dysfunction, arrhythmias, chest pain or tightness. **Respiratory:** *Respiratory arrest, ARDS, respiratory failure, cardiogenic or noncardiogenic pulmonary edema, apnea,*

Bold Italic = life threatening side effect   ■ = black box warning   ✦ = Available in Canada

dyspnea, **bronchospasm**, wheezing, SOB, hypoxemia, tachypnea, hyperventilation, abnormal chest sounds, pneumonia, pneumonitis. **Dermatologic:** Rash, urticaria, pruritus, erythema, flushing, diaphoresis, **Stevens-Johnson syndrome**. **GI:** N&V, diarrhea, abdominal pain, **bowel infarction, GI hemorrhage**. **Hematologic:** Pancytopenia, **aplastic anemia**, neutropenia, leukopenia, thrombocytopenia, lymphopenia, leukocytosis, lymphadenopathy, **arterial and venous thrombosis of allografts and other vascular beds (heart, lung, brain, bowel), disturbances of coagulation**. **Musculoskeletal:** Arthralgia, arthritis, myalgia, stiffness, aches and pain. **Hepatic:** Hepatomegaly, splenomegaly, hepatitis (usually secondary to viral infection or lymphoma). **GU:** Anuria, oliguria, delayed graft function, abnormal urinary cytology (including exfoliation of damaged lymphocytes, collecting ducts, and cellular casts). **Ophthalmic:** Blindness, blurred vision, diplopia, photophobia, conjunctivitis. **Otic:** Hearing loss, otitis media, tinnitus, vertigo, nasal and ear stuffiness. **Body as a whole:** Fever, chills, rigors, flu-like syndrome, fatigue, malaise, generalized weakness, anorexia. **Miscellaneous:** Palsy of cranial nerve VI, **increased risk of developing neoplasms**.

LABORATORY TEST CONSIDERATIONS
↑ AST, ALT. Transient and reversible ↑ in BUN and serum creatinine.

OD **OVERDOSE MANAGEMENT**
Symptoms: Hyperthermia, myalgia, severe chills, diarrhea, vomiting, edema, oliguria, pulmonary edema, acute renal failure. *Treatment:* Observe client carefully and provide symptomatic and supportive treatment.

DRUG INTERACTIONS
Azathioprine, corticosteroids, cyclosporine / Psychosis, infections, malignancies, seizures, encephalopathy, and thrombosis when taken with muromonab-CD3
H *Echinacea* / Do not give with muromonab-CD3
Indomethacin / Encephalopathy and other CNS effects

HOW SUPPLIED
Injection: 1 mg/mL.

DOSAGE
• **IV BOLUS**
Reverse acute allograft rejection in kidney transplants.
Adults: 5 mg/day for 10–14 days, beginning treatment once acute renal rejection is diagnosed.
Cardiac/hepatic allograft rejection, steroid-resistant.
5 mg/day for 10–14 days with treatment beginning after determination that corticosteroids will not reverse the rejection.

NURSING CONSIDERATIONS

ADMINISTRATION/STORAGE
IV 1. Give methylprednisolone sodium succinate, 8 mg/kg IV, 1–4 hr before dose to decrease incidence of first-dose reactions. Acetaminophen and antihistamines, given together, may reduce early reactions.
2. Initiate treatment as soon as acute renal rejection is diagnosed.
3. Give the dose in less than 1 min.
4. Do not give the drug by IV infusion or with any other drug solutions.
5. If the body temperature is 37.8°C (100°F), do not initiate drug therapy.
6. Draw the solution (which is a protein) into a syringe through a 0.2- or 0.22-μm filter; discard the filter and attach a 20-gauge needle.
7. Do not add or infuse other drugs through the same IV line. If the same IV line is used for sequential infusion of different drugs, flush the line with saline before and after infusion of muromonab-CD3.
8. The appearance of a few translucent particles of protein does not affect the potency of the preparation.
9. Use ampule immediately after opening; no bacteriostatic agent in product. Discard any unused drug.
10. Decrease dose of other immunosuppressant drugs as follows during muromonab-CD3 use: Prednisone, 0.5 mg/kg/day; azathioprine, 25 mg/day. Cyclosporine should be discontinued. Maintenance doses of these drugs can

M

be resumed approximately 3 days prior to termination of muromonab-CD3.

11. Store at 2–8°C (36–46°F); do not freeze or shake.

ASSESSMENT

1. Note transplant type (heart, liver, renal), any early adverse effects, and characteristics of S&S.

2. Determine any seizure history, past use, and assess closely for evidence of antibodies. For one course only. If second course of therapy attempted, may develop drug antibodies leading to loss of effectiveness and adverse reactions. Note any sensitivity to murine derivatives.

3. Obtain CXR before therapy. Monitor CBC, LFTs, and T-cell assays with CD_3 antigen daily.

INTERVENTIONS

1. Anticipate pretreatment administration of an antihistamine, antipyretic, and methylprednisolone/hydrocortisone succinate posttreatment to minimize intensity of side effects.

2. Monitor I&O and weights; assess for a positive fluid balance and report rapid weight gain, rash, itching. rapid heart rate, SOB, or difficulty swallowing.

3. Obtain CXR, assess lung sounds, and report evidence of congestion.

4. Take temperature q 4 hr; if above 37.7°C (100°F), withhold drug until temperature drops.

5. Monitor for a decrease in urine volume and C_{CR}; these are S&S of transplant rejection.

6. Administer acetaminophen for flu-like symptoms/febrile reaction.

7. Symptoms of aseptic meningitis are usually evident within 3 days characterized by fever, headache, nuchal rigidity, and photophobia.

8. Avoid crowds, vaccinations and contact with persons with infections or those who have received oral polio vaccine as this drug suppresses the immune system.

CLIENT/FAMILY TEACHING

1. Drug used to prevent transplant rejection.

2. Chills, fever, SOB, and fatigue are 1st/2nd-dose symptoms that should diminish with therapy.

3. Report any persistent SOB, swelling of extremities, weight gain, chest pain, N&V, or fever/infection. Under side effects note cytokine release syndrome (CRS); report if evident.

4. Perform frequent, careful oral care to minimize oral inflammation.

5. Avoid vaccinia, crowds, and persons with known infections.

6. Continue to practice reliable birth control for 12 weeks following therapy.

OUTCOMES/EVALUATE

- Reversal of kidney transplant rejection and improved organ function
- Prevention of allograft rejection

Mycophenolate mofetil ■ IV

(**my**-koh-**FEN**-oh-layt)

CLASSIFICATION(S):
Immunosuppressant
PREGNANCY CATEGORY: C
Rx: CellCept.

Mycophenolate sodium

CLASSIFICATION(S):
Immunomodulator
PREGNANCY CATEGORY: C
Rx: Myfortic.

USES

Mycophenolate mofetil. With cyclosporine and corticosteroids to prevent organ rejection in those receiving allogeneic renal, heart, or liver transplants. May be used in children with renal transplants. The IV product is an alternative to PO forms for those unable to take PO medication. *Investigational:* In combination with previous corticosteroid, cyclosporine, or tacrolimus therapy to treat refractory uveitis. In combination with prednisolone to treat diffuse proliferative lupus nephritis. Secondary therapy for Churg-Strauss syndrome.

Bold Italic = life threatening side effect   ■ = black box warning   ✦ = Available in Canada

Mycophenolate sodium. With cyclosporine and corticosteroids for prophylaxis of organ rejection in clients receiving allogeneic renal transplants.

ACTION/KINETICS

Action

Is hydrolyzed to the active mycophenolic acid (MPA). MPA has potent cytostatic effects on lymphocytes. Inhibits proliferative responses of T- and B-lymphocytes to both mitogenic and allospecific stimulation. MPA also suppresses antibody formation of B-lymphocytes. MPA may also inhibit recruitment of leukocytes into sites of inflammation and graft rejection.

Pharmacokinetics

Rapidly absorbed after PO administration. The enteric-coated delayed-release tablets do not release mycophenolic acid under a pH of 5 (e.g., in the stomach) but is highly soluble in neutral pH of the intestine. Food has no effect on absorption of the mofetil salt but decreases C_{max} of the sodium salt. Metabolized in the liver by glucuronyl transferase. **t½, MPA:** 17.9 hr. MPA and additional metabolites excreted mainly in the urine (93%). **Plasma protein binding:** Mycophenolic acid (MPA) at clinical doses: 97%.

CONTRAINDICATIONS

Hypersensitivity to mycophenolate, mycophenolic acid, or polysorbate 80 (Tween; IV only). Use in those with rare hereditary deficiency of hypoxanthine-guanine phosphoribosyl transferase, such as Lesch-Nyhan and Kelley-Seegmiller syndrome. Lactation.

SPECIAL CONCERNS

■ Increased susceptibility to infection and possible development of lymphoma may result from immunosuppression. Only providers experienced in immunosuppressive therapy and management of renal, hepatic, or cardiac transplant clients should use mycophenolate. Manage those receiving the drug in facilities equipped and staffed with adequate lab and supportive medical resources. The provider responsible for maintenance therapy should have complete information requisite for the follow-up of the client.■ Higher blood levels are seen in those with severe impaired renal function. Use with caution in active serious digestive system disease. The elderly are particularly prone to certain infections, including CMV tissue invasive disease and possibly GI hemorrhage and pulmonary edema. Use the oral suspension with caution in those with phenylketonuria as the product contains aspartame, a source of phenylalanine. Avoid the use of live, attenuated vaccines during treatment; vaccinations may be less effective. Clients receiving immunosuppressants involving combinations of drugs, including mycophenolate, are at an increased risk of developing lymphomas and other malignancies, especially of the skin. Safety and efficacy have not been determined in children.

SIDE EFFECTS

Most Common

Hypertension, constipation, diarrhea, N&V, UTI, anemia, leukopenia, peripheral edema, infection, abdominal pain, fever, headache, infections (viral, fungal), pain, asthenia, back/chest pain.

Hematologic: Severe neutropenia, anemia, leukopenia, thrombocytopenia, hypochromic anemia, leukocytosis, ecchymosis, *hemorrhage*, polycythemia, pancytopenia, coagulation disorder, petechiae, *thrombosis (after IV)*. **GI:** *GI tract bleeding/hemorrhage/perforations*, diarrhea, abdominal pain, constipation, N&V, dyspepsia, flatulence, enlarged abdomen, anorexia, cholangitis, hepatitis, cholestatic jaundice, oral/GI moniliasis, esophagitis, gastritis, gastroenteritis, *GI hemorrhage*, gingivitis, gum hyperplasia, ileus, infection, mouth ulceration, rectal disorder, GI disorder, liver damage, dysphagia, jaundice, stomatitis, thirst, melena, stomach ulcer, periotonitis, colitis, pancreatitis. **CNS:** Headache, tremor, insomnia, anxiety, paresthesia, hypertonia, depression, agitation, somnolence, confusion, nervousness, dizziness, emotional lability, neuropathy, convulsions, hallucinations, abnormal thinking, vertigo, delirium, dry mouth, hypesthesia, psychosis. **GU:** UTI, hematuria, abnormal kidney function, oliguria, kidney tubular necrosis, dysuria, al-

M

---

buminuria, hydronephrosis, impotence, pain, pyelonephritis, urinary frequency, nocturia, kidney failure, urine abnormality, urinary incontinence, prostate disorder, urinary retention, urinary tract disorder, dysuria, acute kidney failure, scrotal edema, hernia. **CV:** Hypertension, hypotension, CV disorder, tachycardia, arrhythmia, bradycardia, pericardial effusion, *cardiac failure, angina pectoris*, atrial fibrillation, palpitation, peripheral vascular disorder, postural hypotension, thrombosis, vasodilation, ventricular extrasystole, CHF, supraventricular tachycardia, ventricular tachycardia, atrial flutter, pulmonary hypertension, *cardiac arrest, arterial thrombosis*, increased venous pressure, syncope, supraventricular extrasystoles, extrasystoles, pallor, vasospasm, phlebitis. **Respiratory:** Infection, dyspnea, increased cough, pharyngitis, lung disorder, sinusitis, rhinitis, pleural effusion, asthma, atelectasis, pneumonia, lung edema, hiccough, pneumothorax, increased sputum, epistaxis, apnea, voice alteration, pain, hemoptysis, *neoplasm*, respiratory acidosis, bronchitis, respiratory disorder, hyperventilation, respiratory moniliasis, *fatal pulmonary fibrosis*. **Dermatologic:** Alopecia, fungal dermatitis, hirsutism, benign skin neoplasm, skin hypertrophy, skin ulcer, hemorrhage, skin carcinoma, vesiculobullous rash. **Metabolic/Endocrine:** Peripheral edema, edema, weight gain, diabetes mellitus, parathyroid disorder, Cushing's syndrome, hypothyroidism. **Musculoskeletal:** Leg cramps, myasthenia, myalgia, arthralgia, joint disorder, osteoporosis. **Ophthalmic:** Cataract, conjunctivitis, abnormal vision, lacrimation disorder, eye hemorrhage, amblyopia. **Otic:** Ear pain, deafness, ear disorder, tinnitus. **Body as a whole:** Pain, fever, *sepsis, infection (may be fatal),* asthenia, accidental injury, chills, ascites, flu syndrome, malaise, cellulitis (with IV), abnormal healing, abscess, gout. **Miscellaneous:** Increased incidence of lymphoma/lymphoproliferative disease, nonmelanoma skin carcinoma, and other malignancies. Increased incidence of opportunistic infections, including herpes simplex, CMV, herpes zoster, *Candida, Aspergillus/Mucor* invasive disease, and *Pneumocystis carinii*. **Life-threatening infections, including meningitis and infectious endocarditis**. Tuberculosis, atypical mycobacterial infection, enlarged abdomen, cyst, facial edema, chest pain, back pain, pelvic pain, neck pain, weight gain.

LABORATORY TEST CONSIDERATIONS
↑ Creatinine, BUN, LDH, AST, ALT, alkaline phosphatase, GGT, prothrombin, thromboplastin. Hypophosphatemia, hypo-/hyperkalemia, hypo-/hyperglycemia, bilirubinemia, hypervolemia, hyperuricemia, hypomagnesemia, acidosis, hyponatremia, hyperlipemia, hypo-/hypercalcemia, hypochloremia, hypoproteinemia. Abnormal LFTs.

OD **OVERDOSE MANAGEMENT**
Symptoms: Nausea, vomiting, diarrhea, hematologic abnormalities, especially neutropenia. *Treatment:* Reduce dose of the drug. Removal of MPA by bile acid sequestrants (e.g., cholestyramine).

DRUG INTERACTIONS
Acyclovir / ↑ Plasma levels of both drugs R/T competition for renal tubular excretion
Antacids containing Al/ Mg / ↓ Absorption of mycophenolate
Azathioprine / Avoid concomitant use R/T lack of clinical studies
Cholestyramine / ↓ Absorption of mycophenolate; do not use together
Cyclosporine / ↓ Mycophenolic acid levels
H *Echinacea* / Do not give with mycophenolate
Ganciclovir / ↑ Plasma levels of both drugs R/T competition for renal tubular excretion
Iron / ↓ Mycophenolate absorption; do not use together
Levonorgestrel (including oral contraceptives containing levonorgestrel) / Significant ↓ in levonorgestrel AUC; consider additional birth control measures
Metronidazole & Norfloxacin / ↓ Mycophenolic acid and mycophenolic acid glucuronide AUC
Phenytoin / ↓ Plasma protein binding of phenytoin → ↑ free phenytoin lev-

---

Bold Italic = life threatening side effect   ■ = black box warning   ✛ = Available in Canada els

Probenecid / Significant ↑ plasma levels of MPA

Rifampin / Possible ↓ mycophenolic acid levels in lung transplant clients

Salicylates / ↑ Free fraction of MPA

Sirolimus / Possible ↑ mycophenolic acid levels and ↓ WBCs

Theophylline / ↓ Plasma protein binding of theophylline → ↑ free theophylline levels

Vaccines, life attenuated / Vaccinations may be less effective

HOW SUPPLIED

Mycophenolate mofetil *Capsules:* 250 mg; *Powder for Injection, Lyophilized:* 500 mg; *Powder for Oral Suspension:* 200 mg/mL; *Tablets:* 500 mg.

Mycophenolate sodium *Tablets, Delayed-Release:* 180 mg, 360 mg.

DOSAGE

MYCOPHENOLATE MOFETIL

• **CAPSULES; IV; ORAL SUSPENSION; TABLETS**

Renal transplantation.

Adults: 1 gram twice a day (a dose of 1.5 grams twice a day is also safe and effective). Give IV dose over 2 hr. **Children:** 600 mg/m^2 twice a day, up to a maximum daily dose of 2 grams/10 mL oral suspension. Those with a body surface area of 1.25–1.5 m^2 may be dosed with mycophenolate capsules, 750 mg twice a day. Clients with a body surface area greater than 1.5 m^2 may be dosed with capsules or tablets, 1 gram twice a day.

Cardiac transplantation.

Adults: 1.5 grams twice a day. Give IV dose over 2 hr or more.

Hepatic transplantation.

1 gram twice a day IV given over 2 hr or 1.5 grams twice a day PO.

MYCOPHENOLATE SODIUM

• **TABLETS, DELAYED-RELEASE**

Renal transplantation.

Adults: 720 mg twice a day (1,440 total daily dose) on an empty stomach, 1 hr before or 2 hr after food. For the elderly, give no more than 720 mg twice daily. **Children:** 400 mg/m^2 twice a day in stable pediatric clients, up to a maximum of 720 mg twice a day. Clients with a body surface area (BSA) of 1.19

to 1.58 m^2 may be dosed with either three 180 mg extended-release tablets or one 180 mg extended-release tablet plus one 360 mg extended-release tablet twice a day. Clients with a BSA of more than 1.58 m^2 may be dosed with either four 180 mg extended-release tablets or two 360 mg extended-release tablets. Pediatric doses for clients with a BSA less than 1.19 m^2 cannot be accurately given the drug using currently available extended-release formulations.

NURSING CONSIDERATIONS

ADMINISTRATION/STORAGE

1. For PO dosage forms, start therapy asap following transplantation.

2. Give on an empty stomach. In stable renal transplant clients, may be given with food if necessary.

3. The oral suspension may be given via a nasogastric tube with a minimum size of 8 French catheter.

4. Avoid doses of 1 gram twice a day in CRF (i.e., GFR <25 mL/min/1.73 m^2) outside the immediate posttreatment period.

5. Mycophenolate is teratogenic; do not open or crush capsules. Avoid inhalation or direct contact with the skin or mucous membranes; wash area thoroughly with soap and water if contact occurs. Rinse eyes with plain water.

6. Dispense tablets in light-resistant containers, i.e., manufacturer's original container.

7. To prepare oral suspension tap the closed bottle several times to loosen the powder. Measure 94 mL water and add one half the total amount of water to the bottle and shake well for about 1 min. Add the remainder of the water and shake the closed bottle well for about 1 min. Remove child-resistant cap and push the bottle adapter into the neck of bottle. Close bottle with child-resistant cap tightly to ensure proper seating of the bottle adapter and the child-resistant status of the cap.

8. If neutropenia develops (ANC <1.3 x 10^3/mcL), interrupt or reduce dose; perform appropriate diagnostic tests and manage appropriately.

9. Store capsules, dry powder for oral suspension, or tablets from 15–30°C (59–86°F). Store constituted suspension from 15–30°C (59–86°F) for up to 60 days; may also be stored from 2–8°C (36–46°F). Do not freeze. Discard any unused portion 60 days after reconstitution.

IV 10. Give IV over 2 or more hours by a peripheral or central vein. Do not give by rapid or IV bolus. IV recommended for those unable to take capsules, oral suspension, or tablets.

11. Begin 24 or fewer hours after transplantation and give for 14 days or fewer; switch to PO mycophenolate as soon as PO medication can be tolerated.

12. Reconstitute each vial with 14 mL of D5W. Solution is slightly yellow. Discard if particulate matter or discoloration is seen. Further dilute the contents of 2 reconstituted vials into 140 mL of D5W for a 1 gram dose or of 3 reconstituted vials into 210 mL of D5W for a 1.5 gram dose. The final concentration of both solutions is 6 mg/mL. Use within 4 hr of reconstitution and dilution.

13. Do not mix or give IV mycophenolate via the same infusion catheter with any other IV drugs or infusion admixtures.

14. Because the drug is teratogenic in animals, use caution in handling and preparing IV solutions. If contact occurs, wash thoroughly with soap and water; rinse eyes with plain water.

ASSESSMENT

1. Note date/type of transplant, other procedures trialed/agents used and outcome.

2. Document a negative pregnancy test 1 week prior to initiating therapy in all women of childbearing age.

3. Monitor renal and LFTs, and hematologic profiles and observe closely for severe neutropenia (day 31 to day 180) posttransplant. If ANC is less than 1.3 × 10^3, then drug therapy must be interrupted or decreased.

CLIENT/FAMILY TEACHING

1. Take exactly as directed on an empty stomach twice a day; taken with cyclosporine and steroids. Must take for life to prevent transplant rejection.

2. Do not remove from manufacturer's original container. Do not break/crush, chew, or open capsules as powder may be teratogenic if inhaled or contact with skin/mucus membranes. Wash immediately with soap and water and rinse with plain water if contact occurs.

3. With increased immunosuppression the susceptibility to infection and the risk of lymphoproliferative disease and other malignancies may be increased. Report any new/unusual side effects or fever/infection. Avoid crowds and contact with persons with contagious disease or infection.

4. Practice two reliable forms of contraception simultaneously before, during, and for 6 weeks following therapy.

5. Report for all scheduled labs to evaluate response to therapy and to identify potential problems. Need CBC weekly during first month, twice monthly for the second and third months, and then monthly thereafter for the first year.

OUTCOMES/EVALUATE

Prevention of transplant rejection; improved organ function

N

Nabumetone ■
(nah-**BYOU**-meh-tohn)

CLASSIFICATION(S):
Nonsteroidal anti-inflammatory drug
PREGNANCY CATEGORY: B
✦**Rx:** Apo-Nabumetone, Gen-Nabumetone, Rhoxal-nabumetone.

SEE ALSO NONSTEROIDAL ANTI-INFLAMMATORY DRUGS.
USES
Acute and chronic treatment of osteoarthritis and rheumatoid arthritis.
ACTION/KINETICS
Action
Anti-inflammatory effect is due to inhibition of the enzyme cyclo-oxygenase. Inhibition of cyclo-oxygenase results in decreased prostaglandin synthesis. Prostaglandin will cause inflammation. Effective in reducing joint swelling, pain, and morning stiffness and increases mobility in those with inflammatory disease.
Pharmacokinetics
Greater than 80% is bioavailable. **Time to peak plasma levels:** 2.5–4 hr. **Peak effect:** 9–12 hr. **t½ of active metabolite:** 22.5–30 hr. Excreted mainly (80%) in the urine. **Plasma protein binding:** More than 99%.
CONTRAINDICATIONS
Lactation.
SPECIAL CONCERNS
■ (1) NSAIDs may cause an increased risk of serious CV thrombotic events, MI, and stroke, which can be fatal. This risk may increase with duration of use. Clients with CV disease or risk factors for CV disease may be at greater risk. (2) Nabumetone is contraindicated to treat perioperative pain in the setting of coronary artery bypass graft surgery. (3) NSAIDs cause an increased risk of serious GI side effects including inflammation, bleeding, ulceration, and perfora-

tion of the stomach or intestines, which can be fatal. These events can occur at any time during use and without warning symptoms. Elderly clients are at greater risk for serious GI events.■ Safety and efficacy have not been determined in children.
SIDE EFFECTS
Most Common
Headache, diarrhea, nausea, dizziness, rash, pruritus, constipation, flatulence, edema, tinnitus.
See *Nonsteroidal Anti-Inflammatory Drugs* for a complete list of possible side effects.
HOW SUPPLIED
Tablets: 500 mg, 750 mg.
DOSAGE————————
• **TABLETS**
  Osteoarthritis, rheumatoid arthritis.
Adults, initial: 1,000 mg as a single dose; **maintenance:** 1,500–2,000 mg/day as either a single or twice-daily dosage. Doses greater than 2,000 mg/day have not been studied.

NURSING CONSIDERATIONS
ADMINISTRATION/STORAGE
1. May be taken with or without food.
2. Use the lowest effective dose for the shortest duration consistent with individual treatment goals.
3. Do not exceed a starting dose of 500 mg once daily in severe renal insufficiency or 750 mg once daily in moderate renal insufficiency. If needed, the dose can be increased to 1,000 mg/day in severe renal insufficiency or 1,500 mg/day in moderate renal insufficiency.
4. Store from 20–25°C (68–77°F).
ASSESSMENT
1. List reasons for therapy, onset, characteristics of S&S, other agents trialed, outcome; rate pain level.
2. Note swelling, pain, inflammation, trauma, decreased ROM.
3. Assess for conditions that may preclude therapy, i.e., ulcer hx, pregnancy, HTN, CAD, recent CABG, intestinal hemorrhage or perforation.

 = see color insert   = Herbal   = Intravenous   ℚ = sound alike drug

4. Monitor CBC, renal, LFTs; reduce dose with dysfunction.

CLIENT/FAMILY TEACHING

1. Take as directed; may take with food if GI upset. Report adverse effects or lack of response.

2. Review side effects that require immediate reporting: persistent headaches, altered vision, rash, severe stomach or back pain, extremity swelling, black tarry stools, dark vomiting.

3. Avoid tasks that require mental alertness until drug effects realized; may cause dizziness or drowsiness. Avoid alcohol and aspirin-containing products; may potentiate effects/bleeding.

4. Avoid prolonged sun exposure, use sunscreen and protective clothing, may cause reaction. Keep all F/U appointments.

OUTCOMES/EVALUATE

- Relief of pain
- Improved mobility; ↑ ROM

Nadolol ©
(NAY-doh-lohl)

CLASSIFICATION(S):
Beta-adrenergic blocking agent
PREGNANCY CATEGORY: C
Rx: Corgard.
♣Rx: Apo-Nadol, Novo-Nadolol, ratio-Nadolol.

SEE ALSO *BETA-ADRENERGIC BLOCKING AGENTS.*

USES

(1) Hypertension, either alone or with other drugs (e.g., thiazide diuretic). (2) Long-term management of angina pectoris. *Investigational:* Prophylaxis of migraine, ventricular arrhythmias, aggressive behavior, essential tremor, tremors associated with lithium or parkinsonism, antipsychotic-induced akathisia, rebleeding of esophageal varices, reduce intraocular pressure.

ACTION/KINETICS

Action
Manifests both beta$_1$/beta$_2$-adrenergic blocking activity. Has no membrane stabilizing or intrinsic sympathomimetic activity. Low lipid solubility.

Pharmacokinetics
Peak serum concentration: 3–4 hr. **t½:** 20–24 hr (permits once-daily dosage). **Duration:** 17–24 hr. Absorption variable, averaging 30%; steady plasma level achieved after 6–9 days of administration. Excreted unchanged by the kidney.

CONTRAINDICATIONS
Use in bronchial asthma or bronchospasm, including severe COPD.

SPECIAL CONCERNS
Dosage has not been established in children.

SIDE EFFECTS
Most Common
Nausea, decreased libido, impotence, insomnia, malaise, anxiety, nervousness. See *Beta-Adrenergic Blocking Agents* for a complete list of possible side effects.

HOW SUPPLIED
Tablets: 20 mg, 40 mg, 80 mg, 120 mg, 160 mg.

DOSAGE

- **TABLETS**

  Hypertension.
  Initial: 40 mg once daily; **then,** dose may be increased in 40 to 80 mg increments until optimum response obtained. **Maintenance:** 40–80 mg once daily, although up to 240–320 mg/day may be needed.

  Angina.
  Initial: 40 mg once daily; **then,** increase dose in 40 to 80 mg increments every 3–7 days until optimum response obtained or there is a pronounced slowing of HR. **Maintenance:** 40–80 mg once daily, although up to 160–240 mg/day may be needed.

  Aggressive behavior.
  40–160 mg/day.

  Antipsychotic-induced akathisia.
  40–80 mg/day.

  Essential tremor.
  120–240 mg/day.

  Lithium-induced tremors.
  20–40 mg/day.

  Tremors associated with parkinsonism.
  80–320 mg/day.

  Prophylaxis of migraine.
  40–80 mg/day.

Bold Italic = life threatening side effect   ■ = black box warning   ♣ = Available in Canada

Rebleeding of esophageal varices.
40–160 mg/day.
Ventricular arrhythmias.
10–640 mg/day.
Reduction of intraocular pressure.
10–20 mg twice a day.

NURSING CONSIDERATIONS

Ⓡ Do not confuse Corgard with Coreg (an alpha/beta adrenergic blocking agent).

ADMINISTRATION/STORAGE

1. Adjust dose as follows in clients with renal impairment: If C_{CR} is >50 mL/min/1.73 m^2, use a dosing interval of 24 hr. If C_{CR} is 31–50 mL/min/1.73 m^2, use a dosing interval of 24–36 hr. If C_{CR} is 10–30 mL/min/1.73 m^2, use a dosing interval of 24–48 hr. If C_{CR} is <10 mL/min/1.73 m^2, use a dosing interval of 40–60 hr.
2. Store tablets at room temperature protected from light and excessive heat. Keep bottle tightly closed.

ASSESSMENT

1. Note reasons for therapy, medical history, characteristics of S&S, other agents trialed.
2. List baseline VS, labs, ECG.
3. Assess for asthma, severe COPD; reduce dose with renal dysfunction, see under administration.

CLIENT/FAMILY TEACHING

1. Take only as directed; do not stop abruptly.
2. Report any rapid weight gain, increased SOB, or extremity swelling.
3. Do not perform tasks that require mental alertness until drug effects realized; may cause dizziness/drowsiness. Change positions slowly to prevent sudden drop in BP.
4. May cause increased sensitivity to cold; dress appropriately.
5. Keep log of BP and HR for provider review. Hold dose and report if HR <50 or BP <80, or as directed.

OUTCOMES/EVALUATE

- ↓ BP, ↓ HR
- ↓ Frequency/intensity of angina

Nafarelin acetate
(**NAF**-ah-rel-in)

CLASSIFICATION(S):
Gonadotropin-releasing hormone
PREGNANCY CATEGORY: X
Rx: Synarel.

USES

(1) Endometriosis (including reduction of endometriotic lesions) in clients aged 18 or older (400 mcg/day is clinically comparable to 3.75 mg/month of Lupon Depot). (2) Central precocious puberty in children of both sexes.

ACTION/KINETICS

Action
Produced through biotechnology; differs by only one amino acid from naturally occurring GnRH. Stimulates the release of LH and FSH from the adenohypophysis. Causes estrogen and progesterone synthesis in the ovary, resulting in the maturation and subsequent release of an ovum. With repeated use of the drug, however, the pituitary becomes desensitized and no longer produces endogenous LH and FSH; thus endogenous estrogen is not produced, leading to a regression of endometrial tissue, cessation of menstruation, and a menopausal-like state.

Pharmacokinetics
Broken down by the enzyme peptidase.
Peak serum levels: 10–40 min. **t½:** 3 hr.
Plasma protein binding: 80%.

CONTRAINDICATIONS

Hypersensitivity to GnRH or analogs. Abnormal vaginal bleeding of unknown origin. Pregnancy or possibility of becoming pregnant. Lactation.

SPECIAL CONCERNS

Rule out pregnancy before initiating therapy. Safety and effectiveness have not been established in children.

SIDE EFFECTS

Most Common
Hot flashes, decreased libido, vaginal dryness, headaches, emotional lability, acne, myalgia, reduced breast size, nasal irritation.

Due to hypoestrogenic effects: Hot flashes, decreased libido, vaginal dryness, headaches, emotional lability, insomnia. **Due to androgenic effects:** Acne, myalgia, reduced breast size, edema, seborrhea, weight gain, increased libido, hirsutism. **Musculoskeletal:** Decrease in vertebral trabecular bone density and total vertebral bone mass. **Miscellaneous:** Nasal irritation, depression, weight loss.

LABORATORY TEST CONSIDERATIONS

↑ Cholesterol and triglyceride levels, plasma phosphorus, eosinophils. ↓ Serum calcium, WBCs.

HOW SUPPLIED

Nasal Spray: 2 mg/mL (200 mcg/inh).

DOSAGE

- **NASAL SPRAY**
  Endometriosis.
200 mcg into one nostril in the morning and 200 mcg into the other nostril at night (400 mcg twice a day may be required for some women).
  Central precocious puberty.
400 mcg (2 sprays) into each nostril in the morning (i.e., 4 sprays) and in the evening (total of 8 sprays/day). If adequate suppression is not achieved, 3 sprays (600 mcg) into alternating nostrils 3 times per day (i.e., a total of 9 sprays/day).

NURSING CONSIDERATIONS

ADMINISTRATION/STORAGE

1. Initiate therapy between days 2 and 4 of the menstrual cycle.
2. Use no longer than 6 months; not recommended R/T the lack of safety data.
3. Store at room temperature in an upright position protected from light.

ASSESSMENT

1. Note reasons for therapy. Perform history, noting any osteoporosis, alcohol, tobacco, or corticosteroid use; major risk factors for bone mineral loss that would preclude any repeated courses.
2. With central precocious puberty review history and physical exam and ensure complete endocrinologic exam. Obtain testosterone or estradiol levels, adrenal steroid level, GnRH stimulation

test, beta human chorionic gonadotropin level, pelvic/testicular/adrenal US and CT of the head; monitor after 6 weeks of therapy and then every 3–6 months during therapy.
3. Note description of menstrual cycles and any abnormal vaginal bleeding of unknown origin; drug contraindicated. Document abdominal/vaginal assessments and ultrasound findings.
4. Determine if pregnant; drug is teratogenic.

CLIENT/FAMILY TEACHING

1. With endometriosis, begin treatment between the second and fourth day of the menstrual cycle. Keep accurate records of menstrual patterns and cycles.
2. Use spray upon arising and just before bedtime, alternating nostrils to decrease mucosal irritation. If a topical nasal decongestant is required during treatment, use at least 30 min after nafarelin to prevent interference with drug absorption
3. Menses should cease while on therapy; report if regular menses continues. Breakthrough bleeding may occur if successive doses are missed.
4. Use nonhormonal contraception; drug may cause fetal harm.
5. May cause hypoestrogenic and androgenic side effects; report as a change in dosage or therapy may be indicated. May experience hot flashes.
6. With central precocious puberty use 2 sprays to each nostril in am and 2 to each nostril in pm with the 1600 mcg/day dose. With 1800 mcg/day dosing use 3 sprays into each nostril three times daily.
7. May experience signs of puberty during the first mo of therapy (vaginal bleeding, breast enlargement; should resolve after the first mo. Drug is discontinued when puberty onset is desired.
8. Keep all F/U appointments to evaluate response to therapy.

OUTCOMES/EVALUATE

- Restoration of pituitary-gonadal function in 4–8 weeks
- ↓ Number/size of endometriotic lesions
- Inhibition of early puberty

Naftifine hydrochloride
(**NAF**-tih-feen)

CLASSIFICATION(S):
Antifungal
PREGNANCY CATEGORY: B
Rx: Naftin.

SEE ALSO *ANTI-INFECTIVE DRUGS.*

USES
Tinea cruris (jock itch), tinea pedis (athlete's foot), and tinea corporis (ringworm) caused by *Trichophyton rubrum, T. mentagrophytes, T. tonsurans,* and *Epidermophyton floccosum.*

ACTION/KINETICS
Action
Synthetic antifungal agent with a broad spectrum of activity. Thought to inhibit squalene 2, 3-epoxidase, which is responsible for synthesis of sterols. The decreased levels of sterols (especially ergosterol) and the accumulation of squalene in cells result in fungicidal activity. The drug penetrates the stratum corneum to inhibit the growth of dermatophytes.

Pharmacokinetics
Although used topically, approximately 6% of the drug is absorbed. Naftifine and its metabolites are excreted via the feces and urine. **t½:** 2–3 days.

CONTRAINDICATIONS
Ophthalmic use.

SPECIAL CONCERNS
Use with caution during lactation. Safety and efficacy in children have not been determined.

SIDE EFFECTS
Most Common
Burning, stinging, itching, dryness.
TOPICAL. Cream: Burning, stinging, dryness, itching, local irritation, erythema. **Gel:** Burning, stinging, itching, rash, tenderness, erythema.

HOW SUPPLIED
Topical Cream: 1%; *Topical Gel/Jelly:* 1%.

DOSAGE————————————
• **TOPICAL CREAM; TOPICAL GEL/JELLY**

Massage into affected area and surrounding skin once daily if using the cream and twice daily (morning and evening) if using the gel.

NURSING CONSIDERATIONS
ASSESSMENT
Note reasons for therapy, characteristics of S&S, onset, location, clinical presentation, cultures, other agents trialed, outcome.
CLIENT/FAMILY TEACHING
1. Wash hands before and after use. Gently massage into area containing fungal infection as directed.
2. Avoid contact with eyes, nose, mouth, or other mucous membranes; for external use only.
3. Do not cover area; avoid occlusive dressings, diapers, or wrappings. Report any excessive itching, dryness, burning or irritation.
4. Beneficial effects are usually observed within 1 week; treatment should be continued for 1–2 weeks after symptoms diminish. Report if no beneficial effects after 4 weeks of treatment.
OUTCOMES/EVALUATE
Negative cultures; clinical improvement

Nalmefene hydrochloride
(**NAL**-meh-feen)

CLASSIFICATION(S):
Narcotic antagonist
PREGNANCY CATEGORY: B
Rx: Revex.

SEE ALSO *NARCOTIC ANTAGONISTS.*

USES
(1) Complete or partial reversal of the effects of opioid drugs, including respiratory depression, induced by either natural or synthetic opioids. (2) Management of known or suspected overdose of opioids.

ACTION/KINETICS
Action
Prevents or reverses respiratory depression, sedation, and hypotension due to

opioids, including propoxyphene, nalbuphine, pentazocine, and butorphanol. Has a significantly longer duration of action than naloxone. Does not produce respiratory depression, psychotomimetic effects, or pupillary constriction (i.e., it has no intrinsic activity). Also, tolerance, physical dependence, or abuse potential have not been noted.

Pharmacokinetics
Onset, after IV: 2 min. **Duration:** Up to 8 hr. **t½, after IV:** 41 min (redistribution) and 10.8 hr (terminal elimination). Metabolized by the liver primarily by glucuronide metabolism and excreted in the urine.

SPECIAL CONCERNS
Will precipitate acute withdrawal symptoms in those who have some degree of tolerance and dependence on opioids. Use with caution during lactation, in high-risk CV clients, or in those who have received potentially cardiotoxic drugs. Reversal of buprenorphine-induced respiratory depression may be incomplete; therefore, artificial respiration may be necessary. Safety and effectiveness have not been determined in children.

SIDE EFFECTS
Most Common
N&V, tachycardia, hypertension, postoperative pain, fever, dizziness.

CV: Tachycardia, hypertension, hypotension, vasodilation, bradycardia, arrhythmia. **GI:** N&V, diarrhea, dry mouth. **CNS:** Dizziness, somnolence, depression, agitation, nervousness, tremor, confusion, withdrawal syndrome, myoclonus. **Body as a whole:** Fever, headache, chills, postoperative pain. **Miscellaneous:** Pharyngitis, pruritus, urinary retention.

LABORATORY TEST CONSIDERATIONS
↑ AST.

HOW SUPPLIED
Injection: 100 mcg/mL, 1 mg/mL.

DOSAGE————————
• **IV**
Reversal of postoperative depression due to opiates.
Use the 100 mcg/mL dosage strength (blue label). **Adults:** Titrate in 0.25

mcg/kg incremental doses at 2–5 min intervals until the desired degree of reversal is achieved (i.e., adequate ventilation and alertness without significant pain or discomfort). If client is at increased CV risk, use an incremental dose of 0.1 mcg/kg (the drug may be diluted 1:1 with saline or sterile water). A total dose greater than 1 mcg/kg does not provide additional effects.

Management of known or suspected overdose of opiates.
Use the 1 mg/mL dosage strength (green label). **Adults, initial:** 0.5 mg/70 kg for nonopioid-dependent clients; **then,** 1 mg/70 kg 2–5 min later, if needed. Doses greater than 1.5 mg/70 kg do not increase the beneficial effect. If there is a reasonable suspicion of dependence on opiates, give a challenge dose of 0.1 mg/70 kg first; if there is no evidence of withdrawal in 2 min, give the recommended dose.

NURSING CONSIDERATIONS
ADMINISTRATION/STORAGE
1. May give SC or IM at doses of 1 mg if IV access is lost or not readily obtainable. One mg doses are effective in 5–15 min.
[IV] 2. Treatment should follow, not precede, establishment of patent airway, ventilatory assistance, oxygen, and circulatory access.
3. Nalmefene is longest acting of the available parenteral opioid antagonists. If respiratory depression recurs, titrate dose again to clinical effect using incremental doses to avoid over-reversal.
4. In renal failure, give incremental doses slowly (over 60 sec) to minimize possible hypertension and dizziness.
5. If clients known to be at increased cardiac risk, may be desirable to dilute nalmefene 1:1 with saline or sterile water and use smaller initial and incremental doses of 0.1 mcg/kg.
6. Nalmefene is supplied in two concentrations—ampules containing 1 mL (blue label) at a concentration suitable for postoperative use (100 mcg) and ampules containing 2 mL (green label) suitable for management of overdose (1 mg/mL), i.e., **10 times as concentra-**

ted. Follow specific guidelines, as indicated.

ASSESSMENT

1. List type and amount of agent used; when administered/ingested.

2. Note any opioid dependence; may induce acute withdrawal S&S. Perform challenge test if opioid dependency suspected.

3. Identify high CV risk or if received cardiotoxic drugs; increases risk for cardiac complications.

4. Observe carefully for recurrent respiratory depression. Compared to naloxone (1.1 hr) the half-life of nalmefene is much longer (10.8 hr). Overdose with long-acting opiates (e.g., methadone, LAAM) may cause recurrence of respiratory depression.

5. With renal failure, if more than one dose required, administer incremental doses slowly (over 60 sec) to prevent dizziness and hypertension.

CLIENT/FAMILY TEACHING

1. Drug works by blocking opiate receptor sites, which reverses or prevents toxic effects of narcotic (opioid) analgesics. Usually injected in hospital or clinic.

2. May experience N&V, fever, headaches, chills, pain, dizziness, tachycardia and withdrawal symptoms if narcotic dependent.

3. Do not perform activities that require mental alertness until drug effects realized; may cause dizziness, drowsiness.

4. If you experience a return of symptoms (i.e., drowsiness or difficulty breathing) report immediately.

OUTCOMES/EVALUATE

Reversal of opioid-induced drug effects; ↓ Risk of renarcotization

Naloxone hydrochloride

(nal-**OX**-ohn)

CLASSIFICATION(S):
Narcotic antagonist
PREGNANCY CATEGORY: B
Rx: Narcan.

SEE ALSO NARCOTIC ANTAGONISTS.

USES

(1) Respiratory depression induced by natural and synthetic narcotics, including butorphanol, cyclazocine, methadone, nalbuphine, and pentazocine. Not effective in acute toxicity due to levopropoxyphene. Drug of choice when nature of depressant drug is not known. (2) Diagnosis of acute opiate overdosage. Not effective when respiratory depression is induced by hypnotics, sedatives, or anesthetics and other nonnarcotic CNS depressants. *Investigational:* Treatment of Alzheimer's dementia, alcoholic coma, and schizophrenia.

ACTION/KINETICS

Action

Combines competitively with opiate receptors and blocks or reverses the action of narcotic analgesics. Since the duration of action of naloxone is shorter than that of the narcotic analgesics, the respiratory depression may return when the narcotic antagonist has worn off. In usual doses, has virtually no pharmacologic effects in the absence of opioids. When given to a client with opioid dependence, withdrawal symptoms will appear in minutes and subside in about 2 hr.

Pharmacokinetics

Onset, IV: 2 min; **SC, IM:** <5 min. **Time to peak effect:** 5–15 min. **Duration:** Dependent on dose and route of administration but may be as short as 45 min. **t½:** 60–100 min. Metabolized in the liver to inactive products; eliminated through the kidneys.

CONTRAINDICATIONS

Sensitivity to drug. Narcotic addicts (drug may cause severe withdrawal symptoms). Use in neonates.

SPECIAL CONCERNS

If given during labor, may cause severe hypertension in the mother with mild to moderate hypertension. Absorption after IM or SC use in neonates and children may be erratic. Safe use during lactation and in children is not established.

SIDE EFFECTS
Most Common
Virtually no pharmacologic effects in the absence of opioids.

N&V, sweating, hypertension, tremors, sweating due to reversal of narcotic depression. If used postoperatively, excessive doses may cause ***VT and fibrillation***, hypo-/hypertension, pulmonary edema, and ***seizures*** (infrequent).

HOW SUPPLIED
Injection: 0.02 mg/mL, 0.4 mg/mL.

DOSAGE
- **IM; IV; SC**

    Narcotic overdose.

Initial: 0.4–2 mg IV; if necessary, additional IV doses may be repeated at 2- to 3-min intervals. If no response after 10 mg, reevaluate diagnosis. Higher doses may be needed to reverse buprenophine-induced respiratory depression. **Pediatric, initial:** 0.01 mg/kg IV; **then,** 0.1 mg/kg IV, if needed. The SC or IM route may be used if an IV route is not available.

To reverse postoperative narcotic depression.

Adults, initial, 0.1 to 0.2 mg increments at 2- to 3-min intervals; **then,** repeat at 1- to 2-hr intervals if necessary. Supplemental IM dosage increases the duration of reversal. **Children, initial:** 0.005–0.01 mg IV at 2- to 3-min intervals until desired response is obtained.

Reverse narcotic-induced depression in neonates.

Initial: 0.01 mg/kg IV, IM, or SC. May be repeated using adult administration guidelines.

NURSING CONSIDERATIONS
Ⓒ Do not confuse naloxone with naltrexone (also a narcotic antagonist).

ADMINISTRATION/STORAGE
[IV] 1. May administer undiluted at a rate of 0.4 mg over 15 sec with narcotic overdosage. May reconstitute 2 mg in 500 mL of NSS or D5W to provide a 4 mcg/mL (0.004 mg/mL) concentration. Administration rate varies with client response.

2. Do not mix with preparations containing bisulfite, metabisulfite, long-chain or high molecular weight anions, or alkaline pH solutions.

3. When mixed with other solutions, use within 24 hr.

ASSESSMENT
1. Identify opiod addiction. Note agent, duration, half-life.

2. List cardiopulmonary and neurologic assessments.

3. Make appropriate referrals for those requiring substance-abuse counseling.

INTERVENTIONS
1. Duration of narcotic may exceed naloxone (the antagonist). Therefore, more than one dose may be necessary to counteract the effects of the narcotic.

2. Monitor VS at 5-min intervals, then every 30 min once stabilized.

3. Titrate to avoid interfering with pain control or readminister narcotic at a lower dosage to maintain pain control.

CLIENT/FAMILY TEACHING
1. Drug works by blocking opiate receptor sites, which reverses or prevents toxic effects of narcotic (opioid) analgesics. Administered by injection in hospital setting.

2. May experience N&V, fever, headaches, chills, pain, dizziness, tachycardia and withdrawal symptoms if narcotic dependent.

3. Do not perform activities that require mental alertness until drug effects realized; may cause dizziness, drowsiness.

4. If you experience a return of symptoms (i.e., drowsiness or difficulty breathing) report immediately.

OUTCOMES/EVALUATE
Reversal of narcotic-induced respiratory depression

Naltrexone ■
(nal-**TREX**-ohn)

CLASSIFICATION(S):
Narcotic antagonist
PREGNANCY CATEGORY: C
Rx: Depade, ReVia.

SEE ALSO *NARCOTIC ANTAGONISTS.*

Bold Italic = life threatening side effect   ■ = black box warning   ✚ = Available in Canada

USES

PO. (1) Blockade of the effects of exogenously given opioids. Has not been shown to produce any therapeutic benefit except as part of an appropriate plan of management for opioid dependence. *NOTE:* Use of naltrexone does not eliminate or diminish the alcohol withdrawal syndrome. (2) Treatment of alcohol dependence. *Investigational:* Treat eating disorders and postconcussional syndrome not responding to other approaches.

IM. Treatment of alcohol dependence in those who are able to abstain from alcohol in an outpatient setting prior to initiation of naltrexone treatment. Clients should not be actively drinking at the time of beginning naltrexone. Treatment with naltrexone should be part of a comprehensive management program that includes psychosocial support.

ACTION/KINETICS

Action

A pure opioid antagonist that competitively binds to opiate receptors, thereby reversing or preventing the effects of narcotics. Has few, if any, intrinsic effects besides its ability to block opioid receptors. The drug will precipitate withdrawal if given to an individual physically dependent on a narcotic. The blockade to naltrexone is surmountable; attempts by clients to overcome blockade by taking opioids is dangerous and may lead to a fatal overdose.

Pharmacokinetics

Peak plasma levels: 1 hr after PO; 2 hr after IM for first peak and 2–3 days for second peak. **Duration:** 24–72 hr after PO. Significant first-pass metabolism; thus, PO bioavailability ranges from 5–40%. Metabolized in the liver; a major metabolite—6-beta-naltrexol—is active. **Peak serum levels, after 50 mg PO: naltrexone,** 8.6 ng/mL; **6-beta-naltrexol,** 99.3 ng/mL. **t½, after PO: naltrexone,** approximately 4 hr; **6-beta-naltrexol,** 13 hr. **t½, terminal, after IM, naltrexone:** 5–10 days; **6-beta-naltrexol:** 5–10 days. Naltrexone and its metabolites are excreted mainly in the urine. **Plasma protein binding:** About 21%.

CONTRAINDICATIONS

Those taking narcotic analgesics, dependent on narcotics (including those maintained on methadone), in acute withdrawal from narcotics, failed naloxone challenge, positive urine screen for opioids, or history of hypersensitivity to naltrexone. Liver failure, acute hepatitis. Parenteral product not recommended during lactation.

SPECIAL CONCERNS

■ (1) Naltrexone has the capacity to cause hepatocellular injury when given in excessive doses. It is contraindicated in acute hepatitis or liver failure. Carefully consider its use in clients with active liver disease in light of its hepatotoxic effects. (2) The margin of separation between the apparently safe dose of naltrexone and the dose causing hepatic injury appears to be only 5-fold or less. Naltrexone does not appear to be a hepatotoxin at the recommended doses. (3) Warn clients of the risk of hepatic injury and advise them to stop the use of naltrexone and seek medical attention if they experience symptoms of acute hepatitis.■ Use with caution during lactation if used PO. If using IM, administer with caution to those with thrombocytopenia or any coagulation disorder (e.g., hemophilia, severe hepatic failure). Use with caution in those with imparied renal or hepatic function. There may be unintended precipitation of abstinence; ensure client is opioid-free for 7–10 days before starting naloxone. Safety in children under 18 years of age has not been established.

SIDE EFFECTS

Most Common

Naltrexone, in opioid-free individuals produces almost no side effects. Effects seen are due to narcotic withdrawal.

High doses of naltrexone may produce hepatotoxicity. **Effects due to narcotic withdrawal or alcohol dependence.** A severe narcotic withdrawal syndrome may be precipitated if naltrexone is administered to a dependent individual. The syndrome may begin within 5 min and may last for up to 2 days. **CNS:**

Insomnia, anxiety, somnolence, nervousness, 'feeling down,' irritability, agitation, dizziness, depression, paranoia, fatigue, headache, restlessness, confusion, euphoria, disorientation, abnormal thinking, hallucinations, nightmares, bad dreams, **suicidality (suicidal ideation, suicide attempts, completed suicides)**. **GI:** N&V, abdominal pain, anorexia, diarrhea, constipation, increased thirst, excessive gas, hemorrhoids, ulcer, dry mouth, hepatitis. **Musculoskeletal:** Joint/muscle pain, painful shoulders/legs/knees, tremors, twitching, chest pain, hyperkinesia, myalgia. **CV:** Nosebleeds, phlebitis, edema, hypertension, nonspecific ECG changes, palpitations, tachycardia. **Respiratory:** Nasal congestion, itching, rhinorrhea, sneezing, sore throat, excess mucus/phlegm, sinus trouble, heavy breathing, hoarseness, cough, shortness of breath, dyspnea. **GU:** Delayed ejaculation, increased frequency of or discomfort during urination, increased/decreased libido. **Dermatologic:** Skin rash, oily skin, pruritus, acne, athlete's foot, cold sores, alopecias, hot flushes. **Ophthalmic:** Blurred vision, burning, light sensitivity, swollen/aching/strained eyes. **Otic:** Aching/clogged ears, tinnitus. **Body as a whole:** Low or high energy, chills, fever, swollen glands, asthenia, malaise, tremor, increased sweating. **Miscellaneous:** Increased appetite, anorexia, weight loss/gain, yawning, head 'pounding,' inguinal pain, cold feet, 'hot spells.' NOTE: Death has resulted from ultra rapid opiate detoxification.

LABORATORY TEST CONSIDERATIONS

↑ Eosinophil counts (returned to normal over several months). ↑ AST, ALT, CPK, bilitrubin. ↓ Platelet count. Abnormal hepatic function.

DRUG INTERACTIONS

Opioid-containing products (e.g., cough/cold, antidiarrheals, opioid analgesics) / No beneficial effect may be obtained due to blockade of opioid effect by naltrexone

Thioridazine / Possible lethargy and somnolence

HOW SUPPLIED

Suspension for Injection, Extended-Release: 380 mg/vial; Tablets: 50 mg.

DOSAGE

- **TABLETS**

  Blockade of opiate actions.

  Initial: 25 mg followed by an additional 25 mg in 1 hr if no withdrawal symptoms occur. **Maintenance:** 50 mg/day. **Alternate dosing schedule**: The weekly dose of 350 mg may be given as: (a) 50 mg/day on weekdays and 100 mg on Saturday; (b) 100 mg/48 hr; (c) 100 mg every Monday and Wednesday and 150 mg on Friday; or, (d) 150 mg q 72 hr.

  Alcoholism.

  50 mg once daily for up to 12 weeks. Treatment for longer than 12 weeks has not been studied.

- **IM**

  Alcohol dependence.

  380 mg IM q 4 weeks or once a month.

NURSING CONSIDERATIONS

ADMINISTRATION/STORAGE

1. Never initiate therapy until determined that client is not dependent on narcotics (i.e., a naloxone challenge test should be completed).
2. Client should be opiate free for at least 7–10 days before beginning therapy.
3. When initiating therapy, begin with 25 mg PO and observe for 1 hr for any signs of narcotic withdrawal.
4. The blockade produced by naltrexone may be overcome by taking large doses of narcotics; such doses may be fatal.
5. Clients taking naltrexone may not respond to preparations containing narcotics for use in coughs, diarrhea, or pain.
6. When used parenterally, give as an IM gluteal injection, alternating buttocks, using the components provided. Do not give IV.
7. If an IM dose is missed, give as soon as possible. Pretreatment with PO naltrexone is not required before using parenteral naltrexone.
8. To prepare the IM injection, suspend only in the diluent provided in the car-

---

Bold Italic = life threatening side effect   ■ = black box warning   ✤ = Available in Canada

ton; give only with the needle supplied. All components (i.e., microspheres, diluent, preparation needle, and administration needle) are required for administration. Do not substitute any other components.

9. Inspect the product for particulate matter and discoloration prior to administration. A properly mixed suspension will be milky white, will not contain clumps, and will move freely down the wall of the vial.

10. Store the entire IM dose pack from 2–8°C (36–46°F). Unrefrigerated, can be stored for no more than 7 days at temperatures not exceeding 25°C (77°F). Do not freeze.

ASSESSMENT

1. Note if opiate addicted and when last dose was ingested; must be opiate free for 7–10 days before initiating therapy. Check urine to confirm absence of opiates; note naloxone challenge test results.

2. Assess for hepatitis; monitor LFTs, ECG, and VS. Report if respirations severely lowered or client has difficulty breathing.

3. Obtain LFTs; monitor monthly during the first 6 months of therapy.

4. A non-opiod analgesic should be used when analgesia is necessary. Consider alternative maintenance plan for those with compliance problems.

CLIENT/FAMILY TEACHING

1. This drug blocks the effects of narcotics and opiates. It also may help to prevent alcohol consumption. Taking an opiate with this therapy may prove fatal as the amount needed to overcome the blockade is quite high.

2. May take with food or milk to diminish GI upset. Request list of nonopiod drugs that may be used for pain, cough, or diarrhea.

3. Headaches, restlessness, and irritability may be caused by naltrexone.

4. Report loss of appetite, unusual fatigue, yellowing of skin or sclera, or itching. Abdominal pain or difficulty with bowel function may warrant a dosage reduction.

5. Remain drug free; identify individuals, agencies, and support groups that may assist you in remaining drug free. Attend support groups and behavioral therapy sessions.

6. Always carry/wear medical ID to alert medical personnel that you take naltrexone.

OUTCOMES/EVALUATE

Maintenance of narcotic-free state in detoxified addicts

Naproxen ■
(nah-**PROX**-en)

CLASSIFICATION(S):
Nonsteroidal anti-inflammatory drug
PREGNANCY CATEGORY: B
Rx: EC-Naprosyn, Naprosyn.
✤**Rx:** Apo-Naproxen, Apo-Naproxen SR, Gen-Naproxen EC, Novo-Naprox, Novo-Naprox EC, Novo-Naprox SR, Nu-Naprox, ratio-Naproxen.

Naproxen sodium
PREGNANCY CATEGORY: B
OTC: Aleve, Midol Extended Relief.
Rx: Anaprox, Anaprox DS, Naprelan.
✤**Rx:** Apo-Napro-Na, Apo-Napro-Na DS, Novo-Naprox Sodium, Novo-Naprox Sodium DS.

SEE ALSO NONSTEROIDAL ANTI-INFLAMMATORY DRUGS.

USES

Rx: (1) Mild to moderate pain. (2) Musculoskeletal and soft-tissue inflammation including rheumatoid arthritis, osteoarthritis, bursitis, tendinitis, ankylosing spondylitis. (3) Primary dysmenorrhea. (4) Acute gout. (5) Juvenile rheumatoid arthritis (naproxen only). NOTE: The delayed-release or enteric-coated products are not recommended for initial treatment of pain because, compared to other naproxen products, absorption is delayed. Investigational: Antipyretic in cancer clients, sunburn, acute migraine (sodium salt only), prophylaxis of migraine, migraine due to menses, PMS (sodium salt only). Lower risk of Alzheimer's disease (long-term use).

OTC. (1) Relief of minor aches and pains due to the common cold, headache, toothache, muscular aches, backache, minor arthritis pain, pain due to menstrual cramps. (2) Antipyretic.

ACTION/KINETICS
Action
Anti-inflammatory effect is likely due to inhibition of cyclo-oxygenase. Inhibition of cyclo-oxygenase results in decreased prostaglandin synthesis. Effective in reducing joint swelling, pain, and morning stiffness, as well as to increase mobility in those with inflammatory disease. Does not alter the course of the disease, however. The antipyretic action occurs by decreasing prostaglandin synthesis in the hypothalamus resulting in an increase in peripheral blood flow and heat loss, as well as promoting sweating.

Pharmacokinetics
95% is bioavailable. **Peak serum levels of naproxen:** 2–4 hr; **for sodium salt:** 1–2 hr. **t½ for naproxen:** 12–15 hr; **for sodium salt:** 12–13 hr. **Onset, immediate release for analgesia:** 1–2 hr. **Duration, analgesia:** Approximately 7 hr. **Onset (both immediate and delayed release):** 30 min; **duration:** 24 hr. **Onset, anti-inflammatory effects:** Up to 2 weeks; **duration:** 2–4 weeks. Food delays the rate but not the amount of drug absorbed. 95% excreted in the urine. **Plasma protein binding:** More than 99%.

CONTRAINDICATIONS
Simultaneous use of naproxen and naproxen sodium. Lactation. Use of delayed-release product for initial treatment of acute pain.

SPECIAL CONCERNS
■ (1) NSAIDs may cause an increased risk of serious CV thrombotic events, MI, and stroke, which can be fatal. This risk may increase with duration of use. Clients with CV disease or risk factors for CV disease may be at a greater risk. (2) Naproxen is contraindicated (except for controlled-released tablets) for treatment of perioperative pain in the setting of coronary artery bypass graft surgery. (3) NSAIDs cause an increased risk of serious GI adverse events including bleeding, ulceration, and perforation of the stomach or intestines, which can be fatal. These events can occur at any time during use and without warning symptoms. Elderly clients are at greater risk for serious GI events.■ Safety and effectiveness of naproxen have not been determined in children less than 2 years of age; the safety and effectiveness of naproxen sodium have not been established in children. Geriatric clients may manifest increased total plasma levels of naproxen. Higher doses and use in those at risk of developing Alzheimer's disease may increase the risk of strokes and heart attacks.

SIDE EFFECTS
Most Common
Headache, dizziness, drowsiness, pruritus, skin eruptions, constipation, dyspepsia/indigestion, ecchymoses, edema, dyspnea, tinnitus.

See *Nonsteroidal Anti-Inflammatory Drugs* for a complete list of possible side effects.

LABORATORY TEST CONSIDERATIONS
Naproxen may increase urinary 17-ketosteroid values. Both forms may interfere with urinary assays for 5-HIAA.

DRUG INTERACTIONS
Alendronate / ↑ Risk of gastric ulcers
Methotrexate / Possibility of a fatal interaction
Probenecid / ↓ Plasma clearance of naproxen

HOW SUPPLIED
Naproxen: *Oral Suspension:* 125 mg/mL; *Tablets:* 250 mg, 375 mg, 500 mg; *Tablets, Delayed-Release:* 375 mg, 500 mg.

Naproxen Sodium: OTC: Capsules, Liquid Gel: 220 mg; *Tablets:* 220 mg; **Rx:** *Tablets:* 275 mg, 550 mg; *Tablets, Controlled-Release:* 412.5 mg, 550 mg.

DOSAGE
Naproxen, Naproxen Sodium
• RX: ORAL SUSPENSION; TABLETS; TABLETS, CONTROLLED-RELEASE; TABLETS, DELAYED-RELEASE

Rheumatoid arthritis, osteoarthritis, ankylosing spondylitis, pain, dysmenorrhea, acute tendinitis, bursitis.

Naproxen Tablets: 250–500 mg twice a day. May increase to 1.5 grams for short periods of time. **Naproxen Suspension:** 250 mg (10 mL), 375 mg (15 mL), or 500 mg (20 mL) twice a day. **Naproxen, Delayed-Release (EC-Naprosyn):** 375–500 mg twice a day. **Naproxen Sodium:** 275–500 mg twice a day. May increase to 1.65 grams/day for limited periods. **Naproxen sodium, Controlled-Release (Naprelan):** 750 mg or 1,000 mg once daily, not to exceed 1,500 mg/day. Do not exceed 1.25 grams naproxen (1.375 grams naproxen sodium) per day. If no improvement is seen within 2 weeks, consider an additional 2-week course of therapy.

Acute gout.

Naproxen, adults, initial: 750 mg; **then,** 250 mg q 8 hr until symptoms subside. **Naproxen sodium, adults, initial:** 825 mg; **then,** 275 mg q 8 hr until symptoms subside. **Naproxen, Controlled-Release (Naprelan):** 1,000–1,500 mg once daily on the first day; **then,** 1,000 mg once daily until symptoms subside.

Juvenile rheumatoid arthritis.

Naproxen only: 10 mg/kg/day in two divided doses. If the suspension is used, the following dosage can be used: **13 kg (29 lb):** 2.5 mL twice a day; **25 kg (55 lb):** 5 mL twice a day; **38 kg (84 lb):** 7.5 mL twice a day.

Mild to moderate pain, primary dysmenorrhea, acute tendinitis, bursitis.

Naproxen, initial: 500 mg; **then,** 500 mg q 12 hr or 250 mg q 6–8 hr, not to exceed 1.25 grams/day. Thereafter, do not exceed 1,000 mg/day. **Naproxen sodium, initial:** 550 mg; **then,** 550 mg q 12 hr or 275 mg q 6–8 hr, not to exceed 1.375 grams/day. Thereafter, do not exceed 1,100 mg/day. **Naproxen sodium, Controlled-Release (Naprelan):** 1,000 mg once daily. For a limited time, 1,500 mg/day may be used. Thereafter, do not exceed 1,000 mg/day.

• **OTC: CAPSULES, LIQUID GEL; TABLETS**

Analgesic, antipyretic.

Adults: 220 mg q 8–12 hr with a full glass of liquid. For some clients, 440 mg initially followed by 220 mg 12 hr later will provide better relief. Do not exceed 660 mg in a 24-hr period. Do not exceed 220 mg q 12 hr for geriatric clients. Not for use in children less than 12 years of age unless directed by provider.

NURSING CONSIDERATIONS

ADMINISTRATION/STORAGE

1. Naproxen tablets, naproxen delayed-release tablets, naproxen sodium tablets, and naproxen suspension are recommended for the treatment of rheumatoid arthritis, osteoarthritis, anklyosing spondylitis, and juvenile arthritis. Naproxen suspension is recommended for juvenile rheumatoid arthritis. Naproxen tablets, naproxen sodium tablets, naproxen suspension are also indicated to treat tendonitis, bursitis, acute gout, and to manage pain and primary dysmenorrhea.

2. Do not use naproxen delayed-release tablets for initial treatment of acute pain because absorption is delayed compared with other naproxen-containing products.

3. To be taken in the morning and in the evening. The doses do not have to be equal.

4. Do not give to children under age 2.

5. Delayed-release naproxen is not recommended for acute pain.

6. Do not use the OTC product for more than 10 days for pain or 3 days for fever unless prescribed.

ASSESSMENT

1. List reasons for therapy, onset, characteristics of S&S. Rate pain level using a pain-rating scale. Note any joint swelling, pain, trauma, inflammation, or decreased ROM.

2. Assess for GI bleeding or ulcer hx; use GI protectant if needed. Enteric-coated product (EC-Naprosyn) reduces GI side effects.

3. Monitor CBC, renal and LFTs with chronic therapy.

CLIENT/FAMILY TEACHING

1. Take with food and a full glass of water to ↓ GI upset; in the morning and evening for optimal effects. Do not break, chew, or crush delayed-release tablets.

2. Those consuming 3 or more alcoholic drinks per day should consult their provider for advice on when and how to take naproxen and other pain relievers.

3. May cause dizziness or drowsiness; avoid activities that require mental alertness until effects realized.

4. Report lack of response, worsening of symptoms, unusual bruising/bleeding, persistent abdominal pain, sore throat, fever, rash, altered vision, joint pain, edema, or dark-colored stools. May need periodic eye exams with prolonged therapy.

5. Avoid alcohol, aspirin, corticosteroids and all other OTC agents without approval.

6. Use protection when exposed to prolong sun light; may have sensitivity reaction.

7. NSAIDs have been associated with serious, possibly fatal, heart and blood vessel risks such as heart attack and stroke.

OUTCOMES/EVALUATE

- Improved joint pain and mobility
- Relief of headaches/pain
- ↓ Uterine cramping

Naratriptan hydrochloride

(**NAR**-ah-trip-tan)

CLASSIFICATION(S):

Antimigraine drug
PREGNANCY CATEGORY: C
Rx: Amerge.

USES

Acute treatment of migraine attacks in adults with or without aura.

ACTION/KINETICS

Action

Binds to serotonin 5-HT$_{1D}$ receptors. Activation of these receptors located on intracranial blood vessels, including those on arteriovenous anastomoses, leads to vasoconstriction and thus relief of migraine. Also possible that activation of these receptors on sensory nerve endings in trigeminal system causes inhibition of pro-inflammatory neuropeptide release.

Pharmacokinetics

Well absorbed from GI tract. Bioavailability is 74%. **Time to onset:** 1 hr. **Time to peak effect:** 2–3 hr. Unchanged drug and metabolites are primarily eliminated in urine. t½: 5.5 hr. Excretion is decreased in moderate liver or renal impairment. **Plasma protein binding:** About 28%.

CONTRAINDICATIONS

Use for prophylaxis of migraine, for management of hemiplegic or basilar migraine, in those with ischemic bowel disease. Use in clients with ischemic cardiac, cerebrovascular, or peripheral vascular syndromes; coronary artery vasospasm, uncontrolled hypertension. Use in severe renal impairment (C$_{CR}$ less than 15 mL/min); severe hepatic impairment (Child-Pugh grade C); within 24 hr of treatment with another 5-HT$_1$ agonist, dihydroergotamine, or methysergide. Concurrent use with a MAO inhibitor or within 2 weeks of discontinuing a MAOI.

SPECIAL CONCERNS

Safety and efficacy have not been determined for use in cluster headaches (usually in older males) or for use in children. Use with caution during lactation and with diseases that may alter the absorption, metabolism, or excretion of drugs, such as impaired renal or hepatic function.

SIDE EFFECTS

Most Common

Paresthesia, dizziness, drowsiness, malaise, fatigue, nausea, throat and neck symptoms, pain and pressure sensation.

Side effects that occurred in 0.1% to 1% of clients. GI: Hyposalivation, vomiting, dyspeptic symptoms, diarrhea, GI discomfort and pain, gastroenteritis, constipation. **CNS:** Vertigo, tremors, cognitive function disorders, sleep disorders, disorders of equilibrium, anxiety, depression, detachment. **CV:** Palpitations, increased BP, tachyarrhythmias, syncope, abnormal ECG (PR prolongation, QTc prolongation, ST/T wave abnormalities, premature ventricular contractions, atrial flutter, or atrial fibrillation). **Musculoskeletal:** Muscle pain, arthralgia, articular rheumatism, muscle cramps and spasms, joint and muscle stiffness, tightness, and rigidity. **Dermatologic:** Sweating, skin rashes, pruritus, urticaria. **GU:** Bladder inflammation, polyuria, diuresis. **Body as a whole:** Chills, fever, descriptions of odor or taste, edema and swelling, allergies, allergic reactions, warm/cold temperature sensations, feeling strange, burning/stinging sensation. **Respiratory:** Bronchitis, cough, pneumonia. **Ophthalmic:** Photophobia, blurred vision. **ENT:** Ear, nose, and throat infections; phonophobia, sinusitis, upper respiratory inflammation, tinnitus. **Endocrine/Metabolic:** Thirst, polydipsia, dehydration, fluid retention. **Hematologic:** Increased WBCs.

OD OVERDOSE MANAGEMENT
Symptoms: Increased BP, chest pain. *Treatment:* Standard supportive treatment. Possible use of antihypertensive therapy. Monitor ECG if chest pain presents.

DRUG INTERACTIONS
Dihydroergotamine / Prolonged vasospastic reaction; effects additive
Methysergide / Prolonged vasospastic reaction; effects additive
Oral contraceptives / ↑ Mean plasma levels of naratriptan
SSRIs / Possible weakness, hyperreflexia, and incoordination
Serotonin 5-HT$_1$ agonists / Additive effects
Sibutramine / Possible serotonin syndrome, including CNS irritability, motor weakness, shivering, myoclonus, and altered consciousness

HOW SUPPLIED
Tablets: 1 mg, 2.5 mg.

DOSAGE
• **TABLETS**
Migraine headaches.
Adults: Single doses of 1 mg or 2.5 mg taken with fluid. If headache returns or client has had only partial response, dose may be repeated once after 4 hr, for maximum of 5 mg in a 24-hr period. Doses of 5 mg/24 hr do not provide greater relief than 2.5 mg/24 hr.

NURSING CONSIDERATIONS
ADMINISTRATION/STORAGE
1. A dose of 2.5 mg is usually more effective than 1 mg but causes more side effects. Choice of dose made on individual basis, weighing possible benefit of 2.5-mg dose with greater risk for side effects.
2. Safety of treating, on average, more than four headaches in 30-day period has not been established.
3. In clients with mild-to-moderate renal or hepatic impairment, do not exceed a dose of 2.5 mg over a 24-hr period. Consider lower starting dose.
4. Store medication at controlled room temperature away from light.

ASSESSMENT
1. Note onset, frequency, duration, characteristics of migraines. Assess for neuro documentation of migraine: drug is not intended for preventing migraines or treating basilar migraines, cluster or hemiplegic headaches.
2. List all drugs consumed to ensure none interact.
3. Monitor BP, ECG, renal, LFTs; assess for dysfunction/dosage adjustment. In mild to moderate renal or hepatic impairment, do not exceed a dose of 2.5 mg over a 24-hr period. Consider lower initial dose.
4. Assess baseline cardiac function. Drug may cause coronary vasospasm, elevated BP; avoid with CAD, risk factors for CAD, HTN, arrhythmias.

CLIENT/FAMILY TEACHING
1. Take exactly as directed to relieve headache. Will not reduce or prevent number of attacks experienced.
2. Review package insert; do not use with other similar headache medications. Practice reliable contraception.
3. May repeat once every 4 hr if headache returns or if only partial response attained. Do not exceed 5 mg/24 hr.

4. Report any unusual side effects including chest pain, SOB, palpitations, lack of response.

5. Attempt to identify migraine triggers. Keep a headache diary (identifying factors surrounding each headache) for provider review. Continue other remedies (i.e., noise reduction, reduced lighting, bed rest) that assist to control S&S.

OUTCOMES/EVALUATE
Relief of migraine headache

Natalizumab [IV]
(na-ta-**LIZ**-u-mab)

CLASSIFICATION(S):
Immunomodulator
PREGNANCY CATEGORY: C
Rx: Tysabri.

USES
(1) Treatment of relapsing forms of multiple sclerosis to reduce the frequency of clinical exacerbations. (2) Treatment of Crohn disease in those who cannot control their symptoms with other therapies.

NOTE: Natalizumab is on a special restricted distribution program due to possible progressive multifocal leukoencephalopathy.

ACTION/KINETICS
Action
Natalizumab is a recombinant, humanized IgG4$_k$ monoclonal antibody. The specific mechanism for its effects in multiple sclerosis are not known. However, the effect may be secondary to blockade of the molecular interaction of α4β1-integrin expressed by inflammatory cells on vascular endothelial cells and with CS-1 and/or osteopontin expressed by parenchymal cells in the brain. The drug increases the number of circulating leukocytes due to inhibition of transmigration out of the vascular space; it does not affect the number of circulating neutrophils.

Pharmacokinetics
Maximum serum level, after repeat IV administration: 98 mcg/mL. **Mean, average steady-state levels:** 30 mcg/mL. **t½:** About 11 days.

CONTRAINDICATIONS
Hypersensitivity to the drug or any of its components. Use with other MS medications. Lactation.

SPECIAL CONCERNS
Safety and efficacy have not been established in those with chronic, progressive multiple sclerosis. Safety and efficacy have not been evaluated in combination with other immunosuppressive agents. Safety and efficacy have not been determined in children less than 18 years of age.

SIDE EFFECTS
Most Common
Headache, fatigue, UTI, depression, lower respiratory tract infection, joint pain, abdominal discomfort, arthralgia.

Hypersensitivity reactions: Urticaria, dizziness, fever, rash, rigors, pruritus, nausea, flushing, hypotension, dyspnea, chest pain, *anaphylaxis*. **Infusion-related reactions:** Headache, dizziness, fatigue, hypersensitivity, urticaria, pruritus, rigors. **GI:** Cholelithiasis, abdominal discomfort, gastroenteritis. **CNS:** Depression, including *suicidal ideation;* headache, tremor. **Respiratory:** Lower respiratory tract infection, tonsillits. **GU:** UTI, vaginitis, urinary urgency/frequency, irregular menstruation, amenorrhea, dysmenorrhea. **Dermatologic:** Rash, dermatitis, pruritus. **Body as a whole:** Pneumonia, fatigue, rigors, arthralgia, syncope, presence of anti-natalizumab antibodies. **Miscellaneous:** Chest discomfort, local bleeding.

LABORATORY TEST CONSIDERATIONS
↑ Circulating lymphocytes, monocytes, eosinophils, basophils, and nucleated RBCs; increases are reversible and return to baseline levels within 16 weeks after the last dose.

DRUG INTERACTIONS
Interferon beta-1a / ↓ Natalizumab clearance by about 30%.

HOW SUPPLIED
Injection Concentrate: 300 mg/15 mL.

DOSAGE
- **IV INFUSION**
  Relapsing multiple sclerosis.
  300 mg q 4 weeks.

NURSING CONSIDERATIONS

ADMINISTRATION/STORAGE

[IV] 1. To prepare the infusion, withdraw 15 mL of natalizumab concentrate from the vial using a sterile needle and syringe. Inject the concentrate into 100 mL of 0.9% NaCl injection. No other IV diluents may be used to prepare the infusion. Invert solution gently to mix, do not shake.

2. Infuse over about 1 hr. After the infusion is complete, flush with 0.9% NaCl injection.

3. Do not administer as an IV push or bolus injection.

4. Do not inject other drugs into the infusion set side ports or mix other drugs with natalizumab.

5. Infuse the prepared diluted infusion solution immediately or refrigerate from 2–8°C (36–46°F) and use within 8 hr of preparation. If refrigerated, allow the solution to warm to room temperature prior to infusion. Do not shake or freeze. Protect from light.

ASSESSMENT

1. Note disease onset, other therapies trialed, outcome. Drug is reserved for those with inadequate response or intolerance to alternative therapies for MS.

2. Observe during infusion and for 1–2 hr after infusion complete. Promptly discontinue infusion with any S&S associated with a hypersensitivity reaction. Do not attempt to retreat those who have experienced an allergic reaction as they may have antibodies to natalizumab.

3. Obtain MRI scan prior to starting therapy. Drug increases the risk of progressive multifocal leukoencephalopathy (PML) a viral infection of the brain that causes severe disability or death. Any suggestive symptoms warrants a repeat MRI with gadolinium and/or if indicated CSF for JC viral DNA.

4. Only providers, infusion centers, pharmacies associated with infusion centers will be permitted to prescribe, distribute or infuse this product through a restricted distribution program: Touch Prescribing Program. Signed permission by client is required.

They must be enrolled in the program and meet all the requirements to be eligible for this therapy. Touch Prescribing Program 1-800-456-2255.

5. Evaluate at 3 months and 6 months after first infusion, and every 6 months thereafter. Will be checked every 6 months to determine if treatment should be reauthorized. Questionnaire and Reauthorization forms are required for treatment.

CLIENT/FAMILY TEACHING

1. Drug is administered intravenously to reduce the frequency of exacerbations of relapsing MS. It is used after other therapies have been proven ineffective or client intolerant.

2. Report any dizziness, itching, fever, rash, chills, nausea, flushing, SOB or chest pain (S&S allergic reaction) immediately.

3. May experience depression, infections, and gall stones; report esp. if suicidal ideations occur.

4. Drug requires authorization and acceptance into the Touch Prescribing Program. There have been reports of increased risk of a viral brain infection. This requires that client understand all the benefits and risks of therapy.

5. A scan of the brain is required as well as careful review of the Medication guide before beginning therapy. A signed permit will be required if therapy is to be administered. Review risks of therapy before considering infusion.

6. Must F/U with provider at 3 months, and 6 months after first infusion and every 6 months thereafter.

7. Call with any questions, problems or adverse side effects immediately.

OUTCOMES/EVALUATE

↓ Frequency of relapsing MS exacerbations

Nateglinide
(nah-**TEG**-lin-eyed)

CLASSIFICATION(S):
Antidiabetic agent, oral
PREGNANCY CATEGORY: C
Rx: Starlix.

N

SEE ALSO *ANTIDIABETIC AGENTS: HYPOGLYCEMIC AGENTS.*

USES

Type 2 diabetes: (1) **Monotherapy:** To lower BG in clients whose hyperglycemia cannot be controlled adequately by diet and physical exercise and who have not been treated chronically with other antidiabetic drugs and (2) **Combination Therapy:** In clients whose hyperglycemia is inadequately controlled with metformin or after a therapeutic response to a thiazolidinedione, nateglinide may be added to, but not substituted for, metformin. Do not switch clients to nateglinide when hyperglycemia is not adequately controlled with glyburide or other insulin secretagogues; do not add nateglinide to their treatment.

ACTION/KINETICS

Action

Lowers blood glucose and reduces post-mealtime glucose spikes by stimulating insulin secretion from the pancreas. Action depends on functioning beta-cells in pancreatic islets. Interacts with the ATP-sensitive potassium (K^+_{ATP}) channel on pancreatic beta cells causing depolarization of the beta cells. This opens the calcium channel producing calcium influx and insulin secretion. Drug is highly tissue selective with a low affinity for heart and skeletal muscle.

Pharmacokinetics

Peak plasma levels: 1 hr with a fall to baseline by 4 hr after dosing. Extent of absorption unaffected by food but there is a delay in the rate of absorption. Peak plasma levels are significantly reduced if administered 10 min prior to a liquid meal. Metabolized in the liver by CYP2C9 and CYP3A4 with most excreted through the urine. **$t\frac{1}{2}$, elimination:** About 1.5 hr.

CONTRAINDICATIONS

Use in type 1 diabetes or diabetic ketoacidosis. Lactation.

SPECIAL CONCERNS

Use with caution in chronic liver disease or moderate to severe liver disease. Transient loss of glycemic control with fever, infection, trauma, surgery; insulin therapy may be required during these times. Safety and efficacy have not been determined in children.

SIDE EFFECTS

Most Common

URTI, back pain, bronchitis, flu symptoms, diarrhea.

Metabolic: Hypoglycemia. **Respiratory:** URTI, bronchitis, coughing. **Hypersensitivity (rare):** Rash, itching, urticaria. **Miscellaneous:** Diarrhea, arthropathy, dizziness, flu symptoms, back pain, accidental trauma.

LABORATORY TEST CONSIDERATIONS

↑ Mean uric acid levels.

OD OVERDOSE MANAGEMENT

Symptoms: Hypoglycemia, including coma, seizure, neurological symptoms. *Treatment:* Treat severe symptoms with IV glucose.

DRUG INTERACTIONS

Beta-adrenergic blocking agents, nonselective / Possible potentiation of hypoglycemic effect

Corticosteroids / Possible reduction of hypoglycemic effect

Fluconazole / ↑ Nateglinide AUC and t½ R/T inhibition of CYP2C9 metabolism

NSAIDs / Possible potentiation of hypoglycemic effect

MAO inhibitors / Possible potentiation of hypoglycemic effect

Rifamycins (rifampin) / ↓ Nateglinide plasma levels and pharmacologic effects

Salicylates / Possible potentiation of hypoglycemic effect

Sulfinpyrazone / ↑ Nateglinide AUC R/T ↓ metabolism by CYP2C9

Sympathomimetics / Possible reduction of hypoglycemic effect

Thiazides / Possible reduction of hypoglycemic effect

Thyroid products / Possible reduction of hypoglycemic effect

HOW SUPPLIED

Tablets: 60 mg, 120 mg.

DOSAGE

- **TABLETS**

  Type 2 diabetes mellitus, monotherapy or combination with metformin or a thiazolidinedione.

Bold Italic = life threatening side effect   ■ = black box warning   ✦ = Available in Canada

Initial: 120 mg 3 times per day before meals, with or without metformin. Use the 60 mg dose, alone or with metformin, in those who are near their HbA1c goal when treatment is initiated.

NURSING CONSIDERATIONS

ADMINISTRATION/STORAGE

Store at 15–30°C (59–86°F). Dispense in a tight container.

ASSESSMENT

1. Note disease onset/type of symptoms, HbA1c range, BMI, and all therapies trialed.
2. Obtain VS, baseline labs noting any liver dysfunction and uric acid level; monitor throughout therapy.
3. Assess understanding of disease and refer for diabetes, nutrition, and exercise education.

CLIENT/FAMILY TEACHING

1. Food delays absorption. Take 1–30 min before meals. Do not take while eating, as drug will cause hypoglycemia. May take extra dose with extra meal; may skip dose if meal missed, thus reducing the risk of hypoglycemia.
2. Avoid activities that require mental alertness until drug effects realized.
3. Drug helps to control blood sugar by stimulating the pancreas to release insulin. Must continue diet, exercise, and lifestyle changes conducive to diabetes control.
4. Report unusual side effects, GI upset, or lack of glucose control. Check finger sticks regularly; bring glucometer to all visits.
5. Drug is generally used initially when diet and exercise fail. May be added to metformin therapy but not in those whose DM is not adequately controlled with glyburide or other related agents.
6. Do not take aspirin or use alcohol while taking this drug unless provider approved.
7. Use reliable form of contraception other than oral contraceptives. If pregnant, use insulin during pregnancy.
8. Keep regular F/U appointments to evaluate response to therapy and need for dosage adjustments.

OUTCOMES/EVALUATE

Control of blood sugar; HbA1c <7

Nebivolol
(ne-**BIV**-oh-lol)

CLASSIFICATION(S):
Beta-adrenergic blocking agent
PREGNANCY CATEGORY: C
Rx: Bystolic.

SEE ALSO BETA-ADRENERGIC BLOCKING AGENTS.

USES

Alone or in combination with other drugs to treat hypertension.

ACTION/KINETICS

Action

At doses of 10 mg in extensive metabolizers (most of the population), nebivolol is β-1 selective. In poor metabolizers and at higher doses, the drug inhibits both β-1 and β-2 adrenergic receptors. The mechanism for the antihypertensive effect is not known but may include (1) decreased HR; (2) decreased cardiac contractility; (3) decreased tonic sympathetic outflow to the periphery from cerebral vasomotor centers; (4) suppression of renin activity; and, (5) vasodilation and decreased peripheral resistance.

Pharmacokinetics

Mean peak plasma levels: 1.5-4 hr. Metabolized to the active d-nebivolol and other metabolites by CYP2D6 and by N-dealkylation. Food does not affect the pharmacokinetics. $t\frac{1}{2}$, **active metabolite:** 12 hr in extensive metabolizers and 19 hr in poor metabolizers. Excreted in both the feces and urine. **Plasma protein binding:** Approximately 98%.

CONTRAINDICATIONS

Severe bradycardia, greater than first degree heart block, cardiogenic shock, decompensated cardiac failure, sick sinus syndrome (unless a permanent pacemaker is in place), severe hepatic impairment (Child-Pugh >8), bronchospastic disease, in clients hypersensitive to any component of the product. Use not recommended during lactation.

SPECIAL CONCERNS

Use with caution in severe renal impairment, moderate hepatic impairment, in those with compensated CHF (beta blockade may result in further depression of myocardial contractility and cause more severe failure), and in peripheral vascular disease (possible precipitation or aggravation of symptoms of arterial insufficiency). Nebivolol may mask some manifestations of hypoglycemia or thyrotoxicosis, especially tachycardia. Safety and efficacy have not been determined in children 18 years of age and younger.

SIDE EFFECTS

Most Common

Headache, nausea, diarrhea, bradycardia, fatigue dizziness.

See also *Beta-Adrenergic Blocking Agents* for a complete list of possible side effects. **CNS:** Headache, dizziness, insomnia, paresthesia. **GI:** Nausea, diarrhea, abdominal pain. **CV:** Bradycardia. **Body as a whole:** Fatigue, asthenia. **Miscellaneous:** Chest pain, dyspnea, rash, peripheral edema, anaphylaxis in those with a history of such.

LABORATORY TEST CONSIDERATIONS

↑ BUN, uric acid, triglycerides. ↓ HDL, cholesterol, platelets. Hypercholesterolemia, hyperuricemia.

OD OVERDOSE MANAGEMENT

SEE ALSO *BETA-ADRENERGIC BLOCKING AGENTS.*

DRUG INTERACTIONS

NOTE: Drugs that inhibit (e.g., fluoxetine, paroxetine, propafenone, quinidine) or induce CYP2D6 can be expected to alter plasma levels of nebivolol. Monitor clients closely; adjust the nebivolol dose according to the BP response.

Cimetidine / ↑ Nebivolol plasma levels by 23%

Clonidine / Discontinue nebivolol several days before gradually tapering the dose of clonidine

Cyclopropane / ↑ Risks of general anesthesia R/T additive depression of myocardial function

Digitalis glycosides / Both slow AV conduction → ↑ risk of bradycardia

Diltiazem / Significant negative inotropic and chronotropic effects; monitor ECG and BP

Disopyramide / Significant negative inotropic and chronotropic effects; monitor ECG and BP

Fluoxetine / ↑ Nebivolol AUC by 8-fold and C_{max} by 3-fold

Guanethidine / Possible reduction of sympathetic activity

Insulin / Potential to ↑ insulin-induced hypoglycemia and delay recovery of serum glucose levels

Sildenafil / ↓ Sildenafil AUC by 21% and C_{max} by 23%

Trichloroethylene / ↑ Risks of general anesthesia R/T additive depression of myocardial function

Verapamil / Significant negative inotropic and chronotropic effects; monitor ECG and BP

HOW SUPPLIED

Tablets: 2.5 mg, 5 mg, 10 mg.

DOSAGE

• **TABLETS**

  Hypertension.

Individualize dose. **Adults, initial:** 5 mg once daily, with or without food, as monotherapy or in combination with other drugs. Dose can be increased at 2-week intervals up to 40 mg in those requiring further reduction in BP. In those with C_{CR} <30 mL/min or moderate hepatic impairment, the initial dose is 2.5 mg once daily; undertake upward titration cautiously.

NURSING CONSIDERATIONS

ADMINISTRATION/STORAGE

1. In those with known or suspected pheochromocytoma, an alpha-blocker should be given prior to use of any beta-blocker.
2. Store from 20–25°C (68–77°F). Dispense in a tight, light-resistant container.

ASSESSMENT

1. Note onset, other agents trialed and outcome. List drugs prescribed to ensure none interact.
2. Identify any conditions that may preclude therapy i.e., >1° AVB, severe liver failure, marked bradycardia, decompensated cardiac failure or SSS without permanent pacemaker.

Bold Italic = life threatening side effect　　■ = black box warning　　✤ = Available in Canada

3. Monitor BP, HR, renal, and LFTS; reduce dose with dysfunction.

4. Assess for pulmonary or CAD, diabetes, thyroid disease, or peripheral vascular disease.

CLIENT/FAMILY TEACHING

1. May be taken with or without food. If dose missed, take only the next scheduled dose (i.e., do not double the dose).

2. Those with coronary artery disease should not stop nebivolol therapy abruptly.

3. Avoid activities that require mental alertness until drug effects realized.

4. Report any breathing difficulty, weight gain >2 lb day or >5 lb/week, SOB, or excessive slow heart rate.

5. Those on insulin or oral hypoglycemic agents, should be aware that β-blockers may mask S&S of hypoglycemia, esp. tachycardia. Monitor FS closely.

6. Keep log of BP and HR for provider review.

7. Report any adverse side effects or lack of response. Keep all F/U appointments and labs.

OUTCOMES/EVALUATE

• Desired BP reduction
• BP <130/80

Nedocromil sodium
(neh-**DAH**-kroh-mill)

CLASSIFICATION(S):
Antiasthmatic drug
PREGNANCY CATEGORY: B
Rx: Alocril, Tilade.

USES
Systemic. Maintenance therapy in adults and children (age six and older) with mild to moderate bronchial asthma. **Ophthalmic.** Itching associated with allergic conjunctivitis in adults and children over 3 years old.

ACTION/KINETICS
Action
Is a mast cell stabilizer. Thus, inhibits the release of various mediators, such as histamine, leukotriene C_4, and prostaglandin D_2, from a variety of cell types associated with asthma. Has no intrinsic bronchodilator, antihistamine, or glucocorticoid activity; also, systemic bioavailability is low.

Pharmacokinetics
$t^{1}/_{2}$: 3.3 hr. Excreted unchanged. Only about 4% of the ophthalmic product is absorbed systemically. **Plasma protein binding:** About 89%.

CONTRAINDICATIONS
Use for the reversal of acute bronchospasms, especially status asthmaticus.

SPECIAL CONCERNS
Use with caution during lactation. Safety and efficacy have not been established in children less than 6 years of age. Has not been shown to be able to substitute for the total dose of corticosteroids.

SIDE EFFECTS
Most Common
After systemic use: Coughing, bronchospasm, unpleasant taste, pharyngitis, rhinitis, URTI, headache.
After ophthalmic use: Headache, nasal congestion, ocular burning/irritation/stinging, unpleasant taste.

After systemic use (metered dose inhaler). Respiratory: Coughing, bronchospasm, pharyngitis, rhinitis, URTI, increased sputum, bronchitis, dyspnea, sinusitis, respiratory disorder, pneumonitis with eosinophilia (PIE syndrome), *bronchospasm*. **GI:** Unpleasant taste, N&V, dyspepsia, abdominal pain, dry mouth, diarrhea. **CNS:** Headache (may be severe), dizziness, dysphonia. **Skin:** Rash, sensation of warmth. **Body as a whole:** Chest pain, fatigue, arthritis, fever, tremor, *anaphylaxis*. **Miscellaneous:** Viral infection.

After ophthalmic use (solution): Headache, ocular burning, irritation, stinging, unpleasant taste, nasal congestion, asthma, conjunctivitis, eye redness, photophobia, rhinitis.

LABORATORY TEST CONSIDERATIONS
↑ ALT.

HOW SUPPLIED
Metered Dose Inhaler: 1.75 mg/inh; *Ophthalmic Solution:* 2%.

DOSAGE
• **METERED DOSE INHALER**
  Bronchial asthma.

Adults and children over 12 years of age: Two inhalations 4 times per day at regular intervals in order to provide 14 mg/day. If client under good control on 4 times per day dosing (i.e., requiring inhaled or oral beta agonist no more than twice a week or no worsening of symptoms occur with respiratory infections), a lower dose can be tried. In such instances reduce the dose to 10.5 mg/day (i.e., used 3 times per day). Then, after several weeks with good control, the dose can be reduced to 7 mg/day (i.e., used twice a day).

• **OPHTHALMIC SOLUTION**

Allergic conjunctivitis.

1 or 2 gtt in each eye twice a day. Continue treatment until pollen season is over or until exposure to allergen is terminated.

NURSING CONSIDERATIONS

ADMINISTRATION/STORAGE

1. Each actuation releases 1.75 mg.
2. Must be used regularly, even during symptom-free period, in order to achieve beneficial effects.
3. Teach the proper method of use of the drug. An illustrated pamphlet is included in each pack of nedocromil.
4. Add nedocromil to existing treatment (e.g., bronchodilators). When clinical response is seen and asthma under good control, a gradual decrease in the concomitant medication can be tried.
5. If systemic or inhaled corticosteroid therapy is reduced in clients receiving nedocromil, careful monitoring is required.
6. Store metered dose inhaler between 2–30°C (36–86°F) and do not freeze.
7. Store ophthalmic solution between 2–25°C (36–77°F). Keep tightly closed; out of the reach of children.

ASSESSMENT

1. Note reasons for therapy, type, onset, characteristics of S&S, triggers. List other agents trialed; outcome.
2. Assess respiratory status thoroughly; not for use with status asthmaticus or for reversal of acute bronchospasm. Monitor peak flow/vital capacity measurements (PFTs).

3. List systemic and inhaled steroid therapy accurately. When reduction in progress, nedocromil cannot substitute for total steroid dose/requirements.
4. Review drug usage/time between prescriptions to ensure proper use.

CLIENT/FAMILY TEACHING

1. Review procedure for administration; use the step-by-step instructions provided with the drug.
2. Use eye solution as directed throughout pollen season. Report adverse effects/lack of response.
3. Beneficial *preventative* effects will not be obtained if incorrectly administered by topical lung application. Drug is an inhaled anti-inflammatory that reduces lung inflammation. Continue to monitor peak flows and report loss of lung function or drop in readings.
4. Do not stop inhaler therapy during symptom-free periods; must be taken at regular intervals. Continue to use with other prescribed therapies.
5. Report any persistent headaches, unpleasant taste in mouth that interferes with nutrition, severe nausea, or chest pain. If any coughing, wheezing, or bronchospasm is noted following use, stop drug and report. Have lungs assessed, and substitute an alternative therapy. Keep all F/U to evaluate response to therapy.

OUTCOMES/EVALUATE

• ↓ Severity/frequency of asthmatic episodes.
• ↓ Eye itching/irritation

Nefazodone hydrochloride ■
(nih-**FAY**-zoh-dohn)

CLASSIFICATION(S):
Antidepressant, miscellaneous
PREGNANCY CATEGORY: C
✤**Rx:** Apo-Nefazodone, Lon-Nefazodone, Serzone-5HT₂.

USES
Treatment of depression.

ACTION/KINETICS

Action

Exact antidepressant mechanism not known. Inhibits neuronal uptake of serotonin and norepinephrine and antagonizes central 5-HT$_2$ receptors and alpha-1-adrenergic receptors (which may cause postural hypotension). Produces none to slight anticholinergic effects, moderate sedation, and slight orthostatic hypotension.

Pharmacokinetics

Rapidly and completely absorbed. **Peak plasma levels:** 1 hr. **t½:** 2–4 hr. **Time to reach steady state:** 4–5 days. Extensively metabolized by the liver with less than 1% excreted unchanged in the urine. Food delays the absorption of nefazodone and decreases the bioavailability by approximately 20%.

CONTRAINDICATIONS

Use with pimozide, carbamazepine, or triazolam. In combination with an MAO inhibitor or within 14 days of discontinuing MAO inhibitor therapy. Use in active liver disease, elevated baseline serum transaminases, or those who were withdrawn from nefazodone due to evidence of liver injury. Clients hypersensitive to nefazodone or other phenylpiperazine antidepressants.

SPECIAL CONCERNS

■ (1) Life-threatening hepatic failure has occurred. The reported rate in the U.S. is about 1 case of liver failure resulting in death or transplant per 250,000 to 300,000 client-years of nefazodone treatment. (2) Ordinarily, do not initiate treatment in those with active liver disease or with elevated baseline serum transaminases. There is no evidence that pre-existing liver disease increases the likelihood of developing liver failure; however baseline abnormalities can complicate client monitoring. (3) Advise clients to be alert for signs and symptoms of liver dysfunction (e.g., jaundice, anorexia, GI complaints, malaise) and to report them to their provider immediately if they occur. (4) Discontinue if clinical signs or symptoms suggest liver failure. Those who develop evidence of hepatocellular injury, such as increased serum AST or serum ALT levels greater than 2 times ULN should be withdrawn from the drug. These clients should be presumed to be at increased risk for liver injury if nefazodone is reintroduced. Do not consider such clients for retreatment. (5) Antidepressants, including nefazodone, have the ability to increase the risk of suicidal thinking and behavior in children and adolescents with major depressive disorder and other psychiatric disorders. Anyone considering the use of nefazodone or any other antidepressant in a child or adolescent must balance this risk with the clinical need. Clients who are started on therapy should be observed closely for clinical worsening, suicidality, or unusual changes in behavior. Families and caregivers should be advised of the need for close observation and communication with the prescriber. Nefazodone is not approved for use in pediatric clients. (6) Placebo-controlled trials in children and adolescents with major depressive disorder, obsessive-compulsive disorder, or other psychiatric disorders revealed a greater risk of adverse reactions representing suicidal thinking or behavior (suicidality) during the first few months of treatment in those receiving antidepressants. The average risk of such reactions in those receiving antidepressants was 4%, twice the placebo risk of 2%. No suicides occurred in these trials.■ Use with caution in clients with known CV or cerebrovascular disease (e.g., history of MI, angina, ischemic stroke), conditions that predispose to hypotension (e.g., dehydration, hypovolemia, antihypertensive medications), or a history of mania. Use with caution during lactation. Safety and efficacy have not been determined in individuals below 18 years of age. There is a possibility of a suicide attempt in depression that may persist until significant remission occurs. From 2 weeks to 6 months may elapse between the time from liver injury to liver failure, resulting in death or transplant. Suicide attempts and suicidal thinking have occurred in pediatric clients taking antidepressant drugs for major depressive disorder. Both adult and pediatric clients may experience worsening of their depression.

SIDE EFFECTS

Most Common

Somnolence, dizziness, insomnia, dry mouth, nausea, constipation, headache, asthenia, dyspepsia, diarrhea, abnormal/blurred vision, infection.

CNS: Dizziness, insomnia, agitation, somnolence, light-headedness, activation of mania/hypomania, confusion, memory impairment, paresthesia, abnormal dreams, decreased concentration, ataxia, incoordination, psychomotor retardation, tremor, hypertonia, decreased/increased libido, vertigo, twitching, depersonalization, hallucinations, *suicide thoughts/attempt*, apathy, euphoria, hostility, abnormal gait/thinking, decreased attention, derealization, neuralgia, paranoid reaction, dysarthria, myoclonus, hyperkinesia, hyperesthesia, hypotonia, increased libido, *suicide, neuroleptic malignant syndrome (rare)*. **CV:** Postural hypotension, hypo-/hypertension, sinus bradycardia, tachycardia, syncope, ventricular extrasystoles, angina pectoris, AV block, CHF, hemorrhage, varicose vein, pallor, *CVA* (rare). **GI:** Nausea, dry mouth, constipation, dyspepsia, diarrhea, increased appetite, vomiting, eructation, periodontal abscess, gingivitis, colitis, gastritis, mouth ulceration, stomatitis, esophagitis, glossitis, hepatitis, hepatotoxicity, dysphagia, *GI hemorrhage*, oral moniliasis, ulcerative colitis, peptic ulcer, rectal hemorrhage, gastroenteritis, *hepatic failure*. **Dermatologic:** Pruritus, dry skin, acne, alopecia, urticaria, maculopapular/vesiculobullous rash, eczema. **Musculoskeletal:** Arthralgia, arthritis, tenosynovitis, muscle stiffness, bursitis, tendinous contracture. **Respiratory:** Pharyngitis, increased cough, dyspnea, bronchitis, asthma, pneumonia, laryngitis, voice alteration, epistaxis, hiccups, hyperventilation, yawn. **Hematologic:** Ecchymosis, anemia, leukopenia, lymphadenopathy. **Ophthalmic:** Blurred vision, scotoma, visual trails, abnormal vision/accommodation, visual field defect, dry eye, eye pain, diplopia, conjunctivitis, mydriasis, keratoconjunc-

tivitis, photophobia, night blindness, glaucoma, ptosis. **Otic:** Ear pain, hyperacusis, deafness, tinnitus. **GU:** Urinary frequency/retention/urgency/incontinence, UTI, vaginitis, breast pain, cystitis, metrorrhagia, amenorrhea, polyuria, vaginal/uterine hemorrhage, breast enlargement, menorrhagia, abnormal ejaculation, hematuria, nocturia, kidney calculus, enlarged uterine fibroids, anorgasmia, oliguria, impotence, priaprism (rare). **Body as a whole:** Headache, asthenia, infection, flu syndrome, chills, fever, neck rigidity, allergic reaction, malaise, photosensitivity, facial edema, hangover effect, enlarged abdomen, hernia, pelvic pain, halitosis, cellulitis, weight loss, gout, dehydration. **Miscellaneous:** Peripheral edema, thirst, taste loss.

LABORATORY TEST CONSIDERATIONS

↑ AST, ALT, LDH. ↓ Hematocrit. Hypercholesterolemia, hypoglycemia. Abnormal LFTs.

OD OVERDOSE MANAGEMENT

Symptoms: N&V, somnolence, increased incidence of severity of any of the reported side effects. *Treatment:* Symptomatic and supportive in the cases of hypotension or excessive sedation. Gastric lavage with a large-bore orogastric tube with appropriate airway protection may be used; induction of emesis is not recommended. Ensure an adequate airway, oxygenation, and ventilation. Monitor cardiac rhythm and vital signs. Administer activated charcoal.

DRUG INTERACTIONS

Alprazolam / ↑ Alprazolam levels R/T inhibition of metabolism by CYP3A4

Anesthetics, general / Discontinue nefazodone for as long as clinically feasible before using general anesthetics since little is known about potential interactions

Atorvastatin / ↑ Atorvastatin levels R/T inhibition of metabolism by CYP3A4; ↑ risk of rhabdomyolysis

Benzodiazepines / Possible ↑ CNS depression

Buspirone / ↑ Levels of both drugs R/T inhibition of metabolism by CYP3A4; ↑ risk of light-headedness, somnolence, dizziness, asthenia

Carbamazepine / ↑ Carbamazepine plasma levels → ↑ side effects

Cyclosporine / ↑ Cyclosporine levels → ↑ toxicity

Digoxin / ↑ Digoxin plasma levels; monitor digoxin plasma levels

Ethanol / Do not use together in depressed clients

HMG-CoA reductase inhibitors / ↑ Risk of rhabdomyolysis and myositis

MAO inhibitors / Serious and possibly fatal reactions including symptoms of hyperthermia, rigidity, myoclonus, autonomic instability with possible rigid fluctuations of VS, and mental status changes that may include extreme agitation progressing to delirium and coma

Methylprednisolone / ↑ Methylprednisolone AUC and t½ R/T inhibition of metabolism

Pimozide / ↑ Plasma levels of pimozide resulting in QT prolongation and possible serious CV events, including death due to ventricular tachycardia of the torsades de pointes type

Propranolol / ↓ Propranolol plasma levels

H *St. John's wort* / ↑ Sedative-hypnotic effects

Sibutramine / Serotonin syndrome, including CNS irritability, motor weakness, shivering, myoclonus, and altered consciousness

Simvastatin / ↑ Simvastatin levels R/T inhibition of metabolism by CYP3A4; ↑ risk of rhabdomyolysis

Sumatriptan / Possible serotonin syndrome, including CNS irritability, increased muscle tone, shivering myoclonus, and altered consciousness

Trazodone / Serotonin syndrome, including CNS irritability, motor weakness, shivering, myoclonus, and altered consciousness

Triazolam / ↑ Triazolam plasma levels; reduce initial triazolam dosage by 75% if used together; avoid coadministration for most clients, including the elderly

HOW SUPPLIED

Tablets: 50 mg, 100 mg, 150 mg, 200 mg, 250 mg.

DOSAGE

• **TABLETS**

Depression.

Adults, initial: 200 mg/day given in two divided doses. Increase dose in increments of 100–200 mg/day at intervals of no less than 1 week. Continue treatment for 6 or more months. The effective dose range is 300–600 mg/day. The initial dose for elderly or debilitated clients is 100 mg/day given in two divided doses.

NURSING CONSIDERATIONS

ADMINISTRATION/STORAGE

1. May take several weeks for full beneficial effect to be observed.

2. Although long-term use has not been studied, it is usually recommended that the drug be given for a period of 6 months or longer.

3. At least 14 days should elapse between discontinuation of an MAO inhibitor and initiation of therapy with nefazodone; also, at least 7 days should elapse after stopping nefazodone and before starting an MAO inhibitor.

4. Store at room temperature below 40°C (104°F); dispense in a tight container.

ASSESSMENT

1. Note reasons for therapy, characteristics of S&S, any precipitating factors/triggers, clinical presentation, behavioral manifestations. Assess depression regularly, record mood changes; note any evidence of suicidal ideations.

2. Before initiating treatment, adequately screen those with depressive symptoms to determine if at risk for bipolar disorder.

3. Evaluate for history of drug abuse and follow clients closely, observing for signs of misuse or abuse.

4. List any seizure history, drugs currently prescribed to ensure none interact unfavorably. Assess for CAD, recent MI, or conditions requiring digoxin administration.

5. Monitor VS, CBC, ECG, renal and LFTs. If AST or ALT increase to levels >3 x ULN, stop drug and do not restart.

CLIENT/FAMILY TEACHING

1. Take before meals; food may inhibit absorption.

N

🖭 = see color insert   H = Herbal   IV = Intravenous   ℭ = sound alike drug

2. Do not perform activities that require mental alertness or coordination until drug effects realized; may cause dizziness, drowsiness, confusion, incoordination, decreased concentration/response time. Change positions slowly to prevent drop in BP.

3. Avoid all OTC agents, alcohol and any other CNS depressants. Use reliable birth control.

4. Avoid prolonged or excessive exposure to direct or artificial sunlight.

5. May take several weeks (2–4) before any effects are realized; do not become discouraged.

6. Report any unusual sensations or side effects, rash, memory problems, S&S of liver dysfunction (stomach pain, yellowing of skin, loss of appetite or fatigue), increased depression, or suicidal thoughts/behavior.

7. Keep all F/U visits to evaluate response and for lab review.

OUTCOMES/EVALUATE

Symptomatic improvement; ↓ depression, improved sleeping and eating patterns, ↓ fatigue, and ↑ social interaction

---

Nelfinavir mesylate ©
(nel-**FIN**-ah-veer)

CLASSIFICATION(S):
Antiviral, protease inhibitor
PREGNANCY CATEGORY: B
Rx: Viracept.

SEE ALSO *ANTIVIRAL DRUGS.*

USES
HIV infections in combination with other antiretroviral drugs. *Investigational:* Part of a 3-drug regimen for occupational HIV postexposure prophylaxis where there is an increased risk of transmission. For HIV infection in neonates. Twice-daily dosing in children over age 6 with HIV infection.

ACTION/KINETICS
Action
HIV-1 protease inhibitor, resulting in prevention of cleavage of gagpol polyprotein resulting in production of immature, noninfectious viruses. Activity is increased when used with didanosine, lamivudine, stavudine, zalcitabine, or zidovudine.

Pharmacokinetics
Peak plasma levels: 2–4 hr. **Steady-state plasma levels:** 3–4 mcg/mL. Food increases plasma levels 2–3 fold. **$t\frac{1}{2}$, terminal:** 3.5–5 hr. Metabolites (one of which is as active as parent compound) and unchanged drug excreted mainly in feces.

CONTRAINDICATIONS
Use with drugs that are highly dependent on CYP3A4 for metabolism and for which elevated plasma levels are associated with serious and/or life-threatening events. Drugs include amiodarone, ergot derivatives, lovastatin, midazolam, pimozide, quinidine, simvastatin, and triazolam. Lactation.

SPECIAL CONCERNS
Use with caution with hepatic impairment. Safety and efficacy have not been determined in children less than 2 years of age. Increased bleeding in those with hemophilia type A and B in clients treated with protease inhibitors.

SIDE EFFECTS
Most Common
Diarrhea, nausea, flatulence, rash, anemia, leukopenia.
NOTE: Side effects were determined when used in combination with other antiviral drugs. **GI:** N&V, diarrhea, flatulence, abdominal pain, anorexia, dyspepsia, epigastric pain, GI bleeding, hepatitis, mouth ulcers, pancreatitis. **CNS:** Anxiety, depression, dizziness, emotional lability, hyperkinesia, insomnia, migraine, paresthesia, *seizures*, sleep disorder, somnolence, *suicide ideation.* **CV:** Prolongation of QTc; *torsade de pointes.* **Hematologic:** Anemia, leukopenia, thrombocytopenia. **Respiratory:** Dyspnea, rhinitis, sinusitis, pharyngitis. **GU:** Kidney calculus, sexual dysfunction, urine abnormality. **Ophthalmic:** Eye disorder, acute iritis. **Musculoskeletal:** Arthralgia, arthritis, cramps, myalgia, myasthenia, myopathy. **Dermatologic:** Dermatitis, folliculitis, fungal dermatitis, maculopapular rash, pruritus, urticaria, sweating. **Hy-**

---

persensitivity: **Bronchospasm,** moderate to severe rash, fever, edema, jaundice. **Miscellaneous:** Asthenia, dehydration, allergic reaction, back pain, fever, headache, malaise, pain, accidental injury, new-onset diabetes mellitus or exacerbation of pre-existing diabetes mellitus, hyperglycemia.

LABORATORY TEST CONSIDERATIONS

↑ ALT, AST, creatine CPK, alkaline phosphatase, amylase, LDH, GGT. Hyperlipidemia, hyperuricemia, hypoglycemia, bilirubinemia, metabolic acidosis. Abnormal LFTs.

OD OVERDOSE MANAGEMENT

Symptoms: See Side Effects. *Treatment:* Emesis or gastric lavage, followed by activated charcoal.

DRUG INTERACTIONS

Amiodarone / Possible inhibition of metabolism via CYP3A4 isoenzyme; do not give together

Anticonvulsants / Possible ↓ nelfinavir plasma levels

Azithromycin / ↓ AUC and C_{max} of nelfinavir and ↑ AUC and C_{max} of azithromycin

Azole antifungal drugs / Possible inhibition of metabolism of nelfinavir

Benzodiazepines / Possible severe sedation and respiratory depression R/T ↓ metabolism

Didanosine / ↓ Absorption of nelfinavir; give on an empty stomach

Delavirdine / ↑ AUC and C_{max} of nelfinavir and a ↓ AUC and C_{max} of delavirdine

Efavirenz / ↑ AUC and C_{max} of nelfinavir and a ↓ AUC and C_{max} of efavirenz

Ergot alkaloids / Possible inhibition of metabolism of ergot alkaloids via CYP3A4 isoenzyme; do not give together due to possible severe side effects, including peripheral vasospasm and ischemia of the extremities and other tissues

Felodipine / Possible leg edema and orthostatic hypotension R/T ↓ nelfinavir metabolism by CYP3A4

Fentanyl / Possible ↓ fentanyl metabolism; monitor and adjust dose if needed

HMG-CoA reductase inhibitors / ↑ in C_{max}; potential for serious reactions, such as ↑ risk of myopathy including

rhabdomyolysis

Indinavir / Significant ↑ AUC of nelfinavir and indinavir

Interleukins / Possible inhibition of nelfinavir metabolism; dosage adjustment may be needed

Lamivudine / ↑ Lamivudine AUC and C_{max}

Methadone / ↓ Methadone plasma levels → possible withdrawal S&S

Nevirapine / ↑ Hepatic metabolism of nelfinavir; monitor levels and adjust dose if needed

Oral contraceptives / ↓ Drug effects; use other contraceptive measures

Phenytoin / ↓ Phenytoin AUC and C_{max} dosage adjustment may be needed

Pimozide / Do not give together due to potential for serious or life-threatening reactions, including cardiac arrhythmias

Quinidine / Possible inhibition of metabolism via CYP3A4 isoenzyme; do not give together

Rifabutin / ↑ Rifabutin levels; reduce rifabutin dose one-half; also, ↓ nelfinavir AUC

Rifampin / Significant ↓ in nelfinavir levels; do not coadminister

Ritonavir / Significant ↑ nelfinavir AUC

Saquinavir / ↑ In both nelfinavir and saquinavir AUCs

Sildenafil / ↓ Sildenafil metabolism; coadminister carefully; do not exceed a maximum single dose of sildenafil of 25 mg/48 hr

Sirolimus / ↑ Sirolimus plasma levels; monitor carefully with possible dosage adjustment

H *St. John's wort* / ↑ Nelfinavir metabolism by CYP3A4 → loss of virologic response

Tacrolimus / ↑ Tacrolimus plasma levels; monitor carefully with possible dosage adjustment

Zidovudine / ↓ Zidovudine AUC

HOW SUPPLIED

Oral Powder: 50 mg/1 gram; *Tablets, Film-Coated:* 250 mg, 625 mg.

DOSAGE

- **ORAL POWDER; TABLETS, FILM-COATED**

  HIV

Adults: 1,250 mg (five 250 mg tablets or two 625 mg tablets) twice a day or 750

N

mg (three 250 mg tablets) 3 times per day in combination with nucleoside analogs. **Children, 2 to 13 years:** 20–30 mg/kg/dose 3 times/day. Doses as high as 45 mg/kg q 8 hr have been used.

NURSING CONSIDERATIONS

Do not confuse nelfinavir with nevirapine (also an antiviral drug).

ASSESSMENT

1. Note disease onset, characteristics of S&S, other agents trialed.
2. List drugs prescribed/consumed to ensure none interact unfavorably.
3. Monitor CBC, for any evidence/history of increased bleeding tendencies, CD_4 counts, viral load, renal, LFTs.

CLIENT/FAMILY TEACHING

1. Drug is not a cure but helps to manage disease symptoms; unless postexposure prophylaxis.
2. Take as prescribed with snack or light meal to enhance absorption. Must take drug with other nucleoside analogs as prescribed.
3. Do not reconstitute powder with water in its original container. Mix powder with small amount of water, milk, formula, soy formula/milk or dietary supplement. Once mixed, consume entire amount for full dose or may be refrigerated for up to 6 hr. Do not mix with acidic foods or juice (e.g., orange or apple juice, applesauce) due to their bitter taste.
4. Report any evidence of increased bruising/bleeding, severe headache/fatigue/lethargy, N&V, rash, breathing problems, or changes in stool/urine color. Diarrhea may be controlled with loperamide.
5. Oral contraceptives may be ineffective; use barrier contraception. Men may experience adverse effects with Viagra, use cautiously and do not exceed 25 mg of Viagra in a 48 hr period.
6. Drug does not prevent disease transmission; practice safe sex. Avoid OTC agents without approval.

OUTCOMES/EVALUATE

Control of HIV symptoms; ↓ viral load, Improved CD_4 count

Neomycin sulfate
(nee-oh-**MY**-sin)

CLASSIFICATION(S):
Antibiotic, aminoglycoside
PREGNANCY CATEGORY: D
Rx: Mycifradin Sulfate, Neo-Tabs, Neo-fradin.

SEE ALSO *ANTI-INFECTIVE DRUGS* AND *AMINOGLYCOSIDES*.

USES
PO: (1) Hepatic coma. (2) Sterilization of gut prior to surgery. (3) Inhibition of ammonia-forming bacteria in GI tract in hepatic encephalopathy. (4) Therapy of intestinal infections due to pathogenic strains of *Escherichia coli*, primarily in children. *Investigational:* Hypercholesterolemia.

ACTION/KINETICS
Pharmacokinetics
Peak plasma levels: PO, 1–4 hr; **therapeutic serum level:** 5–10 mcg/mL. **t½:** 2–3 hr.

ADDITIONAL CONTRAINDICATIONS
Intestinal obstruction (PO). Use of topical products in or around the eyes.

SPECIAL CONCERNS
Safe use during pregnancy has not been determined. Use with caution in clients with extensive burns, trophic ulceration, or other conditions where significant systemic absorption is possible.

SIDE EFFECTS
Most Common
N&V, diarrhea, skin rashes.

See *Anti-Infective Drugs* and *Aminoglycosides* for a complete list of possible side effects. Also, N&V, ototoxicity, skin rashes, nephrotoxicity. Sprue-like syndrome with steatorrhea, malabsorption, and electrolyte imbalance.

ADDITIONAL DRUG INTERACTIONS
Digoxin / ↓ Digoxin effect R/T ↓ GI tract absorption
Penicillin V / ↓ PCN effect R/T ↓ GI tract absorption
Procainamide / ↑ Muscle relaxation produced by neomycin

Bold Italic = life threatening side effect   ■ = black box warning   ✦ = Available in Canada

HOW SUPPLIED

Oral Solution: 125 mg/5 mL; *Tablets:* 500 mg.

DOSAGE

- **ORAL SOLUTION; TABLETS**
  Preoperatively in colorectal surgery.

1 gram each of neomycin and erythromycin base for a total of three doses: the first two doses 1 hr apart the afternoon before surgery and the third dose at bedtime the night before surgery.

Hepatic coma, adjunct.

Adults, 4–12 grams/day in divided doses for 5–6 days; **children:** 50–100 mg/kg/day in divided doses for 5–6 days.

NURSING CONSIDERATIONS

ASSESSMENT

1. List reasons for therapy; note any experience with this drug. Include clinical presentation, abdominal assessments, and symptom characteristics.
2. Check all drugs prescribed to ensure none interact.
3. Note fluid and electrolyte status, renal function, C&S.
4. Assess hearing before and after therapy.

CLIENT/FAMILY TEACHING

1. Take as directed. Consume 2–3 L/day of fluids to prevent dehydration.
2. Carefully follow procedure to prepare the GI tract for surgery.
3. Expect slight laxative effect produced by PO neomycin. Withhold and report with S&S of intestinal obstruction.
4. Report any hearing changes such as loss, ringing, roaring, or dizziness.
5. Anticipate low-residue diet for preoperative disinfection and a laxative immediately preceding PO administration of neomycin sulfate.

OUTCOMES/EVALUATE

- Improved level of consciousness
- Bowel sterilization before surgery

Nepafenac

(ne-pa-**FEN**-ak)

CLASSIFICATION(S):
Ophthalmic nonsteroidal anti-inflammatory drug.
PREGNANCY CATEGORY: C
Rx: Nevanac.

USES

Treatment of pain and inflammation associated with cataract surgery.

ACTION/KINETICS

Action

A topical nonsteroidal anti-inflammatory and analgesic prodrug. Nepafenac penetrates the cornea and is converted by ocular tissue hydrolases to amfenac, a nonsteroidal anti-inflammatory drug. Amfenac is believed to inhibit the action of prostaglandin cyclooxygenase, an enzyme required for prostaglandin production. The drug has no effect on intraocular pressure.

Pharmacokinetics

Low plasma levels 2–3 hr post-dose are reached after ocular administration.

CONTRAINDICATIONS

Hypersensitivity to any component of the product or to other NSAIDs. Avoid use during late pregnancy.

SPECIAL CONCERNS

Use with caution in individuals who have previously exhibited sensitivity to aspirin, phenylacetic acid derivatives, or other NSAIDs. May slow or delay healing. Due to an increased risk for corneal side effects (that may be sight-threatening), use with caution in those with complicated ocular surgeries, corneal denervation, corneal epithelial defects, diabetes mellitus, ocular surface diseases (e.g., dry eye syndrome), rheumatoid arthritis, or repeat ocular surgeries within a short period of time. Use with caution in those with known bleeding tendencies or who are receiving medications that may prolong bleeding time. Safety and efficacy have not been determined in children below 10 years of age.

SIDE EFFECTS
Most Common
Capsular opacity, decreased visual acuity, foreign body sensation, increased intraocular pressure, sticky sensation.

Ophthalmic: Capsular opacity, decreased visual acuity, foreign body sensation, increased intraocular pressure, sticky sensation, epithelial breakdown, corneal thinning/erosion, corneal ulceration/perforation, keratitis, conjunctival edema, corneal edema, dry eye, lid margin crusting, ocular discomfort, ocular hyperemia/pain/pruritus, photophobia, tearing, vitreous detachment. **Miscellaneous:** Headache, hypertension, N&V, sinusitis. *NOTE:* Some of the ophthalmic side effects may be a consequence of the cataract surgical procedure.

HOW SUPPLIED
Ophthalmic Suspension: 0.1%.

DOSAGE
- **OPHTHALMIC SUSPENSION**
  Pain and inflammation associated with cataract surgery.

One drop applied to the affected eye(s) three times per day beginning 1 day before surgery, continued on the day of surgery, and throughout the first 2 weeks postsurgery.

NURSING CONSIDERATIONS
ADMINISTRATION/STORAGE
1. Use more than 1 day before surgery or beyond 14 days post surgery may increase the risk for occurrence and severity of corneal side effects.
2. Do not administer while wearing contact lenses.
3. May be given concomitantly with other topical ophthalmic medications, including beta-blockers, carbonic anhydrase inhibitors, alpha-adrenergic agonists, cycloplegics, and mydriatics.
4. Store from 2–25°C (36–77°F).

ASSESSMENT
1. Note reasons for therapy; date of surgery, other agents prescribed/trialed.
2. Ensure ophthalmic post op report reviewed.
3. List any allergies. Start drops 1 day before surgery and for the first two weeks following surgery.

CLIENT/FAMILY TEACHING
1. Drug is an anti-inflammatory medicine used in the eye to relieve pain and inflammation or too much fluid in the eye that occurs after eye surgery.
2. Wash hands, tilt the head back and, press your finger gently on the skin just beneath the lower eyelid, pull the lower eyelid away from the eye to make a space. Drop the medicine into this space. Let go of the eyelid and gently close the eyes. Do not blink. Keep eyes closed and apply pressure to the inner corner of the eye with your finger for 1 or 2 minutes to allow the medicine to be absorbed by the eye.
3. Wash hands after administering to remove any medicine that may be on them.
4. Do not touch applicator tip to any surface (including the eye). Keep container tightly closed.
5. Do not wear contact lenses during treatment with nepafenac; severe irritation (redness and itching) has occurred.
6. May experience change/decrease in vision; feeling of foreign object in eye; loss of vision; sticky sensation of eyelids, blurred vision; report if persistent or bothersome.
7. Any sparks, spots, floaters or cuts in vision require immediate attention.
8. Keep all F/U appointments to evaluate response to therapy/lack of desired effects.

OUTCOMES/EVALUATE
Relief of ocular pain/inflammation after surgery

Nesiritide
(nih-**SIR**-ih-tide)

CLASSIFICATION(S):
Vasodilator, peripheral
PREGNANCY CATEGORY: C
Rx: Natrecor.

USES
IV treatment of acutely decompensated CHF in those who have dyspnea at rest or with minimal activity.

ACTION/KINETICS

Action
Nesiritide is a human B-type natriuretic peptide (hBNP) that binds to the particulate guanylate cyclase receptor in vascular smooth muscle and endothelial cells, leading to increased intracellular levels of guanosine 3'5'-cyclic monophosphate (cGMP) and smooth muscle cell relaxation. Cyclic GMP serves as a second messenger to dilate veins and arteries. In acutely decompensated CHF, the drug reduces pulmonary capillary wedge pressure and improves dyspnea.

Pharmacokinetics
$t^{1/2}$, initial elimination: About 2 min; $t^{1/2}$, mean terminal, elimination: About 18 min. Human BNP is cleared from the circulation by three mechanisms: (1) Binding to cell surface clearance receptors with subsequent cellular internalization and lysosomal proteolysis; (2) Proteolytic cleavage of the peptide by endopeptidases, such as neutral endopeptidase (present on the vascular lumenal surface); and (3) renal filtration.

CONTRAINDICATIONS
Use as primary therapy for those with cardiogenic shock or in those with a systolic BP <90 mm Hg. Hypersensitivity to any of the product components. Use in those suspected of having, or known to have, low cardiac filling pressures. Use in those for whom vasodilating agents are not appropriate, including valvular stenosis, restrictive or obstructive cardiomyopathy, constrictive pericarditis, pericardial tamponade, or other conditions in which cardiac output is dependent on venous return.

SPECIAL CONCERNS
Use with caution during lactation. Increased risk of death. Safety and efficacy have not been determined in children.

SIDE EFFECTS

Most Common
Hypotension (both symptomatic and asymptomatic), ventricular tachycardia, nonsustained ventricular tachycardia, ventricular extrasystole, headache, insomnia, dizziness, anxiety, N&V, angina pectoris, abdominal pain, back pain.

CV: Hypotension (symptomatic, asymptomatic), *ventricular tachycardia*, nonsustained ventricular tachycardia, ventricular extrasystoles, angina pectoris, bradycardia, tachycardia, atrial fibrillation, AV node conduction abnormalities. **CNS:** Headache, insomnia, dizziness, anxiety, confusion, paresthesia, somnolence, tremor. **GI:** N&V, abdominal pain. **Dermatologic:** Sweating, pruritus, rash. **Respiratory:** Increased cough, hemoptysis, apnea. **Miscellaneous:** Back pain, abdominal pain, hypersensitivity reactions, catheter pain, fever, injection site reaction, leg cramps, amblyopia, anemia, *worsened renal function (may be fatal), increased risk of death.*

LABORATORY TEST CONSIDERATIONS
↑ Creatinine.

DRUG INTERACTIONS
↑ Symptomatic hypotension when used with ACE inhibitors.

HOW SUPPLIED
Powder for Injection, Lyophilized: 1.58 mg.

DOSAGE
- **IV ONLY**

  Acutely decompensated CHF.
  IV bolus of 2 mcg/kg, followed by a continuous IV infusion of 0.01 mcg/kg/min.

NURSING CONSIDERATIONS

ADMINISTRATION/STORAGE
[IV] 1. Do not start nesiritide higher than the recommended dose.

2. Prime IV tubing with an infusion of 5 mL before connecting to the client's vascular access port and prior to giving the bolus or starting the infusion.

3. After preparing the infusion bag, withdraw bolus volume and give over about 60 seconds through an IV port in the tubing. Immediately following the bolus, infuse nesiritide at a flow rate of 0.1 mL/kg/hr (this will deliver an infusion dose of 0.01 mcg/kg/min).

4. To calculate the appropriate bolus volume and infusion flow rate to deliver 0.01 mcg/kg/min dose, use the following formulas: Bolus volume (mL) = 0.33 x client weight (kg). Infusion flow rate (mL/hr) = 0.1 x client weight (kg).

5. To prepare infusion, use the following procedure:

- Reconstitute one 1.5 mg vial by adding 5 mL of diluent removed from a prefilled 250 mL plastic IV bag containing the diluent of choice (D5W/0.9% NaCl, D5W/0.45% NaCl, or D5W/0.2% NaCl).
- Do not shake vial but rock gently so that all surfaces, including the stopper, are in contact with diluent to ensure complete reconstitution. Use only a clear, essentially colorless solution.
- Withdraw entire contents of the reconstituted vial and add to the 250 mL plastic IV bag. This will yield a solution with a nesiritide concentration of about 6 mcg/mL. Invert the IV bag several times to ensure complete mixing of the solution.
- Use the reconstituted solution within 24 hr, as there are no preservatives in the product. Inspect visually for particulate matter and discoloration prior to use.

6. If hypotension occurs during administration, reduce or discontinue the dose and begin other measures to support BP (e.g., IV fluids, changes in body position). The drug may be restarted at a dose that is reduced by 30% (with no bolus given). Hypotension may be prolonged; thus, before restarting the drug, a period of observation may be needed.

7. Nesiritide is physically and chemically incompatible with injections of heparin, insulin, ethacrynate sodium, bumetanide, enalaprilat, hydralazine, and furosemide. Do not give these drugs as infusions in the same IV catheter as nesiritide.

8. Do not give injectable drugs that contain sodium metabisulfate in the same infusion line; incompatible with nesiritide. Flush catheter between administration of nesiritide and incompatible drugs.

9. Nesiritide binds to heparin. Thus, **do not** give through a central line heparin-coated catheter.

10. Store at controlled room temperature between 20–25°C (68–77°F) or refrigerated at 2–8°C (36–46°F). Reconstituted vials may be left at controlled room temperature or refrigerated for 24 hr or less. Keep in carton until time of use.

ASSESSMENT

1. Note reasons for therapy, other agents trialed, ejection fraction, NYHA class, S&S, clinical presentation.

2. For IV use only; avoid infusing through central line heparin-coated catheters.

3. Review list of drugs not compatible for co-administration.

4. Monitor cardiac status, renal function, VS; if SBP <90 mm Hg, reduce dose or stop infusion and report.

5. Administer in a closely monitored environment by trained individuals; monitor heart pressures and assess closely for arrhythmias.

CLIENT/FAMILY TEACHING

Report any pain at IV site. May experience dizziness, blurred vision, lightheadedness or sweating; report if evident.

OUTCOMES/EVALUATE

Improved exercise tolerance; ↓ PACWP; ↓ SOB with mild exertion and at rest

Nevirapine   ■ ⓒ
(neh-**VYE**-rah-peen)

CLASSIFICATION(S):
Antiviral, non-nucleoside reverse transcriptase inhibitor
PREGNANCY CATEGORY: C
Rx: Viramune.

SEE ALSO ANTIVIRAL DRUGS.

USES

In combination with nucleoside analogues (e.g., zidovudine, lamivudine, didanosine, zalcitabine) or protease inhibitors (e.g., saquinavir, indinavir, nelfinavir, aritonavir) for HIV-1 infections in adults who have experienced clinical and immunologic deterioration. Always use in combination with at least one other antiretroviral agent, as resistant viruses emerge rapidly when nevirapine is used alone. *NOTE: Use of antiretrovi-*

ral drugs (nonoccupational, postexposure) for prophylaxis of HIV should be restricted to treatment no more than 72 hr after high-risk exposure with a person known to be HIV-infected.

ACTION/KINETICS

Action
A nonnucleoside reverse transcriptase inhibitor. By binding tightly to reverse transcriptase, nevirapine prevents viral RNA from being converted into DNA. In combination with a nucleoside analogue, it reduces the amount of virus circulating in the body and increases CD4+ cell counts.

Pharmacokinetics
Readily absorbed, with peak plasma levels occurring 4 hr after a 200-mg dose. Extensively metabolized in the liver. Excreted through both the urine (about 90%) and the feces (about 10%). Induces hepatic CYP3A4 and CYP2B6; also, induces its own metabolism. Following chronic use the half-life decreases from about 45 hr following a single dose to 25 to 30 hr following multiple dosing with 200 or 400 mg daily.

CONTRAINDICATIONS
Severe hepatic impairment. Beginning therapy in women with CD4+ counts greater than 250 cells/mm^3 or men with counts greater than 400 cells/mm^3 unless benefits outweigh risks. Lactation.

SPECIAL CONCERNS
■ (1) Severe, life-threatening and, in some cases, fatal hepatotoxicity, including fulminant and cholestatic hepatitis, hepatic necrosis, and hepatic failure, has been reported in clients treated with nevirapine. In some cases, clients presented with nonspecific prodromal signs or symptoms of hepatitis and progressed to hepatic failure. These events are often associated with rash. Women and clients with higher CD4 counts are at increased risk of hepatic events. Women with CD4 counts greater than 250 cells/mm^3, including pregnant women receiving chronic treatment for HIV infection, are at considerably higher risk for these events. Advise clients with signs or symptoms of hepatitis to discontinue nevirapine and seek medical evaluation immediately. (2) Severe, life-threatening skin reactions, including fatal cases, have occurred in clients treated with nevirapine. These have included cases of Stevens-Johnson syndrome, toxic epidermal necrolysis, and hypersensitivity reactions characterized by rash, constitutional findings, and organ dysfunction. Clients developing signs or symptoms of severe skin reactions or hypersensitivity must seek medical evaluation immediately. (3) It is essential that clients be monitored intensively during the first 18 weeks of nevirapine therapy to detect potentially life-threatening hepatotoxicity or skin reactions. The greatest risk of severe rash or hepatic events (often associated with rash) occurs in the first 6 weeks of therapy. However, the risk of any hepatic event, with or without rash, continues past this period and monitoring should continue at frequent intervals. In some cases, hepatic injury has progressed despite discontinuation of treatment. Do not restart nevirapine following severe hepatic, skin, or hypersensitivity reactions. In addition, strictly follow the 14-day lead-in period with 200 mg/day nevirapine dosing.■ Is not a cure for HIV infections; clients may continue to experience illnesses associated with HIV infections, including opportunistic infections. Has not been shown to reduce the risk of transmitting HIV to others through sexual contact or blood contamination. Use with caution in moderately impaired renal or hepatic function. Women who received single-dose nevirapine during labor and delivery to prevent prenatal potential transmission of HIV-1 are more likely to manifest virologic failure if nevidrapine is prescribed within 6 months of labor; delaying the use of nevdirapine for 6 months may improve control.

SIDE EFFECTS

Most Common
Rash, fever, nausea, headache, abnormal LFTs, diarrhea.

GI: Nausea, diarrhea, abdominal pain, ulcerative stomatitis, hepatitis, *severe, life-threatening (sometimes fatal) he-*

patotoxicity, including fulminant and cholestatic hepatitis, necrosis, and failure (especially during the first 12 weeks of therapy), abnormal LFTs. **CNS:** Headache, fatigue, paresthesia, somnolence. **Hematologic:** Granulocytopenia (occurs more in children), anemia, esosinophilia, neutropenia. **Dermatologic:** Angioedema, bullous eruptions, ulcerative stomatitis, urticaria. Possible *severe, life-threatening skin reactions, including Stevens-Johnson syndrome, toxic epidermal necrolysis, and hypersensitivity reactions.* **Hypersensitivity:** Severe rash or rash accompanied by fever, general malaise, fatigue, muscle or joint aches, blisters, oral lesions, conjunctivitis, facial edema, hepatitis, eosinophilia, granulocytopenia, lymphadenopathy, renal dysfunction. **Miscellaneous:** Fever, peripheral neuropathy, myalgia, arthralgia. Redistribution/accumulation of body fat, including central obesity, dorsocervical fat enlargement, peripheral wasting, breast enlargement, and 'cushingoid appearance.'

LABORATORY TEST CONSIDERATIONS
↑ ALT, AST, GGT, alkaline phosphatase, amylase, total bilirubin. ↓ Hemoglobin, neutrophils, platelets. Abnormal LFTs.

DRUG INTERACTIONS
Clarithromycin / ↓ Clarithromycin exposure and ↑ levels of active metabolite
Efavirenz / ↓ Efavirenz plasma levels
Fluconazole / ↑ Nevirapine levels
Ketoconazole / Significant ↓ ketoconazole levels; do not use together
Methadone / ↓ Methadone levels R/T ↑ metabolism; ↑ methadone dose
Oral contraceptives / ↓ OC levels → ↓ effect
Protease inhibitors / ↓ Levels of protease inhibitors
Rifabutin / ↓ Nevirapine trough concentrations
Rifampin / ↓ Nevirapine AUC and peak plasma levels
H *St. John's Wort* / ↓ Nelfinavir levels R/T ↑ hepatic metabolism
Warfarin / Possible ↓ anticoagulant activity
Zidovudine / ↓ Zidovudine AUC and C_{max}

HOW SUPPLIED
Suspension: 50 mg/5 mL; *Tablets:* 200 mg.

DOSAGE
• **SUSPENSION; TABLETS**
HIV-1 infections.
Adults, initial: 200 mg/day for 14 days; use this lead-in period to lessen the frequency of rash. **Maintenance:** 200 mg twice a day (e.g., 7:00 a.m. and 7:00 p.m.) in combination with a nucleoside analogue antiretroviral agent. **Children, 8 years and over:** 4 mg/kg once daily for 2 weeks followed by 4 mg/kg twice a day thereafter; **Children, 2 months up to 8 years:** 4 mg/kg once daily for the first 14 days followed by 7 mg/kg twice a day thereafter. Do not exceed a total daily dose of 400 mg for any client.

NURSING CONSIDERATIONS
 Do not confuse nevirapine with nelfinavir (also an antiviral drug).

ADMINISTRATION/STORAGE
1. If nevirapine dosing interrupted for more than 7 days, should restart therapy using one 200-mg tablet daily (4 mg/kg for children) for the first 14 days, followed by 200 mg twice a day (4 or 7 mg/kg twice a day, according to age, for children).
2. Discontinue if severe rash or rash accompanied by constitutional findings noted. Clients experiencing rash during the 14-day lead-in period should have their nevirapine dose decreased until the rash has resolved.
3. Shake suspension gently prior to administration. Give entire measured dose of suspension by using an oral dosing syringe or dosing cup. If dosing cup used, thoroughly rinse with water and give rinse to client.
4. An additional dose of nevirapine, 200 mg, is given following each dialysis treatment. Clients with a C_{CR} of 20 mL/min or greater do not require any adjustment in nevirapine dosage.
5. Use caution in selecting doses for the elderly due to greater frequency of decreased hepatic, renal, or cardiac function and of concomitant disease or other drug therapy.

Bold Italic = life threatening side effect　　■ = black box warning　　♣ = Available in Canada

6. Store tablets and suspension in a tightly closed bottle at 15–30°C (59–86°F).

ASSESSMENT

1. Note disease onset, symptom characteristics, other agents trialed, outcome. List drugs currently prescribed to ensure none interact unfavorably.

2. Monitor CBC, CD4 counts, viral load, renal and LFTs. Most serious hepatic side effects occur during the first 12 weeks of therapy. Perform LFTs at least monthly during the first 12 weeks, especially at baseline, before, and 2 weeks after a dose increase. Monitor liver function frequently thereafter. Stop drug and do not resume at the first sign of liver toxicity.

CLIENT/FAMILY TEACHING

1. Drug is not a cure but helps control disease symptoms.

2. Can be taken with or without food. If dose skipped, take the next dose as soon as possible; do not double dose.

3. Take exactly as directed. Should be taken with other HIV drugs and antiretroviral agent to prevent emergence of resistant viruses.

4. A rash may occur in the first few weeks of therapy; do not increase dosage until rash subsides. Any severe rash or rash accompanied by flu-like symptoms warrants immediate reporting.

5. Drug does not prevent transmission through sexual contact or blood contamination. Practice barrier contraception and nonhormonal form of birth control.

OUTCOMES/EVALUATE

Improved CD4 cell counts; ↓ viral load

Niacin (Nicotinic acid)

(**NYE**-ah-sin, nih-koh-**TIN**-ick **AH**-sid)

CLASSIFICATION(S):
Vitamin B complex

PREGNANCY CATEGORY: C (if used in doses above the RDA),

OTC: Slo-Niacin.

Rx: Niacor, Niaspan.

Niacinamide (Nicotinamide)

(nye-ah-**SIN**-ah-myd)

PREGNANCY CATEGORY: C

USES

Niacin. OTC: Treatment of niacin deficiency. **Rx:** (1) Adjunct therapy in adults with very high serum triglycerides (Types IV and V hyperlipidemia) who are at risk of pancreatitis and who do not respond adequately to diet. (2) Niaspan: Used in combination with lovastatin as an adjunct to exercise and diet to treat adults with dyslipidemia. **Niacinamide.** Prophylaxis and treatment of pellagra. *Investigational:* Treatment of various dermatologic disorders.

ACTION/KINETICS

Action

Niacin (nicotinic acid) and niacinamide are water-soluble, heat-resistant vitamins prepared synthetically. Niacin (after conversion to the active niacinamide) is a component of the coenzymes nicotinamide-adenine dinucleotide and nicotinamide-adenine dinucleotide phosphate, which are essential for oxidation-reduction reactions involved in lipid metabolism, glycogenolysis, and tissue respiration. Deficiency of niacin results in pellagra, the most common symptoms of which are dermatitis, diarrhea, and dementia. In high doses niacin also produces vasodilation. Niacin, but not nicotinamide, reduces total and LDL cholesterol, triglycerides, and VLDL, and increases HDL cholesterol. Mechanism is unknown but may involve a decrease in esterification of hepatic triglycerides.

Pharmacokinetics

Niacin is rapidly absorbed from the GI tract. **Peak serum levels:** 30–60 min, after 1 gram; $t^{1/2}$, **elimination:** 20–45 min. About 88% of a PO dose of niacin is eliminated by the kidneys unchanged or as nicotinuric acid.

N

CONTRAINDICATIONS

Severe hypotension, arterial bleeding, liver dysfunction, active peptic ulcer. Use of the extended-release tablets and capsules in children.

SPECIAL CONCERNS

Extended-release niacin may be hepatotoxic. Use with caution in diabetics, clients with gall bladder disease, in those who consume a large amount of alcohol, and clients with gout. Those with heart disease (especially those who have recurrent chest pain or angina) or who recently suffered a MI, should take niacin only under the supervision of a health care provider. There is no evidence to support the use of nicotinic acid to treat schizophrenia. Safety and efficacy have not been determined in children in doses that exceed the RDA.

SIDE EFFECTS

Most Common

Niacin: Flushing, pruritus, GI distress.

Niacin. GI: N&V, diarrhea, peptic ulcer activation, abdominal pain, GI distress, severe hepatic toxicity (including **fluminating hepatic necrosis** with high doses). **Dermatologic:** Flushing (begins 20 min after ingestion and lasts 30–60 min), warm feeling, skin rash, pruritus, dry skin, itching and tingling feeling, keratosis nigricans. **Miscellaneous:** Hypotension, orthostasis, headache, atrial fibrillation, cystoid macular edema, toxic amblyopia, decreased glucose tolerance, rhabdomyolysis (rare). NOTE: Megadoses are accompanied by serious toxicity including the symptoms listed in the preceding as well as liver damage, hyperglycemia, hyperuricemia, arrhythmias, tachycardia, and dermatoses. **Niacinamide.** Liver dysfunction at high doses.

LABORATORY TEST CONSIDERATIONS

↑ Uric acid.

DRUG INTERACTIONS

Chenodiol / ↓ Effect of chenodiol
HMG-CoA Reductase Inhibitors / ↑ Risk of myopathy and rhabdomyolysis
Probenecid / Niacin may ↓ uricosuric effect of probenecid
Sulfinpyrazone / Niacin ↓ uricosuric effect of sulfinpyrazone

Sympathetic blocking agents / Additive vasodilating effects → postural hypotension

HOW SUPPLIED

OTC: Niacin (Nicotinic acid): *Capsules, Extended-Release:* 250 mg, 400 mg; *Capsules, Sustained-Release:* 125 mg, 500 mg; *Capsules, Timed-Release:* 250 mg, 500 mg; *Tablets:* 50 mg, 100 mg, 250 mg, 500 mg; *Tablets, Controlled-Release:* 250 mg, 500 mg, 750 mg; *Tablets, Sustained-Release:* 500 mg; *Tablets, Timed-Release:* 250 mg, 500 mg.

Niacinamide (Nicotinamide): *Tablets:* 100 mg, 500 mg.

Rx: Niacin (Nicotinic acid) *Tablets:* 500 mg; *Tablets, Extended-Release:* 500 mg, 750 mg, 1000 mg.

DOSAGE

NIACIN

- **OTC: CAPSULES, EXTENDED-RELEASE; CAPSULES, SUSTAINED RELEASE; CAPSULES, TIMED-RELEASE; TABLETS; TABLETS, CONTROLLED-RELEASE; TABLETS, SUSTAINED-RELEASE; TABLETS, TIMED-RELEASE**

    RDA for niacin.

Adult males: 15–20 mg; **adult females:** 13–15 mg.

- **RX: TABLETS; TABLETS, EXTENDED-RELEASE**

    Hyperlipidemia.

Immediate-Release. Adults: 1–2 grams 2–3 times per day. Individualize the dose depending on client response. Initiate at 250 mg as a single dose following the evening meal. The frequency of dosing and total daily dose may be increased q 4–7 days until the desired LDL or triglyceride level is reached or the first-level therapeutic dose of 1.5–2 grams/day is reached. If hyperlipidemia is not controlled adequately after 2 months at this level, increase dosage at 2- to 4-week intervals to 1 gram 3 times per day. Do not exceed 6 grams/day.

Extended-Release. 500 mg at bedtime for 1–4 weeks; **then,** 1,000 mg at bedtime during weeks 5 to 8. After week 8, titrate to client tolerance and response. If response to 1,000 mg/day is inadequate, increase dose to 1,500 mg/day; may then increase to 2,000 mg/day (maximum). Do not increase the daily dose more than 500 mg in a 4-week period.

NIACINAMIDE

- **OTC: TABLETS**
    Pellagra.

Adults: 100–500 mg/day. **Pediatric:** Up to 300 mg/day.

NURSING CONSIDERATIONS
ADMINISTRATION/STORAGE
1. Do not substitute sustained-release niacin products for equivalent doses of immediate-release niacin.
2. Niacin, 100 mg/day, plus a statin may increase HDL levels.

ASSESSMENT
1. Note reasons for therapy, other agents trialed, outcome. Monitor glucose, HbA1c, LFTs, CK, plasma lipid levels.
2. Note any history of CAD, PUD, liver or gallbladder dysfunction.
3. Assess diet, exercise, and lifestyle changes necessary to decrease coronary risk factors.
4. If and when used with statins, monitor LFTs closely; both utilize same metabolic pathway.
5. When using regular-strength tablets for hyperlipidemia, start low and go slow to enhance client tolerance. With the extended-release tablets, titrate up and advise to take at bedtime with an ASA or small snack to diminish side effects (flushing/hot flashes).

CLIENT/FAMILY TEACHING
1. Take nicotinic acid PO only with cold water (no hot beverages). Can be taken with meals if GI upset occurs.
2. May experience a warm flushing in the face and ears within 2 hr after taking. To prevent/reduce, take one aspirin (325 mg) or a small low-fat snack 30–60 min prior to dosing. Hot showers, exercise, hot/spicy foods, and alcohol may increase these effects.
3. Lie down if feeling weak and dizzy after taking niacin (until this feeling passes), avoid activities that require mental alertness and report if feeling persists.
4. Identify food sources high in niacin (dairy products, meats, tuna, and eggs); assess consumption. No unsupervised

excessive vitamin ingestion; high doses may impair liver function.
5. With diabetes, avoid niacin unless specifically ordered; monitor BS levels closely for hyperglycemia; monitor urine for ketonuria and glucosuria. Antidiabetic agents may require adjustment.
6. Report any skin color changes or yellowing of the sclera. Avoid alcohol.
7. Clients predisposed to gout may experience flank, joint, or stomach pains; report immediately.
8. If blurred vision or skin lesions occur, remain out of direct sunlight.
9. Report as scheduled for regular labs and F/U.

OUTCOMES/EVALUATE
- ↓ Triglyceride levels
- Relief of symptoms of pellagra and niacin deficiency

Nicardipine hydrochloride
(nye-**KAR**-dih-peen)

CLASSIFICATION(S):
Calcium channel blocker
PREGNANCY CATEGORY: C
Rx: Cardene, Cardene IV, Cardene SR.

SEE ALSO *CALCIUM CHANNEL BLOCKING AGENTS.*

USES
Immediate release: Chronic stable angina (effort-associated angina) alone or in combination with beta-adrenergic blocking agents.

   Immediate and sustained release: Hypertension alone or in combination with other antihypertensive drugs.

   IV: Short-term treatment of hypertension when PO therapy is not desired or possible.

   Investigational: CHF.

ACTION/KINETICS
Action
Moderately increases CO and HR and significantly decreases peripheral vascular resistance. Slight increase in QT interval and slight to no decrease in

myocardial contractility. No effect on QRS complex or PR interval.

Pharmacokinetics

Nearly 100% absorbed. **Onset of action:** 20 min. **Maximum plasma levels:** 30–120 min. Significant first-pass metabolism. Food (especially fats) will decrease the amount of drug absorbed from the GI tract. Steady-state plasma levels are reached after 2–3 days of therapy. **Therapeutic serum levels:** 0.028–0.050 mcg/mL. **t½, at steady state:** 8.6 hr. **Maximum BP-lowering effects, immediate release:** 1–2 hr; **maximum BP-lowering effects, sustained release:** 2–6 hr. **Duration:** 8 hr. Metabolized by the liver with excretion through both the urine and feces. **Plasma protein binding:** More than 95%.

CONTRAINDICATIONS

Use in advanced aortic stenosis due to the effect on reducing afterload. During lactation.

SPECIAL CONCERNS

Safety and efficacy in children less than 18 years of age have not been established. Use with caution in clients with CHF, especially in combination with a beta blocker due to the possibility of a negative inotropic effect. Use with caution in clients with impaired liver function, reduced hepatic blood flow, or impaired renal function. Initial increase in frequency, duration, or severity of angina.

SIDE EFFECTS

Most Common

Flushing, increased angina, hypotension, palpitations, tachycardia, vasodilation, anxiety, dizziness, lightheadedness, headache, N&V.

CV: Pedal edema, flushing, increased angina, palpitations, vasodilation, tachycardia, other edema, abnormal ECG, hypotension, postural hypotension, syncope, *MI, AV block*, ventricular extrasystoles, PVD. **CNS:** Dizziness, lightheadedness, headache, somnolence, malaise, nervousness, insomnia, abnormal dreams, vertigo, depression, confusion, amnesia, anxiety, weakness, psychoses, hallucinations, paranoia. **GI:** N&V, dyspepsia, dry mouth, constipation, sore throat. **Neuromuscular:**

Asthenia, myalgia, paresthesia, hyperkinesia, arthralgia. **Miscellaneous:** Rash, dyspnea, SOB, nocturia, polyuria, allergic reactions, abnormal LFTs, hot flashes, impotence, rhinitis, sinusitis, nasal congestion, chest congestion, tinnitus, equilibrium disturbances, abnormal or blurred vision, infection, atypical chest pain.

OD OVERDOSE MANAGEMENT

Symptoms: Marked hypotension, bradycardia, palpitations, flushing, drowsiness, confusion, and slurred speech following PO overdose. Lethal overdose may cause systemic hypotension, bradycardia (following initial tachycardia) and progressive AV block.
Treatment:

- Treatment is supportive. Monitor cardiac and respiratory function.
- If client is seen soon after ingestion, emetics or gastric lavage should be considered, followed by cathartics.
- *Hypotension:* IV calcium, dopamine, isoproterenol, metaraminol, or norepinephrine. Also, provide IV fluids. Place client in Trendelenburg position.
- *Ventricular tachycardia:* IV procainamide or lidocaine; cardioversion may be necessary. Also, provide slow-drip IV fluids.
- *Bradycardia, asystole, AV block:* IV atropine sulfate (0.6–1 mg), calcium gluconate (10% solution), isoproterenol, norepinephrine; also, cardiac pacing may be indicated. Provide slow-drip IV fluids.

DRUG INTERACTIONS

Beta-blockers / Additive or synergistic effects; possible ↓ metabolism of certain beta-blockers
Cimetidine / ↑ Bioavailability of nicardipine → ↑ plasma levels
Cyclosporine / ↑ Plasma levels of cyclosporine possibly leading to renal toxicity
Grapefruit juice / ↑ Bioavailability of nicardipine R/T ↓ liver metabolism of nicardipine in the gut wall
Ranitidine / ↑ Bioavailability of nicardipine
Rifampin / ↓ Nicardipine effects

Bold Italic = life threatening side effect ■ = black box warning ✦ = Available in Canada

HOW SUPPLIED

Capsules, Extended-Release: 30 mg, 45 mg, 60 mg; *Capsules, Immediate-Release:* 20 mg, 30 mg; *Injection:* 2.5 mg/mL.

DOSAGE

- **CAPSULES, EXTENDED-RELEASE**
  Hypertension

Initial: 30 mg twice a day (range: 30–60 mg twice a day). *NOTE:* Initial dose in renal impairment: 20 mg 3 times per day. Initial dose in hepatic impairment: 20 mg twice a day.

- **CAPSULES, IMMEDIATE-RELEASE**
  Angina, Hypertension.

Initial, usual: 20 mg 3 times per day (range: 20–40 mg 3 times per day). Wait 3 days before increasing dose to ensure steady-state plasma levels.

- **IV**
  Hypertension.

Individualize dose. Initial: 5 mg/hr; the infusion rate may be increased to a maximum of 15 mg/hr (by 2.5-mg/hr increments q 15 min). For a more rapid reduction in BP, initiate at 5 mg/hr but increase the rate q 5 min in 2.5-mg/hr increments until a maximum of 15 mg/hr is reached. **Maintenance:** 3 mg/hr. The IV infusion rate to produce an average plasma level similar to a particular PO dose is as follows: 20 mg q 8 hr is equivalent to 0.5 mg/hr; 30 mg q 8 hr is equivalent to 1.2 mg/hr; and 40 mg q 8 hr is equivalent to 2.2 mg/hr.

NURSING CONSIDERATIONS

Do not confuse nicardipine with nimodipine or nifedipine (also calcium channel blocker). Also, do not confuse Cardene with Cardura or Cardizem (also calcium channel blocker).

ADMINISTRATION/STORAGE

1. When used for treating angina, may be given safely along with SL nitroglycerin, prophylactic nitrates, or beta blockers.

2. When used to treat hypertension, may be given safely along with diuretics or beta blockers.

3. During initial therapy and when dosage is increased, may experience an increase in frequency, duration, or severity of angina.

4. If transfer to PO antihypertensives other than nicardipine is planned, initiate therapy after discontinuing infusion. If PO nicardipine is used at a dosage regimen of three times daily, give the first dose 1 hr prior to discontinuing infusion.

IV 5. Ampules must be diluted before infusion. Acceptable diluents are D5W, D5W/0.45% NaCl, D5W with 40 mEq potassium, 0.45% NaCl, and 0.9% NaCl. Nicardipine is incompatible with 5% NaHCO$_3$ and RL solution.

6. The infusion concentration is 0.1 mg/mL. The diluted product is stable at room temperature for 24 hr.

7. Store ampules at room temperature; freezing does not affect the product. Protect ampules from light and elevated temperatures.

ASSESSMENT

1. Note reasons for therapy, other agents prescribed, outcome.

2. Assess for CHF, if beta blockers prescribed; monitor closely.

3. Monitor ECG, renal and LFTs; note any dysfunction.

4. Monitor VS. When the immediate-release product is used for hypertension, maximum lowering of BP occurs 1–2 hr after dosing. Evaluate BP at trough (8 hr after dosing). When the sustained-release product is used, maximum lowering of BP occurs 2–6 hr after dosing. Monitor BP frequently during and following IV infusion. Avoid too rapid or excessive decrease in BP and discontinue infusion if significant hypotension or tachycardia.

CLIENT/FAMILY TEACHING

1. Take at the same time each day.

2. Report any persistent/bothersome side effects such as dizziness, flushing, increased chest pain, SOB, weight gain, or swelling of extremities. Avoid activities that require mental alertness until drug effects realized.

3. Maintain proper intake of fluids to avoid constipation. Avoid alcohol; limit caffeine.

4. May experience impotence.

5. Avoid prolonged sun exposure; wear protective clothing when exposed.

---

6. Anginal attacks may persist up to 30 min following drug ingestion due to reflex tachycardia; use nitrates as prescribed.

7. Report any change in psychologic state—depression, anxiety, sleep problems, or decreased mental acuity. Particularly important when working with elderly clients since there is a tendency to misdiagnose as senility.

OUTCOMES/EVALUATE
• Control of hypertension
• ↓ Frequency/intensity of anginal attacks
• Therapeutic drug levels (0.028–0.050 mcg/mL)

Nicotine inhalation system

(**NIK**-oh-teen)

CLASSIFICATION(S):
Smoking deterrent
PREGNANCY CATEGORY: D
Rx: Nicotrol Inhaler.

Nicotine nasal spray

CLASSIFICATION(S):
Smoking deterrent
PREGNANCY CATEGORY: D
Rx: Nicotrol NS.

SEE ALSO *NICOTINE POLACRILEX*
USES
As an aid in smoking cessation for the relief of nicotine withdrawal symptoms. Both products are to be used as part of a comprehensive behavioral smoking cessation program.

ACTION/KINETICS
Action
The nicotine from the inhalation system or spray provides blood levels of niotine approximating those produced by smoking cigarettes.

Pharmacokinetics
Time to peak levels, inhalation system or nasal spray: 15 min. **Peak plasma levels, inhalation system:** 6 ng/mL; **nasal spray:** 12 ng/mL. **t½, in-**

halation system: Not determined; **nasal spray:** 1–2 hr. Nicotine is rapidly and extensively metabolized by the liver; excreted in the urine.

CONTRAINDICATIONS
Not recommended for use during lactation even though nicotine levels in breast milk are lower with inhaler or spray therapy, when used as directed, compared with cigarette smoking. Use of the nasal spray in severe reactive airway disease (e.g., asthma, bronchospasm).

SPECIAL CONCERNS
Use the inhaler with caution in those with bronchospastic disease. Safety and efficacy have not been evaluated in children/adolescents less than 18 years of age who smoke.

SIDE EFFECTS
Most Common
Use of the inhaler: Irritation of mouth/throat, coughing, rhinitis, dyspepsia, headache.
Use of the nasal spray: Irritation of mouth/throat, headache, back pain, dyspnea, nausea, arthralgia, menstrual disorder, palpitations, flatulence, tooth/gum disorder.
• INHALER
Respiratory: Irritation of mouth/throat, coughing, rhinitis, sinusitis. **GI:** Dyspepsia, taste/tooth disorders, flatulence, nausea, diarrhea, hiccough. **CNS:** Headache, paresthesia. **Miscellaneous:** Pain in jaw/neck/back, flu-like symptoms, fever, allergy. **Withdrawal from nicotine:** Dizziness, anxiety, sleep disorder, depression, drug dependence, fatigue, myalgia. **Smoking-related symptoms:** Chest discomfort, bronchitis, hypertension.
• NASAL SPRAY
Respiratory: Irritation of mouth/throat, dyspnea, bronchitis, bronchospasm, increased sputum. **GI:** Nausea, flatulence, tooth/gum disorder, abdominal pain, dry mouth, hiccough, diarrhea. **CNS:** Headache, confusion, aphasia, amnesia, migraine, numbness, calming. **CV:** Palpitations, peripheral edema. **Musculoskeletal:** Arthralgia, myalgia, back pain. **Miscellaneous:** Menstrual disorder, pain, allergy, purpura, rash, abnormal

---

vision, feelings of dependence. **Withdrawal from nicotine:** Anxiety, irritability, restlessness, cravings, dizziness, impaired concentration, emotional lability, somnolence, fatigue, increased weight/appetite/dreaming/sweating, insomnia, confusion, depression, apathy, tremor, incoordination. **Smoking-related symptoms:** Chest tightness, dyspepsia, paresthesia in limbs, constipation, stomatitis.

HOW SUPPLIED

Nicotine inhalation system. *Inhaler:* 4 mg delivered (10 mg/cartridge).
Nicotine nasal spray. *Spray Pump:* 0.5 mg/actuation (10 mg/mL).

DOSAGE

NICOTINE INHALATION SYSTEM
• **INHALER**
 Smoking deterrent.

Individualize initial dose; clients may self-titrate to the level of nicotine they require. **Usual:** Between 6 and 16 cartridges/day. The best effect occurs by frequent continuous puffing (20 minutes). **Recommendation duration:** 3 months, after which clients may be weaned from the inhaler by gradual reduction of the daily dose over 6–12 weeks. *NOTE:* The goal of inhaler therapy is complete abstinence. If a client is unable to stop smoking by the fourth week of therapy, discontinue use of the inhaler.

NICOTINE NASAL SPRAY
• **SPRAY PUMP**
 Smoking deterrent.

Each actuation delivers a metered 50 mcL spray containing 0.5 mg nicotine; one dose is 1 mg of nicotine (2 sprays, 1 in each nostril). **Initial dose:** 1 or 2 doses/hr, which may be increased up to a maximum recommended dose of 40 mg (80 sprays) per day. Clients should use at least the recommended minimum of 8 doses/day, as less is likely to be ineffective. **Maximum duration of treatment:** 3 months with a maximum of 5 doses/hr and 40 doses/day. *NOTE:* Clients should stop smoking completely when they begin using the spray. If the client is unable to stop smoking by the fourth week of therapy, discontinue use of the nasal spray.

NURSING CONSIDERATIONS

ADMINISTRATION/STORAGE
INHALER:
1. Encourage clients to use at least 6 cartridges/day for the first 3–6 weeks of treatment. Regular use of the inhaler during the first week of treatment may help clients adapt to the irritant effects of the product.
2. With the inhaler, some clients may exhibit S&S of nicotine withdrawal or excess that will require dosage adjustment.
3. After using the inhaler, carefully separate the mouthpiece, remove the used cartridge, and throw it away, out of the reach of children and pets. Store the mouthpiece in the plastic storage case for further use. Clean mouthpiece regularly with soap and water.
4. Store the inhaler at room temperature not to exceed 25°C (77°F). Protect from light.
NASAL SPRAY:
1. No tapering strategy has been developed for the nasal spray. Recommended procedure for discontinuation of use include: Use only half a dose (1 spray at a time); use the spray less frequently; keep a tally of daily usage; try to meet a steadily reducing usage target; skip a dose by not medicating every hour; and, set a planned 'quit date' for stopping use of the spray.
2. Regular use of the spray during the first week of treatment may help clients adapt to the irritant effects.
3. Those who are successfully abstinent on the nasal spray should be treated at the selected dosage for up to 8 weeks; then, discontinue the spray over the next 4–6 weeks. Safety of the spray has not been established for more than 6 months of use.
4. If the spray pump is dropped and breaks, clean up the spill immediately with an absorbent cloth/paper towel. Avoid contact of the solution with the skin; wash the area several times. Should even a small amount of the solution come in contact with the skin, lips, mouth, eyes, or ears, immediately rinse the affected area with water.

N

---

5. Dispose of used bottles in a way so as to prevent access by children or pets.

6. Store the nasal spray at room temperature not to exceed 30°C (86°F).

ASSESSMENT

1. Note onset/duration of addiction, amount consumed, other agents trialed, outcome.

2. Assess for any conditions that may preclude therapy: severe COPD/CAD, recent MI, severe chest pain/arrhythmia.

3. Have formal smoking cessation program available to provide support and encouragement to ensure success.

CLIENT/FAMILY TEACHING

1. For nasal spray: Instruct not to sniff, swallow, or inhale through the nose as the spray is being administered. Administer spray with the head tilted back slightly.

2. Use Nicotine Spray in your nose whenever you feel the urge to smoke. Do not sniff, swallow, or inhale through the nose while the spray is being used.

3. Do not use more than 1 spray in each nostril for a dose without approval.

4. Do not exceed 5 doses per hour or 40 doses per day.

5. With inhaler, therapy consists of a mouthpiece and a plastic cartridge delivering 4 mg of nicotine from a porous plug containing 10 mg nicotine. The cartridge is inserted into the mouthpiece prior to use.

6. Clean mouthpiece regularly with soap and water.

7. Stop smoking completely when initiating Nicotrol Inhaler or spray therapy; if smoking continues, may experience adverse effects due to peak nicotine levels higher than those experienced from smoking alone. If clinically significant increase in cardiovascular or other effects attributable to nicotine, stop treatment. Other medications may also need dosage adjustment

8. May experience mild irritation of the mouth or throat and cough when you first use the Nicotrol Inhaler; should subside with use. Stomach upset may occur.

9. Do not use more than 16 cartridges each day unless provider directed.

10. Do not use longer than 6 months.

11. Store cartridges at room temperature, not to exceed 77°F (25°C). If you keep cartridges in car, use care as interiors heat up quickly. Protect from light.

12. Store spray and cartridges away from children or pets; dispose of properly.

OUTCOMES/EVALUATE

Smoking cessation aid; control of S&S nicotine withdrawal symptoms

---

Nicotine polacrilex (Nicotine Resin Complex)
(**NIK**-oh-teen)

CLASSIFICATION(S):
Smoking deterrent
PREGNANCY CATEGORY: C
OTC: Commit, Nicorette, Nicotine Gum.
❧OTC: Nicorette Plus.

USES

Adjunct with behavioral modification in smokers wishing to give up the smoking habit in those 18 years and older. Is considered only as an initial aid, with the ultimate goal being abstention from all forms of nicotine. Most likely to benefit are individuals with the following characteristics: (a) smoke brands of cigarettes containing more than 0.9 mg nicotine; (b) smoke more than 15 cigarettes daily; (c) inhale cigarette smoke deeply and frequently; (d) smoke most frequently during the morning; (e) smoke the first cigarette of the day within 30 min of arising; (f) indicate cigarettes smoked in the morning are the most difficult to give up; (g) smoke even if the individual is ill and confined to bed; (h) find it necessary to smoke in places where smoking is not allowed. *NOTE:* Nicotine may be effective in improving the course of difficult-to-treat ulcerative colitis.

ACTION/KINETICS

Action

Following chewing, nicotine is released from an ion exchange resin in the gum product, providing blood nicotine levels approximating those produced by smoking cigarettes.

Pharmacokinetics

The amount of nicotine released depends on the rate and duration of chewing. **Time to peak levels:** 15–30 min. **Peak plasma levels:** 5–10 ng/mL. If the gum is swallowed, only a minimum amount of nicotine is released. **t½:** 3–4 hr. Metabolized mainly by the liver, with about 10–20% excreted unchanged in the urine.

CONTRAINDICATIONS

Pregnancy, lactation, nonsmokers, serious arrhythmias, angina, vasospastic disease, MI, active temporomandibular joint disease. Use in individuals less than 18 years of age.

SPECIAL CONCERNS

Safety and effectiveness in children and adolescents who smoke have not been determined. Use with caution in hypertension, PUD, oral or pharyngeal inflammation, gastritis, stomatitis, hyperthyroidism, IDDM, and pheochromocytoma.

SIDE EFFECTS

Most Common

Sore mouth/throat, nausea, salivation, dizziness.

CNS: Dizziness, irritability, headache. **GI:** N&V, indigestion, GI upset, salivation, eructation. **Miscellaneous:** Sore mouth or throat, hiccoughs, sore jaw muscles.

OD OVERDOSE MANAGEMENT

Symptoms: **GI:** N&V, diarrhea, salivation, abdominal pain. **CNS:** Headache, dizziness, confusion, weakness, fainting, *seizures*. **Respiratory:** Labored breathing, *respiratory paralysis (cause of death)*. **Other:** Cold sweat, disturbed hearing and vision, hypotension, and rapid, weak pulse. *Treatment:* Institute gastric lavage and/or activated charcoal. Avoid syrup of ipecac. Maintenance of respiration, maintenance of CV function.

DRUG INTERACTIONS

Caffeine / Possibly ↓ caffeine blood levels R/T ↑ rate of liver breakdown
Catecholamines / ↑ Catecholamine levels
Cortisol / ↑ Cortisol levels
Furosemide / Possible ↓ diuretic effect of furosemide
Imipramine / Possibly ↓ imipramine blood levels R/T ↑ rate of liver breakdown
Pentazocine / Possibly ↓ pentazocine blood levels R/T ↑ rate of liver breakdown
Theophylline / Possibly ↓ theophylline blood levels R/T ↑ rate of liver breakdown

HOW SUPPLIED

Gum: 2 mg/square, 4 mg/square; *Lozenges:* 2 mg/lozenge, 4 mg/lozenge.

DOSAGE

- **GUM**

    Smoking deterrent.

If the client smokes less than 25 cigarettes/day, start with the 2 mg nicotine gum. If the client smokes more than 25 cigarettes/day, start with the 4 mg nicotine gum. **Weeks 1–6:** 1 piece of gum q 2 hr; **Weeks 7–9:** 1 piece of gum q 2–4 hr; **Weeks 10–12:** 1 piece of gum q 4–8 hr.

- **LOZENGES**

    Smoking deterrent.

If first cigarette is smoked more than 30 min after waking, start with the 2 mg lozenge. If the first cigarette is smoked within 30 min of waking, start with the 4 mg lozenge. **Weeks 1–6:** 1 lozenge q 2 hr; **Weeks 7–9:** 1 lozenge q 2–4 hr; **Weeks 10–12:** 1 lozenge q 4–8 hr.

NURSING CONSIDERATIONS

ADMINISTRATION/STORAGE

1. All products are over-the-counter.
2. Client must stop smoking completely when beginning to use the gum.
3. Those who smoke more than 25 cigarettes/day should be started on the 4-mg dose.
4. Have client chew gum slowly until it tingles; then, park it between the cheek and gum. When the tingle is gone, have client begin chewing again until the tingle returns. Repeat the process until

most of the tingle is gone (about 30 min).

5. Advise client to place the lozenge in the mouth and allow it to dissolve slowly (20–30 min). Minimize swallowing. Client should not chew or swallow the lozenge. A warm or tingling sensation may be felt. Advise to occasionally move the lozenge from one side of the mouth to the other.

6. Advise client not to eat or drink for 15 min before chewing the nicotine gum or while using the lozenge.

7. To improve chances of quitting, have client chew at least 9 pieces/day for the first 6 weeks. If there are strong and frequent cravings, use a second piece within the hour. Do not have client use continuously 1 piece after the other as hiccoughs, heartburn, nausea, and other side effects may occur.

8. Do not use more than 24 pieces/day. Stop using nicotine gum at the end of 12 weeks.

9. After gum has been chewed, place used chewing pieces in a wrapper and dispose so that children or pets can not obtain them.

10. If the lozenge must be removed, wrap in paper and dispose in the trash. Lozenges have enough nicotine to make pets and children ill.

ASSESSMENT

1. Note nicotine profile: type and brand (cigarettes, chewing tobacco, or cigars), amount used per day, when used, and what triggers/increases usage.

2. List any temporomandibular joint syndrome or cardiac arrhythmia; precludes gum therapy.

CLIENT/FAMILY TEACHING

1. Must want to stop smoking and be willing to do so immediately.

2. Avoid activities, persons, and locations that stimulate the desire to smoke (i.e. drinking, bars, smokers).

3. Use gum only as directed. When the urge to smoke occurs, chew one piece slowly for about 30 min. If a slight tingling becomes evident, stop chewing until sensation subsides.

4. Acidic beverages, such as coffee, juices, soft drinks, and wine, interfere with buccal absorption of nicotine;

thus, avoid eating and drinking 15 min before and during chewing.

5. Gum will not stick to dentures or appliances. Gradually decrease the number of pieces chewed per day; may take up to 3 mo to be completely free of nicotine.

6. Dispose of unit carefully and keep out of the reach of children. May be harmful to pregnant woman and/or fetus.

7. Identify individuals and local support groups that can help with smoking cessation and provide emotional and psychologic support throughout the endeavor. Participate in formal smoking program.

OUTCOMES/EVALUATE

Control of nicotine withdrawal symptoms with smoking cessation

Nicotine transdermal system
(**NIK**-oh-teen)

CLASSIFICATION(S):
Smoking deterrent

PREGNANCY CATEGORY: D

OTC: Nicoderm CQ Step 1, Step 2, and Step 3., Nicotine Transdermal System Step 1, Step 2, and Step 3., Nicotrol Step 1, Step 2, and Step 3.

USES

As an aid to stopping smoking for the relief of nicotine withdrawal symptoms in those 18 years and older. Should be used in conjunction with a comprehensive behavioral smoking cessation program.

ACTION/KINETICS

Action

Nicotine transdermal system is a multilayered film that provides systemic delivery of varying amounts of nicotine over a 24-hr period after applying to the skin. Nicotine's reinforcing activity is due to stimulation of the cortex (via the locus ceruleus), producing increased alertness and cognitive performance and a 'reward' effect due to an action in the limbic system. At low doses the stimulatory effects predominate, whereas at high doses the reward effects predominate. The nicotine transdermal system produces an initial (first day of use) increase in BP, an increase in HR (3%–7%), and a decrease in SV after 10 days.

Pharmacokinetics
Time to peak levels: 2–12 hr. **Peak plasma levels:** 5–17 ng/mL. **t½:** 3–4 hr. Metabolized in the liver to a large number of metabolites, all of which are less active than nicotine.

CONTRAINDICATIONS
Hypersensitivity or allergy to nicotine or any components of the therapeutic system. Use in children and during pregnancy, labor, delivery, and lactation. Use in those with heart disease, hypertension, a recent MI, severe or worsening angina pectoris, those taking certain antidepressants or antiasthmatic drugs, or in severe renal impairment.

SPECIAL CONCERNS
Encourage pregnant smokers to try to stop smoking using educational and behavioral interventions before using the nicotine transdermal system. Use during pregnancy only if the potential benefit outweighs the potential risk of nicotine to the fetus. The use of nicotine transdermal systems for longer than 3 months has not been studied. Before use, screen clients with coronary heart disease (history of MI and/or angina pectoris), serious cardiac arrhythmias, or vasospastic diseases (e.g., Buerger's disease, Prinzmetal's variant angina) carefully. Use with caution in clients with hyperthyroidism, pheochromocytoma, IDDM (nicotine causes the release of catecholamines), in active peptic ulcers, in accelerated hypertension, and during lactation.

SIDE EFFECTS
Most Common
Erythema, pruritus, or burning at site of application; headache.
NOTE: The incidence of side effects is complicated by the fact that clients manifest effects of nicotine withdrawal or by concurrent smoking. **Dermatologic:** Erythema, pruritus, or burning at the site of application; cutaneous hypersensitivity, sweating, rash at application site. **Body as a whole:** Allergy, back pain. **GI:** Diarrhea, dyspepsia, dry mouth, abdominal pain, constipation, N&V. **Musculoskeletal:** Arthralgia, myalgia. **CNS:** Abnormal dreams, somnolence, dizziness, impaired concentration, headache, insomnia. **CV:** Tachycardia, hypertension. **Respiratory:** Increased cough, pharyngitis, sinusitis. **GU:** Dysmenorrhea.

OD OVERDOSE MANAGEMENT
Symptoms: Pallor, cold sweat, N&V, abdominal pain, salivation, diarrhea, headache, dizziness, disturbed hearing and vision, mental confusion, weakness, tremor. Large overdoses may cause prostration, hypotension, *respiratory failure, seizures, and death.* Treatment: Remove the transdermal system immediately. The surface of the skin may be flushed with water and dried; soap should not be used, as it may increase the absorption of nicotine. Diazepam or barbiturates may be used to treat seizures, and atropine can be given for excessive bronchial secretions or diarrhea. Respiratory support for respiratory failure and fluid support for hypotension and CV collapse. If transdermal systems are ingested PO, activated charcoal should be given to prevent seizures. If the client is unconscious, the charcoal should be administered by an NGT. A saline cathartic or sorbitol added to the first dose of activated charcoal may hasten GI passage of the system. Doses of activated charcoal should be repeated as long as the system remains in the GI tract as nicotine will continue to be released for many hours.

HOW SUPPLIED
Nicoderm CQ Step 1, Step 2, Step 3 and Nicotine Transdermal System Step 1, Step 2, Step 3: *Film, Extended-Release:* Amount absorbed/24 hr: 21 mg/24 hr (Step 1), 14 mg/24 hr (Step 2), 7 mg/24 hr (Step 3).
Nicotrol Step 1, Step 2, Step 3: *Patch, Extended-Release:* Amount absorbed/16 hr: 15 mg/16 hr (Step 1), 10 mg/16 hr (Step 2), 5 mg/16 hr (Step 3).

N

DOSAGE

NICODERM CQ, NICOTINE TRANSDERMAL SYSTEM

• **TRANSDERMAL SYSTEM**
  Smoking deterrent.

21 mg/day for the first 6 weeks, 14 mg/day for the next 2 weeks, and 7 mg/day for the last 2 weeks. Total course of therapy: 8–10 weeks. Start with 14 mg/day for 6 weeks for those who smoke less than 10 cigarettes/day. Decrease dose to 7 mg/day for the final 2 weeks.

NICOTROL

• **TRANSDERMAL SYSTEM**
  Smoking deterrent.

15 mg/16 hr for the first 6 weeks, 10 mg/16 hr for the next 2 weeks, and 5 mg/16 hr for the last 2 weeks. Total course of therapy: 10 weeks.

NURSING CONSIDERATIONS

ADMINISTRATION/STORAGE

1. All products are over-the-counter.
2. There will be differences in the duration and length of therapy, depending on the product selected.
3. The goal of therapy with nicotine transdermal systems is complete abstinence. If still smoking by the fourth week of therapy, discontinue treatment.
4. Do not store Nicotrol above 30°C (86°F). Store Nicoderm CQ at 20–25°C (68–77°F).

ASSESSMENT

1. Detail nicotine profile: type and brand (cigarettes, chewing tobacco, or cigars), amount used per day, when used, and what increases usage. Determine any CAD, liver or renal dysfunction.
2. List medications currently prescribed. Cessation of smoking, with or without nicotine replacement, may alter the response to certain drugs.
3. Note any skin disorders; nicotine transdermal systems may be irritating with skin disorders such as atopic or eczematous dermatitis.

CLIENT/FAMILY TEACHING

1. Follow manufacturer's guidelines for proper system application. Review information sheet that comes with the product for instructions on how to use and dispose of the transdermal systems.
2. Use extreme caution during application; remove old patch first then immediately apply the new one to a non-hairy, dry skin site. Avoid eye contact. These systems can be a skin irritant and cause contact dermatitis. Report any persistent skin irritations such as redness, swelling, or itching at the application site as well as any generalized skin reactions such as large red skin elevations, or a generalized rash; remove system.
3. Stop smoking completely. If smoking continues, may experience adverse side effects due to higher nicotine levels in the body. Nicotine in any form can be toxic and addictive; transdermal systems may lead to dependence. To minimize this risk, withdraw system gradually after 4–8 weeks of use.
4. Participate in a formal smoking program. The success or failure of smoking cessation depends on the quality, intensity, and frequency of supportive care.
5. Symptoms of nicotine withdrawal include craving, nervousness, restlessness, irritability, mood lability, anxiety, drowsiness, sleep disturbances, impaired concentration, increased appetite, headache, myalgia, constipation, fatigue, and weight gain; report as dosage may require adjustment.
6. Change site of application daily; do not reuse same site for 1 week. With Nicotrol, remove patch at bedtime and apply upon arising.
7. Keep all products (used and unused) away from children and pets; sufficient nicotine is still present in used systems to cause toxicity.
8. Apply the transdermal system promptly after its removal from the protective pouch to prevent loss of nicotine due to evaporation. Only use systems where the pouch is intact.
9. Apply system once daily to a non-hairy, clean, and dry site on the trunk or upper, outer arm. Hold for 10 seconds. Wash hands thoroughly after application. Do not wear more than 1 patch at a time. Do not cut the patch in half or in smaller pieces.

---

10. For Nicoderm CQ, remove the used system after 16–24 hr and apply a new system to alternate skin site. Do not leave the patch on for more than 24 hr as skin irritation may occur and potency is lost. Apply at the same time each day. If vivid dreams or other sleep disturbances, patch may be removed at bedtime and a new patch applied in the morning.

11. For Nicotrol, apply a new system each day upon waking and remove at bedtime. If forget to remove patch at bedtime, vivid dreams or other sleep disturbances may result. Do not wear patch more than 16 hr.

12. When a used system is removed, fold over and place in the protective pouch from the new system. Dispose of the used system to prevent access by children or pets.

13. If therapy is unsuccessful after 4 weeks, discontinue and identify reasons for failure so that a later attempt may be more successful.

OUTCOMES/EVALUATE

Smoking cessation; control of nicotine withdrawal symptoms

Nifedipine
(nye-**FED**-ih-peen)

CLASSIFICATION(S):
Calcium channel blocker
PREGNANCY CATEGORY: C
Rx: Adalat CC, Afeditab CR, Nifediac CC, Nifedical XL, Procardia, Procardia XL.
♣Rx: Adalat XL, Apo-Nifed, Apo-Nifed PA, Novo-Nifedin, Nu-Nifed, Nu-Nifedipine-PA.

SEE ALSO *CALCIUM CHANNEL BLOCKING AGENTS.*

USES

(1) Vasospastic (Prinzmetal's or variant) angina (except Adalat CC). (2) Chronic stable angina without vasospasm (except Adalat CC), including angina due to increased effort (especially in clients who cannot take beta blockers or nitrates or who remain symptomatic following clinical doses of these drugs). (3)

Essential hypertension (sustained-release only). *Investigational:* PO, sublingually, or chewed in hypertensive emergencies. Also prophylaxis of migraine headaches, primary pulmonary hypertension, severe pregnancy-associated hypertension, esophageal diseases, Raynaud's phenomenon, CHF, asthma, premature labor, biliary and renal colic, and cardiomyopathy. To prevent strokes and to decrease the risk of CHF in geriatric hypertensives.

ACTION/KINETICS

Action

Inhibits the influx of calcium through the cell membrane, resulting in a depression of automaticity and conduction velocity leading to a depression of contraction. Also dilates coronary vessels in both normal and ischemic tissues and inhibits spasms of coronary arteries. Decreases total peripheral resistance thus reducing energy and oxygen requirements of the heart. Variable effects on AV node effective and functional refractory periods. CO is slightly increased while peripheral vascular resistance is significantly decreased. Slight to no increase in HR and slight to no decrease in myocardial contractility.

Pharmacokinetics

Onset: 20 min. **Peak plasma levels:** 30 min (up to 4 hr for extended-release). $t\frac{1}{2}$: 2–5 hr. **Therapeutic serum levels:** 0.025–0.1 mcg/mL. **Duration:** 4–8 hr (12 hr for extended-release). Low-fat meals may slow the rate but not the extent of absorption. Metabolized in the liver to inactive metabolites with 60–80% excreted in the urine and 15% excreted in the feces. **Plasma protein binding:** 92–95%.

CONTRAINDICATIONS

Hypersensitivity. Lactation.

SPECIAL CONCERNS

Use with caution in impaired hepatic or renal function and in elderly clients. Initial increase in frequency, duration, or severity of angina (may also be seen in clients being withdrawn from beta blockers and who begin taking nifedipine).

SIDE EFFECTS

Most Common

Flushing, headache, fatigue/lethargy, edema, peripheral edema, weakness, muscle cramps, dizziness/lightheadedness, disturbed equilibrium.

CV: Peripheral and pulmonary edema, MI, hypotension, palpitations, syncope, CHF (especially if used with a beta blocker), decreased platelet aggregation, arrhythmias, tachycardia. Increased frequency, length, and duration of angina when beginning nifedipine therapy. **GI:** Nausea, diarrhea, constipation, flatulence, abdominal cramps, dysgeusia, vomiting, dry mouth, eructation, gastroesophageal reflux, melena. **CNS:** Dizziness, light-headedness, giddiness, nervousness, sleep disturbances, headache, weakness, depression, migraine, psychoses, hallucinations, disturbances in equilibrium, somnolence, insomnia, abnormal dreams, malaise, anxiety. **Dermatologic:** Rash, dermatitis, urticaria, pruritus, photosensitivity, erythema multiforme, **Stevens-Johnson syndrome**. **Respiratory:** Dyspnea, cough, wheezing, SOB, respiratory infection; throat, nasal, or chest congestion. **Musculoskeletal:** Muscle cramps or inflammation, joint pain or stiffness, arthritis, ataxia, myoclonic dystonia, hypertonia, asthenia. **Hematologic:** Thrombocytopenia, leukopenia, purpura, anemia. **Miscellaneous:** Fever, chills, sweating, weakness, fatigue/lethargy, blurred vision, sexual difficulties, flushing, transient blindness, hyperglycemia, hypokalemia, gingival hyperplasia, allergic hepatitis, hepatitis, tinnitus, gynecomastia, polyuria, nocturia, erythromelalgia, weight gain, epistaxis, facial and periorbital edema, hypoesthesia, gout, abnormal lacrimation, breast pain, dysuria, hematuria.

ADDITIONAL DRUG INTERACTIONS

Anticoagulants, oral / Possibility of ↑ PT
Barbiturates / ↓ Nifedipine effects
Cimetidine / ↑ Bioavailability of nifedipine
Cyclosporine / ↑ Cyclosporine levels and toxicity
Digoxin / ↑ Effect of digoxin by ↓ excretion by kidney
Diltiazem / ↑ Plasma levels of both nifedipine and diltiazem
H *Ginkgo biloba* / ↑ Nifedipine plasma levels R/T inhibition of nifedipine CYP3A4 metabolism
Grapefruit juice / ↑ Nifedipine plasma levels R/T ↓ metabolism
Itraconazole / ↑ Nifedipine serum levels
Mg sulfate / ↑ Neuromuscular blockade and hypotension
Melatonin / Melatonin may ↓ antihypertensive effect
Nafcillin / Significant ↓ nifedipine plasma levels
Quinidine / Possible ↓ quinidine effect R/T ↓ plasma levels; ↑ risk of hypotension, bradycardia, AV block, pulmonary edema, and VT
Quinupristin/Dalfopristin / ↑ Nifedipine plasma levels
Ranitidine / ↑ Nifedipine bioavailability
Rifampin ↑ Nifedipine effects
H *St. John's wort* / ↓ Nifedipine plasma levels R/T ↑ metabolism
Tacrolimus / ↑ Tacrolimus levels → ↑ toxicity
Theophylline / Possible ↑ effect of theophylline
Vincristine / ↑ Vincristine levels → ↑ toxicity

LABORATORY TEST CONSIDERATIONS

↑ Alkaline phosphatase, CPK, LDH, AST, ALT. Positive Coombs' test.

HOW SUPPLIED

Capsules: 10 mg, 20 mg; *Tablets, Extended-Release:* 30 mg, 60 mg, 90 mg.

DOSAGE

• **CAPSULES**

Angina.

Individualized. Initial: 10 mg 3 times per day (range: 10–20 mg 3 times per day); **maintenance:** 10–30 mg 3–4 times per day. Those with coronary artery spasm may respond better to 20–30 mg 3–4 times per day. Doses greater than 120 mg/day are rarely needed while doses greater than 180 mg/day are not recommended.

• **TABLETS, EXTENDED-RELEASE**

Angina, essential hypertension.

Initial: 30 or 60 mg once daily for Nifedical XL or Procardia XL and 30 mg once daily for Adalat CC. Titrate over a

7- to 14-day period. Dosage can be increased as required and as tolerated to a maximum of 120 mg/day for Nifedical XL or Procardia XL and 90 mg/day for Adalat CC.

Investigational: Hypertensive emergencies.

10–20 mg given PO (capsule is punctured several times and then chewed). This is not recommended.

NURSING CONSIDERATIONS

@ Do not confuse nifedipine with nicardipine (also a calcium channel blocker).

ADMINISTRATION/STORAGE

1. Do not exceed a single dose (other than sustained-release) of 30 mg.
2. Before increasing dose, carefully monitor BP.
3. Use only the sustained-release tablets to treat hypertension.
4. Sublingual nitroglycerin and long-acting nitrates may be used concomitantly with nifedipine.
5. Concomitant therapy with beta-adrenergic blocking agents may be used. In these cases, note any potential drug interactions.
6. Clients withdrawn from beta blockers may manifest symptoms of increased angina which cannot be prevented by nifedipine; in fact, nifedipine may increase the severity of angina in this situation.
7. Clients with angina may be switched to the sustained-release product at the nearest equivalent total daily dose. Use doses greater than 90 mg/day with caution.
8. No rebound effect noted when nifedipine discontinued. If drug to be discontinued, decrease dosage gradually with supervision.
9. Protect capsules from light and moisture; store at room temperature in original container.
10. During initial therapy and when dosage increased, may experience increase in frequency, duration, or severity of angina.
11. Food may decrease rate but not extent of absorption; can be taken without regard to meals.

ASSESSMENT

1. List reasons for therapy, other agents trialed/outcome, any sensitivity to calcium channel blockers.
2. Note pulmonary edema, ECG abnormalities, or palpitations. Document K+ levels, BP, and cardiopulmonary assessment findings.

INTERVENTIONS

1. During titration period, note any hypotensive response, increased HR that result from peripheral vasodilation; may precipitate angina.
2. Although beta-blocking drugs may be used concomitantly with chronic stable angina, the combined drug effects cannot be predicted (esp with compromised LV function or cardiac conduction abnormalities). Pronounced hypotension, heart block, and CHF may occur.
3. If therapy with a beta blocker is to be discontinued, gradually decrease dosage to prevent withdrawal syndrome.

CLIENT/FAMILY TEACHING

1. May take with or without food. Sustained-release tablets should not be chewed, crushed, or divided. Grapefruit juice may cause increased serum drug levels.
2. Avoid activities that require mental alertness until drug effects realized; may cause dizziness or lightheadedness.
3. Maintain fluid intake of 2–3 L/day to avoid constipation. No cause for concern if a tablet coating appears in the stool.
4. Do not switch brands; Adalat CC and Procardia XL are not interchangeable; not equivalent.
5. Do not use OTC agents unless approved; avoid alcohol and caffeine.
6. Report persistent headache, flushing, nausea, palpitations, weight gain, dizziness, rash, palpitations, or lack of response.
7. Brush teeth and floss regularly to reduce swelling and tenderness of your gums.
8. Keep log of BPs. Perform weekly weights, note any extremity swelling. This may result from arterial vasodila-

N

tion precipitated by nifedipine, or the swelling may indicate increasing ventricular dysfunction and should be reported.

9. If also receiving beta-adrenergic blocking agents, report any evidence of hypotension, exacerbation of angina, or evidence of heart failure. Once beta-blocking agents have been discontinued, report increased anginal pain.

OUTCOMES/EVALUATE

- ↓ Frequency and intensity of anginal episodes ↓ BP
- Improved peripheral circulation
- Prevention of strokes and ↓ risk of CHF in geriatric hypertensives

Nilotinib hydrochloride ■
(nye-**LOE**-tih-nib)

CLASSIFICATION(S):
Protein-tyrosine kinase inhibitor
PREGNANCY CATEGORY: D
Rx: Tasigna.

USES

Chronic- and accelerated-phase Philadelphia chromosome-positive chronic myelogenous leukemia in adults resistant to or intolerant to prior therapy that included imatinib. The major hematologic response rate was 31% in clients younger than 65 years of age and 15% in those 65 years of age and older.

ACTION/KINETICS

Action

Nilotinib binds to and stabilizes the inactive conformation of the kinase domain of Ab1 protein. Thus, proliferation is inhibited of cells from Philadelphia chromosome-positive CML.

Pharmacokinetics

Peak levels: 3 hr. Steady-state levels are reached within 8 days. Bioavailability is increased when the drug is given with a meal. Metabolized by oxidation and hydroxylation in the liver. **t½, elimination:** 17 hr. About 93% of the parent drug and metabolites are excreted in

the feces. **Plasma protein binding:** Approximately 98%.

CONTRAINDICATIONS

Hypokalemia, hypomagnesemia, or long QT syndrome. Lactation. Use not recommended in those with galactose intolerance, severe lactase deficiency, or glucose-galactose malabsorption.

SPECIAL CONCERNS

■ QT prolongation and sudden deaths. Nilotinib prolongs the QT interval. Sudden deaths have been reported in clients receiving nilotinib. Do not use nilotinib in clients with hypokalemia, hypomagnesemia, or long QT syndrome. Hypokalemia or hypomagnesemia must be corrected prior to nilotinib administration and should be periodically monitored. Avoid drugs known to prolong the QT interval and strong CYP3A4 inhibitors. Clients should avoid food 2 hr before and 1 hr after taking a nilotinib dose. Use with caution in clients with hepatic function impairment. Obtain ECGs to monitor the QTc baseline, 7days after initiation, and periodically thereafter, as well as following any dose adjustments.■ Safety and efficacy have not been established in children.

SIDE EFFECTS

Most Common

Constipation, diarrhea, fatigue, headache, N&V, pruritus, rash, neutropenia, thrombocytopenia, arthralgia, myalgia, cough, nasopharyngitis.

Listed are side effects with an incidence of 0.1% or more. **GI:** N&V, diarrhea, constipation, abdominal pain/discomfort/distention, dyspepsia, flatulence, dry mouth, gastroenteritis, gastroesophageal reflux, *GI hemorrhage*, melena, mouth ulceration, pancreatitis, stomatitis, hepatitis. **CNS:** Headache, fatigue, asthenia, dizziness, insomnia, paresthesia, anxiety, depression, hyperesthesia, hypoesthesia, *intracranial hemorrhage*, migraine, tremor. **CV:** ECG QT prolonged, flushing, hypertension, palpitations, angina pectoris, atrial fibrillation, bradycardia, *cardiac failure*, cardiac murmur, cardiomegaly, CAD, hematoma, *hemorrhagic shock*, *hypertensive crisis*, pericardial effusion, *torsades*

Bold Italic = life threatening side effect   ■ = black box warning   ✚ = Available in Canada

de pointes. **Dermatologic:** Rash, pruritus, alopecia, dry skin, eczema, erythema, hyperhidrosis, night sweats, urticaria, ecchymosis, exfoliative rash, facial swelling. **Musculoskeletal:** Arthralgia, myalgia, pain in extremity, muscle spasms, back/chest/bone pain, musculoskeletal pain, muscle weakness. **Respiratory:** Cough, nasopharyngitis, dyspnea, dysphonia, exertional dyspnea, epistaxis, interstitial lung disease, pharyngitis, pharyngolaryngeal pain, pleural effusion, pleurisy, pleuritic pain, pneumonia, pulmonary edema, throat irritation. **GU:** Breast pain, dysuria, erectile dysfunction, gynecomastia, micturition urgency, nocturia, pollakiuria, UTI. **Hematologic:** Neutropenia, thrombocytopenia, anemia, febrile neutropenia, pancytopenia. **Metabolic:** Anorexia, weight loss/gain, decreased/increased appetite, dehydration. **Ophthalmic:** Conjunctivitis, dry eye, eye irritation/hemorrhage, periorbital edema, reduced visual acuity. **Body as a whole:** Pyrexia, peripheral edema, chills, flu-like illness, malaise. **Miscellaneous:** Hyperthyroidism, vertigo, gravitational edema, *sudden death.*

LABORATORY TEST CONSIDERATIONS

↑ Alkaline phosphatase, ALT, AST, total bilirubin, creatinine, lipase, phosphokinase, GGT, blood glucose. ↓ Albumin, blood glucose. Hyperglycemia, hyper-/hypokalemia, hypocalcemia, hyponatremia, hypophosphatemia.

DRUG INTERACTIONS

Atazanavir / Avoid concomitant use; if coadministration needed, nilotinib dose should be ↓ to half of the original daily dose

Carbamazepine / Avoid concomitant use; if coadministration needed, nilotinib dose may need to be ↑

Clarithromycin / Avoid concomitant use; if coadministration needed, nilotinib dose should be ↓ to half the original daily dose

Cyclosporine / Use caution when giving nilotinib with drugs that are substrates of P-glycoprotein; ↑ levels of substrates likely

Dexamethasone / Avoid concomitant use; if coadministration needed, nilotinib dose may need to be ↑

Grapefruit juice / ↑ Nilotinib levels; do not use together

Indinavir / Avoid concomitant use; if coadministration needed, nilotinib dose should be ↓ to half the original daily dose

Itraconazole / Avoid concomitant use; if coadministration needed, nilotinib dose should be ↓ to half the original daily dose

Ketoconazole / Avoid concomitant use; if coadministration needed, nilotinib dose should be ↓ to half the original daily dose

Midazolam / ↑ Midazolam exposure by 30%; use together with caution

Nefazodone / Avoid concomitant use; if coadministration needed, nilotinib dose should be ↓ to half the original daily dose

Nelfinavir / Avoid concomitant use; if coadministration needed, nilotinib dose should be ↓ to half the original daily dose

P-glycoprotein inhibitors / Nilotinib is a substrate of P-glycoprotein; If coadministered → ↑ nilotinib levels

Phenobarbital / Avoid concomitant use; if coadministration needed, nilotinib dose may need to be ↑

Phenytoin / Avoid concomitant use; if coadministration needed, nilotinib dose may need to be ↑

Pimozide / Use caution when giving nilotinib with drugs that are substrates of P-glycoprotein; ↑ levels of substrates likely

Rifabutin/Rifampin/Rifapentine / Avoid concomitant use; if coadministration needed, nilotinib dose may need to be ↑

Ritonavir / Avoid concomitant use; if coadministration needed, nilotinib dose should be ↓ to half the original daily dose

Saquinavir / Avoid concomitant use; if coadministration needed, nilotinib dose should be ↓ to half the original daily dose

H *St. John's wort* / Avoid concomitant use; if coadministration needed, nilotinib dose may need to be ↑

Telithromycin / Avoid concomitant use; if coadministration needed, nilotinib dose should be ↓ to half the original daily dose

N

Voriconazole / Avoid concomitant use; if coadministration needed, nilotinib dose should be ↓ to half of the original daily dose

Warfarin / Avoid concurrent use if possible since warfarin is metabolized by CYP3A4 and CYP2C9

HOW SUPPLIED
Capsules: 200 mg.

DOSAGE
• **CAPSULES**
Chronic myelogenous leukemia.

Adults: 400 mg twice a day. Continue treatment as long as the client does not show evidence of progression or unacceptable toxicity.

NURSING CONSIDERATIONS
ADMINISTRATION/STORAGE

1. If a dose is missed, client should not take a make-up dose but should resume taking the next prescribed daily dose.

2. May be given in combination with erythropoietin or granulocyte-stimulating factor if clinically indicated.

3. May be given with hydroxyurea or anagrelide if clinically indicated.

4. Use the following guidelines for dosage adjustments if ECGs indicate a QTc >480 msec:

• Withhold nilotinib and measure serum K^+ and Mg^+. If below the lower limit of normal, correct with supplements to within normal limits. Concomitant medication usage must be reviewed.

• Resume within 2 weeks at prior dose if QTcF (Fredericia correction of QT interval) returns to <450 msec and to within 20 msec of baseline.

• If QTcF is between 450 and 480 msec after 2 weeks, reduce dose to 400 mg once a day.

• If QTcF returns to >480 msec following dose reduction to 400 mg once a day, discontinue nilotinib.

• An ECG should be repeated approximately 7 days after any dose adjustment.

5. Use the following guidelines for dosage adjustment for hematological toxicity (e.g., neutropenia, thrombocytopenia) that are not related to underlying leukemia. Dose of nilotinib is 400 mg twice a day to treat chronic-phase or accelerated-phase chronic myelogenous leukemia. If the absolute neutrophil count (ANC) is <1 x 10^9/L and/or platelet counts are <50 x 10^9/L, stop nilotinib and monitor blood cell counts. Resume drug within 2 weeks at prior dose if ANC is >1 x 10^9/L and platelet counts are >50 x 10^9/L. If blood cell counts remain low for >2 weeks, reduce the dose to 400 mg once a day.

6. Use the following guidelines for dosage adjustments for elevations of lipase, amylase, bilirubin, and/or hepatic transaminases.

• If serum lipase or amylase are elevated to less than or equal to grade 3, withhold nilotinib and monitor serum lipase or amylase.

• If bilirubin is elevated to greater than or equal to grade 3, withhold nilotinib and monitor bilirubin. Resume treatment at 400 mg once a day if bilirubin returns to less than or equal to grade 1.

• If hepatic transaminases are elevated to greater than or equal to grade 3, withhold nilotinib and monitor hepatic transaminases. Resume treatment at 400 mg once a day if hepatic transaminases return to less than or equal to grade 1.

7. Avoid the use of strong CYP3A4 inhibitors. If treatment with any of these drugs is required, therapy with nilotinib should be interrupted. If clients must be coadministered a strong CYP3A4 inhibitor with nilotinib, reduce dose of nilitinib to 400 mg once a day. If the strong inhibitor is discontinued, allow a washout period before adjusting the nilotinib dose upward. Closely monitor for prolongation of the QT interval in those who cannot avoid strong CYP3A4 inhibitors.

8. Avoid use of strong CYP3A4 inducers. If clients must be given a strong CYP3A4 inducer, nilitinib dose may need to be increased, depending on client tolerability. If the strong inducer is discontinued, reduce the nilitinib dose.

9. Store from 15–30°C (59–86°F).

Bold Italic = life threatening side effect   ■ = black box warning   ✦ = Available in Canada

ASSESSMENT

1. Note reasons for therapy, disease onset, phase of disease, other therapies trialed/failed (when resistant/intolerant to prior therapy that included imatinib).

2. List any exposure to ionizing radiation which could trigger this chromosome abnormality or treatment of a previous cancer.

3. List drugs prescribed; avoid drugs known to prolong the QT interval and strong CYP3A4 inhibitors.

4. Monitor LFTs, amylase, lipase, bilirubin, potassium and magnesium levels before and during therapy. Must correct any K^+ or Mg^+ deficiencies prior to starting therapy. Avoid drug with hepatic failure.

5. Assess for history or evidence of prolonged QT syndrome. Obtain ECG to monitor QTc at baseline, seven days after initiation, and periodically thereafter, as well as with any dose adjustments.

6. Obtain CBC every two weeks for the first two months and then monthly thereafter. Assess for enlarged spleen and counsel to avoid contact sports or rough activities.

7. Follow administration guidelines carefully; dose is adjusted for various phases of disease, as well as altered renal/liver function, neutropenia/thrombocytopenia.

CLIENT/FAMILY TEACHING

1. Take twice a day (at 12 hr intervals) on an empty stomach, at least 2 hours before or 1 hour after a meal.

2. Swallow capsules whole with water-do not open capsules. No food should be consumed for at least one hour after the dose is taken.

3. Avoid grapefruit, grapefruit juice, and/or any supplements containing grapefruit extract during therapy; increases blood drug levels in your body.

4. Do not take any OTC agents, vitamins, herbals or other prescription drugs without consulting provider. Many products may inhibit CYP3A4 and create toxic drug levels.

5. Report any unexplained bruising/bleeding, new onset weakness, or any blood in the urine or stools.

6. Yellow skin and eyes may indicate liver failure; report immediately.

7. Any swelling of the hands or feet or face, sudden weight gain, new onset SOB require medical attention.

8. Sudden stomach pain with nausea and vomiting may indicate pancreas inflammation; report immediately.

9. Review potential adverse effects including sudden death R/T prolonged QT syndrome preceded by irregular heart beat and fainting; low blood counts, liver damage, pancreatitis, or lack of desired response.

10. Females should practice reliable contraception; will harm fetus.

11. May be required to have periodic bone marrow aspirations done to eval. response to therapy.

12. Keep all F/U appointments for labs, regular EKGs (before starting, 7 days after starting therapy and with any dose increase) and provider review.

OUTCOMES/EVALUATE

- ↓ WBCs with hematologic stabilization of CML
- Control of malignant cell proliferation

Nilutamide ■
(nye-**LOO**-tah-myd)

CLASSIFICATION(S):
Antineoplastic, hormone
PREGNANCY CATEGORY: C
Rx: Nilandron.
🍁**Rx:** Anadron.

SEE ALSO *ANTINEOPLASTIC AGENTS.*

USES

In combination with surgical castration to treat metastatic prostate cancer (Stage D_2).

ACTION/KINETICS

Action

Antiandrogen with no estrogen, progesterone, mineralocorticoid, or glucocorticoid effects. Binds to the androgen receptor, thus blocking effects of testosterone and preventing the normal androgenic response.

📷 = see color insert   Ⓗ = Herbal   Ⓘⓥ = Intravenous   © = sound alike drug

Pharmacokinetics

Rapidly and completely absorbed from the GI tract. Extensively metabolized by the liver; one of the five metabolites is active. Excreted mainly in the urine. **t½, elimination:** Approximately, 41–49 hr. **Plasma protein binding:** Moderately bound.

CONTRAINDICATIONS

Severe hepatic impairment, severe respiratory deficiency, hypersensitivity to nilutamide or any product components. Use in women.

SPECIAL CONCERNS

■ (1) Interstitial pneumonitis has been reported. Have been rare reports of interstitial changes, including pulmonary fibrosis that led to hospitalization and death. Symptoms included exertional dyspnea, cough, chest pain, and fever. X-rays revealed interstitial or alveolo-interstitial changes; pulmonary function tests showed a restricted pattern with decreased carbon monoxide diffusion in the lung (DLCO). Most cases occurred within the first 3 months of treatment and most reversed if the drug was discontinued. (2) Perform a routine chest x-ray prior to starting treatment. Baseline pulmonary function tests may be considered. Instruct clients to report any new or worsening shortness of breath that they experience while on the drug. If symptoms occur, discontinue nilutamide immediately until it can be determined if the symptoms are drug-related. Hepatitis may occur. Many experience a delay in adaptation to the dark ranging from a few seconds to a few minutes. Safety and efficacy have not been determined in children.■

SIDE EFFECTS

Most Common

When used with leuprolide: Hot flushes, impaired adaptation to dark, pain, insomnia, headache, dizziness, nausea, constipation, testicular atrophy, gynecomastia, dyspnea, asthenia, back pain.

CV: Hypertension, angina, *heart failure*, syncope. **GI:** Nausea, constipation, diarrhea, dry mouth, GI disorder, *GI hemorrhage*, melena, hepatotoxicity, *hepatitis* (rare). **CNS:** Dizziness, nervousness,

paresthesia. **Respiratory:** Increased cough, interstitial pneumonitis, lung disorder, rhinitis, dyspnea. **Ophthalmic:** Cataract, photophobia, impaired adaptation to dark, abnormal vision, colored vision. **Metabolic/Nutritional:** Edema, weight loss, intolerance to alcohol. **Miscellaneous:** UTI, malaise, arthritis, pruritus, hot flashes, leukopenia, aplastic anemia (rare).

LABORATORY TEST CONSIDERATIONS

↑ Haptoglobin, alkaline phosphatase, BUN, creatinine, AST, ALT. Hyperglycemia.

DRUG INTERACTIONS

Phenytoin / Possible phenytoin delayed elimination and ↑ serum t½ → toxic levels

Theophylline / Possible theophylline delayed elimination and ↑ serum t½ → toxic levels

Vitamin K antagonists / Possible vitamin K antagonist delayed elimination and ↑ serum t½ → toxic levels

HOW SUPPLIED

Tablets: 50 mg.

DOSAGE

- **TABLETS**

  Metastatic prostate cancer.

  300 mg (six 50-mg tablets) once daily for 30 days followed by 150 mg (three 50-mg tablets) once daily.

NURSING CONSIDERATIONS

ADMINISTRATION/STORAGE

1. To ensure maximum beneficial effects, initiate treatment on the same day as or the day after surgical castration.

2. Protect from light and store at room temperature at 15–30°C (59–86°F).

ASSESSMENT

1. Note prostate cancer onset, other agents/therapies trialed, outcome. Anticipate first dosing on or the day after surgical castration.

2. Obtain CBC, LFTs, and CXR. Assess cardiopulmonary status closely; may cause interstitial pneumonitis. Monitor VS, PSA, PFTs, ECG.

CLIENT/FAMILY TEACHING

1. Take daily as directed, with or without food. Do not stop or interrupt dose without provider approval.

Bold Italic = life threatening side effect   ■ = black box warning   ♣ = Available in Canada

2. May experience difficulty driving at night or through tunnels (delayed dark adaptation); tinted glasses may alleviate this effect.

3. Immediately report any symptoms of chest pain, cough with fever, jaundice, dark urine, fatigue, SOB or unusual side effects.

4. Avoid alcohol, especially if intolerance of alcohol is experienced following nilutamide use.

OUTCOMES/EVALUATE

Control of malignant cell proliferation

Nimodipine
(nye-**MOH**-dih-peen)

CLASSIFICATION(S):

Calcium channel blocker

PREGNANCY CATEGORY: C

Rx: Nimotop.

♣Rx: Nimotop I.V.

SEE ALSO *CALCIUM CHANNEL BLOCKING AGENTS.*

USES

Improvement of neurologic deficits due to spasm following subarachnoid hemorrhage (SAH) from ruptured congenital intracranial aneurysms irrespective of the postictus neurological condition. *Investigational:* Migraine headaches and cluster headaches.

ACTION/KINETICS

Action

Has a greater effect on cerebral arteries than arteries elsewhere in the body (probably due to its highly lipophilic properties). Mechanism to reduce neurologic deficits following subarachnoid hemorrhage not known.

Pharmacokinetics

Peak plasma levels: 1 hr. **t½:** 1–2 hr; **t½, elimination:** 8–9 hr. Undergoes first-pass metabolism in the liver; metabolites excreted through the urine. **Plasma protein binding:** More than 95%.

CONTRAINDICATIONS

Lactation.

SPECIAL CONCERNS

Safety and efficacy have not been established in children. Use with caution in clients with impaired hepatic function and reduced hepatic blood flow. The half-life may be increased in geriatric clients.

SIDE EFFECTS

Most Common

Hypotension, headache, rash, diarrhea, nausea, flushing.

CV: Hypotension, peripheral edema, CHF, ECG abnormalities, tachycardia, bradycardia, palpitations, rebound vasospasm, hypertension, hematoma, *DIC, DVT*. **GI:** Nausea, dyspepsia, diarrhea, abdominal discomfort, cramps, *GI hemorrhage*, vomiting. **CNS:** Headache, depression, light-headedness, dizziness. **Hepatic:** Abnormal LFT, hepatitis, jaundice. **Hematologic:** Thrombocytopenia, anemia, purpura, ecchymosis. **Dermatologic:** Rash, dermatitis, pruritus, urticaria. **Miscellaneous:** Dyspnea, muscle pain or cramps, acne, itching, flushing, diaphoresis, wheezing, hyponatremia.

ADDITIONAL DRUG INTERACTIONS

Cimetidine / ↑ Nimodipine serum levels
Valproic acid / ↑ AUC of nimodipine

LABORATORY TEST CONSIDERATIONS

↑ Nonfasting BS, LDH, alkaline phosphatase, ALT. ↓ Platelet count.

HOW SUPPLIED

Capsules, Liquid-Filled: 30 mg.

DOSAGE

- **CAPSULES, LIQUID-FILLED**

Neurological deficits due to subarachnoid hemorrhage.

Adults: 60 mg (two 30 mg capsules) q 4 hr beginning within 96 hr after subarachnoid hemorrhage and continuing for 21 consecutive days. Reduce the dose to 30 mg q 4 hr in clients with hepatic impairment.

NURSING CONSIDERATIONS

ADMINISTRATION/STORAGE

If unable to swallow capsule (e.g., unconscious or at time of surgery), make a hole in both ends of the capsule (soft gelatin) with an 18-gauge needle and withdraw the contents into a syringe. This may be administered into the NG tube and washed down with 30 mL of NSS. Do not administer the contents of the capsule by IV injection or any other parenteral route.

ASSESSMENT

1. Note reasons for therapy, characteristics of S&S. Initiate therapy within 96 hr of subarachnoid hemorrhage.
2. Obtain baseline labs, determine if pregnant; reduce dose with hepatic dysfunction.
3. Perform baseline neurologic scores and thoroughly document deficits. Monitor BP, I&O, and weights.

CLIENT/FAMILY TEACHING

1. Take the drug on time; sleep must be interrupted to give the medication q 4 hr ATC for 21 days.
2. Report any side effects such as nausea, light-headedness, irregular heartbeat, low BP, dizziness, muscle cramps/pain or swelling of extremities. Change positions slowly to prevent dizziness.
3. Wear protective clothes and sunscreen to prevent photosensitivity reactions.
4. Avoid activities that require mental alertness until drug effects realized.
5. Report ↑ SOB, the need to take deep breaths on occasion, or wheezing. Keep all F/U visits.

OUTCOMES/EVALUATE

- ↓ Neurologic deficits R/T venospasm after subarachnoid hemorrhage
- Termination of migraine and cluster headaches

Nisoldipine ©
(NYE-sohl-dih-peen)

CLASSIFICATION(S):
Calcium channel blocker
PREGNANCY CATEGORY: C
Rx: Sular.

USES
Hypertension alone or in combination with other antihypertensive drugs.

ACTION/KINETICS

Action
Inhibits the transmembrane influx of calcium into vascular smooth muscle and cardiac muscle, resulting in dilation of arterioles. Has greater potency on vascular smooth muscle than on cardiac muscle. Chronic use results in a sustained decrease in vascular resistance and small increases in stroke index and LV ejection fraction. Weak diuretic effect and no clinically important chronotropic effects.

Pharmacokinetics
Well absorbed following PO use; however, absolute bioavailability is low due to presystemic metabolism in the gut wall. Foods high in fat result in a significant increase in peak plasma levels. **Maximum plasma levels:** 6–12 hr. **$t^{1/2}$, terminal:** 7–12 hr. Metabolized in the liver and excreted through the urine. **Plasma protein binding:** Almost completely bound.

CONTRAINDICATIONS
Use with grapefruit juice as it interferes with metabolism, resulting in a significant increase in plasma levels of the drug. Use in those with known hypersensitivity to dihydropyridine calcium channel blockers. Lactation.

SPECIAL CONCERNS
Geriatric clients may show a two- to three-fold higher plasma concentration; use caution in dosing. Use with caution and at lower doses in those with hepatic insufficiency. Use with caution in clients with CHF or compromised ventricular function, especially in combination with a beta blocker.

SIDE EFFECTS

Most Common
Peripheral edema, headache, dizziness/lightheadedness, palpitations, chest pain, vasodilation, rash, nausea, pharyngitis, sinusitis, flushing.

CV: Increased angina and/or MI in clients with CAD. Initially, excessive hypotension, especially in those taking other antihypertensive drugs. Vasodilation, palpitations, atrial fibrillation, **CVA, MI**, CHF, first-degree AV block, hyper-/hypotension, JVD, migraine, ventricular extrasystoles, SVT, syncope, systolic ejection murmur, T-wave abnormalities on ECG, venous insufficiency. **Body as a whole:** Peripheral edema, cellulitis, chills, facial edema, fever, flu syndrome, malaise. **GI:** Anorexia, nausea, colitis, diarrhea, dry mouth, dyspepsia, dysphagia, flatulence, gastritis, **GI hemorrhage**,

---

Bold Italic = life threatening side effect   ■ = black box warning   ✦ = Available in Canada

gingival hyperplasia, glossitis, hepatomegaly, increased appetite, melena, mouth ulceration. **CNS:** Headache, dizziness/lightheadedness, abnormal dreams/thinking and confusion, amnesia, anxiety, ataxia, cerebral ischemia, decreased libido, depression, hypesthesia, hypertonia, insomnia, nervousness, paresthesia, somnolence, tremor, vertigo. **Musculoskeletal:** Arthralgia, arthritis, leg cramps, myalgia, myasthenia, myositis, tenosynovitis. **Hematologic:** Anemia, ecchymoses, leukopenia, petechiae. **Respiratory:** Pharyngitis, sinusitis, asthma, dyspnea, end-inspiratory wheeze and fine rales, epistaxis, increased cough, laryngitis, pleural effusion, rhinitis. **Dermatologic:** Acne, alopecia, dry skin, exfoliative dermatitis, fungal dermatitis, herpes simplex/zoster, maculopapular rash, pruritus, pustular rash, skin discoloration/ulcer, sweating, urticaria. **GU:** Dysuria, hematuria, impotence, nocturia, urinary frequency, vaginal hemorrhage, vaginitis. **Metabolic:** Gout, hypokalemia, weight gain/loss. **Ophthalmic:** Abnormal vision, amblyopia, blepharitis, conjunctivitis, glaucoma, watery/itchy eyes, keratoconjunctivitis, retinal detachment, temporary unilateral loss of vision, vitreous floater. **Miscellaneous:** Flushing, diabetes mellitus, thyroiditis, chest/ear pain, otitis media, tinnitus, taste disturbance.

LABORATORY TEST CONSIDERATIONS
↑ Serum creatine kinase, NPN, BUN, serum creatinine. Abnormal LFTs.

OD OVERDOSE MANAGEMENT
Symptoms: Pronounced hypotension. *Treatment:* Active CV support, including monitoring of CV and respiratory function, elevation of extremities, judicious use of calcium infusion, pressor agents, and fluids. Dialysis is not likely to be beneficial, although plasmapheresis may be helpful.

DRUG INTERACTIONS
Azole antifungals / ↑ Nisoldipine levels; avoid coadministration
Cimetidine / Significant ↑ nisoldipine levels
Ketoconazole / ↑ Nisoldipine levels R/T ↓ liver metabolism

Phenytoin / ↑ Nisoldipine pharmacologic effects
Quinidine / ↑ AUC of nisoldipine but not peak concentration

HOW SUPPLIED
Tablets, Extended-Release: 10 mg, 20 mg, 30 mg, 40 mg.

DOSAGE
• **TABLETS, EXTENDED-RELEASE**
Hypertension.
Dose must be adjusted to the needs of each person. **Initial:** 20 mg once daily; **then,** increase by 10 mg/week or longer intervals to reach adequate BP control. **Usual maintenance:** 20–40 mg once daily. Doses beyond 60 mg once daily are not recommended. **Initial dose, clients over 65 years and those with impaired renal function:** 10 mg once daily.

NURSING CONSIDERATIONS
@ Do not confuse nisoldipine with nicardipine or nifedipine (also calcium channel blockers).

ADMINISTRATION/STORAGE
1. Closely monitor dosage adjustments in clients over age 65 and those with impaired liver/renal function.
2. Store at controlled room temperature of 20–25°C (68–77°F) protected from light and moisture. Should be dispensed in tight, light-resistant containers.

ASSESSMENT
1. Note reasons for therapy, characteristics of S&S, agents trialed, outcome.
2. List drugs prescribed to ensure none interact unfavorably. Reduce dosage in the elderly and with liver/renal dysfunction.
3. Obtain baseline VS and ECG; monitor BP closely and note any history/evidence of CHF, CAD, or compromised LV function.

CLIENT/FAMILY TEACHING
1. Swallow tablets whole; do not chew, divide, or crush. Do not take with grapefruit juice or a high-fat meal.
2. Headaches, extremity swelling, and dizziness may occur; use caution and report if persistent.
3. Report as scheduled for BP evaluation during titration period. Maintain

N

BP log and report any new/adverse side effects or loss of BP control.

OUTCOMES/EVALUATE
↓ BP

Nitazoxanide
(**nye**-tah-**ZOX**-ah-nyde)

CLASSIFICATION(S):
Antiprotozoal
PREGNANCY CATEGORY: B
Rx: Alinia.

SEE ALSO *ANTI-INFECTIVE DRUGS.*

USES
(1) Diarrhea due to *Giardia lamblia* in clients 12 years and older (tablets) and children 1–11 years of age (PO suspension). (2) Diarrhea due to *Cryptosporidium parvum* in clients 1–11 years of age and for those 12 years and older who are not infected with HIV. *Investigational:* Treatment of rotavirus diarrhea.

ACTION/KINETICS
Action
Action is due to interference with the pyruvate: feredoxin oxidoreductase enzyme-dependent electron transfer reaction which is required for anaerobic energy metabolism.

Pharmacokinetics
Rapidly metabolized to the active tizoxanide and tizoxanide glucuronide. **Maximum plasma levels, active metabolites:** 1–4 hr. The oral suspension is not bioequivalent to the tablets; the relative bioavailability of the suspension compared with the tablets is 70%. Food increases the AUC of both the tablets and suspension. Excreted in the urine, bile, and feces. **Plasma protein binding:** Tizoxanide (active metabolite): more than 99%.

CONTRAINDICATIONS
Use in prior hypersensitivity to nitazoxanide.

SPECIAL CONCERNS
Safety and efficacy of the oral suspension have not been determined in children less than 1 year of age, in children greater than 11 years of age, in adults, in HIV-positive clients, or those with immunodeficiency. Use with caution in those with hepatic and biliary disease, in renal disease, and in those with combined renal and hepatic disease. Use with caution during lactation.

SIDE EFFECTS
Most Common
Abdominal pain, diarrhea, N&V, headache.
Due to oral suspension. GI: Anorexia, increased appetite, enlarged salivary glands, flatulence, nausea. **CNS:** Dizziness. **GU:** Discolored urine. **Respiratory:** Rhinitis. **Ophthalmic:** Eye discoloration (pale yellow). **Miscellaneous:** Fever, infection, malaise.
Due to tablets. GI: Anorexia, constipation, dry mouth, dyspepsia, flatulence, thirst, vomiting. **CNS:** Dizziness, hypesthesia, insomnia, somnolence, tremor. **CV:** Hypertension, syncope, tachycardia. **GU:** Amenorrhea, discolored urine, dysuria, edema labia, kidney pain, metrorrhagia. **Respiratory:** Epistaxis, lung disease, pharyngitis. **Musculoskeletal:** Leg cramps, myalgia, spontaneous bone fracture. **Dermatologic:** Pruritus, rash. **Hematologic:** Anemia, leukocytosis. **Ophthalmic:** Eye discoloration. **Miscellaneous:** Allergic reaction, asthenia, chills, fever, flu syndrome, pain, pelvic pain, earache.

LABORATORY TEST CONSIDERATIONS
Oral suspension: ↑ ALT, creatinine.
Tablets: ↑ ALT.

DRUG INTERACTIONS
Since tizoxanide is highly bound to plasma proteins, use caution when giving together with other highly plasma protein-bound drugs (especially those with narrow therapeutic ranges) as competition for binding sites may occur.

HOW SUPPLIED
Powder for Oral Suspension: 100 mg/5 mL (after reconstitution); *Tablets, Film-Coated:* 500 mg.

DOSAGE
● **ORAL SUSPENSION; TABLETS, FILM-COATED**
Diarrhea due to Giardia lamblia.
Children, 1–3 years: 5 mL (100 mg) of the oral suspension q 12 hr with food for 3 days. **Children, 4–11 years:** 10 mL

Bold Italic = life threatening side effect   ■ = black box warning   ✦ = Available in Canada

(200 mg) of the oral suspension q 12 hr with food for 3 days. **Adults and children over 12 years:** 1 tablet (500 mg) or 25 mL (500 mg) of the oral suspension q 12 hr with food for 3 days.

Diarrhea due to C. parvum.
Children, 1–3 years: 5 mL (100 mg) of the oral suspension q 12 hr with food for 3 days. **Children, 4–11 years:** 10 mL (200 mg) of the oral suspension q 12 hr with food for 3 days. **Adults and children over 12 years:** 1 tablet (500 mg) q 12 hr with food for 3 days.

NURSING CONSIDERATIONS
ADMINISTRATION/STORAGE
1. To prepare suspension, tap bottle until all powder flows freely. Add about one-half of the total amount (48 mL) of water required for reconstitution and shake vigorously to suspend powder. Add remainder of water and shake vigorously.
2. After reconstitution, keep bottle tightly closed and shake well before each use. Suspension may be stored for 7 days; discard any unused portion after this period.
3. Store the tablets, unsuspended powder, and the reconstituted oral suspension from 15–30°C (59–86°F).

ASSESSMENT
1. Note onset and characteristics of S&S. May be transmitted by travelers to endemic areas or through contact with stools which are highly infectious.
2. Confirm flagellate in pediatric clients. Cysts or trophozites are evident in the stools. Flagellate may cause explosive diarrhea and abdominal cramps. In immunocompromised child who becomes malnourished, response rate may be impaired or death may ensue.
3. Drug is highly protein bound; use cautiously with other therapies as primary binding site competition may exist.
4. Monitor CBC, renal, LFTs; assess stool cultures.

CLIENT/FAMILY TEACHING
1. Shake well before each use. Administer with food. Suspension is pink and strawberry flavored. Inform diabetic clients and caregivers that oral suspension contains 1.48 grams of sucrose/5 mL. May store container tightly closed at room temperature for 7 days; discard any unused portions.
2. Dose is based on age and given every 12 hr x 3 days.
3. May experience GI upset: N&V, abdominal pain, headaches, and diarrhea. Also may discolor urine and give eyes a pale yellow discoloration. Report any lack of response, bloody stools, or worsening of S&S.
4. Prevent dehydration, ensure adequate hydration and fluid replacement to compensate for fluid loss through liquid stools. Handle stools carefully utilizing Universal Precautions, as they are highly infectious, especially to immunocompromised individuals.

OUTCOMES/EVALUATE
- Control/relief of watery explosive diarrhea R/T protozoa infection
- Three consecutive negative stool samples for cysts or trophozites with *Giardia lamblia*

Nitrofurantoin
(**nye**-troh-fyour-**AN**-toyn)

CLASSIFICATION(S):
Urinary anti-infective
PREGNANCY CATEGORY: B
Rx: Capsules (as macrocrystals): Macrodantin. **Capsules (as monohydrate/macrocrystals):** Macrobid. **Oral Suspension:** Furadantin.
✤**Rx:** Apo-Nitrofurantoin, Novo-Furantoin.

SEE ALSO *ANTI-INFECTIVE DRUGS.*

USES
UTIs due to susceptible strains of *Escherichia coli, Staphylococcus aureus,* Enterococci, and certain strains of *Enterobacter* and *Klebsiella*. Not indicated to treat pyelonephritis or perinephric abscesses. *NOTE:* Nitrofurantoin monohydrate/macrocrystals is indicated only for treatment of uncomplicated UTIs (e.g., acute cystitis) caused by susceptible strains of

N

E. coli or *Staphylococcus saprophyticus* in clients 12 years of age and older.

ACTION/KINETICS

Action

Nitrofurantoin is reduced by bacterial flavoproteins to reactive intermediates that inactivate or alter bacterial ribosomal proteins and other macromolecules. As a result, vital biochemical processes of protein synthesis, aerobic energy metabolism, DNA and RNA synthesis, and cell wall synthesis are inhibited. Is bactericidal in urine at therapeutic doses. Development of resistance has not been a significant problem.

Pharmacokinetics

Absorption of macrocrystals is slower when compared with the oral suspension (which is readily absorbed from the GI tract). Each monohydrate/macrocrystal capsule contains two forms of nitrofurantoin: 25% is macrocrystalline, which has slower dissolution and absorption than the monohydrate, and 75% is the monohydrate. Upon exposure to gastric and intestinal fluids the monohydrate forms a gel matrix that releases nitrofurantoin over time. Bioavailability is increased by food. $t^{1/2}$: 20 min (60 min in anephric clients). **Urine levels:** 50–250 mcg/mL. The oral suspension is rapidly excreted in urine while excretion of macrocrystals and the monohydrate/macrocrystals is somewhat less.

CONTRAINDICATIONS

Anuria, oliguria, and clients with impaired renal function (C_{CR} below 40 mL/min), and clinically significant elevated serum creatinine. Also, during pregnancy, especially near term; during labor; infants less than 1 month of age; and lactation.

SPECIAL CONCERNS

Use with extreme caution in anemia, diabetes, electrolyte imbalance, avitaminosis B, or a debilitating disease. There may be a higher proportion of pulmonary reactions, including fatalities, in the elderly (See *Side Effects*). Safety and efficacy of the monohydrate/macrocrystals in children less than 12 years of age have not been determined.

SIDE EFFECTS

Most Common

Headache, dizziness, N&V, anorexia, diarrhea, drowsiness, rust-colored or brownish urine.

Nitrofurantoin is a potentially toxic drug with many side effects. **GI:** Abdominal pain, anorexia, diarrhea, emesis, N&V, ***pancreatitis***, sialadenitis, pseudomembranous colitis. **Hepatic:** Hepatitis, cholestatic jaundice, chronic active hepatitis, ***hepatic necrosis***. **CNS:** Asthenia, confusion, depression, dizziness, drowsiness, headache, nystagmus, psychotic reactions, vertigo. **CV:** Benign intracranial hypertension (pseudotumor cerebri), nonspecific ST/T wave changes, bundle branch block (in association with pulmonary reactions). **Pulmonary, acute (usually within first week of treatment):** Fever, chills, cough, chest pain, dyspnea, pulmonary infiltration with consolidation or pleural effusion on x-ray, eosinophilia. **Pulmonary, subacute use:** Fever and eosinophilia occur less often. **Pulmonary, chronic use (6 months or longer):** Malaise, dyspnea on exertion, cough, altered pulmonary function, diffuse interstitial pneumonitis or fibrosis (or both). **Dermatologic:** Erythema multiforme (including ***Stevens-Johnson syndrome***), exfoliative dermatitis (rare), alopecia. **Hypersensitivity:** Angioedema, arthralgia, chills, drug fever, anaphylaxis, lupus-like syndrome (associated with pulmonary reactions), myalgia, pruritus, urticaria; eczematous, erythematous, or maculopapular eruptions. **Hematologic:** Hemolytic anemia (similar to the primaquine-sensitivity type), agranulocyosis, eosinophilia, glucose-6-phosphate dehydrogenase deficiency anemia, granulocytopenia, hemolytic anemia, leukopenia, megaloblastic anemia, thrombocytopenia, ***aplastic anemia*** (rare). **Ophthalmic:** Optic neuritis (rare). **Miscellaneous:** Peripheral neuropathy, super infections caused by resistant organisms, rust-colored or brownish urine.

Monohydrate/macrocrystals. GI: Nausea, flatulence, abdominal pain, constipation, diarrhea, dyspepsia, emesis.

Bold Italic = life threatening side effect   ■ = black box warning   ✚ = Available in Canada

CNS: Headache, amblyopia, drowsiness, dizziness. **Dermatologic:** Alopecia. **Respiratory:** Acute pulmonary hypersensitivity reactions (see above). **Miscellaneous:** Chills, fever, malaise.

LABORATORY TEST CONSIDERATIONS
↑ ALT, AST, serum phosphorus. ↓ Hemoglobin. False + glucose using Benedict and Fehling solutions.

OD OVERDOSE MANAGEMENT
Symptoms: Vomiting (most common). *Treatment:* Induce emesis. High fluid intake to promote urinary excretion. The drug is dialyzable.

DRUG INTERACTIONS
Anticholinergics / ↑ Nitrofurantoin bioavailability R/T delaying gastric emptying and increasing absorption
Magnesium salts / Delay or ↓ nitrofurantoin absorption
Uricosurics / High doses of probenecid ↓ nitrofurantoin renal clearance and ↑ serum levels → possible toxicity

HOW SUPPLIED
Nitrofurantoin: *Oral Suspension*: 25 mg/5 mL.
Nitrofurantoin Macrocrystals: *Capsules*: 25 mg, 50 mg, 100 mg.
Nitrofurantoin Monohydrate/Macrocrystals: *Capsules*: 100 mg.

DOSAGE————————
• **CAPSULES (MACROCRYSTALS), ORAL SUSPENSION**
UTIs.
Adults: 50–100 mg 4 times per day, not to exceed 600 mg/day. The lower dose is for uncomplicated UTIs. **Children, 1 month of age and older:** 5–7 mg/kg/day given in 4 divided doses. The following dosages in children, using the oral suspension, are based on average weight in each range receiving 5–6 mg/kg/day given in 4 divided doses: **7–11 kg (15–26 lb):** 2.5 mL 4 times per day; **12–21 kg (27–46 lb):** 5 mL 4 times per day; **22–30 kg (47–68 lb):** 7.5 mL 4 times per day; **31–41 kg (69–91 lb):** 10 mL 4 times per day.
Long-term suppressive therapy.
Adults: 50–100 mg at bedtime may be sufficient. **Children:** 1 mg/kg per day, given in a single dose or in 2 divided doses, may be adequate.

• **CAPSULES (MONOHYDRATE/MACROCRYSTALS)**
Uncomplicated UTIs (cystitis).
Adults: 100 mg q 12 hr for 7 days. **Pediatric, 1 month of age and over:** 5–7 mg/kg/day in four equal doses.

NURSING CONSIDERATIONS
ADMINISTRATION/STORAGE
1. Continue therapy for UTIs for 1 week or for at least 3 days after urine sterility obtained.
2. Avoid exposure of oral suspension to strong light (may darken drug). Is stable when stored from 20–25°C (68–77°F). Protect from freezing. Dispense in glass amber bottles.
3. Store capsules from 15–30°C (59–86°F). Dispense in a tight container using child-resistant closures.

ASSESSMENT
1. Note reasons for therapy. Monitor CBC, urine C&S, renal, LFTs, also CXR and PFTs with chronic therapy.
2. Observe for acute or delayed-onset anaphylactic reaction.
3. Monitor for recurrent UTI symptoms; urinary superinfections may occur.
4. Blacks and ethnic groups of Mediterranean and Near Eastern origin should be assessed for symptoms of anemia (G6PD).

CLIENT/FAMILY TEACHING
1. Do not crush or chew tablets; swallow whole.
2. Take with food or milk to minimize gastric irritation and enhance absorption; complete full course of therapy to prevent bacterial resistance. Avoid alcohol.
3. Increase fluid intake; drink at least 2 qt/day of water. Acidic foods (prunes, cranberry juice, plums) enhance drug action whereas alkaline foods (milk products) minimize drug action.
4. May turn urine a dark yellow or brown color.
5. Report persistent/bothersome side effects or lack of response. May cause dizziness or drowsiness. Breathing problems require immediate help.
6. Any numbness and tingling of extremities or flu-like symptoms must be reported; indications for drug with-

N

---

drawal as condition may worsen and become irreversible.

7. Report persistent N&V, diarrhea; may be symptoms of a GI superinfection. Keep all F/U appointment to evaluate response to therapy.

OUTCOMES/EVALUATE
- Negative urine culture results
- Resolution of infection
- Symptomatic improvement (↓ dysuria, frequency)

Nitroglycerin IV IV ©
(nye-troh-**GLIH**-sir-in)

CLASSIFICATION(S):
Vasodilator, coronary
PREGNANCY CATEGORY: C
Rx: Nitroglycerin in 5% Dextrose.

SEE ALSO *ANTIANGINAL DRUGS— NITRATES/NITRITES.*

USES
(1) Perioperative hypertension. (2) CHF associated in the setting of acute MI. (3) Angina unresponsive to sublingual nitroglycerin and beta-adrenergic blocking agents. (4) Induction of intraoperative hypotension. *Investigational:* Management of an acute MI; treatment of hypertensive emergencies; with vasopressin to treat variceal bleeding; treat cocaine-induced acute coronary syndrome; management of Prinzmetal's angina that occurs in those without coronary heart disease.

ACTION/KINETICS
Pharmacokinetics
Onset: 1–2 min; **duration:** 3–5 min (dose-dependent).

SPECIAL CONCERNS
Dosage has not been established in children.

SIDE EFFECTS
Most Common
Headache (may be severe and persistent), lightheadedness, hypotension. See *Antianginal Drugs—Nitrates/Nitrites* for a complete list of possible side effects.

HOW SUPPLIED
Injection: 100 mcg/mL, 200 mcg/mL, 400 mcg/mL; *Solution for Injection:* 5 mg/mL (requires dilution).

DOSAGE
- **IV INFUSION ONLY**
  All uses.
Initial: When using a nonabsorbing infusion set, start with 5 mcg/min delivered through an infusion pump capable of exact and constant delivery of the drug. May be increased by 5 mcg/min q 3–5 min until response is seen. If no response seen at 20 mcg/min, dose can be increased by 10 or even 20 mcg/min until response noted. Monitor titration continuously until client reaches desired level of response. Then, reduce the dose and lengthen the interval between increments.

NURSING CONSIDERATIONS
© Do not confuse nitroglycerin with nitroprusside (drug for hypertensive emergencies).

ADMINISTRATION/STORAGE
IV 1. There is no fixed optimum dose due to variations in responsiveness. Thus, titrate to the desired level of hemodynamic function. Continuously monitor BP, HR, and other measurements to achieve the correct dosage. Maintain adequate systemic blood and coronary perfusion pressures.
2. Not for direct IV use; must first be diluted. Transfer contents of 1 nitroglycerin vial (containing nitroglycerin 25 or 50 mg, i.e., 5 mg/mL) into a 500 mL glass bottle of either D5W or 0.9% NaCl. This yields a final concentration of 50 mcg/mL or 100 mcg/mL.
3. After the initial dosage titration, the concentration of the solution may be increased to limit the volume of fluids given. Do not exceed a nitroglycerin concentration of 400 mcg/mL.
4. Use glass IV bottle only and administration set provided by the manufacturer; is readily absorbed onto many plastics. Avoid adding unnecessary plastic to IV system.
5. Aspirate medication into a syringe and then inject immediately into a glass bottle (or polyolefin bottle) to minimize

contact with plastic. Greater absorption occurs with low flow rates, high concentrations, and long tubing.

6. If the concentration is adjusted, the infusion set must be flushed or replaced before a new concentration is used. If the set is not flushed or replaced, it may take minutes to hours (depending on flow rate and the dead space of the set), for new concentration to reach the client.

7. Do not administer with any other medications in the IV system.

8. Do not interrupt IV nitroglycerin for administration of a bolus of any other medication.

9. Administer solution with infusion device (volumetric) in a closely monitored environment.

10. Store from 15–30°C (59–86°F). Discard unused portion. Do not freeze. Protect from light.

11. The premixed nitroglycerin with dextrose can be stored at room temperature (25°C). Brief exposure up to 40°C does not affect potency. Avoid excessive heat and protect from freezing.

ASSESSMENT

1. Note reasons/goals of therapy. Assess VS, ECG, history, cardiopulmonary assessments.

2. Assess and rate pain, noting location, onset, duration, and any precipitating factors.

INTERVENTIONS

1. Obtain written parameters for BP and pulse; monitor during therapy. Note any evidence of hypotension, N&V, or sweating. Monitor CVP/PA pressure as ordered; document presence of tachycardia or bradycardia:

- Elevate the legs to restore BP.
- Reduce the rate of flow or administer additional IV fluids.

2. Assess for thrombophlebitis at the IV site; remove if reddened.

3. After the initial positive response to therapy, dosage increments will be smaller and made at longer intervals.

4. Sinus tachycardia may occur in client with angina receiving a maintenance dose of nitroglycerin (HR of 80 beats/min or less reduces myocardial demand).

5. Check that topical, PO, or SL doses are adjusted/held if on concomitant IV nitroglycerin.

6. Wean from IV nitroglycerin by gradually decreasing doses to avoid posttherapy CV distress. Usually initiated when the client is receiving the peak effect from PO or topical vasodilators; monitor for hypertension and angina.

7. Administer nonnarcotic analgesic (usually acetaminophen) because headache is a common side effect of drug therapy.

CLIENT/FAMILY TEACHING

1. Drug is used to lower BP, control chest pain, and/or reduce cardiac workload.

2. Report pain and level so dose may be adjusted to control.

3. Report any headaches so medications to relieve them can be administered.

4. Change to upright position slowly and if dizzy lie down.

5. Keep all F/U visits to evaluate response to therapy.

OUTCOMES/EVALUATE

- Resolution/control of angina
- ↓ BP; ↑ activity tolerance
- ↓ LVEDP (preload) and ↓ systemic vascular resistance (afterload)
- Improvement in S&S of CHF (↑ output, ↓ rales, ↓ CVP)

Nitroglycerin sublingual

(nye-troh-**GLIH**-sir-in)

CLASSIFICATION(S):
Vasodilator, coronary
PREGNANCY CATEGORY: C
Rx: NitroQuick, NitroTab, Nitrostat.

SEE ALSO *ANTIANGINAL DRUGS–NITRATES/NITRITES.*

USES

Acute relief or prophylaxis of angina pectoris caused by coronary artery disease.

ACTION/KINETICS

Action

Relax vascular smooth muscle by stimulating production of intracellular cyclic guanosine monophosphate. Dilation of postcapillary vessels decreases venous return to the heart due to pooling of blood; thus, LV end-diastolic pressure (preload) is reduced. Relaxation of arterioles results in a decreased systemic vascular resistance and arterial pressure (afterload).

Pharmacokinetics

Rapidly absorbed. Absolute bioavailability is 40% (but is variable). **Onset:** 1–3 min; **mean peak plasma levels:** 6–7 min. **duration:** 30–60 min. **t½, elimination:** About 2–3 min. Rapidly metabolized to dinitrates and mononitrates by a liver reductase enzyme. Also metabolized by red blood cells and vascular walls.

SPECIAL CONCERNS

Dosage has not been established in children.

SIDE EFFECTS

Most Common

Headache (may be severe and persistent), dizziness, palpitations vertigo, weakness, postural hypotension, syncope.

See *Antianginal Drugs—Nitrates/Nitrites* for a complete list of possible side effects.

ADDITIONAL DRUG INTERACTIONS

Tadalafil ↑ The hypotensive effect of sublingual nitroglycerin for 24 hr after tadalafil administration.

HOW SUPPLIED

Tablets, Sublingual: 0.3 mg, 0.4 mg, 0.6 mg.

DOSAGE

• TABLETS, SUBLINGUAL

Dissolve 1 tablet under the tongue or in the buccal pouch at first sign of attack; may be repeated in 5 min if necessary (no more than 3 tablets should be taken within 15 min). For prophylaxis, tablets may be taken 5–10 min prior to activities that may precipitate an attack.

NURSING CONSIDERATIONS

ADMINISTRATION/STORAGE

Store sublingual tablets from 15–30°C (59–86°F).

ASSESSMENT

1. Note reasons for therapy, characteristics of S&S, cardiac history/assessments.
2. Assess for anemia, heart failure, overactive thyroid, recent head trauma, recent heart attack or stroke; list drugs prescribed to ensure none interact.

CLIENT/FAMILY TEACHING

1. Sit down and place sublingual tablet under the tongue and allow to dissolve; do not swallow until entirely dissolved. May sting when it comes in contact with the mucosa.
2. Take 5–10 min *before* stressful activity, i.e., exercise, sex. Check with provider, may consider additional dose before anticipated stressful activity or if chest pain at night.
3. Report immediately if pain is not controlled with prescribed dosage (usually 1 tab q 5 min x 3). Call 911 or for an ambulance as directed by provider if relief not attained.
4. Date sublingual container upon opening. Keep medicine tightly closed in original glass bottle; discard cotton once bottle is opened. Protect from moisture. Discard unused tablets if 6 months has elapsed since the original container opened.
5. Encourage family members to learn CPR.

OUTCOMES/EVALUATE

- Angina prophylaxis
- Termination of anginal attack

Nitroglycerin sustained-release capsules

(nye-troh-**GLIH**-sir-in)

CLASSIFICATION(S):
Vasodilator, coronary
PREGNANCY CATEGORY: C
Rx: Nitro-Time.

USES

Prophylaxis and long-term treatment of recurrent angina. Onset of effect of capsules is not sufficiently rapid to be useful in aborting an acute anginal attack.

ACTION/KINETICS

Pharmacokinetics

Sustained-release. Onset: 20–45 min; **duration:** 3–8 hr.

SPECIAL CONCERNS

Dosage has not been established in children.

SIDE EFFECTS

Most Common

Headache (may be severe and persistent), lightheadedness, hypotension.

See *Antianginal Drugs–Nitrates/Nitrites* for a complete list of possible side effects.

HOW SUPPLIED

Capsules, Sustained-Release: 2.5 mg, 6.5 mg, 9 mg.

DOSAGE

• **CAPSULES, SUSTAINED-RELEASE**

Angina pectoris, prophylaxis.

Initial: 2.5–6.5 mg 3–4 times per day. Titrate upward to an effective dose until side effects limit dose. Upward dose titration in 2.5–6.5 mg increments 2–4 times per day over a period of days or weeks can be attempted. Doses as high as 26 mg given 4 times per day have been effective. However, give the smallest effective dose 2–4 times per day.

NURSING CONSIDERATIONS

ASSESSMENT

Note reasons for therapy, onset, characteristics of S&S, cardiac history/assessments.

CLIENT/FAMILY TEACHING

1. Drug is used to control/prevent chest pain.

2. Do not chew or crush sustained-release capsules-swallow whole; not intended for sublingual use.

3. Take smallest effective dose 2–4 times per day with a glass of water. Report if tolerance/lack of response evident.

4. Avoid alcohol during therapy.

5. Keep all F/U visits to evaluate response to therapy.

OUTCOMES/EVALUATE

Angina prophylaxis

Nitroglycerin topical ointment @

(nye-troh-**GLIH**-sir-in)

CLASSIFICATION(S):
Vasodilator, coronary

PREGNANCY CATEGORY: C

Rx: Nitro-Bid.

USES

Prophylaxis and treatment of angina pectoris due to CAD. *NOTE:* Onset of action of the ointment is not rapid enough to be used to abort an acute anginal attack. *Investigational:* Management of acute MI; treat chronic anal fissure pain; erectile dysfunction; Raynaud disease; management of Prinzmetal angina that occurs in clients without CAD.

ACTION/KINETICS

Pharmacokinetics

Onset: 30–60 min; **duration:** 2–12 hr (depending on amount used per unit of surface area).

SPECIAL CONCERNS

Dosage has not been established in children.

SIDE EFFECTS

Most Common

Headache (may be severe and persistent), flushing, dizziness, weakness, hypotension, paresthesia.

See *Antianginal Drugs–Nitrates/Nitrites* for a complete list of possible side effects.

HOW SUPPLIED

Ointment: 2%.

DOSAGE

• **OINTMENT;**

Two daily ½ inch (7.5 mg) doses; apply one on rising in morning and apply one 6 hr later. The dose can be doubled and even doubled again in those tolerating this dose but failing to respond to it.

NURSING CONSIDERATIONS

⚕ Do not confuse Nitro-Bid with Nitro-Tab (also a nitroglycerin product).

ADMINISTRATION/STORAGE

Store from 15-30°F (59-86°F).

ASSESSMENT

Note reasons for therapy, characteristics of S&S, cardiac history/assessments, EKG.

CLIENT/FAMILY TEACHING

1. Squeeze ointment carefully onto dose-measuring application papers (packaged with the medicine). Use applicator to spread ointment or fold paper in half and rub back and forth. Clean around tube opening and tightly cap tube after use.

2. Use the paper to spread the ointment onto a nonhairy area of skin. Application to the chest may be psychologically helpful, but may be applied to other nonhairy areas. Avoid distal extremities or any cut, callused, or irritated skin area.

3. Rotate sites to prevent irritation. Keep a record of areas used to avoid unnecessary repetitive use of sites.

4. Apply ointment in a thin, even layer covering an area of skin 3–6 inches in diameter; remove last dose. Date and tape the application paper over the area, or cover the area with a piece of plastic wrap-type material. A clear plastic cover causes less leakage of ointment, decreases skin irritation, increases absorption, and prevents clothing stains.

5. Once the dose is established, use the same type of covering to ensure that the same amount of drug is absorbed during each application.

6. To prevent systemic absorption, protect skin from contact with ointment. Prevent contact with hands and wash hands thoroughly after application to avoid headache.

7. Remove at bedtime or as directed to prevent tolerance or loss of drug effect. Remember to reapply upon awakening the next morning. Report adverse effects and lack of response.

8. Cellegesic may help to avoid the risk of surgery of anal fissures by gently relaxing the sphincter muscle. Follow provider guidelines for administration.

OUTCOMES/EVALUATE

- Termination/prevention of anginal episodes
- Relief of chronic anal fissure pain

Nitroglycerin transdermal system
(nye-troh-**GLIH**-sir-in)

CLASSIFICATION(S):
Vasodilator, coronary

PREGNANCY CATEGORY: C

Rx: Minitran 0.1 mg/hr, 0.2 mg/hr, 0.4 mg/hr, and 0.6 mg/hr., Nitrek 0.2 mg/hr, 0.4 mg/hr, and 0.6 mg/hr., Nitro-Dur 0.1 mg/hr, 0.2 mg/hr, 0.3 mg/hr, 0.4 mg/hr, 0.6 mg/hr, and 0.8 mg/hr.

SEE ALSO *ANTIANGINAL DRUGS – NITRATES/NITRITES.*

USES

Prophylaxis of angina pectoris due to CAD. The onset of action is not sufficiently rapid to be used in aborting an acute anginal attack. *Investigational:* Management of acute MI; erectile dysfunction; Raynaud disease; management of Prinzmetal angina that occurs in those without coronary heart disease.

ACTION/KINETICS

Pharmacokinetics

Onset: 30–60 min; **duration:** 8–24 hr. The amount released each hour is indicated in the name.

SPECIAL CONCERNS

Dosage has not been established in children.

SIDE EFFECTS

Most Common

Headache (may be severe and persistent), lightheadedness, hypotension.

See *Antianginal Drugs—Nitrates/Nitrites* for a complete list of possible side effects.

HOW SUPPLIED

Transdermal Patch (Extended-Release): To release: 0.1 mg/hr, 0.2 mg/hr, 0.3 mg/hr, 0.4 mg/hr, 0.6 mg/hr, 0.8 mg/hr.

Bold Italic = life threatening side effect ■ = black box warning ♣ = Available in Canada

DOSAGE

• TRANSDERMAL PATCH (EXTENDED-RELEASE)

Angina pectoris, prophylaxis.

Initial: 0.2–0.4 mg/hr (initially the smallest available dose in the dosage series) applied each day to skin site free of hair and free of excessive movement (e.g., chest, upper arm). Doses between 0.4 and 0.8 mg/hr are effective for 10–12 hr/day for at least 1 month of intermittent administration. A nitrate-free interval of 10–12 hr is sufficient. Thus, an appropriate dosing schedule would include a daily 'patch-on' period of 10–12 hr and a 'patch-off' period of 10–12 hr. **Maintenance:** Additional systems or strengths may be added depending on the clinical response. *NOTE:* Tolerance is a major limiting factor to efficacy when the system is used constantly for more than 12 hr/day.

NURSING CONSIDERATIONS

ADMINISTRATION/STORAGE

1. Follow instructions for specific products on package insert.
2. Remove patch before defibrillating, as patch may explode.
3. The various products differ in the mechanism for the delivery system; the most important factor is the amount of drug released per hour. A wide range of client variability will be noted. Variables in the absorption rate include skin, physical exercise, and elevated ambient temperature.
4. Store from 15–30°C (59–86°F). Avoid extremes of temperature/humidity. Do not refrigerate or store outside of protective package.

ASSESSMENT

Note reasons for therapy, onset, characteristics of S&S, EKG, cardiac history/assessments.

CLIENT/FAMILY TEACHING

1. Apply as directed at the same time each day. Dry skin completely before applying to a hair-free site; apply immediately upon removal from the package. *Do not change brands or attempt to trim or cut system.*
2. Rotate application sites each day to avoid skin irritation. Do not apply to distal extremities or to skin that is irritated, abraded, or scarred. Date patch as a reminder that drug has been administered. Once applied, do not disturb or open patch. Do not stop abruptly.
3. Remove at bedtime or as directed to prevent a diminished response (tolerance) to the drug. Remember to reapply a new system upon awakening the next morning.
4. Report adverse effects or breakthrough pain. Bathing or swimming should not interfere with therapy.
5. When terminating therapy, gradually reduce the dose and frequency of application over 4–6 weeks.
6. Remove patch before defibrillating, as patch may explode. Have family/significant other learn CPR.

OUTCOMES/EVALUATE

Control/prevention of anginal episodes

Nitroglycerin translingual spray

(nye-troh-**GLIH**-sir-in)

N

CLASSIFICATION(S):

Vasodilator, coronary
PREGNANCY CATEGORY: C
Rx: Nitrolingual, Nitromist.

SEE ALSO ANTIANGINAL DRUGS—NITRATES/NITRITES.

USES

(1) Terminate an acute anginal attack due to coronary artery disease. (2) Prophylactically 10–15 min before beginning activities that can cause an acute anginal attack due to coronary artery disease.

ACTION/KINETICS

Pharmacokinetics
Onset: 2 min; **duration:** 30–60 min.

SPECIAL CONCERNS

Dosage has not been established in children.

SIDE EFFECTS

Most Common
Headache (may be severe and persistent), flushing, dizziness, weakness, hypotension, paresthesia.

📷 = see color insert   H = Herbal   IV = Intravenous   © = sound alike drug

See *Antianginal Drugs—Nitrates/Nitrites* for a complete list of possible side effects. Also, **hypersensitivity:** N&V, pallor, perspiration, restlessness, weakness, collapse. **Dermatologic:** Rash, exfoliative dermatitis. **Miscellaneous:** Abdominal pain, asthenia, dyspnea, peripheral edema, pharyngitis, rhinitis, vasodilation.

HOW SUPPLIED
Aerosol Spray, Lingual: 0.4 mg (400 mcg)/metered dose (spray).

DOSAGE
- **AEROSOL SPRAY, LINGUAL**
  Termination of acute attack.

One to two metered doses (400–800 mcg) on or under the tongue q 5 min as needed; no more than three metered doses should be administered within a 15-min period.

  Prophylaxis of angina.

One to two metered doses (400–800 mcg) 5–10 min before beginning activities that might precipitate an acute attack.

NURSING CONSIDERATIONS
ADMINISTRATION/STORAGE
1. Each metered spray delivers 48 mg of solution containing 400 mcg nitroglycerin, after an initial priming of 1 spray. The container will remain adequately primed for 6 weeks.
2. If the product is not used within 6 weeks, reprime with 1 spray.
3. There are 60–200 doses/bottle. The total number of available sprays depends on the number of sprays per use (1 or 2 sprays) and the frequency of repriming.
4. Store from 15–30°C (59–86°F).

ASSESSMENT
Note reasons for therapy, onset, characteristics of S&S, EKG, cardiac history/assessments.

CLIENT/FAMILY TEACHING
1. Hold container vertically with the valve head uppermost and the spray orifice as close to the mouth as possible. Preferably spray onto the tongue by pressing the button firmly; the mouth should be closed immediately after each dose. Do not inhale the spray.

2. Spray under or on the tongue 5–10 min before anticipated activity or when pain is experienced. Wait 10 sec and then swallow.
3. Sit upright during application.
4. Seek immediate medical attention if chest pain persists.
5. Have family/significant other learn CPR.

OUTCOMES/EVALUATE
Control/prevention of acute anginal episodes

Nitroprusside sodium
(nye-troh-**PRUS**-eyed)

CLASSIFICATION(S):
Antihypertensive, peripheral vasodilator
PREGNANCY CATEGORY: C
Rx: Nitropress.

USES
(1) Hypertensive crisis to reduce BP immediately. (2) To produce controlled hypotension during anesthesia to reduce bleeding. (3) Acute CHF. *Investigational:* In combination with dopamine for acute MI. Left ventricular failure with coadministration of oxygen, morphine, and a loop diuretic.

ACTION/KINETICS
Action
Direct action on vascular smooth muscle, leading to peripheral vasodilation of arteries and veins. Acts on excitation-contraction coupling of vascular smooth muscle by interfering with both influx and intracellular activation of calcium. No effect on smooth muscle of the duodenum or uterus and is more active on veins than on arteries. May also improve CHF by decreasing systemic resistance, preload and afterload reduction, and improved CO. Caution must be exercised as nitroprusside injection can result in toxic levels of cyanide. However, when used briefly or at low infusion rates, the cyanide produced reacts with thiosulfate to pro-

duce thiocyanate, which is excreted in the urine.

Pharmacokinetics

Onset (drug must be given by IV infusion): 0.5–1 min; **peak effect:** 1–2 min; **t½:** 2 min; **duration:** Up to 10 min after infusion stopped. Reacts with hemoglobin to produce cyanmethemoglobin and cyanide ion.

CONTRAINDICATIONS

Compensatory hypertension where the primary hemodynamic lesion is aortic coarctation or AV shunting. Use to produce controlled hypotension during surgery in clients with known inadequate cerebral circulation or in moribund clients. Clients with congenital optic atrophy or tobacco amblyopia (both of which are rare). Acute CHF associated with decreased peripheral vascular resistance (e.g., high-output heart failure that may be seen in endotoxic sepsis). Lactation.

SPECIAL CONCERNS

■ (1) After reconstitution, nitroprusside is not suitable for direct injection. The reconstituted solution must be further diluted in D5W before infusion. (2) Can cause a precipitous drop in BP. In clients not properly monitored, these decreases can lead to irreversible ischemic injuries or death. Use only when available equipment and personnel allow BP to be monitored continuously. (3) Nitroprusside injection gives rise to important quantities of cyanide except when used briefly or at low (less than 2 mcg/kg/min) infusion rates. This can lead to toxic and potentially lethal levels. The usual dose rate is 0.5–10 mcg/kg/min, but infusion at the maximum rates should never last beyond 10 minutes. If BP has not been adequately controlled after 10 min of infusion at the maximum rate, terminate administration immediately. (4) Monitor acid-base balance and venous oxygen levels; they may indicate cyanide toxicity but these tests provide imperfect guidance.■ Use with caution in hypothyroidism, liver or kidney impairment, during lactation, and in the presence of increased ICP. Geriatric clients may be more sensitive to the hypotensive effects of nitroprusside; also, a decrease in dose may be necessary in these clients due to age-related decreases in renal function.

SIDE EFFECTS

Most Common

Excessive hypotension, dizziness, nausea, restlessness, headache, sweating, palpitations, abdominal pain, muscle twitching, retrosternal discomfort.

Large doses may lead to cyanide toxicity. Following rapid BP reduction: Dizziness, nausea, restlessness, headache, sweating, muscle twitching, palpitations, abdominal pain, apprehension, retching, retrosternal discomfort. **Other side effects:** Bradycardia, tachycardia, ECG changes, venous streaking, rash, vomiting or skin rash, methemoglobinemia, decreased platelet aggregation, flushing, ileus, irritation at injection site, hypothyroidism. **Symptoms of thiocyanate toxicity:** Blurred vision, tinnitus, confusion, hyperreflexia, seizures. **CNS symptoms (transitory):** Restlessness, agitation, increased ICP, and muscle twitching.

OD OVERDOSE MANAGEMENT

Symptoms: Excessive hypotension, cyanide toxicity, thiocyanate toxicity.

Treatment:

• Measure cyanide levels and blood gases to determine venous hyperoxemia or acidosis.
• To treat cyanide toxicity, discontinue nitroprusside and give sodium nitrite, 4–6 mg/kg (about 0.2 mL/kg) over 2–4 min (to convert hemoglobin into methemoglobin); follow by sodium thiosulfate, 150–200 mg/kg (about 50 mL of the 25% solution). This regimen can be given again, at half the original doses, after 2 hr.

DRUG INTERACTIONS

Concomitant use of other antihypertensives, volatile liquid anesthetics, or certain depressants ↑ nitroprusside response.

HOW SUPPLIED

Powder for Injection: 50 mg/vial.

DOSAGE

• **IV INFUSION ONLY**
  Hypertensive crisis.

 = see color insert   = Herbal   = Intravenous   @ = sound alike drug

Adults: Average, 3 mcg/kg/min. **Range:** 0.3–10 mcg/kg/min. Smaller dose is required for clients receiving other antihypertensives. **Pediatric:** 1.4 mcg/kg/min adjusted slowly depending on the response.

Monitor BP and use as guide to regulate rate of administration to maintain desired antihypertensive effect. Do not exceed a rate of administration of 10 mcg/kg/min.

NURSING CONSIDERATIONS

℃ Do not confuse nitroprusside with nitroglycerin (a coronary vasodilator).

ADMINISTRATION/STORAGE

IV 1. Dissolve contents of the vial (50 mg) in 2–3 mL of D5W. Must be further diluted in 250–1,000 mL D5W.

2. If protected from light, reconstituted solution is stable for 24 hr. Discard solutions that are any color but light brown.

3. Do not add any other drug or preservative to solution.

4. Protect dilute solutions during administration by wrapping bag and tubing with opaque material such as aluminum foil or foil-lined bags; change setup every 24 hr. Explain that covering the IV bag protects the medication from light and maintains drug stability. Administer IV solution with an electronic infusion device in a monitored environment.

5. Cyanide toxicity is possible if more than 500 mcg/kg nitroprusside is given faster than 2 mcg/kg/min. To reduce this possibility, sodium thiosulfate can be co-infused with nitroprusside at rates of 5–10 times that of nitroprusside.

6. Protect drug from heat, light, and moisture. Store at 15–30°C (59–86°F).

ASSESSMENT

1. Note onset and etiology of hypertensive crisis, S&S, other therapies trialed, outcome.

2. Note any hypothyroidism or B_{12} deficiency. Assess for any increased ICP, electrolyte disturbance, liver or renal dysfunction or conditions that would preclude drug therapy (i.e., AV shunt, coarctation of aorta, etc.).

3. Monitor VS, I&O, ECG, CBC, electrolytes, ABGs, PAWP, renal, and LFTs.

INTERVENTIONS

1. Monitor BP closely and titrate infusion. Administer only in a continuously monitored environment by trained personnel.

2. Observe for symptoms of thiocyanate toxicity. Evaluate thiocyanate levels daily with prolonged infusions of >3 mcg/kg, min or in anuric clients and q 48–72 hr otherwise. Levels should be <100 mcg thiocyanate/mL or 3 μmol cyanide/mL. Metabolic acidosis may precede cyanide toxicity.

3. With cyanide toxicity, administer sodium nitrite 4–6 mg/kg over 2–4 min (as a 3% solution). Then use sodium thiosulfate 150–200 mcg/kg as a 25% or 50% solution to convert cyanide to thiocyanate so the body can eliminate it.

CLIENT/FAMILY TEACHING

1. Drug is given in a monitored environment to rapidly lower BP and to reduce the workload of the heart.

2. Aluminum foil or foil-lined bags are used to protect solutions from light during administration and to maintain drug stability.

3. Report any ringing in the ears, headache, dizziness or blurred vision as well as any other adverse side effects or pain at injection site immediately.

OUTCOMES/EVALUATE

- ↓ BP; ↓ Preload/afterload
- Improved S&S of refractory CHF

Nizatidine
(nye-**ZAY**-tih-deen)

CLASSIFICATION(S):
Histamine H_2 receptor blocking drug
PREGNANCY CATEGORY: B
OTC: Axid AR.
Rx: Axid, Axid Pulvules.
♣**Rx:** Apo-Nizatidine, Novo-Nizatidine, PMS-Nizatidine.

SEE ALSO *HISTAMINE H$_2$ ANTAGONISTS.*

USES

Rx: (1) Treatment of acute duodenal ulcer (up to 8 weeks) and maintenance following healing of a duodenal ulcer. (2) GERD, including erosive and ulcerative esophagitis and associated heartburn. Has been used for up to 12 weeks in adults and 8 weeks in children 12 years and older. (3) Short-term (up to 8 weeks) treatment of benign gastric ulcer.

OTC: Prevention and relief of heartburn, acid indigestion, and sour stomach due to certain foods and beverages.

Investigational: Prevention of olanzapine-induced weight gain. Prevention of NSAID-induced gastroduodenal ulcer. In combination with amoxicillin and clarithromycin for *Helicobacter pylori* infection.

ACTION/KINETICS

Action

Decreases gastric acid secretion by blocking the effect of histamine on histamine H_2 receptors. Does not affect the P-450 and P-448 drug metabolizing enzymes.

Pharmacokinetics

Greater than 70% bioavailable. **Onset:** 30 min. **Peak plasma levels:** 0.5–3 hr after a PO dose. **Time to peak effect:** 0.5–3 hr. **Duration, nocturnal:** Up to 12 hr; **basal:** Up to 8 hr. **t½:** 1–2 hr. Approximately 60% of a PO dose is excreted unchanged in the urine. Clients with moderate to severe renal impairment manifest a significant prolongation of t½ with decreased clearance. **Plasma protein binding:** About 35%.

CONTRAINDICATIONS

Hypersensitivity to H_2 receptor antagonists. Cirrhosis of the liver, impaired renal or hepatic function. Lactation.

SPECIAL CONCERNS

Use oral solution and OTC tablets only for those 12 years of age and older.

SIDE EFFECTS

Most Common

Headache, dizziness, insomnia, agitation/anxiety, somnolence, fatigue, rash, nausea, diarrhea.

CNS: Headache, fatigue, somnolence, insomnia, dizziness, abnormal dreams, agitation/anxiety, nervousness, confusion (rare). **GI:** N&V, diarrhea, pancreatitis, constipation, abdominal discomfort, flatulence, dyspepsia, anorexia, dry mouth. **Dermatologic:** Rash, exfoliative dermatitis, erythroderma, pruritus, urticaria, erythema multiforme. **CV:** Asymptomatic VT; *rarely, cardiac arrhythmias or arrest following rapid IV use.* **Respiratory:** Rhinitis, pharyngitis, sinusitis, cough. **Body as a whole:** Asthenia, back/chest pain, infection, fever, myalgia. **Miscellaneous:** Impotence, loss of libido, thrombocytopenia, sweating, gynecomastia, hyperuricemia, eosinophilia, gout, and cholestatic or hepatocellular effects (resulting in increased AST, ALT, or alkaline phosphatase).

LABORATORY TEST CONSIDERATIONS

False + test for urobilinogen.

DRUG INTERACTIONS

Antacids containing Al and Mg hydroxides / ↓ Nizatidine absorption by about 10%

Aspirin, high doses / ↑ Salicylate levels
Simethicone / ↓ Nizatidine absorption by about 10%

HOW SUPPLIED

Capsules (Rx): 150 mg, 300 mg; *Oral Solution (Rx):* 15 mg/mL; *Tablets (OTC):* 75 mg.

DOSAGE

AXID, AXID PULVULES

• **RX: CAPSULES, ORAL SOLUTION**
  Acute therapy for duodenal ulcer.

Adults: Either 300 mg once daily at bedtime or 150 mg 2 times per day. Most heal within 4 weeks. **Maintenance therapy:** 150 mg once daily at bedtime.
  Treatment of benign gastric ulcer.

Adults: Either 150 mg twice a day or 300 mg once daily at bedtime
  GERD, including erosive and ulcerative esophagitis.

Adults and children 12 years and older: 150 mg twice a day.

AXID AR

• **OTC: TABLETS**
  Heartburn, acid indigestion, sour stomach.

For relief of symptoms: 1 tablet with a full glass of water. To prevent symptoms: 1 tablet with a full glass of water before eating or up to 60 minutes be-

---

fore consuming foods and beverages that cause heartburn. *NOTE:* Can be used up to two times per day (i.e., 2 tablets in 24 hr).

NURSING CONSIDERATIONS

ADMINISTRATION/STORAGE

1. Use the following doses for moderate to severe renal insufficiency for treating active duodenal ulcer, GERD, or benign gastric ulcer: If the C_{CR} is 20–50 mL/min: 150 mg/day and 150 mg every other day for maintenance; if C_{CR} <20 mL/min: 150 mg every other day and 150 mg every 3 days for maintenance.
2. Maintain treatment for active duodenal ulcer for up to 8 weeks.
3. Gastric malignancy may be present even though a clinical response to nizatidine has occurred.
4. Doses of 150 and 300 mg can be mixed with commercial juices (apple juice, *Gatorade, Ocean Spray,* and others); such preparations are stable for 48 hr when refrigerated. However, a 10% loss in potency is seen if mixed with *V8* or *Cran-Grape* juices.
5. Store capsules from 20–25°C (68–77°F) in tightly closed container. Store solution from 15–30°C (59–86°F).

ASSESSMENT

1. List type, onset, characteristics of S&S, other agents trialed, outcome.
2. Note any experience/intolerance to H_2 receptor antagonists. Document abdominal assessment.
3. Monitor hepatic and renal function studies; reduce dosage with renal insufficiency. *NOTE: H. pylori* results and diagnostic findings, i.e., radiographic/endoscopic.

CLIENT/FAMILY TEACHING

1. Take at bedtime if sedative effects noted. Continue to take as ordered even if symptoms subside to ensure adequate healing. With erosive esophagitis expect prolonged therapy.
2. OTC use: To relieve heartburn, take 1 tablet (75 mg) with a full glass of water. To prevent heartburn, take 1 tablet with a full glass of water just before eating or up to 60 min before consuming food/beverages that cause heartburn.

3. Use caution when performing tasks that require mental alertness until drug effects realized.
4. Report any rashes, flaking of skin, extreme sleepiness, blood in stool/vomit, or lack of response.
5. Avoid alcohol, caffeine, spicy foods, and aspirin-containing products. Do not smoke, as this aggravates condition by increasing gastric acid secretion.
6. Keep all F/U appointments to evaluate response to therapy.

OUTCOMES/EVALUATE

Improvement in ulcer pain/irritation with healing; ↓ GERD S&S

Norepinephrine bitartrate (Levarterenol) ■ IV

(nor-ep-ih-**NEF**-rin)

CLASSIFICATION(S):
Sympathomimetic
PREGNANCY CATEGORY: C
Rx: Levophed.

SEE ALSO *SYMPATHOMIMETIC DRUGS.*

USES

(1) Hypotensive states caused by septicemia, blood transfusions, drug reactions, spinal anesthesia, poliomyelitis, sympathectomy, MI, and pheochromocytomectomy. (2) Adjunct to treatment of cardiac arrest and profound hypotension. Used during cardiac resuscitation after cardiac arrest to restore and maintain an adequate BP after an effective heartbeat and ventilation have been established.

ACTION/KINETICS

Action

Norepinephrine is a powerful peripheral vasoconstrictor due to stimulation of alpha-adrenergic receptors; it is also a potent inotropic agent due to its action on B_1 receptors in the heart. Coronary vasodilation occurs secondary to enhanced myocardial contractility. The result is an increase in systemic BP and coronary artery blood flow. Cardiac out-

---

Bold Italic = life threatening side effect   ■ = black box warning   ✦ = Available in Canada

put changes vary but is usually increased in hypotension when BP is raised to optimal levels. Venous return is increased and the heart tends to have a more normal rate and rhythm compared with the hypotensive state. Minimal hyperglycemic effect.

Pharmacokinetics

Onset: immediate; **duration:** 1–2 min after discontinuation of the infusion. Metabolized in liver and other tissues by the enzymes MAO and catechol-O-methyltransferase; however, the pharmacologic activity is terminated by uptake and metabolism in sympathetic nerve endings. Metabolites excreted in urine.

CONTRAINDICATIONS

Use in hypotension due to blood volume deficits, except as an emergency measure to maintain coronary and cerebral artery perfusion until blood volume replacement therapy can be completed. Use in clients with mesenteric or peripheral vascular thrombosis (due to increased risk of ischemia and extending the area of infarction) unless use is necessary as a life-saving procedure. Use during cyclopropane and halothane anesthesia or in those with profound hypoxia or hypercarbia (due to risk of producing ventricular tachycardia or fibrillation).

SPECIAL CONCERNS

■ Antidote for extravasation ischemia. To prevent sloughing and necrosis in areas in which extravasation has taken place, the area should be infiltrated as soon as possible with 10 mL to 15 mL of saline solution containing from 5 mg to 10 mg of phentolamine, an adrenergic blocking agent. A syringe with a fine hypodermic needle should be used, with the solution being infiltrated liberally throughout the area, which is easily identified by its cold, hard, and pallid appearance. Sympathetic blockade with phentolamine causes immediate and conspicuous local hyperemic changes if the area is infiltrated within 12 hours. Therefore, phentolamine should be given as soon as possible after the extravasation is noted.■ Use is not a substitute for replacement of blood, plasma, fluids, and electrolytes. Some products contain sulfites that may cause allergic effects, including anaphylaxis or life-threatening or less severe asthmatic episodes. Use with caution during lactation. Select doses carefully in the elderly. Safety and efficacy have not been demonstrated in children.

SIDE EFFECTS

Most Common

Bradycardia, headache, anxiety.

CV: Bradycardia (probably as a reflex due to a rise in BP), arrhythmias. **CNS:** Headache (may be a symptom of overdosage and severe hypertension), transient headache, anxiety. **Miscellaneous:** Ischemic injury due to potent vasoconstriction and tissue hypoxia, respiratory difficulty, extravasation necrosis at injection site, gangrene (when infused into an ankle vein). *NOTE:* Prolonged administration may result in plasma volume depletion which should be continuously corrected by appropriate fluid and electrolyte replacement. If plasma volume is not corrected, hypotension may recur when norepinephrine injection is discontinued.

OD **OVERDOSE MANAGEMENT**

Symptoms: Dangerously high BP, headache, reflex bradycardia, marked increase in peripheral resistance, decreased cardiac output. Prolonged administration may result in plasma volume depletion. *Treatment:* Appropriate fluid and electrolyte replacement. If plasma volumes are not corrected, hypotension may result when norepinephrine is discontinued or BP may be maintained at the risk of severe peripheral vasoconstriction with diminution of blood flow and tissue perfusion.

DRUG INTERACTIONS

Anesthetics, halogenated hydrocarbon (e.g., halothane) / Sensitization of heart to the effects of norepinephrine → possible ventricular tachycardia and fibrillation; do not use together

Bretylium / Potentiation of action of vasopressors on adrenergic receptors → possible arrhythmias

Guanethidine / ↑ Pressor response of norepinephrine → possible severe hypertension

Monoamine oxidase inhibitors / Possible severe, prolonged hypertension; use together with extreme caution

Oxytocic drugs / In obstetrics, if norepinephrine is used either to correct hypotension or added to the local anesthetic solution → possible severe persistent hypertension

Tricyclic antidepressants / Potentiation of pressor response; use together with caution

HOW SUPPLIED

Injection: 1 mg (as base)/mL.

DOSAGE

- **IV INFUSION ONLY**

    Restoration of BP in acute hypotensive states.

Correct blood volume as much as possible before giving any vasopressor. In emergency situations when intra-aortic pressures must be maintained to prevent cerebral or coronary artery ischemia, give norepinephrine before and concurrently with blood volume replacement.

Effect on BP determines dosage, initial: 8–12 mcg base/min or 2–3 mL of a 4-mcg/mL solution. Adjust the rate of flow to establish and maintain a low normal BP (usually 80–100 mm Hg systolic). In previously hypertensive clients, raise the BP no more than 40 mm Hg below the pre-existing systolic pressure. **Average maintenance:** 2–4 mcg base/min with the dose determined by client response.

NURSING CONSIDERATIONS

ADMINISTRATION/STORAGE

[IV] 1. Norepinephrine is a potent, concentrated drug that must be diluted in dextrose solution before infusion.

2. Monitor BP q 2 min from the time administration is started until desired BP is obtained; then, monitor q 5 min if administration is continued. Constantly watch flow rate. Never leave client unmonitored during infusion.

3. Whenever possible, infuse into a large vein, particularly an antecubital or femoral vein to minimize necrosis from overlying skin and prolonged vasoconstriction.

4. If extravasation occurs, infiltrate as soon as possible with 10–15 mL of saline solution containing 5–10 mg phentolamine to prevent sloughing and necrosis. Infiltrate liberally, using a syringe with a fine needle, throughout the ischemic area.

5. Avoid a catheter tie-in technique because obstruction to blood flow around the tubing may cause stasis and increased local concentration of the drug.

6. Avoid leg veins in elderly clients or in those suffering from such disorders due to an increased risk of atherosclerosis, arteriosclerosis, diabetic endarteritis, or Buerger's disease.

7. If large fluid volumes are needed at a flow rate involving an excessive dose of the drug per unit of time, use a solution more diluted than 4 mcg/mL. When large fluid volumes are undesirable, a higher concentration may be given.

8. Continue the norepinephrine infusion until adequate BP and tissue perfusion are maintained without therapy. Reduce infusion gradually, avoiding abrupt withdrawal.

9. When used to restore BP in hypotensive states, add 4 mL of the solution to 1,000 mL D5W in water or saline solution for a concentration of 4 mcg base/mL. Do not use saline solution alone.

10. Do not administer through the same tube as blood products. However, a Y-tube and individual flasks may be used.

11. Store at room temperature protected from light. Discard solutions that are brown or that have a precipitate.

ASSESSMENT

1. Note reasons for therapy; ensure adequately hydrated.

2. Administer in a monitored environment Monitor BP by arterial line or electronically continously until stable then q 5 min during drug therapy. Assess I&O, ECG, VS, CVP, and PA wedge pressures.

3. Observe infusion site frequently for extravasation; ischemia and sloughing may occur. Blanching along the course of the vein may indicate permeability of the vein wall, which could allow leakage to occur. If evident, change IV site

and give phentolamine at extravasation site.

4. Withdraw drug gradually; may experience an initial rebound drop in BP. Extra fluids parenterally may diminish rebound hypotension and help stabilize BP during withdrawal. Keep atropine on hand for reflex bradycardia, and propranol for arrhythmias.

CLIENT/FAMILY TEACHING

Drug is given by infusion in a closely monitored environment. Report any pain or discomfort at IV site or difficulty breathing immediately.

OUTCOMES/EVALUATE

- ↑ BP/CO
- Improved tissue perfusion

Norfloxacin ⓒ
(nor-**FLOX**-ah-sin)

CLASSIFICATION(S):
Antibiotic, fluoroquinolone
PREGNANCY CATEGORY: C
Rx: Noroxin.
✤Rx: Apo-Norflox, Noroxin Ophthalmic Solution, Novo-Norfloxacin, Riva-Norfloxacin.

SEE ALSO *ANTI-INFECTIVE DRUGS* AND *FLUOROQUINOLONES.*

USES

(1) Uncomplicated UTIs (including cystitis) caused by *Escherichia coli, Klebsiella pneumoniae, Enterobacter cloacae, Proteus mirabilis, P. vulgaris, Pseudomonas aeruginosa, Citrobacter freundii, Staphylococcus aureus, S. epidermidis, Enterococcus faecalis, Enterobacter aerogenes, S. saprophyticus,* and *S. agalactiae.* (2) Complicated UTIs caused by *Enterococcus faecalis, E. coli, K. pneumoniae, P. mirabilis, P. aeruginosa,* or *Serratia marcescens.* (3) Urethral gonorrhea and endocervical gonococcal infections due to penicillinase- or non–penicillinase-producing *Neisseria gonorrhoeae.* (4) Prostatitis due to *E. coli.*

ACTION/KINETICS

Action

Active against gram-positive and gram-negative organisms by inhibiting bacterial DNA synthesis. Not effective against obligate anaerobes.

Pharmacokinetics

Peak plasma levels: 1.4–1.6 mcg/mL after 1–2 hr following a dose of 400 mg and 2.5 mcg/mL 1–2 hr after a dose of 800 mg. **t½:** 3–4.5 hr. Food decreases the absorption of norfloxacin. Approximately 30% excreted unchanged in the urine and 30% through the feces.

CONTRAINDICATIONS

Hypersensitivity to nalidixic acid, cinoxacin, or norfloxacin. Lactation, infants, and children.

SPECIAL CONCERNS

Use with caution in clients with a history of seizures and in impaired renal function. Geriatric clients eliminate norfloxacin more slowly.

SIDE EFFECTS

Most Common

Headache, dizziness, N&V, diarrhea, dyspepsia/heartburn, eosinophilia, neutropenia.

See *Fluoroquinolones* for a complete list of possible side effects. **GI:** N&V, diarrhea, abdominal pain/discomfort, dry/painful mouth, dyspepsia/heartburn, flatulence, constipation, pseudomembranous colitis, stomatitis. **CNS:** Headache, dizziness, fatigue, malaise, drowsiness, depression, insomnia, confusion, psychoses. **Hematologic:** Decreased hematocrit, eosinophilia, leukopenia, neutropenia, increased/decreased platelets. **Dermatologic:** Photosensitivity, rash, pruritus, exfoliative dermatitis, *toxic epidermal necrolysis,* erythema, erythema multiforme, *Stevens-Johnson syndrome.* **Miscellaneous:** Paresthesia, hypersensitivity, fever, visual disturbances, hearing loss, crystalluria, cylindruria, candiduria, myoclonus (rare), hepatitis, pancreatitis, arthralgia.

ADDITIONAL DRUG INTERACTIONS

Metronidazole and Mycophenolate / ↓ Mycophenolic and mycophenolic acid glucuronide when all three taken together
Nitrofurantoin / ↓ Norfloxacin antibacterial effect

LABORATORY TEST CONSIDERATIONS

↑ AST, ALT, alkaline phosphatase, BUN, serum creatinine, and LDH.

HOW SUPPLIED
Tablets: 400 mg.

DOSAGE

- **TABLETS**
  Uncomplicated UTIs due to E. coli, K. pneumoniae, or P. mirabilis.
  400 mg q 12 hr for 3 days.
  Uncomplicated UTIs due to other organisms.
  400 mg q 12 hr for 7–10 days.
  Complicated UTIs.
  400 mg q 12 hr for 10–21 days. Maximum dose for UTIs should not exceed 800 mg/day.
  Uncomplicated gonorrhea.
  800 mg as a single dose.
  Impaired renal function, with C_{CR} equal to or less than 30 mL/min/1.73 m².
  400 mg/day for appropriate duration for infection present.
  Prostatis due to E. coli.
  400 mg q 12 hr for 28 days.

NURSING CONSIDERATIONS

© Do not confuse Noroxin with Floxin (also a fluoroquinolone) or Neurontin (an anticonvulsant).

ASSESSMENT

1. Note reasons for therapy, characteristics of S&S, other agents trialed, outcome. List drugs prescribed to ensure none interact unfavorably.
2. List any seizure disorder or impaired renal/liver function; reduce dose with impaired function.
3. Assess CBC and culture results. Determine if pregnant.

CLIENT/FAMILY TEACHING

1. Take 1 hr before or 2 hr after meals, with a glass of water; food decreases drug absorption. Antacids should not be taken with or for 2 hr after dosing. Take drug at evenly spaced intervals, generally every 12 hr.
2. To prevent crystalluria, consume 2–3 L/day of fluids.
3. Use caution if operating equipment or driving a motor vehicle; may cause dizziness.
4. Avoid prolonged sun exposure, wear sunscreen and protective clothing if exposed.
5. Females of childbearing age should practice reliable contraception.
6. Keep all F/U appointments. Report any new or unusual side effects or lack of response.

OUTCOMES/EVALUATE

- Negative culture reports
- Symptomatic improvement

Nortriptyline hydrochloride ■ ©

(nor-**TRIP**-tih-leen)

CLASSIFICATION(S):
Antidepressant, tricyclic
PREGNANCY CATEGORY: C
Rx: Aventyl, Pamelor.
✿Rx: Apo-Nortriptyline, Gen-Nortriptyline, Novo-Nortriptyline, Nu-Nortriptyline, PMS-Nortriptyline, ratio-Nortriptyline.

SEE ALSO *ANTIDEPRESSANTS, TRICYCLIC.*

USES
Treatment of symptoms of depression. Endogenous depressions are more likely to be helped than other depressive illnesses.

ACTION/KINETICS

Action
Causes adaptive changes in the serotonin and norepinephrine receptor systems, resulting in changes in the sensitivities of both presynaptic and postsynaptic receptor sites. The overall effect is a re-regulation of the abnormal receptor neurotransmitter relationship. Manifests moderate anticholinergic and sedative effects but slight orthostatic hypotensive effects.

Pharmacokinetics
Well absorbed; significant first-pass effect. Long serum t½ (thus once daily dosing may suffice). **Effective plasma levels:** 50–150 ng/mL. **t½:** 18–44 hr. **Time to reach steady state:** 4–19 days. Partially metabolized in the liver; primarily excreted in the urine.

CONTRAINDICATIONS
Use in children (safety and efficacy have not been determined).

Bold Italic = life threatening side effect   ■ = black box warning   ✿ = Available in Canada

SPECIAL CONCERNS

■ (1) Antidepressants increased the risk of suicidal thinking and behavior (suicidality) in short-term studies in children and adolescents with major depressive disorder and other psychiatric disorders. Anyone considering the use of nortriptyline or any other antidepressant in a child or adolescent must balance this risk with the clinical need. Clients who are started on therapy should be observed closely for clinical worsening, suicidality, or unusual changes in behavior. Families and caregivers should be advised of the need for close observation and communication with the prescriber. Nortriptyline is not approved for use in pediatric clients. (2) Short-term placebo-controlled trials of 9 antidepressant drugs in children and adolescents with major depressive disorder, obsessive-compulsive disorder, or other psychiatric disorders revealed a greater risk of adverse reactions during the first few months of treatment. The average risk of such reactions in clients receiving antidepressants was 4%, twice the placebo risk of 2%. No suicides occurred in these trials.■

SIDE EFFECTS

Most Common

Tachycardia, blurred vision, urinary retention, dry mouth, weight gain/loss, orthostatic hypotension.

See *Antidepressants, Tricyclic* for a complete list of possible side effects.

LABORATORY TEST CONSIDERATIONS

↓ Urinary 5-HIAA.

HOW SUPPLIED

Capsules: 10 mg, 25 mg, 50 mg, 75 mg; *Oral Solution:* 10 mg base/5 mL.

DOSAGE

- **CAPSULES; ORAL SOLUTION**
  Depression.

Adults: 25 mg 3–4 times per day. Dose individualized; begin at a low dosage and increase as needed. **Doses above 150 mg/day are not recommended. Adolescent and elderly clients:** 30–50 mg/day in divided doses or total daily dose may be given once a day.

NURSING CONSIDERATIONS

@ Do not confuse nortriptyline (Aventyl, Pamelor) with amitriptyline or norpramin, each of which is a tricyclic antidepressant. Do not confuse Pamelor with Tambocor (an antiarrhythmic).

ADMINISTRATION/STORAGE

1. The total daily dose may be given at bedtime.
2. Monitor plasma levels if doses greater than 100 mg/day are given. Maintain plasma levels in the range of 50–150 ng/mL.
3. Store at controlled room temperatures.

ASSESSMENT

1. List reasons for therapy, clinical presentation, onset, age, characteristics of S&S, other agents trialed. Identify causative factors; rate pain if indicated.
2. Monitor CBC, liver, renal function studies. Reduce dose with dysfunction, elderly debilitated clients.
3. Stop several days before surgery to prevent hypertensive episodes; reduce dose if psychosis occurs/increases.

CLIENT/FAMILY TEACHING

1. Take after meals and at bedtime to minimize GI upset. May take several weeks before beneficial effects noted. Do not stop suddenly after long term use.
2. Take entire dose at bedtime with chronic pain conditions to minimize daytime sedation. Avoid activities that require mental alertness until drug effects realized. Move slowly, may experience drop in BP with sudden changes in position.
3. Report unusual/intolerable side effects. May require dosage adjustment or change in therapy. Report visual changes; ensure regular eye exams.
4. May experience sun sensitivity, use sunscreen and protective clothing.
5. Avoid alcohol, and CNS depressants; may potentiate effects. May experience dry mouth; use sugar free candy/gum, frequent sips of water/ice chips to offset.

N

OUTCOMES/EVALUATE
- Control of symptoms of depression ($\downarrow$ fatigue, improved sleeping/eating patterns, effective coping)
- $\downarrow$ Nocturnal pruritus
- Control of chronic neurogenic pain

Nystatin
(nye-**STAT**-in)

CLASSIFICATION(S):
Antifungal

PREGNANCY CATEGORY: C (A for vaginal use),

Rx: Lozenges: Mycostatin Pastilles. **Oral Suspension**: Mycostatin, Nilstat, Nystex. **Tablets**: Mycostatin. **Topical Cream/Ointment**: Mycostatin, Nilstat, Nystex. **Topical Powder**: Mycostatin, Nystop, Pedi-Dri. **Vaginal Tablets**: Mycostatin.

❧**Rx**: Candistatin, Nyaderm, PMS-Nystatin, ratio-Nystatin.

SEE ALSO *ANTI-INFECTIVE DRUGS*.

USES
Candida infections of the skin, mucous membranes, GI tract, vagina, and mouth (thrush). The drug is too toxic for systemic infections although it can be given PO for intestinal moniliasis infections, as it is not absorbed from the GI tract.

ACTION/KINETICS
Action
Binds to fungal cell membranes (sterols), resulting in altered cellular permeability and leakage of potassium and other essential intracellular components. Is both fungistatic and fungicidal against all species of *Candida*.

Pharmacokinetics
Poorly absorbed from the GI tract; unabsorbed nystatin is excreted in the feces.

CONTRAINDICATIONS
Use for systemic mycoses. Use of topical products in or around the eyes.

SPECIAL CONCERNS
Do not use occlusive dressings when treating candidiasis. Do not use lozenges in children less than 5 years of age.

SIDE EFFECTS
Most Common
GI upset, N&V, diarrhea, rash.
Nystatin has few toxic effects.
GI: Epigastric distress, GI upset, N&V, diarrhea. **Dermatologic:** Rash (including urticaria), *Stevens-Johnson syndrome* (rare). **Miscellaneous:** Tachycardia, bronchospasm, facial swelling, nonspecific myalgia (rare).

HOW SUPPLIED
Cream: 100,000 units/gram; *Lozenge/Troche:* 200,000 units; *Ointment:* 100,000 units/gram; *Powder, Topical:* 100,000 units/gram; *Oral Suspension:* 100,000 units/mL; *Tablets, Oral:* 500,000 units; *Tablets, Vaginal:* 100,000 units.

DOSAGE
- **LOZENGES; ORAL SUSPENSION; TABLETS, ORAL**
  Intestinal candidiasis.
Tablets, 500,000–1,000,000 units 3 times per day; continue treatment for 48 hr after cure to prevent relapse.
  Oral candidiasis.
Oral Suspension, adults and children: 400,000–600,000 units 4 times per day ($\frac{1}{2}$ dose in each side of mouth, held as long as possible before swallowing); **infants:** 200,000 units 4 times/day (same procedure as with adults); **premature or low birth weight infants:** 100,000 units 4 times per day. **Lozenge, adults and children:** 200,000–400,000 units 4–5 times per day, up to 14 days. *NOTE:* Lozenges should not be chewed or swallowed.
- **TABLETS, VAGINAL**
  Vaginal candidiasis.
100,000 units (1 tablet) inserted high in the vagina once each day for 2 weeks. Improvement may occur in a few days; however, continue the full course of treatment.
- **TOPICAL CREAM; TOPICAL OINTMENT; TOPICAL POWDER**
  Cutaneous or mucocutaneous Candida infections.
Apply to affected areas 2–3 times per day, or as indicated, until healing is complete.

Bold Italic = life threatening side effect ■ = black box warning ❧ = Available in Canada

NURSING CONSIDERATIONS

ADMINISTRATION/STORAGE

1. Powder for extemporaneous compounding of oral suspension is available. To reconstitute, add ⅛ tsp of the powder (about 500,000 units) to approximately ½–1 cup water and stir well. Administer this product immediately after mixing. Suspension can be stored for 7 days at room temperature or 10 days in the refrigerator without loss of potency.

2. Protect drug from heat, light, moisture, and air.

3. For *Candida* infections of the feet, powder can be freely dusted on feet as well as in socks and shoes.

4. The cream is generally used in *Candida* infections involving intertriginous areas; treat moist lesions with powder.

5. If irritation occurs, stop drug treatment.

6. Store vaginal tablets from 15–30°C (59–86°F).

ASSESSMENT

1. Note onset, location, clinical presentation. List precipitating factors/triggers.

2. Assess carefully, monitor recovery; severe oral candidiasis especially after XRT may include esophagus and require systemic therapy as opposed to topical applications.

CLIENT/FAMILY TEACHING

1. Review method and technique for administration. Use as directed for amount of time designated to ensure desired results; usually 2 days after symptoms disappear to prevent reinfection. Works best if it is taken at the same time every day.

2. Do not mix oral suspension in foods; inactivates drug. Remove food from mouth. Drop 1 mL of oral suspension in each side of mouth or apply with a swab to treat oral moniliasis. Swish around and keep in the mouth as long as possible before swallowing.

3. For pediatric use, 250,000 units of cherry flavor nystatin has been frozen in the form of popsicles. If unavailable may swab suspension on oral mucosa.

4. Do not use mouthwash with oral candidiasis; may alter normal flora and promote infections. Ensure properly fitting dentures and good oral hygiene to promote healing/prevention. Report increased irritation of oral cavity; drug may need to be stopped/evaluated.

5. Vaginal tablets may be taken by mouth for candidiasis. Suck on these as a lozenge and do not chew or swallow (for prolonged contact with oral mucosa).

6. Insert vaginal tablets high in vagina with applicator. Continue using vaginal tablets even when menstruating; continue for 2 weeks. Avoid tampons.

7. Continue vaginal tablets in gravid client for 3–6 weeks before term to reduce incidence of thrush in the newborn.

8. Stop and report if vaginal tablets cause irritation, redness, or swelling. May stain; sanitary pads may help protect clothing and linens. Regular hygiene and wipe perineal area from front to back.

9. Apply cream or ointment to mycotic lesions with a swab or wear gloves to avoid direct contact with hands; contact dermatitis may ensue.

10. To prevent reinfection, avoid intercourse during therapy or use condoms. Advise partner to seek treatment if symptomatic. Report lack of response, worsening of symptoms, or adverse side effects.

OUTCOMES/EVALUATE

• Negative culture results
• Improvement in skin and mucous membrane irritation/lesions with less discomfort and itching

Ofloxacin

(oh-**FLOX**-ah-sin)

CLASSIFICATION(S):
Antibiotic, fluoroquinolone
PREGNANCY CATEGORY: C
Rx: Floxin, Floxin Otic, Ocuflox.
✽**Rx:** Apo-Oflox.

SEE ALSO *ANTI-INFECTIVE DRUGS AND FLUOROQUINOLONES.*

USES

Systemic: (1) Pneumonia or acute bacterial exacerbations of chronic bronchitis or community-acquired pneumonia due to *Haemophilus influenzae* or *Streptococcus pneumoniae.* Not a drug of first choice in the treatment of presumed or confirmed pneumococcal pneumonia. Not effective for syphilis. (2) Acute, uncomplicated urethral and cervical gonorrhea due to *Neisseria gonorrhoeae;* nongonococcal urethritis, and cervicitis due to *Chlamydia trachomatis.* Mixed infections of the urethra and cervix due to *N. gonorrhoeae* and *C. trachomatis.* (3) Mild to moderate skin and skin structure infections due to *Staphylococcus aureus, Streptococcus pyogenes,* or *Proteus mirabilis.* (4) Uncomplicated cystitis due to *Citrobacter diversus, Enterobacter aerogenes, Escherichia coli, Klebsiella pneumoniae, Proteus mirabilis,* or *Pseudomonas aeruginosa.* (5) Complicated UTIs due to *E. coli, K. pneumoniae, P. mirabilis, C. diversus,* or *P. aeruginosa.* (6) Prostatitis due to *E. coli.* (7) Monotherapy for PID due to *C. trachomatis* or *N. gonorrhoeae.* (8) Tuberculosis in adults.

Ophthalmic: (1) Treatment of conjunctivitis caused by *S. aureus, Staphylococcus epidermidis, S. pneumoniae, Enterobacter cloacae, H. influenzae, P. mirabilis,* and *P. aeruginosa.* (2) Corneal ulcers caused by *S. aureus, S. epidermidis, S. pneumoniae, P. aeruginosa,* and *S. marcescens.*

Otic: (1) Otitis externa due to *S. au-reus, E. coli,* and *P. aeruginosa* in clients six months of age and older. (2) Acute otitis media with tympanostomy tubes due to *S. aureus, S. pneumoniae, H. influenzae, Moraxella catarrhalis,* and *P. aeruginosa* (from age one and older). (3) Chronic suppurative otitis media due to *S. aureus, P. mirabilis,* and *P. aeruginosa* in in those 12 years and older who have perforated tympanic membranes.

ACTION/KINETICS

Action

Effective against a wide range of gram-positive and gram-negative aerobic and anaerobic bacteria. Penicillinase has no effect on the activity of ofloxacin.

Pharmacokinetics

Widely distributed to body fluids. **Maximum serum levels:** 1–2 hr. **t½, first phase:** 5–7 hr; **second phase:** 20–25 hr. **Peak serum levels at steady state, after PO doses:** 1.5 mcg/mL after 200-mg doses, 2.4 mcg/mL after 300-mg doses, and 2.9 mcg/mL after 400-mg doses. Between 70% and 80% is excreted unchanged in the urine.

CONTRAINDICATIONS

Hypersensitivity to quinolone antibacterial agents. Use during lactation. Use for syphilis (ineffective). Ophthalmic use in dendritic keratitis, vaccinia, varicella, mycobacterial infections of the eye, fungal diseases of the eye, and with steroid combinations after uncomplicated removal of a corneal foreign body.

SPECIAL CONCERNS

Safety and effectiveness of the systemic forms have not been established in children, adolescents under the age of 18 years, pregnant women, and lactating women. Safety and effectiveness of the ophthalmic form have not been established in children less than 1 year of age. Use with caution in clients with known or suspected CNS disorders such as severe cerebral atherosclerosis, epilepsy, or factors that predispose to seizures.

Bold Italic = life threatening side effect   ■ = black box warning   ✽ = Available in Canada

SIDE EFFECTS
Most Common
After systemic use: N&V, abdominal pain/discomfort, diarrhea, dry/painful mouth, constipation, flatulence, headache, dizziness, fatigue/malaise, depression, insomnia, rash, pruritus, fever, vaginitis, visual disturbances.

After ophthalmic use: Transient irritation/burning/stinging, itching, inflammation.

After otic use: Pruritus, application site reaction, dizziness, earache, vertigo.

See *Fluoroquinolones* for a complete list of possible side effects. **GI:** N&V, diarrhea, abdominal pain/discomfort, dry/painful mouth, dyspepsia, flatulence, constipation, flatulence, pseudomembranous colitis, dysgeusia, decreased appetite. **CNS:** Headache, dizziness, fatigue, malaise, somnolence, depression, insomnia, seizures, sleep disorders, nervousness, anxiety, cognitive change, dream abnormality, euphoria, hallucinations, vertigo. **CV:** Chest pain, edema, hypertension, palpitations, vasodilation. **Hypersensitivity reactions:** Dyspnea, *anaphylaxis*. **GU:** External genital pruritus in women, vaginitis, vaginal discharge; burning, irritation, pain, and rash of the female genitalia; glucosuria, proteinuria, hematuria, pyuria, dysmenorrhea, menorrhagia, metrorrhagia, urinary frequency or pain. **Respiratory:** Cough, rhinorrhea. **Dermatologic:** Diaphoresis, vasculitis, photosensitivity, rash, pruritus. **Hematologic:** Leukocytosis, lymphocytopenia, eosinophilia. **Musculoskeletal:** Asthenia, extremity pain, arthralgia, myalgia, possibility of osteochondrosis. **Miscellaneous:** Fever, chills, malaise, syncope, hyperglycemia or hypoglycemia, whole body pain, thirst, weight loss, photophobia, trunk pain, paresthesia, visual disturbances, hypersensitivity, hearing loss, superinfection.

After ophthalmic use: Visual disturbances, transient ocular burning or discomfort, stinging, redness, itching, photophobia, tearing, and dryness.

After otic use: Pruritus, application site reaction, dizziness, earache, vertigo, taste perversion, paresthesia, rash, diarrhea, otorrhagia, dry mouth, headache, tinnitus, fever, N&V.

HOW SUPPLIED
Ophthalmic Solution: 0.3% (3 mg/mL); *Otic Solution:* 0.3% (3 mg/mL); *Tablets:* 200 mg, 300 mg, 400 mg.

DOSAGE
- **TABLETS**

  Pneumonia, exacerbation of chronic bronchitis.

400 mg q 12 hr for 10 days.

Acute uncomplicated urethral or cervical gonorrhea.

One 400-mg dose. The Centers for Disease Control also recommend adding doxycycline or azithromycin.

Cervicitis/urethritis due to C. trachomatis *or* N. gonorrhoeae.

300 mg q 12 hr for 7 days.

Mild to moderate skin and skin structure infections.

400 mg q 12 hr for 10 days.

Uncomplicated cystitis due to E. coli *or* K. pneumoniae.

200 mg q 12 hr for 3 days.

Uncomplicated cystitis due to other organisms.

200 mg q 12 hr for 7 days.

Complicated UTIs.

200 mg q 12 hr for 10 days.

Prostatitis due to E. coli.

300 mg q 12 hr for 6 weeks.

Chlamydia.

300 mg PO twice a day for 7 days.

Epididymitis.

300 mg PO twice a day for 10 days.

PID, outpatient.

400 mg PO twice a day for 14 days plus metronidazole.

Tuberculosis.

Adults: 600–800 (maximum) mg/day. *NOTE:* The dose should be adjusted in clients with a C_{CR} of 50 mL/min or less. If the C_{CR} is 10–50 mL/min, the dosage interval should be q 24 hr, and if C_{CR} is <10 mL/min, the dose should be half the recommended dose given q 24 hr.

- **OPHTHALMIC SOLUTION, (0.3%)**

  Conjunctivitis.

Initial: 1–2 gtt in the affected eye(s) q 2–4 hr for the first 2 days; **then,** 1–2 gtt 4 times per day for 7 additional days.

Bacterial corneal ulcer.

1–2 gtt q 30 min while awake. Awaken at about 4 and 6 hr after retiring and instill 1–2 gtt. **Then,** instill 1–2 gtt hourly while awake for days 3 through 7–9; for days 7–9 through treatment completion, instill 1–2 gtt 4 times per day.

• OTIC SOLUTION (0.3%)

Otitis externa.

Adults and children over 13 years: 0.5 mL (10 drops) of the 0.3% solution instilled once daily for 7 days. **Children, six months to 13 years:** 0.25 mL (5 drops) of the 0.3% solution instilled once daily for 7 days.

Acute otitis media in children with tympanostomy tubes.

Children 1–12 years: 0.25 mL (5 drops) in the affected ear twice a day for 10 days.

Chronic suppurative otitis media with perforated tympanic membranes.

Children, 12 years and older: 0.5 mL (10 drops) twice a day for 14 days.

NURSING CONSIDERATIONS

℗ Do not confuse Ocuflox with Ocufen (an ophthalmic NSAID).

ADMINISTRATION/STORAGE

1. Do not take with food.
2. Do not exceed a daily PO dose of 400 mg in those with a Child-Pugh score of 10-15.
3. Do not inject the ophthalmic solution subconjunctivally and do not introduce directly into the anterior chamber of the eye.
4. Do not confuse the ophthalmic and otic dosage forms; they are not interchangeable.
5. Store tablets in tightly closed containers at a temperature <30°C (86°F). Store otic solution from 15–30°C (59–86°F); protect from light.

ASSESSMENT

1. Note reasons for therapy, characteristics of S&S, any sensitivity to quinolone derivatives.
2. Monitor CBC, cultures, renal and LFTs; reduce dose with renal dysfunction. Review other prescribed agents; probenecid may block renal tubular excretion.

3. Assess for any CNS disorders. Report tremors, restlessness, confusion, hallucinations; may need to stop therapy.

CLIENT/FAMILY TEACHING

1. Do not take with food. Take oral form 1 hr before or 3 hr after meals. Drink 2–3 L/day of fluids to assist in drug elimination.
2. Avoid vitamins, iron or mineral combinations, Al- or Mg-based antacids 2 hr before and 2 hr after ingestion of ofloxacin.
3. Do not perform activities that require mental alertness until drug effects realized; may cause drowsiness and lightheadedness.
4. Wash hands before and after use. Avoid contamination of the eye or ear applicator tip with material from the eye, ear, or fingers. Do not confuse eye and ear dosage forms; not interchangeable.
5. Before using, warm ear drops by rolling the bottle in hands; instillation of cold drops may cause dizziness.
6. When used in the ear, lie with the affected ear upward. Instill drops and maintain this position for 5 min to ensure penetration of the drops into the ear canal. If ordered, repeat for the opposite ear.
7. May experience burning, stinging, itching, or tearing after eye use; should subside.
8. Side effects include N&V and diarrhea; report adverse effects, tendon pain, or lack or response.
9. Avoid direct sunlight; photosensitivity reaction may occur. If exposed, wear sunglasses, protective clothing, and sunscreen.
10. Those with diabetes should monitor sugars closely as extreme variations may occur. Keep all F/U appointments to eval. response to therapy; report adverse side effects.

OUTCOMES/EVALUATE

Negative culture reports; symptomatic improvement

Bold Italic = life threatening side effect   ■ = black box warning   ✦ = Available in Canada

Olanzapine ■ Ⓒ📷
(oh-**LAN**-zah-peen)

CLASSIFICATION(S):
Antipsychotic
PREGNANCY CATEGORY: C
Rx: Zyprexa, Zyprexa IntraMuscular, Zyprexa Zydis.

USES

PO: (1) Short- and long-term management (including maintenance of treatment response) of schizophrenia. (2) As monotherapy to treat acute mixed, or manic episodes associated with bipolar I disorder and for maintenance monotherapy of bipolar disorder. (3) In combination with lithium or valproate for the short-term treatment of acute mixed or manic episodes associated with bipolar I disorder.

IM: Agitation associated with schizophrenia and bipolar I mania.

Investigational: Dementia related to Alzheimer's disease.

ACTION/KINETICS

Action

A thienobenzodiazepine antipsychotic believed to act by antagonizing dopamine D_{1-4} and serotonin ($5HT_2$) receptors. Also binds to muscarinic, histamine H_1, and alpha$_1$-adrenergic receptors, which can explain many of the side effects. Some effect on the QTc interval may result in sudden cardiac death and torsades de pointes. Moderate incidence of sedation, anticholinergic effects, and orthostatic hypotension. High incidence of weight gain.

Pharmacokinetics

Well absorbed from the GI tract. **Peak plasma levels:** 6 hr after PO dosing. Undergoes significant first-pass metabolism with about 40% metabolized before it reaches the systemic circulation; about 60% bioavailable. Food does not affect the rate or extent of absorption. Metabolized in the liver through glucuronidation and oxidation by CYP1A2 and CYP2D6. **t½:** 21–54 hr. Unchanged drug and metabolites are excreted through both the urine and feces. **Plasma protein binding:** About 93%.

CONTRAINDICATIONS

Lactation. IV or SC use of the parenteral product.

SPECIAL CONCERNS

■ Elderly clients with dementia-related psychosis treated with atypical antipsychotic drugs are at an increased risk of death compared with placebo. Analyses of placebo-controlled trials (modal duration of 10 weeks) in these clients revealed a risk of death in the drug-treated clients between 1.6–1.7 times that seen in placebo-treated clients. Over the course of a typical 10-week controlled trial, the rate of death in drug-treated clients was about 4.5%, compared with a rate of about 2.6% in the placebo group. Although the causes of death were varied, most of the deaths appeared to be either cardiovascular (e.g., heart failure, sudden death) or infectious (e.g., pneumonia) in nature. Olanzapine is not approved for the treatment of clients with dementia-related psychosis.■ Use with caution in geriatric clients, as the drug may be excreted more slowly in this population. Use with caution in impaired hepatic function and in those where there is a chance of increased core body temperature (e.g., strenuous exercise, exposure to extreme heat, concomitant anticholinergic drug administration, dehydration). Due to anticholinergic side effects, use with caution in clients with significant prostatic hypertrophy, narrow-angle glaucoma, or a history of paralytic ileus. Maximal dosing of IM olanzapine (e.g., 3 doses of 10 mg given 2 to 4 hr apart) may be associated with significant orthostatic hypotension. There is an increased risk of hyperglycemia and diabetes. Safety and efficacy have not been determined in children less than 18 years of age.

SIDE EFFECTS

Most Common

Asthenia, dizziness, drowsiness/sedation/somnolence, constipation, dry mouth, dyspepsia, weight gain, increased cough, hypotension.

O

Neuroleptic malignant syndrome: Hyperpyrexia, muscle rigidity, altered mental status, irregular pulse/BP, tachycardia, diaphoresis, cardiac dysrhythmia, rhabdomyolysis, *acute renal failure, death*. **GI:** Dysphagia, constipation, dry mouth, dyspepsia, increased appetite/salivation, N&V, thirst, aphthous stomatitis, eructation, esophagitis, rectal incontinence, flatulence, gastritis, gastroenteritis, gingivitis, glossitis, hepatitis, melena, mouth ulceration, oral moniliasis, periodontal abscess, *rectal hemorrhage*, tongue edema. **CNS:** Tardive dyskinesia, seizures, somnolence, drowsiness, asthenia, agitation, insomnia, nervousness, hostility, dizziness, anxiety, personality disorder, akathisia, hypertonia, tremor, amnesia, impaired articulation, euphoria, stuttering, *suicide*, abnormal gait, alcohol misuse, antisocial reaction, ataxia, CNS stimulation, coma, delirium, depersonalization, hypesthesia, hypotonia, incoordination, decreased libido, obsessive-compulsive symptoms, phobias, somatization, stimulant misuse, stupor, vertigo, withdrawal syndrome. **CV:** Tachycardia, orthostatic/postural hypotension, *CVA, hemorrhage, heart arrest*, migraine, palpitation, vasodilation, ventricular extrasystoles. **Body as a whole:** Headache, fever, abdominal/chest pain, neck rigidity, intentional injury, flu syndrome, chills, facial edema, hangover effect, malaise, moniliasis, neck/pelvic pain, photosensitivity. **Respiratory:** Rhinitis, increased cough, pharyngitis, dyspnea, apnea, asthma, epistaxis, hemoptysis, hyperventilation, voice alteration. **GU:** PMS, hematuria, metrorrhagia, urinary incontinence, UTI, abnormal ejaculation, priapism, amenorrhea, breast pain, cystitis, decreased/increased menstruation, dysuria, female lactation, impotence, menorrhagia, polyuria, pyuria, urinary retention/frequency, impaired urination, enlarged uterine fibroids. **Hematologic:** Leukocytosis, lymphadenopathy, thrombocytopenia. **Metabolic/nutritional:** Weight gain/loss, peripheral/lower extremity edema, dehydration, hypo/hyperglycemia, hypo/hyperkalemia, hyperuricemia, hypona-tremia, ketosis, water intoxication. **Musculoskeletal:** Joint/extremity pain, twitching, arthritis, back/hip pain, bursitis, leg cramps, myasthenia, rheumatoid arthritis. **Dermatologic:** Vesiculobullous rash, alopecia, contact dermatitis, dry skin, eczema, hirsutism, seborrhea, skin ulcer, urticaria. **Ophthalmic:** Amblyopia, blepharitis, corneal lesion, cataract, diplopia, dry eyes, eye hemorrhage, eye inflammation/pain, ocular muscle abnormality. **Otic:** Deafness, ear pain, tinnitus. **Miscellaneous:** DM, goiter, cyanosis, taste perversion, sleepwalking (rare).

LABORATORY TEST CONSIDERATIONS ↑ ALT, AST, GGT, alkaline phosphatase, serum prolactin, eosinophils, CPK. Hyperprolactinemia.

OD **OVERDOSE MANAGEMENT**
Symptoms: Drowsiness, slurred speech. Possible obtundation, seizures, dystonic reaction of the head and neck. CV symptoms, arrhythmias. *Treatment:* Establish and maintain an airway and ensure adequate oxygenation and ventilation. Gastric lavage followed by activated charcoal and a laxative can be considered, although dystonic reaction may cause aspiration with induced emesis. Begin CV monitoring immediately with continuous ECG monitoring to detect possible arrhythmias. Hypotension and circulatory collapse are treated with IV fluids or sympathomimetic agents. Do not use epinephrine, dopamine, or other sympathomimetics with beta-agonist activity, as beta stimulation may worsen hypotension.

DRUG INTERACTIONS
Antihypertensive agents / ↑ Antihypertensive effect
Carbamazepine / ↑ Olanzapine clearance R/T ↑ metabolism
CNS depressants / ↑ CNS depressant effect
Divalproex / ↑ Hepatic enzyme levels to a greater degree than either drug used alone
Fluoxetine / ↑ Olanzapine peak levels
Fluvoxamine / ↑ Olanzapine plasma levels R/T inhibition of CYP1A2
Levodopa and Dopamine agonists / May antagonize the effects of levodopa and

---

Bold Italic = life threatening side effect   ■ = black box warning   ✦ = Available in Canada

dopamine agonists
Probenecid / ↑ Olanzapine rate of absorption, AUC, and peak plasma level
Ritonavir / ↑ Olanzapine oral clearance and ↓ systemic exposure R/T ↑ metabolism
H *St. John's wort* / Possible ↓ olanzapine plasma levels R/T ↑ metabolism
Smoking / ↓ Olanzapine effect R/T ↑ liver metabolism by CYP1A2

HOW SUPPLIED
Powder for Injection: 10 mg; *Tablets:* 2.5 mg, 5 mg, 7.5 mg, 10 mg, 15 mg, 20 mg; *Tablets, Oral Disintegrating:* 5 mg, 10 mg, 15 mg, 20 mg.

DOSAGE

• **TABLETS; TABLETS, ORAL DISINTEGRATING**
Schizophrenia.
Adults, initial: 5–10 mg once daily without regard to meals. Goal is 10 mg daily within several days of initiation. Adjust dosage, if needed, at 5 mg/day increments or decrements in intervals of not less than 1 week. Doses higher than 10 mg daily are recommended only after clinical assessment and should not be greater than 20 mg/day. The recommended initial dose is 5 mg in those who are debilitated, who have a predisposition to hypotensive reactions, who may have factors that cause a slower metabolism of olanzapine (e.g., nonsmoking female clients over 65 years of age), or who may be more sensitive to the drug. It is recommended that clients who respond to the drug be continued on it at the lowest possible dose to maintain remission with periodic evaluation to determine continued need for the drug.
Bipolar mania, monotherapy.
Initial: 10–15 mg/day without regard to meals. Adjust dose, if needed, at 5 mg increments in intervals not less than 24 hr, if needed. **Dose range:** 5–20 mg/day for short-term (3 to 4 weeks) use. The safety of doses above 20 mg/day has not been determined.
Maintenance: 5–20 mg/day, after reaching an effective dose for an average duration of 2 weeks. Periodically reevaluate in those taking the drug for extended periods.

Bipolar mania when combined with lithium or valproate.
Initial: 10 mg once daily without regard to meals; **then** 5–20 mg/day.
Behavioral symptoms in Alzheimer's disease.
10 mg/day.
• **IM ONLY**
Agitation associated with schizophrenia and bipolar I mania.
Usual recommended: 10 mg; a lower dose of 5 or 7.5 mg may be given when clinical factors warrant. If agitation warrants, additional IM doses up to 10 mg may be given (efficacy of repeated doses has not been evaluated systematically). Consider a dose of 5 mg/injection for geriatric clients or when other clinical factors indicate. Consider a dose of 2.5 mg/injection for those who otherwise might be debilitated, predisposed to hypotensive reactions, or more sensitive to olanzapine. Maximal dosing (e.g., three 10 mg doses given 2 to 4 hr apart) may cause significant orthostatic hypotension.

NURSING CONSIDERATIONS

Do not confuse Zyprexa with Zyrtec (an antihistamine) or Celexa (an antidepressant). Do not confuse olanzapine with olsalazine (an anti-inflammatory).

ADMINISTRATION/STORAGE
1. The safety of parenteral total daily doses greater than 30 mg, or 10 mg given more frequently than every 2 hr after the initial dose and 4 hr after the second dose have not been evaluated.
2. If ongoing olanzapine is indicated after IM therapy, PO olanzapine may be initiated at doses from 5–20 mg/day.
3. To prepare for IM use, dissolve the contents of the vial with 2.1 mL of sterile water for injection (results in a solution containing about 5 mg/mL olanzapine). The solution should be clear and yellow. Use within 1 hr after reconstitution and discard any unused portion. Do **not** give by IV or SC routes.
4. IM injection volumes: If the olanzapine dose is 10 mg, withdraw the total contents of the reconstituted drug; if the dose is 7.5 mg, withdraw 1.5 mL; if

---

🔳= see color insert   H = Herbal   IV = Intravenous   ℂ= sound alike drug the dose is 5 mg, withdraw 1 mL; and, if the dose is 2.5 mg, withdraw 0.5 mL.

5. Do not combine in a syringe with diazepam injection as a precipitation will occur. Also, do not use lorazepam injection to reconstitute olanzapine injection as this combination results in a delayed reconstitution time. Do not combine olanzapine injection with haloperidol injection because the resulting low pH will degrade olanzapine over time.

6. Protect tablets from light and moisture and store at a controlled room temperature of 20–25°C (68–77°F). Orally disintegrating tablets contain phenylalanine.

7. Protect the injection from light; do not freeze. Before reconstitution and up to 1 hr after reconstitution, store from 20–25°C (68–77°F). Discard any unused portion of reconstituted olanzapine.

ASSESSMENT

1. Note onset, duration, characteristics of S&S, presenting behaviors, reasons for therapy; list agents trialed and outcome.

2. Monitor VS, ECG, CBC, renal and LFTs. Temperature regulation may be impaired especially with strenuous exercise or if exposed to extreme heat. Assess carefully for dehydration especially in the elderly. Voiding before drug administration may decrease anticholinergic effects of urinary retention.

3. Assess for S&S of diabetes mellitus. If neuroleptic malignant syndrome occurs, stop therapy immediately. After prolonged use, monitor for tardive dyskinesia which may occur months or years after therapy and may persist for lifetime or disappear suddenly, despite stopping therapy.

CLIENT/FAMILY TEACHING

1. To take disintegrating tablets, peel back foil on blister; do not push tablet through foil. Using dry hands, remove from foil and place entire tablet in the mouth; will disintegrate with or without liquid in about 2 min.

2. Take only as directed; do not share medications; do not exceed prescribed dosage.

3. Avoid activities or situations where overheating may occur, e.g., strenuous exercise, hot baths. Heat exposure may impair ability to reduce core body temperatures.

4. Do not drive or perform activities that require mental alertness until drug effects realized; may experience drowsiness, trouble in thinking, trouble in controlling movements, or trouble in seeing clearly.

5. Avoid changing positions suddenly, especially from lying to standing position R/T low BP effects.

6. Avoid prolonged/excessive exposure to direct or artificial light.

7. Report any suicidal ideations, abnormal bleeding, sudden muscle pain/weakness, irregular heartbeat.

8. Avoid alcohol, CNS depressants or OTC agents.

9. Practice reliable birth control.

10. Report as scheduled for medication renewals, therapy sessions, and evaluation of drug effectiveness.

OUTCOMES/EVALUATE

Improved patterns of behavior with ↓ agitation, ↓ hostility, and fewer delusions.

Olmesartan medoxomil

(ohl-meh-SAR-tan)

CLASSIFICATION(S):

Antihypertensive agent–angiotensin II receptor antagonist

PREGNANCY CATEGORY: C

Rx: Benicar.

SEE ALSO ANGIOTENSIN II RECEPTOR ANTAGONISTS

USES

Hypertension, alone or in combination with other antihypertensives.

ACTION/KINETICS

Action

Selectively blocks the binding of angiotensin II to the AT_1 receptor in vascular smooth muscle, resulting in a decrease in BP. Angiotensin II is a pressor agent causing vasoconstriction, stimulation of

---

the synthesis of and release of aldosterone, cardiac stimulation, and renal reabsorption of sodium.

Pharmacokinetics
Rapid and complete conversion of olmesartan medoxomil to olmesartan occurs during absorption from the GI tract. Olmesartan itself is not further metabolized. Is about 26% bioavailable. **Peak plasma levels:** 1–2 hr. Food does not affect bioavailability. **Steady-state levels:** Within 3 to 5 days, with no drug accumulation following once-daily dosing. **t½, terminal:** 13 hr. Excreted through the urine (35%–50%) and feces (50%–65%). **Plasma protein binding:** More than 99%.

CONTRAINDICATIONS
Hypersensitivity to the drug or any component of the product. Lactation.

SPECIAL CONCERNS
■ Use of drugs during the second and third trimesters of pregnancy that act directly on the renin-angiotensin system can cause injury and even death to the developing fetus. When pregnancy is detected, discontinue as soon as possible.■ Safety and efficacy have not been determined in children.

SIDE EFFECTS
Most Common
Dizziness, diarrhea, GI upset, insomnia, headache.
CV: Hypotension, especially in volume- and/or salt-depleted clients, tachycardia. **GI:** Diarrhea, abdominal pain, dyspepsia, gastroenteritis, GI upset, nausea. **CNS:** Dizziness, headache, vertigo, insomnia. **GU:** Oliguria, progressive azotemia, hematuria, *acute renal failure (rare)*. **Musculoskeletal:** Arthralgia, arthritis, myalgia, skeletal pain. **Respiratory:** Bronchitis, pharyngitis, rhinitis, sinusitis, URTI. **Body as a whole:** Inflicted injury, flu-like symptoms, fatigue, pain, peripheral edema, rash. **Miscellaneous:** Back/chest pain, facial edema, angioedema.

LABORATORY TEST CONSIDERATIONS
↑ CPK. Slight ↓ H&H. Hyperglycemia, hypertriglyceridemia, hypercholesterolemia, hyperlipemia, hyperuricemia.

OD OVERDOSE MANAGEMENT
Symptoms: Hypotension, tachycardia. *Treatment:* If needed, supportive treatment for symptomatic hypotension.

HOW SUPPLIED
Tablets: 5 mg, 20 mg, 40 mg.

DOSAGE
• **TABLETS**
Hypertension.
Individualize dosage. **Initial:** 20 mg once daily when used as monotherapy in those not volume-depleted. After 2 weeks of therapy, if further reduction in BP is required, dose may be increased to 40 mg. Doses above 40 mg appear not to have a greater effect. Consider a lower starting dose, with close monitoring, in those who are volume- and salt-depleted (e.g., those treated with diuretics, especially clients with impaired renal function).

NURSING CONSIDERATIONS

℗ Do not confuse Benicar (olmesartan alone) with Benicar HCT (olmesartan combined with hydrochlorothiazide).

ADMINISTRATION/STORAGE
1. Twice-daily dosing has no advantage over once-daily dosing.
2. No initial dosage adjustment is recommended for the elderly or those with moderate to severe renal or hepatic dysfunction.
3. May be given with or without food.
4. If BP is not controlled with olmesartan alone, a diuretic or other antihypertensive drugs may be added.
5. Store from 20–25°C (68–77°F).

ASSESSMENT
1. Note disease onset, reasons for therapy, risk factors, all medical conditions, other agents trialed, outcome. List drugs prescribed to ensure none interact.
2. Monitor BP, hydration status, CBC, electrolytes, renal, LFTs; reduce dose with dysfunction/dehydration.

CLIENT/FAMILY TEACHING
1. May take with or without food and with other prescribed BP medications.
2. Change positions slowly and avoid dehydration to prevent sudden drop in BP and dizziness. Consume plenty of fluids to ensure adequate hydration.

3. Practice reliable contraception; report if pregnancy suspected- drug may cause fetal death.

4. Continue low-fat, low-sodium diet, regular exercise, weight loss, smoking and alcohol cessation, and stress weight reduction to regain BP control.

5. May experience headaches, altered glucose readings with diabetes, coughing, diarrhea, nausea, and joint aches; report if persistent.

6. Practice reliable contraception.

7. Keep all F/U appointments and log of BP readings for provider review.

OUTCOMES/EVALUATE

↓ BP

—— *COMBINATION DRUG* ——

Olmesartan medoxomil and Hydrochlorothiazide

(**ohl**-meh-**SAR**-tan, hy-droh-klor-oh-**THIGH**-ah-zyd)

CLASSIFICATION(S):
Antihypertensive combination drug
PREGNANCY CATEGORY: C (first trimester), **D** (second and third trimesters).
Rx: Benicar HCT.

SEE ALSO *OLMESARATN MEDOXOMIL* AND *HYDROCHLOROTHIAZIDE*.

USES
Treatment of hypertension. Not indicated for initial therapy; begin combination therapy only after a client has failed to achieve the desired effect with monotherapy.

CONTENT
Each Benicar HCT 20 mg/12.5 mg tablet contains: Olmesartan medoxomil, 20 mg (angiotensin II receptor antagonist) and Hydrochlorothiazide, 12.5 mg (thiazide diuretic). Each Benicar HCT 40 mg/ 12.5 mg tablet contains: Olmesartan medoxomil, 40 mg and Hydrochlorothiazide, 12.5 mg. Each Benicar HCT 40 mg/25 mg tablet contains: Olmesartan medoxomil, 40 mg and Hydrochlorothiazide, 25 mg.

ACTION/KINETICS
Action
Olmesartan selectively blocks the binding of angiotensin II to the AT_1 receptor in vascular smooth muscle, resulting in a decrease in BP. Angiotensin II is a pressor agent causing vasoconstriction, stimulation of the synthesis of and release of aldosterone, cardiac stimulation, and renal reabsorption of sodium. Hydrochlorothiazide promotes the excretion of sodium and chloride, and thus water, by the distal renal tubule. Also increases excretion of potassium and to a lesser extent bicarbonate. The antihypertensive activity is thought to be due to direct dilation of the arterioles, as well as to a reduction in the total fluid volume of the body and altered sodium balance.

Pharmacokinetics
Olmesartan. Absolute bioavailability is about 26%; food does not affect bioavailability. Olmesartan medoxomil is rapidly and completely bioactivated by ester hydrolysis to olmesartan during absorption from the GI tract. **Peak plasma levels:** 1–2 hr. **t½, elimination, terminal:** 13 hr. Steady state levels reached within 3–5 days; no accumulation in plasma occurs with once-daily dosing. Olmesartan is excreted in both the urine (35–50%) and feces (50–65%). **Hydrochlorothiazide. t½, plasma:** 5.6–14.8 hr. **Onset of diuresis:** 2 hr; **peak:** About 4 hr; **duration:** 6–12 hr. Not metabolized; eliminated rapidly by the kidney (61% within 24 hr). **Plasma protein binding:** Olmesartan: 99% bound to plasma proteins.

CONTRAINDICATIONS
Hypersensitivity to any component of the product. Clients with anuria or hypersensitivity to other sulfonamide-derived drugs. Use during lactation is not recommended.

SPECIAL CONCERNS
■ Use of drugs during the second and third trimesters of pregnancy that act directly on the renin-angiotensin system can cause injury and even death to the fetus. When pregnancy is detected,

---

Bold Italic = life threatening side effect   ■ = black box warning   ✦ = Available in Canada

discontinue as soon as possible.■ In clients who are volume- or salt-depleted, symptomatic hypotension may occur after beginning treatment with Benicar HCT. Use with caution in those with impaired hepatic function, progressive liver disease (minor alterations of fluid and electrolyte balance in these clients may precipitate hepatic coma) or severe renal disease. Hypersensitivity reactions to hydrochlorothiazide may occur in those with or without a history of allergy or bronchial asthma (but are more likely in those with such a history). Safety and efficacy have not been established in children.

SIDE EFFECTS
Most Common
Dizziness, URTI, nausea, hyperuricemia, headache, UTI.
See *Olmesartan medoxomil* and *Diuretics, Thiazides* for a complete list of possible side effects. **GU:** Oliguria and/or progressive azotemia with acute renal failure and/or death (rare). **Miscellaneous:** Thiazides may cause exacerbation or activation of systemic lupus erythematosus.

LABORATORY TEST CONSIDERATIONS
↑ Cholesterol, triglycerides, creatinine, BUN. ↓ H&H. ↓ Urinary calcium and ↑ serum calcium. Possible hypokalemia, hyponatremia, hypochloremic alkalosis, hyperuricemia, hypomagnesemia.

OD **OVERDOSE MANAGEMENT**
Symptoms: Olmesartan: Hypotension, tachycardia, bradycardia (if vagal stimulation occurs). Hydrochlorothiazide: Electrolyte depletion and dehydration. *Treatment:* Institute supportive treatment.

DRUG INTERACTIONS
See Drug Interactions for *Olmesartan medoxomil* and *Diuretics, Thiazides*. *NOTE:* Olmesartan is not metabolized by the cytochrome P450 system and has no effects on P450 enzymes; thus, interactions with drugs that inhibit, induce, or are metabolized by those enzymes are not expected.

HOW SUPPLIED
See Content.

DOSAGE
• TABLETS

Hypertension.
Once daily dosing with either 20 mg/12.5 mg, 40 mg/12.5 mg, or 40 mg/25 mg. Individualize dosage based on BP response. Titrate in 2–4 week intervals.

NURSING CONSIDERATIONS
ℂ Do not confuse Benicar (olmesartán alone) with Benicar HCT (olmesartan and hydrochlorothiazide).

ADMINISTRATION/STORAGE
1. In diabetics, the dosage of insulin or oral hypoglycemics may need to be increased due to hyperglycemia.
2. For those with possible depletion of intravascular volume, initiate Benicar HCT under close medical supervision. Consider use of a lower starting dose.
3. No initial dosage adjustment is recommended for elderly clients, for those with marked renal impairment (C_{CR} <40 mL/min), or with moderate to marked hepatic dysfunction.

ASSESSMENT
1. Note reasons for therapy, disease onset, other agents trialed, outcome.
2. List medications prescribed to ensure none interact.
3. Assess for any drug allergies.
4. Monitor electrolytes, VS, renal, LFTs; may need to reduce dose with dysfunction.

CLIENT/FAMILY TEACHING
1. May take on an empty stomach or with food.
2. Can cause dizziness or drowsiness, avoid activities that require mental alertness until drugs effects realized.
3. Take even though you may feel tired or run down. Avoid alcohol and OTC drugs without provider approval.
4. Consume plenty of fluids to ensure well hydrated. Avoid strenuous exercise in hot weather or situations that may predispose to high fluid loss.
5. May experience abdominal/stomach pain, cough, diarrhea, dizziness, headache, unusual tiredness; report if persistent or bothersome.
6. Practice reliable contraception. If pregnancy suspected or desired, notify provider.

O

7. Keep all F/U appointments to assess drug response. Bring BP log for provider review.
OUTCOMES/EVALUATE
Desired BP control

Olopatadine hydrochloride
(oh-loh-**PAT**-uh-deen)

CLASSIFICATION(S):
Antihistamine, ophthalmic
PREGNANCY CATEGORY: C
Rx: Pataday, Patanol.

SEE ALSO *ANTIHISTAMINES (H₁ BLOCKERS).*

USES
Temporary prevention of itching of the eye due to allergic conjunctivitis.
ACTION/KINETICS
Action
Selective histamine H_1 receptor antagonist that inhibits histamine release from mast cells.
Pharmacokinetics
Little is absorbed into the systemic circulation. $t\frac{1}{2}$, **plasma:** About 3 hr. Excreted through the urine.
CONTRAINDICATIONS
Not to be injected. Not to be instilled while the client is wearing contact lenses.
SPECIAL CONCERNS
Use with caution during lactation. Safety and efficacy have not been determined for children less than 3 years of age.
SIDE EFFECTS
Most Common
Headaches, burning/stinging of the eye.
Ophthalmic: Burning or stinging, dry eye, foreign body sensation, hyperemia, keratitis, lid edema, pruritus, blurred vision. **Nose/throat:** Pharyngitis, rhinitis, sinusitis. **Miscellaneous:** Headache, asthenia, cold syndrome, taste perversion, hypersensitivity, nausea.
HOW SUPPLIED
Solution: 0.1%, 0.2%.
DOSAGE
• **SOLUTION (0.1%)**

Allergic conjunctivitis.
Adults and children over 3 years of age: 1–2 drops in each affected eye twice a day at an interval of 6–8 hr.
• **SOLUTION, 0.2%**
Allergic conjunctivitis.
1 gtt in each affected eye once a day.

NURSING CONSIDERATIONS
ADMINISTRATION/STORAGE
Store at 4–30°C (39–86°F).
ASSESSMENT
Document indications for therapy; note onset, duration, occurrence, and characteristics of symptoms. Identify triggers.
CLIENT/FAMILY TEACHING
1. Wash hands before and after administration; do not let the dropper tip touch the eyelids or surrounding areas to prevent contamination.
2. Burning and stinging, swelling, redness, and foreign body sensation may occur; report if persistent.
3. Remove contact lens before instilling eye drops.
4. Review potential triggers and how to avoid and reduce contact to prevent increased irritation. Report adverse effects or lack of response.
OUTCOMES/EVALUATE
Relief of allergic ocular manifestations.

Olsalazine sodium ©
(ohl-**SAL**-ah-zeen)

CLASSIFICATION(S):
Anti-inflammatory drug
PREGNANCY CATEGORY: C
Rx: Dipentum.

USES
Maintain remission of ulcerative colitis in clients who cannot take sulfasalazine.
ACTION/KINETICS
Action
A salicylate that is converted by bacteria in the colon to 5-PAS (5-para-aminosalicylate), which exerts an anti-inflammatory effect for the treatment of ulcerative colitis. 5-PAS is slowly absorbed resulting in a high concentration of

---

drug in the colon. The anti-inflammatory activity is likely due to inhibition of synthesis of prostaglandins in the colon.

Pharmacokinetics

After PO use the drug is only slightly absorbed (2.4%) into systemic circulation where it has a short half-life (<1 hr). **Plasma protein binding:** More than 99%.

CONTRAINDICATIONS

Hypersensitivity to salicylates.

SPECIAL CONCERNS

Use with caution during lactation. Safety and efficacy have not been established in children. May cause worsening of symptoms of colitis.

SIDE EFFECTS

Most Common

Diarrhea, pain/cramps, headache, nausea, dyspepsia, rash.

GI: Diarrhea, pain or cramps, nausea, dry mouth, dyspepsia, bloating, anorexia, vomiting, stomatitis. **CNS:** Headache, drowsiness, lethargy, fatigue, dizziness, vertigo. **Ophthalmic:** Dry eyes, watery eyes, blurred vision. **Miscellaneous:** Arthralgia, rash, itching, upper respiratory tract infection. NOTE: The following symptoms have been reported on withdrawal of therapy: Diarrhea, nausea, abdominal pain, rash, itching, headache, heartburn, insomnia, anorexia, dizziness, light-headedness, rectal bleeding, depression.

LABORATORY TEST CONSIDERATIONS

↑ ALT, AST.

OD **OVERDOSE MANAGEMENT**

Symptoms: Diarrhea, decreased motor activity. *Treatment:* Treat symptoms.

HOW SUPPLIED

Capsules: 250 mg.

DOSAGE

- **CAPSULES**

  Maintain remission of ulcerative colitis.

Adults: Total of 1 gram/day in two divided doses.

NURSING CONSIDERATIONS

✅ Do not confuse olsalazine with olanzapine (an antipsychotic).

ASSESSMENT

1. Note reasons for therapy, type, onset, characteristics of S&S (stools). List

sensitivity to salicylates/intolerance to sulfasalazine, other agents trialed, outcome.

2. With renal disease, monitor urinalysis, BUN, creatinine. With chronic therapy, monitor CBC, renal function studies.

3. Review radiographic/endoscopic findings; assess abdomen.

CLIENT/FAMILY TEACHING

1. Drug works by reducing inflammation of the colon by possibly preventing the production of substances that cause inflammation.

2. Take with food and in evenly divided doses.

3. Report any persistent diarrhea, lethargy, pain, fatigue, fever, blood in the stools, or lack of desired response.

OUTCOMES/EVALUATE

Symptom remission with ulcerative colitis; ↓ mucus in stools ↓ abdominal pain

Omalizumab ■
(oh-mah-lye-**ZOO**-mab)

O

CLASSIFICATION(S):

Monoclonal antibody-antiasthmatic

PREGNANCY CATEGORY: B

Rx: Xolair.

USES

Moderate to severe persistent asthma in adults and adolescents 12 years and older who have a positive skin test or in vitro reactivity to a perennial aeroallergen with symptoms not adequately controlled with inhaled corticosteroids. Safety and efficacy have not been determined for other allergic conditions. *Investigational:* Seasonal allergic rhinitis.

ACTION/KINETICS

Action

Omalizumab is a recombinant monoclonal antibody that binds selectively to human IgE. Omalizumab inhibits binding of IgE to the high affinity IgE receptor on the surface of mast cells and basophils. Reduction in the surface-bound IgE on IgE receptor-bearing cells limits the degree of release of mediators of the allergic response. The drug also reduces the number of IgE receptors on basophils in atopic clients. After the drug was discontinued, the increase in total IgE and decrease in free IgE receptor levels were reversible but did not return to pretreatment levels for up to 1 year after discontinuing omalizumab.

Pharmacokinetics
About 62% of the drug is bioavailable but it is slowly absorbed; **peak serum levels:** 7–8 days. Drug is metabolized in the liver and excreted in the bile. **$t^{1/2}$, elimination:** 26 days.

CONTRAINDICATIONS
Severe hypersensitivity to omalizumab. Use to treat acute bronchospasm or status asthmaticus.

SPECIAL CONCERNS
■ Anaphylaxis, presenting as bronchospasm, hypotension, syncope, urticaria, and/or angioedema of the throat or tongue, has been reported to occur after administration of omalizumab. Anaphylaxis has occurred as early as after the first dose of omalizumab but also has occurred beyond 1 year after beginning regularly administered treatment. Because of the risk of anaphylaxis, closely observe clients for an appropriate period of time after omalizumab administration, and be prepared to manage anaphylaxis that can be life-threatening. Also inform clients of the signs and symptoms of anaphylaxis and instruct them to seek immediate medical care if symptoms occur.■ Use with caution during lactation. Safety and efficacy have not been determined in children younger than 12 years of age.

SIDE EFFECTS
Most Common
Injection site reactions, viral infections, URTI, headache, sore throat, pharyngitis, sinusitis.

Respiratory: URTI, sinusitis, pharyngitis, sore throat, cold symptoms. **CNS:** Dizziness, fatigue. **Dermatologic:** Pruritus, dermatitis, hair loss. **Musculoskeletal:** Arthralgia, leg/arm pain, fracture. **Injection Site:** Bruising, redness, warmth, burning, stinging, itching, hive formation, pain, indurations, mass, and inflammation. **Hematologic:** Severe thrombocytopenia. **Hypersensitivity:** Urticaria, dermatitis, pruritus, *anaphylaxis*. **Miscellaneous:** Leg/arm/ear pain, earache, viral infections, headache, cold symptoms, possible parasitic (helminth) infections. Most serious side effects include malignancies and *anaphylaxis*.

HOW SUPPLIED
Injection, Lyophilized Powder for Solution: 129.6 mg (delivers 75 mg/0.6 mL after reconstitution), 202.5 mg (delivers 150 mg/1.2 mL after reconstitution).

DOSAGE
• **SC**
Moderate to severe persistent asthma.
Adults and adolescents 12 years and older: 150–375 mg q 2–4 weeks. Doses and dosing frequency are determined by serum total immunoglobulin E (IgE) level (units/mL), measured before starting treatment and body weight (kg). See package insert for appropriate dose assignment.

NURSING CONSIDERATIONS
ADMINISTRATION/STORAGE
1. The injection may take 5–10 seconds to administer because solution is slightly viscous.
2. Doses of more than 150 mg are divided among more than 1 injection site; no more than 150 mg should be given in any one site.
3. Total IgE levels are elevated during treatment and remain elevated for up to 1 year after termination of therapy. Thus, retesting of IgE levels during treatment cannot be used as a guide for dose determinations. Base dose determinations after treatment interruptions lasting <1 year on serum IgE levels obtained at the initial dose determination.
4. Total serum IgE levels may be retested for dose determination if treatment with omalizumab has been interrupted for 1 year or more.
5. Adjust doses for significant changes in body weight.
6. Prepare omalizumab for SC use as follows:
• Use only sterile water for injection.

Bold Italic = life threatening side effect   ■ = black box warning   ♣ = Available in Canada

- Draw 1.4 mL sterile water for injection into a 3 mL syringe equipped with a 1 inch 18-gauge needle.
- Inject sterile water directly into product.
- Keeping vial upright, gently swirl vial for about 1 min to evenly wet powder. Do not shake.
- Gently swirl vial for 5–10 sec about every 5 min to dissolve any remaining solids. There should be no visible gel-like particles in the solution. Some vials may take longer than 20 min to dissolve completely. Do not use if contents do not dissolve completely by 40 min.
- Invert vial for 15 sec to allow the solution to drain toward the stopper. Using a new 3 mL syringe equipped with a 1 inch 18-gauge needle, insert needle into the inverted vial. Before removing needle from vial, pull plunger all the way back to the end of the syringe barrel in order to remove all of the solution from the inverted vial.
- Replace 18-gauge needle with a 25-gauge needle for SC injection.
- Expel air, large bubbles, and any excess solution to obtain the required 1.2 mL dose

7. A vial delivers 1.2 mL (150 mg) of omalizumab. For a 75 mg dose, draw up 0.6 mL into the syringe and discard the remaining product. For doses higher than 150 mg, use the following: Dose of 225 mg: Inject 1.8 mL (2 injections); dose of 300 mg: Inject 2.4 mL (2 injections); dose of 375 mg: Inject 3 mL (3 injections).

8. Store omalizumab under refrigeration from 2–8°C (36–46°F).

9. Omalizumab is for single use only as it contains no preservatives. Solution may be used SC within 8 hr following reconstitution when stored in the vial from 2–8°C (36–46°F) or within 4 hr of reconstitution when stored at room temperature. Protect reconstituted vials from direct sunlight.

10. Do not abruptly discontinue systemic or inhaled corticosteroids when starting omalizumab therapy. Perform decreases (may need to be done gradually) in corticosteroids under direct provider supervision.

ASSESSMENT

1. Note reasons for therapy, onset, clinical presentation, characteristics of S&S, other agents trialed, outcome.
2. Assess lungs; document PFTs, CXR, breath sounds.
3. Dose is determined by total IgE level (international units/mL) which is measured before therapy and by body weight (kg). Doses >150 mg should be divided and administered into different injection sites.

CLIENT/FAMILY TEACHING

1. Drug administered once every 2 to 4 weeks SC after dosage determined by wt and IgE level.
2. To self-administer, follow written guidelines after injection demonstration and practice. Solution is thick so may take 5 to 10 sec to administer. May experience bruising, burning/stinging, itching, redness, warmth, and induration at injection site. Usually occurs within 1 hr of injection and lasts less than 8 days; should decrease with repeated use.
3. Do not decrease dose or stop other systemic or inhaled antiasthmatics unless directed by provider.
4. Use peak flow meter to evaluate breathing patterns and to identify volumes to call for medication adjustment and for hospitalization. Identify triggers; practice avoidance.
5. Not for use with acute bronchospasms or acute asthma attack. Report lack of desired response and adverse side effects. Keep all F/U appointments.

OUTCOMES/EVALUATE

Improved breathing patterns; control of asthma

Omeprazole   © 📷

(oh-**MEH**-prah-zohl)

CLASSIFICATION(S):
Proton pump inhibitor
PREGNANCY CATEGORY: C
OTC: Prilosec OTC.

Rx: Prilosec.
✦Rx: Losec.

USES

Rx. (1) Short-term treatment of active duodenal ulcer. (2) With clarithromycin to treat duodenal ulcer associated with *H. pylori*. (3) Short-term (4–8 weeks) treatment of erosive esophagitis diagnosed by endoscopy. Maintain healing of erosive esophagitis. (4) Short-term (4–8 weeks) treatment of active benign gastric ulcer. (5) Long-term treatment of hypersecretory conditions (e.g., Zollinger-Ellison syndrome, multiple endocrine adenomas, systemic mastocytosis). (6) Treatment of heartburn and other symptoms associated with GERD. *Investigational:* GERD-related laryngitis. GERD in infants and children. In combination with amoxicillin/clarithromycin to eradicate *H. pylori* in children with *H. pylori*-induced gastritis. Improve pancreatic enzyme absorption in cystic fibrosis clients with intestinal malabsorption.

OTC. Frequent heartburn occurring 2 or more days/week. Not intended for immediate relief.

ACTION/KINETICS

Action

Thought to be a gastric pump inhibitor in that it blocks the final step of acid production by inhibiting the H^+/K^+ ATPase system at the secretory surface of the gastric parietal cell. Both basal and stimulated acid secretions are inhibited. Serum gastrin levels are increased during the first 1 or 2 weeks of therapy and are maintained at such levels during the course of therapy.

Pharmacokinetics

Because omeprazole is acid-labile, the product contains an enteric-coated granule formulation; however, absorption is rapid. Bioavailability is 30–40%. **Peak plasma levels:** 0.5–3.5 hr. **Onset:** Within 1 hr. **t½:** 0.5–1 hr. **Duration:** Up to 72 hr (due to prolonged binding of the drug to the parietal H^+/K^+ ATPase enzyme). Metabolized in the liver and inactive metabolites are excreted through the urine. Consider dosage adjustment in Asians. **Plasma protein binding:** About 95%.

CONTRAINDICATIONS

Lactation. Use as maintenance therapy for duodenal ulcer disease. OTC use in those who have trouble or pain swallowing food, are vomiting blood, or excreting bloody or black stools.

SPECIAL CONCERNS

Bioavailability may be increased in geriatric clients. Use with caution during lactation. Symptomatic effects with omeprazole do not preclude gastric malignancy. Safety and effectiveness have not been determined in children.

SIDE EFFECTS

Most Common

Headache, abdominal pain, diarrhea, N&V, URTI, dizziness, rash.

CNS: Headache, dizziness. Possibly, anxiety disorders, abnormal dreams, vertigo, insomnia, nervousness, apathy, paresthesia, somnolence, depression, aggression, hallucinations, hemifacial dysesthesia, tremors, confusion. **GI:** Diarrhea, N&V, abdominal pain/swelling, constipation, flatulence, anorexia, fecal discoloration, esophageal candidiasis, mucosal atrophy of the tongue, dry mouth, irritable colon, gastric fundic gland polyps, gastroduodenal carcinoids. **Hepatic:** *Pancreatitis.* Overt liver disease, including hepatocellular, cholestatic, or mixed hepatitis; *liver necrosis, hepatic failure,* hepatic encephalopathy. **CV:** Angina, chest pain, tachycardia, bradycardia, palpitation, peripheral edema, elevated BP. **Respiratory:** URTI, pharyngeal pain, bronchospasms, cough, epistaxis. **Dermatologic:** Rash, severe generalized skin reaction including *toxic epidermal necrolysis, Stevens-Johnson syndrome*; erythema multiforme, skin inflammation, urticaria, pruritus, alopecia, dry skin, hyperhidrosis. **GU:** UTI, acute interstitial nephritis, urinary frequency, hematuria, proteinuria, glycosuria, testicular pain, microscopic pyuria, gynecomastia. **Hematologic:** Pancytopenia, thrombocytopenia, anemia, leukocytosis, neutropenia, hemolytic anemia, *agranulocytosis.* **Musculoskeletal:** Asthenia, back pain, myalgia, joint/leg pain, muscle cramps,

---

Bold Italic = life threatening side effect   ■ = black box warning   ✦ = Available in Canada

muscle weakness. **Otic:** Anterior ischemic optic neuropathy, blurred vision, double vision, dry eye syndrome, ocular irritation, optic atrophy/neuritis. **Miscellaneous:** Rash, angioedema, fever, pain, gout, fatigue, malaise, weight gain, tinnitus, alteration in taste; allergic reactions, including **anaphylaxis** (rare), fever, pain, malaise. When used with clarithromycin the following *additional* side effects were noted: Tongue discoloration, rhinitis, pharyngitis, and flu syndrome. NOTE: Data are lacking on the effect of long-term hypochlorhydria and hypergastrinemia on the risk of developing tumors.

LABORATORY TEST CONSIDERATIONS

↑ ALT, AST, alkaline phosphatase, bilirubin, serum creatinine, GGTP. Hyponatremia, hypoglycemia.

OD **OVERDOSE MANAGEMENT**

Symptoms: Confusion, drowsiness, blurred vision, tachycardia, nausea, diaphoresis, flushing, headache, dry mouth. *Treatment:* Symptomatic and supportive. Omeprazole is not readily dialyzable.

DRUG INTERACTIONS

Ampicillin (esters) / Possible ↓ absorption of ampicillin esters R/T ↑ stomach pH

Calcium / Possible ↓ Fractional calcium absorption from calcium carbonate

Clarithromycin / Possible ↑ plasma levels of both drugs

Cyanocobalamin / ↓ Cyanocobalamin absorption R/T ↑ gastric pH

Diazepam / ↑ Diazepam plasma levels R/T ↓ rate of liver metabolism

Escitalopram / ↑ Escitalopram AUC and t½ R/T inhibition of metabolism

H *Ginkgo biloba* / ↑ Omeprazole metabolism by CYP2C19

Iron salts / Possible ↓ absorption of iron salts R/T ↑ stomach pH

Ketoconazole / Possible ↓ ketoconazole absorption R/T ↑ stomach pH

Phenytoin / ↑ Plasma phenytoin levels R/T ↓ rate of liver metabolism

Sucralfate / ↓ Omeprazole absorption; take 30 min before sucralfate

Tacrolimus / ↓ Tacrolimus dose/weight normalized trough levels in renal transplant clients

Tolterodine / ↑ Peak concentration of tolterodine R/T ↑ gastric pH due to omeprazole administration

Warfarin / Prolonged rate of warfarin elimination R/T ↓ rate of liver metabolism

HOW SUPPLIED

RX *Capsules, Delayed-Release (as omeprazole magnesium):* 10 mg, 20 mg, 40 mg.

OTC. *Tablets, Delayed-Release:* 20 mg.

DOSAGE

• **CAPSULES, DELAYED-RELEASE (RX)**

Active duodenal ulcer.

Adults, 20 mg/day for 4–8 weeks.

Erosive esophagitis.

Adults: 20 mg/day for 4–8 weeks. Maintenance of healing erosive esophagitis. 20 mg/day. Controlled studies do not exceed 1 year.

GERD without esophageal lesions.

Adults: 20 mg/day for up to 4 weeks. **Children:** For treatment of GERD or other acid-related disorders in children 2 years and older: Give 10 mg for clients weighing less than 20 kg and 20 mg for clients weighing 20 kg or more. Note: On a per kg basis, the doses of omeprazole needed to heal erosive esophagitis are greater for children than for adults.

GERD with erosive esophagitis.

20 mg/day for 4–8 weeks. In the occasional client not responding to 8 weeks of treatment, an additional 4 weeks of therapy may help. If there is a recurrence of erosive esophagitis or GERD, an additional 4–8 week course may be considered.

Treatment of H. pylori.

The following regimens may be used: **Triple Therapy:** Omeprazole, 20 mg, plus clarithromycin, 500 mg, plus amoxicillin, 1,000 mg, each given twice daily for 10 days. If an ulcer is present at the beginning of therapy, continue omeprazole, 20 mg once daily, for an additional 18 days. **Dual Therapy:** Omeprazole, 40 mg once daily plus clarithromycin, 500 mg, 3 times per day for 14 days. If an ulcer is present at the beginning of therapy, continue omeprazole, 20 mg daily, for an additional 14 days.

Pathologic hypersecretory conditions.

Adults, initial: 60 mg/day; then, dose individualized although doses up to 120 mg 3 times/day have been used. Daily doses greater than 80 mg should be divided. Continue treatment for as long as needed.

Gastric ulcers.

Adults: 40 mg once daily for 4–8 weeks.

• **TABLETS, DELAYED-RELEASE (OTC)**

Frequent heartburn, greater than 2 or more days/week.

20 mg tablet taken with a full glass of water once daily before the first meal of the day, every day, for 14 days. **Maximum daily dose:** 20 mg. Takes 1 to 4 days for the full effect. The 14-day course may be repeated q 4 months.

NURSING CONSIDERATIONS

Do not confuse Prilosec with Prozac (an antidepressant) or Prinivil (ACE inhibitor).

ADMINISTRATION/STORAGE

1. Efficacy for more than 8 weeks has not been determined. However, if a client does not respond to 8 weeks of therapy, an additional 4 weeks may help. If there is a recurrence of erosive or symptomatic GERD poorly responsive to usual treatment, an additional 4 to 8 weeks of therapy may be tried.

2. Consider dosage adjustment in Asian clients or in those with impaired hepatic function especially when used for maintaining clients with erosive esophagitis.

3. Can repeat OTC therapy once every 4 months.

4. Store capsules from 15–30°C (59–86°F) in a tight container protected from light and moisture. Store tablets from 20–25°C (68–77°F) protected from high heat, humidity, and moisture.

ASSESSMENT

1. List reasons for therapy, triggers, frequency, characteristics of S&S, other agents trialed.

2. Record abdominal assessments, radiographic/endoscopic findings, and *H. pylori* results.

3. Monitor U/A, CBC, and LFTs; adjust dosage with hepatic dysfunction.

4. Determine if pregnant.

CLIENT/FAMILY TEACHING

1. Take capsule at least 1 hr before eating and swallow whole; do not open, chew, or crush. Antacids can be administered with omeprazole.

2. For those who have difficulty swallowing capsules, add 1 tablespoon of applesauce to an empty bowl. Open omeprazole capsule and empty pellets onto applesauce. Mix pellets with the applesauce and swallow immediately. Do not heat or chew the applesauce and do not chew or crush the pellets. Do not store mixture for future use.

3. Take oral suspension on an empty stomach at least 1 hr before a meal. To prepare the oral suspension, empty the contents of a packet into a small cup containing 1 or 2 tablespoons of water. Do not use other liquids or foods. Stir well and drink immediately. Refill cup with water and drink.

4. Report any changes in urinary elimination, pain, discomfort or persistent diarrhea.

5. Avoid alcohol and OTC agents as well as foods known to cause GI upset/irritation.

6. Avoid activities that require mental alertness until drug effects realized; may cause dizziness.

7. Do not use OTC product for more than 14 days unless directed by provider.

8. For short-term use only, drug inhibits total gastric acid secretion. Side effects of prolonged therapy and suppression of acid secretion alter bacterial colonization and lead to hypochlorhydria and hypergastrinemia which may cause an increased risk for gastric tumors.

OUTCOMES/EVALUATE

Promotion of ulcer healing; relief of pain; ↓ gastric acid production

---

Bold Italic = life threatening side effect ■ = black box warning ✦ = Available in Canada

Ondansetron hydrochloride

(on-**DAN**-sih-tron)

CLASSIFICATION(S):
Antiemetic
PREGNANCY CATEGORY: B
Rx: Zofran, Zofran ODT.

USES

Oral: (1) Prevent N&V resulting from initial and repeated courses of cancer chemotherapy, including cisplatin, greater than 50 mg/m². (2) Prevent N&V associated with initial and repeat courses of moderately emetogenic cancer chemotherapy. (3) Prevent N&V associated with radiotherapy in clients receiving either total body irradiation, single high-dose fraction to the abdomen, or daily fractions to the abdomen. (4) Prevent posoperative N&V. Routine prophylaxis is not recommended if there is little chance N&V will occur postoperatively. (5) Postoperatively in clients in whom N&V must be avoided, even when the incidence of postoperative N&V is low. Use oral solution, oral disintegrating tablets, or tablets. *Investigational:* Reduce alcohol consumption/effects; treat vomiting associated with N-acetylcysteine use.

   Parenteral: (1) Prevent N&V associated with initial and repeat courses of emetogenic cancer chemotherapy, including high-dose cisplatin. Efficacy of the 32 mg single dose beyond 24 hr has not been determined. (2) Prevention of N&V postoperatively for those in whom nausea and/or vomiting must be avoided, even when the incidence of postoperative N&V is low. For those who do not receive prophylactic ondansetron injection and experience nausea and/or vomiting postoperatively, the injection may be given to prevent further episodes. *Investigational:* Prevent and/or treat opioid-induced pruritus; post-anesthetic shivering; treat radiation-induced N&V; reduction in alcohol consumption and/or alcohol intoxication.

ACTION/KINETICS

Action

Cytotoxic chemotherapy is thought to release serotonin from enterochromaffin cells of the small intestine. The released serotonin may stimulate the vagal afferent nerves through the 5-HT$_3$ receptors, thus stimulating the vomiting reflex. Ondansetron, a 5-HT$_3$ antagonist, blocks this effect of serotonin. Whether the drug acts centrally and/or peripherally to antagonize the effect of serotonin is not known.

Pharmacokinetics

Time to peak plasma levels, after PO: 1.7–2.1 hr. **t½, after IV use:** 3.5–4.7 hr; **after PO use:** 3.1–6.2 hr, depending on the age. A decrease in clearance and increase in half-life are observed in clients over 75 years of age, although no dosage adjustment is recommended. Clients less than 15 years of age show a shortened plasma half-life after IV use (2.4 hr). Significantly metabolized with 5% of a dose excreted unchanged in the urine.

SPECIAL CONCERNS

Use with caution during lactation. Safety and effectiveness in children 3 years of age and younger are not known.

SIDE EFFECTS

Most Common

Diarrhea, headache, dizziness, malaise/fatigue, constipation, bradycardia, hypotension, drowsiness/sedation, anxiety/agitation, gynecological disorder, urinary retention, hypoxia, pruritus, pyrexia, shivers.

GI: Diarrhea, constipation, xerostomia, abdominal pain. **CNS:** Headache, dizziness, drowsiness, sedation, malaise, fatigue, anxiety, agitation, extrapyramidal syndrome, ***clonic-tonic seizures***. **CV:** Tachycardia, chest pain, hypotension, ECG alterations, angina, bradycardia, syncope, vascular occlusive events. **Dermatologic:** Pain, redness, and burning at injection site; cold sensation, pruritus, paresthesia. **Hypersensitivity (rare):** ***Anaphylaxis, bronchospasm, shock***, SOB, hypotension, angioedema, urticaria. **Miscellaneous:** Rash, ***bronchospasm***, transient blurred vision, hypokalemia, weakness, fever, musculo-

O

skeletal pain, shivers, dysuria, postoperative carbon-dioxide-related pain, akathisia, acute dystonic reactions, gynecologic disorder, urinary retention, wound problem.

LABORATORY TEST CONSIDERATIONS
↑ AST, ALT.

DRUG INTERACTIONS
Rifampin ↓ ondansetron plasma levels R/T ↑ liver metabolism.

HOW SUPPLIED
Ondansetron (as hydrochloride dihydrate): *Injection:* 2 mg/mL, 4 mg/mL, 40 mg/20 mL (multiple dose), 32 mg/50 mL (premixed); *Oral Solution:* 4 mg/5 mL; *Tablets:* 4 mg, 8 mg, 16 mg, 24 mg. Ondansetron (as base): *Tablets, Orally Disintegrating:* 4 mg, 8 mg.

DOSAGE
• **IM; IV**
  Prevention of N&V due to chemotherapy.
Adults: A single 32 mg dose or three 0.15 mg/kg doses. A single 32 mg dose is infused over 15 min beginning 20 min prior to the start of emetogenic chemotherapy. For the 3-dose regimen, the first dose is infused over 15 min starting 30 min before the start of chemotherapy; the second and third doses are given 4 hr and 8 hr, respectively, after the first dose. **Children, 6 months–18 years:** Three 0.15 mg/kg doses. The first dose is infused over 15 min starting 30 min before the start of chemotherapy; the second and third doses are given 4 hr and 8 hr, respectively, after the first dose.
  Prevent postoperative N&V.
Adults: 4 mg IV undiluted over 2–5 min immediately before induction of anesthesia or postoperatively as needed. Alternatively, 4 mg undiluted may be given IM as a single injection. **Children, 1 month–12 years, less than 40 kg:** 0.1 mg/kg IV over 2–5 min, but not less than 30 seconds. **Children, 2 to 12 years weighing over 40 kg:** 4 mg IV over 2–5 min, but not less than 30 seconds. For children, give immediately prior to or following anesthesia induction, or postoperatively as needed.
• **ORAL SOLUTION; TABLETS; TABLETS, ORAL DISINTEGRATING**

  Prevent N&V associated with moderately emetogenic cancer chemotherapy.
Adults and children over 12 years of age: One 8 mg tablet or orally disintegrating tablet or 10 mL (equivalent to 8 mg ondansetron) oral solution twice a day. Give the first dose 30 min before treatment followed by a second 8-mg dose 8 hr after the first dose; **then,** 8 mg twice a day for 1–2 days after chemotherapy. **Children, 4–11 years:** One 4 mg tablet or orally disintegrating tablet or 5 mL (equivalent to 4 mg ondansetron) oral solution 3 times/day. The first dose is given 30 min before chemotherapy with subsequent doses 4 and 8 hr after the first dose. **Then,** 4 mg q 8 hr for 1–2 days after completion of chemotherapy.
  Prevent N&V associated with highly emetogenic cancer chemotherapy.
Adults: 24 mg once a day given 30 min before the start of single-day highly emetogenic chemotherapy, including cisplatin greater than or equal to 50 mg/m^2.
  Prevention of N&V associated with radiotherapy.
One-8 mg tablet or orally disintegrating tablet or 10 mL (equivalent to 8 mg ondansetron) oral solution 3 times per day. For total body irradiation give the above dose 1–2 hr before each fraction of radiotherapy administered each day.
  Prevention of N&V in single high-dose fraction radiotherapy to the abdomen.
One-8 mg tablet or orally disintegrating tablet of 10 mL (equivalent to 8 mg ondansetron) oral solution 1–2 hr before radiotherapy, with subsequent doses 8 hr after the first dose for each day radiotherapy is given.
  Prevention of postoperative N&V.
Adults: 16 mg given as a single dose of two-8 mg tablets or orally disintegrating tablets or 20 mL (equivalent to 16 mg ondansetron) 1 hr before induction of anesthesia. There is no experience giving ondansetron to children to prevent postoperative N&V.

NURSING CONSIDERATIONS

@ Do not confuse Zofran with Zoloft (an antidepressant), Zosyn (an antibiotic), or Zantac (an H₂ receptor blocker).

ADMINISTRATION/STORAGE

1. With impaired hepatic function, do not exceed 8 mg PO or 8 mg IV daily infused over 15 min, 30 min prior to starting chemotherapy.

2. Tablets may be used to prepare a liquid product with cherry syrup, Syrpalta, Ora Sweet, or Ora Sweet Sugar Free. The concentration is 4 mg/5 mL and is stable for 42 days at 4°C (39°F).

3. Suppositories can be made by adding pulverized tablets to a melted fatty acid base, mixing thoroughly, and pouring into suppository molds. They are stable for 30 or more days if stored in light-resistant containers under refrigeration.

4. Store tablets and orally disintegrating tablets from 2–30°C (36–86°F). Protect the 4 mg tablets from light. Store blisters in cartons. Store oral solution from 15–30°C (59–86°F) protected from light. Store upright in cartons.

IV 5. When used to prevent chemotherapy-induced N&V, dilute the 2 mg/mL injection in 50 mL of D5W or 0.9% NaCl injection and infuse over 15 min. The 32 mg premixed injection in 50 mL D5W requires no dilution.

6. Ondansetron injection, 2 mg/mL, requires no dilution for administration for postoperative N&V.

7. Do not use flexible plastic containers in series connections.

8. Inspect visually for particulate matter and discoloration before administration.

9. Do not mix the premixed solutions for which physical and chemical compatibility have not been established. In particular, this applies to alkaline solutions as a precipitate may form.

10. The diluted drug is stable at room temperature, with normal lighting, for 48 hr after dilution with 0.9% NaCl, D5W, D5W/0.9% NaCl, D5/0.45% NaCl, and 3% NaCl injection.

11. Store the premixed injection between 2–30°C (36–86°F). Protect from light. Avoid excessive heat; do not freeze.

ASSESSMENT

1. Note reasons for therapy, characteristics of S&S, agents trialed, outcome.

2. Assess for dehydration, electrolyte imbalance with diarrhea/N&V, monitor I&O, adjust dose as needed.

3. Monitor LFTs; adjust dosage with liver dysfunction.

CLIENT/FAMILY TEACHING

1. Drug is used to prevent N&V. It is to be given exactly as prescribed q 8 h RTC in order to ensure desired results. May be continued 1–2 days following radiation/chemotherapy to ensure prevention of N&V.

2. May cause drowsiness or dizziness. Do not perform activities that require mental alertness until drug effects realized. Using Ondansetron Solution alone, with certain other medicines, or with alcohol may lessen your ability to drive or perform other potentially dangerous tasks.

3. Report any rash, diarrhea, constipation, altered respirations (bronchospasms), or loss of response.

OUTCOMES/EVALUATE

• Prevention/control of chemotherapy-induced N&V

• Prophylaxis/relief of postoperative N&V

Oprelvekin ■
(Interleukin 11, IL-11)
(oh-**PREL**-veh-kin)

CLASSIFICATION(S):
Interleukin, human recombinant
PREGNANCY CATEGORY: C
Rx: Neumega.

USES

Prevention of severe thrombocytopenia and the need for platelet transfusions following myelosuppressive chemotherapy in adult clients with nonmyeloid malignancies who are at high risk

O

of severe thrombocytopenia. *Investigational:* Crohn's disease.

ACTION/KINETICS
Action
Produced by DNA recombinant technology. Interleukin 11 is a thrombopoietic growth factor that directly stimulates proliferation of hematopoietic stem cells and megakaryocyte progenitor cells and induces megakaryocyte maturation. This results in increased platelet production.
Pharmacokinetics
Absolute bioavailability is greater than 80%. **Peak serum levels:** 3.2 hr. **t½, terminal:** 6.9 hr. Metabolized and excreted through urine.

CONTRAINDICATIONS
Use following myeloablative chemotherapy. Lactation.

SPECIAL CONCERNS
■ Oprelvekin has caused allergic or hypersensitivity reactions, including anaphylaxis. Permanently discontinue administration of oprelvekin in any client who develops an allergic or hypersensitivity reaction.■ Use with caution in CHF or those who may be susceptible to developing CHF, and in those with history of heart failure who are well compensated and receiving appropriate medical therapy. Use with caution in those with history of atrial arrhythmia, in preexisting papilledema or with tumors involving CNS. Safety and efficacy have not been determined for chronic use or in children.

SIDE EFFECTS
Most Common
N&V, edema, neutropenic fever, mucositis, diarrhea, headache, dizziness, insomnia, dyspnea, rhinitis, tachycardia, increased cough, pharyngitis, rash, conjunctival injection, palpitations, atrial arrhythmias, pleural effusions.
Body as a whole: Edema, neutropenic fever, headache, fever, conjunctival infection, asthenia, chills, pain, infection, flu-like symptoms, fluid retention (may be serious and cause peripheral edema, dyspnea on exertion, pulmonary edema, capillary leak syndrome, atrial arrhythmias, and worsening of preexisting pleural effusions), hypersensitivity reactions (including **anaphylaxis**). **GI:** N&V, mucositis, diarrhea, oral moniliasis, abdominal pain, constipation, dyspepsia. **CV:** Tachycardia, vasodilation, palpitations, syncope, atrial fibrillation or flutter, *CHF, ventricular arrhythmias*, thrombocytosis, thrombotic events. **CNS:** Dizziness, headache, insomnia, nervousness. **Respiratory:** Dyspnea, rhinitis, increased cough, pharyngitis, pleural effusion, pneumonia, pulmonary edema, rhinitis. **Dermatologic:** Rash, alopecia. **Injection site reactions:** Dermatitis, pain, discoloration. **Ophthalmic:** Conjunctival injection, mild visual blurring (transient), blindness, optic neuropathy. **Miscellaneous:** Anorexia, ecchymosis, myalgia, bone pain, papilledema (more common in children 12 years and younger), renal failure.

In children: The following side effects occurred more commonly in children than in adults: Tachycardia, conjunctival injections, radiographic and echocardiographic evidence of cardiomegaly, and periosteal changes.

In cancer clients: The following side effects occurred more commonly in cancer clients: Amblyopia, dehydration, exfoliative dermatitis, eye hemorrhage, paresthesia, skin discoloration.

LABORATORY TEST CONSIDERATIONS
↑ Fibrinogen. ↓ H& H, RBCs, serum albumin, transferrin, gamma globulins (all due to expansion of plasma volume), calcium.

OD OVERDOSE MANAGEMENT
Symptoms: Increased incidence of cardiovascular events if doses greater than 50 mcg/kg are given. *Treatment:* Discontinue drug and observe for signs of toxicity.

HOW SUPPLIED
Powder for Injection, Lyophilized: 5 mg.

DOSAGE
- **SC INJECTION**
  Prevent thrombocytopenia.
Adults: 50 mcg/kg once daily SC either in the abdomen, thigh, or hip. The dose in adults with severe impaired renal function (C_{CR} <30 mL/min) is 25 mcg/kg. The mean AUC for children receiving 50 mcg/kg was about one-half

---

Bold Italic = life threatening side effect   ■ = black box warning   ♣ = Available in Canada

that achieved in healthy adults receiving 50 mcg/kg.

NURSING CONSIDERATIONS

ADMINISTRATION/STORAGE

1. Initiate dosing 6 to 24 hr after completion of chemotherapy. Continue until post-nadir platelet count is 50,000 cells/mcL or more. Duration of dosing is usually 10 to 21 days; beyond 21 days is not recommended.

2. Discontinue treatment 2 or more days before starting next planned cycle of chemotherapy.

3. Reconstitute with 1 mL of sterile water for injection without preservative. Direct water at side of vial and swirl gently. Avoid excessive or vigorous shaking.

4. Reconstituted solution contains 5 mg/mL and is clear, colorless, and isotonic with a pH of 7. Use within 3 hr as there is no preservative. Store vial either in refrigerator or at room temperature. Do not shake or freeze reconstituted solution.

5. Do not re-enter or reuse single-use vial. Discard unused portion.

6. Store lyophilized drug and diluent at 2–8°C (36–46°F). Protect from light; do not freeze.

ASSESSMENT

1. Note reasons for therapy, onset, duration, clinical manifestations.

2. Monitor I&O, electrolytes, CBC, platelet counts.

3. List chemotherapy agent and platelet nadir; initiate therapy 6–24 hr after chemotherapy completed. Stop oprelvekin at least 2 days before next round of chemotherapy.

CLIENT/FAMILY TEACHING

1. Review administration and dosage guidelines. Use as directed, SC, into abdomen, thigh, or hip; rotate sites.

2. Drug is used to prevent chemotherapy-induced low platelets by stimulating bone marrow to increase platelet production. Low platelets may cause increased bleeding.

3. Report any unusual side effects, SOB, swelling of extremities, fatigue/weakness, irregular heartbeat, blurred vision, or increased bruising/bleeding.

OUTCOMES/EVALUATE

Thrombocytopenia prophylaxis; ↑ platelet production

Orlistat
(**OR**-lih-stat)

CLASSIFICATION(S):
Antiobesity drug
PREGNANCY CATEGORY: B
OTC: Alli.
Rx: Xenical.

USES

OTC. Weight loss in overweight adults 18 years of age and older along with a reduced calorie, low-fat diet.

Rx. (1) Management of obesity, including weight loss and weight maintenance when used with a reduced-calorie diet. (2) To reduce risk for weight regain after prior weight loss. Orlistat is indicated for obese clients with an initial body mass index of 30 kg/m^2 or more, or 27 kg/m^2 or more in the presence of risk factors such as hypertension, diabetes, dyslipidemia.

ACTION/KINETICS

Action

Reversible inhibitor of lipases resulting in inhibition of absorption of dietary fats. Acts in the lumen of the stomach and small intestine to form a covalent bond with the active serine residue site of gastric and pancreatic lipases. Inactivated enzymes are not available to hydrolyze dietary fat, in the form of triglycerides, into absorbable free fatty acids and monoglycerides. At therapeutic doses, it inhibits dietary fat absorption by about 30%. Effect on absorption of lipids seen as soon as 24–48 hr after dosing. Weight loss was seen within 2 weeks of starting therapy and continued for 6–12 months.

Pharmacokinetics

Systemic absorption is not needed for activity, although a small amount is absorbed. Metabolism occurs mainly in the GI wall. Unabsorbed drug is excreted through the feces. Weight loss caused by orlistat delayed the onset of

---

type 2 diabetes in obese clients with impaired glucose tolerance.

CONTRAINDICATIONS
Use in chronic malabsorption syndrome or cholestasis; known hypersensitivity to the drug. Lactation.

SPECIAL CONCERNS
Exclude organic causes of obesity (e.g., hypothyroidism) before prescribing. GI side effects may increase when taken with a high-fat diet. Potential exists for misuse (e.g., in those with anorexia nervosa or bulimia). Use with caution in those with a history of hyperoxaluria or calcium oxalate nephrolithiasis. Safety and effectiveness have not been determined in children aged 12 to 16 and has not been studied in children less than 12 years of age.

SIDE EFFECTS
Most Common
Headache, oily spotting, flatus with discharge, fecal urgency, fatty/oily stool, oily evacuation, increased defecation, abdominal pain/discomfort, influenza, URTI.

GI: Oily spotting, flatus with discharge, fecal urgency, fatty/oily stool, oily evacuation, increased defecation, fecal incontinence, abdominal pain or discomfort, N&V, infectious diarrhea, rectal pain or discomfort, tooth disorder, gingival disorder. **CNS:** Headache, dizziness, psychiatric anxiety, depression. **Respiratory:** Influenza, URTI, lower respiratory infection, ENT symptoms. **Musculoskeletal:** Back pain, arthritis, myalgia, joint disorder, lower extremity pain, tendonitis. **Dermatologic:** Rash, dry skin. **GU:** Menstrual irregularity, vaginitis, UTI. **Hypersensitivity (rare):** Pruritus, rash, urticaria, angioedema, ***anaphylaxis***. **Miscellaneous:** Fatigue, sleep disorder, otitis, pedal edema,

DRUG INTERACTIONS
Beta-carotene / 30% ↓ absorption of beta-carotene supplement
Cyclosporine / ↓ Cyclosporine levels R/T ↓ absorption
Pravastatin / Additive lipid-lowering effects
Vitamin A / Possible malabsorption of Vitamin A
Vitamin D / Possible malabsorption of

Vitamin D
Vitamin E / 60% ↓ absorption of vitamin E acetate supplement
Vitamin K / Possible ↓ vitamin K absorption
Warfarin / Possible ↑ INR following chronic orlistat dosing

HOW SUPPLIED
Capsules: 60 mg (OTC), 120 mg (Rx).

DOSAGE
• **OTC: CAPSULES**
Management of obesity.
Adults, 18 years and older: 60 mg 3 times per day with each meal containing fat, not to exceed 3 capsules/day.
• **RX: CAPSULES**
Management of obesity.
120 mg (1 capsule) 3 times per day with each main meal containing fat; give during or up to 1 hr after the meal. Doses greater than 120 mg 3 times per day have not been shown to produce additional benefit. Safety and effectiveness beyond 2 yr have not been determined.

NURSING CONSIDERATIONS

☙ Do not confuse Zenical with Xeloda (an antineoplastic drug).

ADMINISTRATION/STORAGE
1. When the Rx form is used, the client should be on a nutritionally balanced, reduced-calorie diet that contains about 30% of calories from fat. Distribute over 3 main meals the daily intake of fat, carbohydrate, and protein.
2. To ensure adequate nutrition, clients on either the OTC or Rx product should take a multivitamin containing fat-soluble vitamins and beta-carotene. The supplement should be taken at least 2 hr before or after the administration of orlistat (i.e., at bedtime).
3. Weight lost due to orlistat may be accompanied by improved metabolic control in diabetics; this might require a reduction in dose of oral hypoglycemic drugs or insulin.

ASSESSMENT
1. Note reasons for therapy, length of weight problem, other agents/therapies trialed, and outcome.
2. Assess for history of cholestasis, eating disorders, or malabsorption syn-

drome. Note any thyroid dysfunction or kidney stones (drug may increase urinary oxalate).

3. List medical conditions/risk factors necessitating treatment (i.e, DM, HTN, hyperlipidemia). Obtain baseline BMI, weight, VS, waist and hip circumference.

4. Assess electrolytes, cholesterol profile, BS, urinalysis, renal and LFTs.

CLIENT/FAMILY TEACHING

1. Drug acts by inhibiting absorption of some of the dietary fat intake. Take with or within 1 hr following each main meal. If a meal is occasionally missed or contains no fat, the dose of orlistat can be omitted.

2. In order to be successful in losing weight, follow a nutritionally balanced, reduced-calorie diet containing 30% of calories from fat and perform 20 min of daily exercise. Distribute the daily intake of CHO, protein, and fat over three main meals.

3. Drug may reduce absorption of fat-soluble vitamins (A, D, E) and beta-carotene. Take supplements at least 2 hr after therapy or at bedtime daily.

4. Diabetics should monitor FS; improved metabolic control may require a reduction of the dose of hypoglycemic agents.

5. May cause GI S&S, gas with discharge, fecal urgency/incontinence, oily or spotty discharge, abdominal pain/discomfort, diarrhea. Should subside with continued use; report any persistent side effects.

6. Report as scheduled for assessment of BP, labs, side effects, and weight.

OUTCOMES/EVALUATE

- ↓ Risk of weight gain after prior loss
- ↓ BMI
- Desired weight loss

Oseltamivir phosphate
(oh-sell-**TAM**-ih-vir)

CLASSIFICATION(S):
Antiviral
PREGNANCY CATEGORY: C
Rx: Tamiflu.

USES
(1) Prophylaxis of influenza A and B in adults and children, 1 year of age and older. (2) Treatment of uncomplicated acute influenza in adults and children over 1 year of age who have been symptomatic for 2 days or less. *NOTE:* Oseltamivir is not a substitute for early vaccination on an annual basis as recommended by the CDC.

ACTION/KINETICS
Action
Hydrolyzed by hepatic esterases to the active oseltamivir carboxylate. May act by inhibiting the flu virus neuraminidase with possible alteration of virus particle aggregation and release. Drug resistance to influenza A virus is possible.

Pharmacokinetics
Readily absorbed from the GI tract and extensively converted to oseltamivir carboxylate. About 75% of an oral dose reaches the systemic circulation as the carboxylate. **t½, oseltamivir:** 1–3 hr; **t½, oseltamivir carboxylate:** 6–10 hr. Over 99% is eliminated in the urine as oseltamivir carboxylate. Children up to 12 years of age clear the prodrug and the active metabolite (carboxylate) faster than adults. **Plasma protein binding:** 42% of oseltamivir but only 3% of oseltamivir carboxylate are bound to plasma proteins.

CONTRAINDICATIONS
Use in children less than 1 year of age.

SPECIAL CONCERNS
Use during lactation only if potential benefits outweigh the potential risk to the infant. Efficacy has not been determined in clients who begin treatment after 40 hr of symptoms, for prophylac-

O

tic use to prevent influenza, for repeated treatment courses, or for use in those with chronic cardiac or respiratory disease. Has not been shown to prevent bacterial infections. Not been shown to prevent complications from serious bacterial infections. Efficacy has not been determined for treatment or prophylaxis in immunocompromised clients. Safety and efficacy have not been determined in children less than 1 year of age or of repeated treatment or prophylaxis.

SIDE EFFECTS
Most Common
When used in adults: N&V, headache, diarrhea, dizziness, abdominal pain, bronchitis.
When used in children: Diarrhea, N&V, abdominal pain, asthma, epistaxis, otitis media.
GI: N&V, diarrhea, abdominal pain, pseudomembranous colitis, dyspepsia, hepatitis. **CNS:** Dizziness, headache, insomnia, vertigo, seizure, confusion; self-injury and delirium, primarily in children. **CV:** Arrhythmia, unstable angina. **Body as a whole:** Fatigue, rash, pyrexia, anemia, aches and pains, allergy. **Respiratory:** Bronchitis, cough, pneumonia, sinusitis, peritonsillar abscess, rhinorrhea, URTI. **Dermatologic:** Dermatitis, eczema, rash, urticaria. Rarely, *toxic epidermal necrolysis, Stevens-Johnson syndrome,* erythema multiforme. **Miscellaneous:** Swelling of face or tongue, anemia, humerus fracture, aggravation of diabetes, hepatitis, abnormal LFTs, *anaphylaxis (rare).* NOTE: For children and adolescents, additional side effects include otitis media, tympanic membrane disorder, aggravated asthma, epistaxis, pneumonia, ear disorder, sinusitis, conjunctivitis, lymphadenopathy, dermatitis.

LABORATORY TEST CONSIDERATIONS
Abnormal LFTs.

DRUG INTERACTIONS
Live attenuated influenza vaccine / Possible inhibition of replication of live vaccine virus; do not give the vaccine within 2 weeks before or 48 hr after oseltamivir administration (unless medically indicated

Probenecid / About a 2-fold ↑ in exposure to oseltamivir carboxylate R/T ↓ in kidney tubular secretion

HOW SUPPLIED
Capsules: 30 mg, 45 mg, 75 mg; *Powder for Oral Suspension:* 12 mg/mL (after reconstitution).

DOSAGE
• CAPSULES; ORAL SUSPENSION
Prophylaxis of influenza.
Adults and children 13 years and older: 75 mg once daily for at least 10 days. The recommended daily dose for prophylaxis during a community outbreak of influenza is 75 mg. For clients with a C_{CR} between 10 and 30 mL/min, reduce dose to 75 mg every other day or 30 mg of the oral suspension every day. Begin treatment within 2 days of exposure to flu. For adults, safety and efficacy have been shown for use for 6 weeks or less.

Children, 1 year of age and older following close contact with an infected individual: 15 kg or less (33 lbs or less): 30 mg (2.4 mL of the suspension) twice a day; **>15–23 kg (>33–51 lbs):** 45 mg (3.6 mL of the suspension) twice a day; **>23–40 kg (>51–88 lbs):** 60 mg (4.8 mL of the suspension) twice a day; **>40 kg (>88 lbs):** 75 mg (6 mL of the suspension) twice a day. Prophylaxis in children has not been evaluated for longer than 10 days duration. Begin therapy within 2 days of exposure.

Treatment of influenza.
Adults and children 13 years and older: 75 mg twice a day for 5 days. For clients with a C_{CR} between 10 and 30 mL/min, reduce dose to 75 mg once daily for 5 days. **Children 1 year and older: 15 kg or less (33 lbs or less):** 30 mg (2.4 mL of the suspension) twice a day; **>15–23 kg (>33–51 lbs):** 45 mg (3.6 mL of the suspension) twice a day; **>23–40 kg (51–88 lbs):** 60 mg (4.8 mL of the suspension) twice a day; **>40 kg (>88 lbs):** 75 mg (6 mL of the suspension) twice a day. Duration: 5 days. Begin treatment within 2 days of onset of flu symptoms.

Bold Italic = life threatening side effect   ■ = black box warning   ✦ = Available in Canada

NURSING CONSIDERATIONS

ADMINISTRATION/STORAGE

1. Prepare the oral suspension as follows:
- Tap the closed bottle several times to loosen powder.
- Measure 23 mL of water into a graduated cylinder.
- Add the total amount of water for reconstitution to the bottle and shake the closed bottle well for 15 seconds.
- Remove child-resistant cap and push bottle adapter into the neck of the bottle.
- Close bottle with child-resistant cap tightly to ensure proper seating of the bottle adapter in the bottle and child-resistant status of the cap.

2. Use the reconstituted solution within 10 days of preparation.

3. Store capsules and the dry powder for suspension from 15–30°C (59–86°F). Store the reconstituted suspension under refrigeration from 2–8°C (36–46°F). Do not freeze.

ASSESSMENT

1. Note onset, characteristics of S&S; if for prevention or treatment of influenza.

2. Assess medical condition, history. Anticipate reduced dose with renal dysfunction.

3. Recently pediatric deaths (Japan), serious skin reactions, and neuropsychiatric events have been reported; use cautiously until further research available.

CLIENT/FAMILY TEACHING

1. Initiate treatment as soon as possible or within 2 days of the first appearance of flu S&S. Drug is used to diminish side effects and duration of illness. An annual flu shot is still required.

2. Do not double up on doses. Take any missed dose as soon as remembered. If the missed dose is remembered within 2 hr of the next scheduled dose, take at the usual time and resume usual schedule.

3. Tolerability may be enhanced if taken with food. May aggravate diabetes control.

4. May cause dizziness or lightheadedness; alcohol, hot weather, exercise, or fever may increase effects. To prevent, sit up or stand slowly, especially in the morning. Sit or lie down at the first sign of these effects.

5. An increased risk of confusion and unusual behavioral changes has been noted. The risk may be greater in children. Report symptoms of confusion or any other unusual behavioral changes.

6. Not for preventive use in children under age 13; must be provider-initiated. May cause more adverse effects than benefits in children.

OUTCOMES/EVALUATE

↓ Intensity/duration of S&S of influenza A and B.

Oxaliplatin ■ IV
(**OX**-al-ee-**plah**-tin)

CLASSIFICATION(S):
Antineoplastic, alkylating
PREGNANCY CATEGORY: D
Rx: Eloxatin.

SEE ALSO ANTINEOPLASTIC AGENTS.

USES

(1) In combination with infusional 5-fluorouracil/leucovorin for adjuvant treatment of stage III colon cancer in those who have undergone complete resection of the primary tumor. (2) In combination with infusional 5-fluorouracil/leucovorin to treat advanced carcinoma of the colon or rectum. *Investigational:* Treat relapsed or refractory non-Hodgkin lymphoma; treat advanced ovarian cancer.

ACTION/KINETICS

Action

Undergoes nonenzymatic conversion to form active derivatives, which bind to macromolecules. Both inter- and intrastrand Pt-DNA crosslinks are formed. These crosslinks inhibit DNA replication and transcription. Cytotoxicity is cell-cycle nonspecific. Plasma levels increase as renal function decreases.

Pharmacokinetics

Undergoes rapid and extensive metabolism. Excreted through the urine. **Plasma protein binding:** More than 90%.

CONTRAINDICATIONS

Hypersensitivity to oxaliplatin or other platinum compounds. Lactation.

SPECIAL CONCERNS

■ (1) Administer oxaliplatin under the supervision of a physician experienced in the area of cancer chemotherapeutic agents. Appropriate management of therapy and complications is possible only when adequate diagnostic and treatment facilities are readily available. (2) Anaphylactic-like reactions to oxaliplatin have been reported, and may occur within minutes of administration. Epinephrine, corticosteroids, and antihistamines have been employed to alleviate symptoms.■ Use the treatment regimen with caution in preexisting renal impairment. Safety and efficacy have not been demonstrated in children.

SIDE EFFECTS

Most Common

Neuropathies, fatigue, paresthesias, skin disorder, N&V, stomatitis, diarrhea, constipation, epistaxis, cough, anorexia, abdominal pain, fever, infection, injection site reaction, alopecia, conjunctivitis, anemia, neutropenia, leukopenia, thrombocytopenia.

CNS: Neuropathies (acute and persistent), fatigue, anxiety, headache, insomnia, depression, somnolence, nervousness, ataxia, dizziness, loss of deep tendon reflexes, dysarthria, cranial nerve palsies, fasciculations, loss of deep tendon reflexes, Lhermitte sign. **GI:** Nausea, vomiting and diarrhea (may be severe, leading to hypokalemia and metabolic acidosis), dry mouth, gingivitis, constipation, anorexia, stomatitis, dyspepsia, taste perversion, flatulence, mucositis, hiccough, gastroesophageal reflux, ileus, enlarged abdomen, intestinal obstruction, pancreatitis, rectal hemorrhage, hemorrhoids, melena, proctitis, tenesmus, colitis (including *Clostridum difficile* diarrhea). **Hepatic:** *Hepatotoxicity*, perisinusoidal fibrosis (rarely progresses), venoocclusive liver disease. **Hematologic:** Anemia, thrombocytopenia, leukopenia, neutropenia, immuno-allergic thrombocytopenia, hemolytic uremic syndrome, febrile neutropenia, immuno-allergic hemolytic anemia. **Dermatologic:** Flushing, rash, alopecia, erythematous rash, increased sweating, dry skin, purpura, hot flashes. Extravasation may cause pain and inflammation that may be severe and lead to necrosis. Injection site reaction, including redness, swelling, and pain. **Respiratory:** Dyspnea, coughing, URTI, rhinitis, pharyngitis, epistaxis, pulmonary fibrosis, interstitial lung diseases, pneumonia. **GU:** Hematuria, dysuria, abnormal micturition frequency, urinary incontinence, vaginal hemorrhage. **Musculoskeletal:** Arthralgia, myalgia, muscle weakness, involuntary muscle contractions. **Hypersensitivity:** May be fatal. Rash, urticaria, erythema, pruritus, angioedema, *bronchospasm, anaphylactic shock*, hypotension. **Ophthalmic:** Decreased visual acuity, visual field disturbance, optic neuritis, abnormal lacrimation, conjunctivitis. **Body as a whole:** Fever, infection, edema, pain, dehydration, peripheral edema, rigors, decreased weight, ascites, pruritus, metabolic acidosis. **Miscellaneous:** Deafness, injection site reaction, abdominal pain, back pain, tachycardia, *thromboembolism*, chest pain, hand-foot syndrome, hemoptysis.

LABORATORY TEST CONSIDERATIONS

Changes in ALT, AST, bilirubin. ↑ Serum creatinine.

DRUG INTERACTIONS

Anticoagulants / Prolonged PT and INR associated with hemorrhage when oxaliplatin used with 5-FU and leucovorin
Fluorouracil (5-FU) / ↑ 5-FU levels by about 20% following doses of 130 mg/m^2 of oxaliplatin q 3 weeks
Nephrotoxic drugs / ↓ Clearance of oxaliplatin

HOW SUPPLIED

Injection: 50 mg, 100 mg, 200 mg.

DOSAGE

* **IV**

    Advanced colorectal cancer (previously treated and untreated); adjuvant treatment of stage III colon cancer.

The following dosage schedule is given every 2 weeks. **Day 1:** Oxaliplatin, 85 mg/m^2 by IV infusion in 250–500 mL D5W and leucovorin, 200 mg/m^2 by IV infusion in D5W, both given over 120 min at the same time in separate bags using a Y-line. Followed by 5-FU, 400 mg/m^2 IV bolus given over 2–4 min, followed by 5-FU, 600 mg/m^2 IV infusion in 500 mL D5W recommended as a 22-hr continuous infusion. **Day 2:** Leucovorin, 200 mg/m^2 by IV infusion over 120 min, followed by 5-FU, 400 mg/m^2 by IV bolus given over 2–4 min, followed by 5-FU, 600 mg/m^2 by IV infusion in 500 mL D5W recommended as a 22-hr continuous infusion. Repeat every 2 weeks.

NURSING CONSIDERATIONS

ADMINISTRATION/STORAGE

[IV] 1. Premedicate with antiemetics, including 5-HT$_3$ blockers with or without dexamethasone. Prehydration is not required.

2. Increasing the infusion time from 2 to 6 hr decreases the C_{max} and may decrease acute toxicity. Infusion times for leucovorin or 5-FU do not need to be changed.

3. Adjuvant treatment in clients with stage III colon cancer is recommended for a total of 6 months (i.e., 12 cycles, each cycle given every 2 weeks).

4. **When used as adjuvant therapy in stage III colon cancer:** For those who manifest persistent Grade 2 neurosensory effects that do not resolve, consider reducing the dose of oxaliplatin to 75 mg/m^2. For those with persistent Grade 3 neurosensory effects, consider terminating therapy. The infusional 5-FU/leucovorin regimen need not be altered.

5. **When used as adjuvant therapy in stage III colon cancer:** Consider a dose reduction of oxaliplatin to 75 mg/m^2 and infusional 5-FU by 20% (to 300 mg/m^2 bolus and 500 mg/m^2 22 hr-infusion) in clients after recovery from Grade 3/4 GI (despite prophylactic treatment) or Grade 3/4 hematologic toxicity (neutrophils less than 1.5 x 10^9/L and platelets less than 100 x 10^9/L). Delay the next dose until neutrophils

are 1.5 x 10^9/L or more and platelets are 75 x 10^9/L or more.

6. **When used for advanced colorectal cancer (previously untreated or treated):** For those who experience persistent grade 2 neurosensory events that do not resolve, consider a dose reduction of oxaliplatin to 65 mg/m^2. For those with persistent grade 3 neurosensory events, consider discontinuing therapy. The 5-FU/leucovorin regimen need not be altered.

7. **When used for advanced colorectal cancer (previously untreated or treated):** A dose reduction of oxaliplatin to 65 mg/m^2 and 5-FU by 20% (to 300 mg/m^2 and 500 mg/m^2 22-hr infusion) is recommended for clients after recovery from grade 3/4 GI (despite prophylactic treatment), grade 4 neutropenia, or grade 3/4 thrombocytopenia. Delay next dose until neutrophils are greater than or equal to 1.5 x 10^9/L and platelets are greater than or equal to 75 x 10^9/L.

8. Do not reconstitute or make a final dilution with any solution containing chloride.

9. Reconstitute by adding 10 mL (for the 50 mg vial) or 20 mL (for the 100 mg vial) of water for injection or D5W. This solution *must* be further diluted in an infusion solution of 250–500 mL of D5W.

10. After initial reconstitution the solution may be stored up to 24 hr under refrigeration. After final dilution with 250–500 mL D5W, can keep for 6 hr at room temperature or up to 24 hr in the refrigerator. Drug is not light sensitive.

11. Oxaliplatin is incompatible in solution with alkaline drugs or media (e.g., basic solutions of 5-FU). Do not mix or give simultaneously through the same infusion line. Flush infusion line with D5W before giving any concomitant drug.

12. Do not use Al-containing needles or IV administration sets containing parts that may come into contact with the drug. Al may degrade platinum compounds.

13. Exercise care in preparing and handling infusion solution; use gloves. If so-

lution comes in contact with the skin, wash immediately and thoroughly with soap and water. If oxaliplatin comes in contact with mucous membranes, flush thoroughly with water.

14. Store from 15–30°C (59–86°F); do not freeze and protect from light. After dilution with 250–500 mL D5W, the shelf life is 6 hr at room temperature or up to 24 hr when refrigerated. After final dilution, protection from light is not needed.

ASSESSMENT

1. Note reasons for therapy, occurrence/recurrence, other agents trialed. Given with leucovorin and 5-FU; assess appropriately.

2. Assess/monitor cardiac, neuro, and pulmonary status.

3. Ensure premedication with antiemetics and dexamethasone to minimize side effects. Assess for anaphylactic reaction with infusion.

4. Monitor CBC, electrolytes, renal, and LFTs; adjust dosage with dysfunction.

CLIENT/FAMILY TEACHING

1. Drug is used in combination with other agents to treat metastatic/recurrent colon/rectal cancer.

2. May experience significant neurosensory deficits, such as numbness or tingling in any body parts. Cold temperatures/objects (ice) may worsen these side effects. Report immediately as may be acute (reversible) or persistent (long-term) peripheral neuropathy.

3. Causes reduced blood counts; report any S&S of infection, fever, or diarrhea. Avoid crowds and persons with known infections.

4. No immunizations without provider approval. Avoid persons who have taken oral polio vaccine within the last several months. If unable to avoid contact, wear protective mask that covers face and nose.

5. Avoid cold drinks or ice cubes in drinks. Cover skin if you must go out in cold temperatures. Do not put ice or ice packs on your body. Do not breathe deeply when exposed to cold air. Do not take things from the freezer or refrigerator without wearing gloves. Do not run air conditioner at high levels in the house or in the car in hot weather.

6. Take care to avoid contact sports or other situations where bruising or injury could occur.

7. Be careful when using a regular toothbrush, dental floss, or toothpick. Use soft brush or gauze to clean teeth and gums. Avoid dental work unless cleared by provider.

8. Practice reliable contraception; identify if candidate for egg/sperm harvesting.

9. Keep regular F/U visits and report any adverse SE or injection site reaction.

OUTCOMES/EVALUATE

Inhibition of malignant cell proliferation

Oxaprozin, Oxaprozin Potassium ■
(**ox**-ah-**PROH**-zin)

CLASSIFICATION(S):
Nonsteroidal anti-inflammatory drug

PREGNANCY CATEGORY: C

Rx: Daypro, Daypro ALTA.

✢Rx: Apo-Oxaprozin, Rhoxal-oxaprozin.

SEE ALSO *NONSTEROIDAL ANTI-INFLAMMATORY DRUGS.*

USES

Acute and chronic management of rheumatoid arthritis and osteoarthritis.

ACTION/KINETICS

Pharmacokinetics

Is 95% bioavailable. **Peak effect:** 3–5 hr. **t½:** 42–50 hr. Excreted in the urine (65%) and feces (35%). **Plasma protein binding:** More than 99%.

CONTRAINDICATIONS

Use in clients who have had asthma, urticaria, or an allergic-type reaction after taking aspirin or other NSAIDs. Treatment of perioperative pain in coronary artery bypass graft.

SPECIAL CONCERNS

■ (1) NSAIDs may cause an increased risk of serious cardiovascular thrombotic events, MI, and stroke, which can be

---

fatal. This risk may increase with duration of use. Clients with cardiovascular disease or risk factors for cardiovascular disease may be at greater risk. (2) Oxaprozin is contraindicated for treatment of perioperative pain in the setting of coronary artery bypass graft surgery. (3) NSAIDs cause an increased risk of serious GI adverse events including bleeding, ulceration, and perforation of the stomach or intestines, which can be fatal. These events can occur at any time during use and without warning symptoms. Elderly clients are at greater risk for serious GI events. ■

SIDE EFFECTS
Most Common
Rash, diarrhea, N&V, constipation, dyspepsia/indigestion, anorexia, dysuria, urinary frequency, tinnitus.

See *Nonsteroidal Anti-Inflammatory Drugs* for a complete list of possible side effects. Also, weight changes and nephrotic syndrome.

HOW SUPPLIED
Caplets: 600 mg; *Tablets:* 600 mg (oxaprozin); 678 mg (oxaprozin potassium - equivalent to 600 mg oxaprozin).

DOSAGE
- **CAPLETS; TABLETS**
  Rheumatoid arthritis.
Adults: 1,200 mg once daily. For those unable to tolerate once-daily dosing, 600 mg twice a day may be tried. Lower and higher doses may be required in certain clients.
  Osteoarthritis.
Adults, initial: 600 mg once a day.
Usual daily dose: 1,200 mg once daily. For clients with a lower body weight or with a milder disease, 600 mg/day may be appropriate. Maximum daily dose for either rheumatoid arthritis or osteoarthritis: 1,800 mg (or 26 mg/kg, whichever is lower) given in divided doses.

NURSING CONSIDERATIONS
ADMINISTRATION/STORAGE
1. Regardless of the use, individualize and use the lowest effective dose to minimize side effects.
2. Reserve doses greater than 1,200 mg/day for those who weigh more than 50 kg, have normal renal and hepatic function, are at low risk of peptic ulcer, and whose disease severity justifies maximal therapy.
3. Store below 25°C (77°F) in tightly closed bottles. Protect the unit dose from light.

ASSESSMENT
1. Note reasons for therapy, characteristics of S&S, pain level, quality of life. List other agents used, outcome.
2. Assess involved joint(s), baseline ROM, extent of inflammation and functionality.
3. List any history of diabetes, stomach or bowel problems (eg, bleeding, perforation, ulcers), peripheral edema, asthma, nasal polyps, mouth inflammation; may preclude drug therapy.
4. Monitor BP, CBC, renal and LFTs; adjust dose with dysfunction.

CLIENT/FAMILY TEACHING
1. Take exactly as directed with a full glass of water to enhance absorption; do not share medications. May take with food or milk if GI upset occurs.
2. May cause dizziness or drowsiness; assess effects before driving or performing activities that require alertness. Report any evidence of unusual bruising/bleeding, blurred vision, ringing or roaring in ears (may indicate toxicity).
3. Report S&S of kidney problems: Wt gain, edema, increased joint pain, fever, blood in the urine.
4. Avoid prolonged sun exposure; use protection when exposed to prevent reaction.
5. If surgery scheduled should stop 2 weeks before surgery.
6. May take up to one month to note positive effects; report lack of response.

OUTCOMES/EVALUATE
Relief of joint pain/inflammation with improved mobility

O

Oxcarbazepine
(ox-kar-**BAY**-zeh-peen)

CLASSIFICATION(S):
Anticonvulsant, miscellaneous
PREGNANCY CATEGORY: C
Rx: Trileptal.

SEE ALSO *ANTICONVULSANTS.*

USES
(1) Adjunctive therapy or monotherapy to treat partial seizures in adults. (2) Monotherapy to treat partial seizures in children 4 years of age and older. (3) Adjunctive therapy to treat partial seizures in children 2 years of age and older. *Investigational:* Alternative treatment for bipolar disorder. Diabetic neuropathy.

ACTION/KINETICS
Action
Anticonvulsant mechanism not known with certainty but effect is primarily through the active 10-monohydroxy metabolite. May block voltage-sensitive sodium channels, resulting in stabilization of hyperexcited neural membranes, inhibition of repetitive neuronal firing, and decreased propagation of synaptic impulses. These effects thought to be important in preventing seizure spread. Also, increased potassium conductance and modulation of high-voltage activated calcium channels may contribute to the anticonvulsant effects.

Pharmacokinetics
Oxcarbazepine (active) is completely absorbed and extensively metabolized to the active 10-monohydroxy metabolite (MHD). Maximum plasma levels are higher in geriatric clients. **Peak levels:** 4.5 hr for oxcarbazepine and 6 hr for MHD. Steady-state plasma levels reached in 2–3 days. MHD is further metabolized to inactive compounds. $t^{1/2}$, **oxcarbazepine:** About 2 hr; $t^{1/2}$, **MHD:** About 9 hr. MHD and inactive metabolites are excreted mainly in the urine.

CONTRAINDICATIONS
Hypersensitivity to the drug or any of its components. Lactation.

SPECIAL CONCERNS
About 25–30% of clients who experience hypersensitivity reactions to carbamazepine will experience hypersensitivity to oxcarbazepine. Clinically significant hyponatremia may occur usually during the first 3 months of treatment. Use with caution in severe hepatic impairment.

SIDE EFFECTS
Most Common
Adults: Headache, dizziness, somnolence, ataxia, N&V, abdominal pain, dyspepsia, diplopia, abnormal vision, fatigue, abnormal gait, tremor.
Children: Headache, somnolence, dizziness, ataxia, nystagmus, N&V, rhinitis, diplopia, abnormal vision, fatigue.
Side effects listed include those clients on adjunctive therapy treated with oxcarbazepine, monotherapy previously treated with other antiepileptic drugs, and those on monotherapy not previously treated with other antiepileptic drugs. **CNS:** Psychomotor slowing, concentration difficulty, somnolence, fatigue, speech/language problems, abnormal coordination (ataxia, gait disturbances), headache, dizziness, anxiety, ataxia, vertigo, abnormal gait, nystagmus, insomnia, tremor, amnesia, ***aggravated convulsions***, emotional lability, hypoesthesia, nervousness, agitation, abnormal coordination, abnormal EEG, speech disorder, confusion, dysmetria, abnormal thinking, vertigo, aggressive reaction, anguish, apathy, aphasia, aura, delirium, delusion, dysphonia, dystonia, depressed level of consciousness, euphoria, extrapyramidal disorder, feeling 'drunk,' hemiplegia, hyperkinesia, hyperreflexia, hypesthesia, hypokinesia, hyporeflexia, hypotonia, hysteria, decreased or increased libido, mania, migraine, nervousness, neuralgia, panic disorder, paralysis, paroniria, personality disorder, psychosis, stupor. **GI:** N&V, abdominal pain, anorexia, dry mouth, ***rectal hemorrhage***, toothache, diarrhea, dyspepsia, constipation, gastritis, increased appetite, blood in stool, cholelithiasis, colitis, duodenal ulcer, dysphagia, enteritis, eructation, esophagitis, flatulence, gastric ulcer, gingival

---

Bold Italic = life threatening side effect   ◼ = black box warning   ✤ = Available in Canada bleeding, gum hyperplasia, hematemesis, hemorrhoids, hiccough, biliary pain, retching, right hypochondrium pain, sialoadenitis, stomatitis, ulcerative stomatitis. **CV:** Bradycardia, *cardiac failure, cerebral hemorrhage*, hypertension, postural hypotension, palpitations, syncope, tachycardia. **Respiratory:** Rhinitis, URTI, coughing, bronchitis, pharyngitis, epistaxis, chest infection, sinusitis, rhinitis, pneumonia, asthma, dyspnea, laryngismus, pleurisy. **GU:** UTI, frequent urination, vaginitis, dysuria, hematuria, intermenstrual bleeding, leukorrhea, menorrhagia, renal pain, urinary tract pain, polyuria, priapism, renal calculus. **Hematologic:** Leukopenia, thrombocytopenia. **Dermatologic:** Acne, hot flushes, purpura, rash, alopecia, angioedema, bruising, increased sweating, contact dermatitis, eczema, facial rash, flushing, folliculitis, heat rash, hot flushes, photosensitivity, genital pruritus, psoriasis, purpura, erythematous rash, maculopapular rash, vitiligo, erythema multiforme, urticaria, *Stevens-Johnson syndrome, toxic epidermal necrolysis*. **Musculoskeletal:** Muscle weakness, back pain, sprains, strains, involuntary muscle contractions, tetany, muscle hypertonia. **Ophthalmic:** Diplopia, nystagmus, abnormal vision, abnormal accommodation, oculogyric crisis, ptosis, cataract, conjunctival hemorrhage, eye edema, hemianopia, mydriasis, xerophthalmia, photophobia, scotoma. **Otic:** Earache, ear infection, otitis externa, tinnitus. **Body as a whole:** Fatigue, fever, malaise, allergy, rigors, generalized edema, asthenia, weight increase or decrease, abnormal feeling, falling down, viral infection, infection. **Miscellaneous:** Thirst, precordial chest pain, leg edema, lymphadenopathy, taste perversion, systemic lupus erythematosus. Multiorgan hypersensitivity reaction with symptoms of rash, fever, lymphadenopathy, abnormal LFTs, eosinophilia and arthralgia.

LABORATORY TEST CONSIDERATIONS
↑ GGT, liver enzymes, serum transaminase. ↓ Serum sodium, T_4. Hyponatremia, hypocalcemia, hyper/hypoglycemia, hypokalemia.

DRUG INTERACTIONS
Carbamazepine / ↓ Plasma MHD (oxcarbazepine) levels R/T ↑ liver metabolism
Felodipine / ↓ Felodipine levels
Lamotrigine / ↓ Lamotrigine levels
Oral contraceptives ↓ Plasma levels of both estrogen and progestin
Phenobarbital / ↓ MHD (oxcarbazepine) levels R/T ↑ liver metabolism; ↑ levels of phenobarbital
Phenytoin / ↓ MHD (oxcarbazepine) levels R/T ↑ liver metabolism; ↑ levels of phenytoin
Valproic acid / ↓ MHD (oxcarbazepine) levels
Verapamil / ↓ MHD (oxcarbazepine) levels

HOW SUPPLIED
Oral Suspension: 300 mg/5 mL; *Tablets:* 150 mg, 300 mg, 600 mg.

DOSAGE
• **ORAL SUSPENSION; TABLETS**
Adjunctive therapy for partial seizures in adults.
Adults, initial: 600 mg per day given as a twice daily regimen. If indicated, may increase by a maximum of 600 mg/day at approximately weekly intervals; recommended daily dose is 1,200 mg. Doses greater than 2,400 mg/day are not well tolerated due to CNS effects.
Conversion to monotherapy for partial seizures in adults.
Adults, initial: 300 mg twice a day while simultaneously reducing other anticonvulsant drug(s) over 3–6 weeks. Achieve maximum oxcarbazepine dose in 2–4 weeks. Dose may be increased by a maximum of 600 mg/day at approximately weekly intervals to a maximum daily dose of 2,400 mg.
Initiation of monotherapy for partial seizures in adults.
Adults: 600 mg/day given as a twice daily regimen. May increase by 300 mg/day every third day to a dose of 1,200 mg/day.
Adjunctive therapy for partial seizures in children, 2 to 16 years of age.
Children, aged 4–12 years, initial: 8–10 mg/kg, not to exceed 300 mg twice a day. Achieve target maintenance dose over 2 weeks according to

client weight as follows: **20–29 kg:** 900 mg/day; **29.1–39 kg:** 1,200 mg/day; **over 39 kg:** 1,800 mg/day. **Children, 2–4 years of age, initial:** 8–10 mg/kg, not to exceed 300 mg twice a day. For those weighing less than 20 kg, consider a starting dose of 16–20 mg/kg. Achieve a target maintenance dose over 2 weeks, not to exceed 60 mg/kg/day as a twice daily regimen. *NOTE:* Children 2 to younger than 4 years may require twice the dose of oxcarbazpine per body weight compared with adults and children 4 to 12 years of age may require a 50% higher oxcarbazepine dose per body weight compared with adults.

Conversion to monotherapy in children 4–16 years of age.

Initial: 8–10 mg/kg/day in 2 divided doses while simultaneously reducing the dose of the concomitant antiepileptic drug. The concomitant drug can be completely withdrawn over 3–6 weeks, while oxcarbazepine may be increased, up to a maximum increment of 10 mg/kg/day at approximately weekly intervals to reach the recommended daily dose.

Initiation of monotherapy in children 4–16 years of age.

Initial: 8–10 mg/kg/day in 2 divided doses. Increase the dose by 5 mg/kg/day every third day to the recommended daily maintenance dose as follows: **20 kg:** 600–900 mg/day; **25 kg & 30 kg:** 900–1,200 mg/day. **35 kg & 40 kg:** 900–1,500 mg/day; **45 kg:** 1,200–1,500 mg/day; **50 kg & 55 kg:** 1,200–1,800 mg/day; **60 kg & 65 kg:** 1,200–2,100 mg/day; **70 kg:** 1,500–2,100 mg/day.

NOTE: Initiate therapy at 300 mg/day in those with a C_{CR} less than 30 mL/min. May then increase slowly to achieve the desired response.

NURSING CONSIDERATIONS

ADMINISTRATION/STORAGE

1. Dosage adjustment is recommended for clients with impaired renal function. Initiate therapy at one-half the usual starting dose and increase, if needed, at a slower than usual rate until the desired response is obtained.

2. If withdrawal is needed, do so gradually to prevent increased seizure frequency.

ASSESSMENT

1. Note behaviors, with seizures identify type, onset/frequency, characteristics. Note other agents trialed, outcome.

2. If hypersensitivity reaction to carbamazepine may also have one to oxcarbazepine.

3. Assess neuro status. Monitor electrolytes, renal and LFTs. Assess for hyponatremia; adjust dose with renal dysfunction.

CLIENT/FAMILY TEACHING

1. Take exactly as directed with or without food. Do not double or skip doses.

2. Shake oral suspension well. May mix with water or swallow directly from syringe.

3. May cause dizziness/drowsiness. Do not perform activities that require mental alertness until drug effects realized. Get up slowly to prevent low BP effects.

4. Avoid alcohol; may increase sedative effect.

5. Report adverse effects or seizure recurrence. Do not stop therapy without approval.

6. Practice reliable contraception; hormonal forms may be ineffective.

7. Keep all F/U appointments to evaluate response to drug therapy, and to monitor serum sodium results. Report any S&S of low sodium, i.e., headache, confusion, nausea, malaise, or lethargy.

OUTCOMES/EVALUATE

Absence or ↓ Seizure activity

--- **COMBINATION DRUG** ---

Oxycodone and Acetaminophen ■ ©

(ox-ee-**KOH**-dohn, ah-**SEAT**-ah-**MIN**-oh-fen)

CLASSIFICATION(S):

Analgesic

PREGNANCY CATEGORY: C

Rx: Endocet, Magnacet, Percocet, Perloxx, Roxicet, Roxicet 5/500 Capsules, Roxilox, Tylox, **C-II**

Bold Italic = life threatening side effect   ■ = black box warning   ♣ = Available in Canada

♣Rx: Endocet, Percocet-Demi, ratio-Oxycodan.

SEE ALSO *ACETAMINOPHEN AND NARCOTIC ANALGESICS.*

USES

Relief of moderate to moderately severe pain.

CONTENT

Oxocodone hydrochloride (*Narcotic analgesic*) and Acetaminophen (*Nonnarcotic analgesic*). *NOTE:* The amount of oxycodone hydrochloride is listed first followed by the amount of acetaminophen. **Endocet Tablets:** 5 mg/325 mg, 7.5 mg/325 mg, 10 mg/325 mg, 10 mg/650 mg. **Generic Tablets:** 7.5 mg/325 mg, 7.5 mg/500 mg, 10 mg/325 mg, 10 mg/650 mg. **Magnacet Tablets:** 2.5 mg/400 mg, 5 mg/400 mg, 7.5 mg/400 mg, 10 mg/400 mg. **Percocet Tablets:** 2.5 mg/325 mg, 7.5 mg/325 mg, 7.5 mg/500 mg, 10 mg/325 mg, 10 mg/650 mg. **Perloxx Tablets:** 2.5 mg/300 mg, 5 mg/300 mg, 7.5 mg/300 mg, 10 mg/300 mg. **Roxicet Oral Solution:** 5 mg/325 mg per 5 mL. **Roxicet Tablets:** Oxycodone hydrochloride, 2.5 mg or 5 mg and Acetaminophen, 325 mg. **Roxicet 5/500 Caplets, Roxilox Capsules, Tylox Capsules:** Oxycodone hydrochloride, 5 mg and Acetaminophen, 500 mg.

ACTION/KINETICS

Action

Oxycodone is a semisynthetic opiate that combines with specific receptors located in the CNS to produce various effects. The mechanism is believed to involve decreased permeability of the cell membrane to sodium, which results in diminished transmission of pain impulses and therefore analgesia. Causes mild sedation and little or no antitussive effect. Most effective in relieving acute pain. Acetaminophen may cause analgesia by inhibiting CNS prostaglandin synthesis. Does not cause any anticoagulant effect or ulceration of the GI tract. Antipyretic and analgesic effects are comparable to those of aspirin.

Pharmacokinetics

Oxycodone. Onset: 15–30 min. **Peak effect:** 60 min. **Duration, immediate-release:** 3–4 hr; **controlled-release:** 12 hr. **t½, elimination:** 3.2 hr. Metabolized in the liver (somewhat involves CYP2D6 enzymes); excreted in the urine. **Acetaminophen. Peak plasma levels:** 30–120 min. **t½:** 45 min–3 hr. **Therapeutic serum levels** (analgesia): 5–20 mcg/mL. Metabolized in the liver and excreted in the urine as glucuronide and sulfate conjugates. However, an intermediate hydroxylated metabolite is hepatotoxic following large doses of acetaminophen.

CONTRAINDICATIONS

Hypersensitivity to either oxycodone or acetaminophen.

SPECIAL CONCERNS

■ See Oxycodone hydrochloride.■ Can produce drug dependence and has abuse potential. The respiratory depressant effects of oxycodone can be exaggerated in clients with head injury, other intracranial lesions, or a preexisting increase in intracranial pressure. Use with caution in clients who are elderly, are debilitated, have severely impaired hepatic or renal function, are hyperthyroid, have Addison's disease, have prostatic hypertrophy, or have urethral stricture. Use for acute abdominal conditions may obscure the diagnosis or clinical course. Use with caution during lactation. Safety and efficacy in children have not been established.

SIDE EFFECTS

Most Common

Dizziness, light-headedness, N&V, sedation, sweating, itching, dry mouth, constipation.

See *Acetaminophen* and *Narcotic Analgesics* for a complete list of possible side effects. Above side effects are more common in ambulatory clients than nonambulatory clients. Other side effects include euphoria, dysphoria, skin rash, and pruritus.

DRUG INTERACTIONS

Anticholinergic drugs / Production of paralytic ileus
Antidepressants, tricyclic / ↑ Effect of either the TCAs or oxycodone
CNS depressants (including other narcotic analgesics, phenothiazines, antianxiety drugs, sedative-hypnotics, anesthetics, alcohol) / Additive CNS depression

MAO inhibitors / ↑ Effect of either the MAO inhibitor or oxycodone

HOW SUPPLIED
See Content.

DOSAGE
• **CAPLETS; CAPSULES; ORAL SOLUTION; TABLETS**
Analgesic
Adults: 5 mL of the oral solution q 6 hr or 1 caplet, capsule, or tablet q 6 hr as needed for pain. From 6 to 12 caplets, capsules, or tablets may be taken per day, depending on the strength. *NOTE:* Check strength and maximum daily dose carefully for each dosages form.

NURSING CONSIDERATIONS

℘ Do not confuse Percocet (oxycodone/acetaminophen combination) with Percodan (oxycodone/aspirin combination). Do not confuse Roxicet (oxycodone/acetaminophen combination) with Roxicodone (oxycodone alone). Do not confuse Oxycodone (generic name) with OxyContin (trade name for oxycodone).

ASSESSMENT
1. List reasons for therapy, type, onset, characteristics of S&S. Use a pain-rating scale to rate pain level. List other agents prescribed, outcome.
2. Note VS, x-rays, CNS assessment findings, ROM, level of consciousness, TSH, renal and LFTs.
3. Assess for head injury, increased ICP, drug seeking behaviors.

CLIENT/FAMILY TEACHING
1. Take only as directed; may take with food to decrease GI upset. Do not share drugs, store in a safe place.
2. Drug may cause dizziness and drowsiness; do not perform activities that require mental or physical alertness and do not change positions abruptly.
3. May cause constipation, N&V, dry mouth, rash/itching, and physical dependence (withdrawal S&S include N&V, cramps, fever, fainting, and anorexia); report.
4. Avoid alcohol and any other CNS depressants without provider approval. (*NOTE:* Oral solution contains small amounts of alcohol.)

5. Tolerance may occur; report loss of effectiveness.

OUTCOMES/EVALUATE
Desired pain control

Oxycodone hydrochloride ■ ℘
(ox-ee-**KOH**-dohn)

CLASSIFICATION(S):
Narcotic analgesic
PREGNANCY CATEGORY: C
Rx: Capsules, Immediate-Release: OxyIR. **Solution, Concentrate**: ETH-Oxydose, OxyFAST, Roxicodone Intensol. **Solution, Oral**: Roxicodone. **Tablets, Controlled-Release**: Oxy-Contin. **Tablets, Immediate-Release**: M-oxy, Roxicodone, **C-II**
♣**Rx:** Supeudol.

SEE ALSO *NARCOTIC ANALGESICS.*

USES
Immediate-release: Management of moderate to severe pain.
    Controlled-release: Management of moderate to severe pain when a continuous, around-the-clock analgesic is required for an extended period of time. To be used postoperatively if the client has received the drug prior to surgery or if the postoperative pain is expected to be moderate to severe and last for an extended period of time. Not intended for use as an 'as needed' analgesic. Not for pain in the immediate postoperative period (i.e., first 12–24 hr following surgery) or if the pain is mild or not expected to persist for a long period of time. Individualize treatment moving from parenteral to PO analgesics as appropriate.

ACTION/KINETICS
Action
Semisynthetic opiate that combines with specific receptors located in the CNS to produce various effects. The mechanism is believed to involve decreased permeability of the cell membrane to sodium, which results in diminished transmission of pain impulses and therefore analgesia. Causes mild se-

---

dation and little or no antitussive effect. Most effective in relieving acute pain.

Pharmacokinetics
Onset: 15–30 min. **Peak effect:** 60 min. **Duration, immediate-release:** 3–4 hr; **controlled-release:** 12 hr. **t½, elimination:** 3.2 hr for immediate-release product and 4.5 hr for extended-release. Metabolized in the liver (somewhat involves CYP2D6 enzymes); excreted in the urine. Oxycodone terephthalate is available but only in combination with aspirin (e.g., Percodan) or acetaminophen. **Plasma protein binding:** 45% bound to plasma proteins.

ADDITIONAL CONTRAINDICATIONS
Use in hypercarbia, paralytic ileus, children, or during labor.

SPECIAL CONCERNS
■ (1) Controlled-release oxycodone is an opiate and a Schedule II drug with an abuse liability similar to morphine. (2) Oxycodone can be abused in a manner similar to other opiates, legal or illicit. Consider this when prescribing or dispensing oxycodone controlled-release tablets in situations where there is concern about an increased risk of misuse, abuse, or diversion. (3) Controlled-release tablets are for the management of moderate-to-severe pain when a continuous, around-the-clock analgesic is needed for an extended period of time. (4) Controlled-release tablets are not intended for use as an as-needed analgesic. (5) Oxycodone 80 mg controlled-release tablets are for use in opiate-tolerant clients only. This tablet strength may cause fatal respiratory depression when given to clients not previously exposed to opiates. (6) Controlled-release tablets are to be swallowed whole and are not to be broken, chewed, or crushed. Taking broken, chewed, or crushed oxycodone controlled-release tablets leads to rapid release and absorption of a potentially fatal dose of oxycodone.■ Chewing, snorting, or injecting oxycodone can lead to death. Is a widely abused drug.

SIDE EFFECTS
Most Common
Constipation, dry mouth, N&V, mild itching, drowsiness, lightheadedness, anorexia, weakness.

See *Narcotic Analgesics* for a complete list of possible side effects.

ADDITIONAL DRUG INTERACTIONS
Use with protease inhibitors → ↑ CNS and respiratory depression.

HOW SUPPLIED
Capsules, Immediate-Release: 5 mg; *Oral Solution:* 5 mg/5 mL; *Solution, Concentrate:* 20 mg/mL; *Tablets, Controlled-Release:* 10 mg, 15 mg, 20 mg, 30 mg, 40 mg, 60 mg, 80 mg; *Tablets, Immediate-Release:* 5 mg, 10 mg, 15 mg, 20 mg, 30 mg.

DOSAGE
- **CAPSULES, IMMEDIATE-RELEASE; SOLUTION, CONCENTRATE; TABLETS, CONTROLLED-RELEASE; TABLETS, IM-MEDIATE-RELEASE**

  Analgesia.
  Individualize dose depending on severity of pain, client response, and client size. **Adults:** 10–30 mg q 4 hr (5 mg q 6 hr for OxyIR, oxycodone IR capsules, ETH-Oxydose, and OxyFAST) as needed. More severe pain may require 30 mg or more q 4 hr. If pain increases in severity, analgesia is not adequate, or tolerance occurs, a gradual increase in dosage may be required. **Not recommended for use in children.**

  Analgesia in opioid-naive clients.
  Adults, initial: 5–15 mg q 4–6 hr, as needed for pain. Titrate dose based on client response to the initial dose of IR product. To prevent recurrence of pain, use an around-the-clock regimen for those with chronic pain.

NURSING CONSIDERATIONS
⬩ Do not confuse Roxicodone (oxycodone alone) with Roxicet (oxycodone/acetaminophen combination).

ADMINISTRATION/STORAGE
1. Give around-the-clock dosing with chronic pain. For control of severe chronic pain, give immediate-release products on a regularly scheduled basis, q 4–6 hr at the lowest dose level that will provide adequate analgesia.

---

2. It is critical to individualize the dosing regimen taking into account the client's prior analgesic treatment. Attention must be given to: the daily dose, potency, and characteristics of a pure agonist or mixed agonist/antagonist the client has taken previously; the reliability of the relative potency estimate to calculate the dose of oxycodone required; the degree of opioid tolerance; the general condition and medical status of the client; and, the balance between pain control and side effects.

3. When converting from a fixed-ratio opioid/nonopioid regimen, determine whether or not to continue the nonopioid drug. If the nonopioid drug is to be discontinued, it may be necessary to titrate the dose of immediate-release tablets in response to the level of analgesia and side effects experienced. If the nonpiod drug is to be continued, base the oxycodone starting dose on the most recent dose of opioid as a baseline.

4. If taking opiates prior to taking immediate-release oxycodone, factor the potency of the prior opiate into the selection of the total daily dose of oxycodone.

5. Continuous evaluation of those receiving immediate-release or controlled-release oxycodone is required. Supplemental doses for breakthrough or incident pain and titration of the total daily dose may be required, especially in those with rapidly changing disease states.

6. When client no longer requires therapy with immediate-release or controlled-release tablets, gradually discontinue over time to prevent development of withdrawal symptoms. Generally decrease therapy by 25–50% per day and monitor carefully for signs of withdrawal. If withdrawal symptoms develop, raise the dose to the previous level and titrate down more slowly.

7. For controlled-release tablets, swallow whole; do not break, chew, or crush. Controlled-release tablets are intended for moderate to severe pain when a continuous, around-the-clock analgesic is needed for an extended period of time.

8. For controlled-release tablets, the dosing regimen must be individualized based on prior opioid and nonopioid drug treatment, as well as the general condition and medical status of the client.

9. Follow manufacturer's guidelines carefully for conversion from other opiates.

10. Controlled-release tablets, 80 mg, are for use only in opioid-tolerant clients requiring daily oxycodone equivalent dosages of 160 mg or more for the 80 mg tablets.

11. Oral concentrate solutions (ETH-Oxydose, OxyFAST, and Roxicodone) are highly concentrated solutions. Care must be taken in prescribing and dispensing this solution strength. Fill dropper to the level of the prescribed dose (1 mL = 20 mg; 0.75 mL = 15 mg; 0.5 mL = 10 mg; and, 0.25 mL = 5 mg). Add the dose to approximately 30 mL (1 fl. oz) or more of juice or other liquid. May also be added to applesauce, pudding, or other semi-solid foods. Use the drug-food mixture immediately; do not store for future use.

12. Store from 15–30°C (59–86°F). Discard open bottles of oral solution after 90 days.

ASSESSMENT

1. List reasons for therapy; onset, location, duration of pain, ROM, characteristics of S&S.

2. Use a pain-rating scale to rate pain levels. Note other agents trialed and the outcome.

3. Note ability to function and perform daily activities. Review x-rays, CT/MRIs and hx.

4. Assess carefully for drug seeking behaviors: visits near end of office hours, not making appointments for full exam, emergency calls—severe pain, repeated 'loss' or accidental destruction of drugs. They often doctor shop for multiple prescriptions.

5. Those with severe chronic pain deserve to be medicated and pain controlled appropriately; use opiods accordingly and in doses strong enough

---

Bold Italic = life threatening side effect   ■ = black box warning   ♣ = Available in Canada

to control their pain. Have client keep record of 'break thru pain' so that dosage can be adjusted accordingly; and/or break thru medication provided.

CLIENT/FAMILY TEACHING

1. Take medication with food to minimize GI upset.

2. Swallow controlled-release tablets whole. Ingesting broken, crushed, or chewed extended-release tablets may lead to rapid release/absorption and possibility of toxic effects.

3. Use caution; do not perform activities that require mental alertness. Avoid alcohol in any form.

4. May cause constipation, N&V, dry mouth, and physical dependence (withdrawal S&S include N&V, cramps, fever, fainting and anorexia); report.

5. Do not share medications; store in a safe, protected location. Drug has a high abuse potential. Tolerance may develop; report loss of effectiveness.

6. The extended-release 80 mg tablets should not be used in anyone not currently prescribed opioids. This tablet strength may cause fatal respiratory depression/death.

OUTCOMES/EVALUATE

Relief/control of pain

Oxytocin, parenteral

(ox-eh-**TOE**-sin)

CLASSIFICATION(S):

Oxytocic drug

PREGNANCY CATEGORY: X

Rx: Pitocin, Syntocinon.

USES

(1) *Antepartum:* Induction or stimulation of labor at term. To overcome true primary or secondary uterine inertia. Induction of labor with oxytocin is indicated only under certain *specific* conditions and is not usual because serious toxic effects can occur. Oxytocin is indicated:

• For uterine inertia.

• For induction of labor in cases of erythroblastosis fetalis, maternal diabetes mellitus, preeclampsia, and eclampsia.

• For induction of labor after premature rupture of membranes in last month of pregnancy when labor fails to develop spontaneously within 12 hr.

• To hasten uterine involution.

• To complete inevitable abortions after the 20th week of pregnancy.

(2) *Postpartum:* Produce uterine contractions during the third stage of labor and to control postpartum bleeding or hemorrhage.

ACTION/KINETICS

Action

Acts on smooth muscle of the uterus to stimulate contractions; response depends on the uterine threshold of excitability. Is selective for the uterus, especially toward the end of pregnancy, during labor, and immediately following delivery. Oxytocin stimulates rhythmic contractions of the uterus, increases the frequency of existing contractions, and raises the tone of uterine musculature.

Pharmacokinetics

Onset, IV: Immediate; **Duration:** Within 1 hr after infusion stopped. **IM:** 3–5 min; **Duration:** 2–3 hr. **t½:** 1–6 min. Plasma clearance occurs mainly by the kidney and liver; only small amounts excreted unchanged in the urine.

CONTRAINDICATIONS

Hypersensitivity to drug. Significant cephalopelvic disproportion; unfavorable fetal positions or presentations that are undeliverable without conversion prior to delivery. In obstetric emergencies where the benefit-to-risk ratio for either the mother or fetus favors surgical intervention. Fetal distress where delivery is not imminent, prolonged use in uterine inertia or severe toxemia, hypertonic or hyperactive uterine patterns, when adequate uterine activity does not achieve satisfactory progress. Induction of augmentation of labor where vaginal delivery is contraindicated, including invasive cervical cancer, cord presentation or prolapse, total placenta previa and vasa previa, active herpes genitalis. Also, predisposition to thromboplastin and amniotic fluid embolism (dead fetus, abruptio placentae), history of previous traumatic deliveries, or women with four or more deliveries. Never give oxytocin IV undiluted or in high concentrations.

SPECIAL CONCERNS

■ Oxytocin is indicated for the medical rather than elective induction of labor. Data and information are not available to define the benefit-to-risk consideration for using oxytocin for elective induction.■

SIDE EFFECTS

Most Common

When used in the mother: N&V, cramping, stomach pain, headache, dizziness.

Mother: CV: Cardiac arrhythmia, hypertensive episodes, PVCs. **GI:** N&V, stomach pain, cramping. **CNS:** Headache, dizziness. **GU:** Pelvic hematoma, postpartum hemorrhage. Rupture of the uterus, spasm, tetanic contraction, uterine hypertonicity may occur due to excessive dosage or hypersensitivity to the drug. **Miscellaneous: *Anaphylaxis, fatal afibrinogenemia, subarachnoid hemorrhage, severe water intoxication with seizures, coma, death.***

Fetus: CV: Bradycardia, PVCs, other arrhythmias. **CNS:** Permanent CNS or brain damage, *neonatal seizures*. **Miscellaneous: *Fetal death,*** low Apgar scores at 5 min, neonatal jaundice, neonatal retinal hemorrhage.

OD OVERDOSE MANAGEMENT

Symptoms: Hyperstimulation of the uterus resulting in hypertonic or tetanic contractions. Or, a resting tone of 15–20 cm water between contractions can result in uterine rupture, cervical and vaginal lacerations, tumultuous labor, uteroplacental hypoperfusion, ***postpartum hemorrhage***, and a variable deceleration of fetal heart rate, fetal hypoxia, hypercapnia, or ***death***. Water intoxication with seizures can occur if large doses (40–50 mL/min) of the drug are infused for long periods of time. *Treatment:* Discontinue the drug and restrict fluid intake. Start diuresis and give a

hypertonic saline solution IV. Correct electrolyte imbalance and control seizures with a barbiturate. If the client is comatose, provide special nursing care.

DRUG INTERACTIONS

Sympathomimetic amines / Severe hypertension and possible stroke
Vasoconstrictors/Caudal block anesthesia / Severe hypertension possible

HOW SUPPLIED

Injection: 10 units/mL.

DOSAGE

• **IV INFUSION (DRIP METHOD)**

Induction or stimulation of labor.

Initial: 0.5–2 milliunits/min. Increase dose gradually in increments of no more than 1–2 milliunits/min at 30–60 min intervals until a contraction pattern has been established that is similar to normal labor. Rates exceeding 9–10 milliunits/min are rarely required.

Control of postpartum bleeding.

Add 10–40 units (maximum of 40 units) to 1,000 mL of a nonhydrating diluent and run at a rate needed to control uterine atony.

Treatment of incomplete or inevitable abortion.

Infuse 10 units of oxytocin with 500 mL physiological saline solution or D5W in physiological saline infused at a rate of 10–20 milliunits (20–40 drops/min). Do not exceed 30 units in a 12-hr period due to the risk of water intoxication.

• **IM**

Control of postpartum bleeding.

Give 10 units after delivery of the placenta.

NURSING CONSIDERATIONS

℗ Do not confuse Pitocin (oxytocin) with Pitressin (vasopressin). Do not confuse oxytocin with oxyContin (a narcotic analgesic).

ADMINISTRATION/STORAGE

IV 1. To reconstitute add 1 mL (10 units) to 1,000 mL of 0.9% aqueous NaCl or Ringer's lactate. Solution contains 10 milliunits/mL (0.01 units/mL). 2. Use Y-tubing system, with one bottle containing IV solution and oxytocin, and the other containing only the IV solution. This allows for the discontinuation of the drug while maintaining the

---

Bold Italic = life threatening side effect   ■ = black box warning   ✦ = Available in Canada

patency of the vein when it is decided to change to the drug-free infusion bottle. Use a constant infusion pump to control the rate of infusion accurately.

3. Oxytocin is rapidly broken down by sodium bisulfite. Have Mg sulfate immediately available to relax the uterus in case of tetanic uterine contractions.

4. Have the provider immediately available during drug administration.

ASSESSMENT

1. Note reasons for therapy, onset, characteristics of S&S. Note any sensitivity to drug.

2. Determine fetal maturity (size), pelvic adequacy, fetal presentation/position and lack of complications prior to initiating drug therapy.

3. Provide continuous observation of client checking for dilation, resting uterine tone, characteristics of uterine contractions, e.g., time, duration and frequency. Record maternal/fetal HRs; intrauterine pressures. Assess for any distress.

4. Carefully review history and medical conditions; some may preclude oxytocin therapy.

INTERVENTIONS

For induction and stimulation of labor and/or oxytocin challenge test:

1. Before initiating therapy, inform client of rationale for using oxytocic agents and reassure that this procedure is not unusual. Explain drug will induce contractions that may feel like menstrual cramps initially but can be very painful; analgesics may be given as needed.

2. Remain with client during induction period and throughout the stimulation of labor. Titrate oxytocin to establish uterine contractions that are similar to normal labor; continuously monitor rate and strength of contractions. Monitor VS, check I&O q 15 min.

3. Note resting uterine tone and assess contractions for frequency, duration, and strength. Monitor fetal HR and rhythm at least every 10 min. Document and immediately report any alterations.

4. Prevent uterine rupture and fetal damage by clamping off IV oxytocin, starting medication-free IV fluids, turn-

ing client on left side to prevent fetal anoxia, providing oxygen, and reporting when the following events occur:

- If contractions occur more frequently than every 2 min and last longer than 60–90 sec with no period of uterine relaxation in between.
- If the contractions are excessively strong and/or exceed 50–65 mm Hg or if they stop.
- If resting uterine tone is 15–20 mm Hg or more.
- If the fetal HR indicates bradycardia, tachycardia, or irregularities of rhythm.

5. The fetal heart rate, resting uterine tone, and the frequency, duration, and force of contractions should be monitored.

6. The oxytocin infusion should be discontinued immediately in the event of uterine hyperactivity or fetal distress. Give oxygen to the mother.

7. Assess for water intoxication following prolonged administration; drug has intrinsic antidiuretic effect, acting to increase water reabsorption from the glomerular filtrate. Monitor I&O and serum electrolytes closely. Observe for lethargy, confusion, and stupor. Note any neuromuscular hyperexcitability with increased reflexes and muscular twitching. Report symptoms immediately; convulsions and coma may occur if left untreated. Mg sulfate should be readily available for IV administration. Stop infusion and report any uterine hyperactivity or fetal distress. **During the fourth stage of labor when oxytocin is administered for prevention or control of hemorrhage:**

1. Describe location, size, and firmness of the uterus. Report if uterus is displaced or boggy; follow designated facility protocol.

2. In clients with spinal anesthesia, visually inspect for any evidence of bleeding. Sensation is diminished and hemorrhage may occur insidiously.

3. Note amount and color of lochia. Report bright red lochia, excessive bleeding, or the passage of clots.

4. Monitor VS until stable. Closely monitor I&O. Observe for S&S of water intox-

O

ication; document and report immediately.

CLIENT/FAMILY TEACHING
1. Drug is a uterine stimulant. It works by causing uterine contractions by changing calcium concentrations in the uterine muscle cells.
2. Cramps will feel like strong menstrual cramps but will continue to increase in intensity. Report increased blood/

fluid loss, severe headaches, fever, foul-smelling drainage, or severe abdominal cramps.
3. Review potential adverse effects associated with this therapy.

OUTCOMES/EVALUATE
• Induction of labor with effective uterine contractions
• ↑ Uterine tone with ↓ postpartum bleeding

Paclitaxel
(**PACK**-lih-**tax**-el)

CLASSIFICATION(S):
Antineoplastic, miscellaneous
PREGNANCY CATEGORY: D
Rx: Abraxane, Onxol, Taxol.

SEE ALSO *ANTINEOPLASTIC AGENTS.*

USES
Abraxane. Breast cancer after failure of combination chemotherapy (that should have included an anthracycline, unless contraindicated) for metastatic disease or relapse within 6 months of adjuvant chemotherapy. **Onxol.** (1) Advanced carcinoma of the ovary as subsequent therapy. (2) Breast cancer after failure of combination chemotherapy for metastases (including use of an anthracycline unless contraindicated) or relapse within 6 months of adjuvant chemotherapy. **Taxol.** (1) Advanced carcinoma of the ovary as first-line or subsequent therapy. When used as first-line therapy, combine with cisplatin. (2) Adjuvant treatment of node-positive breast cancer given sequentially to doxorubicin-containing combination therapy. (3) Treatment of breast cancer after failure of combination chemotherapy (including use of an anthracycline unless contraindicated) for metastases or relapse within 6 months of adjuvant chemotherapy. (4) Combined with cis-

platin for first-line treatment of non-small cell lung cancer in those not candidates for potentially curative surgery or radiation therapy. (5) Second-line therapy for AIDS-related Kaposi's sarcoma. *Investigational:* Alone or in combination with other chemotherapeutic drugs for advanced head and neck cancer, small-cell lung cancer, adenocarcinoma of the upper GI tract, hormone-refractory prostate cancer, non-Hodgkin's lymphoma, transitional cell carcinoma of the urothelium, pancreatic cancer, polycystic kidney disease.

ACTION/KINETICS
Action
Naturally occurring antineoplastic agent that promotes the assembly of microtubules from tubulin dimers and stabilizes microtubules by preventing depolymerization. The stabilization results in the inhibition of the normal dynamic reorganization of the microtubule network that is required for vital interphase and mitotic cellular functions. Also induces abnormal "bundles" of microtubules throughout the cell cycle and multiple esters of microtubules during mitosis.

Pharmacokinetics
Following IV administration, there is a biphasic decline in plasma levels. The initial rapid decline is due to distribution to the peripheral compartment and significant elimination, whereas the second phase is due, in part, to a slow efflux of the drug from the peripheral

---

compartment. Both forms (injection and albumin-bound) are metabolized in the liver by CYP2C8 (major) and CYP3A4 (minor). About 70% is excreted through the feces and 14% (including a small amount of unchanged drug) excreted in the urine. The clearance of protein-bound paclitaxel particles is larger (43%) than the clearance of paclitaxel injection.

CONTRAINDICATIONS

Onxol/Taxol: Hypersensitivity to paclitaxel, in those with a hypersensitivity to products containing polyoxymethylated castor oil (Cremophor EL), clients with solid tumors when baseline neutrophil counts are below 1,500 cells/mm^3, and those with AIDS-related Kaposi's sarcoma with baseline neutrophil counts below 1,000 cells/mm^3. **Abraxane:** Use in clients who have baseline neutrophil counts of less than 1,500 cells/mm^3. Lactation (all products).

SPECIAL CONCERNS

■ (1) Give under the supervision of a physician experienced in the use of cancer chemotherapeutic drugs. Appropriate management of complications is possible only when adequate diagnostic and treatment facilities are readily available. (2) Onxol/Taxol. Do not give paclitaxel therapy to those with solid tumors who have baseline neutrophil counts of less than 1,500 cells/mm^3, and do not give to clients with AIDS-related Kaposi sarcoma if the baseline neutrophil count is less than 1,000 cells/mm^3. In order to monitor the occurrence of bone marrow suppression, primarily neutropenia, which may be severe and result in infection, perform frequent peripheral blood cell counts on all clients receiving paclitaxel. (3) Anaphylaxis and severe hypersensitivity reactions characterized by dyspnea and hypotension requiring treatment, angioedema, and generalized urticaria have occurred in 2–4% of clients receiving paclitaxel in clinical trials. Fatal reactions have occurred in clients despite premedication. Pretreat all clients with corticosteroids, diphenhydramine, and H$_2$ antagonists to prevent such reactions. Do not readminister to those who experience severe hypersensitivity reactions. (4) Abraxane. Do not give paclitaxel to those with metastatic breast cancer who have baseline neutrophil counts of less than 1,500 cells/mm^3. In order to monitor the occurrence of bone marrow suppression (primarily neutropenia) which may be severe and result in infection, perform frequent peripheral blood cell counts on all who receive the drug. (5) An albumin form of paclitaxel may substantially affect a drug's functional properties relative to those of drug in solution. Do not substitute for or use with other paclitaxel formulations.■ Use with caution in clients with moderate to severe impaired hepatic function. Safety and efficacy have not been determined in children.

SIDE EFFECTS

Most Common

Alopecia, peripheral neuropathy, N&V, mucositis, diarrhea, anemia, leukopenia, neutropenia, hypersensitivity, abnormal ECG, myalgia/arthralgia, infections.

Onxol/Taxol. GI: N&V, diarrhea, mucositis. Rarely, paralytic ileus, intestinal obstruction, **intestinal perforation, pancreatitis,** ischemic colitis, neutropenic enterocolitis, and dehydration. **CNS:** Peripheral neuropathy, neurotoxicity, neuromotor/sensory toxicity, ataxia, **tonic-clonic seizures** (rare), neuroencephalopathy, syncope. **Hematologic:** Leukopenia, neutropenia, febrile neutropenia, anemia hemoglobin, thrombocytopenia, bleeding, packed cell transfusions, platelet transfusions. **CV:** Abnormal ECG (including nonspecific repolarization abnormalities, sinus tachycardia, premature beats), bradycardia, hypotension, significant CV events (e.g., syncope, rhythm abnormalities, hypertension, venous thrombosis), bradycardia, atrial fibrillation, SVT, **CHF, MI** (rare). **Dermatologic:** Alopecia, transient skin changes, changes in nail pigmentation or discoloration of nail bed. **Musculoskeletal:** Myalgia, arthralgia. **Respiratory:** Rarely, interstitial pneumonia, **lung fibrosis, pulmonary embolism. GU:** Renal insufficiency. **Ophthalmic:** Optic nerve or visual disturbances (e.g., scintillating scotomata), conjunctivitis, increased lacrimation. **Hypersensitivity:** Severe symptoms, including *anaphylaxis*, usually occur during the first hour of therapy and occur during both the first or second course of therapy despite premedication. Severe symptoms include dyspnea, *angioedema*, hypotension, or generalized urticaria all of which require immediate cessation of the drug and aggressive treatment therapy. Symptoms not requiring treatment include milder dyspnea, flushing, skin reactions, hypotension, or tachycardia. **Infections:** Cytomegalovirus, herpes simplex, *Mycobacterium avium intracellulare* infection, *Pneumocystis carinii* infection, esophageal candidiasis, cryptosporidiosis, cryptococcal meningitis. Also, infections of the urinary tract, GI tract (e.g., peritonitis) and upper respiratory tract (e.g., pneumonia), as well as *sepsis due to neutropenia.* **Body as a whole:** Asthenia, malaise, edema, fever without infection. **Injection site reaction:** Erythema, extravasation, tenderness, skin discoloration, swelling. Rarely, phlebitis, cellulitis, induration, skin exfoliation, necrosis, fibrosis. **Accidental inhalation of injection:** Burning eyes, chest pain, dyspnea, nausea, sore throat; tingling, burning, and redness following topical exposure. **Abraxane. GI:** N&V, diarrhea, mucositis. Rarely, intestinal obstruction, *intestinal perforation, pancreatitis,* neutropenic enterocolitis, ischemic colitis, *hepatic necrosis, hepatic encephalopathy leading to death.* **CNS:** Sensory neuropathy. **CV:** Abnormal ECG (including nonspecific repolarization abnormalities, sinus tachycardia, premature beats), hypotension, severe CV events (*cardiac arrest,* chest pain, edema, hypertension, *pulmonary emboli, pulmonary thromboembolism,* SVT, *thrombosis*), bradycardia. Rarely, *cardiac ischemia/infarction.* **Hematologic:** Neutropenia, anemia hemoglobin, thrombocytopenia, febrile neutropenia, bleeding. **Dermatologic:** Alopecia, changes in nail pigmentation or discoloration of nail bed, skin abnormalities related to radiation recall, *toxic epidermal necrolysis.* **Musculoskeletal:** Arthralgia, myalgia. **Respiratory:** Dyspnea, cough. Rarely, pneumothorax. **Ophthalmic:** Conjunctivitis, increased lacrimation, ocular and visual disturbances (e.g., keratitis, blurred vision). **Infections:** Oral candidiasis, respiratory tract infections, pneumonia. **Body as a whole:** Asthenia, fluid retention/edema, infections, injection site reaction. **Miscellaneous:** Ototoxicity (hearing loss, tinnitus).

LABORATORY TEST CONSIDERATIONS
↑ Bilirubin, alkaline phosphatase, ALT, AST, creatinine.

OD **OVERDOSE MANAGEMENT**
Symptoms: **Bone marrow suppression,** peripheral neurotoxicity, mucositis. Accidental inhalation may cause dyspnea, chest pain, burning eyes, sore throat, and nausea. *Treatment:* Treat symptomatically.

DRUG INTERACTIONS
Carbamazepine / ↑ Paclitaxel metabolism by CYP3A4
Cisplatin / More profound myelosuppression when paclitaxel was given after cisplatin than when paclitaxel was given before cisplatin R/T a ⅓ decrease in paclitaxel clearance
Cyclosporine / ↓ Paclitaxel metabolism R/T inhibition of CYP3A4
Diazepam / ↓ Paclitaxel metabolism R/T inhibition of CYP2C8
Doxorubicin / ↑ Levels of doxorubicin and doxorubicinol; also, ↓ paclitaxel metabolism R/T inhibition of CYP2C8 and CYP3A4
Ethinyl estradiol / ↓ Paclitaxel metabolism R/T inhibition of CYP2C8
Felodipine / ↓ Paclitaxel metabolism R/T inhibition of CYP2C8
Gemcitabine / ↓ Gemcitabine clearance and volume distribution → ↑ gemcitabine levels
Ketoconazole / ↓ Paclitaxel metabolism R/T inhibition of CYP2C8 and CYP3A4
Midazolam / ↓ Paclitaxel metabolism R/T inhibition of CYP2C8
Phenobarbital / ↑ Paclitaxel metabolism by CYP3A4
Retinoic acid / ↓ Paclitaxel metabolism R/T inhibition of CYP2C8
Troleandomycin / ↓ Paclitaxel metabo-

lizing enzymes R/T inhibition of drug metabolism

HOW SUPPLIED
Onxol, Taxol: *Injection:* 6 mg/mL.
Abraxane: *Powder for Injection, Lyophilized:* 100 mg (albumin-bound).

DOSAGE

TAXOL

• IV INFUSION
Ovarian cancer.

In clients untreated previously for ovarian cancer, use one of the following regimens given every three weeks: (1) **Adults:** Paclitaxel, 175 mg/m^2 given IV over 3 hr followed by cisplatin, 75 mg/m^2. (2) **Adults:** Paclitaxel, 135 mg/m^2 IV over 24 hr followed by cisplatin, 75 mg/m^2. In clients previously treated with chemotherapy for ovarian cancer, the recommended regimen is paclitaxel, either 135 mg/m^2 or 175 mg/m^2, IV over 3 hr every 3 weeks.

Adjuvant treatment of node-positive breast cancer.

Adults: 175 mg/m^2 given IV over 3 hr q 3 weeks for 4 courses given sequentially to doxorubicin-containing combination therapy. After failure of initial chemotherapy for metastatic disease or relapse within 6 months of adjuvant chemotherapy, paclitaxel, 175 mg/m^2, given IV over 3 hr q 3 weeks has been effective.

Non-small cell lung carcinoma.

135 mg/m^2 over 24 hr followed by cisplatin, 75 mg/m^2, q 3 weeks. Do not repeat courses of Taxol until the neutrophil count is at least 1,500 cells/mm^3 and the platelet count is at least 100,000 cells/mm^3.

AIDS-related Kaposi's sarcoma.

135 mg/m^2 given IV over 3 hr q 3 weeks or 100 mg/m^2 given IV over 3 hr q 2 weeks. The former regimen is more toxic than the latter.

ONXOL

• IV INFUSION
Ovarian cancer.

In clients previously treated with chemotherapy for ovarian cancer, use the following regimen: 135 mg/m^2 or 175 mg/m^2 over 3 hr q 3 weeks.

Breast cancer.

After failure of initial chemotherapy for metastatic disease or relapse within 6 months of adjuvant chemotherapy: 175 mg/m^2 over 3 hr q 3 weeks. Repeat courses; do not give paclitaxel until the neutrophil count is at least 1,500 cells/mm^3 and the platelet count is at least 100,000 cells/mm^3.

ABRAXANE

• IV INFUSION
Metastatic breast cancer or relapse.

After failure of combination chemotherapy for metastatic breast cancer or relapse within 6 months of adjuvant chemotherapy: 260 mg/m^2 of paclitaxel protein-bound particles given over 30 min q 3 weeks.

NURSING CONSIDERATIONS

@ Do not confuse paclitaxel with paroxetine (an antidepressant) or Paxil (trade name for paroxetine). Also, do not confuse Taxol with Taxotere (an antineoplastic) or Paxil.

ADMINISTRATION/STORAGE
IV 1. Do not allow the undiluted concentrate to come in contact with plasticized PVC equipment or devices used to prepare solutions for infusion.

2. Premedicate before use to prevent severe hypersensitivity reactions. Premedication may consist of oral dexamethasone, 20 mg, given 12 and 6 hr before paclitaxel; diphenhydramine (or equivalent), 50 mg IV, 30–60 min before; and cimetidine, 300 mg IV, or ranitidine, 50 mg IV, 30–60 min before paclitaxel.

3. In those with advanced HIV disease, reduce dose of dexamethasone to 10 mg PO; initiate or repeat treatment only if neutrophil count is 1,000 cells/mm^3 or greater; reduce the dose of subsequent courses of paclitaxel 20% for clients who experience severe neutropenia (neutrophil <500 cells/mm^3 for a week or longer); begin concomitant hematopoietic growth factor as needed.

4. Dilute paclitaxel concentrate prior to infusion in 0.9% NSS, D5W, D5W/0.9% NaCl, or D5W/RL to a final concentration of 0.3–1.2 mg/mL. Diluted solutions are stable for up to 24 hr at room temperature.

P

 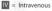

5. Paclitaxel protein-bound particles (Abraxane) is suppled as a sterile lyophilized powder. To reconstitute:

- Asceptically reconstitute each vial by injecting 20 mL of 0.9% NaCl injection.
- Slowly inject the 20 mL of 0.9% NaCl injection over a minimum of 1 min, using sterile syringe to direct solution flow onto inside wall of the vial.
- Do not inject NaCl injection directly onto lyophilized cake; will result in foaming.
- Once injection complete, allow the vial to sit for a minimum of 5 min to ensure proper wetting of lyophilized cake/powder.
- Gently swirl/invert the vial slowly for at least 2 min until complete dissolution of any cake/powder occurs. Avoid generation of foam.
- If foaming or clumping occurs, stand solution for at least 15 min until foam subsides.
- Each mL of the reconstituted formulation will contain paclitaxel, 5 mg/mL.
- The reconstituted product should be milky and homogenous without visible particulates. If particulates or settling are visible, gently invert vial again to ensure complete resuspension prior to use.

6. Administer Taxol or Onxol through an in-line filter with a microporous membrane not greater than 0.22 μm. Use of filter devices, such as IVEX-2 filters that incorporate short inlet and outlet PVC-coated tubing, has not resulted in significant leaching of DEHP.

7. Do not use the Chemo Dispensing Pin device or similar devices with spikes with vials of paclitaxel because they can cause the stopper to collapse, resulting in loss of sterile integrity of the paclitaxel solution.

8. The dilutions may show haziness, which is due to the formulation vehicle. No significant loss of potency has been noted following simulated delivery of the solution through IV tubing containing an in-line (0.22-μm) filter.

9. To minimize client exposure to the plasticizer DHEP which may be leached from PVC infusion bags or sets, store diluted paclitaxel solutions in bottles (glass, polypropylene) or plastic bags (polypropylene, polyolefin) and administer through polyethylene-lined administration sets.

10. Unopened vials of the concentrate are stable when stored under refrigeration, protected from light, in the original package.

11. Do not undertake repeat courses until the neutrophil count is at least 1,500 cells/mm^3 and the platelet count is at least 100,000 cells/mm^3. When using Taxol or Onxol, reduce dose by 20% for subsequent courses in those who experience a neutrophil count <500 cells/mm^3 for 1 week or more or if there is severe peripheral neuropathy during therapy.

12. When using Abraxane, reduce the dose to 220 mg/m^2 for subsequent doses if the neutrophil count is <500 cells/mm^3 for 1 week or longer or severe sensory neuropathy has occurred. For recurrence of severe neutropenia or severe sensory neuropathy, make an additional dose reduction to 180 mg/m^2. For grade 3 sensory neuropathy, hold treatment until resolution to grade 1 or 2, followed by a dose reduction for all subsequent courses of paclitaxel protein-bound particles.

13. Use gloves when handling drug. If solution comes in contact with the skin, wash immediately and thoroughly with soap and water. If the drug comes in contact with mucous membranes, thoroughly flush the membranes with water. Due to possible extravasation, monitor infusion site closely for possible infiltration.

14. *Treatment of Hypersensitivity Reactions:* Stop infusion and treat with bronchodilators (such as albuterol or theophylline), epinephrine, antihistamines, and corticosteroids.

15. Store Onxol/Taxol between 20–25°C (68–77°F) in the original package. Upon refrigeration, components in the vial may precipitate but will redissolve upon reaching room temperature with little or no agitation. If the solution remains cloudy or if an insoluble precipi-

tate is noted, discard the vial. Solutions for infusion prepared as recommended are stable at ambient temperature (25°C, 77°F) and lighting conditions for up to 27 hr.

16. Unopened vials of Abraxane are stable when stored between 20–25°C (68–77°F) in the original package. Use reconstituted Abraxane immediately, although it may be refrigerated at 2–8°C (36–46°F) for a maximum of 8 hr. Ensure complete resuspension by mild agitation before use. Discard reconstituted suspension if precipitates are observed.

ASSESSMENT

1. Note tumor type, location, previous therapy (include agents, dosage, duration), esp. radiation; may enhance myelosuppressive drug effects. Check if client has received this drug and response.

2. Give pretreatment meds. If S&S of severe hypersensitivity reaction (dyspnea, hypotension, angioedema, generalized urticaria) appear, interrupt infusion and report. These reactions usually occur during first hour and despite premedication. Document any severe reaction so that client is *NOT* rechallenged with paclitaxel.

3. Monitor neurologic status, VS, I&O, CBC, renal, LFTs regularly; ensure neutrophil count is 1,500 cells/mm^3 before giving drug (with AIDS-related Kaposi's sarcoma with baseline neutrophil counts >1,000 cells/mm^3) and platelet count at least 100,000 cells/mm^3. Neutrophil nadir: 11 days; platelet nadir 8–9 days.

CLIENT/FAMILY TEACHING

1. Drug is administered every 2–3 weeks IV to inhibit/control rapid cell division of abnormal cells. Anticipate premedication with other agents to prevent hypersensitivity reactions.

2. Anticipate hair loss; should regrow. Avoid crowds and those with infections during therapy.

3. Joint pain and discomfort may be experienced 2–3 days after therapy but should resolve in several days.

4. Report any severe N&V, fever, chills, sore throat, infection, abnormal bruising/bleeding, or numbness and tingling in fingers/toes.

5. Avoid alcohol, aspirin, and NSAIDs.

6. Use reliable contraception during and for 4 months following therapy.

OUTCOMES/EVALUATE

↓ Tumor size and spread

Palifermin   IV

(pal-ee-**FER**-min)

CLASSIFICATION(S):
Keratinocyte growth factor
PREGNANCY CATEGORY: C
Rx: Kepivance.

USES

Decrease the incidence and duration of severe oral mucositis in clients with hematologic malignancies who are receiving myelotoxic therapy requiring hematopoietic stem cell support.

ACTION/KINETICS

Action

Palifermin is a human keratinocyte growth factor (KGF) produced by recombinant DNA technology. KGF is an endogenous protein that binds to the KGF receptor that results in proliferation, differentiation, and migration of epithelial cells, thus decreasing the incidence of mucositis. The KGF receptor is found on epithelial cells in many tissues including the tongue, buccal mucosa, esophagus, stomach, intestine, salivary gland, lung, liver, pancreas, kidney, bladder, mammary gland, skin, and the lens of the eye.

Pharmacokinetics

After IV administration, plasma levels declined rapidly in the first 30 min after dosing. This was followed by a slight increase or plateau at about 1–4 hr and then a terminal decline phase followed. **t½, terminal:** 3.3–5.7 hr in both cancer clients and healthy subjects.

CONTRAINDICATIONS

Hypersensitivity to *E. coli-* derived proteins, palifermin, or any other component of the product. Use within 24 hr before, during infusion of, or within 24

P

hr after administration of myelotoxic chemotherapy.

SPECIAL CONCERNS

Safety and efficacy have not been determined to treat clients with nonhematologic malignancies or in pediatric clients. Use with caution during lactation.

SIDE EFFECTS

Most Common

Skin rash, pruritus, erythema, edema, fever.

GI: Alteration of taste, tongue discoloration, tongue thickening, altered taste. **Dermatologic:** Skin rash, edema, erythema, pruritus. **CNS:** Dysesthesia, including hyperesthesia, hypesthesia, and paresthesia, usually in the perioral region. **CV:** Hypertension. **Musculoskeletal:** Arthralgia. **Body as a whole:** Fever, pain, possible immunogenicity.

LABORATORY TEST CONSIDERATIONS

↑ Serum amylase and lipase.

DRUG INTERACTIONS

Binds to heparin *in vitro*

HOW SUPPLIED

Powder for Injection: 6.25 mg.

DOSAGE

- **IV BOLUS**

  Severe oral mucositis.

60 mcg/kg/day given 3 consecutive days before and 3 consecutive days after myelotoxic therapy for a total of 6 doses. Give the third dose 24–48 hr before myelotoxic therapy. Give the first postmyelotoxic dose after, but on the same day of, hematopoietic stem cell infusion and at least 4 days after the most recent dose of palifermin.

NURSING CONSIDERATIONS

ADMINISTRATION/STORAGE

1. To reconstitute, slowly inject 1.2 mL of sterile water for injection, using aseptic technique, to yield a final concentration of 5 mg/mL. Gently swirl contents during dissolution. Do not shake or vigorously agitate the vial. Dissolution usually takes <3 min.

2. Do not filter reconstituted solution during preparation or administration. The reconstituted solution should be clear and colorless. Visually inspect for discoloration and particulate matter before use; do not administer if observed.

3. The product contains no preservative. After reconstitution, use immediately. If not used immediately, the reconstituted solution may be stored refrigerated (but not frozen) in its carton for up to 24 hr. Prior to injection, allow to reach room temperature for a maximum of 1 hr; protect from light. Discard drug left at room temperature for more than 1 hr.

4. Give by IV bolus injection. If heparin is used to maintain an IV line, use saline to rinse the line prior to and after palifermin administration as the drug has been shown to bind to heparin in vitro.

5. Store palifermin lyophilized powder in its carton and refrigerate at 2–8°C (36–46°F). Protect from light. Keep vials in the pack until use.

ASSESSMENT

1. Note reasons for therapy, timing of myelotoxic chemotherapy to ensure dosing is done accurately: 3 days before and 3 days after therapy.

2. List drugs prescribed to ensure none interact, follow guidelines to ensure heparin is cleared from tubing before and after administration.

3. Identify any hypersensitivity to E. Coli derived products.

4. Note neurologic presentation, status of oral mucosa, VS; monitor during therapy.

5. Avoid infusing within 24 hr before, during, or 24 hr after myelotoxic chemotherapy; may increase severity/duration of oral mucositis.

CLIENT/FAMILY TEACHING

1. Drug is administered IV push 3 days before and 3 consecutive days after chemotherapy to decrease or prevent the development of mouth sores.

2. May experience skin rash, redness and swelling, itching, or numbness in the mouth, alterations in taste, thickening and discoloration of the tongue; report if evident.

3. Palifermin has only been used with hematologic malignancies; in some cell cultures and animal models there was evidence of enhanced rates of nonhe-

---

Bold Italic = life threatening side effect   ■ = black box warning   ♣ = Available in Canada

matopoietic tumor growth. Report all adverse side effects.

OUTCOMES/EVALUATE

↓ Incidence and duration of oral mucositis from myelotoxic therapy in hematologic malignancies

Paliperidone ∎
(pal-ee-**PER**-i-done)

CLASSIFICATION(S):
Antipsychotic
PREGNANCY CATEGORY: C
Rx: Invega.

USES
Acute and maintenance treatment of schizophrenia.

ACTION/KINETICS
Action Paliperidone is the major active metabolite of risperidone. The mechanism of action is unknown but the drug may act through a combination of central dopamine type 2 (D_2) and serotonin type 2 ($5HT_{2A}$) receptor antagonism. It is also an antagonist at α-1, α-2, and histamine H_1 receptors. The drug also has antiemetic effects.

Pharmacokinetics
Absolute bioavailability: 28%. **Peak plasma levels:** 24 hr. A high fat/high caloric meal increases both C_{max} and AUC. Steady state levels reached in 4-5 days. Metabolized to a limited extent by CYP2D6 and CYP3A4. **$t\frac{1}{2}$, terminal:** About 23 hr. Unchanged drug and metabolites are excreted in the urine (80%) and feces (11%).

CONTRAINDICATIONS
Hypersensitivity to paliperidone or risperidone (paliperidone is a metabolite of risperidone). Use with drugs that prolong QTc (see *Drug Interactions*), in those with congenital long QT syndrome, in those with a history of cardiac arrhythmias. Use of alcohol.

SPECIAL CONCERNS
∎ Elderly clients with dementia-related psychosis treated with atypical antipsychotic drugs are at an increased risk of death compared to placebo. Analysis of 17 placebo-controlled trials (modal duration of 10 weeks) in these subjects revealed a risk of death in the drug-treated subjects of between 1.6 to 1.7 times that seen in placebo-treated subjects. Over the course of a typical 10-week controlled trial, the rate of death in drug-treated subjects was about 4.5%, compared to a rate of about 2.6% in the placebo group. Although the causes of death were varied, most of the deaths appeared to be either cardiovascular (e.g., heart failure, sudden death) or infectious (e.g., pneumonia) in nature. Paliperidone is not approved for the treatment of clients with dementia-related psychosis.∎ Dosage adjustment may be needed in elderly clients. Use during pregnancy only if the potential benefit outweighs the potential risk to the fetus. Use with caution during lactation or when used with other CNS drugs and alcohol. Safety and efficacy have not been determined in children less than 18 years of age.

SIDE EFFECTS
Most Common
Headache, tachycardia, extrapyramidal disorder, dizziness, somnolence, akathisia, tremor, hypertonia, dry mouth, upper abdominal pain, orthostatic hypotension, bundle branch block, asthenia, fatigue.

GI: Upper abdominal pain, dry mouth, salivary hypersecretion, abdominal pain, swollen tongue, GI obstruction, dysphagia. **CNS:** Headache, dizziness, somnolence, akathisia, extrapyramidal disorder (dyskinesia, hyperkinesia), tremor, dystonia, hypertonia, Parkinsonism, tardive dyskinesia, *neuroleptic malignant syndrome* (e.g., hyperpyrexia, muscle rigidity, altered mental status, irregular pulse or BP, tachycardia, diaphoresis, cardiac dysrhythmia, acute renal failure), cognitive and motor impairment, *seizures, suicide*. **CV:** Tachycardia, BBB, sinus arrhythmia, first degree AV block, orthostatic hypotension, syncope, bradycardia, palpitations, ischemia, QTc interval prolongation, *CVA/TIA in elderly clients with dementia-related psychosis*. **GU:** Priapism. **Hematologic:** Thrombotic thrombocytopenic purpura. **Metabolic:** Hyperglycemia, di-

P

 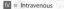

abetes mellitus. **Body as a whole:** Asthenia, fatigue, edema, weight gain (with higher doses). **Miscellaneous:** *Anaphylaxis, increased mortality in elderly clients with dementia-related psychosis,* impaired regulation of body temperature.

LABORATORY TEST CONSIDERATIONS
Hyperprolactinemia. ↑ Sensitivity with Lewy bodies.

OD OVERDOSE MANAGEMENT
Symptoms: Extrapyramidal symptoms, gait unsteadiness, drowsiness, sedation, tachycardia, hypotension, QT prolongation.
Treatment: There is no specific antidote to paliperidone. Use the following approaches:
- Institute supportive measures.
- Provide close medical supervision and monitoring until the client recovers.
- In cases of acute overdosage, establish and maintain an airway; ensure adequate oxygenation and ventilation.
- Begin CV monitoring immediately. If antiarrhythmic therapy is instituted, note that disopyramide, procainamide, and quinidine may add to QT prolongation.
- Treat hypotension and circulatory collapse with IV fluids and/or sympathomimetic agents (do not use epinephrine or dopamine since beta stimulation may worsen hypotension)
- Gastric lavage (after intubation if client is unconscious).
- Consider giving activated charcoal with a laxative.
- In cases of severe extrapyramidal symptoms, give an anticholinergic.

DRUG INTERACTIONS
Amiodarone / Prolongs QTc → possible torsade de pointes; do not use together
Chlorpromazine / Prolongs QTc → possible torsade de pointes; do not use together
Dopamine agonists / Possible antagonism of dopamine agonist effects
Gatifloxacin / Prolongs QTc → possible torsade de pointes; do not use together
Levodopa / Possible antagonism of levodopa effects
Moxifloxacin / Prolongs QTc → possible torsade de pointes; do not use together
Procainamide / Prolongs QTc → possible torsade de pointes; do not use together
Quinidine / Prolongs QTc → possible torsade de pointes; do not use together
Risperidone / Additive effects R/T paliperidone is the major active metabolite of risperidone
Sotalol / Prolongs QTc → possible torsade de pointes; do not use together
Thioridazine / Prolongs QTc → possible torsade de pointes; do not use together

HOW SUPPLIED
Tablets, Extended-Release: 3 mg, 6 mg, 9 mg.

DOSAGE ————————
- **TABLETS, EXTENDED-RELEASE**
  Schizophrenia.
Adults: 6 mg once daily given in the morning. Initial dose titration is not necessary. Some clients may benefit from doses up to 12 mg/day and others from a lower dose of 3 mg/day. Increase the dose above 6 mg/day only after clinical assessment and should occur at intervals of more than 5 days. When dose increases are indicated, small increments of 3 mg/day are recommended. **Maximum dose:** 12 mg/day.

NURSING CONSIDERATIONS

ADMINISTRATION/STORAGE
1. Incidence of side effects is dose-related.
2. For clients with C_{CR} from 50-80 mL/min, the maximum recommended dose is 6 mg once daily. For those with C_{CR} from 10–50 mL/min, the maximum recommended dose is 3 mg once daily.
3. No dosage adjustment is necessary in clients with mild-moderate hepatic impairment (Child-Pugh score of A or B). Paliperidone has not been studied in those with severe hepatic impairment.

ASSESSMENT
1. List reasons for therapy, onset, duration, characteristics of S&S, presenting behavioral manifestations, mental status. Note all drugs prescribed to ensure none interact.

Bold Italic = life threatening side effect   ■ = black box warning   ✦ = Available in Canada

2. Perform appropriate baseline assessments. Electrolyte imbalance, bradycardia, and concomitant administration with drugs that prolong the QT interval may increase risk of torsades de pointes.

3. Reduce dose with renal dysfunction; monitor liver, renal, and cardiac conditions closely.

4. Observe for altered mental status, muscle rigidity, dyskinetic movements, or overt changes in VS. Monitor for S&S of diabetes. **Not** for use with dementia-related psychosis in the elderly.

5. The antiemetic effect of risperidone may mask S&S of overdose with certain drugs or conditions such as intestinal obstruction, Reye's syndrome, brain tumor.

CLIENT/FAMILY TEACHING

1. Take with or without food; do not chew, divide, or crush the extended-release tablets.

2. Since drug is contained with a nonabsorbable shell, the tablet shell is eliminated from the body. Do not be concerned if something that looks like a tablet is noted in the stool.

3. Use caution while driving, riding a bike, or performing other tasks requiring mental alertness until tolerance determined; may cause drowsiness, impaired judgment/thinking skills.

4. Avoid sudden position changes to prevent sudden drop in BP. Rise slowly from a sitting or lying position.

5. During periods of high temperature or humidity avoid strenuous activity to prevent overheating and dehydration.

6. Do not use alcohol while taking paliperidone.

7. Report any adverse side effects or lack of response. Keep all F/U appointments to evaluate response to therapy, labs, and EKG.

OUTCOMES/EVALUATE

- Improved behavior patterns with ↓ agitation, ↓ hyperactivity, and reality orientation
- Improved concentration and self-control

Palivizumab
(**pal**-ih-**VIZ**-you-mab)

CLASSIFICATION(S):
Monoclonal antibody
PREGNANCY CATEGORY: C
Rx: Synagis.

USES
Prevention of serious lower respiratory tract disease due to RSV in pediatric clients at high risk of RSV disease. May be used (1) in children with hemodynamically significant congenital heart disease to prevent hospitalization due to RSV, (2) in infants with bronchopulmonary dysplasia, and (3) infants 35 weeks or less gestational age.

ACTION/KINETICS
Action
Humanized monoclonal antibody that exhibits neutralizing and fusion-inhibitory activity against respiratory syncytial virus (RSV), leading to a reduction in the quantity of RSV in the lower respiratory tract.

Pharmacokinetics
t½, **children:** 20 days.

CONTRAINDICATIONS
Use in adults. Pediatric clients with a history of severe reaction to palivizumab or other components of the product.

SPECIAL CONCERNS
Safety and efficacy have not been determined for treatment of established RSV disease. Rare cases of anaphylaxis have been noted following initial or re-exposure to the drug. Side effects after a sixth or greater dose are similar in character and frequency to those after the initial five doses.

SIDE EFFECTS
Most Common
N&V, fever, URTI, otitis media, rhinitis, rash, pain, hernia, pharyngitis.

Respiratory: URTI, rhinitis, pharyngitis, cough, wheezing, bronchiolitis, pneumonia, bronchitis, asthma, croup, dyspnea, sinusitis, apnea. **GI:** Diarrhea, N&V, gastroenteritis, abnormal liver function, oral monilia. **Dermatologic:** Rash, fun-

P

gal dermatitis, eczema, seborrhea. **Hypersensitivity:** Dyspnea, cyanosis, *respiratory failure*, urticaria, pruritus, angioedema, hypotonia, unresponsiveness. **Miscellaneous:** Otitis media, fever, pain, hernia, failure to thrive, nervousness, injection site reaction, conjunctivitis, viral infection, anemia, flu syndrome, allergic reactions, *anaphylaxis* (rare).

LABORATORY TEST CONSIDERATIONS
↑ AST, ALT.

HOW SUPPLIED
Injection: 100 mg/mL; *Powder for Injection, Lyophilized:* 50 mg, 100 mg.

DOSAGE
* **IM**

 Prevention of RSV disease.
Children: 15 mg/kg per month IM (preferably in the anterolateral part of the thigh) throughout the RSV season. To calculate the monthly dose: [client weight (kg) x 15 mg/kg divided by 100 mg/mL of palivizumab]

NURSING CONSIDERATIONS

ADMINISTRATION/STORAGE
1. Give injection volumes >1 mL in divided doses.
2. To prepare powder for injection for administration, slowly add 0.6 mL of sterile water to the 50 mg vial and 1 mL of sterile water to a 100 mg vial. Swirl gently for 30 seconds to avoid foaming (do not shake vial). Allow reconstituted drug to stand at room temperature for a minimum of 20 min until solution clarifies.
3. The injection does not have to be reconstituted and is available for injection immediately.
4. Reconstituted pavlivizumab does not contain a preservative; administer within 6 hr of reconstitution.
5. Palivizumab is supplied in single-use vials. Do not reenter vial. Give immediately after withdrawal from the vial. Discard any unused portion.
6. Serum levels are decreased after cardiopulmonary bypass. Administer a dose of palivizumab to clients undergoing cardiopulmonary bypass as soon as possible after procedure (even if sooner than 1 mo from previous dose). Thereafter give doses monthly.
7. Prior to reconstitution store between 2–8°C (36–46°F) in its original container. Do not freeze.

ASSESSMENT
1. Note candidates for therapy, i.e., premature infants at 35 weeks or less gestation without BPD and infants with BPD requiring intervention for RSV in the past 6 mo. Assess for congenital defects, coagulation disorders or liver dysfunction.
2. Give monthly doses throughout the RSV season. In the northern hemisphere, the RSV season usually begins in November and lasts through April (may be different in some communities). Give the first dose prior to the beginning of the RSV season to ensure protection.
3. Due to possibility of sciatic nerve damage, do not use the gluteal site routinely as the injection site. Give volumes greater than 1 mL in divided doses and in different sites. Follow dosing guidelines for correct dosage.

CLIENT/FAMILY TEACHING
1. Therapy consists of monthly injections based on body weight, during the RSV season. In the northern hemisphere, the RSV season typically starts in November and lasts through April, but it may begin earlier or last later in certain communities. Drug is used to prevent RSV, not to treat the disease.
2. Protect child from exposure to infection while on therapy, i.e., limit visitors, and avoid infected persons. Providers may need to wear masks and gloves.
3. May experience URI, runny nose, sore throat, ear infections, rash, or pain at injection site; report fever, other infections, and difficulty breathing.

OUTCOMES/EVALUATE
RSV prophylaxis in high risk infants

Bold Italic = life threatening side effect ■ = black box warning ✦ = Available in Canada

Palonosetron hydrochloride

IV

(pal-oh-**NOE**-see-tron)

CLASSIFICATION(S):
Antiemetic, 5-HT$_3$ receptor antagonist

PREGNANCY CATEGORY: B

Rx: Aloxi.

USES

(1) Prevention of acute N&V associated with initial and repeat courses of moderately and highly emetogenic cancer chemotherapy. (2) Prevention of delayed N&V associated with initial and repeat courses of moderately emetogenic cancer chemotherapy.

ACTION/KINETICS

Action

It is believed cancer chemotherapeutic drugs cause N&V by releasing serotonin from the enterochromaffin cells of the small intestine and that released serotonin activates 5-HT$_3$ receptors on vagal afferent nerves to initiate the vomiting reflex. Palonosetron is a selective 5-HT$_3$ receptor antagonist with a strong binding affinity for this receptor. Thus, by blocking serotonin on these receptors, N&V are reduced.

Pharmacokinetics

About 50% of a dose is metabolized in the liver to inactive metabolites. Unchanged drug and metabolites are excreted mainly in the urine. **t½, elimination:** 40 hr. **Plasma protein binding:** About 62%.

CONTRAINDICATIONS

Hypersensitivity to palonosetron or any component of the product. Lactation.

SPECIAL CONCERNS

Use with caution in those who have or may develop prolongation of cardiac conduction intervals (i.e., QTc). These include clients with hypokalemia or hypomagnesia, those taking diuretics with potential for inducing electrolyte abnormalities, those with congenital QT syndrome, those taking anti-arrhythmic drugs or other drugs which lead to QT prolongation, and cumulative high dose anthracycline therapy. Effects are unknown in women undergoing labor or delivery. Safety and efficacy have not been determined in children less than 18 years of age.

SIDE EFFECTS

Most Common

Headache, constipation, dizziness, diarrhea, bradycardia, hypotension, hyperkalemia, weakness.

CNS: Headache, dizziness, insomnia, somnolence, hypersomnia, paresthesia, anxiety, euphoria. **CV:** Non-sustained tachycardia, bradycardia, hypotension, hypertension, myocardial ischemia, extrasystoles, sinus tachycardia, sinus arrhythmia, supraventricular extrasystoles, QT prolongation, vein discoloration, vein distention. **GI:** Constipation, diarrhea, abdominal pain, dyspepsia, dry mouth, hiccups, flatulence. **Body as a whole:** Fatigue, weakness, fever, hot flashes, flu-like syndrome, arthralgia. **Metabolic:** Hyperkalemia, electrolyte fluctuations, hyperglycemia, metabolic acidosis, glycosuria, decreased appetite, anorexia. **Ophthalmic:** Eye irritation, amblyopia. **Otic:** Motion sickness, tinnitus. **Dermatologic:** Allergic dermatitis, rash. **GU:** Urinary retention.

LABORATORY TEST CONSIDERATIONS

↑ ALT, AST, bilirubin.

HOW SUPPLIED

Injection (IV): 0.25 mg/5 mL.

DOSAGE

• **IV**

Prevention of acute and delayed N&V.

Adults: 0.25 mg given as a single dose about 30 min before the start of chemotherapy.

NURSING CONSIDERATIONS

ADMINISTRATION/STORAGE

IV 1. Repeated dosing within a 7 day period is not recommended as safety and efficacy of frequent dosing have not been evaluated.

2. Give over 30 seconds. Flush infusion line with normal saline before and after palonosetron administration.

3. Do not mix with other drugs.

4. Inspect visually for particulate matter and discoloration before administration.

5. Store from 20–25°C (68–77°F). Protect from freezing and light.

ASSESSMENT

1. Note reasons for therapy, chemotherapy prescribed, other agents trialed, outcome.

2. Assess hydration status, lytes, EKG findings.

3. Administer 30 min before chemo on day one of each cycle. Also may need other agents (corticosteroids) to help control N&V especially with highly emetogenic agents. May also require additional antiemetic agents for breakthrough N&V.

CLIENT/FAMILY TEACHING

1. Will receive IV 30 min before chemotherapy. Consume adequate fluids to prevent dehydration.

2. Drug may prolong the QT interval with other agents so report any new drugs prescribed or any cardiac conduction problems.

3. Report if constipation problematic.

4. Take additional prescribed antiemetic for N&V that is not controlled with this therapy. Keep all F/U appointments to evaluate response to therapy and any adverse side effects.

OUTCOMES/EVALUATE

Prevention of chemotherapy induced N&V

Pamidronate disodium

(pah-**MIH**-droh-nayt)

CLASSIFICATION(S):

Bone growth regulator, bisphosphonate

PREGNANCY CATEGORY: D

Rx: Aredia.

USES

(1) In conjunction with hydration to treat moderate to severe hypercalcemia of malignancy associated with breast and lung cancers and multiple myeloma (with or without bone metastases). (2) Moderate to severe Paget's disease. (3) With standard therapy to treat osteolytic bone metastases of breast cancer or osteolytic lesions of multiple myeloma. *Investigational:* Postmenopausal osteoporosis; hyperparathyroidism; prophylaxis of glucocorticoid-induced osteoporosis; reduce bone pain in clients with prostatic carcinoma; treat immobilization-induced hypercalcemia.

ACTION/KINETICS

Action

Inhibits both normal and abnormal bone resorption without inhibiting bone formation and mineralization. Precise mechanism is not known, but the drug may inhibit dissolution of hydroxyapatite crystal or have an effect on bone reabsorbing cells. Causes decreased serum phosphate levels probably due to a decreased release of phosphate from bone and increased renal excretion as parathyroid levels return to normal. Urinary calcium/creatinine and urinary hydroxyproline/creatinine ratios decrease and usually return to normal or below normal after treatment.

Pharmacokinetics

$t^{1/2}$: Biphasic, 1.6 hr (alpha) and 27.3 hr (beta). Approximately 50% of an IV infused dose is excreted unchanged in the urine within 72 hr.

CONTRAINDICATIONS

Hypersensitivity to bisphosphonates.

SPECIAL CONCERNS

Use with caution during lactation. Safety and efficacy have not been determined in children or to treat hypercalcemia associated with hyperparathyroidism or non-tumor-related conditions. Pamidronate has not been tested in clients who have creatinine levels greater than 5 mg/dL.

SIDE EFFECTS

Most Common

N&V, anemia, bone/skeletal pain, dyspnea, fatigue, fever, headache, anorexia, diarrhea, dyspepsia, abdominal pain, headache, insomnia.

Metabolic/Electrolytes: Hypocalcemia, hypokalemia, hypomagnesemia, hypophosphatemia. **Body as a whole:** Slight increase in body temperature, fluid

---

overload, generalized pain, back pain, fatigue, fever, moniliasis. **GI:** N&V, diarrhea, constipation, abdominal pain, dyspepsia, anorexia, *GI hemorrhage*, ulcerative stomatitis. **CNS:** Somnolence, insomnia, dizziness, headache, paresthesia, abnormal vision, slight possibility of *seizures*. **CV:** Hypertension, atrial fibrillation, syncope, tachycardia. **Respiratory:** Dyspnea, rales, rhinitis, URTI. **GU:** UTI. **Musculoskeletal:** Bone/skeletal pain, osteonecrosis of the jaw. **At site of administration:** Redness, swelling or induration, pain on palpation. **Miscellaneous:** Anemia, hypothyroidism, sweating.

HOW SUPPLIED

Injection: 3 mg/mL, 6 mg/mL, 9 mg/mL; *Powder for Injection, Lyophilized:* 30 mg, 90 mg.

DOSAGE

- **IV INFUSION**

  Moderate hypercalcemia (corrected serum calcium of about 12–13.5 mg/dL) of malignancy.

Initial therapy: 60–90 mg given as a single dose over 2–24 hr. Infusions more than 2 hr may reduce the risk for renal toxicity, especially in those with preexisting renal insufficiency.

  Severe hypercalcemia (corrected serum calcium greater than 13.5 mg/dL) of malignancy.

Initial therapy: 90 mg as a single initial infusion given over 2–24 hr. Infusions longer than 2 hr may reduce the risk for renal toxicity, especially in those with preexisting renal insufficiency. If retreatment is necessary, use the same dose as for initial therapy; at least 7 days should elapse before retreatment.

  Moderate to severe Paget's disease.

30 mg/day given as a 4-hr infusion on 3 consecutive days (total dose: 90 mg). If retreatment is necessary, the same dosage schedule is used.

  Osteolytic bone lesions of breast cancer.

90 mg given as a 2-hr infusion q 3–4 weeks.

  Osteolytic bone lesions of multiple myeloma.

90 mg given as a 4-hr infusion every month. Those with marked Bence-Jones

proteinuria and dehydration should receive adequate hydration before infusion of pamidronate.

NOTE: Single doses should not exceed 90 mg due to renal toxicity and potential renal failure.

NURSING CONSIDERATIONS

@ Do not confuse Aredia with Meridia (antiobesity drug) or Adriamycin (antineoplastic).

ADMINISTRATION/STORAGE

 1. Hydrate clients adequately throughout treatment; overhydration, however, must be avoided, especially in those clients who have cardiac failure. Do not use diuretic therapy before correcting hypovolemia.

2. If hypercalcemia recurs, may retreat provided a minimum of 7 days has elapsed to allow full response to initial dose.

3. Reconstitute drug by adding 10 mL sterile water which results in a concentration of 30 mg/10 mL or 90 mg/10 mL with a pH of 6–7.4.

4. For hypercalcemia of malignancy, dilute recommended dose in 1,000 mL of sterile 0.45% or 0.9% NaCl or D5W. This solution stable for 24 hr at room temperature.

5. For treating Paget's disease dilute the daily dose of 30 mg in 500 mL of 0.45% or 0.9% NaCl or D5W; give over a 4-hr period for 3-consecutive days.

6. For treating osteolytic bone lesions of breast cancer, dilute the dose of 90 mg dose in 250 mL of 0.45% or 0.9% NaCl or D5W; give over a 2-hr period every 3-4 weeks.

7. For treating osteolytic bone lesions of multiple myeloma, dilute the dose of 90 mg in 500 mL of sterile 0.45% or 0.9% NaCl or D5W; give over a 4-hr period on a monthly basis.

8. Visually inspect parenteral drug products for particulate matter or discoloration prior to administration.

9. Do not mix with calcium-containing infusion solutions such as Ringer's solution.

10. Infusing over 2 or more hr reduces risk of renal toxicity.

 = see color insert   **H** = Herbal   = Intravenous   @ = sound alike drug

11. Give as single IV solution in a separate line.

12. Do not store above 30°C (86°F). May be stored from 2–8°C (36–46°F) for up to 24 hr when reconstituted with sterile water for injection.

ASSESSMENT

1. Note reasons for therapy, (i.e., hypercalcemia of malignancy, symptomatic Paget's disease, osteolytic bone lesions/pain), onset, presenting symptoms, any biphosphonate hypersensitivity.

2. List any cardiac disease. Monitor x-rays, BMD, ECG, serum Ca, Mg, K, PO_4, CBC, and renal function studies. Those with renal dysfunction are at greater risk for adverse side effects. Replace calcium if needed and ensure aggressive hydration with NSS.

3. Due to possible osteonecrosis of the jaw (primarily in cancer clients who have received bisphosphonates as part of their therapy), consider dental exam before treating with bisphosphonates, esp in those with concomitant risk factors such as cancer, chemotherapy, corticosteroids, or poor oral hygiene. Steroids may increase the risk of jaw bone problems.

INTERVENTIONS

1. Monitor VS and I&O. Ensure adequate fluids to correct hypovolemia/volume deficits before giving diuretics.

2. During drug therapy, vigorous saline hydration should be undertaken for moderate to severe hypercalcemia to restore urine output to about 2 L/day. For less severe hypercalcemia, more conservative approaches can be taken including saline hydration with or without loop diuretics. Overhydration should be avoided, esp with CHF. Weigh daily; observe for edema.

3. Assess for seizure activity; incorporate seizure precautions.

CLIENT/FAMILY TEACHING

1. Drug works to decrease calcium levels with cancer. Review dietary sources of calcium (dark green vegetables, yogurt, cheese, milk, etc.) that should be avoided with hypercalcemia.

2. Avoid activities that require mental alertness; may cause dizziness or drowsiness.

3. May experience transient mild temperature elevations for up to 48 hr following therapy.

4. Maintain adequate hydration; keep a log of I&O.

5. Report any increase in N&V, bone/jaw pain, thirst, or lethargy R/T hypercalcemia.

6. Practice reliable contraception; may cause fetal harm.

OUTCOMES/EVALUATE

- Desired calcium levels
- ↓ Bone pain/instability

Pancrelipase (Lipancreatin)
(pan-kree-**LY**-payz)

CLASSIFICATION(S):
Digestive enzyme

PREGNANCY CATEGORY: C

Rx: Creon 5, 10, or 20 Delayed-Release Capsules; Ku-Zyme HP Capsules; Lipram 4500 Delayed-Release Capsules; Lipram UL12, UL 18, or UL 20 Delayed-Release Capsules; Lipram-PN10, PN-16, or PN-20 Delayed-Release Capsules; PAN-2400 Capsules; Palcaps 10 or 20 Delayed-Release Capsules; Pancrease MT 4, MT 10, MT 16, or MT 20 Capsules; Pancrecarb MS-4, MS-8, or MS-16 Delayed-Release Capsules; Pangestyme CN-10, CN-20, EC, UL 12, UL 18, UL 20 or MT 16 Delayed-Release Capsules; Panocaps Delayed-Release Capsules; Panocaps MT 16 or MT 20 Delayed-Release Capsules; Panocase Tablets; Plaretase 8000 Tablets; Ultrase Capsules; Ultrase MT 12, MT 18, or MT 20 Capsules; Viokase 8 or 16 Tablets; Viokase Powder.

♦Rx: Creon 5, 10, 20, 25 Minimicrospheres; Pancrease MT; Ultrase; Ultrase MT.

USES

(1) Pancreatic deficiency diseases such as chronic pancreatitis, cystic fibrosis of the pancreas, pancreatectomy, ductal obstructions caused by cancer of the pancreas or common bile duct, steatorrhea of malabsorption syndrome, post-

gastrectomy, or postgastrointestinal surgery. (2) Presumptive test for pancreatic function, especially in insufficiency due to chronic pancreatitis.

ACTION/KINETICS

Action
Enzyme concentrate from hog pancreas, which contains lipase, amylase, and protease, enzymes that replace or supplement naturally occurring enzymes. More active at neutral or slightly alkaline pH. Has 12 times the lipolytic activity and 4 times both the proteolytic and amylolytic activity of pancreatin.

Pharmacokinetics
Certain products have an enteric coating that protects the enzymes from deactivation in the stomach.

CONTRAINDICATIONS
Hog protein sensitivity. Acute pancreatitis, acute exacerbation of chronic pancreatic disease.

SPECIAL CONCERNS
Safety for use during lactation and in children less than 6 months of age not established. Methacrylic acid copolymer, which is found in the enteric coating of certain products, may cause fibrosing colonopathy.

SIDE EFFECTS

Most Common
N&V, diarrhea, abdominal cramps (after high doses), flatulence, bloating.

GI: N&V, diarrhea, abdominal cramps (after high doses), colonic strictures, intestinal obstruction, intestinal stenosis, constipation, flatulence, melena, bloating, cramping, perianal irritation. **Miscellaneous:** Dermatitis, weight decrease, pain. Inhalation of the powder is irritating to the skin and mucous membranes and may result in an asthma attack. High doses cause hyperuricemia and hyperuricosuria.

OD OVERDOSE MANAGEMENT
Symptoms: Diarrhea, intestinal upset.

DRUG INTERACTIONS
Calcium carbonate / ↓ Effect of pancreatic enzymes
Folic acid / ↓ Folic acid absorption may → folic acid deficiency
Iron / Response to oral iron may ↓ if given with pancreatic enzymes
Mg hydroxide / ↓ Effect of pancreatic enzymes

HOW SUPPLIED
Capsules, Powder, Tablets: with varying amounts of lipase, protease, and amylase.

DOSAGE

CREON 5
Pancreatic deficiency diseases.

Adults and children over 6 years of age: Usual starting dose is 2–4 capsules per meal or snack. **Children, under 6 years:** Select exact dose based on clinical experience with this age group. Start with 1 to 2 capsules per meal or snack. **Cystic fibrosis clients:** Usual doses are 1,500–3,000 lipase units/kg/meal. Doses in excess of 6,000 lipase units/kg/meal are not recommended.

CREON 10
Pancreatic deficiency diseases.

Adults and children over 6 years: Usual starting dose is 1–2 capsules per meal or snack. **Children, under 6 years:** Usual starting dose is up to 1 capsule per meal or snack. **Cystic fibrosis clients:** Usual doses are 1,500–3,000 lipase units/kg/meal. Doses in excess of 6,000 lipase units/kg/meal are not recommended.

CREON 20
Pancreatic deficiency diseases.

Adults and children over 6 years: Usual starting dose is 1 capsule per meal or snack. **Children under 6 years:** Select the exact dose based on clinical experience with this age group. **Cystic fibrosis clients:** Usual doses are 1,500–3,000 lipase units/kg/meal. Doses in excess of 6,000 units are not recommended.

PANCRECARB, ULTRASE, ULTRASE MT
Pancreatic deficiency diseases.

Initiate with 1 or 2 capsules with each meal or snack.

KU-ZYME HP
Pancreatic deficiency diseases.

1 to 3 capsules with each meal or snack. In severe deficiencies, increase the dose to 8 capsules with meals or increase the frequency to hourly if nausea, cramps, or diarrhea do not occur.

LIPRAM, PANCRELIPASE
Pancreatic deficiency diseases.

P

Children, 6 months to less than 1 year of age: 2,000 lipase units/meal. **Children, 1–6 years:** 4,000–8,000 lipase units with each meal and 4,000 units with snacks. **Children, 7–12 years:** 4,000–12,000 lipase units with each meal and with snacks. **Adults:** 4,000–20,000 lipase units with each meal and with snacks.

PANCREASE, PANCREASE MT4
Pancreatic deficiency diseases.

Infants, up to 12 months: 2,000–4,000 lipase units/120 mL of formula or breast milk. **Children under 4 years of age:** Initiate with 1,000 lipase units/kg/meal, up to a maximum of 2,500 lipase units/kg/meal. **Children over 4 years of age:** Initiate with 400 lipase units/kg/meal, up to a maximum of 2,500 lipase units/kg/meal. Doses greater than 2,500 lipase units/kg/meal should be used with caution and only if they are documented to be effective by 3-day fecal measures.

PANOKASE, PLARETASE, VIOKASE TABLETS
Pancreatic deficiency diseases.

Cystic fibrosis and chronic pancreatitis clients: Dose ranges from 8,000–32,000 lipase units (1–4 tablets of Plaretase, Panokase, or Viokase 8 or 1–2 tablets of Viokase 16). Take with meals. **Pancreatectomy or obstruction of pancreatic ducts:** 1–2 tablets (Plaretase, Panokase, or Viokase 8) or 1 tablet (Viokase 16) q 2 hr.

VIOKASE POWDER
Pancreatic deficiency diseases.
0.7 gram (¼ teaspoon) with meals.

NURSING CONSIDERATIONS

Ⓒ Do not confuse Ultrase with Ultram (an analgesic).

ADMINISTRATION/STORAGE

1. When administering to young children, may sprinkle capsule contents on food.

2. After several weeks of use, adjust dosage according to therapeutic response.

3. Store unopened preparations in tight containers at a temperature not to exceed 25°C (77°F).

4. Do not crush or chew enteric-coated products (i.e., microspheres, microta-

blets). If unable to swallow, the capsule may be opened and shaken on a small amount of soft, cold food (e.g., applesauce, gelatin) that does not require chewing. Swallow immediately without chewing (enzymes may irritate the mucosa). Follow with a glass of juice or water to ensure complete swallowing of the product. Enteric-coated products that come in contact with foods with a pH greater than 5.5 will dissolve.

5. Generally, 300 mg of pancrelipase is required to digest every 17 grams of dietary fat. Products are not bioequivalent; do not interchange without approval.

6. Store Creon, Ultrase, and Ultrase MT from 15–25°C (59–86°F) in a dry place. Protect from high humidity; do not refrigerate.

7. Store Ku-Zyme HP, Lipram, Pancrease, Pancrease MT, Pancrecarb, Pancrelipase, Panokase, Plaretase, and Viokase at room temperature not exceeding 25°C (77°F) in a dry place. Protect from high humidity; store in tight containers. Do not refrigerate.

ASSESSMENT

1. Note reasons for therapy; obtain thorough medical/surgical history.

2. Assess for any sensitivity or allergy to pork, since hog protein is the main constituent of pancrelipase.

3. Perform nutritional assessment noting ht, wt, BMI, muscle tone.

4. Assess abdomen noting tenderness, BS, quality/frequency of stooling (foul-smelling, frothy, fatty, frequency) and pancreatic function tests (amylase, lipase).

CLIENT/FAMILY TEACHING

1. Drug is used to help absorb and digest fat, proteins, and CHO. Review appropriate dietary recommendations (usually low fat, high calorie, high protein); utilize dietitian for dietary counseling/help in meal planning.

2. Take just before or with meals and snacks and with plenty of liquids to prevent oral mucosal irritation. Do not crush or chew enteric-coated capsules; drug will deactivate in acid stomach environment; swallow whole. Avoid inhal-

---

Bold Italic = life threatening side effect   ■ = black box warning   ✦ = Available in Canada

ing powder forms; may cause severe side effects.

3. Report any joint pain/swelling/soreness, significant weight loss, or breathing difficulty. With nausea, cramping, or diarrhea, dosage may need adjustment to control steatorrhea (fat in stool). May experience diarrhea and abdominal discomfort; report if persistent.

OUTCOMES/EVALUATE

- Improved digestion/nutritional status with deficiency states
- Control of diarrhea, ↓ steatorrhea

Pancuronium bromide ■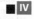

(pan-kyou-**ROH**-nee-um)

CLASSIFICATION(S):
Neuromuscular blocking drug
PREGNANCY CATEGORY: C
Rx: Pavulon.

SEE ALSO *NEUROMUSCULAR BLOCKING AGENTS.*

USES
(1) Adjunct to anesthesia to facilitate tracheal intubation. (2) To provide skeletal muscle relaxation during surgery or mechanical ventilation.

ACTION/KINETICS

Action
Five times as potent as d-tubocurarine. Anticholinesterase agents will reverse effects. Possesses vagolytic activity although it is not likely to cause histamine release.

Pharmacokinetics
Onset: Within 45 sec. **Time to peak effect:** 3–4.5 min (depending on the dose). **Duration:** 35–45 min (increased with multiple doses). **t½, elimination:** 89–161 min. Forty percent is excreted through the urine either unchanged or as metabolites; 10% is excreted through the bile. In clients with renal failure, the t½ is doubled. **Plasma protein binding:** About 87%.

SPECIAL CONCERNS
■ Give in carefully adjusted doses only by, or under the supervision of, experienced clinicians. Do not give unless reversal agents and facilities for intubation, artificial respiration, and oxygen therapy are immediately available. Be prepared to assist or control respiration.■ Children up to 1 month of age may be more sensitive to the effects of pancuronium. Clients with myasthenia gravis or Eaton-Lambert syndrome may have profound effects from small doses.

SIDE EFFECTS
Most Common
Skeletal muscle weakness, prolonged skeletal muscle relaxation, respiratory insufficiency/apnea.

See *Neuromuscular Blocking Agents* for a complete list of possible side effects. Also, **Respiratory: *Apnea, respiratory insufficiency*. CV:** Increased HR and MAP. **Miscellaneous:** Salivation, skin rashes, ***hypersensitivity reactions*** (e.g., ***bronchospasm***, flushing, hypotension, redness, tachycardia).

ADDITIONAL DRUG INTERACTIONS
Azathioprine / Reverses effects of pancuronium
Bacitracin / Additive muscle relaxation
Enflurane / ↑ Muscle relaxation
Isoflurane / ↑ Muscle relaxation
Metocurine / ↑ Muscle relaxation but duration is not prolonged
Phenytoin / Possible pancuronium shorter duration of action or less effective
Quinidine, Quinine / ↑ Effect of pancuronium
Sodium colistimethate / ↑ Muscle relaxation
Succinylcholine / ↑ Intensity and duration of action of pancuronium
Tetracyclines / Additive muscle relaxation
Theophyllines / ↓ Effects of pancuronium; also, possible cardiac arrhythmias
Tricyclic antidepressants with halothane / Administration of pancuronium may cause severe arrhythmias
Tubocurarine / ↑ Muscle relaxation but duration is not prolonged

HOW SUPPLIED
Injection: 1 mg/mL, 2 mg/mL.

DOSAGE
- **IV**
  Muscle relaxation during balanced anesthesia.

P

Adults and children over 1 month of age, initial: 0.04–0.1 mg/kg. Additional doses of 0.01 mg/kg may be administered as required (usually q 20–60 min). **Neonates:** Administer a test dose of 0.02 mg/kg first to determine responsiveness.

ET intubation.
0.06–0.1 mg/kg as a bolus dose. Can undertake intubation in 2 to 3 min.

NURSING CONSIDERATIONS

ASSESSMENT

1. Note reasons for therapy, expected duration, other agents/therapies trialed.
2. Drug should only be used on a short-term basis and in a continuously monitored environment. Drug blocks the effect of acetylcholine at the myoneural junction thus preventing neuromuscular transmission.

INTERVENTIONS

1. Provide ventilatory support.
2. Monitor and record VS, ECG, and I&O. Drug can cause vagal stimulation resulting in bradycardia, hypotension, and cardiac arrhythmias.
3. A peripheral nerve stimulator or train of four may be used to evaluate neuromuscular response and recovery. Before reversing with neostigmine, ensure evidence of spontaneous recovery present.
4. Consciousness and pain threshold are not affected by pancuronium. Explain all procedures and provide emotional support and pain and anxiety medications. Do not conduct any discussions that should not be overheard.
5. With short-term therapy, reassure that client will be able to talk and move once the drug effects are reversed.
6. Muscle fasciculations may cause soreness or injury after recovery. Administer prescribed nondepolarizing agent and reassure that soreness is likely caused by the unsynchronized contractions of adjacent muscle fibers just before the onset of paralysis.
7. Position for comfort and so that the body is in proper alignment. Turn and perform mouth care and eye care frequently (protect eyes and instill liquid tears q 2 hr as blink reflex is suppressed).
8. Assess airway at frequent intervals. Have a suction machine at the bedside.
9. Check to be certain that the ventilator alarms are set and on at all times. *Never* leave client unmonitored.
10. Determine client need and administer medications for anxiety, pain, and/or sedation regularly (valium, morphine). Store this medication away from any other drugs to prevent confusion.

CLIENT/FAMILY TEACHING

1. Drug will make you feel like you are paralyzed; sensation will return once drug is discontinued and wears off.
2. Explain all procedures and events as client may be paralyzed but can hear everything being said and see everything being done. Attempt to allay fears.
3. May experience some burning at IV site. Reassure they will be continuously monitored and will receive medication for anxiety and pain regularly.

OUTCOMES/EVALUATE

- Desired level of paralysis; suppression of twitch response
- Facilitation of ET intubation; tolerance of mechanical ventilation

Panitumumab   ■ IV
(pan-ih-tuh-**MYOO**-mab)

CLASSIFICATION(S):
Monoclonal antibody–antineoplastic drug
PREGNANCY CATEGORY: C
Rx: Vectibix.

USES
Treatment of epidermal growth factor receptor (EGFR)-expressing, metastatic colorectal carcinoma with disease progression or following fluoropyrimidine-, oxaliplatin-, and irinotecan-containing chemotherapy regimens. *NOTE:* Efficacy is based on progression-free survival.

ACTION/KINETICS

Action
A recombinant, human immunoglobulin G2 kappa monoclonal antibody that binds to the human epidermal growth factor receptor (EGFR). EGFR is a mem-

---

Bold Italic = life threatening side effect   ■ = black box warning   ✦ = Available in Canada

ber of a subfamily of type 1 receptor tyrosine kinases. Overexpression of EGFR is detected in many human cancers, including the colon and rectum. Panitumumab binds specifically to EGFR and competitively inhibits the binding of ligands for EGFR. This results in inhibition of cell growth, induction of apoptosis, decreased proinflammatory cytokine and vascular growth factor production, and internalization of EGFR. It is believed panistimumab inhibits growth and survival of selected human tumor cell lines expressing EGFR.

Pharmacokinetics

Drug levels reach steady-state levels by the third infusion. $t^{1/2}$, **elimination:** About 7.5 days (3.6–10.9 days).

CONTRAINDICATIONS

During lactation and for 2 months following the last dose of panitumumab.

SPECIAL CONCERNS

■ (1) Dermatologic toxicity. Dermatologic toxicities, related to panitumumab blockade of epidermal growth factor-binding and subsequent inhibition of epidermal growth factor receptor (EGFR)-mediated signaling pathways were reported in 89% of clients and were severe (NCI Common Toxicity Criteria, grade 3 and higher) in 12% of clients receiving panitumumab monotherapy. The clinical manifestations included, but were not limited to, dermatitis acneiform, pruritus, erythema, rash, skin exfoliation, paronychia, dry skin, and skin fissures. Severe dermatologic toxicities were complicated by infections including sepsis, septic death, and abscesses requiring incisions and drainage. Withhold or discontinue panitumumab and monitor for inflammatory or infectious sequelae in those with severe dermatologic toxicities. (2) Infusion reactions. Severe infusion reactions occurred with the administration of panitumumab in approximately 1% of clients. Severe infusion reactions were identified by reports of anaphylactic reaction, bronchospasm, fever, chills, and hypotension. Although fatal infusion reactions have not been reported with panitumumab, fatalities have occurred with other monoclonal antibody products. Stop the infusion if a severe infusion reaction occurs. Depending on the severity and/or persistence of the reaction, permanently discontinue panitumumab.■ Safety and efficacy have not been determined in children.

SIDE EFFECTS

Most Common

Skin rashes/toxicity, hypomagnesemia, paronychia, fatigue, abdominal pain, nausea, diarrhea, infusion reactions, eye toxicities.

Dermatologic: Skin rashes, erythema, pruritus, acneiform dermatitis, skin exfoliation/fissures, paronychia, other nail disorders, acne, dry skin, growth of eyelashes. **Infusion reactions:** Fever, chills, dyspnea, hypotension, *anaphylactoid reaction*. **GI:** N&V, abdominal pain, constipation, diarrhea, stomatitis, mucositis, mucosal inflammation. **Metabolic :** Hypomagnesemia, peripheral edema. **Respiratory:** Cough, pulmonary fibrosis. **Ophthalmic:** Conjunctivitis, ocular hyperemia, increased lacrimation, eye/eyelid irritation. **Body as a whole:** Fatigue, general deterioration, *sepsis, septic death,* abscesses requiring incisions and drainage, immunogenicity.

HOW SUPPLIED

Solution for Injection: 20 mg/mL.

DOSAGE

* **IV INFUSION**

    EGFR-expressing, metastatic colorectal carcinoma.

6 mg/kg given over 60 min every 14 days. Give doses higher than 1,000 mg over 90 min. For the duration of the infusion, reduce the infusion rate 50% in clients experiencing a mild or moderate (grade 1 or 2) reaction.

NURSING CONSIDERATIONS

ADMINISTRATION/STORAGE

 1. Discontinue immediately and permanently in those experiencing severe (grade 3 or 4) infusion reactions. 2. Withhold for dermatologic toxicities that are grade 3 or higher or are considered intolerable. If toxicity does not improve to grade 2 or lower within 1 month, stop permanently. If dermatologic toxicity improves to grade 2 or lower, and the client is symptomatically

P

improved after withholding up to 2 doses of panitumumab, resume treatment at 50% of the original dose. If toxicities recur, stop permanently. If toxicities do not recur, subsequent doses may be increased by increments of 25% of the original dose until the recommended dose of 6 mg/kg is reached.

3. Do not administer panitumumab as an IV push or bolus. Must be given by an IV infusion pump using a low-protein binding 0.2 or 0.22 mcm in-line filter. Infuse through peripheral line or indwelling catheter.

4. Flush the line before and after panitumumab administration with NaCl 0.9% injection to avoid mixing with other drug products or IV solutions.

5. Do not mix with or administer as an infusion with other drugs.

6. Store in the original carton from 2–6°C (36–46°F) until time of use. Protect from direct sunlight; do not freeze. Discard any unused portion as the product contains no preservatives.

ASSESSMENT
1. List reasons for therapy, onset, other therapies trialed/failed.
2. Monitor VS, I&O, infusion site, Mg, Ca, lytes, renal, and LFTs.
3. Assess skin turgor and condition; monitor for any reaction.

CLIENT/FAMILY TEACHING
1. Drug is used to treat cancer that has metastasized following standard chemotherapy. Panitumumab is a monoclonal antibody. Monoclonal antibodies are made in the laboratory and can locate and bind to cancer cells. Panitumumab binds to the epidermal growth factor receptor (EGFR) and may block tumor cell growth.
2. May experience skin rash, fatigue, abdominal pain, nausea, and diarrhea. Report any skin or eye changes or new onset SOB. Any breathing problems (pulmonary fibrosis), severe skin rash esp. if complicated by infections, infusion reactions, and vomiting should be reported.
3. Skin may be more sensitive to sunlight and may easily burn. Use sunscreen (minimum SPF 15), wear protective clothing if must be out in the sun.

4. May affect female's fertility; consider egg/sperm harvesting prior to therapy. May also cause irregular menstrual periods.

5. Keep all F/U appointments for labs, infusions every 2 weeks, and to evaluate disease and response.

OUTCOMES/EVALUATE
Inhibition of malignant cell proliferation

Pantoprazole sodium
(pan-**TOH**-prah-zohl)

CLASSIFICATION(S):
Proton pump inhibitor
PREGNANCY CATEGORY: B
Rx: Protonix.
♣Rx: Panto IV, Pantoloc.

USES
PO: (1) Short-term treatment (up to 8 weeks) in the healing and symptomatic relief of erosive esophagitis associated with GERD. An additional 8 weeks therapy may be indicated for those who have not healed after the initial 8 weeks of therapy. (2) Maintenance of healing of erosive esophagitis and reduction in relapse rates of day- and night-time heartburn symptoms in those with GERD. (3) Long-term treatment of pathological hypersecretory conditions, including Zollinger-Ellison syndrome. *Investigational:* Treat duodenal ulcer. In combination with antibiotics to treat duodenal ulcer associated with *H. pylori.* Treat gastric ulcer.

IV: (1) Short-term (7–10 days) treatment of GERD associated with a history of erosive esophagitis, as an alternative to PO therapy in those who are unable to continue taking the delayed-release tablets. (2) Pathological hypersecretory conditions associated with Zollinger-Ellison syndrome or other neoplastic conditions.

ACTION/KINETICS
Action
Proton pump inhibitor that suppresses the final step in gastric acid production

by forming a covalent bond to two sites of the H⁺/ K⁺-ATPase enzyme system at the secretory surface of the gastric parietal cell. Results in inhibition of both basal and stimulated gastric acid secretion regardless of the stimulus. Duration greater than 24 hr due to binding to ATPase. Gastrin levels increase.

Pharmacokinetics
About 77% is bioavailable. Absorption begins only after the tablet leaves the stomach although it occurs rapidly. Absorption is not affected by antacids, although food may delay absorption up to 2 hr or longer. **Duration:** Over 24 hr. Extensively metabolized in the liver by the CYP system. **t½:** About 1 hr. Excreted in both the urine (71%) and feces (18%). **Plasma protein binding:** About 98%.

CONTRAINDICATIONS
Hypersensitivity to any component of the formulation. Lactation.

SPECIAL CONCERNS
Safety and efficacy for children or for maintenance therapy (i.e., beyond 16 weeks) have not been established. Safety and efficacy of IV use as initial treatment for GERD not established. Use with caution in severe hepatic impairment as there may be modest drug accumulation when dosed once/day.

SIDE EFFECTS
Most Common
Headache, diarrhea, flatulence, abdominal pain.
Side effects listed are those with an incidence of 1% or more. **GI:** Diarrhea, flatulence, abdominal pain, eructation, constipation, dyspepsia, gastroenteritis, GI disorder, N&V, rectal disorder. **CNS:** Headache, insomnia, anxiety, dizziness, migraine. **Respiratory:** Bronchitis, increased cough, dyspnea, pharyngitis, rhinitis, sinusitis, URTI. **GU:** Urinary frequency, UTI. **Body as a whole:** Rash, asthenia, flu syndrome, infection, pain, arthralgia. **Miscellaneous:** Back/chest/neck pain.

LABORATORY TEST CONSIDERATIONS
↑ SGOT, creatinine. Hyperlipemia, hyperglycemia, hypercholesterolemia, hyperuricemia. Abnormal LFTs.

DRUG INTERACTIONS
Ampicillin esters / ↓ Ampicillin absorption R/T ↓ bioavailability R/T inhibition of gastric acid secretion
Iron salts / ↓ Iron absorption R/T ↓ bioavailability R/T inhibition of gastric acid secretion
Ketoconazole / ↓ Ketoconazole absorption R/T ↓ bioavailability R/T inhibition of gastric acid secretion
Warfarin / Possible ↑ INR and PT; monitor carefully

HOW SUPPLIED
Powder for Injection, Freeze-Dried: 40 mg (as base)/vial; *Tablets, Delayed-Release:* 20 mg (as base), 40 mg (as base).

DOSAGE
• **TABLETS, DELAYED-RELEASE**
Treatment of erosive esophagitis.
Adults: 40 mg once daily for up to 8 weeks; an additional 8 weeks therapy may be considered for those who have not healed after 8 weeks of treatment.
Maintenance of healing of erosive esophagitis.
Adults: 40 mg once daily.
Pathological hypersecretory conditions, including Zollinger-Ellison syndrome.
Adults, initial: 40 mg twice a day Adjust dose as needed as dosage varies with each individual; up to 240 mg/day may be given, if needed. Treatment in some has continued for more than 2 years.
• **IV ONLY**
GERD associated with a history of erosive esophagitis.
Adults: 40 mg once daily for 7–10 days. Safety and efficacy for more than 10 days have not been shown.
Pathological secretory conditions.
Individualize dose. **Adults:** 80 mg q 12 hr. Doses higher than 240 mg or given for more than 6 days have not been evaluated.

NURSING CONSIDERATIONS
ADMINISTRATION/STORAGE
1. Store Delayed-Release Tablets from 15–30°C (59–86°F).
[IV] 2. IV pantoprazole may be given as follows:

P

- *Two minute infusion.* Reconstitute IV pantoprazole with 10 mL of 0.9% NaCl injection for a final concentration of 4 mg/mL. For both uses, give over at least 2 min using the filter provided. Reconstituted solution may be stored for up to 24 hr at room temperature before administration. The solution does not need to be protected from light.
- *Fifteen minute infusion.* If used for GERD associated with a history of erosive esophagitis, reconstitute IV pantoprazole with 10 mL of 0.9% NaCl injection, and further dilute (admix) with 100 mL of D5W injection, 0.9% NaCl injection, or LR injection to a final concentration of about 0.4 mg/mL. The admixed solution may be stored at room temperature and must be used within 24 hr.
- *Fifteen minute infusion.* If used for pathological hypersecretory conditions, reconstitute each vial with 10 mL of 0.9% NaCl injection. Combine the contents of the 2 vials and further dilute (admix) with 80 mL of 5% dextrose, 0.9% NaCl, or lactated Ringer's injection to a total volume of 100 mL, with a final concentration of about 0.8 mg/mL. Give the admixture over about 15 min at a rate of approximately 7 mg/min using the filter provided. The reconstituted solution may be stored for up to 6 hr at room temperature prior to further dilution; the admixed solution may be stored for up to 24 hr at room temperature prior to IV infusion. Give the admixture IV over approximately 15 min at a rate of about 7 mL/min using the filter provided. Do not freeze reconstituted drug. It is not necessary to protect the reconstituted or admixed solutions from light.

3. Give by IV infusion through a dedicated line using the filter provided. The filter must be used to remove precipitate that may form when the drug is reconstituted or mixed with IV solution.
4. If administration is through a Y-site, the in-line filter must be positioned below the Y-site that is closest to the client. Flush the IV line before and after the administration of pantoprazole with either D5W or lactated Ringer's injection.
5. Do not give pantoprazole injection through the same line with other IV solutions.
6. Discontinue IV therapy as soon as able to resume PO therapy with the delayed-release tablets.
7. Store IV product at 2–8°C (36–46°F). Protect from light.
8. Midazolam is incompatible with Y-site administration. Pantoprazole may not be compatible with products containing zinc.
9. Immediately stop use if precipitation or discoloration occurs.

ASSESSMENT
1. Note reasons for therapy, onset, duration, triggers, characteristics of S&S. Record abdominal assessment, skin lesions, urea breath, labs, UGI/endoscopic findings.
2. Assess renal, LFTs; may reduce dose to every other day with dysfunction to prevent drug accumulations.
3. List drugs prescribed to ensure none require acidity for metabolism.
4. There have been reports of false positive screening tests for tetrahydrocannabinol (THC) in those receiving most proton pump inhibitors. May require more selective testing to confirm results.

CLIENT/FAMILY TEACHING
1. Take as directed at the same time each day. Do not split, crush, or chew the delayed release tablets; swallow whole. If unable to swallow a 40-mg tablet, two 20 mg tablets may be taken.
2. May take with or without food in the stomach. Antacid consumption will not affect.
3. Avoid alcohol, aspirin or NSAIDs, and foods that may cause GI irritation.
4. Report abdominal pains, evidence of bleeding (bright blood or black tarry stools) and any unusual side effects, worsening of S&S, or lack of response; keep F/U appointments.
5. Avoid long term consumption; may mask GI malignancies.
6. May cause false positive THC drug test; ask for confirmatory testing.

OUTCOMES/EVALUATE
Reduced gastric acidity with relief of S&S of erosive esophagitis

Paroxetine hydrochloride, Paroxetine mesylate
■ⓒ📷
(pah-**ROX**-eh-teen)

CLASSIFICATION(S):
Antidepressant, selective serotonin reuptake inhibitor
PREGNANCY CATEGORY: D
Rx: Paxil, Paxil CR, Pexeva.

SEE ALSO *SELECTIVE SEROTONIN REUPTAKE INHIBITORS.*

USES
Hydrochloride. Immediate- and Controlled-Release: (1) Treatment of major depressive episodes as defined in the DSM-III (immediate-release) or DSM-IV (controlled-release). (2) Panic disorder with or without agoraphobia (as defined in DSM-IV). (3) Treatment of social anxiety disorder (social phobia) as defined in the DSM-IV. Use does not include Pexeva. **Immediate-Release:** (1) Obsessive-compulsive disorders in clients with OCD (as defined in DSM-IV). (2) Generalized anxiety disorder (as defined in DSM-IV); up to 24 weeks for maintenance therapy. (3) Posttraumatic stress disorder as defined in DSM-IV. **Controlled-Release:** Premenstrual dysphoric disorder as defined in DSM-IV. *Investigational:* Hot flashes.
   Mesylate, Immediate-Release. (1) Treatment of major depressive disorder. Periodically evaluate the long-term usefulness. (2) Treatment of obsessive compulsive disorder as defined in DSM-III-R. (3) Panic disorder as defined in DSM-IV.

ACTION/KINETICS
Action
Antidepressant effect likely due to inhibition of CNS neuronal uptake of serotonin and to a lesser extent norepinephrine and dopamine. Results in increased levels of serotonin in synapses.

Pharmacokinetics
Completely absorbed from the GI tract; bioavailability is 100%. **Time to peak plasma levels:** 5.2 hr for immediate-release and 6–10 hr for controlled-release. **Peak plasma levels:** 61.7 ng/mL for immediate-release and 30 ng/mL for controlled-release. **t½:** 21 hr for immediate-release and 15–20 hr for controlled-release. **Time to reach steady state:** About 10 days for immediate-release and 14 days for controlled-release. Plasma levels are increased in impaired renal and hepatic function as well as in geriatric clients. Extensively metabolized in the liver to inactive metabolites. Approximately two-thirds of the drug is excreted through the urine and one-third is excreted in the feces. *NOTE:* A generic form of paroxetine (Pexeva) is available as paroxetine mesylate, not paroxetine HCl (Paxil). **Plasma protein binding:** About 93–95%.

ADDITIONAL CONTRAINDICATIONS
Use during the first trimester of pregnancy. Use of alcohol. Concomitant use of thioridazine. Use in children and adolescents less than 18 years of age with major depressive disorder due to increased risk of suicidal thoughts and attempts.

SPECIAL CONCERNS
■ (1) Antidepressants increased the risk of suicidal thinking and behavior (suicidality) in short-term studies in children and adolescents with major depressive disorder and other psychiatric disorders. Anyone considering the use of paroxetine or any other antidepressant in a child or adolescent must balance this risk with the clinical need. Clients who are started on therapy should be observed closely for clinical worsening, suicidality, or unusual changes in behavior. Families and caregivers should be advised of the need for close observation and communication with the health care provider. Paroxetine is not approved for use in pediatric clients with major depressive disorder and obsessive-compulsive disorder. (2) Short-term placebo-controlled trials of 9 antidepressant drugs in children and adolescents with major depressive disorder,

P

obsessive-compulsive disorder, or other psychiatric disorders revealed a greater risk of adverse reactions representing suicidal thinking or behavior (suicidality) during the first few months of treatment. The average risk of such reactions in clients receiving antidepressants was 4%, twice the placebo risk of 2%. No suicides occurred in these trials.■ Use with caution and initially at reduced dosage in elderly clients as well as in those with impaired hepatic or renal function, with a history of mania, with a history of seizures, in clients with diseases or conditions that could affect metabolism or hemodynamic responses. Concurrent administration of paroxetine with lithium or digoxin should be undertaken with caution. Allow at least 14 days between discontinuing a monoamine oxidase inhibitor and starting paroxetine or stopping paroxetine and starting a MAOI. Infants exposed to paroxetine during the third trimester of pregnancy may develop complications requiring prolonged hospitalization, respiratory support, and tube feeding. Carefully consider the potential risks and benefits of treating women during their third trimester; consider tapering paroxetine during the third trimester.

SIDE EFFECTS
Most Common
Insomnia, somnolence, nausea, dry mouth, asthenia, headache, dizziness, tremor, excessive sweating, diarrhea/loose stools, constipation, abnormal ejaculation.

The side effects listed were observed with a frequency up to 1 in 1,000 clients. **CNS:** Headache, somnolence, insomnia, agitation, *seizures*, tremor, anxiety, activation of mania/hypomania, dizziness, nervousness, paresthesia, drugged feeling, myoclonus, CNS stimulation, confusion, amnesia, impaired concentration, depression, emotional lability, vertigo, abnormal thinking, akinesia, alcohol abuse, ataxia, *convulsions, possibility of suicide attempt*, depersonalization, hallucinations, hyperkinesia, hypertonia, incoordination, lack of emotion, manic reaction, paranoid reaction. **GI:** Nausea, abdominal pain, diarrhea/loose stools, dry mouth, vomiting, constipation, decreased appetite, flatulence, oropharynx disorder ('lump' in throat, tightness in throat), dyspepsia, increased appetite, bruxism, dysphagia, eructation, gastritis, glossitis, increased salivation, mouth ulceration, *rectal hemorrhage*, abnormal LFTs. **Hematologic:** Anemia, leukopenia, lymphadenopathy, purpura. **CV:** Palpitation, vasodilation, postural hypotension, hypertension, syncope, tachy/bradycardia, conduction abnormalities, abnormal ECG, migraine, peripheral vascular disorder. **Dermatologic:** Sweating, rash, pruritus, acne, alopecia, dry skin, ecchymosis, eczema, furunculosis, urticaria. **Metabolic/Nutritional:** Edema, weight gain/loss, hyperglycemia, peripheral edema, thirst. **Respiratory:** Respiratory disorder (cold symptoms or URI), pharyngitis, yawn, increased cough, rhinitis, asthma, bronchitis, dyspnea, epistaxis, hyperventilation, pneumonia, respiratory flu, sinusitis. **GU:** Abnormal ejaculation (usually delay), erectile difficulties, sexual dysfunction, impotence, decreased libido, urinary frequency/difficulty/hesitancy, anorgasmia in women, difficulty in reaching climax/orgasm in women, abortion, amenorrhea, breast pain, cystitis, dysmenorrhea, dysuria, menorrhagia, nocturia, polyuria, urethritis, urinary incontinence/retention, vaginitis. **Musculoskeletal:** Asthenia, back/neck pain, myopathy, myalgia, myasthenia, arthralgia, arthritis. **Ophthalmic:** Blurred vision, abnormality of accommodation, eye pain, mydriasis. **Otic:** Ear pain, otitis media, tinnitus. **Miscellaneous:** Asthenia, fever, chest pain, trauma, taste perversion/loss, chills, malaise, allergic reaction, *carcinoma*, face edema, moniliasis, anorexia. *NOTE:* Over a 4- to 6-week period, there was evidence of adaptation to side effects such as nausea and dizziness but less adaptation to dry mouth, somnolence, and asthenia.

ADDITIONAL DRUG INTERACTIONS
Antiarrhythmics, Type IC / Possible ↑ effect R/T ↓ liver breakdown
Cimetidine / ↑ Paroxetine effect R/T ↓ liver breakdown

Bold Italic = life threatening side effect   ■ = black box warning   ♣ = Available in Canada

Digoxin / Possible ↓ plasma levels
Phenobarbital / Possible ↓ paroxetine effect R/T ↑ liver breakdown
Phenytoin / Possible ↓ paroxetine effect R/T ↑ liver breakdown; also, ↓ phenytoin levels
Procyclidine / ↓ Procyclidine dose R/T significant anticholinergic effects
Risperidone / ↑ Risperidone levels R/T ↓ metabolism
H *St. John's wort* / Possible CNS depression
Theophylline / ↑ Theophylline levels
Thioridazine / ↑ Thioridazine levels → possible prolongation of QTc interval

OD OVERDOSE MANAGEMENT
Symptoms: N&V, drowsiness, sinus tachycardia, dilated pupils. *Treatment:*
- Establish and maintain an airway.
- Ensure adequate oxygenation and ventilation.
- Induction of emesis, lavage, or both; following evacuation, 20–30 grams activated charcoal may be given q 4–6 hr during the first 24–48 hr after ingestion.
- Take an ECG and monitor cardiac function if evidence of abnormality.
- Provide supportive care with monitoring of VS.

HOW SUPPLIED
Hydrochloride: *Oral Suspension:* 10 mg/5 mL; *Tablets, Immediate-Release:* 10 mg, 20 mg, 30 mg, 40 mg; *Tablets, Controlled-Release:* 12.5 mg, 25 mg, 37.5 mg.
Mesylate: *Tablets, Immediate-Release:* 10 mg, 20 mg, 30 mg, 40 mg.

DOSAGE—————————
• **ORAL SUSPENSION; TABLETS, IMMEDIATE-RELEASE**
Major depressive disorder.
Adults, initial: 20 mg/day, usually given as a single dose in the morning. Some clients not responding to the 20 mg dose may benefit from increasing the dose in 10 mg/day increments, up to a maximum of 50 mg/day. Make dose changes at intervals of at least 1 week. **Maintenance:** Doses average about 30 mg/day.
Panic disorders.
Adults, initial: 10 mg/day usually given in the morning; may be increased by 10

mg increments each week until a dose of 40 mg/day (range is 10–60 mg/day) is reached. Maximum daily dose: 60 mg.
Obsessive-compulsive disorders.
Adults, initial: 20 mg/day; **then,** increase by 10 mg increments a day in intervals of at least 1 week until a dose of 40 mg/kg (range is 20–60 mg/day) is reached. Maximum daily dose: 60 mg.
Social anxiety disorder.
Adults, initial: 20 mg/day, given as a single dose with or without food, usually in the morning. Dose range is 20–60 mg/day.
Generalized anxiety disorder.
Adults, initial: 20 mg/day, given as a single dose with or without food, usually in the morning. Dose range is 20–50 mg/day. Change doses in 10 mg/day increments at intervals of 1 week or more. Doses greater than 20 mg/day do not provide additional benefit. **Maintenance:** Adjust dose to maintain the client on the lowest effective dosage; periodically reassess to determine need for continued treatment. Found to be effective for up to 24 weeks.
Posttraumatic stress disorder.
Adults, initial: 20 mg/day given as a single daily dose with or without food. Usual range: 20–50 mg/day. If needed, can increase dose by 10 mg/day at intervals of 1 week. **Maintenance:** Adjust dose to maintain the client on the lowest effective dosage; periodically reassess to determine need for continued treatment.
Hot flashes.
20 mg/day.
Diabetic neuropathy.
10–60 mg/day.
• **TABLETS, CONTROLLED-RELEASE**
Major depressive disorder.
Adults, initial: 25 mg/day given as a single dose with or without food, usually in the morning. Range: 25–62.5 mg/day. Change doses in increments of 12.5 mg/day, if needed, at intervals of at least 1 week. **Maintenance:** Average of 37.5 mg/day.
Panic disorder.
Adults, initial: 12.5 mg/day given as a single dose with or without food usually in the morning. If needed, increase

P

dose by 12.5 mg/day at 1 week intervals, not to exceed 75 mg/day.

Social anxiety disorder.
Adults, initial: 12.5 mg/day given as a single dose, with or without food, usually in the morning. Usual range is 12.5–37.5 mg/day. If needed, increase dose at intervals of at least 1 week in increments of 12.5 mg/day, up to a maximum of 37.5 mg/day. **Maintenance:** Adjust dose to maintain the client on the lowest effective dosage; periodically reassess to determine need for continued treatment.

Premenstrual dysphoric disorder.
Adults, initial: 12.5 mg/day given as a single daily dose, with or without food, usually in the morning. Paroxetine CR may be given either daily throughout the menstrual cycle or limited to the luteal phase of the menstrual cycle. Usual range is 12.5–25 mg/day. Change doses at intervals of at least 1 week. **Maintenance:** Efficacy exceeding 3 menstrual cycles has not been evaluated systematically.

Hot flashes.
12.5–25 mg/day.
NOTE: Geriatric or debilitated clients, those with severe hepatic or renal impairment, **initial:** 10 mg/day of immediate-release or 12.5 mg/day of controlled-release, up to a maximum of 40 mg/day of immediate-release or 50 mg/day of controlled-release for all uses.

NURSING CONSIDERATIONS

Do not confuse paroxetine with paclitaxel (an antineoplastic). Also, do not confuse Paxil with either paclitaxel (an antineoplastic) or Taxol (an antineoplastic).

ADMINISTRATION/STORAGE

1. Even though beneficial effects may be seen in 1–4 weeks, continue therapy as prescribed. Effectiveness is maintained for up to 1 year with daily doses averaging 30 mg of immediate-release or 37.5 mg of controlled-release.
2. If discontinuing therapy, decrease dose incrementally. Abrupt cessation may cause dizziness, sensory disturbances, agitation, anxiety, nausea, and sweating.
3. Store immediate-release tablets between 15–30°C (59–86°F) and controlled-release tablets and suspension at or below 25°C (77°F).

ASSESSMENT

1. Note reasons for therapy, type, onset, characteristics of S&S, other therapy trialed, outcome. Assess clinical presentation and behavioral manifestations.
2. Document mania, altered metabolic or hemodynamic states, seizures.
3. List drugs currently prescribed to ensure none interact. Avoid use with a MAOI or within 14 days of discontinuing treatment with a MAOI.
4. Monitor weight, VS, ECG, electrolytes, CBC, renal and LFTs; note any dysfunction.
5. Closely monitor infants born to mothers who took paroxetine during pregnancy due to the possibility of a withdrawal syndrome and baby heart defects.
6. During management of overdose, always entertain the possibility of multiple drug involvement.
7. Women who are or who may become pregnant and who are currently taking paroxetine should discuss the risks and benefits of continuing the drug with their provider; alternative therapies should be considered.

CLIENT/FAMILY TEACHING

1. Shake suspension well before using. May be given with or without food. Swallow controlled-release tablet whole; do not crush or chew.
2. Take only as directed. Prescriptions may be for small quantities to ensure compliance and to discourage overdose. Allow up to 4 weeks for therapeutic effects.
3. Do not engage in tasks that require mental alertness until drug effects realized. Avoid alcohol; OTC products without provider approval.
4. Report excessive weight loss/gain and adjust diet and exercise to compensate.
5. Notify provider if pregnancy is suspected or planned. Practice reliable

---

Bold Italic = life threatening side effect   ■ = black box warning   ✦ = Available in Canada

birth control and avoid breastfeeding during therapy.

6. Report any thoughts of suicide or increased suicide ideations. Advise family not to leave severely depressed individuals alone; possibility of a suicide attempt is inherent in depression and may persist until significant remission is observed.

7. Avoid prolonged sun exposure and use protection when exposed.

8. Participate in therapy sessions designed to assist with underlying problems. With prolonged use may require gradual titrated withdrawal.

OUTCOMES/EVALUATE
- ↓ Anxiety/depression
- ↓ Panic attacks; ↓ palpitations; ↓ obsessive repetitive behaviors
- Resolution/control of post menopausal hot flashes

Pegaptanib sodium
(peh-**GAP**-tih-nib)

CLASSIFICATION(S):
Selective vascular endothelial growth factor antagonist
PREGNANCY CATEGORY: B
Rx: Macugen.

USES
Treatment of neovascular (wet) age-related macular degeneration. *Investigational:* Diabetic macular edema.

ACTION/KINETICS
Action
Pegaptanib is a selective vascular endothelial growth factor antagonist. Vascular endothelial growth factor selectively binds and activates its receptors located mainly on the surface of vascular endothelial cells. It induces angiogenesis and increases vascular permeability and inflammation, which are believed to contribute to the progression of the wet form of age-related macular degeneration. Pegaptanib binds to vascular endothelial growth factor thereby inhibiting its binding to receptors, thus decreasing the effect of vascular endothelial growth factor.

Pharmacokinetics
Slowly absorbed into the systemic circulation from the eye. The drug is metabolized by endo- and exonucleases.

CONTRAINDICATIONS
Ocular or periocular infections. Hypersensitivity to the drug or any component of the product.

SPECIAL CONCERNS
Safety and efficacy of pegaptanib therapy administered to both eyes, concurrently, have not been determined. Use with caution during lactation. Safety and efficacy have not been determined in children.

SIDE EFFECTS
Most Common
Anterior chamber inflammation, blurred vision, cataract, conjunctival hemorrhage, corneal edema, eye discharge/irritation/pain, hypertension, increased intraocular pressure, ocular discomfort, punctuate keratitis, reduced visual acuity, visual disturbance, vitreous floaters/opacities.

Ophthalmic: Endophthalmitis, increased intraocular pressure (within 30 min of administration), anterior chamber inflammation, blurred vision, cataract, conjunctival hemorrhage, corneal edema, eye discharge/irritation/pain, ocular discomfort, punctuate keratitis, reduced visual acuity, visual disturbance, vitreous floaters/opacities, blepharitis, conjunctivitis, photopsia, vitreous disorder, allergic conjunctivitis, conjunctival edema, corneal abrasion/deposits, corneal epithelium disorder, endophthalmitis, eye inflammation/swelling, eyelid irritation, mydriasis, periorbital hematoma, retinal edema, vitreous hemorrhage. **CNS:** Dizziness, headache, vertigo. **GI:** Diarrhea, nausea, dyspepsia, vomiting. **CV:** Hypertension, carotid artery occlusion, *CVA*, TIA. **Musculoskeletal:** Arthritis, bone spur. **GU:** UTI, urinary retention. **Miscellaneous:** Bronchitis, chest pain, contact dermatitis, contusion, diabetes mellitus, pleural effusion, hearing loss, meibomianitis, *anaphylaxis/anaphylactoid reactions*, including angioedema.

HOW SUPPLIED
Injection: 0.3 mg.

 = see color insert   **H** = Herbal **IV** = Intravenous   = sound alike drug

DOSAGE

- **INTRAVITREOUS INJECTION**

  Age-related macular degeneration.

0.3 mg once every 6 weeks by intravitreous injection into the eye to be treated.

NURSING CONSIDERATIONS

ADMINISTRATION/STORAGE

1. Inspect visually for particulate matter and discoloration prior to administration.
2. Carry out the injection under controlled aseptic conditions. Adequate anesthesia and a broad-spectrum antibiotic should be given prior to the injection.
3. Administration of the contents of the syringe involves attaching the threaded plastic plunger rod to the rubber stopper inside the syringe barrel. Do not pull back on the plunger. Then remove the syringe needle cap to allow administration of the drug.
4. Store from 2–8°C (36–46°F). Do not freeze or shake vigorously.

ASSESSMENT

1. List reasons for therapy, age at onset, other therapies trialed, outcome.
2. Note clinical presentation, any erythema, drainage, IOP, and level of vision.
3. Ensure that adequate anesthesia and a broad-spectrum microbicide have been administered prior to injection.
4. Drug is only administered by those trained to manage wet AMD. After injection, monitor client's elevation in IOP and for endophthalmitis. May check perfusion of the optic nerve head immediately after injection, tonometry within 30 min of administration and biomicroscopy between 2 and 7 days following injection.

CLIENT/FAMILY TEACHING

1. Drug is administered into the affected eye with a needle once every 6 weeks to prevent blindness from macular degeneration.
2. Seek immediate care from the provider if a change in vision, redness of the eye, or light sensitivity develops.
3. Therapy will require check ups to ensure that no infection develops, and if there is an increase in ocular pressure after the injection, the client may require more frequent monitoring procedures.

OUTCOMES/EVALUATE

Suppression of age-related neovascular (wet) macular degeneration (AMD) progression

Pegaspargase Ⅳ©
(PEG-L-asparaginase)
(peg-**ASS**-pair-gays)

CLASSIFICATION(S):
Antineoplastic, miscellaneous
PREGNANCY CATEGORY: C
Rx: Oncaspar.

SEE ALSO *ANTINEOPLASTIC AGENTS.*

USES

(1) As a component of a multiagent chemotherapeutic regimen for clients with acute lymphoblastic leukemia who have developed hypersensitivity to the native forms of L-asparaginase. (2) As a component of a multiagent chemotherapeutic regimen for the first-line treatment of acute lymphoblastic leukemia.

ACTION/KINETICS

Action

Pegaspargase is a modification of the enzyme L-asparaginase. Some leukemic cells are not able to synthesize asparagine due to a lack of the enzyme asparaginase synthetase and are thus dependent on exogenous asparaginase for survival. Rapid depletion of asparagine, due to administration of asparaginase, kills leukemic cells. Normal cells, which can synthesize their own asparagine, are less affected.

Pharmacokinetics

$t^{1/2}$, elimination: About 5.8 days during the induction.

CONTRAINDICATIONS

History of serious allergic reactions to pegaspargase (e.g., generalized urticaria, bronchospasm, laryngeal edema, hypotension, or other side effects); serious thrombosis, pancreatitis, and/or serious hemorrhagic events with prior L-asparaginase therapy. Lactation.

Bold Italic = life threatening side effect   ■ = black box warning   ✦ = Available in Canada

SPECIAL CONCERNS

Clients taking pegaspargase are at a higher risk for bleeding problems, especially with simultaneous use of other drugs that have anticoagulant properties (e.g., aspirin, NSAIDs). Safety and efficacy have not been determined in clients from 1 to 21 years of age with known previous hypersensitivity to L-asparaginase.

SIDE EFFECTS

Most Common

Chemical hepatoxicity, coagulopathies, hypersensitivity reactions, clinical pancreatitis, hyperglycemia requiring insulin therapy, thrombosis.

Most commonly hypersensitivity reactions, chemical hepatotoxicity, and coagulopathies. **Allergic reactions: Hypersensitivity reactions** (acute or delayed), including **life-threatening anaphylaxis**, may occur during therapy, especially in clients with known hypersensitivity to other forms of L-asparaginase. Also, skin rashes, erythema, edema, pain, fever, chills, urticaria, dyspnea, **bronchospasm**, increased ALT, N&V, malaise, arthralgia, induration, hives, tenderness, swelling, lip edema. **GI:** *Pancreatiti*s (may be severe), GI/abdominal pain, anorexia, diarrhea, constipation, flatulence, indigestion, mucositis, mouth tenderness, severe colitis. **Coagulation disorders:** Decreased anticoagulant effect, **DIC**, decreased fibrinogen, increased thromboplastin, increased coagulation time, prolonged PT/PTTs, **clinical hemorrhage (may be fatal)**, decreased antithrombin III, superficial and deep venous thrombosis, sagittal sinus thrombosis, venous catheter thrombosis, atrial thrombosis, decreased platelet count, purpura, ecchymosis, easy bruaisable. **Hepatic:** Jaundice, abnormal LFTs, fatty liver deposits, hepatomegaly, ascites, **liver failure. CV:** Hypotension (may be severe), tachycardia, thrombosis (including sagittal sinus thrombosis), chest pain, hypertension, subacute bacterial endocarditis, edema. **Hematologic: Hemolytic anemia**, leukopenia, pancytopenia, thrombocytopenia, **agranulocytosis**, anemia. **CNS: Convulsions, sta-** *tus epilepticus*, temporal lobe seizures, headache, paresthesia, mild to severe confusion, thrombosis/hemorrhage, disorientation, dizziness, emotional lability, somnolence, **coma**, mental status changes, Parkinson-like syndrome. **Respiratory:** Dyspnea, **bronchospasm**, increased cough, epistaxis, URI. **Dermatologic:** Injection site hypersensitivity, rash, petechial rash, erythema simplex, pruritus, itching, alopecia, fever blister, hand whiteness, fungal changes, nail whiteness and ridging. **GU:** Hematuria, increased urinary frequency, abnormal kidney function, severe hemorrhagic cystitis, **renal failure**, uric acid nephropathy. **Musculoskeletal:** Arthralgia, myalgia, bone pain, joint disorder, local/diffuse musculoskeletal pain, joint stiffness, cramps. **Miscellaneous:** Pain in the extremities, injection site reaction (including pain, swelling, or redness), night sweats, peripheral edema, increased/decreased appetite, excessive thirst, weight loss, face/lesional edema, **septic shock, sepsis**, infection, malaise, fatigue, metabolic acidosis, glucose intolerance, immunogenicity.

LABORATORY TEST CONSIDERATIONS

↑ AST, ALT, amylase, lipase, gamma-glutamyltranspeptidase, BUN, creatinine. Hyperbilirubinemia, hyperglycemia, hyperuricemia, hypoglycemia, hypoproteinemia, hyperammonemia, hyponatremia, hypoalbuminemia, proteinuria.

DRUG INTERACTIONS

Depletion of serum proteins by pegaspargase may ↑ the toxicity of other drugs which are protein bound. ↑ Predisposition to bleeding when used with warfarin, heparin, dipyridamole, aspirin, or NSAIDs. May ↓ the effect of methotrexate.

HOW SUPPLIED

Injection: 750 units/mL.

DOSAGE

- **IM (PREFERRED); IV**
  Acute lymphoblastic leukemia.

Adults: 2,500 international units/m^2 no more frequently than q 14 days. This dose is also used if the drug is given as a sole agent. **Children with a BSA greater than 0.6 m^2:** 2,500 international units/m^2 no more frequently than q 14 days. **Children with a BSA less than 0.6 m^2:** 82.5 international units/kg no more frequently than q 14 days.

NURSING CONSIDERATIONS

Ⓒ Do not confuse pegaspargase (Oncaspar) with asparaginase (Elspar), each of which is an antineoplastic drugs.

ADMINISTRATION/STORAGE

1. The preferred route of administration is IM due to a lower risk of hepatotoxicity, coagulopathy, and GI and renal disorders.
2. Do not give if there is any indication drug has been frozen; freezing destroys pegaspargase activity.
3. When given IM, do not exceed 2 mL to a single injection site; if more than 2 mL is necessary, use multiple injection sites.
4. When remission is obtained, appropriate maintenance therapy may be instituted.
5. Do not shake; avoid excessive agitation. Do not use if cloudy, if a precipitate is present, or if drug has been stored at room temperature for more than 48 hr.
6. Store at 2–8°C (36–46°F).
7. Use only one dose per vial; do not reenter the vial. Discard any unused portions.
Ⅳ 8. When used IV, administer over a 1- to 2-hr period in 100 mL of NSS or D5W, through an infusion tube of a solution that is already running.

ASSESSMENT

1. List disease onset, characteristics of S&S, other agents trialed/failed.
2. Note previous therapy and outcome. Use the National Cancer Institute Common Toxic Criteria to grade the severity of any hypersensitivity reaction.
3. Anticipate giving with other antineoplastic agents. Monitor continuously for anaphylaxis during the first hour of therapy.
4. Assess for early S&S of infection due to immunosuppressive effects; or pancreatitis (↑ amylase). Ensure adequate hydration to prevent hyperuricemia.

5. IM administration may decrease many of the drug-associated adverse systemic effects.
6. Monitor CBC, uric acid level, renal and LFTs.

CLIENT/FAMILY TEACHING

1. Avoid agents that may increase bleeding (e.g., aspirin/NSAIDs, alcohol). Report bruising or bleeding, and any early S&S of infection.
2. Report any persistent N&V, yellow skin discoloration, difficulty breathing, chest pain, rash, or severe abdominal pain immediately. Report any altered mental status or evidence of seizure activity.
3. Increase fluid intake to 2–3 L/day to prevent urate deposits/calculi formation. Consume diet low in purines to maintain alkaline urine.
4. Drug lowers resistance to infections; avoid situations that may put one at risk (i.e., crowds, persons with infectious diseases, vaccinia).

OUTCOMES/EVALUATE

Improved hematologic parameters; remission of acute lymphoblastic leukemia

Pegfilgrastim
(peg-fill-**GRAH**-stim)

CLASSIFICATION(S):
Hematopoietic agent
PREGNANCY CATEGORY: C
Rx: Neulasta.

USES

Decrease incidence of infection, as demonstrated by febrile neutropenia, in clients with nonmyeloid malignancies who are receiving myelosuppressive anticancer drugs associated with a significant incidence of febrile neutropenia.

ACTION/KINETICS

Action

A colony stimulating factor that binds to specific cell surface receptors of hematopoietic cells resulting in proliferation, differentiation, commitment, and end cell function activation. Has same mechanism of action as filgrastim but has decreased renal clearance and prolonged activity compared with filgrastim.

Pharmacokinetics

A single SC dose will stimulate hematopoiesis for up to 14 days. Clients with higher body weights experienced higher systemic exposure after receiving a dose normalized for body weight. **t½:** 15–80 hr after SC.

CONTRAINDICATIONS

Known hypersensitivity to *Escherichia coli*-derived proteins, pegfilgrastim, filgrastim, or any component of the product. Use of the 6 mg fixed-dose single-use syringe formulation in infants, children, and smaller adolescents weighing less than 45 kg. Use between 14 days before and 24 hr after cytotoxic chemotherapy due to the potential for an increase in sensitivity of rapidly dividing myeloid cells to cytotoxic chemotherapy.

SPECIAL CONCERNS

The possibility that pegfilgrastim can act as a growth factor for any tumor type cannot be excluded. Use with caution during lactation. Safety and efficacy have not been established in children.

SIDE EFFECTS

Most Common

Most side effects appear to be due to the underlying malignancy or cytotoxic chemotherapy. Medullary bone pain.

GI: Nausea, diarrhea, vomiting, constipation, anorexia, taste perversion, dyspepsia, abdominal pain, stomatitis, mucositis, *splenic rupture*. **CNS:** Headache, insomnia, dizziness. **Allergic:** *Anaphylaxis*, skin rash, urticaria. **Body as a whole:** Fatigue, alopecia, fever, skeletal pain, myalgia, arthralgia, generalized weakness, peripheral edema. **Hematologic:** Granulocytopenia, leukocytosis, neutropenic fever. **Miscellaneous:** Medullary bone pain, hypoxia, *ARDS*, sickle cell crisis with sickle cell disease.

LABORATORY TEST CONSIDERATIONS

↑ LDH, alkaline phosphatase, uric acid (all are reversible).

DRUG INTERACTIONS

Lithium may potentiate the release of neutrophils; if used together with pegfilgrastim, monitor neutrophil counts more frequently.

HOW SUPPLIED

Single-Dose Syringe: Preservative-free solution containing 6 mg (0.6 mL) of pegfilgrastim (10 mg/mL).

DOSAGE

* **SC**

    Myelosuppressive chemotherapy.
Single 6 mg dose given once per chemotherapy cycle.

NURSING CONSIDERATIONS

ADMINISTRATION/STORAGE

1. Not to be given during the 14 days preceding a dose of cytotoxic drugs through the first 24 hr afterward.
2. Visually inspect for discoloration and particulate matter before administration. Do not give if discoloration/particulate matter are noted.
3. Refrigerate at 2–8°C (36–46°F) and keep syringes in their carton to protect from light until use.
4. Avoid shaking. May be allowed to reach room temperature for a maximum of 48 hr before use, but protect from light. Discard any drug left at room temperature for more than 48 hr.
5. Avoid freezing. If accidentally frozen, allow to thaw in the refrigerator before administration. Discard if frozen a second time.

ASSESSMENT

1. Note chemotherapeutic agents being used, reasons for therapy.
2. Obtain CBC with platelet count before giving chemotherapy; monitor regularly with alkaline phosphatase, LDH, uric acid.

CLIENT/FAMILY TEACHING

1. Review S&S of allergic drug reactions and appropriate actions to take. Report abdominal pain, shoulder pain, fever, or breathing problems immediately.
2. Ensure product is refrigerated as directed. Do not freeze. Must be compliant with therapy; have regular monitoring of blood counts.
3. May be given at home if instruction on the proper use of the drug is com-

P

pleted. Do not reuse syringes, needles, or drug products and follow proper disposal techniques. May obtain a puncture-resistant container for disposal of used needles and syringes.

4. Immediately report any adverse side effects or high fevers. Potential exists for tumor cell growth with this product.

OUTCOMES/EVALUATE

Reduced incidence of infection during myelosuppressive chemotherapy ↑ WBC

Peginterferon alfa-2a ■

(**peg**-in-ter-**FEAR**-on)

CLASSIFICATION(S):

Immunomodulator
PREGNANCY CATEGORY: C
Rx: Pegasys.

USES

(1) Adults with HbeAg-positive and HbeAg-negative chronic hepatitis B virus infection who have compensated liver disease and evidence of viral replication and liver inflammation. (2) Alone or in combination with ribavirin tablets to treat chronic hepatitis C in adults who have compensated liver disease and have not been treated previously with interferon alfa. (3) Combination of chronic hepatitis C in adults also infected with HIV whose HIV infection is clinically stable. *Investigational:* Renal cell carcinoma, chronic myelogenous leukemia.

ACTION/KINETICS

Action

Interferons bind to specific receptors on the cell surface initiating intracellular signaling via a complex cascade of protein-protein interactions; this leads to rapid activation of gene transcription. Peginterferon alfa-2a stimulates production of effector proteins (e.g., serum neopterin and 2′,5′-oligoadenylate synthetase), raises body temperature, and causes reversible decreases in leukocyte and platelet counts.

Pharmacokinetics

Maximum serum levels: 72–96 hr (sustained for up to 168 hr). **t½, terminal:** 80 hr (range: 50–140 hr). AUC is increased in clients over 62 years of age. Is a 25–45% reduction in clearance in those with end-stage renal disease. Clearance in children is nearly 4-fold lower compared with that in adults.

CONTRAINDICATIONS

Peginterferon alfa-2a alone: Hypersensitivity to peginterferon alfa-2a or any of its components; autoimmune hepatitis; hepatic decompensation (Child-Pugh score greater than 6–class B and C) in cirrhotic hepatitis C clients coinfected with HIV before or during treatment with peginterferon alfa-2a. Use in neonates and infants (contains benzyl alcohol). **Peginterferon alfa-2a with Ribavirin:** Hypersensitivity to ribavirin tablets or to any component; pregnancy; men whose female partners are pregnant; those with hemoglobinopathies (e.g., thalessemia major, sickle-cell anemia). Lactation (alone or with ribavirin).

SPECIAL CONCERNS

■ (1) Alpha interferons, including peginterferon alfa-2a may cause or aggravate fatal or life-threatening neuropsychiatric, autoimmune, ischemic, or infectious disorders. Closely monitor clients with periodic clinical and lab evaluations. Withdraw therapy in those with persistently severe or worsening signs or symptoms of these conditions. In many, but not all, cases these disorders resolve after stopping peginterferon alfa-2a therapy. (2) Ribavirin may cause birth defects and/or death of the fetus. Extreme care must be taken to avoid pregnancy in women taking peginterferon alfa-2a and in female partners of men taking peginterferon alfa-2a. (3) Ribavirin causes hemolytic anemia. The anemia associated with ribavirin therapy may result in a worsening of cardiac disease. (4) Because ribavirin is genotoxic and mutagenic, consider it a potential carcinogen.■ Use with caution in pre-existing cardiac disease, in those with a history of depression, in those with a creatinine clearance less than 50 mL/min, and in those with baseline neutrophil counts under 1,500 cells/mm³, baseline platelet counts less than 90,000/mm³, or baseline hemoglobin less than 10 grams/dL. Product contains benzyl alcohol which is associated with an increased incidence of neurological and other complications in neonates and infants (may be fatal). Side effects may be more severe in elderly clients. Safety and efficacy have not been determined in children under age 18.

SIDE EFFECTS

Most Common

Peginterferon alfa-2a used alone: Depression, dizziness, fatigue/asthenia, headache, insomnia, irritability/anxiety, alopecia, pruritus, abdominal pain, diarrhea, N&V, neutropenia, anorexia, arthralgia, myalgia, injection site reaction, pyrexia, rigors.

NOTE: If used with ribavirin, consult information on that drug as well. **CNS:** Depression, irritability, anxiety, nervousness, headache, insomnia, dizziness, impaired concentration/memory, depressed mood. Neuropsychiatric reactions, including aggressive behavior, psychoses, hallucinations, bipolar disorders, mania, suicidal ideation, *suicide,* homicidal iddeation, depression, relapse of drug addiction, drug overdose. **GI:** N&V, anorexia, diarrhea, abdominal pain, dry mouth, dyspepsia, hepatic dysfunction, fatty liver, cholangitis, peptic ulcer, GI bleeding, *pancreatitis, colitis (hemorrhagic/ischemic)*, exacerbations of hepatitis during hepatitis B therapy. **Hematologic:** Neutropenia, thrombocytopenia, lymphopenia, aplastic anemia (rare). **CV:** Arrhythmia, endocarditis, hypertension, supraventricular arrhythmias, chest pain, *MI, pulmonary embolism, cerebral hemorrhage*. **Dermatologic:** Alopecia, pruritus, increased sweating, dermatitis, rash, dry skin, eczema. **Musculoskeletal:** Myalgia, arthralgia, back pain, myositis. **Respiratory:** Pneumonia, cough, interstitial pneumonitis, dyspnea, pulmonary infiltrates, bronchiolitis obliterans, sarcoidosis. **Body as a whole:** Flu-like symptoms (fatigue, pyrexia, myalgia, headache, rigors), pain, asthenia, autoimmune phenomena, decreased weight, infections, hypo-/hyperglycemia, hypersensitivity reactions (urticaria, angioedema, bronchoconstriction, *anaphylaxis*), bacterial infections (sepsis, osteomyelitis, endocarditis, pyelonephritis). **Ophthalmic:** Corneal ulcer, decrease/loss of vision, macular edema, retinal artery or vein thrombosis, retinal hemorrhage, cotton wool spots, optic neuritis, papilledema. **Miscellaneous:** Injection site reaction, diabetes mellitus, peripheral neuropathy, impaired renal function, coma, aggravation of hypo-/hyperthyroidism. Development of or exacerbation of autoimmune disorders, including hepatitis, idiopathic thrombocytopenia purpura, interstitial nephritis, myositis, psoriasis, rheumatoid arthritis, systemic lupus erythematosus, thrombotic thrombocytopenic purpura, thyroiditis.

LABORATORY TEST CONSIDERATIONS

↑ ALT (transient). ↓ WBC, ANC, platelet counts. Abnormal thyroid lab values.

DRUG INTERACTIONS

Methadone / ↑ (10–15%) Methadone levels after 4 weeks treatment with peginterferon alfa-2a

Nucleoside reverse transcriptase inhibitors (didanosine, stabudine, zidovudine) / ↑ Hematologic toxicity; possible fatal hepatic decomposition

Theophylline / ↑ Theophylline AUC R/T inhibition of CYP1A2; monitor theophylline levels

HOW SUPPLIED

Injection: 180 mcg/mL.

DOSAGE

- **SC**

  Chronic hepatitis C in adults.

Peginterferon alfa-2a monotherapy: 180 mcg once a week for 48 weeks by SC injection in the abdomen or thigh. If dosage reduction is needed due to moderate to severe side effects, reduce dose to 135 mcg; in some cases drug reduction to 90 mcg may be necessary. Following improvement of side effects, re-escalation of dose may be considered. **When combined with ribavirin:** Dose depends on viral genotype. **Genotype 1, 4:** Peginterferon alfa-2a, 180 mcg as above. If weight is less than 75 kg, give ribavirin 1,000 mg/day. If weight is 75 kg or more, give ribavirin 1,200 mg/day. Duration of therapy is 48 weeks. **Genotype 2, 3:** Peginterferon alfa-2a, 180 mcg once a week with ribavirin 800 mg/day for 24 weeks.

Chronic hepatitis C with HIV.

Peginterferon alfa-2a monotherapy: 180 mcg once weekly for 48 weeks by SC injection into the abdomen or thigh. **Combination therapy with ribavirin:** 180 mcg peginterferon alfa-2a weekly and 800 mg ribavirin PO every day for 48 weeks, regardless of genotype.

Chronic hepatitis B.

Peginterferon alfa-2a monotherapy: 180 mcg once weekly for 48 weeks by SC injection in the abdomen or thigh.

NURSING CONSIDERATIONS

ADMINISTRATION/STORAGE

1. Consider discontinuing after 12 weeks if there is no demonstrable response.

2. Consider dose reduction to 135 mcg if the neutrophil count is <750 cells/mm^3. If ANC falls below 500 cells/mm^3, suspend treatment until ANC values return to >1,000 cells/mm^3. Initially reinstitute therapy at 90 mcg and monitor neutrophil count.

3. Reduce dose to 135 mcg in clients with end-stage renal disease requiring hemodialysis.

4. If platelets decrease to <50,000/mm^3, reduce dose to 90 mcg. Discontinue peginterferon alfa-2a if the platelet count decreases to <25,000/mm^3.

5. In chronic hepatitis C clients with progressive ALT increases above baseline values, reduce dose to 135 mcg. Perform more frequent monitoring of liver function. Therapy can be resumed after ALT flares subside.

6. In chronic hepatitis B clients with elevations of ALT >5 times ULN, perform more frequent monitoring of liver function and consider either reducing the dose to 135 mcg or temporarily discontinuing treatment. Therapy can be resumed after ALT flares subside.

7. In hepatitis B clients with persistent, severe ALT values >10 times ULN, consider discontinuing treatment.

8. Check manufacturer's guidelines for modification or discontinuation of peginterferon alfa-2a for clients with depression.

9. Vials are for single use only; discard any unused portion. Prefilled syringes are available for ease of administration.

10. Store in the refrigerator but do not freeze. Do not shake. Protect from light.

ASSESSMENT

1. Note reasons for therapy, disease onset, genotype, liver biopsy results, clinical presentation, other agents trialed, outcome.

2. Assess for CAD, depression, renal failure. Monitor CBC, viral load, uric acid, renal, thyroid, LFTs. Reduce dose as directed for specific deficits under administration/storage and for adverse effects. May increase/reestablish dose once these subside.

3. Review treatment criteria, i.e., platelets >90,000 cells/mm^3; ANC >1,500 cells/mm^3; creatinine <1.5 x ULN and TSH/T$_4$ WNL or controlled function.

4. Obtain baseline labs (hematologic and biochemical) and monitor: CBC q 2 weeks, chemistries q 4 weeks, and TSH every 12 weeks. Progressive increases in ALT and bilirubin require interruption of therapy, as well as do severe depression/suicide ideations.

CLIENT/FAMILY TEACHING

1. Drug is used to prevent progressive liver destruction from the hepatitis C virus. It is not known for sure if treatment will cure hepatitis C or prevent cirrhosis, liver failure, or liver cancer from infection with hepatitis C. It is also not known if the drug will prevent transmission of HCV or HIV infection to others. Use protection and reliable birth control.

2. To minimize flu-like symptoms, administer drug at bedtime once a week. Use antipyretics as needed.

3. Review procedure for storage (refrigeration), preparation, injection, and disposal of drug/equipment. Proper disposal of needles is imperative; do not reuse needles or syringes. A puncture-

resistant container will be supplied for disposal of used needles and syringes at home.

4. Do not perform activities that require mental alertness until drug effects realized. May experience depression, flu-like symptoms, bleeding abnormalities, visual problems, dizziness, disorientation, sleepiness, joint/muscle pains, fever, abdominal pain, bloody diarrhea, breathing problems, chills, and fatigue. Report any unusual/adverse side effects.

5. Must commit to a monitoring program for standard blood testing. Labs are required before beginning therapy and at periodic set intervals in order to continue drug therapy.

6. Schedule activities/work to provide rest periods as fatigue accompanies therapy.

OUTCOMES/EVALUATE

- Inhibition of viral replication/proliferation with hepatitis C
- ↓ HCV/HIV RNA; ↓ liver inflammation/fibrosis

Peginterferon alfa-2b ■

(peg-**in**-ter-**FEER**-on)

CLASSIFICATION(S):
Immunomodulator
PREGNANCY CATEGORY: C
Rx: PEG-Intron.

USES

Chronic hepatitis C, alone or in combination with ribavirin, in adults who have compensated liver disease and have not been treated previously with interferon alfa and are at least 18 years of age. *NOTE:* When used with ribavirin, consult ribavirin information as well.

ACTION/KINETICS

Action

Effect due to the interferon alfa-2b moiety which binds to specific membrane receptors on the cell surface. This initiates a complex series of intracellular effects, including suppression of cell proliferation, enhancement of phagocytic activity of macrophages, augmentation of specific cytotoxicity of lymphocytes for target cells, and inhibition of virus replication in virus-infected cells.

Pharmacokinetics

Maximum serum levels: 15–44 hr; serum levels sustained for 48 hr (or less) to 72 hr. **t½, elimination:** About 40 hr. About 30% excreted in the urine. Clearance is decreased by about one-half in those with impaired renal function.

CONTRAINDICATIONS

Peginterferon alfa-2b: Hypersensitivity to the drug or any component of the product, autoimmune hepatitis, decompensated liver disease. Lactation. **Peginterferon alfa-2b and ribavirin:** Hypersensitivity to the drugs or any component of the product, pregnancy, men whose female partners are pregnant, those with hemoglobinopathies (e.g., thalassemia major, sickle-cell anemia). Lactation. Neonates and infants (product contains benzyl alcohol).

SPECIAL CONCERNS

■ Peginterferon alfa-2b may cause or aggravate fatal or life-threatening neuropsychiatric, autoimmune, ischemic, and infectious disorders. Closely monitor clients with periodic clinical and lab evaluations. Clients with persistently severe or worsening signs or symptoms of these conditions should be withdrawn from therapy. In many (but not all) cases, these disorders resolve after terminating peginterferon alfa-2b.■ Serious, acute hypersensitivity reactions, although rare, may occur. When combined with ribavirin, side effects are common and severe. Use with caution in those with a C_{CR} less than 50 mL/min, in the elderly, and in CV disease. May be development or worsening of autoimmune disorders (e.g., thyroiditis, thrombocytopenia, rheumatoid arthritis, interstitial nephritis, SLE, psoriasis). Safety and efficacy have not been determined in children less than 18 years of age, for the treatment of clients with HCV coinfected with HIV or HBV, or to treat hepatitis C in clients who have received liver or other organ transplants.

P

SIDE EFFECTS

Most Common
Headache, fatigue/asthenia, myalgia, injection site inflammation/reaction, anxiety/irritability, depression, insomnia, alopecia, anorexia, nausea, arthralgia, musculoskeletal pain, fever, rigors, dizziness, impaired concentration, dry skin, pruritus, abdominal pain, pharyngitis, weight loss.

CNS: Headache, depression (may be severe), suicidal behavior (attempt, ideation), anxiety, emotional lability, irritability, insomnia, dizziness, impaired concentration, agitation, nervousness, relapse of drug addiction/overdose, loss of consciousness, aggressive reaction, nerve palsy, psychosis, seizures, vertigo, *life-threatening or fatal neuropsychiatric events (e.g., suicide, homicidal ideation)*. **GI:** Nausea, anorexia, diarrhea, abdominal pain, vomiting, dyspepsia, dry mouth, constipation, gastroenteritis, stomatitis, *fatal/nonfatal ulcerative and hemorrhagic colitis, fatal/nonfatal pancreatitis*. **Respiratory:** Pharyngitis, sinusitis, coughing, dyspnea, rhinitis, pulmonary infiltrates, bronchiolitis obliterans, interstitial pneumonitis, sarcoidosis, pneumonitis, pneumonia, emphysema, pleural effusion. **Dermatologic:** Alopecia, pruritus, dry skin, increased sweating, rash, flushing, aggravated psoriasis, urticaria, vasculitis, phototoxicity, erythema multiforme, *Stevens-Johnson syndrome, toxic epidermal necrolysis*. **Hematologic:** Thrombocytopenia, neutropenia, leukopenia, anemia, autoimmune thrombocytopenia with or without purpura. **CV:** *Cardiomyopathy, MI*, hypotension, arrhythmia, TIA, supraventricular arrhythmias, angina, pericardial effusion, cardiac ischemia. **Ophthalmic:** Retinal hemorrhages, cotton wool spots, retinal artery/vein obstruction, retinal ischemia/artery or vein thrombosis, decrease or loss of vision, blurred vision, conjunctivitis, optic neuritis, papilledema, decreased visual acuity. **Otic:** Impaired hearing, hearing loss. **Body as a whole:** Flu-like symptoms, musculoskeletal pain, myalgia, arthralgia, fatigue, asthenia, malaise, rigors, fever, weight decrease, abscess, lupus-like syndrome, viral infection, infection (abscess, sepsis, cellulitis), rheumatoid arthritis, sarcoidosis, rhabdomyolysis. **Hypersensitivity reaction:** Urticaria, angioedema, bronchoconstriction, *anaphylaxis*. **At injection site:** Bruising, itchiness, irritation, pain, inflammation, alopecia, necrosis. **Miscellaneous:** RUQ pain, hepatomegaly, hypertonia, menstrual disorder, chest pain, fungal infection, taste perversion, hypo-/hyperthyroidism, nerve palsy (facial, oculomotor), development or exacerbation of autoimmune disorders (e.g., thyroiditis, rheumatoid arthritis, interstitial nephritis, lupus erythematosis, psoriasis), gout, hyperglycemia, peripheral neuropathy, renal failure/insufficiency.

LABORATORY TEST CONSIDERATIONS
↑ ALT. ↓ Neutrophils, platelet counts. TSH abnormalities. Appearance of serum neutralizing antibodies. When used with ribavirin: Hyperbilirubinemia, hyperuricemia (with hemolysis).

HOW SUPPLIED
Powder for Injection, Lyophilized: 100 mcg/mL, 160 mcg/mL, 240 mcg/mL, 300 mcg/mL (all strengths are after reconstitution).

DOSAGE

• SC
Chronic hepatitis C.

Monotherapy, initial: Based on weight. Dose of 1 mcg/kg is given once weekly (on the same day of each week) for 1 year. Doses, based on body weight, are: **45 kg or less:** 40 mcg (0.4 mL of the 100 mcg/mL strength); **46–56 kg:** 50 mcg (0.5 mL of the 100 mcg/mL strength); **57–72 kg:** 64 mcg (0.4 mL of the 160 mcg/mL strength); **73–88 kg:** 80 mcg (0.5 mL of the 160 mcg/mL strength); **89–106 kg:** 96 mcg (0.4 mL of the 240 mcg/mL strength); **107–136 kg:** 120 mcg (0.5 mL of the 240 mcg/mL strength); **137–160 kg:** 150 mcg (0.5 mL of the 300 mcg/mL strength).

When used with ribavirin: 1.5 mcg/kg/week. Doses of peginterferon alfa-2b, based on body weight, are: **<40 kg:** 50 mcg (0.5 mL of the 100 mcg/mL strength); **40–50 kg:** 64 mcg (0. 4 mL of the 160 mcg/mL strength); **51–60 kg:**

Bold Italic = life threatening side effect   ■ = black box warning   ♣ = Available in Canada

80 mcg (0.5 mL of the 160 mcg/mL strength): **61–75 kg:** 96 mcg (0.4 mL of the 240 mcg/mL strength); **76–85 kg:** 120 mcg (0.5 mL of the 240 mcg/mL strength); **>85 kg:** 150 mcg (0.5 mL of the 300 mcg/mL strength).

NURSING CONSIDERATIONS

ADMINISTRATION/STORAGE

1. Reconstitute with 0.7 mL of supplied diluent (sterile water for injection). Swirl gently to hasten complete dissolution. Diluent vial is for single use only; discard any remaining diluent. Do not reconstitute with any other diluent.

2. Use immediately after reconstitution as the product contains no preservative; do not freeze.

3. Reconstituted solution should be clear and colorless. Do not use the solution if it is discolored, cloudy, or contains particulate matter.

4. Peginterferon alfa-2b is also available in an easier to use product called Redipen. To reconstitute, hold the Redipen upright (dose button down) and press the two halves of the pen together until there is an audible click. Gently invert the pen to mix the solution; do not shake. Keeping the pen upright, attach the supplied needle and select the appropriate peginterferon alfa-2b dose by pulling back on the dosing button until the dark bands are visible and turning the button until the dark band is aligned with the correct dose. Redipen is for single use only.

5. Do not add other medications to peginterferon alfa-2b solutions.

6. Stop therapy if hepatitis C virus levels remain high after 6 mo of therapy.

7. Consult package insert for dose reduction instructions if adverse reactions develop.

8. Store the vials of unreconstituted drug between 15–30°C (59–86°F). After reconstitution use immediately, but may be stored for 24 hr or less between 2–8°C (36–46°F). Do not freeze.

9. Store Redipen at 2–8°C (36–46°F). After reconstitution, use immediately, but it may be stored up to 24 hr from 2–8°C (36–46°F). The reconstituted solution contains no preservative; it is clear and colorless. Do not freeze.

ASSESSMENT

1. Note reasons for therapy, onset/characteristics of disease, other agents trialed. Assess mental status, history of depression. Note results of liver biopsy.

2. Monitor CBC, eye exams, TSH, renal, LFTs, viral load. Assess clients with impaired renal function for S&S of interferon toxicity; adjust dose accordingly.

3. Ensure adequate hydration, esp. during initial stages of treatment.

4. List any other medical conditions that may require monitoring during therapy; drug may aggravate hypo/hyperthyroidism or diabetes control.

CLIENT/FAMILY TEACHING

1. To minimize flu-like symptoms, administer the drug at bedtime once a week. Use antipyretics as needed.

2. It is not known if treatment will cure hepatitis C or prevent cirrhosis, liver failure, or liver cancer that may result from infection with the hepatitis C virus. It is also not known if the drug will prevent transmission of HCV infection to others.

3. Once reconstituted, may only store in the refrigerator up to 24 hr.

4. Proper disposal of needles is imperative; do not reuse needles or syringes. A puncture-resistant container will be supplied for disposal of used needles and syringes at home.

5. Drug may cause depression, flu-like symptoms, bleeding abnormalities, and autoimmune dysfunction. Report any unusual/adverse side effects.

6. Labs are required before beginning therapy and at periodic set intervals; must comply to continue therapy.

OUTCOMES/EVALUATE

Inhibition of progression of hepatitis C; improved LFTs ↓ HCV RNA

Pegvisomant
(peg-**VIH**-so-mant)

CLASSIFICATION(S):
Drug to treat acromegaly
PREGNANCY CATEGORY: B
Rx: Somavert.

USES

Treat acromegaly in those who have had an inadequate response to surgery/radiation therapy and/or other medical therapies, or if other therapies are not appropriate. The goal is to normalize serum IGF-1 levels.

ACTION/KINETICS

Action

Pegvisomant, a product of recombinant DNA technology, binds selectively to growth hormone (GH) receptors on cell surfaces and subsequently blocks the binding of endogenous GH interfering with GH signal transduction. Inhibition of the action of GH causes decreased serum insulin-like growth factor (IGF-1) levels as well as other GH-responsive serum proteins, including IGF binding protein-3 and the acid-labile subunit.

Pharmacokinetics

Peak serum levels, after SC: 33–77 hr. Clearance of the drug increases with body weight. **t½, mean:** About 6 days after either single or multiple doses. Less than 1% is recovered in the urine; the route of elimination has not been studied.

CONTRAINDICATIONS

Hypersensitivity to the drug or any component of the product. The stopper on the vial contains latex.

SPECIAL CONCERNS

Use caution in selecting the dose for geriatric clients. Use with caution during lactation. Safety and efficacy have not been determined in children. Tumors that secrete GH may expand and cause serious complications; thus, carefully monitor all clients with these tumors, including those receiving pegvisomant. Glucose tolerance may increase in some clients since GH opposes the effects of insulin on carbohydrate metabolism by decreasing insulin sensitivity.

SIDE EFFECTS

Most Common

Pain/redness/itching at injection site, diarrhea, nausea, pain, back pain, flu syndrome.

GI: Diarrhea, nausea. **Body as a whole:** Infection, accidental injury, pain/redness/itching at injection site, pain, flu syndrome, paresthesia. **Miscellaneous:** Abnormal LFTs, chest/back pain, dizziness, peripheral edema, sinusitis, hypertension. Also, development of low titer, nonneutralizing anti-GH antibodies.

LABORATORY TEST CONSIDERATIONS

↑ ALT and AST greater than 10 x ULN is possible. Interference with serum GH measurements by commercially available GH assays. *NOTE:* Even when determined accurately, GH levels usually increase during therapy.

DRUG INTERACTIONS

Insulin / Possible need to decrease dosage of insulin after beginning pegvisomant therapy

Opiates / Possible need to increase serum pegvisomant levels to reach appropriate IGF-1 suppression

Oral hypoglycemics / Possible need to decrease dosage of oral hypoglycemics after beginning pegvisomant therapy

HOW SUPPLIED

Powder for Injection, Lyophilized: 10 mg, 15 mg, 20 mg (all are as protein/vial).

DOSAGE

- **SC**

  Acromegaly.

  Loading dose: 40 mg given under physician supervision. **Then,** instruct client to begin daily SC injections of 10 mg. Measure serum IGF-1 levels q 4–6 weeks; adjust dosage in 5 mg increments if IGF-1 levels are still elevated or 5 mg decrements if IGF-1 levels have decreased below the normal range. Do not exceed a maximum daily dose of 30 mg.

NURSING CONSIDERATIONS

ADMINISTRATION/STORAGE

1. It is not known whether those who remain symptomatic while achieving normalized IGF-1 levels would benefit from an increased dose of pegvisomant.
2. To prepare solution, withdraw 1 mL of sterile water (provided) and inject into the vial aiming stream of liquid against the glass wall. Hold vial between the palms of both hands and gently roll it to dissolve the powder. Do not shake vial as this may cause dena-

---

Bold Italic = life threatening side effect   ■ = black box warning   ✦ = Available in Canada

turation. Discard diluent vial containing the remaining water for injection.

3. After reconstitution, each vial contains 10, 15, or 20 mg of pegvisomant protein in 1 mL of solution.

4. Visually inspect for particulate matter and discoloration prior to administration. The solution should be clear after reconstitution; if cloudy, do not inject.

5. Give only 1 dose from each vial. Give within 6 hr after reconstitution.

6. Do not adjust pegvisomant dosage based on serum GH levels.

7. Prior to reconstitution, store vials in a refrigerator at 2–8°C (36–46°F). Protect from freezing.

ASSESSMENT

1. Note growth charts, all other therapies trialed, outcome. List drugs prescribed to ensure none interact unfavorably.

2. Obtain baseline serum IGF-1, ALT, AST, total bilirubin, and alkaline phosphatase levels before starting pegvisomant therapy. Initiation of therapy based on the results of liver tests:

- Normal baseline liver tests: May treat with pegvisomant. Monitor liver tests every month for the first 6 months, quarterly for the next 6 months, and biannually for the next year.

- If baseline liver tests elevated but less than or equal to 3 times ULN: May treat with pegvisomant; however monitor liver tests monthly for 1 year or more after starting therapy and then biannually for the next year.

- If baseline liver tests >3 times ULN: Do not treat with pegvisomant until a complete workup determines cause of liver dysfunction. Determine if cholelithiasis or choledocholithiasis present. Based on work-up, consider initiation of pegvisomant therapy. If drug used, closely monitor LFTs and clinical symptoms.

3. Continuation of therapy based on results of liver tests:

- If liver tests greater than or equal to 3 x ULN without any S&S of hepatitis or other liver injury, or increase in serum bilirubin: May continue therapy. Monitor liver tests weekly. Perform comprehensive hepatic workup to determine if an alternative cause of liver dysfunction is present.

- If liver tests greater than or equal to 5 x ULN, or transaminase elevations greater than or equal to 3 x ULN associated with any increase in serum bilirubin (with or without signs/symptoms of hepatitis or other liver injury): Discontinue pegvisomant immediately. Perform comprehensive hepatic workup, including serial liver tests, to determine if and when serum levels return to normal. If liver tests normalize, consider cautious reinitiation of therapy with frequent liver test monitoring.

- If there are S&S suggestive of hepatitis or other liver injury: Immediately perform a comprehensive hepatic workup. If liver injury is confirmed, discontinue pegvisomant.

4. Monitor carefully: those with diabetes/tumors and the elderly.

CLIENT/FAMILY TEACHING

1. Drug is administered once a day by a subcutaneous injection. Review how to prepare, and inject drug.

2. Immediately report any evidence of liver problems, i.e., RUQ pain, yellowing of eyes/skin, injection site reaction, or any other adverse side effects.

3. Therapy requires frequent lab studies to evaluate liver function and to adjust drug dosage.

4. May increase glucose tolerance, decrease insulin sensitivity, and require adjustment of diabetes drugs in those with diabetes.

OUTCOMES/EVALUATE

- Control of S&S of acromegaly
- Normalization of IGF-1 levels

Pemetrexed   **IV**
(pem-e-**TREKS**-ed)

CLASSIFICATION(S):
Antineoplastic, folic acid antagonist
PREGNANCY CATEGORY: D
Rx: Alimta.

USES

(1) In combination with cisplatin to treat malignant pleural mesothelioma that is unresectable or for clients who are not candidates for curative surgery. (2) Locally advanced or metastatic non-small cell lung cancer after prior chemotherapy.

ACTION/KINETICS

Action

Pemetrexed acts by disrupting folate-dependent metabolic processes needed for cell replication. The drug is transported into cells by the reduced folate carrier and membrane folate binding protein transport systems. Once inside the cell, the drug is converted to polyglutamate forms by the enzyme folyl polyglutamate synthase. The polyglutamate forms are retained in cells and are inhibitors of thymidylate synthase and glycinamide ribonucleotide formyltransferase. Polyglutamation is a time- and concentration-dependent process that occurs in tumor cells (and to a lesser extent in normal cells). Polyglutamated metabolites have an increased intracellular half life, resulting in prolonged drug activity in malignant cells. Synergistic effects occur when combined with cisplatin.

Pharmacokinetics

Pemetrexed is not metabolized significantly; from 70–90% of a dose is eliminated in the urine within 24 hr. $t^{1/2}$, **elimination:** 3.5 hr in clients with normal renal function. **Plasma protein binding:** About 81%.

CONTRAINDICATIONS

History of severe hypersensitivity to pemetrexed or any ingredient of the formulation. Use in clients whose C_{CR} is less than 45 mL/min. Lactation.

SPECIAL CONCERNS

Use with caution when given concurrently with NSAIDs to clients whose C_{CR} is less than 80 mL/min. Safety and efficacy have not been determined in children.

SIDE EFFECTS

Most Common

N&V, anorexia, fatigue, dyspnea, sensory neuropathy, constipation, diarrhea, stomatitis, pharyngitis, anemia, myalgia, chest pain, edema, fever, infection without neutropenia.

NOTE: Side effects include those manifested when combined with cisplatin. **GI:** N&V, constipation, anorexia, stomatitis, pharyngitis, diarrhea (without colostomy), dehydration, dysphagia, esophagitis, odynophagia. **CNS:** Sensory neuropathy, depression, mood alteration. **Hematologic:** Neutropenia, leukopenia, anemia, thrombocytopenia, febrile neutropenia. **CV:** Hypertension, thrombosis, embolism, *cardiac ischemia*. **Respiratory:** Dyspnea, chest pain. **Dermatologic:** Alopecia, rash (higher incidence in men), desquamation. **Musculoskeletal:** Arthralgia, myalgia. **Body as a whole:** Fatigue, fever, dehydration, edema, infection without neutropenia, infection with grade 3 or 4 neutropenia, other infection, allergic reaction, hypersensitivity, renal failure.

LABORATORY TEST CONSIDERATIONS

↑ ALT, AST, creatinine. ↓ Creatinine clearance.

OD OVERDOSE MANAGEMENT

Symptoms: Neutropenia, anemia, thrombocytopenia, mucositis, rash, bone marrow suppression, infection with or without fever, diarrhea. *Treatment:* Institute general supportive measures. Possibly leucovorin for CTC grade 4 leukopenia lasting at least 3 days, CTC grade 4 neutropenia lasting at least 3 days, and immediately for CTC grade 4 thrombocytopenia, bleeding associated with grade 3 thrombocytopenia, or grade 3 or 4 mucositis. IV dose of leucovorin is 100 mg/m^2 once, followed by 50 mg/m^2 q 6 hr for 8 days.

DRUG INTERACTIONS

NSAIDs / Closely monitor for toxicity, especially myelosuppression, renal, and GI toxicity
Nephrotoxic drugs / Possible delayed clearance of pemetrexed
Probenecid / Possible delayed clearance of pemetrexed

HOW SUPPLIED

Powder for Injection, Lyophilized: 500 mg.

DOSAGE

- **IV INFUSION ONLY**

  Malignant pleural mesothelioma.

Pemetrexed, 500 mg/m^2, infused over 10 min on day 1 of each 21-day cycle plus cisplatin, 75 mg/m^2, infused over 2 hr beginning about 30 min after the end of the pemetrexed administration. See *Administration/Storage* for information on premedication therapy.

Non-small cell lung cancer.
500 mg/m^2 over 10 min on day 1 of each 21-day cycle. See *Administration/ Storage* for information on premedication therapy.

NURSING CONSIDERATIONS

ADMINISTRATION/STORAGE

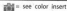 1. The following protocol for premedication therapy is followed for administration of pemetrexed:

- Folic acid, 350–1,000 mg PO. Begin 1 week prior to treatment, continue through treatment, and for 21 days after the last pemetrexed dose.
- Vitamin B$_{12}$, 1,000 mcg IM. Begin 1 week prior to treatment, continue through treatment, and for every 3 cycles thereafter.
- Dexamethasone, 4 mg 2 times per day PO. Give the day before, the day of, and the day after treatment to help prevent skin rash.

2. Reconstitute 500 mg vials with 20 mL 0.9% NaCl injection (preservative-free) to give a solution containing 25 mg/mL pemetrexed. Gently swirl each vial until powder is completely dissolved. The resulting solution is clear and ranges in color from colorless to yellow or green-yellow. The pH of the reconstituted solution ranges from 6.8 to 7.8. Further dilute the appropriate volume of reconstituted solution to 100 mL with 0.9% NaCl injection (preservative-free) and give as an IV infusion over 10 min.

3. Pemetrexed is physically incompatible with diluents containing calcium, including LR injection and Ringer's injection; do not use these diluents. Coadministration with other drugs and diluents not recommended.

4. If a pemetrexed solution contacts the skin, wash skin immediately and thoroughly with soap and water. If contact with mucous membranes occurs, flush thoroughly with water.

5. Be sure clients receive consistent hydration prior to and after receiving cisplatin. Consult cisplatin monograph.

6. Base dosage adjustments at the start of a subsequent cycle on nadir hematologic counts or maximum nonhematologic toxicity from the preceding cycle of therapy. Treatment may be delayed to allow sufficient time for recovery. Do not begin a new cycle of treatment unless the ANC is 1,500 cells/mm^3 or more, the platelet count is 100,000 cells/mm^3, and C$_{CR}$ is 45 mL/min or more.

7. Upon recovery from hematologic toxicity, use the following dose reduction schedule for pemetrexed and cisplatin:

- Give 75% of the previous doses of both drugs if the nadir ANC is <500/mm^3 and nadir platelets are 50,000/mm^3 or more.
- Give 50% of the previous dose of both drugs if the nadir platelets are <50,000/mm^3 regardless of the nadir ANC.

8. If nonhematologic toxicity (excluding neurotoxicity) develops of grade 3 (except grade 3 transaminase elevations) or more, withhold pemetrexed until toxicity resolves to less than or equal to the client's pretherapy value. Resume treatment according to the following guidelines:

- Any grade 3 (except grade 3 transaminase elevations) or 4 toxicities except mucositis: Give 75% (mg/m^2) of the previous doses of both pemetrexed and cisplatin.
- Any diarrhea requiring hospitalization: Give 75% (mg/m^2) of the previous doses of both pemetrexed and cisplatin.
- Grade 3 or 4 mucositis: Give 50% (mg/m^2) of the previous dose of pemetrexed and 100% (mg/m^2) of the previous dose of cisplatin.

9. If neurotoxicity occurs, adjust the doses of pemetrexed and cisplatin as follows:

- If the CTC grade for neurotoxicity is 0 to 1, give 100% (mg/m^2) of the previ-

ous doses of both pemetrexed and cisplatin.
- If the CTC grade for neurotoxicity is 2, give 100% of the previous dose of pemetrexed and 50% of the previous dose of cisplatin.

10. Discontinue pemetrexed therapy if the client shows any hematologic or nonhematologic grade 3 or 4 toxicity after 2 dose reductions (except grade 3 transaminase elevations). Discontinue immediately if grade 3 or 4 neurotoxicity occurs.

11. Avoid giving NSAIDs with short elimination half-lives 2 days before, the day of, and 2 days after pemetrexed. Stop dosing in all clients taking NSAIDs with long elimination half lives for at least 5 days before, the day of, and 2 days after pemetrexed administration.

12. Consider draining the effusion prior to pemetrexed administration in those with clinically significant third space fluid.

13. Store vials from 15–30°C (59–86°F). Reconstituted and infusion solutions may be stored for up to 24 hr from 2–8°C (36–46°F). Discard unused portion as reconstituted and infusion solutions contain no preservatives.

ASSESSMENT

1. Note reasons for therapy, other agents used, when disease determined unresectable, physical status of client.

2. List all drugs prescribed to ensure none interact. Avoid/monitor use carefully with NSAIDs during therapy; may cause myelosuppression, renal and GI toxicity.

3. Ensure corticosteroid is prescribed and taken for 3 days during treatment to reduce skin reactions from pemetrexed. Also ensure that client has folic acid tablets and is scheduled for B_{12} shots.

4. Monitor chemistry, renal, LFTs, CBC during therapy (before each dose and on days 8 and 15 of each cycle). Dosage adjustments at the start of a subsequent cycle are based on nadir hematologic counts or maximum nonhematologic toxicity from the preceding cycle of therapy. Treatment may be delayed to allow sufficient time for recovery. Do not begin a new cycle of treatment unless the ANC is 1,500 cells/mm^3 or more, the platelet count is 100,000 cells/mm^3, and C_{CR} is 45 mL/min or more. Upon recovery from hematologic toxicity, follow dose reduction schedule for pemetrexed and cisplatin as directed.

CLIENT/FAMILY TEACHING

1. Drug is administered IV and used to treat malignant pleural mesothelioma and lung cancer, usually in combination with cisplatin.

2. Take steroid pill for 3 days during therapy to help reduce risk of rash occurrence.

3. To minimize chances of side effects, take folic acid tablets in doses of 350–1,000 mcg for at least 5 of the 7 days prior to starting pemetrexed, daily during treatment, and for 21 days following treatment. Also vitamin B_{12} injections will be administered the week before starting therapy and then about every 9 weeks during therapy.

4. Practice reliable contraception. Drug is fetal toxic; do not nurse during therapy. Identify egg/sperm donor candidates.

5. May experience GI upset, diarrhea, fatigue, mouth/throat/lip sores, appetite loss, low blood cell counts and rash. Report if persistent or bothersome.

6. Avoid all OTC medications, vitamins, and health supplements without provider knowledge/approval. Keep all F/U visits for labs so dose or delay in therapy may be determined.

OUTCOMES/EVALUATE

Inhibition of malignant cell proliferation with pleural mesothelioma/lung cancer

Penbutolol sulfate
(pen-**BYOU**-toe-lohl)

CLASSIFICATION(S):
Beta-adrenergic blocking agent
PREGNANCY CATEGORY: C
Rx: Levatol.

SEE ALSO *BETA-ADRENERGIC BLOCKING AGENTS.*

USES

Alone or in combination with other antihypertensive drugs for mild to moderate arterial hypertension

ACTION/KINETICS

Action

Has both beta$_1$- and beta$_2$-receptor blocking activity. It has no membrane-stabilizing activity but does possess minimal intrinsic sympathomimetic activity.

Pharmacokinetics

High lipid solubility. **t½:** 5 hr. Metabolized in the liver and excreted through the urine. **Plasma protein binding:** 80–98%.

CONTRAINDICATIONS

Bronchial asthma or bronchospasms, including severe COPD.

SPECIAL CONCERNS

Dosage has not been established in children. Geriatric clients may manifest increased or decreased sensitivity to the usual adult dose.

SIDE EFFECTS

Most Common

Nausea, decreased libido, impotence, insomnia, malaise, anxiety, nervousness. See *Beta-Adrenergic Blocking Agents* for a complete list of possible side effects.

HOW SUPPLIED

Tablets: 20 mg.

DOSAGE

• TABLETS

Hypertension.

Initial: 20 mg/day either alone or with other antihypertensive agents. **Maintenance:** Same as initial dose. Doses greater than 40 mg/day do not result in a greater antihypertensive effect.

NURSING CONSIDERATIONS

ADMINISTRATION/STORAGE

Doses of 10 mg/day are effective but full effects are not evident for 4–6 weeks. The full effect of a 20- to 40-mg dose may not be observed for 2 weeks.

ASSESSMENT

1. Note onset, BP log, characteristics of S&S, other agents trialed, outcome.
2. Assess for asthma or COPD history; precludes therapy.

CLIENT/FAMILY TEACHING

1. Avoid activities that require mental alertness until drug effects realized.
2. May cause low BP; to avoid, rise slowly from a sitting or lying position.
3. Take only as prescribed; full effects may not be realized for a month or more.
4. May cause an increased sensitivity to cold; dress appropriately.
5. Avoid alcohol. Do not stop drug suddenly, may exacerbate heart disease.
6. Report low heart rate, breathing problems/wheezing, depression, confusion, rash, fever, dizziness, cold hands/feet, unusual bruising/bleeding, or sore throat. Keep BP log for provider review.

OUTCOMES/EVALUATE

↓ BP

Penciclovir
(pen-**SIGH**-kloh-veer)

CLASSIFICATION(S):

Antiviral
PREGNANCY CATEGORY: B
Rx: Denavir.

SEE ALSO *ANTIVIRAL DRUGS.*

USES

Treatment of recurrent herpes labialis (cold sores) in adults and children, 12 years and older.

ACTION/KINETICS

Action

Active against herpes simplex viruses (HSVs), including HSV-1 and HSV-2. In infected cells, viral thymidine kinase phosphorylates penciclovir to a monophosphate form which then is converted to penciclovir triphosphate by cellular kinases. Penciclovir triphosphate inhibits HSV polymerase competitively with deoxyguanosine triphosphate which inhibits herpes viral DNA synthesis and replication.

Pharmacokinetics

Not absorbed through the skin.

CONTRAINDICATIONS

Lactation. Application of the drug to mucous membranes.

P

SPECIAL CONCERNS

Use with caution if applied around the eyes due to the possibility of irritation. The effect of the drug in immunocompromised clients has not been determined. Safety and efficacy have not been determined in children.

SIDE EFFECTS

Most Common

Application site reaction, hypesthesia, local anesthesia.

Dermatologic: Application site reaction, hypesthesia, local anesthesia, erythematous rash, mild erythema, pruritus, pain, allergic reaction. **Miscellaneous:** Headache, taste perversion.

HOW SUPPLIED

Cream: 1%.

DOSAGE

- **CREAM**

  Cold sores.

  Apply q 2 hr while awake for 4 days.

NURSING CONSIDERATIONS

ADMINISTRATION/STORAGE

1. Start treatment as soon as possible during prodrome or when lesions appear.
2. Use only on the lips and face.

ASSESSMENT

1. Note onset, location, description, extent of lesions.
2. List frequency of occurrence, any triggers or prodrome.

CLIENT/FAMILY TEACHING

1. Wash hands before and after application. Apply q 2 hr while awake for 4 days at first cold sore symptoms.
2. Avoid contact with mucous membranes and eyes; apply to lips and face only.
3. Use sunscreens and lip balms with a sunscreen when sun exposed to prevent recurrence and to diminish intensity of outbreaks.
4. Report if lesions do not improve or if a foul odor or purulent drainage appears.

OUTCOMES/EVALUATE

↓ Intensity/pain; clearing of herpes lesions

Penicillamine

(pen-ih-**SILL**-ah-meen)

CLASSIFICATION(S):

Antirheumatic

PREGNANCY CATEGORY: D

Rx: Cuprimine, Depen.

USES

(1) Wilson's disease. (2) Cystinuria. (3) Rheumatoid arthritis (severe active disease unresponsive to conventional therapy). (4) Heavy metal antagonist. *Investigational:* Primary biliary cirrhosis. Scleroderma.

ACTION/KINETICS

Action A chelating agent for mercury, lead, iron, and copper; forms soluble complexes, thus decreasing toxic levels of the metal (e.g., copper in Wilson's disease). Anti-inflammatory activity may be due to its ability to inhibit T-lymphocyte function and therefore decrease cell-mediated immune response. May also protect lymphocytes from hydrogen peroxide generated at the site of inflammation by inhibiting release of lysosomal enzymes and oxygen radicals. Beneficial effects may not be seen for 2 to 3 months when used for rheumatoid arthritis. In cystinuria, reduces excess cystine excretion, probably by disulfide interchange between penicillamine and cystine. This results in penicillamine-cysteine disulfide, which is a complex that is more soluble than cystine and is thus readily excreted.

Pharmacokinetics

Well-absorbed from the GI tract and excreted in urine. Food decreases the absorption of penicillamine over 50%. **Peak plasma levels:** 1–3 hr. **t½:** Approximately 2 hr. Metabolites excreted through the urine. **Plasma protein binding:** About 80%.

CONTRAINDICATIONS

Pregnancy, lactation, penicillinase-related aplastic anemia or agranulocytosis, hypersensitivity to drug. Clients allergic to penicillin may cross-react with penicillamine. Renal insufficiency or history thereof.

SPECIAL CONCERNS
Use for juvenile rheumatoid arthritis has not been established. Clients older than 65 years may be at greater risk of developing hematologic side effects.

SIDE EFFECTS
Most Common
Anorexia, altered taste perception, epigastric pain, N&V, diarrhea, thrombocytopenia, leukopenia, generalized pruritus, early/late rashes, lupus erythematous-like syndrome, proteinura.

NOTE: This drug manifests a large number of potentially serious side effects. Clients should be carefully monitored. **GI:** Altered taste perception, N&V, diarrhea, anorexia, epigastric pain, stomatitis, oral ulcerations, reactivation of peptic ulcer, glossitis, cheilosis, colitis, gingivostomatitis (rare). **CNS:** Tinnitus, myasthenia gravis, peripheral sensory and motor neuropathies (with or without muscle weakness), reversible optic neuritis, polyradiculopathy (rare). **Hematologic:** Thrombocytopenia, leukopenia, *agranulocytosis, aplastic anemia,* eosinophilia, monocytosis, red cell aplasia, *hemolytic anemia,* leukocytosis, thrombocytosis. **Renal:** Proteinuria, hematuria, nephrotic syndrome, *Goodpasture's syndrome* (a severe and ultimately fatal glomerulonephritis). **Allergic:** Rashes (common), lupus-like syndrome, drug fever, pruritus, pemphigoid-type symptoms (e.g., bullous lesions), arthralgia, lymphadenopathy, dermatoses, urticaria, thyroiditis, hypoglycemia, migratory polyarthralgia, polymyositis, allergic alveolitis. **Respiratory:** Obliterative bronchiolitis, pulmonary fibrosis, pneumonitis, bronchial asthma, interstitial pneumonitis. **Dermatologic:** Increased skin friability, early/late rashes, excessive skin wrinkling, development of small white papules at venipuncture and surgical sites, alopecia or falling hair, lichen planus, dermatomyositis, nail disorders, *toxic epidermal necrolysis,* cutaneous macular atrophy. **Hepatic:** Pancreatitis, hepatic dysfunction, intrahepatic cholestasis, *toxic hepatitis (rare).* **Miscellaneous:** Thrombophlebitis, hyperpyrexia, polymyositis, mammary hyperplasia, renal vasculitis (may be fatal), hot flashes, lupus erythematosus–like syndrome.

LABORATORY TEST CONSIDERATIONS
↑ Serum alkaline phosphatase, LDH. Proteinuria. Positive thymol turbidity test and cephalin flocculation test.

DRUG INTERACTIONS
Antacids / ↓ Effect of penicillamine R/T ↓ absorption from GI tract
Antimalarial drugs / ↑ Risk of blood dyscrasias and adverse renal effects
Cytotoxic drugs / ↑ Risk of blood dyscrasias and adverse renal effects
Digoxin / ↓ Effect of digoxin
Gold therapy / ↑ Risk of blood dyscrasias and adverse renal effects
Iron salts / ↓ Effect of penicillamine R/T ↓ absorption from GI tract
Pyridoxine / ↑ Pyridoxine requirements

HOW SUPPLIED
Capsules: 125 mg, 250 mg; *Tablets, Titratable:* 250 mg.

DOSAGE
• CAPSULES; TABLETS, TITRATABLE
Rheumatoid arthritis.

Adults, individualized, initial: 125–250 mg/day. Dosage may be increased at 1- to 3-month intervals by 125- to 250-mg increments until adequate response is attained. **Maximum:** 500–750 mg/day. Up to 500 mg/day can be given as a single dose; higher dosages should be divided. **Maintenance, individualized. Range:** 500–750 mg/day. If the client is in remission for 6 or more months, a gradual stepwise decrease in dose of 125 or 250 mg/day at about 3-month intervals can be attempted.

Wilson's disease.
Dosage is usually calculated on the basis of the urinary excretion of copper. One gram of penicillamine promotes excretion of 2 mg of copper. **Adults and adolescents, usual, initial:** 250 mg 4 times per day. Dosage may have to be increased to 2 grams/day. A further increase does not produce additional excretion. **Pediatric, 6 months to young children:** 250 mg as a single dose given in fruit juice.

Antidote for heavy metals.

P

 = see color insert   **H** = Herbal   **IV** = Intravenous   = sound alike drug

Adults: 0.5–1.5 grams/day for 1–2 months; **pediatric:** 30–40 mg/kg/day (600–750 mg/m²/day) for 1–6 months.

Cystinuria.

Individualized and based on excretion rate of cystine (100–200 mg/day in clients with no history of stones, below 100 mg with clients with history of stones or pain). Initiate at low dosage (250 mg/day) and increase gradually to minimum effective dosage. **Adult, usual:** 2 grams/day (range: 1–4 grams/day); **pediatric:** 7.5 mg/kg 4 times per day If divided in fewer than four doses, give larger dose at night.

Primary biliary cirrhosis.

Adults: 600–900 mg/day.

NURSING CONSIDERATIONS

Ⓒ Do not confuse penicillamine with penicillin (an antibiotic).

ADMINISTRATION/STORAGE

1. If unable to tolerate dosage for cystinuria, the bedtime dosage should be larger and should be continued.

2. Administer contents of the capsule in 15–30 mL of chilled juice or pureed fruit if unable to swallow capsules or tablets.

3. When treating rheumatoid arthritis, discontinue if doses up to 1.5 grams/day for 2–3 months do not produce improvement.

4. Alternative dosage forms may be prepared if needed. An elixir containing 50 mg/mL may be prepared by dissolving the contents of 48 capsules in 100 mL of water. This is then filtered, and 100 mL of cherry syrup and 30 mL of alcohol stirred in. The volume is then brought up to 240 mL with water. The preparation is shaken well and stored in the refrigerator. Suppositories (750 mg) may be prepared by melting 51 grams of cocoa butter and dissolving the contents of 150 capsules in the cocoa butter; the mixture is poured into a prelubricated suppository mold and then frozen and stored in a refrigerator.

ASSESSMENT

1. Note indications, presenting symptoms, other therapies prescribed, outcome.

2. List any meds consumed with which penicillamine will interact unfavorably; impedes absorption of many drugs. White papules appearing at the site of venipuncture or at surgical sites may indicate sensitivity to penicillamine or presence of infection.

3. Assess CNS/neurologic status. Test hearing to detect any evidence of hearing loss.

4. With arthritis, assess joints for pain, stiffness, erythema, soreness, swelling, and ↓ ROM.

5. Test for pregnancy; drug can cause fetal damage.

6. If to undergo surgery, anticipate dosage reduction to 250 mg/day until wound healing complete.

7. Monitor CBC, LFTs, urinalysis. If WBC falls below 3,500/mm³ or platelet count falls below 100,000/mm³, withhold drug and report. If counts are low for three successive lab tests, a temporary interruption of therapy is indicated.

8. A positive ANA test indicates client may develop a lupus-like syndrome in the future. The drug need not be discontinued.

CLIENT/FAMILY TEACHING

1. Give on an empty stomach 1 hr before or 2 hr after meals; wait 1 hr after ingestion of any other food, milk, or drug. With Wilson's disease take 30–60 min before meals and at bedtime.

2. Take temperature nightly during the first few months of therapy. A fever may indicate a hypersensitivity reaction. Report any evidence of fever, sore throat, chills, skin rash, bruising/bleeding; early S&S of granulocytopenia.

3. If mouth inflammation occurs, report immediately and stop drug. Practice regular oral hygiene i.e., brushing teeth with a soft toothbrush, flossing daily, using alcohol free mouth rinses.

4. Inspect skin surfaces at regular intervals. Skin tends to become friable and susceptible to injury; avoid activities that could injure skin. Elderly should avoid excessive pressure on the shoulders, elbows, knees, toes, and buttocks. Report if ulcers appear and are severe or persistent; may need to reduce drug

---

dose as may interfere with wound healing.

5. Penicillamine increases the body's need for pyridoxine; add pyridoxine (vitamin B_6 25 mg/day PO).

6. A loss of taste perception or a metallic taste may develop; relates to zinc chelation and may last for 2 months or more. With N&V or diarrhea, monitor weight and I&O. Report jaundice or other signs of hepatic dysfunction.

7. If to receive an oral iron preparation, at least 2 hr should elapse between ingestion of penicillamine and dose of therapeutic iron. Iron decreases the copper lowering effects of penicillamine.

8. Report cloudy urine or urine that is smoky brown (signs of proteinuria and hematuria). Practice reliable birth control; report missed menstrual period or other symptoms of pregnancy.

9. With Wilson's disease:

• Eat a diet low in copper. Exclude foods such as chocolate, nuts, shellfish, mushrooms, liver, molasses, broccoli, and copper-enriched cereals.

• Use distilled or demineralized water if drinking water contains more than 0.1 mg/L copper.

• Unless taking iron supplements, take sulfurated potash or Carbo-Resin with meals to minimize the absorption of copper.

• It may take 1–3 months for neurologic improvements to occur. Therefore, continue the therapy even if no improvements seem evident.

• Check any vitamin preparations being used to ensure that they do not contain copper.

10. If excess cystine in urine, do the following:

• Drink large amounts of fluid to prevent the formation of renal calculi. Drink 500 mL of fluid at bedtime and another pint during the night, when the urine tends to be the most concentrated and most acidic. The greater the fluid intake, the lower the required dose of penicillamine.

• Measure urine specific gravity (SG) and determine pH. The urine SG should be maintained at <1.010 and the pH maintained at 7.5–8.0.

• Obtain yearly x-ray of the kidneys to detect presence of renal calculi.

• Eat a diet low in methionine, a major precursor of cystine. Exclude foods high in cystine such as rich meat, soups and broths, milk, eggs, cheeses, and peas.

• If client is pregnant or a child, diets low in methionine are also low in calcium; consider calcium supplementation.

11. With rheumatoid arthritis, continue using other therapies and medications to achieve relief from symptoms; penicillamine may take 4–6 mo to have therapeutic effect. As improvement begins, analgesic drugs and NSAIDs may be slowly tapered.

OUTCOMES/EVALUATE

• ↑ Urinary excretion of copper

• ↓ Cystine excretion and prevention of renal calculi in cystinuria

• ↓ Joint pain, swelling, inflammation, and stiffness with ↑ mobility

Penicillin G Aqueous 〔IV〕ⓒ
(pen-ih-**SILL**-in)

CLASSIFICATION(S):
Antibiotic, penicillin
PREGNANCY CATEGORY: B
Rx: Pfizerpen.

SEE ALSO *ANTI-INFECTIVE DRUGS AND PENICILLINS.*

USES
Streptococci of groups A, C, G, H, L, and M are sensitive to penicillin G. High serum levels are effective against streptococci of the D group.

ACTION/KINETICS
Pharmacokinetics
The first choice for treatment of many infections due to low cost. Rapid onset makes it especially suitable for fulminating infections. Is neither penicillinase resistant nor acid stable. **Peak plasma levels: IM or SC,** 6–20 units/mL after 15–30 min. **t½:** 30 min.

SIDE EFFECTS

Most Common

Hypersensitivity reactions, N&V, diarrhea, abdominal cramps, thrush/yeast infection, sore mouth/tongue.

See *Penicillins* for a complete list of possible side effects. Also, rapid IV administration may cause hyperkalemia and cardiac arrhythmias. Renal damage occurs rarely.

ADDITIONAL DRUG INTERACTIONS

Aspirin, ethacrynic acid, furosemide, indomethacin, sulfonamides, or thiazide diuretics may compete with penicillin G for renal tubular secretion → prolongation of serum $t\frac{1}{2}$ of penicillin

HOW SUPPLIED

Injection (Premix): 1 million units/vial, 2 million units/vial, 3 million units/vial; *Powder for Injection:* 1 million units, 5 million units, 20 million units.

DOSAGE

- **IM; IV, INFUSION (CONTINUOUS)**
  Serious streptococcal infections (empyema, endocarditis, meningitis, pericarditis, pneumonia).

Adults: 5–24 million units/day in divided doses q 4 to 6 hr. **Pediatric:** 150,000 units/kg/day given in equal doses q 4 to 6 hr. **Infants over 7 days of age:** 75,000 units/kg/day in divided doses q 8 hr. **Infants less than 7 days of age:** 50,000 units/kg/day given in divided doses q 12 hr. For group B streptococcus, give 100,000 units/kg/day.

Meningococcal meningitis/septicemia.
Adults: 1–2 million units IM q 2 hr or 20–30 million units/day continuous IV drip for 14 days or until afebrile for 7 days. Or, 200,000–300,000 units/kg/day q 2-4 hr in divided doses for a total of 24 doses.

Meningitis due to susceptible strains of Pneumococcus *or* Meningococcus.
Children: 250,000 units/kg/day divided in equal doses q 4 to 6 hr for 7 to 14 days (maximum total daily dose: 12–20 million units). **Infants over 7 days of age:** 200,000–300,0000 units/kg/day divided into equal doses given q 6 hr. **Infants less than 7 days of age:** 100,000–150,000 units/kg/day.

Anthrax.

Adults: A minimum of 5 million units/day (up to 12–20 million units have been used).

Clostridial infections.
Adults: 20 million units/day in divided doses q 4–6 hr used with an antitoxin.

Actinomycosis.
Adults: *Cervicofacial:* 1–6 million units/day. *Thoracic and abdominal disease:* **Initial,** 10–20 million units/day divided into equal doses given q 4–6 hr IV for 6 weeks followed by penicillin V, PO, 500 mg 4 times/day for 2–3 months.

Rat-bite fever, Haverhill fever.
Adults: 12–20 million units/day q 4 to 6 hr for 3–4 weeks. **Children:** 150,000–250,000 units/kg/day in equal doses q 4 hr for 4 weeks.

Endocarditis due to Listeria.
Adults: 15–20 million units/day q 4 to 6 hr for 4 weeks.

Endocarditis due to Erysipelothrix rhusiopathiae.
Adults: 12–20 million units/day q 4 to 6 hr for 4–6 weeks.

Meningitis due to Listeria.
Adults: 15–20 million units/day q 4 to 6 hr for 2 weeks.

Pasteurella infections causing bacteremia and meningitis.
Adults: 4–6 million units/day q 4 to 6 hr for 2 weeks.

Severe fusospirochetal infections of the oropharynx, lower respiratory tract, and genital area.
Adults: 5–10 million units/day q 4 to 6 hr.

Pneumococcal infections causing empyema.
Adults: 5–24 million units/day in divided doses q 4–6 hr.

Pneumococcal infections causing meningitis.
Adults: 20–24 million units/day for 14 days.

Pneumococcal infections causing endocarditis, pericarditis, peritonitis, suppurative arthritis, osteomyelitis, mastoiditis.
Adults: 12–20 million units/day for 2–4 weeks.

Adjunct with antitoxin to prevent diphtheria.

Adults: 2–3 million units/day in divided doses q 4 to 6 hr for 10–12 days. **Children:** 150,000–250,000 units/kg/day in equal doses q 6 hr for 7–10 days.

Neurosyphilis.

Adults: 18–24 million units/day (3–4 million units q 4 hr) for 10–14 days (can be followed by benzathine penicillin G, 2.4 million units IM weekly for 3 weeks).

Disseminated gonococcal infections.

Adults: 10 million units/day q 4 to 6 hr (for meningococcal meningitis/septicemia, give q 2 hr). **Children, less than 45 kg:** *Arthritis:* 100,000 units/kg/day in 4 equally divided doses for 7 to 10 days. *Endocarditis:* 250,000 units/kg/day in equal doses q 4 hr for 4 weeks. *Meningitis:* 250,000 units/kg/day in equal doses q 4 hr for 10 to 14 days. **Children, over 45 kg:** *Arthritis, endocarditis, meningitis:* 10 million units/day in 4 equally divided doses (duration depends on type of infection).

Syphilis (congenital, neurosyphilis) after the newborn period.

200,000–300,000 units/kg/day (given as 50,000 units/kg q 4–6 hr) for 10–14 days.

Symptomatic or asymptomatic congenital syphilis in infants.

Infants: 50,000 units/kg/dose IV q 12 hr the first 7 days; then, q 8 hr for a total of 10 days. **Children:** 50,000 units/kg q 4–6 hr for 10 days.

NURSING CONSIDERATIONS

𝒞 Do not confuse penicillin with penicillamine (a heavy metal antagonist).

ADMINISTRATION/STORAGE

1. Depending on the route of administration, prepare injections with sterile water, isotonic sodium chloride, or dextrose injection. Penicillin is rapidly inactivated in carbohydrate solutions at alkaline pH.

2. IM administration is preferred; discomfort is minimized by using solutions of up to 100,000 units/mL. Keep the total volume of the IM injection small.

3. Use 1–2% lidocaine solution as diluent for IM (if ordered) to lessen pain at injection site. Do not use procaine as diluent for aqueous penicillin.

4. Electrolyte contents: Pfizerpen contains 0.3 mEq sodium and 1.68 mEq potassium/million units.

5. If penicillin G is to be given by intrapleural or other local infusion and fluid is aspirated, give infusion in a volume equal to ¼ or ½ the amount of fluid aspirated. Otherwise, prepare as for the IM injection.

6. Intrathecal use must be highly individualized and used only with full consideration of possible irritating effects of penicillin when given intrathecally. The preferred route in bacterial meningitis is IV supplemented by IM.

IV 7. Use sterile water, isotonic saline, or D5W and mix with recommended volume for desired strength. When larger doses are needed, give by continuous IV infusion.

8. For intermittent IV administration (q 6 hr) reconstitute with 100 mL of dextrose or saline solution; infuse over 1 hr.

9. Loosen powder by shaking bottle before adding diluent. Hold vial horizontally and rotate slowly while directing the stream of diluent against the vial wall, then shake vigorously.

10. Solutions may be stored at room temperature for 24 hr or in refrigerator for 1 week. Discard remaining solution.

11. The following drugs should *not* be mixed with penicillin during IV administration: Aminophylline, amphotericin B, ascorbic acid, chlorpheniramine, chlorpromazine, gentamicin, heparin, hydroxyzine, lincomycin, metaraminol, novobiocin, oxytetracycline, phenylephrine, phenytoin, polymyxin B, prochlorperazine, promazine, promethazine, sodium bicarbonate, sodium salts of barbiturates, sulfadiazine, tetracycline, tromethamine, vancomycin, vitamin B complex.

12. The dry powder does not require refrigeration. Sterile solutions may be kept in the refrigerator for 1 week. Solutions prepared for IV infusion are stable at room temperature for 24 or more hr.

13. For the premixed, frozen solution, thaw at room temperature or in a refrigerator. Do not force thaw by immersion in water baths or by microwave irradiation. The thawed solution is sta-

ble for 24 hr at room temperature or for 14 days under refrigeration. Do not re-freeze thawed solutions.

ASSESSMENT

1. Note reasons for therapy, onset, characteristics of S&S; check culture results.

2. Assess drug allergies. Order drug by specifying sodium or potassium salt.

3. Monitor I&O. Dehydration decreases drug excretion and may raise blood level of penicillin G to dangerously high levels causing kidney damage. GI disturbances may lead to dehydration. Obtain baseline CBC, renal, LFTs.

4. Very high doses (>20 million units) may cause seizures or platelet dysfunction, especially with impaired renal function.

CLIENT/FAMILY TEACHING

1. With IM dosing, drug must be given by injection into the muscle to clear up infection. May experience pain at injection site; apply ice to relieve pain.

2. Report any unusual bruising, bleeding, N&V, sore mouth, diarrhea, rash, fever, difficulty breathing, adverse side effects, or lack of improvement.

OUTCOMES/EVALUATE

• Symptomatic improvement; negative culture reports

• Resolution of infective process

Penicillin G benzathine, intramuscular   ■ ©

(pen-ih-**SILL**-in, **BEN**-zah-theen)

CLASSIFICATION(S):
Antibiotic, penicillin
PREGNANCY CATEGORY: B
Rx: Bicillin L-A, Permapen.
✤Rx: Penicillin G/Penicillin V.

SEE ALSO *ANTI-INFECTIVE DRUGS AND PENICILLINS.*

USES

(1) URTI (mild to moderate) due to susceptible streptococci. (2) Sexually transmitted diseases, such as syphilis, yaws,

bejel, and pinta. (3) Prophylaxis of rheumatic fever or chorea. (4) Follow-up prophylactic therapy for rheumatic heart disease and acute glomerulonephritis.

ACTION/KINETICS

Action

Penicillin G is neither penicillinase resistant nor acid stable. The product is a long-acting (repository) form of penicillin in an aqueous vehicle; it is administered as a sterile suspension.

Pharmacokinetics

Peak plasma levels, IM: 0.03–0.05 unit/mL.

CONTRAINDICATIONS

IV use. Injection into or near an artery or nerve.

SPECIAL CONCERNS

■ This product is not intended for IV administration.■

SIDE EFFECTS

Most Common

Hypersensitivity reactions, N&V, diarrhea, abdominal cramps, thrush/yeast infection, sore mouth/tongue.

See *Penicillins* for a complete list of possible side effects.

ADDITIONAL DRUG INTERACTIONS

Aspirin, ethacrynic acid, furosemide, indomethacin, sulfonamides, or thiazide diuretics may compete with penicillin G for renal tubular secretion → prolongation of serum $t\frac{1}{2}$ of penicillin

HOW SUPPLIED

Injection (Suspension): 600,000 units/dose; 1,200,000 units/dose; 2,400,000 units/dose.

DOSAGE

• **IM ONLY (SUSPENSION)**

URTI due to Group A streptococcus.

Adults: 1,200,000 units as a single dose; **older children:** 900,000 units as a single dose; **children under 27 kg:** 300,000–600,000 units as a single dose.

Early syphilis (primary, secondary, or latent).

Adults: 2,400,000 units as a single dose. **Children:** 50,000 units/kg, up to the adult dose.

Gummas and cardiovascular syphilis (latent).

P

Bold Italic = life threatening side effect   ■ = black box warning   ✤ = Available in Canada

Adults: 2,400,000 units q 7 days for 3 weeks. **Children:** 50,000 units/kg, up to adult dose.

Neurosyphilis.

Adults: Aqueous penicillin G, 18,000,000–24,000,000 units IV/day (3–4 million units q 4 hr) for 10–14 days followed by penicillin G benzathine, 2,400,000 units IM q week for 3 weeks. An alternative regimen is procaine penicillin G, 2,400,000 units/day plus probenecid, 500 mg PO, 4 times per day, both for 10–14 days. Some recommend benzathine G penicillin, 2.4 million units following completion of this regimen.

Congenital syphilis.

Children less than 2 years of age: 50,000 units/kg. **Children, 2–12 years:** Adjust dose based on adult dosage schedule.

Yaws, bejel, pinta.

1,200,000 units in a single dose.

Prophylaxis of rheumatic fever and glomerulonephritis.

Following an acute attack, 1,200,000 units once a month or 600,000 units q 2 weeks.

NURSING CONSIDERATIONS

@ Do not confuse Bicillin L-A with Bicillin C-R (combination of benzathine and procaine penicillin).

ADMINISTRATION/STORAGE

1. Shake multiple-dose vial vigorously before withdrawing desired dose as drug tends to clump on standing. Check that all medication is dissolved and no residue present at bottom of bottle.

2. Use a 20-gauge needle and do not allow medication to remain in the syringe and needle for long periods of time before administration; needle may become plugged and the syringe 'frozen.'

3. Inject slowly and steadily into muscle; *do not massage* injection site. For adults, use upper outer quadrant of the buttock; for infants and small children, the midlateral aspect of the thigh should be used. Do not administer in the gluteal region in children less than 2 years of age. Rotate and chart site of injections. Divide between two injection sites if dose is large or available muscle mass is small.

4. *Do not administer IV.* Before injection of medication, aspirate to ensure that needle is not in a vein.

5. Bicillin C-R should not be given in place of Bicillin L-A.

6. Refrigerate, but do not freeze.

ASSESSMENT

1. Note reasons for therapy, onset, characteristics of S&S, other agents trialed, outcome.

2. List client history, allergies; review culture results.

CLIENT/FAMILY TEACHING

1. Must return as scheduled for repository penicillin injections.

2. With STDs obtain sexual counseling. Sexual partner(s) should also undergo treatment.

3. Report any unusual side effects, lack of response or worsening of condition.

OUTCOMES/EVALUATE

- Prophylaxis of poststreptococcal rheumatic fever
- Resolution of infection/STD

——COMBINATION DRUG——

Penicillin G ■@ benzathine/Penicillin G procaine

(pen-ih-**SILL**-in, **BEN**-zah-theen, **PROH**-kain)

CLASSIFICATION(S):
Antibiotic, penicillin
PREGNANCY CATEGORY: B
Rx: Bicillin C-R, Bicillin C-R 900/300.

SEE ALSO *ANTI-INFECTIVE DRUGS AND PENICILLINS.*

USES

(1) Moderately severe to severe infections of the upper respiratory tract, skin, soft tissues, and scarlet fever due to susceptible streptococci in groups A, C, G, H, L, and M. (2) Moderately severe pneumonia and otitis media due to susceptible pneumococci. *NOTE:* For severe pneumonia, empyema, bacteremia, per-

icarditis, meningitis, peritonitis, arthritis of pneumococcal etiology, and streptococcal infections with bacteremia, use penicillin G sodium or potassium. Not to be used to treat venereal diseases, including syphilis, gonorrhea, yaws, bejel, and pinta.

CONTENT
Bicillin C-R: *600,000 units/dose:* 300,000 units each of penicillin G benzathine and penicillin G procaine. *1,200,000 units/dose:* 600,000 units each of penicillin G benzathine and penicillin G procaine. *2,400,000 units/dose:* 1,200,000 units each of penicillin G benzathine and penicillin G procaine. **Bicillin C-R 900/300:** 900,000 units of penicillin G benzathine and 300,000 units of penicillin G procaine.

CONTRAINDICATIONS
Use to treat syphilis, gonorrhea, yaws, bejel, and pinta. IV use. Injection into or near an artery or nerve. Use with IV solutions.

SPECIAL CONCERNS
■ This product is not for IV administration. Do not inject IV or admix with other IV solutions. There have been reports of inadvertent IV administration of penicillin G benzathine, which has been associated with cardiorespiratory arrest and death. Prior to administration of this drug, carefully read the labeling.■

SIDE EFFECTS
Most Common
Hypersensitivity reactions, N&V, diarrhea, abdominal cramps, thrush/yeast infection, sore mouth/tongue.
See *Penicillins* for a complete list of possible side effects.

ADDITIONAL DRUG INTERACTIONS
Aspirin, ethacrynic acid, furosemide, indomethacin, sulfonamides, or thiazide diuretics may compete with penicillin G for renal tubular secretion → prolongation of serum $t\frac{1}{2}$ of penicillin

HOW SUPPLIED
See Content

DOSAGE
- **IM ONLY**
  Streptococcal infections.
Bicillin C-R. Adults and children over 27 kg: 2,400,000 units, given at a single session using multiple injection sites or,

alternatively, in divided doses on days 1 and 3 (as long as client cooperation is assured); **children 13.5–27 kg:** 900,000–1,200,000 units; **infants and children under 13.5 kg:** 600,000 units. *NOTE:* A single injection of Bicillin C-R 900/300 is usually sufficient to treat group A streptococcal infections in children.

  Pneumococcal infections, except pneumococcal meningitis.
Bicillin C-R. Adults: 1,200,000 units; **pediatric:** 600,000 units. Give q 2–3 days until temperature is normal for 48 hr. **Bicillin C-R 900/300:** One Tubex cartridge repeated at 2- or 3-day intervals until the temperature is normal for 48 hr. For severe cases, other forms of penicillin may be needed.

NURSING CONSIDERATIONS
Ⓒ Do not confuse Bicillin C-R with Bicillin L-A (benzathine penicillin).

ADMINISTRATION/STORAGE
1. For adults, administer by deep IM injection in the upper outer quadrant of the buttock. For infants and children, use the midlateral aspect of the thigh. Rotate injection sites for repeated doses.
2. Refrigerate. Protect from freezing.

ASSESSMENT
1. Note reasons for therapy, symptom type/onset/location, disease confirmation.
2. Assess for drug allergies, culture results.

CLIENT/FAMILY TEACHING
1. Drug must be given by injection into the muscle to clear up infection. May experience pain at injection site; apply ice to relieve pain.
2. Report any unusual bruising, bleeding, N&V, sore mouth, diarrhea, rash, fever, difficulty breathing, adverse side effects, or lack of improvement.

OUTCOMES/EVALUATE
Resolution of infection

Bold Italic = life threatening side effect   ■ = black box warning   ✦ = Available in Canada

Penicillin G procaine, intramuscular

(pen-ih-**SILL**-in, **PROH**-caine)

CLASSIFICATION(S):
Antibiotic, penicillin
PREGNANCY CATEGORY: B
Rx: Wycillin.

SEE ALSO *ANTI-INFECTIVE DRUGS* AND *PENICILLINS*.

USES
(1) Penicillin-sensitive staphylococci, pneumococci, streptococci, and bacterial endocarditis (for *Streptococcus viridans* and *S. bovis* infections). (2) Gonorrhea and all stages of syphilis. (3) *Prophylaxis*: Rheumatic fever, pre- and postsurgery. (4) Diphtheria, anthrax, fusospirochetosis (Vincent's infection), erysipeloid, rat-bite fever. *NOTE*: Severe pneumonia, empyema, bacteremia, pericarditis, meningitis, peritonitis, and purulent or septic arthritis due to pneumococcus are better treated with aqueous penicillin G during the acute stage.

ACTION/KINETICS
Action
Long-acting (repository) form in aqueous or oily vehicle. Destroyed by penicillinase. Because of slow onset, a soluble penicillin is often administered concomitantly for fulminating infections.

CONTRAINDICATIONS
Use in newborns due to possible sterile abscesses and procaine toxicity. Injection into or near an artery or nerve. IV use.

SIDE EFFECTS
Most Common
Hypersensitivity reactions, N&V, diarrhea, abdominal cramps, thrush/yeast infection, sore mouth/tongue.
See *Penicillins* for a complete list of possible side effects.

ADDITIONAL DRUG INTERACTIONS
Aspirin / May compete with penicillin G for renal tubular secretion → prolongation of serum t½ of penicillin

Ethacrynic acid / May compete with penicillin G for renal tubular secretion → prolongation of serum t½ of penicillin
Furosemide / May compete with penicillin G for renal tubular secretion → prolongation of serum t½ of penicillin
Indomethacin / May compete with penicillin G for renal tubular secretion → prolongation of serum t½ of penicillin
Oral contraceptives / ↓ Effectiveness of oral contraceptives
Sulfonamides / May compete with penicillin G for renal tubular secretion → prolongation of serum t½ of penicillin
Thiazide diuretics / May compete with penicillin G for renal tubular secretion → prolongation of serum t½ of penicillin

HOW SUPPLIED
Injection: 600,000 units/vial, 1,200,000 units/vial.

DOSAGE
- **DEEP IM ONLY**
  Pneumococcal, streptococcal (Group A, including tonsillitis, erysipelas, scarlet fever, URTI, and skin and skin structure infections), staphylococcal infections (moderate to severe of the skin and soft tissues).
Adults, usual: 600,000–1 million units/day for 10–14 days. **Children, less than 27.2 kg:** 300,000 units/day.
  Bacterial endocarditis (only very sensitive S. viridans or S. bovis infections).
Adults: 600,000–1 million units/day.
  Diphtheria carrier state.
300,000 units/day for 10 days.
  Diphtheria, adjunct with antitoxin.
300,000–600,000 units/day for 14 days.
  Anthrax (cutaneous), erysipeloid, rat-bite fever.
600,000 to 1 million units/day.
  Fusospirochetosis: Vincent's gingivitis, pharyngitis.
600,000 to 1 million units/day. Obtain necessary dental care in infections involving gum tissue.
  Gonococcal infections.
4.8 million units divided into at least two doses at one visit and given with 1 gram PO probenecid (given 30 min before the injections).
  Neurosyphilis.

2.4 million units/day for 10 to 14 days (given at two sites) with probenecid 500 mg PO 4 times per day; **then,** benzathine penicillin G, 2.4 million units/week for 3 weeks. *NOTE:* For yaws, bejel, and pinta, treat the same as syphilis in corresponding stage of disease.

Congenital syphilis in children (less than 32 kg), symptomatic and asymptomatic.

50,000 units/kg/day given as a single dose for 10–14 days.

Syphilis: Primary, secondary, latent with negative spinal fluid.

Adults and children over 12 years: 600,000 units/day for 8 days (total of 4.8 million units).

Syphilis: Tertiary, neurosyphilis, latent with positive spinal fluid examination or no spinal fluid examination.

Adults: 600,000 units/day for 10 to 15 days (total of 6 to 9 million units).

Anthrax, cutaneous.

600,000–1,000,000 units/day. Continue prophylaxis until exposure to *Bacillus anthracis* has been excluded. If exposure is confirmed and vaccine is available, continue prophylaxis for 4 weeks and until 3 doses of vaccine have been given, or for 30–60 days if vaccine is not available.

NURSING CONSIDERATIONS

ADMINISTRATION/STORAGE

1. Shake multiple-dose vial thoroughly to ensure uniform suspension before injection. If it is clumped at the bottom of the vial, shake until clump dissolves.
2. Use a 20-gauge needle and aspirate immediately after withdrawing medication from the vial; otherwise needle may become clogged and syringe may 'freeze.' Aspirate to check that the needle is not in a vein.
3. Administer into two sites if dose is large or available muscle mass is small. Inject slowly, deep into the muscle. For IM use only. Rotate and chart injection sites. Do not massage site.
4. Inspect visually for particulate matter and discoloration prior to administration.
5. Store from 2–8°C (36–46°F). Do not freeze.

ASSESSMENT

Note reasons for therapy, onset, characteristics of S&S, any drug allergies, other therapies trialed, culture results.

CLIENT/FAMILY TEACHING

1. Drug can only be given IM. Report a wheal or other skin reactions at injection site, or mental disturbances; may indicate reaction to procaine as well as to penicillin. Report N&V, diarrhea, mouth sores, severe pain at injection site, unusual bruising/bleeding, or difficulty breathing.
2. With STDs obtain sexual counseling; have sexual partner also undergo treatment. Use an additional non-hormonal form of birth control due to decreased effectiveness.
3. With a history of rheumatic fever or congenital heart disease, must remember to use antibiotic prophylaxis prior to any invasive medical/dental procedure. Check with a provider.
4. Report any adverse side effects or lack of response.

OUTCOMES/EVALUATE

- Resolution of infection
- Infection prophylaxis

Penicillin V potassium (Phenoxymethyl-penicillin potassium)
(pen-ih-**SILL**-in)

CLASSIFICATION(S):
Antibiotic, penicillin

PREGNANCY CATEGORY: B

Rx: Penicillin VK, Veetids.

✦**Rx:** Apo-Pen-VK, Nadopen-V, Novo–Pen-VK, Nu-Pen-VK, PVF K, Penicillin G/Penicillin V.

SEE ALSO *ANTI-INFECTIVE DRUGS AND PENICILLINS.*

USES

(1) Mild to moderate upper respiratory tract streptococcal infections, including scarlet fever and erysipelas. (2) Mild to moderate upper respiratory tract pneumococcal infections, including otitis

media. (3) Mild staphylococcal infections of the skin and soft tissue. (4) Mild to moderate fusospirochetosis (Vincent's infection) of the oropharynx, pharyngitis. (5) Prophylaxis of recurrence following rheumatic fever or chorea. *Investigational:* Prophylactic treatment of children with sickle cell anemia or splenectomy to reduce the incidence of *S. pneumoniae* septicemia; actinomycosis; early Lyme disease; postexposure prophylaxis to anthrax (confirmed or suspected). *NOTE:* Streptococci in groups A, C, G, H, L, and M are very sensitive to penicillin. Other groups, including group D (enterococci), are resistant. An increasing number of staphylococcal strains are resistant to penicillin; culture and susceptibility studies are important.

ACTION/KINETICS

Action

Binds to penicillin-binding proteins (PBP-1 and PBP-3) in the cytoplasmic membranes of bacteria, thus inhibiting cell wall synthesis. Cell division and growth are inhibited and often lysis and elongation of susceptible bacteria occur. Related closely to penicillin G. Products are not penicillinase resistant but are acid stable and resist inactivation by gastric secretions.

Pharmacokinetics

Well absorbed from the GI tract and not affected by foods. **Peak plasma levels: PO:** 1–9 mcg/mL after 30–60 min. **t½:** 30 min. Periodic blood counts and renal function tests are indicated during long-term usage.

CONTRAINDICATIONS

PO penicillin V to treat severe pneumonia, empyema, bacteremia, pericarditis, meningitis, and arthritis during the acute stage. Prophylactic uses for GU instrumentation or surgery, sigmoidoscopy, or childbirth.

SPECIAL CONCERNS

More and more strains of staphylococci are resistant to penicillin V, necessitating culture and sensitivity studies.

SIDE EFFECTS

Most Common

Hypersensitivity reactions, N&V, diarrhea, abdominal cramps, thrush/yeast infection, sore mouth/tongue.

See *Penicillins* for a complete list of possible side effects.

ADDITIONAL DRUG INTERACTIONS

Contraceptives, oral / ↓ Effectiveness of oral contraceptives
Neomycin, oral / ↓ Absorption of penicillin V

HOW SUPPLIED

Powder for Oral Solution: 125 mg/5 mL (when reconstituted), 250 mg/5 mL (when reconstituted); *Tablets:* 250 mg, 500 mg.

DOSAGE

- **ORAL SOLUTION; TABLETS**

  Streptococcal infections of the upper respiratory tract, including scarlet fever and mild erysipelas.

  Adults and children over 12 years: 125–250 mg q 6–8 hr for 10 days. **Pharyngitis in children, usual:** 25–50 mg/kg/day divided q 6 hr for 10 days.

  Staphylococcal infections (mild infections of the skin and soft tissue); fusospirochetosis of oropharynx (mild to moderate infections).

  Adults and children over 12 years: 250 mg q 6–8 hr.

  Pneumococcal infections, mild to moderate respiratory tract infections, including otitis media.

  Adults and children over 12 years: 250 mg q 6 hr until afebrile for at least 2 days.

  Prophylaxis of recurrence of rheumatic fever/chorea.

  Adults and children over 12 years: 125–250 mg twice a day, on a continuing basis.

  Prophylactic treatment of children with sickle cell anemia or splenectomy to reduce incidence of S. pneumoniae septicemia.

  Children, 3 months–5 years: 125 mg twice a day. **Children, over 5 years of age:** 250 mg twice a day.

  Actinomycosis.

  Penicillin G, 10–20 mg/kg/day IV for 4–6 weeks; then, Penicillin V, 2–4 grams/day for 6–12 months.

Anthrax, postexposure prophylaxis (confirmed or suspected exposure to B. anthracis).

Adults: 7.5 mg/kg 4 times/day. **Children, less than 9 years of age:** 50 mg/kg/day divided 4 times/day. Continue prophylaxis until exposure to *B. anthracis* has been excluded. If exposure is confirmed and vaccine is available, continue prophylaxis for 4 weeks and until 3 doses of vaccine have been given or for 30–60 days if vaccine is not available.

Early Lyme disease (Borrelia burgdorferi).

Adults and children over 12 years of age: 500 mg 4 times/day for 10–20 days.

NURSING CONSIDERATIONS

Do not confuse penicillin V with penicillin G or with penicillamine (a heavy metal antagonist).

ADMINISTRATION/STORAGE

1. To reconstitute the solution, tap bottle until all powder flows freely. Add about one-half of the total amount of water for reconstitution and shake well to wet powder. Add the remainder of the water and shake well again.
2. Store reconstituted solution in the refrigerator; discard unused portion after 14 days.

ASSESSMENT

Note reasons for therapy, onset, exposures, characteristics of S&S, any drug allergies, other therapies trialed, and culture results. List drugs prescribed to ensure none interact.

CLIENT/FAMILY TEACHING

1. Take without regard to meals. Blood levels may be slightly higher when administered on an empty stomach. Take after meals to enhance absorption. Complete entire prescription to prevent bacterial resistance.
2. Clients with history of rheumatic fever or congenital heart disease need to use and understand the importance of antibiotic prophylaxis prior to any invasive medical or dental procedure.
3. Report lack of response, adverse side effects, bloody stools, severe diarrhea, or stomach cramps/pain or if throat/ear symptoms do not improve after 48 hr of therapy; may need to reevaluate and alter therapy.
4. With oral administration, if reaction is going to occur, you usually see it after the second dose. Seek medical intervention immediately if respiratory distress or skin wheals appear.
5. Use an additional nonhormonal form of birth control if taking oral contraceptives because their effectiveness may be diminished.

OUTCOMES/EVALUATE

- Resolution of symptoms
- Negative C&S reports
- Infection prophylaxis

Pentamidine isethionate IV

(pen-**TAM**-ih-deen)

CLASSIFICATION(S):

Antibiotic, miscellaneous
PREGNANCY CATEGORY: C
Rx: NebuPent, Pentacarinate, Pentam 300.

USES

Parenteral: Pneumonia caused by *Pneumocystis carinii.* **Inhalation:** Prophylaxis of *P. carinii* in high-risk HIV-infected clients defined by one or both of the following: (a) a history of one or more cases of pneumonia caused by *P. carinii* and/or (b) a peripheral CD4+ lymphocyte count <200/mm^3. *Investigational:* Trypanosomiasis, visceral leishmaniasis.

ACTION/KINETICS

Action

Inhibits synthesis of DNA, RNA, phospholipids, and proteins, thereby interfering with cell metabolism. May also interfere with folate transformation.

Pharmacokinetics

Plasma levels following inhalation are significantly lower than after a comparable IV dose. About one-third of the dose excreted unchanged in the urine.

Bold Italic = life threatening side effect　　■ = black box warning　　✦ = Available in Canada

CONTRAINDICATIONS

Anaphylaxis to inhaled or parenteral pentamidine.

SPECIAL CONCERNS

Use with caution in clients with hepatic or kidney disease, hyper-/hypotension, hyper-/hypoglycemia, hypocalcemia, leukopenia, thrombocytopenia, anemia, ventricular tachycardia, pancreatitis, Stevens-Johnson syndrome.

SIDE EFFECTS

Most Common

When used parenterally: Sterile abscess/pain/induration at IM injection site, leukopenia, nausea, anorexia, hypotension, fever, hypoglycemia, rash, bad taste in mouth, confusion, hallucinations.

When used as aerosol: Fatigue, metallic taste, shortness of breath, decreased appetite, dizziness, rash, cough, N&V, pharyngitis, chest pain/congestion, night sweats, chills, bronchospasm.

Parenteral. CV: Hypotension, *ventricular tachycardia*, phlebitis. **GI:** Nausea, anorexia, bad taste in mouth. **Hematologic:** Leukopenia, thrombocytopenia, anemia. **Electrolytes/glucose:** Hypoglycemia, hypocalcemia, hyperkalemia. **CNS:** Dizziness without hypotension, confusion, hallucinations. **Miscellaneous:** Acute renal failure, *Stevens-Johnson syndrome*, elevated serum creatinine, elevated LFTs, fever, sterile abscess/pain/induration at IM injection site, rash, neuralgia.

Inhalation. Most frequent include the following: **GI:** Decreased appetite, N&V, metallic taste, diarrhea, abdominal pain. **CNS:** Fatigue, dizziness, headache. **Respiratory:** SOB, cough, pharyngitis, chest pain/congestion, *bronchospasm*, pneumothorax. **Miscellaneous:** Rash, night sweats, chills, myalgia, headache, anemia, edema.

HOW SUPPLIED

Aerosol (for Inhalation): 300 mg; *Injection:* 300 mg; *Powder for Injection, Lyophilized:* 300 mg.

DOSAGE

- **IM, (DEEP); IV**
  Pneumonia due to Pneumocystis carinii.

Adults and children: 4 mg/kg/day for 14 days. Dosage should be reduced in renal disease.

- **INHALATION AEROSOL**
  Prevention of P. carinii *pneumonia.*
300 mg q 4 weeks given via the Respirgard II nebulizer.

NURSING CONSIDERATIONS

ADMINISTRATION/STORAGE

1. For use in the nebulizer, reconstitute by dissolving vial contents in 6 mL sterile water for injection. Avoid saline solution as it causes the drug to precipitate. Do not mix with other medications in the nebulizer chamber.

2. Deliver the dose using the nebulizer until the chamber is empty (30–45 min). The suggested flow rate is 5–7 L/min from a 40- to 50-psi (pounds per square inch) air or oxygen source.

3. When used for nebulization, do not mix with any other drug. The solution for nebulization is stable at room temperature for 48 hr if protected from light.

4. To prepare IM solution, dissolve one vial in 3 mL of sterile water for injection.

IV 5. To prepare IV solution, dissolve one vial in 3–5 mL of sterile water for injection or D5W. The drug is then further diluted in 50–250 mL of D5W. Infuse slowly over 60 min.

6. IV solutions in concentrations of 1 and 2.5 mg/mL in D5W are stable for 48 hr at room temperature.

ASSESSMENT

1. Note reasons for therapy, onset, S&S; assess extent of infection.

2. Check for history of kidney disease, hypertension, past blood disorders. Monitor cultures, CBC, lytes, glucose, calcium, CD_4 counts, renal, LFTs.

3. List results of TB skin test. Auscultate lungs; document VS, CXR, respiratory assessment findings.

INTERVENTIONS

1. Observe for S&S of hypoglycemia, hypocalcemia, hyperkalemia.

2. During IV therapy monitor BP (q 15 min during therapy and q 2 hr after therapy until stable), VS and I&O. Obtain apical pulse; auscultate for evidence of arrhythmia.

P

3. During administration of aerosolized pentamidine, follow precautions to protect health care worker. Do not administer if pregnant; remove contact lenses. Administer with the Respirgard II nebulizer. Document worker exposure(s) and report any persistent or unusual symptoms, especially chronic URIs. Wear:

- Eye protection with side shields
- Disposable gowns
- Respiratory protective equipment such as an organic dust-mist respirator unless client is under hood stalls or in a ventilated booth
- Gloves

4. Follow appropriate institutional guidelines and Occupational Safety and Health Administration (OSHA) standards for administration of drug/exposure. Incorporate Standard Precautions.

CLIENT/FAMILY TEACHING

1. Parenteral drug therapy must be given every day (IV/IM). Use warm soaks for IM site pain. Inhalation therapy must be used once every 4 weeks. Use aerosol device until chamber is empty. Follow appropriate guidelines for administration.

2. Report any blood in urine/stools, or unusual bruising/bleeding. Expect frequent blood tests and BP checks. Consume 2–3 L/day of fluids.

3. Avoid aspirin-containing compounds, alcohol, IM injections, or rectal thermometers. Use a soft toothbrush, electric razor, and night light to prevent injury and falls.

4. Be alert for S&S of low sugar level (which may be severe). Report early signs of Stevens-Johnson syndrome (characterized by high fever, severe headaches, mouth, eye, nose or penis inflammation or swelling).

5. Rise from a prone position slowly and dangle legs before standing as drug may cause dizziness and low BP.

6. During inhalation, a metallic taste and GI upset may be experienced. Eat small, frequent meals and perform regular mouth care to offset. Report any breathing difficulty or adverse side effects immediately.

OUTCOMES/EVALUATE

- (Parenteral) Improvement in symptoms of PCP
- (Inhalation) PCP prophylaxis

Perphenazine
(per-**FEN**-ah-zeen)

CLASSIFICATION(S):
Antipsychotic, phenothiazine
PREGNANCY CATEGORY: C
❦**Rx:** Apo-Perphenazine.

SEE ALSO *ANTIPSYCHOTIC AGENTS, PHENOTHIAZINES.*

USES
(1) Psychotic disorders (tablets). (2) Manifestations of psychotic disorders (oral concentrate). (3) Control severe N&V in adults. (4) Relief of intractable hiccoughs.

ACTION/KINETICS

Action
Resembles chlorpromazine. Moderate incidence of extrapyramidal effects and sedation; strong antiemetic effects; low incidence of anticholinergic effects and orthostatic hypotension.

Pharmacokinetics
About 20% bioavailable. T_{max}: 1–3 hr. Metabolized in the liver, including by CYP2D6. $t\frac{1}{2}$: 9–12 hr.

CONTRAINDICATIONS
Use in children less than 12 years of age.

SPECIAL CONCERNS
Use during pregnancy only if benefits clearly outweigh risks. Geriatric, emaciated, or debilitated clients usually require a lower initial dose as they are particularly sensitive to the side effects.

SIDE EFFECTS

Most Common
Decreased sweating, dry mouth, constipation, blurred vision, drowsiness, tremor, difficult urination, decreased libido, dizziness, increased appetite, menstrual irregularities, swollen breasts.
See *Antipsychotic Agents, Phenothiazines* for a complete list of possible side effects.

HOW SUPPLIED
Oral Concentrate: 16 mg/5 mL; *Tablets:* 2 mg, 4 mg, 8 mg, 16 mg.

DOSAGE
- **ORAL CONCENTRATE; TABLETS**

  Moderately disturbed, nonhospitalized clients with schizophrenia.

  4–8 mg 3 times per day. Reduce as soon as possible to minimum effective dosage.

  Hospitalized clients with schizophrenia.

  8–16 mg 2 to 4 times per day. Avoid doses greater than 64 mg/day.

  Severe N&V.

  Adults: 8–16 mg daily in divided doses; up to 24 mg may be needed. Reduce dosage as soon as possible.

NURSING CONSIDERATIONS
Ⓒ Do not confuse perphenazine with prochlorperazine (Compazine).

ADMINISTRATION/STORAGE
1. Geriatric clients are particularly sensitive to the side effects of perphenazine. Start on lower doses and observe closely.
2. Children over 12 years may receive the lowest limit of the adult dose.
3. Protect from light and store solutions in an amber-colored container. Shake well before using.
4. Avoid skin contact with oral solution; may cause contact dermatitis.
5. Store tablets from 15–30°C (59–86°F). Dispense in a tight, light-resistant container. Store the oral concentrate from 2–30°C (36–86°F); protect from light. Dispense concentrate in amber bottles; shake well before using.

ASSESSMENT
1. Note reasons for therapy; describe behavioral manifestations, onset, characteristics of S&S. List other agents prescribed, duration of therapy, outcome.
2. Monitor VS closely; may cause hypotension, tachy/bradycardia. Supervise activity until drug effects realized. Assess for dehydration. Obtain baseline CBC, ECG, LFTs.
3. Observe for tardive dyskinesia and other extrapyramidal symptoms; requires a dosage reduction/discontinuation.

CLIENT/FAMILY TEACHING
1. May dilute each 5 mL of oral concentrate with 60 mL of water, homogenized milk, saline, carbonated orange drink, or orange, pineapple, apricot, prune, tomato, and grapefruit juice. Avoid skin contact with drug solution.
2. Do not mix with caffeinated beverages (e.g., tea, coffee, cola), grape juice, or apple juice as precipitates form. Avoid alcohol/CNS depressants.
3. Change positions slowly to avoid sudden drop in BP. May cause drowsiness/dizziness; avoid activities that require mental alertness.
4. Report any rash, fever, constipation, or urinary retention as well as tardive dyskinesia (fine tongue movements) and extrapyramidal symptoms (tremors, jerking movements).
5. Wear protective clothes and sunscreen when sunlight exposure necessary; may discolor skin a bluish color.
6. Drug impairs body temperature regulation; dress appropriately and avoid temperature extremes. May discolor urine pinkish brown. Report any problems with bowels or urination.

OUTCOMES/EVALUATE
- ↓ Agitation/excitability or withdrawn behaviors
- Control of severe N&V/intractable hiccoughs

P

Phenazopyridine hydrochloride
(Phenylazodiamino-pyridine HCl)
(fen-**AY**-zoh-**PEER**-ih-deen)

CLASSIFICATION(S):
Urinary tract drug
PREGNANCY CATEGORY: B
OTC: Azo-Standard, Baridium, Prodium.
Rx: Geridium, Pyridiate, Pyridin, Pyridium, Pyridium Plus, UTI Relief, Urodine, Urogesic.
✤**Rx:** Phenazo.

USES
Relief of pain, urgency, frequency, burning, and other discomforts due to irrita-

tion of the lower urinary tract mucosa caused by infection, trauma, surgery, endoscopic procedures, or passage of sounds or catheters. Use may eliminate the need for systemic analgesics or narcotics. The drug treats painful symptoms but does not treat the source or cause of the disorder causing the pain.

ACTION/KINETICS

Action

An azo dye with local analgesic effect on the urinary tract mucosa. Mechanism of action is unknown.

Pharmacokinetics

Rapidly excreted by the urine; 65% excreted unchanged within 24 hr.

CONTRAINDICATIONS

Renal insufficiency. Use in children less than 12 years of age. Chronic use to treat undiagnosed pain of the urinary tract.

SPECIAL CONCERNS

No information is available on the effect of phenazopyridine on lactation.

SIDE EFFECTS

Most Common

Headache, itching, rash, GI upset.

GI: Nausea, GI upset, indigestion, stomach cramps/pain. **CNS:** Headache, dizziness, confusion. **Hematologic:** Methemoglobinemia, hemolytic anemia (especially in clients with G6PD deficiency). **Respiratory:** SOB, chest tightness, wheezing, troubled breathing. **Dermatologic:** Yellowish tinge of the skin or sclerae may indicate accumulation of drug due to renal insufficiency, blue or blue-purple skin color, pruritus, rash, itching. **Body as a whole:** Fever, unusual tiredness or weakness, weight gain. **Miscellaneous:** Renal and hepatic toxicity, anaphylactoid reaction, staining of contact lenses, sudden decrease in amount of urine; swelling of face, fingers, feet, and/or lower legs.

LABORATORY TEST CONSIDERATIONS

Ehrlichs test for urine urobilinogen, phenolsulfonphthalein excretion test for kidney function, urine bilirubin, Clinistix or Tes-Tape, colorimetric laboratory test procedures (e.g., urine ketone tests, urine protein tests, urine steroid determinations).

Symptoms: Methemoglobinemia following massive overdoses. Hemolysis due to G6PD deficiency. *Treatment:* Methylene blue, 1–2 mg/kg IV or 100–200 mg PO of ascorbic acid to treat methemoglobinemia.

HOW SUPPLIED

OTC: Tablet: 95 mg, 100 mg; **Rx:** Tablet: 97.2 mg, 100 mg, 150 mg, 200 mg.

DOSAGE

- **TABLETS**

  Symptomatic relief of pain, burning, urgency, frequency, discomfort.

  Adults: 200 mg 3 times per day after meals for not more than 2 days when used together with an antibacterial agent for UTI. **Pediatric, 6–12 years:** 4 mg/kg 3 times per day with food for 2 days.

NURSING CONSIDERATIONS

ADMINISTRATION/STORAGE

Do not use for more than 2 days; there is no evidence that combined administration of phenazopyridine and an antibacterial provides greater benefit than administration of the antibacterial alone after 2 days.

ASSESSMENT

1. Note reasons for therapy, type, onset, characteristics of S&S, other agents used.
2. Review culture results; assess for G-6-PD, liver/renal dysfunction.

CLIENT/FAMILY TEACHING

1. Take with or after meals to prevent GI upset. Consume 2–3 L/day of fluids.
2. Generally used for only 2 days when taken together with an antibacterial agent for UTIs; complete entire prescription.
3. With diabetes, check finger sticks regularly.
4. May cause staining of contact lenses; do not wear during therapy.
5. Drug turns urine orange-red; may stain fabrics. Wear a sanitary napkin to avoid staining garments. A 0.25% sodium dithionate or sodium hydrosulfite solution, available from a pharmacy, will remove these stains.
6. Report itching/yellowing of skin/eyes, blueish skin hue, or lack of re-

sponse. Keep all F/U appointments to evaluate response to therapy.

OUTCOMES/EVALUATE
Relief of pain and discomfort with UTI

Phenobarbital IV ©
(fee-no-**BAR**-bih-tal)

CLASSIFICATION(S):
Sedative-hypnotic, barbiturate
PREGNANCY CATEGORY: D
Rx: Bellatal, Solfoton, **C-IV**

Phenobarbital sodium
PREGNANCY CATEGORY: D
Rx: Luminal Sodium, **C-IV**

USES
PO: (1) Sedative or hypnotic (short-term). (2) Anticonvulsant (partial and generalized tonic-clonic or cortical focal seizures). (3) Emergency control of acute seizure disorders due to status epilepticus, meningitis, tetanus, eclampsia, toxicity of local anesthetics.
　　Parenteral: (1) Sedative or hypnotic (short-term). (2) Preanesthetic. (3) Anticonvulsant (generalized tonic-clonic and cortical focal seizures). (4) Emergency control of acute seizure disorders (e.g., tetanus, eclampsia, status epilepticus).

ACTION/KINETICS
Action
Depressant and anticonvulsant effects may be related to its ability to increase and/or mimic the inhibitory activity of GABA on nerve synapses. Is not an analgesic; not to be given to relieve pain.
Pharmacokinetics
Onset: 30 to more than 60 min. **Duration:** 10–16 hr. **Anticonvulsant therapeutic serum levels:** 15–40 mcg/mL. **Time for peak effect, after IV:** Up to 15 min. Distributed more slowly than other barbiturates due to lower lipid solubility. Long-acting. **t½:** 53–140 hr. Twenty-five percent eliminated unchanged in the urine. **Plasma protein binding:** 50–60%.

CONTRAINDICATIONS
Hypersensitivity to barbiturates, severe trauma, pulmonary disease when dyspnea or obstruction is present, edema, uncontrolled diabetes, history of porphyria, and impaired liver function and for clients in whom they produce an excitatory response. Also, clients who have been addicted previously to sedative-hypnotics.

SPECIAL CONCERNS
Use with caution during lactation and in clients with CNS depression, hypotension, marked asthenia (characteristic of Addison's disease, hypoadrenalism, and severe myxedema), porphyria, fever, anemia, hemorrhagic shock, cardiac, hepatic or renal damage, and a history of alcoholism in suicidal clients. Geriatric clients usually manifest increased sensitivity to barbiturates, as evidenced by confusion, excitement, mental depression, and hypothermia. Reduce the dose in geriatric and debilitated clients, as well as those with impaired hepatic or renal function. When given in the presence of pain, restlessness, excitement, and delirium may result.

SIDE EFFECTS
Most Common
Somnolence, headache, agitation, confusion, ataxia, dizziness.
CNS: Sleepiness, drowsiness, agitation, confusion, hyperkinesia, ataxia, CNS depression, nightmares, nervousness, psychiatric disturbances, hallucinations, insomnia, anxiety, dizziness, headache, abnormal thinking, vertigo, lethargy, hangover, excitement, appearance of being inebriated. Irritability and hyperactivity in children. **Musculoskeletal:** Localized or diffuse myalgic, neuralgic, or arthritic pain, especially in psychoneurotic clients. Pain is often most intense in the morning and is frequently located in the neck, shoulder girdle, and arms. **Respiratory:** Hypoventilation, *apnea*, *respiratory depression*. **CV:** Bradycardia, hypotension, syncope, *circulatory collapse*. **GI:** N&V, constipation, liver damage (especially with chronic use of phenobarbital). **Allergic:** Skin rashes, *angioedema*, exfoliative dermatitis (including *Stevens-Johnson*

P

syndrome and toxic epidermal necro-lysis). Allergic reactions are most common in clients who have asthma, urticaria, angioedema, and similar conditions. Symptoms include localized swelling (especially of the lips, cheeks, or eyelids) and erythematous dermatitis.

• **AFTER IV USE**
CV: Circulatory depression, thrombophlebitis, *peripheral vascular collapse, seizures with cardiorespiratory arrest, myocardial depression, cardiac arrhythmias.* **Respiratory:** *Apnea, laryngospasm, bronchospasm,* dyspnea, rhinitis, sneezing, coughing. **CNS:** Emergence delirium, headache, anxiety, prolonged somnolence and recovery, restlessness, *seizures.* **GI:** N&V, abdominal pain, diarrhea, cramping. **Hypersensitivity:** *Acute allergic reactions,* including erythema, pruritus, *anaphylaxis.* **Miscellaneous:** Pain or nerve injury at injection site, salivation, hiccups, skin rashes, shivering, skeletal muscle hyperactivity, *immune hemolytic anemia with renal failure,* and radial nerve palsy.

• **AFTER IM USE**
Pain at injection site.
NOTE: Although barbiturates can induce physical and psychologic dependence if high doses are used regularly for long periods of time, the incidence of dependence on phenobarbital is low. Withdrawal symptoms usually begin after 12–16 hr of abstinence. Manifestations of withdrawal include anxiety, weakness, N&V, muscle cramps, delirium, and even tonic-clonic seizures. Chronic use may result in headache, fever, and megaloblastic anemia.

LABORATORY TEST CONSIDERATIONS
Interference with test method: ↑ 17-Hydroxycorticosteroids. ↑ CPK, alkaline phosphatase, serum transaminase, serum testosterone (in certain women), urinary estriol, porphobilinogen, coproporphyrin, uroporphyrin. ↓ PT in clients on coumarin. ↑ or ↓ Bilirubin. False + lupus erythematosus test.

OD OVERDOSE MANAGEMENT
Symptoms: Acute Toxicity: Characterized by cortical and *respiratory depression;*

anoxia; *peripheral vascular collapse;* feeble, rapid pulse; pulmonary edema; decreased body temperature; clammy, cyanotic skin; depressed reflexes; stupor; and *coma.* After initial constriction the pupils become dilated. *Death results from respiratory failure or arrest followed by cardiac arrest.* Symptoms: *Chronic Toxicity:* Prolonged use of barbiturates at high doses may lead to physical and psychological dependence, as well as tolerance. Symptoms of dependence are similar to those associated with chronic alcoholism, and withdrawal symptoms are equally severe. Withdrawal symptoms usually last for 5–10 days and are terminated by a long sleep.
Treatment: Acute Toxicity:
• Maintenance of an adequate airway, oxygen intake, and carbon dioxide removal are essential.
• After PO ingestion, gastric lavage or gastric aspiration may delay absorption. Emesis should not be induced once the symptoms of overdosage are manifested, as the client may aspirate the vomitus into the lungs. Also, if the dose of barbiturate is high enough, the vomiting center in the brain may be depressed.
• Absorption following SC or IM administration of the drug may be delayed by the use of ice packs or tourniquets.
• Maintain renal function.
• Removal of the drug by peritoneal dialysis or an artificial kidney should be carried out.
• Supportive physiologic methods have proven superior to use of analeptics.
Treatment: Chronic Toxicity: Cautious withdrawal of the hospitalized addict over a 2–4-week period. A stabilizing dose of 200–300 mg of a short-acting barbiturate is administered q 6 hr. The dose is then reduced by 100 mg/day until the stabilizing dose is reduced by one-half. The client is then maintained on this dose for 2–3 days before further reduction. The same procedure is repeated when the initial stabilizing dose has been reduced by three-quarters. If a

mixed spike and slow activity appear on the EEG, or if insomnia, anxiety, tremor, or weakness is observed, the dosage is maintained at a constant level or increased slightly until symptoms disappear.

DRUG INTERACTIONS

General Considerations: Phenobarbital stimulates the activity of enzymes responsible for the metabolism of a large number of other drugs by a process known as *enzyme induction*. As a result, when phenobarbital is given to clients receiving such drugs, their therapeutic effectiveness may be markedly reduced or even abolished.

The CNS depressant effect of the barbiturates is potentiated by many drugs. Concomitant administration may result in coma or fatal CNS depression. Barbiturate dosage should either be reduced or eliminated when other CNS drugs are given. Barbiturates also potentiate the toxic effects of many other agents.

Acetaminophen / ↑ Risk of hepatotoxicity when used with large or chronic doses of barbiturates

Alcohol / Potentiation or addition of CNS depressant effects. Concomitant use may lead to drowsiness, lethargy, stupor, respiratory collapse, coma, or death

Anesthetics, general / See *Alcohol*

Anorexiants / ↓ Effect of anorexiants R/T opposite effects

Antianxiety drugs / See *Alcohol*

Anticoagulants, oral / ↓ Effect of anticoagulants R/T ↓ GI tract absorption and ↑ liver breakdown

Antidepressants, tricyclic / ↓ Antidepressant effects R/T ↑ liver breakdown

Antidiabetic agents / Prolong the effects of barbiturates

Antihistamines / See *Alcohol*

Beta-adrenergic agents / ↓ Beta blockade R/T ↑ liver breakdown

Carbamazepine / ↓ Carbamazepine levels may occur

Charcoal / ↓ Absorption of barbiturates from the GI tract

Chloramphenicol / ↑ Effect of barbiturates R/T ↓ liver breakdown and ↓ effect of chloramphenicol by ↑ liver breakdown

Clonazepam / Barbiturates may ↑ excretion of clonazepam → loss of efficacy

Clozapine / ↓ Clozapine levels R/T ↑ liver metabolism

CNS depressants / See *Alcohol*

Corticosteroids / ↓ Effect of corticosteroids R/T ↑ liver breakdown

Doxorubicin / ↓ Effect of doxorubicin R/T ↑ excretion

Doxycycline / ↓ Effect of doxycycline R/T ↑ liver breakdown (effect may last up to 2 weeks after barbiturates are discontinued)

Estrogens / ↓ Effect of estrogen R/T ↑ liver breakdown

Felodipine / ↓ Felodipine levels → ↓ effect

Fenoprofen / ↓ Bioavailability of fenoprofen

Furosemide / ↑ Risk or intensity of orthostatic hypotension

Griseofulvin / ↓ Effect of griseofulvin R/T ↓ absorption from GI tract

Haloperidol / ↓ Effect of haloperidol R/T ↑ liver breakdown

H *Indian snakeroot* / Additive CNS depression

H *Kava kava* / Potentiation of CNS depression

MAO inhibitors / ↑ Effect of barbiturates R/T ↓ liver breakdown

Meperidine / CNS depressant effects may be prolonged

Methadone / ↓ Effect of methadone

Methoxyflurane / ↑ Kidney toxicity R/T ↑ liver breakdown of methoxyflurane to toxic metabolites

Metronidazole / ↓ Effect of metronidazole

Narcotic analgesics / See *Alcohol*

Oral contraceptives / ↓ Effect of contraceptives R/T ↑ liver breakdown

Phenothiazines / ↓ Effect of phenothiazines R/T ↑ liver breakdown; also see *Alcohol*

Phenytoin / Effect variable and unpredictable; monitor carefully

Procarbazine / ↑ Effect of barbiturates

Quinidine / ↓ Effect of quinidine R/T ↑ liver breakdown

Rifampin / ↓ Effect of barbiturates R/T ↑ liver breakdown

Sedative-hypnotic, nonbarbiturate / See Alcohol

Theophyllines / ↓ Effect of theophyllines R/T ↑ liver breakdown

Valproic acid / ↑ Effect of barbiturates R/T ↓ liver breakdown

Verapamil / ↑ Excretion of verapamil → ↓ effect

Vitamin D / Barbiturates may ↑ requirements for vitamin D R/T ↑ liver breakdown

HOW SUPPLIED

Phenobarbital: *Capsules:* 16 mg; *Elixir:* 15 mg/5 mL, 20 mg/5 mL; *Tablets:* 15 mg, 16 mg, 16.2 mg, 30 mg, 60 mg, 90 mg, 100 mg.

Phenobarbital sodium: *Injection:* 30 mg/mL, 60 mg/mL, 65 mg/mL, 130 mg/mL.

DOSAGE

PHENOBARBITAL, PHENOBARBITAL SODIUM

• **CAPSULES; ELIXIR; TABLETS**

Sedation.

Adults: 30–120 mg/day in two to three divided doses. Or, a single dose of 30–120 mg may be given at intervals; frequency is determined by response, but no more than 400 mg per day. **Pediatric:** 8–32 mg.

Hypnotic.

Adults: 100–200 mg at bedtime. **Pediatric:** Dose should be determined by provider, based on age and weight.

Anticonvulsant.

Adults: 60–200 mg/day in single or divided doses. **Pediatric:** 3–6 mg/kg/day in single or divided doses. In infants and children, a loading dose of 15–20 mg/kg achieves blood levels of about 20 mcg/mL shortly after administration. To reach therapeutic blood levels of 10–25 mcg/mL, higher doses per kilogram are generally necessary compared with adults.

• **IM; IV**

Sedation.

Adults: 30–120 mg/day IM or IV in two to three divided doses.

Preoperative sedation.

Adults: 100–200 mg IM only, 60–90 min before surgery. **Pediatric:** 1–3 mg/kg IM or IV 60–90 min prior to surgery.

Hypnotic.

Adults: 100–320 mg IM or IV.

Acute convulsions.

Adults: 200–320 mg IM or IV; may be repeated in 6 hr if needed. **Pediatric:** 4–6 mg/kg/day for 7–10 days to achieve a blood level of 10–15 mcg/mL (or 10–15 mg/kg/day, IV or IM).

Status epilepticus.

Adults: 15–20 mg/kg IV (given over 10–15 min); may be repeated if needed. **Pediatric:** 15–20 mg/kg given over a 10 to 15 min period. *NOTE:* Use the minimal amount required and wait for the anticonvulsant effect to occur before giving a second dose.

NURSING CONSIDERATIONS

Ⓒ Do not confuse phenobarbital with pentobarbital (a shorter-acting barbiturate).

ADMINISTRATION/STORAGE

1. Use parenterally only when PO use is impossible or impractical.

2. Reduce dose in the elderly, debilitated, or those with impaired hepatic or renal function.

3. When used for seizures, give major part of the dose according to when seizures are likely to occur (i.e., on arising for daytime seizures; at bedtime when seizures occur at night).

4. When used IM, inject into large muscle (e.g., gluteus maximus, vastus lateralis). Injection into/near peripheral nerves may cause permanent neurologic deficit.

5. In most cases, when used for epilepsy, drug must be taken regularly to avoid seizures, even when no seizures are imminent. Give lowest dose possible to avoid adding to the depression that may follow seizures.

IV 6. Reserve IV use for conditions when other routes are not feasible. There is the possibility of overdose, including respiratory depression, even with slow injection of fractional doses.

7. In convulsive states, minimize dosage to avoid compounding the depression that may follow seizures. Make the injection slowly.

8. Administer preferably into a larger vein to minimize the possibility of

---

Bold Italic = life threatening side effect   ■ = black box warning   ✦ = Available in Canada

thrombosis. Do not give into varicose veins due to slowed circulation.

9. Inadvertant injection into or adjacent to an artery may cause gangrene requiring amputation of the extremity or portion thereof. Aspirate to avoid inadvertent intra-arterial injection.

10. Freshly prepare aqueous solution for injection and inject slowly at a rate of 50 mg/min.

11. Some ready-dissolved solutions for injection are available; the vehicle is propylene glycol, water, and alcohol.

12. Avoid any extravasation as tissue damage and necrosis may result.

ASSESSMENT

1. List reasons for therapy, type, onset, characteristics of S&S/seizures, other agents trialed. Note clinical presentation; list drugs prescribed to ensure none interact.

2. Assess VS, CBC, renal, and LFTs. Reduce dose with dysfunction and in debilitated/elderly clients.

CLIENT/FAMILY TEACHING

1. Take as directed. Store away from bedside and out of child's reach.

2. May initially cause drowsiness; assess effects before performing tasks that require mental alertness.

3. Phenobarbital may require an increase in vitamin D consumption; consume foods high in vitamin D. May also contribute to folate deficiency requiring supplemental folic acid and vitamin D.

4. Drug decreases effects of oral contraceptives; practice other nonhormonal forms of birth control. Avoid alcohol, CNS depressants, and OTC agents without approval.

5. Do not stop abruptly following long term use; may precipitate seizures. Tolerance may develop and require dosage adjustment.

6. Report any loss of effects, adverse effects or fever, sore throat, rash or bruising/bleeding. Brush teeth frequently and carefully to prevent gingivitis.

7. Keep all F/U appointments to evaluate response and blood levels.

OUTCOMES/EVALUATE

• Sedation; control of seizures

• Therapeutic anticonvulsant drug levels (10–40 mcg/mL)

Phentermine hydrochloride
(**FEN**-ter-meen)

CLASSIFICATION(S):
Anorexiant
PREGNANCY CATEGORY: C
Rx: Adipex-P, Ionamin, **C-IV**

USES

Short-term (few weeks) treatment for weight reduction with exercise, behavioral modification, and caloric restriction in the management of exogenous obesity in clients with an initial body mass of 30 kg/m^2 or more or 27 mg/m^2 or more in the presence of other risk factors (e.g., hypertension, diabetes, hyperlipidemia).

ACTION/KINETICS

Action

Phentermine is a sympathomimetic amine with similar actions as amphetamine, including increase in BP and CNS stimulation. Tachyphylaxis and tolerance can occur.

CONTRAINDICATIONS

Advanced arteriosclerosis, CV disease, moderate to severe hypertension, hyperthyroidism, glaucoma, or known hypersensitivity to sympathomimetic amines. Also, agitated states, those with a history of drug abuse, during or within 14 days following the administration of MAO inhibitors (hypertensive crisis may occur). Use with other drugs for weight loss, as well as with selective serotonin reuptake inhibitors is not recommended. Lactation. Use in children less than 16 years of age.

SPECIAL CONCERNS

Abuse of phentermine and development of intense psychological dependence and severe social dysfunction are possible. Abrupt discontinuation following administration of high doses results in extreme fatigue and mental depression. Use with caution even in

P

those with mild hypertension. Insulin requirements in diabetes mellitus may be altered. Safety and efficacy have not been determined in children.

SIDE EFFECTS

Most Common

Dizziness, constipation, dry mouth, headache, false sense of well being, N&V, nervousness, insomnia, tremors.

CNS: Overstimulation, restlessness, nervousness, dizziness, insomnia, euphoria, dysphoria, tremor, headache, exaggerated feelings of depression or elation, false sense of well being, psychotic episodes (rare). **GI:** Dry mouth, unpleasant taste, diarrhea, constipation, GI disturbances. **CV:** Palpitation, tachycardia, throbbing heartbeat, increased BP, *primary pulmonary hypertension, regurgitant cardiac valvular disease*. **Miscellaneous:** Urticaria, impotence, changes in libido, tremors.

OD OVERDOSE MANAGEMENT

Symptoms: **Acute overdose: CNS:** Restlessness, tremor, hyperreflexia, rapid respiration, confusion, assaultiveness, hallucinations, panic states. Fatigue and depression follow the central stimulation. **CV:** Arrhythmias, hypertension or hypotension, *circulatory collapse*. **GI:** N&V, diarrhea, abdominal cramps. Fatal poisoning usually terminates in *convulsions and coma*. **Chronic intoxication:** Severe dermatoses, marked insomnia, irritability, hyperactivity, personality changes, psychosis (indistinguishable from schizophrenia).

Treatment: **Acute overdose:**
* Largely symptomatic.
* Gastric lavage.
* Sedation with a barbiturate.
* Acidification of the urine (increases phentermine excretion).
* Phentolamine, IV for acute, severe hypertension.

DRUG INTERACTIONS

Alcohol / Adverse drug reaction possible

Dexfenfluramine / Possible primary pulmonary hypertension (rare); also, possible serious regurgitant cardiac valvular disease (primarily affecting the mitral, aortic, and/or tricuspid valves)

Fenfluramine / Possible primary pulmonary hypertension (rare); also, possible serious regurgitant cardiac valvular disease (primarily affecting the mitral, aortic, and/or tricuspid valves)

Guanethidine / ↓ Guanethidine hypotensive effect

MAO inhibitors / Possible significant ↑ BP

HOW SUPPLIED

Capsules: 18.75 mg, 30 mg, 37.5 mg; *Capsules (resin):* 15 mg, 30 mg; *Tablets:* 8 mg, 37.5 mg.

DOSAGE

* **CAPSULES; TABLETS**
  Exogenous obesity.

Adipex-P: One capsule or tablet (37.5 mg) once daily, given before breakfast or 1–2 hr after breakfast. For some, ½ tablet (i.e., 18.75 mg) daily may be adequate. Or, for some, give ½ tablet two times/day. **Ionamin:** One capsule or tablet (various doses) once daily, given before breakfast or 2 hr after breakfast. For some, ½ tablet may be adequate Take capsules 10–14 hr before bedtime.

NURSING CONSIDERATIONS

ADMINISTRATION/STORAGE

1. Tolerance to the anorectic effect usually occurs within a few weeks. Do not exceed the recommended dose in an attempt to increase the effect; rather, discontinue the drug.
2. Store at room temperature.

ASSESSMENT

1. List reasons for therapy, risk factors, BMI, other agents trialed, outcome.
2. List medical conditions that may require weight loss. Identify those that preclude therapy: advanced arteriosclerosis/CAD, hyperthyroidism, glaucoma, drug abuse history, extreme agitation.
3. Monitor VS, renal and LFTs, BMI. Assess for tolerance.

CLIENT/FAMILY TEACHING

1. Take only as directed. Avoid late evening administration due to the possibility of insomnia. Swallow Ionamin capsules whole.
2. If a dose is missed, skip the missed dose completely; take the next dose at the regularly scheduled time.

Bold Italic = life threatening side effect   ■ = black box warning   ♣ = Available in Canada

3. Do not perform activities that require mental alertness until drug effects realized; may experience cognitive impairment.

4. Continue calorie restrictions and regular daily exercise to ensure weight loss.

5. Drug may cause pulmonary hypertension which is fatal. Shortness of breath is the first symptom but other symptoms include: chest pain (angina pectoris), syncope, or lower extremity edema. Report immediately any S&S or deterioration in exercise tolerance and stop therapy.

6. Drug may cause psychological dependence and social isolation. Do not increase dose and do not stop abruptly after prolonged therapy. Severe side effects may occur. Store safely out of the reach of children.

7. Monitor FS. Insulin requirements may be altered with the use of Ionamin and the recommended dietary regimen.

8. With hypertension, monitor BP closely. Drug may cause significant increases in BP.

9. Keep all F/U appointments to monitor VS, labs, and drug response.

OUTCOMES/EVALUATE
Desired weight loss

Phenylephrine hydrochloride Ⅳ Ⓒ
(fen-ill-**EF**-rin)

CLASSIFICATION(S):
Sympathomimetic
PREGNANCY CATEGORY: C
OTC: Nasal Solution: 4-Way Fast Acting, Afrin Children's Pump Mist, Little Colds for Infants & Children, Little Noses Gentle Formula (Infants & Children), Neo-Synephrine 4-Hour Extra Strength, Neo-Synephrine 4-Hour Mild Formula, Neo-Synephrine 4-Hour Regular Strength, Rhinall, Vicks Sinex Ultra Fine Mist. **Ophthalmic Solution:** Altafrin, Relief. **Strips:** Sudafed PE Quick-Dissolve. **Tablets:** Sudafed PE.
Rx: Ophthalmic Solution: AK-Di-late, Altafrin, Mydfrin 2.5%, Neofrin. **Parenteral:** Neo-Synephrine. **Tablets, Chewable:** AH-chew D. **Tablets, Oral Disintegrating:** Nasop.

SEE ALSO *SYMPATHOMIMETIC DRUGS.*

USES
Parenteral: (1) Maintenance of an adequate level of BP during spinal and inhalation anesthesia. (2) Treatment of vascular failure in shock, shock-like states, drug-induced hypotension, or hypersensitivity. (3) To overcome paroxysmal SVT. (4) Prolong spinal anesthesia. (5) Vasoconstrictor in regional anesthesia.

Oral: (1) Temporary relief of nasal congestion due to the common cold, hay fever, or other upper respiratory allergies. (2) Nasal congestion associated with sinusitis. (3) Promote nasal or sinus drainage.

Nasal: Nasal congestion due to allergies, sinusitis, common cold, hay fever, or other upper respiratory allergies.

Ophthalmic, 0.12%: Temporary relief of redness of the eye associated with colds, hay fever, wind, dust, sun, smog, smoke, contact lens and as a lubricant to prevent further irritation or to relieve dryness of the eye.

Ophthalmic, 2.5% and 10%: (1) Decongestant, mydriatic, and vasoconstrictor. (2) Pupillary dilation in uveitis to prevent or aid in the disruption of posterior synechia formation. (3) Open-angle glaucoma. (4) Refraction without cycloplegia, ophthalmoscopic examination, funduscopy, prior to surgery (2.5%).

ACTION/KINETICS
Action
Stimulates alpha-adrenergic receptors (with little or no effect on beta receptors in the heart), producing pronounced vasoconstriction and hence an increase in both SBP and DBP; reflex bradycardia results from increased vagal activity. Also acts on alpha receptors producing vasoconstriction in the skin, mucous membranes, and the mucosa as well as mydriasis by contracting the dilator muscle of the pupil. Resembles

P

epinephrine, but it has more prolonged action and few cardiac effects.

Pharmacokinetics

IV, Onset: immediate; **duration:** 15–20 min. **IM, SC, Onset:** 10–15 min; **duration:** 0.5–2 hr for IM and 50–60 min for SC. **Nasal decongestion (topical), Onset:** 15–20 min; **duration:** 30 min–4 hr. **Ophthalmic, time to peak effect for mydriasis:** 15–60 min for 2.5% solution and 10–90 min for 10% solution. **Duration:** 0.5–1.5 hr for 0.12%, 3 hr for 2.5%, and 5–7 hr with 10% (when used for mydriasis). Excreted in urine.

CONTRAINDICATIONS

Parenteral use in severe hypertension, VT. Use as a decongestant in children less than 6 years of age. Ophthalmic, 10%, in infants and 2.5% in low-birth weight neonates and infants; also, ophthalmic in those with anatomically narrow angles or narrow-angle glaucoma.

SPECIAL CONCERNS

Use with extreme caution in geriatric clients, severe arteriosclerosis, bradycardia, partial heart block, myocardial disease, hyperthyroidism and during pregnancy and lactation. Systemic absorption with nasal or ophthalmic use. Use of the 2.5% or 10% ophthalmic solutions in children may cause hypertension and irregular heart beat. In geriatric clients, chronic use of the 2.5% or 10% ophthalmic solutions may cause rebound miosis and a decreased mydriatic effect.

SIDE EFFECTS

Most Common

When used parenterally: Headache, reflex bradycardia, excitability, restlessness.

When used for nasal decongestion: Burning/stinging/dryness inside of nose, headache, dizziness.

When used ophthalmically: Blurred vision, stinging on instillation, mydriasis, increased redness/irritation, lacrimation.

Parenteral use: Reflex bradycardia, arrhythmias (rare), headache, excitability, restlessness. **Nasal use:** Burning/stinging/dryness inside of nose, headache, dizziness, insomnia, nervousness, increased runny/stuffy nose, increased

sweating, tremor, paleness, fast/irregular/pounding heart beat. **Ophthalmic use:** Rebound miosis and decreased mydriatic response in geriatric clients, blurred vision, stinging on instillation, mydriasis, increased redness, irritation, discomfort, blurring, punctuate keratitis, lacrimation, increased intraocular pressure, transient pigment floaters in older clients in the aqueous humor 30 to 45 min after instillation, rebound miosis and decreased mydriatic response in older clients. The 10% solution may cause serious CV reactions, including ventricular arhythmias and ***MI***.

ADDITIONAL DRUG INTERACTIONS

Anesthetics, halogenated hydrocarbon / May sensitize myocardium → serious arrhythmias; includes ophthalmic use
Atropine / Concomitant ophthalmic use → ↑ pressor effects of phenylephrine and cause tachycardia
Bretylium / ↑ Effect of phenylephrine → possible arrhythmias
Guanethidine / Possible ↑ pressor effect of phenylephrine → severe hypertension, including phenylephrine ophthalmic use
MAO inhibitors / Ophthalmic use with or up to 21 days after discontinuing MAOIs → exaggerated adrenergic effects or a severe hypertensive crisis
Methyldopa / Coadministration ophthalmically → potentiation of phenylephrine pressor effects
Oxytocic drugs / Possible severe persistent hypertension
Tricyclic antidepressants / Possible ↑ or ↓ sensitivity to IV phenylephrine; phenylephrine ophthalmic use → potentiation of pressor response

OD OVERDOSE MANAGEMENT

Symptoms: Ventricular extrasystoles, short paroxysms of ventricular tachycardia, sensation of fullness in the head, tingling of extremities. *Treatment:* Administer an alpha-adrenergic blocking agent (e.g., phentolamine).

HOW SUPPLIED

Nasal Solution: *Drops/Spray:* 0.125%, 0.25%, 0.5%, 1%.
Oral: *Strips:* 10 mg; *Tablets:* 10 mg; *Tablets, Chewable:* 10 mg; *Tablets, Oral Dis-*

Bold Italic = life threatening side effect　　■ = black box warning　　✦ = Available in Canada

integrating: 14 mg total (10 mg hydro-chloride and 4 mg base).
Ophthalmic: *Solution:* 0.12%, 2.5%, 10%.
Parenteral: *Injection:* 1% (10 mg/mL).

DOSAGE

- **IM; IV; SC**

    Vasopressor, mild to moderate hypotension.

Adults: 2–5 mg (range: 1–10 mg) IM or SC, not to exceed an initial dose of 5 mg repeated no more often than q 10–15 min; or, 0.2 mg (range: 0.1–0.5 mg) IV, not to exceed an initial dose of 0.5 mg repeated no more often than q 10–15 min. *NOTE:* A 5 mg IM dose should raise BP for 1–2 hr; a 0.5 mg IV dose should raise BP for about 15 min.
Pediatric: 0.1 mg/kg (3 mg/m^2) IM or SC repeated in 1–2 hr if needed.

Vasopressor, severe hypotension and shock (including drug-related hypotension).

Correct blood volume before any vasopressor is given. **Adults, initial:** 10 mg (1 mL of 1% solution) added to 500 mL dextrose injection or NaCl injection. To raise BP rapidly, start the infusion at about 100 mcg/min to 180 mcg/min (based on 20 gtt/mL; this is 100–180 gtt/min) by continuous IV infusion. If a prompt initial response is not obtained, additional increments of 10 mg or more are added to the infusion bottle. Adjust the rate of flow until the desired BP is obtained. Avoid hypertension.

Prophylaxis and treatment of hypotension during spinal anesthesia.

Adults: 2–3 mg IM or SC 3–4 min before anesthetic given; subsequent doses should not exceed the previous dose by more than 0.1–0.2 mg. No more than 0.5 mg should be given in a single dose. **Pediatric:** 0.044–0.088 mg/kg IM or SC.

Hypotensive emergencies during spinal anesthesia.

Adults, initial: 0.2 mg IV; dose can be increased by no more than 0.1–0.2 mg for each subsequent dose not to exceed 0.5 mg/dose.

Prolongation of spinal anesthesia.

2–5 mg added to the anesthetic solution increases the duration of action up to 50% without increasing side effects or complications.

Vasoconstrictor for regional anesthesia.

Add 1 mg to every 20 mL (1:20,000 of phenylephrine) of local anesthetic solution. If more than 2 mg phenylephrine is used, pressor reactions can be expected.

Paroxysmal SVT.

Initial: 0.5 mg (maximum) given by rapid IV injection (over 20–30 seconds). Subsequent doses are determined by BP and should not exceed the previous dose by more than 0.1–0.2 mg and should never be more than 1 mg.

- **NASAL DROPS; NASAL SPRAY**

Adults and children over 12 years of age: 2–3 gtt of the 0.25% or 0.5% solution into each nostril q 3–4 hr as needed. In resistant cases, the 1% solution can be used but no more often than q 4 hr. **Children, 6–12 years of age:** 2–3 gtt of the 0.25% solution not more often than q 4 hr. **Children, 2–less than 6 years of age:** Do not use.

- **STRIPS**

    Decongestant.

Adults: 1 strip (10 mg) q 4 hr, up to 6 strips/day. **Children, <12 years of age:** Check with provider.

- **TABLETS, CHEWABLE; TABLETS, ORAL DISINTEGRATING**

    Nasal congestion.

Adults: 1–2 tablets (10–20 mg) q 4 hr. **Children, 6 to <12 years of age:** 1 tablet (10 mg) q 4 hr.

- **OPHTHALMIC SOLUTION, 0.12%**

    Minor eye irritations.

1–2 gtt of the 0.12% solution in the eye(s) up to 4 times per day as needed.

- **OPHTHALMIC SOLUTION, 2.5%, 10%**

    Vasoconstriction, pupillary dilation.

1 gtt of the 2.5% or 10% solution on the upper limbus a few minutes following 1 gtt of topical anesthetic (prevents stinging and dilution of solution by lacrimation). An additional drop may be needed 1 hr after the use of a topical anesthetic.

Uveitis.

1 gtt of the 2.5% or 10% solution with atropine. To free recently formed poste-

P

rior synechiae, 1 gtt of the 2.5% or 10% solution to the upper surface of the cornea; dose may be repeated as needed, but not to exceed three applications. Continue treatment the following day, if needed. In the interim, apply hot compresses for 5–10 min 3 times per day using 1 gtt of 1% or 2% atropine sulfate solution before and after each series of compresses.

Glaucoma.
1 gtt of 10% solution on the upper surface of the cornea as needed to reduce intraocular tension temporarily. Both the 2.5% and 10% solutions may be used with miotics in clients with open-angle glaucoma.

Surgery.
2.5% or 10% solution 30–60 min before surgery for short-term wide dilation of the pupil.

Refraction.
Adults: 1 gtt of a cycloplegic (homatropine HBr, atropine sulfate, cyclopentolate, tropicamide HCl, or a combination of homatropine and cocaine HCl) in each eye followed in 5 min with 1 gtt of 2.5% phenylephrine solution and in 10 min with another drop of cycloplegic. The eyes are ready for refraction in 50–60 min. **Children:** 1 gtt of atropine sulfate, 1%, in each eye followed in 10–15 min with 1 gtt of phenylephrine solution, 2.5%, and in 5–10 min with a second drop of atropine sulfate, 1%. The eyes are ready for refraction in 1–2 hr.

Ophthalmoscopic examination.
1 gtt of 2.5% solution in each eye. The eyes are ready for examination in 15–30 min and the effect lasts for 1–3 hr.

NURSING CONSIDERATIONS

Ⓒ Do not confuse Sudafed PE (contains phenylephrine) with Sudafed (contains pseudoephedrine).

ADMINISTRATION/STORAGE
1. Store drug in a brown bottle and away from light.
2. Instill a drop of local anesthetic before administering the 10% ophthalmic solution.
3. Store ophthalmic products from 20–25°C (68–77°F); store Neofrin in the

refrigerator. Protect from light and excessive heat. Prolonged exposure to air or strong light may cause oxidation and discoloration. Do not use solution if it is brown or contains a precipitate.

IV 4. For intermittent IV administration, dilute each 1 mL (1 mg) of the 1% solution with 9 mL of sterile water. Further dilution of 10 mg in 500 mL of dextrose, Ringer's, or saline solution may be titrated to client response.
5. Monitor infusion site closely to avoid extravasation. If evident, administer SC phentolamine locally to prevent tissue necrosis.
6. Prolonged exposure to air or strong light may result in oxidation and discoloration. Do not use solution if it changes color, becomes cloudy, or contains a precipitate.
7. The injection is for single use only; discard any unused portion.
8. Store the injection from 15–30°C (59–86°F). Protect from light.

ASSESSMENT
1. Note reasons for therapy, type, onset, characteristics of S&S, clinical presentation; note goals of therapy.
2. During IV dosing monitor cardiac rhythm, BP continuously until stabilized; note any evidence of bradycardia or arrhythmias.
3. With IV extravasation infiltrate site using a fine gauge needle with 10–15 mL of NSS that contains 5–10 mg of phentolamine.

CLIENT/FAMILY TEACHING
1. Review frequency, method of administration, and care of containers.
2. Ophthalmic instillations and nasal decongestants may produce systemic sympathomimetic effects; chronic excessive use may cause rebound congestion.
3. Wear sunglasses in bright light. Report if symptoms of photosensitivity and blurred vision persist after 12 hr. Blurred vision should decrease with repeated use.
4. With ophthalmic solution, report if there is no relief of symptoms within 5 days. Remove contact lens as some solutions may stain.

Bold Italic = life threatening side effect   ■ = black box warning   ✦ = Available in Canada

5. When using for nasal decongestion, blow nose before administering; report if no relief of symptoms within 3 days. Rebound nasal congestion may occur with prolonged therapy.

OUTCOMES/EVALUATE

- ↑ BP
- Termination of paroxysmal SVT
- Relief of nasal congestion
- ↓ Conjunctivitis/allergic S&S
- Dilatation of pupils

Phenytoin IV ©
(**FEN**-ih-toyn)

CLASSIFICATION(S):
Antiarrhythmic, Class IB; anticonvulsant, hydantoin
PREGNANCY CATEGORY: C
Rx: Dilantin Infatab, Dilantin-125.
♣Rx: Dilantin-30 Pediatric.

Phenytoin sodium, extended
PREGNANCY CATEGORY: C
Rx: Dilantin Kapseals, Phenytek.

Phenytoin sodium, parenteral
PREGNANCY CATEGORY: C
Rx: Dilantin Sodium.

Phenytoin sodium prompt
PREGNANCY CATEGORY: C
Rx: Diphenylan Sodium.

SEE ALSO *ANTICONVULSANTS* AND *ANTIARRHYTHMIC DRUGS.*

USES
(1) Chronic epilepsy, especially of the tonic-clonic, psychomotor type. Not effective against absence seizures and may even increase the frequency of seizures in this disorder. (2) **Parenteral:** Status epilepticus and to control seizures during neurosurgery. IV for PVCs and tachycardia. Particularly useful for arrhythmias produced by digitalis overdosage. (3) **PO:** Certain PVCs. *Investigational:* Paroxysmal choreoathetosis; to treat blistering and erosions in clients with recessive dystrophic epidermolysis bullosa; episodic dyscontrol; trigeminal neuralgia; as a muscle relaxant in neuromyotonia, myotonia congenita, or myotonic muscular dystrophy; to treat cardiac symptoms in overdosage of tricyclic antidepressants. Severe preeclampsia.

ACTION/KINETICS

Action
Acts in the motor cortex of the brain to reduce the spread of electrical discharges from the rapidly firing epileptic foci in this area. This is accomplished by stabilizing hyperexcitable cells possibly by affecting sodium efflux. Also, phenytoin decreases activity of centers in the brain stem responsible for the tonic phase of grand mal seizures. Has few sedative effects.

Pharmacokinetics
Phenytoin extended is designed for once-a-day dosage. It has a slow dissolution rate—no more than 35% in 30 min, 30–70% in 60 min, and less than 85% in 120 min. Absorption is variable following PO dosage. **Peak serum levels, PO:** 4–8 hr. Since the rate and extent of absorption depend on the particular preparation, the same product should be used for a particular client. **Peak serum levels, IM:** 24 hr (wide variation). **Therapeutic serum levels:** 5–20 mcg/mL. **t½:** 8–60 hr (average: 20–30 hr). **Steady state:** 7–10 days after initiation. Biotransformed in the liver. Both inactive metabolites and unchanged (less than 5%) drug are excreted in the urine. As an antiarrhythmic, phenytoin increases the electrical stimulation threshold of heart muscle, although it is less effective than quinidine, procainamide, or lidocaine. It also decreases the QT interval. **Onset:** 30–60 min. **Duration:** 24 hr or more. **t½:** 22–36 hr. **Therapeutic serum level:** 10–20 mcg/mL. **Plasma protein binding:** 87–93%.

P

CONTRAINDICATIONS

Hypersensitivity to hydantoins, exfoliative dermatitis, sinus bradycardia, second- and third-degree AV block, clients with stokes-Adams syndrome, SA block. Lactation.

SPECIAL CONCERNS

Use with caution in acute, intermittent porphyria. Administer with extreme caution to clients with a history of asthma or other allergies, impaired renal or hepatic function, and heart disease (hypotension, severe myocardial insufficiency). Abrupt withdrawal may cause status epilepticus. Combined drug therapy is required if petit mal seizures are also present.

SIDE EFFECTS

Most Common

Ataxia, drowsiness, slurred speech, confusion, N&V, rash, constipation/diarrhea, gingival hyperplasia.

CNS: Drowsiness, ataxia, dysarthria, confusion, insomnia, nervousness, irritability, depression, tremor, numbness, headache, psychoses, slurred speech, *increased seizures*. Choreoathetosis following IV use. **GI:** Gingival hyperplasia, N&V, either diarrhea or constipation. **Dermatologic:** Various dermatoses including a measles-like rash (common), scarlatiniform, maculopapular, and urticarial rashes. Rarely, drug-induced lupus erythematosus, *Stevens-Johnson syndrome*, exfoliative or purpuric dermatitis, and *toxic epidermal necrolysis*. Alopecia, hirsutism. Skin reactions may necessitate withdrawal of therapy. **Hematopoietic:** Leukopenia, granulocytopenia, thrombocytopenia, pancytopenia, *agranulocytosis*, macrocytosis, megaloblastic anemia, leukocytosis, monocytosis, eosinophilia, simple anemia, *aplastic anemia, hemolytic anemia*. **Hepatic:** Liver damage, *toxic hepatitis*, hypersensitivity reactions involving the liver including hepatocellular degeneration and *fatal hepatocellular necrosis*. **Ophthalmic:** Diplopia, nystagmus, conjunctivitis. **Miscellaneous:** Hyperglycemia, chest pain, edema, fever, photophobia, weight gain, *pulmonary fibrosis*, lymph node hyperplasia, gynecomastia, periarteritis nodosa, depression of IgA, soft tissue injury at injection site, coarsening of facial features, Peyronie's disease, enlarged lips.

Rapid parenteral administration may cause serious CV effects, including hypotension, arrhythmias, CV collapse, and heart block, as well as CNS depression. Many clients have a partial deficiency in the ability of the liver to degrade phenytoin, and as a result, toxicity may develop after a small PO dose. Liver and kidney function tests and hematopoietic studies are indicated prior to and periodically during drug therapy.

OD OVERDOSE MANAGEMENT

Symptoms: Initially, ataxia, dysarthria, and nystagmus followed by unresponsive pupils, hypotension, and coma. Plasma levels greater than 40 mcg/mL result in significant decreases in mental capacity. *Treatment:* Treat symptoms. Hemodialysis may be effective. In children, total-exchange transfusion has been used.

DRUG INTERACTIONS

Acetaminophen / ↓ Acetaminophen effect R/T ↑ liver breakdown; hepatotoxicity may &arrowup.

Alcohol, ethyl / ↓ Phenytoin effect in alcoholics R/T ↑ liver breakdown

Allopurinol / ↑ Phenytoin effect R/T ↓ liver breakdown

Amiodarone / ↑ Phenytoin or amiodarone effect R/T ↓ liver breakdown

Antacids / ↓ Phenytoin effect R/T ↓ GI absorption

Anticoagulants, oral / ↑ Phenytoin effect R/T ↓ liver breakdown. Also, possible ↑ anticoagulant effect R/T ↓ plasma protein binding

Antidepressants, tricyclic / ↑ Risk of epileptic seizures or ↑ phenytoin effect by ↓ plasma protein binding

Barbiturates / Phenytoin effect may be ↑, ↓, or not changed; possible ↑ effect of barbiturates

Benzodiazepines / ↑ Phenytoin effect R/T ↓ liver breakdown

Carbamazepine / ↓ Phenytoin or carbamazepine effect R/T ↑ liver breakdown

Charcoal / ↓ Phenytoin effect R/T ↓ absorption from GI tract

Bold Italic = life threatening side effect　　■ = black box warning　　♣ = Available in Canada

Chloramphenicol / ↑ Phenytoin effect R/T ↓ liver breakdown

Chlorpheniramine / ↑ Phenytoin effect

Cimetidine / ↑ Phenytoin effect R/T ↓ liver breakdown

Clonazepam / ↓ Plasma levels of clonazepam or phenytoin; ↑ risk of phenytoin toxicity

Contraceptives, oral / Estrogen-induced fluid retention may precipitate seizures; also, ↓ effect of contraceptives R/T ↑ liver breakdown

Corticosteroids / ↓ Corticosteroid effect R/T ↑ liver breakdown; also, corticosteroids may mask hypersensitivity reactions due to phenytoin

Cyclosporine / ↓ Cyclosporine effect R/T ↑ liver breakdown

Diazoxide / ↓ Phenytoin effect R/T ↑ liver breakdown

Dicumarol / ↓ Dicumarol effect R/T ↑ liver breakdown

Digitalis glycosides / ↓ Digitalis effect R/T ↑ liver breakdown

Disopyramide / ↓ Disopyramide effect R/T ↑ liver breakdown

Disulfiram / ↑ Phenytoin effect R/T ↓ liver breakdown

Dopamine / IV phenytoin → hypotension and bradycardia; also, ↓ dopamine effect

Doxycycline / ↓ Doxycycline effect R/T ↑ liver breakdown

Estrogens / See *Contraceptives, oral*

Fluconazole / ↑ Phenytoin effect R/T ↓ liver breakdown

Folic acid / ↓ Phenytoin effect

Furosemide / ↓ Furosemide effect R/T ↓ absorption

Haloperidol / ↓ Haloperidol effect R/T ↑ liver breakdown

Ibuprofen / ↑ Phenytoin effect

Irinotecan / ↓ AUC and ↑ clearance of irinotecan R/T ↑ metabolism

Isoniazid / ↑ Phenytoin effect R/T ↓ liver breakdown

Itraconazole / Possible ↓ itraconazole plasma levels

Levodopa / ↓ Levodopa effect

Levonorgestrel / ↓ Levonorgestrel effect

Lithium / ↑ Risk of lithium toxicity

Lopinavir/Ritonavir / Phenytoin ↓ lopinavir plasma levels R/T induction of CYP3A4 and lopinavir/ritonavir ↓ phenytoin plasma levels R/T induction of CYP2C9

Loxapine / ↓ Phenytoin effect

Mebendazole / ↓ Mebendazole effect

Meperidine / ↓ Meperidine effect R/T ↑ liver breakdown; toxic effects of meperidine may ↑ due to accumulation of active metabolite (normeperidine)

Methadone / ↓ Methadone effect R/T ↑ liver breakdown

Metronidazole / ↑ Phenytoin effect R/T ↓ liver breakdown

Metyrapone / ↓ Metyrapone effect R/T ↑ liver breakdown

Mexiletine / ↓ Mexiletine effect R/T ↑ liver breakdown

Miconazole / ↑ Phenytoin effect R/T ↓ liver breakdown

H *Milk thistle /* Helps prevent liver damage from phenytoin

Mirtazapine / ↓ Plasma mirtazapine levels R/T ↑ metabolism

Nitrofurantoin / ↓ Phenytoin effect

Omeprazole / ↑ Phenytoin effect R/T ↓ liver breakdown

Phenothiazines / ↑ Phenytoin effect R/T ↓ liver breakdown

Primidone / Possible ↑ primidone effect

Pyridoxine / ↓ Phenytoin effect

Quetiapine / ↓ Peak and trough quetiapine levels R/T ↑ liver metabolism

Quinidine / ↓ Quinidine effect R/T ↑ liver breakdown

Rifampin / ↓ Phenytoin effect R/T ↑ liver breakdown

Salicylates / ↑ Phenytoin effect R/T ↓ plasma protein binding

Sucralfate / ↓ Phenytoin effect R/T ↓ absorption from GI tract

Sulfonamides / ↑ Phenytoin effect R/T ↓ liver breakdown

Sulfonylureas / ↓ Sulfonylurea effect

Theophylline / ↓ Effect of both drugs R/T ↑ liver breakdown

Trimethoprim / ↑ Phenytoin effect R/T ↓ liver breakdown

Valproic acid / ↑ Phenytoin effect R/T ↓ liver breakdown and ↓ plasma protein binding; phenytoin may also ↓ effect of valproic acid R/T ↑ liver breakdown

P

📷 = see color insert   **H** = Herbal   **IV** = Intravenous   ©̶ = sound alike drug

HOW SUPPLIED

Phenytoin: *Tablets, Chewable:* 50 mg; *Oral Suspension:* 125 mg/5 mL.

Phenytoin sodium, extended: *Capsules, Extended-Release:* 30 mg, 100 mg, 200 mg, 300 mg.

Phenytoin sodium, parenteral: *Injection:* 50 mg/mL.

Phenytoin sodium prompt: *Capsules:* 100 mg.

DOSAGE

• ORAL SUSPENSION; TABLETS, CHEWABLE

Seizures.

Adults, initial: 100 mg (125 mg of the suspension) 3 times per day; adjust dosage at 7- to 10-day intervals until seizures are controlled; **usual, maintenance:** 300–400 mg/day, although 600 mg/day (625 mg of the suspension) may be required in some. **Pediatric, initial:** 5 mg/kg/day in two to three divided doses; **maintenance,** 4–8 mg/kg (up to maximum of 300 mg/day). Children over 6 years may require up to 300 mg/day. **Geriatric:** 3 mg/kg initially in divided doses; **then,** adjust dosage according to serum levels and response. Once dosage level has been established, the extended capsules may be used for once-a-day dosage.

• CAPSULES; CAPSULES, EXTENDED-RELEASE

Seizures.

Adults, initial: 100 mg 3 times per day; adjust dose at 7- to 10-day intervals until control is achieved. An initial loading dose of 12–15 mg/kg divided into two to three doses over 6 hr followed by 100 mg 3 times per day on subsequent days may be preferred if seizures are frequent. **Pediatric:** See dose for Oral Suspension and Chewable Tablets.

Arrhythmias.

Adults: 200–400 mg/day.

• IV

Status epilepticus.

Adults, loading dose: 10–15 mg/kg at a rate not to exceed 50 mg/min; **then,** 100 mg PO or IV q 6–8 hr. **Pediatric, loading dose:** 15–20 mg/kg in divided doses of 5–10 mg/kg given at a rate of 1–3 mg/kg/min.

Arrhythmias.

Adults: 100 mg q 5 min up to maximum of 1 gram.

• IM

Neurosurgery.

Dose should be 50% greater than the PO dose. 100–200 mg q 4 hr during and after surgery (during first 24 hr, administer no more than 1,000 mg; after first day, give maintenance dosage).

NURSING CONSIDERATIONS

Ⓒ Do not confuse Dilantin with Dilaudid (a narcotic analgesic). Do not confuse phenytoin with fosphenytoin or mephyton (also anticonvulsants).

ADMINISTRATION/STORAGE

1. Full effectiveness of PO administered hydantoins is delayed and may take 6–9 days to be fully established. A similar period of time will elapse before effects disappear completely.

2. When hydantoins are substituted for or added to another anticonvulsant medication, their dosage is gradually increased, while dosage of the other drug is decreased proportionally.

3. Avoid IM, SC, or perivascular injections. Pain, inflammation, and necrosis may be caused by the highly alkaline solutions.

4. If receiving tube feedings of Isocal or Osmolite, the PO absorption of phenytoin may be decreased. Do not administer together.

5. Due to potential differences in bioavailability between PO products, do not interchange brands. Also, when switching from extended to prompt products, dosage adjustments may be required.

IV 6. Use of IV infusion is not recommended, as the drug is poorly soluble and may form a precipitate. Inject slowly and directly into a large vein through a large-gauge needle or IV catheter.

7. For parenteral preparations:
• Use only a clear solution.
• Dilute with special diluent supplied by manufacturer.
• Shake the vial until the solution is clear. It may take about 10 min for the drug to dissolve.

Bold Italic = life threatening side effect   ■ = black box warning   ✤ = Available in Canada

- To hasten the process, warm the vial in warm water after adding the diluent.
- The drug is incompatible with acid solutions.

8. *Do not* add phenytoin to an already running IV solution.

9. If IV infusion is used, a rate of 50 mg/min should not be exceeded in adults or 1–3 mg/kg/min in neonates.

10. Following IV administration, administer NSS through the same needle or IV catheter to avoid local irritation of the vein due to alkalinity of the solution. Do not use dextrose solutions.

11. For treatment of status epilepticus, inject IV slowly at a rate not to exceed 50 mg/min. May repeat the dose 30 min after the initial administration if needed.

ASSESSMENT

1. List reasons for therapy, onset, characteristics of S&S, clinical presentation, blood levels, other agents trialed, outcome.

2. Note history and nature of seizures, addressing location, frequency, duration, causes/characteristics, triggers and EEG findings.

3. Determine if hypersensitive to hydantoins or has exfoliative dermatitis. Consider fosphenytoin in those unable to tolerate phenytoin. Do not breastfeed following delivery.

4. Monitor ECG, VS, CBC, liver, and renal function studies. May lower serum Mg, folate, calcium and vitamin D. Avoid with sinus bradycardia, sino-atrial block, second and third degree A-V block.

INTERVENTIONS

1. During IV administration, monitor VS and for hypotension.

2. Monitor serum drug levels because the serum concentrations of phenytoin increase disproportionately as the dosage is increased:

- Seven to 10 days may be required to achieve recommended serum levels. Drug is highly protein bound; may order free and bound drug levels to better assess response. Drug is metabolized much slower by the elderly; thus most may be managed with once a day dosing.
- If receiving drugs that interact with hydantoins or with impaired liver function, obtain level more frequently. Dilantin induces hepatic microsomal enzymes for drug metabolism.3. Oral form has variable absorption; do not administer with tube feedings. Administer separately, flush, and clamp tube for 20 min to ensure absorption.

CLIENT/FAMILY TEACHING

1. May take with food to minimize GI upset. Do not take antacids within 1 hr of ingestion. Do not chew or crush; take tablets whole.

2. Use care when performing tasks that require mental alertness. Drug may cause drowsiness, dizziness, and blurred vision.

3. Do not substitute products or exchange brands; bioavailability of phenytoin may vary. Seizure control may be lost or toxic blood levels may develop with substitutions.

4. Prompt-release forms cannot be substituted for another unless the dosage is also adjusted.

- If taking phenytoin extended, do not substitute chewable tablets for capsules. Medication strengths are not equal.
- If taking phenytoin extended, check bottle carefully. Chewable tablets are never extended form.
- With extended release, take only a single dose daily; take only as directed and only in the brand prescribed.

5. If dose is missed, take as soon as remembered. Then resume the usual schedule. Do not double up to make up for the missed dose. If the doses of drug are scheduled throughout the day, and one of the doses is missed, take the drug as soon as it is realized unless it's within 4 hr of the next dose. In that case, omit unless otherwise instructed.

6. Do not take any other agents. Hydantoins interact with many other medications and may require adjustment of the anticonvulsant dose. Avoid alcohol in any form and CNS depressants.

7. With diabetes, monitor FS and report changes; may have to adjust insulin dosage and/or diet.

8. May cause urine to appear pink, red, or brown; do not be alarmed.

9. To minimize bleeding from the gums and prevent gingival hyperplasia, practice good oral hygiene. Brush teeth with a soft toothbrush, massage the gums, and floss every day. Advise dentist of therapy.

10. Hydantoin has an androgenic effect on the hair follicle. Acne may develop; practice good skin care. Report any excessive hair growth on the face and trunk and any discolorations or skin rash; may require dermatologist referral.

11. Complaints of weakness, ease of fatigue, headaches, or feeling faint may be signs of folic acid deficiency or megaloblastic anemia. Dietitian evaluation as well as hematologic evaluations may be indicated.

12. Report for lab studies as ordered, including CBC, drug levels, and renal and liver function studies. Drug may alter thyroid function results. If thyroid studies are conducted, for ensured accuracy, they should be repeated 10 days after therapy has been discontinued.

13. Do not stop abruptly. Report all bothersome side effects because these may be dose-related.

14. Practice reliable birth control; drug may decrease effectiveness of oral contraceptives.

OUTCOMES/EVALUATE

- Control of seizures
- Termination of ventricular arrhythmias; stable cardiac rhythm
- Therapeutic drug levels (5–20 mcg/mL)

Phytonadione (Vitamin K₁)

(fye-toe-nah-**DYE**-ohn)

CLASSIFICATION(S):
Vitamin K derivative
PREGNANCY CATEGORY: C
Rx: Mephyton.

USES
Coagulation disorders due to faulty formation of factors II, VII, IX, and X when caused by vitamin K deficiency or interference with vitamin K activity.

PO. (1) Anticoagulant-induced PT deficiency due to coumarin or indandione derivatives. (2) Hypoprothrombinemia secondary to antibacterial therapy or salicylates. (3) Secondary to obstructive jaundice and biliary fistulas (use only if bile salts are given together with phytonadione so phytonadione will be absorbed).

Parenteral. (1) Anticoagulant-induced prothrombin deficiency caused by coumarin or indandione derivatives. (2) Hypoprothrombinemia secondary to conditions limiting absorption or synthesis of vitamin K (e.g., obstructive jaundice, biliary fistula, sprue, ulcerative colitis, celiac disease, intestinal resection, cystic fibrosis of the pancreas, regional enteritis). (3) Drug-induced hypoprothrombinemia due to interference with vitamin K metabolism (e.g., salicylates, antibacterial therapy). (4) Prophylaxis and therapy of hemorrhagic disease in newborns.

ACTION/KINETICS

Action
Vitamin K is essential for the hepatic synthesis of factors II, VII, IX, and X, all of which are essential for blood clotting. Vitamin K deficiency causes an increase in bleeding tendency, demonstrated by ecchymoses, epistaxis, hematuria, GI bleeding, and postoperative and intracranial hemorrhage. Phytonadione is similar to natural vitamin K. GI absorption occurs only via intestinal lymphatics and requires the presence of bile salts. Vitamin K is not effective in reversing the anticoagulant effect of heparin. Frequent determinations of PT are indicated during therapy.

Pharmacokinetics
IM, Onset: 1–2 hr. **Control of bleeding:** Parenteral, 3–6 hr. **Normal PT:** 12–14 hr. **PO, Onset:** 6–10 hr.

CONTRAINDICATIONS
Severe liver disease.

Bold Italic = life threatening side effect   ■ = black box warning   ✦ = Available in Canada

SPECIAL CONCERNS

■ IV or IM use. Severe reactions, including death, have occurred during and immediately after IV injection, even with precautions to dilute the injection and to avoid rapid infusion. Severe reactions, including fatalities, have also been reported following IM administration. These severe reactions have resembled hypersensitivity or anaphylaxis, including shock and cardiac or respiratory arrest. Some clients exhibit these severe reactions on receiving vitamin K for the first time. Thus, restrict the IV route to those situations where other routes are not feasible and the serious risk involved is considered justified.■ Use with caution in clients with sulfite sensitivity and during lactation as phytonadione is excreted in breast milk. Safety and efficacy have not been determined in children. Benzyl alcohol, contained in some preparations, may cause toxicity in newborns.

SIDE EFFECTS

Most Common

After PO use: N&V, stomach upset, headache, transient flushing of face, sweating, chills, fever.

After parenteral use: Flushing, sweating, hypotension, dizziness, pain/swelling/tenderness at injection site.

May be transient flushing of the face, sweating, a sense of constriction of the chest, and weakness. Cramp-like pain, weak and rapid pulse, convulsive movements, chills and fever, hypotension, cyanosis, or hemoglobinuria has been reported occasionally. *Shock and cardiac and respiratory failure may be observed.* **Allergic:** Rash, urticaria, anaphylaxis.

After PO use: N&V, stomach upset, headache.

After parenteral use: Flushing, alteration of taste, sweating, hypotension, dizziness, rapid and weak pulse, dyspnea, cyanosis, delayed skin reactions. Pain, swelling, and tenderness at injection site. *IV administration may cause severe reactions (e.g., shock, cardiac or respiratory arrest, anaphylaxis) leading to death.* These effects may occur when receiving vitamin K for the

first time. **Newborns:** *Fatal kernicterus,* hemolysis, jaundice, hyperbilirubinemia (especially in premature infants).

DRUG INTERACTIONS

Antibiotics / May inhibit vitamin K production → bleeding; give vitamin K supplements

Anticoagulants, oral / Antagonizes anticoagulant effect

Cholestyramine / ↓ Phytonadione effect R/T ↓ GI tract absorption

Colestipol / ↓ Phytonadione effect R/T ↓ GI tract absorption

Hemolytics / ↑ Potential for toxicity

Mineral oil / ↓ Phytonadione effect R/T ↓ GI tract absorption

Quinidine, Quinine / ↑ Requirement for vitamin K

Salicylates / High doses → ↑ vitamin K requirements

Sulfonamides / ↑ Requirements for vitamin K

Sucralfate / ↓ Phytonadione effect R/T ↓ GI tract absorption

HOW SUPPLIED

Injection, Aqueous Colloidal Solution: 2 mg/mL, 10 mg/mL; *Tablets:* 5 mg.

DOSAGE

- **IM, IV, SC; TABLETS**

  Hypoprothrombinemia, anticoagulant-induced (coumarin or indandione derivatives).

Adults: 2.5–10 mg (up to 25 mg). Dose may be repeated after 6–8 hr (parenteral use) or 12–48 hr (PO use) if PT has not been shortened sufficiently.

  Hypoprothrombinemia due to other causes (antibiotics, salicylates or other drugs, factors limiting absorption or synthesis).

Adults, PO: 2.5–25 mg (rarely up to 50 mg). If possible, discontinue or reduce the dose of drugs interfering with coagulation mechanisms that is an alternative to administering concurrent phytonadione. Amount and route of administration depend on severity of condition and client response. Avoid PO route when condition would prevent proper absorption.

  Hemorrhagic disease of the newborn.

Prophylaxis: Single IM dose of 0.5–1 mg within 1 hr of birth. **Treatment:** 1 mg SC or IM (higher doses may be nec-

P

---

essary) if the mother has been receiving PO anticoagulants.

NURSING CONSIDERATIONS
ADMINISTRATION/STORAGE
1. Whenever possible, give by SC injection.
2. Store tablets from 15–30°C (59–86°F). Protect from light.
3. Heparin may be used to reverse effects from overdosage.
IV 4. If IV use is unavoidable, inject very slowly, not exceeding 1 mg/min.
5. May be diluted with 0.9% NaCl, D5W, or D5W/NaCl injection. All the diluents should be preservative-free. Do not use other diluents.
6. When dilutions are indicated, begin administration immediately after mixing with the diluent and discard any unused portion of the dilution, as well as unused contents of the ampule.
7. The product contains aluminum that may be toxic with prolonged parenteral administration if kidney function is impaired. Premature neonates are particularly at risk as their kidneys are immature and they require large amounts of calcium and phosphate solutions, which contain aluminum.
8. Protect vitamin K from light. Store injectable emulsion or colloidal solutions in cool, 5–15°C (41–59°F), dark place. Do not freeze.

ASSESSMENT
1. Note reasons for therapy, other agents trialed, outcome; assess for any sensitivity to sulfites.
2. List drugs prescribed to ensure none interact.
3. Monitor PT/PTT, liver, B_{12}, hematologic values; determine history or lab evidence of advanced liver disease. This results in loss of protein synthesis and is not responsive to vitamin K.
4. It takes a minimum of 1–2 hr for measurable improvement in the PT after phytonadione is given.

INTERVENTIONS
1. Note any frank bleeding. Test stools, urine, and GI drainage for occult blood.
2. Observe hospitalized clients with poor nutrition (receiving TPN), uremia, recent surgery, and multiple antibiotic

therapy for vitamin K deficiency. Administer slowly. Rapid parenteral administration can produce dyspnea, chest and back pain, and even death.
3. With decreased bile secretion, administer bile salts to ensure absorption of PO phytonadione. If receiving bile acid–binding resins such as colestipol or cholestyramine, monitor PT and assess carefully for malabsorption of vitamin K.

CLIENT/FAMILY TEACHING
1. Take only as directed. Dietary sources high in vitamin K include dairy products, meats, and green leafy vegetables. The dietary requirement is low since it is also synthesized by colonized bacteria in the intestine.
2. Report any evidence of unusual bruising or bleeding. Use a soft toothbrush, electric razor, and a night light at night. Wear shoes and avoid IM shots and flossing to prevent injury with bleeding.
3. If possible, discontinue or reduce the dose of drugs interfering with coagulation mechisms (e.g., salicylates, antibiotics).
4. Avoid alcohol, aspirin, and ibuprofen compounds (NSAIDs) as well as any other OTC preparations. Report any adverse effects.

OUTCOMES/EVALUATE
- Prevention/control of bleeding
- Prophylaxis of hypoprothrombinemia during prolonged TPN
- Prevention of hemorrhagic disease in the newborn

Pilocarpine hydrochloride ©
(pie-low-**CAR**-peen)

CLASSIFICATION(S):
Cholinergic agonist
PREGNANCY CATEGORY: C
Rx: Adsorbocarpine, Isopto Carpine, Pilocar, Piloptic-½, -1, -2, -3, -4, and -6, Pilostat, Salagen.
✦Rx: Pilopine HS.

USES

HCl: (1) Chronic simple glaucoma (especially open-angle). Chronic angle-closure glaucoma, including after iridectomy. Acute angle-closure glaucoma (alone or with other miotics, epinephrine, beta-adrenergic blocking agents, carbonic anhydrase inhibitors, or hyperosmotic agents). (2) To reverse mydriasis (i.e., after cycloplegic and mydriatic drugs). (3) Pre- and postoperative intraocular tension. (4) Salagen (tablet) for treatment of radiation-induced dry mouth in head and neck cancer clients, as well as in Sjögen's (dry mouth) syndrome. *Investigational:* Hydrochloride used to treat xerostomia in clients with malfunctioning salivary glands.

ACTION/KINETICS

Action When used to treat dry mouth due to radiotherapy in head and neck cancer clients, pilocarpine stimulates residual functioning salivary gland tissue to increase saliva production.

Pharmacokinetics

Gel/Solution: Onset: 10–30 min; **duration:** 4–8 hr. Rate of absorption is decreased when taken with a high-fat meal.

CONTRAINDICATIONS

Inflammatory eye disease, acute-angle glaucoma, history of retinal detachment, ocular hypotension, asthma, epilepsy, parkinsonism, gangrene, diabetes, CV disease, GI or GU tract obstruction, spastic GI conditions, vasomotor instability, severe bradycardia or hypotension, recent MI, lactation, in those receiving choline esters or depolarizing neuromuscular blocking drugs.

SPECIAL CONCERNS

Use with caution in those with narrow angles (angle closure may result), in those with known or suspected cholelithiasis or biliary tract disease, and in clients with controlled asthma, chronic bronchitis, or COPD. Safety and efficacy have not been established in children.

SIDE EFFECTS

Most Common

When used ophthalmically: Transient burning/stinging, tearing, blurred vision, headache.

When used orally: Sweating, headache, urinary frequency, nausea, flushing, flu syndrome, rhinitis, diarrhea, dyspepsia, dizziness, chills, asthenia.

Ophthalmic use. Transient burning/stinging, tearing, ciliary spasm, conjunctival vascular congestion, temporal/peri-/or supra-orbital headache, superficial keratitis, induced myopia (especially in younger clients who have just begun therapy), blurred vision, poor dark adaptation, reduced visual acuity in poor illumination in older clients and in those with lens opacity, subtle corneal granularity (with gel), lens opacity with prolonged use, retinal detachment (rare).

Oral use (tablets). Dermatologic: Sweating, flushing, rash, pruritus. **GI:** N&V, dyspepsia, diarrhea, abdominal pain, taste perversion, anorexia, increased appetite, esophagitis, tongue disorder, salivation. **CV:** Hypertension, tachycardia, bradycardia, ECG abnormality, palpitations, syncope. **CNS:** Dizziness, asthenia, headache, tremor, anxiety, confusion, depression, abnormal dreams, hyperkinesia, hypesthesia, nervousness, paresthesias, speech disorder, twitching. **Respiratory:** Sinusitis, rhinitis, bronchiolar spasm, pulmonary edema, pharyngitis, epistaxis, increased sputum, stridor, yawning. **Ophthalmic:** Lacrimation, amblyopia, conjunctivitis, abnormal vision, eye pain, glaucoma. **GU:** Urinary frequency, dysuria, metrorrhagia, urinary impairment. **Body as a whole:** Chills, sweating, edema, body odor, hypothermia, mucous membrane abnormality. **Miscellaneous:** Dysphagia, voice alteration, myalgias, seborrhea.

OD **OVERDOSE MANAGEMENT**

Treatment: Titrate with atropine (0.5–1 mg SC or IM) and supportive measures to maintain circulation and respiration. If there is severe cardiovascular depression or bronchoconstriction, epinephrine (0.3–1 mg SC or IV) may be used.

DRUG INTERACTIONS

Anticholinergics / Antagonism of anticholinergic drug effects
Beta blockers / Possible conduction disturbances; use together with caution

---

HOW SUPPLIED

Pilocarpine hydrochloride: *Ophthalmic Gel:* 4%; *Ophthalmic Solution:* 0.25%, 0.5%, 1%, 2%, 3%, 4%, 5%, 6%, 8%, 10%; *Tablets:* 5 mg, 7.5 mg.

DOSAGE

PILOCARPINE HYDROCHLORIDE

- **OPHTHALMIC GEL, 4%**
  Glaucoma.

Adults and adolescents: ½ in ribbon in the lower conjunctival sac of the affected eye(s) once daily at bedtime.

- **OPHTHALMIC SOLUTION, 0.25%, 0.5%, 1%, 2%, 3%, 4%, 5%, 6%, 8%, 10%**
  Doses listed are all for adults and adolescents.
  Chronic glaucoma.

1–2 gtt of a 0.5–4% solution 2–4 times per day.
Acute angle-closure glaucoma.

1 gtt of a 1% or 2% solution q 5–10 min for three to six doses; then, 1 gtt q 1–3 hr until pressure is decreased.
Miotic, to counteract sympathomimetics.

1 gtt of a 1% solution.
Miosis, prior to surgery.

1 gtt of a 2% solution q 4–6 hr for one or two doses before surgery.
Miosis before iridectomy.

1 gtt of a 2% solution for four doses immediately before surgery.

- **TABLETS**
  Dry mouth due to radiotherapy in head and neck cancer.

Initial: 5 mg 3 times per day. Adjust dose based on therapeutic response.
Usual dose range: 15–30 mg/day, not to exceed 10 mg/dose. At least 12 weeks of uninterrupted therapy may be needed to assess beneficial effect.
Sjögren's syndrome.

5 mg 4 times per day. Efficacy may take up to 6 weeks.

NURSING CONSIDERATIONS

Ⓒ Do not confuse Salagen with selegiline (an antiparkinson drug).

ADMINISTRATION/STORAGE

1. Start with 5 mg twice a day and increase as tolerated in clients with a Child-Pugh score of 7–9. Pilocarpine is not recommended for clients with a Child-Pugh score of 10–15.

2. Concentrations greater than 4% of pilocarpine HCl may be more effective in clients with dark pigmented eyes; however, the incidence of side effects increases.

3. For acute, narrow-angle glaucoma, give pilocarpine in the unaffected eye to prevent angle-closure glaucoma.

4. Store the solution, protected from light, at 8–30°C (46–86°F). Refrigerate the gel at 2–8°C (36–46°F) until dispensed. Do not freeze gel; discard any unused portion after 8 weeks.

ASSESSMENT

1. Note reasons for therapy, eye exam findings, other agents trialed, outcome, client ability to use system.

2. Those with acute infectious conjunctivitis or keratitis should be carefully evaluated before use of the pilocarpine ocular system.

CLIENT/FAMILY TEACHING

1. If other glaucoma medication (i.e., drops) used with the gel at bedtime, instill drops at least 5 min before the gel.

2. Report for periodic eye pressure readings to evaluate drug effectiveness.

3. Use only as directed. Report lack of response/adverse effects. Refrigerate gel.

OUTCOMES/EVALUATE

- ↓ IOP; pupillary constriction
- ↑ Saliva production; relief of radiation-induced or Sjögen's syndrome dry mouth

Pimecrolimus ■
(pim-e-**KROE**-lih-mus)

CLASSIFICATION(S):
Immunomodulator, topical
PREGNANCY CATEGORY: C
Rx: Elidel.

USES

Second-line therapy for short-term and noncontinuous chronic treatment of mild to moderate atopic dermatitis in nonimmunocompromised clients 2

Bold Italic = life threatening side effect   ■ = black box warning   ✦ = Available in Canada

years of age and older who have failed to respond adequately to other topical medications or when such treatments are not advisable.

ACTION/KINETICS

Action

The mechanism of action is not known. Pimecrolimus binds with high affinity to macrophilin-12 and inhibits the calcium-dependent phosphatase, calcineurin. It thus inhibits T-cell activation by blocking the transcription of early cytokines. Specifically, pimecrolimus inhibits interleukin-2 and interferon gamma and interleukin-4 and interleukin-10 cytokine synthesis in human T-cells. The drug also prevents the release of inflammatory cytokines and mediators from mast cells, in vitro, after stimulation by antigen/immunoglobulin E.

Pharmacokinetics

Some of the drug is absorbed into the systemic circulation.

CONTRAINDICATIONS

Hypersensitivity to pimecrolimus or any component of the product. Use in Netherton syndrome or other skin diseases in which there is the potential of increased systemic absorption of pimecrolimus. Use on malignant or premalignant skin conditions, such as cutaneous T-cell lymphoma. Lactation. Use in children younger than 2 years of age.

SPECIAL CONCERNS

■ Long-term safety of topical calcineurin inhibitors has not been established. Although a causal relationship has not been established, rare cases of malignancy (e.g., skin malignancy, lymphoma) have been reported in clients treated with topical calcineurin inhibitors including pimecrolimus. Therefore, (1) avoid continuous, long-term use of topical calcineurin inhibitors, including pimecrolimus, in any age group, and limit application to areas of involvement with atopic dermatitis; (2) pimecrolimus is not indicated for use in children younger than 2 years of age.■ The safety has not been determined for use in generalized erythroderma or beyond 1 year of noncontinuous use.

SIDE EFFECTS

Most Common

Application site burning, headache, skin infection, diarrhea, conjunctivitis, asthma, bronchitis, cough, nasopharyngitis, rhinitis, URTI, hypersensitivity, sore throat.

Local reactions: Burning sensation, erythema, stinging, soreness, pruritus. **CNS:** Headache. **Dermatologic:** Acne, folliculitis, herpes simplex dermatitis, impetigo, molluscum contagiosum, skin infection/papilloma, warts, urticaria, photosensitivity, skin flushing associated with alcohol use. **GI:** Abdominal pain (including upper pain), constipation, diarrhea, gastroenteritis, loose stools N&V. **GU:** Dysmenorrhea. **Respiratory:** Aggravated asthma, acute bronchitis, bronchitis, cough, dyspnea, epistaxis, influenza, nasal congestion, pharyngitis, naso-/streptococcal pharyngitis, pneumonia, rhinitis, rhinorrhea, sinus congestion, sinusitis, sore throat, tonsillitis, URTI (including viral), wheezing. **Hematologic:** Lymphadenopathy. **Musculoskeletal:** Arthralgias, back pain. **Ophthalmic:** Conjunctivitis, eye infection, ocular irritation after application to the eyelids or near the eyes. **Otic:** Ear infection, earache, otitis media. **Infections:** Increased risk of chickenpox, shingles, herpes simplex virus infection, eczema herpeticum, bacterial (including staphylococcal) infections. **Carcinomas:** Basal cell/squamous cell carcinoma, lymphomas, malignant melanoma. **Miscellaneous:** Hypersensitivity, laceration, pyrexia, toothache, **anaphylaxis**, angioneurotic/facial edema. NOTE: May cause an increased risk of infections, lymphomas, and skin malignancies after prolonged use.

DRUG INTERACTIONS

Use with caution in clients with widespread or erythrodermic disease when coadministering pimecrolimus with CYP3A inhibitors, including calcium channel blockers, cimetidine, erythromycin, fluconazole, itraconazole, or ketoconazole.

HOW SUPPLIED

Cream: 1%.

DOSAGE

- **CREAM**

Atopic dermatitis.

Apply a thin layer of the cream to the affected area two times per day. If S&S persist >6 weeks, re-examine and confirm the diagnosis of atopic dermatitis.

NURSING CONSIDERATIONS

ADMINISTRATION/STORAGE

1. Stop using medication when S&S (e.g., itch, rash, redness) resolve.
2. Do not use occlusive dressing with pimecrolimus as safety has not been evaluated.
3. Store from 15–30°C (59–86°F). Do not freeze.

ASSESSMENT

1. Note reasons for therapy, onset, duration, and characteristics of S&S. List other agents trialed/failed.
2. Identify any form of light therapy (phototherapy, UVA or UVB) being utilized.
3. List any other type of skin treatments in use.
4. Determine if pregnant or planning to become pregnant. Elidel not for use during pregnancy.

CLIENT/FAMILY TEACHING

1. Drug used to clear up red, itchy, skin conditions unresponsive to usual therapy. Apply a thin layer of pimecrolimus cream and rub it in well to cover the affected areas.
2. Do not use this medicine in the eyes and do not swallow it. Wash hands thoroughly after applying cream, unless hands are part of the area for treatment.
3. Use of this medicine may cause reactions at the site of application such as a mild to moderate feeling of warmth/sensation of burning. Report if severe or persists for more than 1 week.
4. If S&S skin condition go away, stop cream and report. If skin condition reoccurs, consult provider.
5. Do not use any occlusive dressings (a dressing that seals the area that is being treated such as a plastic exercise suit or plastic wraps used to store foods).
6. Do not bathe, shower, or swim right after applying; could wash off cream.
7. For atopic dermatitis apply cream to skin that is clean and dry twice a day. Stop using when S&S of eczema, such as itching, rash, and redness go away, as directed.
8. Minimize or avoid exposure to natural or artificial sunlight (tanning beds or UVA/B treatment) while using Elidel Cream.
9. Report any S&S of adverse reactions to provider.
10. If no improvement in the atopic dermatitis is seen following 6 weeks of treatment stop therapy and report.
11. Drug has been associated with carcinogenic side effects with long term therapy.

OUTCOMES/EVALUATE

Relief of S&S atropic dermatitis (eczema)

Pioglitazone hydrochloride

(**pie**-oh-**GLIT**-ah-zohn)

CLASSIFICATION(S):

Antidiabetic, oral; thiazolidinedione

PREGNANCY CATEGORY: C

Rx: Actos.

SEE ALSO *ANTIDIABETIC AGENTS: HYPOGLYCEMIC AGENTS.*

USES

(1) Type 2 diabetes as monotherapy as an adjunct to diet and exercise. (2) Type 2 diabetes in combination with a sulfonylurea, metformin, or insulin as an adjunct to diet and exercise. Used when diet and exercise plus the single drug does not adequately control blood glucose.

ACTION/KINETICS

Action

Depends on the presence of insulin to act. Decreases insulin resistance in the periphery and liver resulting in increased insulin-dependent glucose disposal and decreased hepatic glucose output. It is not an insulin secretagogue. Is an agonist for peroxisome

---

Bold Italic = life threatening side effect   ■ = black box warning   ✤ = Available in Canada

proliferator-activated receptor (PPAR) gamma, which is found in adipose tissue, skeletal muscle, and liver. Activation of these receptors modulates the transcription of a number of insulin responsive genes that control glucose and lipid metabolism. Reduces fasting plasma glucose 39–65 mg/dL from placebo and HbA1c 1–1.6% from placebo.

Pharmacokinetics
After PO, steady state serum levels are reached within 7 days. **Peak levels:** 2 hr; food slightly delays the time to peak serum levels to 3–4 hr, but does not change the extent of absorption. Metabolized by CYP2C8, CYP3A4, and CYP1A1 to both active and inactive metabolites. Unchanged drug and metabolites are excreted in the urine (15–30%) and feces. **t½:** 3–7 hr (pioglitazone); 16–24 hr (total pioglitazone). **Plasma protein binding:** Over 99%.

CONTRAINDICATIONS
In type 1 diabetes, diabetic ketoacidosis, active liver disease, with ALT levels that exceed 2.5 times ULN, in clients with NYHA Class III or IV heart failure, lactation, or in pediatric clients less than 18 years of age.

SPECIAL CONCERNS
■ (1) Thiazolidinediones, including pioglitazone, cause or exacerbate CHF in some clients. After initiation of pioglitazone, and after dose increases, observe clients carefully for signs and symptoms of heart failure (including excessive, rapid weight gain, dyspnea, and/or edema). If these signs and symptoms develop, the heart failure should be managed according to the current standards of care. Furthermore, discontinuation or dose reduction of pioglitazone must be considered. (2) Pioglitazone is not recommended in clients with symptomatic heart failure. Initiation of pioglitazone in clients with established NYHA Class III or IV heart failure is contraindicated.■ Treatment may result in resumption of ovulation in premenopausal anovulatory clients with insulin resistance. Increased risk for hypoglycemia when combined with insulin or other oral hypoglycemics. May cause

osteoporosis. Safety and efficacy have not been determined in children.

SIDE EFFECTS
Most Common
URTI, headache, sinusitis, hypoglycemia, aggravated diabetes mellitus, tooth disorder, pharyngitis, myalgia, edema.
Metabolic: Hypoglycemia, aggravation of diabetes mellitus, weight gain (dose-related). **Respiratory:** URTI, sinusitis, pharyngitis. **CV:** Fluid retention leading to heart failure (especially when used as monotherapy or with insulin), usually in those with underlying cardiac disease or a history of CV conditions. **Miscellaneous:** Headache, myalgia, tooth disorder, anemia, edema, increased risk of bone fracture (more common in women), osteoporosis.

LABORATORY TEST CONSIDERATIONS
↑ ALT, HDL cholesterol, creatine phosphokinase (sporadic and transient); ↓ H&H.

DRUG INTERACTIONS
Atorvastatin / ↑ Serum levels of both drugs
Gemfibrozil / ↑ Pioglitazone AUC R/T inhibition of CYP2C8 isoenzyme
Ketoconazole / ↑ Pioglitazone AUC and C_{max} R/T significant inhibition of pioglitazone metabolism
Midazolam / Possible ↓ midazolam C_{max} and AUC
Nifedipine (extended release) / ↑ Nifedipine levels
Oral contraceptives (containing ethinyl estradiol/norethindrone) / ↓ Plasma levels of both hormones; possible loss of contraception

HOW SUPPLIED
Tablets: 15 mg, 30 mg, 45 mg.

DOSAGE
• **TABLETS**
Type 2 diabetes as monotherapy.
Adults: 15 mg or 30 mg once daily in clients not adequately controlled with diet and exercise. Initial dose can be increased in increments up to 45 mg once daily for those who respond inadequately. Consider combination therapy for those not responding adequately to monotherapy.
Type 2 diabetes as combination therapy.

P

If combined with a sulfonylurea: Initiate pioglitazone at 15 or 30 mg once daily. The current sulfonylurea dose can be continued unless hypoglycemia occurs; then, reduce the sulfonylurea dose.

If combined with metformin: Initiate pioglitazone at 15 or 30 mg once daily. The current metformin dose can be continued; it is unlikely the metformin dose will have to be adjusted due to hypoglycemia.

If combined with insulin: Initiate pioglitazone at 15 or 30 mg once daily. The current insulin dose can be continued unless hypoglycemia occurs or plasma glucose levels decrease to less than 100 mg/dL; then, decrease the insulin dose by 10 to 25%. Individualize further dosage adjustments based on glucose-lowering response.

NOTE: Daily dose of pioglitazone should not exceed 45 mg.

NURSING CONSIDERATIONS

  Do not confuse Actos with Actonel (bone growth regulator).

ADMINISTRATION/STORAGE

1. It is recommended that clients be treated with pioglitazone for a period of time (3 months) adequate to evaluate changes in HbA1c unless glycemic control deteriorates.

2. Do not initiate if there is clinical evidence of active liver disease or increased ALT levels more than 2.5 ULN at the start of therapy.

3. Discontinue if signs of heart failure emerge.

4. Store at 15–30°C (59–86°F) in a tightly closed container protected from moisture and humidity.

ASSESSMENT

1. List reasons for therapy, onset, characteristics of disease, other agents trialed, outcome. List drugs prescribed to ensure none interact.

2. Obtain BP, CBC, HbA1c, microalbumin, renal and LFTs. Ensure clients undergo periodic monitoring of liver enzymes. Evaluate ALT prior to initiation of therapy, every two months for the first year of therapy, and periodically thereafter. Obtain LFTs if symptoms suggest hepatic dysfunction.

Discontinue if jaundice noted and if elevated LFTs.

3. Review diet, exercise, and other life style changes to ensure good glucose control.

4. Ensure no evidence of heart failure or NYHA III or IV disease. May cause fluid accumulation and worsening of failure.

CLIENT/FAMILY TEACHING

1. Take once daily without regard to meals. Follow dietary guidelines, perform regular exercise, weight loss, dietary restrictions and other lifestyle changes consistent with controlling diabetes.

2. May cause swelling of extremities, resumption of ovulation (in premenopausal, anovulatory women), and hypoglycemia. Report if dark urine, abdominal pain, fatigue or unexplained N&V occur.

3. Immediately report onset of an unusually rapid increase in weight or extremity swelling, SOB, or other symptoms of heart failure.

4. Practice reliable non-hormonal contraception to prevent pregnancy.

5. Monitor FS at different times during the day and maintain log for provider review. Keep all lab appointments to ensure LFTs WNL and desired glycemic control.

OUTCOMES/EVALUATE

- Control of NIDDM by ↓ insulin resistance
- Normalization of glucose and HbA1c <7

—— *COMBINATION DRUG* ——

Piperacillin sodium and Tazobactam sodium

IV

(pie-**PER**-ah-**sill**-in, tay-zoh-**BAC**-tam)

CLASSIFICATION(S):
Antibiotic, penicillin

PREGNANCY CATEGORY: B

Rx: Zosyn.

✦**Rx:** Tazocin.

SEE ALSO *PENICILLINS* AND *PIPERACILLIN SODIUM*.

USES

(1) Appendicitis complicated by rupture or abscess and peritonitis caused by piperacillin-resistant, beta-lactamase-producing strains of *Escherichia coli, Bacteroides fragilis, B. ovatus, B. thetaiotaomicron,* or *B. vulgatus.* (2) Uncomplicated and complicated skin and skin structure infections (including cellulitis, cutaneous abscesses, and ischemic/diabetic foot infections) caused by piperacillin-resistant, beta-lactamase-producing strains of *Staphylococcus aureus.* (3) Postpartum endometritis or PID caused by piperacillin-resistant, beta-lactamase-producing strains of *E. coli.* (4) Community-acquired pneumonia of moderate severity caused by piperacillin-resistant, beta-lactamase-producing strains of *Haemophilus influenzae.* (5) Moderate to severe nosocomial pneumonia caused by piperacillin-resistant, beta-lactamase-producing strains of *S. aureus* and by susceptible strains of *Acinetobacter baumanii, H. influenzae, K. pneumoniae,* and *Pseudomonas aeruginosa* (in combination with an aminoglycoside). (6) Infections caused by piperacillin-susceptible organisms for which piperacillin is effective may also be treated with this combination. NOTE: The treatment of mixed infections caused by piperacillin-susceptible organisms and piperacillin-resistant, beta-lactamase-producing organisms susceptible to this combination does not require addition of another antibiotic. The exception is treatment of *P. aeruginosa* in nosocomial pneumonia which should be treated in combination with an aminoglycoside.

ACTION/KINETICS

Action

A combination of piperacillin sodium and tazobactam sodium, a beta-lactamase inhibitor. Tazobactam inhibits beta-lactamases, thus ensuring activity of piperacillin against beta-lactamase-producing microorganisms. Thus, tazobactam broadens the antibiotic spectrum of piperacillin to those bacteria normally resistant to it.

Pharmacokinetics

Peak plasma levels: Attained immediately after completion of an IV infusion. $t\frac{1}{2}$, piperacillin and tazobactam: 0.7–1.2 hr. Both drugs are eliminated through the kidney with piperacillin and tazobactam both excreted unchanged and as inactive metabolites. The $t\frac{1}{2}$ of both drugs is increased in clients with renal impairment and in hepatic cirrhosis (dose adjustment not required).

CONTRAINDICATIONS

Hypersensitivity to penicillins, cephalosporins, or beta-lactamase inhibitors.

SPECIAL CONCERNS

Use with caution during lactation. Safety and efficacy have not been determined in children less than 12 years of age.

SIDE EFFECTS

Most Common

Diarrhea, constipation, N&V, dyspepsia, headache, rash, rhinitis, dyspnea, abdominal pain.

See *Penicillins* for a complete list of possible side effects. The highest incidence of side effects include the following: **GI:** Diarrhea, constipation, N&V, dyspepsia, stool changes, abdominal pain. **CNS:** Headache, insomnia, fever, agitation, dizziness, anxiety. **Dermatologic:** Rash, including maculopapular, bullous, urticarial, and eczematoid; pruritus. **Hematologic:** Thrombocytopenia, eosinophilia, leukopenia, neutropenia, hemolytic anemia. **Miscellaneous:** Pain, moniliasis, hypertension, chest pain, edema, rhinitis, dyspnea.

LABORATORY TEST CONSIDERATIONS

↓ H&H. Transient ↑ AST, ALT, alkaline phosphatase, and bilirubin. ↑ Serum creatinine, BUN. Prolonged PT and PTT. Positive direct Coombs' test. Proteinuria, hematuria, pyuria, abnormalities in electrolytes (↑ and ↓ sodium, potassium, calcium), hyperglycemia. ↓ Total protein or albumin.

DRUG INTERACTIONS

Heparin / Possible ↑ heparin effect
Oral anticoagulants / Possible ↑ anticoagulant effect

Tobramycin / ↓ AUC, renal clearance, and urinary recovery of tobramycin
Vecuronium / Prolongation of neuromuscular blockade

HOW SUPPLIED
Injection, Solution: 2 grams–0.25 gram, 3 grams–0.375 gram, 4 grams–0.5 gram (first number refers to amount of piperacillin sodium); *Injection, Powder for Solution:* 2 grams–0.25 gram; 3 grams–0.375 gram; 4 grams–0.5 gram; 36 grams–4.5 grams (first number refers to amount of piperacillin sodium).

DOSAGE
• IV INFUSION
  Susceptible infections.

Adults: 12 grams/day piperacillin and 1.5 grams/day tazobactam, given as 3.375 grams (i.e., 3 grams piperacillin and 0.375 gram tazobactam) q 6 hr for 7–10 days. In clients with renal insufficiency, the IV dose is adjusted depending on the extent of impaired function. If C_{CR} is 20–40 mL/min, the dose is 8 grams/day piperacillin and 1 gram/day tazobactam in divided doses of 2.25 grams q 6 hr. If the C_{CR} <20 mL/min, the dose is 6 grams/day piperacillin and 0.75 gram/day tazobactam in divided doses of 2.25 grams q 8 hr. In hemodialysis clients or continuous ambulatory peritoneal dialysis, give 2.25 grams q 12 hr; give 0.75 gram following each hemodialysis session on hemodialysis days.

  Moderate to severe nosocomial pneumonia due to piperacillin-resistant, beta-lactamase-producing S. aureus.

Adults: 4.5 grams piperacillin q 6 hr with an aminoglycoside for 7 to 14 days. Adjust the dose as follows in clients with impaired renal function: If C_{CR} is 20–40 mL/min, give 3.375 grams q 6 hr; if C_{CR} <20 mL/min, give 2.25 grams q 6 hr. If the client is on hemodialysis or continuous ambulatory peritoneal dialysis, give 2.25 grams q 8 hr; give 0.75 gram following each hemodialysis session on hemodialysis days.

  Children, 2 months and older, with appendicitis and/or peritonitis, weighing up to 40 kg, and with healthy renal function.

Children, 9 months and older: 100 mg piperacillin/12.5 mg of tazobactam/kg q 8 hr. **Children, 2–9 months:** 80 mg piperacillin/10 mg tazobactam/kg q 8 hr. Children weighing more than 40 kg with healthy renal function should receive the adult dose.

NURSING CONSIDERATIONS
Ⓒ Do not confuse Zosyn with Zofran (an antiemetic).

ADMINISTRATION/STORAGE
Ⅳ 1. For IV administration or by infusion, reconstitute the powder for injection with 5 mL suitable diluent/gram piperacillin. IV diluents that can be used include 0.9% NaCl, sterile water for injection, dextran 6% in saline, D5W, KCl 40 mEq, bacteriostatic saline/parabens, bacteriostatic water/parabens, bacteriostatic saline/benzyl alcohol, bacteriostatic water/benzyl alcohol. *LR is not compatible.* After the diluent is added, shake vial well until the powder is dissolved. May further dilute to the desired final volume with the diluent.

2. A formulation contains edetate disodium dihydrate and the buffer sodium citrate; it is compatible with lactated Ringer's injection and, under certain conditions, with amikacin or gentamicin.

3. If intermittent IV infusion is used, the 5 mL diluent/gram piperacillin is further diluted to a volume of at least 50 mL. Give the infusion over a period of 30 min. During the infusion, discontinue the primary infusion solution.

4. To prevent unintental overdose, do not use piperacillin/tazobactam in Galaxy containers for children who require less than the full adult dose.

5. If concomitant therapy with aminoglycosides is indicated, give piperacillin/tazobactam and the aminoglycoside separately, as penicillin can inactivate the aminoglycoside if they are mixed.

6. Use single-dose vials immediately after reconstitution. Discard any unused drug after 24 hr if stored at room temperature or after 48 hr if stored in the refrigerator at 2–8°C (36–46°F).

7. After reconstitution, is stable in glass and plastic syringes, IV bags, and tub-

ing. Is stable in IV bags for up to 24 hr at room temperature and up to 1 week in the refrigerator. Is stable in an ambulatory IV infusion pump for 24 hr at room temperature.

ASSESSMENT

1. Note reasons for therapy, type, location, characteristics of S&S.
2. List any sensitivity to penicillins, cephalosporins, beta-lactamase inhibitors, or other allergens.
3. List drugs prescribed to ensure none interact unfavorably. Use of heparin and oral anticoagulants may require dosage adjustments.
4. Monitor C&S, lytes, urinalysis, hematologic, coagulation profile, renal, LFTs; reduce dosage with renal impairment.

CLIENT/FAMILY TEACHING

Report any pain at injection site, fever/chills, rash, diarrhea, GI upset, lack of response or worsening of condition.

OUTCOMES/EVALUATE

Resolution of infection

Pirbuterol acetate

(peer-**BYOU**-ter-ohl)

CLASSIFICATION(S):
Sympathomimetic
PREGNANCY CATEGORY: C
Rx: Maxair Autohaler.

SEE ALSO *SYMPATHOMIMETIC DRUGS.*

USES

Alone or with theophylline or steroids in clients 12 years and older for prophylaxis and treatment of bronchospasm in asthma and other conditions with reversible bronchospasms, including exercise-induced bronchospasm, bronchitis, emphysema, bronchiectasis, obstructive pulmonary disease.

ACTION/KINETICS

Action

Causes bronchodilation by stimulating $beta_2$-adrenergic receptors. Has minimal effects on $beta_1$ receptors. Also inhibits histamine release from mast cells, causes vasodilation, and increases ciliary motility.

Pharmacokinetics

Onset, inhalation: Approximately 5 min. **Time to peak effect:** 30–60 min. **Duration:** 5 hr.

CONTRAINDICATIONS

Cardiac arrhythmias due to tachycardia; tachycardia caused by digitalis toxicity.

SPECIAL CONCERNS

Safety and efficacy have not been determined in children less than 12 years of age.

SIDE EFFECTS

Most Common

Palpitations, tachycardia, tremor, dizziness/vertigo, nervousness/shakiness, headache, N&V, diarrhea, dry mouth, cough.

See *Sympathomimetic Drugs* for a complete list of possible side effects. **CV:** Palpitations, tachycardia, PVCs, hypotension. **CNS:** Dizziness/vertigo, nervousness, shakiness, hyperactivity, headache, hyperkinesia, anxiety, confusion, depression, fatigue, syncope. **GI:** N&V, diarrhea, dry mouth, anorexia, loss of appetite, bad taste or taste change, abdominal pain/cramps, stomatitis, glossitis. **Dermatologic:** Rash, edema, pruritus, alopecia, bruising. **Miscellaneous:** Cough, flushing, numbness in extremities, weight gain.

HOW SUPPLIED

Autoinhaler: 200 mcg/actuation.

DOSAGE

• **AUTOINHALER**
  Bronchodilation.

Adults and children over 12 years, usual: 2 inhalations (400 mcg) q 4–6 hr, not to exceed 12 inhalations (2,400 mcg) daily. Some may benefit from one inhalation (200 mcg) q 4–6 hr.

NURSING CONSIDERATIONS

ADMINISTRATION/STORAGE

1. For optimal results, the canister should be at room temperature (15–30°C; 59–86°F) before use. Failure to use the prodcut at room temperature may result in improper dosing. Shake well before using.
2. Exposure to a temperature above 120°F may cause bursting.
3. The light blue plastic actuator supplied with the aerosol should not be

used with any other product canisters. Also, actuators from other products shouuld not be used with pirbuterol acetate inhalation canisters.

ASSESSMENT
1. Note reasons for therapy, onset, duration, characteristics of S&S.
2. Assess lungs; note ECG, CXR, oxygen saturation, PFTs/spirometry readings.

CLIENT/FAMILY TEACHING
1. Review methods, frequency, and reasons for therapy. Shake well and prime the unit by releasing three test sprays into the air before using for the first time or resuming use after 2 or more weeks of nonuse. Use a spacer (chamber) to enhance dispersion. Wash in warm water and dry equipment after use and rinse mouth to prevent fungal infections. Do not exceed prescribed dosage.
2. If a previously effective dose does not provide relief, seek medical advice immediately as this is often a sign of seriously worsening asthma.
3. Report if condition or peak flows deteriorate, bronchospasm increases after treatment, or if inhaler is ineffective in relieving symptoms at prescribed dosage. Avoid triggers.
4. If using more than one corticosteroid inhaler, use the pirbuterol first, wait 5 min and then use the other inhaler. If more than one inhalation prescribed, wait at least 2 min before the next inhalation. Keep all F/U appointments to evaluate response to therapy.

OUTCOMES/EVALUATE
Improved airway exchange; ↓ airway resistance; ↓ bronchospasm

Piroxicam ■
(peer-**OX**-ih-kam)

CLASSIFICATION(S):
Nonsteroidal anti-inflammatory drug

PREGNANCY CATEGORY: C
Rx: Feldene.
✦Rx: Apo-Piroxicam, Gen-Piroxicam, Novo–Pirocam, Nu-Pirox.

SEE ALSO *NONSTEROIDAL ANTI-INFLAMMATORY DRUGS.*

USES
Acute and chronic treatment of rheumatoid arthritis and osteoarthritis. *Investigational:* Juvenile rheumatoid arthritis, primary dysmenorrhea, sunburn.

ACTION/KINETICS
Action
May inhibit prostaglandin synthesis. Effect is comparable to that of aspirin, but with fewer GI side effects and less tinnitus. May be used with gold, corticosteroids, and antacids.

Pharmacokinetics
Peak plasma levels: 1.5–2 mcg/mL after 3–5 hr (single dose). **Steady-state plasma levels** (after 7–12 days): 3–8 mcg/mL. **t½:** 50 hr. **Analgesia, onset:** 1 hr; **duration:** 2–3 days. **Anti-inflammatory activity, onset:** 7–12 days; **duration:** 2–3 weeks. Metabolites and unchanged drug excreted in urine and feces. **Plasma protein binding:** 98.5%.

CONTRAINDICATIONS
Safe use during pregnancy has not been determined. Use in children less than 14 years old. Lactation.

SPECIAL CONCERNS
■ (1) NSAIDs may cause an increased risk of serious cardiovascular thrombotic events, MI, and stroke, which can be fatal. This risk may increase with duration of use. Clients with cardiovascular disease or risk factors for cardiovascular disease may be at greater risk. (2) Piroxicam is contraindicated for treatment of perioperative pain in the setting of coronary artery bypass graft surgery. (3) NSAIDs cause an increased risk of serious GI adverse events including bleeding, ulceration, and perforation of the stomach or intestines, which can be fatal. These events can occur at any time during use and without warning symptoms. Elderly clients are at greater risk for serious GI events.■ Safety and efficacy have not been established in children. Increased plasma levels and elimination half-life may be observed in geriatric clients (especially women).

Bold Italic = life threatening side effect   ■ = black box warning   ✦ = Available in Canada

SIDE EFFECTS
Most Common
Headache, dizziness, rash, pruritus, abdominal pain/cramps, diarrhea, N&V, constipation, flatulence, dyspepsia/indigestion, heartburn, gross bleeding/perforation, peptic ulcer, impaired renal function, anemia, abnormal LFTs, increased bleeding time, edema, tinnitus.

See *Nonsteroidal Anti-Inflammatory Drugs* for a complete list of possible side effects.

ADDITIONAL DRUG INTERACTIONS
Ritonavir may ↑ piroxicam levels and possibly toxicity R/T inhibition of metabolism

LABORATORY TEST CONSIDERATIONS
Reversible ↑ BUN.

HOW SUPPLIED
Capsules: 10 mg, 20 mg.

DOSAGE
- **CAPSULES**
  Rheumatoid arthritis, osteoarthritis.
Adults: 20 mg/day in one or more divided doses. Do not assess the effect of therapy for 2 weeks.

NURSING CONSIDERATIONS
ADMINISTRATION/STORAGE
1. Steady-state plasma levels may not be reached for 2 weeks.
2. Clients over 70 years of age generally require one-half the usual adult dose of medication.

ASSESSMENT
1. Note reasons for therapy, symptom characteristics, other agents prescribed, outcome. Rate pain level and quality of life.
2. Assess involved joints, note ROM, erythema, swelling/warmth, pain, spasm.
3. Monitor CBC, renal, LFTs as well as auditory function with prolonged therapy.

CLIENT/FAMILY TEACHING
1. Take as directed with food or milk to decrease GI upset. A stomach protectant (i.e., Cytotec, or H2 blocker) may be prescribed for those with a history of ulcer disease.
2. Take at anti-inflammatory dose to prevent further joint destruction during acute exacerbations. Therapeutic effects of the medication cannot be evaluated fully for at least 2–4 weeks after treatment onset.
3. Avoid activities that require mental alertness until drug effects realized, may experience dizziness/drowsiness.
4. Aspirin decreases the effectiveness of piroxicam and may increase the occurrence of side effects. Avoid concomitant aspirin, ethanol, other NSAIDs, and OTC products. Report any increased abdominal pain, abnormal bruising or bleeding, malaise, or changes in the color of the stool immediately.
5. Avoid prolonged sun exposure; use protection if exposed.
6. Drug side effects may not be evident for 7–10 days. Report for scheduled labs; report lack of response or adverse side effects.

OUTCOMES/EVALUATE
↓ Joint pain and inflammation with improved mobility

Polymyxin B sulfate, parenteral ■IV
(pol-ee-**MIX**-in)

CLASSIFICATION(S):
Antibiotic, polymyxin
PREGNANCY CATEGORY: C

Polymyxin B sulfate, sterile ophthalmic
PREGNANCY CATEGORY: C

SEE ALSO *ANTI-INFECTIVE DRUGS.*

USES
Systemic: (1) Acute infections of the urinary tract and meninges, septicemia caused by *Pseudomonas aeruginosa.* (2) Meningeal infections caused by *Haemophilus influenzae,* UTIs caused by *Escherichia coli,* bacteremia caused by *Enterobacter aerogenes* or *Klebsiella pneumoniae.* (3) Combined with neomycin for irrigation of the urinary bladder to prevent

---

bacteriuria and bacteremia from in-dwelling catheters.

Ophthalmic: Conjunctival and corneal infections (e.g., conjunctivitis, keratitis, keratoconjunctivitis, corneal ulcers, blepharitis, blepharoconjunctivitis, acute meibomianitis, dacryocystitis) due to susceptible strains of *Pseudomonas aeruginosa*.

ACTION/KINETICS
Action
Bactericidal against most gram-negative organisms; rapidly inactivated by alkali, strong acid, and certain metal ions. Increases the permeability of the plasma cell membrane of the bacterium (i.e., similar to detergents), causing leakage of essential metabolites and ultimately inactivation.

Pharmacokinetics
Peak serum levels: IM, 2 hr. **t½:** 4.3–6 hr. Longer in presence of renal impairment. Sixty percent of drug excreted in urine. Virtually unabsorbed from the GI tract except in newborn infants. Remains in plasma after parenteral administration.

CONTRAINDICATIONS
Hypersensitivity. A potentially toxic drug to be reserved for the treatment of severe, resistant infections in hospitalized clients. Not indicated for clients with severely impaired renal function or nitrogen retention. Use with nephro- or neurotoxic drugs. Ophthalmic use in dendritic keratitis, vaccinia, varicella, mycobacterial infections/fungal diseases of the eye, use with steroid combinations after uncomplicated removal of a foreign body from the cornea. Ophthalmic use in deep-seated infections or in those likely to become systemic infections.

SPECIAL CONCERNS
■ (1) When given IM or intrathecally, give only to hospitalized clients to provide constant physician supervision. (2) Carefully determine renal function; reduce dosage in those with renal damage and nitrogen retention. Clients with nephrotoxicity due to polymyxin B sulfate usually show albuminuria, cellular casts, and azotemia. Diminishing urine output and a rising BUN are indications to discontinue therapy. (3) Neurotoxic reactions may be manifested by irritability, weakness, drowsiness, ataxia, perioral paresthesia, numbness of the extremities, and blurring of vision. These are usually associated with high serum levels found in those with impaired renal function or nephrotoxicity. Avoid concurrent use of other nephrotoxic and neurotoxic drugs, especially colistin, gentamicin, kanomycin, neomycin, paromomycin, streptomycin, and tobramycin. (4) Neurotoxicity can result in respiratory paralysis from neuromuscular blockade, especially when the drug is given soon after anesthesia or muscle relaxants.■ Safe use during pregnancy has not been established.

SIDE EFFECTS
Most Common
When used parenterally: N&V, diarrhea, nephrotoxicity, facial flushing, dizziness, paresthesias, drowsiness, abdominal cramps.
When used ophthalmically: Burning, stinging, irritation, inflammation, itching.

Nephrotoxic: Albuminuria, cylindruria, azotemia, hematuria, proteinuria, leukocyturia, electrolyte loss. **Neurologic:** Dizziness, flushing of face, mental confusion, irritability, nystagmus, muscle weakness, drowsiness, paresthesias, blurred vision, slurred speech, ataxia, *coma, seizures. Neuromuscular blockade may lead to respiratory paralysis.* **GI:** N&V, diarrhea, abdominal cramps. **Miscellaneous:** Fever, urticaria, skin exanthemata, eosinophilia, *anaphylaxis*.

Intrathecal use: Meningeal irritation with fever, stiff neck, headache, increase in leukocytes and protein in the CSF. Nerve-root irritation may result in neuritic pain and urine retention.

IM use: Irritation, severe pain.

IV use: Thrombophlebitis.

Ophthalmic use: Burning, stinging, irritation, inflammation, angioneurotic edema, itching, urticaria, vesicular and maculopapular dermatitis.

LABORATORY TEST CONSIDERATIONS
False + or ↑ levels of urea nitrogen and creatinine. Casts and RBCs in urine.

Bold Italic = life threatening side effect   ■ = black box warning   ✦ = Available in Canada

DRUG INTERACTIONS

Aminoglycoside antibiotics / Additive nephrotoxic effects

Anesthetics / Additive muscle relaxation → respiratory paralysis

Cephalosporins / ↑ Risk of renal toxicity

Phenothiazines / ↑ Risk of respiratory depression

Skeletal muscle relaxants (surgical) / Additive muscle relaxation → respiratory paralysis

HOW SUPPLIED

Powder for Injection: 500,000 units; *Powder for Ophthalmic Solution:* 500,000 units.

DOSAGE

- **IV**
  Infections.

Adults and children: 15,000–25,000 units/kg/day (maximum) in divided doses q 12 hr. **Infants,** up to 40,000 units/kg/day.

- **IM (NOT USUALLY RECOMMENDED DUE TO PAIN AT INJECTION SITE)**
  Infections.

Adults and children: 25,000–30,000 units/kg/day in divided doses q 4–6 hr. **Infants,** up to 40,000 units/kg/day. Both IV and IM doses should be reduced in renal impairment.

- **INTRATHECAL**
  Meningitis.

Adults and children over 2 years: 50,000 units/day for 3–4 days; **then,** 50,000 units every other day until 2 weeks after cultures are negative; **children under 2 years,** 20,000 units/day for 3–4 days or 25,000 units once every other day; dosage of 25,000 units should be continued every other day for 2 weeks after cultures are negative.

- **OPHTHALMIC SOLUTION**
  Pseudomonal aeruginosa infections of the eye.

1 to 3 gtt q hr using a concentration of 0.1% to 0.25% (10,000–25,000 units/mL). Increase the interval between administration as response indicates. Subconjunctival injection of up to 10,000 units/day may be used to treat *P. aeruginosa* infections of the cornea and conjunctiva. Avoid total ophthalmic instillation of over 25,000 units/day.

NURSING CONSIDERATIONS

ADMINISTRATION/STORAGE

1. Store and dilute as directed on package insert.

2. Lessen pain on IM injection by reducing drug concentration as much as possible. It is preferable to give drug more frequently in more dilute doses. If ordered, procaine hydrochloride (2 mL of a 0.5–1.0% solution per 5 units of dry powder) may be used for mixing the drug for IM injection.

3. Only give intrathecally for meningeal infections.

4. For ophthalmic use, dissolve 500,000 units of polymyxin B in 20–50 mL sterile water for injection or NaCl injection for a 10,000-25,000 units/mL concentration.

5. Before reconstitution of the ophthalmic product, store from 15–30°C (59–86°F) protected from light. After reconstitution, solution must be stored under refrigeration between 2–8°C (36–46°F); discard any unused portion after 72 hr.

IV 6. For IV administration, reconstitute 500,000 units with 300–500 mL of D5W and infuse over 60–90 min.

ASSESSMENT

1. Note reasons for therapy, onset, characteristics of S&S, C&S results.

2. Assess respiratory function; note any prior problems/conditions.

3. Observe for any muscle weakness and early signs of muscle paralysis R/T neuromuscular blockade. Assess for evidence of respiratory paralysis; withhold drug and report. Ambulatory or bedridden clients with neurologic disturbances require supervision.

4. Monitor I&O; reduce dose with impaired renal function; observe for nephrotoxicity, characterized by albuminuria, urinary casts, nitrogen retention, and hematuria.

CLIENT/FAMILY TEACHING

1. Avoid hazardous tasks until drug effects realized; may cause dizziness, vertigo, and gait problems.

2. Consume at least 2 L/day of fluids.

3. Report any neurologic disturbances, i.e., dizziness, blurred vision, irritability,

---

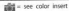

circumoral and peripheral numbness and tingling, weakness, and ataxia; usually gone 24–48 hr after drug discontinued; associated with high drug levels.

4. Anticipate a prolonged regimen of topical application of solution because drug is not toxic when used in wet dressings. Provider may wish to prevent emergence of resistant strains. Wash hands.

5. When used in the eye(s), tilt the head back and place the medication in the conjunctival sac. Light finger pressure should be applied on the lacrimal sac for 1 min. To avoid contamination, do not allow the tip of the container to touch any surface. Report any itching or burning.

OUTCOMES/EVALUATE

Negative cultures; resolution of infection; symptomatic improvement

---

Posaconazole
(**POE**-sah-**KON**-ah-zole)

CLASSIFICATION(S):
Antifungal, triazole
PREGNANCY CATEGORY: C
Rx: Noxafil.

USES
(1) Prophylaxis of invasive *Aspergillus* and *Candida* infections in clients 13 years and older who are at high risk of developing these infections because of being severely immunocompromised, such as hematopoietic stem cell transplant recipients with graft-versus-host disease or those with hematologic malignancies with prolonged neutropenia from chemotherapy. (2) Oropharyngeal candidiasis, including oropharyngeal candidiasis refractory to itraconazole and/or fluconazole.

ACTION/KINETICS
Action
Posaconazole blocks the synthesis of ergosterol, a key component of the fungal cell membrane, inhibiting the enzyme lanosterol 14α-demethylase and accumulation of methylated sterol precursors.

Pharmacokinetics
T_{max}: 3–5 hr. AUC and C_{max} are about 4 times higher when the drug is given with a high-fat meal (about 50 grams of fat) and about 3 times higher when given with a liquid nutritional supplement (14 grams of fat). Metabolized by glucuronidation. Metabolites and parent drug excreted through the feces (71%) and urine (13%). **$t\frac{1}{2}$, elimination:** 35 hr. **Plasma protein binding:** Greater than 98% bound to plasma proteins (mainly albumin).

CONTRAINDICATIONS
Use with drugs that prolong the QTc interval. Lactation.

SPECIAL CONCERNS
Closely monitor clients with severe impaired renal function for breakthrough fungal infections. Use with caution in impaired hepatic function, in those with potential proarrhythmic conditions, or in those hypersensitive to other azoles. Safety and efficacy have not been determined in children less than 13 years of age.

SIDE EFFECTS
Most Common
Fever, N&V, diarrhea, hypokalemia, headache, abdominal pain, constipation, anemia, febrile neutropenia, neutropenia, thrombocytopenia, rigors, coughing, dyspnea, hypertension, fatigue, insomnia, rash, mucositis, bilirubinemia, hepatocellular damage.

CV: Hyper-/hypotension, tachycardia, QT/QTc prolongation. **CNS:** Headache, fatigue, insomnia, dizziness, anxiety, weakness, tremor. **GI:** Diarrhea, N&V, abdominal pain, dry mouth, constipation, mucositis, dyspepsia, anorexia, hepatocellular damage, clinical hepatitis, abnormal hepatic function, hepatomegaly, jaundice. **Dermatologic:** Rash, pruritus, increased sweating. **GU:** Vaginal hemorrhage, acute renal failure. **Hematologic:** Febrile neutropenia, thrombocytopenia, anemia, neutropenia, petechiae, thrombotic thrombocytopenia (rare), hemolytic uremic syndrome (rare). **Musculoskeletal:** Rigors, musculoskeletal pain, arthralgia, myalgia, back pain, rigors. **Respiratory:** Coughing, dyspnea, epistaxis, pharyngitis, URTI,

---

Bold Italic = life threatening side effect   ■ = black box warning   ♣ = Available in Canada

pneumonia, **pulmonary embolus (rare)**. **Body as a whole:** Fever, bacteremia, asthenia, cytomegalovirus infection, edema, dehydration, weight decrease, allergic/**hypersensitivity reactions**. **Miscellaneous:** Herpes simplex, edema in legs, taste perversion, blurred vision, adrenal insufficiency, oral candidiasis, allergic/**hypersensitivity reactions**.

LABORATORY TEST CONSIDERATIONS

↑ ALT, AST, GGT, hepatic enzymes, alkaline phosphatase, bilirubin, blood creatine, total bilirubin. Bilirubinemia, hypokalemia, hypomagnesemia, hyperglycemia, hypocalcemia.

DRUG INTERACTIONS

Calcium channel blockers metabolized by CYP3A4 (e.g., felodipine) / Monitor frequently for side effects and toxicity; dose reduction of CCB may be needed

Cimetidine / ↓ (39%) Posaconazole C_{max} and AUC; avoid use together unless benefit outweighs risk

Cyclosporine / ↑ Cyclosporine levels → possible nephrotoxicity, leukoencephalopathy, and death; reduce cyclosporine dose by three fourths; monitor plasma levels

Ergot alkaloids (ergotamine, dihydroergotamine) / ↑ Ergot alkaloid plasma levels → possible ergotism; do not use together

Glipizide / ↓ Glucose levels; monitor glucose concentrations

HMG-CoA reductase inhibitors metabolized by CYP3A4 (e.g., atorvastatin) / ↑ Statin levels → possible rhabdomyolysis; consider statin dose reduction

Midazolam / ↑ Midazolam AUC (83%); monitor and consider midazolam dose reduction

Phenytoin / ↓ Posaconazole C_{max} (41%) and AUC (50%) and ↑ (16%) phenytoin C_{max} and AUC; avoid use together unless benefit outweighs risk and monitor frequently

Quinidine / ↑ Quinidine levels → QT prolongation and rarely torsade de pointes; do not use together

Rifabutin / ↓ Posaconazole C_{max} (43%) and AUC (49%) and ↑ rifabutin C_{max} (31%) and AUC (72%); avoid use together unless benefit outweighs risk and

monitor frequently

Sirolimus / ↑ Sirolimus plasma levels → possible serious side effects; monitor sirolimus blood levels frequently

Tacrolimus / ↑ Tacrolimus plasma levels → possible serious side effects; reduce tacrolimus dose by one-third and monitor frequently

Vinca alkaloids (vinblastine, vincristine) / ↑ Vinca alkaloids plasma levels → neurotoxicity. consider alkaloid dosage adjustment

HOW SUPPLIED

Oral Suspension: 40 mg/mL.

DOSAGE

• **ORAL SUSPENSION**

Prophylaxis of invasive Aspergillus *or* Candida *fungal infection.*

Adults and children, 13 years and older: 200 mg (5 mL) three times per day. Duration is based on recovery from neutropenia or immunosuppression.

Oropharyngeal candidiasis.

Loading dose: 100 mg (2.5 mL) twice the first day; **then,** 100 mg (2.5 mL) once daily for 13 days.

Oropharyngeal candidiasis refractory to itraconazole and/or fluconazole.

400 mg (10 mL) twice a day. Base duration of therapy on the severity of the client's underlying disease and clinical response.

NURSING CONSIDERATIONS

ADMINISTRATION/STORAGE

1. Use the following guidelines to enhance oral absorption and optimize plasma levels:

• Give each dose with a full meal or liquid nutritional supplement. For those who cannot eat a full meal or tolerate an oral nutritoinal supplement, consider alternative antifungal therapy or monitor closely for breakthrough fungal infections.

• Those who have severe diarrhea or vomiting should be monitored closely for breakthrough fungal infections.

• Coadministration of drugs that can decrease the plasma levels of posaconazole should be avoided unless the benefit outweighs the risk. If such drugs are required, monitor

P

🎨 = see color insert   H = Herbal   IV = Intravenous   ℂ = sound alike drug closely for breakthrough fungal infections.

2. Store from 15–30°C (59–86°F). Do not freeze.

ASSESSMENT

1. Note reasons for therapy, onset, duration, characteristics of S&S, other agents trialed, cultures, outcome.

2. List drugs, herbals consumed to ensure none interact.

3. Assess lytes, renal and LFTs; note any diarrhea or vomiting.

CLIENT/FAMILY TEACHING

1. Shake well before each use and measure dose with enclosed measuring spoon. Take each dose with food or nutritional supplement. Rinse spoon with water after each use and before storage.

2. Take on regular schedule to get the most benefit (at the same times each day). Continue to take even if you feel well. Do not miss any doses; do not take 2 doses at once.

3. May cause dizziness or blurred vision. May be worse if taken with alcohol or certain medicines. Do not drive or perform other possibly unsafe tasks until drug effects realized.

4. Drug only works against fungi; it does not treat viral infections; complete full course of treatment. The fungus could become less sensitive to this or other medicines making the infection harder to treat in the future. May experience secondary infections; report if evident. Report severe diarrhea or vomiting.

5. Birth control pills may not work as well while using Posaconazole Suspension. To prevent pregnancy, use additional non hormonal form of BC (e.g., condoms).

6. With diabetes, check blood sugar levels closely.

7. Use with extreme caution in CHILDREN younger than 13 years old; safety and effectiveness have not been confirmed.

8. Not known if Posaconazole Suspension can cause harm to the fetus. Report if pregnant, planning to become pregnant, or breast-feeding.

9. Keep all F/U appointments to evaluate response to therapy and adverse side effects.

OUTCOMES/EVALUATE

Resolution of fungal infection

Potassium Salts IV ©

CLASSIFICATION(S):
Electrolyte

Potassium acetate, parenteral

PREGNANCY CATEGORY: C

Potassium acetate, Potassium bicarbonate, and Potassium citrate (Trikates)

Rx: Oral Solution: Tri-K.

Potassium bicarbonate

Rx: Tablets, Effervescent: K+ Care ET.

Potassium bicarbonate and Potassium chloride

Rx: Tablets, Effervescent: K-Lyte/Cl, K-Lyte/Cl 50, Klor-Con/EF, Klorvess.

✚**Rx: Granules, Effervescent**: Neo-K. **Tablets, Effervescent**: Potassium-Sandoz.

Potassium bicarbonate and Potassium citrate

Rx: Tablets, Effervescent: Effer-K, K-Lyte.

Bold Italic = life threatening side effect   ■ = black box warning   ✚ = Available in Canada

Potassium chloride

Rx: Capsules, Extended Release: Micro-K 10 Extencaps, Micro-K Extencaps. **Injection**: Potassium Chloride for Injection Concentrate. **Oral Solution**: Cena-K 10% and 20%, Kaon-Cl 20% Liquid, Klorvess 10% Liquid, Potasalan. **Powder for Oral Solution**: Gen-K, K+ Care, K-Lor, K-Lyte/Cl Powder, Klor-Con Powder, Klor-Con/25 Powder, Mirco-K LS. **Tablets, Extended-Release**: K+ 10, K-Dur 10 and 20, K-Tab, Kaon-Cl, Kaon-Cl-10, Klor-Con 8 and 10, Klor-Con M10, M15, and M20, Klotrix, Ten-K.

✢**Rx: Oral Solution**: K-10, KCl 5%, Kaochlor-10 and -20. **Tablets, Extended-Release**: Apo-K, K-Long, K-Lyte/Cl, Slow-K.

Potassium chloride, Potassium bicarbonate, and Potassium citrate

Rx: Granules, Effervescent: Klorvess Effervescent Granules.

Potassium gluconate

Rx: Elixir: K-G Elixir, Kaon, Kaylixir.

Potassium gluconate and Potassium chloride

Rx: Oral Solution and Powder for Oral Solution: Kolyum.

USES

PO: (1) Treat hypokalemia due to digitalis intoxication, diabetic acidosis, diarrhea and vomiting, attacks of familial periodic paralysis, certain cases of uremia, hyperadrenalism, starvation and debilitation, and corticosteroid or diuretic therapy. (2) Hypokalemia with or without metabolic acidosis and following surgical conditions accompanied by nitrogen loss, vomiting and diarrhea, suction drainage, and increased urinary excretion of potassium. (3) Prophylaxis of potassium depletion when dietary intake is not adequate in the following conditions: Clients on digitalis and diuretics for CHF, hepatic cirrhosis with ascites, excess aldosterone with normal renal function, significant cardiac arrhythmias, potassium-losing nephropathy, and certain states accompanied by diarrhea. *Investigational:* Mild hypertension. *NOTE:* Use potassium chloride when hypokalemia is associated with alkalosis; potassium bicarbonate, citrate, acetate, or gluconate should be used when hypokalemia is associated with acidosis.

IV: (1) Prophylaxis and treatment of moderate to severe potassium loss when PO therapy is not feasible. (2) Potassium acetate is used as an additive for preparing specific IV formulas when client needs cannot be met by usual nutrient or electrolyte preparations. (3) Potassium acetate is also used in the following conditions: Marked loss of GI secretions due to vomiting, diarrhea, GI intubation, or fistulas; prolonged parenteral use of potassium-free fluids (e.g., dextrose or NSS); diabetic acidosis, especially during treatment with insulin and dextrose infusions; prolonged diuresis; metabolic alkalosis; hyperadrenocorticism; primary aldosteronism; overdose of adrenocortical steroids, testosterone, or corticotropin; attacks of hereditary or familial periodic paralysis; during the healing phase of burns or scalds; and cardiac arrhythmias, especially due to digitalis glycosides.

GENERAL STATEMENT

Potassium is the major cation of the body's intracellular fluid. It is essential for the maintenance of important physiologic processes, including cardiac, smooth, and skeletal muscle function, acid-base balance, gastric secretions, renal function, protein and carbohydrate metabolism. Symptoms of hypokalemia include weakness, cardiac arrhythmias, fatigue, ileus, hyporeflexia or areflexia, tetany, polydipsia, and, in severe cases, flaccid paralysis and inability to concentrate urine. Loss of potassium is usually

P

accompanied by a loss of chloride resulting in hypochloremic metabolic alkalosis. The usual adult daily requirement of potassium is 40–80 mg. In adults, the normal extracellular concentration of potassium ranges from 3.5 to 5 mEq/L with the intracellular levels being 150–160 mEq/L. Extracellular concentrations of up to 5.6 mEq/L are normal in children. Both hypokalemia and hyperkalemia, if uncorrected, can be fatal; thus, potassium must always be administered cautiously.

ACTION/KINETICS

Action

Potassium is required to maintain intracellular tonicity; for transmission of nerve impulses; contraction of cardiac, skeletal, and smooth muscle; and, maintenance of normal renal function. Potassium participates in carbohydrate utilization and protein synthesis. It is critical in regulating nerve conduction and muscle contraction, especially the heart.

Potassium is readily and rapidly absorbed from the GI tract. Though a number of salts can be used to supply the potassium cation, potassium chloride is the agent of choice since hypochloremia frequently accompanies potassium deficiency. Dietary measures can often prevent and even correct potassium deficiencies. Potassium-rich foods include most meats (beef, chicken, ham, turkey, veal), fish, beans, broccoli, brussels sprouts, lentils, spinach, potatoes, milk, bananas, dates, prunes, raisins, avocados, watermelon, cantaloupe, apricots, and molasses.

Pharmacokinetics

From 80 to 90% of potassium intake is excreted by the kidney and is partially reabsorbed from the glomerular filtrate. A deficit of either potassium or chloride will lead to the deficit of the other.

CONTRAINDICATIONS

Severe renal function impairment with azotemia or oliguria, postoperatively before urine flow has been reestablished, early postoperative oliguria except during GI drainage. Crush syndrome, Addison's disease, hyperkalemia from any cause, anuria, heat cramps, acute dehydration, severe hemolytic reactions, adynamia episodica hereditaria, clients receiving potassium-sparing diuretics or aldosterone-inhibiting drugs, renal failure and conditions in which potassium retention is present. Solid dosage forms in clients in whom there is a reason for delay or arrest in passage of tablets through the GI tract.

SPECIAL CONCERNS

Safety during lactation, pregnancy (give during pregnancy only if clearly needed), and in children has not been established. Geriatric clients are at greater risk of developing hyperkalemia due to age-related changes in renal function. Administer with caution in the presence of cardiac disease, especially in digitalized clients, or in the presence of renal disease; metabolic acidosis; Addison's disease, acute dehydation, prolonged or severe diarrhea, familial periodic paralysis, hypoadrenalism, hyperkalemia, hyponatremia, and, myotonia congenita. Potassium loss is often accompanied by an obligatory loss of chloride resulting in hypochloremic metabolic alkalosis; thus, the underlying cause of the potassium loss should be treated.

SIDE EFFECTS

Most Common

N&V, diarrhea, flatulence, abdominal discomfort.

GI: N&V, diarrhea, flatulence, abdominal discomfort, GI obstruction, GI bleeding, GI ulceration or perforation. **Nutritional:** Hyperkalemia. **Dermatologic:** Skin rash.

Symptoms of hyperkalemia. CNS: Mental confusion, listlessness, weakness. **Musculoskeletal:** Paresthesias of extremities, flaccid paralysis, muscle or respiratory paralysis, areflexia, weakness and heaviness of legs. **CV:** Hypotension, cardiac arrhythmias, heart block, ECG abnormalities (e.g., disappearance of P waves, spreading and slurring of QRS complex with development of a biphasic curve), *cardiac arrest*.

Effects due to solution or IV technique used: Fever, infection at injection site, venous thrombosis, phlebitis extending from injection site, extravasation, venospasm, hypervolemia, hyperkalemia.

OD **OVERDOSE MANAGEMENT**
Symptoms: Mild (5.5–6.5 mEq/L) to moderate (6.5–8 mEq/L) hyperkalemia (may be asymptomatic except for ECG changes). ECG changes include progression in height and peak of T waves, lowering of the R wave, decreased amplitude and eventually disappearance of P waves, prolonged PR interval and QRS complex, shortening of the QT interval, *ventricular fibrillation, death. Muscle weakness that may progress to flaccid quadriplegia and respiratory failure,* although dangerous cardiac arrhythmias usually occur before onset of complete paralysis. *Treatment: (plasma potassium levels greater than 6.5 mEq/L):* All measures must be monitored by ECG. Measures consist of actions taken to shift potassium ions from plasma into cells by:

- **Sodium bicarbonate:** IV infusion of 50–100 mEq over period of 5 min. May be repeated after 10–15 minutes if ECG abnormalities persist.
- **Glucose and insulin:** IV infusion of 3 grams glucose to 1 unit regular insulin to shift potassium into cells.
- **Calcium gluconate or other calcium salt** (only for clients not on digitalis or other cardiotonic glycosides): IV infusion of 0.5–1 grams (5–10 mL of a 10% solution) over period of 2 min. Dosage may be repeated after 1–2 min if ECG remains abnormal. When ECG is approximately normal, the excess potassium should be removed from the body by administration of polystyrene sulfonate, hemodialysis, or peritoneal dialysis (clients with renal insufficiency) or other means.
- **Sodium polystyrene sulfonate, hemodialysis, peritoneal dialysis:** To remove potassium from the body.

DRUG INTERACTIONS
ACE inhibitors / May cause potassium retention → hyperkalemia in certain clients
Digitalis glycosides / Possible cardiac arrhythmias
Potassium-sparing diuretics / Severe hyperkalemia with possibility of cardiac arrhythmias or arrest

HOW SUPPLIED
Potassium acetate, parenteral: *Injection:* 2 mEq/mL, 4 mEq/mL.
Potassium acetate, potassium bicarbonate, and potassium citrate: *Liquid:* 45 mEq/15 mL.
Potassium bicarbonate: *Tablets, Effervescent:* 25 mEq, 650 mg.
Potassium bicarbonate and potassium citrate: *Tablets, Effervescent:* 25 mEq.
Potassium bicarbonate and potassium chloride: *Granule for Reconstitution:* 20 mEq; *Tablets, Effervescent:* 25 mEq, 50 mEq.
Potassium chloride: *Capsules, Extended-Release:* 8 mEq, 10 mEq; *Injection:* 1.5 mEq/mL, 2 mEq/mL, 10 mEq/50 mL, 10 mEq/100 mL, 20 mEq/50 mL, 20 mEq/100 mL, 30 mEq/100 mL, 40 mEq/100 mL, 100 mEq/L, 200 mEq/L; *Liquid:* 20 mEq/15 mL, 30 mEq/15 mL, 40 mEq/15 mL; *Powder for Reconstitution:* 20 mEq, 25 mEq, 200 mEq; *Tablets:* 180 mg; *Tablets, Extended-Release:* 8 mEq, 10 mEq, 15 mEq, 20 mEq.
Potassium gluconate: *Elixir:* 20 mEq/15 mL; *Tablets:* 486 mg, 500 mg, 550 mg, 595 mg, 610 mg, 620 mg; *Tablets, Extended-Release:* 595 mg.
Potassium gluconate and potassium citrate: *Liquid:* 20 mEq/15 mL.

DOSAGE————————
Highly individualized. Oral administration is preferred because the slow absorption from the GI tract prevents sudden, large increases in plasma potassium levels. Dosage is usually expressed as mEq/L of potassium. The bicarbonate, chloride, citrate, and gluconate salts are usually administered PO. The chloride, acetate, and phosphate may be administered by **slow IV** infusion.
- **IV INFUSION**
  Serum K less than 2.0 mEq/L.
400 mEq/day at a rate not to exceed 40 mEq/hr. Use a maximum concentration of 80 mEq/L.
  Serum K more than 2.5 mEq/L.
200 mEq/day at a rate not to exceed 20 mEq/hr. Use a maximum concentration of 40 mEq/L. **Pediatric:** Up to 3 mEq

P

potassium/kg (or 40 mEq/m^2) daily. Adjust the volume administered depending on the body size.

• **CAPSULES, EXTENDED-RELEASE; ELIXIR; GRANULES, EFFERVESCENT; GRANULES, EXTENDED-RELEASE; ORAL SOLUTION; POWDER FOR ORAL SOLUTION; TABLETS; TABLETS, EFFERVESCENT; TABLETS, EXTENDED-RELEASE**

Prophylaxis of hypokalemia.
16–24 mEq/day.

Potassium depletion.
Usual additive dilution of potassium chloride is 40–80 mEq/L of IV fluid. If serum K$^+$ is >2.5 mEq/L, the maximum infusion rate is 10 mEq/hr, the maximum concentration is 40 mEq/L and the maximum 24 hour dose is 200 mEq. If serum K$^+$ is <2 mEq/L, the maximum infusion rate is 40 mEq/hr, the maximum concentration is 80 mEq/L, and the maximum 24 hr dose is 400 mEq.
Children: 3 mEq/kg or 40 mEq/m^2/day; adjust volume of administered fluids to body size.

NOTE: Usual dietary intake of potassium is 40–250 mEq/day. For clients with accompanying metabolic acidosis, use an alkalizing potassium salt (potassium bicarbonate, potassium citrate, potassium acetate, or potassium gluconate).

NURSING CONSIDERATIONS

℃ Do not confuse K-Phos Neutral with Neutra-Phos-K.

ADMINISTRATION/STORAGE

1. Give PO doses 2–4 times per day. Correct hypokalemia slowly over a period of 3–7 days to minimize risk of hyperkalemia.
2. With esophageal compression, administer dilute liquid solutions of potassium rather than tablets.
IV 3. Do not administer potassium IV undiluted. Usual method is to administer by slow IV infusion in dextrose solution at a concentration of 40–80 mEq/L and at a rate not to exceed 10–20 mEq/hr.
4. Do not infuse rapidly; high plasma levels of potassium may result in death due to cardiac depression, arrhythmias, or arrest.

5. IV administration can cause fluid or solute overloading resulting in dilution of serum electrolyte levels, overhydration, congested states, or pulmonary edema.
6. Avoid "layering" by inverting container during addition of potassium solution and properly agitating the prepared IV solution. Squeezing the plastic container will not prevent KCl from settling to the bottom. Never add potassium to an IV bottle that is hanging.
7. Check site of administration frequently for pain and redness because drug is extremely irritating.
8. Discontinue administration if signs of renal insufficiency develop during infusions.
9. In critical clients, KCl may be given slow IV in a solution of saline (unless contraindicated) since dextrose may lower serum potassium levels by producing an intracellular shift.
10. Administer all concentrated potassium infusions and riders with an infusion control device.
11. Have sodium polystyrene sulfonate (Kayexalate) available for oral or rectal administration in the event of hyperkalemia.

ASSESSMENT

1. Identify reasons for therapy; document electrolytes and ECG. List all drugs and OTC agents consumed.
2. Note any impaired renal function. Assess for adequate urinary flow before administering; dysfunction can lead to hyperkalemia.

INTERVENTIONS

1. Withhold and report: abdominal pain, distention, or GI bleeding.
2. Complaints of weakness, fatigue, or the presence of cardiac arrhythmias may be S&S of hypokalemia indicating a low *intracellular* potassium level, although serum level may appear to be WNL.
3. Monitor I&O. Withhold drug and report oliguria, anuria, or azoturia.
4. Observe for S&S of adrenal insufficiency or extensive tissue breakdown.
5. Report complaints of weakness or heaviness of the legs, the presence of a gray pallor, cold skin, listlessness, men-

---

Bold Italic = life threatening side effect　　■ = black box warning　　✦ = Available in Canada

tal confusion, flaccid paralysis, hypotension, or cardiac arrhythmias (S&S of hyperkalemia).

6. Monitor serum potassium levels during parenteral therapy; normal level is 3.5–5.0 mEq/L.

CLIENT/FAMILY TEACHING

1. Dilute or dissolve PO liquids, effervescent tablets, or soluble powders in 3–8 oz of cold water, fruit or vegetable juice, or other suitable liquid and drink slowly. Chill to improve taste. Take all products with plenty of water.

2. If GI upset occurs, products can be taken after meals or with food- with a full glass of water.

3. Swallow enteric-coated tablets and extended-release capsules and tablets; do not chew or dissolve in the mouth.

4. Do not use salt substitutes concomitantly with potassium preparations.

5. If receiving potassium-sparing diuretics, such as spironolactone or triamterene, do not take potassium supplements or eat foods high in potassium.

6. Identify high-potassium sources in the diet: Spinach, potatoes, collards, brussel sprouts, beet greens, tomato juice, celery. Once parenteral potassium is discontinued, ingest potassium-rich foods such as citrus juices, bananas, apricots, raisins, and nuts. The daily adult requirement is usually 40–80 mg. A dietitian may assist with meal planning.

7. Avoid self-prescribed enemas, and large amounts of licorice.

8. Report adverse effects; keep all F/U visits for labs and evaluation of response to therapy.

OUTCOMES/EVALUATE

Correction of potassium deficiency; potassium levels within desired range

---

Pramipexole
(prah-mih-**PEX**-ohl)

CLASSIFICATION(S):
Antiparkinson drug
PREGNANCY CATEGORY: C
Rx: Mirapex.

USES
(1) Signs and symptoms of idiopathic Parkinson's disease. (2) Moderate to severe restless legs syndrome.

ACTION/KINETICS

Action
Thought to act by stimulating dopamine (especially D_3) receptors in striatum.

Pharmacokinetics
Rapidly absorbed. **Peak levels:** 2 hr. Food increases time for maximum levels to occur. **t½, terminal:** About 8 hr (12 hr in geriatric clients). Excreted mainly unchanged in urine. Clearance decreases with age.

CONTRAINDICATIONS
Lactation.

SPECIAL CONCERNS
Possible sudden, overwhelming urge to sleep. Safety and efficacy have not been determined in children.

SIDE EFFECTS

Most Common
Postural hypotension, dyskinesia, extrapyramidal syndrome, insomnia, dizziness, hallucinations, abnormal dreams, confusion, constipation, dry mouth, accidental injury, asthenia.

CNS: Hallucinations (especially in elderly), dyskinesia, extrapyramidal syndrome, dizziness, somnolence, insomnia, abnormal dreams, confusion, amnesia, hypesthesia, dystonia, akathisia, abnormal thinking, decreased libido, myoclonus, abnormal gait/hypokinesia, hypertonia, amnesia, tremor, akathisia, paranoid reaction, delusions, sleep disorders, sudden uncontrolled sedation.
GI: Nausea, constipation, anorexia, dysphagia, dry mouth. **CV:** Postural hypotension. **GU:** Urinary frequency/infection/incontinence. **Musculoskeletal:** Arthritis, twitching, bursitis, myasthenia, chest pain. **Respiratory:** Dyspnea, rhinitis, pneumonia. **Ophthalmic:** Abnormal accommodation, vision abnormalities, diplopia. **Body as a whole:** Asthenia, general edema, malaise, fever. **Miscellaneous:** Accidental injury, impotence, peripheral edema, decreased weight, skin disorders.

P

DRUG INTERACTIONS

Butyrophenones / Possible ↓ effect of pramipexole

Cimetidine / ↑ Levodopa levels and half-life

CNS depressants / Additive CNS depression

Levodopa / ↑ Levodopa levels; also, may cause or worsen pre-existing dyskinesia

Metoclopramide / Possible ↓ effect of pramipexole

Phenothiazines / Possible ↓ effect of pramipexole

Thioxanthines / Possible ↓ effect of pramipexole

HOW SUPPLIED

Tablets: 0.125 mg, 0.25 mg, 0.5 mg, 1 mg, 1.5 mg.

DOSAGE

• **TABLETS**

Parkinsonism.

Week 1: 0.125 mg 3 times per day. **Week 2:** 0.25 mg 3 times per day. **Week 3:** 0.5 mg 3 times per day. **Week 4:** 0.75 mg 3 times per day. **Week 5:** 1 mg 3 times per day. **Week 6:** 1.25 mg 3 times per day. **Week 7:** 1.5 mg 3 times per day. **Maintenance:** 1.5–4.5 mg/day in equally divided doses 3 times per day with or without concomitant levodopa (about 800 mg/day).

Impaired renal function: C_{CR} >60 mL/min: Start with 0.125 mg 3 times per day, up to maximum of 1.5 mg 3 times per day. **C_{CR} 35–59 mL/min:** Start with 0.125 mg twice/day, up to maximum of 1.5 mg twice/day. **C_{CR} 15–34 mL/min:** Start with 0.125 mg once daily, up to maximum of 1.5 mg once daily. **C_{CR} <15 mL/min and hemodialysis clients:** Pramipexole not adequately studied in this group.

Restless legs syndrome.

Initial: 0.125 mg once daily 2–3 hr before bedtime. For those requiring additional relief, the dose may be increased as follows after the initial dose is given for 4–7 days: 0.25 mg for 4–7 days followed by 0.5 mg for 4–7 days. Increase the duration between titration steps to 14 days in those with severe and moderate impaired renal function (C_{CR} from 20–60 mL/min).

NURSING CONSIDERATIONS

ADMINISTRATION/STORAGE

1. Gradually titrate dosage; increase the dose to reach a maximum therapeutic effect, balanced against the main side effects of dyskinesia, hallucinations, somnolence, and dry mouth.

2. Consider a decrease in levodopa dose if taken with pramipexole.

3. Do not increase dosage more frequently than every 5–7 days.

4. Discontinue pramipexole over a 1 week period.

5. Store from 15–30°C (59–86°F). Protect from light.

ASSESSMENT

1. Note disease onset, extent of motor function, reflexes, gait, strength of grip, rigidity, amount of tremor.

2. With tremor, assess for muscle weakness, muscle rigidity, difficulty walking, or changing directions.

3. Use very low dose for control of RLS symptoms.

4. Monitor mental status, neurologic evaluations, VS, ECG, renal, LFTs; reduce dose with dysfunction.

CLIENT/FAMILY TEACHING

1. Take only as prescribed; may take with food to decrease nausea.

2. Rise slowly from sitting or lying position to prevent drop in BP.

3. Do not drive or perform activities that require mental/motor alertness until stabilized on drug. May cause dizziness, fainting, blackouts, hypotension, sudden urge to sleep, and sedative effects.

4. Practice reliable contraception.

5. Report lack of response, worsening of condition, or any vision problems; obtain regular eye exams.

6. May cause hallucinations; report if evident.

7. Do not stop abruptly; must do so over one week period.

8. Avoid alcohol and any other CNS depressants, may exaggerate drowsiness and dizziness.

9. Keep all F/U visits to eval. response to therapy.

OUTCOMES/EVALUATE

- Control of Parkinsonian symptoms (e.g., improvement in motor function, reflexes, gait, strength of grip, and amount of tremor)
- Relief of RLS S&S

Pramlintide acetate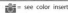
(**PRAM**-lin-tide)

CLASSIFICATION(S):
Antidiabetic, amylin analog
PREGNANCY CATEGORY: C
Rx: Symlin.

USES

(1) Adjunct treatment in type 1 diabetes mellitus in clients who use mealtime insulin therapy and who have failed to achieve desired glucose control despite optimal insulin therapy. (2) Adjunct treatment in type 2 diabetes mellitus in clients who use mealtime insulin therapy and who have failed to achieve desired glucose control despite optimal insulin therapy, with or without a concurrent sulfonylurea agent and/or metformin. *NOTE:* Proper client selection is critical to safe and effective use of pramlintide.

ACTION/KINETICS

Action

Pramlintide is a synthetic analog of human amylin, a naturally occurring neuroendocrine hormone synthesized by pancreatic beta cells; it contributes to glucose control during the postprandial period. Amylin is stored with insulin in secretory granules and cosecreted with insulin by pancreatic beta cells in response to food intake. Amylin affects the rate of postprandial glucose appearance through a variety of mechanisms. It slows gastric emptying without altering the overall absorption of nutrients. Also, amylin suppresses glucagon secretion which leads to suppression of endogenous glucose output from the liver. It also regulates food intake caused by centrally-mediated modulation of appetite. Thus, pramlintide, by acting as an amylinomimetic agent, has the following effects: (1) modulation of gastric emptying; (2) prevention of the postprandial rise in plasma glucagon; and, (3) satiety leading to decreased caloric intake and potential weight loss.

Pharmacokinetics

The bioavailability of a SC dose is about 30–40%. Not extensively bound to plasma proteins. Metabolized primarily by the kidneys; the primary metabolite is biologically active. **t½, parent drug and active metabolite:** 48 min.

CONTRAINDICATIONS

Hypersensitivity to pramlintide acetate or any of its components, including metacresol. Diagnosis of gastroparesis. Hypoglycemia.

SPECIAL CONCERNS

■ Pramlintide is used with insulin and has been associated with an increased risk of insulin-induced severe hypoglycemia, particularly in clients with type 1 diabetes. When severe hypoglycemia associated with pramlintide use occurs, it is seen within 3 hr following a pramlintide injection. If severe hypoglycemia occurs while operating a motor vehicle, heavy machinery, or while engaging in other high-risk activities, serious injuries may occur. Appropriate client selection, careful client instruction, and insulin dose adjustments are critical elements for reducing this risk.■ Pramlintide has the potential to delay the absorption of coadministered PO drugs; when the rapid onset of a PO coadministered drug is a critical determinant of effectiveness (e.g., analgesics), administer the drug at least 1 hr prior to or 2 hr after pramlintide injection. Give during lactation only if the potential benefit outweighs the potential risk to the infant. Safety and efficacy have not been determined in children.

SIDE EFFECTS

Most Common

Hypoglycemia, headache, N&V, abdominal pain, anorexia, inflicted injury, fatigue, coughing.

Side effects listed are associated with administration of pramlintide with insulin. **GI:** N&V, abdominal pain, anorexia. **CNS:** Headache, dizziness. **Respiratory:**

P

Coughing, pharyngitis. **At injection site:** Redness, swelling, itching. **Body as a whole:** Fatigue, *systemic allergic reaction*. **Miscellaneous:** *Hypoglycemia (may be severe),* inflicted injury, arthralgia. *NOTE:* Pramlintide alone does not cause hypoglycemia but when mixed with insulin, the risk of hypoglycemia is increased.

OD OVERDOSE MANAGEMENT
Symptoms: Hypoglycemia, severe nausea. *Treatment:* Severe hypoglycemia treatment may include glucagon injection, IV glucose, hospitalization, paramedic assistance, or ER visit.

DRUG INTERACTIONS
Alpha-glucosidase inhibitors / Do not use together with pramlintide due to effects on gastric emptying
Anticholinergic drugs, including atropine / Do not use together with pramlintide due to effects on gastric emptying
Insulins / ↑ Risk of hypoglycemia
Sulfonylureas / ↑ Risk of hypoglycemia

HOW SUPPLIED
Solution for Injection: 0.6 mg/mL.

DOSAGE
• **SC**
Type 1 diabetes mellitus.
Initial: 15 mcg; **then,** titrate at 15 mcg increments to a maintenance dose of 30 or 60 mcg, as tolerated. Increase the pramlintide dose to the next increment (30, 45, or 60 mcg) when no clinically significant nausea has occurred for at least 3 days.
Type 2 diabetes mellitus.
Initial: 60 mcg; **then,** increase the dose, as tolerated, to 120 mcg. Increase the pramlintide dose to 120 mcg when no clinically significant nausea has occurred for 3–7 days. If significant nausea persists at the 120 mcg dose, decrease the dose to 60 mcg.

NURSING CONSIDERATIONS
ADMINISTRATION/STORAGE
1. When used for type 1 diabetes, reduce preprandial, rapid-acting, or short-acting insulin dosages, including fixed-mix insulins (e.g. 70/30) by 50%.
2. If significant nausea persists at the 45 or 60 mcg dose when used for type 1 diabetics, decrease the dose to 30

mcg. If the 30 mcg dose is not tolerated, consider discontinuing pramlintide.
3. Both type 1 and type 2 diabetics should only make pramlintide dose adjustments as directed by their provider.
4. Both type 1 and type 2 diabetics should adjust insulin doses to optimize glycemic control once the target dose of pramlintide is achieved and nausea has subsided. Only make insulin dose changes as directed by the provider.
5. Administer pramlintide SC immediately prior to each major meal (250 or more kcal or containing 30 grams or more of carbohydrate). If a pramlintide dose is missed, the client should not be give an additional injection.
6. To give SC, use a U-100 insulin syringe (preferably a 0.3 mL) size for optimal accuracy. Check package insert for conversion of pramlintide dose to insulin unit equivalents.
7. SC administration should be into the abdomen or thigh. The arm is not recommended because of variable absorption. Rotate injection sites. The injection site should be distinct from the site chosen for any concomitant insulin injection.
8. Clients should always use a new syringe and needle to give pramlintide and insulin injections.
9. Pramlintide and insulin should always be given as separate injections. Mixing may alter the pharmacokinetic parameters.
10. Discontinue pramlintide if any of the following occur:
• Recurrent unexplained hypoglycemia that requires medical assistance.
• Persistent clinically significant nausea.
• Noncompliance with self-monitoring of blood glucose concentrations.
• Noncompliance with insulin dose adjustments.
• Noncompliance with scheduled health care professional contacts or recommended clinic visits.
11. Store unopened (not in-use) vials in the refrigerator at 2–8°C (36–46°F) protected from light. Do not freeze; if a vial has been frozen or overheated, discard it. Keep opened (in-use) vials refrigerat-

---

ed or at room temperature for up to 28 days as long as the temperature is not more than 25°C (77°F). Discard after 28 days.

ASSESSMENT

1. Note reasons for therapy, onset and characteristics of disease, other agents trialed, outcome.

2. Monitor weight, VS, A1c, glucose monitoring results, insulin or antihypoglycemic regimen followed and client compliance.

3. Assess for conditions that would preclude drug therapy: gastroparesis, poor compliance or HbA1c >9%, hypoglycemia unawareness, hospitalized with hypoglycemia in past 6 mo, requires drug to stimulate gastric motility, poor compliance with insulin administration or blood sugar monitoring, or a child.

4. Monitor A1c, CBC, renal and LFT's, microalbuminuria, eye and foot exams.

CLIENT/FAMILY TEACHING

1. Drug administered by injection under the skin to help better control blood sugar. It cannot be administered or mixed with insulin and cannot be injected within 2 inches of the insulin administration site. Generally it should be injected into the abdomen or thigh and not the arm

2. Injections are given at meal times and do not replace the daily or more frequent insulin injections, but may lower the amount of insulin or antihypoglycemic agent required.

3. Avoid activities that require mental alertness until drug effects realized. May significantly lower blood glucose levels especially if adequate food and carbohydrates not consumed.

4. Most frequent side effect is nausea and can be managed with reduction in dosage.

5. May experience profound hypoglycemia. Early S&S include: hunger, headaches, sweating, tremor, irritability, difficulty concentrating. These S&S may vary or be less noticeable with long history of diabetes, diabetic nerve disease, or when on certain drugs such as clonidine, or beta blockers.

6. Follow and refer to pramlintide Medication Guide for additional information

and guidelines for things such as omitted dose, inadequate food intake, missed meals or accidental excess dose of insulin.

7. Must monitor finger sticks regularly and follow schedule for meal times, injections, caloric consumption, and exercise.

8. Avoid alcohol, may cause increase in low blood sugar and associated symptoms.

9. Keep all F/U visits to assess response to therapy, monitor labs and review side effects.

OUTCOMES/EVALUATE

Control of blood glucose with HbA1c <7

Pravastatin sodium

(prah-vah-**STAH**-tin)

CLASSIFICATION(S):

Antihyperlipidemic, HMG-CoA reductase inhibitor

PREGNANCY CATEGORY: X

Rx: Pravachol.

✦**Rx:** Apo-Pravastatin, Lin-Pravastatin, Nu-Pravastatin.

SEE ALSO *ANTIHYPERLIPIDEMIC-HMG-COA REDUCTASE INHIBITORS*

USES

(1) Adjunct to diet for reducing elevated total and LDL cholesterol and triglyceride levels in clients with primary hypercholesterolemia (type IIa and IIb) and mixed dyslipidemia when the response to a diet with restricted saturated fat and cholesterol has not been effective. Treat elevated serum triglyceride levels (Fredrickson Type IV) and primary dysbetalipoproteinemia (Fredrickson Type III). Reduction of apolipoprotein B serum levels. (2) Reduce the risk of recurrent MI in those with previous MI and normal cholesterol levels; reduce risk of undergoing myocardial revascularization procedures; reduce risk of stroke or TIA. (3) Reduce risk of MI in hypercholesterolemia without evidence of coronary heart disease; reduce

 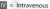

risk of CV mortality with no increase in death from noncardiovascular causes. (4) Slow the progression of coronary atherosclerosis and reduce risk of acute coronary events in hypercholesterolemia with clinically evident CAD, including prior MI. (5) Adjunct to diet and lifestyle modification to treat heterozygous familial hypercholesterolemia in children and adolescents 8 years of age and older if after an adequate trial of diet the following are present: LDL-C remains 190 mg/dL or greater or LDL-C remains 160 mg/dL and there is a positive family history of premature CV disease or 2 or more other cardiovascular disease factors are present. *Investigational:* To lower cholesterol levels in those with heterozygous familial hypercholesterolemia, familial combined hyperlipidemia, diabetic dyslipidemia in non-insulin-dependent diabetics, hypercholesterolemia secondary to nephrotic syndrome, homozygous familial hypercholesterolemia in those not completely devoid of LDL receptors but who have a decreased level of LDL receptor activity.

ACTION/KINETICS

Action

Competitively inhibits HMG-CoA reductase; this enzyme catalyzes the early rate-limiting step in the synthesis of cholesterol. Thus, cholesterol synthesis is inhibited/decreased. Decreases total cholesterol, triglycerides, LDL, and VLDL and increases HDL. Drug increases survival in heart transplant recipients.

Pharmacokinetics

Rapidly absorbed from the GI tract; absolute bioavailability is 17%. **Peak plasma levels:** 1–1.5 hr. Significant first-pass extraction and metabolism in the liver, which is the site of action of the drug; thus, plasma levels may not correlate well with lipid-lowering effectiveness. **t½, elimination:** 77 hr (including metabolites). Metabolized in the liver; excreted in the urine (about 20%) and feces (70%). Potential accumulation of drug with renal or hepatic insufficiency. **Plasma protein binding:** About 50%.

ADDITIONAL CONTRAINDICATIONS

To treat hypercholesterolemia due to hyperalphaproteinemia.

SPECIAL CONCERNS

Use with caution in clients with a history of liver disease or renal insufficiency.

SIDE EFFECTS

Most Common

Localized pain, N&V, diarrhea, abdominal cramps/pain, constipation, flatulence, fatigue, flu syndrome, common cold, rhinitis, rash/pruritus, cardiac chest pain, dizziness, headache.

Musculoskeletal: Rhabdomyolysis with renal dysfunction secondary to myoglobinuria, myalgia, myopathy, arthralgias, localized pain, muscle cramps, leg cramps, bursitis, tenosynovitis, myasthenia, tendinous contracture, myositis. **CNS:** CNS vascular lesions characterized by *perivascular hemorrhage*, edema, and mononuclear cell infiltration of perivascular spaces; headache, dizziness, psychic disturbances. Dizziness, vertigo, memory loss, anxiety, insomnia, somnolence, abnormal dreams, emotional lability, incoordination, hyperkinesia, torticollis, psychic disturbances. **GI:** N&V, diarrhea, abdominal pain, cramps, constipation, flatulence, heartburn, anorexia, gastroenteritis, dry mouth, rectal hemorrhage, esophagitis, eructation, glossitis, mouth ulceration, increased appetite, stomatitis, cheilitis, duodenal ulcer, dysphagia, enteritis, melena, gum hemorrhage, stomach ulcer, tenesmus, ulcerative stomach. **CV:** Palpitation, vasodilation, syncope, migraine, postural hypotension, phlebitis, arrhythmia. **Hepatic:** Hepatitis (including chronic active hepatitis), fatty change in liver, cirrhosis, *fulminant hepatic necrosis, hepatoma,* pancreatitis, cholestatic jaundice, biliary pain. **GU:** Gynecomastia, erectile dysfunction, loss of libido, cystitis, hematuria, impotence, dysuria, kidney calculus, nocturia, epididymitis, fibrocystic breast, albuminuria, breast enlargement, nephritis, urinary frequency, incontinence, retention and urgency, abnormal ejaculation, vaginal or uterine hemorrhage, menorrhagia, UTI. **Ophthalmic:** Progression of cataracts, lens opacities, ophthalmoplegia. **Hy-**

persensitivity reaction Vasculitis, purpura, polymyalgia rheumatica, *angioedema*, lupus erythematosus–like syndrome, thrombocytopenia, *hemolytic anemia*, leukopenia, positive ANA, arthritis, arthralgia, urticaria, asthenia, ESR increase, fever, chills, photosensitivity, malaise, dyspnea, *toxic epidermal necrolysis*, *Stevens-Johnson syndrome*. **Dermatologic:** Alopecia, pruritus, rash, skin nodules, discoloration of skin, dryness of skin and mucous membranes, changes in hair and nails, contact dermatitis, sweating, acne, urticaria, eczema, seborrhea, skin ulcer. **Neurologic:** Dysfunction of certain cranial nerves resulting in alteration of taste, impairment of extraocular movement, and facial paresis; paresthesia, peripheral neuropathy, tremor, vertigo, memory loss, peripheral nerve palsy. **Respiratory:** Common cold, rhinitis, cough. **Hematologic:** Anemia, transient asymptomatic eosinophilia, thrombocytopenia, leukopenia, ecchymosis, lymphadenopathy, petechiae. **Miscellaneous:** Cardiac chest pain, localized pain, fatigue, influenza.

ADDITIONAL DRUG INTERACTIONS
Bile acid sequestrants / ↓ Bioavailability of pravastatin
Clofibrate / ↑ Risk of myopathy

LABORATORY TEST CONSIDERATIONS
↑ CPK, AST, ALT, alkaline phosphatase, bilirubin. Abnormalities in thyroid function tests.

HOW SUPPLIED
Tablets: 10 mg, 20 mg, 40 mg, 80 mg.

DOSAGE
• **TABLETS**
Antihyperlipidemic.
Adults, initial: 40 mg once daily (at any time of the day) with or without food. A dose of 80 mg/day can be used if the 40 mg dose does not achieve desired results. Use a starting dose of 10 mg/day at bedtime in renal/hepatic dysfunction, in those taking concomitant immunosuppressants, and in the elderly (maximum maintenance dose for these clients is 20 mg/day). **Children, 8–13 years of age (inclusive):** 20 mg once daily. Doses greater than 20 mg have not been studied in this population.

Adolescents, 14–18 years of age, initial: 40 mg once daily. Doses greater than 40 mg have not been studied in this population.

NURSING CONSIDERATIONS

@ Do not confuse Pravachol with Prevacid (proton pump inhibitor) or propranolol (a beta-adrenergic blocking agent).

ADMINISTRATION/STORAGE
1. In clients taking immunosuppressants (e.g., cyclosporine), begin pravastatin therapy at 10 mg/day at bedtime and titrate to higher doses with caution. Usual maximum dose is 20 mg/day.
2. Place on a standard cholesterol-lowering diet for 3–6 months before beginning pravastatin and continue during therapy, unless >3 risk factors.
3. Drug may be taken without regard to meals.
4. The lipid-lowering effects are enhanced when combined with a bile-acid binding resin. When given with a bile-acid binding resin (e.g., cholestyramine, colestipol), give pravastatin either 1 hr or more before or 4 or more hr after the resin. Only use this combination if further changes in lipid levels are likely to outweigh the increased risk of the drug combination.
5. The maximum effect is seen within 4 weeks during which time periodic lipid determinations should be undertaken.

ASSESSMENT
1. Note reasons for therapy, other agents trialed/outcome. Rule out secondary causes for hypercholesterolemia; these include hypothyroidism, poorly controlled diabetes mellitus, dysproteinemias, obstructive liver disease, nephrotic syndrome, alcoholism, other drug therapy.
2. Determine if pregnant or planning pregnancy.
3. Assess for liver disease, if alcohol abused, before initiating therapy, before increasing the dose, and as clinically indicated.
4. Document all CAD risk factors. Initiate therapy during hospitalization for MI/angioplasty procedure to improve clinical outcomes.

P

📷 = see color insert   Ⓗ = Herbal   IV = Intravenous   @ = sound alike drug

5. Monitor cholesterol profile, CBC, renal and LFTs.

INTERVENTIONS

1. Obtain LFTs prior to therapy and 6 weeks after starting therapy and with any dose increases; if WNL may monitor at 6-month intervals.

2. Pravastatin should be discontinued if markedly elevated CPK levels occur or myopathy is diagnosed.

3. Stop pravastatin temporarily in clients experiencing an acute or serious condition (e.g., sepsis, hypotension, major surgery, trauma, uncontrolled epilepsy, or severe metabolic, endocrine, or electrolyte disorders) predisposing to the development of renal failure R/T rhabdomyolysis.

CLIENT/FAMILY TEACHING

1. Take as directed at bedtime.

2. Review the prescribed dietary recommendations (restricted cholesterol and saturated fats); continue diet during drug therapy.

3. Continue regular exercise program; strive to attain recommended weight loss.

4. Report unexplained muscle pain, tenderness, or weakness, especially if accompanied by malaise or fever.

5. Practice reliable barrier contraception; report if pregnancy is suspected as drug therapy is hazardous to a developing fetus.

6. Report severe GI upset, unusual bruising/bleeding, vision changes, dark urine or light colored stools.

7. Avoid prolonged or excessive exposure to direct or artificial sunlight.

8. Keep all F/U visits to evaluate lipid panel and liver function.

OUTCOMES/EVALUATE

↓ Serum cholesterol and LDL levels; MI prophylaxis in those with atherosclerosis and hypercholesterolemia

Praziquantel
(pray-zih-**KWON**-tell)

CLASSIFICATION(S):
Anthelmintic
PREGNANCY CATEGORY: B
Rx: Biltricide.

USES

(1) Schistosomal infections due to *Schistosoma japonicum, S. mansoni, S. mekongi,* and *S. hematobium.* (2) Liver flukes (*Clonorchis sinensis, Opisthorchis viverrini*). *Investigational:* Neurocysticercosis, other tissue flukes, and intestinal cestodes. Low doses of oxamniquine and praziquantel as a single-dose treatment of schistosomiasis.

ACTION/KINETICS

Action
Causes increased cell permeability in the helminth, resulting in a loss of intracellular calcium with massive contractions, and paralysis of musculature with breakdown of the integrity of the organism. Also causes vacuolization and disintegration of phagocytes to the parasite, resulting in death.

Pharmacokinetics
Maximum serum levels: 1–3 hr. **t½:** 0.8–1.5 hr. Levels in the CSF are approximately 14–20% of the total amount of the drug in the plasma. Significant first-pass effect. Excreted primarily in the urine.

CONTRAINDICATIONS

Ocular cysticercosis. Lactation.

SPECIAL CONCERNS

Safety in children less than 4 years of age not established. When schistosomiasis or fluke infection is associated with cerebral cysticercosis, hospitalize client for treatment duration.

SIDE EFFECTS

Most Common
Malaise, headache, dizziness, abdominal discomfort.

GI: Nausea, abdominal discomfort. **CNS:** Malaise, headache, dizziness, drowsiness. **Miscellaneous:** Fever, urticaria (rare). *NOTE:* These side effects may also be due to the helminth infection itself.

P

Bold Italic = life threatening side effect   ■ = black box warning   ♥ = Available in Canada

OD **OVERDOSE MANAGEMENT**

Symptoms: Extension of side effects. *Treatment:* Administer a fast-acting laxative.

DRUG INTERACTIONS

Grapefruit juice / ↑ Praziquantel C_{max} and AUC

H-2 Antagonists / ↑ Plasma praziquantel levels → ↑ effectiveness and side effects

Hydantoins / Possible ↓ serum praziquantel levels

HOW SUPPLIED

Tablets: 600 mg.

DOSAGE

- **TABLETS**

    Schistosomiasis.

Three doses of 20 mg/kg as a 1-day treatment with an interval between doses not less than 4 hr or more than 6 hr.

    Chonorchiasis and opisthorchiasis.

Three doses of 25 mg/kg as a 1-day treatment with an interval between doses not less than 4 hr or more than 6 hr.

NURSING CONSIDERATIONS

ASSESSMENT

1. Note reasons for therapy, onset/duration, characteristics of S&S, source of infestation.

2. Assess if schistosomiasis or fluke infection is accompanied by cerebral cysticercosis; if so, hospitalize for treatment.

3. Note any liver dysfunction; reduce dosage.

4. List drugs currently prescribed to ensure none interact unfavorably or deactivate drug (i.e., hydantoins).

CLIENT/FAMILY TEACHING

1. Swallow tablets unchewed with liquid during meals. Keeping the tablets in the mouth may cause gagging or vomiting; do not chew the tablets as their bitter taste can cause retching and vomiting.

2. Use caution while driving or performing tasks requiring alertness; may cause dizziness/drowsiness.

3. Do not nurse baby on treatment day and for 3 days following.

4. With schistosomiasis, larvae enter through the skin and are usually acquired by swimming in cercaria-infested water found in many parts of the world especially Africa and the Middle East. Schistosomal worms usually die 7 days following treatment.

5. Report any high fever or sustained headaches with cestode infection. May require corticosteroids for treatment of cerebral cysticerosis caused by the pork tapeworm.

OUTCOMES/EVALUATE

Eradication of parasitic infestation; negative cultures

Prazosin hydrochloride

(**PRAY**-zoh-sin)

CLASSIFICATION(S):

Antihypertensive, alpha-1-adrenergic blocking drug

PREGNANCY CATEGORY: C

Rx: Minipress.

✤**Rx:** Apo-Prazo, Novo-Prazin, Nu-Prazo.

SEE ALSO *ALPHA-1-ADRENERGIC BLOCKING AGENTS* **AND** *ANTIHYPERTENSIVE AGENTS.*

USES

Mild to moderate hypertension alone or in combination with other antihypertensive drugs. *Investigational:* CHF refractory to other treatment. Raynaud's disease, BPH.

ACTION/KINETICS

Action

Produces selective blockade of postsynaptic alpha-1-adrenergic receptors. Dilates arterioles and veins, thereby decreasing total peripheral resistance and decreasing DBP more than SBP. CO, HR, and renal blood flow are not affected. Can be used to initiate antihypertensive therapy; most effective when used with other agents (e.g., diuretics, beta-adrenergic blocking agents).

Pharmacokinetics

Onset: 2 hr. Absorption not affected by food. **Maximum effect:** 2–3 hr; **dura-**

📷 = see color insert   **H** = Herbal   **IV** = Intravenous   ℂ = sound alike drug tion: 6–12 hr. t½: 2–3 hr. Full therapeutic effect: 4–6 weeks. Metabolized extensively; excreted primarily in feces.

SPECIAL CONCERNS

Safe use in children has not been established. Use with caution during lactation. Geriatric clients may be more sensitive to the hypotensive and hypothermic effects; may be necessary to decrease the dose due to age-related decreases in renal function.

SIDE EFFECTS

Most Common

Dizziness, drowsiness, headache, lack of energy, weakness, palpitations, nausea.
First-dose effect: *Marked hypotension* and syncope 30–90 min after administration of initial dose (usually 2 or more mg), increase of dosage, or addition of other antihypertensive agent. **CNS:** Dizziness, drowsiness, headache, fatigue, paresthesias, depression, vertigo, nervousness, hallucinations. **CV:** Palpitations, syncope, tachycardia, orthostatic hypotension, aggravation of angina. **GI:** N&V, diarrhea or constipation, dry mouth, abdominal pain, pancreatitis. **GU:** Urinary frequency/incontinence, impotence, priapism. **Respiratory:** Dyspnea, nasal congestion, epistaxis. **Musculoskeletal:** Arthralgia, myalgia. **Dermatologic:** Pruritus, rash, sweating, alopecia, lichen planus. **Body as a whole:** Lack of energy, weakness, asthenia, edema. **Miscellaneous:** Symptoms of lupus erythematosus, blurred vision, tinnitus, reddening of sclera, eye pain, conjunctivitis, edema, fever.

LABORATORY TEST CONSIDERATIONS

↑ Urinary metabolites of norepinephrine, VMA.

OD OVERDOSE MANAGEMENT

Symptoms: Hypotension, shock. *Treatment:* Keep client supine to restore BP and HR. If shock is manifested, use volume expanders and vasopressors; maintain renal function.

DRUG INTERACTIONS

Antihypertensives (other) / ↑ Antihypertensive effect
Beta-adrenergic blocking agents / Enhanced acute postural hypotension after first dose of prazosin

Clonidine / ↓ Antihypertensive effect
Diuretics / ↑ Antihypertensive effect
Indomethacin / ↓ Effect of prazosin
Nifedipine / ↑ Hypotensive effect
Propranolol / Especially pronounced additive hypotensive effect
Verapamil / ↑ Hypotensive effect; ↑ sensitivity to prazosin-induced postural hypotension

HOW SUPPLIED

Capsules: 1 mg, 2 mg, 5 mg.

DOSAGE

* **CAPSULES**
  Hypertension.

Individualized: Initial, 1 mg 2–3 times per day; **maintenance:** if necessary, increase gradually to 6–15 mg/day in two to three divided doses. Do not exceed 20 mg/day, although some clients have benefitted from doses of 40 mg daily. If used with diuretics or other antihypertensives, reduce dose to 1–2 mg 3 times per day. **Pediatric, less than 7 years of age, initial:** 0.25 mg 2–3 times per day adjusted according to response. **Pediatric, 7–12 years of age, initial:** 0.5 mg 2–3 times per day adjusted according to response.

NURSING CONSIDERATIONS

ADMINISTRATION/STORAGE

Reduce dose to 1 or 2 mg 3 times per day if a diuretic or other antihypertensive agent is added to the regimen and then re-titrate client.

ASSESSMENT

1. Note reasons for therapy, other agents trialed, outcome.
2. Assess cardiopulmonary status, VS, and renal function.

CLIENT/FAMILY TEACHING

1. Take the first dose at bedtime. Also, take the first dose of each increment at bedtime to reduce the incidence of syncope.
2. Do not drive or operate machinery for 24 hr after the first dose; may cause dizziness and drowsiness.
3. Food may delay absorption and minimize side effects of the drug.
4. Avoid rapid changes in body position that may precipitate weakness, dizziness, and syncope. Lie down or sit

---

Bold Italic = life threatening side effect   ■ = black box warning   ♣ = Available in Canada

down and put head below knees to avoid fainting if a rapid heartbeat is felt.

5. Avoid dangerous situations that may lead to fainting.

6. Report any bothersome side effects because reduction in dosage may be indicated. Use sips of water and sugarless gum or candies for dry mouth effects.

7. Do not stop medication unless directed.

8. Avoid cold, cough, and allergy medications. The sympathomimetic component of such medications will interfere with the action of prazosin.

9. Comply with prescribed drug regimen; full drug effect may not be evident for 4–6 weeks.

OUTCOMES/EVALUATE

↓ BP; ↓ symptoms of refractory CHF

Prednisolone [IV] ©
(pred-**NISS**-oh-lohn)

CLASSIFICATION(S):
Glucocorticoid
PREGNANCY CATEGORY: C
Rx: Syrup: Prelone. **Tablets:** Delta-Cortef.

Prednisolone acetate
PREGNANCY CATEGORY: C

Rx: Ophthalmic Suspension: Econopred Plus, Pred Forte Ophthalmic, Pred Mild Ophthalmic, Prednisolone Acetate Ophthalmic. **Parenteral:** Predcor-50.

✤Rx: Ophthalmic Suspension: ratio-Prednisolone.

Prednisolone sodium phosphate
PREGNANCY CATEGORY: C

Rx: Ophthalmic Solution: Prednisol. **Oral Liquid/Solution:** Pediapred. **Oral Solution:** Orapred. **Tablets, Orally Disintegrating:** Orapred ODT.

Prednisolone tebutate
PREGNANCY CATEGORY: C
Rx: Prednisol TPA.

SEE ALSO CORTICOSTEROIDS.

ACTION/KINETICS

Action

Intermediate-acting. Is five times more potent than hydrocortisone and cortisone. Minimal side effects except for GI distress. Moderate mineralocorticoid activity.

Pharmacokinetics
Plasma t½: over 200 min.

CONTRAINDICATIONS

Lactation.

SPECIAL CONCERNS

Use with particular caution in diabetes.

SIDE EFFECTS

Most Common

Insomnia, N&V, GI upset, fatigue, dizziness, muscle weakness, increased hunger/thirst, joint pain, decreased diabetic control.

See *Corticosteroids* for a complete list of possible side effects.

HOW SUPPLIED

Prednisolone: *Syrup:* 15 mg/5 mL; *Tablets:* 5 mg.

Prednisolone acetate: *Injection:* 25 mg/mL, 50 mg/mL; *Ophthalmic Suspension:* 0.12%, 1%.

Prednisolone sodium phosphate: *Ophthalmic Solution:* 1%; *Oral Liquid/Solution:* 5 mg/5 mL, 6.7 mg/5 mL, 15 mg (base)/5 mL; *Tablets, Orally Disintegrating:* 10 mg, 15 mg, 30 mg.

Prednisolone tebutate: *Injection:* 20 mg/mL.

DOSAGE

PREDNISOLONE
• **SYRUP; TABLETS**

Most uses.

5–60 mg/day, depending on disease being treated.

Multiple sclerosis (exacerbation).

200 mg/day for 1 week; **then,** 80 mg on alternate days for 1 month.

Pleurisy of tuberculosis.

0.75 mg/kg/day (then taper) given concurrently with antituberculosis therapy.

PREDNISOLONE ACETATE
• **IM**

4–60 mg/day. **Not for IV use.**

Multiple sclerosis (exacerbation).
See *Prednisolone.*

• **INJECTION, SOFT TISSUE; INTRA-ARTICULAR; INTRALESIONAL**
4–100 mg (larger doses for large joints).

• **OPHTHALMIC SUSPENSION (0.12%, 0.125%, 1%)**
Instill 1–2 gtt into the conjunctival sac 2–4 times per day. During the first 24 to 48 hr, the frequency of dosing may be increased if necessary.

PREDNISOLONE SODIUM PHOSPHATE

• **ORAL LIQUID/SOLUTION**
Most uses.
5–60 mg/day in single or divided doses.

Adrenocortical insufficiency.
Pediatric: 0.14 mg/kg (4 mg/m²) daily in three to four divided doses.

Other pediatric uses.
0.5–2 mg/kg (15–60 mg/m²) daily in three to four divided doses.

• **OPHTHALMIC SOLUTION (0.125%, 1%)**
1–2 gtt into the conjunctival sac q hr during the day and q 2 hr during the night; **then,** after response obtained, decrease dose to 1 gtt q 4 hr and then later 1 gtt 3–4 times per day.

• **TABLETS, ORALLY DISINTEGRATING**
10–60 mg/day (prednisolone base).

PREDNISOLONE TEBUTATE

• **INJECTION, SOFT TISSUE; INTRA-ARTICULAR; INTRALESIONAL**
4–30 mg, depending on site and severity of disease. Doses higher than 40 mg are not recommended.

NURSING CONSIDERATIONS

🕭 Do not confuse prednisolone with prednisone (also a corticosteroid).

ADMINISTRATION/STORAGE

1. Before administering, check spelling and dose carefully; frequently confused with prednisone.

2. Check if provider wants PO form administered with an antacid.

3. Prednisolone sodium phosphate oral solution produces a 20% higher peak plasma level than tablets.

4. Shake suspension well before using.

IV 5. The IV form (sodium phosphate) may be administered at a rate not to exceed 10 mg/min.

ASSESSMENT

1. Note reasons for therapy, onset, characteristics of S&S, any previous experiences with this drug, outcome.

2. Monitor VS, CBC, lytes, blood sugar, weight, mental status.

CLIENT/FAMILY TEACHING

1. Take as directed and do not stop suddenly without provider approval; adrenal crisis may occur.

2. May take with food to decrease GI upset. Report any loss of effect; dose may need adjustment.

3. Avoid exposure to infected persons and crowds.

4. Report nausea, anorexia, fatigue, joint pain, weakness, dizziness, or SOB; S&S of adrenal insufficiency.

5. With joint injections, do not overuse joint after therapy despite improvement in ROM and pain.

6. Assess for weight gain, swelling of extremities, and adjust diet/salt intake and exercise to control.

OUTCOMES/EVALUATE

• Replacement therapy during adrenocortical hypofunction

• Symptomatic relief of allergic, immune, and inflammatory manifestations

---

Prednisone
(**PRED**-nih-sohn)

CLASSIFICATION(S):
Glucocorticoid

PREGNANCY CATEGORY: C

Rx: Oral Solution: Prednisone Intensol Concentrate. **Syrup**: Liquid Pred. **Tablets**: Deltasone, Meticorten, Orasone, Panasol-S, Prednicen-M, Sterapred, Sterapred DS.

✤**Rx: Tablets**: Apo-Prednisone, Winpred.

SEE ALSO *CORTICOSTEROIDS*.

USES

See *Corticosteroids.* Also, (1) COPD. (2) Ophthalmopathy due to Graves' disease. (3) Duchenne's muscular dystrophy.

Bold Italic = life threatening side effect   ▮ = black box warning   ✤ = Available in Canada

ACTION/KINETICS

Action

The anti-inflammatory effect is due to inhibition of prostaglandin synthesis. The drug also inhibits accumulation of macrophages and leukocytes at sites of inflammation and inhibits phagocytosis and lysosomal enzyme release.

Pharmacokinetics

Three to five times as potent as cortisone or hydrocortisone. May cause moderate fluid retention. Metabolized in the liver to prednisolone, the active form.

SPECIAL CONCERNS

Dose must be highly individualized.

SIDE EFFECTS

Most Common

Insomnia, N&V, GI upset, fatigue, dizziness, muscle weakness, increased hunger/thirst, joint pain, decreased diabetic control.

See *Corticosteroids* for a complete list of possible side effects.

HOW SUPPLIED

Oral Solution: 5 mg/5 mL; *Syrup:* 5 mg/5 mL; *Tablets:* 1 mg, 2.5 mg, 5 mg, 10 mg, 20 mg, 50 mg.

DOSAGE

- **ORAL SOLUTION; SYRUP; TABLETS**
  Acute, severe conditions.

Initial: 5–60 mg/day in four equally divided doses after meals and at bedtime. Decrease gradually by 5–10 mg q 4–5 days to establish minimum maintenance dosage (5–10 mg) or discontinue altogether until symptoms recur.

Replacement.
Pediatric: 0.1–0.15 mg/kg/day.

COPD.
30–60 mg/day for 1–2 weeks; then taper.

Ophthalmopathy due to Graves' disease.
60 mg/day; **then,** taper to 20 mg/day.

Duchenne's muscular dystrophy.
0.75–1.5 mg/kg/day (used to improve strength).

NURSING CONSIDERATIONS

Ⓒ Do not confuse prednisone with prednisolone (also a corticosteroid).

ASSESSMENT

1. Note reasons for therapy, type, onset, characteristics of S&S, clinical presentation. List other agents trialed/prescribed, outcome.
2. Monitor CBC, ESR, electrolytes, BP, blood sugar, weights, and mental status.
3. With chronic back pain, titrate dose to assess for relief; if relief attained may send for trigger point injections. Generally, if pain is diffuse/severe or involves joints other than spine, trigger point injections are usually not effective. Titrate to lowest dose possible to control symptoms and to ensure adequate physical functioning level. Address benefits versus risks with client/family.
4. With asthma/COPD provide rescue doses and instruct client how and when to use, i.e., during acute exacerbation when sputum is clear to white and no fever. May suggest 30 mg to start and decrease by 5 mg/day until down to 5 mg and continue for 5 days then off. If no relief, advise to call for instructions or seek hospitalization depending on severity of symptoms/peak flow readings.

CLIENT/FAMILY TEACHING

1. Take in the morning to prevent insomnia and with food to decrease GI upset.
2. Do not stop abruptly with long-term therapy. Take as directed and wean as directed.
3. Report any S&S of adrenal insufficiency (N&V, confusion, appetite loss, low BP), loss of effectiveness.
4. Avoid alcohol and OTC agents.
5. With weight gain, adjust caloric intake and exercise to control.
6. Avoid live vaccines, crowds and infected persons when on suppressive therapy; more susceptible to illnesses.
7. With long term therapy may experience cataracts, glaucoma, eye infections, bone weakening which may lead to osteoporosis, elevation in BP, diabetes, salt and water retention, and increased potassium loss. Consume adequate calcium and vitamin D supplements. Keep all F/U visits and report any unusual side effects. Once stabi-

lized, every other day dosing may assist to reduce adverse effects.

OUTCOMES/EVALUATE
• Relief of allergic, immune, and inflammatory manifestations
• Control of pain

Pregabalin
(pre-**GAB**-a-lin)

CLASSIFICATION(S):
Anticonvulsant, miscellaneous
PREGNANCY CATEGORY: C
Rx: Lyrica, **C-V**

USES
(1) Management of neuropathic pain associated with diabetic peripheral neuropathy. (2) Adjunctive therapy for adults with partial-onset seizures. (3) Management of postherpetic neuralgia. (4) Management of fibromyalgia. *Investigational:* Generalized anxiety disorder.

ACTION/KINETICS
Action
Binds with high affinity to the alpha$_2$-delta site (subunit of voltage-gated calcium channels) in CNS tissues. Binding may be involved in pregabalin's antinociceptive and antiseizure effects.

Pharmacokinetics
Well absorbed after PO use; rate of absorption is decreased when given with food. **Peak plasma levels:** 1.5 hr. Is more than 90% bioavailable; does not bind to plasma proteins. **Steady state:** 24–48 hr. Excreted mainly in the urine unchanged. t½: About 6.3 hr.

CONTRAINDICATIONS
Hypersensitivity to any component of the product, including lactose. Lactation.

SPECIAL CONCERNS
Dosage reduction may be needed in geriatric clients with age-related decreased renal function. Withdraw the drug gradually in those with seizure disorders to minimize the potential of increased seizure frequency or symptoms such as insomnia, nausea, headache, and diarrhea. Use with caution in those with CHF. Discontinue if myopathy is diagnosed or suspected or if markedly elevated creatine kinase levels occur. Safety and efficacy have not been determined in children.

SIDE EFFECTS
Most Common
Dizziness, somnolence, dry mouth, peripheral edema, asthenia, ataxia, confusion, headache, blurred vision, diplopia, flu syndrome, infection, pain, amnesia, incoordination, speech disorder, abnormal thinking, tremor, twitching, constipation, weight gain.

Side effects most commonly resulting in discontinuation: Dizziness, somnolence, asthenia, ataxia, blurred vision, confusion, incoordination, peripheral edema, abnormal thinking. **The following side effects have a frequency of more than 0.1%. CNS:** Dizziness, somnolence, neuropathy, vertigo, headache, ataxia, abnormal gait, confusion, abnormal thinking, amnesia, myoclonus, euphoria, speech disorder, incoordination, tremor, twitching, nervousness, anxiety, depersonalization, hypertonia, hypesthesia, decreased/increased libido, paresthesia, stupor, twitching, abnormal dreams, agitation, apathy, aphasia, circumoral paresthesia, dysarthria, hallucinations, hostility, hyperalgesia, hyperesthesia, hyperkinesis, hypokinesia, hypotonia, myoclonus, neuralgia. **GI:** Dry mouth, constipation, flatulence, vomiting, increased appetite, abdominal pain, gastroenteritis, cholecystitis, cholelithiasis, colitis, dysphagia, esophagitis, gastritis, *GI hemorrhage,* melena, mouth ulceration, *pancreatitis, rectal hemorrhage,* tongue edema. **CV:** Deep thrombophlebitis, *heart failure,* hypotension, postural hypotension, retinal vascular disorder, syncope, prolonged PR interval. **Respiratory:** Dyspnea, bronchitis. **Dermatologic:** Pruritus, alopecia, dry skin, eczema, hirsutism, skin ulcer, urticaria, vesiculobullous rash. **GU:** Anorgasmia, impotence, urinary frequency/incontinence/retention, abnormal ejaculation, amenorrhea, dysmenorrhea, dysuria, hematuria, kidney calculus, leukorrhea, menorrhagia, metrorrhagia, nephritis, oliguria. **Musculoskeletal:** Myasthenia, arthralgia, leg

---

Bold Italic = life threatening side effect   ■ = black box warning   ♣ = Available in Canada

cramps, myalgia. **Hematologic/Lymphatic:** Ecchymosis, anemia, eosinophilia, hypochromic anemia, leukocytosis, leukopenia, lymphadenopathy, thrombocytopenia. **Metabolic/Nutritional:** Peripheral edema, weight gain, edema. **Ophthalmic:** Blurred/abnormal vision, diplopia, conjunctivitis, abnormal accommodation, blepharitis, dry eyes, eye hemorrhage/disorder, photophobia, retinal edema, nystagmus. **Otic:** Otitis media, tinnitus. **Hypersensitivity:** Blisters, dyspnea, hives, rash, red skin, wheezing, angioedema. **Body as a whole:** Asthenia, accidental injury, flu syndrome, infection, pain, *allergic reaction*, abscess, cellulitis, chills, malaise, photosensitivity reaction. **Miscellaneous:** Back/chest pain, facial edema, urinary incontinence, hyperacusis, taste loss/perversion, weight gain, suicide attempt, neck rigidity, pelvic pain.

LABORATORY TEST CONSIDERATIONS
↑ Creatine kinase. ↓ Platelet count. Albuminuria.

OD OVERDOSE MANAGEMENT
Symptoms: Similar to usual side effects. *Treatment:* There is no specific antidote. Elimination of unabsorbed drug may be attempted by emesis or gastric lavage. Use general supportive care, including monitoring of vital signs and observation of the clinical status.

DRUG INTERACTIONS
Antidiabetic drugs, thiazolidinedione class / Weight gain and/or fluid retention can exacerbate or lead to heart failure; use together with caution
Ethanol / Additive effects on cognition and gross motor function
Lorazepam / Additive effects on cognition and gross motor function
Oxycodone / Additive effects on cognition and gross motor function

HOW SUPPLIED
Capsules: 25 mg, 50 mg, 75 mg, 100 mg, 150 mg, 200 mg, 225 mg, 300 mg.

DOSAGE————————
• **CAPSULES**
Neuropathic pain associated with diabetic peripheral neuropathy.
Adults, initial: 50 mg 3 times per day; may be increased to 300 mg/day within 1 week based on efficacy and tolerability. **Maximum dose:** 100 mg 3 times per day provided clients have a C_{CR} of at least 60 mL/min.

Partial-onset seizures.
Adults, initial: 75 mg twice a day or 50 mg 3 times per day. Based on individual client response and tolerability, may be increased to a maximum dose of 600 mg/day in 2 or 3 divided doses.

Postherpetic neuralgia.
Adults, initial: 75 mg twice a day or 50 mg 3 times per day in those with a C_{CR} of at least 60 mL/min. Based on efficacy and tolerability, dose may be increased in 1 week to 75–150 mg twice a day or 50–100 mg 3 times per day. **Maximum daily dose:** 300 mg/day. Clients whose pain is not relieved following 2–4 weeks of treatment with 300 mg/day and who are able to tolerate pregabalin, may be given up to 300 mg twice a day or 200 mg 3 times per day (i.e., total of 600 mg/day).

Fibromyalgia.
Adults, initial: 75 mg two times a day; may increase to 150 mg two times a day (300 mg/day) within 1 week. **Maximum dose:** 225 mg two times a day (450 mg/day). Doses greater than 450 mg/day offered no additional benefit and side effects were increased.

P

NURSING CONSIDERATIONS
ADMINISTRATION/STORAGE
1. Adjust dosage, as follows, in clients with impaired renal function:
• For a C_{CR} between 30 to 60 mL/min, give 75 to 300 mg/day in 2 or 3 divided doses.
• For a C_{CR} between 15 to 30 mL/min, give 25–150 mg/day in a single daily dose or 2 divided doses.
• For a C_{CR} less than 15 mL/min, give 25–75 mg/day in a single daily dose.
2. For clients undergoing hemodialysis, the daily dose should be adjusted based on renal function. In addition to the daily dose adjustment, a supplemental dose should be given immediately following every 4-hr hemodialysis treatment. For clients on the 25 mg single daily dose regimen, give 1 supplemental dose of 25 or 50 mg. For clients on the 25–50 mg single daily dose regi-

men, give 1 supplemental dose of 50 or 75 mg. For clients on the 75 mg single daily dose regimen, give 1 supplemental dose of 100 or 150 mg.

3. A dosage decrease may be needed in those who have age-related compromised renal function.

4. When discontinuing, taper gradually over a minimum of 1 week.

5. Store from 15–30°C (59–86°F).

ASSESSMENT

1. Note reasons for therapy, onset, characteristics of S&S, other agents trialed, outcome. Document clinical presentation; rate pain level.

2. Monitor VS, weight, HbA1c, liver, CK, CBC, and renal function studies; adjust dose with dysfunction. May note decrease in platelet counts.

3. Note medical history, esp Seizures, CAD. Assess ECG, note NYHA class; avoid or use cautiously with NYHA class III and IV.

4. Assess for history of drug abuse. Drug is schedule V. Observe for evidence or S&S of pregabalin misuse or abuse (i.e., tolerance development, drug-seeking behavior, dose escalation).

CLIENT/FAMILY TEACHING

1. May take with or without food as directed. Do not stop drug abruptly; may experience insomnia, nausea, headache, or diarrhea.

2. Drug is used to help manage nerve pain with diabetes or for pain after shingles outbreak. It is also used with other seizure medicine to help control partial seizures. Do not stop suddenly, may precipitate seizure activity.

3. Review patient information pamphlet prior to taking drug.

4. Do not perform activities that require mental alertness until drug effects realized; may cause dizziness, blurred vision, and sleepiness.

5. May experience weight gain and swelling of extremities. If already taking another antidiabetic thiaglitazone agent may increase effects of swelling and weight gain and with heart conditions, may increase risk of heart failure.

6. Report any unexplained muscle pain, weakness, or tenderness esp if accompanied by fever or increased tiredness. Report any changes in vision, significant weight gain, or trouble concentrating.

7. Avoid alcohol and CNS depressants as these may potentiate sedation and impairment of motor skills. If CNS depressants prescribed, expect additive side effects such as sleepiness.

8. Practice reliable contraception; report if pregnancy suspected. Males intending to father a child should be advised of risk of male mediated teratogenicity.

9. With diabetes, special attention to skin integrity should be maintained. Report any ulcerations or rashes.

10. Keep all F/U visits and report any adverse side effects or lack of desired response.

OUTCOMES/EVALUATE

- Control of partial seizures
- Relief of post herpetic neuralagia
- Control of neuropathic pain in diabetics

Primaquine phosphate
(**PRIM**-ah-kwin)

CLASSIFICATION(S):
Antimalarial, 8-aminoquinolone
PREGNANCY CATEGORY: C

USES
(1) Radical cure of *Plasmodium vivax* malaria. (2) Prophylaxis of relapse in *P. vivax* malaria. (3) Following the termination of chloroquine phosphate suppressive therapy in areas where *P. vivax* is endemic.

ACTION/KINETICS

Action
Mechanism of action not known, but the drug binds to and may alter the properties of DNA leading to decreased protein synthesis. Both the gametocyte and exoerythrocyte forms are inhibited. Some gametocytes are destroyed while others cannot undergo maturation division in the gut of the mosquito.

Pharmacokinetics

Well absorbed from GI tract. **Peak plasma levels:** 1–3 hr. Poorly distributed in body tissues. **t½, elimination:** 4 hr. Rapidly metabolized.

CONTRAINDICATIONS

Concomitant use with quinacrine. In clients with rheumatoid arthritis or lupus erythematosus who are acutely ill or who have a tendency to develop granulocytopenia. Concomitant use with other bone marrow depressants or hemolytic drugs.

SPECIAL CONCERNS

Use during pregnancy only when benefits outweigh risks.

SIDE EFFECTS

Most Common

N&V, abdominal cramps, epigastric distress, leukopenia.

GI: Abdominal cramps, epigastric distress, N&V. **Hematologic:** Leukopenia. Methemoglobinemia in NADH-methemoglobin reductase deficient individuals. Blacks and members of certain Mediterranean ethnic groups (Sardinians, Sephardic Jews, Greeks, Iranians) manifest a high incidence of G6PD deficiency and as a result have a low tolerance for primaquine. These individuals manifest *marked hemolytic anemia* following primaquine administration. **Miscellaneous:** Headache, pruritus, interference with visual accommodation, *cardiac arrhythmias*, hypertension.

OD OVERDOSE MANAGEMENT

Symptoms: Abdominal cramps, vomiting, burning and epigastric distress, cyanosis, methemoglobinemia, anemia, moderate leukocytosis or leukopenia, CNS and CV disturbances. Granulocytopenia and *acute hemolytic anemia* in sensitive clients. *Treatment:* Treat symptoms.

DRUG INTERACTIONS

Bone marrow depressants, hemolytic drugs / Additive side effects
Quinacrine / ↓ Metabolic degradation of primaquine → ↑ effects. **Do not give primaquine** to clients who are receiving or have received quinacrine within the past 3 months

HOW SUPPLIED

Tablets: 26.3 mg.

DOSAGE

• **TABLETS**

Acute attack of vivax malaria, clients with parasitized RBCs.

26.3 mg (15 mg base) daily for 14 days together with chloroquine phosphate (to destroy erythrocytic parasites).

Suppression of malaria.

Adults: 26.3 mg (15 mg base) daily for 14 days or 78.9 mg once a week for 8 weeks; **children:** 0.5 mg/kg/day (0.3 mg/kg base) for 14 days.

NURSING CONSIDERATIONS

ADMINISTRATION/STORAGE

1. Store in tightly closed containers.
2. For suppression therapy, initiate during the last 2 weeks of or after suppressive therapy with chloroquine or a similar drug.

ASSESSMENT

1. Note reasons for therapy, other agents trialed, history of rheumatoid arthritis or lupus.
2. List other drugs prescribed to ensure no unfavorable interactions.
3. Determine if pregnant. Do not give during first trimester and preferably not until after delivery.
4. Obtain hematologic profile and cultures. Monitor for indications to withdraw drug: dark urine may indicate hemolysis.
5. Assess dark-skinned clients closely. Because of a possible inborn deficiency of G6PD, these clients are particularly susceptible to hemolytic anemia while on primaquine.

CLIENT/FAMILY TEACHING

1. Take immediately before or after meals or with antacids to minimize gastric irritation.
2. For suppressive therapy, take drug on same day each week.
3. Monitor color of urine; report darkening or brown discoloration.
4. Must complete a full course of therapy for effective results.
5. If visual disturbances experienced avoid driving or hazardous activities.
6. Report any GI, neurologic, and cardiovascular disturbances; symptoms of overdose. Keep all F/U visits to ensure desired response.

P

📷 = see color insert   H = Herbal   IV = Intravenous   © = sound alike drug

OUTCOMES/EVALUATE
Termination of acute malarial attacks; suppression of malarial symptoms.

Primidone
(PRIH-mih-dohn)

CLASSIFICATION(S):
Anticonvulsant, miscellaneous
PREGNANCY CATEGORY: D
Rx: Mysoline.
♣Rx: Apo-Primidone.

USES
Alone or with other anticonvulsants to treat psychomotor, focal, or tonic-clonic seizures (including those refractory to anticonvulsant regimens). *Investigational:* Benign familial tremor (essential tremor).

ACTION/KINETICS
Action
Closely related to the barbiturates; however, the anticonvulsant mechanism is unknown. Produces a greater sedative effect than barbiturates when used for seizure treatment. Side effects usually subside with use.

Pharmacokinetics
Rapidly and almost completely absorbed after PO. **Peak plasma levels:** 3 hr. Primidone is converted in the liver to two active metabolites, phenobarbital and phenylethylmalonamide (PEMA). **Peak plasma levels (PEMA):** 7–8 hr. **t½ (primidone):** 5–15 hr; **t½ (PEMA):** 10–18 hr; **t½ (phenobarbital):** 53–140 hr. The appearance of phenobarbital in the plasma may be delayed several days after initiation of therapy. **Therapeutic plasma levels, primidone:** 5–12 mcg/mL; **phenobarbital,** 15–40 mcg/mL. Primidone and metabolites are excreted through the kidneys, although 40% of primidone is excreted unchanged.

CONTRAINDICATIONS
Porphyria. Hypersensitivity to phenobarbital. Lactation.

SPECIAL CONCERNS
Safe use during pregnancy has not been determined. Use during lactation may result in drowsiness in the neonate. Children and geriatric clients may react to primidone with restlessness and excitement. Abrupt withdrawal may precipitate status epilepticus. Neonatal hemorrhage, with coagulation defect resembling vitamin K deficiency, may occur in newborns whose mothers were taking primidone.

SIDE EFFECTS
Most Common
Ataxia, vertigo, fatigue, N&V, anorexia, hyperirritability.
CNS: Drowsiness, ataxia, vertigo, fatigue, hyperirritability, emotional disturbances, personality disturbances with mood changes and paranoia. **GI:** N&V, anorexia, painful gums. **Hematologic:** Megaloblastic anemia, thrombocytopenia; rarely granulocytopenia, agranulocytosis, and red-cell hyperplasia. **Ophthalmic:** Diplopia, nystagmus. **Miscellaneous:** Impotence, morbilliform and maculopapular skin rashes. Occasionally has caused hyperexcitability, especially in children. *Postpartum hemorrhage and hemorrhagic disease of the newborn.* Symptoms of SLE.

DRUG INTERACTIONS
SEE ALSO *BARBITURATES*
Acetazolamide / ↓ Effect of primidone R/T ↓ levels
Carbamazepine / ↓ Levels of primidone and phenobarbital and ↑ levels of carbamazepine
Doxycycline / ↓ Doxycycline t½ and serum levels with possible ↓ effect; may persist for weeks following primidone discontinuation; consider an alternate tetracycline
Ethanol / Impaired hand-eye coordination, additive CNS effects, and possible death upon acute ingestion; avoid concomitant use
Felodipine / ↓ Effects of felodipine; may need ↑ felodipine doses if used chronically
Hydantoins / ↑ Levels of primidone, phenobarbital, and PEMA
Isoniazid / ↑ Effect of primidone R/T ↓ liver breakdown
Methadone / ↓ Methadone effects; those on chronic methadone therapy may experience withdrawal symptoms

---

Bold Italic = life threatening side effect   ■ = black box warning   ♣ = Available in Canada

Metronidazole / Possible metronidazole therapeutic failure; higher metronidazole doses may be needed

Nicotinamide / ↑ Effect of primidone R/T ↓ rate of clearance from body

Nifedipine / Possible ↓ nifedipine serum levels → ↓ efficacy; titrate dose according to response

Oral contraceptives / ↓ Levels of estrogens → contraceptive failure; consider use of alternative contraceptive

Prednisone / ↓ Effect of prednisone; avoid concomitant use

Propranolol / ↓ Effect of propranolol; may need to ↑ propranolol dose

Quinidine / ↓ Quinidine levels and elimination t½

Succinimides / ↓ Levels of primidone and phenobarbital

Theophylline / ↓ Theophylline levels → ↓ therapeutic effect; may need to ↑ theophylline dose

Valproic acid / ↑ Primidone levels → ↑ pharmacologic and side effects; in some, decreased primidone dose may be needed

Warfarin ↓ Effect of warfarin; monitor warfarin dose and adjust dose as needed

HOW SUPPLIED
Tablets: 50 mg, 250 mg.

DOSAGE
- **TABLETS**

Seizures, in clients on no previous anticonvulsant medication.

Adults and children over 8 years, initial: Days 1–3, 100–125 mg at bedtime; days 4–6, 100–125 mg twice a day (morning and evening); days 7–9, 100–125 mg 3 times per day (morning, noon, and evening); day 10 to maintenance: 250 mg 3 to 4 times per day (morning, noon, evening). **Usual maintenance:** 250 mg 3–4 times daily. Dose may be increased to 250 mg 5–6 times per day, not to exceed 500 mg 4 times per day. **Children under 8 years, initial:** Days 1–3, 50 mg at bedtime; days 4–6, 50 mg twice a day; days 7–9, 100 mg twice a day; day 10 to maintenance: 125 mg twice a day to 250 mg 3 times per day. **Usual maintenance:** 125–250 mg 3 times daily or 10–25 mg/kg in divided doses.

Seizures, in clients receiving other anticonvulsants.

Initial: 100–125 mg at bedtime; **then,** increase to maintenance levels as other drug is slowly withdrawn (transition should take at least 2 weeks).

Benign familial tremor.

750 mg/day.

NURSING CONSIDERATIONS

ADMINISTRATION/STORAGE
1. Pregnant women should receive prophylactic vitamin K therapy for 1 month prior to and during delivery.
2. Due to bioequivalence problems, brand interchange is not recommended unless bioavailability data are available.

ASSESSMENT
1. Note age at seizure onset, frequency/characteristics of seizures, and cause if known. Note other agents trialed, outcome.
2. List other agents prescribed to ensure none interact unfavorably.
3. Monitor CBC, renal, LFTs; assess for dysfunction.

CLIENT/FAMILY TEACHING
1. May be taken with food if GI upset occurs.
2. Do not stop abruptly as withdrawal symptoms may occur.
3. Avoid alcohol, OTC agents, and CNS depressants. Do not perform activities that require mental alertness until drug effects realized; may cause dizziness and drowsiness.
4. Review the following conditions that should be reported:
- Hyperexcitability in children
- Excessive loss of hair
- Edema of eyelids and legs
- Visual disturbances
- Mental status changes
- Impotence
- Loss of seizure control
- Lack of response/adverse side effects
5. Vitamin K may be prescribed during the last month of pregnancy to prevent postpartum hemorrhage in the mother and hemorrhagic disease of the newborn.

OUTCOMES/EVALUATE
- Control of refractory seizures

P

- Therapeutic drug levels (5–12 mcg/mL)

Probenecid
(proh-**BEN**-ih-sid)

CLASSIFICATION(S):
Antigout drug, uricosuric
PREGNANCY CATEGORY: B
Rx: Benemid.
✤**Rx:** Benuryl.

USES
(1) Hyperuricemia in chronic gout and gouty arthritis. (2) Adjunct in therapy with penicillins or cephalosporins to elevate and prolong plasma antibiotic levels.

ACTION/KINETICS
Action
A uricosuric agent that increases the excretion of uric acid by inhibiting the tubular reabsorption of uric acid; this results in a decreased serum level of uric acid. Also inhibits the renal secretion of penicillins and cephalosporins; this effect is often taken advantage of in the treatment of infections because concomitant administration of probenecid will increase plasma levels of antibiotics.

Pharmacokinetics
Peak plasma levels: 2–4 hr. **Time to peak effect, uricosuric:** 0.5 hr; **for suppression of penicillin excretion:** 2 hr. **Therapeutic plasma levels for inhibition of antibiotic secretion:** 40–60 mcg/mL; **therapeutic plasma levels for uricosuric effect:** 100–200 mcg/mL. **t½:** Approximately 5–8 hr. **Duration for inhibition of penicillin excretion:** 8 hr. Metabolized in the liver to active metabolites; excreted in urine (5–10% unchanged). Excretion is increased in alkaline urine.

CONTRAINDICATIONS
Hypersensitivity to drug, blood dyscrasias, uric acid, and kidney stones. Use for hyperuricemia in neoplastic disease or its treatment. Use in children less than 2 years of age. Concomitant use of salicylates or use with penicillin in renal impairment.

SPECIAL CONCERNS
Use with caution in renal disease, porphyria, G6PD deficiency, history of allergy to sulfa drugs, and peptic ulcer.

SIDE EFFECTS
Most Common
Headache, dizziness, anorexia, N&V, diarrhea, constipation, skin rash, abdominal discomfort, urinary frequency.
CNS: Headaches, dizziness. **GI:** Anorexia, N&V, diarrhea, constipation, and abdominal discomfort. **Allergic:** Skin rash, dermatitis, pruritus, drug fever, and rarely **anaphylaxis**. **GU:** Nephrotic syndrome, uric acid stones with or without hematuria, urinary frequency, renal colic, or costovertebral pain. **Miscellaneous:** Flushing, **hemolytic anemia (possibly related to G6PD deficiency)**, anemia, sore gums, **hepatic necrosis**, **aplastic anemia**. Initially, the drug may increase frequency of acute gout attacks due to mobilization of uric acid.

DRUG INTERACTIONS
Acyclovir / ↓ Renal excretion of acyclovir
Allopurinol / Additive effects to ↓ uric acid serum levels
Benzodiazepines / More rapid onset and longer duration of benzodiazepine effects
Carbamazepine / ↑ Carbamazepine metabolism R/T induction of CYP2C8 and CYP3A4
Cephalosporins / ↑ Cephalosporin effect R/T ↓ kidney excretion
Ciprofloxacin / 50% ↑ in systemic levels of ciprofloxacin
Clofibrate / ↑ Clofibric acid (active) levels → ↑ effects
Dapsone / ↑ Dapsone effects
Dyphylline / ↑ Dyphylline effect R/T ↓ kidney excretion
Fexofenadine / ↑ Fexofenadine AUC and ↓ renal clearance R/T inhibition of P-glycoprotein transport
Methotrexate / ↑ Methotrexate effect and toxicity R/T ↓ kidney excretion
Niacin / ↓ Uric acid-lowering effects of probenecid
NSAIDs / ↑ NSAID effects R/T ↓ kidney excretion

Bold Italic = life threatening side effect   ■ = black box warning   ✤ = Available in Canada

Olanzapine / ↑ AUC, peak plasma levels, and rate of olanzapine absorption R/T inhibition of olanzapine metabolism
Pantothenic acid / ↑ Pantothenic acid effects
Penicillamine / ↓ Penicillamine effects
Penicillins / ↑ Penicillin effects R/T ↓ kidney excretion
Pyrazinamide / Inhibits hyperuricemia produced by pyrazinamide
Rifampin / ↑ Rifampin effects R/T ↓ kidney excretion
Salicylates / Inhibits uricosuric activity of probenecid
Sulfinpyrazone / ↑ Sulfinpyrazone effects R/T ↓ kidney excretion
Sulfonamides / ↑ Sulfonamide effects R/T ↓ plasma protein binding
Sulfonylureas, oral / ↑ Sulfonylurea effect → ↑ hypoglycemia
Thiopental / ↑ Thiopental effects
Zidovudine (AZT) / ↑ Bioavailabilit of AZT; possible malaise, myalgia, fever

HOW SUPPLIED
Tablets: 500 mg.

DOSAGE

- **TABLETS**

    Gout.
Adults, initial: 250 mg twice a day for 1 week. **Maintenance:** 500 mg twice a day. Dosage may have to be increased further (by 500 mg/day q 4 weeks to maximum of 2 grams) until urate excretion <700 mg in 24 hr. Colbenemid, a combination tablet containing colchicine (0.5 mg) and probenecid (500 mg), is also available.

    Adjunct to penicillin or cephalosporin therapy.
Adults: 500 mg 4 times per day. Dosage is decreased for elderly clients with renal damage. **Pediatric, 2–14 years, initial:** 25 mg/kg (or 700 mg/m²); **maintenance,** 10 mg/kg 4 times per day (or 300 mg/m² 4 times per day). **For children 50 kg or more:** Give adult dosage.

    Gonorrhea, uncomplicated.
Adults: 1 gram (as a single dose) 30 min before 4.8 million units of penicillin G procaine aqueous; **pediatric, less than 45 kg:** 25 mg/kg (up to a maximum of 1 gram) with appropriate antibiotic therapy.

    Neurosyphilis.
Adults: 0.5 gram 4 times per day with penicillin G procaine aqueous, 2.4 million units/day IM, both for 10–14 days.

    Pelvic inflammatory disease.
Adults: 1 gram (as a single dose) plus cefoxitin, 2 grams IM given concurrently.

NURSING CONSIDERATIONS

ADMINISTRATION/STORAGE

1. Do not start therapy until acute gouty attack has subsided. If an acute attack is precipitated during therapy, continue drug.
2. To prevent kidney stones, take at least 6 to 8 (8-oz) glasses of water.
3. Maintain an alkaline urine by taking sodium bicarbonate, 3–7.5 grams/day, or potassium citrate, 7.5 grams/day.

ASSESSMENT

1. Note reasons for therapy, onset, characteristics of S&S, other agents trialed, triggers if evident.
2. List any PUD, G6PD deficiency, uricemia R/T neoplastic disease, kidney stones, sulfa allergy, blood dyscrasia.
3. Assess involved joints, noting pain, inflammation, heat, swelling, deformity, tophaceous deposits, ROM.
4. Monitor CBC, uric acid, renal and LFTs. Note urate excretion levels, urine alkalinity; urates crystalize in acid urine.
5. Hypersensitivity reactions may occur more frequently with intermittent therapy.
6. Assess for toxic plasma antibiotic levels if excretion inhibited by probenecid; adjust dosage.

CLIENT/FAMILY TEACHING

1. Take with food or milk to minimize gastric irritation. Report gastric intolerance so dosage may be corrected without loss of therapeutic effect.
2. Take a liberal amount of fluid (2.5–3 L/day) to prevent the formation of sodium urate stones. Avoid cranberry juice or vitamin C preparations, which acidify urine. Sodium bicarbonate may be used to maintain an alkaline urine to prevent urates from crystallizing and forming kidney stones.
3. Acute gout attacks may initially be more frequent due to mobilization of

uric acid. Report increase in the number of acute attacks at initiation of therapy since colchicine may need to be added. Continue to take during acute attacks with colchicine unless otherwise specified.

4. Report any unexplained fever, fatigue, skin rash, persistent GI upset, flushing, increased sweating, headaches, or dizziness.

5. Do not take salicylates or use caffeine or alcohol during uricosuric therapy. Acetaminophen preparations may be used for analgesia.

6. Monitor FS closely; drug may increase hypoglycemic effects of PO antidiabetic agents.

OUTCOMES/EVALUATE

- ↓ Uric acid levels; ↓ gout attacks
- ↓ Joint pain/swelling
- Elevated/prolonged antibiotic (penicillin or cephalosporin) levels

Procainamide hydrochloride
■ IV
(proh-**KAYN**-ah-myd)

CLASSIFICATION(S):
Antiarrhythmic, Class IA
PREGNANCY CATEGORY: C
Rx: Procanbid, Pronestyl.
♣Rx: Apo-Procainamide, Procan SR.

SEE ALSO *ANTIARRHYTHMIC DRUGS.*

USES
Documented ventricular arrhythmias (e.g., sustained ventricular tachycardia) that may be life threatening in clients where benefits of treatment clearly outweigh risks. *NOTE:* Antiarrhythmic drugs have not been shown to improve survival in clients with ventricular arrhythmias. *Investigational:* Atrial fibrillation/flutter.

ACTION/KINETICS
Action
Produces a direct cardiac effect to prolong the refractory period of the atria and to a lesser extent the bundle of His-Purkinje system and ventricles. Large

doses may cause AV block. Some anticholinergic and local anesthetic effects.

Pharmacokinetics
Onset, PO: 30 min; **IV:** 1–5 min. **Time to peak effect, PO:** 90–120 min; **IM:** 15–60 min; **IV:** Immediate. **Duration:** 3 hr. **t½:** 2.5–4.7 hr. **Therapeutic serum level:** 4–8 mcg/mL. **Toxic serum levels:** Over 16 mcg/mL. From 40–70% excreted unchanged. Metabolized in the liver (16–21% by slow acetylators and 24–33% by fast acetylators) to the active N-acetylprocainamide (NAPA); has antiarrhythmic properties with a longer half-life than procainamide. **Plasma protein binding:** 14–23%.

CONTRAINDICATIONS
Hypersensitivity to drug, complete AV heart block, lupus erythematosus, torsades de pointes, asymptomatic ventricular premature depolarizations. Lactation.

SPECIAL CONCERNS
■ (1) Prolonged use of procainamide often leads to development of a positive antinuclear antibody (ANA) test, with or without symptoms of lupus erythematosus-like syndrome. If a positive ANA titer develops, assess the benefit/risk ratio related to continued procainamide therapy. (2) Use should be reserved for those with life-threatening ventricular arrhythmias. (3) Agranulocytosis, bone marrow depression, neutropenia, hypoplastic anemia, and thrombocytopenia have been reported. Most cases occurred after recommended dosage. Fatalities have occurred (usually with agranulocytosis). Because most of these events occur during the first 12 weeks of therapy, it is recommended that CBC, including WBC, differential, and platelet counts be performed weekly for the first 3 months of therapy and periodically thereafter. Perform CBC promptly if the client develops any signs of infection (e.g., fever, chills, sore throat, stomatitis), bruising, or bleeding. If any of these hematologic disorders occur, discontinue therapy. Blood counts usually return to normal within 1 month after discontinuation. Use caution in those with pre-existing bone marrow failure or cytopenia of

any type.■ There is an increased risk of death in those with non-life-threatening arrhythmias. Although used in children, safety and efficacy have not been established. Use with extreme caution in clients for whom a sudden drop in BP could be detrimental, in CHF, acute ischemic heart disease, or cardiomyopathy. Also, use with caution in clients with liver or kidney dysfunction, preexisting bone marrow failure or cytopenia of any type, development of first-degree heart block while on procainamide, myasthenia gravis, and those with bronchial asthma or other respiratory disorders. May cause more hypotension in geriatric clients; also, in this population, the dose may have to be decreased due to age-related decreases in renal function.

SIDE EFFECTS
Most Common
Dizziness, fatigue, bitter taste, GI upset, nausea, anorexia, diarrhea, headache, blurred vision, giddiness, depression.
CV: Following IV use: Hypotension, *ventricular asystole or fibrillation, partial or complete heart block*. Rarely, second-degree heart block after PO use. **GI:** N&V, diarrhea, anorexia, bitter taste, GI upset, abdominal pain. **Hematologic:** Thrombocytopenia, *agranulocytosis*, neutropenia, hypoplastic anemia. Rarely, hemolytic anemia. **Dermatologic:** Urticaria, pruritus, angioneurotic edema, flushing, maculopapular rash. **CNS:** Depression, headache, dizziness, weakness, giddiness, psychoses with hallucinations. *Body as a whole:* Lupus erythematosus–like syndrome especially in those on maintenance therapy and who are slow acetylators. Symptoms include arthralgia, pleural or abdominal pain, arthritis, pleural effusion, pericarditis, fever, chills, myalgia, skin lesions, hematologic changes. **Miscellaneous:** Granulomatous hepatitis, weakness, fever, chills, blurred vision.

LABORATORY TEST CONSIDERATIONS
May affect LFTs. False + ↑ in serum alkaline phosphatase. Positive ANA test. High levels of lidocaine and meprobamate may inhibit fluorescence of procainamide and NAPA.

OD OVERDOSE MANAGEMENT
Symptoms: Plasma levels of 10–15 mcg/mL are associated with toxic symptoms. Progressive widening of the QRS complex, prolonged QT or PR intervals, lowering of R and T waves, increased AV block, increased ventricular extrasystoles, *ventricular tachycardia or fibrillation*. IV overdose may result in hypotension, CNS depression, tremor, respiratory depression.
Treatment:
- Induce emesis or perform gastric lavage followed by administration of activated charcoal.
- To treat hypotension, give IV fluids and/or a vasopressor (dopamine, phenylephrine, or norepinephrine).
- Infusion of ⅙ molar sodium lactate IV reduces the cardiotoxic effects.
- Hemodialysis (but not peritoneal dialysis) is effective in reducing serum levels.
- Renal clearance can be enhanced by acidification of the urine and with high flow rates.
- A ventricular pacing electrode can be inserted as a precaution in the event AV block develops.

DRUG INTERACTIONS
Acetazolamide / ↑ Procainamide effect R/T ↓ kidney excretion
Amiodarone / ↑ Procainamide levels
Antiarrhythmics (e.g., lidocaine, disopyramide, quinidine) / Additive effects on the heart; quinidine may also ↑ procainamide and metabolite levels
Anticholinergic agents, atropine / Additive antivagal effects on AV conduction
Antihypertensive agents / Additive hypotensive effect
Cholinergic agents / Anticholinergic activity of procainamide antagonizes effect of cholinergic drugs
Cimetidine / ↑ Procainamide effect R/T ↓ renal clearance
Disopyramide / ↑ Risk of enhanced prolongation of conduction or depression of contractility and hypotension
Ethanol / Effect of procainamide may be altered, but because the main metabolite is active as an antiarrhythmic, specific outcome not clear

P

H *Henbane leaf* / ↑ Anticholinergic effects

Kanamycin / ↑ Kanamycin-induced muscle relaxation

Lidocaine / Additive cardiodepressant effects

Mg salts / ↑ Mg-induced muscle relaxation

Neomycin / ↑ Neomycin-induced muscle relaxation

Ofloxacin / See *Quinolones;* also, possible ↑ procainamide levels

Propranolol / ↑ Serum procainamide levels

Quinidine / ↑ Risk of enhanced prolongation of conduction or depression of contractility and hypotension

Quinolones / ↑ Risk of life-threatening cardiac arrhythmias, including torsades de pointes

Ranitidine / ↑ Procainamide effect R/T ↓ renal clearance

Sodium bicarbonate / ↑ Procainamide effect R/T ↓ kidney excretion

Succinylcholine / ↑ Succinylcholine-induced muscle relaxation

Thioridazine / Possible synergistic or additive prolongation of the QTc interval and ↑ risk for life-threatening cardiac arrhythmias, including torsades de pointes

Trimethoprim / ↑ Procainamide effect R/T ↑ serum levels

Ziprasidone / Possible synergistic or additive prolongation of the QTc interval and ↑ risk for life-threatening cardiac arrhythmias, including torsades de pointes

HOW SUPPLIED

Capsules: 250 mg, 375 mg, 500 mg; *Injection:* 500 mg/mL; *Tablets, Extended-Release:* 250 mg, 500 mg, 750 mg, 1000 mg; *Tablets, Immediate-Release:* 250 mg, 375 mg, 500 mg.

DOSAGE

• **CAPSULES; TABLETS, EXTENDED-RELEASE; TABLETS, IMMEDIATE-RELEASE**

Adults, initial: Up to 50 mg/kg/day in divided doses q 3 hr. **Usual, 40–50 kg:** 250 mg q 3 hr or 500 mg q 6 hr of immediate release; 500 mg q 6 hr of sustained-release; or, 1 gram q 12 hr of Procanbid; **60–70 kg:** 375 mg q 3 hr or

750 mg q 6 hr of immediate release; 750 mg q 6 hr of sustained-release; or, 1.5 grams q 12 hr of Procanbid; **80–90 kg:** 500 mg q 3 hr or 1 gram q 6 hr of immediate release; 1 gram q 6 hr of sustained-release; or, 2 grams q 12 hr of Procanbid; **over 100 kg:** 625 mg q 3 hr or 1.25 grams q 6 hr of immediate release; 1.25 grams q 6 hr of sustained-release; or, 2.5 grams q 12 hr of Procanbid.

• **IM**

Ventricular arrhythmias.

Adults, initial: 50 mg/kg/day divided into fractional doses of ⅛–¼ given q 3–6 hr until PO therapy is possible. If more than 3 injections are given, assess client factors as age, renal function, clinical response, and blood procainamide and n-acetylprocainamide levels in adjusting further doses.

Arrhythmias associated with surgery or anesthesia.

Adults: 100–500 mg.

• **IV**

Ventricular arrhythmias.

Initial loading infusion: Slowly inject into a vein or tubing at a rate not to exceed 50 mg/min; doses of 100 mg may be given q 5 min until arrhythmia is suppressed or until 500 mg has been given. Wait at least 10 min to allow for more distribution into tissues before resuming. Alternatively, a loading infusion containing 20 mg/mL (1 gram diluted to 50 mL with D5W) may be given at a constant rate of 1 mL/min for 25–30 min to deliver 500–600 mg. Maximum dosage either by repeated bolus injections or loading infusion is 1 gram. **Maintenance infusion:** 2–6 mg/min.

NURSING CONSIDERATIONS

ADMINISTRATION/STORAGE

1. Extended-release tablets are not recommended for use in children or for initiating treatment.

2. IM therapy may be used as an alternative to PO in clients with less threatening arrhythmias but who are nauseated or vomiting, who cannot take anything PO (e.g., preoperatively), or who have malabsorptive problems.

Bold Italic = life threatening side effect   ■ = black box warning   ♣ = Available in Canada

3. If more than three IM injections are required, assess the age, renal function, and blood levels of procainamide and NAPA; adjust dosage accordingly.

IV 4. Reserve IV use for emergency situations.

5. For IV initial therapy, dilute the drug with D5W; give a maximum of 1 gram slowly to minimize side effects by one of the following methods:

- Direct injection into a vein or into tubing of an established infusion line at a rate not to exceed 50 mg/min. Dilute either the 100- or 500-mg/mL vials prior to injection to facilitate control of the dosage rate. Doses of 100 mg may be given q 5 min until arrhythmia is suppressed or until 500 mg has been given (then wait 10 or more min before resuming administration).

- Loading infusion containing 20 mg/mL (1 gram diluted with 50 mL of D5W) given at a constant rate of 1 mL/min for 25–30 min to deliver 500–600 mg.

6. For IV maintenance infusion, dose is usually 2–6 mg/min. Administer with electronic infusion device.

7. Discard solutions that are darker than light amber or otherwise colored. Solutions that have turned slightly yellow on standing may be used. Consult pharmacist if unsure.

ASSESSMENT

1. Note reasons for therapy, type, onset, characteristics of S&S. List other agents prescribed, outcome.

2. Assess cardiopulmonary status and note findings. List any sensitivity to tartrazine, pregnancy, or heart block.

3. Monitor VS, ECG, CBC, lytes, ANA titers, renal, LFTs.

INTERVENTIONS

1. Place supine during IV infusion and monitor BP. Discontinue if SBP falls 15 mm Hg or more during administration or if increased SA or AV block noted.

2. Reduce dose with liver or renal dysfunction, or if client <120 lb.

3. Assess for symptoms of SLE, manifested by polyarthralgia, arthritis, pleuritic pain, fever, myalgia, and skin lesions. ANA titer may become positive in 60% of those taking this drug without lupus—like S&S; may progress to SLE if drug is not discontinued.

CLIENT/FAMILY TEACHING

1. Take with a full glass of water to lessen GI symptoms. Take either 1 hr before or 2 hr after meals.

2. If GI symptoms are severe and persistent may take with meals or with a snack to ensure adherence.

3. Sustained-release preparations should be swallowed whole. They should not be crushed, broken, or chewed. The wax matrix of sustained-release tablets may be evident in the stool and is considered normal.

4. Report any sore throat, fever, rash, chills, bruising, diarrhea or increased palpitations. With long term use may note loss of effectiveness.

5. Do not take any OTC drugs, do not stop suddenly. Report any adverse side effects, i.e., irregular pulse, anxiety, sudden fatigue.

OUTCOMES/EVALUATE

- Termination of arrhythmias with restoration of stable cardiac rhythm
- Therapeutic drug levels (4–8 mcg/mL)

P

Procarbazine hydrochloride (PCB, MIH, N-Methylhydrazine)
(pro-**KAR**-bah-zeen)

CLASSIFICATION(S):
Antineoplastic, miscellaneous
PREGNANCY CATEGORY: D
Rx: Matulane.

SEE ALSO *ANTINEOPLASTIC AGENTS.*

USES

Adjunct in the treatment of Hodgkin's disease (stage III and stage IV) as part of MOPP (nitrogen mustard, vincristine, procarbazine, prednisone) or ChlVPP (chlorambucil, vinblastine, procarbazine, prednisone) therapies. *Investigational:* Non-Hodgkin's lymphomas, malignant melanoma, primary brain tumors, lung cancer.

ACTION/KINETICS

Action

May inhibit synthesis of protein, RNA, and DNA and inhibit transmethylation of methyl groups of methionine into t-RNA. Absence of t-RNA could result in cessation of protein synthesis and subsequently DNA and RNA synthesis. Also, hydrogen peroxide formed during auto-oxidation of the drug may attack protein sulfhydryl groups found in residual protein that is tightly bound to DNA.

Pharmacokinetics

Rapidly and completely absorbed from GI tract. Drug quickly equilibrates between plasma and CSF (peak CSF levels occur within 30–90 min and peak plasma levels occur within 60 min). **t½, after IV:** 10 min. Metabolized in the liver and kidneys to cytotoxic products. About 70% eliminated in urine, mostly as metabolites, after 24 hr.

CONTRAINDICATIONS

Inadequate bone marrow reserve as shown by bone marrow aspiration (i.e., in clients with leukopenia, thrombocytopenia, or anemia). Lactation. Hypersensitivity to drug.

SPECIAL CONCERNS

Use with caution in impaired kidney or liver function. Due to the possibility of tremors, convulsions, and coma, close monitoring is necessary when used in children.

SIDE EFFECTS

Most Common

N&V, constipation, dry mouth, difficulty swallowing, fatigue, weakness, drowsiness, dizziness, darkening of skin, muscle twitching, insomnia, temporary alopecia.

GI: N&V, anorexia, stomatitis, dry mouth, dysphagia, difficulty swallowing, abdominal pain, hematemesis, melena, diarrhea, constipation. **CNS:** Paresthesias, neuropathies, headache, dizziness, depression, apprehension, nervousness, insomnia, nightmares, hallucinations, falling, weakness, fatigue, lethargy, drowsiness, unsteadiness, ataxia, foot drop, decreased reflexes, tremors, confusion, *coma, convulsions*. **CV:** Hypotension, tachycardia, syncope. **Respiratory:** Pleural effusion, pneumonitis, cough. **Hematologic:** Leukopenia, anemia, thrombocytopenia, pancytopenia, eosinophilia, *hemolytic anemia*, petechiae, purpura, epistaxis, hemoptysis. **GU:** Hematuria, urinary frequency, nocturia. **Dermatologic:** Dermatitis, pruritus, rash, urticaria, herpes, hyperpigmentation, flushing, alopecia (temporary). **Ophthalmic:** Retinal hemorrhage, nystagmus, photophobia, diplopia, inability to focus, papilledema. **Hepatic:** Jaundice, hepatic dysfunction. **Miscellaneous:** Gynecomastia in prepubertal and early pubertal boys, muscle twitching, pain, myalgia and arthralgia, pyrexia, diaphoresis, chills, intercurrent infections, edema, hoarseness, generalized allergic reactions, hearing loss, slurred speech, second nonlymphoid malignancies (including AML, malignant myelosclerosis) and azoospermia in those treated with procarbazine combined with other chemotherapy or radiation.

OD OVERDOSE MANAGEMENT

Symptoms: N&V, diarrhea, enteritis, hypotension, tremors, seizures, coma, hematologic and hepatic toxicity. *Treatment:* Induce vomiting or undertake gastric lavage. IV fluids. Perform frequent blood counts and LFTs.

DRUG INTERACTIONS

Alcohol / Antabuse-like reaction
Antihistamines / Additive CNS depression
Antihypertensive drugs / Additive CNS depression
Barbiturates / Additive CNS depression
Chemotherapy / Depressed bone marrow activity
Digoxin / ↓ Digoxin levels
Guanethidine / Excitation and hypertension
Hypoglycemic agents, oral / ↑ Hypoglycemic effect
Insulin / ↑ Hypoglycemic effect
Levodopa / Flushing and hypertension within 1 hr of administration
MAO inhibitors / Possibility of hypertensive crisis

Methotrexate / ↑ Methotrexate nephrotoxicity; wait 72 hr after the last dose of procarbazine and first dose of methotrexate infusion

Methyldopa / Excitation and hypertension

Narcotics / Significant CNS depression → possible deep coma/death

Phenothiazines / Additive CNS depression; possible hypertensive crisis

Sympathomimetics, indirectly acting / Possibility of hypertensive crisis

Tricyclic antidepressants / Possible toxic and fatal reactions, including excitability, fluctuations in BP, seizures, and coma

Tyramine-containing foods / Possibility of hypertensive crisis

HOW SUPPLIED

Capsules: 50 mg.

DOSAGE

- **CAPSULES**

    When used alone for Hodgkin's disease.

Adults: 2–4 mg/kg/day for first week; **then,** 4–6 mg/kg/day until leukocyte count falls below 4,000/mm³ or platelet count falls below 100,000/mm³. If toxic symptoms appear, discontinue drug until satisfactory recovery, and resume treatment at rate of 1–2 mg/kg/day; **maintenance:** 1–2 mg/kg/day. **Children, highly individualized:** 50 mg/m²/day for first week; then 100 mg/m² (to nearest 50 mg) until maximum response obtained or until leukopenia or thrombocytopenia occurs. When maximum response is reached, maintain the dose at 50 mg/m²/day.

    When used in combination with other antineoplastic drugs (e.g., MOPP or ChIVPP therapies) for Hodgkin's disease.

100 mg/m² for 14 days.

NURSING CONSIDERATIONS

ASSESSMENT

1. Note reasons for therapy, other agents/treatments prescribed.
2. Assess cardiopulmonary, neurologic status.
3. Monitor CBC, hemoglobin, uric acid, renal, LFTs. May cause granulocyte and platelet suppression. Nadir: 14 days; recovery: 21–28 days.
4. Discontinue if any CNS S&S (paresthesias, neuropathies, seizures) occur, if stomatitis or diarrhea with frequent bowel movements or watery stools occur, or if there is hemorrhage or bleeding tendencies.

CLIENT/FAMILY TEACHING

1. Consult provider before taking any other medication because procarbazine has MAO inhibitory activity. Avoid sympathomimetic drugs and foods with a high tyramine content (yeasts, yogurt, caffeine, chocolate, aged cheese, liver, smoked or pickled fish, fermented sausage, etc.) during and for 2 weeks after completing therapy; may precipitate a hypertensive crisis.
2. Do not drive or perform tasks that require mental alertness until drug effects realized.
3. Consume adequate fluids (2–3 L/day) to prevent dehydration.
4. Drug increases effect of insulin and oral hypoglycemic agents; report symptoms as medication adjustment may be necessary.
5. Avoid exposure to sun or to ultraviolet rays because a photosensitive skin reaction may occur. Wear sunscreen, sunglasses, and protective clothing if exposure is necessary.
6. Avoid alcohol; a disulfiram-type reaction may occur.
7. Practice reliable contraception.
8. Avoid crowds and persons with known infections.
9. Report fever, rash, chills, SOB, abnormal bruising/bleeding, persistent constipation (esp if diet, increased fluids, and bulk are ineffective); laxatives may be needed.

OUTCOMES/EVALUATE

Suppression of malignant cell proliferation

P

Prochlorperazine 〔IV〕ⓒ

(proh-klor-**PAIR**-ah-zeen)

CLASSIFICATION(S):

Antipsychotic, phenothiazine

PREGNANCY CATEGORY: C

Rx: Compazine, Compro Suppositories.

✤**Rx:** Stemetil Suppositories.

Prochlorperazine edisylate

PREGNANCY CATEGORY: C

Rx: Compazine.

Prochlorperazine maleate

PREGNANCY CATEGORY: C

Rx: Compazine.

✤**Rx:** Apo-Prochlorazine.

SEE ALSO *ANTIPSYCHOTIC AGENTS, PHENOTHIAZINES.*

USES

(1) Schizophrenia. (2) Short-term treatment of generalized nonpsychotic anxiety (not drug of choice). (3) Severe N&V. *Investigational:* Migraine headache.

ACTION/KINETICS

Action

Prochlorperazine causes a high incidence of extrapyramidal and antiemetic effects, moderate sedative effects, and a low incidence of anticholinergic effects and orthostatic hypotension.

Pharmacokinetics

t½: 3.5 hr after PO and 6.9 hr after IV.

CONTRAINDICATIONS

Use in clients who weigh less than 44 kg or who are under 2 years of age.

SPECIAL CONCERNS

Safe use during pregnancy has not been established. Geriatric, emaciated, and debilitated clients usually require a lower initial dose.

SIDE EFFECTS

Most Common

Drowsiness, dizziness, amenorrhea, blurred vision, skin reactions, hypotension, extrapyramidal reactions.

See *Antipsychotic Agents, Phenothiazines* for a complete list of possible side effects.

HOW SUPPLIED

Prochlorperazine: *Suppositories:* 2.5 mg, 5 mg, 25 mg.

Prochlorperazine edisylate: *Injection:* 5 mg/mL; *Syrup:* 5 mg/5 mL.

Prochlorperazine maleate: *Capsules, Sustained-Release:* 30 mg; *Tablets:* 5 mg, 10 mg, 25 mg.

DOSAGE

• **EDISYLATE SYRUP; MALEATE SUSTAINED-RELEASE CAPSULES; MALEATE TABLETS**

Schizophrenia.

Adults and adolescents: 5 or 10 mg 3 or 4 times per day for mild conditions. For moderate to severe conditions, for hospitalized, or adequately supervised clients: 10 mg 3 or 4 times per day. Dose can be increased gradually q 2–3 days as needed and tolerated. For extended-release capsules, up to 100–150 mg/day can be given for severe conditions. **Pediatric, 2–12 years:** 2.5 mg 2–3 times per day. Do not give more than 10 mg on the first day. For children, aged 2–5 years, the usual daily dose does not exceed 20 mg; for children, aged 6–12 years, the usual daily dose does not exceed 25 mg.

Anxiety, nonpsychotic.

Adults and adolescents: 5 mg 3–4 times per day on arising. Or, 15 mg sustained release on arising or 10 mg sustained release q 12 hr. Do not give more than 20 mg/day for more than 12 weeks. Do not use in pediatric clients under 20 lb or under 2 years old.

N&V.

Adults and adolescents: 5–10 mg 3–4 times per day (up to 40 mg/day). For extended-release capsules, the dose is 15–30 mg once daily in the morning (or 10 mg q 12 hr, up to 40 mg/day). **Pediatric, 18–39 kg:** 2.5 mg (base) 3 times per day (or 5 mg twice a day), not to exceed 15 mg/day; **14–17 kg:** 2.5 mg

---

Bold Italic = life threatening side effect   ▮ = black box warning   ✤ = Available in Canada

(base) 2–3 times per day, not to exceed 10 mg/day; **9–13 kg:** 2.5 mg (base) 1–2 times per day, not to exceed 7.5 mg/day. The total daily dose for children should not exceed 10 mg the first day; on subsequent days, the total daily dose should not exceed 20 mg for children 2–5 years of age or 25 mg for children 6–12 years of age.

- **IM, EDISYLATE INJECTION**
  Psychotic disorders, for immediate control of severely disturbed clients.
Adults and adolescents, initial: 10–20 mg; dose can be repeated q 2–4 hr as needed (usually up to three or four doses). If prolonged therapy is needed: 10–20 mg q 4–6 hr. **Children, less than 12 years of age:** 0.03 mg/kg by deep IM injection. After control is achieved (usually after 1 injection), switch to PO at same dosage level or higher.
  N&V.
Adults and adolescents: 5–10 mg; repeat the dose q 3–4 hr as needed, not to exceed 40 mg/day. **Pediatric, 2–12 years:** 0.132 mg/kg by deep IM.
  N&V during surgery.
Adults and adolescents: 5–10 mg (base) given 1–2 hr before induction of anesthesia; may be repeated once in 30 min. Also, to control acute symptoms during and after surgery (may repeat once).

- **RECTAL SUPPOSITORY**
Adults: 25 mg twice a day. **Pediatric, 2–12 years:** 2.5 mg 2–3 times per day with no more than 10 mg given on the first day. Then no more than 20 mg/day for children 2–5 years of age and 25 mg/day for children 6–12 years of age.

- **IV**
  Severe N&V.
Injection: 5–10 mg, 15–30 min before induction of anesthesia, or to control symptoms during or after surgery. Repeat once if needed. Do not exceed 5 mg/mL/min. Do not use bolus injection.
Infusion: 20 mg/L of isotonic solution.

NURSING CONSIDERATIONS

𝒞 Do not confuse prochlorperazine with chlorpromazine or promethazine, both of which are also antipsychotics.

ADMINISTRATION/STORAGE

1. Use doses in the lower range for the elderly, as they are more susceptible to hypotension and neuromuscular reactions.
2. Store all forms of the drug in tight-closing amber-colored bottles; store suppositories below 37°C (98.6°F).
3. Due to local irritation, do not give SC.
4. Do not mix with other agents in a syringe.
5. Do not dilute with any material containing the preservative parabens.
6. When given IM to children for N&V, the duration of action may be 12 hr.
7. Parenteral prescribing limits are 20 mg/day for children 2–5 years of age and 25 mg/day for children 6–12 years of age.

ASSESSMENT

1. Note reasons for therapy, onset/characteristics of S&S, clinical presentation, any triggers evident.
2. Assess mental status; note behavioral presentation/manifestations.
3. Monitor CBC, LFTs, ECG.

INTERVENTIONS

1. Monitor I&O and VS. Auscultate bowel sounds; assess function.
2. Incorporate safety precautions during treatment of overdose. If taking spansules, continue treatment until all signs of overdosage are no longer evident. Saline laxatives may hasten the evacuation of pellets that have not yet released their medication.

CLIENT/FAMILY TEACHING

1. Do not exceed prescribed dose. Avoid skin contact with solution. Do not crush or chew sustained release tablets.
2. Withhold drug and report if child shows signs of restlessness and excitement. Report symptoms of extrapyramidal effects and tardive dyskinesia (tremor, involuntary twitching).
3. Do not drive or operate machinery until drug effects are realized; drowsiness or dizziness may occur.
4. Consume adequate fluids to prevent dehydration; use precautions in hot weather. When in the sun, use protection to prevent photosensitivity reaction. Avoid high temperature expo-

P

---

sures; may precipitate heat stroke. Urine may be pink to reddish-brown.
5. Rise and change positions slowly to prevent low BP effects.
6. Report adverse side effects, fever, sore throat, rashes, tremors, dark urine, pale stools, impaired vision, or lack of response.

OUTCOMES/EVALUATE
- Control of N&V
- Reduction in agitation, excitability, withdrawn behaviors

Progesterone gel
(pro-**JES**-ter-ohn)

CLASSIFICATION(S):
Progesterone
Rx: Crinone, Prochieve.

SEE ALSO PROGESTERONE AND PROGESTINS

USES
(1) Progesterone supplementation or replacement as part of assisted reproductive technology treatment for infertile women with progesterone deficiency. (2) Secondary amenorrhea. The 4% gel is to treat secondary amenorrhea and the 8% gel is for women who have failed to respond to treatment with the 4% gel.

ACTION/KINETICS
Pharmacokinetics t½, **absorption:** 25–50 hr. t½, **elimination:** 5–20 min. Metabolized in liver; excreted through urine and feces. **Plasma protein binding:** Extensively bound.

CONTRAINDICATIONS
Undiagnosed vaginal bleeding, liver disease or dysfunction, known or suspected malignancy of breast or genital organs, missed abortion, active thrombophlebitis or thromboembolic disease (or history of such). Concurrent use with other local intravaginal therapy.

SPECIAL CONCERNS
See *Progesterone and Progestins.* Safety and efficacy have not been determined in children.

SIDE EFFECTS
Most Common
Breast enlargement, somnolence, constipation, nausea, headache, perineal pain, nervousness, depression, abdominal pain, decreased libido.
See *Progesterone and Progestins* for a complete list of possible side effects.

HOW SUPPLIED
Vaginal Gel/Jelly: 45 mg/1.125 grams (Crinone 4%, Prochieve 4%), 90 mg/ 1.125 grams (Crinone 8%, Prochieve 8%).

DOSAGE
CRINONE 8% OR PROCHIEVE 8%
- VAGINAL GEL/JELLY
  Assisted reproductive technology.
90 mg once daily for women who require progesterone supplementation. Administer 90 mg twice a day in women with partial or complete ovarian failure who require progesterone replacement. If pregnancy occurs, treatment may be continued until placental autonomy has been achieved (up to 10–12 weeks).
CRINONE 4% OR PROCHIEVE 4%
- VAGINAL GEL/JELLY
  Secondary amenorrhea.
45 mg every other day up to total of 6 doses. For women who fail to respond, the 8% gel (90 mg) may be given every other day up to total of 6 doses.

NURSING CONSIDERATIONS
ADMINISTRATION/STORAGE
1. Dosage increase from 4% gel can only be accomplished by using 8% gel. Increasing volume of gel does not increase amount absorbed.
2. If other local intravaginal therapy is to be used, wait at least 6 hr before or after Crinone administration.
3. Store at controlled room temperature below 25°C (77°F).

ASSESSMENT
1. Note reasons for therapy, physical and gynecologic findings.
2. Assess for liver disease, breast or genital malignancy, undiagnosed vaginal bleeding, or history of thromboembolic disease; precludes drug therapy.

CLIENT/FAMILY TEACHING

1. Review product information sheet on how to use product; use only as directed.

2. Do not use with other intravaginal products; if concurrent therapy prescribed, wait for 6 hr.

3. May experience breast enlargement, constipation, headaches, sleepiness, and perineal pain.

4. Report any adverse symptoms, lack of desired response, or depression.

OUTCOMES/EVALUATE

Progesterone replacement/supplementation

Promethazine hydrochloride ■ IV ©

(proh-METH-ah-zeen)

CLASSIFICATION(S):

Antihistamine, first generation, phenothiazine

PREGNANCY CATEGORY: C

Rx: Phenadoz, Phenergen.

SEE ALSO *ANTIHISTAMINES* AND *ANTIEMETICS*.

USES

PO, Rectal. (1) Perennial and seasonal allergic rhinitis; vasomotor rhinitis. (2) Allergic conjunctivitis due to inhalant allergens and foods. (3) Mild, uncomplicated allergic skin manifestations of urticaria and angioedema. (4) Relief of allergic reactions to blood or plasma. (5) Dermatographism. (6) Adjunct to epinephrine and other measures to treat anaphylactic reactions after acute symptoms have been controlled. (7) Preoperative, postoperative, or obstetric sedation. (8) Prevention and control of N&V associated with certain types of anesthesia and surgery. (9) Adjunct to meperidine or other analgesics to control postoperative pain. (10) Sedation in both children and adults. (11) Relief of apprehension and production of light sleep from which the client can be easily aroused. (12) Active and prophylactic treatment of motion sickness. (13) Antiemetic in postoperative clients.

Parenteral. (1) Adjunct to control postoperative pain. (2) Prevention and control of N&V associated with certain types of anesthesia and surgery and in postoperative clients. (3) Type I hypersensitivity reactions, including perennial and seasonal allergic rhinitis; vasomotor rhinitis; allergic conjunctivitis due to inhalant allergens and foods; mild, uncomplicated allergic skin reactions of urticaria and angioedema; amelioration of allergic reactions due to blood or plasma; dermatographism; adjunctive anaphylactic therapy. (4) Preoperative, postoperative, or obstetric sedation. (5) Relief of apprehension and production of light sleep. Use parenteral therapy when PO therapy is impossible or contraindicated.

ACTION/KINETICS

Action

Antiemetic effects are likely due to inhibition of the CTZ. Effective in vertigo by its central anticholinergic effect which inhibits the vestibular apparatus and the integrative vomiting center as well as the CTZ. May cause severe drowsiness. Significant anticholinergic and antiemetic effects.

Pharmacokinetics

Onset, PO, IM, PR: 20 min; **IV:** 3–5 min. **Duration, antihistaminic:** 6–12 hr; **sedative:** 2–8 hr. Slowly eliminated through urine and feces.

CONTRAINDICATIONS

Lactation. Comatose clients, CNS depression due to drugs (including barbituates, general anesthetics, tranquilizers, alcohol, narcotics), previous phenothiazine idiosyncrasy or hypersensitivity, acutely ill or dehydrated children (due to greater susceptibility to dystonias). Children up to 2 years of age. Treatment of uncomplicated vomiting in children. Use in children whose signs and symptoms may suggest Reye's syndrome or other hepatic diseases. SC or intra-arterial use due to tissue necrosis and gangrene. Use in the treatment of lower respiratory tract symptoms, including asthma.

SPECIAL CONCERNS

■ (1) Do not use promethazine in children younger than 2 years of age be-

---

cause of the potential for fatal respiratory depression. (2) Postmarketing cases of respiratory depression, including fatalities, have been reported with use of promethazine in children younger than 2 years of age. A wide range of weight-based doses of promethazine have resulted in respiratory depression in these clients. (3) Exercise caution when administering promethazine to children 2 years of age and older. It is recommended that the lowest effective dose of promethazine be used in children 2 years of age and older and that concomitant administration of other drugs with respiratory depressant effects should be avoided.■ Safe use during pregnancy has not been established. Use in children may cause paradoxical hyperexcitability and nightmares. Geriatric clients are more likely to experience confusion, dizziness, hypotension, and sedation. The extrapyramidal symptoms that can occur following promethazine use may be confused with the CNS signs of undiagnosed primary diseases such as encephalopathy or Reye's syndrome.

SIDE EFFECTS

Most Common
Drowsiness, dizziness, confusion, blurred vision, dry mouth, tinnitus, N&V, photosensitivity.

CNS: Drowsiness, sedation, somnolence, dizziness, confusion, disorientation, extrapyramidal symptoms, lassitude, incoordination, fatigue, euphoria, nervousness, insomnia, tremors, *seizures,* excitation, catatonic-like states, hysteria, hallucinations. **CV:** Increased or decreased BP, tachycardia, bradycardia, faintness. **GI:** Dry mouth, N&V, jaundice. **Dermatologic:** Dermatitis, photosensitivity, urticaria. **Hematologic:** Leukopenia, thrombocytopenia, thrombocytopenic purpura, *agranulocytosis*. **Respiratory:** Asthma, nasal stuffiness, *respiratory depression*, *apnea*. **Ophthalmic:** Blurred vision, diplopia. **Miscellaneous:** Tinnitus, angioneurotic edema, *neuroleptic malignant syndrome*, hyperexcitability, abnormal movements.

HOW SUPPLIED

Injection: 25 mg/mL, 50 mg/mL (IM only); *Suppositories:* 12.5 mg, 25 mg, 50 mg; *Syrup:* 6.25 mg/5 mL; *Tablets:* 12.5 mg, 25 mg, 50 mg.

DOSAGE

- **SUPPOSITORIES; SYRUP; TABLETS**
  Allergies.

Adults and children over 2 years of age: 25 mg at bedtime (usual dose); 12.5 mg before meals and at bedtime may be given, if needed. Single 25 mg doses at bedtime or 6.25–12.5 mg taken 3 times per day will usually suffice. Adjust dose to the smallest amount needed to relieve symptoms. If given rectally, resume PO administration as soon as possible if continued therapy is needed.
  Sedation.

Adults: 25–50 mg at bedtime. **Children, over 2 years of age:** 12.5–25 mg at bedtime. *NOTE:* If used for preoperative sedation, give the night before surgery to relieve apprehension and to produce quiet sleep.
  Antiemetic.

Adults: 25 mg (usual dose); doses of 12.5–25 mg may be repeated q 4–6 hr as needed for prophylaxis or treatment of active N&V. **Children, over 2 years of age:** 25 mg or 0.5 mg/lb (usual dose); doses of 12.5–25 mg may be repeated q 4–6 hr as needed for prophylaxis and treatment of active N&V. Adjust dose to the age, weight, and severity of the condition of the client. Limit use to prolonged vomiting of known etiology.
  Motion sickness.

Adults: 25 mg twice a day (usual dose); take first dose 30–60 min before anticipated travel. Repeat 8–12 hr later if needed. On successive travel days, take 25 mg on rising and again before the evening meal. **Children, over 2 years of age:** 12.5–25 mg twice a day.
  Pre- and postoperative use.

Adults: 50 mg preoperatively given with an appropriately reduced dose of narcotic or barbiturate and the required amount of an atropine-like drug. Give 25–50 mg for postoperative sedation and adjunctive use with analgesics. **Children, over 2 years of age:** 0.5 mg/

---

lb (1.2 mg/kg) preoperatively in combination with an appropriately reduced dose of narcotic or barbiturate and the appropriate dose of an atropine-like drug. Give 12.5–25 mg for postoperative sedation and adjunctive use with analgesics. To produce quiet sleep and to relieve apprehension, give 12.5–25 mg the night before surgery.

- **IM (PREFERRED); IV**
  Hypersensitivity reactions, Type I.
  Adults: 25 mg; may repeat dose within 2 hr, if needed. Resume PO therapy as soon as possible. **Children, 2 years and older:** Do not exceed one-half the adult dose.

  Sedation.
  Adults: 25–50 mg at bedtime for night-time sedation. Doses of 50 mg provide sedation and relieve apprehension during early stages of labor. When labor is definitely established, may give 25–75 mg (usual is 50 mg) IM or IV with an appropriately reduced dose of any desired narcotic. If needed, promethazine with a reduced dose of analgesic may be repeated once or twice at 4-hr intervals, not to exceed 100 mg/24 hr for clients in labor. **Children, 2–12 years of age:** Do not exceed one-half the adult dose.

  Antiemetic.
  Adults: 12.5–25 mg; may repeat q 4 hr as needed. If used postoperatively, reduce dose of concomitant analgesics or barbiturate accordingly. **Children, 2–12 years of age:** Do not exceed one-half the adult dose. Do not use when etiology of vomiting is unknown.

  Pre- and postoperative use.
  Adults: 25–50 mg in combination with an appropriately reduced dose of analgesics, hypnotics, and atropine-like drugs. **Children, 2–12 years of age:** 0.5 mg/lb (1.2 mg/kg) in combination with appropriately reduced doses of narcotic or barbiturate and atropine-like drugs.

NURSING CONSIDERATIONS

Ⓒ Do not confuse promethazine with chlorpromazine or with prochlorperazine, both of which are antipsychotics.

ADMINISTRATION/STORAGE

1. The extrapyramidal symptoms that can occur secondary to promethazine administration may be confused with the CNS signs of undiagnosed primary disease (e.g., encephalopathy, Reye syndrome). Avoid promethazine in such situations.
2. Decrease dosage in dehydrated or oliguric clients.
3. Store tablets at controlled room temperature from 20–25°C (68–77°F). Protect from light and dispense in a tight, light-resistant container.
4. Store syrup at controlled room temperature from 15–25°C (59–77°F).
5. Refrigerate suppositories between 2–8°C (36–46°F). Dispense in well-closed container.
6. Store injection at controlled room temperature from 20–25°C (68–77°F). Protect from light. Keep covered in carton until used. Do not use if solution has developed color or contains a precipitate.
7. Ampules may contain sulfite. Inject IM deep into large muscle mass rotating sites. Not for SC or intra-arterial administration; may cause tissue necrosis.
ⅣⅤ 8. If given correctly, IV doses are well tolerated; however IV use is associated with increased risks. Do not exceed a concentration of 25 mg/mL at a rate of greater than 25 mg/min.

ASSESSMENT

1. List reasons for therapy, onset/characteristics of S&S, triggers, other agents trialed.
2. Note age; avoid in those under 2 years of age; older clients may manifest more adverse side effects. Assess for respiratory depression and level of sedation following dosing.
3. May experience tremors, drooling, shuffling gait, dysphagia (parkinsonism like effects); restlessness (akathisia) or muscle spasms and twisting like motions (dystonia). Hold drug and report if any of these S&S become evident.
4. With chronic therapy, may experience blood dyscrasias; monitor CBC.
5. Stop drug 48 hr prior to scheduled myelogram and do not resume for 24

---

hr following procedure or may risk seizure activity.

6. When used as adjunct to analgesics be aware it has no analgesic ability only sedative effects; which may be pronounced.

CLIENT/FAMILY TEACHING

1. Take only as directed and do not exceed dose; cardiac arrhythmias may occur. May take with food or milk to decrease GI upset.

2. When used to prevent motion sickness, take 30–60 min before travel. On successive travel days, take on rising and again before the evening meal.

3. Avoid activities requiring mental alertness until drug effects realized; may cause sedation.

4. Do not consume alcohol. CNS depressants, or OTC agents unless provider approved.

5. Drug may alter skin testing; stop 72 hr before testing.

6. Consume adequate fluids to prevent dehydration; use caution in hot weather to prevent heat stroke.

7. Avoid prolonged sun exposure; may cause photosensitivity reaction. Wear sunscreen and protection if exposed.

8. Report any involuntary muscle movements. Keep all F/U appointments.

OUTCOMES/EVALUATE

- Prevention of vertigo/motion sickness
- Relief of N&V
- Sedation
- Control of allergic manifestations

Propafenone hydrochloride

(proh-pah-**FEN**-ohn)

CLASSIFICATION(S):
Antiarrhythmic, Class IC
PREGNANCY CATEGORY: C
Rx: Rythmol, Rythmol SR.
✣Rx: Apo-Propafenone.

USES

Immediate-Release. (1) Prolong the time to recurrence of paroxysmal atrial fibrillation/flutter associated with disabling symptoms in clients without structural heart disease. (2) To prolong the time to recurrence of paroxysmal supraventricular tachycardia associated with disabling symptoms in clients without structural heart disease. (3) Treatment of ventricular arrhythmias, such as sustained ventricular tachycardia, that are life-threatening.

Extended-Release. Prolong the time to recurrence of symptomatic atrial fibrillation in clients without structural heart disease. *NOTE:* Antiarrhythmic drugs have not been shown to improve survival in clients with ventricular arrhythmias.

Investigational: Arrhythmias associated with Wolff-Parkinson-White syndrome.

ACTION/KINETICS

Action

Manifests local anesthetic effects and a direct stabilizing action on the myocardium. Reduces upstroke velocity (Phase O) of the monophasic action potential, reduces the fast inward current carried by sodium ions in the Purkinje fibers, increases diastolic excitability threshold, and prolongs the effective refractory period. Also, spontaneous activity is decreased. Slows AV conduction and causes first-degree heart block. Has slight beta-adrenergic blocking activity.

Pharmacokinetics

Almost completely absorbed after PO administration. **Peak plasma levels:** 3.5 hr. **Therapeutic serum levels:** 0.06–1 mcg/mL. Significant first-pass effect. Most metabolize rapidly ($t^{1/2}$: 2–10 hr) to two active metabolites: 5-hydroxypropafenone and N-depropylpropafenone. However, approximately 10% (as well as those taking quinidine) metabolize the drug more slowly ($t^{1/2}$: 10–32 hr). Less than 1% excreted unchanged. Because the 5-hydroxy metabolite is not formed in slow metabolizers and because steady-state levels are reached after 4–5 days in all clients, the recommended

---

dosing regimen is the same for all clients. **Plasma protein binding:** 97%.

CONTRAINDICATIONS

Uncontrolled CHF, cardiogenic shock, sick sinus node syndrome or AV block in the absence of an artificial pacemaker, bradycardia, marked hypotension, bronchospastic disorders, electrolyte disorders, hypersensitivity to the drug. MI more than 6 days but less than 2 years previously. Use to control ventricular rate during atrial fibrillation. Use with lesser ventricular arrhythmias, even if clients are symptomatic. Lactation.

SPECIAL CONCERNS

■ The National Heart, Lung, and Blood Institute's Cardiac Arrhythmia Suppression Trial (CAST) reported that in clients with asymptomatic non-life-threatening ventricular arrhythmias who had an MI more than 6 days but less than 2 years previously, an increased rate of death or reversed cardiac arrest rate was seen in clients treated with encainide or flecainide (Class 1C antiarrhythmics) compared with that seen in those receiving a placebo. The applicability of the CAST results to other populations (e.g., those without recent MI) or other antiarrhythmic drugs is uncertain, but at present, it is prudent to consider any 1C antiarrhythmic to have a significant risk in clients with structural heart disease. Given the lack of any evidence that these drugs improve survival, antiarrhythmic drugs should generally be avoided in those with non-life-threatening ventricular arrhythmias, even if the clients are experiencing unpleasant, but not life-threatening symptoms or signs.■ May cause new or worsened arrhythmias or CHF. Use with caution during labor and delivery. Safety and effectiveness have not been determined in children. Use with caution in clients with impaired hepatic or renal function. Geriatric clients may require lower dosage. Monitor clients taking propafenone and an inhibitor of CYP1A2, CYP2D6, or CYP3A4 metabolizing enzymes; dosage adjustment may be necessary.

SIDE EFFECTS
Most Common

Dizziness, N&V, unusual taste, constipation, blurred vision, angina, CHF, palpitations, proarrhythmia, fatigue, headache, dyspnea, rash, weakness.

CV: *New or worsened arrhythmias*. First-degree AV block, intraventricular conduction delay, palpitations, PVCs, proarrhythmia, bradycardia, atrial fibrillation, angina, syncope, CHF, ***ventricular tachycardia, second-degree AV block***, increased QRS duration, chest pain, hypotension, bundle branch block. Less commonly, atrial flutter, AV dissociation, flushing, hot flashes, sick sinus syndrome, sinus pause or arrest, SVT, prolongation of the PR and QRS interval, ***cardiac arrest***. **CNS:** Dizziness, headache, anxiety, drowsiness, fatigue, loss of balance, ataxia, insomnia. Less commonly, abnormal speech/dreams/vision, confusion, depression, memory loss, ***apnea***, psychosis/mania, vertigo, ***seizures, coma***, numbness, paresthesias. **GI:** Unusual taste, constipation, nausea and/or vomiting, dry mouth, anorexia, flatulence, abdominal pain, cramps, diarrhea, dyspepsia. Less commonly, gastroenteritis and liver abnormalities (cholestasis, hepatitis, elevated enzymes). **Hematologic: *Agranulocytosis***, increased bleeding time, anemia, granulocytopenia, bruising, leukopenia, purpura, thrombocytopenia. **Miscellaneous:** Blurred vision, dyspnea, weakness, rash, edema, tremors, diaphoresis, joint pain, possible decrease in spermatogenesis. Less commonly, tinnitus, unusual smell sensation, alopecia, eye irritation, hyponatremia, inappropriate ADH secretion, impotence, increased glucose, kidney failure, lupus erythematosus, muscle cramps or weakness, nephrotic syndrome, pain, pruritus, exacerbation of myasthenia gravis.

LABORATORY TEST CONSIDERATIONS
↑ ANA titers, alkaline phosphatase, AST, ALT.

OD OVERDOSE MANAGEMENT

Symptoms: Bradycardia, hypotension, IA and intraventricular conduction disturbances, somnolence. ***Rarely, high-grade ventricular arrhythmias and sei-***

---

zures. *Treatment:* To control BP and cardiac rhythm, defibrillation and infusion of dopamine or isoproterenol. If seizures occur, diazepam, IV, can be given. External cardiac massage and mechanical respiratory assistance may be required.

DRUG INTERACTIONS
Drugs that inhibit CYP2D6, CYP1A2, and CYP3A4 may lead to increased plasma levels of propafenone; monitor such situations carefully.

Beta-adrenergic blockers / ↑ Levels of beta blockers metabolized by the liver
Cimetidine / ↓ Propafenone levels → ↑ effects
Cyclosporine / ↑ Cyclosporine trough levels; ↓ renal function
Desipramine / ↑ Desipramine levels
Digoxin / ↑ Digoxin levels → ↓ digoxin dose
Local anesthetics / May ↑ risk of CNS side effects
Mexiletine / ↓ Metabolic clearance of mexiletine in extensive metabolizers → no differences between extensive and poor metabolizers
Quinidine / ↑ Propafenone levels in rapid metabolizers → possible ↑ effect
Rifamycins / ↓ Propafenone effect R/T ↑ clearance
Ritonavir / Large ↑ in propafenone levels; do not use together
SSRIs / Certain SSRIs may inhibit the metabolism (by CYP2D6) of propafenone
Theophylline / ↑ Theophylline levels → possible toxicity
Warfarin / May ↑ warfarin levels; ↓ warfarin dose

HOW SUPPLIED
Capsules, Extended-Release: 225 mg, 325 mg, 425 mg; *Tablets, Immediate-Release:* 150 mg, 225 mg, 300 mg.

DOSAGE
- **CAPSULES, EXTENDED-RELEASE**
  Sympatomatic atrial fibrillation without structural heart disease.
  Individualize dosage based on response and tolerance. **Initial:** 225 mg q 12 hr; increase in 5 day or more intervals to 325 mg q 12 hr. Increase to 425 mg q 12 hr if needed.
- **TABLETS, IMMEDIATE-RELEASE**

Titrate on basis of response and tolerance. **Adults, initial:** 150 mg q 8 hr; dose may be increased at a minimum of q 3–4 days to 225 mg q 8 hr and, if necessary, to 300 mg q 8 hr. The safety and efficacy of doses exceeding 900 mg/day have not been established.

NURSING CONSIDERATIONS
ADMINISTRATION/STORAGE
1. Always initiate therapy in a hospital setting.
2. Consider dose reduction in those in whom significant widening of the QRS complex or second- or third-degree AV block occurs. Consider dose reduction in those with hepatic impairment.
3. Increase the dose of the immediate-release tablets more gradually during the initial treatment phase in the elderly or in those with marked previous myocardial damage.
4. There is no evidence that the use of propafenone affects the survival or incidence of sudden death with recent MI or SVT.

ASSESSMENT
1. List reasons for therapy noting ECG and baseline arrhythmias; note any cardiac problems, list drugs prescribed.
2. Monitor CBC, lytes, renal, LFTs. Assess for renal or hepatic disease.
3. Report any significant widening of the QRS complex, any evidence of second- or third-degree AV block. May induce new or more severe arrhythmias; titrate dose based on client response and tolerance.
4. Increase dose more gradually in elderly clients as well as those with previous myocardial damage.
5. Evaluate hematologic studies for anemia, agranulocytosis, leukopenia, thrombocytopenia, altered prothrombin and coagulation times.

CLIENT/FAMILY TEACHING
1. Drink adequate quantities of fluid (2–3 L/day) and add bulk to the diet to avoid constipation.
2. The sustained-release capsules can be taken with or without food. Do not crush or further divide the contents of the capsule.

Bold Italic = life threatening side effect   ■ = black box warning   ♣ = Available in Canada

3. May experience dizziness or unusual taste in the mouth; report if interferes with walking, eating, or nutritional status.

4. Report increased chest pain, SOB, blurred vision, palpitations, unusual bruising/bleeding, or S&S of liver failure such as yellow eyes, dark-yellow urine, or yellow skin.

5. Report any urinary tract problems, decreased urinary output, or adverse side effects.

6. Record BP and pulse readings for provider review.

OUTCOMES/EVALUATE

- Termination of life-threatening VT; restoration of stable rhythm
- Therapeutic drug levels (0.5–3 mcg/mL)

Propoxyphene hydrochloride
(proh-**POX**-ih-feen)

CLASSIFICATION(S):
Narcotic analgesic
PREGNANCY CATEGORY: C
Rx: Darvon Pulvules, **C-IV**
✤**Rx:** 642 Tablets.

Propoxyphene napsylate
PREGNANCY CATEGORY: C
Rx: Darvon-N, **C-IV**

USES
Relief of mild to moderate pain. *Investigational:* Suppress the withdrawal syndrome from narcotics (napsylate).

ACTION/KINETICS
Action
Resembles narcotics with respect to its mechanism and analgesic effect; it is one-half to one-third as potent as codeine. Is devoid of antitussive, anti-inflammatory, or antipyretic activity. When taken in excessive doses for long periods, psychologic dependence and occasionally physical dependence and tolerance will be manifested.

Pharmacokinetics
Peak plasma levels: Hydrochloride: 2–2.5 hr; **Napsylate:** 3–4 hr. **Analgesic onset:** 30–60 min. **Peak analgesic effect:** 2–2.5 hr. **Duration:** 4–6 hr. **Therapeutic serum levels:** 0.05–0.12 mcg/mL. **t½, propoxyphene:** 6–12 hr; **norpropoxyphene:** 30–36 hr. Extensive first-pass effect; metabolites are excreted in the urine.

CONTRAINDICATIONS
Hypersensitivity to drug. Use in children or in those who are suicidal or addiction-prone.

SPECIAL CONCERNS
■ (1) Do not prescribe propoxyphene for clients who are suicidal or addiction prone. (2) Prescribe with caution for clients taking tranquilizers or antidepressants and for those who use alcohol in excess. (3) Tell clients not to exceed the recommended dose and to limit alcohol intake. (4) Propoxyphene products in excessive doses, either alone or in combination with other CNS depressants (including alcohol), are a major cause of drug-related deaths. Fatalities within the first hour of overdosage are common. In a survey of deaths due to overdosage conducted in 1975, in approximately 20% of fatal cases, death occurred within the first hour (5% within 15 minutes). Propoxyphene should not be taken in higher doses than those recommended by the health care provider. (5) Judicious prescribing is essential for safety. Consider nonnarcotic analgesics for depressed or suicidal clients. (6) Caution clients about the concomitant use of propoxyphene products and alcohol because of potentially fatal CNS additive effects of these agents. Because of added CNS depressant effects, cautiously prescribe with concomitant sedatives, tranquilizers, muscle relaxants, antidepressants, or other CNS-depressant drugs. Advise clients of the additive depressant effects of such combinations. (7) Many propoxyphene-related deaths have occurred in those with histories of emotional disturbances, suicidal ideation or attempts, or misuse of tranquilizers, alcohol, and other CNS-active drugs.

P

Deaths have occurred as a consequence of the accidental ingestion of excessive quantities of propoxyphene alone or in combination with other drugs. Do not exceed the recommended dosage.■ Safe use during pregnancy has not been established. Use with caution during lactation and in those taking tranquilizers, antidepressants, and who use excess alcohol.

SIDE EFFECTS

Most Common

Dizziness, dysphoria, euphoria, hallucinations, headache, lightheadedness, somnolence, weakness, rash, abdominal pain, constipation, N&V.

GI: N&V, constipation, abdominal pain. **CNS:** Sedation, somnolence, dizziness, lightheadedness, headache, weakness, euphoria, dysphoria, hallucinations. **Miscellaneous:** Skin rashes, visual disturbances, weakness. Propoxyphene can produce psychologic dependence, as well as physical dependence and tolerance.

OD **OVERDOSE MANAGEMENT**

Symptoms: Stupor, respiratory depression, **apnea,** hypotension, pulmonary edema, **circulatory collapse, cardiac arrhythmias,** conduction abnormalities, **coma, seizures,** respiratory-metabolic acidosis. *Treatment:* Maintain an adequate airway, artificial respiration, and naloxone, 0.4–2 mg IV (repeat at 2- to 3-min intervals) to combat respiratory depression. Gastric lavage or administration of activated charcoal may be helpful. Correct acidosis and electrolyte imbalance. Acidosis due to lactic acid may require IV sodium bicarbonate.

DRUG INTERACTIONS

Alcohol, antianxiety drugs, antipsychotic agents, narcotics, sedative-hypnotics / Concomitant use → drowsiness, lethargy, stupor, respiratory depression, and coma

Carbamazepine / ↑ Carbamazepine effects R/T ↓ liver breakdown

Charcoal / ↓ Propoxyphene absorption from GI tract

CNS depressants / Additive CNS depression

Orphenadrine / Concomitant use → confusion, anxiety, and tremors

Phenobarbital / ↑ Phenobarbital effects R/T ↓ liver breakdown

Protease inhibitors / Do not use together

Skeletal muscle relaxants / Additive respiratory depression

Smoking / ↓ Propoxyphene analgesia and side effects R/T ↑ hepatic metabolism; smokers may need a higher dose

Warfarin / ↑ Warfarin hypoprothrombinemic effects

HOW SUPPLIED

Hydrochloride: *Capsules:* 65 mg. **Napsylate:** *Tablets:* 100 mg.

DOSAGE

HYDROCHLORIDE

• **CAPSULES**

  Analgesia.

Adults: 65 mg q 4 hr, not to exceed 390 mg/day.

NAPSYLATE

• **TABLETS**

  Analgesia.

Adults: 100 mg q 4 hr, not to exceed 600 mg/day.

NURSING CONSIDERATIONS

☙ Do not confuse Darvon-N with Darvocet (combination analgesic that contains propoxyphene and acetaminophen).

ADMINISTRATION/STORAGE

1. Because of differences in molecular weight, 100 mg of propoxyphene napsylate is required to supply the propoxyphene equivalent of 65 mg of the hydrochloride.

2. Consider a reduced total daily dose in those with hepatic or renal impairment.

3. Consider an increased dosing interval in the elderly due to reduced metabolic rate.

4. Store from 15–30°C (59–86°F).

ASSESSMENT

1. Note reasons for therapy, onset, duration, pain characteristics. Use a pain-rating scale to assess pain. List other agents prescribed, outcome.

2. Assess for opiate or alcohol dependency. Use with caution in elderly; review drug profile to ensure other prescribed agents do not cause additive CNS effects.

Bold Italic = life threatening side effect ■ = black box warning ♣ = Available in Canada

3. Monitor renal, LFTs; reduce dose with dysfunction.

4. Determine if smoker; smoking reduces drug effect by increasing metabolism.

5. The propoxyphene hydrochloride 65 mg is comparable to 100 mg of propoxyphene napsylate.

CLIENT/FAMILY TEACHING

1. Take only as directed. Do not share medications or take for conditions other than prescribed. Store out of reach of children.

2. May take with food/milk to decrease GI upset.

3. Avoid activities that require mental alertness; may cause dizziness/drowsiness.

4. Report lack of response, any unusual side effects, or loss of effectiveness. Tolerance may develop over time.

5. Do not smoke (induces liver enzymes that rapidly metabolize propoxyphene), avoid alcohol, or any OTC agents without approval. Drug may become habit forming.

OUTCOMES/EVALUATE
Relief of pain

—— COMBINATION DRUG ——

Propoxyphene napsylate and Acetaminophen

(pro-**POX**-ih-feen **NAP**-syl-ate, ah-**SEAT**-ah-**MIN**-oh-fen)

CLASSIFICATION(S):
Narcotic and nonnarcotic analgesic combination

Rx: Darvocet A500, Darvocet-N 100, Darvocet-N 50, Propacet 100, Trycet, **C-IV**

SEE ALSO *ACETAMINOPHEN.*

USES
Relief of mild to moderate pain, either when pain is present alone or when accompanied by fever.

CONTENT
Each **Darvocet-N 50** tablet contains: Propoxyphene napsylate *(narcotic analgesic),* 50 mg, and acetaminophen *(non-narcotic analgesic),* 325 mg. Each **Darvocet A500** tablet contains: propoxyphene napsylate, 100 mg, and acetaminophen, 500 mg. Each **Darvocet-N 100** tablet or **Propacet 100** tablet contains: propoxyphene napsylate, 100 mg, and acetaminophen, 650 mg. Each **Trycet** tablet contains propoxyphene napsylate, 100 mg, and acetaminophen, 325 mg.

ACTION/KINETICS
Action
Propoxyphene is a centrally-acting narcotic analgesic related to methadone. The potency of propoxyphene is from two-thirds to equal that of codeine. Acetaminophen may cause analgesia by inhibiting CNS prostaglandin synthesis; however, due to minimal effects on peripheral prostaglandin synthesis, acetaminophen has no anti-inflammatory or uricosuric effects. Decreases fever by (1) a hypothalamic effect leading to sweating and vasodilation and (2) inhibits the effect of pyrogens on the hypothalamic heat-regulating centers. The combination of propoxyphene and acetaminophen produces greater analgesia than either drug administered alone.

Pharmacokinetics
Propoxyphene. Peak plasma levels: 2–2.5 hr. Metabolized in the liver to norpropoxyphene which has significantly less CNS depressant effect than propoxyphene. **t½, propoxyphene:** 6–12 hr; **t½, norpropoxyphene:** 30–36 hr. **Acetaminophen.** Peak plasma levels: 30–120 min. **t½:** 2–3 hr. **Therapeutic serum levels** (analgesia): 5–20 mcg/mL. Metabolized in the liver and excreted in the urine as glucuronide and sulfate conjugates. However, an intermediate hydroxylated metabolite is hepatotoxic following large doses of acetaminophen.

CONTRAINDICATIONS
Hypersensitivity to propoxyphene or acetaminophen. Use in those who are suicidal or addiction-prone. Use in preg-

nancy unless potential benefits outweigh possible risks.

SPECIAL CONCERNS

■ (1) Propoxyphene products in excessive doses, either alone or in combination with other CNS depressants, including alcohol, are a major cause of drug-related deaths. Fatalities within the first hour of overdosage are not uncommon. In a survey of deaths due to overdosage in approximately 20% of the fatal cases, death occurred within the first hour (5% occurred within 15 minutes). Propoxyphene should not be taken in doses higher than those recommended by the provider. The judicious prescribing of propoxyphene is essential to the safe use of this drug. With clients who are depressed or suicidal, consideration should be given to the use of nonnarcotic analgesics. Clients should be cautioned about the concomitant use of propoxyphene products and alcohol because of potentially serious CNS-additive effects of these agents. Because of the additive depressant effect, propoxyphene should be prescribed with caution for those clients whose medical condition requires the concomitant administration of sedatives, tranquilizers, muscle relaxants, antidepressants, or other CNS-depressant drugs. Clients should be advised of the additive depressant effects of these combinations. (2) Many of the propoxyphene-related deaths have occurred in clients with previous histories of emotional disturbances or suicidal ideation or attempts, as well as histories of misuse of tranquilizers, alcohol, and other CNS-active drugs. Some deaths have occurred as a consequence of the accidental ingestion of excessive quantities of propoxyphene alone or in combination with other drugs. Clients taking propoxyphene should be warned not to exceed the dosage recommended by the physician.■ Propoxyphene, when taken in higher-than-recommended doses over long periods can produce psychological dependence and, less frequently, physical dependence and tolerance. The abuse liability is comparable to codeine. Use with caution in those with impaired hepatic or renal function. Safety and efficacy have not been determined in children.

SIDE EFFECTS

Most Common

Drowsiness, dizziness, N&V, sedation.
See *Acetaminophen* for a complete list of possible side effects. **GI:** Constipation, abdominal pain, liver dysfunction, cholestatic jaundice, ***hepatic necrosis***. **CNS:** Lightheadedness, headache, euphoria, dysphoria, hallucinations. **GU:** Renal papillary necrosis (following chronic acetaminophen use). **Miscellaneous:** Weakness, minor visual disturbances, skin rashes, subacute painful myopathy.

LABORATORY TEST CONSIDERATIONS

Abnormal LFTs.

OD OVERDOSE MANAGEMENT

Symptoms: **Propoxyphene.** Similar to narcotic overdosage. Somnolence, stupor, coma, respiratory depression, decreased ventilatory rate and/or tidal volume (results in cyanosis and hypoxia). Also, pinpoint pupils (initially) followed by dilation. Cheyne-Stokes respiration, apnea, decreased BP, pulmonary edema, ***circulatory collapse***. Cardiac arrhythmias and conduction delay, combined respiratory-metabolic acidosis. ***Death***.

Acetaminophen. Initially and for 24 hr: Anorexia, N&V, diaphoresis, general malaise, abdominal pain. Liver dysfunction becomes evident within 72 hr after ingestion with elevated serum transaminase and lactic dehydrogenase levels, increased serum bilirubin levels, and prolonged PT. Acute renal failure. ***Death from hepatic failure*** may occur 3–7 days after ingestion of the overdose.

Treatment: **Propoxyphene.**
- Establish a patent airway to restore ventilation. Mechanically-assisted ventilation, with or without oxygen, may be required. Positive pressure respiration may be desirable if pulmonary edema is present.
- Naloxone, 0.4–2 mg IV, to reverse respiratory depression. Can be repeated in 2- to 3-min intervals. The duration of action of naloxone may

be brief, requiring additional doses. Naloxone may also be given by continuous IV administration. For children, the dose of naloxone is 0.01 mg/kg IV. If this dose does not result in the desired improvement, a subsequent dose of 0.1 mg/kg may be given. If an IV route is not available, can be given IM or SC in divided doses. Can be diluted with sterile water for injection.

- Monitor blood gases, pH, and electrolytes to determine if acidosis and/or electrolyte imbalance are present. Prompt correction of hypoxia, acidosis, and electrolyte disturbances will minimize cardiac problems.
- Have available CPR measures should cardiac arrhythmias be present.
- Electrocardiographic monitoring is essential.
- Careful titration with an anticonvulsant may be needed to control seizures. Do not use caffeine or amphetamine to control CNS depression, as they are likely to precipitate seizures.
- General supportive measures, when necessary, include IV fluids, vasopressor-inotropic compounds, and anti-infective drugs.
- Gastric lavage may be helpful. Activated charcoal can adsorb significant amounts of propoxyphene.
- Determine if other agents (e.g., alcohol, barbiturates, tranquilizers, or other CNS depressants) were also ingested.

Treatment: **Acetaminophen.**
- Undertake liver function tests initially and at 24-hr intervals since hepatic toxicity may not be evident for 48–72 hr.
- Obtain serum acetaminophen levels as soon as possible, but no sooner than 4 hr after ingestion.
- Gastric lavage or induction of emesis.
- For best results, N-acetylcysteine should be given as early as possible and within 16 hr of the overdose.

DRUG INTERACTIONS
See also *Acetaminophen.*

Anticonvulsants / ↑ Anticonvulsant pharmacologic and toxic effects R/T inhibition of metabolism
Antidepressants / ↑ Antidepressant pharmacologic and toxic effects R/T inhibition of metabolism
CNS depressants (including alcohol, antidepressants, muscle relaxants, sedatives, tranquilizers) / Additive CNS depression
Warfarin / ↑ Warfarin pharmacologic and toxic effects R/T inhibition of metabolism

HOW SUPPLIED
See Content.

DOSAGE————————————
- **TABLETS**
  Mild-to-moderate pain with or without fever.

Adults, usual: 100 mg propoxyphene napsylate and 650 mg acetaminophen q 4 hr, not to exceed 600 mg propoxyphene per day.

NURSING CONSIDERATIONS

ADMINISTRATION/STORAGE
1. Consideration should be given to reducing the dose of propoxyphene in geriatric clients and in those with renal or hepatic impairment.
2. Store from 15–30°C (59–86°F).

ASSESSMENT
1. Note reasons for therapy, location, characteristics of S&S, other agents trialed, outcome; rate pain level.
2. List drugs prescribed to ensure none interact.
3. Assess for depression, suicide ideations, excessive alcohol use, drug addiction prone; precludes drug use.
4. Monitor ROM, VS, renal, LFTs; reduce dose with dysfunction.

CLIENT/FAMILY TEACHING
1. Take only as directed, do not exceed prescribed dose.
2. Do not perform activities that require mental alertness until drug effects realized; may cause dizziness or drowsiness.
3. May cause nausea, vomiting, dizziness. Lie down and rest if these effects occur to relieve symptoms.
4. Avoid alcohol and CNS depressants during therapy.

---

5. Practice reliable contraception; report if pregnancy suspected.

6. Drug may cause dependence. Store safely away from the bedside and out of reach of children.

7. Keep all F/U appointments to assess response to drug therapy and evaluate all side effects and lab results.

OUTCOMES/EVALUATE
Relief of pain

Propranolol hydrochloride   **IV** ©
(proh-**PRAN**-oh-lohl)

CLASSIFICATION(S):
Beta-adrenergic blocking agent
PREGNANCY CATEGORY: C
Rx: Inderal, Inderal LA, InnoPran XL, Propranolol Intensol.
✚**Rx:** Apo-Propranolol, Nu-Propranolol.

SEE ALSO *BETA-ADRENERGIC BLOCKING AGENTS.*

USES
(1) Hypertension, alone or in combination with other antihypertensive agents. (2) Angina pectoris when caused by coronary atherosclerosis (except Innopran XL). (3) Hypertrophic subaortic stenosis (especially to treat exercise or other stress-induced angina, palpitations, and syncope); except Innopran XL. (4) MI (except extended-release forms). (5) Adjunctive treatment of pheochromocytoma after primary therapy with an alpha-adrenergic blocker (except extended-release forms). (6) Prophylaxis of migraine (except Innopran XL). (7) Essential tremor (familial or hereditary); except extended-release forms. (8) Cardiac arrhythmias, including supraventricular, ventricular, tachyarrhythmias of digitalis intoxication and resistant tachyarrhythamias due to excessive catecholamines during anesthesia (except extended-release forms). *Investigational:* Schizophrenia, tremors due to parkinsonism, aggressive behavior, antipsychotic-induced akathisia, rebleeding due to esophageal varices, si-tuational anxiety, acute panic attacks, gastric bleeding in portal hypertension, vaginal contraceptive, anxiety, alcohol withdrawal syndrome, winter depression.

ACTION/KINETICS
Action
Combines reversibly with beta-adrenergic receptors to block the response to sympathetic nerve impulses, circulating catecholoamines, or adrenergic drugs. Manifests both $beta_1$- and $beta_2$-adrenergic blocking activity. Is also an antiarrhythmic, type II. Antiarrhythmic action is due to both beta-adrenergic receptor blockade and a direct membrane-stabilizing action on the cardiac cell; decreases HR. Has no intrinsic sympathomimetic activity and has high lipid solubility.

Pharmacokinetics
Bioavailability is 30% for immediate-release and 9–18% for the long-acting product. **Onset, PO:** 30 min; **IV:** immediate. **Maximum effect:** 1–1.5 hr. **Duration:** 3–5 hr. **t½:** 2–3 hr (8–11 hr for long-acting). **Therapeutic serum level, antiarrhythmic:** 0.05–0.1 mcg/mL. Completely metabolized by liver and excreted in urine. Although food increases bioavailability, absorption may be decreased. **Plasma protein binding:** 90–95%.

CONTRAINDICATIONS
Bronchial asthma, bronchospasms including severe COPD.

SPECIAL CONCERNS
It is dangerous to use propranolol for pheochromocytoma unless an alpha-adrenergic blocking agent is already in use.

SIDE EFFECTS
Most Common
Insomnia, anxiety, impotence, nervousness, fatigue, dizziness, drowsiness, lightheadedness, diarrhea, vision problems.

See *Beta-Adrenergic Blocking Agents* for a complete list of possible side effects. Also, psoriasis-like eruptions, skin necrosis, SLE (rare).

ADDITIONAL DRUG INTERACTIONS
Gabapentin / Possible paroxysmal dystonic movements in the hands

---

Haloperidol / Severe hypotension
Hydralazine / ↑ Effect of both agents
Methimazole / May ↑ propranolol effects
Phenobarbital / ↓ Propranolol effect R/T ↑ liver breakdown
Propylthiouracil / May ↑ Propranolol effects
Rifampin / ↓ Propranolol effect R/T ↑ liver breakdown
Rizatriptan / ↑ AUC and peak rizatriptan levels R/T ↓ rizatriptan metabolism
Smoking / ↓ Serum levels and ↑ clearance of propranolol R/T ↑ hepatic metabolism

LABORATORY TEST CONSIDERATIONS
↑ Blood urea, serum transaminase, alkaline phosphatase, LDH. Interference with glaucoma screening test.

HOW SUPPLIED
Capsules, Extended-Release: 60 mg, 80 mg, 120 mg, 160 mg; *Injection:* 1 mg/mL; *Oral Solution:* 4 mg/mL, 8 mg/mL; *Oral Solution, Concentrated:* 80 mg/mL; *Tablets:* 10 mg, 20 mg, 40 mg, 60 mg, 80 mg, 90 mg.

DOSAGE

- **CAPSULES, EXTENDED-RELEASE; ORAL SOLUTION; ORAL SOLUTION, CONCENTRATED; TABLETS**
  Hypertension.
Initial: 40 mg twice a day or 80 mg of extended-release once a day; **then,** increase dose to maintenance level of 120–240 mg/day given in two to three divided doses or 80–160 mg of extended-release medication once daily. Do not exceed 640 mg/day. **Pediatric, initial:** 0.5 mg/kg twice a day; dose may be increased at 3- to 5-day intervals to a maximum of 16 mg/kg/day. Calculate the dosage range by weight and not by body surface area.
  Angina.
Initial: 80–320 mg 2–4 times per day; or, 80 mg of extended-release once daily. **Dose range:** 80–320 mg 2-, 3-, or 4 times per day or 80–160 mg extended release once daily (gradually increase initial dose at 3–7 day intervals until optimum response is obtained). Do not exceed 320 mg/day.
  Arrhythmias.

10–30 mg 3–4 times per day given after meals and at bedtime.
  Hypertrophic subaortic stenosis.
20–40 mg 3–4 times per day before meals and at bedtime or 80–160 mg of extended-release medication given once daily.
  MI prophylaxis.
180–240 mg/day given in three to four divided doses. Do not exceed 240 mg/day.
  Pheochromocytoma, preoperatively.
60 mg/day for 3 days before surgery, given concomitantly with an alpha-adrenergic blocking agent.
  Pheochromocytoma, inoperable tumors.
30 mg/day in divided doses.
  Migraine.
Initial: 80 mg extended-release medication given once daily or in divided doses; **then,** increase dose gradually to maintenance of 160–240 mg once daily or in divided doses. If a satisfactory response has not been observed after 4–6 weeks, discontinue the drug and withdraw gradually.
  Essential tremor.
Initial: 40 mg twice a day; **then,** 120 mg/day up to a maximum of 320 mg/day.
  Aggressive behavior.
80–300 mg/day.
  Antipsychotic-induced akathisia.
20–80 mg/day.
  Tremors associated with Parkinson's disease.
160 mg/day.
  Rebleeding from esophageal varices.
20–180 mg twice a day
  Schizophrenia.
300–5,000 mg/day.
  Acute panic symptoms.
40–320 mg/day.
  Anxiety.
80–320 mg/day.
  Intermittent explosive disorder.
50–1,600 mg/day.
  Nonvariceal gastric bleeding in portal hypertension.
24–480 mg/day.
- **IV**
  Life-threatening arrhythmias or those occurring under anesthesia.

P

1–3 mg not to exceed 1 mg/min; a second dose may be given after 2 min, with subsequent doses q 4 hr. Begin PO therapy as soon as possible. Although use in pediatrics is not recommended, investigational doses of 0.01–0.1 mg/kg/dose, up to a maximum of 1 mg/dose (by slow push), have been used for arrhythmias.

NURSING CONSIDERATIONS

℘ Do not confuse propranolol with Pravachol (antihyperlipidemic). Also, do not confuse Inderal with Inderide (an antihypertensive) or with Isordil (a coronary vasodilator).

ADMINISTRATION/STORAGE

1. Do not administer for a minimum of 2 weeks after MAO drug use.

2. Protect products from light, moisture, freezing, and excessive heat. Store in tight, light-resistant containers.

IV 3. Reserve IV use for life-threatening arrhythmias or those occurring during anesthesia.

4. If signs of serious myocardial depression occur, slowly infuse isoproterenol (Isuprel) IV.

5. Dilute 1 mg in 10 mL of D5W and administer IV over at least 1 min. May be further reconstituted in 50 mL of dextrose or saline solution and infused IVPB over 10–15 min.

6. After IV administration, have emergency drugs and equipment available to combat hypotension or circulatory collapse.

ASSESSMENT

1. List reasons for therapy, onset, duration, characteristics of S&S, other agents trialed, outcome.

2. Note ECG, and cardiopulmonary findings. Assess for pulmonary disease, bronchospasms, bradycardia, heart block, depression; may preclude therapy.

3. Report rash, fever, and/or purpura; S&S of hypersensitivity reaction.

4. Monitor glucose, renal/LFTs, TSH, VS, I&O. Observe for S&S of CHF (e.g., SOB, rales, edema, and weight gain).

CLIENT/FAMILY TEACHING

1. May cause drowsiness; assess drug response before performing activities that require mental alertness.

2. Sustained-release products are usually taken at bedtime. It is recommended that InnoPran XL be taken about 10 p.m. on an empty stomach or with food.

3. Mix the concentrated oral solution with liquid or semi-solid food (e.g., water, juices, soda or soda-like beverages, applesauce, and puddings). Draw into dropper the amount prescribed for a single dose; squeeze the dropper contents into the liquid or semi-solid food. Stir for a few seconds. Consume the entire amount of the mixture immediately. Do not store for future use.

4. Do not smoke; smoking decreases serum levels and interferes with drug clearance.

5. May mask signs of low blood sugar, such as a rapid heartbeat; monitor FS carefully.

6. Keep log of BP and pulse for provider review; report significant changes.

7. Do not stop abruptly; may precipitate hypertension, myocardial ischemia, or cardiac arrhythmias.

8. Dress appropriately; may cause increased sensitivity to cold.

9. Avoid alcohol and any OTC agents containing alpha-adrenergic stimulants or sympathomimetics.

10. Report persistent side effects, e.g., skin rashes, abnormal bleeding, unusual crying, or feelings of depression.

OUTCOMES/EVALUATE

- ↓ BP, ↓ HR
- ↓ Angina; prophylaxis of myocardial reinfarction
- Migraine prophylaxis
- Control of tachyarrhythmias
- Therapeutic drug levels as an antiarrhythmic (0.05–0.1 mcg/mL)

Bold Italic = life threatening side effect   ■ = black box warning   ♣ = Available in Canada

Propylthiouracil

(proh-pill-thigh-oh-**YOUR**-ah-sill)

CLASSIFICATION(S):
Antithyroid drug
PREGNANCY CATEGORY: D
✤**Rx:** Propyl-Thyracil.

USES
(1) Hyperthyroidism prior to surgery or radiotherapy. (2) Adjunct in treatment of thyrotoxicosis or thyroid storm. (3) Reduce mortality due to alcoholic liver disease.

ACTION/KINETICS

Action
Inhibits (partially or completely) the production of thyroid hormones by the thyroid gland by preventing the incorporation of iodide into tyrosine and coupling of iodotyrosines. Does not affect release or activity of preformed hormone; thus, it may take several weeks for the therapeutic effect to become established. May be preferred for treatment of thyroid storm, as it inhibits peripheral conversion of thyroxine to triiodothyronine.

Pharmacokinetics
Rapidly absorbed from the GI tract. **Duration:** 2–3 hr. **t½:** 1–2 hr. **Onset:** 10–20 days. **Time to peak effect:** 2–10 weeks. Metabolized by the liver and excreted through the kidneys. **Plasma protein binding:** 80%.

CONTRAINDICATIONS
Lactation (may cause hypothyroidism in infant).

SPECIAL CONCERNS
Incidence of vasculitis is increased. Use with caution in the presence of CV disease. Monitor PT due to possible hypoprothrombinemia and bleeding.

SIDE EFFECTS

Most Common
Rash, itching, urticaria, N&V, heartburn, loss of taste, swelling, joint/muscle aches, headache, numbness.

Hematologic: *Agranulocytosis*, thrombocytopenia, granulocytopenia, hypoprothrombinemia, *aplastic anemia*, leukopenia. **GI:** N&V, taste loss, epigastric pain, sialadenopathy. **CNS:** Headache, paresthesia, drowsiness, vertigo, depression, CNS stimulation. **Dermatologic:** Skin rash, urticaria, alopecia, skin pigmentation, pruritus, exfoliative dermatitis, erythema nodosum. **Miscellaneous:** Jaundice, arthralgia, myalgia, neuritis, edema, lymphadenopathy, vasculitis, lupus-like syndrome, drug fever, periarteritis, hepatitis, nephritis, interstitial pneumonitis, insulin autoimmune syndrome resulting in hypoglycemic coma.

OD OVERDOSE MANAGEMENT
Symptoms: N&V, headache, fever, pruritus, epigastric distress, arthralgia, pancytopenia, *agranulocytosis* (most serious). Rarely, exfoliative dermatitis, hepatitis, neuropathies, CNS stimulation or depression. *Treatment:* Maintain a patent airway and support ventilation and perfusion. Very carefully monitor and maintain VS, blood gases, and serum electrolytes. Monitor bone marrow function.

DRUG INTERACTIONS
Propylthiouracil may produce hypoprothrombinemia, adding to the effect of anticoagulants

HOW SUPPLIED
Tablets: 50 mg.

DOSAGE
- **TABLETS**
  Hyperthyroidism.

Adults, initial: 300 mg/day, usually given in 3 divided doses about 8 hr apart. In those with severe hyperthyroidism, very large goiters or both, the initial dose is usually 400 mg/day; occasionally a client will require 600–900 mg/day. **Maintenance, usual:** 100–150 mg/day. **Pediatric, 6–10 years, initial:** 50–150 mg/day in three equal doses about 8 hr apart; **over 10 years, initial:** 150–300 mg/day in 3 equal doses about 8 hr apart. Maintenance for all pediatric use is based on response. **Alternative dose for children, initial:** 5–7 mg/kg/day (150–200 mg/m²/day) in divided doses q 8 hr; **maintenance:** ⅓–⅔ the initial dose when the client is euthyroid.
  Thyrotoxic crisis.

P

Adults: 200–400 mg q 4 hr during the first day as an adjunct to other treatments.

NURSING CONSIDERATIONS
ASSESSMENT
1. Note onset, symptoms experienced, physical presentation, any underlying cause.
2. Check if pregnant; may require reduced dosage as pregnancy progresses.
3. Monitor VS, I&O, and weights; PT, CBC, ECG, and thyroid function studies.
4. Assess thyroid gland noting any enlargement, pain, asymmetry, nodules, or bruits.
5. Check children every 6 months for appropriate growth and development; plot on a graph.

CLIENT/FAMILY TEACHING
1. It takes 6–12 weeks for the drug to produce full effect. Take regularly and exactly as directed q 8 hr around the clock. Hyperthyroidism may recur if not taken properly. Regularly record heart rate and weight.
2. Report symptoms of hyperthyroidism or thyrotoxicosis (palpitations, increased HR, nervousness, sleeplessness, sweating, diarrhea, weight loss, fever). Report symptoms of hypothyroidism (weak, listless, tired, headache, dry skin, cold intolerance, constipation) as dosage may require adjustment.
3. Any sore throat, skin eruptions, enlargement of the cervical lymph nodes, GI disturbances, fever, skin rashes, itching, or jaundice should be reported; may require either a dosage reduction or withdrawal of the drug.
4. Report symptoms of iodism (cold symptoms, skin lesions, stomatitis, GI upset, metallic taste)
5. Identify dietary sources of iodine (iodized salt, shellfish, turnips, cabbage, kale) that may need to be omitted from the diet.
6. Report unusual bleeding, alopecia, nausea, loss of taste, or epigastric pain.
7. When drug is taken for 1 year, more than half the clients achieve a permanent remission. Those who relapse are usually treated with radioiodine.

8. Carry ID listing medical problems and currently prescribed medications.
9. Read labels carefully for sources of iodine. Avoid all OTC agents without approval. Report as scheduled for evaluation and labs.

OUTCOMES/EVALUATE
- Normal metabolism; control of S&S ($\uparrow$ weight, $\downarrow$ sweating, $\downarrow$ HR)
- Suppression of thyroid hormones ($\downarrow$ T_3, T_4); thyroid function studies within desired range (euthyroid)

Protamine sulfate [IV]
(**PROH**-tah-meen)

CLASSIFICATION(S):
Heparin antagonist
PREGNANCY CATEGORY: C

USES
Only for treatment of heparin overdose.

ACTION/KINETICS
Action
A strong basic polypeptide that complexes with strongly acidic heparin to form an inactive stable salt. The complex has no anticoagulant activity. Heparin is neutralized within 5 min after IV protamine.

Pharmacokinetics
Duration: 2 hr (but depends on body temperature). The $t\frac{1}{2}$ of protamine is shorter than heparin; thus, repeated doses may be required. Upon metabolism, the complex may liberate heparin (heparin rebound).

CONTRAINDICATIONS
Previous intolerance to protamine. Use to treat spontaneous hemorrhage, postpartum hemorrhage, menorrhagia, or uterine bleeding. Administration of over 50 mg over a short period.

SPECIAL CONCERNS
Use with caution during lactation. Safety and efficacy have not been determined in children. Rapid administration may cause severe hypotension and anaphylaxis.

SIDE EFFECTS

Most Common

Sudden fall in BP, bradycardia, transitory flushing, warm feeling, dyspnea, N&V, lassitude.

CV: Sudden fall in BP, bradycardia, transitory flushing, warm feeling, *acute pulmonary hypertension, circulatory collapse (possibly irreversible) with myocardial failure* and decreased CO. Pulmonary edema in clients on cardiopulmonary bypass undergoing CV surgery. **Anaphylaxis:** Severe respiratory distress, capillary leak, and noncardiogenic pulmonary edema. **GI:** N&V. **CNS:** Lassitude. **Miscellaneous:** Dyspnea, back pain in conscious clients undergoing cardiac catheterization, hypersensitivity reactions.

OD OVERDOSE MANAGEMENT

Symptoms: Bleeding. Rapid administration may cause dyspnea, bradycardia, flushing, warm feeling, severe hypotension, hypertension. In assessing overdose, there may be the possibility of multiple drug overdoses leading to drug interactions and unusual pharmacokinetics. *Treatment:* Replace blood loss with blood transfusions or fresh frozen plasma. Fluids, epinephrine, dobutamine, or dopamine to treat hypotension

HOW SUPPLIED

Injection: 10 mg/mL.

DOSAGE

- **SLOW IV**

  Heparin overdose.

Give no more than 50 mg of protamine sulfate in any 10-min period. One mg of protamine sulfate can neutralize about 90 USP units of heparin derived from lung tissue or about 115 USP units of heparin derived from intestinal mucosa.

NOTE: The dose of protamine sulfate depends on the amount of time that has elapsed since IV heparin administration. For example, if 30 min has elapsed, one-half the usual dose of protamine sulfate may be sufficient because heparin is cleared rapidly from the circulation.

NURSING CONSIDERATIONS

ADMINISTRATION/STORAGE

IV 1. Incompatible with several penicillins and with cephalosporins.

2. To minimize side effects, give slowly over 10 min. May also be diluted in 50 mL of D5W or saline solution and administered at a rate of 50 mg over 10–15 min. Do not store diluted solutions.

3. Refrigerate at 2–8°C (36–46°F).

ASSESSMENT

1. Note amount, time of overdose, source to ensure appropriate antidote dosing.

2. Request type and crossmatch; assess need for fresh frozen plasma or whole blood.

3. Coagulation studies should be performed 5–15 min after protamine has been administered; repeat in 2–8 hr to assess for heparin rebound (increased bleeding, lowered BP, and/or shock).

4. Monitor VS, I&O; assess for sudden fall in BP, bradycardia, dyspnea, transitory flushing, or sensations of warmth.

CLIENT/FAMILY TEACHING

Drug is administered IV to offset the effects of too much heparin which can lead to hemorrhage shock due to fluid volume loss.

OUTCOMES/EVALUATE

Stable H&H; control of heparin-induced hemorrhage

Pseudoephedrine hydrochloride ©

(soo-doh-eh-**FED**-rin)

CLASSIFICATION(S):

Sympathomimetic

PREGNANCY CATEGORY: B

OTC: Capsules: Sinustop. **Capsules, Soft Gel:** Dimetapp Maximum Strength Non-Drowsy Liqui-Gels. **Drops:** Dimetapp Decongestant Pediatric, Kid Kare, Nasal Decongestant Oral, PediaCare Decongestant Infants'. **Liquid/Syrup:** Cenafed Syrup, Decofed Syrup, ElixSure Children's Congestion, Simply Stuffy, Sudafed Children's

Non-Drowsy, Triaminic Allergy Congestion, Unified. **Tablets:** Cenafed, Congestaid, Genaphed, Medi-First Sinus Decongestant, Simply Stuffy, Sudafed Non-Drowsy Maximum Strength, Sudodrin. **Tablets, Chewable:** Sudafed Children's Non-Drowsy, Triaminic Allergy Congestion Softchews. **Tablets, Controlled Release or Extended-Release:** Dimetapp Maximum Strength 12-Hour Non-Drowsy Extentabs, Efidac 24 Pseudoephedrine, Sudafed Non-Drowsy 12 Hour Long-Acting, Sudafed Non-Drowsy 24 Hour Long-Acting.
✦**OTC:** Balminil Decongestant Syrup, Contac Cold 12 Hour Relief Non Drowsy, Eltor 120, PMS-Pseudoephedrine, Triaminic Oral Pediatric Drops.

Pseudoephedrine sulfate

PREGNANCY CATEGORY: B
OTC: Drixoral 12 Hour Non-Drowsy Formula.
✦**OTC:** Drixoral Day, Drixoral N.D.

SEE ALSO *SYMPATHOMIMETIC DRUGS.*

USES
Temporary relief of nasal congestion due to hay fever, common cold, or other upper respiratory allergies associated with sinusitis.

ACTION/KINETICS
Action
Produces direct stimulation of both alpha-(pronounced) and beta-adrenergic receptors, as well as indirect stimulation through release of norepinephrine from storage sites. Results in decongestant effect on the nasal mucosa. Systemic administration eliminates possible damage to the nasal mucosa.

Pharmacokinetics
Onset: 15–30 min. **Time to peak effect:** 30–60 min. **Duration:** 3–4 hr. **Extended-release, duration:** 8–12 hr. Urinary excretion slowed by alkalinization, causing reabsorption of drug.

ADDITIONAL CONTRAINDICATIONS
Lactation. Not recommended for use in children less than 6 years of age. Use of

sustained-release products in children less than 12 years of age.

SPECIAL CONCERNS
Geriatric clients may be more prone to age-related prostatic hypertrophy. *NOTE:* Pseudoephedrine products must be kept behind the counter in pharmacies, thus requiring clients to ask for the product.

SIDE EFFECTS
Most Common
Somnolence, insomnia, nervousness, excitability, dizziness, anxiety, skin rashes, nausea, gastric irritation.
See *Sympathomimetic Drugs* for a complete list of possible side effects

HOW SUPPLIED
Pseudoephedrine hydrochloride: *Capsules:* 60 mg; *Capsules, Soft Gel:* 30 mg; *Drops:* 7.5 mg/0.8 mL; *Liquid/Syrup:* 15 mg/5 mL, 30 mg/5 mL; *Tablets:* 30 mg, 60 mg; *Tablets, Chewable:* 15 mg; *Tablets, Controlled-Release:* 240 mg (60 mg immediate-release and 180 mg controlled-release); *Tablets, Extended-Release:* 120 mg.
Pseudoephedrine sulfate: *Tablets, Extended-Release:* 120 mg.

DOSAGE
PSEUDOEPHEDRINE HYDROCHLORIDE
• **CAPSULES; CAPSULES, SOFT GEL; DROPS; LIQUID/SYRUP; TABLETS; TABLETS, CHEWABLE**
Decongestant.
Adults, and children over 12 years: 60 mg q 4–6 hr, not to exceed 240 mg in 24 hr. **Pediatric, 6–12 years:** 30 mg using the drops, liquid, syrup or chewable tablets q 4–6 hr, not to exceed 120 mg in 24 hr; **2–6 years:** Use not recommended.
• **TABLETS, CONTROLLED-RELEASE (24 HR); TABLETS, EXTENDED-RELEASE (12 HR)**
Decongestant.
Adults and children over 12 years: 120 mg of the sustained-release q 12 hr or 240 mg of the controlled-release q 24 hr. Do not exceed 240 mg/24 hr.
PSEUDOEPHEDRINE SULFATE
• **TABLETS, EXTENDED-RELEASE**
Decongestant.
Adults and children over 12 years: 120 mg q 12 hr, not to exceed 240 mg/

24 hr. Use is not recommended for children less than 12 years of age.

NURSING CONSIDERATIONS

🕮 Do not confuse Sudafed (containing pseudoephedrine) with Sudafed PE (containing phenylephrine). Also, do not confuse Sudafed with Sotalol (an antiarrhythmic drug).

ASSESSMENT

1. Note reasons for therapy, onset, characteristics of S&S.
2. Assess ENT, lung/heart sounds, BP, HR; note allergy history and any triggers.

CLIENT/FAMILY TEACHING

1. Drug acts by constricting (shrinking)blood vessels (veins and arteries) in the nose, lungs, and other mucus membranes.
2. Avoid taking near bedtime; stimulation may produce insomnia.
3. With hypertension, report headaches, dizziness, or increased BP. Any extreme restlessness or sensitivity reactions should be reported.
4. Take exactly as directed. Do not crush or chew extended-release products. Continuous use or excessive dosing may cause rebound congestion.
5. Avoid OTC medications; may also contain ephedrine or other sympathomimetic amines and intensify drug action.
6. Report if symptoms do not improve after 3–5 days or worsen. Identify triggers and practice avoidance especially with seasonal allergies.

OUTCOMES/EVALUATE

Relief of nasal, sinus, or eustachian tube congestion

Psyllium hydrophilic muciloid

(**SILL**-ee-um hi-droh-**FILL**-ik)

CLASSIFICATION(S):

Laxative, bulk-forming

OTC: Fiberall Natural Flavor, Fiberall Orange Flavor, Fiberall Tropical Fruit Flavor, Fiberall Wafers, Genfiber, Genfiber Orange Flavor, Hydrocil Instant, Konsyl, Konsyl Easy Mix Formula, Konsyl-D, Konsyl-Orange, Metamucil, Metamucil Lemon-Lime Flavor, Metamucil Orange Flavor, Metamucil Orange Flavor-Original Texture, Metamucil Orange Flavor-Smooth Texture, Metamucil Original Texture, Metamucil Sugar Free, Metamucil Sugar Free Orange Flavor, Metamucil Sugar Free-Orange Flavor-Smooth Texture, Metamucil Sugar Free-Smooth Texture, Modane, Natural Fiber Laxative, Natural Psyllium Fiber, Natural Psyllium Fiber-Orange, Perdiem Fiber Therapy, Reguloid, Reguloid Orange, Reguloid Sugar Free Orange, Reguloid Sugar Free Regular, Serutan, Syllact.

SEE ALSO *LAXATIVES.*

USES

(1) Prophylaxis of constipation in clients who should not strain during defecation. (2) Short-term treatment of constipation; useful in geriatric clients with diminished colonic motor response and during pregnancy and postpartum to reestablish normal bowel function. (3) To soften feces during fecal impaction.

ACTION/KINETICS

Action

The powder forms a gelatinous mass with water, which adds bulk to the stools and stimulates peristalsis. Also has a demulcent effect on an inflamed intestinal mucosa. Products may also contain dextrose, sodium bicarbonate, monobasic potassium phosphate, citric acid, and benzyl benzoate.

Pharmacokinetics

Laxative effects usually occur in 12–24 hr. The full effect may take 2–3 days. Dependence may occur.

CONTRAINDICATIONS

Severe abdominal pain or intestinal obstruction.

SIDE EFFECTS

Most Common

Diarrhea, N&V, perianal irritation, bloating, flatulence, cramps.

GI: Diarrhea, N&V, perianal irritation, bloating, flatulence, cramps. Obstruction of the esophagus, stomach, small intestine, and rectum. **CNS:** Fainting.

DRUG INTERACTIONS

Do not use concomitantly with salicylates, nitrofurantoin, or cardiac glycosides (e.g., digitalis)

HOW SUPPLIED

Caplets, Capsules: 0.5 gram, 0.52 gram; *Effervescent Powder; Granules; Powder; Wafers:*

DOSAGE

Dose depends on the product. General information on adult dosage follows.

- **GRANULES; POWDER**
  Laxative.

Adults: 1–2 teaspoons 1–3 times per day; spread on food or take with a 8 oz of water or other liquid.

- **EFFERVESCENT POWDER**
  Laxative.

Adults: 1 packet in water 1–3 times per day.

- **WAFERS**

Adults: 2 wafers followed by a glass of water 1–3 times per day.

NURSING CONSIDERATIONS

ASSESSMENT

Note reasons for therapy, characteristics of S&S, abdominal/rectal assessment, other agents trialed, outcome.

CLIENT/FAMILY TEACHING

1. Mix powder with 8 oz of liquid just prior to administering; otherwise, the mixture may become thick and difficult to drink. Wash down with another glass of water/juice.

2. The powder may be noxious and irritating when removing from the packets or canister. Open in a well-ventilated area and avoid inhaling particulate matter.

3. Take exactly as directed. Report lack of response, severe stomach pain, N&V, or intolerable side effects.

4. May take 12–24 hrs for desired response or up to 3 days. If taken before meals may reduce appetite. Check contents- some contain sugar.

5. Ensure adequate fluid intake and consume other dietary sources of fiber such as bran, cereals with this listed, fresh fruits and vegetables.

OUTCOMES/EVALUATE

Prophylaxis/relief of constipation

Pyrantel pamoate
(pie-**RAN**-tell)

CLASSIFICATION(S):

Anthelmintic

PREGNANCY CATEGORY: C

OTC: Pin-Rid, Pin-X, Reese's Pinworm.

♣**Rx:** Combantrin.

USES

(1) Pinworm (enterobiasis) and roundworm (ascariasis) infestations. (2) Multiple helminth infections, as it is also effective against roundworm and hookworm.

ACTION/KINETICS

Action

Has neuromuscular blocking effect which paralyzes the helminth, allowing it to be expelled through the feces. Also inhibits cholinesterases.

Pharmacokinetics

Poorly absorbed from GI tract. **Peak plasma levels:** 0.05–0.13 mcg/mL after 1–3 hr. Partially metabolized in liver. Fifty percent is excreted unchanged in feces and less than 15% excreted unchanged in urine.

CONTRAINDICATIONS

Pregnancy. Hepatic disease.

SPECIAL CONCERNS

Use with caution in presence of liver dysfunction. Safe use in children less than 2 years of age has not been established.

SIDE EFFECTS

Most Common

Anorexia, N&V, diarrhea, headache, dizziness.

GI: Anorexia, N&V, abdominal cramps, diarrhea. **Hepatic:** Transient elevation of AST. **CNS:** Headache, dizziness, drowsiness, insomnia. **Miscellaneous:** Skin rashes.

DRUG INTERACTIONS

Use with piperazine for ascariasis results in antagonism of the effect of both drugs

---

HOW SUPPLIED

Capsules, Soft Gel: 180 mg (equivalent to 62.5 mg pamoate base); *Liquid:* 50 mg (as pamoate)/mL; *Oral Suspension:* 50 mg (as pamoate)/mL; *Tablets:* 180 mg (equivalent to 62.5 mg pyrantel base); *Tablets, Chewable:* 720.5 mg (equivalent to 250 mg pyrantel base).

DOSAGE

• **CAPSULES, SOFT GEL; LIQUID; ORAL SUSPENSION; TABLETS**

Pinworm, other helminth infections.

Adults and children: One dose of 11 mg/kg (maximum). **Maximum total dose:** 1.0 gram.

NURSING CONSIDERATIONS

ASSESSMENT

1. Note reasons for therapy, symptom characteristics, and stool culture results.
2. Identify close contacts; assess for hepatic dysfunction.

CLIENT/FAMILY TEACHING

1. May be taken without regard to food intake. Can take with milk or fruit juices.
2. Dizziness or drowsiness may occur; do not engage in activities that require mental alertness.
3. Purging is not required. Report rash, severe headaches/GI upset, joint pain, or prolonged dizziness.
4. When treating pinworms, review client/family precautions R/T transmission:

• Strict handwashing and hygiene measures with daily cleansing of perianal area and cleaning of finger nails
• Wash hands before meals and after each bm carefully
• Do not prepare food for others when infested
• Change underwear and pajamas daily
• Launder undergarments, bed linens, sleep clothes in hot water daily
• Disinfect toilet facilities and bathroom floors daily
• Wet mop bedroom floors to prevent egg spread
• Do not share towels or wash clothes
• Treat all family members

OUTCOMES/EVALUATE

Resolution of infection; negative stool and perianal swabs

Pyridoxine hydrochloride (Vitamin B₆)

(peer-ih-**DOX**-een)

IV

CLASSIFICATION(S):

Vitamin B complex

PREGNANCY CATEGORY: A (C for doses that exceed the RDA)

OTC: Aminoxin, Vitelle Nestrex.

Rx: Pyridoxine HCl Injection.

USES

Pyridoxine deficiency including poor diet, drug-induced (e.g., oral contraceptives, isoniazid), and inborn errors of metabolism. *Investigational:* Hydrazine poisoning, PMS, high urine oxalate levels, N&V due to pregnancy, carpal tunnel syndrome, tardive dyskinesia due to antipsychotic drugs.

ACTION/KINETICS

Action

A water-soluble, heat-resistant vitamin that is destroyed by light. Acts as a coenzyme in the metabolism of protein, carbohydrates, and fat. As the amount of protein increases in the diet, the pyridoxine requirement increases. However, pyridoxine deficiency alone is rare.

Pharmacokinetics

Recommended RDAs, adult males: 1.7–2 mg; **adult females:** 1.4–1.6 mg. **t½:** 2–3 weeks. Metabolized in the liver and excreted through the urine.

SPECIAL CONCERNS

Safety and effectiveness have not been established in children for doses that exceed the RDA.

SIDE EFFECTS

Most Common

Paresthesia, numbess of feet, perioral numbness, unstable gait.

CNS: Unstable gait; decreased sensation to touch, temperature, and vibration; paresthesia, sleepiness; numbness of feet; awkwardness of hands; perioral numbness, photoallergic reaction, ataxia. *NOTE:* Abuse and dependence have been noted in adults administered 200 mg/day.

OD OVERDOSE MANAGEMENT
Symptoms: Ataxia, severe sensory neuropathy. *Treatment:* Discontinue pyridoxine; allow up to 6 months for CNS sensation to return.

DRUG INTERACTIONS
Chloramphenicol / ↑ Pyridoxine requirements
Contraceptives, oral / ↑ Pyridoxine requirements
Cycloserine / ↑ Pyridoxine requirements
Ethionamide / ↑ Pyridoxine requirements
Hydralazine / ↑ Pyridoxine requirements
Immunosuppressants / ↑ Pyridoxine requirements
Isoniazid / ↑ Pyridoxine requirements
Levodopa / Doses exceeding 5 mg/day pyridoxine antagonize the therapeutic effect of levodopa
Penicillamine / ↑ Pyridoxine requirements
Phenobarbital / ↓ Serum phenobarbital levels
Phenytoin / ↓ Serum phenytoin levels

HOW SUPPLIED
Injection: 100 mg/mL; *Tablets:* 25 mg, 50 mg, 100 mg, 250 mg, 500 mg.

DOSAGE————————
• **TABLETS**
  Dietary supplement.
Adults: 10–20 mg/day for 2 weeks; **then,** 2–5 mg/day as part of a multivitamin preparation for several weeks. **Pediatric,** 2.5–10 mg/day for 3 weeks; **then,** 2–5 mg/day as part of a multivitamin preparation for several weeks.
  Isoniazid-induced deficiency.
Adults, prophylaxis: 6–100 mg/day for isoniazid. **Adults, treatment:** 50–200 mg/day for 3 weeks followed by 25–100 mg/day to prevent relapse. **Adults, alcoholism:** 50 mg/day for 2–4 weeks; if anemia responds, continue pyridoxine indefinitely.
  PMS.
40–500 mg/day.
  High urine oxalate levels.

25–300 mg/day.
  Carpal tunnel syndrome.
100–200 mg/day for 12 or more weeks.
  Tardive dyskinesia due to antipsychotic drugs.
100 mg/day for 4 weeks.
• **IM; IV**
  Isoniazid-induced deficiency.
Adults: 50–200 mg/day for 3 weeks followed by 25–100 mg/day as needed.
  Cycloserine poisoning.
Adults: 300 mg/day.
  Isoniazid poisoning.
Adults: 1 gram for each gram of isoniazid taken.

NURSING CONSIDERATIONS

ADMINISTRATION/STORAGE
1. If receiving levodopa, avoid preparations of vitamins containing B$_6$ as this decreases the availability of levodopa to the brain.
IV 2. May be administered by direct IV or placed in infusion solutions.

ASSESSMENT
1. Note reasons for therapy, e.g., to prevent toxicity (peripheral neuropathy) with long term isoniazid or contraceptive therapy, to replace vitamin B$_6$ with inborn errors of metabolism or with poor nutrition, or other conditions, characteristics of S&Ss, nutritional status.
2. Take a complete dietary/drug history. Report cycloserine, isoniazid, or oral contraceptive use as these increase pyridoxine requirements.
3. Monitor uric acid levels, renal, LFTs; assess for dysfunction.

CLIENT/FAMILY TEACHING
1. Foods high in vitamin B$_6$ include potatoes, lima beans, broccoli, bananas, chicken breast, liver, yeast, wheat germ, whole-grain cereals. Well-balanced diets are the best source of vitamins.
2. If prescribed levodopa, avoid vitamin supplements containing vitamin B$_6$. More than 5 mg of the vitamin antagonizes levodopa effect. At the same time, concomitant carbidopa administration will prevent effects of vitamin B$_6$ on levodopa.
3. If taking phenobarbital and/or phenytoin, obtain serum drug levels rout-

P

---

inely, as pyridoxine alters serum concentrations.

4. Pyridoxine may inhibit lactation. Protein rich diet increases pyridoxine needs. Usual RDA for adults is 2.2 mg; in pregnancy/lactation, 2.6 mg.

5. Do not take OTC vitamin preparations without provider approval.

OUTCOMES/EVALUATE

• Relief of symptoms of pyridoxine deficiency

• Prophylaxis of drug-induced deficiency; ↓ toxic drug side effects

Q

Quetiapine fumarate

(kweh-**TYE**-ah-peen)

CLASSIFICATION(S):
Antipsychotic
PREGNANCY CATEGORY: C
Rx: Seroquel, Seroquel XR.

USES

(1) Treatment of schizophrenia. (2) Short-term treatment of acute manic episodes associated with bipolar I disorder either as monotherapy or adjunct therapy with divalproex or lithium. (3) Treatment of depressive episodes associated with bipolar disorder.

ACTION/KINETICS

Action

Mechanism unknown but may act as an antagonist at dopamine D_2 and serotonin $5HT_2$ receptors. Side effects may be due to antagonism of other receptors (e.g., histamine H_1, dopamine D_1, adrenergic $alpha_1$ and $alpha_2$, serotonin $5HT_{1A}$).

Pharmacokinetics

Rapidly absorbed. Bioavailability is 73% or more. **Peak plasma levels:** 1.5 hr. Metabolized by liver by CYP3A4 and sulfoxidation and oxidation and excreted through urine (about 73%) and feces (about 20%). **$t\frac{1}{2}$, terminal:** About 6 hr.

CONTRAINDICATIONS

Lactation.

SPECIAL CONCERNS

■ (1) Elderly clients with dementia-related psychosis treated with atypical antipsychotic drugs are at an increased risk of death compared with placebo. Analyses of placebo-controlled trials (modal duration of 10 weeks) in these clients revealed a risk of death in the drug-treated clients between 1.6–1.7 times that seen in placebo-treated clients. Over the course of a typical 10-week controlled trial, the rate of death in drug-treated clients was about 4.5%, compared with a rate of about 2.6% in the placebo group. Although the causes of death were varied, most of the deaths appeared to be either cardiovascular (e.g., heart failure, sudden death) or infectious (e.g., pneumonia) in nature. Olanzapine is not approved for the treatment of clients with dementia-related psychosis. (2) Antidepressants increased the risk of suicidal thinking and behavior (suicidality) in short-term studies in children and adolescents with major depressive disorder and other psychiatric disorders. Anyone considering the use of quetiapine or any other antidepressant in a child or adolescent must balance this risk with the clinical need. Closely observe clients who are started on therapy for clinical worsening, suicidality, or unusual changes in behavior. Advise families and caregivers of the need for close observation and communication with the prescriber. Quetiapine is not approved for use in children. (3) Pooled analysis of short-term (4 to 16 weeks) placebo-controlled trials of 9 antidepressant drugs (selective serotonin reuptake inhibitors and others) in children and adolescents with major depressive disorder, obsessive-compulsive disorder, or other psychiatric disorders have revealed a greater risk of adverse reactions representing suicidal thinking or behavior (suicidality) during the first few months of treatment in those receiving antidepressants. The average risk of such reactions in clients receiving antidepressants was 4%, twice the placebo risk of 2%. No suicides occurred in these trials.■ Use with caution in liver disease, in those at risk for aspiration pneumonia, and in those with history of seizures or conditions that lower seizure threshold (e.g., Alzheimer's). There is an increased risk of hyperglycemia and diabetes associated with quetiapine. Use with caution in geriatric clients, as the drug may be excreted more slowly in this population (rate of death due to CV events or infections is higher in clients with dementia). Safety and efficacy have not been determined in children.

SIDE EFFECTS

Most Common

Headache, drowsiness/somnolence, dizziness, hypotension, tachycardia, constipation, dry mouth, dyspepsia.

Side effects with an incidence of 1% or more are listed. **Body as a whole:** Asthenia, rash, fever, weight gain, back pain, flu syndrome. **CNS:** Headache, drowsiness/somnolence, dizziness, hypertonia, dysarthria. **GI:** Constipation, dry mouth, dyspepsia, anorexia, abdominal pain. **CV:** Orthostatic hypotension, syncope, tachycardia, palpitation, possible prolongation of QTc interval that may result in **sudden cardiac death and torsades de pointes**. **Respiratory:** Pharyngitis, rhinitis, increased cough, dyspnea. **Miscellaneous:** Peripheral edema, hyperprolactinemia, sweating, leukopenia, ear pain, diabetes. NOTE: **Neuroleptic malignant syndrome and seizures**, although rare, may occur.

LABORATORY TEST CONSIDERATIONS

↑ ALT during initial therapy, AST, total cholesterol, triglycerides.

OD OVERDOSE MANAGEMENT

Symptoms: Drowsiness, sedation, tachycardia, hypotension, dystonic reaction of the head and neck, seizures, obtun-

dation. *Treatment:* Cardiovascular monitoring for arrhythmias. If antiarrhythmic therapy is used, disopyramide, procainamide, and quinidine increase risk of prolongation of QT. Treat hypotension and circulatory shock with IV fluids or sympathomimetic drugs (do not use epinephrine or dopamine as they may worsen hypotension). Use anticholinergic drugs to treat severe extrapyramidal symptoms.

DRUG INTERACTIONS

Barbiturates / ↓ Quetiapine effect R/T ↑ liver breakdown; higher maintenance doses may be needed

Carbamazepine / ↓ Quetiapine effect R/T ↑ liver breakdown; higher maintenance doses may be needed

Dopamine agonists / Quetiapine antagonizes effect

Erythromycin / ↑ Quetiapine peak plasma levels, AUC, and t½ R/T inhibition of metabolism by CYP3A4

Glucocorticoids / ↓ Quetiapine effect R/T ↑ liver breakdown

Levodopa / Quetiapine antagonizes effect

Phenytoin / ↓ Quetiapine effect R/T ↑ liver breakdown; higher maintenance doses may be needed

Rifampin / ↓ Quetiapine effect R/T ↑ liver breakdown

Thioridazine / ↑ Quetiapine clearance

HOW SUPPLIED

Tablets: 25 mg, 50 mg, 100 mg, 200 mg, 300 mg, 400 mg; *Tablets, Extended-Release:* 200 mg, 300 mg, 400 mg.

DOSAGE

• **TABLETS; TABLETS, EXTENDED-RELEASE**

   Schizophrenia.

Initial: 25 mg 2 times per day, with increases of 25 to 50 mg 2–3 times per day on the second and third day, as tolerated. Target dose range, by fourth day, is 300 to 400 mg divided into 2 or 3 doses. Further dosage adjustments can occur at intervals of two or more days. The antipsychotic dose range is 150 to 750 mg/day. If dosage adjustments are needed, increments/decrements of 25–50 mg twice daily are recommended. Consider a slower rate of dose titration and a lower target dose in the elderly, in those with hepatic impairment, debilitated clients, or in those with a predisposition to hypotensive reactions.

Bipolar disorder.

When used as either monotherapy or adjunct therapy (with lithium or divalproex), begin quetiapine with a total of 100 mg/day on day 1 (given in 2 doses); increase to 400 mg/day on day 4 in increments of up to 100 mg/day in 2–3 divided doses daily. Further dosage adjustments, up to 800 mg/day by day 6, should be in increments of no more than 200 mg/day. The majority of clients respond at doses between 400 and 800 mg/day. The safety of doses above 800 mg/day has not been evaluated.

Depressive episodes.

Adults, Day 1: 50 mg; **Day 2:** 100 mg; **Day 3:** 200 mg; **Day 4:** 300 mg. Those receiving 600 mg increased from 300 to 400 mg on day 5 and to 600 mg on day 8 (week 1). No additional benefit was observed at doses of 600 mg.

NURSING CONSIDERATIONS

Ⓒ Do not confuse Seroquel with Serzone (an antidepressant).

ADMINISTRATION/STORAGE

1. Once daily therapy may be possible if using the extended-release tablets.
2. Continue clients who respond to quetiapine using the lowest dose needed to maintain remission. Periodically reassess.
3. Start clients with impaired hepatic function on 25 mg/day. Increase the dose daily by 25–50 mg/day to an effective dosage, depending on the clinical response and client tolerability.
4. Consider a slower rate of titration and a lower target dose in elderly, debilitated clients, or in those who have a predisposition to hypotensive reactions.
5. Titration is not required when restarting clients who have had an interval of less than one week off quetiapine. Initial titration schedule is followed if clients have been off drug for more than one week.
6. The period of overlapping antipsychotic drugs should be minimized.

When switching clients from depot antipsychotics, if medically appropriate, start quetiapine therapy in place of the next scheduled injection. Periodically reevaluate clients.

7. Store from 15–30°C (59–86°F). Protect from moisture.

ASSESSMENT

1. List reasons for therapy, clinical presentation, behavioral manifestations. List other agents prescribed.
2. Note any predisposition to hypotensive reactions if debilitated; if hepatic impairment present.
3. Document ophthalmic exam initially, and at 6 month intervals, to assess for cataract formation.
4. Assess for S&S of Alzheimer's disease, history of seizures, cardiovascular disease; note VS, ECG, renal, glucose, LFTs. Use cautiously in the elderly; do not clear drug normally and have increased mortality with dementia-related psychosis.

CLIENT/FAMILY TEACHING

1. May take with or without food.
2. Total daily dose is divided and given two or three times a day unless using the extended-release tablets.
3. Do not perform activities that require mental alertness until after titration period and until drug effects realized; may impair judgement and motor skills, and cause sleepiness. Change positions slowly to prevent low BP effects.
4. Avoid alcohol and any OTC agents without approval. May induce or aggravate diabetes control; report for scheduled labs.
5. Use reliable contraception; report if pregnancy suspected. Do not breastfeed.
6. Report any evidence of tardive dyskinesia (involuntary movements) and extrapyramidal symptoms (tremors, jerking movements).
7. Avoid situations where overheating or dehydration may occur.
8. Long-term usefulness must be evaluated periodically while on lowest dose to maintain remission. Keep all F/U appointments to evaluate response to therapy.

📖 = see color insert   Ⓗ = Herbal   Ⓘⓥ = Intravenous   Ⓒ = sound alike drug

OUTCOMES/EVALUATE
- Control of S&S of psychotic disorders i.e., ↓ Paranoia/ delusions/hallucinations/emotional lability
- Control of bipolar mania/depression

Quinapril hydrochloride
(**KWIN**-ah-prill)

CLASSIFICATION(S):
Antihypertensive, ACE inhibitor
PREGNANCY CATEGORY: D
Rx: Accupril.

SEE ALSO ANGIOTENSIN-CONVERTING ENZYME INHIBITORS.

USES
(1) Alone or in combination with a thiazide diuretic for the treatment of hypertension. (2) Adjunct with a diuretic or digitalis to treat CHF in those not responding adequately to diuretics or digitalis.

ACTION/KINETICS
Action
Inhibits angiotensin-converting enzyme resulting in decreased plasma angiotensin II, which leads to decreased vasopressor activity and decreased aldosterone secretion. Also appears to improve endothelial function, an early marker of coronary atherosclerosis.

Pharmacokinetics
Onset: 1 hr. **Time to peak serum levels:** 1 hr. **Peak effect:** 2–4 hr. Bioavailability is about 60%. Metabolized to quinaprilat, the active metabolite. t½, **quinaprilat:** 2–3 hr. **Duration:** 24 hr. Significantly bound to plasma proteins. Food reduces absorption. Metabolized with approximately 60% excreted through the urine and 40% excreted in the feces. **Plasma protein binding:** About 97%.

SPECIAL CONCERNS
■ When used in pregnancy during the second and third trimesters, ACE inhibitors can cause injury and even death to the developing fetus. When pregnancy is detected, discontinue as soon as possible.■ Use with caution during lacta-tion. Safety and effectiveness have not been determined in children. Geriatric clients may be more sensitive to the effects of quinapril and manifest higher peak quinaprilat blood levels.

SIDE EFFECTS
Most Common
Dizziness, headache, fatigue, chest pain, hypotension, dyspnea, N&V.
CV: Vasodilation, tachycardia, **heart failure**, palpitations, chest pain, hypotension, **MI, CVA, hypertensive crisis**, angina pectoris, orthostatic hypotension, **cardiac rhythm disturbances, cardiogenic shock**. **GI:** Dry mouth or throat, constipation, diarrhea, N&V, abdominal pain, hepatitis, pancreatitis, **GI hemorrhage**. **CNS:** Somnolence, vertigo, insomnia, sleep disturbances, paresthesias, nervousness, depression, headache, dizziness, fatigue. **Hematologic: Agranulocytosis**, bone marrow depression, thrombocytopenia. **Dermatologic: Angioedema of the lips, tongue, glottis, and larynx**; sweating, pruritus, exfoliative dermatitis, photosensitivity, dermatopolymyositis, flushing, rash. **Body as a whole:** Malaise, edema, back pain. **GU:** Oliguria and/or progressive azotemia and rarely **acute renal failure and/or death in severe heart failure**. Impotence. Worsening renal failure. **Respiratory:** Pharyngitis, cough, asthma, bronchospasm, dyspnea. **Musculoskeletal:** Myalgia, arthralgia. **Miscellaneous:** Oligohydramnios in fetuses exposed to the drug in utero. Syncope, hyperkalemia, amblyopia, viral infection.

OD OVERDOSE MANAGEMENT
Symptoms: Commonly, hypotension. *Treatment:* IV infusion of normal saline to restore blood pressure.

DRUG INTERACTIONS
Potassium-containing salt substitutes / ↑ Risk of hyperkalemia
Potassium-sparing diuretics / ↑ Risk of hyperkalemia
Potassium supplements / ↑ Risk of hyperkalemia
Tetracyclines / ↓ Absorption R/T high Mg^+ content of quinapril tablets

HOW SUPPLIED
Tablets: 5 mg, 10 mg, 20 mg, 40 mg.

DOSAGE

- **TABLETS**

Hypertension, client not on diuretics.
Initial: 10 or 20 mg once daily; **then,** adjust dosage based on BP response at peak (2–6 hr) and trough (predose) blood levels. The dose should be adjusted at 2-week intervals. **Maintenance:** 20, 40, or 80 mg daily as a single dose or in two equally divided doses; usual dose is 10–40 mg/day. With impaired renal function, the maximal initial dose should be 10 mg if the C_{CR} is greater than 60 mL/min, 5 mg if the C_{CR} is between 30 and 60 mL/min, and 2.5 mg if the C_{CR} is between 10 and 30 mL/min. If the initial dose is well tolerated, the drug may be given the following day as a twice a day regimen.

Hypertension, client on diuretics.
Initial: 5 mg with careful supervision for several hr until BP stabilizes.

CHF.
Initial: 5 mg twice a day. If this dose is well tolerated, titrate clients at weekly intervals until an effective dose, usually 20–40 mg daily in two equally divided doses, is attained. Undesirable hypotension, orthostasis, or azotemia may prevent this dosage level from being reached.

NURSING CONSIDERATIONS

ⓡ Do not confuse Accupril with Accutane (antiacne drug) or with Aciphex (proton pump inhibitor).

ADMINISTRATION/STORAGE

1. If taking a diuretic, discontinue diuretic 2–3 days prior to beginning quinapril. If BP is not controlled, reinstitute the diuretic. If the diuretic cannot be discontinued, the initial dose should be 5 mg.
2. If the antihypertensive effect decreases at the end of the dosing interval with once-daily therapy, consider either twice-daily administration or increasing the dose.
3. If the initial dose is well tolerated for treating CHF, quinapril may be given as a twice a day regimen. In the absence of excessive hypotension or significant renal function deterioration, the dose may be increased at weekly intervals, based on clinical and hemodynamic responses.
4. The antihypertensive effect may not be observed for 1–2 weeks.
5. Store from 15–30°C (59–86°F).

ASSESSMENT

1. Note reasons for therapy, all medical conditions, other agents trialed.
2. Observe infants exposed to quinapril in utero for the development of hypotension, oliguria, and hyperkalemia.
3. If angioedema occurs, stop drug, assess airway, and observe until swelling resolved. Antihistamines may help relieve symptoms.
4. Monitor VS, I&O, weights, electrolytes, CBC, microalbumin, renal and LFTs. Agranulocytosis and bone marrow depression seen more often with renal impairment, esp. if collagen vascular disease (e.g., SLE, scleroderma) present. Check BP before and 2–6 hr after therapy to assess BP control.
5. Clients with unilateral or bilateral renal artery stenosis may manifest increased BUN and creatinine if given quinapril. Assess renal function closely esp. during first few weeks of therapy; reduce dose with dysfunction. Monitor renal function and serum K^+ during therapy.

CLIENT/FAMILY TEACHING

1. Take as directed; 1–2 hr before food or antacids as they will reduce absorption. Avoid foods high in potassium/potassium supplements. Consume adequate fluids to prevent dehydration; hot weather and exercise may increase loss.
2. Avoid activities that require mental alertness until drug effects realized; may cause dizziness or drowsiness. Change positions slowly to prevent sudden low BP.
3. Report unusual bruising/bleeding, fever, sore throat, cough, or persistent side effects.
4. Any increased SOB, palpitations, swelling, or persistent nonproductive cough should be evaluated as well as rash and altered taste perception. Immediately report any sudden breathing difficulty, swelling of eyes, tongue, lips or face.

Q

---

5. Keep a log of BP and HR readings at different times during the day for provider review.

6. Practice reliable contraception; report if pregnancy suspected.

7. Some OTC drugs may affect the action of quinapril; consult provider before taking OTC drugs. Keep all F/U appointments.

OUTCOMES/EVALUATE

↓ BP

Quinidine gluconate

IV ©

(**KWIN**-ih-deen)

CLASSIFICATION(S):
Antiarrhythmic, Class IA
PREGNANCY CATEGORY: C
Rx: Quinidine Gluconate Injection.

Quinidine sulfate

PREGNANCY CATEGORY: C
❧**Rx:** Apo-Quinidine.

SEE ALSO ANTIARRHYTHMIC AGENTS.

USES
(1) Premature atrial, AV junctional, and ventricular contractions. (2) Treatment and control of atrial flutter, established atrial fibrillation, paroxysmal atrial tachycardia, paroxysmal AV junctional rhythm, paroxysmal and chronic atrial fibrillation, paroxysmal ventricular tachycardia not associated with complete heart block. (3) Maintenance therapy after electrical conversion of atrial flutter or fibrillation. The parenteral route is indicated when PO therapy is not feasible or immediate effects are required. *Investigational:* Gluconate salt for life-threatening *Plasmodium falciparum* malaria.

ACTION/KINETICS
Action
Reduces the excitability of the heart and depresses conduction velocity and contractility. Prolongs the refractory period and increases conduction time. It

also decreases CO and possesses anticholinergic, antimalarial, antipyretic, and oxytocic properties.

Pharmacokinetics
PO: Onset: 0.5–3 hr. **Maximum effects, after IM:** 30–90 min. **t½:** 6–7 hr. **Time to peak levels, PO:** 3–5 hr for gluconate salt and 1–1.5 hr for sulfate salt. **IM:** 1 hr. **Therapeutic serum levels:** 2–6 mcg/mL. **Duration:** 6–8 hr for tablets/capsules and 12 hr for extended-release tablets. Metabolized by liver. Urine pH affects rate of urinary excretion (10–50% excreted unchanged). **Plasma protein binding:** 60–80%.

CONTRAINDICATIONS
Hypersensitivity to drug or other cinchona drugs. Myasthenia gravis, history of thrombocytopenic purpura associated with quinidine use, digitalis intoxication evidenced by arrhythmias or AV conduction disorders. Also, complete heart block, left bundle branch block, or other intraventricular conduction defects manifested by marked QRS widening or bizarre complexes. Complete AV block with an AV nodal or idioventricular pacemaker, aberrant ectopic impulses and abnormal rhythms due to escape mechanisms. History of drug-induced torsades de pointes or long QT syndrome.

SPECIAL CONCERNS
Safety in children and during lactation has not been established. Use with extreme caution in clients in whom a sudden change in BP might be detrimental or in those suffering from extensive myocardial damage, subacute endocarditis, bradycardia, coronary occlusion, disturbances in impulse conduction, chronic valvular disease, considerable cardiac enlargement, frank CHF, and renal or hepatic disease. Use with caution in acute infections, hyperthyroidism, muscular weakness, respiratory distress, and bronchial asthma. The dose in geriatric clients may have to be reduced due to age-related changes in renal function.

SIDE EFFECTS
Most Common
Diarrhea, anorexia, bitter taste in mouth, dizziness, headache, tinnitus,

blurred vision, GI upset, fever, rash, arrhythmias, N&V, asthenia, cerebral ischemia.
CV: Widening of QRS complex, hypotension, *cardiac asystole*, ectopic ventricular beats, *ventricular tachycardia/flutter or fibrillation, torsades de pointes*, paradoxical tachycardia, *arterial embolism*, ventricular extrasystoles (one or more every 6 beats), prolonged QT interval, cerebral ischemia, *complete AV block*. **GI:** N&V, GI upset, abdominal pain, anorexia, diarrhea, urge to defecate as well as urinate, bitter taste in mouth, esophagitis (rare). **CNS:** Syncope, headache, dizziness, confusion, excitement, vertigo, apprehension, delirium, dementia, ataxia, depression. **Dermatologic:** Rash, urticaria, exfoliative dermatitis, photosensitivity, flushing with intense pruritus, eczema, psoriasis, pigmentation abnormalities. **Musculoskeletal:** Arthritis, myalgia, increase in serum skeletal muscle CPK. **Allergic:** Acute asthma, angioneurotic edema, *respiratory arrest*, dyspnea, fever, *vascular collapse*, purpura, vasculitis, hepatic dysfunction (including granulomatous hepatitis), *hepatic toxicity*. **Hematologic:** Hypoprothrombinemia, *acute hemolytic anemia*, thrombocytopenic purpura, *agranulocytosis*, thrombocytopenia, leukocytosis, neutropenia, shift to left in WBC differential. **Ophthalmic:** Blurred vision, mydriasis, alterations in color perception, decreased field of vision, double vision, photophobia, optic neuritis, night blindness, scotomata. **Miscellaneous:** Fever, asthenia, liver toxicity including hepatitis, lupus nephritis, tinnitus, decreased hearing acuity, lupus erythematosus.

LABORATORY TEST CONSIDERATIONS
False + or ↑ PSP, 17-ketosteroids, PT.

OD OVERDOSE MANAGEMENT
Symptoms: **CNS:** Lethargy, confusion, *coma, seizures, respiratory depression or arrest*, headache, paresthesia, vertigo. CNS symptoms may be seen after onset of CV toxicity. **GI:** Vomiting, diarrhea, abdominal pain, hypokalemia, nausea. **CV:** Sinus tachycardia, *ventricular tachycardia or fibrillation, tor-* *sades de pointes, depressed automaticity and conduction* (including bundle branch block, sinus bradycardia, SA block, prolongation of QRS and QTc, sinus arrest, AV block, ST depression, T inversion), syncope, *heart failure*. Hypotension due to decreased conduction and CO and vasodilation. **Miscellaneous:** Cinchonism, visual and auditory disturbances, hypokalemia, tinnitus, acidosis.
Treatment:
- Perform gastric lavage, induce vomiting, and administer activated charcoal if ingestion is recent.
- Monitor ECG, blood gases, serum electrolytes, and BP.
- Institute cardiac pacing, if necessary.
- Acidify the urine.
- Use artificial respiration and other supportive measures.
- Infusions of ⅙ molar sodium lactate IV may decrease the cardiotoxic effects.
- Treat hypotension with metaraminol or norepinephrine after fluid volume replacement.
- Use phenytoin or lidocaine to treat tachydysrhythmias.
- Hemodialysis is effective but not often required.

DRUG INTERACTIONS
Acetazolamide, Antacids / ↑ Quinidine effect R/T ↓ renal excretion
Amiodarone / ↑ Quinidine levels with possible fatal cardiac dysrhythmias
Anticholinergic agents, Atropine / Additive effect on blockade of vagus nerve action
Anticoagulants, oral / Additive hypoprothrombinemia with possible hemorrhage
Barbiturates / ↓ Quinidine effect R/T ↑ liver breakdown
H *Belladonna leaf/root /* Increased anticholinergic effect
Cholinergic agents / Quinidine antagonizes effect of cholinergic drugs
Cimetidine / ↑ Quinidine effect R/T ↓ liver breakdown
Digoxin / ↑ Symptoms of digoxin toxicity
Disopyramide / Either ↑ disopyramide levels or ↓ quinidine levels

Guanethidine / Additive hypotensive effect

Grapefruit juice / ↓ Quinidine absorption and inhibition of quinidine metabolism; effects on the QTc interval delayed and reduced

H *Henbane leaf* / ↑ Anticholinergic effects

Itraconazole / ↑ Risk of tinnitus and ↓ hearing

H *Lily-of-the-valley* / ↑ Effect and side effects of quinidine

Methyldopa / Additive hypotensive effect

Metoprolol / ↑ Metoprolol effect in fast metabolizers

Neuromuscular blocking agents / ↑ Respiratory depression

Nifedipine / ↓ Quinidine effect

H *Pheasant's eye herb* / ↑ Effect and side effects of quinidine

Phenobarbital, Phenytoin / ↓ Quinidine effect R/T ↑ rate of liver metabolism

Potassium / ↑ Quinidine effect

Procainamide / ↑ Procainamide effects with possible toxicity

Propafenone / ↑ Serum propafenone levels in rapid metabolizers

Propranolol / ↑ Propranolol effect in fast metabolizers

Rifampin / ↓ Quinidine effect R/T ↑ liver breakdown

H *Scopolia root* / ↑ Quinidine effect

Skeletal muscle relaxants / ↑ Skeletal muscle relaxation

Sodium bicarbonate / ↑ Quinidine effect R/T ↓ renal excretion

H *Squill* / ↑ Effect and side effects of quinidine

Sucralfate / ↓ Serum quinidine levels → ↓ effect

Thiazide diuretics / ↑ Quinidine effect R/T ↓ renal excretion

Tricyclic antidepressants / ↑ TCA effect R/T ↓ clearance

Verapamil / ↓ Verapamil clearance → ↑ hypotension, bradycardia, AV block, VT, and pulmonary edema

HOW SUPPLIED

Quinidine gluconate. *Injection:* 80 mg/mL; *Tablets, Extended-Release:* 324 mg.

Quinidine sulfate. *Tablets:* 200 mg, 300 mg; *Tablets, Extended-Release:* 300 mg.

DOSAGE

QUINIDINE SULFATE

- **TABLETS**

  Premature atrial and ventricular contractions.

  Adults: 200–300 mg 3–4 times per day.

  Paroxysmal SVTs.

  Adults: 400–600 mg q 2–3 hr until the paroxysm is terminated.

  Conversion of atrial flutter.

  Adults: 200 mg q 2–3 hr for five to eight doses; daily doses can be increased until rhythm is restored or toxic effects occur.

  Conversion of atrial flutter, maintenance therapy.

  Adults: 200–300 mg 3–4 times per day. Large doses or more frequent administration may be required in some clients.

QUINIDINE GLUCONATE AND QUINIDINE SULFATE

- **TABLETS, EXTENDED-RELEASE**

  All uses.

  Adults: 300–600 mg q 8–12 hr.

QUINIDINE GLUCONATE INJECTION

- **IM; IV**

  Acute tachycardia.

  Adults, initial: 600 mg IM; **then,** 400 mg IM repeated as often as q 2 hr.

  Arrhythmias.

  Adults: 330 mg IM or less IV (as much as 500–750 mg may be required).

  P. falciparum malaria.

  Two regimens may be used. (1) *Loading dose:* 15 mg/kg in 250 mL NSS given over 4 hr; **then,** 24 hr after beginning the loading dose, institute 7.5 mg/kg infused over 4 hr and given q 8 hr for 7 days or until PO therapy can be started. (2) **Loading dose:** 10 mg/kg in 250 mL NSS infused over 1–2 hr followed immediately by 0.02 mg/kg/min for up to 72 hr or until parasitemia decreases to less than 1% or PO therapy can be started.

NURSING CONSIDERATIONS

© Do not confuse quinidine with quinine (an antimalarial) or with clonidine (an antihypertensive).

ADMINISTRATION/STORAGE

1. A preliminary test dose may be given. **Adults:** 200 mg quinidine sulfate or quinidine gluconate administered PO or

---

Bold Italic = life threatening side effect   ■ = black box warning   ♣ = Available in Canada

IM. **Children:** Test dose of 2 mg/kg of quinidine sulfate.

2. The extended-release forms are not interchangeable.

3. Prepare IV solution by diluting 10 mL of quinidine gluconate injection (800 mg) with 50 mL of D5W; give at a rate of 1 mL/min.

4. Use only colorless clear solution for injection. Light may cause quinidine to crystallize, which turns solution brownish.

ASSESSMENT

1. Note any allergic reactions to antiarrhythmic drugs or tartrazine, which is found in some formulations. Perform a test dose; observe for hypersensitivity reactions and check for intolerance.

2. List reasons for therapy, onset, characteristics S&S, other agents/therapies trialed, outcome.

3. Obtain CXR; monitor lytes, CBC, renal and LFTs.

4. Assess VS, ECG, cardiopulmonary findings.

INTERVENTIONS

1. Report any increased AV block, prolonged PR or QT intervals, cardiac irritability, or rhythm suppression during IV administration and stop drug therapy.

2. Monitor I&O, VS; observe for ↓ BP. Drug induces urinary alkalization. Report any persistent diarrhea.

3. Report any neurologic deficits/sensory impairment (i.e., numbness, confusion, psychosis, depression, or involuntary movements).

4. Among the elderly, there is a higher risk of toxicity, reduced CO, and unpredictable drug effects.

5. Clients with long-standing atrial fibrillation or CHF with atrial fibrillation run a risk of embolization from mural thrombi when converting to sinus rhythm. Assess echocardiogram and ensure antiocoagulated to prevent thromboembolism.

6. Monitor LFTs, PT/INR to ensure no adverse drug side effects.

CLIENT/FAMILY TEACHING

1. Take with food to minimize GI effects.

2. Avoid activities that require mental alertness until drug effects realized; may cause dizziness or blurred vision.

3. Add fruit and grain to diet. A high intake of fruits and vegetables (alkaline-ash foods) may prolong drug half-life. However, avoid grapefruit juice if taking quinidine sulfate extended-release tablets. Intake of salt may increase the plasma levels of quinidine.

4. Report any of the following adverse effects:
- Severe skin rash, hives, or itching
- Severe headache
- Unexplained fever
- Ringing in the ears, buzzing, or hearing loss
- Unusual bruising or bleeding
- Blurred vision
- Irregular heart beat, palpitations, or faintness
- Continued diarrhea

5. Wear dark glasses if light sensitive.

6. Report for labs, ECG, PFTs, eye exams as scheduled.

OUTCOMES/EVALUATE
- Restoration of stable rhythm
- Therapeutic drug levels (2–6 mcg/mL)
- Malaria treatment

Quinine sulfate
(**KWYE**-nine)

CLASSIFICATION(S):
Antimalarial
PREGNANCY CATEGORY: X
Rx: Qualaquin.
♣Rx: Quinine-Odan.

USES

(1) Alone or in combination with pyrimethamine and a sulfonamide or a tetracycline for chloroquine-resistant forms of *Plasmodium falciparum*. (2) As alternative therapy for chloroquine-sensitive stains of *P. falciparum, P. malariae, P. ovale,* and *P. vivax*. Mefloquine and clindamycin may also be used with quinine, depending on where the malaria was acquired. *Investigational:* Preven-

tion and treatment of nocturnal recumbency leg cramps.

ACTION/KINETICS

Action

Natural alkaloid having antimalarial, antipyretic, analgesic, and oxytocic properties. Antimalarial mechanism not known precisely; quinine does affect DNA replication and may raise intracellular pH. Eradicates the erythrocytic stages of plasmodia. Increases the refractory period of skeletal muscle, decreases the excitability of the motor end-plate region, and affects the distribution of calcium within the muscle fiber, thus making it useful for nocturnal leg cramps. Is oxytocic and may cause congenital malformations.

Pharmacokinetics

Rapidly and completely absorbed from the upper small intestine; widely distributed in body tissues. **Peak plasma levels:** 1–3 hr; **plasma levels following chronic use:** 7 mcg/mL. **t½:** 4–5 hr. Metabolized in the liver with about 5% excreted unchanged in urine. Small amounts found in saliva, bile, feces, and gastric juice. Acidifying the urine increases the rate of excretion. Pharmacokinetics of quinine are affected by malaria, with a decrease in volume of distribution and systemic clearance. **Plasma protein binding:** 70–85%. Protein binding increases to more than 90% in clients with cerebral malaria, in pregnancy, and in children.

CONTRAINDICATIONS

Use with tinnitus, G6PD deficiency, optic neuritis, history of blackwater fever, and thrombocytopenia purpura associated with previous use of quinine. Pregnancy.

SPECIAL CONCERNS

Use with caution in clients with cardiac arrhythmias and during lactation. Hemolysis, with a potential for hemolytic anemia, may occur in clients with G6PD deficiency; use in these clients only if essential and under close supervision. Tinnitus and impaired hearing may occur at plasma quinine levels >10 mcg/mL (a level not normally reached with 260–530 mg/day of quinine) but in a hypersensitive client, as little as 300 mg may produce tinnitus.

SIDE EFFECTS

Most Common

Headache, vasodilation, sweating, nausea, tinnitus, impaired hearing, vertigo/dizziness, blurred vision, disturbed color perception.

Use of quinine may result in a syndrome referred to as cinchonism. Mild cinchonism is characterized by tinnitus, headache, nausea, slight visual disturbances. Larger doses, however, may cause severe CNS, CV, GI, or dermatologic effects. **Allergic:** Flushing, cutaneous rashes (papular, scarlatinal, urticarial), fever, facial edema, pruritus, dyspnea, tinnitus, sweating, asthmatic symptoms, visual impairment, gastric upset. **GI:** N&V, epigastric pain, hepatitis, GI disturbance. **Ophthalmologic:** Blurred vision with scotomata, photophobia, diplopia, night blindness, decreased visual fields, impaired color vision and perception, amblyopia, mydriasis, optic atrophy. **CNS:** Headache, confusion, restlessness, vertigo, syncope, fever, apprehension, excitement, delirium, hypothermia, dizziness, ***convulsions***. **Otic:** Tinnitus, deafness. **Hematologic:** Acute hemolysis, hemolytic anemia, thrombocytopenic purpura, agranulocytosis, hypoprothrombinemia. **CV:** Symptoms of angina, ventricular tachycardia, conduction disturbances, vasculitis. **Miscellaneous:** Sweating, hypoglycemia, lichenoid photosensitivity.

OD OVERDOSE MANAGEMENT

Symptoms: Dizziness, intestinal cramping, skin rash, tinnitus. With higher doses, symptoms include apprehension, confusion, fever, headache, vomiting, and seizures.

Treatment:
- Induce vomiting or undertake gastric lavage.
- Maintain BP and renal function.
- If necessary, provide artificial respiration.
- Sedatives, oxygen, and other supportive measures may be required.
- Give IV fluids to maintain fluid and electrolyte balance.

- Treat angioedema or asthma with epinephrine, corticosteroids, and antihistamines.
- Urinary acidification will hasten excretion; however, in the presence of hemoglobinuria, acidification of the urine will increase renal blockade.

DRUG INTERACTIONS

Acetazolamide / ↑ Blood levels with potential for quinine toxicity R/T ↓ rate of elimination

Al-containing antacids / ↓ Or delayed quinine absorption

Anticoagulants, oral / Additive hypoprothrombinemia R/T ↓ synthesis of vitamin K–dependent clotting factors

Cimetidine / ↑ Quinine effect R/T ↓ rate of excretion (↑ elimination t½)

Digoxin / ↑ Digoxin serum levels; periodically monitor digoxin levels

Heparin / ↓ Heparin effect

Mefloquine / ↑ Risk of ECG abnormalities or cardiac arrest; also, ↑ risk of convulsions. **Do not** use together; delay mefloquine administration at least 12 hr after the last dose of quinine.

Neuromuscular blocking agents (depolarizing and nondepolarizing) / ↑ Neuromuscular blockade → Respiratory depression and apnea

Rifabutin, Rifampin / ↑ Hepatic clearance of quinine R/T induction of hepatic microsomal enzymes; can persist for several days after discontinuing rifampin

Smoking / Significantly greater quinine clearance R/T ↑ hepatic metabolism

Sodium bicarbonate/urinary alkalinizers / ↑ Quinine blood levels with potential for quinine toxicity R/T ↓ elimination rate

Succinylcholine / ↓ Succinylcholine metabolism rate due to ↓ plasma cholinesterase activity

HOW SUPPLIED

Capsules: 200 mg, 260 mg, 324 mg, 325 mg; *Tablets:* 260 mg.

DOSAGE————————

- **CAPSULES; TABLETS**
  Chloroquine-resistant malaria.

Adults: 650 mg q 8 hr for at least 3 days (7 days in Southeast Asia) along with pyrimethamine, 25 mg twice a day for the first 3 days and sulfadiazine, 2

grams/day for the first 5 days. There are two alternative regimens: (1) quinine, 650 mg q 8 hr for at least 3 days (7 days in Southeast Asia) along with a tetracycline, 250 mg q 6 hr for 10 days or (2) quinine, 650 mg q 8 hr for 3 days with sulfadoxine, 1.5 grams and pyrimethamine, 75 mg as a single dose

  Chloroquine-sensitive malaria.

Adults: 260–650 mg q 8 hr for 6–12 days. **Pediatric:** 10 mg/kg q 8 hr for 5–7 days.

NURSING CONSIDERATIONS

⦿ Do not confuse quinine with quinidine (an antiarrhythmic).

ADMINISTRATION/STORAGE

1. Rule out clients at risk for G-6PD deficiency before breastfeeding.
2. Dispense in a light-resistant and child-resistant container; store at controlled room temperatures of 15–30°C (59–86°F).
3. The parenteral form is available from the Centers for Disease Control if client unable to take PO.

ASSESSMENT

1. List reasons for therapy, onset, duration, symptoms, travel dates, other agents trialed.
2. Note any history or evidence of cardiac arrhythmias or CAD.
3. Obtain baseline LFTs, CBC, and eye exam; monitor status.

CLIENT/FAMILY TEACHING

1. Do not take with antacids. Take with food or after meals with a full glass of water to minimize GI irritation. Stop smoking.
2. Do not drive a car or operate machinery until drug effects realized; may cause dizziness or blurred vision.
3. Use sunglasses to protect from photophobia.
4. Avoid tonic water and OTC agents, especially cold remedies. If also taking cimetidine or digoxin, may require dosage adjustment; report side effects.
5. Females should use non-hormonal contraception; drug may harm fetus.
6. Report adverse effects, lack of response, ringing in the ears, blurring of vision, and headache, which may be followed by digestive disturbances, confu-

Q

sion, and delirium. May indicate intolerance or overdosage and requires immediate medical intervention.

OUTCOMES/EVALUATE
• Termination of acute malarial attack/ control of malaria symptoms

——COMBINATION DRUG——

Quinupristin/ Dalfopristin ■ IV

(**kwin**-oo-**PRIS**-tin, **DAL**-foh-**pris**-tin)

CLASSIFICATION(S):
Antibiotic, streptogramin
PREGNANCY CATEGORY: B
Rx: Synercid.

USES
(1) Serious or life-threatening infections associated with vancomycin-resistant *Enterococcus faecium* bacteremia. (2) Complicated skin and skin structure infections caused by *Staphylococcus aureus* (methicillin-sensitive) or *Streptococcus pyogenes*.

ACTION/KINETICS
Action
A sterile, lyophilized product of two semisynthetic pristinamycin derivatives—quinupristin (30 parts) and dalfopristin (70 parts). The two act synergistically so the microbiologic activity is greater than each individually. Metabolites of the two are also active. The drugs act at the bacterial ribosome: Dalfopristin inhibits the early phase of protein synthesis while quinupristin inhibits the late phase of protein synthesis. Vancomycin-resistant infections may also be resistant to this product.

Pharmacokinetics
$t\frac{1}{2}$, **quinupristin and metabolites:** 3.07 hr; $t\frac{1}{2}$, **dalfopristin and metabolites:** 1.04 hr. Both can interfere with the metabolism of other drugs that are associated with QTc prolongation; however, they do not themselves induce QTc prolongation. Excreted through the feces (about 75% for both drugs) and urine (about 17% for both drugs).

CONTRAINDICATIONS
Hypersensitivity to quinupristin/dalfopristin or prior hypersensitivity to other streptogramins. Use with drugs metabolized by the CYP3A4 enzyme system that may prolong the QTc interval.

SPECIAL CONCERNS
■ This drug was approved through FDA's accelerated approval regulations for serious or life-threatening infections associated with vancomycin-resistant *Enterococcus faecium* bacteremia. Approval is based on a demonstrated effect on a surrogate endpoint that is likely to predict clinical benefit. Clearance of vancomycin-resistant *E. faecium* from the bloodstream with clearance of bacteremia is considered to be a surrogate endpoint. No results from well-controlled clinical studies confirm the validity of this surrogate marker, although such studies are underway.■ Use with caution during lactation. Although sometimes used for emergencies in children, safety and efficacy have not been determined in clients less than 16 years of age.

SIDE EFFECTS
Most Common
Inflammation/pain/edema at infusion site, N&V, diarrhea, rash, thrombophlebitis, pain, arthralgia, myalgia, pruritus.
At infusion site: Inflammation, pain, edema, infusion site reaction. **GI:** Pseudomembranous colitis (mild to life-threatening), N&V, diarrhea, constipation, dyspepsia, oral moniliasis, pancreatitis, stomatitis. **CNS:** Headache, anxiety, confusion, dizziness, hypertonia, insomnia, leg cramps, paresthesia. **CV:** Thrombophlebitis, palpitation, phlebitis, vasodilation. **Dermatologic:** Rash, pruritus, maculopapular rash, sweating, urticaria. **Musculoskeletal:** Arthralgia, myalgia, myasthenia. **GU:** Hematuria, vaginitis. **Respiratory:** Dyspnea, pleural effusion. **Miscellaneous:** Pain, abdominal pain, worsening of underlying illness, allergic reaction, chest pain, fever, infection, superinfection.

LABORATORY TEST CONSIDERATIONS
↑ AST, ALT, bilirubin, conjugated bilirubin, LDH, alkaline phosphatase, GGT,

---

Bold Italic = life threatening side effect   ■ = black box warning   ✚ = Available in Canada

CPK, creatinine, BUN, hematocrit. ↓ Hemoglobin. ↑ or ↓ Blood glucose, bicarbonates, CO_2, sodium, potassium, platelets. Hyperbilirubinemia.

DRUG INTERACTIONS
Quinupristin/dalfopristin may cause increased plasma levels of drugs primarily metabolized by the CYP3A4 enzyme system. These drugs include: Carbamazepine, cisapride, cyclosporine, delavirdine, diazepam, diltiazem, disopyramide, docetaxel, HMG-CoA reductase inhibitors, indinavir, lidocaine, methylprednisolone, midazolam, nevirapine, nifedipine, paclitaxel, quinidine, ritonavir, tacrolimus, verapamil, vinca alkaloids.

HOW SUPPLIED
Injection, Lyophilized: 500 mg (150 mg quinupristin and 350 mg dalfopristin)/ 10 mL.

DOSAGE
- **IV INFUSION**
  Vancomycin-resistant Enterococcus faecium *infections.*
7.5 mg/kg q 8 hr. Base treatment duration on the site and severity of the infection.
  Complicated skin and skin structure infections.
7.5 mg/kg q 12 hr for 7 days.

NURSING CONSIDERATIONS
ADMINISTRATION/STORAGE
IV 1. Give by IV infusion in D5W over a 60-min period.
2. Central venous access may be used to decrease venous irritation.
3. Use infusion pump/device to control infusion rate.
4. Prepare and give as follows:
- Reconstitute the single dose vial by slowly adding 5 mL D5W or sterile water for injection under strict aseptic conditions (e.g., laminar flow hood).
- To ensure dissolution, gently swirl the vial by manual rotation without shaking (limits foam formation).
- Allow solution to sit for a few minutes until all the foam has disappeared. Solution should be clear. Concentration is 100 mg/mL. Further dilution is required before administration; dilute within 30 min of reconstitution.
- According to the client's weight, add the reconstituted solution to 250 mL of D5W (about 2 mg/mL). An infusion volume of 100 mL may be used for central line infusions.
- If moderate-to-severe venous irritation occurs following peripheral administration, consider increasing the infusion volume to 500 or 750 mL, changing the infusion site, or inserting a central venous catheter.
5. Do not dilute/flush with saline solution because the drugs are incompatible.
6. Do not mix with or physically add these drugs to other drugs except for the following: Aztreonam (20 mg/mL), ciprofloxacin (1 mg/mL), fluconazole (2 mg/mL), haloperidol (0.2 mg/mL), metoclopramide (5 mg/mL), and potassium chloride (40 mEq/L).
7. With intermittent infusion of these drugs and other drugs through a common IV line, flush the line before and after administration with D5W.
8. Before reconstitution, refrigerate vials at 2–8°C (36–46°F).
9. Prior to infusion, diluted solution stable for 5 hr at room temperature or 54 hr if refrigerated. Do not freeze the solution.

ASSESSMENT
1. Note reasons for therapy, characteristics of infection, culture and sensitivity results. Obtain blood cultures to verify *E. faecium* and not *E. faecalis.*
2. If these drugs are used with drugs that are CYP3A4 substrates (see drug interactions) and possess a narrow therapeutic index, monitor liver function and client carefully.
3. If client develops diarrhea, test for *C. difficile* colitis.
4. Isolate client and take special precautions to identify source and to prevent spread of organism.

CLIENT/FAMILY TEACHING
1. Drug is given parenterally to clear up infection that is resistant to vancomycin (VRE). May require isolation and care to prevent transmission throughout facility.

Q

---

2. Report any pain redness or irritation at injection site, diarrhea, pain in joints/muscles. With persistent muscle and joint pains, may reduce severity by re-ducing the dosing interval to every 12 hrs. If S&S worsen, report.

OUTCOMES/EVALUATE
Resolution of VRE infection

R

Rabeprazole sodium

(rah-**BEP**-rah-zohl)

CLASSIFICATION(S):
Proton pump inhibitor
PREGNANCY CATEGORY: B
Rx: Aciphex.
♣Rx: Pariet.

USES
(1) Short-term (4–8 weeks) treatment in the healing and symptomatic relief of erosive or ulcerative gastroesophageal reflux disease (GERD). (2) Maintenance of healing and reduction in relapse rates of heartburn symptoms in clients with erosive or ulcerative GERD. (3) Short-term (up to 4 weeks) treatment in healing and symptomatic relief of duodenal ulcers. (4) Long-term treatment of pathological hypersecretory symptoms, including Zollinger-Ellison syndrome. (5) Daytime and nighttime heartburn and other symptoms of GERD. *Investigational:* Treatment of gastric ulcer.

ACTION/KINETICS

Action
Suppresses gastric secretion by inhibiting gastric H^+/K^+ ATPase at the secretory surface of parietal cells; it is a gastric proton-pump inhibitor. Blocks the final step of gastric acid secretion.

Pharmacokinetics
Is about 52% bioavailable. **Peak plasma levels:** 2–5 hr. **$t\frac{1}{2}$, plasma:** 1–2 hr. **Onset:** Less than 1 hr. **Duration:** Over 24 hr. Extensively metabolized in the liver by CYP3A4 and CYP2C19. Excreted mainly in the urine. **Plasma protein binding:** More than 96%.

CONTRAINDICATIONS
Known sensitivity to rabeprazole or substituted benzimidazoles. Lactation.

SPECIAL CONCERNS
Safety and efficacy have not been determined in children. Greater sensitivity in some geriatric clients is possible. Symptomatic response to therapy does not preclude presence of gastric malignancy. Use with caution in severe hepatic impairment.

SIDE EFFECTS
Most Common
Headache, GI upset, diarrhea, insomnia, nervousness, rash, itching.
GI: Diarrhea, N&V, abdominal pain, GI upset, dyspepsia, flatulence, constipation, dry mouth, eructation, gastroenteritis, *rectal hemorrhage*, melena, anorexia, cholelithiasis, mouth ulceration, stomatitis, dysphagia, gingivitis, cholecystitis, increased appetite, abnormal stools, colitis, esophagitis, glossitis, pancreatitis, proctitis. **Hepatic:** Hepatic encephalopathy, hepatitis, hepatoma, liver fatty deposit. **CNS:** Insomnia, headache, anxiety, dizziness, depression, nervousness, somnolence, hypertonia, neuralgia, vertigo, *convulsions*, abnormal dreams, decreased libido, neuropathy, paresthesia, tremor, coma, disorientation, delirium. **CV:** Hypertension, *MI*, abnormal EEG, migraine, syncope, angina pectoris, bundle branch block, palpitation, sinus bradycardia, tachycardia. **Musculoskeletal:** Myalgia, arthritis, leg cramps, bone pain, arthrosis, twitching, bursitis, neck rigidity, *rhabdomyolysis*. **Respiratory:** Dyspnea, asthma, epistaxis, laryngitis, apnea, hiccough, hyper-/hypoventilation, interstitial pneumo-

---

Bold Italic = life threatening side effect   ■ = black box warning   ♣ = Available in Canada

nia. **Dermatologic:** Rash, pruritus, sweating, urticaria, alopecia, jaundice, bullous and other skin eruptions, erythema multiforme, **toxic epidermal necrolysis, Stevens-Johnson syndrome**. **GU:** Cystitis, urinary frequency, dysmenorrhea, dysuria, kidney calculus, metorrhagia, polyuria, breast enlargement, hematuria, impotence, menorrhagia, orchitis, urinary incontinence, urine abnormality, interstitial nephritis. **Endocrine:** Hyper/hypothyroidism. **Hematologic:** Anemia, ecchymosis, lymphadenopathy, hypochromic anemia, agranulocytosis, hemolytic anemia, leukopenia, pancytopenia, thrombocytopenia. **Metabolic:** Peripheral/facial edema, edema, weight gain/loss, gout, dehydration. **Body as a whole:** Asthenia, fever, allergic reaction, chills, malaise, thirst, substernal chest pain, photosensitivity reaction, hangover effect, jaundice, **sudden death**. **Ophthalmic:** Cataract, amblyopia, glaucoma, dry eyes, abnormal/blurred vision, corneal opacity, diplopia, eye pain, retinal degeneration, strabismus. **Otic:** Tinnitus, otitis media, deafness. **Miscellaneous:** **Anaphylaxis,** angioedema.

LABORATORY TEST CONSIDERATIONS
↑ CPK, AST, ALT, TSH, PSA. Abnormal platelets, erythrocytes, LFTs, urine, WBCs. Albuminuria, hypercholesterolemia, hyperglycemia, hyperlipemia, hypokalemia, hyponatremia, leukocytosis, leukorrhea, hyperammonemia.

DRUG INTERACTIONS
Digoxin / ↑ Plasma levels of digoxin R/T changes in gastric pH
Ketoconazole / ↓ Plasma levels of ketoconazole R/T changes in gastric pH
Warfarin / ↑ PT and INR

HOW SUPPLIED
Tablets, Delayed-Release: 20 mg.

DOSAGE

• **TABLETS, DELAYED-RELEASE**
Healing of erosive or ulcerative GERD.
Adults: 20 mg once daily for 4–8 weeks. An additional 8 weeks of therapy may be considered for those who have not healed.
Maintenance of healing of erosive or ulcerative GERD.
Adults: 20 mg once daily.

Healing of duodenal ulcers.
Adults: 20 mg once daily after the morning meal for up to 4 weeks. A few clients may require additional time to heal.
Treatment of pathological hypersecretory conditions.
Individualized. Adults, initial: 60 mg once a day. Adjust dosage to individual client needs (doses up to 100 mg/day and 60 mg 2 times per day have been used). Continue as long as clinically needed.
Heartburn and other symptoms related to GERD.
20 mg once daily for 4 weeks. If symptoms do not resolve after 4 weeks, an additional course of treatment may be considered.

NURSING CONSIDERATIONS

 ℮ Do not confuse Aciphex with Accupril (ACE inhibitor) or with Aricept (drug for Alzheimer's disease).

ADMINISTRATION/STORAGE
1. No dosage adjustment is needed in elderly clients, those with renal disease, or in mild to moderate hepatic impairment.
2. Protect tablets from moisture.
3. Store from 15–30°C (59–86°F).

ASSESSMENT
1. List reasons for therapy, characteristics of S&S, other agents tried, outcome. List drugs prescribed to ensure none interact.
2. Note UGI/endoscopy findings/biopsies, abdominal assessment, LFTs.

CLIENT/FAMILY TEACHING
1. Take as directed. Swallow tablets whole with or without food; do not crush, chew, or split tablets.
2. Report unusual bleeding, acid reflux, abdominal pain, severe light-headedness, diarrhea, rash, or lack of effectiveness.
3. Avoid alcohol, NSAIDs, and salicylates; may increase GI upset.
4. Do not perform activities that require mental alertness until drug effects realized.
5. Keep all F/U appointments to evaluate drug response. Prolonged therapy may mask GI malignancies.

R

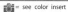 = see color insert   **H** = Herbal   **IV** = Intravenous   ℮ = sound alike drug

OUTCOMES/EVALUATE
- ↓ Intraesophageal acid exposure
- Healing of duodenal ulcers; symptomatic improvement

Raloxifene hydrochloride

(ral-**OX**-ih-feen)

CLASSIFICATION(S):
Estrogen receptor modulator
PREGNANCY CATEGORY: X
Rx: Evista.

USES
Prevention and treatment of osteoporosis in postmenopausal women. Not effective in reducing hot flashes or flushes associated with estrogen deficiency. *Investigational:* Reduce risk of breast cancer in high risk postmenopausal women.

ACTION/KINETICS
Action
Selective estrogen receptor modulator that reduces bone resorption and decreases overall bone turnover. Considered an estrogen antagonist that acts by combining with estrogen receptors. Has not been associated with endometrial proliferation, breast enlargement, breast pain, increased risk of breast cancer, or increased risk of heart attack and other heart problems. Also decreases total and LDL cholesterol levels.

Pharmacokinetics
Absorbed rapidly after PO; significant first-pass effect. $t\frac{1}{2}$: 32.5 hr (multiple doses). Excreted primarily in feces with small amounts excreted in urine.

CONTRAINDICATIONS
In women who are or who might become pregnant, active or history of venous thromboembolic events (e.g., DVT, pulmonary embolism, retinal vein thrombosis). Use in premenopausal women, during lactation, or in pediatric clients. Concurrent use with systemic estrogen or hormone replacement therapy.

SPECIAL CONCERNS
Use with caution with highly protein-bound drugs, including clofibrate, diazepam, diazoxide, ibuprofen, indomethacin, and naproxen. Effect on bone mass density beyond 2 years of treatment is not known.

SIDE EFFECTS
Most Common
Hot flashes, weight gain, nausea, dyspepsia, arthralgia, myalgia, sinusitis, pharyngitis, infection, flu syndrome.
CV: Hot flashes, migraine, venous thromboembolic events (e.g., pulmonary embolism, DVT), syncope, migraine. **Body as a whole:** Infection, flu syndrome, headache, chest pain, fever, weight gain, peripheral edema, infection. **CNS:** Depression, insomnia, vertigo, neuralgia, hypesthesia. **GI:** N&V, dyspepsia, diarrhea, flatulence, GI disorder, gastroenteritis, abdominal pain. **GU:** Vaginitis, UTI, cystitis, leukorrhea, endometrial disorder, uterine disorder, vaginal hemorrhage, urinary tract disorder, breast pain. **Respiratory:** Sinusitis, rhinitis, pharyngitis, bronchitis, increased cough, pneumonia, laryngitis. **Musculoskeletal:** Arthralgia, myalgia, leg cramps, arthritis, tendon disorder. **Dermatologic:** Rash, sweating. **Miscellaneous:** Conjunctivitis.

LABORATORY TEST CONSIDERATIONS
↑ Apolipoprotein A1, steroid-binding globulin, thyroxine-binding globulin, corticosteroid-binding globulin. ↓ Total cholesterol, LDL cholesterol, fibrinogen, apolipoprotein B, lipoprotein.

DRUG INTERACTIONS
Cholestyramine / ↓ Raloxifene absorption
Diazepam / Use with caution R/T both drugs highly protein bound
Diazoxide / Use with caution R/T both drugs highly protein bound
Levothyroxine / ↓ Levothyroxine absorption
Lidocaine / Use with caution R/T both drugs highly protein bound
Warfarin / ↓ PT

HOW SUPPLIED
Tablets: 60 mg.

DOSAGE
- **TABLETS**

Prevention and treatment of osteoporosis in postmenopausal women.
Adults: 60 mg once daily.

NURSING CONSIDERATIONS

🕮 Do not confuse Evista with Avinza (an extended-release morphine sulfate).

ADMINISTRATION/STORAGE
1. May be taken without regard for meals.
2. Take supplemental calcium and vitamin D if daily dietary intake is inadequate.

ASSESSMENT
1. Note reasons for therapy; bone mineral density, onset of menopause, any history of chronic steroid therapy.
2. Assess for history/evidence of CHF, active cancer, ↑ risk of breast cancer in high risk postmenopausal women, blood clots in legs, lungs, or eyes.
3. Monitor bone density, lipids, LFTs; assess for any dysfunction.

CLIENT/FAMILY TEACHING
1. Take as directed once daily. If dietary calcium and vitamin D intake is inadequate, take supplements. May take without regard to food.
2. Drug is used by women after menopause to prevent bones from becoming weak and thin when bone mineral density is very low.
3. Avoid prolonged immobilization and movement restrictions as with travel due to increased risk of blood clots. Stop 3 days prior to and during prolonged immobilization as with surgery or prolonged bed rest.
4. Drug is not effective in reducing hot flashes or flushes associated with low estrogen; does not stimulate breast or uterus.
5. Regular weight-bearing exercises as well as tobacco cessation and alcohol modification should be practiced.
6. Report pain in calves or swelling in legs, fever, insomnia, acute migraines, emotional distress, unexplained uterine bleeding, breast abnormalities, sudden chest pain, SOB, or coughing up blood, as well as any vision changes.

OUTCOMES/EVALUATE
• Treatment of postmenopausal osteoporosis

• Reduction in bone turnover/resorption
• Reduce risk of breast cancer in high risk postmenopausal women

Ramelteon
(ram-**EL**-tee-on)

CLASSIFICATION(S):
Sedative-hypnotic, non-barbiturate
PREGNANCY CATEGORY: C
Rx: Rozerem.

USES
Insomnia due to difficulty with sleep onset.

ACTION/KINETICS

Action
Ramelteon is a melatonin receptor agonist with high affinity for melatonin MT_1 and MT_2 receptors. The activity at melatonin receptors is thought to contribute to its sleep-promoting properties, as these receptors are thought to be involved in the maintenance of the circadian rhythm underlying the normal sleep-wake cycle.

Pharmacokinetics
Rapidly absorbed. **Median peak levels:** 0.75 hr (0.5–1.5 hr) after fasting PO administration. Significant first-pass metabolism is primarily oxidation to hydroxyl and carbonyl derivatives by CYP1A2. Excreted mainly in the urine. Repeated once-daily administration does not result in significant accumulation because of the short elimination $t\frac{1}{2}$ (about 1–2.6 hr).

CONTRAINDICATIONS
Hypersensitivity to the drug or any component of the product. Use with severely impaired hepatic function. Use in clients with severe sleep apena or chronic COPD as the drug has not been evaluated in these populations. Lactation.

SPECIAL CONCERNS
Use with caution in moderate impaired hepatic function. Give with caution to those taking less strong CYP1A2 inhibitors.

R

SIDE EFFECTS
Most Common
Somnolence, dizziness, nausea, diarrhea, fatigue, headache, insomnia.
CNS: Somnolence, dizziness, headache, insomnia, depression. **GI:** Diarrhea, nausea, dysgeusia. **Respiratory:** URTI. **Body as a whole:** Fatigue, influenza, myalgia, arthralgia.

DRUG INTERACTIONS
Alcohol / Additive CNS depressant effects
Azole antifungals (e.g., fluconazole, ketoconazole) / Significant ↑ ramelteon AUC and C_{max}
Fluvoxamine / Significant (190-fold) ↑ ramelteon AUC; do not use together
Rifampin / ↓ Ramelteon AUC and C_{max}

HOW SUPPLIED
Tablets: 8 mg.

DOSAGE
- **TABLETS**
  Insomnia due to difficulty with sleep onset.
  Adults: 8 mg taken within 30 min of going to bed.

NURSING CONSIDERATIONS
ADMINISTRATION/STORAGE
1. Should not be taken with or immediately after a high-fat meal.
2. Store from 15–30°C (59–86°F). Protect from moisture and humidity; keep container tightly closed.

ASSESSMENT
1. Note reasons for therapy, onset, characteristics of S&S, contributing factors, other agents trialed, outcome.
2. Assess for any history of breathing problems (bronchitis, emphysema, sleep apnea), psychiatric illness, or liver disease; may preclude drug therapy.
3. List drugs prescribed to ensure none interact unfavorably.
4. If GU dysfunction or problems with fertility surface, consider reviewing prolactin/testosterone levels.

CLIENT/FAMILY TEACHING
1. Take drug as prescribed within 30 min of going to bed; confine activities to those for sleep preparation. Never attempt to engage in hazardous activities (i.e., operate machinery or drive a car).

2. Ramelteon acts like a natural substance called melatonin that is produced by your body. It helps regulate your sleep-wake cycle (circadian rhythm).
3. Avoid alcohol and do not consume ramelteon with or immediately after consuming a high fat meal; fat may interfere with drug action.
4. May experience sedation; avoid activities that require mental alertness upon awakening.
5. Report any problems with menses or breast drainage, decreased libido, or fertility problems. Also advise provider of any adverse side effects, behavioral changes, or worsening of insomnia.

OUTCOMES/EVALUATE
- Ability to get to sleep
- Relief of insomnia

Ramipril
(**RAM**-ih-prill)

CLASSIFICATION(S):
Antihypertensive, ACE inhibitor
PREGNANCY CATEGORY: D
Rx: Altace.

SEE ALSO ANGIOTENSIN-CONVERTING ENZYME INHIBITORS.

USES
(1) Alone or in combination with other antihypertensive agents (especially thiazide diuretics) for the treatment of hypertension. (2) Treatment of CHF following MI to decrease risk of CV death and decrease the risk of failure-related hospitalization and progression to severe or resistant heart failure. (3) Reduce risk of stroke, MI, and death from CV causes in clients over 55 years with a history of CAD, stroke, peripheral vascular disease, or with diabetes and one other risk factor (e.g., elevated total cholesterol, cigarette smoking, hypertension, low HDL levels, documented microalbuminuria). Can be used in addition to other therapy, including antihypertensive, antiplatelet, or lipid-lowering therapy. *Investigational:* Reduce

---

Bold Italic = life threatening side effect   ■ = black box warning   ♣ = Available in Canada

progression of nondiabetic nephropathy.

ACTION/KINETICS

Action

Inhibits angiotensin-converting enzyme resulting in decreased plasma angiotensin II, which leads to decreased vasopressor activity and decreased aldosterone secretion.

Pharmacokinetics

Onset: 1–2 hr. From 50–60% bioavailable. **Time to peak serum levels:** 1 hr (1–2 hr for ramiprilat, the active metabolite). **Peak effect:** 3–6 hr. Ramiprilat has approximately six times the ACE inhibitory activity than ramipril. **t½:** 1–2 hr (9–18 hr for ramiprilat); prolonged in impaired renal function. **Duration:** 24 hr. Metabolized in the liver with 60% excreted through the urine and 40% in the feces. Food decreases the rate, but not the extent, of absorption of ramipril. **Plasma protein binding:** Ramipril: about 73%; ramiprilat: 56%.

CONTRAINDICATIONS

Lactation.

SPECIAL CONCERNS

■ When used in pregnancy during the second and third trimesters, ACE inhibitors can cause injury and even death to the developing fetus. When pregnancy is detected, discontinue as soon as possible.■ Geriatric clients may manifest higher peak blood levels of ramiprilat. May cause hyperkalemia, especially when used with salt substitutes.

SIDE EFFECTS

Most Common

Hypotension, headache, dizziness, N&V, cough.

CV: Hypotension, chest pain, palpitations, angina pectoris, orthostatic hypotension, *MI, CVA, arrhythmias.* **GI:** N&V, abdominal pain, diarrhea, dysgeusia, anorexia, constipation, dry mouth, dyspepsia, enzyme changes suggesting pancreatitis, dysphagia, gastroenteritis, increased salivation, jaundice, *hepatic failure, fatal fulminant hepatic necrosis.* **CNS:** Headache, dizziness, fatigue, insomnia, sleep disturbances, somnolence, depression, nervousness, malaise, vertigo, anxiety, amnesia, *convulsions,* tremor. **Respiratory:** Cough, dyspnea,

URI, asthma, *bronchospasm.* **Hematologic:** Leukopenia, anemia, eosinophilia. Rarely, decreases in hemoglobin or hematocrit. **Dermatologic:** Diaphoresis, photosensitivity, pruritus, rash, dermatitis, purpura, alopecia, erythema multiforme, urticaria. **Body as a whole:** Paresthesias, angioedema, asthenia, syncope, fever, muscle cramps, myalgia, arthralgia, arthritis, neuralgia, neuropathy, influenza, edema. **Miscellaneous:** Impotence, tinnitus, hearing loss, vision disturbances, epistaxis, weight gain, proteinuria, angioneurotic edema, edema, flu syndrome.

ADDITIONAL DRUG INTERACTIONS

Hypoglycemic drugs, oral / Possible hypoglycemia
Insulin / Possible hypoglycemia

LABORATORY TEST CONSIDERATIONS

↓ H&H.

HOW SUPPLIED

Capsules: 1.25 mg, 2.5 mg, 5 mg, 10 mg.

DOSAGE

• CAPSULES

Hypertension.

Initial: 2.5 mg once daily in clients not taking a diuretic; **maintenance:** 2.5–20 mg/day as a single dose or two equally divided doses.

CHF following MI.

Initial: 2.5 mg twice a day. Clients intolerant of this dose may be started on 1.25 mg twice a day. The target maintenance dose is 5 mg twice a day.

Reduce risk of MI, stroke, death in clients 55 and over with risk factors.

Initial: 2.5 mg/day for 1 week followed by 5 mg/day for the next 3 weeks. **Maintenance:** 10 mg/day. If the client is hypertensive or post-MI, the dose can be divided.

NOTE: In clients with a C_{CR} of 40 mL/min/m² or less, doses of 25% of those normally used should cause full therapeutic levels of ramiprilat. For use in hypertension, start with 1.25 mg once daily; dose may be titrated upward until BP is controlled or to a maximum of 5 mg/day. For use in heart-failure post-MI, start with 1.25 mg once daily. Dose may be increased to 1.25 mg twice a day, up to a maximum of 2.5

R

mg twice a day, depending on response and tolerability.

NURSING CONSIDERATIONS

🖉 Do not confuse Altace with Artane (cholinergic blocking agent).

ADMINISTRATION/STORAGE

1. If antihypertensive effect decreases at the end of the dosing interval with once-daily dosing, consider either twice-daily administration or an increase in dose.
2. If taking diuretic, discontinue 2–3 days prior to beginning ramipril. If BP is not controlled, reinstitute diuretic. If the diuretic cannot be discontinued, consider an initial dose of ramipril of 1.25 mg.

ASSESSMENT

1. Note reasons for therapy, other agents trialed, outcome.
2. Monitor BP, K$^+$, microalbumin, CBC, renal, and LFTs to ensure no abnormality; adjust dose with dysfunction.
3. Assess for other medical conditions that may preclude therapy; renal artery stenosis, severe autoimmune disease, lupus, scleroderma, or bone marrow depression.

CLIENT/FAMILY TEACHING

1. For ease of swallowing, may mix contents of the capsule with water, apple juice, or apple sauce.
2. Use caution; drug may cause drowsiness or dizziness and low BP effects with sudden changes in position.
3. Report persistent, dry, nonproductive cough, increased SOB, edema, significant weight gain, unusual bruising/bleeding or other adverse effects.
4. Record BP at different times of day/night for provider review.
5. Practice reliable birth control; report if pregnancy suspected or desired as drug will need to be stopped.
6. Do not take OTC agents, including potassium/potassium-based salt supplements without approval.

OUTCOMES/EVALUATE

- ↓ BP
- ↓ Mortality with AMI/DM

Ranibizumab
(ran-ih-**BIZ**-oo-mab)

CLASSIFICATION(S):
Selective vascular endothelial growth factor antagonist.
PREGNANCY CATEGORY: C
Rx: Lucentis.

USES
Neovascular (wet) age-related macular degeneration.

ACTION/KINETICS

Action
Binds to the receptor-binding site of active forms of vascular endothelial growth factor A (VEGF-A). VEGF-A causes neovascularization and leakage and is thought to contribute to the progression of the neovascular form of age-related macular degeneration. The binding of ranibizumab to VEGF-A prevents the interaction of VEGF-A with its receptors on the surface of endothelial cells, reducing endothelial cell proliferation, vascular leakage, and new blood vessel formation.

Pharmacokinetics
Small amounts are absorbed systemically. **t½, vitreous elimination:** 9 days.

CONTRAINDICATIONS
Ocular or periocular infections. Hypersensitivity to any component of the product.

SPECIAL CONCERNS
Use with caution during lactation. Safety and efficacy have not been determined in children.

SIDE EFFECTS

Most Common
Conjunctival hemorrhage, eye irritation/pain, foreign body sensation in eyes, intraocular inflammation, increased intraocular pressure, retinal hemorrhage, blurred/decreased visual acuity, vitreous detachment/floaters, headache, arthralgia, nasopharyngitis, URTI, hypertension.

Ophthalmic: Blepharitis, cataract, conjunctival hemorrhage, dry eye, eye irritation, eye pain, eye pruritus, foreign body sensation in eyes, intraocular in-

---

flammation, increased lacrimation, maculopathy, ocular discomfort, ocular hyperemia, posterior capsule opacification, retinal exudates, retinal hemorrhage, subretinal fibrosis, blurred/decreased visual acuity, visual disturbance, vitreous detachment, vitreous floaters, increased intraocular pressure, endophthalmitis, retinal detachments. **CNS:** Headache, dizziness. **GI:** Nausea, constipation. **CV:** Hypertension/elevated BP, arterial thromboembolic reactions, possible increased risk of stroke. **Musculoskeletal:** Arthralgia, arthritis, back pain. **Respiratory:** Bronchitis, cough, nasopharyngitis, sinusitis, URTI. **Miscellaneous:** Anemia, influenza, UTI.

DRUG INTERACTIONS
When used adjunctively with verteporfin photodynamic therapy, possible serious intraocular inflammation

HOW SUPPLIED
Injection, Ophthalmic: 10 mg/mL.

DOSAGE
- **INTRAVITREAL INJECTION ONLY**
  Neovascular (wet) age-related macular degeneration.
Administer 0.5 mg (0.05 mL) by intravitreal injection once a month. Although less effective, treatment may be reduced to 1 injection every 3 months after the first 4 injections, if monthly injections are not feasible.

NURSING CONSIDERATIONS
ADMINISTRATION/STORAGE
1. For ophthalmic intravitreal injection only.
2. Using aseptic technique, all (0.2 mL) of the ranibizumab vial contents are withdrawn through a 5-micron, 19-gauge filter needle attached to a 1 mL tuberculin syringe. Discard filter needle after withdrawal from the vial; do not use for intravitreal injection. Replace filter needle with a sterile 30-gauge x $\frac{1}{2}$-inch needle for the intravitreal injection. Expel the contents until plunger tip is aligned with the line that marks 0.05 mL on the syringe.
3. Carry out intravitreal injection under controlled aseptic conditions, including use of sterile gloves, sterile drape, and a sterile eyelid speculum. Give adequate anesthesia and a broad-spectrum microbicide prior to the injection.
4. Use each vial only to treat a single eye. If the contralateral eye requires treatment, use a new vial. Change the sterile field, syringe, gloves, drapes, eyelid speculum, filter, and injection needles.
5. Refrigerate from 2–8°C (36–46°F). Do not freeze; protect from light.

ASSESSMENT
1. Note onset, symptoms, history, baseline vision level.
2. List drugs prescribed to ensure none interact.
3. Assess eye area to ensure infection free.
4. Add daily supplement of vitamins A, C, and E, along with beta-carotene, zinc, and copper.
5. Identify agencies and support groups that can assist with low vision.

CLIENT/FAMILY TEACHING
1. Drug is injected into eye by retinal Dr to maintain or improve vision with macular degeneration (wet). Will have a post-injection exam before leaving office. Have a friend or family member accompany you so they can drive you home after your injection. Bring sunglasses or a hat to wear after your injection, as you may be sensitive to light for a while. (eyes were dilated).
2. May experience red eye, eye pain, small specks in vision, sensation of something in your eye, and increased tears. Other side effects may include high blood pressure, nose and throat infection, and headache.
3. Can track progress in-between visits (using an Amsler grid). By using an Amsler grid once a week, you may be able to see changes to your vision. Ask retinal Dr for one or download one from www.lucentis.com.
4. Macular degeneration is usually seen in white females over 55 years old that have a family history, are obese, smoke, consume a diet low in minerals such as zinc, and vitamins A, C, and E and have cardiovascular disease.
5. Generally the injections are given once a month. Keep all F/U visits to evaluate progress, maintain/improve vi-

R

sion, and to assess for any adverse side effects.

OUTCOMES/EVALUATE
Maintenance/improvement in vision with macular degeneration

Ranitidine hydrochloride ⅣⒸ
(rah-**NIH**-tih-deen)

CLASSIFICATION(S):
Histamine H₂ receptor blocking drug

PREGNANCY CATEGORY: B

OTC: Zantac 150 Maximum Strength Acid Reducer, Zantac 75 Acid Reducer.

Rx: Zantac, Zantac EFFERdose.

✦Rx: Apo-Ranitidine, Gen-Ranitidine, Novo-Ranitidine, Nu-Ranit, PMS-Ranitidine, Rhoxal-ranitidine, ratio-Ranitidine.

SEE ALSO *HISTAMINE H₂ ANTAGONISTS.*

USES
Rx: (1) Short-term (4–8 weeks) and maintenance treatment of duodenal ulcer. (2) Pathologic hypersecretory conditions such as Zollinger-Ellison syndrome and systemic mastocytosis. (3) Short-term treatment of active, benign gastric ulcers and maintenance treatment after healing of the acute ulcer. (4) Treatment of GERD. (5) Treatment of endoscopically diagnosed erosive esophagitis and for maintenance of healing of erosive esophagitis. (6) IV in some hospitalized clients with pathological hypersecretory conditions or intractable duodenal ulcers, or as an alternative to PO doses for short-term use in those who are unable to take PO medication. *Investigational:* **PO or IM/IV.** As part of a multidrug regimen to eradicate *Helicobacter pylori* in the treatment of peptic ulcer; perioperatively to suppress gastric acid secretion, prevent stress ulcers, and prevent aspiration pneumonitis; in combination with H₁ histamine antagonists to treat certain types of urticaria; and, as prophylaxis to reduce the incidence of NSAID-induced duodenal ulcers.

IV. Prevent paclitaxel hypersensitivity; reduce the incidence of GI hemorrhage associated with stress-related ulcers.

OTC: (1) Relief of heartburn associated with acid indigestion and sour stomach. (2) Prophylaxis of heartburn associated with acid indigestion and sour stomach due to certain foods and beverages.

ACTION/KINETICS
Action
Competitively inhibits gastric acid secretion by blocking the effect of histamine on histamine H₂ receptors. Both daytime and nocturnal basal gastric acid secretion, as well as food- and pentagastrin-stimulated gastric acid are inhibited. Weak inhibitor of cytochrome P-450 (drug-metabolizing enzymes); thus, drug interactions involving inhibition of hepatic metabolism are not expected to occur.

Pharmacokinetics
Bioavailability is 50% after PO administration and 90–100% after IM. Food increases the bioavailability. **Peak effect, PO:** 2–3 hr; **IM; IV:** 15 min. **t½:** 2.5–3 hr. **Duration, nocturnal:** 13 hr; **basal:** 4 hr. **Serum level to inhibit 50% stimulated gastric acid secretion:** 36–94 ng/mL. From 30% to 35% of a PO dose and from 68% to 79% of an IV dose excreted unchanged in urine. **Plasma protein binding:** 15% is bound to plasma proteins.

CONTRAINDICATIONS
Cirrhosis of the liver, impaired renal or hepatic function.

SPECIAL CONCERNS
Use with caution during lactation, in the elderly, and in clients with decreased hepatic or renal function. Safety and efficacy not established in children.

SIDE EFFECTS
Most Common
Headache, abdominal pain, constipation, diarrhea, N&V.

GI: Constipation, N&V, diarrhea, abdominal pain, pancreatitis (rare). **CNS:** Headache, dizziness, malaise, insomnia, verti-

---

Bold Italic = life threatening side effect   ■ = black box warning   ✦ = Available in Canada

go, confusion, anxiety, agitation, depression, fatigue, somnolence, hallucinations. **CV:** Bradycardia or tachycardia, premature ventricular beats following rapid IV use (especially in clients predisposed to cardiac rhythm disturbances), vasculitis, **cardiac arrest. Hematologic:** Thrombocytopenia, granulocytopenia, leukopenia, pancytopenia (sometimes with marrow hypoplasia), **agranulocytosis, autoimmune hemolytic or aplastic anemia. Hepatic:** Hepatotoxicity, jaundice, hepatitis, increase in ALT. **Dermatologic:** Erythema multiforme, rash, alopecia. **Allergic: Bronchospasm, anaphylaxis,** angioneurotic edema (rare), rashes, fever, eosinophilia. **Miscellaneous:** Arthralgia, gynecomastia, impotence, loss of libido, blurred vision, pain at injection site, local burning or itching following IV use.

LABORATORY TEST CONSIDERATIONS
False + test for urine protein using Multistix.

DRUG INTERACTIONS
Antacids / May ↓ ranitidine absorption
Cyanocobalamin / ↓ Cyanocobalamin absorption R/T ↑ gastric pH
Diazepam / ↓ Diazepam effects R/T ↓ GI tract absorption
Glipizide / ↑ Glipizide effects
Procainamide / ↓ Procainamide excretion → possible ↑ effect
Smoking / ↓ Rate of ulcer healing
Theophylline / Possible ↑ theophylline pharmacologic and toxicologic effects
Warfarin / May ↑ warfarin hypoprothrombinemic effects

HOW SUPPLIED
Rx: *Capsules:* 150 mg, 300 mg; *Injection:* 1 mg/mL (premixed), 25 mg/mL; *Syrup:* 15 mg/mL; *Tablets:* 150 mg, 300 mg; *Tablets, Effervescent:* 25 mg, 150 mg. **OTC:** *Tablets:* 75 mg, 150 mg.

DOSAGE
• **RX: CAPSULES; SYRUP; TABLETS; TABLETS, EFFERVESCENT**
Duodenal ulcer, short-term.
Adults: 150 mg twice a day or 300 mg after the evening meal or at bedtime. A dose of 100 mg twice daily is as effective as the 150 mg dose in inhibiting gastric acid secretion. **Maintenance:** 150 mg at bedtime. **Children:** 2–4

mg/kg/day given twice a day, up to a maximum of 300 mg/day. For maintenance in children, 2–4 mg/kg once daily, up to a maximum of 150 mg/day.
Pathologic hypersecretory conditions.
Adults: 150 mg twice a day (up to 6 grams/day has been used in severe cases). **Children:** 5–10 mg/kg/day, usually in 2 divided doses.
Benign gastric ulcer.
Adults: 150 mg twice a day for active ulcer. **Maintenance:** 150 mg at bedtime. **Children:** 2–4 mg/kg/day given twice a day, up to a maximum of 300 mg/day. For maintenance in children, 2–4 mg/kg once daily, up to a maximum of 150 mg/day.
Gastroesophageal reflux disease.
Adults: 150 mg twice a day. **Children:** 5–10 mg/kg/day, usually given as 2 divided doses.
Erosive esophagitis.
Adults: 150 mg 4 times per day.
Maintenance of healing of erosive esophagitis.
Adults: 150 mg twice a day. **Maintenance:** 150 mg twice a day. **Children:** 5–10 mg/kg/day, usually in 2 divided doses.

• **IM; IV**
Treatment and maintenance for duodenal ulcer, hypersecretory conditions, gastroesophageal reflux.
Adults, IM: 50 mg q 6–8 hr. **Intermittent bolus:** 50 mg q 6–8 hr (dilute 50 mg in 0.9% NaCl or other compatible IV solution to a concentration no greater than 2.5 mg/mL [20 mL]). Inject at a rate no greater than 4 mL/min (5 minutes). **Intermittent IV infusion:** 50 mg q 6–8 hr. Dilute 50 mg in 5% dextrose injection or other compatible IV solution to a concentration no greater than 0.5 mg/mL (100 mL) and infuse at a rate no greater than 5–7 mL/min (15–20 min) or use 50 mL of 1 mg/mL premixed solution and infuse over 15–20 min. Do not exceed 400 mg/day. **Continous IV infusion:** Add the injection to 5% dextrose injection or other compatible IV solution. Give at a rate of 6.25 mg/hr (e.g., 150 mg ranitidine injection in 250 mL of 5% dextrose injection at 10.7 mL/hr).

📷 = see color insert   Ⓗ = Herbal   Ⅳ = Intravenous   ©ᵉ = sound alike drug

Children, IV: 2–4 mg/kg/day in divided doses q 6–8 hr, up to a maximum of 50 mg q 6–8 hr.

Zollinger-Ellison clients.

Continuous IV infusion: Dilute ranitidine in 5% dextrose injection or other compatible IV soution to a concentration no greater than 2.5 mg/mL with an initial infusion rate of 1 mg/kg/hr. If after 4 hr the client shows a gastric acid output of greater than 10 mEq/hr or if symptoms appear, increase the dose by 0.5 mg/kg/hr increments and measure the acid output. Doses up to 2.5 mg/kg/hr may be necessary.

- **OTC: TABLETS**
  Treat heartburn.

Treatment: 75 mg or 150 mg with a glass of water. **Maintenance:** Use up to 2 times per day (up to 2 tablets in 24 hr).

Prevent heartburn.

75 mg or 150 mg with a glass of water 30–60 min before eating food or drinking beverages that cause heartburn.

NURSING CONSIDERATIONS

℗ Do not confuse Zantac with Xanax (an antianxiety drug) or with Zyrtex (an H_1 receptor blocker). Do not confuse ranitidine with rimantadine (an antiviral).

ADMINISTRATION/STORAGE

1. If the C_{CR} is less than 50 mL/min, give 50 mg PO q 24 hr or 50 mg parenterally q 18–24 hr. Parenteral dosing may be increased to q 12 hr or further with caution.

2. Give antacids concomitantly for gastric pain although they may interfere with ranitidine absorption.

3. Dissolve EFFERdose tablets and granules in 6–8 oz of water before taking. The 25 mg EFFERdose tablets (for use in infants) are dissolved in at least 5 mL of water; solution may be given with dosing cup, medicine dropper, or oral syringe.

4. About one-half of clients may heal completely within 2 weeks; thus, endoscopy may show no need for further treatment.

5. No dilution is required for IM use.

6. Store tablets from 15–30°C (59–86°F) in a dry place protected from light. Store effervescent tablets and granules from 2–30°C (36–86°F). Store the syrup from 4–25°C (39–77°F). Dispense in a light-resistant container.

Ⅳ 7. The premixed injection does not require dilution; give by slow IV drip over 15–20 min. Do not introduce additives into the solution. If used with a primary IV fluid system, discontinue primary solution during drug infusion.

8. Drug is stable for 48 hr at room temperature when mixed with 0.9% NaCl, 5% or 10% dextrose injection, RL, or 5% $NaHCO_3$ injection.

9. Undiluted ranitidine injection tends to manifest a yellow color that may intensify over time without adversely affecting potency.

10. Visually inspect parenteral drug product for particulate matter and discoloration before administration.

11. Premixed ranitidine injection (50 mg/50 mL), in 0.45% NaCl, is available as a sterile, premixed solution for IV use in single-dose, flexible plastic containers. The product does not contain preservatives.

12. Store the premixed injection from 2–25°C (36–77°F) and the injection from 4–25°C (39–77°F) protected from light.

ASSESSMENT

1. List reasons for therapy, onset/characteristics of S&S, other agents used, anticipated treatment period.

2. Assess stomach pain, noting characteristics, frequency of occurrence, triggers, things that alter/relieve.

3. Obtain CBC; assess for infections, renal, LFTs.

4. Note *H. pylori,* UGI, or endoscopy findings. Determine if pregnant.

5. Skin tests using allergens may elicit false negative results; stop drug 24–72 hr prior to testing.

CLIENT/FAMILY TEACHING

1. Take as directed with or immediately following meals. Wait 1 hr before taking an antacid. For EFFERdose tablets and granules, dissolve each dose in 6–8 oz of water before drinking. A liquid (syrup) is available if you cannot swallow

pills. Those who have feeding tubes may use this preparation.

2. Do not drive or operate machinery until drug effects are realized; dizziness or drowsiness may occur.

3. Avoid alcohol, aspirin-containing products, and beverages that contain caffeine (tea, cola, coffee); these increase stomach acid. Avoid things that may aggravate symptoms, i.e., alcohol, aspirin, NSAIDs, caffeine, chocolate, and black pepper. Avoid herbals such as garlic, ginseng, ginkgo, or vitamin E with ulcer.

4. Do not smoke; interferes with healing and drug's effectiveness.

5. Report any evidence of yellow discoloration of skin or eyes, or diarrhea. Maintain adequate hydration. Report any confusion/disorientation, unusual bruising or bleeding, black tarry stools, diarrhea or rash immediately.

6. Symptoms of breast tenderness will usually disappear after several weeks; report if persistent and evaluate need to stop drug.

7. Report as scheduled to determine extent of healing and expected length of therapy.

OUTCOMES/EVALUATE

- ↓ Gastric acid production
- ↓ Abdominal pain/discomfort
- Endoscopic/radiographic evidence of duodenal ulcer healing

Ranolazine
(rah-**NOH**-la-zeen)

CLASSIFICATION(S):
Antianginal drug
PREGNANCY CATEGORY: C
Rx: Ranexa.

USES
Treat chronic angina. Use in combination with amlodipine, beta-blockers, or nitrates. *NOTE:* Ranolazine prolongs the QT interval; thus, reserve use in those who have not achieved an adequate response with other antianginal drugs.

ACTION/KINETICS
Action
Mechanism is not known. The drug has antianginal and anti-ischemic effects that do not depend on decreases in HR or BP. The drug does not increase the rate-pressure product, a measure of myocardial work at maximal exercise.
Pharmacokinetics
Absorption is highly variable. **Peak plasma levels:** Between 2–5 hr. Bioavailability is 76%. Food has no significant effect on C_{max} or AUC. **t½, terminal:** 7 hr. Metabolized rapidly and extensively in the liver (mainly by CYP3A and CYP2D6) and intestine. Excreted in the urine (75%) and feces (25%). **Plasma protein binding:** About 62%.

CONTRAINDICATIONS
Use in pre-existing QT prolongation, in impaired hepatic function (Child-Pugh classes A, B, or C), in severe impaired renal function, if on QT-prolonging drugs, and if on potent and moderately potent CYP3A inhibitors (e.g., diltiazem, HIV protease inhibitors, ketoconazole, macrolide antibiotics, verapamil). Lactation.

SPECIAL CONCERNS
Safety and efficacy have not been determined in children.

SIDE EFFECTS
Most Common
Dizziness, headache, constipation, nausea, lightheadedness.
CV: Palpitations, bradycardia, hypotension, orthostatic hypotension, prolongation of QTc interval. **GI:** N&V, constipation, abdominal pain, dry mouth. **CNS:** Dizziness, headache, lightheadedness, vertigo, hypesthesia, paresthesia, tremor. **Respiratory:** Dyspnea. **Ophthalmic:** Blurred vision. **Otic:** Tinnitus. **Miscellaneous:** Peripheral edema, hematuria.

LABORATORY TEST CONSIDERATIONS
Small, reversible ↑ BUN and serum creatinine. Small, mean ↓ hematocrit. Transient esosinophilia.

OD OVERDOSE MANAGEMENT
Symptoms: Expected symptoms include confusion, diplopia, dizziness, N&V, paresthesia, syncope with prolonged loss of consciousness. *Treatment:* Continuous ECG monitoring (due to increase in

---

QTc interval). Initiate general supportive measures. Complete clearance by hemodialysis is not likely.

DRUG INTERACTIONS

Digoxin / ↑ Digoxin levels 1.5 fold; may need to ↓ digoxin dose

Diltiazem / ↑ Ranolazine steady-state levels by about 1.8–2.3 fold R/T inhibition of metabolism by CYP3A; do not use together

Grapefruit juice / ↑ Ranolazine levels and QTc prolongation R/T inhibition of metabolism by CYP3A

Ketoconazole / ↑ Ranolazine steadstate levels 3.2 fold R/T inhibition of metabolism by CYP3A; do not use together

Macrolide antibiotics (e.g., erythromycin) / ↑ Ranolazine levels and QTc prolongation R/T inhibition of metabolism by CYP3A; do not use together

Paroxetine / ↑ Ranolazine steady-state plasma levels 1.2 fold

Protease inhibitors / ↑ Ranolazine levels and QTc prolongation R/T inhibition of metabolism by CYP3A; do not use together

Quinidine / ↑ QTc prolongation; do not use together

Simvastatin / ↑ Levels of simvastatin and its active metabolites; may need to ↓ simvastatin dose

Sotalol / ↑ QTc prolongation; do not use together

Thioridazine / ↑ QTc prolongation; do not use together

Verapamil / ↑ Ranolazine steady-state levels by about 2 fold R/T inhibition of metabolism by CYP3A; do not use together

Ziprasidone / ↑ QTc prolongation; do not use together

HOW SUPPLIED

Tablets, Extended-Release: 500 mg, 1,000 mg.

DOSAGE

• TABLETS, EXTENDED-RELEASE

Chronic angina.

Adults, initial: 500 mg two times a day; increase to a maximum of 1,000 mg two times a day, as needed based on clinical symptoms. Dosage adjustments are usually not needed on the basis of age, gender, in those with CHF (NYHA, class I-IV), or diabetes mellitus.

NURSING CONSIDERATIONS

ADMINISTRATION/STORAGE

1. For the elderly, use caution when selecting the dose; start at the low end of the dosage range.

2. Store from 15–30°C (59–86°F).

ASSESSMENT

1. Ranexa is only for those not responding adequately to other antianginal drugs; list all other therapies, procedures, and outcomes.

2. Check baseline EKG and monitor; may cause QTc interval prolongation. Assess for any personal or family history of QTc prolongation, congenital long QT syndrome, or proarrhythmic conditions such as hypokalemia.

3. List drugs prescribed; note if receiving drugs that prolong the QTc interval such as Class Ia (e.g., quinidine) or Class III (e.g., dofetilide, sotalol) antiarrhythmic agents, erythromycin, and certain antipsychotics (e.g., thioridazine, ziprasidone)

4. If receiving drugs that are potent or moderately potent inhibitors of CYP3A, i.e., ketoconazole, HIV protease inhibitors, macrolide antibiotics, diltiazem, and verapamil do not use this drug.

5. Avoid using doses of Ranexa higher than 1,000 mg twice a day and in the elderly.

6. Generally used in combination with another medicine (i.e., amlodipine, beta-blockers, nitrates).

7. Monitor EKG, lytes, renal and LFTs; avoid use with renal/liver dysfunction, QT prolongation.

CLIENT/FAMILY TEACHING

1. May take with or without meals. Grapefruit juice or grapefruit products should be avoided.

2. Swallow tablets whole; do not crush, break, or chew tablets. Drug is used with others such as amlodipine, beta-blockers, nitrates to control angina symptoms.

3. Avoid activities that require mental alertness, may cause dizziness, lightheadedness, or fainting. Alcohol, hot weather, exercise, and fever can in-

crease these effects. To prevent, sit up or stand slowly, esp. in the morning. Report any palpitations or fainting spells.

4. If dose of drug is missed, take the next dose at the next scheduled time. The next dose should not be doubled.

5. Ranexa will not stop an acute angina episode; use other therapy for acute angina and notify provider.

6. Keep all F/U appointments to evaluate response to therapy and development of adverse side effects.

OUTCOMES/EVALUATE

Control of resistant angina

Rasagiline

(rah-**SA**-jih-leen)

CLASSIFICATION(S):
Antiparkinson drug.
PREGNANCY CATEGORY: C
Rx: Azilect.

USES

Treat signs and symptoms of idiopathic Parkinson's disease as initial monotherapy and as adjunct therapy to levodopa.

ACTION/KINETICS

Action

Rasagiline is a potent, irreversible monoamine oxidase (MAO) inhibitor of MAO type B. The precise mechanism in treating parkinsonism is not known but may include an increase in extracellular levels of dopamine in the striatum. Elevated dopamine levels and subsequent increased dopaminergic activity likely mediate rasagiline's beneficial effects.

Pharmacokinetics

Rapidly absorbed. **Peak plasma levels:** 1 hr. Absolute bioavailability is about 36%. Food does not affect the time to reach T_{max}, although T_{max} and AUC are decreased by about 60% and 20%, respectively when the drug is taken with a high-fat meal. Undergoes almost complete metabolism in the liver mainly by CYP1A2. Excreted in the urine (62%) and feces (7%).

CONTRAINDICATIONS

Hypersensitivity to any component of the product. Tyramine-rich foods, beverages, or dietary supplements and amines (from OTC cough/cold medications) to prevent a possible hypertensive crisis. Pheochromocytoma. Coadministration with meperidine, methadone, propoxyphene, tramadol, dextromethorphan, St. John's wort, mirtazapine, cyclobenzaprine, sympathomimetic amines (including amphetamines, nasal and oral decongestants, cold products, and weight-reducing products), other MAO inhibitors, cocaine, and local or general anesthetics. Moderate or severe impaired hepatic function.

SPECIAL CONCERNS

Use with caution during lactation. Safety and efficacy have not been determined in children.

SIDE EFFECTS

Most Common

When used as monotherapy: Headache, dyspepsia, flu syndrome, depression, fall, dyspepsia, arthralgia, gastroenteritis, rhinitis, fever.

When used as an adjunct to levodopa therapy: Dyskinesia, accidental injury, weight loss, postural hypotension, N&V, anorexia, arthralgia, abdominal pain, constipation, dry mouth, rash, ecchymosis, somnolence, paresthesia.

Monotherapy. CNS: Hallucinations, depression, headache, malaise, paresthesia, vertigo, dizziness, hallucinations, syncope. **GI:** Dyspepsia, gastroenteritis, diarrhea, anorexia, vomiting. **CV:** Angina pectoris. **Musculoskeletal:** Arthralgia, arthritis. **Respiratory:** Rhinitis, asthma. **Dermatologic:** Ecchymosis, alopecia, skin carcinoma, vesiculobullous rash. **GU:** Impotence, decreased libido. **Hematologic:** Leukopenia. **Miscellaneous:** Fall, flu syndrome, conjunctivitis, fever, neck/chest pain, allergic reaction.

Adjunct to levodopa therapy. CNS: Hallucinations, dyskinesia, somnolence, paresthesia, headache, ataxia, dystonia, amnesia, confusion, abnormal gait, anxiety, hyperkinesia, neuropathy, tremor, agitation, aphasia, circumoral paresthesia, convulsions, delusions, de-

R

---

mentia, dysarthria, dysautonomia, dysesthesia, emotional lability, facial paralysis, foot drop, hemiplegia, hypesthesia, incoordination, manic reaction, migraine, myoclonus, neuritis, neurosis, paranoid reaction, personality disorder, psychosis, wrist drop, apathy, delirium, hostility, manic depressive reaction, myelitis, neuralgia, psychotic depression, stupor. **GI:** Diarrhea, N&V, anorexia, abdominal pain, constipation, dry mouth, dyspepsia, gingivitis, dysphagia, *GI hemorrhage*, colitis, esophageal ulcer, esophagitis, fecal incontinence, intestinal obstruction, mouth ulceration, stomach ulcer, stomatitis, tongue edema, hematemesis, *hemorrhagic gastritis, intestinal perforation*, intestinal stenosis, jaundice, *large intestine perforation*, megacolon, melena. **CV:** Postural hypotension, hemorrhage, *CVA*, bundle branch block, deep thrombophlebitis, *heart failure, MI*, phlebitis, ventricular tachycardia, *arterial thrombosis*, atrial arrhythmia, complete AV block, second degree AV block, bigeminy, *cerebral hemorrhage*, cerebral ischemia, *ventricular fibrillation*. **Hematologic:** Anemia, macrocytic anemia, purpura, thrombocythemia. **Respiratory:** Dyspnea, epistaxis, increased cough, apnea, emphysema, laryngismus, pleural effusion, pneumothorax, interstitial pneumonia, *larynx edema*, lung fibrosis. **Musculoskeletal:** Arthralgia, tenosynovitis, myasthenia, arthritis, bursitis, leg cramps, bone necrosis, muscle atrophy, arthrosis. **Dermatologic:** Rash, ecchymosis, sweating, skin carcinoma/ulcer, pruritus, eczema, urticaria, exfoliative dermatitis, leukoderma, increased risk of melanoma. **GU:** Hernia, hematuria, urinary incontinence, abnormal sexual function, acute kidney failure, dysmenorrhea, dysuria, kidney calculus, nocturia, polyuria, scrotal edema, urinary retention, impaired urination, vaginal hemorrhage, vaginal moniliasis, vaginitis, abnormal ejaculation, amenorrhea, anuria, epididymitis, gynecomastia, hydroureter, leukorrhea, priapism. **Ophthalmic:** Blepharitis, diplopia, eye hemorrhage, eye pain, glaucoma, keratitis, ptosis, retinal degeneration, visual field defect, blindness, retinal detachment, retinal hemorrhage, strabismus. **Otic:** Deafness, vestibular disorder. **Body as a whole:** Weight loss, infection, asthenia, chills, photosensitivity. **Miscellaneous:** Accidental injury/falls, hernia, neck pain, taste perversion, parosmia, photophobia, taste loss.

LABORATORY TEST CONSIDERATIONS
Monotherapy: Albuminuria, leukopenia. **Adjunct to levodopa therapy:** Albuminuria. hypocalcemia.

OD OVERDOSE MANAGEMENT
Symptoms: Possible symptoms include drowsiness, dizziness, faintness, irritability, hyperactivity, agitation, severe headache, hallucinations, trismus, opisthotonos, *convulsions, coma,* rapid and irregular pulse, hypertension, hypotension, *vascular collapse,* precordial pain, respiratory depression/failure, hyperpyrexia, diaphoresis, cool/clammy skin. *Treatment:* Treatment is symptomatic and supportive. Support respiration, including management of the airway, supplemental oxygen, and mechanical ventilatory assistance, if needed. Monitor body temperature closely. Intensive management of hyperpyrexia may be required. Maintain fluid and electrolyte balance.

DRUG INTERACTIONS
Anesthetics / Do not use together; discontinue rasagiline at least 14 days prior to elective surgery
Antidepressants (e.g., tricyclic antidepressants, mirtazapine, SNRIs, SSRIs) / Severe CNS toxicity with hyperpyrexia and death; at least 14 days should elapse between discontinuing rasagiline and beginning an antidepressant.
Ciprofloxacin / ↑ Rasagiline AUC by 83%
Cocaine / Possible hypertensive crisis; do not use together
Cyclobenzaprine / Do not use together as cyclobenzaprine is structurally related to tricyclic antidepressants
CYP1A2 inhibitors (e.g., atazanavir, mexiletine, tacrine) / Possible 2-fold ↑ in rasagiline plasma levels → ↑ side effects
Dextromethorphan / Possible brief episodes of psychosis and bizarre behavior; do not use together

---

Bold Italic = life threatening side effect   ■ = black box warning   ✤ = Available in Canada

Fluoxetine / Possible CNS toxicity with hyperpyrexia and death; at least 5 weeks should elapse between discontinuing fluoxetine and beginning rasagiline

Levodopa / Possible potentiation of dopaminergic side effects and exacerbation of dyskinesia; possibly reduce levodopa dose

MAO inhibitors / Possible hypertensive crisis; at least 14 days should elapse between discontinuing rasagiline and starting MAO inhibitors

Meperidine / Possible coma, severe hypertension or hypotension, severe respiratory depression, convulsions, death; at least 14 days should elapse between discontinuing rasagiline and beginning meperidine

Methadone / Possible coma, severe hypertension or hypotension, severe respiratory depression, convulsions, death

Propoxyphene / Possible coma, severe hypertension or hypotension, severe respiratory depression, convulsions, death

H *St. John's wort* / Do not use together

Sympathomimetic (e.g., amphetamines, cold products, anorexiants) / Possible severe hypertensive reactions

Tramadol / Possible coma, severe hypertension or hypotension, severe respiratory depression, convulsions, death

Tyramine-containing foods/beverages / Possible severe hypertensive crisis

HOW SUPPLIED
Tablets: 0.5 mg (as base), 1 mg (as base).

DOSAGE
• **TABLETS**
 Idiopathic Parkinson's disease.
Monotherapy: 1 mg once daily. **Adjunctive therapy, initial:** 0.5 mg once daily; if satisfactory response is not obtained, may increase the dose to 1 mg once daily.

NURSING CONSIDERATIONS
ADMINISTRATION/STORAGE
1. When used wtih levodopa, consider a decrease in the levodopa dosage, depending on individual client response.
2. Use a dose of 0.5 mg in clients with mild impaired hepatic function. Do not give rasagiline to those with moderate or severe impaired hepatic function.
3. Plasma levels of rasagiline may double in those taking concomitant ciprofloxacin or other CYP1A2 inhibitors. Thus, in such clients, use rasagiline, 0.5 mg/day.
4. Store form 15–30°C (59–86°F).

ASSESSMENT
1. Note onset, duration and reasons for therapy, other agents trialed, outcome.
2. List drugs prescribed to ensure none interact especially, SSRI antidepressants, sympathomimetic amine drugs, Ciprofloxacin inhibits the enzymes in the liver that eliminate rasagiline, thereby increasing blood levels and possibly adverse SE of rasagiline.
3. With PD note range of motion, rigidity, tremor, gait, and facial expressions.
4. Belongs to a class of drugs called monoamine oxidase inhibitors (MAO) that also includes selegiline and tranylcypromine. Use cautiously especially with other drugs.

CLIENT/FAMILY TEACHING
1. Used alone or in combination with levodopa to treat S&S of Parkinson's disease. If you miss a dose of this drug, take it as soon as possible.
2. Hypertensive crisis may occur if foods high in tyramine are consumed while taking rasagilin.
3. Use caution, do not drive or perform other tasks that require mental alertness until drug effects realized.
4. May cause dizziness, drowsiness, lightheadedness, or fainting; alcohol, hot weather, exercise, or fever may increase these effects. To prevent them, sit up or stand slowly, esp. in the a.m. Sit or lie down at the first sign of any of these effects.
5. Eating foods high in tyramine (eg, aged cheeses, red wines, beer, certain meats and sausages, liver, sour cream, soy sauce, raisins, bananas, avocados) while you use an MAOI may cause severe high blood pressure. This could occur for up to 2 weeks after you stop taking an MAOI. Do not eat foods high in tyramine while you take Rasagiline. Ask your health care provider for a complete list of foods you should avoid.

R

Seek medical attention at once if symptoms of severe high blood pressure occur. These may include severe headache, fast or irregular heartbeat, sore or stiff neck, nausea, vomiting, sweating, enlarged pupils, or sensitivity to light.

6. Avoid medicines that contain dextromethorphan, pseudoephedrine, phenylephrine, or ephedrine while using Rasagiline.

7. Rasagiline should be discontinued at least 14 days before elective surgery.

8. If advised to stop taking Rasagiline, you will need to wait at least 14 days before beginning to take certain other medicines (eg, medicines for depression, anxiety, pain, cough, congestion, weight loss, Parkinson disease; muscle relaxants). Confirm when you should start to take your new medicines after you have stopped taking Rasagiline.

9. Rasagiline may increase your risk of developing skin cancer. Ask if you should have skin exams while taking Rasagiline. Report any skin changes (eg, change in color or thickness).

10. Keep all F/U appointments for skin exams, labs, and to evaluate response to therapy and adverse side effects.

OUTCOMES/EVALUATE
Relief of S&S of Parkinsons disease

Rasburicase ■Ⅳ©
(ras-**BYOUR**-ih-kase)

CLASSIFICATION(S):
Antimetabolite, purine analog
PREGNANCY CATEGORY: C
Rx: Elitek.

USES
Initial treatment to reduce plasma uric acid levels in children with leukemia, lymphoma, and solid tumor malignancies who are receiving anticancer therapy expected to cause tumor lysis and thus increases in plasma uric acid.

ACTION/KINETICS
Action
A recombinant urate-oxidase enzyme that catalyzes enzymatic oxidation of uric acid into an inactive and soluble metabolite (allantoin), thus decreasing plasma levels.

Pharmacokinetics
$t^{1}\!/_{2}$, **terminal:** 18 hr. No accumulation of drug has been noted.

CONTRAINDICATIONS
Use in G6PD deficient clients, known history of anaphylaxis or hypersensitivity reactions, hemolytic reactions, methemoglobinemia reactions to rasburicase. Lactation.

SPECIAL CONCERNS
■ (1) May cause hypersensitivity reactions, including anaphylaxis. Discontinue immediately and permanently in any client developing clinical evidence of a serious hypersensitivity reaction. (2) Can cause severe hemolysis if given to clients with glucose-6-phosphate dehydrogenase (G6PD) deficiency. Discontinue immediately and permanently in any client developing hemolysis. It is recommended that clients at higher risk for G6PD deficiency (e.g., those of African or Mediterranean ancestry) be screened prior to starting rasburicase. (3) Use has been associated with methemoglobinemia. Discontinue immediately and permanently in any client who develops methemoglobinemia. (4) Will cause enzymatic degradation of the uric acid within blood samples left at room temperature, resulting in spuriously low uric acid levels. To ensure accurate measurements, blood must be collected into prechilled tubes containing heparin and immediately immersed and maintained in an ice water bath; plasma samples must be assayed within 4 hr of sample collection.■ Safety and efficacy have been established only for a single course of treatment once daily for 5 days. Children less than 2 years of age had a lower rate of success by 48 hr after treatment and also experienced more toxicity.

SIDE EFFECTS
Most Common
N&V, fever, headache, abdominal pain, constipation, diarrhea, mucositis, rash.
Allergic reaction: Chest pain, dyspnea, hypotension, urticaria, *anaphylaxis*.
Hematologic: Hemolysis, methemoglobinemia, neutropenia with fever, neu-

---

Bold Italic = life threatening side effect   ■ = black box warning   ♣ = Available in Canada

tropenia, pancytopenia. **GI:** N&V, diarrhea, ileus, intestinal obstruction, abdominal pain, constipation. **CNS: Convulsions**, headache. **CV:** Arrhythmia, **cardiac failure/arrest, MI**, cerebrovascular disorder, hot flushes, **hemorrhage**, thrombosis, thrombophlebitis. **Respiratory:** Respiratory distress, pneumonia, pulmonary edema, **pulmonary hypertension. Miscellaneous:** Rash, fever, mucositis, acute renal failure, cellulitis, chest pain, cyanosis, dehydration, infection, paresthesia, retinal hemorrhage, rigors.

LABORATORY TEST CONSIDERATIONS
At room temperature, rasburicase causes enzymatic degradation of uric acid in blood, plasma, or serum samples that may cause low plasma uric acid assay readings.

HOW SUPPLIED
Powder for Injection, Lyophilized: 1.5 mg/vial, 7.5 mg/vial.

DOSAGE
• **IV**
 Decrease plasma uric acid in children treated for cancer.
Children: Either 0.15 or 0.2 mg/kg as a single daily dose for 5 days.

NURSING CONSIDERATIONS

🕮 Do not confuse Elitek with Elidel (a drug for atopic dermatitis.

ADMINISTRATION/STORAGE
[IV] 1. Begin chemotherapy 4–24 hr after the first rasburicase dose.
2. Give as an IV infusion over 30 min; **do not give as bolus infusion.** Do not use filters for infusion.
3. Infuse through a different line than that used for other drugs. If use of a separate line not possible, flush line with at least 15 mL of saline solution before and after infusion with rasburicase.
4. Determine number of vials of drug required based on weight and dose/kg. Must reconstitute with the diluent provided. Add 1 mL of the diluent to each vial and mix by swirling gently. Do not shake or vortex.
5. Visually inspect for particulate matter and discoloration before administer-

ing. Discard if particulate matter visible or if there is discoloration.
6. After reconstitution, remove dose to be given and inject into an infusion bag containing an amount of 0.9% NaCl to achieve a final volume of 50 mL.
7. IV hydration of clients is needed to manage plasma uric acid in those at risk for tumor lysis syndrome.
8. There are no preservatives in the product; thus, give within 24 hr of reconstitution. The reconstituted or diluted solution can be stored at 2–8°C (36–46°F) up to 24 hr. Do not freeze; protect from light. Discard any unused product.

ASSESSMENT
1. Note age, onset, type of cancer/chemotherapy regimen. Monitor VS.
2. Alert lab to collect blood in prechilled tubes containing heparin. Immediately immerse in ice water bath; specimen must be analyzed within 4 hr of draw; otherwise results not reliable.
3. Assess for G6PD; screen those of African or Mediterranean ancestry prior to therapy; prone to hemolysis. Assess all recipients carefully for allergic reaction, hemolysis and methoglobinemia. If evident stop drug and never reuse in this client.
4. Monitor oral/auxilliary temperature, serum uric acid level, lytes, renal and LFTs.
5. Assess GI symptoms; N&V, severe diarrhea may signal toxicity. Ensure well hydrated and administer antiemetic 1 hr before therapy and as needed.

CLIENT/FAMILY TEACHING
1. Drug is given to child to lower the uric acid levels from tumor breakdown during chemotherapy.
2. Generally given once daily IV x 5 days.
3. Report any temperature elevation, unusual bruising/bleeding, N&V, diarrhea or adverse side effects immediately.

OUTCOMES/EVALUATE
↓ Uric acid levels R/T chemotherapy

R

Remifentanil hydrochloride
IV

(rem-ih-**FEN**-tah-nil)

CLASSIFICATION(S):
Narcotic analgesic
PREGNANCY CATEGORY: C
Rx: Ultiva, **C-II**

SEE ALSO NARCOTIC ANALGESICS.

USES
(1) As an analgesic during the induction and maintenance of general anesthesia for inpatient and outpatient procedures and for continuation as an analgesic in the immediate postoperative period. (2) Analgesic component of monitored anesthesia care. *NOTE:* Not indicated as the sole agent for general anesthesia because loss of consciousness cannot be guaranteed and also due to a high incidence of apnea, muscle rigidity, and tachycardia.

ACTION/KINETICS
Action
Narcotic analgesic that binds with mu-opioid receptors. Depresses respiration in a dose-dependent manner and causes muscle rigidity.

Pharmacokinetics
Rapidly metabolized by nonspecific blood and tissue esterases; not metabolized appreciably by the liver or lung. **Onset:** 1 min. **Peak effect:** 1 min. **t½, elimination:** 10–20 min. **Recovery:** Within 5–10 min. Metabolized in the liver by hydrolysis by esterases. Excreted in the urine.

CONTRAINDICATIONS
Epidural or intrathecal use due to the presence of glycine in the formulation. Hypersensitivity to fentanyl analogues. Use as the sole agent in general anesthesia because LOC cannot be ensured and due to a high incidence of apnea, muscle rigidity, and tachycardia.

SPECIAL CONCERNS
Use with caution in obese clients and during lactation. Respiratory depression and other narcotic effects may be seen in newborns whose mothers are given remifentanil shortly before delivery. Geriatric clients are twice as sensitive as younger clients to the effects of the drug.

Not studied in children less than one year of age; also, has not been studied in children for use in the immediate postoperative period or for use as a component of monitored anesthesia care. Possible intraoperative awareness in clients less than 55 years old when given with propofol infusion rates of 75 or less mcg/kg/min.

SIDE EFFECTS
Most Common
Hypotension, apnea, headache, itching/pruritus, dizziness, shivering, sweating, N&V, muscle rigidity, flank pain.

GI: N&V, constipation, abdominal discomfort, xerostomia, gastroesophageal reflux, dysphagia, diarrhea, heartburn, ileus. **CNS:** Shivering, fever, dizziness, headache, agitation, chills, warm sensation, anxiety, involuntary movement, prolonged emergence from anesthesia, tremors, disorientation, dysphoria, nightmares, hallucinations, paresthesia, nystagmus, twitch, sleep disorder, seizures, amnesia. **CV:** Hypo-/hypertension, brady-/tachycardia, atrial and ventricular arrhythmias, *heart block*, ECG change consistent with myocardial ischemia, syncope. **Musculoskeletal:** Muscle rigidity/stiffness, flank pain, musculoskeletal chest pain, delayed recovery from neuromuscular block. **Respiratory:** Respiratory depression, *apnea*, hypoxia, cough, dyspnea, *bronchospasm, laryngospasm,* rhonchi, stridor, nasal congestion, pharyngitis, pleural effusion, hiccoughs, pulmonary edema, rales, bronchitis, rhinorrhea. **Dermatologic:** Pruritus, itching, rash, urticaria, erythema, sweating, flushing, pain at IV site. **GU:** Urine retention/incontinence, oliguria, dysuria. **Hematologic:** Anemia, lymphopenia, leukocytosis, thrombocytopenia. **Metabolic:** Abnormal liver function, hyperglycemia, electrolyte disorders. **Miscellaneous:** Decreased body temperature, *anaphylactic reaction*, visual disturbances, postoperative pain.

Bold Italic = life threatening side effect   ■ = black box warning   ✚ = Available in Canada

LABORATORY TEST CONSIDERATIONS

↑ CPK-MB levels.

OD **OVERDOSE MANAGEMENT**

Symptoms: Apnea, chest-wall rigidity, seizures, hypoxemia, hypotension, bradycardia. *Treatment:* Discontinue administration, maintain a patent airway, initiate assisted or controlled ventilation with oxygen, and maintain adequate CV function. A neuromuscular blocking agent or a mu-opiate receptor antagonist may be used to treat muscle rigidity. IV fluids, vasopressors, and other supportive measures are indicated to treat hypotension. Bradycardia or hypotension may also be treated with atropine or glycopyrrolate. IV naloxone is used to treat respiratory depression or muscle rigidity. Reversal of the opioid effects may lead to acute pain and sympathetic hyperactivity.

DRUG INTERACTIONS

Remifentanil is synergistic with other anesthetics. Doses of thiopental, propofol, isoflurane, and midazolam have been reduced by up to 75% with the coadministration of remifentanil.

HOW SUPPLIED

Powder for Injection: 1 mg (as base), 2 mg (as base), 5 mg (as base).

DOSAGE

• **CONTINUOUS IV INFUSION**

Induction of anesthesia through intubation.

0.5–1 mcg/kg/min given with a hypnotic or volatile agent. If endotracheal intubation is to occur less than 8 min after the start of the infusion of remifentanil, the initial dose of 1 mcg/kg may be given over 30 to 60 sec.

Maintenance of nitrous oxide (66%) anesthesia.

The dose of remifentanil is 0.4 mcg/kg/min by continuous IV infusion (dose range for IV infusion is 0.1–2 mcg/kg/min). A supplemental IV bolus dose of 1 mcg/kg may be given q 2-5 min in response to light anesthesia or transient episodes of intense surgical stress.

Maintenance of isoflurane (0.4 to 1.5 MAC) or propofol (100–200 mcg/kg/min) anesthesia.

The dose of remifentanil is 0.25 mcg/kg/min by continuous IV infusion (dose range is 0.05–2 mcg/kg/min). A supplemental IV bolus dose of 1 mcg/kg may be given.

Continuation as an analgesic into the immediate postoperative period.

0.1 mcg/kg/min (range of 0.025–0.2 mcg/kg/min). The infusion rate may be adjusted every 5 min in 0.025-mcg/kg/min increments to balance the client's level of analgesia and respiratory rate. Infusion rates more than 0.2 mcg/kg/min are associated with respiratory depression (less than 8 breaths/min). The use of bolus injections to treat pain during the postoperative period is not recommended.

Analgesic component of monitored anesthesia care.

Adults only. Single IV dose: 1 mcg/kg administered over 30 to 60 sec and given 90 sec before the local anesthetic. If remifentanil is given with midazolam (2 mg), the dose is 0.5 mcg/kg given over 30–60 sec. **Continuous IV infusion:** 0.1 mcg/kg beginning 5 min before the local anesthetic. After the local anesthetic, the dose of remifentanil is 0.05 mcg/kg/min (range 0.025–0.2 mcg/kg/min) at 5-min intervals in order to balance the level of analgesia and respiratory rate. If remifentanil is given with midazolam (2 mg), the dose is 0.025 mcg/kg/min (range 0.025–0.2 mcg/kg/min).

Coronary artery bypass surgery.

Induction of anesthesia through intubation: 1 mcg/kg/min by continuous IV infusion. **Maintenance of anesthesia:** 1 mcg/kg/min (range: 0.125–4 mcg/kg/min) by continuous IV infusion. A supplemental bolus dose of 0.5–1 mcg/kg may be given. **Continuation as an analgesic into ICU:** 1 mcg/kg/min (range: 0.05–1 mcg/kg/min) by continuous IV infusion.

Pediatric clients, 1 year of age and older, with physical status of I, II, or III.

Maintenance of anesthesia (given with halothane, 0.3–1.5 MAC; sevoflurane, 0.3–1.5 MAC; or, isoflurane, 0.4–1.5 MAC): 0.25 mcg/kg/min (range: 0.05–3 mcg/kg/min) by continuous IV

R

infusion. A supplemental IV bolus dose of 1 mcg/kg may be given. *NOTE:* Remifentanil was given with nitrous oxide or nitrous oxide in combination with halothane, sevoflurane, or isoflurane.

NURSING CONSIDERATIONS

ADMINISTRATION/STORAGE

[IV] 1. Individualize choice of anesthetic and need for preanesthetic drugs.

2. Use under the direct supervision of an anesthesia practitioner in a postoperative anesthesia care unit or intensive care setting.

3. Decrease starting dose by 50% in clients over age 65. Cautiously titrate to desired effect.

4. In obese clients (i.e., greater than 30% over ideal body weight [IBW]) base the starting dose on IBW.

5. The need for premedication and the choice of anesthetic agents must be individualized.

6. Give continuous infusions only by an infusion device. Have the injection site close to the venous cannula.

7. Give IV bolus injections only during the maintenance of general anesthesia.

8. Do not give remifentanil into the same IV tubing with blood.

9. Due to the rapid onset and short duration, administration during anesthesia can be titrated upward in 25% to 100% increments or downward in 25% to 50% decrements every 2 to 5 min to attain the desired opiate effect. With light anesthesia or transient periods of intense surgical stress, supplemental bolus doses of 1 mcg/kg may be given q 2–5 min.

10. Administer under close anesthesia supervision into the immediate postoperative period. Infusion rates greater than 0.2 mcg/kg/min are associated with respiratory depression. Manage respiratory depression by decreasing the rate of infusion by 50% or discontinue the infusion temporarily.

11. When infusion is discontinued, clear the IV tubing to prevent inadvertant administration at a later time.

12. Due to its short duration, no opioid activity will be present within 5–10 min of discontinuation.

13. Stable for 24 hr at room temperature after reconstitution and further dilution to concentrations of 20–250 mcg/mL. Dilute with sterile water for injection, D5W, D5W/0.9% NaCl, 0.9% NaCl, 0.45% NaCl injection, or lactated Ringer's/D5W. Is stable for 4 hr at room temperature after reconstitution and further dilution to concentrations of 20–250 mcg/mL with lactated Ringer's injection.

14. Compatible with propofol when coadministered into a running IV administration set.

15. Store at 2–25°C (36–77°F).

ASSESSMENT

1. Note reasons for therapy and expected duration. Determine if pain is acute or chronic in nature; describe distinguishing characteristics; use a pain-rating scale to rate pain perception.

2. Monitor renal and LFTs. Observe closely for progressive respiratory depression. Assess level of consciousness, VS, I&O and for any evidence of allergic reaction.

3. Have resuscitative and intubation equipment readily available. Monitor oxygen sats during therapy.

4. Manage respiratory depression in spontaneously breathing clients by decreasing rate of Ultiva infusion by 50% or by temporarily discontinuing the infusion.

CLIENT/FAMILY TEACHING

1. Drug is administered in a monitored environment to ensure no adverse side effects.

2. Call caregiver for assistance. Do not perform activities that require mental alertness for 24 hr; drug causes dizziness, drowsiness, and impaired physical and mental performance.

3. Avoid alcohol and any other CNS depressants for 24 hr after procedure.

4. Change positions slowly to prevent postural effects (low BP).

OUTCOMES/EVALUATE

Pain control; maintenance of anesthesia

Repaglinide ©
(re-**PAY**-glin-eyed)

CLASSIFICATION(S):
Antidiabetic, oral; meglitinide
PREGNANCY CATEGORY: C
Rx: Prandin.
♣Rx: GlucoNorm.

SEE ALSO *ANTIDIABETIC AGENTS: HYPOGLYCEMIC AGENTS.*

USES
(1) Adjunct to diet and exercise in type 2 diabetes mellitus where hyperglycemia cannot be controlled by diet and exercise alone. (2) In combination with metformin, pioglitazone or rosiglitazone to lower blood glucose where hyperglycemia cannot be controlled by exercise, diet, or metformin, sulfonylureas, repaglinide, or thiazolidinediones used alone.

ACTION/KINETICS
Action
Lowers blood glucose by stimulating release of insulin from the pancreas. Action depends on functioning beta cells in pancreatic islets. Drug closes ATP-dependent potassium channels in beta-cell membrane due to binding at sites. Blockade of potassium channel depolarizes beta cells, which leads to opening of calcium channels. This causes calcium influx which induces insulin secretion. Is highly tissue selective with low affinity for heart and skeletal muscle.

Pharmacokinetics
Rapidly and completely absorbed from GI tract, although food decreases mean C_{max} and AUC. Mean absolute bioavailability is 56%. **Peak plasma levels:** 1 hr. **t½:** 1 hr. Completely metabolized in liver with 90% excreted in feces and 8% excreted in the urine.

CONTRAINDICATIONS
Lactation. Diabetic ketoacidosis, with or without coma. Type 1 diabetes. Known hypersensitivity to any component of the product. Use in combination with NPH insulin.

SPECIAL CONCERNS
Use with caution in impaired hepatic function. Oral hypoglycemics are associated with increased CV mortality compared with diet alone or diet plus insulin. It may be necessary to discontinue repaglinide and give insulin if the client is exposed to stress (e.g., fever, trauma, infection, surgery); known as secondary failure. Safety and efficacy have not been determined in children.

SIDE EFFECTS
Most Common
Hypoglycemia, headache, paresthesia, N&V, diarrhea, constipation, dyspepsia, back pain, arthralgia, bronchitis, rhinitis, sinusitis, URTI, chest pain, tooth disorder, UTI, allergy.

CNS: Headache, paresthesia. **CV:** Chest pain, angina, ischemia, hypertension, abnormal EKG, arrhythmias, palpitations, *MI*. **GI:** N&V, diarrhea, constipation, dyspepsia, *pancreatitis*, severe hepatic dysfunction. **Hematologic:** Thrombocytopenia, leukopenia, hemolytic anemia. **Respiratory:** URTI, sinusitis, rhinitis, bronchitis. **Musculoskeletal:** Arthralgia, back pain. **Miscellaneous:** Hypoglycemia, chest pain, UTI, tooth disorder, allergy, alopecia, *Stevens-Johnson syndrome, anaphylaxis*.

OD OVERDOSE MANAGEMENT
Symptoms: Hypoglycemia. Symptoms of severe hypoglycemia include coma, seizure, or other neurologic impairment; this is a medical emergency. *Treatment:* Oral glucose. Also adjust drug dosage or meal patterns. For severe hypoglycemia, give a rapid IV injection of 50% glucose solution followed by a continuous infusion of more dilute (10%) glucose solution at a rate that will maintain BG at a level above 100 mg/dL.

DRUG INTERACTIONS
See *Antidiabetic Agents: Hypoglycemic Agents.*

Beta blockers / Potentiation of repaglinide action, including by drugs highly protein bound
Calcium channel blockers / Calcium channel blockers cause hyperglycemia → loss of glycemic control
Chloramphenicol / Potentiation of repaglinide action, including by drugs high-

---

ly protein bound

Clarithromycin / Possible ↑ peak plasma levels and t½ of repaglinide

Corticosteroids / Corticosteroids cause hyperglycemia → loss of glycemic control

Coumarins / Potentiation of repaglinide action, including by drugs highly protein bound

Cyclosporine / ↑ Repaglinide plasma levels R/T inhibition of metabolism by CYP3A4

CYP3A4 inducers (e.g., barbiturates, carbamazepine, rifampin) / ↓ Repaglinide AUC and plasma levels R/T induction of its metabolism

CYP3A4 inhibitors (e.g., ketoconazole, macrolide antibiotics, miconazole) / ↑ Repaglinide AUC and plasma levels R/T inhibition of its metabolism

Estrogens / Estrogens cause hyperglycemia → loss of glycemic control

Gemfibrozil / Enhanced and prolonged BG lowering effects of repaglinide R/T inhibition of metabolism → ↑ repaglinide blood levels; repaglinide dosage adjustment may be needed

Gemfibrozil/Itraconazole / Combination has a synergistic metabolic inhibitory effect on repaglinide; do not take itraconazole with repaglinide and gemfibrozil

Isoniazid / Isoniazid cause hyperglycemia → loss of glycemic control

Levonorgestrel/ethinyl estradiol / 20% ↑ in repaglinide, levonorgestrel, and ethinyl estradiol C$_{max}$; also 20% ↑ in ethinyl estradiol AUC

Nicotinic acid / Nicotinic acid causes hyperglycemia → loss of glycemic control

MAOIs / Potentiation of repaglinide action, including by drugs highly protein bound

NSAIDs / Potentiation of repaglinide action, including by drugs highly protein bound

Oral contraceptives / Oral contraceptives cause hyperglycemia → loss of glycemic control

Phenothiazines / Phenothiazines cause hyperglycemia → loss of glycemic control

Phenytoin / Phenytoin cause hyperglycemia → loss of glycemic control

Probenecid / Potentiation of repaglinide action, including by drugs highly protein bound

Rifampin / ↓ Plasma levels and effects of repaglinide R/T ↑ liver metabolism

Salicylates / Potentiation of repaglinide action, including by drugs highly protein bound

Simvastatin / ↑ Repaglinide C$_{max}$ by 26%

Sulfonamides / Potentiation of repaglinide action, including by drugs highly protein bound

Sympathomimetics / Sympathomimetics cause hyperglycemia → loss of glycemic control

Thiazides (and other diuretics) / Thiazides and other diuretics cause hyperglycemia → loss of glycemic control

Thyroid drugs / Thyroid drugs cause hyperglycemia → loss of glycemic control

HOW SUPPLIED

Tablets: 0.5 mg, 1 mg, 2 mg.

DOSAGE

- **TABLETS**

  Diabetes mellitus, type 2.

Individualize dosage as there is no fixed dosage. **Initial:** In those not previously treated or whose HbA1c is less than 8%, give 0.5 mg with each meal. For those previously treated or whose HbA1c is 8% or more, give 1 or 2 mg before each meal. **Dose range:** 0.5–4 mg taken with meals. May also be dosed preprandially 2, 3, or 4 times a day in response to changes in the client's meal pattern. **Maximum daily dose:** 16 mg. Start those with severe renal impairment at 0.5 mg taken with meals.

NURSING CONSIDERATIONS

Ⓒ Do not confuse Prandin with Avandia (also an oral hypoglycemic).

ADMINISTRATION/STORAGE

1. Usually taken within 15 min of meal but time may vary from immediately preceding meal to as long as 30 min before meal.

2. In renal impairment, initial dose adjustments not required. Make subsequent increases in dose carefully in impaired renal function or in renal failure requiring hemodialysis.

---

3. When used to replace another oral hypoglycemic, may be started the day after the last dose of other drug. Observe carefully for hypoglycemia as drug effects may overlap. When transferring from a longer-acting sulfonylurea (e.g., chlorpropamide), monitor for up to 1 week or longer.

4. If combined with metformin, starting dose and dose adjustments are the same as if repaglinide was used alone.

5. If glucose control has not been achieved after a suitable trial of combination therapy, consider discontinuing these drugs and starting insulin.

6. Fever, trauma, infection, or surgery may result in loss of glycemic control (known as secondary failure). At these times, it may be necessary to discontinue repaglinide and administer insulin.

7. Do not store above 25°C (77°F). Protect from moisture.

ASSESSMENT

1. Note onset, duration, characteristics of disease, other agents/methods tried, outcome.

2. Monitor VS, HbA1c, microalbumin, renal, LFTs.

CLIENT/FAMILY TEACHING

1. Take as prescribed within 15 min of the meal up to as long as 30 min before the meal for glucose control. Do not take if meal is skipped.

2. Continue regular exercise, diabetic diet, and lifestyle modifications to control BS and prevent organ damage.

3. Record FS for provider review; report any unusual side effects or lack of response. Have regular foot and eye exams. Strive for BP and weight control.

4. Report fever, sore throat, unusual bruising/bleeding, severe abdominal pain, or lack of effectiveness. Attend diabetic education classes and dietary instruction.

OUTCOMES/EVALUATE

HBA1c <7, control of BS

Respiratory Syncytial Virus Immune Globulin Intravenous (RSV-IGIV) (Human)   [IV]

CLASSIFICATION(S):
Immunosuppressant
PREGNANCY CATEGORY: C
Rx: RespiGam.

USES
Prevention of serious lower respiratory tract infection caused by RSV in children, less than 24 months old with bronchopulmonary dysplasia or a history of premature birth (less than 35 weeks gestation). *Investigational:* In place of IGIV during the RSV season in immunocompromised children who get IGIV monthly.

ACTION/KINETICS

Action
Is an IgG containing neutralizing antibody to RSV. The immunoglobulin is obtained and purified from pooled adult human plasma that has been selected for high titers of neutralizing antibody against RSV. Each milliliter contains 50 mg of immunoglobulin, primarily IgG with trace amounts of IgA and IgM.

CONTRAINDICATIONS
History of a severe prior reaction associated with administration of RSV-IGIV or other human immunoglobulin products. Clients with selective IgA deficiency who have the potential for developing antibodies to IgA and which could cause anaphylaxis or allergic reactions to blood products that contain IgA.

SPECIAL CONCERNS
Safety and efficacy have not been determined in children with congenital heart disease. Give close attention to the infusion rate as side effects may be related to the rate of administration. Since RSV-IGIV is made from human plasma, there is the possibility for transmission of blood-borne pathogenic organisms, although the risk is considered

to be low due to screening of donors and viral inactivation and removal steps in the manufacturing process.

SIDE EFFECTS

Most Common

Fever, respiratory distress, vomiting, wheezing, diarrhea, rales, fluid overload, tachycardia, rash, hypertension, hypoxia, tachypnea, gastroenteritis, injection site reaction.

Infusion of RSV-IGIV may cause fluid overload, especially in children with bronchopulmonary dysplasia. Aseptic meningitis syndrome has been reported within several hours to 2 days following RSV-IGIV treatment. Symptoms include severe headache, drowsiness, fever, photophobia, painful eye movements, muscle rigidity, nausea, and vomiting. The CSF shows pleocytosis, predominately granulocytic, as well as elevated protein levels. **Allergic:** Hypotension, *anaphylaxis, angioneurotic edema*, respiratory distress. **CNS:** Fever, pyrexia, sleepiness. **Respiratory:** Respiratory distress, wheezing, rales, tachypnea, cough. **GI:** Vomiting, diarrhea, gagging, gastroenteritis. **CV:** Tachycardia, increased pulse rate, hypertension, hypotension, heart murmur. **Dermatologic:** Rash, pallor, cyanosis, eczema, cold and clammy skin. **Miscellaneous:** Hypoxia, hypoxemia, inflammation at injection site, edema, rhinorrhea, conjunctival hemorrhage. Reactions similar to other immunoglobulins may occur as follows. **Body as a whole:** Dizziness, flushing, *immediate allergic, anaphylactic, or hypersensitivity reactions*. **CV:** Blood pressure changes, palpitations, chest tightness. **Miscellaneous:** Anxiety, dyspnea, abdominal cramps, pruritus, myalgia, arthralgia.

OD OVERDOSE MANAGEMENT

Symptoms: Symptoms due to fluid volume overload. *Treatment:* Administration of diuretics and reduce the infusion rate.

DRUG INTERACTIONS

Antibodies found in immunoglobulin products may interfere with the immune response to live virus vaccines, including those for mumps, rubella, and measles. Also, the antibody response to

diphtheria, tetanus, pertussis, and *Haemophilus influenzae* may be lower in RSV-IGIV recipients.

HOW SUPPLIED

Injection: 50 +/- 10 mg immunoglobulin/mL.

DOSAGE

- **INJECTION (IV)**

  Prevention of RSV infections.

Infusion rate of 1.5 mL/kg/hr for 0–15 min. If the clinical condition of the client allows, the rate can be increased to 3.6 mL/kg/hr for the remainder of the infusion. *Do not exceed these rates of infusion.* **Maximum dose/monthly infusion:** 750 mg/kg.

NURSING CONSIDERATIONS

ADMINISTRATION/STORAGE

IV 1. Enter single-use vial only once. Initiate infusion within 6 hr and complete within 12 hr of removal from the vial.

2. Do not use if solution is turbid.

3. Give separately from other drugs or medications.

4. Give through an IV line (preferably a separate line) using an infusion pump. Administration may be "piggy-backed" into an existing line if that line contains one of the following dextrose solutions (with or without NaCl): 2.5%, 5%, 10%, or 20% dextrose in water. If a preexisting line must be used, do not dilute RSV-IGIV more than 1:2 with one of the above solutions. Do not predilute RSV-IGIV before infusion.

5. Although use of filters is not necessary, an in-line filter with a pore size greater than 15 μm may be used.

6. Store the injection at 2–8°C (36–46°F). Do not freeze or shake (to prevent foaming).

ASSESSMENT

1. Note reasons for therapy, any previous experiences with this drug, outcome. Note any IgA deficiency.

2. Assess VS, I&O, and heart/lung/breathing status: prior to infusion, before each rate increase, and thereafter at 30-min intervals until 30 min following infusion completion.

3. Observe for fluid overload (increased HR, increased respiratory rate, crackles,

---

retractions), esp. in infants with BPD (bronchopulmonary dysplasia). A loop diuretic (e.g., furosemide or bumetanide) should be available for management of fluid overload.

CLIENT/FAMILY TEACHING

1. The first dose of RSV-IGIV should be given prior to the beginning of the RSV season and monthly throughout the RSV season (in the Northern Hemisphere, from Nov–April) to maintain protection.

2. Drug is derived from human plasma; review potential risks related to bloodborne pathogens.

3. Report any severe headaches, painful eye movements, drowsiness, fever, N&V, or muscle rigidity (symptoms of aseptic meningitis); must be evaluated to rule out other causes of meningitis.

4. If virus vaccines are given during or within 10 months after RSV-IGIV infusion, reimmunization is recommended.

OUTCOMES/EVALUATE

RSV prophylaxis; ↓ severity of RSV illness

Retapamulin
(ree-teh-**PAM**-you-lin)

CLASSIFICATION(S):
Antibiotic, topical
PREGNANCY CATEGORY: B
Rx: Altabax.

USES

Topical treatment of impetigo due to *Staphylococcus aureus* (methicillin-susceptible isolates only) or *Streptococcus pyogenes* in adults and children 9 months of age and older.

ACTION/KINETICS

Action

An antibacterial agent that is a semisynthetic derivative of pleuromutilin.

Pharmacokinetics

Low systemic absorption. Extensively metabolized to numerous metabolites by CYP3A4. **Plasma protein binding:** 94%.

CONTRAINDICATIONS

Oral, intranasal, ophthalmic, or intravaginal use.

SPECIAL CONCERNS

Use with caution during lacatation. Safety and efficacy has not been established in children less than 9 months of age.

SIDE EFFECTS

Most Common

Application-site irritation/pruritus.

GI: Diarrhea, nausea. **CNS:** Headache. **Dermatologic:** Application site irritation/pruritus/pain, eczema, pruritus, contact dermatitis, erythema. **Respiratory:** Nasopharyngitis. **Miscellaneous:** Pyrexia.

DRUG INTERACTIONS

Coadministration with ketoconazole ↑ retapamulin mean AUC and C_{max}.

HOW SUPPLIED

Ointment: 10 mg/gram.

DOSAGE
- **OINTMENT**
  Impetigo.

Apply a thin layer to the affected area (up to 100 cm^2 in total area) in adults or 2% total body surface area in children 9 months of age and older. Give twice a day for 5 days. The treated area may be covered with a sterile bandage or gauze dressing.

NURSING CONSIDERATIONS

ADMINISTRATION/STORAGE

1. Use of retapamulin in the absence of a proven or strongly suspected bacterial infection is not likely to be of benefit and it increases the risk of development of drug-resistant bacteria.

2. In the event of severe local irritation due to the drug, discontinue use, wipe off the ointment, and use alternative therapy

3. Store from 15–30°C (59–86°F).

ASSESSMENT

1. Note reasons for therapy, onset, characteristics of area requiring treatment, VS, culture results.

2. Assess for any other medicines prescribed or cleansers on skin; advise to hold until therapy completed.

3. Advise that repeated use of Retapamulin Ointment may cause a second

---

 = see color insert   = Herbal   **IV** = Intravenous   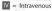 = sound alike drug infection and require alternative therapy.

CLIENT/FAMILY TEACHING

1. Use as directed for entire time prescribed even if symptoms have improved or resolved. Apply a thin layer of ointment to the affected area twice daily for 5 days.

2. Wash hands before and immediately after using Retapamulin Ointment unless they are part of the treated area.

3. Drug is not intended for ingestion or oral, nasal, eye, or vaginal use, or for use on mucosal surfaces (i.e., lips, mouth, or inside nose). Rinse with cool water at once if any contact occurs.

4. May cover treatment area with a sterile bandage or gauze dressing, if desired. Useful when treating children or infants over 9 mo old to protect the area and to help prevent them from getting the medicine on other areas (i.e., eyes, nose, mouth).

5. Notify provider if no improvement in S&S within 3 to 4 days of starting treatment.

6. Report any irritation, redness, itching, burning, swelling, blistering, or oozing worsens in the treatment area.

7. Keep all F/U appointments to evaluate response to therapy and effectiveness of therapy.

OUTCOMES/EVALUATE

Resolution of bacterial skin infection (impetigo)

Reteplase recombinant Ⅳ

(**REE**-teh-place)

CLASSIFICATION(S):

Thrombolytic, tissue plasminogen activator

PREGNANCY CATEGORY: C

Rx: Retavase.

USES

Acute MI in adults for improvement of ventricular function, reduction of the incidence of CHF, and reduction of mortality. *Investigational:* Clearance of occluded venous catheters, thrombolytic treatment of acute and chronic DVT, treatment of massive pulmonary embolism with a double bolus, with heparin and percutaneous transluminal angioplasty to treat thrombosed polytetrafluoroethylene hemodialysis arteriovenous grafts.

ACTION/KINETICS

Action

Plasminogen activator that catalyzes the cleavage of endogenous plasminogen to generate plasmin. Plasmin, in turn, degrades the matrix of the thrombus, causing a thrombolytic effect.

Pharmacokinetics

$t\frac{1}{2}$: 13 to 16 min. Cleared primarily by the liver and kidney.

CONTRAINDICATIONS

Active internal bleeding; history of CVA; recent intracranial or intraspinal surgery or trauma; intracranial neoplasm, arteriovenous malformation, or aneurysm; known bleeding diathesis; severe uncontrolled hypertension.

SPECIAL CONCERNS

Use with caution during lactation. Safety and efficacy have not been determined in children.

SIDE EFFECTS

Most Common

Bleeding disorders.

See *NOTE* below. **Bleeding disorders:** From internal bleeding sites, including intracranial, retroperitoneal, GI, GU, or respiratory. *Hemorrhage may occur* from superficial bleeding sites, including venous cutdowns, arterial punctures, sites of recent surgery. **CV:** *Cholesterol embolism,* coronary thrombolysis resulting in arrhythmias associated with perfusion (no different from those seen in the ordinary course of acute MI), *cardiogenic shock,* sinus bradycardia, accelerated idioventricular rhythm, ventricular premature depolarizations, SVT, ventricular *tachycardia/fibrillation,* AV block, pulmonary edema, *heart failure, cardiac arrest, recurrent ischemia, myocardial rupture, cardiac tamponade, venous thrombosis or embolism, electromechanical dissociation, mitral regurgitation, pericardial effusion, pericarditis.* **Hypersensitivity:** Serious

---

Bold Italic = life threatening side effect   ■ = black box warning   ♣ = Available in Canada

allergic reactions. *NOTE:* Many of the CV side effects listed are frequent sequelae of MI and may or may not be attributable to reteplase recombinant.

LABORATORY TEST CONSIDERATIONS
↓ Plasminogen, fibrinogen. Degradation of fibrinogen in blood samples removed for analysis.

DRUG INTERACTIONS
Use with abciximab, aspirin, dipyridamole, heparin, or vitamin K antagonists may increase the risk of bleeding.

HOW SUPPLIED
Powder for Injection, Lyophilized: 10.4 international units (18.1 mg).

DOSAGE———————————
* **IV ONLY**
  Acute MI.
Adults: 10 + 10 unit double-bolus injection. Each bolus is given over 2 min, with the second bolus given 30 min after initiation of the first bolus injection.

NURSING CONSIDERATIONS

ADMINISTRATION/STORAGE
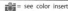 1. Initiate treatment as soon as possible after symptom onset.
2. Have available antiarrhythmic therapy for bradycardia and/or ventricular irritability.
3. Give each bolus by an IV line in which no other medication is being simultaneously infused/injected. Do not add any other medication to the reteplase solution. If drug is to be given through an IV line containing heparin, flush normal saline or D5W through the line prior to and following reteplase injection.
4. Reconstitution is performed using the diluent, syringe, needle, and dispensing pin provided with the drug as follows:
* Remove the flip-cap from one vial of sterile water (preservative free), and, with the syringe provided, withdraw 10 mL of the sterile water.
* Open the package containing the dispensing pin. Remove the needle from the syringe and discard. Remove the protective cap from the spike end of the dispensing pin and connect the syringe to the dispens-

ing pin. Remove the protective flip-cap from one vial of reteplase.
* Remove the protective cap from the spike end of the dispensing pin, and insert the spike into the vial of reteplase. Transfer the 10 mL of sterile water through the dispensing pin into the vial.
* With the dispensing pin and syringe still attached to the vial, gently swirl the vial to dissolve the reteplase. *Do not shake.*
* Withdraw the 10 mL of reconstituted reteplase back into the syringe (a small amount will remain due to overfill).
* Detach the syringe from the dispensing pin, and attach the sterile 20-gauge needle provided. The solution is ready to administer.
5. Since reteplase contains no antibacterial preservatives, reconstitute just prior to use. When reconstituted as directed, the solution may be used within 4 hr when stored at 2–30°C (36–86°F).
6. Keep the kit sealed until use and store at 2–25°C (36–77°F).

ASSESSMENT
1. Note reasons for therapy, onset, pain level, characteristics of chest pain.
2. List drugs currently prescribed to ensure none interact unfavorably.
3. Note evidence of CVA, internal bleeding, trauma, neurosurgery, or bleeding disorders.
4. Obtain CBC, type/cross, coagulation times, cardiac enzyme panel, renal and LFTs.
5. Note cardiopulmonary assessments, ECG.

INTERVENTIONS
1. During administration, continuously monitor cardiac rhythm. Have medications available for management of arrhythmias. Record VS every 15 min during infusion and for 2 hr following.
2. Administer first dose over 2 min, the second dose 30 min later if no serious bleeding is observed. In the event of any uncontrolled bleeding, terminate heparin infusion and withhold second dose.
3. Avoid: unnecessary client handling, IM injections, and invasive procedures.

R

Observe all puncture sites and areas for evidence of bleeding. Arterial sticks require 30 min of manual pressure followed by application of a pressure dressing.

4. Assess for reperfusion reactions such as:

- Arrhythmias usually of short duration, which may include bradycardia or ventricular tachycardia
- Reduction of chest pain
- Return of elevated ST segment and smaller Q waves

5. Maintain bed rest and observe for S&S of abnormal bleeding (hematuria, hematemesis, melena, CVA, cardiac tamponade).

CLIENT/FAMILY TEACHING

1. Review goals of therapy and inherent risks of drug therapy during acute coronary artery occlusion.

2. To be effective, initiate therapy as soon as possible after symptom onset.

3. Encourage family members to learn CPR.

OUTCOMES/EVALUATE

Improved ventricular function; ↓ incidence of CHF, and ↓ mortality with AMI

$Rh_o(D)$ Immune Globulin $(Rh_o[D]$ IGIM) $(Rh_o[D]$ IGIM) ■ IV

CLASSIFICATION(S):
Immunosuppressant
Rx: BayRho-D Full Dose, RhoGAM.

$Rh_o(D)$ Immune Globulin IV $(RH_o[D]$ IGIV) $(Rh_o[D]$ IGIV)

(roh (dee) im-**MYOUN GLOH**-byou-lin)

PREGNANCY CATEGORY: C
Rx: Rhophylac, WinRho SDF.

USES

$Rh_o(D)$ IGIM: BayRho-D Full Dose, RhoGAM. (1) Prevention of Rh hemolytic disease of the newborn (given to the $Rh_o(D)$ negative mother 72 hr after birth of a $Rh_o(D)$ positive infant) if the following criteria are met: The mother must be $Rh_o(D)$ negative and must not already be sensitized to the $Rh_o(D)$ factor and her child must be $Rh_o(D)$ positive and should have a negative direct antiglobulin test. Give within 72 hr to all nonimmunized $Rh_o(D)$ negative women who have undergone spontaneous or induced abortion, following ruptured tubal pregnancy, amniocentesis or abdominal trauma unless the blood group of the fetus or the father is known to be $Rh_o(D)$ negative. If the fetal blood group cannot be determined, assume that it is $Rh_o(D)$ positive, and $Rh_o(D)$ immune globulin should be given to the mother. (2) Prevent isoimmunization in $Rh_o(D)$ negative persons who have been transfused with $Rh_o(D)$ positive RBCs or blood components containing RBCs.

Investigational (controversial): Prior to external version attempts for breech presentation (due to induced fetomaternal hemorrhage) and following tubal ligation after delivery of a $Rh_o D$ positive infant (to prevent problems should sterilization fail or subsequent tubal reanastomoses occur).

$Rh_o(D)$ IGIV: Rhophylac, WinRho SDF. (1) Non-splenectomized, $Rh_o(D)$ positive children with chronic or acute immune thrombocytopenic purpura (ITP), adults with chronic ITP, or children and adults with ITP secondary to HIV infection, in situations requiring an increase in platelet count to prevent excessive hemorrhage. Safety and efficacy have not been determined for use in non-ITP causes of thrombocytopenia or in previously splenectomized clients or in those who are $Rh_o(D)$ negative. (2) **Rhophylac:** Suppression of Rh isoimmunization in nonsensitized $Rh_o(D)$-negative women with an Rh-incompatible pregnancy, including routine antepartum and postpartum Rh prophylaxis and Rh prophylaxis in cases of obstetric

---

complications (e.g., miscarriage, abortion, threatened abortion, ectopic pregnancy or hydatidiform mole, transplacental hemorrhage resulting from antepartum hemorrhage), invasive procedures during pregnancy (e.g., amniocentesis, chorionic biopsy), or obstetric manipulative procedures (e.g., external version, abdominal trauma). An Rh-incompatible pregnancy is assumed if the fetus/baby is either Rho(D)-positive or Rho(D)-unknown, or if the father is either Rho(D)-positive or Rho(D)-unknown. (3) **WinRho SDF:** Suppression of Rh isoimmunization in nonsensitized Rh$_o$(D)-negative women within 72 hr after spontaneous or induced abortions, amniocentesis, chorionic villus sampling, ruptured tubal pregnancy, abdominal trauma or transplacental hemorrhage, or in the normal course of pregnancy unless the blood type of the fetus or father is known to be Rh$_o$(D)-negative. In the case of maternal bleeding due to threatened abortion, give as soon as possible. Suppression of Rh isoimmunization decreases the likelihood of hemolytic disease in an Rh$_o$(D)-positive fetus in present and future pregnancies. Do not give to infants born to Rh-incompatible mothers. (4) Suppression of Rh isoimmunization in Rh$_o$(D)-negative female children and female adults in their childbearing years transfused with Rh$_o$(D)-positive RBCs or blood components containing Rh$_o$(D)-positive RBCs. Initiate treatment within 72 hr of exposure. Give treatment (without preceding exchange transfusion) only if the transfused Rh$_o$(D)-positive blood represents less than 20% of the total circulating red cells. A 300 mcg (1,500 units) dose will suppress the immunizing potential of about 17 mL of Rh$_o$(D)-positive RBCs.

ACTION/KINETICS

Action

Sterile, freeze-dried gamma globulin (IgG) fraction containing antibodies to Rh$_o$(D) derived from human plasma. The manufacturing process is effective in inactivating lipid-enveloped viruses, including hepatitis B and C and HIV. Contains approximately 2 mcg IgA/

1,500 international units (300 mcg). It suppresses the immune response of nonsensitized Rh$_o$(D) antigen-negative individuals following Rh$_o$(D) antigen-positive red blood cell exposure. Mechanism for ITP may be due to formation of anti-Rh$_o$(D) (anti-D) coated RBC complexes resulting in Fc receptor blockade; this spares antibody-coated platelets. Suppression of Rh isoimmunization decreases the possibility of hemolytic disease in an Rh$_o$(D) antigen-positive fetus in present and future pregnancies.

Pharmacokinetics

For Rh$_o$(D) IGIV, **Peak levels, after IV:** 2 hr; **after IM:** 5–10 days. **t$^{1}\!/_{2}$, after IV:** 24 days; **after IM:** 30 days.

CONTRAINDICATIONS

History of anaphylactic or severe systemic reaction to human globulin (i.e., due to the presence of trace amounts of IgA). Administration to Rh$_o$(D) antigen-negative or splenectomized individuals, as efficacy has not been shown. Use in Rh$_o$(D) antigen-negative clients who are Rh immunized (Rh antibody-positive), as evidenced by standard manual Rh antibody screening tests. Use in infants. IV use of Rh$_o$(D) IGIM.

SPECIAL CONCERNS

■ These products have been associated with renal dysfunction, acute renal failure, osmotic nephrosis, and death. Clients predisposed to acute renal failure include those with any degree of preexisting renal insufficiency, diabetes mellitus, those over 65 years of age, volume depletion, sepsis, paraproteinemia, or those receiving known nephrotoxic drugs. IGIV should be given in such clients at the minimum concentration available and the minimum rate of infusion practical. While reports of renal dysfunction and acute renal failure have been associated with many of the IGIV products, those containing sucrose as a stabilizer account for a disproportionate share of the total number.■ Use with extreme caution in those with a hemoglobin level less than 8 grams/dL due to the possibility of increasing the severity of anemia. There is a risk of transmitting infectious agents since products are made from human plasma.

R

SIDE EFFECTS

Most Common

Rh₀(D) IGIM: Headache, muscle aches/pains, pain/tenderness at injection site. **Rh₀(D) IGIV:** Fever, chills, wheezing, muscle aches/pains, back pain, pain/tenderness at injection site.

Side effects are infrequent. At injection site: Pain/tenderness at injection site, discomfort and slight swelling at the injection site. **CNS:** Headache. **Musculoskeletal:** Muscle aches/pains, back pain. **GU:** Symptoms following IGIV include anuria, acute renal failure, acute tubular necrosis, proximal tubular nephropathy, osmotic nephrosis. **Hematologic:** Decreased hemoglobin. **Body as a whole:** Fever, chills, wheezing, *anaphylaxis*. NOTE: Immune thrombocytopenic clients positive for Rho antigen D-(positive) may show symptoms of intravascular hemolysis, clinically compromising anemia, and renal insufficiency.

HOW SUPPLIED

BayRho-D Full Dose (IGIM): *Solution for Injection:* 15–18% protein.

RhoGAM (IGIM): *Solution for Injection:* 5% +/- 1% gamma globulin.

Rhophylac (IGIV): *Injection Solution:* 1,500 units (300 mcg).

WinRho SDF (IGIV): *Liquid Injection:* 600 units (120 mcg); 1,500 units (300 mcg); 2,500 units (500 mcg); 5,000 units (1,000 mcg); 15,000 units (3,000 mcg).

DOSAGE

BayRho-D Full Dose, RhoGAM.

- **IM ONLY**

Postpartum prophylaxis.

Give 1 vial or syringe (300 mcg) preferably within 72 hr of delivery. Dosage requirements vary with full-term deliveries depending on magnitude of fetomaternal hemorrhage. One 300 mcg dose provides sufficient antibody to prevent Rh sensitization if the RBC volume that has entered the circulation is 15 mL or less. If more than 15 mL is suspected or if the dose calculation results in a fraction, give the next higher whole number of vials or syringes.

Antenatal prophylaxis.

One 300 mcg vial or syringe given at about 28 weeks, gestation. Must be followed by another 300 mcg dose, preferably within 72 hr after delivery if infant is Rh positive.

Following threatened abortion at any stage of gestation with continuation of pregnancy.

Give 300 mcg. If more than 15 mL RBCs is suspected due to fetomaternal hemorrhage, give a dose as described under postpartum prophylaxis.

Following miscarriage, abortion, or termination of ectopic pregnancy at or beyond 13 weeks' gestation.

Give 300 mcg. If more than 15 mL RBCs is suspected due to fetomaternal hemorrhage, give a dose as described under postpartum prophylaxis. If pregnancy is terminated pror to 13 weeks gestation, where licensed, a single dose of Rh₀(D) IG micro-dose (about 50 mcg) may be used instead of Rh₀(D) IGIM.

Following amniocentesis at either 15–18 weeks gestation or during the third trimester, or following abdominal trauma in the second or third trimester.

Give 300 mcg of Rh₀(D) immune globulin (human). If there is fetomaternal hemorrhage in excess of 15 mL of RBCs, give a dose as described under postpartum prophylaxis. If these conditions occur at 13–18 weeks gestation, give another 300 mcg at 26–28 weeks. A dose should be given within 72 hr after delivery if the baby is Rh positive. If delivery occurs within 3 weeks after the last dose, the postpartum dose may be withheld unless there is fetomaternal hemorrhage in excess of 15 mL of RBCs.

Transfusion of Rh₀(D)-positive red cells to an Rh₀(D)-negative recipient.

Determine the volume of Rh₀(D)-positive red cells given to an Rh₀(D)-negative recipient. Then, multiply the volume of Rh-positive whole blood given by the hematocrit of the donor unit. The volume of RBCs is divided by 15 to determine the number of vials or syringes of Rh₀(D) IGIM to give. If the dose calculated results in a fraction, give the next higher whole number of vials or syringes. Give as soon as possible after the incompatible transfusion, but within 72 hr.

Bold Italic = life threatening side effect   ■ = black box warning   ♣ = Available in Canada

RHOPHYLAC
- **IM, IV**
  ITP.

50 mcg (250 units)/kg given as a single IV injection given at a rate of 2 mL/15—60 seconds. Use the following formula to calculate the amount of Rhophylac to administer:

dose (units) x body weight (kg) = total units/1,500 units per syringe = number of syringes.

Suppression of Rh isoimmunization.

Routine antepartum prophylaxis: 300 mcg (1,500 units) IM or IV at weeks 28 to 30 of gestation.

Postpartum prophylaxis (only if the newborn is Rh$_o$(D)-positive): 300 mcg (1,500 units) IM or IV within 72 hr of birth.

Obstetric complications: 300 mcg (1,500 units) IM or IV within 72 hr of the complication.

Invasive procedures during pregnancy: 300 mcg (1,500 units) IM or IV within 72 hr of procedure.

Excessive fetomaternal hemorrhage (>15 mL): 300 mcg (1,500 units) IM or IV within 72 hr of complication plus 20 mcg (100 units)/mL fetal RBC's in excess of 15 mL if excess transplacental bleeding is quantified OR an additional 300 mcg (1,500 units) if excess transplacental bleeding cannot be quantified.

Incompatible transfusions: 20 mcg (100 units)/2 mL of transfused blood OR per 1 mL of erythrocyte concentrate within 72 hr of exposure. Give IM or IV.

WINRHO SDF
- **IV ONLY**
  ITP.

Initial after confirming the client is Rh$_o$(D) positive: 50 mcg/kg (250 units/kg) body weight, given as a single injection. The initial dose may be given in 2 divided doses given on separate days, if desired. If the client has a hemoglobin level that is less than 10 grams/dL, a reduced dose of 25–40 mcg/kg (125–200 units/kg) should be given to minimize the risk of increasing the severity of anemia. If subsequent dosing is required to elevate platelet counts, give an IV dose of 25–60 mcg/kg (125–300 units/kg) body weight. Deter-mine the frequency and dose used in maintenance therapy by the clinical response by assessing platelet counts, RBC counts, hemogblobin, and reticulo-cyte levels. **Maintenance:** If the client responded to the initial dose with a sat-isfactory response in platelets, a main-tenance dose of 25–60 mcg/kg (125–300 units/kg) is individualized based on platelet and hemoglobin lev-els. If the client did not respond to the initial dose, give a subsequent dose based on hemoglobin levels. If hemo-globin is between 8–10 grams/dL, re-dose from 25–40 mcg/kg (125–200 units/kg). If hemoglobin is greater than 10 grams/dL, redose from 50–60 mcg/kg (250–300 mcg/kg). If hemoglo-bin is less than 8 grams/dL, use with caution.

- **IM OR IV**
  Pregnancy.

300 mcg (1,500 units) given IM or IV at 28 weeks gestation. If WinRho SDF is given early in the pregnancy, give at 12-week intervals to maintain an adequate level of passively acquired anti-Rh.

Give 120 mcg (600 units) IM or IV as soon as possible after delivery of a con-firmed Rh$_o$(D)-positive baby and nor-mally no later than 72 hr after delivery. If the Rh status of the baby is unknown at 72 hr, give WinRho SDF to the moth-er at 72 hr after delivery. If more than 72 hr have passed, do not withhold WinRho SDF but give as soon as possi-ble up to 28 days after delivery.

Other obstetric conditions.

Postpartum (if newborn is Rh$_o$(D)-positive: 120 mcg (600 units) IMor IV within 72 hr.

Abortion, amniocentesis, or any other manipulation after 24 weeks' gestation: 120 mcg (600 units) IM or IV within 72 hr.

Twenty-eight weeks gestation: 300 mcg (1,500 units) IM or IV.

Threatened abortion at any time: 300 mcg (1,500 units) IM or IV as soon as possible.

Amniocentesis and chorionic villus sampling before 34 weeks' gestation: 300 mcg (1,500 units) IM or IV. Repeat

R

every 12 weeks while the woman is pregnant.

Transfusion.

IM. 12 mcg (60 units)/mL blood if exposed to Rh$_o$(D)-positive whole blood. Or, 24 mcg (120 units)/Ml cells if exposed to Rh$_o$(D)-positive RBCs. Administer 1,200 mcg (6,000 units) q 12 hr IM until the total calculated dose is given.

IV. 9 mcg (45 units)/mL blood if exposed to Rh$_o$(D)-positive whole blood. Or, 18 mcg (90 units)/mL cells if exposed to Rh$_o$(D)-positive RBCs. Administer 600 mcg (3,000 units) q 8 hr IV until the total calculated dose is given.

NURSING CONSIDERATIONS

ADMINISTRATION/STORAGE

1. Never inject Rh$_o$(D) IGIM IV.

2. Do not give Rh$_o$(D) IGIM or IGIV to a neonate.

3. If Rh$_o$(D) IGIM is given antepartum, it is essential that the mother receive another dose of Rh$_o$(D) IGIM after delivery of a Rh$_o$(D)-positive infant. If the father can be determined to be Rh$_o$(D)-negative, RH$_o$(D) IGIM need not be given.

4. Administer Rh$_o$(D) IGIM preferably in the anterolateral aspects of the upper thigh and the deltoid muscle of the upper arm. Do not use the gluteal area routinely due to possible injury to the sciatic nerve. If used, only the upper, outer quadrant should be used.

5. When using a single vial or syringe of Rh$_o$(D) IGIM, give the entire amount. If using multiple vials or syringes, calculate total number of vials or syringes needed. The total volume can be given in divided doses at different sites at 1 time or the total dose may be divided and given at intervals, provided the total dose is given within 72 hr of the fetomaternal hemorrhage or transfusion.

6. Use the following administration procedure for a syringe containing Rh$_o$(D) IGIM:

• Remove the prefilled syringe from the package. Lift by the barrel, not the plunger.

• Twist the plunger rod clockwise until the threads are seated.

• With the rubber needle shield secured on the syringe tip, push the plunger rod forward a few millimeters to break any friction seal between the rubber stopper and the glass syringe barrel.

• Remove needle shield and expel air bubbles.

• Proceed with puncture with the needle.

• Aspirate prior to injection to ensure needle is not in an artery or vein.

• Inject the drug. Withdraw the needle and destroy it.

7. For IM use of Rh$_o$(D) IGIV, reconstitute the 600 international units and the 1,500 international units product aseptically with 1.25 mL of 0.9% NaCl injection and the 5,000 international units product with 8.5 mL 0.9% NaCl, using the same method as for IV use. Administer into the deltoid muscle of the upper arm or the anterolateral aspects of the upper thigh. Do not use the gluteal region routinely, due to the risk of sciatic nerve injury; if used, give only in the upper, outer quadrant.

8. Reduce dose (125–200 international units/kg) of Rh$_o$(D) IGIV if hemoglobin level is less than 10 grams/dL, to reduce the risk of increasing the severity of anemia.

This information is for Rh$_o$(D) IGIV:

IV 9. The drug must be given IV for treating ITP, as the SC or IM routes are not effective.

10. The following formulas are to be used to calculate the dose and number of vials needed to treat immune thrombocytopenic purpura:

• weight in lbs/2.2083 = weight in kg
• weight in kg x selected mcg (units) dosing level = dose
• dosage/vial size = number of vials needed

11. Rhophylac Preparation for Administration: Bring to room temperature before use. If more than 5 mL is required and IM injection is chosen, give in divided doses at different sites. Give IV at a rate of 2 mL/15 to 60 seconds for ITP clients.

12. WinRho SDF Preparation for Administration: No reconstitution is required.

Bold Italic = life threatening side effect   ■ = black box warning   ✤ = Available in Canada

Remove the entire contents of the vial to obtain the labeled dosage. If partial vials are required for dosage calculation, the entire contents of the vial should be withdrawn to ensure accurate calculation of the required dose. For IV administration, the entire dose may be injected into a suitable vein as rapidly as over 3 to 5 min; give separately from other drugs. For IM administration, give into the deltoid muscle of the upper arm or the anterolateral aspects of the upper thigh. Due to the possibility of sciatic nerve injury, do not use the gluteal region as a routine injection site. If the gluteal region is used, use only the upper outer quadrant. If using the Liquid for IV or IM injection, reconstitution is not required.

13. Store IGIM and IGIV products from 2–8°C (36–46°F); do not freeze. Discard any unused portion.

ASSESSMENT

1. Note reasons and condition requiring therapy. Review history of Rh-positive exposure in Rh-negative client, any reactions to immunizations and allergies.

2. Determine Rh factor to ensure client is not antibody positive. Obtain blood sample for type and cross from mother and the neonate's cord. The neonate should be $Rh_o(D)$ positive and the mother must be $Rh_o(D)$ negative and (D^u) negative. A large fetomaternal hemorrhage late in pregnancy or following delivery may cause a weak mixed field positive (D^u) test result. Assess for a large fetomaternal hemorrhage and adjust the dose of $Rh_o(D)$ immune globulin accordingly. Give drug if there is any doubt about the blood type of the mother.

3. Reduce dose if hemoglobin is <10 or there is evidence of a large fetomaternal hemorrhage.

4. When used to treat ITP, monitor clinical response by assessing platelet counts, red cell counts, hemoglobin, and reticulocyte levels.

5. Monitor Rh_o clients for S&S of intravascular hemolysis, clinically compromising anemia, and renal insufficiency.

CLIENT/FAMILY TEACHING

1. When an Rh-negative mother carries an Rh-positive fetus, the fetal RBCs cross the placenta and enter the mother's circulation, evoking maternal antibody production against the Rh factor. When these antibodies cross to the fetal circulation, they destroy fetal RBCs, hence the need for monitoring and administration with all subsequent pregnancies. The medication prevents sensitization of an Rh-negative mother by an Rh-positive fetus, ultimately preventing hemolytic disease of the newborn.

2. Avoid immunizations with live-virus vaccines for at least 3 months after receiving drug.

OUTCOMES/EVALUATE

- Suppression of Rh isoimmunization
- Prevention of hemolytic disease of the newborn
- ↑ Platelets

Ribavirin
(rye-bah-**VYE**-rin)

CLASSIFICATION(S):
Antiviral
PREGNANCY CATEGORY: X
Rx: Copegus, Rebetrol, RibaPak, Ribaspheres, Ribatab, Virazole.

R

SEE ALSO ANTIVIRAL DRUGS.

USES

Aerosol (Virazole): Hospitalized pediatric clients (including infants) with severe lower respiratory tract infections (viral pneumonia including bronchiolitis) due to RSV. Underlying conditions, such as prematurity or cardiopulmonary disease, may increase the severity of the RSV infection. Ribavirin is intended to be used along with standard treatment (including fluid management) for such clients with severe lower respiratory tract infections.

Capsules (Rebetol, Ribaspheres, Ribatab): (1) In combination with interferon alfa-2b to treat chronic hepatitis C in those with compensated liver disease previously untreated with alpha interferon or who have relapsed following alpha interferon therapy. (2) In combination with peginterferon alfa-2b to treat chronic hepatitis C in those with compensated liver disease who have not been previously treated with interferon alpha and who are at least 18 years of age.

Oral Solution (Rebetol): In combination with interferon alfa-2b to treat chronic hepatitis C in clients 3 years and older with compensated liver disease who have not been treated previously with alpha interferon.

Tablets (Copegus): In combination with peginterferon alfa-2a to treat adults with chronic hepatitis C virus infections who have compensated liver disease and have not been treated previously with interferon alpha. Is effective in those with compensated liver disease and histological evidence of cirrhosis (Child-Pugh Class A).

Investigational: Treatment of viral hemorrhagic fevers such as Lassa fever or hemorrhagic fever with renal syndrome.

NOTE: Ribavirin capsules, oral solution, or tablets as monotherapy are not effective to treat chronic HCV infection.

ACTION/KINETICS
Action
Has antiviral activity against respiratory syncytial virus (RSV), influenza virus, and HSV. Precise mechanism not known; may act as a competitive inhibitor of cellular enzymes that act on guanosine and xanthosine.

Pharmacokinetics
Ribavirin is distributed to the plasma, respiratory tract, and RBCs and is rapidly taken up by cells. The capsules are rapidly and extensively absorbed but due to first-pass metabolism the bioavailability averages 64%. Ribavirin tablets reach C_{max} in 2 hr. Steady state is reached in about 4 weeks using capsules. **t½ of tablets:** 120–170 hr; **of capsules:** 298 hr. Eliminated through both the urine and feces.

CONTRAINDICATIONS
Capsules/Oral Solution / Tablets: Women who are pregnant or in men whose female partners are pregnant. Clients with hemoglobinopathies (e.g., thalessemia major or sickle-cell anemia). As monotherapy to treat chronic hepatitis C. Lactation. **Aerosol:** Pregnancy or the potential for pregnancy during drug exposure.

Capsules, Tablets, and Aerosol: Lactation. In those with hemoglobinopathies (e.g., thalassemia major, sickle-cell anemia) or pancreatitis. Use in those with a history of significant or unstable cardiac disease. **Tablets:** Use in clients with a C_{CR} <50 mL/min. **Capsules/Oral Solution and peginterferon alfa-2b:** Autoimmune hepatitis. **Tablets and peginterferon alfa-2a:** Clients with autoimmune hepatitis and hepatic decompensation (Child-Pugh class B and C) before or during treatment.

SPECIAL CONCERNS
■ Capsules/Tablets/Oral Solution. (1) Ribavirin monotherapy is not effective to treat chronic hepatitis C virus infection. Do not use alone for this condition. (2) The primary toxicity of ribavirin is hemolytic anemia. The anemia may result in worsening of cardiac disease and has led to fatal and nonfatal MIs. Do not treat clients with a history of significant or unstable cardiac disease with ribavirin. (3) Significant teratogenic or embryocidal effects have been shown in all animal species exposed to ribavirin. Also, ribavirin has a multiple-dose half-life of 12 days and may persist in nonplasma compartments for as long as 6 months. Thus, ribavirin therapy is contraindicated in women who are pregnant and in the male partners of women who are pregnant. Extreme care must be taken to avoid pregnancy during therapy and for 6 months after completion of therapy in both female clients and in female partners of male clients who are taking ribavirin. At least 2 reliable forms of effective contraception must be used during treatment and during the 6-month posttreatment period. Aerosol. (1) Use of aerosolized ribavirin in those requiring mechanical ventilator assistance should be undertaken only by health care providers and support staff familiar with the specific ventilator being used and this mode of ad-

ministration of the drug. Strict attention must be paid to procedures that minimize the accumulation of drug precipitate that can result in mechanical ventilator dysfunction and associated increased pulmonary pressure. (2) Sudden deterioration of respiratory function has been associated with initiation of aerosolized ribavirin use in infants. Carefully monitor respiratory function during treatment. If initiation of aerosolized ribavirin treatment seems to produce sudden deterioration of respiratory function, stop treatment and reinstitute only with extreme caution, continuous monitoring, and consideration of concomitant administration of bronchodilators. (3) Ribavirin aerosol is not indicated for use in adults. Ribavirin has been shown to produce testicular lesions in rodents and to be teratogenic in all animal species in which adequate studies have been conducted.■ Use of capsules or oral solution in the elderly cause a higher frequency of anemia; use with caution in the elderly. Use the tablets with caution in those with preexisting cardiac disease. Safety and efficacy of the tablets have not been determined in children less than 18 years of age. Safety and efficacy of ribavirin and interferon alfa-2b or peginterferon alfa-2a combination therapy for hepatitis C have not been determined in clients coinfected with HIV or HBV or in those who have received liver or other organ transplants. The safety and efficacy of ribavirin and peginterferon alfa-2a, interferon alfa-2b, and peginterferon alfa-2b combination therapy have not been established to treat HIV infection, adenovirus RSV, parainfluenza, or influenza infections.

SIDE EFFECTS

Most Common

When used with interferon alfa-2b or peginterferon alfa-2b: Alopecia, pruritus, rash, dry skin, anorexia, diarrhea, N&V, neutropenia, arthralgia, myalgia, musculoskeletal pain, viral infection, coughing, dyspnea, pharyngitis, fever, injection site inflammation/reaction, decreased weight.

Aerosol. Respiratory: Worsening of respiratory status, pneumothorax, apnea, bacterial pneumonia, dependence on ventilator, *bronchospasm*, pulmonary edema, hypoventilation, cyanosis, dyspnea, atelectasis. **CV:** Hypotension, *cardiac arrest*, manifestations of digitalis toxicity, bradycardia, bigeminy, tachycardia. **Hematologic:** Anemia (with IV or PO ribavirin), hemolytic anemia that may worsen cardiac disease leading to nonfatal and *fatal MI*, reticulocytosis. **Miscellaneous:** Conjunctivitis, rash, *seizures*, asthenia. NOTE: The following symptoms were noted in health care workers exposed to the aerosol: Headache, conjunctivitis, rhinitis, nausea, rash, dizziness, pharyngitis, lacrimation, bronchospasm and/or chest pain, damage to contact lenses after prolonged close exposure.

Capsules or Oral Solution in combination with interferon alfa-2a, interferon alfa-2b, or peginterferon alfa-2b. CNS: Headache, dizziness, agitation, anxiety, emotional lability, irritability, impaired concentration, depression (may be severe), insomnia, nervousness, *suicidal ideation*. **GI:** N&V, anorexia, dyspepsia, constipation, abdominal pain, diarrhea, dry mouth, hepatomegaly, pancreatitis. **CV:** Nonfatal and *fatal MI*. **Musculoskeletal:** Myalgia, arthralgia, musculoskeletal pain. **Hematologic:** Hemolytic anemia, anemia, leukopenia, neutropenia, thrombocytopenia, suppression of bone marrow function. **Respiratory:** Dyspnea, sinusitis, coughing, pharyngitis, rhinitis, pulmonary infiltrates, pneumonitis, pneumonia, pulmonary dysfunction. **Dermatologic:** Alopecia, injection site inflammation/reaction, pruritus, rash, flushing, dry skin, increased sweating. **Ophthalmic:** Conjunctivitis, blurred vision. **Body as a whole:** Fungal or viral infection, asthenia, fatigue, fever, flu-like symptoms, rigors, malaise, decreased weight, diabetes. **Miscellaneous:** Chest pain, taste perversion, menstrual disorder, hypothyroidism, right upper quadrant pain, autoimmune and infectious disorders.

R

Tablets in combination with peginterferon alfa-2a. **CNS:** Depression (may be severe), *suicide*, relapse of drug abuse/overdose, irritability, anxiety, impaired concentration, dizziness (including vertigo), headache, insomnia, nervousness, impaired memory, altered mood. **Hematologic:** Neutropenia, thrombocytopenia, anemia, lymphopenia, hemolytic anemia, suppression of bone marrow function. **GI:** N&V, anorexia, diarrhea, decreased weight, abdominal pain, dyspepsia, dry mouth, pancreatitis. **CV:** Nonfatal and *fatal MI.* **Dermatologic:** Alopecia, injection site reaction, pruritus, dermatitis, dry skin, rash, increased sweating, eczema. **Musculoskeletal:** Myalgia, arthralgia, back pain. **Respiratory:** Dyspnea, cough, exertional dyspnea, pneumonitis, pneumonia, pulmonary dysfunction. **Body as a whole:** Fatigue, asthenia, pyrexia, rigors, fever, overall resistance mechanism disorder, pain, flu-like symptoms (e.g., fatigue, pyrexia, myalgia, headache, rigors), bacterial infection (e.g., sepsis, osteomyelitis, endocarditis, pyelonephritis, pneumonia), autoimmune disorders, diabetes. **Miscellaneous:** Hypothyroidism, blurred vision.

LABORATORY TEST CONSIDERATIONS
↑ Bilirubin, uric acid. ↓ Hemoglobin. When combined with interferon alfa-2b: Alterations in hemoglobin, leukocytes, neutrophils, ALT, platelets and total bilirubin.

OD OVERDOSE MANAGEMENT
Symptoms: Following overdose of the capsules: Hepatic enzyme abnormalities, renal failure, hemorrhage, MI. *Treatment:* No specific antidote; hemodialysis and peritoneal dialysis are not effective.

DRUG INTERACTIONS
Al- or Mg-containing products / ↓ Mean ribavirin AUC using ribavirin capsules or oral solution
Didanosine / Possible fatal hepatic failure or peripheral neuropathy, pancreatitis, and symptomatic hyperlactatemia/ lactic acidosis; do not use together
Simethacone / ↓ Mean ribavirin AUC
Stavudine / Ribavirin tablets inhibit phosphorylation which could lead to ↓ antiretroviral activity. Avoid concomitant use
Zidovudine / Ribavirin tablets inhibit phosphorylation which could lead to ↓ antiretroviral activity. Avoid concomitant use

HOW SUPPLIED
Capsules: 200 mg; *Lyophilized Powder for Aerosol Reconstitution:* 6 grams/100 mL vial; *Oral Solution:* 40 mg/mL; *Tablets:* 200 mg, 400 mg, 600 mg; *Tablets, Film-Coated:* 200 mg, 400 mg, 600 mg.

DOSAGE
• **AEROSOL ONLY, TO AN INFANT OXYGEN HOOD USING THE SMALL PARTICLE AEROSOL GENERATOR-2 (SPAG-2)**
Severe lower respiratory tract infections due to RSV in infants.
The concentration administered is 20 mg/mL and the average aerosol concentration for a 12-hr period is 190 mcg/L of air. Treatment is continued for 12–18 hr a day for 3 (minimum)–7 days (maximum). See *Administration/Storage.*
• **CAPSULES; ORAL SOLUTION**
Chronic hepatitis C.
Body weight, 75 kg or less: 2 x 200 mg capsules in the a.m. and 3 x 200 mg capsules in the p.m. daily. **Body weight, over 75 kg:** 3 x 200 mg capsules in the a.m. and 3 x 200 mg capsules in the p.m. daily. Give for 24–48 weeks in those previously untreated with interferon. If combination therapy of ribavirin capsules and peginterferon alfa-2b is used, the recommended dose of ribavirin capsules is 800 mg/day in 2 divided doses (2 x 200 mg capsules in the morning with food and 2 x 200 mg capsules in the evening with food).
• **TABLETS**
Chronic hepatitis C.
800–1,200 mg/day in 2 divided doses with food for 24–48 weeks (for clients previously untreated with ribavirin and interferon). Individualize doses depending on baseline disease characteristics (e.g., genotype, response to therapy, and tolerability of the regimen).
RIBAVIRIN WITH PEGINTERFERON ALFA-2A
• **TABLETS**
Chronic hepatitis C.

Genotype 1, 4: Peginterferon alfa-2a, 180 mcg/week and ribavirin tablets in those <75 kg, 1,000 mg/day, and for those weighing 75 or more kg, 1,200 mg/day. Therapy is continued for 48 weeks. **Genotype 2, 3:** Peginterferon alfa-2a, 180 mcg/week and ribavirin tablets, 800 mg/day. Therapy is continued for 24 weeks. If severe side effects or lab abnormalities develop, modify or discontinue the dose, if appropriate, until side effects abate. If tolerance persists, discontinue both drugs.

RIBAVIRIN WITH PEGINTERFERON ALFA-2B
• **CAPSULES ORAL SOLUTION**
  Chronic hepatitis C.
Children, 25–36 kg: Ribavirin, 1 x 200 mg capsule in the a.m. and 1 x 200 mg capsule in the p.m. each day plus peginterferon alfa-2b injection, 3 million units/m^2 3 times weekly SC. **Children, 37–49 kg:** Ribavirin, 1 x 200 mg capsule in the a.m. and 2 x 200 mg capsules in the p.m. each day plus peginterferon alfa-2b injection, 3 million units/m^2 3 times weekly SC. **Children, 50–61 kg:** Ribavirin, 2 x 200 mg capsules in the a.m. and 2 x 200 mg capsules in the p.m. each day plus peginterferon alfa-2b injection, 3 million units/m^2 3 times weekly SC. **Children, >61 kg:** Use adult dose.

NURSING CONSIDERATIONS

Do not confuse ribavirin with riboflavin (vitamin B$_2$).

ADMINISTRATION/STORAGE

1. Treatment is most effective if initiated within the first 3 days of the RSV that causes lower respiratory tract infections.
2. Administer ribavirin aerosol using only the SPAG-2 aerosol generator.
3. Do *not* institute therapy in clients requiring artificial respiration.
4. Do not give any other aerosolized medications if using ribavirin aerosol.
5. Reconstitute with a minimum of 75 mL sterile water (USP) for injection or inhalation in the original 100-mL vial. Shake well and transfer the solution to the SPAG-2 reservoir utilizing a sterilized 500-mL wide-mouth Erlenmeyer flask and further dilute to a final volume of 300 mL with sterile water. Use water that has no antimicrobial agent or other substance added.
6. Replace solutions in the SPAG-2 reservoir daily. Also, if the liquid level is low, discard before new drug solution is added.
7. The dose and administration schedule for infants who require mechanical ventilation are the same as for those who do not.
8. For nonmechanically ventilated infants, the aerosol is delivered to an infant oxygen hood from the SPAG-2 aerosol generator. If a hood cannot be used, the aerosol is given by face mask or oxygen tent. However, due to the larger size of a tent, the delivery dynamics may be altered.
9. Store reconstituted solutions at room temperature up to 24 hr.
10. Women of childbearing age are not to administer the drug. *Post* this advisement so they do not come in contact with the drug.
11. Once ribavirin tablets have been withheld because of a lab abnormality or clinical manifestation, the drug may be restarted at 600 mg/day with a further increase to 800 mg/day, depending on the provider's judgment. It is not recommended that ribavirin tablets be increased to the original assigned dose of 1,000–1,200 mg/day.
12. Dosage modification guidelines for ribavirin tablets are:
• If hemoglobin with no cardiac disease is <10 grams/dL, reduce only the ribavirin tablet dose to 600 mg/day (1 x 200 mg tablet in the morning and 2 x 200 mg tablets in the evening). If hemoglobin is <8.5 grams/dL, discontinue ribavirin tablets.
• If there is a 2 or more grams/dL decrease in hemoglobin during any 4-week treatment period in clients with a history of stable cardiac disease, reduce only the ribavirin tablet dose to 600 mg/day (1 x 200 mg tablet in the morning and 2 x 200 mg tablets in the evening). If hemoglobin <12 grams/dL despite 4

R

weeks at a reduced ribavirin dose, discontinue ribavirin tablets.

13. Store capsules and tablets between 15–30°C (59–86°F) and store lyophilized drug powder for the aerosol from 15–25°C (59–78°F). Store reconstituted solutions under sterile conditions at room temperature for 24 hr or less.

ASSESSMENT

1. Note reasons for therapy, onset, characteristics of S&S, any experience with this drug, outcome. Document laboratory confirmation of RSV infection.

2. When using the aerosol, carefully monitor respiratory function. If sudden deterioration occurs, stop drug and restart only with extreme caution. When restarted, consider concurrent therapy with bronchodilators.

3. With hepatitis C document genotype, viral load, CBC, renal, LFTs. Document weight, clinical presentation; assess carefully for anemia with therapy-may require transfusion.

INTERVENTIONS

1. Health care workers administering aerosolized drug should use goggles and respirator to protect mucous membranes; remove contact lens, and monitor exposure times. Review drug-related side effects.

2. It is essential that constant monitoring be undertaken for both the fluid and respiratory status of the client. For ventilator-assisted clients be sure to drain tubing often to prevent obstruction and impaired ventilation.

3. Assess frequently for evidence of respiratory distress; stop therapy and report if distress occurs. Do not leave child unattended and unstimulated in the tent for long periods.

4. Monitor and record VS and I&O and H&H, esp. in the elderly.

5. Anticipate limited use in infants and adults with COPD or asthma.

6. With prolonged therapy assess for anemia; monitor VS and CBC values.

CLIENT/FAMILY TEACHING

1. Drug is an antiviral that has been used to successfully treat a variety of conditions. The aerosol form is used for infections caused by the RSV.

2. Oral agents have been used in combination with other drugs to treat chronic hepatitis C infections.

3. For children weighing 25 kg or less or who cannot swallow capsules, use ribavirin oral solution. For children weighing more than 25 kg, give either the 200 mg capsule or the oral solution.

4. Practice reliable contraception; report immediately if pregnancy suspected.

5. Keep all meds stored safely out of reach. Do not share with anyone.

6. Report any unusual fatigue, SOB, wt loss or other adverse side effects.

OUTCOMES/EVALUATE

- Improved airway exchange; resolution of RSV pneumonia
- Improved liver condition with Hepatitis C; ↓ HCVRNA

Rifabutin
(**rif**-ah-**BYOU**-tin)

CLASSIFICATION(S):
Antitubercular drug
PREGNANCY CATEGORY: B
Rx: Mycobutin.

USES
Prevention of disseminated *Mycobacterium avium* complex (MAC) disease in clients with advanced HIV infection. *Investigational:* Eradicate *H. pylori* as part of a triple-therapy (amoxicillin, pantoprazole, rifabutin), 10-day regimen.

ACTION/KINETICS

Action
Inhibits DNA-dependent RNA polymerase in susceptible strains of *Escherichia coli* and *Bacillus subtilis*.

Pharmacokinetics
Rapidly absorbed from the GI tract. **Peak plasma levels after a single dose:** 3.3 hr. **Mean terminal t½:** 45 hr. High-fat meals slow the rate, but not the extent, of absorption. About 30% of a dose is excreted in the feces and 53% in the urine, primarily as metabolites. The 25-O-desacetyl metabolite is equal in activity to rifabutin. **Plasma protein binding:** About 85%.

CONTRAINDICATIONS
Hypersensitivity to rifabutin or other rifamycins (e.g., rifampin). Use in active tuberculosis. Lactation.

SPECIAL CONCERNS
Safety and efficacy have not been determined in children, although the drug has been used in HIV-positive children.

SIDE EFFECTS
Most Common
Discolored urine, rash, abdominal pain, diarrhea, N&V, dyspepsia, eructation, headache, taste perversion.

GI: Anorexia, abdominal pain, diarrhea, dyspepsia, eructation, flatulence, N&V, taste perversion. **Respiratory:** Chest pain, chest pressure or pain with dyspnea. **CNS:** Insomnia, *seizures*, paresthesia, aphasia, confusion. **Musculoskeletal:** Asthenia, myalgia, arthralgia, myositis. **Body as a whole:** Fever, headache, generalized pain, flu-like syndrome. **Dermatologic:** Rash, skin discoloration. **Hematologic:** Neutropenia, leukopenia, anemia, eosinophilia, thrombocytopenia. **Miscellaneous:** Discolored urine, nonspecific T wave changes on ECG, hepatitis, hemolysis, uveitis.

LABORATORY TEST CONSIDERATIONS
↑ AST, ALT, alkaline phosphatase.

OD OVERDOSE MANAGEMENT
Symptoms: Worsening of side effects. *Treatment:* Gastric lavage followed by instillation into the stomach of an activated charcoal slurry.

DRUG INTERACTIONS
Although less potent than rifampin, rifabutin induces liver enzymes and may be expected to have similar interactions as does rifampin.
Amprenavir / ↓ Rifabutin clearance; ↓ rifabutin dose by 50%
Oral contraceptives / May ↓ OC effectiveness
Saquinavir / ↓ AUC and peak levels of saquinavir (after giving soft-gelatin capsules) and ↑ AUC and peak levels of rifabutin
Zidovudine (AZT) / ↓ AZT steady-state plasma levels after repeated rifabutin dosing

HOW SUPPLIED
Capsules: 150 mg.

DOSAGE
- **CAPSULES**
  Prophylaxis of MAC disease in clients with advanced HIV infection.
  Adults: 300 mg/day.

NURSING CONSIDERATIONS
ASSESSMENT
1. Note reasons for therapy, type, onset, characteristics of S&S.
2. Monitor CBC for neutropenia/thrombocytopenia.
3. Ensure CXR, PPD, and sputum AFB cultures have been performed to rule out active tuberculosis. Clients who develop active TB during therapy must be covered with appropriate antituberculosis medications.

CLIENT/FAMILY TEACHING
1. Take as directed and do not interrupt therapy. If N&V or other GI upset occurs, may take doses of 150 mg twice a day with food.
2. Urine, feces, saliva, sputum, perspiration, tears, skin, and mucous membranes may be colored brown-orange. Soft contact lenses may be permanently stained.
3. Report any S&S of muscle or eye pain, irritation, or inflammation as well as any persistent vomiting or abnormal bruising/bleeding.
4. Avoid crowds and those with infections.
5. Practice nonhormonal form of birth control.

OUTCOMES/EVALUATE
Prevention of disseminated *Mycobacterium avium* complex (MAC) with advanced HIV

Rifampin   IV ©
(rih-**FAM**-pin)

CLASSIFICATION(S):
Antitubercular drug
PREGNANCY CATEGORY: C
Rx: Rifadin, Rimactane.
✚Rx: Rofact.

R

USES

(1) All types of tuberculosis. Must be used in conjunction with at least one other tuberculostatic drug (such as isoniazid, ethambutol, pyrazinamide) but is the drug of choice for retreatment. (2) Treatment of asymptomatic meningococcal carriers to eliminate *Neisseria meningitis*. *Investigational:* Used in combination for infections due to *Staphylococcus aureus* and *S. epidermidis* (endocarditis, osteomyelitis, prostatitis); Legionnaire's disease; in combination with dapsone for leprosy; prophylaxis of meningitis due to *Haemophilus influenzae* and gram-negative bacteremia in infants.

ACTION/KINETICS

Action

Suppresses RNA synthesis by binding to the beta subunit of DNA-dependent RNA polymerase. This prevents attachment of the enzyme to DNA and blockade of RNA transcription. Both bacteriostatic and bactericidal; most active against rapidly replicating organisms.

Pharmacokinetics

Well absorbed from the GI tract; widely distributed in body tissues. **Peak plasma concentration:** 4–32 mcg/mL after 2–4 hr. **t½:** 1.5–5 hr (higher in clients with hepatic impairment). In normal clients t½ decreases with usage. Metabolized in liver; 60% is excreted in feces.

CONTRAINDICATIONS

Hypersensitivity; not recommended for intermittent therapy.

SPECIAL CONCERNS

Safe use during lactation has not been established. Safety and effectiveness not determined in children less than 5 years of age. Use with extreme caution in clients with hepatic dysfunction. Use with caution, if at all, with pyrazinamide in a 2 month regimen to treat latent tuberculosis in those not infected with human immunodeficiency virus.

SIDE EFFECTS

Most Common

Diarrhea, N&V, dizziness, headache, drowsiness, anorexia, sore mouth/tongue, flushing.

GI: N&V, diarrhea, anorexia, pseudomembranous colitis, pancreatitis, sore mouth and tongue, cramps, heartburn, flatulence. **CNS:** Headache, drowsiness, fatigue, ataxia, dizziness, confusion, generalized numbness, fever, difficulty in concentrating. **Hepatic:** Jaundice, hepatitis, *severe/fatal liver injury when used with pyrazinamide.* Increases in AST, ALT, bilirubin, alkaline phosphatase. **Hematologic:** Thrombocytopenia, eosinophilia, hemolysis, leukopenia, *hemolytic anemia.* **Allergic:** Flu-like symptoms, dyspnea, wheezing, SOB, purpura, pruritus, urticaria, skin rashes, sore mouth and tongue, conjunctivitis. **Renal:** Hematuria, hemoglobinuria, renal insufficiency, acute renal failure. **Miscellaneous:** Visual disturbances, flushing, muscle weakness or pain, arthralgia, decreased BP, osteomalacia, menstrual disturbances, edema of face and extremities, adrenocortical insufficiency, increases in BUN and serum uric acid. *NOTE:* Urine, saliva, tears, sweat, and feces may be red-orange to red-brown in color.

OD OVERDOSE MANAGEMENT

Symptoms: Shortly after ingestion, N&V, and lethargy will occur. Followed by severe hepatic involvement (liver enlargement with tenderness, increased direct and total bilirubin, change in hepatic enzymes) with unconsciousness. Also, brownish red or orange discoloration of urine, saliva, tears, sweat, skin, and feces. *Treatment:* Gastric lavage followed by activated charcoal slurry introduced into the stomach. Antiemetics to control N&V. Forced diuresis to enhance excretion. If hepatic function is seriously impaired, bile drainage may be required. Extracorporeal hemodialysis may be necessary.

DRUG INTERACTIONS

Acetaminophen / ↓ Acetaminophen effects R/T ↑ liver breakdown
Aminophylline / ↓ Aminophylline effects R/T ↑ liver breakdown
Amiodarone / ↓ Amiodarone serum levels R/T ↑ liver breakdown
Aminosalicylic acid / ↓ Rifampin effect; give 2 agents 8–12 hr apart
Amprenavir / Significant ↑ amprenavir clearance; do not use together
Anticoagulants, oral / ↓ Anticoagulant

Bold Italic = life threatening side effect   ■ = black box warning   ✦ = Available in Canada

effects R/T ↑ liver breakdown

Antidiabetics, oral / ↓ Antidiabetic effects R/T ↑ liver breakdown

Barbiturates / ↓ Barbiturate effects R/T ↑ liver breakdown

Benzodiazepines / ↓ Benzodiazepine effects R/T ↑ liver breakdown

Beta-adrenergic blocking agents / ↓ Beta-blocking effects R/T ↑ liver breakdown

Buspirone / ↓ Buspiron effect R/T ↑ liver metabolism

Chloramphenicol / ↓ Chloramphenicol effects R/T ↑ liver breakdown

Clofibrate / ↓ Clofibrate effects R/T ↑ liver breakdown

Contraceptives, oral / ↓ OC effects R/T ↑ liver breakdown

Corticosteroids / ↓ Corticosteroid effects R/T ↑ liver breakdown

Cyclosporine / ↓ Cyclosporine effects R/T ↑ liver breakdown

Delaviridine / ↓ Delaviridine effect R/T ↑ liver metabolism

Digoxin / ↓ Digoxin serum levels

Disopyramide / ↓ Disopyramide effects R/T ↑ liver breakdown

Doxycycline / ↓ Doxycycline serum level and t½ possible; ↓ effect

Enalapril / ↓ Enalapril effect

Estrogens / ↓ Estrogen effects R/T ↑ liver breakdown

Fluconazole / Rifampin ↑ fluconazole metabolism

Fluoroquinolones / Possible ↑ fluoroquinolone liver metabolism

Haloperidol / ↓ Haloperidol plasma levels and effect

Halothane / ↑ Risk of hepatotoxicity and hepatic encephalopathy

Hydantoins / ↓ Hydantoin effects R/T ↑ liver breakdown

Imatinib / ↓ Imatinib peak plasma levels and AUC R/T ↑ metabolism by CYP3A4

Isoniazid / ↑ Risk of hepatotoxicity

Ketoconazole / Rifampin ↑ ketoconazole metabolism; ketoconazole ↓ rifampin absorption → ↓ effect of both drugs

Lamotrigine / ↓ Lamotrigine AUC and t½ due to ↑ liver metabolism

Linezolid / ↓ Linezolid serum levels after IV use R/T induction of P-glycoprotein which may increase linezolid secretion into the intestine

Losartan / Rifampin may ↑ losartan liver metabolism

Macrolide antibiotics (e.g., clarithromycin) / Possible ↑ clarithromycin liver metabolism and ↓ rifamycin liver metabolism

Methadone / ↓ Methadone effects R/T ↑ liver breakdown

Mexiletine / ↓ Mexiletine effects R/T ↑ liver breakdown

Morphine / ↓ Morphine analgesia

Nevirapine / ↓ AUC and peak plasma nevirapine levels in HIV-infected clients

Nifedipine / ↓ Nifedipine effects

Ondansetron / ↓ Ondansetron plasma levels R/T ↑ liver breakdown

Propafenone / ↓ Propafenone serum levels R/T ↑ liver breakdown

Protease inhibitors (e.g., indinavir, nelfinavir, ritonavir) / Possible ↓ liver metabolism of both drugs

Pyrazinamide / Possible severe hepatitis

Quinine / ↑ Quinine liver metabolism

Quinidine / ↓ Quinidine effects R/T ↑ liver breakdown

Repaglinide / ↓ Repaglinide plasma levels and effects R/T ↑ liver metabolism

Rosiglitazone / ↓ Rosiglitazone AUC, peak plasma levels, and elimination t½ R/T ↑ rosiglitazone metabolism by CYP2C8

Sertraline / ↓ Sertraline effect R/T ↑ liver metabolism

Sulfapyridine / ↓ Sulfapyridine plasma levels

Sulfones / ↓ Sulfone effects R/T ↑ liver breakdown

Tacrolimus / ↓ Tacrolimus immunosuppressant effects

Theophylline / ↓ Theophylline effects R/T ↑ liver breakdown

Thyroid hormones / TSH levels may ↑ → hypothyroidism

Tocainide / ↓ Tocainide effects R/T ↑ liver breakdown

Tricyclic antidepressants / ↓ TCA levels R/T ↑ liver breakdown

Trimethoprim/Sulfamethoxazole / ↓ AUC and serum levels of trimethoprim and sulfamethoxazole

Verapamil / ↓ Verapamil effects R/T ↑

R

---

liver breakdown
Zidovudine / ↓ Zidovudine effect R/T ↑ liver metabolism
Zolpidem / ↓ Zolpidem plasma levels and effect

HOW SUPPLIED
Capsules: 150 mg, 300 mg; *Powder for Injection:* 600 mg.

DOSAGE

- **CAPSULES; IV**
  Pulmonary tuberculosis.
  Adults: 10 mg/kg in a single daily dose, not to exceed 600 mg/day; **children over 5 years:** 10–20 mg/kg/day, not to exceed 600 mg/day.

  Meningococcal carriers.
  Adults: 600 mg q 12 hr for 2 days; **children, over 1 month:** 10–20 mg/kg q 12 hr for four doses, not to exceed 600 mg/day.

NURSING CONSIDERATIONS

℘ Do not confuse rifampin with rifabutin (also an antitubercular drug) or with rifaximin (drug for traveler's diarrhea).

ADMINISTRATION/STORAGE
1. Give capsules once daily 1 hr before or 2 hr after meals to ensure maximum absorption.
2. A PO suspension (10 mg/mL) may be prepared as follows: The contents of either four 300-mg rifampin capsules or eight 150-mg capsules are emptied into a 4-oz amber glass bottle. Add 20 mL of simple syrup; shake vigorously; then add 100 mL of simple syrup and shake again. The suspension is stable for 4 weeks when stored at room temperature or in the refrigerator.
3. Check to ensure there's a desiccant in the bottle containing capsules of rifampin because these are relatively moisture sensitive.
4. If administered concomitantly with PAS, give drugs 8–12 hr apart; the acid interferes with the absorption of rifampin.
5. When used for tuberculosis, continue therapy for 6–9 months.
IV 6. IV use is restricted for initial treatment and retreatment of tuberculosis when the drug cannot be taken PO.

7. Reconstitute the 600-mg vial using 10 mL of sterile water for injection; swirl gently to dissolve. The resultant solution contains 60 mg/mL rifampin; stable at room temperature for 24 hr.
8. Add the volume of reconstituted solution needed to 500 mL of D5W and infuse over 3 hr, or may be added to 100 mL D5W and infused over 30 min. Sterile saline may be used when dextrose is contraindicated; however, the stability of rifampin is slightly less.
9. Use diluted solution within 4 hr or drug may precipitate from solution.
10. Injectable solution appears dark reddish brown.

ASSESSMENT
1. Note reasons for therapy, type, onset, characteristics of S&S. List drugs prescribed to ensure none interact; note any previous therapy, outcome.
2. Monitor CBC, cultures, renal, LFTs; note any dysfunction.
3. Assess for GI disturbances or auditory nerve impairment.
4. Obtain baseline CXR; auscultate and describe lung sounds/characteristics of sputum. Note PPD skin test results.

CLIENT/FAMILY TEACHING
1. Take drug on an empty stomach 1 hr before or 2 hr after meals; report if GI upset occurs.
2. Must take daily for months to effectively treat tuberculosis. Do not stop or skip doses of medication or relapse may occur.
3. Avoid alcohol; increases risk of liver toxicity.
4. Headache, drowsiness, confusion, fever, muscle/joint aches may occur during the first few weeks of therapy; report if symptoms persist or increase in intensity.
5. Rifampin may impart a red-orange color to urine, feces, saliva, sputum, and tears; may *permanently* discolor contact lenses.
6. Practice alternative birth control since oral contraceptives are not effective; drug has teratogenic properties.

OUTCOMES/EVALUATE
- Adjunct in treating tuberculosis

- Prophylaxis of meningitis due to *H. influenzae* and gram-negative bacteremia in infants

Rifapentine
(rih-fah-**PEN**-teen)

CLASSIFICATION(S):
Antitubercular drug
PREGNANCY CATEGORY: C
Rx: Priftin.

USES
Pulmonary tuberculosis. Must be used with at least one other antituberculosis drug.

ACTION/KINETICS
Action
Similar activity to rifampin. Inhibits DNA–dependent RNA polymerase in susceptible strains of *Mycobacterium tuberculosis*, but not in mammalian cells. Is bactericidal against both intracellular and extracellular organisms.

Pharmacokinetics
Food increases amount absorbed. **Maximum levels:** 5–6 hr. **Steady state conditions:** 10 days after 600 mg/day. Metabolized to the active 25–desacetyl rifapentine. **t½:** 13.2 hr for parent drug, 13.4 hr for active metabolite. Excreted in the feces (70%) and the urine (17%). **Plasma protein binding:** Both the parent drug and active metabolite are significantly bound to plasma proteins.

CONTRAINDICATIONS
Hypersensitivity to other rifamycins (e.g., rifampin or rifabutin). Porphyria, lactation.

SPECIAL CONCERNS
Experience is limited in HIV-infected clients. Organisms resistant to other rifamycins are likely to be resistant to rifapentine. Use only if necessary and with caution in clients with abnormal liver tests or liver disease. Use caution in dose selection for elderly clients. Use during pregnancy only if the potential benefit justifies the potential risk to the fetus. Safety and efficacy have not been determined in children less than 12 years of age.

SIDE EFFECTS
Most Common
When combined with other antituberulosis drugs: Hyperuricemia, lymphopenia, proteinuria, hematuria, pyuria, urinary casts, pruritus, rash, anorexia, N&V, anemia, neutropenia, arthralgia, pain.
Side effects listed occurred in 1% or more of clients and were seen when rifapentine was used in combination with other antituberculosis drugs (e.g., isoniazid, pyrazinamide, ethambutol). **GI:** N&V, anorexia, dyspepsia, diarrhea, hemoptysis, pseudomembranous colitis, constipation, esophagitis, gastritis, hepatitis, *pancreatitis*. **CNS:** Headache, dizziness, aggressive reaction, fatigue. **GU:** Pyuria, proteinuria, hematuria, urinary casts. **Dermatologic:** Rash, acne, maculopapular rash, pruritus, skin discoloration, urticaria. **Hematologic:** Neutropenia, lymphopenia, anemia, leukopenia, thrombocytosis, hematoma, leukocytosis, neutrophilia, purpura, thrombocytopenia. **Musculoskeletal:** Arthrosis, gout, arthralgia. **Miscellaneous:** Hyperuricemia (probably due to pyrazinamide), hyperbilirubinemia, hypertension, pain, red coloration of body tissues and fluids, peripheral edema.

LABORATORY TEST CONSIDERATIONS
↑ ALT, AST, alkaline phosphatase, LDH. Hyperkalemia, hypovolemia. Inhibition of standard microbiological assays for serum folate and vitamin B_{12}.

DRUG INTERACTIONS
Cytochrome P450 / Rifapentine is an inducer of certain cytochromes P450 → reduced activity of a number of drugs (See *Rifampin*). Dosage adjustment may be required
Indinavir / Three fold ↑ in clearance of indinavir

HOW SUPPLIED
Tablets: 150 mg.

DOSAGE
- **TABLETS**
   Tuberculosis, intensive phase.
600 mg (four 150 mg tablets) twice weekly with an interval of 72 hr or more between doses; continue for 2 months.
   Tuberculosis, continuation phase.

R

Continue rifapentine therapy once weekly for 4 months in combination with isoniazid or another antituberculosis drug. If the client is still sputum-, smear-, or culture-positive, if resistant organisms are present, or if the client is HIV-positive, follow ATS/CDC treatment guidelines.

NURSING CONSIDERATIONS

ADMINISTRATION/STORAGE
1. Give rifapentine in combination as part of a regimen that includes other antituberculosis drugs, especially on days when rifapentine is not given.
2. For the elderly, start at the low end of the dosage range.
3. Store from 15–30°C (59–87°F) protected from heat and humidity.

ASSESSMENT
1. Note onset, duration, S&S of disease. List medical history, other attempts at treatment, outcome.
2. Obtain chemistries, CBC, and LFTs; assess sputum culture. Monitor LFTs every two to four weeks during therapy.
3. List other drugs prescribed to ensure none interact.
4. Give concomitant pyridoxine in the malnourished, those predisposed to neuropathy (e.g., alcoholics, diabetics), and in adolescents.

CLIENT/FAMILY TEACHING
1. Take exactly as directed. May take with food if stomach upset, nausea, or vomiting occurs.
2. Vitamin B$_6$ is prescribed for those malnourished or predisposed to neuropathy, and in adolescents.
3. May stain body fluids/tissues (tears, urine, saliva, sweat, skin, feces, tongue) a red-orange color.
4. Drug is administered less frequently and in conjunction with other antitubercular agents. During the two-month intensive phase, drug is taken every three days. Following this phase, rifapentine is given once a week for four months in combination with isoniazid or other agent for susceptible organisms called the continuation phase for TB. A more frequent dosing pattern is used in HIV infected clients. Adherence to prescribed regimen is of utmost importance.
5. Report any unusual tiredness/fatigue, SOB, N&V, fever, darkened urine, pain or swelling of the joints, or yellow discolorations of the skin and eyes. Avoid crowds and persons with infections.
6. Practice nonhormonal method of contraception. Keep all F/U visits.

OUTCOMES/EVALUATE
- Treatment of pulmonary TB
- Negative sputum cultures

Rifaximin
(rif-AX-i-min)

CLASSIFICATION(S):
Drug for traveler's diarrhea
PREGNANCY CATEGORY: C
Rx: Xifaxan.

USES
Treatment of traveler's diarrhea due to noninvasive strains of *Escherichia coli* in clients 12 years of age and older.

ACTION/KINETICS

Action
Rifaximin binds to the beta subunit of bacterial DNA-dependent RNA polymerase causing inhibition of bacterial RNA synthesis.

Pharmacokinetics
Less than 0.4% is absorbed; thus, it is not useful for treating systemic bacterial infections. Rifaximin induces CYP3A4. Excreted mainly in the feces predominantly as unchanged drug.

CONTRAINDICATIONS
Use in those with diarrhea complicated by fever, blood in the stool, or diarrhea caused by pathogens other than *E. coli.* Hypersensitivity to rifaximin, any of the rifamycin antimicrobial drugs, or any components of the product. Lactation.

SPECIAL CONCERNS
Use of rifaximin may promote development of superinfection. Safety and efficacy have not been determined in children less than 12 years of age.

R

SIDE EFFECTS
Most Common
Dizziness, headache, N&V, abdominal pain, flatulence, constipation, defecation urgency, rectal tenesmus, fever, rash.
GI: Flatulence, rectal tenesmus, abdominal pain, defecation urgency, N&V, constipation, abdominal distension, anorexia, blood in stool, diarrhea, dry lips, dry throat, fecal abnormality, gingival disorder, inguinal hernia, stomach discomfort, loss of taste, dysentery. **CNS:** Headache, abnormal dreams, dizziness, insomnia, migraine, syncope. **Respiratory:** Dyspnea, irritated nasal passages, nasopharyngitis, pharyngitis, pharyngolaryngeal pain, RTI, rhinitis, rhinorrhea, URTI, chest pain. **Dermatologic:** Clamminess, rash, sunburn, increased sweating. **Hematologic:** Lymphocytosis, monocytosis, neutropenia. **GU:** Blood in urine, choluria, dysuria, hematuria, polyuria, proteinuria, urinary frequency. **Musculoskeletal:** Arthralgia, muscle spasms, myalgia, neck pain. **Otic:** Ear pain, tinnitus. **Hypersensitivity:** Allergic dermatitis, angioneurotic edema, pruritus, rash, urticaria. **Body as a whole:** Fever, motion sickness, fatigue, hot flashes, malaise, pain, weakness, dehydration, weight loss.

LABORATORY TEST CONSIDERATIONS
↑ Aspartate aminotransferase.

OD OVERDOSE MANAGEMENT
Symptoms: Similar to side effects. *Treatment:* Discontinue the drug. Treat symptomatically and institute supportive care as needed.

HOW SUPPLIED
Tablets: 200 mg.

DOSAGE
- **TABLETS**
  Traveler's diarrhea.
Adults and children over 12 years: 200 mg 3 times per day for 3 days given with or without food.

NURSING CONSIDERATIONS
Ⓡ Do not confuse rifaximin with rifampin (an antituberculosis drug).
ASSESSMENT
1. Note reasons for therapy, onset/characteristics of S&S, culture results.

2. Attempt to identify source of infection; note all travel areas.
CLIENT/FAMILY TEACHING
1. Drug may be taken with or without food.
2. Stop drug and report if blood noted in stools, fever develops, or if diarrhea worsens or persists for more than 24 to 48 hr.
OUTCOMES/EVALUATE
Relief of *E. coli* traveler's diarrhea

Riluzole
(**RIL**-you-zohl)

CLASSIFICATION(S):
Drug for amyotropic lateral sclerosis
PREGNANCY CATEGORY: C
Rx: Rilutek.

USES
Amyotropic lateral sclerosis to extend both survival and time to tracheostomy.
ACTION/KINETICS
Action
Mechanism not known. Possible effects include (a) inhibition of glutamate release, (b) inactivation of voltage-dependent sodium channels, and (c) interference with intracellular events that follow transmitter binding at excitatory amino acid receptors.
Pharmacokinetics
Well absorbed following PO use; high-fat meals decrease absorption. $t\frac{1}{2}$, **elimination, after repeated doses:** 12 hr. Extensively metabolized, mainly in the liver, and excreted in the urine. **Plasma protein binding:** About 96%.
CONTRAINDICATIONS
Lactation.
SPECIAL CONCERNS
Use with caution in hepatic and renal impairment due to decreased excretion and higher plasma levels. Use with caution in the elderly, as age-related changes in renal and hepatic function may cause a decreased clearance. Clearance of riluzole in Japanese clients is 50% lower compared with Caucasians; clearance may also be lower in women.

Safety and efficacy have not been determined in children.

SIDE EFFECTS

Most Common

Hypertension, tachycardia, hypertonia, depression, dizziness, dry mouth, insomnia, vertigo, circumoral paresthesia, pruritus, eczema, N&V, dyspepsia, anorexia, diarrhea, flatulence, UTI, weight loss, peripheral edema, decreased lung function, rhinitis, increased cough, asthenia, headache, abdominal pain, arthralgia, back pain.

Side effects listed occurred at a frequency of 0.1% or more. **GI:** N&V, diarrhea, anorexia, abdominal pain, dyspepsia, flatulence, dry mouth, stomatitis, tooth disorder, oral moniliasis, dysphagia, constipation, increased appetite, intestinal obstruction, fecal impaction, *GI hemorrhage*, GI ulceration, gastritis, fecal incontinence, jaundice, hepatitis, glossitis, *gum hemorrhage, pancreatitis*, tenesmus, esophageal stenosis. **Body as a whole:** Asthenia, malaise, weight loss/gain, peripheral edema, flu syndrome, abscess, *sepsis*, photosensitivity reaction, cellulitis, facial edema, hernia, peritonitis, reaction at injection site, chills, *attempted suicide*, enlarged abdomen, neoplasm. **CNS:** Dizziness (more common in women), vertigo, somnolence, circumoral paresthesia, headache, aggravation reaction, hypertonia, depression, insomnia, agitation, tremor, hallucination, personality disorders, abnormal thinking, coma, paranoid reaction, manic reaction, ataxia, extrapyramidal syndrome, hypokinesis, emotional lability, delusions, apathy, hypesthesia, incoordination, confusion, *convulsion*, amnesia, increased libido, stupor, subdural hematoma, abnormal gait, delirium, depersonalization, facial paralysis, hemiplegia, decreased libido, hostility. **CV:** Hypertension, tachycardia, phlebitis, palpitation, postural hypotension, *heart arrest, heart failure*, syncope, hypotension, migraine, PVD, angina pectoris, *MI*, ventricular extrasystoles, *cerebral hemorrhage*, atrial fibrillation, BBB, CHF, pericarditis, lower extremity embolus, *myocardial ischemia, shock*. **Hematologic:** Neutropenia, anemia, leukocytosis, leukopenia, ecchymosis. **Respiratory:** Decreased lung function, pneumonia, rhinitis, increased cough, sinusitis, apnea, bronchitis, dyspnea, respiratory disorder, increased sputum, hiccup, pleural disorder, asthma, epistaxis, hemoptysis, yawn, hyperventilation, lung edema, hypoventilation, *lung carcinoma*, hypoxia, laryngitis, pleural effusion, pneumothorax, respiratory moniliasis, stridor. **Musculoskeletal:** Arthralgia, back pain, leg cramps, dysarthria, myoclonus, arthrosis, myasthenia, *bone neoplasm*. **GU:** Urinary retention/urgency/incontinence, urine abnormality, kidney calculus, hematuria, impotence, *prostate carcinoma*, kidney pain, menorrhagia, priapism. **Dermatologic:** Pruritus, eczema, alopecia, exfoliative dermatitis, skin ulceration, urticaria, psoriasis, seborrhea, skin disorder, fungal dermatitis. **Metabolic:** Gout, respiratory acidosis, edema, thirst, hypokalemia, hyponatremia. **Ophthalmic:** Amblyopia, ophthalmitis. **Miscellaneous:** Accidental or intentional injury, *death*, diabetes mellitus, thyroid neoplasia.

LABORATORY TEST CONSIDERATIONS

↑ GGT, alkaline phosphatase, gamma globulins. Abnormal LFTs, positive direct Coombs' test.

DRUG INTERACTIONS

Amitriptyline / ↓ Elimination of riluzole → higher plasma levels
Caffeine / ↓ Elimination of riluzole → higher plasma levels
Charcoal-broiled foods / ↑ Elimination of riluzole → lower plasma levels
Omeprazole / ↑ Elimination of riluzole → lower plasma levels
Quinolones / ↓ Elimination of riluzole → higher plasma levels
Rifampin / ↑ Elimination of riluzole → lower plasma levels
Smoking (cigarettes) / ↑ Elimination of riluzole → lower plasma levels
Theophyllines / ↓ Elimination of riluzole → higher plasma levels

HOW SUPPLIED

Tablets: 50 mg.

DOSAGE

• **TABLETS**

  Treatment of ALS.

---

50 mg q 12 hr. Higher daily doses will not increase the beneficial effect but will increase the incidence of side effects.

NURSING CONSIDERATIONS
ADMINISTRATION/STORAGE
Protect from bright light.

ASSESSMENT
1. Note symptom onset, characteristics, ethnic background, familial associations. Note clinical presentation and respiratory assessment.
2. Assess renal, LFTs. Elevations of several liver functions, especially bilirubin, should preclude drug use.
3. Monitor LFTs. measure SGPT levels q month for first 3 months of therapy, q 3 months for the remainder of the first year, and then periodically.
4. Review potential side effects R/T therapy with client.

CLIENT/FAMILY TEACHING
1. Take 1 hr before or 2 hr after meals to maintain drug bioavailability.
2. Take at the same time each day. Do not double up if dose is missed or forgotten, take the next tablet as originally planned.
3. Report any febrile illnesses. Severe dry mouth symptoms may require use of Salagen.
4. Drug may cause dizziness, drowsiness, or vertigo. Do not perform activities that require mental alertness until drug effects realized.
5. Do not smoke. Avoid alcohol; may potentiate liver toxicity.
6. Keep all F/U appointments and report any adverse effects.

OUTCOMES/EVALUATE
↑ Survival/time to tracheostomy with ALS

Rimantadine hydrochloride ⓒ
(rih-**MAN**-tih-deen)

CLASSIFICATION(S):
Antiviral
PREGNANCY CATEGORY: C
Rx: Flumadine.

SEE ALSO *ANTIVIRAL DRUGS* AND *AMANTADINE HYDROCHLORIDE.*

USES
Adults: Prophylaxis and treatment against strains of influenza A virus. **Children:** Prophylaxis against influenza A virus. *NOTE:* Recommendations for prophylaxis: High risk clients vaccinated after flu outbreak has begun. Consider prophylaxis until immunity from the flu vaccine has developed (up to 2 weeks).

Caretakers of those at high risk: Consider prophylaxis for unvaccinated caretakers of high-risk clients durng peak flu activity.

Clients with immune deficiency: Consider prophylaxis for high-risk clients who are expected to have inadequate antibody response to flu vaccine (e.g., HIV).

Consider prophylaxis in high-risk clients who should not be vaccinated. Prophylaxis may be offered to those who desire to avoid the flu.

ACTION/KINETICS
Action
May act early in the viral replication cycle, possibly by inhibiting the uncoating of the virus. A virus protein specified by the virion M_2 gene may play an important role in the inhibition of the influenza A virus by rimantadine. Has little or no activity against influenza B virus.

Pharmacokinetics
Syrup and tablet equally absorbed after PO use. Plasma trough levels following 100 mg twice a day for 10 days range from 118 to 468 ng/mL; however, levels are higher in clients over the age of 70 years. **Time to peak levels:** About 6 hr. Metabolized in the liver, and both unchanged drug (25%) and metabolites excreted through the urine. **Plasma protein binding:** About 40% bound to plasma proteins.

CONTRAINDICATIONS
Hypersensitivity to amantadine, rimantadine, or other drugs in the adamantane class. Lactation.

SPECIAL CONCERNS
Use with caution in clients with renal or hepatic insufficiency. An increased incidence of seizures is possible in clients with a history of epilepsy who have re-

R

ceived amantadine. Influenza A virus strains resistant to rimantadine can emerge during treatment and be transmitted, causing symptoms of influenza. Safety and efficacy of rimantadine in the treatment of symptomatic influenza infections in children have not been established. Safety and efficacy for prophylaxis of infections have not been determined in children less than 1 year of age. The incidence of side effects in geriatric clients is higher than in other clients.

SIDE EFFECTS

Most Common

Insomnia, nervousness, impaired concentration, dizziness, asthenia, nervousness, N&V, anorexia, dry mouth, abdominal pain.

GI: N&V, anorexia, dry mouth, abdominal pain, diarrhea, dyspepsia, constipation, dysphagia, stomatitis. **CNS:** Insomnia, dizziness, headache, nervousness, fatigue, asthenia, impaired concentration, ataxia, somnolence, agitation, depression, gait abnormality, euphoria, hyperkinesia, tremor, hallucinations, confusion, **convulsions**, agitation, diaphoresis, hypesthesia. **Respiratory:** Dyspnea, **bronchospasm**, cough. **CV:** Pallor, palpitation, hypertension, **cerebrovascular disorder, cardiac failure**, pedal edema, heart block, tachycardia, syncope. **Miscellaneous:** Tinnitus, taste loss or change, parosmia, eye pain, rash, nonpuerperal lactation, increased lacrimation, increased frequency of micturition, fever, rigors. *NOTE:* Geriatric clients experience more GI and CNS side effects, including dizziness, anxiety, headache, asthenia, fatigue, N&V, and abdominal pain.

OD OVERDOSE MANAGEMENT

Symptoms: Extensions of side effects including the possibility of agitation, hallucinations, **cardiac arrhythmias, and death.** *Treatment:* Supportive therapy. IV physostigmine at doses of 1–2 mg IV in adults and 0.5 mg in children, not to exceed 2 mg/hr, has been reported to be beneficial in treating overdose for amantadine (a related drug).

DRUG INTERACTIONS

Acetaminophen / ↓ Rimantadine peak concentration and AUC
Aspirin / ↓ Rimantadine peak plasma levels and AUC
Cimetidine / ↓ Rimantadine clearance of rimantadine

HOW SUPPLIED

Syrup: 50 mg/5 mL; *Tablets:* 100 mg.

DOSAGE

• SYRUP; TABLETS

Prophylaxis of influenza A virus.

Adults and children over 10 years of age: 100 mg twice a day. In clients with severe hepatic dysfunction (C_{CR} <10 mL/min) and in elderly nursing home clients, reduce the dose to 100 mg/day.
Children, less than 10 years of age: 5 mg/kg once daily, not to exceed a total dose of 150 mg/day.

Treatment of influenza A virus.

Adults: 100 mg twice a day. In clients with severe hepatic dysfunction and in elderly nursing home clients, reduce the dose to 100 mg/day.

NURSING CONSIDERATIONS

Ⓒ Do not confuse rimantadine with ranitidine (a H-2 receptor blocker), amantadine (an antiviral drug), or Flumadine with Flutamide (an antineoplastic).

ADMINISTRATION/STORAGE

1. For treatment of influenza A virus infections, initiate therapy as soon as possible, preferably within 48 hr after onset of S&S. Continue treatment for approximately 7 days from the initial onset of symptoms.
2. Store syrup and tablets between 15–30°C (59–86°F).

ASSESSMENT

1. Note reasons for therapy, onset, duration of symptoms/exposure. Determine when immunized/exposed.
2. List other drugs prescribed to ensure none interact unfavorably. With epilepsy; assess for loss of seizure control.
3. Assess renal, LFTs to note any dysfunction; reduce dosage with severe renal/hepatic dysfunction and with elderly nursing home clients.

CLIENT/FAMILY TEACHING

1. Take only as directed; do not share medications. Taking several hours be-

fore bedtime may help minimize insomnia.

2. Initiate within 48 hr of when symptoms appear and continue for 7 days after S&S noted. Still able to spread disease so use care.

3. Drug may cause dizziness; avoid activities that require mental alertness until drug effects realized. Report any adverse side effects or psychosis.

4. Early annual vaccination is the method of choice for influenza prophylaxis. The 2- to 4-week time frame required to develop an antibody response can be managed with rimantadine.

OUTCOMES/EVALUATE

Prevention/ ↓ severity of influenza A virus

Risedronate sodium ©

(rih-**SEH**-droh-nayt)

CLASSIFICATION(S):

Bone growth regulator, bisphosphonate

PREGNANCY CATEGORY: C

Rx: Actonel.

USES

(1) Treatment of Paget's disease in men and women who (a) have a serum alkaline phosphatase level at least two times the ULN, (b) are symptomatic, or (c) are at risk for future complications from the disease. (2) Prophylaxis and treatment of postmenopausal osteoporosis. The drug increases bone mineral density and reduces the incidence of vertebral fractures and a composite end point of nonvertebral osteoporosis-related fractures. (3) Prophylaxis and treatment of glucocorticoid-induced osteoporosis in men and women taking the daily dosage equivalent of 7.5 mg or more of prednisone for chronic diseases. Adequate amounts of calcium and vitamin D must be given as well. (4) To increase bone mass in men with osteoporosis. *Investigational:* Reduce the chance of spine fractures in clients on long-term steroid therapy.

ACTION/KINETICS

Action

Binds to bone hydroxyapatite and inhibits osteoclast activity, thereby preventing bone resorption. Appears to reduce fracture risk and reverse the progression of osteoporosis. Does not inhibit bone mineralization.

Pharmacokinetics

Rapidly absorbed; food decreases absorption. $t\frac{1}{2}$, **initial:** 1.5 hr; **terminal:** 220 hr. Excreted unchanged in the urine.

CONTRAINDICATIONS

Use in those with C_{CR} less than 30 mL/min. Hypocalcemia. Lactation.

SPECIAL CONCERNS

May cause upper GI disorders, including dysphagia, esophagitis, esophageal ulcer, or gastric ulcer. Use with caution in those with a history of upper GI disorders. Safety and efficacy have not been determined in children.

SIDE EFFECTS

Most Common

Infection, hypertension, chest pain, dizziness, headache, rash, abdominal pain, constipation, diarrhea, nausea, arthralgia, pharyngitis, edema, pain

GI: Diarrhea, abdominal pain, nausea, constipation, belching, colitis. **CNS:** Headache, dizziness. **Body as a whole:** Flu syndrome, chest pain, pain, asthenia, infection, neoplasm. **Musculoskeletal:** Arthralgia, bone pain, leg cramps, myasthenia, osteonecrosis. **Respiratory:** Sinusitis, bronchitis. **Ophthalmic:** Amblyopia, dry eye. **Miscellaneous:** Peripheral edema, pharyngitis, skin rash, tinnitus, hypertension.

OD **OVERDOSE MANAGEMENT**

Symptoms: Hypocalcemia. *Treatment:* Gastric lavage to remove unabsorbed drug. Milk or antacids to bind risedronate. IV calcium.

DRUG INTERACTIONS

Antacids, calcium-containing / ↓ Absorption of risedronate

Bone imaging agents / Risedronate interferes with these agents

Calcium / ↓ Absorption of risedronate

NSAIDs / Possible additive GI side effects

HOW SUPPLIED
Tablets: 5 mg, 30 mg, 35 mg, 75 mg.

DOSAGE

• **TABLETS**
Paget's disease.

Adults: 30 mg once daily for 2 months. Retreatment may be considered following posttreatment observation for at least 2 months if relapse occurs or if treatment fails to normalize serum alkaline phosphatase. For retreatment, the dose and duration of therapy are the same as for initial treatment.

Prevention and treatment of postmenopausal osteoporosis.

5 mg once daily or one 35 mg tablet taken once weekly or 75 mg taken on 2 consecutive days for a total of 2 tablets per month.

Prevention and treatment of glucocorticoid-induced osteoporosis.

5 mg once daily.

Osteoporosis in men.

35 mg once per week.

NURSING CONSIDERATIONS
Do not confuse Actonel with Actos (oral hypoglycemic).

ADMINISTRATION/STORAGE
1. Before starting therapy, treat hypocalcemia, other disturbances of bone and mineral metabolism.
2. Dosage adjustment is not necessary in clients with a C_{CR} 30 mL/min or greater.
3. Store from 20–25°C (68–77°F).

ASSESSMENT
1. Note reasons for therapy, onset, characteristics of disease; list other agents trialed. Assess for GI disease/dysfunction.
2. Obtain chemistries, alkaline phosphatase, phosphorus, Ca, lipids, renal and LFT; assess for dysfunction, avoid if C_{CR} <30 mL/min.
3. Assess nutritional status, vitamin D, calcium intake. Assess bone density (BMD), for low bone mass, evidence of fracture on x-ray, history of osteoporotic fracture, height loss or kyphosis indicative of vertebral fracture.

CLIENT/FAMILY TEACHING
1. Take dose sitting or standing with a full glass of water at least 30 min before the first food or drink of the day. To facilitate delivery to the stomach and minimize esophageal irritation, take in an upright position with 6 to 8 oz of water. Avoid lying down for 30 min after taking drug. Mark calendar to ensure weekly dosing not missed.
2. If dietary intake inadequate, consume supplemental calcium and vitamin D. Antacids and calcium may interfere with drug; take them at different times during the day with food.
3. May experience nausea, diarrhea, bone pain, headache, and rash. Report so appropriate analgesics and skin care may be prescribed.
4. Regular weight bearing exercise and cessation of alcohol and tobacco is advised.
5. Report any swallowing difficulty, GI bleeding, throat/abdominal pain, muscle spasms, or dark-colored urine. Keep all F/U appointments to assess bone mineral density and drug response.

OUTCOMES/EVALUATE
• ↓ Bone resorption, ↓ pain, ↓ alkaline phosphatase levels, ↑ bone mass
• Inhibition of bone resorption/progression of osteoporosis

Risperidone
(ris-**PAIR**-ih-dohn)

CLASSIFICATION(S):
Antipsychotic
PREGNANCY CATEGORY: C
Rx: Risperdal, Risperdal Consta, Risperdal M-Tab.

USES
PO. (1) Monotherapy for short-term treatment of acute manic or mixed episodes associated with bipolar I disorder, as defined in DSM-IV. (2) In combination with lithium or valproate for the short-term treatment of acute manic or mixed episodes associated with bipolar I disorder, as defined in DSM-IV. (3) Irritability associated with autistic disorder in children and adolescents, including symptoms of aggression toward others,

deliberate self—injuriousness, temper tantrums, and quickly changing moods.

PO and IM. Treatment of schizophrenia. *NOTE:* Has not been shown to be safe or effective to treat dementia-related psychosis.

Investigational: Severe behavioral problems in children (with or without autism); improve severely disruptive behavior in children with subaverage intelligence; treat clients with OCD refractory to selective serotonin reuptake inhibitors; psychosis in clients with Parkinson's disease; treat tics in clients with Tourette syndrome.

ACTION/KINETICS

Action

Mechanism may be due to a combination of antagonism of dopamine (D_2) and serotonin (5-HT$_2$) receptors. Also has high affinity for the alpha$_1$-, alpha$_2$-, and histamine$_1$ receptors.

Pharmacokinetics

Metabolized significantly in the liver to the active metabolite 9-hydroxyrisperidone, which has equal receptor-binding activity as risperidone. Thus, the effect is likely due to both the parent compound and the metabolite. Food does not affect either the rate or extent of absorption. Bioavailability is 70%. The ability to convert risperidone to 9-hydroxyrisperidone is subject to genetic variation. A low percentage of Asians have the ability to metabolize the drug. **Peak plasma levels, risperidone:** 1 hr; **peak plasma levels, 9-hydroxyrisperidone:** 3 hr for extensive metabolizers and 17 hr for poor metabolizers. **t$_{1/2}$, risperidone and 9-methylrisperidone:** 3 and 20 hr, respectively, for extensive metabolizers and 20 and 30 hr, respectively, for poor metabolizers. Metabolized by CYP2D6 and by N-dealkylation. Excreted in the feces (about 66%) and urine (about 14%). Clearance is decreased in geriatric clients and in clients with hepatic and renal impairment. The orally disintegrating tablets are bioequivalent to the original-formulation tablets.

CONTRAINDICATIONS

Lactation.

SPECIAL CONCERNS

■ Elderly clients with dementia-related psychosis treated with atypical antipsychotic drugs are at an increased risk of death compared with placebo. Analyses of placebo-controlled trials (modal duration of 10 weeks) in these clients revealed a risk of death in the drug-treated clients between 1.6–1.7 times that seen in placebo-treated clients. Over the course of a typical 10-week controlled trial, the rate of death in drug-treated clients was about 4.5%, compared with a rate of about 2.6% in the placebo group. Although the causes of death were varied, most of the deaths appeared to be either cardiovascular (e.g., heart failure, sudden death) or infectious (e.g., pneumonia) in nature. Risperidone is not approved for the treatment of clients with dementia-related psychosis.■ Use with caution in clients with known CV disease (including history of MI or ischemia, heart failure, conduction abnormalities), cerebrovascular disease, and conditions that predispose the client to hypotension (e.g., dehydration, hypovolemia, use of antihypertensive drugs). Use with caution in clients who will be exposed to extreme heat or when taken with other CNS drugs or alcohol. Greater risk of orthostatic hypotension, aspiration pneumonia, and toxic effects in geriatric clients with impaired renal function. The effectiveness of risperidone for more than 6–8 weeks has not been studied. Safety and effectiveness have not been established for children.

SIDE EFFECTS

Most Common

Agitation, anxiety, extrapyramidal symptoms, headache, insomnia, constipation, dyspepsia, weight gain, rhinitis. **Neuroleptic malignant syndrome.** Hyperpyrexia, muscle rigidity, altered mental status, autonomic instability (i.e., irregular pulse or BP, tachycardia, diaphoresis, cardiac dysrhythmia), elevated CPK, rhabdomyolysis, *acute respiratory failure, death.* **CNS:** Tardive dyskinesia (especially in geriatric clients), somnolence, insomnia, agitation, anxiety, aggressive reaction, extra-

R

---

pyramidal symptoms, headache, dizziness, ↑ dream activity, ↓ sexual desire, nervousness, impaired concentration, depression, apathy, catatonia, euphoria, ↑ libido, amnesia, ↑ duration of sleep, dysarthria, vertigo, stupor, paresthesia, confusion. **GI:** Constipation, nausea, dyspepsia, vomiting, abdominal pain, ↑ or ↓ salivation, toothache, anorexia, flatulence, diarrhea, ↑ appetite, stomatitis, melena, dysphagia, hemorrhoids, gastritis. **CV:** Prolongation of the QT interval that might lead to *torsades de pointes and sudden cardiac death*. Orthostatic hypotension, tachycardia, palpitation, hyper-/hypotension, *AV block, MI, stroke or ischemic attacks in elderly clients with dementia*. **Respiratory:** Rhinitis, coughing, URTI, sinusitis, pharyngitis, dyspnea. **Body as a whole:** Arthralgia, back/chest pain, fever, fatigue, rigors, malaise, edema, flu-like symptoms, ↑ or ↓ in weight. **Hematologic:** Purpura, anemia, hypochromic anemia. **GU:** Polyuria, polydipsia, urinary incontinence, hematuria, dysuria, menorrhagia, orgasmic dysfunction, dry vagina, erectile dysfunction, nonpuerperal lactation, amenorrhea, female breast pain, leukorrhea, mastitis, dysmenorrhea, female perineal pain, intermenstrual bleeding, *vaginal hemorrhage*, failure to ejaculate. **Dermatologic:** Rash, dry skin, seborrhea, ↑ pigmentation, ↑ or ↓ sweating, acne, alopecia, hyperkeratosis, pruritus, skin exfoliation. **Ophthalmic:** Abnormal vision/accommodation, xerophthalmia. **Miscellaneous:** ↑ Prolactin, photosensitivity, increased risk of diabetes mellitus, thirst, myalgia, epistaxis.

LABORATORY TEST CONSIDERATIONS
↑ CPK, serum prolactin, AST, ALT. Hyponatremia.

OD OVERDOSE MANAGEMENT
Symptoms: Exaggeration of known effects, especially drowsiness, sedation, tachycardia, hypotension, and extrapyramidal symptoms.
Treatment: Establish and secure airway, and ensure adequate oxygenation and ventilation. Follow gastric lavage with activated charcoal and a laxative. Moni-

tor CV system, including continuous ECG readings. Provide general supportive measures. Treat hypotension and circulatory collapse with IV fluids or sympathomimetic drugs; however, do not use epinephrine and dopamine, as beta stimulation may worsen hypotension due to risperidone-induced alpha blockade. Anticholinergic drugs can be given for severe extrapyramidal symptoms.

DRUG INTERACTIONS
Carbamazepine / ↑ Risperidone clearance R/T ↑ metabolism; titrate dosage accordingly
Clozapine / ↓ Risperidone clearance following chronic use of clozapine
Fluoxetine / ↑ Risperidone levels; titrate dose of risperidone accordingly
Levodopa / Risperidone antagonizes the effects of levodopa and dopamine agonists
Maprotiline / ↑ Maprotiline levels R/T ↓ metabolism
Paroxetine / Significant ↑ in risperidone levels R/T ↓ liver metabolism; titrate dose of risperidone accordingly
Phenobarbital / ↑ Risperidone clearance R/T ↑ metabolism; titrate dosage accordingly
Phenytoin / ↑ Risperidone clearance R/T ↑ metabolism; titrate dosage accordingly
Rifampin / ↑ Risperidone clearance R/T ↑ metabolism; titrate dosage accordingly
Thioridazine / ↑ Risperidone levels and ↓ 9-hydroxyrisperidone levels R/T inhibition of CYP2D6

HOW SUPPLIED
Oral Solution: 1 mg/mL; *Powder for Solution (Injection), Extended—Release:* 12.5 mg, 25 mg, 37.5 mg, 50 mg; *Tablets:* 0.25 mg, 0.5 mg, 1 mg, 2 mg, 3 mg, 4 mg; *Tablets, Oral Disintegrating:* 0.5 mg, 1 mg, 2 mg, 3 mg, 4 mg.

DOSAGE
• **ORAL SOLUTION; TABLETS; TABLETS, ORAL DISINTEGRATING**
Schizophrenia.
Adults, initial: 1 mg twice a day. Once daily dosing can also be used. Can be increased by 1 mg twice a day on the second and third days, as tolerated, to

reach a dose of 3 mg twice a day by the third day. Further increases in dose should occur at intervals of about 1 week. Is safe and effective up to 8 mg once daily. **Maximal effect:** 4–8 mg/day. Doses greater than 6 mg/day were not shown to be more effective and were associated with greater incidence of side effects. Safety of doses greater than 16 mg/day have not been studied. **Maintenance:** Use lowest dose that will maintain remission; doses from 2–8 mg/day have been shown to be effective for longer-term therapy.

Bipolar mania.
Initial: 2–3 mg/day. If needed, adjust dose at intervals of not less than 24 hr in increments/decrements of 1 mg/day. There are no data to support use for more than 3 weeks with a dose range from 1–6 mg/day.

Irritability associated with autistic disorder.
Individualize dose according to response and client tolerability. **Initial:** 0.25 mg/day for those weighing less than 20 kg and 0.5 mg/day for those at least 20 kg. After a minimum of 4 days, the dose may be increased to the recommended dose of 0.5 mg/day for those weighing less than 20 kg and 1 mg/day for those at least 20 kg. Maintain these doses for a minimum of 14 days. In those not achieving a sufficient response, the dose may be increased at intervals of at least 2 weeks in increments of 0.25 mg/day for those weighing less than 20 kg or 0.5 mg/day for those at least 20 kg. Use caution for smaller children who weigh less than 15 kg. The total daily dose can be given once daily or half the total daily dose can be given twice daily. For those experiencing somnolence, the dose can be given once daily at bedtime. **Maintenance:** Once a satisfactory response has been obtained, consider lowering the dose gradually to acheive the optimal balance of safety and efficacy. *NOTE:* The safety and efficacy in children younger than 5 years of age with autistic disorder have not been determined.
• **IM**

Schizophrenia.
25 mg q 2 weeks by deep IM injection. Some not responding to 25 mg may benefit from doses of 37.5 mg or 50 mg. Do not exceed a dose of 50 mg q 2 weeks. Do not make upward dosage adjustments more frequently than q 4 weeks. Periodically reassess to determined need for continued therapy. For the elderly, the recommended dosage is 25 mg IM q 2 weeks. Treat clients with hepatic or renal impairment with titrated doses of PO risperidone prior to beginning risperidone injections. **Initial PO dose:** 0.5 mg twice daily during the first week; can be increased to 1 mg twice daily or 2 mg once daily during the second week. If a dose of PO risperidone, 2 mg, is well tolerated, an injection of risperidone, 25 mg, can be given q 2 weeks. PO supplementation should be continued for 3 weeks after the first injection until the main release of risperidone from the injection site has begun.

NURSING CONSIDERATIONS
ⓒ Do not confuse Risperdal with Restoril (a hypnotic).

ADMINISTRATION/STORAGE
1. The initial dose is 0.5 mg twice a day for clients who are elderly or debilitated, those with severe renal or hepatic impairment, and those predisposed to hypotension or in whom hypotension would pose a risk. Dosage increases in these clients should be in increments of 0.5 mg twice a day. Dosage increases above 1.5 mg twice a day should occur at intervals of about 1 week. The PO solution may ease administration to geriatric clients and those in an acute-care setting.
2. When restarting clients who have had an interval of risperidone, follow the initial 3-day dose titration schedule.
3. If switching from other antipsychotic drugs to risperidone, stop other antipsychotic drug when starting risperidone therapy. When switching from a depot antipsychotic injection, initiate risperidone in place of the next scheduled injection.

4. For those who have never taken PO risperidone, establish tolerability with PO risperidone before beginning treatment with the injectable form.

5. Coadministration of carbamazepine and other enzyme inducers (e.g., phenobarbital, phenytoin, rifampin) with risperidone will likely cause decreases in plasma levels of both risperidone and its active metabolite; this could result in decreased efficacy of risperidone treatment. Titrate the dose of risperidone accordingly in this situation.

6. Give PO risperidone or another antipsychotic drug with the first risperidone injection and continue for 3 weeks (then discontinue) to ensure adequate therapeutic plasma levels are maintained prior to the main release phase of risperidone from the injection site.

7. For IM use, suspend only in the diluent provided in the dose pack; doses must be given using the needle supplied in each dose pack. Do not substitute any components of the dose pack. Remove the dose pack from the refrigerator and allow to come to room temperature prior to reconstitution.

8. After reconstitution, it is recommended to use immediately. However, the suspension must be used within 6 hr. Resuspension will be necessary prior to administration as settling will occur over time. Keeping the vial upright, shake vigorously back and forth for as long as it takes to resuspend the microspheres.

9. IM injections should be given by a healthcare provider using the safety needle provided. Alternate injections between the 2 buttocks. Do not give IV. Do not combine 2 different dosage strengths of risperidone in a single administration.

10. Store tablets, orally disintegrating tablets, and solution between 15–25°C (59–77°F) away from children. Protect from light and freezing.

11. Refrigerate entire injection dose pack from 2–8°C (36–46°F) and protect from light. If refrigeration is not available, store at temperatures not exceeding 25°C (77°F) for no more than 7 days prior to use. Once in suspension, do not expose to temperatures above 25°C (77°F); use within 6 hr.

ASSESSMENT

1. List reasons for therapy, onset, duration, characteristics of S&S, presenting behavioral manifestations, mental status. Note history of drug dependency.

2. Perform appropriate baseline assessments. Electrolyte imbalance, bradycardia, and concomitant administration with drugs that prolong the QT interval may increase risk of torsades de pointes.

3. Reduce dose with severe liver, cardiac, or renal dysfunction; monitor closely.

4. Observe for altered mental status, muscle rigidity, dyskinetic movements, or overt changes in VS. Monitor for S&S of diabetes.

5. The antiemetic effect of risperidone may mask S&S of overdose with certain drugs or conditions such as intestinal obstruction, Reye's syndrome, brain tumor.

6. With Phenylketonuria-Risperidone Orally Disintegrating Tablets contains phenylalanine.

CLIENT/FAMILY TEACHING

1. May mix oral solution with water, coffee, orange juice, or lowfat milk; do not mix with cola or tea—drug is incompatible. Take only as directed; do not share medications or stop abruptly.

2. Do not open blister containing orally disintegrating tablets until ready to administer. For single tablet removal, separate 1 of the 4 blister units by tearing apart at the perforation. Bend the corner where indicated and peel back foil to expose the tablet. Do not push tablet through the foil as this could damage the tablet. Using dry hands, remove tablet from blister unit and immediately place entire tablet on the tongue. Consume tablet immediately; cannot be stored once removed from the blister unit. Tablets disintegrate in the mouth within seconds and can be subsequently swallowed with or without liquid. Do not split or chew tablet.

3. Drug may cause drowsiness and impair judgment, motor skills, and thinking and cause blurred vision; determine

drug effects before engaging in activities that require mental alertness. Rise slowly from a lying to a sitting position, dangle legs before standing; may cause drop in BP.

4. Wear protective clothing, sunscreen, hat, and sunglasses when sun exposure is necessary; may cause a photosensitivity reaction. Avoid prolonged or excessive exposure to direct or artificial sunlight. May alter temperature regulation; avoid exposure to extreme heat or overheating in hot weather; heatstroke may occur

5. Report abnormal bruising/bleeding, yellow skin discoloration, or adverse effects. Avoid alcohol, CNS depressants or OTC agents.

6. If any muscle problems with your arms; legs; or your tongue, face, mouth, or jaw (eg, tongue sticking out, puffing of cheeks, mouth puckering, chewing movements) occurs report may become irreversible.

7. Practice reliable birth control; report if pregnancy suspected/desired.

8. Risperidone elevates serum prolactin levels evidenced by unusual breast milk production, missed menstrual period, decreased sexual ability, decreased ability to produce sperm, or enlarged breasts. The potential relationships of prolactin and human breast cancer development are being explored; report evidence/history of breast cancer.

9. Fever, stiff muscles, confusion, abnormal thinking, fast or irregular heartbeat, and sweating may be S&S of neuroleptic malignant syndrome; seek help immediately.

10. Report any suicide ideations or bizarre behavior immediately. Due to the possibility of suicide attempts with schizophrenia, close supervision of high-risk clients is necessary and prescriptions will be written for the smallest quantity of tablets. Close F/U is required.

OUTCOMES/EVALUATE
- Improved behavior patterns with ↓ agitation, ↓ hyperactivity, and reality orientation
- Improved concentration and self-control

- ↓ Irritability, mood swings, aggressiveness, temper tantrums associated with autistic disorder

Ritonavir ■
(rih-**TOH**-nah-veer)

CLASSIFICATION(S):
Antiviral, protease inhibitor
PREGNANCY CATEGORY: B
Rx: Norvir.
✤**Rx:** Norvir Sec.

SEE ALSO *ANTIVIRAL DRUGS.*

USES
In combination with other antiretroviral drugs to treat HIV infection. Use of ritonavir may result in a reduction in both mortality and AIDS-defining clinical events. Clinical benefit has not been determined for periods longer than 6 months.

ACTION/KINETICS
Action
A peptidomimetic inhibitor of both the HIV-1 and HIV-2 proteases. Inhibition of HIV protease results in the enzyme incapable of processing the 'gag-pool' polyprotein precursor that leads to production of noninfectious immature HIV particles.

Pharmacokinetics
Peak concentrations after 600 mg of the solution: 2 hr after fasting and 4 hr after nonfasting. $t\frac{1}{2}$: 3–5 hr. Metabolized by both CYP3A and CYP2D6. Metabolites and unchanged drug are excreted through both the feces and urine. The pharmacokinetic profile has not been determined in children less than 2 years of age. **Plasma protein binding:** 98–99% bound to plasma proteins.

CONTRAINDICATIONS
Use of ritonavir concurrently with any of the following drugs because competition for the drug-metabolizing system CYP3A by ritonavir may result in inhibition of metabolism, creating the potential for serious or life-threatening side effects (e.g., cardiac arrhythmias, prolonged or increased sedation, respira-

tory depression): Alfuzosin hydrochloride, amiodarone, bepridil, dihydroergotamine, ergonovine, ergotamine, flecainide, methylergonovine, midazolam, pimozide, propafenone, quinidine, triazolam. Lactation.

SPECIAL CONCERNS

■ Coadministration of ritonavir with certain nonsedating antihistamines, sedative hypnotics, antiarrhythmics, or ergot alkaloid products may result in potentially serious or life-threatening adverse effects due to possible effects of ritonavir on the hepatic metabolism of certain drugs. The following drugs are contraindicated with ritonavir: Alfuzosin, amiodarone, astemizole, bepridil, cisapride, dihydroergotamine, ergonovine, ergotamine, flecainide, methylergonovine, midazolam, pimozide, propafenone, quinidine, terfenadine, triazolam, voriconazole.■ Not considered a cure for HIV infection; clients may continue to manifest illnesses associated with advanced HIV infection, including opportunistic infections. Also, therapy with ritonavir has not been shown to decrease the risk of transmitting HIV to others through sexual contact or blood contamination. Use with caution in those with pre-existing liver diseases, liver enzyme abnormalities, hepatitis, and impaired hepatic function. Hemophiliacs treated with protease inhibitors may manifest spontaneous bleeding episodes. Varying degrees of cross resistance have been noted among protease inhibitors. For the elderly, start at the low end of the dosing range. Safety and efficacy have not been determined in children less than 2 years of age.

SIDE EFFECTS

Most Common

N&V, diarrhea, anorexia, abdominal pain, taste perversion, circumoral/peripheral paresthesias, dizziness, headache, insomnia, somnolence, sweating, malaise, asthenia.

Side effects listed are those with a frequency of 2% or greater or which are serious and must be monitored. **GI:** N&V, diarrhea, taste perversion, anorexia, flatulence, constipation, abdominal pain, dyspepsia, local throat irritation, fecal incontinence, *pancreatitis*, impaired hepatic function. **CNS:** Anxiety, circumoral paresthesia, confusion, depression, dizziness, headache, insomnia, paresthesia, peripheral paresthesia, somnolence, abnormal thinking. **CV:** Syncope, vasodilation. Increased bleeding, including spontaneous skin hematomas and hemarthrosis in those with hemophilia type A and B. **Hypersensitivity:** Urticaria, mild skin eruptions, *bronchospasms*, angioedema. Rarely, *anaphylaxis, Stevens-Johnson syndrome*. **Body as a whole:** Asthenia, headache, malaise, fever, weight loss, redistribution/accumulation of body fat (e.g., central obesity, dorsocervical fat enlargement, peripheral wasting, breast enlargement, 'cushingoid' appearance). **Musculoskeletal:** Arthralgia, myalgia. **Dermatologic:** Sweating, rash. **Respiratory:** Pharyngitis. **Metabolic:** New onset or exacerbation of existing diabetes mellitus, hyperglycemia. **Miscellaneous:** Hyperlipidemia, pharyngitis, nocturia, unspecified pain, immune reconstitution syndrome.

LABORATORY TEST CONSIDERATIONS

↑ Triglycerides, cholesterol, AST, ALT, GGT, CPK, uric acid. ↓ Hematocrit, hemoglobin, neutrophils, RBCs, WBCs.

OD **OVERDOSE MANAGEMENT**
Symptoms: Extension of side effects. *Treatment:* General supportive measures, including monitoring of VS and observing the clinical status. Elimination of unabsorbed drug may be assisted by emesis or gastric lavage, with attention given to maintaining a patent airway. Activated charcoal may also help in removing any unabsorbed drug. Dialysis is not likely to be of benefit in removing the drug from the body.

DRUG INTERACTIONS

(1) Ritonavir is expected to produce large *increases* in the plasma levels of a number of drugs, including amiodarone, amlodipine, bupropion, carbamazepine, clozapine, cyclosporine, dexamethasone, diltiazem, dronabinol, ethosuximide, methamphetamine, metoprolol, nefazodone, nifedipine, perphenazine, pimozide, piroxicam, prednisone, quinine, risperidone, sirolimus,

R

tacrolimus, thioridazine, timolol, tricyclic antidepressants, trimethoprim, verapamil, and zolpidem. This may lead to an increased risk of arrhythmias, hematologic complications, seizures, or other serious adverse effects. (2) Ritonavir may produce a *decrease* in the plasma levels of the following drugs: Atovaquone, clofibrate, daunorubicin, diphenoxylate, divalproex, lamotrigine, metoclopramide, olanzapine, phenytoin, sedative/hypnotics, sulfamethoxazole, and zidovudine. (3) Coadministration of ritonavir with the following drugs may cause extreme sedation and respiratory depression and thus should **not** be combined: Alprazolam, clonazepam, clorazepate, diazepam, estazolam, flurazepam, midazolam, triazolam, and zolpidem.

Aldesleukin / ↑ Ritonavir levels → ↑ risk of toxicity; adjust ritonavir dose as needed

Alfuzosin / ↑ Alfuzosin blood levels → ↑ pharmacologic & side effects (e.g., hypotension); do not use together

Antiarrhythmics (e.g., amiodarone, bepridil, disopyramide, flecainide, lidocaine, mexiletine, propafenone, quinidine) / ↑ Plasma level of antiarrhythmic → serious and/or life-threatening cardiac arrhythmias

Astemizole / Potential serious and/or life-threatening reactions (e.g., cardiac arrhythmias); use together contraindicated

Atovaquone / ↓ Atovaquone levels; dosage ↑ may be needed

Azole antifungals (fluconazole, itraconazole, ketoconazole) / ↑ Ritonavir plasma levels → ↑ risk of toxicity

Bupropion / Possible ↓ bupropion dose needed; monitor levels

Buspirone / ↑ Buspirone levels; ↓ buspirone dose may be needed

Calcium channel blockers (e.g, diltaizem, nifedipine, verapamil) / Possible ↑ level of calcium channel blocker; use with caution/monitor; possible ↓ blocker dose may be needed

Carbamazepine / ↑ Carbamazepine levels; ↓ dose may be needed

Cetirizine / ↑ Cetirizine AUC, elimination t½ , and volume of distribution

Cisapride / ↑ Risk of cardiac arrhythmias; do not use together

Clarithromycin / ↑ Clarithromycin and ritonavir levels; reduce clarithromycin dose by 50% in those with C_{cr} 30–60 mL/min and by 75% in those with C_{CR} <30 mL/min

Clonazepam / ↑ Clonazepam levels; ↓ dose may be needed

Clorazepate / ↑ Clorazepate levels; ↓ dose may be needed

Clozapine/ ↑ Clozapine serum levels → ↑ toxicity

Corticosteroids (e.g., dexamethasone, predinsone) / ↑ Steroid levels; dose ↓ may be needed

Cyclosporine / ↑ Cyclosporine levels; monitor levels

Delavirdine / ↑ Ritonavir AUC and C_{max}; appropriate doses of the combination not established

Desipramine / Significant ↑ desipramine AUC (145%) and C_{max} (32%); reduce desipramine dose and monitor levels

Diazepam / ↑ Diazepam levels; ↓ dose may be needed

Didanosine / ↓ Didanosine AUC and C_{max}; separate dosing by 2.5 hr

Digoxin / ↑ Digoxin levels → ↑ risk of toxicity; monitor digoxin levels closely and adjust dose as needed

Disopyramide / Possible ↑ disopyramide plasma levels → cardiac arrhythmias

Disulfiram / Ritonavir products contain alcohol → disulfiram-like serious reactions

Divalproex / ↓ Divalproex levels; dose ↑ may be needed

Dronabinol / ↑ Dronabinol levels; ↓ dose may be needed

Efavirenz / ↑ Ritonavir AUC and C_{max}; appropriate doses of the combination not established

Eplerenone / ↑ Eplerenone levels → ↑ risk for hyperkalemia and associated arrhythmias; use together contraindicated

Ergot derivatives (dihydroergotamine, ergonovine, ergotamine, methylergonovine) / ↑ Plasma levels of ergot derivatives → ↑ risk of ergot toxicity (e.g., vasospasm, ischemia of extremities and other tissues); use together contraindicated

Estazolam / ↑ Estazolam levels; ↓ dose may be needed

Ethinyl estradiol / ↓ Ethinyl estradiol levels; use alternative contraceptive

Ethosuximide / ↑ Ethosuximide levels; ↓ dose may be needed

Fentanyl / ↑ Plasma levels of fentanyl → ↑ risk of fentanyl-induced respiratory depression due to ↓ liver metabolism; dose ↓ may be needed

Fluoxetine / Possible ↓ fluoxetine dose needed; monitor levels; also, ↑ ritonavir levels

Flurazepam / ↑ Flurazepam levels; ↓ dose may be needed

Fluticasone / ↑ Fluticasone (using nasal spray) AUC by 350-fold and C_{max} by 25-fold and a significant ↓ of 86% in plasma cortisol AUC; do not use together

HMG-CoA reductase inhibitors (e.g., atorvastatin, lovastatin, pravastatin, simvastatin) / ↑ Plasma levels of HMG-CoA reductase inhibitor → ↑ risk of myopathy, including rhabdomyolysis; do not use ritonavir with lovastatin or simvastatin; start with lowest dose and monitor

HMG-CoA reductase inhibitors + Saquinavir / Coadministered with ritonavir → ↑ AUC of atorvastatin and simvastatin and ↓ AUC of pravastatin

Indinavir / ↑ Indinavir plasma levels → ↑ toxicity

Interleukins / ↑ Ritonavir plasma levels → ↑ risk of toxicity

Itraconazole / ↑ Ritonavir plasma levels → ↑ risk of toxicity; also, ↑ itraconazole plasma levels

Lamotrigine / ↓ Lamotrigine levels; dose ↑ may be needed

Levothyroxine / ↑ Thyroxine levels → hyperthyroidism; monitor when starting or stopping ritonavir

Lidocaine / Possible ↑ lidocaine plasma levels → cardiac arrhythmias

Loperamide / ↑ Loperamide AUC and peak plasma levels and ↓ clearance R/T ↓ metabolism

Meperidine / ↓ Plasma meperidine levels but ↑ plasma levels of normeperidine → ↑ risk of neurologic toxicity; do not use together

Methadone / ↓ Plasma levels of methadone; consider ↑ dose

Methamphetamine / ↑ Methamphetamine levels; dose ↓ may be needed

Metoprolol / ↑ Metoprolol levels; ↓ metoprolol dose may be needed; use together with caution and monitor

Metronidazole / Ritonavir products contain alcohol → serious disulfiram-like reactions

Mexiletine / Possible ↑ mexiletine plasma levels → cardiac arrhythmias

Midazolam / ↑ Risk of prolonged or increased sedation or respiratory depression; use together contraindicated

Nefazodone / Possible ↓ nefazodone dose needed; monitor levels

Nevirapine / ↑ Ritonavir AUC and C_{max}; appropriate doses of the combination not established

Olanzapine / ↑ Oral clearance and ↓ systemic olanzapine levels R/T ↑ metabolism; adjust dose as needed

Oral contraceptives or patch (ethinyl estradiol) / ↓ Ethinyl estradiol AUC by 40% and C_{max} by 32%; consider dosage increase or alternate contraceptives

Phenothiazines (e.g., perphenazine, thioridazine) / ↑ Phenothiazine levels; dose ↓ may be needed

Phenytoin / ↓ Phenytoin levels; dose ↑ may be needed

Pimozide / ↑ Potential for cardiac arrhythmias; use together contraindicated

Propoxyphene / ↑ Propoxyphene plasma levels → ↑ risk of toxicity; dose ↓ may be needed

Quinine / ↑ Quinine levels; dose ↓ may be needed

Rifamycins (Rifabutin, Rifampin) / ↓ Ritonavir serum levels → loss of virologic response; also, ↑ rifabutin serum levels; reduce rifabutin dose by 75% or more

Risperidone / ↑ Risperidone levels; dose ↓ may be needed

H *St. John's wort* / ↓ Ritonavir plasma levels R/T ↑ hepatic metabolism by CYP3A4 → loss of virologic response; do not use together

Saquinavir / Significant ↑ in saquinavir blood levels; do not coadminister saquinavir/ritonavir with rifampin due to ↑

risk of severe hepatotoxicity

Selective serotonin reuptake inhibitors (e.g., fluoxitine) / Possible ↓ SSRI dose; needed monitor levels

Sildenafil / ↑ Sildenafil levels → severe and potentially fatal hypotension; do not exceed a dose of 25 mg of sildenafil within 48 hr

Sirolimus / ↑ Sirolimus levels; monitor levels

Sulfamethoxazole / Coadministration of ritonavir with sulfamethoxazole/trimethoprim ↓ sulfamethoxazole AUC

Tacrolimus / ↑ Tacrolimus levels; monitor levels

Tadalafil / Possible hypotension; do not exceed a dose of 10 mg of tadalafil every 72 hr

Terfenadine / Potential serious and/or life-threatening reactions (e.g., cardiac arrhythmias); use together contraindicated

Theophylline / ↓ Theophylline AUC by 43% and C_{max} by 32%; monitor theophylline levels and consider increased dosage

Timolol / ↑ Timolol levels; ↓ timolol dose may be needed; use together with caution and monitor

Tramadol / ↑ Tramadol plasma levels → ↑ risk of toxicity; dose ↓ may be needed

Trazodone / ↓ Clearance, prolonged $t\frac{1}{2}$, and ↑ peak plasma levels of trazodone R/T ↓ metabolism; consider ↓ trazodone dosage

Triazolam / ↑ Risk of prolonged or increased sedation or respiratory depression; use together contraindicated

Tricyclic antidepressants (TCA's) / Possible ↓ TCA dose needed; monitor levels

Vardenafil / Possible hypotension; do not exceed a dose of 2.5 mg vardenafil every 72 hr

Voraconazole / ↑ Ritonavir plasma levels → ↑ risk of toxicity; also, ↓ voraconazole plasma levels; do not give together

Warfarin / ↓ or ↑ Warfarin anticoagulant effect; monitor INR frequently

Zidovudine / ↓ Zidovudine AUC 25% and C_{max} 27%

Zolpidem / ↑ Zolpidem levels → possible severe sedation and respiratory depression

HOW SUPPLIED

Capsules, Soft Gelatin: 100 mg; *Oral Solution:* 80 mg/mL.

DOSAGE

- **CAPSULES; ORAL SOLUTION**

  HIV infection.

Adults: 600 mg twice a day. Use of a dose titration schedule may help reduce treatment-emergent side effects while maintaining appropriate ritonavir plasma levels. Do not start with less than 300 mg twice a day; increase at 2- to 3-day intervals by 100 mg twice daily. If nausea is experienced upon initiation of therapy, dose escalation may be tried as follows: 300 mg twice a day for 1 day, 400 mg twice a day for 2 days, 500 mg twice a day for 1 day, and then 600 mg twice a day thereafter.

Children: 400 mg/m^2 twice a day, PO, not to exceed 600 mg/day. Start with 250 mg/m^2 and increase at 2- to 3-day intervals by 50 mg/m^2 twice a day. Check the package insert for pediatric dosage guidelines. If 400 mg/m^2 is not tolerated, give the highest tolerated dose for maintenance in combination with other antiretroviral drugs; alternate therapy may also be considered.

NURSING CONSIDERATIONS

ⓒ Do not confuse ritonavir with Retrovir (zidovudine, also an antiviral drug). Also do not confuse Norvir (the trade name for ritonavir) with Retrovir or Norvasc (a calcium channel blocker).

ADMINISTRATION/STORAGE

1. Mild to moderate GI disturbances and paresthesias may decrease as therapy continues. Clients prescribed combination regimens with nucleoside analogues may improve GI tolerance by starting therapy with ritonavir alone and then adding the nucleoside before completing 2 weeks of ritonavir monotherapy.

2. If saquinavir and ritonavir are used together, reduce the dose of saquinavir to 400 mg twice a day. The optimum dosage level of ritonavir (400 or 600 mg twice a day), in combination with saquinavir has not been determined. How-

R

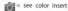

ever, this combination is better tolerated in those who received ritonavir, 400 mg twice a day.

3. Until dispensed, store soft gelatin capsules in refrigerator at 2–8°C (36–46°F) and protect from light. Capsule refrigeration is recommended after dispensing; however, this is not necessary if used within 30 days, and kept below 25°C (77°F).

4. Store the solution at room temperature between 20–25°C (68–77°F). Do not refrigerate. Shake well before each use. Store and dispense in the original container and keep cap tightly closed. Avoid exposure to excessive heat.

ASSESSMENT

1. Note onset S&S, serum confirmation of diagnosis, other agents trialed, outcome.

2. Monitor CBC, T-lymphocytes (CD_4), viral load, and LFTs. Note impaired liver function; drug hepatically metabolized via cytochrome P450 system.

3. List other agents prescribed to ensure none interact unfavorably; esp. note if using viagra because side effects may be enhanced and may cause severe drop in BP; advise against or not to exceed 25 mg every 2 days.

CLIENT/FAMILY TEACHING

1. Take with food, if possible. Taste may be improved by mixing with chocolate milk, Ensure, or Advera within 1 hr of dosing. Give the pediatric dose using a calibrated dosage syringe.

2. Take each day as prescribed. Do not alter dosage or discontinue without approval. If dose is missed, take the next dose as soon as possible; if dose is skipped, do not double the next dose.

3. Use reliable birth control and barrier protection; drug does not reduce the risk of transmitting disease through sexual contact or blood contamination.

4. Drug is not a cure for HIV; illnesses associated with advanced HIV infection may still occur, including opportunistic infections.

5. Keep all F/U appointments to evaluate response to therapy and disease progression.

OUTCOMES/EVALUATE

Inhibition of disease progression and early death with HIV infection

Rituximab
(rih-**TUK**-sih-mab)

CLASSIFICATION(S):

Antineoplastic, monoclonal antibody

PREGNANCY CATEGORY: C

Rx: Rituxan.

SEE ALSO *ANTINEOPLASTIC AGENTS.*

USES

(1) Relapsed or refractory low-grade or follicular, CD20 positive, B-cell non-Hodgkin's lymphoma. Used in combination with cyclophosphamide, doxorubicin, vincristine, and prednisone or other anthracycline-based chemotherapy regimens. (2) With methotrexate to reduce signs and symptoms of moderate-to-severe rheumatoid arthritis in adult clients who have had an inadequate response to one or more tissue necrosis factor antagonist therapies. *Investigational:* Relapsed or refractory chronic lymphocytic leukemia, relapsed or refractory Waldenstrom macroglobinemia, thrombocytopenic purpura.

ACTION/KINETICS

Action

A chimeric murine/human monoclonal antibody which binds specifically to CD20 antigen found on the surface of normal and malignant B lymphocytes causing cell lysis. Cell lysis may result due to complement-dependent cytotoxicity and antibody-dependent cellular cytotoxicity. Circulating B cells are almost completely depleted for up to 9 months. CD20 regulates early steps in the activation process for cell cycle initiation and differentiation and possibly functions as a calcium ion channel.

Pharmacokinetics

Causes significant decreases in both IgM and IgG serum levels from months 5 to 11. **Mean serum $t^{1}\!/_{2}$:** 76.3 hr after first infusion and 205.8 hr after fourth

---

Bold Italic = life threatening side effect   ■ = black box warning   ✤ = Available in Canada

infusion. **Mean terminal t½, elimination:** 19 days.

CONTRAINDICATIONS

Use in known IgE-mediated hypersensitivity or anaphylactic reactions to murine proteins or any component of product. Use not recommended in those with rheumatoid arthritis who have no prior inadequate response to one or more tissue necrosis factor antagonists. Lactation.

SPECIAL CONCERNS

■ (1) Deaths within 24 hr of rituximab infusion have been reported. These fatal reactions followed an infusion reaction complex that included hypoxia, pulmonary infiltrates, acute respiratory distress syndrome, MI, ventricular fibrillation, or cardiogenic shock. About 80% of fatal infusion reactions occurred in association with the first infusion. Those who develop severe infusion reactions should have the infusion discontinued and receive medical treatment. (2) Acute renal failure requiring dialysis with instances of fatal outcome has been reported following tumor lysis syndrome following rituximab therapy. (3) Severe mucocutaneous reactions, some with fatal outcome, have been reported in association with rituximab treatment.■ Use with caution in preexisting cardiac conditions, including arrhythmias and angina. Infusion-related symptoms may occur from 30 to 120 min at beginning of first infusion and with less frequency with subsequent infusions. Use is associated with severe infusion and hypersensitivity reactions. Possible reactivation of hepatitis B virus with fulminant hepatitis, hepatic failure, and death. Safety of immunization with any vaccine, especially live viral vaccines, has not been studied. Geriatric clients are more likely to experience cardiac side effects (especially supraventricular arrhythmias) and serious pulmonary side effects (e.g., pneumonia, pneumonitis). Safety and efficacy have not been determined in children.

SIDE EFFECTS

Most Common

Infusion reactions, fever, chills, infection, asthenia, headache, hypo-/hyper-tension, night sweats, rash, pruritus, N&V, diarrhea, lymphopenia, leukopenia, neutropenia, thrombocytopenia, angioedema, myalgia, arthralgia, increased cough, rhinitis, abdominal/back pain, pain.

Infusion-related events: Fever, chills, and rigors are most common. Also, nausea, urticaria, fatigue, headache, pruritus, bronchospasm, hypotension, angioedema, dyspnea, rhinitis, vomiting, flushing, pain at disease sites, hypoxia, pulmonary infiltrates, *acute respiratory distress syndrome, MI, ventricular fibrillation, cardiogenic shock, anaphylactic/anaphylactoid events*. **Retreatment events:** Asthenia, throat irritation, flushing, tachycardia, anorexia, leukopenia, thrombocytopenia, anemia, peripheral edema, dizziness, depression, respiratory symptoms, night sweats, pruritus. (General side effects). **CV:** Arrhythmias, including VT and SVTs; trigeminy, angina, hypo-/hypertension, tachycardia, postural hypotension, bradycardia, cardiac disorder, *cardiac failure.* **Hematologic:** Thrombocytopenia (up to 30 days following last dose), severe anemia, neutropenia (including late onset), leukopenia, lymphopenia, anemia, coagulation disorder, marrow hypoplasia, prolonged pancytopenia, hyperviscosity syndrome in Waldenstrom macroglobulinemia. **Body as a whole:** Asthenia, pain, fever, infections (bacterial, viral, fungal), chills, malaise, viral infections, *severe mucocutaneous reactions, hypersensitivity reactions* (e.g., hypotension, *bronchospasm*, angioedema), systemic vasculitis, serum sickness. **GI:** Abdominal pain (including upper abdominal pain), N&V, diarrhea, dyspepsia, throat irritation, taste perversion, *bowel obstruction/perforation*. **Hepatic:** Reactivation of hepatitis B with related fulminant hepatitis. **CNS:** Headache, dizziness, paresthesia, anxiety, agitation, insomnia, hypesthesia, nervousness, migraine, paresthesia. Reactivation of hepatitis B virus with fulminant hepatitis, *hepatic failure, and death.* **Respiratory:** *Bronchospasm*, increased cough, rhinitis, dyspnea, bronchiolitis obliterans, hypoxia,

R

---

asthma, sinusitis, respiratory disorder, bronchitis, lung disorder, pneumonitis (including interstitial), URTI, pleuritis. **Musculoskeletal:** Myalgia, arthralgia, polyarticular arthritis and vasculitis with rash. **Dermatologic:** Pruritus, rash, urticaria, flushing, night sweats, *mucocutaneous skin reactions (rare).* **GU:** Acute renal failure (may require dialysis). **Ophthalmic:** Optic neuritis, conjunctivitis, uveitis. **Miscellaneous:** Angioedema, lacrimation disorder, chest/back/tumor pain, peripheral edema, anorexia, abdominal enlargement, pain at injection site, hypertonia, immunogenicity, lupus-like syndrome, increase in fatal infections in HIV-associated lymphoma, multifocal leukoencephalopathy. *Tumor lysis syndrome with acute renal failure requiring dialysis,* as well as hyperkalemia, hypocalcemia, hyperuricemia, hyperphosphatemia.

LABORATORY TEST CONSIDERATIONS
↑ LDH. Hyperglycemia, hypocalcemia.

DRUG INTERACTIONS
Biologic agents / Closely observe for signs of infection
Cisplatin / Renal toxicity
Vaccines, live virus / Vaccination with live viruses is not recommended

HOW SUPPLIED
Injection: 10 mg/mL.

DOSAGE

• **IV INFUSION**
Relapsed or refractory, low-grade or follicular, CD20-positive B cell non-Hodgkin's lymphoma.
Initial: 375 mg/m^2 as IV infusion once a week for 4 or 8 doses. Progressive disease may be retreated at the same dose, once weekly for 4 doses. **Retreatment:** 375 mg/m^2 by IV infusion once weekly for 4 doses in responding clients who developed progressive disease after previous rituximab therapy. **Do not administer as IV push or bolus.**
Diffuse, large B cell non-Hodgkin's lymphoma.
375 mg/m^2 by IV infusion on day 1 of each cycle of chemotherapy, for up to 8 infusions.
With methotrexate to treat moderate to severe rheumatoid arthritis.

Adults: A single treatment course of two infusions of rituximab, 1,000 mg each, on days 1 and 15 combined with stable doses of methotrexate. To reduce the incidence of infusion reactions, also give methylprednisolone, 100 mg IV (or its equivalent) 30 min prior to each infusion.
Rituximab as part of the ibritumomab tiuxetan therapeutic regimen.
Rituximab, 250 mg/m^2, infused within 4 hr prior to the administration of indium IN 11 ibritumomab tiuxetan and within 4 hr prior to the administration of yttrium Y-90-ibritumomab tiuxetan. Administration of rituximab and indium IN 111 ibritumomab tiuxetan should precede rituximab and Y-90-ibritumomab tiuxetan by 7–9 days.

NURSING CONSIDERATIONS
ADMINISTRATION/STORAGE
IV 1. To prepare for administration, withdraw necessary amount of rituximab and dilute to final concentration of 1 to 4 mg/mL into infusion bag containing either 0.9% NaCl or D5W. Discard any unused portion left in vial.
2. Premedicate with acetaminophen and diphenhydramine to attenuate infusion reactions. IV saline and vasopressors may also be used to slow or interrupt an infusion reaction. Consider withdrawaing antihypertensive medication 12 hr prior to rituximab infusion due to rituximab-induced transient hypotension.
3. For first infusion, give at initial rate of 50 mg/hr. If hypersensitivity or infusion-related events do not occur, escalate infusion rate in 50 mg/hr increments every 30 min to maximum of 400 mg/hr. If hypersensitivity or infusion-related events occur, temporarily slow or interrupt infusion; infusion can continue at one-half previous rate until symptoms improve. Subsequent infusions can be given at initial rate of 100 mg/hr, and increased by 100 mg/hr increments at 30 min intervals to maximum of 400 mg/hr (as long as tolerated).
4. Do not administer as an IV push or bolus.

Bold Italic = life threatening side effect   ■ = black box warning   ✦ = Available in Canada

5. Do not mix or dilute with other drugs.

6. Protect vials from direct sunlight.

7. Solutions for infusion are stable at 2–8°C (36–46°F) for 24 hr and at room temperature for an additional 12 hr.

ASSESSMENT

1. Note any cardiac disease and assess for arrhythmias.

2. Screen persons at high risk for hepatitis B viral infections before initiation of therapy. Monitor for S&S of hepatitis B virus in carriers during therapy and for several months following therapy.

3. Therapy usually consists of once-weekly infusions for four doses. Due to the possibility of transient hypotension during infusion, consider withholding antihypertensive medication 12 hr prior to rituximab. Infusion-related reaction consisting of fever and chills/rigors may occur with first infusion.

4. Due to the potential of hypersensitivity reactions, consider premedication with acetaminophen and diphenhydramine. Interrupt infusion if severe reaction occurs; may resume infusion at 50% initial rate once symptoms resolved. Also, institute supportive care (IV fluids, vasopressors, oxygen, bronchodilators, diphenhydramine, acetaminophen).

5. Monitor CBC, CD20 positive B lymphocytes, BP, and EKG.

CLIENT/FAMILY TEACHING

1. Drug is administered IV once a week for about 4–8 weeks to eradicate the cancer cells.

2. Practice reliable contraception during and for up to 12 months following therapy.

3. Report any adverse reactions.

OUTCOMES/EVALUATE

- Control of malignant cell proliferation
- Depletion of B lymphocytes

Rivastigmine tartrate
(rih-vah-**STIG**-meen)

CLASSIFICATION(S):
Treatment of Alzheimer's disease
PREGNANCY CATEGORY: B
Rx: Exelon.

USES

PO, Transdermal: (1) Mild to moderate dementia of the Alzheimer's type. (2) Mild to moderate dementia associated with Parkinson's disease. *Investigational:* Treat behavioral effects in Lewy-body dementia.

ACTION/KINETICS

Action

Probably acts by enhancing cholinergic function by increasing levels of acetylcholine through reversible inhibition of its hydrolysis by acetylcholinesterase. There is no evidence that the drug alters the course of the underlying disease.

Pharmacokinetics

After PO, is rapidly and completely absorbed. Absolute bioavailability is 40% (after 3 mg). Absorption from the patch is greatest from the back, chest, or upper arm. Administration with food delays absorption by 90 min, lowers C_{max} by about 30%, and increases AUC by about 30%. **Peak plasma levels, after PO:** 1 hr; **from the patch:** 8 hr. Is rapidly and extensively metabolized by cholinesterase-mediated hydrolysis. **t½, elimination:** About 1.5 hr. Excreted mainly in the urine. **Plasma protein binding:** 40%.

CONTRAINDICATIONS

Hypersensitivity to rivastigmine or other carbamate derivatives, or other components of the product.

SPECIAL CONCERNS

Use with caution during lactation; it is not known if rivastigmine is excreted in breast milk. Use with caution in clients with a history of asthma or obstructive pulmonary disease. Drugs that increase cholinergic activity may have vagotonic effects on the heart, cause urinary obstruction, and may cause seizures. Safe-

R

ty and efficacy have not been determined in children.

SIDE EFFECTS

Most Common

N&V, dizziness, headache, diarrhea, anorexia, weight loss, abdominal pain, insomnia, confusion, asthenia, dyspepsia, accidental trauma, fatigue, UTI, tremor. Side effects listed are those with a frequency of 1% or greater. Significant GI side effects may occur. **GI:** N&V, diarrhea, anorexia, weight loss, abdominal pain (including upper), peptic ulcers, GI bleeding (active or occult), dyspepsia, constipation, flatulence, eructation, fecal incontinence, gastritis. **CNS:** Dizziness, headache, insomnia, confusion, depression, anxiety, somnolence, hallucination, tremor, aggressive reaction, syncope, abnormal gait, ataxia, paresthesia, agitation, nervousness, delusion, **convulsions**, paranoid reaction, confusion, vertigo, worsening of Parkinson's disease, bradykinesia, dyskinesia, restlessness. **CV:** Hypotension, postural hypotension, hypertension, **cardiac failure, MI**, atrial fibrillation, bradycardia, palpitation, angina pectoris, TIA. **Body as a whole:** Accidental trauma, fatigue, asthenia, malaise, increased sweating, flu-like symptoms, syncope, dehydration, fever, edema, allergy, hot flushes, general infection, pain. **Dermatologic:** Rashes, including maculopapular, eczema, bullous, exfoliative, psoriaform, erythematous; pruritus. **GU:** UTI, urinary obstruction, hematuria, urinary incontinence. **Musculoskeletal:** Arthritis, leg cramps, myalgia, back pain, arthralgia, bone fracture. **Respiratory:** Rhinitis, epistaxis, URTI, coughing, pharyngitis, nasopharyngitis, bronchitis, dyspnea, pneumonia. **Miscellaneous:** Anemia, hypokalemia, tinnitus, cataract, rigors, chest pain, peripheral edema.

LABORATORY TEST CONSIDERATIONS

Hematuria, hypokalemia.

OD OVERDOSE MANAGEMENT

Symptoms: Cholinergic crisis, including symptoms of severe nausea, vomiting, salivation, sweating, bradycardia, hypotension, respiratory depression, collapse, seizures. Increasing muscle weakness with possible death if respiratory muscles are involved. *Treatment:* General supportive measures. Treat severe nausea and vomiting with antiemetics.

DRUG INTERACTIONS

Anticholinergics / Rivastigmine interferes with anticholinergic activity
Bethanechol / Synergistic effect
Neuromuscular blocking agents / Synergistic effect
Nicotine / ↑ PO clearance of rivastigmine by 23%
NSAIDs / Rivastigmine ↑ gastric acid secretion; monitor for active or occult GI bleeding
Succinylcholine / Exaggeration of succinylcholine-induced muscle relaxation during anesthesia

HOW SUPPLIED

Capsules: 1.5 mg, 3 mg, 4.5 mg, 6 mg; *Oral Solution:* 2 mg/mL (all concentrations as the base); *Transdermal Patch:* 4.6 mg/24 hr, 9.5 mg/24 hr.

DOSAGE

- **CAPSULES; ORAL SOLUTION**
  Mild-to-moderate dementia due to Alzheimer's disease.

Initial: 1.5 mg twice a day to minimize GI side effects. If the dose is well tolerated after a minimum of 2 weeks, may increase dose to 3 mg twice a day. Attempt subsequent increases to 4.5 mg and 6 mg twice a day only after a minimum of 2 weeks at the previous dose. If side effects are intolerable, discontinue treatment for several doses and then restart at the same or next lower dose level. If treatment is interrupted for longer than several days, reinitiate treatment with the lowest daily dose and titrate as described above. **Maximum dose:** 6 mg twice a day.
  Dementia associated with Parkinson's disease.
Initial: 1.5 mg twice a day; **then,** the dose may be increased to 3 mg twice a day and further to 4.5 mg twice a day and 6 mg twice a day, based on tolerability. There should be a minimum of 4 weeks at each dose. **Dose range:** 1.5–6 mg twice a day.

- **TRANSDERMAL PATCH**
  Dementia due to Alzheimer's disease or Parkinsons' disease.

Initial: 4.6 mg/24 hr. After a minimum of 4 weeks and if well tolerated, the dose should be increased to 9.5 mg/24 hr (the recommended effective dose). **Maintenance:** Increase doses only after a minimum of 4 weeks at the previous dose and only if the previous dose has been well tolerated. The maximum recommended dose is 9.5 mg/24 hr; higher doses offer no significant additional benefit but there is a significant increase in side effects.

NURSING CONSIDERATIONS

ADMINISTRATION/STORAGE

1. If side effects develop during treatment, discontinue treatment for several doses; restart at the lowest daily dose (to prevent severe vomiting) and titrate back to the maintenance dose.
2. The capsules and oral solution may be interchanged at equal doses.
3. Clients with a body weight less than 50 kg may experience more side effects using the transdermal patch. Use particular caution in titrating these clients above the recommended maintenance dose of 9.5 mg/24 hr.
4. Clients on capsules or oral solution may be switched to the transdermal patch as follows: (a) a client who is on a total daily dose of less than 6 mg PO can be switched to the 4.6 mg/24 hr patch; (b) A client who is on a total daily dose of 6–12 mg PO may be directly switched to the 9.5 mg/24 hr transdermal patch. Apply the first transdermal patch on the day following the last PO dose.
5. Store the oral solution, tablets, and transdermal patches from 15–30°C (59–86°F). Store solution in an upright position; protect from freezing. When combined with cold fruit juice or soda, the mixture is stable at room temperature for up to 4 hr. Keep patches in the individually sealed pouches until use.

ASSESSMENT

1. Note onset, characteristics of S&S, performance of ADLs, other agents trialed, outcome. Identify caregiver and start therapy as soon as diagnosed.
2. Describe clinical presentation, cognitive functioning, mini mental exam score or similar test of cognitive ability.
3. Note history of asthma, seizures, BPH, or COPD.
4. Obtain baseline weight, VS, ECG, lytes and metabolic panel, B12, CBC, RPR, U/A, and BS; monitor.

CLIENT/FAMILY TEACHING

1. Take with food in divided doses in the morning and evening. Establish reasonable expectations.
2. If using the oral solution, remove the oral dosing syringe provided and withdraw the correct amount of drug from the container. Each dose of rivastigmine may be swallowed directly from the syringe or first mixed with a small glass of water, cold fruit juice, or soda. When mixed with fruit juice or soda, the mixture is stable for 4 hr or less.
3. Apply the transdermal patch once a day to clean, dry, hairless, intact healthy skin in a location that will not be rubbed by tight clothing. Press down on the patch firmly until the edges stick well. The patch can be used in situations that include bathing and hot wetaher. Do not apply to a skin area where cream, lotion, or powder has been applied recently.
4. The upper or lower back is recommended for patch placement since the client is less likely to remove the patch. When sites on the back are not accessible, the patch can be applied to the upper arm or chest. Do not apply patch to skin that is red, irritated, or cut. Change the site of the transdermal patch application daily to avoid potential irritation, although consecutive patches can be applied to the same anatomic site (i.e., another site on the upper back). Do not use the same site within 14 days.
5. Used patches should be folded, with the adhesive surfaces pressed together; discard safely.
6. Drug may cause a high incidence of (GI effects) N&V; monitor weight and report if loss significant so therapy can be reassessed. Stop drug and report any evidence of seizures, urinary obstruction, dizziness, and low heart rate.

R

---

7. Dosage may be gradually increased by provider if drug is tolerated and desired effects not evident. Report lack of response, intolerance, evidence of behavioral disturbances or psychosis and agitation.

OUTCOMES/EVALUATE
- Improved daily and cognitive functioning with Alzheimer's disease
- Reduced caregiver time and reduced institutionalization

Rizatriptan benzoate
(rise-ah-**TRIP**-tan)

CLASSIFICATION(S):
Antimigraine drug
PREGNANCY CATEGORY: C
Rx: Maxalt, Maxalt-MLT.
✤Rx: Maxalt RPD.

USES
Acute treatment of migraine attacks in adults with or without aura.

ACTION/KINETICS
Action
Binds to $5-HT_{1B/1D}$ receptors, resulting in cranial vessel vasoconstriction, inhibition of neuropeptide release, and reduced transmission in trigeminal pain pathways.

Pharmacokinetics
Completely absorbed after PO use; rate of absorption of Maxalt-MLT is somewhat slower. 40% is bioavailable. **Time to onset of action:** 45 min. **Peak plasma levels, Maxalt:** 1–1.5 hr; **Maxalt-MLT:** 1.6–2.5 hr. Food has no effect on bioavailability, but will delay time to reach peak levels by one hr. **t½:** 2–3 hr. Metabolized by MAO-A; most is excreted through the urine. Is a significant first-pass effect. **Plasma protein binding:** About 14%.

CONTRAINDICATIONS
Use in children less than 18 years of age, as prophylactic therapy of migraine, or use in the management of hemiplegic or basilar migraine. Use in those with ischemic heart disease or vasospastic coronary artery disease, uncontrolled hypertension, within 24 hr of treatment with another $5-HT_1$ agonist or an ergotamine-containing or ergot-type medication (e.g., dihydroergotamine, methysergide). Use concurrently with MAO inhibitors or use of rizatriptan within 2 weeks of discontinuing an MAO inhibitor. Strongly recommended the drug not be given in unrecognized coronary artery disease (CAD) predicted by the presence of risk factors, including hypertension, hypercholesterolemia, smoking, obesity, diabetes, strong family history of CAD, female with surgical or physiological menopause, or males over 40, unless a CV evaluation reveals the client is free from CAD or ischemic myocardial disease.

SPECIAL CONCERNS
Safety and efficacy have not been determined for use in cluster headache or in children. Use with caution during lactation, with diseases that may alter the absorption, metabolism, or excretion of drugs; in dialysis clients, and in moderate hepatic insufficiency. Maxalt-MLT tablets contain phenylalanine; may be of concern to phenylketonurics. Serious cardiac events may occur within a few hours after giving Maxalt. The safety of treating more than 4 headaches in a 30-day period has not been established.

SIDE EFFECTS
Most Common
Palpitations, dizziness, fatigue, headache, somnolence, chest tightness/pressure/heaviness, neck/throat/jaw heaviness, dry mouth, N&V, hypesthesia, decreased mental acuity, euphoria, tremor, flushing, diarrhea, hot flashes, dsypnea, warm/cold sensations.
CV: *Acute MI, coronary artery vasospasm, life-threatening disturbances in cardiac rhythm (VT, ventricular fibrillation), death, cerebral hemorrhage, subarachnoid hemorrhage, stroke, hypertensive crisis.* Also, transient myocardial ischemia, peripheral vascular ischemia, colonic ischemia with abdominal pain and bloody diarrhea, palpitations, tachycardia, cold extremities, hypertension, arrhythmia, bradycardia.
GI: N&V, diarrhea, dry mouth, abdominal distention, dyspepsia, thirst, acid regurgitation, dysphagia, constipation,

---

flatulence, tongue edema. **CNS:** Somnolence, headache, dizziness, paresthesias, hypesthesia, decreased mental acuity, euphoria, tremor, nervousness, vertigo, insomnia, anxiety, depression, disorientation, ataxia, dysarthria, confusion, dream abnormality, abnormal gait, irritability, impaired memory, agitation, hypesthesia. **Pain and pressure sensations:** Chest tightness/pressure/heaviness; pain, tightness, or pressure in the precordium, neck, throat, jaw; regional pain, tightness, pressure, or heaviness; or unspecified pain. **Musculoskeletal:** Muscle weakness, stiffness, myalgia, muscle cramps, musculoskeletal pain, arthralgia, muscle spasm. **Respiratory:** Dyspnea, pharyngitis, nasal irritation, nasal congestion, dry throat, URI, yawning, dry nose, epistaxis, sinus disorder. **GU:** Urinary frequency, polyuria, menstrual disorder. **Dermatologic:** Flushing, sweating, pruritus, rash, urticaria. **Body as a whole:** Asthenia, fatigue, chills, heat sensitivity, hangover effect, warm/cold sensations, dehydration, hot flashes. **Ophthalmic:** Blurred vision, dry eyes, burning eye pain, eye irritation, tearing. **Miscellaneous:** Facial edema, tinnitus, ear pain.

DRUG INTERACTIONS
Dihydroergotamine / Additive vasospastic reactions; do not use within 24 hr of each other
MAO Inhibitors / ↑ Rizatriptan plasma levels; do not use together
Methysergide / Additive vasospastic reactions; do not use within 24 hr of each other
Propranolol / ↑ Rizatriptan levels
Selective serotonin reuptake inhibitors / Possible weakness, hyperreflexia, and incoordination
Sibutramine / Possible serotonin syndrome, including CNS irritability, motor weakness, shivering, myoclonus, and altered consciousness

HOW SUPPLIED
Tablets: 5 mg, 10 mg; *Tablets, Oral Disintegrating:* 5 mg, 10 mg.

DOSAGE
- **TABLETS; TABLETS, ORAL DISINTEGRATING**
  Acute treatment of migraine.

Adults: Single dose of 5 mg or 10 mg of Maxalt or Maxalt-MLT. Doses should be separated by at least 2 hr, with no more than 30 mg taken in any 24-hr period.

NURSING CONSIDERATIONS
ADMINISTRATION/STORAGE
1. In clients receiving propranolol, use the 5 mg dose of Maxalt, up to a maximum of 3 doses in any 24-hr period.
2. There is little evidence that the 10 mg dose provides a greater effect than the 5 mg dose. Individualize dose, weighing the potential benefits of the 10 mg dose with the potential risks.
3. Store Maxalt and Maxalt-MLT tablets at room temperature (15–20°C or 59–86°F).

ASSESSMENT
1. Note characteristics of migraines, when diagnosed, neurologist findings, other agents trialed, outcome.
2. List any evidence of CAD, uncontrolled HTN, DM, or allergies. Assess risk factors for CAD. Clients over age 40 should be carefully screened for CAD.
3. List all medications consumed to ensure none interact. Reduce dose if prescribed propranolol.

CLIENT/FAMILY TEACHING
1. For Maxalt-MLT, do not remove the blister from the outer pouch until just before dosing. Peel open the blister (do not push through the blister) with dry hands, and place the orally disintegrating tablet on the tongue. It will dissolve in the saliva and be swallowed; fluids are not needed, which eases administration.
2. May cause dizziness, drowsiness, or pressure sensation in the upper chest; do not operate equipment or drive until effects realized.
3. Do not take within 24 hr of any other prescription drug used to treat headaches or depression.
4. Review 'patient information sheet' provided for side effects; report if persistent or intolerable. May experience rebound headaches if taken >2–3 times per week.
5. If headache returns or only a partial response is attained, may repeat dose after waiting at least 2 hr. Taking with

R

📷 = see color insert   🅗 = Herbal   Ⅳ = Intravenous   📖 = sound alike drug food may delay drug onset. Do not exceed 30 mg in a 24-hr period.

6. Use alternative birth control if oral contraceptives prescribed. Report if pregnancy suspected.

7. Prevent photosensitivity by using sunscreen and protective clothing.

8. Keep a headache diary and attempt to identify triggers.

9. Inform phenylketonuric clients that each 5 mg of the oral disintegrating tablets contain 1.05 mg phenylalanine.

OUTCOMES/EVALUATE

Relief of migraine headache

Rocuronium bromide ■ IV
(**roh**-kyou-**ROH**-nee-um)

CLASSIFICATION(S):
Neuromuscular blocking drug
PREGNANCY CATEGORY: B
Rx: Zemuron.

SEE ALSO NEUROMUSCULAR BLOCKING AGENTS.

USES

(1) As an adjunct to general anesthesia to facilitate rapid sequence and routine tracheal intubation. (2) To cause relaxation of skeletal muscle during surgery or mechanical ventilation.

ACTION/KINETICS

Action

A nondepolarizing neuromuscular blocking agent that acts by competing with acetylcholine for receptors at the motor end-plate. Causes histamine release in a small number of clients. Use must be accompanied by adequate anesthesia or sedation, as the drug has no effect on consciousness, pain threshold, or cerebration.

Pharmacokinetics

Depending on the dose, it has a rapid to intermediate onset and an intermediate duration of action. $t\frac{1}{2}$, **rapid distribution phase:** 1–2 min; $t\frac{1}{2}$, **slower distribution phase:** 14–18 min. Metabolized by the liver.

SPECIAL CONCERNS

■ The drug should be given by adequately trained individuals familiar with its actions, characteristics, and hazards.■ Use with caution in clients with pulmonary hypertension, valvular heart disease, or significant hepatic disease. Burn clients may develop resistance to nondepolarizing neuromuscular blocking agents. Elderly clients may exhibit a slightly prolonged medical clinical duration of action. Small doses of nondepolarizing neuromuscular blocking drugs have profound effects in clients with either myasthenia gravis or Eaton-Lambert syndrome. Use in children less than 3 months of age and older than 14 years of age has not been studied.

SIDE EFFECTS

Most Common
Transient hypotension and hypertension.

CV: Arrhythmias, abnormal ECG, transient hypotension and hypertension, tachycardia. **GI:** N&V. **Respiratory:** Symptoms of asthma, including ***bronchospasm***, wheezing, rhonchi; hiccup. **Dermatologic:** Rash, edema at injection site, pruritus. **Miscellaneous:** Malignant hyperthermia, severe allergic reactions, including ***anaphylaxis, anaphylactoid reactions, and shock***.

OD **OVERDOSE MANAGEMENT**
Symptoms: Neuromuscular blockade longer than needed for anesthesia and surgery. *Treatment:* Careful monitoring of client. Artificial respiration may be required.

DRUG INTERACTIONS

Anesthetics, inhalation (enflurane, halothane, isoflurane) / ↑ Neuromuscular blockade

Antibiotics (aminoglycosides, bacitracin, colistin, polymyxin, sodium colistimethate, tetracycles, vancomycin) / ↑ Neuromuscular blocking action of rocuronium

Azathioprine / Reversal of neuromuscular blocking effects

Carbamazepine / Shorter duration of action of rocuronium

Diuretics / Diuretics may cause electrolyte imbalance which may modify neuromuscular blockade

---

Ketamine / ↑ Neuromusclar blockade → profound and severe respiratory depression

Mg sulfate / Potentiation of the effects of rocuronium

Phenytoin / Shorter duration or less effectiveness of rocuronium

Quinidine / Possibility of recurrent paralysis

Succinylcholine / ↑ Rocuronium blockade and duration of action

Theophyllines / Dose-dependent reversal of neuromuscular blockade *Verapamil* / Possible enhanced effects of rocuronium → prolonged respiratory depression

HOW SUPPLIED

Injection: 10 mg/mL.

DOSAGE

- **IV ONLY**

  Rapid sequence intubation.

0.6–1.2 mg/kg in appropriately premedicated and adequately anesthetized clients will result in good intubating conditions in less than 2 min.

  Tracheal intubation.

Initial, regardless of anesthetic technique: 0.6 mg/kg. Maximum blockade is noted in less than 3 min with a mean duration of 31 min. However, a dose of 0.45 mg/kg may also be used with maximum blockade in less than 4 min with a mean duration of 22 min. Initial doses of 0.6 mg/kg in children under halothane anesthesia produce good intubating conditions within 1 min with a mean duration of 41 min in children 3 months to 1 year and 27 min in children 1–2 years of age. Maintenance doses in children of 0.075–0.125 mg/kg, given upon return of T_1 of 25% of control provide muscle relaxation for 7–10 min.

  Maintenance doses.

0.1, 0.15, and 0.2 mg/kg, given at 25% recovery of control T_1 (defined as three twitches of train-of-four), provide a median of 12, 17, and 24 min of duration under opioid/nitrous oxide/oxygen anesthesia. Do not administer the dose until recovery of neuromuscular function is evident.

  Continuous infusion.

Initial: 0.01–0.02 mg/kg/min only after early evidence of spontaneous recovery from an intubating dose. Upon reaching the desired level of neuromuscular blockade, the infusion must be individualized for each client; adjust the rate based on the twitch response (monitored with the use of a peripheral nerve stimulator) of the client. **Maintenance, usual:** 0.004–0.016 mg/kg/min.

NURSING CONSIDERATIONS

ADMINISTRATION/STORAGE

IV 1. In obese clients, base the initial dose of 0.6 mg/kg on the client's actual body weight.

2. Inhalation anesthetics (especially enflurane or isoflurane) may enhance the effects of rocuronium. When inhalation anesthetics are used, it may be necessary to reduce the rate of infusion by 30–50% 45–60 min after the intubating dose.

3. In myasthenia gravis or Lambert-Eaton syndrome clients, a peripheral nerve stimulator and use of a small test dose may be of value in monitoring the response to muscle relaxants as these clients are very sensitive to nondepolarizing neuromuscular blockers.

4. Prepare solutions for infusion by mixing with D5W or RL solution. Drug is also compatible with 0.9% NaCl solution, sterile water for injection, and D5W/NSS. Use solution within 24 hr after mixing; discard any unused solutions.

5. Spontaneous recovery occurs at about the same rate in children 3–12 months as in adults, but is more rapid in children 1–12 years old.

6. Do not mix rocuronium, which has an acid pH, with alkaline solutions (e.g., barbiturates) in the same syringe or give at the same time during infusion through the same needle.

7. Store at 2–8°C (36–46°F); do not freeze.

ASSESSMENT

1. Note reasons for therapy, other agents trialed. Monitor ECG, renal, LFTs. Those with liver disease may require a higher dosage to desired response and may have prolonged drug effects.

2. In the critically ill, intubate prior to rocuronium administration. Use a pe-

R

ripheral nerve stimulator/train of four to assess neuromuscular function and to confirm recovery from neuromuscular blockade.

3. Medicate for pain and anxiety as drug does not affect these conditions and client may be unable to convey. Reassure that once drug is stopped client may resume breathing, moving, and talking again.

INTERVENTIONS

1. Provide ventilatory support. Monitor and record VS, ECG, and I&O. Drug can cause vagal stimulation resulting in bradycardia, hypotension, and cardiac arrhythmias. A peripheral nerve stimulator/train of four monitoring may be used to evaluate neuromuscular response and recovery.

2. Consciousness is not affected by drug. Provide analgesics for pain and antianxiety agents for anxiety. Explain all procedures and provide emotional support. Do not conduct any discussions that should not be overheard. Reassure that client will be able to talk and move once drug effects reversed. Determine client need and administer medications for anxiety, pain, and/or sedation regularly (valium, morphine).

3. Muscle fasciculations may cause soreness or injury after recovery. Administer prescribed nondepolarizing agent and reassure that soreness likely caused by the unsynchronized contractions of adjacent muscle fibers just before the onset of paralysis.

4. Position for comfort and so that the body is in proper alignment. Turn and perform mouth care and eye care frequently (protect eyes and instill liquid tears q 2 hr as blink reflex is suppressed).

5. Assess airway at frequent intervals. Have a suction machine at the bedside. Check to be certain that the ventilator alarms are set and on at all times. *Never* leave client unmonitored.

CLIENT/FAMILY TEACHING

1. Reassure that once the drug is discontinued, they will regain use of body, and be able to walk and talk again.

2. Explain all procedures and exams as consciousness is not affected by rocuro-

nium. Reassure that they will be medicated for pain and anxiety.

OUTCOMES/EVALUATE

- Desired level of skeletal muscle relaxation/paralysis
- Control of breathing during mechanical ventilation

Ropinirole hydrochloride
(roh-**PIN**-ih-roll)

CLASSIFICATION(S):
Antiparkinson drug
PREGNANCY CATEGORY: C
Rx: Requip.

SEE ALSO *ANTIPARKINSON AGENTS*.

USES
(1) Signs and symptoms of idiopathic Parkinson's disease (PD), both as initial therapy and adjunctive therapy with levodopa. (2) Moderate to severe restless legs syndrome.

ACTION/KINETICS

Action
Mechanism is not known but believed to involve stimulation of postsynaptic D_2 dopamine receptors in caudate-putamen in brain. Causes decreases in both systolic and diastolic BP at doses above 0.25 mg.

Pharmacokinetics
Rapidly absorbed. **Peak plasma levels:** 1–2 hr. Food reduces maximum concentration. $t\frac{1}{2}$, **elimination:** 6 hr. First pass effect; extensively metabolized in liver.

CONTRAINDICATIONS
Lactation.

SPECIAL CONCERNS
Safety and efficacy have not been determined in children.

SIDE EFFECTS

Most Common
Dyskinesia, dizziness, somnolence, headache, hallucinations, falls, N&V, abdominal pain, pneumonia, fatigue, viral infection, increased sweating, edema, confusion.

R

Bold Italic = life threatening side effect   ▮ = black box warning   ✤ = Available in Canada

CNS: Hallucinations, cause and/or exacerbate preexisting dyskinesia, dizziness, somnolence, headache, abnormal dreams, confusion, falls, abnormal gait/hypokinesia, amnesia, tremor/twitching, nervousness, paresthesia, paresis, sudden uncontrolled sedation. **GI:** N&V, constipation, abdominal pain, diarrhea, dysphagia, flatulence, increased salivation, dry mouth, anorexia, flatulence. **CV:** Syncope (sometimes with bradycardia), postural hypotension. **GU:** UTI, urinary incontinence, pyuria, impotence. **Musculoskeletal:** Arthritis, twitching. **Respiratory:** Pharyngitis, rhinitis, sinusitis, bronchitis, dyspnea, pneumonia. **Ophthalmic:** Abnormal vision, eye abnormality, xerophthalmia. **Body as a whole:** Asthenia, fatigue, viral infection, pain, edema, malaise. **Miscellaneous:** Increased sweating, anemia, decreased weight, peripheral edema, chest pain, peripheral ischemia.

OD OVERDOSE MANAGEMENT
Symptoms: Agitation, increased dyskinesia, grogginess, sedation, orthostatic hypotension, chest pain, confusion, N&V. *Treatment:* General supportive measures. Maintain vital signs. Gastric lavage.

DRUG INTERACTIONS
Ciprofloxacin / Significant ↑ ropinirole levels
Estrogens / ↓ Oral clearance of ropinirole

HOW SUPPLIED
Tablets: 0.25 mg, 0.5 mg, 1 mg, 2 mg, 3 mg, 4 mg, 5 mg.

DOSAGE
• **TABLETS**
  Parkinson's disease.
Week 1: 0.25 mg 3 times per day. **Week 2:** 0.5 mg 3 times per day. **Week 3:** 0.75 mg 3 times per day. **Week 4:** 1 mg 3 times per day. After week 4, daily dose, if necessary, may be increased by 1.5 mg/day on weekly basis up to dose of 9 mg/day. This may be followed by increases of up to 3 mg/day weekly to total dose of 24 mg/day.
  Restless legs syndrome.
Days 1 and 2: 0.25 mg. **Days 3–7:** 0.5 mg. **Week 2:** 1 mg. **Week 3:** 1.5 mg. **Week 4:** 2 mg. **Week 5:** 2.5 mg. **Week 6:** 3 mg. **Week 7:** 4 mg. *NOTE:* Dose is to be taken once daily 1–3 hr before bedtime.

NURSING CONSIDERATIONS
ADMINISTRATION/STORAGE
1. If taken with L-dopa, decrease dose of L-dopa gradually, as tolerated.
2. When discontinued, do so gradually over 7-day period. Reduce frequency of administration to twice daily for 4 days. For remaining 3 days, reduce frequency to once daily prior to complete withdrawal.
3. Titrate dose with caution in clients with impaired hepatic function.
4. Store from 20–25°C (68–77°F). Protect from light and moisture.

ASSESSMENT
1. Note reasons for therapy (PD, restless leg syndrome, periodic limb movements of sleep), disease onset, symptom occurrence, extent of motor function, stiffness, reflexes, gait, strength of grip, amount of tremor. Assess clinical presentation.
2. Note neurological, mental status. With tremor, note extent, muscle weakness/rigidity, difficulty walking or changing direction.
3. Monitor VS, weight, ECG, renal, LFTs. With long-term therapy obtain CXR, eye exams.

CLIENT/FAMILY TEACHING
1. May be taken with or without food. Drug will be gradually increased at weekly intervals to control symptoms.
2. Change positions slowly to prevent sudden drop in BP. Avoid tasks that require mental alertness until drug effects realized. May cause dizziness, use caution; report if persists.
3. Report any loss of effectiveness or worsening of condition. Avoid alcohol during therapy.
4. Practice reliable birth control and do not nurse. Report if pregnancy suspected.
5. Do not stop abruptly. Drug must be gradually withdrawn over seven-day period.
6. Report as scheduled for periodic lab tests, CXR, eye and medical evaluations.

R

OUTCOMES/EVALUATE

- Control of tremor, bradykinesia, and rigidity in PD
- Improvement in periodic limb movements of sleep (PLMD) and restless leg syndrome (RLS) resulting in improved sleep efficiency

Rosiglitazone maleate

(**roh**-sih-**GLIH**-tah-zohn)

CLASSIFICATION(S):

Antidiabetic, oral; thiazolidinedione

PREGNANCY CATEGORY: C

Rx: Avandia.

SEE ALSO *ANTIDIABETIC AGENTS: HYPOGLYCEMIC AGENTS.*

USES

(1) Monotherapy as an adjunct to diet and exercise to improve glycemic control in type 2 diabetes. (2) In combination with a sulfonylurea, insulin, or metformin in clients with type 2 diabetes when diet and exercise and either single agent does not achieve adequate control. In clients inadequately controlled with a maximum dose of a sulfonylurea or metformin, add rosiglitazone to the regimen, rather than substitute for the sulfonylurea or metformin. (3) In combination with a sulfonylurea plus metformin when diet, exercise, and both agents do not result in adequate glycemic control. *Investigational:* Increased ovulation frequency in women with polycystic ovary syndrome; reduced in-stent restenosis in clients with diabetes.

ACTION/KINETICS

Action

Improves blood glucose levels by improving insulin sensitivity in type II diabetes insulin resistance. Active only in the presence of insulin. A highly selective and potent agonist for the peroxisome proliferator-activated receptor (PPAR)-gamma which is found in adipose tissue, skeletal muscle, and liver. Activation of these receptors regulates the transcription of insulin-responsive genes involved in the control of glucose production, transport, and use. The genes also participate in regulation of fatty acid metabolism. Fasting blood glucose decreases from 31–64 mg/dL from placebo and HbA1c decreases from 0.8–1.5% from placebo.

Pharmacokinetics

Peak plasma levels: 1 hr (over 99% bioavailable). Food decreases the rate of absorption but not the total amount absorbed. $t^{1/2}$, **elimination:** 3–4 hr. Extensively metabolized in the liver by CYP2C8 and CYP2C9; excreted in the urine (64%) and feces (23%). The drug does not inhibit any of the major P450 enzymes at clinical doses. *NOTE:* A product called Avandamet is available that contains 1 gram metformin with either 2 or 4 mg rosiglitazone. **Plasma protein binding:** Approximately 99.8%.

CONTRAINDICATIONS

Type 1 diabetes, diabetic ketoacidosis, use with metformin in renal impairment, active liver disease, if serum ALT levels are 2.5 times ULN, in clients with NYHA Class III and IV heart failure, during lactation, and in children less than 18 years of age.

SPECIAL CONCERNS

■ (1) Thiazolidinediones, including rosiglitazone, cause or exacerbate CHF in some clients. After initiation of rosiglitazone, and after dose increases, observe clients carefully for signs and symptoms of heart failure (including excessive, rapid weight gain, dyspnea, and/or edema). If these signs and symptoms develop, the heart failure should be managed according to current standards of care. Furthermore, discontinuation or dose reduction of rosiglitazone must be considered. (2) Rosiglitazone is not recommended in clients with symptomatic heart failure. Initiation of rosiglitazone in such clients with established NYHA Class III or IV heart failure is contraindicated. (3) A meta-analysis of 42 clinical studies, most of which compared rosiglitazone (Avandia) with placebo, showed rosiglitazone to be associated with an increased risk of myocardial ischemic events, such as angina or MI. Three other studies comparing rosiglita-

---

Bold Italic = life threatening side effect   ■ = black box warning   ♣ = Available in Canada

zone (Avandia) to some other approved PO antidiabetic agents or placebo, have not confirmed or excluded this risk. In their entirety, the available data on the risk of myocardial ischemia are inconclusive.■ Treatment may result in resumption of ovulation in premenopausal anovulatory clients with insulin resistance. Use with caution in clients with edema, at risk for heart failure, or hepatic impairment. There is an increased risk of MI and CV events, especially in long-term users of insulin and those taking nitrates. May cause osteoporosis. Safety and efficacy have not been determined in clients less than 18 years of age.

SIDE EFFECTS
Most Common
Headache, edema, back pain, injury, URTI, hyperglycemia, fatigue, sinusitis, diarrhea, anemia.

CV: Cardiac failure, cardiac effects, fluid retention that may worsen or cause CHF, increased risk of **MI, death from CV causes**. **Respiratory:** URTI, sinusitis. **Metabolic:** Hypoglycemia/hyperglycemia, dose-related weight gain. **Miscellaneous:** Injury, headache, back pain, fatigue, diarrhea, anemia, edema, hepatitis, hepatic enzyme elevations, osteoporosis.

LABORATORY TEST CONSIDERATIONS
↑ ALT, total cholesterol, LDL, HDL. ↓ H&H, free fatty acids. Hyperbilirubinemia.

DRUG INTERACTIONS
Gemfibrozil / ↑ Rosiglitazone AUC R/T inhibition of CYP2C8 isoenzyme
Ketoconazole / ↑ Rosiglitazone AUC, peak plasma levels, prolongation in t½, and ↓ PO clearance R/T inhibition of metabolism by CYP2C8 and CYP2C9
Trimethoprim / ↑ Rosiglitazone plasma levels R/T inhibition of metabolism by CYP2C8

HOW SUPPLIED
Tablets: 2 mg, 8 mg.

DOSAGE
• **TABLETS**
Type 2 diabetes, monotherapy.
Adults, initial: 4 mg once daily or in divided doses twice a day. If the response is inadequate after 8–12 weeks,

the dose can be increased to 8 mg as a single dose once daily or in divided doses twice a day. A dose of 4 mg twice a day resulted in the greatest decrease in fasting blood glucose and HbA1c.

Type 2 diabetes, combination therapy with sulfonylurea, insulin, or metformin.
Adults, initial: 4 mg once daily or in divided doses twice a day. If the response is inadequate after 12 weeks, the dose can be increased to 8 mg (maximum daily dose) as a single dose once daily or in divided doses twice a day.

NURSING CONSIDERATIONS
℞ Do not confuse Avandia with Coumadin (an anticoagulant) or with Prandin (also an oral hypoglycemic drug).

ADMINISTRATION/STORAGE
1. Metformin is contraindicated in clients with renal impairment, as is co-administration with rosiglitazone. However, no dosage adjustment is required when rosiglitazone is used as monotherapy in those with renal impairment.
2. Doses of rosiglitazone higher than 4 mg daily in combination with insulin are not recommended. It is recommended that the insulin dose be decreased 10–25% if the client reports hypoglycemia or if the FBS concentrations decrease to less than 100 mg/dL. Make further adjustments based on glucose-lowering response.
3. Store between 15–30°C (59–86°F) in a tight, light-resistant container.

ASSESSMENT
1. Note disease onset, degree of control, other agents trialed, dietary/exercise adherence.
2. List any history of macular edema, CAD, CHF; NYHA class as drug may aggravate. List agents prescribed to ensure none interact.
3. Monitor LFTs following initiation of therapy, every 2 months during first year of use, and periodically thereafter. If ALT increase to 3x ULN at any time, recheck LFTs as soon as possible. If ALT levels remain >3x ULN, stop therapy.

R

4. Monitor BS, microalbumin, HbA1c levels regularly.

5. Assess for S&S of heart failure (SOB, swelling of lower extremities). Stop drug if symptoms appear.

CLIENT/FAMILY TEACHING

1. Take once or twice daily as prescribed with meals (may also be taken without regard to meals). If dose missed may be taken at next meal.

2. May cause swelling of extremities, resumption of ovulation in premenopausal women, and hypoglycemia.

3. Report if dark urine, abdominal pain, fatigue, or unexplained N&V occur. Also report any fever, sore throat, unusual bleeding/bruising, rash, or hypoglycemic reactions.

4. Practice reliable barrier contraception if using hormonal contraception and pregnancy is not desired.

5. Follow dietary guidelines, perform regular daily exercise, weight loss, and other life style changes consistent with controlling diabetes. Ensure annual foot exam and eye exam and keep SBP below 130 and DBP below 80; LDL below 100 and TG below 150. Record BP and monitor FS at different times during the day and maintain log for provider review.

6. Report any new onset visual changes, SOB, chest pain, significant weight gain or swelling of extremities.

7. Advise there is an increased risk of MI and CV events, especially in long—term users of insulin and those taking nitrates.

8. Must report as scheduled for regular monitoring of renal and LFTs q 2 mo and A1C, as well as BP, foot and eye exams.

OUTCOMES/EVALUATE

- Control of NIDDM by ↓ insulin resistance
- HbA1c <7

Rosuvastatin calcium 📷

(roe-**SUE**-vuh-stah-tin)

CLASSIFICATION(S):
Antihyperlipidemic, HMG-CoA reductase inhibitor
PREGNANCY CATEGORY: X
Rx: Crestor.

SEE ALSO ANTIHYPERLIPIDEMIC AGENTS, HMG-COA REDUCTASE INHIBITOR.

USES

(1) As an adjunct to diet in heterozygous familial and nonfamilial hypercholesterolemia. (2) Adjunct to diet in mixed dyslipidemia (Fredrickson Type IIa and IIb). (3) Adjunct to diet in elevated serum triglyceride levels (Fredrickson type IV). (4) Reduce LDL-C, total-C, and Apo-B in homozygous familial hypercholesterolemia (as an adjunct to other lipid-lowering treatments).

ACTION/KINETICS

Action

Competitively inhibits HMG-CoA reductase; this enzyme catalyzes the early rate-limiting step in the synthesis of cholesterol. Thus, cholesterol synthesis is inhibited/decreased. Reduces total cholesterol, LDL-C, ApoB, and non–HDL-C in clients with homozygous and heterozygous familial hypercholesterolemia, nonfamilial forms of hypercholesterolemia, and mixed dyslipidemia. Also, reduces triglycerides and increases HDL-C.

Pharmacokinetics

Peak plasma levels: 3–5 hr. Absolute bioavailability is about 20%. About 10% metabolized by CYP2C9 to N-desmethyl rosuvastatin which has some activity. Excreted primarily (90%) in the feces. **$t\frac{1}{2}$, elimination:** About 19 hr. Severe renal or hepatic insufficiency significantly increase plasma levels. **Plasma protein binding:** About 95%.

CONTRAINDICATIONS

Pregnancy and lactation. Use in clients with active liver disease or with unex-

---

Bold Italic = life threatening side effect   ■ = black box warning   ♣ = Available in Canada

plained persistent elevations of serum transaminases.

SPECIAL CONCERNS

Use with caution in clients who consume substantial amounts of alcohol and/or have a history of liver disease. Use with caution in those 65 years and older, in hypothyroidism, and renal insufficiency (all predispose clients to myopathy). Cases (rare) of rhabomyolysis with acute renal failure secondary to myoglobinuria have been reported.

SIDE EFFECTS

Most Common

Myalgia, constipation, asthenia, abdominal pain, N&V, headache, diarrhea, dyspepsia, back pain, flu syndrome, UTI.
Musculoskeletal: Rhabdomyolysis with acute renal failure, myalgia, muscle aches/weakness, arthritis, arthralgia, pathological fracture, myasthenia, myositis. **CNS:** Headache, dizziness, insomnia, hypertonia, paresthesia, depression, anxiety, vertigo, neuralgia. **GI:** Diarrhea, dyspepsia, abdominal pain/cramps, N&V, constipation, gastroenteritis, flatulence, periodontal abscess, gastritis, hepatitis, pancreatitis, tooth disorder. **Respiratory:** Pharyngitis, rhinitis, sinusitis, bronchitis, common cold, increased cough, dyspnea, pneumonia, asthma. **CV:** Hypertension. **Dermatologic:** Ecchymosis, rash, pruritus. **Body as a whole:** Asthenia, flu syndrome, accidental injury, infection, pain, peripheral edema, syncope. **CV:** Hypertension, angina pectoris, vasodilation, palpitation, arrhythmia. **Hypersensitivity:** Facial edema, thrombocytopenia, leukopenia, vesiculobullous rash, urticaria, angioedema. **Miscellaneous:** Back/neck/pelvic pain, chest pain, UTI, diabetes mellitus, anemia, kidney damage/failure, organ failure, photosensitivity reaction.

LABORATORY TEST CONSIDERATIONS

↑ Serum transaminases (up to 3 or more times ULN), creatine kinase, bilirubin, glutamyl transpeptidase. Proteinuria, microscopic hematuria, hyperglycemia. Thyroid function abnormalities.

DRUG INTERACTIONS

Amiodarone / Possible ↑ serum transaminase levels

Antacids, Al/Mg combination / ↓ Rosuvastatin levels; give antacid 2 hr after rosuvastatin

Cyclosporine / Significant ↑ of rosuvastatin C_{max} and AUC → ↑ risk of myopathy

Gemfibrozil / Significant ↑ of rosuvastatin C_{max} and AUC → ↑ risk of myopathy

Oral contraceptives / ↑ Levels of ethinyl estradiol and norgestrel

Warfarin / Significant ↑ INR

HOW SUPPLIED

Tablets: 5 mg, 10 mg, 20 mg, 40 mg (all as base).

DOSAGE

- **TABLETS**

Heterozygous familial and nonfamilial hypercholesterolemia, mixed dyslipidemia (Fredrickson Type IIa and IIb).
Individualize therapy. **Initial:** 10 mg once daily (use 5 mg once daily for those requiring less aggressive LDL-C reductions or who have predisposing factors for myopathy). For clients with marked hypercholesterolemia (LDL-C >190 mg/dL) and aggressive lipid targets, consider a 20-mg starting dose. After initiation and/or upon titration, analyze lipid levels within 2 to 4 weeks; adjust dosage accordingly. Reserve the 40-mg dose for those who have not achieved goal LDL-C at 20 mg.

Homozygous familial hypercholesterolemia.
Initial: 20 mg once daily. **Maximum recommended dose:** 40 mg daily. Use as an adjunct to other lipid-lowering treatments. Use rosuvastatin as an adjunct to other lipid-lowering treatments (e.g., LDL apheresis) or if other treatments are not available. *NOTE:* For clients with severe renal impairment (C_{CR} less than 30 mL/min/1.73 m^2 not on hemodialysis), use an initial dose of 5 mg once daily; dosage should not exceed 10 mg once daily in these clients.

NURSING CONSIDERATIONS

ADMINISTRATION/STORAGE

1. Temporarily withhold rosuvastatin in clients with an acute, serious condition suggestive of myopathy or predisposing to the development of renal failure secondary to rhabdomyolysis (e.g., sep-

R

---

sis, hypotension, major surgery, trauma, uncontrolled seizures and severe metabolic, endocrine, and electrolyte disorders).

2. Due to the possibility of myopathy and rhabodmyolysis, reserve 40 mg dose for clients who have not achieved their goal for LDL cholesterol with the 20-mg regimen.

3. Before beginning rosuvastatin therapy, try to control hypercholesterolemia with appropriate diet and exercise, weight reduction in obese clients, and treatment of underlying medical problems. Continue cholesterol-lowering diet during drug treatment.

4. In clients taking cyclosporine, limit the rosuvastatin dose to 5 mg once daily.

5. The effect of rosuvastatin on LDL-C and total cholesterol may be enhanced if used with a bile acid binding resin such as gemfibrozil. If gemfibrozil is used with rosuvastatin, limit the dose of rosuvastatin to 10 mg once daily.

6. In Asian clients, initiate therapy with 5 mg once daily.

7. Consider dose reduction in clients on 40 mg rosuvastatin therapy with unexplained persistent proteinuria during routine urinalysis.

8. Store at controlled room temperature (20–25°C; 68–77°F) protected from moisture.

ASSESSMENT

1. Note reasons for therapy: plaque stability or elevated TG/LDL cholesterol in CAD. Review risk factors and family history.

2. Monitor CBC, lipid profile, TSH, renal, CPK, and LFTs. Schedule LFTs at the beginning of therapy, in 3 mo and semi-annually for the first year of therapy. Special attention should be paid to elevated serum transaminase and CK levels.

3. List all medications prescribed to ensure none interact unfavorably.

4. Assess adherence to weight reduction, exercise, cholesterol-lowering diet and BP/BS control. Note any alcohol abuse; liver or renal dysfunction.

CLIENT/FAMILY TEACHING

1. Take once daily with or without food as directed. Do not use antacid for 2 hr after consuming drug.

2. Report any S&S of infections, unexplained muscle pain, tenderness/weakness (especially if accompanied by fever or malaise), surgery, trauma, or metabolic disorders as drug should be stopped.

3. Review importance of following a low-cholesterol diet, regular exercise, low alcohol consumption, and not smoking in the overall plan to reduce serum cholesterol levels and inhibit progression of CAD.

4. Not for use during pregnancy; use barrier contraception.

5. Report for F/U labs and to assess drug response.

OUTCOMES/EVALUATE

↓ Total and LDL cholesterol

Rotigotine

(roe-**TIG**-oh-teen)

CLASSIFICATION(S):

Antiparkinson drug.

PREGNANCY CATEGORY: C

Rx: Neupro.

USES

Treat signs and symptoms of early-stage idiopathic Parkinson's disease.

ACTION/KINETICS

Action

Rotigotine is a dopamine agonist. Mechanism is unknownn but is thought to be due to stimulation of dopamine D_2 receptors within the caudate-putamen in the brain.

Pharmacokinetics

About 45% of the drug from the patch is released within 24 hr. When a 40 cm^2 system is applied, about 3 hr elapses before drug is detected in the plasma. $t\frac{1}{2}$, **initial:** 3 hr; **terminal:** 5–7 hr. T_{max}: 15–18 hr range: 4-27 hr) post-dose. Steady-state plasma levels reached in 2–3 days. Application to the shoulder shows the highest bioavailability. Extensively metabolized in the liver and primarily excreted in the urine.

CONTRAINDICATIONS

Hypersensitivity to rotigotine or components of the transdermal system (e.g., metasulfite). Lactation. Use in pregnancy unless the potential benefits outweigh the potential risk to the fetus.

SPECIAL CONCERNS

No dosage adjustment is needed in clients with moderately impaired hepatic function or in those with severe renal impairment not on dialysis. Levels may be higher in older clients due to skin changes with aging. Falling asleep may occur with no warning signs (e.g., excessive drowsiness) that may occur as late as one year after initiation of treatment; clients believed they were alert immediately prior to the event. Safety and efficacy have not been demonstrated in children.

SIDE EFFECTS

Most Common

N&V, application site reaction, somnolence, dizziness, headache, insomnia.

CNS: Somnolence (e.g., falling asleep while engaged in activities of daily living), dizziness, headache, insomnia, hallucinations, dyskinesia, vertigo, abnormal dreaming, depression, tremor, anxiety, hyper-/hypoesthesia, paresthesia, confusion, ataxia, abnormal gait, neuralgia, hypertonia, paranoid reaction, psychosis, **convulsions** (rare). **GI:** N&V, dry mouth, constipation, dyspepsia, anorexia, diarrhea, abdominal pain, increased salivation/appetite. **CV:** Postural hypotension, edema of the extremities, hypertension, syncope, increased HR/BP, AV block, BBB, atrial fibrillation, purpura, **cardiac failure** (rare), **ventricular tachycardia**/arrhythmia (rare). **Musculoskeletal:** Back/leg pain, arthralgia, chest pain, myalgia. **Respiratory:** Sinusitis, rhinitis, URTI, coughing. **Dermatologic:** Increased sweating, erythematous rash, contact dermatitis, flushing, hot flushes, pruritus, melanoma (may be due to the disease). **GU:** UTI, micturition frequency, urinary incontinence, impotence. **Hematologic:** Thrombocytopenia (rare). **Application site reactions:** Localized erythema, edema, pruritus, allergic rash. **Ophthalmic:** Abnormal vision, photopsia. **Body as a whole:** Fatigue, accidents, weight gain/loss, fluid retention, asthenia, flu-like symptoms, malaise, fever, rigors, **allergic reaction. Miscellaneous:** Falls, tinnitus.

LABORATORY TEST CONSIDERATIONS

↑ BUN. ↓ Prolactin secretion (may inhibit lactation), hemoglobin, blood glucose.

DRUG INTERACTIONS

Antipsychotic drugs (i.e., dopamine antagonists) / Possible ↓ effectiveness of rotigotine

Metoclopramide / Possible ↓ effectiveness of rotigotine

HOW SUPPLIED

Transdermal System: 10 cm^2 (releases 2 mg/24 hr), 20 cm^2 (releases 4 mg/24 hr), 30 cm^2 (releases 6 mg/24 hr).

DOSAGE

- **TRANSDERMAL SYSTEM**
  Parkinson's disease.

Initial: 2 mg/24 hr. Based on client response and tolerance, dose may be increased weekly by 2 mg/24 hr. The lowest effective dose is 4 mg/24 hr; the highest recommended dose is 6 mg/24 hr.

NURSING CONSIDERATIONS

ADMINISTRATION/STORAGE

1. Daily rotation of application sites reduces the incidence of application site reactions.

2. To avoid skin burns due to the aluminum backing layer of the product, remove the patch before magnetic resonance imaging or cardioversion.

3. Although neuroleptic malignant syndrome has not been seen with rotigotine, taper dose at the end of rotigotine treatment as a prophylactic measure.

4. If dose reduction is necessary, discontinue gradually. Reduce the daily dose by 2 mg/24 hr with a dose reduction preferably every other day until complete withdrawal of the drug.

5. Store from 15–30°C (59–86°F). Store in the original pouch.

ASSESSMENT

1. Note onset, assess condition and document baseline rigidity, tremors,

 = see color insert   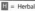 = Herbal   **IV** = Intravenous   = sound alike drug motor function, and involuntary movements r/t Parkinson's disease. Note mental status.

2. Drug contains sodium metabisulfite; may cause allergic-type reactions

3. Check BP; monitor for S&S postural hypotension, esp. during dose increases.

4. Monitor for melanoma.

CLIENT/FAMILY TEACHING

1. Apply the patch immediately upon removal from the pouch. Do not cut or damage the patch. Press system in place for 20 to 30 seconds.

2. Wash hands after applying patch; avoid touching eyes.

3. Wear patch continuously for 24 hr and apply at the same time each day. Do not apply creams, lotions, ointments, oils, or powders to skin area where applying patch.

4. Apply the adhesive side of the transdermal system to clean, dry, intact skin on the front of the abdomen, thigh, hip, flank, shoulder, or upper arm. Avoid applying on skin folds. If applying patch to a hairy area, must shave area at least 3 days prior to application. Do not apply to skin that is oily, irritated, or damaged, or where it will rub against tight clothing.

5. Rotate site on a daily basis, do not use the same site more than once every 14 days.

6. While showering/bathing, or during physical activity take care to avoid dislodging patch. If it becomes dislodged or you forget to replace patch, apply another for remainder of the day.

7. Remove patch prior to MRI or cardioversion; may cause skin burn.

8. Use caution while driving, operating machinery, or working at heights; drug had sedative effects. Some have reported suddenly falling asleep while engaged in activities of daily living, including operation of motor vehicles.

9. Heat application increases the absorption of rotigotine several fold. Avoid exposing patch to external sources of direct heat, such as heating pads, electric blankets, heat lamps, saunas, hot tubs, heated water beds, and prolonged direct sunlight.

10. When changing positions use care to prevent sudden drop in BP.

11. Report any changes in color or size of moles; melanoma has occurred and requires skin monitoring.

12. Keep all F/U appointments to evaluate response to therapy and for any adverse effects.

OUTCOMES/EVALUATE

Control of parkinsonian symptoms (e.g., improvement in motor function, physical mobility, reflexes, gait, strength of grip, and amount of tremor)

Salmeterol xinafoate

(sal-**MET**-er-ole)

CLASSIFICATION(S):
Sympathomimetic
PREGNANCY CATEGORY: C
Rx: Serevent Diskus.

SEE ALSO SYMPATHOMIMETIC DRUGS.

USES

(1) Long-term (twice daily) maintenance treatment of asthma or in the prevention of bronchospasm in clients 4 years and older with reversible obstructive airway disease. Includes those with symptoms of nocturnal asthma. (2) Chronic maintenance (twice daily) treatment of bronchospasms associated with COPD, including emphysema and chronic bronchitis. (3) Prevention of exercise-induced bronchospasm in clients 4 years of age and older.

Bold Italic = life threatening side effect   ■ = black box warning   ✦ = Available in Canada

ACTION/KINETICS

Action

Selective for beta$_2$-adrenergic receptors located in the bronchi and heart. Acts by stimulating intracellular adenyl cyclase, the enzyme that converts ATP to cyclic AMP. Increased AMP levels cause relaxation of bronchial smooth muscle and inhibition of release of mediators of immediate hypersensitivity, especially from mast cells.

Pharmacokinetics

Onset: Within 20 min. **Duration:** 12 hr. Cleared by hepatic metabolism. **Plasma protein binding:** Significantly bound.

CONTRAINDICATIONS

Use in clients who can be controlled by short-acting, inhaled beta$_2$-agonists or in those whose asthma can be successfully managed by inhaled corticosteroids or other controller medications, along with occasional use of inhaled, short-acting beta$_2$ agonists. Use to treat acute symptoms of asthma or in those who have worsening or deteriorating asthma. Lactation.

SPECIAL CONCERNS

■ Long-acting beta$_2$-adrenergic agonists, such as salmeterol, may increase the risk of asthma-related death. Therefore, when treating clients with asthma, salmeterol should only be used as additional therapy for clients not adequately controlled on other asthma-controller medications (e.g., low-to medium-dose inhaled corticosteroids) or whose disease severity clearly warrants initiation of treatment with two maintenance therapies, including salmeterol.■ Not a substitute for PO or inhaled corticosteroids. The safety and efficacy of using salmeterol with a spacer or other devices has not been studied adequately. Use with caution in impaired hepatic function; with cardiovascular disorders, including coronary insufficiency, cardiac arrhythmias, and hypertension; with convulsive disorders or thyrotoxicosis; and in clients who respond unusually to sympathomimetic amines. Because of the potential of the drug interfering with uterine contractility, use of salmeterol during labor should be restricted to those in whom benefits clearly outweigh risks. Safety and efficacy have not been determined in children less than 12 years of age.

SIDE EFFECTS

Most Common

Palpitations, tachycardia, tremor, dizziness/vertigo, nervousness, headache, N&V, heartburn, diarrhea, cough, dry/irritated throat, pharyngitis.

Respiratory: *Paradoxical bronchospasms*, upper or lower respiratory tract infection, nasopharyngitis, nasal cavity/sinus disease, dry/irritated throat, sinus headache, cough, pharyngitis, allergic rhinitis, rhinitis, laryngitis, tracheitis, bronchitis, *increased risk of severe, fatal asthma episodes*. **Allergic:** *Immediate hypersensitivity reactions*, including urticaria, rash, and *bronchospasm*. **CV:** Palpitations, chest pain, increased BP, tachycardia. **CNS:** Headache, sinus headache, tremors, nervousness, malaise, fatigue, dizziness/vertigo, giddiness. **GI:** N&V, diarrhea, heartburn, stomach ache, viral gastroenteritis. **Dermatologic:** Skin eruption, urticaria, rash. **Musculoskeletal:** Joint/back pain, muscle cramps/contractions/soreness, myalgia, myositis. **Miscellaneous:** Flu, dental pain, dysmenorrhea.

LABORATORY TEST CONSIDERATIONS

↓ Serum potassium.

OD OVERDOSE MANAGEMENT

Symptoms: Tachycardia, arrhythmia, tremors, headache, muscle cramps, hypokalemia, hyperglycemia. *Treatment:* Supportive therapy. Consider judicious use of a beta-adrenergic blocking agent, although these drugs can cause bronchospasms. Cardiac monitoring is necessary. Dialysis is not an appropriate treatment of overdosage.

DRUG INTERACTIONS

Diuretics / Worsening of diuretic-induced ECG changes and hypokalemia
MAO Inhibitors / ↑ Salmeterol effect
Tricyclic antidepressants / ↑ Salmeterol effect

HOW SUPPLIED

Powder for Inhalation: 50 mcg (base)/inhalation.

DOSAGE

• **POWDER FOR INHALATION**

Bronchospasm, asthma, including nocturnal asthma.

Adults and children 4 years and over:
1 inhalation (50 mcg) twice a day (morning and evening, approximately 12 hr apart). If a previously effective dose fails to provide the usual response, seek medical advice immediately as this is often a sign of destabilization of asthma. If symptoms arise in the period between doses, use a short-acting, inhaled beta₂-agonist for immediate relief.

COPD.

Adults: One inhalation (50 mcg) of the powder twice a day in the morning and evening (about 12 hr apart).

Prevention of exercise-induced bronchospasms.

Adults and children over 4 years of age: 1 inhalation (50 mcg) at least 30 min before exercise. Protection may last up to 9 hr in adolescents and adults and up to 12 hr in those 4–11 years of age. Additional doses should not be used for 12 hr. In those who are receiving salmeterol twice daily, do not use additional salmeterol for prevention of exercise-induced bronchospasm.

NURSING CONSIDERATIONS

⊚ Do not confuse Serevent with Serentil (an antipsychotic).

ADMINISTRATION/STORAGE

1. Ensure doses are spaced 12 hr apart. Side effects are more likely to occur with higher doses or more frequent administration.

2. The safety of more than 8 inhalations per day of short-acting beta₂-agonists with salmeterol has not been established. If a previously effective dose fails to provide the usual response, contact provider immediately.

3. Do not exhale into the inhalation device; only activate and use the inhalation device in a level, horizontal position. Do not use a spacer.

4. Store the inhalation powder from 20–25°C (68–77°F) in a dry place away from direct heat or sunlight. Keep the mouthpiece dry and never wash the mouthpiece or any part of the device.

5. For the inhalation of powder (Diskus), a built-in dose counter shows the number of doses remaining. The inhalation device is not reusable; discard after every blister has been used or 6 weeks after removal from the moisture-protective foil overwrap, whichever comes first.

ASSESSMENT

1. Note onset, duration, characteristics of S&S; list agents trialed, outcome.

2. Assess for cardiac/liver dysfunction, thyrotoxicosis, hypertension, seizure disorders; may preclude therapy.

3. Review CXR and cardiopulmonary findings. Monitor VS, lung sounds, liver enzymes, lytes, PFTs (ABGs, FEV).

CLIENT/FAMILY TEACHING

1. Review proper use (with actuator) and obtain instruction. Shake well. Use the inhalation device in a level, horizontal position. Do not use a spacer. Record peak flows and identify critical zones.

2. Use only as directed; do not exceed prescribed dosage and administration frequency (drug effects last 12 hr).

3. Do not use drug during an acute asthma attack.

4. Review procedure for use of the short-acting beta₂-agonist (i.e., albuterol) prescribed to treat symptoms of asthma that occur between the salmeterol dosing schedule. Increased utilization warrants medical evaluation.

5. May experience palpitations, chest pain, headaches, tremors, nervousness, dizziness, drowsiness as side effects. Report immediately if chest pain, fast pounding irregular heartbeat, hives, increased wheezing, or difficulty breathing occurs.

6. Acetaminophen or other analgesic may relieve drug related headaches.

7. Take 30–60 min before activity to prevent acute bronchospasms. If already prescribed twice daily, do not take additional dose before exercise.

8. Salmeterol does not replace inhaled or systemic steroids; do not stop prescribed steroid therapy abruptly without approval.

9. Identify appropriate support groups that may assist to cope and live a normal life with asthma.

10. Stop smoking; avoid smoky environments and any other triggers that

---

Bold Italic = life threatening side effect   ▋ = black box warning   ♣ = Available in Canada may aggravate breathing condition. Keep all F/U appointments.

OUTCOMES/EVALUATE

- Prevention/control of bronchospasm with COPD and asthma (e.g., decreased wheezing, dyspnea, orthopnea, and cough)
- Prevention of exercise-induced bronchospasms

Saquinavir mesylate
(sah-**KWIN**-ah-veer)

CLASSIFICATION(S):
Antiviral, protease inhibitor
PREGNANCY CATEGORY: B
Rx: Fortovase, Invirase.

SEE ALSO *ANTIVIRAL DRUGS.*

USES

Combined with ritonavir and other antiretroviral drugs to treat HIV infections in selected clients. *NOTE:* Use only combined with ritonavir which significantly inhibits metabolism of saquinavir, thus providing saquinavir plasma levels at least equal to those achieved with saquinavir soft gelatin capsules. (Fortovase [soft gelatin capsules] has been withdrawn from the market.)

ACTION/KINETICS

Action

HIV protease cleaves viral polyprotein precursors to form functional proteins in HIV-infected cells. Cleavage of viral polyprotein precursors is required for maturation of the infectious virus. Saquinavir inhibits the activity of HIV protease and prevents the cleavage of viral polyproteins.

Pharmacokinetics

Has a low bioavailability after PO use, probably due to incomplete absorption and first-pass metabolism. A high-fat meal or high-calorie meal increases the amount of drug absorbed. Women have a higher AUC than men. About 87% metabolized in the liver mainly by the CYP3A4. Saquinavir is also a substrate for P-glycoprotein; thus drugs that affect CYP3A4 or P-glycoprotein may change the pharmacokinetics of

saquinavir. Both metabolites and unchanged drug are excreted mainly through the feces. **Plasma protein binding:** More than 98%.

CONTRAINDICATIONS

Hypersensitivity to saquinavir or any component of the product. Use in severe hepatic impairment. Use with antiarrhythmics (amiodarone, flecainide, propafenone, or quinidine), ergot derivatives (ergonovine, ergotamine, dihydroergotamine, or methylergonovine), rifampin, pimozide, midazolam, triazolam. Lactation.

SPECIAL CONCERNS

Photoallergy or phototoxicity may occur; take protective measures against exposure to ultraviolet or sunlight until tolerance is assessed. Use with caution in those with hepatic insufficiency and in the elderly. Hemophiliacs treated with protease inhibitors for HIV infections may manifest spontaneous bleeding episodes. Cross resistance is possible among protease inhibitors. Safety and efficacy have not been determined in HIV-infected children or adolescents less than 16 years of age. Fortovase is not interchangeable with Invirase.

SIDE EFFECTS

Most Common

N&V, fatigue, diarrhea, abdominal pain, pneumonia, pruritus, rash, fever, hyperglycemia, bronchitis, influenza, sinusitis.
GI: N&V, constipation, diarrhea, abdominal pain, dry mouth, dyspepsia, dysphagia, esophagitis, eructation, flatulence, gastralgia, gastritis, GI inflammation, gingivitis, glossitis, rectal hemorrhage, hemorrhoids, infectious diarrhea, melena, bloodstained feces, frequent bowel movements, cheilitis, abdominal colic, pelvic pain, painful defecation, pancreatitis, parotid disorder, salivary glands disorder, stomach upset, stomatitis, toothache, tooth disorder. **Hepatic:** Hepatitis, hepatomegaly, hepatosplenomegaly, jaundice, liver enzyme disorder. **CNS:** Agitation, amnesia, anxiety, depression, excessive dreaming, euphoria, hallucinations, insomnia, decreased intellectual ability, irritability, lethargy, libido disorder, psychosis, somnolence, speech disorder, *suicide*

S

attempt, ataxia, confusion, convulsions, dysarthria, dysesthesia, facial numbness, hyperesthesia, hyper-/hyporeflexia, lightheadedness, myelopolyradiculoneuritis, paresis, poliomyelitis, prickly sensation, progressive multifocal leukoencephalopathy, spasms, tremor, unconsciousness. **CV:** Cyanosis, heart murmur, heart rate/heart valve disorder, hyper-/hypotension, syncope, vein distended. **Dermatologic:** Acne, dry lips/skin, pruritus, rash, alopecia, chalazion, dermatitis, eczema, erythema, folliculitis, furunculosis, hair changes, hot flushes, maculopapular rash, nail disorder, papillomatosis, photosensitivity reaction, seborrheic dermatitis, skin disorder/nodule/pigment changes, skin ulceration, increased sweating, urticaria, verruca, xeroderma. **GU:** Impotence, enlarged prostate, vaginal discharge. **Musculoskeletal:** Arthralgia, arthritis, back pain, leg cramps, facial pain, generalized weakness, muscle cramps, musculoskeletal disorders, stiffness, tissue changes, trauma. **Respiratory:** Bronchitis, cough, dyspnea, epsitaxis, hemoptysis, laryngitis, pharyngitis, pneumonia, pulmonary disease, respiratory disorder, rhinitis, sinusitis, URTI. **Hematologic:** Thrombocytopenia, anemia, leukopenia, neutropenia, dermal bleeding, microhemorrhages, pancytopenia, splenomegaly. **Metabolic:** Dehydration, diabetes mellitus, hyperglycemia, weight decrease/increase, lipodystrophy. **Ophthalmic:** Blepharitis, dry eye syndrome, eye irritation, visual disturbance, xerophthalmia. **Otic:** Decreased hearing, earache, ear pressure, otitis, tinnitus. **Body as a whole:** Allergic reaction, edema, fatigue, influenza, fever, intoxication, shivering, wasting syndrome. **Miscellaneous:** Taste alteration, anorexia, chest pain, external parasites, night sweats, redistribution/accumulation of body fat, retrosternal pain.

LABORATORY TEST CONSIDERATIONS

↑ ALT, AST, GGT, TSH, amylase, lactic dehydrogenase, creatine phosphokinase. Hyper-/hypoglycemia, hypertriglyceridemia, hypocalcemia, hypophosphatemia, hyper-/hypokalemia, hyper-/hyponatremia, hyperbilirubinemia.

DRUG INTERACTIONS

Aldesleukin / ↑ Saquinavir levels; ↑ risk of toxicity

Amiodarone / Use together contraindicated due to potential for serious and/or life-threatening side effects

Amitriptyline / ↑ Amitriptyline levels; monitor

Atorvastatin / ↑ Atorvastatin AUC when given with ritonavir and saquinavir

Benzodiazepines (alprazolam, clorazepate, diazepam, flurazepam) / ↑ Benzodiazepine levels; ↓ dose may be needed

Bepridil / Use together contraindicated due to potential for serious and/or life-threatening side effects

Calcium channel blockers (all) / ↑ Calcium channel blocker levels; use caution and monitor

Carbamazepine / ↓ Saquinavir blood levels R/T ↑ metabolism

Cimetidine / ↑ Saquinavir AUC and peak plasma levels R/T inhibition of CYP3A4 metabolism

Clarithromycin / ↑ Blood levels of both drugs and ↓ levels of 14-OH clarithromycin (active); no dosage adjustment needed when given together for a limited time

Cyclosporine / Significant ↑ cyclosporine blood levels; monitor levels

Delaviridine / Significant ↑ in saquinavir plasma AUC

Dexamethasone / ↓ Saquinavir blood levels; use with caution

Efavirenz / ↓ Saquinavirs and efavirenz blood levels

Ergot derivatives (dihydroergotamine, ergonovine, ergotamine, methylergonovine) / Possibility of serious and life-threatening reactions, including acute ergot toxicity (peripheral vasospasm and ischemia of the extremities and other tissues)

Fentanyl / ↑ Fentanyl plasma levels → ↑ risk of side effects, including respiratory depression

Flecainide / Use together contraindicated due to potential for serious and/or life-threatening side effects

Fluconazole / ↑ Saquinavir plasma levels R/T ↓ metabolism

Bold Italic = life threatening side effect   ■ = black box warning   ♣ = Available in Canada

H *Garlic (capsules)* / ↓ Saquinavir plasma levels; do not use if taking saquinavir as the sole protease inhibitor
Grapefruit juice / ↑ Bioavailability and blood levels of saquinavir R/T inhibition of metabolism by CYP3A4
HMG-CoA reductase inhibitors / Potential for serious side effects (↑ risk of myopathy, including rhabdomyolysis); do not use together
Imipramine / ↑ Imipramine levels; monitor
Indinavir / ↑ Saquinavir blood levels
Itraconazole / ↑ Saquinavir blood levels R/T ↓ metabolism
Ketoconazole / ↑ Saquinavir blood levels R/T ↓ metabolism
Levothyroxine / ↑ Thyroxine levels → hyperthyroidism
Lidocaine / ↑ Lidocaine levels; use with caution and monitor levels
Loperamide / ↑ Loperamide plasma levels and ↓ saquinavir plasma levels R/T ↓ saquinavir absorption
Methadone / ↓ Methadone levels; may need to ↑ methadone dosage when given with saquinavir/ritonavir
Midazolam / Possible serious and/or life-threatening side effects, such as prolonged or increased sedation or respiratory depression; do not use together
Nelfinavir / ↑ Saquinavir and nelfinavir blood levels
Nevirapine / ↓ Saquinavir blood levels
Oral contraceptives containing ethinyl estradiol / ↓ Ethinyl estradiol levels; use alternative or additional contraception
Phenobarbital / ↓ Saquinavir blood levels R/T ↑ metabolism
Phenytoin / ↓ Saquinavir blood levels R/T ↑ metabolism
Pravastatin / ↓ Pravastatin AUC when given with ritonavir and saquinavir
Propafenone / Use together contraindicated due to potential for serious and/or life-threatening side effects
Quinidine / Use together contraindicated due to potential for serious and/or life-threatening side effects
Rifabutin / ↓ Saquinavir and rifabutin levels; do not use together
Rifampin / ↓ Saquinavir blood levels and ↑ rifampin levels. Also, ↑ risk of hepatitis; rifampin is contraindicated in those

taking ritonavir, 100 mg/saquinavir, 1,000 mg twice daily
Risperidone / ↑ Risperidone plasma levels; ↑ risk of toxicity
Ritonavir / ↑ Saquinavir blood levels R/T inhibition of metabolism; must be used together
Sildenafil / ↑ Sildenafil plasma levels; use sildenafil with caution at ↓ doses of 25 mg q 48 hr; monitor
Simvastatin / ↑ Simvastatin AUC when given with ritonavir and saquinavir
H *St. John's wort* / ↓ Saquinavir plasma levels R/T ↑ CYP3A4 metabolism; do not use together
Tadalafil / ↑ Tadalafil plasma levels; use tadalafil with caution at ↓ doses of no more than 10 mg q 72 hr; monitor
Tacrolimus / ↑ Tacrolimus levels; monitor levels
Trazodone / ↑ Trazodone levels
Triazolam / Possible serious and/or life-threatening side effects, such as prolonged or increased sedation or respiratory depression; do not use together
Vardenafil / ↑ Vardenafil plasma levels; use vardenafil with caution at ↓ doses of 2.5 mg q 72 hr; monitor
Warfarin / Warfarin levels may be affected; monitor INR

HOW SUPPLIED
Capsules: 200 mg (as mesylate); *Tablets:* 500 mg (as mesylate).

DOSAGE————————————
* **CAPSULES; TABLETS**
  HIV infection, saquinavir given with ritonavir.
Adults, age 16 years and older: Saquinavir 1,000 mg twice a day (5 x 200 mg capsules) in combination with ritonavir 100 mg twice a day. Take ritonavir at the same time as saquinavir and within 2 hr of a meal.

NURSING CONSIDERATIONS
ADMINISTRATION/STORAGE
1. Take within 2 hr of a full meal. If taken without food, blood levels may not be sufficiently high to exert an antiviral effect.
2. Doses less than 200 mg 3 times per day are not recommended; lower doses have not shown antiviral activity.

S

3. Interrupt therapy for serious toxicities associated with saquinavir mesylate. Base dosage adjustments on the known toxicity profile of the individual agent and the pharmacokinetic interaction between saquiniavir and the coadministered drug. Doses of saquinavir mesylate less than 1,000 mg with ritonavir 100 mg twice a day are not recommended since lower doses do not have antiviral activity.

4. Store Invirase from 15–30°C (59–86°F) in tightly closed bottles.

ASSESSMENT

1. Note onset, duration, characteristics of S&S.

2. Monitor CBC, T-lymphocytes/viral load, renal and LFTs.

3. List drugs currently prescribed; drug is metabolized hepatically via cytochrome P450 system.

4. If serious or severe toxicity occurs, stop therapy until cause determined or toxicity resolves. Monitor for opportunistic infections; treat appropriately.

CLIENT/FAMILY TEACHING

1. Take only as prescribed and within 2 hr of a full meal; blood levels markedly reduced when taken without food. Invirase and fortanase are not interchangeable; dosage differs.

2. Drug is not a cure for HIV infections. It does not prevent the occurrence or decrease the frequency of opportunistic infections associated with HIV but may prolong life.

3. Avoid sun exposure; take protective measures against UV or sunlight until tolerance assessed.

4. Continue to use barrier contraception and safe sex; drug does not inhibit disease transmission.

5. Long-term drug effects still unknown; report side effects. May use analgesics, antidiarrheal, or antiemetics as prescribed/needed. Avoid any unprescribed or OTC agents; viagra may cause adverse side effects, visual changes, and low BP. If needed use once every 2 days and in doses not exceeding 25 mg.

OUTCOMES/EVALUATE

Control of progression of HIV infections

Sargramostim   IV
(sar-**GRAM**-oh-stim)

CLASSIFICATION(S):
Granulocyte colony-stimulating factor, human
PREGNANCY CATEGORY: C
Rx: Leukine.

USES
(1) Increase myeloid recovery in clients with non-Hodgkin's lymphoma, ALL, and Hodgkin's disease undergoing autologous bone marrow transplantation. (2) Bone marrow transplantation failure or engraftment delay. (3) Shorten recovery time to neutrophil recovery and to decrease the incidence of severe and life-threatening infections in older adult clients with AML. Safety and efficacy have not been determined in those less than 55 years of age. (4) Mobilize hematopoietic progenitor cells into peripheral blood collection by leukapheresis. (5) Acceleration of myeloid recovery in allogeneic bone marrow transplantation from human lymphocyte antigen-matched related donors. *Investigational:* Increase WBC counts in clients with myelodysplastic syndrome and in AIDS clients taking AZT; correct neutropenia in clients with aplastic anemia; decrease the nadir of leukopenia secondary to myelosuppressive chemotherapy and decrease myelosuppression in preleukemic clients; and, decrease organ system damage following transplantation, especially in the liver and kidney.

ACTION/KINETICS
Action
A granulocyte-macrophage colony-stimulating factor (rhu GM-CSF) that stimulates the proliferation and differentiation of hematopoietic progenitor cells. It stimulates partially committed progenitor cells to divide and differentiate in the granulocyte-macrophage pathways. Division, maturation, and activation are induced through GM-CSF binding to specific receptors located on the surface of target cells. Also activates mature granulocytes and macrophages.

Bold Italic = life threatening side effect   ■ = black box warning   ♣ = Available in Canada

Increases the cytotoxicity of monocytes toward certain neoplastic cell lines as well as activates polymorphonuclear neutrophils, thus inhibiting the growth of tumor cells. Sargramostim differs from the naturally occurring GM-CSF by one amino acid and by a different carbohydrate moiety.

Pharmacokinetics

Peak levels: 2–3 hr, depending on the dose. **t½, initial:** 12–17 min; **t½, terminal:** 1.6–2.6 hr, depending on the dose. Neutralizing antibodies have been detected in a small number of clients.

CONTRAINDICATIONS

Use in more than 10% leukemic myeloid blasts in the bone marrow or peripheral blood. Known hypersensitivity to GM-CSF, yeast-derived products, or any component of the product. Simultaneous use with cytotoxic chemotherapy or radiotherapy or use within 24 hr preceding or following chemotherapy or radiotherapy.

SPECIAL CONCERNS

Use with caution in clients with preexisting cardiac disease and hypoxia and during lactation. Safety and effectiveness have not been determined in children although it appears the drug is no more toxic in children than in adults. May aggravate fluid retention in clients with preexisting peripheral edema, or pleural or pericardial effusion. Insufficient data on effectiveness of sargramostim in increasing myeloid recovery after peripheral blood stem cell transplantation. It is possible that sargramostim can act as a growth factor for any tumor type, especially myeloid malignancies; thus, use with caution in any malignancy with myeloid characteristics.

SIDE EFFECTS

Most Common

Hypertension, hemorrhage, headache, rash, alopecia, N&V, diarrhea, abdominal pain, bone pain, GI disorder, stomatitis, anorexia, GI hemorrhage, blood dyscrasias, dyspnea, fever, mucous membrane disorder, malaise, weight loss, chills, asthenia, edema, myalgia, increased glucose.

First-dose effects (rare): Respiratory distress, hypoxia, flushing, hypotension, syncope, tachycardia. **CV:** Hyper-/hypotension, *hemorrhage*, edema, peripheral edema, cardiac event, tachycardia, pericardial effusion, pleural effusion, *capillary leak syndrome*, transient supraventricular arrhythmia, tachycardia, thrombosis. **GI:** N&V, diarrhea, abdominal pain, GI disorder, stomatitis, dyspepsia, anorexia, hematemesis, dysphagia, *GI hemorrhage*, constipation, abdominal distension, liver damage. **CNS:** Neuroclinical, neuromotor, neuropsychiatric, and neurosensory side effects. Paresthesia, headache, CNS disorder, insomnia, anxiety, fainting, dizziness. **Respiratory:** Pulmonary event, pharyngitis, lung disorder, epistaxis, dyspnea, rhinitis. **Hematologic:** Blood dyscrasias, thrombocytopenia, leukopenia, petechia, agranulocytosis, coagulation disorders, eosinophilia. **Musculoskeletal:** Bone pain, arthralgia. **Dermatologic:** Rash, alopecia, pruritus, sweating. **GU:** Urinary tract disorder, hematuria, abnormal kidney function. **Body as a whole:** Asthenia, fever, infection, malaise, weight loss/gain, chills, pain, allergy, edema, mucous membrane disorder, metabolic disorder, *sepsis, hypersensitivity reactions including anaphylaxis*. **Miscellaneous:** Chest/back/joint pain, eye hemorrhage, peripheral edema, injection site reactions.

LABORATORY TEST CONSIDERATIONS

↑ Glucose, BUN, cholesterol, bilirubin, serum creatinine, ALT, alkaline phosphatase. ↓ Albumin, calcium. Hypomagnesemia. Transient liver function abnormalities.

OD OVERDOSE MANAGEMENT

Symptoms: Dyspnea, malaise, nausea, fever, rash, sinus tachycardia, chills, headache. *Treatment:* Discontinue therapy. Monitor for increases in WBCs and for respiratory symptoms.

DRUG INTERACTIONS

Drugs such as corticosteroids and lithium may ↑ the myeloproliferative effects of sargramostim. The effect of sargramostim may be limited in those who have received alkylating agents, anthracycline antibiotics, or antimetabolites.

S

📷 = see color insert   H = Herbal   IV = Intravenous   ℂ = sound alike drug

HOW SUPPLIED

Injection: 500 mcg/mL; *Powder for Injection, Lyophilized:* 250 mcg.

DOSAGE

- **IV INFUSION; SC**

  Myeloid reconstitution after autologous or allogenic bone marrow transplantation.

250 mcg/m²/day as a 2-hr infusion beginning 2–4 hr after the autologous bone marrow infusion and greater than 24 hr after the last dose of chemotherapy and 12 hr after the last dose of radiotherapy. Do not give drug until the postmarrow infusion absolute neutrophil count (ANC) is less than 500 cells/mm³. Continue until ANC is >1,500 cells/mm³ for 3 consecutive days. To avoid complications of excessive leukocytosis, a CBC with differential is recommended twice weekly during therapy; interrupt or reduce the dose by 50% if the ANC >20,000 cells/mm³.

  Bone marrow transplantation failure or engraftment delay.

250 mcg/m²/day for 14 days as a 2-hr IV infusion. If engraftment has not occurred, therapy may be repeated after 7 days off therapy. A third course of 250 mcg/m²/day may be undertaken after another 7 days off therapy. However, if no response occurs after three courses, it is unlikely the drug will be beneficial. To avoid complications of excessive leukocytosis, a CBC with differential is recommended twice weekly during therapy; interrupt or reduce the dose by 50% if the ANC >20,000 cells/mm³.

  Neutrophil recovery following chemotherapy in acute myelogenous leukemia.

250 mcg/m²/day given over a 4-hr period starting at about day 11 or 4 days following completion of induction chemotherapy. Use if the day 10 bone marrow is hypoplastic with less than 5% blasts. If a second cycle of therapy is needed, give about 4 days after the completion of chemotherapy if the bone marrow is hypoplastic with less than 5% blasts. Continue therapy until an absolute neutrophil count >1,500/mm³ is noted for 3 consecutive days or a maximum of 42 days. If a severe ad-

verse reaction occurs, decrease the dose by 50% or discontinue temporarily until the drug reaction is reduced. To avoid complications of excessive leukocytosis, a CBC with differential is recommended twice weekly during therapy; interrupt or reduce the dose by 50% if the ANC >20,000 cells/mm³.

  Mobilization of peripheral blood progenitor cells (PBPCs).

250 mcg/m²/day IV over 24 hr or SC once daily. Use this dose throughout the PBPC collection period. If the WBC count is >50,000 cells/mm³, reduce the dose by 50%. If sufficient numbers of progenitor cells are not collected, use other mobilization therapy.

  Postperipheral blood progenitor cell transplantation.

250 mcg/m²/day IV over 24 hr or SC once daily beginning immediately after infusion of progenitor cells and continuing until an absolute neutrophil count >1,500 is reached for 3 consecutive days.

NURSING CONSIDERATIONS

ADMINISTRATION/STORAGE

1. Use for SC injection with no further dilution.

IV 2. Give daily dosage as a 2-hr IV infusion beginning 2–4 hr after the autologous bone marrow infusion. Ensure at least 24 hr have elapsed after last dose of chemotherapy and 12 hr elapsed since the last dose of XRT.

3. Reduce dose or discontinue if severe adverse reactions occur; may resume once reactions abate.

4. Reconstitute lyophilized powder with 1 mL of sterile water for injection without preservatives. Direct sterile water at the side of the vial, followed by a gentle swirling of the contents to avoid foaming. Avoid excessive or vigorous agitation. Reconstituted solutions are clear, colorless, and isotonic with a pH of 7.4.

5. Dilute for IV infusion in 0.9% NaCl injection. If the final concentration is less than 10 mcg/mL, add human albumin at a final concentration of 0.1% to the saline prior to the addition of sargramostim (prevents adsorption of the

drug delivery system). For a final concentration of 0.1% human albumin, add 1 mg human albumin/1 mL of 0.9% NaCl (use 1 mL of 5% human albumin) in 50 mL 0.9% NaCl injection.

6. Do not use an in-line membrane filter for IV infusion. Do not add other drugs to sargramostim infusion.

7. Do not reenter or reuse the vial; discard unused portion.

8. Contains no preservatives; thus, give as soon as possible, but within 6 hr, following reconstitution or dilution for IV infusion. Store the sterile powder, reconstituted solution, and dilution solution in the refrigerator at 2–8°C (36–46°F). Do not freeze or shake solutions or use beyond the expiration date on the vial.

9. Sargramostim liquid may be stored for up to 20 days at 2–8°C (36–46°F). Do not freeze or shake.

ASSESSMENT

1. Note sensitivity to yeast-derived products. List any cardiac disease, hypoxia, peripheral edema, pleural or pericardial effusion, or myeloid-type malignancy. Drug can act as tumor growth factor with myeloid cancers.

2. Monitor CBC (ANC and platelets twice weekly during therapy- examine for blast cells), renal, LFTs.

3. List any therapy with drugs or radiation. Drug should *not* be administered 24 hr before or after cytotoxic chemotherapy or within 12 hr preceding or following radiation therapy. Give within 2–4 hr of bone marrow infusion.

INTERVENTIONS

1. Monitor I&O, VS, and weight; assess for fluid retention or edema.

2. Assess for respiratory symptoms during or immediately following infusion, especially with preexisting lung disease. Reduce rate of infusion by one-half if dyspnea occurs.

3. Monitor hematologic response with a CBC twice weekly. If the ANC exceeds 20,000/mm^3 or the platelet count exceeds 500,000/mm^3 or a severe reaction occurs, stop therapy and reduce dose by one-half. Excessive blood counts have returned to normal levels within

3–7 days following termination of therapy.

4. Renal and hepatic function should be monitored every 2 weeks with hepatic/renal dysfunction.

5. Drug effectiveness may be limited in clients who, before autologous bone marrow transplantation, received extensive radiotherapy in the chest or abdomen to treat the primary disease; effectiveness is also limited in those who have received multiple myelotoxic agents such as antimetabolites, alkylating agents, or anthracycline antibiotics.

CLIENT/FAMILY TEACHING

Drug is administered by injection to improve recovery time with transplant or chemotherapy. Report any unusual or adverse side effects immediately.

OUTCOMES/EVALUATE

• Inhibition of tumor cell growth
• Improved hematologic parameters; neutrophil recovery
• Mobilization of peripheral blood progenitor cells

Scopolamine hydrobromide (Hyoscine hydrobromide) **IV**

(scoh-**POLL**-ah-meen)

CLASSIFICATION(S):
Cholinergic blocking drug; antiemetic

PREGNANCY CATEGORY: C
Rx: Isopto Hyoscine Ophthalmic, Scopace.

Scopolamine transdermal therapeutic system

PREGNANCY CATEGORY: C
Rx: Transderm-Scop.
✤**Rx:** Transderm-V.

SEE ALSO CHOLINERGIC BLOCKING AGENTS.

S

USES

Ophthalmic: (1) For cycloplegia and mydriasis in diagnostic procedures. (2) Preoperatively and postoperatively in the treatment of iridocyclitis. (3) Dilate the pupil in treatment of uveitis or posterior synechiae. *Investigational:* Prophylaxis of synechiae, treatment of iridocyclitis.

Oral: (1) Prevention of motion sickness. (2) Inhibits excessive motility and hypertonus of the GI tract, including conditions such as irritable bowel syndrome, mild dysentery, diverticulitis, pylorospasm, and cardiospasm.

Parenteral: (1) Preanesthetic sedation and obstetric amnesia in conjunction with analgesics. (2) Calming delirium.

Transdermal: In adults for prevention of N&V associated with motion sickness or recovery from anesthesia and surgery.

ACTION/KINETICS

Action

Anticholinergic with CNS depressant effects; produces amnesia when given with morphine or meperidine. Inhibits excessive motility and hypertonus of the GI tract. In the presence of pain, delirium may be produced. Causes pupillary dilation and paralyzes the muscle required to accommodate for close vision (cycloplegia). This enables the physician to examine the inner structure of the eye, including the retina, as well as to examine refractive errors of the lens without automatic accommodation by the client. Tolerance may develop if scopolamine is used alone.

Pharmacokinetics

When used for refraction: **Peak for mydriasis:** 20–30 min; **peak for cycloplegia:** 30–60 min; **duration:** 24 hr (residual cycloplegia and mydriasis may last for 3–7 days). Recovery time can be reduced by using 1–2 gtt pilocarpine (1% or 2%). To reduce absorption, apply pressure over the nasolacrimal sac for 2–3 min. The transdermal therapeutic system contains 1.5 mg scopolamine, which is slowly released from a mineral oil–polyisobutylene matrix. Approximately 0.5 mg is released from the system per day.

ADDITIONAL CONTRAINDICATIONS

Use of the transdermal system in children or lactating women. Ophthalmic use in glaucoma or infants less than 3 months of age. Use for prophylaxis of excess secretions in children less than 4 months of age.

SPECIAL CONCERNS

Use with caution in children, infants, geriatric clients, diabetes, hypo- or hyperthyroidism, narrow anterior chamber angle.

SIDE EFFECTS

Most Common

When used systemically: Dizziness, drowsiness, dry mouth, flushing, blurred vision, headache, nausea.

When used ophthalmically: Transient stinging/burning, increased intraocular pressure, blurred vision, light sensitivity, dry mouth, dizziness, drowsiness.

See *Cholinergic Blocking Agents* for a complete list of possible side effects. Disorientation, delirium, increased HR, decreased respiratory rate. **Ophthalmic:** Blurred vision, stinging, increased intraocular pressure. Long-term use may cause irritation, photophobia, conjunctivitis, hyperemia, or edema. **Transdermal:** Frequently, dry mouth, drowsiness, blurred vision, dilation of pupils. Infrequently, disorientation, memory disturbances, dizziness, restlessness, hallucinations, confusion, difficulty urinating, rashes or erythema, narrow-angle glaucoma; dry, itchy, or red eyes.

ADDITIONAL DRUG INTERACTIONS

Grapefruit juice / ↑ Scopolamine bioavailability and time to reach peak plasma levels

HOW SUPPLIED

Scopolamine hydrobromide: *Injection:* 0.3 mg/mL, 0.4 mg/mL, 0.86 mg/mL, 1 mg/mL; *Ophthalmic Solution:* 0.25%; *Tablets, Soluble:* 0.4 mg.

Scopolamine transdermal therapeutic system: *Film, Extended-Release, Transdermal:* 1.5 mg (delivers about 1 mg over 3 days).

DOSAGE

- **OPHTHALMIC SOLUTION**
  Cycloplegia/mydriasis.

Bold Italic = life threatening side effect   ■ = black box warning   ✤ = Available in Canada

Adults: 1–2 gtt of the 0.25% solution in the conjunctiva 1 hr prior to refraction. **Children:** 1 gtt of the 0.25% solution twice a day for 2 days prior to refraction.

Uveitis.

Adults and children: 1 gtt of the 0.25% solution in the conjunctiva 1–4 times per day, depending on the severity of the condition.

Treatment of posterior synechiae.

Adults and children: 1 gtt of the 0.25% solution q min for 5 min (1 gtt of either a 2.5% or 10% solution of phenylephrine instilled q min for 3 min will enhance the effect of scopolamine.)

Postoperative mydriasis.

Adults: 1 gtt of the 0.25% solution once daily. For dark brown irides, administration 2 or 3 times per day may be required.

Pre- or postoperative iridocyclitis.

Adults and children: 1 gtt of the 0.25% solution 1–4 times per day as required. Individualize the pediatric dose based on age, weight, and severity of the inflammation.

• **IM; IV; SC**

Anticholinergic, antiemetic.

Adults: 0.3–0.6 mg (single dose). **Pediatric:** 0.006 mg/kg (0.2 mg/m^2) as a single dose. Maximum dose: 0.3 mg.

Prophylaxis of excessive salivation and respiratory tract secretions in anesthesia.

Adults: 0.2–0.6 mg 30–60 min before induction of anesthesia. **Pediatric (given IM): 8–12 years:** 0.3 mg; **3–8 years:** 0.2 mg; **7 months–3 years:** 0.15 mg; **4–7 months:** 0.1 mg. Not recommended for children under 4 months of age.

Adjunct to anesthesia, sedative-hypnotic.

Adults: 0.6 mg 3–4 times per day

Adjunct to anesthesia, amnesia.

Adults: 0.32–0.65 mg.

• **TABLETS, SOLUBLE**

Prevent motion sickness. Excessive GI tract motility and hypertonus.

0.4–0.8 mg.

• **TRANSDERMAL SYSTEM**

Antiemetic, antivertigo.

Adults: 1 transdermal system placed on the postauricular skin to deliver 1 mg over 3 days (apply at least 4 hr before antiemetic effect is required). The Canadian product should be applied about 12 hr before the antiemetic effect is desired.

NURSING CONSIDERATIONS

ADMINISTRATION/STORAGE

1. Give drops into the conjunctival sac followed by digital pressure for 2–3 min after instillation.
2. Do not give alone for pain because it may cause delirium; use an analgesic or sedative as needed.
3. Protect solution from light.

ASSESSMENT

1. Note reasons for therapy, onset, characteristics of S&S. List any conditions that may preclude therapy.
2. With eye drops, check for angle-closure glaucoma; may precipitate glaucoma crisis.
3. Some clients may experience toxic delirium with therapeutic doses. Observe closely and have physostigmine available to reverse effects.

CLIENT/FAMILY TEACHING

1. Use exactly as directed. Take oral agents 30 min before meals. Do not share; store safely out of reach of children.
2. Do not drive or operate dangerous machinery until drug effects realized; may cause drowsiness, confusion, disorientation, and, with eye drops, blurred vision and dilated pupils.
3. Wash hands before and after use. Do not permit dropper to come in contact with eye. If other eye drops prescribed, wait 5 min before instilling.
4. Wear dark glasses if photosensitivity occurs; report if eye pain occurs. May temporarily impair vision.
5. With the transdermal system:
• Wash hands before and after application
• Apply at least 4 hr before desired effect
• Apply to a clean, nonhairy site, behind the ear
• To minimize exposure to the newborn baby, apply 1hr prior to cesarean section

- Use pressure to apply the patch to ensure contact with the skin
- Replace with a new system on another site if patch becomes dislodged
- System is waterproof so bathing and swimming are permitted
- System effects last for 3 days
- NOT for use in children
- Wear only one patch at the time; do not cut the patch
- After applying on dry skin behind the ear, wash hands thoroughly with soap and water and dry. Discard the removed patch and wash hands and old application site thoroughly with soap and water. May cause pupillary dilation if eye is touched and hand contaminated with drug.

6. Report any unusual movements, urinary retention, constipation and lack of response. Increase fluids and bulk to prevent constipation and ensure adequate hydration. Avoid hot temperatures; may become heat intolerant.

7. Avoid alcohol and any other CNS depressants. Use gum, sugarless candies, and frequent mouth rinses to alleviate symptoms of dry mouth.

OUTCOMES/EVALUATE
- Control of vomiting
- Preoperative sedation; postoperative amnesia
- Desired mydriasis
- Prevention of motion sickness

Sertaconazole nitrate
(sir-tah-**KON**-ah-zohl)

CLASSIFICATION(S):
Topical antifungal
PREGNANCY CATEGORY: C
Rx: Ertaczo.

USES
Topical treatment of interdigital tinea pedis due to *Trichophyton rubrum, T. mentagrophytes,* and *Epidermophyton floccosum* in immunocompetent clients 12 years and older.

ACTION/KINETICS
Action
Exact mechanism not known. Is believed the drug acts primarily to inhibit the cytochrome P450-dependent synthesis of ergosterol. Ergosterol is the key component of the cell membrane of fungi; lack of this compound leads to fungal cell injury primarily by leakage of key components into the cytoplasm of the cell.

CONTRAINDICATIONS
Hypersensitivity to the drug, any of its components, or to other imidazoles. Ophthalmic, oral, or intravaginal use.

SPECIAL CONCERNS
Use with caution in those known to be sensitive to imidazole antifungals due to the possibility of cross-reactivity. Use with caution during lactation. Safety and efficacy have not been determined in children less than 12 years of age.

SIDE EFFECTS
Most Common
Contact dermatitis, dry skin, burning skin, application site reaction, skin tenderness.

Dermatologic: Application-site reaction, burning skin, contact dermatitis, dry skin, skin tenderness, desquamation, erythema, hyperpigmentation, pruritus, vesiculation, redness, severe itching, blistering.

HOW SUPPLIED
Cream: 2%.

DOSAGE
- **CREAM**
  Interdigital tinea pedis.
Apply twice a day to the affected areas between the toes and the adjacent healthy skin for 4 weeks. If no improvement is seen after 2 weeks, review the diagnosis.

NURSING CONSIDERATIONS
ADMINISTRATION/STORAGE
1. Apply a sufficient amount to cover the affected areas between the toes and the immediately surrounding healthy skin.
2. Store from 15–30°C (59–86°F).
3. If irritation or sensitivity develop, discontinue treatment and begin appropriate therapy.

Bold Italic = life threatening side effect   ■ = black box warning   ✦ = Available in Canada

ASSESSMENT
Describe onset, clinical presentation, characteristics of S&S of rash.

CLIENT/FAMILY TEACHING
1. Wash and dry affected area before applying cream. Wash hands before and after use; avoid contact with eyes, nose, or mouth.
2. Do not apply a dressing unless specifically directed.
3. Report any increased oozing, itching, odor, blistering, redness, or swelling, as well as lack of response.
4. Complete entire therapy as prescribed; do not stop if S&S subside or improve.

OUTCOMES/EVALUATE
Resolution of fungal foot infection

Sertraline hydrochloride
(**SIR**-trah-leen)

CLASSIFICATION(S):
Antidepressant, selective serotonin reuptake inhibitor
PREGNANCY CATEGORY: C
Rx: Zoloft.
✤Rx: Apo-Sertraline, Gen-Sertraline, Novo-Sertraline, Rhoxal-sertraline, ratio-Sertraline.

SEE ALSO *SELECTIVE SEROTONIN REUPTAKE INHIBITORS.*

USES
(1) Major depressive disorder as defined in the DSM-III. (2) Obsessive-compulsive disorders in adults and children as defined in DSM-III-R. (3) Panic disorder, with or without agoraphobia, as defined in DSM-IV. (4) Long-term use for posttraumatic stress disorder in men and women as defined in the DSM-III-R. (5) Premenstrual dysphoric disorder as defined in the DSM-III-R/IV. (6) Acute and chronic treatment of social anxiety disorder (social phobia) as defined in the DSM-IV.

ACTION/KINETICS
Action
Antidepressant effect likely due to inhibition of CNS neuronal uptake of serotonin and to a less extent norepinephrine and dopamine. Results in increased levels of serotonin in synapses.

Pharmacokinetics
Steady-state plasma levels are usually reached after 1 week of once-daily dosing but is increased to 2–3 weeks in older clients. May cause slight sedation. **Time to peak plasma levels:** 4.5–8.4 hr. **Peak plasma levels:** 20–55 ng/mL. **Time to reach steady state:** 7 days. **Terminal elimination t½:** 1–4 days (including active metabolite). Washout period is 7 days. Food decreases the time to reach peak plasma levels. Undergoes significant first-pass metabolism. Excreted through the urine (40–45%) and feces (40–45%). Metabolized to N-desmethylsertraline, which has minimal antidepressant activity. **Plasma protein binding:** 98%.

CONTRAINDICATIONS
Use with pimozide or MAO inhibitors due to increased risk of QT prolongation.

SPECIAL CONCERNS
■ (1) Antidepressants increased the risk of suicidal thinking and behavior (suicidality) in short-term studies in children and adolescents with major depressive disorder and other psychiatric disorders. Anyone considering the use of sertraline or any other antidepressant in a child or adolescent must balance this risk with the clinical need. Clients who are started on therapy should be observed closely for clinical worsening, suicidality, or unusual changes in behavior. Families and caregivers should be advised of the need for close observation and communication with the prescriber. Sertraline is not approved for use in pediatric clients with major depressive disorder and obsessive-compulsive disorder. (2) Short-term placebo-controlled trials of 9 antidepressant drugs in children and adolescents with major depressive disorder, obsessive-compulsive disorder, or other psychiatric disorders revealed a greater risk of adverse reactions during the first few months of treatment. The average risk of such reactions in clients receiving antidepressants was 4%, twice the place-

S

---

bo risk of 2%. No suicides occurred in these trials.■ Use with caution in hepatic or renal dysfunction, and with seizure disorders. Plasma clearance may be lower in elderly clients. Neonates exposed to sertraline late in the third trimester have developed serious complications requiring prolonged hospitalization, respiratory support, and tube feeding; when treating pregnant women with sertraline during the third trimester, carefully consider the potential risks and benefits. The possibility of a suicide attempt is possible in depression and may persist until significant remission occurs.

SIDE EFFECTS
Most Common
Nausea, diarrhea/loose stools, headache, insomnia, somnolence, rash, dry mouth, dizziness, anorexia, abnormal ejaculation.

A large number of side effects is possible; listed are those side effects with a frequency of 0.1% or greater. **GI:** Nausea, diarrhea/loose stools, dry mouth, constipation, dyspepsia, vomiting, flatulence, anorexia, abdominal pain, thirst, increased salivation/appetite, gastroenteritis, dysphagia, eructation, taste perversion/change, teeth-grinding. **CV:** Palpitations, hot flushes, edema, hyper-/hypotension, peripheral ischemia, postural hypotension or dizziness, syncope, tachycardia. **CNS:** Headache, insomnia, somnolence, agitation, nervousness, activation of mania/hypomania, *seizures*, anxiety, dizziness, tremor, fatigue, impaired concentration, yawning, paresthesia, hyper-/hypoesthesia, twitching, hypertonia, confusion, ataxia or abnormal coordination/gait, hyper-/hypokinesia, abnormal dreams, aggressive reaction, amnesia, apathy, delusion, depersonalization, depression, aggravated depression, emotional lability, euphoria, hallucinations, neurosis, paranoid reaction, *suicidal ideation or attempt*, abnormal thinking, migraine, nystagmus, vertigo. **Dermatologic:** Rash, acne, excessive sweating, alopecia, pruritus, cold/clammy skin, facial edema, erythematous rash, maculopapular rash, dry skin. **Musculoskeletal:** Myalgia, arthralgia, arthrosis, dystonia, muscle cramps/weakness. **GU:** Urinary frequency/incontinence, UTI, abnormal ejaculation, micturition/menstrual disorders, dysmenorrhea, dysuria, painful menstruation, intermenstrual bleeding, sexual dysfunction and decreased libido, nocturia, polyuria, dysuria. **Respiratory:** Rhinitis, pharyngitis, bronchospasm, coughing, dyspnea, epistaxis. **Ophthalmic:** Blurred/abnormal vision, abnormal accommodation, conjunctivitis, diplopia, eye pain, xerophthalmia. **Otic:** Tinnitus, earache. **Body as a whole:** Asthenia, fever, chest/back pain, chills, weight loss/gain, generalized edema, malaise, flushing, hot flashes, rigors, lymphadenopathy, purpura.

ADDITIONAL DRUG INTERACTIONS
Because sertraline is highly bound to plasma proteins, its use with other drugs that are also highly protein bound may lead to displacement, resulting in higher plasma levels of the drug and possibly increased side effects.

Alcohol / Concurrent use is not recommended in depressed clients
Benzodiazepines / ↓ Clearance of benzodiazepines metabolized by hepatic oxidation
Carbamazepine / Possible ↓ sertraline effect R/T ↑ liver metabolism
Cimetidine / ↑ Half-life and blood levels of sertraline
Clozapine / ↑ Serum clozapine levels
Diazepam / ↑ Levels of desmethyldiazepam (significance not known)
Erythromycin / Possibility of 'Serotonin Syndrome'
Hydantoins / Possible ↑ hydantoin levels
MAO inhibitors / ↑ Risk of QT prolongation; do not use together
Pimozide / ↑ Pimozide levels → QT prolongation; do not use together
Rifampin / Possible ↓ sertraline levels

LABORATORY TEST CONSIDERATIONS
↑ AST or ALT, total cholesterol, triglycerides. ↓ Serum uric acid. Altered platelet function. Hyponatremia.

OD OVERDOSE MANAGEMENT
Symptoms: Intensification of side effects.

Treatment:

- Establish and maintain an airway, ensuring adequate oxygenation and ventilation.
- Activated charcoal, with or without sorbitol, may be as or more effective than emesis or lavage.
- Monitor cardiac and vital signs.
- Provide general supportive measures and symptomatic treatment.
- Since sertraline has a large volume of distribution, it is unlikely that dialysis, forced diuresis, hemoperfusion, or exchange transfusion will benefit.

HOW SUPPLIED

Solution, Oral Concentrate: 20 mg/mL (as base); *Tablets:* 25 mg, 50 mg, 100 mg (all as base).

DOSAGE————————————

- **SOLUTION, ORAL CONCENTRATE; TABLETS**

Major depressive disorder.

Adults, initial: 50 mg once daily either in the morning or evening. Clients not responding to a 50 mg dose may benefit from doses ranging from 50–200 mg/day (average: 70 mg/day).

Obsessive-compulsive disorder.

Adults: 50 mg once daily either in the morning or evening; up to 200 mg/day may be required in some. **Children, 6 to 12 years, initial:** 25 mg once a day; **adolescents, 13 to 17 years, initial:** 50 mg once a day. Those not responding may require doses up to a maximum of 200 mg/day.

Panic disorder.

Adults, initial: 25 mg/day for the first week; **then,** increase the dose to 50 mg once daily. Up to 200 mg/day have been used.

Post-traumatic stress syndrome.

Adults, initial: 25 mg once daily. After 1 week, increase dose to 50 mg once daily. **Dose range:** 50–200 mg/day.

Premenstrual dysphoric disorder.

Adults, initial: 50 mg/day either daily throughout the menstrual cycle or limited to the luteal phase, depending on provider assessment. **Dose range:** 50–150 mg/day.

Social anxiety disorder.

Adults, initial: 25 mg once daily. After 1 week, increase to 50 mg once daily.

Dose range: 50–200 mg/day. *NOTE:* Lower the dose or space dose frequency in those with hepatic or renal impairment.

NURSING CONSIDERATIONS

🔊 Do not confuse Zoloft with Zocor (an antihyperlipidemic).

ADMINISTRATION/STORAGE

1. It is generally recognized that acute periods of depression and other disorders require several months or longer of sustained drug therapy. Periodically reassess clients to determine the need for maintenance therapy.

2. Due to the long elimination t½, do not increase dosage at intervals of less than 1 week.

3. Beneficial effects may not be observed for 2–4 weeks after starting.

4. Use for more than 12 weeks for panic attacks has not been studied.

5. Give a lower or less frequent dose in those with hepatic impairment.

6. If used in pregnant women, consider tapering the dose in the third trimester.

7. At least 14 days should elapse between discontinuing a monoamine oxidase inhibitor and starting sertraline therapy. Also, allow at least 14 days after discontinuing sertraline and starting an MAOI.

8. When discontinuing sertraline, a gradual reduction in dose rather than abrupt cessation is recommended whenever possible.

9. The oral concentrate is contraindicated with disulfiram due to the alcohol content of the concentrate.

10. Store tablets and oral concentrate at controlled room temperature from 15–30°C (59–86°F).

ASSESSMENT

1. Note reasons for therapy, onset, triggers, symptom/behavioral characteristics/presentation, other agents/therapies trialed. List drugs prescribed to ensure none interact/compete.

2. Assess lifestyle, i.e., recent loss (death of loved one), stress, job change/loss, alcohol/drug use, or other factors that may contribute to symptoms.

3. Monitor ECG, renal, LFTs; reduce dose with dysfunction/elderly. Assess

S

for hepatitis, alcohol overuse, seizure disorder.

4. Determine if at risk for bipolar disorder; assess detailed psychiatric history, including a family history of suicide, bipolar disorder, and depression.

CLIENT/FAMILY TEACHING

1. Take only as directed, do not share medications, store safely, and remain under close medical supervision. May take with/without food and in the evening if sedation is noted.

2. Prior to use of the oral concentrate, dilute with 4 oz of water, ginger ale, lemon/lime soda, lemonade, or orange juice only. Take immediately after mixing; do not mix in advance. Dropper may contain latex avoid using if allergic.

3. Do not perform activities that require mental and physical alertness until drug effects are realized.

4. Review side effects, noting those that require immediate medical attention, esp yellow eyes/skin, abd pain, N&V, or light stool color.

5. Loss of appetite, persistent nausea, and diarrhea with excessive weight loss should be reported.

6. Report any suicidal thoughts or aggression. Attend counseling and maintain contact with provider so drug utilization can be assessed, as the risk of suicide is tantamount in a depressive phase. May take 2–4 weeks to work.

7. Avoid OTC agents, alcohol, and any other CNS depressants. If alcohol consumed wait and take dose in the am.

8. Use reliable contraception; report if pregnancy suspected.

9. Keep all F/U appointments to determine response to therapy.

OUTCOMES/EVALUATE

- Improved symptoms of depression/OCD/PTSD/panic disorder
- ↓ Levels of agitation and anxiety

Sibutramine hydrochloride monohydrate

(sih-**BYOU**-trah-meen)

CLASSIFICATION(S):
Antiobesity drug
PREGNANCY CATEGORY: C
Rx: Meridia, **C-IV**

USES

Management of obesity, including weight loss and maintenance of weight loss. Recommended for obese clients with initial body mass index of 30 kg/m^2 or more or 27 kg/m^2 in presence of hypertension, diabetes, or dyslipidemia. Use in conjunction with reduced-calorie diet. Safety and efficacy have not been determined for more than 2 years.

ACTION/KINETICS

Action

Main effect is likely due to primary and secondary amine metabolites of sibutramine. Inhibits reuptake of norepinephrine (NE) and serotonin (5HT), resulting in enhanced NE and 5HT activity and reduced food intake. Significant improvement in serum uric acid.

Pharmacokinetics

Rapidly absorbed from GI tract. Extensive first-pass metabolism in liver. **Peak plasma levels of active metabolites:** 3–4 hr. **t½, sibutramine:** 1.1 hr; **t½, active metabolites:** 14–16 hr. Excreted in urine and feces.

CONTRAINDICATIONS

Lactation. Use in clients receiving MAO inhibitors, who have anorexia nervosa, those taking centrally acting appetite suppressant drugs, those with history of coronary artery disease, CHF, arrhythmias, or stroke. Use in severe renal impairment or hepatic dysfunction. Use with serotonergic drugs, such as fluoxetine, fluvoxamine, paroxetine, sertraline, venlafaxine, sumatriptan, and dihydroergotamine; also, use with dextromethorphan, meperidine, pentazocine, fentanyl, lithium, or tryptophan.

SPECIAL CONCERNS

Use with caution in geriatric clients. Safety and efficacy have not been determined in children less than 16 years of age. Use with caution in narrow angle glaucoma, history of seizures, or with drugs that may raise BP (e.g., phenylpropanolamine, ephedrine, pseudoephedrine). Exclude organic causes (e.g., untreated hypothyroidism) before use.

SIDE EFFECTS

Most Common

Headache, dry mouth, insomnia, nervousness, anorexia, constipation, increased appetite, nausea, dyspepsia, arthralgia, rhinitis, pharyngitis, sinusitis, back pain, flu syndrome, asthenia.

Body as a whole: Headache, back pain, flu syndrome, injury/accident, asthenia, chest/neck pain, allergic reaction. **GI:** Dry mouth, anorexia, abdominal pain, constipation, N&V, rectal disorder, increased appetite, dyspepsia, gastritis, diarrhea, flatulence, gastroenteritis, tooth disorder. **CNS:** Insomnia, dizziness, paresthesia, nervousness, anxiety, depression, somnolence, CNS stimulation, emotional lability, agitation, hypertonia, abnormal thinking, seizures. **CV:** Increased blood pressure and pulse, tachycardia, vasodilation, migraine, palpitation. **Dermatologic:** Sweating, rash, herpes simplex, acne, pruritus, ecchymosis. **Musculoskeletal:** Arthralgia, myalgia, tenosynovitis, joint disorder, arthritis. **Respiratory:** Rhinitis, pharyngitis, sinusitis, increased cough, laryngitis, bronchitis, dyspnea. **GU:** Dysmenorrhea, UTI, vaginal monilia, menorrhagia, menstrual disorder. **Otic:** Ear disorder/pain. **Miscellaneous:** Thirst, generalized edema, taste perversion, fever, amblyopia, leg cramps.

DRUG INTERACTIONS

Alcohol / Do not use excess alcohol if taking sibutramine
Dextromethorphan / Possible life-threatening serotonin syndrome
Dihydroergotamine / Possible life-threatening serotonin syndrome
Ephedrine / ↑ BP and HR
Fentanyl / Possible life-threatening serotonin syndrome
Isocarboxazid / Possible life-threatening serotonin syndrome
Lithium / Additive serotonergic effects
Meperidine / Possible life-threatening serotonin syndrome
Pentazocine / Possible life-threatening serotonin syndrome
Phenelzine / Possible life-threatening serotonin syndrome
Pseudoephedrine / ↑ BP and HR
SSRIs / Possible life-threatening serotonin syndrome
Selegiline / Possible life-threatening serotonin syndrome
Sumatriptan / Possible life-threatening serotonin syndrome
L-Tryptophan / Possible life-threatening serotonin syndrome
Tranylcypromine / Possible life-threatening serotonin syndrome
Zolmitriptan / Possible life-threatening serotonin syndrome

HOW SUPPLIED

Capsules: 5 mg, 10 mg, 15 mg.

DOSAGE

- **CAPSULES**

Obesity.

Adults, initial: 10 mg once daily (usually in morning) with or without food. Use the 5 mg dose for those who do not tolerate 10 mg. If there is inadequate weight loss, dose may be titrated after 4 weeks to a total of 15 mg once daily. Do not exceed 15 mg daily.

NURSING CONSIDERATIONS

ADMINISTRATION/STORAGE

1. May take with or without food.
2. Reevaluate therapy if client has not lost at least 4 pounds in first 4 weeks of treatment.
3. Allow at least 2 weeks to elapse between discontinuation of an MAO inhibitor and initiation of sibutramine and between discontinuation of sibutramine and initiation of an MAO inhibitor.
4. Store at controlled room temperature. Protect from heat and moisture and dispense in tight, light-resistant container.

ASSESSMENT

1. Note reasons for therapy, BMI, length of weight problem, other agents/therapies trialed, outcome.

S

2. Assess for anorexia nervosa and MAOI use.

3. List drugs prescribed as may require adjustment.

4. Monitor ECG, Wt., VS and labs; assess for increased BP or increased HR.

CLIENT/FAMILY TEACHING

1. Take only as directed with or without food. Do not exceed prescribed dosage.

2. Continue regular exercise, weight counseling, and low-calorie diet during therapy.

3. Review package insert before starting therapy and review with each refill.

4. Report any signs of allergic reaction including rash or hives.

5. Practice reliable nonhormonal form of birth control; may harm fetus.

6. Avoid alcohol and OTC agents and report all prescribed medications to prevent interactions.

7. Report regularly for F/U visits and lab work; record BP and pulse for provider review.

OUTCOMES/EVALUATE

Desired weight loss

Sildenafil citrate
(sill-**DEN**-ah-fill)

CLASSIFICATION(S):

Drug for erectile dysfunction; drug for pulmonary arterial hypertension

PREGNANCY CATEGORY: B

Rx: Revatio, Viagra.

USES

(1) **Viagra:** Erectile dysfunction. Has no effect in the absence of sexual stimulation. (2) **Revatio:** Pulmonary arterial hypertension (World Health Organization Group 1) to improve ability to exercise. *Investigational:* Female sexual dysfunction.

ACTION/KINETICS

Action

Nitric oxide activates the enzyme guanylate cyclase, which causes increased levels of guanosine monophosphate (cGMP) and subsequently smooth muscle relaxation in the corpus cavernosum allowing inflow of blood. Sildenafil en-

hances effect of nitric oxide by inhibiting phosphodiesterase type 5 which is responsible for degradation of cGMP in the corpus cavernosum. When sexual stimulation causes local release of nitric oxide, inhibition of phosphodiesterase type 5 by sildenafil causes increased levels of cGMP in the corpus cavernosum and thus smooth muscle relaxation and inflow of blood resulting in an erection. Drug has no effect in absence of sexual stimulation.

Pharmacokinetics

Rapidly absorbed after PO use; about 40% is bioavailable. Absorption is decreased when taken with high-fat meal. Increased plasma levels will occur in clients older than 65 years (40% increase in AUC), hepatic impairment (e.g., cirrhosis, 80% increase), severe renal impairment (C_{CR} under 30 mL/min, 100% increase), and concomitant use of potent cytochrome CYP 3A4 inhibitors (see Drug Interactions); in these clients, start with a 25 mg dose. T_{max}: 0.5–2 hr. **Onset:** About 30 min. **Duration:** 4 or more hr. Metabolized in liver by CYP3A4 (major) and CYP2C9 (minor). Is converted to active metabolite (N-desmethyl sildenafil). $t\frac{1}{2}$, **sildenafil and metabolite:** 4 hr. Excreted mainly in feces (80%) with about 13% excreted in urine. Reduced clearance is seen in geriatric clients. **Plasma protein binding:** About 96%.

CONTRAINDICATIONS

Concomitant use with organic nitrates (potentiate hypotensive effects) in any form or with other treatments for erectile dysfunction. Use in men for whom sexual activity is not advisable due to underlying cardiovascular status. Use in newborns, children, or women. Severe hepatic impairment (Child-Pugh score from 10–15).

SPECIAL CONCERNS

Use with caution in clients with anatomical deformation of penis, in those with predisposition to priapism (e.g., sickle cell anemia, multiple myeloma, leukemia), in bleeding disorders or active peptic ulceration, and in those with genetic disorders of retinal phosphodiesterases. Drug is potentially hazardous

---

Bold Italic = life threatening side effect   ■ = black box warning   ♣ = Available in Canada

in those with acute coronary ischemia but not on nitrates; have CHF, borderline low BP, or borderline low volume status; are on complicated antihypertensive therapy with several drugs; are taking erythromycin or cimetidine; or have impaired hepatic or renal function. Is said to be safe in those with stable coronary artery disease managed without nitrites.

SIDE EFFECTS
Most Common
Headache, flushing, dyspepsia, nasal congestion, UTI, abnormal vision, diarrhea, dizziness, rash.

CNS: Headache, dizziness, ataxia, hypertonia, neuralgia, neuropathy, paresthesia, tremor, vertigo, depression, insomnia, somnolence, abnormal dreams, decreased reflexes, hypesthesia, migraine, seizures, anxiety. **GI:** Dyspepsia, diarrhea, vomiting, glossitis, colitis, dysphagia, gastritis, gastroenteritis, esophagitis, stomatitis, dry mouth, rectal hemorrhage, gingivitis. **CV:** Hypertension, TIA, *MI, sudden cardiac death, ventricular arrhythmia, CVA, subarachnoid and intracerebral hemorrhage, pulmonary hemorrhage*, especially with preexisting CV risk factors. Also, angina pectoris, AV block, syncope, tachycardia, palpitation, hypotension, postural hypotension, myocardial ischemia, cerebral thrombosis, *cardiac arrest, heart failure, cardiomyopathy*, abnormal ECG. **Dermatologic:** Flushing, rash, urticaria, herpes simplex, pruritus, sweating, skin ulcer, contact dermatitis, exfoliative dermatitis. **GU:** UTI, cystitis, nocturia, urinary frequency/incontinence, abnormal ejaculation, genital edema and anorgasmia, prolonged erection, priaprism, hematuria, breast enlargement. **Ophthalmic:** Mild and transient predominantly color tinge to vision, increased sensitivity to light, blurred vision, mydriasis, conjunctivitis, photophobia, eye pain, eye hemorrhage, cataract, dry eyes, diplopia, sudden vision loss (related to nonarteritic anterior ischemic optic neuropathy especially in those with underlying anatomic or vascular risk factors), temporary vision loss, ocular redness/burning/swelling/pressure or bloodshot appearance, increased intraocular pressure, retinal vascular disease or bleeding, vitreous detachment/traction, paramacular edema. **Otic:** Tinnitus, deafness, ear pain. **Respiratory:** Nasal congestion, respiratory tract infection, asthma, dyspnea, laryngitis, pharyngitis, sinusitis, bronchitis, increased sputum, increased cough. **Musculoskeletal:** Arthritis, arthrosis, arthralgia, myalgia, tendon rupture, tenosynovitis, bone pain, myasthenia, synovitis. **Metabolic:** Thirst, edema, gout, unstable diabetes, hyperglycemia, peripheral edema, hyperuricemia, hypoglycemic reaction, hypernatremia. **Miscellaneous:** Flu syndrome, facial edema, shock, asthenia, pain, chills, accidental fall/injury, back/abdominal pain, allergic reaction, chest pain, anemia, leukopenia. *NOTE:* Death has occurred in some clients following use of the drug.

LABORATORY TEST CONSIDERATIONS
Abnormal LFTs.

OD OVERDOSE MANAGEMENT
Symptoms: Extension of side effects. *Treatment:* Standard supportive measures.

DRUG INTERACTIONS
Alcohol (substantial amount) / ↓ BP, postural dizziness, and orthostatic hypotension

Alpha-adrenergic blockers / Symptomatic hypotension

Amlodipine / Additional ↓ in BP in clients with pulmonary arterial hypertension R/T induction of CYP3A4 metabolism

Cimetidine / ↑ Sildenafil levels by 56%

Diuretics, loop or potassium-sparing / ↑ Sildenafil AUC by 62%

Erythromycin / Significant ↑ sildenafil levels R/T inhibition of sildenafil first-pass metabolism

Fluvoxamine / ↑ Sildenafil levels and t½ R/T inhibition of CYP3A4 first-pass metabolism

Grapefruit juice / ↑ Sildenafil levels R/T ↓ metabolism

Indinavir / ↑ Sildenafil levels → severe and possibly fatal hypotension

Itraconazole / ↑ Sildenafil levels R/T ↓ CYP3A4 metabolism

S

Ketoconazole / ↑ Sildenafil levels R/T ↓ CYP3A4 metabolism

Mibefradil / ↑ Sildenafil levels

Nitrites / Potentiation of vasodilatory effects → significant and potential fatal ↓ BP; do not use together

Rifampin / ↓ Sildenafil clearance

Ritonavir / ↑ Sildenafil levels → severe and possibly fatal hypotension

Saquinavir / ↑ Sildenafil levels → severe and possibly fatal hypotension

Tacrolimus / ↑ Tacrolimus AUC, peak levels, and prolonged t½ R/T inhibition of metabolism

Thiazide diuretics / ↓ BP

HOW SUPPLIED

Viagra: *Tablets:* 25 mg, 50 mg, 100 mg.
Revatio: *Tablets:* 20 mg.

DOSAGE

- **TABLETS**

Treat erectile dysfunction.

Viagra: For most clients, 50 mg no more than once daily, as needed, about 1 hr before sexual activity. Take anywhere from 0.5 hr to 4 hr before sexual activity. Depending on tolerance and effectiveness, dose may be increased to maximum of 100 mg or decreased to 25 mg. The maximum recommended dosing frequency is once daily.

Pulmonary arterial hypertension.

Revatio: 20 mg 3 times per day. Take doses about 4–6 hr apart with or without food. Doses higher than 20 mg 3 times per day are not recommended.

NURSING CONSIDERATIONS

ADMINISTRATION/STORAGE

1. Consider starting dose of 25 mg in the following situations associated with higher plasma levels of sildenafil: Over 65 years of age, mild hepatic impairment (Child-Pugh score of 5 or 6), severe renal impairment (C_{CR} <30 mL/min), and concomitant use of cytochrome CYP3A4 inhibitors (including erythromycin, itraconazole, ketoconazole, and saquinavir).

2. Do not exceed a maximum single dose of 25 mg sildenafil in a 48 hr period with concomitant use of protease inhibitors (e.g., ritonavir) for HIV disease.

3. Do not take 50 or 100 mg of sildenafil within 4 hr of alpha-blocker administration. A 25 mg dose may be taken at any time.

4. Store from 15–30°C (59–86°F).

ASSESSMENT

1. List reasons for therapy, onset/cause of erectile dysfunction, i.e., organic, psychogenic, or combined; pulmonary artery pressure, distance able to walk.

2. Assess cardiovascular status; get ECG. Clients using nitrates should not use this drug; should be nitrate free for 24 hr prior to use.

3. List drugs prescribed; some may potentiate drug effects.

4. Assess for any retinal, bleeding disorders, active ulcers.

5. Ensure client aware of potential for sudden visual loss.

6. Check for conditions that may predispose to priapism, i.e., multiple myelomas, sickle cell anemia, or leukemia.

7. Assess for any anatomical deformation of penis (Peyronie's disease, angulation, or cavernosal fibrosis).

8. Drug for pulmonary hypertension will be a different color.

CLIENT/FAMILY TEACHING

1. Take only as directed on an empty stomach 1–3 hr prior to intercourse; high-fat meal may slow drug absorption. May split drug if dose is adequate.

2. Plan some form of sexual stimulation after ingestion to ensure desired erection obtained.

3. May experience headache, flushing, upset stomach, stuffy nose, dizziness (from drop in BP) drowsiness, or abnormal vision (esp blue/green color discrimination); report any unusual, persistent or bothersome effects.

4. Do not use any other agent for erections with this therapy. Effects may be evident the day after therapy; assess before taking additional drug. Do not use more than once a day. Erections lasting more than 4 hr or painful erections lasting more than 6 hr require immediate care; penile damage may result.

5. Report all medications currently prescribed to ensure none alter effects. Stop smoking; may inhibit drug effect. If

S

taking meds for BP or prostate be aware may cause lowered BP; also alpha blockers should be taken 4 hr apart from viagra.

6. Practice safe sex; drug does not prevent disease transmission.

7. Do not share medications or prescriptions due to potential for adverse interactions and effects. *Never* use this drug if taking nitrates in any form.

8. When used for pulmonary hypertension drug is called revatio and is produced in a different shape, color and dosage. This vascular disease is characterized by fatigue, shortness of breath on exertion, chest pain, and dizziness. If untreated, median survival time after diagnosis may be as short as three years.

OUTCOMES/EVALUATE
- Improvement in S&S of ED
- ↓ Pulmonary artery pressure; improved exercise tolerance

Simvastatin ©
(**sim**-vah-**STAH**-tin)

CLASSIFICATION(S):
Antihyperlipidemic, HMG-CoA reductase inhibitor
PREGNANCY CATEGORY: X
Rx: Zocor.

SEE ALSO *ANTIHYPERLIPIDEMIC AGENTS, HMG–COA REDUCTASE INHIBITORS.*

USES
(1) Adjunct to diet to reduce elevated total and LDL cholesterol, apoprotein B, and triglyceride levels in hypercholesterolemia and mixed dyslipidemia (Fredrickson types IIa and IIb) when the response to diet and other approaches has been inadequate. (2) To increase HDL cholesterol in primary hypercholesterolemia and mixed dyslipidemia (Fredrickson types IIa and IIb)s. (3) Treatment of isolated hypertriglyceridemia (Frederickson type IV) and dysbetalipoproteinemia (Fredrickson type III). (4) In coronary heart disease and hypercholesterolemia to reduce risk of total mortality by reducing coronary death; to reduce the risk of nonfatal MI; to reduce the risk for undergoing myocardial revascularization procedures; to reduce the risk of stroke or TIAs. (5) As an adjunct to diet to reduce total and LDL cholesterol and Apo-B levels in adolescent boys and girls who are at least 1 year postmenarche, 10–17 years of age, with heterozygous familial hypercholesterolemia. Given if after an adequate trial of diet therapy, LDL cholesterol remains 190 mg/dL or greater or LDL cholesterol remains 160 mg/dL or greater and there is a positive family history of premature CV disease or 2 or more other CV disease risk factors are present in the adolescent client. *Investigational:* Heterozygous familial hypercholesterolemia, familial combined hyperlipidemia, diabetic dyslipidemia in NIDDM, hyperlipidemia secondary to the nephrotic syndrome, and homozygous familial hypercholesterolemia in clients with defective LDL receptors. *NOTE:* Simvastatin reduces risks of fatal and nonfatal heart attacks and strokes, as well as reduces the need for bypass surgery and angioplasty.

ACTION/KINETICS
Action
Competitively inhibits HMG-CoA reductase; this enzyme catalyzes the early rate-limiting step in the synthesis of cholesterol. Thus, cholesterol synthesis is inhibited/decreased. Decreases cholesterol, triglycerides, VLDL, LDL, and increases HDL. Does not reduce basal plasma cortisol or testosterone levels or impair renal reserve.

Pharmacokinetics
Peak therapeutic response: 4–6 weeks. Approximately 85% absorbed; significant first-pass effect with less than 5% of a PO dose reaching the general circulation. $t\frac{1}{2}$: 3 hr. Metabolites excreted in the feces (60%) and urine (13%). Increased levels seen in those with hepatic and severe renal insufficiency. Plasma protein binding: About 95%.

CONTRAINDICATIONS
Use if pregnant, planning to become pregnant, or while breastfeeding.

S

SPECIAL CONCERNS
Use with caution in clients who have a history of liver disease/consume large quantities of alcohol or with drugs that affect steroid levels or activity. Higher plasma levels may be observed in clients with hepatic and severe renal insufficiency. Safety and efficacy have not been determined in children less than 18 years of age.

SIDE EFFECTS

Most Common
Headache, abdominal pain/cramps, constipation, URTI, flatulence, diarrhea, asthenia, N&V, dyspepsia, myalgia, rash/pruritus.

Musculoskeletal: ***Rhabdomyolysis*** with renal dysfunction secondary to myoglobinuria, myopathy, arthralgias, myalgia. **GI:** N&V, diarrhea, abdominal pain, constipation, flatulence, dyspepsia, ***pancreatitis***, anorexia, stomatitis. **Hepatic:** Hepatitis (including chronic active hepatitis), cholestatic jaundice, cirrhosis, fatty change in liver, ***fulminant hepatic necrosis, hepatoma***. **Neurologic:** Dysfunction of certain cranial nerves resulting in alteration of taste, impairment of extraocular movement, and facial paresis. Paresthesia, peripheral neuropathy, peripheral nerve palsy. **CNS:** Headache, tremor, vertigo, memory loss, anxiety, insomnia, depression. **Hypersensitivity reactions:** Although rare, the following symptoms have been noted: ***Angioedema, anaphylaxis***, lupus erythematous–like syndrome, vasculitis, purpura, thrombocytopenia, leukopenia, ***hemolytic anemia***, polymyalgia rheumatica, positive ANA, ESR increase, arthritis, arthralgia, asthenia, urticaria, photosensitivity, chills, fever, flushing, malaise, dyspnea, ***toxic epidermal necrolysis, erythema multiforme (including Stevens-Johnson syndrome)***. **GU:** Gynecomastia, loss of libido, erectile dysfunction. **Ophthalmic:** Lens opacities, ophthalmoplegia. **Hematologic:** Transient asymptomatic eosinophilia, anemia, thrombocytopenia, leukopenia. **Miscellaneous:** URTI, asthenia, alopecia, edema, rash/pruritus.

ADDITIONAL DRUG INTERACTIONS
Amiodarone / Possibility of myopathy, muscle weakness, and rhabdomyolysis; if used together, do not give client more than 20 mg/day of simvastatin
Bosentan / ↓ Simvastatin levels R/T ↑ metabolism
Carbamazepine / ↓ Simvastatin AUC, peak levels, and shortened $t\frac{1}{2}$ R/T ↑ metabolism by CYP3A4
Clarithromycin / ↑ Risk of severe myopathy and rhabdomyolysis
Diltiazem ↑ Risk of myopathy R/T ↑ simvastatin levels
Erythromycin / ↑ Risk of severe myopathy and rhabdomyolysis
Grapefruit juice / Chronic use of grapefruit juice ↑ simvastatin levels R/T ↓ liver metabolism
Nefazodone / ↑ Risk of myopathy
Protease inhibitors (e.g., nelfinavir, ritonavir) / ↑ Simvastatin levels → ↑ risk of myopathy
H *St. John's wort* / ↓ Simvastatin levels → ↓ efficacy
Verapamil / ↑ Risk of myopathy
Warfarin / ↑ INR

LABORATORY TEST CONSIDERATIONS
↑ CPK, AST, ALT.

HOW SUPPLIED
Tablets: 5 mg, 10 mg, 20 mg, 40 mg, 80 mg.

DOSAGE
• **TABLETS**
Hyperlipidemia, coronary heart disease.

Adults, initially: 20–40 mg once daily in the evening; **maintenance:** 5–80 mg/day as a single dose in the evening. Consider a starting dose of 5 mg/day for clients on immunosuppressants (e.g., cyclosporine), those with LDL less than 190 mg/dL, or in those with severe renal insufficiency. Consider a starting dose of 10 mg/day for clients with LDL greater than 190 mg/dL. Consider a starting dose of 40 mg as an alternative for those who require a reduction of more than 45% in their LDL cholesterol (most often those with CAD). For geriatric clients, the starting dose should be 5 mg/day with maximum LDL reductions seen with 20 mg or less daily. Do not exceed 10 mg/day if used in combination with fibrates or niacin.

Homozygous familial hypercholesterolemia.

Adults: 40 mg/day in the evening or 80 mg/day in 3 divided doses of 20 mg, 20 mg, and an evening dose of 40 mg. Use as an adjunct to other lipid-lowering treatments (e.g., LDL apheresis) or if such treatments are unavailable.

Adolescents 10–17 years of age with heterozygous familial hypercholesterolemia.

Initial: 10 mg once a day in the evening. **Dose range:** 10–40 mg/day (maximum). Individualize dose. Adjust at intervals of 4 weeks or more.

NURSING CONSIDERATIONS

ℂ Do not confuse Zocor with Cozaar (an antihypertensive) or with Zoloft (an antidepressant).

ADMINISTRATION/STORAGE

1. If no more than two risk factors, place on a standard cholesterol-lowering diet for 3–6 months before starting simvastatin; continue diet during drug therapy.

2. May give without regard to meals.

3. Dosage may be adjusted at intervals of at least 4 weeks.

4. In clients taking cyclosporine or danazol together with simvastatin, begin therapy with 5 mg/day of simvastatin; do not exceed 10 mg/day simvastatin.

5. In clients taking amiodarone or verapamil together with simvastatin, the dose of simvastatin should not exceed 20 mg/day.

6. In clients with severely impaired renal function, start at 5 mg/day simvastatin; monitor closely.

7. Simvastatin is effective alone or together with bile acid sequestrants. Avoid use of simvastatin with gemfibrozil, other fibrates, or lipid-lowering doses (1 gram/day or more) of niacin unless the benefit of further alteration in lipid levels is likely to outweigh the increased risk of the drug combination. However, if simvastatin is used together with fibrates or niacin, monitor carefully; do not exceed 10 mg/day of simvastatin.

8. Store from 5–30°C (41–86°F).

ASSESSMENT

1. Note reasons for therapy: plaque stability or elevated TG/LDL cholesterol in CAD.

2. Monitor CBC, lipid profile, CPK, renal, LFTs; reduce dose with dysfuction. Schedule LFTs at the beginning of therapy and semiannually for the first year of therapy. LFTs should be done before dose is increased to 80 mg, three months after the change, and twice a year thereafter. Special attention should be paid to elevated serum transaminase levels.

3. List all medications prescribed; ensure none interact. Reduce dose with certain drug combinations. Identify/list risk factors for CHD.

4. Assess level of adherence to weight reduction, regular exercise, cholesterol-lowering diet, BP, BS control. Note any alcohol abuse.

5. Assess for any secondary causes for hypercholesterolemia (e.g., hypothyroidism, nephrotic syndrome, dysproteinemias, obstructive liver disease, other drug therapy, alcoholism).

CLIENT/FAMILY TEACHING

1. Take once or twice daily as directed. More preferable in evening.

2. A low-cholesterol diet must be followed during drug therapy. Consult dietitian for assistance in meal planning and food preparation. Do not take with grapefruit juice. May enjoy grapefruit juice at other times during the day.

3. Report any S&S of infections, unexplained muscle pain, tenderness/weakness (especially if accompanied by fever or malaise), surgery, trauma, or metabolic disorders. Report as scheduled for lab tests, eye exam, and F/U.

4. Review importance of regular exercise, low alcohol consumption, smoking abstinence, and following a low-cholesterol diet in the overall plan to reduce serum cholesterol levels and inhibit progression of CAD.

5. Not for use during pregnancy; use barrier contraception.

6. May experience sun sensitivity; take precautions to avoid sun or use sun protection.

7. Keep all F/U appointments to assess response to therapy and if at goal.

OUTCOMES/EVALUATE

↓ Elevated total-C, LDL-C, Apo B, and TG ↑ HDL; cardiovascular risk reduction

---

Sirolimus ∎

(sir-oh-**LIH**-mus)

CLASSIFICATION(S):
Immunosuppressant
PREGNANCY CATEGORY: C
Rx: Rapamune.

USES

Use with corticosteroids and cyclosporine to prevent organ rejection in renal transplants, including for cyclosporine-sparing immunosuppression in those with kidney transplants who are at low or moderate risk of organ rejection. Use only in clients 13 years of age and older. *Investigational:* Treat psoriasis.

ACTION/KINETICS

Action
Inhibits both T-lymphocyte activation and proliferation that occurs in response to antigenic and interleukin IL-2, IL-4, and IL-15 stimulation. Also inhibits antibody production.

Pharmacokinetics
Rapidly absorbed after PO use. **Peak levels:** About 1 hr in healthy clients and about 2 hr in renal transplant clients. High-fat meals increase C_{max}, T_{max}, and AUC. The majority of the drug is sequestered in erythrocytes resulting in much higher blood levels compared with plasma levels. A high-fat meal alters the bioavailability of sirolimus. Extensively metabolized by CYP3A4 and P-glycoprotein in the liver and gut wall. Over 90% is excreted in the feces. Adjust dosage for mild-to-moderate hepatic impairment. $t\frac{1}{2}$, **terminal, after multiple dosing in renal transplant clients:** About 62 hr. **Plasma protein binding:** Approximately 92%.

CONTRAINDICATIONS

Hypersensitivity to sirolimus, its derivatives, or any component of the drug product. Use as an immunosuppressant in liver or lung transplants. Lactation.

SPECIAL CONCERNS

∎ (1) Increased susceptibility to infection and possible development of lymphoma may result from immunosuppression. Only health care providers experienced in immunosuppressive therapy and management of renal transplant clients should use sirolimus. Manage those receiving the drug in facilities equipped and staffed with adequate lab and supportive medical resources. The physician responsible for maintenance therapy should have complete information needed for the follow-up of the client. (2) Liver transplantation. The use of sirolimus in combination with tacrolimus was associated with excess mortality and graft loss in de novo liver transplant recipients. Many had evidence of infection at or near the time of death. (3) The use of sirolimus with cyclosporine or tacrolimus was associated with an increase in hepatic artery thrombosis; most cases occurred within 30 days after transplantation and most led to graft loss or death. The safety and efficacy of sirolimus as immunosuppressive therapy have not been established in liver transplant clients; therefore, use is not recommended in these clients. (4) Cases of bronchial anastomotic dehiscence, most fatal, have been reported in de novo lung transplant clients when sirolimus was used as part of an immunosuppressive regimen. The safety and efficacy of sirolimus as immunosuppressive therapy have not been established in lung transplant clients; therefore, use is not recommended in these clients. ∎ Use with caution in those with impaired renal function or when used with drugs that impair renal function (e.g., aminoglycosides, amphotericin B). Safety and efficacy have not been determined in combination with other immunosuppressant drugs or in pediatric clients less than 13 years of age. Increased susceptibility to infection and possible development of lymphoma due to immunosuppression.

Bold Italic = life threatening side effect   ∎ = black box warning   ✤ = Available in Canada

SIDE EFFECTS

Most Common

Peripheral edema, tremor, acne, diarrhea, N&V, hypercholesterolemia/hyperlipidemia, asthenia, hypertension, headache, constipation, abdominal pain, anemia, edema, weight gain, dyspnea, URTI, fever, pain, arthralgia, UTI.

GI: Diarrhea, N&V, constipation, abdominal pain, dyspepsia, anorexia, dysphagia, eructation, esophagitis, flatulence, gastritis, gastroenteritis, gingivitis, gum hyperplasia, ileus, mouth ulceration, oral moniliasis, stomatitis, rectal disorder, *pancreatitis, fatal hepatic necrosis.* **CNS:** Tremor, headache, insomnia, anxiety, confusion, depression, dizziness, emotional lability, hyper-/hypotonia, hypesthesia, insomnia, neuropathy, paresthesia, somnolence. **CV:** Hyper-/hypotension, atrial fibrillation, CHF, *hemorrhage,* hypervolemia, palpitation, peripheral vascular disorder, postural hypotension, syncope, tachycardia, thrombophlebitis, thrombosis, vasodilation, venous thromboembolism (including DVT), *hepatic artery thrombosis.* **Dermatologic:** Acne, rash, fungal dermatitis, hirsutism, pruritus, skin hypertrophy, skin ulcer, sweating, photosensitivity, skin cancer. **Respiratory:** Dyspnea, URTI, pharyngitis, asthma, atelectasis, bronchitis, increased cough, epistaxis, hypoxia, lung edema, pleural effusion, pneumonia, rhinitis, sinusitis, interstitial lung disease, *pulmonary embolism.* **Hematologic:** Anemia, thrombocytopenia, ecchymosis, leukopenia, leukocytosis, lymphadenopathy, polycythemia, lymphoma, lymphoproliferative disease, thrombotic thrombocytopenic purpura (*hemolytic uremic syndrome*), pancytopenia (rare), lymphedema (rare). **GU:** UTI, bladder pain, dysuria, hematuria, hydronephrosis, impotence, kidney pain, kidney tubular necrosis, nocturia, oliguria, pyuria, scrotal edema, testis disorder, pyelonephritis, *toxic nephrotoxicity,* impaired renal function urinary frequency/incontinence/retention, menorrhagia, metrorrhagia, polyuria. **Musculoskeletal:** Arthralgia, arthrosis, bone necrosis, leg cramps, myalgia, osteoporosis, tetany.

Endocrine: Cushing's syndrome, diabetes mellitus, glycosuria. **Ophthalmic:** Abnormal vision, cataract, conjunctivitis. **Otic:** Deafness, ear pain, otitis media, tinnitus. **Body as a whole:** Asthenia, fever, dehydration, abnormal healing, weight loss/gain, abscess, cellulitis, chills, flu syndrome, generalized edema, infection, malaise, hypersensitivity reactions, mycobacterial infections, Epstein-Barr viral infections, *sepsis.* **Miscellaneous:** Peripheral edema, pain (abdominal, pelvic, back, chest), enlarged abdomen, ascites, facial edema, hernia, lymphocele, herpes simplex, acidosis, *peritonitis,* increased susceptibility to infection (including *Pneumocystis carinii*) and possible development of lymphoma.

LABORATORY TEST CONSIDERATIONS

↑ Alkaline phosphatase, BUN, CPK, LDH, ALT, AST, serum cholesterol, triglycerides, serum creatinine. ↓ Mean GFR, platelets, hemoglobin. Abnormal LFTs. Acidosis, albuminuria, hyper-/hypophosphatemia, hyper-/hypocalcemia, hyper-/hypoglycemia, hyper-/hypokalemia, hyperlipemia, hypomagnesemia, hyponatremia.

OD OVERDOSE MANAGEMENT

Symptoms: Symptoms due to overdosage are consistent with those listed under *Side Effects. Treatment:* Institute general supportive measures. Sirolimus is not dialyzable to any extent.

DRUG INTERACTIONS

Angiotensin-converting enzyme (ACE) inhibitors / Possibile angioneurotic edema-type reactions

Azole antifungal drugs / ↑ Sirolimus levels → ↑ toxicity

Bromocriptine / ↑ Sirolimus levels R/T ↓ metabolism

Carbamazepine / ↓ Sirolimus levels R/T ↑ metabolism

Cimetidine / ↑ Sirolimus levels R/T ↓ metabolism

Clarithromycin / ↑ Sirolimus levels R/T ↓ metabolism

Clotrimazole / ↑ Sirolimus levels R/T ↓ metabolism

Cyclosporine / ↑ Risk of hepatic artery thrombosis → graft loss or death; also, ↑ sirolimus levels → ↑ toxicity (give

S

sirolimus 4 hr after cyclosporine)

Danazol / ↑ Sirolimus levels R/T ↓ metabolism

Diltiazem / ↑ Sirolimus levels

Erythromycin / ↑ Sirolimus levels R/T ↓ metabolism

Fluconazole / ↑ Sirolimus levels R/T ↓ metabolism

Grapefruit juice / ↓ CYP3A4-mediated metabolism of sirolimus; do not give together

HIV-protease inhibitors / ↑ Sirolimus levels R/T ↓ metabolism

Itraconazole / ↑ Sirolimus levels R/T ↓ metabolism

Ketoconazole / Significant ↑ sirolimus levels; do not use together

Metoclopramide / ↑ Sirolimus levels R/T ↓ metabolism

Mycophenolate / ↑ Mycophenolic acid exposure and ↓ WBC compared with coadministration of cyclosporine

Nicardipine / ↑ Sirolimus levels R/T ↓ metabolism

Phenobarbital / ↓ Sirolimus levels R/T ↑ metabolism

Phenytoin / ↓ Sirolimus levels R/T ↑ metabolism

Protease inhibitors (e.g., indinavir, ritonavir) / ↑ Sirolimus levels R/T ↓ metabolism

Rifabutin / ↓ Sirolimus levels R/T ↑ metabolism

Rifampin / ↓ Sirolimus levels R/T ↑ metabolism

Rifapentine / ↓ Sirolimus levels R/T ↑ metabolism

[H] *St. John's wort* / ↓ Sirolimus levels R/T ↑ metabolism

Tacrolimus / ↑ Risk of hepatic artery thrombosis → graft loss or death; ↓ tacrolimus AUC and peak plasma levels in pediatric renal transplant clients

Troleandomycin / ↑ Sirolimus levels R/T ↓ metabolism

Vaccines / Vaccines may be less effective

Verapamil / ↑ Sirolimus levels R/T ↓ metabolism

HOW SUPPLIED

Oral Solution: 1 mg/mL; *Tablets:* 1 mg, 2 mg.

DOSAGE

• **ORAL SOLUTION; TABLETS**

Prophylaxis of rejection following kidney transplantation.

Loading dose, initial: 6 mg; **maintenance dose:** 2 mg/day. Or, **Loading dose, initial:** 15 mg; **maintenance:** 5 mg/day (this regimen not shown to be any more effective than the lower dosage regimen). **Clients, 13 years and older weighing <40 kg:** Adjust the initial dose based on body surface area to 1 mg/m²/day. The loading dose should be 3 mg/m². Reduce the maintenance dose by about 33% in clients with impaired hepatic function; it is not necessary to reduce the initial loading dose. At 2–4 months after transplantation, cyclosporine should be discontinued progressively over 4–8 weeks; the dosage of sirolimus should be adjusted to obtain whole blood trough levels within the range of 12–24 ng/mL (using chromatographic method). Therapeutic drug monitoring should not be the only basis for adjusting sirolimus dosage. Pay careful attention to clinical signs/symptoms, tissue biopsy, and lab parameters.

Because cyclosporine inhibits the metabolism of sirolimus, the dose of sirolimus must be increased approximately 4-fold after cyclosporine withdrawal. Once the sirolimus maintenance dose is adjusted, retain clients on the new maintenance dose for 7-14 days before adjusting the dose further. In most clients, dosage adjustments can be based on the following:

New sirolimus dose =
current dose x target
concentration/current concentration.

A loading dose should be considered in addition to a new maintenance dose when it is necessary to increase significantly the sirolimus trough levels. The following formula can be used:

Sirolimus loading dose =
3 x (new maintenance dosage –
current maintenance dosage).

Maximum daily sirolimus dosage should not exceed 40 mg. If an estimated daily dose exceeds 40 mg, give the loading dose over 2 days.

Bold Italic = life threatening side effect   ■ = black box warning   ✦ = Available in Canada

NURSING CONSIDERATIONS

ADMINISTRATION/STORAGE

1. Use sirolimus with cyclosporine and corticosteroids. Give sirolimus 4 hr after cyclosporine. Give initial dose of sirolimus as soon as possible after transplantation.

2. Reduce the dose by one-third in those with mild to severe abnormal hepatic function.

3. Note that 2 mg of oral solution is equivalent to 2 mg oral tablets, making them interchangeable on a mg-to-mg basis. It is not known if higher doses of oral solutions are clinically equivalent to higher doses of tablets on a mg-to-mg basis.

4. To reduce dosing errors, read the label carefully. The strength of the liquid is 1 mg/mL but it is available in 1 mL, 2 mL, and 5 mL quantities. Thus a 2 mL vial contains 2 mg of the drug.

5. Take consistently with or without food. Grapefruit juice reduces CYP3A4-mediated metabolism; do not give sirolimus with grapefruit juice.

6. After dilution, use the product immediately. Discard syringe after 1 use.

7. In those at low to moderate immunological risk, withdraw cyclosporine 2–4 months after transplantation; increase sirolumus dose to reach recommended blood concentrations.

8. Dilute and administer oral solution in *bottles* as follows:

- Use the amber oral dose syringe to withdraw the prescribed amount of solution from the bottle.
- Empty the correct amount from the syringe into a glass or plastic (only) container containing at least 2 ounces of water or orange juice. No other liquids (including grapefruit juice) should be used for the dilution.
- Stir vigorously and drink at once.
- Refill the container with an additional volume (minimum of 4 ounces) of water or orange juice, stir vigorously, and drink at once.

9. Dilute and administer the oral solution in *pouches* as follows:

- Squeeze the entire contents of the pouch into a glass or plastic (only) container holding at least 2 ounces of water or orange juice. No other liquids, including grapefruit juice, should be used for the dilution.
- Stir vigorously and drink at once.
- Refill container with an additional volume (minimum of 4 ounces) of water or orange juice, stir vigorously, and drink at once.

10. Protect the oral solution bottles and pouches from light. Refrigerate at 2–8° C (36–46° F). The oral solution is stable for 24 months under these storage conditions. Use the contents within 1 month once the bottle has been opened. If necessary, both the pouches and bottles may be stored at room temperature (25°C; 77°F) for no more than 24 hr. If the oral solution in bottles develops a slight haze when refrigerated, allow to stand at room temperature and shake gently until haze disappears. Haze does not affect the quality of the product.

ASSESSMENT

1. Note date of transplant and for what reasons required. Ensure F/U provided by transplant center as drugs require careful monitoring for adverse effects (especially with liver/lung transplants if used at all or in combination therapy).

2. Monitor sirolimus levels closely in pediatric clients, in those with impaired hepatic function, during concurrent administration of strong CYP3A4 inhibitors and inducers, and if cyclosporine is markedly reduced or discontinued.

3. Assess VS, ensure BP well controlled. Due to immunosuppressant effect, assess for infections and development of lymphoma.

4. Monitor CBC, renal, and LFTs as well as cyclosporine and sirolimus drug levels.

CLIENT/FAMILY TEACHING

1. Take sirolimus as prescribed with cyclosporine and corticosteroids. Take sirolimus 4 hr after cyclosporine to prevent variations in sirolimus levels. Follow directions carefully for storage, dilution, and dosing of drug.

---

2. Initial dose of sirolimus will be given asap after transplantation. Review drug insert carefully.

3. Report any unusual side effects including rash, fever, chills, sore throat, diarrhea, or infections. Do not permit solution to touch skin or eyes; if contact occurs rinse eyes with plain water and wash skin with soap and water.

4. Take consistently with or without food. Grapefruit juice reduces metabolism; do not give sirolimus with grapefruit juice. Use water or orange juice and rinse glass to ensure entire dose consumed.

5. If the oral solution in bottles develops a slight haze when refrigerated, allow to stand at room temperature and shake gently until haze disappears. Haze does not affect the quality of the product.

6. May also be prescribed antibiotics for one year to prevent *P. carinii* and CMV prophylaxis for 3 months post transplant.

7. Females must use reliable contraception before, during and for 12 weeks after therapy has been discontinued.

8. Avoid prolonged sun exposure; use protective sun screen, clothing and glasses if exposed.

9. While receiving immunosuppressive drugs, one may be more susceptible to infections and possibly lymphoma. Avoid crowds, infected persons and report any unusual side effects or symptoms of illness. Keep regularly scheduled visits at transplant center to evaluate labs and organ status.

OUTCOMES/EVALUATE
- Prophylaxis of renal transplant rejection
- Therapeutic serum drug levels

Sitagliptin phosphate
(**SI**-tah-glip-tin)

CLASSIFICATION(S):
Antidiabetic agent, dipeptidyl peptidase-4 inhibitor
PREGNANCY CATEGORY: B
Rx: Januvia.

USES
Adjunct to diet and exercise to improve glycemic control in type 2 diabetes mellitus either as monotherapy or in combination with metformin or a thiazolidinedione.

ACTION/KINETICS
Action
Incretin hormones are released by the intestine throughout the day; levels increase in response to a meal. The incretins are involved in the physiologic regulation of glucose homeostasis. When blood glucose levels are normal or elevated, incretins increase insulin synthesis and release from pancreatic beta cells. One of the incretins also lowers glucagon secretion from pancreatic alpha cells, leading to reduced hepatic glucose production. The incretins are normally rapidly inactivated by the enzyme, dipeptidyl peptidase-4. Sitagliptin is a specific inhibitor of dipeptidyl peptidase–4 and acts by slowing inactivation of incretin hormones. By increasing and prolonging active incretin levels, sitagliptin increases insulin release and decreases glucagon levels in the circulation in a glucose-dependent manner.

Pharmacokinetics
Rapidly absorbed; **peak plasma levels:** 1–4 hr. Absolute bioavailability is about 87%. About 79% excreted unchanged in the urine with metabolites excreted in the urine and feces. The primary enzyme responsible for the limited metabolism is CYP3A4 with some contribution from CYP2C8. **$t^1\!/_2$, terminal:** 12.4 hr. **Plasma protein binding:** 38%.

CONTRAINDICATIONS
Use in type 1 diabetes mellitus or to treat diabetic ketoacidosis as the drug is not effective for these conditions.

SPECIAL CONCERNS
Use with caution during lactation. Safety and efficacy have not been established in children less than 18 years of age.

SIDE EFFECTS
Most Common
Headache, nasopharyngitis, URTI.
GI: Abdominal pain, nausea, diarrhea. **CNS:** Headache. **Respiratory:** Naso-

---

Bold Italic = life threatening side effect   ■ = black box warning   ✦ = Available in Canada

pharyngitis, URTI. **Metabolic:** Hypoglycemia.

LABORATORY TEST CONSIDERATIONS
Small ↑ WBCs and serum creatinine.

HOW SUPPLIED
Tablets: 25 mg, 50 mg, 100 mg.

DOSAGE

* **TABLETS**
  Type 2 diabetes mellitus.
100 mg once daily either as monotherapy or in combination with metformin or a thiazolidinedione.

NURSING CONSIDERATIONS

ADMINISTRATION/STORAGE
1. Give a dose of 50 mg once daily for those with moderately impaired renal function: C_{CR} greater than or equal to 30 mL/min to <50 mL/min, approximately corresponding to serum creatinine levels less than or equal to 1.7 mg/dL in men and less than or equal to 1.5 mg/dL in women.
2. Give a dose of 25 mg once daily for severely impaired renal function: C_{CR} <30 mL/min, corresponding to serum creatinine levels of >3 mg/dL in men and >2.5 mg/dL in women or with end stage renal disease requiring hemodialysis or peritoneal dialysis. Sitagliptin can be given without regard to the timing of hemodialysis.
3. Store from 15–30°C (59–86°F).

ASSESSMENT
1. Note reasons for therapy, onset, characteristics of S&S, other agents trialed, outcome.
2. Assess renal function in the elderly before initiating sitagliptin therapy; reduce dose with renal dysfunction.
3. List risk factors, wt, lipid profile, BP, eye and foot exam findings. Assess for organ damage, neuropathy or other diabetes related problems.
4. Monitor renal/lipid profile, HbA1c, microalbum.

CLIENT/FAMILY TEACHING
1. Can be taken with or without food.
2. May experience upper respiratory tract infection, stuffy or runny nose, sore throat, and headache; report if persistent or bothersome.

3. Drug is used alone or with other agents to control blood sugar in addition to diet and exercise.
4. Record finger sticks to share with provider.
5. Keep all F/U appointments to evaluate response to therapy and dosage adjustments.

OUTCOMES/EVALUATE
Control of diabetes; HbA1c <7

Sodium bicarbonate   IV

(**SO**-dee-um bye-**KAR**-bon-ayt)

CLASSIFICATION(S):
Alkalinizing agent, Antacid, Electrolyte
PREGNANCY CATEGORY: C
OTC: Arm and Hammer Pure Baking Soda, Bell/ans, Citrocarbonate, Soda Mint.
Rx: Neut.

USES
(1) Treatment of hyperacidity. (2) Severe diarrhea (where there is loss of bicarbonate). (3) Alkalization of the urine to treat drug toxicity (e.g., due to barbiturates, salicylates, methanol). (4) Treatment of acute mild to moderate metabolic acidosis due to shock, severe dehydration, anoxia, uncontrolled diabetes, renal disease, cardiac arrest, extracorporeal circulation of blood, severe primary lactic acidosis. (5) Prophylaxis of renal calculi in gout. (6) During sulfonamide therapy to prevent renal calculi and nephrotoxicity. (7) Neutralizing additive solution to decrease chemical phlebitis and client discomfort due to vein irritation at or near the site of infusion of IV acid solutions. *Investigational:* Sickle cell anemia.

ACTION/KINETICS
Action
The antacid action is due to neutralization of hydrochloric acid by forming sodium chloride and carbon dioxide (1 gram of sodium bicarbonate neutralizes

S

12 mEq of acid). Provides temporary relief of peptic ulcer pain and of discomfort associated with indigestion. Although widely used by the public, sodium bicarbonate is rarely prescribed as an antacid because of its high sodium content, short duration of action, and ability to cause alkalosis (sometimes desired). Is also a systemic and urinary alkalinizer by increasing plasma and urinary bicarbonate, respectively.

CONTRAINDICATIONS

Chloride loss due to vomiting or from continuous GI suction. With diuretics known to produce a hypochloremic alkalosis. Metabolic and respiratory alkalosis. Hypocalcemia in which alkalosis may cause tetany. Hypertension, convulsions, CHF, and other situations where administration of sodium can be dangerous. As a systemic alkalinizer when used as a neutralizing additive solution. As an antidote for strong mineral acids because carbon dioxide is formed, which may cause discomfort and even perforation.

SPECIAL CONCERNS

Use with caution in impaired renal function, toxemia of pregnancy, with oliguria or anuria, during lactation, in edema, CHF, liver cirrhosis, with low-salt diets, and in geriatric or postoperative clients with renal or CV insufficiency with or without CHF.

SIDE EFFECTS

Most Common
Rebound hyperacidity, milk-alkali syndrome.

GI: Rebound hyperacidity, gastric distention. **Milk-alkali syndrome:** Hypercalcemia, metabolic alkalosis (dizziness, cramps, thirst, anorexia, N&V, hyperexcitability, tetany, diminished breathing, *seizures*), renal dysfunction. **Miscellaneous:** Systemic alkalosis after prolonged use. **Following rapid infusion:** Hypernatremia, alkalosis, hyperirritability, tetany, fluid or solute overload. Extravasation following IV use may manifest ulceration, sloughing, cellulitis, or tissue necrosis at the site of injection.

OD **OVERDOSE MANAGEMENT**

Symptoms: Severe alkalosis that may be accompanied by tetany or hyperirritability. *Treatment:* Discontinue sodium bicarbonate. Reverse symptoms of alkalosis by rebreathing expired air from a paper bag or using a rebreathing mask. Use an IV infusion of ammonium chloride solution, 2.14%, to control severe cases. Treat hypokalemia by IV sodium chloride or potassium chloride. Calcium gluconate will control tetany.

DRUG INTERACTIONS

Amphetamines / ↑ Amphetamine effect by ↑ renal tubular reabsorption
Antidepressants, tricyclic / ↑ TCA effect by ↑ renal tubular reabsorption
Benzodiazepines / ↓ Benzodiazepine effect R/T ↑ urine alkalinity
Chlorpropamide / ↑ Chlorpropamide excretion rate R/T urine alkalinization
Ephedrine / ↑ Ephedrine effect by ↑ renal tubular reabsorption
Erythromycin / ↑ Erythromycin effect in urine R/T ↑ urine alkalinity
Flecainide / ↑ Flecainide effect R/T ↑ urine alkalinity
Iron products / ↓ Iron effects R/T ↑ urine alkalinity
Ketoconazole / ↓ Ketoconazole effect R/T ↑ urine alkalinity
Lithium carbonate / Excretion of lithium proportional to amount of sodium ingested. If client on sodium-free diet, may develop lithium toxicity R/T ↓ lithium excreted
Mecamylamine / ↓ Mecamylamine excretion R/T alkalinization of the urine
Methenamine compounds / ↓ Methenamine effect R/T ↑ urine alkalinity
Methotrexate / ↑ Renal methotrexate excretion R/T alkalinization of the urine
Nitrofurantoin / ↓ Nitrofurantoin effect R/T ↑ urine alkalinity
Procainamide / ↑ Procainamide effect R/T ↓ kidney excretion
Pseudoephedrine / ↑ Pseudoephedrine effect R/T ↑ tubular reabsorption
Quinidine / ↑ Quinidine effect by ↑ renal tubular reabsorption
Salicylates / ↑ Rate of salicylate excretion R/T alkalinization of the urine
Sulfonylureas / ↓ Sulfonylurea effect R/T ↑ urine alkalinity
Sympathomimetics / ↓ Sympathomimetic renal excretion R/T alkalinization of the urine

Tetracyclines / ↓ Tetracycline effect R/T
↑ kidney excretion

HOW SUPPLIED

Injection: 4%, 4.2%, 5%, 7.5%, 8.4%;
Powder; Tablets: 325 mg, 520 mg, 650 mg.

DOSAGE

• **EFFERVESCENT POWDER**
  Antacid.
Adults: 3.9–10 grams in a glass of cold water after meals. **Geriatric and pediatric, 6–12 years:** 1.9–3.9 grams after meals.

• **ORAL POWDER**
  Antacid.
Adults: ½ teaspoon in a glass of water q 2 hr; adjust dosage as required.
  Urinary alkalinizer.
Adults: 1 teaspoon in a glass of water q 4 hr; adjust dosage as required. Dosage not established for this form for children.

• **TABLETS**
  Antacid.
Adults: 0.325–2 grams 1–4 times per day; **pediatric, 6–12 years:** 520 mg; may be repeated once after 30 min.
  Urinary alkalinizer.
Adults, initial: 0.325–2 grams up to 4 times per day; **then,** maximum of 15 grams in those under age 60 and 8 grams in those over age 60.

• **IV**
  Cardiac arrest.
Adults: 200–300 mEq given rapidly as a 7.5% or 8.4% solution. In emergencies, 300–500 mL of a 5% solution given as rapidly as possible without overalkalinizing the client. **Infants, less than 2 years of age, initial:** 1–2 mEq/kg/min given over 1–2 min; **then,** 1 mEq/kg q 10 min of arrest. Do not exceed 8 mEq/kg/day.
  Severe metabolic acidosis.
90–180 mEq/L (about 7.5–15 grams) at a rate of 1–1.5 L during the first hour. Adjust to needs of client.
  Less severe metabolic acidosis.
Add to other IV fluids. **Adults and older children:** 2–5 mEq/kg given over a 4 to 8 hr period.
  Neutralizing additive solution.
One vial of neutralizing additive solution added to 1 L of commonly used

parenteral solutions, including dextrose, NaCl, and Ringer's.

NURSING CONSIDERATIONS

ADMINISTRATION/STORAGE

Ⅳ 1. Hypertonic solutions must be administered by trained personnel. Avoid extravasation as tissue irritation or cellulitis may result.

2. Determine IV dose by arterial blood pH, pCO_2, and base deficit; may be given IV push in arrest situation or diluted in dextrose or saline solution and given over 4–8 hr.

3. Administer isotonic solutions slowly; too rapid administration may result in death due to cellular acidity. Check rate of flow frequently.

4. If only the 7.5% or 8.4% solution is available, dilute 1:1 with D5W when used in infants for cardiac arrest.

5. Do not exceed a rate of administration of 8 mEq/kg/day in infants with cardiac arrest to guard against hypernatremia, induction of intracranial hemorrhage, and decreasing CSF pressure.

6. In the event of severe alkalosis or tetany, have available a parenteral solution of calcium gluconate and 2.14% ammonium chloride.

7. Do not add to calcium-containing solutions, except where compatibility has been established.

8. Norepinephrine and dobutamine are incompatible with $NaHCO_3$.

ASSESSMENT

1. Note reasons for therapy, any history of renal impairment or CHF.

2. Assess for edema, which may indicate inability to utilize $NaHCO_3$. May try potassium bicarbonate (sodium content is 27%).

3. If on low continuous or intermittent NG suctioning or vomiting, assess for evidence of excessive chloride loss.

4. Record I&O. Observe for dry skin/mucous membranes, polydipsia, polyuria, and air hunger; may indicate a reversal of metabolic acidosis. With acidosis, assess relief of dyspnea and hyperpnea.

5. If prescribed to counteract metabolic acidosis, monitor electrolytes and ABGs (pH, pCO_2, and HCO_3). For urine, test q

S

4–8 hr with nitrazine paper to determine if becoming alkaline (pH >7).

CLIENT/FAMILY TEACHING

1. Chew tablets thoroughly and take only as prescribed. Follow with a full glass of water. Do not take with milk or yogurt; will fizz up.

2. If routinely taking excessive PO preparations of sodium bicarbonate to relieve gastric distress, a rebound reaction may occur, resulting either in an increased acid secretion or systemic alkalosis. Persistent symptoms of gastric distress esp. with chest pain, SOB, diarrhea or dark tarry BMs require medical care.

3. Continuous, routine ingestion of sodium bicarbonate may cause formation of phosphate crystals in the kidney, kidney stones and fluid retention.

4. Consuming sodium bicarbonate with milk or calcium may result in a milk-alkali syndrome. Report immediately if anorexia, N&V, or mental confusion occurs.

5. Avoid OTC preparations that contain sodium bicarbonate, such as Alka/Bromo-Seltzer, Gaviscon, or Fizrin.

OUTCOMES/EVALUATE

- Reversal of metabolic acidosis
- ↑ Urinary and serum pH
- ↓ Gastric discomfort

Sodium chloride IV

(**SO**-dee-um **KLOR**-eyed)

CLASSIFICATION(S):
Electrolyte
PREGNANCY CATEGORY: C
OTC: Ophthalmic: AK-NaCl, Adsorbonac Ophthalmic, Hypersal 5%, Muro-128 Ophthalmic, Muroptic-5. **Tablets:** Slo-Salt. **Nasal Solution/ Nasal Spray:** Ayr Saline, HuMIST Saline Nasal, NaSal Saline Nasal, Ocean Mist, Ocean for Kids, Salinex Nasal Mist.

Rx: Parenteral: Concentrated Sodium Chloride Injection (14.6%, 23.4%), Sodium Chloride Diluent (0.9%), Sodium Chloride IV Infusions (0.45%, 0.9%, 3%, 5%), Sodium Chloride Injection for Admixtures (50, 100, 625 mEq/vial).

♣**OTC:** Bacteriostatic Sodium Chloride Diluent for Inhalation, Minims Sodium Chloride, Rhinaris Saline Pediatric Drops/Saline Spray.

USES

PO: (1) Prophylaxis of heat prostration or muscle cramps. (2) Chloride deficiency due to diuresis or salt restriction. (3) Prevention or treatment of extracellular volume depletion.

Parenteral: 0.9% (Isotonic) NaCl. (1) Restore sodium and chloride losses. (2) Dilute or dissolve drugs for IV, IM, or SC use or for inhalation. (3) Flushing of IV catheters. (4) Extracellular fluid replacement. (5) Priming solution for hemodialysis. (6) Initiate and terminate blood transfusions so RBCs will not hemolyze. (7) Metabolic alkalosis when there is fluid loss and mild sodium depletion.

0.45% (Hypotonic) NaCl. (1) Fluid replacement when fluid loss exceeds depletion of electrolytes. (2) Hyperosmolar diabetes when dextrose should not be used (need for large volume of fluid but without excess sodium ions). (3) Dissolve drugs for IM, IV, or SC injection or for inhalation.

0.45% and 0.9% Flexible plastic containers. Parenteral replenishment of fluid and NaCl as required by the clinical condition of the client.

3% or 5% (Hypertonic) NaCl. (1) Hyponatremia and hypochloremia due to electrolyte losses. (2) Dilute body water significantly following excessive fluid intake. (3) Emergency treatment of severe salt depletion.

Concentrated NaCl (14.6%). Electrolyte replenisher in parenteral fluid therapy. Serves as a sodium supplement in hyponatremia or low salt syndrome, as an additive for TPN, and as an additive for carbohydrate-containing IV fluids.

Concentrated NaCl (23.4%). Additive in parenteral fluid therapy for those who have special problems of sodium electrolyte intake or excretion.

Bacteriostatic NaCl. Used only to dilute or dissolve drugs for IM, IV, or SC injection.

Nasal Topical: (1) Relief of inflamed, dry, or crusted nasal membranes. (2) Irrigating solution.

Ophthalmic: (1) Hypertonic solutions to decrease corneal edema due to bullous keratitis. (2) An aid to facilitate ophthalmoscopic examination in gonioscopy, biomicroscopy, and funduscopy.

ACTION/KINETICS

Action

Sodium is the major cation of the body's extracellular fluid. It plays a crucial role in maintaining the fluid and electrolyte balance. Excess retention of sodium results in overhydration (edema, hypervolemia), which is often treated with diuretics. Abnormally low levels of sodium result in dehydration. Normally, the plasma contains 136–145 mEq sodium/L and 98–106 mEq chloride/L. The average daily requirement of salt is approximately 5 grams.

CONTRAINDICATIONS

Congestive heart failure, severely impaired renal function, hypernatremia, fluid retention. Use of the 3% or 5% solutions in elevated, normal, or only slightly depressed levels of plasma sodium and chloride. Use of bacteriostatic NaCl injection in newborns.

SPECIAL CONCERNS

Use with caution in CV, cirrhotic, or renal disease; in presence of hyperproteinemia, hypervolemia, urinary tract obstruction, and CHF; in those with concurrent edema and sodium retention and in clients receiving corticosteroids or corticotropin; and during lactation. Use with caution in geriatric or postoperative clients with renal or CV insufficiency with or without CHF. Safety and efficacy of NaCl injection have not been determined in children, although 0.45% and 0.9% flexible plastic containers are used in children. In neonates or very small infants, the volume of fluid may affect fluid and electrolyte balance. Only preservative-free NaCl solution should be used in newborns.

SIDE EFFECTS

Most Common

When used IV: Reactions at site of IV administration, hypernatremia, local pain/irritation from too rapid infusion.

Hypernatremia: Excessive NaCl may lead to hypopotassemia and acidosis. Hypokalemia due to excessive administration of potassium-free solutions. Fluid and solute overload leading to dilution of serum electrolyte levels, CHF, overhydration, *acute pulmonary edema* (especially in clients with CV disease or in those receiving corticosteroids or other drugs that cause sodium retention). Too rapid administration may cause local pain and venous irritation. Ion excess or deficit due to ions present/not present in the solution. Sodium overload can result from administration of concentrated NaCl solutions. **Postoperative intolerance of NaCl:** Cellular dehydration, weakness, asthenia, disorientation, anorexia, nausea, oliguria, increased BUN levels, distention, deep respiration.

Symptoms due to solution or administration technique: Fever, abscess, tissue necrosis, infection at injection site, venous thrombosis or phlebitis extending from injection site, local tenderness, extravasation, hypervolemia. *Inadvertent administration of concentrated NaCl (i.e., without dilution) will cause sudden hypernatremia with the possibility of CV shock, extensive hemolysis, CNS problems, necrosis of the cortex of the kidneys, local tissue necrosis (if given extravascularly).*

OD OVERDOSE MANAGEMENT

Symptoms: Irritation of GI mucosa, N&V, abdominal cramps, diarrhea, edema. Hypernatremia symptoms include: irritability, restlessness, *weakness, seizures,* coma, tachycardia, hypertension, fluid accumulation, *pulmonary edema, respiratory arrest. Treatment:* Supportive measures, including gastric lavage, induction of vomiting, provide adequate airway and ventilation, maintain vascular volume and tissue perfusion. Mg sulfate given as a cathartic.

DRUG INTERACTIONS
Use solutions containing sodium with caution in clients receiving corticosteroids or corticotropin.

HOW SUPPLIED
Injection: 0.45%, 0.9%, 2.5%, 3%, 5%, 14.6%, 23.4%; *Inhalation Solution:* 0.45%, 0.9%, 3%, 10%; *Irrigation Solution:* 0.45%, 0.9%; *Nasal Solution/Nasal Spray:* 0.4%, 0.65%, 0.75%; *Ophthalmic Ointment:* 5%; *Ophthalmic Solution:* 0.44%, 2%, 5%; *Tablets:* 600 mg, 1 gram, 2.25 grams; *Tablets, Slow Release:* 600 mg; *Powder for Reconstitution.*

DOSAGE
- **TABLETS; TABLETS, SLOW RELEASE**
  Heat cramps/dehydration.
0.5–1 gram with 8 oz water up to 10 times/day; total daily dose should not exceed 4.8 grams.
- **IV**
Individualized. Daily requirements of sodium and chloride can be met by administering 1 L of 0.9% NaCl.
To calculate sodium deficit. Amount of sodium to be given to raise serum sodium to the desired level:
Total body water (TBW): sodium deficit (mEq) = TBW × (desired plasma Na – observed plasma Na).
- **OPHTHALMIC SOLUTION 2% OR 5%**
1–2 gtt in eye q 3–4 hr.
- **OPHTHALMIC OINTMENT**
A small amount (approximately ¼ in.) to the inside of the affected eye(s) (i.e., by pulling down the lower eyelid) q 3–4 hr.

NURSING CONSIDERATIONS
ADMINISTRATION/STORAGE
IV 1. Give hypertonic injections of NaCl slowly through a small-bore needle placed well within the lumen of a large vein (to minimize irritation). Avoid infiltration.
2. Concentrated NaCl injection must be diluted before use.
3. Flush IV catheters before and after the medications are given using 0.9% NaCl for injection.
4. Incompatibilities may occur when mixing NaCl injection with other additives; inspect the final product for cloudiness or a precipitate immediately after mixing, before administration, and periodically during administration. Do not store these mixtures.

ASSESSMENT
1. Note reasons for therapy; monitor electrolytes, ECG, renal, LFTs. Note level of consciousness; assess heart and lung sounds.
2. Monitor VS and I&O. Assess urine specific gravity and serum sodium levels. Report if urine specific gravity is above 1.020 and serum sodium level is above 146 mEq/L.
3. When administering IV the 0.45% NaCl is hypotonic, the 0.9% NaCl is isotonic, and the 3% and 5% NaCl solutions are hypertonic.
4. Observe for S&S of hypernatremia: flushed skin, elevated temperature, rough dry tongue, and edema. S&S of hyponatremia include N&V, muscle cramps, dry mucous membranes, increased HR, and headaches.

CLIENT/FAMILY TEACHING
1. Review form of drug prescribed and when and how to use. May take tablet with a glass of water.
2. Report lack of response, swelling of extremities, or other adverse side effects.

OUTCOMES/EVALUATE
- Prophylaxis of heat prostration during exposure to high temperatures or during increased activity
- Prevention of chloride deficiency R/T excessive diuresis or salt restriction or excessive sweating

Solifenacin succinate
(sol-i-**FEN**-a-cin)

CLASSIFICATION(S):
Cholinergic blocking drug
PREGNANCY CATEGORY: C
Rx: Vesicare.

SEE ALSO *CHOLINERGIC BLOCKING AGENTS.*

USES
Treatment of overactive bladder with symptoms of urge urinary incontinence, urgency, and urinary frequency.

ACTION/KINETICS
Action
Solifenacin is a competitive muscarinic receptor antagonist. Muscarinic receptors play an important role in contraction of urinary bladder smooth muscle. Thus, blockade of such receptors will decrease an overactive bladder.

Pharmacokinetics
Peak plasma levels: 3–8 hr. Absolute bioavailability is about 90%. Is extensively metabolized by CYP3A4 isoenzymes. About 70% is excreted in the urine and 22.5% in the feces. **t½, elimination:** 45–68 hr. **Plasma protein binding:** About 98%,.

CONTRAINDICATIONS
Use in those with urinary retention, gastric retention, uncontrolled narrow-angle glaucoma, severe hepatic impairment (Child-Pugh score 10–15), and in those with hypersensitivity to the drug or any components of the product. Lactation.

SPECIAL CONCERNS
Use with caution in those with reduced renal and hepatic function and in those with clinically significant bladder outflow obstruction, GI obstructive disorders or decreased GI motility, or in clients being treated for narrow-angle glaucoma. Use with caution in those with a known history of QT prolongation or in those who are taking medications known to prolong the QT interval. Safety and efficacy have not been determined in children.

SIDE EFFECTS
Most Common
Dry mouth, constipation, blurred vision, influenza, UTI, upper abdominal pain, dizziness.

GI: Dry mouth, constipation, N&V, upper abdominal pain, dyspepsia. **CNS:** Dizziness, depression. **GU:** UTI, urinary retention. **Respiratory:** Pharyngitis, cough. **Ophthalmic:** Blurred vision (accommodation abnormalities), dry eyes. **Body as a whole:** Fatigue, influenza. **Miscellaneous:** Lower limb edema, hypertension.

OD OVERDOSE MANAGEMENT
Symptoms: **Acute:** Severe anticholinergic effects. **Chronic:** Intolerable anti-cholinergic side effects, including fixed and dilated pupils, blurred vision, failure of heel-to-toe exam, tremors, dry skin. *Treatment:* Gastric lavage. Appropriate supportive measures.

DRUG INTERACTIONS
CYP3A4 inducers / May alter the pharmacokinetics of solifenacin
CYP3A4 inhibitors / May alter the pharmacokinetics of solifenacin
Ketoconazole / ↑ Solifenacin AUC and C_{max}

HOW SUPPLIED
Tablets: 5 mg, 10 mg.

DOSAGE
• TABLETS
Overactive bladder.
5 mg once daily. If the 5 mg dose is well tolerated, the dose may be increased to 10 mg once daily.

NURSING CONSIDERATIONS
ADMINISTRATION/STORAGE
1. Do not exceed a dose of 5 mg daily in clients with severe renal impairment (C_{CR} <30 mL/min), with moderate hepatic impairment (Child-Pugh score 7 to 9), or when administered with therapeutic doses of ketoconazole or other CYP3A4 inhibitors.
2. Store from 15–30°C (59–86°F).

ASSESSMENT
1. Note reasons for therapy, other agents trialed, urologic findings.
2. List drugs prescribed to ensure none interact. Monitor renal and LFTs.
3. Review urinary patterns and voiding diary noting triggers.
4. Note history of CAD, urinary/gastric retention, ulcerative colitis, BPH, narrow angle glaucoma, myasthenia gravis or severe liver/renal disease; may preclude drug therapy.

CLIENT/FAMILY TEACHING
1. Read the 'Patient Information Leaflet' before using solifenacin and each time you get a refill.
2. Take by mouth, with or without food, usually once a day, as directed. Swallow tablet whole with a full glass of liquid.
3. Take at the same time each day. Do not increase dose or take more often without approval.

---

4. Avoid activities that require mental alertness until drug effects realized; may experience dizziness and blurred vision.

5. Dry mouth, constipation, stomach upset/pain, dry eyes, or unusual tiredness/weakness may occur. Report if side effects persistent or bothersome.

6. To relieve dry mouth, suck on (sugarless) hard candy or ice chips, chew (sugarless) gum, drink water or use a saliva substitute.

7. Avoid strenuous activities in hot weather; avoid overheating.

8. Maintain a diet adequate in fiber, drink plenty of water, and exercise to prevent constipation. If constipated, may need stimulant-type laxative with stool softener.

9. Practice reliable contraception report if pregnancy suspected or desired as drug may cause fetal harm.

10. Report if condition does not improve or worsens. Keep all F/U visits.

OUTCOMES/EVALUATE

Control of urination with ↓ frequency and ↓ urgency

Somatropin Ⓒ
(so-mah-**TROH**-pin)

PREGNANCY CATEGORY: C
(B: Genotropin, Saizen, Serostim, Zorbtive. **C:** Humatrope, Norditropin, Nutropin, Nutropin AQ)

Rx: Genotropin, Genotropin Miniquick, Humatrope, Norditropin, Nutropin, Nutropin AQ, Omnitrope, Saizen, Serostim, Serostim LQ, Zorbtive.

USES

Genotropin. (1) Long-term treatment in children who have growth failure due to inadequate secretion of endogenous growth hormone, growth failure due to Prader-Willi syndrome, or who are born small for gestation age and who fail to manifest catch-up growth by age 2. (2) Long-term replacement therapy in adults with growth hormone deficiency of either childhood- or adult-onset etiology. **Humatrope.** (1) Long-term treat-ment of children who have growth failure due to inadequate secretion of normal endogenous growth hormone. (2) Treatment of short stature associated with Turner syndrome in those whose epiphyses have not closed. (3) Long-term treatment of idiopathic short stature. (4) Replacement of endogenous growth hormone in adults with growth hormone deficiency who meet **both** of the following two criteria: Those who have growth hormone deficiency either alone, or with multiple hormone deficiencies as a result of pituitary disease, hypothalamic disease, surgery, radiation therapy, or trauma **and** those who were growth hormone-deficient during childhood who have growth hormone deficiency as an adult before replacement therapy with Humatrope is started. **Norditropin and Saizen.** Long-term treatment of children with growth failure due to inadequate secretion of endogenous growth hormone. **Nutropin and Nutropin AQ.** (1) Long-term treatment of growth failure due to a lack of adequate endogenous growth hormone secretion. (2) Treatment of growth failure associated with chronic renal insufficiency up to the time of renal transplantation. Use in conjunction with optimal management of chronic renal insufficiency. (3) Long-term treatment of short stature associated with Turner syndrome. (4) Replacement of endogenous growth hormone in clients with adult growth hormone deficiency who meet **both** of the following two criteria: Biochemical diagnosis of adult growth hormone deficiency by means of a subnormal response to a standard growth hormone stimulation test **and** those who have adult growth hormone deficiency either alone or with multiple hormone deficiencies (hypopituitarism) as a result of pituitary disease, hypothalamic disease, surgery, radiation therapy, or trauma; or childhood onset (those who were growth hormone deficient during childhood, confirmed as an adult before replacement therapy with Nutropin or Nutropin AQ is started). **Serostim.** Treatment of HIV clients with wasting or cachexia to increase lean body mass and body weight, and improve physical endurance. Must use with antiretroviral therapy. **Serostim LQ.** Indicated for AIDS wasting or cachexia. **Zorbtive.** Treatment of short bowel syndrome in those receiving specialized nutritional support. Should use with optimal management of short bowel syndrome.

ACTION/KINETICS

Action

Derived from recombinant DNA technology. Somatropin has the identical sequence of amino acids as does human growth hormone of pituitary origin. The drug stimulates linear growth by increasing somatomedin-C serum levels, which, in turn, increases the incorporation of sulfate into proteoglycans, thereby stimulating skeletal growth. It also increases the number and size of muscle cells, increases synthesis of collagen, increases protein synthesis, and increases internal organ size. Serum insulin levels increase (indicative of insulin resistance), and there is acute mobilization of lipid.

Pharmacokinetics

The various products have different pharmacokinetic properties. Check the package insert carefully.

CONTRAINDICATIONS

Known hypersensitivity to growth hormone. In clients in whom epiphyses have closed. Use if there is any evidence of active malignancy; antimalignancy treatment must be complete with evidence of remission prior to beginning somatropin therapy. Treatment of clients with acute critical illness due to complications following open heart or abdominal surgery, multiple accidental trauma, or in those having acute respiratory failure (due to increased risk of mortality). When reconstituted with bacteriostatic water for injection in clients with a known sensitivity to benzyl alcohol. Use in hypopituitary children who have evidence of actively growing intracranial tumors; discontinue if there is evidence of recurrent tumor growth. Reconstitution of Humatrope with the supplied diluent for use by those with a known sensitivity to

either metacresol or glycerin. Use of Genotropin in those with Prader-Willi syndrome who are severely obese or have severe respiratory impairment.

SPECIAL CONCERNS

Use with caution during lactation. Concomitant use of glucocorticoids may decrease the response to growth hormone.

SIDE EFFECTS

NOTE: Due to the large number of somatropin products with varying side effects, each product will be listed separately.

Genotropin. Body as a whole: Development of antibodies to the protein, edema, fluid retention, peripheral swelling, fatigue. **Injection site reactions:** Pain/burning on injection, fibrosis, nodules, rash, inflammation, pigmentation, bleeding. **CNS:** Headache, aggressiveness, paresthesia, hypoesthesia, central precocious puberty. **Musculoskeletal:** Arthralgia, myalgia, jaw prominence, aggravation of preexisting scoliosis, pain and stiffness of the extremities, back pain, carpal tunnel syndrome. **Respiratory:** URTI. **Miscellaneous:** Lipoatrophy, hematuria, hair loss in children, benign intracranial hypertension, hypothyroidism, mild hyperglycemia, leukemia in children, diabetes mellitus.

Humatrope. Body as a whole: Development of antibodies to the protein, edema (conjunctival, nonspecific, facial, peripheral), lymphedema, weakness, pain, flu syndrome, asthenia. **Injection site reactions:** Pain. **GI:** Gastritis, pancreatitis (rare). **CNS:** Headache, paresthesia, hypesthesia. **CV:** Hypertension. **Musculoskeletal:** Bone disorder, scoliosis, aching joints, hip/muscle/joint/back pain, joint disorder, arthralgia, arthrosis, myalgia, localized muscle pain, carpal tunnel syndrome. **Respiratory:** Increased cough, rhinitis, respiratory tract disorder, pharyngitis. **GU:** Gynecomastia. **Otic:** Otitis media, ear disorders. **Miscellaneous:** Leukemia, hyperglycemia, acne, glucosuria, hyper-/hypothyroidism, hyperlipidemia, increased nevi (possible malignant transformation), changes in mean fasting insulin levels,

S

increases in serum insulin-like growth factor-1, increased ALT and AST.

Norditropin. Body as a whole: Development of antibodies to the protein, weakness, fluid retention, peripheral edema. **CNS:** Headache. **Musculoskeletal:** Localized muscle pain. **Miscellaneous:** Mild hyperglycemia, glucosuria, leukemia in children.

Nutropin, Nutropin AQ. Body as a whole: Development of antibodies to the protein, peripheral edema (mild, transient), edema. **At injection site:** Discomfort, pain. **GI:** Pancreatitis. **Musculoskeletal:** Arthralgia, carpal tunnel syndrome, joint disorders. **Dermatologic:** Increased growth of pre-existing nevi (rare but possible malignant transformation). **GU:** Renal osteodystrophy, gynecomastia. **Miscellaneous:** Increased median fasting insulin, leukemia.

Saizen. Body as a whole: Development of antibodies to the protein, disturbances in fluid balance. **Injection site reactions:** Pain, numbness, redness, swelling. **CNS:** *Seizures.* **Miscellaneous:** Hypothyroidism, hypoglycemia, leukemia, exacerbation of preexisting psoriasis.

Serostim. Body as a whole: Edema (generalized, peripheral, dependent, periorbital), fatigue, rigors, fever, night sweats, pain, flu-like syndrome, asthenia. **GI:** Diarrhea, nausea, abdominal pain, anorexia, constipation, dyspepsia, gastroenteritis, vomiting. **CNS:** Insomnia, paresthesia, hypesthesia, headache, peripheral neuropathy, dizziness, hypertonia, depression, anxiety, somnolence. **CV:** Hypertension, tachycardia. **Musculoskeletal:** Increased tissue turgor (swelling, especially of the hands and feet), musculoskeletal discomfort (pain, swelling, stiffness), carpal tunnel syndrome, arthralgia, myalgia, arthrosis, back/leg/chest pain, arthropathy. **Respiratory:** Rhinitis, URTI, bronchitis, cough, sinusitis, pharyngitis, pneumonia. **Dermatologic:** Folliculitis, rash, verruca, maculopapular rash. **GU:** Gynecomastia, renal calculus, UTI, male breast neoplasm. **Hematologic:** Lymphadenopathy. **Ophthalmic:** Conjunctivitis.

Miscellaneous: Elevated glucose and triglycerides, glucose intolerance, new onset diabetes mellitus, diabetic ketoacidosis, *diabetic coma,* herpes simplex, moniliasis, viral infection.

Zorbtive. Body as a whole: Dehydration, thirst, edema (peripheral, facial, generalized, periorbital), pain, fever, flu-like disorder, malaise, fatigue, rigors, allergic reaction. **GI:** Abdominal pain, flatulence, N&V, constipation, pancreatitis, tenesmus, hemorrhoids, dry mouth, enlarged abdomen, aggravated Crohn disease, gastric ulcer, GI fistula, melena, *rectal hemorrhage,* mouth disorder, steatorrhea, abnormal hepatic function. **Injection site reactions:** Pain, injection site disorders, inflammation, reaction pain. **CNS:** Dizziness, headache, hypesthesia, depression, insomnia, paresthesia, phantom pain. **CV:** Vascular disorder, vasodilation, tachycardia. **Dermatologic:** Rash, pruritus, increased sweating, nail disorder, skin disorder, increased sweating, alopecia, bullous eruption. **Respiratory:** Rhinitis, laryngitis, pharyngitis, bronchospasm, dyspnea, respiratory tract disorder/infection. **Musculoskeletal:** Increased tissue turgor (swelling, especially of the hands and feet), musculoskeletal discomfort (pain, swelling, stiffness), carpal tunnel syndrome, arthralgia, myalgia, chest/back pain, arthritis, arthropathy, bursitis, cramps. **GU:** Pyelonephritis, breast pain/enlargement (females), vaginal fungal infection, renal calculus, dysuria, UTI, abnormal urine, vaginal fungal infection. **Hematologic:** Purpura, decreased prothrombin. **Ophthalmic:** Visual field defect. **Otic:** Hearing/ear problems. **Miscellaneous:** Infection (bacterial, viral, fungal), moniliasis, hypomagnesemia, *sepsis.*

OD **OVERDOSE MANAGEMENT**
Symptoms: In acute overdose, hypoglycemia followed by hyperglycemia. Long-term overdose can result in S&S of acromegaly or gigantism.

DRUG INTERACTIONS
Drugs metabolized by P450 liver enzymes / Possible alteration of clearance of such drugs; monitor carefully

---

Bold Italic = life threatening side effect   ■ = black box warning   ♣ = Available in Canada

Glucocorticoids / Inhibition of the effect of somatrem on growth

HOW SUPPLIED

Genotropin: *Powder for Injection, Lyophilized:* 5.8 mg (about 17.4 units)/vial, 13.8 mg (about 41.4 units)/vial;.

Genotropin Miniquick: *Powder for Injection, Lyophilized:* 0.2 mg/vial, 0.4 mg/vial, 0.6 mg/vial, 0.8 mg/vial, 1 mg/vial, 1.2 mg/vial, 1.4 mg/vial, 1.6 mg/vial, 1.8 mg/vial, 2 mg/vial.

Humatrope: *Powder for Injection, Lyophilized:* 5 mg (about 15 units)/vial, 6 mg (18 units)/cartridge, 12 mg (36 units)/cartridge, 24 mg (72 units)/cartridge.

Norditropin: *Injection:* 5 mg/1.5 mL, 10 mg/1.5 mL, 15 mg/1.5 mL; *Powder for Injection, Lyophilized:* 4 mg (about 12 units)/vial, 8 mg (about 24 units)/vial.

Nutropin: *Powder for Injection, Lyophilized:* 5 mg (about 15 units)/vial, 10 mg (about 30 units)/vial.

Nutropin AQ: *Injection:* 10 mg (about 30 units)/vial.

Omnitrope: *Powder for Injection, Lyophilized:* 1.5 mg (about 4.5 units), 5.8 mg (about 17.4 units).

Saizen: *Powder for Injection, Lyophilized:* 5 mg (about 15 units)/vial.

Serostim: *Powder for Injection, Lyophilized:* 4 mg (about 12 units)/vial, 5 mg (about 15 units)/vial, 6 mg (about 18 units)/vial, 8.8 mg (about 26.4 units)/vial.

Serostim LQ: *Injection:* 6 mg (about 18 units)/0.5 mL.

Zorbtive: *Powder for Injection:* 4 mg (about 12 units)/vial, 5 mg (about 15 units)/vial, 6 mg (about 18 units)/vial, 8.8 mg (about 26.4 units)/vial.

DOSAGE————————

GENOTROPIN

• **SC**

Adult growth hormone deficiency.

Individualize. Initial: No more than 0.04 mg/kg/week. Divide the weekly dose into 6 or 7 SC injections. May increase dose at 4- to 8–week intervals according to client response, up to a maximum of 0.08 mg/kg/week.

Pediatric growth hormone deficiency.

Usual: 0.16–0.24 mg/kg/week divided into 6–7 SC injections.

Pediatric Prader-Willi syndrome.

Usual: 0.24 mg/kg/week divided into 6–7 SC injections.

Pediatric small for gestational age.

Usual: 0.48 mg/kg/week divided into 6–7 SC injections.

HUMATROPE

• **IM; SC**

Growth hormone-deficient children.

Individualize. Usual: 0.18 mg/kg/week (0.54 international units/kg/week), up to a maximum of 0.3 mg/kg/week (0.90 international units/kg/week). Divide weekly dose into equal doses given either on 3 alternate days, 6 times per week, or daily. SC is preferred.

Turner syndrome.

Usual: 3.75 mg/kg/week (1.125 international units/kg/week) SC. Divide into equal doses given daily or on 3 alternate days.

Idiopathic short stature.

Usual: Up to 0.37 mg/kg/week SC. Divide into equal doses given 6–7 times per week.

Growth hormone-deficient adults.

Initial: No more than 0.006 mg/kg/day (0.0198 international units/day) SC. Dose may be increased, depending on individual requirements, to a maximum of 0.0125 mg/kg/day (0.0375 international units/kg/day). Titrate dose based on side effects or to maintain the insulin-like growth factor response below the ULN levels matched for age and gender. Dose reductions may be needed in clients with advancing age or excessive body weight.

NORDITROPIN

• **SC**

All uses.

Individualize. Usual: 0.024–0.034 mg/kg 6 to 7 times per week. Give injections in the thighs; vary injection site in the thigh on a rotating basis.

NUTROPIN, NUTROPIN AQ

• **SC**

Growth hormone deficiency in adults or children.

Adults, initial: Not more than 0.006 mg/kg/day, up to a maximum of 0.025 mg/kg/day in those less than 35 years of age and to a maximum of 0.0125 mg/kg/day in those over 35 years of

S

---

age. Lower doses may be needed in older or overweight clients. Decrease dose if needed due to side effects or excessive IGF-I levels. **Children:** Up to 0.3 mg/kg/week divided into daily SC injections. In pubertal children, a dose of 0.7 mg/kg/week divided daily may be used.

Chronic renal insufficiency.
Up to 0.35 mg/kg/week divided into daily SC injections. May continue therapy up to renal transplantation. Hemodialysis clients should receive their injection at night just prior to going to sleep or at least 3–4 hr after their hemodialysis to prevent hematoma formation due to the heparin. Chronic cyclic peritoneal dialysis clients should receive their injection in the morning after they have completed dialysis. Chronic ambulatory peritoneal dialysis clients should receive their injection in the evening at the time of the overnight exchange.

Turner syndrome.
0.375 mg/kg/week or less divided into equal doses 3–7 times per week SC.

SAIZEN
• **IM; SC**
Growth hormone inadequacy.
Individualize. Usual: 0.06 mg/kg (about 0.18 international units/kg) 3 times weekly. Discontinue when epiphyses fuse. Evaluate those who fail to respond to determine the cause.

SEROSTIM
• **SC**
HIV clients with wasting or cachexia.
Initial: 0.1 mg/kg daily, up to 6 mg, given at bedtime. Use the following dosage recommendations: **Weight >55 kg:** 6 mg daily SC; **45–55 kg:** 5 mg daily SC ; **35–45 kg:** 4 mg daily SC; **less than 35 kg:** 0.1 mg/kg. Give daily dose at bedtime. Giving Serostim every other day (0.1 mg/kg) produced fewer side effects with similar improvement in work output compared with 0.1 mg/kg daily. Effects on work output and lean body mass usually apparent after 12 weeks of therapy. Dosage can be maintained for an additional 12 weeks. Rotate injection sites.

ZORBTIVE
• **SC**

Short-bowel syndrome.
About 0.1 mg/kg/day, up to 8 mg/day, for 4 weeks. Rotate injection sites. Monitor for side effects. Treat moderate fluid retention and arthralgias symptomatically or reduce dose by 50%. Discontinue Zorbtive for up to 5 days for severe toxicity. Upon resolution of symptoms, resume at 50% of the original dose. Permanently discontinue treatment if severe toxicity recurs and does not disappear within 5 days. Safety and efficacy have not been determined in children with short bowel syndrome.

NURSING CONSIDERATIONS

※ Do not confuse Somatrem with Somatropin (human growth hormone) or Sumatriptan (an antimigraine agent).

ADMINISTRATION/STORAGE

1. Somatrem should be prescribed only by a physician experienced in the diagnosis and treatment of pituitary disorders.

2. Due to the development of insulin resistance, evaluate for possible glucose intolerance.

3. If used in newborns, reconstitute somatrem with water for injection because benzyl alcohol can be toxic to newborns.

4. Inject only reconstituted somatrem solution that is clear and without particulate matter.

5. Be sure needle used for injection is at least 1 inch so that the injection reaches muscle layer.

6. Use reconstituted somatrem within 7 days; do not freeze.

7. The following information is applicable to *Genotropin*:

• Store the lyophilized powder under refrigeration from 2–8°C (36–46°F). Do not freeze. Protect from light.

• *Genotropin* is supplied in a two-chamber cartridge with the drug in the front chamber and the diluent in the rear chamber. Use a reconstitution device to co-mix the drug and diluent following the directions on the package. Gently tip the cartridge upside down a few times until com-

---

Bold Italic = life threatening side effect   ■ = black box warning   ♣ = Available in Canada

plete dissolution occurs. Do not shake.

- The 1.5-mg cartridge may be refrigerated for 24 hr or less because it contains no preservative. Use once and discard any remaining solution. The 5.8- and 13.8-mg cartridges contain a preservative and may be stored under refrigeration for up to 14 days.
- Refrigerate the *Genotropin Miniquick* delivery device before dispensing; may be stored below 25°C (77°F) for up to 3 months after dispensing. The product contains no preservative. After reconstitution, may be stored refrigerated for 24 hr before use. Use only once and then discard.

8. The following information is applicable to *Humatrope:*

- Reconstitute by adding 1.5–5 mL of the diluent for *Humatrope* supplied for each 5-mg vial. Inject the diluent into the vial by aiming the stream of liquid against the glass wall. Following reconstitution, swirl the vial with a gentle rotary motion until contents are completely dissolved. Do not shake the vial. Do not give the reconstituted solution if it is cloudy or contains particulate material. Use a small enough syringe to ensure accuracy when the solution is withdrawn from the vial.
- Vials are stable for 14 days or less after reconstitution with diluent for *Humatrope* or bacteriostatic water for injection when stored in a refrigerator.
- After reconstitution with sterile water, use only one dose/ *Humatrope* vial and discard the unused portion.
- If the solution is not used immediately, refrigerate at 2–8°C (36–46°F) and use within 24 hr.
- The cartridge allows the dosage volume to be dialed in increments of 0.048 mL per click of the dosage knob; the maximum dosage volume that can be injected is 0.576 mL (based on a 12 click maximum). After reconstitution, cartridges of *Humatrope* are stable for up to 28 days when reconstituted with diluent for

Humatrope and stored in a refrigerator. Avoid freezing.

- Store the *HumatroPen* with the *Humatrope* cartridge attached in the refrigerator until the time of the next injection.

9. The following information is applicable to *Norditropin:*

- Give in the thighs and vary injection site on the thigh on a rotating basis.
- When using the cartridges, use the corresponding color-coded Nordipen injection pen (sold separately). The 5 mg/1.5 mL cartridge uses the orange pen, the 10 mg/1.5 mL cartridge uses the blue pen, and the 15 mg/1.5 mL cartridge uses the green pen.
- Reconstitute each 4 or 8 mg vial with the 2 mL diluent.
- Before and after reconstitution, refrigerate. Do not freeze; avoid direct light.
- Use reconstituted vials within 14 days after dissolution.
- After the *Norditropin* cartridge has been inserted into the *NordiPen* injector, it must be stored in the pen in the refrigerator and used within 4 weeks.

10. The following information is applicable to *Nutropin, Nutropin AQ:*

- To reconstitute *Nutropin*, add 1–5 mL bacteriostatic water for injection (benzyl alcohol preserved) per each 5 mg vial and 1–10 mL bacteriostatic water per each 10 mg vial.
- Before reconstitution, refrigerate *Nutropin* and bacteriostatic water for injection. Avoid freezing. Reconstituted vials are stable for up to 14 days when refrigerated.
- For *Nutropin AQ*, vials are stable for 28 days after initial use when stored in the refrigerator. Avoid freezing. Protect from light; store the vial and the cartridge refrigerated in a dark place when they are not in use.
- Follow guidelines in the package insert carefully for reconstitution and administration.

11. The following information is applicable to *Saizen:*

- Reconstitute the 5 mg vial with 1–3 mL bacteriostatic water for injection (benzyl alcohol preserved). Reconstitute the 8.8 mg vial with 2–3 mL of bacteriostatic water for injection. About 10% mechanical loss can be expected with reconstitution and multi-dose administration.
- To reconstitute, inject the diluent into the vial, aiming the liquid against the glass vial wall. Swirl with a gentle rotary motion until contents are completely dissolved. Do not shake. Ensure the solution is clear immediately after reconstitution.
- Do not inject *Saizen* if reconstituted product is cloudy immediately after reconstitution or refrigeration. On occasion, small colorless particles may be present after refrigeration; this is not unusual.
- Benzyl alcohol may cause toxicity in newborns; if giving somatropin (rDNA origin) to newborns, reconstitute with sterile water for injection. Use only 1 dose per vial and discard any unused portion.
- Before reconstitution store at room temperature. Reconstituted solutions are stable for up to 14 days when refrigerated. Avoid freezing reconstituted vials.

12. The following information is applicable to *Serostim, Serostim LQ*:

- Each vial of *Serostim* 4, 5, or 6 mg is reconstituted with 0.5–1 mL sterile water for injection. Vials are single use.
- To reconstitute, inject the diluent into the vial aiming the liquid against the glass vial wall. Swirl the vial with a gentle rotary motion until contents are completely dissolved. The solution should be clear immediately after reconstitution.
- Do not inject if the reconstituted product is cloudy immediately after reconstitution or after refrigeration for up to 14 days. On occasion, after refrigeration, small colorless particles may be present; this is not unusual.
- Before reconstitution, store vials and diluent at room temperature. After

reconstitution, use immediately; discard any unused portion.
- Store *Serostim LQ* under refrigeration; protect from light and avoid freezing cartridges.

13. The following information is applicable to *Zorbtive*:

- Reconstitute each 4, 5, or 6 mg vial with 0.5–1 mL sterile water for injection. Reconstitute the 8.8 mg vial with 1–2 mL bacteriostatic water for injection (benzyl alcohol preserved). About 10% mechanical loss can be expected with reconstitution and administration from multidose vials.
- To reconstitute, inject the diluent into the vial, aiming the liquid against the glass vial wall. Swirl the vial with a gentle rotary motion until the contents are completely dissolved. The solution should be clear immediately after reconstitution.
- Do not inject if the reconstituted product is cloudy immediately after reconstitution or after refrigeration (except the 8.8 mg product). The 8.8 mg product can be refrigerated for up to 14 days. On occasion, small colorless particles may be present after refrigeration; this is not unusual.
- Allow refrigerated solution to come to room temperature prior to administration.
- Use a standard insulin-type syringe for administration.
- Benzyl alcohol can cause toxicity in newborns. Thus, when giving somatropin (rDNA origin) injection to newborns reconstitute with sterile water for injection. Use only 1 dose per vial; discard any unused portion.
- Before reconstitution, store at room temperature.
- After reconstitution with sterile water for injection, use immediately; discard any unused portion.
- After reconstitution with bacteriostatic water for injection, store under refrigeration for up to 14 days. Avoid freezing reconstituted solution.

ASSESSMENT

1. Note reasons for therapy, age of client, other therapy trialed.

---

2. Determine that x-ray evidence of bone growth (wrists, hands) has been conducted. Record height and weight monthly. Generally a growth increase of 2 cm/year should be attained in order for treatment to be continued.

3. If growth slow in absence of rising antibody titers, hypopituitarism should be ruled out; untreated hypothyroidism or excessive glucocorticoid replacement can impair growth.

4. Monitor blood sugar and thyroid function studies; assess for diabetes or hypothyroidism. With diabetes, assess for hyperglycemia and acidosis.

5. Note any limps or knee/hip pain because a slipped capital epiphysis may occur.

CLIENT/FAMILY TEACHING

1. Keep and review drug literature with guidelines for administration, drug preparation, name, and storage, after instructed by provider. Somatrem is usually given once a week whereas somatropin is given more often.

2. Keep a growth record and report as scheduled for F/U.

3. Report any adverse effects or any limping or knee or hip pain. May experience sudden growth spurts with increased appetite.

4. The cost per year depends on the amount of drug used, which is based on client's weight and typically runs $10,000–$30,000 or more.

OUTCOMES/EVALUATE

Desired skeletal growth; (growth hormone replacement with deficiency)

Sorafenib

(sor-ah-**FEE**-nib)

CLASSIFICATION(S):

Antineoplastic, multikinase inhibitor
PREGNANCY CATEGORY: D
Rx: Nexavar.

USES

Treatment of advanced renal cell carcinoma.

ACTION/KINETICS

Action

A multikinase inhibitor that decreases tumor cell proliferation. Sorafenib interacts with multiple intracellular and cell surface kinases, several of which are thought to be involved in angiogenesis.

Pharmacokinetics

Mean relative bioavailability is 38–49%. Bioavailability is reduced by 29% following a high-fat meal. Japanese clients (limited study) show a 45% lower systemic exposure compared with white clients. **Steady-state plasma levels:** 7 days. **Peak plasma levels:** 3 hr. Metabolized primarily in the liver by CYP3A4, as well as glucuronidation. One of the metabolites is as active as sorafenib. About 77% is excreted in the feces and 19% in the urine. Unchanged sorafenib (51%) is excreted in the feces but none in the urine. **t½, elimination:** 25–48 hr. **Plasma protein binding:** About 99.5%.

CONTRAINDICATIONS

Severe hypersensitivity to sorafenib or any component of the product. Lactation.

SPECIAL CONCERNS

Use with caution with drugs that are metabolized/eliminated predominantly by glucuronidation mediated by UGT1A9. Greater sensitivity of the drug in the elderly is possible. Safety and efficacy in children have not been determined.

SIDE EFFECTS

Most Common

Rash, hand-foot skin reaction, hypertension, alopecia, pruritus, diarrhea, N&V, fatigue, sensory neuropathy, anorexia, asthenia, pain, constipation, hemorrhage (all sites), dyspnea, cough.

GI: Diarrhea, N&V, anorexia, constipation, abdominal pain, dyspepsia, dysphagia, mucositis, stomatitis, glossodynia, dry mouth, gastritis, GI reflux, pancreatitis. **CNS:** Sensory neuropathy, headache, depression, tinnitus. **CV:** Hypertension, increased risk of bleeding, *myocardial ischemia/infarction, hypertensive crisis,* arrhythmia, *cardiac failure, cerebral hemorrhage,* TIA, thromboembolism. **Dermatologic:** Rash/desquamation, hand-foot skin re-

S

---

action, alopecia, pruritus, dry skin, erythema, acne, exfoliative dermatitis, flushing, eczema, erythema multiforme, folliculitis. **Respiratory:** Dyspnea, cough, hoarseness, rhinorrhea. **GU:** Erectile dysfunction, gynecomastia, acute renal failure. **Musculoskeletal:** Arthralgia, myalgia. **Hematologic:** Hemorrhage (all sites), leukopenia, lymphopenia, anemia, neutropenia, thrombocytopenia, abnormal INR. **Body as a whole:** Fatigue, joint pain, weight loss, hypersensitivity reaction including skin reactions and urticaria, dehydration, asthenia, pyrexia, infection. **Miscellaneous:** Pain (including mouth/bone/muscle pain), decreased appetite, flu-like illness.

LABORATORY TEST CONSIDERATIONS
↑ Lipase, amylase, transaminases (transient), bilirubin, alkaline phosphatase (transient). Hypophosphatemia, hyponatremia, hypothyroidism.

OD **OVERDOSE MANAGEMENT**
Symptoms: Diarrhea, dermatologic events. *Treatment:* Withhold sorafenib and institute supportive treatment.

DRUG INTERACTIONS
Carbamazepine / ↓ Sorafenib levels R/T ↑ metabolism by CYP3A4
Dexamethasone / ↓ Sorafenib levels R/T ↑ metabolism by CYP3A4
Doxorubicin / ↑ Doxorubin AUC by 21%; use together with caution
Drugs metabolized by CYP2B6 / Possible ↑ in levels of drugs metabolized by CYP2B6 R/T inhibition by sorafenib
Drugs metabolized by CYP2C6 / Possible ↑ in levels of drugs metabolized by CYP2C6 R/T inhibition by sorafenib
Irinotecan / Use together with caution as both drugs are metabolized by a similar pathway
Phenobarbital / ↓ Sorafenib levels R/T ↑ metabolism by CYP3A4
Phenytoin / ↓ Sorafenib levels R/T ↑ metabolism by CYP3A4
Rifampin / ↓ Sorafenib levels R/T ↑ metabolism by CYP3A4
H *St. John's wort /* ↓ Sorafenib levels R/T ↑ metabolism by CYP3A4
Warfarin / Infrequent bleeding events or ↑ INR; monitor regularly for changes in PT, INR, or clinical bleeding episodes

HOW SUPPLIED
Tablets: 200 mg.

DOSAGE
• **TABLETS**
Advanced renal cell carcinoma.
400 mg (2–200 mg tablets) twice a day, at least 1 hr before or 2 hr after eating. Continue treatment until the client is no longer benefiting from the drug or until unacceptable side effects occur. When dose reduction is necessary, due to side effects, reduce dose to 400 mg once daily. If additional dose reduction is needed, reduce to a single 400 mg dose every other day.

NURSING CONSIDERATIONS
ADMINISTRATION/STORAGE
1. Temporary interruption of therapy and/or dose reduction may be necessary for side effects. For skin toxicity, the following dose modifications are recommended:
• **Grade 1:** Any occurrence of numbness, paresthesia, dysesthesia, tingling, painless swelling, erythema, discomfort of the hands or feet that do not disrupt normal living. Continue treatment and consider topical therapy for symptomatic relief.
• **Grade 2:** First occurrence of painful erythema and swelling of the hands or feet and/or discomfort affecting normal activities. Continue treatment and consider topical therapy for symptomatic relief. If no improvement in 7 days (or if there is a second or third occurrence), interrupt treatment until toxicity resolves to grade 0 or 1. When resuming treatment, decrease dose by one dose level (400 mg per day or 400 mg every other day). If a fourth occurrence occurs, discontinue sorafenib.
• **Grade 3:** First or second occurrence of moist desquamation, ulceration, blistering, or severe pain of the hands or feet, or severe discomfort that causes inability to work or perform activities of daily living. Interrupt treatment until toxicity resolves to 0 or 1. When resuming treatment, decrease dose by one dose level (400 mg per day or 400 mg every other

---

Bold Italic = life threatening side effect   ■ = black box warning   ✣ = Available in Canada day). For a third occurrence, discontinue sorafenib.

2. Consider temporary or permanent discontinuation of sorafenib in those who develop cardiac ischemia or infarction.

3. Temporary interruption of therapy is recommended in those undergoing major surgical procedures. Base the decision on when to resume sorafenib therapy on a judgment of adequate wound healing.

ASSESSMENT

1. Note reasons for therapy, disease onset, stage, other agents/therapies trialed, outcome.

2. Monitor BP, EKG, CBC, renal and LFTs; reduce dose with dysfunction.

3. List any bleeding disorders, HTN, kidney, liver or heart disease; may preclude drug therapy.

CLIENT/FAMILY TEACHING

1. Drug used to treat advanced kidney cancer. Take as directed 1 hr before or 2 hr after meals with a full glass of water.

2. Use reliable contraception in both male and females during and for a least 2 weeks after completing therapy. May cause birth defects or fetal loss.

3. May develop hand-foot skin reaction and rash during treatment. Follow guidelines for skin toxicity under Administration/Storage.

4. Elevated BP may develop during treatment, especially during the first 6 weeks; monitor regularly during treatment.

5. Report any episodes of bleeding; drug increases risk and may even cause GI perforation.

6. May experience ischemia to the heart or heart attack during treatment; immediately report any chest pain or SOB.

7. If diarrhea, flushing, impaired wound healing, increased sweating, suppressed skin test reaction or thin fragile skin evident-report.

8. Keep all F/U appointments to evaluate response to therapy or any adverse side effects.

OUTCOMES/EVALUATE

Inhibition of malignant cell proliferation

Sotalol hydrochloride ■ ⓒ
(**SOH**-tah-lol)

CLASSIFICATION(S):
Antiarrhythmic, class III beta-adrenergic blocking agent
PREGNANCY CATEGORY: B
Rx: Betapace, Betapace AF, Sotalol HCl AF.
✤Rx: Apo-Sotalol, Gen-Sotalol, Lin-Sotalol, Novo-Sotalol, Nu-Sotalol, PMS-Sotalol, Rhoxal-sotalol, Sotacor, ratio-Sotalol.

SEE ALSO *BETA-ADRENERGIC BLOCKING AGENTS.*

USES
(1) Treatment of documented ventricular arrhythmias such as life-threatening sustained VT. (2) Betapace AF is used for maintenance of normal sinus rhythm in those with symptomatic atrial fibrillation/atrial flutter who are in sinus rhythm; since Betapace AF can cause life-threatening ventricular arrhythmias, reserve use for those who are highly symptomatic. *Do not substitute Betapace for Betapace AF.*

ACTION/KINETICS
Action
Blocks both $beta_1$- and $beta_2$-adrenergic receptors; has no membrane-stabilizing activity or intrinsic sympathomimetic activity. Has both Group II and Group III antiarrhythmic properties (dose dependent). Significantly increases the refractory period of the atria, His-Purkinje fibers, and ventricles. Also prolongs the QTc and JT intervals and decreases heart rate.

Pharmacokinetics
t½: 12 hr. Not metabolized; excreted unchanged in the urine.

CONTRAINDICATIONS
Use in asymptomatic PVCs or supraventricular arrhythmias due to the proarrhythmic effects of sotalol. Congenital or acquired long QT syndromes. Use in clients with hypokalemia or hypomagnesemia until the imbalance is corrected, as these conditions aggravate the

---

degree of QT prolongation and increase the risk for torsades de pointes.

SPECIAL CONCERNS

■ (1) To minimize the risk of induced arrhythmia, those initiated or reinitiated on Betapace or Betapace AF should be placed for a minimum of 3 days (on their maintenance dose) in a facility that can provide cardiac resuscitation, continuous electrocardiographic monitoring, and calculations of creatinine clearance. Consult the package insert for detailed instructions regarding dose selection and special cautions for those with renal impairment. (2) Do not substitute Betapace for Betapace AF because of significant differences in labeling (e.g., patient package insert, dosing administration, and safety information).■ Clients with sustained ventricular tachycardia and a history of CHF appear to be at the highest risk for serious proarrhythmia. Dose, presence of sustained ventricular tachycardia, females, excessive prolongation of the QTc interval, and history of cardiomegaly or CHF are risk factors for torsades de pointes. Use with caution in clients with chronic bronchitis or emphysema and in asthma if an IV agent is required. Use with extreme caution in clients with SSS associated with symptomatic arrhythmias due to the increased risk of sinus bradycardia, sinus pauses, or sinus arrest. Reduce dosage in impaired renal function. Safety and efficacy in children have not been established. Do *not* interchange Betapace and Betapace AF due to significant differences in dosage and safety, although clients can be transferred to Betapace AF from Betapace.

SIDE EFFECTS

Most Common

Angina, abnormal ECG, diarrhea, N&V, fatigue, hyperhidrosis, weakness, musculoskeletal pain, dizziness, headache, dyspnea, fever, insomnia, URTI, tracheobronchitis.

See *Beta-Adrenergic Blocking Agents* for a complete list of possible side effects.

CV: New or worsened ventricular arrhythmias, including sustained VT or ventricular fibrillation that might be fatal. Torsades de pointes.

HOW SUPPLIED

Betapace: *Tablets:* 80 mg, 120 mg, 160 mg, 240 mg.

Betapace AF: *Tablets:* 80 mg, 120 mg, 160 mg.

Sotalol HCl: : 80 mg, 120 mg, 160 mg, 240 mg.

DOSAGE

BETAPACE

• **TABLETS**

Ventricular arrhythmias.

Adults, initial: 80 mg twice a day. The dose may be increased to 240 or 320 mg/day after appropriate evaluation. **Usual:** 160–320 mg/day given in two or three divided doses. Clients with life-threatening refractory ventricular arrhythmias may require doses ranging from 480 to 640 mg/day (due to potential proarrhythmias, use these doses only if the potential benefit outweighs the increased risk of side effects). Use the following doses in clients with impaired renal function: 80 mg twice a day if C_{CR} is greater than 60 mL/min, 80 mg once daily if the C_{CR} is between 30 and 59 mL/min, and 80 mg every 36–48 hr if the CCR is between 10 and 29 mL/min. Individualize dose if the C_{CR} is less than 10 mL/min.

BETAPACE AF

• **TABLETS**

Maintenance of normal sinus rhythm in those with symptomatic atrial fibrillation/flutter who are in sinus rhythm.

Dose individualized according to calculated creatinine clearance. Initial: 80 mg. **Maintenance:** 80 mg twice a day if C_{CR} is greater than 60 mL/min and 80 mg once daily if the C_{CR} is between 40 and 60 mL/min. Do not use in clients with a C_{CR} less than 40 mL/min. Can be titrated upward to 120 mg during initial hospitalization or after discharge on 80 mg in the event of recurrence, by rehospitalization and repeating the same steps used during initiation of therapy. An increase in dose to 160 mg twice a day or daily can be considered if the 120 mg dose does not reduce the frequency of early relapse of AFIB/AF and is tolerated without excessive QT interval prolongation. Doses higher than 160 mg twice a day are associated with an

---

Bold Italic = life threatening side effect   ■ = black box warning   ✦ = Available in Canada

increased incidence of torsade de pointes.

NURSING CONSIDERATIONS

ⓒ Do not confuse Sotalol with Sorbitol (GU irrigant), Stadol (opioid analgesic), or Sudafed (pseudoephedrine).

ADMINISTRATION/STORAGE

1. Adjust dosage gradually, allowing 2–3 days between increments in dosage. This allows steady-state plasma levels to be reached and QT intervals to be monitored.

2. Undertake dosage initiation and increases in a hospital with facilities for cardiac rhythm monitoring. Dosage must be individualized only after appropriate clinical assessment.

3. Proarrhythmias can occur during initiation of therapy and with each dosage increment.

4. In clients with impaired renal function, alter the dosing interval as follows: If C_{CR} is 30–60 mL/min, the dosing interval is 24 hr; if C_{CR} is 10–30 mL/min, the dosing interval should be 36–48 hr. If C_{CR} <10 mL/min, dose must be individualized. Undertake dosage adjustments with impaired renal function only after five to six doses at the intervals described.

5. Before initiating sotalol, withdraw previous antiarrhythmic therapy with careful monitoring for a minimum of 2–3 plasma half-lives if condition permits.

6. Do not initiate sotalol after amiodarone is discontinued until the QT interval is normalized.

Initiation and Maintenance of Betapace AF Therapy

1. Determine the QT interval prior to initiation of therapy using an average of 5 beats. If the baseline QT is greater than 450 msec (JT equal to or greater than 330 msec if QRS over 100 msec), do not use Betapace AF.

2. Calculate the creatinine clearance.

3. Initiate correct dose of Betapace AF, depending on the creatinine clearance (see Dosage).

4. Begin continuous ECG monitoring with QT interval measurements 2–4 hr after each dose.

5. If the 80 mg dose is tolerated and QT interval remains <500 msec after at least 3 days (after 5 or 6 doses if client receiving once daily dosing), client can be discharged. Alternatively, during hospitalization, the dose can be increased to 120 mg twice a day if the 80 mg dose does not reduce the frequency and relapses of AFIB/AFL. Once again, client is followed for 3 days on this dose (or 5 or 6 doses if receiving once daily dosing).

6. If the 120 mg dose twice a day or daily does not reduce the frequency of early relapses of AFIB/AFL and is tolerated without excessive QT interval prolongation (520 msec or longer), Betapace AF can be increased to 160 mg twice a day or daily, provided appropriate monitoring is undertaken.

7. Re-evaluate renal function and QT regularly if medically warranted. If QT is 520 msec or greater (JT 430 msec or greater if QRS >100 msec), reduce dose of Betapace AF and monitor carefully until QT returns to <520 msec.

8. If the QT interval is 520 msec or greater while on the lowest maintenance dose (80 mg), discontinue drug.

9. If renal function decreases, reduce daily dose in half and administer drug once daily.

10. If a dose is missed, the next dose should not be doubled. The next dose should be taken at the usual time.

11. Before starting Betapace AF, withdraw previous antiarrhythmic therapy, with careful monitoring, for a minimum of 2 or 3 plasma half-lives if the clinical condition permits.

12. Do not initiate Betapace AF after amiodarone until the QT interval is normalized.

ASSESSMENT

1. Perform nursing history; note any cardiomegaly or CHF.

2. Obtain ECG, document QT interval (must be (,450 msec) note symptoms associated with arrhythmia. Monitor q2–4hr and report if QTc interval >500 msec; reduce/stop therapy.

3. Administer in a closely monitored environment with VS and ECG moni-

---

tored during initiation and adjustment of sotalol.

4. Monitor VS, I&O, electrolytes, Mg$^+$, renal, LFTs.

CLIENT/FAMILY TEACHING

1. Take on an empty stomach; food decreases absorption.

2. Take exactly as directed, do not stop abruptly; drug controls symptoms but does not cure condition. Betapace and Betapace AF are not interchangeable.

3. Avoid activities that require mental alertness until drug effects realized; may cause dizziness/drowsiness.

4. Report increased chest pain/SOB, night cough, swelling of feet and ankles, increased fatigue, low heart rate, or unsteady gait.

5. Continue dietary and exercise guidelines as prescribed and healthy lifestyle changes. Avoid alcohol and OTC agents.

6. Keep all F/U appointments to evaluate EKG and response to therapy.

OUTCOMES/EVALUATE

Control/conversion of life-threatening arrhythmias to stable cardiac rhythm

Spironolactone ■ⓒ
(speer-oh-no-**LAK**-tohn)

CLASSIFICATION(S):
Diuretic, potassium-sparing
PREGNANCY CATEGORY: D
Rx: Aldactone.
♣Rx: Novo-Spiroton.

SEE ALSO *DIURETICS, THIAZIDES*.

USES

(1) Primary hyperaldosteronism, including diagnosis, short-term preoperative treatment, long-term maintenance therapy for those who are poor surgical risks and those with bilateral micronodular or macronodular adrenal hyperplasia. (2) Edema when other approaches are inadequate or ineffective (e.g., CHF, cirrhosis of the liver, nephrotic syndrome). (3) Essential hypertension (usually in combination with other drugs). (4) Prophylaxis of hypokalemia in clients taking digitalis. *Investigational:* Hirsutism, treat symptoms of PMS, with testolactone to treat familial male precocious puberty (short-term treatment), acne vulgaris. In severe heart failure with recommended therapies to reduce mortality.

ACTION/KINETICS

Action

Mild diuretic that acts on the distal tubule to inhibit sodium exchange for potassium, resulting in increased secretion of sodium and water and conservation of potassium. An aldosterone antagonist. Manifests a slight antihypertensive effect. Interferes with synthesis of testosterone and may increase formation of estradiol from testosterone, thus leading to endocrine abnormalities.

Pharmacokinetics

Onset: Urine output increases over 1–2 days. **Peak:** 2–3 days. **Duration:** 2–3 days, and declines thereafter. Metabolized to an active metabolite (canrenone). **t½:** 13–24 hr for canrenone. Canrenone is excreted through the urine (primary) and the bile. **Plasma protein binding:** Almost completely bound.

CONTRAINDICATIONS

Acute renal insufficiency, progressive renal failure, hyperkalemia, and anuria. Clients receiving potassium supplements, amiloride, or triamterene.

SPECIAL CONCERNS

■ Spironolactone has been shown to be tumorigenic in chronic toxicity studies in rats. Use only in those conditions described under *Uses*. Avoid unnecessary use of the drug.■ Use during pregnancy only if benefits clearly outweigh risks. Use with caution in impaired renal function. Geriatric clients may be more sensitive to the usual adult dose.

SIDE EFFECTS

Most Common

Dizziness, blurred vision, N&V, fatigue, anorexia, insomnia, nasal congestion, gynecomastia.

Electrolyte: Hyperkalemia, hyponatremia (characterized by lethargy, dry mouth, thirst, tiredness). **GI:** Diarrhea, cramps, ulcers, gastritis, gastric bleeding, N&V, anorexia. **CNS:** Drowsiness, dizziness, ataxia, lethargy, mental confusion, headache, fatigue, insomnia. **Endocrine:** Gynecomastia, menstrual irregularities, impotence, bleeding in postmenopausal women, deepening of voice, hirsutism. **Dermatologic:** Maculopapular or erythematous cutaneous eruptions, urticaria. **Miscellaneous:** Blurred vision, nasal congestion, drug fever, breast carcinoma, gynecomastia, hyperchloremic metabolic acidosis in hepatic cirrhosis (decompensated), *agranulocytosis.* NOTE: Spironolactone has been shown to be tumorigenic in chronic rodent studies.

DRUG INTERACTIONS

ACE inhibitors / Significant hyperkalemia
Anesthetics, general / Additive hypotension
Anticoagulants, oral / Inhibited by spironolactone
Antihypertensives / ↑ Hypotensive effect of both agents; ↓ dosage, especially of ganglionic blockers, by one-half
Captopril / ↑ Risk of significant hyperkalemia
Digoxin / ↑ Half-life of digoxin → ↓ clearance. Spironolactone may ↓ inotropic effect of digoxin
Diuretics, others / Often given together R/T potassium-sparing effect of spironolactone. Possible severe hyponatremia; monitor closely
Lithium / ↑ Risk of lithium toxicity R/T ↓ renal clearance
Norepinephrine / ↓ NE effect
Potassium salts / Hyperkalemia R/T spironolactone conserving potassium excessively. Rarely used together
Salicylates / Large doses may ↓ spironolactone effects
Triamterene / Possible hazardous hyperkalemia

HOW SUPPLIED

Tablets: 25 mg, 50 mg, 100 mg.

DOSAGE

• TABLETS

Edema.

Adults, initial: 100 mg/day (range: 25–200 mg/day) in 2 to 4 divided doses for at least 5 days; **maintenance:** 75–400 mg/day in 2 to 4 divided doses. **Pediatric:** 3.3 mg/kg/day as a single dose or as 2 to 4 divided doses.

Antihypertensive.

Adults, initial: 50–100 mg/day as a single dose or as 2 to 4 divided doses—

give for at least 2 weeks; **maintenance:** adjust to individual response. **Pediatric:** 1–2 mg/kg in a single dose or in 2 to 4 divided doses.

Hypokalemia.

Adults: 25–100 mg/day as a single dose or 2 to 4 divided doses.

Diagnosis of primary hyperaldosteronism.

Adults: 400 mg/day for either 4 days (short-test) or 3–4 weeks (long-test).

Hyperaldosteronism, prior to surgery.

Adults: 100–400 mg/day in 2 to 4 doses prior to surgery.

Hyperaldosteronism, chronic-therapy.

Use lowest possible dose.

Hirsutism.

50–200 mg/day.

Symptoms of PMS.

25 mg 4 times per day beginning on day 14 of the menstrual cycle.

Familial male precocious puberty, short-term.

Spironolactone, 2 mg/kg/day, and testolactone, 20–40 mg/kg/day, for at least 6 months.

Acne vulgaris.

100 mg/day.

Reduce mortality in severe CHF.

25–50 mg/day with other therapies (e.g., ACE inhibitor, loop diuretic).

NURSING CONSIDERATIONS

℞ Do not confuse Aldactone with Aldactazide (combination antihypertensive/diuretic).

ADMINISTRATION/STORAGE

1. When used as sole drug to treat edema, maintain initial dose for at least 5 days. After that, adjustments may be made. If dosage not effective, a second diuretic may be added, especially one that acts in the proximal tubules.

2. When administered to small children, tablets may be crushed and given as a suspension in cherry syrup.

3. Food may increase absorption of spironolactone.

4. Protect drug from light.

ASSESSMENT

1. Note reasons for therapy, other agents prescribed, outcome.

2. Monitor ABGs, ECG, CBC, blood sugar, uric acid, serum electrolytes, renal,

LFTs. With cardiac disease, be alert for hypokalemia. Record VS, I&O, weights.

3. If client develops dysuria, urinary frequency, or renal spasm, obtain a urinalysis and urine culture.

4. Assess for drug tolerance characterized by edema/reduced urine output. Ensure client informed that studies show drug tumorigenic in rats.

CLIENT/FAMILY TEACHING

1. Take as directed with a snack/meal to minimize GI upset. Report if nausea, bloating, anorexia, vomiting, or diarrhea persist. Take early in day to prevent frequent nighttime urination.

2. Avoid foods or salt substitutes high in potassium; drug is potassium-sparing. Record BP and weight twice a week for provider review. Report any increased swelling of extremities or weight gain of more than 5 lb (2.2 kg) weekly.

3. Do not drive/operate dangerous machinery until drug effects realized; may cause drowsiness or unsteady gait.

4. Drug may cause breast swelling and diminished sex drive by reducing testosterone levels.

5. Report if deep, rapid respirations, headaches, or mental slowing occurs; may indicate hyperchloremic metabolic acidosis.

6. Drug is metabolized in the liver. Report jaundice, tremors, or mental confusion; may develop hepatic encephalopathy with liver disease. Avoid alcohol.

OUTCOMES/EVALUATE

- Enhanced diuresis with ↓ edema
- ↓ BP
- Antagonism of high levels of aldosterone
- Prevention of hypokalemia
- Reduced mortality in CAD with CHF

Stavudine ■
(STAH-vyou-deen)

CLASSIFICATION(S):
Antiviral, nucleoside reverse transcriptase inhibitor

PREGNANCY CATEGORY: C
Rx: Zerit XR.

SEE ALSO ANTIVIRAL AGENTS.

USES

(1) Adults with advanced HIV infection who cannot tolerate approved therapies or who have experienced significant clinical or immunologic deterioration while receiving such therapies (or for whom such therapies are contraindicated). (2) With didanosine, as well as either a protease inhibitor or nonnucleoside analog, as first-line therapy for HIV-1 infections.

ACTION/KINETICS

Action

The drug causes antiviral activity and inhibition of HIV replication by two known mechanisms: (1) Inhibition of HIV reverse transcriptase by competing with the natural substrate deoxythymidine triphospate and (2) Inhibition of viral DNA synthesis by its incorporation into viral DNA, causing DNA chain elongation termination (because stavudine lacks the 3'-hydroxyl group necessary for DNA elongation). Stavudine triphosphate also inhibits cellular DNA polymerase beta and gamma, and markedly decreases mitochondrial DNA synthesis.

Pharmacokinetics

Rapidly absorbed. **Peak plasma levels:** 1 hr or less. **t½, terminal:** Approximately 1.4 hr after PO use in adults and 0.96 hr in children. About 40% of the drug is eliminated through the kidney.

CONTRAINDICATIONS

Lactation.

SPECIAL CONCERNS

■ (1) Lactic acidosis and severe hepatomegaly with steatosis, including fatal cases, have been reported for nucleoside analogs used alone or in combination, including stavudine and other antiretrovirals. (2) Fatal lactic acidosis has been reported in pregnant women who received stavudine and didanosine with other antiretroviral drugs. Use the combination of stavudine and didanosine with caution during pregnancy; use is recommended only if the potential benefit clearly outweighs the potential risk. (3) Fatal and nonfatal pancreatitis have occurred during therapy when stavudine was combined with didanosine with or without hydroxyurea, in both treatment-naive and treatment-experienced clients, regardless of the degree of immunosuppression.■ The effect of stavudine on the clinical progression of HIV infection, such as incidence of opportunistic infections or survival, has not been determined. Early signs of lactic acidosis include fatigue, nausea, respiratory symptoms, and neurologic symptoms (including motor weakness). HIV clients have a significantly increased risk for developing symptomatic sensory neuropathies.

SIDE EFFECTS

Most Common
When used in combination therapy: Dizziness, peripheral neurologic symptoms/neuropathy, abnormal dreams, diarrhea, nausea, headache, rash, somnolence, insomnia.

Neurologic: Peripheral neuropathy, including numbness, tingling, or pain in feet or hands. **CNS:** Insomnia, abnormal dreams, headache, anxiety, depression, nervousness, dizziness, confusion, migraine, somnolence, tremor, neuralgia, dementia. **GI:** Diarrhea, N&V, anorexia, dyspepsia, constipation, ulcerative stomatitis, aphthous stomatitis, *pancreatitis and severe hepatomegaly with steatosis, hepatic failure.* **Body as a whole:** Lactic acidosis (especially in pregnancy when combined with didanosine with other antiretroviral drugs), headache, chills, fever, asthenia, abdominal/back pain, malaise, weight loss, *allergic reactions*, flu syndrome, lymphadenopathy, pelvic pain, myalgia, ascending neuromuscular weakness, *neoplasms, death.* **CV:** Chest pain, vasodilation, hypertension, peripheral vascular disorder, syncope. **Hematologic:** Anemia, leukopenia, thrombocytopenia. **GU:** Dysuria, genital pain, dysmenorrhea, vaginitis, urinary frequency, hematuria, impotence, urogenital neoplasm. **Respiratory:** Dyspnea, pneumonia, asthma. **Dermatologic:** Rash, sweating, pruritus, maculopapular rash, benign skin neoplasm, urticaria, exfoliative dermatitis. **Ophthalmic:** Conjunctivitis, abnormal vision.

LABORATORY TEST CONSIDERATIONS
↑ AST, ALT, amylase, bilirubin, GGT, lipase.

DRUG INTERACTIONS
Didanosine / ↑ Risk for lactic acidosis, hepatotoxicity, pancreatitis, or peripheral neuropathy
Doxorubicin / Inhibition of phosphorylation of stavudine; coadminister with caution
Hydroxyurea / ↑ Risk for lactic acidosis, hepatotoxicity, pancreatitis, or peripheral neuropathy
Methadone / ↓ AUC and peak drug levels of stavudine
Ribavirin / Inhibition of phosphorylation of stavudine; coadminister with caution
Zidovudine / Competitive inhibition of intracellular phosphorylation of stavudine; do not use together

HOW SUPPLIED
Capsules, Extended-Release: 37.5 mg, 50 mg, 75 mg, 100 mg.

DOSAGE
- **CAPSULES, EXTENDED-RELEASE**
  HIV infections.
Adults: 100 mg once daily for clients weighing 60 kg or more and 75 mg once daily for clients weighing <60 kg. Extended-release capsules have not been studied for use in children or in those with renal impairment. *NOTE:* Dosage adjustment, as follows, is required in those with peripheral neuropathy: **Clients weighing 60 kg or greater:** 50 mg once daily of the extended-release capsules. **Clients weighing <60 kg:** 37.5 mg once daily of the extended-release capsules.

NURSING CONSIDERATIONS
ADMINISTRATION/STORAGE
1. If peripheral neuropathy recurs after resumption of stavudine, consider permanent discontinuation.
2. Store extended-release capsules in tightly closed containers from 15–30°C (59–86°F).

ASSESSMENT
1. List symptom onset, other agents trialed/prescribed, date confirmed; note intolerance. List drugs prescribed to ensure none interact.

---

2. Note clinical presentation, other medical problems, any history of neuropathy while prescribed other drugs for this condition or if undergoing chemotherapy with cytotoxic drugs.

3. Obtain baseline CBC, CD_4 counts/viral load, PT/PTT, renal, LFTs. Reduce dose with impaired renal function and peripheral neuropathy.

4. Assess closely for S&S of lactic acidosis, pancreatitis, infections, or peripheral neuropathy during therapy.

CLIENT/FAMILY TEACHING

1. May be taken without regard to meals. Take exactly as prescribed q 12hr RTC, do not exceed prescribed dose, do not share medications.

2. Shake container with oral solution vigorously before measuring each dose. Store, tightly closed, in the refrigerator. Discard any unused portion after 30 days.

3. Drug is not a cure, but alleviates/manages the symptoms of HIV infections and may help prolong life. May continue to acquire illnesses associated with AIDS or ARC, including opportunistic infections; must remain under close medical supervision.

4. The risk of transmission of HIV to others through blood or sexual contact is not reduced with drug therapy. Review the criteria and precautions for safe sex and do not share needles.

5. Report any S&S of infection (i.e., sore throat, swollen glands, fever). Abdominal pain, N&V, weight loss and fatty material in stool may indicate pancreatitis; fatigue, sob or faster breathing may signal lactic acidosis, pain, burning, feeling of pins and needles in hands/feet may indicate peripheral neuropathy and should all be reported immediately as drug will need to be stopped. Symptoms may temporarily worsen following cessation of drug therapy but, once resolved, drug may be reintroduced at a lower dose.

6. Insomnia and GI upset usually resolve after 3–4 weeks of therapy. Report for all scheduled lab studies and follow-up visits to assess response to therapy and to identify any adverse drug effects.

7. Identify local support groups that may assist client/family to understand and cope with this disease.

OUTCOMES/EVALUATE

Clinical/immunologic improvement with AIDS and ARC

Streptokinase   IV
(strep-toe-**KYE**-nayz)

CLASSIFICATION(S):
Thrombolytic enzyme
PREGNANCY CATEGORY: C
Rx: Streptase.

USES

(1) DVT. (2) Arterial thrombosis and embolism. (3) Acute evolving transmural MI. (4) Pulmonary embolism. (5) Clearing of occluded arteriovenous and IV cannulae. *Investigational:* Chronic arterial occlusions, retinal vessel thrombosis, hemolytic-uremic syndrome, renal artery thrombosis, renal cortical necrosis.

ACTION/KINETICS

Action

Streptokinase acts with plasminogen to produce an "activator complex," which enhances the conversion of plasminogen to plasmin. Plasmin then breaks down fibrinogen, fibrin clots, and other plasma proteins, promoting the dissolution (lysis) of the insoluble fibrin trapped in intravascular emboli and thrombi. Also, inhibitors of streptokinase, such as alpha-2-macroglobulin, are rapidly inactivated by streptokinase.

Pharmacokinetics

Onset: rapid; **duration:** 12 hr. **t½, activator complex:** 23 min.

CONTRAINDICATIONS

Any condition presenting a risk of hemorrhage, such as recent surgery or biopsies, delivery within 10 days, ulcerative disease. Arterial emboli originating from the left side of the heart. Also, hepatic or renal insufficiency, tuberculosis, recent cerebral embolism, thrombosis, hemorrhage, SBE, rheumatic valvular disease, thrombocytopenia. Streptokinase resistance in excess of 1 mil-

---

Bold Italic = life threatening side effect   ■ = black box warning   ♣ = Available in Canada

lion international units. Use to restore patency to IV catheters.

SPECIAL CONCERNS
The use of streptokinase in septic thrombophlebitis may be hazardous. History of significant allergic response. Safety in children has not been established. Geriatric clients have an increased risk of bleeding during therapy. Serious reactions, including hypotension, hypersensitivity, apnea, and bleeding have been associated with using streptokinase for restoring catheter patency.

SIDE EFFECTS
Most Common
Minor bleeding at invaded or disturbed sites, major bleeding, fever, shivering in acute MI.

CV: Superficial bleeding, minor bleeding at invaded or disturbed sites, *severe and internal bleeding, involving GI, GU, retroperitoneal, or intracerebral sites*. **Allergic:** Nausea, headache, breathing difficulties, *fever, shivering in acute MI, bronchospasm, angioneurotic edema*, urticaria, itching, flushing, musculoskeletal pain, vasculitis, interstitial nephritis, periorbital swelling, *delayed hypersensitivity reactions* (e.g., vasculitis, interstitial nephritis). **Miscellaneous:** Respiratory depression, back pain, possible development of Guillain-Barré syndrome, development of antistreptokinase antibody (i.e., streptokinase may be ineffective if administered between 5 days and 6 months following prior use of streptokinase or following streptococcal infections).

LABORATORY TEST CONSIDERATIONS
↓ Fibrinogen, plasminogen. ↑ Thrombin time, PT, and activated PTT.

DRUG INTERACTIONS
Anticoagulants and drugs that alter platelet function (e.g., aspirin, NSAIDs, dipyridamole, GP IIb/IIIa inhibitors) ↑ the risk of serious bleeding when given with streptokinese

HOW SUPPLIED
Powder for Injection: 250,000 international units, 750,000 international units, 1.5 million international units.

DOSAGE
NOTE: Most clients have a natural resistance to streptokinase that must be overcome with the loading dose before the drug becomes effective.

- **IV INFUSION**
  DVT, Pulmonary embolism, Arterial thrombosis or embolism.
Loading dose: 250,000 international units over 30 min (use the 1,500,000 international units vial diluted to 90 mL); **maintenance:** 100,000 international units/hr for 24–72 hr for arterial thrombosis or embolism, 72 hr for deep vein thrombosis, and 24 hr (72 hr if deep vein thrombosis is suspected) for pulmonary embolism.
  Acute evolving transmural MI.
1,500,000 international units within 60 min (use the 1,500,000 international units vial diluted to a total of 45 mL).
  Arteriovenous cannula occlusion.
Before using, try to clear cannula using heparinized saline solution (syringe technique). If adequate flow does not occur, slowly instill 250,000 international units in 2-mL IV solution into each occluded limb of cannula and clamp off; **then**, after 2 hr aspirate cannula limbs, flush with saline, and reconnect cannula.

- **INTRACORONARY INFUSION**
  Acute evolving transmural MI.
20,000 international units by bolus; **then**, 2,000 international units/min for 60 min (total dose of 140,000 international units). Use the 250,000 international units vial diluted to 125 mL.

NURSING CONSIDERATIONS
ADMINISTRATION/STORAGE
[IV] 1. NaCl injection USP or D5W is the preferred diluent for IV use.
2. For AV cannulae, dilute 250,000 units with 2 mL of NaCl injection or D5W.
3. Reconstitute gently, as directed, without shaking vial.
4. Use within 24 hr of reconstitution.
5. Use an electronic infusion device to administer streptokinase and do not add any other medications to the line. Note any redness and/or pain at the site of infusion; may need to further dilute to prevent phlebitis.

S

---

6. Have emergency drugs and equipment available. Have corticosteroids and aminocaproic acid available for excessive bleeding.

7. Do not add other medication to streptokinase.

ASSESSMENT

1. Note reasons for therapy, type, onset, characteristics of S&S.

2. List history of SBE, ulcerative disease, recent surgery/trauma/CVA, TB, or streptococcal infection.

3. Assess for bleeding tendency, heart disease, allergic drug reactions.

4. Identify other drugs taking such as aspirin or NSAIDs that could increase bleeding times.

5. Clients with high allergy potential or high streptokinase antibody titer may benefit by skin testing prior to starting therapy (100 international units intradermal; if erythema and wheal develop within 20 min then allergic). Drug may not be effective if administered within 5 days to 6 months of a strep infection or if previous streptokinase use during acute event.

6. Obtain baseline lab studies; ensure that bleeding studies, type and cross-match, and streptokinase resistance have been completed before initiation of therapy as dose is based on these parameters.

7. Monitor VS, circulation (color, warmth, pulses), I&O, sensation, and for any bleeding sites.

INTERVENTIONS

1. Observe in a continuously monitored environment; document rhythm strips and VS.

2. Check access sites for evidence of bleeding. Test stool, urine, and emesis for occult blood.

3. During IV therapy, arterial sticks require 30 min of manual pressure followed by application of a pressure dressing. To prevent bruising, avoid unnecessary handling of client, procedures and injections. If IM injections necessary, apply pressure after withdrawing needle to prevent hematoma and bleeding from puncture site. Observe injection sites and postoperative wounds for bleeding during therapy

4. If excessive bleeding develops from invasive procedure, stop therapy and call for packed RBCs and plasma expanders *other than dextran.*

5. To prevent new thrombus formation, or rethrombosis, IV heparin and oral anticoagulants are used when therapy is concluded.

6. Note allergic reactions, ranging from anaphylaxis to moderate and mild reactions. These usually can be controlled with antihistamines and corticosteroids. Aminocaproic acid may help control bleeding.

7. Fever reaction may be treated with acetaminophen.

8. Following recanalization of an occluded coronary artery, clients may develop reperfusion reactions; these may include:

- Reperfusion arrhythmias (accelerated idioventricular rhythm, sinus bradycardia) usually of short duration.
- Reduction of chest pain
- Return of elevated ST segment to near baseline levels

CLIENT/FAMILY TEACHING

1. Review inherent benefits and risks of drug therapy.

2. Drug is used to break down clots and to reestablish blood flow. To be effective, therapy should be instituted within 4–6 hr of onset of symptoms of acute MI.

3. Report any evidence of bleeding or side effects immediately.

4. Encourage family members or significant other to learn CPR.

OUTCOMES/EVALUATE

- Lysis of emboli/thrombi with restoration of normal blood flow
- ↓ Myocardial infarct size; improved ventricular function
- Catheter patency in previously occluded AV or IV cannulae

Streptozocin ■

(strep-toe-**ZOH**-sin)

CLASSIFICATION(S):
Antineoplastic, alkylating
PREGNANCY CATEGORY: C
Rx: Zanosar.

SEE ALSO *ANTINEOPLASTIC AGENTS* AND *ALKYLATING AGENTS*.

USES

Metastatic islet cell pancreatic carcinomas (functional and nonfunctional) in clients with symptomatic or progressive metastases. *Investigational:* Malignant carcinoid tumors.

ACTION/KINETICS

Action

Cell-cycle nonspecific although it does inhibit progression out of the G_2 phase of cell division. Forms methylcarbonium ions that alkylate or bind with intracellular substances such as nucleic acids. Also cytotoxic by virtue of cross-linking of DNA strands resulting in inhibition of DNA synthesis. May cause hyperglycemia.

Pharmacokinetics

Does not penetrate the blood-brain barrier well, although within 2 hr after administration, metabolites do and produce levels similar to those in plasma. $t\frac{1}{2}$, **unchanged drug, initial:** 35 min. $t\frac{1}{2}$, **metabolites, initial:** 6 min; **intermediate:** 3.5 hr; **terminal:** 40 hr. Unchanged drug and metabolites excreted in urine.

CONTRAINDICATIONS

Lactation.

SPECIAL CONCERNS

■ Hospitalization is not necessary but clients should have access to a facility with lab and supportive resources sufficient to monitor drug tolerance and to protect and maintain the client compromised by drug toxicity. Renal toxicity is dose-related and cumulative and may be severe or fatal. Other major toxicities are N&V, which may be severe and, at times, treatment limiting. In addition, liver dysfunction, diarrhea, and hematological changes have been observed. Judge the possible benefit against the known toxic effects.■ Dosage has not been determined for children.

SIDE EFFECTS

Most Common
N&V, diarrhea, renal toxicity, depression, hypoglycemia.

See *Antineoplastic Agents* for a complete list of possible side effects. **GI:** N&V, diarrhea, sore mouth/lips/throat, bleeding, duodenal ulcer, hepatic toxicity, jaundice. **CNS:** Confusion, lethargy, depression. **GU:** Renal toxicity (up to two-thirds of clients) manifested by anuria, azotemia, glycosuria, hypophosphatemia, and renal tubular acidosis. *Toxicity is dose-related and cumulative and may be fatal.* **Miscellaneous:** Glucose intolerance (reversible) or insulin shock with hypoglycemia.

LABORATORY TEST CONSIDERATIONS

↑ AST, LDH. Hypoalbuminemia.

HOW SUPPLIED

Powder for Injection: 1 gram (100 mg/mL).

DOSAGE

• **IV**
Pancreatic carcinomas.
Daily schedule: 500 mg/m^2 for 5 consecutive days q 6 weeks (until maximum benefit is achieved or toxicity occurs). Do not increase dose. **Weekly schedule: Initial:** 1,000 mg/m^2/week for 2 weeks; **then,** if no response or no toxicity, dose can be increased, not to exceed a single dose of 1,500 mg/m^2. Expect a response in 17–35 days.

NURSING CONSIDERATIONS

ADMINISTRATION/STORAGE

 1. Reconstitute with 9.5 mL dextrose or 0.9% NaCl injection. Reconstituted solution is pale gold in color and contains 100 mg/mL streptozocin. This may be further diluted. Administer slowly over 1–2 hr.
2. Total storage time for reconstituted drug is 12 hr, as there are no preservatives present. The ampule is not multiple dose.
3. Observe caution (wear gloves) in handling the drug.

S

4. Drug is a vesicant. Infiltration may result in tissue ulceration and necrosis.

ASSESSMENT
1. Note reasons for therapy, characteristics of S&S, other agents trialed.
2. Premedicate with antiemetic; may cause severe N&V.
3. Monitor I&O, lab studies, weight. Encourage 3 L/day of fluids to reduce the risk of renal damage; if urine output decreases- streptozocin can cause anuria.
4. Monitor blood sugar, CBC, uric acid, renal, LFTs. Drug may cause lymphocyte and platelet suppression. Nadir: 10 days; recovery: 14–17 days. Assess carefully for renal toxicity.

CLIENT/FAMILY TEACHING
1. Drug can cause permanent renal damage or toxicity resulting in death. Report any S&S of dysfunction, i.e., decreased urine output, changes in color, early protein in urine. Keep all F/U visits for labs and evaluation.
2. Consume 2–3 L fluid/day to ensure adequate hydration.
3. Report any unusual bruising/bleeding, blood in urine, ↑ nose bleeds or S&S anemia (SOB, easy fatigue, rapid pulse, paleness).

OUTCOMES/EVALUATE
↓ Tumor size and spread; suppression of malignant cell proliferation

Succinylcholine chloride ■
(suck-sin-ill-**KOH**-leen)

CLASSIFICATION(S):
Neuromuscular blocking drug, depolarizing
PREGNANCY CATEGORY: C
Rx: Anectine, Anectine Flo-Pack, Quelicin.

SEE ALSO *NEUROMUSCULAR BLOCKING AGENTS.*

USES
Adjunct to general anesthesia to facilitate ET intubation and to induce relaxation of skeletal muscle during surgery or mechanical ventilation. *Investigation-al:* Reduce intensity of electrically induced seizures or seizures due to drugs.

ACTION/KINETICS
Action
Initially excites skeletal muscle by combining with cholinergic receptors preferentially to acetylcholine. Subsequently, it prevents the muscle from contracting by prolonging the time during which the receptors at the neuromuscular junction cannot respond to acetylcholine. The order of paralysis is levator muscles of the eyelid, mastication muscles, limb muscles, abdominal muscles, glottis muscles, the intercostals, the diaphragm, and all other skeletal muscles. Prolonged use may change from a depolarizing neuromuscular block (phase I block) to a block that resembles a nondepolarizing block (phase II block). This may be associated with prolonged respiratory depression and apnea. No effect on pain threshold, cerebration, or consciousness; use with sufficient anesthesia. Effects are not blocked by anticholinesterase drugs and may even be enhanced by them. May cause a change in myocardial rhythm due to vagal stimulation due to surgical procedures (especially in children) and from potassium-mediated alterations in electrical conductivity (enhanced by halogenated anesthetics).

Pharmacokinetics
Onset, IV: 30–60 sec; **duration:** 4–6 min; **recovery:** 8–10 min. **Onset, IM:** 2–3 min; **duration:** 10–30 min. Metabolized by plasma pseudocholinesterase to succinylmonocholine, which is a nondepolarizing muscle relaxant, and then to succinic acid and choline. About 10% excreted unchanged in the urine.

CONTRAINDICATIONS
Use in genetically determined disorders of plasma pseudocholinesterase. Personal or family history of malignant hyperthermia. Myopathies associated with elevated CPK values. Acute narrow-angle glaucoma or penetrating eye injuries. Use of IV infusion in children due to the risk of malignant hyperpyrexia.

SPECIAL CONCERNS
■ Use only if skilled in the management of artificial respiration and when facili-

ties are instantly available for tracheal intubation and for providing adequate ventilation of the client, including the administration of oxygen under positive pressure and the elimination of carbon dioxide. The clinician must be prepared to assist or control ventilation.■ Use with caution during lactation. Pediatric clients may be especially prone to myoglobinemia, myoglobinuria, and cardiac effects. Use with caution in clients with severe liver disease, severe anemia, malnutrition, impaired cholinesterase activity, fractures. Also, use with caution in CV, pulmonary, renal, or metabolic diseases. Use with great caution in those with severe burns, electrolyte imbalance, hyperkalemia, those receiving quinidine, and those who are digitalized or recovering from severe trauma, as serious cardiac arrhythmias or cardiac arrest may result. Clients with myasthenia gravis may show resistance to succinylcholine. Those with fractures or muscle spasms may manifest additional trauma due to succinylcholine-induced muscle fasciculations.

SIDE EFFECTS

Most Common

Respiratory depression, bradycardia, hypo-/hypertension, salivation, postoperative muscle pain.

Skeletal muscle: May cause *severe, persistent respiratory depression or apnea*. Muscle fasciculations, postoperative muscle pain. **CV:** Hyper-/hypotension, brady-/tachycardia, *arrhythmias, cardiac arrest*. **Respiratory:** *Apnea, respiratory depression*. **Miscellaneous:** Fever, salivation, hyperkalemia, *anaphylaxis*, myoglobinemia, myoglobinuria, skin rashes, increased intraocular pressure, myalgia, jaw rigidity, perioperative dreams in children, *rhabdomyolysis* with possible myoglobinuric acute renal failure. Repeated doses may cause *tachyphylaxis*. *Malignant hyperthermia:* Muscle rigidity (especially of the jaw), tachycardia, tachypnea unresponsive to increased depth of anesthesia, increased oxygen requirement and carbon dioxide production, increased body temperature, metabolic acidosis.

OD **OVERDOSE MANAGEMENT**

Symptoms: Skeletal muscle weakness, decreased respiratory reserve, low tidal volume, apnea. *Treatment:* Maintain a patent airway and respiratory support until normal respiration is ensured.

DRUG INTERACTIONS

Aminoglycoside antibiotics / Additive skeletal muscle blockade
Amphotericin B / ↑ Succinylcholine effect R/T induced electrolyte imbalance
Antibiotics, nonpenicillin / Additive skeletal muscle blockade
Beta-adrenergic blocking agents / Additive skeletal muscle blockade
Chloroquine / Additive skeletal muscle blockade
Cimetidine / Inhibits pseudocholinesterase
Clindamycin / Additive skeletal muscle blockade
Cyclophosphamide / ↑ Succinylcholine effect by ↓ breakdown by plasma pseudocholinesterase
Cyclopropane / ↑ Risk of bradycardia, arrhythmias, sinus arrest, apnea, and malignant hyperthermia
Diazepam / ↓ Succinycholine effect
Digitalis glycosides / ↑ Risk of cardiac arrhythmias, including VF; possible ↑ in toxic effects of both drugs
Echothiophate iodide / ↑ Succinylcholine effect by ↓ breakdown by plasma pseudocholinesterase
Furosemide / ↑ Skeletal muscle blockade
Halothane / ↑ Risk of bradycardia, arrhythmias, sinus arrest, apnea, and malignant hyperthermia
Isoflurane / Additive skeletal muscle blockade
Lidocaine / Additive skeletal muscle blockade
Lincomycin / Additive skeletal muscle blockade
Lithium carbonate / ↑ Skeletal muscle blockade
Mg salts / Additive skeletal muscle blockade
Muscle relaxants, nondepolarizing / Possible synergistic or antagonistic effect of succinylcholine
Narcotics / ↑ Risk of bradycardia and sinus arrest

S

Nitrous oxide / ↑ Risk of bradycardia, arrhythmias, sinus arrest, apnea, and malignant hyperthermia

Oxytocin / ↑ Succinylcholine effect

Phenelzine / ↑ Succinylcholine effect

Phenothiazines / ↑ Succinylcholine effect

Polymyxin / Additive skeletal muscle blockade

Procainamide / ↑ Succinylcholine effect

Procaine / ↑ Succinylcholine effect by inhibiting plasma pseudocholinesterase

Promazine / ↑ Succinylcholine effect

Quinidine / Additive skeletal muscle blockade

Quinine / Additive skeletal muscle blockade

Tacrine / ↑ Succinylcholine effect

Thiazide diuretics / ↑ Succinylcholine effect due to induced electrolyte imbalance

Thiotepa / ↑ Succinylcholine effect by ↓ breakdown by plasma pseudocholinesterase

Trimethaphan / ↑ Succinylcholine effect by inhibiting plasma pseudocholinesterase

HOW SUPPLIED

Injection: 20 mg/mL, 50 mg/mL, 100 mg/mL; *Powder for Infusion:* 500 mg, 1 gram.

DOSAGE

- **IM; IV**

    Short or prolonged surgical procedures.

Adults, IV, initial: 0.3–1.1 mg/kg (average: 0.6 mg/kg); **then,** repeated doses can be given based on client response. **Adults, IM:** 3–4 mg/kg, not to exceed a total dose of 150 mg.

    Electroshock therapy.

Adults, IV: 10–30 mg given 1 min prior to the shock (individualize dosage). **IM:** Up to 2.5 mg/kg, not to exceed a total dose of 150 mg.

    ET intubation.

Pediatric, IV: 1–2 mg/kg; if necessary, dose can be repeated. **IM:** 3–4 mg/kg, not to exceed a total dose of 150 mg.

- **IV INFUSION (PREFERRED)**

    Prolonged surgical procedures.

Adults: Average rate ranges from 2.5 to 4.3 mg/min. Most commonly used are 0.1–0.2% solutions in D5W, sodium

chloride injection, or other diluent given at a rate of 0.5–10 mg/min depending on client response and degree of relaxation desired, for up to 1 hr.

- **IV, INTERMITTENT**

    Prolonged muscle relaxation.

Initial: 0.3–1.1 mg/kg; **then,** 0.04–0.07 mg/kg at appropriate intervals to maintain required level of relaxation.

NURSING CONSIDERATIONS

ADMINISTRATION/STORAGE

[IV] 1. Give an initial test dose of 0.1 mg/kg to assess sensitivity and recovery time; if no or transient respiratory depression lasting less than 5 min, may give drug.

2. Do not mix with anesthetic. To reduce salivation, premedicate with atropine or scopolamine.

3. For IV infusion, use 1 or 2 mg/mL solution of drug in D5W, 0.9% NaCl, or other suitable IV solution; not compatible with alkaline solutions.

4. Refrigerate drug at 2–8°C (36–46°F). Multidose vials stable for 14 days or less at room temperature without significant loss of potency.

ASSESSMENT

1. List reasons for therapy, agents currently prescribed to ensure that none interact unfavorably. Note if taking digitalis products or quinidine; these clients sensitive to the release of intracellular potassium.

2. Obtain baseline ECG, electrolytes, renal, LFTs. Those with low plasma pseudocholinesterase levels are sensitive to the effects of succinylcholine and require lower doses.

3. Note any evidence/history of MS, malignant hyperthermia, CPK myopathy, acute glaucoma, or eye injury; drug generally contraindicated.

4. Medicate for pain and anxiety as drug does not affect these symptoms; client unable to speak. Reassure they will regain function once therapy completed.

INTERVENTIONS

1. A peripheral nerve stimulator/train of four should be used to assess neuromuscular response and recovery. The order of paralysis is levator muscles of

the eyelid, mastication muscles, limb muscles, abdominal muscles, glottis muscles, the intercostals, the diaphragm, and all other skeletal muscles. This is reversed with recovery. Tests of muscle strength indicate recovery, such as return of hand grip, head lift, and ability to cough.

2. Monitor VS and ECG; can cause vagal stimulation resulting in bradycardia, hypotension, and cardiac arrhythmias, especially in children.

3. Muscle fasciculations may cause the client to be sore and injured after recovery. Administer prescribed nondepolarizing agent (i.e., tubocurarine) and reassure that the soreness is likely caused by unsynchronized contractions of adjacent muscle fibers just before onset of paralysis.

4. Observe for excessive, transient increase in intraocular pressure. Monitor for evidence of malignant hyperthermia, unresponsive tachycardia, jaw spasm, or lack of laryngeal relaxation.

5. Drug should be used only on a short-term basis in a continuously monitored environment by those trained in its use. Prolonged use may change from a depolarizing neuromuscular block (phase I block) to a block that resembles a nondepolarizing block (phase II block) which may be associated with prolonged respiratory depression and apnea.

6. Client is fully conscious and aware of surroundings/conversations. Drug does not affect pain or anxiety. Explain all procedures and provide emotional support. Do not conduct any discussions that should not be overheard. Reassure will be able to talk and move once drug effects reversed. Determine client need and administer medications for anxiety, pain, and/or sedation regularly (valium, morphine).

7. When used for seizures, ensure that serum level of anticonvulsant agent is therapeutic. Succinylcholine does not cross the blood-brain barrier and will only suppress peripheral manifestations of seizures, not the central process.

CLIENT/FAMILY TEACHING
1. Reassure will be continuously monitored and protected and procedures/tests explained.
2. Once drug withdrawn will regain ability to move and talk again. May feel stiff and sore but should soon subside.
3. Medication for anxiety and pain will also be given, as this drug does not affect consciousness or alter pain threshold.

OUTCOMES/EVALUATE
- Muscle relaxation/paralysis
- Suppression of the twitch response
- Facilitation of ET intubation; control of breathing during mechanical ventilation
- ↓ Muscle contractions with drug/electroshock induced seizures

Sucralfate ©
(sue-**KRAL**-fayt)

CLASSIFICATION(S):
Antiulcer drug
PREGNANCY CATEGORY: B
Rx: Carafate.
✦Rx: Apo-Sucralfate, Novo-Sucralate, Nu-Sucralfate, PMS-Sucralfate, Sulcrate, Sulcrate Suspension Plus.

USES
(1) Short-term treatment (up to 8 weeks) of active duodenal ulcers. (2) Maintenance for duodenal ulcer at decreased dosage after healing of acute ulcers (tablets only). *Investigational:* Hasten healing of gastric ulcers, chronic treatment of gastric ulcers. Treatment of reflux and peptic esophagitis. Treatment of aspirin- and NSAID-induced GI symptoms; prevention of stress ulcers and GI bleeding in critically ill clients. The suspension has been used to treat oral and esophageal ulcers due to chemotherapy, radiation, or sclerotherapy.

ACTION/KINETICS
Action
Thought to form an ulcer-adherent complex with albumin and fibrinogen at the site of the ulcer, protecting it

S

from further damage by gastric acid. May also form a viscous, adhesive barrier on the surface of the gastric mucosa and duodenum.

Pharmacokinetics

Minimally absorbed from the GI tract; 95% remains in the GI tract. It adsorbs pepsin, thus inhibiting its activity. May be used in conjunction with antacids. Approximately 90% excreted in the feces. **Duration:** 5 hr.

SPECIAL CONCERNS

Safety for use in children and during lactation has not been fully established. A successful course resulting in healing of ulcers will not alter posthealing frequency or severity of duodenal ulceration.

SIDE EFFECTS

Most Common

Constipation, nausea, upset stomach, diarrhea, dizziness, sleepiness, back pain, pruritus.

GI: Constipation, N&V, upset stomach, diarrhea, indigestion, flatulence, dry mouth, gastric discomfort. **Hypersensitivity:** Urticaria, *angioedema, respiratory difficulty, laryngospasm*, facial swelling, rhinitis. **Dermatologic:** Rash, pruritus. **Miscellaneous:** Back pain, headache, dizziness, sleepiness, insomnia, vertigo.

DRUG INTERACTIONS

Antacids containing Al / ↑ Total body burden of Al

Anticoagulants / ↓ Warfarin hypoprothrombinemic effect

Cimetidine / ↓ Cimetidine absorption R/T binding to sucralfate

Ciprofloxacin / ↓ Ciprofloxacin absorption R/T binding to sucralfate

Diclofenac / ↓ Diclofenac effects

Digoxin / ↓ Digoxin absorption R/T binding to sucralfate

Ketoconazole / ↓ Ketoconaozle bioavailability

Levothyroxine / ↓ Therapeutic effect of levothyroxine due to ↓ GI absorption

Norfloxacin / ↓ Norfloxacin absorption R/T binding to sucralfate

Penicillamine / ↓ Penicillamine effects

Phenytoin / ↓ Phenytoin absorption R/T binding to sucralfate

Quinidine / ↓ Quinidine levels → ↓ effect

Quinolones / ↓ Quinolone bioavailability; giving 2 hr before sucralfate may eliminate the interaction

Ranitidine / ↓ Ranitidine absorption R/T binding to sucralfate

Tetracycline / ↓ Tetracycline absorption R/T binding to sucralfate

Theophylline / ↓ Theophylline absorption R/T binding to sucralfate

HOW SUPPLIED

Suspension: 1 gram/10 mL; *Tablets:* 1 gram.

DOSAGE

• **SUSPENSION, TABLETS**

Active duodenal ulcer.

Adults, usual: 1 gram 4 times per day on an empty stomach (10 mL of the suspension) 1 hr before meals and at bedtime (it may also be taken 2 hr after meals). Take for 4–8 weeks unless x-ray films or endoscopy have indicated significant healing. **Maintenance (tablets only):** 1 gram twice a day.

NURSING CONSIDERATIONS

Ⓒ Do not confuse Carafate with Cafergot (combination analgesic drug).

ASSESSMENT

1. Note reasons for therapy, onset, characteristics of S&S, other agents trialed, outcome.

2. Reconstitute tablets prior to administering through NGT. When placed in a cup with a small amount of water and left for 10–15 min, the tablets will dissolve completely.

3. Assess and monitor gastric pH; maintain pH >5.

4. Monitor CBC, serum phosphate levels. Drug binds phosphate and may lead to hypophosphatemia.

CLIENT/FAMILY TEACHING

1. Take on an empty stomach 1 hr before or 2 hr after meals. Do not crush or chew tablets or skip doses. If antacids are used, take 30 min before or after.

2. Avoid large meals within 2 hr of bedtime and elevate head of bed to prevent reflux S&S.

3. Take exactly as prescribed. It binds to proteins at the site of the lesions to create a protective barrier that prevents

---

Bold Italic = life threatening side effect   ■ = black box warning   ♣ = Available in Canada

diffusion of hydrogen ions at a normal gastric pH. Do not stop if feeling better, must complete entire course to ensure healing has occurred.

4. May cause constipation; increase fluids/bulk and perform regular exercise.

5. Avoid smoking, alcohol, chocolate, spicy foods, and caffeine to prevent a recurrence of ulcers. Even though healing of ulcers may result, the frequency or severity of subsequent attacks is not altered.

6. Report as scheduled for follow-up, upper GI/endoscopy, and labs.

OUTCOMES/EVALUATE
- ↓ Abdominal pain/discomfort
- Prophylaxis of GI bleeding
- Healing of duodenal ulcers

Sulfacetamide sodium
(sul-fah-**SEAT**-ah-myd)

CLASSIFICATION(S):
Sulfonamide, topical

Rx: AK-Sulf, Bleph-10, Carmol Scalp Treatment, Cetamide, Isopto-Cetamide, Klaron 10%, Ocusulf-10, Seb-Prev, Sebizon, Sodium Sulamyd, Storz Sulf, Sulf-10, Sulster.

SEE ALSO SULFONAMIDES.

USES
(1) Topically for conjunctivitis, corneal ulcer, and other superficial ocular infections. (2) Adjunct to systemic sulfonamides to treat trachoma.

CONTRAINDICATIONS
Use in infants less than 2 months of age. Use in the presence of epithelial herpes simplex keratitis, vaccinia, varicella, and other viral diseases of the cornea and conjunctiva. Mycobacterial or fungal infections of the ocular structures. After uncomplicated removal of a corneal foreign body.

SPECIAL CONCERNS
Safe use during pregnancy and lactation or in children less than 12 years of age has not been established. Use with caution in clients with dry eye syndrome. Ophthalmic ointments may retard corneal wound healing.

SIDE EFFECTS
Most Common
Itching, local irritation, headache, burning, transient stinging, redness, swelling

Ophthalmic: Itching, local irritation, redness, swelling, periorbital edema, burning and transient stinging, headache, bacterial or fungal corneal ulcers.
CNS: Headache. *NOTE:* Sulfonamides may cause serious systemic side effects, including **severe hypersensitivity reactions**. Symptoms include fever, skin rash, GI disturbances, bone marrow depression, **Stevens-Johnson syndrome, toxic epidermal necrolysis**, exfoliative dermatitis, photosensitivity. Fatalities have occurred.

DRUG INTERACTIONS
Preparations containing silver are incompatible.

HOW SUPPLIED
Lotion: 10%; *Ophthalmic Ointment:* 10%; *Ophthalmic Solution:* 1%, 10%, 15%, 30%; *Suspension, Topical:* 10%.

DOSAGE
- **OPHTHALMIC SOLUTION**
  Conjunctivitis or other superficial ocular infections.

For all strengths, 1–2 gtt in the conjunctival sac q 1–4 hr. Doses may be tapered by increasing the time interval between doses as the condition improves.

  Trachoma.

2 gtt q 2 hr with concomitant systemic sulfonamide therapy.

- **OPHTHALMIC OINTMENT**
  Conjunctivitis, corneal ulcer, and other superficial ocular infections.

Apply approximately ¼ inch into the lower conjunctival sac 3–4 times per day and at bedtime. Alternatively, ½–1 in. is placed in the conjunctival sac at bedtime along with use of drops during the day.

- **LOTION**
  For cutaneous infections.

Apply locally (10%) to affected area 2–4 times per day

  Seborrheic dermatitis.

Apply 1–2 times per day (for mild cases, apply overnight).

  Cutaneous bacterial infections.

S

Apply 2–4 times per day until infection clears.

NURSING CONSIDERATIONS

ADMINISTRATION/STORAGE
Solutions will darken in color if left standing for long periods; discard these products.

ASSESSMENT
1. Note reasons for therapy, onset, duration, characteristics of S&S.
2. List other agents prescribed, outcome.
3. Note any allergy to sulfa drugs.

CLIENT/FAMILY TEACHING
1. Use only as directed. Wash hands before and after instillation.
2. Ophthalmic products may cause sensitivity to bright light; wear sunglasses to minimize.
3. Report lack of response and any purulent eye drainage as this inactivates sulfacetamide.
4. If prescribed additional eye drops, wait 5 min after sulfacetamide instillation.
5. Do not wear contact lenses until infection is resolved.
6. Discard any cloudy or dark solutions. Do not let dropper/tip touch any part of eye so as to prevent contamination of bottle/tube contents.

OUTCOMES/EVALUATE
Resolution of inflammation/infection

Sulfadiazine ©
(sul-fah-**DYE**-ah-zeen)

CLASSIFICATION(S):
Antibiotic, sulfonamide
PREGNANCY CATEGORY: C
Rx: Microsulfon.

SEE ALSO *SULFONAMIDES*.

USES
(1) UTIs caused by *Escherichia coli, Klebsiella, Enterobacter, Staphylococcus aureus, Proteus mirabilis,* and *Proteus vulgaris.* (2) Chancroid. (3) Inclusion conjunctivitis. (4) Adjunct to treat chloroquine-resistant strains of *Plasmodium falciparum.* (5) Meningitis caused by *Haemophilus influenzae,* meningococcal meningitis for sulfonamide-sensitive group A strains. (6) Nocardiosis. (7) With penicillin to treat acute otitis media caused by *H. influenzae.* (8) Rheumatic fever prophylaxis. (9) Adjunct with pyrimethamine for toxoplasmosis in selected immunocompromised clients (e.g., those with AIDS, neoplastic disease, or congenital immune compromise). (10) Trachoma.

ACTION/KINETICS
Pharmacokinetics
Short-acting; often combined with other anti-infectives.

CONTRAINDICATIONS
Use in infants less than 2 months of age unless combined with pyrimethamine to treat congenital toxoplasmosis.

SPECIAL CONCERNS
Safe use during pregnancy has not been established.

SIDE EFFECTS
Most Common
Diarrhea, dizziness, headache, insomnia, rash, anorexia, stomach pain, tinnitus, myalgia.

See *Sulfonamides* for a complete list of possible side effects.

HOW SUPPLIED
Tablets: 500 mg.

DOSAGE
- **TABLETS**
  General use.

Adults, loading dose: 2–4 grams; **maintenance:** 2–4 grams/day in 3 to 6 divided doses; **infants over 2 months, loading dose:** 75 mg/kg/day (2 grams/m^2); **maintenance:** 150 mg/kg/day (4 grams/m^2/day) in 4 to 6 divided doses, not to exceed 6 grams/day.
  Rheumatic fever prophylaxis.

Under 30 kg: 0.5 gram/day; **over 30 kg:** 1 gram/day.
  As adjunct with pyrimethamine in congenital toxoplasmosis.

Infants less than 2 months: 25 mg/kg 4 times per day for 3 to 4 weeks. **Children >2 months:** 25–50 mg/kg 4 times per day for 3 to 4 weeks.

NURSING CONSIDERATIONS
© Do not confuse sulfadiazine with sulfasalazine (also a sulfonamide).

Bold Italic = life threatening side effect   ■ = black box warning   ✦ = Available in Canada

ASSESSMENT

1. Note reasons for therapy, onset, duration, characteristics of S&S.
2. Obtain appropriate labs/cultures.

CLIENT/FAMILY TEACHING

1. Take as directed with a full glass of water to prevent dehydration and crystalluria. Do not share medications; complete entire prescription.
2. Avoid prolonged sun exposure and use protection; may cause photosensitivity reaction.
3. No OTC medications especially aspirin or vitamin C without provider approval.
4. Report any unusual bruising/bleeding, rash, fever, sore throat, or lack of effectiveness.

OUTCOMES/EVALUATE

- Negative culture reports
- Infection prophylaxis

Sulfasalazine   ©

(sul-fah-**SAL**-ah-zeen)

CLASSIFICATION(S):

Antibiotic, sulfonamide

PREGNANCY CATEGORY: B

Rx: Azulfidine, Azulfidine EN-Tabs.

♥Rx: Salazopyrin, Salazopyrin En-Tabs, ratio-Sulfasalazine.

SEE ALSO *SULFONAMIDES.*

USES

Tablets and Delayed-Release Tablets.
(1) Mild-to-moderate ulcerative colitis.
(2) Adjunctive in severe ulcerative colitis. (3) Prolongation of the remission period between acute attacks of ulcerative colitis. **Delayed-Release Tablets.** (1) Treat rheumatoid arthritis in adults who have responded inadequately to salicylates or other NSAIDs. (2) Pediatric clients with polyarticular-course juvenile rheumatoid arthritis who have responded inadequately to salicylates or other NSAIDs. *Investigational:* Ankylosing spondylitis, granulomatous colitis, Crohn's disease, regional enteritis.

ACTION/KINETICS

Pharmacokinetics

Bioavailability is less than 15% for the parent drug. The drug passes to the colon, where it is split to 5-aminosalicylic acid (5-ASA) and sulfapyridine. The drug does not affect the microflora. Peak plasma levels of both sulfasalazine and 5-aminosalicylic acid occur after about 10 hr. Sulfapyridine is metabolized by acetylation. **Mean plasma t½, fast acetylators:** 10.4 hr; **mean plasma t½, slow acetylators:** 14.8 hr. 5-ASA is metabolized by the liver and intestine. Absorbed sulfapyridine and 5-ASA and their metabolites are excreted primarily in the urine. However, the majority of 5-ASA remains in the colon and is excreted with the feces.

ADDITIONAL CONTRAINDICATIONS

Children below 2 years. In persons with marked sulfonamide, salicylate, or related drug hypersensitivity. Intestinal or urinary obstruction.

SPECIAL CONCERNS

Use with caution during lactation and in those with severe allergy or bronchial asthma. Observe closely those with glucose-6-phosphate dehydrogenase deficiency for signs of hemolytic anemia (reaction is frequently dose-related). Safety and efficiency have not been determined in children less than 2 years of age with ulcerative colitis.

SIDE EFFECTS

Most Common

Anorexia, headache, N&V, dyspepsia, gastric distress, rash, reversible oligospermia.

GI: Anorexia, N&V, dyspepsia, gastric distress, stomatitis, diarrhea, hepatitis, pancreatitis, bloody diarrhea, impaired folic acid absorption, impaired digoxin absorption, abdominal pain, neutropenic enterocolitis, hepatotoxicity, jaundice, cholestatic jaundice, cirrhosis, *liver necrosis, liver failure.* **CNS:** Headache, dizziness, transverse myelitis, *convulsions, meningitis,* transient lesions of the posterior spinal column, cauda equina syndrome, Guillain-Barre syndrome, peripheral neuropathy, mental depression, vertigo, hearing loss, insomnia, ataxia, hallucinations, tinnitus,

S

drowsiness. **Dermatologic:** Pruritus, urticaria, skin rash/discoloration. **GU:** Oligospermia (reversible), infertility in men, toxic nephrosis with oliguria and anuria, nephritis, nephrotic syndrome, hematuria, crystalluria, proteinuria, hemolytic-uremic syndrome, urine discoloration. **Hematologic: *Agranulocytosis, aplastic anemia,*** leukopenia, thrombocytopenia, suppression of immunoglobulin, megaloblastic anemia, purpura, hypoprothrombinemia, methemoglobinemia, congenital neutropenia, myelodysplastic syndrome. **Hypersensitivity: *Stevens-Johnson syndrome,*** exfoliative dermatitis, epidermal necrolysis with corneal damage, ***anaphylaxis,*** serum sickness syndrome, pneumonitis with or without eosinophilia, vasculitis, fibrosing alveolitis, pleuritis, ***pericarditis with or without tamonade,*** allergic myocarditis, polyarteritis nodosa, lupus erythematosus-like syndrome, hepatitis, ***hepatic necrosis with or without immune complexes,*** fulminant hepatitis (possible liver transplant necessary), parapsoriasis, varioliformis acute, rhabdomyolysis, photosensitivity, arthralgia, periorbital edema, conjunctival and scleral injection, alopecia. **Miscellaneous:** Fever, Heinz body anemia, ***hemolytic anemia,*** cyanosis. *NOTE:* Symptoms of sore throat, fever, pallor, purpura or jaundice may be signs of serious blood disorders.

LABORATORY TEST CONSIDERATIONS

↑ AST, ALT, GGT, lactic dehydrogenase, alkaline phosphatase, bilirubin. Abnormal LFTs.

OD OVERDOSE MANAGEMENT

Symptoms: N&V, gastric distress, abdominal pain, drowsiness, convulsions.
Treatment:
- Gastric lavage or emesis plus catharsis.
- Alkalinize the urine to hasten excretion.
- Force fluids if kidney function is normal.
- If anuria is present, restrict fluids and salt and treat appropriately.

- Catherization of the ureters may be indicated for complete renal blockage by crystals.
- The low molecular weight of sulfasalazine and its metabolites may help their removal by dialysis.

DRUG INTERACTIONS

Azathioprine / High rate of leukopenia and ↑ whole blood 6-thioguanine in Crohn's disease clients
Cyclosporine / ↓ Cyclosporine levels; ↑ risk of nephrotoxicity
Digoxin / ↓ Digoxin absorption
Folic acid / ↓ Folic acid absorption; folic acid dosage adjustment may be needed
Mercaptopurine / High rate of leukopenia and ↑ whole blood 6-thioguanine in Crohn's disease clients
Methotrexate / ↑ Risk of methotrexate-induced bone marrow suppression R/T displacement of methotrexate from plasma protein binding sites; also, ↑ GI side effects, especially nausea
Sulfonylureas (e.g., glipizide) / ↑ Sulfonylurea levels R/T impaired hepatic metabolism or altered plasma protein binding; monitor and possibly decrease sulfonylurea dose
Warfarin / ↑ Warfarin anticoagulant effect; monitor carefully

HOW SUPPLIED

Tablets: 500 mg; *Tablets, Delayed-Release*: 500 mg.

DOSAGE ─────────────────

- **TABLETS; TABLETS, DELAYED-RELEASE**
  Ulcerative colitis.

Adults, initial: 3–4 grams/day in evenly divided doses with dosage intervals not exceeding 8 hr. A lower initial dosage (1–2 grams/day) may decrease side effects; **maintenance:** 500 mg 4 times per day. Doses greater than 4 grams/day increase the risk of toxicity. **Pediatric, over 6 years of age, initial:** 40–60 mg/kg/day in 3 to 6 equally divided doses; **maintenance:** 30 mg/kg/day in 4 divided doses.
  Adult rheumatoid arthritis.
Delayed-Release Tablets: To reduce GI intolerance, **initial:** 0.5 gram in the evening for the first week, increased to 0.5 gram in the morning and evening the

---

Bold Italic = life threatening side effect   ■ = black box warning   ✤ = Available in Canada

S

second week, 0.5 gram in the morning and 1 gram in the evening the third week; then, beginning week 4, 1 gram in the morning and evening. Consider increasing the daily dose to 3 grams if the clinical response after 12 weeks is inadequate. Monitor closely for doses over 2 grams/day.

Juvenile rheumatoid arthritis, polyarticular course.

Children, 6 years and older: 30–50 mg/kg daily in 2 evenly divided doses (maximum 2 grams/day). To reduce GI intolerance, begin with a quarter to a third of the planned maintenance dose and increase weekly until reaching the maintenance dose at 1 month.

Collagenous colitis.

2–3 grams/day.

Psoriasis.

3–4 grams/day.

Psoriatic arthritis.

2 grams/day.

NURSING CONSIDERATIONS

◎ Do not confuse sulfasalazine with salsalate, sulfisoxazole, or sulfadiazine (also a sulfonamide).

ADMINISTRATION/STORAGE

1. Adjust dose individually to each client's response and tolerance.

2. The enteric-coated delayed-release tablets are indicated particularly for those clients with ulcerative colitis who can not take uncoated sulfasalazine tablets due to GI intolerance (e.g., N&V with the first few doses, clients in whom a reduction in dosage does not alleviate the adverse GI effects).

3. Rest and physiotherpy should be continued in adults and children with rheumatoid arthritis.

4. The delayed-release tablets do not produce an immediate response. Concurrent treatment with analgesics or NSAIDs is recommended, at least until the effect of sulfasalazine delayed-release tablets is apparent.

5. When used for rheumatoid arthritis, a therapeutic response has been seen as early as 4 weeks after initiating treatment with delayed-release tablets; however, treatment for 12 weeks may be needed in some before a clinical benefit is noted. Give consideration to increasing the daily dose of the delayed-release tablets to 3 grams if the clinical response after 12 weeks is inadequate; monitor carefully.

6. It is possible, in isolated instances, for delayed-release tablets to be excreted undisintegrated. If this occurs, discontinue the delayed-release tablets immediately.

7. Store from 15–30°C (59–86°F).

ASSESSMENT

1. Note ireasons for therapy, onset, characteristics of S&S. List other agents trialed; outcome.

2. List frequency, quantity, and consistency of stool production; assess abdominal pain with ulcerative colitis.

3. Note joint deformity, pain, ROM, inflammation, and swelling with rheumatoid arthritis.

4. Monitor CBC, folate, renal function studies, and urinalysis; and with colitis, also send stool for analysis.

CLIENT/FAMILY TEACHING

1. Take exactly as ordered at the same time each day; even if using intermittent therapy (2 weeks on, 2 weeks off). Take with or after meals at evenly spaced intervals to reduce GI upset.

2. Take at least 2–3 L/day of water to decrease incidence of dehydration and crystalluria/stone formation. Drug may discolor urine or skin a yellow-orange color. May permanently discolor soft contact lenses.

3. Avoid prolonged exposure to sunlight; may increase sensitivity. Wear protective clothing, sunglasses, and sunscreen.

4. Report any unusual bruising/bleeding, rash, fever, sore throat, intact tablet in stool, or lack of response. Keep all F/U visits so dose and response can be assessed.

OUTCOMES/EVALUATE

- ↓ Frequency of loose stools; ↓ abdominal pain; ↓ colon inflammation
- Relief of pain from joint deformity, swelling, and inflammation

S

Sulfinpyrazone
(sul-fin-**PEER**-ah-zohn)

CLASSIFICATION(S):
Antigout drug, uricosuric
Rx: Anturane.
♣Rx: Apo-Sulfinpyrazone, Nu-Sulfinpyrazone.

USES
Chronic and intermittent gouty arthritis. Not effective during acute attacks of gout and may even increase the frequency of acute episodes during the initiation of therapy. However, do not discontinue during acute attacks. Concomitant administration of colchicine during initiation of therapy is recommended. *Investigational:* To decrease sudden death during first year after MI.

ACTION/KINETICS
Action
Inhibits tubular reabsorption of uric acid, thereby increasing its excretion. Also exhibits antithrombotic and platelet inhibitory actions.

Pharmacokinetics
Peak plasma levels: 1–2 hr. **Therapeutic plasma levels:** Up to 160 mcg/mL following 800 mg/day for uricosuria. **Duration:** 4–6 hr (up to 10 hr in some). **t½:** 3–8 hr. Metabolized by the liver. Approximately 45% of the drug is excreted unchanged by the kidney, and a small amount is excreted in the feces.

CONTRAINDICATIONS
Active peptic ulcer or symptoms of GI inflammation or ulceration. Blood dyscrasias. Sensitivity to pyrazoles. Use to control hyperuricemia secondary to treatment of malignancies.

SPECIAL CONCERNS
Use with caution in pregnant women. Dosage has not been established in children. Use with extreme caution in clients with impaired renal function and in those with a history of peptic ulcers.

SIDE EFFECTS
Most Common
Upper GI disturbances, N&V, skin rash.
GI: N&V, abdominal discomfort, upper GI disturbances. May reactivate peptic ulcer. **Hematologic:** Leukopenia, *agranulocytosis*, anemia, thrombocytopenia, *aplastic anemia*. **Miscellaneous:** Skin rash (which usually disappears with usage), *bronchoconstriction in aspirin-induced asthma.* Acute attacks of gout may become more frequent during initial therapy. Give concomitantly with colchicine at this time.

OD OVERDOSE MANAGEMENT
Symptoms: N&V, diarrhea, epigastric pain, labored respiration, ataxia, *seizures*, coma. *Treatment:* Supportive measures.

DRUG INTERACTIONS
Acetaminophen / ↓ Effect of acetaminophen; ↑ risk of hepatotoxicity
Anticoagulants / ↑ Anticoagulant effect R/T ↓ plasma protein binding
Nateglinide / ↑ Nateglinide AUC R/T inhibition of metabolism by CYP2C9
Niacin / ↓ Uricosuric effect of sulfinpyrazone
Salicylates / Inhibit uricosuric effect of sulfinpyrazone
Theophylline / ↓ Theophylline effect R/T to ↑ plasma clearance
Tolbutamide / ↑ Risk of hypoglycemia
Verapamil / ↓ Verapamil effect R/T ↑ plasma clearance

HOW SUPPLIED
Capsules: 200 mg; *Tablets:* 100 mg.

DOSAGE
- **CAPSULES; TABLETS**
  Gout.

Adults, initial: 200–400 mg/day in two divided doses with meals or milk. Clients who are transferred from other uricosuric agents can receive full dose at once. **Maintenance:** 100–400 mg twice a day. Maintain full dosage without interruption even during acute attacks of gout.

Following MI.

Adults: 300 mg 4 times/day or 400 mg twice a day.

NURSING CONSIDERATIONS
ASSESSMENT
1. Note reasons for therapy, onset, characteristics of S&S. List other agents trialed, outcome.
2. List any ulcer disease or recent bleeding/surgery/stroke.

Bold Italic = life threatening side effect   ■ = black box warning   ♣ = Available in Canada

3. Assess joint(s) for pain, deformity, ROM, mobility, swelling, and inflammation.

4. Monitor I&O, CBC, renal function, and uric acid levels.

CLIENT/FAMILY TEACHING

1. If GI upset occurs, take with food, milk, or antacids. May still reactivate peptic ulcer.

2. Consume at least ten to twelve 8-oz glasses of fluid daily to prevent the formation of uric acid stones. Avoid cranberry juice or vitamin C preparations, as these acidify urine; acidification may cause formation of uric acid stones.

3. Sodium bicarbonate may be ordered to alkalinize the urine to prevent urates from crystallizing in acid urine and forming kidney stones.

4. Avoid alcohol and aspirin; may interfere with drug effectiveness.

5. During *acute* attacks of gout, concomitant administration of colchicine is indicated.

6. Report any unusual side effects or lack of desired response.

OUTCOMES/EVALUATE

- ↓ Pain/stiffness in joints; ↑ ROM
- ↓ Frequency/intensity of gout attacks
- ↓ Serum uric acid levels

Sulindac
(sul-**IN**-dak)

CLASSIFICATION(S):
Nonsteroidal anti-inflammatory drug

Rx: Clinoril.

❋Rx: Apo-Sulin, Novo–Sundac, Nu-Sulindac.

SEE ALSO *NONSTEROIDAL ANTI-INFLAMMATORY DRUGS.*

USES
Acute or chronic use for the relief of signs and symptoms of the following: (1) Rheumatoid arthritis. *NOTE:* Safety and efficacy have not been determined for those designated by the American Rheumatism Association classification as Functional Class IV. (2) Osteoarthritis.

(3) Anklyosing spondylitis. (4) Acute painful shoulder (acute subacromial bursitis/supraspinatus tendinitis). (5) Acute gouty arthritis.

ACTION/KINETICS

Pharmacokinetics
Bioavailability is 90%. Biotransformed in the liver to a sulfide, the active metabolite. **Peak plasma levels of sulfide:** After fasting, 2 hr; after food, 3–4 hr. **Onset, anti-inflammatory effect:** Within 1 week; **duration, anti-inflammatory effect:** 1–2 weeks. $t\frac{1}{2}$ of sulindac: 7.8 hr; of metabolite: 16.4 hr. Excreted in both urine (50%) and feces (25%). **Plasma protein binding:** More than 93%.

CONTRAINDICATIONS
Use with active GI lesions or a history of recurrent GI lesions.

SPECIAL CONCERNS
■ (1) Cardiovascular risk. NSAIDs may cause an increased risk of serious cardiovascular thrombotic events, MI, and stroke, which can be fatal. This risk may increase with duration of use. Clients with cardiovascular disease or risk factors for cardiovascular disease may be at greater risk. (2) Sulindac is contraindicated for treatment of perioperative pain in the setting of coronary artery bypass graft surgery. (3) GI risk. NSAIDs cause an increased risk of serious GI adverse events including bleeding, ulceration, and perforation of the stomach or intestines, which can be fatal. These events can occur at any time during use and without warning symptoms. Elderly clients are at greater risk for serious GI events.■ Safety and efficacy have not been established for children. Safe use during pregnancy has not been established. Use with caution during lactation.

SIDE EFFECTS

Most Common
Headache, dizziness, rash, abdominal pain, diarrhea, nausea, constipation.

See *Nonsteroidal Anti-Inflammatory Drugs* for a complete list of possible side effects. Also, hypersensitivity, pancreatitis, GI pain (common), maculopapular rash. Stupor, ***coma,*** hypotension, and diminished urine output.

ADDITIONAL DRUG INTERACTIONS
Sulindac ↑ Warfarin effect R/T ↓ plasma protein binding

HOW SUPPLIED
Tablets: 150 mg, 200 mg.

DOSAGE
• **TABLETS**
  Osteoarthritis, rheumatoid arthritis, ankylosing spondylitis.
Adults, initial: 150 mg twice a day. Individualize dosage based on response, but not to exceed 400 mg/day.
  Acute painful shoulder, acute gouty arthritis.
Adults: 200 mg twice a day. In acute painful shoulder, usual therapy is for 7–14 days; for acute gouty arthritis, therapy for 7 days is usually adequate.

NURSING CONSIDERATIONS
℮ Do not confuse Clinoril with Clozaril (an antipsychotic).

ADMINISTRATION/STORAGE
1. A response within 1 week can be expected in about one-half of clients with osteoarthritis, rheumatoid arthritis, or ankylosing spondylitis.
2. For acute conditions, reduce dosage when satisfactory response is attained.

ASSESSMENT
1. Note type, onset, characteristics of S&S.
2. List baseline ROM; describe location, inflammation, swelling; rate pain level, note functional class of arthritis.
3. Monitor CBC, uric acid, renal, LFTs; reduce dose with renal dysfunction.

CLIENT/FAMILY TEACHING
1. Take with food to decrease GI upset; consume plenty of water. A stomach protectant (i.e., misoprostol) may be prescribed with history of ulcer disease.
2. Drug may cause dizziness/drowsiness; assess response prior to any activity requiring mental alertness or driving.
3. Do not take aspirin because plasma levels of sulindac will be reduced. Avoid alcohol.
4. Record BP for provider review; BP may increase due to drug induced sodium retention.
5. Report changes in urine pattern, weight gain, swelling of extremities, fever or any incidence of unexplained bleeding (oozing of blood from the gums, nosebleeds, or excessive bruising), blurred vision, or ringing/noise in ears.
6. When used for arthritis, a favorable response usually occurs within 1 week; report lack of response.

OUTCOMES/EVALUATE
↓ Pain and inflammation with ↑ mobility

Sumatriptan succinate
(**soo**-mah-**TRIP**-tan)

CLASSIFICATION(S):
Antimigraine drug
PREGNANCY CATEGORY: C
Rx: Imitrex.

USES
(1) Acute migraine attacks with or without aura. Photophobia, phonophobia, N&V associated with migraine attacks are also relieved. Intended to relieve migraine, but not to prevent or reduce the number of attacks experienced. (2) Acute treatment of cluster headaches (injection only). *Investigational:* Relieve persistent headaches in head and neck cancer clients despite standard drug therapy.

ACTION/KINETICS
Action
Selective agonist for a vascular $5\text{-}HT_1$ receptor subtype (probably $5\text{-}HT_{1D}$) located on cranial arteries, on the basilar artery, and the vasculature of the dura mater. Activates the $5\text{-}HT_1$ receptor, causing vasoconstriction and therefore relief of migraine. Transient increases in BP may be observed. Weak activity against $5\text{-}HT_{1A}$, $5\text{-}HT_{5A}$, and $5\text{-}HT_7$ receptors. No significant activity at $5\text{-}HT_2$ or $5\text{-}HT_3$ receptor subtypes.

Pharmacokinetics
Bioavailablity ranges from 14–19% after PO, nasal, or rectal use and 96% after SC administration. **Time to onset after SC:** 10 min after a 6 mg SC dose; **time to onset after PO:** 30 min; **time to onset**

S

after intranasal: 15 min. **Time to peak effect after SC:** 12 min; **time to peak effect after PO:** 2.5 hr; **time to peak effect after intranasal:** 1–1.5 hr. **t½ distribution, after SC:** 15 min; **terminal t½:** 2.5 hr. Approximately 22% of a SC dose is excreted in the urine as unchanged drug and 38% as metabolites. Rapidly absorbed after PO administration, although bioavailability is low due to incomplete absorption and a first-pass effect (bioavailability may be significantly increased in those with impaired liver function). **PO, elimination t½:** About 2.5 hr. About 60% of a PO dose is excreted through the urine and 40% in the feces. **Plasma protein binding:** 14–21%.

CONTRAINDICATIONS

Hypersensitivity to sumatriptan. Tablets and spray for prophylactic therapy of migraine or for cluster headache. IV use due to the possibility of coronary vasospasm. SC use in clients with ischemic heart disease, history of MI, documented silent ischemia, Prinzmetal's angina, or uncontrolled hypertension. Concomitant use with ergotamine-containing products or MAO inhibitor therapy (or within 2 weeks of discontinuing an MAO inhibitor). Use in clients with hemiplegic or basilar migraine. Use in women who are pregnant, think they may be pregnant, or are trying to get pregnant.

SPECIAL CONCERNS

Use with caution during lactation, in clients with impaired hepatic or renal function, and in clients with heart conditions. Clients with risk factors for CAD (e.g., men over 40, smokers, postmenopausal women, hypertension, obesity, diabetes, hypercholesterolemia, family history of heart disease) should be screened before initiating treatment. Safety and efficacy have not been determined for use in children.

SIDE EFFECTS

Most Common

Paresthesia, warm/cold sensation, chest pain/tightness, vertigo, malaise/fatigue, neck/throat/jaw pain or pressure, N&V, headache, dizziness.

Side effects listed are for either SC or PO use of the drug.

CV: Coronary vasospasm in clients with a history of CAD. **Serious and/or life-threatening arrhythmias, including atrial fibrillation, ventricular fibrillation, ventricular tachycardia, MI, marked ischemic ST elevations**, chest and arm discomfort representing angina pectoris. Flushing, pallor, hyper/hypotension, brady/tachycardia, palpitations, pulsating sensations, ECG changes (including nonspecific ST- or T-wave changes, prolongation of PR or QTc intervals, sinus arrhythmia, nonsustained ventricular premature beats, isolated junctional ectopic beats, atrial ectopic beats, and delayed activation of the right ventricle), syncope, abnormal pulse, vasodilatation, atherosclerosis, cerebral ischemia, CV lesion, **heart block,** peripheral cyanosis, thrombosis, transient myocardial ischemia, vasodilation, Raynaud's syndrome. **Injection site:** Pain, redness. **Atypical sensations:** Sensation of warmth, cold, tingling, or paresthesia. Localized or generalized feeling of pressure, burning, numbness, and tightness. Feeling of heaviness, feeling strange, tight feeling in head. **CNS:** Fatigue, dizziness, drowsiness, vertigo, sedation, headache, anxiety, malaise, confusion, euphoria, agitation, relaxation, chills, tremor, shivering, prickling or stinging sensations, phonophobia, depression, euphoria, facial pain, heat sensitivity, incoordination, monoplegia, sleep disturbances, shivering. **EENT:** Throat discomfort, discomfort in nasal cavity or sinuses. Vision alterations, eye irritation, photophobia, lacrimation, otalgia, feeling of fullness in ear, disorders of sclera, mydriasis. **GI:** Abdominal discomfort, N&V, dysphagia, discomfort of mouth and tongue, gastroesophageal reflux, diarrhea, peptic ulcer, retching, flatulence, eructation, gallstones, taste disturbances, GI bleeding, hematemesis, melena. **Respiratory:** Dyspnea, diseases of the lower respiratory tract, hiccoughs, influenza, asthma. **Dermatologic:** Erythema, pruritus, skin rashes/eruptions/tenderness, dry/scaly skin, tightness/wrinkling of

S

skin. **GU:** Dysuria, dysmenorrhea, urinary frequency, renal calculus, breast tenderness, increased urination, intermenstrual bleeding, nipple discharge, abortion, hematuria. **Musculoskeletal:** Weakness, neck pain/stiffness, myalgia, muscle cramps, joint disturbances (pain, stiffness, swelling, ache), muscle stiffness, need to flex calf muscles, backache, muscle tiredness, swelling of the extremities, tetany. **Endocrine:** Elevated TSH levels, galactorrhea, hyper/hypoglycemia, hypothyroidism, weight gain/loss. **Miscellaneous:** Chest, jaw, or neck tightness. Sweating, thirst, polydipsia, chills, fever, dehydration.

LABORATORY TEST CONSIDERATIONS
Disturbance of LFTs.

OD OVERDOSE MANAGEMENT
Symptoms: Tremor, **convulsions,** inactivity erythema of extremities, reduced respiratory rate, cyanosis, ataxia, mydriasis, injection site reactions (desquamation, hair loss, scab formation), paralysis. *Treatment:* Continuous monitoring of client for at least 10 hr and especially when signs and symptoms persist.

DRUG INTERACTIONS
Ergot drugs / Prolonged vasospastic reactions
MAO inhibitors / ↑ t½ of sumatriptan
Selective serotonin reuptake inhibitors (SSRIs) / Rarely, weakness, hyperreflexia, and incoordination
Sibutramine / Possible serotonin syndrome, including CNS irritability, motor weakness, shivering, myoclonus, and altered consciousness

HOW SUPPLIED
Injection: 4 mg/0.5 mL (as part of STATdose System); 12 mg/mL; *Nasal Spray:* 5 mg, 20 mg; *Tablets:* 25 mg, 50 mg, 100 mg.

DOSAGE
• **SC**
  Migraine headaches.
Adults: 6 mg. A second injection may be given if symptoms of migraine come back but no more than two injections (6 mg each) should be taken in a 24-hr period and at least 1 hr should elapse between doses.
• **TABLETS**
  Migraine headaches.

Adults: A single dose of 25 mg, 50 mg, or 100 mg with fluids as soon as symptoms of migraine appear. Doses of 50 mg or 100 mg may provide a greater effect than 25 mg. A second dose may be taken if symptoms return but no sooner than 2 hr following the first dose. **Maximum recommended dose:** 100 mg, with no more than 200 mg taken in a 24-hr period.
• **NASAL SPRAY**
  Migraine headaches.
A single dose of 5, 10, or 20 mg given in one nostril. The 20 mg dose increases the risk of side effects, although it is more effective. The 10 mg dose may be given as a single 5 mg dose in each nostril. If the headache returns, repeat the dose once after 2 hr, not to exceed a total daily dose of 40 mg. The safety of treating an average of more than 4 headaches in a 30 day period has not been studied.

NURSING CONSIDERATIONS
ADMINISTRATION/STORAGE
1. No increased beneficial effect found with administration of a second 6-mg dose SC in clients not responding to the first injection.
2. If side effects are dose limiting, a dose lower than 6 mg SC may be given; in such cases, use the single-dose 6 mg vial. An autoinjection device can be used to deliver the drug.
3. Consideration should be given to administering the first dose of sumatriptan in the provider's office due to the possibility (although rare) of coronary events R/T undiagnosed CAD.
4. Is equally effective at whatever stage of the attack given; advisable to take as soon as possible after the onset of migraine attack.
5. Store away from heat (no higher than 30°C; 86°F) and light.

ASSESSMENT
1. Note headache characteristics of S&S; onset/duration, frequency. Rate pain levels, other agents used/outcome.
2. Assess neurologic exam/findings; review headache diary, triggers.
3. Monitor ECG, renal, LFTs, VS; expect transient increases in BP.

Bold Italic = life threatening side effect　　■ = black box warning　　♣ = Available in Canada

4. Parenteral form for SC use only- may see erythema at injection site. IV use may cause coronary vasospasm, MI.

5. Check for cardiac problems/disease, ischemic CV disease, history of stroke or TIAs, PVD, Raynaud syndrome, or if BP not controlled; precludes therapy.

CLIENT/FAMILY TEACHING

1. Review appropriate method for administration. Drug is used to terminate headaches not to prevent them. Take with plenty of water. With SC form, administer first dose in office to assess response and administration technique.

2. Printed instructions concerning how to load the autoinjector, administer the medication, and remove the syringe, are enclosed and provided by the manufacturer. The injection is given just below the skin as soon as migraine symptoms appear or any time during the attack. A second injection may be administered 1 hr later if migraine symptoms return; do *not* exceed two injections in 24 hr. Report lack of response or loss of effectiveness. Practice safe handling, storage, and disposal of syringes. Pain and tenderness may be evident at injection site for up to an hour after administration.

3. For tablets, take a single dose with fluids as soon as symptoms appear; a second dose may be taken if symptoms return, but no sooner than 2 hr after the first dose. If there is no response to the first tablet, do not take a second tablet without consulting provider.

4. With nasal spray, use one spray in one nostril at onset of symptoms; may repeat in 2 hr if headache returns but not if pain persists after initial dose.

5. Check expiration date before use and discard all outdated drugs.

6. Report if chest, jaw, throat, and neck pain occur after injection; this should be medically evaluated before using more Imitrex. Severe chest pain or tightness, wheezing, palpitations, facial swelling, or rashes/hives should be immediately reported.

7. Symptoms of flushing, tingling, heat and heaviness, as well as dizziness or drowsiness may occur and should be reported before taking more sumatriptan.

8. Practice barrier contraception and do not use Imitrex if pregnancy is suspected.

9. Avoid prolonged or excessive exposure to direct or artificial sunlight.

10. Keep a headache diary to share at each F/U visit and attempt to identify triggers.

11. Use caution, may cause coronary artery vasospasm. If angina occurs following dosing report so the presence of CAD or a predisposition to Prinzmetal variant angina may be assessed before additional therapy. Other S&S suggestive of decreased arterial flow, such as ischemic bowel syndrome or Raynaud syndrome following therapy should also be evaluated for atherosclerosis by provider.

OUTCOMES/EVALUATE

Termination of acute migraine attack with relief of symptoms

Sunitinib maleate
(soo-**NI**-tih-nib)

CLASSIFICATION(S):
Antineoplastic, protein-tyrosine kinase inhibitor
PREGNANCY CATEGORY: D
Rx: Sutent.

S

USES
(1) Treatment of GI stromal tumor after disease progression on or intolerance to imatinib. (2) Treatment of advanced renal cell carcinoma.

ACTION/KINETICS

Action
Inhibits multiple receptor tyrosine kinases, some of which are implicated in tumor growth, pathologic angiogenesis, and metastatic progression of cancer. The primary metabolite exhibits similar potency to the parent compound. Sunitinib inhibits tumor growth or tumor regression and/or inhibited metastases.

Pharmacokinetics

Maximum plasma levels: 6–12 hr. Food has no effect on the bioavailability; thus the drug may be taken with or without food. Metabolized primarily by CYP3A4 to a primary active metabolite, which is further metabolized by CYP3A4. **Steady state:** 10–14 days. Excreted primarily by the feces (61%) with a smaller amount in the urine (16%). $t^{1/2}$, **terminal:** 40–60 hr for sunitinib and 80–110 hr for the primary active metabolite.

CONTRAINDICATIONS

Hypersensitivity to sunitinib or any component of the product. Lactation.

SPECIAL CONCERNS

Safety and efficacy have not been determined in children.

SIDE EFFECTS

Most Common

Fatigue, skin discoloration, altered taste, anorexia, diarrhea, N&V, dyspepsia, mucositis, stomatitis, constipation, abdominal pain, asthenia, headache, rash, hypertension, arthralgia, dyspnea.

GI: Altered taste, abdominal pain, anorexia, diarrhea, dyspepsia, flatulence, N&V, mucositis, stomatitis, oral pain, constipation, abdominal pain, glossodynia, *GI perforation*. **CNS:** Fatigue, headache, dizziness. **CV:** Hypertension, peripheral edema, left ventricular dysfunction, bleeding events (including epistaxis; rectal, gingival, upper GI, genital, and wound bleeding), *tumor-related hemorrhage*. **Hematologic:** Neutropenia, thormbocytopenia, lymphopenia, anemia. **Dermatologic:** Skin discoloration, rash, hand-foot syndrome, hair color changes, alopecia, dry skin. **Musculoskeletal:** Arthralgia, back pain, myalgia, limb pain. **Respiratory:** Dyspnea, cough. **Body as a whole:** Asthenia, fever, bleeding (all sites), dehydration.

LABORATORY TEST CONSIDERATIONS

↑ ALT, AST, alkaline phosphatase, total bilirubin, indirect bilirubin, amylase, lipase, creatinine, uric acid, pancreatic enzymes. Hypokalemia, hyperkalemia, hypernatremia, hyponatremia, hypophosphatemia. ↑ LFTs.

DRUG INTERACTIONS

Atazanavir / Possible ↑ sunitinib levels R/T inhibition of metabolism by CYP3A4

Carbamazepine / Possible ↓ sunitinib levels R/T ↑ metabolism by CYP3A4

Clarithromycin / Possible ↑ sunitinib levels R/T inhibition of metabolism by CYP3A4

Dexamethasone / Possible ↓ sunitinib levels R/T ↑ metabolism by CYP3A4

Grapefruit / Possible ↑ sunitinib plasma levels

Indinavir / Possible ↑ sunitinib levels R/T inhibition of metabolism by CYP3A4

Itraconazole / Possible ↑ sunitinib levels R/T inhibition of metabolism by CYP3A4

Ketoconazole / Possible ↑ sunitinib levels R/T inhibition of metabolism by CYP3A4

Nefazodone / Possible ↑ sunitinib levels R/T inhibition of metabolism by CYP3A4

Nelfinavir / Possible ↑ sunitinib levels R/T inhibition of metabolism by CYP3A4

Phenobarbital / Possible ↓ sunitinib levels R/T ↑ metabolism by CYP3A4

Phenytoin / Possible ↓ sunitinib levels R/T ↑ metabolism by CYP3A4

Rifabutin, Rifampin, Rifapentine / Possible ↓ sunitinib levels R/T ↑ metabolism by CYP3A4

Ritonavir / Possible ↑ sunitinib levels R/T inhibition of metabolism by CYP3A4

Saquinavir / Possible ↑ sunitinib levels R/T inhibition of metabolism by CYP3A4

H *St. John's wort* / Possible ↓ sunitinib levels R/T ↑ metabolism by CYP3A4

Telithromycin / Possible ↑ sunitinib levels R/T inhibition of metabolism by CYP3A4

Voriconazole / Possible ↑ sunitinib levels R/T inhibition of metabolism by CYP3A4

HOW SUPPLIED

Capsules: 12.5 mg (as base), 25 mg (as base), 50 mg (as base).

DOSAGE

- **CAPSULES**

  GI stromal tumor, advanced renal cell carcinoma.

  One-50 mg capsule once daily on a schedule of 4 weeks on treatment followed by 2 weeks off. Dose increases or

---

Bold Italic = life threatening side effect   ■ = black box warning   ✦ = Available in Canada

reductions of 12.5 mg increments is recommended based on individual safety and tolerability.

NURSING CONSIDERATIONS

ADMINISTRATION/STORAGE

1. Consider a dosage increase to a maximum of 87.5 mg/day if the drug must be coadministered with a CYP3A4 inducer (see *Drug Interactions*). If dose increased, monitor carefully for toxicity.

2. Consider a dosage reduction of sunitinib to a minimum of 37.5 mg/day if the drug must be coadministered with a strong CYP3A4 inhibitor (see *Drug Interactions*). If the dose is increased, monitor carefully for toxicity.

3. Store from 15–30°C (59–86°F).

ASSESSMENT

1. Note reasons for therapy, characteristics of S&S, other agents trialed/failed. Identify disease progression, or intolerance to imatinib.

2. Assess for active bleeding, history of heart problems (eg, congestive heart failure, angina), blood vessel disease, bleeding problems, high blood pressure, adrenal gland problems, blood clot in the lung, or an underactive thyroid; had a heart attack or stroke, or are at risk for heart problems.

3. Identify if any severe infection, have recently been injured, or will be having surgery.

4. List drugs prescribed to ensure none interact. Avoid all OTC agents without approval.

5. Monitor baseline: VS, labs, lytes, CBC, renal and LFTs.

CLIENT/FAMILY TEACHING

1. May be taken with or without food. Eating grapefruit or drinking grapefruit juice may affect the amount of Sunitinib in your blood.

2. Sunitinib may cause dizziness. Avoid activities that require mental alertness until drug effects realized.

3. Avoid OTC drugs and alcohol; may lessen cognitive functioning.

4. Drug may reduce number of clot-forming cells (platelets) in your blood. To prevent bleeding, avoid situations in which bruising or injury may occur. Report any unusual bleeding, bruising, blood in stools, or dark, tarry stools.

5. Avoid contact with people with colds or other infections. Report any signs of infection, including fever, sore throat, rash, or chills.

6. Skin or hair discoloration may occur while using Sunitinib.

7. Practice reliable contraception; may cause fetal harm.

8. Keep all F/U visits to eval. response to therapy, labs, and heart function tests.

9. Report adverse side effects, for F/U visits and for lack of response.

OUTCOMES/EVALUATE

Inhibition of malignant cell proliferation

T

Tacrolimus ■ IV
(tah-**KROH**-lih-mus)

CLASSIFICATION(S):
Immunosuppressant
PREGNANCY CATEGORY: C
Rx: Prograf, Protopic.

USES

Systemic: Prophylaxis of organ rejection in allogeneic liver, heart, and kidney transplants; usually used with corticosteroids. In heart transplants, use in conjunction with azathioprine or mycophenolate mofetil. *Investigational:* Prevention and treatment of acute graft vs. host disease following hematopoietic stem cell transplantation. Also, rheumatoid arthritis, Crohn's disease.

Topical: Second-line therapy for short-term and intermittent long-term therapy to treat moderate to severe atopic dermatitis in nonimmunocompromised adults and children unable to take traditional agents or who do not respond to conventional therapy. *Investigational:* Vitiligo in children; facial, flexural, and intertriginous psoriasis.

ACTION/KINETICS

Action

Mechanism of action for either systemic or topical use is not known but it inhibits T-lymphocyte activation by first binding to FKBP-12 (an intracellular protein). A complex of tacrolimus-FKBP-12, calcium, calmodulin, and calcineurin is formed leading to inhibition of phosphatase activity of calcineurin. This effect prevents dephosphorylation and translocation of nuclear factor of activated T-cells (NF-AT) which is a nuclear component thought to initiate gene transcription to form lymphokines. Tacrolimus also inhibits transcription for genes that encode factors involved in the early states of T-cell activation. The net result is inhibition of T-lymphocyte activation (i.e., immunosuppression).

Pharmacokinetics

Absorption from the GI tract is variable; absorption is greatest under fasting conditions. Minimally absorbed after topical use. Absolute bioavailability ranges from 17–23%. **$t\frac{1}{2}$, terminal elimination:** 11.7 hr in liver transplant clients, 18.8 hr in kidney transplant clients, 23.6 hr in heart transplant clients, and 34 hr in healthy volunteers. The $t\frac{1}{2}$ is increased significantly in those with hepatic impairment. Food decreases both the absorption and bioavailability of tacrolimus. Extensively metabolized by the liver by CYP3A enzymes and excreted mainly through the feces (about 93%). **Plasma protein binding:** Approximately 99% bound to plasma proteins.

CONTRAINDICATIONS

Hypersensitivity to tacrolimus or HCO-60 polyoxyl 60 hydrogenated castor oil (vehicle used for the injection). Lactation. Concomitant use with cyclosporine. Use of the ointment in Netherton syndrome or other skin diseases where there is an increased potential for systemic absorption of tacrolimus. Use in children younger than 2 years of age. Use in children or adults with weakened or compromised immune systems.

SPECIAL CONCERNS

■ (1) Increased susceptibility to infection and possible development of lymphoma may result from immunosuppression. Only health care providers experienced in immunosuppressive therapy and management of organ transplant clients should prescribe tacrolimus. Manage those receiving the drug in facilities equipped and staffed with adequate lab and supportive medical resources. The physician responsible for maintenance therapy should have complete information necessary for follow-up of the client. (2) Long-term safety of topical calcineurin inhibitors has not been determined. Although a causal relationship has not been established, rare cases of malignancy (i.e., skin cancer and lymphoma) have been reported in those treated with topical calcineurin inhibitors, including tacrolimus. Therefore, (a) avoid continuous long-term use of topical calcineurin inhibitors, including tacrolimus ointment, in any age group, and limit application to areas of involvement with atopic dermatitis; (b) tacrolimus ointment is not indicated for use in children younger than 2 years of age. Only tacrolimus 0.03% ointment is indicated for use in children 2–15 years of age.■ Safety and efficacy of the ointment to treat infected atopic dermatitis have not been studied. With ointment, clients are predisposed to superficial skin infections, including eczema herpeticum, chicken pox or shingles, and herpes simplex virus infection. There is a potential cancer risk with use of tacrolimus; thus, use only as indicated in clients who have failed treatment with other therapies. Should only be used for short periods of time, not continuously as the long-term safety is not known. Safety and efficacy have not been established for concomitant use with sirolimus.

SIDE EFFECTS

Most Common

After systemic use, liver transplants: Tremor, headache, diarrhea, hypertension, nausea, abnormal renal function, hyperglycemia.

After systemic use, kidney transplants: Infection, tremor, hypertension, abnormal renal function, constipation, diarrhea, headache, abdominal pain, insomnia.

After systemic use, heart transplants: Abnormal renal function, hypertension, diabetes mellitus, CMV infection, tremor, hyperglycemia, leukopenia, infection, hyperlipemia.

After topical use: Skin burning/erythema, flu-like symptoms, allergic reaction, headache, acne, folliculitis, rash, dysmenorrhea, peripheral edema, asthma, sinusitis, fever.

After Systemic Use. Listed are the more common and/or more serious side effects. **CNS:** Headache, tremor, insomnia, paresthesia, *seizures, coma,* delirium, abnormal dreams, anxiety, agitation, confusion, depression, dizziness, emotional lability, hallucinations, hypertonia, incoordination, myoclonus, nervousness, psychosis, somnolence, abnormal thinking, cerebral infection, hemiparesis, leukoencephalopathy, mental disorder, mutism, quadriplegia, speech disorder, syncope. **Neurotoxicity:** Changes in motor/sensory function, and mental status; tremor, headache. **GI:** Diarrhea, nausea, abdominal pain, constipation, anorexia, vomiting, dyspepsia, dysphasia, flatulence, *GI hemorrhage/perforation,* ileus, increased appetite, oral moniliasis, colitis, enterocolitis, gastroenteritis, GERD, impaired gastric emptying, mouth/stomach ulceration. **Hepatic:** Hepatitis, cholangitis, cholestatic jaundice, jaundice, liver damage, bile duct stenosis, abnormal LFTs, hepatic cytolysis, hepatotoxicity, fatty liver, venoocclusive liver disease, *hemorrhagic pancreatitis, necrotizing pancreatitis, hepatic necrosis.* **CV:** Chest pain, abnormal ECG, *hemorrhage, QT-interval prolongation, torsades de pointes,* hyper-/hypotension, tachycardia, myocardial hypertrophy, pericardial effusion, atrial fibrillation/flutter, cardiac arrhythmia, *cardiac arrest,* ECG T-wave abnormality, MI, myocardial ischemia, pericardial effusion, deep limb venous thrombosis, ventricular extrasystoles, *ventricular fibrillation.* **Hematologic:** Anemia, thrombocytopenia, leukocytosis, coagulation disorder, ecchymosis, hypochromic anemia, leukopenia, decreased prothrombin, disseminated intravascular coagulation, neutropenia, pancytopenia, thrombocytopenic purpura, thrombotic thrombocytopenic purpura. **GU:** Abnormal kidney function, nephrotoxicity, UTI, oliguria, hematuria, hemorrhagic cystitis, hemolytic uremic syndrome, micturition disorder, *kidney failure (acute).* **Metabolic:** Hyper-/hypokalemia, hyperglycemia, hypomagnesemia, acidosis, alkalosis, hyperlipemia, hyperuricemia, hypocalcemia, hyper-/hypoproteinemia, hypophosphatemia, hyponatremia, bilirubinemia, diabetes mellitus (insulin-dependent), glycosuria. **Respiratory:** Pleural effusion, atelectasis, dyspnea, asthma, bronchitis, increased cough, pulmonary edema, pharyngitis, pneumonia, lung/respiratory disorder, rhinitis, sinusitis, alteration in voice, acute respiratory distress syndrome, lung infiltration, *respiratory distress/failure.* **Musculoskeletal:** Arthralgia, leg cramps, myalgia, myasthenia, osteoporosis, generalized spasm, carpal tunnel syndrome. **Dermatologic:** Pruritus, rash, alopecia, herpes simplex, sweating, skin disorder, hot flushes, *Stevens-Johnson syndrome, toxic epidermal necrolysis.* **Ophthalmic:** Abnormal vision, amblyopia, blindness, cortical blindness. **Otic:** Hearing loss including deafness, tinnitus. **Body as a whole:** Hypersensitivity reactions (including anaphylaxis), increased incidence of malignancies, lymphoma, pain, fever, asthenia, ascites, abscess, chills, edema, photosensitivity, abnormal healing, decreased weight, photophobia, feeling hot and cold, feeling jittery. **Miscellaneous:** Peripheral edema, back/abdominal pain, enlarged abdomen, hernia, peritonitis, lymphoproliferative disorder related to Epstein-Barr virus infection,

 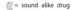

CMV infection, primary graft dysfunction, **multiorgan failure**.

After Topical Use: Dermatologic: Phototoxicity, herpes simplex, skin erythema/burning/infection, pruritus, eczema herpeticum, pustular/ maculopapular/vesiculobullous rash, folliculitis, urticaria, fungal dermatitis, acne, alopecia, cellulitis, sunburn, skin disorder/tingling, dry skin, benign skin neoplasm, contact dermatitis, eczema, exfoliative dermatitis, varicella zoster/herpes zoster. **GI:** N&V, diarrhea, abdominal pain, gastroenteritis, dyspepsia. **Respiratory:** Increased cough, asthma, pharyngitis, rhinitis, sinusitis, bronchitis, pneumonia. **CNS:** Headache, insomnia, asthenia, depression, paresthesia. **GU:** Dysmenorrhea, UTI, acute renal failure (rare). **Musculoskeletal:** Arthralgia, back pain, myalgia. **Miscellaneous:** Flu-like symptoms, allergic reaction, headache, fever, infection, accidental injury, otitis media, ear pain, alcohol intolerance, conjunctivitis, pain, herpes simplex, lymphadenopathy, facial/peripheral edema, hyperesthesia, asthenia, periodontal abscess, tooth disorder, cyst.

LABORATORY TEST CONSIDERATIONS
↑ Alkaline phosphatase, AST, ALT, BUN, creatinine, GGT.

DRUG INTERACTIONS
Al-Mg hydroxide combinations / ↑ Tacrolimus levels
Aminoglycosides / Additive or synergistic impairment of renal function
Amphotericin B / Additive or synergistic impairment of renal function
Antifungal drugs (clotrimazole, fluconazole, itraconazole, voriconazole) / ↑ Tacrolimus levels → ↑ risk of toxicity
Bromocriptine / ↑ Tacrolimus levels → ↑ risk of toxicity
Calcium channel blockers (e.g., diltiazem, nicardipine, nifedipine, verapamil) / ↑ Tacrolimus levels → ↑ risk of toxicity
Carbamazepine / ↓ Tacrolimus levels → ↑ risk of organ transplant rejection
Caspofungin / ↓ Tacrolimus levels → ↑ risk of organ transplant rejection
Chloramphenicol / ↑ Tacrolimus levels → ↑ risk of toxicity
Cimetidine / ↑ Tacrolimus levels → ↑ risk of toxicity

Cisapride / ↑ Tacrolimus levels → ↑ risk of toxicity
Cisplatin / Additive or synergistic impairment of renal function
Clarithromycin / ↑ Tacrolimus levels → ↑ risk of toxicity
Corticosteroids / Higher tacrolimus doses required
Cyclosporine / Additive or synergistic nephrotoxicity; also, ↑ tacrolimus blood levels; give the first tacrolimus dose no sooner than 24 hr after the last cyclosporine dose
Danazol / ↑ Tacrolimus levels → ↑ risk of toxicity
Diltiazem / ↑ Tacrolimus levels
Diuretics, potassium-sparing / Tacrolimus causes hyperkalemia; avoid using potassium-sparing diuretics
 Echinacea / Do not give with tacrolimus
Erythromycin / ↑ Tacrolimus levels → ↑ risk of toxicity
Ethinyl estradiol / ↑ Tacrolimus levels → ↑ risk of toxicity
Fosphenytoin / ↓ Tacrolimus levels → ↑ risk of organ transplant rejection
Grapefruit juice / ↑ Tacrolimus trough levels in liver transplant clients; do not use together
Methylprednisolone / ↑ Tacrolimus levels → ↑ risk of toxicity
Metoclopramide / ↑ Tacrolimus levels → ↑ risk of toxicity
Metronidazole / ↑ Tacrolimus levels → ↑ risk of toxicity
Mycophenolate mofetil / ↑ Mycophenolate trough levels → ↑ risk of side effects
Nefazodone / ↑ Tacrolimus levels → ↑ risk of toxicity
Nelfinavir / ↑ Tacrolimus levels probably due to ↓ liver metabolism; monitor in liver-transplant clients
Omeprazole / ↑ Tacrolimus levels → ↑ risk of toxicity
Phenobarbital / ↓ Tacrolimus levels → ↑ risk of organ transplant rejection
Phenytoin / ↓ Tacrolimus levels → ↑ risk of organ transplant rejection; also, ↑ phenytoin levels
Prednisone/Prednisolone / ↓ Tacrolimus levels → ↑ risk of organ transplant rejection

---

Bold Italic = life threatening side effect   ■ = black box warning   ✦ = Available in Canada

Protease inhibitors / ↑ Tacrolimus levels → ↑ risk of toxicity

Rifamycins / ↓ Tacrolimus levels → ↑ risk of organic transplant rejection

H *St. John's wort* / ↓ Tacrolimus levels R/T induction of CYP3A4

Sildenafil / ↑ Sildenafil AUC, peak levels, and half-life

Sirolimus / ↓ Tacrolimus levels; do not use together or ↑ tacrolimus dose

Troleandomycin / ↑ Tacrolimus levels → ↑ risk of toxicity

Vaccines / ↓ Effectiveness of vaccines; avoid use of live vaccines

Ziprasidone / ↑ Risk of life-threatening cardiac arrhythmias, including torsades de pointes

Voriconazole / ↑ Tacrolimus levels

HOW SUPPLIED

Capsules: 0.5 mg, 1 mg, 5 mg; *Injection:* 5 mg/mL; *Ointment:* 0.03%, 0.1%.

DOSAGE

• CAPSULES

Heart transplantation.

Initial: 0.075 mg/kg/day given q 12 hr in 2 divided doses. **Typical whole blood trough levels, month 1–3:** 10–20 ng/mL; **month 4 and beyond:** 5–15 ng/mL. If possible initiate therapy with tacrolimus capsules. If IV therapy is necessary, convert from IV to PO tacrolimus as soon as PO therapy can be tolerated (usually 2–3 days). Give the initial dose no sooner than 6 hr after transplantation. If using an IV infusion, the first PO dose should be given 8–12 hr after discontinuing the IV infusion. Base dosing on clinical assessment of rejection and tolerance. Lower doses may be sufficient as maintenance therapy. Adjunct therapy with corticosteroids is recommended early after transplantation.

Kidney transplantation.

Initial: 0.2 mg/kg/day given q 12 hr in 2 divided doses. **Whole blood trough levels, month 1–3:** 7–20 ng/mL; **month 4–12:** 5–15 ng/mL. The initial dose may be given within 24 hr of transplantation but should be delayed until renal function has recovered. Black clients may require higher doses to achieve comparable blood levels.

Liver transplantation.

Initial, adults: 0.1–0.15 mg/kg/day given in 2 divided doses q 12 hr. **Initial, children:** 0.15–0.2 mg/kg/day given in 2 divided doses q 12 hr. **Whole blood trough levels, adults/children, month 1–12:** 5–20 ng/mL. If possible initiate therapy with tacrolimus capsules. If IV therapy is necessary, convert from IV to PO tacrolimus as soon as PO therapy can be tolerated (usually 2–3 days). Give the initial dose no sooner than 6 hr after transplantation. If using an IV infusion, the first PO dose should be given 8–12 hr after discontinuing the IV infusion.

• IV INFUSION

Heart, liver, kidney transplantation.

In those unable to take capsules, therapy may be initiated with the injection. Give the initial dose no sooner than 6 hr after transplantation. **Initial, adults, heart transplants:** 0.01 mg/kg/day; **initial, adults, kidney/liver transplants:** 0.03–0.05 mg/kg/day. For children, start at 0.03–0.05 mg/kg/day; dosage adjustments may be needed. Concomitant corticosteroid therapy is recommended early posttransplantation.

• OINTMENT (0.03%, 0.1%)

Atopic dermatitis.

Adults: Apply a thin layer of either the 0.03% or 0.1% ointment to the affected skin areas twice a day. **Children, 2–15 years of age:** Apply a thin layer of only the 0.03% ointment to the affected skin areas twice a day. Stop when signs and symptoms of atopic dermatitis resolve. If signs and symptoms (e.g., itch, rash, redness) do not improve within 6 weeks, reassess to confirm the diagnosis of atopic dermatitis.

NURSING CONSIDERATIONS

ADMINISTRATION/STORAGE

1. The safety of using tacrolimus ointment with occlusive dressings has not been evaluated; thus, do not use with occlusive dressings.

2. Store ointment from 15–30°C (59–86°F).

IV 3. IV therapy may be started if unable to take capsules. Continue IV therapy only until client can be switched to PO therapy (usually within 2–3 days).

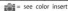

Give the first PO dose 8–12 hr after stopping the IV infusion.

4. Use the minimum amount of tacrolimus to control client symptoms; the risk of cancer increases with increased exposure to the drug.

5. For both IV and PO administration, give doses for adult clients at the lower end of the dosage range. Initiate doses for pediatric clients at the higher end of the dosage range (i.e., 0.03–0.05 mg/kg/day for IV use and 0.15–0.2 mg/kg/day for PO use).

6. Give the initial dose no sooner than 6 hr after implantation.

7. Children receiving liver transplants generally require higher doses of tacrolimus to maintain blood trough levels similar to those of adults.

8. Prior to use dilute with either 0.9% NaCl or D5W to a concentration between 0.004 and 0.02 mg/mL. Where more dilute solutions are needed (e.g., children), polyvinyl chloride-free tubing should be used to minimize significant drug adsorption onto the tubing.

9. Do not mix with solutions of pH 9 or greater (e.g., acyclovir, ganciclovir).

10. With renal or hepatic impairment administer at the lowest level of the dosage range.

11. Do not use tacrolimus and cyclosporine simultaneously unless specifically ordered; discontinue either agent at least 24 hr before initiating the other.

12. Store the diluted solution for infusion in glass or polyethylene containers and discard after 24 hr. Do not use PVC containers for storage due to decreased stability and the possibility of extraction of phthalates.

ASSESSMENT

1. Note reasons for use and form prescribed; assess clinical condition.

2. Identify time of transplantation; monitor in facilities equipped and staffed with adequate lab and supportive medical resources.

3. Injection contains castor oil derivatives; note any sensitivity.

4. Monitor serum lytes, CBC, uric acid, blood sugar, renal and LFTs. Monitor VS, for tremors or changes in mental and CV status and I&O. Anticipate higher dosages in children to maintain trough levels and reduced dosage with impaired renal function.

5. During IV therapy, observe continuously for the first 30 min and at frequent intervals until infusion completed; interrupt infusion if S&S of anaphylaxis occur.

6. Monitor tacrolimus levels; helpful in clinical evaluation of rejection and toxicity.

CLIENT/FAMILY TEACHING

1. Review risk of therapy associated with neoplasia (lymphomas and other malignancies).

2. Must follow written guidelines for medication therapy explicitly. Call with questions or if problems arise. Drug must be taken throughout one's lifetime to prevent transplant rejection.

3. Because this drug is so important in preventing rejection, a written list of all possible side effects and how to identify which side effects need to be reported will be provided.

4. Perform daily weights and I&O. Take BP and keep a log of these values for provider review. Report any persistent diarrhea, N&V and other adverse effects.

5. Report as scheduled to specialist/transplant center for assessment and labs to evaluate drug effectiveness, since dosage is based on clinical assessments of rejection and tolerability.

6. Avoid crowds, infections, and those with infections. Report any S&S of infection or if injury occurs.

7. With skin disorders, rub in the ointment gently and completely and report adverse effects. Do not use with occlusive dressings.

8. Limit exposure to sunlight and UV light due to the potential to increase risk of malignant skin changes.

9. Keep all F/U appointments to evaluate dose, labs, and response to therapy.

OUTCOMES/EVALUATE

- Prophylaxis of organ rejection
- Immune suppression
- Median trough blood concentrations of 9.8–19.4 ng/mL
- Improvement in atopic dermatitis presentation (topically)

Tadalafil

(tah-**DA**-la-fil)

CLASSIFICATION(S):
Drug for erectile dysfunction
PREGNANCY CATEGORY: B
Rx: Cialis.

USES

Treat erectile dysfunction.

ACTION/KINETICS

Action

During sexual stimulation, nitric oxide is released from nerve endings and endothelial cells in the corpus cavernosum of the penis. Nitric oxide activates the enzyme guanylate cylase causing an increased synthesis of cyclic guanosine monophosphate (cGMP) in the smooth muscle cells of the corpus cavernosum. The cGMP in turn causes smooth muscle relaxation, allowing increased blood flow to the penis, resulting in erection. Tissue levels of cGMP are regulated by both the rate of synthesis and degradation via phosphodiesterases (PDEs). The most abundant PDE in the human corpus cavernosum is the cGMP-specific phosphodiesterase type 5 (PDE5). Thus, tadalafil, which is a selective inhibitor of PDE5, enhances erectile function by increasing the amount of cGMP.

Pharmacokinetics

Onset: About 30 min. **Maximum plasma levels:** 0.5–6 hr. **Duration:** 36 hr. Rate and extent of absorption are not affected by food. Predominantly metabolized by CYP3A4. **$t\frac{1}{2}$, terminal:** 17.5 hr. Excreted mainly as metabolites in the feces (61%) and urine (36%). **Plasma protein binding:** About 94%.

CONTRAINDICATIONS

Use in those with severe hepatic impairment. Use, either regularly or intermittently, in those taking any form of nitrates (due to potential for severe hypotension) or in those taking alpha-adrenergic blockers (except 0.4 mg daily of tamsulosin). Use in men for whom sexual activity is inadvisable due to their underlying CV status. Use in those with MI within the last 90 days, unstable angina or angina occurring during sexual intercourse, those with NYHA Class 2 or greater heart failure in the last 6 months, uncontrolled arrhythmias, hypotension, uncontrolled hypertension, those with a stroke within the last 6 months, and hereditary degenerative retinal disorders (including retinitis pigmentosa). Use in women or children. Lactation.

SPECIAL CONCERNS

Older clients or those with significant left ventricular outflow obstruction or severely impaired autonomic control of BP may be more sensitive to the drug. Use with caution in conditions that might predispose clients to priapism (e.g., such as sickle cell anemia, multiple myeloma, or leukemia) or anatomical deformation of the penis (e.g., angulation, cavernosal fibrosis, Peyronie's disease). Use in clients with bleeding disorders or significant active peptic ulcerations should be based on a careful risk to benefit assessment and caution. Safety and efficacy have not been determined in clients less than 18 years of age.

SIDE EFFECTS

Most Common
Headache, dyspepsia, nasal congestion, back pain, flushing, limb pain, myalgia, hypotension.

CV: Chest pain, hypotension, hypertension, *angina pectoris*, *MI*, palpitations, syncope, tachycardia. **GI:** Dyspepsia, diarrhea, dry mouth, dysphagia, esophagitis, gastroesophageal reflux, gastritis, loose stools, N&V, upper abdominal pain. **CNS:** Headache, dizziness, hypesthesia, insomnia, paresthesia, somnolence, vertigo. **Musculoskeletal:** Back pain, myalgia, arthralgia, neck pain, pain in limb. **Respiratory:** Nasal congestion, dyspnea, epistaxis, pharyngitis. **Dermatologic:** Flushing, pruritus, rash, sweating. **Ophthalmic:** Impaired blue/green color discrimination, blurred vision, conjunctivitis (including conjunctival hyperemia), eye pain, increased lacrimation, swelling of eyelids, sudden loss of vision, vision loss related to nonarteritic anterior ischemic optic neuropathy (especially in those with

T

---

underlying anatomic or vascular risk factors). **GU:** Prolonged erections (more than 4 hr), priapism (greater than 6 hr), spontaneous penile erection. **Body as a whole:** Asthenia, facial edema, fatigue, pain.

LABORATORY TEST CONSIDERATIONS
↑ GGTP. Abnormal LFTs.

DRUG INTERACTIONS
Alcohol / Possible ↓ BP with postural dizziness and orthostatic hypotension

Alpha-adrenergic blockers / Possible significant hypotension; do not use together

Al-Mg antacids / ↓ Tadalafil absorption

Amlodipine / ↑ Hypotensive effect

Angiotensin II receptor blockers / ↑ Hypotensive effect

Antacids, Mg- or calcium-containing / Possible ↓ rate of tadalafil absorption

Doxazosin / Significant ↓ BP

Enalapril / Mean ↓ of supine BP

Erythromycin / Possible ↑ tadalafil levels R/T ↓ hepatic metabolism

Grapefruit juice / Possible ↑ tadalafil levels R/T ↓ hepatic metabolism

Indinavir / ↑ Tadalafil levels R/T ↓ hepatic metabolism; possible severe (or even fatal) hypotension

Itraconazole / Possible ↑ tadalafil levels R/T ↓ hepatic metabolism

Ketoconazole / ↑ Tadalafil plasma levels R/T ↓ hepatic metabolism

Nitrates / Possible severe hypotension; **do not use together**

Rifampin / ↓ Tadalafil levels R/T ↑ hepatic metabolism

Ritonavir / ↑ Tadalafil levels R/T ↓ hepatic metabolism; possible severe (or even fatal) hypotension

Saquinavir / ↑ Tadalafil levels R/T ↓ hepatic metabolism; possible severe (or even fatal) hypotension

HOW SUPPLIED
Tablets: 5 mg, 10 mg, 20 mg.

DOSAGE
- **TABLETS**
  Erectile dysfunction.
Adults, initial: 10 mg taken prior to anticipated sexual activity. Dose may be increased to 20 mg or decreased to 5 mg based on individual efficacy and tolerability. The maximum recommended dosing frequency is once per day for most clients.

NURSING CONSIDERATIONS
ADMINISTRATION/STORAGE
1. Tadalafil improves erectile function up to 36 hr following dosing.
2. May be taken without regard to food.
3. Although clients 65 years and older may be more sensitive to the drug, no dosage adjustment is necessary.
4. The maximum daily dose should not exceed 10 mg in clients with mild or moderate hepatic impairment.
5. The maximum daily dose should not exceed 5 mg in clients with severe renal insufficiency or end-stage renal disease. A starting dose of 5 mg not more than once daily is recommended for those with moderate renal insufficiency (C_{CR} 31–50 mL/min); the maximum recommended dose is 10 mg not more than once every 48 hr. For severe renal insufficiency (C_{CR} <30 mL/min), maximum recommended dose is 5 mg.
6. At least 48 hr should elapse between the last dose of tadalafil and beginning nitrate therapy; administer nitrates under close medical observation with appropriate hemodynamic monitoring.
7. The dose should be limited to 10 mg no more than once every 72 hr in those taking potent inhibitors of CYP3A4 (i.e., itraconazole, ketoconazole, ritonavir).
8. Store from 15–30°C (59–86°F) and away from children.

ASSESSMENT
1. Note onset, cause of erectile dysfunction, i.e., organic, psychogenic, or combined, any contributing factors.
2. Assess cardiovascular status; obtain ECG. List drugs prescribed; some may potentiate drug effects.
3. Note conditions that may predispose client to priapism, i.e., multiple myelomas, sickle cell anemia, leukemia.
4. Assess for anatomical deformation of penis (Peyronie's disease, angulation, or cavernosal fibrosis).
5. Monitor testosterone initially, renal, LFT; reduce dose with dysfunction.

Bold Italic = life threatening side effect   ■ = black box warning   ✚ = Available in Canada

CLIENT/FAMILY TEACHING

1. Take as directed approximately 1 hr before anticipated act. Plan some form of sexual stimulation after ingestion to ensure desired erection obtained.

2. May experience headache, flushing, stuffy nose, GI upset, back/limb pain or muscle pains, dizziness (from drop in BP) drowsiness, or abnormal vision; report any unusual, persistent or bothersome effects. If chest pain experienced seek medical care.

3. Report all medications currently prescribed to ensure none alter effects. Avoid OTC agents, alcohol in large amounts and stop smoking; may inhibit drug effect. Allow at least 4 hr between alpha blocker use.

4. Practice safe sex; drug does not prevent disease transmission.

5. Effects may be evident the day after therapy; assess before taking additional drug dose. Do not use more than once a day. Erections lasting more than 4 hr or painful erections lasting more than 6 hr require immediate medial care; penile damage may result.

6. Do not share medications or prescriptions due to potential for adverse interactions and effects. *Never* use this drug if currently taking nitrates in any form; may cause significant drop in BP and increase the risk of heart attack or stroke.

7. Keep F/U appointment; report lack of response, sudden change in vision or adverse effects.

OUTCOMES/EVALUATE

Desired erection

Tamoxifen citrate ■
(tah-**MOX**-ih-fen)

CLASSIFICATION(S):

Antiestrogen
PREGNANCY CATEGORY: D
Rx: Soltamox.
✚**Rx:** Apo-Tamox, Gen-Tamoxifen, Nolvadex-D, Novo–Tamoxifen, PMS-Tamoxifen, Tamofen.

SEE ALSO *ANTINEOPLASTIC AGENTS.*

USES

(1) Adjuvant treatment of axillary node-negative or node-positive breast cancer in women following total or segmental mastectomy, axillary dissection, and breast irradiation. *NOTE:* The estrogen receptor and progesterone receptor values may help to predict whether adjuvant tamoxifen therapy is likely to be beneficial. (2) Metastatic breast cancer in premenopausal women as an alternative to oophorectomy or ovarian irradiation (especially in women with estrogen-positive tumors). (3) Reduce risk of invasive breast cancer following breast surgery and radiation in women with ductal carcinoma in situ. (4) Advanced metastatic breast cancer in men. (5) To reduce the incidence of breast cancer in high-risk women, taking into account age, previous breast biopsies, age at first live birth, number of first-degree relatives with breast cancer, age at first menstrual period, and a history of lobular carcinoma in situ. *NOTE:* See the package insert for examples of combinations of factors in various age groups predicting a 5-year risk greater than or equal to 1.67%. *Investigational:* Mastalgia, sympatomatic gynecomastia (to treat pain and size), malignant carcinoid tumor and carcinoid syndrome. Migraine associated with menstruation, metastatic malignant melanoma, oligozoospermia, McCune-Albright syndrome in pediatric females (in combination with other drugs), metastatic melanoma, desmoid tumors. Stimulate ovulation in certain anovulatory women desiring pregnancy, especially those with amenorrhea or oligomenorrhea who previously took oral contraceptives.

ACTION/KINETICS

Action

Antiestrogen believed to compete with estrogen for estrogen-binding sites in target tissue (breast); also blocks uptake of estradiol.

Pharmacokinetics

The rate and extent of absorption of the oral solution is bioequivalent to that of the tablets under fasting conditions. **Steady-state plasma levels (after 10 mg twice a day for 3 months):** 120 ng/mL for tamoxifen and 336 ng/mL for N-desmethyltamoxifen (active metabolite). **Steady-state levels, tamoxifen:** About 4 weeks; **for N-desmethyltamoxifen:** About 8 weeks. **t½ for metabolite:** about 14 days. Tamoxifen is metabolized by CYP3A4, CYP2C9, and CYP2D6; tamoxifen and metabolites are excreted mainly through the feces. Objective response may be delayed 4–10 weeks with bone metastases.

CONTRAINDICATIONS

Lactation. Concomitant coumarin anticoagulant therapy or women with a history of deep vein thrombosis or pulmonary embolus.

SPECIAL CONCERNS

■ (1) Serious and life-threatening events associated with tamoxifen in the risk-reduction setting (women at high risk for cancer and women with ductal carcinoma in situ) include uterine malignancies, stroke, and pulmonary embolism. Incidence rates for these events were estimated from the National Surgical Adjuvant Breast and Bowel Project P-1 trial. Uterine malignancies consist of both endometrial adenocarcinoma (incidence rate per 1,000 women years of 2.2 for tamoxifen verses 0.71 for placebo) and uterine sarcoma (incidence rate per 1,000 women years of 0.17 for tamoxifen versus 0.4 for placebo). (2) For stroke, the incidence rate per 1,000 women years was 1.43 for tamoxifen versus 1 for placebo. For pulmonary embolism, the incidence rate per 1,000 women years was 0.75 for tamoxifen versus 0.25 for placebo. Some of the strokes, pulmonary embolisms, and uterine malignancies were fatal. (3) Discuss the potential benefits versus the potential risks of these serious events with women at high risk of breast cancer and with women with ductal carcinoma in situ considering tamoxifen to reduce their risks of developing breast cancer. (4) The benefits of tamoxifen outweigh its risks in women already diagnosed with breast cancer.■ Use with caution in clients with leukopenia or thrombocytopenia. Women should not become pregnant while taking tamoxifen. Safety and efficacy in girls 2–10 years of age with McCune-Albright syndrome and precocious puberty have not been studied beyond 1 year of treatment.

SIDE EFFECTS

Most Common

Flushing/hot flashes, altered/irregular menses, amenorrhea, vaginal discharge/bleeding, skin changes, fluid retention, mood changes.

GI: N&V, distaste for food, anorexia, diarrhea, abdominal cramps, constipation, pancreatitis. **CV:** Peripheral edema, flushing, superficial phlebitis, DVT, *pulmonary embolism*, *thromboembolic disorders* (especially when tamoxifen is combined with other cytotoxic agents). **CNS:** Depression, dizziness, lightheadedness, headache, fatigue, mood changes. **Hepatic:** Rarely, fatty liver, cholestasis, hepatitis, liver cancer, *hepatic necrosis*. **GU:** Hot flashes, vaginal bleeding/discharge discharge, menstrual irregularities, amenorrhea, altered menses, oligomenorrhea, vaginal dryness, pruritus vulvae, ovarian cysts, hyperplasia of the uterus, polyps, endometrial cancer and uterine sarcoma. **Dermatologic:** Flushing/hot flashes, skin rash, skin changes, hair thinning or partial loss, alopecia. Rarely, erythema multiforme, *Stevens-Johnson syndrome*, bullous pemphigoid. **Respiratory:** Coughing, throat irritation, interstitial pneumonitis (rare). **Musculoskeletal:** Bone pain, musculoskeletal pain. **Ophthalmic:** Corneal changes, cataracts, decrease in color vision perception, retinal vein thrombosis, retinopathy. **Hematologic:** Leukopenia, thrombocytopenia, neutropenia, pancytopenia, anemia. **Miscellaneous:** Hypercalcemia, edema, pain, hyperlipidemia, weight gain/loss, increased bone/tumor pain, fluid retention, allergy, hypersensitivity (including angioedema), infection/*sepsis*. In men, may be loss of libido and impotence after discontinuing therapy.

Bold Italic = life threatening side effect   ■ = black box warning   ✦ = Available in Canada

LABORATORY TEST CONSIDERATIONS

↑ Serum calcium (transient), thyroid-binding globulin and thyroxine in postmenopausal women, BUN, AST, alkaline phosphatase, bilirubin, creatinine, serum triglycerides. ↓ Platelet count in breast cancer clients. Hyperlipidemias (rare). In oligospermic men: ↑ LH, FSH, testosterone, estrogen.

DRUG INTERACTIONS

Aminoglutethimide / ↓ Tamoxifen and N-desmethyltamoxifen levels R/T ↑ metabolism by CYP3A4

Anticoagulants / ↑ Hypoprothrombinemic effect; carefully monitor PT

Bromocriptine / ↑ Serum tamoxifen and N-desmethyltamoxifen levels

Cytotoxic drugs / ↑ Risk of thromboembolic event

Letrozole / ↓ Plasma letrozole levels by 37%

Medroxyprogesterone / ↓ Plasma N-desmethyltamoxifen levels but not tamoxifen levels

Rifamycins / ↓ Plasma tamoxifen levels R/T ↑ metabolism by CYP3A4; may need to ↑ dose

HOW SUPPLIED

Oral Solution: 10 mg/5 mL; *Tablets:* 10 mg, 20 mg.

DOSAGE

- **ORAL SOLUTION; TABLETS**
  Breast cancer.

10–20 mg twice/day (morning and evening) or 20 mg daily. If using the oral solution, give 10 mL for a 20 mg dose. Doses of 10 mg 2–3 times per day for 2 years and 10 mg twice a day for 5 or more years have been used. There is no evidence that doses greater than 20 mg daily are more effective.

  Reduction in incidence of breast cancer in high-risk women.

20 mg/day for 5 years. There are no data to support use beyond 5 years.

  Ductal carcinoma in situ.

20 mg/day for 5 years.

  Mastalgia.

10 mg/day for 10 months.

NURSING CONSIDERATIONS

ADMINISTRATION/STORAGE

1. Initiate tamoxifen during menses in sexually active women of child-bearing age. In those with menstrual irregularities, a negative B-hCG just before starting therapy is sufficient.

2. If hypercalcemia occurs (may occur in breast cancer with bone metastases), take appropriate measures; if severe, discontinue tamoxifen.

3. Store tablets from 20–25°C (68–77°F) in a well-closed, light-resistant container. Do not store the oral solution above 25°C (77°F); store in the original container protected from light. Use within 3 months of opening; do not freeze or refrigerate the oral solution.

ASSESSMENT

1. Note onset, duration, characteristics of S&S, surgery, biopsy results. List other therapies received. With increased pain, administer adequate analgesics and ensure adequate hydration.

2. The effect of the steroid and osteolytic metastases may result in hypercalcemia. Monitor calcium level and report symptoms of hypercalcemia (insomnia, lethargy, anorexia, N&V, coma, and vascular collapse).

3. Assess lipid panel, hematologic profile; monitor. Drug may cause granulocyte suppression. Nadir: 14 days; recovery: 21 days.

CLIENT/FAMILY TEACHING

1. Review side effects that should be reported; a reduction in dosage or discontinuation may be indicated.

2. Increased bone and lumbar pain or local disease flares should subside; take analgesics as needed. Continue to have regular gyn exam to assess for any evidence of uterine cancer and regular mammograms.

3. Consume 2–3 L/day of fluids to minimize hypercalcemia. Exercise to reduce calcium levels, improve circulation, and prevent thrombophlebitis. (Perform ROM exercises if bedridden.) Record weights weekly; report excessive weight gain or evidence of extremity swelling.

4. May experience 'hot flashes'; stay in cool environment. Wear protective clothing, sunscreens, and sunglasses to prevent photosensitivity reactions.

5. Obtain regular GYN exams; report menstrual irregularities, abnormal vagi-

nal bleeding, change in discharge, or pelvic pain/pressure.

6. Practice safe, barrier or nonhormonal methods of contraception during and for 1 month following therapy.

7. Report headaches or decreased visual acuity; may be irreversible. Have regular eye exams, especially if higher than usual dosage.

8. Although the risk of breast cancer is significantly lowered, there is also an increased risk of endometrial cancer, pulmonary embolism, and DVT. Report any redness or tenderness in extremity, increased SOB, chest pain, mental confusion, or sleepiness to ensure no stroke or blood clot. Avoid smoking.

OUTCOMES/EVALUATE

- Suppression of tumor growth and malignant cell proliferation
- Relief of breast pain
- Prophylaxis of breast cancer in high-risk women

Tamsulosin hydrochloride

(tam-**SOO**-loh-sin)

CLASSIFICATION(S):
Alpha-adrenergic blocking drug
PREGNANCY CATEGORY: B
Rx: Flomax.

USES
Signs and symptoms of BPH. Rule out prostatic carcinoma before using tamsulosin. *Investigational:* Adjunctive therapy to manage ureteral stones.

ACTION/KINETICS

Action
Blockade of alpha$_1$-receptors (probably alpha$_{1A}$) in the prostate results in relaxation of smooth muscles in the bladder neck and prostate; thus, urine flow rate is improved and there is a decrease in symptoms of BPH.

Pharmacokinetics
Food interferes with the rate of absorption. **t½, elimination:** 5–7 hr. Extensively metabolized in liver; excreted through urine and feces. **Plasma protein binding:** Significantly bound.

CONTRAINDICATIONS
Use to treat hypertension, with other alpha-adrenergic blocking agents, or in women or children.

SPECIAL CONCERNS
Use with caution with concurrent administration of warfarin. Possible development of intraoperative floppy iris syndrome during phacoemulsification cataract surgery.

SIDE EFFECTS
Most Common
Headache, dizziness, pharyngitis/rhinitis, abnormal ejaculation, shoulder/neck/back/extremity pain, asthenia, diarrhea, chest pain.

Body as a whole: Headache, infection, asthenia, back/chest pain. **CV:** Postural hypotension, syncope. **GI:** Diarrhea, nausea, tooth disorder. **CNS:** Dizziness, vertigo, somnolence, insomnia, decreased libido. **Respiratory:** Rhinitis, pharyngitis, increased cough, sinusitis. **GU:** Abnormal ejaculation. **Miscellaneous:** Amblyopia.

OD OVERDOSE MANAGEMENT
Symptoms: Hypotension. *Treatment:* Keep client in supine position to restore BP and normalize HR. If this is inadequate, consider IV fluids. Vasopressors may also be used; monitor renal function.

DRUG INTERACTIONS
Cimetidine → Significant ↓ in clearance of tamsulosin.

HOW SUPPLIED
Capsules: 0.4 mg.

DOSAGE
- **CAPSULES**
  Benign prostatic hypertrophy.
Adult males: 0.4 mg once daily given about 30 min after same meal each day. If, after 2 to 4 weeks, clients have not responded, dose can be increased to 0.8 mg daily.

NURSING CONSIDERATIONS
Do not confuse Flomax with Fosamax (a bisphosphonate), Flonase (a corticosteroid), or Volmax (a sympathomimetic).

Bold Italic = life threatening side effect   ■ = black box warning   ✦ = Available in Canada

ADMINISTRATION/STORAGE

1. If dose is discontinued or interrupted for several days after either the 0.4 mg or 0.8 mg dose, start therapy again with 0.4 mg dose.
2. Store at 20–25°C (68–77°F).

ASSESSMENT

1. List reasons for therapy, onset, characteristics/frequency of symptoms. Note BPH score, prostate size, voiding diary.
2. Identify drugs prescribed to ensure none interact; esp. cimetidine and coumadin.
3. Monitor CBC, I&O, VS, weight, urodynamic studies.
4. Note PSA levels, results of digital rectal exam.

CLIENT/FAMILY TEACHING

1. Take as directed, do not chew, crush, or open capsule. May take 30 minutes after the same meal each day to decrease GI upset. Report any loss of effectiveness or increased nighttime voiding.
2. Do not perform activities that require mental/physical alertness until drug effects realized; may cause dizziness, drowsiness, and syncope. Change positions slowly to prevent sudden drop in BP.
3. Stop fluid intake at least 4 hr before bedtime.
4. Do not stop suddenly after prolonged use. Avoid OTCs without provider approval. Keep F/U visit to evaluate response.

OUTCOMES/EVALUATE

Improvement in BPH symptoms; decreased nocturia

Telbivudine ■
(tel-**BIV**-yoo-deen)

CLASSIFICATION(S):
Antiviral drug, nucleoside reverse transcriptase inhibitor
PREGNANCY CATEGORY: B
Rx: Tyzeka.

USES
Treatment of chronic hepatitis B in adults with evidence of viral replication and either evidence of persistent elevations in serum ALT or AST or histologically active disease.

ACTION/KINETICS
Action
Telbivudine is phosphorylated by cellular kinases to the active telbivudine triphosphate. The triphosphate inhibits hepatitis B virus DNA polymerase (reverse transcriptase) by competing with the natural substrate, thymidine 5'-triphosphate. Incorporation of telbivudine 5-triphosphate into viral DNA causes DNA chain termination, resulting in inhibition of hepatitis B viral replication.

Pharmacokinetics
Steady-state peak plasma levels: 1–4 hr. **Steady state:** About 5–7 days. $t^{1/2}$: About 15 hr. Food does not affect absorption. $t^{1/2}$, **terminal:** 40–49 hr. Eliminated primarily by renal excretion of unchanged drug. Cross-resistance has been observed among hepatitis B nucleoside analogs. **Plasma protein binding:** About 3.3%.

CONTRAINDICATIONS
Hypersensitivity to telbivudine or any component of the product. Lactation.

SPECIAL CONCERNS
■ Lactic acidosis and severe hepatomegaly with steatosis, including fatal cases, have been reported with the use of nucleoside analogs alone or in combination with antiretrovirals. Severe acute exacerbations of hepatitis B have been reported in clients who have discontinued anti-hepatitis B therapy, including telbivudine. Closely monitor hepatic function with clinical and laboratory follow-up for at least several months in clients who discontinue anti-hepatitis B therapy. If appropriate, resumption of antihepatitis B therapy may be warranted.■ Exacerbations of hepatitis B are possible in those who have discontinued antihepatitis B therapy. Use with caution in elderly clients. Safety and efficacy have not been determined in children.

SIDE EFFECTS

Most Common

URTI, abdominal pain, fatigue, malaise, headache, nasopharyngitis, cough, diarrhea/loose stools, flu/flu-like symptoms, N&V, post-procedural pain.

CNS: Fatigue, malaise, headache, dizziness, insomnia. **GI:** Abdominal pain, diarrhea/loose stools, gastritis, N&V, dyspepsia. **Musculoskeletal:** Fibromyalgia, arthralgia, back pain, myalgia, myopathy, muscle cramps, musculoskeletal chest pain, pain in extremity, tenderness. **Respiratory:** Cough, URTI, nasopharyngitis, pharyngolaryngeal pain. **Hematologic:** Neutropenia, thrombocytopenia. **Dermatologic:** Rash. **Body as a whole:** Flu and flu-like symptoms, pyrexia, pain. **Miscellaneous:** Post-procedural pain.

LABORATORY TEST CONSIDERATIONS

↑ CPK, creatine kinase, ALT, AST, lipase, amylase, total bilirubin.

DRUG INTERACTIONS

Telbivudine is excreted mainly by renal excretion; coadministration with drugs that alter renal function may alter plasma levels of telbivudine.

HOW SUPPLIED

Tablets: 600 mg.

DOSAGE

- **TABLETS**

  Chronic hepatitis B.

Adults and children, 16 years and older: 600 mg once daily, with or without food. Adjustment of dosage, as follows, is necessary in those with C_{CR} less than 50 mL/min: **C_{CR} 30–49 mL/min:** 600 mg once every 48 hr; **C_{CR} <30 mL/min, not requiring dialysis:** 600 mg q 72 hr; **end-stage renal disease on hemodialysis:** 600 mg once q 72 hr.

NURSING CONSIDERATIONS

ASSESSMENT

1. Note reasons for therapy, disease onset, other agents trialed, outcome.
2. List drugs prescribed to ensure none interact.
3. Monitor renal and LFTs; reduce dose with dysfunction. Assess for lactic acidosis.
4. Note liver biopsy date/findings and disease stage.

CLIENT/FAMILY TEACHING

1. Take as directed with or without food to control progression of HBV.
2. Practice reliable contraception; drug does not reduce risk of transmission of HBV to others through blood contamination or sexual contact.
3. May experience muscle aches/pain, fatigue, fever, abdominal pain, diarrhea, headaches; report if persistent or bothersome.
4. Do not stop drug suddenly, may cause exacerbation of HBV.
5. Keep all F/U appointments to evaluate drug response and labs for any adverse side effects.

OUTCOMES/EVALUATE

- ↓ HBV viral load
- ↑ Virological suppression

Telithromycin   ■
(tel-ith-roe-**MYE**-sin)

CLASSIFICATION(S):
Antibiotic, ketolide
PREGNANCY CATEGORY: C
Rx: Ketek.

USES

Mild to moderate community acquired pneumonia due to *S. pneumoniae* (including multidrug resistant *S. pneumoniae* isolates, including isolates known as penicillin-resistant *S. pneumoniae* and isolates resistant to two or more of the following: penicillin, second-generation cephalosporins, macrolides, tetracyclines, and trimethoprim/sulfamethoxazole), *H. influenzae, M. catarrhalis, Chlamydophila pneumoniae,* or *Mycoplasma pneumoniae.*

ACTION/KINETICS

Action

A ketolide antibiotic structurally related to the macrolide family of antibiotics. Telithromycin blocks protein synthesis by binding to domains II and V of 23S rRNA of the 50S ribosomal subunit. By binding at domain II, the drug retains activity against gram-positive cocci in the presence of resistance caused by methylases that alter the domain V

---

binding site of telithromycin. May also inhibit the assembly of nascent ribosomal units.

Pharmacokinetics

Maximum plasma levels: About 1 hr. Absolute bioavailability of 57%. Rate and extent of absorption not affected by food. **t½, terminal:** 9.8 hr (after multiple doses). About 50% metabolized in the liver by CYP3A4 and 50% of metabolism is CYP450-independent. Excreted in the feces and urine. **Plasma protein binding:** About 60–70% (mainly albumin).

CONTRAINDICATIONS

History of hypersensitivity to telithromycin and/or any components of the product or any macrolide antibiotic. Coadministration with cisapride or pimozide. Use with congenital prolongation of the QTc interval, in those with uncorrected hypokalemia or hypomagnesemia, clinically significant bradycardia, and in those receiving Class IA (quinidine and procainamide) or Class III (dofetilide) antiarrhythmics. Use to treat less serious bacterial infections, such as bronchitis and sinusitis. Use in myasthenia gravis, previous history of hepatitis and/or jaundice associated with the use of telithromycin or any macrolide antibiotic.

SPECIAL CONCERNS

■ Telithromycin is contraindicated in clients with myasthenia gravis. There have been reports of fatal and life-threatening respiratory failure in clients with myasthenia gravis associated with the use of telithromycin.■ Due to potential severe liver problems, use of the drug is restricted to treating pneumonia. Elderly clients may be more sensitive to the drug. Use with caution during lactation. Safety and efficacy have not been determined in children.

SIDE EFFECTS

Most Common

Diarrhea, N&V, dizziness, headache, dysgeusia, loose stools.

GI: Diarrhea, N&V, dysgeusia, loose/watery stools, abdominal distention/pain, anorexia, constipation, dyspepsia, flatulence, gastritis, gastroenteritis, GI upset, glossitis, oral candidiasis, stomatitis, upper abdominal pain, dry mouth, pseudomembranous colitis, *Clostridium difficile-* associated diarrhea, pancreatitis. **Hepatic:** Hepatitis with or without jaundice, hepatic dysfunction including increased liver enzymes, hepatocellular and/or cholestatic hepatitis with or without jaundice, *fatal liver toxicity*. **CNS:** Dizziness, headache, insomnia, anxiety, somnolence, vertigo, paresthesia, loss of consciousness. **CV:** Bradycardia, hypotension, atrial arrhythmias, prolongation of QTc interval (may lead to ventricular arrhythmias), palpitations. **Dermatologic:** Rash, increased sweating, eczema, erythema multiforme, flushing, pruritus, urticaria. **Hypersensitivity:** Facial edema, *angioedema*, *anaphylaxis*. **Musculoskeletal:** Muscle cramps, exacerbation of myasthenia gravis (rare). **GU:** Vaginal candidiasis, vaginitis, fungal vaginosis. **Ophthalmic:** Blurred vision, diplopia, difficulty focusing. **Body as a whole:** Fatigue.

LABORATORY TEST CONSIDERATIONS

↑ AST, ALT, blood alkaline phosphatase, eosinophil count, platelets, blood bilirubin.

DRUG INTERACTIONS

Antiarrhythmic drugs (amiodarone, bretylium, disopyramide, dofetilide, procainamide, quinidine, sotalol) / ↑ Risk of life-threating cardiac arrhythmias, including torsade de pointes; do not use telithromycin with class 1A and class III antiarrhythmics

Buspirone / ↑ Telithromycin plasma levels → ↑ pharmacologic and toxicologic effects

Cabergoline / ↑ Telithromycin plasma levels → ↑ pharmacologic and toxicologic effects

Carbamazepine / ↓ Telithromycin C_{max} and AUC → subtherapeutic levels R/T induction of CYP3A4 metabolism; ↑ or prolongation of the therapeutic and/or side effects of carbamazepine

Cisapride / ↑ Cisapride plasma levels → significant ↑ in the QTc interval; do not use together

Colchicine / ↑ Colchicine levels (possible toxicity) R/T inhibition of CYP3A4

Cyclosporine / ↑ Cyclosporine serum levels → ↑ or prolongation of therapeutic and/or side effects

Digoxin / ↑ Digoxin peak and trough levels by 73% and 21% respectively; monitor digoxin levels

Ergot alkaloids / Possible severe peripheral vasospasm and dysesthesia; do not use together

Hexobarbital / ↑ Hexobarbital serum levels → ↑ or prolongation of therapeutic and/or side effects

HMG-CoA Reductase Inhibitors (atorvastatin, lovastatin, simvastatin) / ↑ C_{max} and AUC of HMG-CoA reductase inhibitors; do not use together

Itraconazole / ↑ Telithromycin C_{max} and AUC by 22% and 54% respectively

Ketoconazole / ↑ Telithromycin C_{max} and AUC by 51% and 95% respectively

Metoprolol / ↑ Metoprolol C_{max} and AUC by 38%. use together with caution

Midazolam / ↑ Midazolam AUC R/T inhibition of metabolism by CYP3A4

Oral contraceptives containing ethinyl estradiol/levonorgestrel / ↑ Levonorgestrel steady state AUC by 50%

Phenobarbital / ↓ Telithromycin C_{max} and AUC → subtherapeutic levels R/T induction of CYP3A4 metabolism

Phenytoin / ↓ Telithromycin C_{max} and AUC → subtherapeutic levels R/T induction of CYP3A4 metabolism; ↑ or prolongation of the therapeutic and/or side effects of phenytoin

Pimozide / ↑ Pimozide plasma levels; do not use together

Ranolazine / ↑ Telithromycin plasma levels → ↑ pharmacologic and toxicologic effects

Repaglinide / ↑ Telithromycin plasma levels → ↑ pharmacologic and toxicologic effects

Rifampin / ↓ Telithromycin C_{max} and AUC by 79% and 86% respectively → subtherapeutic levels; do not use together

Sirolimus / ↑ Sirolimus serum levels → ↑ or prolongation of therapeutic and/or side effects

Sotalol / ↑ Risk of life-threating cardiac arrhythmias, including torsade de pointes; do not use telithromycin with class 1A and class III antiarrhythmics; also, ↓ sotalol C_{max} and AUC by 35% and 20% respectively

Tacrolimus / ↑ Tacrolimus serum levels → ↑ or prolongation of therapeutic and/or side effects

Theophylline / ↑ Theophylline C_{max} and AUC → worsening of N&V; give 1 hr apart

Triazolam / Possible ↑ triazolam levels R/T inhibition of metabolism by CYP3A4

Verapamil / ↑ Risk of cardiotoxicity; monitor closely

Warfarin / ↑ Warfarin anticoagulant effect; hemorrhage has occurred; monitor PT and INR

HOW SUPPLIED

Tablets: 300 mg 400 mg.

DOSAGE

• **TABLETS**

Community acquired pneumonia.

Adults and adolescents over 18 years of age: 800 mg (2 x 400 mg) once daily for 7–10 days without regard to food. In the presences of severe renal failure (e.g., C_{CR} <30 mL/min), including those who need dialysis, reduce the dose to 600 mg once daily. In those undergoing hemodialysis, give after the dialysis sesson on dialysis days. In the presence of severe impaired renal function with coexisting impaired hepatic function, reduce the dose to 400 mg once a day.

NURSING CONSIDERATIONS

ADMINISTRATION/STORAGE

Store at 25°C (77°F); limited time storage permitted to 15°–30°C (59°–86°F) for excursions.

ASSESSMENT

1. Note reasons for therapy, S&S of infections, culture results. List drugs prescribed to ensure none interact. Avoid use with Class 1A (i.e., quinidine, procanamide) or Class III (i.e., dofetilide) antiarrhythmics. Stop statins (simvastatin, lovastatin and atorvastatin) during the course of treatment.

2. Monitor VS, renal, LFTs; assess for dysfunction and report. Check EKG for any QT prolongation; precludes drug therapy.

3. Assess for any history/evidence of myasthenia gravis, family history of QT prolongation or arrhythmias, clinically significant bradycardia, or hypokalemia.

Bold Italic = life threatening side effect   ■ = black box warning   ✦ = Available in Canada

4. This drug belongs to a new class of antibiotics called ketolides and is structurally similar to the macrolides. Has caused fatal liver failure in some clients; monitor carefully.

CLIENT/FAMILY TEACHING

1. Drug is used to treat pneumonia and should not be used to treat less serious bacterial infections or be used with viral conditions. Take as directed with or without food. Complete entire prescription even if feeling better to prevent drug resistant organisms.

2. If visual difficulties are experienced (blurred/double vision, difficulty focusing) during therapy, avoid driving a motor vehicle, operating dangerous equipment, or performing hazardous activities; avoid quick changes to view distant and close objects to minimize these effects. Usually noted with first or second doses but may recur. Report if persistent or interferes with daily activities.

3. Drug may cause EKG changes; report any fainting or dizziness during therapy.

4. Report if S&S do not improve or worsen during therapy. Keep all F/U visits.

OUTCOMES/EVALUATE

Resolution of infection

Telmisartan ■

(**tell**-mih-**SAR**-tan)

CLASSIFICATION(S):
Antihypertensive, angiotensin II receptor blocker

PREGNANCY CATEGORY: C (first trimester), **D** (second and third trimesters).

Rx: Micardis.

SEE ALSO *ANGIOTENSIN II RECEPTOR ANTAGONISTS* AND *ANTIHYPERTENSIVES.*

USES

Hypertension alone or in combination with other antihypertensives.

ACTION/KINETICS

Pharmacokinetics

Control of BP in blacks is less than in whites. Is from 42–58% bioavailable

(depending on dose). **Time to maximum levels:** 30–60 min. **t½, terminal:** About 24 hr. Excreted mainly in the feces by way of the bile. **Plasma protein binding:** Over 99.5%.

SPECIAL CONCERNS

■ When used in pregnancy during the second and third trimesters, drugs that act directly on the renin-angiotensin system can cause injury and even death to the developing fetus. When pregnancy is detected, discontinue telmisartan as soon as possible.■ Use with caution in impaired hepatic function or in biliary obstructive disorders. Clients on dialysis may develop orthostatic hypotension.

SIDE EFFECTS

Most Common

URTI, diarrhea, pain, sinusitis, dizziness, fatigue, N&V, abdominal pain, myalgia, cough, pharyngitis, UTI, flu-like symptoms.

GI: Diarrhea, dyspepsia, heartburn, N&V, abdominal pain. **CNS:** Dizziness, headache, fatigue, anxiety, nervousness, insomnia. **Musculoskeletal:** Pain, including back/neck pain; myalgia, arthralgia. **Respiratory:** URTI, sinusitis, cough, rhinitis, pharyngitis, influenza, bronchitis. **Miscellaneous:** Chest pain, UTI, peripheral edema, rash, tachycardia, hypertension, flu-like symptoms.

LABORATORY TEST CONSIDERATIONS

↑ Creatinine (in small number of clients). ↓ Hemoglobin.

OD OVERDOSE MANAGEMENT

Symptoms: Hypotension, dizziness, tachycardia or bradycardia. *Treatment:* Supportive for hypotension.

DRUG INTERACTIONS

↑ Digoxin peak plasma and trough levels

HOW SUPPLIED

Tablets: 20 mg, 40 mg, 80 mg.

DOSAGE

• **TABLETS**

Antihypertensive.

Individualize dose. **Adults, initial:** 40 mg/day. **Maintenance:** 20–80 mg/day. If additional BP reduction is desired beyond that achieved with 80 mg/day, add a diuretic.

NURSING CONSIDERATIONS

ADMINISTRATION/STORAGE
1. May be taken with or without food.
2. Correct depletion of intravascular volume or begin therapy under close supervision.
3. Most of the antihypertensive effect occurs within 2 weeks with maximal reduction of BP within 4 weeks.
4. Clients on dialysis may develop orthostatic hypotension; monitor BP closely.
5. Begin treatment under close medical supervision in those with biliary obstructive disorders.
6. Store from 15–30°C (59–86°F). Do not remove tablets from blisters until just before use.

ASSESSMENT
1. Note onset, duration of disease, other agents trialed, outcome.
2. Symptomatic hypotension may occur in clients who are volume- or salt-depleted. Correct prior to using telmisartan, use a lower starting dose and monitor closely.
3. With renal dialysis may develop orthostatic hypotension; monitor BP closely.
4. Monitor VS, ECG, electrolytes, H&H, renal, and LFTs. With hepatic or renal dysfunction, use cautiously.

CLIENT/FAMILY TEACHING
1. Take as directed at the same time daily with or without food.
2. Do not remove tablets from blisters until just before administration.
3. Use caution may experience dizziness R/T low BP. Change positions slowly and report if persistent or bothersome.
4. Regular exercise, low-salt diet, and life-style changes (i.e., no smoking, low alcohol, low-fat diet, low stress, adequate rest) contribute to enhanced BP control.
5. Use effective contraception; report pregnancy as drug use during second and third trimesters is associated with fetal injury and morbidity. Report drop in urine output.

OUTCOMES/EVALUATE
↓ BP

Temazepam ©
(teh-**MAZ**-eh-pam)

CLASSIFICATION(S):
Sedative-hypnotic, benzodiazepine
PREGNANCY CATEGORY: X
Rx: Restoril, **C-IV**
♣**Rx:** Apo-Temazepam, Gen-Temazepam, Novo-Temazepam, Nu-Temazepam, PMS-Temazepam.

SEE ALSO *TRANQUILIZERS/ ANTIMANIC DRUGS/HYPNOTICS.*

USES
Insomnia in clients unable to fall asleep, with frequent awakenings during the night, and/or early morning awakenings.

ACTION/KINETICS
Action
Benzodiazepine derivative. Believed to potentiate GABA neuronal inhibition. The hypnotic action involves GABA receptors located in the CNS. The drug decreases sleep latency, the number of awakenings, and the time spent in the awake stage. Disturbed nocturnal sleep may occur the first one or two nights following discontinuance of the drug. Prolonged administration is not recommended because physical dependence and tolerance may develop. See also *Flurazepam.*

Pharmacokinetics
Peak blood levels: 1.2–1.6 hr. **t½:** 10–17 hr. **Steady-state plasma levels:** 382 ng/mL (2.5 hr after 30-mg dose). Accumulation of the drug is minimal following multiple dosage. Metabolized in the liver to inactive metabolites. **Plasma protein binding:** 98%.

CONTRAINDICATIONS
Pregnancy.

SPECIAL CONCERNS
Use with caution in severely depressed clients. Use during lactation may cause sedation and feeding problems in the infant. Geriatric clients may be more sensitive to the effects of temazepam.

SIDE EFFECTS
Most Common
Drowsiness, dizziness, lightheadedness, incoordination.

Bold Italic = life threatening side effect   ■ = black box warning   ♣ = Available in Canada

CNS: Drowsiness, dizziness, lightheadedness, incoordination, lethargy, confusion, euphoria, weakness, ataxia, lack of concentration, hallucinations. In some clients, paradoxical excitement (less than 0.5%), including stimulation and hyperactivity, occurs. **GI:** Anorexia, diarrhea. **Miscellaneous:** Tremors, horizontal nystagmus, falling, palpitations. Rarely, **_blood dyscrasias_**.

HOW SUPPLIED
Capsules: 7.5 mg, 15 mg, 22.5 mg, 30 mg.

DOSAGE
- **CAPSULES**
  Insomnia.
Individualize. **Adults, usual:** 15–30 mg at bedtime (7.5 mg may be sufficient for some to improve sleep latency). **In elderly or debilitated clients, initial:** 7.5–15 mg until individual response is determined.

NURSING CONSIDERATIONS
ⓒ Do not confuse temazepam with flurazepam (a benzodiazepine hypnotic) or terazosin (an antihypertensive). Do not confuse Restoril with Vistaril (nonbenzodiazepine anti-anxiety drug) or Risperdal (an antipsychotic).

ADMINISTRATION/STORAGE
Store from 15–25°C (68–77°F) in a well-closed, light-resistant container.

ASSESSMENT
1. Note reasons for therapy, onset, duration, characteristics of S&S, other agents trialed, outcome.
2. Assess sleep patterns, diet, lifestyle, routines; identify factors/triggers contributing to insomnia. With long term use, monitor renal and LFTs.
3. Determine any depression, or addiction history.

CLIENT/FAMILY TEACHING
1. Take only as directed; do not increase dose. May take several days before effects evident.
2. May cause daytime drowsiness. Avoid activities that require mental alertness until drug effects realized.
3. Avoid alcohol and CNS depressants; may increase CNS depression. Avoid tobacco; decreases drug's effect.

4. No daytime napping. May still have difficulty getting to sleep but once asleep will have increased rest. Keep diary listing routines, exercise time (do at least 4 hr before bedtime), use of caffeine, chocolate, alcohol, medications taking, distractions in bedroom.
5. Review nonpharmacologic methods of sleep induction (i.e., white noise, warm milk, camomile tea, soft music).
6. Practice reliable birth control; drug may cause fetal harm.
7. For short-term use only. Long-term use can cause dependence and withdrawal symptoms. After more than 3 weeks of continuous use; may experience rebound insomnia.

OUTCOMES/EVALUATE
Improved sleeping patterns; ↓ awakenings

Temozolomide
(tem-oh-**ZOHL**-oh-myd)

CLASSIFICATION(S):
Antineoplastic, miscellaneous
PREGNANCY CATEGORY: D
Rx: Temodar.
✦**Rx:** Temodal.

USES
(1) Refractory anaplastic astrocytoma in adults, i.e., those at first relapse whose disease has progressed on a drug regimen containing a nitrosourea and procarbazine. (2) With radiotherapy to treat adults with newly diagnosed glioblastoma multiforme concomitantly with radiotherapy and then as maintenance treatment. *Investigational:* Metastatic melanoma.

ACTION/KINETICS
Action
Temozolomide is a prodrug that is hydrolyzed, nonenzymatically, at physiologic pH to the reactive 3-methyl-(triazen-1-yl) imidazole-4-carboxamide (MTIC). MTIC methylates specific guanine-rich areas of DNA that initiate transcription, leading to cytotoxicity and antiproliferative effects.

Pharmacokinetics

Rapidly and completely absorbed after PO use. **Peak plasma levels:** 1 hr. Food reduces the rate and extent of absorption. Metabolized by hydrolysis. Excreted mainly in the urine. **t½:** 1.8 hr.

CONTRAINDICATIONS

Hypersensitivity to dacarbazine (DTIC) because it is also metabolized to MTIC. Lactation.

SPECIAL CONCERNS

Use with caution in the elderly and in those with severe renal or hepatic impairment. Safety and efficacy have not been determined in children.

SIDE EFFECTS

Most Common

N&V, headache, fatigue, constipation, diarrhea, abnormal coordination, amnesia, asthenia, convulsions, dizziness, hemiparesis, insomnia, peripheral edema, fever, viral infection.

Hematologic: Thrombocypenia, neutropenia, *myelodysplastic syndrome (rare), myeloid leukemia.* **CNS: Convulsions,** hemiparesis, dizziness, abnormal coordination, amnesia, insomnia, paresthesia, somnolence, paresis, ataxia, anxiety, dysphasia, depression, abnormal gait, confusion, impaired memory. **GI:** N&V, constipation, diarrhea, abdominal pain, anorexia, stomatitis, dysphasia. **Dermatologic:** Rash, pruritus, alopecia, dry skin, erythema, erythema multiforme. **Respiratory:** URTI, pharyngitis, sinusitis, dyspnea, coughing. **GU:** Urinary incontinence, UTI, increased micturition, frequency. **Ophthalmic:** Diplopia, blurred vision, visual deficit/changes/troubles. **Body as a whole:** Fatigue, asthenia, fever, viral infection, weight increase, myalgia, weakness, allergic reaction (rarely, *anaphylaxis*), rarely opportunistic infections (including *P. carinii* pneumonia). **Miscellaneous:** Headache, peripheral edema, back pain, adrenal hypercorticism, female breast pain, blurred vision, taste perversion, arthralgia, radiation injury.

OD OVERDOSE MANAGEMENT

Symptoms: Neutropenia, thrombocytopenia. *Treatment:* Hematologic evaluation. Supportive measures, as necessary.

DRUG INTERACTIONS

Valproic acid ↓ PO clearance of temozolomide

HOW SUPPLIED

Capsules: 5 mg, 20 mg, 100 mg, 140 mg, 180 mg, 250 mg.

DOSAGE

• **CAPSULES**

Anaplastic astrocytoma.

Adults, initial: 150 mg/m^2 once daily for 5 consecutive days per 28-day treatment cycle; the dose may be increased to 200 mg/m^2/day for 5 days. During treatment, obtain a CBC on day 22 (21 days after the first dose) or within 48 hr of that day, and weekly. Modify the dose as follows: If the ANC <1 x 10^9/L (1,000/mcL) or the platelet count <50 x 10^9/L (50,000/mcL), postpone therapy until ANC is >1.5 x 10^9/L (1,500/mcL) and the platelet count exceeds 100 x 10^9 (100,000/mcL); reduce dose by 50 mg/m^2/day for subsequent cycles. If ANC is 1,000–1,500/mcL or platelets are 50,000–100,000/mcL, postpone therapy until the ANC is >1,500/mcL and platelets are >100,000/mcL; maintain initial dose. If the ANC is >1,500/mcL and platelets are >100,000/mcL, increase dose to, or maintain dose at, 200 mg/m^2/day x 5 days for subsequent cycles.

Glioblastoma multiforme.

Concomitant phase, adults: 75 mg/m^2 daily for 42 days concomitant with focal radiotherapy followed by maintenance temozolomide for 6 cycles. No dose reductions are recommended during the concomitant phase; however, dose interruptions or discontinuation may occur based on toxicity. The dose should be continued throughout the 42-day concomitant period, up to 49 days, if all of the following conditions are met: ANC count greater than or equal to 1.5 x 10^9/L; platelet count greater than or equal to 100 x 10^9/L; common toxicity criteria nonhematological toxicity less than or equal to grade 1 (except for alopecia, N&V). Obtain a CBC weekly. **Maintenance phase, cycle 1:** Temozolomide is given for an additional 6 cycles of maintenance treatment 4 weeks after completing the temozolomide plus radiotherapy phase. Dosage in cy-

---

Bold Italic = life threatening side effect   ■ = black box warning   ♦ = Available in Canada cle 1 (maintenance) is 150 mg/m^2 once daily for 5 days followed by 23 days without treatment. **Cycles, 2–6:** At the start of cycle 2, the dose is increased to 200 mg/m^2 if the common toxicity criteria nonhematologic toxicity for cycle 1 is less than or equal to grade 2 (except for alopecia, N&V), ANC is greater than or equal to 1.5 x 10^9/L, and the platelet count is greater than or equal to 100 x 10^9/L. The dosage remains at 200 mg/m^2/day for the first 5 days of each subsequent cycle, except if toxicity occurs. If the dose is not escalated in cycle 2, escalation should not occur in subsequent cycles.

NURSING CONSIDERATIONS
ADMINISTRATION/STORAGE
1. Therapy can be continued until disease progression; optimum duration is not known.
2. Consult package insert for dosage calculations based on BSA and suggested capsule combinations to achieve required daily dose.
3. Follow institutional procedures for proper handling and disposal of antineoplastic agents.
4. Prophylaxis of *Pneumocystis carinii* pneumonia is required during the concomitant phase when used to treat gliobastoma multiforme.
5. The following guidelines are followed for temozolomide interruption or discontinuation during concomitant radiotherapy:
- Interrupt temozolomide therapy if ANC is greater than or equal to 0.5 and <1.5 x 10^9/L. Discontinue temozolomide if ANC is <0.5 x 10^9/L.
- Interrupt temozolomide if platelet count is greater than or equal to 10 and <100 x 10^9/L. Discontinue temozolomide if platelet count is <10 x 10^9/L.
- Interrupt temozolomide if common toxicity criteria (CTC) nonhematological toxicity (except for alopecia, N&V) is CTC grade 2. Discontinue temozolomide if CTC is grade 3 or 4.
6. Apply dose reductions during the maintenance phase according to the following:

- During treatment, a CBC should be obtained on day 22 (21 days after the first dose of temozolomide) or within 48 hr of that day and weekly until the ANC is about 1.5 x 10^9/L and the platelet count exceeds 100 x 10^9/L. The next cycle of temozolomide should not be started until the ANC and platelet count exceed these levels. Dose reductions during the next cycle should be based on the lowest blood counts and worst nonhematologic toxicity during the previous cycle.
7. Apply dose reductions or discontinuations during the maintenance phase according to the following:
- Reduce temozolomide by 1 dose level (i.e., to 100 mg/m^2/day) if ANC <1 x 10^9/L. Discontinue if dose reduction to <100 mg/m^2/day is required or if the same grade 3 nonhematological toxicity recurs after dose reduction.
- Reduce temozolomide by 1 dose level (i.e., to 100 mg/m^2/day) if the platelet count <50 x 10^9/L. Discontinue if dose reduction to <100 mg/m^2/day is required or if the same grade 3 nonhematological toxicity recurs after dose reduction.
- Reduce temozolomide by 1 dose level (i.e., to 100 mg/m^2/day) if CTC nonhematological toxicity (except for alopecia, N&V) is CTC grade 3. Discontinue temozolomide if the CTC grade is 4.

ASSESSMENT
1. Note disease onset, previous drug regimen, date of relapse or other condition requiring treatment.
2. Determine BSA–daily dosage dependent on calculations; see package insert. Temozolomide capsule combinations based on daily dose/BSA.
3. Obtain CBC 21 days after first dose and weekly until recovery (ANC >1.5 x 10^9/L). If ANC <1 x 10^9/L or platelet count <50 x 10^9/L during any cycle reduce dose as directed under dosage. Nadir 21–40 days for platelets and 1–44 days for neutrophils.
4. Follow dosage guidelines for glioblastoma with radiotherapy treatments.

Monitor VS, CBC, renal, and LFTs. Assess for bleeding, infection or dehydration.

CLIENT/FAMILY TEACHING
1. Do not open or chew capsules; swallow whole with a glass of water. If capsules are accidentally opened or damaged, take serious precautions to avoid inhalation or contact with the skin or mucous membranes.
2. To reduce N&V, take on an empty stomach, preferably at bedtime.
3. May experience nausea, vomiting, fatigue, and headaches. Antiemetic therapy may be given before or after temozolomide administration. Report S&S infection, skin rash/discoloration, bleeding, dizziness, or other adverse effects.
4. Avoid activities that require mental alertness until drug effects realized. Practice reliable birth control.
5. Store away from children and pets.

OUTCOMES/EVALUATE
↓ Tumor size and spread

Temsirolimus   **IV**

(**TEM**-sir-**OH**-lih-mus)

CLASSIFICATION(S):
Antineoplastic, protein-tyrosine kinase inhibitor
PREGNANCY CATEGORY: D
Rx: Torisel.

USES
Treatment of advanced renal cell carcinoma.

ACTION/KINETICS
Action Temsirolimus binds to an intracellular protein (FKBP-12); this protein-drug complex inhibits the activity of the target that controls cell division.

Pharmacokinetics
CYP3A4 is the major isoenzyme responsible for temsirolimus metabolites. Sirolimus is an active metabolite of temsirolimus. Temsirolimus inhibits CYP2D6 and CYP3A4 isoenzymes. Excreted mainly in the feces (78%) with a small amount (4.6%) excreted in the urine. **t½, mean:** 17.3 hr for temsirolimus and 54.6 hr for sirolimus.

CONTRAINDICATIONS
Avoid concomitant use of strong CYP3A4 inhibitors (e.g., atazanavir, clarithromycin, indinavir, itraconazole, ketoconazole, nefazodone, nelfinavir, ritonavir, saquinavir, telithromycin, voriconazole). Avoid concomitant use of strong CYP3A4 inducers (e.g., carbamazepine, dexamethasone, phenobarbital, phenytoin, rifampin, rifabutin, rifampicin). Lactation.

SPECIAL CONCERNS
Avoid the use of live vaccine and close contact with those who have received live vaccines (e.g., intranasal influenza, measles, mumps, rubella, oral polio, Bacille Calmette-Guerin, yellow fever, varicella, and TY21a typhoid vaccines). Safety and efficacy have not been determined in children.

SIDE EFFECTS
Most Common
Anorexia, asthenia, edema, mucositis, N&V, rash, dysgeusia, diarrhea, back pain, dyspnea, cough, pain, pyrexia.
CNS: Dysgeusia (includes taste loss/perversion), headache, insomnia, depression. **GI:** Mucositis (includes aphthous stomatitis, glossitis, mouth ulceration, stomatitis), N&V, anorexia, diarrhea, abdominal pain, constipation, *fatal bowel perforation.* **CV:** Hypertension, *DVT, pulmonary embolism,* thrombophlebitis, *intracerebral hemorrhage.* **Dermatologic:** Rash (includes eczema, exfoliative dermatitis, maculopapular/pruritic/pustular/vesiculobullous rash), pruritus, nail disorder, dry skin, acne. **Musculoskeletal:** Back pain, arthralgia, myalgia, chest pain. **Respiratory:** Dyspnea, cough, epistaxis, pharyngitis, rhinitis, pneumonia, URTI, *interstitial lung disease* (rarely fatal). **Hematologic:** Anemia, leukopenia, lymphopenia, thrombocytopenia. **GU:** Cystitis, dysuria, hematuria, urinary frequency, UTI, renal failure. **Hypersensitivity:** Dyspnea, flushing, chest pain, *anaphylaxis.* **Ophthalmic:** Conjunctivitis, lacrimation disorder. **Body as a whole:** Asthenia, edema (includes facial/peripheral edema), pain, pyrexia, infections (includes abscess, bronchitis, cellulitis, herpes

simplex/zoster), weight loss, chills, impaired wound healing.

LABORATORY TEST CONSIDERATIONS
↑ Alkaline phosphatase, AST, serum creatinine, glucose, total bilirubin, total cholesterol, triglycerides. ↓ Phosphorus, potassium, hemoglobin, leukocytes, lymphocytes, neutrophils, platelets. Hyperglycemia, hyperlipemia, hypertriglyceridemia, hypophosphatemia,

DRUG INTERACTIONS
Azole antifungals (fluconazole, itraconazole, ketoconazole, posaconazole, voriconazole) / ↑ Temsirolimus levels R/T inhibition of CYP3A4; monitor temsirolimus levels and adjust dose if needed
Clarithromycin / ↑ Temsirolimus levels R/T inhibition of CYP3A4; monitor temsirolimus levels and adjust dose if needed
Cyclosporine / ↑ Sirolimus (active metabolite of temsirolimus) levels → ↑ toxicity
Dexamethasone / ↓ Temsirolimus levels R/T induction of CYP3A4; if concomitant use necessary, consider ↑ temsirolimus dose to 50 mg/week
Diltiazem / ↑ Temsirolimus levels R/T inhibition of CYP3A4; monitor temsirolimus levels and adjust dose if needed; also, ↑ sirolimus (active metabolite of temsirolimus) levels → ↑ toxicity
Grapefruit juice / ↑ Temsirolimus levels; do not use together
Hydantoins (e.g., phenytoin) / ↓ Temsirolimus levels R/T induction of CYP3A4; if concomitant use necessary, consider ↑ temsirolimus dose to 50 mg/week
Mycophenolate / ↑ Mycophenolic acid trough levels → ↑ risk of toxicity
Phenobarbital / ↓ Temsirolimus levels R/T induction of CYP3A4; monitor temsirolimus levels and adjust dose if needed
Protease inhibitors (e.g., atazanavir, indinavir, nelfinavir, ritonavir, saquinavir) / ↑ Temsirolimus levels R/T inhibition of CYP3A4; monitor temsirolimus levels and adjust dose if needed
Rifamycins (e.g., rifabutin, rifampin, rifapentin) / ↓ Temsirolimus levels R/T induction of CYP3A4; consider ↑ temsirolimus dose to 50 mg/week

 St. John's wort / ↓ Temsirolimus levels R/T induction of CYP3A4; do not use together
Sunitinib / Dose-limiting toxicity (e.g., grade 3/4 erythematous maculopapular rash, gout/cellulitis requiring hospitalization)
Tacrolimus / ↓ Tacrolimus trough levels due to sirolimus (active metabolite) → ↓ pharmacologic effect; frequently monitor tacrolimus trough levels and adjust dose if needed

HOW SUPPLIED
Injection Solution, Concentrate: 25 mg/mL.

DOSAGE

• **IV INFUSION**
Advanced renal cell carcinoma.
25 mg infused over a 30- to 60-minute period once a week. Continue treatment until disease progression or unacceptable toxicity occurs.

NURSING CONSIDERATIONS

ADMINISTRATION/STORAGE
IV 1. Do not add undiluted temsirolimus injection to infusion solutions; will cause the drug to precipitate. Always combine temsirolimus injection with the diluent provided before adding to infusion solutions. It is recommended that after the diluent is added, the drug should be given in 0.9% NaCl injection.
2. Avoid adding other drugs or nutrients to admixtures of temsirolimus in NaCl injection.
3. Premedicate with prophylactic diphenhydramine, 25-50 mg IV (or similar antihistamine) about 30 min before the start of each infusion of temsirolimus.
4. If a hypersensitivity reaction occurs during temsirolimus infusion, stop infusion and observe client for at least 30-60 min. At the discretion of the HCP, treatment may be resumed with the administration of an H-1 receptor antagonist (e.g., diphenhydramine) if not given previously and/or an H-2 receptor antagonist (e.g., famotidine, 20 mg IV or ranitidine, 50 mg IV) approximately 30 min before restarting the temosirolimus infusion. The infusion may then be resumed at a slower rate (up to 60 min).

5. Interrupt dosage if the absolute neutrophil count is <1,000/mm³, platelet count is <75,000/mm³, or for National Cancer Institute Common Terminology Criteria for Adverse Events grade 3 or greater adverse reactions. Once toxicities have resolved to grade 2 or less, temsirolimus may be restarted with the dose reduced by 5 mg weekly to a dose no lower than 15 mg/week.

6. Avoid concomitant use of strong CYP3A4 inhibitors (see *Contraindications* and *Drug Interactions*). If concomitant use is necessary, consider reducing the temsirolimus dose to 12.5 mg/week. If the strong inhibitor is discontinued, a washout period of about 1 week should be allowed before adjusting the temsirolimus dose back to the dose used prior to starting the strong CYP3A4 inhibitor.

7. Avoid concomitant use of strong CYP3A4 inducers (See *Contraindications* and *Drug Interactions*). If concomitnat use is necessary, consider increasing the dose of temsirolimus to 50 mg/week. If the strong inducer is discontinued, the temsirolimus dose should be returned to the dose used prior to starting the strong CYP3A4 inducers.

8. Store the final temsirolimus dilution for infusion in polypropylene or glass bottles or polypropylene or polyolefin plastic bags. If polyvinyl chloride bags are used, the plasticizer di-2-ethylhexylphthalate may be leached from these bags.

9. Protect temsirolimus from excessive room light and sunlight.

10. Store from 2-8°C (36-46°F). The 10 mg/mL diluent/solution mixture is stable for up to 24 hr at controlled room temperature.

ASSESSMENT

1. Note disease onset, radiographic findings, other therapies trialed/failed.

2. List drugs prescribed to ensure none interact.

3. Assess for other conditions i.e., brain tumor, infections/wounds, or recent surgery. CNS tumors and anticoagulant therapy may increase risk of life-threatening intracerebral bleeding.

4. Monitor renal and LFTs, cholesterol, glucose levels, and CBC. May require starting or increasing dose of lipid-lowering agents.

5. Check for diabetes, hyperlipidemia, liver problems, bone marrow problems, low WBC/platelet levels, or a weakened immune system. Follow administration guidelines R/T adverse events or lowered ANC/platelet count.

CLIENT/FAMILY TEACHING

1. Administered IV for advanced kidney cancer. Will receive premedication with an antihistamine (benadryl) 30 min prior to therapy to help prevent allergic reactions.

2. Do not eat grapefruit or drink grapefruit juice while receiving this drug.

3. Report any facial swelling, breathing difficulty, increased abdominal pain, blood in stools, S&S of infection i.e., fever, sore throat, rash, or chills, excessive thirst or urinary frequency.

4. May be more susceptible to infections, abnormal wound healing, interstitial lung disease—a severe and possibly fatal reaction, bowel perforation, kidney failure, or elevated triglycerides/cholesterol during therapy (may require therapy to control).

5. Vaccinations may not be as effective during therapy; avoid live vaccines and close contact with those who recently received a live vaccine.

6. Men with partners of childbearing potential should use reliable contraception throughout treatment and for 3 months after the last dose. Women should avoid pregnancy during and for 3 months following therapy; may cause fetal damage.

7. May increase blood sugar; report if confused, drowsy, or thirsty. May also cause flushing, fast breathing, or fruit-like breath odor; report if evident.

8. Keep all F/U appointments for weekly therapy, labs and to evaluate tumor response.

OUTCOMES/EVALUATE

Inhibition of malignant cell proliferation

Tenecteplase
(teh-**NECK**-teh-plays)

CLASSIFICATION(S):
Thrombolytic, tissue plasminogen activator
PREGNANCY CATEGORY: C
Rx: TNKase.

USES
Reduce mortality due to acute myocardial infarction (AMI).

ACTION/KINETICS
Action
A tissue plasminogen activator produced by recombinant DNA. It binds to fibrin and converts plasminogen to plasmin. In the presence of fibrin, tenecteplase conversion of plasminogen to plasmin is increased relative to conversion in the absence of fibrin. Following the drug there are decreases in circulating fibrinogen.
Pharmacokinetics
t$\frac{1}{2}$, **initial disposition:** 20–24 min; **terminal disposition:** 90–130 min. Metabolized in the liver.

CONTRAINDICATIONS
Active internal bleeding, history of CVA, within 2 months of intracranial or intraspinal surgery or trauma, intracranial neoplasm, arteriovenous malformation or aneurysm, known bleeding diathesis, severe uncontrolled hypertension. IM use.

SPECIAL CONCERNS
The following high risk conditions warrant an assessment of the risk of therapy versus the anticipated benefits: Recent major surgery (e.g., CABG, OB delivery, organ biopsy); previous puncture of noncompressible vessels; CV disease; recent GI or GU bleeding; recent trauma; hypertension (systolic BP equal to or greater than 180 mm Hg or diastolic BP equal to or greater than 110 mm Hg); high likelihood of left heart thrombus (e.g. mitral stenosis with atrial fibrillation); acute pericarditis; subacute bacterial endocarditis; hemostatic defects (including those secondary to severe hepatic or renal disease); severe hepatic dysfunction; pregnancy; diabetic hemorrhagic retinopathy or other hemorrhagic ophthalmic conditions; septic thrombophlebitis or occluded AV cannula at seriously infected site; advanced age; clients receiving PO anticoagulants (e.g., warfarin sodium); recent administration of GP IIB/IIIa inhibitors; and, any other condition in which bleeding constitutes a significant hazard or would be particularly difficult to manage because of its location. There is the possibility of cholesterol embolization and arrhythmias associated with reperfusion. Use with caution in the elderly, weighing the benefits versus risks, including bleeding. Use with caution during lactation. Safety and efficacy have not been determined in children.

SIDE EFFECTS
Most Common
Bleeding is the most common side effect (see below).
Bleeding. Most common side effect. Major bleeding includes hematoma, GI tract, urinary tract, puncture site (including cardiac catheterization site), retroperitoneal, respiratory tract. Minor bleeding includes hematoma, urinary tract, puncture site (including cardiac catheterization site), pharyngeal, GI tract, and epistaxis. **CV:** Cardiogenic shock, arrhythmias e.g., sinus bradycardia, accelerated idioventricular rhythm, ventricular premature depolarization, ventricular tachycardia), AV block, *heart failure*, *cardiac arrest*, recurrent myocardial ischemia, *myocardial reinfarction/rupture*, *cardiac tamponade*, pericarditis, pericardial effusion, mitral regurgitation, thrombosis, embolism, electromechanical dissociation. **Miscellaneous:** Pulmonary edema, N&V, hypotension, fever, *serious allergic or anaphylactic reactions.*

LABORATORY TEST CONSIDERATIONS
Results of coagulation tests or measures of fibrinolytic activity may be unreliable; specific precautions must be taken to prevent in vitro artifacts. Degradation of fibrinogen in blood samples removed for analysis is possible.

DRUG INTERACTIONS

Heparin, vitamin K antagonists, aspirin, dipyridamole, and GP IIb/IIIa inhibitors may increase the risk of bleeding if given prior to, during, or after tenecteplase therapy.

HOW SUPPLIED

Powder for Injection, Lyophilized: 50 mg.

DOSAGE

- **IV ONLY**
  AMI.

Dose is based on client weight, but not to exceed 50 mg. Given as a single bolus dose over 5 sec. **Less than 60 kg:** 30 mg (6 mL); **60 kg–less than 70 kg:** 35 mg (7 mL); **70 kg–less than 80 kg:** 40 mg (8 mL); **80 kg–less than 90 kg:** 45 mg (9 mL); **90 kg and over:** 50 mg (10 mL).

NURSING CONSIDERATIONS

ADMINISTRATION/STORAGE

 1. Initiate treatment as soon as possible after onset of symptoms of MI.
2. Reconstitute and administer as follows:

- Aseptically withdraw 10 mL sterile water from that supplied. Use the red hub cannula syringe filling device. Do not discard the shield assembly. Do *not* use bacteriostatic water for injection.
- Inject entire contents of the syringe (10 mL) into the tenecteplase vial. Direct the stream into the powder. Slight foaming may occur; any large bubbles will dissipate if allowed to stand undisturbed for several minutes.
- Swirl contents gently until completely dissolved. Do not shake. The reconstituted product is colorless to pale yellow and is transparent with a concentration of 5 mg/mL and pH of about 7.3.
- Determine appropriate dose of tenecteplase and withdraw correct volume (in mL) from the reconstituted vial with the syringe. Discard any unused portion.
- With correct dose in the syringe, stand the shield vertically on a flat surface with the green side down

and passively recap the red hub cannula.

- Remove the entire shield assembly, including the red hub cannula by twisting counter clockwise. The shield assembly also contains the clear-ended blunt plastic cannula; retain for split septum IV access.
- Administer as a single IV bolus over 5 sec.

3. Tenecteplase contains no preservatives; thus, reconstitute immediately before use.
4. If given in an IV line with dextrose, precipitation may occur. Flush dextrose-containing lines with a saline-containing solution prior to and following single bolus administration of tenecteplase.
5. Store lyophilized tenecteplase at controlled temperatures not to exceed 30°C (86°F) or under refrigeration at 2–8°C (36–46°F).
6. If reconstituted drug is not used immediately, refrigerate tenecteplase vial at 2–8°C (36–46°F) and use within 8 hr.

ASSESSMENT

1. Note reasons for therapy identifying symptom onset and site of infarct.
2. Do not use with active internal bleeding, history of CVA, recent: intracranial bleed, spinal surgery, trauma, neoplasm, AV malformation, aneurysm, or uncontrolled HTN.
3. Obtain baseline cardiac enzymes, weight, CBC, bleeding times, type and crossmatch. Monitor for S&S active bleeding, stop heparin infusion and report.
4. Assess for reperfusion arrhythmias after therapy which may include accelerated idioventricular rhythm, sinus bradycardia of short duration, and return of elevated ST segment to near baseline.

CLIENT/FAMILY TEACHING

1. Review inherent benefits and risks of drug therapy. Maintain bed rest during therapy.
2. To be effective, the therapy should be instituted as soon as possible after symptom onset of AMI.

Bold Italic = life threatening side effect   ■ = black box warning   ♣ = Available in Canada

3. Report any adverse side effects i.e. sudden severe headache or active bleeding immediately.
4. Encourage family members or significant other to learn CPR.

OUTCOMES/EVALUATE
↓ Mortality with AMI

Teniposide (VM-26)

■ IV

(teh-**NIP**-ah-side)

CLASSIFICATION(S):
Antineoplastic, miscellaneous
PREGNANCY CATEGORY: D
Rx: Vumon.

SEE ALSO *ANTINEOPLASTIC AGENTS.*

USES
(1) In combination with other antineoplastic agents for induction therapy in clients with refractory childhood acute lymphoblastic leukemia (ALL). (2) Relapsed ALL.

ACTION/KINETICS
Action
Acts in the late S or early G_2 phase of the cell cycle, preventing cells from entering mitosis. Inhibits type II topoisomerase activity resulting in both single- and double-stranded breaks in DNA and DNA: protein cross-links. Active against sublines of certain murine leukemias that have developed resistance to amsacrine, cisplatin, daunorubicin, doxorubicin, mitoxantrone, or vincristine.

Pharmacokinetics
Terminal $t^1/_2$: 5 hr. Metabolized in the liver and excreted mainly through the urine (4–12% unchanged) with small amounts excreted in the feces. **Plasma protein binding:** More than 99%.

CONTRAINDICATIONS
Hypersensitivity to teniposide, etoposide, or the polyoxyethylated castor oil present in teniposide products. Lactation.

SPECIAL CONCERNS
■ (1) Severe myelosuppression with resulting infection or bleeding may occur. (2) Hypersensitivity reactions, including anaphylaxis-like symptoms, may occur with initial or repeated dosing. Epinephrine with or without corticosteroids and antihistamines, has been used to alleviate symptoms.■ Clients with both Down syndrome and leukemia may be especially sensitive to myelosuppressive chemotherapy; thus, reduce initial dosing. Use with caution in clients with impaired hepatic function. Contains benzyl alcohol associated with a fatal 'gasping' syndrome in premature infants.

SIDE EFFECTS
Most Common
Thombocytopenia, neutropenia, anemia, leukopenia, nonspecified myelosuppression, mucositis, N&V, diarrhea, infection.
Hematologic: *Severe myelosuppression*, leukopenia, neutropenia, thrombocytopenia, anemia, nonspecified myelosuppression. **Hypersensitivity reactions: *Anaphylaxis*** manifested by chills, fever, ***bronchospasm***, dyspnea, facial flushing, hypertension or hypotension, tachycardia. **CV:** Hypotension. **GI:** Mucositis, N&V, diarrhea. **Dermatologic:** Alopecia (reversible), rash, hepatic dysfunction/toxicity, peripheral neurotoxicity, infection, bleeding, renal dysfunction, metabolic abnormalities.

OD OVERDOSE MANAGEMENT
Symptoms: Myelosuppression, hypotension, anaphylaxis.
Treatment: Anaphylaxis or Overdose:
- Treat anaphylaxis promptly with antihistamines, corticosteroids, epinephrine, IV fluids, and other supportive measures. If a client who manifested a hypersensitivity reaction must be retreated, undertake pretreatment with corticosteroids and antihistamines; carefully observe client during and after the infusion.
- If hypotension occurs, stop the infusion and give fluids. Undertake other supportive therapy as needed.
- Myelosuppression may be treated with supportive care including blood products and antibiotics.

T

 = see color insert   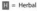 = Herbal   IV = Intravenous   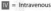 = sound alike drug

DRUG INTERACTIONS

Antiemetic drugs / Acute CNS depression and hypotension in clients receiving high doses of teniposide and pretreated with antiemetics

Methotrexate / ↑ Plasma clearance of methotrexate

Sodium salicylate / ↑ Teniposide effect R/T displacement from plasma protein binding sites

Sulfamethizole / ↑ Teniposide effect R/T displacement from plasma protein binding sites

Tolbutamide / ↑ Teniposide effect R/T displacement from plasma protein binding sites

HOW SUPPLIED

Injection: 10 mg/mL.

DOSAGE

- **IV INFUSION**

  Regimen 1 for childhood ALL clients failing induction therapy with cytarabine.

  Teniposide, 165 mg/m², and cytarabine, 300 mg/m² IV twice weekly for eight to nine doses.

  Regimen 2 for childhood ALL refractory to vincristine/prednisone-containing regimens.

  Teniposide, 250 mg/m², and vincristine, 1.5 mg/m², IV weekly for 4–8 weeks, and prednisone, 40 mg/m² orally for 28 days. *NOTE:* Dosage adjustment may be needed for clients with significant renal or hepatic dysfunction.

NURSING CONSIDERATIONS

ADMINISTRATION/STORAGE

 1. Give over 30–60 min or longer; do not give by rapid IV infusion, as hypotension may occur.

2. The IV catheter or needle must be in the proper position and functional prior to infusion. Improper administration may cause extravasation resulting in local tissue necrosis or thrombophlebitis. Also, occlusion of central venous access devices has occurred during 24-hr infusion at concentrations of 0.1–0.2 mg/mL.

3. Dilute with either D5W or 0.9% NaCl injection to give a final concentration of 0.1, 0.2, 0.4, or 1 mg/mL.

4. Contact of undiluted teniposide with plastic equipment/devices used to prepare IV infusions may result in softening, cracking, and possible drug leakage. To prevent extraction of plasticizer DEHP, prepare and give solutions in non-DEHP-containing LVP containers such as glass or polyolefin plastic bags or containers. Avoid PVC containers.

5. Lipid administration sets or low DEHP-containing nitroglycerin sets will keep exposure to DEHP at low levels and can be used. Diluted solutions are chemically/physically compatible with the recommended IV administration sets and LVP containers for up to 24 hr at ambient room temperature and lighting conditions.

6. Use caution in handling and preparing the solution as skin reactions may occur with accidental exposure and drug is cytotoxic. Use of gloves is recommended; if the solution comes in contact with the skin, wash immediately with soap and water. If the drug comes in contact with mucous membranes, flush thoroughly with water.

7. Heparin solution can cause precipitation of teniposide, flush administration apparatus thoroughly with D5W or 0.9% NaCl injection before and after administration.

8. Unopened ampules are stable until the date indicated if stored at 2–8°C (36–46°F) in the original package (protected from light).

9. Give solutions containing 1 mg/mL within 4 hr of preparation to reduce the potential for precipitation. Refrigeration of solutions is not recommended.

10. Precipitation of teniposide may occur at the recommended concentrations, especially if the diluted solution is agitated more than recommended during preparation. Also, minimize storage time prior to administration; take care to avoid contact of the diluted solution with other drugs or fluids.

11. Not for use in premature infants; contains benzyl alcohol.

ASSESSMENT

1. Note any sensitivity to product derivatives, especially polyoxyethylated ca-

---

Bold Italic = life threatening side effect   ■ = black box warning   ✢ = Available in Canada stor oil. Product also contains benzyl alcohol.

2. Premedicate with antiemetics; observe for enhanced CNS effects. If S&S of anaphylaxis occur (chills, fever, tachycardia, chest pain, dyspnea, or altered BP), interrupt infusion and report. May use corticosteroids and antihistamines in these clients if retreatment considered.

3. Reduce dose with Down syndrome, liver or renal dysfunction.

4. Monitor BP, hematologic profile, uric acid, renal and LFTs. May cause granulocyte and platelet suppression. Withhold if BP <90 systolic and platelet count <50,000/mm^3 or ANC <500/mm^3 do not resume treatment until hematologic recovery is evident. Nadir: 14 days; recovery: 21 days.

CLIENT/FAMILY TEACHING
1. Drug is a 'possible carcinogen'; review risk of developing secondary acute nonlymphocytic leukemia with intensive therapy schedules (1–2 times per week during remission).

2. Report promptly if fever, chills, rapid heartbeat, infusion site pain, or difficulty breathing occurs.

3. N&V and hair loss are frequent drug side effects.

4. Avoid those with infections and crowds to prevent any infections.

5. Drug will cause fetal harm; use reliable contraceptive measures during treatment.

OUTCOMES/EVALUATE
Remission with relapsed or refractory ALL

Tenofovir disoproxil fumarate (PMPA)   ■
(teh-**NOFF**-oh-veer)

CLASSIFICATION(S):
Antiviral, nucleoside reverse transcriptase inhibitor
PREGNANCY CATEGORY: B
Rx: Viread.

USES
In combination with other antiretroviral drugs to treat HIV-1 infection.

ACTION/KINETICS
Action
Tenofovir disoproxil fumarate requires initial diester hydrolysis for conversion to tenofovir and subsequent phosphorylation to form tenofovir diphosphate. Tenofovir diphosphate inhibits HIV reverse transcriptase activity by competing with the natural substrate deoxyadenosine 5'-triphosphate and, after incorporation into DNA, by DNA chain termination.

Pharmacokinetics
Bioavailability is about 25%. **Maximum serum levels:** About 1 hr. High fat meals increase the PO bioavailability with an increase in C_{max} of about 14% and AUC of about 40%. About 70–80% excreted unchanged in the urine by a combination of glomerular filtration and active tubular secretion. Impairment of renal or hepatic function affects the pharmacokinetics. **t½, terminal:** 17 hr.

CONTRAINDICATIONS
Hypersensitivity to tenofovir or any component of the product. Use in pregnancy only if clearly needed. Lactation.

SPECIAL CONCERNS
■ (1) Lactic acidosis and severe hepatomegaly with steatosis, including fatalities, may occur with the use of nucleoside analogs alone or in combination with other antiretrovirals. A majority of such cases have been in women. Obesity and prolonged nucleoside exposure may be risk factors. Use particular caution when giving nucleoside analogs to any client with known risk factors for liver disease. Cases have also been observed in those with no known risk factors. Suspend treatment in anyone who develops clinical or lab findings suggestive of lactic acidosis or prolonged hepatotoxicity, which may include hepatomegaly and steatosis, even in the absence of marked transaminase elevations. (2) Tenofovir is not indicated for the treatment of chronic hepatitis B virus infection, and the safety and efficacy of tenofovir have not been estab-

lished in clients coinfected with hepatitis B virus and HIV. Severe acute exacerbations of hepatitis B have been reported in clients who are coinfected with hepatitis B virus and HIV and have discontinued tenofovir. Closely monitor hepatic function with both clinical and laboratory follow-up for at least several months in clients who discontinue tenofovir and are coinfected with hepatitis B virus and HIV. If appropriate, initiation of anti-hepatitis B therapy may be warranted.■ A high rate of virologic failure and emergence of nucleoside reverse transcriptase inhibitor resistance may occur in clients receiving a regimen containing didanosine enteric-coated beadlets, lamivudine, and tenofovir. Use with caution in the elderly. Safety and efficacy have not been determined in children.

SIDE EFFECTS
Most Common
Asthenia, N&V, depression, headache, diarrhea, rashes, pain.
GI: N&V, diarrhea, flatulence, abdominal pain, anorexia, dyspepsia, pancreatitis. **CNS:** Headache, depression, insomnia, dizziness, abnormal dreams, paresthesia. **Dermatologic:** Rash, pruritus, maculopapular rash, urticaria, vesiculobullous rash, pustular rash, sweating. **GU:** Renal toxicity, renal insufficiency/failure, proximal tubulopathy, acute renal failure, acute tubular necrosis. **Body as a whole:** Asthenia, peripheral neuritis, neuropathy, pain, myalgia, arthralgia, fever, weight loss, pneumonia, allergic reaction. **Miscellaneous:** *Lactic acidosis, severe hepatomegaly with steatosis*, virologic failure, redistribution and accumulation of body fat, dyspnea, back pain, chest pain, Fanconi syndrome, bone toxicity (decreased bone density).

LABORATORY TEST CONSIDERATIONS
↑ AST, ALT, creatine kinase, creatinine, triglycerides, serum amylase, urine/serum glucose. ↓ Neutrophils. Hypophosphatemia. Proteinuria, hematuria.

DRUG INTERACTIONS
Abacavir / ↑ Abacavir C_{max}
Acyclovir / ↑ Levels of tenofovir R/T competition for tubular secretion
Atazanavir / ↓ Atazanavir levels; possible loss or lack of response; ↑ tenofovir AUC and C_{max}
Cidofovir / ↑ Levels of tenofovir R/T competition for tubular secretion
Didanosine / ↑ Maximum concentration and AUC of didanosine (buffered or enteric coated formulations
Ganciclovir / ↑ Levels of tenofovir R/T competition for tubular secretion
Indinavir / ↑ Tenofovir C_{max}; ↓ indinavir C_{max}
Lamivudine / ↓ Lamivudine C_{max}
Lopinavir/Ritonavir / ↑ Tenofovir C_{max} and AUC; ↓ lopinavir and ritonavir C_{max} and AUC
Valacyclovir / ↑ Tenofovir levels R/T competition for tubular secretion
Valganciclovir / ↑ Tenofovir levels R/T competition for tubular secretion

HOW SUPPLIED
Tablets: 300 mg (equivalent to 245 mg tenofovir disoproxil).

DOSAGE
- **TABLETS**
  HIV-1 infection.
300 mg once daily taken PO without regard to food. Adjust the dose as follows in renal impairment: **C_{CR}, 30–49 mL/min:** 300 mg q 48 hr; **C_{CR}, 10–29 mL/min:** 300 mg twice a week; **hemodialysis clients:** 300 mg q 7 days or after a total of about 12 hr of dialysis. *NOTE:* No dosing recommendation is available for those with C_{CR} <10 mL/min.

NURSING CONSIDERATIONS
ADMINISTRATION/STORAGE
Store from 15–30°C (59–86°F).

ASSESSMENT
1. Note reasons for therapy, disease onset, other therapies trialed. List drugs prescribed to ensure none interact.
2. Assess for evidence of liver/renal disease, hepatitis B coinfection, bone abnormalities, and acidosis. Monitor CBC, viral loads, renal and LFTs; anticipate reduced dose with renal dysfunction.

CLIENT/FAMILY TEACHING
1. When taken with didanosine, take the tenofovir 2 hr before or 1 hr after didanosine administration.

---

2. Take once a day as prescribed with a meal to enhance drug bioavailability.

3. May experience changes in body fat, N&V, diarrhea, and gas; report if intolerable.

4. Report any yellowing of skin or eyes, abdominal pain, muscle aches/pains; stop drug therapy.

5. Keep all F/U visits for labs and clinical evaluation

OUTCOMES/EVALUATE
Control of progression of tenofovir susceptible HIV infection

Terazosin   ©
(ter-**AY**-zoh-sin)

CLASSIFICATION(S):
Antihypertensive, alpha$_1$-adrenergic blocking drug

PREGNANCY CATEGORY: C
Rx: Hytrin.

❤Rx: Apo-Terazosin, Novo-Terazosin, Nu-Terazosin, PMS-Tarazosin, ratio-Terazosin.

USES
(1) Hypertension, alone or in combination with diuretics or beta-adrenergic blocking agents. (2) Symptoms of benign prostatic hyperplasia.

ACTION/KINETICS
Action
Blocks postsynaptic alpha$_1$-adrenergic receptors, leading to a dilation of both arterioles and veins, and ultimately, a reduction in BP. Both standing and supine BPs are lowered with no reflex tachycardia. Also relaxes smooth muscle of the prostate and bladder neck. Usefulness in BPH is due to alpha$_1$-receptor blockade, which relaxes the smooth muscle of the prostate and bladder neck and relieves pressure on the urethra.

Pharmacokinetics
Bioavailability is not affected by food. **Onset:** 15 min. **Peak plasma levels:** 1–2 hr. **t½:** 9–12 hr. **Duration:** 24 hr. Excreted unchanged and as inactive metabolites in both the urine and feces.

SPECIAL CONCERNS
Use with caution during lactation. Safety and efficacy have not been determined in children. Geriatric clients may be more sensitive to the hypotensive and hypothermic effects of terazosin.

SIDE EFFECTS
Most Common
Asthenia, dizziness, headache, somnolence, flu symptoms, nasal congestion, pharyngitis/rhinitis.

First-dose effect: Marked postural hypotension and syncope. **CV:** Palpitations, tachycardia, postural hypotension, syncope, *arrhythmias*, chest pain, vasodilation, atrial fibrillation. **CNS:** Dizziness, headache, somnolence, drowsiness, nervousness, paresthesia, depression, anxiety, insomnia, vertigo. **Respiratory:** Nasal congestion, dyspnea, sinusitis, epistaxis, bronchitis, *bronchospasm*, cold or flu symptoms, increased cough, pharyngitis, rhinitis. **GI:** Nausea, constipation, diarrhea, dyspepsia, dry mouth, vomiting, flatulence, abdominal discomfort or pain. **Musculoskeletal:** Asthenia, arthritis, arthralgia, myalgia, joint disorders, back pain, pain in extremities, neck and shoulder pain, muscle cramps. **Miscellaneous:** Peripheral edema, weight gain, blurred vision, impotence, chest pain, fever, gout, pruritus, rash, sweating, urinary frequency, UTI, tinnitus, conjunctivitis, abnormal vision, edema, facial edema, thrombocytopenia, priapism.

LABORATORY TEST CONSIDERATIONS
↓ H&H, WBCs, albumin.

OD OVERDOSE MANAGEMENT
Symptoms: Hypotension, drowsiness, *shock.* *Treatment:* Restore BP and HR. Client should be kept supine; vasopressors may be indicated. Volume expanders can be used to treat shock.

DRUG INTERACTIONS
When used with finasteride → ↑ finasteride plasma levels.

HOW SUPPLIED
Capsules: 1 mg, 2 mg, 5 mg, 10 mg.

DOSAGE
• **CAPSULES**
Hypertension.
Individualized, initial: 1 mg at bedtime (this dose is not to be exceeded);

then, increase dose slowly to obtain desired response. **Range:** 1–5 mg/day; doses as high as 20 mg may be required in some clients. Doses greater than 20 mg daily do not provide further BP control.

Benign prostatic hyperplasia. **Initial:** 1 mg/day; dose should be increased to 2 mg, 5 mg, and then 10 mg once daily to improve symptoms and/or urinary flow rates. Doses greater than 20 mg daily have not been studied.

NURSING CONSIDERATIONS

Ⓒ Do not confuse terazosin with temazepam (a sedative-hypnotic).

ADMINISTRATION/STORAGE

1. The initial dosing regimen must be carefully observed to minimize severe hypotension.
2. Monitor BP 2–3 hr after dosing and at end of dosing interval to ensure BP control maintained.
3. Consider an increase in dose or twice a day dosing if BP control is not maintained at 24-hr interval.
4. To prevent dizziness or fainting due to a drop in BP, take the initial dose at bedtime; the daily dose can be given in the morning.
5. If terazosin must be discontinued for more than a few days, reinstitute the initial dosing regimen if restarted.
6. Due to additive effects, use caution when combined with other antihypertensive agents.
7. When treating BPH, a minimum of 4–6 weeks of 10 mg/day may be needed to determine if a beneficial effect has occurred.

ASSESSMENT

1. Note onset, duration, characteristics of S&S, other agents trialed.
2. Assess BP, prostate gland, PSA level, BPH score.
3. A gradual increase in dose until symptom control, i.e., 1 mg/day for 7 days, then 2 mg/day for 7 days, then 3 mg/day for 7 days, then 4 mg/day for 7 days, and then 5 mg/day, may assist to diminish adverse effects and enhance compliance, especially in the elderly.

CLIENT/FAMILY TEACHING

1. Take initial dose at bedtime to minimize side effects. Do not stop abruptly or titration must restart. Use caution when performing activities that require mental alertness until drug effects realized; may cause dizziness or drowsiness.
2. Do not drive or undertake hazardous tasks for 12 hr after the first dose and after increasing dose or reinstituting therapy.
3. Avoid symptoms of dizziness (drop in BP) by rising slowly from a sitting or lying position and waiting until symptoms subside.
4. Do not take within 2 hr of meds used for erectile dysfunction.
5. Record BP, weight twice a week; report persistent side effects, excessive weight gain, low BP or extremity swelling.
6. Report if nighttime urinary frequency increases or does not improve after 2 months of therapy. Keep F/U visits for DRE and labs.

OUTCOMES/EVALUATE

- Improvement in BPH symptoms
- ↓ BP

Terbinafine hydrochloride ■ Ⓒ
(ter-**BIN**-ah-feen)

CLASSIFICATION(S):
Antifungal
PREGNANCY CATEGORY: B
OTC: DesenexMax, Lamisil AT.
Rx: Lamisil.
✿Rx: Apo-Terbinafine, Gen-Terbinafine, Novo-Terbinafine, PMS-Terbinafine.

USES
Topical use: (1) Interdigital tinea pedis (athlete's foot), tinea cruris (jock itch), or tinea corporis (ringworm) due to *Epidermophyton floccosum, Trichophyton mentagrophytes,* or *T. rubrum.* (2) Plantar tinea pedis. (3) Tinea versicolor due to *Malassezia furfur. Investigational:* Cutaneous candidiasis and tinea versicolor.

Bold Italic = life threatening side effect   ■ = black box warning   ✿ = Available in Canada

Oral use: Onychomycosis of the toenail or fingernail due to dermatophytes (tinea unguium).

ACTION/KINETICS

Action

Inhibits squalene epoxidase, a key enzyme in the sterol biosynthesis in fungi. Results in ergosterol deficiency and a corresponding accumulation of squalene leading to fungal cell death.

Pharmacokinetics

Approximately 75% of cutaneously absorbed drug is excreted in the urine, mostly as metabolites. Well absorbed following PO administration, with bioavailability after first-pass metabolism being about 40%. **Peak plasma levels:** 1 mcg/mL within 2 hr. Food enhances absorption. Slowly excreted from adipose tissue and skin. Inhibits CYP2D6-mediated metabolism. Extensively metabolized, with about 70% of the dose eliminated in the urine. Renal or hepatic disease decreases clearance from the body. **Plasma protein binding:** More than 99%.

CONTRAINDICATIONS

Ophthalmic or intravaginal use. PO use in chronic or active liver disease or renal impairment (C_{CR} less than 50 mL/min). Lactation.

SPECIAL CONCERNS

■ Rare cases of hepatic failure, some leading to death or liver transplant, have occurred with terbinafine use for the treatment of onychomycosis in those with and without preexisting liver disease. In the majority of such cases, clients had serious underlying systemic conditions and an uncertain causal relationship with terbinafine. Terbinafine is not recommended for those with chronic or active liver disease. Before prescribing, assess preexisting liver disease. Hepatotoxicity may occur in those with and without pre-existing liver disease. Pretreatment serum ALT and AST tests are advised for all those before taking terbinafine.■ Safety and efficacy have not been determined in children less than 12 years of age.

SIDE EFFECTS

Most Common

Following oral use: Headache, rash, diarrhea, dyspepsia, pruritus, nausea, taste disturbance.

Following topical use: Irritation, burning, itching, dryness.

Following oral use. GI: Diarrhea, dyspepsia, abdominal pain, nausea, flatulence, vomiting, taste disturbance, rarely taste loss, *rarely, severe and fatal liver failure.* **Dermatologic:** Rash, pruritus, urticaria, *Stevens-Johnson syndrome, toxic epidermal necrolysis.* **Body as a whole:** Malaise, fatigue, arthralgia, myalgia. **Miscellaneous:** Headache, taste or visual disturbances (changes in the ocular lens or retina), hair loss. Rarely, symptomatic idiosyncratic hepatobiliary dysfunction (including cholestatic hepatitis), severe neutropenia, thrombocytopenia, allergic reactions (including *anaphylaxis*). **Following topical use. Dermatologic:** Irritation, burning, itching, dryness.

LABORATORY TEST CONSIDERATIONS

Liver enzyme abnormalities that are two or more times the upper limit of the normal range. ↓ Absolute neutrophil counts.

DRUG INTERACTIONS

Beta blockers / ↓ Metabolism of beta blockers by CYP2D6; possible ↑ pharmacologic and toxic effects

Caffeine / ↑ Clearance of IV caffeine

Cimetidine / Terbinafine clearance is ↓ by one-third

Cyclosporine / ↑ Cyclosporine clearance

Dextromethorphan / ↑ Dextromethorphan levels R/T ↓ liver metabolism by CYP2D6

MAOIs type B / ↓ Metabolism MAOIs, type B by CYP2D6; possible ↑ pharmacologic and toxic effects

Rifampin / ↑ Terbinafine clearance (100%)

Selective serotonin reuptake inhibitors (SSRIs) / ↓ Metabolism of SSRIs by CYP2D6; possible ↑ pharmacologic and toxic effects

Tricyclic antidepressants / ↓ Metabolism of tricyclic antidepressants by

CYP2D6; possible ↑ pharmacologic and toxic effects
Warfarin / Altered PT

HOW SUPPLIED

Cream: 1%; Gel: 1%; Spray: 1%; Tablets: 250 mg.

DOSAGE

- **CREAM; GEL**

    Interdigital tinea pedis.

Apply to cover the affected and immediately surrounding areas twice a day for 1 week. The cream is OTC.

    Tinea cruris or tinea corporis.

Apply to cover the affected and immediately surrounding areas 1–2 times per day for 1 week.

- **SPRAY**

    Tinea pedis, Tinea versicolor.

Spray twice a day for one week.

    Tinea corporis, Tinea cruris.

Spray once daily for one week.

- **TABLETS**

    Onychomycosis.

Fingernail(s): 250 mg/day for 6 weeks. *Toenail(s):* 250 mg/day for 12 weeks. Alternatively, intermittent dosing may be used: 500 mg daily for 1 week each month (use 2 months for fingernails and 4 months for toenails). The optimal clinical effect is observed several months after mycologic cure and cessation of treatment due to slow period for outgrowth of healthy nails.

NURSING CONSIDERATIONS

℃ Do not confuse Lamisil with Lamictil (an anticonvulsant).

ADMINISTRATION/STORAGE

1. Avoid contact of cream with eyes, nose, mouth, or other mucous membranes.

2. Avoid occlusive dressings.

3. For topical use, many clients treated for 1–2 weeks continue to improve during the 2–4 weeks after drug therapy has been completed. Do not consider clients therapeutic failures until they have been observed for a period of 2–4 weeks off therapy.

4. Store the cream between 5–30°C (41–86°F). Protect tablets from light; store below 25°C (77°F).

ASSESSMENT

1. Note clinical presentation; list location, onset, duration, and characteristics of symptoms.

2. If presentation unclear, use infected tissue scrapings to confirm diagnosis.

3. Obtain baseline AST and ALT; note any liver or renal dysfunction.

CLIENT/FAMILY TEACHING

1. Cream for topical dermatologic use only; review application method.

2. Wash hands before and after topical application. Use a clean towel and washcloth; avoid sharing.

3. Avoid contact of cream with mouth, nose, eyes, and other mucous membranes; do not cover treated areas with occlusive dressing.

4. Take tablets with food to ensure maximal absorption.

5. Report symptoms of increased irritation or possible sensitization such as redness, itching, burning, blistering, swelling, or oozing.

6. Use for prescribed time; do not skip or double up on doses.

7. Continued improvement in skin condition and/or mycotic nails may be noted for 2–4 weeks after therapy.

OUTCOMES/EVALUATE

- Improvement in dermatologic condition

- Clearing/healing of mycotic nail beds

Terbutaline sulfate ©
(ter-**BYOU**-tah-leen)

CLASSIFICATION(S):
Sympathomimetic, direct-acting
PREGNANCY CATEGORY: B
Rx: Brethine.

SEE ALSO *SYMPATHOMIMETIC DRUGS*.

USES

Prophylaxis and treatment of bronchospasm in clients 12 years and older with asthma and reversible bronchospasms associated with bronchitis and emphysema. *Investigational:* Tocolytic agent to treat preterm labor.

Bold Italic = life threatening side effect   ■ = black box warning   ♣ = Available in Canada

ACTION/KINETICS
Action
Specific beta-2 receptor stimulant, resulting in bronchodilation and relaxation of peripheral vasculature. Minimum beta-1 activity. Action resembles that of isoproterenol.

Pharmacokinetics
PO, Onset: 30 min; **maximum effect:** 2–3 hr; **duration:** 4–8 hr. **SC, Onset:** 5–15 min; **maximum effect:** 30 min–1 hr; **duration:** 1.5–4 hr. **Inhalation, Onset:** 5–30 min; **time to peak effect:** 1–2 hr; **duration:** 3–6 hr.

CONTRAINDICATIONS
Lactation.

SPECIAL CONCERNS
Large IV doses may aggravate preexisting diabetes and ketoacidosis. Safe use in children less than 12 years of age not established.

SIDE EFFECTS
Most Common
Palpitations, tremor, dizziness/vertigo, nervousness/tension, N&V, PVCs/arrhythmias, drowsiness, headache.

See *Sympathomimetic Drugs* for a complete list of possible side effects. Also, **CV:** PVCs, ECG changes (e.g., atrial premature beats, ventricular premature beats, AV block, sinus pause, ST-T wave depression, T-wave inversion, sinus bradycardia, atrial escape beat (with aberrant conduction), tachycardia. **Respiratory:** Wheezing. **Miscellaneous:** *Hypersensitivity reactions* (including vasculitis), flushing, sweating, bad taste or taste change, muscle cramps, CNS stimulation, pain at injection site, elevation in liver enzymes.

LABORATORY TEST CONSIDERATIONS
↑ Liver enzymes.

HOW SUPPLIED
Injection: 1 mg/mL; *Tablets:* 2.5 mg, 5 mg.

DOSAGE
- **TABLETS**
  Bronchodilation.

Adults and children over 15 years: 5 mg 3 times per day q 6 hr during waking hours, not to exceed 15 mg q 24 hr. If disturbing side effects are observed, dose can be reduced to 2.5 mg 3 times per day without loss of beneficial effects. Anticipate use of other therapeutic measures if client fails to respond after second dose. **Children 12–15 years:** 2.5 mg 3 times per day, not to exceed 7.5 mg q 24 hr.

- **SC ONLY**
  Bronchodilation.

Adults: 0.25 mg into the lateral deltoid area. May be repeated 1 time after 15–30 min if no significant clinical improvement is noted. If client does not respond to the second dose, undertake other measures. Do not exceed a dose of 0.5 mg over 4 hr.

NURSING CONSIDERATIONS
 Do not confuse terbutaline with terbinafine (antifungal) or tolbutamide (an oral hypoglycemic).

ADMINISTRATION/STORAGE
1. Discard unused portion after single client use.
2. Do not use if solution is discolored.
3. Store tablets and injection, protected from light, from 15–30°C (59–86°F).

ASSESSMENT
1. Note type, onset, characteristics of S&S.
2. Auscultate and document lung assessments and PFTs. Observe respiratory client for evidence of drug tolerance and rebound bronchospasm.
3. Note frequency/consistency/duration of contractions, fetal HR with preterm labor. With SC administration the lateral deltoid is often used.
4. Observe mother for headache, tremor, anxiety, palpitations, symptoms of pulmonary edema, and tachycardia. Assess fetus for distress; report increased contractions. Monitor both for symptoms of hypoglycemia and mother for hypokalemia. A mild analgesic may be used for drug-induced headaches.

CLIENT/FAMILY TEACHING
1. Take oral medication with meals to minimize GI upset.
2. Review and demonstrate appropriate method for administration.
3. Report any persistent or bothersome side effects. Do not increase dose or frequency if symptoms are not relieved. Report so dose can be reevaluated.

---

4. May use analgesic to relieve headache, use deltoid area for injections and if bronchospasm occurs with inhaltion therapy report immediately.

5. Increase fluid intake to help liquefy secretions.

6. With preterm labor, notify provider immediately if labor resumes or unusual side effects are noted.

OUTCOMES/EVALUATE
• Improved airway exchange
• Inhibition of premature labor

Terconazole nitrate
(ter-**KON**-ah-zohl)

CLASSIFICATION(S):
Antifungal
PREGNANCY CATEGORY: C
Rx: Terazol 3, Terazol 7, Zazole.
✤**Rx:** Terazol.

USES
Vulvovaginitis caused by *Candida*. Ineffective in infections due to *Trichomonas* or *Haemophilus vaginalis*.

ACTION/KINETICS
Action
May exert its antifungal activity by disrupting cell membrane permeability leading to loss of essential intracellular materials. Also inhibits synthesis of triglycerides and phospholipids, as well as inhibiting oxidative and peroxidative enzyme activity. When used for *Candida*, terconazole inhibits transformation of blastospores into the invasive mycelial form.

SPECIAL CONCERNS
During lactation, consider discontinuing nursing or the drug. Safety and efficacy have not been established in children.

SIDE EFFECTS
Most Common
Headache, dysmenorrhea, pain of the female genitalia, abdominal pain, vulvovaginal burning/irritation.
GU: Vulvovaginal burning, irritation, or itching; dysmenorrhea, pain of the female genitalia. **Miscellaneous:** Headache, body pain, photosensitivity, abdominal pain, chills, fever.

HOW SUPPLIED
Vaginal Cream: 0.4%, 0.8%; *Vaginal Suppositories:* 80 mg.

DOSAGE
• **VAGINAL CREAM**
Vulvovaginitis due to Candida.
One applicator full (5 grams) intravaginally, once daily at bedtime for 7 consecutive days for the 0.4% cream and for 3 consecutive days for the 0.8% cream.

• **VAGINAL SUPPOSITORIES**
Vulvovaginitis due to Candida.
One 80-mg suppository once daily at bedtime for 3 consecutive days.

NURSING CONSIDERATIONS
ASSESSMENT
1. Obtain a thorough nursing history because recurrent candidiasis may be caused by oral contraceptives, antibiotics, or diabetes whereas intractable candidiasis may be the result of undetected diabetes mellitus or reinfection.

2. Prior to a second course of therapy, the diagnosis should be confirmed to rule out other pathogens associated with vulvovaginitis.

CLIENT/FAMILY TEACHING
1. Review the appropriate method for administration and cleansing (the cream should be inserted high into the vagina using the applicator). After suppositories administered remain lying down for 30 min. Sitz baths and vaginal douches may also be used.

2. Discontinue use and report if any burning, irritation, fever, chills, or pain occurs.

3. May stain clothes; use sanitary napkins during therapy and change frequently because damp sanitary napkins may harbor infecting organisms. Avoid tampons during therapy.

4. To avoid reinfection, refrain from sexual intercourse. Advise partner to use a condom as med may also irritate partner; use care as drug may interact with diaphragm and latex condoms.

5. Use for prescribed time frame even if symptoms subside.

Bold Italic = life threatening side effect   ■ = black box warning   ✤ = Available in Canada

6. Effect not affected by menses. Thus, continue to use during menses to ensure a full course of therapy.

OUTCOMES/EVALUATE
Resolution of fungal infections; symptomatic improvement

Testolactone
(tes-toe-**LACK**-tohn)

CLASSIFICATION(S):
Antineoplastic, hormone
PREGNANCY CATEGORY: C
Rx: Teslac, **C-III**

SEE ALSO *TESTOSTERONE.*

USES
Palliative treatment of advanced disseminated breast cancer in postmenopausal women or in premenopausal ovariectomized clients. Is effective in only 15% of clients.

ACTION/KINETICS
Action
Synthetic steroid related to testosterone. May act to reduce synthesis of estrone from adrenal androstenedione by inhibiting steroid aromatase activity. Does not cause virilization.

Pharmacokinetics
Well absorbed from the GI tract. Metabolized in the liver and unchanged drug and metabolites are excreted through the urine.

CONTRAINDICATIONS
Breast cancer in men. Lactation. Premenopausal women with intact ovaries.

SPECIAL CONCERNS
Safety and efficacy have not been determined in children.

SIDE EFFECTS
Most Common
N&V, anorexia, glossitis, inflammation/irritation at injection site, alopecia.
See *Antineoplastic Agents* for a complete list of possible side effects. Also, **GI:** N&V, glossitis, anorexia. **CNS:** Numbness or tingling of fingers, toes, face. **Miscellaneous:** Inflammation and irritation at injection site; increased BP. Hypercalcemia. Maculopapular erythema, alopecia, aches and edema of the extremities, nail growth disturbances.

LABORATORY TEST CONSIDERATIONS
↑ Plasma calcium, urinary excretion of creatine (24 hr) and 17-ketosteroids. ↓ Estradiol levels using radioimmunoassays.

DRUG INTERACTIONS
Testolactone may ↑ effect of oral anticoagulants

HOW SUPPLIED
Tablets: 50 mg.

DOSAGE
• **TABLETS**
  Advanced disseminated breast cancer.
  250 mg 4 times per day. Continue therapy for 3 months unless there is active progression of the disease.

NURSING CONSIDERATIONS
ASSESSMENT
Note onset of breast cancer, duration of symptoms, other agents or therapies trialed. Monitor fluid and electrolytes and calcium levels.

INTERVENTIONS
1. Reduce dose of anticoagulants with concomitant therapy and monitor INR.
2. The effect of the steroid and osteolytic metastases may result in hypercalcemia. Monitor calcium levels and assess for symptoms of hypercalcemia (insomnia, lethargy, anorexia, N&V). Encourage high fluid intake (2–3 L/day) to minimize hypercalcemia. Assess need for diuretics if edema persists.
3. Monitor BP and report any significant increases >20 mm Hg DBP.
4. Perform ROM exercises if bedridden and encourage others to exercise to reduce calcium levels, improve circulation, and prevent thrombophlebitis.

CLIENT/FAMILY TEACHING
1. Drug is usually given for a minimum of 3 months. After 6–12 weeks, may assess for desired clinical response:
• Decrease in size of tumor
• Nonosseous lesion reduction by 50%
2. Ensure at least 2 L fluid intake daily to prevent dehydration and elevated calcium levels.
3. Report all adverse side effects; keep regularly scheduled followup appointments.

 = see color insert   = Herbal   **IV** = Intravenous   = sound alike drug

OUTCOMES/EVALUATE
↓ Tumor size and spread

Testosterone ©
(tess-**TOSS**-ter-ohn)

CLASSIFICATION(S):
Androgen, naturally-occurring
PREGNANCY CATEGORY: X
Rx: Buccal System: Striant. **Gel:** AndroGel 1%, Testim. **Pellets:** Testopel, **C-III**

Testosterone cypionate in oil
PREGNANCY CATEGORY: X
Rx: Depo-Testosterone, **C-III**
✦**Rx:** Depo-Testosterone Cypionate.

Testosterone enanthate in oil
PREGNANCY CATEGORY: X
Rx: Delatestryl, **C-III**

Testosterone transdermal system
PREGNANCY CATEGORY: X
Rx: Androderm, **C-III**

USES
Parenteral: (1) Congenital or acquired primary hypogonadism. (2) Congenital or acquired hypogonadotropic hypogonadism. (3) Delayed puberty (use testostatic enanthate only). (4) Metastatic mammary cancer in females (use testosterone enanthate only) who are 1–5 years postmenopausal. *Investigational:* Male contraceptive (testosterone enanthate).
Buccal/Gel: (1) Congenital or acquired primary hypogonadism. (2) Congenital or acquired hypogonadotropic hypogonadism.
Pellets: (1) Congenital or acquired primary hypogonadism. (2) Congenital

or acquired hypogonadotropic hypogonadism. (3) Stimulation of puberty in carefully selected males with clearly delayed puberty.
Transdermal products: (1) Acquired or congenital primary hypogonadism. (2) Acquired or congenital secondary hypogonadotropic hypogonadism.

ACTION/KINETICS
Action
Testosterone, the primary male androgen, is produced naturally by the Leydig cells of the testes. In many tissues, the action of testosterone is due to the active metabolite, dihydrotestosterone, which binds to cytosol receptors. The steroid-receptor complex is transported to the nucleus where it initiates transcription and other cellular changes. Exogenous testosterone administration results in inhibition of endogenous testosterone release due to negative feedback of pituitary LH. Large doses of exogenous testosterone may suppress spermatogenesis through feedback inhibition of pituitary FSH.

Pharmacokinetics
Oral testosterone is metabolized in the gut and 44% is cleared by the liver in the first pass. Thus, the parenteral, transdermal, and gel forms are used. Testosterone esters (cypionate or enanthate) are slowly absorbed after IM use. The $t\frac{1}{2}$ of testosterone varies over a wide range (10–100 min). $t\frac{1}{2}$, **testosterone cypionate after IM:** 8 days. Following use of Androderm to nonscrotal skin, there is continual absorption over 24 hr. Ninety percent is excreted through the urine as metabolites and 6% is excreted through the feces. **Plasma protein binding:** About 98%.

CONTRAINDICATIONS
Serious renal, hepatic, or cardiac disease due to edema formation. Known or suspected prostatic or breast carcinoma in males. Use in pregnancy (masculinization of female fetus) and lactation. Discontinue if hypercalcemia occurs.

SPECIAL CONCERNS
Prolonged use of high doses associated with development of potentially life-threatening peliosis hepatitis, hepatic

---

neoplasms, cholestatic hepatitis, jaundice, and hepatocellular carcinoma. Use with caution in young males who have not completed their growth (because of premature epiphyseal closure). Androgens may also cause virilization in females or precocious sexual development in males. Geriatric clients may manifest an increased risk of prostatic hypertrophy or prostatic carcinoma. Androgen therapy occasionally seems to accelerate metastatic breast carcinoma in women. Use of the gel has not been evaluated in women. Use with caution in children.

SIDE EFFECTS

Most Common

When used systemically or by implant: Headache, anxiety, depression, generalized paresthesia, acne, hirsutism, nausea, cholestatic jaundice, libido increased/decreased.

When used transdermally: Pruritus, application site itching/erythema, headache, dizziness/vertigo, burn-like blister under system.

Hepatic: Liver toxicity is the most serious side effect. Jaundice, cholestasis, alterations in BSP retention, AST, and ALT. Rarely, *hepatic necrosis*, *hepatocellular neoplasms*, peliosis hepatitis, acute intermittent porphyria in clients with this disease. **GI:** N&V, diarrhea, anorexia, symptoms of peptic ulcer. **CNS:** Headache, anxiety, increased or decreased libido, insomnia, excitation, paresthesias, sleep apnea syndrome, *CNS hemorrhage*, chills, choreiform movements, habituation, confusion (toxic doses). **GU:** Testicular atrophy with inhibition of testicular function (e.g., oligospermia), impotence, epididymitis, irritable bladder, prepubertal phallic enlargement, gynecomastia, hypercalcemia in breast cancer. **Electrolyte:** Retention of sodium, chloride, calcium, potassium, phosphates. Edema, with or without CHF. **Miscellaneous:** Acne, flushing, suppression of clotting factors (II, V, VII, X), polycythemia, leukopenia, rashes, dermatitis, *anaphylaxis (rare)*, muscle cramps, hypercholesterolemia, male-pattern baldness, acne, seborrhea, hirsutism. Hypercalcemia, especially in im-

mobilized clients or those with metastatic breast carcinoma. Virilization in women.

In females: Menstrual irregularities (including amenorrhea), virilization, clitoral enlargement, hirsutism, increased libido, baldness (male pattern), virilization of external genitalia of female fetus.

In males: Decreased ejaculatory volume, oligospermia (high doses), gynecomastia, increased frequency and duration of penile erections.

In children: Disturbances of growth, premature closure of epiphyses, precocious sexual development. Inflammation and pain at site of IM or SC injection.

NOTE: Side effects of the cypionate and enanthate products are not readily reversible due to the long duration of action of these dosage forms. The patch may cause itching, irritation, erythema, or discomfort on skin areas where applied (Androderm). Potentially, small amounts of testosterone may be transferred to a sex partner.

LABORATORY TEST CONSIDERATIONS

Altered thyroid function tests, including ↓ levels of throxine-binding globulin causing decreased total T_4 serum levels and ↑ resin uptake of T_3 and T_4. False + or ↑ BSP, alkaline phosphatase, bilirubin, cholesterol, and acid phosphatase (in women). Alteration of glucose tolerance tests.

DRUG INTERACTIONS

Anticoagulants, oral / ↑ Anticoagulant effect

Antidiabetic agents / Additive hypoglycemia

Barbiturates / ↓ Androgenic effect R/T ↑ breakdown by liver

Corticosteroids, ACTH / ↑ Chance of edema

Insulin / In diabetics, ↓ blood glucose → ↓ insulin requirements

Propranolol / ↑ Propranolol clearance if used with testosterone cypionate

H *Saw palmetto* / Antiandrogenic effect may ↓ testosterone activity

HOW SUPPLIED

Testosterone buccal system: 30 mg.

Testosterone cypionate: *Injection:* 100 mg/mL, 200 mg/mL.
Testosterone enanthate: *Injection:* 200 mg/mL.
Testosterone gel: *Gel:* 1%; *Metered Dose Pump:* 1%.
Testosterone pellets: *Pellets:* 75 mg.
Testosterone transdermal system: *Film, Extended-Release:* 2.5 mg/24 hr, 4 mg/24 hr, 5 mg/24 hr, 6 mg/24 hr.

DOSAGE

TESTOSTERONE ENANTHATE AND CYPIONATE.
• **IM ONLY**
Male hypogonadism, replacement therapy.
50–400 mg q 2–4 weeks.
Delayed puberty, males.
50–200 mg q 2–4 weeks for no more than 4–6 months.
Palliation of inoperable breast cancer in women (testosterone enanthate only).
200–400 mg q 2–4 weeks. Monitor closely as androgen therapy may accelerate the disease.
• **BUCCAL SYSTEM**
Primary hypogonadism, Hypogonadotropic hypogonadism.
Apply 1 buccal system (30 mg) to the gum region twice a day, morning and evening (i.e., about 12 hr apart).
• **GEL**
Primary hypogonadism, Hypogonadotropic hypogonadism.
Apply 5 grams (50 mg testosterone) once daily (preferable in the morning) to clean, dry, intact skin of the shoulders, upper arms, and/or abdomen. Do not apply Testim to the abdomen.
• **PELLETS**
Replacement therapy.
150–450 mg SC q 3–6 months.
Delayed puberty.
Often a lower dose range is used than for replacement and for a limited time duration (e.g., 4–6 months). The number of pellets to be implanted for all uses depends on the minimum daily requirement of testosterone determined by a gradual reduction of the amount given parenterally. The usual ratio is to implant two-75 mg pellets for each 25 mg testosterone propionate required weekly. About ⅓ of the material is absorbed during the first month, ¼ the second month, and ⅙ the third month.
• **TRANSDERMAL SYSTEM**
Replacement therapy (congenital or acquired primary hypogonadism, congenital or acquired hypogonadotropic hypogonadism).
Testoderm and Testoderm with Adhesive: One 6-mg patch applied daily on clean, dry scrotal skin that has been dry-shaved to remove hair. Clients with a smaller scrotum can use a 4-mg patch. Are designed to be applied to scrotal skin only. The patch should be worn for 22–24 hr/day for 6–8 weeks. *Androderm:*
Initial dose, usual: One 5-mg system or two 2.5-mg systems applied nightly for 24 hr providing a total dose of 5 mg/day. The systems are applied to a clean, dry area of the skin on the back, abdomen, upper arms, or thighs. Do not apply to the scrotum. *NOTE:* For the nonvirilized client, dosing may be started with one 2.5 mg system applied nightly.

NURSING CONSIDERATIONS

Ⓒ Do not confuse testosterone with testolactone (antineoplastic drug).

ADMINISTRATION/STORAGE
1. The following information is applicable to testosterone cypionate and/or testosterone enanthate:
• Do not use testosterone enanthate interchangeably with testosterone cypionate R/T differences in duration of action.
• Redissolve crystals of testosterone enanthate or cypionate by warming and shaking the vial.
• If needle or syringe is wet, product may become cloudy; this does not affect potency.
• Warm unopened vial in warm water to decrease the viscosity of the oil. Vigorously rotate vial to resuspend drug in the oil. A film may appear on the sides of the vial. When no more suspended particles are observed on the bottom or sides of the vial, the drug has been suspended appropriately. Administer deep into the muscle; give slowly.

Bold Italic = life threatening side effect　■ = black box warning　✦ = Available in Canada

- Continue therapy for at least 2 months for satisfactory response and 5 months for objective response.
- When used for delayed puberty, consider the chronological and skeletal ages when determining initial and subsequent doses. Use is for a limited time (e.g., 4–6 months).

2. The following information is applicable to testosterone gel:
- When using the gel, squeeze the entire contents of the packet onto the palm of the hand and apply immediately to the application site. Allow the site to dry for a few minutes prior to dressing. Wash hands with soap and water after application. Do not apply gel to the genitals.
- After applying the gel, wait 5–6 hr or more before showering or swimming.
- Measure serum testosterone levels 14 days after beginning therapy with the gel. If the desired serum testosterone levels are below the normal range or if the desired effect has not been reached, the dose may be increased from 5 to 7.5 grams and from 7.5 to 10 grams.
- Testosterone from the gel will be transferred from males to female partners. Washing the area of contact on the other person as soon as possible with soap and water will remove residual testosterone from the skin surface.

3. Store testosterone pellets in a cool place.

4. The following information is applicable to *Testoderm* and *Testoderm with Adhesive* transdermal systems:
- Dry-shave scrotal hair for optimal skin contact. Do not use chemical depilatories.
- If the system comes off after it has been worn for more than 12 hr and it cannot be reapplied, the client may wait until it is time for the next routine application to apply a new system.
- To determine serum total testosterone, draw blood 2–4 hr after system application after 3–4 weeks of daily system use.

- If clients have not achieved desired results by the end of 6–8 weeks, consider another form of testosterone replacement therapy.
- Prior to sexual activity, remove the Testoderm patch from the scrotum and wash the scrotal area to remove residue.

5. The following information is applicable to *Androderm* transdermal system:
- Do not apply the Androderm patch to bony areas such as the shoulders or hips; it is *not* to be applied to the scrotum.
- Sites of application should be rotated, with an interval of 7 days between applications to the same site. Areas should not be oily, damaged, or irritated.
- The system does not have to be removed during sexual intercourse or while taking a shower or bath.
- Apply Androderm immediately after opening the pouch and removing protective liner. Press the system firmly in place, making sure there is good contact with the skin, especially around the edges of the patch.

6. For all transdermal products, do not use damaged patches. Excessive heat or pressure can cause drug reservoir to burst. Discard systems safely to prevent accidental application or ingestion by children, pets, or others.

7. The following information is applicable to testosterone buccal:
- Place buccal product in a comfortable position just above the incisor tooth on either side of the mouth. With each application, rotate to alternate sides of the mouth.
- After opening the packet, place the rounded side surface of the buccal system against the gum and hold firmly in place with a finger over the lip and against the product for 30 seconds to ensure adhesion. The system is designed to stay in place until removed.
- If the buccal system fails to adhere to the gum or should fall out of position within 4 hr before the next dose, apply a new buccal system; it may

remain in place until the time of the next regularly scheduled dosing.

- Take care to avoid dislodging the buccal system and check to see that it is still in place following tooth-brushing, use of mouthwash, or consumption of food/beverages.
- Do not chew or swallow the buccal system.
- To remove the system, gently slide it downwards from the gum toward the tooth to avoid scratching the gum.
- Store from 20–25°C (68–77°F). Protect from light and moisture. Dispose of buccal systems in a manner that prevents accidental application or ingestion by children or pets.

8. Due to variability in analytical values among various diagnostic labs, have testosterone levels analyzed at the same lab so results can be compared more easily.

ASSESSMENT
1. Note reasons for therapy, type, onset, characteristics of S&S.
2. Assess for any cardiac, renal, or hepatic dysfunction. List neurologic status, BP, respirations, heart sounds, and GU function.
3. Note hair distribution and skin texture.
4. Check prescribed medications for any drugs that may interact unfavorably (i.e., anticoagulants, hypoglycemic agents, and mineralocorticoids).
5. Determine if pregnant. Monitor CBC, serum glucose, calcium, electrolytes, cholesterol, liver and renal function studies.
6. Treatment with aplastic anemia has resulted in several cases of hepatocellular carcinoma.

INTERVENTIONS
1. Monitor for signs of mental depression such as insomnia, lack of interest in personal appearance, and withdrawal from social contacts.
2. Monitor weight, BP, pulse, and serum electrolytes. Auscultate lung sounds and note any JVD. Report edema, as sodium retention and edema can be easily treated with diuretics.

3. Assess for relaxation of the skeletal muscles and pain deep in the bones. The discomfort in the bones is caused by a honeycombing; often caused by increased calcium levels.
4. Flank pain may be caused by kidney stones from excessively high serum calcium levels. Administer large amounts of fluids to prevent renal calculi. If hypercalcemia is the result of metastases, initiate other appropriate therapy.
5. Observe for jaundice, malaise, complaints of RUQ pain, pruritus, or a change in the color/consistency of stools. Document LFTs.
6. Observe for easy bruising, bleeding, S&S sore throat or fever. Obtain CBC to rule out polycythemia and leukopenia.
7. With a child, monitor closely for growth retardation and development of precocious puberty. Use with caution as the effect on the CNS in developing children is still being explored.

- Review therapy with parents; often intermittent to allow for periods of normal bone growth.
- Regular x-rays to monitor bone maturation and effects on epiphyseal centers; obtain q 6 months.
- Record height/weight regularly.

8. If female, report the signs of virilization, (except in those with gender disorder requesting such changes) such as deepening of the voice, hirsuitism, acne, menstrual irregularity, and clitoral enlargement. Usually only evident with doses exceeding 200–300 mg/month.
9. Increased libido in females may be early sign of drug toxicity.
10. Report if acne is severe; may be necessary to change dose.
11. May alter serum lipid levels enhancing susceptibility to arteriosclerotic heart disease in women; monitor thyroid and lipid panel.

CLIENT/FAMILY TEACHING
1. Review method for administration/application, dosage, frequency of administration, site preparation, and time of application for the transdermal patch.
2. Apply testoderm on clean, dry scrotal skin; may need to have scrotal hair to ensure adherence. Apply to clean dry

skin; Androderm to back, abdomen, upper arms or thighs and Testoderm TTS to back, arm, or upper buttocks. May be reapplied after swimming or bathing.

3. The buccal system should be placed in a comfortable position just above the incisor tooth on either side of the mouth. Rotate to alternate sides of the mouth with each application. To apply the buccal system, place the rounded side surface against the gum and hold firmly in place with a finger over the lip and against the product for 30 seconds to ensure adhesion. If the system fails to adhere properly to the gum or should fall off during the 12-hr dosing interval, remove the old system and apply a new one. If the system falls out of position within 4 hr before the next dose, apply a new system; it may remain in place until the time of the next regularly scheduled dosing. To remove the system, gently slide it downwards from the gum toward the tooth to avoid scratching the gum. Take care to avoid dislodging the buccal system and check to see it is still in place after toothbrushing, use of mouthwash or consumption of food or beverages. Do not chew or swallow the buccal system.

4. Report any unusual incidents of bleeding/bruising. Androgens suppress clotting factors (II, V, VII, and X); polycythemia and leukopenia may occur.

5. If drug received via pellets, sloughing can occur; report.

6. In older males, urinary obstruction may occur as a result of enlarged prostate.

7. Parents of children receiving testosterone should record weight twice a week and height every 2–3 months. X-rays will be performed periodically on prepubertal children to assess effect on bone growth.

8. Women with metastatic breast cancer need lab tests of serum and urine calcium levels, alkaline phosphatase, and serum cholesterol. If the serum cholesterol level is high, the dosage of drug may need to be changed. Follow a low-cholesterol diet and see dietitian for further assistance with diet. Facial hair and acne in females are reversible once drug withdrawn.

9. Drug may cause irregularities in the menstrual cycle; in postmenopausal women may cause withdrawal bleeding.

10. Use reliable birth control during and for several weeks after therapy withdrawn. Report if pregnancy suspected; increased risk of fetal abnormalities with this drug.

11. Males should report breast swelling or sustained erections; may necessitate drug withdrawal (at least temporarily).

12. Report any tingling of the fingers and toes or loss of appetite.

13. Follow a diet high in calories, proteins, vitamins, minerals, and other nutrients. Restrict sodium to reduce extremity swelling. Perform regular daily exercise to maintain weight and muscle mass.

14. With diabetes, hypoglycemia may occur. Report extreme variations as diet and/or dose of antidiabetic agents may require modification.

15. In females with gender disorder, monitor testosterone levels and assess CBC, thyroid and lipid panels regularly (4 months).

16. Review potential for drug abuse. High doses of androgens for enhancement of athletic performance can result in serious irreversible side effects/permanent physical damage.

OUTCOMES/EVALUATE

- Replacement therapy with control of S&S of androgen deficiency
- Male contraceptive agent
- Suppression of breast tumor size and spread
- Desired gender reassignment

Tetracycline hydrochloride

(teh-trah-**SYE**-kleen)

CLASSIFICATION(S):
Antibiotic, tetracycline
PREGNANCY CATEGORY: D
Rx: Capsules: Sumycin '250' and '500'. **Dental Fiber:** Actisite. **Syrup:** Sumycin Syrup.

♣Rx: Apo-Tetra, Novo-Tetra, Nu-Tetra.

SEE ALSO *TETRACYCLINES*.

USES

PO: (1) Gram-negative organisms, including *Haemophilus ducreyi* (chancroid), *Francisella tularensis* (tularemia), *Yersinia pestis* (plague), *Bartonella bacilliformis* (bartonellosis), *Campylobacter fetus, Vibrio cholerae* (cholera), *Brucella* species (in conjunction with streptomycin), *Calymmatobacterium granulomatis* (granuloma inguinale). (2) Infections caused by: *Rickettsiae* (Rocky Mountain spotted fever, typus fever and the typus group, Q fever, rickettsialpox, tick fevers); *Mycoplasma pneumoniae* (respiratory tract infections), *Chlamydia trachomatis* (lymphogranuloma venerum, trachoma, inclusion conjunctivitis, uncomplicated urethral, endocervical or rectal infections), *Chlamydia psittaci* (psittacosis), *Borellia* species (relapsing fever), *Ureaplasma urealyticum* (nongonoccal urethritis) (3) Following susceptibility testing (resistance has been noted) for the following: *Escherichia coli, Enterobacter aerogenes, Acinetobacter* species, *Haemophilus influenzae* (URTI), *Klebsiella* species (respiratory and UTI), *Streptococcus pneumoniae* (upper respiratory infections), *Streptococcus pyogenes, S. pneumoniae, Mycoplasma pneumoniae, Klebsiella* species (lower respiratory tract infections), *Staphylococcus aureus, S. pyogenes* (skin and skin structure infections), *Bacteroides* and *Shigella* species. (4) Alternative therapy for the following when penicillin is contraindicated: Uncomplicated gonorrhea due to *Neisseria gonorrhoeae*, syphilis due to *Treponema pallidum*, yaws due to *Treponema pertenue, Listeria monocytogenes*, anthrax due to *Bacillus anthracis*, Vincent's infection due to *Fusobacterium fusiforme*, actinomycosis due to *Actinomyces* species, *Clostridium* species. (5) Adjunct with amebicides for acute intestinal amebiasis. (6) Adjunct therapy for severe acne. (7) Part of combination therapy to eradicate *Helicobacter pylori* infections. *Investigational:* Pleural sclerosing agent in malignant pleural effu-

sions (administered by chest tube); in combination with gentamicin for *Vibrio vulnificus* infections due to wound infection after trauma or by eating contaminated seafood.

ACTION/KINETICS

Pharmacokinetics

From 60–80% absorbed. **Time to maximum levels:** 2–4 hr. **t½, serum:** 6–12 hr. From 40 to 70% excreted unchanged in urine. Always express dose as the hydrochloride salt. **Plasma protein binding:** 20–65%.

CONTRAINDICATIONS

Use of the topical ointment in or around the eyes. Use of PO products for streptococcal disease unless organism has been shown to be susceptible. Tetracyclines are not the drugs of choice to treat any type of staphylococcal infections.

SIDE EFFECTS

Most Common

Anorexia, N&V, diarrhea, dizziness, headache, rashes.

See *Tetracyclines* for a complete list of possible side effects. **Use of the tetracycline fiber:** Oral candidiasis, glossitis, staining of the tongue, severe gingival hyperplasia, minor throat irritation, pain following placement in an abscessed area, throbbing pain, *hypersensitivity reactions*.

HOW SUPPLIED

Capsules: 250 mg, 500 mg; *Dental Fiber:* 12.7 mg; *Syrup:* 125 mg/5 mL.

DOSAGE

• **CAPSULES; SYRUP**

Mild to moderate infections.

Adults, usual: 500 mg twice a day or 250 mg 4 times per day.

Severe infections.

Adult: 500 mg 4 times per day. **Children over 8 years:** 25–50 mg/kg/day in four equal doses.

Eradication of H. pylori.

The following regimens may be used: (1) Tetracycline, 500 mg 4 times per day for 2 weeks, plus metronidazoloe, 250 mg 4 times per day for 2 weeks, plus bismuth subsalicylate, 525 mg 4 times per day for 2 weeks, plus a H_2 receptor antagonist for 28 days. (2) Clarithromycin, 500 mg twice a day for 2 weeks, plus ranitidine bismuth citrate, 400 mg twice a day for 4 weeks, plus either metronidazole, 500 mg twice a day, or amoxicillin, 1 gram twice a day, or tetracycline, 500 mg twice a day for 2 weeks. (3) Tetracycline, 500 mg 4 times per day for 2 weeks, plus metronidazole, 500 mg 3 times per day for 2 weeks, plus bismuth subsalicylate, 525 mg 4 times per day for 2 weeks, plus either lansoprazole, 30 mg once daily or omeprazole, 20 mg once daily, for 2 weeks.

Brucellosis.

500 mg 4 times per day for 3 weeks with 1 gram streptomycin IM twice a day for first week and once daily the second week.

Syphilis.

Sumycin only: Total of 30–40 grams over 10–15 days. **All products except Sumycin:** Early (<1 year): 500 mg 4 times per day for 15 days; >1 year duration: 500 mg 4 times per day for 30 days.

Uncomplicated gonorrhea.

500 mg q 6 hr for 7 days.

Uncomplicated urethral, endocervical, or rectal infections in adults due to Chlamydia trachomatis.

500 mg 4 times per day for minimum of 7 days.

Severe acne, long-term therapy.

Initially, 1 gram/day in divided doses; **then,** 125–500 mg/day (long-term). Alternate-day for intermittent therapy may be adequate in some clients.

• DENTAL FIBER

All uses.

Insert a sufficient number of fibers to fill the periodontal pocket. Secure fibers with cyanoacrylate adhesive and leave for 10 days.

NURSING CONSIDERATIONS

ADMINISTRATION/STORAGE

1. Treat streptococcal infections for at least 10 days.
2. Decrease recommended doses and/or extend dosing intervals in those with renal impairment.
3. Food, some dairy products, and antacids containing Al, Ca, or Mg interfere with tetracycline absorption.

4. In renal impairment, decrease the dose or extend dosing intervals.
5. Under no circumstances should outdated tetracyclines be given; degradation products of tetracyclines are highly nephrotoxic and may cause a Fanconi-like syndrome.
6. Store products below 30°C (86°F) protected from light and excessive heat.

ASSESSMENT

1. Note reasons for therapy, type, onset, characteristics of S&S.
2. Monitor cultures, CBC, liver and renal function studies; anticipate reduced dose or dosing intervals with renal dysfunction.

CLIENT/FAMILY TEACHING

1. Take PO form 1 hr before or 2 hr after meals and 1 hr before bedtime with a full glass of water. Avoid dairy products, antacids, or iron preparations for 2–3 hr of ingestion; reduces drug effectiveness.
2. May cause photosensitivity reaction; avoid exposure to sunlight and wear protective clothing and sunscreen when exposed.
3. Drug may cause increased yellow-brown discoloration and softening of teeth and bones. *Not* advised for children under 8 years old.
4. Use additional nonhormonal form of contraception to prevent pregnancy.
5. Check expiration date; degraded drug is very nephrotoxic and may cause kidney damage.
6. Report any new onset diarrhea, severe headache, visual disturbances, or lack of effectiveness.

OUTCOMES/EVALUATE

• Resolution of infection; symptomatic improvement
• ↓ Acne lesions

Thalidomide ■
(thah-**LID**-ah-myd)

CLASSIFICATION(S):
Immunomodulator
PREGNANCY CATEGORY: X
Rx: Thalomid.

USES

(1) Acute treatment of moderate to severe erythema nodosum leprosum (ENL). Not indicated for monotherapy for ENL in the presence of moderate to severe neuritis. (2) Maintenance therapy for prevention and suppression of the cutaneous symptoms of erythema nodosum leprosum recurrence. (3) In combination with dexamethasone to treat newly diagnosed multiple myeloma. *Investigational:* Prostate cancer in combination with docetaxel; graft vs. host disease after bone marrow transplantation; refractory multiple myeloma; primary brain tumors; appetite stimulant for cachexia in advanced cancer; aphthous ulcers.

ACTION/KINETICS

Action

Immunomodulatory drug; mechanism of action not known. Possesses immunomodulatory, antiinflammatory, and antiangiogenic properties. Drug may suppress excessive tumor necrosis factor–alpha (TNF–α) production and down–modulation of selected cell surface adhesion molecules involved in leukocyte migration. When used to treat multiple myeloma, there is an increase in the number of circulating natural killer cells and an increase in plasma levels of interleukin-2 and interferon-gamma (associated with cytotoxic activity).

Pharmacokinetics

Peak plasma levels: 2.9–5.7 hr. High fat meals increase the time to peak plasma levels to about 6 hr. **t½, elimination:** 5–7 hr. Appears to undergo nonenzymatic hydrolysis in the plasma. Excreted in the urine. **Plasma protein binding:** Approximately 60%.

CONTRAINDICATIONS

Never to be used in pregnancy or in those who could become pregnant while taking the drug (even a single 50 mg dose can cause severe birth defects). Use in males unless the client meets several conditions (see package insert). Use during heterosexual sexual contact. Use as monotherapy for ENL in the presence of moderate to severe neuritis. Lactation.

SPECIAL CONCERNS

■ (1) If taken during pregnancy, thalidomide can cause severe birth defects or death to a fetus. Thalidomide should never be used by women who are pregnant or who could become pregnant while taking the drug. Even a single dose (one 50, 100, or 200 mg capsule) taken by a pregnant woman can cause severe birth defects. Because of this toxicity and in an effort to make the chance of fetal exposure as negligible as possible, thalidomide is approved for marketing only under a special restricted distribution program approved by the FDA. This program is called the 'System for Thalidomide Education and Prescribing Safety' (S.T.E.P.S.) Under this restricted distribution program, only prescribers and pharmacists registered with the program are allowed to prescribe and dispense the product at one month intervals. In addition, clients must be advised of, agree to, and comply with the requirements of the S.T.E.P.S. program in order to receive the product.

(2) Prescribers: Thalidomide is prescribed only by licensed prescribers who are registered in the S.T.E.P.S. program and understand the risk of teratogenicity of thalidomide if used during pregnancy. The following major human fetal abnormalities related to thalidomide given during pregnancy have been documented:

- Absence of bones, absence of limbs (amelia), congenital heart defects, external ear abnormalities (including anotia, micropinna, small or absent external auditory canals), eye abnormalities (anophthalmos, microphthalmos), facial palsy, hypoplasticity of the bones, and phcomelia (short limbs).
- Alimentary tract, urinary tract, and genital malformations have also been documented.
- Mortality at or shortly after birth has been reported at about 40%.

Effective contraception must be used for at least 1 month before beginning thalidomide, during therapy, and for 1 month following discontinuation of therapy. Reliable contraception is indi-

---

Bold Italic = life threatening side effect   ■ = black box warning   ♣ = Available in Canada

cated even where there has been a history of infertility, unless the patient has had a hysterectomy or has been postmenopausal for at least 24 months. Two reliable forms of contraception must be used simultaneously unless continuous abstinence from heterosexual sexual intercourse is the chosen method. Refer women of childbearing potential to a qualified provider of contraceptive methods, if needed. Sexually mature women who have not undergone a hysterectomy or who have not been postmenopausal for at least 24 consecutive months (i.e., who have had menses at some time in the preceding 24 consecutive months) are considered to be women of childbearing potential. Before starting treatment, administer a pregnancy test (sensitivity at least 50 milliunits/mL) to women of childbearing potential. Perform the test with the 24 hours prior to beginning therapy. A prescription for thalidomide for a woman of childbearing potential must not be issued until a written report of a negative pregnancy test has been obtained by the prescriber. Once treatment has been started, test for pregnancy weekly during the first 4 weeks of use, then repeat pregnancy testing at 4 weeks in women with regular menstrual cycles. If menstrual cycles are irregular, test for pregnancy every 2 weeks. Perform pregnancy testing and counseling if a client misses her period or if there is any abnormality in menstrual bleeding. If pregnancy occurs during thalidomide treatment, discontinue the drug immediately. Report any suspected fetal exposure to thalidomide to the FDA immediately via MedWatch at 1-800-FDA-1088 and also to the manufacturer. Refer the client to an obstetrician/gynecologist experienced in reproductive toxicity for further evaluation and counseling.

(3) Men: Because thalidomide is present in the semen of patients receiving the drug, males receiving thalidomide must always use a latex condom during any sexual contact with women of childbearing potential even if he has undergone a successful vasectomy. Thalido-

mide is contraindicated in sexually mature men unless the client meets ALL of the following conditions:
• He understands and can reliably carry out instructions.
• He is capable of complying with the mandatory contraceptive measures that are appropriate for men, client registration, and client survey as described in the S.T.E.P.S. program.
• He has received both oral and written warnings of the hazards of taking thalidomide and exposing a fetus to the drug.
• He has received both oral and written warnings of the risk of possible contraception failure and of the presence of thalidomide in semen. He has been instructed that he must always use a latex condom during any sexual contact with women of childbearing potential, even if he has undergone a successful vasectomy.
• He acknowledges, in writing, his understanding of these warnings and of the need to use a latex condom during any sexual contact with women of childbearing potential, even if has undergone a successful vasectomy, when having sexual intercourse with women of childbearing potential. Sexually mature women who have not undergone a hysterectomy or who have not been postmenopausal for at least 24 consecutive months (i.e., who have had menses at some time in the preceding 24 consecutive months) are consider to be women of childbearing potential.
• If the client is between 12 and 18 years of age, his parents or legal guardian must have read this material and agreed to ensure compliance.
(4) Women: Thalidomide is contraindicated in women of childbearing potential unless alternative therapies are considered inappropriate and the client meets ALL of the following conditions (i.e., essentially she is unable to become pregnant while on thalidomide therapy):
• She understands and can reliably carry out instructions.
• She is capable of complying with the

mandatory contraceptive measures, pregnancy testing, patient registration, and patient survey as described in the S.T.E.P.S. program.

• She has received both oral and written warnings of the hazards of taking thalidomide during pregnancy and of exposing a fetus to the drug.

• She has received both oral and written warnings of the risk of possible contraception failure and of the need to use 2 reliable forms of contraception simultaneously, unless continuous abstinence from reproductive heterosexual intercourse is the chosen method. Sexually mature women who have not undergone a hysterectomy or who have not been postmenopausal for at least 24 consecutive months (i.e., who have had menses at some time in the preceding 24 consecutive months) are considered to be women of childbearing potential.

• She acknowledges, in writing, her understanding of these warnings and of the need for using 2 reliable methods of contraception for 4 weeks prior to starting thalidomide therapy, during thalidomide therapy, and for 4 weeks after stopping thalidomide therapy.

• She has had a negative pregnancy test with a sensitivity of at least 50 milli-international units/mL, within the 24 hr prior to beginning therapy.

• If the patient is between 12 and 18 years of age, her parent or legal guardian must have read this material and agreed to ensure compliance.

(5) Venous thromboembolic effects: The use of thalidomide in multiple myeloma results in an increased risk of venous thromboembolic events, such as deep venous thrombosis and pulmonary embolus. This risk increases significantly when thalidomide is used in combination with standard chemotherapeutic agents, including dexamethasone. In one controlled trial, the rate of venous thromboembolic events was 22.5% in clients receiving thalidomide in combination with dexamethasone, compared with 4.9% in clients receiving dexamethasone alone. Clients and health care providers are advised to be observant for the signs and symptoms of thromboembolism. Instruct clients to seek medical care if they develop symptoms such as arm or leg swelling, chest pain, or shortness of breath. Preliminary data suggest that clients who are appropriate candidates may benefit from concurrent prophylactic anticoagulation or aspirin treatment. ■ Clients with Hansen disease may have an increased bioavailability of thalidomide. Safety and efficacy have not been determined in children less than 12 years of age.

SIDE EFFECTS
Most Common
Dizziness, somnolence, orthostatic hypotension, acne, rash/desquamation, maculopapular rash, hematuria, leukopenia, fever, headache, neuropathy, dry mouth, flatulence, peripheral edema, pharyngitis, sinusitis, infection, constipation, dyspnea, edema.

NOTE: Only the most common side effects and possible serious side effects are listed. Included are common and/or serious side effects noted when combined with dexamethasone. **GI:** Constipation, dry mouth, flatulence, diarrhea, nausea, oral moniliasis, tooth pain, abdominal pain, anorexia, dyspepsia, N&V. **CNS:** Drowsiness, somnolence, dizziness, confusion, tremor, vertigo, headache, anxiety, agitation, depression, lightheadedness, insomnia, paresthesia, seizures (including *generalized tonic-clonic*). **Neurologic:** Peripheral sensory/motor neuropathy (may be permanent). **CV:** Orthostatic hypotension, bradycardia (may require medical intervention), hyper-/hypotension, embolism. Increased incidence of pulmonary embolism, DVT, thrombophlebitis, or thrombosis. **Respiratory:** Pharyngitis, rhinitis, sinusitis, dyspnea, cough. **Hematologic:** Neutropenia, leukopenia. **Hypersensitivity:** Erythematous macular rash, fever, tachycardia, hypotension. **Dermatologic:** Photosensitivity, rash (maculopapular, exfoliative, purpuric, bullous), dermatitis, desquamation, fungal nail disorder, pruritus, *Stevens-Johnson syndrome*, *toxic epidermal necrolysis* . **Musculoskeletal:** Back/neck/bone pain, neck rigidity, muscle

---

Bold Italic = life threatening side effect　　■ = black box warning　　✚ = Available in Canada

weakness, arthralgia, myalgia. **Body as a whole:** Peripheral edema, accidental injury, infection (with/without neutropenia), weight gain/loss, asthenia, chills, malaise, pain, fatigue, fever. **Miscellaneous: *Human teratogenicity*.** HIV viral load increase, hematuria, impotence, facial edema.

LABORATORY TEST CONSIDERATIONS
↑ Alkaline phosphatase, AST, bilirubin. ↓ Hemoglobin, leukocytes, neutrophils, platelets. Hyperglycemia, hyper-/hypokalemia, hypocalcemia, hyponatremia.

DRUG INTERACTIONS
Alcohol / Enhanced sedative effects
Barbiturates / Enhanced sedative effects
Chlorpromazine / Enhanced sedative effects
Isoniazid / Enhanced symptoms of peripheral neuropathy
Metronidazole / Enhanced symptoms of peripheral neuropathy
Vincristine / Enhanced symptoms of peripheral neuropathy

HOW SUPPLIED
Capsules: 50 mg, 100 mg, 200 mg.

DOSAGE————————
• **CAPSULES**
Cutaneous ENL, initial therapy.
Adults, initial: 100–300 mg once daily with water, preferably at bedtime and at least 1 hr after the evening meal. Clients weighing less then 50 kg should be started at the low end of the dose range. In those with severe cutaneous ENL or who have required higher doses previously, dosing may be started at doses up to 400 mg once daily at bedtime or in divided doses with water 1 hr after meals. Continue initial dosing until signs and symptoms of active reaction have been eliminated (usually at least 2 weeks). Following this, taper clients off medication in 50 mg decrements q 2 to 4 weeks.
Maintenance therapy for prevention and suppression of ENL recurrence.
Maintain the minimum dose (see initial therapy) necessary to control the reaction. Attempt tapering of medication q 3 to 6 months, in decrements of 50 mg q 2 to 4 weeks.
Multiple myeloma.

Thalidomide, 200 mg, once daily with water preferably at bedtime, and at least 1 hr after the evening meal *plus* dexamethasone, 40 mg daily given PO on days 1–4, 9–12, 17–20 every 28 days.

NURSING CONSIDERATIONS
ADMINISTRATION/STORAGE
1. The product is supplied only to pharmacists registered with the S.T.E.P.S. program. The drug is dispensed in no more than a 1-month supply and only on presentation of a new prescription written within the previous 14 days and client signature. Pharmacists are required to obtain a confirmation number for each prescription and record that number on the prescription.
2. Specific informed consent and compliance with the mandatory client registry and survey are required of all male and female clients prior to dispensing the drug. The drug must not be repackaged.
3. Cutaneous absorption or inhalation of the drug, especially from handling the capsules or being exposed to body fluids of a thalidomide-user is possible. Wash exposed areas with soap and water.
4. Continue dosing until signs and symptoms of active reaction have subsided (usually 2 weeks). Clients may then be tapered off medication in 50 mg decrements q 2–4 weeks.
5. In clients with moderate to severe neuritis associated with a severe erythema nodosum leprosum reactions, corticosteroids may be given along with thalidomide. Steroid doses can be tapered and discontinued when the neuritis has improved.
6. Discontinue if a rash occurs. Do not resume therapy if the rash is exfoliative, purpuric, or bullous, or if Stevens-Johnson syndrome or toxic epidermal necrolysis is suspected.
7. Concomitant use with carbamazepine, griseofulvin, HIV-protease inhibitors, modafinil, penicillins, phenytoin, rifabutin, rifampin, or certain herbal supplements (e.g., St. John's wort) with hormonal contraceptive drugs may decrease effectiveness of contraception

T

———————————
📷 = see color insert   Ⓗ = Herbal   Ⓘ = Intravenous   Ⓡ = sound alike drug

for up to 1 month after discontinuing these therapies. Women requiring treatment with 1 or more of these drugs must use 2 other effective or highly effective methods of contraception, or abstain from heterosexual contact while taking thalidomide.

8. Store from 15–30°C (59–86°F). Protect from light.

ASSESSMENT

1. Note reasons for therapy. With leprosy, note characteristics including number of painful skin nodules and any systemic manifestations (fever, neuritis, malaise). With multiple myeloma note protein levels and steroid failures. List other agents trialed and outcome.

2. Obtain negative pregnancy test. Drug is teratogenic; even one dose taken during pregnancy can cause severe birth defects. Pregnancy tests will be performed weekly during the first month of therapy and then monthly thereafter with regular menses and every two weeks with irregular menses.

3. Drug will only be dispensed under a restricted distribution program (S.T.E.P.S.) requiring written consent. With relapsed MM client must still sign consent and agree to required monitoring.

4. If HIV-seropositive, monitor viral load the first and third month of treatment and then every 3 months.

CLIENT/FAMILY TEACHING

1. Take as prescribed at least one hr after evening meal or at bedtime unless otherwise directed.

2. May cause dizziness/drowsiness; avoid activities that require mental acuity. Avoid alcohol and CNS depressants.

3. Women of child bearing age must practice two methods of reliable birth control or abstain continuously from heterosexual intercourse. Males must always wear a latex condom when engaging in sexual intercourse with women of childbearing age, despite successful vasectomy. During therapy do not donate blood or sperm.

4. Report any numbness, tingling, pain, or burning in the hands or feet. Peripheral neuropathy may occur and may be irreversible.

5. Drug is continued until S&S of active reaction subsides (approx. 2 weeks). The dosage may then be tapered by provider every 2–4 weeks.

6. Drug will only be dispensed in a one month supply, and only upon presentation of a valid prescription written within past 14 days. Drug therapy requires informed consent and compliance with the mandatory patient registry (MD must call company with drug ID number) and survey prior to dispensing and clinical monitoring during therapy (S.T.E.P.S. -system for thalidomide education and prescribing safety program).

OUTCOMES/EVALUATE

- Suppression of cutaneous manifestations with ENL
- Inhibition of malignant cell proliferation

Theophylline
(thee-**OFF**-ih-lin)

CLASSIFICATION(S):
Antiasthmatic, xanthine derivative
PREGNANCY CATEGORY: C
Rx: Capsules, Extended-Release or Timed-Release: Slo-Bid Gyrocaps, Theo-24. **Capsules, Immediate-Release:** Bronkodyl, Elixophyllin. **Elixir:** Asmalix, Elixophyllin, Lanophyllin. **Syrup:** Accurbron. **Tablets, Extended-Release or Timed-Release:** T-Phyl, Theochron, Theolair-SR, Theophylline Extended-Release, Theophylline SR, Uniphyl.
✤**Rx:** Apo-Theo LA, Novo-Theophyl SR, Quibron-T/SR.

USES

(1) Prophylaxis and treatment of bronchial asthma. (2) Reversible bronchospasms associated with chronic bronchitis and emphysema. *Investigational:* Apnea and bradycardia of prematurity. Essential tremor. Improve pulmonary function and dyspnea in COPD.

ACTION/KINETICS

Action

Theophylline stimulates the CNS, directly relaxes the smooth muscles of the bronchi (relieve bronchospasms) and

---

Bold Italic = life threatening side effect   ■ = black box warning   ✤ = Available in Canada

pulmonary blood vessels, produces diuresis, inhibits uterine contractions, stimulates gastric acid secretion, and increases the rate and force of contraction of the heart. Although the exact mechanism is not known, theophyllines may alter the calcium levels of smooth muscle, blocking adenosine receptors, inhibiting the effect of prostaglandins on smooth muscle, and inhibiting the release of slow-reacting substance of anaphylaxis and histamine.

Pharmacokinetics
Well absorbed PO liquids. **Time to peak serum levels, oral solution:** 1 hr; **extended-release capsules and tablets:** 4–7 hr. **Therapeutic plasma levels:** 10–20 mcg/mL. **t½:** 3–15 hr in nonsmoking adults, 4–5 hr in adult heavy smokers, 1–9 hr in children, and 20–30 hr for premature neonates. An increased t½ may be seen in individuals with CHF, alcoholism, liver dysfunction, or respiratory infections. Because of great variations in the rate of absorption (due to dosage form, food, dose level) as well as its extremely narrow therapeutic range, theophylline therapy is best monitored by determination of the serum levels. 85% to 90% metabolized in the liver to various metabolites, including the active 3-methylxanthine. Theophylline is metabolized partially to caffeine in the neonate. The premature neonate excretes 50% unchanged theophylline and may accumulate the caffeine metabolite. Excretion is through the kidneys (about 10% unchanged in adults). **Plasma protein binding:** Healthy adults: about 60%; Neonates: 36%.

CONTRAINDICATIONS
Hypersensitivity to any xanthine, peptic ulcer, seizure disorders (unless on medication), hypotension, CAD, angina pectoris.

SPECIAL CONCERNS
Use during lactation may result in irritability, insomnia, and fretfulness in the infant. Use with caution in premature infants due to the possible accumulation of caffeine. Xanthines are not usually tolerated by small children because of excessive CNS stimulation. Geriatric clients may manifest an increased risk of toxicity. Use with caution in the presence of gastritis, alcoholism, acute cardiac diseases, hypoxemia, severe renal and hepatic disease, severe hypertension, severe myocardial damage, hyperthyroidism, glaucoma.

SIDE EFFECTS
Most Common
N&V, diarrhea, headache, insomnia, irritability.
Side effects are uncommon at serum theophylline levels less than 20 mcg/mL. At levels greater than 20 mcg/mL, 75% of individuals experience side effects including N&V, diarrhea, irritability, insomnia, and headache. At levels of 35 mcg/mL or greater, individuals may manifest *cardiac arrhythmias*, hypotension, tachycardia, hyperglycemia, *seizures, brain damage, or death.* **GI:** N&V, diarrhea, anorexia, epigastric pain, hematemesis, dyspepsia, rectal bleeding, gastroesophageal reflux during sleep or while recumbent. **CNS:** Headache, insomnia, irritability, fever, dizziness, lightheadedness, vertigo, reflex hyperexcitability, *seizures*, depression, speech abnormalities, alternating periods of mutism and hyperactivity, *brain damage, death.* **CV:** Hypotension, *life-threatening ventricular arrhythmias*, palpitations, tachycardia, *peripheral vascular collapse*, extrasystoles. **Renal:** Proteinuria, excretion of erythrocytes and renal tubular cells, dehydration due to diuresis, urinary retention (men with PPH). **Miscellaneous:** Tachypnea, *respiratory arrest*, fever, flushing, hyperglycemia, antidiuretic hormone syndrome, leukocytosis, rash, alopecia.

LABORATORY TEST CONSIDERATIONS
↑ Plasma free fatty acids, bilirubin, urinary catecholamines, ESR. Interference with uric acid tests and tests for furosemide and probenecid.

OD OVERDOSE MANAGEMENT
Symptoms: Agitation, headache, nervousness, insomnia, tachycardia, extrasystoles, anorexia, N&V, fasciculations, tachypnea, tonic-clonic seizures. The first signs of toxicity may be seizures or ventricular arrhythmias. Toxicity is usually associated with parenteral adminis-

T

tration but can be observed after PO administration, especially in children.

Treatment:

- Have gastric lavage equipment, and cathartics available to treat overdose if the client is conscious and not having seizures. Otherwise a mechanical ventilator, oxygen, diazepam, and IV fluids may be necessary for the treatment of overdosage.
- For postseizure coma, maintain an airway and oxygenate the client. To remove the drug, perform only gastric lavage and give the cathartic and activated charcoal by a large-bore gastric lavage tube. Charcoal hemoperfusion may be necessary.
- Treat atrial arrhythmias with verapamil and treat ventricular arrhythmias with lidocaine or procainamide.
- Use IV fluids to treat acid-base imbalance, hypotension, and dehydration. Hypotension may also be treated with vasopressors.
- To treat hyperpyrexia, use a tepid water sponge bath or a hypothermic blanket.
- Treat apnea with artificial respiration.
- Monitor serum levels of theophylline until they fall below 20 mcg/mL as secondary rises of theophylline may occur, especially with sustained-release products.

DRUG INTERACTIONS

Allopurinol / ↑ Theophylline levels
Aminogluthethimide / ↓ Theophylline levels
Barbiturates / ↓ Theophylline levels
Benzodiazepines / Sedative effect may be antagonized by theophylline
Beta-adrenergic agonists / Additive effects
Beta-adrenergic blocking agents / ↑ Theophylline levels
Calcium channel blocking drugs / ↑ Theophylline levels
Carbamazepine / Either ↑ or ↓ theophylline levels
Charcoal / ↓ Theophylline levels R/T ↑ metabolism
Cimetidine / ↑ Theophylline levels
Ciprofloxacin / ↑ Theophylline plasma levels; ↑ possibility of side effects
Corticosteroids / ↑ Theophylline levels

Digitalis / ↑ Digitalis toxicity
Disulfiram / ↑ Theophylline levels
Ephedrine and other sympathomimetics / ↑ Theophylline levels
Erythromycin / ↑ Theophylline effect R/T ↓ liver metabolism
Ethacrynic acid / Either ↑ or ↓ theophylline levels
Furosemide / Either ↑ or ↓ theophylline levels
Halothane / ↑ Risk of cardiac arrhythmias
Interferon / ↑ Theophylline levels
Isoniazid / Either ↑ or ↓ theophylline levels
Ketamine / Seizures of the extensor-type
Ketoconazole / ↓ Theophylline levels
Lithium / ↓ Lithium effect R/T ↑ rate of excretion
Loop diuretics / ↓ Theophylline levels
Mexiletine / ↑ Theophylline levels
Muscle relaxants, nondepolarizing / ↓ Muscle relaxation
Oral contraceptives / ↑ Theophylline effect R/T ↓ liver metabolism
Phenytoin / ↓ Theophylline levels
Propofol / ↓ Propofol sedative effect
Quinolones / ↑ Theophylline levels
Rifampin / ↓ Theophylline levels
Smoking / ↑ Metabolism (including second—hand smoke exposure) of theophylline R/T induction of CYP1A2 → ↓ t½ ; monitor levels
H *St. John's wort* / Possible ↓ theophylline plasma levels R/T ↑ metabolism
Sulfinpyrazone / ↓ Theophylline levels
Sympathomimetics / ↓ Theophylline levels
Tetracyclines / ↑ Risk of theophylline toxicity
Thiabendazole / ↑ Theophylline levels
Thyroid hormones / ↓ Theophylline levels in hypothyroid clients
Tobacco smoking / ↓ Theophylline effect R/T ↑ liver metabolism; consider dosage ↑
Troleandomycin / ↑ Theophylline effect R/T ↓ liver metabolism
Verapamil / ↑ Theophylline effect
Zafirlukast / Possible ↑ theophylline levels

Bold Italic = life threatening side effect   ■ = black box warning   ♣ = Available in Canada

HOW SUPPLIED

Capsules, Extended-Release or Timed-Release: 50 mg, 75 mg, 100 mg, 125 mg, 200 mg, 300 mg, 400 mg; *Capsules, Immediate-Release:* 100 mg, 200 mg; *Elixir:* 80 mg/15 mL; *Syrup:* 150 mg/15 mL; *Tablets, Extended-Release or Timed-Release:* 100 mg, 200 mg, 250 mg, 300 mg, 400 mg, 450 mg, 500 mg, 600 mg.

DOSAGE

• **CAPSULES, IMMEDIATE-RELEASE; ELIXIR; SYRUP**

Bronchodilator, acute attacks, in clients not currently on theophylline.

Children, 1–9 years of age, PO loading dose: 5 mg/kg; **maintenance:** 4 mg/kg q 6 hr. **Children 9–16 years of age and young adult smokers, PO loading dose:** 5 mg/kg; **maintenance:** 3 mg/kg q 6 hr. **Healthy non-smoking adults, PO loading dose:** 5 mg/kg; **maintenance:** 3 mg/kg q 8 hr. **Older clients, clients with cor pulmonale, PO loading dose:** 5 mg/kg; **maintenance:** 2 mg/kg q 8 hr. **Clients with CHF, PO loading dose:** 5 mg/kg; **maintenance:** 1–2 mg/kg q 12 hr.

Infants, premature, initial maintenance dose, 24 or less days postnatal: 1 mg/kg q 12 hr; **more than 24 day postnatal:** 1.5 mg/kg q 12 hr. **Infants, 6–52 weeks of age, initial maintenance dose:** Calculate as follows: ([0.2 x age in weeks] + 5) x kg = 24 hr dose in mg.

For those 26 weeks of age or less, divide into q 8 hr dosing and for those 26–52 weeks of age, divide into q 6 hr dosing. Guide final dosage by serum levels after reaching steady state.

Bronchodilator, acute attacks, in clients currently receiving theophylline.

Adults and children up to 16 years of age: If possible, a serum theophylline level should be obtained first. Then, base loading dose on the premise that each 0.5 mg theophylline/kg lean body weight will increase in serum theophylline levels about 1 mcg/mL. If immediate therapy is needed and a serum level cannot be obtained, a single dose of the equivalent of 2.5 mg/kg of anhydrous theophylline in a rapidly absorbed form will raise serum levels by about 5 mcg/mL. If the client is not experiencing theophylline toxicity, this dose is unlikely to result in dangerous side effects.

Chronic therapy, based on anhydrous theophylline.

Adults and children, initial: 16 mg/kg/24 hr, up to a maximum of 400 mg/day in three to four divided doses at 6–8-hr intervals; **then,** dose can be increased in 25% increments at 2–3 day intervals up to a maximum, as follows: **Adults and children over 16 years of age:** 13 mg/kg, not to exceed 900 mg/day; **12–16 years:** 18 mg/kg/day; **9–12 years:** 20 mg/kg/day; **1–9 years:** 24 mg/kg/day.

• **CAPSULES, EXTENDED RELEASE OR TIMED-RELEASE; TABLETS, EXTENDED-RELEASE OR TIMED-RELEASE**

Bronchodilator, chronic therapy, based on equivalent of anhydrous theophylline.

Adults, initial: 6–8 mg/kg up to a maximum of 400 mg/day in three to four divided doses at 6–8-hr intervals; **then,** dose may be increased, if needed and tolerated, by increments of 25% at 2–3 day intervals up to a maximum of 13 mg/kg/day or 900 mg/day, whichever is less, without measuring serum theophylline. **Pediatric, over 12 years of age, initial:** 4 mg/kg q 8–12 hr; **then,** dose may be increased by 2–3 mg/kg/day at 3-day intervals up to the following maximum doses (without measuring serum levels): **16 years and older:** 13 mg/kg/day or 900 mg/day, whichever is less; **12–16 years:** 18 mg/kg/day.

• **ELIXIR; SYRUP**

Neonatal apnea.

Loading dose: Using the equivalent of anhydrous theophylline administered by NGT, 5 mg/kg; **maintenance:** 2 mg/kg/day in two to three divided doses given by NGT.

NURSING CONSIDERATIONS

ADMINISTRATION/STORAGE

1. Individualize chronic dosage to maintain serum levels of 10–20 mcg/mL. Adjust dose following serum theophylline determinations as follows:

📷 = see color insert   H = Herbal   IV = Intravenous   © = sound alike drug

- If serum theophylline is too low (5–10 mcg/mL), increase dose by about 25% at 3-day intervals until either the desired clinical effect or serum levels are reached.
- If serum theophylline is within the desired range (10–20 mcg/mL), maintain dosage if tolerated. Check serum theophylline levels at 6–12 month intervals.
- If serum theophylline is too high (20–25 mcg/mL), decrease doses by about 10%; recheck serum theophylline levels after 3 days. If serum levels are from 25–30 mcg/mL, skip the next dose and decrease subsequent doses by about 25%; recheck serum theophylline levels after 3 days. If serum levels >30 mcg/mL, skip the next 2 doses and decrease subsequent doses by about 50%; recheck serum theophylline levels after 3 days.

2. Calculate dosage based on lean body weight (theophylline does not distribute to body fat). Once stabilized on a dosage, serum levels tend to remain constant.

3. Review list of agents with which theophylline derivatives interact.

4. Monitor serum theophylline levels in chronic therapy, especially if the maximum maintenance doses are used or exceeded. Obtain the serum sample at the time of peak absorption (1–2 hr) after administration for immediate-release products and 5–9 hr after the morning dose for sustained-release products (as long as the client has not missed doses during the previous 48 hr).

5. The extended-release tablets or capsules are not recommended for children less than age 6. Dosage for once-a-day products has not been established in children less than 12 years old.

6. Serum levels may vary significantly following brand interchange.

7. When converting from an immediate release to an extended release product, keep the total daily dose the same; only the dosing interval is adjusted.

ASSESSMENT

1. Note reasons for therapy, type, onset, characteristics of S&S. Assess for hypersensitivity to xanthine compounds. List experience with this class of drugs.

2. List any hypotension, CAD, angina, PUD, or seizure disorders; avoid drug or use very cautiously with these conditions.

3. Assess for cigarette/marijuana use; induces hepatic metabolism of drug and may require increase in dosage from 50% to 100%.

4. Check for diet habits which can influence the excretion of theophylline. A high-protein and/or low-carbohydrate diet will cause an increased drug excretion. A low-protein and/or high-carbohydrate diet will decrease excretion of drug.

5. Assess lung fields closely. Note characteristics of sputum and cough; assess CXR, ABGs, and PFTs.

6. Check levels; obtain serum sample at time of peak absorption (1–2 hr after administration for immediate release and 5–9 hr after the morning dose or sustained release products). The client must not have missed doses during the previous 48 hr and the dosing intervals must have been reasonably typical during this time.

CLIENT/FAMILY TEACHING

1. To avoid epigastric pain, take with a snack or with meals. Take ATC and only as prescribed; more is *not* better. Do not crush, dissolve, chew, or break slow-release forms of the drug.

2. May cause dizziness, evaluate drug effects before performing activities that require mental alertness. Report S&S of toxicity such as N&V, anorexia, insomnia, restlessness/irritability, hyperexcitability; will need drug levels and ECG to assess for arrhythmias.

3. Do not smoke; may aggravate underlying medical conditions as well as interfere with drug absorption. Attend smoking cessation program. Do not take any OTC cough, cold, or breathing preparations without provider approval.

4. Protect from acute exacerbations of illness by avoiding crowds, dressing warmly in cold weather, obtaining the

---

Bold Italic = life threatening side effect ■ = black box warning ✚ = Available in Canada

pneumonia vaccine and seasonal flu shot, covering mouth and nose so cold air is not directly inhaled, staying in air conditioning during excessively hot and humid weather, maintaining proper diet and nutrition, exercising daily, and consuming adequate fluids.

5. Report S&S of infections, adverse drug effects, difficulty breathing, and significant peak flow readings.

6. Avoid caffeine- and xanthine-containing beverages and foods (chocolate, coffee, colas) and daily intake of char-broiled foods; increases drug side effects.

7. When secretions become thick and tacky, increase intake of fluids as these thin secretions and assist in their removal. (Avoid milk/milk products.)

8. Learn to pace activity and avoid overexertion at all times.

9. Hold medication and report side effects or excessive CNS depression/stimulation in children and infants (unable to report side effects).

10. Identify local support groups that may assist in understanding and coping with chronic respiratory disease/dysfunction.

OUTCOMES/EVALUATE

- Knowledge/understanding of disease management; compliance with prescribed regimen
- Improved airway exchange and breathing patterns; ↓ wheezing
- Therapeutic drug levels (10–20 mcg/mL)
- Stimulation of respirations in the neonate

Thiabendazole
(thigh-ah-**BEN**-dah-zohl)

CLASSIFICATION(S):
Anthelmintic
PREGNANCY CATEGORY: C
Rx: Mintezol.

USES
(1) Primarily for threadworm infections, cutaneous larva migrans, visceral larva migrans when these infections occur also one or if pinworm is also present. (2) Use for hookworm, whipworm, or large roundworm only if specific therapy is not available or cannot be used or if a second drug is desirable. (3) Reduce symptoms of trichinosis during the invasive phase.

ACTION/KINETICS
Action
Exact mechanism is unknown; interferes with the enzyme fumarate reductase, which is specific to several helminths.
Pharmacokinetics
Readily absorbed from the GI tract. **Peak plasma levels:** 1–2 hr. **t½:** 0.9–2 hr. Metabolized almost completely and most excreted within 24 hr, mainly through the urine.

CONTRAINDICATIONS
Lactation. Use in mixed infections with ascaris as it may cause worms to migrate.

SPECIAL CONCERNS
Safety and efficacy not established in children less than 13.6 kg. Use with caution in clients with hepatic disease or impaired hepatic function.

SIDE EFFECTS
Most Common
N&V, anorexia, diarrhea, dizziness, drowsiness, headache.

GI: N&V, anorexia, diarrhea, epigastric distress. **CNS:** Dizziness, drowsiness, headache, irritability, weariness, giddiness, numbness, psychic disturbances, collapse, *seizures*. **Allergic:** Pruritus, *angioedema*, flushing of face, chills, fever, skin rashes, *Stevens-Johnson syndrome*, *anaphylaxis*, lymphadenopathy, conjunctival injection, erythema multiforme. **Hepatic:** Jaundice, cholestasis, parenchymal liver damage. **GU:** Crystalluria, hematuria, enuresis, foul odor of urine. **Ophthalmic:** Blurred vision, abnormal sensation in the eyes, yellow appearance of objects, drying of mucous membranes. **Miscellaneous:** Tinnitus, hypotension, hyperglycemia, transient leukopenia, perianal rash, appearance of live Ascaris in nose and mouth.

LABORATORY TEST CONSIDERATIONS
Rarely, ↑ AST and cephalin flocculation.

OD OVERDOSE MANAGEMENT
Symptoms: Psychic changes, transient vision changes. *Treatment:* Induce vomiting or perform gastric lavage. Treat symptoms.

DRUG INTERACTIONS
↑ Serum levels of xanthines to potentially toxic levels R/T ↓ breakdown by liver

HOW SUPPLIED
Oral Suspension: 500 mg/5 mL; *Tablets, Chewable:* 500 mg.

DOSAGE
• **ORAL SUSPENSION; TABLETS, CHEWABLE**
   Anthelmintic.
Over 68 kg: 1.5 grams/dose; **less than 68 kg:** 22 mg/kg/dose. The usual dosage schedule for strongyloidiasis, cutaneous larva migrans, hookworm, whipworm, or roundworm is 2 doses/day for 2 successive days, not to exceed 3 grams/day after meals. For trichinosis, give 2 doses/day for 2–4 successive days and for visceral larva migrans, give 2 doses/day for 7 successive days.

NURSING CONSIDERATIONS
ADMINISTRATION/STORAGE
1. Take with food to reduce stomach upset.
2. Chew chewable tablets before swallowing.
3. Cleansing enemas are not required after drug therapy.

ASSESSMENT
1. Note reasons for therapy, onset/duration, and characteristics of S&S. Determine how and when acquired. Culture stool for ova and parasites.
2. List agents currently prescribed to ensure none interact.

CLIENT/FAMILY TEACHING
1. Administer with food or after meals to decrease stomach upset; chew tablets thoroughly. May drink fruit juice to help remove mucus that intestinal tapeworms burrow in; facilitates expulsion of worms.
2. Do not operate hazardous machinery; drug may cause dizziness and drowsiness. Report any CNS disturbances, including muscular weakness and loss of alertness.

3. May notice a urine odor 24 hr following ingestion; this is normal. Report any evidence of rash, fever, or itching immediately.
4. With pinworms, treat all household members. Practice strict handwashing and hygiene measures, launder all bedlinens, underwear and sleep attire daily in hot water, disinfect toilets daily and bathroom and bedroom floors should be wet mopped; do not share towels and washclothes.

OUTCOMES/EVALUATE
• Negative consecutive stool cultures
• Eradication of infestation

Thioguanine (6-TG, 6-Thioguanine) ■
(thigh-oh-**GWON**-een)

CLASSIFICATION(S):
Antineoplastic, antimetabolite
PREGNANCY CATEGORY: D
Rx: Tabloid.
❧**Rx:** Lanvis.

SEE ALSO *ANTINEOPLASTIC AGENTS.*

USES
For remission, induction, consolidation, and maintenance therapy of acute non-lymphocytic leukemias (usually in combination with other drugs such as cyclophosphamide, cytarabine, prednisone, vincristine). Not recommended for maintenance therapy or long-term continuous treatment due to the high risk of liver toxicity. *NOTE:* Although thioguanine is one of several drugs that have activity in treating the chronic phase of chronic myelogenous leukemia, busulfan is usually regarded as the preferred drug. *Investigational:* Second-line therapy for Crohn's disease and ulcerative colitis. Psoriasis.

ACTION/KINETICS
Action
Purine antagonist that is cell-cycle specific for the S phase of cell division. Converted to 6-thioguanylic acid, which

---

Bold Italic = life threatening side effect   ■ = black box warning   ❧ = Available in Canada in turn interferes with the synthesis of guanine nucleotides by competing with hypoxanthine and xanthine for the enzyme phosphoribosyltransferase (HGPRTase). Ultimately the synthesis of RNA and DNA is inhibited. Resistance to the drug may result from increased breakdown of 6-thioguanylic acid or loss of HGPRTase activity.

Pharmacokinetics
Partially absorbed (30%) from GI tract. **$t_{\frac{1}{2}}$, plasma disappearance:** 80 min. Metabolized by the liver and excreted in the urine. More effective in children than in adults. Cross-resistance with mercaptopurine.

CONTRAINDICATIONS
Resistance to mercaptopurine or thioguanine; there is usually complete cross-resistance between the two. Use for maintenance or long-term continuous therapy due to the high risk of liver toxicity from vascular endothelial damage; liver toxicity is not always associated with elevated liver-enzyme concentrations (signs of portal hypertension may indicate toxicity). Lactation.

SPECIAL CONCERNS
■ Thioguanine is a potent drug. Do not use unless a diagnosis of acute nonlymphocytic leukemia has been adequately established and the responsible physician is knowledgeable in assessing response to chemotherapy.■ Clients having an inherited deficiency of thiopurine methyltransferase are usually sensitive to the myelosuppressive effects of mercaptopurine.

SIDE EFFECTS
Most Common
Myelosuppression (pancytopenia, anemia, leukopenia, thrombocytopenia—or any combination thereof), hyperuricemia.

See *Antineoplastic Agents* for a complete list of possible side effects. **Hematologic:** Myelosuppression (pancytopenia, anemia, leukopenia, thrombocytopenia—or any combination thereof). *hepatoxicity.* **GI:** N&V, anorexia, stomatitis, *intestinal necrosis and perforation. hepatotoxicity* **Miscellaneous:** Loss of vibration sense, unsteadiness of gait, hyperuricemia. Adults tend to

show a more rapid fall in WBC count than children.

LABORATORY TEST CONSIDERATIONS
↑ Uric acid in blood and urine.

OD OVERDOSE MANAGEMENT
Symptoms: N&V, hypertension, malaise, and diaphoresis may be seen immediately, which may be followed by myelosuppression and azotemia. *Severe hematologic toxicity. Treatment:* Induce vomiting if client is seen immediately after an acute overdosage. Treat symptoms. Hematologic toxicity may be treated by platelet transfusions (for bleeding) and granulocyte transfusions. Antibiotics are indicated for sepsis.

DRUG INTERACTIONS
Busulfan / Chronic concomitant therapy → esophageal varices associated with abnormal LFTs and evidence of nodular regenerative hyperplasia
Mesalamine / Exacerbation of rapid bone marrow suppression in clients with thiopurine methyltransferase deficiency
Olsalazine / Exacerbation of rapid bone marrow suppression in clients with thiopurine methyltransferase deficiency
Sulfasalazine / Exacerbation of rapid bone marrow suppression in clients with thiopurine methyltransferase deficiency

HOW SUPPLIED
Tablets: 40 mg.

DOSAGE
• **TABLETS**
Acute nonlymphocytic leukemias.
Individualized. Adults and pediatric, initial: 2 mg/kg/day (or 75–100 mg/m²) given at one time. From 2 to 4 weeks may elapse before beneficial results become apparent. Compute dose to nearest multiple of 20 mg. If no response after 4 weeks, dosage may be increased to 3 mg/kg/day. Dosage of thioguanine does not have to be decreased during administration of allopurinol (to inhibit uric acid production).

NURSING CONSIDERATIONS
ADMINISTRATION/STORAGE
1. Some individuals have an inherited deficiency of thiopurine methyltransferase and who may be unusually sensitive

to the myelosuppressive effects of thio-guanine resulting in rapid bone marrow suppression. Substantial dosage reduction may be needed to avoid the development of life-threatening bone marrow suppression.

2. Store from 15–25°C (59–77°F).

ASSESSMENT

1. Note reasons for therapy, onset, characteristics of S&S; list other agents trialed, outcome.

2. Identify those experiencing loss of vibration sense and with unsteady gaits; (may be unable to rely on canes) may require assistance.

3. Expect hyperuricemia after tumor lysis, which may be reduced with administration of allopurinol, by preventing purine breakdown and excessive uric acid formation.

4. Monitor CBC, uric acid, renal and LFTs. Obtain CBC weekly and LFTs monthly during course of therapy; may cause granulocyte and platelet suppression. Nadir: 10 days; recovery: 21 days.

5. Perform platelet counts weekly; discontinue drug if abnormally large fall in blood count is noted, indicating severe bone marrow depression.

CLIENT/FAMILY TEACHING

1. Take on an empty stomach for best results. Expect maintenance doses to be continued during remissions.

2. Increase fluid intake (2–3 L/day) to minimize uric acid (crystals) in blood and urine.

3. Withhold drug and report yellowing of skin, decreased urine output, diarrhea, S&S of anemia (fatigue, dyspnea), or extremity swelling.

4. Avoid crowds, vaccinia, and persons with infectious diseases. Any sore throat, fever, or flu-like symptoms as well as increased bruising/bleeding require immediate reporting.

5. Practice reliable contraception.

OUTCOMES/EVALUATE

- Suppression of malignant cell proliferation
- Hematologic evidence of leukemia remission

Thiotepa   IV
(thigh-oh-**TEP**-ah)

CLASSIFICATION(S):
Antineoplastic, alkylating agent
PREGNANCY CATEGORY: D
Rx: Thioplex.

SEE ALSO *ANTINEOPLASTIC AGENTS* AND *ALKYLATING AGENTS*.

USES

(1) Adenocarcinoma of the breast or ovary. (2) Control intracavitary effusions secondary to diffuse or localized neoplastic disease of various serosal cavities. (3) Superficial papillary carcinoma of the urinary bladder. (4) Lymphosarcoma and Hodgkin's disease, although other treatments are used more often.

ACTION/KINETICS

Action

Cell-cycle nonspecific; thought to act by causing the release of ethylenimmonium ions that bind or alkylate various intracellular substances such as nucleic acids. Is cytotoxic by virtue of cross-linking of DNA and RNA strands as well as by inhibition of protein synthesis.

Pharmacokinetics

Rapidly cleared from the plasma following IV use. **$t^{1/2}$, elimination:** About 2.3 hr. May be significantly absorbed through the bladder mucosa. Approximately 85% excreted through the urine, mainly as metabolites.

CONTRAINDICATIONS

Lactation. Pregnancy. Renal, hepatic, or bone marrow damage. Acute leukemia. Use with other alkylating agents due to increased toxicity.

SPECIAL CONCERNS

Is both carcinogenic and mutagenic. Use with caution in renal and hepatic dysfunction. Safety and efficacy have not been determined in children.

SIDE EFFECTS

Most Common

N&V, anorexia, urticaria, missed menses, dizziness, headache, blurred vision, alopecia (temporary).

GI: N&V, abdominal pain, anorexia. **CNS:** Dizziness, headache, blurred vi-

---

Bold Italic = life threatening side effect   ■ = black box warning   ✖ = Available in Canada sion, fatigue, weakness, febrile reaction. **Dermatologic:** Contact dermatitis, urticaria, alopecia (temporary), pain at injection site, dermatitis, skin depigmentation following topical use. **GU:** Dysuria, urinary retention, chemical or hemorrhagic cystitis following intravesical use, missed menses, amenorrhea, interference with spermatogenesis. **Hypersensitivity:** Rash, urticaria, wheezing, *laryngeal edema*, asthma, *anaphylactic shock*. **Miscellaneous:** Conjunctivitis, discharge from a SC lesion due to tumor tissue breakdown. Significant toxicity to the hematopoietic system.

OD OVERDOSE MANAGEMENT
Symptoms: **Hematopoietic toxicity.**
Treatment: Transfusions of whole blood, platelets, or leukocytes have been used.

DRUG INTERACTIONS
Alkylating agents / Combination with other alkylating agents ↑ toxicity
Pancuronium / Prolonged muscle paralysis and respiratory depression
Phenytoin / ↑ Thiotepa metabolism by CYP2B6 → possible toxicity due to active metabolites
Succinylcholine / Risk of ↑ apnea

HOW SUPPLIED
Powder for Injection, Lyophilized: 15 mg, 30 mg.

DOSAGE
• **IV (MAY BE RAPID)**
  Adenocarcinoma of the breast or ovary; lymphosarcoma and Hodgkin's disease.
IV (may be rapid): 0.3–0.4 mg/kg at 1- to 4-week intervals by rapid administration or 0.2 mg/kg for 4–5 days q 2–4 weeks.
• **INTRATUMOR OR INTRACAVITARY ADMINISTRATION**
  Intracaviatry effusions secondary to diffuse/localized neoplastic disease.
0.6–0.8 mg/kg q 1–4 weeks through the same tubing used to remove fluid from the cavity.
• **INTRAVESICALLY**
  Bladder cancer.
After dehydrating client with papillary carcinoma of the bladder for 8–12 hr, instill 60 mg thiotepa in 30–60 mL of sterile water for injection in the bladder using a catheter. Retain, if possible, for 2 hr. If it is not possible to retain 60 mL, give the dose in a volume of 30 mL. Reposition client q 15 min for maximum contact area. This dose is given once a week for 4 weeks.

NURSING CONSIDERATIONS
ADMINISTRATION/STORAGE
1. Reconstitute with sterile water (usually 1.5 mL to give a concentration of 5 mg/0.5 mL). Do not use NSS as a diluent. The reconstituted solution can then be mixed with NaCl, dextrose, dextrose and NaCl, Ringer's, or RL injection (i.e., if a large volume is needed for intracavitary use, IV drip, or perfusion). Discard solutions grossly opaque or with precipitate.
2. Minimize pain on injection and retard rate of absorption by simultaneous administration of local anesthetics. Drug may be mixed with procaine HCl 2% or epinephrine HCl 1:1,000, or both, as ordered.
3. Store vials in the refrigerator. Reconstituted solutions may be stored for 5 days in the refrigerator without substantial loss of potency.
4. Since thiotepa is not a vesicant, it may be injected quickly and directly into the vein with the desired volume of sterile water. Usual amount of diluent is 1.5 mL.
5. When used for bladder carcinoma, a second or third course of treatment may be undertaken, although bone marrow depression may be increased.

ASSESSMENT
1. Note reasons for therapy, onset/type of S&S, other agents trialed, any previous therapy with this agent. Note all biopsy results and cystoscopy findings with bladder lesions
2. Monitor CBC, uric acid, renal and LFTs. Drug causes platelet and granulocyte suppression. Nadir: 21 days; recovery: 40–50 days.

CLIENT/FAMILY TEACHING
1. Those who receive drug as bladder instillations should retain fluid for 2 hr and remain NPO for 6 hr to ensure drug retention. Report bloody or painful urination.

T

2. With bladder instillation, change positions q 15 min to ensure maximum bladder area contact.

3. Practice reliable contraception; drug can cause fetal damage or death.

4. Avoid OTC agents without provider approval, especially those containing aspirin.

5. Record temperatures and report any S&S of fever, infection, sore throat, or unusual bruising or bleeding. Keep all F/U visits.

OUTCOMES/EVALUATE

Control of tumor size and malignant cell proliferation

Tiagabine hydrochloride ©

(tye-**AG**-ah-been)

CLASSIFICATION(S):

Anticonvulsant, miscellaneous

PREGNANCY CATEGORY: C

Rx: Gabatril.

SEE ALSO ANTICONVULSANTS.

USES

Adjunctive therapy for partial seizures in adults and children at least 12 years of age.

ACTION/KINETICS

Action

Mechanism not known but activity of GABA, an inhibitory neurotransmitter, may be enhanced. Drug may block uptake of GABA into presynaptic neurons allowing more GABA to bind to postsynaptic cells. This prevents propagation of neural impulses that contribute to seizures due to GABA-ergic action.

Pharmacokinetics

Well absorbed after PO; absolute bioavailability is about 90%. **Peak plasma levels:** About 45 min when fasting. High fat meals decrease rate but not extent of absorption. **Steady-state:** 2 days. Metabolized in liver; excreted in urine and feces. **t½, elimination:** 7–9 hr. Diurnal effect occurs with levels being lower in evening compared with morning. **Plasma protein binding:** 96%.

CONTRAINDICATIONS

Hypersensitivity to tiagabine or any component of the product. Lactation.

SPECIAL CONCERNS

Do not discontinue abruptly due to the possibility of withdrawal seizures. Safety and efficacy have not been determined in children less than 12 years of age.

SIDE EFFECTS

Most Common

Dizziness/lightheadedness, asthenia, somnolence, nausea, nervousness/irritability, tremor, abdominal pain, abnormal/difficulty with concentration/attention.

NOTE: Side effects with an incidence of at least 1% are listed. **CNS:** Asthenia, dizziness/lightheadedness, nervousness, difficulty with concentration/attention, abnormal gait, agitation, ataxia, confusion, depression, difficulty with memory, emotional lability, hostility, insomnia, language problems, nystagmus, paresthesia, somnolence, speech disorder, tremor, twitching, headache, anxiety, incoordination, depersonalization, dysarthria, euphoria, hallucinations, hyperkinesia, hypertonia, hypesthesia, hypokinesia, hypotonia, migraine, myoclonus, paranoid reaction, personality disorder, decreased reflexes, stupor, vertigo. **GI:** N&V, diarrhea, increased appetite, mouth ulceration, constipation, anorexia, dry mouth, flatulence, dyspepsia, gastroenteritis, gingivitis, stomatitis. **CV:** Vasodilation, hypertension, palpitation, syncope, tachycardia. **Dermatologic:** Rash, pruritus, ecchymosis, acne, alopecia, dry skin, sweating. **Musculoskeletal:** Myasthenia, chest/back/neck pain, myalgia, arthralgia. **Respiratory:** Pharyngitis, increased cough, rhinitis, sinusitis, bronchitis, dyspnea, epistaxis, pneumonia. **GU:** UTI, urinary frequency, dysmenorrhea, dysuria, metrorrhagia, urinary incontinence, vaginitis. **Ophthalmic:** Amblyopia, conjunctivitis, diplopia, abnormal vision. **Otic:** Ear pain, otitis media, tinnitus. **Body as a whole:** Unspecified pain, flu syndrome, infection, lymphadenopathy, edema, peripheral edema, weight gain/loss, allergic reaction,

---

Bold Italic = life threatening side effect   ■ = black box warning   ✚ = Available in Canada

chills, malaise, fever. **Miscellaneous:** Abdominal pain, accidental injury, cyst. *NOTE:* There is a risk of new onset seizures and status epilepticus in clients without a history of epilepsy, especially when used for unapproved indications (e.g., bipolar disorder).

OD OVERDOSE MANAGEMENT
Symptoms: Somnolence, impaired consciousness, agitation, confusion, drowsiness, lethargy, speech difficulties, hostility, depression, weakness, myoclonus, seizures (including status epilepticus), coma, ataxia, spike wave stupor, tremors, disorientation, vomiting, temporary paralysis, respiratory depression.
Treatment:
- There is no specific antidote.
- Increase elimination by gastric lavage.
- Maintain the airway.
- Use general supportive care, including monitoring of vital signs and observation of the clinical status.
- Dialysis is not likely to be beneficial.

DRUG INTERACTIONS
Carbamazepine / ↑ Clearance (60%) due to ↑ metabolism
Highly protein-bound drugs / ↑ Possibility of an interaction with other highly-protein bound drugs → ↑ free fractions of either drug
Phenobarbital / ↑ Clearance (60%) due to ↑ metabolism
Phenytoin / ↑ Clearance (60%) due to ↑ metabolism
Primidone / ↑ Clearance (60%) due to ↑ metabolism
Valproate / Significant ↓ tiagabine binding → 40% ↑ free tiagabine; significance is unknown

HOW SUPPLIED
Tablets (Filmtabs): 2 mg, 4 mg, 12 mg, 16 mg.

DOSAGE————————————
- **TABLETS (FILMTABS)**
  Partial seizures in those taking enzyme-inducing antiepileptic drugs.
Adults and children over 18 years, initial: 4 mg once daily. **Week 2:** 8 mg/day in 2 divided doses; **Week 3:** 12 mg/day in 3 divided doses; **Week 4:** 16 mg/day in 2–4 divided doses; **Week 5:** 20–24 mg/day in 2–4 divided doses;

Week 6: 24–32 mg/day in 2–4 divided doses; **usual adult maintenance dose:** 32–56 mg/day in 2–4 divided doses. **Children, 12 to 18 years, initial, week 1:** 4 mg once daily. The total daily dose may be increased by 4 mg at the beginning of week 2. Thereafter, the total daily dose may be increased by 4–8 mg at weekly intervals until a clinical effect is noted or up to 32 mg/day is reached. Give the total daily dose in 2–4 divided doses. Dosages above 32 mg/day have been tolerated for a short period of time in a small number of children.
  Partial seizures in those not taking an enzyme-inducing antiepileptic drug.
12 years and older: The estimated plasma levels in noninduced clients is more than two times that in those receiving enzyme-inducing drugs. Thus, use in noninduced clients requires lower doses of tiagabine and such clients also require a slower titration of tiagabine compared with that of induced clients.

NURSING CONSIDERATIONS

℮ Do not confuse tiagabine with tizanidine (skeletal muscle relaxant).

ADMINISTRATION/STORAGE
1. It is not necessary to modify dose of concomitant anticonvulsant drugs, unless clinically indicated.
2. Those with impaired liver function may require reduced initial and maintenance doses and/or longer dosing intervals compared with those with normal hepatic function.
3. The following recommendations for dosing apply to all clients taking tiagabine:
- Give orally and take with food.
- Do not use a loading dose.
- Do not use rapid dose escalation and/or large dose increments.
- Consider dosage adjustment whenever a change in the client's enzyme-inducing system occurs (i.e., as a result of the addition, discontinuation, or dose change of the enzyme-inducing agent).
4. Store from 20–25°C (68–77°F) protected from light and moisture.

ASSESSMENT

1. Note reasons for therapy, characteristics of seizures, other agents trialed, outcome.
2. Monitor LFTs; decrease dosage or dosing intervals with dysfunction.

CLIENT/FAMILY TEACHING

1. Take with food as directed. Do not stop abruptly; may trigger seizures.
2. Avoid activities requiring mental alertness until drug effects realized; may cause dizziness, sleepiness, or confusion.
3. Report any increased frequency or loss of seizure control, rash, weakness, or visual disturbances.
4. Practice reliable contraception; do not breast feed.
5. Keep all F/U appointments to evaluate response to therapy.

OUTCOMES/EVALUATE

Control of seizures

Ticarcillin disodium   IV

(tie-kar-**SILL**-in)

CLASSIFICATION(S):
Antibiotic, penicillin
PREGNANCY CATEGORY: B
Rx: Ticar.

SEE ALSO *ANTI-INFECTIVE DRUGS AND PENICILLINS.*

USES

Primarily suitable for treatment of gram-negative organisms but also effective for mixed infections. (1) Bacterial septicemia, skin and soft tissue infections, acute and chronic respiratory tract infections caused by susceptible strains of *Pseudomonas aeruginosa, Proteus, Escherichia coli,* and other gram-negative organisms. Combined therapy with gentamicin or tobramycin is sometimes indicated for treatment of *Pseudomonas* infections. (2) GU tract infections (complicated and uncomplicated) due to susceptible strains of *P. aeruginosa, Proteus* (both indole-positive and indole-negative), *E. coli, Enterobacter* and *Streptococcus faecalis.* (3) Anaerobic

bacteria causing empyema, anaerobic pneumonitis, lung abscess, bacterial septicemia, peritonitis, intra-abdominal abscess, skin and soft tissue infections, salpingitis, endometritis, PIP, pelvic abscess. Ticarcillin may be used with infections in which protective mechanisms are impaired such as during use of oncolytic or immunosuppressive drugs or in clients with acute leukemia.

ACTION/KINETICS

Action

A parenteral, semisynthetic antibiotic with an antibacterial spectrum resembling that of carbenicillin.

Pharmacokinetics

Peak plasma levels, IM: 25–35 mcg/mL after 1 hr; **IV:** 15 min. **t½:** 70 min. Elimination complete after 6 hr.

ADDITIONAL CONTRAINDICATIONS

Pregnancy.

SPECIAL CONCERNS

Use with caution in presence of impaired renal function and for clients on restricted salt diets.

ADDITIONAL SIDE EFFECTS

Most Common

Hypersensitivity, N&V, gastritis, stomatitis, diarrhea, skin rashes.

Neurotoxicity and neuromuscular excitability, especially in clients with impaired renal function. **Hematologic:** Neutropenia, leukopenia, thrombocytopenia, anemia. **GI:** N&V, diarrhea, constipation, abdominal pain, stomatitis, anorexia. **Respiratory:** Dyspnea, coughing. **Dermatologic:** Alopecia, rash. **Body as a whole:** Fatigue, fever, headache, pain (body, back, skeletal), asthenia.

ADDITIONAL DRUG INTERACTIONS

Effect of carbenicillin may be enhanced when used in combination with gentamicin or tobramycin for *Pseudomonas* infections.

LABORATORY TEST CONSIDERATIONS

↑ Alkaline phosphatase, AST, ALT.

HOW SUPPLIED

Powder for Injection: 3 grams.

DOSAGE

• **DIRECT IV; IM; IV INFUSION**
    Bacterial septicemia, intra-abdominal infections, skin and soft tissue infections, infections of the female genital

---

system and pelvis, respiratory tract infections.

Adults: 200–300 mg/kg/day by IV infusion in divided doses q 4 or 6 hr (3 grams q 4 hr or 4 grams q 6 hr), depending on the weight and severity of the infection. **Pediatric, less than 40 kg:** 200–300 mg/kg/day by IV infusion q 4 or 6 hr (daily dose should not exceed the adult dose).

UTIs, uncomplicated.

Adults and children: 1 gram IM or direct IV q 6 hr. **Pediatric, <40 kg:** 50–100 mg/kg/day IM or direct IV in divided doses q 6 or 8 hr.

UTIs, complicated.

Adults: 150–200 mg/kg/day by IV infusion in divided doses q 4 or 6 hr (usual dose is 3 grams 4 times per day for a 70-kg client).

Neonates with sepsis due to Pseudomonas, Proteus, *or* E. coli.

Less than 7 days of age and less than 2 kg, 75 mg/kg q 12 hr; **more than 7 days of age and less than 2 kg,** 75 mg/kg q 8 hr; **less than 7 days of age and 2 kg or more,** 75 mg/kg q 8 hr; **more than 7 days of age and 2 kg or more,** 100 mg/kg q 8 hr. Can be given IM or by IV infusion over 10–20 min.

NURSING CONSIDERATIONS

ADMINISTRATION/STORAGE

1. Clients with renal insufficiency should receive a loading dose of 3 grams **IV**, and subsequent doses, as follows by C_{CR}. C_{CR} **>60 mL/min:** 3 grams IV q 4 hr; C_{CR} **from 30–60 mL/min:** 2 grams IV q 4 hr; C_{CR} **from 10–30 mL/min:** 2 grams IV q 8 hr; C_{CR}, **<10 mL/min:** 2 grams IV q 12 hr or 1 gram IM q 6 hr; C_{CR}, **<10 mL/min with hepatic dysfunction:** 2 grams IV q 24 hr or 1 gram IM q 12 hr. **Clients on peritoneal dialysis:** 3 grams IV q 12 hr; **clients on hemodialysis:** 2 grams IV q 12 hr and 3 grams after each dialysis.

2. Clients seriously ill should receive higher doses i.e., serious urinary tract and systemic infections.

3. For IM use, reconstitute each gram with 2 mL sterile water for injection, NaCl injection, or 1% lidocaine HCl (without epinephrine) to prevent pain and induration. Use the reconstituted solution quickly; inject well into a large muscle.

4. Do not administer more than 2 grams of the drug in each IM site.

5. Give adult dose to children weighing over 40 kg.

6. Discard unused reconstituted solutions after 24 hr when stored at room temperature and after 72 hr when refrigerated.

7. For IV use, reconstitute each gram with 4 mL of the desired solution. Administer slowly to prevent vein irritation and phlebitis. A dilution of 1 gram/20 mL (or more) will decrease the chance of vein irritation.

8. For IV infusion, give by continuous or intermittent IV drip. Administer intermittent infusion over a 30 minute–2 hr period in equally divided doses. Concentrations of about 50 mg/mL will reduce vein irritation.

9. For an IV infusion, use 50 or 100 mL *ADD-Vantage* container of either D5W or NaCl injection and give by intermittent infusion over 30–120 min in equally divided doses.

10. Do not mix ticarcillin together with amikacin, gentamicin, or tobramycin in the same IV solution due to the gradual inactivation of these aminoglycosides.

11. Do not use refrigerated solutions longer than 72 hr for multidose purposes. Discard unused solutions after appropriate time period (72 hr if diluted with NaCl injection or D5W injection and 48 hr if diluted with lactated Ringer's injection).

12. After reconstitution and dilution to a concentration of 10–100 mg/mL, the solution can be frozen at -18°C (0°F) for up to 30 days. The thawed solution must be used within 24 hr.

13. Store the dry powder at room temperature or below.

ASSESSMENT

1. Note type, onset, characteristics of S&S; note clinical presentation.

2. Monitor bleeding times, cultures, renal and LFTs. Reduce dosage with liver or renal dysfunction.

---

3. With high doses, monitor for signs of electrolyte imbalance (especially Na and K levels) and seizures.

4. List sodium content of drug (usually 4.75 mEq Na/gram) and calculate accordingly if Na restricted.

CLIENT/FAMILY TEACHING

1. Drug is administered by injection or IV for serious infections.

2. Report any symptoms of bleeding abnormalities, such as small purple spots on skin, easy bruising, or frank bleeding.

3. Extremity swelling, weight gain, or difficulty breathing may be precipitated by drug's large sodium content.

4. Review drug side effects that should be reported if evident. Report persistent diarrhea or lack of improvement.

OUTCOMES/EVALUATE

• Negative cultures
• Symptomatic improvement

———COMBINATION DRUG———

Ticarcillin disodium and Clavulanate potassium   IV

(tie-kar-**SILL**-in, klav-you-**LAN**-ate)

CLASSIFICATION(S):
Antibiotic, penicillin
PREGNANCY CATEGORY: B
Rx: Timentin.

SEE ALSO TICARCILLIN DISODIUM AND PENICILLINS.

USES

(1) Septicemia, including bacteremia, due to β-lactamase producing strains of Klebsiella sp., Staphylococcus aureus, Escherichia coli, and Pseudomonas aeruginosa (and other Pseudomonas species). (2) Lower respiratory tract infections due to β-lactamase producing strains of S. aureus, Haemophilus influenzae, and Klebsiella sp. (3) Bone and joint infections due to β-lactamase producing strains of S. aureus. (4) Skin and skin structure infections due to β-lacta-

mase producing strains of S. aureus, Klebsiella sp., and E. coli. (5) UTIs (complicated and uncomplicated) due to β-lactamase producing strains of E. coli, Klebsiella sp., P. aeruginosa (and other Pseudomonas species), Citrobacter sp., Enterobacter cloacae, Serratia marcescens, and S. aureus. (6) Endometritis due to β-lactamase producing strains of Bacteroides melaninogenicus, Enterobacter sp. (including E. cloacae), E. coli, Klebsiella pneumoniae, S. aureus, and Staphylococcus epidermidis. (7) Peritonitis due to β-lactamase producing strains of E. coli, K. pneumoniae, and Bacteroides fragilis group.

CONTENT

Each vial of the Powder for Injection and the Injection Solution (per 100 mL) contains: Ticarcillin disodium, 3 grams, and clavulanate potassium, 0.1 gram.

ACTION/KINETICS

Action

Contains clavulanic acid, which protects the breakdown of ticarcillin by beta-lactamase enzymes, thus ensuring appropriate blood levels of ticarcillin.

SIDE EFFECTS

Most Common

Hypersensitivity, N&V, gastritis, stomatitis, diarrhea, skin rashes.

See Penicillins and Ticarcillin for a complete list of possible side effects.

HOW SUPPLIED

See Content

DOSAGE————

• IV INFUSION

Systemic Infections and UTIs.

Adults, 60 kg or more: 3.1 grams (containing 0.1 gram clavulanic acid) q 4–6 hr for 10–14 days. **Adults <60 kg:** 200–300 mg ticarcillin/kg/day in divided doses q 4–6 hr for 10–14 days.

Gynecologic infections.

Adults, 60 kg or more, moderate infections: 200 mg/kg/day in divided doses q 6 hr; **severe infections:** 300 mg/kg/day in divided doses q 4 hr. **Adults, less than 60 kg:** 200–300 mg/kg/day in divided doses q 4–6 hr.

Mild to moderate infections in children.

Children, 60 kg or more: 3.1 grams q 6 hr. **Children, less than 60 kg:** 200

Bold Italic = life threatening side effect   ■ = black box warning   ✦ = Available in Canada

mg/kg/day (dosed at 50 mg/kg/dose) q 6 hr.

Severe infections in children.
Children, 60 kg or more: 3.1 grams q 4 hr. **Children, less than 60 kg:** 300 mg/kg/day (dosed at 50 mg/kg/dose) q 4 hr.

NURSING CONSIDERATIONS

ADMINISTRATION/STORAGE
[IV] 1. For renal insufficiency: **Initially,** loading dose of 3 grams ticarcillin and 0.1 gram clavulanic acid; **then,** dose based on C_{CR} as follows. **C_{CR} >60 mL/min:** 3.1 grams q 4 hr; **C_{CR} from 30–60 mL/min:** 2 grams q 4 hr; **C_{CR} from 10–30** mL/min: 2 grams q 8 hr; **C_{CR} <10 mL/min:** 2 grams q 12 hr; **C_{CR} <10 mL/min with hepatic dysfunction:** 2 grams q 24 hr. **Clients on peritoneal dialysis:** 3.1 grams q 12 hr; **clients on hemodialysis:** 2 grams q 12 hr and 3.1 grams after each dialysis.
2. To attain the appropriate dilution for 3 grams ticarcillin and 0.1 gram clavulanic acid, dilute with 13 mL of either NaCl or sterile water for injection. Further dilutions can be undertaken with D5W, RL injection, or NaCl.
3. Administer over a 30-min period, either through a Y-type IV infusion or by direct infusion.
4. Continue treatment for at least 2 days after S&S of infection have disappeared. The usual duration is 10–14 days.
5. This product is incompatible with sodium bicarbonate.
6. Dilutions with NaCl or RL injection may be stored at room temperature for 24 hr or refrigerated for 7 days. Dilutions with D5W are stable at room temperature for 12 hr or for 3 days if refrigerated.
7. If used with another anti-infective agent (e.g., an aminoglycoside), give each drug separately.

ASSESSMENT
1. Note type, onset, characteristics of S&S. Obtain cultures before starting therapy; note clinical presentation.
2. Monitor bleeding times, CBC, cultures, renal and LFTs. Reduce dose with liver or renal dysfunction.

CLIENT/FAMILY TEACHING
1. Drug is administered parenterally to treat serious infections.
2. Report any symptoms of bleeding abnormalities, such as small purple spots on skin, easy bruising, or frank bleeding.
3. Extremity swelling, weight gain, or difficulty breathing may be precipitated by drug's large sodium content.
4. Review drug side effects that should be reported if evident. Report persistent diarrhea or lack of improvement.

OUTCOMES/EVALUATE
Resolution of infection; symptomatic improvement

Ticlopidine hydrochloride ■
(tie-**KLOH**-pih-deen)

CLASSIFICATION(S):
Antiplatelet drug
PREGNANCY CATEGORY: B
Rx: Ticlid.
❧**Rx:** Apo-Ticlopidine, Gen-Ticlopidine, Nu-Ticlopidine, PMS-Ticlopidine, Rhoxal-ticlopidine.

USES
(1) With aspirin to decrease the incidence of subacute stent thrombosis in clients undergoing successful coronary stent implantation. (2) Reduce the risk of fatal or nonfatal thrombotic stroke in clients who have manifested precursors of stroke or who have had a completed thrombotic stroke. Due to the risk of neutropenia or agranulocytosis, reserve for clients who are intolerant to aspirin therapy or who have failed aspirin therapy. *Investigational:* Chronic arterial occlusion, coronary artery bypass grafts, intermittent claudication, open heart surgery, primary glomerulonephritis, subarachnoid hemorrhage, sickle cell disease, uremic clients with AV shunts or fistulas.

ACTION/KINETICS
Action
Irreversibly inhibits ADP-induced platelet-fibrinogen binding and subsequent

---

platelet-platelet interactions. This results in inhibition of both platelet aggregation and release of platelet granule constituents as well as prolongation of bleeding time.

Pharmacokinetics

Peak plasma levels: 2 hr. **Maximum platelet inhibition:** 8–11 days after 250 mg twice a day. **Steady-state plasma levels:** 14–21 days. **t½, elimination:** 4–5 days. After discontinuing therapy, bleeding time and other platelet function tests return to normal within 14 days. Rapidly absorbed; bioavailability is increased by food. Extensively metabolized by the liver with approximately 60% excreted through the kidneys; 23% is excreted in the feces (with one-third excreted unchanged). Clearance of the drug decreases with age. **Plasma protein binding:** 98%.

CONTRAINDICATIONS

Use in the presence of neutropenia and thrombocytopenia, hemostatic disorder, or active pathologic bleeding such as bleeding peptic ulcer or intracranial bleeding. Severe liver impairment. Lactation.

SPECIAL CONCERNS

■ (1) Can cause life-threatening hematological side effects, including neutropenia/agranulocytosis and thrombotic thrombocytopenic purpura. (2) Severe hematological side effects may occur within a few days of starting therapy. The incidence of thrombotic thrombocytopenic purpura peaks after about 3–4 weeks of therapy and neutropenia peaks at about 4–6 weeks with both declining thereafter. Only a few cases have been seen after more than 3 months of therapy. (3) Hematological side effects cannot be reliably predicted by any demographic or clinical characteristics. During the first 3 months of therapy, hematologically and clinically monitor those receiving ticlopidine for evidence of neutropenia or thrombotic thrombocytopenic purpura (TTP). Immediately discontinue if there is any evidence of neutropenia or TTP.■ Use with caution in clients with ulcers (i.e., where there is a propensity for bleeding). Consider reduced dosage in im-

paired renal function. Geriatric clients may be more sensitive to the effects of the drug. Safety and effectiveness have not been established in children less than 18 years of age.

SIDE EFFECTS

Most Common

Diarrhea, N&V, dyspepsia, rash, GI pain, neutropenia, purpura, flatulence, pruritus, dizziness.

Hematologic: Neutropenia, *agranulocytosis*, *thrombotic thrombocytopenia purpura*, thrombocytopenia, pancytopenia, immune thrombocytopenia, *hemolytic anemia with reticulocytosis*. **GI:** Diarrhea, N&V, GI pain, dyspepsia, flatulence, anorexia, GI fullness, peptic ulcer. **Hepatic:** Hepatitis, cholestatic jaundice, hepatocellular jaundice, *hepatic necrosis*. *Bleeding complications:* Ecchymosis, hematuria, epistaxis, conjunctival hemorrhage, *GI bleeding*, perioperative bleeding, posttraumatic bleeding, *intracerebral bleeding (rare)*. **Dermatologic:** Maculopapular or urticarial rash, pruritus, urticaria. Rarely, erythema multiforme, exfoliative dermatitis, *Stevens-Johnson syndrome*. **CNS:** Dizziness, headache. **Neuromuscular:** Asthenia, SLE, peripheral neuropathy, arthropathy, myositis. **Miscellaneous:** Tinnitus, pain, allergic pneumonitis, vasculitis, nephrotic syndrome, renal failure, angioedema, hyponatremia, serum sickness.

LABORATORY TEST CONSIDERATIONS

↑ Alkaline phosphatase, ALT, AST, serum cholesterol, and triglycerides. Abnormal LFTs.

DRUG INTERACTIONS

Antacids / ↓ Ticlopidine plasma levels
Aspirin / ↑ Effect of aspirin on collagen-induced platelet aggregation
Bupropion / ↑ Bupropion AUC and peak plasma levels and ↓ bupropion clearance R/T inhibition of metabolism by CYP2B6
Carbamazepine / ↑ Carbamazepine plasma levels → toxicity
Cimetidine / ↓ Ticlopidine clearance R/T ↓ liver metabolism
Digoxin / Slight ↓ in digoxin plasma levels

H *Evening primrose oil* / Potential for ↑ antiplatelet effect

H *Feverfew* / Potential for ↑ antiplatelet effect

H *Garlic* / Potential for ↑ antiplatelet effect

H *Ginger* / Potential for ↑ antiplatelet effect

H *Ginkgo biloba* / Potential for ↑ antiplatelet effect

H *Ginseng* / Potential for ↑ antiplatelet effect

H *Grapeseed extract* / Potential for ↑ antiplatelet effect

Phenytoin / ↑ Phenytoin plasma levels → somnolence and lethargy

Theophylline / ↑ Theophylline plasma levels R/T ↓ clearance

HOW SUPPLIED

Tablets: 250 mg.

DOSAGE

• **TABLETS**

Reduce risk of thrombotic stroke, Adjunct with aspirin to reduce subacute stent thrombosis.

250 mg twice a day.

NURSING CONSIDERATIONS

ⓒ Do not confuse Ticlid with Tequin (a fluoroquinolone antibiotic).

ADMINISTRATION/STORAGE

1. To increase bioavailability and decrease GI discomfort, take with food or just after eating.

2. If switched from an anticoagulant or fibrinolytic drug to ticlopidine, discontinue the former drug before initiation of ticlopidine therapy.

3. IV methylprednisolone (20 mg) may normalize prolonged bleeding times, usually within 2 hr.

ASSESSMENT

1. Note reasons for therapy; assess for liver disease, bleeding disorders, or ulcer disease. Ascertain aspirin intolerance.

2. See increased use of clopidogrel due to less side effect profile and once daily dosing advantage.

3. List baseline hematologic profile (e.g., CBC, PT, PTT, INR), renal and LFTs. Monitor CBC biweekly to screen for possibly fatal thrombotic thrombocytopenic purpura (↓ platelets and ↓ WBCs).

CLIENT/FAMILY TEACHING

1. Take with food or after meals to minimize GI upset.

2. It may take longer than usual to stop bleeding; report unusual bleeding as severe hematological side effects may occur.

3. Brush teeth with a soft-bristle toothbrush, use an electric razor for shaving, wear shoes when ambulating, use caution and avoid injury, as bleeding times may be prolonged.

4. During the first 3 months of therapy, low white blood count can occur, resulting in an increased risk of infection. Come for scheduled blood tests and report any symptoms of infection (e.g., fever, chills, sore throat).

5. Any severe or persistent diarrhea, SC bleeding, skin rashes, or evidence of cholestasis (e.g., yellow skin or sclera, dark urine, light-colored stools) should be reported.

6. Avoid OTC agents without provider approval. Keep all F/U visits and labs.

OUTCOMES/EVALUATE

Prevention of a complete or recurrent cerebral thrombotic event

Tigecycline   **IV**
(tye-gah-**SYE**-kleen)

CLASSIFICATION(S):
Antibiotic, miscellaneous

PREGNANCY CATEGORY: D

Rx: Tygacil.

USES

(1) Complicated skin and skin structure infections due to *Escherichia coli*, *Enterococcus faecalis* (vancomycin-susceptible isolates only), *Staphylococcus aureus* (methicillin-susceptible and methicillin-resistant isolates), *Streptococcus agalactiae*, *Streptococcus anginosus* group (includes *S. anginosus*, *S. intermedius*, and *S. constellatus*), *Streptococcus pyogenes*, and *Bacteroides fragilis*. (2) Complicated intraabdominal infections due to *Citrobacter freundii*, *Tnerobacter*

cloacae, *E. coli, Klebsiella oxytoca, Klebsiella pneumoniae, E. faecalis* (vancomycin-susceptible isolates only), *S. aureus* (methicillin-susceptible isolates only), *S. anginosus* group (includes *S. anginosus, S. intermedius,* and *S. constellatus*), *B. fragilis, Bacteroides thetaiotaomicron, Bacteroides uniformis, Bacteroides vulgatus, Clostridium perfringens,* and *Peptostreotococcus micros.*

ACTION/KINETICS

Action

Tigecycline is a glycylcycline that inhibits protein translation in bacteria by binding to the 30S ribosomal subunit and blocking entry of amino-acyl tRNA molecules into the A site of the ribosome. This prevents incorporation of amino acid residues into elongating peptide chains. The drug is structurally similar to tetracyclines and may have similar side effects.

Pharmacokinetics

Is not extensively metabolized. Excreted through both the feces (59%) and urine (33%). **t½:** 42.4 hr after multiple doses. **Plasma protein binding:** 71–89%.

CONTRAINDICATIONS

Use during tooth development unless other drugs are not likely to be effective or are contraindicated. Use in children less than 18 years of age.

SPECIAL CONCERNS

To reduce the development of drug-resistant bacteria and maintain efficacy, only use tigecycline to treat infections that are proven or strongly suspected to be caused by susceptible bacteria. Use with caution in severe hepatic impairment, in those with known hypersensitivity to tetracycline class antibiotics, and during lactation. Use during tooth development (last half of pregnancy, infancy, childhood until age 8 years), may cause permanent discoloration of the teeth (yellow-gray-brown). Use caution when considering use in clients with complicated intraabdominal infections secondary to clinically apparent intestinal perforation due to the possibility of sepsis/septic shock. Safety and efficacy have not been determined in children less than 18 years of age.

SIDE EFFECTS

Most Common

N&V, hypertension, headache, diarrhea, anemia, thrombocytopenia, hypoproteinemia, abdominal pain, fever, infection, injection site reaction.

GI: N&V, diarrhea, abdominal pain, dyspepsia, constipation, pseudomembranous colitis, abnormal stools, anorexia, dry mouth, jaundice. **CNS:** Headache, dizziness, insomnia, somnolence. **CV:** Hypertension, hypotension, phlebitis, bradycardia, tachycardia, thrombophlebitis, vasodilation. **Respiratory:** Increased cough, dyspnea, pulmonary physical finding. **GU:** Leukorrhea, vaginal moniliasis, vaginitis. **Hematologic:** Thrombocytopenia, anemia, leukocytosis, eosinophilia. **Body as a whole:** Infection, fever, abnormal healing, asthenia, hypersensitivity/allergic reactions, chills, superinfection (including fungi), *septic shock.* **Miscellaneous:** Abscess, back pain, peripheral edema, taste perversion, infusion-related serious reactions, injection site edema/inflammation/pain, injection site phlebitis.

LABORATORY TEST CONSIDERATIONS

↑ Alkaline phosphatase, BUN, lactic dehydrogenase, AST, ALT, INR. Bilirubinemia, hyper-/hypoglycemia, hypokalemia, hypoproteinemia, hypocalcemia, hyponatremia. Prolonged aPTT and prothrombin.

DRUG INTERACTIONS

Oral contraceptives / Possible ↓ oral contraceptive effectiveness
Warfarin / ↓ Warfarin clearance, ↑ warfarin AUC and C$_{max}$

HOW SUPPLIED

Powder for Injection, Lyophilized: 50 mg.

DOSAGE

- **IV INFUSION**

  Complicated skin/skin structure infections, complicated intraabdominal infections.

Adults, initial: 100 mg; **then,** 50 mg q 12 hr for 5–14 days. Duration of therapy is dependent on the severity and site of the infection and the client's clinical and bacteriological progress. Give IV infusions over about 30–60 min q 12 hr. *NOTE:* In severe hepatic impairment (Child-Pugh class C), the initial dose is

---

Bold Italic = life threatening side effect   ■ = black box warning   ♣ = Available in Canada

100 mg, followed by a reduced maintenance dose of 25 mg q 12 hr.

NURSING CONSIDERATIONS

ADMINISTRATION/STORAGE

IV 1. To prepare the injection, reconstitute each vial with 5.3 mL of 0.9% NaCl injection or D5W injection to achieve a concentration of 10 mg/mL. Gently swirl the vial until the drug dissolves. Immediately withdraw 5 mL of the reconstituted solution and add to 100 mL IV bag for infusion (for a 100 mg dose, reconstitute 2 vials; for a 50 mg dose, reconstitute 1 vial) over 30–60 min. The maximum concentration in the IV bag should be 1 mg/mL. The reconstituted solution should be yellow to orange in color; discard if the solution is not this color. Inspect visually for particulate matter and discoloration (green, black) prior to administration. May be stored in the IV bag at room temperature for up to 6 hr or refrigerated for up to 24 hr.

2. May be given IV through a dedicated line or through a Y-site. If the same IV line is used for sequential infusion of several drugs, flush the line before and after tigecycline infusion with either 0.9% NaCl injection or D5W injection.

3. When given through a Y-site, tigecycline is compatible with the following: Dobutamine, dopamine, RL, lidocaine, KCl, ranitidine, and theophylline.

4. The following drugs should **not** be given simultaneously through the same Y-site as tigecycline: Amphotericin B, chlorpromazine, methylprednisolone, and voriconazole.

ASSESSMENT

1. Note reasons for therapy, onset, characteristics of S&S, culture results, clinical presentation, other agents trialed.

2. Assess for any known hypersensitivity to tetracycline class antibiotics.

3. Monitor CBC, renal and LFTs; reduce dose with liver dysfunction. Use caution with hepatic dysfunction, during lactation and during tooth development (last half of pregnancy, infancy, childhood until age 8 years) may cause permanent discoloration of the teeth (yellow-gray-brown).

CLIENT/FAMILY TEACHING

1. Drug is administered intravenously every 12 hours and used to treat bacterial infections, not viral infections. It should be administered exactly as directed despite feeling better. Skipping doses or not completing the full course of therapy may (a) decrease the effectiveness of the immediate treatment and (b) increase the likelihood that bacteria will develop resistance and will not be treatable by tigecycline or other antibacterial drugs in the future.

2. Use nonhormonal form of birth control as drug may impair effectiveness of these during therapy; avoid pregnancy.

3. Report any adverse or unusual side effects including bruising/bleeding, lack of response or worsening of symptoms, pain and swelling at injection site, diarrhea or vaginal infection, or severe N&V.

OUTCOMES/EVALUATE

Resolution of infection; negative culture results

Tiludronate disodium

(tye-**LOO**-droh-nayt)

CLASSIFICATION(S):
Bone growth regulator, bisphosphonate
PREGNANCY CATEGORY: C
Rx: Skelid.

USES

Paget's disease where the level of serum alkaline phosphatase is at least twice upper limit of normal, in those who are symptomatic, or who are at risk for future complications of disease.

ACTION/KINETICS

Action

Inhibits activity of osteoclasts and decreases bone turnover. Does not interfere with bone mineralization.

Pharmacokinetics

Poorly absorbed from GI tract when fasting and in presence of food. **Peak serum levels:** 2 hr. Not metabolized; excreted in urine. **t½:** About 150 hr.

CONTRAINDICATIONS
Not recommended for those with C_{CR} less than 30 mL/min.

SPECIAL CONCERNS
Use with caution during lactation and in those with dysphagia, symptomatic esophageal disease, gastritis, duodenitis, or ulcers. Safety and efficacy have not been determined in children.

SIDE EFFECTS

Most Common
Pain, diarrhea, dyspepsia, N&V, back pain, rales/rhinitis, sinusitis, URTI, accidental injury, flu-like symptoms.

GI: Diarrhea, N&V, dyspepsia, flatulence, tooth disorder, abdominal pain, constipation, dry mouth, gastritis. **Body as whole:** Pain, back pain, accidental injury, flu-like symptoms, chest pain, asthenia, syncope, fatigue, flushing. **CNS:** Headache, dizziness, paresthesia, vertigo, anorexia, somnolence, anxiety, nervousness, insomnia. **CV:** Dependent edema, peripheral edema, hypertension, syncope. **Musculoskeletal:** Arthralgia, arthrosis, pathological fracture, involuntary muscle contractions. **Respiratory:** Rhinitis, sinusitis, URTI, coughing, pharyngitis, bronchitis. **Dermatologic:** Rash, skin disorder, pruritus, increased sweating, ***Stevens-Johnson type syndrome (rare)***. **Ophthalmic:** Cataract, conjunctivitis, glaucoma. **Miscellaneous:** Hyperparathyroidism, vitamin D deficiency, UTI, infection.

OD OVERDOSE MANAGEMENT
Symptoms: Hypocalcemia. *Treatment:* Supportive.

DRUG INTERACTIONS
Antacids, Al or Mg / Antacids, taken 1 hr before, ↓ tiludronate bioavailability
Aspirin / Aspirin, taken 2 hr after, ↓ tiludronate bioavailability by 50%
Calcium / ↓ Tiludronate bioavailability when taken at same time
Indomethacin / ↑ Tiludronate bioavailability by 2- to 4-fold

HOW SUPPLIED
Tablets: 240 mg (equivalent to 200 mg tiludronic acid).

DOSAGE
- **TABLETS**
  Paget's disease.

Adults: Single 400 mg/day dose (2–240 tablets) taken with 6 to 8 oz of plain water for period of only 3 months.

NURSING CONSIDERATIONS

ADMINISTRATION/STORAGE
1. Allow an interval of 3 months to assess response.
2. Data regarding retreatment are limited, although favorable improvement has been observed.
3. Store from 15–30°C (59–86°F).

ASSESSMENT
1. Note reasons for therapy, other agents trialed, outcome. List clinical presentation and subjective complaints.
2. Monitor electrolytes, mineral panel, calcium, alk phosphatase, renal and LFTs.

CLIENT/FAMILY TEACHING
1. Take with 6 to 8 oz of plain water. Do not take within 2 hr of food. Beverages other than water, food, and some medications reduce absorption of tiludronate.
2. Do not take aspirin, indomethacin, aluminum- or magnesium-containing antacids, or calcium or mineral supplements within 2 hr of taking drug.
3. Do not remove tablets from foil strips until they are to be used.
4. May experience nausea, diarrhea, and GI upset; report if severe.
5. Report any rashes, itching, hives, severe stomach pains, bloody or black tarry stools, flank pain, N&V, or other adverse side effects.

OUTCOMES/EVALUATE
Inhibition of Paget's disease progression; ↓ Bone reabsorption and calcium levels

---

Timolol maleate
(**TIE**-moh-lohl)

CLASSIFICATION(S):
Beta-adrenergic blocking agent
PREGNANCY CATEGORY: C
Rx: Ophthalmic Gel Forming Solution: Timoptic-XE. **Ophthalmic Solution:** Betimol, Istalol, Timoptic. **Tablets:** Blocadren.

✦Rx: Apo-Timol, Apo-Timop, Gen-Timolol, Novo-Timol, Nu-Timolol, PMS-Timolol, Rhoxal-timolol, ratio-Timolol.

SEE ALSO *BETA-ADRENERGIC BLOCKING AGENTS.*

USES

Tablets (Blocadren): (1) Hypertension (alone or in combination with other antihypertensives such as thiazide diuretics). (2) Reduce CV mortality and risk of reinfarction in clinically stable MI survivors. (3) Prophylaxis of migraine. *Investigational:* Ventricular arrhythmias and tachycardias, essential tremors.

Ophthalmic solution (Betimol, Istalol, Timoptic): Lower IOP in chronic open-angle glaucoma, selected cases of secondary glaucoma, ocular hypertension, aphakic (no lens) clients with glaucoma.

Gel-Forming Solution (Timoptic-XE): Reduce elevated IOP in open-angle glaucoma or ocular hypertension.

ACTION/KINETICS

Action

Exerts both $beta_1$- and $beta_2$-adrenergic blocking activity. Has minimal sympathomimetic effects, direct myocardial depressant effects, or local anesthetic action. Does not cause pupillary constriction or night blindness. The mechanism of the protective effect in MI is not known.

Pharmacokinetics

Peak plasma levels: 1–2 hr. **$t\frac{1}{2}$:** 4 hr. Metabolized in the liver. Metabolites and unchanged drug excreted through the kidney. Also reduces both elevated and normal IOP, whether or not glaucoma is present; thought to act by reducing aqueous humor formation and/or by slightly increasing outflow of aqueous humor. Does not affect pupil size or visual acuity. For use in eye: **Onset:** 30 min. **Maximum effect:** 1–2 hr. **Duration:** 24 hr.

CONTRAINDICATIONS

Hypersensitivity to drug. Bronchial asthma or bronchospasm including severe COPD. Use of the ophthalmic solution in those with sinus bradycardia, second- or third-degree AV block or overt cardiac failure, cardiogenic shock.

SPECIAL CONCERNS

Use ophthalmic preparation with caution in clients for whom systemic beta-adrenergic blocking agents are contraindicated. Safe use in children not established.

SIDE EFFECTS

Most Common

When used ophthalmically: Ocular irritation (including conjunctivitis), local hypersensitivity reactions.

When used systemically: Insomnia, malaise/fatigue, anxiety, nervousness, impotence, bradycardia, dizziness, cold hands/feet.

See *Beta-Adrenergic Blocking Agents* for a complete list of possible side effects.

Following use of ophthalmic product: Ocular irritation (including conjunctivitis), blepharitis, keratitis, blepharoptosis, decreased corneal sensitivity, visual disturbances (including refractive changes), diplopia, ptosis, local hypersensitivity reactions, slight decrease in resting HR.

DRUG INTERACTIONS

When used ophthalmically, possible potentiation with systemically administered beta-adrenergic blocking agents.

HOW SUPPLIED

Ophthalmic Gel Forming Solution: 0.25%, 0.5%; *Ophthalmic Solution:* 0.25%, 0.5%; *Tablets:* 5 mg, 10 mg, 20 mg.

DOSAGE

- **TABLETS**

  Hypertension.

  Initial: 10 mg twice a day alone or with a diuretic; **maintenance:** 20–40 mg/day (up to 60 mg/day in two doses may be required), depending on BP and HR. If dosage increase is necessary, wait 7 days.

  MI prophylaxis in clients who have survived the acute phase.

  10 mg twice a day.

  Migraine prophylaxis.

  Initially: 10 mg twice a day. **Maintenance:** 20 mg/day given as a single dose; total daily dose may be increased to 30 mg in divided doses or decreased to 10 mg, depending on the response and client tolerance. If a satisfactory response for migraine prophylaxis is not obtained within 6–8 weeks using the maximum daily dose, discontinue the drug.

Essential tremor.
10 mg/day.

BETIMOL OR TIMOPTIC, EACH 0.25% OR 0.5%

• **OPHTHALMIC SOLUTION**
Glaucoma.
1 gtt of 0.25 or 0.50% solution in each eye twice a day. If the decrease in intraocular pressure is maintained, reduce dose to 1 gtt once a day.

ISTALOL OPHTHALMIC (0.5%)

• **OPHTHALMIC SOLUTION**
Glaucoma.
Initial: 1 gtt per affected eye once daily in the morning. If this does not adequately control intraocular pressure, an agent other than another topical β-adrenergic blocker should be added to the regimen.

TIMOPTIC-XE 0.25% OR 0.5%

• **OPHTHALMIC GEL FORMING SOLUTION**
Glaucoma.
1 gtt once daily.

NURSING CONSIDERATIONS

℃ Do not confuse timolol with atenolol, each of which is a beta-adrenergic blocking drug.

ADMINISTRATION/STORAGE

1. When transferring from another antiglaucoma agent, continue old medication on day 1 of timolol therapy (1 gtt of 0.25% solution). Then, discontinue former therapy. Initiate with 0.25% solution. Increase to 0.50% solution if response is insufficient. Further dosage increases are ineffective.

2. When transferring from several antiglaucoma agents, individualize the dose. If one of the agents is a beta-adrenergic blocking agent, discontinue it before starting timolol. Dosage adjustments should involve one drug at a time at 1-week intervals. Continue the antiglaucoma drugs with the addition of timolol, 1 gtt of 0.25% solution twice a day (if response is inadequate, 1 gtt of 0.5% solution may be used twice a day). The following day, discontinue one of the other antiglaucoma agents while

continuing the remaining agents or discontinue based on client response.

3. Before using the gel, invert the closed container and shake once before each use.

4. Administer other ophthalmics at least 10 min before the gel.

5. The ocular hypotensive effect has been maintained when switching clients from timolol solution given twice a day to the gel once daily.

ASSESSMENT

1. Note reasons for therapy, onset, characteristic of S&S, intraocular pressure readings.

2. Monitor VS, IOPs, renal, and LFTs.

CLIENT/FAMILY TEACHING

1. Review procedure for eye administration.
• Wash hands before and after use
• Instill drops as instructed and prescribed
• Apply finger lightly to lacrimal sac for 1 min following administration. Do not permit container to contact skin.
• Regular intraocular measurements by an eye dr. are required because ocular hypertension may recur without any overt S&S.

2. When tablets used for long-term prophylaxis against MI, do not interrupt therapy; abrupt withdrawal may precipitate reinfarction.

3. Do not perform tasks such as driving or operating machinery until drug effects are realized; may cause dizziness.

4. Report any evidence of rash, dizziness, heart palpitations, SOB, edema, or depression. May cause increased sensitivity to cold; dress appropriate.

5. With diabetes, drug may mask S&S of hypoglycemia. Keep log of FS, pulse, and BP for provider review.

6. Continue lifestyle modifications (i.e., weight reduction, regular exercise, reduced intake of sodium and alcohol, and no smoking) in the overall goal of BP control.

OUTCOMES/EVALUATE

• ↓ BP
• Myocardial reinfarction prophylaxis
• Migraine prophylaxis
• ↓ Intraocular pressures

Bold Italic = life threatening side effect   ■ = black box warning   ✤ = Available in Canada

Tinidazole
(tye-**NI**-dah-zole)

CLASSIFICATION(S):
Antiprotozoal, second generation
PREGNANCY CATEGORY: C
Rx: Tindamax.

USES
(1) Intestinal amebiasis and amebic liver abscess due to *Entamoeba histolytica* in adults and children over 3 years of age. (2) Giardiasis due to *Giardia duodenalis (Giardia lamblia)* in adults and children over 3 years of age. (3) Trichomoniasis due to *Trichomonas vaginalis* in female and male partners.

ACTION/KINETICS
Action
An antiprotozoal drug. The nitro group of tinidazole is reduced by *Trichomonas*. The free nitro group generated may be responsible for the antiprotozoal activity. The mechanism against *Giardia* and *Entamoeba* is not known.

Pharmacokinetics
Rapidly and completely absorbed. **Time to maximum levels:** 1.6 hr. Administration with food delayed the maximum levels by about 2 hr along with a decrease of 10% in C_{max}. Distributed to virtually all tissues and body fluids; crosses the blood brain barrier. Metabolized in the liver, mainly by CYP3A4. **$t\frac{1}{2}$, plasma:** 12–14 hr. Excreted in both the feces and urine. **Plasma protein binding:** 12%.

CONTRAINDICATIONS
Hypersensitivity to tinidazole, any component of the product, or other nitroimidazole derivatives. Use during the first trimester of pregnancy. Lactation (interruption during therapy and for 3 days following the last dose).

SPECIAL CONCERNS
Reserve use for conditions described in *Uses;* avoid unnecessary use. Use with caution in those with evidence of or history of blood dyscrasias. Safety and efficacy have not been demonstrated in children except to treat giardiasis and amebiasis in children over 3 years of age.

SIDE EFFECTS
Most Common
N&V, anorexia, excessive thirst, salivation, metallic/bitter taste, constipation, diarrhea, headache, darkened urine, swollen/sore/discolored tongue.
CNS: Headache, dizziness, seizures, transient peripheral neuropathy (including numbness and paresthesia), ataxia, drowsiness, giddiness, insomnia, vertigo, coma, confusion, depression (rare). **GI:** Metallic/bitter taste, N&V, abdominal pain, dyspepsia, cramps, epigastric discomfort, anorexia, constipation, diarrhea, stomatitis, swollen/sore/discolored tongue, oral candidiasis, excessive thirst, salivation, furry tongue (rare). **Musculoskeletal:** Arthralgias, arthritis, myalgias. **Respiratory:** Bronchospasm, dyspnea, pharyngitis (rare). **GU:** Darkened urine, increased vaginal discharge. **Hematologic:** Transient leukopenia, transient neutropenia, reversible thrombocytopenia (rare). **Hypersensitivity:** Angioedema, burning sensation, dry mouth, fever, flushing, pruritus, rash, salivation, sweating, thirst, urticaria. **Body as a whole:** Weakness, fatigue, malaise. **Miscellaneous:** Candida overgrowth, hepatic abnormalities (including increased transaminase levels), palpitations.

LABORATORY TEST CONSIDERATIONS
Possible interference (values of zero) with serum chemistry values, including AST, ALT, LDH, triglycerides, and hexokinase glucose.

DRUG INTERACTIONS
Alcohol / Possible abdominal cramps, N&V, headaches, and flushing; avoid alcoholic beverages during therapy and for 3 days after discontinuation
Anticoagulants / ↑ Warfarin effect → prolonged PT
Cholestyramine / Possible ↓ tinidazole bioavailability; separate doses of cholestyramine and tinidazole
Cimetidine / ↑ Tinidazole $t\frac{1}{2}$ and ↓ clearance R/T inhibition of metabolism by CYP3A4
Cyclosporine / Possible ↑ cyclosporine levels

 = see color insert   = Herbal   = Intravenous   = sound alike drug

Disulfiram / Possible psychotic reactions; do not give to clients who have taken disulfiram within the past 2 weeks

Fluorouracil / ↓ Fluorouracil clearance → toxicity

Fosphenytoin (IV) / Prolonged phenytoin t½ and ↓ clearance

Ketoconazole / ↑ Tinidazole t½ and ↓ clearance R/T inhibition of metabolism by CYP3A4

Lithium / Possible ↑ serum lithium levels

Oxytetracycline / May antagonize the effect of tinidazole

Phenobarbital / ↑ Tinidazole elimination R/T ↑ metabolism by CYP3A4

Phenytoin / ↑ Tinidazole elimination R/T ↑ metabolism by CYP3A4

Rifampin / ↑ Tinidazole elimination R/T ↑ metabolism by CYP3A4

Tacrolimus / Possible ↑ tacrolimus levels

HOW SUPPLIED
Tablets: 250 mg, 500 mg.

DOSAGE
- **TABLETS**

  Amebic liver abscess.

  Adults: 2 grams/day for 3–5 days. **Children over 3 years:** 50 mg/kg/day (up to 2 grams) for 3–5 days.

  Intestinal amebiasis.

  Adults: 2 grams/day for 3 days. **Children over 3 years:** 50 mg/kg/day (up to 2 grams/day) for 3 days.

  Giardiasis.

  Adults: 2 grams as a single dose. **Children over 3 years:** 50 mg/kg (up to 2 grams) as a single dose.

  Trichomoniasis.

  Adults: 2 grams as a single dose.

NURSING CONSIDERATIONS

ADMINISTRATION/STORAGE
1. Take with food to minimize incidence of epigastric distress and other GI side effects.
2. Because trichomoniasis is a sexually transmitted disease, treat sexual partners with the same dose and at the same time.
3. If tinidazole is given on a day when hemodialysis is performed, give an additional dose of the drug equivalent to one-half the recommended dose after the end of the hemodialysis.
4. An extemporaneous oral suspension may be compounded as follows: Grind 4 x 500 mg tablets to a fine powder using a mortar and pestle. Add about 10 mL of cherry syrup to the powder and mix until smooth. Transfer the suspension to a graduated amber container. Use several small rinses of cherry syrup to transfer any remaining drug in the mortar to the final suspension for a final volume of 30 mL. The suspension in cherry syrup is stable for 7 days at room temperature; shake well before using.
5. Store tablets from 15–30°C (59–86°F) and protect from light.

ASSESSMENT
1. Note reasons for therapy, onset, characteristics of S&S, other agents trialed, culture results. Identify source/causative agent.
2. List drugs prescribed to ensure none interact.
3. Assess for any history/evidence of nervous system diseases or blood dyscrasia.
4. Monitor CBC, renal, and LFTs.

CLIENT/FAMILY TEACHING
1. Take tablets as directed with food.
2. Report any adverse side effects, such as numbness in extremities, chest pain, SOB, dizziness, drowsiness, unusual bruising/bleeding, confusion, or symptoms of infection.
3. Avoid alcohol during and for three days following therapy.
4. Practice reliable contraception and do not breastfeed during therapy.
5. With STD ensure partner is also treated at the same time.

OUTCOMES/EVALUATE
Resolution of infection

Bold Italic = life threatening side effect   ■ = black box warning   ✦ = Available in Canada

Tinzaparin sodium ■
(tin-**ZAH**-pah-rin)

CLASSIFICATION(S):
Anticoagulant, low molecular weight heparin
PREGNANCY CATEGORY: B
Rx: Innohep.

SEE ALSO *HEPARIN, LOW MOLECULAR WEIGHT*

USES
Treat acute symptomatic deep vein thrombosis (DVT) with or without pulmonary embolism when given with warfarin sodium. *Investigational:* Prophylaxis of DVT (which may lead to pulmonary embolism) in clients undergoing moderate risk surgery, orthopedic surgery, hip fracture surgery, or neurosurgery at risk for thromboembolic complications.

ACTION/KINETICS
Pharmacokinetics
Maximum plasma levels: 0.25–0.87 international units/mL within 4 to 5 hr after a single SC dose of 4,500 international units. Metabolized in the liver. $t\frac{1}{2}$: 3–4 hr. Excreted mainly in the urine. Clearance is reduced in impaired renal function.

ADDITIONAL CONTRAINDICATIONS
Use in those with a history of heparin-induced thrombocytopenia (HIT). Sensitivity to heparin, sulfites, benzyl alcohol, or pork products. Mixing with other injections or infusions.

SPECIAL CONCERNS
■ (1) Spinal/Epidural hematomas. When neuraxial anesthesia (spinal/epidural anesthesia) or spinal puncture is used, those anticoagulated or scheduled to be anticoagulated with low molecular weight heparins or heparinoids to prevent thromboembolic complications are at risk of developing a spinal or epidural hematoma that can result in long-term or permanent paralysis. The risk of these events is increased using indwelling epidural catheters for giving analgesics or by the concurrent use of drugs affecting hemostasis, such as NSAIDs, platelet inhibitors, or other anticoagulants. The risk also appears to be increased by traumatic or repeated spinal or epidural puncture. (2) Frequently monitor for signs and symptoms of neurological impairment. If neurological compromise is observed, immediate treatment is required. (3) The physician should consider potential benefits vs risk before neuraxial intervention in clients anticoagulated or to be anticoagulated for thromboprophylaxis.■ Use with caution in pregnancy and only if clearly needed since benzyl alcohol in the product may cross the placenta and cause a fatal 'gasping syndrome' in premature neonates. Use with caution during lactation. Safety and efficacy have not been determined in children.

SIDE EFFECTS
Most Common
Injection site reactions, chest pain, bleeding, constipation, N&V, UTI, epistaxis, dyspnea, pulmonary embolism, back pain, pain, fever, headache.
CV: Bleeding, *hemorrhage (fatal or nonfatal)*, hypo-/hypertension, tachycardia, angina pectoris, deep thrombophlebitis, deep leg thrombophlebitis, cardiac arrhythmias, *MI, coronary thrombosis,* thromboembolism, peripheral ischemia, hemoptysis, ocular hemorrhage, anorectal bleeding, cerebral/intracranial bleeding, hemarthrosis, hemoptysis, *GI hemorrhage, hemopericardium*. **Hematologic:** Thrombocytopenia, anemia, hematoma, agranulocytosis, pancytopenia, granulocytopenia, thrombocythemia. **GI:** N&V, abdominal pain, diarrhea, constipation, flatulence, GI disorder, dyspepsia, cholestatic hepatitis, hematemesis, melena, retroperitoneal/intra-abdominal bleeding, cholestatic hepatitis. **CNS:** Headache, dizziness, insomnia, confusion. **GU:** Priapism, UTI, hematuria, urinary retention, dysuria, *vaginal hemorrhage*. **Respiratory:** *Pulmonary embolism*, dyspnea, epistaxis, pneumonia, respiratory disorder. **Dermatologic:** Rash, erythematous rash, maculopapular rash, pruritus, bullous eruption, skin disorder, necrosis, epidermal necrolysis, ischemic necrosis, urticaria, ecchymosis,

purpura, cellulitis, allergic purpura, **Stevens-Johnson syndrome**. **Injection site:** Mild local irritation, pain, hematoma, ecchymosis, necrosis, abscess, bleeding. **Hypersensitivity:** *Anaphylaxis*, allergic reaction, urticaria, angioedema. **Body as a whole:** Fever, impaired healing, infection, dependent edema, abcess, acute febrile reaction. **Miscellaneous:** Back/chest pain, pain, rash, neonatal hypotonia, congenital anomaly, *fetal death*/distress, fetal/neonatal cutis aplasia of the scalp, ischemic necrosis, necrosis, neoplasm.

ADDITIONAL DRUG INTERACTIONS
Anticoagulants, oral / ↑ Risk of bleeding
Dextran / ↑ Risk of bleeding
Thrombolytics / ↑ Risk of bleeding

HOW SUPPLIED
Injection: 20,000 anti-Factor Xa international units/mL.

DOSAGE
• **SC ONLY**
  Deep vein thrombosis with or without pulmonary embolism.
Adults: 175 anti-Factor IX units/kg once daily for 6 days or until client is adequately anticoagulated with warfarin (INR at least 2.0 for two consecutive days). Initiate warfarin when appropriate (usually 1–3 days after tinzaparin initiation).

NURSING CONSIDERATIONS

ADMINISTRATION/STORAGE
1. Do not give IM or IV.
2. Do not mix with other injections or infusions.
3. To assure withdrawal of the correct volume, use an appropriately calibrated syringe.
4. Inspect visually before administration to ensure there is no particulate matter or discoloration of the vial contents.
5. Position clients either supine or sitting and give by deep SC injection. Alternate injections between left and right anterolateral and left and right posterolateral abdominal wall. Vary the injection site daily. Introduce the entire length of the needle into a skin fold held between the thumb and forefinger; hold the skin fold throughout the

injection. To minimize bruising, do not rub the injection site after completing the injection.
6. Dosage adjustments are not required for the elderly and those with renal impairment.
7. Store between 15–30°C (59–86°F).

ASSESSMENT
1. Assess for any bleeding disorders or active major bleeding, HIT, or any hypersensitivity to heparin sulfite, benzyl alcohol or pork products.
2. Use cautiously with history of recent GI ulcerations, diabetic retinopathy, hemorrhage, uncontrolled HTN, or bleeding diathesis.
3. Confirm PE by segmental lung scan defect and/or DVT by US. Start SC tinzaparin treatment x 6 days; add coumadin on day 2 and titrate to an INR of 2–3.
4. Weigh client; calculate dose for client weight (kg x 0.00875 mL/kg = volume in mL to be administered SC).
5. Monitor PT, INR, platelet count, CBC, renal function and FOB.

CLIENT/FAMILY TEACHING
1. Review indications for therapy, self administration techniques, and importance of site rotation.
2. To administer, lie down or sit and give by deep SC injection only. Alternate sites between the left and right anterolateral and left and right posterolateral abdominal wall as shown. Vary injection site daily.
3. Insert whole length of needle into a skin fold held between the thumb and forefinger. Hold the skin fold throughout the injection.
4. To minimize bruising do not rub site after administering and avoid OTC agents such as NSAIDs or aspirin.
5. Use caution to prevent injury; avoid contact sports, excessive jostling and use soft bristle tooth bush, and use electric razor to prevent bleeding.
6. Report any unusual bruising, bleeding, chest pain, acute SOB, itching, rash, or swelling. Keep F/U appointment to evaluate blood tests and response.

OUTCOMES/EVALUATE
• Anticoagulation and prevention of complications R/T clot formation
• Resolution of DVT

Tioconazole

(tie-oh-**KON**-ah-zohl)

CLASSIFICATION(S):
Antifungal
PREGNANCY CATEGORY: C
OTC: Monistat 1, Vagistat-1.

USES
Vulvovaginal candidiasis, including moniliasis and vaginal yeast infections.

ACTION/KINETICS
Action
Antifungal activity thought to be due to alteration of the permeability of the cell membrane of the fungus, causing leakage of essential intracellular compounds.

Pharmacokinetics
The systemic absorption of the drug in nonpregnant clients is negligible.

CONTRAINDICATIONS
Use of a vaginal applicator during pregnancy may be contraindicated.

SPECIAL CONCERNS
Safety and effectiveness have not been determined during lactation or in children.

SIDE EFFECTS
Most Common
Burning, itching, irritation, vaginal discharge.
GU: Burning, itching, irritation, vulvar edema and swelling, discharge, vaginal pain/swelling/redness, dysuria, dyspareunia, nocturia, difficult or burning urination, desquamation, dryness of vaginal secretions. **Miscellaneous:** Headache, abdominal pain/cramping, URTI.

HOW SUPPLIED
Vaginal Ointment: 6.5%.

DOSAGE————————
• **VAGINAL OINTMENT**
  Vulvovaginal candidiasis.
Single dose of about 4.6 grams (one applicator full) intravaginally at bedtime.

NURSING CONSIDERATIONS
ASSESSMENT
Obtain a thorough nursing and GYN history; carefully evaluate symptoms, clinical presentation, and sources of infection.

CLIENT/FAMILY TEACHING
1. Review appropriate method for administration. Use just prior to bedtime.
2. Report if burning, irritation, or pain occurs. Effectiveness is not altered by menstruation.
3. May stain clothes; use sanitary napkins during therapy and change frequently because damp sanitary napkins may harbor infecting organisms. Avoid tampons during therapy.
4. To avoid reinfection, refrain from sexual intercourse. The ointment base may interact with rubber and latex; avoid condoms or diaphragms for 3 days following treatment.
5. Symptomatic improvement is usually seen within 3 days and complete relief within 7 days.

OUTCOMES/EVALUATE
Resolution of fungal infection; symptomatic improvement

Tiotropium bromide

(tee-oh-**TROE**-pee-um)

CLASSIFICATION(S):
Anticholinergic
PREGNANCY CATEGORY: C
Rx: Spiriva.

USES
Long-term, once daily, maintenance treatment of bronchospasm associated with COPD, including chronic bronchitis and emphysema.

ACTION/KINETICS
Action
Long-acting antimuscarinic (anticholinergic). In the airways it inhibits muscarinic M_3 receptors at the smooth muscle, leading to bronchodilation.

Pharmacokinetics
Since the drug is inhaled, the majority is deposited in the GI tract and, to a lesser extent, the lungs (site of action). The portion metabolized is through the CYP2D6 and CYP3A4 enzyme systems. However, most is excreted unchanged

T

---

through the urine. **t½, terminal:** 5–6 days. **Plasma protein binding:** 72%.

CONTRAINDICATIONS

History of hypersensitivity to atropine or its derivatives, including ipratropium. Use for initial treatment of acute episodes of bronchospasm (rescue therapy). Use with other anticholinergics (e.g., ipratropium).

SPECIAL CONCERNS

As an anticholinergic the drug may worsen signs and symptoms of narrow-angle glaucoma, prostatic hyperplasia, or bladder-neck obstruction; use with caution in these conditions. Immediate hypersensitivity reactions, including angioedema, may result after administration. Use with caution during lactation. Safety and efficacy have not been determined in children.

SIDE EFFECTS

Most Common
URTI, dry mouth, accidents, sinusitis, pharyngitis/rhinitis, abdominal pain, chest pain (non-specific), dependent edema, UTI, dyspepsia.
GI: Dry mouth, dyspepsia, abdominal pain, constipation, vomiting, gastro-esophageal reflux, GI disorder, stomatitis (including ulcerative). **CNS:** Depression, dysphonia, paresthesia. **Respiratory:** URTI, sinusitis, pharyngitis, rhinitis, epistaxis, coughing, laryngitis, paradoxical bronchospasm. **CV:** Angina pectoris (including aggravated angina pectoris), atrial fibrillation, SVT, palpitations. **Musculoskeletal:** Arthritis, skeletal pain, myalgia. **GU:** UTI, urinary retention. **Dermatologic:** Rash, pruritus, urticaria. **Body as a whole:** Accidents, dependent edema, infection, moniliasis, flu-like symptoms, allergic reaction, ***angioedema***. **Miscellaneous:** Herpes zoster, chest pain, leg pain, cataract.

`OD` OVERDOSE MANAGEMENT
Symptoms: High doses cause anticholinergic signs and symptoms. However, acute intoxication by inadvertent PO ingestion is unlikely as the drug is not well absorbed systemically.

HOW SUPPLIED

Capsules, Containing Powder for Inhalation: 18 mcg (as base).

DOSAGE

• **CAPSULES CONTAINING POWDER FOR INHALATION**
 COPD.
Inhale contents of 1 tiotropium capsule once daily using the *HandiHaler* inhalation device.

NURSING CONSIDERATIONS

ADMINISTRATION/STORAGE

1. To administer tiotropium bromide, use the following guidelines:
• Immediately before using the tiotropium dose, peel back the aluminum foil using the tab until 1 capsule is fully visible. Peel back the foil only as far as the 'STOP' line printed on the blister foil in order to prevent exposure of more than 1 capsule. Use the drug immediately after opening the package or its effectiveness may be reduced.
• Open the dust cap of the *HandiHaler* by pulling it upwards; then, open the mouthpiece.
• Place the capsule in the center chamber. It does not matter which end of the capsule is placed in the chamber.
• Firmly close the mouthpiece until a click is heard, leaving the dustcap open.
• Hold the *HandiHaler* device with the mouthpiece upwards; press the piercing button in completely once and release. This makes holes in the capsule and allows the medication to be released.
• Breathe out completely. Do not breathe into the mouthpiece at any time.
• Raise the *HandiHaler* device to the mouth and close lips tightly around the mouthpiece.
• Keep head in an upright position and breath in slowly and deeply but at a rate sufficient to hear the capsule vibrate. Breathe in until lungs are full and then hold breath as long as is comfortable. At the same time, take the *HandiHaler* device out of the mouth and resume normal breathing.
• To ensure getting the entire dose, repeat this once again.

- After finishing the daily dose of tiotropium, open the mouthpiece again. Tip out the used capsule and dispose of it. Close the mouthpiece and dust cap for storage.
2. Tiotropium capsules containing powder for inhalation are to be inhaled using a special device; do not take orally.
3. Store capsules from 15–30°C (59–86°F). Do not expose to extreme temperatures or moisture. Do not store capsules in the *HandiHaler*.

ASSESSMENT
1. List reasons for therapy, characteristics of S&S, other agents trialed, outcome.
2. Note CXR, PFTs, lung sounds, other drugs prescribed, overall physical condition/clinical presentation of client.
3. Assess EKG for QT prolongation, renal dysfunction, inability to self administer drug. Check for BPH, narrow angle glaucoma, bladder neck obstruction; drug may aggravate these conditions.
4. Closely monitor clients with moderate to severe renal impairment (C_{CR} 50 mL/min or less).

CLIENT/FAMILY TEACHING
1. Drug is administered once a day using the *HandiHaler* to control bronchospasms with lung disease. It is not to be used for acute bronchospasms or breathing problems; use rescue medication.
2. Capsules come in sealed blisters. Do not remove until ready to use. If an additional blister is accidently opened, and pill is exposed to air, discard capsule; do not save for next day use.
3. The capsules are to be placed in the *HandiHaler*; do not swallow. Review *Patient's Instructions for Use* pamphlet enclosed with medication to fully understand how to correctly administer capsules after instruction and return demonstration with provider. Contains pictures with step by step instruction. Rinse mouth after each use.
4. Do not use *HandiHaler* with any other capsules or drugs. Clean as directed (usually once a month) and as needed following instructions in the *Patient's Instructions* pamphlet.

5. When using *HandiHaler* do not permit powder to enter the eyes; may cause pupillary dilatation and blurred vision.
6. Report any eye pain/discomfort, colored images, blurred vision or vision halos associated with red eyes. May indicate glaucoma and should be immediately assessed by eye doctor.
7. Keep all F/U visits to evaluate breathing patterns and response. Report adverse side effects, chest pain, ↑ SOB, mental status changes, tremors, abdominal pain, severe constipation, or lack of response.

OUTCOMES/EVALUATE
Improved breathing patterns; long-term control of bronchospasm with COPD, emphysema and chronic bronchitis.

Tipranavir
(tye-**PRAN**-ah-veer)

CLASSIFICATION(S):
Antiviral, protease inhibitor
PREGNANCY CATEGORY: C
Rx: Aptivus.

USES
Given with ritonavir, 200 mg, to treat HIV-1 infected adults with evidence of viral replication who are highly treatment-experienced or have HIV-1 strains resistant to multiple protease inhibitors.

ACTION/KINETICS

Action
Tipranavir is a nonpeptidic HIV-1 protease inhibitor that inhibits the virus-specific processing of the viral Gag and Gag-Pol polyproteins in HIV-1 infected cells, thus preventing formation of mature virions. Development of resistance is possible, as well as cross resistance to other antiviral drugs.

Pharmacokinetics
Absorption is limited. **$t\frac{1}{2}$ for tipranavir/ritonavir (taken for longer than 2 weeks):** 5.5 hr (women) and 6 hr (men); **T_{max}:** 2.9 hr (women) and 3 hr (men). These differences do not warrant a dose adjustment. Bioavailability is increased with a high fat meal. Tipranavir is me-

tabolized in the liver by CYP3A4. Excreted mainly in the feces. **Plasma protein binding:** >99.9%.

CONTRAINDICATIONS

Known hypersensitivity to any of the components of the product. Moderate to severe hepatic insufficiency (Child-Pugh class B and C, respectively). Coadministration of tipranavir and ritonavir with drugs that are highly dependent on CYP3A for clearance and for which elevated plasma levels are associated with serious and/or life-threatening side effects; see Drug Interactions for drugs involved. Lactation.

SPECIAL CONCERNS

■ (1) Tipranavir coadministered with ritonavir, 200 mg, has been associated with reports of fatal and nonfatal intracranial hemorrhage. (2) Tipranavir coadministered with ritonavir, 200 mg, has been associated with reports of clinical hepatitis and hepatic decompensation, including some fatalities. Extra vigilance is warranted in clients with chronic hepatitis B or C coinfection because these individuals have an increased risk of hepatotoxicity.■ Use with caution in the elderly and in those with known sulfonamide allergy. Safety and efficacy have not been determined in children.

SIDE EFFECTS

Most Common

Diarrhea, N&V, pyrexia, headache, fatigue, bronchitis, depression, insomnia, rash, abdominal pain, asthenia.

NOTE: Side effects listed are those for concomitant use of tipranavir and ritonavir. **GI:** N&V, diarrhea, abdominal pain/distension, anorexia, dyspepsia, flatulence, GERD, *pancreatitis*, *hepatitis and hepatic decompensation, with possible fatal outcome*. **CNS:** Headache, depression, insomnia, dizziness, peripheral neuropathy, sleep disorder, somnolence. **CV:** *Intracranial hemorrhage*. **Dermatologic:** Urticarial rash, maculopapular rash, photosensitivity, acquired lipodystrophy, exanthema, lipoatrophy, lipohypertrophy, pruritus. **Respiratory:** Bronchitis, cough, dyspnea. **Musculoskeletal:** Muscle cramps, myalgia. **GU:** Impaired renal function. **Metabolic:** New-onset diabetes mellitus, exacerbation of preexisting diabetes mellitus, hyperglycemia, diabetic ketoacidosis, decreased appetite, dehydration. **Hematologic:** Anemia, neutropenia, thrombocytopenia, hemophilia, including spontaneous skin hematomas and hemarthrosis in those with hemophilia type A and B. Inhibition of platelet aggregation. **Body as a whole:** Pyrexia, fatigue, asthenia, redistribution/accumulation of body fat (including central obesity, dorsocervial fat enlargement, peripheral wasting, facial wasting, breast enlargement, and 'cushingoid appearance'), hypersensitivity, flu-like illness, malaise, weight loss, dehydration, reactivation of herpes simplex and varicella zoster, immune reconstitution syndrome.

LABORATORY TEST CONSIDERATIONS

↑ ALT, AST, amylase, lipase, cholesterol, triglycerides. ↓ WBCs. Abnormal LFTs. Hypercholesterolemia, hyperglycemia.

OD OVERDOSE MANAGEMENT

Symptoms: See *Side Effects. Treatment:* There is no known antidote. Treatment should consist of general supportive measures, including monitoring of vital signs and observation of clinical status. If needed, elimination of unabsorbed tipranavir can be achieved by gastric lavage or activated charcoal. Dialysis is unlikely to be of benefit.

DRUG INTERACTIONS

Al- and Mg-based antacids / ↓ Tipranavir absorption; consider separating dosing

Antiarrhythmics (e.g., amiodarone, bepridil, flecainide, propafenone, quinidine) / Coadministration is contraindicated R/T potential for cardiac arrhythmias secondary to ↑ antiarrhythmic levels

Antihistamines (e.g., astemizole, terfenadine) / Coadministration contraindicated R/T potential for serious and/or life-threatening reactions, including cardiac arrhythmias

Azole antifungals (e.g., fluconazole) / Possible ↑ tipranavir levels; high doses of fluconazole not recommended

Benzodiazepines (e.g., midazolam, triazolam) / Coadministration contraindicated R/T risk of prolonged or increased

sedation or respiratory depression

Calcium channel blockers (e.g., diltiazem, felodipine, nicardipine, nisoldipine, verapamil) / Caution warranted and clinical monitoring recommended

Cisapride / ↑ Risk of arrhythmias; concurrent use contraindicated

Clarithromycin / ↑ Levels of both clarithromycin and tipranavir; for those with C_{CR}, 30–60 mL/min, ↓ clarithromycin dose by 50%; for those with C_{CR}, <30 mL/min, ↓ clarithromycin dose by 75%

Contraceptives, oral (estrogen-containing) / ↓ Ethinyl estradiol levels by 50%; use nonhormonal contraceptives; also, ↑ risk of rash

Desipramine / ↑ Desipramine levels; reduce desipramine dosage and monitor

Didanosine / ↓ Tipranavir levels; separate dosing by at least 2 hr

Disulfiram / Tipranavir capsules contain alcohol → disulfiram-like reaction.

Ergot derivatives / ↑ Risk of ergot toxicity; do not use together

Efavirenz / ↓ Tipranavir levels

Fluticasone / ↑ Fluticasone plasma levels → significant ↓ serum cortisol levels; combination not recommended

HMG-CoA reductase inhibitors (e.g., aorvastatin, lovastatin, simvastatin) / ↑ Risk of myopathy, including rhabdomyolysis; do not use tipranavir with lovastatin or simvastatin but if using atorvastatin, start with the lowest possible dose with careful monitoring

Hypoglycemic drugs (e.g., glimepiride, glipizide, glyburide, pioglitazone, repaglinide, tolbutamide) / Careful glucose monitoring recommended

Immunosuppressants (e.g., cyclosporine, sirolimus, tacrolimus) / Careful drug concentration monitoring recommended

Loperamide / ↓ Levels of both loperamide and tipranavir

Metronidazole / Tipranavir capsules contain alcohol → disulfiram-like reaction

Opioid analgesics (e.g., meperidine, methadone) / Possible ↓ meperidine and methadone levels; levels of normeperidine (metabolite) may be ↑ → ↑ risk for seizures. Do not use increased meperidine doses or use meperidine long-term. May need to ↑ methadone dosage

Oral contraceptives (estrogen-containing) / Possible ↓ ethinyl estradiol levels; use alternate contraceptive methods; also, ↑ risk of rash

Phosphodiesterase type 5 inhibitors (e.g., sildenafil, tadalafil, vardenail) / Use together with caution. Do not exceed sildenafil, 25 mg within 48 hr; tadalafil, 10 mg q 72 hr; or vardenafil, 2.5 mg q 72 hr if taken with tipranavir

Pimozide / ↑ Potential for cardiac arrhythmias; do not use together

Protease inhibitors (e.g., amprenavir, lopinavir, saquinavir) / Possible ↓ protease inhibitor levels; do not use together

Ranolazine / ↑ Ranolazine plasma levels → ↑ risk of dose-related prolongation of QTc interval, torsades de pointes-type arrhythmias and sudden death; do not use together

Rifabutin / Possible loss of virologic response and possible resistance to tipranavir; do not use together. Also, possible ↑ rifabutin levels; reduce rifabutin dose by 75% (e.g., 150 mg q other day)

Rifamycins (e.g., rifampin, rifabutin) / Possible loss of virologic response and resistance to tipranavir; do not use together

 St. John's wort / Loss of virologic response and possible resistance to tipranavir; do not use together

Selective serotonin reuptake inhibitors (e.g., fluoxetine, paroxetine, sertraline) / SSRI dose may need to be adjusted

Tenofovir / ↓ Levels of both drugs

Trazodone / Possible ↑ trazodone levels; use together with caution

Warfarin / Monitor INR frequently

Zidovudine / ↓ Tipranavir levels; separate dosing by at least 2 hr

HOW SUPPLIED

Capsules: 250 mg.

DOSAGE

• **CAPSULES**

HIV-1 infection.

Adults: Tipranavir, 500 mg (2 x 250 mg capsules), coadministered with ritonavir, 200 mg, twice daily.

NURSING CONSIDERATIONS

ADMINISTRATION/STORAGE

1. Tipranavir and ritonavir should be taken with food.

 = see color insert   = Herbal   = Intravenous   ℝ = sound alike drug

2. Bioavailability is increased with a high-fat meal.

3. Failure to administer tipranavir with ritonavir results in reduced plasma levels of tipranavir that will be insufficient to reach the desired antiviral effect; also, some drug interactions will be altered.

4. Prior to opening the bottle, store tipranavir in the refrigerator from 2–8°C (36–46°F). After opening the bottle, capsules may be stored from 15–30°C (59–86°F). Use capsules within 60 days.

ASSESSMENT

1. Note disease onset, characteristics of S&S, other agents trialed, outcome. Assess viral replication, in those who are highly treatment-experienced or have HIV-1 strains resistant to multiple protease inhibitors.

2. List drugs prescribed to ensure none interact unfavorably. Many require a reduction in dose, or discontinuation to prevent reaction or loss of effect.

3. Monitor I&O, VS, weight, CBC, CD4 counts, viral load, renal and LFTs.

4. In those with chronic hepatitis B or C co-infection, monitor carefully for hepatotoxicity. LFTs should be performed prior to initiating therapy and frequently throughout the duration of treatment. Those with chronic hepatitis B or C co-infection or elevations in liver enzymes prior to treatment are at increased risk (approximately 2.5-fold) for developing further liver enzyme elevations or severe liver disease; increased testing is warranted. With moderate to severe liver disease, avoid drug use.

CLIENT/FAMILY TEACHING

1. Swallow tipranavir capsules whole; do not chew. Prior to opening bottle store in refrigerator. After opening, capsules may be stored at room temperature.

2. Drug must be co-administered with 200 mg ritonavir to ensure therapeutic effect. Failure to correctly co-administer tipranavir with ritonavir will result in reduced plasma levels of tipranavir which will not be sufficient to achieve the desired antiviral effect.

3. The 'Patient Package Insert' should be reviewed with each refill as it provides updated written information concerning this drug and therapy.

4. Do not alter the dose or stop therapy without provider approval. If a dose is missed, may take the dose as soon as possible and then return to normal dosing schedule. If a dose is skipped, do not double the next dose.

5. This drug co-administered with 200 mg of ritonavir, has been associated with severe liver disease, and some deaths. Stop drug and report S&S of hepatitis which include fatigue, malaise, nausea, yellow skin or eyes, loss of appetite, change in stools, abdominal tenderness.

6. May experience a mild to moderate rash; report if persistent or bothersome.

7. Women receiving estrogen-based hormonal contraceptives will require an additional or alternative contraceptive measure during therapy. Also may be increased risk of rash when tipranavir is used with hormonal contraceptives.

8. A redistribution or accumulation of body fat may occur; cause and long-term health effects of these conditions are unknown at this time.

9. Drug combination is not a cure for HIV infection; may continue to develop opportunistic infections and other complications associated with this disease. Sustained decreases in plasma HIVRNA have been associated with a reduced risk of progression to AIDS and death.

10. Practice reliable contraception; drug does not reduce the risk of transmitting HIV to others through sexual contact.

11. Report use of any other prescription, nonprescription medication, or herbal products, particularly St. John's wort, as they may cause significant adverse drug interactions.

12. To monitor maternal-fetal outcomes of pregnant women exposed to tipranavir, an antiretroviral pregnancy registry has been developed. Health care providers are encouraged to register clients by calling 1-800-258-4263.

OUTCOMES/EVALUATE

- ↓ HIVRNA
- Control of HIV progression

Tirofiban hydrochloride

(ty-roh-**FYE**-ban)

CLASSIFICATION(S):
Antiplatelet drug
PREGNANCY CATEGORY: B
Rx: Aggrastat.

USES
In combination with heparin for acute coronary syndrome (ACS), including those being treated medically and those undergoing PTCA or atherectomy. Tirofiban decreases the rate of combined endpoint of death, new MI, or refractory ischemia/repeat cardiac procedure.

ACTION/KINETICS
Action
Non–peptide antagonist of the platelet glycoprotein (GP) IIb/IIIa receptor, which is the major platelet surface receptor involved in platelet aggregation. Activation of the receptor leads to binding of fibrinogen and von Willebrand's factor to platelets, and thus aggregation. Tirofiban is a reversible antagonist of fibrinogen binding to the GP IIb/IIIa receptor, thus inhibiting platelet aggregation.

Pharmacokinetics
t½: About 2 hr. Cleared from the plasma mainly unchanged by renal excretion (65%) and feces (25%). Plasma clearance is lower in clients over 65 years of age and is significantly decreased in those with a C_{CR} less than 30 mL/min.

CONTRAINDICATIONS
Active internal bleeding or history of diathesis within the previous 30 days; history of intracranial hemorrhage, intracranial neoplasm, AV malformation, or aneurysm; history of thrombocytopenia following prior use of tirofiban; history of stroke within 30 days or any history of hemorrhagic stroke; major surgical procedure or severe physical trauma within the last month; history, findings, or symptoms suggestive of aortic dissection; severe hypertension (systolic BP greater than 180 mm Hg or diastolic BP greater than 110 mm Hg); concomitant use of another parenteral GP IIb/IIIa inhibitor; acute pericarditis.

SPECIAL CONCERNS
Use with caution in clients with a platelet count less than 150,000/mm³ in hemorrhagic retinopathy or with other drugs that affect hemostasis (e.g., warfarin). Elderly clients have a higher incidence of bleeding complications than younger clients. Safety and efficacy in children less than 18 years of age have not been established. Safety when used in combination with thrombolytic drugs has not been determined.

SIDE EFFECTS
Most Common
Bleeding (see below), bradycardia, coronary artery dissection, pelvic pain, dizziness, leg pain.

CV: Bleeding, including ***intracranial bleeding, retroperitoneal bleeding, major GI and GU bleeding***. Female and elderly clients have a higher incidence of bleeding than male or younger clients. **Miscellaneous:** Nausea, fever, headache, bradycardia, ***coronary artery dissection***, dizziness, edema or swelling, leg/pelvic pain, vasovagal reaction, sweating.

LABORATORY TEST CONSIDERATIONS
↓ H&H, platelets. ↑ Urine and FOB.

OD OVERDOSE MANAGEMENT
Symptoms: Bleeding, including minor mucocutaneous bleeding events and minor bleeding at the site of cardiac catheterization. *Treatment:* Assess clinical condition. Adjust or cease infusion, as appropriate. Can be removed by hemodialysis.

DRUG INTERACTIONS
Aspirin / ↑ Bleeding
H *Evening primrose oil* / Potential for ↑ antiplatelet effect
H *Feverfew* / Potential for ↑ antiplatelet effect
H *Garlic* / Potential for ↑ antiplatelet effect
H *Ginger* / Potential for ↑ antiplatelet effect
H *Ginkgo biloba* / Potential for ↑ antiplatelet effect

H *Ginseng* / Potential for ↑ antiplatelet effect

H *Grapeseed extract* / Potential for ↑ antiplatelet effect

Heparin / ↑ Bleeding

Levothyroxine / ↑ Tirofiban clearance

Omeprazole / ↑ Tirofiban clearance

HOW SUPPLIED

Injection: 50 mcg/mL; *Injection Concentrate:* 250 mcg/mL.

DOSAGE

* **IV**

Acute coronary syndrome.

Initial: 0.4 mcg/kg/min for 30 min; **then,** 0.1 mcg/kg/min. Use half the usual rate in those with severe renal impairment. Consult the package insert for the guide to dosage adjustment by weight in clients with normal renal function and in those with severe renal impairment.

NURSING CONSIDERATIONS

🕲 Do not confuse Aggrastat with Argatroban (anticoagulant) or Aggrenox (antiplatelet drug).

ADMINISTRATION/STORAGE

IV 1. May be given in the same IV line as heparin, dopamine, lidocaine, potassium chloride, and famotidine. Do not give in the same IV line as diazepam.

2. Tirofiban injection (250 mcg/mL) must be diluted to the same strength as tirofiban injection premixed (50 mcg/mL). One of three methods can be used to achieve a final concentration of 50 mcg/mL (mix well prior to use):

* Withdraw and discard 100 mL from a 500 mL bag of either sterile 0.9% NaCl or D5W; replace this volume with 100 mL of tirofiban injection (i.e., from two 50 mL vials).
* Withdraw and discard 50 mL from a 250 mL bag of either sterile 0.9% NaCl or D5W and replace this volume with 50 mL of tirofiban injection (i.e., from two-25 mL vials or one-50 mL vial).
* Add the contents of a 25 mL vial to a 100 mL bag of sterile 0.9% NaCl or D5W.

3. Tirofiban injection premix comes in 500 mL *Intravia* containers with 0.9% NaCl and tirofiban, 50 mcg/mL. To open the *Intravia* container, remove the dust cover. The plastic may be opaque due to moisture absorption during sterilization; the opacity will decrease gradually. Check for leaks by firmly squeezing the inner bag. Lack of sterility may be suspected if leaks are found; discard the solution. Do not use unless the solution is clear and the seal is intact.

4. Do not add other drugs or remove tirofiban from the bag without a syringe.

5. Do not use plastic containers in series connections as an air embolism can result by drawing air from the first container if it is empty.

6. Store both the premixed and concentrated injection from 15–30°C (59–86°F); do not freeze and protect from light.

7. Discard any unused solution 24 hr after start of the infusion.

ASSESSMENT

1. Note reasons for therapy, onset, characteristics of S&S.

2. List any history of intracranial hemorrhage, neoplasm, AV malformation, or aneurysm.

3. Monitor VS, H&H, platelets, PTT initially and 6 hr after loading infusions of tirofiban and heparin, and daily; monitor renal function studies, reduce dosage with dysfunction (C_{CR} <30 mL/min).

4. Avoid excessive handling, sticks and procedures to prevent increased bleeding.

CLIENT/FAMILY TEACHING

1. Drug is used IV with heparin to reduce death and symptoms associated with heart vessel blockage.

2. May experience bleeding so all sites will be carefully assessed and blood work evaluated frequently.

3. May experience dizziness; use caution. If smoking, stop now.

4. Encourage family to learn CPR.

OUTCOMES/EVALUATE

Inhibition of platelet aggregation with ↓ refractory ischemia, MI, and death

---

Bold Italic = life threatening side effect   ■ = black box warning   ✿ = Available in Canada

Tizanidine hydrochloride

(tye-**ZAN**-ih-deen)

CLASSIFICATION(S):
Skeletal muscle relaxant, centrally-acting
PREGNANCY CATEGORY: C
Rx: Zanaflex.

SEE ALSO *SKELETAL MUSCLE RELAXANTS, CENTRALLY ACTING.*

USES
Acute and intermittent management of increased muscle tone associated with muscle spasticity.

ACTION/KINETICS
Action
Acts on central alpha$_2$-adrenergic receptors; reduces spasticity by increasing presynaptic inhibition of motor neurons possibly by reducing release of excitatory amino acids. Greatest effects are on polysynaptic pathways. Also may reduce postsynaptic excitatory transmitter activity, decrease the firing rate of noradrenergic locus ceruleas neurons, and inhibit synaptic transmission of nociceptive stimuli in the spinal pathways.

Pharmacokinetics
Absolute bioavailability is about 40% due to extensive first-pass metabolism in the liver. **Peak effect:** 1–2 hr. **Duration:** 3–6 hr. **t½:** About 2.5 hr. Excreted in urine and feces. Elderly clear drug more slowly.

CONTRAINDICATIONS
Use with α$_2$-adrenergic agonists.

SPECIAL CONCERNS
Use with caution in renal impairment, in elderly, and during laction. Use with extreme caution in hepatic insufficiency and in those with C$_{CR}$ of 25 mL/min or less. Safety and efficacy have not been determined in children.

SIDE EFFECTS
Most Common
Sedation/somnolence, dry mouth, asthenia, dizziness, UTI, infection.
NOTE: Side effects listed are those with a frequency of 0.1% or greater. **CV:** Hypotension, vasodilation, postural hypotension, syncope, migraine, arrhythmia. **GI:** *Hepatotoxicity*, dry mouth, constipation, pharyngitis, vomiting, abdominal pain, diarrhea, dyspepsia, dysphagia, cholelithiasis, fecal impaction, flatulence, *GI hemorrhage* hepatitis, melena. **CNS:** Dizziness, dyskinesia, nervousness, somnolence, sedation, hallucinations, psychotic-like symptoms, depression, anxiety, paresthesia, tremor, emotional lability, seizures, paralysis, abnormal thinking, vertigo, abnormal dreams, agitation, depersonalization, euphoria, stupor, dysautonomia, neuralgia. **GU:** Urinary frequency/urgency, UTI, cystitis, menorrhagia, pyelonephritis, urinary retention, kidney calculus, enlarged uterine fibroids, vaginal moniliasis, vaginitis. **Hematologic:** Ecchymosis, anemia, leukopenia, leukocytosis. **Musculoskeletal:** Myasthenia, back pain, pathological fracture, arthralgia, arthritis, bursitis. **Respiratory:** Sinusitis, pneumonia, bronchitis, rhinitis. **Dermatologic:** Rash, sweating, skin ulcer, pruritus, dry skin, acne, alopecia, urticaria. **Body as a whole:** Flu syndrome, infection, asthenia, weight loss, infection, *sepsis*, *cellulitis*, *death*, allergic reaction, moniliasis, malaise, asthenia, fever, abscess, edema. **Ophthalmic:** Glaucoma, amblyopia, conjunctivitis, eye pain, optic neuritis, retinal hemorrhage, visual field defect. **Otic:** Ear pain, tinnitus, deafness, otitis media. **Miscellaneous:** Speech disorder.

LABORATORY TEST CONSIDERATIONS
↑ ALT. Abnormal LFTs. Hypercholesterolemia, hyperlipemia, hypothyroidism, adrenal cortical insufficiency, hyperglycemia, hypokalemia, hyponatremia, hypoproteinemia.

DRUG INTERACTIONS
Alcohol / ↑ Tizanidine side effects; additive CNS depressant effects
Alpha$_2$-adrenergic agonists / Additive hypotension
Ciprofloxacin / ↑ Tizanidine AUC and peak levels R/T inhibition of metabolism by CYP1A2
Fluvoxamine / ↑ Tizanidine AUC and peak levels R/T inhibition of metabolism by CYP1A2

Oral contraceptives / ↓ Tizanidine clearance

HOW SUPPLIED

Capsules: 2 mg, 4 mg, 6 mg; *Tablets:* 2 mg, 4 mg.

DOSAGE

• **CAPSULES; TABLETS**

Muscle spasticity.

Initial: 4 mg; **then,** increase dose gradually in 2 to 4 mg steps to optimum effect. Dose can be repeated at 6–8-hr intervals, to maximum of 3 doses/24 hr, not to exceed 36 mg/day. There is no experience with repeated, single, daytime doses greater than 12 mg or total daily doses of 36 mg or more.

NURSING CONSIDERATIONS

ADMINISTRATION/STORAGE

1. Food has complex effects on tizanidine pharmacokinetics that differ with the different formulations as follows:
- Switching administration to the tablet between the fed or fasted state.
- Switching administration of the capsule between the fed or fasted state.
- Switching between the tablet and capsule in the fed state.
- Switching between the intact capsule and sprinkling the contents of the capsule on applesauce. These changes may result in increased side effects or delayed/more rapid onset of action.

3. If the drug must be discontinued, especially in those receiving high doses for long periods, decrease the dose slowly to minimize the risk of withdrawal and rebound hypertension, tachycardia, and hypertonia.

4. Store from 25–30°C (59–86°F). Dispense in a tight, light-resistant container with child-resistant closure.

ASSESSMENT

1. Note reasons for therapy, onset characteristics of S&S, other agents trialed, outcome.

2. Assess ROM, pain level, erythema, swelling, muscle spasticity, DTR's, sensory findings, muscle tone and gait.

3. Monitor VS, CBC, liver, and renal function studies; reduce dose with dysfunction.

CLIENT/FAMILY TEACHING

1. Food delays absorption time of drug.

2. Do not perform activities that require mental alertness; drug causes sedation.

3. Report if hallucinations or delusions experienced.

4. May cause drop in BP; avoid sudden changes in position.

5. Avoid alcohol and any other CNS depressants.

6. Report loss of effect, visual problems, ↓ ROM, or worsening of symptoms.

7. With prolonged therapy do not stop suddenly; taper over a 1–2 week period.

8. Use reliable contraception; oral contraceptives may inhibit drug clearance by 50%.

9. Report any adverse effects or unusual events. Keep all F/U appointments to evaluate response to therapy and to monitor renal/LFTs q 3 mo during first year of therapy.

OUTCOMES/EVALUATE

↓ Spasticity; ↑ muscle relaxation

Tobramycin sulfate

(toe-brah-**MY**-sin)

CLASSIFICATION(S):

Antibiotic, aminoglycoside

PREGNANCY CATEGORY: D (B for ophthalmic use)

Rx: Inhalation: TOBI. **Ophthalmic:** AKTob Ophthalmic Solution, Defy Ophthalmic Solution, Tobrex Ophthalmic Ointment or Solution. **Parenteral:** Tobramycin for Injection, Tobramycin in 0.9% Sodium Chloride.

♣**Rx:** PMS-Tobramycin.

SEE ALSO *AMINOGLYCOSIDES.*

USES

Systemic: (1) Complicated and recurrent UTIs due to *Pseudomonas aeruginosa, Proteus, Escherichia coli, Klebsiella, Enterobacter, Serratia, Staphylococcus aureus, Citrobacter,* and *Providencia.* (2) Lower respiratory tract infections due to *P. aeruginosa, Klebsiella, Enterobacter,*

E. coli, Serratia, and S. aureus (penicillinase- and non–penicillinase-producing). (3) Intra-abdominal infections (including peritonitis) due to E. coli, Klebsiella, and Enterobacter. (4) Septicemia in neonates, children, and adults due to P. aeruginosa, E. coli, and Klebsiella. (5) Skin, bone, and skin structure infections due to P. aeruginosa, Proteus, E. coli, Klebsiella, Enterobacter, and S. aureus. (6) Serious CNS infections, including meningitis. Can be used with penicillins or cephalosporins in serious infections when results of susceptibility testing are not yet known.

Ophthalmic: Treat external ocular infections (involving the conjunctiva, or cornea) due to Staphylococcus, S. aureus, Streptococcus, S. pneumoniae, beta-hemolytic streptococci, Corynebacterium, E. coli, Haemophilus aegyptius, H. ducreyi, H. influenzae, H. parainfluenzae, Klebsiella pneumoniae, Neisseria, N. gonorrhoeae, Proteus, Acinetobacter calcoaceticus, Enterobacter, Enterobacter aerogenes, Serratia marcescens, Moraxella, Pseudomonas aeruginosa, and Vibrio.

Inhalation: Management of lung infections (P. aeruginosa) in cystic fibrosis clients. Also improves lung function.

ACTION/KINETICS
Action
Similar to gentamicin and can be used concurrently with carbenicillin.

Pharmacokinetics
Therapeutic serum levels, IM: 4–8 mcg/mL. **$t\frac{1}{2}$:** 2–2.5 hr. **Toxic serum levels:** >12 mcg/mL (peak) and >2 mcg/mL (trough).

CONTRAINDICATIONS
Use with diuretics or nephrotoxic drugs. Ophthalmically to treat dendritic keratitis, vaccinia, varicella, fungal or mycobacterial eye infections, after removal of a corneal foreign body. Lactation.

SPECIAL CONCERNS
■ See Aminoglycosides in Chapter 2.■ Use with caution in premature infants and neonates. Ophthalmic ointment may retard corneal epithelial healing.

SIDE EFFECTS
Most Common
After ophthalmic use: Transient irritation/burning/stinging, itching, inflammation.
After systemic use: N&V, redness/irritation at injection site, dizziness, tinnitus, fatigue, pale skin, weakness.
See Aminoglycosides for a complete list of possible side effects. **Ophthalmic use:** Transient irritation/burning/stinging, itching, inflammation, angioneurotic edema, urticaria, vesicular and maculopapular dermatitis. **Systemic use:** Neurotoxicity, both auditory and vestibular ototoxicity. Nephrotoxicity (reversible).

ADDITIONAL DRUG INTERACTIONS
Carbenicillin or ticarcillin: ↑ Tobramycin effect when used for Pseudomonas infections

OD OVERDOSE MANAGEMENT
Symptoms: Ophthalmic Use: Edema, lid itching, punctuate keratitis, erythema, lacrimation. Treatment: Treat symptomatically.

HOW SUPPLIED
Injection: 10 mg/mL, 40 mg/mL; Injection Solution: 0.8 mg/mL, 1.2 mg/mL, 60 mg/mL; Ophthalmic Ointment: 0.3% (3 mg/mL); Ophthalmic Solution: 0.3% (3 mg/mL); Powder for Injection: 1.2 grams.

DOSAGE
- **IM; IV**
  Non-life-threatening serious infections.
  Adults: 3 mg/kg/day in three equally divided doses q 8 hr. For cystic fibrosis, an initial dosing regimen of 10 mg/kg/day IV in 3–4 equally divided doses is recommended as a guide.
  Life-threatening infections.
  Up to 5 mg/kg/day in three or four equal doses. **Pediatric:** Either 2–2.5 mg/kg q 8 hr or 1.5–1.9 mg/kg q 6 hr; **neonates 1 week of age or less:** Up to 4 mg/kg/day in two equal doses q 12 hr.
  Impaired renal function.
  Initially: 1 mg/kg; **then,** maintenance dose calculated according to information supplied by manufacturer.
- **INHALATION SOLUTION**
  Pseudomonas aeruginosa in cystic fibrosis.

T

Dose using a nebulizer twice a day for 10–15 min in cycles of 28 days on and then 28 days off. See package insert for detailed instructions for administration.

- **OPHTHALMIC OINTMENT (0.3%)**
  Mild to moderate infections.

0.5 in ribbon into the affected eye(s) 2-3 times a day.

Severe infections.

0.5 in ribbon into the affected eye(s) q 3-4 hr until improvement, followed by reduced treatment prior to discontinuation.

- **OPHTHALMIC SOLUTION, (0.3%)**
  Mild to moderate infections.

Instill 1–2 gtt into the affected eye(s) q 4 hr.

Severe infections.

Instill 2 gtt into the eye(s) hourly until improvement; reduce treatment prior to discontinuation.

NURSING CONSIDERATIONS

ADMINISTRATION/STORAGE

1. Use the inhalation solution as close as possible to q 12 hr, but not less than q 6 hr.
2. Do not mix TOBI with dornase alfa in the nebulizer.
3. Store ophthalmic products from 8–27°C (46–80°F).
IV 4. Prepare IV solution by diluting drug with 50–100 mL of dextrose or saline solution; infuse over 30–60 min.
5. Use proportionately less diluent for children than for adults.
6. Do not mix with other drugs for parenteral administration.
7. Discard solution of drug containing up to 1 mg/mL after 24 hr at room temperature.
8. Store drug at room temperature no longer than 2 years.

ASSESSMENT

1. Note reasons for therapy, type, onset, characteristics of S&S.
2. Monitor cultures, CBC, renal and LFTs.
3. Assess for renal, auditory, and vestibular dysfunction during therapy.

CLIENT/FAMILY TEACHING

1. Drink plenty of fluids (2–3 L/day) during parenteral drug therapy.

2. With eye infections, avoid wearing contact lenses until infection is cleared and provider approves.
3. With inhalation therapy the time frame is usually a month of therapy and then a month off. Follow guidelines for proper equipment cleaning and care. Sit and breathe normally through the inhaler mouthpiece to ensure adequate dispersion.
4. Report sore throat, unusual bruising/bleeding, joint pains, bloody diarrhea, furry tongue, if symptoms do not improve or if they worsen after several days of therapy.

OUTCOMES/EVALUATE

- Negative cultures; resolution of infection
- Therapeutic drug levels (peak: 4–8 mcg/mL; trough: <2 mcg/mL)

Tolcapone ■
(**TOHL**-kah-pohn)

CLASSIFICATION(S):
Antiparkinson drug
PREGNANCY CATEGORY: C
Rx: Tasmar.

USES

Adjunct to levodopa and carbidopa for idiopathic Parkinson's disease. Since hepatotoxicity from the drug may be fatal, reserve for Parkinson clients on levodopa/carbidopa with symptom fluctuations who are not satisfactorily responding.

ACTION/KINETICS

Action

Reversible inhibitor of catechol-O-methyltransferase (COMT), resulting in an increase in plasma levodopa. When given with levodopa/carbidopa, plasma levels of levodopa are more sustained, allowing for more constant dopaminergic stimulation of the brain. May also increase side effects of levodopa.

Pharmacokinetics

Rapidly absorbed from the GI tract; **peak levels:** 2 hr. Food given within 1 hr before or 2 hr after PO use decreases bioavailability by 10–20%. **t½, elimina-**

tion: 2–3 hr. Almost completely metabolized in the liver; excreted in the urine (60%) and feces (40%). **Plasma protein binding:** More than 99.9%.

CONTRAINDICATIONS

Use with a nonselective MAO inhibitor. In clients with liver disease, history of nontraumatic rhabdomyolysis or hyperpyrexia, confusion possibly related to the drug, and in those withdrawn from tolcapone due to hepatocellular injury.

SPECIAL CONCERNS

■ (1) Because of the risk of potentially fatal, acute fulminant liver failure, use tolcapone in those with Parkinsonism on levodopa/carbidopa who are experiencing symptom fluctuation and are not responding satisfactorily to, or are not appropriate candidates for other therapies. (2) Because of the risk of liver injury, withdraw clients from tolcapone who fail to show substantial improvement within 3 weeks of initiation of therapy. (3) Do not initiate tolcapone if there is clinical evidence of liver disease or ALT or AST values are greater than twice ULN. Treat those with severe dyskinesia or dystonia with caution. (4) Those who develop evidence of hepatocellular injury and are withdrawn from the drug for any reason may be at increased risk for liver injury if tolcapone is reintroduced. Do not consider such clients for retreatment. (5) Advise a prescriber who elects to use tolcapone in face of the increased risk of liver injury to monitor clients for evidence of emergent liver injury. Instruct clients about the need for self-monitoring for classical signs of liver disease (e.g., clay-colored stools, jaundice) and nonspecific signs (e.g., fatigue, appetite loss, lethargy). (6) Although frequent lab monitoring for evidence of hepatocellular injury is essential, it is not clear that baseline and periodic monitoring of liver enzymes will prevent fulminant liver failure. However, it is believed that early detection of drug-induced hepatic injury with immediate withdrawal of the drug enhances likelihood for recovery. Clients with preexisting hepatic disease are more vulnerable to hepatotoxins; thus, following the liver monitoring program is recommended. (7) Perform appropriate tests to exclude presence of liver disease before starting tolcapone therapy. Determine baseline levels of ALT and AST every 2 weeks for the first year of therapy, every 4 weeks for the next 6 months, and every 8 weeks thereafter. Monitor liver enzymes before increasing the dose to 200 mg 3 times per day and reinitiate at the frequency above. (8) Discontinue tolcapone if ALT or AST exceeds the ULN or if clinical signs and symptoms suggest the onset of hepatic failure (e.g., persistent nausea, fatigue, lethargy, anorexia, jaundice, dark urine, pruritus, and right upper quadrant tenderness).■ Use with caution in severe renal or hepatic impairment, in those with severe dystonia/dyskinesias, and during lactation.

SIDE EFFECTS

Most Common

Dyskinesia, sleep disorder, dystonia, excessive dreaming, somnolence, confusion, dizziness, headache, nausea, anorexia, diarrhea, muscle cramps, orthostatic complaints.

GI: N&V, anorexia, diarrhea, constipation, xerostomia, abdominal pain, dyspepsia, flatulence, *acute fulminant liver failure.* **CNS:** Hallucinations, dyskinesias, sleep disorder, dystonia, excessive dreaming, somnolence, confusion, dizziness, headache, syncope, loss of balance, hyperkinesia, paresthesia, hypokinesia, agitation, irritability, mental deficiency, hyperactivity, panic reaction, euphoria, hypertonia, sudden uncontrolled sedation. **CV:** Orthostatic hypotension, chest pain, hypotension, chest discomfort. **Respiratory:** URTI, dyspnea, sinus congestion. **Musculoskeletal:** Muscle cramps, stiffness, arthritis, neck pain. **GU:** Hematuria, UTIs, urine discoloration, micturition disorder, uterine tumor. **Dermatologic:** Increased sweating, dermal bleeding, skin tumor, alopecia. **Ophthalmic:** Cataract, eye inflammation. **Body as a whole:** Falling, fatigue, influenza, burning, malaise, fever, rhabdomyolysis. *NOTE:* Clients over 75 years of age may develop more hallucinations but less dystonia. Females

may develop somnolence more frequently than males.

LABORATORY TEST CONSIDERATIONS
↑ AST, ALT.

OD OVERDOSE MANAGEMENT
Symptoms: Nausea, vomiting, dizziness,
possibility of respiratory difficulties.
Treatment: Hospitalization is advised.
Give supportive care.

HOW SUPPLIED
Tablets: 100 mg, 200 mg.

DOSAGE

• **TABLETS**
  Adjunct for Parkinsonism.
Initial: 100 mg 3 times per day with/
without food. Use 200 mg 3 times per
day only if anticipated benefit is justified. Do **not** increase the dose to 200
mg 3 times per day in those with moderate to severe liver cirrhosis.

NURSING CONSIDERATIONS
ADMINISTRATION/STORAGE
1. Even though 200 mg 3 times per day
is reasonably well tolerated, the prescriber may start with 100 mg 3 times
per day due to the potential for increased dopaminergic side effects and
the possibility of adjustment of the concomitant levodopa/carbidopa dose.
2. A suggested dosing regimen is to
give the first dose of tolcapone on the
day with the first dose of levodopa/car-
bidopa; subsequent doses of tolcapone
can be given 6 to 12 hr later.
3. Reductions in the daily dose of levodopa may be required.
4. Tolcapone can be used with either
the immediate– or sustained–release
formulations of levodopa/carbidopa.
ASSESSMENT
1. Note reasons for therapy, character-
istics/duration of Parkinson symptoms,
other agents trialed/failed.
2. List drugs currently prescribed to ensure none interact unfavorably.
3. Ensure client aware of potential for
liver toxicity; record informed consent.
4. May cause severe hepatotoxicity. Do
not use with clinical evidence of liver
disease or if ALT or AST 2x ULN. When
used, monitor LFTs q 2 weeks for the
first year of therapy, then q 4 weeks for
the next 6 months and then q 8 weeks

thereafter. Stop drug with any evidence
of liver dysfunction or if no improvement in symptoms after 3–4 weeks of
therapy.
CLIENT/FAMILY TEACHING
1. Take as directed with your levodopa/
carbidopa. Drug increases the action of
levodopa by decreasing its metabolism
in the peripheral tissues. If taken without levodopa there is no treatment
benefit. May experience nausea initially;
should subside.
2. Do not drive or perform activities requiring mental alertness until drug effects realized; may cause sedation.
3. Stop drug and report any evidence
of liver dysfunction: fatigue, loss of appetite, lethargy, yellow skin discoloration, clay colored stools, hallucinations
or diarrhea.
4. Rise slowly from a sitting or lying
position to prevent low BP effects. May
experience nausea initially and an increase in involuntary repetitive movements; these should subside. Six weeks
into therapy may experience diarrhea;
report if persistent or severe. May discolor urine bright yellow.
5. Practice reliable birth control; do not
breastfeed.
6. Report lack of response, tremors or
repetitive movements, or any unusual
symptoms or side effects; labs will be
required frequently during the first year
of therapy to protect from liver toxicity.
OUTCOMES/EVALUATE
Control of S&S Parkinson's disease

Tolmetin sodium ■
(**TOLL**-met-in)

CLASSIFICATION(S):
Nonsteroidal anti-inflammatory
drug
PREGNANCY CATEGORY: C
Rx: Tolectin.

SEE ALSO *NONSTEROIDAL ANTI-
INFLAMMATORY DRUGS.*

USES
(1) Relief of the signs and symptoms of
acute flares and long—term manage-

---

ment of rheumatoid arthritis and osteoarthritis. (2) Juvenile rheumatoid arthritis. *Investigational:* Sunburn.

ACTION/KINETICS
Pharmacokinetics
Peak plasma levels: 30–60 min. **t½:** 2–7 hr. **Therapeutic plasma levels:** 40 mcg/mL. **Onset, anti-inflammatory effect:** Within 1 week; **duration, anti-inflammatory effect:** 1–2 weeks. Inactivated in liver and excreted in urine. **Plasma protein binding:** More than 93%.

SPECIAL CONCERNS
■ (1) Cardiovascular risk. NSAIDs may cause an increased risk of serious CV thrombotic events, myocardial infarction, and stroke, which can be fatal. This risk may increase with duration of use. Clients with CV disease or risk factors for CV disease may be at greater risk. (2) Tolmetin sodium is contraindicated for the treatment of perioperative pain in the setting of coronary artery bypass graft. (3) GI risk. NSAIDs cause an increased risk of serious GI adverse effects, including bleeding, ulceration, and perforation of the stomach or intestines, which can be fatal. These events can occur at any time during use and without warning symptoms. Elderly clients are at greater risk for serious GI events.■ Use with caution during lactation. Safety and efficacy have not been determined in children less than 2 years of age.

SIDE EFFECTS
Most Common
Hypertension, headache, dizziness, asthenia/malaise, diarrhea, N&V, flatulence, abdominal/GI distress, peripheral edema, edema.

See *Nonsteroidal Anti-Inflammatory Drugs* for a complete list of possible side effects.

LABORATORY TEST CONSIDERATIONS
Tolmetin metabolites give a false + test for proteinuria using sulfosalicylic acid.

HOW SUPPLIED
Capsules: 400 mg; *Tablets:* 200 mg, 600 mg.

DOSAGE
• CAPSULES; TABLETS
Rheumatoid arthritis, osteoarthritis.

Adults: 400 mg 3 times per day (including one dose on arising and one at bedtime); adjust dosage according to client response after 1–2 weeks. **Maintenance, rheumatoid arthritis:** 600–1,800 mg/day in 3–4 divided doses; **osteoarthritis,** 600–1,600 mg/day in 3–4 divided doses. Doses larger than 1,800 mg/day for rheumatoid arthritis and osteoarthritis are not recommended.

Juvenile rheumatoid arthritis.

2 years and older, initial: 20 mg/kg/day in 3–4 divided doses to start; **then,** 15–30 mg/kg/day. Doses higher than 30 mg/kg/day are not recommended. Beneficial effects may not be observed for several days to a week.

NURSING CONSIDERATIONS
ADMINISTRATION/STORAGE
Store form 15–30°C (59–86°F). Protect from light.

ASSESSMENT
1. List reasons for therapy; note joint pain/level, deformity, swelling, inflammation, and ROM.
2. Review history for conditions that may preclude therapy.
3. Monitor CBC and renal function studies.

CLIENT/FAMILY TEACHING
1. Doses should be spaced so that one dose is taken in the morning on arising, one during the day, and one at bedtime. The dosage is based on the treatment condition and varies according to indications. Take as directed. It may take several weeks before effects are evident.
2. May administer with meals, milk, a full glass of water, or antacids if gastric irritation occurs. Never administer with sodium bicarbonate. The elderly are particularly susceptible to gastric irritation and should take with milk, meals, an antacid, or stomach protectant if prescribed.
3. Assess response; drug may cause drowsiness or dizziness. Report any unusual bruising or bleeding, weight gain, edema, fever, blood in urine or increased joint pain.

T

4. Avoid alcohol and any OTC medications without approval.

5. Report for labs to evaluate renal function and hematologic parameters.

OUTCOMES/EVALUATE

↓ Joint pain and inflammation; ↑ mobility

Tolnaftate
(toll-**NAF**-tayt)

CLASSIFICATION(S):
Antifungal

OTC: Absorbine Athlete's Foot Cream, Absorbine Footcare, Aftate for Athlete's Foot, Aftate for Jock Itch, Genaspor, Quinsana Plus, Tinactin, Tinactin for Jock Itch, Ting. ♣**OTC:** ZeaSorb AF.

SEE ALSO *ANTI-INFECTIVE DRUGS.*

USES
(1) Tinea pedis, tinea cruris, tinea corporis, and tinea versicolor. (2) Fungal infections of moist skin areas.

ACTION/KINETICS

Action
Exact mechanism not known; is thought to stunt mycelial growth causing a fungicidal effect.

CONTRAINDICATIONS
Scalp and nail infections. Avoid getting into eyes. Use in children less than 2 years of age.

SIDE EFFECTS

Most Common
Mild skin irritation.

Dermatologic: Sensitivity, mild skin irritation.

HOW SUPPLIED
Cream: 1%; *Gel:* 1%; *Powder:* 1%; *Solution:* 1%; *Spray Liquid:* 1%; *Spray Powder:* 1%.

DOSAGE

• **TOPICAL: CREAM; GEL; POWDER; SOLUTION; SPRAY LIQUID; SPRAY POWDER**

Tinea pedia, tinea cruris, tinea corporis, tinea versicolor; fungal infections of moist skin areas.

Apply twice a day for 2–3 weeks although treatment for 4–6 weeks may be necessary in some instances.

NURSING CONSIDERATIONS

ASSESSMENT
1. Note reasons for therapy, location, onset, characteristics of S&S. Inspect source of infection and presentation as the choice of vehicle is important for effective therapy.

• Powders are used in mild conditions as adjunctive therapy.

• For primary therapy and prophylaxis, creams, liquids, or ointments are used, esp. if area is moist.

• Liquids and solutions are used if area is hairy.

2. Assess cultures; use concomitant therapy if bacterial or *Candida* infections also present.

CLIENT/FAMILY TEACHING
1. Skin should be thoroughly cleaned and dried before applying. Use care; do not rub medication into or near the eye.

2. Continue to use as directed, despite improvement of symptoms. Takes 2–6 weeks to clear infection.

3. Report any bothersome side effects; local relief of symptoms should be evident within the first 24–48 hr. Report if no improvement noted within 10 days.

OUTCOMES/EVALUATE
• Symptomatic relief; skin healing

• Eradication of fungal infection

Tolterodine tartrate
(tohl-**TER**-oh-deen)

CLASSIFICATION(S):
Urinary tract drug
PREGNANCY CATEGORY: C
Rx: Detrol, Detrol LA.
♣**Rx:** Unidet.

USES
Overactive bladder with symptoms of urinary frequency, urgency, or urge incontinence.

Bold Italic = life threatening side effect   ▉ = black box warning   ♣ = Available in Canada

ACTION/KINETICS

Action
Acts as a competitive muscarinic receptor antagonist in the bladder to cause increased bladder control.

Pharmacokinetics
Metabolized by first pass effect in the liver to the active 5–hydroxymethyl derivative, which has similar activity as tolterodine. Rapidly absorbed with peak serum levels within 1–2 hr. Food increases bioavailability. Excreted in the urine. **Plasma protein binding:** Highly bound.

CONTRAINDICATIONS
Urinary retention, gastric retention, uncontrolled narrow–angle glaucoma, lactation.

SPECIAL CONCERNS
Use with caution in renal impairment, in bladder outflow obstruction, in GI obstructive disorders (e.g., pyloric stenosis), and in those being treated for narrow–angle glaucoma. Do not give greater than 1 mg twice a day to those with significantly decreased hepatic function. Safety and efficacy have not been determined in children.

SIDE EFFECTS

Most Common
Immediate-Release: Dry mouth, headache, constipation, vertigo/dizziness, abdominal pain, diarrhea, dyspepsia, fatigue.
Extended-Release: Dry mouth, headache, constipation, abdominal pain, somnolence, dyspepsia, xerophthalmia.
GI: Dry mouth, dyspepsia, constipation, abdominal pain, N&V, diarrhea, flatulence. **CNS:** Headache, vertigo, dizziness, somnolence, anxiety, paresthesia, nervousness. **Respiratory:** URTI, bronchitis, coughing, pharyngitis, rhinitis, sinusitis. **Dermatologic:** Rash, erythema, dry skin, pruritus. **GU:** UTI, dysuria, urinary frequency, urinary retention. **Ophthalmic:** Abnormalities with vision, including accommodation, xerophthalmia, dry eyes. **Musculoskeletal:** Arthralgia, back pain, chest pain. **Body as a whole:** Fatigue, flu–like symptoms, infection, fungal infection. **Miscellaneous:** Hypertension, weight gain, fall,

chest pain, tachycardia, peripheral edema, **anaphylactoid reactions.**

OD OVERDOSE MANAGEMENT
Symptoms: Significant anticholinergic symptoms. *Treatment:* Symptomatic. Monitor ECG.

DRUG INTERACTIONS
Clarithromycin / ↑ Tolterodine levels R/T ↓ liver metabolism; do not give tolterodine >1 mg twice a day
Cyclosporine / ↑ Tolterodine levels R/T ↓ liver metabolism; do not give tolterodine >1 mg twice a day
Erythromycin / ↑ Tolterodine levels R/T ↓ liver metabolism; do not give tolterodine >1 mg twice a day
Fluoxetine / ↓ Tolterodine metabolism in EM1, EM2, and poor metabolizers
Itraconazole / ↑ Tolterodine levels R/T ↓ liver metabolism; do not give tolterodine >1 mg twice a day
Ketoconazole / ↑ Tolterodine levels R/T ↓ liver metabolism; do not give tolterodine >1 mg twice a day
Miconazole / ↑ Tolterodine levels R/T ↓ liver metabolism; do not give tolterodine >1 mg twice a day
Omeprazole / ↑ Tolterodine peak levels R/T ↑ rate of drug release from the extended-release product from ↑ gastric pH
Vinblastine / ↑ Tolterodine levels R/T ↓ liver metabolism; do not give tolterodine >1 mg twice a day
Warfarin / Prolonged INR values → possible bleeding

HOW SUPPLIED
Capsules, Extended-Release: 2 mg, 4 mg; *Tablets, Immediate-Release:* 1 mg, 2 mg.

DOSAGE
- **CAPSULES, EXTENDED-RELEASE**
  Overactive bladder.
4 mg once daily taken with liquids and swallowed whole. May lower dose to 2 mg daily based on response and tolerability. For those with significantly decreased hepatic or renal function or who are taking drugs that are inhibitors of CYP3A4, the recommended dose is 1 mg twice a day.
- **TABLETS, IMMEDIATE-RELEASE**
  Overactive bladder.
Initial: 2 mg twice a day. Dose may be lowered to 1 mg twice a day based on

---

T

individual response and side effects. Adjust dose to 1 mg twice a day in those with significantly reduced hepatic function or who are currently taking drugs that are inhibitors of CYP3A4 (see *Drug Interactions*).

NURSING CONSIDERATIONS

ADMINISTRATION/STORAGE
Protect from light.

ASSESSMENT
1. Note reasons for therapy, onset, occurrence/triggers, frequency, characteristics of S&S. Describe daily bladder function (use a voiding diary) and r/o infections and stones.
2. List drugs currently prescribed to ensure none interact or alter dosage. Determine evidence of urinary/gastric retention, GI obstructive disorders, or glaucoma.
3. Monitor renal and LFTs; decrease dose with dysfunction.

CLIENT/FAMILY TEACHING
1. Take as directed with or without food. Avoid alcohol and OTC antihistamines.
2. Drug is used to help reduce the frequency and urgency associated with urination. It is not for stress incontinence or UTI but is for treatment of an overactive bladder.
3. May experience dizziness/drowsiness, headache, blurred vision, dry mouth and light sensitivity; use caution and report if persistent. If eye pain, rapid heart rate, SOB, urinary retention, rash or hives appears notify provider.
4. Dry mouth symptoms may be relieved with sugar free candy/gum, ice/water, or saliva substitute.
5. There is a user support number. Call 1-800-896-8596 to enroll and to receive free information/updates and 24-hr hotline access.

OUTCOMES/EVALUATE
↑ Bladder control with ↓ urinary frequency, urgency, or urge incontinence

Topiramate
(toh-**PYRE**-ah-mayt)

CLASSIFICATION(S):
Anticonvulsant, miscellaneous
PREGNANCY CATEGORY: C
Rx: Topamax.

SEE ALSO *ANTICONVULSANTS*.

USES
(1) Adjunct treatment for partial onset seizures in adults and children, 2–16 years. (2) Adjunct treatment for primary generalized tonic-clonic seizures in adults and children, 2–16 years old. (3) Adjunct treatment of seizures associated with Lennox-Gastaut syndrome in clients 2 years of age and older. (4) Monotherapy in clients 10 years and older to treat partial-onset or primary generalized tonic-clonic seizures. (5) Prophylaxis of migraine headaches in adults. Use in acute treatment of migraines has not been studied. *Investigational:* Alcohol and cocaine dependence, binge eating disorder, bulimia nervosa, cluster headaches, infantile spasms, adjunctive therapy for bipolar disorder, weight loss in obesity, smoking.

ACTION/KINETICS

Action
Precise mechanism not known. The following effects may contribute to the anticonvulsant activity. (1) Action potentials seen repetitively by sustained depolarization of neurons are blocked in a time-dependent manner, suggesting an effect to block sodium channels. (2) Increases the frequency at which GABA activates GABA$_A$ receptors, thus enhancing the ability of GABA to cause a flux of chloride ions into neurons (i.e., enhanced effect of the inhibitory transmitter, GABA$_A$). (3) Antagonizes the ability of kainate to activate the kainate/AMPA subtype of excitatory amino acid aspartate, thus reducing the excitatory effect. (4) Inhibits the carbonic anhydrase enzyme, particularly isozymes II and IV.

Bold Italic = life threatening side effect   ▇ = black box warning   ♣ = Available in Canada

Pharmacokinetics
Rapidly absorbed; **peak plasma levels:** About 2 hr. Bioavailability is about 80%. **t½, elimination:** 21 hr. **Steady state:** About 4 days in those with normal renal function. Excreted mostly unchanged in the urine.

CONTRAINDICATIONS
Lactation.

SPECIAL CONCERNS
Use with caution in impaired hepatic and renal function. Clients taking the drug, especially children, should be monitored for decreased sweating and hyperthermia, especially those exposed to elevated environmental temperatures and/or engaged in vigorous activity. Safety and efficacy have not been determined in children less than 2 years old for adjunctive therapy of partial onset seizures, primary generalized tonic-clonic seizures, or seizures associated with Lennox-Gastaut syndrome.

SIDE EFFECTS
Most Common
Dizziness, paresthesia, ataxia, anxiety, confusion, nervousness, depression, fatigue, somnolence, insomnia, URTI, anorexia, rhinitis, abnormal vision, diplopia, nystagmus, tremor, nausea.
NOTE: Side effects with an incidence of 0.1% or greater are listed. **CNS:** Psychomotor slowing, including difficulty with concentration and speech or language problems. Somnolence, fatigue, dizziness, nervousness, ataxia, nystagmus, paresthesia, nervousness, difficulty with memory/concentration, tremor, confusion, depression, abnormal coordination, agitation, mood problems, aggressive reaction, hypoesthesia, apathy, emotional lability, depersonalization, hypo-/hyperkinesia, hyporeflexia, vertigo, stupor, *clonic/tonic seizures,* hyperkinesia, hypertonia, insomnia, personality disorder, impotence, hallucinations, euphoria, psychosis, decreased libido, *suicide attempt,* hyporeflexia, neuropathy, migraine, apraxia, hyperesthesia, dyskinesia, hyperreflexia, dysphonia, scotoma, dystonia, coma, encephalopathy, upper motor neuron lesion, paranoid reaction, delusion, paranoia, delirium, abnormal dreaming, neuroses, abnormal gait, tremor, vertigo. **GI:** Nausea, dyspepsia, anorexia, abdominal pain, constipation, dry mouth, thirst, gingivitis, glossitis, halitosis, diarrhea, vomiting, fecal incontinence, flatulence, gastroenteritis, GI disorder, gum hyperplasia, hemorrhoids, increased appetite, tooth caries, stomatitis, dysphagia, melena, gastritis, esophagitis, increased saliva, hiccough, gastroesophageal reflux, tongue edema, esophagitis, gall bladder disorder, gingival bleeding, enlarged abdomen, hepatitis, *pancreatitis, hepatic failure (including fatalities).* **CV:** Palpitation, hyper-/hypotension, postural hypotension, AV block, bradycardia, bundle branch block, angina pectoris, *DVT,* abnormal EEG, syncope, vasodilation, phlebitis. **Body as a whole:** Asthenia, flu-like symptoms, infection, viral infections, hot flashes, body odor, edema, rigors, fever, malaise, syncope, enlarged abdomen, hyperthermia (especially in children during vigorous activity or exposure to elevated environmental temperatures). **Respiratory:** URTI, pharyngitis, sinusitis, rhinitis, epistaxis, dyspnea, coughing, bronchitis, asthma, pneumonia, respiratory disorder, *bronchospasm, pulmonary embolism.* **Dermatologic:** Acne, alopecia, dermatitis, nail disorder, folliculitis, dry skin, urticaria, skin discoloration, pallor, eczema, photosensitivity reaction, erythematous rash, flushing, seborrhea, decreased/increased sweating, abnormal hair texture, facial edema, pemphigus, erythema multiforme, *Stevens-Johnson syndrome, toxic dermal necrolysis.* **GU:** Breast pain, renal stone formation, dysmenorrhea, amenorrhea, menstrual disorder, hematuria, intermenstrual bleeding, leukorrhea, menorrhagia, vaginitis, UTI, micturition frequency, urinary incontinence, abnormal urine, dysuria, renal calculus, ejaculation disorder, breast discharge, urinary retention, renal pain, nocturia, albuminuria, polyuria, oliguria, kidney stones, renal tubular acidosis, prostatic disorder. **Musculoskeletal:** Arthralgia, muscle weakness, arthrosis, osteoporosis, myalgia, skeletal pain, leg cramps, involuntary

muscle contractions, back/chest/leg pain. **Metabolic:** Increased/decreased weight, dehydration, xeropthalmia, metabolic acidosis, diabetes mellitus. **Hematologic:** Anemia, leukopenia, lymphadenopathy, eosinophilia, lymphopenia, granulocytopenia, lymphocytosis, thrombocytothemia, purpura, thrombocytopenia, hematoma. **Ophthalmic:** Diplopia, abnormal vision, eye pain, conjunctivitis, abnormal accommodation, photophobia, abnormal lacrimation, strabismus, color blindness, acute myopia, mydriasis, ptosis, xerothalmia, scotoma, visual field defect, acute myopia with secondary angle-closure glaucoma, nystagmus. **Miscellaneous:** Decreased hearing, taste perversion, tinnitus, taste loss, parosmia, goiter, basal cell carcinoma.

LABORATORY TEST CONSIDERATIONS
↑ AST, ALT, gamma-GT, alkaline phosphatase, creatinine. Hypokalemia, hyperglycemia, hyperlipidemia, hyperchloremia, hypernatremia, hypocholesterolemia, hyponatremia, hypophosphatemia.

OD **OVERDOSE MANAGEMENT**
Symptoms: Abdominal pain, abnormal coordination, agitation, blurred vision, convulsions, depression, diplopia, dizziness, drowsiness, hypotension, lethargy, impaired mentation, metabolic acidosis, speech disturbance, stupor.
Treatment: Gastric lavage or induction of emesis if ingestion is recent. Activated charcoal. Supportive treatment. Hemodialysis.

DRUG INTERACTIONS
Alcohol / CNS depression; cognitive and neuropsychiatric side effects
Amitriptyline / ↑ Amytriptyline levels; adjust amitriptyline dose
Anticholinergics / ↑ Risk of heat-related disorders
Carbamazepine / ↓ Topiramate levels by about 40% R/T ↑ metabolism
Carbonic anhydrase inhibitors / ↑ Risk of renal stone formation and heat-related disorders
CNS depressants / CNS depression; cognitive and neuropsychiatric side effects
Digoxin / ↓ Serum digoxin AUC; clinical relevance not established

Estrogens / ↓ Effect of estrogens R/T ↓ estradiol AUC and plasma levels; consider ↑ estrogen dose
Hydantoins / ↓ Topiramate levels R/T ↑ metabolism; also, ↑ phenytoin levels R/T ↓ metabolism
Hydrochlorothiazide / ↑ Topiramate C_{max} and AUC; adjust dose accordingly
Lamotrigine / ↑ Topiramate levels
Lithium / ↓ Lithium AUC and C_{max}
Metformin / ↓ Metformin plasma clearance → ↑ AUC and C_{max}
Oral contraceptives / ↓ Effect of OCs; consider an alternate method of contraception or ↑ estrogen dose
Phenytoin / ↓ Topiramate levels and ↑ phenytoin levels; possible dosage adjustment
Pioglitazone / ↓ Topiramate's active metabolites; monitor carefully; also, ↓ pioglitazone AUC
Risperidone / ↓ Risperidone levels by 25%; monitor closely
Valproic acid / ↓ Levels of both topiramate and valproic acid; possible hyperammonemia with or without encephalopathy

HOW SUPPLIED
Capsules, Sprinkle: 15 mg, 25 mg; *Tablets:* 25 mg, 50 mg, 100 mg, 200 mg.

DOSAGE
• **CAPSULES, SPRINKLE; TABLETS**
Epilepsy, monotherapy.
Adults and children, 10 years and older: 400 mg/day in 2 divided doses. Achieve this dosage using the following titration schedule: **Week 1:** 25 mg in the morning and evening; **Week 2:** 50 mg in the morning and evening; **Week 3:** 75 mg in the morning and evening; **Week 4:** 100 mg in the morning and evening; **Week 5:** 150 mg in the morning and evening; **Week 6:** 200 mg in the morning and evening.
Epilepsy, adjunctive therapy: Partial seizures, primary generalized tonic-clonic seizures, Lennox-Gastaut syndrome.
Adults, 17 years and older, initial: 25–50 mg/day; then, titrate in increments of 25 to 50 mg/week until an effective daily dose is reached. The recommended total daily dose is 200–400 mg/day; doses greater than 1,600

---

mg/day have not been studied. **Children, 2–16 years:** Begin titration at 25 mg or less (based on a range of 1–3 mg/kg/day) nightly for the first week. Then, increase dose at 1- or 2-week intervals by increments of 1–3 mg/kg/day (given in 2 divided doses) to reach optimal clinical response. The recommended total daily dose is 5–9 mg/kg/day in two divided doses.

Migraine prophylaxis.

Week 1, initial: 25 mg at night; **Week 2:** 25 mg in the morning and evening; **Week 3:** 25 mg in the morning and 50 mg in the evening; **Week 4:** 50 mg in the morning and evening. **Maintenance:** 100 mg/day in 2 doses.

NURSING CONSIDERATIONS

℞ Do not confuse Topamax with Toprol-XL (antihypertensive) or with Tegretol and Tegretol-XR (anticonvulsants).

ADMINISTRATION/STORAGE

1. If C_{CR} is <70 mL/1.73 m², use one half of the usual adult dose. These clients will require a longer time to reach steady state at each dose.
2. Plasma levels may be increased in those with hepatic impairment.
3. The sprinkle capsule is bioequivalent to the tablet and thus may be substituted as therapeutically equivalent.
4. Addition of topiramate to phenytoin therapy may require adjustment of the phenytoin dose to achieve an optimal response. The addition or withdrawal of phenytoin and/or carbamazepine during therapy with topiramate may require adjustment of the topiramate dose.
5. If necessary, withdraw topiramate gradually to minimize the risk of increased seizure frequency.
6. A prolonged period of dialysis may result in topiramate levels too low to maintain antiseizure effect. To avoid rapid falls in topiramate plasma levels during hemodialysis, a supplemental topiramate dose may be required.
7. Store tablets from 15–30°C (59–86°F) in a tightly closed container. Store sprinkle capsules at 25°C (77°F) in a tightly closed container. Protect capsules and tablets from moisture.

ASSESSMENT

1. Note reasons for therapy; with seizures note age at onset, type, and characteristics, other agents trialed, outcome.
2. List drugs currently prescribed to ensure none interact or lose effectiveness; MAO inhibitors may promote kidney stones. Monitor CBC, liver, and renal function studies; reduce dose with renal dysfunction.
3. Measure baseline serum bicarbonate and monitor periodically during treatment to assess for metabolic acidosis.
4. Document baseline psychomotor and mental status; assess for psychomotor slowing, speech or expression problems, difficulty concentrating, fatigue, or sleepiness.
5. Evaluate for acute myopia or secondary angle closure glaucoma. Immediately discontinue drug if symptoms present.

CLIENT/FAMILY TEACHING

1. Take exactly as prescribed. Due to the bitter taste of the drug, do not break tablets. Can be taken without regard for meals. Do not stop drug abruptly due to risk of increased seizure frequency.
2. For sprinkle capsules, either swallow whole or carefully open capsule and sprinkle the entire contents on a small amount (teaspoon) of soft food. Swallow the drug/food mixture immediately. Do not chew and do not store for future use.
3. Distinguish if drug affects motor or mental capacity before driving or performing activities that require mental alertness; may cause dizziness, confusion, drowsiness, and altered concentration. Review list of side effects, noting those that require attention. Report any blurred vision or periorbital edema immediately.
4. Increase fluid intake to decrease substance concentration as drug may precipitate renal stone formation by increasing urinary pH and reducing urinary citrate excretion.
5. Avoid strenuous activity in hot weather; decreased sweating and in-

---

 = see color insert   = Herbal   **IV** = Intravenous   ℞ = sound alike drug creased body temperature, especially in hot weather may cause dehydration

6. Use reliable, nonhormonal form of birth control; drug may compromise efficacy of PO contraceptives.

7. Keep all F/U appointments to monitor renal and LFTs and assess drug response.

OUTCOMES/EVALUATE

• Control of seizures
• Migraine prophylaxis

Topotecan hydrochloride ■ IV
(toh-poh-**TEE**-kan)

CLASSIFICATION(S):
Antineoplastic, hormone
PREGNANCY CATEGORY: D
Rx: Hycamtin.

SEE ALSO *ANTINEOPLASTIC AGENTS.*

USES
(1) Metastatic cancer of the ovary after failure of initial or subsequent chemotherapy. (2) Small cell lung cancer sensitive disease after failure of first-line chemotherapy. (3) In combination with cisplatin to treat stage IV-B, recurrent, or persistent carcinoma of the cervix, that is not amenable to curative therapy with surgery and/or radiation therapy. *Investigational:* In combination with paclitaxel to treat advanced non-small cell lung cancer.

ACTION/KINETICS
Action
An inhibitor of topoisomerase I. Topoisomerase I relieves torsional strain in DNA by causing reversible single-strand breaks. Topotecan binds to the topoisomerase I-DNA complex and prevents religation of single-strand breaks. Cytotoxicity thought to be caused by double-strand DNA damage produced during DNA synthesis when replication enzymes interact with the ternary complex formed by topotecan, topoisomerase I, and DNA.

Pharmacokinetics
Hydrolyzed to the active lactone form of the drug. About 30% of the drug is excreted in the urine. $t^{1/2}$, **terminal:** 2 to 3 hr. About 30% of a dose is excreted in the urine. **Plasma protein binding:** About 35%.

CONTRAINDICATIONS
Hypersensitivity to topotecan or any component of the product. Pregnancy, lactation. Severe bone marrow depression, including those with baseline neutrophil counts less than 1,500 cells/mm^3.

SPECIAL CONCERNS
■ (1) Administer under the supervision of a physician experienced in the use of cancer chemotherapeutic drugs. Appropriate management of complications is possible only when adequate diagnostic and treatment facilities are readily available. (2) Do not give topotecan to those with baseline neutrophil counts of less than 1,500 cells/mm^3. In order to monitor the occurrence of bone marrow suppression (primarily neutropenia) that may be severe and result in infection and death, perform frequent peripheral blood cell counts on all clients receiving topotecan.■ Safety and efficacy have not been determined in children.

SIDE EFFECTS
Most Common
Myelosuppression (see below), headache, total alopecia, N&V, diarrhea, constipation, abdominal pain, pyrexia, pain, coughing, dyspnea.

Hematologic: Bone marrow suppression, including neutropenia (grade 4: <500 cells/mm^3), thrombocytopenia (grade 4: <25,000 cells/mm^3), anemia (severe: grade 3/4, leukopenia (<3,000 cells/mm^3), hemoglobin <8 grams/dL), sepsis or fever/infection with grade 4 neutropenia, platelet or RBC infusions, ***severe bleeding in association with thrombocytopenia*** (rare). **GI:** N&V, abdominal pain, constipation, diarrhea, intestinal obstruction, stomatitis, anorexia. **CNS:** Headache, pain, paresthesias, neuropathy. **Musculoskeletal:** Arthralgia, myalgia. **Body as a whole:** Anorexia, fatigue, asthenia, malaise, fever,

---

Bold Italic = life threatening side effect   ■ = black box warning   ✦ = Available in Canada

pain, **sepsis**. **Respiratory:** Dyspnea, coughing, pharyngitis, pneumonia. **Dermatologic:** Total alopecia, rash, severe dermatitis, severe pruritus. **At injection site:** Erythema, bruising. **Miscellaneous:** Chest pain, allergic reactions, ocular disturbances, *anaphylaxis* (rare), *angioedema*.

LABORATORY TEST CONSIDERATIONS
↑ AST, ALT, bilirubin.

DRUG INTERACTIONS
Cisplatin / More severe myelosuppression
Cytotoxic drugs / More severe myelosuppression
Filgrastim / Prolonged duration of neutropenia; do not initiate until 24 hr after completion of topotecan treatment

HOW SUPPLIED
Powder for Injection, Lyophilized: 4 mg (as base).

DOSAGE————————
- **IV INFUSION**
  Metastatic ovarian cancer, small cell lung cancer.

Adults: 1.5 mg/m^2 by IV infusion over 30 min daily for 5 consecutive days, starting on day 1 of a 21-day course of therapy. The median time to response in ovarian cancer is 9–12 weeks and the median time to response in small cell lung cancer is 5–7 weeks. In the absence of tumor progression, a minimum of four courses is recommended. If severe neutropenia occurs, reduce the dose to 1.25 mg/m^2 for subsequent courses. Reduce doses similarly if the platelet count falls below 25,000 cells/mm^3. Also, for severe neutropenia, filgrastim may be given following the subsequent course and before dosage reduction starting from day 6 of the course (i.e., 24 hr after completion of topotecan administration). Reduce the dose to 0.75 mg/m^2 for clients with a C$_{CR}$ of 20–39 mL/min. No dosage reduction is required if the C$_{CR}$ is 40–60 mL/min.

  Cervical cancer.
Topotecan, 0.75 mg/m^2 daily over 30 min on days 1, 2, and 3 followed by cisplatin, 50 mg/m^2 on day 1 repeated every 21 days (i.e., a 21-day course of therapy). If severe febrile neutropenia

(<1,000 cells/mm^3) occurs, reduce the dose of topotecan to 0.6 mg/m^2 for subsequent courses. Also, decrease the dose of topotecan to 0.6 mg/m^2 if the platelet count falls below 10,000/mm^3. Alternatively, in the event of severe febrile neutropenia, filgrastim (granulocyte colony-stimulating factor; G-CSF) can be given following the subsequent course and before reducing the dose. Give G-CSF starting from day 4 of the course (i.e., 24 hr after completion of topotecan dosing regimen). If febrile neutropenia occurs despite the use of G-CSF, reduce the dose of topotecan to 0.45 mg/m^2 for subsequent courses. *NOTE:* See cisplatin for administration and hydration guidelines.

NURSING CONSIDERATIONS
ADMINISTRATION/STORAGE
IV 1. To begin therapy, clients must have a baseline neutrophil count >1,500 cells/mm^3, a platelet count >100,000 cells/mm^3, and a hemoglobin level of 9 mg/dL or higher. Do not retreat until neutrophils are >1,000 cells/mm^3, platelets are >100,000 cells/mm^3, and hemoglobin levels are 9 mg/dL or greater.

2. For those with moderately impaired renal function (C$_{CR}$, 20–39 mL/min), give a dose of 0.75 mg/m^2.

3. Only initiate cisplatin with topotecan if serum creatinine is 1.5 mg/dL or less.

4. Reconstitute the 4 mg topotecan vial with 4 mL of sterile water for injection. This may then be further diluted either with 0.9% NaCl or D5W and administered over 30 min. Because there is no antibacterial preservative in the product, use the reconstituted product immediately.

5. Topotecan is a cytotoxic drug. Prepare under a vertical laminar flow hood while wearing gloves and protective clothing. If topotecan solution contacts the skin, wash immediately and thoroughly with soap and water. If the drug contacts mucous membranes, flush thoroughly with water.

6. Reconstituted vials diluted for infusion are stable at controlled room tem-

---

perature and ambient lighting conditions when stored for 24 hr.

7. Store vials in their original carton, protected from light, at controlled room temperature of 20–25°C (68–77°F).

ASSESSMENT

1. Note reasons for therapy, other agents/therapies trialed, when administered.

2. Monitor CBC, renal and LFTs; reduce dose with C_{CR} of 20–39 mL/m². Ensure baseline neutrophil count above 1,500 cells/mm³ and platelet count at 100,000/mm³. Do not readminister until neutrophils are above 1,000, platelets are 100,000 cells/mm³, and hemoglobin levels are at least 9 mg/dL. Drug causes neutropenia and anemia. Nadir: 15 days.

CLIENT/FAMILY TEACHING

1. Drug is administered IV over 30 min. to stop the growth of cancer cells.

2. Report any evidence of infection: sore throat, fever, chills, unusual bruising /bleeding.

3. Practice reliable contraception; avoid breast feeding.

4. Keep all F/U for evaluation and labs.

OUTCOMES/EVALUATE

Control of malignant cell proliferation in metastatic cancer

Toremifene citrate
(**TOR**-em-ih-feen)

CLASSIFICATION(S):
Antineoplastic, hormone (antiestrogen)

PREGNANCY CATEGORY: D

Rx: Fareston.

SEE ALSO *ANTINEOPLASTIC AGENTS.*

USES
Metastatic breast cancer in postmenopausal women with positive estrogen-receptor (ER) or ER unknown tumors.

ACTION/KINETICS

Action
Antiestrogen that binds to estrogen receptors and may cause estrogenic, an-

tiestrogenic, or both effects, depending on duration of treatment, gender, and endpoint/target organ selected. Antitumor effect is likely due to antiestrogenic effect, i.e., competes for estrogen at receptor and blocks growth-stimulating effects of estrogen in the tumor.

Pharmacokinetics
Well absorbed from GI tract; absorption not affected by food. **Peak plasma levels:** 3 hr. **t½, distribution:** About 4 hr. **t½, elimination:** About 5 days. Extensively metabolized in liver by CYP3A4 and mainly excreted in feces. The elimination half-life is increased in both the elderly and in those with hepatic insufficiency.

CONTRAINDICATIONS
Use with history of thromboembolic disease or in pediatric clients.

SPECIAL CONCERNS
Hypercalcemia and tumor flare in some breast cancer clients with bone metastases during first weeks of treatment. Use with caution during lactation.

SIDE EFFECTS

Most Common
Hot flashes, sweating, N&V, vaginal discharge/bleeding, dizziness, edema.

CV: *Cardiac failure, MI, pulmonary embolism, CVA,* TIA. **GI:** Constipation, N&V. **Hematologic:** Leukopenia, thrombocytopenia. **Dermatologic:** Hot flashes, sweating, skin discoloration, dermatitis, alopecia, pruritus. **Ophthalmic:** Cataracts, dry eyes, abnormal visual fields, corneal keratopathy, glaucoma, reversible corneal opacity. **CNS:** Dizziness, tremor, vertigo, depression. **GU:** Vaginal discharge/bleeding. **Miscellaneous:** Dyspnea, edema, paresis, anorexia, asthenia, jaundice, rigors, tumor flare, hypercalcemia.

LABORATORY TEST CONSIDERATIONS
↑ AST, alkaline phosphatase, bilirubin. Hypercalcemia.

OD OVERDOSE MANAGEMENT
Symptoms: Vertigo, headache, dizziness. Possibly, hot flashes, vaginal bleeding, vertigo, dizziness, ataxia, nausea. *Treatment:* General supportive measures.

DRUG INTERACTIONS
Carbamazepine / ↓ Toremifene blood levels R/T ↑ liver breakdown

---

Clonazepam / ↓ Toremifene blood levels R/T ↑ liver breakdown

Erythromycin / Inhibition of toremifene breakdown

Ketoconazole / Inhibition of toremifene breakdown

Macrolide antibiotics / Inhibition of toremifene breakdown

Phenobarbital / ↓ Toremifene blood levels R/T ↑ liver breakdown

Phenytoin / ↓ Toremifene blood levels R/T ↑ liver breakdown

Warfarin / ↑ PT

HOW SUPPLIED
Tablets: 60 mg.

DOSAGE

- **TABLETS**
  Metastatic breast cancer.
  Adults: 60 mg once daily. Continue until disease progression is observed.

ASSESSMENT
1. Note reasons for therapy, characteristics of S&S, other agents trialed, outcome.
2. List any history/evidence of thromboembolic disorders.
3. Monitor CBC, calcium, renal, and LFTs.

CLIENT/FAMILY TEACHING
1. Take once daily as directed. May take with food to decrease GI upset; do not crush, break or chew enteric coated products.
2. Report any unusual vaginal bleeding, muscle/bone pain, visual changes, or calf pain/tenderness, SOB, or chest pain.
3. May experience 'tumor flare,' syndrome of diffuse musculoskeletal pain and erythema with increased size of tumor lesions that regress later; if accompanied by hypercalcemia must stop drug.
4. Use reliable barrier birth control as drug may induce ovulation.
5. Avoid prolonged sun exposure, use protection if exposure necessary.
6. Hair loss may occur and regrowth may be of a different texture and color.

OUTCOMES/EVALUATE
Control of malignant cell proliferation

Torsemide
(TOR-seh-myd)

CLASSIFICATION(S):
Diuretic, loop
PREGNANCY CATEGORY: B
Rx: Demadex.

SEE ALSO *DIURETICS, LOOP.*
USES
(1) Congestive heart failure. (2) Acute or chronic renal failure. (3) Hepatic cirrhosis. (4) Hypertension.

ACTION/KINETICS
Pharmacokinetics
Onset, IV: Within 10 min; **PO:** Within 60 min. **Peak effect, IV:** Within 60 min; **PO:** 60–120 min. **Duration:** 6–8 hr. **t½:** 210 min. Metabolized by the liver and excreted through the urine. Food delays the time to peak effect by about 30 min, but the overall bioavailability and the diuretic activity are not affected.

CONTRAINDICATIONS
Lactation.

SPECIAL CONCERNS
■ Loop diuretics are potent drugs; excess amounts can lead to a profound diuresis with water and electrolyte depletion. Careful medical supervision is required and dosage must be individualized.■ Clients sensitive to sulfonamides may show allergic reactions to torsemide. Safety and efficacy in children have not been determined.

SIDE EFFECTS
Most Common
Excessive urination, headache, dizziness, asthenia, diarrhea, abnormal ECG, arthralgia, nausea, rhinitis, increased cough.
CNS: Headache, dizziness, asthenia, insomnia, nervousness, syncope. **GI:** Diarrhea, constipation, nausea, dyspepsia, edema, *GI hemorrhage*, rectal bleeding. **CV:** ECG abnormality, chest pain, atrial fibrillation, hypotension, *ventricular tachycardia*, shunt thrombosis. **Respiratory:** Rhinitis, increase in cough. **Musculoskeletal:** Arthralgia, myalgia. **Miscellaneous:** Sore throat, excessive urination, rash.

T

LABORATORY TEST CONSIDERATIONS
Hyperglycemia, hyperuricemia, hypokalemia, hypovolemia

HOW SUPPLIED
Injection: 10 mg/mL; *Tablets:* 5 mg, 10 mg, 20 mg, 100 mg.

DOSAGE

• **IV; TABLETS**
  Congestive heart failure.
  Adults, initial: 10 or 20 mg once daily.
  Chronic renal failure.
  Adults, initial: 20 mg once daily.
  Hepatic cirrhosis.
  Adults, initial: 5 or 10 mg once daily given with an aldosterone antagonist or a potassium-sparing diuretic.
  Hypertension.
  Adults, initial: 5 mg once daily. If this dose does not lead to an adequate decrease in BP within 4–6 weeks, the dose may be increased to 10 mg once daily. If the 10 mg dose is not adequate, an additional antihypertensive agent is added to the treatment regimen.

NURSING CONSIDERATIONS

Do not confuse torsemide with furosemide (also a loop diuretic).

ADMINISTRATION/STORAGE
1. If the response is inadequate for the initial dose used for CHF, chronic renal failure, or hepatic cirrhosis, the dose may be doubled until the desired diuretic response is obtained. Doses greater than 200 mg for CHF or chronic renal failure and greater than 40 mg for hepatic cirrhosis have not been adequately studied.
2. May be given without regard to meals.
3. It is not necessary to adjust the dose for geriatric clients.
4. Give the IV dose slowly over a period of 2 min or as a continuous infusion.
5. Oral and IV doses are therapeutically equivalent; may switch to and from the IV form with no change in dose.

ASSESSMENT
1. Note reasons for therapy, onset, characteristics of S&S. List agents trialed, outcome.
2. Assess pulmonary, renal, and CV systems. List sensitivity to sulfonamides.

3. Monitor VS, weight, I&O, blood sugar, uric acid, BUN, creatinine, and potassium; drug may increase blood sugar and uric acid levels.

CLIENT/FAMILY TEACHING
1. Take only as directed in the am to prevent nighttime awakening to void. May take with food to decrease GI upset.
2. With hypertension, keep a BP log for provider review.
3. Report immediately any chest pain, increased SOB, ringing in the ears, or sudden weight gain with extremity swelling.
4. Drug may cause dizziness, lightheadedness, and fatigue; use caution. Rise slowly from a sitting or lying position to minimize low BP effects.
5. May experience blurred vision, yellowing of vision, or sensitivity to sunlight. Report any unusual, persistent symptoms or lack of response.

OUTCOMES/EVALUATE
• ↓ Edema; ↑ diuresis; ↓ BP
• Reduction of interdialysis weight gain and promotion of Na, Cl, and water excretion

Tramadol hydrochloride
(**TRAM**-ah-dol)

CLASSIFICATION(S):
Analgesic, centrally-acting
PREGNANCY CATEGORY: C
Rx: Ultram, Ultram ER.

USES
Immediate-Release (IR): Management of moderate to moderately severe pain in adults. **Extended-Release (ER):** Moderate to moderately severe chronic pain in adults who require around-the-clock pain therapy for an extended period of time. *Investigational:* Premature ejaculation.

ACTION/KINETICS
Action
A centrally acting analgesic not related chemically to opiates. Precise mecha-

nism is not known. Two complimentary mechanisms may be applicable: It may bind to mu-opioid receptors and inhibit reuptake of norepinephrine and serotonin. The analgesic effect is only partially antagonized by the antagonist naloxone. Causes significantly less respiratory depression than morphine. In contrast to morphine, tramadol does not cause release of histamine. Produces dependence of the mu-opioid type (i.e., like codeine or dextropropoxyphene); however, there is little evidence of abuse. Tolerance occurs but is relatively mild; the withdrawal syndrome is not as severe as with other opiates.

Pharmacokinetics
Rapidly absorbed after PO administration. Food does not affect the rate or extent of absorption. **Onset:** 1 hr. **Peak effect:** 2–3 hr. **Peak plasma levels:** 2 hr. **Duration:** 2 hr for tramadol and 3 hr for the M1 active metabolite. **$t^{1/2}$, plasma:** 6.3 hr for tramadol and 7.4 hr for the M1 active metabolite. Extensively metabolized in the liver by CYP2D6 and CYP3A4. Excreted in the urine, with about 30% excreted unchanged and 60% as metabolites. The M-metabolite is active.

CONTRAINDICATIONS
Hypersensitivity to tramadol. In acute intoxication with alcohol, hypnotics, centrally acting analgesics, opiates, or psychotropic drugs. Use in clients with past or present addiction or opiate dependence or in those with a prior history of allergy to codeine or opiates. Use for obstetric preoperative medication or for postdelivery analgesia in nursing mothers. Use in children less than 16 years of age, as safety and efficacy have not been determined.

SPECIAL CONCERNS
Use with great caution in those taking MAO inhibitors, as tramadol inhibits norepinephrine and serotonin uptake. Dosage reduction is recommended with impaired hepatic or renal function and in clients over 75 years of age. Use with caution in increased intracranial pressure or head injury, in epilepsy, or in clients with an increased risk for seizures, including head trauma, metabolic disorders, alcohol or drug withdrawal, use of certain drugs (e.g., SSRIs, tricyclic compounds, cyclobenzaprine, promethazine), and CNS infections. Seizures may occur in any client, especially if the dose is increased. Tramadol may complicate the assessment of acute abdominal conditions. Has abuse potential for some clients.

SIDE EFFECTS
Most Common
Dizziness, headache, CNS stimulation, ataxia, sedation/somnolence, vertigo, itching/pruritus, constipation, nausea.
CNS: Dizziness, vertigo, headache, somnolence, ataxia, CNS stimulation, anxiety, confusion, incoordination, euphoria, nervousness, sleep disorders, *seizures*, paresthesia, cognitive dysfunction, hallucinations, tremor, amnesia, concentration difficulty, abnormal gait, migraine, development of drug dependence, speech disorders, depression, increased risk of seizures. **GI:** Nausea, constipation, vomiting, dyspepsia, dry mouth, diarrhea, abdominal pain, anorexia, flatulence, GI bleeding, hepatitis, stomatitis, dysgeusia, *liver failure*. **CV:** Vasodilation, syncope, orthostatic hypotension, hypertension, tachycardia, abnormal ECG, myocardial ischemia, palpitations, pulmonary edema/embolism. **Dermatologic:** Pruritus, sweating, rash, itching, urticaria, vesicles, *Stevens-Johnson syndrome*, *toxic epidermal necrolysis*. **Body as a whole:** Asthenia, malaise, allergic reaction, accidental injury, weight loss, *suicidal tendency*. **GU:** Urinary retention/frequency, menopausal symptoms, dysuria, menstrual disorder. **Ophthalmic:** Miosis, visual disturbancers, cataracts. **Miscellaneous:** *Anaphylaxis*, deafness, tinnitus, hypertonia, dyspnea, serotonin syndrome.

LABORATORY TEST CONSIDERATIONS
↑ Creatinine, liver enzymes. ↓ Hemoglobin. Proteinuria.

OD OVERDOSE MANAGEMENT
Symptoms: Extension of side effects, especially *respiratory depression and seizures*. *Treatment:* Naloxone will reverse some, but not all, of the symptoms of overdose. General supportive

treatment, with special attention to maintenance of adequate respiration. Diazepam or barbiturates may help if seizures occur. Hemodialysis is not helpful.

DRUG INTERACTIONS

Alcohol / ↑ Respiratory depression

Anesthetics, general / ↑ Respiratory depression

Carbamazepine / ↓ Tramadol effect R/T ↑ metabolism

CNS depressants / Additive CNS depression

Cyclobenzaprine / ↑ Risk of seizures

Digoxin / ↑ Risk (rare) of digoxin toxicity

MAO Inhibitors / ↑ Risk of seizures

Naloxone / ↑ Risk of seizures if naloxone used for tramadol overdose.

Promethazine / ↑ Risk of seizures

Quinidine / ↑ Levels of tramadol and ↓ levels of M1 R/T inhibition of metabolism

SSRIs / ↑ Risk of seizures and ↑ risk of serotonin syndrome

Tricyclic antidepressants / ↑ Risk of seizures

Warfarin ↑ PT and INR

HOW SUPPLIED

Tablets, Extended-Release: 100 mg, 200 mg, 300 mg; *Tablets, Immediate-Release:* 50 mg.

DOSAGE————————————

• **TABLETS, IMMEDIATE-RELEASE**

Management of pain.

Individualize dose based on lowest effective dose. **Adults:** For those requiring rapid onset of analgesia, 50–100 mg q 4–6 hr, as needed, but not to exceed 400 mg/day. For moderate pain, 50 mg, initially, may be adequate, and for severe pain, 100 mg, initially, is often more effective. For moderate chronic pain not requiring rapid analgesic onset, use 25 mg/day to improve tolerability; titrate in 25 mg increments, as separate doses, q 3 days to 100 mg/day. Can then be titrated by 50 mg q 3 days to 200 mg/day, not to exceed 400 mg/day. For clients over 75 years of age, the recommended dose is no more than 300 mg/day in divided doses. In impaired renal function with a C_{CR} less than 30 mL/min, the dosing interval should be increased to 12 hr, with a maximum daily dose of 200 mg. The recommended dose for clients with cirrhosis is 50 mg q 12 hr. Dialysis clients can receive their regular dose on the day of dialysis.

• **TABLETS, EXTENDED-RELEASE**

Long-term around-the-clock management of pain in adults.

Adults, 18 years and older, initial: 100 mg once daily; titrate up as needed in 100 mg increments q 5 days. Maximum dose: 300 mg/day. Administer with caution to clients 65 years of age and older. Do not use the dosage form in clients with a C_{CR} <30 mL/min or in severely impaired hepatic function.

NURSING CONSIDERATIONS

🖜 Do not confuse Ultram with Ultrase (pancreatic enzymes).

ADMINISTRATION/STORAGE

Store from 15–30°C (59–86°F) in a tight container.

ASSESSMENT

1. List reasons for therapy, location, onset, triggers, characteristics of S&S. Use a pain-rating scale to rate pain.

2. Assess for history of drug addiction, allergy to opiates or codeine, seizures; drug may increase the risk of convulsions.

3. Monitor VS, I&O, renal and LFTs; reduce dose with dysfunction and if over 75 years old.

CLIENT/FAMILY TEACHING

1. Take only as directed. May be taken without regard to meals. Do not exceed doses of tramadol; do not share meds, store safely out of reach of child.

2. Extended-release tablets should not be chewed, crushed, or split; swallow whole.

3. Do not perform activities that require mental alertness; drug may cause drowsiness and impair mental or physical performance. Alcohol may intensify drug effects.

4. Report lack of response. Review list of side effects (nausea, dizziness, somnolence, pruritus, and constipation) that one may experience and report if persistent or intolerable.

Bold Italic = life threatening side effect   ▮ = black box warning   ✤ = Available in Canada

5. Avoid alcohol and CNS depressants. Report if pregnant or seizure activity.

6. May mask abdominal pathology and obscure intracranial pathology due to abnormal pupil contraction. Carry ID of drugs currently prescribed.

7. Keep all F/U appointments to evaluate response to therapy.

OUTCOMES/EVALUATE
Desired pain control

— COMBINATION DRUG —

Tramadol hydrochloride and Acetaminophen

(**TRAM**-ah-dol, ah-**SEAT**-ah-**MIN**-oh-fen)

CLASSIFICATION(S):
Narcotic/nonnarcotic analgesic combination drug
PREGNANCY CATEGORY: C
Rx: Ultracet.

SEE ALSO *TRAMADOL HYDROCHLORIDE* AND *ACETAMINOPHEN*.

USES
Short-term use (5 days or less) for management of acute pain. *NOTE:* Onset of analgesia is less than 1 hr and faster than tramadol alone.

CONTENT
Each Ultracet tablet contains tramadol hydrochloride (*narcotic analgesic*), 37.5 mg and acetaminophen (*nonnarcotic analgesic*), 325 mg.

ACTION/KINETICS
Action
Tramadol is a centrally-acting synthetic opioid analgesic. Its mechanism is not completely known but both tramadol and its active metabolite bind to μ-opioid receptors and they are weak inhibitors of norepinephrine and serotonin reuptake. Tramadol is only partially antagonized by naloxone. Acetaminophen may cause analgesia by inhibiting CNS prostaglandin synthesis, although it has no anti-inflammatory activity.

Pharmacokinetics
Tramadol. Rapidly absorbed after PO administration; absolute bioavailability is about 75%. Food does not affect the rate or extent of absorption. **Onset:** 1 hr. **Peak effect:** 2–3 hr. **Peak plasma levels:** 2 hr. **Duration:** 2 hr for tramadol and 3 hr for the M1 active metabolite. **t½, plasma:** 6.3 hr for tramadol and 7.4 hr for the M1 active metabolite. Extensively metabolized in the liver by CYP2D6 and CYP3A4. Excreted in the urine, with about 30% excreted unchanged and 60% as metabolites. Excretion is reduced in those with C_{CR} <30 mL/min.

Acetaminophen. Peak plasma levels: 30–120 min. **t½:** 2–3 hr. **Therapeutic serum levels** (analgesia): 5–20 mcg/mL. Metabolized in the liver and excreted in the urine as glucuronide and sulfate conjugates. However, an intermediate hydroxylated metabolite is hepatotoxic following large doses of acetaminophen. **Plasma protein binding:** About 20% of tramadol is bound to plasma proteins.

CONTRAINDICATIONS
Not recommended for those with hepatic impairment. Hypersensitivity to any component of the product or to opioids. Use in acute intoxication with alcohol, hypnotics, narcotics, centrally-acting analgesics, opioids, or psychotropic drugs (CNS and respiratory depression may worsen). Not recommended for use during labor and delivery unless potential benefits outweigh risks. Lactation.

SPECIAL CONCERNS
Seizures may occur in those taking tramadol within the recommended dosage range; seizure risk is increased with doses above the recommended range, in those with epilepsy or a history of seizures, and in those with a recognized risk of seizures (e.g., head trauma, metabolic disorders, alcohol and drug withdrawal). Use with caution in those at risk for respiratory depression, in those with increased intracranial pressure or head injury, and in the elderly. Safety

and efficacy have not been determined in children.

SIDE EFFECTS
Most Common
Constipation, somnolence, increased sweating, nausea, diarrhea, anorexia, dizziness, dry mouth, insomnia, pruritus, prostatic disorder.

See *Tramadol* and *Acetaminophen* for a complete list of possible side effects.
Hypersensitivity: Serious (but rarely fatal) *anaphylactoid* reactions, often following the first dose. Also, pruritus, hives, *bronchospasm, angioedema, toxic epidermal necrolysis, Stevens-Johnson syndrome.*

OD OVERDOSE MANAGEMENT
Symptoms: **Tramdol:** Respiratory depression, lethargy, coma, *seizure, cardiac arrest, death.* **Acetaminophen:** Hepatic centrilobular necrosis leading to *hepatic failure and death.* Also, renal tubular necrosis, hypoglycemia, and coagulation defects. Early symptoms include N&V, diaphoresis, and general malaise.
Treatment:
- Maintain adequate ventilation (primary concern).
- Naloxone will reverse some, but not all, symptoms of tramadol overdose but the risk of seizures increases.
- Provide supportive measures.
- For acetaminophen: Initially, induction of emesis, gastric lavage, activated charcoal. Oral N-acetylcysteine is said to reduce or prevent hepatic damage by inactivating acetaminophen metabolites, which cause liver toxicity.

DRUG INTERACTIONS
Acetaminophen-containing products / ↑ Potential for acetaminophen hepatotoxicity; do not use together
Alcohol / Do not use together
Amitriptyline / Possible inhibition of tramadol metabolism R/T inhibition of CYP2D6
Carbamazepine / Significantly ↓ analgesic effect of tramadol R/T ↑ metabolism; R/T ↑ seizure risk, do not use together
Fluoxetine / Possible inhibition of tramadol metabolism R/T inhibition of CYP2D6

MAO inhibitors / ↑ Risk of seizures and serotonin syndrome; use together with great caution
Naloxone / ↑ Risk of seizures if given in tramadol overdose
Neuroleptics / ↑ Risk of seizures
Opioids (other than tramadol) / ↑ Risk of seizures
Paroxetine / Possible inhibition of tramadol metabolism R/T inhibition of CYP2D6
Quinidine / ↑ Levels of tramadol and ↓ levels of the active metabolite R/T inhibition of CYP2D6
Selective serotonin reuptake inhibitors / ↑ Risk of seizures and serotonin syndrome
Tricyclic antidepressants / ↑ Risk of seizures
Warfarin / Rarely, alterations of warfarin effects, including ↑ PT

HOW SUPPLIED
See Content.

DOSAGE
- **TABLETS**
  Management of acute pain.

Adults: 2 tablets q 4–6 hr, as needed for relief of pain, up to a maximum of 8 tablets per day for 5 or fewer days. In those with C_{CR} <30 mL/min, do not exceed 2 tablets q 12 hr.

NURSING CONSIDERATIONS
ADMINISTRATION/STORAGE
1. Do not exceed the recommended dose.
2. Tramadol may cause psychological and physical dependence of the morphine-type. Withdrawal symptoms may occur if Ultracet is discontinued abruptly.
3. Store from 15–30°C (59–86°F).

ASSESSMENT
1. List reasons for therapy, onset, characteristics of S&S, other agents trialed, rate pain level.
2. Assess for history of seizures, alcohol disorder, renal/liver abnormalities; reduce dose with dysfunction.
3. Note drugs prescribed to ensure none interact.
4. Ensure x-ray/CT/MRI performed to assess skeletal damage. Note ROM,

---

carefully assess areas of pain and reduced function.

CLIENT/FAMILY TEACHING

1. Drug is a combination medication used to relive pain; used as directed.

2. Avoid activities that require mental alertness until drug effects realized.

3. Do not take alcohol or OTC agents during therapy.

4. Do not stop suddenly after long term use; withdrawal symptoms (craving/tolerance) may occur which include: anxiety, sweating, insomnia, pain, nausea, tremors, rigors, diarrhea, upper respiratory symptoms and rarely hallucinations-report if evident.

5. Keep all F/U appointments to assess response.

OUTCOMES/EVALUATE

Relief of pain

Trandolapril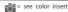
(tran-**DOHL**-ah-pril)

CLASSIFICATION(S):
Antihypertensive, ACE inhibitor
PREGNANCY CATEGORY: C (first trimester), **D** (second and third trimesters).
Rx: Mavik.

SEE ALSO ANGIOTENSIN
CONVERTING ENZYME (ACE)
INHIBITORS.

USES

(1) Hypertension, alone or in combination with other antihypertensives such as hydrochlorothiazide. (2) For stable clients who have left-ventricular systolic dysfunction or who are symptomatic from CHF within the first few days after an acute MI. (3) Heart failure after MI.

ACTION/KINETICS

Pharmacokinetics

Rapidly absorbed; food slows rate, but not amount absorbed. Metabolized in liver to active trandolaprilat. **Onset:** 2–4 hr. Bioavailability is about 10% (70% of trandolaprilat, the active metabolite). Food slows absorption. **Peak plasma levels, trandolapril:** 30–60 min; **trandolaprilat:** 4–10 hr. **t½, trandolapril:** About 5 hr; **t½, trandoprilat:** About 10

hr. **Peak effect:** 4–8 hr. **Duration:** 24 hr. About one-third trandolaprilat is excreted in urine and two-thirds in feces. **Plasma protein binding:** About 80%.

CONTRAINDICATIONS

In those with a history of angioedema with ACE inhibitors.

SPECIAL CONCERNS

■ When used during the second and third trimesters of pregnancy, injury and even death can result in the developing fetus. When pregnancy is detected, discontinue as soon as possible.■ Safety and efficacy have not been determined in children.

SIDE EFFECTS

Most Common

Hypotension, dizziness, dyspepsia, cough, asthenia, syncope, myalgia, gastritis, hypocalcemia, intermittent claudication.

See also *Angiotensin Converting Enzyme Inhibitors* for a complete list of possible side effects. **Hypersensitivity: Angioedema. CNS:** Dizziness, headache, fatigue, insomnia, paresthesias, drowsiness, vertigo, anxiety. **GI:** Diarrhea, dyspepsia, gastritis, abdominal pain, vomiting, constipation, pancreatitis. **CV:** Hypotension, bradycardia, chest pain, ***cardiogenic shock,*** intermittent claudication, stroke. **Respiratory:** Cough, dyspnea, URTI, epistaxis, throat inflammation. **Hepatic:** *Hepatic failure,* including cholestatic jaundice, ***fulminant hepatic necrosis, death.*** **Dermatologic:** Photosensitivity, pruritus, rash. **GU:** UTI, impotence, decreased libido. **Miscellaneous:** Neutropenia, syncope, myalgia, asthenia, muscle cramps, hypocalcemia, intermittent claudication, edema, extremity pain, gout.

LABORATORY TEST CONSIDERATIONS

Hyperkalemia, hypocalcemia. ↑ Serum uric acid, BUN, creatinine.

DRUG INTERACTIONS

Diuretics / Excessive hypotensive effects
Diuretics, potassium-sparing: ↑ Risk of hyperkalemia
Lithium / ↑ Risk of lithium toxicity

HOW SUPPLIED

Tablets: 1 mg, 2 mg, 4 mg.

DOSAGE————————
• **TABLETS**

T

Hypertension.

Initial: 1 mg once daily in nonblack clients (2 mg once daily in black clients) for those not receiving a diuretic. Adjust dosage according to response; usually, adjustments are made at intervals of 1 week. **Maintenance, usual:** 4 mg once daily (twice daily dosing may be needed in some). If BP is still not adequately controlled, diuretic may be added.

Heart failure post–MI/Left ventricular dysfunction post–MI.

Initial: 1 mg/day. Then, increase the dose, as tolerated, to a target dose of 4 mg/day. If 4 mg is not tolerated, continue with the highest tolerated dose. If C_{CR} is less than 30 mL/min or if there is hepatic cirrhosis, initial dose is 0.5 mg daily. Titrate dose to optimal response.

NURSING CONSIDERATIONS

ADMINISTRATION/STORAGE

1. If client is on a diuretic, discontinue 2 to 3 days prior to beginning therapy with trandolapril to reduce likelihood of hypotension. If diuretic can not be discontinued, use an initial trandolapril dose of 0.5 mg. Titrate subsequent dosage.
2. Store tablets from 20–25°C (68–77°F).

ASSESSMENT

1. Note reasons for therapy, disease onset, other agents trialed, outcome.
2. Monitor BP, cardiac status, CBC, electrolytes, renal and LFTs; reduce dosage with impairment.

CLIENT/FAMILY TEACHING

1. Take only as directed.
2. Change positions slowly to prevent sudden drop in BP.
3. May experience cough, dizziness, and diarrhea; report if persistent.
4. Practice reliable contraception; stop drug and report if pregnancy suspected.
5. Continue lifestyle changes (i.e., regular exercise, smoking/alcohol cessation, low fat, low salt diet in overall goal of BP control).
6. Keep log of BP for provider review.

OUTCOMES/EVALUATE

- ↓ BP

- Control of heart failure/ventricular dysfunction after MI

Trastuzumab
(traz-**TOO**-zah-mab)

CLASSIFICATION(S):
Antineoplastic, miscellaneous
PREGNANCY CATEGORY: B
Rx: Herceptin.

SEE ALSO *ANTINEOPLASTIC AGENTS.*

USES

(1) Adjuvant treatment of clients with human epidermal growth factor receptor 2 (HER2)-overexpressing, node-positive breast cancer as part of a regimen including doxorubicin, cyclophosphamide, and paclitaxel. (2) As a single drug to treat metastatic breast cancer in which tumors overexpress the HER2 protein and who have received one or more chemotherapy regimens for their metastatic disease. (3) In combination with paclitaxel to treat metastatic breast cancer in those whose tumors overexpress HER2 protein and who have not received chemotherapy for their metastatic disease.

ACTION/KINETICS

Action

A recombinant DNA-derived humanized monoclonal antibody that selectively binds with high affinity to the extracellular domain of the HER2 protein. Results in inhibition of the proliferation of human tumor cells that overexpress HER2 and mediates antibody-dependent cellular cytotoxicity. The HER2 protein is overexpressed in 25 to 30% of primary breast cancers.

Pharmacokinetics

$t\frac{1}{2}$, **following loading dose of 4 mg/kg and weekly dose of 2 mg/kg:** Average of 5.8 days. Mean serum trough levels of trastuzumab, when given with paclitaxel, were elevated 1.5 fold compared to use in combination with anthracycline plus cyclophosphamide.

Bold Italic = life threatening side effect   ■ = black box warning   ♣ = Available in Canada

CONTRAINDICATIONS

Lactation during therapy and for six months after the last trastuzumab dose.

SPECIAL CONCERNS

■ (1) Cardiomyopathy: Use can result in the development of ventricular dysfunction and CHF. Evaluate left ventricular function in all clients prior to and during treatment. The incidence and severity of left ventricular cardiac dysfunction/CHF was highest in those who received trastuzumab concurrently with anthracycline (doxorubicin or epirubicin)-containing chemotherapy regimens. Discontinue trastuzumab treatment in clients receiving adjuvant therapy for breast cancer and strongly consider terminating therapy in those who develop a clinically significant decrease in left ventricular function. (2) Hypersensitivity reactions: Use can also result in serious infusion reactions and pulmonary toxicity. Rarely, these have been fatal. In most cases, symptoms occurred during or within 24 hr of administration. Interrupt trastuzumab infusion for those experiencing dyspnea or clinically significant hypotension. Monitor clients until S&S completely resolve. Strongly consider terminating therapy for those who develop anaphylaxis, angioedema, pneumonitis, or ARDS.■ Advanced age may increase the incidence of cardiac dysfunction. Use with caution during pregnancy and in those with sensitivity to Chinese hamster ovary proteins. Increased risk for severe pulmonary side effects in those with symptomatic intrinsic pulmonary disease (e.g., asthma, COPD) or those with extensive tumor involvement of the lungs. The product contains benzyl alcohol that has been associated with a fatal 'gasping syndrome' in premature infants. Safety and efficacy have not been determined in children.

SIDE EFFECTS

Most Common

Headache, dizziness, insomnia, rash, abdominal pain, diarrhea, N&V, anorexia, anemia, increased cough, dyspnea, fatigue, pharyngitis, rhinitis, asthenia, back pain, chills, fever, myalgia, headache, infection, pain, peripheral edema, infusion reactions.

CV: Tachycardia, *vascular thrombosis*, pericardial effusion, *heart arrest, hemorrhage, shock arrhythmia,* hypotension, syncope. Cardiomyopathy, including left ventricular dysfunction and CHF. Cardiac dysfunction, including dyspnea, increased cough, paroxysmal nocturnal dyspnea, peripheral edema, S3 gallop, reduced left ventricular ejection fraction. **GI:** Diarrhea, anorexia, N&V, abdominal pain, *hepatic failure,* gastroenteritis, hematemesis, ileus, intestinal obstruction, colitis, esophageal ulcer, stomatitis, pancreatitis, hepatitis. **CNS:** Dizziness, insomnia, headache, paresthesia, peripheral neuritis, depression, neuropathy, convulsion, ataxia, confusion, manic reaction. **Respiratory:** Increased cough, dyspnea, pharyngitis, rhinitis, sinusitis, apnea, pneumothorax, asthma, hypoxia, laryngitis, pulmonary infiltrates, pleural effusions, noncardiogenic pulmonary edema, pulmonary insufficiency, pneumonia, pneumonitis, pulmonary fibrosis, *acute respiratory distress syndrome.* **Dermatologic:** Rash, desquamation, acne, herpes simplex/zoster, skin ulceration, nail changes, hot flashes. **Hematologic:** Anemia, leukopenia, pancytopenia, acute leukemia, coagulation disorder, lymphangiitis, exacerbation of chemotherapy-induced neutropenia, exacerbation of chemotherapy-induced neutropenia, *febrile neutropenia and infection (may be fatal).* **Musculoskeletal:** Arthralgia, myalgia, bone pain/necrosis, pathological fractures, myopathy. **GU:** Hydronephrosis, kidney failure, cervical cancer, hematuria, hemorrhagic cystitis, UTI, pyelonephritis, nephrotic syndrome with glomerulopathy (rare). **Metabolic:** Peripheral edema, edema, hypoglycemia, growth retardation, weight loss. **First-infusion-associated reaction:** Chills, fever, N&V, pain, rigors, bronchospasm, hypoxia, headache, dizziness, dyspnea, severe hyper-/hypotension, rash, asthenia. More serious reactions, occurring infrequently, include bronchospasm, hypoxia, severe hypotension, *death.* **Hypersensitivity reac-**

tions: *Anaphylaxis*, urticaria, *broncho-spasm*, angioedema, hypotension, hypoxia, dyspnea, pulmonary infiltrates, pleural effusions, noncardiogenic pulmonary edema, *acute respiratory distress syndrome*. *Reaction may be fatal*. **Miscellaneous:** Increased incidence of infections, especially of the upper respiratory tract, skin, and urinary tract; abdominal/back pain, accidental injury, allergic reaction, asthenia, chills, fever, flu syndrome, headache, pain, UTI, infection, cellulitis, *extreme respiratory distress*, ascites, hydrocephalus, radiation injury, deafness, amblyopia, hypothyroidism.

LABORATORY TEST CONSIDERATIONS
Hypercalcemia, hypomagnesemia, hyponatremia.

DRUG INTERACTIONS
Paclitaxel / ↑ Trastuzumab serum levels
Warfarin / Hypoprothrombinemia and ↑ risk of bleeding

HOW SUPPLIED
Powder for Injection, Lyophilized: 440 mg.

DOSAGE
- **IV**
  Metastatic breast cancer.
  Initial: 4 mg/kg infused over 90 min; **maintenance:** 2 mg/kg weekly, infused over 30 min if initial dose was tolerated. Give until tumor progression occurs.

NURSING CONSIDERATIONS
ADMINISTRATION/STORAGE
IV 1. Do not give as an IV push or bolus. May give in outpatient setting.
2. Do not coadminister with doxorubicin and cyclophosphamide. Following completion of doxorubicin and cyclophosphamide, give trastuzumab weekly for 52 weeks. During the first 12 weeks, coadminister trastuzumab with paclitaxel.
3. Decrease the rate of infusion for mild or moderate infusion reactions. Interrupt the infusion in those with dyspnea or clinically significant hypotension. Consider permanent discontinuation for severe and life-threatening infusion reactions.

4. Follow carefully the specific guidelines for reconstitution of trastuzumab, including use of the proper diluent, correct amount of diluent, and proper administration.
5. Reconstitute with 20 mL bacteriostatic water, 1.1% benzyl alcohol, as supplied. Resulting solution contains 21 mg/mL.
6. For those with sensitivity to benzyl alcohol, reconstitute with sterile water rather than bacteriostatic water for injection.
7. After reconstitution, immediately label vial in the area marked 'Do not use after' with the date 28 days from the reconstitution date.
8. Shaking the reconstituted solution or causing excessive foaming during the addition of diluent may cause problems with dissolution and the amount of trastuzumab that can be withdrawn from the vial.
9. Do not mix or dilute with other drugs. Do not administer through an IV line containing dextrose.
10. Interrupt trastuzumab infusion in all clients experiencing dyspnea or significant hypotension; initiate medical therapy, that may include epinephrine, corticosteroids, diphenhydramine, bronchodilators, and oxygen. Monitor carefully until complete resolution of all signs and symptoms. Consider permanent discontinuation in all those with severe infusion reactions.
11. Determine dose needed based on an initial dose of 4 mg/kg or a maintenance dose of 2 mg/kg. Calculate the volume needed from the reconstituted vial; withdraw this amount and add it to an infusion bag containing 250 mL of 0.9% NaCl. Gently invert the bag to mix the solution. The reconstituted preparation is a colorless to pale yellow transparent solution.
12. Prior to reconstitution, vials are stable at 2–8°C (36–46°F). When reconstituted with bacteriostatic water for injection, as supplied, is stable for 28 days when stored at 2–8°C and may be preserved for multiple use. If reconstituted with unpreserved sterile water for injection, use immediately and discard any

unused portion. Do not freeze reconstituted drug.

13. Trastuzumab diluted in polyvinyl-chloride or polyethylene bags containing 0.9% NaCl for injection may be stored at 2–8°C (36–46°F) or at room temperature for 24 hr or less. Since this solution contains no effective preservative, refrigeration is recommended.

ASSESSMENT

1. Note breast cancer onset/diagnosis, other therapies trialed, outcome. Determine if first-line therapy or second-or third-line therapy for tumors overexpressing the HER2 protein.

2. During infusion assess for fever, chills, and other infusion-associated symptoms (see *Side Effects*).

3. Assess cardiac function. Obtain ECG, echocardiogram and/or MUGA to evaluate left ventricular function prior to and during therapy.

CLIENT/FAMILY TEACHING

1. Drug is used in combination regimens to treat metastatic disease. It is administered as an IV infusion once a week. May be given in an outpatient setting.

2. Acetaminophen may help with flu-like symptoms after infusion; may also experience diarrhea, anemia, and infections during therapy; report.

3. Immediately report any S&S of ventricular dysfunction and congestive heart failure (SOB, cough, swelling of extremities); may cause cardiac toxicity.

OUTCOMES/EVALUATE

Inhibition of malignant breast cells that overexpress HER2 protein

---

Travoprost
(TRAH-voh-prahst)

CLASSIFICATION(S):
Antiglaucoma drug
PREGNANCY CATEGORY: C
Rx: Travatan, Travatan Z.

USES
Decrease intraocular pressure in open-angle glaucoma or ocular hypertension.

ACTION/KINETICS
Action
A synthetic prostaglandin $F_{2\alpha}$ analog. Believed to act by increasing uveoscleral aqueous humor outflow.

Pharmacokinetics
Onset: About 2 hr. **Maximum effect:** After 12 hr. Is absorbed through the cornea.

CONTRAINDICATIONS
Hypersensitivity to travoprost, benzalkonium chloride, or other ingredients in the product. Use during pregnancy or by women attempting to become pregnant.

SPECIAL CONCERNS
Has not been evaluated for treatment of angle closure, inflammatory, or neovascular glaucoma. May cause increased brown pigmentation of the iris, darkening of the eyelid, and increased pigmentation and growth of eyelashes; changes may be permanent. Use with caution in active intraocular inflammation (e.g., iritis, uveitis), in aphakic or pseudophakic clients with a torn posterior lens capsule, in those with known risk factors for macular edema, and during lactation. Contamination of the product may cause bacterial keratitis. Safety and efficacy have not been determined in children.

SIDE EFFECTS
Most Common
Ocular hyperemia, decreased visual acuity, eye discomfort, foreign body sensation, pain, pruritus, headache.

Ophthalmic: Ocular hyperemia, decreased visual acuity, eye discomfort, foreign body sensation, pain, pruritus, abnormal vision, blepharitis, blurred vision, cataract, cells, conjunctivitis, dry eye, eye disorder, flare, iris discoloration, keratitis, lid margin crusting, photophobia, subconjunctival hemorrhage, tearing, bacterial keratitis. **CV:** Angina pectoris, bradycardia, hypertension, hypotension. **GI:** Dyspepsia, GI disorder. **CNS:** Anxiety, depression, headache. **Body as a whole:** Accidental injury, infection, pain, arthritis. **GU:** Urinary incontinence, UTI, prostate disorder. **Respiratory:** Bronchitis, sinusitis. **Miscella-

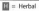

neous: Back pain, chest pain, cold syndrome, hypercholesterolemia.

HOW SUPPLIED

Ophthalmic Solution: 0.004%.

DOSAGE

• **OPHTHALMIC SOLUTION**

Elevated IOP.

1 gtt in the affected eye(s) once daily in the evening.

NURSING CONSIDERATIONS

ADMINISTRATION/STORAGE

Store between 2–25°C (36–77°F). Discard the container within 6 weeks of removing it from the sealed pouch.

ASSESSMENT

1. Note reasons for therapy, other agents trialed, ocular pressure readings. Used with open angle glaucoma or ocular hypertension.

2. Assess eye for inflammation, exudate, pain, level of vision, note iris color.

3. May alter BP, breathing and elimination patterns.

CLIENT/FAMILY TEACHING

1. Use once daily as directed, more frequent use may decrease the IOP-lowering effect.

2. Do not let tip of dropper touch any part of eye or surrounding tissue. Rinse well if contact suspected and do not share eye dropper. Discard the container within 6 weeks of removing it from the sealed pouch.

3. May be used together with other topical ophthalmic drug products to lower IOP. If more than 1 eye drop is used, administer them at least 5 min apart.

4. Do not administer while wearing contact lenses. Remove contact lenses prior to instillation, lenses may be reinserted 15 min after drug administration.

5. May cause irreversible pigmentation changes to iris (brown color) and skin around the eye and lid. May also cause increased eyelash growth which may be of more concern if only one eye is being treated.

6. Report any unusual or intolerable side effects. Keep all F/U appointments to evaluate response to treatment. Do not drive or perform hazardous functions until vision clears.

7. If pregnant or attempting to become pregnant notify provider. If contact made with solution, wash the exposed/contacted area thoroughly with soap and water immediately.

OUTCOMES/EVALUATE

↓ IOP

Trazodone hydrochloride ■

(**TRAYZ**-oh-dohn)

CLASSIFICATION(S):

Antidepressant, miscellaneous

PREGNANCY CATEGORY: C

Rx: Desyrel, Desyrel Dividose.

✤Rx: Apo-Trazodone, Apo-Trazodone D, Gen-Trazodone, Novo-Trazodone, Nu-Trazodone, Nu-Trazodone-D, PMS-Trazodone, ratio-Trazodine, ratio-Trazodone Dividose.

USES

Depression with or without accompanying anxiety. *Investigational:* In combination with tryptophan for treating aggressive behavior. Panic disorder or agoraphobia with panic attacks. Treatment of cocaine withdrawal. In combination with a selective serotonin reuptake inhibitor to treat insomnia. Alcoholism.

ACTION/KINETICS

Action

A novel antidepressant that does not inhibit MAO and is also devoid of amphetamine-like effects. Response usually occurs after 2 weeks (75% of clients), with the remainder responding after 2–4 weeks. May inhibit serotonin uptake by brain cells, therefore increasing serotonin concentrations in the synapse. May also cause changes in binding of serotonin to receptors. Causes moderate sedative and orthostatic hypotensive effects and slight anticholinergic effects.

Pharmacokinetics

Well absorbed. **Peak plasma levels:** 1 hr (empty stomach) or 2 hr (when taken with food). $t^{1/2}$, **initial:** 3–6 hr; **final:** 5–9 hr. **Effective plasma levels:** 800–1,600

Bold Italic = life threatening side effect   ■ = black box warning   ✤ = Available in Canada

ng/mL. **Time to reach steady state:** 3–7 days. Three-fourths of those with a therapeutic effect respond by the end of the second week of therapy. Metabolized in liver and excreted through both the urine and feces.

CONTRAINDICATIONS

During the initial recovery period following MI. Concurrently with electroshock therapy.

SPECIAL CONCERNS

■ (1) Antidepressants increased the risk of suicidal thinking and behavior (suicidality) in short-term studies in children and adolescents with major depressive disorder and other psychiatric disorders. Anyone considering the use of trazodone or any other antidepressant in a child or adolescent must balance this risk with the clinical need. Clients who are started on therapy should be observed closely for clinical worsening, suicidality, or unusual changes in behavior. Families and caregivers should be advised of the need for close observation and communication with the prescriber. Trazodone is not approved for use in pediatric clients with major depressive disorder and obsessive-compulsive disorder. (2) Short-term placebo-controlled trials of 9 antidepressant drugs in children and adolescents with major depressive disorder, obsessive-compulsive disorder, or other psychiatric disorders revealed a greater risk of adverse reactions during the first few months of treatment. The average risk of such reactions in clients receiving antidepressants was 4%, twice the placebo risk of 2%. No suicides occurred in these trials.■ Use with caution during lactation. Safety and efficacy in children less than 18 years of age have not been established. Geriatric clients are more prone to the sedative and hypotensive effects.

SIDE EFFECTS

Most Common

Drowsiness, dizziness/lightheadedness, nervousness, dry mouth, headache, insomnia, headache, hypotension, N&V, blurred vision.

CV: Hypertension or hypotension, syncope, palpitations, tachycardia, SOB, chest pain. **GI:** Diarrhea, N&V, bad taste in mouth, flatulence, dry mouth, constipation, abdominal/gastric disorder. **GU:** Delayed urine flow, priapism, hematuria, increased urinary frequency. **CNS:** Nightmares/vivid dreams, confusion, anger/hostility, excitement, decreased ability to concentrate, dizziness, disorientation, drowsiness, lightheadedness, fatigue, insomnia, nervousness, impaired memory, headache, incoordination, paresthesia, tremors. Rarely, hallucinations, impaired speech, hypomania. **Ophthalmic:** Blurred vision, red eyes, tired/itching eyes. **Body as a whole:** Dermatitis, edema, skeletal muscle aches and pains, weight gain or loss, sweating or clamminess, malaise, full/heavy head. **Miscellaneous:** Decreased libido, decreased appetite, nasal/sinus congestion, tinnitus, anemia, hypersalivation. Rarely, akathisia, muscle twitching, increased libido, impotence, retrograde ejaculation, early menses, missed periods.

LABORATORY TEST CONSIDERATIONS

Low WBC and neutrophil counts (not considered clinically significant).

OD OVERDOSE MANAGEMENT

Symptoms: CNS depression, including **respiratory arrest, seizures,** ECG changes, hypotension, priapism as well as an increase in the incidence and severity of side effects noted above (vomiting and drowsiness are the most common). *Treatment:* Treat symptoms (especially hypotension and sedation). Gastric lavage and forced diuresis to remove the drug from the body.

DRUG INTERACTIONS

Alcohol / ↑ Depressant effects
Antihypertensives / Added hypotension
Barbiturates / ↑ Depressant effects
Carbamazepine / ↑ Carbamazepine levels → ↑ pharmacologic and toxic effects
Clonidine / ↓ Clonidine effects
CNS depressants / ↑ CNS depression
Digoxin / ↑ Digoxin levels; monitor digoxin levels
Indinavir / ↓ Trazodone clearance → ↑ peak plasma levels and t½ R/T ↓ metabolism by CYP3A4
Itraconazole / ↓ Trazodone clearance

→ ↑ peak plasma levels and t½ R/T ↓ metabolism by CYP3A4

Ketoconazole / ↓ Trazodone clearance → ↑ peak plasma levels and t½ R/T ↓ metabolism by CYP3A4

MAO inhibitors / Initiate therapy cautiously if used together

Phenothiazines / ↑ Trazodone levels → ↑ pharmacologic and toxic effects; monitor and adjust dosage as needed

Phenytoin / ↑ Phenytoin levels; monitor phenytoin levels

Ritonavir / ↓ Trazodone clearance → ↑ peak plasma levels and t½ R/T ↓ metabolism by CYP3A4

SSRIs / 'Serotonin syndrome,' including irritability, shivering, myoclonus, increased muscle tone, and altered consciousness

Venlafaxine / 'Serotonin syndrome,' including irritability, shivering, myoclonus, increased muscle tone, and altered consciousness

Warfarin / Either ↑ or ↓ PT; monitor frequently

HOW SUPPLIED

Tablets: 50 mg, 100 mg, 150 mg, 300 mg.

DOSAGE————

● **TABLETS**

Depression.

Adults and adolescents, initial: 150 mg/day in divided doses; **then,** increase by 50 mg/day every 3–4 days to maximum of 400 mg/day in divided doses (outpatients). Inpatients may require up to, but not exceeding, 600 mg/day in divided doses. **Maintenance:** Use lowest effective dose. Therapy may be required for several months. **Geriatric clients:** 75 mg/day in divided doses; dose can then be increased, as needed and tolerated, at 3 to 4 day intervals.

Aggressive behavior.

Trazodone, 50 mg twice a day, with tryptophan, 500 mg twice a day. Dosage adjustments may be required to reach a therapeutic response or if side effects develop.

Panic disorder or agoraphobia with panic attacks.

300 mg/day.

Insomnia.

25–75 mg, often with a selective serotonin reuptake inhibitor.

Alcoholism.

50–100 mg/day.

NURSING CONSIDERATIONS

ADMINISTRATION/STORAGE

1. Initiate dose at the lowest possible level; increase gradually.

2. Beneficial effects may be observed within 1 week with optimal effects seen within 2 weeks.

ASSESSMENT

1. List reasons for therapy, onset, symptoms, associated factors, other agents trialed. Note any history of recent MI.

2. List drugs prescribed to ensure none interact.

3. Monitor VS, ECG, CBC, renal and LFTs.

CLIENT/FAMILY TEACHING

1. Take with food to enhance absorption and minimize dizziness and/or lightheadedness. Take major portion of dose at bedtime to reduce daytime side effects.

2. Use caution when driving or when performing other hazardous tasks; may cause drowsiness/dizziness. Avoid alcohol and CNS depressants. Report any persistent/bothersome side effects.

3. With prolonged or inappropriate penile erection; stop drug and report.

4. Use sugarless gum or candies and frequent mouth rinses to diminish dry mouth effects.

5. Inform surgeon if elective surgery is planned to minimize interaction with anesthetic agent.

6. Encourage family to share responsibility for drug therapy to optimize treatment, prevent overdosage, and observe for any suicidal cues. Clients taking antidepressants and emerging from deepest phases of depression are more prone to suicide.

7. May take 2–4 weeks for full drug effects to be realized. Report any evidence of suicidal thoughts or ideas. Keep all regular F/U visits to evaluate drug response.

Bold Italic = life threatening side effect   ■ = black box warning   ✦ = Available in Canada

OUTCOMES/EVALUATE

- ↓ Depression (e.g., improved sleeping/eating patterns, ↓ fatigue, and ↑ social interactions)
- Control of overwhelming anxiety/panic symptoms
- ↓ Insomnia

Treprostinil sodium 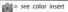 IV
(treh-**PROSS**-tih-nill)

CLASSIFICATION(S):
Antiplatelet drug
PREGNANCY CATEGORY: B
Rx: Remodulin.

USES
(1) As a continuous IV or SC infusion to reduce symptoms associated with exercise in pulmonary arterial hypertension with NYHA Class II through Class IV symptoms. (2) To diminish the rate of clinical deterioration in clients requiring transition from epoprostenol.

ACTION/KINETICS
Action
Causes direct dilation of pulmonary and systemic arterial vascular beds and inhibition of platelet aggregation. Also causes a dose-related negative inotropic and lusitropic effect.

Pharmacokinetics
Rapidly and completely absorbed after SC infusion. Absolute bioavailability is 100%. Steady state levels occurred in about 10 hr. Metabolized in the liver and excreted in the urine (79%) and feces (13%). **t½, terminal:** 2–4 hr. **Plasma protein binding:** 91%.

CONTRAINDICATIONS
Known hypersensitivity to the drug or structurally-related compounds.

SPECIAL CONCERNS
Use with caution in renal or hepatic impairment, during lactation, and in the elderly. Safety and efficacy have not been determined in children.

SIDE EFFECTS
Most Common
Infusion-site pain and reaction (bleeding/bruising, erythema, induration), rash.

Some adverse reactions noted may be due to the underlying disease (e.g., chest pain, dyspnea, fatigue, pallor, right ventricular heart failure). **At site of injection:** Infusion site pain and reaction (bleeding/bruising, erythema, induration), rash, problems with the infusion system. **GI:** Nausea, diarrhea. **CNS:** Headache, dizziness. **CV:** Vasodilation, hypotension. **Dermatologic:** Rash (including macular or papular), pruritus. **Miscellaneous:** Jaw pain, edema, cellulitis.

OD OVERDOSE MANAGEMENT
Symptoms: Extensions of pharmacological effects, including flushing, headache, hypotension, N&V, diarrhea. *Treatment:* Symptoms are usually self-limiting and are treated with reducing or withholding the drug.

DRUG INTERACTIONS
Anticoagulants / ↑ Risk of bleeding especially in clients maintained on anticoagulants
Antihypertensive drugs / Significant BP reduction
Diuretics / Significant BP reduction
Vasodilators / Significant BP reduction

HOW SUPPLIED
Injection: 1 mg/mL, 2.5 mg/mL, 5 mg/mL, 10 mg/mL.

DOSAGE
- **CONTINUOUS SC OR IV INFUSION; IV**

Pulmonary arterial hypertension.
Initial: 1.25 nanograms/kg/min. If this dose can not be tolerated, reduce to 0.625 nanograms/kg/min. Increase the infusion rate in increments of no more than 1.25 nanograms/kg/min per week for the first 4 weeks and then no more than 2.5 nanograms/kg/min per week for the remaining duration of infusion, depending on the response. Doses above 40 nanograms/kg/min have not been studied sufficiently. Avoid abrupt cessation of the infusion. In clients with mild or moderate hepatic insufficiency, decrease the initial dose to 0.625 nanograms/kg/min and increase cautiously. *NOTE:* Dosage is in units of nanograms (ng) per kg per unit of time.

Transition from epoprostenol to treprostinil.

T

Initiate the infusion of trepostinil and increase it while simultaneously reducing the dose of IV epoprostenol. Undertake the transition in a hospital with constant observation. During the transition, initiate treprostinil at a dose of 10% of the current epoprostenol dose; escalate as the epoprostenol dose is decreased. Use the following transition dose changes:

- Step 1: Epoprostenol dose unchanged; give treprostinil at 10% of the starting epoprostenol dose.
- Step 2: 80% of the starting epoprostenol dose; give treprostinil at 30% of the starting epoprostenol dose.
- Step 3: 60% of the starting epoprostenol dose; give treprostinil at 50% of the starting epoprostenol dose.
- Step 4: 40% of the starting epoprostenol dose; give treprostinil at 70% of the starting epoprostenol dose.
- Step 5: 20% of the starting epoprostenol dose; give treprostinil at 90% of the starting epoprostenol dose.
- Step 6: 5% of the starting epoprostenol dose; give treprostinil at 110% of the starting epoprostenol dose.
- Step 7: No epoprostenol given; give treprostinil at 110% of the starting epoprostenol dose + additional 5-10% increments as needed.

NURSING CONSIDERATIONS

ADMINISTRATION/STORAGE

1. Treprostinil should be used only by those experienced in the diagnosis and treatment of pulmonary arterial hypertension. Initiation of therapy must be in a setting with adequate personnel and equipment for physiological monitoring and emergency care.
2. Give only SC or IV.
3. Can be given as supplied or diluted for IV infusion with sterile water for injection or 0.9% NaCl.
4. Use the following formula to calculate infusion rates: Infusion rate (mL/hr) = Dose (ng/kg/min) x weight (kg) x (0.00006/treprostinil dosage strength concentration [mg/mL]). Check the package insert for sample calculations for SC or IV infusion.

5. A single reservoir syringe can be given up to 72 hr at 37°C (99°F). Do not use a single vial for more than 14 days after initial introduction into the vial.
6. Given by continuous SC infusion via a self-inserted SC catheter using an infusion pump designed for SC drug delivery.
7. To avoid interruptions in drug delivery, the client must have available a backup infusion pump and SC infusion sets.
8. To prevent worsening symptoms, avoid abrupt withdrawal or sudden large increases in dosage of the drug.
9. Unopened vials are stable until the date indicated if stored from 15–25°C (59–77°F). Solutions as dilute as 0.004 mg/mL are stable at ambient temperature for up to 48 hr.
IV 10. If used IV, the product must first be diluted with sterile water for injection or 0.9% NaCl injection.

ASSESSMENT

1. Note NYHA stage and symptom characteristics. List other agents trialed and the outcome. Identify if transplant candidate.
2. List cardiopulmonary assessment findings and catherization results. Monitor renal and LFTs, use cautiously with dysfunction.

CLIENT/FAMILY TEACHING

1. Drug is administered as a continuous infusion through a SC catheter with an infusion pump for an extended period of time.
2. Review proper administration techniques, catheter insertion, site care, drug loading and pump maintenance/alarms/care. Refer to home infusion agency for management/support.
3. Report any adverse drug effects i.e., headache, N&V, anxiety/restlessness and infusion site pain so dose can be adjusted to control these effects yet improve present functioning level/exercise tolerance.
4. Keep close contact and all F/U visits to assess status and heart disease progression. May eventually require conversion to IV therapy.

Bold Italic = life threatening side effect   ■ = black box warning   ♣ = Available in Canada

OUTCOMES/EVALUATE
↑ Exercise tolerance ↑ CO with pulmonary artery hypertension

Tretinoin (Retinoic ■ acid, Vitamin A acid)
(**TRET**-ih-noyn)

CLASSIFICATION(S):
Retinoid

PREGNANCY CATEGORY: C (Topical products), **D** (Oral products).

Rx: Capsules: Vesanoid. **Topical Cream, Gel, Liquid**: Altinac, Atralin, Avita, Renova, Retin-A, Retin-A Micro, Tretin-X.

🍁**Rx**: Rejuva-A, Stieva-A.

USES
Dermatologic: *Altinac, Atralin, Avita, Retin-A, Retin-A Micro:* Topical treatment of acne vulgaris. *Renova, 0.02% Cream:* Adjunct for mitigation of fine wrinkles in those who use comprehensive skin care and sun avoidance programs. *Renova, 0.05% Cream:* Adjunct for mitigation of fine wrinkles, mottled hyperpigmentation, and tactile roughness of facial skin for those who do not achieve palliation using comprehensive skin care and sun avoidance programs alone.

Oral: Induce remission in acute promyelocytic leukemia (APL). After induction therapy with tretinoin, give clients a standard consolidation or maintenance chemotherapy regimen for APL, unless contraindicated.

ACTION/KINETICS
Action
Topical tretinoin is believed to decrease microcomedone formation by decreasing the cohesiveness of follicular epithelial cells. Also believed to increase mitotic activity and increase turnover of follicular epithelial cells as well as decrease keratin synthesis. In APL clients, tretinoin produces an initial maturation of the primitive promyelocytes derived from the leukemic clone, followed by a repopulation of the bone marrow and peripheral blood by normal, polyclonal hematopoietic cells.

Pharmacokinetics
After topical use, some systemic absorption occurs (approximately 5% is recovered in the urine). Absorption after PO use is enhanced when the drug is taken with food. **Time to peak levels:** 1–2 hr. **Terminal elimination t½:** 0.5–2 hr in APL clients. Metabolized by the liver by P 450 enzymes, with about two-thirds excreted in the urine and one-third in the feces. **Plasma protein binding:** More than 95% (mainly to albumin).

CONTRAINDICATIONS
Eczema, sunburn. Use if inherently sensitive to sunlight or if taking other drugs that increase sensitivity to sunlight. Use of Renova if client is also taking drugs known to be photosensitizers (e.g., fluoroquinolones, phenothiazines, sulfonamides, tetracyclines, thiazides). Those allergic to parabens (preservative in the gelatin capsules). Use of PO form during lactation. Use around the eyes, mouth, angles of the nose, and mucous membranes.

SPECIAL CONCERNS
■ For Capsules. (1) Clients with acute promyelocytic leukemia (APL) are at high risk and can have severe side effects to tretinoin. Thus, give under the strict supervision of a physician who is experienced in the management of those with acute leukemia and in a facility with lab and supportive services sufficient to monitor drug tolerance and to protect and maintain a client compromised by drug toxicity, including respiratory compromise. Use of tretinoin requires the physician to assess that the possible benefit to the client outweighs the side effects listed below. (2) About 25% of APL clients treated with tretinoin experience a syndrome called the retinoic acid-APL syndrome. Symptoms include fever, dyspnea, weight gain, radiographic pulmonary infiltrates, and pleural or pericardial effusions, edema, and hepatic, renal, and multiorgan failure. Occasionally the syndrome is accompanied by impaired

myocardial contractility and episodic hypotension. The syndrome has been observed with or without concomitant leukocytosis. Endotracheal intubation and mechanical ventilation have been required in some cases due to progressive hypoxia; several clients have died due to multi-organ failure. The syndrome generally occurs during the first month of treatment, with some cases following the first dose. (3) Management of retinoic acid-APL syndrome has not been defined rigorously but includes high-dose steroids at the first suspicion of the syndrome in order to reduce morbidity and mortality. At the first signs suggestive of the syndrome (unexplained fever, dyspnea, weight gain, abnormal chest auscultatory findings, or radiographic abnormalities), immediately start high-dose steroids (e.g., dexamethasone, 10 mg IV q 12 hr for 3 days) or until resolution of symptoms, regardless of leukocyte count. The majority of clients do not require termination of tretinoin therapy during treatment of the retinoic acid-APL syndrome. However, in cases of moderate and severe RA-APL syndrome, consider temporary interruption of tretinoin therapy. (4) During treatment, about 40% of clients will develop rapidly evolving leukocytosis. Those who present with a high WBC at diagnosis (e.g., more than 5 x 10^9/L) have an increased risk of a further rapid increase in WBC counts. Rapidly evolving leukocytosis is associated with a higher risk of life-threatening complications. (5) If signs and symptoms of retinoic acid-APL are present with leukocytosis, begin treatment with high-dose steroids immediately. Some routinely add chemotherapy to tretinoin treatment in cases where clients present with a WBC count more than 5 x 10^9/L or in the case of a rapid increase in WBC count for clients leukopenic at the start of treatment. Consider adding full-dose chemotherapy, including an anthracycline (if not contraindicated) to tretinoin therapy on day 1 or 2 for those presenting with a WBC count of more than 5 x 10^9/L or immediately for those presenting with a WBC count of less than 5 x 10^9/L if the WBC count reaches 6 or more x 10^9/L by day 5, or 10 or more x 10^9/L by day 10, or 15 or more x 10^9/L by day 28. (6) The drug is classified as pregnancy category D. There is a high risk that a severely deformed infant will result if tretinoin is given during pregnancy. If it is determined that tretinoin represents the best available treatment for a pregnant woman or a woman of childbearing age, it must be assured that the client has received full information and warnings of the risk to the fetus if she were pregnant and of the risk of possible contraceptive failure. She must be instructed of the need to use 2 reliable forms of contraception simultaneously during therapy and for 1 month following discontinuation of therapy, unless abstinence is the chosen method. (7) Within 1 week prior to starting tretinoin therapy, the client should have blood or urine collected for a serum or urine pregnancy test with a sensitivity of at least 50 milli-international units. When possible, delay tretinoin therapy until a negative result from this test is obtained. When a delay is not possible, place the client on 2 reliable forms of contraception. Repeat pregnancy testing and contraceptive counseling monthly throughout the treatment period.■ Use topical products with caution during lactation. Safety and effectiveness have not been determined in children. Excessive sunlight and weather extremes (e.g., wind and cold) may be irritating. Use Avita and Renova with caution with concomitant topical medications, medicated or abrasive soaps, shampoos, cleansers, cosmetics with a strong drying effect, permanent wave solutions, electrolysis, hair depilatories or waxes, and products with high concentrations of alcohol, astringents, spices, or lime. Safety and efficacy of Renova have not been determined in children less than 18 years of age, in individuals over the age of 50 years, or in individuals with moderately or heavily pigmented skin. Use of the PO form has resulted in retonoic acid-APL syndrome, especially during the

---

Bold Italic = life threatening side effect   ■ = black box warning   ♣ = Available in Canada

first month of treatment. The safety and efficacy of oral tretinoin at doses less than 45 mg/m²/day have not been evaluated in children.

SIDE EFFECTS

Most Common

After PO use: Headache, fever, weakness, fatigue, arrhythmias, flushing, hypertension, phlebitis, dizziness, anxiety, paresthesia, depression, confusion, GI hemorrhage, abdominal pain, diarrhea, constipation, anorexia, dyspepsia, renal impairment, hemorrhage, disseminated intravascular coagulation, peripheral edema, edema, URTI, dyspnea, respiratory insufficiency, pleural effusion, earache, malaise, shivering, infections, pain, chest discomfort, myalgia.

After topical use: Dry skin, peeling, burning, stinging, erythema, pruritus.

Following topical use: Dermatologic: Red, edematous, crusted, or blistered skin; hyperpigmentation or hypopigmentation, increased susceptibility to sunlight, erythema, peeling, stinging, pruritus, burning, dryness. Excessive application will cause redness, peeling, or discomfort with no increase in results.

Following oral use: Retinoic acid-APL syndrome: Fever, dyspnea, weight gain, radiographic pulmonary infiltrate, pleural or pericardial effusions, edema; hepatic, renal, and multiorgan failure. Occasional impaired myocardial contractility and episodic hypotension; possibility of concomitant leukocytosis. *Progressive hypoxemia with possible fatal outcome.* Respiratory symptoms, including upper respiratory tract disorders, respiratory insufficiency, pneumonia, rales, expiratory wheezing, lower respiratory tract disorders, bronchial asthma, acute respiratory distress, ***pulmonary or larynx edema,*** unspecified pulmonary disease.

Pseudotumor cerebri (especially in children): Papilledema, headache, N&V, visual disturbances. **Typical retinoid toxicity (similar to ingestion of high doses of vitamin A):** Headache, fever, dryness of skin and mucous membranes, bone pain, N&V, rash, mucositis, pruritus, increased sweating, visual disturbances, ocular disorders, alopecia, skin changes, changed visual acuity, bone inflammation, visual field defects. **Body as a whole:** Malaise, shivering, infections, peripheral edema, pain, chest discomfort, anorexia, myalgia, flank pain, pallor, acidosis, hypothermia, ascites. **GI: *GI hemorrhage,*** abdominal pain, various GI disorders, diarrhea, constipation, dyspepsia, abdominal distension, hepatosplenomegaly, hepatitis, ulcer, unspecified liver disorders. **CV:** Arrhythmias, flushing, hypotension, hypertension, phlebitis, ***cardiac failure, cardiac arrest, stroke,*** MI, enlarged heart, heart murmur, ischemia, myocarditis, pericarditis, pulmonary hypertension, secondary cardiomyopathy, thrombosis (venous or arterial) during the first month of treatment involving various sites (e.g., CVA, MI, renal infarct). **CNS:** Dizziness, paresthesias, anxiety, insomnia, depression, confusion, ***cerebral hemorrhage, intracranial hypertension,*** agitation, hallucinations, abnormal gait, agnosia, aphasia, asterixis, cerebellar edema, cerebellar disorders, ***convulsions, coma,*** CNS depression, dysarthria, encephalopathy, facial paralysis, hemiplegia, hyporeflexia, hypotaxia, no light reflex, neurologic reaction, spinal cord disorder, tremor, leg weakness, unconsciousness, dementia, forgetfulness, somnolence, slow speech. **GU:** Renal insufficiency, dysuria, acute renal failure, micturition frequency, renal tubular necrosis, enlarged prostate. **Respiratory:** Upper respiratory tract disorders, dyspnea, respiratory insufficiency, pleural effusion, expiratory wheezing, pneumonia, rales, lower respiratory tract disorders, pulmonary infiltration, bronchial asthma, larynx edema, pulmonary edema, unspecified pulmonary disease. **Dermatologic:** Cellulitis, pallor, genital ulceration, vasculitis (predominantly involving the skin). **Hematologic: *Hemorrhage, disseminated intravascular coagulation,*** lymph disorders, thrombocytosis. **Metabolic:** Peripheral edema, edema, weight increase/decrease, facial edema, fluid imbalance. **Otic:** Earache, feeling of fullness in the ears, hearing loss, unspecified auricular dis-

 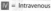

orders, irreversible hearing loss. **Miscellaneous:** Erythema nodosum, basophilia, hyperhistaminemia, Sweet's syndrome, organomegaly, hypercalcemia, pancreatitis, myositis.

LABORATORY TEST CONSIDERATIONS
Abnormal LFTs. Hypercholesterolemia.

DRUG INTERACTIONS
Aminocaproic acid / Rarely, cases of fatal thrombotic complications
Aprotinin / Rarely, cases of fatal thrombotic complications
Benzoyl peroxide / Use with topical tretinoin may cause significant skin irritation
Ketoconazole / Significant ↑ in tretinoin mean plasma AUC if ketoconazole given 1 hr prior to tretinoin
Photosensitizers (fluoroquinolones, phenothiazines, sulfonamides, thiazides) / Possible ↑ phototoxicity
Resorcinol / Use with topical tretinoin may cause significant skin irritation
Salicylic acid / Use with topical tretinoin may cause significant skin irritation
Sulfur / Use with topical tretinoin may cause significant skin irritation
Tetracyclines / ↑ Risk of pseudotumor cerebri and intracranial hypertension; also possible ↑ phototoxicity
Tranexamic acid / Rarely, cases of fatal thrombotic complications
Vitamin A / Possible aggravation of symptoms of hypervitaminosis A

HOW SUPPLIED
Capsules: 10 mg; *Cream:* 0.02%, 0.025%, 0.05%, 0.1%; *Gel:* 0.01%, 0.025%, 0.04%, 0.1%.

DOSAGE
- **CREAM; GEL**
  Acne vulgaris.
Apply lightly over the affected areas once daily at bedtime. Beneficial effects many not be seen for 2–6 weeks.
- **CREAM**
  Palliation for skin conditions.
Apply cream (0.02% or 0.05%) once daily at bedtime, using only enough to lightly cover the entire affected area. Up to 6 months of therapy may be needed before effects are seen.
- **CAPSULES**
  Acute promyelocytic leukemia.

Adults: 45 mg/m²/day given as two evenly divided doses. Given until complete remission is obtained. Discontinue 30 days after achieving complete remission or after 90 days of treatment, whichever comes first.

NURSING CONSIDERATIONS
ADMINISTRATION/STORAGE
1. If after initiation of tretinoin the presence of the t(15;17) translocation is not confirmed by cytogenetics and/or by polymerase chain reaction studies and the client has not responded to tretinoin, alternative therapy appropriate for acute myelogenous leukemia should be considered.
2. Apply the liquid carefully with the fingertip, cotton swab, or gauze pad only to affected areas.
3. Excessive amounts of the gel will cause a 'pilling' effect which minimizes the likelihood of overapplication.
4. Before applying Renova, wash the face gently with a mild soap and pat the skin dry, waiting 20–30 min before applying. When applied, take care to avoid contact with eyes, ears, nostrils, and mouth. Wash hands thoroughly immediately after applying tretinoin.
5. Do not freeze Renova cream.
6. Treatment with Renova for more than 24 weeks does not appear to increase improvement. The results of continued irritation of the skin for more than 48 weeks are not known.

ASSESSMENT
1. Note reasons for therapy, type, onset, characteristics of S&S.
2. With acne, thoroughly describe pretreatment skin condition; obtain photographs to compare with results of therapy.
3. Check if pregnant. Monitor hematologic, renal and LFTs.

CLIENT/FAMILY TEACHING
Topical:
1. Keep away from normal skin, mucous membranes, eyes, ears, mouth, nostrils, and nose angles.
2. Wash with mild soap and warm water and pat skin dry. Wait 20–30 min before applying tretinoin. Do not wash face for 1 hr or more after applying tre-

---

tinoin. Wash hands thoroughly before and after applying tretinoin.

3. On application there will be a transitory feeling of warmth and stinging. May use nonmedicated cosmetics during therapy but remove before treatment. Avoid any additional self treatment with antiacne products.

4. Do not apply another skin care product or cosmetic and do not wash face for at least 1 hr after applying tretinoin. Expect dryness and peeling of skin from the affected areas.

5. May be more sensitive to wind and cold. Do not apply to wind or sunburned skin or to open wounds. Avoid excessive exposure to sunlamps and to the sun. If exposed, use a sunscreen and protective clothing over affected areas.

6. Avoid alcohol-containing preparations such as shaving lotions and creams, perfumes, cosmetics with drying effects, skin cleansers, and medicated soaps.

7. Initially, lesions may worsen, caused by the effect of the drug on deep lesions that had been previously undetected. Report if lesions become severe; discontinue drug until skin integrity restored.

8. Improvement should be evident in 6 weeks but therapy should be continued for at least 3 months.

9. Practice reliable birth control; may cause fetal harm.

Oral:

1. Drug will be administered until complete remission is obtained. It will be stopped 30 days after remission or after 90 days of therapy, whichever comes first. This does not replace standard maintenance chemotherapy for APL.

2. Take with food to enhance absorption. Follow a low fat diet and exercise regularly to reduce drug-induced elevated triglyceride levels.

3. Take exactly as prescribed; do not exceed or skip doses.

4. Review list of potential drug side effects, noting those that require immediate reporting.

5. Do not donate blood while on this therapy; may be harmful to recipient.

6. Avoid pregnancy. Must use two reliable forms of contraception during, and for one month following therapy; may cause fetal harm.

OUTCOMES/EVALUATE

- ↓ Size/number of acne eruptions
- Clearing of skin condition; symptomatic improvement
- Remission with APL

Triamcinolone ∎
(try-am-**SIN**-oh-lohn)

CLASSIFICATION(S):
Glucocorticoid
PREGNANCY CATEGORY: C
Rx: Tablets: Aristocort, Atolone, Kenacort.

Triamcinolone acetonide
PREGNANCY CATEGORY: C
Rx: Dental Paste: Kenalog in Orabase, Oralone Dental. **Inhalation Aerosol**: Azmacort, Nasacort AQ, Nasacort HFA. **Parenteral**: Kenaject-40, Kenalog-10 and -40, Tac-3 and -40, Tri-Kort, Triam-A, Triamonide 40, Trilog. **Topical Spray**: Kenalog. **Topical Lotion/Ointment**: Aristocort, Aristocort A, Delta-Tritex, Flutex, Kenalog, Kenalog-H, Kenonel, Triacet, Triderm.
✚**Rx: Dental Paste**: Oracort.

Triamcinolone hexacetonide
PREGNANCY CATEGORY: C
Rx: Aristospan Intra-Articular, Aristospan Intralesional.

SEE ALSO CORTICOSTEROIDS.
ADDITIONAL USES
(1) Pulmonary emphysema accompanied by bronchospasm or bronchial edema. (2) Diffuse interstitial pulmonary fibrosis. (3) With diuretics to treat refractory CHF or cirrhosis of the liver with ascites. (4) Multiple sclerosis. (5) Inflammation following dental proce-

dures. **Triamcinolone acetonide:** (1) PO inhalation is used for maintenance treatment of chronic asthma (use Azmacort). (2) Intranasal for seasonal and perennial allergic rhinitis in adults and children 6 years and older (use Nasacort AQ or HFA). **Triamcinolone hexacetonide:** Restricted to intra-articular or intralesional treatment of rheumatoid arthritis and osteoarthritis.

ACTION/KINETICS
Action
The anti-inflammatory effect is due to inhibition of prostaglandin synthesis. The drug also inhibits accumulation of macrophages and leukocytes at sites of inflammation and inhibits phagocytosis and lysosomal enzyme release. More potent than prednisone. Intermediate-acting. Has no mineralocorticoid activity.

Pharmacokinetics
Onset: Several hours. **Duration:** One or more weeks. **t½:** Over 200 min. Metabolized by the liver. About 60% excreted in the feces and 40% in the urine. **t½, after intranasal use:** 3.1 hr.

SPECIAL CONCERNS
■ Azmacort Aerosol: Particular care is needed in clients who are transferred from systemically active corticosteroids to triamcinolone inhalation aerosol because deaths due to adrenal insufficiency have occurred in asthmatic clients during and after transfer from systemic corticosteroids to aerosolized steroids in recommended doses. After withdrawal from systemic corticosteroids, a number of months is usually required for recovery of hypothalamic-pituitary-adrenal (HPA) function. For some clients who have received large doses of oral steroids for long periods of time before therapy with triamcinolone is initiated, recovery may be delayed for 1 year or longer. During this period of HPA suppression, clients may exhibit signs and symptoms of adrenal insufficiency when exposed to trauma, surgery, or infections, particularly gastroenteritis or other conditions with acute electrolyte loss. Although triamcinolone may provide control of asthmatic symptoms during these episodes, in recommended doses it supplies only normal physiological amounts of corticosteroid systemically and does not provide the increased systemic steroid that is needed for coping with these emergencies. During periods of stress or severe asthmatic attack, clients who have been recently withdrawn from systemic corticosteroids should be instructed to resume systemic steroids (in large doses) immediately and to contact their physician for further instruction. Instruct these clients to carry a warning card indicating that they may need supplementary systemic steroids during periods of stress or a severe asthma attack.■ Use during pregnancy only if benefits clearly outweigh risks. Use special caution with decreased renal function or renal disease. Dose must be highly individualized.

ADDITIONAL SIDE EFFECTS
Most Common
After nasal/respiratory use: Burning/dryness of nasal passages, nasal/throat irritation, sneezing, epistaxis, cough.
After parenteral use: N&V, acne, diarrhea, constipation, headache, heartburn, restlessness, insomnia, sweating.
After intra-articular, intrasynovial, intrabursal use: Transient flushing, dizziness, local depigmentation, local irritation.

See *Corticosteroids* for a complete list of possible side effects. Exacerbation of symptoms has also been reported. A marked increase in swelling and pain and further restricted joint movement may indicate septic arthritis. Intradermal injection may cause local vesicular ulceration and persistent scarring. Syncope and ***anaphylactoid reactions*** have been reported with triamcinolone regardless of route of administration.

HOW SUPPLIED
Triamcinolone: *Tablets:* 4 mg, 8 mg.
Triamcinolone acetonide: *Aerosol, Oral:* 100 mcg/inh; *Cream:* 0.025%, 0.1%, 0.5%; *Dental Paste:* 0.1%; *Inhaler/Spray (Intranasal):* 55 mcg/inh; *Injection, Suspension:* 3 mg/mL, 10 mg/mL, 40 mg/mL; *Lotion:* 0.025%, 0.1%; *Ointment:* 0.025%, 0.1%, 0.5%; *Topical Spray:* 0.147 mg/gram (to deliver 0.2 mg).

Bold Italic = life threatening side effect   ■ = black box warning   ♣ = Available in Canada

Triamcinolone hexacetonide: *Injection:* 5 mg/mL, 20 mg/mL.

DOSAGE

TRIAMCINOLONE

- **TABLETS**

  Adrenocortical insufficiency (with mineralocorticoid therapy).

  4–12 mg/day.

  Acute leukemias (children).

  1–2 mg/kg.

  Acute leukemia or lymphoma (adults).

  16–40 mg/day (up to 100 mg/day may be necessary for leukemia).

  Edema.

  16–20 mg (up to 48 mg may be required until diuresis occurs).

  Tuberculosis meningitis.

  32–48 mg/day.

  Rheumatic disease, dermatologic disorders, bronchial asthma.

  8–16 mg/day.

  SLE.

  20–32 mg/day.

  Allergies.

  8–12 mg/day.

  Hematologic disorders.

  16–60 mg/day.

  Ophthalmologic diseases.

  12–40 mg/day.

  Respiratory diseases.

  16–48 mg/day.

  Acute rheumatic carditis.

  20–60 mg/day.

TRIAMCINOLONE ACETONIDE

- **IM ONLY (NOT FOR IV USE)**

  2.5–60 mg/day, depending on the disease and its severity.

- **INTRA-ARTICULAR; INTRABURSAL; TENDON SHEATHS**

  Initial: 2.5–5 mg for smaller joints and 5–15 mg for larger joints, although up to 40 mg has been used.

- **INTRADERMAL**

  Initial: 1 mg/injection site (use 3 mg/mL or 10 mg/mL suspension only).

- **CREAM; LOTION; OINTMENT; PASTE (ALL STRENGTHS); TOPICAL AEROSOL**

  Apply sparingly to affected area 2–4 times per day and rub in lightly.

- **AEROSOL, ORAL (AZMACORT)**

  Adults, usual: 2 inhalations (200 mcg) 3–4 times per day or 4 inhalations (400 mcg) twice a day, not to exceed 1,600

mcg/day. High initial doses (1,200–1,600 mcg/day) may be needed in those with severe asthma. **Pediatric, 6–12 years:** 1–2 inhalations (100–200 mcg) 3–4 times per day or 2–4 inhalations (200–400 mcg) twice a day, not to exceed 1,200 mcg/day (i.e., 12 inhalations). Use in children less than 6 years of age has not been determined.

- **INTRANASAL SPRAY (NASACORT AQ, NASACORT HFA)**

  Seasonal and perennial allergic rhinitis.

  For Nasacort AQ, Adults and children over 12 years of age, initial and maximum dose: 2 sprays (110 mcg) in each nostril once daily (total of 220 mcg once daily). **Children, 6–11 years of age:** 1 spray (55 mcg) in each nostril (total of 110 mcg) once daily; maximum recommended dose is 220 mcg/day as 2 sprays/nostril once daily. Not recommended for children less than 6 years of age.

  For Nasacort HFA, Adults, initial: 2 sprays in each nostril once daily (220 mcg/day). If needed, the dose may be increased to 440 mcg/day (55 mcg/spray) either as once-a-day dosage or divided up to 4 times/day. When maximum effect is reached, decrease dose to 110 mcg/day (1 spray in each nostril once/day). **Children, 6–11 years of age:** 220 mcg/day given as 2 sprays (55 mcg/spray) in each nostril once a day. Once maximal effect has been reached, titrate dose to the minimum effective dose. Not recommended for children less than 6 years of age.

TRIAMCINOLONE HEXACETONIDE

- **INTRA-ARTICULAR (NOT FOR IV USE)**

  Small joints (interphalangeal, metacarpophalangeal).

  2–6 mg.

  Large joints (knee, hip, shoulder).

  10–20 mg.

- **INTRALESIONAL; SUBLESIONAL**

  Up to 0.5 mg/sq in of affected area.

NURSING CONSIDERATIONS

ADMINISTRATION/STORAGE

1. Initially, use aerosol concomitantly with a systemic steroid. After 1 week,

initiate a gradual withdrawal of systemic steroid. Make next reduction after 1–2 weeks, depending on response. If symptoms of insufficiency occur, dose of systemic steroid can be increased temporarily. Also, dose of systemic steroid may need to be increased in times of stress or during a severe asthmatic attack.

2. For Nasacort AQ, individualize to the minimum effective dose to reduce the chance of side effects.

3. Do not use the acetonide products if they clump due to exposure to freezing temperatures.

4. Nasacort AQ (triamcinolone acetonide) not recommended for children under age 6.

5. Triamcinolone acetonide nasal spray for allergic rhinitis may be effective as soon as 12 hr after initiation of therapy. Re-evaluate if improvement is not seen within 2–3 weeks.

6. For best results, store Azmacort canister at room temperature and shake well before use. Do not puncture and do not use or store near heat or open flame; exposure to temperatures greater than 48.8°C (120°F) may cause bursting.

7. Nasacort AQ is viscous at rest but a liquid when shaken. This allows the drug to stay in the nasal airways at the site of inflammation for up to 2 hr.

8. Nasacort HFA contains hydrofluoroalkane as the propellant instead of chlorofluorocarbon.

9. Store Nasacort AQ and HFA from 20–25°C (68–77°F). Do not puncture canister or store or use near heat or open flames. Exposure to temperatures above 49°C (120°F) may cause bursting.

ASSESSMENT

1. Note reasons for therapy; type of therapy prescribed; type, onset, and characteristics of S&S, other agents trialed, outcome.

2. Assess area/condition requiring treatment and clinical presentation.

3. Monitor blood sugar, CBC, electrolytes, renal, and LFTs.

CLIENT/FAMILY TEACHING

1. Take at the same time each day. Assess mouth and report any evidence of oral lesions with inhaled therapy.

2. Ingest a liberal amount of protein; with regular use may experience gradual weight loss, associated with anorexia, muscle wasting, and weakness. See dietitian for assistance in meal planning.

3. Lie down if feeling faint; report if episodes persist and interfere with daily activities.

4. Report evidence of abnormal bruising/bleeding, weight gain, swelling of extremities, or SOB.

5. Drug may suppress reactions to skin allergy testing. Do not stop suddenly with long term therapy.

6. With topical therapy, wash hands and apply to clean, slightly moist skin. Report if area does not improve with therapy or if symptoms worsen.

7. With nasal spray or inhaler, review appropriate method of administration and proper care and storage of equipment. Always rinse mouth and equipment after use. If bronchodilator also prescribed, use this first and allow at least 1 min before repeat inhalations.

8. For Nasacort AQ, prime the nasal spray before use by pushing down on the actuator until a fine spray appears (5 pumps). If the pump has not been used for more than 14 days, the pump must be reprimed with 1 spray. For Nasacort HFA, the canister must be primed with 3 actuations prior to the first use or after 3 days of non-use.

9. Store Nasacort AQ or HFA at room temperature. Discard container when the labeled number of actuations has been used, even if the bottle is completely empty. For Nasacort HFA, do not puncture and do not use or store near heat or open flame. Exposure of Nasacort HFA above 120°F may cause the canister to burst; never throw the canister into a fire or incinerator.

10. Report immediately any new onset of depression as well as aggravation of existing depressive symptoms.

Bold Italic = life threatening side effect   ■ = black box warning   ♣ = Available in Canada

11. Keep all F/U visits and labs to evaluate response to therapy; adverse side effects.

OUTCOMES/EVALUATE

- ↓ Immune and inflammatory responses in autoimmune disorders and allergic reactions
- Improved airway exchange
- Restoration of skin integrity
- Relief of pain/inflammation; improved joint mobility
- Control of S&S allergic rhinitis

Triamterene

(try-**AM**-ter-een)

CLASSIFICATION(S):

Diuretic, potassium-sparing
PREGNANCY CATEGORY: B
Rx: Dyrenium.

SEE ALSO *DIURETICS.*

USES

(1) Edema due to CHF. (2) Hepatic cirrhosis. (3) Nephrotic syndrome. (4) Steroid therapy. (5) Secondary hyperaldosteronism. (6) Idiopathic edema. May be used alone or with other diuretics. *Investigational:* Prophylaxis and treatment of hypokalemia, adjunct in the treatment of hypertension.

ACTION/KINETICS

Action

Acts directly on the distal tubule to promote the excretion of sodium—which is exchanged for potassium or hydrogen ions—bicarbonate, chloride, and fluid. It increases urinary pH and is a weak folic acid antagonist.

Pharmacokinetics

Onset: 2–4 hr. **Peak effect:** 6–8 hr. **Duration:** 7–9 hr. **t½:** 3 hr. Metabolized to hydroxytriamterene sulfate, which is also active. About 20% is excreted unchanged through the urine. **Plasma protein binding:** One-half to two-thirds of the drug is bound.

CONTRAINDICATIONS

Hypersensitivity to drug, severe or progressive renal insufficiency, severe hepatic disease, anuria, hyperkalemia, hyperuricemia, gout, history of nephrolithiasis. Lactation.

SPECIAL CONCERNS

Safety and efficacy have not been determined in children.

SIDE EFFECTS

Most Common

N&V, diarrhea, dry mouth, headache, dizziness, malaise.

Electrolyte: Hyperkalemia, electrolyte imbalance. **GI:** Nausea, vomiting (may also be indicative of electrolyte imbalance), diarrhea, dry mouth. **CNS:** Dizziness, drowsiness, fatigue, malaise, weakness, headache. **Hematologic:** Megaloblastic anemia, thrombocytopenia. **Renal:** Azotemia, interstitial nephritis. **Miscellaneous:** *Anaphylaxis*, photosensitivity, hypokalemia, jaundice, muscle cramps, rash.

OD **OVERDOSE MANAGEMENT**

Symptoms: Electrolyte imbalance, especially hyperkalemia. Also, nausea, vomiting, other GI disturbances, weakness, hypotension, reversible acute renal failure. *Treatment:* Immediately induce vomiting or perform gastric lavage. Evaluate electrolyte levels and fluid balance and treat if necessary. Dialysis may be beneficial.

DRUG INTERACTIONS

Amantadine / ↑ Amantadine toxic effects R/T ↓ renal excretion
Angiotensin-converting enzyme inhibitors / Significant hyperkalemia
Antihypertensives / Potentiated by triamterene
Captopril / ↑ Risk of significant hyperkalemia
Cimetidine / ↑ Bioavailability and ↓ clearance of triamterene
Digitalis / Inhibited by triamterene
Indomethacin / ↑ Risk of nephrotoxicity and acute renal failure
Lithium / ↑ Chance of toxicity R/T ↓ renal clearance
Potassium salts / Additive hyperkalemia
Spironolactone / Additive hyperkalemia

HOW SUPPLIED

Capsules: 50 mg, 100 mg.

DOSAGE

- **CAPSULES**
  Diuretic.

T

Adults, initial: 100 mg twice a day after meals; **maximum daily dose:** 300 mg.

NURSING CONSIDERATIONS

☞ Do not confuse triamterene with trimipramine (antidepressant).

ADMINISTRATION/STORAGE

1. Minimize nausea by giving the drug after meals.
2. Dosage is usually reduced by one-half when another diuretic is added to the regimen.

ASSESSMENT

1. Note reasons for therapy, other agents trialed; list agents prescribed to ensure none interact.
2. Assess for alcoholism; megaloblastic anemia may occur because triamterene is a weak antagonist of folic acid.
3. Monitor BP, weight, ECG, CBC, BS, uric acid, electrolytes, I&O, and renal function.

CLIENT/FAMILY TEACHING

1. Take in the a.m. with food to minimize GI upset/nausea. Take care, drug may cause dizziness.
2. Report any sore throat, rash, fever (S&S of blood dyscrasia), or lack of effectiveness.
3. Persistent headaches, drowsiness, vomiting, restlessness, mental wandering, lethargy, and foul breath may be signs of uremia; report.
4. Avoid alcohol and OTC agents. Also avoid potassium supplements, salt substitutes that contain potassium, and foods high in potassium; drug is potassium-sparing.
5. Urine may appear pale fluorescent blue.
6. Avoid direct sunlight for prolonged periods; may cause a photosensitivity reaction. Use sunscreens, sunglasses, hat, long sleeves, and pants when exposed.

OUTCOMES/EVALUATE

↓ Edema; ↑ diuresis; ↓ BP

— **COMBINATION DRUG** —

Triamterene and Hydrochlorothiazide

(try-**AM**-teh-reen, hy-droh-**kloh**-roh-**THIGH**-ah-zyd)

CLASSIFICATION(S):

Antihypertensive, combination drug
PREGNANCY CATEGORY: C
Rx: Dyazide, Maxzide, Maxzide-25 MG.
♣Rx: Apo-Triazide, Novo-Triamzide, Nu-Triazide.

SEE ALSO *HYDROCHLOROTHIAZIDE* AND *TRIAMTERENE.*

USES

Hypertension or edema in clients who manifest hypokalemia on hydrochlorothiazide alone. In clients requiring a diuretic and in whom hypokalemia cannot be risked (i.e., clients with cardiac arrhythmias or those taking digitalis). Usually not the first line of therapy, except for clients in whom hypokalemia should be avoided.

CONTENT

Capsules. Hydrochlorothiazide (*thiazidediuretic*), 25 or 50 mg and Triamterene (*potassium-sparing diuretic*), 37.5, 50, or 100 mg. **Tablets.** Hydrochlorothiazide, 25 or 50 mg and Triamterene, 37.5 or 75 mg. (In Canada the tablets contain 25 mg of hydrochlorothiazide and 50 mg triamterene.)

ACTION/KINETICS

Action

Triamterene acts directly on the distal tubule to promote the excretion of sodium, bicarbonate, chloride, and fluid. It increases urinary pH. Hydrochlorothiazide promotes the excretion of sodium and chloride, and thus water by the distal renal tubule. Also increases excretion of potassium and to a lesser extent bicarbonate. The antihypertensive effect is thought to be due to direct dilation of the arterioles, as well as to a reduction in the total fluid volume of the body and altered sodium balance.

Pharmacokinetics

Triamterene. Onset: 2–4 hr. **Peak effect:** 6–8 hr. **Duration:** 7–9 hr. **t½:** 3 hr. Metabolized to hydroxytriamterene sulfate, which is also active. About 20% is excreted unchanged through the urine. **Hydrochlorothiazide. Onset:** 2 hr. **Peak effect:** 4–6 hr. **Duration:** 6–12 hr. **t½:** 5.6–14.8 hr. Hydrochlorothiazide is not metabolized but is eliminated rapidly by the kidney.

CONTRAINDICATIONS

Clients receiving other potassium-sparing drugs such as amiloride and spironolactone. Use in anuria, acute or chronic renal insufficiency, significant renal impairment, preexisting elevated serum potassium.

SPECIAL CONCERNS

Use with caution during lactation. Geriatric clients may be more sensitive to the hypotensive and electrolyte effects of this combination; also, age-related decreases in renal function may require a decrease in dosage.

SIDE EFFECTS

Most Common

N&V, headache, anorexia, GI upset, diarrhea, flatulence, dizziness, photosensitivity.

See Diuretics, Thiazides and Triamterene for a complete list of possible side effects.

LABORATORY TEST CONSIDERATIONS

Triamterene may impart blue fluorescence to urine, interfering with fluorometric assays (e.g., lactic dehydrogenase, quinidine). ↑ BUN, creatinine. ↑ Serum uric acid in clients predisposed to gouty arthritis.

HOW SUPPLIED

See Content.

DOSAGE

• **CAPSULES**

Hypertension or edema.

Adults: Triamterene/hydrochlorothiazide: 37.5 mg/25 mg to 1–2 capsules given once daily with monitoring of serum potassium and clinical effect. Triamterene/hydrochlorothiazide: 50 mg/25 mg to 1–2 capsules twice a day after meals. Some clients may be controlled using 1 capsule every day or every other day. No more than 4 capsules should be taken daily.

• **TABLETS**

Hypertension or edema.

Adults: Triamterene/hydrochlorothiazide: 37.5 mg/25 mg to 1–2 tablets/day (determined by individual titration with the components). Or, triamterene/hydrochlorothiazide: 75 mg/50 mg to 1 tablet daily.

NURSING CONSIDERATIONS

ADMINISTRATION/STORAGE

Monitor clients who are transferred from less bioavailable formulations of triamterene and hydrochlorothiazide for serum potassium levels following the transfer.

ASSESSMENT

1. Note reasons for therapy, other agents trialed; list agents prescribed to ensure none interact.
2. Assess for alcoholism; megaloblastic anemia may occur because triamterene is a weak antagonist of folic acid.
3. Monitor BP, weight, ECG, CBC, BS, uric acid, electrolytes, I&O, and renal function; reduce dose with dysfunction.

CLIENT/FAMILY TEACHING

1. Drug is used to lower BP and reduce swelling of extremities. Take in the A.M. with food to minimize GI upset/nausea.
2. Report any adverse effects including sore throat, rash, or fever (S&S of blood dyscrasia) or lack of effectiveness.
3. Persistent headaches, drowsiness, vomiting, restlessness, mental wandering, lethargy, and foul breath may be signs of uremia; report.
4. Avoid alcohol and OTC agents. Also avoid potassium supplements, salt substitutes that contain potassium, and foods high in potassium; drug is potassium-sparing.
5. Urine may appear pale fluorescent blue.
6. Avoid direct sunlight for prolonged periods; may cause a photosensitivity reaction. Use sunscreens, sunglasses, hat, and long sleeves and pants when exposed.
7. Use care, drug may cause dizziness. Keep log of BP for provider review; report as scheduled for F/U.

OUTCOMES/EVALUATE
- Control of hypertension
- Resolution of edema

Triazolam
(try-**AYZ**-oh-lam)

CLASSIFICATION(S):
Sedative-hypnotic, benzodiazepine
PREGNANCY CATEGORY: X
Rx: Halcion, **C-IV**
♣Rx: Apo-Triazo, Gen-Triazolam.

SEE ALSO TRANQUILIZERS, ANTIMANIC DRUGS, AND HYPNOTICS.

USES
(1) Insomnia (short-term management, not to exceed 1 month). (2) May be beneficial in preventing or treating transient insomnia from a sudden change in sleep schedule.

ACTION/KINETICS
Action
Decreases sleep latency, increases the duration of sleep, and decreases the number of awakenings.

Pharmacokinetics
Time to peak plasma levels: 0.5–2 hr.
t½: 1.5–5.5 hr. Metabolized in liver; inactive metabolites excreted in the urine.
Plasma protein binding: 90%.

CONTRAINDICATIONS
Use concomitantly with itraconazole, ketoconazole, nefaxodone. Lactation (may cause sedation and feeding problems in infants).

SPECIAL CONCERNS
Safety and efficacy in children under 18 years of age not established. Geriatric clients may be more sensitive to the effects of triazolam.

SIDE EFFECTS
Most Common
Drowsiness, headache, dizziness, nervousness, lightheadedness, coordination disorders/ataxia, N&V.
See *Tranquilizers, Antimanic Drugs, and Hypnotics* for a complete list of possible side effects. **CNS:** Rebound insomnia, anterograde amnesia, headache, ataxia, decreased coordination, "traveler's"

amnesia. Psychologic and physical dependence. **GI:** N&V.

DRUG INTERACTIONS
Azole antifungals / ↑ Triazolam effect R/T ↓ liver metabolism
Clarithromycin / ↑ Triazolam effect R/T ↓ liver metabolism
Erythromycin / ↑ Triazolam effect R/T ↓ liver metabolism
Grapefruit juice / ↑ Triazolam effect R/T ↓ liver metabolism
Modafinil / ↑ Triazolam mean AUC and mean peak plasma levels
Protease inhibitors / ↑ Triazolam effect R/T ↓ liver metabolism
SSRIs / ↑ Triazolam effect R/T ↓ liver metabolism

HOW SUPPLIED
Tablets: 0.125 mg, 0.25 mg.

DOSAGE
- **TABLETS**
  Insomnia.
Adults, initial: 0.25–0.5 mg before bedtime. **Geriatric or debilitated clients, initial:** 0.125 mg; **then,** depending on response, 0.125–0.25 mg before bedtime.

NURSING CONSIDERATIONS
© Do not confuse Halcion with Haldol (antipyschotic).
ASSESSMENT
1. Note reasons for therapy, onset, duration, characteristics of S&S. Assess mental status and note behavioral manifestations.
2. Evaluate sleep patterns; determine underlying cause of insomnia so that source may be removed. With simple insomnia, try nonpharmacologic interventions to induce sleep, such as soft music, guided imagery, no daytime napping, or progressive muscle relaxation.
3. Initiate safety precautions (i.e., side rails, supervised ambulation, frequent observations), especially with elderly and confused clients.
4. Assess for tolerance and for psychologic and physical dependence. Monitor closely for CNS toxic effects especially during prolonged therapy (longer than 2 weeks). Monitor CBC and LFTs.

T

Bold Italic = life threatening side effect   ■ = black box warning   ♣ = Available in Canada

CLIENT/FAMILY TEACHING
1. Take only as directed. Store away from bedside.
2. Use caution when driving or operating machinery until daytime sedative effects evaluated.
3. Drug is for short-term use only; may cause physical and psychological dependence. Try warm baths/milk, and other methods to induce sleep, such as white noise simulator, soft music, guided imagery, or progressive muscle relaxation, rather than become dependent on drugs for insomnia.
4. Avoid alcohol and CNS depressants. Report unusual side effects including hallucinations, nightmares, depression, or periods of confusion.
5. Keep sleep diary noting all foods, drinks, drugs consumed, activities before bedtime for provider review.

OUTCOMES/EVALUATE
Improved sleeping patterns; insomnia relief

Trifluoperazine ©
(try-**flew**-oh-**PER**-ah-zeen)

CLASSIFICATION(S):
Antipsychotic, phenothiazine
PREGNANCY CATEGORY: C
✤**Rx:** Apo-Trifluoperazine.

SEE ALSO *ANTIPSYCHOTIC AGENTS, PHENOTHIAZINES.*

USES
(1) Schizophrenia. (2) Short-term treatment of nonpsychotic anxiety (not the drug of choice).

ACTION/KINETICS
Action
Causes a high incidence of extrapyramidal symptoms and antiemetic effects and a low incidence of sedation, orthostatic hypotension, and anticholinergic side effects.

Pharmacokinetics
Maximum therapeutic effect: Usually 2–3 weeks after initiation of therapy.

SPECIAL CONCERNS
Use during pregnancy only when benefits clearly outweigh risks. Dosage has not been established in children less than 6 years of age. Geriatric, emaciated, or debilitated clients usually require a lower initial dose.

SIDE EFFECTS
Most Common
Drowsiness, dizziness, skin reactions, rash, dry mouth, insomnia, amenorrhea, fatigue, muscle weakness, anorexia, lactation, extrapyramidal reactions.
See *Antipsychotic Agents, Phenothiazines* for a complete list of possible side effects.

HOW SUPPLIED
Tablets: 1 mg, 2 mg, 5 mg, 10 mg.

DOSAGE
• **TABLETS**
Schizophrenia.
Adults and adolescents, initial: 2–5 mg twice a day; **maintenance:** 15–20 mg/day (up to 40 mg/day may be needed in some) in 2–3 divided doses. Use lower doses in small, emaciated, or elderly clients. **Pediatric, 6–12 years:** 1 mg 1–2 times per day; adjust dose as required and tolerated.
Nonpsychotic anxiety.
Adults and adolescents: 1–2 mg twice a day, not to exceed 6 mg/day. Not to be given for this purpose longer than 12 weeks.

NURSING CONSIDERATIONS
© Do not confuse trifluoperazine with trihexyphenidyl (an antiparkinson drug).

ASSESSMENT
1. Note reasons for therapy, onset of symptoms, behavioral manifestations. Assess/note mental status findings.
2. List other agents prescribed; outcome.
3. Monitor CBC, ECG, LFTs.

CLIENT/FAMILY TEACHING
1. Avoid activities that require mental alertness until drug effects realized.
2. Consume plenty of fluids to prevent dehydration; use caution in hot weather to prevent heatstroke.
3. Avoid alcohol and OTC agents. Do not stop drug suddenly.

---

4. Use sunscreen and protective clothing when out and avoid prolonged sun exposure.

5. Report unusual side effects or lack/loss of response. Drug may discolor urine a reddish brown.

6. Report any unusual tremor, movements, tongue protrusion, abdominal pain, urine retention, constipation, or muscle spasms immediately. Keep all F/U appointments/therapies sessions.

OUTCOMES/EVALUATE

- Reduction in paranoid, excitable, or withdrawn behaviors
- ↓ Levels of anxiety, tension, and agitation

Trifluridine
(try-**FLUR**-ih-deen)

CLASSIFICATION(S):
Antiviral
PREGNANCY CATEGORY: C
Rx: Viroptic.

SEE ALSO *ANTI-INFECTIVE DRUGS AND ANTIVIRAL DRUGS.*

USES
(1) Primary keratoconjunctivitis and recurrent epithelial keratitis caused by HSV types 1 and 2. (2) Epithelial keratitis resistant to idoxuridine or if ocular toxicity or hypersensitivity to idoxuridine has occurred. (3) Infections resistant to vidarabine.

ACTION/KINETICS
Action
Closely resembles thymidine; inhibits thymidylic phosphorylase and specific DNA polymerases necessary for incorporation of thymidine into viral DNA. Trifluridine, instead of thymidine, is incorporated into viral DNA, resulting in faulty DNA and the ability to infect or reproduce in tissue. Also incorporated into mammalian DNA. Has activity against herpes simplex virus types 1 and 2 and vaccinia virus.

Pharmacokinetics
$t\frac{1}{2}$: 12–18 min.

CONTRAINDICATIONS
Hypersensitivity or chemical intolerance to drug.

SPECIAL CONCERNS
Safe use during pregnancy not established. Use with caution during lactation.

SIDE EFFECTS
Most Common
Mild, transient burning or stinging when instilled, palpebral edema.

Ophthalmic: Mild, transient burning or stinging when instilled. Palpebral edema, stromal edema, superficial punctuate keratopathy, epithelial keratopathy, hypersensitivity reaction, stomal edema, irritation, keratitis sicca, hyperemia, increased IOP.

HOW SUPPLIED
Ophthalmic Solution: 1%.

DOSAGE

- **SOLUTION**
  Primary keratoconjunctivitis, recurrent epithelial keratitis.
  1 gtt solution q 2 hr onto cornea, up to maximum of 9 gtt/day in each eye during acute stage (presence of corneal ulcer). Following reepithelialization, decrease dosage to 1 gtt/4 hr (or minimum of 5 gtt/day in each eye) for 7 days. Do not use for more than 21 days.

NURSING CONSIDERATIONS
ADMINISTRATION/STORAGE
1. May be used concomitantly in the eye with antibiotics (chloramphenicol, bacitracin, polymyxin B sulfate, erythromycin, neomycin, gentamicin, tetracycline, sulfacetamide sodium), corticosteroids, anticholinergics, epinephrine HCl, and NaCl.
2. Drug is heat-sensitive. Store in refrigerator at 2–8°C (36–46°F).

ASSESSMENT
Note reasons for therapy, onset, characteristics of S&S, ophthalmic findings, and other agents trialed. Recurrent herpetic eye infections may lead to corneal damage with vision loss if not treated completely.

CLIENT/FAMILY TEACHING
1. Use eyedrops exactly as directed.
2. Wash hands before/after using eyedrops.

Bold Italic = life threatening side effect   ■ = black box warning   ♣ = Available in Canada

3. To apply eyedrops:

- Tilt head back slightly and pull down on the lower eyelid. Position the dropper above your eye. Look up and away from the dropper. Squeeze out a drop and close your eye. A mild, transient burning sensation may occur on instillation. Apply gentle pressure to the inside corner of the eye (near the nose) for about 1 minute to prevent the liquid from draining down the tear duct. If you are using more than one drop in the same eye, repeat the process. If you are also using another eye medication in the same eye, wait about 10 minutes between application of the different medications.
- Do not touch the dropper to any surface, including the eyes or hands. The dropper is sterile. If it becomes contaminated, it could cause an infection in the eye.
- Contact provider if symptoms get worse or if no improvement is noted after a few days of use.
- Do not use any eyedrop that is discolored or has particles in it.
- Store trifluridine ophthalmic in the refrigerator. Keep the bottle properly capped.

4. Report any new or bothersome side effects but do not stop medication without specific instructions as herpetic keratitis may recur. Have regular eye exams.

5. Improvement usually occurs within 7 days and healing takes place within 14 days. Thereafter, 7 more days of therapy are necessary to prevent recurrence. Report if no improvement noted within 7 days. Do not administer for more than 21 days because toxicity may occur (discard remaining drug after 21 days). Keep all F/U exams to ensure positive outcome.

OUTCOMES/EVALUATE

- Resolution of infection
- Reepithelialization of herpetic eye lesions

——COMBINATION DRUG——

Trimethoprim and Sulfamethoxazole [IV]

(try-**METH**-oh-prim, sul-fah-meh-**THOX**-ah-zohl)

CLASSIFICATION(S):
Antibiotic, combination
PREGNANCY CATEGORY: C
Rx: Bactrim, Bactrim DS, Bactrim IV, Bactrim Pediatric, Cotrim, Cotrim D.S., Cotrim Pediatric, Septra, Septra DS, Sulfatrim.

SEE ALSO *SULFONAMIDES.*
USES
PO, Parenteral: (1) UTIs due to *Escherichia coli, Klebsiella, Enterobacter, Pseudomonas mirabilis* and *vulgaris,* and *Morganella morganii.* (2) Enteritis due to *Shigella flexneri* or *S. sonnei. (3)* Pneumocystis carinii pneumonitis in children and adults.

PO: (1) Acute otitis media in children due to *Haemophilus influenzae* or *Streptococcus pneumoniae.* (2) Traveler's diarrhea in adults due to *E. coli.* (3) Prophylaxis of *P. carinii* pneumonia in immunocompromised clients (including those with AIDS). (4) Acute exacerbations of chronic bronchitis in adults due to *H. influenzae* or *S. pneumoniae. Investigational:* Cholera, salmonella, nocardiosis, prophylaxis of recurrent UTIs in women, prophylaxis of neutropenic clients with *P. carinii* infections or leukemia clients to decrease incidence of gram-negative rod bacteremia. Treatment of acute and chronic prostatitis. Decrease chance of urinary and blood bacterial infections in renal transplant clients.
CONTENT
These products contain the antibacterial agents sulfamethoxazole and trimethoprim.
Concentrate for injection: Sulfamethoxazole, 80 mg and trimethoprim, 16 mg/mL.
Oral Suspension: Sulfamethoxazole, 200 mg and trimethoprim, 40 mg/5 mL.
Tablets: Sulfamethoxazole, 400 mg and trimethoprim, 80 mg/tablet.

Tablets, Double Strength (DS): Sulfamethoxazole, 800 mg and trimethoprim, 160 mg/tablet.

ACTION/KINETICS

Action

Sulfamethoxazole inhibits bacterial synthesis of dihydrofolic acid by competing with para-aminobenzoic acid. Trimethoprim blocks the production of tetrahydrofolic acid by inhibiting the enzyme dihdrofolate reductase. Thus, this combination blocks two consecutive steps in the bacterial biosynthesis of essential nucleic acids and proteins.

Pharmacokinetics

The combination is rapidly and completely absorbed after PO use. **Peak plasma levels, after PO:** 1–4 hr; **after IV:** 1–1.5 hr. Urine concentrations are considerably higher than serum levels. **Sulfamethoxazole, t½, after PO:** 10–12 hr; after IV: 11.3 hr. **Trimethoprim, t½, after PO:** 8–11 hr; **after IV:** 12.8 hr. t½'s are increased significantly in those with severely impaired renal function. Sulfamethoxazole is metabolized to inactive compounds whereas trimethoprim is metabolized only to a small extent. Both are excreted through the kidneys.

CONTRAINDICATIONS

Infants under 2 months of age. During pregnancy at term. Megaloblastic anemia due to folate deficiency. Lactation.

SPECIAL CONCERNS

Use with caution in impaired liver or kidney function and in clients with possible folate deficiency. AIDS clients may not tolerate or respond to this product.

SIDE EFFECTS

Most Common

N&V, anorexia, rash, urticaria.

GI: Glossitis, anorexia, stomatitis, N&V, emesis, abdominal pain, diarrhea, pseudomembranous enterocolitis, hepatitis (including cholestatic jaundice and **hepatic necrosis**), **pancreatitis**. **CNS:** Headache, mental depression, **seizures**, ataxia, hallucinations, vertigo, insomnia, apathy, nervousness, aseptic meningitis, peripheral neuritis. **Musculoskeletal:** Arthralgia, myalgia. **Respiratory:** Pulmonary infiltrates. **GU:** Renal failure, interstitial nephritis, toxic nephrosis with oliguria nad anuria. **Hematologic:** **Agranulocytosis, aplastic anemia**, hemolytic anemia, megaloblastic anemia, thrombocytopenia, leukopenia, neutropenia, hypoprothrombinemia, eosinophilia, methemoglobinemia. **Hypersensitivity:** Erythema multiforme, **Stevens-Johnson syndrome,** generalized skin eruptions, rash, toxic epidermal necrolysis, urticaria, serum sickness-like syndrome, pruritus, exfoliative dermatitis, anaphylaxis, conjunctival and scleral injection, photosensitivity, allergic myocarditis, angioedema, drug fever, chills, Henoch-Schoenlein purpura, systemic lupus erythematosus, generalized allergic reactions, periarteritis nodosa. **Body as a whole:** Fatigue, weakness. **Miscellaneous:** Tinnitus.

LABORATORY TEST CONSIDERATIONS

↑ Serum transaminase, bilirubin, and creatinine; BUN. Crystalluria. The drugs may interfere with the Jaffe alkaline picrate reaction assay for creatinine, resulting in overestimation by about 10% in the range of normal values.

OD OVERDOSE MANAGEMENT

Symptoms: **Acute:** Anorexia, colic, N&V, dizziness, headache, drowsiness, unconsciousness, pyrexia, hematuria, crystalluria, depression, confusion; blood dyscrasias and jaundice are late manifestations. **Chronic:** Bone marrow depression manifested as thrombocytopenia, leukopenia, or megaloblastic anemia. *Treatment:*
- Usual supportive measures.
- Perform gastric lavage or emesis.
- Force oral fluids and give IV fluids if urine output is low and renal function is normal.
- Acidifying the urine will increase renal elimination of trimethoprim.
- Monitor blood counts and appropriate blood chemistries, including electrolytes.
- If blood dyscrasias or jaundice occur, begin specific therapy, including leucovorin, 5–15 mg/day.
- Peritoneal dialysis is not effective and hemodialysis is only moderately effective in eliminating these drugs.

DRUG INTERACTIONS

Alcohol / Possible disulfiram-like reaction

Cyclosporine / ↓ Cyclosporine effect; ↑ risk of nephrotoxicity

Dapsone / ↑ Effect of both dapsone and trimethoprim

Methotrexate / ↑ Risk of toxicity R/T displacement from plasma protein binding sites

Phenytoin / ↑ Effect R/T ↓ hepatic clearance

Rifampin / ↓ Sulfamethoxazole and trimethoprim AUC and serum levels

Sulfonylureas / ↑ Hypoglycemic effect

Thiazide diuretics / ↑ Risk of thrombocytopenia with purpura in geriatric clients

Warfarin / ↑ PT

Zidovudine / ↑ Zidovudine serum levels R/T ↓ renal clearance

HOW SUPPLIED
See Content.

DOSAGE
• **DOUBLE-STRENGTH TABLETS; ORAL SUSPENSION; TABLETS**
  UTIs, shigellosis, bronchitis, acute otitis media.
Adults: 1 DS tablet, 2 tablets, or 4 teaspoonfuls of suspension q 12 hr for 10–14 days. **Pediatric:** Total daily dose of 8 mg/kg trimethoprim and 40 mg/kg sulfamethoxazole divided equally and given q 12 hr for 10–14 days. (*NOTE:* For shigellosis, give adult or pediatric dose for 5 days.) For clients with impaired renal function the following dosage is recommended: C_{CR} of 15–30 mL/min: One-half the usual regimen and for C_{CR} less than 15 mL/min: Use is not recommended.
  Chancroid.
1 DS tablet twice a day for at least 7 days (alternate therapy: 4 DS tablets in a single dose).
  Pharyngeal gonococcal infection due to penicillinase-producing Neisseria gonorrhoeae.
720 mg trimethoprim and 3,600 mg sulfamethoxazole once daily for 5 days.
  Prophylaxis of P. carinii *pneumonia.*
Adults: 160 mg trimethoprim and 800 mg sulfamethoxazole q 24 hr. **Children:** 150 mg/m^2 of trimethoprim and 750 mg/m^2 sulfamethoxazole daily in equally divided doses twice a day on three consecutive days per week. Do not ex-

ceed a total daily dose of 320 mg trimethoprim and 1,600 mg sulamethoxazole.
  Treatment of P. carinii *pneumonia.*
Adults and children: Total daily dose of 15–20 mg/kg trimethoprim and 100 mg/kg sulfamethoxazole divided equally and given q 6 hr for 14–21 days.
  Prophylaxis of P. carinii *pneumonia in immunocompromised clients.*
1 DS tablet daily
  Traveler's diarrhea.
Adults: 1 DS tablet q 12 hr for 5 days.
  Prostatitis, acute bacterial.
1 DS tablet twice a day until client is afebrile for 48 hr; treatment may be required for up to 30 days.
  Prostatitis, chronic bacterial.
1 DS tablet twice a day for 4–6 weeks.
• **IV**
  UTIs, shigellosis, acute otitis media.
Adults and children: 8–10 mg/kg/day (based on trimethoprim) in two to four divided doses q 6, 8, or 12 hr for up to 14 days for severe UTIs or 5 days for shigellosis.
  Treatment of P. carinii *pneumonia.*
Adults and children: 15–20 mg/kg/day (based on trimethoprim) in 3–4 divided doses q 6–8 hr for up to 14 days.

NURSING CONSIDERATIONS
ADMINISTRATION/STORAGE
IV 1.   Dilute each 5-mL vial to 125 mL with D5W and use within 6 hr. If the amount of fluid should be restricted, each 5 mL can be diluted up to 75 mL with D5W and used within 2 hr. Do not refrigerate the diluted solution.
2. Administer IV infusion over a 60–90 min period.
3. Do not mix the IV infusion with any other drugs or solutions.
4. If the diluted IV infusion is cloudy or precipitates after mixing, discard and prepare a new solution.

ASSESSMENT
1. Note reasons for therapy, onset, characteristics of S&S. Monitor VS, I&O, cultures, CBC, urinalysis, renal and LFTs; reduce dose with dysfunction.
2. Assess for megaloblastic anemia; drug inhibits ability to produce folinic acid. Simultaneous administration of fo-

lic acid (6–8 mg/day) may prevent antifolate drug effects.

3. If infected with AIDS virus may be intolerant to product.

CLIENT/FAMILY TEACHING

1. Take only as directed. Complete entire prescription and do not share.

2. Report any symptoms of persistent fever, inflammation/swelling of veins/lymph glands, N&V, rash, joint pain/swelling, mental disturbances or lack of response.

3. Consume 2.5–3 L of fluids/day to prevent crystalluria and dehydration.

4. May experience dizziness, use caution with activities that require mental alertness.

5. Avoid prolonged sun exposure; use protective clothing, sunglasses, and sunscreen if exposure necessary.

6. Report any adverse side effects or lack of desired results. Keep all F/U visits to evaluate response.

OUTCOMES/EVALUATE

- Resolution of infection
- *P. carinii* pneumonia prophylaxis

Triptorelin pamoate

(**TRIP**-toh-rel-in)

CLASSIFICATION(S):

Antineoplastic, gonadotropin-releasing hormone analog

PREGNANCY CATEGORY: X

Rx: Trelstar Depot, Trelstar LA.

USES

Palliative treatment of advanced prostate cancer when orchiectomy or estrogen therapy are either not indicated or unacceptable.

ACTION/KINETICS

Action

A synthetic decapeptide agonist analog of luteinizing hormone releasing hormone (LHRH or GnRH). Potent inhibitor of gonadotropic secretion when given continuously. Initially, there is a transient surge in circulating LH, FSH, estradiol, and testosterone. However, after 2–4 weeks, a sustained decrease in LH and FSH secretion and marked reduc-

tion of testicular and ovarian steroidogenesis occurs. In men, levels of serum testosterone fall to those seen in surgically castrated men. Thus, tissues and functions that depend on testosterone for maintenance become quiescent. These effects are reversible upon discontinuing therapy.

Pharmacokinetics

IM injection of the depot formulation achieves plasma levels over a 1 month period. **Time to maximum levels:** 1–3 hr for Trelstar Depot and about 2.9 hr for Trelstar LA. Metabolism is unknown but probably involves hepatic microsomal enzymes. Eliminated by the liver and kidneys. Is distributed and eliminated by a 3-compartment model; **$t\frac{1}{2}$:** About 6 min, 45 min, and 3 hr.

CONTRAINDICATIONS

Hypersensitivity to triptorelin, other components of the product, other LHRH agonists, or LHRH. Lactation.

SPECIAL CONCERNS

Initially, due to transient increase in serum testosterone levels, there may be worsening signs and symptoms of prostate cancer during the first few weeks of treatment.

SIDE EFFECTS

Most Common

Hot flushes, hypertension, headache, nausea, impotence, dysuria, skeletal/leg pain, leg edema, injection site pain, pain.

Worsening of signs/symptoms of prostate cancer: Bone pain, neuropathy, hematuria, urethral or bladder outlet obstruction, spinal cord compression with weakness or paralysis of lower extremities.

Side effects due to Trelstar Depot. GI: Vomiting, diarrhea. **CNS:** Headache, insomnia, dizziness, emotional lability. **GU:** Impotence, urinary retention, UTI. **Miscellaneous:** Hypertension, hot flushes, skeletal pain, injection site pain, pain, leg pain, fatigue, anemia, pruritus.

Side effects due to Trelstar LA. CNS: Headache, fatigue, insomnia, dizziness, asthenia. **GI:** Nausea, anorexia, constipation, dyspepsia, diarrhea, abdominal pain. **CV:** Hypertension, chest pain. **GU:** Impotence, dysuria, urinary retention,

---

Bold Italic = life threatening side effect   ■ = black box warning   ✦ = Available in Canada

breast pain, decreased libido, gynecomastia. **Musculoskeletal:** Skeletal pain, arthralgia, leg cramps, myalgia. **Respiratory:** Coughing, dyspnea, pharyngitis. **Miscellaneous:** Rash, hot flushes, leg edema, injection site pain, leg/back pain, dependent edema, conjunctivitis, eye pain, peripheral edema.

LABORATORY TEST CONSIDERATIONS
Suppression of the pituitary-gonadal axis may cause misleading results of diagnostic tests. **Due to Trelstar LA.** ↑ Alkaline phosphatase, glucose, BUN, AST, ALT. ↓ Hemoglobin, RBC. Abnormal hepatic function.

DRUG INTERACTIONS
Do not give hyperprolactinemic drugs together with triptorelin since hyperprolactinemia reduces the number of pituitary GnRH receptors.

HOW SUPPLIED
Microgranules for Injection, Lyophilized: Equivalent to 3.75 mg triptorelin peptide base, and equivalent to 11.25 mg triptorelin peptide base.

DOSAGE
* **IM**
  Advanced prostate cancer.
3.75 mg of Trelstar Depot incorporated in a depot formulation given monthly as a single IM injection. Or, Trelstar LA, 11.25 mg incorporated in a long-acting formulation given q 84 days as a single IM injection given in either buttock.

NURSING CONSIDERATIONS

ADMINISTRATION/STORAGE
1. Alter the IM injection site periodically.
2. Prepare Trelstar Depot as follows:
* Withdraw 2 mL sterile water for injection using a syringe with a sterile 20-gauge needle. Do not use other diluents. Inject into the drug vial.
* Shake well to disperse particles thoroughly and to obtain a uniform suspension. The suspension will appear milky.
* Withdraw contents of the vial into the syringe and inject the reconstituted suspension immediately.
3. Prepare Trelstar LA as follows:
* Withdraw 2 mL sterile water for injection using a syringe with a 20-gauge needle. Do not use other diluents. Inject into the drug vial.
* Shake well to disperse particles thoroughly and to obtain a uniform suspension, which will appear milky.
* Slowly withdraw the entire contents into the syringe.
* Inject in either buttock.
4. Store from 15–30°C (59–86°F).
5. Discard if not used immediately after reconstitution.

ASSESSMENT
1. Note symptom onset, PSA levels, biopsy/staging results, other therapies trialed, outcome.
2. Monitor PSA/free PSA, alkaline phosphatase levels, calcium, cholesterol profile, testosterone levels, renal and LFTs.

CLIENT/FAMILY TEACHING
1. Drug therapy of the depo product consists of monthly IM injections. Must continue to prevent progression of disease.
2. Hot flashes may occur with drug therapy R/T chemical castration.
3. May initially experience worsening of symptoms and/or onset of new symptoms such as bone pain, urine blood/obstruction, and numbness/tingling during the first few weeks of therapy. Immediately report any weakness, numbness, itching/hives/rash, respiratory difficulty or impaired urination.
4. Keep F/U visits with provider and lab to gauge drug response.
5. Identify local support groups that assist in coping with disease.

OUTCOMES/EVALUATE
↓ Prostate tumor size and spread

Trospium chloride
(tros-**PEE**-um)

CLASSIFICATION(S):
Antispasmodic/antimuscarinic drug
PREGNANCY CATEGORY: C
Rx: Sanctura, Sanctura XR.

USES
Treatment of overactive bladder with symptoms of urge urinary incontinence, urgency, and urinary frequency.

ACTION/KINETICS
Action
A quaternary ammonium compound that antagonizes the effect of acetylcholine on muscarinic receptors leading to a reduction in the tone of smooth muscle in the bladder. The drug increases maximum cystometric bladder capacity and volume at first detrusor contraction.

Pharmacokinetics
Less than 10% of a dose is absorbed. **Peak plasma levels:** 5–6 hr. Administration with high fat meals reduces absorption. Metabolized in the liver by ester hydrolysis. Not significantly metabolized by the cytochrome P450 enzyme system. **t½, plasma:** 20 hr. About 85% excreted in the feces. **Plasma protein binding:** 50–85% (dose-dependent).

CONTRAINDICATIONS
Use in clients with urinary retention, gastric retention, or uncontrolled narrow-angle glaucoma, or in those at risk for these conditions. Hypersensitivity to the drug or its ingredients.

SPECIAL CONCERNS
Use with caution in clients with severe hepatic dysfunction, in those with significant bladder outflow obstruction (due to increased risk of urinary retention), in those with GI obstructive disorders (due to risk of gastric retention), ulcerative colitis, intestinal atony, and myasthenia gravis. Use in those with narrow-angle glaucoma or during lactation only if potential benefits outweigh risks. Side effects are greater in those 75 years of age and older. Safety and efficacy have not been determined in children.

SIDE EFFECTS
Most Common
Dry mouth, constipation, upper abdominal pain, headache, fatigue, dry eyes, blurred vision, dizziness, drowsiness.

GI: Dry mouth, constipation, upper abdominal pain, aggravated constipation, flatulence, dyspepsia, gastritis, abdominal distention, vomiting, dysgeusia, dry throat. **CNS:** Headache, dizziness, drowsiness, hallucinations, delirium. **CV:** Tachycardia, palpitations, SVT, syncope, *hypertensive crisis.* **Ophthal-**mic: Dry eyes, blurred vision, abnormal vision. **Dermatologic:** Dry skin, *Stevens-Johnson syndrome.* **Miscellaneous:** Fatigue, urinary retention, chest pain, rhabdomyolysis, *anaphylaxis.*

OD OVERDOSE MANAGEMENT
Symptoms: Severe anticholinergic effects. *Treatment:* Symptomatic and supportive treatment. ECG monitoring is recommended.

DRUG INTERACTIONS
Anticholinergic drugs / ↑ Risk and/or severity of dry mouth, constipation, and other anticholinergic effects

Digoxin / Possible ↑ trospium or digoxin serum levels since both drugs are eliminated by active tubular secretion

Metformin / Possible ↑ trospium or metformin serum levels since both drugs are eliminated by active tubular secretion

Morphine / Possible ↑ trospium or morphine serum levels since both drugs are eliminated by active tubular secretion

Pancuronium / Possible ↑ trospium or pancuronium serum levels since both drugs are eliminated by active tubular secretion

Procainamide / Possible ↑ trospium or procainamide serum levels since both drugs are eliminated by active tubular secretion

Tenofovir / Possible ↑ trospium or tenofovir serum levels since both drugs are eliminated by active tubular secretion

Vancomycin / Possible ↑ trospium or vancomycin serum levels since both drugs are eliminated by active tubular secretion

HOW SUPPLIED
Tablets: 20 mg.

DOSAGE
- **TABLETS**
  Overactive bladder.
  Adults: 20 mg twice a day at least one hr before meals or given on an empty stomach.

NURSING CONSIDERATIONS
ADMINISTRATION/STORAGE
1. For clients with severe renal impairment (C_{CR} <30 mL/min), the recom-

---

mended dose is 20 mg once daily at bedtime.

2. In geriatric clients 75 years and older, the dose may be titrated down to 20 mg once daily based on tolerability.

3. Store from 20–25°C (68–77°F).

ASSESSMENT

1. Note reasons for therapy, characteristics of S&S, other agents trialed, outcome.

2. List drugs prescribed to ensure none interact.

3. Monitor VS, I&O, urine C&S, renal and LFTs. Anticipate reduced dose with renal dysfunction. Review voiding diary and attempt to identify any triggers.

4. Assess for those at risk for urinary/gastric retention, uncontrolled narrow-angle glaucoma and in those with hypersensitivity to the drug or ingredients; precludes drug therapy.

CLIENT/FAMILY TEACHING

1. Take twice a day as directed on an empty stomach or 1 hr before meals for day and night coverage. Taking with meals decreases drug availability by up to 80%.

2. Practice exercises for bladder training, i.e., pelvic floor muscle training, voiding schedules/diary, and urge suppression strategy.

3. Identify and avoid certain potential bladder irritants, i.e., caffeine, artificial sweeteners, citrus fruits, alcohol, and nicotine.

4. Avoid activities that require mental alertness until drug effects realized, may cause dizziness or drowsiness.

5. Drug causes dry mouth; use frequent sips of water, sugar free gum/hard candy, ice, or a saliva substitute to alleviate.

6. Avoid strenuous exercise in hot weather; overheating may result in heat stroke. Avoid alcohol; may increase risk of drowsiness.

7. Report any adverse side effects, lack of response, or urinary/gastric retention.

OUTCOMES/EVALUATE

Treatment of overactive bladder with relief of urinary urge incontinence and frequency

Tubocurarine chloride

(too-boh-kyour-**AR**-een)

CLASSIFICATION(S):

Neuromuscular blocking drug

PREGNANCY CATEGORY: C

Rx: Tubocurarine Cl.

SEE ALSO *NEUROMUSCULAR BLOCKING AGENTS.*

USES

(1) Muscle relaxant during surgery or setting of fractures and dislocations. (2) Spasticity caused by injury to or disease of CNS. (3) Treat seizures electrically induced or induced by drugs. (4) Diagnosis of myasthenia gravis.

ACTION/KINETICS

Action

Cumulative effects may occur. Most likely of the nondepolarizing drugs to cause histamine release. Narrow margin between therapeutic dose and toxic dose.

Pharmacokinetics

Onset, IV: 1 min; **IM:** 15–25 min. **Time to peak effect, IV:** 2–5 min. **Duration, IV:** 20–90 min. **t½:** 1–3 hr. About 43% excreted unchanged in urine.

ADDITIONAL CONTRAINDICATIONS

Clients in whom release of histamine is hazardous.

SPECIAL CONCERNS

Use with caution during pregnancy and lactation and in children. If repeated doses are used before delivery, the newborn may manifest decreased skeletal muscle activity. Children up to 1 month of age may be more sensitive to the effects of tubocurarine. Use with extreme caution in clients with renal dysfunction, liver disease, or obstructive states.

SIDE EFFECTS

Most Common

Skeletal muscle weakness, prolonged skeletal muscle relaxation, respiratory insufficiency/apnea, flushing, increased salivation.

See *Neuromuscular Blocking Agents* for a complete list of possible side effects.

Also, **Allergic reactions:** Excessive histamine secretion and circulatory collapse.

ADDITIONAL DRUG INTERACTIONS

Acetylcholine / Antagonizes effect of tubocurarine

Anticholinesterases / Antagonizes effect of tubocurarine

Calcium salts / ↑ Tubocurarine effect

Diazepam / ↑ Risk of malignant hyperthermia

Potassium / Antagonizes effect of tubocurarine

Propranolol / ↑ Tubocurarine effect

Quinine / ↑ Tubocurarine effect

Succinylcholine chloride / ↑ Relaxant effect of both drugs

OD OVERDOSE MANAGEMENT

Symptoms: Respiratory insufficiency. *Treatment:* Overdosage chiefly treated by artificial respiration, although neostigmine, atropine, and edrophonium chloride should also be on hand.

HOW SUPPLIED

Injection: 3 mg (20 units/mL).

DOSAGE

• **IM; IV**

Adjunct to surgical anesthesia.

Adults, IM, IV, initial: 6–9 mg (40–60 units); **then,** 3–4.5 mg (20–30 units) in 3–5 min if needed. Supplemental doses of 3 mg (20 units) can be given for prolonged procedures. Dosage can be calculated on the basis of 1.1 units/kg. **Pediatric, up to 4 weeks of age, IV, initial:** 0.3 mg/kg; **then,** give subsequent doses in increments of 1/5–1/6 the initial dose. **Infants and children, IV:** 0.6 mg/kg.

Electroshock therapy.

Adults, IV: 0.165 mg/kg (1.1 units/kg) given over 30–90 sec. It is recommended that the initial dose be 3 mg less than the calculated total dose.

Diagnosis of myasthenia gravis.

Adults, IV: 0.004–0.033 mg/kg. A test dose should be given within 2–3 min with IV neostigmine, 1.5 mg, to minimize prolonged respiratory paralysis.

NURSING CONSIDERATIONS

ADMINISTRATION/STORAGE

IV 1. Give IV as a sustained injection over 1–1.5 min. May also be given IM.

2. Give in incremental doses until relaxation is reached.

3. Decrease the initial dose if the inhalation anesthetic used enhances the action of curariform drugs or with compromised renal function.

4. Review the drugs with which tubocurarine interacts.

5. Tubocurarine is incompatible with alkaline solutions and may form a precipitate when mixed with them (e.g., methohexital sodium or thiopental sodium).

6. Have neostigmine methylsulfate available as an antidote.

ASSESSMENT

1. Note reasons for therapy, onset, characteristics of symptoms.

2. Utilize a peripheral nerve stimulator (train of four) to assess neuromuscular response and recovery.

3. Record length of time receiving drug. Should only be used on a short-term basis and in a continuously monitored environment. May experience residual muscle weakness with prolonged therapy.

4. Client may be fully conscious and aware of surroundings and conversations.

5. Drug does not affect pain or anxiety; administer analgesics and antianxiety agents as needed.

6. Continually monitor VS, I&O, ECG, and lab studies. Drug can cause vagal stimulation resulting in bradycardia, hypotension, and cardiac arrhythmias.

CLIENT/FAMILY TEACHING

1. Client will be able to use arms and legs and talk once the drug wears off.

2. Reassure client that they will be carefully monitored during therapy and receive medications for anxiety and pain in addition to this drug.

3. Procedures and activities will be explained at the time of performance.

4. Report any adverse or unusual side effects once medication therapy completed.

OUTCOMES/EVALUATE

• Skeletal muscle relaxation
• Control of drug or electrically induced seizures
• Diagnosis of myasthenia gravis

Bold Italic = life threatening side effect   ■ = black box warning   ✦ = Available in Canada

Valacyclovir hydrochloride ©

(**val**-ah-**SIGH**-kloh-veer)

CLASSIFICATION(S):
Antiviral
PREGNANCY CATEGORY: B
Rx: Valtrex.

SEE ALSO *ANTIVIRAL DRUGS*.

USES
(1) Treatment or suppression of genital herpes in immunocompetent adults and for suppression of recurrent genital herpes in HIV-infected individuals. When used as suppressive therapy in immunocompetent clients with genital herpes, the risk of heterosexual transmission to susceptible partners is reduced. (2) Herpes zoster (shingles) in immunocompetent adults. (3) Treatment of herpes labialis (cold sores). *Investigational:* Prophylaxis to prevent cytomegalovirus disease in those who have undergone stem-cell or renal transplantation from a seropositive donor; use in those with AIDS for CMV prophylaxis is not recommended due to trend of increasing deaths with its use in this group.

ACTION/KINETICS
Action
Rapidly converted to acyclovir, which has inhibitory activity against herpes simplex virus types 1 (HSV-1) and 2 (HSV-2) and varicella-zoster virus. Acts by inhibiting replication of viral DNA by competitive inhibition of viral DNA polymerase, incorporation and termination of the growing viral DNA chain, and inactivation of the viral DNA polymerase.

Pharmacokinetics
Rapidly absorbed after PO administration (absolute bioavailability is about 55%) and is rapidly and nearly completely converted to acyclovir and l-valine by first-pass intestinal or hepatic metabolism. **Time to peak levels:** Approximately 1.5 hr. **Peak plasma levels:** Less than 0.5 mcg/mL of valacyclovir at all doses. **t½, acyclovir, plasma:** 2.5–3.3 hr. Approximately 50% is excreted through the urine. **Plasma protein binding:** 13.5–17.9%.

CONTRAINDICATIONS
Hypersensitivity or intolerance to acyclovir or valacyclovir. Use in immunocompromised individuals. Use in AIDS clients due to increasing deaths associated with use in this population. Lactation.

SPECIAL CONCERNS
Use with caution in renal impairment or in those taking potentially nephrotoxic drugs. Thrombotic thrombocytopenic purpura or hemolytic uremic syndrome has been seen in some clients. Dosage reduction may be necessary in geriatric clients depending on the renal status. Use with caution during lactation. Safety and efficacy have not been determined in prepubertal children Safety and efficacy have not been determined in the following disease states: Immunocompromised clients, other than for the suppression of genital herpes in HIV-infected clients; for suppression of recurrent genital herpes in those with advanced HIV disease (CD4 count less than 100 cells/mm³); to treat genital herpes in HIV-infected clients; and, to treat disseminated herpes zoster.

SIDE EFFECTS
Most Common
Headache, N&V, dizziness, abdominal pain, rash, dysmenorrhea, arthralgia, depression.
GI: N&V, diarrhea, constipation, abdominal pain, anorexia, hepatitis. **CNS:** Headache, dizziness, depression, aggressive behavior, agitation, coma, confusion, ataxia, decreased consciousness, encephalopathy, mania, psychosis, auditory and visual hallucinations, *seizures*, tremors. **CV:** Hypertension,

 = see color insert   **H** = Herbal   **IV** = Intravenous   © = sound alike drug tachycardia. **Hematologic:** Leukopenia, thrombocytopenia, anemia, *aplastic anemia*. **Respiratory:** Nasopharyngitis, URTI. **Dermatologic:** Erythema multiforme, rashes including photosensitivity, alopecia. **Hypersensitivity:** Rash, urticaria, pruritus, dyspnea, angioedema, *anaphylaxis*. **Miscellaneous:** Asthenia, facial edema, visual abnormalities, dysmenorrhea, arthralgia, dysarthria, leukocytoclastic vasculitis, precipitation of acyclovir in renal tubules resulting in acute renal failure and anuria. Thrombotic thrombocytopenic purpura, hemolytic uremic syndrome.

LABORATORY TEST CONSIDERATIONS
↑ Creatinine, AST, ALT, alkaline phosphatase. ↓ Neutrophil and platelet counts. Liver enzyme abnormalities.

OD OVERDOSE MANAGEMENT
Symptoms: Precipitation of acyclovir in renal tubules if the solubility (2.5 mg/mL) is exceeded in the intratubular fluid. *Treatment:* Hemodialysis until renal function is restored. About 33% of acyclovir in the body is removed during a 4-hr hemodialysis session.

DRUG INTERACTIONS
Administration of cimetidine and/or probenecid decreases the rate, but not the extent, of conversion of valacyclovir to acyclovir. Also, the renal clearance of acyclovir decreases.

HOW SUPPLIED
Tablets: 0.5 gram, 1 gram.

DOSAGE
• **TABLETS**
   Herpes zoster (shingles).
Adults: 1 gram 3 times per day for 7 days. *Dosage with renal impairment:* C_{CR}, 30–49 mL/min: 1 gram q 12 hr; C_{CR}, 10–29 mL/min: 1 gram q 24 hr; and, C_{CR}, <10 mL/min: 500 mg q 24 hr.
   Genital herpes, initial episodes.
1 gram twice a day for 10 days. Begin therapy within 72 hr of signs and symptoms. *Dosage with renal impairment:* C_{CR}, 30–40 mL/min: No reduction in dosage; C_{CR}, 10–29 mL/min: 1 gram q 24 hr; C_{CR} <10 mL/min: 500 mg q 24 hr.
   Recurrent genital herpes.
Adults: 500 mg q 12 hr for 3 days. *Dosage with renal impairment:* C_{CR}, 30–49 mL/min: No reduction in dose; C_{CR},

10–29 mL/min: 500 mg q 24 hr; and, C_{CR}, <10 mL/min: 500 mg q 24 hr.
   Suppression of genital herpes.
Adults: 1 gram once daily in those with a healthy immune system (500 mg once daily for those who have 9 or fewer recurrences per year). *Dosage with renal impairment:* C_{CR}, 20–49 mL/min: No reduction in dose; C_{CR}, 10–29 mL/min: 500 mg q 24 hr for those taking 1 gram/24 hr and 500 mg q 48 hr for those taking 500 mg/24 hr; C_{CR}, <10 mL/min: 500 mg q 24 hr for those taking 1 gram/24 hr and 500 mg q 48 hr for those taking 500 mg/24 hr.
   Suppressive therapy in HIV-infected clients with CD4 cell count at least 100 cells/mm^3.
500 mg twice a day for chronic suppressive therapy of recurrent genital herpes (500 mg once daily in those with a history of 9 or fewer recurrence per year). *Dosage for renal impairment:* C_{CR}, 20–40 mL/min: No reduction in dose; C_{CR}, 10–29 mL/min: 500 mg q 24 hr; C_{CR}, <10 mL/min: 500 mg q 24 hr.
   Herpes labialis (cold sores).
2 grams twice a day for 1 day taken about 12 hr apart. Initiate therapy at the earliest symptoms. Therapy beyond one day does not provide additional beneficial effects. *Dosage with renal impairment:* C_{CR}, 30–49 mL/min: 2 x 1 gram doses taken about 12 hr apart; C_{CR}, 10–20 mL/min: 2 x 500 mg doses taken about 12 hr apart; C_{CR}, <10 mL/min: Single 500 mg dose.

NURSING CONSIDERATIONS
Ⓒ Do not confuse valacyclovir with valganciclovir (also an antiviral drug).

ADMINISTRATION/STORAGE
1. Begin therapy as soon as possible after herpes zoster has been diagnosed. The drug is most effective when started within 48 hr after the onset of rash. For recurrent genital herpes, initiate at the first S&S of a flare.
2. Clients requiring hemodialysis should receive the recommended dose after hemodialysis.
3. Store from 15–25°C (59–77°F).

Bold Italic = life threatening side effect   ■ = black box warning   ✦ = Available in Canada

ASSESSMENT

1. List reasons for therapy, onset, characteristics of S&S. With herpes zoster, note dermatone(s) location, characteristics of lesions; most effective if initiated within 48 hr of rash/symptoms.

2. With recurrent genital herpes, note extent of lesions; initiate at first S&S of outbreak.

3. Monitor CBC, renal function studies; reduce dose if C_{CR} <50 mL/min.

CLIENT/FAMILY TEACHING

1. Take exactly as prescribed; do not share medications, skip, or double up on doses. Complete entire course of therapy. May take without regard to meals; food may decrease GI upset.

2. Vesicles usually become red or pustular after 4 or 5 days and by the 7th to 10th day dry up and crust over. The acute phase is completed by approximately 3 weeks, when the scabs slough from the skin.

3. Immunocompromised clients usually experience a more severe case and disease course usually doubles. In clients with AIDS review high risk potential with this drug use.

4. During acute stage, cover area and avoid contact with immunocompromised individuals, pregnant women, or anyone else that has not had the chicken pox virus. If unsure may check titers.

5. Report pain and headaches so appropriate analgesics can be prescribed. May cause drowsiness or dizziness. Report persistent pain once lesions have healed (postherpetic neuralgia may last many months-yrs), if there is eye involvement or any other unusual symptoms or behaviors.

6. With genital herpes, abstain from sexual contact during acute outbreaks to prevent infecting partner; use condoms during all other times.

OUTCOMES/EVALUATE

- ↓ Duration/progression of herpes zoster outbreak with reduced healing time; symptomatic relief
- ↓ Pain, ↓ duration, ↓ intensity ↓ frequency/transmission with genital herpes outbreak

Valganciclovir hydrochloride ■ ©

(**val**-gan-**SIGH**-kloh-veer)

CLASSIFICATION(S):
Antiviral
PREGNANCY CATEGORY: C
Rx: Valcyte.

SEE ALSO *ANTIVIRAL DRUGS.*

USES

(1) Cytomegalovirus (CMV) retinitis in AIDS clients. (2) Prevention of CMV disease in kidney, heart, and kidney-pancreas clients at high risk (Donor CMV seropositive/Recipient CMV seronegative [(D+/R-)]).

ACTION/KINETICS

Action
Is a prodrug that is metabolized to ganciclovir by intestinal and hepatic esterases. In CMV-infected cells, ganciclovir is first phosphorylated to ganciclovir monophosphate and then further phosphorylated to ganciclovir triphosphate. The triphosphate inhibits viral DNA synthesis. Resistant viruses to ganciclovir occur after prolonged treatment with valganciclovir.

Pharmacokinetics
Well absorbed from the GI tract. No other metabolites than ganciclovir have been identified. Excreted by the kidney. **$t\frac{1}{2}$, terminal:** About 4 hr.

CONTRAINDICATIONS

Hypersensitivity to ganciclovir or valganciclovir. Use if the absolute neutrophil count is <500 cells/mm^3, the platelet count is <25,000/mm^3, or the hemoglobin is <8 grams/dL. Use in clients receiving hemodialysis or in liver transplant clients. Lactation.

SPECIAL CONCERNS

■ The clinical toxicity of valganciclovir, which is metabolized to ganciclovir, includes granulocytopenia, anemia, and thrombocytopenia. In animal studies, ganciclovir was carcinogenic, teratogenic, and caused aspermatogenesis.■ Use with caution in pre-existing cytopenias or in those who have received or are receiving myelosuppressive drugs or irradiation. Safety and efficacy have not been determined in other solid organ transplants (e.g., lung) or in children.

SIDE EFFECTS
Most Common
Diarrhea, neutropenia, N&V, headache, anemia, catheter-related infection, abdominal pain, pyrexia, insomnia, retinal detachment, tremors, hypertension. See also *Ganciclovir*. **Hematologic:** Granulocytopenia, anemia, thrombocytopenia, severe leukopenia, neutropenia, pancytopenia, bone marrow depression, *aplastic anemia*. **GI:** Diarrhea, N&V, abdominal pain. **CNS:** Headache, insomnia, paresthesia, convulsions, psychosis, hallucinations, confusion, agitation. **Miscellaneous:** Peripheral neuropathy, local and systemic infections and sepsis, *potential life-threatening bleeding due to thrombocytopenia*, hypersensitivity.

LABORATORY TEST CONSIDERATIONS
↑ Serum creatinine.

DRUG INTERACTIONS
Since valganciclovir is rapidly metabolized to ganciclovir, any drug interactions will be those for ganciclovir. Thus, see *Ganciclovir*

HOW SUPPLIED
Tablets: 450 mg (as base).

DOSAGE
* **TABLETS**
  CMV retinitis.
Induction: 900 mg (2 x 450 mg tablets) twice a day for 21 days with food. **Maintenance:** Following induction or in those with inactive CMV retinitis, give 900 mg (2 x 450 mg tablets) once daily with food.
  Prevention of CMV disease.
900 mg (2–450 mg tablets) once daily with food starting within 10 days of transplantation until 100 days posttransplantation. For all uses, adjust the dose as follows in those with renal impairment: If C_{CR} is 40 to 59 mL/min, give 450 mg twice a day for the induction dose and 450 mg once daily for the maintenance dose, If C_{CR} is 25 to 39 mL/min, give 450 mg once daily for the induc-

tion dose and 450 mg q 2 days for the maintenance dose, If C_{CR} is 10 to 24 mL/min, give 450 mg q 2 days for the induction dose and 450 mg twice weekly for the maintenance dose.

NURSING CONSIDERATIONS
Ⓒ Do not confuse valganciclovir with valacyclovir (also an antiviral drug).

ADMINISTRATION/STORAGE
1. Valganciclovir tablets cannot be substituted for ganciclovir tablets on a one-to-one basis.
2. Use caution in handling valganciclovir tablets. Do not break or crush tablets; is potential teratogen and carcinogen. Avoid direct contact of broken/crushed tablets with the skin or mucous membranes. If contact occurs, wash thoroughly with soap and water; rinse eyes thoroughly with plain water.
3. Cytopenia may occur at any time during treatment and may increase with continued dosing. Cell counts usually begin to recover within 3 to 7 days after stopping the drug.

ASSESSMENT
1. Note reasons for therapy, characteristics of S&S, other agents trialed, outcome. Assess orientation and mentation levels.
2. Determine CMV retinitis by indirect ophthalmoscopy.
3. Review history and assess carefully for pre-existing cytopenias or if have received or are receiving myelosuppressive drugs or irradiation.
4. Drug is converted to ganciclovir but drugs are not interchangeable
5. Monitor CBC, hold and report if ANC is <500 cells/mm^3, the platelet count is <25,000/mm^3, or the hemoglobin is <8 grams/dL. Anticipate reduced dose with renal dysfunction, see dosing guidelines.

CLIENT/FAMILY TEACHING
1. Take with food to maximize bioavailability. Drug is not a cure; it controls symptoms and progression of disease.
2. Follow directions carefully for induction and then maintenance dosing. Valganciclovir *cannot* be substituted for ganciclovir on a mg to mg basis.

---

3. If others must handle the tablets, use caution. Do not break or crush tablets, and do not handle broken tablets. If contact with skin or mucous membranes occurs, wash thoroughly with soapy water and rinse eyes well with plain water.

4. Drug is a potential teratogen and carcinogen. Practice barrier contraception during and for 90 days following therapy.

5. Do not perform activities requiring mental alertness until drug effects realized; may cause dizziness, seizures, altered balance, and confusion.

6. Report any abnormal bruising or bleeding; drug impairs clotting.

7. Avoid crowds, those with active infections and wash hands frequently to reduce chances of infection.

8. See eye doctor q 4–6 weeks as scheduled for eval. and F/U.

OUTCOMES/EVALUATE

↓ Progression of CMV retinitis

Valproic acid ■
(val-**PROH**-ick)

CLASSIFICATION(S):
Anticonvulsant, miscellaneous
PREGNANCY CATEGORY: D
Rx: Depacon, Depakene.
✤**Rx:** Apo-Valproic, Epiject I.V., Gen-Valproic, Novo-Valproic, Nu-Valproic, PMS-Valproic Acid, PMS-Valproic Acid E.C., Rhoxal-valproic, Rhoxal-valproic EC, ratio-Valproic.

Divalproex sodium
(die-val-**PROH**-ex)

PREGNANCY CATEGORY: D
Rx: Depakote, Depakote ER.
✤**Rx:** Apo-Divalproex, Epival, Epival ER, Novo-Divalproex, Nu-Divalproex.

SEE ALSO *ANTICONVULSANTS*.

USES
PO or IV. (1) Alone or in combination with other anticonvulsants for treatment of complex partial seizures in adults and children 10 years of age and older that occur either in isolation or in association with other types of seizures. (2) Use as sole and adjunctive therapy to treat simple and complex absence seizures (petit mal). (3) As an adjunct in multiple seizure patterns that include absence seizures.

PO. (1) Divalproex sodium delayed-release and extended-release tablets used for the acute treatment of acute manic or mixed episodes with or without psychotic features associated with bipolar disorder. (2) Divalproex sodium delayed-release and extended-release tablets for prophylaxis of migraine headaches in adults.

ACTION/KINETICS
Action
The precise anticonvulsant action is unknown; may increase brain levels of the neurotransmitter GABA. Other possibilities include acting on postsynaptic receptor sites to mimic or enhance the inhibitory effect of GABA, inhibiting an enzyme that catabolizes GABA, affecting the potassium channel, or directly affecting membrane stability.

Pharmacokinetics
Absorption is more rapid with the syrup (sodium salt) than capsules. Rapidly dissociates to the valproic ion in the stomach. Rate of absorption of the ion may vary with the formulation (i.e., liquid, solid, or sprinkle), conditions of use (fasting, after food), and the method of administration (i.e., whether sprinkled on food or taken intact). **Peak levels, with syrup:** 15 min–2 hr. Equivalent PO doses of divalproex sodium and valproic acid deliver equivalent amounts of valproate ion to the system. **Peak serum levels, capsules and syrup:** 1–4 hr (delayed if the drug is taken with food); **peak serum levels, enteric-coated tablet (divalproex sodium):** 3–4 hr. **t½:** 9–16 hr, with the lower time usually seen in clients taking other anticonvulsant drugs (e.g., primidone, phenytoin, phenobarbital, carbamazepine). **t½, children less than 10 days:** 10–67 hr; **t½, children over 2 months:** 7–13 hr. **t½, cirrhosis or acute hepatitis:** Up

---

to 18 hr. **Therapeutic serum levels:** 50–100 mcg/mL, although a good correlation has not been established between daily dose, serum level, and therapeutic effect. Metabolized in the liver and inactive metabolites are excreted in the urine; small amounts of valproic acid are excreted in the feces. **Plasma protein binding:** Is concentration dependent; ranges from about 10% to 18.5%.

CONTRAINDICATIONS

Liver disease or dysfunction. Known urea cycle disorders. Lactation.

SPECIAL CONCERNS

■ (1) Hepatotoxicity. Hepatic failure (may be fatal) has occurred. Children less than 2 years of age are at considerably increased risk of developing fatal hepatotoxicity, especially those on multiple anticonvulsants, those with congenital metabolic disorders, those with severe seizure disorders accompanied by mental retardation, and those with organic brain disease. Use valproic acid with extreme caution and as a sole agent in this group. Above this age group, experience in epilepsy has indicated that the incidence of fatal hepatotoxicity decreases considerably in progressively older groups. These incidents have usually occurred during the first 6 months of treatment. Serious or fatal heptotoxicity may be preceded by nonspecific symptoms such as anorexia, facial edema, lethargy, malaise, vomiting, and weakness. In clients with epilepsy, a loss of seizure control may also occur. Closely monitor clients for appearance of such symptoms. Peform LFTs prior to therapy and at frequent intervals thereafter, especially during the first 6 months of therapy. (2) Valproate can produce teratogenic effects such as neural tube defects (e.g., spina bifida). Accordingly, the use of valproate products in women of childbearing potential requires that the benefits of use be weighed against the risk of injury to the fetus. This is especially important when the treatment of a spontaneously reversible condition not ordinarily associated with permanent injury or death (e.g., migraine) is contemplated. An information sheet describing the teratogenic potential of valproate is available for clients. (3) Pancreatitis. Cases of life-threatening pancreatitis have been reported in both children and adults receiving valproate. Some cases have been described as hemorrhagic with a rapid progression from initial symptoms to death. Cases have been reported shortly after initial use as well as after several years of use. Warn clients and caregivers that abdominal pain, N&V, and/or anorexia can be symptoms of pancreatitis that require prompt medical evaluation. If pancreatitis is diagnosed, discontinue valproate. Initiate alternative treatment for the underlying medical condition as clinically indicated.■ Use lower doses in geriatric clients because they may have increased free, unbound valproic acid levels in the serum.

Use with caution in those with a history of hepatic disease; at particular risk are users of multiple anticonvulsants, children, those with metabolic disorders, those with severe seizure disorders accompanied by mental retardation, and those with organic brain disease. Children less than 2 years of age are at a considerably increased risk of developing fatal hepatotoxicity.

Safety and efficacy of divalproex sodium have not been determined for treating acute mania in children less than 18 years of age and for treating migraine in children less than 16 years of age. Safety and efficacy of divalproex sodium ER tablets for the prophylaxis of migraines in children has not been established; also, safety and efficacy of divalproex sodium ER for the treatment of complex partial seizures, simple and complex absence seizures, and multiple seizure types (that include absence seizures) have not been determined in children less than 10 years of age. Use of valproate sodium injection in children less than 2 years of age has not been studied.

SIDE EFFECTS

Most Common

Asthenia, headache, somnolence, dizziness, tremor, insomnia, amnesia, ner-

---

vousness, ataxia, N&V, dyspepsia, diarrhea, abdominal pain, anorexia, flu syndrome, infection, nystagmus, dipolopia, amblyopia/blurred vision, thrombocytopenia, alopecia.

Side effects listed include all uses. CNS: Somnolence, insomnia, sedation, dizziness, tremor, ataxia, emotional lability, abnormal thinking, amnesia, euphoria, headache, hypesthesia, nervousness, paresthesia, insomnia, depression, hallucinations, anxiety, confusion, abnormal gait, hypertonia, hypokinesia, increased reflexes, tardive dyskinesia, incoordination, abnormal dreams, personality disorder, emotional upset, psychosis, aggression, hyperactivity, behavioral deterioration, depression, emotional upset, psychosis, hostility, tremor, vertigo, parkinsonism, agitation, catatonic reaction, confusion, dysarthria, speech disorder, *suicidal ideation*, coma (alone or with phenobarbital—rare), encephalopathy with and without fever (rare), reversible cerebral atrophy, dementia, *hyperammonemic encephalopathy* with urea cycle disorders (including ornithine transcarbamylase deficiency). **GI:** N&V, abdominal pain, dyspepsia, anorexia (with weight loss), dry mouth, stomatitis, tooth disorder, GI disorder, constipation, increased appetite (with weight gain), flatulence, hematemesis, eructation, periodontal abscess, taste perversion, indigestion, fecal incontinence, gastroenteritis, glossitis, acute intermittent porphyria, *acute pancreatitis*. **CV:** Hypertension, palpitation, tachycardia, bradycardia, vasodilation, postural hypotension, hypotension, cutaneous vasculitis. **Hematologic:** Thrombocytopenia, ecchymosis, petechia, bruising, hematoma formation, *frank hemorrhage*, relative lymphocytosis, macrocytosis, hypofibrinogenemia, leukopenia, eosinophilia, anemia (including macrocytic with or without folate deficiency), bone marrow suppression, pancytopenia, *aplastic anemia*, acute intermittent porphyria. **Respiratory:** Infection, flu syndrome, pharyngitis, dyspnea, bronchitis, rhinitis, epistaxis, pneumonia, sinusitis, increased cough. **Musculoskel-**

etal: Arthralgia, arthrosis, leg cramps, myalgia, myasthenia, twitching. **Dermatologic:** Dry skin, rash, pruritus, petechiae, transient hair loss, skin rash, ecchymosis, erythema multiforme, photosensitivity, generalized pruritus, alopecia, sweating, rash, discoid lupus erythematosus, furunculosis, maculopapular rash, seborrhea, *Stevens-Johnson syndrome, toxic epidermal necrolysis (rare)*. **GU:** Amenorrhea, dysmenorrha, urinary frequency, urinary incontinence, vaginitis, irregular menses, secondary amenorrhea, breast enlargement, galactorrhea, dysuria, cystitis, metrorrhagia, vaginal hemorrhage, polycystic ovary disease (rare), enuresis, UTI. **Metabolic:** Hyperammonemia, hyponatremia, inappropriate ADH secretion, Fanconi syndrome (rare; seen mainly in children), decreased carnitine concentrations. **Ophthalmic:** Nystagmus, diplopia, asterixis, 'spots before eyes,' amblyopia/blurred vision, abnormal vision, conjunctivitis, dry eyes, eye pain. **Otic:** Tinnitus, deafness, otitis media, hearing loss (either reversible or irreversible), ear pain, ear disorder. **Body as a whole:** Asthenia, flu syndrome, infection, malaise, weakness, fever, hypothermia, chills, chills and fever, injection site inflammation/pain/reaction, unspecified pain, peripheral edema, infection, viral infection, accidental injury, lupus erythematosis, bone pain, multiorgan hypersensitivity reactions (rare), *anaphylaxis*. **Miscellaneous:** Hyperammonemia, back/chest pain, neck pain/rigidity, facial edema.

LABORATORY TEST CONSIDERATIONS
False + for ketonuria. ↑ AST, ALT, LDH, serum bilirubin, amylase. Altered thyroid or liver function tests. Possible false interpretation of the urine ketone test.

OD OVERDOSE MANAGEMENT
Symptoms: Motor restlessness, asterixis, visual hallucinations, somnolence, heart block, *deep coma*. *Treatment:* Perform gastric lavage if client is seen early enough (valproic acid is absorbed rapidly). Undertake general supportive measures making sure urinary output is maintained. Naloxone has been used to reverse the CNS depression (however, it

 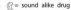

could also reverse the anticonvulsant effect). Hemodialysis and hemoperfusion have been used with success.

DRUG INTERACTIONS

Alcohol / ↑ Incidence of CNS depression

Antacids (Al-Mg hydroxide, Al-Mg trisilicate, calcium carbonate) / ↑ Risk of valproic acid toxicity; monitor carefully

Barbiturates / ↓ Valproic acid hepatic metabolism; may need to ↓ barbiturate dose

Carbamazepine / Variable changes in carbamazepine levels with possible loss of seizure control

Charcoal / ↓ Valproic acid absorption from the GI tract

Chlorpromazine / ↓ Clearance and ↑ elimination t½ of valproic acid → ↑ pharmacologic effects

Cholestyramine / ↓ Valproic acid serum levels with possible loss of seizure control; give valproic acid at least 3 hr before cholestyramine

Cimetidine / ↓ Clearance and ↑ t½ of valproic acid → ↑ pharmacologic effects

Clonazepam / ↑ CNS depression R/T ↓ plasma protein binding and ↓ metabolism; coadministration may induce absence status in those with a history of absence seizures

CNS depressants / ↑ Incidence of CNS depression

Diazepam / ↑ Diazepam effect R/T ↓ plasma protein binding and ↓ metabolism

Erythromycin / ↑ Serum valproic acid levels → valproic acid toxicity

Ethosuximide / ↑ Ethosuximide effect R/T ↓ metabolism; ↓ valproic acid levels

Felbamate / ↑ Mean peak valproate levels

Lamotrigine / ↓ Valproic acid serum levels and ↑ lamotrigine serum levels; reduce dose of lamotrigine

Lorazepam / ↑ Lorazepam effect R/T ↓ plasma protein binding and ↓ metabolism

Olanzapine / ↑ Hepatic enzymes; monitor AST and ALT q 3–4 months during the first year of therapy

Phenobarbital / ↑ Phenobarbital effect R/T ↓ liver breakdown; possible double the clearance of liver breakdown; ↓ effect of valproic acid R/T ↑ metabolism

Primidone / ↑ Primidone effect R/T ↓ liver breakdown; ↓ effect of valproic acid R/T ↑ metabolism

Rifampin / ↑ Valproate oral clearance

Salicylates (aspirin) / Effect of valproic acid in children R/T ↓ plasma protein binding and ↓ metabolism; monitor serum levels

Tolbutamide / Possible ↑ unbound fraction of tolbutamide; relevance not known

Topiramate / Possible ↑ metabolism of both drugs; hyperammonemia with and without encephalopathy

Tricyclic antidepressants / ↑ TCA plasma levels and side effects

Warfarin sodium / ↑ Warfarin effect R/T ↓ plasma protein binding. Also, additive anticoagulant effect

Zidovudine / ↓ Clearance in HIV-seropositive clients

HOW SUPPLIED

Valproic acid: *Capsules:* 250 mg; *Injection, Concentrate:* 100 mg/mL (as sodium valproate); *Syrup:* 250 mg/5 mL (as sodium valproate).

Divalproex sodium: *Capsules, Sprinkle:* 125 mg; *Tablets, Delayed-Release:* 125 mg, 250 mg, 500 mg; *Tablets, Extended-Release:* 250 mg, 500 mg.

DOSAGE

• **CAPSULES; CAPSULES, SPRINKLE; DELAYED-RELEASE AND EXTENDED-RELEASE TABLETS (DIVALPROEX); SYRUP (VALPROIC ACID)**

Complex partial seizures, monotherapy.

Adults and children 10 years and older: 10–15 mg/kg/day for monotherapy. Increase by 5–10 mg/kg/week until seizures are controlled or side effects occur, up to a maximum of 60 mg/kg/day. If a satisfactory response has not been reached, measure plasma levels to determine whether they are in the usually accepted therapeutic range of 50 to 100 mcg/mL. The probability of thrombocytopenia increases significantly at total trough valproate plasma levels about 100 mcg/mL in women and 135 mcg/mL in men. When converting to

---

V

monotherapy, initiate at 10–15 mg/kg/day. Increase the dose by 5–10 mg/kg/week to achieve the optimum clinical effect. Concomitant antiepileptic drug dosage can usually be reduced by approximately 25% every 2 weeks. This reduction may be started at initiation of valproic acid therapy or delayed by 1 to 2 weeks if there is a concern that seizures are likely to occur with a reduction. The speed and duration of withdrawal of the concomitant antiepileptic drug can be highly variable; monitor clients closely during this period for increased seizure frequency.

Complex partial seizures, adjunctive therapy.

Adults and children 10 years and older: Valproic acid may added to the client's regimen at a dose of 10–15 mg/kg/day. The dose may be increased by 5–10 mg/kg/week to achieve the optimum clinical response. Usually, the optimum response is seen at daily doses less than 60 mg/kg/day. If the total daily dose exceeds 250 mg, give in divided doses.

Simple and complex absence seizures.

Initial: 15 mg/kg/day, increasing at 1-week intervals by 5–10 mg/kg/day until seizures are controlled or side effects occur. Usual recommended dose is 60 mg/kg/day. If the total daily dose exceeds 250 mg, give in divided doses. Therapeutic valproate serum levels for most clients with absence seizures are from 50 to 100 mcg/mL.

Acute manic episodes in bipolar disorder (use divalproex sodium delayed- or extended-release tablets).

Initial, using extended-release tablets: 25 mg/kg/day given once daily; increase the dose as rapidly as possible to reach the lowest therapeutic dose that will control symptoms. A trough plasma level between 85 and 125 mcg/mL may be effective. Maximum recommended dose: 60 mg/kg/day. **Initial, using delayed-release tablets:** 250 mg 3 times per day; **then,** increase dose as rapidly as possible to reach the lowest therapeutic dose that will control symptoms. A trough plasma level between 50 and 125 mcg/mL may be

effective. Maximum levels usually reached within 14 days. The maximum dose is 60 mg/kg/day.

Migraine (use divalproex sodium delayed- or extended-release tablets).

Initial, using extended-release: 500 mg once daily for 1 week; **then,** increase to 1,000 mg once daily. **Initial, using delayed-release:** 250 mg twice daily; some may benefit from doses up to 1,000 mg/day. *NOTE:* The ER tablets are not bioequivalent to the delayed-release tablets.

• **IV**

Epilepsy.

Give as a 60 min infusion at 20 mg or less/min with the same frequency as PO products. Use of the injection for more than 14 days has not been studied. Switch to PO valproate products as soon as possible.

NURSING CONSIDERATIONS

ADMINISTRATION/STORAGE

1. Divide daily dosage if it exceeds 250 mg/day.

2. Do not confuse Depakote ER, an extended-release divalproex sodium, with Depakote delayed-release. The two forms can not be substituted for each other. Depakote still requires dosing q 8–12 hr whereas Depakote ER is given once daily.

3. Convert from Depakote to Depakote ER as follows: In adults and children over 10 years of age receiving Depakote, Depakote ER can be given once daily using a dose 8–20% higher than the total daily dose of Depakote. For those whose Depakote total daily dose can not be directly converted to Depakote ER, the client's Depakote total daily dose may be increased to the next higher dosage before converting it to the appropriate daily dose of Depakote ER.

4. To minimize GI irritation, initiate at a lower dose, give with food, or use delayed-release (Depakote).

5. To minimize CNS depression, give at bedtime.

6. Do not administer valproic acid syrup to clients whose *sodium* intake must be restricted. Consult provider if a sodi-

---

 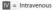

um-restricted client is unable to swallow capsules.

7. With valproic acid therapy, conversion to divalproex sodium can be undertaken at the same total daily dose and dosing schedule.

8. Reduce starting dose in geriatric clients, depending on response. Younger children will require larger maintenance doses, esp. if receiving enzyme-inducing drugs.

9. Do not abruptly discontinue antiepileptic drugs in clients in whom the drug is given to prevent major seizures due to the strong possibility of precipitating status epilepticus with accompanying hypoxia that are life-threatening.

IV 10. Give as a 60 min infusion (not more than 20 mg/min) with the same frequency as PO products. More rapid infusion increases frequency of side effects.

11. When switching from PO to IV, the total daily dose of valproate sodium injection should be equivalent to the total daily dose of PO product. Monitor closely if receiving doses near maximum recommended dose of 60 mg/kg/day. If total daily dose exceeds 250 mg, give in divided doses.

12. The equivalence between injectable and PO products at a steady state is valid in every 6-hr regimen. If given less frequently, trough levels may fall below those of a PO dosage form; closely monitor trough plasma levels.

13. Well tolerated if infused over 5–10 min at rates up to 3 mg/kg/min at doses up to 15 mg/kg.

14. IV use for more than 14 days has not been studied. Switch to PO valproate products as soon as feasible.

15. Injection is compatible and chemically stable with dextrose (5%) injection, NaCl (0.9%), and LR injection for at least 24 hr when stored in glass or polyvinyl chloride bags at controlled room temperature.

ASSESSMENT

1. Note reasons for therapy, type, onset, symptom characteristics. List other agents trialed, outcome.

2. Identify type, frequency, duration of behaviors that warrant therapy; assess mental status. With seizures, document characteristics of seizures, onset, aura, and associated findings.

3. Monitor CBC, bleeding times, and LFTs due to increased potential for hepatoxicity. Follow dosing guidelines carefully.

CLIENT/FAMILY TEACHING

1. Take with or after meals to minimize GI upset and at bedtime to minimize sedative effects. Delayed-release products may reduce irritating GI side effects. Do not chew tablets or capsules; swallow whole to prevent irritation of mouth and throat. Do not take antacids, dairy products, or carbonated drinks with drug; hastens dissolution. Do not confuse ER form with regular form. The syrup may contain a high sodium content; avoid in those salt restricted. Do not mix syrup with carbonated beverages.

2. Sprinkle capsules may be swallowed whole or the capsule opened and the contents sprinkled on a small amount (teaspoonful) of applesauce or pudding. Swallow the mixture immediately; do not chew. Do not store for future use.

3. Take only as directed and do not stop suddenly; may induce seizures. Report any loss of seizure control.

4. Do not drive or perform activities that require mental alertness until drug effects realized and seizure control verified.

5. Report any unexplained fever, sore throat, skin rash, tremors, vision problems, yellow skin discoloration, unusual bruising/bleeding; may have liver toxicity. Abdominal pain, N&V, or anorexia can be symptoms of pancreatitis that require prompt medical evaluation.

6. With diabetes, drug may cause a false positive urine test for ketones. Report symptoms of ketoacidosis (dry mouth, thirst, dry flushed skin).

7. Avoid alcohol, any CNS depressants, or OTC products without approval.

8. Report for periodic CBC, serum glucose/acetone, ammonia, and LFTs.

9. Practice reliable contraception. Do not take if pregnant.

---

10. Store safely out of childs reach. Keep all F/U visits for labs and evaluation.

OUTCOMES/EVALUATE
- Control of seizures
- Migraine headache prophylaxis
- Control of manic episodes
- Therapeutic drug levels (50–100 mcg/mL)

Valrubicin
(val-**ROO**-bih-sin)

CLASSIFICATION(S):
Antineoplastic, antibiotic
PREGNANCY CATEGORY: C
Rx: Valstar.
✦Rx: Valtaxin.

SEE ALSO *ANTINEOPLASTIC AGENTS.*

USES
Intravesical therapy of BCG-refractory carcinoma in situ of the urinary bladder.

ACTION/KINETICS

Action
Related to doxorubicin. Inhibits incorporation of nucleosides into nucleic acids, causes extensive chromosome damage, and arrests cell cycle G_2. Although minimal metabolism occurs when instilled into the bladder, valrubicin metabolites interfere with normal DNA breaking-resealing action of DNA topoisomerase II. It penetrates the bladder wall.

Pharmacokinetics
Almost completely excreted by voiding the instillate.

CONTRAINDICATIONS
Hypersensitivity to anthracyclines or Cremophor EL. Concurrent UTIs, small bladder capacity (i.e., unable to hold 75 mL instillation). Use in those with a perforated bladder or when the integrity of the bladder mucosa has been compromised. IM or IV use. Lactation.

SPECIAL CONCERNS
Use with caution in severe irritable bladder symptoms. Safety and efficacy have not been determined in children.

SIDE EFFECTS
Most Common
Urinary frequency/urgency/incontinence, dysuria, bladder spasm, hematuria, bladder pain, cystitis.
GU: Local bladder symptoms, urinary frequency/urgency/incontinence/retention, dysuria, urinary bladder spasm, hematuria, bladder pain, urinary cystitis, nocturia, local burning symptoms, urethral pain, pelvic pain, UTI, poor urine flow, urethritis. **GI:** Abdominal pain, N&V, diarrhea, flatulence, taste loss. **Metabolic:** Hyperglycemia, peripheral edema. **CNS:** Headache, dizziness. **Dermatologic:** Rash, pruritus, local skin irritation. **Body as a whole:** Asthenia, malaise, fever, myalgia. **Miscellaneous:** Back/chest pain, anemia, vasodilation, pneumonia, tenesmus.

LABORATORY TEST CONSIDERATIONS
↑ NPN.

HOW SUPPLIED
Solution for Intravesical Instillation: 40 mg/mL.

DOSAGE
- **SOLUTION FOR INTRAVESICAL INSTILLATION**
  Bladder cancer.
Adults: 800 mg once a week for 6 weeks.

NURSING CONSIDERATIONS

ADMINISTRATION/STORAGE
1. Use aseptic techniques during administration to avoid introducing contaminants into the GU tract or traumatizing the urinary mucosa.
2. Delay use for 2 or more weeks after transurethral resection or fulguration.
3. Insert a urethral catheter under aseptic conditions, drain bladder, and instill 75 mL valrubicin (diluted) slowly via gravity flow for several minutes. Withdraw catheter and have client retain drug for 2 hr before voiding.
4. Maintain adequate hydration following treatment.
5. Cremophor EL, which contains the valrubicin, may leach a hepatotoxic plasticizer from PVC bags and IV tubing. Thus, prepare and store the drug in glass, polypropylene, or polyolefin containers and tubing.

 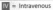

6. Do not mix with other drugs.

7. For each instillation, warm four 5-mL vials to room temperature slowly (do not heat). Withdraw 20 mL from the 4 vials and dilute with 55 mL 0.9% NaCl injection.

8. Valrubicin solution is clear red.

9. Valrubicin diluted in 0.9% NaCl is stable for 12 hr at temperatures up to 25°C (77°F).

10. At temperatures less than 4°C (30°F), Cremophor EL may form a waxy precipitate. If this occurs, warm vial in the hand until the solution is clear. If particulate matter is still seen, do not use.

11. Store unopened vials at 2–8°C (36–46°F). Do not freeze or heat vials.

ASSESSMENT
Note diagnosis/BCG failure; ensure client is unable to undergo, or not a candidate for cystectomy. Monitor VS, for evidence of infection, I&O.

CLIENT/FAMILY TEACHING
1. Drug induces complete response in only about 1 in 5 clients. Delaying cystectomy could lead to metastatic bladder cancer.

2. Drug is administered into the bladder by a catheter once a week for 6 weeks. The catheter is removed and the drug retained in the bladder for 2 hr; then may void.

3. For the first 24–48 hr following instillation, red-tinged urine is typical. Report prolonged blood tinged urine, irritation, pain or other adverse effects.

4. Consume adequate fluids during therapy (2–3 L/day).

5. Men are to refrain from sexual intercourse; use reliable contraception during therapy.

6. Evaluation for recurrence of bladder cancer should be done every 3 months with a biopsy, cystoscopy, and urine cytology.

OUTCOMES/EVALUATE
Control of bladder cancer

Valsartan ■ ©
(val-**SAR**-tan)

CLASSIFICATION(S):
Antihypertensive, angiotensin II receptor blocker

PREGNANCY CATEGORY: C (1st trimester), **D** (2nd and 3rd trimesters).

Rx: Diovan.

SEE ALSO *ANGIOTENSIN II RECEPTOR ANTAGONISTS AND ANTIHYPERTENSIVE AGENTS.*

USES
(1) Alone or in combination with other antihypertensives to treat hypertension. (2) Heart failure (NYHA class II to IV). (3) In clinically stable clients with left ventricular failure or left ventricular dysfunction following a MI; used to reduce CV mortality.

ACTION/KINETICS
Action
Selectively blocks the binding of angiotensin II to the AT_1 receptor in vascular smooth muscle, resulting in a decrease in BP. Angiotensin II is a pressor agent causing vasoconstriction, stimulation of the synthesis of and release of aldosterone, cardiac stimulation, and renal reabsorption of sodium. Also reduces left ventricular hypertrophy.

Pharmacokinetics
About 25% bioavailable. Food decreases absorption. **Peak plasma levels:** 2–4 hr. **t½:** 6 hr. Eliminated mostly unchanged in feces (83%) and urine (about 13%). **Plasma protein binding:** 95%.

SPECIAL CONCERNS
■ When used in pregnancy during the second and third trimesters, drugs that act directly on the renin-angiotensin system can cause injury and even death to the developing fetus. When pregnancy is detected, discontinue valsartan as soon as possible. The use of drugs that act directly on the renin-angiotensin system during the second and third trimesters of pregnancy has been associated with fetal and neonatal injury, including hypotension, neonatal skull hy-

V

Bold Italic = life threatening side effect   ■ = black box warning   ✦ = Available in Canada

poplasia, anuria, reversible or irreversible renal failure, and death. Oligohydramnios has also been reported, presumably resulting from decreased fetal renal function; oligohydramnios in this setting has been associated with fetal limb contractures, craniofacial deformation, and hypoplastic lung development. Prematurity, intrauterine growth retardation, and patent ductus arteriosus have also been reported, although it is not clear whether these occurrences were due to exposure to the drug.■ Use with caution in severe hepatic or renal impaired function. May increase the death rate in clients also taking beta blockers and ACE inhibitors for CHF.

SIDE EFFECTS
Most Common
Dizziness, anxiety, nervousness, abdominal pain, viral infection.
CNS: Headache, dizziness, fatigue, anxiety, insomnia, nervousness, paresthesia, somnolence. **GI:** Abdominal pain, diarrhea, nausea, constipation, dry mouth, dyspepsia, flatulence. **Respiratory:** URTI, cough, rhinitis, sinusitis, pharyngitis, dyspnea. **Body as a whole:** Viral infection, edema, asthenia, allergic reaction, viral infection. **Musculoskeletal:** Arthralgia, back pain, muscle cramps, myalgia. **Dermatologic:** Pruritus, rash. **Miscellaneous:** Palpitations, vertigo, neutropenia, impotence.

LABORATORY TEST CONSIDERATIONS
↓ H&H. ↑ Serum potassium, liver enzymes, serum bilirubin.

DRUG INTERACTIONS
Atenolol / ↑ Antihypertensive effect; no effect on HR
Potassium-sparing diuretics (e.g., amiloride, spironolactone, triamterene) / ↑ Serum potassium; also, ↑ serum creatinine in heart failure clients

HOW SUPPLIED
Tablets: 40 mg, 80 mg, 160 mg, 320 mg.

DOSAGE
- **TABLETS**
  Hypertension.

Adults, initial: 80 or 160 mg once daily as monotherapy in clients who are not volume depleted. A higher dose may be used in those requiring greater reductions. **Dose range:** 80–320 mg once daily. If additional antihypertensive effect is needed, dose may be increased to 160 mg or 320 mg once daily or diuretic may be added (has greater effect when valsartan dose increases beyond 80 mg).
  Heart failure.
Adults, initial: 40 mg twice a day. Increase dose to 80 and 160 mg twice a day as tolerated. **Maximum daily dose:** 320 mg in divided doses. Consider dose reduction of concomitant diuretics. Concomitant use with both an ACE inhibitor and beta-blocker is not recommended.
  Postmyocardial infarction.
Initial: 20 mg twice daily. Dose may be titrated upward within 7 days to 40 mg twice daily, with subsequent titrations to a target maintenance dose of 160 mg twice daily, as tolerated. May be given with other postmyocardial infarction treatment, including aspirin, beta-blockers, thrombolytics, and statins.

NURSING CONSIDERATIONS
🕮 Do not confuse Diovan with Diovan HCT (valsartan plus hydrochlorothiazide).

ADMINISTRATION/STORAGE
1. Give on an empty stomach.
2. Antihypertensive effect is usually seen within 2 weeks with maximum reduction after 4 weeks.
3. Store between 15–30°C (59–86°F) in a tight container protected from moisture.

ASSESSMENT
1. Note reasons for therapy, disease onset, characteristics of S&S, other agents trialed, outcome. List drugs prescribed to ensure none interact.
2. Monitor CBC, electrolytes, renal, LFTs; note dysfunction. Ensure client well hydrated.

CLIENT/FAMILY TEACHING
1. May take with or without food (works better without) and with other prescribed BP medications.
2. Change positions slowly and avoid dehydration to prevent sudden drop in BP and dizziness.

3. Practice reliable contraception; report if pregnancy suspected—may cause fetal death. Do not take if pregnant.

4. Continue low fat, low sodium diet, regular exercise, weight loss, smoking/alcohol cessation, and stress reduction in goal of BP control. Avoid salt replacements that contain potassium.

5. May experience headaches, coughing, diarrhea, nausea, and joint aches; report if persistent.

6. Before taking OTC drugs, obtain medical advice as some may affect the action of valsartan.

7. Keep log of BP and HR for provider review.

OUTCOMES/EVALUATE
- ↓ BP
- Reduced risk of stroke
- ↓ Workload of heart

—COMBINATION DRUG—

Valsartan and Hydrochlorothiazide

(val-**SAR**-tan, **hy**-droh-klor-oh-**THIGH**-ah-zyd)

CLASSIFICATION(S):
Antihypertensive combination drug
PREGNANCY CATEGORY: C (first trimester), **D** (second and third trimesters).
Rx: Diovan HCT.

SEE ALSO VALARTAN AND HYDROCHLOROTHIAZIDE.

USES
Treatment of hypertension. Not indicated for initial therapy.

CONTENT
Each Diovan HCT tablet contains the following amounts of valsartan (*angiotensin II receptor blocker*, listed first) and hydrochlorothiazide (*thiazide diuretic*): 80 mg/12.5 mg, 160 mg/12.5 mg, 160 mg/25 mg, 320 mg/12.5 mg, 320 mg/25 mg.

ACTION/KINETICS

Action
Valsartan selectively blocks the binding of angiotensin II to the AT_1 receptor in vascular smooth muscle, resulting in a decrease in BP. Angiotensin II is a pressor agent causing vasoconstriction, stimulation of the synthesis of and release of aldosterone, cardiac stimulation, and renal reabsorption of sodium. Also reduces left ventricular hypertrophy. Hydrochlorothiazide promotes the excretion of sodium and chloride, and thus water, by the distal renal tubule. Also increases excretion of potassium and to a lesser extent bicarbonate. The antihypertensive activity is thought to be due to direct dilation of the arterioles, as well as to a reduction in the total fluid volume of the body and altered sodium balance.

Pharmacokinetics
Valsartan. About 25% bioavailable. Food decreases absorption. **Peak plasma levels:** 2–4 hr. **t½:** 6 hr. Eliminated mostly unchanged in feces (83%) and urine (about 13%). **Hydrochlorothiazide. Onset:** 2 hr. **Peak effect:** 4–6 hr. **Duration:** 6–12 hr. **t½:** 5.6–14.8 hr. Hydrochlorothiazide is not metabolized but is eliminated rapidly by the kidney. **Plasma protein binding:** Valsartan is about 95% bound to plasma proteins.

CONTRAINDICATIONS
Hypersensitivity to any component of the product. Use in those with anuria or hypersensitivity to other sulfonamide-derived drugs. Lactation.

SPECIAL CONCERNS
■ When used in pregnancy during the second and third trimesters, drugs that act directly on the renin-angiotensin system can cause injury and even death to the developing fetus. When pregnancy is detected, Diovan HCT should be discontinued as soon as possible.■ Use with caution in those with impaired hepatic (including biliary obstructive disorders), or renal function or progressive liver disease (minor alterations of fluid and electrolyte balance may precipitate hepatic coma). Hypersensitivity reactions to hydrochlorothiazide may occur in clients with or without a history of allergy or bronchial asthma but are more likely in those with such a history. May increase the death rate in clients also taking beta blockers and ACE in-

---

hibitors for CHF. Safety and efficacy have not been determined in children.

SIDE EFFECTS

Most Common

Nasopharyngitis, headache, dizziness, orthostatic hypotension, hypokalemia.

See *Valsartan* and *Diuretics, Thiazides* for a complete list of possible side effects. **Miscellaneous:** Thiazides may exacerbate or activate systemic lupus erythematosus.

LABORATORY TEST CONSIDERATIONS

↑ Creatinine, BUN, liver enzymes. ↓ H&H.

OD OVERDOSE MANAGEMENT

Symptoms: Valsartan: Hypotension, tachycardia, bradycardia (if vagal stimulation occurs). Hydrochlorothiazide: Electrolyte depletion and dehydration. *Treatment:* Institute supportive treatment.

DRUG INTERACTIONS

See *Valsartan* and *Diuretics, Thiazides.*

HOW SUPPLIED

See Content.

DOSAGE

* **TABLETS**

    Hypertension.

Adults: Clients whose BP is not controlled using valsartan alone can be switched to Diovan HCT (80/12.5 mg, 160/12.5 mg, or 320/12.5 mg) once daily. If BP remains uncontrolled after 3–4 weeks, increase the dose of valsartan or both components. Clients whose BP is inadequately controlled by hydrochlorothiazide, 25 mg daily or is controlled but experiences hypokalemia, may be switched to Diovan HCT (80/12.5 mg or 160/12.5 mg) once daily. If BP remains uncontrolled after 3–4 weeks, the dose may be increased up to a maximum of 320/25 mg. The maximal antihypertensive effect is reached in about 4 weeks after beginning therapy.

NURSING CONSIDERATIONS

℘ Do not confuse Diovan (valsartan alone) with Diovan HCT (valsartan and hydrochlorothiazide).

ADMINISTRATION/STORAGE

1. It is appropriate to begin combination therapy only after a client has failed to achieve the desired effect with monotherapy.

2. Diovan HCT can be given to clients with impaired renal function as long as the C_{CR} is >30 mL/min. In clients with more severe renal impairment, loop diuretics are preferred to thiazide diuretics.

3. No dosage adjustment is required in those with mild-to-moderate renal or hepatic dysfunction.

4. May be given with other antihypertensive drugs.

5. Store from 15–30°C (59–86°F) protected from moisture.

ASSESSMENT

1. Note reasons for therapy, disease onset, other agents trialed, outcome.

2. List drugs prescribed to ensure none interact.

3. Monitor VS, renal and LFTs; ensure C_{CR} >30 if using combo drug. Use caution with impaired hepatic function or progressive liver disease; minor alterations of fluid and electrolyte balance may precipitate hepatic coma.

4. Assess other medical conditions; ensure all stabilized. Dilutional hyponatremia may occur in edematous clients in hot weather; appropriate therapy is water restriction.

5. Hyperuricemia or frank gout may be precipitated in some receiving thiazide therapy.

6. In diabetics, dosage adjustments of insulin or oral hypoglycemic agents may be required. Hyperglycemia may occur with thiazide diuretics; latent diabetes mellitus may occur during thiazide therapy.

7. Monitor electrolytes, Mg, and calcium. Thiazides have been shown to increase the urinary excretion of magnesium; may decrease urinary calcium excretion. Marked hypercalcemia may be evidence of hidden hyperparathyroidism. Thiazides should be discontinued before carrying out tests for parathyroid function.

8. Increases in cholesterol and triglyceride levels may be associated with thiazide therapy.

CLIENT/FAMILY TEACHING

1. May take with or without food at the same time each day.
2. Use caution with activities that require mental alertness until drug effects realized; may experience dizziness.
3. Change positions slowly to prevent sudden drop in BP (postural hypotension).
4. Ensure adequate fluid intake; especially during high activity, excessive sweating, nausea/vomiting, or in hot weather. May experience excessive drop in BP.
5. Avoid potassium supplements unless specifically prescribed by provider.
6. Keep record of BP for provider review.
7. Report any unusual effects, changes in voiding patterns, or lack of desired response.
8. Practice reliable contraception; stop drug and report if pregnancy suspected.
9. Keep all F/U appointments to evaluate drug response, labs, and to assess adverse effects.

OUTCOMES/EVALUATE

Desired BP control

Vancomycin hydrochloride

(van-koh-**MY**-sin)

CLASSIFICATION(S):

Antibiotic, miscellaneous
PREGNANCY CATEGORY: C (B for capsules only),
Rx: Vancocin, Vancoled.

SEE ALSO *ANTI-INFECTIVE DRUGS.*

USES

PO: (1) Antibiotic-induced pseudomembranous colitis due to *Clostridium difficile.* (2) Staphylococcal enterocolitis. (3) Severe or progressive antibiotic-induced diarrhea caused by *C. difficile* that is not responsive to the causative antibiotic being discontinued; also for debilitated clients.

IV: (1) Severe staphylococcal infections in clients who have not responded to penicillins or cephalosporins, who cannot receive these drugs, or who have resistant infections. Infections include lower respiratory tract infections, bone infections, endocarditis, septicemia, and skin and skin structure infections. (2) Alone or in combination with aminoglycosides to treat endocarditis caused by *Streptococcus viridans* or *S. bovis.* Must combine with an aminoglycoside to treat endocarditis due to *Streptococcus faecalis.* (3) Used with rifampin, an aminoglycoside (or both) to treat early onset prosthetic valve endocarditis caused by *Staphylococcus epidermidis* or other diphtheroids. (4) Prophylaxis of bacterial endocarditis in penicillin-allergic clients who have congenital heart disease, or rheumatic or other acquired or valvular heart disease, if such clients are undergoing dental or surgical procedures of the upper respiratory tract. (5) The parenteral dosage form may be given PO to treat pseudomembranous colitis or staphylococcal enterocolitis due to *C. difficile.*

ACTION/KINETICS

Action

Appears to bind to bacterial cell wall, arresting its synthesis and lysing the cytoplasmic membrane by a mechanism that is different from that of penicillins and cephalosporins. May also change the permeability of the cytoplasmic membranes of bacteria, thus inhibiting RNA synthesis. Bactericidal for most organisms and bacteriostatic for enterococci.

Pharmacokinetics

Poorly absorbed from the GI tract. Diffuses in pleural, pericardial, ascetic, and synovial fluids after parenteral administration. **Peak plasma levels, IV:** 33 mcg/mL 5 min after 0.5 gram dosage. **t½, after PO:** 4–8 hr for adults and 2–3 hr for children; **t½, after IV:** 4–11 hr for adults and ranging from 2–3 hr in children to 6–10 hr for newborns. The half-life is increased markedly in the presence of renal impairment (240 hr has been noted). Primarily excreted in urine unchanged. Auditory and renal function

---

tests are indicated before and during therapy.

CONTRAINDICATIONS

Hypersensitivity. Minor infections. Lactation.

SPECIAL CONCERNS

Use with extreme caution in the presence of impaired renal function or previous hearing loss. Geriatric clients are at a greater risk of developing ototoxicity.

SIDE EFFECTS

Most Common

Ototoxicity (including tinnitus), chills, coughing, drowsiness, anorexia, N&V, weakness, sore throat, fever.

Ototoxicity (may lead to deafness; deafness may progress after drug is discontinued), *nephrotoxicity* (may lead to uremia). **Red-neck syndrome. *Sudden and profound drop in BP*** with or without a maculopapular rash over the face, neck, upper chest, and extremities. **GI:** N&V, anorexia. **CNS:** Vertigo, dizziness, drowsiness. **CV:** Exaggerated hypotension (due to rapid bolus administration), including ***shock and possibly cardiac arrest.*** **GU:** Renal failure (rare), interstitial nephritis (rare). **Respiratory:** Wheezing, dyspnea, coughing, sore throat. **Dermatologic:** Urticaria, pruritus, macular rashes, exfoliative dermatitis, ***Stevens-Johnson syndrome, toxic epidermal necrolysis***, vasculitis. **Allergic:** Drug fever, hypersensitivity, ***anaphylaxis.*** **At injection site:** Tissue irritation, including pain, tenderness, necrosis, thrombophlebitis. **Miscellaneous:** Chills, fever, tinnitus, weakness, eosinophilia, neutropenia (reversible), pseudomembranous colitis.

DRUG INTERACTIONS

Aminoglycosides / ↑ Risk of nephrotoxicity

Anesthetics / ↑ Risk of erythema and histamine-like flushing in children

Methotrexate / Possible ↑ methotrexate serum levels and markedly delayed methotrexate excretion

Muscle relaxants, nondepolarizing / ↑ Neuromuscular blockade

Nephrotoxic/Neurotoxic drugs / Carefully monitor with concurrent or sequential systemic or topical use

HOW SUPPLIED

Capsules: 125 mg, 250 mg; *Powder for Injection:* 500 mg, 1 gram, 5 grams, 10 grams; *Powder for Oral Solution:* 1 gram, 10 grams.

DOSAGE—————————

- **CAPSULES; ORAL SOLUTION**
  All PO uses.

Adults: 0.5–2 grams/day in 3–4 divided doses for 7–10 days. Alternatively, 125 mg 3–4 times per day for *C. difficile* may be as effective as the 500 mg dosage. **Children:** 40 mg/kg/day in 3–4 divided doses for 7–10 days, not to exceed 2 grams/day. **Neonates:** 10 mg/kg/day in divided doses.

- **IV**
  Severe staphylococcal infections.

Adults: 500 mg q 6 hr or 1 gram q 12 hr. **Children:** 10 mg/kg/6 hr. **Infants and neonates, initial:** 15 mg/kg for one dose; **then,** 10 mg/kg q 12 hr for neonates in the first week of life and q 8 hr thereafter up to 1 month of age.

Prophylaxis of bacterial endocarditis in dental, oral, or upper respiratory tract procedures in penicillin-allergic clients.

Adults: 1 gram vancomycin over 1 hr plus 1.5 mg/kg gentamicin (IV or IM), not to exceed 80 mg, 1 hr before the procedure. May repeat once, 8 hr after the initial dose. **Children:** 20 mg/kg vancomycin plus 2 mg/kg gentamicin (IV or IM), not to exceed 80 mg, 1 hr before the procedure. May repeat once, 8 hr after the initial dose.

NURSING CONSIDERATIONS

ADMINISTRATION/STORAGE

1. Reduce dosage in renal disease; see package insert for procedure.

2. The PO solution is prepared by adding 115 mL distilled water to the 10 gram container. The appropriate dose of PO solution may be mixed with 1 oz of water or flavored syrup to improve the taste. The diluted drug may also be given by NGT.

3. The parenteral form may be administered PO by diluting the 1-gram vial with 20 mL distilled or deionized water (each 5 mL contains about 250 mg vancomycin).

IV 4. For IV use, dilute each 500 mg vial with 10 mL of sterile water. This may be further diluted in 200 mL of dextrose or saline solution and infused over 60 min.

5. Intermittent infusion is the preferred route, but continuous IV drip may be used.

6. Avoid rapid IV administration because this may result in hypotension, nausea, warmth, and generalized tingling. Administer over 1 hr in at least 200 mL of NSS or D5W.

7. Avoid extravasation during injections; may cause tissue necrosis.

8. Reduce risk of thrombophlebitis by rotating injection sites or adding additional diluent.

9. Aqueous solution is stable for 2 weeks.

10. Once rubber stopper is punctured, ampule should be refrigerated to maintain stability.

ASSESSMENT

1. Note reasons for therapy, type, onset, characteristics of S&S, culture results.

2. Assess renal and auditory functions (including 8th CN function). Monitor for hearing loss.

3. Monitor VS, I&O, CBC, cultures, urinalysis, and renal function studies; reduce dose with renal dysfunction.

4. Systemic infections require perenteral administration where as pseudomembranous diarrhea (C. difficile) requires oral administration.

INTERVENTIONS

1. Record weight, VS, I&O; ensure adequate hydration.

2. Report adverse drug effects, such as:

- Ototoxicity, demonstrated by tinnitus, progressive hearing loss, dizziness, and/or nystagmus; may occur latently

- Nephrotoxicity, demonstrated by albuminuria, hematuria, anuria, casts, edema, and uremia

3. During IV administration ensure that peak and trough drug levels are performed at the prescribed dosing interval, usually 30 min prior to scheduled IV dose (trough) and 1 hr following IV dose (peak) to accurately assess serum levels.

CLIENT/FAMILY TEACHING

1. Complete entire course of drug therapy as prescribed otherwise infection may recur.

2. Report any fullness/ringing in ears, adverse effects, worsening of symptoms or lack of response.

3. Keep all F/U visits for drug levels and culture results.

OUTCOMES/EVALUATE

- Negative cultures
- Relief of S&S R/T infection
- Serum levels within therapeutic range (trough 1–5 mcg/mL; peak 20–50 mcg/mL)

Vardenafil hydrochloride

(var-**DE**-nah-fil)

CLASSIFICATION(S):

Drug for erectile dysfunction

PREGNANCY CATEGORY: B

Rx: Levitra.

USES

Treatment of erectile dysfunction.

ACTION/KINETICS

Action

During sexual stimulation, nitric oxide is released from nerve endings and endothelial cells in the corpus cavernosum of the penis. Nitric oxide activates the enzyme guanylate cyclase causing an increased synthesis of cyclic guanosine monophosphate (cGMP) in the smooth muscle cells of the corpus cavernosum. The cGMP in turn causes smooth muscle relaxation, allowing increased blood flow to the penis, resulting in erection. Tissue levels of cGMP are regulated by both the rate of synthesis and degradation via phosphodiesterases (PDEs). The most abundant PDE in the human corpus cavernosum is the cGMP-specific phosphodiesterase type 5 (PDE5). Thus, inhibition of PDE5 enhances erectile function by increasing the amount of cGMP. Vardenafil is a selective inhibitor of PDE5.

Pharmacokinetics
Rapidly absorbed with a bioavailability of about 15%. **Maximum plasma levels:** 30–120 min after a single 20 mg dose. Food decreases C_{max} by 18–50%. **Onset:** About 20 min; **maximum effect:** 45–90 min. **Duration:** Less than 5 hr. Eliminated primarily by hepatic metabolism by CYP3A4 and to a minor extent by CYP2C isoforms. The major metabolite, M1, is active. **t$\frac{1}{2}$, terminal:** 4–5 hr for both vardenafil and the M1 metabolite. Excreted mainly in the feces (91–95%) with a small amount in the urine (2–6%). **Plasma protein binding:** About 95%.

CONTRAINDICATIONS
Regular or intermittent use with nitrates due to potentiation of hypotensive effects of nitrates. Concomitant use with alpha-adrenergic blockers. Known hypersensitivity to vardenafil or any component of the product. Use in clients with congenital QT prolongation and those taking Class 1A (quinidine, procainamide) or Class III (amiodarone, sotalol) antiarrhythmic drugs. Use in unstable angina, hypotension, uncontrolled hypertension, recent history of stroke, life-threatening arrhythmia, MI (within the last 6 months), severe cardiac failure, severe hepatic impairment (Child-Pugh score from 10 to 15), end stage renal disease requiring dialysis, known hereditary degenerative retinal disorders (including retinitis pigmentosa).

SPECIAL CONCERNS
Use with caution in clients with bleeding disorders or active peptic ulceration, in those with anatomical deformation (e.g., angulation, cavernosal fibrosis, Peyronie's disease) of the penis, or in those who have conditions that may predispose them to priapism (e.g., sickle cell anemia, multiple myeloma, leukemia). It is not known if vardenafil is excreted into human breast milk.

SIDE EFFECTS
Most Common
Headache, dizziness, dyspepsia, nausea, diarrhea, rhinitis, sinusitis, accidental injury, back pain, flu syndrome, flushing, myalgia, rash, abnormal vision.

CNS: Headache, dizziness, hypertonia, hypesthesia, insomnia, paresthesia, somnolence, vertigo. **CV:** Hypo-/hypertension, *MI, angina pectoris*, chest pain, *myocardial ischemia*, palpitation, postural hypotension, syncope, tachycardia. **GI:** Dyspepsia, N&V, abdominal pain, diarrhea, dry mouth, dysphagia, esophagitis, gastritis, gastroesophageal reflux. **Body as a whole:** Flu syndrome, asthenia, pain, *anaphylaxis (including laryngeal edema)*. **Musculoskeletal:** Arthralgia, back pain, myalgia, neck pain. **Respiratory:** Rhinitis, sinusitis, dyspnea, epistaxis, pharyngitis. **Dermatologic:** Flushing, photosensitivity reaction, pruritus, rash, sweating. **GU:** Abnormal ejaculation, priapism (including prolonged or painful erections). **Ophthalmic:** Abnormal/decreased/blurred vision, sudden vision loss, chromatopsia, changes in color vision, conjunctivitis, dim vision, eye pain, glaucoma, photophobia, watery eyes. **Miscellaneous** Accidental injury, tinnitus.

LABORATORY TEST CONSIDERATIONS
↑ Creatine kinase, GGTP. Abnormal LFTs.

DRUG INTERACTIONS
Alcohol (substantial consumption) / ↓ BP, postural dizziness, and orthostatic hypotension
Alpha-adrenergic blockers / ↑ Risk of significant hypotension
Erythromycin / ↑ Vardenafil levels R/T ↓ metabolism by CYP3A4
Indinavir / ↑ Vardenafil levels R/T ↓ liver metabolism
Itraconazole / ↑ Vardenafil levels R/T ↓ liver metabolism by CYP3A4
Ketoconazole / ↑ Vardenafil levels R/T ↓ liver metabolism by CYP3A4
Nifedipine / Additional ↓ BP
Nitrates / Sudden, severe ↓ in BP → dizziness, syncope, heart attack, stroke; do not use together
Ritonavir / ↑ Vardenafil levels R/T ↓ liver metabolism

HOW SUPPLIED
Tablets: 2.5 mg, 5 mg, 10 mg, 20 mg.

DOSAGE————————————
• **TABLETS**

   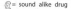

Erectile dysfunction.
Adults, initial: 10 mg about 60 min before sexual activity. Dose may be increased to 20 mg or decreased to 5 mg based on efficacy and side effects. Maximum recommended dosing is once a day. An initial dose of 5 mg should be considered in clients 65 years and older and in those with moderate hepatic impairment.

NURSING CONSIDERATIONS
ADMINISTRATION/STORAGE
1. The initial dose in those with moderate hepatic impairment (Child-Pugh score from 7 to 9) is 5 mg; the maximum dose in those with moderate hepatic impairment should not exceed 10 mg.
2. A single dose of 2.5 mg should not be exceeded in clients taking indinavir or ritonavir. No more than a single 2.5 mg dose should be taken in a 72-hr period in those taking ritonavir.
3. A dose of 2.5 mg daily should not be exceeded in those taking ketoconazole, 400 mg/day, or itraconazole, 400 mg/day. A dose of 5 mg daily should not be exceeded in those taking ketoconazole, 200 mg/day, or itraconazole, 200 mg/day.
4. Can be taken with or without food.
5. Sexual stimulation is required for a response to treatment.
6. Store from 15–30°C (59–86°F).
ASSESSMENT
1. Note onset and cause of erectile dysfunction, i.e., organic, psychogenic, or combined.
2. Assess cardiovascular status and obtain ECG. List drugs prescribed as some may potentiate drug effects.
3. Ensure client aware of potential for visual changes or loss.
4. Note any conditions that may predispose client to priapism, i.e., multiple myelomas, sickle cell anemia, or leukemia.
5. Assess for any anatomical deformation of penis (Peyronie's disease, angulation, or cavernosal fibrosis).
CLIENT/FAMILY TEACHING
1. Take only as directed one hour before anticipated act. Plan some form of

sexual stimulation after ingestion to ensure desired erection obtained.
2. Report all medications currently prescribed to ensure none alter effects. Avoid nitrates and alpha blocking drugs. Stop smoking; may inhibit drug effect.
3. Practice safe sex; drug does not prevent disease transmission.
4. May experience headache, flushing, upset stomach, stuffy nose, dizziness (from drop in BP) drowsiness, or abnormal vision (especially blue/green color discrimination); report any unusual, persistent or bothersome effects.
5. Do not use any other agent for erections with this therapy. Effects may be evident the day after therapy; assess before taking additional drug. Do not use more than once a day. Erections lasting more than 4 hr or painful erections lasting more than 6 hr require immediate ER care; penile damage may result.
6. Do not share medications or prescriptions due to potential for adverse interactions/effects. *Never* use this drug if currently taking nitrates in any form. May be fatal.
OUTCOMES/EVALUATE
Relief of erectile dysfunction; desired erection

Varenicline tartrate
(var-**EN**-ih-kline)

CLASSIFICATION(S):
Smoking deterrent
PREGNANCY CATEGORY: C
Rx: Chantix.

USES
Aid to smoking cessation treatment.

ACTION/KINETICS
Action
Varenicline binds with high affinity and selectivity at α4β2 neuronal nicotinic acetylcholine receptors. The effectiveness in smoking cessation is thought to be due to the drug preventing nicotine from binding to α4β2 receptors. Thus, nicotine cannot stimulate the central

---

nervous mesolimbic dopamine system, believed to be the neuronal mechanism underlying reinforcement and reward experienced by smoking.

Pharmacokinetics
Maximum plasma levels: 3–4 hr. **Steady state levels:** 4 days. Oral bioavailability is not affected by food. **t½, elimination:** 24 hr. Undergoes minimal metabolism with 92% excreted unchanged in the urine. **Plasma protein binding:** 20% or less is bound to plasma proteins.

CONTRAINDICATIONS
Lactation.

SPECIAL CONCERNS
Due to decreased renal function in the elderly, use care in dose selection; consider monitoring renal function. Safety and efficacy have not been determined in children younger than 18 years of age.

SIDE EFFECTS
Most Common
N&V, sleep disturbances, constipation, flatulence, headache, insomnia, abnormal dreams, dysgeusia, upper respiratory tract disorder, hypertension, hyperhidrosis.

CNS: Headache, insomnia, abnormal/frightening dreams, somnolence, lethargy, nightmares, sleep disorder, anxiety, depression, attention disturbances, dizziness, emotional disorder, irritability, restlessness, sensory disturbances, aggression, agitation, amnesia, disorientation, dissociation, decreased libido, migraine, mood swings, parosmia, psychomotor hyperactivity, restless legs syndrome, syncope, abnormal thinking, tremor, balance disorder, bradyphrenia, convulsions, dysarthria, euphoria, facial palsy, hallucinations, mental impairment, multiple sclerosis, impaired psychomotor skills, psychotic disorder *suicidal ideation, suicide*. **GI:** N&V, flatulence, dysgeusia, abdominal pain, constipation, dyspepsia, dry mouth, diarrhea, gingivitis, dysphagia, enterocolitis, eructation, esophagitis, gastritis, *GI hemorrhage,* mouth ulceration, gastric ulcer, intestinal obstruction, gallbladder disorder, *acute pancreatitis*. **CV:** Hypertension, angina pectoris, arrhythmia, bradycardia, hypotension, *MI*, palpitations, peripheral ischemia, tachycardia, *thrombosis*, ventricular extrasystoles, acute coronary syndrome, atrial fibrillation, cardiac flutter, coronary artery disease, cor pulmonale, transient ischemic attack, *CVA*. **Dermatological:** Rash, pruritus, hyperhidrosis, acne, dermatitis, dry skin, eczema, erythema, psoriasis, urticaria, photosensitivity reaction, hot flush. **Respiratory:** Upper respiratory tract disorder, dyspnea, rhinorrhea, epsitaxis, respiratory disorder, asthma, pleurisy, *pulmonary embolism*. **GU:** Menstrual disorder, polyuria, erectile dysfunction, nephrolithiasis, nocturia, urethral syndrome, urine abnormality, sexual dysfunction, urinary retention, acute renal failure. **Musculoskeletal:** Arthralgia, back pain, muscle cramps, musculoskeletal pain, myalgia, arthritis, osteoporosis, myositis, chest pain. **Hematologic:** Anemia, lymphadenopathy, leukocytosis, splenomegaly, thrombocytopenia. **Metabolic:** Decreased/increased appetite, anorexia, increased weight, diabetes mellitus. **Ophthalmic:** Conjunctivitis, dry eye, eye irritation/pain, blurred vision, acquired night blindness, transient blindness, subcapsular cataract, ocular vascular disorder, photophobia, vitreous floaters, nystatmus, visual field defect. **Otic:** Tinnitus, deafness, Meniere syndrome. **Body as a whole:** Fatigue, malaise, asthenia, edema, flu-like illness. **Miscellaneous:** Thyroid gland disorders, vertigo, thirst, chills, pyrexia, chest discomfort, hypersensitivity, drug hypersensitivity.

DRUG INTERACTIONS
Cimetidine / ↑ Varenicline exposure by 29% R/T ↓ renal clearance
Nicotine transdermal / ↑ Incidence of N&V, headache, dizziness, dyspepsia, and fatigue

HOW SUPPLIED
Tablets: 0.5 mg (as base), 1 mg (as base).

DOSAGE
• **TABLETS**
Aid to smoking cessation.
Dosage titration, Days 1–3: 0.5 mg once a day; **days 4–7:** 0.5 mg twice a day. **Day 8 through end of treatment:** 1 mg twice a day. Treat clients for 12

 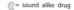

weeks. For those who have successfully stopped smoking at the end of 12 weeks, an additional course of 12 weeks is recommended to increase further the likelihood of long-term abstinence.

NURSING CONSIDERATIONS
ADMINISTRATION/STORAGE
1. Those who cannot tolerate the side effects may have the dose lowered temporarily or permanently.
2. Clients who do not stop smoking during 12 weeks of initial therapy, or who relapse after treatment should be encouraged to make another attempt after identifying and addressing the factors that contributed to the failed attempt.
3. For clients with severe impaired renal function, the recommended initial dose is 0.5 mg once a day. Then titrate as needed to a maximum of 0.5 mg twice a day. For those with end-stage renal disease undergoing hemodialysis, a maximum dosage of 0.5 mg once a day may be given if well tolerated.
4. Store from 15–30°C (59–86°F).

ASSESSMENT
1. Note smoking history, other attempts to quit, activities that trigger desire to smoke.
2. Monitor renal and LFTs; reduce dose with renal dysfunction. Use with caution in the elderly; may be more sensitive to its effects.
3. List all drugs prescribed (eg, theophylline, warfarin, insulin); drug may affect their actions/side effects. May require dosage adjustment.

CLIENT/FAMILY TEACHING
1. Drug works in the brain to block the pleasurable effects of smoking. This helps to decrease your desire to smoke.
2. Set a date to stop smoking. Start varenicline dosing one week before this date.
3. Take after eating and with a full glass of water (8 oz/240 mL).
4. Even if you smoke after your quit date, continue to try to quit. If you miss a dose do not take 2 doses at once.
5. May cause drowsiness or dizziness; may be worse with alcohol or certain medicines. Do not drive or perform activities that require mental alertness until drug effects realized.
6. Do not stop drug suddenly; may cause increased irritability or difficulty sleeping.
7. May experience nausea and insomnia; report if persistent as a dose reduction may be considered.
8. Review provided educational materials and attend counseling to support attempt to quit smoking.
9. Practice reliable contraception. Report if pregnancy suspected.
10. Keep all F/U appointments to evaluate response to therapy and adverse side effects.

OUTCOMES/EVALUATE
• Smoking cessation
• Loss of desire to smoke

Vasopressin
(vay-so-**PRESS**-in)

CLASSIFICATION(S):
Pituitary hormone
PREGNANCY CATEGORY: C
Rx: Pitressin.
♣Rx: Pressyn.

USES
(1) Neurogenic (central) diabetes insipidus (ineffective when diabetes insipidus is of renal origin—nephrogenic diabetes insipidus). (2) Prevention and treatment of postoperative abdominal distention. (3) Dispel interfering gas shadows in abdominal roentgenography. *Investigational:* Acute variceal hemorrhage, treat refractory septic shock (low doses), treat ventricular fibrillation/pulseless ventricular tachycardia, cardiac arrest.

ACTION/KINETICS
Action
Released from the anterior pituitary gland; regulates water conservation by promoting reabsorption of water by increasing the permeability of the collecting ducts in the kidney. Depending on the concentration, the hormone acts directly on both V_1 and V_2 receptors. Also causes contraction of smooth muscle of

---
Bold Italic = life threatening side effect   ■ = black box warning   ♣ = Available in Canada

the GI tract and all parts of the vascular system, especially the capillaries, small arterioles, and venules; has less effect on the small muscle of large veins. Also increases the smooth muscular activity of the bladder, GI tract, and uterus. The direct effect is not antagonized by adrenergic blockers or by vascular denervation.

Pharmacokinetics

Onset, IM, SC: variable; **duration,** 2–8 hr. **t½:** 10–20 min. **Effective plasma levels:** 4.5–6 microunits. Most is metabolized and rapidly destroyed by the kidneys and liver. About 5% excreted unchanged in the urine after 4 hr.

CONTRAINDICATIONS

Anaphylaxis or hypersensitivity to vasopressin or any component of the product. Vascular disease, especially when involving coronary arteries; angina pectoris. Chronic nephritis until reasonable blood nitrogen levels are attained.

SPECIAL CONCERNS

Pediatric and geriatric clients have an increased risk of hyponatremia and water intoxication. Use caution during lactation and in the presence of asthma, epilepsy, migraine, and CHF. Use with extreme caution in CAD as even small doses may precipitate anginal pain and larger doses may cause a MI.

SIDE EFFECTS

Most Common

Nausea, diarrhea, flatulence, pale-colored lips, stomach pain, headache, tremors, abdominal cramps, sweating.

GI: N&V, increased intestinal activity (e.g., belching, cramps, urge to defecate), diarrhea, abdominal cramps, flatulence. **CV:** Circumoral pallor, arrhythmias, decreased cardiac output, *cardiac arrest*, angina, *myocardial ischemia*, peripheral vasoconstriction, gangrene. **CNS:** Tremor, headache, vertigo, 'pounding' in head. **Dermatologic:** Sweating, urticaria, skin blanching, pale-colored lips, cutaneous gangrene. **Miscellaneous:** Tremor, *allergic/hypersensitivity reactions, bronchoconstriction, anaphylaxis, water intoxication* (drowsiness, listlessness, headache, *coma, convulsions*). *NOTE:* Use of vasopressin may result in severe vasocon-

striction and local tissue necrosis if extravasation occurs.

OD **OVERDOSE MANAGEMENT**

Symptoms: Water intoxication. *Treatment:* Withdraw vasopressin until polyuria occurs. If water intoxication is serious, administration of mannitol (i.e., an osmotic diuretic), hypertonic dextrose, or urea alone (or with furosemide) is indicated.

DRUG INTERACTIONS

Alcohol / May decrease antidiuretic effect of vasopressin

Carbamazepine / May potentiate antidiuretic effect of vasopressin

Chlorpropamide / May potentiate antidiuretic effect of vasopressin

Clofibrate / May potentiate antidiuretic effect of vasopressin

Demeclocycline / May decrease antidiuretic effect of vasopressin

Fludrocortisone / May potentiate antidiuretic effect of vasopressin

Ganglionic blocking drugs / May ↑ significantly sensitivity to pressor effects of vasopressin

Heparin / May decrease antidiuretic effect of vasopressin

Lithium / May decrease antidiuretic effect of vasopressin

Norepinephrine / May decrease antidiuretic effect of vasopressin

Tricyclic antidepressants / May potentiate antidiuretic effect of vasopressin

HOW SUPPLIED

Injection: 20 pressor units/mL.

DOSAGE

• **IM; SC**

  Diabetes insipidus.

Adults: 5–10 units 2–3 times per day as needed; **pediatric:** 2.5–10 units 3–4 times per day

  Abdominal distention.

Adults, initial: 5 units IM; **then,** 10 units IM q 3–4 hr; **pediatric:** individualize the dose (usual: 2.5–5 units).

  Abdominal roentgenography.

IM, SC: 2 injections of 10 units every 2 hr and ½ hr before x-rays are taken.

  Esophageal varices.

Initial: 0.2 units/min IV or selective IA; **then,** 0.4 units/min if bleeding continues. The maximum recommended dose is 0.9 units/min.

 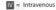

- **INTRANASAL (USING INJECTION SOLUTION)**

Diabetes insipidus.

Individualize the dose using the injection solution on cotton pledgets, by nasal spray, or by dropper.

NURSING CONSIDERATIONS

ADMINISTRATION/STORAGE

1. Administration of 1–2 glasses of water prior to use for diabetes insipidus will reduce side effects such as nausea, cramps, and skin blanching.
2. An enema may be given prior to the first dose when used for abdominal roentgenography.

ASSESSMENT

1. Note reasons for therapy, type, onset, characteristics of S&S.
2. Identify any vascular disease, esp. involving the coronary arteries (e.g., hypertension, CHF, CAD).
3. List any asthma, seizures, or migraine headaches. Assess closely for water intoxication to prevent seizures and coma.

INTERVENTIONS

1. Check skin turgor, mucous membranes, and presence of thirst to assess for dehydration.
2. Monitor BP and I&O; report any excessive BP elevation or lack of response characterized by a ↓ BP.
3. Record weight daily and assess for edema; report rapid gains.
4. Perform urine specific gravity and report if <1.005 or >1.030. Determine urine osmolarity.
5. With abdominal distention, assess/document presence/characteristics of bowel sounds and passage of flatus/stool. A rectal tube may facilitate expulsion of gas.
6. Injection solution may be used as nasal spray or used in a dropper or applied to cotton pledgets for topical administration.

CLIENT/FAMILY TEACHING

1. Lack of vasopressin causes your body to lose too much water.
2. Review appropriate method for administration/instillation. Rotate sites with SC injections. Take with 16 oz water to prevent N&V and cramps.
3. With nasal therapy, insert tube into nasal cavity to administer drug. Follow provider guidelines for administration.
4. Avoid alcohol and OTC agents without approval.
5. Keep a record of intake and output. Report any adverse side effects immediately.

OUTCOMES/EVALUATE

- Prevention of dehydration: ↓ urinary output/osmolarity
- Control of intra-arterial bleeding
- ↓ Abdominal distention/discomfort; elimination of intestinal gas

Vecuronium bromide
(veh-kyour-**OH**-nee-um)

■ **IV**

CLASSIFICATION(S):
Neuromuscular blocking drug, nondepolarizing
PREGNANCY CATEGORY: C
Rx: Norcuron.

SEE ALSO NEUROMUSCULAR BLOCKING AGENTS.

USES
(1) Induce skeletal muscle relaxation during surgery or mechanical ventilation. (2) Facilitate ET intubation. (3) Adjunct to general anesthesia. *Investigational:* To treat electrically induced seizures or seizures induced by drugs.

ACTION/KINETICS

Action
Less likely than other agents to cause histamine release. Effects can be antagonized by anticholinesterase drugs.

Pharmacokinetics
Onset: 2.5–3 min; **peak effect:** 3–5 min; **duration:** 25–40 min using balanced anesthesia. About one-third more potent than pancuronium, but its duration of action is shorter at initial equipotent doses. No cumulative effects noted after repeated administration. **t½, elimination:** 65–75 min; a shortened half-life (35–40 min) has been noted in late pregnancy. Metabolized in liver and excreted through the kidneys and bile. Recovery may be doubled in clients

with cirrhosis or cholestasis; renal failure does not affect recovery time. **Plasma protein binding:** 60–80%.

ADDITIONAL CONTRAINDICATIONS
Use in neonates, obesity. Sensitivity to bromides.

SPECIAL CONCERNS
■ Do not administer unless facilities for intubation, artificial respiration, oxygen therapy, and reversal agents are immediately available. Be prepared to assist or control respiration.■ Those from 7 weeks to 1 year of age are more sensitive to the effects of vecuronium leading to a recovery time up to 1½ times that for adults. The dose for children aged 1–10 years of age must be individualized and may, in fact, require a somewhat higher initial dose and a slightly more frequent supplemental dosing schedule than adults. Those with myasthenia gravis or Eaton-Lambert syndrome may experience profound effects with small doses of vecuronium. Cardiovascular disease, old age, and edematous states result in increased volume of distribution and thus a delay in onset time—the dose should *not* be increased.

SIDE EFFECTS
Most Common
Skin flushing, itching, skeletal muscle weakness, wheezing, bronchial secretions, hives, increased HR, increased mean arterial pressure.
See *Neuromuscular Blocking Agents* for a complete list of possible side effects. Also, moderate to severe skeletal muscle weakness, which may require artificial respiration. *Malignant hyperthermia.*

ADDITIONAL DRUG INTERACTIONS
Bacitracin / High IV or IP bacitracin doses → ↑ muscle relaxation
Sodium colistimethate / High IV or IP sodium colistimethate doses → ↑ muscle relaxation
Tetracyclines / High IV or IP tetracycline doses → ↑ muscle relaxation
Succinylcholine / ↑ Vecuronium effect

HOW SUPPLIED
Powder for Injection: 10 mg, 20 mg.

DOSAGE————————
• **IV**

Intubation.
Adults and children over 10 years of age. 0.08–0.1 mg/kg.
For use after succinylcholine-assisted ET intubation.
0.04–0.06 mg/kg for inhalation anesthesia and 0.05–0.06 mg/kg using balanced anesthesia. *NOTE:* For halothane anesthesia, doses of 0.15–0.28 mg/kg may be given without adverse effects.
For use during anesthesia with enflurane or isoflurane after steady state established.
0.06–0.085 mg/kg (about 15% less than the usual initial dose).
Supplemental use.
IV only: 0.01–0.015 mg/kg given 25–40 min following the initial dose; **then,** given q 12–15 min as needed. **IV infusion:** Initiated after recovery from effects of initial IV dose of 0.08–0.1 mg/kg has started. **Initial:** 0.001 mcg; **then** adjust according to client response and requirements. Average infusion rate: 0.0008–0.0012 mg/kg/min (0.8–1.2 mcg/kg/min). After steady-state enflurane, isoflurane, and possibly halothane anesthesia has been established; reduce IV infusion by 25–60%.

NURSING CONSIDERATIONS

ADMINISTRATION/STORAGE

1. Dosage must be individualized and depends on prior or concomitant use of anesthetics or succinylcholine.
2. May be mixed with saline, D5W alone or with saline, RL solution, and sterile water for injection.
3. Refrigerate after reconstitution. Use within 8 hr of reconstitution.
4. Have neostigmine, pyridostigmine, or edrophonium available to reverse vecuronium; atropine helps counteract muscarinic effects.

ASSESSMENT
1. Note reasons for therapy, anticipated time frame for use.
2. Monitor ECG, VS, CBC, electrolytes, renal, LFTs, and lung assessments.
3. Use a nerve stimulator to determine neuromuscular blockade and muscle strength recovery. Anticholinesterase will reverse neuromuscular blockade

 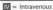

but should not be used until some evidence of spontaneous recovery noted.

INTERVENTIONS

1. Monitor VS and ECG. Can cause vagal stimulation resulting in bradycardia, hypotension, and cardiac arrhythmias.

2. Muscle fasciculations may cause soreness or injury after recovery. Give prescribed nondepolarizing agent and reassure that soreness is likely caused by unsynchronized contractions of adjacent muscle fibers just before onset of paralysis.

3. Monitor closely for any evidence of malignant hyperthermia, unresponsive tachycardia, jaw spasm, or lack of laryngeal relaxation. Stop infusion and report; temperature elevations are late S&S.

4. Drug should only be used on a short-term basis and in a continuously monitored environment.

5. Client is fully conscious and aware of surroundings and conversations. Drug does not affect pain or anxiety; give analgesics and antianxiety agents.

6. Prolonged use, as in an ICU setting, may lead to skeletal muscle weakness and symptoms consistent with muscle disuse atrophy. This may complicate ventilator weaning; some may require extensive physical therapy.

CLIENT/FAMILY TEACHING

1. Reassure that the client will be able to move arms and legs and walk and talk once therapy is discontinued.

2. Reassure the client will be carefully monitored during therapy and medicated for pain and anxiety.

3. Explain all tests and procedures and care to be performed.

OUTCOMES/EVALUATE

- Skeletal muscle relaxation
- Facilitation of intubation; tolerance of mechanical ventilation

Venlafaxine hydrochloride ■ 📷
(ven-lah-**FAX**-een)

CLASSIFICATION(S):
Antidepressant, miscellaneous
PREGNANCY CATEGORY: C
Rx: Effexor, Effexor XR.

USES
(1) Major depressive disorder. (2) Treatment of generalized anxiety disorder. (3) Treatment of social anxiety disorder (social phobia). Use extended-release product. (4) Adults with panic disorder. *Investigational:* Hot flashes. Premenstrual dysphoric disorder. Posttraumatic stress disorder (after no response with a selective serotonin reuptake inhibitor for 8 weeks).

ACTION/KINETICS

Action
Not related chemically to any of the currently available antidepressants. A potent inhibitor of the uptake of neuronal serotonin and norepinephrine in the CNS and a weak inhibitor of the uptake of dopamine. Has no anticholinergic, sedative, or orthostatic hypotensive effects.

Pharmacokinetics
Well absorbed (92%); absolute bioavailability is about 45%. Metabolized in the liver by CYP2D6 and CYP3A4. The major metabolite—O-desmethylvenlafaxine (ODV)—is active. The drug and metabolite are eliminated through the kidneys. $t^{1/2}$, **venlafaxine:** 5 hr; $t^{1/2}$, **ODV:** 11 hr. **Time to reach steady state:** 3–4 days. The half-life of the drug and metabolite are increased in clients with impaired liver or renal function. Food has no effect on the absorption of venlafaxine.

CONTRAINDICATIONS
Use with a MAO inhibitor or within 14 days of discontinuation of a MAO inhibitor. Use of alcohol. Lactation.

SPECIAL CONCERNS
■ (1) Antidepressants increased the risk of suicidal thinking and behavior (suicidality) in short-term studies in children

---

Bold Italic = life threatening side effect   ■ = black box warning   ✦ = Available in Canada

and adolescents with major depressive disorder and other psychiatric disorders. Anyone considering the use of venlafaxine or any other antidepressant in a child or adolescent must balance this risk with the clinical need. Clients who are started on therapy should be observed closely for clinical worsening, suicidality, or unusual changes in behavior. Families and caregivers should be advised of the need for close observation and communication with the prescriber. Venlafaxine is not approved for use in pediatric clients with major depressive disorder and obsessive-compulsive disorder. (2) Short-term placebo-controlled trials of 9 antidepressant drugs in children and adolescents with major depressive disorder, obsessive-compulsive disorder, or other psychiatric disorders revealed a greater risk of adverse reactions during the first few months of treatment. The average risk of such reactions in clients receiving antidepressants was 4%, twice the placebo risk of 2%. No suicides occurred in these trials.■ Use with caution with impaired hepatic (e.g., cirrhosis) or renal (GFR = 10–70 mL/min) function, in clients with a history of mania, and in those with diseases or conditions that could affect the hemodynamic responses or metabolism. Although it is possible for a geriatric client to be more sensitive, dosage adjustment is not necessary. Clinical worsening and suicide risk is possible in both adult and pediatric clients with major depressive disorder. Use for more than 4–6 weeks has not been evaluated. Safety and efficacy of the immediate-release product have not been determined in children less than 18 years of age. Safety and efficacy of the sustained-release product have not been established in children. Infants exposed to venlafaxine during the third trimester of pregnancy may develop complications requiring prolonged hospitalization, respiratory support, and tube feeding; carefully consider the potential risks and benefits of treatment and consider tapering the medication in the third trimester.

SIDE EFFECTS
Most Common
Nausea, headache, somnolence, dizziness, insomnia, nervousness, constipation, asthenia, dry mouth, abnormal ejaculation/orgasm, sweating.

Side effects with an incidence of 0.1% or greater are listed. **CNS:** Anxiety, nervousness, insomnia, mania, hypomania, *seizures, suicide attempts*, dizziness, somnolence, tremors, abnormal dreams, hypertonia, paresthesia, decreased libido, agitation, confusion, abnormal thinking, depersonalization, depression, twitching, migraine, emotional lability, trismus, vertigo, apathy, ataxia, circumoral paresthesia, CNS stimulation, euphoria, hallucinations, hostility, hyperesthesia, hyperkinesia, hyper-/hypotonia, incoordination, increased libido, myoclonus, neuralgia, neuropathy, paranoid reaction, psychosis, psychotic depression, sleep disturbance, abnormal speech, stupor, torticollis. **CV:** Sustained increase in BP (hypertension), vasodilation, tachycardia, postural hypotension, angina pectoris, extrasystoles, hypotension, arrhythmia, peripheral vascular disorder, syncope, thrombophlebitis, peripheral edema. **GI:** Anorexia, N&V, dry mouth, constipation, diarrhea, dyspepsia, flatulence, dysphagia, eructation, colitis, edema of tongue, esophagitis, gastroenteritis, gastritis, bruxism, glossitis, gingivitis, hemorrhoids, *rectal hemorrhage*, melena, stomatitis, stomach ulcer, mouth ulceration. **Body as a whole:** Headache, asthenia, infection, chills, chest pain, trauma, yawn, weight loss, accidental injury, malaise, neck pain, enlarged abdomen, allergic reaction, cyst, facial edema, generalized edema, hangover effect, hernia, intentional injury, neck rigidity, moniliasis, substernal chest pain, pelvic pain, photosensitivity reaction. **Respiratory:** Bronchitis, dyspnea, asthma, chest congestion, epistaxis, hyperventilation, laryngismus, laryngitis, pneumonia, voice alteration, pharyngitis. **Dermatologic:** Acne, alopecia, brittle nails, contact dermatitis, dry skin, herpes simplex, herpes zoster, maculopapular rash, urticaria. **Hematologic:**

Ecchymosis, anemia, leukocytosis, leukopenia, lymphadenopathy, lymphocytosis, thrombocytopenia, thrombocythemia, abnormal WBCs. **Endocrine:** Hypothyroidism, hyperthyroidism, goiter. **Musculoskeletal:** Arthritis, arthrosis, bone pain, bone spurs, bursitis, joint disorder, myasthenia, tenosynovitis. **Ophthalmic:** Blurred vision, mydriasis, abnormal accommodation, abnormal vision, cataract, conjunctivitis, corneal lesion, diplopia, dry eyes, exophthalmos, eye pain, photophobia, subconjunctival hemorrhage, visual field defect. **GU:** Urinary retention, abnormal ejaculation, impotence, urinary frequency, impaired urination, disturbed orgasm, menstrual disorder, anorgasmia (female), dysuria, hematuria, metrorrhagia, vaginitis, amenorrhea, kidney calculus, cystitis, leukorrhea, menorrhagia, nocturia, bladder pain, breast pain, kidney pain, polyuria, prostatitis, pyelonephritis, pyuria, urinary incontinence, urinary urgency, enlarged uterine fibroids, **uterine hemorrhage, vaginal hemorrhage,** vaginal moniliasis. **Miscellaneous:** Sweating, tinnitus, taste perversion, thirst, diabetes mellitus, alcohol intolerance, gout, hypoglycemic reaction, hemochromatosis, ear pain, otitis media. Possible changes in height of children.

LABORATORY TEST CONSIDERATIONS
↑ Alkaline phosphatase, creatinine, AST, ALT. Glycosuria, hyperglycemia, hyperlipemia, bilirubinemia, hyperuricemia, hypercholesterolemia, hypoglycemia, hypo-/hyperkalemia, hyponatremia, hypophosphatemia, hypoproteinemia, uremia, albuminuria.

OD OVERDOSE MANAGEMENT
Symptoms: Extensions of side effects, especially somnolence. Other symptoms include prolongation of QTc, mild sinus tachycardia, and **seizures.** *Treatment:* General supportive measures; treat symptoms. Ensure an adequate airway, oxygenation, and ventilation. Monitor cardiac rhythm and VS. Activated charcoal, induction of emesis, or gastric lavage may be helpful.

DRUG INTERACTIONS
Cimetidine / ↓ First-pass metabolism of venlafaxine
Clozapine / Possible ↑ Clozapine levels → side effects (including seizures)
Cyproheptadine / ↓ Pharmacologic effects of venlafaxine
Desipramine / ↑ Desipramine AUC, C_{max}, and C_{min}
Haloperidol / ↑ Serum AUC and C_{max}
Indinavir / ↓ Indinavir AUC and C_{max}; clinical significance unknown
MAO inhibitors / Serious and possibly fatal reaction, including hyperthermia, rigidity, myoclonus, autonomic instability with rapid changes in VS, extreme agitation, delirium, coma; *do not use together.*
H *St. John's wort* / Possible 'serotonin syndrome,' including shivering, irritability, myoclonus, ↑ muscle tone, and altered consciousness
Sibutramine / Possible 'serotonin syndrome,' including shivering, irritability, myoclonus, ↑ muscle tone, and altered consciousness
Sumatriptan / Possible 'serotonin syndrome,' including shivering, irritability, myoclonus, ↑ muscle tone, and altered consciousness
Trazodone / Possible 'serotonin syndrome,' including shivering, irritability, myoclonus, ↑ muscle tone, and altered consciousness
Warfarin / Possible ↑ PT, PTT, INR

HOW SUPPLIED
Capsules, Extended-Release: 37.5 mg, 75 mg, 150 mg; *Tablets, Immediate-Release:* 25 mg, 37.5 mg, 50 mg, 75 mg, 100 mg.

DOSAGE
- **TABLETS, IMMEDIATE-RELEASE**
  Major depressive disorder.
Adults, initial: 75 mg/day given in two or three divided doses. Depending on the response, the dose can be increased to 150–225 mg/day in divided doses. Make dosage increments up to 75 mg/day at intervals of 4 or more days. Severely depressed clients may require 375 mg/day in divided doses. **Maintenance:** Periodically assess client to determine the need for maintenance treatment and the appropriate dose.
- **CAPSULES, EXTENDED-RELEASE**

Bold Italic = life threatening side effect   ■ = black box warning   ✦ = Available in Canada

Major depressive disorder.
Adults, initial: 75 mg as a single dose once daily in the morning or evening at about the same time each day. For some clients it may be desirable to start at 37.5 mg/day for 4–7 days to allow adjustment to the drug before increasing to 75 mg/day. Dose can be increased by up to 75 mg no more often than every 4 days, to a maximum of 225 mg/day.

Generalized/social anxiety disorder.
Initial, usual: 75 mg/day as a single dose; if necessary, the dose may be increased to 225 mg/day. Increase in increments of up to 75 mg/day at intervals of not less than 4 days. To avoid overstimulation, some may need to start with 37.5 mg/day. Take on a daily basis not on an as-needed basis. **Maintenance:** Periodically reassess the need for continuing the medication.

Hot flushes in otherwise healthy postmenopausal women.
75 mg/day.

NURSING CONSIDERATIONS

ADMINISTRATION/STORAGE
1. Take with food.
2. If switching from the immediate-release to extended-release, use the dosage form at the nearest equivalent dose. Individual dosage adjustments may be needed.
3. Reduce dose by at least 50% in those with severe hepatic impairment; further dose reduction may be needed. Reduce dose by 50% with moderate hepatic impairment and by 25–50% with mild to moderate renal impairment.
4. When discontinuing after 1 week or more of therapy, taper dose to minimize risk of withdrawal syndrome. If drug has been taken for 6 weeks or more, taper dose gradually over a 2-week period.
5. At least 14 days should elapse between discontinuation of a MAO inhibitor and initiation of venlafaxine therapy; at least 7 days should elapse after stopping venlafaxine before starting a MAO inhibitor.

6. Take extended-release form in the morning or evening, but at the same time each day.
7. Abrupt discontinuation or dose reduction of venlafaxine (at various doses) may be associated with the appearance of new symptoms (frequency increased with increased dose level and with longer duration of treatment). Symptoms include agitation, anorexia, anxiety, confusion, impaired coordination, diarrhea, dizziness, dry mouth, dysphoric mood, fasciculation, fatigue, headaches, hypomania, insomnia, nausea, nervousness, nightmares, sensory disturbances (including shock-like electrical sensations), somnolence, sweating, tremor, vertigo, and vomiting.

ASSESSMENT
1. List reasons for therapy, onset, characteristics of S&S, mental status, clinical presentation. Note other agents trialed, outcome.
2. List agents prescribed to ensure none interact.
3. Monitor VS, weight, CBC, lipid panel, renal and LFTs; reduce dose with hepatic/renal impairment.
4. May cause sustained hypertension; monitor HR and BP.
5. Prior to beginning treatment with an antidepressant, adequately screen clients with depressive symptoms to determine if they are at risk for bipolar disorder may cause a mixed/manic episode.

CLIENT/FAMILY TEACHING
1. Do not chew or crush extended-release tablets; swallow whole. Take with food either in the morning or evening at approximately the same time each day. The contents of the capsule may be sprinkled on applesauce and promptly consumed without chewing and followed with a glass of water to ensure complete swallowing of the pellets. Drug may impair appetite and induce weight loss; report if excessive.
2. Take only as directed; *do not* stop abruptly if used for 6 weeks or more— may cause withdrawal syndrome. Taper over a two week period.
3. Do not perform activities that require mental alertness until drug effects

realized; may cause dizziness or drowsiness. Avoid alcohol and any unprescribed or OTC preparations.

4. Report any rash, hives, or other allergic manifestations immediately. May experience anxiety, palpitations, headaches, and constipation; report if persistent or intolerable.

5. Use reliable contraception. Notify provider if pregnant or intend to become pregnant while taking drug.

6. Any suicide ideations or abnormal behaviors should be reported. Due to the possibility of suicide, high-risk clients should be observed closely during initial therapy. Prescriptions should be written for the smallest quantity to reduce the risk of overdose. Family should supervise medication administration with severely depressed clients.

7. May take several weeks to notice any improvement in symptoms; report if no improvement or if symptoms worsen or if intolerable side effects experienced.

OUTCOMES/EVALUATE
- Improvement in symptoms of depression
- ↓ Hot flashes with menopause
- Control of anxiety

Verapamil   Ⅳ ©
(ver-**AP**-ah-mil)

CLASSIFICATION(S):
Calcium channel blocker
PREGNANCY CATEGORY: C
Rx: Calan, Calan SR, Covera-HS, Isoptin SR, Verelan, Verelan PM.
✦**Rx:** Apo-Verap, Chronovera, Gen-Verapamil, Gen-Verapamil SR, Isoptin, Isoptin I.V., Isoptin SR, Novo-Veramil, Novo-Veramil SR, Nu-Verap.

SEE ALSO *CALCIUM CHANNEL BLOCKING AGENTS.*

USES
PO, Immediate-Release: (1) Angina pectoris due to coronary artery spasm (Prinzmetal's variant), chronic stable angina including angina due to increased effort, unstable angina (preinfarction, crescendo). (2) With digitalis to control rapid ventricular rate at rest and during stress in chronic atrial flutter or atrial fibrillation. (3) Prophylaxis of repetitive paroxysmal supraventricular tachycardia. (4) Essential hypertension.

PO, Extended-Release: (1) Essential hypertension (Covera-HS only). (2) Angina (Covera-HS only).

IV: (1) Paroxysmal supraventricular tachyarrhythmias. (2) Atrial flutter or fibrillation. *Investigational:* Manic depression (alternate therapy), exercise-induced asthma, recumbent nocturnal leg cramps, cluster headaches.

ACTION/KINETICS
Action
Slows AV conduction and prolongs effective refractory period. ↓ HR and ↑ PR interval. IV doses may slightly increase LV filling pressure. Moderately decreases myocardial contractility and peripheral vascular resistance. Worsening of heart failure may result if verapamil is given to clients with moderate to severe cardiac dysfunction.

Pharmacokinetics
Onset, PO: 30 min; **IV:** 3–5 min. **Time to peak plasma levels (PO):** 1–2 hr (5–7 hr for extended-release). **t½, PO:** 4.5–12 hr with repetitive dosing; **IV, initial:** 4 min; **final:** 2–5 hr. **Therapeutic serum levels:** 0.08–0.3 mcg/mL. **Duration, PO:** 8–10 hr (24 hr for extended-release); **IV:** 10–20 min for hemodynamic effect and 2 hr for antiarrhythmic effect. Metabolized to norverapamil, which possesses 20% of the activity of verapamil. *NOTE:* Covera HS is designed to deliver verapamil in concert with the 24-hr circadian variations in BP. Verelan PM allows for bedtime dosing and incorporates a 4- to 5-hr delay in drug delivery so there are maximum plasma levels in the morning.

CONTRAINDICATIONS
Severe hypotension, second- or third-degree AV block, cardiogenic shock, severe CHF, sick sinus syndrome (unless client has artificial pacemaker), severe LV dysfunction. Cardiogenic shock and severe CHF unless secondary to SVT that can be treated with verapamil. Lactation. Use of verapamil, IV, with beta-adrenergic blocking agents (as both de-

---

Bold Italic = life threatening side effect   ■ = black box warning   ✦ = Available in Canada

press myocardial contractility and AV conduction). Ventricular tachycardia.

SPECIAL CONCERNS

Infants less than 6 months of age may not respond to verapamil. Use with caution in hypertrophic cardiomyopathy, impaired hepatic and renal function, and in the elderly.

SIDE EFFECTS

Most Common

Infection, flu-like symptoms, URTI, rhinitis, nausea, dyspepsia, diarrhea, constipation, headache, fatigue/lethargy, dizziness, peripheral edema.

CV: CHF, bradycardia, *AV block, asystole*, premature ventricular contractions and tachycardia (after IV use), peripheral and pulmonary edema, hypotension, syncope, palpitations, AV dissociation, *MI, CVA.* **GI:** Nausea, constipation, abdominal discomfort or cramps, dyspepsia, diarrhea, dry mouth. **CNS:** Dizziness, headache, sleep disturbances, depression, amnesia, paranoia, psychoses, hallucinations, jitteriness, confusion, drowsiness, vertigo. IV verapamil may increase intracranial pressure in clients with supratentorial tumors at the time of induction of anesthesia. **Dermatologic:** Rash, dermatitis, alopecia, urticaria, pruritus, erythema multiforme, *Stevens-Johnson syndrome.* **Respiratory:** URTI, rhinitis, nasal or chest congestion, dyspnea, SOB, wheezing. **Musculoskeletal:** Paresthesia, asthenia, muscle cramps or inflammation, decreased neuromuscular transmission in Duchenne's muscular dystrophy. **Body as a whole:** Infection, flu-like symptoms, sweating, flushing, fatigue, lethargy. **Miscellaneous:** Blurred vision, equilibrium disturbances, sexual difficulties, spotty menstruation, rotary nystagmus, gingival hyperplasia, polyuria, nocturia, gynecomastia, claudication, hyperkeratosis, purpura, petechiae, bruising, hematomas, tachyphylaxis.

ADDITIONAL DRUG INTERACTIONS

Amiodarone / Possible cardiotoxicity with ↓ CO; monitor closely

Antihypertensive agents / Additive hypotensive effects

Antineoplastics / ↓ Verapamil absorption by several antineoplastics

Atorvastatin / ↑ Atorvastatin plasma levels

Barbiturates / ↓ Verapamil bioavailability

Buspirone / ↑ Buspirone effects

Calcium salts / ↓ Verapamil effect; can reverse clinical and toxic effects of verapamil

Carbamazepine / ↑ Carbamazepine effect R/T ↓ liver breakdown

Cimetidine / ↑ Verapamil bioavailability

Clarithromycin / Possible severe hypotension and bradycardia

Cyclosporine / ↑ Cyclosporine plasma levels → possible renal toxicity

Digoxin / ↑ Risk of digoxin toxicity R/T ↑ plasma levels

Disopyramide / Additive depressant effects on myocardial contractility and AV conduction

Dofetilide ↑ Dofetilide plasma levels → ↑ risk of ventricular arrhythmias

Ethanol / Prolonged and ↑ ethanol effects

Etomidate / Anesthetic effect may be ↑ with prolonged respiratory depression and apnea

Fexofenadine / ↑ Fexofenadine peak plasma levels and AUC R/T ↑ bioavailability by inhibiting P-glycoprotein transport

Grapefruit juice / ↑ Verapamil plasma levels R/T ↓ liver metabolism

Imipramine / ↑ Imipramine serum levels

Lithium / ↓ Lithium levels; lithium toxicity also observed

Muscle relaxants, nondepolarizing / ↑ Neuromuscular blockade R/T verapamil effect on calcium channels

Prazosin / Acute hypotensive effect

Quinidine / Possibility of bradycardia, hypotension, AV block, VT, and pulmonary edema

Ranitidine/ ↑ Verapamil bioavailability

Rifampin / ↓ Verapamil effect

Risperidone / Significant ↑ plasma risperidone levels R/T ↑ bioavailability through P-glycoprotein inhibition

Sirolimus / ↑ Sirolimus plasma levels

Smoking / ↓ Verapamil and norverapamil AUC and peak plasma levels R/T inhibition of CYP1A2

Sulfinpyrazone / ↑ Verapamil clearance

 = see color insert   = Herbal   = Intravenous   ⓒ = sound alike drug

Tacrolimus / ↑ Tacrolimus plasma levels → ↑ toxicity
Theophylline / ↑ Theophylline effects
Vitamin D / ↓ Verapamil effects
Warfarin / Possible ↑ effect of either drug R/T ↓ plasma protein binding
NOTE: Since verapamil is significantly bound to plasma proteins, interaction with other drugs bound to plasma proteins may occur.

LABORATORY TEST CONSIDERATIONS
↑ Alkaline phosphatase, transaminase.

OD OVERDOSE MANAGEMENT
Symptoms: Extension of side effects. *Treatment:* Beta-adrenergics, IV calcium, vasopressors, pacing, and resuscitation.

HOW SUPPLIED
Capsules, Extended-Release: 100 mg, 120 mg, 180 mg, 200 mg, 240 mg, 300 mg; *Capsules, Sustained-Release:* 120 mg, 180 mg, 240 mg, 360 mg; *Injection:* 2.5 mg/mL; *Tablets, Extended-Release:* 120 mg, 180 mg, 240 mg; *Tablets, Immediate-Release:* 40 mg, 80 mg, 120 mg; *Tablets, Sustained-Release:* 120 mg, 180 mg, 240 mg.

DOSAGE
* **TABLETS, IMMEDIATE-RELEASE**
  Angina at rest and chronic stable angina.
Individualized. Adults, initial: 80–120 mg 3 times per day (40 mg 3 times per day if client is sensitive to verapamil); **then,** increase dose to total of 240–480 mg/day.
  Arrhythmias.
Dosage range in digitalized clients with chronic atrial fibrillation: 240–320 mg/day in divided doses 3–4 times per day.
  Prophylaxis of paroxysmal supraventricular tachycardia.
240–480 mg/day in divided doses 3–4 times per day in nondigitalized clients. Maximum effects: During first 48 hr.
  Essential hypertension.
Initial, when used alone: 80 mg 3 times per day. Doses up to 360–480 mg daily may be used. Effects are seen in the first week of therapy. In the elderly or in people of small stature, initial dose should be 40 mg 3 times per day.
  Prophylaxis of migraine headache.
40–80 mg 3–4 times per day.

* **CAPSULES, EXTENDED RELEASE; CAPSULES, SUSTAINED-RELEASE; TABLETS, EXTENDED-RELEASE; TABLETS, SUSTAINED-RELEASE**
  Essential hypertension.
Covera-HS, initial: 180 mg at bedtime. If an adequate response is not reached, the dose can be increased as follows: 240 mg each evening, 360 mg each evening, or 480 mg each evening. **Verelan PM:** 200 mg/day at bedtime. If an adequate response is not reached, the dose can be increased as follows: 300 mg each evening or 400 mg each evening. **Calan SR or Isoptin SR, initial:** 180 mg in the a.m. with food. If an adequate response is not reached, the dose may be increased as follows: 240 mg each morning, 180 mg each morning plus 180 mg each evening (or 240 mg each morning plus 120 mg each evening), or 240 mg q 12 hr. **Verelan, initial:** 120 mg once daily in the morning. If an adequate response is not reached, the dose may be increased as follows: 180 mg in the morning, 240 mg in the morning (usual dose), 360 mg in the morning, or 480 mg in the morning
* **SLOW IV**
  Supraventricular tachyarrhythmias.
Adults, initial: 5–10 mg (0.075–0.15 mg/kg) as an IV bolus given over 2 min (over 3 min in older clients); **then,** 10 mg (0.15 mg/kg) 30 min later if response is not adequate. **Infants, up to 1 year:** 0.1–0.2 mg/kg (0.75–2 mg) given as an IV bolus over 2 min; **1–15 years:** 0.1–0.3 mg/kg (2–5 mg, not to exceed 5 mg total dose) over 2 min. If response to initial dose is inadequate, it may be repeated after 30 min, but not more than a total of 10 mg should be given to clients from 1 to 15 years of age.

NURSING CONSIDERATIONS
℮ Do not confuse Isoptin with Intropin (a vasopressor), or Covera with Provera (a progestin).

ADMINISTRATION/STORAGE
1. SR tablets (120 mg) may be useful for small stature and elderly clients who require less medication.
2. Take SR tablets with food.

3. Verelan pellet filled capsules may be carefully opened and the contents sprinkled on a spoonful of applesauce. Swallow applesauce immediately without chewing; follow with a glass of cool water to ensure complete swallowing of the pellets. Subdividing the contents of a capsule is not recommended.

 4. Before administration, inspect ampules for particulate matter or discoloration.

5. Administer IV dosage under continuous ECG monitoring with resuscitation equipment readily available.

6. Give as slow IV bolus (5–10 mg) over 2 min (3 min to elderly clients) to minimize toxic effects.

7. Store ampules at 15–30°C (59–86°F), protect from light.

8. Do not give verapamil in an infusion line containing 0.45% NaCl with NaHCO₃; a crystalline precipitate will form.

9. Do not give verapamil by IV push in the same line used for nafcillin infusion because a milky white precipitate will form.

10. Do not mix with albumin, amphotericin B, hydralazine, trimethoprim/sulfamethoxazole, or diluted with sodium lactate in PVC bags.

11. Verapamil will precipitate in any solution with a pH greater than 6.

12. Always individualize dose in the elderly because the pharmacologic effects are more pronounced and more prolonged.

ASSESSMENT

1. Note reasons for therapy, onset, characteristics of S&S. List agents trialed, outcome.

2. Review list of prescribed medications to ensure none interact.

3. Monitor VS, ECG, CBC, renal and LFTs; reduce dose with hepatic or renal impairment, compromised cardiac function, and in those prescribed beta blockers. Assess for conditions that preclude therapy: SSS, 2nd or 3rd degree AV block, hypotension.

INTERVENTIONS

1. Monitor VS; assess for bradycardia and hypotension, symptoms that may indicate overdosage. May lower BP to dangerously low levels if BP already low.

2. *Do not* administer concurrently with IV beta-adrenergic blocking agents.

3. Unless treating verapamil overdosage, withhold drugs that may elevate calcium levels.

4. Clients receiving concurrent digoxin therapy should be assessed for symptoms of toxicity and have digoxin levels checked periodically.

5. If disopyramide is to be used, do not administer for at least 48 hr before to 24 hr after verapamil dose.

6. Administer extended-release tablets with food to minimize fluctuations in serum levels.

CLIENT/FAMILY TEACHING

1. Take SR capsule in a.m. with food; do not cut, crush, or chew; swallow capsules whole.

2. May cause dizziness and sudden drop in BP; use caution until drug effects realized.

3. Keep log of BP and pulse for provider review. Report unusual bruising/bleeding, weight gain, ↑ SOB, swelling of hands or feet, other adverse effects.

4. Avoid alcohol, CNS depressants, and OTC agents without approval.

5. Continue lifestyle modifications (low-fat and low-salt diet, decreased caloric and alcohol consumption, weight loss, no smoking, and regular exercise) in the overall goal of BP control.

6. Avoid prolonged sun exposure; use protection if exposed.

7. Increase fluids and fiber in diet to prevent constipation. With higher doses constipation occurs more frequently. Report if bothersome as psyllium (fiber) may be prescribed or, if severe, drug therapy may be changed.

OUTCOMES/EVALUATE

- ↓ Frequency/severity of anginal attacks
- Control of BP
- Restoration of stable rhythm
- Therapeutic drug levels (0.08–0.3 mcg/mL)

Verteporfin   [IV]
(ver-teh-**POR**-fin)

CLASSIFICATION(S):
Ophthalmic phototherapy
PREGNANCY CATEGORY: C
Rx: Visudyne.

USES
Treatment of predominantely classic subfoveal choroidal neovascularization due to age-related macular degeneration (AMD), pathologic myopia, or presumed ocular histoplasmosis. *Investigational:* Psoriasis, psoriatic arthritis, rheumatoid arthritis, nonmelanoma skin cancers, circumscribed choroidal hemangioma.

ACTION/KINETICS
Action
A light-activated drug that is transported in the plasma, mainly by lipoproteins. Once activated by light in the presence of oxygen, highly reactive, short-lived singlet oxygen and reactive oxygen radicals are activated. Light activation causes local damage to neovascular endothelium, resulting in vessel occlusion. Damaged endothelium releases procoagulant and vasoactive factors through leukotriene and eicosanoids (e.g., thromboxane) pathways, resulting in platelet aggregation, fibrin clot formation, and vasoconstriction. The drug appears to accumulate preferentially in neovasculature, including choroidal neovasculature. The drug may also accumulate in the retina causing collateral damage to retinal structures, including retinal pigmented epithelium and outer nuclear layer of the retina.

Pharmacokinetics
t½: 5–6 hr. Metabolized to a small extent by liver and plasma esterases. Excreted through the feces.

CONTRAINDICATIONS
Use with porphyria or hypersensitivity to any component of the product.

SPECIAL CONCERNS
Use with caution during lactation and in those with moderate-to-severe hepatic impairment. A reduced effect may be seen with increasing age.

SIDE EFFECTS
Most Common
Injection site reactions (extravasation, rashes), blurred vision, decreased visual acuity, visual field defects.
Ophthalmic: Severe vision decrease (equivalent of 4 or more lines) within 7 days after treatment. Blepharitis, blurred vision, decreased visual acuity, visual field defects, cataracts, conjunctivitis/conjunctival injection, diplopia, dry eyes, ocular itching, severe vision loss with or without subconjunctival, subretinal, or vitreous hemorrhage. **At site of infusion:** Injection site reactions, including extravasation and rashes. **CNS:** Hypesthesia, sleep disorder, headaches, vertigo. **CV:** Atrial fibrillation, hypertension, peripheral vascular disorder, varicose veins. **GI:** Constipation, GI cancers, nausea. **Hematologic:** Anemia, decreased or increased WBC count. **Musculoskeletal:** Arthralgia, arthrosis, myasthenia. **Respiratory:** Pharyngitis, pneumonia, cough. **Miscellaneous:** Photosensitivity reactions, decreased hearing, lacrimation disorder, asthenia, back pain (primarily during infusion), eczema, fever, flu syndrome, prostatic disorder.

LABORATORY TEST CONSIDERATIONS
↑ Creatinine. Albuminuria. Elevated LFTs.

[OD] OVERDOSE MANAGEMENT
Symptoms: Overdose of drug or light in the treated eye may cause nonperfusion of normal retinal vessels with possible severe decreased vision that could be permanent. Prolongation of the time during which there is photosensitivity to bright light. *Treatment:* Extend photosensitivity precautions for a time proportional to the overdose.

DRUG INTERACTIONS
Calcium channel blockers, polymyxin B, or radiation might increase the rate of verteporfin uptake by vascular endothelium.

HOW SUPPLIED
Lyophilized cake: 15 mg (reconstituted to 2 mg/mL).

Bold Italic = life threatening side effect   ■ = black box warning   ✦ = Available in Canada

DOSAGE
- **IV**

Age-related macular degeneration.
Treatment consists of two steps—drug (first step) and light (second step). **Step 1:** verteporfin, 6 mg/m². **Step 2:** Initiate 689 nm wavelength laser light delivery 15 min after the start of the 10-min drug infusion with verteporfin.

NURSING CONSIDERATIONS

ASSESSMENT
Note reasons for therapy, age at onset, other therapies trialed, outcome. Assess for liver or renal dysfunction.

CLIENT/FAMILY TEACHING
1. Age-related macular degeneration (AMD) is a progressive disease with no known cure. This therapy consists of a two-step process involving IV administration of the drug followed by light therapy from a laser about 15 min after the start of the infusion.
2. Report any pain or swelling at injection site as extravasation should be avoided.
3. Avoid skin exposure to direct sunlight or bright indoor light for at least 5 days after therapy.
4. Wear protective clothing and dark glasses if it is necessary to go out in daytime. UV sunscreens are not protective due to the skin deposition of drug.
5. May expose skin to low indoor light to help inactivate drug in skin through the process of photobleaching. Avoid complete darkness.
6. Report any adverse reactions or deterioration in baseline vision levels.

OUTCOMES/EVALUATE
Improved vision in those with impairment R/T AMD

Vinblastine sulfate
(vin-**BLAS**-teen)

CLASSIFICATION(S):
Antineoplastic, vinca alkaloid
PREGNANCY CATEGORY: D
Rx: Velban.

SEE ALSO *ANTINEOPLASTIC AGENTS.*

USES
(1) Palliative treatment of generalized Hodgkin's disease (stages III and IV, Ann Arbor modification of Rye staging system). (2) Lymphocytic lymphoma (nodular and diffuse, poorly and well differentiated). (3) Histiocytic lymphoma. (4) Advanced stages of mycosis fungoides. (5) Advanced testicular carcinoma. (6) Kaposi's sarcoma. (7) Letterer-Siwe disease (histiocytosis X). **Less frequently responsive malignancies.** (1) Choriocarcinoma resistant to other chemotherapy. (2) Breast cancer unresponsive to endocrine surgery and hormonal therapy.

Usually given in combination therapy. However, it has been used as a single agent to treat Hodgkin's disease and advanced testicular germinal-cell cancers (embryonal carcinoma, teratocarcinoma, choriocarcinoma), although combination therapy is more effective).

ACTION/KINETICS

Action
Believed to interfere with metabolic pathways of amino acids leading from glutamic acid to the citric acid cycle and urea. Also affects cell energy production needed for mitosis (affects growing cells in metaphase) and interferes with nucleic acid synthesis.

Pharmacokinetics
Rapidly cleared from plasma but poor penetration to the brain. Almost completely metabolized in the liver after IV administration. **t½, triphasic:** initial, 3.7 min; intermediate, 1.6 hr; final, 24.8 hr. Metabolites are excreted in the bile with smaller amounts in the urine. No cross-resistance with vincristine. **Plasma protein binding:** About 75%.

CONTRAINDICATIONS
Leukopenia, significant granulocytopenia (unless it is due to the disease being treated). Bacterial infections. Lactation.

SPECIAL CONCERNS
■ (1) It is extremely important that the needle be positioned properly in the vein before injected. If leakage into surrounding tissue occurs during IV administration, it may cause considerable irri-

---

tation. Immediately discontinue the injection and introduce any remaining portion of the dose into another vein. Local injection of hyaluronidase and the application of moderate heat to the area of leakage will help disperse the drug and may minimize the discomfort and the possibility of cellulitis. (2) The drug is fatal if given intrathecally. It is for IV use only.■

SIDE EFFECTS
Most Common
Fatigue, alopecia, N&V, cough, fever, chills, infection, malaise, shortness of breath, easy bruising, lower back/side pain, painful/difficult urination.

See *Antineoplastic Agents* for a complete list of possible side effects. Toxicity is dose-related and more pronounced in clients over age 65 or in those suffering from cachexia (profound general ill health) or skin ulceration. **GI:** N&V, ileus, rectal bleeding, ***hemorrhagic enterocolitis***, vesiculation of the mouth, ***bleeding from a former ulcer***. **Dermatologic:** Total epilation, skin vesiculation. **Respiratory:** Acute SOB, ***severe bronchospasm***. **Neurologic:** Paresthesias, neuritis, mental depression, loss of deep tendon reflexes, ***seizures***. Extravasation may result in phlebitis and cellulitis with sloughing.

DRUG INTERACTIONS
Bleomycin sulfate and cisplatin / Combination of bleomycin, cisplatin, and vinblastine may produce signs of Raynaud's disease in clients with testicular cancer
Erythromycin / Severe myalgia, neutropenia, and constipation
Glutamic acid / Inhibits effect of vinblastine
Mitomycin C / Severe bronchospasm with SOB
Phenytoin / ↓ Effect of phenytoin due to ↓ plasma levels
Tryptophan / Inhibits effect of vinblastine

HOW SUPPLIED
Injection: 1 mg/mL; *Powder for Injection:* 10 mg.

DOSAGE
- **IV**
  All uses.

Individualized, using WBC count as guide. Administered once every 7 days. **Adults, initial:** 3.7 mg/m^2; **then,** after 7 days, graded doses of 5.5, 7.4, 9.25, and 11.1 mg/m^2 at intervals of 7 days (maximum dose should not exceed 18.5 mg/m^2). Usually the weekly dosage range is 5.5–7.7 mg/m$^{2.}$ Do not increase the dose after the WBC count is reduced to about 3,000 cells/mm^3. **Children, initial:** 2.5 mg/m^2; **then,** after 7 days, graded doses of 3.75, 5.0, 6.25, and 7.5 mg/m^2 at intervals of 7 days (maximum dose should not exceed 12.5 mg/m^2). **Maintenance** doses are calculated based on WBC count—at least 4,000/mm^3. When the dose produces leukopenia of about 3,000 cells/mm^3, give a dose one increment smaller at weekly intervals for maintenance. Even though 7 days have elapsed, do not give the next dose until the WBC count has returned to at least 4,000 cells/mm^3.

NURSING CONSIDERATIONS
❀ Do not confuse vinblastine with vincristine (another vinca alkaloid antineoplastic agent).

ADMINISTRATION/STORAGE
IV 1. Reconstitute under a laminar flow hood; add 10 mL of bacteriostatic NaCl, which is preserved with either benzyl alcohol or phenol for a final concentration of 1 mg/mL.

2. Do not reconstitute with solutions that raise or lower the pH from between 3.5 and 5.5.

3. Inject into tubing of flowing IV infusion or directly into vein and administer over 1 min. May be further diluted in 50–100 mL of NSS and infused over 15–30 min.

4. Assess peripheral IV site for patency to prevent extravasation, local irritation and pain. If extravasation occurs, move infusion to another vein. Treat affected area with hyaluronidase injection and application of moderate heat to decrease local reaction.

5. After reconstitution and removal of a portion from the vial, the remainder may be stored in the refrigerator for 30 days. Unopened vials should be refrig-

V

erated at temperatures of 2–8°C (36–46°F).

6. If drug gets into the eye, immediately wash eye thoroughly with water to prevent irritation and ulceration.

ASSESSMENT

1. Take a thorough drug history; note reasons for therapy. List any neuropathies.

2. Do not increase dose after WBC count is reduced to about 3000 cells/mm³. When the dose causes such a degree of leukopenia, give a dose one increment smaller at weekly intervals for maintenance. Even though 7 days has elapsed, do not give the next dose until the WBC has returned to at least 4000 cells/mm³.

3. Monitor uric acid, renal function, and hematologic profiles. Drug may cause granulocyte and platelet suppression. Nadir: 10 days; recovery: 21 days.

INTERVENTIONS

1. Administer antiemetic for N&V. Monitor I&O. Encourage fluid intake of 2–3 L/day.

2. Observe for cyanosis and pallor of extremities and S&S of Raynaud's disease if also receiving bleomycin and severe bronchospasms if also receiving mitomycin.

3. Check for manifestations of neurotoxicity and report if evident; dosage may need to be adjusted. Monitor neurologic toxicity by checking reflexes and strength of hand grip.

4. Observe for S&S of gout; may use allopurinol empirically.

CLIENT/FAMILY TEACHING

1. Drug is given by injection to interfere with the growth of cancer cells.

2. Report any signs of infection, fever, sore throat/mouth, unusual bruising/bleeding.

3. Practice barrier contraception.

4. Avoid vaccinations and exposure to persons with infectious diseases during therapy

5. To prevent constipation, eat a high-fiber diet, increase intake of fluids, remain active, and take stool softeners as prescribed.

6. Wear protective clothing, sunglasses, and a sunscreen if exposure to sunlight is necessary.

7. Partial hair loss may occur; plan for cosmetic replacement.

8. Report any S&S of neurotoxicity: paresthesias, difficulty walking, and diminished reflexes; indication to discontinue drug therapy.

OUTCOMES/EVALUATE

Control/regression of malignant process

Vincristine sulfate (VCR, LCR)
(vin-**KRIS**-teen)

CLASSIFICATION(S):
Antineoplastic, vinca alkaloid
PREGNANCY CATEGORY: D
Rx: Oncovin, Vincasar PFS.

SEE ALSO *ANTINEOPLASTIC AGENTS.*

USES
Frequently used in combination therapy. (1) ALL in children. (2) Hodgkin's and non-Hodgkin's lymphomas (lymphocytic, mixed-cell, histiocytic, undifferentiated, nodular, and diffuse). (3) Wilms' tumor, neuroblastoma, lymphosarcoma, rhabdomyosarcoma, reticulum cell sarcoma. *Investigational:* ITP; cancer of the breast, ovary, cervix, lung, colorectal area; malignant melanoma, osteosarcoma, multiple myeloma, ovarian germ cell tumors, mycosis fungoides, CLL, CML, Kaposi's sarcoma.

ACTION/KINETICS

Action
Inhibits mitosis at metaphase. The antineoplastic effect is due to interference with intracellular tubulin function by binding to microtubule and spindle proteins in the S phase.

Pharmacokinetics
After IV use, drug is distributed within 15–30 min to tissues. Poorly penetrates blood-brain barrier. **t½, triphasic:** initial, 5 min; intermediate, 2.3 hr; final, 85 hr. Approximately 80% is excreted in the

 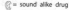

feces and up to 20% in the urine. No cross-resistance with vinblastine.

CONTRAINDICATIONS

Use in demyelinating Charcot-Marie-Tooth syndrome or during radiation therapy. Lactation.

SPECIAL CONCERNS

■ (1) It is extremely important that the IV needle or catheter be properly positioned before injection. Leakage into surrounding tissue may cause considerable irritation. (2) Intrathecal use usually results in death. For IV use only.■ Geriatric clients are more susceptible to the neurotoxic effects.

SIDE EFFECTS

Most Common

Fatigue, abdominal cramps, constipation, diarrhea, peripheral neuropathy, loss of fertility, alopecia, paralytic ileus, N&V, weight loss, rash, bloating.

See *Antineoplastic Agents* for a complete list of possible side effects. **Neurologic:** Paresthesias, depression of DTRs, foot drop, *seizures*, difficulties in gait. **GI:** *Intestinal necrosis or perforation*. Constipation, paralytic ileus. **Renal:** Inappropriate ADH secretion (polyuria or dysuria). Acute uric acid nephropathy. **Ophthalmic:** Blindness, ptosis, diplopia, photophobia. **Miscellaneous:** CNS leukemia, leukopenia or complicating infection, *bronchospasm*, SOB. Less bone marrow depression than vinblastine. Significant tissue irritation if leakage occurs during IV use.

OD OVERDOSE MANAGEMENT

Symptoms: Exaggeration of side effects. *Treatment:*

- Treat side effects due to inappropriate secretion of ADH.
- Use an anticonvulsant (e.g., phenobarbital), if necessary.
- Prevent ileus by use of enemas, cathartics, or decompression of the GI tract.
- Monitor the CV system.
- Monitor blood counts daily to determine risk of infection and whether blood transfusions are necessary.
- Folinic acid, 100 mg IV q 3 hr for 24 hr and then q 6 hr for a minimum of 48 hr, may help with treating the symptoms of overdose.

DRUG INTERACTIONS

L-Asparaginase / ↓ Vincristine renal clearance; give vincristine 12–14 hr before asparaginase
Calcium channel blocking drugs / ↑ Accumulation of vincristine in cells
Digoxin / ↓ Digoxin effect R/T ↓ plasma levels
Glutamic acid / Inhibits effect of vincristine
Itraconazole / ↑ Risk of neurotoxicity R/T ↓ vincristine metabolism
Methotrexate / Possible hypotension
Mitomycin C / Severe bronchospasm and acute SOB
Phenytoin / ↓ Phenytoin effect R/T ↓ plasma levels

HOW SUPPLIED

Injection: 1 mg/mL.

DOSAGE

- **IV ONLY (DIRECT, INFUSION)**
  Individualized for all uses with extreme care as overdose can be fatal.

  Adults, usual, initial: 0.4–1.4 mg/m^2 (or 0.01–0.03 mg/kg) once a week; **children:** 1.5–2 mg/m^2 once a week. **Children <10 kg or with body surface area less than 1 m^2:** 0.05 mg/kg once a week. Hepatic insufficiency: If serum bilirubin is 1.5–3, administer 50% of the dose; if serum bilirubin is more than 3.1 or AST is more than 180, omit the dose.

NURSING CONSIDERATIONS

© Do not confuse vincristine with vinblastine (another vinca alkaloid antineoplastic agent).

ADMINISTRATION/STORAGE

IV 1. Dissolve powder in sterile water or isotonic saline injection to a concentration ranging from 0.01 to 1 mg/mL.
2. Do not mix with anything other than NSS or dextrose in water.
3. Do not mix with any solution that alters the pH outside the range of 3.5–5.5.
4. Inject either directly into a vein or into the tubing of a flowing IV infusion over a period of 1 min.
5. If extravasation occurs, move to another vein. Treat affected area with hyaluronidase injection (150 units/mL in 1 mL NaCl) and apply moderate heat to decrease local reaction.

Bold Italic = life threatening side effect   ■ = black box warning   ✦ = Available in Canada

6. Protect from light exposure.

7. Store in refrigerator. Dry powder is stable for 6 months. Solutions are stable for 2 weeks under refrigeration.

ASSESSMENT

1. Note reasons for therapy, onset, characteristics of S&S, other agents trialed.

2. List neurologic assessment; monitor for early S&S of neurologic and neuromuscular side effects (e.g., sensory impairment, paresthesias) before neuritic pain and motor difficulties are apparent; neuromuscular manifestations are irreversible.

3. Monitor CBC, uric acid, renal, LFTs. May cause granulocyte suppression. Nadir: 10 days; recovery: 21 days.

INTERVENTIONS

1. Drug is administered IV to inhibit cancer cell progression.

2. Premedicate and regularly administer antiemetic to control N&V.

3. Record I&O, weights, and assessment of nutritional/neurologic status.

4. Observe for S&S of gout. May add allopurinol empirically to prevent uric acid nephropathy.

5. Use laxatives and enemas to treat high colon impaction.

6. Absence of bowel sounds is indicative of paralytic ileus; temporarily stop drug.

CLIENT/FAMILY TEACHING

1. Prevent constipation by increased intake of fluids (2–3 L/day), regular exercise, a high-fiber diet, and stool softeners as needed.

2. Report any S&S of neurotoxicity: paresthesias (numbness/tingling), difficulty walking, and diminished reflexes.

3. Avoid vaccinations and persons with infectious diseases.

4. Practice reliable contraception during and for 2 mo following therapy.

5. Report any increased dyspnea, cough, fatigue or unusual bruising or bleeding.

6. Avoid alcohol and OTC agents. Keep all F/U appointments.

OUTCOMES/EVALUATE

Inhibition of malignant cell proliferation

Vinorelbine tartrate

(vin-**OR**-el-been)

CLASSIFICATION(S):
Antineoplastic, vinca alkaloid
PREGNANCY CATEGORY: D
Rx: Navelbine.

USES

Alone or in combination with cisplatin for first-line treatment of ambulatory clients with unresectable, advanced non-small cell lung cancer. In clients with Stage IV non-small cell lung cancer, can be used as a single agent or with cisplatin. In stage II non-small cell lung cancer, vinorelbine is not indicated for use with cisplatin. *Investigational:* Breast cancer, cisplatin-resistant ovarian carcinoma, and Hodgkin's disease.

ACTION/KINETICS

Action

Semisynthetic vinca alkaloid thought to act by inhibiting mitosis at metaphase through the drug's interaction with tubulin. Other possible actions may include interference with (a) amino acid, cyclic AMP, and glutathione metabolism, (b) calmodulin-dependent calcium transport ATPase activity, (c) cellular respiration, and (d) nucleic acid and lipid biosynthesis.

Pharmacokinetics

Following IV use, plasma levels decay in a triphasic manner. The initial rapid decline is due to distribution of the drug to peripheral compartments. The prolonged terminal phase is due to a slow efflux of the drug from peripheral compartments. **Terminal phase, t½:** Averages 27.7–43.6 hr. Metabolized by the liver and excreted through the urine and feces.

CONTRAINDICATIONS

Clients with pretreatment granulocyte counts less than 1,000 cells/mm³. Lactation.

SPECIAL CONCERNS

■ (1) Give under the supervision of a physician experienced in the use of cancer chemotherapeutic agents. For IV use only; intrathecal use of other vinca alkaloids has been fatal. Label syringes containing this product: 'Warning: Vinorelbine for IV use only. Fatal if given intrathecally.' (2) Severe granulocytopenia, resulting in increased susceptibility to infection may occur. Granulocyte counts should be 1,000 or more cells/mm³ prior to giving the drug. Adjust dosage according to CBC with differentials obtained on the day of treatment. (3) It is extremely important that the IV needle or catheter be properly positioned before injection. Improper administration of vinorelbine may result in extravasation causing local tissue necrosis or thrombophlebitis.■ Use with caution in clients with severe hepatic injury or impairment. Use with extreme caution in clients whose bone marrow reserve may have been compromised by chemotherapy or prior to irradiation; also, in those whose bone marrow function is recovering from the effects of previous chemotherapy. Older clients may be more sensitive to the effects of the drug. Safety and efficacy have not been determined in children.

SIDE EFFECTS
Most Common
N&V, constipation, diarrhea, asthenia, injection site reactions/pain, periphreal neuropathy, alopecia, granulocytopenia, leukopenia, anemia.

Hematologic: Granulocytopenia (may require hospitalization), leukopenia, thrombocytopenia, anemia. **GI:** N&V, constipation (may be severe), diarrhea, paralytic ileus, anorexia, stomatitis, intestinal obstruction, *necrosis, perforation*, dysphagia, mucositis. **CNS:** Mild to severe peripheral neuropathy including paresthesia and hypesthesia, loss of DTRs, headache. **CV:** Chest pain, especially in those with a history of CV disease or tumor within the chest; phlebitis, hyper-/hypotension, vasodilation, tachycardia, pulmonary edema. **Respiratory:** SOB (may be severe), dyspnea, interstitial pulmonary changes, pneumonia. **Dermatologic:** Alopecia, flushing, erythema, rash. **At injection site:** Vein discoloration, chemical phlebitis

along the vein proximal to the site of injection, localized rash and urticaria, blister formation, skin sloughing. **Musculoskeletal:** Musculoskeletal aches and pains, back pain, jaw pain, myalgia, arthralgia. **Hypersensitivity:** Pruritus, urticaria, angioedema, *anaphylaxis*. **Miscellaneous:** Asthenia, fatigue, hemorrhagic cystitis, SIADH secretion, vestibular and auditory deficits (especially when used with cisplatin), abdominal pain, pain in tumor-containing tissue, radiation recall events (e.g., dermatitis, esophagitis).

LABORATORY TEST CONSIDERATIONS
↑ Total bilirubin, AST. Transient elevations of liver enzymes.

OD OVERDOSE MANAGEMENT
Symptoms: Bone marrow suppression, peripheral neurotoxicity. *Treatment:* There is no known antidote for vinorelbine. For overdosage, begin general supportive measures together with appropriate blood transfusions and antibiotics, as necessary.

DRUG INTERACTIONS
Cisplatin / ↑ Incidence of granulocytopenia
Mitomycin / Acute pulmonary reactions
Paclitaxel / Possible neuropathy when used together or sequentially

HOW SUPPLIED
Injection: 10 mg/mL.

DOSAGE
• IV ONLY
Non-small-cell lung cancer.
Granulocytes (1,500 or more cells/mm³) on the day of treatment: 30 mg/m² weekly given over 6–10 min into the side port of a free-flowing IV closest to the IV bag followed by flushing with at least 75–125 mL of the solution used to dilute the product. May also be given, at the same dose level, with cisplatin, 120 mg/m² on days 1 and 29 and then q 6 weeks. **Granulocytes (1,000–1,499 cells/mm³) on the day of treatment:** 15 mg/m² weekly given over 6–10 min as described previously. *Breast cancer, Hodgkin's disease.* 30 mg/m²/week.

NURSING CONSIDERATIONS

ADMINISTRATION/STORAGE

IV 1. During therapy, if clients have manifested fever or sepsis while granulocytopenic or had two consecutive weekly doses held due to granulocytopenia, give subsequent doses of vinorelbine as follows: 22.5 mg/m² for granulocytes equal to or >1,500 cells/mm³ or 11.25 mg/m² for granulocytes from 1,000 to 1,499 cells/mm³.

2. Ensure granulocyte counts are equal to or >1,000 cells/mm³ prior to giving vinorelbine. Base dosage on granulocyte counts on the day of drug treatment.

3. If hyperbilirubinemia develops during treatment, adjust the dose of vinorelbine as follows: 30 mg/m² for a total bilirubin of 2 or less mg/dL, 15 mg/m² for a total bilirubin of 2.1–3 mg/dL, and 7.5 mg/m² for a total bilirubin >3 mg/dL.

4. Before any drug is given, properly position the needle or catheter, as leakage into surrounding tissue may cause considerable irritation, local tissue necrosis, or thrombophlebitis. If extravasation occurs, stop the injection immediately and give the remaining dose in another vein. Use institutional guidelines to treat extravasation.

5. Due to the toxicity of vinorelbine, wear gloves and use caution in handling/preparing the solution. If it comes in contact with skin or mucosa, wash the area immediately with soap and water. If the eye is affected, flush with water immediately.

6. Must be diluted in either a syringe or IV bag. If an IV bag is used, dilute the dose to a concentration between 0.5 and 2 mg/mL using one of the following solutions: D5W, 0.45% or 0.9% NaCl, D5W/0.45% NaCl, Ringer's, or RL injection. When dilution in a syringe is used, dilute the dose to a concentration between 1.5 and 3 mg/mL with D5W or 0.9% NaCl.

7. Diluted vinorelbine solutions may be used for up to 24 hr under normal room light when stored in polypropylene syringes or PVC bags at 5–30°C (41–96°F).

Unopened vials are stable until the expiration date indicated if stored under refrigeration at 2–8°C (36–46°F). Protect unopened vials from light and do not freeze. Do not use if particulate matter present.

ASSESSMENT

1. Note reasons for therapy, other agents/therapies prescribed, when administered, outcome.

2. Drug may cause skin irritation with contact; avoid inhaling vapors.

3. Monitor CBC, uric acid, renal, and LFTs. Reduce dose with impaired liver and hematologic function. Do not administer if granulocyte counts are not at least 1,000 cells/mm³. Granulocyte nadir 7–10 days; recovery 7–14 days thereafter.

CLIENT/FAMILY TEACHING

1. Report any fever or chills immediately; drug-induced granulocytopenia (reduction in WBC) makes one much more susceptible to infections.

2. Avoid crowds, persons with infectious diseases, and vaccinations during therapy.

3. Practice reliable contraception during and for several months after therapy.

4. Rinse mouth frequently and brush teeth often to prevent mouth sores; use unwaxed floss. Use multivitamin and nutritious diet to prevent weight loss

5. Antiemetics will be given to prevent N&V; report if persistent. Ensure adequate fluid consumption.

6. Report any S&S of neurotoxicity: numbness/tingling, difficulty walking, and diminished reflexes.

OUTCOMES/EVALUATE

Control of malignant cell proliferation.

Voriconazole **IV**

(**vor**-ih-**KOH**-nah-zohl)

CLASSIFICATION(S):

Antifungal

PREGNANCY CATEGORY: D

Rx: Vfend.

USES

(1) Invasive aspergillosis. (2) Serious fungal infections due to *Scedosporium apiospermum* (asexual form of *Pseudallescheria boydii*) and *Fusarium* species, including *Fusarium solani* in those intolerant of, or refractory to, other therapy. (3) Esophageal candidiasis. (4) Candidemia in those without low WBC counts (nonneutropenic clients) of the following: Disseminated infections in skin and infections in the abdomen, kidney, bladder wall, and wounds.

ACTION/KINETICS

Action

Acts by inhibiting fungal cytochrome P450-mediated 14 alpha-lanosterol demethylation, which is an essential step in fungal ergosterol biosynthesis. Accumulation of 14 alpha-methyl sterols results in the loss of ergosterol in the fungal cell wall and is thought to be responsible for the antifungal activity.

Pharmacokinetics

Maximum plasma levels, after PO: 1–2 hr. Metabolized by hepatic cytochrome P450 enzymes CYP2C19 (major enzyme for metabolism of this drug), CYP2C9, and CYP3A4. Excreted in the urine. Terminal $t\frac{1}{2}$ is dose dependent and thus not useful in predicting accumulation or elimination of the drug. Fifteen to 20% of Asian populations are slow metabolizers compared with 3–5% of Caucasians and Blacks. **Plasma protein binding:** About 58%.

CONTRAINDICATIONS

Known hypersensitivity to the drug or product components or to other azoles. IV voriconazole in moderate or severe renal impairment unless benefit to risk justifies use. Use with CYP3A4 substrates, including pimozide and quinidine, as increased plasma levels may cause QT prolongation and torsades de pointes (rare). Use with barbiturates (long-acting), carbamazepine, efavirenz, ergot alkaloids (ergotamine, dihydroergotamine), rifabutin, rifampin, ritonavir (400 mg q 12 hr), sirolimus. Use in those with galactose intolerance, Lapp lactase deficiency, or glucose-galactose malabsorption. Lactation.

SPECIAL CONCERNS

Accumulation of the IV vehicle (sulfobutyl ether beta-cyclodextrin sodium) in those with moderate to severe renal dysfunction. Use with caution in clients with potential proarrhythmic conditions. Safety and efficacy have not been determined in children under 12 years of age.

SIDE EFFECTS

Most Common

Abnormal vision, tachycardia, hallucinations, headache, abdominal pain, diarrhea, peripheral edema, rash, respiratory disorder, sepsis, visual disturbances, sepsis, N&V, abnormal LFTs, photophobia, chills, fever, cholestatic jaundice, chromatopsia.

Side effects listed are the more common or more serious. **Infusion reactions:** Flushing, fever, sweating, tachycardia, chest tightness, dyspnea, fainting, nausea, pruritus, rash. **Hematologic:** Thrombocytopenia, leukopenia, anemia, pancytopenia. **GI:** N&V, diarrhea, abdominal pain, cholestatic jaundice, dry mouth, abnormal LFTs, ***hepatic toxicity*** (hepatitis, jaundice, cholestasis, ***fulminant hepatic failure***). **CNS:** Headache, hallucinations, dizziness. **Dermatologic:** Serious cutaneous reactions, including ***Stevens-Johnson syndrome***, photosensitivity skin reaction (especially with long-term use), rash, pruritus, maculopapular rash. **CV:** Tachycardia, hyper-/hypotension, vasodilation, prolongation of QT interval (rarely, ***torsades de pointes*** in seriously ill clients with multiple confounding risk factors), ***cardiac arrest***. **GU:** Abnormal kidney function, ***acute kidney failure***. **Ophthalmic:** Visual disturbances, abnormal vision, photophobia, chromatopsia, eye hemorrhage. **Body as a whole:** Fever, sepsis, peripheral edema, chills. **Miscellaneous:** Respiratory disorders, chest pain.

LABORATORY TEST CONSIDERATIONS

↑ Alkaline phosphatase, hepatic enzymes, ALT, AST, creatinine, total bilirubin. Hypokalemia, hypomagnesemia, bilirubinemia.

Bold Italic = life threatening side effect   ■ = black box warning   ✤ = Available in Canada

DRUG INTERACTIONS

Voriconazole is metabolized by CYP2C19, CYP2C9, and CYP3A4; thus, inhibitors or inducers of these 3 enzymes may increase or decrease voriconazole plasma levels. Also, voriconazole inhibits metabolic activity of these three enzymes; thus, there is the potential to increase plasma levels of other drugs metabolized by these CYP450 enzymes.

Amprenavir / Metabolism of amprenavir may be inhibited; ↑ or ↓ metabolism of voriconazole

Barbiturates (long-acting, including mephobarbital, phenobarbital) / Significant ↓ voriconazole levels R/T CYP450 induction; do not use together

Benzodiazepines (alprazolam, midazolam, triazolam) / ↑ Levels of benzodiazepines metabolized by CYP3A4; adjust dose if necessary

Calcium channel blockers (e.g., felodipine) / Inhibition of metabolism of CCBs metabolized by CYP3A4; adjust dose if necessary

Carbamazepine / Significant ↓ voriconazol levels R/T CYP450 induction; do not use together

Cimetidine / ↑ Voriconazole C_{max} and AUC; no dosage adjustment required

Cyclosporine / ↑ Cyclosporine C_{max} and AUC; reduce cyclosporine dose by 50%

Efavirenz / Significant ↓ voraconazole levels; significant ↑ efavirenz levels; do not use together

Ergot alkaloids (ergotamine, dihydroergotamine) / ↑ Ergot levels → possible ergotism

HMG-CoA reductase inhibitors (e.g., lovastatin) / Possible ↑ statin levels metabolized by CYP3A4; consider dosage adjustment

Methadone / ↑ Methadone levels → possible QT prolongation; possibly reduce dose of methadone

Nelfinavir / Metabolism of nelfinavir may be inhibited; &arrowup. or ↓ metabolism of voriconazole

Nonnucleoside reverse transcriptase inhibitors (delavirdine, nevirapine) / Coadministration may ↑ or ↓ voriconazole metabolism; also, possible ↓ metabolism of nonnucleoside reverse transcriptase inhibitors

Omeprazole / ↑ Voriconazole AUC and C_{max}; ↑ omeprazole C_{max} and AUC; reduce dose of omeprazole by 50%

Phenytoin / ↓ Voriconazole C_{max} and AUC R/T ↑ CYP450 induction; ↑ phenytoin C_{max} and AUC up to 2 times

Pimozide / Metabolism of pimozide inhibited → R/T possible QT prolongation and rarely torsades de pointes; do not use together

Prednisolone / ↑ Prednisolone C_{max} and AUC; no dosage adjustment needed

Quinidine / Metabolism of quinidine inhibited → possible QT prolongation and rarely torsades de pointes; do not use together

Rifabutin / Significant ↓ voriconazole levels; ↑ C_{max} and AUC of rifabutin by 3- or 4-fold ; do not use together

Rifampin / Significant ↓ voriconazole levels; do not use together

Ritonavir (400 mg q 12 hr) / Significant ↓ voriconazole levels; do not use together

Saquinavir / Metabolism of saquinavir may be inhibited; ↑ or ↓ metabolism of voriconazole

Sirolimus / Significant ↑ sirolimus C_{max} and AUC; do not use together

Sulfonamides / ↑ Sulfonamide levels; monitor for hypoglycemia

Sulfonylureas / ↑ Sulfonylurea levels; dosage adjustment of the sulfonylurea is recommended

Tacrolimus / Significant ↑ tacrolimus C_{max} and AUC; reduce the dose of tacrolimus to 33% ; frequently monitor tacrolimus levels

Vinca alkaloids (vinblastine, vincristine) ↑ Vinca alkaloid levels → neurotoxicity; consider dosage adjustment of the vinca alkaloid and monitor for toxicity

Warfarin / Significant ↑ maximum PT time; closely monitor; also, voriconazole may ↑ PT in clients receiving other coumarin anticoagulants

HOW SUPPLIED

Powder for Injection, Lyophilized: 200 mg; *Powder for Oral Suspension:* 40 mg/mL (after reconstitution); *Tablets:* 50 mg, 200 mg.

DOSAGE

• IV; ORAL SUSPENSION; TABLETS

 = see color insert   = Herbal   = Intravenous   ℞ = sound alike drug

Candidemia in nonneutropenic clients and other deep tissue Candida *infections.*

Adults, initial, IV loading dose: 6 mg/kg q 12 hr for the first 24 hr; **then,** give an IV maintenance dose of 3–4 mg/kg q 12 hr or PO maintenance dose of 200 mg q 12 hr once the client can tolerate medication given PO. If clients are unable to tolerate 4 mg/kg IV, reduce the IV maintenance dose to 3 mg/kg q 12 hr.

Invasive aspergillosis; scedosporiosis and fusariosis.

Adults, initial, IV loading dose: 6 mg/kg q 12 hr for the first 24 hr; **then,** 4 mg/kg IV q 12 hr or 200 mg q 12 hr PO, once the client can tolerate PO medication. If clients are unable to tolerate 4 mg/kg IV, reduce the IV maintenance dose to 3 mg/kg q 12 hr.

• **ORAL SUSPENSION; TABLETS**
Esophageal candidiasis.

Adults: 200 mg q 12 hr. **Maintenance:** 200 mg q 12 hr for clients weighing 40 kg or more; 100 mg q 12 hr for those weighing 40 kg or less.

NURSING CONSIDERATIONS

ADMINISTRATION/STORAGE

1. Use only the tablets in those with moderate to severe renal dysfunction.
2. In those with mild to moderate hepatic cirrhosis (Child-Pugh Class A and B), the standard loading dose can be used but the maintenance dose should be halved. Use not recommended in those with severe liver impairment.
3. Dosage adjustment: If client response is inadequate, the PO maintenance dose may be increased from 200 mg q 12 hr to 300 mg q 12 hr. For adult clients weighing 40 kg or less, the PO maintenance dose may be increased from 100 mg q 12 hr to 150 mg q 12 hr. If clients are unable to tolerate 300 mg PO q 12 hr, decrease the PO maintenance dose by 50 mg steps to a minimum of 200 mg q 12 hr (or 100 mg q 12 hr for clients weighing 40 kg or less).
4. To reconstitute the oral suspension, tap the bottle to release the powder. Add 46 mL of water to the bottle and shake vigorously for about 1 min. Re-

move the child-resistant cap and push the bottle adaptor into the neck of the bottle; replace the cap. The date of expiration of the reconstituted suspension should be written on the bottle label (shelf-life is 14 days at controlled room temperature).

IV 5. To reconstitute, add 19 mL of water for injection to obtain an extractable volume of 20 mL containing 10 mg/mL. Use a standard 20 mL (nonautomated) syringe to ensure the exact amount of 19 mL of water for injection is used. Discard the vial if a vacuum does not pull the diluent into the vial. Shake the vial until all of the powder is dissolved.

6. Must be infused over 1–2 hr at a concentration of 5 mg/mL or less and at a rate of 3 mg/kg/hr. Thus, the reconstituted solution must be further diluted as follows:

• Calculate the volume of 10 mg/mL of concentrate required based on client weight (see package insert).

• To allow the required volume of voriconazole to be added, withdraw and discard at least an equal amount of diluent from the infusion bag or bottle to be used. The volume of diluent remaining in the bag/bottle should be such that when 10 mg/mL of drug is added, the final concentration is not less than 0.5 mg/mL or more than 5 mg/mL.

• Using an appropriate size syringe and aseptic technique, withdraw the required volume of 10 mg/mL voriconazole from the correct number of vials and add to the infusion bag/bottle. Discard partially used vials; do not use solutions that contain particles.

7. The reconstituted voriconazole (10 mg/mL) may be diluted with 0.9% NaCl, lactated Ringer's, D5W/RL, D5W/0.45% NaCl, D5W, D5W and 20 mEq KCl, 0.45% NaCl, and D5W/NSS. Do *not* dilute with 4.2% sodium bicarbonate infusion as the alkaline solution causes slight degradation of the drug after 24 hr at room temperature.

8. Do not infuse voriconazole into the same line or cannula at the same time

---

Bold Italic = life threatening side effect   ■ = black box warning   ✦ = Available in Canada

with other drug infusions, including parenteral nutrition. Also, do not give infusions of blood products or any electrolyte supplement at the same time as voriconazole.

9. Use the reconstituted concentrate immediately. If not used immediately do not store longer than 24 hr at 2–8°C (37–46°F).

ASSESSMENT

1. Note reasons for therapy, site, where contracted, characteristics of S&S, culture results.

2. List other agents prescribed to ensure none interact/compete.

3. During initial infusion, assess carefully for anaphylactoid–type reactions.

4. Monitor renal and LFTs carefully; reduce dose with dysfunction.

5. With prolonged therapy (>1 mo) ensure that eye exam for visual fields, acuity, and color perception performed.

CLIENT/FAMILY TEACHING

1. Take tablets or oral suspension at least 1 hr before or 1 hr after a meal.

2. Avoid activities that require mental alertness until drug effects realized. Do not drive at night as drug may cause vision changes including blurred vision and light sensitivity.

3. Avoid prolonged sun exposure; photosensitivity reaction may occur.

4. Practice reliable contraception.

5. Report any unusual or adverse side effects. Drug is used for a prolonged period and requires regular lab and medical F/U.

OUTCOMES/EVALUATE

• Resolution of fungal infection
• Symptomatic improvement

Vorinostat
(voh-**RIN**-oh-stat)

CLASSIFICATION(S):
Antineoplastic, histone deacetylase inhibitor
PREGNANCY CATEGORY: D
Rx: Vorinostat.

USES
Treat cutaneous manifestations of cutaneous T-cell lymphoma in those who have progressive, persistent, or recurrent disease on or following two systemic therapies.

ACTION/KINETICS

Action
Vorinostat inhibits activity of the enzymes histone deacetylases; these enzymes catalyze the removal of acetyl groups from the lysine residues of proteins, including histones. In some cancer cells there is an overexpression of histone deactylases or abnormal recruitment of histone acetylases causing hypoacetylation of histones. This leads to transcriptional activity of cancer cells. Vorinostat is believed to induce cell cycle arrest and/or apoptosis of some transformed cancer cells.

Pharmacokinetics
A high fat meal modestly increases the extent of absorption but decreases the rate of absorption of the drug. Metabolized in the liver by glucuronidation and hydrolysis; liver microsomes are negligibly involved in the metabolism. Excreted in the urine; **t½, terminal:** 2 hr.

CONTRAINDICATIONS
Lactation.

SPECIAL CONCERNS
Use with particular caution in those with congenital long QT syndrome or clients taking antiarrhythmics or other drugs that lead to QT prolongation. Greater sensitivity of older clients can not be ruled out. Use with caution in those with impaired renal or hepatic function. Safety and efficacy have not been determined in children.

SIDE EFFECTS

Most Common
Anorexia, diarrhea, constipation, N&V, weight decrease, chills, fatigue, anemia, thrombocytopenia, dry mouth, dysgeusia, alopecia.

CNS: Fatigue, dizziness, headache, syncope, lethargy, spinal cord injury. **GI:** Diarrhea, N&V, dysgeusia, dry mouth, anorexia, constipation, decreased appetite, cholecystitis, *GI hemorrhage.* **CV:** DVT, ischemic stroke, *MI, pulmonary embolism.* **Dermatologic:** Alopecia, pruritus, exfoliative dermatitis. **Hematologic:** Thombocytopenia, anemia, leukopenia, neutropenia. **Musculoskeletal:** Muscle spasms, chest pain. **Respiratory:** Cough, URTI, lobar pneumonia, *pulmonary embolism*. **GU:** Pelvic-ureteric obstruction, ureteric obstruction. **Body as a whole:** Weight decrease, chills, peripheral edema, pyrexia, angioneurotic edema, asthenia, dehydration, infection, *sepsis*, *death*. **Miscellaneous:** Hyperglycemia, enterococcal infection, streptococcal bacteremia, T-cell lymphoma.

LABORATORY TEST CONSIDERATIONS

↑ Serum glucose, serum creatinine. Proteinuria, hypokalemia.

DRUG INTERACTIONS

Valproic acid / Severe thrombocytopenia and GI bleeding; monitor platelet count every 2 weeks for the first 2 months

Warfarin / Prolongation of PT and INR; monitor carefully

HOW SUPPLIED

Capsules: 100 mg.

DOSAGE

- **CAPSULES**

  Cutaneous T-cell lymphoma.

  400 mg once daily with food. Continue treatment as long as there is no evidence of disease progression or unacceptable side effects. If intolerant to therapy, dose may be reduced to 300 mg once daily with food; the dose may be reduced further to 300 mg once daily with food for 5 consecutive days each week.

NURSING CONSIDERATIONS

ADMINISTRATION/STORAGE

1. Avoid direct contact of the powder in the capsules with the skin or mucous membranes. If contact occurs, wash thoroughly.

2. Store from 15–30°C (59–86°F).

ASSESSMENT

1. Note reasons for therapy, other systemic agents trialed with disease progression/recurrence.

2. Obtain EKG monitor for QT prolongation during treatment.

3. Monitor CBC, platelets, chemistry, lytes, glucose, renal and LFTs every 2 weeks during first 2 months of therapy and monthly thereafter.

4. List drugs prescribed. Assess for bleeding, pregnancy, severe N&V; may require antiemetics, fluids, or change in dosage.

5. Assess for conditions that may preclude therapy or require very close monitoring: DM, prolonged QT syndrome, blood clots, pregnancy.

CLIENT/FAMILY TEACHING

1. Do not open or crush vorinostat capsules; if accidentally opened do not touch capsule or powder. Take capsules with food.

2. High glucose may occur; adjustment of diet and/or therapy for increased glucose may be required.

3. Consume at least eight 8-ounce glasses of water per day during therapy to prevent dehydration.

4. May experience N&V, diarrhea; report so antiemetics, antidiarrheals and fluid and electrolyte replacements may be prescribed.

5. Report any sudden SOB or chest pain; may cause pulmonary embolus or DVT.

6. Practice reliable contraception; may cause fetal harm.

7. Keep all F/U appointments to evaluate CBC, EKG, response to therapy and any adverse side effects.

OUTCOMES/EVALUATE

Inhibition of progression of cutaneous T-cell lymphoma (CTCL)

Warfarin sodium
(**WAR**-far-in)

CLASSIFICATION(S):
Anticoagulant, coumarin derivative
PREGNANCY CATEGORY: X
Rx: Coumadin, Jantoven.
♣Rx: Apo-Warfarin, Gen-Warfarin, Taro-Warfarin.

USES
(1) Prophylaxis and treatment of venous thrombosis and its extension. (2) Prophylaxis and treatment of atrial fibrillation with embolization. (3) Prophylaxis and treatment of pulmonary embolism. (4) Prophylaxis and treatment of thromboembolic complications associated with atrial fibrillation. *Investigational:* Adjunct to treat small cell carcinoma of the lung with chemotherapy and radiation. Prophylaxis of recurrent transient ischemic attacks and to reduce the risk of recurrent MI. In combination with aspirin to reduce risk of a second MI.

ACTION/KINETICS
Action
Interferes with synthesis of vitamin K–dependent clotting factors resulting in depletion of clotting factors II, VII, IX, and X. Has no direct effect on an established thrombus although therapy may prevent further extension of a formed clot as well as secondary thromboembolic problems.

Pharmacokinetics
Well absorbed from the GI tract although food affects the rate (but not the extent) of absorption. Suitable for parenteral administration. **Peak activity:** 1.5–3 days; **duration:** 2–5 days. **t½:** 1–2.5 days. Metabolized in the liver and inactive metabolites are excreted through the urine and feces. **Plasma protein binding:** Highly bound.

CONTRAINDICATIONS
Lactation. IM use. Use of a large loading dose (30 mg) is not recommended due to increased risk of hemorrhage and lack of more rapid protection.

SPECIAL CONCERNS
Geriatric clients are at an increased risk for bleeding, thromboembolic events and atrial fibrillation. Anticoagulant use in the following clients leads to increased risk: Trauma, infection, renal insufficiency, sprue, vitamin K deficiency, severe to moderate hypertension, polycythemia vera, severe allergic disorders, vasculitis, indwelling catheters, severe diabetes, anaphylactic disorders, surgery or trauma resulting in large exposed raw surfaces. Use with caution in impaired hepatic and renal function. Safety and efficacy have not been determined in children less than 18 years of age. Careful monitoring and dosage regulation are required during dentistry and surgery.

SIDE EFFECTS
Most Common
Bleeding/hemorrhage (see possible symptoms below).
CV: *Hemorrhage* is the main side effect and may occur from any tissue or organ. Symptoms of hemorrhage include headache, paralysis; pain in the joints, abdomen, or chest; difficulty in breathing or swallowing; SOB, unexplained swelling or shock. **GI:** N&V, diarrhea, sore mouth, mouth ulcers, anorexia, abdominal pain/cramping (including cramping, flatulence, bloating), paralytic ileus, intestinal obstruction (due to intramural or submucosal hemorrhage). **Hepatic:** Hepatitis, cholestatic hepatic injury, jaundice. **Dermatologic:** Rash, dermatitis (including bullous eruptions), exfoliative dermatitis, urticaria, pruritus, alopecia, necrosis or gangrene of the skin and other tissues (due to protein C deficiency). **Body as a whole:** Hypersensitivity/allergic reactions, edema, fever, fatigue, lethargy, malaise, asthenia, pain, headache, dizziness, paresthesia, cold intolerance, paresthesia (including feeling of cold and chills). **Mis-**

 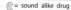

cellaneous: Red-orange urine, priapism, leukopenia, systemic cholesterol microembolization ("purple toes" syndrome), vasculitis, taste perversion, tracheal or tracheobronchial calcification (with long-term therapy).

LABORATORY TEST CONSIDERATIONS

False ↓ levels of serum theophylline determined by Schack and Waxler UV method (warfarin and dicumarol).

OD OVERDOSE MANAGEMENT

Symptoms: Early symptoms include melena, petechiae, microscopic hematuria, oozing from superficial injuries (e.g., nicks from shaving, excessive bruising, bleeding from gums after teeth brushing), excessive menstrual bleeding. *Treatment:* Discontinue therapy. Administer parenteral phytonadione (e.g., 5–25 mg parenterally). In emergency situations, 200–250 mL fresh frozen plasma or commercial factor IX complex. Fresh whole blood may be needed in clients unresponsive to phytonadione.

DRUG INTERACTIONS

Warfarin is responsible for more adverse drug interactions than any other group. Clients on anticoagulant therapy must be monitored carefully each time a drug is added or withdrawn. Monitoring usually involves determination of PT or INR. In general, a lengthened PT or INR means potentiation of the anticoagulant. Since potentiation may mean hemorrhages, a lengthened PT or INR warrants **reduction of the dosage of the anticoagulant.** However, the anticoagulant dosage must again be increased when the second drug is discontinued. A shortened PT or INR means inhibition of the anticoagulant and may require an increase in dosage.

Acetaminophen / ↑ Anticoagulant effect

Alcohol, ethyl / Chronic use ↓ warfarin effect

Aminoglutethimide / ↓ Warfarin effect R/T ↑ liver breakdown

Aminoglycoside antibiotics / ↑ Warfarin effect R/T interference with vitamin K

Amiodarone / ↑ Warfarin effect R/T ↓ liver breakdown

Androgens / ↑ Warfarin effect

Aprepitant / ↓ Warfarin levels and INR R/T increased metabolism by CYP2C9

Ascorbic acid / ↓ Warfarin effect by unknown mechanism

Aspirin / ↑ Risk of major bleeding

H *Avocado* / Possible ↓ warfarin effect (↓ INR)

Barbiturates / ↓ Warfarin effect R/T ↑ liver breakdown

Beta-adrenergic blockers / ↑ Warfarin effect

Bosentan / Possible ↓ INR

H *Bromelain* / ↑ Tendency for bleeding

Capecitabine / ↑ Risk of bleeding and altered coagulation

Carbamazepine / ↓ Warfarin effect R/T ↑ liver breakdown *Celecoxib* / ↑ PT & INR; ↑ risk of upper GI hemorrhage in geriatric clients

Cephalosporins / ↑ Warfarin effect R/T effects on platelet function

Chloral hydrate / ↑ Warfarin effect R/T ↓ plasma protein binding

Chloramphenicol / ↑ Warfarin effect R/T ↓ liver breakdown

Cholestyramine / ↓ Anticoagulant effect R/T binding and ↓ absorption from GI tract

Cimetidine / ↑ Anticoagulant effect R/T ↓ liver breakdown

H *Cinchona bark* / ↑ Anticoagulant effect

Clarithromycin / ↑ Warfarin effect R/T ↓ liver metabolism

Clofibrate / ↑ Anticoagulant effect

Clopidogrel / ↑ Risk of major bleeding

Contraceptives, oral / ↓ Anticoagulant effect R/T ↑ activity of certain clotting factors (VII and X); rarely, the opposite effect of ↑ risk of thromboembolism

Contrast media containing iodine / ↑ Warfarin effect by ↑ PT

Corticosteroids / ↑ Warfarin effect; also ↑ risk of GI bleeding R/T steroids ulcerogenic effect

H *Cranberry* / ↑ Warfarin effect R/T inhibition of cytochrome P450 isoenzymes

Cyclophosphamide / ↑ Anticoagulant effect

H *Danshen* / Possible ↑ warfarin effects

Dextrothyroxine / ↑ Warfarin effect

Bold Italic = life threatening side effect   ■ = black box warning   ✦ = Available in Canada

Dicloxacillin / ↓ Warfarin effect

Diflunisal / ↑ Anticoagulant effect and ↑ risk of bleeding R/T effect on platelet function and GI irritation

Dipyridamole / ↑ Risk of major bleeding

Disulfiram / ↑ Warfarin effect

H *Dong quai* / Potential for ↑ anticoagulant effects

Erythromycin / ↑ Warfarin effect R/T ↓ liver metabolism

Estrogens / ↓ Anticoagulant response by ↑ activity of certain clotting factors; rarely, the opposite effect of ↑ risk of thromboembolism

Etretinate / ↑ Warfarin effect R/T ↑ liver breakdown

H *Evening primrose oil* / Potential to ↓ platelet aggregation

H *Feverfew* / Potential to ↓ platelet aggregation

Fluconazole / ↑ Warfarin effect

H *Garlic* / Potential to ↓ platelet aggregation

Gatifloxacin / ↑ INR values

Gemfibrozil / ↑ Warfarin effect

H *Ginger* / Potential to ↓ platelet aggregation

H *Ginkgo biloba* / Potential to ↓ platelet aggregation; also, ginseng may ↑ warfarin metabolism

H *Ginseng, panax* / Potential to ↓ platelet aggregation

Glucagon / ↑ Warfarin effect

H *Grapeseed extract* / Potential to ↓ platelet aggregation

Griseofulvin / ↓ Warfarin effect

Hydantoins / ↑ Warfarin effect; also, ↑ hydantoin serum levels

Hypoglycemics, oral / ↑ Warfarin effect R/T ↓ plasma protein binding; also, ↑ effect of sulfonylureas

Ifosfamide / ↑ Warfarin effect R/T ↓ liver breakdown and displacement from protein binding sites

Indomethacin / ↑ Warfarin effect R/T effect on platelet function; also, indomethacin is ulcerogenic → GI hemorrhage

Isoniazid / ↑ Warfarin effect

Itraconazole / Anticoagulant effect is enhanced

Ketoconazole / ↑ Warfarin effect

Loop diuretics / ↑ Warfarin effect by displacement from protein binding sites

Lovastatin / ↑ Warfarin effect R/T ↓ liver breakdown

Metronidazole / ↑ Warfarin effect R/T ↓ liver breakdown *Miconazole* / ↑ Bleeding or bruising

Mineral oil / ↑ Hypoprothrombinemia by ↓ absorption of vitamin K from GI tract; also mineral oil may ↓ absorption of warfarin from GI tract

Moricizine / ↑ Warfarin effect

Nafcillin / ↓ Warfarin effect

Nalidixic acid / ↑ Warfarin effect R/T displacement from protein binding sites

Nevirapine / Possible ↓ anticoagulant effect

NSAIDs / ↑ Warfarin effect; ↑ risk of bleeding R/T effects on platelet function and GI irritation; ↑ risk of upper GI hemorrhage in geriatric clients

Omeprazole / ↑ Warfarin effect R/T ↓ liver breakdown

Orlistat / Possible ↑ INR

Oxandrolone / Large ↑ in INR; dose of warfarin may have to be greatly ↓

Penicillins / ↑ Warfarin effect → ↑ risk of bleeding R/T effects on platelet function

Propafenone / ↑ Warfarin effect R/T ↓ liver breakdown

Propoxyphene / ↑ Warfarin effect

Quinidine, quinine / ↑ Warfarin effect R/T ↓ liver breakdown

Quinolones / ↑ Warfarin effect

Rifampin / ↓ Anticoagulant effect R/T ↑ liver breakdown

Ritonavir / Possible ↓ anticoagulant effect

H *St. John's wort* / Possible ↓ warfarin plasma levels R/T ↑ metabolism

Salicylates / ↑ Warfarin effect and ↑ risk of bleeding R/T effect on platelet function and GI irritation

Spironolactone / ↓ Warfarin effect R/T hemoconcentration of clotting factors due to diuresis

Streptokinase / ↑ Warfarin effect

Sucralfate / ↓ Warfarin effect

Sulfamethoxzole and Trimethoprim / ↑ Warfarin effect R/T ↓ liver breakdown

Sulfinpyrazone / ↑ Anticoagulant effect R/T ↓ liver breakdown and inhibition

W

of platelet aggregation

Sulfonamides / ↑ Sulfonamide effects

Sulindac / ↑ Warfarin effect

Tamoxifen / ↑ Warfarin effect

Tetracyclines / ↑ Warfarin effect R/T interference with vitamin K

Thiazide diuretics / ↓ Warfarin effect R/T hemoconcentration of clotting factors due to diuresis

Thioamines / ↑ Warfarin effect

Thiopurines / ↓ Warfarin effect R/T ↑ synthesis or activation of prothrombin

Thyroid hormones / ↑ Anticoagulant effect with ↑ risk of bleeding

Tolterodine / Prolonged INR values

Trazodone / ↓ Warfarin effect

Trastuzumab / ↑ bleeding risk

Urokinase / ↑ Warfarin effect

Vitamin A / Possible ↑ anticoagulant effect if using large doses of Vitamin A

Vitamin C / Slightly prolonged PT

Vitamin E / ↑ Warfarin effect R/T interference with vitamin

Vitamin K / ↓ Warfarin effect

HOW SUPPLIED

Powder for Injection, Lyophilized: 2 mg; *Tablets:* 1 mg, 2 mg, 2.5 mg, 3 mg, 4 mg, 5 mg, 6 mg, 7.5 mg, 10 mg.

DOSAGE

- **IV; TABLETS**

    Induction.

    Adults, initial: 5–10 mg/day for 2–4 days; **then,** adjust dose based on prothrombin or INR determinations. A lower dose should be used in geriatric or debilitated clients or clients with increased sensitivity. Dosage has not been established for children.

    Maintenance.

    Adults: 2–10 mg/day, based on prothrombin or INR.

    Prevent blood clots with prosthetic heart valve replacement.

    2–5 mg daily.

NURSING CONSIDERATIONS

ADMINISTRATION/STORAGE

1. Frequent monitoring of PT/INR is recommended during the first week of therapy, during adjustment periods, and monthly thereafter.

2. Do not change brands; may be differences in bioavailability.

3. To transfer from heparin therapy, give heparin and warfarin together from the first day (delayed onset of oral anticoagulant effects). Alternatively, warfarin may be started on the third to sixth day of heparin therapy.

4. Levels of anticoagulation that are recommended for specific indications by the American College of Chest Physicians and the National Heart, Lung, and Blood Institute should be followed.

5. Protect from light; store at controlled room temperature. Dispense in tight, light-resistant container.

IV 6. Give as slow bolus over 1–2 min into peripheral vein.

7. To reconstitute for IV use: Add 2.7 mL sterile water for injection. Inspect for particulate matter and discoloration.

8. After reconstitution, injection stable for 4 hr at room temperature. There is no preservative; take care to assure sterility of prepared solution.

9. Vial is not for multiple use; discard unused solution.

ASSESSMENT

1. Note reasons for therapy, timeframe (i.e., DVT [initial] 6 months; recurrent/multiple DVT and heart valve replacement—lifetime); identify desired PT/INR range.

2. List drugs prescribed to ensure none interacts unfavorably by increasing or decreasing PT as a result of competition for protein binding at receptor sites.

3. Note any bleeding tendencies. Review PMH for conditions that may preclude therapy: PUD, chronic GI tract ulcerations, alcoholic, severe renal or liver dysfunction, endocardial infections.

4. Determine if pregnant. May cause fetal malformations and neonatal hemorrhage.

5. Monitor ECG, CBC, PT/PTT, INR, renal and LFTs.

6. Some clients may be managed/discharged early on low molecular weight heparin injections and coumadin until desired INR obtained. Adjust oral anticoagulant weekly, especially if receiving one of the many drugs known to interact or compete with warfarin.

Bold Italic = life threatening side effect   ■ = black box warning   ✚ = Available in Canada

7. Have available vitamin K, FFP, or factor IX concentrate for warfarin overdoses.

8. With atrial fibrillation assess echocardiogram and EKG; monitor INR.

INTERVENTIONS

1. Request written parameters noting the desired range for PT or INR, once anticoagulated (orally). It usually takes 36–48 hr for drug to reach steady state; therefore allow time to equilibrate. The INR is the PT ratio (test/control) obtained from human brain thromboplastin and is universally considered most accurate to calculate dosage.

2. Drug inhibits production of factors II, VII, IX, and X; onset in response is delayed because of degradation of clotting factors that have already been synthesized.

3. Question about bleeding (gums, urine, stools, vomit, bruises). If urine discolored, determine cause, i.e., from drug therapy or hematuria. Indanedione-type anticoagulants turn alkaline urine a red-orange color; acidify urine or test for occult blood.

4. Sudden lumbar pain may indicate retroperitoneal hemorrhage.

5. GI dysfunction may indicate intestinal hemorrhage. Test for blood in urine and feces; check H&H to assess for abnormal bleeding.

6. Observe for "purple toes" syndrome related to inhibition of protein C and S.

CLIENT/FAMILY TEACHING

1. Take oral warfarin as prescribed and at the same time each day; must be compliant with therapy. Do not change brands of drug; may alter response. Avoid eating large amounts of grapefruit or drinking grapefruit or cranberry juice.

2. This drug does not dissolve clots but decreases the clotting ability of the blood and helps to prevent the formation of harmful blood clots in the blood vessels and heart valves.

3. Avoid IM shots, activities/contact sports that may cause injury or cuts and bruises. Use a soft toothbrush, electric razor to shave, wear shoes and use a night light to avoid falls at night.

4. Report immediately unusual bruising/bleeding, dark brown or blood-tinged body secretions, injury or trauma, dizziness, abdominal pain or swelling, back pain, severe headaches, and joint swelling and pain.

5. If prescribed, may carry vitamin K for emergency use. (The usual dosage is 5–25 mg parenterally, to be used in the event of excessive bleeding.)

6. Foods high in vitamin K: asparagus, broccoli, cabbage, brussel sprouts, spinach, turnips, milk, cheese. Consistent intake of vitamin K foods should be done to ensure a stable INR as these may alter (lower) results.

7. Use reliable birth control. Menstruation may be prolonged and flow slightly increased. Report if excessive and unusual.

8. Skin eruptions may develop as an allergic reaction; report.

9. Avoid OTC drugs. Check prior to taking any OTC drugs that have anticoagulant-type effects such as salicylates, NSAIDS, steroids, vitamin K, mineral preparations from health food stores, vitamins, herbal teas, herbals, alcohol. Check with provider to see if they intend you to continue your baby aspirin. Should be done with AMI to prevent recurrence.

10. Wear identification and alert all providers of anticoagulant therapy.

11. Avoid smoking; increases dose requirements.

12. Identify social/economic situations that may alter compliance (lack of transportation for testing, inability to distinguish tablets or read directions); identify reliable resources.

13. Report as scheduled for regular labs to evaluate effectiveness of therapy and need for dosage changes. Once dose stabilized, PT/INR once monthly.

14. Unusual hair loss and itching are common with the elderly; advise to report if intolerable or skin break down occurs.

15. Elderly are more prone to developing bleeding complications. Many elderly use multiple pharmacies and shop for value; stress need to know what they are taking and why and to carry

---

the name and dosage of ALL drugs prescribed. Remind not to skip a dose as drug works for only 24 hr and must be readministered in order to be effective. Carry list of all meds/vitamins/herbals prescribed/consumed to all visits to provider/pharmacy.

OUTCOMES/EVALUATE

- PT within desired range (1.5–2 times the control)
- INR within desired range (2.0–3.0 with standard therapy; 2.5–4.0 with high-dose therapy)
- ↓ Risk of thromboembolism with prosthetic heart valves
- Resolution/prophylaxis of DVT

Zafirlukast
(zah-**FIR**-loo-kast)

CLASSIFICATION(S):
Antiasthmatic drug
PREGNANCY CATEGORY: B
Rx: Accolate.

USES
Prophylaxis and chronic treatment of asthma in adults and children 5 years of age and older. *Investigational:* Chronic urticaria.

ACTION/KINETICS
Action
A selective and competitive antagonist of leukotriene receptors D_4 and E_4, which are components of slow-reacting substance of anaphylaxis. It is believed that cysteinyl leukotriene occupation of receptors causes asthma, including airway edema, smooth muscle constriction, and altered cellular activity associated with the inflammatory process. Zafirlukast inhibits bronchoconstriction caused by sulfur dioxide and cold air in clients with asthma. It also attenuates the early- and late-phase reaction in asthmatics caused by inhalation of antigens such as grass, cat dander, ragweed, and mixed antigens.

Pharmacokinetics
Rapidly absorbed after PO use; bioavailability may be decreased when taken with food. **Peak plasma levels:** 3 hr. **$t\frac{1}{2}$, terminal:** About 10 hr. Extensively metabolized in the liver by CYP2C9, with about 90% excreted in the feces and 10% in the urine. Clearance is reduced in clients with cirrhosis. Inhibits certain cytochrome P450 isoenzymes. The C_{max} and AUC are increased in geriatric clients. **Plasma protein binding:** More than 99%.

CONTRAINDICATIONS
Use to terminate an acute asthma attack, including status asthmaticus. Lactation.

SPECIAL CONCERNS
The clearance is reduced in clients 65 years of age and older. Safety and efficacy have not been determined in children less than 5 years of age.

SIDE EFFECTS
Most Common
Headache, N&V, diarrhea, abdominal pain, infection, asthenia, dizziness, fever.
GI: N&V, diarrhea, abdominal pain, dyspepsia. **CNS:** Headache, dizziness. **Hepatic:** Hepatic dysfunction, especially in women and girls. Rarely, symptomatic hepatitis and hyperbilirubinemia. *Hypersensitivity reactions.* Urticaria, angioedema, rashes (with and without blistering). **Hematologic:** Agranulocytosis, systemic eosinophilia with vasculitis consistent with Churg-Strauss syndrome. **Miscellaneous:** Infection (especially in the elderly), generalized pain, asthenia, accidental injury, myalgia, arthralgia, fever, back pain, bleeding, bruising, edema.

LABORATORY TEST CONSIDERATIONS
↑ ALT.

Bold Italic = life threatening side effect   ■ = black box warning   ✦ = Available in Canada

DRUG INTERACTIONS

Aspirin / ↑ Zafirlukast levels by about 45%

Erythromycin / ↓ Zafirlukast levels R/T ↓ zafirlukast bioavailability

Theophylline / ↓ Zafirlukast levels

Warfarin / Significant ↑ PT; closely monitor and adjust dose if needed

HOW SUPPLIED

Tablets: 10 mg, 20 mg.

DOSAGE

- **TABLETS**
  Asthma.

Adults and children aged 12 and older: 20 mg 2 times per day. **Children, 7–11 years:** 10 mg 2 times/day; even during symptom-free periods.

NURSING CONSIDERATIONS

ADMINISTRATION/STORAGE

Protect from light and moisture; store at controlled room temperatures of 20–25°C (68–77°F). Dispense in original air-tight container.

ASSESSMENT

1. Note reasons for therapy, onset, duration, characteristics of S&S. List other agents trialed, outcome.

2. Note cardiopulmonary assessment findings. If liver dysfunction is suspected, discontinue therapy and perform LFTs immediately. If LFTs are consistent with hepatic dysfunction, do not resume therapy.

3. Monitor labs, symptomatic complaints, and PFTs. Reinforce that drug is not for acute bronchospasm during asthma attack.

CLIENT/FAMILY TEACHING

1. Take 1 hr before or 2 hr after meals to prevent loss of bioavailability.

2. Take drug regularly during symptom-free periods. Do not increase or decrease dose without approval.

3. Drug is not appropriate for acute episodes of asthma. Continue all other antiasthma agents as prescribed.

4. Review peak flow meter use and set targets for intervention or additional therapy.

5. Avoid triggers, i.e., dust, chemicals, cigarette smoke, pollutants, pets, and perfumes.

6. Practice reliable birth control; do not breastfeed during therapy.

7. Keep all F/U appointments to evaluate lungs/pulmonary function and response to therapy.

OUTCOMES/EVALUATE

Inhibition of bronchoconstriction; improved breathing patterns

Zalcitabine (Dideoxycytidine, ddC) ■

(zal-**SIGH**-tah-been)

CLASSIFICATION(S):

Antiviral, nucleoside reverse transcriptase inhibitor

PREGNANCY CATEGORY: C

SEE ALSO *ANTIVIRAL DRUGS* AND *ANTI-INFECTIVE DRUGS*.

USES

In combination with antiretroviral drugs to treat HIV infection.

ACTION/KINETICS

Action

Converted in cells to the active metabolite, dideoxycytidine 5′-triphosphate (ddCTP), by cellular enzymes. ddCTP serves as an alternative substrate to deoxycytidine triphosphate for HIV-reverse transcriptase, thereby inhibiting the in vitro replication of HIV-1 and inhibiting viral DNA synthesis. The incorporation of ddCTP into the growing DNA chain leads to premature chain termination. ddCTP serves as a competitive inhibitor of the natural substrate for deoxycytidine triphosphate for the active site of the viral reverse transcriptase, which further inhibits viral DNA synthesis.

Pharmacokinetics

Food reduces the rate of absorption. Does not appear to undergo significant metabolism by the liver. **Elimination** **t½:** 1–3 hr. Approximately 70% of a PO dose is excreted through the kidneys and 10% in the feces. Prolonged elimination (t½ up to 8.5 hr) is observed in clients with impaired renal function.

Z

 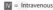

CONTRAINDICATIONS
Lactation.

SPECIAL CONCERNS

■ (1) Use has been associated with significant clinical side effects, some of which may be fatal. Zalcitabine can cause severe peripheral neuropathy; thus, use with extreme caution in those with pre-existing neuropathy. (2) May also cause pancreatitis (rare); immediately stop therapy in those who develop any symptoms suggestive of pancreatitis while using zalcitabine until this diagnosis is excluded. (3) Lactic acidosis and severe hepatomegaly with steatosis, including fatalities, have been reported with the use of antiretroviral nucleoside analogs alone or in combination, including zalcitabine. Also, rare cases of hepatic failure and death, possibly related to underlying hepatitis B and zalcitabine have been reported.■ Use with extreme caution in clients with low CD$_4$ cell counts (<50/mm^3). Use with caution in clients with a history of pancreatitis or known risk factors for the development of pancreatitis. Clients with a C$_{CR}$ less than 55 mL/min may be at a greater risk for toxicity due to decreased clearance. Clients may continue to develop opportunistic infections and other complications of HIV infection. Safety and efficacy have not been determined in HIV-infected children less than 13 years of age. Hypersensitivity. Use with caution in moderate or severe peripheral neuropathy or with drugs that have the potential to cause peripheral neuropathy (see *Drug Interactions*). Severe peripheral neuropathy, pancreatitis (rare), hepatic failure (rare), lactic acidosis, and severe hepatomegaly with steatosis, reported. Caution in elderly. Monitor CBC and clinical chemistry tests before therapy and at appropriate intervals thereafter. Possible redistribution or accumulation of body fat.

SIDE EFFECTS

Most Common

Peripheral neuropathy, abnormal hepatic function, fatigue, rash/pruritus/urticaria, convulsions, headache, abdominal pain, oral lesions/stomatitis, N&V, diarrhea, constipation, fever.

NOTE: The incidence of certain side effects is dependent on the duration of use and the dose of the drug. **Neurologic:** Peripheral neuropathy (may be severe) characterized by numbness and burning dysesthesia involving the distal extremities; this may be followed by sharp shooting pains or severe continuous burning pain if the drug is not withdrawn. The neuropathy may progress to severe pain requiring narcotic analgesics and may be irreversible. **GI:** *Fatal pancreatitis, lactic acidosis and hepatomegaly with steatosis* when given alone or with zidovudine. Esophageal ulcers, oral/esophageal ulcers, N&V, dysphagia, anorexia, abdominal pain, constipation, ulcerative stomatitis, aphthous stomatitis, diarrhea, dry mouth, dyspepsia, glossitis, *rectal hemorrhage*, hemorrhoids, enlarged abdomen, gum disorders, flatulence, anorexia, tongue ulceration, dysphagia, eructation, gastritis, *GI hemorrhage*, left quadrant pain, salivary gland enlargement, esophageal pain, esophagitis, rectal ulcers, melena, painful swallowing, mouth lesion, acute pharyngitis, abdominal bloating or cramps, anal/rectal pain, colitis, dental abscess, epigastric pain, gagging with pills, gingivitis, heartburn, *hemorrhagic pancreatitis*, increased salivation, odynophagia, painful sore gums, rectal mass, sore tongue, sore throat, tongue disorder, toothache, unformed/loose stools. **Dermatologic:** Rash (including erythematous, maculopapular, follicular), pruritus, night sweats, dermatitis, skin lesions, acne, alopecia, bullous eruptions, increased sweating, urticaria, hot flashes, lip blister or lesions, carbuncle/furuncle, cellulitis, dry skin, dry rash desquamation, exfoliative dermatitis, finger inflammation, impetigo, infection, itchy rash, moniliasis, mucocutaneous/skin disorder, nail disorder, photosensitivity, skin fissure, skin ulcer. **CNS:** Headache, convulsions, dizziness, seizures, ataxia, abnormal coordination, Bell's palsy, dysphonia, hyperkinesia, hypokinesia, migraine, neuralgia, neuritis, stupor, aphasia, decreased neurologic function, disequilibrium, facial

---

Bold Italic = life threatening side effect   ■ = black box warning   ✦ = Available in Canada

nerve palsy, focal motor seizures, memory loss, paralysis, speech disorder, *status epilepticus*, tremor, vertigo, hypertonia, hand tremor, twitching, confusion, impaired concentration, insomnia, agitation, depersonalization, hallucinations, emotional lability, nervousness, anxiety, depression, euphoria, manic reaction, dementia, amnesia, somnolence, abnormal thinking, crying, loss of memory, decreased concentration/motivation/sexual desire, acute psychotic disorder, acute stress reaction, mood swings, paranoid states, *suicide attempt*. **Respiratory:** Coughing, dyspnea, respiratory distress, rales/rhonchi, nasal discharge, flu-like symptoms, cyanosis, acute nasopharyngitis, chest/sinus congestion, dry nasal mucosa, hemoptysis, sinus pain, sinusitis, wheezing. **Musculoskeletal:** Myalgia, arthralgia, arthritis, arthropathy, cold extremities, leg cramps, myositis, joint pain or inflammation, weakness in leg muscle, generalized muscle weakness, back pain, backache, bone aches and pains, bursitis, pain in extremities, joint swelling, muscle disorder/stiffness/cramps, arthrosis, myopathy, neck pain, rib pain, stiff neck. **Hepatic:** Exacerbation of hepatic dysfunction, especially in those with preexisting liver disease or with a history of alcohol abuse. Abnormal hepatic function, hepatitis, jaundice, hepatocellular damage, severe hepatomegaly with steatosis, cholecystitis. **CV:** *Cardiomyopathy*, CHF, abnormal cardiac movement arrhythmia, atrial fibrillation, *cardiac failure*, cardiac dysrhythmias, heart racing, hypertension, palpitations, *subarachnoid hemorrhage*, syncope, tachycardia, ventricular ectopy, epistaxis. **Hematologic:** Anemia, leukopenia, thrombocytopenia, alteration of absolute neutrophil count, granulocytosis, eosinophilia, neutropenia, hemoglobinemia, neutrophilia, platelet alteration, purpura, thrombus, unspecified hematologic toxicity, alteration of WBCs. **Hypersensitivity:** Urticaria, *anaphylaxis* (rare). **Endocrine:** Diabetes mellitus, gout, hot flushes, hypoglycemia, hyperglycemia, hypocalcemia, hypophosphatemia, hyper-/hyponatremia, hypomagnesemia, hyperkalemia, hypokalemia, hyperlipidemia, polydipsia. **GU:** Dysuria, toxic nephropathy, polyuria, renal calculi, *acute renal failure*, hyperuricemia, increased frequency of micturition, abnormal renal function, renal cyst, albuminuria, bladder pain, genital lesion/ulcer, nocturia, painful/sore penis, penile edema, testicular swelling, urinary retention, vaginal itch/ulcer/pain, vaginal/cervix disorder. **Ophthalmic:** Abnormal vision, burning or itching eyes, xerophthalmia, eye pain or abnormality, blurred or decreased vision, eye inflammation/irritation, eye redness/hemorrhage, increased tears, mucopurulent conjunctivitis, photophobia, dry eyes, unequal sized pupils, yellow sclera. **Otic:** Ear pain/blockage, fluid in ears, hearing loss, tinnitus. **Body as a whole:** Fatigue, fever, rigors, chest pain or tightness, weight decrease, pain, malaise, asthenia, generalized edema, general debilitation, chills, difficulty moving, facial pain or swelling, flank pain, flushing, pelvic/groin pain. **Miscellaneous:** Lymphadenopathy, taste perversion, decreased taste, parosmia, lactic acidosis.

LABORATORY TEST CONSIDERATIONS

↑ ALT, AST, alkaline phosphatase, CPK, amylase, nonprotein nitrogen. Abnormal gamma-glutamyl transferase, GGT, LDH, lactate dehydrogenase, triglycerides, lipase. Bilirubinemia. ↓ Hematocrit.

DRUG INTERACTIONS

The following drugs have the potential to cause peripheral neuropathy. **Concomitant use is not recommended.** Drugs include: Chloramphenicol, cisplatin, dapsone, didanosine, disulfiram, ethionamide, gold, hydralazine, iodoquinol, isoniazid, metronidazole, nitrofurantoin, phenytoin, ribavirin, vincristine. Drugs such as amphotericin, foscarnet, and aminoglycosides may increase the risk of peripheral neuropathy by interfering with the renal clearance of zalcitabine, thus increasing plasma levels.

Antacids (Mg/Al-containing) / ↓ Zalcitabine absorption
Cimetidine / ↓ Zalcitabine elimination

by ↓ renal tubular secretion

Metoclopramide / ↓ Zalcitabine absorption

Pentamidine / ↑ Risk of fulminant pancreatitis

Probenecid / ↓ Zalcitabine elimination by ↓ renal tubular secretion

HOW SUPPLIED
Tablets: 0.375 mg, 0.75 mg.

DOSAGE

- **TABLETS**

  In combination with antiretroviral drugs (e.g., zidovudine) in advanced HIV infection.

  Adults and children 13 years and older: 0.75 mg q 8 hr given at the same time with 200 mg zidovudine q 8 hr for a total daily dose of 2.25 mg zalcitabine and 600 mg zidovudine.

NURSING CONSIDERATIONS

ADMINISTRATION/STORAGE
1. Greater effect noted when new antiretroviral drugs are started at the same time as zalcitabine.
2. If C_{CR} is 10–40 mL/min, reduce dose to 0.75 mg/12 hr; if C_{CR} <10 mL/min, reduce dose to 0.75 mg/24 hr.
3. Dosage reduction not required for weights down to 30 kg.

ASSESSMENT
1. Clients with a history of pancreatitis or elevated serum amylase should be followed closely while on zalcitabine therapy. Obtain baseline serum amylase and triglyceride levels with history of pancreatitis, increased amylase, those on parenteral nutrition, or those with a history of drug abuse.
2. Frequent monitoring of hematologic indices is recommended to detect serious anemia or granulocytopenia. In clients manifesting hematologic toxicity, decreases in hemoglobin may occur as early as 2–4 weeks after beginning therapy, whereas granulocytopenia may be seen after 6–8 weeks of therapy.
3. Monitor CBC, CD_4 counts/viral loads, liver and renal function studies; adjust dose with renal dysfunction.
4. Assess for symptoms of peripheral neuropathy: pain, numbness, and tingling. If symptoms evident, drug may

be reintroduced at 50% of the initial dose (i.e., 0.375 mg/8 hr) once all symptoms related to the peripheral neuropathy have improved to mild. Permanently discontinue the drug if severe discomfort due to peripheral neuropathy progresses for 1 week or longer.

CLIENT/FAMILY TEACHING
1. Take with or without food (with concurrently prescribed zidovudine, if appropriate) every 8 hr.
2. Drug is not a cure, may prolong life and helps to alleviate and manage the symptoms of HIV infections. May continue to develop opportunistic infections and other complications of HIV infection; remain under close medical supervision.
3. Use reliable contraceptive and practice safe sex.
4. Discontinue and report if symptoms of peripheral neuropathy occur, especially if they are bilateral and progress for more than 72 hr. Symptoms include numbness, tingling, or burning sensation especially in the feet or tips of the toes. Peripheral neuropathy may continue to worsen despite interruption of therapy. If symptoms improve, then drug may be reintroduced at a lower dose.
5. Schedule retinal exams q 6 months to assess for retinal depigmentation.
6. Identify local support groups that may assist client/family to understand and cope with this disease.

OUTCOMES/EVALUATE
Improved CD_4 cell counts, ↓ viral load, ↓ incidence of opportunistic infection, and improved survival rates in clients with advanced HIV infections

Zaleplon
(**ZAL**-leh-plon)

CLASSIFICATION(S):
Sedative-hypnotic, nonbenzodiazepine

PREGNANCY CATEGORY: C

Rx: Sonata, **C-IV**

✤**Rx:** Starnoc.

USES
Treat insomnia for up to 5 weeks.

ACTION/KINETICS
Action
Nonbenzodiazepine hypnotic. However, it interacts with the GABA-benzodiazepine receptor complex. It binds selectively to the brain omega-1 receptor located on the alpha subunit of $GABA_A$ receptor complex and potentiates t-butyl-bicyclophosphorothionate (TBPS) binding. Although it decreases the time to sleep, it does not increase total sleep time or decrease the number of awakenings. Decreased hangover effect.

Pharmacokinetics
Rapidly and almost completely absorbed. **Peak plasma levels:** 1 hr. Undergoes significant first-pass metabolism. A high-fat or heavy meal prolongs absorption. Extensively metabolized to inactive metabolites which are excreted in the urine (70%) and feces (17%). **$t\frac{1}{2}$:** About 1 hr.

CONTRAINDICATIONS
Use with alcohol, severe hepatic impairment, or during lactation.

SPECIAL CONCERNS
Use with caution in diseases or conditions that could affect metabolism or hemodynamic responses, in clients with compromised respiratory function, or in clients showing signs or symptoms of depression. Abuse potential is similar to benzodiazepine and benzodiazepine-like hypnotics. The products contain tartrazine (FD&C yellow #5) which may cause an allergic-type reaction, especially in those with aspirin hypersensitivity. May cause amnesia and dependence.

SIDE EFFECTS
Most Common
Headache, myalgia, nausea, dyspepsia, eye pain, abdominal pain, asthenia, dysmenorrhea, fever, hyperacusis, vertigo, anorexia, abnormal vision, malaise, epistaxis.

Listed are side effects with an incidence of 0.1% or greater. **CNS:** Dizziness, amnesia, somnolence, anxiety, paresthesia, depersonalization, hypesthesia, tremor, hallucinations, vertigo, depression, hypertonia, nervousness, abnormal thinking/concentration, abnormal gait, agitation, apathy, ataxia, circumoral paresthesia, confusion, emotional lability, euphoria, hyperesthesia, hyperkinesia, hypotonia, incoordination, insomnia, decreased libido, neuralgia, nystagmus. **GI:** Nausea, dyspepsia, anorexia, colitis, constipation, dry mouth, eructation, esophagitis, flatulence, gastritis, gastroenteritis, gingivitis, glossitis, increased appetite, melena, mouth ulceration, rectal hemorrhage, stomatitis. **CV:** Migraine, angina pectoris, bundle branch block, hypertension, hypotension, palpitation, syncope, tachycardia, vasodilation, ventricular extrasystoles. **Dermatologic:** Pruritus, rash, acne, alopecia, contact dermatitis, dry skin, eczema, maculopapular rash, skin hypertrophy, sweating, urticaria, vesiculobullous rash. **GU:** Bladder/breast/kidney pain, cystitis, decreased urine stream, dysuria, hematuria, impotence, kidney calculus, menorrhagia, urinary frequency/incontinence/urgency, vaginitis, dysmenorrhea. **Respiratory:** Bronchitis, asthma, dyspnea, laryngitis, pneumonia, snoring, voice alteration. **Musculoskeletal:** Arthritis, arthrosis, bursitis, joint disorder (swelling, stiffness, pain), myasthenia, tenosynovitis. **Hematologic:** Anemia, ecchymosis, lymphadenopathy. **Metabolic:** Edema, gout, hypercholesterolemia, thirst, weight gain. **Ophthalmic:** Eye pain, abnormal vision, conjunctivitis, diplopia, dry eyes, photophobia, watery eyes. **Otic:** Ear pain, hyperacusis, tinnitus. **Body as a whole:** Headache, asthenia, myalgia, fever, malaise, chills, generalized edema. **Miscellaneous:** Abdominal pain, photosensitivity, peripheral edema, epistaxis, back pain, chest pain, substernal chest pain, face edema, hangover effect, neck rigidity, parosmia.

DRUG INTERACTIONS
Cimetidine / Significantly ↑ zaleplon levels

CNS depressants (anticonvulsants, antihistamines, ethanol) / Additive CNS depression

Rifampin / Significantly ↓ zaleplon levels

HOW SUPPLIED
Capsules: 5 mg, 10 mg.

DOSAGE

- **CAPSULES**

Insomnia.

Adults, nonelderly: 10 mg for no more than 7–10 days. Consider 20 mg for the occasional client who does not benefit from the lower dose. Do not exceed a dose of 20 mg. **Mild to moderate hepatic impairment, elderly clients, or low-weight individuals:** 5 mg, not to exceed 10 mg.

NURSING CONSIDERATIONS

© Do not confuse Sonata and Soriatane (for severe psoriasis)

ASSESSMENT
1. Note reasons for insomnia, characteristics of S&S, contributing factors. Note drugs prescribed to ensure none interact; with cimetidine initially reduce zaleplon dose to 5 mg and assess response.
2. List any depression, respiratory dysfunction, alcohol or drug dependence. Drug may cause dependence and amnesia.
3. Contains tartrazine (FD&C yellow #5); note any aspirin hypersensitivity. Monitor renal and LFTs; reduce dose with liver dysfunction.

CLIENT/FAMILY TEACHING
1. Due to its rapid onset, ingest immediately prior to going to bed or after going to bed and experiencing difficulty falling asleep. Store out of the reach of children.
2. Taking zaleplon with or immediately after a heavy, high-fat meal causes slower absorption leading to a reduced effect on sleep latency.
3. Do not engage in activities requiring mental alertness after ingesting drug and during the next day until drug effects realized. Avoid alcohol and CNS depressants.
4. May experience amnesia. Obtain at least 4 hr sleep after ingestion and before activity. If also taking cimetidine, take an initial lowered dose of 5 mg of zaleplon.
5. May experience withdrawal symptoms or worsening of insomnia with abrupt drug discontinuation especially with daily use for an extended period of time.
6. If behavioral changes or unusual thinking occur involving aggressiveness, confusion, loss of personal identity, agitation, hallucinations, increased depression or suicide ideations, report.
7. Identify triggers (caffeine, day time naps) and alternative methods to induce sleep i.e soft music, warm milk, white noise simulator etc.

OUTCOMES/EVALUATE
Relief of insomnia

Zanamivir
(zah-**NAM**-ih-vir)

CLASSIFICATION(S):
Antiviral
PREGNANCY CATEGORY: C
Rx: Relenza.

USES
(1) Treatment of uncomplicated acute illness due to influenza virus A and B (limited) in adults and children 7 years and older who have been symptomatic for 2 or less days. (2) Prophylaxis of influenza in adults and children at least 5 years of age. *NOTE:* There is no evidence that zanamivir is effective in any illness caused by agents other than influenza virus A and B.

ACTION/KINETICS
Action
Selectively inhibits influenza virus neuraminidase. The enzyme allows virus release from infected cells, prevents virus aggregation, and possibly decreases virus inactivation by respiratory mucus. Zanamivir may alter virus particle aggregation and release. There is the possibility of emergence of resistance. Does not prevent complications from bacterial infections.

Pharmacokinetics
About 4–17% is absorbed systemically. **Peak serum levels:** 17–142 ng/mL within 1–2 hr after a 10 mg dose. Readily excreted as unchanged drug in the urine. Unabsorbed drug is excreted in

---

the feces. **t½:** 2.5–5.1 hr after PO inhalation. **Plasma protein binding:** Less than 10%.

CONTRAINDICATIONS

Hypersensitivity to zanamivir or any component of the product. Use in asthma or COPD.

SPECIAL CONCERNS

Use with caution during lactation. It is possible the elderly may be more sensitive to effects of the drug. Safety and efficacy have not been determined for treating influenza in children less than 7 years of age, in clients with underlying chronic pulmonary disease, in those with high-risk underlying medical conditions (e.g., respiratory disease), or in those with severe renal insufficiency. Serious bacterial infections may begin with flu-like symptoms or may coexist with or occur as complications during the course of flu; zanamivir has not been shown to prevent such complications.

SIDE EFFECTS

Most Common

Dizziness, headache, N&V, diarrhea, bronchitis, cough, ENT infections, sinusitis

GI: Diarrhea, N&V, abdominal pain, anorexia, increased/decreased appetite. **Respiratory:** Nasal S&S, bronchitis, ***bronchospasm,*** dyspnea, cough, sinusitis, ENT infections, ***ENT hemorrhages in children***, asthma in children, throat/tonsil discomfort and pain in children, viral respiratory infections in children with chronic respiratory disease, nasal inflammation in children. **CNS:** Dizziness, headache, ***seizures***. **CV:** Arrhythmias, syncope. **Hypersensitivity:** Oropharyngeal edema, serious skin rashes, ***anaphylaxis***. **Musculoskeletal:** Myalgia, arthralgia, muscle pain, articular rheumatism. **Dermatologic:** Facial edema, rash, including serious cutaneous reactions. **Body as a whole:** Malaise, chills, fatigue, fever, urticaria, allergic reactions (including oropharyngeal edema and serious skin rashes), serious bacterial infections with flu-like symptoms or as complications of flu.

LABORATORY TEST CONSIDERATIONS

↑ Liver enzymes, CPK. Lymphopenia, neutropenia.

HOW SUPPLIED

Power for Inhalation, Blisters: 5 mg.

DOSAGE

- **POWDER FOR ORAL INHALATION (BLISTERS)**

Influenza treatment.

Adults and children over 7 years: 2 inhalations (one 5-mg blister per inhalation for a total dose of 10 mg) twice a day for 5 days. Two doses are taken on the first day of treatment whenever possible, provided there are 2 or more hr between doses. On subsequent days, doses are taken about 12 hr apart (i.e., morning and evening) at about the same time each day. Safety and efficacy of repeated treatment courses have not been studied.

Prophylaxis of influenza: household setting.

10 mg once daily for 10 days. The 10 mg dose is obtained by 2 inhalations (one-5 mg blister/inhalation). Administer the dose about the same time each day. There are no data on the efficacy of prophylaxis in a household setting begun more than 1.5 days after the onset of signs and symptoms.

Prophylaxis of influenza: community outbreaks.

10 mg once daily for 28 days. The 10 mg dose is obtained by 2 inhalations (one-5 mg blister/inhalation). Administer the dose at about the same time each day. There are no data on the efficacy of prophylaxis in a community outbreak when started more than 5 days after the outbreak was identified. Safety and efficacy of prophylaxis have not been determined for longer than 28 days' duration.

NURSING CONSIDERATIONS

ADMINISTRATION/STORAGE

1. The drug is given by oral inhalation only, using the Diskhaler provided.
2. Do not puncture the zanamivir blister until taking a dose using the Diskhaler.
3. Store at from 15–30°C (59–86°F).

 = see color insert   = Herbal   = Intravenous   @ = sound alike drug

ASSESSMENT

1. Note reasons for therapy, onset, characteristics of influenza S&S, contact with infected individuals, any other medical conditions; note drug allergies.

2. Not for use in those with asthma or COPD.

3. Monitor CBC, LFTs, lung assessment findings. Stop drug if bronchospasm or decline in peak flows evident.

4. Some pediatric deaths (Japan), and neuropsychiatric events have been reported; use cautiously until further research available.

5. Useful if started within 48 hr of onset of S&S; ensure yearly flu shot.

CLIENT/FAMILY TEACHING

1. Therapy is used to lessen the symptoms of influenza. To be given by oral inhalation only, using the Diskhaler provided. Review/demonstrate use of the delivery system.

2. Do not puncture any Relenza Rotadisk blister until taking a dose using the Diskhaler. Keep Diskhaler level and close lips around the mouth piece. Breath in deep and steadily. Hold breath for a few seconds after inhaling to keep the drug in the lungs, then slowly expire.

3. Continue complete treatment (5 days) despite feeling better. Take oral inhalations twice a day 12 hr apart at approximately the same time each day. Safety and efficacy of repeated treatment courses have not been evaluated.

4. If client is to use an inhaled bronchodilator at the same time as zanamivir, use the bronchodilator before taking zanamivir.

5. Does not reduce the risk of transmission of flu to others. Vaccination is still the primary means to prevent and control influenza. Therapy may or may not improve symptoms and recovery time.

6. Clients with asthma or COPD may experience bronchospasm with zanamivir; weigh risk benefit ratio and have a fast-acting inhaled bronchodilator available, stop zanamivir and contact provider immediately if worsening of respiratory symptoms experienced.

7. An increased risk of confusion and unusual behavioral changes has been noted. The risk may be greater in children. Report symptoms of confusion or any other unusual behavioral changes.

OUTCOMES/EVALUATE

Relief of influenza S&S

Ziconotide ∎

(zye-**KOH**-noh-tide)

CLASSIFICATION(S):
Analgesic
PREGNANCY CATEGORY: C
Rx: Prialt.

USES

Management of severe chronic pain in clients for whom intrathecal therapy is warranted and who are intolerant or refractory to other treatment (e.g., systemic analgesics, adjunctive therapies, or intrathecal morphine).

ACTION/KINETICS

Action

Ziconotide is a conopeptide that binds to N-type calcium channels located on the primary nociceptive (A-sigma and C) afferent nerves in the superficial layers of the dorsal horn of the spinal cord. The mechanism of action is not known but it is believed the drug's binding blocks N-type calcium channels, which leads to a blockade of excitatory neurotransmitter release in the primary afferent nerve terminals resulting in analgesia. Ziconotide is not an opiate and will not prevent or relieve symptoms associated with opiate withdrawal.

Pharmacokinetics

The drug is administered intrathecally. Following passage from the CSF into the systemic circulation during continuous intrathecal administration, the drug is susceptible to proteolytic cleavage by various ubiquitous peptidases/proteases present in most organs (i.e., kidney, liver, lung, muscle). Thus, it is readily degraded to peptide fragments and free amino acids. **t$\frac{1}{2}$, terminal, from CSF:** 4.6 hr; **t$\frac{1}{2}$, plasma:** 1.3 hr.

CONTRAINDICATIONS

Hypersensitivity to ziconotide or any components of the product and in those with any other concomitant treatment or medical condition that would render intrathecal administration hazardous. Preexisting history of psychosis with ziconotide. Presence of infection at the microinfusion injection site, uncontrolled bleeding diathesis, and spinal canal obstruction that impairs circulation of CSF. IV use of the product. Lactation.

SPECIAL CONCERNS

■ Severe psychiatric symptoms and neurological impairment may occur during treatment. Do not treat clients with a pre-existing history of psychosis with ziconotide. Monitor all clients frequently for evidence of cognitive impairment, hallucinations, or changes in mood or consciousness. In the event of serious neurological or psychiatric signs or symptoms, ziconotide therapy can be interrupted or discontinued abruptly without evidence of withdrawal effects.■ Safety and efficacy have not been determined in children.

SIDE EFFECTS

Most Common

Dizziness, asthenia, somnolence, N&V, abnormal gait, ataxia, confusion, headache, hypertonia, impaired memory, diarrhea, anorexia, abnormal vision, pain.

CNS: Dizziness, somnolence, asthenia, confusion, ataxia, abnormal gait, headache, impaired memory, hyper-/hypotonia, anxiety, speech disorder, aphasia, dysesthesia, hallucinations, nervousness, paresthesia, vertigo, abnormal dreams, agitation, anxiety, aphasia, abnormal CSF, confusion, depression, difficulty concentrating, emotional lability, hostility, hyperesthesia, incoordination, insomnia, impaired memory, mental slowing, *meningitis*, nervousness, neuralgia, paranoid reaction, decreased reflexes, speech disorder, stupor, abnormal thinking, tremor, twitching, vertigo, *tonic-clonic seizures*, myoclonus, psychosis, *suicidal ideations, suicide (rare)*. **GI:** N&V, diarrhea, anorexia, dry mouth, abdominal pain, constipation, dyspepsia, GI disorder. **CV:** Hyper-/hypotension, postural hypotension, syncope, tachycardia, vasodilation, atrial fibrillation, *CVA*, abnormal ECG. **Respira-**

tory: Bronchitis, increased cough, dyspnea, lung disorder, pharyngitis, pneumonia, rhinitis, sinusitis, respiratory distress, *fatal aspiration pneumonia (rare)*. **Dermatologic:** Cutaneous surgical complication, dry skin, pruritus, rash, skin disorder, sweating. **Musculoskeletal:** Arthralgia, arthritis, leg cramps, myalgia, myasthenia, myoclonus, rhabdomyolysis. **GU:** Urinary retention, dysuria, urinary incontinence, UTI, impaired urination, acute kidney failure. **Metabolic:** Dehydration, edema, peripheral edema, weight loss. **Ophthalmic:** Abnormal vision, nyastagmus, diplopia, photophobia. **Body as a whole:** Fever, pain, cellulitis, chills, fever, flu syndrome, infection, malaise, viral infection, *sepsis*. **Miscellaneous:** Taste perversion, tinnitus, accidental injury, back pain, catheter complication, catheter-site pain, chest pain, neck pain/rigidity, pump-site complication, pump-site mass/pain.

LABORATORY TEST CONSIDERATIONS

↑ Creatinine phosphokinase.

OD OVERDOSE MANAGEMENT

Symptoms: Overdoses may occur because of pump programming errors or incorrect drug concentration preparations. Symptoms of overdose include ataxia, nystagmus, dizziness, stupor, unresponsiveness, spinal myoclonus, confusion, sedation, hypotension, word-finding difficulties, garbled speech, N&V. *Treatment:* There is no known antidote. Provide general medical supportive measures. Hospitalization may be necessary. The effects are not blocked by opioid antagonists. In the event of an inadvertent IV or epidural administration, hypotension could result; treat with a recumbent posture and BP support, as needed.

DRUG INTERACTIONS

CNS depressants / ↑ Incidence of CNS side effects, including confusion and dizziness

Opioids / Concomitant use with intrathecal opioids has not been studied; use together is not recommended

HOW SUPPLIED

Solution: 25 mcg/mL, 100 mcg/mL.

 = see color insert   = Herbal   IV = Intravenous   = sound alike drug

DOSAGE

- ### INTRATHECAL

Management of severe chronic pain.
Initial: No more than 2.4 mcg/day (0.1 mcg/hr); titrate to client response. Adjust the dose of intrathecal administration according to the client's pain severity, their response to therapy, and the incidence of side effects. The effective dose is variable. The average dose level at the end of the 21-day titration used in clinical trials was 6.9 mcg/day (0.29 mcg/hr); maximum dose was 19.2 mcg/day (0.8 mcg/hr) on day 21.

Doses may be titrated upward by up to 2.4 mcg/day (0.1 mcg/hr) at intervals of no more than 2–3 times per week, up to a maximum of 19.2 mcg/day (0.8 mcg/hr) by day 21. Dose increases in increments of less than 2.4 mcg/day (0.1 mcg/hr) and increases in doses less frequently than 2–3 times per week may be used.

NURSING CONSIDERATIONS

ADMINISTRATION/STORAGE

1. The drug is used undiluted (20 mcg/mL in 20 mL vial) or diluted (100 mcg/mL in 1, 2, or 5 mL vials). Diluted drug is prepared with 0.9% NaCl injection using aseptic procedures to the desired concentration prior to placement in the microinfusion pump. The 100 mcg/mL formulation may be given undiluted once an appropriate dose has been established.

2. Saline solutions containing preservatives are not appropriate for intrathecal drug administration and are not to be used.

3. Refrigerate, but do not freeze, all ziconotide solutions after preparation and begin infusion within 24 hr.

4. Because of the lower incidence of serious side effects and discontinuation for side effects associated with a slower titration, use a faster titration schedule only if there is an urgent need for analgesic that outweighs the risk to the client's safety.

5. Ziconotide is intended for intrathecal delivery using a programmable implanted variable-rate microinfusion device or an external microinfusion device and catheter. Specific instructions and precautions for programming the microinfusion device and/or refilling the reservoir are available from the manufacturer's manual.

6. There is a higher incidence of confusion in elderly clients; dose selection for an elderly person should be cautious, starting at the low end of the dose range.

7. Refrigerate ziconotide during transit. Store from 2–8°C (36–46°F). Once diluted aseptically with saline, the drug may be stored from 2–8°C (36–46°F) for 24 hr. Protect from light. Discard any ziconotide solution if particulate matter or discoloration is observed; discard any unused portion remaining in the vial.

ASSESSMENT

1. Note reasons for therapy, onset, duration, location of pain. Rate pain level; note other agents trialed/failed.

2. Review medical history to ensure no conditions that would preclude drug therapy (e.g., psychosis, severe depression, suicide attempts).

3. This medication will not prevent withdrawal reactions from narcotics.

4. Medication should not be given into a vein (IV) or under the skin. It can cause fainting R/T severe hypotension if accidentally given into a vein. It is for intrathecal use only in those that have not responded to IV or intrathecal morphine, or other opioids for pain control.

5. Assess client ability to perform steps to ensure safe administration. Set up a schedule for refilling pump. Check product visually for particles or discoloration.

6. Determine if using a narcotic (e.g., codeine, hydrocodone, morphine) regularly for more than a few weeks, or if it has been used in high doses; may be dependent on it. Suddenly stopping the narcotic will cause withdrawal reactions, when stopping extended, regular treatment with narcotics, gradually reducing the dosage will help prevent withdrawal reactions.

7. Monitor VS, renal and LFTs. May cause elevated CK levels, monitor for associated side effects.

Bold Italic = life threatening side effect　■ = black box warning　✦ = Available in Canada

Z

CLIENT/FAMILY TEACHING

1. This is a pain reliever that works by blocking the nerves in the spinal cord that send pain signals. It decreases ongoing pain caused by cancer, AIDS, failed back surgery, multiple sclerosis, neuropathy, and other causes that have not responded to other therapies.

2. This medication is injected into the spinal fluid (intrathecal) using a small pump. Treatment is usually started slowly and gradually increased to the dose that works best for you. To prevent infection, you will be taught how to handle the infusion pump, and learn proper care of the injection site. Call your provider/infusion nurse immediately if there is any sign of infection around the injection site (e.g., swelling, redness, tenderness). Must set up a schedule for refilling your pump. Before using, check this product visually for particles or discoloration. If either is present, do not use the liquid. Report if your pain persists or worsens.

3. Do not engage in activities that require mental alertness or coordination while being treated with ziconotide.

4. Avoid alcohol and any other CNS depressant type drugs without provider approval.

5. Report any unusual soreness, worsening muscle pain, weakness and darkened urine.

6. Notify provider immediately of any change in mental status (e.g., lethargy, confusion, disorientation, decreased alertness) or a change in mood, or perception (hallucinations, including unusual tactile sensations in the mouth) or symptoms of depression or suicidal thoughts. Report any nausea, vomiting, seizures, fever, headache, and/or stiff neck, as these may be symptoms of developing meningitis.

7. Keep all F/U visits and report lack or response or adverse side effects.

OUTCOMES/EVALUATE

Relief of intractable pain

Zidovudine ■ IV ©
(Azidothymidine, AZT)

(zye-**DOH**-vyou-deen, ah-**zee**-doh-**THIGH**-mih-deen)

CLASSIFICATION(S):

Antiviral, nucleoside reverse transcriptase inhibitor

PREGNANCY CATEGORY: C

Rx: Retrovir.

♣Rx: Apo-Zidovudine, Novo-AZT.

SEE ALSO *ANTIVIRAL DRUGS* AND *ANTI-INFECTIVE DRUGS*.

USES

PO: (1) Initial treatment of HIV-infected adults who have a CD_4 cell count of $500/mm^3$ or less. Superior to either didanosine or zalcitabine monotherapy for initial treatment of HIV-infected clients who have not had previous antiretroviral therapy. (2) Prevent HIV transmission from pregnant women to their fetuses. (3) HIV-infected children over 3 months of age who have HIV-related symptoms or are asymptomatic with abnormal laboratory values indicating significant immunosuppression. (4) In combination with zalcitabine in selected clients with advanced HIV disease (CD_4 cell count of 300 cells/mm^3 or less).

IV: Selected adults with symptomatic HIV infections who have a history of confirmed *Pneumocystis carinii* pneumonia or an absolute CD_4 (T_4 helper/inducer) lymphocyte count of less than 200 cells/mm^3 in the peripheral blood prior to therapy.

ACTION/KINETICS

Action

The active form of the drug is zidovudine triphosphate, which is derived from zidovudine by cellular enzymes. Zidovudine triphosphate competes with thymidine triphosphate (the natural substrate) for incorporation into growing chains of viral DNA by retroviral reverse transcriptase. Once incorporated, zidovudine triphosphate causes premature termination of the growth of the DNA chain. Delays appearance of AIDS symptoms. Low concentrations of zidovudine also inhibit the activity of *Shigella, Klebsiella, Salmonella, Enterobacter, Escherichia coli,* and *Citrobacter,* although resistance develops rapidly.

Pharmacokinetics
Rapidly absorbed from the GI tract and is distributed to both plasma and CSF. **Peak serum levels:** 0.1–1.5 hr. $t^{1/2}$: Approximately 1 hr. $t^{1/2}$, **clients younger than 3 months of age:** 13 hr. In neonates 14 days of age or less, bioavailability is greater, total body clearance is slower, and half-life was longer than in pediatric clients over 14 days of age. Metabolized rapidly by the liver and excreted through the urine.

CONTRAINDICATIONS
Allergy to zidovudine or its components. Lactation.

SPECIAL CONCERNS
■ (1) Zidovudine has been associated with hematologic toxicity, including neutropenia and severe anemia, especially in clients with advanced HIV disease. (2) Prolonged zidovudine use has been associated with symptomatic myopathy. (3) Lactic acidosis and severe hepatomegaly with steatosis, including fatalities, have been reported with the use of nucleoside analogs alone or in combination, including zidovudine and other antiretrovirals.■ Use with caution in clients who have a hemoglobin level of less than 9.5 grams/dL or a granulocyte count less than 1,000/mm³. Zidovudine is not a cure for HIV; thus, clients may continue to acquire opportunistic infections and other illnesses associated with ARC or HIV. Zidovudine has not been shown to reduce the risk of HIV transmission to others through sexual contact or blood contamination.

SIDE EFFECTS
Most Common
Headache, malaise, N&V, anorexia, constipation, asthenia, abdominal cramps/pain, arthralgia, chills, dyspepsia, fatigue, insomnia, musculoskeletal pain, myalgia, neuropathy.

Adults. Hematologic: Anemia (severe), neutropenia, granulocytopenia, thrombocytopenia, pure red cell aplasia, *aplastic anemia,* hemolytic anemia, leukopenia, lymphadenopathy, pancytopenia with marrow hypoplasia. **Body as a whole:** Headache, asthenia, fever, fatigue, neuropathy, diaphoresis, malaise, body odor, chills, edema of the lip, flu-like syndrome, hyperalgesia, abdominal/chest/back pain. **GI:** N&V, GI pain, diarrhea, anorexia, dyspepsia, constipation, dysphagia, edema of the tongue, eructation, flatulence, bleeding gums, mouth ulcers, oral mucosa pigmentation, abdominal cramps/pain, *rectal hemorrhage.* **Hepatic:** Hepatitis, *hepatomegaly with steatosis,* jaundice, lactic acidosis, *pancreatitis.* **CNS:** Somnolence, dizziness, paresthesia, insomnia, anxiety, confusion, emotional lability, depression, nervousness, vertigo, paresthesia, loss of mental acuity, mania, *seizures.* **CV:** Vasodilation, syncope, vasculitis (rare), *cardiomyopathy.* **Musculoskeletal:** Myalgia, myositis, arthralgia, tremor, twitch, muscle spasm, musculoskeletal pain, myopathy (with chronic use), myositis with pathological changes (similar to that produced by HIV disease), *rhabdomyolysis.* **Respiratory:** Dyspnea, cough, epistaxis, rhinitis, pharyngitis, sinusitis, hoarseness. **Dermatologic:** Rash, pruritus, urticaria, acne, pigmentation changes of the skin and nails, sweating, *Stevens-Johnson syndrome, toxic epidermal necrolysis.* **GU:** Dysuria, polyuria, urinary hesitancy/frequency, gynecomastia. **Ophthalmic:** Anblyopia, photophobia, macular edema. **Miscellaneous:** Hearing loss, taste perversion, hypersensitivity reactions (including *anaphylaxis,* angioedema, vasculitis), hyperbilirubinemia (rare), *seizures.*
Children. The following side effects have been observed in children, although any of the side effects reported for adults can also occur in children. **Body as a whole:** Granulocytopenia, anemia, fever, headache, phlebitis, bacteremia. **GI:** N&V, abdominal pain, diarrhea, weight loss, stomatitis, splenomegaly. **CNS:** Decreased reflexes, ner-

---

Bold Italic = life threatening side effect   ■ = black box warning   ♣ = Available in Canada

vousness, irritability, insomnia, **seizures**. **CV:** Abnormalities in ECG, left ventricular dilation, CHF, generalized edema, **cardiomyopathy**, S_3 gallop. **GU:** Hematuria, viral cystitis

LABORATORY TEST CONSIDERATIONS
↑ ALT, AST, CPK, LDH, lipase, total amylase. Neutropenia, anemia, thrombocytopenia.

OD OVERDOSE MANAGEMENT
Symptoms: N&V. Transient hematologic changes. Headache, dizziness, drowsiness, confusion, lethargy. *Treatment:* Treat symptoms. Hemodialysis will enhance the excretion of the primary metabolite of zidovudine.

DRUG INTERACTIONS
Acetaminophen / ↑ Risk of granulocytopenia; ↓ zidovudine AUC
Adriamycin / ↑ Risk of cytotoxicity, nephrotoxicity, or hematologic toxicity
Atovaquone / ↑ Zidovudine levels
Bone marrow depressants / ↑ Zidovudine's hematologic toxicity
Clarithromycin / Peak serum zidovudine levels may be ↑ or ↓
Cytotoxic drugs / ↑ Zidovudine's hematologic toxicity
Dapsone / ↑ Risk of cytotoxicity, nephrotoxicity, or hematologic toxicity
Doxorubicin / Drugs antagonize each other; do not give together
Fluconazole / ↑ Zidovudine levels
Flucytosine / ↑ Risk of cytotoxicity, nephrotoxicity, or hematologic toxicity
Ganciclovir / ↑ Risk of hematologic toxicity
Interferon alfa / ↑ Risk of hematologic toxicity
Interferon beta-1b / ↑ Zidovudine serum levels
Methadone / ↑ Zidovudine serum levels and AUC → ↑ risk of side effects
Nelfinavir / ↓ Zidovudine AUC
Phenytoin / Levels of phenytoin may ↑, ↓, or remain unchanged; also, ↓ zidovudine excretion
Probenecid / ↓ Biotransformation or renal excretion of zidovudine → flu-like symptoms, including myalgia, malaise or fever, and maculopapular rash
Ribavirin / Possible antagonism of zidovudine against HIV; do not use together
Rifampin / ↓ Zidovudine levels

Ritonavir / ↓ Zidovudine AUC
Stavudine / Possible antagonism of zidovudine against HIV; do not use together
Trimethoprim / ↑ Zidovudine serum levels especially in those with impaired hepatic glucuronidation
Valproic acid / ↑ Zidovudine AUC R/T ↓ metabolism
Vinblastine / ↑ Risk of cytotoxicity, nephrotoxicity, or hematologic toxicity
Vincristine / ↑ Risk of cytotoxicity, nephrotoxicity, or hematologic toxicity

HOW SUPPLIED
Capsules: 100 mg; *Injection:* 10 mg/mL; *Oral Solution:* 50 mg/5 mL; *Syrup:* 50 mg/5 mL; *Tablets:* 300 mg.

DOSAGE
• **CAPSULES; ORAL SOLUTION; SYRUP; TABLETS**
Symptomatic HIV infections.
Adults: 100 mg (one 100-mg capsule or 10-mL syrup) q 4 hr around the clock (i.e., total of 600 mg daily).
Asymptomatic HIV infections.
Adults: 100 mg q 4 hr while awake (500 mg/day); **Pediatric, 6 weeks–12 years, initial:** 160 mg/m² q 8 hr (480 mg/m²/day, not to exceed 200 mg q 8 hr).
Prevent transmission of HIV from mothers to their fetuses (after week 14 of pregnancy).
Maternal dosing: 100 mg 5 times/day until the start of labor. During labor and delivery, zidovudine IV at 2 mg/kg over 1 hr followed by continuous IV infusion of 1 mg/kg/hr until clamping of the umbilical cord. **Infant dosing:** 2 mg/kg PO q 6 hr beginning within 12 hr after birth and continuing through 6 weeks of age. Infants unable to take the drug PO may be given zidovudine IV at 1.5 mg/kg, infused over 30 min q 6 hr.
In combination with zalcitabine.
Zidovudine, 200 mg, with zalcitabine, 0.75 mg, q 8 hr.
• **IV**
HIV infection.
1 mg/kg infused over 1 hr. The IV dose is given 5 to 6 times per day around the clock only until PO therapy can be instituted. The IV dosing regimen equivalent to the PO administration of 100 mg q 4 hr is about 1 mg/kg IV q 4 hr. Avoid

rapid infusion or bolus injection. Dosage adjustment may be necessary due to hematologic toxicity.

Maternal during labor and delivery. 2 mg/kg infused over 1 hr followed by a continuous IV infusion of 1 mg/kg/hr until clamping of the umbilical cord.

NURSING CONSIDERATIONS

Ⓒ Do not confuse Retrovir with ritonavir (also an antiviral drug) or Norvir (also an antiviral drug).

ADMINISTRATION/STORAGE

1. Protect capsules and syrup from light.

2. Dosage adjustment should not be required for clients with a C_{CR} greater than or equal to 15 mL/min.

3. Lamivudine/zidovudine and abacavir/lamivudine/zidovudine are combination products that contain zidovudine. Do not administer zidovudine concomitantly with either of these products.

4. Do not mix with blood products or protein solutions.

5. Remove dose from 20-mL vial and dilute in D5W injection to a concentration not to exceed 4 mg/mL. Administer calculated dose IV at a constant rate over 1 hr.

6. After dilution, the solution is stable at room temperature for 24 hr and if refrigerated (2–8°C, 36–46°F) for 48 hr. To ensure safety from microbial contamination, give within 8 hr if stored at room temperature and 24 hr if refrigerated.

ASSESSMENT

1. Note reasons for therapy, onset, other therapies trialed, baseline CD_4 counts, viral load.

2. Initially monitor SMA-6 and CBC at least q 2 weeks. If lactic acidosis, anemia or granulocytopenia severe, the dose must be adjusted or discontinued. Epoetin alfa recombinant may be administered with iron to stimulate RBC production. A blood transfusion may also be required.

3. Safety and effectiveness of chronic zidovudine therapy are not known, especially in those with a less advanced form of disease.

4. When used to prevent maternal-fetal transmission of HIV, zidovudine should be initiated in pregnant women between 14 and 24 weeks of gestation; also, IV zidovudine should be given during labor up until the cord is clamped, and newborn infants should receive zidovudine syrup. Infected mothers may not breast feed.

CLIENT/FAMILY TEACHING

1. Take with or without food q 4 hr ATC as ordered; sleep must be interrupted to take medication. Do not share and do not exceed the prescribed dose of zidovudine.

2. Report for all labs, especially lytes and CBC, because drug causes lactic acidosis and anemia, and additional medications or blood transfusions may be necessary.

3. Report early S&S of anemia, e.g., SOB, weakness, lightheadedness, palpitations, and increased fatigue as well as muscle aches/pain.

4. Consume 2–3 L/day fluids to ensure adequate hydration. Maintain a record of weights and I&O.

5. Report any S&S of superinfections (e.g., furry tongue, mouth lesions, vaginal/rectal itching, rash).

6. Avoid tylenol and any other unprescribed drugs that may exacerbate the toxicity of zidovudine.

7. Drug is not a cure but helps to alleviate and manage symptoms of HIV infections and prolong life with continuous therapy. May continue to develop opportunistic infections and other complications due to AIDS or ARC.

8. The risk of transmission of HIV to others through blood or sexual contact is not reduced in individuals on zidovudine therapy. Practice safe sex and do not share needles.

9. With pregnancy, zidovudine therapy should start after the 14-week gestation period to help prevent the transmission from mother to infant. Once delivered, do not nurse infant.

10. With accidental needle stick/occupational exposure initiate therapy after incident for best outcome.

---

11. Identify local support groups that may assist one to understand/cope with this disease.

OUTCOMES/EVALUATE

- Control of symptoms of HIV, AIDS, or ARC
- ↑ CD_4 counts; ↓ viral load; enhanced longevity
- ↓ Maternal fetal HIV transmission

Zileuton
(zye-**LOO**-ton)

CLASSIFICATION(S):
Antiasthmatic, leukotriene receptor antagonist
PREGNANCY CATEGORY: C
Rx: Zyflo, Zyflo CR.

USES
Prophylaxis and chronic treatment of asthma in adults and children over 12 years of age.

ACTION/KINETICS
Action
Specific inhibitor of 5-lipoxygenase; thus, inhibits the formation of leukotrienes. Leukotrienes are substances that induce various biological effects including aggregation of neutrophils and monocytes, leukocyte adhesion, increase of neutrophil and eosinophil migration, increased capillary permeability, and contraction of smooth muscle. These effects of leukotrienes contribute to edema, secretion of mucus, inflammation, and bronchoconstriction in asthmatic clients. By inhibiting leukotriene formation, zileuton reduces bronchoconstriction due to cold air challenge in asthmatics.

Pharmacokinetics
Rapidly absorbed from the GI tract; **peak plasma levels:** 1.7 hr. Food affects the C_{max} of extended-release tablets but not immediate-release tablets. Metabolized in liver and mainly excreted through the urine. **t½:** 2.5 hr (immediate-release) and 3.2 hr (extended-release). **Plasma protein binding:** 93%, primarily to albumin.

CONTRAINDICATIONS
Active liver disease or transaminase elevations greater than or equal to three times the ULN. Hypersenstivity to any component of the product. Treatment of bronchoconstriction in acute asthma attacks, including status asthmaticus. Lactation.

SPECIAL CONCERNS
Use with caution in clients who ingest large quantities of alcohol or who have a past history of liver disease. Women 65 years of age or older appear to have an increased risk of ALT elevations. Safety and efficacy have not been determined in children less than 12 years of age.

SIDE EFFECTS
Most Common
Immediate-Release: Headache, dyspepsia, nausea, unspecified pain, abdominal pain, asthenia, accidental injury, myalgia.
Delayed-Release: Sinusitis, pharyngolaryngeal pain, nausea.
Immediate-Release: GI: Dyspepsia, N&V, constipation, flatulence, severe hepatic injury. **CNS:** Headache, dizziness, insomnia, malaise, nervousness, somnolence. **Body as a whole:** Unspecified pain, abdominal pain, chest pain, asthenia, accidental injury, fever. **Musculoskeletal:** Myalgia, arthralgia, neck pain/rigidity. **GU:** UTI, vaginitis. **Dermatologic:** Pruritus, rash, urticaria. **Miscellaneous:** Conjunctivitis, hypertonia, lymphadenopathy.
Delayed-Release: GI: N&V, diarrhea, dyspepsia, upper abdominal pain, hepatotoxicity. **CNS:** Headache. *Respiratory:* Sinusitis, pharyngolyarngeal pain, URTI. **Dermatologic:** Rash. **Musculoskeletal:** Myalgia. **Body as a whole:** Hypersensitivity.

LABORATORY TEST CONSIDERATIONS
↑ LFTs. Low WBC count.

DRUG INTERACTIONS
CYP3A4 agents (calcium channel blockers, cyclosporine, ketoconazole) / Possible interaction; use caution and monitoring if coadministered with zileuton
Propranolol / ↑ Propranolol levels → ↑ effect; adjust propranolol dose as needed and monitor

Z

Theophylline / ↑ Theophylline levels; ↓ theophylline dose by 50% and monitor theophylline levels

Warfarin / ↑ PT; adjust warfarin dose and monitor

HOW SUPPLIED

Tablets: 600 mg.; *Tablets, Extended-Release:* 600 mg.

DOSAGE

• **TABLETS**

Symptomatic treatment of asthma.

Adults and children over 12 years of age: 600 mg 4 times per day; **total daily dose:** 2,400 mg.

• **TABLETS, EXTENDED-RELEASE**

Symptomatic relief of asthma.

Adults and children, 12 years and older: 1,200 mg (two 600 mg tablets) twice daily, within 1 hr after morning and evening meals; **total daily dose:** 2,400 mg

NURSING CONSIDERATIONS

ADMINISTRATION/STORAGE

1. Do not decrease dose or stop taking any other antiasthmatics when taking zileuton.

2. Store tablets from 20–25°C (68–77°F) and extended-release tablets from 15–30°C (59–86°F). Protect from light.

ASSESSMENT

1. Note onset, characteristics of S&S, and severity of disease. List triggers and currently prescribed therapy.

2. Screen for excessive alcohol use and any evidence of liver disease. Monitor CBC, PFTs, and LFTs monthly x 3 mo then every 3 mo during the first year of therapy.

3. Document lung assessments, PFTs, peak flow readings, and CXR findings.

CLIENT/FAMILY TEACHING

1. Take tablets regularly as directed (may take with meals and at bedtime) and continue other antiasthmatic medications as prescribed. Tablets may be swallowed whole or split in half for ease of administration.

2. Take the extended-release tablets within 1 hr of morning and evening meals. Do not chew, cut, or crush extended-release tablets. If a dose is missed, take the next dose at the next scheduled time; do not double the dose.

3. Use caution, may cause dizziness; avoid hazardous activities.

4. Drug will not reverse bronchospasm during acute asthma attack; use bronchodilators and other prescribed therapy. Seek medical attention if symptoms are severe or peak flow readings indicate need. Use peak flow meter readings to monitor airway effectiveness and for medication increases.

5. Drug inhibits formation of those substances that cause bronchoconstrictive symptoms in asthmatics.

6. Report immediately if experiencing RUQ pain, lethargy, itching, jaundice, fatigue, or flu-like symptoms (S&S of liver toxicity).

7. Report for CBC, regularly scheduled LFTs, and evaluation of pulmonary status. Bring record of peak flow readings.

8. Review triggers (i.e., smoke, cold air, and exercise) that may cause increased hyperresponsiveness which can last up to a week. If more than the usual or maximum number of inhalations of short-acting bronchodilator treatment in a 24-hr period are required, notify provider.

9. Avoid alcohol and OTC agents without approval.

10. Keep all F/U appointments to evaluate response to therapy.

OUTCOMES/EVALUATE

Asthma prophylaxis; ↑ airway exchange.

Ziprasidone hydrochloride ■

(zigh-**PRAYZ**-oh-dohn)

CLASSIFICATION(S):
Antipsychotic
PREGNANCY CATEGORY: C
Rx: Geodon.

USES

PO. (1) Treatment of schizophrenia. Due to the possibility of causing prolongation of the QT/QTc interval, other drugs should be considered first. (2) Acute manic or mixed episodes associated with bipolar disorder, with or without psychotic features.

IM. Acute agitation in clients with schizophrenia for whom treatment with ziprasidone is appropriate and who need IM antipsychotic medication for rapid control of agitation.

ACTION/KINETICS

Action

Mechanism unknown but thought to be due to a combination of dopamine (D_2) and serotonin (5-HT_2) receptor antagonism. Causes moderate sedation, extrapyramidal symptoms, and orthostatic hypotension; low incidence of anticholinergic effects.

Pharmacokinetics

Well absorbed; bioavailability is about 60% for PO product. **Peak plasma levels:** 6–8 hr after PO and 1 hr after IM. Absorption increased up to 2-fold in the presence of food. Extensively metabolized in the liver by aldehyde oxidase, methylation, and oxidation by CYP3A4 and CYP1A2. About 20% excreted in the urine and 66% eliminated in the feces. **$t\frac{1}{2}$, terminal:** 7 hr after PO and 2–5 hr after IM administration. **Plasma protein binding:** More than 99%.

CONTRAINDICATIONS

Use with other drugs that prolong the QT interval, including class Ia and III antiarrhythmic drugs, chlorpromazine, dofetilide, dolasetron, droperidol, gatifloxacin, halofantrine, mefloquine, mesoridazine, moxifloxacin, pentamidine, pimozide, probucol, quinidine, sotalol, sparfloxacin, tacrolimus, or thioridazine. Do not use in clients with a known history of QT prolongation, with recent acute MI, with uncompensated heart failure, or cardiac arrhythmia. Lactation.

SPECIAL CONCERNS

■ Elderly clients with dementia-related psychosis treated with atypical antipsychotic drugs are at an increased risk of death compared with placebo. Studies revealed a risk of death in the drug-treated clients between 1.6 and 1.7 times that seen in placebo-treated clients. Over the course of a typical 10-week controlled trial, the rate of death in drug-treated clients was about 4.5%, compared with a rate of about 2.6% in the placebo group. Although causes of death were varied, most of the deaths appeared to either cardiovascular (e.g., heart failure, sudden death) or infectious (e.g., pneumonia) in nature. Ziprasidone is not approved for the treatment of clients with dementia-related psychosis.■ Ziprasidone has a greater capacity to prolong the QT/QTc interval compared with other antipsychotic drugs. Prolongation of the QTc interval is associated with a torsade de pointes-type arrhythmia, which is a potentially fatal ventricular tachycardia. It is not known whether ziprasidone will cause torsade de pointes or increase the rate of sudden death. Use of antipsychotic drugs may cause tardive dyskinesia and/or neuroleptic malignant syndrome. Use with caution in those with a history of MI, ischemic heart disease, heart failure, or conduction abnormalities; in cerebrovascular disease; in conditions that predispose to hypotension; or in those with a history of seizures or conditions that potentially lower the seizure threshold (e.g., Alzheimer's). Use with caution in geriatric clients, as the drug may be excreted more slowly in this population (rate of death due to CV events or infections is higher in clients with dementia). Safety and efficacy have not been established in children.

SIDE EFFECTS

Most Common

Akathisia, asthenia, drowsiness/sedation, extrapyramidal symptoms, headache, insomnia, rash, diarrhea, diverticulitis, dry mouth, dyspepsia, nausea, weight gain, increased cough, rhinitis, abnormal vision, accidental injury.

Mainly listed are side effects with an incidence of 1% or more. **GI:** Nausea, constipation, dyspepsia, diarrhea, dry mouth, anorexia, diverticulitis, *pancreatitis*. **CNS:** *Seizures*, drowsiness/sedation, headache, insomnia, somnolence, *suicide attempts*, akathisia, dizziness, extrapyramidal syndrome, dystonia, hypertonia, tardive dyskinesia, migraine. **CV:** Orthostatic hypotension, tachycardia, *sudden cardiac death, torsades de pointes*. **Respiratory:** Cold symptoms, URTI, rhinitis, increased cough. **Derma-**

Z

tologic: Rash, urticaria, fungal dermatitis. **Body as a whole:** Asthenia, accidental injury, weight gain. **Miscellaneous:** Myalgia, abnormal vision, ***rhabdomyolysis***, diabetes.

LABORATORY TEST CONSIDERATIONS
↑ Prolactin.

OD OVERDOSE MANAGEMENT
Symptoms: Hypotension, ***circulatory collapse***, severe extrapyramidal symptoms. *Treatment:* Establish and maintain an airway and ensure adequate oxygenation and ventilation. Establish IV access. Undertake gastric lavage if necessary and consider activated charcoal with a laxative. Monitor CV status, including continuous ECG monitoring to detect possible arrhythmias. Treat hypotension and circulatory collapse with IV fluids (do not use epinephrine or dopamine). Give anticholinergic drugs to treat severe extrapyramidal symptoms.

DRUG INTERACTIONS
Antihypertensive drugs / Additive hypotension with certain antihypertensive drugs
Carbamazepine / ↓ Ziprasidone levels R/T ↑ liver metabolism
Centrally-acting drugs / Use caution due to CNS effects of ziprasidone
Dopamine agonists / Antagonism of agonist effect
Ketoconazole / ↑ Ziprasidone levels R/T inhibition of metabolism
Levodopa / Antagonism of levodopa effects

HOW SUPPLIED
Capsules: 20 mg, 40 mg, 60 mg, 80 mg; *Powder for Injection:* 20 mg (as mesylate).

DOSAGE
• **CAPSULES**
Schizophrenia.
Initial: 20 mg twice a day with food. Adjust dose based on individual clinical status, up to 80 mg twice a day. If needed, adjust dose at intervals of 2 or more days, as steady state is reached in 1–3 days. **Maintenance:** Efficacy is maintained for 52 weeks or less at a dose of 20–80 mg (maximum) twice a day. The safety of doses above 100 mg twice a day has not been evaluated. Periodical-

ly assess to determine need for continued treatment.

Manic or mixed episodes associated with bipolar disorder (bipolar mania).
Day 1: 40 mg twice daily with food; **Day 2:** 60 or 80 mg twice daily; **then,** 40–80 mg twice daily, depending on client progress and tolerance. There are no data to support the use of ziprasidone beyond 3 weeks for bipolar mania.

• **IM**
Acute agitation in schizophrenics.
10–20 mg IM, up to a maximum of 40 mg/day. Doses of 10 mg may be given q 2 hr and doses of 20 mg may be given q 4 hr, up to 40 mg/day. IM use for more than 3 days has not been evaluated.

NURSING CONSIDERATIONS
ADMINISTRATION/STORAGE
1. If long-term therapy is needed, replace IM administration with PO ziprasidone as soon as possible. Do not coadminister both PO and IM forms.
2. To reconstitute the injection for IM use, add 1.2 mL sterile water for injection and shake vigorously until the drug is dissolved. Each mL of reconstituted solution contains 20 mg ziprasidone. To administer a 10 mg dose, draw up 0.5 mL of the reconstituted solution and to give a 20 mg dose, draw up 1 mL of the reconstituted solution.
3. The product contains no preservative or bacteriostatic agent; thus, use aseptic technique in preparing final solution.
4. Do not mix the reconstituted drug with any other drugs or solvents other than sterile water for injection.
5. Store capsules and the dry form of the injection at 15–30°C (59–86°F). Following reconstitution, injection can be stored, protected from light, for up to 24 hr from 15–30°C (59–86°F) or up to 7 days refrigerated at 2–8°C (36–46°F).

ASSESSMENT
1. Note disease onset, symptom characteristics, presenting behaviors, other agents trialed.
2. Note any history of CAD, abnormal QT interval, arrhythmias, CVA, Alzhei-

---

Bold Italic = life threatening side effect   ■ = black box warning   ✦ = Available in Canada

mer's disease or seizures. If QTc interval >500 msec, do not give drug.

3. List drugs currently prescribed to ensure none interact unfavorably.

4. Monitor CBC, U/A, LFTs, electrolytes, and Mg levels. Those being considered for ziprasidone therapy who are at risk for significant electrolyte disturbances, especially hypokalemia, should have baseline serum K and Mg levels. Hypokalemia and/or hypomagnesemia may increase the risk of QT prolongation and arrhythmias. Also monitor for S&S of diabetes mellitus.

CLIENT/FAMILY TEACHING

1. Take as directed, twice a day with food. Do not stop suddenly; drug should be withdrawn slowly to prevent adverse side effects.

2. Continue regular psychotherapy sessions. Report any changes in behavior, loss of control, increased tremor, or evidence of seizures.

3. Avoid activities that require mental alertness until drug effects realized; dizziness and drowsiness may occur.

4. Change positions slowly to prevent drop in BP. Avoid hot baths/showers, hot tubs as low BP may occur.

5. Do not perform strenuous activities in warm weather, may have heat stroke.

6. Drug may alter electrolyte levels. Report as scheduled for periodic labs.

7. Avoid OTC drugs and alcohol. Report any unusual side effects or lack of response. Monitor weights.

OUTCOMES/EVALUATE

Improved patterns of behavior with less agitation, less hyperactivity, and reality orientation

---

Zoledronic acid [IV]
(ZOH-leh-dron-ick)

CLASSIFICATION(S):
Bone growth regulator, bisphosphonate
PREGNANCY CATEGORY: C
Rx: Reclast, Zometa.

USES
Reclast: (1)Treat Paget's disease of the bone in men and women who have elevations in serum alkaline phosphatase of 2 times or higher the upper limit of the age-specific normal reference range, or in those who are symptomatic, or those at risk for complications from their disease. Goal is to induce remission and normalize serum alkaline phosphatase. (2) Once-yearly dose to treat postmenopausal osteoporosis.
Zometa: (1) Hypercalcemia of malignancy. (2) Multiple myeloma and bone metastases of solid tumors with standard antineoplastic therapy. Prostate cancer should have progressed after treatment with at least 1 hormonal therapy.

ACTION/KINETICS
Action
Hyperactivity of osteoclasts causes excessive bone resorption in hypercalcemia of malignancy. Such hypercalcemia causes polyuria and GI disturbances with progressive dehydration and decreased glomerular filtration rate. Reducing excessive bone resorption and maintaining adequate fluid intake are essential to managing hypercalcemia of malignancy. Zoledronic acid acts to inhibit bone resorption perhaps by inhibiting osteoclastic activity and inducing osteoclast apoptosis. Zoledronic acid also blocks the osteoclastic resorption of mineralized bone and cartilage by binding to bone. It inhibits the increased osteoclastic activity and skeletal calcium release induced by various stimulatory factors released by tumors.
Pharmacokinetics
$t\frac{1}{2}$: 0.23 hr, 1.75 hr, and 167 hr for the distribution, elimination, and terminal elimination, respectively. Is primarily excreted through the urine unchanged.

CONTRAINDICATIONS
Hypersensitivity to zoledronic acid or other bisphosphonates.

SPECIAL CONCERNS
Use with caution in aspirin-sensitive asthma. Safety and efficacy have not been determined in treating hypercalcemia associated with hyperparathyroidism or other non-tumor-related dis-

Z

---

eases. Use with caution during lactation and in the elderly. Safety and efficacy have not been determined in children.

SIDE EFFECTS

Most Common

Anorexia, constipation, diarrhea, N&V, anemia, arthralgia, bone/skeletal pain, myalgia, dyspnea, edema/peripheral edema, fatigue, fever.

GU: *Renal toxicity*, including deterioration of renal function and potential renal failure, UTI. **GI:** N&V, constipation, diarrhea, abdominal pain, anorexia, dysphagia. **CNS:** Insomnia, anxiety, confusion, agitation, headache, somnolence. **CV:** Hypotension. **Body as a whole:** Fever, ***progression of cancer***, flu-like syndrome (fever, chills, bone pain, arthralgias, myalgias), edema/peripheral edema, rash, pruritus, chest pain, nonspecific infection, dehydration, asthenia, leg edema, mucositis, ***metastases***. **Hematologic:** Anemia, granulocytopenia, thrombocytopenia, pancytopenia. **Respiratory:** Dyspnea, coughing, pleural effusion. **Musculoskeletal:** Skeletal pain, myalgia, bone/skeletal pain, arthralgia. **Infusion site reaction:** Redness, swelling. **Miscellaneous:** Moniliasis. Osteonecrosis of the jaw in cancer clients.

LABORATORY TEST CONSIDERATIONS

↑ Creatinine. Hypocalcemia, hypophosphatemia, hypomagnesemia.

DRUG INTERACTIONS

Aminoglycosides / Possible additive effect to lower serum calcium levels for prolonged periods
Diuretics, loop / ↑ Risk of hypocalcemia

HOW SUPPLIED

Injection Solution (Reclast): 5 mg/100 mL; *Injection Solution, Concentrate (Zometa):* 4 mg/5 mL.

DOSAGE

• **IV ONLY**

Hypercalcemia of malignancy.

Maximum recommended dose: 4 mg if albumin-corrected serum calcium is greater than or equal to 12 mg/dL. Give as a single IV infusion over no less than 15 min. Consider retreatment if serum calcium does not return to normal or remain normal after initial treatment.

Allow 7 days to elapse before retreatment.

Multiple myeloma and metastatic bone lesions from solid tumors.

4 mg infused over 15 min q 3 or 4 weeks if C_{CR} is higher than 60 mL/min. **Duration:** At least 15 months for prostate cancer, 12 months for breast cancer and multiple myeloma, and 9 months for other solid tumors. Give PO calcium supplement of 500 mg and a multiple vitamin containing 400 international units vitamin D per day.

RECLAST

• **IV**

Paget disease of bone.

Clients with C_{CR} greater than or equal to 35 mL/min: Infuse the ready made injection (5 mg/100 mL) via a vented infusion line over no less than 15 min at a constant infusion rate. Can be dosed without regard to meals.

Postmenopausal osteoporosis.

5 mg given once yearly as a 15 minute IV infusion.

NURSING CONSIDERATIONS

ADMINISTRATION/STORAGE

IV 1. When used for hypercalcemia of malignancy, initiate vigorous saline hydration promptly and attempt to restore urine output to about 2 L/day throughout treatment. Avoid overhydration.

2. When used for Paget disease of the bone, infusion time must not be less than 15 min given over a constant infusion rate. Retreatment may be considered in those who have relapsed, based on increases in serum alkaline phosphatase, or in those who failed to achieve normalization of their serum alkaline phosphatase, or in clients with symptoms.

3. When used for hypercalcemia of malignancy, due to the risk of significant deterioration of renal function, do not exceed single doses of 4 mg of zoledronic acid with the duration of infusion no less than 15 minutes.

4. To reduce the risk of hypocalcemia, give all clients elemental calcium, 1,500 mg/day in divided doses (e.g., 750 mg twice a day or 500 mg 3 times a day) as

---

Bold Italic = life threatening side effect   ■ = black box warning   ✤ = Available in Canada

well as vitamin D, 800 units/day, especially in the 2 weeks following drug administration.

5. Use the following dosage for mild to moderate impaired renal function: If baseline C_{CR} is 50–60 mL/min, give 3.5 mg zoledronic acid; if baseline C_{CR} is 40–49 mL/min, give 3.3 mg zoledronic acid; if baseline C_{CR} is 30–39 mL/min, give 3 mg zoledronic acid.

6. Use the following criteria in those who experience a decrease in renal function after zoledronic acid:

- If the serum creatinine was normal prior to zoledronic acid and there is an increase of 0.5 mg/dL within 2 weeks of the next dose, withhold zoledronic acid until serum creatinine is at least within 10% of the baseline value.
- If the serum creatinine is abnormal prior to zoledronic acid and there is an increase of 1.0 mg/dL within 2 weeks of the next dose, withhold zoledronic acid until serum creatinine is at least within 10% of the baseline value.

7. After reconstitution, the resulting solution allows for withdrawal of 5 mL containing 4 mg zoledronic acid. Completely dissolve before withdrawing solution. For those with baseline C_{CR} <60 mL/min, the following volumes are withdrawn after reconstitution: 4.4 mL for the 3.5 mg dose; 4.1 mL for the 3.3 mg dose; and, 3.8 mL for the 3 mg dose.

8. Dilute the concentrate in 100 mL sterile 0.9% NaCl or D5W. Give as a single IV infusion over no less than 15 min.

9. Do not mix with calcium-containing solutions, such as lactated Ringer's. Administer in a line separate from all other drugs.

10. Store Reclast from 15–30°C (59–86°F). After opening, the solution is stable for 24 hr at 2-8°C (36-46°F). If refrigerated, allow solution to reach room temperature before administration.

11. Store Zonata from 15–30°C (59–86°F). If not used immediately after reconstitution, refrigerate. The total time between reconstitution, dilution, storage in the refrigerator, and the end of administration must not exceed 24 hr.

ASSESSMENT

1. Note reasons for therapy, source of malignancy, serum Ca levels, other agents/methods trialed.

2. Initiate vigorous NSS hydration to ensure urinary output is 2 L/day during treatment. Avoid diuretics until client is adequately hydrated.

3. Monitor CBC, Ca, PO_4, Mg, and renal function. Ensure albumin corrected calcium level: (cCa, mg/dL= Ca + 0.8). Assess for renal failure and deficiency states, give calcium 500 mg and vitamin D 400 international units daily.

4. Because of the possibility of osteonecrosis of the jaw in cancer clients, undertake a dental exam with appropriate preventive dentistry before beginning therapy (especially in those with risk factors such as cancer, chemotherapy, corticosteroids, or poor oral hygiene).

CLIENT/FAMILY TEACHING

1. This drug is administered IV to reduce high calcium levels which result from tumors that cause increased bone activity and skeletal calcium release which cause your bones to weaken.

2. Report adverse side effects or unusual response to therapy. Nausea, vomiting, pain/redness/swelling at the injection site, or flu-like symptoms (e.g., fever, chills, muscle/joint aches or pains) may occur. Immediately report any changes in urine output, rash, itching, dizziness, weakness, trouble breathing or swallowing, burning or painful urination, mental/mood changes (e.g., agitation, anxiety, confusion) and jaw pain, chest pain, swelling of the legs or mouth, eye or vision problems, persistent sore throat and fever, unusual bruising or bleeding.

3. Take oral calcium replacement of 1,500 mg and 800 international units of vitamin D daily.

4. Avoid invasive dental procedures during therapy.

OUTCOMES/EVALUATE

↓ Serum calcium levels in malignancy
Inhibition of bone resorption

Z

Zolmitriptan
(zohl-mih-**TRIP**-tin)

CLASSIFICATION(S):
Antimigraine drug
PREGNANCY CATEGORY: C
Rx: Zomig, Zomig ZMT.
♣Rx: Zomig Rapimelt.

USES
Treatment of acute migraine in adults with or without aura. Use only when there is clear diagnosis of migraine.

ACTION/KINETICS
Action
Binds to serotonin 5-HT$_{1B/1D}$ receptors on intracranial blood vessels and in sensory nerves of trigeminal system. This results in cranial vessel constriction and inhibition of pro-inflammatory neuropeptide release.

Pharmacokinetics
Well absorbed after PO use. THe PO forms are from 29–46% bioavailable while the nasal form is 100% bioavailable. Orally disintegrating tablets may have a faster onset. **Time to onset of action:** 45 min (15 min for the nasal spray). **Peak plasma levels:** 1.5–3 hr. **t½, elimination:** About 3 hr (for zolmitriptan and active metabolite). Excreted in feces and urine. **Plasma protein binding:** About 25% bound to plasma proteins.

CONTRAINDICATIONS
Prophylaxis of migraine or management of hemiplegic or basilar migraine. Use in angina pectoris, history of MI, documented or silent ischemia, ischemic heart disease, coronary artery vasospasm (including Prinzmetal's variant angina), other significant underlying CV disease. Also use in uncontrolled hypertension, within 24 hr of treatment with another serotonin HT$_1$ agonist or an ergotamine-containing or ergot-type drug (e.g., dihydroergotamine, methysergide). Concurrent use with MAO inhibitor or within 2 weeks of discontinuing MAO inhibitor.

SPECIAL CONCERNS
Use with caution in liver disease and during lactation. A significant increase in BP may occur in those with moderate-to-severe hepatic impairment. Safety and efficacy have not been determined for cluster headache. Safety for treating >3 headaches in a 30-day period has not been determined. Efficacy has not been determined in children, 12–17 years, who have migraine headaches.

SIDE EFFECTS
Most Common
Warm/cold sensation, paresthesia, asthenia, dizziness, somnolence, chest tightness/pressure/heaviness, neck/throat/jaw pain, dry mouth, dyspepsia, nausea, pain.

GI: Dry mouth, dyspepsia, dysphagia, nausea, increased appetite, *tongue edema*, esophagitis, gastroenteritis, abnormal liver function, thirst. **CV:** Palpitations, arrhythmias, hypertension, syncope. **Atypical sensations:** Hypesthesia, paresthesia, warm/cold sensation. **CNS:** Dizziness, somnolence, vertigo, agitation, anxiety, depression, emotional lability, insomnia. **Pain/pressure sensations:** Chest pain, tightness, pressure and/or heaviness. Pain, tightness, or heaviness in the neck, throat, or jaw. Heaviness, pressure, tightness other than in the chest or neck. **Musculoskeletal:** Myalgia, myasthenia, back pain, leg cramps, tenosynovitis. **Respiratory:** Bronchitis, *bronchospasm*, epistaxis, hiccup, laryngitis, yawn. **Dermatologic:** Sweating, pruritus, rash, urticaria, ecchymosis, photosensitivity. **GU:** Hematuria, cystitis, polyuria, urinary frequency/urgency. **Body as a whole:** Asthenia, allergic reaction, chills, facial edema, edema, fever, malaise. **Miscellaneous:** Dry eye, eye pain, hyperacusis, ear pain, parosmia, tinnitus.

DRUG INTERACTIONS
Cimetidine / t½ of zolmitriptan is doubled
Ergot-containing drugs / Prolonged vasospastic reactions
MAO Inhibitors / ↑ Zolmitriptan levels
Oral contraceptives / ↑ Zolmitriptan plasma levels

Bold Italic = life threatening side effect   ■ = black box warning   ♣ = Available in Canada

Z

Selective serotonin reuptake inhibitors / Possible weakness, hyperreflexia, and incoordination

Sibutramine / Possible serotonin syndrome, including weakness, hyperreflexia, and incoordination

HOW SUPPLIED

Nasal Spray: 5 mg; *Tablets:* 2.5 mg, 5 mg; *Tablets, Oral Disintegrating:* 2.5 mg, 5 mg.

DOSAGE

- **NASAL SPRAY**
  Migraine headaches.

Give 1 dose of 5 mg. If headache returns, the dose may be repeated after 2 hr, not to exceed a maximum daily dose of 10 mg in any 24-hr period.

- **TABLETS**
  Migraine headaches.

Adults, initial: 2.5 mg or lower (break tablet in half). Dose of 5 mg may be required. If headache returns, repeat dose after 2 hr, not to exceed 10 mg in 24-hr period.

- **TABLETS, ORAL DISINTEGRATING**
  Migraine headaches.

Single dose of 2.5 mg. If headache returns, repeat dose after 2 hr, not to exceed 10 mg in 24-hr period.

NURSING CONSIDERATIONS

ADMINISTRATION/STORAGE

1. Use doses less than 2.5 mg in those with liver disease. Doses less than 2.5 mg may be obtained by manually breaking 2.5 mg tablet in half.
2. Safety of treating more than 3 headaches in a 30 day period has not been established.
3. Store from 20–25°C (68–77°F) protected from light and moisture.

ASSESSMENT

1. Note headache characteristics, including onset, frequency, type, duration of symptoms. Rate pain levels.
2. Assess neurologic exam, findings; review headache diary and note any triggers. Assess for LOC, N&V, vision changes/blurring, tingling in extremities, and if precedes headache
3. Determine any cardiac problems or ischemic CV disease. Assess ECG, renal and LFTs; reduce dose with dysfunction.

Monitor VS; expect transient increases in BP.

CLIENT/FAMILY TEACHING

1. Take exactly as directed; strictly to relieve migraine headaches, not to prevent them. Do not exceed dosage or dosing intervals of 2 hr apart and total of 10 mg/24 hr.
2. If using the orally disintegrating tablet, remove from the blister just prior to dosing. Place on the tongue where it will dissolve and be swallowed with saliva. Taking a liquid is not necessary. Do not break the orally disintegrating tablet.
3. Do not perform activities that require mental alertness until drug effects realized. Report if chest pain, SOB, chest/throat tightness, wheezing, swelling of face occurs.
4. Practice reliable contraception; report if pregnancy suspected.
5. Attempt to identify triggers. Report any loss of effect, unusual, or adverse side effects.

OUTCOMES/EVALUATE

Relief of migraine headache

Zolpidem tartrate©📷
(**ZOL**-pih-dem)

CLASSIFICATION(S):

Sedative-hypnotic, nonbenzodiazepine

PREGNANCY CATEGORY: B (Immediate-Release), **C** (Extended-Release).

Rx: Ambien, Ambien CR, Tovalt ODT, **C-IV**

USES

Immediate-Release Tablets: Short-term treatment of insomnia (7–10 days of use). Re-evaluate if hypnotics are to be taken for more than 2–3 weeks.

Extended-Release/Orally Disintegrating Tablets: Treatment of insomnia characterized by difficulties with sleep onset and/or sleep maintenance.

ACTION/KINETICS

Action

May act by subunit modulation of the GABA receptor chloride channel macromolecular complex resulting in sedative, anticonvulsant, anxiolytic, and myorelaxant properties. Although unrelated chemically to the benzodiazepines or barbiturates, it interacts with a GABA-benzodiazepine receptor complex and shares some of the pharmacologic effects of the benzodiazepines. Specifically, it binds to the omega-1 receptor preferentially. No evidence of residual next-day effects or rebound insomnia at usual doses; little evidence for memory impairment. Sleep time spent in stage 3 to 4 (deep sleep) was comparable to placebo with only inconsistent, minor changes in REM sleep at recommended doses.

Pharmacokinetics

Rapidly absorbed from the GI tract. **t½, elimination, immediate-release:** About 2.5 hr (increased in geriatric clients and those with impaired hepatic function). **t½ elimination, orally disintegrating:** 3.5 hr (nighttime dosing). **t½, elimination, extended-release:** 2.8 hr. Food decreases the bioavailability of zolpidem. Metabolized in the liver; inactive metabolites are excreted primarily through the urine. **Plasma protein binding:** 92.5%.

CONTRAINDICATIONS

Not recommended for use during lactation.

SPECIAL CONCERNS

Use with caution and at reduced dosage in clients with impaired hepatic function, in compromised respiratory function, in those with impaired renal function, and in clients with S&S of depression. Impaired motor or cognitive performance after repeated use or unusual sensitivity to hypnotic drugs may be noted in geriatric or debilitated clients. Closely observe individuals with a history of dependence on or abuse of drugs or alcohol as drug is habit-forming. Safety and efficacy have not been determined in children less than 18 years of age.

SIDE EFFECTS

Most Common

Immediate-Release/Oral Disintegrating: Dizziness, drowsiness, drugged feeling, headache, nausea, diarrhea, dyspepsia, myalgia, URTI.
Extended-Release: Headache, somnolence, dizziness, nausea, diarrhea, nasopharyngitis. Listed are side effects with an incidence greater than 1%.

Immediate Release/Orally Disintegrating: CNS: Headache, drowsiness, dizziness, depression, drugged feeling, lethargy, lightheadedness, abnormal dreams, amnesia, anxiety, fatigue, nervousness, sleep disorder. **GI:** N&V, dyspepsia, dry mouth, diarrhea, constipation, abdominal pain, anorexia. **CV:** Palpitations. **GU:** UTI. **Musculoskeletal:** Myalgia, arthralgia, back pain. **Respiratory:** URTI, pharyngitis, rhinitis, sinusitis. **Miscellaneous:** Allergy, flu-like symptoms, chest pain, rash, infection, hypersensitivity reactions.

Extended-Release: CNS: Headache, somnolence, dizziness, hallucinations, disorientation, fatigue, memory disorders, depression, anxiety, apathy, balance disorder, depression, disturbed attention, hypoesthesia, psychomotor retardation, ataxia, binge eating, depersonalization, disinhibition, euphoria, mood swings, paresthesia, stress symptoms, tremor, ataxia, confusion, drowsines, euphoria, insomnia, lethargy, vertigo, lightheadedness, burning sensation, postural dizziness. **GI:** N&V, constipation, abdominal discomfort/tenderness, abdominal pain, diarrhea, dyspepsia, hiccup, flatulence, frequent bowel movements, GERD, gastroenteritis. **CV:** Increased BP, palpitations. **GU:** Dysuria, vulvovaginal dryness, menorrhagia. **Dermatologic:** Rash, skin wrinkling, urticaria. **Musculoskeletal:** Back pain, myalgia, arthralgia, muscle cramps, neck pain/injury, involuntary muscle contractions. **Respiratory:** Throat irritation, dry throat, lower RTI, URTI, nasopharyngitis. **Ophthalmic:** Red eyes, visual disturbances, blurred vision, diplopia, altered visual depth perception. **Otic:** Vertigo, labyrinthitis, tinnitus, otitis externa. **Miscellaneous:**

Bold Italic = life threatening side effect   ■ = black box warning   ✦ = Available in Canada

Asthenopia, appetite disorder, allergy, asthenia, increased body temperature, chest discomfort, contusion, pyrexia, flu, flu-like illness, pyrexia, hypersensitivity reactions.

Symptoms of withdrawal: Although there is no clear evidence of a withdrawal syndrome, the following symptoms were noted with zolpidem following placebo substitution: Fatigue, nausea, flushing, lightheadedness, uncontrolled crying, emesis, stomach cramps, panic attack, nervousness, abdominal discomfort.

LABORATORY TEST CONSIDERATIONS
↑ ALT, AST, BUN. Hyperglycemia, hypercholesterolemia, hyperlipidemia, abnormal hepatic function.

OD OVERDOSE MANAGEMENT
Symptoms: Symptoms ranging from somnolence to light coma. Rarely, CV and respiratory compromise. *Treatment:* Gastric lavage if appropriate. General symptomatic and supportive measures. IV fluids as needed. Flumazenil may be effective in reversing CNS depression. Monitor hypotension and CNS depression and treat appropriately. Sedative drugs should not be used, even if excitation occurs. Zolpidem is not dialyzable.

DRUG INTERACTIONS
Alcohol / Additive effect on psychomotor performance
Azole antifungals (fluconazole, itraconazole, ketoconazole) / ↑ Zolpidem levels and therapeutic effects; monitor closely and adjust dose if necessary
Chlorpromazine / Additive ↓ alertness and psychomotor performance
CNS depressants / Additive CNS depression
Flumazenil / Reverses effect of zolpidem
Imipramine / ↓ Peak imipramine levels; additive decreased alertness
Rifamycins (e.g., rifampin) / ↓ Zolpidem levels and therapeutic effects; monitor closely and adjust dose if necessary
Ritonavir / Possible severe sedation and respiratory depression; do not use together
SSRIs / Shortened onset of zolpidem and ↑ effect

HOW SUPPLIED
Tablets, Extended-Release: 6.25 mg, 12.5 mg; *Tablets, Immediate-Release:* 5 mg, 10 mg; *Tablets, Orally Disintegrating:* 5 mg, 10 mg.

DOSAGE
• **TABLETS, IMMEDIATE-RELEASE; TABLETS, ORALLY DISINTEGRATING**
Hypnotic.
Adults, individualized, usual: 10 mg just before bedtime. In the elderly or in hepatic insufficiency, use an initial dose of 5 mg.
• **TABLETS, EXTENDED-RELEASE**
Hypnotic.
Individualize dose. **Adults:** 12.5 mg just before bedtime. For elderly or debilitated clients, give 6.25 mg just before bedtime.

NURSING CONSIDERATIONS

ℰ Do not confuse Ambien with Amen (progestin).

ADMINISTRATION/STORAGE
1. Limit therapy to 7–10 days. Reevaluate if the drug is required for more than 2–3 weeks.
2. Do not prescribe in quantities exceeding a 1-month supply.
3. Do not exceed 10 mg daily of the immediate-release or oral disintegrating tablets or 12.5 mg of the extended-release tablets.
4. Store the immediate-release and orally disintegrating tablets from 20–25°C (68–77°F) and the extended-release from 15–25°C (59–77°F).

ASSESSMENT
1. Note reasons for therapy, onset, symptom characteristics, triggers, other drugs prescribed to ensure none interact.
2. Assess for respiratory dysfunction (sleep apnea), drug or alcohol dependence; assess for symptoms of depression. Monitor CBC, LFTs.
3. Review sleep patterns (trouble falling/staying asleep, early a.m. awakenings) and lifestyle. Identify underlying cause(s) of insomnia (i.e., napping during the daytime, lack of exercise, ↑ stress, fear, loneliness, alcohol/caffeine use, lack of routine).

Z

4. Evaluate mental status, use lower dose in elderly/debilitated client; monitor for impaired motor/cognitive performance.

CLIENT/FAMILY TEACHING

1. Take only as directed, whole, on an empty stomach with a full glass of water just before going to bed. For faster sleep onset, do not administer with or immediately after a meal.

2. If using orally disintegrating tablets, open the blister pack and peel back the foil on the blister. Do not push the tablet through the foil. Remove the tablet and place it in the mouth where it will dissolve in seconds; then swallow with saliva. Can be taken with or without water. Do not chew, break, or split the tablet. Do not give with or immediately after a meal.

3. Swallow the extended-release tablets whole. Do not divide, crush, or chew the extended-release tablets.

4. Do not perform any activities that require mental or physical alertness until drug effects realized. Evaluate response the following day to ensure that no residual effects are present

5. Avoid alcohol, caffeine, chocolate after 4 p.m., and any unprescribed or OTC drugs.

6. Drug is only for short-term use; keep a log and identify factors that may be contributing to insomnia. Review alternative methods for inducing sleep: relaxation techniques, daily early day exercise, soft music, no daytime napping, guided imagery, white noise, dietary changes, special effects simulator.

7. Those with depression are at a higher risk for suicide or intentional overdose. Advise family that these clients warrant closer observation and limited prescriptions and to report any evidence of suicidal thoughts or aggressive behavior.

8. Keep out of reach of children and store in a safe place away from bedside; drug has a high potential for abuse and withdrawal after 2 weeks of use.

9. Do not take if pregnant; use contraception and report if suspected.

OUTCOMES/EVALUATE

Relief of insomnia

Zonisamide
(zoh-**NISS**-ah-myd)

CLASSIFICATION(S):
Anticonvulsant, miscellaneous
PREGNANCY CATEGORY: C
Rx: Zonegran.

USES

Adjunctive therapy to treat partial seizures in adults with epilepsy.

ACTION/KINETICS

Action

Is a sulfonamide. Precise mechanism unknown. May block sodium channels and reduce voltage-dependent, transient inward currents (T-type Ca^{2+} currents), thus stabilizing neuronal membranes and suppressing neuronal hypersynchronization. May bind to the GABA/benzodiazepine receptor ionophore complex.

Pharmacokinetics

Peak plasma levels: 2–5 mcg/mL in 2–6 hr. Food delays time to maximum levels but does not affect bioavailability. Extensively binds to erythrocytes. Due to the long $t\frac{1}{2}$, up to 2 weeks may be needed to achieve steady-state levels. $t\frac{1}{2}$, **elimination:** About 63 hr from plasma and about 105 hr from erythrocytes. Excreted primarily in the urine as unchanged drug and the glucuronide metabolite (mediated by CYP3A4). **Plasma protein binding:** About 40%.

CONTRAINDICATIONS

Hypersensitivity to sulfonamides or zonisamide. Use in those with a glomerular filtration rate <50 mL/min. Lactation.

SPECIAL CONCERNS

Hypersensitivity reactions are possible (zonisamide is a sulfonamide). Use with caution when coadministered with carbonic anhydrase inhibitors and drugs with anticholinergic activity. Use with caution in impaired hepatic or renal dysfunction. Use caution in dose selection in the elderly. Children seem to be at increased risk for zonisamide-associated oligohidrosis and hyperthermia. Abrupt withdrawal may precipitate in-

---

Bold Italic = life threatening side effect   ■ = black box warning   ✚ = Available in Canada

creased seizure frequency or status epilepticus. Safety and efficacy have not been determined in pediatric clients under 16 years of age.

SIDE EFFECTS

Most Common

Somnolence, anorexia, dizziness, headache, agitation/irritability, tiredness, nausea, diplopia, nystagmus, paresthesia, abdominal pain, dyspepsia, diarrhea, speech abnormalities, flu syndrome, rash, weight loss.

CNS-associated side effects are frequent. They can be classified as psychiatric symptoms (including depression and psychosis), psychomotor slowing (difficulty with concentration, speech, language), and somnolence or fatigue. Side effects listed are those with an incidence of 0.1% or more. **Hypersensitivity:** *Stevens-Johnson syndrome, toxic epidermal necrolysis, fulminant hepatic necrosis, agranulocytosis, aplastic anemia.* **CNS:** Somnolence, dizziness, headache, agitation, irritability, tiredness, ataxia, anxiety, confusion, depression, difficulty concentrating, difficulty with memory, speech/language problems, insomnia, mental slowing, paresthesia, nervousness, schizophrenia/schizophrenic behavior, tremor, convulsion, *status epilepticus,* abnormal gait, hyperesthesia, incoordination, hypertonia, twitching, abnormal dreams, vertigo, decreased libido, neuropathy, hyperkinesia, movement disorder, incoordination, disarthria, hypotonia, peripheral neuritis, increased reflexes, euphoria. **GI:** Anorexia, nausea, abdominal pain, diarrhea, dry mouth, taste perversion, dyspepsia, constipation, vomiting, flatulence, gingivitis, gum hyperplasia, gastritis, gastroenteritis, stomatitis, cholelithiasis, glossitis, melena, rectal hemorrhage, ulcerative stomatitis, gastroduodenal ulcer, dysphagia, gum hemorrhage, *pancreatitis.* **CV:** Palpitation, tachycardia, vascular insufficiency, *CVA,* hypertension, hypotension, thrombophlebitis, syncope, bradycardia. **Respiratory:** Pharyngitis, increased cough, dyspnea, rhinitis. **Musculoskeletal:** Leg cramps, myalgia, myasthenia, arthralgia, arthritis. **Dermatologic:** Pruritus, maculopapular rash, acne, alopecia, dry skin, sweating, eczema, ecchymosis, urticaria, hirsutism, pustular rash, vesiculobullous rash, *serious skin reactions (death possible).* **GU:** Urinary frequency, dysuria, urinary incontinence, hematuria, kidney stones, impotence, urinary retention, urinary urgency, amenorrhea, polyuria, nocturia. **Hematologic:** Leukopenia, anemia, immunodeficiency, lymphadenopathy, *aplastic anemia, agranulocytosis.* **Metabolic:** Peripheral edema, weight gain/loss, edema, thirst, dehydration. **Ophthalmic:** Diplopia, nystagmus, amblyopia, conjunctivitis, visual field defect, glaucoma, photophobia, iritis. **Otic:** Tinnitus, deafness. **Body as a whole:** Flu syndrome, accidental injury, asthenia, fatigue, malaise, allergic reaction. **Miscellaneous:** Difficulties in verbal expression, speech abnormalities, parosmia, chest pain, flank pain, facial edema, neck rigidity, *unexplained death.* NOTE: Pediatric clients may get heat stroke, oligohydrosis, decreased sweating, and hyperthermia, especially in warm or hot weather.

LABORATORY TEST CONSIDERATIONS

↑ Serum creatinine, BUN, serum alkaline phosphatase, CPK.

OD OVERDOSE MANAGEMENT

Symptoms: CNS symptoms (see *Side Effects*). *Treatment:* Induce emesis or gastric lavage; protect the airway. Institute general supportive care, including frequent monitoring of vital signs. *NOTE:* Zonisamide has a long $t\frac{1}{2}$.

DRUG INTERACTIONS

Carbamazepine / ↓ Zonisamide $t\frac{1}{2}$ R/T ↑ liver metabolism

Phenobarbital / ↓ Zonisamide $t\frac{1}{2}$ R/T ↑ liver metabolism

Phenytoin / ↓ Zonisamide $t\frac{1}{2}$ R/T ↑ liver metabolism

Sulfonamides / Potentially fatal reactions, including Stevens-Johnson syndrome, toxic epidermal necrolysis, agranulocytosis, aplastic anemia, and other blood dyscrasias

Valproate / ↑ Zonisamide $t\frac{1}{2}$ R/T ↓ liver metabolism

HOW SUPPLIED

Capsules: 25 mg, 50 mg, 100 mg.

Z

DOSAGE

- **CAPSULES**

  Partial seizures.

Adults and those over 16 years of age: Individualize. **Initial:** 100 mg/day. May increase to 200 mg/day after 2 weeks. Additional increases to 300 and 400 mg/day may be made in 2 weeks or longer to achieve steady state. **Effective dose range:** 100–600 mg/day. Administer dosage once or twice daily except for the 100-mg dose

NURSING CONSIDERATIONS

ADMINISTRATION/STORAGE

Store from 15–30°C (59–86°F) in a dry place protected from light.

ASSESSMENT

1. Note type, onset, characteristics of seizures, other agents trialed, outcome. List other drugs prescribed to ensure none interact.

2. Note any sulfonamide allergy/use. Monitor VS, CBC, renal, and LFTs; anticipate reduced dose with dysfunction.

CLIENT/FAMILY TEACHING

1. Take capsules once or twice a day as directed. May take with or without food but should swallow capsules whole.

2. May cause drowsiness; do not perfom tasks that require alertness until drug effects realized and able to determine if drug affects performance. Report any evidence of depression or mental disturbances.

3. Increase fluid intake (8 glasses of water/day) to reduce kidney stone risk. Report increased back or abdominal pain or any blood in urine. Stop drug and report immediately if a rash occurs or seizures worsen.

4. During the summer or hot weather, monitor temperature especially in children under age 17 as abnormally decreased sweating may occur resulting in severe dehydration and heatstroke.

5. Report any new onset fever, sore throat, easy bruising, oral ulcers, or lack of sweating with fever.

6. Practice reliable birth control. Report if pregnancy suspected/anticipated or if breast feeding, as drug should be avoided.

7. Abrupt withdrawal may precipitate increased seizure frequency or status epilepticus. Gradually reduce dose.

8. Keep all F/U appointments to evaluate response to therapy, labs and adverse side effects.

OUTCOMES/EVALUATE

Control of seizures

---

chapter 2
Therapeutic Drug Classifications

Refer to the accompanying website for additional drugs. Note that some drugs have recently been withdrawn from the market. Consult www.fda.gov for more information.

ALKYLATING AGENTS

SEE ALSO THE FOLLOWING INDIVIDUAL ENTRIES:

Busulfan
Carboplatin
Carmustine
Chlorambucil
Cisplatin
Cyclophosphamide
Dacarbazine
Ifosfamide
Lomustine
Mechlorethamine hydrochloride
Melphalan
Mesna
Streptozocin
Thiotepa

ACTION/KINETICS
Action

Alkylating agents donate an alkyl group (carbonium ion) to biologically important macromolecules, such as DNA. The molecule is inactivated bringing *cell division* to a halt. This cytotoxic activity affects replication of cancerous cells and other cells, especially in rapidly proliferating tissues, such as the bone marrow, intestinal epithelium, and hair follicles. The toxic effects are usually cell-cycle nonspecific and become apparent when the cell enters the S phase and cell division is blocked at the G_2 phase (premitotic phase), resulting in cells having a double complement of DNA. Resistance of cancer cells to alkylating agents usually develops slowly and gradually. Resistance seems to be the sum total of several minor adaptations, including decreased permeability of the cells, increased production of noncancer receptors (nucleophilic substances), and increased efficiency of the DNA repair system.

NURSING CONSIDERATIONS
ASSESSMENT

1. Note physical presentation, reasons for therapy; ensure client is well hydrated. Restrict within 4 weeks aft_r full XRT or chemotherapy to prevent critical bone marrow depression.
2. Monitor during therapy for adverse side effects; report. Assess catheter carefully to ensure patency and no extravasation.
3. Review VS, CBC, uric acid, renal, and LFTs.

CLIENT/FAMILY TEACHING

1. Note reasons for therapy, anticipated results, frequency of dosing, and what to expect.
2. Review list of side effects (i.e., N&V, loss of appetite, fatigue) and identify ways to cope (i.e., small frequent meals, dividing dose, and consuming 8-10 glasses of fluid/day.)
3. If infertility a possible side effect; suggest those that are considering families have eggs/sperm harvested prior

---

to therapy. Drug may cause birth defects; practice reliable contraception.

4. Practice good oral hygiene and complete dental work prior to starting therapy or wait until after therapy when blood counts are stabilized.

5. Report unusual side effects, unusual bleeding/bruising, fever, chills, sore throat, cough, SOB, yellowing of skin/eyes, flank or stomach pain, changes in bladder/bowel function.

6. Avoid those with infections; drugs may cause immunosuppression and make one more susceptible to infections.

7. Keep all F/U appointment to evaluate response to therapy and need for dosage adjustments.

OUTCOMES/EVALUATE

Clinical/radiographic evidence of tumor regression and disease stabilization

ALPHA-1-ADRENERGIC BLOCKING AGENTS

SEE ALSO THE FOLLOWING INDIVIDUAL ENTRIES:

Alfuzosin hydrochloride
Doxazosin mesylate
Prazosin hydrochloride
Tamsulosin hydrochloride
Terazosin

USES

(1) Hypertension, alone or in combination with diuretics or beta-adrenergic blocking agents. (2) Doxazocin, terazosin, and tamulosin are used to treat BPH. *Investigational:* Prazosin is used for refractory CHF, management of Raynaud's vasospasm, and to treat BPH. Doxazosin, along with digoxin and diuretics, is used to treat CHF.

ACTION/KINETICS

Action

Selectively block postsynaptic alpha-1-adrenergic receptors. Results in dilation of both arterioles and veins leading to a decrease in supine and standing BP. Diastolic BP is affected the most. Prazosin and terazosin do not produce reflex tachycardia. Terazosin also relaxes smooth muscle in the bladder neck and prostate, making it useful to treat BPH.

Have many undesirable effects which, although not toxic, limit their use. Always start treatment at low doses and increase gradually.

CONTRAINDICATIONS

Hypersensitivity to these drugs (i.e., quinazolines).

SPECIAL CONCERNS

The first few doses may cause postural hypotension and syncope with sudden loss of consciousness. Use with caution in lactation, with impaired hepatic function, or if receiving drugs known to influence hepatic metabolism. Safety and efficacy have not been established in children.

SIDE EFFECTS

The following side effects are common to alpha-1-adrenergic blockers. See individual drugs as well. **CV:** Marked hypotension and/or syncope with sudden loss of consciousness (first-dose effect), palpitations, postural hypotension, hypotension, tachycardia, chest pain, arrhythmia. **GI:** N&V, dry mouth, diarrhea, constipation, abdominal discomfort/pain, flatulence. **CNS:** Dizziness, depression, decreased libido, sexual dysfunction, nervousness, paresthesia, somnolence, anxiety, insomnia, asthenia, drowsiness. **Musculoskeletal:** Pain in the shoulder, neck, or back; gout, arthritis, joint pain, arthralgia. **Respiratory:** Dyspnea, nasal congestion, sinusitis, bronchitis, *bronchospasm,* cold symptoms, epistaxis, increased cough, flu symptoms, pharyngitis, rhinitis. **Ophthalmic:** Blurred vision, abnormal vision, reddened sclera, conjunctivitis, intraoperative floppy iris syndrome during phacoemulsification cataract surgery. **GU:** Impotence, urinary frequency, incontinence, priapism. **Miscellaneous:** Tinnitus, vertigo, pruritus, sweating, alopecia, lichen planus, headache, edema, weight gain, facial edema, fever.

OD OVERDOSE MANAGEMENT

Symptoms: Extension of the side effects, especially on BP. *Treatment:* Keep supine to restore BP and normalize heart rate. Shock may be treated with volume expanders or vasopressors; support renal function.

Bold Italic = life threatening side effect   ■ = black box warning   ♣ = Available in Canada

DRUG INTERACTIONS
Ethanol / ↑ Risk of hypotension; advise clients to avoid alcohol
Clonidine / ↓ Antihypertensive effect of clonidine.

LABORATORY TEST CONSIDERATIONS
↑ Urinary VMA.

DOSAGE
See individual agents.

NURSING CONSIDERATIONS

ADMINISTRATION/STORAGE
Take the first dose of prazosin and terazosin at bedtime to prevent dizziness.

ASSESSMENT
1. Note reasons for therapy, characteristics of S&S. If history of PUD, use drug cautiously.
2. Assess for heart or lung disease; note drugs currently prescribed. Some may cause vasospasm with Prinzmetal or vasospastic angina.
3. Monitor lytes, ECG, VS. Base titration on standing BP R/T postural effects.
4. Use cautiously in older clients; may fall R/T orthostatic hypotension. They may tolerate a slower, more gradual increase in dosage (i.e., terazosin 1 mg/day for 5 days followed by 2 mg/day for 5 days, etc., until desired response).

CLIENT/FAMILY TEACHING
1. May take with milk/meals to minimize GI upset. Do not stop abruptly; with terazosin, will have to re-titrate up to effective dosage if therapy stopped/interrupted.
2. Take at bedtime esp. first dose, to minimize fainting and low BP effects. Do not drive or perform hazardous tasks for 12–24 hr: after first dose, after increasing dose, or following an interruption of dosage. Avoid low BP symptoms by rising slowly from a sitting or lying position and waiting until symptoms subside.
3. Record BP and weight. Report any weight gain or extremity swelling; without a diuretic, may experience retention of salt/water due to vessel dilation.
4. Dizziness, fatigue, headache, and palpitations may occur as well as transient apprehension, fear/anxiety. Report if persistent so dosage may be adjusted.

5. Report for yearly DRE and PSA to ensure prostate lesion free.
6. Avoid alcohol, excess caffeine and OTC agents (esp. cold remedies).
7. Excessive exercise/heat exposure, prolonged standing and alcohol may intensify side effects.
8. Review life-style changes needed for BP control (i.e., dietary restrictions of fat and sodium, weight reduction, regular physical exercise, decreased use of alcohol, stress reduction, and smoking cessation). For BPH control: no fluid intake 4 hr before bedtime, empty bladder before going to sleep, avoid caffeine and alcohol in the evening. Report if no improvement in S&S.

OUTCOMES/EVALUATE
↓ BP ↓ Nocturia, urgency/frequency. Improved stream

AMINOGLYCOSIDES   ■

SEE ALSO THE FOLLOWING INDIVIDUAL ENTRIES:

Amikacin sulfate
Gentamicin sulfate
Neomycin sulfate
Tobramycin sulfate

USES
These are powerful antibiotics that induce serious side effects—**do not use for minor infections.** (1) Gram-negative bacteria causing bone and joint infections, septicemia (including neonatal sepsis), skin and soft tissue infections (including those from burns), respiratory tract infections, postoperative infections, intra-abdominal infections (including peritonitis), UTIs. (2) In combination with clindamycin for mixed aerobic-anaerobic infections. Also, see individual drugs.

Used for gram-positive bacteria only when other less toxic drugs are either ineffective or contraindicated. Use in CNS *Pseudomonas* infections such as meningitis or ventriculitis is questionable.

ACTION/KINETICS

Action
Broad-spectrum antibiotics believed to inhibit protein synthesis by binding ir-

Classifications

reversibly to ribosomes (30S subunit), thereby interfering with an initiation complex between messenger RNA and the 30S subunit. This leads to production of nonfunctional proteins; polyribosomes are split apart and are unable to synthesize protein. Usually bactericidal due to disruption of the bacterial cytoplasmic membrane.

Pharmacokinetics

Poorly absorbed from the GI tract; usually administered parenterally (exceptions: some enteric infections of the GI tract and prior to surgery). Also absorbed from the peritoneum, bronchial tree, wounds, denuded skin, and joints. Distributed in the extracellular fluid. Cross the placental barrier, but not the blood-brain barrier. Penetration of the CSF is increased when the meninges are inflamed.

Rapidly absorbed after IM injection. **Peak plasma levels, after IM:** Usually $\frac{1}{2}$–2 hr. Measurable levels persist for 8–12 hr after a single administration. **t$\frac{1}{2}$:** 2–3 hr (increases sharply in impaired kidney function). Ranges of t$\frac{1}{2}$ from 24 to 110 hr have been observed. Excreted mainly unchanged in urine. Resistance develops slowly.

CONTRAINDICATIONS

Hypersensitivity to aminoglycosides, long-term therapy (except streptomycin for tuberculosis).

SPECIAL CONCERNS

■(1) Aminoglycosides cause significant nephrotoxicity or ototoxicity. They are excreted primarily by glomerular filtration; thus, serum half-life will be prolonged and significant accumulation will occur in clients with impaired renal function. Toxicity may develop even with conventional doses, especially in those with prerenal azotemia or impaired renal function. (2) Neurotoxicity, manifested as both auditory and vestibular ototoxicity can occur with any aminoglycoside. Auditory changes are irreversible, usually bilateral, and may be partial or total. The risk of hearing loss increases with the degree of exposure to either high peak or high trough serum levels and continues to progress after drug withdrawal. The risk is great-

er in clients with renal impairment and with preexisting hearing loss. High frequency deafness usually occurs first and can be detected by audiometric testing. When possible, obtain serial audiograms. There may be no clinical symptoms to warn of developing cochlear damage. Tinnitus or vertigo may occur and are evidence of vestibular injury. Other symptoms of neurotoxicity may include numbness, skin tingling, muscle twitching, and convulsions. Total or partial irreversible bilateral deafness may occur after drug discontinuation. (3) Vestibular toxicity is more predominant with gentamicin and streptomycin; auditory toxicity is more common with kanamycin, amikacin, and netilmicin. Tobramycin affects both functions equally. Relative ototoxicity is streptomycin > kanamycin > amikacin = gentamicin = tobramycin > netilmicin. Kanamycin, amikacin, and streptomycin appear in this relative comparison based on high dose (kanamycin, amikacin) and antituberculosis (streptomycin) therapy. (4) Renal toxicity is characterized by decreased creatinine clearance, cells or casts in the urine, decreased urine specific gravity, oliguria, proteinuria or evidence of nitrogen retention (increasing BUN, NPN, or serum creatinine). Renal damage is usually reversible. The relative nephrotoxicity of aminoglycosides is kanamycin = amikacin = gentamicin = netilmicin > tobramycin > streptomycin. (5) Closely observe all clients treated with aminoglycosides. Monitoring renal and eighth cranial nerve function at onset of therapy is essential for those with known or suspected renal impairment and in those whose renal function is initially normal, but who develop signs of renal dysfunction. (6) Evidence of renal impairment or ototoxicity requires drug discontinuation or appropriate dosage adjustments. When possible, monitor drug serum levels. Avoid concomitant use with other ototoxic, neurotoxic, or nephrotoxic drugs. Other factors which may increase risk of toxicity are dehydration and advanced age.■ Safe use in pregnancy and during lactation not established. Assess

---

premature infants, neonates, and older clients closely; they are particularly sensitive to toxic effects. Considerable cross-allergenicity occurs among the aminoglycosides.

SIDE EFFECTS

Ototoxicity: Both auditory and vestibular damage have been noted. Increased risk with poor renal function and in the elderly. Auditory symptoms include tinnitus and hearing impairment, while vestibular symptoms include dizziness, nystagmus, vertigo, and ataxia. **Renal Impairment:** Characterized by cylindruria, oliguria, proteinuria, azotemia, hematuria, increase/decrease in frequency of urination; increased BUN, NPN, or creatinine; and increased thirst. **Neurotoxicity:** Neuromuscular blockade, headache, tremor, lethargy, paresthesia, peripheral neuritis (numbness, tingling, or burning of face/mouth), arachnoiditis, encephalopathy, acute OBS. CNS depression, characterized by stupor, flaccidity, and rarely, *coma, and respiratory depression in infants.* Optic neuritis with blurred/loss of vision. **GI:** N&V, diarrhea, increased salivation, anorexia, weight loss. **Allergic:** Rash, urticaria, pruritus, burning, fever, stomatitis, eosinophilia. Rarely, *agranulocytosis and anaphylaxis.* Cross-allergy among aminoglycosides has been observed. **Miscellaneous:** Joint pain, *laryngeal edema, pulmonary fibrosis,* superinfection.

OD OVERDOSE MANAGEMENT

Symptoms: Extension of side effects. *Treatment:* Undertake hemodialysis (preferred) or peritoneal dialysis.

DRUG INTERACTIONS

Bumetanide / ↑ Risk of ototoxicity
Capreomycin / ↑ Muscle relaxation
Cephalosporins / ↑ Risk of renal toxicity
Ciprofloxacin HCl / Additive antibacterial activity
Cisplatin / Additive renal toxicity
Colistimethate / ↑ Muscle relaxation
Digoxin / Possible ↑ or ↓ effect
Ethacrynic acid / ↑ Risk of ototoxicity
Furosemide / ↑ Risk of ototoxicity
Methoxyflurane / ↑ Risk of renal toxicity
Penicillins / ↓ Effect of aminoglycosides
Polymyxins / ↑ Muscle relaxation

Skeletal muscle relaxants (surgical) / ↑ Muscle relaxation
Vancomycin / Additive ototoxicity and renal toxicity
Vitamin A / ↓ Effect R/T ↓ absorption from GI tract.

LABORATORY TEST CONSIDERATIONS

↑ BUN, BSP retention, creatinine, AST, ALT, bilirubin. ↓ Cholesterol values.

DOSAGE

See individual drugs.

NURSING CONSIDERATIONS

ADMINISTRATION/STORAGE

1. Check expiration date.
2. Warn if drug being administered stings or causes a burning sensation.
3. During IM administration:
- Inject deep into muscle mass to minimize transient pain.
- Use a Z track method for thin, elderly clients.
- Rotate/document injection sites.
4. With IV administration:
- Dilute with compatible solution.
- Infuse at the rate ordered to prevent excessive serum concentrations.
5. Administer for only 7–10 days. Avoid repeating course of therapy unless serious infection present that does not respond to other antibiotics.
6. Administer ATC to maintain therapeutic drug levels.

ASSESSMENT

1. Note reasons for therapy, other agents trialed, characteristics of S&S. Assess for presence/source(s) of infection. Monitor and document fever, culture/lab reports, and wound characteristics (i.e., color, odor, drainage, temperature) and clinical presentation.
2. Assess for allergies; note history of sensitivity to anti-infectives.
3. Weigh/calculate BMI to ensure correct dosage. For peak drug level determinations, draw blood 1 hr after IM injection and 30 to 60 min after IV infusion in non-heparinized tube. For trough levels, draw just before next dose due. Ensure adequate hydration to prevent renal tubule irritation.
4. Obtain/monitor VS, U/A, C&S, liver, renal, auditory, and vestibular function; assess for oto/nephrotoxicity. Ensure

adequately hydrated before and during therapy.

INTERVENTIONS

1. Monitor VS and I&O; increase fluids to prevent renal tubule irritation.

2. Monitor drug levels (e.g., Amikacin levels >30 mcg/mL are considered toxic).

3. With vestibular dysfunction protect by supervised ambulation and side rails; note (potential for) fall hazard.

4. Assess for ototoxicity with pretreatment audiograms. Hearing loss is a dose-related side effect of drug therapy most commonly associated with amikacin, kanamycin, neomycin, or paromomycin. Tinnitus, dizziness, and loss of balance are also signs of vestibular injury and more commonly seen with gentamicin and streptomycin. Deafness may occur several weeks after discontinuing drug.

5. Do not administer concurrently or sequentially with a topical or systemic nephrotoxic or ototoxic drug (e.g., potent diuretics such as ethacrynic acid or furosemide) unless provider designates benefits outweigh risks.

6. Observe for neuromuscular blockade with muscular weakness leading to apnea, when administered with a muscle relaxant, after anesthesia, or too rapidly during IV infusion. Have calcium gluconate or neostigmine available to reverse blockade.

7. With IM injections select large muscle mass such as gluteal or midlateral thigh and administer deep to prevent tissue damage. May use ice to relieve pain at injection site.

8. Note cells or casts in the urine, oliguria, proteinuria, lowered specific gravity, increasing BUN/creatinine, all of which indicate altered renal function.

CLIENT/FAMILY TEACHING

1. Review goals of therapy and prescribed method of administration. Infuse as prescribed, ATC, until prescription is completed when utilizing home infusion therapy.

2. Follow a well-balanced diet and consume at least 2–3 L/day of fluids. If N&V or loss of appetite occur, try small frequent meals and frequent mouth care.

3. Report S&S of superinfection (black, furry tongue; loose, foul-smelling stools; vaginal itching) or other adverse effects.

4. Report lack of response after 3 days of therapy, alterations in hearing, vision, and/or ambulation. Use safety measures to prevent injury.

5. Keep all F/U appointments. to evaluate response to therapy and need for dosage adjustments.

OUTCOMES/EVALUATE

• Negative culture reports
• Resolution of infection with ↓ WBCs, ↓ fever, symptomatic improvement

AMPHETAMINES AND DERIVATIVES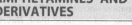

SEE ALSO THE FOLLOWING INDIVIDUAL ENTRIES:

Amphetamine mixtures
Dexmethylphenidate hydrochloride
Dextroamphetamine sulfate
Lisdexamfetamine dimesylate
Methylphenidate hydrochloride

USES

See individual drugs. Uses include: (1) To improve wakefulness in those with excessive daytime sleepiness associated with narcolepsy. (2) As part of a total treatment program for attention deficit disorder with hyperactivity in children 3–16 years of age. (3) Short-term use as an adjunct in a regimen of weight reduction for exogenous obesity. *Investigational:* Dextroamphetamine for treatment of cocaine dependence and to treat autism.

ACTION/KINETICS

Action

Thought to act on the cerebral cortex and reticular activating system (including the medullary, respiratory, and vasomotor centers) by releasing norepinephrine from central adrenergic neurons. High doses cause release of dopamine from the mesolimbic system. The stimulatory effect on the CNS causes an increase in motor activity and mental alertness, a mood-elevating effect, a slight euphoric effect, and an anorexigenic effect. The anorexigenic effect is thought to be produced by direct stimulation of the satiety center in the lateral hypothalamic feeding center of the brain.

Peripheral effects are mediated by alpha- and beta-adrenergic receptors and include increases in both systolic and diastolic BP, respiratory stimulation, and weak bronchodilator activity. Large doses may cause cardiac arrhythmias.

Psychic stimulation is often followed by a rebound effect manifested as fatigue. Tolerance will develop to all drugs of this class. There is a relatively wide margin of safety between the therapeutic and toxic doses of amphetamines. However, both acute and chronic toxicity can occur.

Pharmacokinetics

Readily absorbed from the GI tract and distributed throughout most tissues, with the highest concentrations in the brain and CSF. **Duration of anorexia (PO):** 3–6 hr. Metabolized in liver and excreted by kidneys. Excreted slowly (5–7 days); cumulative effects may occur with continued administration.

CONTRAINDICATIONS

Hyperthyroidism, advanced arteriosclerosis, moderate to severe hypertension, symptomatic CV disease, narrow-angle glaucoma, angina pectoris, CV disease, and individuals with hypersensitivity to these drugs. Use in emotionally unstable persons susceptible to drug abuse, in those with a history of drug abuse, and in agitated states. Use of methamphetamine to combat fatigue or replace rest in normal people. Psychotic children. Lactation. During or within 14 days of MAO inhibitor use (hypertensive crisis may occur). Use not recommended in children less than 3 years of age for attention deficit disorder with hyperactivity.

SPECIAL CONCERNS

■ (1) Amphetamines have a high potential for abuse. Use in weight reduction programs only when alternative therapy has been ineffective. Administration for prolonged periods may lead to drug dependence and must be avoided. Pay particular attention to the possibility of individuals obtaining amphetamines for nontherapeutic use or distribution to others. Prescribe or dispense sparingly. (2) There is an increased risk of cardiovascular effects and adverse psychiatric symptoms. There are reports of sudden death in clients with underlying heart disease and serious heart defects and cases of stroke and MI. Clients with a history of heart disease, depression, or psychosis should not receive these medications.■

Use with caution in clients suffering from hyperexcitability states; in elderly, debilitated, or asthenic clients; and in clients with psychopathic personality traits or a history of homicidal or suicidal tendencies. Prescribe with caution for clients with even mild hypertension. Amphetamines have been significantly abused leading to tolerance, extreme psychological dependence, and severe social disability. Clients may increase the dosage to many times that recommended. Safety and efficacy have not been established for the use of amphetamines as anorectic agents in children less than 12 years of age. Amphetamines may exacerbate symptoms of behavior disturbance and thought disorder in psychotic children and they may exacerbate motor and phonic tics and Tourette's syndrome.

SIDE EFFECTS

CNS: Overstimulation, restlessness, dizziness, insomnia, dyskinesia, euphoria, dysphoria, tremor, headache, changes in libido, psychotic episodes at usual doses (rare). Rarely, psychoses. In children, manifestation of vocal and motor tics and Tourette's syndrome. **GI:** N&V, cramps, diarrhea, dry mouth, constipation, metallic taste, anorexia. **CV:** Arrhythmias, palpitations, dyspnea, pulmonary hypertension, peripheral hyper-/hypotension, precordial pain, fainting, tachycardia, increased BP, reflex decrease in HR, cardiomyopathy after chronic use. **Dermatologic:** Symptoms of allergy including rash, urticaria, erythema, burning. Pallor. **GU:** Urinary frequency, dysuria. **Ophthalmologic:** Blurred vision, mydriasis. **Hematologic:** *Agranulocytosis,* leukopenia. **Endocrine:** Menstrual irregularities, gynecomastia, impotence, changes in libido.

Miscellaneous: Alopecia, increased motor activity, fever, sweating, chills, muscle/chest pain, weight loss, urticaria, impotence. Long-term use results in psychic dependence, as well as high degree of tolerance. Growth inhibition in children after long-term use. *NOTE:* Abrupt cessation following prolonged high doses results in extreme fatigue, mental depression, and changes on the sleep EEG.

OD OVERDOSE MANAGEMENT

Symptoms of Acute Overdose (Toxicity): Restlessness, irritability, insomnia, tremor, hyperreflexia, rhabdomyolysis, rapid respiration, **hyperpyrexia,** assaultiveness, hallucinations, panic states, sweating, mydriasis, flushing, hyperactivity, confusion, hyper-/hypotension, extrasystoles, tachypnea, fever, delirium, self-injury, arrhythmias, **seizures, coma, circulatory collapse, death. Death usually results from CV collapse or convulsions.**

Symptoms of Chronic Toxicity: Chronic use/abuse is characterized by emotional lability, loss of appetite, severe dermatoses, hyperactivity, insomnia, irritability, somnolence, mental impairment, occupational deterioration, a tendency to withdraw from social contact, teeth grinding, continuous chewing, and ulcers of the tongue and lips. Prolonged use of high doses can elicit symptoms of paranoid schizophrenia, including auditory and visual hallucinations and paranoid ideation.

Treatment of Acute Toxicity (Overdosage):

- Symptomatic treatment. After oral ingestion, induce emesis or perform gastric lavage, followed by use of activated charcoal. Acidification of the urine increases the rate of excretion. Give fluids until urine flow is 3–6 mL/kg/hr; furosemide or mannitol may be beneficial.
- Maintain adequate circulation and respiration.
- Treat CNS stimulation with chlorpromazine. Reduce stimuli and maintain in a quiet, dim environment. Treat clients who have ingested an overdose of long-acting products for tox-

icity until all symptoms of overdosage have disappeared.

- IV phentolamine may be used for hypertension, whereas hypotension may be reversed by IV fluids and possibly vasopressors (used with caution).

DRUG INTERACTIONS

Acetazolamide / ↑ Amphetamine effect by ↑ renal tubular reabsorption

Ammonium chloride / ↓ Amphetamine effect by ↑ renal tubular excretion

Anesthetics, general / ↑ Risk of cardiac arrhythmias

Antihypertensives / ↓ Effect

Ascorbic acid / ↓ Amphetamine effect by ↓ renal tubular reabsorption

Furazolidone / ↑ Toxicity of anorexiants R/T MAO activity of furazolidone

Guanethidine / ↓ Guanethidine effect by displacement from its site of action

Haloperidol / ↓ Amphetamine effect by ↓ drug uptake at its site of action

Insulin / Altered requirements

MAO inhibitors / All peripheral, metabolic, cardiac, and central amphetamine effects are potentiated for up to 2 weeks after termination of MAO inhibitor therapy (symptoms include hypertensive crisis with possible intracranial hemorrhage, hyperthermia, convulsions, coma); death may occur. ↓ Amphetamine effect by ↓ drug uptake into its site of action

Methyldopa / ↓ Hypotensive effect by ↑ sympathomimetic activity

Phenothiazines / ↓ Amphetamine effect by ↓ drug uptake at its site of action

SSRIs / ↑ Sensitivity to amphetamines; possible serotonin syndrome; if given together, monitor for increased S&S of CNS effects.

Sodium bicarbonate / ↑ Amphetamine effect by ↑ renal tubular reabsorption

Thiazide diuretics / ↑ Amphetamine effect by ↑ renal tubular reabsorption

Tricyclic antidepressants / ↓ Amphetamine effects.

LABORATORY TEST CONSIDERATIONS

↑ BUN and creatinine (both transient and reversible). ↑ Liver enzymes, plasma corticosteroids, serum bilirubin, uric acid, blood glucose. Small ↑ serum po-

---

tassium. Urinary steroid determinations may be altered.

DOSAGE

See individual drugs. Administer at the lowest effective dose and individualize dosage. Many compounds are timed-release preparations.

NURSING CONSIDERATIONS

ADMINISTRATION/STORAGE

1. If prescribed to suppress appetite, administer 30 min before anticipated meal time.
2. Extended-release amphetamine mixture products are indicated for children 6 years and older.
3. Use a small initial dose; then increase gradually as necessary. Use lowest effective dose.
4. Unless otherwise ordered, give last dose of day at least 6 hr before bedtime.
5. When used for ADD in children, interrupt therapy on occasion to determine necessity for continued therapy.
6. When tolerance develops to the anorectic effect, do not exceed the recommended dose in an attempt to increase the effect; rather, stop the drug.

ASSESSMENT

1. Note reasons for therapy, clinical presentation, characteristics of S&S. List all drugs currently taking.
2. Assess for conditions that would preclude using drugs in this category, i.e., ASHD, HTN, hyperthyroidism, DM, glaucoma. Note age and if debilitated.
3. Monitor lytes, ECG, weight/height to assess for growth inhibition, VS, and CBC.
4. Under the Controlled Substances Act; follow appropriate policy for dispensing/handling to restrict availability and discourage abuse.

INTERVENTIONS

1. If agitated or complains of sleeplessness, reduce dosage of drug. If somnolent or appears mentally or physically impaired, stop the drug. Observe for signs of psychologic dependence and drug tolerance.
2. If receiving MAO inhibitors or received them 7–14 days before amphetamine therapy, assess for hypertensive crisis. Monitor and report fever, marked sweating, excitation, delirium, tremors, or twitching; pad side rails and have suction available.
3. Monitor VS. Assess for arrhythmias, tachycardia, or hypertension. CV changes with psychotic syndrome may indicate toxicity.

CLIENT/FAMILY TEACHING

1. Take only as prescribed, 1 hr before meals and last dose 6 hr before bedtime to ensure adequate rest. Take only as directed; do not share medications. Report S&S of tolerance. Abrupt withdrawal may cause adverse symptoms.
2. When anorexiants are used for weight reduction, their effect lasts only 4–6 weeks; use is short term. Record food intake, BP, and weight daily the first week and then at least once a week. May become anorexic; report any persistent, severe weight loss so therapy can be adjusted. Follow an established dietary and exercise regimen to maintain weight loss and attend a behavioral modification weight control program.
3. Diets high in fiber, fruit, and fluids assist to reduce drugs' constipating effects. See dietitian to discuss weight control and/or reducing diets when weight loss is the goal.
4. Report any changes in attention span and ability to concentrate. May cause a false sense of euphoria and well being and mask extreme fatigue. These may impair judgment and ability to perform potentially hazardous tasks, such as operating a machine or an automobile. Using amphetamines to treat fatigue is inappropriate because rebound effects may be severe.
5. Seek medical assistance if experiencing extreme fatigue and depression once drug is discontinued. Periodic "drug holidays" may be ordered to assess progress and prevent dependence.
6. Avoid OTC agents and ingesting large amounts of caffeine in any form. Read labels for the presence of caffeine since this contributes to CV side effects.
7. Manage dry mouth by frequent rinsing, chewing sugarless gum, or sucking sugarless hard candies.

Classifications

📷 = see color insert   H = Herbal   IV = Intravenous   𝒞 = sound alike drug

8. Store safely out of child's reach. Keep all F/U visits.

OUTCOMES/EVALUATE
- ↑ Attention span/concentration
- Weight reduction
- ↓ Episodes of narcolepsy

ANGIOTENSIN II RECEPTOR ANTAGONISTS ■

SEE ALSO THE FOLLOWING INDIVIDUAL ENTRIES:

Candesartan cilexetil
Eprosartan mesylate
Irbesartan
Losartan potassium
Olmesartan medoxomil
Telmisartan
Valsartan

USES
(1) Hypertension, alone or in combination with other antihypertensive drugs. (2) Nephropathy in type II diabetes mellitus (irbesartan and losartan). (3) Heart failure (NYHA classes II to IV) in those intolerant to ACE inhibitors (valsartan). (4) Reduce risk of stroke in those with hypertension and left ventricular hypertrophy (losartan). *Investigational:* Congestive heart failure. Can be combined with ACE inhibitors to reduce morbidity and mortality in clients with moderate to severe CHF.

ACTION/KINETICS
Action
Angiotensin II, a potent vasoconstrictor, is the primary vasoactive hormone of the renin-angiotensin system; it is involved in the pathophysiology of hypertension. Angiotensin II increases systemic vascular resistance, causes sodium and water retention, and leads to increased HR and vasoconstriction. The angiotensin II receptor antagonists competitively block the angiotensin AT_1 receptor located in vascular smooth muscle and the adrenal glands, thus blocking the vasoconstrictor and aldosterone-secreting effects of angiotensin II. Thus, BP is reduced. No significant effects on HR with minimal orthostatic hypotension and no significant effect on potassium levels. Does not inhibit angiotensin converting enzyme (ACE).

CONTRAINDICATIONS
Hypersensitivity to any component of the products. Lactation.

SPECIAL CONCERNS
■When used during the second and third trimesters of pregnancy, drugs that act directly on the renin-angiotensin system can cause injury and even death to the developing fetus. When pregnancy is detected, discontinue angiotensin II receptor antagonists as soon as possible.■ Symptomatic hypotension may occur in those who are intravascularly volume-depleted. Fetal and neonatal morbidity and death are possible if given to pregnant women. Safety and efficacy have not been determined in children less than 18 years of age.

DOSAGE
See individual drugs.

NURSING CONSIDERATIONS
ASSESSMENT
1. Note reasons for therapy, characteristics of S&S, PMH, other agents trialed.
2. Ensure adequate hydration to prevent severe hypotensive episode.
3. Not for use during pregnancy or lactation. Observe infants exposed in utero for hypotension, oliguria, fetal defects, and ↑ K.
4. Monitor VS, CBC, lytes, and renal function; reduce dose with dysfunction.
5. Assess for allergic reactions, i.e., rash, fever, itching, angioedema.

CLIENT/FAMILY TEACHING
1. Take only as directed usually once daily. May take with or without food.
2. Advise surgeon that ARB is prescribed; blockage of renin-angiotensin system following surgery may be problematic.
3. Avoid activities that cause reduction in fluid volume, i.e., excessive perspiration, vomiting, diarrhea, dehydration; may cause low BP.
4. Dizziness may occur; avoid activities that require mental alertness until drug effects realized. Change positions slowly to prevent sudden drop in BP.

---

5. Continue regular exercise, weight loss, dietary restrictions, including low salt; stop tobacco/alcohol; life style changes needed to lower BP.

6. Practice reliable contraception. Stop drug and report if pregnancy suspected; do not nurse infant.

7. Record BP regularly at different times of day for provider review. Continue regular medical F/U and lab studies as scheduled; report unusual side effects or lack of response.

OUTCOMES/EVALUATE

- Control of BP
- Stabilization of CHF

ANGIOTENSIN-CONVERTING ENZYME (ACE) INHIBITORS

SEE ALSO THE FOLLOWING INDIVIDUAL ENTRIES:

Benazepril hydrochloride
Captopril
Enalapril maleate
Fosinopril sodium
Lisinopril
Perindopril erbumine*
Quinapril hydrochloride
Ramipril
Trandolapril

Drugs marked with an * are available to view in the online database at www.delmarnursesdrughandbook.com/2009.

GENERAL STATEMENT

Guidelines on the evaluation and management of chronic heart failure were updated during 2005. The new guidelines stress the early diagnosis of heart failure, marked by four stages:

1. Stage A: High risk clients with no structural heart disease or symptoms.

2. Stage B: Structural heart disease without signs or symptoms.

3. Stage C: Structural heart disease with prior or current symptoms.

4. Stage D: Refractory heart failure requiring specialized interventions.

These stages complement, but do not replace, the New York Heart Association functional classification for heart failure.

Treatment guidelines for the various stages follow:

1. Stage A: Prevention through treatment of identifiable risk factors for heart failure, including hypertension, diabetes, and atherosclerotic disease. The guidelines recommend the use of ACE inhibitors for preventing heart failure in stage A clients with atherosclerotic vascular disease, diabetes, or hypertension. As an alternate, angiotensin II receptor blockers are recommended.

2. Stage B: Clients with a history of MI and/or reduced left ventricular ejection fraction should be treated with an ACE inhibitor and a beta blocker. Angiotensin II receptor blockers are recommended for those intolerant of ACE inhibitors. Beta blockers recommended are bisoprolol, carvediol, or sustained-release metoprolol succinate (Toprol XL).

3. Stage C: For clients with reduced left ventricular ejection fraction, an aldosterone antagonist (e.g., spironolactone, eplerenone) is recommended in carefully selected clients with either moderate or severe heart failure or left ventricular dysfunction early after MI, has been added as a class I recommendation. Monitor potassium to avoid hyperkalemia.

4. Stage D: Use of a left ventricular assist device as a permanent "destination" therapy should be considered for select clients. Intermittent infusion of positive inotropes are not recommended; continuous infusions of these drugs should be considered only as palliation in end-stage clients.

Therapeutic considerations include the following guidelines:

- All symptomatic clients should be receiving, at a minimum, both an ACE inhibitor and a beta-blocker (unless contraindicated).
- The dose of ACE inhibitor should be titrated to levels found effective in clinical trials.
- The dose of beta-blocker should be started low and titrated gradually to avoid worsening of symptoms.

Classifications

- Those receiving an aldosterone antagonist should be monitored closely for hyperkalemia, which is usually precipitated by renal impairment or concomitant use of potassium supplements, NSAIDs, COX-2 inhibitors, or high doses of ACE inhibitors.
- Clients should not be prescribed drugs that worsen heart failure, such as antiarrhythmic drugs (other than amiodarone and dofetilide), nondihydropyridine calcium-channel blockers, NSAIDs, and thiazolidinediones.

USES

See individual drugs. Uses include, but are not limited to: (1) Hypertension, alone or in combination with other antihypertensive agents (especially thiazide diuretics). Can be used as initial therapy either alone or in combination with thiazide diuretics. (2) CHF often in combination with diuretics and/or digitalis. Use captopril, enalapril, fosinopril, lisinopril, or quinapril. (3) In stable clients who are symptomatic from CHF within the first few days after an acute MI (use ramipril or trandolapril). (4) Asymptomatic left ventricular dysfunction (enalapril). (5) Diabetic nephropathy (captopril). (6) Improve survival following MI in clinically stable clients with left ventricular dysfunction (ejection fraction of 40% or less) and to reduce incidence of overt heart failure and subsequent hospitalizations (captopril). (7) Reduction of risk of MI, stroke, and death from CV causes (ramipril). (8) Improve survival in hemodynamically stable clients within 24 hr of acute MI (lisinopril). (8) Use in stable clients with evidence of left ventricular systolic dysfunction (trandolapril).

ACTION/KINETICS

Action

Believed to act by suppressing the renin-angiotensin-aldosterone system. Renin, synthesized by the kidneys, produces angiotensin I, an inactive decapeptide derived from plasma globulin substrate. Angiotensin I is converted to angiotensin II by ACE. Angiotensin II is a potent vasoconstrictor that also stimulates secretion of aldosterone from the adrenal cortex, resulting in sodium and fluid retention. The ACE inhibitors prevent the conversion of angiotensin I to angiotensin II. This results in a decrease in plasma angiotensin II and subsequently a decrease in peripheral resistance and decreased aldosterone secretion (leading to fluid loss) and therefore a decrease in BP. There may be either no change or an increase in CO. Several weeks of therapy may be required to achieve the maximum effect to reduce BP. Standing and supine BPs are lowered to about the same extent. ACE inhibitors are also antihypertensive in low renin hypertensive clients. ACE inhibitors are additive with thiazide diuretics in lowering blood pressure; however, β-blockers and captopril have less than additive effects when used with ACE inhibitors.

CONTRAINDICATIONS

Hypersensitivity to the products or a history of angioedema due to previous treatment with an ACE inhibitor. Use of enalapril, enalaprilat, or lisinopril in clients with hereditary or idiopathic angioedema. Use of most ACE inhibitors during lactation.

SPECIAL CONCERNS

■Use during the second and third trimesters of pregnancy can result in injury and even death to the developing fetus. When pregnancy is detected discontinue the ACE inhibitor as soon as possible.■ ACE inhibitors may also cause congenital malformations (atrial and ventricular septal defects, patent ductus arteriosus, spina bifida, microcephaly, renal dysplasia) when present during the first trimester of pregnancy. May cause a profound drop in BP following the first dose; initiate therapy under close medical supervision. Use with caution in renal disease (especially renal artery stenosis) as increases in BUN and serum creatinine have occurred. Use with caution in clients with aortic stenosis due to possible decreased coronary perfusion following vasodilator use. It is possible that clients taking an ACE inhibitor and high-dose aspirin (325 mg/day) will have a higher mortality rate than those taking an ACE inhibitor alone or an ACE inhibitor plus

---

Bold Italic = life threatening side effect   ■ = black box warning   ✦ = Available in Canada

low-dose aspirin (less than 160 mg/day). Most are used with caution during lactation. Geriatric clients may show a greater sensitivity to the hypotensive effects of ACE inhibitors although these drugs may preserve or improve renal function and reverse LV hypertrophy. For most ACE inhibitors, safety and effectiveness have not been determined in children. Compliance in taking the medication and inadequate dosage are problems with ACE inhibitors.

SIDE EFFECTS

See individual entries. Side effects common to most ACE inhibitors include the following. **GI:** Abdominal pain, N&V, diarrhea, constipation, dry mouth, dyspepsia, hepatitis, pancreatitis. **CNS:** Sleep disturbances, insomnia, headache, dizziness, nervousness, paresthesias, depression, somnolence, drowsiness, vertigo. **CV:** Hypotension (especially following the first dose or in those volume- or salt-depleted), palpitations, angina pectoris, *MI, CVA, cardiac arrest,* orthostatic hypotension, chest pain, tachycardia. **Dermatologic:** Diaphoresis, sweating, flushing, pemphigus/pemiphigoid, pruritus, rash, urticaria. **Hepatic:** Rarely, cholestatic jaundice progressing to *hepatic necrosis and death.* **Respiratory:** Chronic cough, dyspnea, URTI. **Body as a whole:** Fatigue, malaise, asthenia, fever, photosensitivity. **Miscellaneous:** Impotence, syncope, asthenia, anemia, tinnitus. *Angioedema* of the face, lips, tongue, glottis, larynx, extremities, and mucous membranes. *Anaphylaxis.*

OD OVERDOSE MANAGEMENT

Symptoms: Hypotension is the most common. *Treatment:* Supportive measures. The treatment of choice to restore BP is volume expansion with an IV infusion of NSS. Certain of the ACE inhibitors (captopril, enalaprilat, lisinopril, trandolaprilat) may be removed by hemodialysis.

DRUG INTERACTIONS

Allopurinol / ↑ Risk of hypersensitivity reactions
Anesthetics / ↑ Risk of hypotension if used with anesthetics that also cause hypotension
Antacids / Possible ↓ bioavailability of ACE inhibitors
Capsaicin / May cause or worsen cough associated with ACE inhibitor use
Digoxin / ↑ or ↓ Digoxin levels; monitor levels
Diuretics / Possible excess ↓ BP especially in those with intravascular volume depletion
Hypoglycemic drugs / Possible ↑ hypoglycemia
Indomethacin / ↓ Hypotensive effects of ACE inhibitors, especially in low renin or volume-dependent hypertensive clients
Insulin / Possible ↑ hypoglycemia
Lithium / ↑ Serum lithium levels → ↑ risk of toxicity
Loop diuretics / ↓ Effect of loop diuretics; possible inhibition of angiotensin II production by the ACE inhibitor
NSAIDs / ↓ Hypotensive effect of ACE inhibitors
Phenothiazines / ↑ Effect of ACE inhibitors
Potassium-sparing diuretics / ↑ Potassium levels
Potassium supplements / ↑ Potassium levels
Thiazide diuretics / Additive effect to ↓ BP.

LABORATORY TEST CONSIDERATIONS

↑ BUN and creatinine (both transient and reversible). ↑ Liver enzymes, serum bilirubin, uric acid, blood glucose. Small ↑ serum potassium.

DOSAGE

See individual drugs.

NURSING CONSIDERATIONS

ADMINISTRATION/STORAGE

Do not interrupt or discontinue ACE inhibitor therapy without consulting provider.

ASSESSMENT

1. Note any previous therapy with ACE inhibitors or antihypertensive agents and outcome.
2. Monitor VS (BP—both arms while lying, standing, and sitting), lytes, CBC, renal and LFTs; check urine for protein if negative on urinalysis; check for microalbuminuria especially in diabetics.

3. Document hereditary angioedema (esp. if caused by a deficiency of C1 esterase inhibitor). Report evidence of angioedema (swelling of face, lips, extremities, tongue, mucous membranes, glottis, or larynx) esp. after first dose (but may also see delayed response). Relieve S&S with antihistamines. If involves laryngeal edema, observe for airway obstruction. *Stop* drug; use epinephrine (1:1000 SC).

4. Monitor VS, I&O, weight, K, and renal function studies. Those hypovolemic due to diuretics, GI fluid loss, or salt restriction may exhibit severe hypotension after initial doses; supervise ambulation until drug response evident.

5. Assess for neutropenia (especially with captopril); precludes drug therapy.

6. If undergoing surgery or general anesthesia with drugs that cause hypotension, ACE inhibitors will block angiotensin II formation; correct hypotension with volume expansion.

7. List risk factors and medical problems. Identify life-style changes needed to achieve and maintain lowered BP. Assess motivation and ensure that a trial of "good behavior" with dietary modifications and regular exercise for 3 months has been done unless BP stage >2.

CLIENT/FAMILY TEACHING

1. Take 1 hr before or 2 hr after meals and only as directed. Drugs control but do not cure hypertension; take as prescribed despite feeling better and do not stop abruptly.

2. Review prescribed dietary guidelines; avoid potassium or salt substitutes containing potassium.

3. Do not perform activities that require mental alertness until drug effects realized; initially may cause dizziness, fainting, or lightheadedness. Rise slowly from a lying position and dangle feet before standing; avoid sudden position changes to minimize low BP effects.

4. Take and record BP readings at various times during the day to share with provider.

5. Practice reliable contraception; report if pregnancy suspected. Do not nurse.

6. Report adverse side effects:
- Nonproductive, persistent, cough
- Sore throat, fever, swelling of hands/feet, irregular heartbeat, chest pains, difficulty breathing, or hoarseness
- Excessive perspiration, dehydration, vomiting, and diarrhea
- Itching, joint pain, fever, or skin rash
- Swelling or weight gain of more than 3 lb/day or 5 lb/week

7. With diabetes (with/without hypertension), ACE inhibitors have been shown to reduce proteinuria and renal protection.

8. Avoid excessive amounts of caffeine (e.g., tea, coffee, cola) and OTC agents, esp. cold remedies.

9. NSAIDs and aspirin may impair the BP lowering effects of ACE inhibitors; antacids may decrease bioavailability.

10. Advise surgeon that ACE is being taken.

11. Avoid activities that may lead to a reduction in fluid volume, i.e., excessive perspiration, vomiting, diarrhea, dehydration may all cause drop in BP.

12. Regular exercise, proper diet, weight loss, stress management, and adequate rest in conjunction with medications are needed in the overall management of high BP. Additional interventions such as stopping alcohol/tobacco products, and salt intake may assist in BP control. Keep all F/U appointments to evaluate response to therapy.

OUTCOMES/EVALUATE
- ↓ BP; ↓ Morbidity post-AMI
- Improvement in S&S of CHF
- ↓ Proteinuria/renal damage

ANTIANGINAL DRUGS—NITRATES/NITRITES

SEE ALSO BETA-ADRENERGIC BLOCKING AGENTS, CALCIUM CHANNEL BLOCKING DRUGS, AND THE FOLLOWING INDIVIDUAL ENTRIES:

Isosorbide dinitrate
Isosorbide mononitrate
Nitroglycerin IV
Nitroglycerin sublingual
Nitroglycerin sustained release
    capsules and tablets

Nitroglycerin topical ointment
Nitroglycerin transdermal system
Nitroglycerin translingual spray

USES

(1) Treatment and prophylaxis of acute angina pectoris (use sublingual, transmucosal, or translingual nitroglycerin). (2) First-line therapy for unstable angina. (3) Prophylaxis of chronic angina pectoris (topical, transdermal, translingual, transmucosal), or oral sustained-release nitroglycerin; isosorbide dinitrate and mononitrate. (4) IV nitroglycerin is used to decrease BP in surgical procedures resulting in hypertension, as well as an adjunct in treating hypertension or CHF associated with MI. *Investigational:* Nitroglycerin ointment has been used as an adjunct in treating Raynaud's disease. Also, isosorbide dinitrate with prostaglandin E_1 for peripheral vascular disease. Sublingual and topical nitroglycerin and oral nitrates have been used to decrease cardiac workload in clients with acute MI and in CHF.

ACTION/KINETICS

Action

Nitrates relax vascular smooth muscle by stimulating production of intracellular cyclic guanosine monophosphate. Dilation of postcapillary vessels decreases venous return to the heart due to pooling of blood; thus, LV end-diastolic pressure (preload) is reduced. Relaxation of arterioles results in a decreased systemic vascular resistance and arterial pressure (afterload). The oxygen requirements of the myocardium are reduced and there is more efficient redistribution of blood flow through collateral channels in myocardial tissue. Diastolic, systolic, and mean BP are decreased. Also, elevated central venous and pulmonary capillary wedge pressures, pulmonary vascular resistance, and systemic vascular resistance are reduced. Reflex tachycardia may occur due to the overall decrease in BP. Cardiac index may increase, decrease, or remain the same; those with elevated left ventricular filling pressure and systemic vascular resistance values with a depressed cardiac index are likely to see improvement of the cardiac index.

Pharmacokinetics

The onset and duration depend on the product and route of administration (sublingual, topical, transdermal, parenteral, oral, and buccal). **Onset:** 1 to 3 min for IV, sublingual, translingual, and transmucosal nitroglycerin or sublingual isosorbide dinitrate; 20 to 60 min for sustained-release, topical, and transdermal nitroglycerin or oral isosorbide dinitrate or mononitrate; and up to 4 hr for sustained-release isosorbide dinitrate. **Duration of action:** 3 to 5 min for IV nitroglycerin; 30 to 60 min for sublingual or translingual nitroglycerin; several hours for transmucosal, sustained-release, or topical nitroglycerin and all isosorbide dinitrate products; and up to 24 hr for transdermal nitroglycerin.

CONTRAINDICATIONS

Sensitivity to nitrites, which may result in severe hypotensive reactions, MI, or tolerance to nitrites. Severe anemia, cerebral hemorrhage, recent head trauma, postural hypotension, closed angle glaucoma, impaired hepatic function, hypertrophic cardiomyopathy, hypotension, recent MI. PO dosage forms should not be used in clients with GI hypermotility or with malabsorption syndrome. IV nitroglycerin should not be used in clients with hypotension, uncorrected hypovolemia, inadequate cerebral circulation, constrictive pericarditis, increased ICP, or pericardial tamponade.

SPECIAL CONCERNS

Use with caution during lactation and in glaucoma. Tolerance to the antianginal and vascular effects may occur. Safety and efficacy have not been determined during lactation and in children.

SIDE EFFECTS

SYSTEMIC. CNS: Headaches (most common) which may be severe and persistent, restlessness, dizziness, weakness, apprehension, vertigo, anxiety, insomnia, confusion, nightmares, hypoesthesia, hypokinesia, dyscoordination. **CV:** Postural hypotension (common) with or without paradoxical

Classifications

bradycardia and increased angina, tachycardia, palpitations, syncope, rebound hypertension, crescendo angina, retrosternal discomfort, *CV collapse,* atrial fibrillation, PVCs, *arrhythmias.* **GI:** N&V, dyspepsia, diarrhea, dry mouth, abdominal pain, involuntary passing of feces and urine, tenesmus, tooth disorder. **Dermatologic:** Crusty skin lesions, pruritus, rash, exfoliative dermatitis, cutaneous vasodilation with flushing. **GU:** Urinary frequency, impotence, dysuria. **Respiratory:** URTI, bronchitis, pneumonia. **Allergic:** Itching, wheezing, tracheobronchitis. **Miscellaneous:** Perspiration, muscle twitching, methemoglobinemia, cold sweating, blurred vision, diplopia, *hemolytic anemia,* arthralgia, edema, malaise, neck stiffness, increased appetite, rigors.

TOPICAL. Peripheral edema, contact dermatitis: Tolerance can occur following chronic use. Nitrites convert hemoglobin to methemoglobin, which impairs the oxygen-carrying capacity of the blood, resulting in *anemic hypoxia.* This interaction is dangerous in clients with preexisting anemia.

OD OVERDOSE MANAGEMENT
Symptoms (Toxicity): Severe toxicity is rarely encountered with therapeutic use. Symptoms include hypotension, flushing, tachycardia, headache, palpitations, vertigo, perspiring skin followed by cold and cyanotic skin, visual disturbances, syncope, nausea, dizziness, diaphoresis, initial hyperpnea, dyspnea and slow breathing, slow pulse, *heart block,* vomiting with the possibility of bloody diarrhea and colic, anorexia, and increased ICP with symptoms of confusion, moderate fever, and paralysis. Tissue hypoxia (due to methemoglobinemia) may result in *cyanosis, metabolic acidosis, coma, seizures, and death due to CV collapse.*
Treatment (Toxicity):
- Induction of emesis or gastric lavage followed by activated charcoal (nitrates are usually rapidly absorbed from the stomach). Gastric lavage may be used if the drug has been recently ingested.

- Maintain in a recumbent shock position and keep warm. Give oxygen and artificial respiration if required.
- Monitor methemoglobin levels.
- Elevate legs and administer IV fluids to treat severe hypotension and reflex tachycardia. Phenylephrine or methoxamine may also be helpful.
- Do not use epinephrine and similar drugs as they are ineffective in reversing severe hypotension.

DRUG INTERACTIONS
Acetylcholine / Effects ↓ when used with nitrates
Alcohol, ethyl / Hypotension and CV collapse R/T vasodilator effect of both agents
Antihypertensive drugs / Additive hypotension
Aspirin / ↑ Levels and effects of nitrates
Beta-adrenergic blocking drugs / Additive hypotension
Calcium channel blocking drugs / Additive hypotension, including significant orthostatic hypotension
Dihydroergotamine / ↑ Effect R/T ↑ bioavailability or antagonism → ↓ antianginal effects
Heparin / Possible ↓ effect
Narcotics / Additive hypotensive effect
Phenothiazines / Additive hypotension
Sympathomimetics / ↓ Effect of nitrates; also, nitrates may ↓ effect of sympathomimetics → hypotension.

LABORATORY TEST CONSIDERATIONS
↑ Urinary catecholamines. False negative ↓ in serum cholesterol.

DOSAGE
See individual agents.

NURSING CONSIDERATIONS
ADMINISTRATION/STORAGE
Store tablets and capsules tightly closed in their original container. Avoid exposure to air, heat, and moisture.
ASSESSMENT
1. Note location, intensity, duration, extent, and any precipitating factors (i.e., activity, stress) surrounding anginal pain. Rate pain levels.
2. List any sensitivity to nitrites.
3. If history of anemia, administer with extreme caution.

---

4. Nitrates are contraindicated with elevated intracranial pressure and use of certain drugs for E.D.

5. Note any changes in ECG or elevated cardiac markers, results of echocardiogram, stress test, and/or catheterization.

INTERVENTIONS

1. Assess experience with self-administered medications; note if SL tablets ordered for bedside.

2. While hospitalized, record when consumed so effectiveness can be determined and usage monitored:
- Frequency given
- Duration and intensity of pain (use a pain-rating scale; rate pain initially and 5 min after administration) and if relief is partial or complete
- Time it takes for relief to occur
- Any side effects or EKG changes

3. Monitor VS. Assess for sensitivity to hypotensive effects (N&V, pallor, restlessness, and CV collapse). Monitor for hypotension when on additional drugs; adjust as needed. Supervise activities/ambulation until drug effects realized.

4. Assess for S&S of tolerance that occur following chronic use but may begin several days after starting treatment; manifested by absence of response to the usual dose. (Nitrites may be discontinued temporarily until tolerance is lost, and then reinstituted. During interim, other vasodilators may be used.) Managed by 12 hr nitrate rest.

5. Observe for N&V, drowsiness, headache, or visual disturbances with long-term therapy (may require a change in drug). Note change in activity and response to drug therapy. Determine if less discomfort experienced when performing regular activity.

CLIENT/FAMILY TEACHING

1. Take oral nitrates on an empty stomach with a glass of water. Drug decreases myocardial oxygen demand and reduces workload of the heart.

2. To prevent sudden drop in BP, use inhalation products or take SL tablets while sitting or lying down. Make position changes slowly and rise only after dangling feet for several minutes. The elderly should sit or lie down when taking NTG; may become dizzy and fall.

3. Monitor BP and pulse and keep record for provider review. Some drugs may lower heart rate (calcium channel/beta blockers), and BP.

4. Avoid changing from one brand to another due to differences in effectiveness between different companies.

5. Always carry SL tablets for use in aborting an attack. Check expiration date; replace when needed or every 6 months. A burning sensation under the tongue attests to drug potency. Carry SL tablets in a *glass* bottle, tightly capped. Keep in original container as heat, moisture, and air cause deterioration. Do not use plastic containers; drug deteriorates in plastic; avoid child-proof caps as must get to tablets quickly.

6. If pain is not relieved in 5 min by first SL tablet, may take up to 2 more tablets at 5-min intervals. If pain has not subsided 5 min after third tablet, client should be taken to the emergency room; *do not* drive; call 911.

7. Take SL tablets 5–15 min prior to any situation likely to cause pain (e.g., climbing stairs, sexual intercourse, exposure to cold weather). Record attacks; report any increase in the frequency/intensity of attacks and loss of NTG effectiveness. Schedule frequent rest periods, pace activities, and avoid stressful situations. Use acetaminophen for headaches.

8. Follow instructions on how to apply topical nitroglycerin. Remove at bedtime and apply upon arising; a nitrate-free period of 8 hr may reduce/prevent nitrate tolerance.

9. Avoid alcohol; nitrite syncope, a severe shock-like state, may occur. Inhalation products are flammable; do not use under situations where they might ignite.

10. Do not smoke. Review risks and lifestyle changes necessary to prevent further CAD (i.e., weight control, dietary changes, ↓ salt intake, modified regular exercise program, BP control, DM control, no alcohol/tobacco, and stress reduction).

11. Have family or significant other learn CPR; survival rate is greatly increased when CPR is initiated immedi-

ately. Carry ID with prescribed drugs. Know what you are taking and why.

OUTCOMES/EVALUATE

- ↓ Myocardial oxygen requirements; ↑ activity tolerance
- Improved myocardial perfusion
- Relief of pain/coronary artery spasm

ANTIARRHYTHMIC DRUGS

SEE ALSO THE FOLLOWING INDIVIDUAL ENTRIES:

Adenosine
Amiodarone hydrochloride
Bretylium tosylate
Calcium Channel Blocking Agents
Digoxin
Diltiazem hydrochloride
Dofetilide
Flecainide acetate
Ibutilide fumarate
Lidocaine hydrochloride
Moricizine hydrochloride
Phenytoin
Phenytoin sodium
Procainamide hydrochloride
Propafenone hydrochloride
Propranolol hydrochloride
Quinidine gluconate
Quinidine sulfate
Verapamil

GENERAL STATEMENT

Examples of cardiac arrhythmias are *premature ventricular beats, ventricular tachycardia, atrial flutter, atrial fibrillation, ventricular fibrillation,* and *atrioventricular heart block.* The various antiarrhythmic drugs are classified according to both their mechanism of action and their effects on the action potential of cardiac cells. Importantly, one drug in a particular class may be more effective and safer in an individual client. The antiarrhythmic drugs are classified as follows:

1. Class I. Decrease the rate of entry of sodium during cardiac membrane depolarization, decrease the rate of rise of phase O of the cardiac membrane action potential, prolong the effective refractory period of fast-response fibers, and require that a more negative membrane potential be reached before the membrane becomes excitable (and thus can propagate to other membranes). Class I drugs are further listed in subgroups (according to their effects on action potential duration) as follows:

- Class IA: Depress phase O and prolong the duration of the action potential. Examples: Disopyramide, procainamide, and quinidine.
- Class IB: Slightly depress phase O and are thought to shorten the action potential. Examples: Lidocaine, mexiletine, phenytoin, and tocainide.
- Class IC: Slight effect on repolarization but marked depression of phase O of the action potential. Significant slowing of conduction. Examples: Flecainide, and propafenone. *NOTE:* Moricizine is classified as a Class I agent but it has characteristics of agents in groups IA, B, and C.

2. Class II. Competitively block beta-adrenergic receptors and depress phase 4 depolarization. Examples: Acebutolol, esmolol, and propranolol.

3. Class III. Prolong the duration of the membrane action potential (relative refractory period) without changing the phase of depolarization or the resting membrane potential. Examples: Amiodarone, bretylium, dofetilide, ibutilide, and sotalol.

4. Class IV. Depresses phase 4 depolarization and lengthens phases 1 and 2 of repolarization. Example: Verapamil.

Adenosine and digoxin are also used to treat arrhythmias. Adenosine slows conduction time through the AV node and can interrupt the reentry pathways through the AV node. Digoxin causes a decrease in maximal diastolic potential and duration of the action potential; it also increases the slope of phase 4 depolarization.

SPECIAL CONCERNS

Monitor serum levels of antiarrhythmic drugs since some drugs can cause toxic side effects that can be confused with the purpose for which the drug is used. For example, toxicity from quinidine can result in cardiac arrhythmias. Antiarrhythmic drugs may cause new or worsening of arrhythmias, ranging from an increase in frequency of PVCs to se-

---

vere ventricular tachycardia, ventricular fibrillation, or tachycardia that is more sustained and rapid. Such situations (called proarrhythmic effect) may make it difficult to distinguish the proarrhythmic effect from the underlying rhythm disorder.

DRUG INTERACTIONS

H *Aloe* / Chronic aloe use → ↑ serum potassium loss causing ↑ effect of antiarrhythmics.

H *Buckthorn bark/berry* / Chronic buckthorn use → ↑ serum potassium loss causing ↑ effect of antiarrhythmics.

H *Cascara sagrada bark* / Chronic cascara use → ↑ serum potassium loss causing ↑ effect of antiarrhythmics.

H *Rhubarb root* / Chronic rhubarb use → ↑ serum potassium loss causing ↑ effect of antiarrhythmics.

H *Senna pod/leaf* / Chronic senna use → ↑ serum potassium loss causing ↑ effect of antiarrhythmics.

NURSING CONSIDERATIONS

ASSESSMENT

1. Note reasons for therapy, drug sensitivity, any previous experiences with these drugs. Assess extent of palpitations, fluttering sensations, chest pains, fainting episodes, or missed beats, prolonged QT; obtain ECG/rhythm strips showing arrhythmia.

2. Assess heart sounds, VS, and EF. Use cardiac monitor if administering drugs by IV route; monitor for rhythm changes.

3. Monitor BP and pulse. A HR <50 bpm or >120 bpm should be avoided. Obtain written parameters for BP and pulse limits.

4. Monitor BS, lytes, drug levels, renal and LFTs. Ensure serum pH, electrolytes, pO₂ and/or O₂ sats are WNL. Review EPS, stress test/catherization results and/or holter findings.

5. Assess life-style related to cigarettes and caffeine use, alcohol consumption, and lack of regular exercise. Certain foods, emotional stress, and other environmental factors may also trigger arrhythmias; identify and eliminate before instituting drugs.

CLIENT/FAMILY TEACHING

1. Drugs work by controlling the irregular heart beats so the heart can pump more efficiently. Take as ordered. If dose is missed, do not double up.

2. Avoid activities that require mental alertness until drug effects realized.

3. Follow recommended dietary guidelines, avoiding/limiting salt, and fluids as directed.

4. Avoid OTC products. Eliminate caffeine, cigarettes, salt, and alcohol; these substances alter drug absorption and may precipitate arrhythmias or cause fluid retention with certain agents.

5. Record BP and pulse for provider review; identify specific levels to hold drug, i.e., HR <50. Keep F/U visits so that therapy can be adjusted and evaluated.

6. Report concerns/fears or problems R/T sexual activity and side effects of drug therapy. Always carry list of prescribed medications and condition being treated.

7. Family/significant other should learn CPR and how to use a defibrillator; survival rates are greatly increased when CPR is initiated immediately.

OUTCOMES/EVALUATE

- ECG evidence of arrhythmia control; restoration of stable cardiac rhythm
- Serum drug concentrations within therapeutic range.

ANTICONVULSANTS

SEE ALSO THE FOLLOWING INDIVIDUAL ENTRIES:

Acetazolamide
Acetazolamide sodium
Carbamazepine
Clonazepam
Clorazepate dipotassium
Diazepam
Ethosuximide
Felbamate
Fosphenytoin sodium
Gabapentin
Lamotrigine
Levetiracetam
Magnesium sulfate
Methsuximide*
Oxcarbazepine

📷 = see color insert   H = Herbal   IV = Intravenous   @ = sound alike drug

Classifications

Phenobarbital
Phenobarbital sodium
Phenytoin
Phenytoin sodium extended
Phenytoin sodium parenteral
Phenytoin sodium prompt
Primidone
Tiagabine hydrochloride
Topiramate
Valproic acid/Divalproex sodium
Zonisamide

Drugs marked with an * are available to view in the online database at www.delmarnursesdrughandbook.com/2009.

GENERAL STATEMENT

Therapeutic agents cannot cure convulsive disorders, but do control seizures without impairing the normal functions of the CNS. This is often accomplished by selective depression of hyperactive areas of the brain responsible for the convulsions. Therefore, these drugs are taken at all times (prophylactically) to prevent the occurrence of the seizures. There are several different types of epileptic disorders; consult the International Classification of Epileptic Seizures. No single drug can control all types of epilepsy; thus, accurate diagnosis is important. Drugs effective against one type of epilepsy may not be effective against another. Therapy begins with a small dose of the drug, which is continuously increased until either the seizures disappear or drug toxicity occurs. Monotherapy is preferred but if a certain drug decreases the frequency of seizures but does not completely prevent them, another drug can be added to the dosage regimen and administered concomitantly with the first. Failure of therapy most often results from the administration of doses too small to have a therapeutic effect or from failure to use two or more drugs together. With appropriate diagnosis and selection of drugs, four out of five cases of epilepsy can be controlled adequately, but it may take the provider some time to find the best drug or combination of drugs with which to treat the client.

ACTION/KINETICS

See individual drugs.

USES

See individual drugs. Use is specific to the drug or drug class.

SPECIAL CONCERNS

Many anticonvulsants can significantly lower bone mineral density at fracture-relevant sites; consider use of calcium/vitamin D supplements.

DOSAGE

Dosage is highly individualized. However, trauma or emotional stress may necessitate an increase in drug dosage requirements (e.g., if the client requires surgery and starts having seizures). For details, see individual agents.

NURSING CONSIDERATIONS

ADMINISTRATION/STORAGE

1. Shake oral suspensions thoroughly before pouring to ensure uniform mixing.
2. Drug therapy must be individualized according to client needs.
3. Do not discontinue abruptly unless provider approved. To avoid severe, prolonged convulsions, withdraw over a period of days or weeks.
4. If there is reason to substitute one anticonvulsant drug for another, withdraw the first drug at the same time the dosage of the second drug is being increased.
5. Be prepared, in case of acute oral toxicity, to assist with inducing emesis (provided the client is not comatose) and with gastric lavage, along with other supportive measures such as administration of fluids and oxygen.

ASSESSMENT

1. Check medical history for hypersensitivity to anticonvulsant drugs. Note derivatives to avoid.
2. Assess mental status: orientation to time and place, affect, reflexes, and VS. Check skin, eyes, and mucous membranes.
3. Note seizure classification (partial or generalized); frequency/severity noting location, duration, consciousness, type, frequency and any precipitating factors, i.e. presence of aura, other characteristics. Note EEG, CT/MRI results.

---

4. Check to see if pregnant; may cause fetal abnormalities.

5. Monitor CBC, glucose, uric acid, urinalysis, renal and LFTs.

6. Determine why receiving therapy and when. If not physiologic and no seizures for over 2 years with prophylactic therapy, may consider gradual drug discontinuation after EEG documents lack of irritable foci.

INTERVENTIONS

1. With IV administration, monitor closely for respiratory depression and CV collapse. Note any evidence of CNS side effects, such as blurred/dimmed vision, slurred speech, nystagmus, or confusion; supervise ambulation until resolved.

2. Observe for muscle twitching, loss of muscle tone, episodes of bizarre behavior, subsequent amnesia.

3. With phenytoin, check Ca level; contributes to bone demineralization which can result in osteomalacia in adults and rickets in children. Risk increases with inactivity. May require calcium replacement with vitamin D and periodic dexa scan for BMD.

4. Administer vitamin K to pregnant women 1 month before delivery to prevent postpartum hemorrhage/bleeding in the newborn and mother.

CLIENT/FAMILY TEACHING

1. Take drug as prescribed. Do not increase, decrease, or discontinue without approval; seizures may result. Lessen GI distress by taking with large amounts of fluids or with food. Increase fluid intake and include fruit and other foods with roughage and bulk in the diet.

2. Avoid driving. Many states require certification that one is seizure free for 6 months or more before license granted. May initially cause a decrease in mental alertness, drowsiness, headache, dizziness, and uncoordination. CNS symptoms are dose-related and should subside with continued therapy; avoid hazardous tasks until symptoms resolve.

3. Dosage may change if undergoing physical trauma or emotional distress.

Avoid alcohol and any other CNS depressants.

4. Calcium and Vitamin D may be prescribed to prevent hypocalcemia (4,000 units of vitamin D weekly); folic acid may prevent megaloblastic anemia.

5. Regular oral hygiene is important. With loose gums, intensify oral hygiene, routinely use dental floss, soft tooth brush, massage gums, and get regular dental exams.

6. If slurred speech develops, try to consciously talk slower to avoid the problem. Avoid situations/exposures that result in fever and low sugar and sodium levels; may lower seizure threshold.

7. Report if rash, fever, severe headaches, pain/swelling of mouth, nose, and urinary tract, or balanitis (inflammation of the glans penis) occur; S&S of hypersensitivity; requires change in drug.

8. Report sore throat, easy bruising/bleeding, or nosebleeds: S&S of hematologic toxicity. Jaundice, dark urine, appetite loss, and abdominal pain may indicate liver toxicity. To detect hepatitis, hepatocellular degeneration, and fatal hepatocellular necrosis: labs for LFTs.

9. Practice reliable birth control; may harm fetus. If nursing, observe infant for signs of toxicity.

10. Keep all F/U visits to evaluate drug levels, labs, and response to therapy.

11. Carry ID with the type of seizures and prescribed therapy. Family should learn CPR and how to protect client during a seizure.

12. Identify support groups (Epilepsy Foundation; Brain Injury Association National Help Line: 1-800-444-6443 and Web site: http://www.biausa.org) that may assist you to understand and cope with these disorders.

OUTCOMES/EVALUATE

- ↓ Frequency of seizures; improved seizure control
- Serum drug levels within desired range

ANTIDEPRESSANTS, TRICYCLIC

SEE ALSO THE FOLLOWING INDIVIDUAL ENTRIES:

Amitriptyline hydrochloride

Amoxapine
Desipramine hydrochloride
Doxepin hydrochloride
Imipramine hydrochloride
Imipramine pamoate
Nortriptyline hydrochloride

GENERAL STATEMENT

Drugs with antidepressant effects include the tricyclic antidepressants (TCAs), selective serotonin reuptake inhibitors (SSRIs) i.e., fluoxetine, fluvoxamine, paroxetine, sertraline; and monoamine oxidase inhibitors (MAOIs) i.e., phenelzine, tranylcypromine.

USES

(1) Endogenous and reactive depressions. (2) Drugs with significant sedative effects may be useful in depression associated with anxiety and sleep disturbances. The selective serotonin reuptake inhibitors are the most widely used antidepressants. See also individual drugs.

ACTION/KINETICS

Action

It is now believed that antidepressant drugs cause adaptive changes in the serotonin and norepinephrine receptor systems, resulting in changes in the sensitivities of both presynaptic and postsynaptic receptor sites. These effects may increase the sensitivity of postsynaptic α-1 adrenergic and serotonin receptors and decrease the sensitivity of presynaptic receptor sites. The overall effect is a reregulation of the abnormal receptor neurotransmitter relationship. The tricyclic antidepressants are chemically related to the phenothiazines; thus, they exhibit many of the same pharmacologic effects (e.g., anticholinergic, antiserotonin, sedative, antihistaminic, and hypotensive). The TCAs are less effective for depressed clients in the presence of organic brain damage or schizophrenia. Also, they can induce mania; note when given to clients with manic-depressive psychoses.

Pharmacokinetics

Well absorbed from the GI tract; significant first-pass effect. All have a long serum half-life. Up to 46 days may be required to reach steady plasma levels and maximum therapeutic effects may not be noted for 24 weeks. Because of the long half-life, single daily dosage may suffice. More than 90% bound to plasma protein. Partially metabolized in the liver; some are metabolized to active compounds. Excreted primarily in the urine.

CONTRAINDICATIONS

Severely impaired liver function. Use during acute recovery phase from MI. Concomitant use with MAO inhibitors.

SPECIAL CONCERNS

■(1) Antidepressants increased the risk of suicidal thinking and behavior (suicidality) in short-term studies in children and adolescents with major depressive disorder and other psychiatric disorders. Anyone considering the use of antidepressants in a child or adolescent must balance this risk with the clinical need. Clients who are started on therapy should be observed closely for clinical worsening, suicidality, or unusual changes in behavior. Families and caregivers should be advised of the need for close observation and communication with the prescriber. (2) Short-term placebo-controlled trials of nine antidepressant drugs in children and adolescents with major depressive disorder, obsessive-compulsive disorder, or other psychiatric disorders revealed a greater risk of adverse reactions during the first few months of treatment. The average risk of such reactions in clients receiving antidepressants was 4%, twice the placebo risk of 2%. No suicides occurred in these trials.■ Use of antidepressants in young adults, ages 18-24 years, may also be associated with suicidality; this group should be monitored carefully if they are taking antidepressants to treat depression. Use with caution during lactation and with epilepsy (seizure threshold is lowered), CV diseases (possibility of conduction defects, arrhythmias, CHF, sinus tachycardia, MI, strokes, tachycardia), glaucoma, BPH, suicidal tendencies, a history of urinary retention, and the elderly. Use during pregnancy only when benefits clearly outweigh risks. Generally not recom-

---

Bold Italic = life threatening side effect   ■ = black box warning   ✦ = Available in Canada

mended for children less than 12 years of age. Geriatric clients may be more sensitive to the anticholinergic and sedative side effects. Electroconvulsive therapy may increase the hazards of therapy.

SIDE EFFECTS
Most frequent side effects are sedation and atropine-like reactions. **CNS:** Agitation, akathisia, EEG pattern alterations, ataxia, anxiety, coma, confusion, disorientation, disturbed concentration, dizziness, drowsiness, dysarthria, exacerbation of psychosis, excitement, excessive appetite, extrapyramidal symptoms (including tardive dyskinesia), fatigue, hallucinations, delusions, headache, hyperthermia, hypomania, incoordination, insomnia, mania, nervousness, neuroleptic malignant syndrome, numbness, panic, nightmares, paresthesias of extremities, peripheral neuropathy, tremors, seizures, restlessness, weakness, tingling. **Anticholinergic:** Dry mouth, blurred vision, increased IOP, disturbed accommodation, mydriasis, constipation, paralytic ileus, urinary retention, delayed micturition, urinary tract dilation, hyperpyrexia. **GI:** N&V, abdominal pain or cramps, anorexia, aphthous stomatitis, constipation, diarrhea, epigastric distress, black tongue, dysphagia, increased pancreatic enzymes, flatulence, indigestion, GI disorder, parotid swelling, stomatitis, taste disturbance, peculiar taste, ulcerative stomatitis, hepatitis (rare), jaundice. **CV:** Arrhythmias, ECG changes, flushing, change in AV conduction, *heart block, stroke, sudden death,* hot flushes, hypertension, hypotension, orthostatic hypotension, palpitations, CHF, PVCs, syncope, tachycardia. **Dermatologic:** Skin rashes, urticaria, flushing, pruritus, petechiae, photosensitivity, edema. **GU:** Testicular swelling and gynecomastia in males, increase or decrease in libido, impotence, menstrual irregularities and galactorrhea in females, breast enlargement, impotence, painful ejaculation, nocturia, urinary frequency. **Hematologic:** Agranulocytosis, aplastic anemia, leukopenia, thrombocytopenia, purpura, eosinophilia. **Hypersensitivity:** Drug fever, edema (generalized or of face/tongue), itching, petechiae, photosensitivity, pruritus, rash, urticaria, vasculitis. **Metabolic:** Increase or decrease in blood sugar, inappropriate ADH secretion. **Miscellaneous:** Sweating, alopecia, fever, hyperthermia, proneness to falling, weight gain or loss, nasal congestion, abnormal lacrimation, tinnitus, chills, worsening of asthma.

High dosage increases the frequency of seizures in epileptic clients and may cause epileptiform attacks in normal subjects.

OD OVERDOSE MANAGEMENT
Symptoms: CNS symptoms include agitation, confusion, hallucinations, hyperactive reflexes, choreoathetosis, *seizures, coma.* Anticholinergic symptoms include dilated pupils, dry mouth, flushing, and *hyperpyrexia.* CV toxicity includes depressed myocardial contractility, decreased HR, decreased coronary blood flow, tachycardia, intraventricular block, *complete AV block, re-entry ventricular arrhythmias, PVCs, ventricular tachycardia or fibrillation, sudden cardiac arrest,* hypotension, pulmonary edema.
Treatment: Admit client to hospital and monitor ECG closely for 3 to 5 days.
- Empty stomach in alert clients by inducing vomiting followed by gastric lavage and charcoal administration **after insertion of cuffed ET tube.** Maintain respiration and avoid the use of respiratory stimulants.
- Normal or half-normal saline to prevent water intoxication.
- To reverse the CV effects (e.g., hypotension and cardiac dysrhythmias), give hypertonic sodium bicarbonate. The usual dose is 0.52 mEq/kg by IV bolus followed by IV infusion to maintain the blood at pH 7.5. If hypotension is not reversed by bicarbonate, vasopressors (e.g., dopamine) and fluid expansion may be needed. If the cardiac dysrhythmias do not respond to bicarbonate, lidocaine or phenytoin may be used.
- Isoproterenol may be effective in controlling bradyarrhythmias and torsades de pointes ventricular

Classifications

tachycardia. Use propranolol, 0.1 mg/kg IV (up to 0.25 mg by IV bolus), to treat life-threatening ventricular arrhythmias in children.

- Treat shock and metabolic acidosis with IV fluids, oxygen, bicarbonate, and corticosteroids.
- Control hyperpyrexia by external means (ice pack, cool baths, spongings).
- To reduce possibility of convulsions, minimize external stimulation. If necessary, use diazepam or phenytoin to control convulsions. Avoid barbiturates if MAO inhibitors have been used recently.

DRUG INTERACTIONS

Acetazolamide / ↑ Effect of tricyclics by ↑ renal tubular reabsorption

Alcohol, ethyl / Concomitant use may lead to ↑ GI complications and ↓ performance on motor skill tests; death has been reported

Ammonium chloride / ↓ Effect of tricyclics by ↓ renal tubular reabsorption

Anticholinergic drugs / Additive anticholinergic side effects

Anticoagulants, oral / ↑ Hypoprothrombinemia R/T ↓ liver breakdown

Anticonvulsants / TCAs may ↑ incidence of epileptic seizures

Antihistamines / Additive anticholinergic side effects

Ascorbic acid / ↓ TCA effects by ↓ renal tubular drug reabsorption

Barbiturates / Additive depressant effects; also, may ↑ liver breakdown of antidepressants.

■ *Belladonna leaf/root* / Additive anticholinergic effects

Benzodiazepines / TCAs ↑ effect of benzodiazepines

Beta-adrenergic blocking agents / TCAs ↓ effect of the blocking agents

Carbamazepine / ↓ Serum TCA levels; ↑ serum carbamazepine levels → ↑ pharmacologic/toxic effects

Charcoal / ↓ Absorption of TCAs → ↓ effectiveness (or toxicity)

Chlordiazepoxide / Concomitant use may cause additive sedative effects and/or additive atropine-like side effects

Cimetidine / ↑ Effect of TCAs (especially serious anticholinergic symptoms) R/T ↓ liver breakdown

Clonidine / Dangerous ↑ BP and hypertensive crisis

Diazepam / Concomitant use may cause additive sedative effects and/or additive atropine-like side effects

Dicumarol / TCAs may ↑ the t ½ of dicumarol → ↑ anticoagulation effects

Disulfiram / ↑ Levels of TCAs; also, possibility of acute organic brain syndrome

Ephedrine / TCAs ↓ effects of ephedrine by preventing uptake at its site of action

Estrogens / Depending on the dose, estrogens may ↑ or ↓ the effects of TCAs.

■ *Evening primrose oil* / May worsen temporal lobe epilepsy or schizophrenia when taken with TCAs

Fluoxetine / ↑ Pharmacologic and toxic effects of TCAs (effect may persist for several weeks after fluoxetine discontinued)

Furazolidone / Toxic psychoses possible

Grepafloxacin / ↑ Risk of life-threatening cardiac arrhythmias, including torsades de pointes

Guanethidine / TCAs ↓ antihypertensive effect of guanethidine by preventing uptake at its site of action

Haloperidol / ↑ TCA effects R/T ↓ liver breakdown.

■ *Henbane leaf* / ↑ Anticholinergic effects

Histamine H-2 antagonists / ↑ Serum TCA levels.

■ *Kava Kava* / Additive effects

Levodopa / ↓ Effect of levodopa R/T ↓ absorption

MAO inhibitors / Concomitant use may result in hyperpyretic crisis, excitation, hyperthermia, delirium, tremors, DIC, severe convulsions, coma, flushing, confusion, tachycardia, tachypnea, headache, mydriasis, and death although combinations have been used successfully

Meperidine / TCAs enhance narcotic-induced respiratory depression; also, additive anticholinergic side effects

Methyldopa / TCAs may block hypotensive effects of methyldopa

Methylphenidate / ↑ TCA effects R/T ↓

liver breakdown

Narcotic analgesics / TCAs enhance narcotic-induced respiratory depression; also, additive anticholinergic effects

Oral contraceptives / ↑ TCA plasma levels R/T ↓ liver breakdown

Oxazepam / Concomitant use may cause additive sedative effects and/or atropine-like side effects

Phenothiazines / Additive anticholinergic side effects; also, phenothiazines ↑ TCA effects R/T ↓ liver breakdown

Procainamide / Additive cardiac effects

Quinidine / Additive cardiac effects

Quinolone antibiotics / ↑ Risk of life-threatening cardiac arrhythmias, including torsade de pointes

Rifamycins / ↓ Serum TCA levels.

H *Scopolia root* / ↑ TCA effects

SSRIs / ↑ Pharmacologic/toxic effects of TCAs; symptoms may persist for at least 5 weeks

Sodium bicarbonate / ↑ TCA effects by ↑ renal tubular drug reabsorption

Sparfloxacin / ↑ Risk of life-threatening cardiac arrhythmias, including torsade de pointes

Sympathomimetics / Potentiation of sympathomimetic effects→ hypertension or cardiac arrhythmias

Tobacco (smoking) / ↓ Serum TCA levels R/T ↑ liver breakdown

Thyroid preparations / Mutually potentiating effects observed

Valproic acid / ↑ Plasma TCA levels → ↑ side effects

Vasodilators / Additive hypotensive effect.

LABORATORY TEST CONSIDERATIONS
↑ Alkaline phosphatase, transaminase, prolactin, bilirubin; ↑ or ↓ blood glucose. False + or ↑ urinary catecholamines. Altered LFTs.

DOSAGE
See individual drugs. Dosage levels vary greatly in effectiveness from one client to another; therefore, carefully individualize dosage regimens.

NURSING CONSIDERATIONS
ADMINISTRATION/STORAGE
1. In adolescents and elderly clients, use lower initial dosage than in adults; gradually increase dose as needed.

2. Individualize dose according to age, weight, physical, mental condition, and response to the therapy. Clients show the largest relative improvement during the first weeks of treatment.

3. For maintenance therapy, a single daily dose may suffice.

4. Dose usually administered at bedtime, so any anticholinergic and/or sedative effects will not impact ADL.

5. To reduce incidence of sedation and anticholinergic effects, start with small doses and then gradually increase to desired dosage levels.

ASSESSMENT
1. Note reasons for therapy, behavioral manifestations, symptom onset, and causative factors. Identify if receiving electroshock therapy; hazardous combination.

2. Monitor mental status. Assess for dysphoric mood, suicide ideations, and excessive appetite/weight changes. Note sleep disturbances, lethargy, apathy, physical hygiene, impaired thought processes, or lack of responses.

3. List drugs currently prescribed; some that may intensify depressive reactions include antihypertensives (i.e., reserpine, methyldopa, beta blockers), antiparkinsonians, hormones, steroids, anticancer agents, and antituberculins (cycloserine) as well as barbiturates and alcohol.

4. Monitor CBC, renal and LFTs. Record ECG, assess heart sounds, note any CAD, and evaluate neurologic functioning. Assess for tachycardia and increase in anginal attacks; may precede MI or stroke.

5. Note eye exam; report visual changes, headaches, halos, eye pain, dilated pupils, or nausea. May need to change, esp with glaucoma.

6. Monitor I&O; report abdominal distention, urinary retention, and absence of bowel sounds (i.e. paralytic ileus).

7. Differentiate type of depression based on diagnostic features related to reactive, major depressive, or bipolar affective disorders. Review symptoms to determine if affective, somatic, psychomotor, or psychological.

INTERVENTIONS

1. Note S&S of allergic response, i.e., rash, alopecia, and eosinophilia. Sore throat, fever, easy bruising, unusual bleeding, presence of petechiae or purpura may be S&S of blood dyscrasias. Check for evidence of agranulocytosis, esp among elderly women and during the second month of therapy.

2. Assess for adverse endocrine disturbances such as increased/decreased libido, gynecomastia, testicular swelling, and impotence. With hyperthyroidism, assess for arrhythmias precipitated by TCAs. May alter blood sugar levels and require adjustment of hypoglycemic agent.

3. Report symptoms of cholestatic jaundice and biliary tract obstruction such as high fever, yellowing of the skin, mucous membranes and sclera, pruritus, and upper abdominal pain.

4. Discontinue TCAs several days prior to surgery; may adversely affect BP. Withdraw therapy slowly to avoid any withdrawal symptoms.

5. Assess for epileptiform seizures precipitated by the drug.

CLIENT/FAMILY TEACHING

1. Take sedating medications at bedtime to minimize daytime sedation; take those that cause insomnia in the a.m. or upon arising.

2. Use caution when performing tasks requiring mental alertness or physical coordination; may cause drowsiness or uncoordination. Rise slowly from a lying position; do not remain standing in one place for any length of time. If feeling faint, lie down to minimize low BP effects.

3. GI complaints of anorexia, N&V, epigastric distress, diarrhea, blackened tongue, or a peculiar taste require a dosage adjustment. Take with or immediately following meals to reduce gastric irritation.

4. Increase oral hygiene, take frequent sips of water, suck on hard candy, or chew sugarless gum to maintain a moist mouth. A high-fiber diet, increased fluid intake, exercise, and stool softeners may prevent constipation. May affect carbohydrate metabolism;

an adjustment of diabetes agent and diet may be indicated.

5. Avoid prolonged sun exposure, use sunscreen and protection if exposure necessary, may cause changes in skin pigmentation and skin burning.

6. May alter libido or reproductive function. Practice reliable birth control; report if pregnancy suspected. May consider sperm/egg harvesting prior to starting therapy.

7. Report alterations in perceptions, i.e., hallucinations, blurred vision, excessive stimulations. Watch those recovering from depression for suicidal tendencies; remove firearms/weapons from the home.

8. May take 4–6 weeks to realize a maximum clinical response; stay on treatment regimen. Will see provider more often the first 2–3 weeks; prescriptions will be for only small amounts to ensure compliance and to prevent an overdose; excess consumption can be lethal. Obtain number to call for help.

9. Do not stop abruptly, may experience withdrawal S&S. Avoid other drugs and alcohol during and for 2 weeks following TCA therapy.

10. Review when and how to take medications, reportable side effects, and importance of regular participation in psychotherapy programs (when indicated).

OUTCOMES/EVALUATE

- Understand/accept illness, need for counselling, drug therapy/medical supervision
- ↓ Depression evidenced by improved appetite, renewed interest in outside activities, ↑ socialization, improved sleeping patterns, ↑ energy
- ↓ Anxiety; improved coping skills
- Control of chronic pain syndromes

ANTIDIABETIC AGENTS: HYPOGLYCEMIC AGENTS

SEE ALSO ANTIDIABETIC AGENTS: INSULINS. SEE ALSO THE FOLLOWING INDIVIDUAL ENTRIES:

Acarbose
Exanatide
Glimepiride

Bold Italic = life threatening side effect   ■ = black box warning   ✦ = Available in Canada

Glipizide
Glyburide
Metformin hydrochloride
Miglitol
Pioglitazone hydrochloride
Pramlintide acetate
Rosiglitazone maleate
Sitagliptin phosphate
Tolbutamide sodium*
Tolbutamide*

Drugs marked with an * are available to view in the online database at www.delmarnursesdrughandbook.com/2009.

GENERAL STATEMENT

The American Diabetes Association has developed standards for treating clients with diabetes. If followed, these standards will enable clients to decrease their blood glucose levels closer to normal; this will reduce the risk of complications, including blindness, kidney disease, heart disease, and amputations. The goals of these standards include establishing specific targets for control of blood glucose (usually between 80 and 120 mg/dL before meals and between 100 and 140 mg/dL at bedtime) and increased emphasis on educating clients for self-management of their disease. Targets for BP and lipid levels are also provided. If the guidelines are followed, it is estimated that the risk of development or progression of retinopathy, nephropathy, and neuropathy can be reduced by 50–75% in clients with insulin-dependent (type 1) diabetes. The guidelines suggest the following treatment modalities:

- Frequent monitoring of blood glucose.
- Regular exercise.
- Close attention to meal planning; consult a registered dietitian.
- For Type 1 diabetics, either continuous SC insulin infusion or multiple daily insulin injections; for Type 2 diabetics, consider insulin administration in certain situations, although dietary modification, exercise, and weight reduction are the cornerstone of treatment.

- Instruction in the prevention and treatment of hypoglycemia and other complications (both acute and chronic) of diabetes.
- Development of a process for ongoing support and continuing education for the client.
- Routine assessment of treatment goals.
- Control of BP.

USES

(1) Non-insulin-dependent diabetes mellitus (type 2) that does not respond to diet management and exercise alone. (2) Concurrent use of insulin and an oral hypoglycemic for type 2 diabetics who are difficult to control with diet and sulfonylurea therapy alone. One method used is the BIDS system: bedtime insulin (usually NPH) with daytime (morning only or morning and evening) oral hypoglycemic.

Guidelines for oral hypoglycemic therapy include onset of diabetes generally in clients over 40 years of age (but is being noted more in children that are overweight and inactive, with poor dietary habits), duration of diabetes less than 5 years, absence of ketoacidosis, client is obese or has normal body weight, fasting serum glucose of 200 mg/dL or less, elevated glucose tolerance test, normal or high C-Peptide, and hepatic and renal function is normal.

ACTION/KINETICS

Action

Oral hypoglycemic drugs are classified as either first or second generation. *Generation* refers to structural changes in the basic molecule. Second-generation oral hypoglycemic drugs are more lipophilic and, as such, have greater hypoglycemic potency. Also, second-generation drugs are bound to plasma protein by covalent bonds, whereas first-generation drugs are bound to plasma protein by ionic bonds. The implication is that the second-generation drugs are potentially less susceptible to displacement from plasma protein by drugs such as salicylates and oral anticoagulants. The oral hypoglycemics bind to plasma membranes of functional beta

Classifications

cells in the pancreas causing a decrease in potassium permeability and membrane depolarization. This leads to an increase in intracellular calcium and subsequent release from insulin-containing secretory granules. The sulfonylureas enhance beta-cell response rather than change the sensitivity of beta-cells to glucose. To be effective, the client must have some ability for endogenous insulin production. Differences in oral hypoglycemic drugs are mainly in their pharmacokinetic properties and duration of action. Sulfonylureas are well absorbed after PO use.

CONTRAINDICATIONS

Stress before and during surgery, ketosis, severe trauma, fever, infections, pregnancy, diabetes complicated by recurrent episodes of ketoacidosis or coma; juvenile, growth-onset, insulin-dependent, or brittle diabetes; impaired endocrine, renal, or liver function. Use in diabetics who can be controlled by diet alone. Relapse may occur with the sulfonylureas in undernourished clients. Long-acting products in geriatric clients.

SPECIAL CONCERNS

Use with caution in debilitated and malnourished clients, during lactation since hypoglycemia may occur in the infant, and in those with impaired renal or hepatic function. Safety and effectiveness in children have not been established. Geriatric clients may be more sensitive to oral hypoglycemics and hypoglycemia may be more difficult to recognize in these clients. Use of sulfonylureas has been associated with an increased risk of CV mortality compared to treatment with either diet alone or diet plus insulin. There may be loss of blood glucose control if the client experiences stress such as infection, fever, surgery, or trauma or develops Syndrome X (insulin resistance or metabolic syndrome).

SIDE EFFECTS

Hypoglycemia is the most common side effect. **GI:** Nausea, heartburn, epigastric fullness, diarrhea, GI pain, constipation, dyspepsia, gastralgia, vomiting, proctocolitis, hunger, flatulence. **CNS:** Fatigue, dizziness, drowsiness, nervousness, asthenia, insomnia, tremor, anxiety, depression, chills, hypesthesia, hypertonia, somnolence, confusion, abnormal gait, decreased libido, migraine, anorexia, myalgia, arthralgia, weakness, paresthesia, vertigo, malaise, headache, confusion, abnormal gait, pain. **Hepatic:** Cholestatic jaundice, aggravation of hepatic porphyria, hepatitis. **CV:** Arrhythmia, hypertension, vasculitis. **Dermatologic:** Skin rashes, urticaria, erythema multiforme, pruritus, eczema, photophobia, morbilliform/maculopapular eruptions, allergic skin rash, exfoliative dermatitis, sweating, lichenoid reactions, porphyria cutanea tarda. **GU:** Polyuria, dysuria. **Respiratory:** Pharyngitis, dyspnea. **Hematologic:** Thrombocytopenia, leukopenia, ***agranulocytosis, aplastic/hemolytic anemia,*** pancytopenia, eosinophilia. **Endocrine:** Inappropriate secretion of ADH resulting in excessive water retention, hyponatremia, low serum/high urine osmolality. **CV:** Arrhythmia, flushing, hypertension, vasculitis. **Ophthalmic:** Eye pain, blurred vision, conjunctivitis, retinal hemorrhage. **Miscellaneous:** Tinnitus, disulfiram-like reaction if taken with alcohol, rhinitis, polyuria, trace blood in stool, thirst, edema, leg cramps, syncope, resistance to drug action develops in a small percentage of clients.

OD OVERDOSE MANAGEMENT

Symptoms: Hypoglycemia. The following symptoms of hypoglycemia are listed in their general order of appearance: Tingling of lips and tongue, hunger, nausea, decreased cerebral function (lethargy, yawning, confusion, agitation, nervousness), increased sympathetic activity (tachycardia, sweating, tremor), seizures, stupor, coma.

Treatment: Mild hypoglycemia is treated with PO glucose and adjusting the dose of the drug or meal patterns. Severe hypoglycemia requires hospitalization. Concentrated (50%) dextrose is given by rapid IV and is followed by continuous infusion of 10% dextrose at a rate that will maintain blood glucose above 100 mg/dL. Client should be monitored for at least 24–48 hr as hypoglycemia

---

Bold Italic = life threatening side effect   ■ = black box warning   ✤ = Available in Canada

may recur (clients with chlorpropamide toxicity should be monitored for 3–5 days due to the long duration of action of this drug).

DRUG INTERACTIONS

Alcohol / Possible Antabuse-like syndrome, especially flushing of face and SOB. Also, ↓ effect of oral hypoglycemic R/T to ↑ liver breakdown

Androgens/anabolic steroids / ↑ Hypoglycemic effect

Anticoagulants, oral / ↑ Oral hypoglycemic effects by ↓ liver breakdown and ↓ plasma protein binding

Azole antifungals ↑ Oral hypoglycemic effect

Beta-adrenergic blocking agents / ↓ Hypoglycemic effect; also, symptoms of hypoglycemia may be masked.

H *Bilberry* / Possible potentiation of antidiabetic agents

Calcium channel blockers / ↓ Hypoglycemic effect

Charcoal / ↓ Hypoglycemic effect R/T ↓ GI tract absorption

Chloramphenicol / ↑ Effect R/T ↓ liver breakdown and ↓ renal excretion

Cholestyramine / ↓ Hypoglycemic effect

Clarithromycin / Possible severe hypoglycemia in clients with moderately impaired renal function after taking sulfonylureas

Clofibrate / ↑ Hypoglycemic effect R/T ↓ plasma protein binding

Corticosteroids / ↓ Hypoglycemic effect

Diazoxide / ↓ Effects of both drugs

Digitalis glycosides / Possibly ↑ Digitalis serum levels

Estrogens / ↓ Hypoglycemic effect

Fenfluramine / ↑ Hypoglycemic effect

Fluconazole / ↑ Hypoglycemic effect

Gatifloxacin / Possible severe and persistent hypoglycemia refractory to IV dextrose after taking gatifloxacin

Gemfibrozil / ↑ Hypoglycemic effect.

H *Ginseng* / ↑ Hypoglycemic effect

Histamine H$_2$ antagonists / ↑ Hypoglycemic effect R/T ↓ liver breakdown

Hydantoins / ↓ Effect of sulfonylureas R/T ↓ insulin release

Isoniazid / ↓ Hypoglycemic effect

Itraconazole / Possible hypoglycemia; monitor BG

Magnesium salts / ↑ Hypoglycemic effect

MAO inhibitors / ↑ Hypoglycemic effect R/T ↓ liver breakdown

Methyldopa / ↑ Hypoglycemic effect R/T ↓ liver breakdown

Niacin, Nicotinic acid / ↓ Hypoglycemic effect

NSAIDs / ↑ Hypoglycemic effect of oral antidiabetics

Oral contraceptives / ↓ Hypoglycemic effect

Phenothiazines / ↓ Hypoglycemic effect

Probenecid / ↑ Hypoglycemic effect

Rifampin / ↓ Effect of sulfonylureas R/T ↑ liver breakdown

Salicylates / ↑ Effect of oral hypoglycemics by ↓ plasma protein binding

Sulfinpyrazone / ↑ Hypoglycemic effect

Sulfonamides / ↑ Effect of oral hypoglycemics by ↓ plasma protein binding and ↓ liver breakdown

Sympathomimetics / ↓ Hypoglycemic effect

Thiazides / ↓ Hypoglycemic effect

Thyroid products / ↓ Hypoglycemic effect

Tricyclic antidepressants / ↑ Hypoglycemic effect

Urinary acidifiers / ↑ Hypoglycemic effect R/T ↓ renal excretion

Urinary alkalinizers / ↓ Hypoglycemic effect R/T ↑ renal excretion

LABORATORY TEST CONSIDERATIONS

↑ BUN, serum creatinine, AST, LDH, alkaline phosphatase. Elevated LFTs. Hyponatremia.

DOSAGE

• **PO**

See individual preparations. Adjust dosage according to needs of client. Exercise, weight loss, and diet are of primary importance in the control of diabetes.

NURSING CONSIDERATIONS

ADMINISTRATION/STORAGE

1. To decrease the incidence of gastric upset, take PO drugs with food.

2. If ketonuria, acidosis, increased glycosuria, or serious side effects occur, withdraw the medication.

3. Transfer from insulin:

= see color insert   H = Herbal   IV = Intravenous   © = sound alike drug

- If receiving 20 units or less of insulin daily, initiate oral hypoglycemic therapy and discontinue insulin abruptly.
- For clients receiving 20–40 units of insulin daily, initiate oral hypoglycemic therapy and reduce insulin dose by 25–50%. Discontinue insulin gradually, using the absence of glucose in the urine as a guide. With glyburide, insulin may be discontinued abruptly.
- For clients receiving more than 40 units of insulin daily, initiate PO therapy and reduce insulin by 20%. Discontinue insulin gradually, using glucose in the urine or finger sticks as a guide. It may be advisable to hospitalize clients on such high doses of insulin while they are being transferred to oral hypoglycemic agents.

4. Transfer from one oral hypoglycemic agent to another:

- Except for chlorpropamide, no transition period is necessary. When transferring from chlorpropamide, use caution for 1–2 weeks due to the long chlorpropamide half-life.
- Mild symptoms of hyperglycemia may appear during the transfer period. Perform finger sticks and test urine for ketones regularly (1–3 times daily) during the transfer period. Positive results must be reported.

5. Be prepared to treat if client develops severe hypoglycemia.

6. Review prescribed drugs to ensure none interact.

7. Type 2 diabetics who do not respond to the sulfonylureas are said to be *primary failures*. Responses to the sulfonylureas during the initial months of therapy followed by failure to respond are referred to as *secondary failures*. A Glucophage trial or combination therapy with insulin and/or up to three oral agents may be useful in these clients.

ASSESSMENT

1. Obtain a thorough nursing history. Assess mental functions to determine if able to understand the complexities of the monitoring and adjustment of medications, when and how to take prescribed agents.

2. If unsure of type of diabetes, may differentiate I and II with C-Peptide levels. Many younger children that are obese and inactive are developing type 2 diabetes at a very early age.

3. Note any previous experience with sulfonylureas and the outcome. Determine metformin and/or thiazolidinedione trial and the outcome; elderly do better with a slower metformin titration (i.e., increase dose weekly or increase by ½ tablet instead of a whole tablet).

4. Document any stress. Clients about to undergo surgical procedures, who have suffered severe trauma, who have a fever and infection, or who are pregnant should generally not be placed on oral hypoglycemic agents.

5. Note effectiveness lessened by oral hypoglycemic agents.

6. Diabetics benefit from ACE and ASA therapy. Assess for metabolic syndrome or insulin resistance, i.e., obesity, HTN, ASHD, dyslipidemia, hyperinsulinemia and type 2 diabetes.

7. Monitor VS, ECG, lipid panel, electrolytes, CBC, HbA1c, and urine for microalbumin. Strive for tight control or HbA1c <7.

8. Routinely review eye and foot exams and labs for evidence of problems or loss of control.

CLIENT/FAMILY TEACHING

1. Type 2 diabetes is a disease of metabolic dysfunction related to excessive weight gain, eating the wrong foods, and physical inactivity. This disease may be reversed with weight loss, exercise, and changes in eating/lifestyle.

2. Record blood sugar (and if directed urine for ketones) at different times during the day and night for provider review. (Urine testing is not an accurate reflection of true serum glucose levels and should not be used to modify treatment.)

3. With hypoglycemic episodes, check finger stick at the time of the reaction. Then drink 4 oz of juice (fast-acting CHO), followed by a longer acting CHO (approximately 10 grams) such as half a meat sandwich or several peanut butter crackers, and recheck finger stick in 15 min. If glucose is <100, repeat the pro-

---

Bold Italic = life threatening side effect   ■ = black box warning   ✦ = Available in Canada

cess, i.e., juice and a CHO and another finger stick. Report frequency.

4. Medication helps to control high BS but does not cure diabetes; therapy is usually long term. Must adhere to prescribed diet if drug is to be effective; most secondary failures are due to poor dietary compliance; see dietitian as needed. Regular exercise, diet, and weight control/loss are imperative.

5. Insulin may be necessary if complications occur or sugar not well controlled. Review administration of insulin and how to rotate sites. Do not change brands of insulin or syringes. Review equipment use, methods of storage and how to discard used syringes.

6. Report illness or if unusual itching, skin rash, jaundice, dark urine, fever, sore throat, nausea/vomiting, or diarrhea occurs.

7. With thyroid scans- advise lab-sulfonylureas interfere with the uptake of radioactive iodine.

8. Avoid alcohol; a disulfuram-like reaction may occur. Do not take any OTC agents without approval.

9. Need close medical supervision for the first 6 weeks and periodic lab tests until control attained; oral agents may cause blood dyscrasias, acidosis, or liver dysfunction.

10. Carry ID, a list of prescribed drugs, juice, and hard candy (such as Lifesavers®) or a fast-acting CHO (candy bar) at all times.

OUTCOMES/EVALUATE

- Knowledge/control of diabetes; adherence to exercise/drug/diet therapy
- ↓ Hypo/hyperglycemic episodes
- HbA1c within desired range <7
- Prevention of target organ damage

ANTIDIABETIC AGENTS: INSULINS

SEE ALSO ANTIDIABETIC AGENTS: HYPOGLYCEMIC AGENTS. AND ALSO THE FOLLOWING INDIVIDUAL ENTRIES:

Insulin aspart
Insulin detemir
Insulin glargine
Insulin glulisine
Insulin injection (Regular insulin)
Insulin injection concentrated
Insulin lispro injection
Insulin zinc suspension (Lente)
Insulin zinc suspension, Extended (Ultralente)
Isophane insulin suspension/Insulin injection 70/30, 50/50
Isophane insulin suspension (NPH)

GENERAL STATEMENT

Insulin preparations with different times of onset, peak activity, and duration of action have been developed. Such products are prepared by precipitating insulin in the presence of zinc chloride to form zinc insulin crystals and/or by combining insulin with a protein such as protamine. Based on these modifications, insulin products are classified as fast-acting, intermediate-acting, and long-acting. These preparations permit the provider to select the preparation best suited to the lifestyle of the client.

RAPID-ACTING INSULINS

1. Insulin aspart
2. Insulin glulisine
3. Insulin injection (Regular insulin)
4. Insulin lispro injection

INTERMEDIATE-ACTING INSULINS

1. Insulin zinc suspension (Lente)
2. Isophane insulin suspension (NPH)

LONG-ACTING INSULIN

1. Insulin detemir
2. Insulin glargine

NOTE: Insulin preparations with various times of onset and duration of action are often mixed to obtain optimum control in diabetic clients.

USES

Human insulins are being used almost exclusively.

1. Replacement therapy in type 1 diabetes.
2. Diabetic ketoacidosis or diabetic coma (use regular insulin).
3. Type 2 diabetes when other measures have failed (e.g., diet, exercise, weight reduction), blood sugars are significantly elevated, or with surgery, trauma, infection, fever, endocrine dysfunction, pregnancy, gangrene, Ray-

---

naud's disease, kidney or liver dysfunction.

4. Glucose and regular insulin to treat hyperkalemia.

5. Insulin and oral hypoglycemic drugs have been used in type 2 diabetics who are difficult to control with diet and PO therapy alone.

6. Single component and human insulins for cases of local insulin allergy, immunologic insulin resistance, injection-site lipodystrophy, temporary insulin use (e.g., surgery, acute stress type 2 diabetes, gestational diabetes), and newly diagnosed diabetics.

ACTION/KINETICS

Action

Following combination with insulin receptors on cell plasma membranes, insulin facilitates the transport of glucose into cardiac and skeletal muscle and adipose tissue. It also increases synthesis of glycogen in the liver. Insulin stimulates protein synthesis and lipogenesis and inhibits lipolysis and release of free fatty acids from fat cells. This latter effect prevents or reverses the ketoacidosis sometimes observed in the type 1 diabetic. Insulin also causes intracellular shifts in magnesium and potassium.

Pharmacokinetics

Since insulin is a protein, it is destroyed in the GI tract. Thus, it must be administered SC so that it is readily absorbed into the bloodstream and distributed throughout the extracellular fluid. Metabolized mainly by the liver.

DIET

The dietary control of diabetes is as important as medication with appropriate drugs. The role of the nurse and dietitian in teaching the client how to eat properly cannot be underestimated. They must teach the client how to calculate exchange values of various foods. Food lists and food-exchange values published by the American Diabetes Association and the American Dietetic Association are valuable teaching aids.

Diabetic clients should adhere to a regular meal schedule. The frequency of meals and the overall caloric intake vary with the type of drug taken and individual client needs. Close attention to meal frequency and meal planning is imperative and a registered dietitian should be consulted. Diabetic children may be on a less restricted diet, adjusting the insulin dosage according to blood and urine glucose readings. Children with negative urine glucose tend to become hypoglycemic rapidly with exercise or decrease in appetite, and many providers allow for glucose spilling.

CONTRAINDICATIONS

Hypersensitivity to insulin. During episodes of hypoglycemia in clients sensitive to any component of the product.

SPECIAL CONCERNS

Pregnant diabetic clients often manifest decreased insulin requirements during the first half of pregnancy and increased requirements during the latter half. Inadequate or excessive insulin treatment of diabetic mothers inhibits milk production.

SIDE EFFECTS

Hypoglycemia: Due to insulin overdose, delayed or decreased food intake, too much exercise in relationship to insulin dose, or when transferring from one preparation to another. Even carefully controlled clients occasionally develop signs of insulin overdosage characterized by one or more of the following: Hunger, weakness, fatigue, nervousness, pallor or flushing, profuse sweating, headache, palpitations, numbness of mouth, tingling in the fingers, tremors, blurred and double vision, hypothermia, excess yawning, mental confusion, incoordination, tachycardia, loss of sensitivity, and loss of consciousness. Level of awareness is markedly diminished after an attack. Symptoms of hypoglycemia may mimic those of psychic disturbances. Severe prolonged hypoglycemia may cause brain damage, and in the elderly, may mimic stroke. **Allergic:** Urticaria, angioedema, lymphadenopathy, bullae, anaphylaxis. Occurs mostly following intermittent insulin therapy or IV administration of large doses to insulin-resistant clients. Antihistamines or corticosteroids may be used to treat these symptoms. **At site of injection:** Swell-

---

Bold Italic = life threatening side effect   ■ = black box warning   ✦ = Available in Canada

ing, stinging, redness, itching, warmth. These symptoms often disappear with continued use. Lipoatrophy or lipodystrophy of subcutaneous fat tissue (minimize by rotating site of injection). **Insulin resistance:** Usual cause is obesity. Acute resistance may occur following infections, trauma, surgery, emotional disturbances, or other endocrine disorders. **Ophthalmic:** Blurred vision, transient presbyopia. Occurs mainly during initiation of therapy or in clients who have been uncontrolled for a long period of time.

Hypokalemia: Hyperglycemic rebound (Somogyi effect): Usually in clients who receive chronic overdosage.

DIFFERENTIATION BETWEEN HYPERGLYCEMIA (DIABETIC COMA) AND HYPOGLYCEMIC REACTION (INSULIN SHOCK)

Coma in diabetes may be caused by uncontrolled diabetes (high sugar content in blood or urine, ketoacidosis) or by too much insulin (insulin shock, hypoglycemia). Hyperglycemia is usually precipitated by the client's failure to take insulin. Hypoglycemia is often precipitated by the client's unpredictable response, excess exertion, stress due to illness or surgery, errors in calculating dosage, or failure to eat.

TREATMENT OF HYPERGLYCEMIA (DIABETIC COMA OR SEVERE ACIDOSIS)

Administer 30–60 units of regular insulin. This is followed by doses of 20 units or more q 30 min. To avoid a hypoglycemic state, 1 gram dextrose is administered for each unit of insulin given. Treatment is often supplemented by electrolytes and fluids. Urine samples are collected for analysis, and VS are monitored regularly.

TREATMENT OF HYPOGLYCEMIA (INSULIN SHOCK)

Mild hypoglycemia can be relieved by PO administration of CHO such as orange juice, candy, or a lump of sugar. If comatose, adults may be given 10–30 mL of 50% dextrose solution IV; children should receive 0.5–1 mL/kg of 50% dextrose solution. Epinephrine, hydrocortisone, or glucagon may be used

in severe cases to cause an increase in blood glucose.

DRUG INTERACTIONS

ACE Inhibitors / ↑ Hypoglycemic effect of insulin

Acetazolamide / ↓ Hypoglycemic effect of insulin

AIDS antiviral drugs / ↓ Hypoglycemic effect of insulin

Albuterol / ↓ Hypoglycemic effect of insulin

Alcohol, ethyl / ↑ Hypoglycemia → low blood sugar and shock

Anabolic steroids / ↑ Hypoglycemic effect of insulin

Antidiabetics, oral / ↑ Hypoglycemic effect of insulin

Asparaginase / ↓ Hypoglycemic effect of insulin

Beta-adrenergic blocking agents / ↑ Hypoglycemic effect of insulin

Calcitonin / ↓ Hypoglycemic effect of insulin

Calcium / ↑ Hypoglycemic effect of insulin

Chloroquine / ↑ Hypoglycemic effect of insulin

Chlorthalidone / ↓ Hypoglycemic effect of antidiabetics

Clofibrate / ↑ Hypoglycemic effect of insulin

Clonidine / ↑ Hypoglycemic effect of insulin

Clozapine / ↓ Hypoglycemic effect of insulin

Contraceptives, oral / ↑ Dosage of antidiabetic R/T impairment of glucose tolerance; ↓ Hypoglycemic effect of insulin

Corticosteroids / ↓ Effect of insulin R/T corticosteroid-induced hyperglycemia

Cyclophosphamide / ↓ Hypoglycemic effect of insulin

Danazol / ↓ Hypoglycemic effect of insulin

Dextrothyroxine / ↓ Effect of insulin R/T dextrothyroxine-induced hyperglycemia

Diazoxide / Diazoxide-induced hyperglycemia → ↓ diabetic control

Digitalis glycosides / Use with caution, as insulin affects serum potassium levels

Diltiazem / ↓ Hypoglycemic effect of

Classifications

insulin

Disopyramide / ↑ Hypoglycemic effect of insulin

Diuretics / ↓ Hypoglycemic effect of insulin

Dobutamine / ↓ Hypoglycemic effect of insulin

Epinephrine / ↓ Effect of insulin due to epinephrine-induced hyperglycemia

Estrogens / ↓ Effect of insulin due to impairment of glucose tolerance

Ethacrynic acid / ↓ Hypoglycemic effect of insulin

Fenfluramine / Additive hypoglycemic effects

Fibrates / ↑ Hypoglycemic effect of insulin

Fluoxetine / ↑ Hypoglycemic effect of insulin

Furosemide / ↓ Hypoglycemic effect of antidiabetics

H *Ginseng* / Possible additive hypoglycemic effects

Glucagon / Glucagon-induced hyperglycemia → ↓ effect of antidiabetics

Guanethidine / ↑ Hypoglycemic effect of insulin

Isoniazid / ↓ Hypoglycemic effect of insulin

Lithium carbonate / ↑ or ↓ Hypoglycemic effect of insulin

MAO inhibitors / MAO inhibitors ↑ and prolong hypoglycemic effect of antidiabetics

Mebendazole / ↑ Hypoglycemic effect of insulin

Morphine sulfate / ↓ Hypoglycemic effect of insulin

Niacin / ↓ Hypoglycemic effect of insulin

Nicotine / ↓ Hypoglycemic effect of insulin

Octreotide / ↑ Hypoglycemic effect of insulin

Olanzapine / ↓ Hypoglycemic effect of insulin

Oxytetracycline / ↑ Effect of insulin

Pentamidine / ↑ Hypoglycemic effect of insulin; may be followed by hyperglycemia

Pentoxifylline / ↑ Hypoglycemic effect of insulin

Phenothiazines / ↓ Hypoglycemic effect of insulin R/T phenothiazine-in-duced hyperglycemia

Phenytoin / Phenytoin-induced hyperglycemia → ↓ diabetic control

Propoxyphene / ↑ Hypoglycemic effect of insulin

Propranolol / Inhibits rebound of blood glucose after insulin-induced hypoglycemia

Protease inhibitors / ↓ Hypoglycemic effect of insulin.

H *Psyllium seed/ Blonde psyllium seed husk* / Possible need to ↓ insulin dose

Pyridoxine / ↑ Hypoglycemic effect of insulin

Salicylates / ↑ Hypoglycemic effect of insulin

Somatropin / ↓ Hypoglycemic effect of insulin

Smoking / ↑ Insulin requirements in heavy smokers R/T ↓ SC insulin absorption; smoking may release endogenous substances that cause insulin resistance

Sulfinpyrazone / ↑ Hypoglycemic effect of insulin

Sulfonamides / ↑ Hypoglycemic effect of insulin

Terbutaline / ↓ Hypoglycemic effect of insulin

Tetracyclines / ↑ Hypoglycemic effect of insulin

Thiazide diuretics / ↓ Hypoglycemic effect of antidiabetics

Thyroid preparations / ↓ Effect of antidiabetic due to thyroid-induced hyperglycemia

Triamterene / ↓ Hypoglycemic effect of antidiabetic.

LABORATORY TEST CONSIDERATIONS
Hypoglycemia, hypokalemia. Alters liver function tests and thyroid function tests. False + Coombs' test, ↑ serum protein. ↓ Serum amino acids, calcium, cholesterol, and urine amino acids.

DOSAGE
Dosage highly individualized. Usually administered SC. Insulin injection (regular insulin) is the **only** preparation that may be administered IV. Give IV only for clients with severe ketoacidosis or diabetic coma. Dosage for insulin is always expressed in USP units. **Adults and children, usual dose:** 0.5-1 unit/kg/day. Dosage is established and mon-

itored by blood glucose (often using glucose monitoring machines in the home), urine glucose, and acetone tests. Furthermore, since requirements may change with time, dosage must be checked at regular intervals. It may be advisable to hospitalize some clients while their daily insulin and caloric requirements are being established. The main goal is to control the blood sugar and send the client home to fine tune as generally the home environment is more reliable for determining drug requirements.

In elderly clients, initial dosing, dosing increments, and maintenance dosing should be conservative to avoid hypoglycemic reactions, which may be difficult to recognize in the elderly.

In pregnancy, insulin requirements may increase suddenly during the last trimester. After delivery, requirements may suddenly drop to prepregnancy levels. To prevent the development of hypoglycemia, insulin is often discontinued on the day of delivery and glucose is administered IV.

The various insulin preparations can be mixed to obtain the combination best suited for the individual client. However, mixing must be done according to the directions received from the physician/provider and/or pharmacist.

NURSING CONSIDERATIONS

Also includes general applications for all clients with diabetes controlled by medication (whether it be insulin or an oral hypoglycemic agent).

ADMINISTRATION/STORAGE

1. Read product information and any important notes inserted into the insulin package.
2. Color has been added to insulin packages to differentiate between products and prevent dispensing errors.
3. Lactating women may require adjustments in insulin dose and diet.
4. Discard open vials not used for several weeks or whose expiration date has passed.
5. Refrigerate stock supply of insulin but avoid freezing. Freezing destroys

the manner in which insulin is suspended in the formulation.
6. Store vial in a cool place, avoiding extremes of temperature or exposure to sunlight.
7. Use the following guidelines with respect to mixing the various insulins:
- Regular insulin may be mixed with NPH or Lente insulins. However, to avoid transfer of the longer-acting insulin into the regular insulin vial, withdraw regular insulin into the syringe first.
- Give a mixture of regular insulin with NPH or Lente insulin within 15 min of mixing due to binding of regular insulin by excess protamine and/or zinc in the longer-acting preparations.
- Lente or Ultralente insulins may be mixed with each other in any proportion; however, do not mix these with NPH insulins.
- When used in an insulin infusion pump, insulin may be mixed in any proportion with either 0.9% NaCl injection or water for injection. Due to stability changes, use such mixtures within 24 hr of their preparation. Buffered insulin is usually the form prescribed and utilized in pumps.
8. Change insulins cautiously and under medical supervision. Changes in purity, strength, brand, type or species source may require dosage adjustment.
9. Store compatible insulin mixtures for no longer than 1 month at room temperature or 3 months at 2–8°C (36–46°F); bacterial contamination may occur.
10. To ensure a constant amount of precipitate in each dose, invert the vial several times to mix before withdrawing the material. Avoid vigorous shaking and frothing of the material. (Regular and globin insulin are the only two insulins that do not have a precipitate.)
11. Discard any vial in which the precipitate is clumped or granular in appearance or which has formed a solid deposit of particles on the side of the vial.
12. To prevent dosage error, do not alter the order of mixing insulins or

---

change the model or brand of syringe or needle.

13. Administer at a 90° angle with a 28- or 29-gauge needle. Syringes come in 0.3 mL (30-units), 0.5 mL (50-units) and 1 mL (100-units) sizes. Get the smallest syringe with the smallest needles to enhance dosage validity (e.g., if client is prescribed <30 units of insulin, advise to obtain the 0.3 mL syringe).

14. Provide an automatic injector for clients fearful of injections.

15. Assist visually impaired clients to obtain information and devices for self-administration by consulting their local diabetes association or by writing to the American Diabetes Association, 149 Madison Avenue, New York, NY 10016 (telephone: 1-800-DIABETES or 1-800-342-2383), for their buyer's guide, which lists numerous products for diabetics. Clients may also contact The Lighthouse, Inc., 800 Second Avenue, New York, NY 10017 for additional information on visual impairments.

16. Lipoatrophy may occur. This may appear as mild dimpling of the skin or as deep pits in young girls and women and lipodystrophy, appearing as well-developed muscle on the anterior and lateral thighs of young boys and men. To prevent, rotate injection sites.

- Make a chart indicating the injection sites.
- Allow 3–4 cm between sites.
- Do not inject in the same site for at least 1–2 weeks.
- Avoid injecting within 1 cm around the umbilicus because of the high vascularity in this area.
- Avoid injections around the waistline because of the sensitive nerve supply to this area and the potential for fabric irritation.
- Use insulin at room temperature to prevent lipodystrophy.

17. Rotation of injection sites may lead to differences in blood levels of insulin. The abdomen is considered the best site due to constant insulin peak times with better gradual absorption. Apply gentle pressure after injection but do not massage since this may alter rate of absorption.

18. If insulin has been refrigerated, allow it to remain at room temperature for at least 1 hr before using.

19. If breakfast is delayed for lab tests, check for dosage adjustment.

ASSESSMENT

1. Obtain thorough history and physical exam. Note any first-degree relatives with disease.

2. Assess for S&S of hyperglycemia: thirst, polydipsia, polyuria, drowsiness, blurred vision, loss of appetite, fruity odor to the breath, and flushed dry skin.

3. Assess for S&S of hypoglycemia: drowsiness, chills, confusion, anxiety, cold sweats, cool pale skin, excessive hunger, nausea, headache, irritability, shakiness, rapid pulse, and unusual weakness or tiredness.

4. Identify first noted changes in physical condition and what these changes were.

5. Weigh to determine amount of agent needed.

6. Monitor electrolytes, lipid profile, thyroid studies, BS, phosphate, Mg, CBC, HbA1c, and urinalysis. Assess for microalbuminuria.

7. Monitor glucose levels carefully, especially in the elderly and those with hepatic or renal impairment.

8. Assess psychologic state, including disease acceptance, readiness to learn, support system, evidence of depression, or need for additional counseling.

9. During physical exam assess DTRs; check extremities (use monofilament) to assess sensation and for evidence of neuropathy. Review proper foot care with each visit.

10. Consider ACE therapy to prevent/preserve renal function and inhibit organ damage and baby aspirin for cardio-protection.

11. Assess injection sites, monitor VS, plot growth and weight every 3–4 months.

12. Schedule yearly eye exams if >12 years old or if client has had the disease for >5 years.

INTERVENTIONS

1. For a *hyperglycemic reaction:*
- Have regular insulin available.

- Obtain BS or finger stick.
- Monitor after giving insulin for further signs of hyperglycemia such as SOB, facial flushing, air hunger, and acetone breath.

2. Assess for S&S of *hypoglycemia,* such as easy fatigue, hunger, headache, cold, clamminess, drowsiness, nausea, lassitude, and tremulousness. Most likely to occur before meals, during or after exercise, and at insulin peak action times (i.e., 3 a.m. with evening dosing).

- Weakness, sweating, tremors, and/or nervousness may occur later.
- Excessive restlessness and profuse sweating at night.
- Obtain BS or finger stick; promptly give 4 oz of juice and a CHO, if conscious.
- If conscious and taking long-acting insulin, also give a slowly digestible CHO, such as bread with corn syrup or honey. Give additional CHO such as crackers and milk for the next 2 hr.
- If unconscious, apply honey or Karo syrup to the buccal membrane or give glucagon.
- If hospitalized, minimally responsive, or unconscious, give 10–20% IV dextrose solution.

3. A Somogyi effect is often mistaken as client not following the prescribed therapy. This occurs when hypoglycemia triggers the release of epinephrine and glucocorticoids, which stimulates glycogenesis and results in a higher a.m. BS level. Reduction in bedtime insulin dosage is necessary to stabilize. If treated for hypoglycemia, check 3 a.m. BS; if normal and then BS rises between 3 a.m. and 7 a.m., this is related to growth hormone release—termed the Dawn Phenomenon. To control, give long-acting insulin at bedtime instead of at dinnertime.

4. Juveniles with type 1 diabetes demand closer attention and observation for infection or emotional disturbances and hypoglycemia. They are more susceptible to insulin shock and have a more limited response to glucagon. Determine if managed with intensive or conventional insulin therapy; adjust for hypoglycemia unawareness (when client passes out due to loss of catecholamine response). Assess for insulin pump placement for better control.

5. For the newly diagnosed elderly client, start insulin doses low and gradually increase.

6. The usual dose of NPH insulin is 0.8–1.5 units/kg; give two-thirds of dose in a.m. and one-third of dose in p.m. If using regular insulin, try 1:2 in a.m. and 1:1 in p.m. with NPH.

7. Identify BS goals, i.e., young child 80–150 mg/dL premeal and 100–150 mg/dL at bedtime; adolescent 70–150 mg/dL premeal and 100–150 mg/dL at bedtime; adult 70–150 mg/dL premeal and 100–150 mg/dL at bedtime. Adjust as symptoms and condition dictate.

CLIENT/FAMILY TEACHING

1. Medications assist to control diabetes but do not cure it. Type 1 diabetes is usually early onset when the pancreas makes little or no insulin; individuals with type 1 diabetes must take insulin injections or they will die. Type 2 diabetes is usually later onset and the pancreas still makes insulin, but the body cannot use it (termed insulin resistance); individuals with type 2 diabetes can use either oral hypoglycemic agents or insulin to lower their blood sugar or a combination of different oral agents to help them utilize their own insulin better. Elevated C-Peptide lab test may help with differentiation between type 1 and type 2.

2. In type 1 diabetics, urine ketones indicate that there is not enough insulin present to get the body's sugar into the cells so it is burning body fat as an alternative and producing ketones as waste products; may lead to ketoacidosis, a life-threatening condition. Test urine for ketones with a "dip-and-read" product when:

- Finger sticks >240 mg/dL
- Pregnant
- Experiencing severe stress
- Vomiting or sick to stomach
- Sick with flu/cold or virus infection
- Experiencing symptoms of hyperglycemia (unusual fatigue, vision difficulty, increased thirst and/or hunger, polydipsia, unusually tired or sleepy,

stomach pain, increased nausea, fruity odor to breath, rapid respirations, weight loss without altering food intake or activity patterns)

3. Perform finger sticks to monitor glucose levels. Review instructions for technique, calibration, operation, and device maintenance. Bring in periodically to double check machine accuracy and to review data bank to ensure values coincide with client log. Some general principles may be followed.

• Rotate sites.
• Cleanse area with soap and water or alcohol prior to stabbing.
• Use a lancet and lancet device to access sample
• Stab finger outside, by nail, where the capillaries are abundant and let a bead of blood form.
• Wipe off with a cotton ball.
• Let blood bead re-form and apply to the test strip.
• Use proper test strips for designated machine; check expiration date
• Follow specific guidelines for the device in use.
• When battery change occurs, reset machine date.

4. Regimens are specific to the individual, based on age, severity of diabetes, weight, any other medical problems they have, as well as the philosophy of the health care team.

5. If not planning to eat then do not take antihypoglycemic agents. Take insulin 30 min before a meal (exception is Humalog, which can be taken at meal time). Administer at a 90° angle with a 28- or 29-gauge needle. Syringes come in 0.3 mL (30-units), 0.5 mL (50-units) and 1 mL (100-units) sizes. Purchase the smallest syringe with the smallest needles to enhance dosage validity (e.g., if prescribed less than 30 units of insulin, obtain the 0.3 mL syringe). May reuse disposable insulin syringes; based on comfort and perceived dullness. Review cleaning procedures to ensure adequately cleaned.

6. Use a chart to document and rotate injection sites to avoid lipohypertrophy of injection sites (lumps from scar tissue after many injections). Avoid these ar-

eas due to unreliable absorption. Warm refrigerated/cold insulin to room temperature and then roll between your palms to prevent lipodystrophy from injecting cold insulin.

7. For self-injection, may brace the arm against a hard surface such as the wall or a chair.

• Cleanse the area thoroughly with alcohol and allow to dry. Then, depending on the condition of the skin, either pinch between the thumb and forefinger of one hand, or spread the skin using the thumb and fingers of one hand.
• Insert into the subcutaneous tissue and aspirate to be sure needle is not in a blood vessel.
• Inject insulin and withdraw the needle.

8. Review use and care of equipment, proper storage and disposal of needles and syringes, and provision and storage of drug.

9. *Always* check expiration dates; have an extra vial and equipment on hand for traveling, away from home, or when detained or hospitalized.

10. Have regular insulin for emergency use.

11. Must balance food, insulin, and exercise. Exercise increases the utilization of CHO and increases CHO needs. Have snacks available; 5–8 Lifesavers®, juice, or hard candy helps counteract hypoglycemia.

12. Adhere to prescribed diet, weight control, and ingestion of food relative to the peak action of insulin being used. Record weekly weights; reduce intake of animal fats and salt; select a variety of foods to meet starch and sugar, protein, and fat requirements (usual recommendation, CHO 50%; protein 20%; fat 30%). Consume the kinds of fiber that help lower BS and fat levels (breads, cereals, and crackers made from whole grains, such as whole wheat and brown rice, fresh vegetables and fruits, dried beans, and peas), low cholesterol and polyunsaturated and monosaturated fats.

13. Confer with dietitian for assistance in shopping, food selection/exchanges,

---

diet, and meal planning. Consume pre-meal snacks in the a.m., midday, and at bedtime.

14. If ill and a meal is omitted because of fever, nausea, or vomiting, replace solid foods that contain starch and sugar, such as bread and fruit, with liquids that contain sugar (fruit juice, regular sodas) and follow designated sliding scale for "sick days." Do not omit insulin or hypoglycemic agents unless instructed. Perform finger sticks q 4 hr, and with Type 1, also test urine for ketones; report if moderate or high.

15. Blurred vision may occur at beginning of insulin therapy; should subside in 6–8 weeks. The effect is caused by fluctuation of blood glucose levels, which produce osmotic changes in the lens of the eye and within the ocular fluids. If it does not clear up in 8 weeks, consult eye doctor.

16. May experience allergic responses: Itching, redness, swelling, stinging, or warmth may occur at the injection site and usually disappears after a few weeks of therapy. Report as purified or human insulins are used for local allergy and lipohypertrophy at injection site.

17. Failure to take insulin will result in ketoacidosis. Adjust insulin based on BS and guidelines for insulin administration during sick days. Identify soft foods and liquids to consume for sick days (i.e., regular soda, apple juice, clear broth, cream soups, puddings, apple sauce, popsicle, ice cream).

18. If ill, notify provider. To prevent coma, maintain adequate hydration by drinking 1 cup or more of noncaloric fluids such as coffee, tea, water, or broth every hour. Test finger sticks and urine more. Identify when to go to the emergency room.

19. If there is no insulin/equipment to administer, decrease food intake by one-third and drink plenty of noncaloric fluids. Obtain supplies as soon as possible and return to prescribed diet and insulin dosage.

20. Follow good hygienic practices to prevent infection. Bathe daily with mild soap and lukewarm water. Use lotion to prevent skin dryness. Avoid injury from punctures. Avoid scratches; wear gloves when working with the hands. Always protect feet and wear shoes. Use sunscreen and protective clothing to avoid sunburn, and dress appropriately for the weather; prevent frostbite.

21. Establish a daily routine of checking and caring for the feet (use a mirror if unable to bend over). Wear comfortable shoes (leather or canvas) and stockings (no garters or elastic tops) and do exercises. Clip toenails (straight across); do not undertake any self-treatment for ingrown toenails, corns, warts, or calluses. Do not use any heat treatments, hot water bottles, or heating pads, and do not smoke, as this decreases blood flow to the feet. Obtain annual foot screen and periodic foot care as needed.

22. Hyperglycemia compounds the risk for tooth and gum problems; brush after meals, floss, and see dentist regularly.

23. Diabetes can damage the small blood vessels to the eye; obtain yearly eye exams. Eye damage has no symptoms in the early, treatable stage. Report blurred or double vision, narrowed visual fields, increased difficulty seeing in dim light, pressure or pain in the eye, or seeing dark spots.

24. May experience decreased sensation in feet, legs, and hands; use care when handling hot or cold items, wear shoes to protect feet, and dress appropriately for the weather.

25. Carry ID noting "diabetic" and list of medications, who to notify, and what to do if unable to respond.

26. Avoid alcohol; causes hypoglycemia. Excessive intake may require a reduction of insulin; also causes a disulfiram-type reaction with oral hypoglycemic agents and increases peripheral neuropathy.

27. Carry all medications, syringes, glucagon, and blood testing equipment in carry-on luggage when traveling. Always carry diabetes ID. Keep to the usual meal, exercise, and medication routines as closely as possible. Carry food and fast-acting sugar in the event meals are delayed. Request medications for

vomiting/diarrhea and plan ahead for mealtimes when crossing two or more time zones. Protect insulin and test strips from extremes in heat or cold (keeping between 15–30°C or 59–86°F).

28. Use only the insulin prescribed; check for correct origin (human or pork), brand name (Lispro, Humulin, etc.), and type (Regular, Lente, NPH, etc.).

29. Check vials before each dose is taken. Regular and Buffered Regular insulin (for pumps) should be clear and colorless, whereas other forms may be cloudy except for the new long acting form.

30. Two kinds of insulin can be mixed in the same syringe:
- Regular insulin can be mixed with any other insulin.
- Lente forms can be mixed with other Lente insulins but cannot be mixed with other insulins except regular insulin.
- Do not mix the fast acting lispro with other agents
- A single form of insulin in a syringe can be stable for weeks or a month.
- Except for the commercially prepared mixtures, mixtures of insulin are not stable and should be administered within 5 min of preparation.
- When mixed, regular (unmodified) insulin should always be drawn up in the syringe first.

31. Impotence may be caused by damaged nerves and reduced blood flow related to diabetes; see urologist to find cause and best treatment.

32. Silent heart attacks may occur. Identify risk factors and alter life-style to prevent CAD (i.e., regular exercise, low-fat, low-salt, low-cholesterol diet, no tobacco or alcohol, stress/weight reduction and BP and cholesterol LDL control).

33. Identify local diabetic educator and support groups to assist in understanding and coping with this disease. The American Diabetes Association (telephone: 1-800-342-2383 and email: AskADA@diabetes.org) and local diabetes support groups offer additional information and support.

OUTCOMES/EVALUATE
- Understanding/acceptance of DM
- Positive lifestyle changes to control DM
- BS, renal and LFTs WNL; HbA1c <7
- Healthy skin at injection sites
- Prevent target organ damage

ANTIEMETICS

SEE ALSO THE FOLLOWING INDIVIDUAL ENTRIES:

Aprepitant
Dimenhydrinate
Diphenhydramine hydrochloride
Granisetron hydrochloride
Hydroxyzine hydrochloride
Hydroxyzine pamoate
Meclizine hydrochloride
Nabilone*
Ondansetron hydrochloride
Palonosetron hydrochloride
Prochlorperazine
Prochlorperazine edisylate
Prochlorperazine maleate
Scopolamine hydrobromide
Trimethobenzamide hydrochloride

Drugs marked with an * are available to view in the online database at www.delmarnursesdrughandbook.com/2009.

GENERAL STATEMENT
Nausea and vomiting can be caused by a variety of conditions, such as infections, drugs, radiation, motion, organic disease, or psychologic factors. The underlying cause of the symptoms must be elicited before emesis is corrected. Many drugs used for other conditions, such as the antihistamines, phenothiazines, barbiturates, and scopolamine, have antiemetic properties and can be used. However, CNS depression make their routine use undesirable.

DRUG INTERACTIONS
Because of their antiemetic and antinauseant activity, the antiemetics may mask overdosage caused by other drugs.

NURSING CONSIDERATIONS
ASSESSMENT
1. Determine if nausea is an unusual occurrence or a recurring phenomenon;

Classifications

establish onset, duration, and associated factors such as vertigo, chemotherapy, or illness. Note past use of antiemetics and response.

2. Evaluate physiologic mechanism triggering N&V. Generally, if centrally mediated to the CTZ, would see nausea without vomiting, whereas if the vomiting center were triggered directly, then may see retching with vomiting.

3. Assess for other effects; antiemetics may mask signs of underlying pathology or overdosage of other drugs. Ensure no intestinal obstruction, drug overdose, or increased ICP. Monitor I&O; observe for dehydration. Offer liquids and advance to regular foods as tolerated.

4. With prolonged activity, monitor for electrolyte disturbance and replace as needed.

CLIENT/FAMILY TEACHING

1. Take exactly as directed. Drug may cause dizziness/drowsiness; avoid driving or other hazardous tasks until drug effects evaluated.

2. Practice measures to decrease nausea when possible, such as ice chips, sips of water, nongreasy foods, removal of irritating stimuli (odors or materials), and frequent mouth rinsing with water and oral hygiene. Advance diet only as tolerated.

3. Dangle legs before standing; rise slowly to prevent symptoms of low BP. Consume adequate fluids to prevent dehydration.

4. Avoid alcohol and any other nonprescribed CNS depressants.

5. Report any adverse effects, unresponsive N&V or abdominal pain. Keep all F/U appointments to assess response and review labs.

OUTCOMES/EVALUATE

Control of N&V; prevention of dehydration/electrolyte imbalance. Improved nutritional status with weight gain/ ↑ caloric intake

ANTIHISTAMINES (H₁ BLOCKERS)

SEE ALSO THE FOLLOWING INDIVIDUAL ENTRIES:

FIRST GENERATION:
Brompheniramine tannate*
Chlorpheniramine maleate
Cyproheptadine hydrochloride*
Diphenhydramine hydrochloride
Hydroxyzine hydrochloride
Hydroxyzine pamoate
Meclizine hydrochloride
Promethazine hydrochloride*

SECOND GENERATION:
Cetirizine hydrochloride
Desloratadine
Fexofenadine hydrochloride
Levocetirizine
Loratidine

OPHTHALMIC ANTIHISTAMINES:
Emedastine difumarate
Epinastine hydrochloride*
Levocabastine hydrochloride*
Olapatidine hydrochloride*

Drugs marked with an * are available to view in the online database at www.delmarnursesdrughandbook.com/2009.

USES

PO: (1) Vasomotor, perennial, or seasonal allergic rhinitis and allergic conjunctivitis. (2) Angioedema, urticarial transfusion reactions, urticaria, pruritus. (3) Atopic dermatitis, contact dermatitis, pruritus ani, pruritus vulvae, insect bites. (4) Sneezing and rhinorrhea due to the common cold. (5) Anaphylactic reactions. (6) Parkinsonism, drug-induced extrapyramidal reactions. (7) Vertigo. (8) Prophylaxis and treatment of motion sickness, including N&V. (9) Nighttime sleep aid.

Parenteral: (1) Relief of allergic reactions due to blood or plasma. (2) Adjunct to epinephrine in treating anaphylaxis. (3) Uncomplicated allergic conditions when PO therapy is not possible.

ACTION/KINETICS

Action

Compete with histamine at H₁ histamine receptors (reversible competitive inhibition), thus preventing or reversing the effects of histamine. First-generation antihistamines bind to central and peripheral H₁ receptors and can cause CNS depression or stimulation. Second-generation antihistamines are selective for peripheral H_1 receptors and cause less sedation. Antihistamines do not prevent the release of histamine, antibody production, or antigen-antibody interactions. Antihistamines prevent or reduce increased capillary permeability (i.e., decrease edema, itching) and bronchospasms. Allergic reactions unrelated to histamine release are not affected by antihistamines. Certain of the first-generation antihistamines also have anticholinergic, antiemetic, antipruritic, or antiserotonin effects. Clients unresponsive to a certain antihistamine may regain sensitivity by switching to a different antihistamine. From a chemical point of view, the antihistamines can be divided into the following classes.

FIRST GENERATION:

1. **Alkylamines.** Among the most potent antihistamines. Minimal sedation, moderate anticholinergic effects, and no antiemetic effects. Paradoxical excitation may also occur. Examples: Brompheniramine, chlorpheniramine, dexchlorpheniramine.

2. **Ethanolamine Derivatives.** Moderate to high sedative, anticholinergic, and antiemetic effects. Low incidence of GI side effects. Examples: Clemastine, diphenhydramine.

3. **Phenothiazines.** High antihistaminic, sedative, and anticholinergic effects; very high antiemetic effect. Example: Promethazine.

4. **Piperazine.** High antihistaminic, sedative, and antiemetic effects; moderate anticholinergic effects. Example: Hydroxyzine.

5. **Piperidines.** Moderate antihistaminic and anticholinergic effects; low to moderate sedation; no antiemetic effects. Examples: Azatadine, cyproheptadine, phenindamine.

SECOND GENERATION:

1. **Phthalazinone.** High antihistaminic effect; low to no sedative and anticholinergic effects; no antiemetic effect. Example: Azelastine.

2. **Piperazine.** Moderate to high antihistaminic effect; low to no sedation or anticholinergic effects; no antiemetic activity. Example: Cetirizine, Levocetirizine.

3. **Piperidines.** Moderate to high antihistaminic activity; low to no sedation and anticholinergic activity; no antiemetic action. Examples: Desloratadine, fexofenadine, loratidine.

Pharmacokinetics

The kinetics of most first-generation antihistamines are similar. **Onset:** 15–30 min; **peak:** 1–2 hr; **duration:** 4–6 hr (piperidines have a longer duration). Many antihistamines are available as timed-release preparations. Most first-generation antihistamines are metabolized by the liver and excreted in the urine. The pharmacokinetics of the second-generation antihistamines vary; consult individual drugs.

CONTRAINDICATIONS

First-generation antihistamines. Hypersensitivity to the drug. Pregnancy or possibility thereof (some agents), lactation, premature and newborn infants, use with MAO inhibitors. The phenothiazine-type antihistamines are contraindicated in CNS depression from any cause, bone marrow depression, jaundice, dehydrated or acutely ill children, and in comatose clients. Use to treat lower respiratory tract symptoms such as asthma, emphysema, chronic bronchitis (due to anticholinergic effects that may thicken secretions and impair expectoration).

Second-generation antihistamines. Hypersensitivity to specific or chemically-related antihistamines.

SPECIAL CONCERNS

Antihistamines have varying degrees of atropine-like effects; use with caution in those with a predisposition to urinary retention, history of bronchial asthma, increased intraocular pressure, hyperthyroidism, CV disease, or hypertension.

Also, use with caution in clients with convulsive disorders, respiratory disease, narrow-angle glaucoma, stenosing peptic ulcer, pyloroduodenal obstruction, symptomatic prostatic hypertrophy, bladder neck obstruction. Use phenothiazine antihistamines with caution in clients with CV disease, liver dysfunction, narrow-angle glaucoma, pros-

---

Bold Italic = life threatening side effect   ■ = black box warning   ♣ = Available in Canada

tatic hypertrophy, stenosing peptic ulcer, pyloroduodenal obstruction, and bladder-neck obstruction. May diminish mental alertness in children and may occasionally cause excitation; larger doses may cause hallucinations, convulsions, and death in infants and children. Use in geriatric clients may result in dizziness, excessive sedation, syncope, toxic confusional states, and hypotension.

SIDE EFFECTS

SYSTEMIC. CNS: Sedation ranging from mild drowsiness to deep sleep. Dizziness, incoordination, faintness, fatigue, confusion, lassitude, restlessness, excitation, nervousness, tremor, ***tonic-clonic seizures,*** headache, irritability, insomnia, euphoria, paresthesias, oculogyric crisis, torticollis, catatonic-like states, hallucinations, disorientation, tongue protrusion (usually with IV use or overdosage), disturbing dreams, nightmares, pseudoschizophrenia, weakness, diplopia, vertigo, hysteria, neuritis, paradoxical excitation, epileptiform seizures in clients with focal lesions. Extrapyramidal reactions include opisthotonus, dystonia, akathisia, dyskinesia, and parkinsonism. **CV:** Postural hypotension, palpitations, bradycardia, tachycardia, reflex tachycardia, extrasystoles, increased or decreased BP, ECG changes (including blunting of T waves and prolongation of the Q-T interval), ***cardiac arrest.*** **GI:** Epigastric distress, anorexia, increased appetite and weight gain, N&V, diarrhea, constipation, change in bowel habits, stomatitis. **GU:** Urinary frequency, dysuria, urinary retention, gynecomastia, inhibition of ejaculation, decreased libido, impotence, early menses, induction of lactation. **Hematologic:** Hypoplastic anemia, ***aplastic anemia, hemolytic anemia,*** thrombocytopenia, leukopenia, pancytopenia, ***agranulocytosis,*** thrombocytopenic purpura. **Respiratory:** Thickening of bronchial secretions, wheezing, nasal stuffiness, chest tightness, sore throat, ***respiratory depression;*** dry mouth, nose, and throat. **Ophthalmic:** Blurred vision, diplopia. **Miscellaneous:** Tinnitus, photosensitivity, hypersensitivity reactions, acute labyrinthitis, ob-structive jaundice, erythema, high or prolonged glucose tolerance curves, glycosuria, elevated spinal fluid proteins, increased plasma cholesterol, increased perspiration, chills; tingling, heaviness, and weakness of the hands.

TOPICAL. Prolonged use may result in local irritation and allergic contact dermatitis.

NASAL SPRAY. GI: Glossitis, ulcerative and aphthous stomatitis, bitter taste, epistaxis, paroxysmal sneezing, rhinitis, conjunctivitis, eye abnormality, eye pain, nasal burning, taste loss, watery eyes, temporomandibular dislocation.

OD OVERDOSE MANAGEMENT

Symptoms (Acute Toxicity): Although antihistamines have a wide therapeutic range, overdosage can nevertheless be fatal. Children are particularly susceptible. Early toxic effects may be seen within 30–120 min and include drowsiness, dizziness, blurred vision, tinnitus, ataxia, and hypotension. Symptoms range from CNS depression (sedation, ***coma,*** decreased mental alertness) to ***CV collapse*** and CNS stimulation (insomnia, hallucinations, tremors, or ***seizures***). Also, ***profound hypotension, respiratory depression, coma, and death*** may occur. Anticholinergic effects include flushing, dry mouth, hypotension, fever, ***hyperthermia*** (especially in children), and fixed, dilated pupils. Body temperature may be as high as 107°F. In children, symptoms include hallucinations, toxic psychosis, delirum tremens, ataxia, incoordination, muscle twitching, excitement, athetosis, ***hyperthermia, seizures,*** and hyperreflexia followed by postictal depression and ***cardiorespiratory arrest.***
Treatment:

- Treat symptoms and provide supportive care.
- Administer a slurry of activated charcoal and a cathartic. Gastric lavage within 3 hr after ingestion and even later if large amounts were taken.
- Hypotension can be treated with a vasopressor such as norepinephrine, dopamine, or phenylephrine (do not use epinephrine).

Classifications

- For convulsions, use only short-acting depressants (e.g., diazepam). IV physostigmine can be used to treat centrally mediated convulsions.
- Ice packs and a cool sponge bath are effective in reducing fever in children.
- Take precautions to protect against aspiration, especially in infants and children.
- Severe cases of overdose can be treated by hemoperfusion.

DRUG INTERACTIONS
SEE ALSO *DRUG INTERACTIONS* FOR *PHENOTHIAZINES.*
Alcohol, ethyl / See *CNS depressants*
Antidepressants, tricyclic / Additive anticholinergic side effects
CNS depressants, antianxiety agents, barbiturates, narcotics, phenothiazines, procarbazine, sedative-hypnotics / Potentiation or addition of CNS depressant effects. Concomitant use may lead to drowsiness, lethargy, stupor, respiratory depression, coma, and possibly death.
H *Henbane leaf* / Enhanced anticholinergic effects
Heparin / Antihistamines may ↓ the anticoagulant effects
MAO inhibitors / Intensification and prolongation of anticholinergic and sedative side effects; use with phenothiazine antihistamine → hypotension and extrapyramidal reactions.

LABORATORY TEST CONSIDERATIONS
Discontinue antihistamines 4 days before skin testing to avoid false-negative result.

DOSAGE
- **Usually PO**
Parenteral administration is seldom used because of irritating nature of drugs. Topical usage is also limited because antihistamines often cause hypersensitivity reactions. When given for motion sickness, antihistamines are usually given 30–60 min before anticipated travel. See individual drugs.

NURSING CONSIDERATIONS

ADMINISTRATION/STORAGE
1. Inject IM preparations deep into the muscle; irritating to tissues.

2. Swallow sustained-release preparations whole. May break scored tablets before swallowing. If difficulty swallowing capsules, may open and put contents into soft food for ingestion.
3. Do not apply topical preparations to raw, blistered, or oozing areas of the skin.
4. Do not apply to the eyes, around the genitalia, or to mucous membranes.

ASSESSMENT
1. Note any drug sensitivity; identify known allergens and all medications prescribed. Avoid with ulcers, glaucoma, or pregnancy.
2. List type, onset, characteristics of symptoms; note triggers. Stop antihistamines 2–4 days prior to skin testing to avoid false negative results.
3. Monitor VS, I&O, CV status, lung sounds/status and characteristics of secretions. Determine any urinary retention, frequency or pain.
4. Describe extent and characteristics of any rash, if present. Monitor CBC with long term therapy; hemolytic anemia may rarely occur.

CLIENT/FAMILY TEACHING
1. Take before or at the onset of symptoms; cannot reverse reactions but may prevent them. Oral products may cause gastric irritation; administer with meals, milk, or a snack.
2. Do not drive or operate equipment until drug effects realized or drowsiness wears off. Sedative effects may disappear after several days or may not occur at all.
3. For motion sickness, take 30-60 min before travel time. May alter skin testing results; stop several days before anticipated testing.
4. Report sore throat, fever, unexplained bruising, bleeding, or petechiae; may cause blood dyscrasia.
5. May cause sensitivity to sun or ultraviolet light; avoid long exposures, use sunscreen, sunglasses, and protective clothing when exposed.
6. Severe CNS depression is a symptom of overdosage. Report dizziness or weakness; avoid other CNS depressants.
7. Reduce symptoms of dry mouth by frequent rinsing with warm water, good

---

Bold Italic = life threatening side effect   ■ = black box warning   ♣ = Available in Canada

oral hygiene, and sugarless gum or candies. Avoid overuse of mouthwash as it may destroy normal flora and worsen dryness.

8. Ensure adequate hydration. If bronchial secretions are thick, increase fluids and humidify air to decrease secretion viscosity; avoid milk temporarily. If problems with urination, void prior to taking the drug.

9. Exercise regularly; consume 2 L fluids/day and fruits, fruit juices, and dietary fiber to prevent constipation. Use stool softeners as needed.

10. Recurrent reactions may be referred to an allergist. Protect self from exposure and create an allergen-free living area.

11. Antihistamines raise BP, use with high BP only if medically supervised. Avoid Alcohol or OTC agents without approval.

12. Children may manifest excitation rather than sedation. Clinical effectiveness may diminish with continued usage; switching to another class may restore drug effectiveness.

13. To ensure accurate skin testing, stop agent 4 days prior to testing.

14. Family/significant other should learn CPR; survival is greatly increased when CPR is initiated immediately.

OUTCOMES/EVALUATE

- ↓ Frequency/intensity of allergic manifestations; ↓ itching/swelling
- Prevention of motion sickness
- Effective nighttime sedation

ANTIHYPERLIPIDEMIC AGENTS—HMG-COA REDUCTASE INHIBITORS

SEE ALSO THE FOLLOWING INDIVIDUAL ENTRIES:

Atorvastatin calcium
Fluvastatin sodium
Lovastatin
Pravastatin sodium
Rosuvastatin calcium
Simvastatin

GENERAL STATEMENT

The National Cholesterol Education Program Expert Panel on Detection, Evaluation, and Treatment of High Blood Cholesterol in Adults has developed guidelines for the treatment of high cholesterol and LDL in adults. High risk clients are defined as those with a greater than 20% risk for cardiovascular heart disease in the next 10 years. Cardiovascular heart disease includes a history of MI, unstable and stable angina, angioplasty, cardiac bypass surgery, or evidence of clinically significant myocardial ischemia. Risk factors include cigarette smoking, hypertension, low high-density lipoprotein cholesterol (HDL-C) less than 40 mg/dL, family history of premature cardiovascular heart disease, and gender (men more than 45 years of age; women greater than 55 years of age). Moderately high-risk clients have two or more risk factors and a 10-20% risk for cardiovascular heart disease in the next 10 years. A client with moderate risk also has two or more risk factors, but the 10-year cardiovascular heart disease risk is less than 10%. A low risk person has 0-1 risk factor with a ten-year cardiovascular heart disease risk at less than 10%.

The goals for treatment are as follows:

1. For high-risk clients with LDL-C >100 mg/dL, an LDL-lowering drug is indicated along with therapeutic lifestyle changes. The threshold for LDL-lowering therapy has been lowered from >130 mg/dL, with drug therapy now optional for LDL-C levels between 100–129 mg/dL. Also, in high-risk clients with a pretreatment LDL-C of >100 mg/dL, initiation of an LDL-lowering drug to reach a treatment goal of <70 mg/dL is considered as an evidence-based therapeutic option.

2. For high-risk clients with high triglycerides or low LDL-C, it is recommended adding a fibrate or nicotonic acid to an LDL-lowering drug regimen. When triglycerides are >200 mg/dL, non-HDL-C is a secondary target of therapy, with a goal of 30 mg/dL higher than the previously identified LDL-C goal.

3. For moderately-high risk clients, an LDL-C treatment goal of <130 mg/dL is still recommended. However, a treat-

---

ment goal of LDL <100 mg/dL is considered an evidence-based therapeutic option. If the LDL is >130 mg/dL, therapeutic lifestyle changes should be started. If the LDL level remains >130 mg/dL after implementation of therapeutic lifestyle changes, initiation of LDL-lowering drug therapy should be considered to achieve and sustain an LDL-C goal of <130 mg/dL. For those with an LDL level between 100–129 mg/dL, at baseline or after therapeutic lifestyle change implementation, beginning LDL-lowering drug therapy to reach an LDL level of <100 mg/dL is a therapeutic option.

4. For clients at moderately high or high risk, LDL-lowering drug therapy, if used, should achieve at least a 30–40% reduction in LDL-C levels. Therapeutic lifestyle changes should also be started, regardless of the clients' LDL level, if the client has lifestyle related risk factors, such as obesity, physical inactivity, elevated triglycerides, low LDL, or metabolic syndrome.

USES
See individual drugs. Uses include: (1) Heterozygous familial hypercholesterolemia in adolescents. (2) Homozygous familial hyperlipidemia. (3) Hypertriglyceridemia, including Fredrickson type IV. Not indicated in such clients with low or normal LDL, despite elevated total cholesterol. (4) Mixed dyslipidemia, including Fredrickson types IIa and IIb. (5) Primary dysbetalipoproteinemia, including Fredrickson type III. (6) Primary hypercholesterolemia, including heterozygous familial and nonfamilial hypercholesterolemia. (7) Primary prevention of coronary events. (8) Secondary prevention of CV events. *Investigational:* Treatment of osteoporosis. Lower risk of developing type 2 diabetes and stroke when taken to reduce cholesterol. Lower cholesterol in women.

ACTION/KINETICS
Action
The HMG-CoA reductase inhibitors competitively inhibit HMG-CoA reductase; this enzyme catalyzes the early rate-limiting step in the synthesis of cholesterol. HMG-CoA reductase inhibi-

tors increase HDL cholesterol and decrease LDL cholesterol, total cholesterol, apolipoprotein B, VLDL cholesterol, and plasma triglycerides. The mechanism to lower LDL cholesterol may be due to both a decrease in VLDL cholesterol levels and induction of the LDL receptor, leading to reduced production or increased catabolism of LDL cholesterol. The maximum therapeutic response is seen in 4–6 weeks. Statins may help prevent infections in clients with diabetes. Statins cause a significant reduction in CV events.

CONTRAINDICATIONS
Active liver disease or unexplained persistent elevated liver function tests. Pregnancy, lactation. Use in children.

SPECIAL CONCERNS
Use with caution in those who ingest large quantities of alcohol or who have a history of liver disease. May cause photosensitivity. Safety and efficacy have not been established in children less than 18 years of age.

SIDE EFFECTS
The following side effects have been reported for HMG-CoA reductase inhibitors. Also see individual drugs. **GI:** N&V, diarrhea, constipation, abdominal cramps or pain, flatulence, dyspepsia, heartburn. Anorexia, biliary pain, cheilitis, cholestatic jaundice, cirrhosis, colitis, duodenal ulcer, dysphagia, enteritis, eructation, eosphagitis, fatty changes in liver, ***fulminant hepatic necrosis***, gastritis, glossitis, gum hemorrhage, ***hemorrhage***, hepatitis (including chronic active hepatitis), hepatoma, increased appetite, melena, pancreatitis, periodontal abscess, rectal mouth ulceration, stomach ulcer, stomatitis, tenesmus, ulcerative stomach. **CNS:** Headache, dizziness, dysfunction of certain cranial nerves (e.g., alteration of taste, facial paresis, impairment of extraocular movement), tremor, vertigo, memory loss, paresthesia, anxiety, insomnia, depression, mental decline, aggressive behavior, ***suicide attempts***. Abnormal dreams, emotional lability, hyperkinesia, hypertonia, hypesthesia, incoordination, migraine, peripheral nerve palsy, peripheral neuropathy, psychic distur-

---

bances, somnolence, torticollis. **CV:** Cardiac chest pain, angina pectoris, arrhythmia, palpitations, phlebitis, postural hypotension, syncope, vasodilation. **Dermatologic:** Acne, rash, alopecia, contact dermatitis, eczema, seborrhea, skin ulcer, pruritus, sweating, urticaria, skin nodules/discoloration, dryness of skin/mucous membranes, changes in hair/nails. **Musculoskeletal:** Localized pain, bursitis, myalgia, muscle cramps or pain, myopathy, rhabdomyolysis, arthralgia, myasthenia, myopathy, myositis, pathological fracture, neck rigidity/pain, pelvic pain. **Respiratory:** URI, rhinitis, cough, asthma, dyspnea, epistaxis, pneumonia. **GU:** Abnormal ejaculation, albuminuria, breast enlargement, cystitis, dysuria, epididymitis, erectile dysfunction, fibrocystic breast, gynecomastia, hematuria, impotence, kidney calculus, loss of libido, metorrhagia, nocturia, nephritis, renal failure, urinary frequency, incontinence, urinary retention/urgency, vaginal or uterine hemorrhage. **Hematologic:** Anemia, ecchymosis, lymphadenopathy, petechiae, thrombocytopenia. **Metabolic:** Diabetes mellitus, gout, hyperglycemia, hypoglycemia, weight gain. **Ophthalmic:** Progression of cataracts (lens opacities), ophthalmoplegia, amblyopia, dry eyes, eye hemorrhage, glaucoma. **Otic:** Deafness, tinnitus. **Hypersensitivity: *Anaphylaxis, angioedema,*** vasculitis, purpura, thrombocytopenia, leukopenia, ***hemolytic anemia,*** lupus erythematosus-like syndrome, polymyalgia rheumatica, positive ANA, ESR increase, arthritis, arthralgia, eosinophilia, urticaria, photosensitivity, fever, chills, flushing, malaise, dyspnea, ***toxic dermal necrolysis, Stevens-Johnson syndrome.*** **Body as a whole:** Fatigue, influenza, edema, fever, malaise, generalized edema, photosensitivity reaction. **Miscellaneous:** Parosmia, taste loss/perversion, facial edema.

DRUG INTERACTIONS

See also individual drugs. *NOTE:* Drugs that are inhibitors of P450 enzymes (especially CYP3A4) increase serum levels of several HMG-CoA reductase inhibitors.

Amiodarone / ↑ Levels of HMG-CoA inhibitors R/T ↓ metabolism → ↑ risk of rhambomyolysis

Antifungals, Azole (e.g., itraconazole, ketoconazole) / ↑ Levels of HMG-CoA inhibitors R/T ↓ metabolism; may ↑ risk of rhambomyolysis

Clarithromycin / ↑ Levels of HMG-CoA inhibitors R/T ↓ metabolism → ↑ risk of rhambomyolysis

Clopidogrel / ↓ Clopidogrel effects on platelet function with atorvastatin or simvastatin

Cyclosporine / ↑ Risk of severe myopathy or rhabdomyolysis

Digoxin / Slight ↑ in digoxin levels

Diltiazem / ↑ Levels of HMG-CoA inhibitors R/T ↓ metabolism → ↑ risk of rhambomyolysis

Erythromycin / ↑ Risk of severe myopathy or rhabdomyolysis R/T ↓ metabolism of the statin

Gemfibrozil / ↑ Plasma levels of statins → possibility of severe myopathy or rhabdomyolysis

Grapefruit juice / Possible ↑ AUC, C_{max}, and elimination t ½ of certain HMG-CoA reductase inhibitors → ↑ risk of rhambomyolysis

Itraconazole / ↑ Levels of HMG-CoA inhibitors

Nefazodone / ↑ Levels of HMG-CoA inhibitors R/T ↓ metabolism → ↑ risk of rhambomyolysis

Niacin, Nicotinic acid / Possibility of myopathy or severe rhabdomyolysis

Propranolol / ↓ Antihyperlipidemic activity

Protease inhibitors / ↑ Levels of HMG-CoA inhibitors R/T ↓ metabolism

Verapamil / ↑ Levels of HMG-CoA inhibitors R/T ↓ metabolism → ↑ risk of rhambomyolysis

Warfarin / ↑ Anticoagulant effect of warfarin.

LABORATORY TEST CONSIDERATIONS

↑ AST, ALT, CPK, alkaline phosphatase, bilirubin, gamma-glutamyl transpeptidase. Abnormal thyroid and liver function tests.

DOSAGE

See individual drugs.

Classifications

NURSING CONSIDERATIONS

ADMINISTRATION/STORAGE

1. Lovastatin should be taken with meals; fluvastatin, pravastatin, and simavastatin may be taken without regard to meals.

2. Step-down therapy (e.g., pravastatin) may decrease medication effectiveness.

ASSESSMENT

1. Review lifestyle, risk factors, attempts to control with diet, exercise, and weight reduction. Also review PMH, ROS, and physical exam; document risk factors. List other drugs trialed and drugs prescribed to ensure no adverse effects.

2. Note any alcohol abuse or liver disease. Monitor LFTs as recommended. Transaminase levels 3 times normal may precipitate severe hepatic toxicity. If CK elevated, assess renal function as rhabdomyolsis with myoglobinuria could cause renal shutdown. Stop drug therapy and clearly mark chart and advise client not to take.

3. Note nutritional analysis by dietitian; assess cholesterol profile (HDL, LDL, cholesterol, and triglycerides) after 3–6 months of exercise and diet therapy if risk factors do not require immediate drug therapy. With diabetes and coronary heart disease a more aggressive drug approach should be instituted in addition to diet therapy with goals of reducing LDL way below 100.

CLIENT/FAMILY TEACHING

1. Take only as directed. Drug is used to lower cholesterol levels and stabilize plaques in order to prevent CAD and control coronary risk factors.

2. Report any pain in skeletal muscles or unexplained muscle pain, tenderness, or weakness promptly, especially with fever or malaise. Stop drug with any major trauma, surgery, or serious illness.

3. May cause photosensitivity; avoid prolonged sun or UV light exposure. Use sunscreens, sunglasses, and protective clothing when exposed.

4. Continue life-style modifications that include low-fat, low-cholesterol, and low-sodium diets, weight reduction with obese clients, smoking cessation, reduction of alcohol consumption, and regular aerobic exercise in the overall goal of cholesterol reduction.

5. Avoid OTC agents. May use niaspan (SR form of niacin) with careful monitoring. Use a fibrate cautiously; lower statin dose is used and LFTs monitored. Report regularly for labs to prevent liver toxicity and to assess drug response.

OUTCOMES/EVALUATE

• ↓ LDL, triglycerides, and total cholesterol levels; ↓ risk of placque rupture and death

ANTIHYPERTENSIVE AGENTS

SEE ALSO THE FOLLOWING DRUG CLASSES AND INDIVIDUAL DRUGS:

Agents Acting Directly on Vascular Smooth Muscle
Diazoxide IV
Nitroprusside sodium

Alpha-1-Adrenergic Blocking Agents
Alfuzosin hydrochloride
Doxazosin mesylate
Prazosin hydrochloride
Tamsulosin hydrochloride*
Terazosin

Angiotensin-II Receptor Blockers
Candesartan cilexetil
Eprosartan mesylate
Irbesartan
Losartan potassium
Olmesartan medoxomil
Telmisartan
Valsartan

Angiotensin-Converting Enzyme Inhibitors
Benazepril hydrochloride
Captopril
Enalapril maleate
Fosinopril sodium
Lisinopril
Moexipril hydrochloride*
Perindopril erbumine*
Quinapril hydrochloride
Ramipril
Trandolapril

Bold Italic = life threatening side effect   ■ = black box warning   ✦ = Available in Canada

Beta-Adrenergic Blocking Agents
Atenolol
Betaxolol hydrochloride
Bisoprolol fumarate
Metoprolol succinate
Metoprolol tartrate
Nadolol
Nebivolol
Penbutolol sulfate
Propranolol hydrochloride
Timolol maleate

Calcium Channel Blocking Agents
Amlodipine
Bepridil hydrochloride*
Diltiazem hydrochloride
Felodipine
Isradipine
Nicardipine hydrochloride
Nifedipine
Nimodipine
Nisoldipine
Verapamil

Centrally-Acting Agents
Clonidine hydrochloride
Guanfacine hydrochloride
Methyldopa
Methyldopate hydrochloride

Combination Drugs Used for Hypertension
Amlodipine/Benazepril
  hydrochloride
Atenolol/Chlorthalidone
Bisoprolol fumarate/
  Hydrochlorothiazide
Irbesartan/Hydrochlorothiazide
Lisinopril/Hydrochlorothiazide
Losartan potassium/
  Hydrochlorothiazide
Olmesartan medoxomil/
  Hydrochlorothiazide
Triamterene/Hydrochlorothiazide
Valsartan/Hydrochlorothiazide

Miscellaneous Agents
Aliskiren
Ambrisentan
Bosentan
Carvedilol
Epoprostenol sodium
Labetalol hydrochloride
Minoxidil, oral

Drugs marked with an * are available to view in the online database at www.delmarnursesdrughandbook.com/2009.

GENERAL STATEMENT
The Seventh Report of the Joint National Committee on Prevention, Detection, Evaluation and Treatment of High Blood Pressure classifies BP for adults aged 18 and over as follows: **Normal** as <120/<80 mm Hg, **Prehypertension** as 120–139/80–89 mm Hg, **Stage 1 Hypertension** as 140–159/90–99 mm Hg, and **Stage 2 Hypertension** as > or equal to 160/> or equal to 100 mm Hg. Drug therapy is recommended depending on the BP and whether certain risk factors (e.g., smoking, dyslipidemia, diabetes, age, gender, target organ damage, clinical CV disease) are present. Lifestyle modification is an important component of treating hypertension, including weight reduction, diet, reduction of sodium intake, aerobic physical exercise, cessation of smoking, and moderate alcohol intake.

The risk of cardiovascular disease begins to increase when either the SPB exceeds 115 mm Hg or the DBP is greater than 75 mm Hg. Beyond 115/75 the risk of CV disease doubles with each advance of 20/10 mm Hg. In clients over 50 years of age, SBPs greater than 140 mm Hg are more important determinants of CV disease than are elevated DBPs. Generally speaking, the primary agents for initial monotherapy of Stage 1 hypertension to treat uncomplicated hypertension are thiazide diuretics; one may also consider ACE inhibitors, angiotensin receptor blockers, calcium channel blockers, and beta-adrenergic blocking agents. It should be noted that diet, exercise, and other life modifications are often sufficient to prevent or reduce hypertension. To treat Stage 2 hypertension, two drug combinations should be considered, i.e., usually a thiazide diuretic and an ACE inhibitor, or angiotensin receptor blocker, or a beta blocker, or a calcium channel blocker.

= see color insert   H = Herbal   IV = Intravenous   = sound alike drug

DRUG INTERACTIONS
See Individual Drugs.

H *Black cohosh* / May potentiate antihypertensive drugs.

H *Garlic* / May potentiate antihypertensive drugs.

H *Hawthorn* / Cardioactive, hypotensive, and coronary vasodilator action of hawthorn may affect antihypertensive effect; monitor.

NURSING CONSIDERATIONS

ASSESSMENT
1. Note reasons for therapy, other agents trialed, family history of hypertension, stroke, CVD, CHD, MI, dyslipidemia, diabetes.
2. Assess baseline pulse rate, and BP before starting antihypertensive therapy. To ensure accuracy of baseline readings, take BP in both (bared and supported) arms (lying, standing, and sitting) 2 min apart (30 min after last cigarette or caffeine consumption) at least three times during one visit and on two subsequent visits. Document BMI (body mass index), height, weight and risk factors.
3. Ascertain life-style modifications (weight reduction, ↓ alcohol intake, regular exercise, reduced sodium/fat intake, stress reduction, and smoking cessation) needed to achieve lowered BP. Offer a trial following these modifications and reassess in 3 months before starting therapy unless BP in severe range or >2 risk factors.
4. Monitor ECG, electrolytes, CBC, uric acid, urinalysis, lipid panel, LFTs; always check for proteinuria.
5. Note funduscopic and neurologic exam findings. Assess for thyroid enlargement and presence of target organ damage. If difficult to control, assess for renal artery stenosis or secondary causes of HTN and refer for 24-hr ambulatory BP monitoring.

CLIENT/FAMILY TEACHING
1. Drugs control but do not cure hypertension. Take medications despite feeling fine and do not stop abruptly; may cause rebound hypertension. Drugs only provide protection/control of BP for the day in which they are taken.

They must be taken daily as prescribed to ensure control. If dose missed, do not double up or take two doses close together.
2. Avoid activities that require mental alertness until drug effects realized.
3. There are generally no S&S of high blood pressure. When S&S become evident is when organ damage has already occurred. Keep a record of BP readings at different times during the day and evening to share with provider.
4. Adhere to a low-sodium, low-fat diet; see dietitian as needed for education, meal planning, and food selections. Avoid excessive amounts of caffeine (tea, coffee, chocolate, or colas).
5. Weakness, dizziness, and fainting may occur with rapid changes of position from lying to standing (postural hypotension). Rise slowly from a lying or sitting position and dangle legs for several minutes before standing to minimize low BP effects. Exercising in hot weather may worsen these effects. Do not become dehydrated.
6. Report any swelling in hands or feet, sudden weight gain, increased SOB, chest pain, or changes in urination, i.e., pain, frequency or reduced amounts. Have yearly eye exams to detect early retinal changes from ↑ BP.
7. Avoid agents that may lower BP (e.g., alcohol, barbiturates, CNS depressants) or that could elevate BP (e.g., OTC cold remedies, oral contraceptives, steroids, NSAIDs, appetite suppressants, tricyclic antidepressants, MAO inhibitors). Sympathomimetic amines in products used to treat asthma, colds, and allergies must be used with extreme caution
8. Report if sexual dysfunction occurs as medication can usually be changed to minimize symptoms or other options for sexual dysfunction explored.
9. Identify holistic interventions/lifestyle modifications necessary for BP control: dietary restrictions of fat and sodium (2–3 grams/day), weight reduction, ↓ alcohol (i.e., less than 24 oz beer or less than 8 oz of wine or less than 2 oz of 100-proof whiskey per day), tobacco cessation, ↑ physical ac-

---

tivity, regular exercise programs, proper rest, and methods to reduce and deal with stress.

10. Keep all F/U visits to assess BP and labs; keep log of BP and HR for provider review.

OUTCOMES/EVALUATE

- Understanding of disease/compliance with prescribed therapy
- ↓ BP (SBP <130 and DBP <80 mm Hg)
- Control/prevent target organ damage, stroke, MI, and/or death

ANTI-INFECTIVE DRUGS

SEE ALSO THE FOLLOWING INDIVIDUAL DRUGS AND DRUG CLASSES:

Aminoglycosides
Antiviral Drugs
Bacitracin
Becaplermin
Butenafine hydrochloride
Cephalosporins
Chloramphenicol
Chloroquine hydrochloride
Chloroquine phosphate
Daptomycin
Drotrecogin alfa
Erythromycins
Fluoroquinolones
Imipenem-Cilastatin sodium
Macrolides
Penicillins
Pentamidine isethionate
Praziquantel
Pyrantel pamoate
Quinupristin/Dalfopristin
Sulfonamides
Telithromycin
Tetracyclines
Thiabendazole
Tigecycline
Vancomycin hydrochloride

GENERAL STATEMENT

The following general guidelines apply to the use of most anti-infective drugs:

1. Anti-infective drugs can be divided into those that are *bacteriostatic,* that is, arrest the multiplication and further development of the infectious agent, or *bactericidal,* that is, kill and thus eradicate all living microorganisms. Both time of administration and length of therapy may be affected by this difference.

2. Some anti-infectives halt the growth of or eradicate many different microorganisms and are termed *broad-spectrum antibiotics.* Others affect only certain specific organisms and are termed *narrow-spectrum antibiotics.*

3. Some of the anti-infectives elicit a hypersensitivity reaction in some persons. Penicillins cause more severe and more frequent hypersensitivity reactions than any other drug.

4. Because of differences in susceptibility of infectious agents to anti-infectives, the sensitivity of the microorganism to the drug ordered should be determined before treatment is initiated. Several sensitivity tests are commonly used for this purpose.

5. Certain anti-infective agents have marked side effects, some of the more serious of which are neurotoxicity, including ototoxicity, and nephrotoxicity. Care must be taken not to administer two anti-infectives with similar side effects concomitantly, or to administer these drugs to clients in whom the side effects might be damaging (e.g., a nephrotoxic drug to a client suffering from kidney disease). The choice of anti-infective also depends on its distribution in the body (i.e., whether it passes the blood-brain barrier).

6. Anti-infective drugs can also eradicate the normal intestinal flora necessary for proper digestion, synthesis of vitamin K, and control of fungi that may gain access to the GI tract (superinfection).

USES

See individual drugs. The choice of the anti-infective depends on the nature of the illness to be treated, the sensitivity of the infecting agent, and the client's previous experience with the drug. Hypersensitivity and allergic reactions may preclude the use of the agent of choice. Labeling advises providers to prescribe antibiotics only to treat infections thought to be caused by bacteria and

---

to counsel clients on the proper use of these drugs.

ACTION/KINETICS

Action

The mechanism of action of the anti-infectives varies. The following modes of action have been identified.* Note the considerable overlap among these mechanisms:

1. Inhibition of synthesis of or activation of enzymes that disrupt bacterial cell walls leading to loss of viability and possibly cell lysis (e.g., penicillins, cephalosporins, cycloserine, bacitracin, vancomycin, miconazole, ketoconazole, clotrimazole).

2. Direct effect on the microbial cell membrane to affect permeability and leading to leakage of intracellular components (e.g., polymyxin, colistimethate, nystatin, amphotericin).

3. Effect on the function of 30S and 50S bacterial ribosomes to cause a reversible inhibition of protein synthesis (e.g., chloramphenicol, tetracyclines, erythromycin, clindamycin).

4. Bind to the 30S ribosomal subunit that alters protein synthesis and leads to cell death (e.g., aminoglycosides).

5. Effect on bacterial nucleic acid metabolism which inhibits DNA-dependent RNA polymerase (e.g., rifampin) or inhibition of gyrase (e.g., fluoroquinolones).

6. Antimetabolites that block essential enzymes of folate metabolism.

7. Antiviral drugs that halt viral replication. Classes include (a) nucleic acid analogs such as acyclovir or gancyclovir that selectively inhibit viral DNA polymerase; (b) nucleic acid analogs such as lamivudine or zidovudine, that inhibit reverse transcriptase; (c) nonnucleoside reverse transcriptase inhibitors, such as efavirenz or nevirapine; and, (d) inhibitors of HIV protease or influenza neuraminidase.

CONTRAINDICATIONS

Hypersensitivity or allergies to the drug.

SIDE EFFECTS

The antibiotics and anti-infective agents have few direct toxic effects. Kidney and liver damage, deafness, and blood dyscrasias are occasionally observed.

The following undesirable manifestations, however, occur frequently: (1) Suppression of the normal flora of the body, which in turn keeps certain pathogenic microorganisms, such as *Candida albicans, Proteus,* or *Pseudomonas,* from causing infections. If the flora is altered, superinfections (monilial vaginitis, enteritis, UTIs), which necessitate the discontinuation of therapy or the use of other antibiotics, can result. (2) Incomplete eradication of an infectious organism. Casual use of anti-infectives favors the emergence of *resistant* strains insensitive to a particular drug. To minimize the chances for the development of resistant strains, anti-infectives are usually given at specified doses for a prescribed length of time after acute symptoms have subsided.

OD OVERDOSE MANAGEMENT

Treatment: Discontinue the drug and treat symptomatically. Supportive measures should be instituted as needed. Hemodialysis may be used although its effectiveness is questionable, depending on the drug and the status of the client (i.e., more effective in impaired renal function).

LABORATORY TEST CONSIDERATIONS

The bacteriologic sensitivity of the infectious organism to the anti-infective (especially the antibiotic) should be tested by the lab before initiation of therapy and during treatment.

GENERAL NURSING CONSIDERATIONS FOR ALL ANTI-INFECTIVES

ADMINISTRATION/STORAGE

1. Check expiration date.
2. Store according to recommended storage method.
3. Mark date and time of reconstitution, your initials, and the solution

---

*Section VIII Chemotherapy of Antimicrobial Diseases. In *Goodman and Gilman's The Pharmacological Basis of Therapeutics,* 11th ed. Edited by Brunton, Laurence, Lazo, John, and Parker, Keith. New York, McGraw-Hill, 2006.

Bold Italic = life threatening side effect   ■ = black box warning   ✦ = Available in Canada

strength. Mark expiration date; store under appropriate conditions.

4. Complete infusion (or as ordered) before the drug loses potency; check drug info.

ASSESSMENT

1. Note onset, characteristics of S&S, clinical presentation, location and source of infection (if known).

2. List any unusual reaction/sensitivity with any anti-infectives (usually penicillin).

3. Obtain cultures before administering empiric therapy. Use correct procedure for obtaining, storing, and transporting specimens. Monitor VS, cultures, CBC, renal and LFTs.

INTERVENTIONS

1. Conspicuously mark allergy: in red on the chart, medication record, ID band, care plan, pharmacy record, computerized record, and bed. Note if observed or reported by client.

2. Monitor VS, I&O; ensure adequate hydration. Assess for hives, rashes, or difficulty breathing, which may indicate a hypersensitivity or allergic response.

3. If drug mainly excreted by the kidneys, reduce dose with renal dysfunction. Nephrotoxic drugs are usually contraindicated with renal dysfunction because toxic drug levels are rapidly attained.

4. Verify orders when two or more anti-infectives are ordered for the same client, esp. if they have similar side effects, such as nephro/neurotoxicity. Electronic entry prevents confusion.

5. Assess for superinfections, particularly of fungal origin, characterized by black furred tongue, nausea, and/or diarrhea. *Prevent superinfections by:*

- Limiting exposure to persons suffering from an active infectious process
- Rotating IV site q 72–96 hr; changing IV tubing q 48 hr
- Providing/emphasizing good hygiene
- Washing hands carefully before and after contact with client
- Screening visitors and having them wash hands before contact

6. Schedule administration throughout 24-hr period to maintain therapeutic drug levels. Administration schedule is determined by the drug half-life (t $\frac{1}{2}$), severity of infection, evidence of organ dysfunction, and client's need for sleep. Assess drug levels (peak and trough) to determine dosing and to assess adequacy of levels.

CLIENT/FAMILY TEACHING

1. Take at prescribed intervals even if feeling better.

2. Use only under supervision. Do not share with friends or family members.

3. Prevent recurrence by completing entire prescription, despite feeling well. This ensures that the organism is eradicated and diminishes the emergence of drug-resistant bacterial strains. Incomplete therapy and indiscriminate use may render client unresponsive to the antibiotic with the next infection.

4. Report any unusual bruising or bleeding, e.g., bleeding gums, blood in stool, urine, or other secretions; S&S of allergic reactions, including rash, fever, itching, and hives or superinfections such as pain, swelling, redness, drainage, perineal itching, diarrhea, rash/sore throat or rash/joint pain/swelling as in serum sickness, or a change in S&S.

5. Report adverse side effects, lack of response, excessive diarrhea, or worsening of condition after 48-72 hr of therapy. Keep all F/U appointments.

6. Take antipyretics as prescribed ATC for fever reduction as needed. Discard any unused drug after therapy completed.

7. Keep all F/U appointments to evaluate response to therapy, adverse effects and desired organism eradication.

OUTCOMES/EVALUATE

- Prevention/resolution of infection
- ↓ Fever, WBCs; ↑ appetite
- Negative culture reports
- Therapeutic serum drug levels

ANTINEOPLASTIC AGENTS

SEE ALSO THE FOLLOWING INDIVIDUAL ENTRIES:

Aldesleukin
Alemtuzumab
Altretamine

Classifications

Amifostine
Anastrozole
Asparaginase
Azacitidine
BCG Intravesical
Bevacizumab
Bicalutamide
Bleomycin sulfate
Bortezomib
Busulfan
Capecitabine
Carboplatin
Carmustine
Cetuximab
Chlorambucil
Cinacalcet hydrochloride
Cisplatin
Cladribine injection*
Clofarabine
Cyclophosphamide
Cytarabine*
Cytarabine, liposomal
Dacarbazine
Dactinomycin
Dasatinib
Daunorubicin hydrochloride
Daunorubiun citrate liposomal
Decitabine
Denileukin diftitox
Docetaxel
Doxorubicin hydrochloride
    conventional
Doxorubicin hydrochloride
    liposomal
Epirubicin hydrochloride
Erlotinib
Estramustine phosphate sodium*
Etoposide
Exemestane
Floxuridine
Fludarabine phosphate
Fluorouracil
Flutamide
Fulvestrant
Gefitinib
Gemcitabine hydrochloride
Gemtuzumab ozogamicin
Goserelin acetate
Hydroxyurea
Ibritumomab tiuxetan
Idarubicin hydrochloride
Ifosfamide
Imatinib mesylate
Interferon alfa-2a recombinant

Interferon alfa-2b recombinant
Interferon alfa-n3
Irinotecan hydrochloride
Ixabepilone
Lapatinib
Letrozole
Leuprolide acetate
Lomustine
Mechlorethamine hydrochloride
Megestrol acetate
Melphalan
Mercaptopurine
Mesna
Methotrexate
Methotrexate sodium
Mitomycin
Mitotane*
Mitoxantrone hydrochloride
Nelarabine*
Nilotinib hydrochloride
Nilutamide
Oxaliplatin
Paclitaxel
Panitumumab
Pegaspargase
Pemetrexed*
Plicamycin*
Porfimer sodium
Procarbazine hydrochloride
Rituximab
Sorafenib
Streptozocin
Sunitinib maleate
Tamoxifen citrate
Temozolomide
Temsirolimus
Teniposide
Testolactone
Thioguanine
Thiotepa
Topotecan hydrochloride
Toremifene citrate
Trastuzumab
Triptorelin pamoate
Valrubicin
Vinblastine sulfate
Vincristine sulfate
Vinorelbine tartrate
Vorinostat

Drugs marked with an * are available to view in the online database at www.delmarnursesdrughandbook.com/ 2009.

Bold Italic = life threatening side effect   ■ = black box warning   ✚ = Available in Canada

Classifications

GENERAL STATEMENT

The choice of the chemotherapeutic agent(s) depends both on the cell type of the tumor and on its site of growth. All antineoplastic agents are cytotoxic (i.e., cell poisons) and therefore interfere with normal as well as neoplastic cells. However, neoplastic cells are more active and multiply more rapidly than normal cells and are thus more affected by the antineoplastic agents. Normal, rapidly growing tissue cells, such as those of the bone marrow, the GI mucosal epithelium, and hair follicles, are particularly susceptible to antineoplastic agents. The margin between the dose of antineoplastic drug needed to destroy the neoplastic cells and that needed to cause bone marrow damage, for example, is narrow. Since WBCs or platelets show the effect of an overdose more rapidly than do erythrocytes, the platelet and WBC counts are often used as a guide to dosage. If a blood or marrow test indicates a precipitous fall in the WBC or platelet count, the antineoplastic agent may have to be discontinued or the dosage modified significantly. Drugs are frequently withheld when the WBC count falls below 2,000/mm^3 and the platelet count falls below 100,000/mm^3. With the advent of granulocyte colony-stimulating factors, providers may now utilize this to support large dosing on an aggressive cancer, thus preventing postponement of therapy until recovery of the client's hematologic parameters. Sometimes the effect of the antineoplastic drugs on the bone marrow is cumulative, with the depression of WBCs and platelets occurring weeks or months after initiation of therapy.

GI tract toxicity is manifested by development of oral ulcers, intestinal bleeding, nausea, vomiting, loss of appetite, and diarrhea. Finally, alopecia often results from antineoplastic drug therapy.

USES

See individual drugs. Most of the drugs discussed in this section are used exclusively for neoplastic disease. A few are used on an experimental basis for some of the rheumatic diseases.

ACTION/KINETICS

Action

During division, cells go through a number of stages during which they may be susceptible to various chemotherapeutic agents (see *Action/Kinetics* of various drugs).

CONTRAINDICATIONS

Hypersensitivity to drug. Some antineoplastic agents may be contraindicated for up to 4 weeks after radiation therapy or chemotherapy with similar drugs. During first trimester of pregnancy.

SPECIAL CONCERNS

Use with caution, and at reduced dosages, in clients with preexisting bone marrow depression, malignant infiltration of bone marrow or kidney, liver dysfunction, or previous recent chemotherapy usage. The safe use of these drugs during pregnancy has not been established.

SIDE EFFECTS

Bone marrow depression (leukopenia, thrombocytopenia, ***agranulocytosis,*** anemia) is the major danger of antineoplastic therapy. ***Bone marrow depression can sometimes be irreversible.*** *It is mandatory that the client have frequent total blood counts and periodic bone marrow examinations. Precipitous falls must be reported to a physician.* **Other side effects include: GI:** N&V (may be severe), anorexia, diarrhea (may be hemorrhagic), stomatitis, mucositis, enteritis, abdominal cramps, intestinal ulcers. **Hepatic:** Hepatic toxicity including jaundice and changes in liver enzymes. **Dermatologic:** Dermatitis, erythema, various dermatoses including maculopapular rash, alopecia (reversible), pruritus, staining of vein path with some drugs, urticaria, cheilosis. **Immunologic:** Immunosuppression with increased susceptibility to viral, bacterial, or fungal infections. **CNS:** Depression, lethargy, confusion, dizziness, headache, fatigue, malaise, fever, weakness. **GU:** ***Acute renal failure,*** reproductive abnormalities including amenorrhea and azoospermia. *NOTE:* Alkylating agents, in particular, may be both carcinogenic and mutagenic.

GENERAL NURSING CONSIDERATIONS FOR ANTINEOPLASTIC AGENTS

ADMINISTRATION/STORAGE

1. Antineoplastic drugs should be prepared only by trained personnel; avoid if pregnant.

2. Cytotoxic exposure may be through inhalation, ingestion, and absorption during preparation; prepare under a laminar flow (biologic) hood.

- If not available, prepare in a separate room in a work area away from cooling or heating vents and away from other people. Cover work table area with a disposable plastic liner.
- Use latex gloves (if not allergic) to protect the skin when reconstituting; do not use gloves made of PVC since these are permeable to some cytotoxic drugs. Good handwashing before and after preparation is essential. Prevent drug contact with skin or mucous membranes; document occurrence and wash area immediately with copious amounts of water.
- Wear disposable, nonpermeable gown with closed front and knit cuffs completely covering wrists.
- Wear goggles. Should material enter eyes, wash well with isotonic saline eyewash (or water if isotonic saline is unavailable) and consult ophthalmologist.

3. Start infusion with a solution not containing the chemotherapy drug. Avoid dorsum of the hand, wrist, or antecubital fossa as infusion site.

4. Use disposable Luer-Lok fittings, protected needles, syringes, and connectors.

- If drug is to be reconstituted from a vial, vent the vial at the beginning of the procedure. Venting lowers internal pressure and reduces risk of spilling/spraying (aerosolization) solution when needle is withdrawn.
- Use sterile alcohol wipe around needle and vial top when withdrawing drug and when expelling air.

5. Wipe external surfaces of syringes and bottles once prepared. Place all disposable equipment in a separate plastic bag specifically marked for incineration.

6. Wear latex gloves when disposing of vomitus, urine, or feces.

7. Record all exposure times during preparation, administration, cleanup, and spills. Follow appropriate institutional guidelines governing exposures allowed, extravasation, spills, and periodic lab determinations.

ASSESSMENT

1. Assess infusion sites for evidence of infection, infiltration, or adverse reactions.

2. Monitor CBC, renal and LFTs carefully. Assess I&O, VS, skin integrity/color, and for evidence of bruising/bleeding, infection, fever, changes in bowel or urinary patterns, and mentation changes.

3. Assess client/family understanding of: illness, as well as risks of therapy, importance of living will, and emotional support needs.

OUTCOMES/EVALUATE

- Understanding of illness, therapy options, drug side effects, and goals of therapy
- Intolerance to therapy evidenced by tumor growth, acute renal failure, and liver/lung/cardiac toxicities
- N&V, pain, anorexia, or diarrhea may indicate inadequate levels of appropriate prescribed agents to control
- Presence and extent of psychologic depression, lethargy, or other mental status changes requiring therapy/intervention
- Prevention of adverse drug side effects
- Control of pain/fear
- Control/inhibition of malignant cell proliferation
- Hair regrowth
- Desired cure

NURSING CONSIDERATIONS DURING INITIATION OF CHEMOTHERAPY

ASSESSMENT

1. Identify condition requiring therapy (onset, location, type, and S&S) and any

---

previous radiation, surgery, or chemotherapy treatments.

2. Note any hypersensitivity to drugs or foods.

3. Determine nutritional status; note height, weight, and VS; doses are based on BSA (m^2) calculations (square root of HT x WT divided by 3600).

4. Perform physical exam noting all findings and any deficiency. Examine carefully for abnormalities/problems including oral cavity and skin integrity.

5. Monitor bone marrow function (CBC with differential), platelets, liver and renal function.

6. Note prescribed route of administration: oral, IV, IM, or directly at the tumor site (intracavity, intrapleural, intrathecal, intravesical, intraperitoneal, intra-arterial, or topical).

7. Depending on the route, length of therapy, frequency of access, venous integrity, and client preference, determine need/location/type of access device.

8. Rate pain using a pain rating scale. Assess pain control regimen to ensure pain is well controlled.

9. Premedicate (antiemetic, antihistamine, and/or anti-inflammatory) 30–60 min before therapy and as needed.

10. Assess emotional status; evaluate need for antidepressant therapy and support groups.

INTERVENTIONS

1. Monitor VS, I&O. Report any pain, redness, or edema near injection site during or after treatment. If extravasation occurs, stop infusion and follow institutional protocol for minimizing effects. General guidelines for managing an extravasation include:

- Document/report.
- Aspirate drug through cannula with small syringe (tuberculin size).
- Administer antidote as indicated.
- Remove catheter/needle and apply ice (heat if vinca alkaloids).
- Assess closely until site is healed.

2. Chart antineoplastic drugs on the medication administration record (MAR), electronic record, and according to the established protocol. Record therapy on the MAR:

- Day 1: first day of the first dose.
- Number each day after that in sequence, even though may not receive drug daily.
- Indicate when nadir (the time of most severe physiologic depression) is likely to occur so that possible complications, such as infection and bleeding, can be anticipated and treated early; note recovery time.
- When repeating drug regimen, first day of therapy is charted as day 1.

3. Establish interventions to promote client adherence. Keep informed and interpret complicated terminology/therapy/test results, treat symptoms, support client/family and help distinguish/understand unconventional emotions/anger.

4. Identify references, information centers, web sites, and support groups to assist in coping with illness, understanding complex therapy, and emotional upset within the family unit.

CLIENT/FAMILY TEACHING

1. Comply with all aspects of the therapeutic regimen.

2. Ensure reliable contraception. Determine if egg/sperm harvesting is indicated in young persons desiring a family.

3. Review information/literature R/T condition requiring treatment. The American Cancer Society provides many free booklets on cancers, chemotherapy, and how to deal with the side effects of treatments. Go to the library, internet, local cancer society, and provider with unanswered questions. May also call 1-800-4-CANCER, the Cancer Information Service at the National Cancer Institute (at http://www.cancer.gov/), or access other sites through the Internet or library.

4. Review drug side effects that may occur and a means for coping with these diseases and adverse effects.

5. Identify community support groups that assist to cope with these illnesses.

6. Identify who to call to report adverse side effects or to request clarification of instructions.

7. When antineoplastic agents are prepared and administered in the home, advise families how to dispose of urine,

---

feces, vomitus, and equipment and how to handle spills and associated side effects.

NURSING CONSIDERATIONS FOR BONE MARROW DEPRESSION (MYELOSUPPRESSION)

LEUKOPENIA

ASSESSMENT

1. Assess for granulocytopenia or decreased WBCs (normal values: 5,000–10,000/mm^3).
2. Review differential (normal values: neutrophils 60–70%, lymphocytes 25–30%, monocytes 2–6%, eosinophils 1–3%, basophils 0.25–0.5%).
3. Note any sudden sharp drop in WBC count or a reduction below 2,000/mm^3; may require a dosage reduction, withdrawal of drug, protective isolation, and a granulocyte colony stimulating factor.
4. Determine nadir (time the blood count reaches its lowest point after chemotherapy) for prescribed agent (generally 7–14 days); assists to predict, monitor, and respond to effects of bone marrow depression.
5. Report fever above 38°C (100°F); limited resistance to infection due to leukopenia and immunosuppression. Assess for early S&S of infection: check oral cavity for sores/ulcerated areas and urine for odor or particulate matter. With reduced/absent granulocytes, local abscesses do not form with pus; infection becomes systemic.
6. Increased weakness or fatigue may indicate anemia or electrolyte imbalance. Fatigue is a significant side effect of therapy. With cytobines, e.g., interferon, fatigue may be overwhelming.

INTERVENTIONS

1. *Prevent infection* by using strict medical asepsis and frequent handwashing.
2. Provide frequent, meticulous, physical hygiene; maintain clean environment.
3. Cleanse and dry rectal area after each bowel movement. Apply ointment if irritated; use Tucks® and/or Nupercainal® for discomfort.
4. Use a gentle antiseptic to wash if tendency for skin eruptions.

5. Provide mouth care q 4–6 hr; otherwise mucosal deterioration occurs. Avoid lemon or glycerin; these tend to reduce saliva production and change pH of the mouth.
6. If WBC falls below 1,500–2,000/mm^3, may protect with:
- Private room; explain reasons
- Universal precautions; use gloves, masks, and gowns
- Avoid indwelling urinary catheters
- Frequent handwashing
- Limit articles brought into room
- Provide private bathroom or bedside commode
- Minimize traffic in and out of room
- Screen visitors for infection before they enter room; limit visitations
- Avoid exposure to dust, sprays, contaminated medical equipment
- Avoid deodorants; blocks sebaceous gland secretion
- Keep fresh fruits, vegetables, cut flowers, and any source of stagnant water (water pitcher, humidifiers, flower vases) away from client
- Review/stress kitchen hygiene and food safety at home
- Dogs, cats, birds, and other pets may carry infection; avoid contact
- Assess orders for granulocyte colony-stimulating factors and ensure availability

7. Prevent nosocomial infections from invasive procedures by:
- Washing hands before and after any contact
- Frequent assessment of skin integrity and all catheter sites
- Cleansing skin with antiseptic before procedure
- Changing IV tubing q 24 hr
- Changing IV site q 48 hr, if no implanted device or other designated catheter for long-term use
- Practice strict asepsis with all contacts, treatments and dressing changes

THROMBOCYTOPENIA

ASSESSMENT

1. Obtain platelet count (normal values: 150,000–400,000/mm^3). If below 50,000/mm^3 monitor closely.

---

2. Inspect skin for petechiae/bruising; assess all orifices for bleeding.

3. May hemorrhage spontaneously, transfuse if platelets <20,000.

INTERVENTIONS

1. Minimize SC or IM injections; apply pressure for 3–5 min to prevent leakage or hematoma.

2. Do not apply BP cuff or other tourniquet for excessive periods.

3. Avoid rectal temps and constipation; test all urine, GI secretions, and stool for occult blood.

4. Use safety precautions to avoid falls.

5. *Control bleeding*

- With epistaxis: pinch nose for 10 min and apply pressure to upper lip to stop; in severe cases, small sponges saturated with neosynephrine ¼ % gently inserted into nare, or nasal packing, may be needed.

- With transfusions, monitor VS before and 15 min after transfusion started and after completed. Assess for histo-incompatibility, indicated by chills, fever, and urticaria. Stop transfusion, provide supportive care, and follow appropriate institutional protocol for transfusion reaction.

6. Advise client to *prevent bleeding* by:

- Not picking or forcefully blowing their nose

- Avoiding contact sports and any activities that may cause injury

- Reporting any severe frontal headaches

- Using an electric razor for shaving rather than a blade

- Using a soft-bristled toothbrush or massaging gums with fingers or a cotton ball and avoiding dental floss to limit irritation

- Avoiding rectal irritation by contact with enemas, suppositories, or thermometers

- Using a water-based lubricant before intercourse

- Consuming plenty of fluids, increasing activity, and taking stool softeners to prevent constipation

- Rearranging furniture so that area for ambulation is unimpeded and also to prevent bumping into furniture at night when getting out of bed to go to the bathroom

- Having a night light to permit visualization during the night

- Wearing shoes or slippers when ambulating

ANEMIA

ASSESSMENT

1. Monitor CBC, reticulocyte count, MCV and hemoglobin (normal values: men, 13.5–18.0 g/dL blood; women, 11.5–15.5 g/dL blood), and hematocrit (normal values: men, 40–52%; women, 35–46%), and iron panel.

2. Assess for pallor, lethargy, dizziness, ↑ SOB, ↑ fatigue, ↓ BP or tilting.

INTERVENTIONS

1. *Minimize anemia* by:

- Providing nutritious tolerable diet

- Taking vitamins/iron supplements

2. *Assist with treatment of anemia* by :

- Administering diet high in iron

- Giving vitamins with minerals

- Administering erythropoietin (Procrit) to stimulate RBC production

- Administering blood transfusions

- Spacing/scheduling activities to permit frequent rest periods

- Positioning to facilitate ventilation; teaching breathing/relaxation techniques and administering oxygen

- Controlling room temperature for comfort. Providing emotional support

---

NURSING CONSIDERATIONS FOR GI TOXICITY

NAUSEA AND VOMITING; ANOREXIA

ASSESSMENT

1. N&V may be due to either a CNS effect on the CTZ or direct irritation to the GI tract. With radiation therapy, N&V may be attributed to the accumulation of toxic waste products of cell destruction and localized damage to the lining of the throat, stomach, and intestine.

2. Anticipatory N&V is a conditioned response of unknown origin prior to chemotherapy which does respond to premedication.

3. Determine if refusing food or fluids or experiencing anorexia.

---

4. Monitor nutritional status and weights.

5. Examine the frequency, character, and amount of vomitus. List antiemetics prescribed and results.

INTERVENTIONS

1. *To prevent N&V:*
- Antiemetics 30–60 min before or just after drug therapy.
- Therapy on empty stomach, with meals, or at bedtime
- Antiemetic suppository
- Ice chips at onset of nausea
- Avoid carbonated beverages
- Ingest dry carbohydrates such as toast/dry crackers before any activity
- Wait for N&V to pass before serving food
- Small, nutritious snacks; plan meal schedules to coincide with best tolerance time
- Cold foods and salads with little cooking aroma to minimize N&V
- Nourishing foods client likes
- Consume a high-protein diet
- Freeze and serve dietary supplements like ice cream; ↑ palatability
- Avoid foods with overpowering aroma
- Chew foods well
- Good oral hygiene before and after meals (try 1 tsp baking soda in a glass of warm water for rinsing mouth)
- Eat favorite foods
- Eat meals with others, preferably at a table. Sharing encourages eating.

2. Antiemetics that have different actions/pharmacokinetics may be administered concurrently in an effort to control severe N&V.

3. *To treat N&V:*
- Administer antiemetic(s). Report all vomiting; may require a change in therapy or dose or need for electrolyte correction.
- Give other medications after meals
- Offer simple foods: rice, toast, noodles, bananas, scrambled eggs, mashed potatoes, custards, ice cream
- Offer salty foods (pretzels, crackers)
- Avoid solid and liquid foods at the same meal

- Eliminate any room odors; avoiding malodorous foods (e.g., cabbage, sauerkraut, etc.)
- Keep as comfortable, clean, and free from odor as possible
- Try another or concurrent antiemetic agents
- Correct electrolytes; provide hyperalimentation p.r.n.
- Screen visitors/calls until client ready

4. *For anorexia:*
- Provide small, frequent meals q 2 or 3 hr on schedule
- Maximize caloric intake by offering nutrient-dense snacks and drinks (yogurt, cheese and crackers, peanut butter and jelly sandwiches, cereal, dried fruit, fruit nectars, and instant breakfast drink mixes)
- Make nutrient-dense supplements with whole milk
- Suggest a walk or activity before eating to boost appetite
- Concentrate on obtaining favorite foods
- Megace may stimulate appetite with certain forms of cancer while GI/colon cancers may require marinol therapy.

5. *To increase caloric intake and protein consumption:*
- Add high-calorie foods such as mayonnaise, butter, and gravy to foods
- Use whole milk in puddings, cream soups, custards
- Make double-strength milk—add powdered milk to whole milk for gravies, hot cereals, mashed potatoes, eggs, casseroles, baked things, etc.
- Add whipped cream to frosting and desserts
- Offer milkshakes, nectar, and eggnog when thirsty
- Offer peanut butter on crackers, bagels with cream cheese, trail mix, and nuts and seeds for snacks
- Cut up meats and cheeses and add to salads, soups, scrambled eggs, etc.

BOWEL DYSFUNCTION (DIARRHEA/ABDOMINAL CRAMPING)

ASSESSMENT

1. Note frequency and severity of cramping caused by hypermotility.

Bold Italic = life threatening side effect ■ = black box warning ✦ = Available in Canada

2. Document frequency, color, consistency, and amount of diarrhea; indicates tissue destruction. C&S stool.

3. Assess for dehydration and acidosis indicating electrolyte imbalance; monitor I&O and skin integrity on buttocks.

INTERVENTIONS

1. *To prevent diarrhea/abdominal cramping:*
- Provide small, frequent meals on a schedule
- Identify factors that aggravate/increase incidence
- Use constipating foods, i.e., hard cheeses

2. *To treat diarrhea:*
- Administer antidiarrheal and narcotic agent (i.e., codeine, tincture of opium, Imodium, or Lomotil). Report S&S as a change in therapy or electrolyte correction may be needed.
- Increase fluids/avoid dehydration
- Provide foods to correct sodium and potassium losses, e.g., bananas, potatoes, fish and meat, apricot nectar, tomato juice, and sports drinks with "electrolytes," of pedialyte®
- Avoid high-fiber foods that contain "insoluble fiber," such as wheat bran, brown rice, popcorn
- Administer bulk-forming agents (i.e., Metamucil)
- Offer "soluble-fiber" foods, i.e., white rice, oatmeal, applesauce, mashed potatoes, and pears
- Avoid fried/greasy foods
- Avoid excessive sweets; may aggravate diarrhea due to sorbitol, found in many gums and candies
- Use alumimum-containing antacids
- Avoid gas-forming foods, such as broccoli, corn, onion, garlic, lentils, and kidney beans
- Avoid dairy products during acute episodes; consider lactose-free products or Lact-Aid®, which facilitates digestion of lactose
- Restrict intake to rest the bowel if necessary
- Provide good skin care, especially to perianal area to prevent skin breakdown. Apply A&D ointment for perianal tenderness. Change gown and bed linens frequently; use special

mattresses, frequent position changes, and room deodorizers as needed.

3. *To prevent constipation:*
- Provide a high-fiber diet
- Give stool softeners and bulk-forming agents
- Increase fluid intake
- Increase activity levels
- Monitor frequency, consistency, and amount of stool

4. *To prevent obstruction:*
- Aggressively manage constipation using lactose, sennosides, and softeners
- Assess for early S&S such as abdominal pain, N&V, and diminished or absent bowel sounds
- Keep NPO, using NG suction to relieve before referring for surgical intervention.

STOMATITIS (MUCOSAL ULCERATION)

ASSESSMENT

1. Assess for mouth dryness, erythema, soreness, painful swallowing, and white patchy areas of oral mucosa.

2. Symptom onset usually 5 days to 2 weeks after starting therapy; assess regularly.

INTERVENTIONS

1. *To prevent stomatitis:*
- Assess oral cavity 3 times/day and report bleeding gums or burning sensation when acid liquids such as fruit juice are ingested
- Set up a regular schedule for oral preventive care
- Provide good mouth care
- Apply lubricant (Vaseline) to lips 3 times/day

2. *To treat stomatitis:*
- Provide regular oral care
- Apply topical viscous anesthetic, such as benzocaine 20%, or a swish and gargle anesthetic such as dyclonine hydrochloride 0.5%, or a swish, swallow/discard agent such as lidocaine 2% (Xylocaine), before meals or as needed to anesthetize oral mucosa. May swallow lidocaine after swishing it around oral cavity but encourage to expectorate it.

- Puncture a vitamin E capsule and apply to painful lesions to promote healing
- Offer "Magic Mouthwash," which consists of 4 grams (approx. ⅛ teaspoon) baking soda, 30 mL viscous xylocaine, 30 mL Benedryl elixir, and 30 mL Maalox (optional) in 1 L NSS; swish and spit out q 1–2 hr as needed
- Provide allopurinol mouthwash for fluorouracil-related stomatitis; or try sucking ice chips ½ hr before and during treatment
- Offer small, frequent meals of bland foods at medium temperatures
- Administer nystatin solution or clotrimazole troches orally for fungal infections

3. Administer medications (antifungals, antivirals) to prevent general infections.
4. Systemic antifungals may be required. If no relief investigate alternative therapies, i.e, neupogen, etc. Do NOT let client continue to suffer as this is very painful and impairs recovery.

NURSING CONSIDERATIONS FOR NEUROTOXICITY

ASSESSMENT

1. Identify agents causing or having the potential to cause neurotoxic effects; further administration once symptoms have become prominent may be life threatening/non-reversible.
2. Involve neurology; report symptoms of minor neuropathies, i.e., tingling in hands and feet; loss of deep tendon reflexes. Use a tuning fork or monofilament to measure progressive loss of sensation. Report serious neuropathies, i.e., weakness of hands, ataxia, loss of coordination, foot drop, wrist drop, or paralytic ileus and hold therapy until evaluation completed.

INTERVENTIONS

1. *To prevent functional loss due to neurotoxicity:*
- Identify neuropathies early so drug regimen can be adjusted/changed
- Practice/teach seizure precautions
2. *To treat neuropathies:*
- Use safety measures with functional losses

- Maintain good body alignment by frequent and anatomically correct repositioning; ROM exercises.
- Provide stool softeners/laxatives as needed
- Identify causative agent and stop
- Administer agents to help control pain
- Use aids to prevent injury/falls i.e., cane, walker
- Wear shoes to prevent injury, puncture, burn
- Adjust water temperatures, wear protection when handling hot pots, bowls etc.

NURSING CONSIDERATIONS FOR OTOTOXICITY

ASSESSMENT

1. Assess for hearing difficulties before initiating therapy and monitor periodically during therapy.
2. Identify prescribed agents that may contribute to loss.

INTERVENTIONS

1. Report tinnitus or new onset hearing impairment.
2. Perform audiometry testing p.r.n. during therapy.

NURSING CONSIDERATIONS FOR HEPATOTOXICITY

ASSESSMENT

1. Obtain/assess the following LFTs:
- Total serum bilirubin (normal values: 0.1–1.0 mg/dL); elevations may indicate liver disease or increased rate of RBC hemolysis.
- AST (normal: 8–33 units/L). Elevations indicative of changes in liver, skeletal muscles, lungs, pancreas, and heart. Hepatitis produces striking elevations in the AST.
- ALT (normal: 8–20 units/L). Elevations may precede hepatic necrosis.
- LDH (normal: 70–250 units/L). Elevations may indicate hepatitis, pulmonary infarction, and CHF.

2. Assess for liver involvement, i.e., abdominal pain, high fever, diarrhea, and yellowing of skin/sclera. Screen for other sources of liver destruction, i.e., alcohol ingestion, heavy acetaminophen use, hepatitis B or C.

---

3. Identify prescribed agents that may contribute to liver dsyfunction or medication combinations that may predispose one to progressive liver failure. Monitor LFTs regularly during therapy.

INTERVENTIONS

1. Prevent further hepatotoxicity by reporting LFT elevations and signs of liver involvement so drug regimen can be adjusted/changed.

2. Assist with treatment for hepatotoxicity by providing supportive nursing care for pain, fever, diarrhea, and jaundice associated symptoms.

3. Educate client on mechanism of disease and how to protect self from progressive liver destruction i.e. avoid alcohol, avoid OTC agents without provider approval.

NURSING CONSIDERATIONS FOR RENAL TOXICITY

ASSESSMENT

1. Assess the following renal function tests:

- Protein (normal urine: negative)
- BUN (normal: 5–20 mg/dL)
- Serum uric acid (normal: men, 3.5–7.0 mg/dL; women, 2.4–6.0 mg/dL)
- C_{CR} (normal: women, 0.8–1.7 grams/24 hr; men, 1.0–1.9 grams/24 hr)
- Quantitative uric acid (normal: 250–750 mg/day)

2. Report stomach pain, swelling of feet or lower legs, shakiness, reduced output, unusual body movements, or stomatitis.

INTERVENTIONS

1. Monitor I&O. Test pH and alkalinize urine as indicated.

2. Limit hyperuricemia with extra fluids to speed excretion of uric acid and to decrease hazard of crystal and urate stone formation. Administer uricosuric agents (i.e., probenecid) or antigout agents (i.e., allopurinol, colchicine) to lower uric acid levels.

3. Monitor and control BP. Educate client concerning disease and how to protect self from progressive renal destruction i.e. avoid elevated BP/BS, avoid OTC agents without provider approval.

4. Consult nephrology for additional recommendations.

NURSING CONSIDERATIONS FOR IMMUNOSUPPRESSION

ASSESSMENT

1. Assess for the presence of fever, chills, muscle aches, rigors, or sore throat.

2. Note changes in CBC, skin integrity, drainage or other S&S R/T infections.

INTERVENTIONS

1. To treat immunosuppression:

- Prevent infection as noted under bone marrow depression
- Delay active immunization for several months after therapy is completed; may experience a hypo- or hyperactive response
- Avoid contact with children who have recently taken the oral polio vaccine or are visibly sick
- Avoid live vaccinia including zoxtrix
- Avoid crowds and persons with known infections
- May be administered granulocyte colony-stimulating factor to boost immune system

2. Educate client to early S&S of infection and importance of early reporting. Regular frequent hand washing.

3. Review food safety (e.g., storage, handling, washing, cook meats thoroughly, avoid raw eggs) and stress importance of kitchen hygiene when preparing meals at home.

NURSING CONSIDERATIONS FOR GU ALTERATIONS

ASSESSMENT

1. Assess for altered GU function. Most S&S, such as amenorrhea, cease after medication is discontinued.

2. Review risks; sterility may be a permanent result of therapy. Identify those that may be candidates for egg/sperm harvesting prior to therapy.

3. Determine baseline function, assess regularly during therapy.

CLIENT/FAMILY TEACHING

1. Certain drugs may render individuals sterile. Advise that egg/sperm harvesting may be performed prior to therapy

to accommodate future pregnancies/desired offspring.

2. To prevent fetal abnormalities/death, client and partner should use reliable contraceptive measures to avoid pregnancy, both during and for several months as directed after therapy.

3. Report any change in elimination patterns, new onset incontinence, pregnancy, or sexual dysfunction.

4. Keep regularly scheduled preventative appointments to evaluate function and to assess any adverse side effects.

NURSING CONSIDERATIONS FOR ALOPECIA

CLIENT/FAMILY TEACHING

1. Hair loss is a normal occurrence during chemotherapy. Treatment disrupts the mitotic activity of the hair follicle which weakens the hair shaft, causing it to break off. This includes all hair, i.e., eyebrows, body, and pubic hair.

2. Alopecia (hair loss) may occur within 2-3 weeks after the initial treatment. Assist to understand, be prepared for, and expect this as normal with chemotherapy. People respond differently; some may lose hair with a certain agent, others may not.

3. Hair usually will grow back but may be of a different texture or color. It should start to grow in again about 8 weeks after therapy is completed.

4. If receiving more than 4,500 rad to the cranium, hair loss may be permanent.

5. To manage hair loss:
- Shop for a wig before hair loss begins
- Wear a bandana or hat to cover head, and take special care to protect the bare head from sun exposure
- Shave head, if hair starts to fall out in large clumps, and use a wig or scarf until scalp hair regrows
- Wear a night cap at bedtime so hair that falls out during the night will be collected in one place and not all over the bed in the morning.
- Attend support groups to share feelings related to changes in self-image and identify with others undergoing same

- Report any loss of skin integrity or adverse effects

NURSING CONSIDERATIONS FOR ALTERATIONS IN SKIN

ASSESSMENT

1. Document skin color, turgor and integrity. Slight changes in skin color may occur during therapy.

2. Skin destruction R/T XRT requires aggressive treatment and care to prevent infection, pain, and further skin breakdown. Steroid therapy and topical creams may assist to reduce skin desquamation, scarring and disfigurement.

3. Identify additional stress that may contribute to skin changes, i.e. sun over-exposure, chemical contact dermatitis, systemic drug reactions.

INTERVENTIONS

1. Maintain cleanliness of skin through bathing with oilated soaps in tepid water and frequent linen changes.

2. Prevent dryness and replenish skin moisture with regular application of emollient lotions and humidified air. Ensure adequate fluid and nutritional intake

3. Prevent excessive exposure to sun or artificial ultraviolet light; use sunscreen and protective clothing when exposed.

4. Use a special mattress or bed to redistribute weight on bony prominences and to minimize pressure and friction on pressure points. Establish and document a schedule for repositioning, massaging, and assessing skin condition.

5. If using wheelchair have special seat cushion to off set wt. and encourage to change positions frequently and to lie on belly on occasion to redistribute weight for a period of time.

6. With itching, attempt to stop scratching as this may impair skin integrity. Use antihistamines, corticosteroids, nonirritating moisturizers, and cool/ice compresses as needed.

7. Use analgesics to control pain as needed.

8. Refer for assistance with makeup application to enhance self esteem and if needed plastic surgery once therapy completed.

OUTCOMES/EVALUATE

- Inhibition of malignant cell proliferation
- Preservation of nerve function and hearing
- Knowledge of reproductive options
- Organ preservation
- Freedom from long term effects R/T adverse drug effects
- Self esteem intact
- Desired cure

ANTIPARKINSON AGENTS

SEE ALSO THE FOLLOWING INDIVIDUAL ENTRIES:

Amantadine hydrochloride
Apomorphine hydrochloride
Benztropine mesylate
Biperiden hydrochloride
Carbidopa
Carbidopa/Levodopa
Diphenhydramine hydrochloride
Entacapone
Levodopa
Pramipexole
Rasagiline
Ropinirole hydrochloride
Rotigotine
Tolcapone

GENERAL STATEMENT

Parkinson's disease is a progressive disorder of the nervous system, affecting mostly people over the age of 50. Parkinsonism is a frequent side effect of certain antipsychotic drugs, including prochlorperazine and chlorpromazine. Drug-induced symptoms usually disappear when the responsible agent is discontinued. The cause of Parkinson's disease is unknown; however, it is associated with a depletion of the neurotransmitter dopamine in the nervous system. Treatment focuses on administration of dopaminergic agents and/or anticholinergic drugs. Administration of levodopa—the precursor of dopamine—relieves symptoms in 75–80% of the clients. Most of the newer antiparkinsonian drugs must be given with levodopa. Anticholinergic agents also have a beneficial effect by reducing tremors and rigidity and improving mobility, muscular coordination, and motor performance. They are often administered together with levodopa. Certain antihistamines, notably diphenhydramine (Benadryl), are also useful in the treatment of parkinsonism. Clients suffering from Parkinson's disease need emotional support and encouragement because the debilitating nature of the disorder often causes depression. Comprehensive treatment also includes physical therapy.

SPECIAL CONCERNS

Clients taking dopamine agonists for parkinsonism may experience narcoleptic-sleep attacks.

NURSING CONSIDERATIONS

See Nursing Considerations for individual drugs.

ASSESSMENT

1. Note onset, characteristics of S&S, clinical presentation/impairment, PMH, family history of PD, disease progression, other agents/procedures trialed, and outcome.
2. List drugs prescribed. Determine if S&S are drug induced i.e., Haldol, phenothiazines) or are vascular forms (i.e., stroke induced), or atypical forms (i.e., multiple system atrophy, corticobasal degeneration and progressive supranuclear palsy). These forms can be differentiated from classic PD by different brain scans, blood tests and/or a thorough review of the history by a movement disorder specialist.
3. Monitor VS, I&O, and mental status. Assess for depression, affect, mood, behavioral changes, and suicide ideations.
4. Identify involvement in exercise, diet, PT/OT, and support groups; stress importance of these to improve mobility, flexibility, balance, range of motion and for preventing many of the disease's secondary symptoms such as depression and constipation.
5. Determine if surgical candidate for deep brain stimulation (DBS); most effective for those who experience disabling tremors, wearing-off spells and drug-induced dyskinesias.

Classifications

CLIENT/FAMILY TEACHING

1. Parkinson's disease is a movement disorder that occurs when a group of cells in the substantia nigra (area of brain) begin to malfunction and die. These cells produce a chemical called dopamine which is a neurotransmitter (chemical messenger) that sends information to the parts of the brain that control movement and coordination. When dopamine-producing cells begin to die and the amount of dopamine produced in the brain decreases then these messages are sent/delivered more slowly thus leaving one incapable of initiating and controlling movements in a normal way.

2. It is thought that a combination of genetic and environmental factors contribute to this disease.

3. Drug therapy is aimed at restoring normal balances of cholinergic and dopaminergic influences in the brain (basal ganglia) to control tremor and permit desired activity.

4. Take only as prescribed; some agents have many adverse side effects. Taking with food may help to minimize GI upset. If stopped abruptly may induce parkinsonian crisis.

5. Close neurologic follow-up is imperative; some drugs may lose effectiveness and changes or additional therapy may be needed.

6. Avoid activities that require mental alertness and coordination until drug effects realized.

7. May use ice chips, fluids or sugarless candy/gum to relieve dry mouth symptoms. Increase fluids and fiber in diet, and activity to prevent constipation.

8. Avoid alcohol and any CNS depressants without provider approval. Report any adverse/unusual effects and lack of response. Keep all F/U visits.

9. Since several drugs will be taken at different times of the day as the disease progresses. Talking systems, beeping watches, PDA's and multi-alarm timers will help remind you when you need to take certain meds before wearing off and loss of function occur.

10. For more information and updates refer to the Parkinson's disease foundation website http://www.pdf.org/.

OUTCOMES/EVALUATE

- ↓ Drooling, ↓ rigidity, ↓ tremors, ↓ slow movements
- Improved gait, posture, balance and coordination

ANTIPSYCHOTIC AGENTS, PHENOTHIAZINES

SEE ALSO THE FOLLOWING INDIVIDUAL ENTRIES:

Chlorpromazine hydrochloride
Fluphenazine decanoate
Fluphenazine hydrochloride
Perphenazine
Prochlorperazine
Prochlorperazine edisylate
Prochlorperazine maleate
Trifluoperazine

GENERAL STATEMENT

Antipsychotic drugs do not cure mental illness, but they calm the intractable client, relieve the despondency of the severely depressed, activate the immobile and withdrawn, and make some clients more accessible to psychotherapy.

Most phenothiazines induce some sedation, especially during the initial phase of the treatment. Medicated clients can, however, be easily roused. In this manner, the phenothiazines differ markedly from the narcotic analgesics and sedative hypnotics. However, phenothiazines potentiate the analgesic properties of opiates and prolong the action of CNS depressant drugs. These drugs also cause sedation, decrease spontaneous motor activity, and many lower BP.

According to their detailed chemical structure, the phenothiazines belong to three subgroups:

1. **Aliphatic compounds.** Moderate to high sedative, anticholinergic, and orthostatic hypotensive effects. Moderate extrapyramidal symptoms. Often the first choice for clients in acute excitatory states. Examples: Chlorpromazine, promazine, trifluopromazine.

Bold Italic = life threatening side effect   ■ = black box warning   ♣ = Available in Canada

2. **Piperazine compounds.** Act most selectively on the subcortical sites. Low to moderate sedative effects; low anticholinergic and orthostatic hypotensive effects; high incidence of extrapyramidal symptoms. Greatest antiemetic effects because they specifically depress the CTZ of the vomiting center. Examples: Fluphenazine, perphenazine, prochlorperazine, trifluoperazine.

3. **Piperidine compounds.** Low incidence of extrapyramidal effects; high sedative and anticholinergic effects; low to moderate orthostatic hypotensive effect. Examples: Mesoridazine, thioridazine.

USES

(1) Psychoses, especially if excessive psychomotor activity manifested. Involutional, toxic, or senile psychoses. Used in combination with MAO inhibitors in depressed clients manifesting anxiety, agitation, or panic (use with caution). (2) With lithium in acute manic phase of manic-depressive illness. (3) As an adjunct in alcohol withdrawal to reduce anxiety, tension, depression, nausea, and/or vomiting. (4) For severe behavioral problems in children, manifested by hyperexcitable and/or combative behavior; also, for short-term use in hyperactive children who exhibit excess motor activity and conduct disorders. (5) Prophylaxis and control of severe N&V due to cancer chemotherapy, radiation therapy, postoperatively. Intractable hiccoughs, intermittent porphyria, tetanus (as adjunct). (6) As preoperative and/or postoperative medications. (7) Some phenothiazines are antipruritics. See also individual drugs.

ACTION/KINETICS

Action

It has been postulated that excess amounts of dopamine in certain areas of the CNS cause psychoses. Phenothiazines are thought to act by blocking postsynaptic mesolimbic dopamine receptors, leading to a reduction in psychotic symptoms. Phenothiazines block both D_1 and D_2 dopamine receptors. The antiemetic effects are thought to be due to inhibition or blockade of dopamine (D_2) receptors in the chemoreceptor trigger zone in the medulla as well as by peripheral blockade of the vagus nerve in the GI tract. Relief of anxiety is manifested as a result of an indirect decrease in arousal and increased filtering of internal stimuli to the brain stem reticular system. Alpha-adrenergic blockade produces sedation. Phenothiazines also raise pain threshold and produce amnesia due to suppression of sensory impulses. In addition, these drugs produce anticholinergic and antihistaminic effects and depress the release of hypothalamic and hypophyseal hormones. Peripheral effects include anticholinergic and alpha-adrenergic blocking properties.

Pharmacokinetics

Peak plasma levels: 2–4 hr after PO administration. Widely distributed throughout the body. $t\frac{1}{2}$ **(average):** 10–20 hr. Most metabolized in the liver and excreted by the kidney.

CONTRAINDICATIONS

Severe CNS depression, coma, clients with subcortical brain damage, bone marrow depression, lactation. In clients with a history of seizures and in those on anticonvulsant drugs. Geriatric or debilitated clients, hepatic or renal disease, CV disorders, glaucoma, prostatic hypertrophy. Contraindicated in children with chickenpox, CNS infections, measles, gastroenteritis, dehydration due to increased risk of extrapyramidal symptoms.

SPECIAL CONCERNS

Use with caution in clients exposed to extreme heat or cold and in those with asthma, emphysema, or acute respiratory tract infections. Certain phenothiazines (e.g., mesoridazine and thioridazine) may cause sudden cardiac death due to drug-prolonged QTc intervals. Use during pregnancy only when benefits outweigh risks. Children may be more sensitive to the neuromuscular or extrapyramidal effects (especially dystonias); those especially at risk include children with chickenpox, CNS infections, measles, dehydration, or gastroenteritis. Thus, generally, phenothiazines are not recommended for use in children less than 12 years of age. Geriatric clients often manifest higher plasma levels due to decreases in lean body mass, total body water, and albumin and an increase in total body fat. Also, geriatric clients may be more likely to manifest orthostatic hypotension, anticholinergic effects, sedative effects, and extrapyramidal side effects. Also, geriatric clients may have an increased risk of death.

SIDE EFFECTS

CNS: Depression, drowsiness, dizziness, lethargy, fatigue. Extrapyramidal effects, Parkinson-like symptoms including shuffling gait or tic-like movements of head and face, tardive dyskinesia (see what follows), akathisia, dystonia. *Seizures,* especially in clients with a history thereof. *Neuroleptic malignant syndrome (rare).* **CV:** Orthostatic hypotension, increase or decrease in BP, tachycardia, fainting. **GI:** Dry mouth, anorexia, constipation, paralytic ileus, diarrhea. **Endocrine:** Breast engorgement, galactorrhea, gynecomastia, increased appetite, weight gain, hyper-/hypoglycemia, glycosuria. Delayed ejaculation, increased or decreased libido. **GU:** Menstrual irregularities, loss of bladder control, urinary difficulty. **Dermatologic:** Photosensitivity, pruritus, erythema, eczema, exfoliative dermatitis, pigment changes in skin (long-term use of high doses). **Hematologic:** *Aplastic anemia,* leukopenia, *agranulocytosis,* eosinophilia, thrombocytopenia. **Ophthalmic:** Deposition of fine particulate matter in lens and cornea leading to blurred vision, changes in vision. **Respiratory:** *Laryngospasm, bronchospasm, laryngeal edema,* breathing difficulties. **Miscellaneous:** Fever, muscle stiffness, decreased sweating, muscle spasm of face, neck, or back; obstructive jaundice, nasal congestion, pale skin, mydriasis, systemic lupus-like syndrome.

Tardive dyskinesia has been observed with all classes of antipsychotic drugs, although the precise cause is not known. The syndrome is most commonly seen in older clients, especially women, and in individuals with organic brain syndrome. It is often aggravated or precipitated by the sudden discontinuance of antipsychotic drugs and may persist indefinitely after the drug is discontinued. Early signs of tardive dyskinesia include fine vermicular movements of the tongue and grimacing or tic-like movements of the head and neck. Although there is no known cure for the syndrome, it may not progress if the dosage of the drug is slowly reduced. Also, a few drug-free days may unmask the symptoms of tardive dyskinesia and help in early diagnosis.

OD OVERDOSE MANAGEMENT

Symptoms: CNS depression including deep sleep and *coma,* hypotension, extrapyramidal symptoms, agitation, restlessness, seizures, hypothermia, *hyperthermia,* autonomic symptoms, *cardiac arrhythmias,* ECG changes.

Treatment: Emetics are not to be used as they are of little value and may cause a dystonic reaction of the head or neck that may result in aspiration of vomitus.

- Hypotension: Volume replacement; norepinephrine or phenylephrine may be used (do not use epinephrine).
- Ventricular arrhythmias: Phenytoin, 1 mg/kg IV, not to exceed 50 mg/min; may be repeated q 5 min up to 10 mg/kg.
- Seizures or hyperactivity: Diazepam or pentobarbital.
- Extrapyramidal symptoms: Antiparkinsonian drugs, diphenhydramine, barbiturates.

DRUG INTERACTIONS

Alcohol, ethyl / Potentiation or addition of CNS depressant effects. Concomitant use may lead to drowsiness, lethargy, stupor, respiratory collapse, coma, or death

Aluminum salts (antacids) / ↓ Absorption from GI tract

Amphetamine / ↓ Drug effect by ↓ drug uptake to the action site

Anesthetics, general / See *Alcohol*

Antacids, oral / ↓ Effect of phenothiazines R/T ↓ GI tract absorption

Antianxiety drugs / See *Alcohol*

Anticholinergic drugs / Additive anticholinergic side effects and/or ↓ antipsychotic effect

Antidepressants, tricyclic / Additive anticholinergic side effects; also, ↑ TCA serum levels

Barbiturate anesthetics / ↑ Chance of tremor, involuntary muscle activity, and hypotension

Barbiturates / See *Alcohol;* also, barbiturates may ↓ effect R/T ↑ liver breakdown

Bromocriptine / Phenothiazines ↓ effect

Charcoal / ↓ Effect of phenothiazines R/T ↓ GI tract absorption

CNS depressants / See *Alcohol;* also, ↓ effect of phenothiazines R/T ↑ liver breakdown

Colistimethate / Additive respiratory depression

Diazoxide / Additive hyperglycemic effect.

H *Evening primrose oil* / May worsen temporal lobe epilepsy or schizophrenia when used with phenothiazines.

H *Ginseng* / Do not use with antipsychotics

Guanethidine / ↓ Drug effect by ↓ drug uptake at action site.

H *Henbane leaf* / Additive anticholinergic effects

Hydantoins / ↑ Risk of hydantoin toxicity

Lithium carbonate / ↑ Risk of extrapyramidal symptoms, disorientation, or unconsciousness

MAO inhibitors / ↑ Effect of phenothiazines R/T ↓ liver breakdown

Meperidine / ↑ Risk of hypotension and sedation

Metrizamide / ↑ Risk of seizures during subarachnoid administration of metrizamide.

H *Milk thistle* / Helps prevent liver damage from phenothiazines

Narcotics / See *Alcohol*

Phenytoin / ↑ or ↓ Serum levels of phenytoin

Pimozide / Additive effect on QT interval; do not use together

Propranolol / ↑ Plasma levels of both drugs

Sedative-hypnotics, nonbarbiturate / See *Alcohol*

LABORATORY TEST CONSIDERATIONS

False-positive: Bile (urine dipstick), ferric chloride, pregnancy tests, urinary porphobilinogen, urinary steroids, urobilinogen (urine dipstick). *False-negative*: Inorganic phosphorus, urinary steroids. *Caused by pharmacologic effects:* ↑ Alkaline phosphatase, bilirubin, serum transaminases, serum cholesterol, urinary catecholamines. ↓ Glucose tolerance, serum uric acid, 5-HIAA, FSH, growth hormone, LH, vanillylmandelic acid.

DOSAGE

See individual drugs. Effective over a wide dosage range. Dosage is usually increased gradually over 7 days to minimize side effects until the minimal effective dose is attained. Dosage is increased more gradually in elderly or debilitated clients because they are more susceptible to the effects and side effects of drugs. After symptoms are controlled, dosage is gradually reduced to maintenance levels. It is usually desirable to keep chronically ill clients on maintenance levels indefinitely. Medication, especially in clients on high dosages, should not be discontinued abruptly.

NURSING CONSIDERATIONS

ADMINISTRATION/STORAGE

1. Do not interchange brands of PO form of drug or suppositories; may differ in bioavailability.

2. To lessen injection pain, dilute commercially available injectable solutions in saline or local anesthetic. When administering IM, inject drug deeply into the muscle. Massage area of injection site after IM administration to reduce pain.

IV 3. Do not use pink or markedly discolored solutions. When preparing or administering parenteral solutions, nurse and client should avoid contact of drug with skin, eyes, and clothing to prevent contact dermatitis.

4. Do not mix antipsychotic drugs with other drugs in the same syringe. Order a specific flow rate when administering parenteral solutions. Prevent extravasation of the IV solution.

5. Store solutions in a cool dry place in amber-colored containers.

ASSESSMENT

1. Take a complete medical and drug history; note any drug hypersensitivity or genetic predisposition. (These agents are referred to as neuroleptics in Europe.)

2. Assess for any history of asthma, emphysema, or seizures; this class of drugs may lower seizure threshold. Use caution in the elderly.

3. Note reasons for therapy. Assess baseline mental status, noting mood, behavior, reflexes, gait, coordination, sleeping problems, clinical presentation, and any reported depression.

4. If administering to children, note extent of hyperexcitability. Assess child for chickenpox, measles or other illness that may preclude drug therapy.

5. Monitor VS; assess BP in both arms in a reclining position, standing position, and sitting position, 2 min apart.

6. Monitor hematologic profile, liver and renal function studies, urinalysis, ECG, and ocular findings.

INTERVENTIONS

1. If administered IV, monitor flow rate and BP. Keep recumbent for at least 1 hr after IV completed, then slowly elevate HOB and observe for tachycardia, faintness, or dizziness; supervise ambulation.

2. If hospitalized, ensure that drug has been swallowed. May give a liquid preparation to permit better control over drug taking and to improve compliance.

3. Measure I&O; report abdominal distention and urinary retention. May need to reduce dosage, add antispasmodics, or change therapy.

4. Note any changes in carbohydrate metabolism (e.g., glycosuria, weight loss, polyphagia, increased appetite, or excessive weight gain); may require a change in diet/drug therapy and can be significant in those with diabetes.

5. Some may develop a hypersensitivity reaction with fever, asthma, laryngeal edema, angioneurotic edema, and anaphylactic reaction. *Stop* medication, notify provider, and treat symptomatically.

6. The antiemetic effects of phenothiazines may mask other pathology such as toxicity to other drugs, intestinal obstruction, or brain lesions; assess carefully.

7. If receiving barbiturates to relieve anxiety, reduce barbiturate dose. If administered as an anticonvulsant, do not reduce dosage.

8. Discontinue drug gradually to minimize severe GI disturbances or tardive dyskinesia. With evidence of EPS, such as akathisia, pseudoparkinsonism or tardive dyskinesia, notify provider. May require antiparkinsonian agent or discontinuation of therapy.

CLIENT/FAMILY TEACHING

1. There are many different types of psychotic disorders. They comprise serious illnesses that affect the mind by altering one's ability to think clearly, make good judgments, respond emotionally, communicate effectively, understand reality and behave appropriately. When these symptoms are severe, one has difficulty staying in touch with reality and often is unable to meet the ordinary demands of daily life. It is extremely important to take the prescribed medications in order to better function in society and to decrease the mental and physical toll on those who care for and about these clients.

2. May take meds with food or milk to minimize GI upset. Take as directed; may be weeks or months before the full effects will be noticed; do not stop taking abruptly. Abrupt cessation of high doses of phenothiazines can cause N&V, tremors, sensations of warmth and cold, sweating, tachycardia, headache, and insomnia.

3. Avoid driving a car or operating heavy machinery or engaging in any activities that require mental alertness until drug effects realized; consult provider prior to resuming.

4. Report distress when in a hot or cold room; may affect heat-regulating mechanism.

- Provide extra blankets if cold.
- Bathe in tepid water if too warm.
- Do *NOT* use heating pads or hot water bottles if feeling cold.

Bold Italic = life threatening side effect   ▬ = black box warning   ✦ = Available in Canada

- Avoid hot tubs, hot baths/showers; low BP may occur from vasodilation.

5. Report if excessively active or depressed. Spasms of face, neck, back, or tongue may be treated with antihistamines, or drug discontinuation.

6. Report S&S of blood dyscrasias: ↑ body temperature, weakness, easy bruising, or sore throat. May cause menstrual irregularity and false positive pregnancy tests; may develop engorged breasts and begin lactating. Keep accurate record of periods and report if pregnant.

7. Take slow, deep breaths if respiratory S&S occur; may depress cough reflex.

8. Males may experience decreased libido and develop breast enlargement. Report so drug can be adjusted.

9. May develop photosensitivity reactions; wear protective clothing, sunglasses, sunscreen, and avoid sunbathing or prolonged sun exposure.

10. Drug may discolor the urine pink or reddish brown. With long-term therapy may develop a yellow-brown skin reaction that may turn grayish purple.

11. Long-term therapy may affect vision; schedule regular eye exams. Report blurred vision and avoid driving.

12. Report evidence of early (cholestatic) jaundice, such as high fever, upper abdominal pain, nausea, diarrhea, itching, and rash. Withhold drug and report if yellowing of the sclera, skin, or mucous membranes occurs; may indicate biliary obstruction.

13. To prevent dry mouth, rinse mouth frequently, increase fluid intake, chew sugarless gum/hard candies. Increase fluids and bulk in diet to minimize constipation; may need laxatives. Report any urinary retention or persistent constipation. If administered to a child, note any reactions, especially if dehydrated or has an acute infection making child more susceptible to side effects.

14. Rise slowly from a lying or sitting position; dangle legs before standing to avoid low BP symptoms. Avoid alcohol, OTC drugs, and any other CNS depressants without approval.

15. With the elderly, be particularly observant for symptoms of tardive dyskinesia. May exhibit puffing of the cheeks or tongue; may develop chewing movements and involuntary movements of the tongue, head, extremities, and body.

16. Report for periodic labs and follow-up care to evaluate response and adjust drug dosage.

OUTCOMES/EVALUATE

- ↓ Excitable, withdrawn, agitated, or paranoid behaviors.
- Orientation to time and place, and an understanding of illness.
- Adherence to prescribed drug regimen

ANTIVIRAL DRUGS

SEE ALSO THE FOLLOWING INDIVIDUAL ENTRIES:

Antiviral, antiherpes
Acyclovir
Famciclovir
Valacyclovir hydrochloride

Antiviral, antiretroviral fusion inhibitor
Enfuvirtide

Antiviral, general
Adefovir dipivoxil
Amantadine hydrochloride
Cidofovir
Foscarnet sodium
Ganciclovir sodium
Oseltamivir phosphate
Penciclovir
Ribavirin
Rimantadine hydrochloride
Trifluridine
Valganciclovir hydrochloride
Zanamivir

Antiviral, nucleoside analog
Entecavir

Antiviral, nonnucleoside reverse transcriptase inhibitor
Delavirdine mesylate
Efavirenz
Etravirine
Nevirapine

Antiviral, nucleoside reverse transcriptase inhibitor
Abacavir sulfate
Didanosine
Emtricitabine
Lamivudine
Lamivudine/Zidovudine
Stavudine
Zalcitabine
Zidovudine

Antiviral, nucleotide analog reverse transcriptase inhibitor
Tenofovir disoproxil fumarate

Antiviral, protease inhibitor
Amprenavir
Atazanavir sulfate
Darunavir ethanolate
Fosamprenavir calcium
Indinavir sulfate
Nelfinavir mesylate
Ritonavir
Saquinavir mesylate
Tipranavir

USES

HIV infection. Guidelines suggest five different combinations as initial therapy: (1) one protease inhibitor plus two nucleoside reverse transcriptase inhibitors; (2) two nucleoside reverse transcriptase inhibitors and a nonnucleoside reverse transcriptase inhibitor; (3) two protease inhibitors with or without nucleoside reverse transcriptase inhibitors; (4) a nucleoside reverse transcriptase inhibitor, a nonnucleoside reverse transcriptase inhibitor, and a protease inhibitor; or, (5) three nucleoside reverse transcriptase inhibitors.

ACTION/KINETICS

Action

To maintain their growth and reproduce, viruses must enter living cells. Thus, it is difficult to find a drug that is specific for the virus and that does not interfere with the function of the host cell. However, there are enzymes and replicative mechanisms that are unique to viruses and an increasing number of drugs with specific antiviral activity have been developed. The antiviral drugs currently marketed act by one of the following mechanisms:

1. Inhibition of enzymes required for DNA synthesis. Example: Idoxuridine.
2. Inhibition of viral nucleic acid synthesis by interacting directly with herpes virus DNA polymerase or HIV reverse transcriptase. Example: Foscarnet.
3. Inhibition of viral DNA or protein synthesis. Examples: Acyclovir, cidofovir, famciclovir, fomivirsen, ganciclovir, penciclovir, trifluridine, valacyclovir, vidarabine.
4. Prevent penetration of the virus into cells by inhibiting uncoating of the RNA virus. Examples: Amantadine, rimantadine.
5. Protease inhibitors resulting in release of immature, noninfectious viral particles. Examples: Indinavir, nelfinavir, ritonavir, saquinavir.
6. Reverse transcriptase inhibitors (nucleoside and non-nucleoside) resulting in inhibition of replication of the virus. Examples of nucleoside inhibitors: Abacavir, didanosine, lamivudine, stavudine, zalcitabine, zidovudine. Examples of non-nucleoside inhibitors: Efavirenz, delavirdine, nevirapine.

It is often necessary to combine two antiviral drugs that have the same or different mechanisms of action in order to treat HIV infections and to minimize development of resistant viruses.

DOSAGE

See individual drugs. Many antiviral drugs are used in combination therapy to treat HIV disease.

NURSING CONSIDERATIONS

ASSESSMENT

1. Note reasons for therapy, type/onset of S&S, exposure characteristics, and other agents trialed.
2. Identify clinical presentation, mental status and any underlying medical conditions that may preclude drug therapy.
3. List other agents prescribed to ensure none interact unfavorably. Monitor CBC, renal and LFTs; also viral loads/T cells as indicated. Adjust dosage with renal dysfunction.
4. Assess support systems and client adherence potential.

5. Determine need for antiemetic and antidiarrheal to control any adverse side effects.

CLIENT/FAMILY TEACHING

1. Review method and frequency for drug administration. Stress importance of adherence to multidrug regimens and how to take exactly as directed even if feeling better; do not share medications.

2. Identify specific measures to decrease/halt disease spread. Continuous therapy without interruption has been shown to prolong life.

3. Maintain adequate nutrition; consume 2–3 L/day of fluids to prevent crystalluria.

4. Report any rashes or unusual drug side effects or if symptoms do not improve or worsen after specified time frame.

5. Close medical supervision/follow-up required during therapy; keep all F/U visits and lab appointment.

OUTCOMES/EVALUATE

- Prophylaxis of viral infections
- Reduction in length and severity of symptoms of viral infections
- ↓ Resistant viruses
- Increased recovery with HIV/Hep B, C infections

BETA-ADRENERGIC BLOCKING AGENTS

SEE ALSO ALPHA-1-ADRENERGIC BLOCKING AGENTS AND THE FOLLOWING INDIVIDUAL AGENTS:

Atenolol
Betaxolol hydrochloride
Bisoprolol fumarate
Esmolol hydrochloride
Levobunolol hydrochloride
Metipranolol hydrochloride
Metoprolol succinate
Metoprolol tartrate
Nadolol
Penbutolol sulfate
Propranolol hydrochloride
Sotalol hydrochloride
Timolol maleate

USES

See individual drugs. Depending on the drug uses include, but are not limited to (1) Hypertension. (2) Angina pectoris. (3) MI. Are important in clients who have survived a first MI. (4) Migraine. (5) Part of the standard therapy for CHF. (6) May increase survival if taken prior to coronary artery bypass surgery. *NOTE:* See *Angiotensin Converting Enzyme (ACE) Inhibitors* for guidelines for the evaluation and management of chronic heart failure.

ACTION/KINETICS

Action

Combine reversibly with beta-adrenergic receptors to block the response to sympathetic nerve impulses, circulating catecholamines, or adrenergic drugs. Beta-adrenergic receptors are classified as beta-1 (predominantly in the cardiac muscle) and beta-2 (mainly in the bronchi and vascular musculature). Blockade of beta-1 receptors decreases HR, myocardial contractility, and CO; in addition, AV conduction is slowed. These effects lead to a decrease in BP, as well as a reversal of cardiac arrhythmias. Blockade of beta-2 receptors increases airway resistance in the bronchioles and inhibits the vasodilating effects of catecholamines on peripheral blood vessels. The various beta-blocking agents differ in their ability to block beta-1 and beta-2 receptors (see individual drugs); also, certain of these agents have intrinsic sympathomimetic action. Certain of these drugs (betaxolol, carteolol, levobunolol, metipranolol, and timolol) are used for glaucoma; act by reducing production of aqueous humor; metipranolol and timolol may also increase outflow of aqueous humor. Drugs have little or no effect on the pupil size or on accommodation.

CONTRAINDICATIONS

Sinus bradycardia, second- and third-degree AV block, cardiogenic shock, CHF unless secondary to tachyarrhythmia treatable with beta blockers, overt cardiac failure. Most are contraindicated in chronic bronchitis, bronchial asthma or history thereof, bronchospasm, emphysema, severe COPD.

SPECIAL CONCERNS

Use with caution in diabetes, thyrotoxicosis, cerebrovascular insufficiency, and impaired hepatic and renal function. Withdrawing beta blockers before major surgery is controversial. Safe use during pregnancy and lactation and in children has not been established. May be absorbed systemically when used for glaucoma; thus, there is the potential for an additive effect with beta blockers used systemically. Certain of the products for use in glaucoma contain sulfites, which may result in an allergic reaction. Also, see individual agents.

SIDE EFFECTS

CV: Bradycardia, hypotension (especially following IV use), CHF, cold extremities, claudication, worsening of angina, strokes, edema, syncope, arrhythmias, chest pain, peripheral ischemia, flushing, SOB, sinoatrial block, pulmonary edema, vasodilation, increased HR, palpitations, conduction disturbances, **first-, second-, and third-degree heart block,** worsening of AV block, **thrombosis of renal or mesenteric arteries,** precipitation/worsening of Raynaud's phenomenon. Sudden withdrawal of large doses may cause angina, **ventricular tachycardia, fatal MI, sudden death,** or **circulatory collapse. GI:** N&V, diarrhea, flatulence, dry mouth, constipation, anorexia, cramps, bloating, gastric pain, dyspepsia, distortion of taste, weight gain/loss, retroperitoneal fibrosis, ischemic colitis. **Hepatic:** Hepatomegaly, acute pancreatitis, elevated liver enzymes, liver damage (especially with chronic use of phenobarbital). **Respiratory:** Asthma-like symptoms, **bronchospasms, bronchial obstruction, laryngospasm with respiratory distress,** wheezing, worsening of cold, dyspnea, cough, nasal stuffiness, rhinitis, pharyngitis, rales. **CNS:** Dizziness, fatigue, lethargy, vivid dreams, depression, hallucinations, delirium, psychoses, paresthesias, insomnia, nervousness, nightmares, headache, vertigo, disorientation of time/place, hypo-/hyperesthesia, decreased concentration, short-term memory loss, change in behavior, emotional lability, slurred speech, lightheadedness. In the elderly, paranoia, disorientation, and combativeness have occurred. **Hematologic: Agranulocytosis,** thrombocytopenia. **Allergic:** Fever, sore throat, respiratory distress, rash, pharyngitis, **laryngospasm, anaphylaxis. Skin:** Pruritus, rashes, increased skin pigmentation/irritation, sweating, dry skin, alopecia, psoriasis (reversible). **Musculoskeletal:** Joint/back/muscle pain, arthritis, arthralgia, muscle cramps, muscle weakness when used in clients with myasthenic symptoms. **GU:** Impotence, decreased libido, dysuria, UTI, nocturia, urinary retention/frequency, pollakiuria. **Ophthalmic:** Visual disturbances, eye irritation, dry/burning eyes, blurred vision, conjunctivitis.

When used ophthalmically: Keratitis, blepharospasm, diplopia, ptosis, and visual disturbances including refractive changes. **Other:** Hyper-//hypoglycemia, lupus-like syndrome, Peyronie's disease, tinnitus, increase in symptoms of myasthenia gravis, facial swelling, decreased exercise tolerance, rigors, speech disorders. **Systemic effects due to ophthalmic beta-1 and beta-2 blockers:** Headache, depression, arrhythmia, heart block, CVA, syncope, CHF, palpitation, cerebral ischemia, nausea, localized and generalized rash, **bronchospasm** (especially in those with preexisting bronchospastic disease), **respiratory failure,** masked symptoms of hypoglycemia in IDDM, keratitis, visual disturbances (including refractive changes), blepharoptosis, ptosis, diplopia.

OD OVERDOSE MANAGEMENT

Symptoms: CV symptoms include bradycardia, hypotension, CHF, **cardiogenic shock,** intraventricular conduction disturbances, **AV block, pulmonary edema, asystole,** and tachycardia. Also, overdosage of pindolol may cause hypertension and overdosage of propranolol may result in ↑ systemic vascular resistance. CNS symptoms include respiratory depression, decreased consciousness, **coma,** and **seizures.** Miscellaneous symptoms include **bronchospasm** (especially in clients with COPD), hyperkalemia, and hypoglycemia.

Bold Italic = life threatening side effect   ■ = black box warning   ♣ = Available in Canada

Treatment:

- To improve blood supply to the brain, place client in a supine position and raise the legs.
- Measure blood glucose and serum potassium. Monitor BP and ECG continuously.
- Provide general supportive treatment such as inducing emesis or gastric lavage and artificial respiration.
- Seizures: Give IV diazepam or phenytoin.
- Excessive bradycardia: If hypotensive, give atropine, 0.6 mg; if no response, give q 3 min for a total of 2–3 mg. Cautious administration of isoproterenol may be tried. Also, glucagon, 5–10 mg rapidly over 30 sec, followed by continuous IV infusion of 5 mg/hr may reverse bradycardia. Transvenous cardiac pacing may be needed for refractory cases.
- Cardiac failure: Digitalis, diuretic, and oxygen; if failure is refractory, IV aminophylline or glucagon may be helpful.
- Hypotension: Place client in Trendelenburg position. IV fluids unless pulmonary edema is present; also vasopressors such as norepinephrine (may be drug of choice), dobutamine, dopamine with monitoring of BP. If refractory, glucagon may be helpful. In intractable cardiogenic shock, intra-aortic balloon insertion may be required.
- Premature ventricular contractions: Lidocaine or phenytoin. Disopyramide, quinidine, and procainamide should be avoided as they depress myocardial function further.
- Bronchospasms: Give a beta-2-adrenergic agonist, epinephrine, or theophylline.
- Heart block, second or third degree: Isoproterenol or transvenous cardiac pacing.

DRUG INTERACTIONS

Aluminum salts / ↓ Bioavailability of certain beta-blockers → ↓ effect

Ampicillin / ↓ Bioavailability of certain beta-blockers → ↓ effect

Anesthetics, general / Additive depression of myocardium

Anticholinergic agents / Counteract bradycardia produced by beta-adrenergic blockers

Antihypertensives / Additive hypotensive effect

Barbiturates / ↓ Bioavailability of certain beta-blockers → ↓ effect

Benzodiazepines / ↑ Effect of certain benzodiazepines by lipophilic beta-blockers

Calcium channel blockers / ↑ Effect of certain beta-blockers

Calcium salts / ↓ Bioavailability of certain beta-blockers → ↓ effect

Chlorpromazine / Additive beta-adrenergic blocking action

Cholestyramine / ↓ Bioavailability of certain beta-blockers → ↓ effect

Cimetidine / ↑ Effect of beta blockers R/T ↓ liver breakdown

Clonidine / Paradoxical hypertension; also, ↑ severity of rebound hypertension

Colestipol / ↓ Bioavailability of certain beta-blockers → ↓ effect

Diphenhydramine / ↑ Plasma levels and CV effects of certain beta-blockers R/T ↓ metabolism

Disopyramide / ↑ Effect of both drugs

Epinephrine / Beta blockers prevent beta-adrenergic action of epinephrine but not alpha-adrenergic action → ↑ SBP/DBP and ↓ HR

Ergot alkaloids / ↑ Risk of peripheral ischemia R/T ergot alkaloid-mediated vasoconstriction and peripheral effects of beta-blockers

Flecainide / Possible ↑ bioavailability of either drug → ↑ effects

Furosemide / ↑ Beta-adrenergic blockade

Haloperidol / ↑ Risk of hypotensive episodes

Hydralazine / ↑ Effect of both beta-blockers and hydralazine

Hydroxychloroquine / ↑ Plasma levels and CV effects of certain beta-blockers R/T ↓ metabolism

Indomethacin / ↓ Effect of beta blockers possibly due to inhibition of prostaglandin synthesis

Insulin / Beta blockers ↑ hypoglycemic effect of insulin

Lidocaine / ↑ Drug effect R/T ↓ liver

Classifications

breakdown

Methyldopa / Possible ↑ BP to alpha-adrenergic effect

Muscle relaxants, nondepolarizing / Beta-blockers may potentiate, counteract, or have no effect on action of nondepolarizing muscle relaxants

NSAIDs / ↓ Effect of beta blockers, possibly R/T inhibition of prostaglandin synthesis

Ophthalmic beta blockers / Additive systemic beta-blocking effects if used with oral beta blockers

Oral contraceptives / ↑ Effect of beta blockers R/T ↓ liver breakdown

Phenformin / ↑ Hypoglycemia

Phenobarbital / ↓ Effect of beta blockers R/T ↑ liver breakdown

Phenothiazines / ↑ Effect of both drugs

Phenytoin / Additive depression of myocardium; also ↓ effect of beta blockers R/T ↑ liver breakdown

Prazosin / ↑ First-dose effect of prazosin (acute postural hypotension)

Propafenone / ↑ Plasma levels of certain beta-blockers R/T ↓ liver metabolism

Quinidine / ↑ Plasma levels of beta-blockers in extensive metabolizers → ↑ effects

Quinolone antibiotics / ↑ Bioavailability of beta-blockers metabolized by the cytochrome P450 system

Rifampin / ↓ Effect of beta blockers due to ↑ breakdown by liver

Ritodrine / Beta blockers ↓ effect of ritodrine

Salicylates / ↓ Effect of beta blockers, possibly R/T inhibition of prostaglandin synthesis

SSRIs / Possible excessive beta-blockade R/T ↓ metabolism

Smoking / ↓ Antihypertensive and heart rate effects possibly R/T nicotine-mediated sympathetic activation; smokers may need ↑ dosages

Succinylcholine / Beta blockers ↑ effects of succinylcholine

Sulfonylureas / ↓ Effect of sulfonylureas

Sympathomimetics / Reverse effects of beta blockers

Theophylline / Beta blockers reverse the effect of theophylline; also, beta blockers ↓ renal drug clearance

Thioamines / ↑ Effects of beta-blockers

Thyroid hormones / Effects of certain beta-blockers may be ↓ when hypothyroid client is converted to euthyroid state

Tubocurarine / Beta blockers ↑ effects of tubocurarine

Verapamil / Possible side effects since both drugs ↓ myocardial contractility or AV conduction; bradycardia and asystole when beta blockers are used ophthalmically.

LABORATORY TEST CONSIDERATIONS
↓ Serum glucose.

DOSAGE
See individual drugs.

NURSING CONSIDERATIONS

ADMINISTRATION/STORAGE

1. Sudden cessation of beta blockers may precipitate or worsen angina.

2. Lowering of intraocular pressure (IOP) may take a few weeks to stabilize when using betaxolol or timolol.

3. Due to diurnal variations in IOP, the response to twice a day therapy is best assessed by measuring IOP at different times during the day.

4. If IOP is not controlled using beta blockers, add additional drugs to the regimen, including pilocarpine, dipivefrin, or systemic carbonic anhydrase inhibitors.

ASSESSMENT

1. Note reasons for therapy, symptom characteristics, other agents trialed. List any history of depression; assess mental status. Review drugs currently prescribed to ensure none interact.

2. Check for any history of asthma, diabetes, or impaired renal function. With asthma, avoid nonselective beta antagonists due to beta-2 receptor blockade which may lead to increased airway resistance. With heart failure, weigh regularly, and with diabetes assess for hypoglycemia.

3. Determine HR and BP in both arms lying, sitting, and standing. Monitor EKG, glucose, CBC, electrolytes, renal and LFTs. Note MUGA, echocardiogram, and/or stress test results.

INTERVENTIONS

1. Monitor HR and BP; obtain written parameters for holding (e.g., for SBP <90 or HR <50).

2. When assessing respirations note rate and quality; may cause dyspnea and bronchospasm.

3. Monitor I&O and daily weights. Observe for increasing dyspnea, coughing, difficulty breathing, Wt gain, chest pain, fatigue, or edema—symptoms of CHF, may require digitalization, diuretics, and/or drug discontinuation.

4. Complaints of cold S&S, easy fatigue, or feeling lightheaded may require a drug change.

5. With diabetics watch for S&S of hypoglycemia, such as hypotension or tachycardia; S&S may be masked.

6. During IV administration, monitor EKG (may slow AV conduction and increase PR interval) and activities closely until drug effects evident.

CLIENT/FAMILY TEACHING

1. When prescribed for BP control, drug helps control BP but does not cure it. Must continue to take despite feeling better. With heart attack, drug is prescribed to prevent remodeling of the heart and to decrease sudden death after heart attack.

2. Record BP and take pulse immediately prior to first dose each day so medication can be adjusted. Review instructions for when to call provider, i.e., if HR <50 beats/min or SBP <80 mm Hg or as specified by provider.

3. Review lifestyle changes for BP control: regular exercise, weight loss, low-fat and reduced-calorie diet, decreased salt and alcohol intake, smoking cessation, and relaxation techniques.

4. Always consult provider before interrupting therapy; stopping abruptly may cause chest pain, heart attack, or ↑ BP. A 2-week taper is generally used.

5. May cause blurred vision, dizziness, or drowsiness; avoid activities that require mental alertness until drug effects realized.

6. Rise from a sitting or lying position slowly and dangle legs before standing to avoid S&S of sudden drop in BP. Elastic support hose may help decrease symptoms.

7. Dress warmly during cold weather. Diminished blood supply to extremities may cause cold sensitivity; check extremities for warmth.

8. Avoid excessive intake of alcohol, coffee, tea, or cola. Avoid OTC agents without approval.

9. If diabetic, monitor FS and report S&S of low sugar <60. With heart failure, check weight daily and report unusual weight gain (>2 lb per day or 5 lb per week), increased SOB, or chest pain.

10. Report any asthma-like symptoms, cough, or nasal stuffiness; may be symptoms of heart failure. Report any bothersome side effects or changes, especially new-onset depression or marked fatigue. Keep all F/U appointments to evaluate response to therapy.

OUTCOMES/EVALUATE

- ↓ BP; ↓ IOP; ↓ Remodeling
- ↓ Frequency/severity of anginal attacks; improved exercise tolerance
- ↓ Anxiety levels; ↓ tremors
- Migraine prophylaxis

CALCIUM CHANNEL BLOCKING AGENTS

SEE ALSO THE FOLLOWING INDIVIDUAL ENTRIES:

Amlodipine
Bepridil hydrochloride
Diltiazem hydrochloride
Felodipine
Isradipine
Nicardipine hydrochloride
Nifedipine
Nimodipine
Nisoldipine
Verapamil

USES

See individual drugs. Uses include, but are not limited to: (1) Angina pectoris (chronic stable, unstable, vasospastic). (2) Hypertension. (3) Subarachnoid hemorrhage. (4) Atrial fibrillation/flutter. (5) Paroxysmal supraventricular tachycardia. *Investigational:* (1) Prevention of migraine headaches (diltiazem, verapamil). (2) Pulmonary hypertension

Classifications

(amlodipine, diltiazem, felodipine, nifedipine). (3) Raynaud's phenomenon (amlodipine, diltiazem, felodipine, isradipine, nifedipine). (4) Preterm labor (nifedipine). (5) Hypertrophic cardiomyopathy (verapamil).

ACTION/KINETICS

Action

For contraction of cardiac and smooth muscle to occur, extracellular calcium must move into the cell through openings called *calcium channels*. The calcium channel blocking agents (also called *slow channel blockers* or *calcium antagonists*) inhibit the influx of calcium through the cell membrane, resulting in a depression of automaticity and conduction velocity in both smooth and cardiac muscle. This leads to a depression of contraction in these tissues. Drugs in this class have different degrees of selectivity on vascular smooth muscle, myocardium, and conduction and pacemaker tissues. In the myocardium, these drugs dilate coronary vessels in both normal and ischemic tissues and inhibit spasms of coronary arteries. They also decrease total peripheral resistance, thus reducing energy and oxygen requirements of the heart. Also effective against certain cardiac arrhythmias by slowing AV conduction and prolonging repolarization. In addition, they depress the amplitude, rate of depolarization, and conduction in atria.

CONTRAINDICATIONS

Sick sinus syndrome, second- or third-degree AV block (except with a functioning pacemaker). Use of bepridil, diltiazem, or verapamil for hypotension <90 mm Hg systolic pressure). Lactation.

SPECIAL CONCERNS

Abrupt withdrawal may result in increased frequency and duration of chest pain. Hypertensive clients treated with calcium channel blockers have a higher risk of heart attack than clients treated with diuretics or beta-adrenergic blockers. May also be an increased risk of heart attacks in diabetics (only nisoldipine studied). Safety and effectiveness of bepridil, diltiazem, felodi-

pine, and isradipine have not been established in children.

SIDE EFFECTS

Side effects vary from one calcium channel blocker to another; refer to individual drugs.

OD OVERDOSE MANAGEMENT

Symptoms: Nausea, weakness, drowsiness, dizziness, slurred speech, confusion, marked and prolonged hypotension, bradycardia, junctional rhythms, *second- or third-degree block.*
Treatment:

- Treatment is supportive. Monitor cardiac and respiratory function.
- If client is seen soon after ingestion, emetics or gastric lavage should be considered followed by cathartics.
- *Hypotension:* IV calcium, dopamine, isoproterenol, metaraminol, norepinephrine. Also, provide IV fluids. Place client in Trendelenburg position.
- *Ventricular tachycardia:* IV procainamide or lidocaine; also, cardioversion may be necessary. Also, provide slow-drip IV fluids.
- *Bradycardia, asystole, AV block:* IV atropine sulfate (0.6–1 mg), calcium gluconate (10% solution), isoproterenol, norepinephrine; also, cardiac pacing may be indicated. Provide slow-drip IV fluids.

DRUG INTERACTIONS

Anesthetics / Potentiation of cardiac effects and vascular dilation associated with anesthetics; possible severe hypotension
Beta-adrenergic blocking agents / Beta blockers may cause depression of myocardial contractility and AV conduction
Cimetidine / ↑ Effect of CCBs R/T ↓ first-pass metabolism.
H *Dong quai* / Possible additive effect
Fentanyl / Severe hypotension or ↑ fluid volume requirements.
H *Ginger* / May alter CCBs effect R/T ↑ calcium uptake by heart muscle
Grapefruit juice / ↑ Serum levels of most calcium channel blockers
Itraconazole / Edema when used with amlodipine or nifedipine
Ranitidine / ↑ Effect of CCBs R/T ↓ first-pass metabolism.

Bold Italic = life threatening side effect ■ = black box warning ✦ = Available in Canada

DOSAGE

See individual drugs.

NURSING CONSIDERATIONS

ASSESSMENT

1. Note reasons for therapy, onset, characteristics of S&S. List other agents used and outcome. Note any experience with these agents and the response. List drugs prescribed to ensure none interact.

2. Assess CV and mental status. These drugs cause peripheral vasodilation. Any excessive hypotensive response and increased HR may precipitate angina. Record VS, weight, ECG and BP in both arms while lying, sitting, and standing. Assess for CHF (weight gain, peripheral edema, dyspnea, crackles, jugular vein distention).

3. Monitor BS, lytes, I&O, renal and LFTs.

CLIENT/FAMILY TEACHING

1. These agents block the entry of calcium into the muscle cells of the heart and the arteries. Calcium causes the heart to contract and the arteries to narrow so by blocking entry, it decreases contraction of the heart and dilate (widen) the arteries.

2. Take with meals to ↓ GI upset. Do not stop therapy suddenly.

3. Review goals of therapy (e.g., ↓ DBP by 10 mm Hg, ↓ HR by 20 beats/min). Record pulse and BP at least twice a week as well as weights; review instructions regarding when to hold medications and notify provider as directed.

4. Do not perform activities that require mental alertness until drug effects realized. Report adverse effects such as dizziness, vertigo, unusual flushing, facial warmth, edema, nausea, constipation. Toxic drug effects are swelling of the hands or feet, pronounced dizziness, chest pain accompanied by sweating, SOB, or severe headaches.

5. If dizziness occurs (drop in BP), change positions slowly, especially when standing from a lying position. Sit down immediately if lightheadedness occurs. Move slowly from a lying to a sitting or standing position.

6. Avoid long periods of standing, excessive heat, hot showers or baths, and ingestion of alcohol; may worsen drop in BP.

7. Review lifestyle changes for BP control, i.e., regular exercise, weight loss, low-fat, low-cholesterol, reduced-calorie diet, decreased salt and alcohol consumption, smoking cessation, and stress reduction.

8. Keep a log of BP and HR for provider review.

OUTCOMES/EVALUATE

- Control of BP; ↓ HR
- ↓ Frequency/intensity of angina
- Stable cardiac rhythm
- Migraine headache prophylaxis

CALCIUM SALTS

SEE ALSO THE FOLLOWING INDIVIDUAL ENTRIES:

Calcium carbonate
Calcium chloride
Calcium gluconate

USES

IV: (1) Acute hypocalcemic tetany secondary to renal failure. (2) Hypoparathyroidism. (3) Premature delivery. (4) Maternal diabetes mellitus in infants. (5) Poisoning due to magnesium, oxalic acid, radiophosphorus, carbon tetrachloride, fluoride, phosphate, strontium, and radium. (6) Treat depletion of electrolytes. (7) During cardiac resuscitation when epinephrine or isoproterenol have not improved myocardial contraction (may also be given into the ventricular cavity for this purpose). (8) To reverse cardiotoxicity or hyperkalemia.

IM or IV: (1) Reduce spasms in renal, biliary, intestinal, or lead colic. (2) Relieve muscle cramps due to insect bites. (3) Decrease capillary permeability in various sensitivity reactions.

PO: (1) Osteoporosis, osteomalacia. (2) Chronic hypoparathyroidism. (3) Rickets. (4) Latent tetany. (5) Hypocalcemia secondary to use of anticonvulsant drugs. (6) Myasthenia gravis. (7) Eaton-Lambert syndrome. (8) Supplement for pregnant, postmenopausal, or nursing

Classifications

women. (9) Prophylactically for primary osteoporosis. *Investigational:* As an infusion to diagnose Zollinger-Ellison syndrome and medullary thyroid carcinoma. To antagonize neuromuscular blockade due to aminoglycosides.

ACTION/KINETICS

Action

Calcium is essential for maintaining normal function of nerves, muscles, the skeletal system, and permeability of cell membranes and capillaries. The normal serum calcium concentration is 9–10.4 mg/dL (4.5–5.2 mEq/L). Hypocalcemia is characterized by muscular fibrillation, twitching, skeletal muscle spasms, leg cramps, tetanic spasms, cardiac arrhythmias, smooth muscle hyperexcitability, mental depression, and anxiety states. Excessive, chronic hypocalcemia is characterized by brittle, defective nails, poor dentition, and brittle hair. Calcium is well absorbed from the upper GI tract; Vitamin D is required for calcium absorption and increases the capability of the absorptive mechanisms. Food increases calcium absorption. Severe low-calcium tetany is best treated by IV administration of calcium gluconate. The hormone of the parathyroid gland is necessary for the regulation of the calcium level. Recommended daily allowances for men and women, age 19–24 years is 1,200 mg/day; and, for men and women, 25 years of age and older is 800 mg/day. Dietary reference intakes for men and women, 19–50 years of age is 1,000 mg/day; for men and women over 51 years of age is 1,200 mg/day; and, for pregnant and breastfeeding women is 1,000 mg/day.

Pharmacokinetics

Calcium is excreted mainly through the feces (as much as 250–300 mg/day in healthy adults eating a regular diet).

CONTRAINDICATIONS

Digitalized clients, sarcoidosis, renal or cardiac disease, ventricular fibrillation. Cancer clients with bone metastases. Renal calculi, hypophosphatemia, hypercalcemia.

SPECIAL CONCERNS

Calcium requirements decrease in geriatric clients; thus, dose may have to be adjusted. Also, low levels of active vitamin D metabolites may impair calcium absorption in older clients. Use with caution in cor pulmonale, sarcoidosis, cardiac or renal disease, or in those receiving cardiac glycosides. May be irritating to the GI tract when given PO and may cause constipation.

SIDE EFFECTS

Following PO use: GI irritation, constipation.

Following IV use: Venous irritation, tingling sensation, feeling of oppression or heat, chalky taste. Rapid IV administration may result in vasodilation, decreased BP and HR, ***cardiac arrhythmias***, syncope, or ***cardiac arrest.***

Following IM use: Burning feeling, necrosis, tissue sloughing, cellulitis, soft tissue calcification. *NOTE:* If calcium is injected into the myocardium rather than into the ventricle, ***laceration of coronary arteries, cardiac tamponade, pneumothorax,*** and ***ventricular fibrillation*** may occur.

Symptoms due to excess calcium (hypercalcemia): Lassitude, fatigue, GI symptoms (anorexia, N&V, abdominal pain, dry mouth, thirst), polyuria, depression of nervous and neuromuscular function (emotional disturbances, confusion, skeletal muscle weakness, and constipation), confusion, delirium, stupor, ***coma,*** impairment of renal function (polyuria, polydipsia, and azotemia), renal calculi, arrhythmias, and bradycardia.

OD OVERDOSE MANAGEMENT

Symptoms: Systemic overloading from parenteral administration can result in an acute hypercalcemic syndrome with symptoms including markedly increased plasma calcium levels, lethargy, intractable N&V, weakness, ***coma,*** and ***sudden death.***

Treatment: Discontinue therapy and lower serum calcium levels by giving an IV infusion of sodium chloride plus a potent diuretic such as furosemide. Consider hemodialysis.

DRUG INTERACTIONS

Atenolol / ↓ Drug effect R/T ↓ bioavailability and plasma levels

Cephalocin / Incompatible with calcium

Bold Italic = life threatening side effect   ■ = black box warning   ♣ = Available in Canada

salts

Corticosteroids / Interfere with absorption of calcium from GI tract

Digitalis / ↑ Digitalis arrhythmias and toxicity. Death has resulted from combination of digitalis and IV calcium salts

Iron salts / ↓ Absorption of iron from the GI tract.

H *Lily-of-the-valley herb* / ↑ Effectiveness and side effects of calcium

Milk / Excess of either may cause hypercalcemia, renal insufficiency with azotemia, alkalosis, and ocular lesions

Norfloxacin / ↓ Drug bioavailability.

H *Pheasant's eye herb* / ↑ Effectiveness and side effects of calcium

Sodium polystyrene sulfonate / Metabolic alkalosis and ↓ binding of resin to potassium with renal impairment.

H *Squill* / ↑ Effectiveness and side effects of calcium

Tetracyclines / ↓ Tetracycline effect R/T ↓ GI tract absorption

Thiazide diuretics / Hypercalcemia R/T thiazide-induced renal tubular reabsorption of calcium and bone release of calcium

Verapamil / Calcium antagonizes the effect of verapamil

Vitamin D / Enhances intestinal absorption of dietary calcium.

DOSAGE
See individual agents.

NURSING CONSIDERATIONS
ASSESSMENT
1. Perform a thorough nursing history, noting clinical presentation, indications for therapy and any precipitating causes. List drugs prescribed, especially if receiving digitalis products; drug may be contraindicated.
2. Monitor calcium levels and renal function; assess for renal or parathyroid disease. Vitamin D facilitates absorption.
3. Identify any conditions that may preclude drug therapy, i.e., cancer, sarcoidosis, etc.
4. Assess for S&S of hypercalcemia, i.e., fatigue and CNS depression. With hypocalcemic tetany, protect client from injury.

5. Note bone mineral density and fracture history.

CLIENT/FAMILY TEACHING
1. General calcium requirements are best met by dietary sources (including milk in the diet) before menopause. Supplements need vitamin D to facilitate absorption. Consult dietitian to assist with proper food selection and meal planning and preparation.
2. Multivitamin and mineral preparations are expensive and do not contain sufficient calcium to meet daily requirements. Usual prescribed replacement regimen:
- Post-menopausal women: 1000–1500 mg
- Pregnant or breast-feeding females: 1200 mg
- Adults and adolescents: 800–1200 mg
- Children 1–10 years old: 500–800 mg
3. Report adverse side effects, lack of desired response, and keep all F/U appointments to evaluate drug response and dosage adjustments to prevent hypercalcemia and hypercalciuria.

OUTCOMES/EVALUATE
- Resolution of hypocalcemia
- Relief of muscle cramps
- Osteoporosis prophylaxis
- Serum calcium levels within desired range (8.8–10.4 mg/dL)

CEPHALOSPORINS

SEE ALSO THE FOLLOWING INDIVIDUAL ENTRIES:

Cefaclor
Cefadroxil monohydrate
Cefdinir
Cefditoren pivoxil
Cefepime hydrochloride
Cefixime oral
Cefoperazone sodium*
Cefotaxime sodium
Cefoxitin sodium
Cefpodoxime proxetil
Cefprozil
Ceftazidime*
Ceftibuten
Ceftizoxime sodium
Ceftriaxone sodium
Cefuroxime axetil

📷 = see color insert   H = Herbal   IV = Intravenous   ⓒ = sound alike drug

Cefuroxime sodium
Cephalexin
Loracarbef

Drugs marked with an * are available to view in the online database at www.delmarnursesdrughandbook.com/2009.

GENERAL STATEMENT

Cephalosporins are broad-spectrum antibiotics classified as first-, second-, and third-generation drugs.

First-Generation Cephalosporins: Cefadroxil, cefazolin, cephalexin, cephapirin, cephradine.

Second-Generation Cephalosporins: Cefaclor, cefmetazole, cefonicid, cefotetan, cefoxitin, cefprozil, cefuroxime, and loracarbef.

Third-Generation Cephalosporins: Cefdinir, cefepime, cefixime, cefoperazone, cefotaxime, cefpodoxime, ceftazidime, ceftibuten, ceftizoxime, ceftriaxone.

The difference among generations is based on pharmacokinetics and antibacterial spectra. Generally, third-generation cephalosporins have more activity against gram-negative organisms and resistant organisms and less activity against gram-positive organisms than first-generation drugs. Third-generation cephalosporins are also stable against beta-lactamases. Cephalosporins can be destroyed by cephalosporinase.

USES

See individual drugs.

ACTION/KINETICS

Action

The cephalosporins interfere with a final step in the formation of the bacterial cell wall (inhibition of mucopeptide biosynthesis), resulting in unstable cell membranes that undergo lysis (same mechanism of actions as penicillins). Also, cell division and growth are inhibited. The cephalosporins are most effective against young, rapidly dividing organisms and are considered bactericidal.

Pharmacokinetics

Cephalosporins are widely distributed to most tissues and fluids. First- and second-generation drugs do not enter the CSF well but third-generation drugs enter inflamed meninges readily. Rapidly excreted by the kidneys.

CONTRAINDICATIONS

Hypersensitivity to cephalosporins or related antibiotics.

SPECIAL CONCERNS

Safe use in pregnancy and lactation has not been established (pregnancy category: B). Use with caution in the presence of impaired renal or hepatic function, together with other nephrotoxic drugs, and in clients over 50 years of age. Perform C_{CR} on all clients with impaired renal function who receive cephalosporins. If hypersensitive to penicillin, may occasionally cross-react to cephalosporins.

SIDE EFFECTS

GI: N&V, diarrhea, constipation, abdominal cramps or pain, dyspepsia, glossitis, heartburn, sore mouth or tongue, dysgeusia, anorexia, flatulence, cholestasis, thirst, abdominal pain, oral candidiasis and moniliasis, flatulence, heartburn, gastritis, stomach cramps, eructation, melena, **bleeding peptic ulcer**, ileus, gall bladder sludge, colitis (including pseudomembranous colitis). **Hepatic:** Hepatomegaly, hepatitis, jaundice, cholestasis, cholestatic jaundice, **hepatic failure. CNS:** Headache, malaise, fatigue, vertigo, dizziness, lethargy, confusion, paresthesia, anxiety, hyperactivity, nervousness, insomnia, hypertonia, somnolence, precipitation of **seizures** (especially in clients with impaired renal function). **CV:** Hypotension, palpitations, chest pain, vasodilation, syncope. **Dermatologic:** Urticaria, diaphoresis, flushing, cutaneous moniliasis. **GU:** Pyuria, dysuria, vaginitis, vaginal discharge, genito-anal pruritus, genital candidiasis and moniliasis, reversible interstitial nephritis, hematuria, nephropathy, acute renal failure (rare). **Musculoskeletal:** Myalgia, arthralgia, rhabomyolysis. **Respiratory:** Asthma, **laryngeal edema,** dyspnea, interstitial pneumonitis, bronchitis, bronchospasm, pneumonia, **respiratory failure. Hypersensitivity:** Urticaria, rashes (maculopapular, morbilliform, or erythematous), pruritus (in-

---

Bold Italic = life threatening side effect   ■ = black box warning   ♣ = Available in Canada

cluding anal/genital areas), fever, chills, erythema, **angioedema**, serum sickness, joint pain, exfoliative dermatitis, chest tightness, myalgia, erythema multiforme, edema, itching, numbness, chills, **Stevens-Johnson syndrome, anaphylaxis.**

NOTE: Cross-allergy may be manifested between cephalosporins and penicillins. **Hematologic:** Leukopenia, leukocytosis, lymphocytosis, neutropenia (transient), eosinophilia, thrombocytopenia, thrombocythemia, **agranulocytosis,** granulocytopenia, bone marrow depression, anemia, **hemolytic anemia,** pancytopenia, decreased platelet function, **aplastic anemia,** hypoprothrombinemia (may lead to bleeding), **hemorrhage**, thrombocytosis (transient), lymphopenia, monocytosis. **Miscellaneous:** Superinfection including oral candidiasis and enterococcal infections, hypotension, sweating, flushing, dyspnea, interstitial pneumonitis.

NOTE: IV or IM use may result in local swelling, inflammation, cellulitis, paresthesia, burning, phlebitis, thrombophlebitis. IM use may also cause pain and induration, tenderness, increased temperature. Sterile abscesses have been observed following SC use. Nephrotoxicity (↑ BUN with and without ↑ serum creatinine) may occur in clients over 50 and in young children. Intrathecal use may result in hallucinations, nystagmus, or **seizures.**

OD OVERDOSE MANAGEMENT
Symptoms: Parenteral use of large doses of cephalosporins may cause **seizures,** especially in clients with impaired renal function.
Treatment: If seizures occur, discontinue the drug immediately and give anticonvulsant drugs. Hemodialysis may also be effective in cases of overwhelming overdosage.

DRUG INTERACTIONS
Alcohol / Antabuse-like reaction if used with cefazolin, cefmetazole, cefoperazone, or cefotetan
Aminoglycosides / ↑ Risk of renal toxicity with certain cephalosporins; monitor renal function closely

Antacids / ↓ Plasma levels of cefaclor, cefdinir, or cefpodoxime
Anticoagulants / ↑ Hypoprothrombinemic effects with cefazolin, cefmetazole, cefoperazone, or cefotetan
Colistimethate / ↑ Risk of renal toxicity; monitor renal function
Colistin / ↑ Risk of renal toxicity; monitor renal function
Ethacrynic acid / ↑ Risk of renal toxicity; monitor renal function
Furosemide / ↑ Risk of renal toxicity; monitor renal function
H$_2$ antagonists / ↓ Plasma levels of cefpodoxime or cefuroxime
Polymyxin B / ↑ Risk of renal toxicity; monitor renal function
Probenecid / ↑ Effect of cephalosporins by ↓ excretion by kidneys
Vancomycin / ↑ Risk of renal toxicity.

LABORATORY TEST CONSIDERATIONS
↑ AST, ALT, total bilirubin, GGTP, LDH, alkaline phosphatase, neutrophil count (slight), PT (due to disturbances in vitamin K-dependent clotting function), platelets. ↓ H&H, False + for urinary glucose with Benedict's solution, Fehling's solution, or Clinitest tablets. Enzyme tests (Clinistix, Tes-Tape) are unaffected. False + Coombs' test and urinary 17-ketosteroids.

DOSAGE
See individual drugs.

NURSING CONSIDERATIONS
ADMINISTRATION/STORAGE
IV 1. Parenteral solutions infused too rapidly may cause pain and irritation; dilute and infuse over 30 min unless otherwise indicated and assess site.
2. Continue therapy for at least 2–3 days after symptoms of infection have disappeared.
3. For group A beta-hemolytic streptococcal infections, continue therapy for at least 10 days to prevent the development of glomerulonephritis or rheumatic fever.

ASSESSMENT
1. Note reasons for therapy, physical presentation, S&S of infection; list other agents trialed and baseline culture results.

---

2. List allergy history. With hypersensitivity reactions to penicillin, assess for cross-sensitivity to cephalosporins.

3. Monitor CBC, platelets, PT, BS, lytes, renal and LFTs. With renal impairment reduce dose; for dialysis clients, administer after treatment. May cause false positive Coombs' test.

INTERVENTIONS

1. The cephalosporins all have similar sounding and similarly spelled names. Use care when transcribing orders for administration and request clarification as needed.

2. Pseudomembranous colitis may occur. If diarrhea develops, report any fevers. Monitor VS, I&O, stool C&S, and electrolytes.

3. Those prescribed sodium salts of cephalosporins may have fluid retention; report if condition precludes this side effect.

4. If also prescribed other antibiotic give cephalosporins 1 hr before bacteroistatic antibiotics (erythromycins, tetracylcines and chloramphenicol) as these keep bacteria from growing by decreasing cephalosporin uptake by bacterial cell walls.

5. Persistent temperature elevations may be drug-induced fever.

CLIENT/FAMILY TEACHING

1. Oral medications should be taken on an empty stomach, but, if GI upset occurs, may be administered with meals. Take as directed and complete entire prescription despite feeling better.

2. Report any S&S that may necessitate drug withdrawal, such as vaginal itching/drainage, fever, or diarrhea. Immediately report any abnormal bleeding or bruising.

3. Yogurt or buttermilk (4 oz) may be prescribed daily for diarrhea related to intestinal superinfections (to restore intestinal flora); consult provider. Report signs of superinfection (black furry tongue, vaginal itching or discharge, and loose, foul-smelling stools). Nystatin may be ordered for secondary infections.

4. May cause false positive Coombs' test. Would be of concern if being cross-matched for blood transfusions or in newborn where the mother used cephalosporins during pregnancy.

5. Avoid alcohol and alcohol-containing products during and for 3 days following completion of therapy, as a disulfiram-type reaction may occur.

6. Report adverse side effects, lack of response or inability to complete prescription. Keep all F/U visits and lab studies.

OUTCOMES/EVALUATE

- Negative C&S reports
- Resolution of infection
- Symptomatic improvement, i.e., ↓ WBCs, ↓ fever, improved appetite, wound healing

CHOLINERGIC BLOCKING AGENTS

SEE ALSO THE FOLLOWING INDIVIDUAL ENTRIES:

Atropine sulfate
Benztropine mesylate
Biperiden hydrochloride
Dicyclomine hydrochloride
Ipratropium bromide
Scopolamine hydrobromide
Scopolamine transdermal
     therapeutic system

USES
See individual drugs.

ACTION/KINETICS

Action
Cholinergic blocking agents prevent the neurotransmitter acetylcholine from combining with receptors on the postganglionic parasympathetic nerve terminal (muscarinic site). Effects include reduction of smooth muscle spasms, blockade of vagal impulses to the heart, decreased secretions (e.g., gastric, salivation, bronchial mucus, sweat glands), production of mydriasis and cycloplegia, and various CNS effects. In therapeutic doses, these drugs have little effect on transmission of nerve impulses across ganglia (nicotinic sites) or at the neuromuscular junction. Several anticholinergic drugs abolish or reduce the S&S of Parkinson's disease, such as tremors and rigidity, and result in some improvement in mobility, muscular

coordination, and motor performance. These effects may be due to blockade of the effects of acetylcholine in the CNS.

CONTRAINDICATIONS

Glaucoma, adhesions between iris and lens of the eye, tachycardia, myocardial ischemia, unstable CV state in acute hemorrhage, partial obstruction of the GI and biliary tracts, prostatic hypertrophy, renal disease, myasthenia gravis, hepatic disease, paralytic ileus, pyloroduodenal stenosis, pyloric obstruction, intestinal atony, ulcerative colitis, obstructive uropathy. Cardiac clients, especially when there is danger of tachycardia; older persons suffering from atherosclerosis or mental impairment. Lactation.

SPECIAL CONCERNS

Use with caution in pregnancy. Infants and young children are more susceptible to the toxic side effects of anticholinergic drugs. Use in children when the ambient temperature is high may cause a rapid increase in body temperature due to suppression of sweat glands. Geriatric clients are particularly likely to manifest anticholinergic side effects and CNS effects, including agitation, confusion, drowsiness, excitement, glaucoma, and impaired memory. Use with caution in hyperthyroidism, CHF, cardiac arrhythmias, hypertension, Down syndrome, asthma, spastic paralysis, blonde individuals, allergies, and chronic lung disease.

SIDE EFFECTS

These are desirable in some conditions and undesirable in others. Thus, the anticholinergics have an antisalivary effect that is useful in parkinsonism. This same effect is unpleasant when the drug is used for spastic conditions of the GI tract. Most side effects are dose-related and decrease when dosage decreases. **GI:** N&V, dry mouth, dysphagia, constipation, heartburn, change in taste perception, bloated feeling, paralytic ileus, epigastric distress, acute suppurative parotiditis, dilation of the colon, development of duodenal ulcer. **CNS:** Dizziness, drowsiness, nervousness, disorientation, headache, weakness, insom-

nia, fever (especially in children). Large doses may produce CNS stimulation including tremor and restlessness. **Anticholinergic psychoses:** Ataxia, euphoria, confusion, disorientation, loss of short-term memory, decreased anxiety, fatigue, insomnia, hallucinations, dysarthria, agitation. **CV:** Palpitations, tachycardia, hypotension, postural hypotension. **GU:** Urinary retention or hesitancy, dysuria, impotence. **Ophthalmic:** Blurred vision, dilated pupils, diplopia, increased intraocular tension, angle-closure glaucoma, photophobia, cycloplegia, precipitation of acute glaucoma. **Dermatologic:** Urticaria, skin rashes, other dermatoses. **Musculoskeletal:** Muscle weakness, muscle cramping. **Other:** *Anaphylaxis,* flushing, decreased sweating, nasal congestion, numbness of fingers, suppression of glandular secretions including lactation. Heat prostration (fever and heat stroke) in presence of high environmental temperatures due to decreased sweating.

OD OVERDOSE MANAGEMENT

Symptoms ("Belladonna Poisoning"): Infants and children are especially susceptible to the toxic effects of atropine and scopolamine. Poisoning (dose-dependent) is characterized by the following symptoms: Dry mouth, burning sensation of the mouth, difficulty in swallowing and speaking, blurred vision, photophobia, dilated and sluggish pupils, rash, tachycardia, *circulatory collapse, cardiac arrest,* increased respiration, *increased body temperature* (up to 109°F, 42.7°C), restlessness, irritability, confusion, anxiety, ataxia, hyperactivity, combativeness, toxic psychosis, anhidrosis, muscle incoordination, dilated pupils, hot dry skin, dry mucous membranes, dysphagia, foul-smelling breath, decreased bowel sounds, *respiratory depression and paralysis,* tremors, *seizures,* hallucinations, and *death.* *Treatment ("Belladonna Poisoning"):*
- Gastric lavage or induction of vomiting followed by activated charcoal. General supportive measures.
- Anticholinergic effects can be reversed by physostigmine (Eserine), 1–3 mg IV (effectiveness uncertain;

thus use other agents if possible). Neostigmine methylsulfate, 0.5–2 mg IV, repeated as necessary.

- If there is excitation, diazepam, a short-acting barbiturate, IV sodium thiopental (2% solution), or chloral hydrate (100–200 mL of a 2% solution by rectal infusion) may be given.
- For fever, cool baths may be used. Keep client in a darkened room if photophobia is manifested.
- Artificial respiration should be instituted if there is paralysis of respiratory muscles.

DRUG INTERACTIONS

Amantadine / Additive anticholinergic side effects

Antacids / ↓ Absorption of anticholinergics from GI tract

Antidepressants, tricyclic / Additive anticholinergic side effects

Antihistamines / Additive anticholinergic side effects

Atenolol / Anticholinergics ↑ effects of atenolol

Benzodiazepines / Additive anticholinergic side effects

Corticosteroids / Additive ↑ intraocular pressure

Digoxin / ↑ Drug effect R/T ↑ GI tract absorption

Disopyramide / Potentiation of anticholinergic side effects

Guanethidine / Reversal of inhibition of gastric acid secretion caused by anticholinergics

Haloperidol / Possible worsening of schizophrenic symptoms, ↓ haloperidol serum levels, and development of tardive dyskinesia

Histamine / Reversal of inhibition of gastric acid secretion caused by anticholinergics

Levodopa / Possible ↓ drug effect R/T ↑ breakdown of levodopa in stomach (R/T delayed gastric emptying time)

MAO inhibitors / ↑ Effect of anticholinergics R/T ↓ liver breakdown

Meperidine / Additive anticholinergic side effects

Methylphenidate / Potentiation of anticholinergic side effects

Metoclopramide / Anticholinergics block action of metoclopramide

Nitrates, nitrites / Potentiation of anticholinergic side effects

Nitrofurantoin / ↑ Bioavailability of nitrofurantoin

Orphenadrine / Additive anticholinergic side effects

Phenothiazines / Additive anticholinergic side effects; also, ↓ phenothiazine effects

Primidone / Potentiation of anticholinergic side effects

Procainamide / Additive anticholinergic side effects

Quinidine / Additive anticholinergic side effects

Sympathomimetics / ↑ Bronchial relaxation

Thiazide diuretics / ↑ Bioavailability of thiazide diuretics

Thioxanthines / Potentiation of anticholinergic side effects.

DOSAGE

See individual drugs.

NURSING CONSIDERATIONS

ADMINISTRATION/STORAGE

Dosage is often small. To prevent overdosage, check dose and measure exactly.

ASSESSMENT

1. Note reasons for therapy and clinical presentation. Assess for asthma, glaucoma, or duodenal ulcer (precludes therapy). Note any renal disease, cardiac problems, or hepatic disease.

2. List age; elderly clients, especially those with mental impairment or atherosclerosis, should not receive these drugs. Assess for constipation, urinary retention, and tolerance.

3. Monitor VS and ECG. Assess for any hemodynamic changes and intraventricular conduction blocks. Note palpitations.

4. With eye therapy, determine any experience with these drugs and eye exam results. Document IOP; assess accommodation and pupillary response.

5. With GI therapy, document UGI and/or endoscopy findings.

6. With GU therapy, note PVR, cystoscopy and prostate exam results.

7. Drugs such as atropine may suppress thermoregulatory sweating; counsel client concerning activity (especially in

---

Bold Italic = life threatening side effect   ■ = black box warning   ✦ = Available in Canada

hot weather) and appropriate clothing. Also, children and infants may exhibit "atropine fever.".

CLIENT/FAMILY TEACHING

1. May take with food or milk to ↓ GI upset. Do not stop suddenly.
2. Avoid activities that require mental alertness until drug effects realized.
3. Certain side effects are to be expected, such as dry mouth or blurred vision, and may have to be tolerated because of the overall beneficial effects of drug therapy. Report if persistent or bothersome; provider may reduce dose or temporarily stop drug.
4. With GI therapy, take early enough before a meal (at least 20 min) so that it will be effective when needed. Review printed information related to the prescribed diet; see dietitian for assistance in meal planning.
5. Gastric emptying times may be prolonged and intestinal transit time lengthened. Drug-induced intestinal paralysis is temporary and should resolve after 1–3 days of therapy.
6. With parkinsonism, do not withdraw abruptly. If the medication is changed, one drug should be withdrawn slowly and the other started in small doses.
7. Avoid prolonged heat exposure; may cause heat stoke.
8. May use ice, sips of fluids or sugar free candy/gum to relieve dry mouth effects.
9. Avoid OTC cough and cold remedies with alcohol and antihistamines unless specifically directed by provider.
10. With eye administration review methods for instillation of drops or ointment and frequency. Wash hands and do not permit container to come in contact with eye tissue. Vision will be affected by the medications; temporary stinging and blurred vision will occur. Assess response and plan activities for safety. Night vision may be impaired. Photophobia, which may occur, can be relieved by wearing dark glasses.
11. Report any marked changes in vision, eye irritation, eye pain after instillation, or persistent headaches immediately.
12. With large doses, tears may diminish; may experience dry/sandy eyes that would benefit with liquid tears.
13. Report urinary retention; may be more pronounced in elderly men with BPH. Report if bladder distended; may need catheterization if no urine output >8 hr.
14. Consult with provider for medication adjustment if impotence occurs; may be drug-related.

OUTCOMES/EVALUATE

Mydriasis and cycloplegia ↓ Heart rate ↓ Secretion production ↓ Tremors and rigidity

CORTICOSTEROIDS ■

SEE ALSO THE FOLLOWING INDIVIDUAL ENTRIES:

Beclomethasone dipropionate
Betamethasone
Betamethasone dipropionate
Betamethasone sodium phosphate
Betamethasone sodium phosphate and Betamethasone acetate
Betamethasone valerate
Budesonide
Cortisone acetate
Cosyntropin*
Dexamethasone
Dexamethasone acetate
Dexamethasone sodium phosphate
Flunisolide
Fluticasone propionate
Hydrocortisone
Hydrocortisone acetate
Hydrocortisone butyrate
Hydrocortisone cypionate
Hydrocortisone probutate
Hydrocortisone sodium phosphate
Hydrocortisone sodium succinate
Hydrocortisone valerate
Loteprednol etabonate
Methylprednisolone
Methylprednisolone acetate
Methylprednisolone sodium succinate
Mometasone furoate monohydrate
Prednisolone
Prednisolone acetate
Prednisolone sodium phosphate
Prednisolone tebutate
Prednisone

Triamcinolone
Triamcinolone acetonide
Triamcinolone hexacetonide

Drugs marked with an * are available to view in the online database at www.delmarnursesdrughandbook.com/2009.

USES

When used for anti-inflammatory or immunosuppressant therapy, the corticosteroid should possess minimal mineralocorticoid activity. Therapy with glucocorticoids is not curative and in many situations should be considered as adjunctive rather than primary therapy. The following list is not inclusive but provides examples of the physiologic and pharmacologic uses of corticosteroids.

1. **Replacement therapy.** Acute and chronic adrenal insufficiency, including Addison's disease. For replacement therapy, drugs must possess both glucocorticoid and mineralocorticoid effects. Also, used for adrenal hyperplasia, nonsuppurative thyroiditis.

2. **Rheumatic disorders,** including rheumatoid arthritis (including juvenile), ankylosing spondylitis, acute and subacute bursitis, acute nonspecific tenosynovitis, acute gouty arthritis, psoriatic arthritis, post-traumatic osteoarthritis, synovitis of osteoarthritis, epicondylitis.

3. **Collagen diseases,** including SLE, acute rheumatic carditis, polymyositis.

4. **Allergic diseases,** including control of severe allergic conditions, such as serum sickness, drug hypersensitivity reactions, anaphylaxis.

5. **Respiratory diseases,** including prophylaxis and treatment of chronic bronchial asthma (including status asthmaticus), seasonal or perennial rhinitis, symptomatic sarcoidosis, Loeffler's syndrome (not manageable by other means), berylliosis, fulminating or disseminated pulmonary tuberculosis (also use tuberculostatic drugs), aspiration pneumonitis. Regular use of inhaled steroids in children could be a life-saving treatment.

6. **Ocular diseases,** including severe acute and chronic allergic and inflammatory conditions such as allergic conjunctivitis, keratitis, allergic corneal marginal ulcers, herpes zoster ophthalmicus, iritis and iridocyclitis, chorioretinitis, diffuse posterior uveitis and choroiditis, optic neuritis, sympathetic ophthalmia and anterior segment inflammation, superficial punctate keratitis, herpes zoster keratitis, selected infective conjunctivitis, vernal conjunctivitis, anterior uveitis, postoperative inflammation following ocular surgery. Corneal injury from chemical, radiation, or thermal burns or penetration of foreign bodies.

7. **Dermatologic diseases,** including angioedema or urticaria, contact dermatitis, atopic dermatitis, severe erythema multiforme (Stevens-Johnson syndrome), pemphigus, dermatitis herpetiformis, mycosis fungoides, severe psoriasis, exfoliative or seborrheic dermatitis, acne rosacea.

8. **Diseases of the intestinal tract,** including chronic ulcerative colitis, regional enteritis, intractable sprue.

9. **Nervous system,** including acute exacerbations of multiple sclerosis.

10. **Malignancies,** including leukemias and lymphomas in adults and acute leukemia in children, hypercalcemia associated with cancer.

11. **Nephrotic syndrome,** including that due to lupus erythematosus or of the idiopathic type.

12. **Hematologic diseases,** including acquired hemolytic anemia, RBC anemia, idiopathic and secondary thrombocytopenic purpura in adults (IV only), congenital hypoplastic anemia.

13. **Intra-articular or soft tissue administration,** including acute episodes of synovitis of osteoarthritis, rheumatoid arthritis, acute gouty arthritis, acute and subacute bursitis, epicondylitis, acute nonspecific tenosynovitis, post-traumatic osteoarthritis.

14. **Intralesional administration,** including keloids; localized hypertrophic, infiltrated, inflammatory lesions of lichen planus; psoriatic plaques, granuloma annulare, neurodermatitis, necro-

---

Bold Italic = life threatening side effect   ■ = black box warning   ♣ = Available in Canada

biosis lipoidica diabeticorum, alopecia areata, discoid lupus erythematosus. Possibly effective in cystic tumors of an aponeurosis or tendon.

15. **Miscellaneous:** Tuberculosis meningitis with subarachnoid block or impending block when accompanied by appropriate tuberculostatic drugs; trichosis with neurologic or myocardial involvement.

Lotions are considered best for weeping eruptions, especially in areas subject to chafing (axilla, feet, and groin). Creams are suitable for most inflammations; ointments are preferred for dry, scaly lesions.

ACTION/KINETICS

Action

The hormones of the adrenal gland influence many metabolic pathways and all organ systems and are essential for survival. These processes include carbohydrate metabolism (e.g., glycogen deposition in the liver and conversion of glycogen to glucose), protein metabolism (e.g., gluconeogenesis, protein catabolism), fat metabolism (e.g., deposition of fatty tissue), and water and electrolyte balance (e.g., fluid retention, excretion of potassium, calcium, and phosphorus). According to their chemical structure and chief physiologic effect, the corticosteroids fall into two subgroups, which have considerable functional overlap. First are those, like cortisone and hydrocortisone, that mainly regulate the metabolic pathways involving protein, carbohydrate, and fat. This group is often referred to as *glucocorticoids*. In the second group are those, like aldosterone and desoxycorticosterone, that are more specifically involved in electrolyte and water balance. These are often referred to as *mineralocorticoids*. Hormones, such as cortisone and hydrocortisone, although classified as glucocorticoids, possess significant mineralocorticoid activity. Therapeutically, a distinction must be made between physiologic doses used for replacement therapy and pharmacologic doses used to treat inflammatory and other disease states.

The hormones have a marked anti-inflammatory effect because of their ability to inhibit prostaglandin synthesis. These agents also inhibit accumulation of macrophages and leukocytes at sites of inflammation as well as inhibit phagocytosis and lysosomal enzyme release. They aid the organism in coping with various stressful situations (trauma, severe illness). The immunosuppressant effect is thought to be due to a reduction of the number of T lymphocytes, monocytes, and eosinophils. Corticosteroids also decrease binding of immunoglobulin to receptors on the cell surface and inhibit the synthesis and/or release of interleukins which, in turn, decrease T-lymphocyte blastogenesis and reduce the primary immune response.

CONTRAINDICATIONS

Suspected infection as these drugs may mask infections. Also peptic ulcer, psychoses, acute glomerulonephritis, herpes simplex infections of the eye, vaccinia or varicella, the exanthematous diseases, Cushing's syndrome, active tuberculosis, myasthenia gravis. Recent intestinal anastomoses, CHF or other cardiac disease, hypertension, systemic fungal infections, open-angle glaucoma. Also, hyperlipidemia, hyperthyroidism or hypothyroidism, osteoporosis, myasthenia gravis, tuberculosis, otitis media with effusion in children. Lactation (if high doses are used). Inhalation products to relieve acute bronchospasms.

Topically in the eye for dendritic keratitis; fungal diseases of ocular structures; vaccinia, varicella and most other viral diseases of the cornea and conjunctiva; ocular tuberculosis; hypersensitivity; after uncomplicated removal of a superficial corneal foreign body; mycobacterial eye infection; acute, purulent, untreated eye infections that may be masked or enhanced by the presence of steroids.

Topically in the ear in aural fungal infections and perforated eardrum. Topically in tuberculosis of the skin, herpes simplex, vaccinia, varicella, and

Classifications

infectious conditions in the absence of anti-infective agents.

Inhalation products for relief of acute bronchospasms, primary treatment of status asthmaticus, or other acute episodes of asthma.

SPECIAL CONCERNS

■(1) Deaths due to adrenal insufficiency have occurred in asthmatic clients during and after transfer from systemic corticosteroids to inhaled corticosteroids. After withdrawal from systemic corticosteroids, several months are needed for recovery of hypothalamic-pituitary-adrenal (HPA) function. During this time of HPA suppression, clients may exhibit symptoms of adrenal insufficiency when exposed to trauma, surgery, or infections (especially gastroenteritis or other conditions with acute electrolyte loss). Although inhaled glucocorticoids may control asthmatic symptoms during these episodes, they do not provide the necessary mineralocorticoids for the treatment of these emergencies. Clients previously maintained on 20 mg/day or more of prednisone (or equivalent) may be most susceptible, especially when their systemic corticosteroids have been almost completely withdrawn. (2) During periods of stress or a severe asthmatic attack, have clients who have been withdrawn from systemic corticosteroids resume them (in large doses) immediately; contact a physician. Have clients carry a warning card indicating that they may need supplementary systemic corticosteroids during such periods. To assess the risk of adrenal insufficiency in emergency situations, periodically perform routine adrenal cortical function tests, including measurement of early morning resting cortisol levels in all clients. An early morning resting cortisol level may be accepted as normal only if it falls at or near the normal mean level.■ Use with caution in diabetes mellitus, hypertension, chronic nephritis, thrombophlebitis, convulsive disorders, infectious diseases, renal or hepatic insufficiency, pregnancy. Use of orally inhaled or intranasal products may inhibit the growth and development of children or adolescents, although this may only be temporary. Prolonged used of ophthalmic products may result in glaucoma, elevated intraocular pressure, optic nerve damage, defects in visual acuity and fields of vision, posterior subcapsular cataract formation or secondary ocular infections from pathogens liberated from ocular tissues. Pediatric clients are also at greater risk for developing cataracts, osteoporosis, avascular necrosis of the femoral heads, and glaucoma. Geriatric clients are more likely to develop hypertension and osteoporosis (especially postmenopausal women). Use inhalation products with caution in children less than 6 years of age.

SIDE EFFECTS

Small physiologic doses given as replacement therapy or short-term high-dosage therapy during emergencies rarely cause side effects. Prolonged therapy may cause a Cushing-like syndrome with atrophy of the adrenal cortex and subsequent adrenocortical insufficiency. A steroid withdrawal syndrome may occur following prolonged use; symptoms include anorexia, N&V, lethargy, headache, fever, joint pain, desquamation, myalgia, weight loss, hypotension.

SYSTEMIC USE

Fluid and electrolyte: Edema, hypokalemic alkalosis, hypokalemia, hypocalcemia, hypotension or shock-like reaction, hypertension, CHF. **Musculoskeletal:** Muscle wasting, muscle pain/weakness, osteoporosis, spontaneous fractures including vertebral compression fractures and fractures of long bones, tendon rupture, aseptic necrosis of femoral and humeral heads. **GI:** N&V, anorexia or increased appetite, diarrhea or constipation, abdominal distention, pancreatitis, gastric irritation, ulcerative esophagitis. Development or exacerbation of peptic ulcers with the possibility of perforation and hemorrhage; *perforation of the small and large bowel,* especially in inflammatory bowel disease. **Endocrine:** Cushing's syndrome (e.g., central obesity, moonface, buffalo hump, enlargement of supraclavicular fat pads), amenorrhea, postmenopausal bleeding, menstrual irregularities, decreased glucose tolerance, hyperglycemia, glycosuria, increased insulin or sulfonylurea requirement in diabetics, development of diabetes mellitus, negative nitrogen balance due to protein catabolism, suppression of growth in children, secondary adrenocortical and pituitary unresponsiveness (especially during periods of stress). **CNS/Neurologic:** Headache, vertigo, insomnia, restlessness, increased motor activity, ischemic neuropathy, EEG abnormalities, *seizures*, pseudotumor cerebri. Also, euphoria, mood swings, depression, anxiety, personality changes, psychoses. **CV:** Thromboembolism, thrombophlebitis, ECG changes (due to potassium deficiency), fat embolism, necrotizing angiitis, cardiac arrhythmias, *myocardial rupture following recent MI,* syncopal episodes. **Dermatologic:** Impaired wound healing, skin atrophy and thinning, petechiae, ecchymoses, erythema, purpura, striae, hirsutism, urticaria, *angioneurotic edema,* acneiform eruptions, allergic dermatitis, lupus erythematosus-like lesions, suppression of skin test reactions, perineal irritation. **Ophthalmic:** Glaucoma, posterior subcapsular cataracts, increased IOP, exophthalmos. **Miscellaneous:** Hypercholesterolemia, atherosclerosis, aggravation or masking of infections, leukocytosis, increased/decreased motility and number of spermatozoa. **In children:** Suppression of linear growth; reversible pseudobrain tumor syndrome characterized by papilledema, oculomotor or abducens nerve paralysis, visual loss, or headache.

PARENTERAL USE
Sterile abscesses, Charcot-like arthropathy, subcutaneous and cutaneous atrophy, burning or tingling (especially in the perineal area following IV use), scarring, inflammation, paresthesia, induration, hyper-/hypopigmentation, blindness when used intralesionally around the face and head (rare), transient or delayed pain or soreness, nystagmus, ataxia, muscle twitching, hiccoughs, *anaphylaxis with or without circulatory collapse, cardiac arrest, bronchospasm,* arachnoiditis

after intrathecal use, foreign body granulomatous reactions.

INTRA-ARTICULAR USE
Postinjection flare, Charcot-like arthropathy, tendon rupture, skin atrophy, facial flushing, osteonecrosis. Due to reduction in inflammation and pain, clients may overuse the joint.

INTRASPINAL USE
Aseptic, bacterial, chemical, cryptococcal, or tubercular meningitis; adhesive arachnoiditis, conus medullaris syndrome.

INTRAOCULAR USE
Increased ocular pressure, thereby inducing or aggravating simple glaucoma. Stinging, burning, dendritic keratitis (herpes simplex), corneal perforation (especially when the drugs are used for diseases that cause corneal thinning). Posterior subcapsular cataracts, especially in children. Exophthalmos, secondary fungal or viral eye infections.

TOPICAL USE
When used over large areas, when the skin is broken, or with occlusive dressings, may cause atrophy of the epidermis, drying of the skin, or atrophy of the dermal collagen. When used on the face, diffuse thinning and homogenization of the collagen, epidermal thinning, and striae formation. Occasionally, sensitization reaction may occur, which necessitates discontinuation of the drug.

INHALATION
In addition to systemic side effects, inhaled corticosteroids may cause hoarseness, oropharyngeal candidiasis, cough, dermatitis, thirst, and tongue hypertrophy.

OD OVERDOSE MANAGEMENT
Symptoms (Continued Use of Large Doses)—Cushing's Syndrome: Acne, hypertension, moonface, striae, hirsutism, central obesity, ecchymoses, myopathy, sexual dysfunction, osteoporosis, diabetes, hyperlipidemia, increased susceptibility to infection, peptic ulcer, electrolyte and fluid imbalance. Acute toxicity or death is rare.
Treatment of Chronic Overdose: Gradually taper the dose of the steroid and frequently monitor lab tests. During periods of stress, steroid supplementation is necessary. Dose should be reduced to the lowest one that will control the

Classifications

symptoms (or discontinue the steroid completely). Recovery of normal adrenal and pituitary function may take up to 9 months. Large, acute overdoses may be treated with gastric lavage, emesis, and general supportive measures.

DRUG INTERACTIONS

Acetaminophen / ↑ Risk of hepatotoxicity R/T ↑ rate of formation of hepatotoxic acetaminophen metabolite

Alcohol / ↑ Risk of GI ulceration or hemorrhage.

H *Aloe* / Hypokalemia related to both drugs could potentiate the effect of digoxin

Amphotericin B / Corticosteroids ↑ K depletion caused by amphotericin B

Aminoglutethimide / ↓ Adrenal response to corticotropin

Anabolic steroids / ↑ Risk of edema

Antacids / ↓ Effect of corticosteroids R/T ↓ GI tract absorption

Antibiotics, broad-spectrum / Concomitant use may result in emergence of resistant strains, → severe infection

Anticholinergics / Combination ↑ IOP; aggravates glaucoma

Anticholinesterases / Anticholinesterase effects may be antagonized when used for myasthenia gravis

Anticoagulants, oral / ↓ Effect of anticoagulants by ↓ hypoprothrombinemia; also ↑ risk of hemorrhage R/T vascular effects of corticosteroids

Anticholinesterases / Corticosteroids may ↓ effect of anticholinesterases when used in myasthenia gravis

Antidiabetic agents / Hyperglycemic effect of corticosteroids may necessitate ↑ antidiabetic dose

Asparaginase / ↑ Hyperglycemic drug effect and the risk of neuropathy and disturbances in erythropoiesis

Barbiturates / ↓ Effect of corticosteroids R/T ↑ liver breakdown

Bumetanide / ↑ Potassium loss R/T potassium-losing properties of both drugs

Carbonic anhydrase inhibitors / Corticosteroids ↑ K depletion caused by carbonic anhydrase inhibitors

Cholestyramine / ↓ Effect of corticosteroids R/T ↓ GI tract absorption

Colestipol / ↓ Effect of corticosteroids R/T ↓ GI tract absorption

Contraceptives, oral / Estrogen ↑ anti-inflammatory effect of hydrocortisone by ↓ liver breakdown

Cyclophosphamide / ↑ Effect of cyclophosphamide R/T ↓ liver breakdown

Cyclosporine / ↑ Effect of both drugs R/T ↓ liver breakdown

CYP 3A4 inhibitors (itraconazole, ketoconazole, miconazole, protease inhibitors) / ↑ Risk of serious side effects if used with budesonide or fluticasone

Digitalis glycosides / ↑ Chance of digitalis toxicity (arrhythmias) R/T hypokalemia

Ephedrine / ↓ Effect of corticosteroids R/T ↑ liver breakdown

Estrogens / ↑ Anti-inflammatory effect of hydrocortisone by ↓ liver breakdown

Ethacrynic acid / Enhanced potassium loss R/T potassium-losing properties of both drugs

Folic acid / Requirements may ↑

Furosemide / ↑ Potassium loss R/T potassium-losing properties of both drugs.

H *Ginseng* / Possible additive effects; do not use together

Heparin / Ulcerogenic effects of corticosteroids may ↑ risk of hemorrhage

Hydantoins / ↑ Corticosteroid clearance → ↓ effects

Immunosuppressant drugs / ↑ Risk of infection

Indomethacin / ↑ Chance of GI ulceration

Insulin / Hyperglycemic effect of corticosteroids may necessitate ↑ antidiabetic dose

Isoniazid / ↓ Effect of isoniazid R/T ↑ liver breakdown and ↑ excretion

Ketoconazole / ↑ Corticosteroid availability and ↓ clearance → possible toxicity.

H *Licorice* / ↑ Levels of corticosteroids.

H *Lily-of-the-valley* / ↑ Effectiveness and side effects of chronic glucocorticoid therapy

Mexiletine / ↓ Effect of mexiletine R/T ↑ liver breakdown

Mitotane / ↓ Response of adrenal gland to corticotropin

Muscle relaxants, nondepolarizing / Effect of muscle relaxants may be ↑, ↓,

---

or not changed

Neuromuscular blocking agents / ↑ Risk of prolonged respiratory depression or paralysis

NSAIDs / ↑ Risk of GI hemorrhage or ulceration.

H *Pheasant's eye herb* / ↑ Effectiveness and side effects of chronic glucocorticoid therapy

Phenobarbital / ↓ Effect of corticosteroids R/T ↑ liver breakdown

Phenytoin / ↑ Effect of corticosteroids R/T ↑ liver breakdown

Potassium supplements / ↓ Plasma levels of potassium

Potassium depleting drugs (e.g., diuretics) / Possible hypokalemia; monitor

Rifampin / ↓ Effect of corticosteroids R/T ↑ liver breakdown

Ritodrine / ↑ Risk of maternal edema

Salicylates / Both are ulcerogenic; also, corticosteroids may ↓ blood salicylate levels

Smoking / ↓ Response to inhaled corticosteroids in smokers

Somatrem, Somatropin / Glucocorticoids may inhibit effect of somatrem.

H *Squill* / ↑ Effectiveness and side effects of chronic glucocorticoid therapy

Streptozocin / ↑ Risk of hyperglycemia

Tacrolimus / Higher tacrolimus doses needed for renal transplant clients also receiving corticosteroids

Theophyllines / Changes in effects of either drug may occur

Thiazide diuretics / ↑ Potassium loss R/T potassium-losing properties of both drugs

Tricyclic antidepressants / ↑ Risk of mental disturbances

Vitamin A / Topical vitamin A can reverse impaired wound healing in clients receiving corticosteroids

LABORATORY TEST CONSIDERATIONS
↑ Urine glucose, serum cholesterol, serum amylase. ↓ Serum potassium, triiodothyronine, serum uric acid. Alteration of electrolyte balance.

DOSAGE
See individual drugs. Corticosteroids are administered by a variety of routes.

NURSING CONSIDERATIONS
ADMINISTRATION/STORAGE
ADMINISTRATION OF ORAL CORTICOSTEROIDS
1. Administer PO forms of drug with food to minimize ulcerogenic effect. Discontinue gradually if used chronically.
2. At frequent intervals, reduce the dose gradually to determine if symptoms of the disease can be effectively controlled by smaller drug dose.
3. When treating clients with conditions such as asthma, ulcerative colitis, and rheumatoid arthritis, corticosteroids, given every other day, provide the beneficial effect of the steroid while minimizing pituitary-adrenal suppression. With this therapy, twice the usual daily dose of an intermediate-acting steroid is given every other morning.
4. Local administration of corticosteroids is preferred over systemic therapy to minimize systemic side effects.
5. Use the lowest effective dose in children and monitor routinely to avoid reduced rate of growth.

ADMINISTRATION OF TOPICAL CORTICOSTEROIDS
1. Cleanse area before applying the medication. Wash hands, wear gloves, apply sparingly, and rub gently into the area.
2. When prescribed, apply an occlusive dressing (not to be used if an infection is present) to promote hydration of the stratum corneum and increase the absorption of the medication. The following are two methods of applying an occlusive type dressing:
- Apply a large amount of medication to the cleansed area. Cover with a thin, pliable, nonflammable plastic film, which is then sealed to the surrounding tissue with skin tape or held in place with gauze. Change the dressing q 3–4 days.
- Apply a small amount of medication to the area and cover with a damp cloth. Then cover with a thin, pliable, nonflammable plastic film and seal to the surrounding tissue with tape, or

Classifications

hold in place with gauze. Change dressing twice a day.

ASSESSMENT

1. Note reasons for therapy, type, onset, characteristics of S&S; assess underlying cause: adrenal or nonadrenal disorder and clinical presentation. Check for any allergic reactions to corticosteroids or tartrazine.

2. List medications taking; identify if any may interact with corticosteroids. These include antidiabetic agents, cardiac glycosides, oral contraceptives, anticoagulants, and drugs influenced by liver enzymes.

3. Assess mental status (i.e., mood, affect, aggression, behavioral changes, depression) and neurological function.

4. Monitor ECG, electrolytes, BS, urinalysis, renal and LFTs (usually see elevated BS and low K+). If female, determine if pregnant.

5. Monitor VS, I&O, and weight. Obtain CXR and PPD if therapy prolonged, assessing for infection. Note childhood illnesses and immunization status.

6. In conditions requiring long term therapy determine if other agents (e.g., methotrexate) can be used to spare long term harmful steroid effects.

7. With trigger point injections, determine if oral trial effective in reducing pain levels before referral.

INTERVENTIONS

TOPICAL CORTICOSTEROIDS

1. Note site of therapy e.g., size, color, location, depth, odor, swelling, drainage and nature of infection. Assess for local sensitivity reaction at site of application.

2. Absorption varies regionally with highest absorption in scrotal skin and lowest on the foot. Inflamed skin increases absorption several-fold. Better action has been noted with the ointment bases than with the lotion or cream vehicles.

3. Observe for S&S of infections since corticosteroids tend to mask. Avoid occlusive dressing when an infection is present. With large occlusive dressing, take temperatures q 4 hr. Report if elevated and remove the dressing.

4. Assess for evidence of systemic absorption. Protracted use of large quantities of potent topical corticosteroids to large BSAs may precipitate iatrogenic Cushing's syndrome. Symptoms may include edema and transient inhibition of pituitary-adrenal cortical function as manifested by muscular pain, lassitude, depression, hypotension, and weight loss.

5. Advise client when applying topical ointment, to wash hands and to wear gloves or to apply with a sterile applicator (e.g., tongue blade). Report redness, dilated blood vessels, purple discolorations, bruising, pustules, and depressed shiny, wrinkled skin. Prolonged use of potent topical corticosteroids may increase incidence of systemic side effects.

ORAL CORTICOSTEROIDS

1. When first placed on corticosteroids, check BP twice a day until maintenance dose established.

2. Short-term oral therapy (e.g., 60 mg PO for 5 days) does not require divided doses or titration. With long-term therapy, monitor for symptoms of adrenal insufficiency, which include hypotension, confusion, restlessness, lethargy, weakness, N&V, anorexia, and weight loss; titrate dose to withdraw.

3. Evaluate for increased sodium and fluid retention. Monitor weight and observe for edema. If noted, adjust to low-sodium, high-potassium diet. Anticipate a small weight gain due to increased appetite, but sudden increases are probably due to edema. Edema occurs most frequently with cortisone or desoxycorticosterone acetate and less frequently with the synthetic agents.

4. Assess for SOB, distended neck veins, edema, and easy fatigue; S&S of CHF. Obtain CXR and ECG.

5. Monitor serum glucose, electrolytes, and platelet counts with long-term therapy. Report any unusual bleeding, bruising, presence of petechiae, symptoms of diabetes, and any other skin changes.

6. Assess muscles for weakness and wasting; signs of a negative nitrogen balance. Report changes in appearance,

---

Bold Italic = life threatening side effect   ▪ = black box warning   ✦ = Available in Canada especially those resembling Cushing's syndrome (such as rounding of the face, hirsutism, presence of acne, and thinning of the hair and nails) so dosage can be adjusted.

7. With diabetes, may develop hyperglycemia necessitating a change in diet and insulin dosage.

8. Assess for signs of depression, lack of interest in personal appearance, insomnia or anorexia.

9. GI bleeding may occur; periodically test stools for occult blood and monitor hematologic profile. Discuss potential for menstrual difficulties and amenorrhea related to long-term therapy.

10. Observe for S&S of other illnesses; these drugs tend to mask their severity.

CLIENT/FAMILY TEACHING

1. Corticosteroids include both mineralocorticoids and glucocorticoids. Mineralocorticoids maintain salt and fluid balance in the body while glucocorticoids have metabolic and anti-inflammatory effects and are mediators of the stress response.

2. Take the oral medication with food in the early morning and report any symptoms of gastric distress. To prevent gastric irritation, may use antacids and eat frequent small meals. If the symptoms persist, diagnostic x-rays may be indicated. High doses of glucocorticoids stimulate the stomach to produce excess acid and pepsin and may cause peptic ulcers. Antacids 3–4 times/day may relieve epigastric distress. Report any unusual bruising/bleeding or dark stools.

3. Eat a diet high in protein to compensate for the loss due to protein breakdown from gluconeogenesis. Identify foods high in potassium and low in sodium to prevent electrolyte disturbances. Supplement diet with potassium-rich foods such as citrus juices, collard greens, or bananas. Read labels of canned or processed foods and consult dietician for assistance in shopping and meal preparation.

4. Obtain weight daily at the same time, wearing clothing of approximately the same weight, and using the same scales. Consistent weight gain may reflect fluid retention; initiate caloric management to prevent obesity.

5. Exercise daily and consume foods high in calcium to decrease possibility of osteoporosis (due to catabolic bone effects). Consume adequate protein, calcium, and vitamin D to minimize bone loss. On-going bone resorption with depressed bone formation is the cause of osteoporosis.

6. Report changes in mood or affect or insomnia. Take early in the day to mimic circadian rhythm and prevent insomnia. Avoid falls and accidents. Steroids may cause osteoporosis, which makes the bones more susceptible to fractures. Use a night light and a hand rail or other device for support if need to get up at night.

7. Corticosteroids can cause a loss of contraceptive action with oral contraceptives. Keep accurate menstrual records and consider alternative methods of birth control. May also have an adverse effect on sperm production and count. Weight gain, acne, and excess hair growth may occur.

8. With dosage reduction, flare-ups may occur caused by the reduction. Need to gradually withdraw the medication when therapy has exceeded 7 consecutive days. This should proceed slowly so that the adrenal cortex will gradually be reactivated and take over the production of hormones. Sudden withdrawal may be life-threatening. Any sudden change will provoke symptoms of adrenal insufficiency.

9. With arthritis, do not overuse the joint once injected and painless. Permanent joint damage may result from overuse, because underlying pathology is still present.

10. With diabetes, monitor glucose levels frequently and report changes as insulin dose and diet may require adjustment.

11. Wounds may heal slowly because steroid therapy causes a delay in development of granulation tissue, increasing potential for infection. Observe any healing process for signs of infection and report any injury or postoperative separation of wound or suture line.

Classifications

Classifications

12. Delay any vaccinations, immunizations, or skin testing while receiving corticosteroid therapy because there is limited immune response. These drugs mask symptoms of infection and cause immunosuppression. Because antibody production is decreased by corticosteroids, clients are at risk for infection. Must maintain general hygiene and scrupulous cleanliness to avoid infection. Report if sore throat, cough, fever, malaise, or an injury that does not heal occurs. Avoid contact with persons with contagious diseases.

13. Clients on long-term eye therapy are prone to developing cataracts, exophthalmos, and increased IOP. Schedule routine eye exams and report any visual changes.

14. Avoid OTC medications, including aspirin and ibuprofen compounds, as well as alcohol, since these may aggravate gastric irritation and bleeding.

15. Check child's height and weight regularly and graph; growth suppression may occur with corticosteroid therapy; not prevented by growth hormone administration. Large doses of glucocorticoids in children may increase intracranial pressure (pseudotumor cerebri); report symptoms: vertigo, headache, and convulsions. These should disappear once therapy discontinued.

16. Carry ID, listing drugs and dosage, condition being treated, and who to contact in the event of an emergency. Periods of increased stress may require dosage increase temporarily.

OUTCOMES/EVALUATE

• Healing/clearing of dermatitis
• Chronic pain control
• Suppression of inflammatory/immune responses or disease manifestation in allergic reactions, autoimmune diseases, organ transplants
• Serum cortisol levels within desired range in adrenal deficiency states (8 a.m. level 110–520 nmol/L)

DIURETICS, LOOP ■

SEE ALSO DIURETICS, THIAZIDES, AND THE FOLLOWING INDIVIDUAL ENTRIES:

Bumetanide

Ethacrynate sodium
Ethacrynic acid
Furosemide
Torsemide

USES
See individual drugs.

ACTION/KINETICS

Action
Loop diuretics inhibit reabsorption of sodium and chloride in the proximal and distal tubules and the loop of Henle.

Pharmacokinetics
Metabolized in the liver and excreted primarily through the urine. Significantly bound to plasma protein.

CONTRAINDICATIONS
Hypersensitivity to loop diuretics or to sulfonylureas. In hepatic coma or severe electrolyte depletion (until condition improves or is corrected). Lactation.

SPECIAL CONCERNS
■Loop diuretics are potent drugs; excess amounts can lead to a profound diuresis with water and electrolyte depletion. Careful medical supervision is required and dosage must be individualized.■ Sudden alterations of electrolytes in hepatic cirrhosis and ascites may precipitate hepatic encephalopathy and coma. SLE may be activated or worsened. Ototoxicity is most common with rapid injection, in severe renal impairment, with doses several times the usual dose, and with concurrent use of other ototoxic drugs. The risk of hospitalization is doubled in geriatric clients who take diuretics and NSAIDs. Safety and efficacy of most loop diuretics have not been determined in children or infants.

SIDE EFFECTS
See individual drugs. Excessive diuresis may cause dehydration with the possibility of *circulatory collapse and vascular thrombosis or embolism.* Ototoxicity including tinnitus, hearing impairment, deafness (usually reversible), and vertigo with a sense of fullness are possible. Electrolyte imbalance, especially in clients with restricted salt intake. Photosensitivity. Changes include hypo-

---

Bold Italic = life threatening side effect   ■ = black box warning   ✦ = Available in Canada

kalemia, hypomagnesemia, and hypocalcemia.

OD **OVERDOSE MANAGEMENT**
Symptoms: Acute profound water loss, volume and electrolyte depletion, dehydration, decreased blood volume, and **circulatory collapse with possibility of fascicular thrombosis and embolism.** *Treatment:* Replace fluid and electrolyte loss. Carefully monitor urine and plasma electrolyte levels. Emesis and gastric lavage may be useful. Supportive measures may include oxygen or artificial respiration.

DRUG INTERACTIONS
Aminoglycosides / ↑ Ototoxicity with hearing loss
Anticoagulants / ↑ Drug activity
Chloral hydrate / Transient diaphoresis, hot flashes, hypertension, tachycardia, weakness and nausea
Cisplatin / Additive ototoxicity
Digitalis glycosides / ↑ Risk of arrhythmias R/T diuretic-induced electrolyte disturbances
Lithium / ↑ Plasma levels of lithium → toxicity
Muscle relaxants, nondepolarizing / Effect of muscle relaxants either ↑ or ↓, depending on diuretic dose
Nonsteroidal anti-inflammatory drugs / ↓ Effect of loop diuretics
Probenecid / ↓ Effect of loop diuretics
Salicylates / Diuretic effect may be ↓ with cirrhosis and ascites
Sulfonylureas / Loop diuretics may ↓ glucose tolerance
Theophyllines / Action of theophyllines may be ↑ or ↓
Thiamine / High doses of loop diuretics → thiamine deficiency
Thiazide diuretics / Additive effects with loop diuretics → profound diuresis and serious electrolyte abnormalities.

DOSAGE
See individual drugs.

NURSING CONSIDERATIONS
ASSESSMENT
1. Note reasons for therapy. List other agents trialed and outcome. Identify sensitivity to sulfonamides; may exhibit cross-reactivity with furosemide.

2. Monitor BP, weight, CBC, lytes, Mg, Ca, BS, uric acid, renal and LFTs; reduce dose with dysfunction.
3. Determine presence of SLE; drug may worsen condition.
4. Assess auditory function carefully when large doses are anticipated or when used concurrently with other ototoxic agents. Ototoxicity is dose related and generally reversible.

INTERVENTIONS
1. Record VS, weights, I&O; keep bedpan or urinal within reach. Report absence/decrease in diuresis and note changes in lung sounds. Diuretics potentiate the effects of antihypertensive agents; monitor BP.
2. When ambulatory, check for edema in the extremities; if on bed rest, check for edema in the sacral area.
3. Monitor for serum electrolyte levels, pH, and the following *signs of electrolyte imbalance:*
- *Hyponatremia* (low-salt syndrome)—characterized by muscle weakness, leg cramps, dryness of mouth, dizziness, and GI upset.
- *Hypernatremia* (excessive sodium retention)—characterized by CNS disturbances, i.e., confusion, loss of sensorium, stupor, and coma. ↓ Skin turgor and postural hypotension not as prominent as with combined sodium and water deficits.
- *Water intoxication*(caused by defective water diuresis)—characterized by lethargy, confusion, stupor, and coma. Neuromuscular hyperexcitability with ↑ reflexes, muscular twitching, and convulsions if acute.
- *Metabolic acidosis*—characterized by weakness, headache, malaise, abdominal pain, and N&V. Hyperpnea occurs in severe metabolic acidosis. S&S of volume depletion: poor skin turgor, soft eyeballs, and dry tongue may be observed.
- *Metabolic alkalosis*—characterized by irritability, neuromuscular hyperexcitability, tetany if severe.
- *Hypokalemia (potassium deficiency)*—characterized by muscular weakness, peristalsis failure, postural hypoten-

---

📷 = see color insert   **H** = Herbal   **IV** = Intravenous   ⓡ = sound alike drug sion, respiratory embarrassment, and cardiac arrhythmias.

- *Hyperkalemia (excess potassium)*—characterized by early signs of irritability, nausea, intestinal colic, and diarrhea; and by later signs of weakness, flaccid paralysis, dyspnea, dysphagia, and arrhythmias.

4. Hyper-/hypokalemia associated with diuretic therapy may potentiate the toxic effects of digitalis and precipitate arrhythmias.

5. With high doses monitor for hyperlipidemia and hyperuricemia; precipitating a gout attack. Assess for sore throat, skin rash, and yellowing of the skin or sclera; may be blood dyscrasias.

6. With liver dysfunction, assess for electrolyte imbalances, which could cause stupor, coma, and death.

7. If receiving EC potassium tablets, assess for abdominal pain, distention, or GI bleeding; can cause small bowel ulceration. Check stool for intact tablets.

8. May precipitate symptoms of diabetes with latent or mild diabetes. Test urine or perform finger sticks and monitor labs closely.

CLIENT/FAMILY TEACHING

1. Take with food or milk to decrease GI upset. May cause frequent, copious voiding. Plan activities/travel; take in the a.m. to prevent sleep disruption.

2. These drugs help rid your body of sodium and water. They make your kidneys excrete more sodium in the urine which takes water with it from your blood. That decreases the amount of fluid going through your blood vessels, which reduces pressure on the walls of your arteries.

3. Include foods high in potassium, such as citrus, grape, cranberry, apple, pear, and apricot juices; bananas; meat, fish- salmon, melons, almonds, potatoes and spinach. This is preferable to taking potassium chloride supplements but potassium supplements are usually prescribed with non-potassium-sparing diuretics. Unless conditions such as gastric ulcer or diabetes exist, drink a large glass of orange juice daily. Consult dietitian as needed for assistance in selecting and preparing foods.

4. Weakness and/or dizziness may occur. Rise slowly from bed and sit down or lie down if evident. Use caution in driving a car or operating other hazardous machinery until drug effects apparent. The use of alcohol, standing for prolonged periods, and exercise in hot weather may enhance/lower BP.

5. Ensure adequate fluids; monitor BP and weight. Report excessive weight loss, loss of skin turgor or if dizziness, nausea, muscle weakness, cramps, SOB, chest, back, or leg pain, excessive weight gain, or tingling of the extremities occur.

6. Wear protective clothing, sunscreens, and sunglasses to prevent photosensitivity reactions. Avoid tanning booths and drink plenty of water when out in the sun. Avoid all OTC preparations without approval.

7. Keep all F/U appointments to evaluate response to therapy and lab reports to assess for electrolyte problems.

OUTCOMES/EVALUATE

- Symptomatic relief ($\downarrow$ weight, $\downarrow$ swelling/edema, $\uparrow$ diuresis)
- Clinical improvement in S&S associated with CHF and renal failure
- $\downarrow$ BP

DIURETICS, THIAZIDES

SEE ALSO THE FOLLOWING INDIVIDUAL ENTRIES:

Hydrochlorothiazide
Indapamide

USES

See individual drugs, (1) Edema due to CHF, nephrosis, nephritis, renal failure, PMS, hepatic cirrhosis, corticosteroid or estrogen therapy. (2) Hypertension. Hydrochlorothiazide is a component of a large number of combination drugs used to treat hypertension. (3) Premenstrual tension. *Investigational:* Thiazides are used alone or in combination with allopurinol (or amiloride) for prophylaxis of calcium nephrolithiasis. Nephrogenic diabetes insipidus.

ACTION/KINETICS

Action

Thiazides promote diuresis by decreasing the rate at which sodium and chloride are reabsorbed by the distal renal tubules of the kidney. By increasing the excretion of sodium and chloride, they force excretion of additional water. They also increase the excretion of potassium and, to a lesser extent, bicarbonate, as well as decrease the excretion of calcium and uric acid. Sodium and chloride are excreted in approximately equal amounts. Thiazides do not affect the glomerular filtration rate. Thiazides also have an antihypertensive effect which is attributed to direct dilation of the arterioles, as well as to a reduction in the total fluid volume of the body and altered sodium balance. The thiazide diuretics are related chemically to the sulfonamides. Although devoid of anti-infective activity, the thiazides can cause the same hypersensitivity reactions as the sulfonamides.

Pharmacokinetics

A large fraction is excreted unchanged in urine.

CONTRAINDICATIONS

Hypersensitivity to drug, anuria, renal decompensation. Impaired renal function and advanced hepatic cirrhosis. Do not use indiscriminately in clients with edema and toxemia of pregnancy, even though they may be therapeutically useful, because the thiazides may have adverse effects on the newborn (thrombocytopenia and jaundice).

SPECIAL CONCERNS

Geriatric clients may manifest an increased risk of hypotension and changes in electrolyte levels. The risk of hospitalization is doubled in geriatric clients who take diuretics and NSAIDs. Administer with caution to debilitated clients or to those with a history of hepatic coma or precoma, gout, diabetes mellitus, or during pregnancy and lactation. Particular care must be exercised when thiazides are administered concomitantly with drugs that also cause potassium loss, such as digitalis, corticosteroids, and some estrogens. Clients with advanced heart failure, renal disease, or hepatic cirrhosis are most likely to develop hypokalemia. May activate or worsen SLE.

SIDE EFFECTS

The following side effects may be observed with most drugs. See also individual drugs. **Electrolyte imbalance:** Hypokalemia (most frequent) characterized by cardiac arrhythmias. Hyponatremia characterized by weakness, lethargy, epigastric distress, N&V. Hypokalemic alkalosis. **GI:** Anorexia, epigastric distress or irritation, N&V, cramping, bloating, abdominal pain, diarrhea, constipation, jaundice, pancreatitis. **CNS:** Dizziness, lightheadedness, headache, vertigo, xanthopsia, paresthesias, weakness, insomnia, restlessness. **CV:** Orthostatic hypotension, MIs in elderly clients with advanced arteriosclerosis, especially if the client is also receiving therapy with other antihypertensive agents. **Hematologic:** *Agranulocytosis, aplastic or hypoplastic anemia, hemolytic anemia,* leukopenia, thrombocytopenia. **Dermatologic:** Purpura, photosensitivity, dermatitis, rash, urticaria, necrotizing angiitis, vasculitis, cutaneous vasculitis. **Metabolic:** Neutropenia, hemolytic anemia. **Endocrine:** Hyperglycemia, glycosuria, hyperuricemia. **Miscellaneous:** Blurred vision, impotence, reduced libido, fever, muscle cramps, muscle spasm, respiratory distress.

OD OVERDOSE MANAGEMENT

Symptoms: Symptoms of plasma volume depletion, including orthostatic hypotension, dizziness, drowsiness, syncope, electrolyte abnormalities, hemoconcentration, hemodynamic changes. Signs of potassium depletion, including confusion, dizziness, muscle weakness, and GI disturbances. Also, N&V, GI irritation, GI hypermotility, CNS effects, cardiac abnormalities, *seizures, hypotension, decreased respiration, and coma.* *Treatment:*
- Induce emesis or perform gastric lavage followed by activated charcoal. Undertake measures to prevent aspiration.
- Electrolyte balance, hydration, respiration, CV, and renal function must be maintained. Cathartics should be

avoided, as use may enhance fluid loss.

- Although GI effects are usually of short duration, treatment may be required.

DRUG INTERACTIONS

Allopurinol / ↑ Risk of hypersensitivity reactions to allopurinol.

[H] *Aloe* / Hypokalemia as both drugs could potentiate effects of digoxin

Amphotericin B / Enhanced loss of electrolytes, especially potassium

Anesthetics / Thiazides may ↑ effects of anesthetics

Anticholinergic agents / ↑ Effect of thiazides R/T ↑ amount absorbed from GI tract

Anticoagulants, oral / Anticoagulant effects may be decreased

Antidiabetic agents / Thiazides antagonize hypoglycemic drug effects

Antigout agents / Thiazides may ↑ uric acid levels; thus, ↑ dose of antigout drug may be necessary

Antihypertensive agents / Thiazides potentiate drug effects

Antineoplastic agents / Thiazides may prolong drug-induced leukopenia

Calcium salts / Hypercalcemia R/T renal tubular reabsorption or bone release of calcium may be ↑ by exogenous calcium

Cholestyramine / ↓ Effect of thiazides R/T ↓ GI tract absorption

Colestipol / ↓ Effect of thiazides R/T ↓ GI tract absorption

Corticosteroids / Enhanced potassium loss R/T potassium-losing properties of both drugs

Diazoxide / Enhanced hypotensive effect. Also, ↑ hyperglycemic response

Digoxin / Thiazides produce ↑ K and Mg loss with ↑ chance of digitalis-induced arrhythmias

Ethanol / Additive orthostatic hypotension

Fenfluramine / ↑ Antihypertensive effect of thiazides

Furosemide / Profound diuresis and electrolyte loss

Guanethidine / Additive hypotensive effect

Indomethacin / ↓ Effect of thiazides, possibly by inhibition of prostaglandins

Insulin / ↓ Effect R/T thiazide-induced hyperglycemia

[H] *Licorice root* / Potassium loss R/T thiazides and licorice → ↑ sensitivity to digitalis glycosides

Lithium / ↑ Risk of lithium toxicity R/T ↓ renal excretion; may be used together but monitored carefully

Loop diuretics / Additive effect to cause profound diuresis and serious electrolyte losses

Methenamine / ↓ Effect of thiazides R/T alkalinization of urine by methenamine

Methyldopa / ↑ Risk of hemolytic anemia (rare)

Muscle relaxants, nondepolarizing / ↑ Effect of muscle relaxants R/T hypokalemia

Norepinephrine / Thiazides ↓ arterial response to norepinephrine

Quinidine / ↑ Effect of quinidine R/T ↑ renal tubular reabsorption

Sulfonamides / ↑ Effect of thiazides R/T ↓ plasma protein binding

Sulfonylureas / ↓ Effect R/T thiazide-induced hyperglycemia

Tetracyclines / ↑ Risk of azotemia

Tubocurarine / ↑ Muscle relaxation and ↑ hypokalemia

Vasopressors (sympathomimetics) / Thiazides ↓ responsiveness of arterioles to vasopressors

Vitamin D / ↑ Effect of vitamin D R/T thiazide-induced hypercalcemia.

LABORATORY TEST CONSIDERATIONS

Hypokalemia, hypercalcemia, hyponatremia, hypomagnesemia, hypochloremia, hypophosphatemia, hyperuricemia. ↑ BUN, creatinine, glucose in blood and urine. ↓ Serum PBI levels (no signs of thyroid disturbance). Initial ↑ total cholesterol, LDL cholesterol, and triglycerides.

DOSAGE

See individual drugs.

NURSING CONSIDERATIONS

ADMINISTRATION/STORAGE

1. Clients resistant to one type of thiazide may respond to another.
2. Liquid potassium preparations are bitter. Administer with fruit juice or milk to enhance palatability.
3. To minimize electrolyte imbalance, thiazides may be taken every other day or on a 3- to 5-day basis for treatment of edema.
4. To prevent excess hypotension, reduce dose of other antihypertensive agents when beginning therapy.

ASSESSMENT

1. Note reasons for therapy and any previous use of these drugs. List any drug hypersensitivity.

2. Monitor BP, weight, CBC, uric acid, glucose, lytes, Ca, Mg, renal and LFTs. Identify extent of edema; assess skin turgor, mucous membranes, extremities, and lung fields.

3. Note any history of heart disease or gout; check uric acid levels. With cirrhosis, avoid K$^+$ depletion and hepatic encephalopathy.

INTERVENTIONS

1. Stop drug at least 48 hr before surgery. Thiazide inhibits pressor effects of epinephrine.

2. Potassium supplements should be given only when dietary measures are inadequate. If required, use liquid preparations to avoid ulcerations that may be produced by potassium salts in the solid dosage form. Exceptions include slow-K forms (potassium salt imbedded in a wax matrix) and micro-K forms (microencapsulated potassium salt).

CLIENT/FAMILY TEACHING

1. Take with food or milk if GI upset occurs. Consume in the morning so that major diuretic effect occurs before bedtime.

2. Eat a diet high in potassium. Include orange juice, bananas, citrus fruits, broccoli, spinach, tomato juice, cucumbers, beets, dried fruits, and apricots. Avoid large amounts of black licorice; may precipitate severe hypokalemia.

3. Rise slowly and dangle legs before standing to minimize low BP effects. Sit or lie down if feeling faint or dizzy. Record weight; report gains >2 lb/day or 5 lb/week and swelling of extremities.

4. With gout, avoid foods that precipitate attacks and continue antigout agents as prescribed. With diabetes, monitor finger sticks more frequently; may need adjustment of insulin or oral hypoglycemic agent.

5. Avoid alcohol; causes severe drop in BP. Do not take any other medication (including OTC drugs for asthma, cough and colds, hay fever, weight control) unless approved.

6. Report any severe weight loss/gain, muscle weakness, cramps, dizziness, or fatigue. Skin rashes may occur but severe symptoms R/T allergic reactions include acute SOB (pulmonary edema), abdominal pain (acute pancreatitis), easy bruising/bleeding (thrombocytopenia), yellowing of skin/eyes; itching (cholestatic jaundice); and pale, weak/dizzy (hemolytic anemia); report immediately.

7. Keep all F/U appointments to evaluate response to therapy and lab reports.

OUTCOMES/EVALUATE

- Control of hypertension; ↓ BP ↑
- Urine output; ↓ edema; ↓ weight
- Normal electrolyte levels and fluid balance

ESTROGENS ▪

SEE ALSO THE FOLLOWING INDIVIDUAL ENTRIES:

Esterified estrogens
Estradiol gel
Estradiol hemihydrate
Estradiol transdermal system
Estrogens conjugated, oral
Estrogens conjugated, parenteral
Estrogens conjugated, synthetic (A & B)
Estrogens conjugated, vaginal
Estropipate
Oral Contraceptives

USES

See individual drugs. Uses include, but are not limited to: (1) Hormone replacement therapy in postmenopausal women to relieve moderate to severe vasomotor symptoms and decrease the risk of osteoporosis. (2) Component of combination oral contraceptives and other forms for contraception. (3) Used vaginally for vulvar/vaginal atrophy (alternative therapies should be tried first), atrophic vaginitis, and treatment of moderate to severe vasomotor symptoms associated with menopause. (4) Less commonly used for palliative treatment of select breast or prostate cancer clients with advanced disease. *NOTE:* Guidelines have been established for the routine use of combined estrogen and progestin hormone replacement therapy in women. Use of hormone replacement therapy carries both benefits and risks; overall risks are likely to exceed benefits. Thus, a D recommendation rating has been established for the routine use of combined estrogen and progestin in postmenopausal women and for the routine use of unopposed estrogen in postmenopausal women with hysterectomy for the prevention of chronic conditions. *Investigational:* Turner syndrome (estrogen replicates the events of puberty).

ACTION/KINETICS

Action

The three primary estrogens in the human female are estradiol 17–β, estrone, and estriol, which are steroids. Estrogens combine with receptors in the cytoplasm of the cell, resulting in an increase in protein synthesis. For example, estrogens are required for development of secondary sex characteristics, development and maintenance of the female genital system, and breasts. They also produce effects in the pituitary and hypothalamus. In adult women, estrogens participate in bone maintenance by aiding the deposition of calcium in the protein matrix of bones. They increase elastic elements in the skin, tend to cause sodium and fluid retention, and produce an anabolic effect by enhancing the turnover of dietary nitrogen and other elements into protein. Furthermore, they tend to keep plasma cholesterol at relatively low levels.

Pharmacokinetics

Natural estrogens have a significant first-pass effect; thus, they are given parenterally. Synthetic derivatives can be given PO and are rapidly absorbed, distributed, and excreted. Estrogens are metabolized in the liver and excreted in urine (major portion) and feces. When given transdermally, the skin metabolizes estradiol only to a small extent.

CONTRAINDICATIONS

Known or suspected breast cancer, except in those clients being treated for metastatic disease. Cancer of the genital tract and other estrogen-dependent neoplasms. Undiagnosed abnormal genital bleeding. Active deep vein thrombosis or history of such. Active or recent (within the past year) arterial thromboembolic disease, including active thrombophlebitis, thrombosis, or thromboembolic disorders. History of thrombophlebitis, thrombosis, or thromboembolic disorders associated with previous estrogen use, except when used to treat breast or prostatic malignancy. Known or suspected pregnancy. Prolonged therapy in women who plan to become pregnant. Porphyria (estradiol vaginal tablets only). Use during lactation. May be contraindicated in clients with blood dyscrasias, hepatic disease, or thyroid dysfunction.

SPECIAL CONCERNS

■(1) Estrogens have been reported to increase the risk of endometrial cancer in postmenopausal women exposed for more than 1 year. Incidence depends on duration of treatment and dose. When estrogens are used to treat menopausal symptoms, use the lowest dose and discontinue as soon as possible. When prolonged treatment is indicated, reassess the client at least semiannually by endometrial sampling to determine the need for continued therapy. (2) Close clinical surveillance of women taking estrogens is important. Adequate diagnostic measures, including endometrial sampling when indicated, should be undertaken to rule out malignancy in all cases of undiagnosed persistent or recurring abnormal vaginal bleeding. (3) There is no evidence that natural estrogens are more or less hazardous than synthetic estrogens at equiestrogenic doses. (4) Do not use estrogens during pregnancy as such use is associated with increased risk of congenital defects in the reproductive organs of the fetus and possibly other birth defects. There is no indication for estrogen therapy during pregnancy or during the immediate postpartum period. Estrogens are ineffective for the prevention and treatment of threatened or habitual abortion. Estrogens are not indicated for the prevention of postpartum breast engorgement. If estrogens

---

are used during pregnancy, or if the client becomes pregnant while taking estrogens, inform her of the potential risks to the fetus. (5) Do not use estrogens with or without progestins for the prevention of CV disease. There is an increased risk of MI, stroke, invasive breast cancer, pulmonary emboli, and DVT in postmenopausal women during 5 years of treatment with conjugated equine estrogens (0.625 mg) combined with medroxyprogesterone acetate (2.5 mg) relative to placebo. Because of these risks, estrogens with or without progestins should be prescribed at the lowest effective doses and for the shortest duration consistent with treatment goals and risks for the individual woman. (6) It has been reported that estrogens increase the risk of developing probable dementia in postmenopausal women 65 years or older during 4 years of treatment with conjugated estrogens plus medroxyprogesterone acetate compared with placebo. It is not known whether this is also true in younger postmenopausal women or women taking estrogen alone therapy.■ Use with caution, if at all, in those with asthma, epilepsy, migraine, cardiac failure, renal insufficiency, diseases involving calcium or phosphorous metabolism, or a family history of mammary or genital tract cancer. Safety and effectiveness have not been determined in children and should be used with caution in adolescents in whom bone growth is incomplete.

SIDE EFFECTS
SYSTEMIC USE
Side effects to estrogens are dose dependent. **CV:** Potentially, the most serious side effects involve the CV system. *Venous thromboembolism, deep and superficial venous thrombosis,* thrombophlebitis, *MI, pulmonary embolism,* retinal thrombosis, *mesenteric thrombosis, subarachnoid hemorrhage, postsurgical thromboembolism.* Hypertension, edema, *stroke.* **GI:** N&V, diarrhea, constipation, abdominal cramps/pain, dyspepsia, flatulence, gastritis, gastroenteritis, enlarged abdomen, hemorrhoids, bloating, cholestatic jaundice, colitis, *acute pancreatitis,* changes in appetite, increased risk of gallbladder disease requiring surgery. **Dermatologic:** Most common are chloasma or melasma. Also, erythema multiforme, erythema nodosum, hemorrhagic eruptions, urticaria, dermatitis, photosensitivity, skin hypertrophy, loss of scalp hair, hirsutism, pruritus, rash, pruritus ani, acne. **Hepatic:** Cholestatic jaundice, aggravation of porphyria, benign (most common) or malignant liver tumors, including hepatic adenoma. **GU:** Breakthrough bleeding, spotting, changes in amount/duration of menstrual flow, amenorrhea during/after use, dysmenorrhea, UTI, leukorrhea, vaginitis, premenstrual-like syndrome, change in cervical eversion and degree of cervical secretion, cystitis-like syndrome, vaginal discomfort/pain, vaginal hemorrhage, asymptomatic genital bacterial growth, hemolytic uremic syndrome, endometrial cystic hyperplasia, increased incidence of *Candida* vaginitis, genital moniliasis, cystitis, dysuria, frequent micturition, urethral disorder, vaginosis fungal, vaginal discharge, genital pruritus, urinary incontinence, endometrial hyperplasia, possible link between long-term use of estrogens after menopause and ovarian cancer, increase in size of pre-existing uterine leiomyomata. **CNS:** Mental depression, dizziness, changes in libido, chorea, insomnia, headache, sinus /tension headache, aggravation of migraine headaches, fatigue, nervousness, anxiety, emotional lability, mood disturbances, irritability, worsening of epilepsy, *convulsions.* **Ocular:** Steepening of corneal curvature resulting in intolerance of contact lenses. Optic neuritis or retinal vascular thrombosis, resulting in sudden or gradual, partial or complete loss of vision, double vision, papilledema. **Respiratory:** URTI, sinusitis, rhinitis, bronchitis, pharyngitis, nasopharyngitis, cough, nasal congestion, pharyngolaryngeal pain, exacerbation of asthma. **Musculoskeletal:** Arthritis, arthralgia, skeletal pain. **Hematologic:** Increase in prothrombin and blood coagulation factors VII, VIII, IX, and X. Decrease in

---

antithrombin III. **Local:** Pain at injection site, sterile abscesses, postinjection flare, redness/irritation at site of application of transdermal system. **Body as a whole:** Edema, reduced carbohydrate tolerance, pain, hypersensitivity reactions, flu-like symptoms, allergy, infection, accidental injury, asthenia, anemia, paresthesia, anaphylactoid/anaphylactic reactions (including urticaria and angioedema), fluid retention. **Miscellaneous:** Aggravation of porphyria, back pain, hot flushes, chest pain, leg edema, otitis media, toothache, tooth disorder, leg cramps, neck pain, neck rigidity, candidal infection, fungal infection, herpes simplex. Breast tenderness, enlargement, or secretions; galactorrhea, fibrocystic breast changes, breast cancer. Premature closure of epiphyses in children. Increased frequency of benign or malignant tumors of the cervix, uterus, vagina, and other organs. Increase or decrease in weight. Increased risk of congenital abnormalities. Hypercalcemia in clients with metastatic breast carcinoma. In males, estrogens may cause gynecomastia, loss of libido, decreased spermatogenesis, testicular atrophy, and feminization. Prolonged use of high doses may inhibit the function of the anterior pituitary. Estrogen therapy affects many laboratory tests.

VAGINAL USE
GU: Vaginal bleeding/discharge, endometrial withdrawal bleeding, serious bleeding in ovariectomized women with endometriosis. **Miscellaneous:** Breast tenderness.

DRUG INTERACTIONS
Anticoagulants, oral / ↓ Anticoagulant response by ↑ activity of certain clotting factors
Anticonvulsants / Estrogen-induced fluid retention may precipitate seizures. Also, contraceptive steroids ↑ drug effects by ↓ liver breakdown and ↓ plasma protein binding
Antidiabetic agents / Estrogens may impair glucose tolerance and thus change requirements for antidiabetic agent
Barbiturates / ↓ Effect of estrogen or changes in uterine bleeding profile by ↑ liver breakdown

H *Black cohosh* / May interfere with estrogen effects
Carbamazepine / ↓ Effect of estrogen or changes in uterine bleeding profile by ↑ liver breakdown
Corticosteroids / ↑ Pharmacologic/toxicologic effects of corticosteroids R/T inactivation of hepatic P450 enzyme.
H *Ginseng* / Additive effects; avoid concomitant use
Grapefruit juice / Possible ↑ estrogen plasma levels
Hydantoins / Breakthrough bleeding, spotting, and pregnancy are possible; also, loss of seizure control R/T fluid retention
Itraconazole / ↑ Plasma estrogen levels → side effects
Ketoconazole / ↑ Plasma estrogen levels → side effects
Macrolide antibiotics / ↑ Plasma estrogen levels → side effects
Rifampin / ↓ Effect of estrogen or changes in uterine bleeding profile by ↑ liver breakdown
Ritonavir / ↑ Plasma estrogen levels → side effects.
H *Saw palmetto* / ↓ Effect of hormones R/T antiestrogen effect.
H *St. John's wort* / ↓ Effect of estrogen or changes in uterine bleeding profile by ↑ liver breakdown
Succinylcholine / Estrogens may ↑ drug effects
Thyroxine, thyroid hormone / Possible ↑ need for thyroxine, thyroid hormone
Topiramate / ↑ Estrogen metabolism → ↓ efficacy
Tricyclic antidepressants / Possible ↑ effects of both drugs (dose-dependent); possible ↑ incidence of toxic effects.

LABORATORY TEST CONSIDERATIONS
Altered LFTs and thyroid function tests. False + urine glucose test. ↓ Serum cholesterol, total serum lipids, pregnanediol excretion, serum folate, antithrombin III, antifactor Xa. ↑ Serum triglyceride levels, thyroxine-binding globulin, sulfobromophthalein retention. ↑ PT, PTT, platelet aggregation time, platelet count, fibrinogen, plasminogen, norepinephrine-induced platelet aggregatability, and factors II, VII, IX, X, XI, VII-X complex, II-VII-X complex,

and β–thromboglobulin. Impaired glucose tolerance, reduced response to metyrapone.

DOSAGE

• PO, IM, SC, vaginal, topical, or by implantation

The dosage of estrogens is highly individualized and is aimed at the minimal effective amount.

NURSING CONSIDERATIONS

ADMINISTRATION/STORAGE

1. Most PO administered estrogens are metabolized rapidly and must be administered daily.

2. Parenterally administered estrogens are released more slowly from aqueous suspensions or oily solutions; give slowly and deeply.

3. To avoid continuous stimulation of reproductive tissue, cyclic therapy consisting of 3 weeks on and 1 week off is usually recommended for most uses.

ASSESSMENT

1. Note reasons for therapy, type/onset of symptoms. List other agents prescribed and outcome.

2. List history of thromboembolic problems as estrogens enhance blood coagulability; avoid use in smoker.

3. Assess mental status; note any history of depression, migraine headaches, or suicide attempts.

4. Identify any undiagnosed genital bleeding, liver disease, asthma, migraines, epilepsy, or cancer of the endometrium or breast (estrogen-dependent neoplasms), as these preclude drug therapy.

5. Monitor ECG, VS, BS, triglycerides, electrolytes, renal and LFTs.

CLIENT/FAMILY TEACHING

1. These are a group of hormones that primarily influence the female reproductive tract in sexual development, function (i.e., breast development, menstrual cycle) and maturation. In women, estrogens are produced mainly in the ovaries and in the placenta during pregnancy with smaller amounts produced by the adrenal glands. In men, small amounts are produced by the adrenal glands and testicles. Also, small amounts of estrone are made through-

out the body in most tissues, especially fat and muscle. This is the major source of estrogen in women who have gone through menopause.

2. Taking oral agents with meals or a light snack will prevent gastric irritation and may eliminate nausea. Review the dose, form, and frequency of prescribed agent. With once-a-day therapy, taking at bedtime may eliminate problems. Nausea, bloating, abdominal cramping, changes in appetite, and vomiting may occur and usually disappear with continued therapy.

3. With cyclical therapy, take medications for 3 weeks and then omit for 1 week. Menstruation may then occur, but pregnancy will not because ovulation is suppressed. Keep a record of periods and problems, such as missed period, unusual vaginal bleeding, spotting, or irregularity. Report if pregnancy suspected.

4. Breast tenderness, enlargement, or secretion may occur. Perform BSE monthly (usually 2 weeks after menses) and report changes.

5. Report immediately: leg pains, sudden onset of chest pain, dizziness, SOB, weakness of the arms or legs, or any numbness (S&S of thromboembolic problems). Report any alterations in mental attitude: depression or withdrawal, insomnia or anorexia, or a lack of attention to personal appearance

6. Changes in the curvature of the cornea may make it difficult to wear contact lenses; consult ophthalmologist. Report any changes, such as hair loss or skin discoloration. Males may develop feminine characteristics or suffer from impotence; usually resolves once therapy completed.

7. May alter glucose tolerance. Monitor sugars and report increases; antidiabetic dose may need to be changed.

8. Insert suppositories high into the vault. Apply vaginal preparations at bedtime. Wear a sanitary napkin and avoid the use of tampons. Store suppositories in the refrigerator. Report if estrogen ointments cause systemic reactions.

---

9. If pregnant and planning to breast-feed, do not take estrogens. Consult provider for alternative forms of contraception; breast-feeding does not provide contraception.

10. *Do not smoke.* Attend formal smoking cessation programs.

11. Some potential risks, related to endometrial/breast cancer, have been associated with estrogen therapy. Close medical follow-up required.

OUTCOMES/EVALUATE

• Control of estrogen imbalance
• Effective contraceptive agent
• Relief of menopausal S&S
• Control of tumor size/spread in metastatic breast and prostate cancer

FLUOROQUINOLONES

SEE ALSO THE FOLLOWING INDIVIDUAL ENTRIES:

Ciprofloxacin hydrochloride
Gatifloxacin
Gemifloxacin mesylate
Levofloxacin
Lomefloxacin hydrochloride
Moxifloxacin hydrochloride
Norfloxacin
Ofloxacin
Sparfloxacin*

Drugs marked with an * are available to view in the online database at www.delmarnursesdrughandbook.com/2009.

USES

See individual drugs. Used for a large number of gram-positive and gram-negative infections.

ACTION/KINETICS

Action

Synthetic, broad-spectrum antibacterial agents. The fluorine molecule confers increased activity against gram-negative organisms as well as broadens the spectrum against gram-positive organisms. Are bactericidal agents by interfering with DNA gyrase and topoisomerase IV. DNA gyrase is an enzyme needed for the replication, transcription, and repair of bacterial DNA. Topoisomerase IV plays a key role in the partitioning of chromosomal DNA during bacterial cell division. Ciprofloxacin, levofloxacin, ofloxacin, and trovafloxacin may be given IV; all fluoroquinolones may be given PO.

Pharmacokinetics

Food may delay the absorption of ciprofloxacin, lomefloxacin, and norfloxacin.

CONTRAINDICATIONS

Hypersensitivity to the quinolone group of antibiotics, including cinoxacin and nalidixic acid. Tendinitis or tendon rupture associated with quinolone use. Clients receiving disopyramide and amiodarone or other drugs (e.g., quinidine, procainamide, sotalol) that prolong the QTc interval and which may cause torsade de pointes. Lactation. Use in children less than 18 years of age. Gatifloxacin with diabetes mellitus.

SPECIAL CONCERNS

Use lower doses in impaired renal function. There may be differences in CNS toxicity between the various fluoroquinolones. Use may increase the risk of Achilles and other tendon inflammation and rupture. Several fluoroquinolones cause phototoxicity. May exacerbate the signs of myasthenia gravis and lead to life-threatening weakness of the respiratory muscles.

SIDE EFFECTS

See individual drugs. The following side effects are common to each of the fluoroquinolone antibiotics. **GI:** N&V, diarrhea, abdominal pain or discomfort, dry or painful mouth, heartburn, dyspepsia, flatulence, constipation, pseudomembranous colitis. **CNS:** Headache, dizziness, malaise, lethargy, fatigue, drowsiness, somnolence, depression, insomnia, *seizures,* paresthesia. **Dermatologic:** Rash, photosensitivity, pruritus (except for ciprofloxacin). **Hypersensitivity reactions:** Facial or *pharyngeal edema,* dyspnea, urticaria, itching, tingling, loss of consciousness, *CV collapse.* **Other:** Visual disturbances and ophthalmic abnormalities, hearing loss, superinfection, phototoxicity, eosinophilia, crystalluria, Achilles and other tendon inflammation and rupture. Fluoroquinolones, except norfloxacin, may also cause vaginitis, syncope, chills, and edema.

OD **OVERDOSE MANAGEMENT**
Symptoms: Extension of side effects. *Treatment:* For acute overdose, vomiting should be induced or gastric lavage performed. The client should be carefully observed and, if necessary, symptomatic and supportive treatment given. Hydration should be maintained. Hemodialysis or peritoneal dialysis may help to remove ciprofloxacin but not other fluoroquinolones.

DRUG INTERACTIONS
Antacids / ↓ Serum fluoroquinolone levels R/T ↓ GI tract absorption
Anticoagulants / ↑ Anticoagulant effects
Cimetidine / ↓ Elimination of fluoroquinolones
Cyclosporine / ↑ Risk of nephrotoxicity
Didanosine / ↓ Serum fluoroquinolone levels R/T ↓ GI tract absorption due to Mg and Al buffers present in didanosine tablets
Iron salts / ↓ Serum fluoroquinolone levels R/T ↓ GI tract absorption
NSAIDs / ↑ Risk of CNS stimulation and seizures
Probenecid / ↑ Serum fluoroquinolone levels R/T ↓ renal clearance
Sucralfate / ↓ Serum fluoroquinolone levels R/T ↓ GI tract absorption
Theophylline / ↑ Theophylline plasma levels and ↑ drug toxicity R/T ↓ clearance
Zinc salts / ↓ Serum fluoroquinolone levels R/T ↓ GI tract absorption.

LABORATORY TEST CONSIDERATIONS
↑ ALT, AST. False + opiate results in urinary assays. See also individual drugs.

DOSAGE————————
See individual drugs.

NURSING CONSIDERATIONS
ASSESSMENT
1. Note reasons for therapy, symptom characteristics, clinical presentation, and culture results. List any previous experiences with these antibiotics. Discontinue at first sign of rash or other allergic manifestations. Hypersensitivity reactions may occur latently.

2. Assess soft tissue/extremity injury; note instability, pain, swelling, erythema, and discharge. Assess Achilles tendon for drug-induced injury.
3. Monitor VS, I&O, CBC, cultures, renal and LFTs; reduce dose with renal dysfunction.
4. If receiving anticoagulants and theophyllines, monitor closely; quinolones can cause increased drug levels with toxic drug effects i.e., bleeding or seizures.

CLIENT/FAMILY TEACHING
1. Take only as directed. Avoid mineral supplements (i.e., iron or zinc) or antacids containing magnesium or aluminum simultaneously or 4 hr before or 2 hr after dosing with fluoroquinolones.
2. Do not perform hazardous tasks until drug effects realized; may experience dizziness, drowsiness, lightheadedness, or ↓ alertness.
3. Report any bothersome symptoms; N&V and diarrhea are most frequently reported side effects. Symptoms of superinfection include furry tongue, vaginal or rectal itching, diarrhea.
4. Hypersensitivity reactions may occur, even after the first dose. Stop drug at first sign of skin rash or other allergic reaction.
5. Consume >2.5 L/day of fluids to ensure adequate hydration.
6. Wear protective clothing and sunscreens; avoid excessive sunlight or artificial UV light. Even brief exposure to sun can cause a severe sunburn or rash. Use a lip balm containing sun block and avoid the use of tanning beds, tanning booths, or sunlamps. Photosensitivity reactions may occur up to several weeks after stopping therapy.
7. Some fluoroquinolones may weaken the tendons in the shoulder, hand, or heel, making these fibrous bands of tissue more likely to tear. Stop drug and report any new onset tendon/extremity pain or inflammation as tendon rupture may occur.
8. Keep all F/U appointments to evaluate response to therapy, labs, and for any adverse side effects.

OUTCOMES/EVALUATE
• Symptomatic improvement

📷 = see color insert   **H** = Herbal   **IV** = Intravenous   @ = sound alike drug

Classifications

- Resolution of infection (↓ WBCs, ↓ temperature, ↑ appetite)
- Negative culture reports

HEPARINS, LOW MOLECULAR WEIGHT ■

SEE ALSO THE FOLLOWING INDIVIDUAL ENTRIES:

Dalteparin sodium
Enoxaparin
Tinzaparin sodium

USES

See individual drugs. Uses include, but are not limited to: (1) Prophylaxis of DVT. (2) Prophylaxis of ischemic complications in unstable angina and non-Q-wave MI when given together with aspirin. (3) With warfarin for inpatient treatment of acute DVT with and without pulmonary embolism or for outpatient treatment of acute DVT without pulmonary embolism.

ACTION/KINETICS

Action

As antithrombotic drugs they enhance the inhibition of Factor Xa and thrombin by binding to and accelerating antithrombin II activity. They potentiate the inhibition of Factor Xa preferentially; slightly affect thrombin and clotting time or activated partial thromboplastin time.

Pharmacokinetics

Primarily metabolized in the liver to lower molecular weight compounds with significantly less activity.

CONTRAINDICATIONS

Hypersensitivity to heparin, pork products, methylparaben, sulfites, or benzyl alcohol. Active major bleeding. Thrombocytopenia with positive in vitro tests for antiplatelet antibody in presence of a low molecular weight heparin. IM or IV use.

SPECIAL CONCERNS

■(1) When spinal/epidural anesthesia or spinal puncture is used, those anticoagulated or scheduled to be anticoagulated with low molecular weight heparins or heparinoids to prevent thromboembolic complications are at risk of developing a spinal or epidural hematoma that can result in long-term or permanent paralysis. Risk is increased using indwelling epidural catheters for giving analgesics or by the concurrent use of drugs affecting hemostasis, such as NSAIDs, platelet inhibitors, or other anticoagulants. Risk also appears to increase by traumatic or repeated spinal or epidural puncture. (2) Frequently monitor for signs and symptoms of neurologic impairment. If observed, immediate treatment is required. (3) The physician should consider potential benefits vs risk before neuraxial intervention in clients anticoagulated or to be anticoagulated for thromboprophylaxis.■ Cannot be used interchangeably (unit for unit) with other low molecular weight heparins or with unfractionated heparin. Use with extreme caution in clients with a history of heparin-induced thrombocytopenia. Use with caution in clients with an increased risk of hemorrhage, including those with severe uncontrolled hypertension, bacterial endocarditis, congenital or acquired bleeding disorders, active ulceration and angiodysplastic GI disease, or hemorrhagic stroke or shortly after brain, spinal, or ophthalmic surgery. Also, use with caution in clients with bleeding diathesis, severe liver or kidney disease, hypertensive or diabetic retinopathy, and recent GI bleeding. Use with caution during lactation. Safety and efficacy have not been determined in children.

SIDE EFFECTS

See individual drugs. **Hemorrhagic side effects: *Clinically significant bleeding (fatal or nonfatal)* from any tissue or organ, hemorrhage, injection site hematoma, wound hematoma. Hemorrhagic complications:** Paralysis, paresthesia, headache, pain (chest, abdomen, joint, muscle, or other), dizziness, shortness of breath, difficulty breathing or swallowing, swelling, weakness, hypotension, *shock, coma*.

OD OVERDOSE MANAGEMENT

Symptoms: Hemorrhagic complications. *Treatment:* Slow IV protamine sulfate (1%) at a dose of 1 mg for every 100 anti-Xa international units of dalteparin or 1 mg for every 1 mg of enoxaparin. A second infusion of protamine sulfate, 0.5 mg per 100 anti-Xa international units of dalteparin or per 1 mg of enoxaparin may be given if the aPTT measured 2–4 hr after the first infusion of protamine sulfate remains prolonged. Take care not to give an overdose of protamine.

DRUG INTERACTIONS

Aspirin / ↑ Risk of bleeding.

H *Bromelain* / ↑ Risk of bleeding

Clopidogrel ↑ Risk of bleeding

Dextran / ↑ Risk of bleeding

Dipyridamole / ↑ Risk of bleeding.

H *Feverfew* / Possible additive antiplatelet effect.

H *Garlic* / Possible additive antiplatelet effect.

H *Ginger* / Possible additive antiplatelet effect

Ketorolac tromethamine / ↑ Risk of bleeding

NSAIDs / ↑ Risk of bleeding

Sulfinpyrazone / ↑ Risk of bleeding

Thrombolytics / ↑ Risk of bleeding

Ticlopidine / ↑ Risk of bleeding.

LABORATORY TEST CONSIDERATIONS

Asymptomatic ↑ AST, ALT.

DOSAGE————————————

See individual drugs.

NURSING CONSIDERATIONS

ASSESSMENT

1. Note reasons for therapy (prophylaxis/treatment), other agents trialed, outcome. Assess for any sensitivity to heparin, sulfite, methylparaben, or pork products.

2. Review list of special concerns that may preclude client receiving drugs. Those who received spinal anesthesia or taps require special monitoring to assess for neurologic S&S and spinal/epidural hematoma formation which may cause permanent paralysis.

3. List any evidence of active bleeding, bleeding disorders, or thrombocytopenia. Assess carefully for masked bleeding. Drug does not usually affect PT/PTT values yet client may be hemorrhaging. Monitor VS, I&O, mental status, H&H,

U/A, electrolytes, renal and LFTs; routinely check all potential bleeding sites. Any unexplained fall in BP or HCT should lead to a search for a bleeding site.

CLIENT/FAMILY TEACHING

1. Many clients are treated with low molecular weight heparins (LMWH)at home. Indications for therapy, self administration techniques, length/frequency of therapy, and site rotation are important concerns. SC injection techniques and recognizing signs of complications are important. To minimize bruising do not rub site after administering.

2. LMWHs are defined as heparin salts produced by depolymerization of unfractionated heparin, rendering them smaller and more bioavailable than heparin. There is less binding to plasma proteins and less inactivation by platelet factor 4.

3. Due to LMWH predictable effects, they do not require the regular laboratory monitoring to ensure adequate anticoagulation and dose adjustment as does heparin.

4. Avoid aspirin, NSAIDs, and all OTC agents. Report any unusual effects, i.e., bruising, bleeding, chest pain, acute SOB, itching, rash, or swelling.

5. Keep all F/U appointments to evaluate response to therapy and for any adverse side effects.

OUTCOMES/EVALUATE

Thromboembolism prophylaxis

HERBS

SEE TABLE 1.

GENERAL STATEMENT

Herbs are medicinal plants, also called botanicals or phytomedicines. Herbal therapy is the use of plants or plant extracts for medicinal purposes (especially plants that are not part of the normal diet). Phytomedicines are medicinal products that contain plant material as their pharmacologically active component. They are often complex mixtures

(continues on page 1866)

TABLE 1: Commonly Used Herbal Products

The following table presents some of the commonly used herbal products. It is not intended to be an extensive listing of information for each product. Rather, the table contains important information regarding use(s), dose, side effects, and other information. Importantly, labels for herbal products vary significantly in the quality and quantity of the information. Also, there is wide variation in plant part ingredients and recommended daily doses.

Name(s)	Use(s)	Dose	Contraindications	Side Effects	Other Information
Aloe juice/latex, Aloe gel	**PO:** *Juice/latex:* Laxative, cathartic. **Topical:** *Gel:* Promote burn or wound healing. Treat cold sores. Cosmetic products.	**Laxative:** 100–200 mg aloe, 50 mg extract, or 1–8 oz of the juice. **Topical:** Apply gel liberally.	PO in intestinal obstruction, Crohn's disease, ulcerative colitis, appendicitis, abdominal pain of unknown origin. Children under 12 years. Pregnancy, lactation.	Abdominal pain, cramps. Diarrhea with long-term use. Potassium loss, albuminura, hematuria, heart disturbances, weight loss, muscle weakness.	Do not use for more than 1–2 weeks without medical advice. Potassium loss can be increased by simultaneous use of corticosteroids, licorice, or thiazides. May interact with cardiac glycosides and antiarrhythmic drugs.

Bold Italic = life threatening side effect   ▮ = black box warning   ✦ = Available in Canada

Name(s)	Use(s)	Dose	Contraindications	Side Effects	Other Information
Bilberry fruit/leaf	**PO:** *Fruit:* Acute diarrhea. Improve visual acuity, including night vision. **Topical:** Mild for inflammation of the mouth and throat mucous membranes. *Leaf:* Diabetes, arthritis, gout, dermatitis, hemorrhoids, poor circulation, heart problems and prevention and treatment of GI, kidney, and urinary tract symptoms.	Dried ripe berries: 20–60 grams/day. *Decoction:* 5–10 grams in cold water; bring to boil and simmer 10 min; strain. Extract: 160 mg 2 times per day for retinopathy. **Topical:** Apply as a 10% concoction. *Leaf:* Drink as a tea: 1–2 tsp. finely chopped dried leaf in 150 mL boiling water for 5–10 min; strain.	Chronic use of the leaf may cause anemia, jaundice, acute excitatory states, disturbance of muscle contraction.	Leaves contain high levels of chromium (may lower blood glucose). Avoid prolonged use of the tea. The leaf may interact with anti-diabetic drugs and disulfiram.	
Cascara sagrada	**PO:** Most commonly as a laxative. Also for gallstones, liver ailments, and cancer. Used to make some sunscreens.	**Capsules, Syrup, Tablets:** 20–30 mg hydroxyanthracene derivatives/day, calculated as cascaroside A. *Fluid extract:* 2–5 mL 3 times per day. May also be used as a tea (2 grams finely chopped bark in 150 mL of boiling water for 5–10 min; strain).	Intestinal obstruction, Crohn's disease, colitis, appendicitis, abdominal pain of unknown origin, ulcers. Pregnancy. Lactation (may cause diarrhea).	Mild abdominal discomfort, colic, cramps. Chronic use: Potassium depletion, albuminuria, hematuria, disturbed heart function, muscle weakness, finger clubbing, and cachexia. Improperly aged bark can cause severe vomiting.	Use with caution, if at all in children less than 2 years old. Potassium loss increased with concomitant use of corticosteroids, licorice, or thiazides. May interfere with absorption of some drugs due to reduced transit time through the GI tract. Increases side effects of cardiac glycosides (e.g., digoxin).

📷 = see color insert   H = Herbal   IV = Intravenous   ℗ = sound alike drug

Name(s)	Use(s)	Dose	Contraindications	Side Effects	Other Information
Cat's Claw	**PO:** Diverticulitis, peptic ulcers, colitis, gastritis, hemorrhoids, parasites, leaky bowel syndrome. With zidovudine (AZT) for HIV positive clients.	**Capsules, Tablets:** 500–1,000 mg 1 to 3 times per day. *Tea:* Simmer 1 gram of root bark in 150 mL boiling water for 5–10 min; strain. Consume tea 3 times per day.	Pregnancy, lactation.	Diarrhea (high doses), hypotension. May contribute to unusual bruising or bleeding gums.	Use with caution if taking antihypertensives. Get up slowly to avoid dizziness. Avoid confusing cat's claw with devil's claw.
Chamomile, German Chamomile	**PO:** Flatulence, travel sickness, nasal mucous membrane inflammation, nervous diarrhea, restlessness, GI spasms, GI inflammatory disease, menstrual cramps. **Topical:** Hemorrhoids, mastitis, leg ulcers; inflammation of skin, anogenital, and mucous membranes, including the mouth and gums.	**PO:** 2–8 grams of the dried flower heads 3 times per day or 1 cup of tea 3 to 4 times per day. Prepare tea by steeping 3 grams of dried flower heads in 150 mL boiling water for 5–10 min; strain. *Liquid extract (1:1 in 45% alcohol):* 1–4 mL 3 times per day. **Topical:** Prepared tea (4 tsp. of dried flower heads in 1.5 cups boiling water for 15 min; strain. **Ointment/Gel (both 3 to 10%):** For external use only.	Pregnancy (may be a teratogen). Lactation.	Highly concentrated tea can cause vomiting. Allergic reactions, including contact dermatitis, severe hypersensitivity reactions, and anaphylaxis. Can be irritating if used near the eyes. May exacerbate asthma.	Cautious use in those with allergies to ragweed, asters, chrysanthemums, or other members of the Asteraceae family. Use with benzodiazepines and other CNS depressants may cause additive effects. May interfere with anticoagulant therapy. Do not confuse with Roman chamomile.

Bold Italic = life threatening side effect   ▇ = black box warning   ✤ = Available in Canada

Name(s)	Use(s)	Dose	Contraindications	Side Effects	Other Information
Chondrotin sulfate	**PO:** Osteoarthritis. Ischemic heart disease, osteoporosis, hyperlipidemia. **IM:** Osteoarthritis. **Topical:** Dry eyes, as a viscoelastic agent in cataract surgery, medium for preservation of corneas used for transplantation. With other agents for osteoarthritis.	**PO:** 200–400 mg 2 to 3 times per day or 1,200 mg as a single daily dose for osteoarthritis. **IM:** 50–100 mg/day in 1 or 2 daily injections. Injection not available in the US.	Pregnancy, lactation. Use in those with clotting disorders.	**PO:** Epigastric pain, nausea, diarrhea, constipation, eyelid edema, lower limb edema, alopecia, estrasystoles. Allergic reactions. **Ophthalmic use:** Intraocular hypertension, discomfort, corneal edema after cataract surgery.	Possible increased risk of bleeding when used with antiplatelet or anticoagulant drugs. No evidence that use of chondroitin sulfate with glucosamine sulfate has a greater beneficial effect than either product alone.
Comfrey	**Topical:** Ulcers, wounds and fractures. Above ground parts used for bruises and sprains. Gargle for gum disease and pharyngitis. **PO:** Tea for ulcers, excessive menstrual flow, diarrhea, bloody urine, persistent cough, rheumatism, pleuritis, bronchitis, cancer, angina.	**Topical:** Ointments and other external products made with 5 to 20% comfrey. Daily use should not exceed 100 mcg of the pyrrolizidine alkaloids. Apply externally only on unbroken skin.	Use of above ground parts during pregnancy and lactation.	Acute veno-occlusive disease, including symptoms of anorexia, lethargy, and a dull, dragging ache in the right upper abdomen with marked abdominal distention (may also be reduced urine output).	Use for no more than 10 days; maximum use is 4 to 6 weeks/year. Unsafe when the root or above ground parts are used PO due to potential for acute or chronic liver toxicity. Teas contain lesser levels of alkaloids but regular use can lead to toxicity. Dietary products are not required to list the amount of product; thus, all products used PO should be considered potentially dangerous.

📷 = see color insert   H = Herbal   IV = Intravenous   ℚ = sound alike drug

Name(s)	Use(s)	Dose	Contraindications	Side Effects	Other Information
Cranberry	**PO:** Prevention and treatment of urinary tract infections. As a urinary deodorizer for incontinent persons. Berries are used in foods, including juices, jelly, and sauce.	**PO: juice:** 3 oz (33% pure cranberry) daily for preventing UTIs and 12–32 oz daily to treat UTIs. **Capsules:** 6/day of dried cranberry powder (equivalent to 3 oz) juice. Or, 300 to 400 mg concentrated juice capsules 2 times per day.	Avoid using amounts greater than consumed in food during pregnancy and lactation.	No side effects. Consuming more than 3–4 L/day can cause diarrhea and other GI symptoms.	Might increase absorption of dietary vitamin B_{12} in clients taking proton pump inhibitors. Do not confuse with highbush cranberry.
Dong quai	**PO:** Root used for menstrual cramps, irregularity, retarded flow, weakness during menses, and menopausal symptoms. Treatment of skin pigmentation and psoriasis.	**PO: women:** 3 to 4 grams/day in divided doses with meals. Sometimes prepared as a tea. Dose of the extract is 1 mL (20 to 40 drops) 3 times per day.	Pregnancy due to uterine stimulant and relaxant effects. Lactation.	Severe photosensitivity and photodermatitis. Potentially carcinogenic and mutagenic.	Increased risk of bleeding if used with antiplatelet drugs or warfarin.

Bold Italic = life threatening side effect   ■ = black box warning   ✦ = Available in Canada

Name(s)	Use(s)	Dose	Contraindications	Side Effects	Other Information
Echinacea	**PO:** Treat or prevent colds and other upper respiratory tract infections. Also as an antiseptic, antiviral immune stimulant, UTIs, peripheral vasodilator, yeast infections. **Topical:** Skin wounds, chronic skin ulcers, psoriasis, herpes simplex.	**PO, tablets:** 500 mg 3 times per day on day 1; then, 250 mg 4 times per day for up to 10 days. For prophylaxis, take for 3 consecutive weeks and then not take for one week. **Juice:** 6–9 mL/day of juice from fresh above the ground parts for a maximum of 8 weeks. **Topical:** A semi-solid product containing at least 15% pressed juice of Echinacea purpura above ground parts.	Pregnancy and lactation. Use with tuberculosis, leukosis, collagenosis, multiple sclerosis, collagen disorders or other progressive systemic diseases due to potential for stimulating the autoimmune response. Use with AIDS, HIV infection, autoimmune disorders.	Allergic reactions, including acute asthma, urticaria, angioedema, and anaphylaxis. Fever, N&V. High doses may reduce male and female fertility.	Individuals sensitive to ragweed, marigolds, daisies, chrysanthemums, and many other herbs are more likely to experience an allergic reaction to echinacea. Use with caution in those with renal disease or who are immunocompromised. May interfere with immunosuppressant therapy. Clients with atopy are more likely to experience an allergic reaction. Induces CYP3A4; thus carefully monitor those receiving echinacea and CYP3A4 (as well as CYP1A2) substrates with a narrow therapeutic index.
Evening primrose oil	**PO:** Premenstrual syndrome, hot flashes, mastalgia, endometriosis. Also, atopic eczema, psoriasis, acne, rheumatoid arthritis, Raynaud's phenomenon, multiple sclerosis, and Sjögren's syndrome.	**PO:** 3–4 grams/day for mastalgia; 2–4 grams/day for PMS. From 0.54–2.8 grams/day for rheumatoid arthritis. From 6–8 grams/day for atopic eczema. Children take 2–4 grams/day.	Pregnancy.	Indigestion, nausea, headache, soft stools, Large doses can cause loose stools and abdominal pain. May increase risk for pregnancy complications.	May worsen temporal lobe epilepsy or schizophrenia if used with phenothiazines or tricyclic antidepressants.

Name(s)	Use(s)	Dose	Contraindications	Side Effects	Other Information
Feverfew	**PO:** Fever, headache, migraines, menstrual irregularities, stomach ache, N&V. **Topical:** Antiseptic, insecticide, toothache.	**PO:** 2.5 leaves/day for migraine prophylaxis (with or without food). The dose of freeze-dried leaf is 50–125 mg/day with or without food.	Pregnancy, lactation, and in children less than 2 years of age.	Mouth ulceration, tongue irritation, inflammation (with chewed leaves), abdominal pain, indigestion, diarrhea, N&V, flatulence. Post-feverfew syndrome: Nervousness, tension headaches, insomnia, joint pain or stiffness, tiredness. **Topical:** Allergic contact dermatitis.	Allergic reactions can occur in those sensitive to ragweed, crysanthemums, daisies, marigolds, and many other herbs. May increase effect of anticoagulant and antiplatelet drugs. May decrease effectiveness of NSAIDs.
Garlic	**PO:** Decrease BP, prevent coronary heart disease, prevent age-related vascular changes and atherosclerosis, reduce reinfarction, and mortality rate post-MI. Treat earaches and menstrual disorders. **Topical:** Oil is used for tinea pedis, tinea corporis, tinea cruris, and onychomycosis.	**PO:** 600–900 mg per day in 3 divided doses for hyperlipidemia and hypertension. Some use fresh garlic (1 clove or 4 grams/day). **Topical:** 0.4% cream and 0.6% gel for tinea infections.	PO use of large amounts during pregnancy and lactation (data vary). Topical use of large amounts.	Breath odor, mouth and GI burning or irritation, heartburn, flatulence, N&V, diarrhea. Possible changes in intestinal flora. Dermatitis when fresh garlic used topically.	Increased effects when used with warfarin (INR). Possible increased effects when used with aspirin, clopidogrel, enoxaparin, and others. Possible increased effects and toxicity when used with insulin or oral hypoglycemics. Can prolong bleeding time; discontinue 1–2 weeks before surgery.

Bold Italic = life threatening side effect   ■ = black box warning   ✦ = Available in Canada

Name(s)	Use(s)	Dose	Contraindications	Side Effects	Other Information
Ginger (African, Black, Cochin, Jamaica, Race)	**PO:** Motion sickness, colic, dyspepsia, flatulence, rheumatoid arthritis, post-surgical N&V, anorexa, URTI, cough, bronchitis. As a flavoring agent in foods/beverages. **Topical:** Juice used for thermal burns.	**PO:** 0.25–1 gram 3 times per day or 1 cup of tea (0.5–1 gram in 150 mL boiling water 5–10 min; strain) 3 times per day. Maximum daily dose: 4 grams. For morning sickness: 250 mg 4 times per day. Prevent post-operative N&V: 1 gram powdered root 1 hr before induction of anesthesia. Antiemetic: 2 grams freshly powdered root with water.	Use in those with gallstones until after medical evaluation.	Dermatitis in sensitive persons. CNS depression, cardiac arrhythmias, or hypoglycemia after high doses.	Use with herbs that have coumarin constituents or affect platelet aggregation thoretically increase the risk of bleeding. May enhance effect of barbiturates. May interfere with BP drug therapy or with diabetes therapy. May prevent cyclophosphamide-induced vomiting.

Name(s)	Use(s)	Contraindications	Dose	Side Effects	Other Information
Ginkgo biloba	*Leaf extract:* **PO:** Dementia syndromes or cerebral vascular insufficiency (memory loss, vertigo, dizziness, difficulty concentrating, mood disturbances, hearing disorders). Intermittent claudication. Reverse sexual dysfunction due to SSRI depressants, attention deficit-hyperactivity disorder, premenstrual syndrome. Prevent acute mountain sickness. Various CV problems **Topical:** Wound dressings.	Use in couples wishing to become pregnant.	**PO:** Dementia syndromes or claudication: 120–240 mg/day in 2 or 3 divided doses. Reverse sexual dysfunction due to SSRI's: 60 mg 2 times per day, up to 240 mg 2 times per day. For vertigo or tinnitus disorders: 120–160 mg/day in 2 or 3 divided doses. Prevent altitude sickness: 160 mg 2 times per day.	Mild GI complaints, headache, dizziness, palpitations, allergic skin reactions. Large doses: N&V, restlessness, diarrhea, weakness, lack of muscle tone. Bleeding disorders (rare). Possible seizures. Gingko pollen is strongly allergenic.	Increased risk of bleeding if used with anticoagulants or antiplatelet drugs. May increase BP if used with thiazide diuretics. May prevent cyclosporine-induced nephrotoxicity; however, may also increase bioavailability, AUC, and peak cyclosporine levels. Increased risk of bleeding if used with herbs that have coumarin constituents or affect platelet aggregation. Cross-reactivity possible with gingko fruit in those allergic to poison ivy, poison oak, poison sumac, mango rind, or cashew shell oil. May also interact with alprazolam, aspirin, haloperidol, ibuprofen, nifedipine, omeprazole, and trazodone.

Bold Italic = life threatening side effect   ■ = black box warning   ✦ = Available in Canada

Name(s)	Use(s)	Dose	Contraindications	Side Effects	Other Information
Ginseng, panax	**PO:** General tonic to improve well-being and to stimulate immune function. To improve physical or athletic stamina, cognitive function, concentration, and work efficiency. To soothe irritated or inflamed tissues, as a diuretic, and an antidepressant. Improve psychological function in post-menopausal women.	**PO:** *Cut or powdered root:* 0.6–3 grams 1–3 times per day or 1 cup tea (3 grams of root in 150 mL of boiling water for 10–15 min or 1 ginseng tea bag usually containing 1,500 mg of the root) 1–3 times per day for 3–4 weeks. *Capsules:* 200–600 mg/day. Usual length of ingestion: 3 weeks to 3 months. A panax-free period of 2 weeks is recommended between consecutive courses.	Use in cases of hemorrhage or thrombosis.	Insomnia, mastalgia, vaginal bleeding, tachycardia, mania, cerebral arteritis, Stevens-Johnson syndrome, edema, amenorrhea, decreased appetite, hyperpyrexia, pruritus, rose spots, hypotension, headache, vertigo, palpitations, euphoria, neonatal death. Diarrhea and allergic skin reactions after high doses. May prolong aPTT or PT. May reduce INR and PT in those treated with warfarin.	Use with herbs that affect platelet aggregation may increase the risk of bleeding. May interfere with effect of antipsychotic drugs. If used with digoxin, synergistic effects possible. May enhance BG lowering effects of anti-diabetic drugs. May interfere with MAO inhibitor therapy. May potentiate the effects of stimulants, including caffeine in tea/coffee. Use with caution in cardiac disorders. Increased risk of hypoglycemia in diabetics.

📷 = see color insert   H = Herbal   IV = Intravenous   Ⓒ = sound alike drug

Name(s)	Use(s)	Dose	Contraindications	Side Effects	Other Information
Goldenseal	**PO:** Urinary tract infections, inflammation of vaginal and ureteral mucous membranes, hemorrhoids, gastritis, anorexia, peptic ulcers, colitis, postpartum hemorrhage, menorrhagia, dysmenorrhea, internal hemorrhage. **Topical:** Eczema, itching, acne, dandruff, ringworm, wounds.	**PO:** *Dried root or rhizome:* 0.5–1 gram 3 times per day. Prepare tea: Simmer 0.5–1 gram in 150 mL boiling water for 5–10 min; strain. *Liquid extract:* 0.3–1 mL 3 times per day. *Tincture:* 2–4 mL 3 times per day **Topical:** Use as mouthwash 3–4 times per day; prepare by steeping 6 grams of dried herb in 150 mL boiling water for 5–10 min; strain and cool.	Use in infectious or inflammatory GI conditions and in newborns.	Prolonged PO use: Digestive disorders, constipation, excitation, delirium (rare), hallucinations. Fresh plant may cause mucosal irritation. Use during pregnancy, lactation, or in newborns may cause kernicteris (may be fatal). Prolonged use: Decrease B vitamin absorption. Increased bilirubin levels.	Enhanced therapeutic and adverse effects if used with herbs with sedative effects. May interfere with antacids, sucralfate, H-2 antagonists, and proton-pump inhibitors. May inhibit anticoagulant effects of heparin. Berberine in the herb may displace highly protein-bound drugs.
Grape seed extract (Muskat)	**PO:** Venous insufficiency, varicose veins, atherosclerosis, peripheral vascular disease, edema associated with injury or surgery, MI, cerebral infarction.	**PO:** Extract as capsules/tablets: 75–300 mg/day for 3 weeks; then, maintenance dose of 40–80 mg/day. For chronic venous insufficiency: Extract procyanidin doses of 150–300 mg/day.	Pregnancy, lactation (avoid amounts greater than in food).	None reported.	May increase the effect of warfarin and the risk of bleeding.

Bold Italic = life threatening side effect   ▮ = black box warning   ♣ = Available in Canada

Name(s)	Use(s)	Dose	Contraindications	Side Effects	Other Information
Green tea	**PO:** Stomach disorders, vomiting, diarrhea, headaches, diuretic, improve cognitive performance, Crohn's disease. Reduce risk of prostate cancer and colon cancer. Protect against heart disease, prevent kidney stones and dental caries. **Topical:** Wash to soothe sunburn, poultice for bags under the eyes, as a compress for headache or tired eyes, stop bleeding in tooth sockets.	**PO:** No reliable information; ranges between 1–10 cups daily. **Topical:** No typical dosage.	Use in infants, lactation. Use in those with gastric/duodenal ulcers.	GI upset and constipation. High doses: Side effects due to caffeine (the active constituent). May induce cardiac arrhythmias in sensitive individuals.	Increased CNS stimulation when used with caffeine-containing products or ephedrine. Many possible drug interactions, including warfarin. Grapefruit juice can increase caffeine levels and increase risk of side effects. Milk may bind the antioxidants in tea and reduce beneficial effects. Possible prolonged bleeding time.

📷 = see color insert   H = Herbal   IV = Intravenous   ℂ = sound alike drug

Name(s)	Use(s)	Dose	Contraindications	Side Effects	Other Information
Hawthorn fruit, flower	**PO, Leaf:** Coronary circulation problems, improve perfusion of myocardium, chronic arrhythmias, hypotension. **Flower:** Improve heart function, coronary insufficiency, angina, cardiac neurasthenia, arrhythmias, cardiac asthma, sedation. **Topical, Leaf:** Poultice for boils, sores, ulcers.	Leaf used as a water extract, a water-alcohol extract, wine tea, and fresh juice. Dosage not available.	Use with cardiac glycoside-containing products (increased risk of toxicity). Pregnancy.	Nausea, GI complaints, fatigue, rash on hands, sweating, palpitations, headache, dizziness, sleeplessness, agitation, circulatory disturbances.	Additive effects when used with vasodilators or CNS depressants. May potentiate effects of digoxin (may need to decrease dose). May potentiate or interfere with conventional cardiovascular drug therapy.
Kava	**PO:** Anxiety disorders, stress, insomnia, restlessness, epilepsy, psychosis, depression.	**PO:** *Extract:* 100 mg (70 mg kava-lactones) 3 times per day. For nervous anxiety, stress, restlessness: 60–120 mg kava-lactones/day. *Tea:* 1 cup up to 3 times per day. To prepare tea: Simmer 2–4 grams of the root in 150 mL boiling water for 5–10 min; strain.	Endogenous depression. Lactation.	After PO: GI complaints, headache, dizziness, enlarged pupils, disturbances of oculomotor equilibrium and accommodation, allergic skin reactions (rare). Mouth numbness if chewed. Drowsiness and impaired motor reflexes may affect ability to drive or operate machinery.	Possible additive effects if used with CNS depressants, including alcohol. Do not use more than 3 months without medical advice.

Bold Italic = life threatening side effect   ▪ = black box warning   ♣ = Available in Canada

Name(s)	Use(s)	Dose	Contraindications	Side Effects	Other Information
Licorice (Glycyrrhiza, Licorice root)	**PO:** Inflammation of upper respiratory tract mucous membranes. Gastric and duodenal ulcers, bronchitis, chronic gastritis, colic, primary adrenocortical insufficiency, dry cough, arthritis, lupus, cholestatic liver disorders, hyperkalemia, hypotonia.	**PO:** *Powdered root:* 1–4 grams. *Tea:* 1 cup 3 times per day. To prepare tea: Simmer 1–4 grams of powdered root in 150 mL boiling water for 5–10 min; strain.	Pregnancy, lactation. Use in diabetes, CHF, hypertension, cholestatic liver disorders, liver cirrhosis, hypokalemia, severe renal insufficiency, hypersensitivity to licorice.	Amenorrhea. High doses or chronic use: Pseudoaldosteronism (hypertension, lethargy, headache, sodium/water retention, edema). Decrease serum testosterone and increase 17-hydroxyprogesterone: May cause decreased libido and sexual dysfunction in men. Hypokalemia.	Increased risk of cardiac toxicity due to potassium depletion. Increased risk of bleeding if used with anticoagulants or antiplatelet drugs. Grapefruit juice may enhance mineralocorticoid activity. Increased potassium loss if used with thiazides.
Melatonin	**PO:** Insomnia, especially to treat jet lag, sleep disorders, shift-work disorder. Many other uses.	**PO:** 0.3–5 mg at bedtime. For jet lag: 5 mg at bedtime for one week beginning 3 days before the flight.	Pregnancy, lactation. Use with immunosuppressive drug therapy.	Headache, transient depressive symptoms, daytime fatigue, drowsiness, dizziness, abdominal cramps, reduced alertness, irritability. Worsen dysphoria in depressed clients.	Additive effects if used with CNS depressants. Do not drive or use machinery for 4–5 hr after taking melatonin. Use with caution in children.

📷 = see color insert   H = Herbal   IV = Intravenous   🔊 = sound alike drug

Name(s)	Use(s)	Dose	Contraindications	Side Effects	Other Information
Milk thistle (Lady's Thistle)	**PO:** *Fruit/Seeds:* Dyspeptic liver complaints, liver protectant, treat toxic liver damage due to chemicals, amanita mushroom poisoning, hepatic cirrhosis, chronic inflammatory liver disease, chronic hepatitis. *Above ground parts:* Treat and stimulate dysfunction of the liver and gallbladder. Jaundice, pleurisy, spleen diseases.	**PO:** *Fruit/Seeds:* 200–400 mg/day calculated as silibinin. Or, 12–15 grams of the dried fruit or seeds/ day. *Above ground parts:* 1 cup of tea 2–3 times per day. Prepare tea by steeping 1/2 tsp. of the above grounds parts in 150 mL boiling water for 5–10 min; strain.	All parts of the plant during pregnancy and lactation.	*Fruit/Seeds:* Laxative effect. Mild allergic reactions.	All parts of the plant can cause an allergic reaction in those sensitive to ragweed, chrysanthemums, marigolds, daisies, and other herbs. May prevent liver damage due to cisplatin. Chemicals causing liver damage that may be treated with the herb include butyrophenones, phenytoin, phenothiazines, alcohol, acetaminophen, and halothane.
Saw palmetto	**PO:** Benign prostatic hypertrophy. Mild diuretic, sedative, antiseptic, anti-inflammatory.	**PO:** For BPH: 1–2 grams of whole berries or 320 mg of a lipophilic extract. Antiseptic, 1.5 mL. Tea: 0.5–1 gram dried berry in 150 mL boiling water for 5–10 min; strain. Tea may not have sufficient levels of active ingredients.	Pregnancy, lactation.	Headache, stomach problems (rare), nausea, dizziness.	May interfere with oral contraceptive or hormone therapy. No significant effect on serum prostate-specific antigen (PSA) levels. Due to lack of proven efficacy, the FDA has banned all OTC products to treat BPH.

Bold Italic = life threatening side effect   ■ = black box warning   ♣ = Available in Canada

Name(s)	Use(s)	Dose	Contraindications	Side Effects	Other Information
Senna	**PO:** *Leaf, fruit:* Laxative for constipation, hemorrhoids, after anorectal surgery, to evacuate the GI tract to facilitate diagnostic tests.	**PO:** 15–30 mg hydroxyanthracene derivatives/day calculated as sennoside B. *Tea:* 1 cup in the a.m. or p.m. To make tea: Steep 0.5–2 grams finely chopped leaf in warm, but not boiling water, for 10 min; strain. A cold water tea may have fewer GI side effects. To make a cold water tea: Steep 0.5–2 grams finely chopped leaf in cold water for 10–12 hr; strain. *Liquid leaf extract:* 0.5–2 mL (frequency not specified).	Pregnancy, lactation. Use in those with abdominal pain, intestinal obstruction, acute intestinal inflammation, including Crohn's disease, ulcerative colitis, appendicitis, stomach inflammation, anal prolapse, hemorrhoids, undiagnosed abdominal pain. Use in those with dehydration, diarrhea, or loose stools.	Abdominal discomfort, colic, cramps. Chronic use: Potassium deficiency, albuminuria, hematuria, "sluggish" colon, laxative-dependency syndrome. Possible senna-tea induced hepatitis (rare).	Loss of potassium may potentiate effect of cardiac glycosides, diuretics, and corticosteroids on heart function. Use with other stimulant laxatives increases the risk of potassium depletion.

📷 = see color insert   H = Herbal   IV = Intravenous   ℞ = sound alike drug

Name(s)	Use(s)	Dose	Contraindications	Side Effects	Other Information
St. John's Wort	**PO:** Depression, dysthymic disorder. Secondary symptoms due to depression, including fatigue, loss of appetite, insomnia, anxiety. OCD, migraine headache, neuralgia, diuretic, vitiligo, cancer. **Topical:** Treat bruises, abrasions, muscle pain, first degree burns, hemorrhoids, anti-inflammatory.	**PO:** For depression: 300 mg 3 times per day of extract standardized to 0.3% hypericin. OCD: 450 mg twice a day of extract standardized to 0.3% hypericin. *Crude drug:* 2–4 grams of above ground parts/day. *Liquid extract:* 2–4 mL/day. *Tincture:* 2–4 mL/day.	Pregnancy, lactation. Use with MAOIs, SSRIs, and tricyclic antidepressants due to potentiation of effects.	Insomnia, vivid dreams, anxiety, agitation, irritability, GI discomfort, fatigue, dry mouth, dizziness, PT/INR, headache, delayed hypersensitivity, paresthesias. Also, hypomania or mania in depressed clients. Photosensitivity. Possible withdrawal symptoms similar to those seen with other antidepressants.	Questionable efficacy in treating depression. Large number of potential drug interactions. Large doses may cause a hypertensive crisis. Can decrease results if used with warfarin. May cause breakthrough bleeding and irregular menstrual bleeding if used with oral contraceptives. Induces CYP3A4; ↓ serum imatinib levels.
Valerian	**PO:** Insomnia, anxiety, stress, depression, epilepsy.	**PO:** 1 cup of tea several times per day. To prepare: Steep 2–3 grams of the root in 150 mL boiling water for 5–10 min; strain. Maximum dose of root/day: 15 grams. *Tincture:* 1–3 mL once to several times per day. *Extract:* 400–900 mg up to 2 hr before bedtime for up to 14 days.	Pregnancy, lactation.	Headache, excitability, cardiac disturbances, insomnia, uneasiness. Morning drowsiness; possible impaired alertness and information processing.	Warn clients not to drive or operate machinery after taking valerian. Additive effect when taken with other CNS depressants, including alcohol. Do not confuse with Valium.

Bold Italic = life threatening side effect   ■ = black box warning   ♣ = Available in Canada

Name(s)	Use(s)	Dose	Contraindications	Side Effects	Other Information
Yohimbe	**PO:** Impotence, aphrodisiac, exhaustion, angina, hypertension, diabetic neuropathy, postural hypotension.	Available in 5.4 mg tablets as a prescription drug with no FDA approval. Products are labeled with a standardized 15 mg yohimbine content.	Pregnancy, lactation. Use in angina, BPH, diabetes, depression, hypertension, hypotension, kidney or liver disease, prostate inflammation. Use with alpha-2 adrenergic blockers or phenothiazines due to possible increased alpha-adrenergic blockade.	Excitation, tremor, insomnia, anxiety, hypertension, tachycardia, N&V, salivation, irritability, fluid retention, Psychosis in people predisposed to it.	Use with caffeine, ephedra, MAOIs, sympathomimetics, tyramine-containing foods, or vasopressors may cause a hypertensive crisis. May interfere with antihypertensive drugs or antidiabetics.

📷 = see color insert   🅗 = Herbal   Ⅳ = Intravenous   © = sound alike drug of compounds that generally do not exert a strong, immediate action. Consumers use herbal products as therapeutic agents for the treatment/cure of illness/disease symptoms and prophylactically to prevent disease and to maintain health and wellness.

Consumer use of herbs and medicinal products over the past two decades has risen dramatically. These agents are found in retail pharmacies, grocery stores, health food shops, corner markets, and other large outlet stores as well as mail order and TV/Internet sales.

Some major health insurance companies are including coverage for herbs under "alternative therapies" and many more are considering this coverage. Herbs are regulated as Dietary Supplements under the Dietary Supplement Health and Education Act of 1994 (DSHEA).

Extracts are concentrated preparations of a liquid, powdered, or viscous consistency that are usually made from dried plant parts by maceration or percolation. Tincture is an alcoholic or hydroalcoholic solution prepared from botanicals. Plant juices are formed from the freshly harvested plant parts macerated in water and pressed. Herbal teas are potable infusions made from infusion (pour boiling water over the herb), decoction (cover herb with cold water and bring to a boil and simmer for 5-10 min), or cold maceration (place herb in tap water and let stand at room temperature for 6-8 hr).

Always ask about herbs, vitamins, teas or other remedies that client may be using for a problem or to maintain health/wellness. Clients generally do not consider these significant or as medicines and often fail to mention them during a drug history. Many of these have the potential to interact or interfere with traditional drug therapies precribed by the provider. Thus the importance of doing a careful drug history documenting all OTC therapies consumed (medication reconciliation). Herbals are not regulated by the FDA; they do not test or authorize any supplement. These may contain a variety of

agents and some have been found not to contain any of the agent it portrays. Natural does not mean that it is safe. Agents approved by the APhA (American Pharmacists Association) or U.S.P. which indicates the manufacturer followed standards established by the U.S. Pharmacopoeia should be those that the consumer purchases to ensure some degree of reliability of the product.

HISTAMINE H2 ANTAGONISTS

SEE ALSO THE FOLLOWING INDIVIDUAL ENTRIES:

Cimetidine
Famotidine
Nizatidine
Ranitidine hydrochloride

USES

See individual drugs. Uses include: **Rx.** (1) Short-term treatment of benign gastric ulcer. Maintenance therapy after healing of acute ulcer (ranitidine). (2) Short-term treatment of active duodenal ulcer and maintenance therapy after the healing of the active ulcer. (3) GERD, including erosive or ulcerative disease diagnosed by endoscopy. (4) Prevention of upper GI bleeding in critically ill clients (IV cimetidine only). (5) Pathological hypersecretory conditions, including Zollinger-Ellison syndrome, systemic mastocytosis, multiple endocrine adenomas. (6) As part of combination therapy to treat *Helicobacter pylori*– associated duodenal ulcer and maintenance therapy after healing of the active ulcer.

OTC. (1) Relief of heartburn associated with acid indigestion and sour stomach. (2) Prevention of heartburn associated with acid indigestion and sour stomach due to certain foods and beverages.

ACTION/KINETICS

Action

Histamine H2 antagonists are competitive blockers of histamine. As such they inhibit all phases of gastric acid secretion including that caused by histamine, gastrin, and muscarinic agents.

Bold Italic = life threatening side effect   ■ = black box warning   ✤ = Available in Canada

Both fasting and nocturnal acid secretion are inhibited. In addition, the volume and hydrogen ion concentration of gastric juice are decreased. These drugs provide rapid symptomatic relief and accelerate ulcer healing when used with antibiotics for *Helicobacter pylori*. Cimetidine, famotidine, and ranitidine have no effect on gastric emptying; cimetidine and famotidine have no effect on lower esophageal pressure. Fasting or postprandial serum gastrin is not affected by famotidine, nizatidine, or ranitidine. Cimetidine is known to affect the cytochrome P450 drug metabolizing system for other drugs. Ranitidine also affects the P450 enzyme system, but its effect on elimination of other drugs is not significant. Famotidine and nizatidine do not affect the P450 enzyme system.

CONTRAINDICATIONS
Hypersensitivity. Use of cimetidine, famotidine, and nizatidine during lactation.

SPECIAL CONCERNS
Use with caution in impaired hepatic and renal function. Symptomatic response to these drugs does not preclude gastric malignancy. Elderly blacks have a greater risk of cognitive impairment if they have used these drugs for 2 or more years. Use ranitidine with caution during lactation. Safety and effectiveness have not been established for use in children. Use of cimetidine in children less than 16 years of age unless benefits outweigh risks.

SIDE EFFECTS
The following side effects are common to all or most of the H$_2$-histamine antagonists. See individual drugs for complete listing. **GI:** N&V, abdominal discomfort, diarrhea, constipation, hepatocellular effects. **CNS:** Headache, fatigue, somnolence, dizziness, confusion, hallucinations, insomnia. **Dermatologic:** Rash, urticaria, pruritus, alopecia (rare), erythema multiforme (rare). **Hematologic:** Rarely, thrombocytopenia, agranulocytosis, granulocytopenia. **Other:** Gynecomastia, impotence, loss of libido, arthralgia, bronchospasm, transient pain at injection site, cardiac arrhythmias following rapid IV use (rare), arthralgia (rare), hypersensitivity reactions (bronchospasm, rash, eosinophilia, *laryngeal edema, rarely anaphylaxis*).

OD OVERDOSE MANAGEMENT
Symptoms: No experience is available for deliberate overdose.
Treatment: Induce vomiting or perform gastric lavage to remove any unabsorbed drug. Monitor the client and undertake supportive therapy.

DRUG INTERACTIONS
See individual drugs.
Cephalosporins / Possible ↓ availability of certain cephalosporins (e.g., cefpodoxime, cefuroxime, cephalexin)
Ethanol / Possible ↑ ethanol plasma levels
Itraconazole / ↓ Itraconazole plasma levels due to changes in gastric pH
Ketoconazole / ↑ Gastric pH may inhibit ketoconazole absorption.

DOSAGE
See individual drugs.

NURSING CONSIDERATIONS
ADMINISTRATION/STORAGE
Dosage may need to be reduced in impaired renal function.

ASSESSMENT
1. Note onset, duration, intensity, other associated S&S, and previous treatments. Assess frequency of reflux occurrences. Chronic treatment usually initiated after two to three recurrences.
2. Perform CNS assessment noting level of orientation.
3. Check results of radiographic/endoscopic procedures; document *H. pylori* results and if/when treated.
4. Monitor CBC, renal and LFTs; reduce dose with renal dysfunction. Determine gastric pH; maintain >5.

CLIENT/FAMILY TEACHING
1. May take without regard to meals; food prolongs drug effect and may help ↓ nausea, diarrhea and/or abdominal pain. Stagger doses of antacids, i.e., 1 hr before or 1 hr after cimetidine or ranitidine. Take as prescribed; do not stop if pain subsides or if "feeling better" as drug is necessary to inhibit gastric acid secretion so ulcer can heal.
2. Do not chew, break or crush SR tabs. If unable to swallow may open and

sprinkle on applesauce or yogurt but must be swallowed immediately.

3. These agents reduce the secretion of gastric acid and are usually prescribed for 4–8 weeks initially to control symptoms and promote ulcer healing.

4. Avoid activities that require mental alertness until drug effects realized. Report any confusion or disorientation immediately. Any blood-tinged emesis or dark tarry stools as well as dizziness or rash, bruising, fatigue, and malaise, require immediate reporting. Avoid alcohol, caffeine, aspirin-containing products (cough and cold products), and foods that may cause GI irritation, i.e., harsh spices, black pepper.

5. Do not take maximum dose of OTC products for more than 2 weeks without medical supervision. Prolonged use may contribute to depletion of intrinsic factor, necessary for vitamin B12 absorption esp. in those >50 y.o.

6. Stop 24–72 hr before skin testing begins; may cause false negative response in tests with allergen extracts. May cause painful swelling of breast tissue and impotence, report as these are reversible.

7. Smoking may interfere with drug's action. Stop smoking and do not smoke after last dose of day.

8. Review GERD instructions, i.e., ↑ HOB, avoid lying down for at least 2 hr after eating, and dietary restrictions.

9. Report for all scheduled follow-up studies; a response to these agents does not preclude gastric malignancy.

OUTCOMES/EVALUATE

Duodenal ulcer healing ↓ Gastric irritation/bleeding ↓ Abdominal pain/discomfort. Gastric pH >5

LAXATIVES

SEE ALSO THE FOLLOWING INDIVIDUAL ENTRIES:

Docusate calcium
Docusate sodium
Magnesium sulfate
Psyllium hydrophilic muciloid

USES

See individual agents. (1) Short-term treatment of constipation. (2) Prophylaxis in clients who should not strain during defecation, i.e., following anorectal surgery or after MI (use fecal softeners or lubricant laxatives). (3) Evacuate the colon for rectal and bowel examinations (certain lubricant, saline, and stimulant laxatives). (4) In conjunction with surgery. (5) With anthelmintic therapy. (6) With chronic opioid therapy. NOTE: The underlying cause of constipation should be determined since a marked change in bowel habits may be a symptom of a pathologic condition.

ACTION/KINETICS

Action

Laxatives act locally, either by stimulating the smooth muscles of the bowel or by changing the bulk or consistency of the stools. Laxatives can be divided into seven categories.

1. *Stimulant laxatives:* Substances that directly stimulate the smooth muscles of the bowel to increase contractions. Also alter water and electrolyte secretion. Examples: Bisacodyl, cascara, casanthranol, and senna.

2. *Saline laxatives:* Substances that cause water retention, and therefore increased intraluminal increased pressure of the intestine. Also cause cholecystokinin release. Examples: Magnesium salts and sodium phosphates.

3. *Bulk-forming laxatives:* Nondigestible substances that increase the bulk of the stools, thereby stimulating peristalsis; they form an emollient gel. Examples: Methylcellulose, polycarbophil, and psyllium.

4. *Emollient laxatives:* Agents that soften hardened feces and facilitate their passage through the lower intestine. Examples: Mineral oil.

5. *Fecal softener:* Facilitates admixture of fat and water to soften the stool. Example: Docusate.

6. *Hyperosmotic:* Glycerin causes local irritation and has a hyperosmotic action. Lactulose has an osmotic effect causing fluid retention in the colon,

---

lowering the pH and increases colonic peristalsis.

7. *Miscellaneous:* Castor oil has a direct action on the intestinal mucosa or nerve plexus; it alters water and electrolyte secretion.

CONTRAINDICATIONS

Severe abdominal pain or N&V that *might* be caused by appendicitis, enteritis, ulcerative colitis, diverticulitis, intestinal obstruction, fecal impaction, undiagnosed abdominal pain. Laxative use in these conditions may cause rupture of the abdomen or intestinal hemorrhage. Undiagnosed abdominal pain. Children under the age of 2.

SIDE EFFECTS

GI: Excess activity of the colon resulting in nausea, diarrhea, griping, or vomiting. Perianal irritation, bloating, flatulence. **Electrolyte balance:** Dehydration, disturbance of the electrolyte balance. **Miscellaneous:** Dizziness, fainting, weakness, sweating, palpitations.

Bulk laxatives: Obstruction in the esophagus, stomach, small intestine, or rectum.

Stimulant laxatives: Chronic abuse may lead to malfunctioning colon.

Mineral oil: Large doses may cause anal seepage resulting in itching, irritation, hemorrhoids, and perianal discomfort.

Chronic use of laxatives may cause laxative dependency and result in chronic constipation and other intestinal disorders because the client may start to depend on the psychologic effect and physical stimulus of the drug rather than on the body's own natural reflexes.

DRUG INTERACTIONS

Anticoagulants, oral / ↓ Absorption of vitamin K from GI tract induced by laxatives may ↑ effects of anticoagulants and result in bleeding

Digitalis / Cathartics may ↓ absorption of digitalis

Tetracyclines / Laxatives containing Al, Ca, or Mg may ↓ effect of tetracyclines R/T ↓ GI tract absorption.

DOSAGE

See individual drugs.

NURSING CONSIDERATIONS

ADMINISTRATION/STORAGE

1. When administering a laxative, note the length of time it takes for the laxative to take effect and give it so that the result of the laxative will not interfere with the client's rest or digestion and absorption of nutrients.

2. Administer liquid laxatives at an agreeable temperature.

3. If laxative is administered in a liquid, select one palatable to client.

4. If ordered to prepare for a diagnostic exam, check directions carefully to ensure accurate administration.

ASSESSMENT

1. Note reasons for therapy, length of use and underlying causes; identify type taking and effectiveness. Determine stool characteristics and frequency. Client's definition of constipation may determine if, in fact, constipation exists.

2. With abdominal pain and discomfort, note location, triggers, and type of discomfort. R/O other intestinal disorders/obstruction where laxatives should not be used.

3. Note age, state of health, activity level, and general nutritional status. Identify recent life-style changes that may contribute to problem. Note any special restriction or limitation due to illness; may include fluid/sodium restrictions.

4. List other drugs that may contribute to constipation (i.e., diuretics, anticholinergics, antihistamines, antidepressants, narcotic analgesics, iron products, and some antihypertensive agents, especially verapamil).

CLIENT/FAMILY TEACHING

1. Take only as directed. Have a regular schedule for defecation; keep record of bowel function and response to all laxatives taken. Laxatives reduce the amount of time other drugs remain in the intestine and may diminish effectiveness.

2. If taken as preparation for a diagnostic study, review instructions. If unable to read, find someone to review directions to ensure an accurate test.

📷 = see color insert   **H** = Herbal   **IV** = Intravenous   @ = sound alike drug

3. Review techniques that facilitate elimination; sitting with legs slightly elevated and leaning forward to increase abdominal pressure often encourages elimination. If ill at home, consider a commode at the bedside. This will promote better bowel function by encouraging client to move about and ensure privacy.

4. Bowel tone will be lost with long-term use of laxatives; bowel movements do not have to occur daily. Use diet to achieve same purpose; two or three prunes a day are preferable to laxatives. Frequent use of any type of enemas may cause damage to the rectum and small bowel as well as inhibit bowel tone and may cause electrolyte abnormalities.

5. Review importance of diet high in fiber foods (and juices such as prune) and daily exercise in maintaining proper bowel function. Include bulk foods and sufficient fluids in diet to enhance elimination. Increase water consumption at least 6-8 8oz glasses per day. Consult dietitian for assistance in meal planning/preparation and food selections.

6. If pregnant, consult with provider before taking any laxatives to treat constipation. Nursing mothers should avoid laxatives unless prescribed as many are excreted in breast milk and can cause infant diarrhea.

7. Daily exercise will enhance regular elimination.

8. Report N&V, abdominal pain or if constipation persists because there could be a physiologic problem that requires attention.

OUTCOMES/EVALUATE
- Relief of constipation; evacuation of a soft, formed stool
- Effective colon preparation for diagnostic procedures (no stool in bowel)

NARCOTIC ANALGESICS

SEE ALSO THE FOLLOWING INDIVIDUAL ENTRIES:

Alfentanil hydrochloride
Buprenorphine hydrochloride
Butorphanol tartrate
Codeine sulfate
Fentanyl citrate
Fentanyl transdermal system
Fentanyl transmucosal system
Hydrocodone bitartrate and Acetaminophen
Hydromorphone hydrochloride
Meperidine hydrochloride
Methadone hydrochloride
Morphine sulfate
Oxycodone hydrochloride
Oxycodone hydrochloride and Acetaminophen
Propoxyphene hydrochloride
Propoxyphene napsylate
Remifentanil hydrochloride
Tramadol hydrochloride
Tramadol hydrochloride and Acetaminophen

USES
See individual drugs. Uses include: (1) Treat pain due to various causes (e.g., MI, carcinoma, surgery, burns, postpartum). (2) Preanesthetic medication. (3) Adjunct to anesthesia. (4) Acute vascular occlusion. (5) Diarrhea. (6) Antitussive.

ACTION/KINETICS

Action

Narcotic analgesics are classified as agonists, mixed agonist-antagonists, or partial agonists depending on their activity at opiate receptors. The narcotic analgesics attach to specific receptors located in the CNS (cortex, brain stem, and spinal cord) resulting in various CNS effects. The mechanism is believed to involve decreased permeability of the cell membrane to sodium, which results in diminished transmission of pain impulses. Five categories of opioid receptors have been identified: mu, kappa, sigma, delta, and epsilon. Narcotic analgesics are believed to exert their activity at mu, kappa, and sigma receptors. Mu receptors are thought to mediate supraspinal analgesia, euphoria, and respiratory and physical depression. Pentazocine-like spinal analgesia, miosis, and sedation are mediated by kappa receptors while sigma receptors mediate dysphoria and hallucinations, as well as respiratory and vasomotor

---

Bold Italic = life threatening side effect   ■ = black box warning   ♣ = Available in Canada

stimulation (caused by drugs with antagonist activity). In addition to an alteration of pain perception (analgesia), the drugs, especially at higher doses, induce euphoria, drowsiness, changes in mood, mental clouding, and deep sleep.

The narcotic analgesics also produce a large number of secondary pharmacologic effects. These include: (1) Depressed tidal volume and respiratory rate due to decreased sensitivity of the respiratory center to carbon dioxide. Death by overdosage is almost always the result of respiratory arrest. (2) Nausea and emesis due to direct stimulation of the CTZ. (3) Depression of the cough reflex by a direct effect on the medullary cough center. (4) Orthostatic hypotension and fainting due to peripheral vasodilation (when client stands), reduced peripheral resistance, and inhibition of baroreceptors. Little effect on BP when the client is in a supine position. (5) Pruritus, flushing, and red eyes due to histamine release. (6) Decrease in gastric motility leading to prolonged gastric emptying time and possible esophageal reflux. (7) In the small intestine decrease in biliary, pancreatic, and intestinal secretions causing delays in digestion of food. Increase in resting tone and periodic spasms occur. (8) Decreased propulsive peristalsis in the large intestine with an increase in tone to spasm. Causes severe constipation. (9) Constriction of the sphincter of Oddi causing epigastric distress or biliary colic. (10) Increased smooth muscle tone in the urinary tract can cause spasms with urinary urgency and difficulty with urination. (11) Pupillary constriction caused by certain narcotic analgesics is a sign of use/dependence. See also individual agents.

CONTRAINDICATIONS

Asthma, emphysema, kyphoscoliosis, severe obesity, convulsive states as in epilepsy, delirium tremens, tetanus and strychnine poisoning, diabetic acidosis, myxedema, Addison's disease, hepatic cirrhosis, and children under 6 months.

SPECIAL CONCERNS

Use with caution in clients with head injury or after head surgery because of morphine's capacity to elevate ICP and mask the pupillary response. Use with caution in the elderly, in the debilitated, in young children, in individuals with increased ICP, in obstetrics, and with clients in shock or during acute alcoholic intoxication.

Use morphine with extreme caution in pulmonary heart disease (cor pulmonale). Deaths following ordinary therapeutic doses have been reported. Use cautiously in prostatic hypertrophy, because it may precipitate acute urinary retention. Use cautiously in clients with reduced blood volume, such as in hemorrhaging clients who are more susceptible to the hypotensive effects of morphine.

Since the drugs depress the respiratory center, give early in labor, at least 2 hr before delivery, to reduce the danger of respiratory depression in the newborn. When given before surgery, give at least 1–2 hr preoperatively so that the danger of maximum depression of respiratory function will have passed before anesthesia is initiated. These drugs may need to be withheld prior to diagnostic procedures so that the physician can use pain to locate dysfunction.

Rapid IV injection increases the likelihood or respiratory depression, hypotension, apnea, circulatory collapse, cardiac arrest, and anaphylactoid reactions.

SIDE EFFECTS

See individual drugs. The following side effects are common to most narcotic analgesics. **Respiratory:** *Respiratory depression, apnea.* **CNS:** Dizziness, lightheadedness, sedation, lethargy, headache, euphoria, mental clouding, fainting. Idiosyncratic effects including excitement, restlessness, tremors, delirium, insomnia. **GI:** N&V, vomiting, constipation, increased pressure in biliary tract, dry mouth, anorexia. **CV:** Flushing, changes in HR and BP, circulatory collapse. **Allergic:** Skin rashes including pruritus and urticaria. Sweating, *laryn-*

Classifications

gospasm, edema. **Miscellaneous:** Urinary retention, oliguria, reduced libido, changes in body temperature. Narcotics cross the placental barrier and depress respiration of the fetus or newborn.

DEPENDENCE AND TOLERANCE

All drugs of this group are addictive. Psychologic and physical dependence and tolerance develop even when clients use clinical doses. Tolerance is characterized by the fact that the client requires shorter periods of time between doses or larger doses for relief of pain. Tolerance usually develops faster when the narcotic analgesic is administered regularly and when the dose is large.

OD OVERDOSE MANAGEMENT

Symptoms (Acute Toxicity): Severe toxicity is characterized by ***profound respiratory depression, apnea, deep sleep, stupor or coma, circulatory collapse, seizures, cardiopulmonary arrest, and death.*** Less severe toxicity results in symptoms including CNS depression, miosis, respiratory depression, deep sleep, flaccidity of skeletal muscles, hypotension, bradycardia, hypothermia, pulmonary edema, pneumonia, shock. The respiratory rate may be as low as 2–4 breaths/min. The client may be cyanotic. Urine output is decreased, the skin feels clammy, and body temperature decreases. If death occurs, it almost always results from ***respiratory depression.***

Symptoms (Chronic Toxicity): The problem of chronic dependence on narcotics occurs not only as a result of "street" use but is often found among those who have easy access to narcotics (physicians, nurses, pharmacists). All the principal narcotic analgesics (morphine, opium, heroin, codeine, meperidine, and others) have, at times, been used for nontherapeutic purposes.

The nurse must be aware of the problem and be able to recognize signs of chronic dependence. These are constricted pupils, GI effects (constipation), skin infections, needle scars, abscesses, and itching, especially on the anterior surfaces of the body, where the client may inject the drug.

Withdrawal signs appear after drug is withheld for 4–12 hr. They are characterized by intense craving for the drug, insomnia, yawning, sneezing, vomiting, diarrhea, tremors, sweating, mental depression, muscular aches and pains, chills, and anxiety. Although the symptoms of narcotic withdrawal are uncomfortable, they are rarely life-threatening. This is in contrast to the withdrawal syndrome from depressants, where the life of the individual may be endangered because of the possibility of tonic-clonic seizures.

Treatment (Acute Overdose): Initial treatment is aimed at combating progressive respiratory depression by maintaining a patent airway and by artificial respiration. Gastric lavage and induced emesis are indicated in case of oral poisoning. The narcotic antagonist naloxone (Narcan), 0.4 mg IV, is effective in the treatment of acute overdosage. Respiratory stimulants (e.g., caffeine) should not be used to treat depression from the narcotic overdosage.

DRUG INTERACTIONS

Alcohol, ethyl / Potentiation or addition of CNS depressant effects; concomitant use may lead to drowsiness, lethargy, stupor, respiratory collapse, coma, or death

Anesthetics, general /See *Alcohol*

Antianxiety drugs /See *Alcohol*

Anticholinergics / ↑ Risk of urinary retention and/or severe constipation which may lead to paralytic ileus

Antidepressants, tricyclic / ↑ Narcotic-induced respiratory depression

Antihistamines /See *Alcohol*

Barbiturates /See *Alcohol*

Cimetidine / ↑ CNS toxicity (e.g., disorientation, confusion, respiratory depression, apnea, seizures)

CNS depressants /See *Alcohol*

MAO inhibitors / Possible potentiation of either MAO inhibitor (excitation, hypertension) or narcotic (hypotension, coma) effects; death has resulted

Methotrimeprazine / Potentiation of CNS depression

Narcotic analgesics, mixed agonist/antagonists (buprenorphine, butorphanol, nalbuphine, pentazocine) / May precipitate withdrawal symptoms in dependent clients

Phenothiazines / Analgesic effect of narcotics may be potentiated; however, there is an ↑ incidence of side effects

Sedative-hypnotics, nonbarbiturate /See *Alcohol*

Skeletal muscle relaxants (surgical) / ↑ Respiratory depression/muscle relaxation.

LABORATORY TEST CONSIDERATIONS
Altered liver function tests. False + or ↑ urinary glucose test (Benedict's). ↑ Plasma amylase or lipase.

DOSAGE
See individual drugs.

NURSING CONSIDERATIONS

ADMINISTRATION/STORAGE
1. Review list of drugs prescribed and with which opioids interact and effects.
2. Request orders be rewritten at timed intervals as required for continued administration.
3. Record amount of opioid used on the controlled inventory sheet, noting drug, date, time, dose, and to whom, or if the drug was wasted; include appropriate witness as necessary, addressing all requirements for documentation.
IV 4. Give by very slow IV injection, preferably as a diluted solution, with the client lying down. Do not give IV unless a narcotic antagonist and facilities for assisted or controlled respiration are available.

ASSESSMENT
1. Note reasons for therapy, type, onset, characteristics of symptoms; differentiate acute vs. chronic syndromes and rate pain levels. Note prior experience with opioids and any adverse reactions.
2. Identify cause and document amount of pain or discomfort, its location, intensity, duration, frequency of occurrence, and what therapy/drug was effective in the past. Use a pain rating scale (e.g., 0–10) to assess pain quantitatively so clients can accurately describe their level of pain and measure effectiveness of therapy.
3. Identify clinical conditions that may precipitate pain syndromes, i.e., cancer,

neuropathic, postherpetic neuralgia, or musculoskeletal injury. Document amount of time elapsed between doses for relief from recurring pain. Note precipitating factors as well as the impact of the pain on the client's ability to function and perform ADLs.
4. Obtain baseline VS; generally, if the respiratory rate <12/min or the SBP <90 mm Hg, an opiod should not be administered unless there is ventilatory support or specific written guidelines, with parameters for administration. Note weight, age, and general body size. Too large a dosage for the client's weight and age can result in serious consequences.
5. Note asthma or other conditions that alter respirations. Determine if pregnant. Opioids cross the placental barrier and depress fetal respirations.
6. Monitor CBC, lytes, renal and LFTs. Assess for dependence, drug seeking behaviors, over use/consumption of prescription and identify those on long-term therapy so opioid agreement can be completed. Periodic drug testing may support proper use.

INTERVENTIONS
1. Explore source of pain; use nonopioid analgesics when possible. Coadministration (as with NSAIDs) may increase analgesic effects and permit lower opioid doses. Determine need for pain management referrals. Administer when needed; *prolonging until the maximum amount of pain experienced reduces drugs' effectiveness.*
2. Determine when to use supportive measures, such as relaxation techniques, repositioning, alternative therapies, and reassurance to assist in relieving pain.
3. Monitor VS and mental status. During parenteral therapy:
- Monitor for ↓ respirations.
- Opioids depress cough reflex. Turn q 2 hr; cough and deep breathe to prevent atelectasis. Splinting incisions and painful areas may assist in compliance. Administer opioid at least 30–60 min prior to activities or painful procedures.
- Monitor for hypotension.

- Report if HR below 50 beats/min in the adult or 110 beats/min in infant.
- Observe for decrease in BP, deep sleep, or constricted pupils.
- Assess during meals to prevent choking and aspiration.
- Monitor closely when administered as sedation for a procedure.
- Note effects on mental status. One who has experienced pain, fear, or anxiety may become euphoric and excited. Note dizziness, drowsiness, pupil reactions, or hallucinations.

4. Report if N&V occurs; may need an antiemetic or change in therapy. A snack or milk may decrease gastric irritation and lessen nausea when taken orally.

5. Monitor bowel function; opioids, esp. morphine, can have a depressant effect on the GI tract and may promote constipation. Increase fluid intake to 2.5–3 L/day; consume fruit juices, fruits, and fiber. Increase level and frequency of exercise. Take stool softeners as directed.

6. Opioids may cause urinary retention. Monitor I&O; palpate abdomen for distention; empty bladder q 3–4 hr. Question about difficulty voiding, pain in the bladder area, sensation of not fully emptying the bladder, dysuria, or any unusual odors.

7. Monitor mental status. If bedridden, use side supports and safety measures; assist with ambulation, bathroom, and transfers to prevent falls. Note difficulty with vision. Check pupillary response to light; report if pupils remain constricted.

8. Reassure that flushing and a feeling of warmth may occur with therapeutic doses. May perspire profusely; be prepared to bathe; change clothes and linens frequently.

9. Assess for evidence of tolerance and addiction with ATC therapy. With terminal diseases and chronic debilitating pain, dependence on drug therapy is not a consideration, whereas *adequate pain control is of the utmost concern.*

CLIENT/FAMILY TEACHING

1. Chronic pain is a multifaceted and complex syndrome, which adversely affects one's physical, emotional, socioeconomic, and spiritual foundations. In order to restore a sense of well-being and desire for one to "go on" to it has been identified that pain problem identification and adequate pain control is imperative.

2. Oral drug formulations of extended-release, controlled-release or sustained-release products are not made to be chewed, crushed, or dissolved.

3. One may never be totally pain free. The intent of therapy is to lower the pain level to one in which activities can be performed R/T daily care, and those that are of interest and concern to the client including holding down a job and going to work every day; not to encourage one to sleep throughout the day. Education concerning chronic pain and its many facets will be provided in classes and information sheets to better prepare one for this chronic disease state.

4. Drug may become habit forming; alternative methods for pain control will be explored and utilized. With chronic debilitating pain, addiction is not a concern whereas functionality is of concern. Take as prescribed before the pain becomes too severe. During prolonged usage, do not stop abruptly; withdrawal symptoms may occur. Providers may expect clients to sign opioid agreements for not only client education but for protection from liability and misuse issues.

5. Can cause drowsiness and dizziness esp. initially and with dose adjustments; use caution when operating a motor vehicle or performing other tasks that require mental alertness. Rise slowly from a lying to sitting position and dangle before standing, to minimize orthostatic effects.

6. Determine extent of relief achieved with each dosage (e.g., pain level decreased from a level 5 to a level 2, 20 min after administration of medication). Keep a record of opioid use for breakthrough pain so that maintenance dose can be reviewed and adjusted.

7. Review techniques to enhance pain relief such as relaxation techniques, ice/

---

heat applications, splinting incision, supporting painful areas, and taking medication before strenuous activities and before pain becomes severe.

8. Do not take OTC agents without approval. Many contain small amounts of alcohol and some may interact unfavorably with the prescribed drug. Avoid alcohol in any form.

9. For fecal impaction, use preventive actions, such as increased fluid intake, increased use of fruit and fruit juices, and a stool softener.

10. Store all drugs in a safe place, out of the reach of children and away from the bedside to prevent accidental overdosage. When used as sedation for outpatient procedures, someone must accompany client. Expect a recovery period (to assess for adverse effects) up to several hours before release.

11. Identify appropriate support groups for assistance with understanding, accepting, and managing chronic pain. Seek locale of regional pain management center for nonresponders with chronic pain syndromes.

12. For those with terminal diseases, identify local support groups to provide contact with those experiencing similar symptoms and treatments and local hospice program.

13. For the elderly, blood levels of opioid may be higher, resulting in longer periods of pain relief. Assess physical parameters and client complaints carefully before readministering opioid for short-term pain control on the prescribed as-needed frequency.

14. Keep all F/U appointments to evaluate response to therapy, adverse side effects, labs, and refills thru prescriptions.

OUTCOMES/EVALUATE
- Control of pain without altered hemodynamics or impaired level of consciousness
- Reduction in pain level on pain rating scale
- Ability to perform ADLs and desired activities that are of client importance

- Absence of acute toxicity, tolerance, or addiction, during short-term therapy

NARCOTIC ANTAGONISTS

SEE ALSO THE FOLLOWING INDIVIDUAL ENTRIES:

Nalmefene hydrochloride
Naloxone hydrochloride
Naltrexone

ACTION/KINETICS
Action
Narcotic antagonists competitively block the action of narcotic analgesics by displacing previously given narcotics from their receptor sites or by preventing narcotics from attaching to the opiate receptors, thereby preventing access by the analgesic. Not effective in reversing the respiratory depression induced by barbiturates, anesthetics, or other nonnarcotic agents. These drugs almost immediately induce withdrawal symptoms in narcotic addicts and are sometimes used to unmask dependence.

NURSING CONSIDERATIONS
ASSESSMENT
1. Note reasons for therapy, when and what agents consumed, and expected time frame for action. Determine etiology of respiratory depression. Narcotic antagonists do not relieve the toxicity of nonnarcotic CNS depressants.

2. Assess/monitor LOC, mental status, clinical presentation, and VS.

INTERVENTIONS
1. Note agent being reversed. If opioid is long acting or sustained release, repeated doses will be required in order to continue to counteract drug effects. Monitor VS and respirations closely after duration of action of antagonist; additional doses may be necessary.

2. Observe for symptoms of airway obstruction; if comatose, turn frequently and position on side to prevent aspiration. Maintain a safe, protective environment. Use side rails, supervise ambulation, and use soft supports as needed.

3. Observe for appearance of withdrawal symptoms characterized by restlessness, crying out due to sudden loss of pain control, lacrimation, rhinorrhea, yawning, perspiration, vomiting, diarrhea, sweating, writhing, anxiety, pain, chills, and an intense craving for the drug. If used to diagnose opioid use or dependence, observe for initial dilation of the pupils, followed by constriction.

4. Anticipate readministration of smaller doses of opioid (once depressant symptoms reversed) with terminal pain and conditions that warrant narcotic pain management.

CLIENT/FAMILY TEACHING

Drug is used to reverse the effects of too much opiod. It may need to be readministered in order to attain this effect of increasing level of consciousness and reversing respiratory depression.

OUTCOMES/EVALUATE

- Reversal of toxic opioid analgesia evidenced by ↑ level of consciousness and improved breathing patterns
- Confirmation of opioid dependence

NEUROMUSCULAR BLOCKING AGENTS

SEE ALSO THE FOLLOWING INDIVIDUAL ENTRIES:

Atracurium besylate
Cisatracurium besylate
Pancuronium bromide
Rocuronium bromide
Succinylcholine chloride
Tubocurarine chloride
Vecuronium bromide

USES

See individual agents. Uses include, but are not limited to: (1) Adjunct to general anesthesia to cause muscle relaxation. (2) Reduce the intensity of skeletal muscle contractions in either drug-induced or electrically-induced convulsions. (3) Assist in the management of mechanical ventilation.

ACTION/KINETICS

Action

These drugs are categorized as competitive (nondepolarizing) and depolarizing agents, both of which act peripherally. Competitive agents include all of the above listed drugs *except* succinylcholine. They compete with acetylcholine for the receptor site in the muscle cells. The depolarizing agent—succinylcholine—initially excites skeletal muscle and then prevents the muscle from contracting by prolonging the time during which the receptors at the end plate cannot respond to acetylcholine (depolarization during refractory time). The muscle paralysis caused by the neuromuscular blocking agents is sequential in the following order: heaviness of eyelids, difficulty in swallowing/talking, diplopia, progressive weakening of extremities and neck, followed by relaxation of the trunk and spine. The diaphragm (respiratory paralysis) is affected last. They do not affect consciousness, and their use, in the absence of adequate levels of general anesthesia, may be frightening to the client. There is a narrow margin of safety between a therapeutically effective dose causing muscle relaxation and a toxic dose causing respiratory paralysis. **The neuromuscular blocking agents are always administered initially by a trained provider.** The nurse must be prepared to maintain and monitor respiration until the effect of the drug subsides.

Pharmacokinetics

After IV infusion, flaccid paralysis occurs within a few minutes with maximum effects within about 6 min. Maximal effects last 35–60 min and effective muscle paralysis may last for 25–90 min with complete recovery taking several hours.

CONTRAINDICATIONS

Allergy or hypersensitivity to any of these drugs.

SPECIAL CONCERNS

Use with caution in myasthenia gravis; renal, hepatic, endocrine, or pulmonary impairment; respiratory depression; during lactation; and in elderly, pediatric, or debilitated clients. The action may be altered in clients by electrolyte imbalances (especially hyperkalemia), some carcinomas, body temperature,

---

dehydration, renal disease, and in those taking digitalis.

SIDE EFFECTS

Respiratory paralysis. Severe and prolonged muscle relaxation. CV: Cardiac arrhythmias, bradycardia, hypotension, cardiac arrest. These side effects are more frequent in neonates and premature infants. **GI:** Excessive salivation during light anesthesia. **Miscellaneous: *Bronchospasms, hyperthermia,*** hypersensitivity (rare). See also individual agents.

OD OVERDOSE MANAGEMENT

Symptoms: Decreased respiratory reserve, extended skeletal muscle weakness, prolonged apnea, low tidal volume, sudden release of histamine, *CV collapse.*

Treatment: There are no known antidotes.

- Use a peripheral nerve stimulator to monitor and assess client's response to the neuromuscular blocking medication.
- Have anticholinesterase drugs, such as edrophonium, pyridostigmine, or neostigmine available to counteract respiratory depression due to paralysis of skeletal muscles. These drugs decrease the body's breakdown of acetylcholine. To minimize the muscarinic cholinergic side effects, give atropine.
- Correct BP, electrolyte imbalance, or circulating blood volume by fluid and electrolyte therapy. Vasopressors can be used to correct hypotension due to ganglionic blockade.

DRUG INTERACTIONS

The following drug interactions are for nondepolarizing skeletal muscle relaxants. See also succinylcholine.

Aminoglycoside antibiotics / Additive muscle relaxation, including prolonged respiratory depression

Amphotericin B / ↑ Muscle relaxation

Anesthetics, inhalation / Additive muscle relaxation

Carbamazepine / ↓ Duration or effect of muscle relaxants

Clindamycin / Additive muscle relaxation, including prolonged respiratory depression

Colistin / ↑ Muscle relaxation

Corticosteroids / ↓ Effect of muscle relaxants

Furosemide / ↑ or ↓ Effect of skeletal muscle relaxants (may be dose-related)

Hydantoins / ↓ Duration or effect of muscle relaxants

Ketamine / ↑ Muscle relaxation, including prolonged respiratory depression

Lincomycin / ↑ Muscle relaxation, including prolonged respiratory depression

Lithium / ↑ Recovery time of muscle relaxants → prolonged respiratory depression

Magnesium salts / ↑ Muscle relaxation, with prolonged respiratory depression

Methotrimeprazine / ↑ Muscle relaxation

Narcotic analgesics / ↑ Respiratory depression and ↑ muscle relaxation

Nitrates / ↑ Muscle relaxation, including prolonged respiratory depression

Phenothiazines / ↑ Muscle relaxation

Pipercillin / ↑ Muscle relaxation, including prolonged respiratory depression

Polymyxin B / ↑ Muscle relaxation

Procainamide / ↑ Muscle relaxation

Procaine / ↑ Muscle relaxation by ↓ plasma protein binding

Quinidine / ↑ Muscle relaxation

Ranitidine / Significant ↓ effect of muscle relaxants

Theophyllines / Reversal of effects of muscle relaxant (dose-dependent)

Thiazide diuretics / ↑ Muscle relaxation due to hypokalemia

Verapamil / ↑ Muscle relaxation, with prolonged respiratory depression.

DOSAGE

See individual drugs.

NURSING CONSIDERATIONS

ASSESSMENT

1. Note reasons for therapy, desired outcome, and anticipated length of use.

2. List other drugs receiving. Clients requiring neuromuscular blocking agents are often receiving other drugs that may prolong response to neuromuscular blocking agent.

3. Question client concerning changes in vision, ability to chew or move the fingers. Note age and condition; elderly

---

and debilitated clients should not receive drugs in this category.

4. Monitor CBC, lytes, CXR, ECG, renal and LFTs.

5. Note initial selective paralysis in the following sequence: levator muscles of the eyelids, mastication muscles, limb muscles, abdominal muscles, glottis muscles, intercostal muscles, and the diaphragm muscles; neuromuscular recovery occurs in the reverse order.

INTERVENTIONS

1. Administer in a closely monitored environment and generally only when client is intubated. Neuromuscular blocking agents are generally used in the ICU setting for 3 reasons: (1) to eliminate spontaneous breathing and promote mechanical ventilation (i.e., eliminate urge to fight the vent. (2) Cause a pharmacologic restraint so clients do not harm themselves. (3) To decrease oxygen consumption.

2. Prevent overdosage during infusions by frequent evaluations with a peripheral nerve stimulator (train-of-four) to document antagonism of neuromuscular blockade and recovery of muscle function and strength.

3. Whenever a paralytic agent is used, the Train of Four (TOF) is the test used to measure the degree of neuromuscular blockade. Do a baseline measurement before paralytic agent is started to determine what current is necessary to obtain twitch. Generally 20 mA may be enough. Complete and document until TOF to 2/4.

Instructions for use of Train of Four:

- Explain to client exactly what you are doing, that it will not hurt, and why you are performing this test
- Attach 2 electrodes along the course of the ulnar nerve. (Temporal may be used.)
- Connect the lead to the peripheral nerve stimulator by inserting the jacks into the Proximal (red) and Distal (black) output jacks. Connect the other end to the client electrodes.
- Turn stimulator on. Select the current necessary (usually 20) for that client to twitch when the stimuli is applied.

- Press TOF once. It will deliver a train of four pulses where each is 0.5 seconds apart. Do NOT use the other buttons on the stimulator!
- Count the number of twitches the client had out of four (0/4, 1/4, 2/4, 3/4, 4/4.) Adjust the medication as ordered. Goal is 1/4 to 2/4 twitches.

4. Perform frequent neurovascular assessments. Prolonged use of neuromuscular blocking agents may cause profound weakness and paralysis; may precipitate an acute myopathy.

5. Monitor VS frequently and pulmonary status continuously. Cardiac monitor and ventilator alarms should be set and checked frequently. Observe for excessive bronchial secretions or respiratory wheezing; suction to maintain patent airway.

6. Consciousness and pain thresholds are not affected by neuromuscular blocking agents; clients can still hear, feel, and see while receiving these agents. Avoid discussions that should not be overheard. Explain all contacts, injections, therapies, and procedures. Adequate anxiolytic therapy and analgesics should be administered for pain and/or fear with procedures and situation requiring this therapy.

7. Clients requiring prolonged ventilatory therapy should be adequately sedated with analgesics and benzodiazepines. Anxiety levels may be very high, but client cannot communicate this. Observe for drug interactions which may potentiate muscular relaxation and prove fatal.

8. Administer eye drops and patches to protect corneas during prolonged therapy; explain why this is done (i.e., blink reflex suppressed). Avoid corticosteroids during prolonged neuromuscular blockade unless benefits far outweigh the risks.

9. Perform passive range of motion to prevent loss of function and contractures with prolonged therapy. Assess skin condition and turn frequently to prevent prolonged pressure on any one area as client unable to feel so unable to communicate discomfort.

Bold Italic = life threatening side effect   ■ = black box warning   ✦ = Available in Canada

Classifications

CLIENT/FAMILY TEACHING

1. Drug is used to paralyze so that procedures or controlled ventilation can occur.

2. Will be constantly monitored and cared for. Medication will be administered for pain and anxiety as needed.

3. Client will regain the ability to move and talk once therapy is discontinued.

OUTCOMES/EVALUATE

- Skeletal muscle paralysis (pharmacologic restraint)
- Insertion of ET tube/tolerance of mechanical ventilation.
- Suppression of twitch response
- ↓ Oxygen consumption

NONSTEROIDAL ANTI-INFLAMMATORY DRUGS

SEE ALSO THE FOLLOWING INDIVIDUAL ENTRIES:

Celecoxib
Diclofenac potassium
Diclofenac sodium
Diflunisal
Etodolac
Fenoprofen calcium
Flurbiprofen
Flurbiprofen sodium
Ibuprofen
Ibuprofen lysine
Indomethacin
Indomethacin sodium trihydrate
Ketoprofen
Ketorolac tromethamine
Meloxicam
Nabumetone
Naproxen
Naproxen sodium
Oxaprozin
Oxaprozin potassium
Piroxicam
Sulindac
Tolmetin sodium

USES

See individual drugs. **Systemic.** Uses include, but are not limited to: (1) Inflammatory disease, including rheumatoid arthritis, osteoarthritis, ankylosing spondylitis, gout, and other musculoskeletal diseases. (2) Nonrheumatic inflammatory conditions including bursitis, acute painful shoulder, synovitis, tendinitis, or tenosynovitis. (3) Mild to moderate pain including primary dysmenorrhea, episiotomy pain, strains and sprains, post extraction dental pain. (4) Primary dysmenorrhea. **Ophthalmic.** (1) Ophthalmically to inhibit intraoperative miosis. (2) Postoperative inflammation after cataract surgery. (3) Ocular itching due to seasonal allergic conjunctivitis. *Investigational:* Reduce risk of prostate cancer. Reduce risk of Alzheimer's disease (high doses).

ACTION/KINETICS

Action

The anti-inflammatory effect is likely due to inhibition of the enzyme cyclooxygenase (COX). There are two COX isoenzymes—COX-1 and COX-2. Depending on the NSAID, either COX-1 or COX-2 or both enzymes may be inhibited. Inhibition of cyclooxygenase results in decreased prostaglandin synthesis. Effective in reducing joint swelling, pain, and morning stiffness, as well as in increasing mobility in individuals with inflammatory disease. They do not alter the course of the disease, however. Their anti-inflammatory activity is comparable to that of aspirin. The analgesic activity is due, in part, to relief of inflammation. Other mechanisms that contribute to the anti-inflammatory effect include reduction of superoxide radicals, induction of apoptosis, inhibition of adhesion molecule expression, decrease of nitric oxide synthase, decrease of proinflammatory cytokine levels, modification of lymphocyte activity, and alteration of cellular membrane functions. Rheumatoid factor production may also be inhibited. The antipyretic action occurs by decreasing prostaglandin synthesis in the hypothalamus, resulting in an increase in peripheral blood flow and heat loss as well as promoting sweating. NSAIDs also inhibit miosis induced by prostaglandins during the course of cataract surgery; thus, these drugs are useful for a number of ophthalmic inflammatory conditions.

Pharmacokinetics

The NSAIDs differ from one another with respect to their rate of absorption, length of action, anti-inflammatory activity, and effect on the GI mucosa. Most are rapidly and completely absorbed from the GI tract; food delays the rate, but not the total amount, of drug absorbed. These drugs are metabolized in the kidney and are excreted through the urine, mainly as metabolites.

CONTRAINDICATIONS

Most for children under 14 years of age. Lactation. Individuals in whom aspirin, NSAIDs, or iodides have caused hypersensitivity, including acute asthma, rhinitis, urticaria, nasal polyps, bronchospasm, angioedema or other symptoms of allergy or anaphylaxis. Use in hepatic porphyria.

SPECIAL CONCERNS

Clients intolerant to one of the NSAIDs may be intolerant to others in this group. Use with caution in clients with a history of GI disease, reduced renal function, in geriatric clients, in clients with intrinsic coagulation defects or those on anticoagulant therapy, in compromised cardiac function, in hypertension, in conditions predisposing to fluid retention, and in the presence of existing controlled infection. The risk of hospitalization is doubled in geriatric clients taking NSAIDs and diuretics. Regular use of NSAIDs may hamper aspirin's prevention of first heart attacks; the risk of MI may be increased in new and current users of NSAIDs. The safety and efficacy of most NSAIDs have not been determined in children or in functional class IV rheumatoid arthritis (i.e., clients incapacitated, bedridden, or confined to a wheelchair). Use during pregnancy increases the risk of pulmonary hypertension in newborns. Products must carry a warning about the possibility of stomach bleeding in clients who consume three or more alcoholic drinks per day.

There is the potential for stomach bleeding in the following groups: Persons over age 60, those who have had prior ulcers or bleeding, persons who take a blood thinner, those taking more than one product containing an NSAID, and those taking a NSAID longer than prescribed.

SIDE EFFECTS

GI (most common): Peptic or duodenal ulceration and GI bleeding, intestinal ulceration with obstruction and stenosis, reactivation of preexisting ulcers. Heartburn, dyspepsia, N&V, anorexia, diarrhea, constipation, increased or decreased appetite, indigestion, stomatitis, epigastric pain, abdominal cramps or pain, gastroenteritis, paralytic ileus, salivation, dry mouth, glossitis, pyrosis, icterus, rectal irritation, gingival ulcer, occult blood in stool, hematemesis, gastritis, proctitis, eructation, sore or dry mucous membranes, ulcerative colitis, rectal bleeding, melena, *perforation and hemorrhage of esophagus, stomach, duodenum, small or large intestine.* **CNS:** Dizziness, drowsiness, vertigo, headaches, nervousness, migraine, anxiety, mental confusion, aggravation of parkinsonism and epilepsy, lightheadedness, paresthesia, peripheral neuropathy, akathisia, excitation, tremor, *seizures*, myalgia, asthenia, malaise, insomnia, fatigue, drowsiness, confusion, emotional lability, depression, inability to concentrate, psychoses, hallucinations, depersonalization, amnesia, *coma*, syncope, aseptic meningitis. **CV:** CHF, hypo-/hypertension, arrhythmias, peripheral edema and fluid retention, vasodilation, exacerbation of angiitis, palpitations, tachycardia, chest pain, sinus bradycardia, peripheral vascular disease, peripheral edema. **Respiratory:** *Bronchospasm, laryngeal edema*, rhinitis, dyspnea, pharyngitis, hemoptysis, SOB, eosinophilic pneumonitis. **Hematologic:** Bone marrow depression, neutropenia, leukopenia, pancytopenia, eosinophila, thrombocytopenia, granulocytopenia, *agranulocytosis, aplastic anemia, hemolytic anemia,* decreased H&H, anemia, hypocoagulability, epistaxis. **Ophthalmic:** Amblyopia, visual disturbances, corneal deposits, retinal hemorrhage, scotomata, retinal pigmentation changes or degeneration, blurred vision, photophobia, diplopia, iritis, loss of color vision (reversible), optic neuritis, cataracts, swollen, dry, or irritated eyes. **Dermatologic:** Pruritus, skin eruptions, sweating, erythema, eczema, hyperpigmentation, ecchymoses, petechiae, rashes, urticaria, purpura, onycholysis, vesiculobullous eruptions, cutaneous vasculitis, *toxic epidermal necrolysis, angioneurotic edema,* erythema nodosum, *Stevens-Johnson syndrome,* exfoliative dermatitis, photosensitivity, alopecia, skin irritation, peeling, erythema multiforme, desquamation, skin discoloration. **GU:** Menometrorrhagia, menorrhagia, impotence, menstrual disorders, hematuria, cystitis, azotemia, nocturia, proteinuria, UTIs, polyuria, dysuria, urinary frequency, oliguria, pyuria, anuria, renal insufficiency, nephrosis, nephrotic syndrome, glomerular/interstitial nephritis, urinary casts, acute renal failure in clients with impaired renal function, renal papillary necrosis. **Metabolic:** Hyper-/hypoglycemia, glycosuria, hyperkalemia, hyponatremia, diabetes mellitus. **Other:** Tinnitus, hearing loss/disturbances, ear pain, deafness, metallic or bitter taste in mouth, thirst, chills, fever, flushing, jaundice, sweating, breast changes, gynecomastia, muscle cramps, dyspnea, involuntary muscle movements, muscle weakness, facial edema, pain, serum sickness, aseptic meningitis, hypersensitivity reactions including asthma, acute respiratory distress, *shock-like syndrome, angioedema,* angiitis, dyspnea, *anaphylaxis.*

Following ophthalmic use: Transient burning and stinging upon installation, ocular irritation.

OD OVERDOSE MANAGEMENT
Symptoms: CNS symptoms include dizziness, drowsiness, mental confusion, lethargy, disorientation, intense headache, paresthesia, and *seizures.* GI symptoms include N&V, gastric irritation, and abdominal pain. Miscellaneous symptoms include tinnitus, sweating, blurred vision, increased serum creatinine and BUN, and acute renal failure.
Treatment: There are no antidotes; treatment includes general supportive

measures. Since the drugs are acidic, it may be beneficial to alkalinize the urine and induce diuresis to hasten excretion.

DRUG INTERACTIONS
ACE inhibitors / Possible ↓ antihypertensive effect of ACE inhibitors
Acetaminophen / ↑ Risk of hypertension in women
Aminoglycosides / ↑ Aminoglycoside levels in premature infants due to ↓ glomerular filtration rate
Anticoagulants / Concomitant use results in ↑ PT
Aspirin / ↓ Effect of NSAIDs R/T ↓ blood levels; also, ↑ risk of adverse GI effects
Beta-adrenergic blocking agents / ↓ Antihypertensive effects R/T NSAID inhibition of prostaglandin synthesis, thus allowing unopposed pressor systems to potentiate hypertension
Bisphosphonates / ↑ Risk of gastric ulceration
Cholestyramine / ↓ GI absorption of NSAIDs → ↓ effect
Cimetidine / ↑ or ↓ Plasma levels of NSAIDs
Cyclosporine / ↑ Risk of nephrotoxicity of both drugs
Diuretics / ↓ Diuretic effects
H *Gingko biloba* / Additive effect on platelet aggregation → ↑ risk of bleeding
H *Ginseng* / Avoid concomitant use or monitor carefully
Lithium / ↑ Serum lithium levels
Loop diuretics / ↓ Drug effects
Methotrexate / ↑ Risk of methotrexate toxicity (i.e., bone marrow suppression, nephrotoxicity, stomatitis)
Phenobarbital / ↓ Effect of NSAIDs R/T ↑ liver breakdown
Phenytoin / ↑ Phenytoin pharmacologic and toxic effects R/T ↓ plasma protein binding
Probenecid / ↑ Levels and possibly toxicity of NSAIDs
Salicylates / Plasma levels of NSAIDs may be ↓ ; also, ↑ risk of GI side effects
SSRIs / ↑ Risk of significant GI side effects; do not use together
Sulfonamides / ↑ Drug effects R/T ↓ plasma protein binding
Sulfonylureas / ↑ Drug effects R/T ↓

Classifications

plasma protein binding
Warfarin / ↑ Risk of upper GI hemorrhage.

DOSAGE

See individual drugs.

NURSING CONSIDERATIONS

ADMINISTRATION/STORAGE

1. Do not take alcohol or aspirin together with NSAIDs. If GI upset occurs, take with food, milk, or antacids.
2. NSAIDs may have an additive analgesic effect when administered with narcotic analgesics, thus permitting lower narcotic dosages.
3. Clients who do not respond clinically to one NSAID may respond to another.

ASSESSMENT

1. Note reasons for therapy, onset, location, intensity, characteristics, and type of pain/swelling experienced. Rate pain level. Assess joint mobility/stability and ROM. Note other agents trialed and outcome.
2. Review indications and dosage prescribed. For anti-inflammatory effects, high doses are required whereas analgesia and pain relief may be achieved with much lower dosages. Metastatic bone pain responds effectively to NSAIDs but not as well to opioids.
3. Note allergic responses to aspirin or other anti-inflammatory agents. Asthma or nasal polyps may be exacerbated by NSAIDs. Children under age 14 generally should not receive drugs in this category.
4. Monitor CBC, renal and LFTs; reduce dose with renal dysfunction. These drugs cause platelet inhibition which is reversible in 24–48 hr, whereas aspirin requires 4–5 days to reverse antiplatelet effects. COX-1 NSAIDs may inhibit the cardioprotective effects of aspirin. Separate dosing intervals.

INTERVENTIONS

1. Explain that the major effect of all NSAIDs is to decrease the synthesis of prostaglandins. This is achieved by reversibly inhibiting cyclooxygenase (COX), an enzyme which catalyzes the formation of prostaglandins and thromboxanes from arachidonic acid (the precursor). This is in contrast to salicylates, which irreversibly bind to COX and inhibit production for the entire life of the cell. Prostaglandins enhance the inflammatory response and renal blood flow, and offer cytoprotection of GI mucosa.
2. Make sure that client understands importance of not self medicating or taking other agents in this class of drug at the same time without provider approval.
3. Monitor VS, H&H, stool for Occult blood.

CLIENT/FAMILY TEACHING

1. Take NSAIDs with a full glass of water or milk, with meals, or with a prescribed antacid and remain upright 30 min following administration to reduce gastric irritation or ulcer formation. Regular intake of drug needed to sustain anti-inflammatory effects. If not obtained, another NSAID may provide desired response.
2. Consume 2–3 L/day of water. Report any changes in stool consistency or symptoms of GI irritation. Sustained GI effects may require stomach protectant.
3. Use caution in operating machinery or in driving a car; may cause dizziness or drowsiness.
4. Avoid alcohol, aspirin, and any other OTC preparations; may cause GI bleeding. Report any episodes of bleeding, eye symptoms, ringing in ears, skin rashes, bruising, weight gain, swelling of limbs, decreased urine output, fever, or increased joint pain.
5. Record weights periodically and report any significant changes. NSAIDs cause sodium and water retention; avoid with CHF.
6. Diabetics need to be aware of the lowered blood sugar effect of NSAIDs on hypoglycemic agents. Dosage adjustments may be required.
7. Notify all providers of medications being taken to avoid unfavorable drug interactions.
8. Keep all F/U appointments to evaluate response to therapy, for any adverse side effects and/or lack of desired response.

OUTCOMES/EVALUATE

- ↑ Joint mobility and ROM
- ↓ Discomfort/pain and swelling

Bold Italic = life threatening side effect   ■ = black box warning   ✤ = Available in Canada

- Improvement in S&S
- Improved pain scores

ORAL CONTRACEPTIVES: ■ ESTROGEN-PROGESTERONE COMBINATIONS

SEE TABLE 2.

GENERAL STATEMENT

There are three types of combination (i.e., both an estrogen and progestin in each tablet) oral contraceptives: (1) monophasic—contain the same amount of estrogen and progestin in each tablet; (2) biphasic—usually contain the same amount of estrogen in each tablet but the progestin content is lower for the first part of the cycle and higher for the last part of the cycle; (3) triphasic—the estrogen content may be the same or may vary throughout the medication cycle; the progestin content may be the same or varies, depending on the part of the cycle. The purpose of the biphasic and triphasic products is to provide hormones in a manner similar to that occurring physiologically. This is said to decrease breakthrough bleeding during the medication cycle. The other type of oral contraceptive is the progestin-only ("mini-pill") product, which contains a small amount of a progestin in each tablet.

Also available are emergency contraceptive kits (Plan B or Preven) containing just four tablets of ethinyl estradiol and levonorgestrel (Preven) or just two tablets of levonorgestrel (Plan B). These products are intended to be used after unprotected intercourse or known or suspected contraceptive failure.

USES

(1) Prevention of pregnancy. (2) Prevent pregnancy after unprotected intercourse or a known or suspected contraceptive failure (Plan B and Preven only). (3) Moderate acne vulgaris in females aged 15 and older who have no contraindications to oral contraceptive therapy, have reached menarche, desire contraception, and who are unrespon-sive to topical antiacne drugs (Estrostep and Ortho Tri-Cyclen only).

ACTION/KINETICS

Combination oral contraceptives. Act by inhibiting ovulation due to an inhibition (through negative-feedback mechanism) of LH and FSH, which are required for development of ova. These products also alter the cervical mucus so that it is not conducive to sperm penetration and render the endometrium less suitable for implantation of the blastocyst should fertilization occur. The estrogen used in combination oral contraceptives is either ethinyl estradiol or mestranol. Ethinyl estradiol is rapidly absorbed; **peak levels:** 2 hr. Mestranol is demethylated to ethinyl estradiol in the liver. **t ½:** 6–20 hr. Several different progestins are used in combination oral contraceptives: Desogestrel, drospire-none, ethynodiol diacetate, levonorgestrel, norethindrone, norethindrone acetate, norgestimate, or norgestrel. Terminal t ½'s for progestins vary over a wide range.

Progestin-only oral contraceptives. These products inhibit ovulation in about 50% of users. However, these products also alter the cervical mucus, render the endometrium unsuitable for implantation, lower midcycle LH and FSH peaks, and slow the movement of the ovum through the fallopian tubes. These products contain either norethindrone or norgestrel. This method of contraception is less reliable than combination therapy.

NOTE: Although oral contraceptives may be associated with serious side effects, a number of noncontraceptive health benefits have been confirmed. These include increased regularity of the menstrual cycle, decreased incidence of dysmenorrhea, decreased blood loss, decreased incidence of functional ovarian cysts and ectopic pregnancies, and decreased incidence of diseases such as fibroadenomas, fibrocystic disease, acute pelvic inflammatory disease, endometrial cancer, and ovarian cancer. OC use has also been

Classifications

Table 2 Hormone Contraceptive Preparations Available in the United States

TRADE NAME	ESTROGEN	MONOPHASIC	PROGESTIN
Alesse (28-Day)	Ethinyl estradiol (20 mcg)		Levonorgestrel (0.1 mg)
Apri (28-Day)	Ethinyl estradiol (30 mcg)		Desogestrel (0.15 mg)
Aviane (28-Day)	Ethinyl estradiol (20 mcg)		Levonorgestrel (0.1 mg)
Balziva (28-Day)	Ethinyl estadiol (35 mcg)		Norethindrone (0.4 mg)
Brevicon (28-Day)	Ethinyl estradiol (35 mcg)		Norethindrone (0.5 mg)
Cryselle (21- and 28-Day)	Ethinyl estradiol (30 mcg)		Norgestrel (0.3 mg)
Demulen 1/35 (21- and 28-Day)	Ethinyl estradiol (50 mcg)		Ethynodiol diacetate (1 mg)
Desogen (28 Day)	Ethinyl estradiol (30 mcg)		Desogestrel (0.15 mg)
Femcon Fe (28-Day) Chewable Tablets	Ethinyl estadiol (35 mcg)		Norethindrone (0.4 mg)
Jolessa (1 hormone-containing tablet/day for 84 days followed by one inert tablet/day for 7 days)	Ethinyl estadiol (30 mcg)		Levonorgestrel (0.15 mg)
Junel 21 Day 1/20	Ethinyl estradiol (20 mcg)		Norethindrone acetate (1 mg)
Junel 21 Day 1.5/30	Ethinyl estradiol (30 mcg)		Norethindrone acetate (1.5 mg)
Junel Fe 1/20 (28-Day)	Ethinyl estradiol (20 mcg)		Norethindrone (1 mg)
Junel Fe 1.5/30 (28-Day)	Ethinyl estradiol (30 mcg)		Norethindrone (1.5 mg)
Kariva*	Ethinyl estradiol (20 mcg and 10 mcg)		Desogestrel (0.15 mg)
Kelnor 1/35	Ethinyl estradiol (35 mcg)		Ethynodiol diacetate (1 mg)
Lessina (21- and 28-Day)	Ethinyl estradiol (20 mcg)		Levonorgestrel (0.1 mg)
Levlen (28-Day)	Ethinyl estradiol (30 mcg)		Levonorgestrel (0.15 mg)
Levlite (28-Day)	Ethinyl estradiol (20 mcg)		Levonorgestrel (0.1 mg)
Levora 0.15/30 (28-Day)	Ethinyl estradiol (30 mcg)		Levonorgestrel (0.15 mg)
Loestrin 21 1/20	Ethinyl estradiol (20 mcg)		Norethindrone acetate (1 mg)
Loestrin 21 1.5/30	Ethinyl estradiol (30 mcg)		Norethindrone acetate (1.5 mg)
Loestrin 24 Fe (28-Day: four iron-containing tablets)	Ethinyl estradiol (20 mcg)		Norethindrone acetate (1 mg)
Loestrin Fe 1/20 (28 Day)	Ethinyl estradiol (20 mcg)		Norethindrone acetate (1 mg)

Bold Italic = life threatening side effect   ■ = black box warning   ♣ = Available in Canada

TRADE NAME	ESTROGEN	PROGESTIN
	MONOPHASIC	
Loestrin Fe 1.5/30 (28 Day)	Ethinyl estradiol (30 mcg)	Norethindrone acetate (1.5 mg)
Lo/Ovral (21- and 28-Day)	Ethinyl estradiol (30 mcg)	Norgestrel (0.3 mg)
Low-Ogestrel (28-Day)	Ethinyl estradiol (20 mcg)	Norgestrel (0.3 mg)
Lutera (28-Day)	Ethinyl estradiol (20 mcg)	Levonorgestrel (0.1 mg)
Lybrel (28 tablets/pack; 1 hormone-containing tablet everyday without any tablet-free interval)	Ethinyl estadiol (20 mcg)	Levonorgestrel (90 mcg)
Microgestin Fe 1/20 (28-Day)	Ethinyl estradiol (20 mcg)	Norethindrone acetate (1 mg)
Microgestin Fe 1.5/30 (28-Day)	Ethinyl estradiol (30 mcg)	Norethindrone acetate (1.5 mg)
Mircette*	Ethinyl estradiol (20 mcg and 10 mcg)	Desogestrel (0.15 mg)
Modicon (28-Day)	Ethinyl estradiol (35 mcg)	Norethindrone (0.5 mg)
MonoNessa (28 Day)	Ethinyl estradiol (35 mcg)	Norgestimate (0.25 mg)
Necon 0.5/35 (21- and 28-Day)	Ethinyl estradiol (35 mcg)	Norethindrone (0.5 mg)
Necon 1/35 (21- and 28-Day)	Ethinyl estradiol (35 mcg)	Norethindrone (1 mg)
Necon 1/50 (21- and 28-Day)	Mestranol (50 mcg)	Norethindrone (1 mg)
Nordette (21- and 28-Day)	Ethinyl estradiol (30 mcg)	Levonorgestrel (0.15 mg)
Norinyl 1 + 35 (21- and 28-Day)	Ethinyl estradiol (35 mcg)	Norethindrone (1 mg)
Norinyl 1 + 50 (28-Day)	Mestranol (50 mcg)	Norethindrone (1 mg)
Nortrel 0.5/35 (21- and 28-Day)	Ethinyl estradiol (35 mcg)	Norethindrone (0.5 mg)
Nortrel 1/35 (21- and 28-Day)	Ethinyl estradiol (35 mcg)	Norethindrone (1 mg)
Ogestrel 0.5/50 (28-Day)	Ethinyl estradiol (50 mcg)	Norgestrel (0.5 mg)
Ortho-Cept (21- and 28-Day)	Ethinyl estradiol (30 mcg)	Desogestrel (0.15 mg)
Ortho-Cyclen (28-Day)	Ethinyl estradiol (35 mcg)	Norgestimate (0.25 mg)
Ortho-Novum 1/35 (28-Day)	Ethinyl estradiol (35 mcg)	Norethindrone (1 mg)
Ortho Novum 1/50 (28-Day)	Mestranol (50 mcg)	Norethindrone (1 mg)
Ovcon 25 Fe (21-Day) Chewable Tablets	Ethinyl estadiol (35 mcg)	Norethindrone (0.4 mg)
Ovcon-50 (28-Day)	Ethinyl estradiol (50 mcg)	Norethindrone (1 mg)
Ovral (23- and 28-Day)	Ethinyl estradiol (50 mcg)	Norgestrel (0.5 mg)
Portia (21- and 28-Day)	Ethinyl estradiol (30 mcg)	Levonorgestrel (0.15 mg)

📷 = see color insert   H = Herbal   IV = Intravenous   ℗ = sound alike drug

TRADE NAME	ESTROGEN	PROGESTIN
	MONOPHASIC	
Quasense (1 hormone-containing tablet/day for 84 days followed by one inert tablet/day for 7 days)	Ethinyl estradiol (30 mcg)	Levonorgestrel (0.15 mg)
Reclipsen (28-Day)	Ethinyl estradiol (30 mcg)	Desogestrel (0.15 mg)
Seasonale*	Ethinyl estradiol (30 mcg)	Levonorgestrel (0.15 mg)
Seasonique*	Ethinyl estradiol (30 mcg—in 84 tablets and 10 mcg in 7 tablets	Levonorgestrel (0.15 mg—in 84 tablets
Solia (28-Day)	Ethinyl estradiol (30 mcg)	Desogestrel (0.15 mg)
Sprintec (28 Day)	Ethinyl estradiol (35 mcg)	Norgestimate (0.25 mg)
Sronyx (28-Day)	Ethinyl estradiol (20 mcg)	Levonorgestrel (0.1 mg)
Yasmin (28-Day)	Ethinyl estradiol (30 mcg)	Drospirenone (3 mg)
Zenchent (28-Day)	Ethinyl estradiol (35 mcg)	Norethindrone (0.4 mg)
Zovia 1/35 (21- and 28-Day)	Ethinyl estradiol (35 mcg)	Ethynodiol diacetate (1 mg)
Zovia 1/50 (21- and 28-Day)	Ethinyl estradiol (50 mcg)	Ethynodiol diacetate (1 mg)
	BIPHASIC	
Necon 10/11 (28-Day)	Ethinyl estradiol (35 mcg in each tablet)	Norethindrone (10 tablets of 0.5 mg followed by 11 tablets of 1 mg)
Ortho-Novum 10/11 (28-Day)	Ethinyl estradiol (35 mcg in each tablet)	Norethindrone (10 tablets of 0.5 mg followed by 11 tablets of 1 mg)
	TRIPHASIC	
Aranelle (28-Day)	Ethinyl estradiol (35 mcg in each tablet for 21 tablets)	Norethindrone (0.5 mg the first 7 days, 1 mg the next 9 days, and 0.5 mg the last 5 days)
Cesia (28-Day)	Ethinyl estradiol (25 mcg in each tablet for 21 days)	Desogestrel (0.1 mg the first 7 days, 0.125 mg the next 7 days, and 0.15 the last 7 days)
Cyclessa (28-Day)	Ethinyl estradiol (25 mcg in each tablet for 21 days)	Desogestrel (0.1 mg the first 7 days, 0.125 mg the next 7 days, and 0.15 mg the last 7 days)

Bold Italic = life threatening side effect   ▪ = black box warning   ♣ = Available in Canada

TRADE NAME	ESTROGEN	PROGESTIN
	MONOPHASIC	
Enpresse (28-Day)	Ethinyl estradiol (30 mcg the first 6 days, 40 mcg the next 5 days, and 30 mcg the last 10 days)	Levonorgestrel (0.05 mg the first 6 days, 0.075 mg the next 5 days, and 0.125 mg the last 10 days)
Estrostep 21 (21-Day) and Estrostep Fe (28-Day)	Ethinyl estradiol (20 mcg the first 5 days, 30 mcg the next 7 days, and 35 mcg the last 9 days)	Norethindrone (1 mg in each tablet)
Leena (28-Day)	Ethinyl estradiol (35 mcg in each tablet for 21 days)	Norethindrone (0.5 mg the first 7 days, 1 mg the next 9 days, and 0.5 mg the last 5 days)
Necon 7/7/7 (28-Day)	Ethinyl estradiol (35 mcg in each tablet)	Norethindrone (0.5 mg the first 7 days, 0.75 mg the next 7 days, and 1 mg the last 7 days)
Ortho-Novum 7/7/7 (28-Day)	Ethinyl estradiol (35 mcg in each tablet)	Norethindrone (0.5 mg the first 7 days, 0.75 mg the next 7 days, and 1 mg the last 7 days)
Ortho Tri-Cyclen (28-Day)	Ethinyl estradiol (35 mcg in each tablet)	Norgestimate (0.18 mg the first 7 days, 0.215 mg the next 7 days, and 0.25 mg the last 7 days)
Ortho Tri-Cyclen Lo (28-Day)	Ethinyl estradiol (25 mcg in each tablet)	Norgestimate (0.18 mg the first 7 days, 0.215 mg the next 7 days, and 0.25 mg the last 7 days)

TRADE NAME	ESTROGEN	PROGESTIN
	TRIPHASIC	
Tri-Levlen (28-Day)	Ethinyl estradiol (30 mcg the first 6 days, 40 mcg the next 5 days, and 30 mcg the last 10 days)	Levonorgestrel (0.05 mg the first 6 days, 0.075 mg the next 5 days, and 0.125 mg the last 10 days)
TriNessa (28-Day)	Ethinyl estradiol (35 mcg in each tablet)	Norgestimate (0.18 mg the first 7 days, 0.215 mg the next 7 days, and 0.25 mg the last 7 days)
Tri-Norinyl (28-Day)	Ethinyl estradiol (35 mcg in each tablet)	Norethindrone (0.5 mg the first 7 days, 1 mg the next 9 days, and 0.5 mg the last 5 days)
Triphasil (21- and 28-Day)	Ethinyl estradiol (30 mcg the first 6 days, 40 mcg the next 5 days, and 30 mcg the last 10 days)	Levonorgestrel (0.05 mg the first 6 days, 0.075 mg the next 5 days, and 0.125 mg the last 10 days)

= see color insert   H = Herbal   IV = Intravenous   = sound alike drug

TRADE NAME	ESTROGEN	PROGESTIN
		TRIPHASIC
Tri-Previfem (28-day)	Ethinyl estradiol (35 mcg in each tablet for 21 days)	Norgestimate (0.18 mg the first 7 days, 0.215 mg the next 7 days, and 0.25 mg the last 7 days)
Tri-Sprintec (28-Day)	Ethinyl estradiol (35 mcg in each tablet)	Norgestimate (0.18 mg the first 7 days, 0.215 mg the next 7 days, and 0.25 mg the last 7 days)
Trivora (28-Day)	Ethinyl estradiol (30 mcg the first 6 days, 40 mcg the next 5 days, and 30 mcg the last 10 days	Levonorgestrel (0.05 mg the first 6 days, 0.075 mg the next 5 days, and 0.125 mg the last 10 days)
Velivet (28-Day)	Ethinyl estradiol (25 mcg in each tablet)	Desogestrel (0.1 mg the first 7 days, 0.125 mg the next 7 days, and 0.15 mg the last 7 days)
		CONTRACEPTIVE PATCH
ClimaraPro	Estradiol (45 mcg)	Levonorgestrel (0.015 mg)
		PROGESTIN-ONLY PRODUCTS**
Camila	Norethindrone (0.35 mg)	Norethindrone (0.35 mg)
Errin		Norethindrone (0.35 mg)
Nora-BE		Norethindrone (0.35 mg)
Ortho-Micronor		Norgestrel (0.075 mg)
Ovrette		
		EMERGENCY CONTRACEPTIVES
Plan B	No estrogen	Levonorgestrel (0.75 mg)
A total of 2 tablets containing levonorgestrel		

NOTE: Plan B is OTC for those 18 years and older but Rx for those younger than 18 years of age.

Bold Italic = life threatening side effect   ■ = black box warning   ✚ = Available in Canada

TRADE NAME	ESTROGEN	PROGESTIN
TRIPHASIC		
Preven A total of 4 tablets containing the hormones listed	Ethinyl estradiol (50 mcg)	Levonorgestrel (0.25 mg)

*See Administration for special dosage/administration information.
**All progestin-only products contain 28 tablets/pack.
***28-Day products either 7 inert tablet or 7 iron-containing tablets.

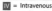

📷 = see color insert   Ⓗ = Herbal   Ⅳ = Intravenous   ⓒ = sound alike drug associated with a reduction in colorectal cancer and positive effects on bone mineral density.

CONTRAINDICATIONS

Thrombophlebitis, history of deep-vein thrombophlebitis, thromboembolic disorders, cerebral vascular disease, CAD, MI, current or past angina, known or suspected breast cancer or estrogen-dependent neoplasm, endometrial carcinoma, hepatic adenoma or carcinoma, undiagnosed abnormal genital bleeding, known or suspected pregnancy, cholestatic jaundice of pregnancy, jaundice with prior tablet use, acute liver disease. Smoking. Lactation.

NOTE: Yasmin may cause hyperkalemia in high-risk clients. Do not use in clients with conditions that predispose to hyperkalemia (e.g., renal insufficiency, hepatic dysfunction, adrenal insufficiency).

SPECIAL CONCERNS

■Cigarette smoking increases the risk of cardiovascular side effects from use of oral contraceptives. This risk increases with age and with heavy smoking (15 or more cigarettes per day) and is marked in women over 35 years of age. Women who use OCs should not smoke.■ There is an increased risk of thromboembolism, stroke, MI, hypertension, hepatic neoplasia, and gallbladder disease. The risk of CV and circulatory disease in OC users is significantly increased in women 35 years and older with other risk factors (e.g., smoking, uncontrolled hypertension, hypercholesterolemia, obesity, diabetes).

Use with caution in clients with a history of hypertension, preexisting renal disease, hypertension-related diseases during pregnancy, familial tendency to hypertension or its consequences, a history of excessive weight gain or fluid retention during the menstrual cycle; these individuals are more likely to develop elevated BP. Use with caution in clients with asthma, epilepsy, migraine, diabetes, metabolic bone disease, renal or cardiac disease, and a history of mental depression. Use with drugs (e.g., barbiturates, hydantoins, rifampin) that increase the hepatic metabolism of oral contraceptives may result in breakthrough bleeding and an increased risk of pregnancy. The risk of becoming pregnant may be increased in overweight women.

Progestin-only products do not appear to have any adverse effects on breastfeeding performance or on the health, growth, or development of the infant.

SIDE EFFECTS

The oral contraceptives have wide-ranging side effects. These are particularly important, since the drugs may be given for several years to healthy women. Many authorities have voiced concern about the long-term safety of these agents. Some advise discontinuing therapy after 18–24 months of continuous use. The majority of side effects of oral contraceptives are due to the estrogen component. **CV:** *Mesenteric thrombosis, MI, thrombophlebitis, venous thrombosis with* or *without embolism, pulmonary embolism, coronary thrombosis, cerebral thrombosis, arterial thromboembolism, mesenteric thrombosis, thrombotic* and *hemorrhagic strokes, postsurgical thromboembolism, subarachnoid hemorrhage, cerebral hemorrhage,* elevated BP, hypertension. **CNS:** Onset or exacerbation of migraine headaches, depression, headaches, dizziness. **GI:** N&V, bloating, diarrhea, abdominal cramps. **Ophthalmic:** Optic neuritis, retinal thrombosis, steepening of the corneal curvature, contact lens intolerance. **Hepatic:** *Benign and malignant hepatic adenomas,* focal nodular hyperplasia, *hepatocellular carcinoma,* gallbladder disease, cholestatic jaundice. **GU:** Breakthrough bleeding, spotting, amenorrhea during and after treatment, change in menstrual flow, change in cervical erosion and cervical secretions, *invasive cervical cancer,* bleeding irregularities (more common with progestin-only products), vaginal candidiasis, *ectopic pregnancies in contraceptive failures, increase in size of pre-existing uterine fibroids,* temporary infertility after discontinuation, breast tenderness, breast enlargement, breast secretion. **Dermatologic:**

Bold Italic = life threatening side effect   ■ = black box warning   ✦ = Available in Canada

Melasma (may persist), allergic rash, hirsutism (rare). **Miscellaneous:** Acute intermittent porphyria, photosensitivity, congenital anomalies, melasma, edema, increase or decrease in weight, decreased carbohydrate tolerance, increased incidence of cervical *Chlamydia trachomatis*, decrease in the quantity and quality of breast milk.

DRUG INTERACTIONS

Acetaminophen / ↓ Effect of acetaminophen R/T ↑ liver metabolism

Acitretin / Acitretin interferes with effect of progestin-only products

Anticoagulants, oral / ↓ Effect of anticoagulants by ↓ levels of certain clotting factors (however, an ↑ effect of anticoagulants has also been noted in some clients)

Antidepressants, tricyclic / ↑ Effect of antidepressants R/T ↓ liver metabolism

Atorvastatin / ↑ AUC of steroid hormones

Barbiturates / ↓ OC effectiveness R/T ↑ liver metabolism

Benzodiazepines / ↑ Effect of alprazolam, chlordiazepoxide, diazepam, and triazolam R/T ↓ in liver breakdown; ↓ Effect of lorazepam, oxazepam, and temazepam R/T ↑ liver breakdown

Beta-adrenergic blockers / ↑ Effect of beta blockers R/T ↓ liver metabolism

H *Black cohosh* / Interferes with effect of oral contraceptives

Caffeine / ↑ Effect of caffeine R/T ↓ liver metabolism

Carbamazepine / ↓ Effect of OCs R/T ↑ liver metabolism

Corticosteroids / ↑ Effect of corticosteroids R/T ↓ liver metabolism

Cyclosporine / ↑ Risk of cyclosporine toxicity R/T ↓ liver metabolism

Dexamethasone ↓ Effect of OCs R/T ↑ liver metabolism

Ethosuximide / ↓ Effect of OCs R/T ↑ liver metabolism

Felbamate / ↓ Effect of OCs R/T ↑ liver metabolism

Griseofulvin / ↓ Effect of OCs R/T altered steroid gut metabolism; also, ↓ OC effectiveness R/T ↑ liver metabolism

Hydantoins / ↓ OC effectiveness R/T ↑ liver metabolism

Hypoglycemics / ↓ Effect of hypoglycemics R/T OC effect on carbohydrate metabolism

Insulin / OCs may ↑ insulin requirements

Lamotrigine / ↓ Lamotrigine plasma levels R/T ↑ liver metabolism

Modafinil / ↓ OC effectiveness R/T ↑ liver metabolism

Nevirapine / ↓ Effect of OCs R/T ↑ liver metabolism

Oxcarbazepine / ↓ OC effectiveness R/T ↑ liver metabolism

Penicillins, oral / ↓ Effect of OCs R/T altered steroid gut metabolism

Phenobarbital / ↓ Effect of OCs R/T ↑ liver metabolism

Phenytoin / ↓ Effect of OCs R/T ↑ liver metabolism

Primidone / ↓ Effect of OCs R/T ↑ liver metabolism

Protease inhibitors / ↓ Effect of OCs R/T ↑ liver metabolism

Pyridoxine / Comcomitant use may ↑ pyridoxine requirements

Rifabutin, Rifampin, Rifapentine / ↓ Effect of contraceptives R/T ↑ liver metabolism

Ritonavir / ↓ Effect of contraceptives R/T ↑ liver breakdown of ethinyl estradiol

H *Saw palmetto* / ↓ OCs effect R/T antiestrogenic activity

Selegeline / ↑ Selegeline plasma levels R/T ↓ metabolism

Smoking / Possible ↓ OC effectiveness R/T ↑ metabolism of hormones in OC's

H *St. John's wort* / ↑ Risk of breakthrough bleeding and contraceptive failure R/T ↑ liver metabolism of OC hormones

Tetracyclines / ↓ Effect of contraceptives R/T altered steroid gut metabolism

Theophyllines / ↑ Effect of theophyllines R/T ↓ liver breakdown

Troleandomycin / ↑ Chance of jaundice

Valproic acid / Possible ↑ seizure frequency R/T ↑ metabolism of valproic acid

Warfarin / ↑ Risk of clotting.

LABORATORY TEST CONSIDERATIONS

↑ Prothrombin, Factors VII, VIII, IX, X; fibrinogen; thyroid-binding globulin (causes ↑ total thyroid hormones as

---

🍶 = see color insert   H = Herbal   IV = Intravenous   @ = sound alike drug measured by PBI, T_4 by column or radio-immunoassay); corticosteroids; triglycerides and phospholipids; aldosterone; amylase; gamma-glutamyltranspeptidase; iron-binding capacity; sex hormone-binding globulins; transferrin; prolactin; renin activity; vitamin A.

↓ Antithrombin III; free T_3 resin uptake; response to metyrapone test; folate; glucose tolerance; albumin; cholinesterase; haptoglobin; tissue plasminogen activator; zinc, vitamin B_{12}; sex-hormone-binding globulin.

Progestin-only products ↓ thyroxine due to ↓ thyroid-binding globulin. Some progestins may ↑ LDL and ↓ HDL.

DOSAGE

- **TABLETS**

    Contraception.

See *Administration/Storage.* Use only low dose tablets; rarely is there a need for tablets containing more than 50 mcg of estrogen.

   Emergency contraception.

Take the initial 1 (Plan B) or 2 (Preven) tablets as soon as possible but within 72 hr of unprotected intercourse. A second dose of 1 (Plan B) or 2 (Preven) tablets is taken 12 hr later. Can be used any time during the menstrual cycle.

   Acne vulgaris.

Ortho Tri-Cyclen: Take 1 hormone-containing tablet daily for 21 days followed by 1 inert tablet daily for 7 days. After 28 tablets have been taken, a new course is started the next day.

NURSING CONSIDERATIONS

ADMINISTRATION/STORAGE

1. For combination oral contraceptive products:

- *Sunday start.* If the product is to be started on Sunday, the first tablet should be taken the Sunday following the beginning of menses; if menses begins on Sunday, the first tablet should be taken that day.
- *21-Day regimen.* Count the first day of menstrual bleeding as Day 1. Take 1 tablet per day for 21 days. No tablets are taken for 7 days. Whether menstrual flow has stopped or not, a new 21-day course of therapy is

started. This schedule is followed whether flow occurs as expected or whether spotting or breakthrough bleeding occurs during the cycle.

- *28-Day regimen.* To eliminate the necessity to count the days between cycles, many products contain 7 inert or iron-containing tablets. Hormone-containing tablets are taken for the first 21 days followed by 7 days of inert or iron-containing tablets, i.e., a tablet is taken every day of the year.
- *Biphasic and Triphasic products.* The biphasic and triphasic products have varying amounts of estrogen and/or progestin, depending on the stage of the cycle; the client should understand fully how these preparations are to be taken and which tablets are to be taken at various times during the medication cycle. Often tablets are different shapes and/or colors to help with compliance.

2. Certain combination oral contraceptive products consist of chewable tablets.

3. *Progestin-only products.* The first tablet is taken on the first day of menses; thereafter, 1 tablet is taken daily every day of the year with no interruption between tablet packs.

4. Ovcon 35 (norethindrone/ethinyl estradiol) is available as a chewable, oral, spearmint-flavored contraceptive tablet. The tablet may also be swallowed whole. If chewed, the woman should drink a full glass of water immediately after to ensure the full dose reaches the stomach.

5. Four of the monophasic oral contraceptive products are taken differently than other products. They are:

- Kariva or Mircette. Each product contains ethinyl estradiol and desogestrel. Take 1 20-mcg ethinyl estradiol/0.15 mg desogestrel tablet per day for 21 days followed by 1 inert tablet per day for 2 days and then 1 10-mcg ethinyl estradiol tablet per day for 5 days.
- Seasonale (ethinyl estradiol and levonorgestrel). Take 1 hormone-containing tablet per day for 84 days followed by 7 days of inert tablets (i.e., a

total of 91 days per cycle). Although women have menstrual periods only 4 times per year, there are more instances of unplanned bleeding and spotting between menstrual cycles, especially in the first few cycles of use.

- Seasonique is an extended-cycle oral contraceptive containing ethinyl estradiol (30 mcg) and levonorgestrol (0.15 mg) in the first 84 tablets and ethinyl estradiol (10 mcg) in the last 7 tablets. The 91-day cycle results in 4 menstrual periods per year (which occurs when the client is taking the 7 tablets containing 10 mcg ethinyl estradiol. Take the first tablet in a package on the first Sunday after the period begins, even if bleeding is still occurring. If the period starts on Sunday, take the first tablet that day. Another form of birth control should be used for the first 7 days after beginning Seasonique. Take one tablet every day at the same time, without interruption. After taking the last tablet containing 10 mcg ethinyl estradiol (white tablet), the client starts a new pack the very next day; no days are to be skipped.

6. Take tablets at approximately the same time each day.

7. Spotting or breakthrough bleeding may occur for the first 1–2 cycles; report if it continues past this time.

8. Side effects seen during the first few cycles may be transient. If they continue, dosage adjustment may be required as many of the side effects are related to the potency of the estrogen or progestin in the product.

9. For the initial cycle, use an **additional** form of contraception the first week.

10. For emergency contraception:

- Preven also contains a pregnancy test which can be used prior to taking the tablets. If a positive pregnancy test is obtained, the client is not to take the tablets in the kit.

- If vomiting occurs within 1 hr of taking either dose of the medication, the provider should be contacted to discuss whether or not to repeat the

dose or take an antinausea medication.

- Emergency contraception tablets are not to be used for ongoing pregnancy protection and are not to be used as a routine form of contraception by women.

11. If it is necessary to switch from combination therapy to progestin-only therapy, take the first progestin-only tablet the day after the last hormone-containing combination therapy tablet is finished. None of the 7 inactive tablets are to be taken. If switching from progestin-only to combination therapy, take the first hormone-containing combination therapy tablet on the first day of menses, even if the progestin-only pack is not finished. If switching to another brand of progestin-only products, start the new brand any time.

12. Non-nursing mothers may begin oral contraceptive therapy at the first postpartum exam (i.e., 4–6 weeks), regardless of whether spontaneous menstruation has occurred. Nursing mothers should not take oral contraceptives until the infant is weaned. Start no earlier than 4–6 weeks after a midtrimester pregnancy termination. Immediate postpartum use increases the risk of thromboembolism.

13. If the woman is fully breastfeeding (i.e., not giving the baby any food or formula), start the client on progestin-only products 6 weeks after delivery. If partially breastfeeding (giving the baby some food or formula), the client should start taking progestin-only products 3 weeks after delivery.

14. In the nonlactating mother, Seasonale may be started no earlier than day 28 postpartum because of the increased risk of thromboembolism. Advise the client to use a nonhormonal backup method for the first 7 days of tablet-taking. However, if intercourse has already occurred, consider the possibility of ovulation and conception prior to beginning the medication. Seasonale may be started immediately after a first-trimester abortion; if the client starts Seasonale immediately, addition-

al contraceptive measures are not needed.

ASSESSMENT

1. Note annual physical/internal exams, mammography, and Pap smears. List any previous experience with these agents and results.

2. Report any family history of breast or uterine cancer or any existing medical condition that may preclude this drug therapy; assess smoking history.

3. Identify any abnormal vaginal bleeding. Assess contraceptive needs and check to ensure not pregnant.

INTERVENTIONS

1. Explain that hormones (synthetic) that mimic natural estrogens and/or progesterones attempt to "trick" the female reproductive system. They accomplish this by providing constant levels of these hormones in the blood and thus suppressing the release of FSH and LH. Follicle stimulating hormone (FSH) suppression inhibits the maturation of the egg in the ovary. While Leutinizing hormone (LH) inhibits the release of the egg from the ovary. With a constant level of estrogen and progestin in the body the endometrium will not be able to thicken sufficiently in order for the egg to attach.

2. A thick, opaque mucus is produced as a result of circulating progestins which prevents sperm from passing through and it also causes changes in the fallopian tubes that can impede the movement of the egg towards the uterus.

3. A combination of estrogen and progestin may interfere with the muscle contraction in the tubes and uterus thus interfering with implantation. All of which contribute to preventing pregnancy.

4. Reinforce that in no way do these hormones provide any protection against sexually transmitted diseases and protection must be used with each encounter.

CLIENT/FAMILY TEACHING

1. Take tablets or apply patches exactly as prescribed to prevent pregnancy. Take oral contraceptives with food.

However, avoid taking with grapefruit juice.

2. If you vomit within 1 hr of taking either Plan B or Preven for emergency contraception, contact your provider to determine whether or not to repeat that dose or take an antinauseant.

3. There is little likelihood that ovulation will occur if only 1 tablet is missed; however the possibility of spotting or bleeding is increased. The possibility of ovulation occurring increases with each successive day that scheduled hormone-containing tablets are missed. The following guidelines can be followed for missed tablets:

- If 1 combination therapy tablet is missed, take as soon as remembered or take 2 tablets the next day. As an alternative, take 1 tablet, discard the other missed tablet, and continue as scheduled. Use another form of contraception until menses.

- If 2 combination therapy tablets are missed, take 2 tablets as soon as remembered with the next tablet at the usual time; or, take 2 tablets daily for the next 2 days and then resume the regular schedule. Use an additional form of contraception for the remainder of the cycle. If 2 hormone-containing tablets are missed in a row in the third week and the client is on a Sunday start regimen, take 1 tablet every day until Sunday. On Sunday, the rest of the pack is discarded and a new pack of tablets started that same day. If 2 hormone-containing tablets are missed in a row in the third week and the client is a Day 1 starter, discard the rest of the pack and a new pack is started on that day. Menses may not occur during this month; this is expected. If menses does not occur 2 months in a row, contact the provider as pregnancy is possible.

- If 3 combination therapy tablets are missed and the client is a Sunday starter, she should keep taking 1 tablet per day until Sunday. On Sunday, the rest of the pack is discarded and a new pack started that same day. If the client is a Day 1 starter, the rest of the pack is discarded and a new pack is started that same day. Menses may not occur during this month; this is expected. If menses does not occur 2 months in a row, contact the provider as pregnancy is possible. Pregnancy may occur during the 7 days after tablets are missed; thus, use another method of birth control as a back-up for those 7 days.

- If the client is more than 3 hr late or misses 1 or more progestin-only tablets, she should take the missed tablet as soon as remembered. Then, take tablets at the regular time. A back-up contraception method must be used every time she has intercourse for the 48 hr following the late or missed tablet. Report any missed menstrual periods. If two consecutive periods are missed, discontinue therapy until pregnancy ruled out.

4. Report pain in the legs or chest, respiratory distress, unexplained cough, severe headaches, dizziness, blurred vision, or partial loss of sight; stop therapy and notify provider immediately.

5. Oral contraceptives decrease the viscosity of cervical mucus, increasing the susceptibility to vaginal infections which are difficult to treat; regular careful hygienic practice is essential.

6. Report if persistent nausea, swelling, and skin eruptions develop and last beyond the four cycles; a dose adjustment or different combination may be needed.

7. Any changes in thought processes, depression, or fatigue should be reported; preparations with less progesterone may be needed.

8. Androgenic effects, such as weight gain, increased oiliness of the skin, acne, or ↑ hairiness may require a change in medication or dosage.

9. Do not take longer than 18 months without medical consultation. Report for yearly Pap smear testing, and physical examination; perform regular BSE (1 week after or 2 weeks before menstrual cycle) and report any changes/findings.

10. Practice another form of contraception if receiving ampicillin, anticonvul-

sants, phenylbutazone, rifampin, or tetracycline. These may cause intermittent bleeding and interactions could result in pregnancy.

11. Contraceptives interfere with the elimination of caffeine. Limit caffeine consumption to prevent insomnia, irritability, tremors, and cardiac irregularities.

12. If breastfeeding infant, another form of contraception should be used until lactation is well established.

13. **Do not smoke.** Attend formal smoking cessation program.

14. Avoid prolonged or excessive exposure to direct or artificial sunlight.

15. Oral contraceptives do not provide any protection against STDs; use appropriate barrier protection with intercourse.

OUTCOMES/EVALUATE

- Desired contraception
- ↓ Acne
- ↓ Severity of endometriosis
- Menstrual regularity
- ↓ Blood loss (hypermenorrhea) with hormone imbalances

PENICILLINS

SEE ALSO THE FOLLOWING INDIVIDUAL ENTRIES:

Amoxicillin
Amoxicillin and Potassium clavulanate
Ampicillin oral
Ampicillin sodium, parenteral
Ampicillin sodium/Sulbactam sodium
Oxacillin sodium*
Penicillin G aqueous
Penicillin G benzathine and procaine combined, intramuscular
Penicillin G benzathine, intramuscular
Penicillin G procaine, intramuscular
Penicillin V potassium
Piperacillin sodium and Tazobactam sodium
Piperacillin sodium*
Ticarcillin disodium
Ticarcillin disodium and Clavulanate potassium

📷 = see color insert   Ⓗ = Herbal   Ⅳ = Intravenous   ℚ = sound alike drug

Drugs marked with an * are available to view in the online database at www.delmarnursesdrughandbook.com/2009.

GENERAL STATEMENT

Penicillins may be classified as: (1) Natural: Penicillin G, Penicillin V. (2) Aminopenicillins: Amoxicillin, Amoxicillin/potassium clavulanate, Ampicillin, Ampicillin/sulbactam, Bacampicillin. (3) Penicillinase-resistant: Cloxacillin, Dicloxacillin, Nafcillin, Oxacillin. (4) Extended spectrum: Carbenicillin, Mezlocillin, Piperacillin, Piperacillin/Tazobactam sodium, Ticarcillin, Ticarcillin/Potassium clavulanate.

USES

See individual drugs. Effective against a variety of gram-positive, gram-negative, and anaerobic organisms.

ACTION/KINETICS

Action

The bactericidal action of penicillins depends on their ability to bind penicillin-binding proteins (PBP-1 and PBP-3) in the cytoplasmic membranes of bacteria, thus inhibiting cell wall synthesis. Some penicillins act by acylation of membrane-bound transpeptidase enzymes, thereby preventing cross-linkage of peptidoglycan chains, which are necessary for bacterial cell wall strength and rigidity. Cell division and growth are inhibited and often lysis and elongation of susceptible bacteria occur. Penicillin is most effective against young, rapidly dividing organisms and has little effect on mature resting cells. Depending on the concentration of the drug at the site of infection and the susceptibility of the infectious microorganism, penicillin is either bacteriostatic or bactericidal.

Pharmacokinetics

Penicillins are distributed throughout most of the body and pass the placental barrier. They also pass into synovial, pleural, pericardial, peritoneal, ascitic, and spinal fluids. Although normal meninges and the eyes are relatively impermeable to penicillins, they are better absorbed by inflamed meninges and eyes. **Peak serum levels, after PO:** 1 hr. **t ½:** 30–110 min; protein binding: 20–98% (see individual agents). Excreted largely unchanged by the urine as a result of glomerular filtration and active tubular secretion.

CONTRAINDICATIONS

Hypersensitivity to penicillins, imipenem, β–lactamase inhibitors, and cephalosporins. PO use of penicillins during the acute stages of empyema, bacteremia, pneumonia, meningitis, pericarditis, and purulent or septic arthritis. Use with a history of amoxicillin/clavulanate–associated cholestatic jaundice or hepatic dysfunction. Lactation.

SPECIAL CONCERNS

Use of penicillins during lactation may lead to sensitization, diarrhea, candidiasis, and skin rash in the infant. Use with caution in clients with a history of asthma, hay fever, or urticaria. Clients with cystic fibrosis have a higher incidence of side effects with broad spectrum penicillins. Safety and effectiveness of carbenicillin, piperacillin, and the beta-lactamase inhibitor/penicillin combinations (e.g., amoxicillin/potassium clavulanate, ticarcillin/potassium clavulanate) have not been determined in children less than age 12. The incidence of resistant strains of staphylococci to penicillinase-resistant penicillins is increasing. Use of prolonged therapy may lead to superinfection (i.e., bacterial or fungal overgrowth of nonsusceptible organisms). Cystic fibrosis clients have a higher incidence of side effects if given extended spectrum penicillins.

SIDE EFFECTS

Penicillins are potent sensitizing agents; it is estimated that up to 10% of the US population is allergic to the antibiotic. Hypersensitivity reactions are reported to be on the increase in pediatric populations. Sensitivity reactions may be immediate (within 20 min) or delayed (as long as several days or weeks after initiation of therapy).

Allergic: Skin rashes (including maculopapular and exanthematous), exfoliative dermatitis, erythema multiforme (rarely, **Stevens-Johnson syndrome**), hives, pruritus, wheezing, **anaphylaxis,** fever, eosinophilia, hypersensitivity myo-

---

carditis, **angioedema,** serum sickness, **laryngeal edema, laryngospasm, prostration, angioneurotic edema, bronchospasm,** hypotension, **vascular collapse, death. GI:** Diarrhea (may be severe), abdominal cramps or pain, N&V, bloating, flatulence, increased thirst, bitter/unpleasant taste, glossitis, gastritis, stomatitis, dry mouth, sore mouth/tongue, furry tongue, black "hairy" tongue, bloody diarrhea, rectal bleeding, enterocolitis, pseudomembranous colitis. **CNS:** Dizziness, insomnia, hyperactivity, fatigue, prolonged muscle relaxation. Neurotoxicity including lethargy, neuromuscular irritability, **seizures,** hallucinations following large IV doses (especially in clients with renal failure). **Hematologic:** Thrombocytopenia, leukopenia, **agranulocytosis,** anemia, thrombocytopenic purpura, **hemolytic anemia,** granulocytopenia, neutropenia, bone marrow depression. **Renal:** Oliguria, hematuria, hyaline casts, proteinuria, pyuria (all symptoms of interstitial nephritis), nephropathy. Electrolyte imbalance following IV use. **Miscellaneous:** Hepatotoxicity (cholestatic jaundice), superinfection, swelling of face and ankles, anorexia, hyperthermia, transient hepatitis, vaginitis, itchy eyes. IM injection may cause pain and induration at the injection site, ecchymosis, and hematomas. IV use may cause vein irritation, deep vein thrombosis, and thrombophlebitis.

OD OVERDOSE MANAGEMENT

Symptoms: Neuromuscular hyperexcitability, **convulsive seizures.** Massive IV doses may cause agitation, asterixis, hallucinations, confusion, stupor, multifocal myoclonus, **seizures,** coma, hyperkalemia, and encephalopathy.

Treatment (Severe Allergic or Anaphylactic Reactions): Administer epinephrine (0.3–0.5 mL of a 1:1,000 solution SC or IM, or 0.2–0.3 mL diluted in 10 mL saline, given slowly by IV). Corticosteroids should be on hand. In those instances where penicillin is the drug of choice, the physician may decide to use it even though the client is allergic, adding a medication to the regimen to control the allergic response.

DRUG INTERACTIONS

Aminoglycosides / Penicillins ↓ effect of aminoglycosides, although they are used together

Antacids / ↓ Effect of penicillins R/T ↓ GI tract absorption

Antibiotics (chloramphenicol, erythromycins, tetracyclines) / ↓ Effect of penicillins, although synergism has also been seen

Anticoagulants / ↑ Bleeding risk by prolonging bleeding time if used with parenteral penicillins

Aspirin / ↑ Effect of penicillins by ↓ plasma protein binding

Chloramphenicol / Either ↑ or ↓ effects

Erythromycins / Either ↑ or ↓ effects

Heparin / ↑ Risk of bleeding following parenteral penicillins

Oral contraceptives / ↓ Effect of OCs

Probenecid / ↑ Effect of penicillins by ↓ excretion

Tetracyclines / ↓ Effect of penicillins

LABORATORY TEST CONSIDERATIONS

↓ Hematocrit, hemoglobin, WBC lymphocytes, serum potassium, albumin, total proteins, uric acid. ↑ Basophils, lymphocytes, monocytes, platelets, serum alkaline phosphatase, serum sodium. ↑ AST, ALT, bilirubin, LDH following semisynthetic penicillins.

DOSAGE

See individual drugs. Penicillins are available in a variety of dosage forms for PO, parenteral, inhalation, and intrathecal administration. PO doses must be higher than IM or SC doses because a large fraction of penicillin given PO may be destroyed in the stomach.

NURSING CONSIDERATIONS

ADMINISTRATION/STORAGE

1. IM and IV administration of penicillin causes a great deal of local irritation; thus, inject slowly.

2. IM injections are made deeply into the gluteal muscle. IV injections are usually diluted with an IV infusion.

ASSESSMENT

1. Note reasons for therapy, symptom characteristics, other agents trialed/outcome, culture results.

2. Assess for allergic reactions; if reaction occurs, stop drug immediately. Allergic reactions are more likely to occur with a history of asthma, hay fever, urticaria, or allergy to cephalosporins.

3. Monitor VS, CBC, cultures, renal and LFTs.

INTERVENTIONS

1. Penicillins were the first antibiotics discovered as natural products from the mold Penicillium. They produce their bacteriocidal effects by inhibition of bacterial cell wall synthesis.

2. Detain in an ambulatory care site for at least 20 min after administering to assess for anaphylaxis. Approximately 300-500 people die each year from penicillin-induced anaphylaxis. In these individuals, the beta-lactam ring binds to serum proteins, initiating an IgE-mediated inflammatory response. There is a 10% cross reactivity with cephalosporins.

3. Long-acting types of penicillin are for IM use only; may cause emboli, CNS/cardiac pathology if administered IV. Do not massage repository (long-acting) penicillin products after injection; rate of absorption should not be increased.

4. Rapid administration of IV penicillin may cause local irritation and may precipitate convulsions. With some agents, high-dose therapy may precipitate aplastic anemia; monitor CBC.

5. The elderly may be more sensitive to the effects of penicillin than younger people. Calculate dose based on weight and height.

6. Most penicillins are excreted in breast milk and should be prescribed cautiously to nursing mothers.

CLIENT/FAMILY TEACHING

1. Take as directed. Oral penicillins may cause GI upset. Take with a glass of water 1 hr before or 2 hr after meals to minimize binding to foods. Review drugs prescribed, method/ frequency of dosing, side effects, and time frame for therapy.

2. Complete the entire prescribed course of therapy, even if feeling well. Incomplete therapy will predispose client to development of resistant bacterial strains. With α-hemolytic *Strepto-*

coccus infection, must take for a minimum of 10 days, and preferably 14 days, to prevent development of rheumatic fever or kidney infection.

3. Stop medication and report any S&S of allergic reactions, i.e., rashes, fever, joint swelling, face/lip swelling, intense itching, and respiratory distress (during therapy and in some cases 7–12 days after therapy).

4. Return for repository penicillin injections as scheduled.

5. Report S&S of superinfections (furry tongue, vaginal or rectal itching, diarrhea). Call provider if S&S do not improve or worsen after 48–72 hr of therapy.

6. Keep all F/U appointments to evaluate response to therapy, labs/cultures, and adverse side effects.

OUTCOMES/EVALUATE
- Symptomatic improvement
- Resolution of infection (↓ fever, ↓ WBCs, ↑ appetite, negative cultures)

PROGESTERONE AND PROGESTINS ■

SEE ALSO THE FOLLOWING INDIVIDUAL ENTRIES:

Medroxyprogesterone acetate
Megestrol acetate
Oral contraceptives
Progesterone gel

USES
(1) Abnormal uterine bleeding. (2) Primary or secondary amenorrhea (used with an estrogen). (3) Endometriosis. (4) Alone or with an estrogen for contraception. (5) In combination with an estrogen for endometriosis and hypermenorrhea. (6) Certain types of cancer. (7) AIDS wasting syndrome (megestrol acetate). (8) Infertility (progesterone gel). *NOTE:* Not to be used to prevent habitual abortion or to treat threatened abortion. *Investigational:* Medroxyprogesterone has been used to treat menopausal symptoms.

ACTION/KINETICS

Action
Progesterone is the primary endogenous progestin. Progesterone inhibits,

---

Bold Italic = life threatening side effect   ■ = black box warning   ♣ = Available in Canada

through positive feedback, the secretion of pituitary gonadotropins; in turn, this prevents follicular maturation and ovulation or alternatively promotes it for the "primed" follicle. It is required to prepare the endometrium for implantation of the embryo. Once implanted, progesterone is required to maintain pregnancy. Progestins inhibit spontaneous uterine contractions; certain progestins may cause androgenic or anabolic effects.

Pharmacokinetics

Progestins given PO are rapidly absorbed and quickly metabolized in the liver. **Peak levels, after PO:** 1–2 hr. $t^{1/2}$, **after PO:** 2–3 hr during the first 6 hr after ingestion; thereafter, 8–9 hr. **After IM,** effective levels can be maintained for 3–6 months with a $t^{1/2}$ of about 10 weeks. $t^{1/2}$, **elimination, gel:** 5–20 min. A major portion is excreted in the urine with a small amount in the bile and feces.

CONTRAINDICATIONS

Carcinoma of the breast or genital organs, thromboembolic disease, thrombophlebitis, vaginal bleeding of unknown origin, impaired liver function, cerebral hemorrhage or clients with a history of such, missed abortion, as a diagnostic test for pregnancy. Pregnancy, especially during the first 4 months.

SPECIAL CONCERNS

■(1) Progestins have been used beginning with the first trimester of pregnancy to prevent habitual abortion or treat threatened abortion. However, there is no adequate evidence that such use is effective. There is evidence of potential harm to the fetus when given during the first 4 months of pregnancy. Thus, the use of such drugs during the first 4 months of pregnancy is not recommended. (2) The cause of abortion is generally a defective ovum, which progestational agents could not be expected to influence. Also, progestational agents have uterine relaxant effects that may cause a delay in spontaneous abortion when given to clients with fertilized defective ova. (3) Several reports indicate an association between intrauterine exposure to progestational drugs in the first trimester of pregnancy and genital abnormalities in male and female fetuses, and congenital anomalies, including congenital heart defects and limb-reduction defects. There are insufficient data to quantify the risk to exposed female fetuses, but because some of the more androgenic types of these drugs induce mild virilization of the external genitalia of the female fetus, and because of the increased association of hypospadias in the male fetus, it is prudent to avoid use of these drugs during the first trimester. (4) If the client is exposed to progestational drugs during the first 4 months of pregnancy or if the woman becomes pregnant while taking progestins, apprise her of the potential risks to the fetus.■ Due to possible fluid retention, use with caution in asthma, epilepsy, depression, migraine, and cardiac or renal dysfunction. Use with caution in those who have a history of psychic depression.

SIDE EFFECTS

See also individual drugs. Occasionally noted with short-term dosage, frequently observed with prolonged high dosage. **CNS:** Depression, insomnia, somnolence. **GU:** Breakthrough bleeding, spotting, amenorrhea, changes in amount and/or duration of menstrual flow, changes in cervical secretions and cervical erosion, breast tenderness or secretions. **Dermatologic:** Allergic rashes with and without pruritus, acne, melasma, chloasma, photosensitivity, local reactions at the site of injection. *NOTE:* Progesterone is especially irritating at the site of injection, especially aqueous products. **Miscellaneous:** Weight gain or loss, cholestatic jaundice, masculinization of the female fetus, nausea, edema, precipitation of acute intermittent porphyria, pyrexia, hirsutism.

LABORATORY TEST CONSIDERATIONS

Progestins may affect laboratory test results of hepatic function, thyroid, pregnanediol determination, and endocrine function. ↑ Prothrombin and Factors VII, VIII, IX, and X. ↓ Glucose tolerance (especially in diabetics).

DOSAGE

See individual drugs. The usual schedule of administration for *functional uterine bleeding, amenorrhea, infertility, dysmenorrhea, premenstrual tension, and contraception* is days 5 through 25 of the menstrual cycle, with day 1 being the first day of menstrual flow.

NURSING CONSIDERATIONS

ASSESSMENT

1. Note reasons for therapy and any prior experience with this drug. Assess for any conditions i.e., thrombophlebitis, pulmonary embolism, cardiac, liver, or renal dysfunction, cerebral hemorrhage, breast or genital cancers that may preclude therapy.
2. Monitor VS, ECG, weight, and labs.
3. Identify any history of psychic depression or diabetes mellitus. Review family history. Document last menstrual period and absence of pregnancy.

INTERVENTIONS

1. Explain that progesterone works as part of hormone replacement therapy by decreasing the amount of estrogen in the uterus. Where estrogen can cause abnormal thickening of the lining of the uterus and increase the risk of developing uterine cancer, progesterone helps prevent this thickening and decreases the risk of developing uterine cancer. Hence the reluctance to give unopposed estrogen in women that still have a uterus.
2. Progesterone is also used to bring on menstruation in women of childbearing age who have had normal periods and then stopped menstruating. Low-dose progestins for contraception are used to prevent pregnancy.

CLIENT/FAMILY TEACHING

1. Take as directed at the same time each day. To avoid gastric irritation and nausea, take with a light snack, in the evening. GI upset usually subsides after first few cycles of drug; report if S&S persist.
2. Stop smoking; enroll in a formal smoking cessation program. Report any symptoms of blood clot disorders such as pains in the legs, sudden onset of chest pain, SOB, and coughing. Report any unusual bruising/bleeding.
3. Weigh twice weekly and report any unusual weight gain/swelling of extremities.
4. Yellowing of the skin or eyes (jaundice) may necessitate discontinuation of the medication, evaluation of LFTs, and possibly a dosage change; advise provider.
5. Progestins may reactivate or worsen psychic depression. Report any mental status changes and circumstance of the depression.
6. With diabetes, progesterone may alter glucose tolerance and the antidiabetic dosage may need to be adjusted.
7. Report early symptoms of eye pathology, such as headaches, dizziness, blurred vision, or partial loss of vision; obtain thorough eye exam.
8. With birth control, injections must be administered every 3 mo to ensure adequate protection. Progestin-only oral contraceptives may be used as early as 3 weeks after delivery in women who partially breast feed and within 6 weeks after delivery in women who fully breast feed.

OUTCOMES/EVALUATE

- Control of abnormal menstrual bleeding; menstrual regularity
- Weight gain with AIDS clients
- Effective contraceptive agent
- ↓ Size/resolution of ovarian cyst(s); ↓ Severity of endometriosis

PROTON PUMP INHIBITORS

SEE ALSO THE FOLLOWING INDIVIDUAL ENTRIES:

Esomeprazole magnesium
Lansoprazole
Omeprazole
Pantoprazole sodium
Rabeprazole sodium

USES

See individual drugs. (1) Short-term treatment of active duodenal ulcer. Lansoprazole is also used to maintain healing of duodenal ulcer. (2) Treatment of duodenal ulcer associated with *H. pylori*

---

infection. Used in combination with other drugs. (3) Short-term treatment of active benign gastric ulcer. Lansoprazole is used for the healing and reducing the risk of NSAID-associated gastric ulcers. (4) Treatment of heartburn and other symptoms associated with GERD. (5) Long-term treatment of pathological hypersecretory conditions (e.g., Zollinger-Ellison syndrome, multiple endocrine adenomas, systemic mastocytosis). *Investigational: H. pylori* astritis in children (lansoprazole, omeprazole), GERD in children (lansoprazole, omeprazole), GERD-related laryngitis (omeprazole), improve pancreatic enzyme absorption in cystic fibrosis clients with intestinal malabsorption (lansoprazole, omeprazole).

ACTION/KINETICS

Action

Act to suppress gastric acid secretion by specifically inhibiting the H^+/K^+ ATPase enzyme system at the secretory surface of gastric parietal cells. This enzyme is the "acid (proton) pump" within the gastric mucosa. Thus, these drugs are classified as proton pump inhibitors as they block the final step of acid production. Both basal and stimulated acid secretion are inhibited. These agents also increase serum pepsinogen levels and decrease pepsin activity.

Pharmacokinetics

Most of these drugs contain enteric-coated granules; absorption is rapid and begins only after the granules leave the stomach. Extensively metabolized in the liver. **$t\frac{1}{2}$, elimination:** Less than 2 hr; however, the acid inhibitory effect lasts more than 24 hr (probably due to prolonged binding to the parietal H^+/K^+ ATPase enzyme.

CONTRAINDICATIONS

Lactation.

SPECIAL CONCERNS

Symptomatic relief does not preclude gastric malignancy. There is an increased risk of hip fracture (especially in those with comorbid conditions and in men) if given in high doses for over one year. Safety and efficacy have not been determined in children.

SIDE EFFECTS

See individual drugs. Side effects common to most proton pump inhibitors follow. **CV:** Chest pain, angina, palpitation, hypertension, tachycardia. **CNS:** Anxiety, apathy, confusion, depression, hallucinations, aggravated hostility, nervousness, paresthesia. **Dermatologic:** Rash, urticaria, pruritus, alopecia. **GI:** Anorexia, fecal discoloration, dry mouth, flatulence, gastric fundic gland polyps. **GU:** Hematuria, glycosuria, gynecomastia, acute interstitial nephritis. **Hematologic:** Anemia, hemolysis. **Metabolic:** Hypoglycemia, gout, weight gain. **Musculoskeletal:** Arthralgia, myalgia. **Miscellaneous:** Epistaxis, taste perversion, tinnitus, fever, malaise.

DRUG INTERACTIONS

See individual drugs. Because of the profound and long-lasting inhibition of gastric acid secretion, these drugs may interfere with absorption of drugs where gastric pH is an important factor in bioavailability (e.g., ampicillin, cyanocobalamin, digoxin, iron salts, ketoconazole).

LABORATORY TEST CONSIDERATIONS

↑ AST, ALT, alkaline phosphatase, bilirubin.

DOSAGE

See individual drugs.

NURSING CONSIDERATIONS

ADMINISTRATION/STORAGE

1. Take with meals.
2. Antacids may be used with proton pump inhibitors.

ASSESSMENT

1. Note reasons for therapy, characteristics of S&S, other agents trialed. List drugs prescribed to ensure none interact or require acidity for metabolism.
2. Record abdominal assessments, x-ray (UGI, US, barium enema), CT/MRI, or endoscopic findings and *H. pylori* results.
3. Assess LFTs; may reduce dose of some to every 4 days with dysfunction to prevent drug accumulations.
4. Identify what may be contributing to symptoms, i.e., tomato-based dishes, peppermint, consumption of alcohol and tobacco, lying down after eating,

---

Classifications

wearing tight waisted pants, Barretts, H. pylori infection etc. Determine if pregnant.

CLIENT/FAMILY TEACHING

1. Take as directed with meals. Swallow tablets whole; do not open, crush, chew, or split tablets.

2. Do not perform activities that require mental alertness until drug effects realized. Report unusual bleeding, acid reflux, abdominal pain, severe light-headedness/diarrhea, rash, worsening of symptoms or lack of effectiveness. Review drug associated side effects; report if diarrhea persists.

3. Avoid alcohol, NSAIDs, and salicylates; may increase GI upset. Report any changes in urinary elimination, pain or discomfort.

4. Follow prescribed diet and activities to control S&S of GERD. Drug should be withdrawn once condition cleared/resolved and new eating behaviors and lifestyle changes in effect.

5. Generally these drugs are for short-term use only as they inhibit total gastric acid secretion. Side effects of prolonged therapy and suppression of acid secretion alter bacterial colonization and lead to hypochlorhydria and hypergastrinemia which may cause an increased risk for gastric tumors.

6. Keep all scheduled visits to ensure accurate dosing and drug for symptom control and the need to continue therapy.

OUTCOMES/EVALUATE

- ↓ Intraesophageal acid exposure
- Promotion of ulcer/esophageal tissue healing; relief of pain
- ↓ Gastric acid production

SELECTIVE SEROTONIN ■ REUPTAKE INHIBITORS

SEE ALSO THE FOLLOWING INDIVIDUAL ENTRIES:

Citalopram hydrobromide
Fluoxetine hydrochloride
Fluvoxamine maleate
Paroxetine hydrochloride
Paroxetine mesylate
Sertraline hydrochloride

USES

See individual entries. Depending on the drug, uses include: (1) Depression. (2) Obsessive-compulsive disorder. (3) Panic disorder. (4) Bulimia nervosa. (5) Generalized anxiety disorder. (6) Premenstrual dysphoric disorder. (7) Post-traumatic stress disorder. (8) Social anxiety disorder. *Investigational:* Enuresis.

ACTION/KINETICS

Action

Antidepressant effect probably due to inhibition of CNS neuronal reuptake of serotonin and to a lesser extent to norepinephrine and dopamine neuronal reuptake. Not related chemically to tricyclic, tetracyclic, or other antidepressants. Slight to no anticholinergic, sedative, or orthostatic hypotensive effects.

Pharmacokinetics

All are extensively metabolized by the liver. The mean maximum plasma levels are higher in geriatric clients and the elimination half-life is delayed in these clients.

CONTRAINDICATIONS

Hypersensitivity to any SSRI or any components of the products. Use in combination with a monoamine oxidase inhibitor (MAOI) or within 14 days of stopping a MAOI. Lactation.

SPECIAL CONCERNS

■Antidepressants increased the risk of suicidal thinking and behavior (suicidality) in short-term studies in children and adolescents with major depressive disorder and other psychiatric disorders. Anyone considering the use of a SSRI or any other antidepressant in a child or adolescent must balance this risk with the clinical need. Clients who are started on therapy should be observed closely for clinical worsening, suicidality, or unusual changes in behavior. Families and caregivers should be advised of the need for close observation and communication with the prescriber. Some SSRIs are not approved for use in pediatric clients. Studies have shown a greater risk of adverse reactions representing suicidal thinking or behavior during the first few months of treatment in those receiving antidepressants. The average risk of such reactions in those receiving antidepressants is 4%, twice the placebo risk of 2%. No suicides occurred in these trials.■ Use with caution in clients with severe hepatic impairment. Use during pregnancy only if clearly needed; possible neonatal withdrawal and/or seizures may occur when therapy is used during pregnancy. Efficacy has not been determined for long-term use in OCD, panic disorder, or bulimia. SSRIs may be associated with an increased risk of fractures in those 50 years and older. Safety and efficacy have not been determined in children less than 18 years of age, other than pediatric clients with OCD and the use of fluoxetine in major depressive disorder.

SIDE EFFECTS

See individual drugs. The following side effects (listed alphabetically) have been observed with several of the selective serotonin reuptake inhibitors (SSRIs): **CNS:** Abnormal dreams, abnormal thinking, agitation, amnesia, anxiety, apathy, confusion, depersonalization, depression, dizziness, emotional lability, headache, hypertonia, hypoesthesia, hypo- or hyperkinesia, impaired concentration, insomnia, libido decrease, myoclonus, nervousness, paresthesia, somnolence, suicide ideation/attempts, tremor, vertigo. **CV:** Chest pain, hypertension, palpitations, postural hypotension, syncope, tachycardia, vasodilation. **GI:** Abdominal pain, anorexia, constipation, diarrhea, dry mouth, dyspepsia, dysphagia, flatulence, gastroenteritis, increased appetite, nausea, tooth disorder/caries, vomiting. **Dermatologic:** Acne, pruritus, rash, sweating (excessive). **GU:** Abnormal ejaculation, anorgasmia, impotence, sexual dysfunction, urinary frequency, UTI, urination disorder/retention. **Musculoskeletal:** Arthralgia, myalgia, myasthenia, myopathy. **Respiratory:** Bronchitis, cough, dyspnea, rhinitis, sinusitis, yawn. **Body as a whole:** Accidental injury/trauma, allergic reaction, asthenia, chills, edema, fever, flu syndrome, malaise, weight gain or loss. **Miscellaneous:** Hyponatremia, taste perversion, tinnitus, vision (blurred/abnormal/disturbed).

DRUG INTERACTIONS

See individual drugs. The following drug interactions are possible with any of the SSRIs.

Alcohol / Possible increased impairment of mental and motor skills; do not use together

Aspirin / ↑ Risk of GI bleeding

Benzodiazepines / Possible ↓ clearance of benzodiazepines metabolized by hepatic oxidation (e.g., alprazolam, fluoxetine, fluvoxamine)

Beta adrenergic blockers / Certain SSRIs may ↓ metabolism of certain beta blockers

Lithium / Possible ↓ serotonergic effects of SSRIs

L-Tryptophan / Both central (headache, sweating, dizziness, agitation, restlessness) and peripheral (GI distress, N&V) toxicity is possible

MAO inhibitors / Serious (and possibly fatal) reactions, including hyperthermia, rigidity, myoclonus, autonomic instability, mental status changes

Metoclopramide / Possible serotonin syndrome (e.g., CNS irritability, shivering, myoclonus, altered consciousness), especially if used with sertraline

NSAIDs / ↑ Risk of GI bleeding and significant other GI side effects; do not use together

H *St. John's wort* / Possible mild serotonin syndrome

Sibutramine / Possible serotonin syndrome (e.g., CNS irritability, shivering, myoclonus, altered consciousness)

Sumatriptan / Weakness, hyperreflexia, incoordination

Sympathomimetics / ↑ Sympathomimetic effects and ↑ risk of serotonin syndrome

Tramadol / Possible serotonin syndrome (e.g., CNS irritability, shivering, myoclonus, altered consciousness)

Tricyclic antidepressants / Possible ↑ TCA plasma levels

Warfarin / Altered anticoagulant effects.

DOSAGE

See individual drugs.

NURSING CONSIDERATIONS

ADMINISTRATION/STORAGE

Clients show the largest relative improvement during the first weeks of treatment.

ASSESSMENT

1. Note reasons for therapy, behavioral manifestations, symptom onset/characteristics, and contributing factors. List other drugs prescribed to ensure none interact; note agents trialed and outcome.

2. Differentiate type of depression based on diagnostic features related to reactive, major depressive, or bipolar affective disorders. Assess for dysphoric mood, suicidal ideations, and excessive appetite/weight changes. Include behavioral health review.

3. Note sleep disturbances, lethargy, apathy, impaired thought processes, or lack of response.

4. Monitor ECG, CBC, renal and LFTs; use caution with liver dysfunction.

5. Carefully monitor adults and children, esp at the beginning of treatment, for worsening depression or emerging suicidal ideation.

6. A major depressive episode may be the initial symptom of bipolar disorder. Prior to initiating treatment with an antidepressant, adequately screen clients with depressive symptoms to determine if they are at risk for bipolar disorder.

CLIENT/FAMILY TEACHING

1. May take with or without food as directed. Avoid other unprescribed or OTC agents and alcohol during therapy.

2. Use caution when performing tasks requiring mental alertness or physical coordination until drug effects realized. May cause drop in BP. Rise slowly from a lying or sitting position to minimize effects.

3. Increase oral hygiene, take frequent sips of water, suck on hard candy, or chew sugarless gum to maintain a moist mouth. A high-fiber diet, increased fluid intake, exercise, and stool softeners may prevent constipation.

4. May alter libido and sexual function. Practice reliable birth control; report if pregnancy suspected.

5. Report any alterations in perceptions, i.e., hallucinations, blurred vision, or excessive stimulations. Watch those recovering from depression for suicidal tendencies; remove firearms from the home and encourage support group therapy.

6. May take 1–4 weeks to notice any change in emotional state; stay on the treatment regimen. Will see provider more often the first 2–3 months; prescriptions will be for a small dosage to start and to prevent adverse side effects. Obtain number from provider to call for help or report adverse effects.

7. Do not stop abruptly at higher dosages; may experience withdrawal S&S. Review when and how to take medications, reportable side effects, especially rash or S&S of liver dysfunction (yellow skin, RUQ abdominal pain, itching, fatigue and change in stool color) and importance of regular participation in psychotherapy programs as prescribed.

OUTCOMES/EVALUATE

• Understand illness and need for counselling, drug therapy/medical supervision

• ↓ Depression evidenced by improved appetite, renewed interest in outside activities, ↑ socialization, improved sleeping patterns, ↑ energy

• ↓ Anxiety; improved coping skills

SEROTONIN 5-HT₁ RECEPTOR AGONISTS (ANTIMIGRAINE DRUGS)

SEE ALSO THE FOLLOWING INDIVIDUAL ENTRIES:

Almotriptan maleate
Eletriptan hydrobromide
Frovatriptan succinate
Naratriptan hydrochloride
Rizatriptan benzoate
Sumatriptan succinate
Zolmitriptan

USES

See individual drugs. Uses include: (1) Acute treatment of migraine with or without aura. Use only when a clear diagnosis of migraine has been determined. Drugs are not intended to prevent or reduce the number of migraine attacks. (2) Acute treatment of cluster headache episodes (sumatriptan injection only).

ACTION/KINETICS

Action

These drugs are selective 5-HT$_1$ receptor agonists. This receptor is present on human basilar arteries and in the vasculature of the dura mater. It is believed that symptoms of migraine are due to local cranial vasodilation or to the release of vasoactive and proinflammatory peptides from sensory nerve endings in an activated trigeminal system. Depending on the drug, the selective 5-HT$_1$ agonists have a high affinity for and combine with 5-HT$_{1B}$, 5-HT$_{1D}$, or 5-HT$_{1F}$ receptors on the extracerebral, intracranial blood vessels that become dilated during a migraine attack. Activation of the receptors causes cranial vessel vasoconstriction, inhibition of neuropeptide release, and reduced transmission in trigeminal pain pathways.

CONTRAINDICATIONS

IV use of injectable products (due to possibility of coronary vasospasm). Use in ischemic bowel disease, angina pectoris, history of MI, strokes, TIAs, documented silent ischemia, Prinzmetal's variant angina, in those with signs and symptoms of ischemic heart disease or coronary artery vasospasm, coronary artery disease (or in presence of risk factors for CAD), uncontrolled hypertension. Concurrent use (or within 24 hr of use) of ergotamine-containing products, dihydroergotamine, methysergide; also, MAO inhibitor therapy (or within 2 weeks of discontinuing an MAOI). Within 24 hr of another 5-HT$_1$ agonist. Use to manage hemiplegic or basilar migraine.

SPECIAL CONCERNS

Increased risk of myocardial ischemia or MI and other adverse cardiac events, including life-threatening disturbances of cardiac rhythm and death, cerebral hemorrhage, subarachnoid hemorrhage, stroke, coronary artery vasospasm, peripheral vascular ischemia, colonic ischemia with abdominal pain, bloody diarrhea, and significant increases in BP. Use with caution during lactation and in those with diseases that may alter the absorption, metabolism, or excretion of drugs. Safety and efficacy have not been determined in children.

SIDE EFFECTS

See individual drugs. Most common side effects include paresthesia, asthenia, nausea, dizziness, fatigue, pain, somnolence, warm sensation, dry mouth, headache, flushing, hot or cold sensation, chest pain, and chest, jaw, or neck tightness or heaviness. More serious side effects follow: **CV:** *Acute MI, life-threatening disturbances of cardiac rhythm,* and *death* within a few hours following use. *Cerebral hemorrhage, subarachnoid hemorrhage, stroke, myocardial ischemia.* Vasospastic reactions, including coronary artery vasospasm; peripheral vascular ischemia, colonic ischemia with abdominal pain and bloody diarrhea, hypertension, *hypertensive crisis.* **Respiratory:** Nasal and throat irritation, burning, numbness, paresthesia, discharge, pain, soreness (all after using nasal spray). **Hypersensitivity:** *Severe anaphylaxis/anaphylactoid reactions.* **Miscellaneous:** Chest, jaw, or neck tightness; pain, tightness, pressure, or heaviness over the precordium. Photosensitivity, long-term ophthalmic effects.

OD OVERDOSE MANAGEMENT

Symptoms: Hypertension and other more serious CV symptoms.
Treatment: There are no specific antidotes. Consider gastric lavage followed by activated charcoal in clients with suspected overdose. Begin standard supportive measures. If chest pain or other symptoms of angina are present, perform ECG monitoring for evidence of ischemia. Continue monitoring clients after an overdose for at least 10–20 hr depending on the drug.

DRUG INTERACTIONS

Ergot alkaloids / ↑ Risk of vasospastic reactions; do not use within 24 hr of each other

---

MAO inhibitors / Do not use 5-HT₁ agonists within 2 weeks following discontinuation of an MAO inhibitor

SSRIs / Possible weakness, hyperreflexia, incoordination

Serotonin 5-HT₁ agonists / ↑ Risk of vasospastic reactions when two 5-HT₁ agonists are given within 24 hr of each other; use together is contraindicated

Sibutramine / Possible "serotonin syndrome," including symptoms of CNS irritability, motor weakness, shivering, myoclonus, and altered consciousness.

DOSAGE
See individual drugs.

NURSING CONSIDERATIONS

ADMINISTRATION/STORAGE
1. Take a single PO dose with fluids as soon as symptoms of migraine appear. A second dose may be taken if symptoms return, but no sooner than 2 or 4 hours (depending on the drug) following the first dose.
2. If there is no response to the first dose, do not take a second dose without consulting provider.

ASSESSMENT
1. Note reasons for therapy, family history, characteristics of S&S; ensure not hemiplegic or basilar type of migraine headaches. List other drugs prescribed to ensure none interact and other agents trialed/outcome.
2. Review neurologic exam and CT/MRI results. A clear diagnosis of migraine should be made; the drug should not be given for headaches due to other neurologic events.
3. Assess for any CAD, CABG, uncontrolled HTN, circulation problems, IBD, or history of CVA/TIAs. With increased CAD risk factors give first dose in the office and assess client for adverse effects or have men undergo a stress test and women a thallium stress test.
4. Review EKG, renal and LFTs; evaluate for dysfunction. Monitor VS; expect transient increases in BP.
5. Review headache diary and assess for triggers or agents that may cause headaches, i.e., tetracycline, niacin, nitrates, magnesium sulfate, red wines,

Nutrasweet, caffeine, conjugated estrogens, etc.

CLIENT/FAMILY TEACHING
1. Take exactly as directed; strictly for migraine headaches. Do not exceed dosage or dosing intervals, do not share medications with others regardless of symptoms; do not use for other types of headaches.
2. Use caution if driving or performing activities that require mental alertness; may cause dizziness or drowsiness. Report any chest pain, SOB, chest tightness, or wheezing.
3. Drug acts to shrink swollen blood vessels surrounding the brain that cause migraine headaches. Keep a headache diary and identify factors/foods/events that surround migraine headaches. Continue other remedies (i.e., noise reduction, reduced lighting, and bed rest) that assist to control S&S. Avoid known triggers, i.e., chocolate, cheese, citrus fruit, caffeine, alcohol, missing sleep/meals.
4. Review package insert and do not use with other similar headache medications.
5. Practice reliable contraception; report if pregnancy suspected.
6. Store away from heat, light, and moisture; store in a safe place. Report any unusual side effects, intolerance, or lack of response.
7. Keep all F/U appointments to evaluate response to therapy, adverse effects, and need for adjustment in dose/drug.

OUTCOMES/EVALUATE
Termination of migraine headaches

SKELETAL MUSCLE RELAXANTS, CENTRALLY ACTING

SEE ALSO THE FOLLOWING INDIVIDUAL ENTRIES:

Baclofen
Cyclobenzaprine hydrochloride
Diazepam
Methocarbamol
Tizanidine hydrochloride

USES

See individual drugs. Uses include: (1) Musculoskeletal and neurologic disorders associated with muscle spasms, hyperreflexia, and hypertonia, including parkinsonism, tetanus, tension headaches, acute muscle spasms caused by trauma, and inflammation (e.g., low back syndrome, sprains, arthritis, bursitis). (2) Management of cerebral palsy and multiple sclerosis.

ACTION/KINETICS

Action

These drugs decrease muscle tone and involuntary movement. Many relieve anxiety and tension as well. Although the precise mechanism of action is unknown, most of these agents depress spinal polysynaptic reflexes. Their beneficial effects may also be attributable to their antianxiety activity. Several of the drugs in this group also manifest analgesic properties.

SIDE EFFECTS

See individual drugs.

OD OVERDOSE MANAGEMENT

Symptoms: Often extensions of the side effects. Stupor, **coma, shock-like syndrome, respiratory depression,** loss of muscle tone, and impaired deep tendon reflexes may also occur.
Treatment: Symptomatic. Emesis or gastric lavage (followed by activated charcoal). If necessary, artificial respiration, oxygen administration, pressor agents, and IV fluids may be used. It may be possible to increase the rate of excretion of selected drugs by diuretics (including mannitol), peritoneal dialysis, or hemodialysis.

DRUG INTERACTIONS

CNS depressants (e.g., alcohol, barbiturates, sedatives and hypnotics, and antianxiety agents) / ↑ Sedative and respiratory depressant effects
H *Kava Kava /* Additive effects.

DOSAGE

See individual drugs.

NURSING CONSIDERATIONS

ADMINISTRATION/STORAGE

1. If unable to swallow, crush tablets or empty capsules into a small amount of fruit juice.

2. If skeletal muscle relaxant is to be discontinued after long-term use, taper dose to prevent rebound spasticity, hallucinations, or other withdrawal symptoms.

3. Determine lowest dosage to treat symptoms.

ASSESSMENT

1. Note reasons for therapy, onset, and characteristics of S&S. List agents trialed/outcome.

2. Assess extent of musculoskeletal/ neurologic disorders associated with muscle spasm. Note muscle tone, stiffness, pain, pain level, and extent of ROM.

3. Review baseline mental status. Note any seizures/history; may cause loss of seizure control.

INTERVENTIONS

1. Monitor BP q 4 hr. Supervise ambulation/transfers and ensure safe environment. If sedentary or immobilized, client is more prone to hypotension upon ambulation.

2. Monitor urinary output; evaluate need for drugs to ↑ excretion rate.

3. Assess level of mobility (ROM) and comfort (pain level) prior to and following drug administration. Check muscle responses and DTRs for evidence of drug overdose.

CLIENT/FAMILY TEACHING

1. Take as directed with meals to reduce GI upset. If unable to swallow, crush tablets or empty capsules into a small amount of fruit juice.

2. These drugs may impair mental alertness; do not operate dangerous machinery or drive a car until drug effects realized. Avoid alcohol and any other CNS depressants. Antihistamines may cause an additive depressant effect.

3. Review additional therapies that may be prescribed for muscle spasm (heat, rest, exercise, physical therapy) and importance of adhering to prescribed regimen.

4. Increase fluids and bulk in diet to prevent constipation. Report if the urine becomes dark, the skin or sclera appears yellow, or skin itching develops.

5. Report persistent nausea, anorexia, or changes in taste perception, as nutritional state may become impaired.

6. Do not stop drug abruptly after prolonged use; may precipitate withdrawal symptoms, rebound spasticity, and hallucinations.

7. Report as scheduled for all lab and medical visits so therapy and symptoms can be evaluated and drug dosage/need assessed.

OUTCOMES/EVALUATE

- ↓ Muscle spasm and pain
- ↑ ROM with measurable improvement in muscle tone, mobility, and involuntary movements
- Relief of tension headaches

SULFONAMIDES

SEE ALSO THE FOLLOWING INDIVIDUAL ENTRIES:

Mafenide acetate*
Sulfacetamide sodium
Sulfadiazine
Sulfasalazine
Trimethoprim and
  Sulfamethoxazole

Drugs marked with a * are available to view in the online database at www.delmarnursesdrughandbook.com/2009.

USES

PO, Parenteral. See individual drugs. Uses include, but are not limited to: (1) Urinary tract infections. (2) Chancroid. (3) Meningitis caused by *Hemophilus influenzae*, meningococcal meningitis. (4) Rheumatic fever. (5) Nocardiosis. (6) Trachoma. (7) With pyrimethamine for toxoplasmosis. (8) With quinine sulfate and pyrimethamine for chloroquine-resistant *Plasmodium falciparum.* (9) With penicillin for otitis media. (10) Sexually transmitted diseases, including lymphogranuloma venereum and *Chlamydia trachomatis* infections.

Ophthalmic. (1) Conjunctivitis, corneal ulcer, and other superficial ocular infections due to susceptible organisms. (2) Adjunct to systemic sulfonamides to treat trachoma. (3) Inclusion conjunctivitis.

ACTION/KINETICS

Action

Structurally related to PABA and, as such, competitively inhibit the enzyme dihydropteroate synthetase, which is responsible for incorporating PABA into dihydrofolic acid. Thus, the synthesis of dihydrofolic acid is inhibited, resulting in a decrease in tetrahydrofolic acid, which is required for synthesis of DNA, purines, and thymidine. Are bacteriostatic.

Pharmacokinetics

Readily absorbed from the GI tract. Distributed throughout all tissues, including the CSF, where concentrations attain 50–80% of those found in the blood. Metabolized in the liver and primarily excreted by the kidneys. Small amounts are found in the feces, bile, breast milk, and other secretions.

CONTRAINDICATIONS

Hypersensitivity reactions to sulfonamides and chemically related drugs (e.g., thiazides, sulfonylureas, loop diuretics, carbonic anhydrase inhibitors, local anesthetics, PABA-containing sunscreens). Use in infants less than 2 years of age, except with pyrimethamine to treat congenital toxoplasmosis. Use at term during pregnancy. Use in premature infants who are nursing or those with hyperbilirubinemia or G6PD deficiency. Group A beta-hemolytic streptococcal infections.

SPECIAL CONCERNS

Use with caution, and in reduced dosage, in clients with impaired liver or renal function, intestinal or urinary tract obstructions, blood dyscrasias, allergies, asthma, and hereditary G6PD deficiency. Use with caution if exposed to sunlight or ultraviolet light as photosensitivity may occur. Superinfection is a possibility. Use ophthalmic products with caution in clients with dry eye. Safety and efficacy of ophthalmic use in children have not been determined.

SIDE EFFECTS

Systemic. GI: N&V, diarrhea, abdominal pain, glossitis, stomatitis, anorexia, pseudomembranous enterocolitis, pancreatitis, hepatitis, ***hepatocellular necrosis.*** **Allergic:** Rash, pruritus, photo-

---

Bold Italic = life threatening side effect   ■ = black box warning   ✦ = Available in Canada

sensitivity, erythema nodosum or multiforme, generalized skin eruptions, **Stevens-Johnson syndrome,** conjunctivitis, rhinitis, balanitis. Serum sickness, urticaria, pruritus, exfoliative dermatitis, **anaphylaxis, toxic epidermal necrolysis** with or without corneal damage, periorbital edema, conjunctival and scleral injection, allergic myocarditis, decreased pulmonary function with eosinophilia, disseminated lupus erythematosus, periarteritis nodosa, arteritis. **CNS:** Headaches, mental depression, **seizures,** hallucinations, vertigo, insomnia, apathy, ataxia, drowsiness, restlessness. **Renal:** Crystalluria, toxic nephrosis with oliguria and anuria, elevated creatinine. **Hematologic: Aplastic anemia,** leukopenia, neutropenia, **agranulocytosis,** thrombocytopenia, hemolytic anemia, methemoglobinemia, purpura, hypoprothrombinemia. **Neurologic:** Peripheral neuropathy, polyneuritis, neuritis, optic neuritis. **Miscellaneous:** Jaundice, tinnitus, arthralgia, superinfection, hearing loss, drug fever, pyrexia, chills, lupus erythematosus phenomenon, transient myopia. By killing the intestinal flora, the sulfonamides also reduce the bacterial synthesis of vitamin K. This may result in **hemorrhage.** Administration of vitamin K to clients on long-term sulfonamide therapy is recommended.

Ophthalmic. Headache, browache. Blurred vision, eye irritation, itching, transient epithelial keratitis, reactive hyperemia, conjunctival edema, burning and transient stinging. Rarely, **Stevens-Johnson syndrome,** exfoliative dermatitis, **toxic epidermal necrolysis,** photosensitivity, fever, skin rash, GI disturbances, and bone marrow depression.

`OD` OVERDOSE MANAGEMENT
Symptoms: N&V, anorexia, colic, dizziness, drowsiness, headache, unconsciousness, vertigo, toxic fever. More serious manifestations include **acute hemolytic anemia, agranulocytosis,** acidosis, maculopapular dermatitis, hepatic jaundice, sensitivity reactions, toxic neuritis, **death** (several days after the first dose).

Treatment: Immediately discontinue the drug.
- Induce emesis or perform gastric lavage, especially if large doses were taken.
- To hasten excretion, alkalinize the urine and force fluids (if kidney function is normal). If there is renal blockage due to sulfonamide crystals, catheterization of the ureters may be needed.
- In the event of agranulocytosis, antibiotic therapy is needed to combat infection.
- To treat severe anemia or thrombocytopenia, blood or platelet transfusions are required.

DRUG INTERACTIONS
Anticoagulants, oral / ↑ Drug effects R/T ↓ plasma protein binding
Antidiabetics, oral / ↑ Hypoglycemic effect R/T ↓ plasma protein binding
Cyclosporine / ↓ Effect of cyclosporine and ↑ nephrotoxicity
Diuretics, thiazide / ↑ Risk of thrombocytopenia with purpura
Indomethacin / ↑ Effect of sulfonamides R/T ↓ plasma protein binding
Methenamine / ↑ Chance of sulfonamide crystalluria due to acid urine
Methotrexate / ↑ Risk of drug-induced bone marrow suppression
Phenytoin / ↑ Drug effect R/T ↓ liver breakdown
Probenecid / ↑ Effect of sulfonamides R/T ↓ plasma protein binding
Salicylates / ↑ Effect of sulfonamides R/T ↓ plasma protein binding
Silver products / Incompatible with ophthalmic products
Uricosuric agents / Potentiation of uricosuric action.

LABORATORY TEST CONSIDERATIONS
False + or ↑ LFTs (amino acids, bilirubin, BSP), renal function (BUN, NPN, C_{CR}), blood counts, PT, Coombs' test. False + or ↑ urine glucose (copper reduction methods, such as Benedict's solution or Clinitest), protein, urobilinogen.

DOSAGE
See individual drugs.

NURSING CONSIDERATIONS

ADMINISTRATION/STORAGE

1. Do not use ophthalmic solutions if they have darkened or contain a precipitate.
2. Take care to avoid contamination of ophthalmic products.

ASSESSMENT

1. Obtain a thorough nursing and drug history. Note previous sulfonamide therapy/response.
2. Note reasons for therapy, type, onset, characteristics of S&S, culture results. List other agents trialed; outcome.
3. Question concerning any conditions that may preclude drug therapy, i.e., intestinal problems, urinary tract obstructions, G6PD deficiency (may precipitate hemolysis), or allergies and explore further.
4. Check if pregnant; drug may be harmful to developing fetus. Monitor VS, CBC, BS, bleeding times, cultures, renal, and LFTs.

INTERVENTIONS

1. During drug therapy, assess for any of the following reactions that may require drug withdrawal:
- Skin rashes, abdominal pain, anorexia, mouth irritation or tingling of extremities
- Blood dyscrasias (characterized by sore throat, fever, pallor, purpura, jaundice, or weakness)
- Serum sickness (characterized by eruptions of purpuric spots and swelling/pain in limbs and joints); onset 7–10 days after initiation of therapy.
- Early S&S of Stevens-Johnson syndrome (characterized by high fever, severe headaches, stomatitis, conjunctivitis, rhinitis, urethritis, and balanitis [inflammation of the tip of the penis])
- Jaundice, indicating hepatic involvement; onset 3–5 days after initiation of therapy
- Renal involvement (characterized by renal colic, oliguria, anuria, hematuria, and proteinuria)
- Ecchymosis and hemorrhage (caused by decreased synthesis of vitamin K by intestinal bacteria)
- Hemolytic anemia especially in the elderly
- Behavioral changes or acute mental disturbances

2. Monitor I&O; ensure adequate fluid intake to prevent crystalluria. Check urinalysis for crystals. Minimum urine output should be 1.5 L/day. Test urine pH for excess acidity. Administration of a particularly insoluble sulfonamide may require urine alkalinization (i.e., NaHCO$_3$).
3. If administering long-acting sulfonamides, adequate fluid intake must be maintained for 24–48 hr after the drug has been discontinued.

CLIENT/FAMILY TEACHING

1. Take on time and as prescribed despite feeling better. Take with 6–8 oz (180–240 mL) of water and maintain adequate fluid intake for 24–48 hr after therapy. May take with food if GI upset.
2. Do not perform activities that require mental alertness until drug effects realized.
3. May cause N&V and loss of appetite. Monitor I&O; consume >2.5 L/day of fluids.
4. May color urine orange-red or brown; not cause for alarm but report.
5. Test urine pH and report changes in acidity as additional drug therapy may be necessary. Avoid Vitamin C; may make the urine more acidic and contribute to crystal formation.
6. If also taking anticoagulants, report increased bleeding tendencies.
7. Avoid prolonged exposure to sunlight; may cause a photosensitivity reaction. Wear protective clothing, sunglasses, and sunscreen.
8. Report any changes in vision or hearing. With ophthalmic use, report if no improvement in 5–7 days, if condition worsens, or if pain, redness, itching, or eye swelling occurs.
9. Vaginal intercourse should be avoided when using vaginal products.
10. Report for labs as scheduled; notify provider if symptoms do not improve or worsen after 48–72 hr.

Bold Italic = life threatening side effect   ■ = black box warning   ✦ = Available in Canada

OUTCOMES/EVALUATE

- Negative C&S results (note any organism resistance to sulfonamide)
- Resolution of infection; symptomatic improvement

SYMPATHOMIMETIC DRUGS

SEE ALSO THE FOLLOWING INDIVIDUAL ENTRIES:

Albuterol
Bitolterol mesylate
Brimonidine tartrate
Dobutamine hydrochloride
Dopamine hydrochloride
Ephedrine sulfate
Epinephrine
Epinephrine bitartrate
Epinephrine borate
Epinephrine hydrochloride
Formoterol
Isoproterenol hydrochloride
Isoproterenol sulfate
Metaproterenol sulfate
Phenylephrine hydrochloride
Pirbuterol acetate
Pseudoephedrine hydrochloride
Pseudoephedrine sulfate
Salmeterol xinafoate
Terbutaline sulfate

USES

See individual drugs.

ACTION/KINETICS

Action

Adrenergic drugs act: (1) by mimicking the action of norepinephrine or epinephrine by combining with alpha and/or beta receptors (directly acting sympathomimetics) or (2) by causing or regulating the release of the natural neurohormones from their storage sites at the nerve terminals (indirectly acting sympathomimetics). Some drugs exhibit a combination of both effects. Adrenergic stimulation of receptors will manifest the following general effects:

- *Alpha-1-adrenergic:* / Vasoconstriction, decongestion, constriction of the pupil of the eye, contraction of splenic capsule, contraction of the trigone-sphincter muscle of the urinary bladder.

- *Alpha-2-adrenergic:* / Presynaptic to regulate amount of transmitter released; decrease tone, motility, and secretory activity of the GI tract (possibly involved in hypersecretory response also); decrease insulin secretion.

- *Beta-1-adrenergic:* / Myocardial contraction (inotropic), regulation of heartbeat (chronotropic), improved impulse conduction, ↑ lipolysis.

- *Beta-2-adrenergic:* / Peripheral vasodilation, bronchial dilation; ↓ tone, motility, and secretory activity of the GI tract; ↑ renin secretion.

Beta adrenergic drugs stimulate adenyl cyclase which catalyzes the formation of cyclic AMP from ATP. The formed cyclic AMP inhibits release of mediators from mast cells and basophils that cause hypersensitivity reactions. The increase in cyclic AMP leads to activation of protein kinase A, which inhibits phosphorylation of myosin and lowers intracellular ionic calcium levels causing smooth muscle relaxation.

CONTRAINDICATIONS

Tachycardia due to arrhythmias; tachycardia or heart block caused by digitalis toxicity. See individual drugs.

SPECIAL CONCERNS

Use with caution in hyperthyroidism, diabetes, prostatic hypertrophy, seizures, degenerative heart disease, especially in geriatric clients or those with asthma, emphysema, or psychoneuroses. Also, use with caution in clients with coronary insufficiency, CAD, ischemic heart disease, CHF, cardiac arrhythmias, hypertension, or history of stroke. Asthma clients who rely heavily on inhaled beta-2-agonist bronchodilators may increase their chances of death. Thus, use to "rescue" clients but do not prescribe for regular long-term use. Beta-2 agonists may inhibit uterine contractions. Long-acting beta-2 adrenergic agonists (e.g., formoterol, salmeterol) have been associated with an increased risk of severe asthma episodes and death.

SIDE EFFECTS

See individual drugs; side effects common to most sympathomimetics are listed. **CV:** Tachycardia, arrhythmias, palpitations, BP changes, anginal pain, precordial pain, pallor, skipped beats, chest tightness, hypertension. **GI:** N&V, heartburn, anorexia, altered taste or bad taste, GI distress, dry mouth, diarrhea. **CNS:** Restlessness, anxiety, tension, insomnia, hyperkinesis, drowsiness, weakness, vertigo, irritability, dizziness, headache, tremors, general CNS stimulation, nervousness, shakiness, hyperactivity. **Respiratory:** Cough, dyspnea, dry throat, pharyngitis, *paradoxical bronchospasm,* irritation, *severe asthma episodes.* **Miscellaneous:** Flushing, sweating, *allergic reactions.*

OD OVERDOSE MANAGEMENT
Symptoms: **Following inhalation:** Exaggeration of side effects resulting in anginal pain, hypertension, hypokalemia, *seizures.* **Following systemic use:** CV symptoms include bradycardia, tachycardia, palpitations, extrasystoles, *heart block,* elevated BP, chest pain, hypokalemia. CNS symptoms include anxiety, insomnia, tremor, delirium, *convulsions, collapse,* and *coma.* Also, fever, chills, cold perspiration, N&V, mydriasis, and blanching of the skin.
Treatment: **For overdosage due to inhalation:** General supportive measures with sedatives given for restlessness. Use metoprolol or atenolol cautiously as they may induce an asthmatic attack in clients with asthma. **For systemic overdose:** Discontinue or decrease dose. General supportive measures. For overdose due to PO agents, emesis, gastric lavage, or charcoal may be helpful. In severe cases, propranolol may be used but this may cause airway obstruction. Phentolamine may be given to block strong alpha-adrenergic effects.

DRUG INTERACTIONS
Ammonium chloride / ↓ Effect of sympathomimetics R/T ↑ kidney excretion
Anesthetics / Halogenated anesthetics sensitize heart to adrenergics—causes cardiac arrhythmias
Anticholinergics / Concomitant use aggravates glaucoma
Antidiabetics / Hyperglycemic effect of epinephrine may necessitate ↑ dosage of insulin or oral hypoglycemic agents
Beta-adrenergic blocking agents / Inhibit

adrenergic stimulation of the heart and bronchial tree; cause bronchial constriction; hypertension, asthma, not relieved by adrenergic agents
Corticosteroids / Chronic use with sympathomimetics may result in or aggravate glaucoma; aerosols containing sympathomimetics and corticosteroids may be lethal in asthmatic children
Digitalis glycosides / Combination may cause cardiac arrhythmias
Furazolidone / ↑ Effects of mixed-acting sympathomimetics
Guanethidine / Direct-acting sympathomimetics ↑ drug effects, while indirect-acting sympathomimetics ↓ effects of guanethidine; also reversal of hypotensive drug effects
H *Indian snakeroot* / Initial significant ↑ BP
Lithium / ↓ Pressor effect of direct-acting sympathomimetics
MAO inhibitors / All effects of sympathomimetics are potentiated; symptoms include hypertensive crisis with possible intracranial hemorrhage, hyperthermia, convulsions, coma; death may occur
Methyldopa / ↑ Pressor response
Methylphenidate / Potentiates pressor effect of sympathomimetics; combination hazardous in glaucoma
Oxytocics / ↑ Chance of severe hypertension
Phenothiazines / ↑ Risk of cardiac arrhythmias
Sodium bicarbonate / ↑ Effect of sympathomimetics R/T ↓ kidney excretion
Theophylline / Enhanced toxicity (especially cardiotoxicity); also ↓ drug levels
Thyroxine / Potentiation of pressor response of sympathomimetics
Tricyclic antidepressants / ↑ Effect of direct-acting sympathomimetics and ↓ effect of indirect-acting sympathomimetics.

DOSAGE
See individual drugs.

NURSING CONSIDERATIONS
ADMINISTRATION/STORAGE
Discard colored solutions.
ASSESSMENT
1. Note reasons for therapy, contributing factors/triggers, clinical presenta-

---

tion, and desired response. Identify any sensitivity/previous use of adrenergic drugs/drugs in this class and outcome.
2. List history of CAD, tachycardia, endocrine disturbances, or respiratory tract problems.
3. Obtain baseline data regarding general physical condition, hemodynamic status including ECG, VS, labs, oxygen saturation, smoking history, work history with any exposure to chemicals/asbestos. Monitor PFTs and lab data including folate levels.

CLIENT/FAMILY TEACHING
1. Take exactly as directed. Do not increase dosage or take more frequently than prescribed. Consult provider if symptoms progress. Take early in the day to prevent insomnia.
2. Review prescribed drug therapy and potential side effects. Feelings/symptoms of fear or anxiety may be evident; these drugs mimic body's stress response. Avoid all OTC preparations.
3. Stop smoking to preserve current lung function. Attend formal smoking cessation classes.

SPECIAL NURSING CONSIDERATIONS FOR ADRENERGIC BRONCHODILATORS

ASSESSMENT
1. Obtain history and PE prior to starting therapy. Note any experience with this class of drugs.
2. Monitor VS; assess CV response. Evaluate cardiac function and note ejection fraction.
3. Document lung assessment, ABGs (or O_2 saturation), and PFTs. Note characteristics of cough and sputum production.

INTERVENTIONS
1. Observe effects on CNS; if pronounced, adjust dosage/frequency of administration.
2. With status asthmaticus and abnormal ABGs, continue to provide oxygen and ventilatory assistance even though the symptoms appear to be relieved by the bronchodilator. To prevent depression of respiratory effort, administer oxygen based on client's clinical symptoms and ABGs or O_2 saturations.

3. If three to five aerosol treatments of the same agent have been administered within the last 6–12 hr, with no relief, further evaluation is warranted. If dyspnea worsens after repeated excessive use of the inhaler, paradoxical airway resistance may occur. Be prepared to assist with alternative therapy and respiratory support.

CLIENT/FAMILY TEACHING
1. Review technique for use/care of inhalers and respiratory equipment. Rinsing of equipment and mouth after use is imperative to prevent oral fungal infections. Maintain record of peak flow readings and seek medical attention as directed.
2. To improve lung ventilation and reduce fatigue during eating, start inhalation therapy upon arising in the morning and before meals.
3. Regular, consistent use of the drug is essential for maximum benefit, but overuse can be life-threatening. If using inhalable medications and bronchodilators, use the bronchodilator first and wait 5 min before using the other medication.
4. A single aerosol treatment is usually enough to control an asthma attack. Overuse of adrenergic bronchodilators may result in reduced effectiveness, paradoxical reaction, and death from cardiac arrest. Consult provider if more than three (or prescribed number) aerosol treatments in a 24-hr period are required for relief.
5. With postural drainage, review how to cough productively and show family how to clap and vibrate the chest and position client to promote good respiratory hygiene.
6. Increased fluid intake will aid in liquefying secretions and removal. Consult provider if dizziness or chest pain occurs, or if there is no relief when the usual dose is used.
7. Avoid OTC preparations and any other unprescribed adrenergic medications.
8. **Stop smoking,** avoid crowds during "flu seasons," dress warmly in cold weather and cover mouth with scarf to filter cold air, receive the pneumonia

vaccine and seasonal flu shot, and stay in air conditioning during hot, humid days to prevent exacerbations of illness. Identify triggers and practice avoidance. Have family/significant other learn CPR.

OUTCOMES/EVALUATE

- Improved airway exchange with ↓ dyspnea/wheezing
- ↑ Exercise tolerance
- ↑ BP/cardiac output
- ↓ Nasal congestion

TETRACYCLINES

SEE ALSO THE FOLLOWING INDIVIDUAL ENTRIES:

Doxycycline calcium
Doxycycline hyclate
Doxycycline monohydrate
Tetracycline hydrochloride

USES
See individual drugs. Uses include: (1) Infections caused by *Rickettsiae* (Rocky Mountain spotted fever, typhus fever and the typhus group, Q fever, rickettsial pox, and tick fevers); *Mycoplasma pneumonia*; agents of psittacosis and ornithosis; agents of lymphogranuloma venereum and granuloma inguinale; *Borrelia recurrentis*. (2) Gram-negative infections caused by *Haemophilus ducreyi* (chancroid); *Yersinia pestis* (plague) and *Francisella tularensis* (tularemia). *Bartonella bacilliformis, Bacteroides* species, *Campylobacter fetus, Vibrio cholerae* (cholera), *Brucella* species (with streptomycin). (3) Infections due to *Chlamydia trachomatis* (lymphogranuloma venereum, trachoma, inclusion conjunctivitis, uncomplicated urethral, endocervical, or rectal infections), *Chlamydia psittaci* (psittacosis), *Borrelia* species (relapsing fever), *Ureaplasma urealyticum* (nongonococcal urethritis). (4) Infections caused by the following microorganisms when testing indicates appropriate susceptibility: *Escherichia coli, Enterobacter aerogenes, Shigella* species, *Acinetobacter calcoaceticus, H. influenzae* (respiratory infections), *Klebsiella* species (respiratory and urinary infections). *Streptococcus* species, including

S. pneumoniae. S. pyogenes (skin and skin structure infections). *Mycoplasma pneumoniae*, and *Klebsiella* species (lower respiratory tract infections), *Staphylococcus aureus, Bacteroides*, and *Shigella* species. (NOTE: Up to 44% of *S. pyogenes* strains and 74% of *S. faecalis* strains are resistant to tetracyclines). (5) As part of combination therapy (e.g., with three or more of the following: Bismuth subsalicylate, metronidazole, omeprazole or lansoprazole, clarithromycin, amoxicillin, H_2-receptor antagonist) to provide symptomatic relief and accelerated ulcer healing for *Helicobacter pylori* eradication. (6) Treatment of trachoma, although the infectious agent is not always eliminated. (7) When penicillin is contraindicated, including infections caused by *Neisseria gonorrhoeae, Treponema pallidum* and *T. pertenue* (syphilis and yaws). Also, *Listeria monocytogenes, Clostridium* species, *Bacillus anthracis, Fusobacterium fusiforme, Actinomycetes* species, *N. meningitis* (IV only). (8) Acute intestinal amebiasis due to *Entamoeba histolytica*. (9) PO in adults to treat uncomplicated urethral, endocervical, or rectal infections due to *Chlamydia trachomatis*. (10) PO as adjunctive therapy to treat severe acne. (11) PO with topical agents to treat inclusion conjunctivitis.

ACTION/KINETICS

Action
Tetracyclines inhibit protein synthesis by microorganisms by binding to the ribosomal 30S subunit, thereby interfering with protein synthesis. They block the binding of aminoacyl transfer RNA to the messenger RNA complex. Cell wall synthesis is not inhibited. Are mostly bacteriostatic and are effective only against multiplying bacteria.

Pharmacokinetics
Adequately, but incompletely, absorbed from the GI tract. Well distributed throughout all tissues and fluids and diffuse through noninflamed meninges and the placental barrier. Are deposited in the fetal skeleton and calcifying teeth. $t\frac{1}{2}$: 7–18.6 hr (see individual agents); increased in the presence of renal impairment. They bind to serum

---

Bold Italic = life threatening side effect   ▪ = black box warning   ♣ = Available in Canada

protein (range: 20–93%; see individual agents). Concentrated in the liver in the bile; excreted mostly unchanged in the urine and feces.

CONTRAINDICATIONS

Hypersensitivity. Use during tooth development stage (last trimester of pregnancy, neonatal period, during breast-feeding, and during childhood up to 8 years) because tetracyclines interfere with enamel formation and dental pigmentation. May be used in children under 8 years of age who have anthrax (including inhalational) only if other drugs are not likely to be effective or are contraindicated. Never administer intrathecally.

SPECIAL CONCERNS

Use with caution and at reduced dosage in clients with impaired kidney function.

SIDE EFFECTS

See individual drugs. **GI:** Anorexia, N&V, diarrhea, glossitis, dysphagia, enterocolitis, inflammatory lesions (with monilial overgrowth) in the anogenital region, esophageal ulcerations, pancreatitis, dyspepsia, stomatitis, enamel hypoplasia, pseudomembranous colitis, esophagitis, bulky loose stools, sore throat, black hairy tongue, hoarseness. **CNS:** Dizziness, headache, bulging fontanel, pseudotumor cerebri, convulsions, hypesthesia, paresthesia, sedation, vertigo. **Dermatologic:** Maculopapular and erythematous rashes, photosensitivity, fixed drug eruptions, balanitis, erythema multiforme, *Stevens-Johnson syndrome, toxic epidermal necrolysis,* skin and mucous membrane pigmentation, alopecia, erythema nodosum, hyperpigmentation of the nails, pruritus, vasculitis, exfoliative dermatitis (rare). **Hematologic:** Anemia, hemolytic anemia, thrombocytopenia, neutropenia, eosinophilia. **Hepatic:** Hepatic toxicity, hepatic cholestasis, *hepatic failure,* hepatitis (rare). **Hypersensitivity:** Urticaria, angioneurotic edema, pericarditis, *anaphylaxis,* anaphylactoid purpura, exacerbation of systemic lupus erythematosus, polyarthralgia, pulmonary infiltrates with eosinophilia. **Musculoskeletal:** Arthralgia, arthritis, bone discoloration, myalgia, joint stiffness, swelling. **GU:** Acute renal failure, interstitial nephritis, vulvovaginitis. **Respiratory:** Cough, dyspnea, bronchospasm, exacerbation of asthma. **Miscellaneous:** Brown-black microscopic discoloration of thyroid glands after prolonged therapy, tooth discoloration, lupus-like syndrome, fever, discolored secretions, tinnitus, decreased hearing, serum sickness-like syndrome.

IV administration may cause thrombophlebitis. IM injections are painful and may cause induration at the injection site.

Use of deteriorated tetracyclines may result in *Fanconi-like* syndrome characterized by N&V, acidosis, proteinuria, glycosuria, aminoaciduria, polydipsia, polyuria, hypokalemia.

OD OVERDOSE MANAGEMENT

Symptoms: The most common effects are dizziness and N&V.

Treatment: Discontinue the drug. Begin symptomatic treatment and supportive measures. Tetracyclines are not significantly removed by hemodialysis or peritoneal dialysis.

DRUG INTERACTIONS

Aluminum salts / ↓ Effect of tetracyclines R/T ↓ GI tract absorption

Antacids, oral / ↓ Effect of tetracyclines R/T ↓ GI tract absorption

Anticoagulants, oral / IV tetracyclines ↑ hypoprothrombinemia; also, ↑ action of PO anticoagulants R/T elimination of vitamin K-producing gut bacteria by tetracyclines

Bismuth salts / ↓ Effect of tetracyclines R/T ↓ GI tract absorption; give bismuth 2 hr after the tetracycline

H *Bromelain /* ↑ Plasma tetracycline levels

Bumetanide / ↑ Risk of kidney toxicity

Calcium salts / ↓ Effect of tetracyclines R/T ↓ GI tract absorption

Cholestyramine/Colestipol / ↓ or Delayed absorption of tetracyclines → ↓ plasma levels

Cimetidine / ↓ Effect of tetracyclines R/T ↓ GI tract absorption

Digoxin / ↑ Bioavailability of digoxin

Diuretics, thiazide / ↑ Risk of kidney toxicity

Classifications

Ethacrynic acid / ↑ Risk of kidney toxicity

Furosemide / ↑ Risk of kidney toxicity

Insulin / Potentiation of ability of insulin to produce hypoglycemia; monitor BG closely and alter insulin regimen as needed

Iron preparations / ↓ Effect of tetracyclines R/T ↓ GI tract absorption

Isotretinoin / ↑ Incidence of pseudotumor cerebi; avoid concomitant use

Magnesium salts / ↓ Effect of tetracyclines R/T ↓ GI tract absorption

Methoxyflurane / ↑ Risk of kidney toxicity

Oral contraceptives / ↓ OC efficacy R/T interference with enterohepatic recirculation of certain contraceptive steroids by tetracyclines

Penicillins / Tetracyclines may interfere with the bactericidal activity of penicillins

Potassium citrate / ↑ Tetracycline excretion and ↓ serum levels

Sodium bicarbonate / ↓ Effect of tetracyclines R/T ↓ GI tract absorption

Sodium lactate / ↑ Tetracycline excretion and ↓ serum levels

Theophyllines / ↑ Incidence of theophylline side effects

Zinc salts / ↓ Effect of tetracyclines R/T ↓ GI tract absorption.

LABORATORY TEST CONSIDERATIONS
False + or ↑ urinary catecholamines and urinary protein (degraded); ↑ coagulation time. False – or ↓ urinary urobilinogen, glucose tests (see *Nursing Considerations*). Prolonged use or high doses may change liver function tests and WBC counts.

DOSAGE————————
See individual drugs.

NURSING CONSIDERATIONS

ADMINISTRATION/STORAGE

1. Do not use outdated or deteriorated drugs as a Fanconi-like syndrome may occur (see *Side Effects*).
2. Administer IM into large muscle mass to avoid extravasation into subcutaneous or fatty tissue.
3. Continue treatment for 24–48 hr after symptoms and fever subside. Treat all infections due to group A

β–hemolytic streptococci for 10 or more days.

[IV] 4. Avoid rapid IV administration.
5. Prolonged IV use may cause thrombophlebitis.
6. Reserve IV use for situations where PO therapy is not indicated/tolerated. Institute PO therapy asap.

ASSESSMENT
1. Note reasons for therapy, onset, characteristics of S&S, clinical presentation, culture results. List other agents trialed and outcome.
2. Identify any drug allergens or sensitivity. IM form contains procaine HCl; assess for reactions.
3. Assess for colitis or other bowel problems. If pregnant, document trimester.
4. Monitor VS, weight, CBC, BUN, creatinine, lytes, and cultures. Assess for impaired kidney function.

INTERVENTIONS
1. Monitor VS and I&O. Maintain adequate I&O as renal dysfunction may result in drug accumulation, leading to toxicity. With impaired renal function assess for increased BUN, acidosis, anorexia, N&V, weight loss, and dehydration; latent symptoms. Assess for altered level of consciousness or other CNS disturbances with impaired hepatic or renal function; may cause toxicity.
2. To prevent/treat pruritus ani, cleanse anal area with water several times a day and/or after each bowel movement. Observe for S&S of enterocolitis, such as diarrhea, pyrexia, abdominal distention, and scanty urine; may need to stop and try another antibiotic.
3. If GI disturbances occur, avoid antacids that contain calcium, magnesium, or aluminum. May take with a light meal or reduce dose but increase administration frequency to reduce distress.
4. Assess with IV therapy for N&V, chills, fever, and hypertension resulting from too rapid administration or an excessively high dose; slow rate/report. Observe infant for bulging fontanel, which may be caused by a too rapid infusion rate.
5. Side effects such as sore throat, dysphagia, fever, dizziness, hoarseness, and

---

inflammation of mucous membranes or candidal superinfections may occur. May cause onycholysis (loosening or detachment of the nail from the nail bed) or discoloration.

CLIENT/FAMILY TEACHING

1. Take on an empty stomach at least 1 hr before or 2 hr after meals. Withhold antacids, iron salts, dairy foods, and other foods high in calcium for at least 2 hr after PO administration. Do not take with milk, cheese, ice cream or yogurt.

2. Zinc tablets or vitamin preparations containing zinc may interfere with drug absorption. Food sources high in zinc that should be avoided include oysters, fresh and raw; cooked lobster; dry oat flakes; steamed crabs; veal; and liver.

3. Avoid direct or artificial sunlight, which can cause a severe sunburn-like reaction; report if erythema occurs. Wear protective clothing, sunglasses, and sunscreen for up to 3 weeks following therapy.

4. Tetracyclines interfere with formation of tooth enamel and dental pigmentation from the third trimester of pregnancy through age 8.

5. Prevent/treat rectal itching by cleansing anal area with water several times a day and/or after each bowel movement.

6. Use alternative method of birth control, as drug may interfere with oral contraceptives; may also cause a vaginal infection.

7. Take only as directed and complete full prescription. Discard any unused capsules to prevent reaction from deteriorated drugs. Report loss of effectiveness or lack of response.

8. Keep all F/U appointments to evaluate response to therapy, labs, and for adverse effects.

OUTCOMES/EVALUATE

- Resolution of infection (↓ temperature, ↓ WBCs, ↑ appetite)
- Symptomatic improvement
- Negative culture reports

THYROID DRUGS ∎

SEE ALSO THE FOLLOWING INDIVIDUAL ENTRIES:

Levothyroxin sodium

Liothyronine sodium

Liotrix

USES

(1) Replacement or supplemental therapy in hypothyroidism due to all causes except transient hypothyroidism during the recovery phase of subacute thyroiditis. (2) Treat or prevent euthyroid goiters, including thyroid nodules, subacute or chronic lymphocytic thyroiditis, multinodular goiter, and to manage thyroid cancer. (3) With antithyroid drugs for thyrotoxicosis (to prevent goiter or hypothyroidism). (4) Diagnostically to differentiate suspected hyperthyroidism from euthyroidism. (5) Myxedema coma and precoma. The treatment of choice for hypothyroidism is usually T_4 because of its consistent potency and its prolonged duration of action although it does have a slow onset and its effects are cumulative over several weeks.

ACTION/KINETICS

Action

The thyroid manufactures two active hormones: Thyroxine and triiodothyronine, both of which contain iodine. Thyroid hormones are released into the bloodstream where they are bound to protein. Synthetic derivatives include liothyronine (T_3), levothyroxine (T_4), and liotrix (a 4:1 mixture of T_4 and T_3). Thyroid hormones regulate growth by controlling protein synthesis and regulating energy metabolism by increasing the resting or basal metabolic rate. This increases respiratory rate, body temperature, CO, oxygen consumption, HR, blood volume, enzyme system activity, rate of fat, carbohydrate and protein metabolism, and growth and maturation. Excess thyroid hormone causes a decrease in TSH, and a lack of thyroid hormone causes an increase in the production and secretion of TSH. Normally, the ratio of T_4 to T_3 released from the thyroid gland is 20:1 with about 35% of T_4 being converted in the periphery (e.g., kidney, liver) to T_3.

Pharmacokinetics

More than 99% of circulating hormone is bound to serum proteins. Thyroid

Classifications

hormones are primarily excreted through the kidney, with about 20% eliminated in the feces.

CONTRAINDICATIONS

Uncorrected adrenal insufficiency, acute MI, hyperthyroidism, and untreated thyrotoxicosis. When hypothyroidism and adrenal insufficiency coexist unless treatment with adrenocortical steroids is initiated first. To treat obesity or infertility. Levothyroxine use in those with unrelated subclinical suppressed serum TSH with normal T_3 and T_4 levels and in acute MI.

SPECIAL CONCERNS

■Drugs with thyroid hormone activity, alone or with other drugs, have been used to treat obesity. In euthyroid clients, doses within the range of daily hormonal requirements are ineffective for weight reduction. Larger doses may produce serious or even life-threatening toxic effects, especially when given in association with sympathomimetic amines (e.g., those used for their anorectic effects).■ Geriatric clients and those with myxedema may be more sensitive to the usual adult dosage of these hormones. Use with extreme caution in the presence of angina pectoris, hypertension, and other CV diseases, renal insufficiency, and ischemic states. Use with caution during lactation and in clients with nontoxic diffuse goiter or nodular thyroid disease (i.e., to prevent thyrotoxicosis). Safety and efficacy have not been determined in children.

SIDE EFFECTS

Thyroid preparations have cumulative effects, and overdosage (e.g., symptoms of hyperthyroidism) may occur. **CV:** Arrhythmias, palpitations, angina, increased BP and pulse pressure, CHF, tachycardia, *MI, cardiac arrest,* aggravation of CHF. **GI:** Abdominal cramps, diarrhea, N&V, appetite changes. **CNS:** Headache, nervousness, mental agitation, irritability, insomnia, tremors, hyperactivity, anxiety, emotional lability, seizures (rare). **Hypersensitivity:** Urticaria, pruritus, skin rash, flushing, angioedema, abdominal pain, N&V, diarrhea, fever, arthralgia, serum sickness, wheezing, allergic skin reactions (rare).

Miscellaneous: Weight loss, hyperhidrosis, excessive warmth, irregular menses, heat intolerance, fatigue, fever, muscle weakness, dyspnea, hair loss, impaired fertility. Decreased bone density in pre- and postmenopausal women following long-term use of levothyroxine. *NOTE:* Pseudotumor cerebri and slipped capital femoral epiphysis seen in children receiving levothyroxine. Overtreatment may cause craniosynostosis in infants and premature closure of the epiphyses in children leading to compromised adult height.

OD OVERDOSE MANAGEMENT

Symptoms: Signs and symptoms of hyperthyroidism including headache, irritability, sweating, tachycardia, nervousness, increased bowel motility, palpitations, vomiting, psychosis, menstrual irregularities, *seizures,* fever. Production or aggravation of angina or CHF, *shock, arrhythmias, cardiac failure.*
Treatment: Reduce dose or temporarily discontinue therapy. Reinstitute therapy at a lower dosage.

DRUG INTERACTIONS

Amiodarone / ↓ T_3 levels
Antacids, Al- and Mg-containing / ↓ Thyroid absorption from the GI tract
Anticoagulants / ↑ Effect of anticoagulants by ↑ hypoprothrombinemia
Antidepressants, tricyclic or tetracyclic / ↑ Therapeutic and toxic effects of both antidepressants and thyroid drugs
Antidiabetic agents / Hyperglycemic effect of thyroid preparations may necessitate ↑ in dose of both insulin or oral hypoglycemics
Beta-adrenergic blockers / ↓ Effect of beta blockers when the hypothyroid state is converted to the euthyroid state
Calcium salts / ↓ Thyroid absorption from the GI tract
Carbamazepine / ↑ Liver metabolism of levothyroxine → ↑ levothyroxine requirements
Cholestyramine / ↓ Effect of thyroid hormone R/T ↓ GI tract absorption
Colestipol / ↓ Effect of thyroid hormone R/T ↓ GI tract absorption
Corticosteroids / Thyroid preparations ↑ tissue demands for corticosteroids. Adrenal insufficiency must be corrected

---

Bold Italic = life threatening side effect   ■ = black box warning   ✦ = Available in Canada

with corticosteroids before administering thyroid hormones. In clients already treated for adrenal insufficiency, dosage of corticosteroids must be increased when initiating therapy with thyroid drug

Digitalis compounds / ↓ Digitalis glycoside levels; ↓ therapeutic effects

Epinephrine / CV effects ↑ by thyroid preparations; ↑ risk of coronary insufficiency

Estrogens / May ↑ requirements for thyroid hormone

Growth hormone (somatrem, somatropin) / Excessive use of thyroid and growth hormone may accelerate epiphyseal closure

Iron salts / ↓ Absorption of thyroid from the GI tract

Ketamine / Concomitant use may result in severe hypertension and tachycardia

Levarterenol / CV effects ↑ by thyroid preparations; ↑ risk of coronary insufficiency

Oral contraceptives / May ↑ requirements for thyroid hormone

Phenobarbital / ↑ Liver metabolism of levothyroxine → ↑ levothyroxine requirements

Phenytoin / ↑ Liver metabolism of levothyroxine → ↑ levothyroxine requirements

Rifamycins / ↑ Liver metabolism of levothyroxine → ↑ levothyroxine requirements

Salicylates / Salicylates compete for thyroid-binding sites on protein

Simethicone / ↓ Thyroid absorption from the GI tract

Sodium polystyrene sulfonate / ↓ Thyroid absorption from the GI tract

H *Soy* / ↓ Absorption of supplemental thyroid hormones; space doses 2 hr apart

Sucralfate / ↓ Thyroid absorption from the GI tract

Theophylline / ↓ Theophylline clearance in hypothyroid client is returned to normal when euthyroid state is reached.

LABORATORY TEST CONSIDERATIONS
Alter thyroid function tests. ↑ PT. ↓ Serum cholesterol. A large number of drugs alter thyroid function tests.

DOSAGE
See individual hormone products.

NURSING CONSIDERATIONS
ADMINISTRATION/STORAGE
1. Initiate treatment with small doses that are gradually increased.
2. A child's dosage may be the same as the dosage for an adult.
3. Differences between brands of a drug mean that brand interchange is not recommended without consulting with provider or pharmacist. Use caution to prevent overdosage or relapse.
4. Store in a cool, dark place away from moisture and light.

ASSESSMENT
1. Perform a thorough history, documenting onset and characteristics of S&S and thyroid function tests (TFTs).
2. Review all medications currently receiving to be sure none interacts with antithyroid drug; especially antidiabetic or anticoagulant therapy.
3. Assess clinical presentation noting S&S consistent with hypothyroidism (i.e., fatigue, lethargy, weight gain, puffy face and eyelids, large tongue, thyroid nodules, cold intolerance, hair loss, and cardiomegaly).
4. Assess general physical condition (age, weight, disease severity/duration) and note angina, cardiac or other health problems. Obtain/monitor ECG, labs, and TFTs.

INTERVENTIONS
1. Note agent prescribed; thyroid extracts from hog or sheep do not have as predictable a response as the synthetic agents, may see more reactions. Animal derivatives are less stable and will degrade with exposure to moisture. Monitor thyroid function studies closely (for reduced T_3, T_4; ↑ radioimmunoassay of TSH).
2. Observe for drug side effects; report complaints of headache, insomnia, and tremors. Note general response to therapy. Complaints of abdominal cramps, weight gain, edema, dyspnea, palpitations, angina, fatigue, or ↑ pallor may indicate cardiac problems.
3. With anticoagulant therapy observe for purpura or ↑ bleeding. Monitor PT/

Classifications

PTT/INR closely; anticoagulant potentiated by thyroid preparations.

4. Report any S&S or history of CAD. Monitor VS and cardiac rhythms; report if HR >100 bpm. Monitor weights. Observe for heat intolerance and excessive weight loss.

5. Stop drug therapy 4 weeks before radioimmunoassay.

CLIENT/FAMILY TEACHING

1. Drug must be taken only under medical supervision and must be taken for life. Take in a single morning dose, at the same time each day, to reduce the likelihood of insomnia.

2. Side effects may not appear for 4–6 weeks after the start of therapy or when dosage increased. Do not substitute or change brands without approval.

3. Record BP, pulse, and weight for review at each visit, to evaluate effectiveness of drug therapy. Any excessive weight loss, palpitations, leg cramps, nervousness, or insomnia requires immediate reporting, as dosage may be too high.

4. Carefully monitor child's growth and chart. Children may experience temporary hair loss.

5. With diabetes, thyroid preparations may require adjustment of insulin dosage. Monitor BS closely and report changes.

6. Certain foods, such as cabbage, turnips, pears, and peaches, are goitrogenic and may alter the requirements for thyroid hormone. Consult dietitian to discuss diet and assist with selecting foods according to increased energy demands resulting from the therapy. Thyroid hormones increase toxicity to iodine. Avoid foods high in iodine (dried kelp, iodized salt, saltwater fish/shellfish), multivitamins, dentifrices, and other nonprescription medications containing iodine.

7. Thyroid preparations potentiate the action of anticoagulants; if receiving anticoagulant therapy, report excessive bleeding. Keep a record of menstrual cycles and report changes.

8. After several weeks of therapy, report if irritability, nervousness, and excitability occur; may indicate overdosage.

9. Report as scheduled for follow-up visits to evaluate response to therapy, lab tests and for adverse side effects.

OUTCOMES/EVALUATE

• TFTs within desired range
• Normal metabolism evidenced by ↑ mental alertness, improvement in hair and skin condition, ↓ fatigue, ↓ panic attacks, normal growth/development, normal HR, regular bowel function

TRANQUILIZERS/ ANTIMANIC DRUGS/ HYPNOTICS

SEE ALSO THE FOLLOWING INDIVIDUAL ENTRIES:

Alprazolam
Buspirone hydrochloride
Chlordiazepoxide
Clorazepate dipotassium
Diazepam
Estazolam*
Eszopiclone
Flurazepam hydrochloride*
Hydroxyzine hydrochloride
Hydroxyzine pamoate
Lithium carbonate
Lithium citrate
Lorazepam
Midazolam hydrochloride
Ramelteon
Temazepam
Triazolam
Zaleplon
Zolpidem tartrate

Drugs marked with an * are available to view in the online database at www.delmarnursesdrughandbook.com/2009.

USES

See individual drugs. Depending on the drug, used as antianxiety agents, hypnotics, anticonvulsants, and muscle relaxants. Many drugs also have special uses (see individual drugs).

Bold Italic = life threatening side effect   ■ = black box warning   ♣ = Available in Canada

Classifications

ACTION/KINETICS

Action

Benzodiazepines are the major antianxiety agents. They are thought to affect the limbic system and reticular formation to reduce anxiety by increasing or facilitating the inhibitory neurotransmitter activity of GABA. Two benzodiazepine receptor subtypes have been identified in the brain—BZ_1 and BZ_2. Receptor subtype BZ_1 is believed to be associated with sleep mechanisms, whereas receptor subtype BZ_2 is associated with memory, motor, sensory, and cognitive function. When used for 3–4 weeks for sleep, certain benzodiazepines may cause REM rebound when discontinued. The benzodiazepines also possess varying degrees of anticonvulsant activity, skeletal muscle relaxation, and the ability to alleviate tension. The benzodiazepines generally have long half-lives (1–8 days); thus cumulative effects can occur. Several of the benzodiazepines are metabolized to active metabolites in the liver, which prolongs their duration of action.

Pharmacokinetics

Benzodiazepines are widely distributed throughout the body. Approximately 70–99% of an administered dose is bound to plasma protein. Metabolites of benzodiazepines are excreted through the kidneys. All tranquilizers have the ability to cause psychologic and physical dependence. Benzodiazepines have a wide margin of safety between therapeutic and toxic doses.

CONTRAINDICATIONS

Hypersensitivity, acute narrow-angle glaucoma, psychoses, primary depressive disorder, psychiatric disorders in which anxiety is not a significant symptom.

SPECIAL CONCERNS

Use with caution in impaired hepatic or renal function and in the geriatric or debilitated client. Use during lactation may cause sedation, weight loss, and possibly feeding difficulties in the infant. Geriatric clients may be more sensitive to the effects of benzodiazepines; symptoms may include oversedation, dizziness, confusion, or ataxia. Increased risk of hip fracture with benzodiazepine use in the elderly, especially during the first 2 weeks. When used for insomnia, rebound sleep disorders may occur following abrupt withdrawal of certain benzodiazepines.

SIDE EFFECTS

CNS: Drowsiness, fatigue, confusion, ataxia, sedation, dizziness, vertigo, depression, apathy, lightheadedness, delirium, headache, lethargy, disorientation, hypoactivity, crying, anterograde amnesia, slurred speech, stupor, *coma,* fainting, difficulty in concentration, euphoria, nervousness, irritability, akathisia, hypotonia, vivid dreams, "glassy-eyed," hysteria, *suicide attempt,* psychosis. Paradoxical excitement manifested by anxiety, acute hyperexcitability, increased muscle spasticity, insomnia, hallucinations, sleep disturbances, rage, and stimulation. **GI:** Increased appetite, constipation, diarrhea, anorexia, N&V, weight gain or loss, dry mouth, bitter or metallic taste, increased salivation, coated tongue, sore gums, difficulty in swallowing, gastritis, fecal incontinence. **Respiratory:** *Respiratory depression and sleep apnea,* especially in clients with compromised respiratory function. **Dermatologic:** Urticaria, rash, pruritus, alopecia, hirsutism, dermatitis, edema of ankles and face. **Endocrine:** Increased or decreased libido, gynecomastia, menstrual irregularities. **GU:** Difficulty in urination, urinary retention, incontinence, dysuria, enuresis. **CV:** Hypertension, hypotension, bradycardia, tachycardia, palpitations, edema, *CV collapse.* **Hematologic:** Anemia, *agranulocytosis,* leukopenia, eosinophilia, thrombocytopenia. **Ophthalmic:** Diplopia, conjunctivitis, nystagmus, blurred vision. **Miscellaneous:** Joint pain, lymphadenopathy, muscle cramps, paresthesia, dehydration, lupus-like symptoms, sweating, SOB, flushing, hiccoughs, fever, hepatic dysfunction. **Following IM use:** Redness, pain, burning. **Following IV use:** Thrombosis and phlebitis at site.

OD OVERDOSE MANAGEMENT

Symptoms: Severe drowsiness, confusion with reduced or absent reflexes,

---

Classifications

tremors, slurred speech, staggering, hypotension, SOB, labored breathing, **respiratory depression,** impaired coordination, **seizures,** weakness, slow HR, **coma.** *NOTE:* Geriatric clients, debilitated clients, young children, and clients with liver disease are more sensitive to the CNS effects of benzodiazepines.

Treatment: Supportive therapy. In the event of an overdose of a benzodiazepine, have a benzodiazepine antagonist (flumazenil) readily available. Gastric lavage, provided that an ET tube with an inflated cuff is used to prevent aspiration of vomitus. Emesis only if drug ingestion was recent and client is fully conscious. Activated charcoal and saline cathartic may be given after emesis or lavage. Maintain adequate respiratory function. Reverse hypotension by IV fluids, norepinephrine, or metaraminol. **Do not** treat excitation with barbiturates.

DRUG INTERACTIONS

Alcohol / Potentiation or addition of CNS depressant effects; concomitant use may lead to drowsiness, lethargy, stupor, respiratory collapse, coma, or death

Anesthetics, general / See *Alcohol*

Antacids / ↓ Rate of absorption of benzodiazepines

Antidepressants, tricyclic / Concomitant use with benzodiazepines may cause additive sedative effect and/or atropine-like side effects

Antihistamines / See *Alcohol*

Barbiturates / See *Alcohol*

Cimetidine / ↑ Effect of benzodiazepines R/T ↓ liver breakdown

CNS depressants / See *Alcohol*

Digoxin / Benzodiazepines ↑ serum digoxin levels

Disulfiram / ↑ Effect of benzodiazepines by ↓ liver breakdown

Erythromycin / ↑ Effect of benzodiazepines by ↓ liver breakdown

Fluoxetine / ↑ Effect of benzodiazepines R/T ↓ liver breakdown

Grapefruit juice / ↑ Bioavailability of certain benzodiazepines (e.g., midazolam)

Isoniazid / ↑ Effect of benzodiazepines R/T ↓ liver breakdown

H *Kava kava* / Additive CNS depressant effect

Ketoconazole / ↑ Effect of benzodiazepines R/T ↓ liver breakdown

Levodopa / Effect may be ↓ by benzodiazepines

Metoprolol / ↑ Effect of benzodiazepines R/T ↓ liver breakdown

Narcotics / See *Alcohol*

Neuromuscular blocking agents / Benzodiazepines may ↑, ↓, or have no effect on the action of neuromuscular blocking agents

Oral contraceptives / ↑ Effect of benzodiazepines R/T ↓ liver breakdown; or, ↑ rate of clearance of benzodiazepines that undergo glucuronidation (e.g., lorazepam, oxazepam)

Phenothiazines / See *Alcohol*

Phenytoin / Concomitant use with benzodiazepines may cause ↑ effect of phenytoin R/T ↓ liver breakdown

Probenecid / ↑ Effect of selected benzodiazepines R/T ↓ liver breakdown

Propoxyphene / ↑ Effect of benzodiazepines R/T ↓ liver breakdown

Propranolol / ↑ Effect of benzodiazepines R/T ↓ liver breakdown

Ranitidine / May ↓ absorption of benzodiazepines from the GI tract

Rifampin / ↓ Effect of benzodiazepines R/T ↑ liver breakdown

Sedative-hypnotics, nonbarbiturate / See *Alcohol*

Smoking / ↓ Benzodiazepine-induced sedation and drowsiness possibly R/T nicotine stimulation of the CNS

Theophyllines / ↓ Sedative effect of benzodiazepines

H *Valerian* / Additive CNS depressant effect

Valproic acid / ↑ Effect of benzodiazepines R/T ↓ liver breakdown.

LABORATORY TEST CONSIDERATIONS

↑ AST, ALT, LDH, alkaline phosphatase.

DOSAGE

See individual drugs.

NURSING CONSIDERATIONS

ADMINISTRATION/STORAGE

1. Persistent drowsiness, ataxia, or visual disturbances may require dosage adjustment.

---

2. Lower dosage is usually indicated for older clients. For example, diazepam, 3 mg or more equivalents/day, increases the risk of hip fracture in the elderly.

3. GI effects are decreased when drugs are given with meals or shortly afterward.

4. Withdraw drugs gradually.

ASSESSMENT

1. Note reasons for therapy, onset of symptoms, behavioral manifestations/clinical presentation. Assess manner in which client responds to questions/problems. Identify any prior treatments, what was used, for how long, and the outcome.

2. List drugs currently prescribed to ensure none interact unfavorably. Check for any adverse reactions to this class of drugs. Review physical exam, reflexes, CNS findings and history for any contraindications to therapy.

3. Assess lifestyle and general level of health; note any situations that may contribute to these symptoms.

4. Monitor VS, I&O, CBC, renal, and LFTs; assess for blood dyscrasias or impaired function.

INTERVENTIONS

1. Administer the lowest possible effective dose, esp if elderly or debilitated. Note any symptoms consistent with overdosage.

2. Report complaints of sore throat (other than those caused by NG or ET tubes), fever, or weakness and assess for blood dyscrasias; check CBC.

3. Monitor BP before and after IV dose of antianxiety medication. Keep recumbent for 2–3 hr after IV. When hospitalized and given PO, remain until swallowed.

4. If client exhibits ataxia, or weakness or lack of coordination when ambulating, provide supervision/assistance. Use side rails once in bed and identify clients at risk for falls; utilize alarms to prevent falls.

5. Note any S&S of cholestatic jaundice: nausea, diarrhea, upper abdominal pain, or the presence of high fever or rash; check LFTs. Report if yellowing of sclera, skin, or mucous membranes evident (late sign of cholestatic jaundice

and biliary tract obstruction); hold if overly sleepy/confused or becomes comatose.

6. With suicidal tendencies, anticipate drug will be prescribed in small doses/quanities. Report signs of increased depression immediately.

7. If history of alcoholism or if taking excessive quantities of drug, carefully supervise amount prescribed and dispensed. Note any evidence of physical or psychologic dependence. Assess for manifestations of ataxia, slurred speech, and vertigo (symptoms of chronic intoxication and that client may be exceeding dose).

CLIENT/FAMILY TEACHING

1. Take most of daily dose at bedtime, with smaller doses during the waking hours to minimize mental/motor impairment. These drugs may reduce ability to handle potentially dangerous equipment, such as cars and machinery especially during the first 2 weeks of therapy; may decrease over time.

2. Rise slowly from a supine position and dangle legs over side of the bed before standing. If feeling faint sit/lie down immediately and lower the head. Allow extra time to prepare for daily activities; take precautions before arising, to reduce one source of anxiety and stress. Identify/practice relaxation techniques that may assist in lowering anxiety levels.

3. Avoid alcohol while taking antianxiety agents. Alcohol potentiates the depressant effects of both the alcohol and the medication. Do not take any unprescribed or OTC medications without approval.

4. Do not stop taking drug suddenly. Any sudden withdrawal after prolonged therapy or after excessive use may cause a recurrence of the preexisting symptoms of anxiety. It may also cause a withdrawal syndrome, manifested by increased anxiety, anorexia, insomnia, vomiting, ataxia, muscle twitching, confusion, and hallucinations. May also develop seizures and convulsions.

5. These drugs are generally for short-term therapy; follow-up is imperative to evaluate response and the need for

continued therapy. Report any adverse side effects and lack of response.

6. Avoid prolonged sun exposure and use protection if exposed. Do not over exert during hot weather, drink plenty of water and remain cool; may cause heat stroke.

7. Attend appropriate counselling sessions as condition and length of therapy dictate.

8. Keep all F/U appointments to evaluate response to therapy, labs, adequate dose, and any adverse side effects.

OUTCOMES/EVALUATE

- ↓ Anxiety/tension episodes; ↑ coping ability
- ↓ Frequency/intensity of muscle spasms/tremor; seizure control
- Improved sleeping patterns
- Control of alcohol withdrawal symptoms

VACCINES

SEE TABLES 3, 4, AND 5.

GENERAL STATEMENT

Vaccines have played an important role in the health and life span of our population. They have been in use over 200 years, but since World War II, once the importance of disease prevention became evident, research into the area of vaccine development exploded.

More recently, the population has been exposed to the threat of biological warfare. This involves the use of a biologic microorganism in a bioterrorist attack. This may include radiation and dirty bombs, occupational health, food and water security. Much discussion has been entertained as to how to deal with this threat, including mass immunizations and post-exposure prophylaxis. To this point, this question has not been resolved.

Most recently the fear of Avian flu or the H5N1 influenza virus in migratory birds from Asia to Eastern Europe has raised the fear of a potential pandemic. Since 2003 this virus or "bird flu" has infected 169 people and resulted in 91 deaths according to the WHO.

At present there is no evidence to support that the virus can be easily spread from person to person.

Use of a vaccine (or actually contracting the disease) usually imparts a temporary or permanent resistance to an infectious disease. The human immune system has a memory. As the body is exposed to a disease-producing organism, the lymphocytes (immune cells) are activated and, by cell division, reproduce and attack the offending organism. Some of these lymphocytes remain in the body indefinitely with memory cells. Vaccines and toxoids promote the type of antibody production one would see if they had experienced the natural infection. This active immunization involves the direct administration of antigens to the host by intentionally exposing the immune system to a foreign infectious agent so it forms a memory of that agent. This causes the individual to produce the desired antibodies and cell-mediated immunity. These agents may consist of live attenuated agents or killed (inactivated) agents, or agents that alter the hosts' genetic structure. Immunizations confer resistance without actually producing disease.

Some vaccines are in short supply due to the push for immunization and are reserved for those individuals who have direct contact with the organism in the laboratory, military personnel deployed to an area with high risk for exposure to the organism, or other at risk individuals. Some organisms (anthrax) can be managed effectively with antibiotics in post-exposure prophylaxis. Passive immunization occurs when immunologic agents are administered. Immunoglobulins and antivenins only offer passive short-term immunity and are usually administered for a specific exposure.

There has been controversy surrounding some childhood vaccines. Some parents have claimed that their child was developing normally until they received their vaccinations. Many parents who have children with autism are attributing this to the thimerosal

---

preservatives found in vaccines (influenza, DTP), which metabolizes into ethylmercury.

The use of thimerosal has diminished since 1977, after recommendations by medical authorities, but trace amounts of thimerosal remain in many vaccines and in some vaccines, thimerosal has not yet been phased out despite recommendations. Some states have enacted laws banning the use of thimerosal in childhood vaccines.

Aggressive pediatric immunization programs have helped reduce preventable infections and death in children worldwide. Vaccines have contributed to the eradication of one of the most contagious and deadly diseases known to man, smallpox. Other diseases such as rubella, polio, chickenpox, measles, mumps, and typhoid are nowhere near as common as they were just one hundred years ago. As long as a vast majority are vaccinated, it is much more difficult for a disease outbreak to occur, let alone spread. A recent publicized measles outbreak was related to lack of immunization. Polio, which is transmitted only between humans, has been targeted by an extensive campaign of eradication that has seen endemic polio restricted to only parts of four countries. Difficulty in reaching all children has caused the eradication date to be missed twice by 2006. This focus should continue and should be expanded to the adult population, many of whom have missed the natural infection and past immunizations. Some adults were never vaccinated as children. Also, some of the newer vaccines were not available when some adults were children. Immunity can begin to fade over time so as we age, we become more susceptible to serious disease caused by common infections (e.g., flu, pneumococcus). A careful immunization history should be documented for every client, regardless of age. When in doubt or if disease/infection or immunization

status is unknown, appropriate serologic evidence/titers may be drawn.

Shingles is caused by the varicella-zoster virus, the same virus that causes chickenpox. After an attack of chickenpox, the virus lies dormant in certain nerve tissue. As we age, the virus can reappear in the form of shingles. It is characterized by clusters of blisters that can cause severe pain that may last for weeks, months, or years. Zostavax is a live virus vaccine recently released that is given as a single injection under the skin (upper arm) to adults over age 60.

Vaccines remain one of the most powerful tools we have for disease prevention. Advances in biotechnology have ushered in a new era in vaccine development that holds even more promise for improving public health. Currently scientists are pursuing many promising new strategies in vaccine development and exploring novel ways to administer vaccines that may provide safer, more effective ways to fight disease. Table 3 lists some of the more common or currently discussed diseases, the general recommended schedule to confer immunization, and the length of immunity conferred; Table 4 outlines the active childhood immunization schedule, while Table 5 identifies an active Adult Immunization Schedule. For more information:

American Academy of Pediatrics: http://www.aap.org
National Immunization Program: http://www.cdc.gov/nip/default.htm
Infectious Diseases Society of America: http://www.idsociety.org
Immunization Action Coalition: http://www.immunize.org
National Network for Immunization Information (offers vaccination requirements by state): http://www.immunizationinfo.org
John Hopkins Center for Public Health Preparedness: http://jhsph.edu/preparedness

---

Table 3 Common Diseases, General Recommended Immunization Schedule, and Length of Immunity

DISEASE	IMMUNIZATION SCHEDULE	LENGTH OF IMMUNITY
Anthrax	3 SC shots q 2 weeks followed by 3 additional SC shots given at 6, 12, and 18 months	1-year boosters (not available to public yet)
BCG vaccine (TB)	Adult/child >1 month: 0.2–0.3 mL; child <1 month ↓ dose by 50% following guidelines	TB post-exposure
Botulism	Pentavalent toxoid (types A,B,C,D,E) 0.5 mL SC (available from USAMRIID)	Post-exposure
Cholera	Two doses 1 week to 1 month apart (0.5 mL)	6 months
Diphtheria	Given as *DTaP; four doses at ages 2, 4, 6, and 15–18 months; booster at 4–6 years.	10 years
*Haemophilus influenzae (Hib)	Four doses at ages 2, 4, 6, and 15 months	Unknown (check titers)
*Hepatitis A	Initial dose with booster given at 6 months	10 yrs
*Hepatitis B	Three doses: At birth (or initial dose), 1 month later, and 6 months after second dose	Unknown (check titers)
Human Papillomavirus vaccine (HPV)	Three dose schedule with the second and third dose given 2 and 6 months after the first dose. Females age 11–12; as young as 9 years; catchup aged 13–26 years old if no previous vaccination or did not complete series	Lifetime
*Influenza (flu)	One dose (or two doses of split virus if under 13 years). All children 6–59 months	1–3 years
Measles	Given as *MMR at ages 12–15 months and 4–6 years	Lifetime
*Meningococcal meningitis	One dose (antibody response requires 5 days); 11 years for MCV4; 2 years for MPSV4; MCV4 at age 11–12 and at HS entry; antibiotic prophylaxis (rifampin 600 mg or 10 mg/kg q 12 hr for four doses should be given to all contacts per exposure)	?Lifetime; not consistently effective in those <2 years of age
Mumps	Given as *MMR at ages 12–15 months and 4–6 years	Lifetime
Pertussis	Given as *DTaP; four doses at ages 2, 4, 6, and 15–18 months	10 years
*Pneumococcal (PCV)	One dose (0.5 mL) before age 5 years and not after age 5	Approx. 5–10 years
Poliovirus (OPV)	Four doses at ages 2, 4, and 6 months, then at age 4–6 years	Lifetime
*Poliovirus (IPV)	If all IPV or all OPV doses given before age 4, a fourth dose is not necessary. If both given in the series, a total of four doses should be given.	Lifetime

Bold Italic = life threatening side effect   ■ = black box warning   ♣ = Available in Canada

DISEASE	IMMUNIZATION SCHEDULE	LENGTH OF IMMUNITY
Rabies	Postexposure: five doses on days 0, 3, 7, 14, and 28 with the rabies immune globulin; pre-exposure: two doses 1 week apart, third dose 2–3 weeks later	Approx. 2 years
*Rotavirus (Rota) G1, G3, G4, G9 strains	Given as three doses at ages 2, 4, and 6 months; do not start after age 12 weeks and do not give after age 32 weeks.	Unknown
Rubella	Given as *MMR at ages 12–15 months and 4–6 years	Lifetime
Smallpox	One dose; this vaccine available at CDC and local public health departments (critical in less than 4 days of exposure); vaccinia immune globulin in special cases, call USAMRIID	3–10 years
*Tetanus	Given initially as *DTaP; four doses at ages 2, 4, 6, and 15–18 months	10 years; a tetanus booster is required every 10 years; 5 years if trauma
Typhoid	CPS vaccine	IM 2 years; capsules 5 years
*Varicella vaccine	One dose (0.5 mL) age 12–15 months and a second dose (0.5 mL) at age 4–6 years	Unknown (check titers)
Varicella Zoster (shingles)	Zostavax (Zoster vaccine live)—SC—one dose	Lifetime
Yellow fever	One dose	10 years

*Recommended immunizations
Centers for Disease Control and Prevention. Recommended immunization schedules for persons aged 0-18 years – United States, 2007. *MMWR* 2006;55(51&52):Q1-Q4.
State Mandates on Immunization and Vaccine—Preventable Diseases www.immunize.org/laws

= see color insert   H = Herbal   IV = Intravenous   = sound alike drug

Table 4 Active Childhood Immunization Schedule

	First	Second	Third	Fourth
DTaP	2 months	4 months	6 months	15–18 months
Hepatitis A	2 doses between 12 and 23 months			
Hepatitus B	birth or initial dose	1 month after first dose	6 months or more after second dose	
Hib (*Haemophilus influenzae* type b)	2 months	4 months	6 months	12–15 months
IPV (inactivated poliovirus vaccine)	2 months	4 months	6-18 months	4–6 years
MMR	12–18 months	4 years		
OPV (oral poliovirus vaccine)	2 months	4 months	~	~
Pneumococcal, influenza	12–15 months		6 months	4–6 years
	At age 6 months and older—yearly			
Rotavirus	2 months	4 months	6 months	
Varicella	2 doses between 12–18 months; and 4–6 years			

Check with the CDC for catch up schedule: www.cdc.gov/vaccines

Table 5 Active Adult Immunization Schedule

HPV	3 doses for females through age 26	
Influenza	Every year	
Tetanus (Td/Tdap)	Tetanus booster every 10 years; with injury obtain one in 5 years	
Pneumococcus	One dose after age 65	
Zostavax	One dose after age 60	

Bold Italic = life threatening side effect   ▮ = black box warning   ✦ = Available in Canada

VITAMINS

SEE TABLES 6, 7, AND 8.

GENERAL STATEMENT

Vitamins are essential, carbon-containing, noncaloric substances that are required for normal metabolism. They are organic compounds the body can not produce but are produced by living materials such as plants and animals and they are generally obtained from the diet. They may also be referred to as nutrients. Vitamin D is synthesized in the body to a limited extent and Vitamin B–12 is synthesized in the intestinal tract by bacterial flora.

Vitamins are essential for promoting growth, health, vitality, life, general well being, and for the prevention and cure of many health problems and diseases. They are necessary for the metabolic processes responsible for transforming foods into tissue or energy. Vitamins are also involved in the formation and maintenance of blood cells, chemicals supporting the nervous system, hormones, and genetic materials. Vitamins do not provide energy because they contain no calories. Yet, some do help convert the calories in fats, carbohydrates, and proteins into usable body energy. Many misinformed people think vitamins can replace food. In fact, vitamins can not be assimilated without ingesting food. That is why they should be taken with a meal. Vitamins regulate metabolism, help convert fat and carbohydrates into energy, and assist in forming bone and tissue.

Disease states caused by severe nutritional deficiencies prompted the discovery of vitamins because scientists were able to reverse the signs and symptoms of these disease states with vitamins. Severe deficiencies include scurvy, rickets, pellagra, pernicious anemia, xerophthalmia, beriberi, osteomalacia, infantile hemolytic anemia, and hemorrhagic diseases of the newborn. Moderate vitamin deficiencies may also produce symptoms of impaired health.

Environmental factors and genetic predisposition may influence individual requirements for specific vitamins. Disease processes, growth, hormone balance, and drugs may also alter the dietary requirements and function of vitamins.

Many deficiency states can be traced to special circumstances such as pernicious anemia after gastrectomy; pellagra in corn–eating populations, and scurvy in the elderly subsisting on soft foods (e.g., eggs, bread, milk) while neglecting citrus fruits. Generally, although not common in the United States, vitamin deficiency usually involves multiple rather than single deficiencies and usually can be attributed to poor lifestyle choices and poor dietary habits with an inadequate intake of many nutrients, including all vitamins. Since vitamins are required in such small amounts, deficiencies are rare in industrialized nations. Vitamin toxicity/excess may occur and is more often the problem due to the ready availability of nutritional supplements.

There are two categories of vitamins: fat soluble and water soluble, depending on how the intestines absorb them. Fat soluble vitamins A, D, E, and K are found in the fat or oil of foods and require digestible fat and bile salts for absorption in the small intestine. The water-soluble vitamins, C and B complex (B-1, B-2, niacin, B-6, folic acid, B-12, pantothenic acid, and biotin) are found in the watery portion of foods and are well absorbed by the GI tract. They are easily lost through overcooking and do not require fat for absorption. Water soluble vitamins mix easily in the blood, are excreted by the kidneys, and only small amounts are stored in the tissues, so regular daily intake is essential. Fat soluble vitamins are stored in the body after binding to specific plasma globulins in fat parts of the body. In high doses they may accumulate in the body and cause adverse reactions.

Recommended Dietary Allowances (RDAs) are the recommended human vitamin and mineral intake requirements. These were developed by the Food and Nutrition Board, National Research Council of the National Academy of Sciences and have evolved over the past 50 years and are updated every 5 years. They are based on age, height, weight, and gender. These are only estimates of nutrient needs; each client and the surrounding factors warrant individualized evaluation when replacement is being considered. Pregnant and breast feeding women, and children require more of some vitamins than most adults. The elderly seem more prone to deficiencies due to poor absorption during the aging process and due to decreased sun exposure, as their skin is not able to absorb enough to produce active forms of vitamin D. In fact, vitamin D deficiency is underdiagnosed and undertreated in our older population today. Clients with impaired liver function should not take large amounts of fat soluble vitamins (i.e., A, D, E, K) unless specifically prescribed due to the toxicity potential from cumulative effects.

The National Academy of Sciences Commission On Life Sciences has published the RDA for healthy people. RDAs are based on various kinds of evidence: 1) studies of subjects maintained on diets containing low or deficient levels of a nutrient, followed by correction of the deficit with measured amounts of the nutrient; 2) nutrient balance studies that measure nutrient status in relation to intake; 3) biochemical measurements of tissue saturation or adequacy of molecular function in relation to nutrient intake; 4) nutrient intakes of fully breastfed infants and of apparently healthy people from their food supply; 5) epidemiological observations of nutrient status in population in relation to intake; 6) in some cases, extrapolation of data from animal experiments. In practice there are only limited data on which estimates of nutrient requirements can be based. These are the elements that the advisory counsel has identified that has led their recommendations.

The HHS and USDA developed the Dietary Guidelines for Americans 2005. The Sixth Edition of *Dietary Guidelines for Americans* was released on January 12, 2005. The *Guidelines* must be issued at least every 5 years by law. (Public Law 101-445, Title III, 7 U.S.Code 301). This is available for view on line at http://www.health.gov/dietaryguidelines/

These guidelines recommended:
- We meet key intakes by adopting a balanced eating pattern, such as the U.S. Department of Agriculture (USDA) Food Guide or the Dietary Approaches to Stop Hypertension (DASH) Eating Plan.
- Consume a variety of nutrient-dense foods and beverages within and among the basic food groups while choosing foods that limit the intake of saturated and trans fats, cholesterol, added sugars, salt, and alcohol.
- Meet recommended intakes within energy needs by adopting a balanced eating pattern, such as the USDA Food Guide or the DASH Eating Plan.

Additionally, it was recommended that people over age 50 should consume vitamin B-12 in its crystalline form (i.e., fortified foods or supplements)

For women of childbearing age who may become pregnant: Eat foods high in heme-iron and/or consume iron-rich plant foods or iron-fortified foods with an enhancer of iron absorption, such as vitamin C-rich foods.

Women of childbearing age who may become pregnant and those in the first trimester of pregnancy: Consume adequate synthetic folic acid daily (from fortified foods or supplements) in addition to food forms of folate from a varied diet.

For older adults, people with darker pigmented skin, and people exposed to insufficient ultraviolet band radiation (i.e., sunlight): Consume extra vitamin D from vitamin D-fortified foods and/or supplements.

NURSING CONSIDERATIONS
ASSESSMENT
1. Document indications for therapy, clinical presentation, and deficiency states. Have a full nutritional assess-

ment done by a registered dietician as needed.

2. Assess metabolic panel and vitamin levels as indicated.

3. Determine client use and knowledge on the utilization of nutrients. Many overtake these agents and waste money on products of little use or that may even cause toxicity.

4. List agents prescribed to ensure none interact or impact vitamin absorption.

5. Identify if vegetarian. There is no vitamin B-12 in any plant product. Also ↓ vitamin B-12 absorption in the elderly. Use caution as folate administered to one deficient in vitamin B-12 may result in subacute spine degeneration with paralysis.

6. With replacement, monitor levels as indicated to ensure requirements are met and levels are as desired (i.e., vitamin D, test-25-OH).

7. Review *Dietary Guidelines for Americans 2005* with client to ensure they have this information available for their review and understand updates and recommendations.

CLIENT/FAMILY TEACHING

1. Comply with dietary recommendations. The best source of vitamins is a well-balanced diet with foods from the basic food groups. Some require vitamin supplementation to replace those lost with continued drug use, certain conditions i.e. pregnancy, elderly, or certain disease states.

2. Take with food for best absorption and utilization.

3. Avoid self-medicating with vitamin supplements that exceed the RDA. Megadoses of vitamins (nutrients) for various medical conditions is unproven and may cause adverse side effects and toxicity. The fat soluble vitamins (A, D, E, K) may accumulate and cause toxicity. At the least it will be a huge waste of money due to the fact that many vitamins in excess of body requirements are excreted.

4. Store away from heat in tight, light-resistant containers, out of childrens' reach. Regularly check for expiration dates and discard if expired.

5. With deficiency states, keep all F/U appointments to evaluate response to therapy, lab levels, and any adverse side effects.

6. Utilize reliable resources to expand knowledge of nutrient/vitamin use and always check with provider before adding to prescribed regimen. These should always be listed on medication lists and updated at each visit during medication reconciliation.

OUTCOMES/EVALUATE

- Prevention/decrease of symptoms of vitamin deficiencies
- Normal healthy functioning of body
- Prevention/cure of related health problems/diseases

Table 6   Common Vitamin Requirements

Vitamin	RDA	Physiologic Effects Essential for:
A (retinol, retinaldehyde, retonic acid)	Men: 5,000; Women: 4,000 international units	Growth and development; epithelial tissue maintenance; reproduction; prevents night blindness; stimulates production/ activity of WBCs, takes part in remodeling bone
B complex:		Increasing intake of folic acid, vitamin B-6, and vitamin B-12 decreases homocysteine levels
B-1 (thiamine)	0.5 mg/ 1,000 kcal	Energy metabolism; normal nerve function
B-2 (riboflavin)	1.2–1.8 mg	Reactions in energy cycle that produce ATP; oxidation of amino acids and hydroxy acids; oxidation of purines
B-3 Niacin (nicotinic acid, nicotinamide)	13–20 mg	Synthesis of fatty acids and cholesterol; blocks FFA; conversion of phenylalanine to tyrosine
B-6 (pyridoxine, pyridoxal, pyridoxamine)	2 mg	Amino acid metabolism; glycogenolysis, RBC/Hb synthesis; formation of neurotransmitters; formation of antibodies
Folacin (folic acid, pteroylglutamic acid)	400 mcg	DNA synthesis, formation of RBCs in bone marrow with cyanocobalamin; prevention of neural tube defects
Pantothenic acid (calcium pantothenate, dexpanthenol)	4–7 mg	Synthesis of sterols, steroid hormones, porphyrins; synthesis and degradation of fatty acids; oxidative metabolism of carbohydrates, gluconeogenesis
B-12 (cyanocobalamin, hydroxocobalamin, extrinsic factor)	6 mcg	DNA synthesis in bone marrow; RBC production with folacin; nerve tissue maintenance; prevents pernicious anemia
B-7 (Biotin)	100–300 mcg	Synthesis of fatty acids, generation of tricarboxylic acid cycle; formation of purines Coenzyme in CHO metabolism

Bold Italic = life threatening side effect   ■ = black box warning   ♣ = Available in Canada

Table 6   Common Vitamin Requirements

Vitamin	RDA	Physiologic Effects Essential for:
C (ascorbic acid, ascorbate)	Men: 90 mg; Women: 75 mg; Extra 35 mg for smokers, alcoholics	Formation of collagen; conversion of cholesterol to bile acids; protects A and E and polyunsaturated fats from excessive oxidation; absorption and utilization of iron; converts folacin to folinic acid; some role in clotting, adrenocortical hormones, and resistance to cancer and infections; powerful antioxidant that can neutralize harmful free radicals
D (calcitriol, cholecalciferol, dihydrotachysterol, ergocalciferol, viosterol)	2,000 international units, or 5 mcg	Intestinal absorption and metabolism of calcium and phosphorus as well as renal reabsorption; release of calcium from bone and resorption
E (tocopherol, retinol)	Tocopherol: 22–33 international units; Retinol: 8–12 mcg (retinol equivalents)	May oppose destruction of Vitamin A and fats by oxygen fragments called free radicals; antioxidant; may affect production of prostaglandins which regulate a variety of body processes
K (menadione, phytonadione)	Men: 80 mcg; Women: 65 mcg	Formation of prothrombin and other clotting proteins by the liver; blood coagulation

Table 7 Vitamin Food Sources

Vitamin	Food Source
A (retinoic acid)	Eggs, liver, green leafy vegetables, milk, butter, colorful fruits and vegetables (carrots, tomatoes, sweet potatoes) some fish
B-3 (Niacin)	Pork, cereals (wheat, rye, corn), green vegetables, meat, fruits, legumes, milk
B-2 (Riboflavin)	Meat, liver, fish, green vegetables, milk products
B-6 (Pyridoxine)	Milk, cereals, meat, some vegetables, beans, fortified grains
B-12	Liver, kidney, meat, dairy products, fortified cereals (vegetarians most at risk for deficiency)
C (Ascorbic acid)	Citrus fruits, juices, other fruits and vegetables, tomatoes
D	Cheese, eggs, fortified milk, butter, fish liver oils
E	Vegetable oils, widely available in a variety of foods
K	Made by bacteria inside intestines; green leafy vegetables, cabbage, potatoes, and liver
Folic Acid	Meats, kidney, liver, vegetables, beans, fortified cereals, fruits, dark green vegetables
Biotin	Available in many food sources; made by intestinal bacteria
Panthothenic Acid	Widely available in many different food sources

Table 8   Vitamin Deficiency States

Vitamin	Deficiency	Signs and Symptoms
A	Xerophthalmia	Progressive eye changes: Night blindness to xerosis of conjunctiva and cornea with scarring
	Keratomalacia	Degeneration of epithelial cells with hardening and shrinking
B-1	Beriberi	Nerve damage, edema, CHF, Wernicke-Korsakoff syndrome
B-3	Biotin deficiency	Hair loss, scaly red rash around eye, nose, mouth, and genital area; depression, lethargy, unusual facial fat distribution; numbness/tingling in extremities
B-6	Rare—usually seen with multiple B deficiencies	Fatigue, weight loss, weakness, irritability; headaches, insomnia, peripheral neuropathy, CHF, cardiomyopathy
Niacin	Pellagra	Depression, anorexia, beefy red glossitis, cheilosis, dermatitis
B-12	Pernicious anemia	Macrocytic, megaloblastic anemia; progressive neuropathy R/T demyelination
C	Scurvy	Joint pain, growth retardation, anemia, poor wound healing with increased susceptibility to infection; petechial hemorrhages
D	Osteomalacia (adult), Rickets (child)	Demineralization of bones and teeth with bone pain and skeletal muscle deformities
E	Hemolytic anemia in low birth weight infants	Macrocytic anemia; increased hemolysis of RBCs and increased capillary fragility
K	Hemorrhagic disease in newborns	Increase tendency to hemorrhage

appendix 1

Commonly Used Abbreviations and Symbols

A1C	hemoglobin A1C
ABG	arterial blood gas
ABI	ankle/brachial systolic pressure index
ACE	angiotensin-converting enzyme
ACLS	advanced cardiac life support
ACS	acute coronary syndrome
ACT	activated clotting time
ACTH	adrenocorticotropic hormone
ADA	adenosine deaminase
ADD	attention deficit disorder
ADH	antidiuretic hormone
ADHD	attention deficit hyperactivity disorder
ADL	activities of daily living
ad lib	as desired, at pleasure
ADP	adenosine diphosphate
AF	atrial fibrillation
AFB	acid fast bacillus
AHF	antihemophilic factor
AIDS	acquired immune deficiency syndrome
ALL	acute lymphocytic leukemia
ALS	amyotrophic lateral sclerosis
ALT	alanine aminotransferase
a.m., A.M.	morning
AMD	age-related macular degeneration
AMI	acute myocardial infarction
AML	acute myelogenous leukemia
AMP	adenosine monophosphate
ANA	antinuclear antibody
ANC	absolute neutrophil count
ANS	autonomic nervous system
APL	acute promyelocytic leukemia
aPTT	activated partial thromboplastin time
ARB	angiotensin receptor blocker
ARC	AIDS-related complex
ARDS	adult respiratory distress syndrome
ASA	aspirin (acetylsalicylic acid)
ASAP, asap	as soon as possible
ASHD	arteriosclerotic heart disease
AST	aspartate aminotransferase
ATC	around the clock
ATP	adenosine triphosphate

ATS	American Thoracic Society
ATU	antithrombin unit
ATX	antibiotics
AUC	area under the curve
AV	atrioventricular
AVB	abnormal vaginal bleeding, AV block
BBB	bundle branch block
BCG	Bacille Calmette-Guerin
BG	blood glucose
BIDS	bedtime insulin, daytime sulfonylurea
BK	below the knee
BMD	bone mineral density
BMI	body mass index
BMR	basal metabolic rate
BMT	bone marrow transplant
BP	blood pressure
BPD	bronchopulmonary dysplasia
BPH	benign prostatic hypertrophy
bpm	beats per minute
BS	blood sugar, bowel sounds
BSA	body surface area
BSE	breast self-exam
BSP	Bromsulphalein
BUN	blood urea nitrogen
C	Celsius/Centigrade
CABG	coronary artery bypass graft
CAD	coronary artery disease
CAP	community-acquired pneumonia
CBC	complete blood count
CCB	calcium channel blocker
C_{CR}	creatinine clearance
CD_4	helper T4 lymphocyte cells
C&DB	cough and deep breathe
CDC	Centers for Disease Control and Prevention
CF	cystic fibrosis
CFU	colony forming units
CHB	complete heart block
CHF	congestive heart failure
CHO	carbohydrate
CIS	carcinoma in situ
CJD	Creutzfeldt-Jakob disease
CK	creatine kinase
CLL	chronic lymphocytic leukemia
CLS	capillary leak syndrome
cm	centimeter
C_{max}	maximum serum concentration
CML	chronic myelocytic leukemia
CMV	cytomegalovirus
CN	cranial nerve
CNS	central nervous system
CO	cardiac output
COMT	catechol-O-methyltransferase
COLD	chronic obstructive lung disease
COPD	chronic obstructive pulmonary disease

CP	cardiopulmonary
CPAP	continuous positive airway pressure
CPB	cardiopulmonary bypass
CPK	creatine phosphokinase
CPR	cardiopulmonary resuscitation
CRF/CRI	chronic renal failure/chronic renal insufficiency
CRS	cytokine release syndrome
C&S	culture and sensitivity
CSF	cerebrospinal fluid
CSID	congenital sucrase-isomaltase deficiency
CT	computerized tomography
CTC	common toxicity criteria (from the National Cancer Institute)
CTS	carpal tunnel syndrome
CTZ	chemoreceptor trigger zone
CV	cardiovascular
CVA	cerebrovascular accident
CVP	central venous pressure
CXR	chest x-ray
dATP	deoxyadenosine triphosphate
DBP	diastolic blood pressure
ddATP	dideoxyadenosine triphosphate
DEA	Drug Enforcement Agency
DEXA	dual energy x-ray absorptiometry
DI	diabetes insipidus
DIC	disseminated intravascular coagulation
dL	deciliter (one-tenth of a liter)
DM	diabetes mellitus
DMARD	disease-modifying antirheumatic drug
DNA	deoxyribonucleic acid
DOE	dyspnea on exertion
DPT	diphtheria, pertussis, tetanus
dr.	dram (0.0625 ounce)
DRE	digital rectal examination
DSM-IV-TR	Diagnostic and Statistical Manual of Mental Disorders, Fourth Edition, Text Revision
DT	delirium tremens
DTR	deep tendon reflex
DVT	deep vein thrombosis
EC	enteric-coated
ECB	extracorporeal cardiopulmonary bypass
ECG, EKG	electrocardiogram, electrocardiograph
ED	erectile dysfunction
EDTA	ethylenediaminetetra-acetic acid
EEG	electroencephalogram
EENT	eye, ear, nose, and throat
EF	ejection fraction
e.g.	for example
ENL	erythema nodosum leprosum
ENT	ear, nose, throat
EPS	electrophysiologic studies, extrapyramidal symptoms
ER	extended release
ESR	erythrocyte sedimentation rate

ESRD	end-stage renal disease
ET	endotracheal
ET-1	Endothelin-1 (neurohormone)
ETOH	alcohol
F	Fahrenheit, fluoride
FBS	fasting blood sugar
FDA	Food and Drug Administration
FEV	forced expiratory volume
FFP	fresh frozen plasma
FOB	fecal occult blood
FS	finger stick
FSH	follicle-stimulating hormone
F/U	follow-up
FUO	fever of unknown origin
FVC	forced vital capacity
fx	fracture
GABA	gamma-aminobutyric acid
G-CSF	granulocyte colony-stimulating factor
GERD	gastroesophageal reflux disease
GFR	glomerular filtration rate
GGT	gamma-glutamyl transferase
GGTP	gamma-glutamyl transpeptidase
GH	growth hormone
gi, GI	gastrointestinal
GnRH	gonadotropin-releasing hormone
GP	glycoprotein
G6PD	glucose-6-phosphate dehydrogenase
gtt	a drop, drops
GU	genitourinary
h, hr	hour
HA, HAL	hyperalimentation
HbA1c	glycosylated hemoglobin (hemoglobin marker)
HBV	hepatitis B virus
HCG, hCG	human chorionic gonadotropin
HCM	hypercalcemia of malignancy
HCP	health care provider
HCT	hematocrit
HCV	hepatitis C virus
HDL	high density lipoprotein
HFN	high flow nebulizer
Hg	mercury
H&H	hematocrit and hemoglobin
HIT	heparin-induced thrombocytopenia
HIV	human immunodeficiency virus
HLA	human leukocyte antigens
HJR	hepatojugular reflux
HMG-CoA	3-hydroxy-3-methyl-glutaryl-coenzyme A
HOB	head of bed
HPA	hypothalamic-pituitary-adrenal axis
HPG	hypothalamus-pituitary-gonadal axis
HR	heart rate
HRT	hormone replacement therapy
HSE	herpes simplex encephalitis
HSV	herpes simplex virus

ht	height
5-HT	5-hydroxytryptamine
HTN	hypertension
IA	intra-arterial
IBD	inflammatory bowel disease
IBS	irritable bowel syndrome
IBW	ideal body weight
ICP	intracranial pressure
ICU	intensive care unit
IDDM	insulin dependent diabetes mellitus
Ig	immunoglobulin
IGF	insulin-like growth factor
im, IM	intramuscular
IMV	intermittent mandatory ventilation
inh	inhalation
INR	international normalized ratio
I&O	intake and output
IOP	intraocular pressure
IP	intraperitoneal
IPPB	intermittent positive pressure breathing
IR	immediate release
ITP	idiopathic thrombocytopenia purpura
IUD	intrauterine device
iv, IV	intravenous
IVPB	IV piggyback, a secondary IV line
JVD	jugular venous distention
kg	kilogram (2.2 lb)
KVO	keep vein open
L	liter (1,000 mL)
lb	pound
LBBB	left bundle branch block
LDH	lactic dehydrogenase
LDL	low density lipoprotein
LFTs	liver function tests
LHRH	luteinizing hormone-releasing hormone
LOC	level of consciousness/loss of consciousness
LV	left ventricular
LVED	left ventricular end diastolic
LVEF	left ventricular ejection fraction
LVH	left ventricular hypertrophy
M	mix
m^2	square meter
m	meter
MAC	Mycobacterium avium complex
MAOI	monoamine oxidase inhibitor
MAP	mean arterial pressure
MAR	medication administration record
max	maximum
mcg	microgram
μ	micro
μCi	microcurie
μL	microliter
μm	micrometer
μM	micromolar

MCH	mean corpuscular hemoglobin
mCi	millicurie
mcL	microliter
mcm	micrometer
MCV	mean corpuscular volume
MDI	metered-dose inhaler
MDRSP	multidrug resistant *Streptococcus pneumoniae*
mEq	milliequivalent
mg	milligram
MI	myocardial infarction
MIC	minimum inhibitory concentration
min	minute, minim
mL	milliliter
mm^3	cubic millimeter
MM	multiple myeloma
MME	mini mental exam
MMSE	mini mental state (status) examination
MRI	magnetic resonance imaging
MS	multiple sclerosis
MTX	methotrexate
MU	million units
MUGA	multigated radionuclide angiography
NaCl	sodium chloride
ng	nanogram
NG	nasogastric
NGT	nasogastric tube
NIDDM	non-insulin dependent diabetes mellitus
NKA	no known allergies
NKDA	no known drug allergies
NMS	neuroleptic malignant syndrome
NPN	nonprotein nitrogen
NPO	nothing by mouth
NR	do not refill (e.g., a prescription)
NSCLC	non-small cell lung cancer
NSAID	nonsteroidal anti-inflammatory drug
NSR	normal sinus rhythm
NSS	normal saline solution
NTG	nitroglycerin
NYHA	New York Heart Association
N&V	nausea and vomiting
O$_2$	oxygen
OBS	organic brain syndrome
OC	oral contraceptive
OCD	obsessive-compulsive disorder
OOB	out of bed
OR	operating room
O$_2$ sat	oxygen saturation
OTC	over the counter
oz	ounce
PA	pulmonary artery
PABA	para-aminobenzoic acid
PAC	premature atrial contraction
PACWP	pulmonary arterial capillary wedge pressure
PAF	paroxysmal atrial fibrillation or flutter

PAS	paraaminosalicylate
PBI	protein-bound iodine
p.c.	after meals
PCA	patient-controlled analgesia
PCI	percutaneous coronary intervention
PCN	penicillin
PCP	*Pneumocystis carinii* pneumonia; phencyclizine psychosis
PCWP	pulmonary capillary wedge pressure
PDT	photodynamic therapy
PE	pulmonary embolus, pulmonary embolism; physical exam
PEEP	positive end expiratory pressure
per	by, through
PFTs	pulmonary function tests
pg	picogram
pH	hydrogen ion concentration
PID	pelvic inflammatory disease
PMH	past medical history
PMI	point of maximal intensity
PMS	premenstrual syndrome
PND	paroxysmal nocturnal dyspnea
po, p.o., PO	by mouth
PPAR	peroxisome proliferator-activated receptor
PPD	purified protein derivative
PR	by rectum
p.r.n., PRN	when needed or necessary
PSA	prostatic specific antigen
PSP	phenolsulfonphthalein
PSVT	paroxysmal supraventricular tachycardia
PT	prothrombin time; physical therapy
PTCA	percutaneous transluminal coronary angioplasty
PTH	parathyroid hormone
PTSD	post traumatic stress disorder
PTT	partial thromboplastin time
PUD	peptic ulcer disease
PUVA	psoralen and ulraviolet A
PVC	premature ventricular contraction; polyvinyl chloride
PVD	peripheral vascular disease
PVR	peripheral vascular resistance
q.h.	every hour
q 2 hr	every two hours
q 3 hr	every three hours
q 4 hr	every four hours
q 6 hr	every six hours
q 8 hr	every eight hours
qhs	every night
q.s.	as much as needed, quantity sufficient
RA	right atrium; rheumatoid arthritis
RAIU	radioactive iodine uptake
RBBB	right bundle branch block
RBC	red blood cell
RDA	recommended daily allowance

REM	rapid eye movement
RICE	rest, ice, compression and elevation
RNA	ribonucleic acid
R/O	rule out
ROM	range of motion
ROS	review of systems
RRMS	relapsing-remitting multiple sclerosis
RSV	respiratory syncytial virus
R/T	related to
RTC	round the clock
RV	right ventricular
RUQ	right upper quadrant
Rx	symbol for a prescription
SA	sinoatrial; sustained-action
SAH	subarachnoid hemorrhage
SARS	severe acute respiratory syndrome
SBE	subacute bacterial endocarditis
SBP	systolic BP
sc, SC	subcutaneous
SCI	spinal cord injury
SCID	severe combined immunodeficiency disease
SGGT	serum gamma-glutamyl transpeptidase
SGOT	serum glutamic-oxaloacetic transaminase
SGPT	serum glutamic-pyruvic transaminase
S., Sig.	mark on the label
SI	sacroiliac
SIADH	syndrome inappropriate antidiuretic hormone
SIMV	synchronized intermittent mandatory ventilation
SL	sublingual
SLE	systemic lupus erythematosus
SOB	shortness of breath
sol	solution
sp.	species
SR	sustained release
ss	one-half
SSNRI	selective serotonin norepinephrine reuptake inhibitor
SSRI	selective serotonin reuptake inhibitor
SSS	sick sinus syndrome
S&S	signs and symptoms
stat	immediately
STD	sexually transmitted disease
SV	stroke volume
SVT	supraventricular tachycardia
syr	syrup
sz	seizure
t ½	half-life
tab	tablet
TB	tuberculosis
TCA	tricyclic antidepressant
TENS	transcutaneous electric nerve stimulation
TG	triglycerides
THR	total hip replacement
TIA	transient ischemic attack

TIBC	total iron binding capacity
TKR	total knee replacement
T_{max}	maximum threshold; time of maximum concentration
TNF	tumor necrosis factor
TPN	total parenteral nutrition
TSH	thyroid stimulating hormone
TURP	transurethral resection of the prostate
U/A	urinalysis
UD	unit dose
UGI	upper gastrointestinal
ULN	upper limit of normal
UO	urine output
URTI	upper respiratory tract infection
US	ultrasound
USP	U. S. Pharmacopeia
UTI	urinary tract infection
UV	ultraviolet
UVB	ultraviolet B (portion of ultraviolet radiation spectrum)
VAD	venous access device
VF	ventricular fibrillation
VLDL	very low density lipoprotein
VMA	vanillylmandelic acid
V. O.	verbal order
VS	vital signs
VT	ventricular tachycardia
WBC	white blood cell
WHO	World Health Organization
WNL	within normal limits
Wt	weight
XRT	radiation therapy
y.o.	years old
&	and
°	degree
>	greater than
<	less than
↑	increased, higher
↓	decreased, lower
-	negative, minus
/	per
%	percent
+	positive, plus
×	times, frequency

Please note that many abbreviations have double meanings or can be misread. It is better to write out the recommendations, especially when ordering specific procedures or specific directions for drug administration. See appendix 2.

appendix 2
Medication Errors: Importance of Reporting

Much news media coverage has been directed to the unnecessary loss of life due to medication errors, many of which were preventable. It is estimated that adverse drug reactions to prescription and over-the-counter medications kill at least 100,000 Americans and seriously injure an additional 2.1 million each year. Staff must understand the potential for medication errors and the importance of the health care facility processes/procedures in place to prevent the errors. Encourage staff to report problems and make suggestions for improvements. Take the fear out of reporting errors by making the system non-punitive and removing the deterrent for not reporting errors. If errors go unreported then facilities have no means of correcting a situation that created the error. For a variety of reasons, some staff members have difficulty admitting their mistakes; however, they must be encouraged to report and participate in the correction of the process(es) that caused the error.

Some of the more common types of errors are:

- Drugs with similar sounding names
- Inappropriate abbreviations
- Poor handwriting; misplaced decimals and zeroes
- Confusion of metric and other dosing units
- Environmental factors such as noise, distractions, lighting, fatigue
- Poor communication
- Lack of complete patient data on allergies, medical conditions, and so forth

Last year, United States Pharmacopeia received more than 2,000 voluntary reports of medication reconciliation errors, and a 1999 Institute of Medicine report estimated that more than 7,000 deaths occur each year in hospitals alone due to medication errors. The Joint Commission's Sentinel Event Database also identifies medication errors as one of the most frequently occurring threats to patient safety. This Database reveals that 63% of the reported medication errors resulting in death or serious injury were due to breakdowns in communication, and approximately half of those would have been avoided through effective medication reconciliation. A 2005 patient safety goal was to initiate medication reconciliation at each facility.

The National Coordinating Council for Medication Error Reporting and Prevention (http://www.nccmerp.org) defines a medication error as "any preventable event that may cause or lead to inappropriate medication use or patient harm while the medication is in the control of the health care professional, patient, or consumer. Such events may be related to professional practice, health care products, procedures, and systems including prescribing; order communication; product labeling; packaging; and nomenclature; compounding; dispensing; distribution; administration; education; monitoring; and use." (Copyright 1998-2002 NCC MERP. All rights reserved.)

The FDA maintains a site for medication errors:
http://www.fda.gov/cder/MedErrors

The FDA began monitoring reports of medication errors in 1992. They reviewed reports that were sent to the FDA from the United States Pharmacopeia (USP) and the Institute for Safe Medication Practices (ISMP). The Med Watch reports were also reviewed. The Division of Medication Errors and Technical Support includes a medication error prevention program. This is staffed with pharmacists and support personnel so they can review the medication error reports sent to the USP-ISMP Medication Errors Reporting Program (MERP) and Med Watch. Since many patient errors are related to medication errors, it is felt that if they share the knowledge gained, this information may lead to patient safety.

The FDA maintains other searchable safety databases related to medical devices, including: biologic products, recalls, drug shortages, vaccine safety, and dietary supplements. All reports are voluntary and without penalty. Forms are easily downloaded for completion or can be completed on line.

All medication error reports should be filed with the MERP. Observed errors may be reported confidentially.

1-800-23-ERROR
http://www.usp.org

The website alerts the health care professional about the need for practice changes. It also alerts industry and regulatory professionals about pharmaceutical labeling, packaging, and nomenclature that may foster error by their design. When you report errors, you are asked for your recommendations. Links are also maintained to the ISMP, USP, and FDA (for adverse drug reports). They also maintain international reporting links. Dual sites for health care professionals and consumers are also available on the web: www.safemedication.com

FDA's Medwatch Program and Online Reporting Forms:
http://www.fda.gov/medwatch and
http://www.fda.gov/medwatch/index.html
1-800-332-1088

Gain information and voluntarily report medication errors and/or fill out Form 3500, which you can download from the site, and return by mail or fax. You can also report the error by phone. This information allows the FDA to require labeling changes, withdraw a drug from market, and distribute safety information to other providers.

Center for Drug Error Reporting (FDA)
http://www.fda.gov/cder

This site offers highlights of new drugs, new safety information, drugs recently approved, and generic and OTC products.

Initiatives to reduce medication error include improving medication systems through bar coding medications/patients (wrist bands), individual dose bins, and computer programs that screen for dosage problems, interactions, and allergies.

Another step is to provide additional warnings for certain medications with greater potential for harm, such as anticoagulants, potassium chloride, opiates, and insulin. Methods to prevent interruptions of health care providers administering medications are of utmost importance, as well as multi-professional team approaches.

The Joint Commission approved a minimum list of dangerous abbreviations. The following abbreviations have been identified as those which promote medication errors and should no longer be used:

Eliminate	Use instead
U	unit
IU	international unit
qd	every day
qod	every other day
trailing zero	eliminate zero after a decimal point
MS	morphine sulfate
MSO$_4$	morphine sulfate
MgSO$_4$	magnesium sulfate

Other abbreviations that have been eliminated from the 2009 edition of the Nurse's Drug Handbook for safety reasons include:

Eliminate	Use instead
b.i.d	twice a day
t.i.d	3 times/day
gm	gram

A secondary list of suggested abbreviations to eliminate in the future has also been created. Visit http://www.jointcommission.org for more information.

Health care professionals are urged to voluntarily report medication errors to the **USP Medication Errors Reporting Program** (1-800-233-7767). In addition, serious adverse events (including those resulting from medication errors) may be reported to the FDA MedWatch Program (1-800-FDA-1088). The USP Medication Errors Reporting Program is a partner in the FDA MedWatch Program and is presented in cooperation with the Institute for Safe Medication Practices.

appendix 3

Controlled Substances in the United States and Canada

Controlled Substances Act—United States

The U.S. Federal Controlled Substances Act of 1970 placed drugs controlled by the Act into five categories or schedules based on their potential to cause psychologic and/or physical dependence as well as on their potential for abuse. The schedules are defined as follows:

Schedule I [C-I]: Includes substances for which there is a high abuse potential and no current approved medical use (e.g., heroin, marijuana, LSD, other hallucinogens, certain opiates and opium derivatives).

Schedule II [C-II]: Includes drugs that have a high ability to produce physical or psychologic dependence and for which there is a current approved or acceptable medical use (e.g. narcotics, certain CNS stimulants).

Schedule III [C-III]: Includes drugs for which there is less potential for abuse than drugs in Schedule II and for which there is a current approved medical use and moderate dependence liability. Certain drugs in this category are preparations containing limited quantities of codeine and nonbarbiturate sedatives. Anabolic steroids are classified in Schedule III.

Schedule IV [C-IV]: Includes drugs for which there is less abuse potential than for Schedule III, for which there is a current approved medical use, and that have limited dependence liability (e.g., some sedatives, antianxiety drugs, nonnarcotic analgesics).

Schedule V [C-V]: Drugs in this category have limited abuse potential and consist mainly of preparations containing limited amounts of certain narcotic drugs for use as antitussives and antidiarrheals. Federal law provides that limited quantities of these drugs (e.g., codeine) may be bought without a prescription by an individual at least 18 years of age if allowed under state statutes. The product must be purchased from a pharmacist, who must keep appropriate records. However, state laws vary, and in many states such products require a prescription.

NOTE: Generally, prescriptions for Schedule II (high abuse potential) drugs cannot be transmitted over the phone and they cannot be refilled. Prescriptions for Schedule III, IV, and V drugs may be refilled up to five times within 6 months. Schedule II drugs are not necessarily "stronger" than drugs in Schedules III, IV, or V; Schedule II drugs are classified as such due to their high abuse potential. Drugs that are not controlled are indicated by an asterisk (*).

Controlled Substances—Canada

In Canada, there are eight schedules. They are:

I Some of the more common groups include opium derivatives and salts (e.g., codeine, morphine, hydrocodone, oxycodone, oxymorphone); coca derivatives and salts (e.g., cocaine); phenylpiperidines and derivatives and salts (e.g., difenoxin, diphenoxylate, pethidine); phenazepines and salts (e.g., ethoheptazine); amidones and salts (e.g., methadone); phenalkoxams and salts (e.g., dextropropoxyphene); morphinans and salts (e.g., buprenorphine, levorphanol); benzazocines and salts (e.g., pentazocine); phencyclidine and salts; and, fentanyls and salts (alfentanil, fentanyl, remifentanil, sufentanil). Note: The above list is not inclusive.

II Cannabis and derivatives (e.g., marijuana, cannabinol).

III Amphetamines, their salts and derivatives (e.g., amphetamine, benzphetamine). Also, methylphenidate, psilocin, psilocybin, mescaline.

IV Barbiturates and their salts and thiobarbiturates and salts. Also, anabolic steroids, benzodiazepines, chlorphentermine, diethylpropion, phendimetrazine, phentermine, butorphanol, nalbuphine, glutethimide, ethchlorvynol, maxindol, meprobamate, methyprylon.

V Phenylpropanolamine and propylhexedrine.

VI Ephedrine, ergotamine, LSD, pseudoephedrine.

VII Specific amounts of cannabis (3 kg), and cannabis resin (3 kg).

VIII Specific amounts of cannabis (30 g) and cannabis resin (1 g).

| | Drug Schedule | |
Drug	United States	Canada
Alfentanil	II	I
Alprazolam	IV	IV
Amobarbital sodium	II	IV
Amphetamine sulfate	II	III
Aprobarbital	III	IV
Benzphetamine HCl	III	III
Buprenorphine HCl	III	I
Butabarbital sodium	III	IV
Butorphanol tartrate	IV	IV
Chloral hydrate	IV	*
Chlordiazepoxide	IV	IV
Clonazepam	IV	IV
Clorazepate dipotassium	IV	IV
Cocaine	II	I
Codeine	II	I
Dexmethylphenidate HCl	II	Not available
Dextroamphetamine sulfate	II	III
Dextropropoxyphene		
Bulk	II	I

Drug	Drug Schedule	
	United States	Canada
Dosage Forms	IV	I
Diazepam	IV	IV
Diethylpropion HCl	IV	IV
Difenoxin products (0.5 mg/25 mcg atropine sulfate)	V	I
Diphenoxylate products (2.5 mg/25 mcg atropine sulfate)	V	I
Dronabinol	III	*
Estazolam	IV	IV
Ethchlorvynol	IV	IV
Fentanyl	II	I
Fluoxymesterone	III	IV
Flurazepam HCl	IV	IV
Glutethimide	II	IV
Halazepam	IV	IV
Hydrocodone	Not available alone (usually C-III in combination drugs)	I
Hydromorphone HCl	II	I
Ketamine	III	*
Levorphanol tartrate	II	I
Lorazepam	IV	IV
Mazindol	IV	IV
Meperidine HCl	II	I
Mephobarbital	IV	IV
Meprobamate	IV	IV
Methadone HCl	II	I
Methamphetamine HCl	II	III
Methandrostenolone	III	IV
Methylphenidate HCl	II	III
Methyltestosterone	III	IV
Midazolam	IV	IV
Modafinil	IV	*
Morphine sulfate	II	I
Nandrolone decanoate	III	IV
Opium	II	I
Opium products (100 mg/100 mL or grams)	V	I
Oxandrolone	III	IV
Oxazepam	IV	IV
Oxycodone HCl	II	I
Oxymetholone	III	IV
Oxymorphone HCl	II	I
Paraldehyde	IV	*
Paregoric	III	I
Pemoline	IV	*
Pentazocine	IV	I

(continues)

	Drug Schedule	
Drug	United States	Canada
Pentobarbital sodium		
PO	II	IV
Rectal	III	IV
Phencyclidine	II	I
Phendimetrazine tartrate	III	IV
Phenobarbital	IV	IV
Phentermine HCl	IV	IV
Prazepam	IV	IV
Quazepam	IV	IV
Remifentanil HCl	II	-
Secobarbital sodium	II	IV
Sibutramine HCl	IV	-
Stanolone	III	IV
Stanozolol	III	IV
Sufentanil citrate	II	I
Temazepam	IV	IV
Testosterone (all forms)	III	IV
Thiopental	III	IV
Triazolam	IV	IV
Zaleplon	IV	-
Zolpidem tartrate	IV	-

appendix 4

Pregnancy Categories: FDA Assigned

The U.S. Food and Drug Administration's use-in-pregnancy rating system weighs the degree to which available information has ruled out risk to the fetus against the drug's potential benefit to the patient. The ratings, and their interpretation, are as follows:

Category	Interpetation
A	**CONTROLLED STUDIES SHOW NO RISK.** Adequate, well-controlled studies in pregnant women have failed to demonstrate a risk to the fetus in any trimester of pregnancy.
B	**NO EVIDENCE OF RISK IN HUMANS.** Either animal studies show risk but human findings do not, or if no adequate human studies have been done, animal findings are negative.
C	**RISK CANNOT BE RULED OUT.** Human studies are lacking, and animal studies are either positive for fetal risk or lacking. However, potential benefits may justify the potential risks.
D	**POSITIVE EVIDENCE OF RISK.** Investigational or post-marketing data show risk to the fetus. However, potential benefits may outweigh the potential risks. If needed in a life-threatening situation or serious disease, the drug may be acceptable if safer drugs cannot be used or are ineffective.
X	**CONTRAINDICATED IN PREGNANCY.** Studies in animals or humans, or investigational or post-marketing reports, have demonstrated positive evidence of fetal abnormalities or risk which clearly outweigh any possible benefit to the patient.

appendix 5

Calculating Body Surface Area and Body Mass Index

Body Surface Area (BSA) Calculator

Use the following formulas to calculate the body surface area (BSA) for drug administration. These formulas replace the BSA Nomogram.

BSA (metric) = $\sqrt{(\text{ht [cm]} \times \text{wt [kg]})/3600}$

BSA (English) = $\sqrt{(\text{ht [in]} \times \text{wt [lb]})/3131}$

Body Mass Index (BMI) Calculator

You may calculate your BMI to assess if you are overweight

1. Multiply your weight in pounds by 703

2. Multiply your height in inches times itself

3. Divide the first number by the second to give your BMI

For example:
You weigh 190 lb and are 5'5" (65") tall

1. 190 x 703 = 133,579

2. 65 x 65 = 4,225

3. 133,579 divided by 4,225 = 31.6

Your BMI is 31.6

A BMI under 18.5 indicates that you are underweight
A BMI between 18.5 and 24.9 is considered a healthy weight
If the BMI is between 25 and 29.9 you are moderately overweight
If the BMI is 30 or more you are extremely obese

A precalculated BMI chart is available in most provider offices.

A precalculated BMI chart is available from the National Institutes of Health at: http://www.nhlbi.nih.gov/guidelines/obesity/bmi_tbl.htm

appendix 6

Elements of a Prescription

To safely communicate the exact elements desired on a prescription, the following items should be addressed:

A. **The prescriber:** Name, address, phone number, and associated practice/specialty

B. **The client:** Name, age/birthdate, address and any allergies of record.

C. **The prescription itself:** Name of the medication (generic or trade); dosage form and quantity to be dispensed (e.g., number of tablets or capsules, 1 vial, 1 tube, volume of liquid); the strength of the medication (e.g., 125-mg tablets, 250 mg/5 mL, 80 mg/1 mL, 10%); and directions for use (e.g., 1 tablet PO 3 times per day; 2 gtt to each eye 4 times per day; 1 teaspoonful PO q 8 hr for 10 days; apply a thin film to lesions twice a day for 14 days)

D. **Other elements:** Date prescription is written, signature of the provider, number of refills; provider number: state license number and Drug Enforcement Agency (DEA) number (when applicable); and brand-product-only indication (when applicable)

A typical prescription as follows:

A.   **Julia Bryan, MSN, RN, CPNP**
Pediatric Associates
1611 Kirkwood Highway
Wilmington, DE 19805
302-645-8261

                     Date: July 10, 20XX

B.   **For: Kathryn Woods, Age 8**
         27 East Parkway
         Lewes, DE 19958
Rx   **Amoxicillin susp. 250 mg/5 mL**
         Disp. 150 mL
         Sig: 1 teaspoon PO q 8 hr x 10 days

Refills: 0   **Provider signature**
                  Provider/State license number

Interpretation of prescription: The above prescription is written by Certified Pediatric Nurse Practitioner Julia Bryan for Kathryn Woods and is for amoxicillin suspension. The concentration desired is 250 mg/5 mL. The directions for taking the medication are 1 teaspoon (i.e., 5 mL) by mouth every 8 hr for 10 days. The prescriber wants 150 mL dispensed and no refills are allowed.

appendix 7

Easy Formulas for IV Rate Calculation

To calculate the continuous drip rate for an IV infusion, the following information is necessary:

    a.   amount of solution to be infused
    b.   time for infusion to be administered
    c.   *drop factor (found in the tubing package)

$$\frac{\text{Total volume to be infused}}{\text{Total hours for infusion}} \times \frac{\text{*drop factor}}{60 \text{ min/hr}} = \text{gtt/min}$$

*if drop factor is: 60 gtt/min, then use 1 in the formula
    10 gtt/min, then use $1/6$ in the formula
    15 gtt/min, then use $1/4$ in the formula
    20 gtt/min, then use $1/3$ in the formula

This gives you $\frac{\text{gtt}}{\text{min}}$.

Example: Infuse 1,000 cc over 8 hr using tubing with a drop factor of 10 gtt/min.

$$\frac{1,000 \text{ mL}}{8 \text{ hr}} \times \frac{1}{6} = 20.8 \text{ or } 21 \frac{\text{gtt}}{\text{min}}$$

Complete equation is:

$$\frac{1,000 \text{ mL}}{8 \text{ hr}} \times \frac{10 \text{ gtt/min}}{60 \text{ min/1 hr}} = \frac{1,000 \text{ mL}}{8 \text{ hr}} \times \frac{10 \text{ gtt}}{\text{mL}} \times \frac{1 \text{ hr}}{60 \text{ min}} = 21 \frac{\text{gtt}}{\text{min}}$$

To get $\frac{\text{mL}}{\text{hr}}$ invert drop factor and multiply by $\frac{\text{gtt}}{\text{min}}$, or:

$$\frac{6}{1} \times 21 \frac{\text{gtt}}{\text{min}} = 126 \frac{\text{mL}}{\text{hr}}$$

When administering intermittent infusions, as with antibiotic therapy, use the following formula:

$$\text{Total volume to be infused} \div \frac{\text{minutes to administer}}{60 \text{ min/hr}} = \frac{\text{mL}}{\text{hr}}$$

Example: Administer 3 g Zosyn in 100 mL of D5W over 45 min

$$100 \div \frac{45}{60} \text{ (invert to multiply)}$$

or

$$100 \times \frac{60}{45} = 133.3 \text{ or } 134 \frac{\text{mL}}{\text{hr}}$$

appendix 8
Commonly Used Combination Drugs

NOTE: Please consult individual drugs for more extensive information. Table entries are alphabetized by generic name.

Accuretic (quinapril hydrochloride and hydrochlorothiazide)
ActoPlus Met (pioglitazone hydrochloride, metformin)
Advicor (niacin and lovastatin)
Aggrenox (aspirin and dipyridamole)
Aldactazide (spironolactone and hydrochlorothiazide)
Angeliq (drospirenone and estradiol)
Arthrotec (diclofenac sodium and misoprostol)
Atacand HCT (candesartan cilexetil and hydrochlorothiazide)
Atripla (efavirenz, emtricitabine, tenofovir disodium fumarate)
Avalide (irbesartan and hydrochlorothiazide)
Avandamet (rosiglitazone maleate and metformin hydrochloride)
Avandaryl (rosiglitazone and glimepiride)
Axocet (butalbital and acetaminophen)
Balacet 325 (acetaminophen and propoxyphene napsylate)
Brontex (codeine phosphate and guaifenesin)
Caduet (amlodipine besylate and atorvastatin calcium)
Claritin-D, Claritin-D 24 Hour Extended (loratidine and pseudoephedrine)
Codeprex (codeine polistirex and chlorpheniramine)
Combunox (oxycodone hydrochloride and ibuprofen)
Cosopt (dorzolamide hydrochloride and timolol maleate)
Darvocet-N 50, Darvocet N-100 (acetaminophen and propoxyphene napsylate)
Donnatal (atropine sulfate, hyoscyamine sulfate, scopolamine hydrobromide, and phenobarbital)
Duetact (pioglitazone and glimepiride)
Dyazide, Maxzide, Maxide-25 MG (triamterene and hydrochlorothiazide)
Empirin with Codeine #3 and #4 (aspirin and codeine phosphate)
Epzicom (abacavir and lamivudine)
Equagesic (aspirin and meprobamate)
Exforge (amlodipine and valsartan)
Fiorinal (aspirin, butalbital and caffeine)
Fiorinal with codeine (aspirin, butalbital, caffeine, and codeine phosphate)
Fosamax Plus D (alendronate sodium and cholecalciferol)
Hycodan (hydrocodone bitartrate and homatropine methylbromide)
Inderide, Inderide LA (propranolol hydrochloride and hydrochlorothiazide)
IsonaRif (rifampin and isoniazid)
Janumet (sitagliptin and metformin hydrochloride)
Kaletra (lopinavir and ritonavir)
Librax (chlordiazepoxide and clidinium bromide)
Lotensin HCT (benazepril hydrochloride and hydrochlorothiazide)

Lotrisone (clotrimazole and betamethasone propionate)
Malarone (atovaquone and proguanil hydrochloride)
Metaglip (glipizide and metformin hydrochloride)
Micardis HCT (telmisarten and hydrochlorothiazide)
Moduretic (amiloride and hydrochlorothiazide)
Pediazole (erythromycin ethylsuccinate and sulfisoxazole)
Prevacid NapraPAC (lansoprazole and naproxen)
Quinaretic (quinapril hydrochloride and hytrochlorothiazide)
Rifamate, Rimactane/INH (rifampin and isoniazid)
Rifater (rifampin, isoniazid and pyrazinamide)
Roxicet (acetaminophen and oxycodone)
Stalevo (carbidopa, levodopa, and entacapone)
Suboxone (buprenorphine hydrochloride and naloxone)
Symbicort (budesonide and formoterol fumarate dehydrate)
Symbyax (olanzapine and fluoxetine hydrochloride)
Synalgos-DC (dihydrocodeine bitartrate, aspirin, and caffeine)
Talwin NX (pentazocine hydrochloride and naloxone hydrochloride)
Tevetan HCT (eprosartan and hydrochlorothiazide)
Triavil (amitriptyline hydrochloride and perphenazine)
Trizivir (abacavir sulfate, lamivudine, zidovudine)
Truvada (emtricitabine and tenofovir disoproxil fumarate)
Uniretic (moexipril hydrochloride and hydrochlorothiazide)
Vaseretic (enalapril maleate and hydrochlorothiazide)
Vicoprofen (hydrocodone bitartrate and ibuprofen)
Zylet (loteprednol etabonate and tobramycin)

Generic Name (Content)	Trade Name	Use	Dose
Abacavir (600 mg), Lamivudine (300 mg)	Epzicom (Rx)	In combination with other antiretroviral agents to treat HIV-1 infections.	**Adults:** 1 tablet daily with other antiretroviral drugs. May be taken without regard to food. Do not give to those with a C_{CR} <50 mL/min or hepatic impairment.
Abacavir sulfate (300 mg), Lamivudine (150 mg), Zidovudine (300 mg)	Trizivir (Rx)	Alone or with other antiretroviral drugs to treat HIV-1 infections.	**Adults and adolescents, 40 kg or more:** 1 tablet twice a day (not for use in those weighing less than 40 kg or if creatinine clearance is 50 mL/min or less due to it being a fixed-dose tablet). May be taken without regard to food.
Acetaminophen (325 mg/tablet or 5 mL), Oxycodone (5 mg/tablet or 5 mL)	Roxicet	Analgesic	1 tablet or 5 mL q 6 hr.
Acetaminophen (325 or 650 mg), Propoxyphene napsylate (50 or 100 mg)	Balacet 325, Darvocet-N 50, Darvocet-N 100 (Rx, C-IV)	Mild to moderate pain (may be used if fever is present)	2-Darvocet-N 50 tablets or 1-Darvocet-100 tablet q 4 hr, not to exceed 600 mg propoxyphene napsylate/day. Reduce dose in impaired renal/hepatic function. 1-Balacet 325 tablet q 4 hr, up to 6 tablets/day

(continues)

Generic Name (Content)	Trade Name	Use	Dose
Alendronate sodium (70 mg), Cholecalciferol (2,800 units)	Fosamax Plus D (Rx)	Increase bone mass in men with osteoporosis. Treat osteoporosis in postmenopausal women to increase bone mass and reduce incidence of fractures.	Once tablet weekly. Do not use in clients with C_{CR} less than 30 mL/min.
Amiloride (5 mg), Hydrochlorothiazide (50 mg)	Moduretic (Rx)	Hypertension or CHF, especially when hypokalemia occurs. May be used with other antihypertensives.	**Initial:** 1 tablet per day; **then,** can increase to 2 tablets per day.
Amitriptyline HCl (10, 25, or 50 mg), Perphenazine (2 or 4 mg)	Triavil 2–10, 2–25, 4–10, 4–25, 4–50 (Rx)	Depression with moderate to severe anxiety and/or agitation (including those with chronic physical disease). Schizophrenia with symptoms of depression.	**Initial:** 1 Triavil 2–25 or 4–25 tablet 3–4 times per day or 1 Triavil tablet 4–50 twice a day (for schizophrenia, use 2 Triavil 4–50 3 times per day with a fourth dose at bedtime if needed). **Maintenance:** 1 Triavil 2–25 or 4–25 2–4 times per day or 1 Triavil 4–50 twice a day.

Generic Name (Content)	Trade Name	Use	Dose
Amlodipine (2.5, 5, or 10 mg), Atorvastatin calcium (10, 20, 40, or 80 mg)	Caduet (Rx)	Hypertension and hypercholesterolemia	Individualize dose. Select dose based on the dosage of the drug being continued and the recommended starting initial dose for the new drug. Maximum amlodipine daily dose: 10 mg. Maximum atorvastatin daily dose: 80 mg.
Amlodipine (5 or 10 mg), Valsartan (160 or 320 mg)	Exforge (Rx)	Antihypertensive	Four strengths are available: 5/160, 10/160, 5/320, 10/320. Begin Exforge therapy only after failure to achieve the desired effect with one or the other as monotherapy.
Aspirin (325 mg), Butalbital (50 mg), Caffeine (40 mg)	Fiorinal (Rx, C-III)	Tension headaches	1–2 tablets or capsules q 4 hr, not to exceed 6 tablets or capsules/day.
Aspirin (325 mg), Butalbital (50 mg), Caffeine (40 mg), Codeine phosphate (7.5 mg, 15 mg, or 30 mg)	Fiorinal with Codeine (Rx, C-III)	Analgesic for all types of pain	**Initial:** 1–2 capsules; then, dose may be repeated, if necessary, up to maximum of 6 capsules/day.
Aspirin (325 mg), Codeine phosphate (15, 30, or 60 mg)	Empirin with Codeine #3, Empirin with Codeine #4 (Rx, C-III)	Analgesic	Tablets with 15 or 30 mg, codeine: 1 or 2 q 4 hr. Tablets with 60 mg codeine: 1 q 4 hr.

(continues)

Generic Name (Content)	Trade Name	Use	Dose
Aspirin (325 mg), Meprobamate (200 mg)	Equagesic (Rx, C-IV)	Short-term treatment of pain due to musculoskeletal disease accompanied by anxiety and tension.	**Adults:** 1-2 tablets 3-4 times per day.

Generic Name (Content)	Trade Name	Use	Dose
Atovaquone (250 mg/tablet or 62.5 mg/pediatric tablet), Proguanil hydrochloride (100 mg/tablet or 25 mg/pediatric tablet)	Malarone Malarone Pediatric	Prophylaxis of *Plasmodium falciparum* malaria including areas where chloroquine resistance seen. Treatment of acute, uncomplicated *P. falciparum*, even in areas where resistance to other drugs seen.	*Prophylaxis.* **Adults:** 1 adult tablet per day. **Children, 11–20 kg:** 1 pediatric tablet per day; **21–30 kg:** 2 pediatric tablets per day as a single dose; **31–40 kg:** 3 pediatric tablets per day as a single dose; **>40 kg:** 1 adult strength tablet per day as a single daily dose. *Treatment.* **Adults:** 4 adult strength tables per day as a single dose per day for 3 consecutive days. **Children, 5–8 kg:** 2 pediatric tablets per day for 3 consecutive days; **9–10 kg:** 3 pediatric tablets per day for 3 consecutive days; **11–20 kg:** 1 adult strength tablet per day for 3 consecutive days; **21–30 kg:** 2 adult strength tablets per day for 3 consecutive days; **31–40 kg:** 3 adult strength tablets per day for 3 consecutive days; **>40 kg:** Use adult dose. Take daily dose at same time each day with food or a milky drink. Those with severe renal impairment should receive the product only if the benefits outweigh the potential risks of 3-day therapy. *(continues)*

Generic Name (Content)	Trade Name	Use	Dose
Atropine sulfate (0.0194 mg), Hyoscyamine sulfate (0.1037 mg), Scopolamine HBr (0.0065 mg), Phenobarbital (16.2 mg) in each tablet, capsule, or 5 mL elixir	Donnatal (Rx)	Adjunct to treat irritable bowel.	**Adults, usual:** 1–2 tablets or capsules 3–4 times per day or 1-Extentab q 12 hr, or 5–10 mL elixir 3–4 times per day. **Pediatric:** Use elixir as follows: **4.5–9.0 kg:** 0.5 mL q 4 hr or 0.75 mL q 6 hr. **9.1–13.5 kg:** 1.0 mL q 4 hr or 1.5 mL q 6 hr; **13.6–22.6 kg:** 1.5 mL q 4 hr or 2.0 mL q 6 hr; **22.7–33.9 kg:** 2.5 mL q 4 hr or 3.75 mL q 6 hr; **34.0–45.3 kg:** 3.75 mL q 4 hr or 5 mL q 6 hr; **45.4 kg:** 5 mL q 4 hr or 7.5 mL q 6 hr.
Benazepril hydrochloride (5, 10, 20 mg), Hydrochlorothiazide (6.25, 12.5, 25 mg)	Lotensin HCT (Rx)	Hypertension	**Usual, initial:** One 10/12.5 or 20/25 tablet/day.
Budesonide (80 or 160 mcg), Formoterol fumarate dehydrate (4.5 mcg)	Symbicort	Long-term maintenance treatment of asthma in clients 12 years and older.	Two inhalations twice a day (in the morning and evening). For those on high doses of inhaled corticosteroids, start with the 160/4.5 product. The maximum daily dose is budesonide/formoterol 640 mcg/18 mcg given as 2 inhalations of 160 mcg/4.5 mcg for

Generic Name (Content)	Trade Name	Use	Dose
Buprenorphine hydrochloride, Naloxone (2 mg Buprenorphine base/0.5 mg Naloxone and 8 mg/2 mg)	Suboxone (Rx)	Treat opioid dependence	12 to 16 mg Buprenorphine per day given sublingually.
Butalbital (50 mg), Acetaminophen (650 mg)	Axocet (Rx)	Tension headaches	1 Capsule q 4 hr, not to exceed 6 capsules/day.
Candesartan cilexetil (16 mg or 32 mg), Hydrochlorothiazide (12.5 mg)	Atacand HCT 16–12.5 or Atacand HCT 32–12.5 (Rx)	Hypertension (not for initial treatment)	**Initial:** 1 tablet of Atacand HCT 16-12.5. Depending on response, can increase to Atacand 32-12.5
Carbidopa (12.5 mg, 25 mg, or 37.5 mg), Levodopa (50 mg, 100 mg, or 150 mg), Entacapone (200 mg)	Stalevo 50, 100, and 150 (Rx)	Idiopathic Parkinson's disease	Individualize optimum daily dose. 1 tablet at each dosing administration not to exceed 8 tablets/day.
Chlordiazepoxide (5 mg), Clidinium Br (2.5 mg)	Librax (Rx)	Adjunct in the treatment of irritable colon, spastic colon, mucous colitis, and acute enterocolitis	**Adults, individualized, usual:** 1–2 capsules 3–4 times per day before meals and at bedtime.

(continues)

Generic Name (Content)	Trade Name	Use	Dose
Clotrimazole (10 mg) and Betamethasone dipropionate (0.5 mg) per gram of cream	Lotrisone cream or lotion (Rx)	Symptomatic inflammatory tinea pedis, tinea cruris, and tinea corporis due to *Epidermophyton rubrum, Trichophyton metagrophytes,* or *T. rubrum.*	Gently massage cream or lotion into the affected skin areas twice a day in the morning and evening.
Codeine phosphate (10 mg/tablet or 20 mL), Guaifenesin (300 mg/tablet or 20 mL)	Brontex (Rx, C-III)	Relief of cough due to cold or inhaled irritants. Loosen mucus and thin bronchial secretions	**Adults and children over 12 years:** 1 tablet or 20 mL q 4 hr. **Children, 6–12 years:** 10 mL q 4 hr.
Codeine polistirex (20 mg/5 mL), Chlorpheniramine (4 mg/5 mL)	Codeprex (Rx, C-III)	Temporary relief of cough, runny nose, sneezing, itching of the nose or throat, and itchy watery eyes due to hay fever, other allergies affecting the upper respiratory tract, or allergic rhinitis	**Age at least 12 years:** 10 mL q 12 hr; **children at least 6 years old but younger than 12 years:** 5 mL q 12 hr.

Generic Name (Content)	Trade Name	Use	Dose
Diclofenac sodium (50 or 75 mg), Misoprostol (200 mcg)	Arthrotec 50, Arthrotec 75 (Rx)	Osteoarthritis or rheumatoid arthritis in those at high risk of developing NSAID-induced gastric and duodenal ulcers	*Osteoarthritis:* 1-Arthrotec 50 tablet with food 3 times per day. If intolerance occurs, give Arthrotec 50 or Arthrotec 75 twice a day, although this dose is less effective in preventing ulcers. *Rheumatoid arthritis:* 1-Arthrotec 50 tablet with food 3–4 times per day. If intolerance occurs, give Arthrotec 50 or Arthrotec 75 twice a day, although this dose is less effective in preventing ulcers.
Dihydrocodeine bitartrate (16 mg), Aspirin (356.4 mg), Caffeine (30 mg)	Synalgos-DC (Rx)	Moderate to moderately severe pain	**Usual:** 2 capsules q 4 hr. Adjust dose to severity of pain.
Dipyridamole (200 mg extended-release), Aspirin (25 mg)	Aggrenox (Rx)	Reduce risk of stroke in those who have had TIAs or complete ischemic stroke due to thrombosis.	One capsule twice a day (in the morning and evening). Do not interchange with individual components of aspirin and dipyridamole tablets.

(continues)

Generic Name (Content)	Trade Name	Use	Dose
Dorzolamide HCl (2%), Timolol maleate (0.5%)	Cosopt (Rx)	Reduce elevated IOP in open-angle glaucoma or ocular hypertension in those inadequately controlled with beta blockers	**Adults:** 1 gtt in the affected eye(s) twice a day.
Drospirenone (0.5 mg), Estradiol (1 mg)	Angeliq (Rx)	Moderate to severe vasomotor symptoms. Moderate to severe vulvar and vaginal atrophy associated with menopause.	One tablet daily. Those already taking an estrogen should stop taking that product before starting Angeliq.
Efavirenz (600 mg), Emtricitabine (200 mg), Tenofovir disodium fumarate (300 mg)	Atripla (Rx)	Alone or with other antiretroviral drugs to treat HIV-1 infections in adults.	One tablet daily on an empty stomach. Contraindicated in those with a C_{CR} <50 mL/min. Not recommended for clients younger than 18 years of age.
Emtricitabine (200 mg), Tenofovir disoproxil fumarate (300 mg)	Truvada (Rx)	With other antiretroviral drugs (e.g., non-nucleoside reverse transcriptase inhibitors or protease inhibitors) to treat HIV disease.	One tablet once daily with or without food. Give one tablet q 48 hr if creatinine clearance is 30 to 49 mL/min. Do not use if creatinine clearance is less than 30 mL/min or if client is on hemodialysis.

Generic Name (Content)	Trade Name	Use	Dose
Enalapril maleate (5 mg or 10 mg), Hydrochlorothiazide (12.5 or 25 mg)	Vaseretic (Rx)	Hypertenstion	**Adults:** 1–2 tablets once daily.
Eprosartan (600 mg), Hydrochlorothiazide (12.5 mg or 25 mg)	Teveten HCT (Rx)	Hypertension	600 mg Eprosartan 1–2 times per day.
Erythromycin ethylsuccinate (200 mg) and Sulfisoxazole (600 mg) in 5 mL of oral suspension.	Pediazole (Rx)	Acute otitis media in children due to *Haemophilus influenzae*.	**Usual:** Equivalent of 50 mg/kg/day of erythromycin and 150 mg/kg/day of sulfisoxazole, up to a maximum of 6 grams/day. **Over 45 kg:** 10 mL q 6 hr; **24 kg:** 7.5 mL q 6 hr; **16 kg:** 5 mL q 6 hr; **8 kg:** 2.5 mL q 6 hr; **less than 8 kg:** Calculate dose according to body weight.

(continues)

Generic Name (Content)	Trade Name	Use	Dose
Glipizide (2.5 mg or 5 mg), Metformin hydrochloride (250 mg or 500 mg). Available as 2.5 mg/ 250 mg, 2.5 mg/500 mg, 5 mg/ 500 mg.	Metaglip (Rx)	Initial or second-line therapy for Type 2 diabetes	Individualize dosage. **Initial:** Glipizide, 2.5 mg / Metformin, 250 mg once a day with a meal. If fasting blood glucose is 280 to 320 mg/dL, start with 2.5 mg/500 mg twice a day. Increase dosage to achieve control in increments of 1 tablet/day q 2 weeks up to a maximum of 10 mg/1,000 mg or 10 mg/2,000 mg/day in divided doses. **Secondary therapy:** Start with 2.5/500 mg or 5 mg/500 mg twice a day with a.m. and p.m. meals. Titrate daily dose in increments of no more than 5 mg/ 500 mg up to a maximum dose of 20 mg/2,000 mg/day
Hydrocodone bitartrate (5 mg), Homatropine methylbromide (1.5 mg) in each tablet or 5 mL	Hycodan (Rx, C-III)	Relief of symptoms of cough	**Adults and children over 12 years:** 1 tablet or 5 mL q 4–6 hr, not to exceed 6 tablets or 30 mL in 24 hr. **Children, 6–12 years:** ½ tablet or 2.5 mL q 4–6 hr, as needed, not to exceed 3 tablets or 15 mL in 24 hr.
Ibuprofen (200 mg), Hydroco-	Vicoprofen (Rx, C-III)	Mild to moderate pain	One tablet q 4–6 hr up to 5 tablets/ day

Generic Name (Content)	Trade Name	Use	Dose
Irbesartan (150 or 300 mg), Hydrochlorothiazide (12.5 or 25 mg)	Avalide (Rx)	Antihypertensive	**Initial:** 150 mg irbesartan and 12.5 mg hydrochlorothiazide. Increase doses if needed. Begin Avalide therapy only after failure to achieve the desired effect with one or the other as monotherapy.
Lansoprazole (15 mg), Naproxen (375 or 500 mg)	Prevacid NapraPAC 375 and 500 (Rx)	Reduce risk of NSAID-associated gastric ulcers in clients requiring use of an NSAID to treat rheumatoid arthritis, osteoarthritis, and ankylosing spondylitis and who have a history of gastric ulcers.	Each daily dose consists of 1–15 mg lansoprazole capsule and 2 of either 375 or 500 mg naproxen. Take the lansoprazole capsule and 1 of the naproxen tablets before eating in the morning with a glass of water. Take the second naproxen tablet in the evening with a glass of water.

(continues)

Generic Name (Content)	Trade Name	Use	Dose
Lopinavir (80 mg/mL solution, 200 mg/tablet), Ritonavir (20 mg/mL solution, 80 mg/tablet)	Kaletra (Rx)	With other antiretroviral drugs to treat HIV infections	**Adults, therapy-naïve:** 5 mL solution taken with food or 2 tablets taken with or without food twice a day. Or, 10 mL solution taken with food or 4 tablets with or without food once daily. **Adults, therapy-experienced:** 5 mL taken with food or 2 tablets taken with or without food twice daily. **Children, 6 month–12 years, oral solution:** 12/3 mg/kg for those weighing 7 to less than 15 kg and 10/2.5 mg/kg for those 15–40 kg (about equal to 230/57.5 mg/m² twice daily with food, up to a maximum of 400/100 mg in children greater than 40 kg [5 mL or 2 tablets] twice daily).
Loratidine (5 mg), Pseudoephedrine (120 mg)	Claritin-D (Rx)	Relieve symptoms of seasonal allergic rhinitis, including asthma	**Adults and children over 12 years:** 1 tablet q 12 hr on an empty stomach. Give 1 tablet/day in those with a GFR less than 30 mL/min.
Loratidine (10 mg), Pseudoephedrine (240 mg)	Claritin-D 24 Hour Extended-Release (Rx)	Relieve symptoms of seasonal allergic rhinitis, including asthma	**Adults:** 1 tablet daily.

(continues)

Generic Name (Content)	Trade Name	Use	Dose
Loteprednol etabonate (0.5%), Tobramycin (0.3%)	Zylet (Rx)	Treat corticosteroid responsive inflammatory conditions in which there is superficial bacterial ocular infection or a risk of bacterial ocular infection	1–2 gtt instilled into the conjunctival sac of the affected eye(s) q 4–6 hr. May be given as often as q 1–2 hr during the first 24–48 hr of therapy.
Moexipril hydrochloride (7.5 or 15 mg), Hydrochlorothiazide (12.5 or 25 mg)	Uniretic 7.5/12.5, 15/12.5, or 15/25 (Rx)	Hypertension	Moexipril, 7.5–30 mg/day with Hydrochlorothiazide, 12.5–25 mg/day given 1–2 times per day 1 hr before meals.
Niacin Extended-Release (500 mg, 750 mg, or 1,000 mg), Lovastatin (20 or 40 mg)	Advicor Extended-Release Tablets (Rx)	Primary hypercholesterolemia, Mixed dyslipidemia	**Initial for niacin:** 500 mg at bedtime. Titrate the niacin dose by no more than 500 mg q 4 weeks, up to a maximum of 2,000 mg/day. **Initial for lovastatin:** 20 mg once a day; make dosage adjustments at intervals of 4 weeks or more.

Generic Name (Content)	Trade Name	Use	Dose
Olanzapine (3, 6 or 12 mg), Fluoxetine hydrochloride (25 or 50 mg)	Symbyax (Rx)	Depressive episodes associated with bipolar disorder	Give once daily in the evening, usually starting with the 6 mg/25 mg capsule. Adjust dosage as needed. Efficacy ranges from 6–12 mg olanzapine and 25–50 mg fluoxetine. Use a starting dose of 6 mg/25 mg for those with a predisposition to hypotension, with hepatic impairment, and in females, the elderly, or nonsmokers. Do not use with thoridazine or a MAO inhibitor or within 14 days of stopping an MAO inhibitor (wait 5 weeks after stopping Symbyax before starting therapy with either drug). Not studied in clients younger than 18 years of age or those over the age of 65 years.
Oxycodone hydrochloride (5 mg), Ibuprofen (400 mg)	Combunox (Rx, C-II)	Short-term (no more than 7 days) management of acute, moderate to severe pain	1 tablet, with no more than 4 tablets in a 24-hr period.
Pentazocine HCl (50 mg), Naloxone HCl (0.5 mg)	Talwin NX (Rx, C-IV)	Moderate to severe pain	**Adults:** 1 tablet q 3–4 hr, up to 2 tablets q 3–4 hr. Daily dose should not exceed 600 mg pentazocine.

Generic Name (Content)	Trade Name	Use	Dose
Pioglitazone hydrochloride (30 mg), Glimepiride (2 or 4 mg)	Duetact (Rx)	Type 2 diabetes	Base initial dose on current regimen of pioglitazone and/or sulfonylurea. **Initial if currently on glimepiride:** 30 mg/2 mg or 30 mg/4 mg once a day. **Initial if currently on pioglitazone:** 30 mg/2 mg once a day. Maximum recommended dose is pioglitazone, 45 mg/day, and glimepiride, 8 mg/day.
Pioglitazone hydrochloride (15 mg), Metformin hydrochloride (500 or 850 mg)	ActoPlus Met	Adjunct to diet and exercise to improve glycemic control in type 2 diabetes.	Select initial dose based on client's current regimen of these drugs. Do not exceed a daily dose of pioglitazone, 45 mg and metformin, 2,550 mg. Recommended starting dose is pioglitazone 15 mg and metformin 500 mg once or twice daily or pioglitazone 15 mg and metformin 850 mg once or twice daily.

(continues)

Generic Name (Content)	Trade Name	Use	Dose
Propranolol HCl (40, 80, 120, or 160 mg), Hydrochlorothiazide (25 or 50 mg)	Inderide 40/25, Inderide 80/25, Inderide LA 80/50, Inderide LA 120/50, Inderide LA 160/50 (Rx)	Hypertension (not for initial therapy)	*Inderide Tablets*: 1–2 tablets twice a day, up to 320 mg propranolol/day. *Inderide LA Capsules*: 1 capsule per day.
Quinapril hydrochloride (10 mg or 20 mg), Hydrochlorothiazide (12.5 mg or 25 mg)	Accuretic, Quinaretic (Rx)	Hypertension (not for initial treatment)	One 10/12.5 or 20/12.5 tablet/day if BP not controlled by quinapril alone. Also for those whose BP adequately controlled by 25 mg hydrochlorothiazide but have significant potassium loss. Those adequately treated with 20 mg quinapril and 25 mg hydrochlorothiazide may switch to 20/25 dosage form.
Rifampin (300 mg), Isoniazid (150 mg)	IsonaRif, Rifamate, Rimactane/INH Dual Pack (Rx)	Pulmonary tuberculosis following completion of initial therapy. In malnourished clients, adolescents, or those predisposed to neuropathy, also treat with pyridoxine	Two capsules once daily.

Generic Name (Content)	Trade Name	Use	Dose
Rifampin (120 mg), Isoniazid (50 mg), Pyrazinamide (300 mg)	Rifater (Rx)	Initial phase of the short course (2 months) treatment of pulmonary tuberculosis. If resistance is high, add streptomycin or ethambutol. In malnourished clients, adolescents, or those predisposed to neuropathy, also treat with pyridoxine. Follow the 2 month course of treatment with Rifamate	**Weight less than 44 kg:** 4 tablets/day given at the same time; **45–54 kg:** 5 tablets/day given at the same time; **Over 55 kg:** 6 tablets/day given at the same time.
Rosiglitazone (4 or 8 mg), Glimepiride (1, 2, or 4 mg)	Avandaryl	Adjunct to diet and exercise in type 2 diabetes in those already treated with a combination of rosiglitazone and a sulfonylurea or who are not adequately controlled on a sulfonylurea alone	Give once daily with the first meal of the day. Usual starting dose is rosiglitazone/glimepiride 4 mg/1 mg or 4 mg/2 mg (in those already treated with a sulfonylurea or thiazolidinedione). Adjust does as needed but not to exceed a total daily dose of 8 mg rosiglitazone and 4 mg glimepiride.

(continues)

Generic Name (Content)	Trade Name	Use	Dose
Rosiglitazone maleate (1, 2, or 4 mg), Metformin hydrochloride (500 or 1,000 mg)	Avandamet (Rx)	Adjunct to diet and exercise to treat type 2 diabetes who are not adequately controlled with metformin alone	Starting dose based on total daily dose of prior therapy. If prior metformin daily dose was 1,000 mg/day, use Avandamet, 2 mg/500 mg (1 tab twice a day); if prior metformin daily dose was 2,000 mg/day, use 1 mg/500 mg (2 tabs twice a day). If prior Rosiglitazone daily dose was 4 mg/day, use Avandamet, 2 mg/500 mg (1 tab twice a day); if prior Rosiglitazone daily dose was 8 mg/day, use Avandamet, 4 mg/500 mg (1 tab twice a day).
Sitagliptin (50 mg), Metformin hydrochloride (500 or 1,000 mg)	Janumet (Rx)	Type 2 diabetes	Base initial dose on current regimen. The following doses are available: 50/500 mg and 50/1,000 mg. Give twice a day with meals.
Spironolactone (25 or 50 mg), Hydrochlorothiazide (25 or 50 mg)	Aldactazide 25 and 50 (Rx)	CHF, essential hypertension, nephrotic syndrome. Edema and/or ascites in cirrhosis of the liver	*Edema.* **Adults, usual:** 100 mg of each drug daily (range 25–200 mg) given as single or divided doses. **Children, usual:** Equivalent to 1.65–3.3 mg/kg spironolactone. *Essential hypertension.* **Adults, usual:** 50–100 mg of each drug daily in single or divided doses.

Generic Name (Content)	Trade Name	Use	Dose
Telmisartan (40 or 80 mg), Hydrochlorothiazide (12.5 or 25 mg)	Micardis HCT (Rx)	Hypertension (second-line treatment)	**Initial:** 40 mg of telmisartan once a day (range: 20–80 mg). Effective dose of hydrochlorothiazide is 12.5–50 mg once daily. Not for use in those with severe hepatic impairment.
Triamterene (37.5 or 75 mg for capsules or tablets), Hydrochlorothiazide (25 mg for capsules, 25 or 50 mg for tablets)	Dyazide, Maxzide, Maxide-25 MG (Rx)	Hypertension or edema in clients who manifest hypokalemia on hydrochlorothiazide alone. Not first-line therapy, except in those in whom hypokalemia should be avoided	Triamterene/Hydrochlorothiazide: **37.5 mg/25 mg:** 1 or 2 capsules/tablets daily; **50 mg/25 mg:** 1 or 2 capsules twice a day after meals; **75 mg/50 mg:** 1 tablet daily.

appendix 9
Drug/Food Interactions

A. DRUGS THAT SHOULD BE TAKEN WHILE FASTING

Alendronate
Ampicillin
AzoGantanol/Gantrisin
Bacampicillin
Bethanechol (may experience N&V)
Bisacodyl
Calcium carbonate
Captopril
Carbenicillin
Castor oil
Chloramphenicol
Claritin
Cyclosporine gel caps only (avoid fatty meals)
Demeclocycline (avoid high calcium foods/dairy products)
Dicloxacillin
Digoxin (avoid high fiber cereals and oatmeal)
Disopyramide
Digitalis preparations (not with high fiber foods)
Erythromycin base/estolate
Etidronate
Ferrous salts (not with tea, coffee, egg, cereals, fiber, or milk)
Fexofenadine
Flavoxate
Furosemide
Isoniazid
Isosorbide dinitrate
Ketoprofen (if GI distress occurs, may take with food)
Lansoprazole
Levodopa (not with high protein foods; meals delay absorption
    and peak plasma concentration; avoid caffeine)
Lisinopril
Lomustine (empty stomach will reduce nausea)
Methotrexate (milk, cream, or yogurt may decrease absorption)
Methyldopa (not with high protein foods; meals delay absorption
    and peak plasma concentration; avoid caffeine)
Nafcillin (inactivated by stomach acid; absorption variable with/
    without food)
Nalidixic acid
Naltrexone
Norfloxacin (milk, cream, or yogurt may decrease absorption)
Oxytetracycline (avoid dairy products and foods high in calcium)
Penicillamine (antacids, iron and food decreases absorption)
Penicillin
Phenytoin (if GI distress occurs, may take with food; food effect
    depends on preparation)

Propantheline
Rifampicin
Sotalol
Sulfamethoxazole
Tetracycline (avoid dairy products and foods high in calcium)
Theophylline (absorption of controlled release varies by preparation)
Thyroid hormone preparations (limit foods containing goitrogens)
Terbutaline sulfate
Trientine (antacids, iron, and food reduces absorption)
Trimethoprim
Zyrtec

B. DRUGS THAT SHOULD BE TAKEN WITH FOOD

Allopurinol (after meal)
Atovaquone
Augmentin
Aspirin
Amiodarone
Baclofen
Bromocriptine
Buspirone
Carbamazepine (erratic absorption)
Carvedilol
Cefpodoxime
Chloroquine
Chlorothiazide
Cimetidine
Clofazimine
Diclofenac
Divalproex
Doxycyline
Felbamate
Fenofibrate (TriCor)
Fiorinal
Fludrocortisone
Fenoprofen
Gemfibrozil
Glyburide
Griseofulvin (high fat meals)
Hydrocortisone
Hydroxychloroquine (Plaquenil)
Indomethacin
Iron products
Isotretinoin
Itraconazole capsules
Ketorolac
Labetalol
Lithium
Lovastatin
Mebendazole
Methenamine
Methylprednisolone

Metoprolol
Metronidazole
Misoprostol
Metoprolol
Naltrexone
Naproxen
Nelfinavir (Viracept)
Niacin
Nifedipine (grapefruit juice increases bioavailability)
Nitrofurantoin
Olsalazine
Oxcarbazepine
Pentoxifylline
Pergolide
Piroxicam
Potassium salts
Prednisone
Probucol (high fat meals)
Procainamide
Propranolol
Ritonavir
Salsalate
Saquinavir
Sevelamer
Spironolactone
Sulfasalazine
Sulfinpyrazone
Sulindac
Ticlopidine
Tolmetin
Trazodone
Verapamil SR (absorption varies by manufacturer; too rapid absorption may cause heart block)

C.   CONSTIPATING AGENTS

Antacids
Anticholinergic drugs
Anticonvulsants
Antihistamines
Antiparkinsonian drugs
BP meds (calcium channel blockers)
Clonidine
Corticosteroids
Diuretics
Ganglionic blocking agents
Iron supplements
Laxatives (when abused)
Lithium
MAO Inhibitors
Muscle relaxants
NSAIDs
Octreotide
Opioids

Phenothiazines
Prostaglandin synthesis inhibitors
Tranquilizers
Tricyclic antidepressants

D. DIARRHEAL AGENTS

Adrenergic neuron blockers: reserpine, guanethidine
Antacids (Mg containing) H_2 receptor antagonists (i.e., ranitidine)
   PPIs (i.e, Omeprazole)
Antiarrhythmics (i.e., quinidine)
Antibiotics (especially broad spectrum agents)
Antihypertensives (beta blockers, ACE Inhibitors)
Anti-inflammatory drugs (NSAIDs, colchicine)
Chemotherapy agents
Cholinergic agonists and cholinesterase inhibitors
Glucophage
Metoclopramide
Misoprostol
Osmotic and stimulant laxatives
Theophylline

E. TYRAMINE CONTAINING FOODS

Moderate amounts of tyramine:
Banana peel
Broad beans
Cheese (all except cream cheese and cottage cheese)
Chianti, vermouth
Concentrated yeast extracts/Brewer's yeast
Fermented cabbage products: sauerkraut, kimchee
Fermented soy products: fermented bean curd, soya bean paste,
   miso soup
Hydrolyzed protein extracts for sauces, soups, gravies
Imitation cheese
Liquid and powdered protein supplements
Meat extracts
Nonalcoholic beers
Prepared meats (sausage, chopped liver, pate, salami, mortadella)
Raspberries
Some non-United States brands of beer
Yeast products

Significant amounts of tyramine:
Avocado
Chocolate
Cream from fresh pasteurized milk
Distilled spirits
Peanuts
Red and white wines, port wines
Soy sauce
Yogurt

F.   FOODS CONTAINING GOITROGENS

Asparagus
Brocolli
Brussels sprouts
Cabbage
Cauliflower
Kale
Lettuce
Millet
Mustard
Other leafy green vegetables
Peaches
Peanuts
Peas
Radishes
Rutabaga
Soy beans
Spinach
Strawberries
Turnip greens
Watercress

G.   COUMARIN ANTICOAGULANTS AND DIETARY EFFECTS

Consumption of vitamin K-enriched foods may counteract the effects of anticoagulants since the drugs act through antagonism of vitamin K. Advise client on anticoagulants to maintain a steady, consistent intake of vitamin K-containing foods. The drug monograph for warfarin clearly lists these foods. Additionally, certain herbal teas (green tea, buckeye, horse chestnut, Woodruff, tonka beans, melitot) contain natural coumarins that can potentiate the effects of coumadin and should be avoided. Large amounts of avocado also potentiate the drug's effects. Brussels sprouts, broccoli, spinach, kale, turnip greens, and other cruciferous vegetables increase the catabolism of warfarin thereby decreasing its anticoagulant activities. Caffeinated beverages (i.e., cola, coffee, tea, hot chocolate, chocolate milk) can affect therapy. Alcohol intake of more than three drinks per day can affect clotting times. Herbal supplements can also affect bleeding time: Coenzyme Q10 is structurally similar to vitamin K, feverfew, garlic, and ginseng. Avoid herbal medications while on warfarin therapy.

H.   GENERAL DRUG CLASS RECOMMENDATIONS

ACE inhibitors: Take captopril and moexipril 1 hr before or 2 hr after meals; food decreases absorption. Avoid high potassium foods as ACE increases K$^+$.

Analgesic/Antipyretic: Take on an empty stomach as food may slow the absorption.

Antacids: Take 1 hr after or between meals. Avoid dairy foods as the protein in them can increase stomach acid.

Anti-anxiety agents: Caffeine may cause excitability, nervousness, and hyperactivity lessening the anti-anxiety drug effects.

Antibiotics: Penicillin generally should be taken on an empty stomach; may take with food if GI upset occurs. Do not mix with acidic foods: coffee, citrus fruits, and tomatoes; the acid interferes with absorption of penicillin, ampicillin, erythromycin and cloxacillin.

Anticoagulants: High vitamin K produces blood-clotting substance and may reduce drug effectiveness. Vitamin E >400 IU may prolong clotting time and increase bleeding risk.

Antidepressant drugs: May be taken with or without food.

Antifungals: Avoid taking with dairy products; avoid alcohol.

Antihistamines: Take on an empty stomach to increase effectiveness.

Bronchodilators with theophylline: High-fat meals may increase bio-availability while high-carbohydrate meals may decrease it. Food increases absorption of Theo-24 and Uniphyl which may cause increased N&V, headache and irritability.

Cephalosporins: Take on an empty stomach 1 hr before or 2 hr after meals. May take with food if GI upset occurs.

Diuretics: Vary in interactions; some cause loss of potassium, calcium, and magnesium. Avoid salty food and natural black licorice as these increase K and Mg losses. Large doses of vitamin D can elevate blood pressure.

H_2 blockers: May take with or without regard to food.

HMG-CoA reductase inhibitors: Take lovastatin with the evening meal to enhance absorption.

Laxatives: Avoid dairy foods as calcium can decrease absorption.

Macrolides: Take on an empty stomach 1 hr before or 2 hr after meals. May take with food for GI upset.

MAO inhibitors: Have many dietary restrictions, so follow dietary guidelines as prescribed. Foods or alcoholic beverages containing tyramine may cause a fatal increase in BP.

Narcotic analgesics: Avoid alcohol as it may increase sedative effects.

Nitroimadazole (metronidazole): Avoid alcohol or food prepared with alcohol for at least three days after finishing the medicine. Alcohol may cause nausea, abdominal cramps, vomiting, headaches, and flushing.

NSAIDs: Take with food or milk to prevent irritation of the stomach.

Quinolones: Take on an empty stomach 1 hr before or 2 hr after meals. May take with food for GI upset but avoid calcium containing foods such as milk, yogurt, vitamins/minerals containing iron and antacids because they decrease drug concentrations. Caffeine containing products may lead to excitability and nervousness.

Sulfonamides: Take on an empty stomach 1 hr before or 2 hr after meals. May take with food if GI upset occurs.

Tetracyclines: Take on an empty stomach 1 hr before or 2 hr after meals. May take with food but avoid dairy products, antacids, and vitamins containing iron with tetracycline.

appendix 10

Drugs Whose Effects Are Modified by Grapefruit Juice

Increasing numbers of drugs have been identified whose effects are modified by short-term or chronic use of grapefruit juice. This effect is likely due to furanocoumarins that are present in grapefruit juice. The following is a representative list of those drugs, including the mechanism for the altered drug effect. The most frequent result is an increase in plasma levels of the drug, which may increase the risk of side effects.

Drug	Mechanism for Altered Effect
Albendazole	↑ Plasma albendazole levels and peak plasma concentration
Amiodarone	↑ Plasma amiodarone levels R/T inhibition of amiodarone metabolism
Amlodipine	↑ Plasma amlodipine levels R/T ↓ liver metabolism
Amprenavir	↓ Amprenavir peak levels and ↑ time to reach peak concentration
Atorvastatin	↑ Plasma atorvastatin levels
Bexarotene	↑ Plasma bexarotene levels R/T ↓ liver metabolism
Budesonide	↑ Plasma budesonide levels
Buspirone	↑ AUC and peak plasma buspirone levels and time to reach peak levels
Calcium channel blockers	↑ Serum levels of calcium channel blockers
Carbamazepine	↑ Peak plasma carbamazepine levels
Cilostazol	↑ Plasma cilostazol levels R/T ↓ liver metabolism
Clarithromycin	Avoid taking with grapefruit juice

Drug	Mechanism for Altered Effect
Cyclosporine	↑ Plasma cyclosporine levels R/T ↓ liver metabolism
Dextromethorphan	↑ Bioavailability of dextromethorphan
Digoxin	↑ Plasma digoxin levels
Dofetilide	Possible ↑ dofetilide plasma levels
Ergot alkaloids	↑ Serum levels of ergotamine derivatives
Erythromycin	↑ Plasma erythromycin levels R/T ↓ metabolism in the small intestine
Estrogens	↑ Plasma levels of 17-beta estradiol/estrone combination
Etoposide	↓ Etoposide AUC and bioavailability
Felodipine	↑ Plasma felodipine levels R/T ↓ liver metabolism
Fexofenadine	↓ Fexofenadine absorption and thus pharmacological effects
Fluvoxamine	↑ Fluvoxamine mean AUC and C_{max}
Indinavir	Delay in indinavir absorption and time to reach peak plasma levels
Itraconzole	↓ Itraconzole bioavailability R/T inhibition of absorption
Ixabepilone	↑ Ixabepilone plasma levels
Lapatinib	↑ Lapatinib plasma levels
Losartan	↓ Liver metabolism to losartan's active form
Lovastatin	↑ Plasma lovastatin levels R/T ↓ liver metabolism
Methylprednisolone	↑ Plasma methylprednisolone levels R/T ↓ liver metabolism
Midazolam	↑ PO midazolam plasma levels R/T ↓ liver metabolism
Mifepristone	↑ Plasma mifepristone levels R/T ↓ liver metabolism

Drug	Mechanism for Altered Effect
Nicardipine	↑ Plasma nicardipine levels R/T ↓ liver metabolism
Nifedipine	↑ Plasma nifedipine levels R/T ↓ liver metabolsim
Nilotinib	↑ Nilotinib plasma levels
Nisoldipine	↑ Plasma nisoldipine levels R/T ↓ liver metabolism
Pimozide	↑ Pimozide plasma levels; possible QTc prolongation and increased risk of life-threatening cardiac arrhythmias. Do not use together.
Praziquantel	↑ Praziquantal AUC and C_{max}
Quinidine	↓ Quinidine absorption and ↓ quinidine metabolism to its major metabolite; effect on QTc interval delayed
Saquinavir	↑ Plasma saquinavir levels R/T ↓ liver metabolism
Scopolamine	↑ Scopolamine bioavailability and ↑ time to reach peak plasma levels
Sildenafil	↑ Plasma sildenafil levels R/T ↓ liver metabolism
Simvastatin	↑ Plasma simvastatin levels R/T ↓ liver metabolism
Sirolimus	↑ Plasma sirolimus levels R/T ↓ liver metabolism
Temsirolimus	↑ Temsirolimus plasma levels
Triazolam	↑ Plasma triazolam levels R/T ↓ liver metabolism
Verapamil	↑ Plasma verapamil levels R/T ↓ liver metabolism

appendix 11
Drugs That Should Not Be Crushed

As a rule of thumb, any sustained-release or extended-release formulation should never be crushed. Instead, attempt to get a liquid formulation of the product so that it can be administered in that form. Coated products should also not be crushed. They were coated for a specific purpose, e.g., to prevent stomach irritation by the product, to prevent destruction of the product by stomach acid, to prevent an unwanted reaction, or to produce a prolonged or extended effect.

These are some of the drugs that should not be crushed:

Accutane
Aciphex
Adalat cc SR
Advicor ER
Afrinol Repetab
Allerest capsule
Allegra D
Aminodur Duratab
Artane Sequel
Arthrotec
ASA E.C.
ASA Enseal
Augmentin XR
Azulfadine Entab
Betaphen-VK
Biaxin XL
Biscodyl EC
Calan SR
Cardizem LA, SR
Ceclor CD
Ceftin
Chlortrimeton SR
Choledyl SR
Cipro XR
Claritin-D
Colace
Colestid
Compazine Spansule
Concerta SR
Creon EC
Depakote ER
Desyrel
Dexedrine SR
Diamox Sequel

Dilacor XR
Dimetapp SR
Ditropan XL
Donnatal Extentab
Drixoral tablet
Ecotrin tablet
Effexor XR
E-Mycin tablet
Entex LA
Erythromycin EC
Feldene
Feosol Spansule
Feosol tablet
Ferro Grad-500 tablet
Flomax
Glucophage XR
Glucatrol XL
Humibid DM, LA
Imdur SR, LA
Indocin SR
Isoptin SR
Isordil sublingual
Isordil Tembids, Dinitrate
Kaon tablet
K-Dur, K-tab
Klor-Con
Levbid SR
Lithobid SR
Macrobid SR
Mestinon Timespans
Metadate CD, SR
MS Contin
Mucinex
Nexium

Niaspan
Nitroglycerin tablet
Nitrospan capsule
Norpace CR
Ornade Spansule
OxyContin
Pancrease EC, MT
Paxil CR
Pentosa
Phazyme
Plendil SR
Prevacid
Prilosec SR
Procardia XL
Protonix
Proventil Repetabs
Prozac weekly
Quinaglute Duratab
Quinidex Extenutab
Slow K tablet; Slow Mag, Slow Fe
Sorbitrate
Sudafed SA capsule

Tegretol XR
Teldrin capsule
Tenuate Dospan
Tessalon Perles
Theobid Duracaps
Theolair SR
Thorazine Spansules
Tiazac SR
Toprol XL
Trental SR
Tylenol ER
Uniphyl SR
Verelan PM
Volmax SR
Voltaren EC
Voltaren SR
Wellbutrin SR
Xanax SR
Zerit XR
Zomig ZMT
Zyban
Zyrtec-D

appendix 12
Patient Safety Goals

The Joint Commission Goals for Health Care Settings 2008

Goal 1: Improve the accuracy of patient identification

1a. Reliably identify the individual as the person for whom the care, treatment, or service is intended and also match the care, treatment, or service to that individual. Patient specific identifiers must be directly associated with the medication, blood products, specimen tubes etc. Two patient identifiers must be used whenever collecting specimens or administering medications or blood products. The patient's room number is not acceptable. A wristband that includes the patient's name and unique ID number to identify them correctly is acceptable, the name and the unique ID number may be considered as two separate pieces of information.

1b. Prior to the start of any invasive procedures such as biopsies require a "time-out" process. At this time a final verification process should be conducted to confirm the correct patient, procedure, and site using active, not passive, communication techniques.

Goal 2: Improve the effectiveness of communication among care givers

2a. All completed orders or critical test results provided verbally must be verified by having the receiver "read back" the complete order or test results.

2b. The organization is required to standardize all abbreviations, acronyms, symbols, and dose designations that are not to be used in the facility or throughout the organization.

2c. A process must be established to assess and measure and if appropriate take action to improve the organization's performance R/T the timeliness of reporting/receipt of critical test results and values to the responsible licensed care giver.

2d. Health care organizations must establish how their laboratories, working with clinicians, will identify critical values, and how they will provide this information in an appropriate and timely way directly to the responsible licensed care giver and/or an alternative care giver.

2e. Implement a standardized approach to "hand off" communications, including an opportunity to ask and respond to questions.

Goal 3: Improve the safety of using medications

3a. Remove concentrated electrolytes from patient care units/areas. (i.e. potassium chloride, potassium phosphate, sodium chloride >0.9%, etc.)

3b. Standardize and limit the number of drug concentrations available in the organization.

3c. Identify, and at a minimum, annually review a list of look alike/sound alike drugs used by the organization and take action to prevent errors involving interchange of these drugs.

3d. Label all medications, medication containers (e.g., syringes, medicine cups, basins), or other solutions on and off the sterile field.

3e. Reduce the likelihood of patient harm associated with the use of anticoagulation therapy.

Goal 4: Eliminate wrong-site, wrong patient, wrong procedure surgery

4a. Create and use a preoperative verification process, such as a check list, to confirm that appropriate documents are available

4b. Implement a process to mark the surgical site and involve the patient in the marking process.

Goal 5: Improve the safety of using infusion pumps

Ensure free-flow protection on all general use and patient-controlled analgesia intravenous infusion pumps used in the organization.

Goal 6: Improve the effectiveness of clinical alarm systems

6a. Implement regular preventive maintenance and testing of alarm systems.

6b. Assure that alarms are activated with appropriate settings and are sufficiently audible.

Goal 7: Reduce the risk of healthcare associated infections

7a. Comply with current World Health Organization (WHO) Hand Hygiene Guidelines or Centers for Disease Control and Prevention (CDC) hand hygiene guidelines.

7b. Manage all identified cases of unanticipated death or major permanent loss of function associated with a healthcare-acquired infection as sentinel events.

Goal 8: Accurately and completely reconcile medications across the continuum of care

8a. There is a process for comparing the patient's current medications with those ordered for the patient while under the care of the organization.

8b. A complete list of the patient's medications is communicated to the next provider of service when a patient is referred or transferred to another setting, service, practitioner, or level of care within or outside the organization. The complete list of medications is also provided to the patient on discharge from the facility.

Goal 9: Reduce the risk of patient harm resulting from falls

9b. Implement a fall reduction program including an evaluation of the effectiveness of the program.

Goal 10: Reduce the risk of influenza and pneumococcal diseases in older adults

10a. Develop and implement a protocol for: administration and documentation of the flu vaccine and

10b. pneumococcus vaccine

10c. Develop and implement a protocol for identifying new cases of influenza and to manage an outbreak.

Goal 11: Reduce the risk of surgical fires

11a. Educate staff, including operating licensed independent practitioners and anesthesia providers, on how to control heat sources and manage fuels with enough time for patient preparation, and establish guidelines to minimize oxygen concentration under drapes.

Goal 12: Implementation of applicable National Patient Safety Goals and associated requirements by components and practitioner sites.

12a. Inform and encourage components and practitioner sites to implement the applicable National Patient Safety Goals and associated requirements.

Goal 13: Encourage patients' active involvement in their own care as a patient safety strategy.

13a. Define and communicate the means for patients and their families to report concerns about safety and encourage them to do so.

Goal 14: Prevent health care-associated pressure ulcers (decubitus ulcers).

Assess and periodically reassess each resident's risk for developing a pressure ulcer (decubitus ulcer) and take action to address any identified risks.

Goal 15 The organization identifies safety risks inherent in its patient population.

15a. The organization identifies patients at risk for suicide.

15b. The organization identifies risks associated with long-term oxygen therapy such as home fires.

Goal 16: Improve recognition and response to changes in a patient's condition.

16a. The organization selects a suitable method that enables health care staff members to directly request additional assistance from a specially trained individual(s) when the patient's condition appears to be worsening.

References

www.jointcommission.org/PatientSafety/NationalPatientSafetyGoals/
o8_npsg_facts

Other Resources

www.patientsafety.gov
www.jointcommission.org

appendix 13
Cultural Aspects of Medicine Therapy

As the diversity of the population increases, it has become clearer that health and medication administration practices should continually be reassessed. Culture and language are central to the process by which the health care provider tries to obtain information and learn from clients what their concerns, worries, and thoughts about their heath condition encompass. This enables the provider to be able to make appropriate assessments, diagnoses, treatment plans, medication selection, and identification of potential side effects. Both providers and clients are guided by their respective cultural norms. Providers may find difficulties in inducing changes in health-related behaviors that conflict with the typical cultural practices of these clients. Providers need to be able to assess the cultural differences in health beliefs and practices in the context of their individual social conditions to prevent confusing their individuality with national or other group stereotypes. Clinical care needs to be a private, yet, personalized situation where these clients can present their problems and complaints. The health care environment and interaction with front desk and other staff also influence the client's response to care. This is most important when there are language and cultural barriers in communication between providers and clients since accurate and honest communication between each is essential to the delivery of quality health services. Common approaches for dealing with communication problems include working with an interpreter, including bilingual family members for interpretation, and identifying those in the facility (employee, visitor, etc.) who are bilingual/bicultural.

Use an approach that is persuasive, but not confrontational or offensive. One can resolve conflict by developing trust, and understanding the social context helps. Elderly clients are especially sensitive about being corrected by younger individuals, so you may consider an older interpreter and one of the same sex as the client. Providers need to make sure that the information that they are giving to the client is understood, accepted, and applied as advised. This requires rewording or conversion of technical medical language into language that is culturally meaningful and that enhances the emotional support that the clients may need. Increased linguistic, racial, and cultural diversity of the population require increased sensitivity and culturally relevant approaches to disease control and health promotion. There is a sociomedical need to remove language and cultural barriers between providers and clients to reduce misunderstandings, inefficiencies, increase rapport with clients, and to prevent negative legal, ethical, and economic consequences. Clients need to be instructed on accessing timely, needed and appropriate health care. They may have a misunderstanding from culturally inappropriate and misleading translations such as verbal and gesture misinterpretation, physical distance and touching. They may experience distrust, fear of discrimination, of being stereotyped and misunderstood, and they may be burdened by unaffordable out of pocket costs.

There are medicine cultures within cultures: 1) Folk medicine: sacred, magic, and empirical. e.g., reading astrological signs, rituals, prayer, sacrifices, herbs, etc. and the provider is referred to as: shaman or priest, spiritualist, herbalist, witch, 2) Popular medicine: horoscopes, cards, magic by "readers" and salespersons on interpersonal basis or using radio, TV, daily press, books, and magazines. This also includes advice by family, friends, coworkers, neighbors, and casual acquaintances (e.g., in subways, buses, sidewalks, waiting rooms, stores, salespersons, etc.). Popular medical practices include sharing prescriptions; taking patented medicines, injections, herbs, and controlled substances brought from abroad, and 3) biomedicine: science based medical care. The client views the quality of care on the basis of his own values and preferences and these are guided and modified by his cultural orientation.

Cultural competence includes knowledge, attitudes, sensitivity, awareness, behaviors, and empathy. The provider must be knowledgeable and capable of managing the communication interplay between the culture and language of medical practice and the client's culturally-oriented health-related values, norms, beliefs and practices. Knowledge is the acquisition of accurate and unbiased information and understanding of the functioning norms, values, belief systems and the common understanding that prevails in one's community of service in relation to health and illness. Cultural awareness is the recognition that the ways of life, behaviors, meanings, and values of individuals are influenced by the social understandings within their communities or social groups. Cultural sensitivity is the ability to recognize similarities and differences in norms, standards of behavior, and conventions between, within and among populations and communities. Cultural sensitivity is expressed by the provider by empathy and respect for cultural differences. With increased diversification of the population, communication barriers have led to misinformation and misunderstandings that have contributed to increases in medical care errors, medication errors, lack of adherence, and lack of health improvement, thus indicating that providers need to reassess their communication skills in providing care.

There are public policies and professional guidelines to eliminate barriers between providers and clients. Among the federal laws and regulation is The Hill Burton Act of 1946 which requires meaningful access to health care as a condition of capital financing. It also requires that providers implement policies and procedures to document the conduct of periodic staff training, issue notices of the right of clients to translation and to oral language assistance, and take responsibility for monitoring these activities. Title VI of the Civil Rights Act of 1964 prohibits discrimination based on race, color, or national origin under any program or activity that receives federal aid. Under Medicare, Medicaid, and the Emergency Medical Treatment and Active Labor Act (EMTALA) guidelines for facilitating access to care have been issued. A variety of federal guidelines have been issued for services to persons of limited English proficiency. According to CLAS guidelines, staff members of a facility are expected to provide effective, understandable, and respectful care that is compatible with their clients' cultural health beliefs and practices and preferred language. There are numerous other national and state councils, medical societies, nursing associations and accreditation bodies that have also issued guidelines supporting the inclusion of cultural competence and language proficiency as tools for effective health care delivery services.

appendix 14

Common Spanish Phrases and Terms Used in a Health Care Setting

Hello/Hi	Hola
Yes	Si
No	No
My name is	Me llamo
What can I do for you today?	¿Que puedo hacer yuo para usted hoy?
How are you feeling?	¿como se siente usted?
Do you take any medications?	¿Toma medicinas?
What are the names of the medications you are taking?	¿Cómo se llaman las medicinas que usted toma?
How old are you?	¿Cuantos anos tiene?
Are you allergic to anything?	¿Usted es alérgico a algo?
Do you have any medical problem?	¿Tiene usted algún problemamédico?
Are you having any pain?	¿Tiene usted aigu'n dolor?
Where is your pain located?	¿Dónde está su dolor localizado?
How long have you had it?	¿Cuán largo lo ha tenido usted?
Have you ever had this pain before?	¿Ha tenido jamás usted este dolor antes?
Are you pregnant?	¿Está embarazada?
How many months?	¿Cuántos meses?
Have you vomited?	¿Vomito?
Diarrhea	diarrea
constipation	estreñimiento
Have a cough?	¿Tiene una tos?
Have a fever?	¿Tiene una fiebre?
Please lie down	Acuestese, por favor
Relax	Rela'jese
What	Que
Where	Donde
When	Cuando
How long	Por cuanto tiempo
Please repeat	Repita, por favor

Numbers

one	uno
two	dos
three	tres
four	cuatro
five	cinco
six	seis
seven	siete
eight	ocho
nine	nueve
ten	diez
twenty	veinte
thirty	treinta
forty	cuarenta
fifty	cincuenta
One Hundred	Cien

Days of the Week

Monday	Lunes
Tuesday	Martes
Wednesday	Miercoles
Thursday	Jueves
Friday	Viernes
Saturday	Sabado
Sunday	Domingo

Colors

red	rojo
green	verde
blue	azul
black	negro
yellow	amarillo
brown	café
white	blanco
gray	gris

appendix 15

Medication Reconciliation

Medication reconciliation is a process by which you obtain a complete and accurate list of the current medications from all sources that a patient is taking. This is performed at all points of contact by verifying the names and dosages of all medications to help reduce medication errors. It is done to prevent errors such as omission, duplications, dosing errors, or drug interactions. This process was developed to try and address the greater than 1.3 million adverse events, many related to medication.

Almost half of all medication errors occur at transition points such as transfer between units, upon admission and upon hospital discharge. One quarter of all medication errors occur in the outpatient setting. Over 350 errors have been identified over the past several years, resulting in major injury or death. Children are three times more at risk than adults for drug errors.

Generally, verification can be accomplished by asking the patient to bring all the medications he is taking to the visit so you can review them. Almost one third of the time there is a difference between the medication orders and the information from the patient about what he is actually taking compared to what the medication label reads.

On January 1, 2007 hospitals were to have implemented medication reconciliation processes to collect and compare patient medication information or risk losing their accreditation from the Joint Commission. Nearly a year after the deadline, at least 25% of hospitals have not yet complied with the patient safety requirement. To comply, hospitals must have processes in place for the five steps of medication reconciliation. These are:

- Developing a list of patients' current medications
- Developing a list of medications that will be prescribed
- Comparing the two lists
- Making clinical decisions based on the comparison
- Communicating the new list to patients and caregivers

The list of current medications must include over-the-counter agents and herbals that the patient is consuming. It is much easier to generate and update the list on a computer-based operating system for patient orders, notes, and medications. This list is provided to patients so they can carry it to all providers and medical points of contact to ensure that the list is accurate, up-to-date, and followed by the patient.

The Joint Commission National Patient Safety Goals for 2008 include:

Goal 8 Accurately and completely reconcile medications across the continuum of care.

> 8a. There is a process for comparing the patient's current medications with those ordered for the patient while under the care of the organization [Ambulatory, Assisted Living, Behavioral Health Care, Critical Access Hospital, Disease-Specific Care, Home Care, Hospital, Long Term Care, Office-Based Surgery].

> 8b. A complete list of the patient's medications is communicated to the next provider of service when a patient is referred or transferred to another setting, service, practitioner, or level of care within or outside the organizations. The complete list of medications is also provided to the patient on discharge from the facility [Ambulatory, Assisted Living, Behavioral Health Care, Critical Access Hospital, Disease-Specific Care, Home Care, Hospital, Long Term Care, Office-Based Surgery].

The Medication Form should:

- List all of the medicines the patient is currently taking, including prescription and over-the-counter medications such as aspirin, vitamins, and herbals such as ginkgo, grape seed extract, ginseng, and glucosamine.

- List medications that are taken only as needed, such as Advil and nitroglycerin.

- Include the patient name identifying information

- Document that you have reviewed the list of medications with the patient; that the patient understands the form will be updated to include future prescriptions ordered/taken; and that this form will be shared with all of the patient's providers and the pharmacist.

Medication reconciliation should be performed at every care transition:

- On admission

- Before surgery

- After surgery

- With any inter-ward transfer

- Upon discharge

- At each visit

- With any change in therapy

- Changes in setting, service, provider, or level of care

A series of interventions, including medication reconciliation can successfully reduce the number of medication errors and patient deaths in this country.

Boldface = generic drug name   CAPITALS = combination drugs

Boldface = generic drug name   CAPITALS = combination drugs

Boldface = generic drug name   CAPITALS = combination drugs

Index

Boldface = generic drug name   CAPITALS = combination drugs

Boldface = generic drug name   CAPITALS = combination drugs

Boldface = generic drug name   CAPITALS = combination drugs

Boldface = generic drug name   CAPITALS = combination drugs

Boldface = generic drug name   CAPITALS = combination drugs

Boldface = generic drug name   CAPITALS = combination drugs

Boldface = generic drug name   CAPITALS = combination drugs

Boldface = generic drug name   CAPITALS = combination drugs

Boldface = generic drug name   CAPITALS = combination drugs

Boldface = generic drug name   CAPITALS = combination drugs

Boldface = generic drug name   CAPITALS = combination drugs

Boldface = generic drug name   CAPITALS = combination drugs

Boldface = generic drug name   CAPITALS = combination drugs

Boldface = generic drug name   CAPITALS = combination drugs

Boldface = generic drug name   CAPITALS = combination drugs

Boldface = generic drug name   CAPITALS = combination drugs

Boldface = generic drug name   CAPITALS = combination drugs

Boldface = generic drug name   CAPITALS = combination drugs